KV-658-687

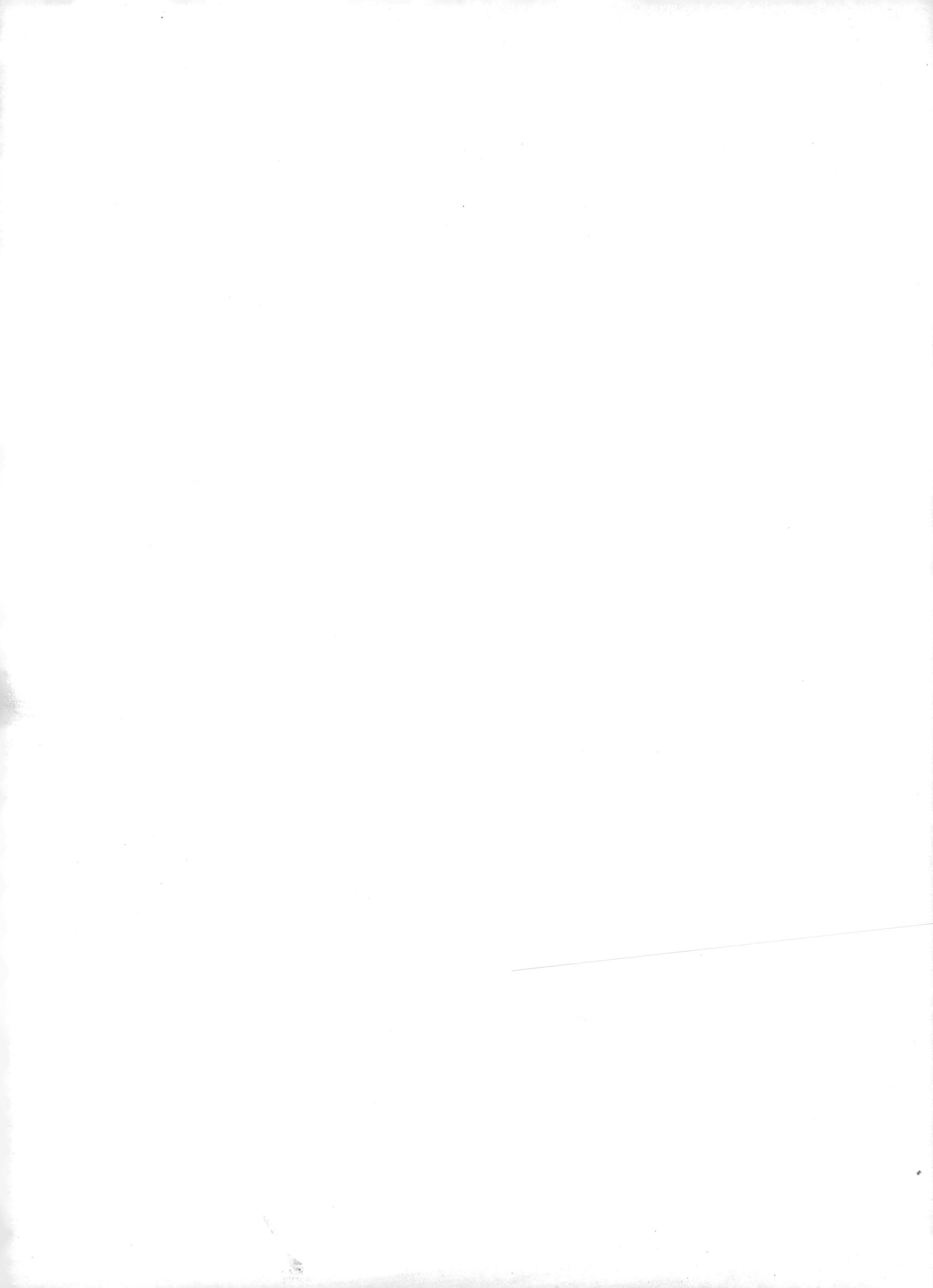

PEDIATRIC INFECTIOUS DISEASES

PRINCIPLES AND PRACTICE

SECOND EDITION

Edited by

Hal B. Jenson, MD
Professor, Departments of Pediatrics and Microbiology
Chief, Division of Pediatric Infectious Diseases
University of Texas Health Science Center at San Antonio
Attending Physician, University Hospital and CHRISTUS Santa Rosa Children's Hospital
San Antonio, Texas

Robert S. Baltimore, MD
Professor, Departments of Pediatrics and of Epidemiology and Public Health
Yale University School of Medicine
Associate Hospital Epidemiologist
Yale–New Haven Hospital
Attending Physician, Yale–New Haven Children's Hospital
New Haven, Connecticut

W.B. SAUNDERS COMPANY
A Harcourt Health Sciences Company
Philadelphia London New York St. Louis Sydney Toronto

W.B. SAUNDERS COMPANY

A Harcourt Health Sciences Company

The Curtis Center
Independence Square West
Philadelphia, Pennsylvania 19106

Library of Congress Cataloging-in-Publication Data

Pediatric infectious diseases: principles and practice / [edited by] Hal B. Jenson, Robert S. Baltimore.—Rev. ed.
p. ; cm.
Includes bibliographical references.
ISBN 0-7216-8121-2
1. Communicable diseases in children. I. Jenson, Hal B. II. Baltimore, Robert S.
[DNLM: 1. Communicable Diseases—Child. 2. Communicable Diseases—Infant.
WC 100 P372 2002]
RJ401 .P426 2002
618.92'9—dc21

2001032283

PEDIATRIC INFECTIOUS DISEASES: PRINCIPLES AND PRACTICE ISBN 0-7216-8121-2

Printed in the United States of America

Last digit is the print number: 9 8 7 6 5 4 3 2 1

To our wives—Polly and Katalin—
and our children—
Casey and LiAnne, and Gwen and Richard

Contributors

Stuart P. Adler, MD

Professor, Virginia Commonwealth University, and Chair, Division of Pediatric Infectious Diseases, Medical College of Virginia Hospitals, Richmond, Virginia
Intrauterine Infections

Stephen C. Aronoff, MD

Professor and Chairman, Department of Pediatrics, Temple University School of Medicine, and Chief Medical Officer, Temple University Children's Medical Center, Philadelphia, Pennsylvania
Osteomyelitis; Infectious Arthritis; Diskitis

David P. Ascher, MD

Professor of Pediatrics, Uniformed Services University of the Health Sciences; Chairman, Department of Pediatrics, Lackland Air Force Base, Texas; and Clinical Professor of Pediatrics, University of Texas Health Science Center at San Antonio, San Antonio, Texas
Mediastinitis; Esophagitis

M. Douglas Baker, MD

Professor of Pediatrics, Yale University School of Medicine, and Chief, Pediatric Emergency Medicine, Yale–New Haven Children's Hospital, New Haven, Connecticut
Fever and Occult Bacteremia in Infants and Young Children

Robert S. Baltimore, MD

Professor, Departments of Pediatrics and of Epidemiology and Public Health, Yale University School of Medicine, Associate Hospital Epidemiologist, Yale–New Haven Hospital, and Attending Physician, Yale–New Haven Children's Hospital, New Haven, Connecticut
Normal Microbial Flora; Laboratory Evaluation of the Inflammatory Response; Prophylaxis of Infectious Diseases; Bronchitis, Bronchiolitis, and Pertussis Syndrome; Pneumonia; Pleural Effusion, Empyema, and Lung Abscess; Infective Endocarditis; Perinatal Bacterial and Fungal Infections

Louis M. Bell, MD

Associate Professor of Pediatrics, University of Pennsylvania School of Medicine; Chief, Division of General Pediatrics, and Attending Physician, Infectious Diseases, The Children's Hospital of Philadelphia, Philadelphia, Pennsylvania
Middle Respiratory Tract Infections

Albert W. Biglan, MD

Adjunct Associate Professor, University of Pittsburgh School of Medicine, and Ophthalmologist, Children's Hospital of Pittsburgh, Pittsburgh, Pennsylvania
Bacterial and Viral Conjunctivitis; Keratitis; Infections of the Eyelids and Ocular Adnexa; Endophthalmitis; Uveitis and Retinitis

Jeffrey L. Blumer, MD, PhD

Professor of Pediatrics and Pharmacology, Case Western Reserve University School of Medicine, and Chief, Division of Pediatric Pharmacology and Critical Care, Rainbow Babies and Children's Hospital, Cleveland, Ohio
Anti-infective Therapy

Kenneth M. Boyer, MD

Professor of Pediatrics, Rush Medical College; Acting Chairman, Department of Pediatrics, and Director, Section of Infectious Diseases, Rush Children's Hospital, Chicago, Illinois
Pediatric Implications of Maternal Infection

John S. Bradley, MD

Associate Professor of Pediatrics, University of California San Diego School of Medicine, and Director, Division of Infectious Diseases, Children's Hospital San Diego, San Diego, California
Cellulitis; Wound and Deep-Tissue Infections; Burn Wound Infections; Bite-Wound Infections

Rebecca C. Brady, MD

Instructor of Pediatrics, University of Cincinnati College of Medicine and Children's Hospital Medical Center, Division of Infectious Diseases, Cincinnati, Ohio
Perinatal Viral Infections

Joseph M. Campos, PhD

Professor, Departments of Pediatrics, Pathology, and Microbiology/Tropical Medicine, George Washington University Medical Center, and Director, Microbiology Laboratory and Laboratory Informatics, Department of Laboratory Medicine, Children's National Medical Center, Washington, DC
Diagnostic Microbiology; Diagnostic Parasitology; Diagnostic Virology; Serologic Diagnosis of Infectious Diseases

Michael Cappello, MD

Associate Professor, Departments of Pediatrics and of Epidemiology and Public Health, Yale University School of Medicine, and Attending Physician, Yale–New Haven Children's Hospital, New Haven, Connecticut
Acute Myocarditis; Acute Pericarditis

John C. Christenson, MD

Professor of Pediatrics and Chief, Division of Infectious Diseases and Geographic Medicine, Department of Pediatrics, University of Utah School of Medicine, and Medical Director, Hospital Epidemiology Program, Primary Children's Medical Center, Salt Lake City, Utah
Epidemiology of Infectious Diseases; Rocky Mountain Spotted Fever; Other Zoonoses and Vectorborne Infections

Celia D.C. Christie, MBBS, DM Pediatrics, MP

Professor and Chair in Pediatrics, University of the West Indies, and Consultant Pediatrician and Specialist in Pediatric Infectious Diseases, University Hospital of the West Indies, Mona, Kingston, Jamaica

Stomatitis; Parotitis and Sialadenitis

Theodore J. Cieslak, MD

Associate Professor of Pediatrics, Uniformed Services University of the Health Sciences, Bethesda, Maryland, and Chief, Division of Operational Medicine, U.S. Army Medical Research Institute of Infectious Diseases, Fort Detrick, Maryland

Dental Infections

Dennis A. Conrad, MD

Associate Professor of Pediatrics, Division of Pediatric Infectious Diseases, University of Texas Health Science Center at San Antonio, and Attending Physician and Director of Medical Education, CHRISTUS Santa Rosa Children's Hospital, San Antonio, Texas

Patients with Cancer; Transplant Recipients; The Vulnerable Host

Toni Darville, MD

Associate Professor of Pediatrics and Microbiology/Immunology, Arkansas Children's Hospital and University of Arkansas for Medical Sciences, Little Rock, Arkansas

Lymphadenopathy, Lymphadenitis, and Lymphangitis

Terence I. Doran, MD, PhD

Associate Professor, University of Texas Health Science Center at San Antonio, and Attending Physician, CHRISTUS Santa Rosa Children's Hospital, San Antonio, Texas

Human Immunodeficiency Virus and Acquired Immunodeficiency Syndrome

Gerald W. Fischer, MD

Professor of Pediatrics, Uniformed Services University of the Health Sciences, Bethesda, Maryland

Immunotherapy and Immunomodulation

Margaret C. Fisher, MD

Professor of Pediatrics, MCP Hahnemann University School of Medicine, Philadelphia, Pennsylvania, and Chair, Department of Pediatrics, Monmouth Medical Center, Long Branch, New Jersey

Nosocomial Infections and Infection Control; Infections Involving Intravascular Devices

Michael A. Gerber, MD

Professor of Pediatrics, University of Cincinnati College of Medicine, and Attending Physician, Division of Infectious Diseases, Children's Hospital Medical Center, Cincinnati, Ohio

Rheumatic Fever and Poststreptococcal Glomerulonephritis

Charles W. Gross, MD

Professor of Otolaryngology, Head and Neck Surgery, and Pediatrics, University of Virginia School of Medicine, Charlottesville, Virginia

Infections of the Deep Fascial Spaces of the Neck

Margaret R. Hammerschlag, MD

Professor of Pediatrics and Medicine and Director, Division of Pediatric Infections Diseases, State University of New York Downstate Medical Center, Brooklyn, New York

Sexually Transmitted Infections

Scott E. Harrison, MD

Otolaryngologist, Department of Pediatrics, University of Mississippi School of Medicine and Mississippi Baptist Medical Center, Jackson, Mississippi

Infections of the Deep Fascial Spaces of the Neck

Gregory F. Hayden, MD

Professor of Pediatrics, University of Virginia, and Attending Pediatrician, University of Virginia Health System, Charlottesville, Virginia

The Common Cold; Pharyngitis

Peter J. Hotez, MD, PhD

Professor and Chair, Department of Microbiology and Tropical Medicine, The George Washington University Medical Center, Washington, DC

Nematode Infections; Trematode Infections; Cestode Infections

Anthony J. Infante, MD, PhD

Professor, Department of Pediatrics, Head, Division of Hematology/Oncology/Immunology, Interim Director, Children's Cancer Research Center, and Associate Dean for Research, Medical School, University of Texas Health Science Center at San Antonio, and Director, Children's Immunology Clinic, CHRISTUS Santa Rosa Children's Hospital, San Antonio, Texas

Host Defenses Against Infection; Evaluation of Immune Function; Primary Immune Deficiency Disorders

Richard F. Jacobs, MD

Horace C. Cabe Professor of Pediatrics and Chief, Section of Infectious Diseases, University of Arkansas for Medical Sciences and Arkansas Children's Hospital, Little Rock, Arkansas

Lymphadenopathy, Lymphadenitis, and Lymphangitis

Jerri Ann Jenista, MD

Pediatrician, Departments of Pediatrics and Emergency Medicine, St. Joseph Mercy Hospital, Ann Arbor, Michigan

The Immigrant, Refugee, or Internationally Adopted Child; The International Child Traveler

Hal B. Jenson, MD

Professor, Departments of Pediatrics and Microbiology, and Chief, Pediatric Infectious Diseases, University of Texas Health Science Center at San Antonio, and Attending Physician, University Hospital and CHRISTUS Santa Rosa Children's Hospital, San Antonio, Texas

Normal Microbial Flora; Infectious Agents and Oncogenesis; Laboratory Evaluation of the Inflammatory Response; Serologic Diagnosis of Infectious Diseases; Measles; Rubella; Roseola; Erythema Infectiosum (Fifth Disease); Chickenpox and Zoster; Mumps; Infectious Mononucleosis; Chronic Fatigue Syndrome; Gastritis; Viral Hepatitis; Hepatic Abscess; Infections of the Biliary Tract; Acute Pancreatitis; Bacterial and Viral Conjunctivitis; Keratitis; Infections of the Eyelids and Ocular Adnexa; Endophthalmitis; Uveitis and Retinitis

Candice E. Johnson, MD, PhD

Professor of Pediatrics, University of Colorado School of Medicine, University of Colorado Health Sciences Center, and Attending Pediatrician, The Children's Hospital, Denver, Colorado

Otitis Media

Naynesh Kamani, MD

Professor, Department of Pediatrics, George Washington University School of Medicine and Health Sciences, and Director, Immunology and Stem Cell Transplantation, Children's National Medical Center, Washington, DC

Evaluation of Immune Function; Primary Immune Deficiency Disorders

Peter J. Krause, MD

Professor of Pediatrics, University of Connecticut School of Medicine, Farmington, Connecticut, and Director of Pediatric Infectious Diseases, Connecticut Children's Medical Center, Hartford, Connecticut
Human Ehrlichiosis; Malaria; Babesiosis

Mary L. Kumar, MD

Professor of Pediatrics and Pathology, Case Western Reserve University School of Medicine, and Chief, Pediatric Infectious Diseases, Metrohealth Medical Center, Cleveland, Ohio
Immunizations

Charles T. Leach, MD

Associate Professor, Department of Pediatrics, Division of Infectious Diseases, The University of Texas Health Science Center at San Antonio, and Attending Physician, University Hospital and CHRISTUS Santa Rosa Children's Hospital, San Antonio, Texas
Measles; Rubella; Roseola; Erythema Infectiosum (Fifth Disease); Chickenpox and Zoster; Mumps

Marc H. Lebel, MD, FREPC

Clinical Associate Professor, Division of Infectious Diseases, Department of Pediatrics, University of Montreal, and Attending Physician, Hôpital Sainte Justine, Montreal, Quebec, Canada
Bacteremia, Sepsis, and Septic Shock; Toxic Shock Syndrome

Colin D. Marchant, MD

Associate Professor of Pediatrics, Boston University School of Medicine and Tufts University School of Medicine, and Attending Pediatrician, Divisions of Pediatric Infectious Diseases, Boston Medical Center and New England Medical Center, Boston, Massachusetts
Immunizations

Richard I. Markowitz, M.D.

Professor of Radiology, University of Pennsylvania School of Medicine, and Radiologist, Children's Hospital of Philadelphia, Philadelphia, Pennsylvania
Diagnostic Imaging

Paul L. McCarthy, MD

Professor of Pediatrics, Yale University School of Medicine, and Head, General Pediatrics, Yale–New Haven Children's Hospital, New Haven, Connecticut
Approach to the Child with Fever; Fever and Occult Bacteremia in Infants and Young Children; Fever of Unknown Origin

Kathryn S. Moffett, MD

Assistant Professor of Pediatrics, West Virginia University School of Medicine, Morgantown, West Virginia
Osteomyelitis; Infectious Arthritis; Diskitis

Claudia P. Molina, MD

Fellow in Clinical Microbiology and Infectious Disease Pathology, University of Texas Medical Branch, Galveston, Texas
Diagnostic Pathology of Infectious Diseases

M. Susan Moyer, MD

Professor of Pediatrics and Chief, Section of Pediatric Gastroenterology/Hepatology, Yale University School of Medicine, and Attending Physician in Pediatrics, Yale–New Haven Children's Hospital, New Haven, Connecticut
Gastritis; Viral Hepatitis; Hepatic Abscess; Infections of the Biliary Tract; Acute Pancreatitis

Edward J. O'Rourke, MD

Assistant Professor of Pediatrics, Harvard Medical School, Boston, Massachusetts
Intra-abdominal and Retroperitoneal Infections

Gary D. Overturf, MD

Professor of Pediatrics, University of New Mexico School of Medicine, and Director of Pediatric Infectious Diseases, Children's Hospital of New Mexico, Albuquerque, New Mexico
Urinary Tract Infections; Infections of the Lower Genitourinary Tract

Sheral S. Patel, MD

Instructor, Division of Pediatric Infectious Diseases and Division of Geographic Medicine, Case Western Reserve University, and Instructor, Division of Pediatric Infectious Diseases, Department of Pediatrics, Rainbow Babies and Children's Hospital, Cleveland, Ohio
Brain and Parameningeal Abscess

Sarah A. Rawstron, MBBS

Assistant Professor of Pediatrics and Medicine, State University of New York Downstate Medical Center, and Attending (Pediatrics), Kings County Hospital Medical Center, Brooklyn, New York
Vulvovaginitis; Sexually Transmitted Infections

Michael D. Reed, PharmD

Professor of Pediatrics, Case Western Reserve University School of Medicine, and Director, Pediatric Clinical Pharmacology and Toxicology, Rainbow Babies and Children's Hospital, Cleveland, Ohio
Anti-infective Therapy

William J. Rodriguez, MD, PhD

Professor Emeritus of Pediatrics, George Washington Medical School, and Science Director for Pediatrics, Pediatric Team, Center for Drug Evaluation and Research, U.S. Food and Drug Administration, Washington, DC
Acute Enteritis

Anne H. Rowley, MD

Associate Professor of Pediatrics, Microbiology/Immunology, Northwestern University Medical School, and Attending Physician, Division of Pediatric Infectious Diseases, Children's Memorial Hospital, Chicago, Illinois
Kawasaki Syndrome

Tod S. Russell, MD

Assistant Professor of Pediatrics, Uniformed Services University of the Health Sciences, Bethesda, Maryland, and Chief, Pediatric Infectious Diseases, Wilford Hall Medical Center, San Antonio, Texas
Mediastinitis; Esophagitis

John R. Schreiber, MD, MPH

Professor of Pediatrics and Pathology, Case Western Reserve University School of Medicine, and Chief, Division of Pediatric Infectious Diseases, Rainbow Babies and Children's Hospital, Cleveland, Ohio
Brain and Parameningeal Abscesses

Kathryn Schwarzenberger, MD

Associate Professor of Dermatology and Medicine, Medical University of South Carolina, Charleston, South Carolina
Cutaneous Signs of Systemic Infections; Superficial Cutaneous Infections

Eugene D. Shapiro, MD

Professor, Departments of Pediatrics and of Epidemiology and Public Health, and of the Investigative Medicine Program, Yale University School of Medicine, and Attending Pediatrician, Yale–New Haven Children's Hospital and the Children's Clinical Research Center, New Haven, Connecticut

Lyme Disease

Stanford T. Shulman, MD

Professor of Pediatrics, Northwestern University Medical School, and Chief, Division of Infectious Diseases, Children's Memorial Hospital, Chicago, Illinois

Kawasaki Syndrome

Paul A. Shurin, MD

Associate Professor of Pediatrics, Albert Einstein College of Medicine, and Associate Pediatrician, Montefiore Medical Center, Bronx, New York

Otitis Externa; Otitis Media

Robert Sidbury, MD

Acting Assistant Professor, Department of Pediatrics and Dermatology, Children's Hospital and Regional Medical Center, University of Washington School of Medicine, Seattle, Washington

Cutaneous Signs of Systemic Infections; Superficial Cutaneous Infections

Nalini Singh, MD, MPH

Professor of Pediatrics, Epidemiology, and International Health, George Washington University Schools of Medicine and Public Health, Washington, DC

Acute Enteritis

Michael B. Smith, MD

Assistant Professor of Pathology and Associate Director of Clinical Microbiology and Information Systems, Department of Pathology, University of Texas Medical Branch, Galveston, Texas

Diagnostic Pathology of Infectious Diseases

Janet Squires, MD

Associate Professor of Pediatrics, University of Texas Southwestern Medical Center of Dallas, and Director, Pediatric Human Immunodeficiency Virus Program, Children's Medical Center of Dallas, Dallas, Texas

Human Immunodeficiency Virus and Acquired Immunodeficiency Syndrome

Lawrence R. Stanberry, MD, PhD

Chairman, Department of Pediatrics, Director, Center for Vaccine Development, and John Sealy Distinguished Chair and Professor, University of Texas Medical Branch, Galveston, Texas

Perinatal Viral Infections

Jeffrey R. Starke, MD

Associate Professor of Pediatrics, Baylor College of Medicine, and Chief of Pediatrics and Director, Children's Tuberculosis Clinic, Ben Taub General Hospital, Houston, Texas

Tuberculosis

Bruce Tapiero, MD, FRCP(C)

Assistant Professor of Pediatrics, University of Montreal Division of Infectious Diseases and Hôpital Sainte-Justine, Montreal, Quebec, Canada

Bacteremia, Sepsis, and Septic Shock; Toxic Shock Syndrome

Sam R. Telford III, DSc

Lecturer in Tropical Public Health, Harvard School of Public Health, and Adjunct Assistant Professor of Medicine, Tufts University School of Medicine, Boston, Massachusetts

Human Ehrlichiosis

James K. Todd, MD

Professor of Pediatrics, Microbiology, and Preventive Medicine, University of Colorado School of Medicine, and Director of Epidemiology and Clinical Microbiology, The Children's Hospital, Denver, Colorado

Microbial Virulence Factors

Philip Toltzis, MD

Associate Professor of Pediatrics, Case Western Reserve University School of Medicine, and Attending Pediatrician, Rainbow Babies and Children's Hospital, Cleveland, Ohio

Infectious Encephalitis; Peripheral Neuropathy and Myelopathy

Ronald B. Turner, MD

Professor of Pediatrics, University of Virginia, Charlottesville, Virginia

The Common Cold; Pharyngitis

Ellen R. Wald, MD

Professor of Pediatrics, University of Pittsburgh School of Medicine, and Chief, Division of Allergy, Immunology and Infectious Diseases, Children's Hospital of Pittsburgh, Pittsburgh, Pennsylvania

Sinusitis; Infections in Daycare Environments

A. Brian West, MD, FRCPath

Professor of Pathology and Director of Anatomic Pathology, New York University School of Medicine, New York, New York

Diagnostic Pathology of Infectious Diseases

Ram Yogev, MD

Professor of Pediatrics, Northwestern University Medical School, Associate Division Head, Division of Infectious Diseases, and Director, Section of Pediatric and Maternal Human Immunodeficiency Virus Infection, Children's Memorial Hospital, Chicago, Illinois

Meningitis; Central Nervous System Shunt-Related Infections

Kenneth M. Zangwill, MD

Associate Professor of Pediatrics, University of California at Los Angeles School of Medicine, Los Angeles, California, and Harbor–University of California at Los Angeles Medical Center, Torrance, California

Cat-Scratch Disease

Preface

This book is written for practitioners in pediatrics and family medicine and for consultants in pediatric infectious diseases. Our objective has been to make this a practical and useful resource for those involved in the clinical care of infants, children, and adolescents in office, clinic, and hospital settings.

This edition has been extensively revised from the first edition. New chapters have been added on cat-scratch disease, ehrlichiosis, and infections associated with central nervous system shunts and intravascular devices to reflect the increasing importance of these infections in pediatric medicine. Existing chapters have all been thoroughly updated, rewritten, and condensed to provide easier access to essential information while maintaining a comprehensive approach.

We have chosen a primarily syndrome-oriented organization of the discipline of pediatric infectious diseases, which reflects the problems that confront practitioners. To provide consistency among chapters and to facilitate access to desired information, authors of syndrome-oriented chapters have organized their topics within the framework of a common outline. The emphasis of this book is on diagnosis, treatment, and prevention. Ancillary information such as microbiology and pathogenesis is presented to enhance understanding of the logic of management. We have attempted to avoid the bulk of encyclopedic texts, extensive reference lists, and the fragmentation and separation of related information that results from duplicate approaches to infectious disease topics (syndrome-oriented and organism-oriented), which impedes the ability to readily find usable information to guide management. Broadly applicable information related to pathogenesis, normal flora, epidemiology, immunology, diagnostic methods, anti-infective therapy, immunotherapy, prophylaxis, immunizations, and fever are found in separate chapters that provide additional depth of information. Keywords and terms are indicated in bold in the text, and selected citations to reviews and key references to the most important studies are listed for each topic. Additional references including updated references for each chapter are regularly posted at http://www.pedid.uthscsa.edu.

The scope of this book is infectious diseases and related issues faced by practitioners who provide care for infants and children, with an emphasis on diseases endemic in North America. Tropical diseases such as malaria and certain helminth infections that are occasionally imported by travelers and new residents are included. This text may be complemented by specialty texts of microbiology and tropical medicine.

All of the contributors are actively engaged in the practice of medicine, have academic affiliations, and are recognized for their expertise in pediatric infectious diseases or in related areas including immunology, diagnostic microbiology, pathology, diagnostic imaging, dermatology, gastroenterology, and ophthalmology. Contributors have been given latitude in presenting their own views where there are differences of opinion in the community of experts in infectious diseases. There may be slight differences between different chapters in the recommended use of diagnostic tests and treatment for similar disease. This reflects the range of opinion in our specialty and the lack of definitive clinical studies of some infections. It has, however, been our intention to keep such differences to a minimum.

This text represents the efforts of 71 contributors who have enthusiastically shared their knowledge and judgment and who have patiently and cheerfully complied with our requests. Many contributors have selflessly contributed figures and provided editorial assistance for chapters other than their own. We sincerely and gratefully acknowledge the hard work and diligent efforts of the contributors and also the expert assistance provided by our new publishers, W.B. Saunders Co., especially Dolores Meloni, Lisette Bralow, Faith Voit, Joan Sinclair, and Mary Espenschied, editorial supervisor.

Finally, we thank Polly Jenson and Katalin Baltimore for their patience and understanding, without which this book and many other wonderful parts of our lives would not have been possible.

Hal B. Jenson, MD
Robert S. Baltimore, MD

NOTICE

Contents

MICROBIAL PATHOGENESIS

1. Microbial Virulence Factors, 1
James K. Todd

2. Normal Microbial Flora, 6
Robert S. Baltimore and Hal B. Jenson

3. Epidemiology of Infectious Diseases, 11
John C. Christenson

4. Infectious Agents and Oncogenesis, 23
Hal B. Jenson

HOST DEFENSES

5. Host Defenses Against Infection, 31
Anthony J. Infante

6. Evaluation of Immune Function, 51
Anthony J. Infante and Naynesh Kamani

DIAGNOSTIC METHODS

7. Diagnostic Microbiology, 57
Joseph M. Campos

8. Diagnostic Parasitology, 80
Joseph M. Campos

9. Diagnostic Virology, 84
Joseph M. Campos

10. Laboratory Evaluation of the Inflammatory Response, 92
Robert S. Baltimore and Hal B. Jenson

11. Serologic Diagnosis of Infectious Diseases, 99
Joseph M. Campos and Hal B. Jenson

12. Diagnostic Pathology of Infectious Diseases, 116
Claudia P. Molina, Michael B. Smith, and A. Brian West

13. Diagnostic Imaging, 126
Richard I. Markowitz

THERAPY AND PROPHYLAXIS OF INFECTIOUS DISEASES

14. Anti-infective Therapy, 147
Michael D. Reed and Jeffrey L. Blumer

Antibacterial Drugs, 153
Antifungal Drugs, 190
Antiviral Drugs, 196
Antiretroviral Drugs, 202
Antimycobacterial Drugs, 205
Antiparasitic Drugs, 208
Antiprotozoal Drugs, 208
Anthelmintic Drugs, 209
Antimalarial Drugs, 211

15. Immunotherapy and Immunomodulation, 216
Gerald W. Fischer

16. Prophylaxis of Infectious Diseases, 225
Robert S. Baltimore

IMMUNIZATIONS

17. Immunizations, 232
Colin D. Marchant and Mary L. Kumar

FEVER

18. Approach to the Child with Fever, 263
Paul L. McCarthy

19. Fever and Occult Bacteremia in Infants and Young Children, 268
M. Douglas Baker and Paul L. McCarthy

Children Older than 8 Weeks of Age, 268
Infants Younger than 8 Weeks of Age, 272

20. Fever of Unknown Origin 275
Paul L. McCarthy

SYSTEMIC INFECTIONS

Bacteremia and Shock

21. Bacteremia, Sepsis, and Septic Shock, 279
Marc H. Lebel and Bruce Tapiero

22. Toxic Shock Syndrome, 296
Bruce Tapiero and Marc H. Lebel

Systemic Infections Characterized Primarily by Rash

23. Measles, 306
Charles T. Leach and Hal B. Jenson

24. Rubella, 316
Charles T. Leach and Hal B. Jenson

25. Roseola, 321
Charles T. Leach and Hal B. Jenson

26. Erythema Infectiosum (Fifth Disease), 325
Charles T. Leach and Hal B. Jenson

27. Chickenpox and Zoster, 331
Hal B. Jenson and Charles T. Leach

Zoonoses and Vectorborne Infections

28. Cat-Scratch Disease, 343
Kenneth M. Zangwill

29. Lyme Disease, 348
Eugene D. Shapiro

30. Rocky Mountain Spotted Fever, 354
John C. Christenson

31. Human Ehrlichiosis, 359
Sam R. Telford III and Peter J. Krause

32. Malaria, 363
Peter J. Krause

33. Babesiosis, 375
Peter J. Krause

34. Other Zoonoses and Vectorborne Infections, 379
John C. Christenson

Brucellosis, 379
Tularemia, 382
Plague, 383
Leptospirosis, 385
Relapsing Fever, 387
Murine Typhus, 388
Q Fever, 390
Rickettsialpox, 391
Dengue Fever, 392
Colorado Tick Fever, 393

Other Systemic Infections

35. Tuberculosis, 396
Jeffrey R. Starke

36. Mumps, 420
Hal B. Jenson and Charles T. Leach

37. Infectious Mononucleosis, 426
Hal B. Jenson

38. Human Immunodeficiency Virus and Acquired Immunodeficiency Syndrome, 437
Terence I. Doran and Janet Squires

39. Kawasaki Syndrome, 479
Anne H. Rowley and Stanford T. Shulman

40. Rheumatic Fever and Poststreptococcal Glomerulonephritis, 486
Michael A. Gerber

Rheumatic Fever, 486
Poststreptococcal Glomerulonephritis, 493

41. Chronic Fatigue Syndrome, 497
Hal B. Jenson

HELMINTH INFECTIONS

42. Nematode Infections, 504
Peter J. Hotez

Hookworm Infection, 504
Trichuriasis, 507
Ascariasis, 508
Toxocariasis and Baylisascariasis (Visceral and Ocular Larva Migrans), 511
Strongyloidiasis, 512
Enterobiasis (Pinworm), 514
Trichinellosis (Trichinosis), 515
Angiostrongyliasis, 517
Filariasis, 518

43. Trematode Infections, 521
Peter J. Hotez

Schistosomiasis, 521

44. Cestode Infections, 525
Peter J. Hotez

Cysticercosis, 525
Echinococcosis, 527
Adult Tapeworm Infections, 530

SKIN AND SOFT TISSUE INFECTIONS

45. Cutaneous Signs of Systemic Infections, 533
Kathryn Schwarzenberger and Robert Sidbury

46. Superficial Cutaneous Infections, 544
Robert Sidbury and Kathryn Schwarzenberger

Bacterial Infections, 544
- Impetigo, 544
- Folliculitis, Furuncles, and Carbuncles, 545
- Acne Vulgaris, 547
- Erythrasma, 549
- Pitted Keratolysis, 549
- Blistering Distal Dactylitis, 549
- Perianal Dermatitis, 550
- Decubitus Ulcers, 550
- Anthrax, 551

Mycobacterial Infections, 552
- Leprosy, 552
- Cutaneous Nontuberculous Mycobacterial Infections, 555

Fungal Infections, 556
- Tinea Capitis, 556
- Cutaneous Dermatophyte Infections, 558
- Tinea Versicolor, 560
- Cutaneous and Oral Candidiasis, 560
- Sporotrichosis, 563

Viral Infections, 564
- Herpes Simplex Virus, 564
- Human Papillomaviruses, 566
- Molluscum Contagiosum, 568

Parasitic Infections, 569
- Cutaneous Larva Migrans, 569
- Cutaneous Leishmaniasis, 570

Infestations, 571
- Myiasis, 571
- Scabies, 571
- Other Mite Infestations, 573
- Pediculosis (Lice), 573

47. Cellulitis, 578
John S. Bradley
Cellulitis of the Extremities and Trunk, 578
Cellulitis of the Head and Neck, 581

48. Wound and Deep-Tissue Infections, 587
John S. Bradley

49. Burn Wound Infections, 596
John S. Bradley

50. Bite-Wound Infections, 602
John S. Bradley

51. Lymphadenopathy, Lymphadenitis, and Lymphangitis, 610
Toni Darville and Richard F. Jacobs
Generalized Lymphadenopathy, 611
Inguinal Lymphadenopathy and Lymphadenitis, 615
Cervical Lymphadenopathy and Lymphadenitis, 619
Lymphangitis, 626

NERVOUS SYSTEM INFECTIONS

52. Meningitis, 630
Ram Yogev

53. Central Nervous System Shunt-Related Infections, 651
Ram Yogev

54. Brain and Parameningeal Abscesses 657
Sheral S. Patel and John R. Schreiber
Brain Abscess, 657
Subdural Empyema and Cranial Epidural Abscess, 664
Spinal Epidural Abscess, 665

55. Infectious Encephalitis, 669
Philip Toltzis
Herpes Simplex Virus Encephalitis, 670
Arboviruses, 673
Arboviruses in the United States, 674
Arboviruses Outside the United States, 675
Enteroviruses, 676
Lymphocytic Choriomeningitis Virus, 677
Rabies, 678
Systemic Infections Occasionally Associated with Encephalitis, 680
Slow Infections of the Central Nervous System, 682
Human Immunodeficiency Virus Infection, 683
Subacute Sclerosing Panencephalitis, 684
Progressive Rubella Encephalitis, 685
Progressive Multifocal Leukoencephalopathy, 685
Transmissible Spongiform Encephalopathies, 685
Reye's Syndrome, 687

56. Peripheral Neuropathy and Myelopathy, 692
Philip Toltzis
Peripheral Neuropathies, 692
Tetanus, 692
Botulism, 695
Poliomyelitis, 698
Guillain-Barré Syndrome, 701
Neuropathies Associated with Multisystem Infections, 703
Diphtheria, 703
Leprosy, 703
Lyme Disease, 704
Human Immunodeficiency Virus Infection, 704
Myelopathy, 704
Human T-Cell Leukemia/Lymphoma Virus Type I Infection, 704

OROPHARYNGEAL INFECTIONS

57. The Common Cold, 707
Ronald B. Turner and Gregory F. Hayden

58. Pharyngitis, 711
Gregory F. Hayden and Ronald B. Turner

59. Infections of the Deep Fascial Spaces of the Neck, 721
Charles W. Gross and Scott E. Harrison

60. Stomatitis, 728
Celia D.C. Christie

61. Dental Infections, 734
Theodore J. Cieslak

62. Parotitis and Sialadenitis, 741
Celia D.C. Christie

EAR AND PARANASAL SINUS INFECTIONS

63. Otitis Externa, 745
Paul A. Shurin

64. Otitis Media, 748
Candice E. Johnson and Paul A. Shurin

65. Sinusitis, 760
Ellen R. Wald

LOWER RESPIRATORY TRACT AND CHEST INFECTIONS

66. Middle Respiratory Tract Infections, 771
Louis M. Bell
Acute Laryngotracheobronchitis, 771
Epiglottitis, 774
Bacterial Tracheitis, 777

67. Bronchitis, Bronchiolitis, and Pertussis Syndrome, 779
Robert S. Baltimore
Bronchitis, 780
Bronchiolitis, 784
Pertussis Syndrome (Whooping Cough), 788

68. Pneumonia, 794
Robert S. Baltimore
Initial Approach to Pneumonia, 794

Bacterial Pneumonia, 803
Streptococcus pneumoniae Pneumonia, 803
Legionellosis, 805
Mycoplasma pneumoniae Pneumonia, 807
Chlamydial Pneumonia, 809
Chlamydia trachomatis Pneumonia, 809
Chlamydia psittaci Pneumonia, 810
Chlamydia pneumoniae Pneumonia, 811
Fungal Pneumonias, 812
Histoplasmosis, 813
Aspergillosis, 814
Cryptococcal Pneumonia, 815
Coccidioidomycosis, 816
Blastomycosis, 816
Candida Pneumonia, 817
Viral Pneumonias, 817
Respiratory Syncytial Virus, 818
Parainfluenza Virus, 818
Adenovirus, 819
Influenza Virus, 819
Enterovirus, 822
Hantavirus Cardiopulmonary Syndrome, 822
Pneumocystis carinii Pneumonia, 824
Aspiration Pneumonia and "Foreign Body" Pneumonia, 826
Nosocomial Pneumonia Including Ventilator-Associated Pneumonia (VAP), 829

69. Pleural Effusion, Empyema, and Lung Abscess, 832
Robert S. Baltimore
Pleural Effusion and Empyema, 832
Lung Abscess, 837

70. Mediastinitis, 842
Tod S. Russell and David P. Ascher

CARDIOVASCULAR INFECTIONS

71. Infective Endocarditis, 845
Robert S. Baltimore

72. Acute Myocarditis, 857
Michael Cappello

73. Acute Pericarditis, 863
Michael Cappello

GASTROINTESTINAL AND ABDOMINAL INFECTIONS

74. Esophagitis, 869
Tod S. Russell and David P. Ascher

75. Gastritis, 872
M. Susan Moyer and Hal B. Jenson

76. Acute Enteritis, 878
Nalini Singh and William J. Rodriguez
Dysenteric Syndromes, 879
Nontyphoidal *Salmonella,* 879
Salmonella typhi (Typhoid Fever), 882
Shigella, 885
Yersinia enterocolitica, 887
Campylobacter, 888
Aeromonas, 890
Amebiasis, 891
Enterotoxigenic Syndromes, 893
Vibrio cholerae (Cholera), 893
Escherichia coli Syndromes, 895
Viral Enteritis, 898
Rotavirus, 898
Enteric Adenoviruses, 900
Norwalk Virus, 900
Astroviruses, 901
Coronaviruses, 901
Chronic Infectious Diarrhea, 901
Giardiasis, 901
Dientamoeba fragilis, 902
Intestinal Spore-forming Coccidian Protozoa, 904
Travelers' Diarrhea, 906
Foodborne and Waterborne Infections, 908
Toxin-associated Illness, 911
Clostridium difficile–Associated Diarrhea, 912
Hemolytic Uremic Syndrome, 913
Whipple's Disease, 916
Supportive Treatment of Acute Enteritis, 916

77. Intra-abdominal and Retroperitoneal Infections, 921
Edward J. O'Rourke
Intra-abdominal and Pelvic Abscesses, 923
Peritonitis, 928
Acute Appendicitis, 931
Splenic Abscess, 936
Retroperitoneal and Psoas Infections, 938
Anorectal Abscess, 940

HEPATOBILIARY AND PANCREATIC INFECTIONS

78. Viral Hepatitis, 943
M. Susan Moyer and Hal B. Jenson

79. Hepatic Abscess, 963
M. Susan Moyer and Hal B. Jenson

80. Infections of the Biliary Tract, 970
M. Susan Moyer and Hal B. Jenson
Cholecystitis, 970
Cholangitis, 972

81. Acute Pancreatitis, 977
M. Susan Moyer and Hal B. Jenson

GENITOURINARY TRACT INFECTIONS

82. Urinary Tract Infections, 983
Gary D. Overturf

83. Infections of the Lower Genitourinary Tract, 992
Gary D. Overturf
Prostatitis, 992
Epididymitis, 993
Orchitis, 994
Urethritis, 995
Meatitis, 996
Balanitis, 996

84. Vulvovaginitis, 998
Sarah A. Rawstron

85. Sexually Transmitted Infections, 1009
Margaret R. Hammerschlag and Sarah A. Rawstron
Initial Approach to Sexually Transmitted Diseases, 1009
Urethritis and Cervicitis, 1010
Gonorrhea, 1010
Chlamydia trachomatis Infection, 1016
Genital Ulcers, 1019
Syphilis, 1019
Herpes Simplex Virus Infection, 1023
Chancroid, 1025
Donovanosis, 1026
Lymphogranuloma Venereum, 1027
Vaginal Discharge, 1027
Trichomoniasis, 1027
Human Papillomavirus Infection, 1029
Sexually Transmitted Infections and Sexual Assault, 1030

SKELETAL INFECTIONS

86. Osteomyelitis, 1034
Kathryn S. Moffett and Stephen C. Aronoff

87. Infectious Arthritis, 1044
Kathryn S. Moffett and Stephen C. Aronoff

88. Diskitis, 1051
Kathryn S. Moffett and Stephen C. Aronoff

OCULAR INFECTIONS

89. Bacterial and Viral Conjunctivitis, 1055
Albert W. Biglan and Hal B. Jenson
Neonatal Conjunctivitis, 1055
Bacterial and Viral Conjunctivitis, 1058

90. Keratitis, 1063
Albert W. Biglan and Hal B. Jenson

91. Infections of the Eyelids and Ocular Adnexa, 1069
Albert W. Biglan and Hal B. Jenson
Blepharitis, 1069
Hordeolum, 1070
Dacryocystitis, 1072

92. Endophthalmitis, 1074
Albert W. Biglan and Hal B. Jenson

93. Uveitis and Retinitis, 1080
Albert W. Biglan and Hal B. Jenson
Uveitis, 1080
Retinitis, 1082

INFECTIONS IN SPECIAL HOSTS

Infections of the Fetus and Newborn Infant

94. Pediatric Implications of Maternal Infection, 1085
Kenneth M. Boyer

95. Intrauterine Infections, 1099
Stuart P. Adler
Treponema pallidum, 1102
Cytomegalovirus, 1107
Herpes Simplex Virus, 1109
Varicella-Zoster Virus, 1110
Rubella Virus, 1111
Human Parvovirus B19, 1113
Lymphocytic Choriomeningitis Virus, 1113
Toxoplasma gondii, 1114

96. Perinatal Bacterial and Fungal Infections, 1119
Robert S. Baltimore
Sepsis, 1119
Focal Bacterial Infections, 1129
Necrotizing Enterocolitis, 1130
Fungal Infections, 1132

97. Perinatal Viral Infections, 1135
Rebecca C. Brady and Lawrence R. Stanberry
Herpes Simplex Virus, 1136
Varicella-Zoster Virus, 1140
Enteroviruses, 1143

Primary Immune Deficiencies

98. Primary Immune Deficiency Disorders, 1148
Anthony J. Infante and Naynesh Kamani
Nonspecific Causes of Increased Susceptibility to Infection, 1148
Primary Immune Deficiency Diseases, 1149

Secondary Immune Deficiencies

99. Patients with Cancer, 1156
Dennis A. Conrad

100. Transplant Recipients, 1168
Dennis A. Conrad

101. The Vulnerable Host, 1181
Dennis A. Conrad

Infections in Special Populations

102. Infections in Daycare Environments, 1187
Ellen R. Wald

103. The Immigrant, Refugee, or Internationally Adopted Child, 1194
Jerri Ann Jenista

104. The International Child Traveler, 1207
Jerri Ann Jenista

NOSOCOMIAL INFECTIONS AND INFECTION CONTROL

105. Nosocomial Infections and Infection Control, 1221
Margaret C. Fisher
Nosocomial Infections, 1223
Prevention of Nosocomial Infections, 1232
Employee Health, 1240

106. Infections Involving Intravascular Devices, 1246
Margaret C. Fisher

Index, 1253

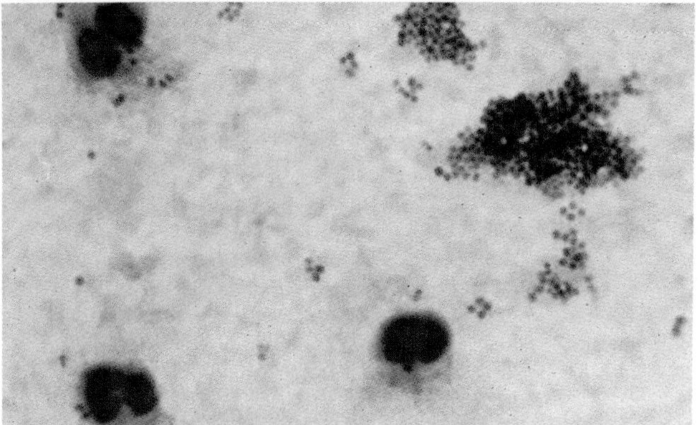

Plate 1A. Gram-stained smear of pus containing *Staphylococcus aureus.* (Courtesy Joseph M. Campos.)

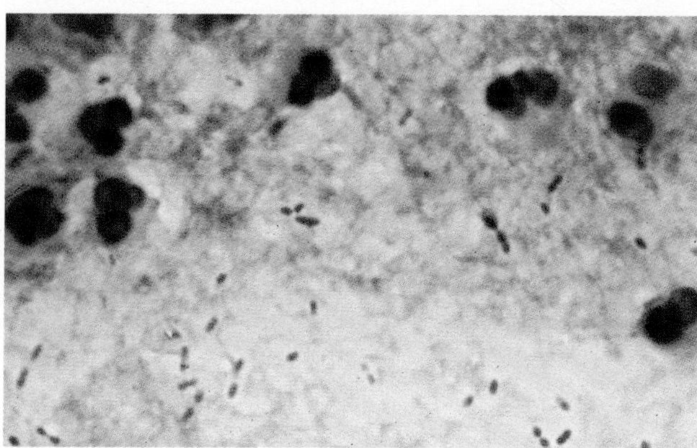

Plate 1B. Gram-stained smear of sputum containing *Streptococcus pneumoniae* (pneumococcus). (Courtesy Joseph M. Campos.)

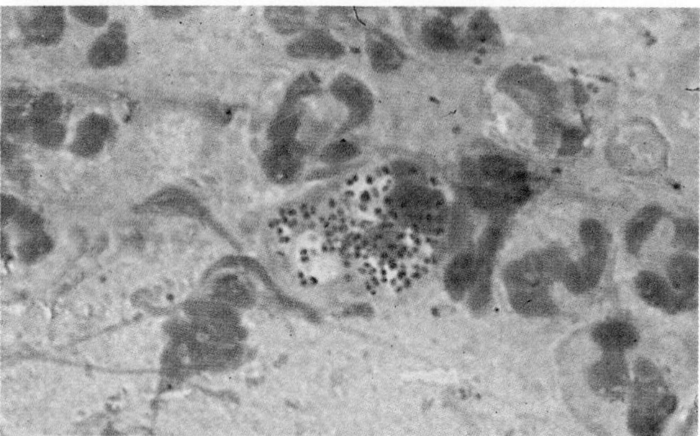

Plate 1C. Gram-stained smear of urethral discharge containing *Neisseria gonorrhoeae* (gonococcus). (Courtesy Joseph M. Campos.)

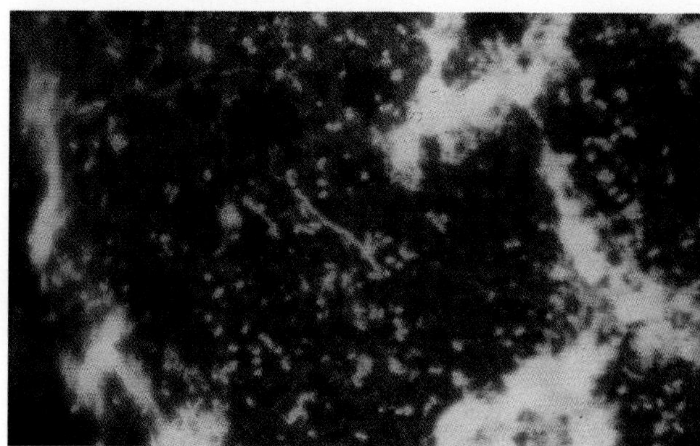

Plate 1D. Acridine-orange-stained smear of cerebrospinal fluid containing *Haemophilus influenzae* type b. (Courtesy Joseph M. Campos.)

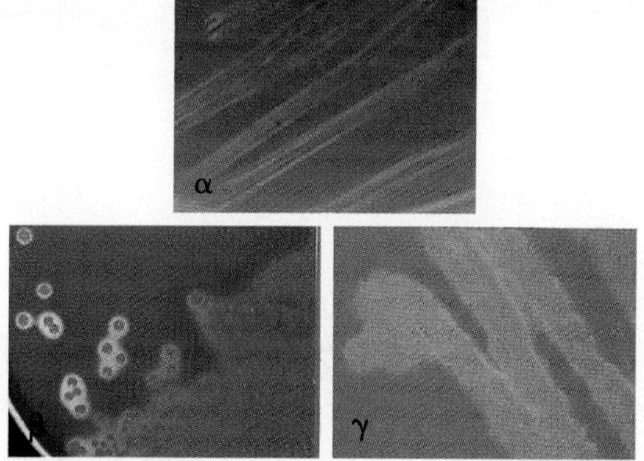

Plate 1E. Blood agar culture plate showing growth of bacteria demonstrating incomplete (α), complete (β), and absent (γ) hemolysis. (Courtesy Joseph M. Campos.)

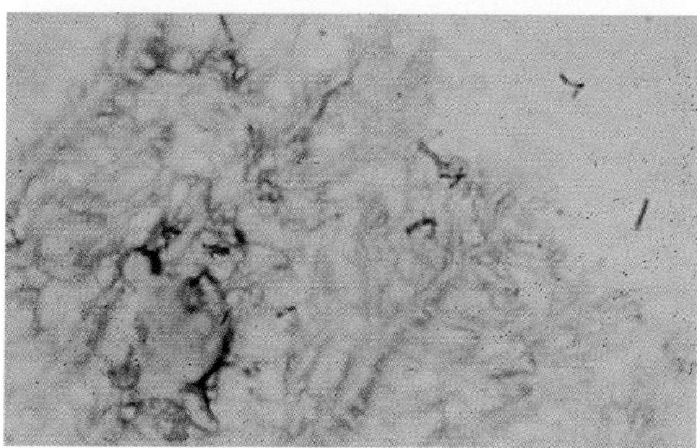

Plate 1F. Kinyoun-stained smear of sputum containing *Mycobacterium tuberculosis.* (Courtesy Joseph M. Campos.)

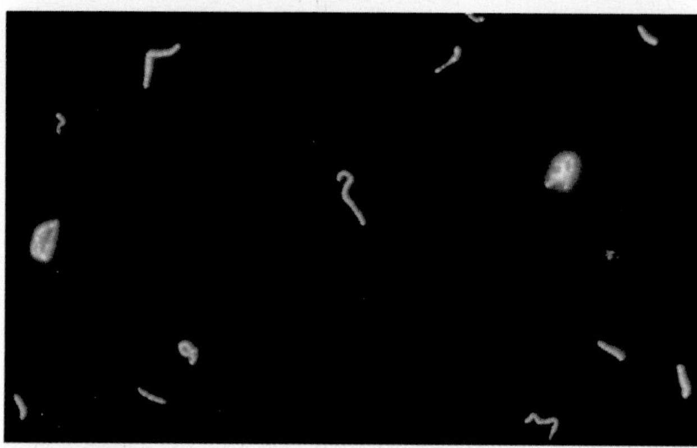

Plate 1G. Fluorochrome-stained smear of wound exudate containing *Mycobacterium kansasii.* (Courtesy Gerri S. Hall.)

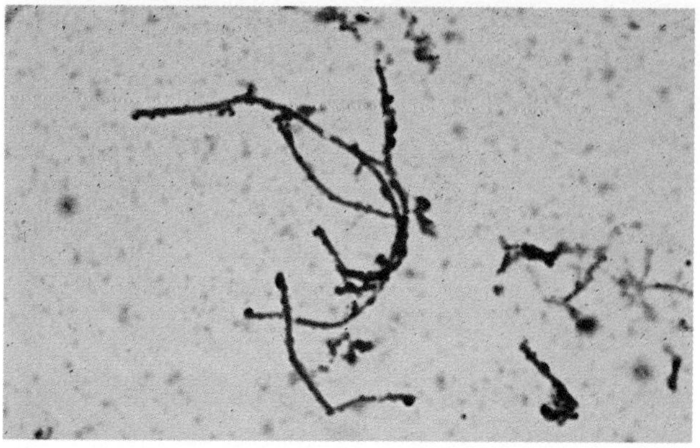

Plate 1H. Modified Kinyoun-stained smear of sputum containing *Nocardia* species. (Courtesy Joseph M. Campos.)

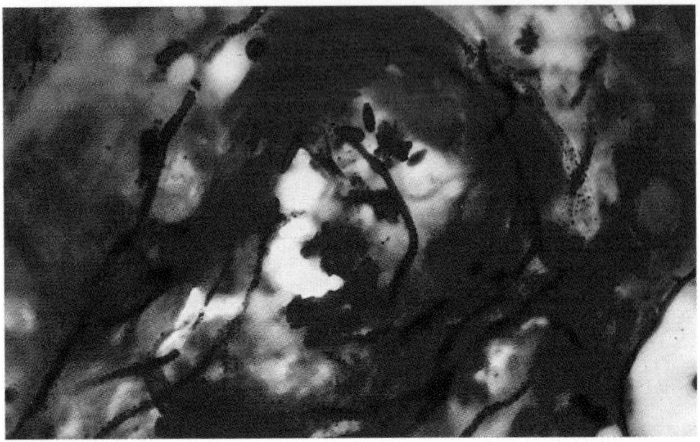

Plate 2A. Gram-stained smear of vaginal discharge containing *Candida albicans.* (Courtesy Joseph M. Campos.)

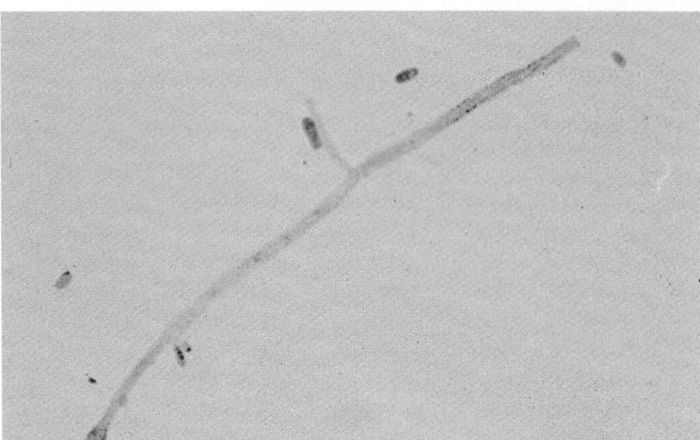

Plate 2B. Methylene-blue-stained smear of vaginal discharge containing *Candida albicans.* (Courtesy Joseph M. Campos.)

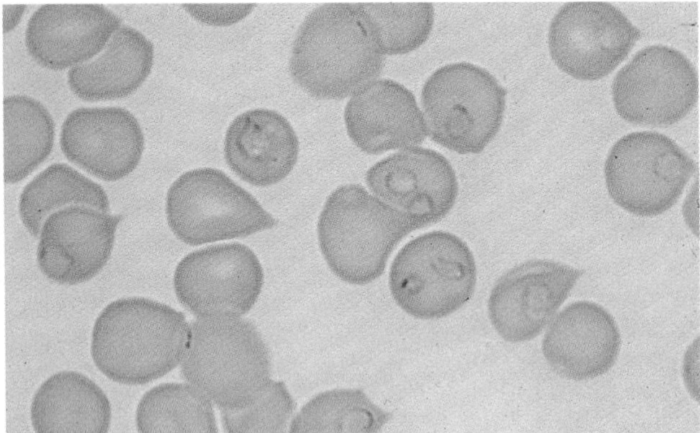

Plate 2C. Wright-stained smear of blood containing *Plasmodium falciparum* trophozoites. (Courtesy Joseph M. Campos.)

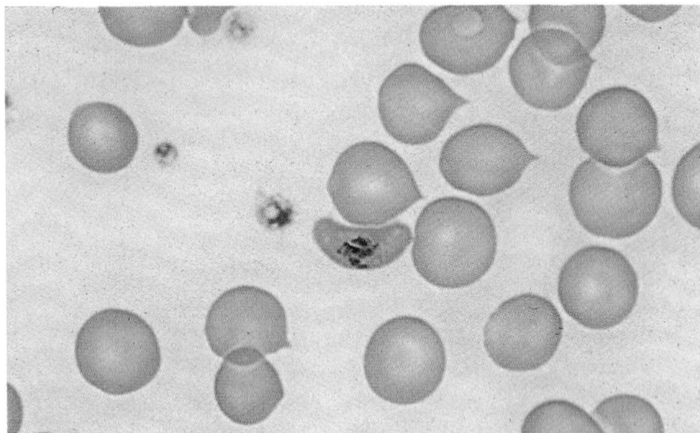

Plate 2D. Wright-stained smear of blood containing *Plasmodium falciparum* gametocyte. (Courtesy Joseph M. Campos.)

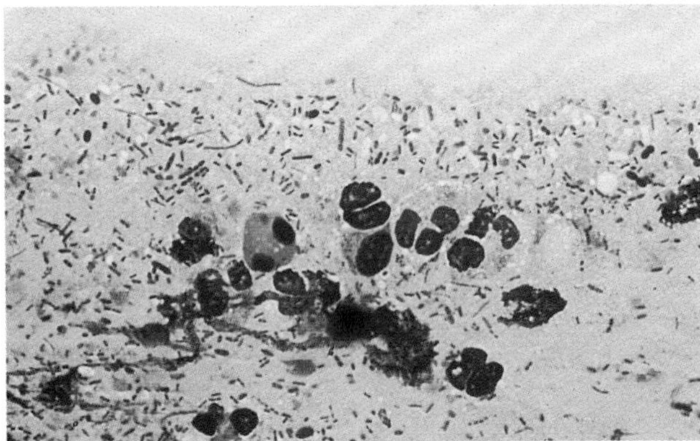

Plate 2E. Wright-stained smear of stool containing fecal leukocytes. (Courtesy Joseph M. Campos.)

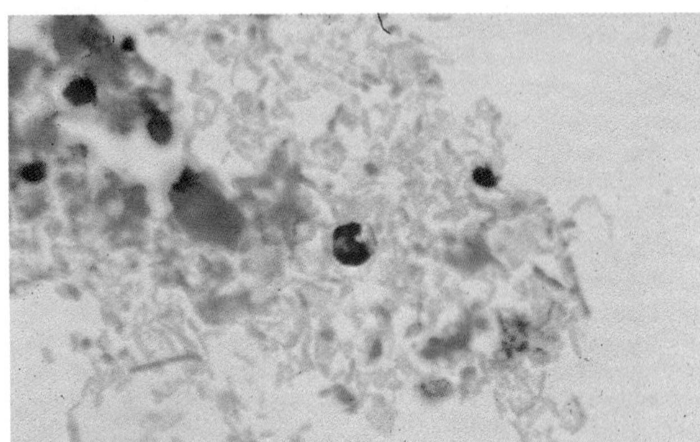

Plate 2F. Modified Kinyoun-stained smear of stool showing *Cryptosporidium parvum.* (Courtesy Joseph M. Campos.)

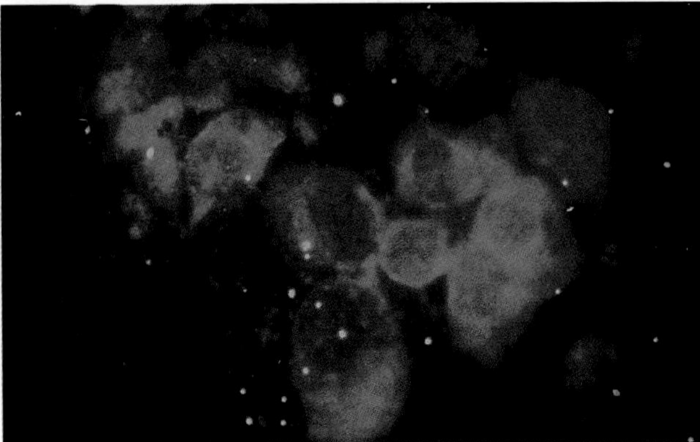

Plate 2G. Immunofluorescent staining of cervical smear containing extracellular elementary bodies (green objects) of *Chlamydia trachomatis.* (Courtesy Syva Company.)

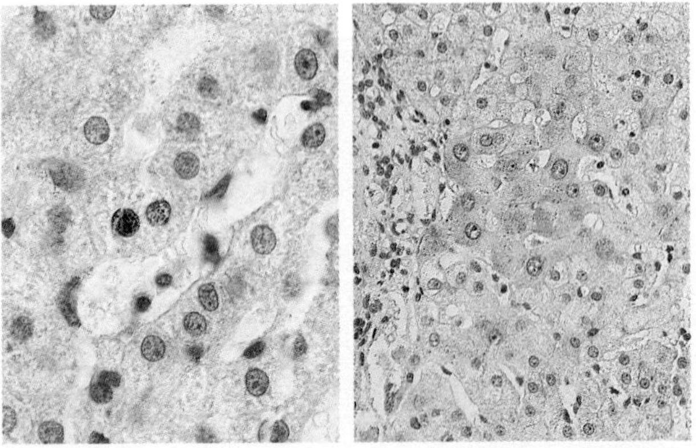

Plate 2H. Immunohistochemical stains of liver with hepatitis B for HBcAg (nuclear) and HBsAg (cytoplasmic). (Courtesy A. Brian West.)

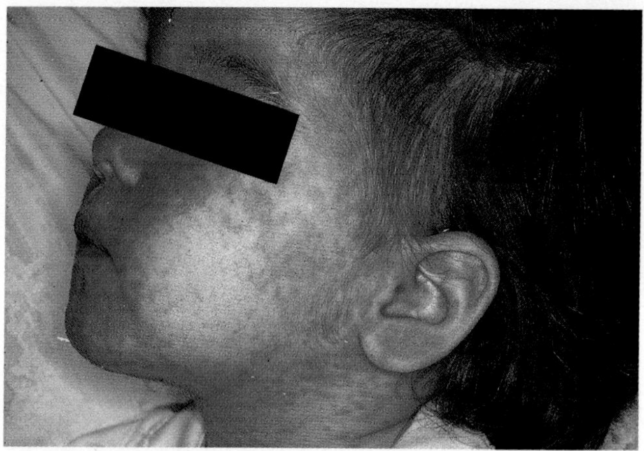

Plate 3A. Measles rash (rubeola). (Courtesy Warren A. Andiman.)

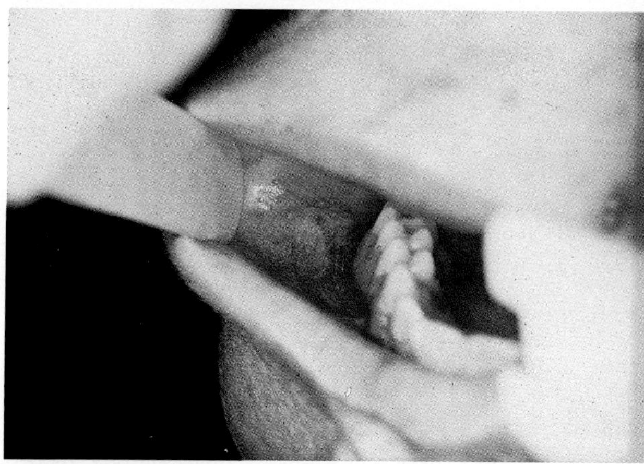

Plate 3B. Koplik spots in a patient with measles (rubeola). (Courtesy Warren A. Andiman.)

Plate 3C. Rubella rash (german measles). (Courtesy Warren A. Andiman.)

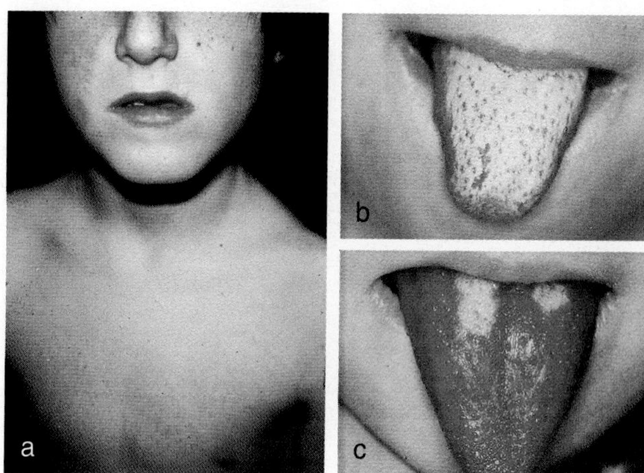

Plate 3D. Scarlet fever rash *(a)* and two variations of strawberry tongue—white strawberry tongue *(b)* and red strawberry tongue *(c)* caused by group A *Streptococcus.* (Courtesy Peter J. Krause.)

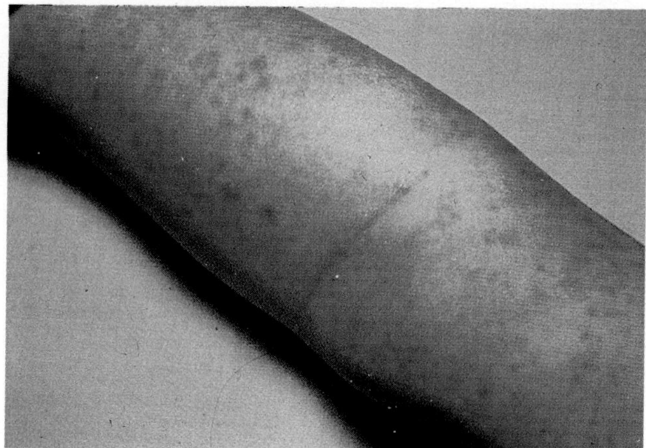

Plate 3E. Roseola rash (roseola infantum or exanthem subitum). (Courtesy Neil S. Prose.)

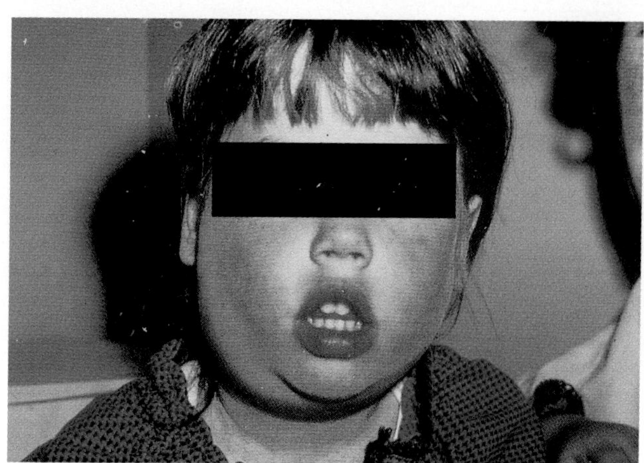

Plate 3F. Parotid swelling of mumps. (Courtesy James W. Bass.)

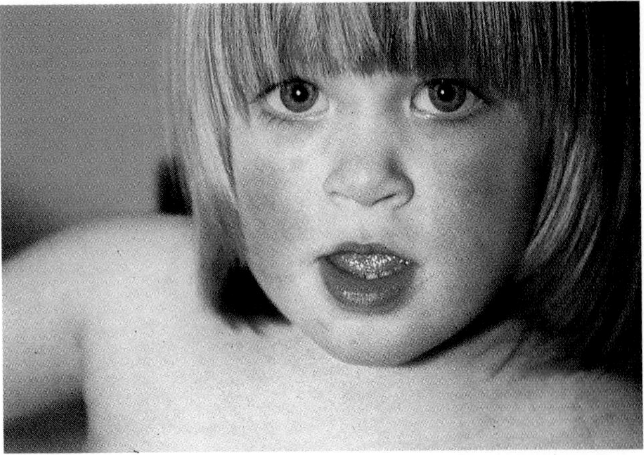

Plate 4A. Erythema infectiosum (fifth disease) facial rash ("slapped cheeks") on the first day of illness. (Courtesy Henry M. Feder, Jr.)

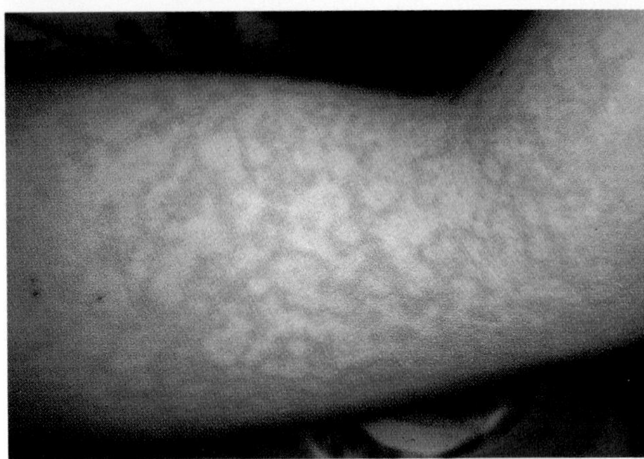

Plate 4B. Erythema infectiosum (fifth disease) reticular or lacelike rash on third day of illness, showing reticulated papules on the extremities. (Courtesy Kathryn Schwarzenberger.)

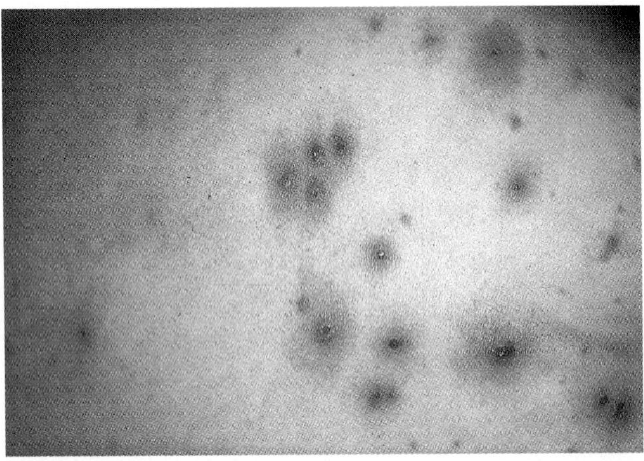

Plate 4C. Chickenpox (varicella) rash. (Courtesy Warren A. Andiman.)

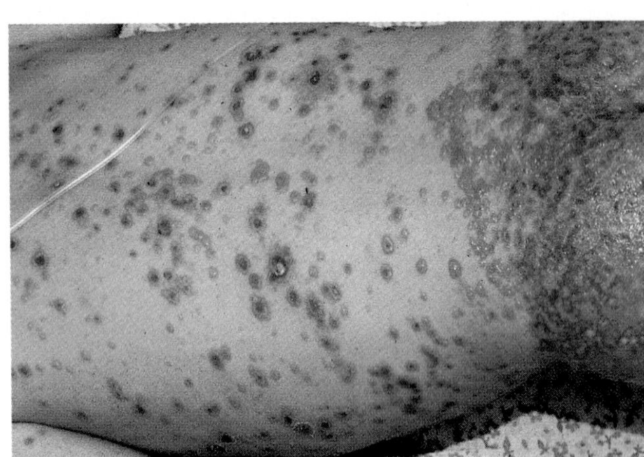

Plate 4D. Progressive varicella rash in an immunocompromised child. (Courtesy Hal B. Jenson.)

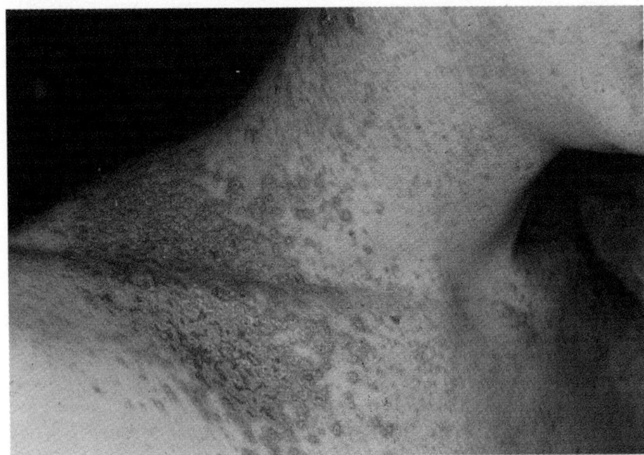

Plate 4E. Eczema herpeticum rash (Kaposi varicelliform eruption), caused by herpes simplex virus. (Courtesy Warren A. Andiman.)

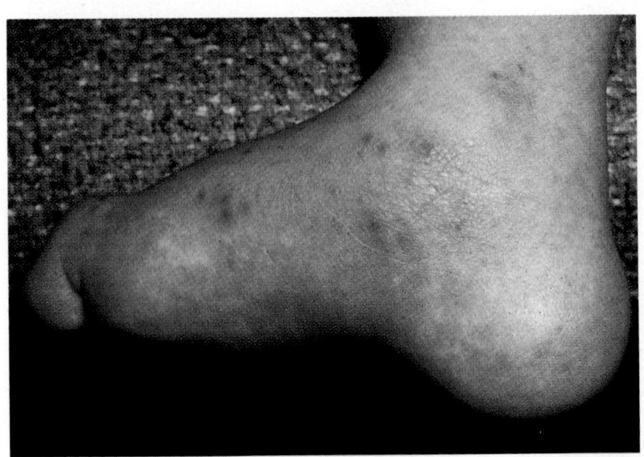

Plate 4F. Hand, foot, and mouth disease vesicular rash on the foot. (Courtesy Neil S. Prose.)

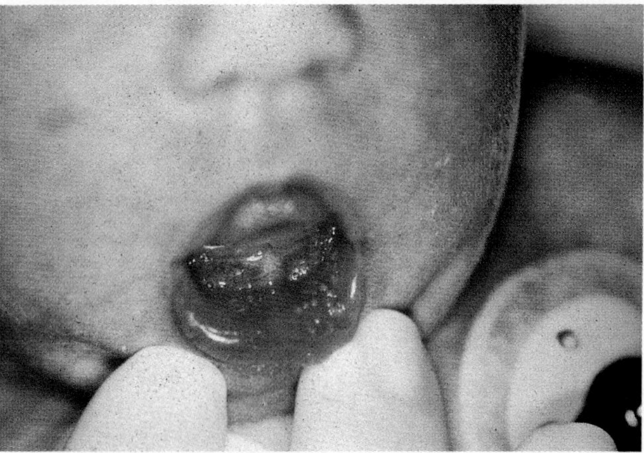

Plate 5A. Neonatal herpes simplex virus infection with vesicles on the oral mucosa. (Courtesy Beverly Connelly.)

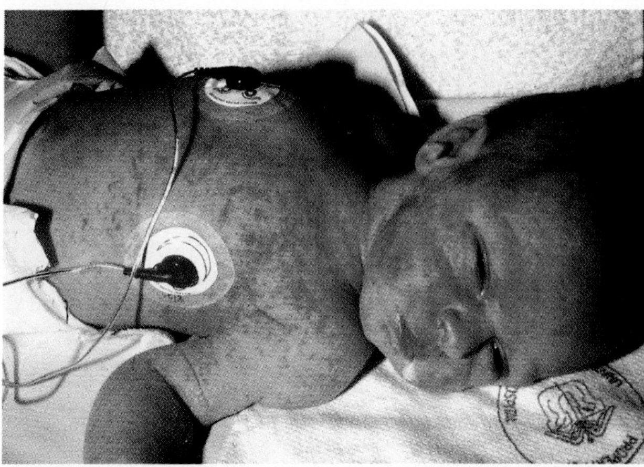

Plate 5B. Neonatal echovirus 11 infection rash. (Courtesy Lawrence R. Stanberry. From Stanberry LR, Glasgow LA: Viral infections of the fetus and newborn. In Stringfellow DA [editor]: *Virology.* Kalamazoo, Mich., Upjohn, 1988, p 102.)

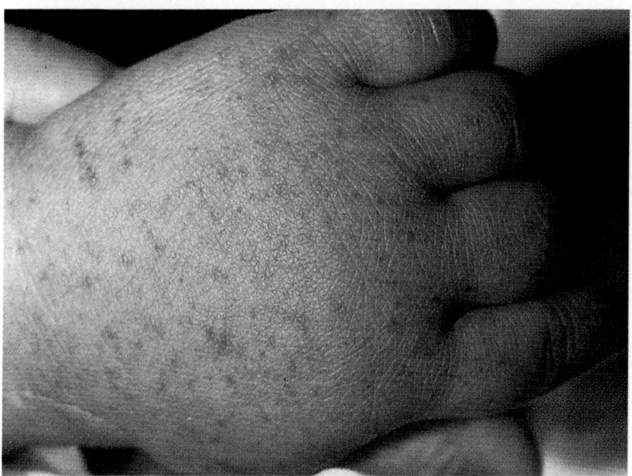

Plate 5C. Rocky Mountain spotted fever peripheral edema and rash. (Courtesy Neil S. Prose.)

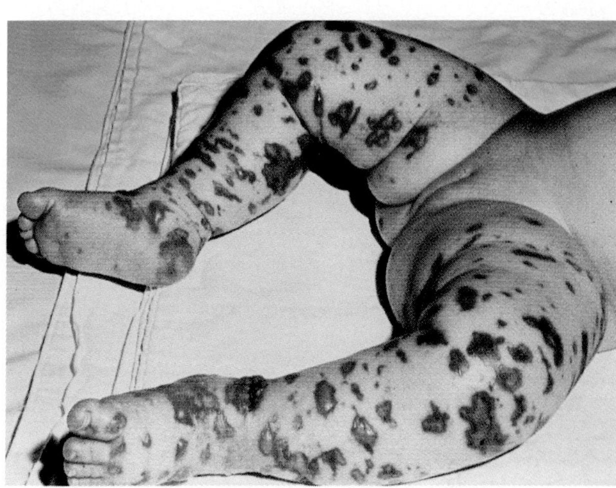

Plate 5D. Meningococcemia rash. (Courtesy Michel L. Weber.)

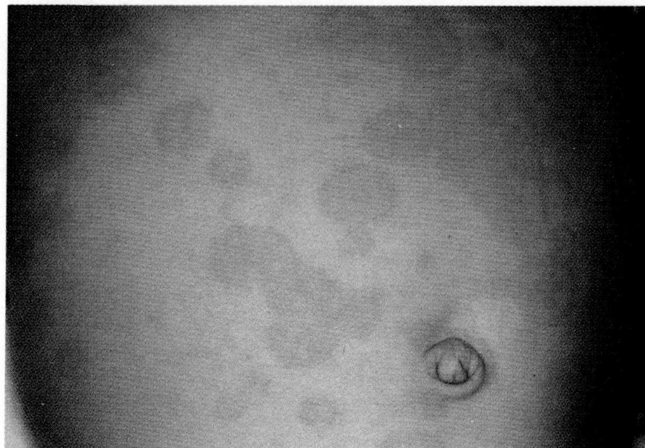

Plate 5E. An erythema multiforme–like rash, which may be observed in some cases of Kawasaki syndrome. (Courtesy Stanford T. Shulman.)

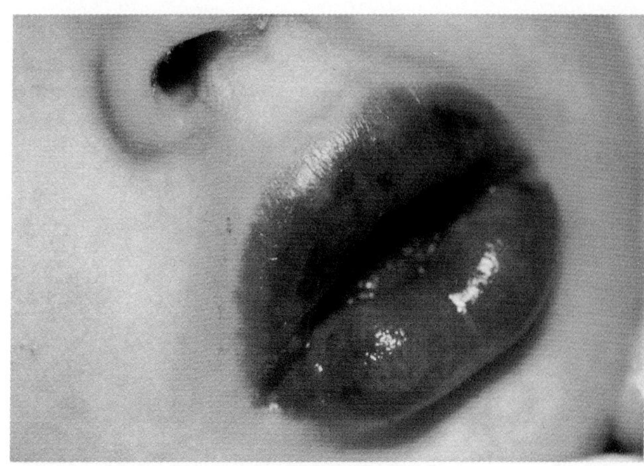

Plate 5F. Kawasaki syndrome strawberry tongue and red, dry, fissured lips. (Courtesy Stanford T. Shulman.)

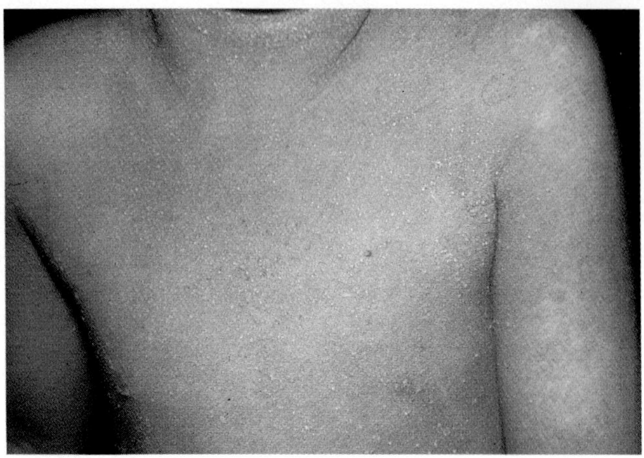

Plate 6A. Toxic shock syndrome rash. (Courtesy Teresita Laude.)

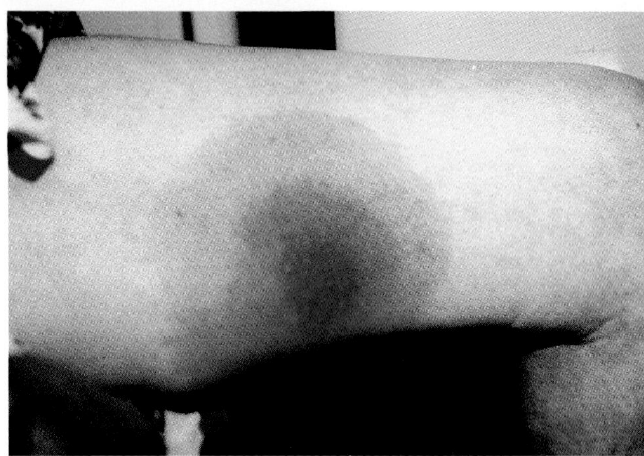

Plate 6B. Lyme disease rash (erythema migrans). (Courtesy Henry M. Feder, Jr.)

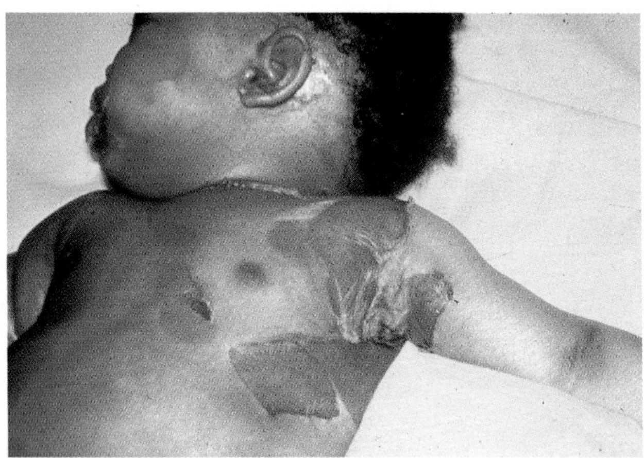

Plate 6C. Peeling skin in a child with staphylococcal scalded skin syndrome. (Courtesy Teresita Laude.)

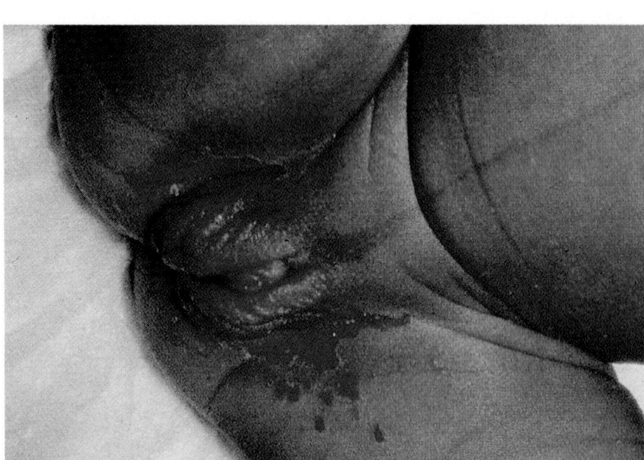

Plate 6D. Diaper dermatitis caused by *Candida albicans.* (Courtesy Neil S. Prose.)

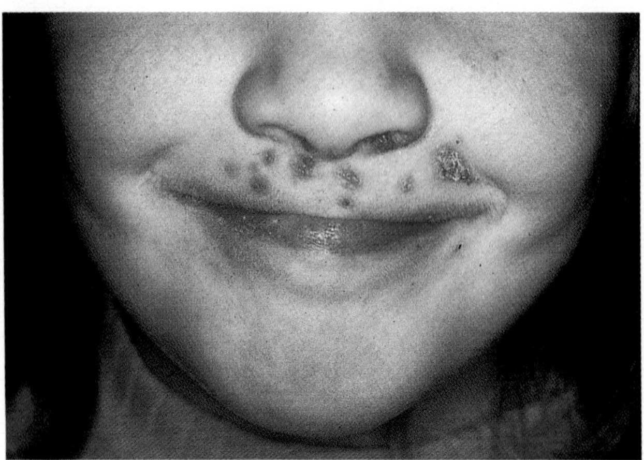

Plate 6E. Impetigo. (Courtesy Warren A. Andiman.)

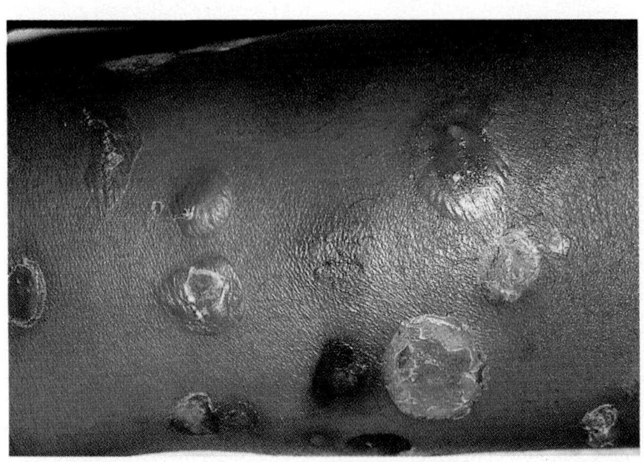

Plate 6F. Bullous impetigo. (Courtesy Ilona Frieden.)

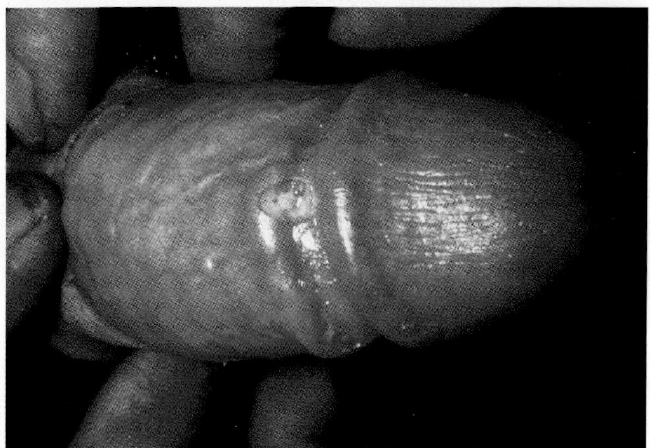

Plate 7A. Primary syphilis chancre, caused by *Treponema pallidum.* (Courtesy Neil S. Prose.)

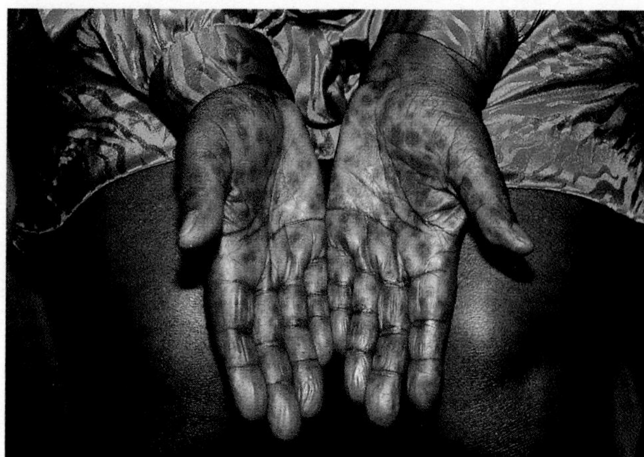

Plate 7B. Secondary syphilis rash, caused by *Treponema pallidum.* (Courtesy Neil S. Prose.)

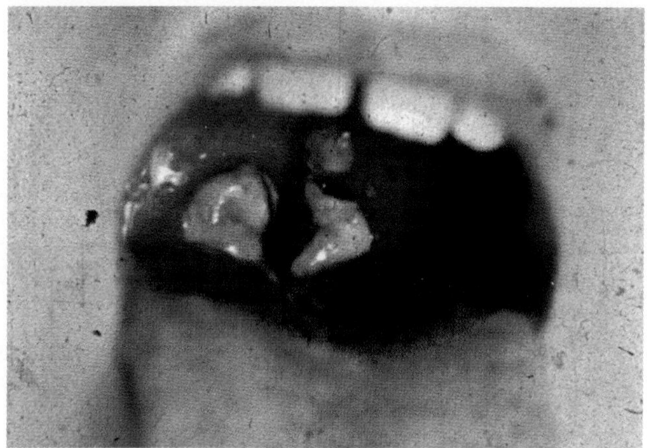

Plate 7C. Laryngeal diphtheria membrane, caused by *Corynebacterium diphtheriae.* (Courtesy Jean Klig.)

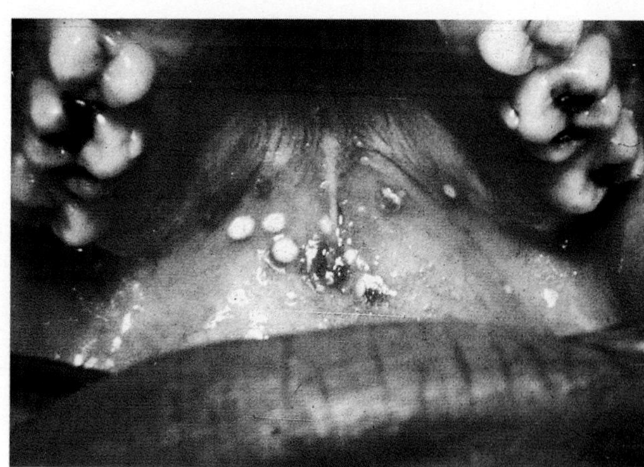

Plate 7D. Herpangina, caused by coxsackieviruses. (Courtesy Ronald C. Hansen.)

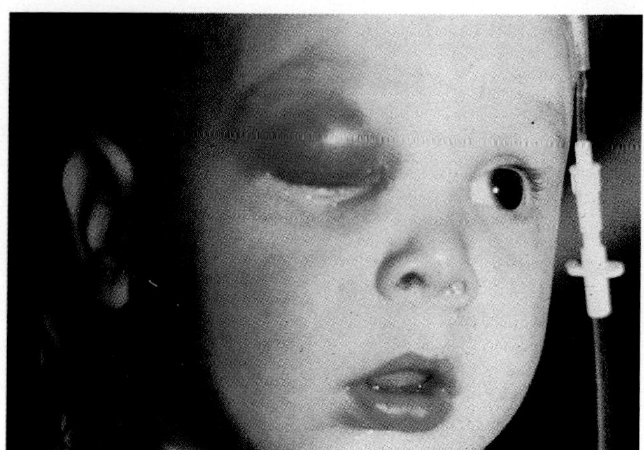

Plate 7E. Periorbital cellulitis. (Courtesy John S. Bradley.)

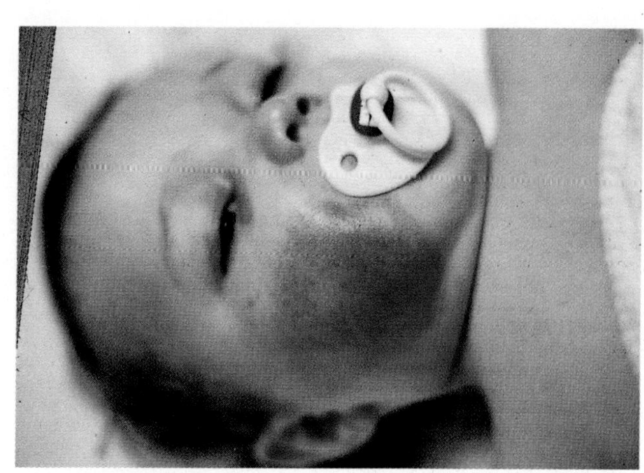

Plate 7F. Buccal cellulitis. (Courtesy John S. Bradley.)

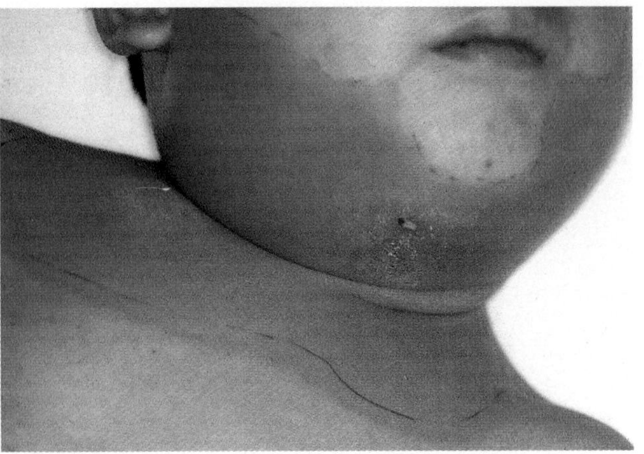

Plate 8A. Erysipelas caused by group A *Streptococcus.* The ink line was drawn 2 hours before this photograph was taken. (Courtesy John S. Bradley.)

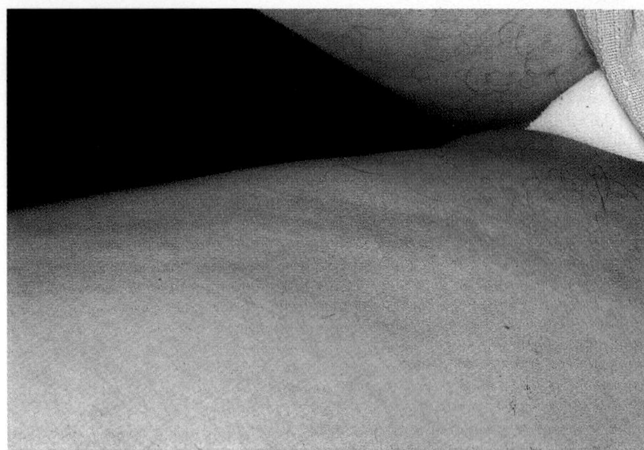

Plate 8B. Lymphangitis. (Courtesy Ronald C. Hansen.)

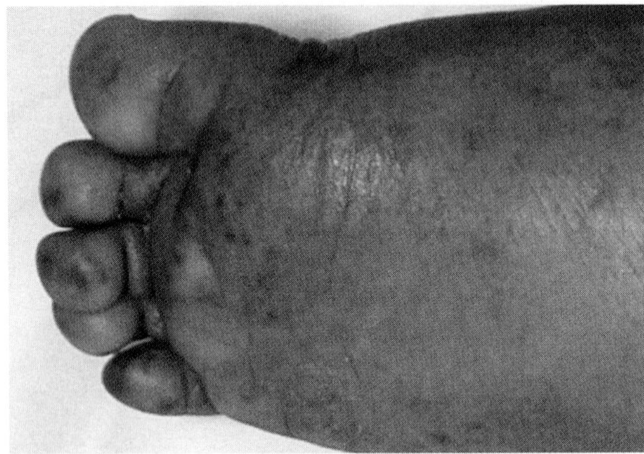

Plate 8C. Janeway lesions on the sole of the foot of a child with infective endocarditis. (Courtesy Hal B. Jenson.)

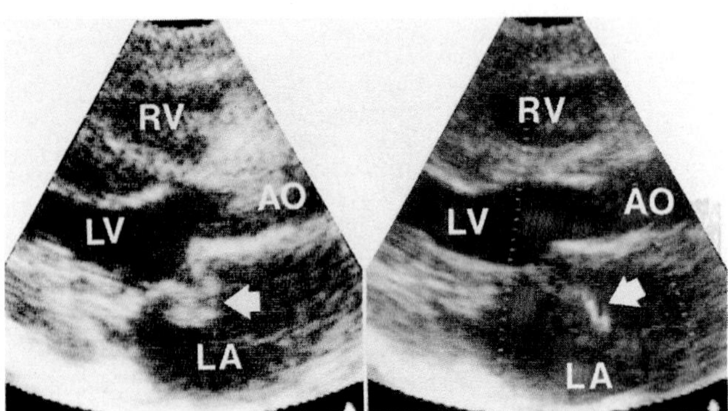

Plate 8D. Infective endocarditis with vegetation on the mitral valve *(arrows)* and disturbance of blood flow demonstrated by color echocardiography. (Courtesy Myung K. Park.)

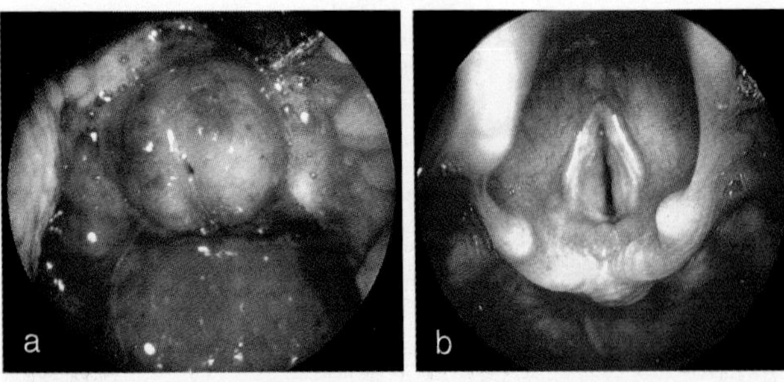

Plate 8E. Epiglottis *(a)* and croup *(b)* shown by laryngoscopy. (Courtesy Bruce Benjamin. From Benjamin B: *A Colour Atlas of Pediatric Otorhinolaryngology.* Philadelphia, Martin Dunitz Publishers/JB Lippincott, 1995, pp 291–2.)

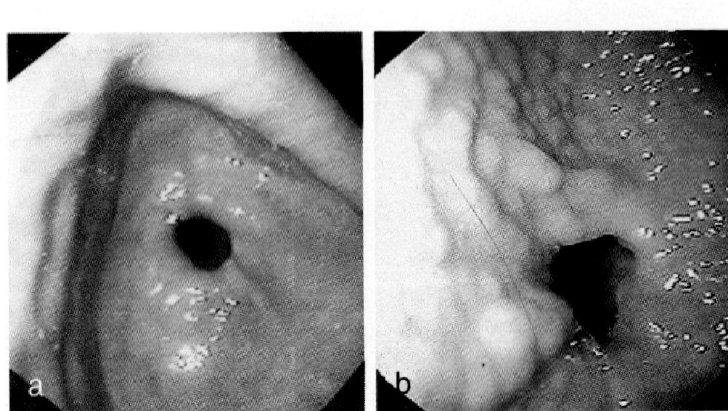

Plate 8F. Normal gastric mucosa *(a)* and gastritis caused by *Helicobacter pylori (b)* shown by endoscopy. (Courtesy Colston F. McEvoy.)

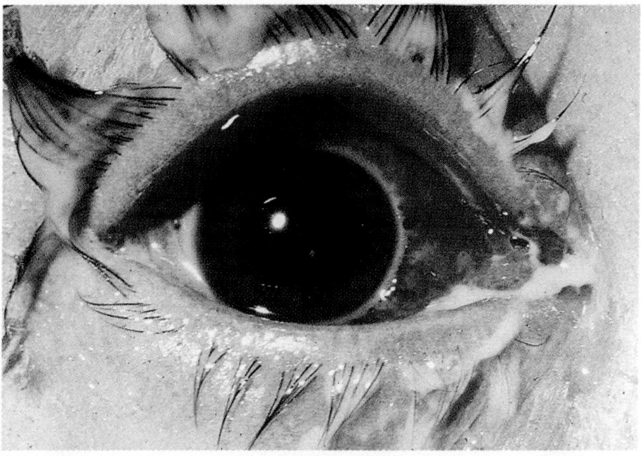

Plate 9A. Bacterial conjunctivitis. (From Farrar WE, Wood MJ, Innes JA, Tubbs H: *A Slide Atlas of Infectious Diseases.* London, Gower Medical Publishing. Times Mirror International Publishers Ltd., 1992.)

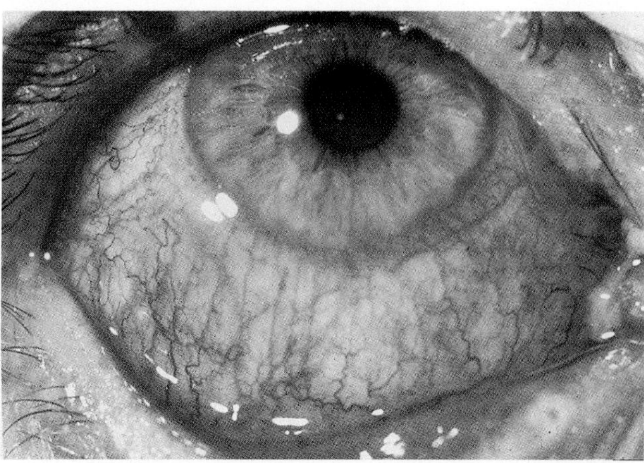

Plate 9B. Viral conjunctivitis. (Adapted with permission of American Academy of Ophthalmology from Young SE: *Managing the Red Eye.* San Francisco, American Academy of Ophthalmology, 1994.)

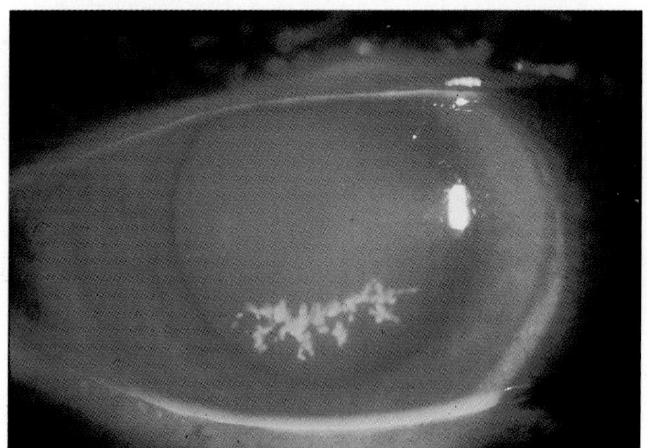

Plate 9C. Dendritic lesion of herpes simplex virus keratitis shown by Woods' lamp examination. (Adapted with permission of American Academy of Ophthalmology from Young SE: *Managing the Red Eye.* San Francisco, American Academy of Ophthalmology, 1994.)

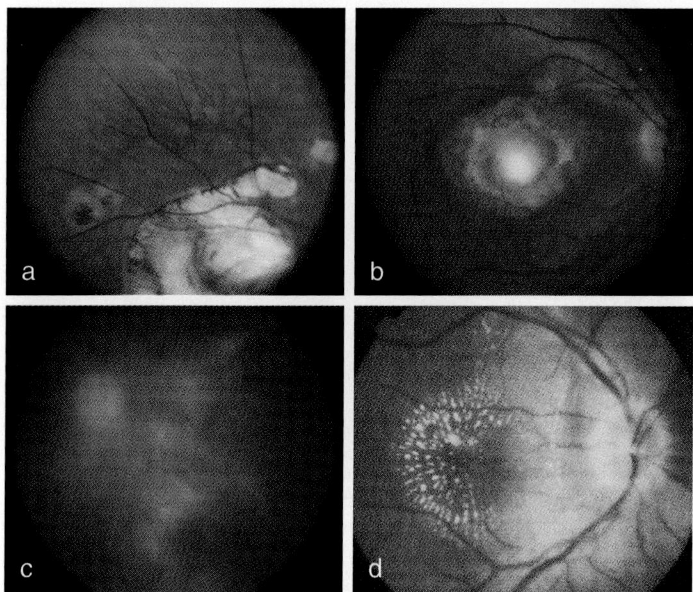

Plate 9D. Chorioretinitis caused by *Toxoplasma gondii* (*a* and *b*), cytomegalovirus *(c)*, and *Bartonella henselae,* which causes the stellate retinopathy of cat-scratch disease *(d).* (Courtesy Albert W. Biglan and David P. Ascher.)

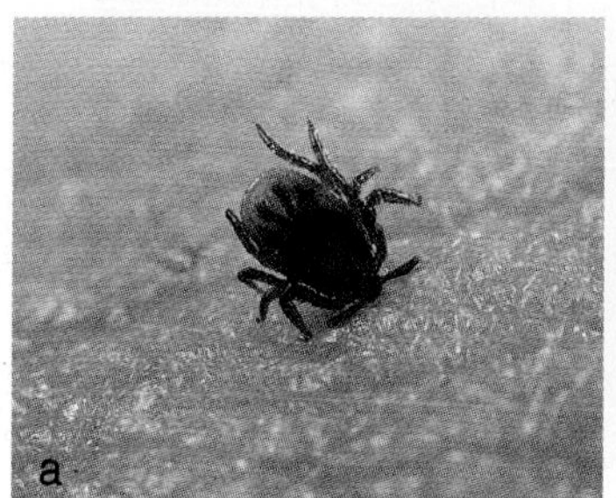

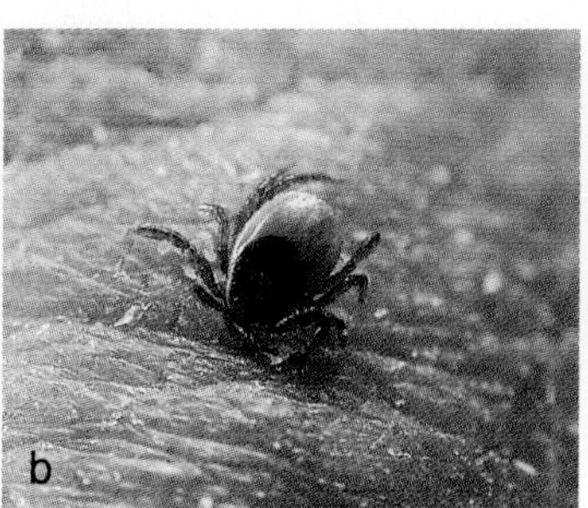

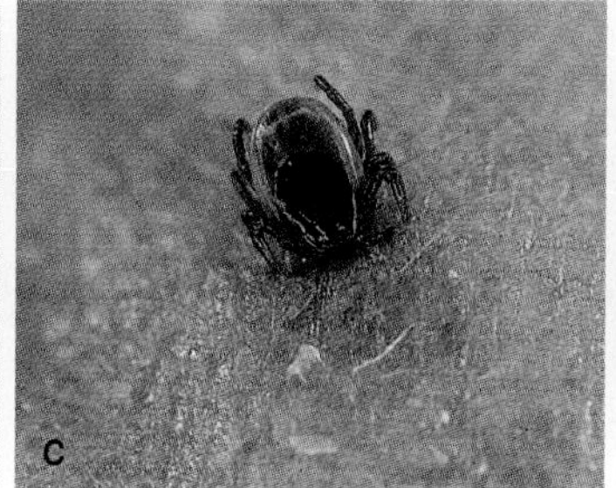

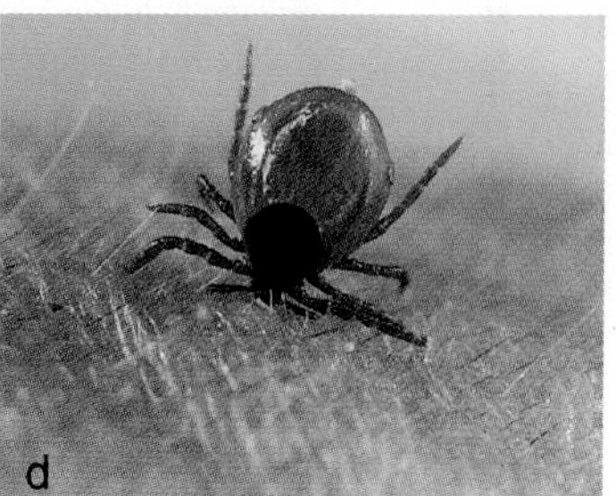

Plate 9E. A feeding nymphal *Ixodes scapularis* (the vector for Lyme disease, babesiosis, and human granulocytic ehrlichiosis) as seen through a hand-held magnifying lens, after 12 hours *(a),* 1 day *(b),* 2 days *(c),* and 4 days *(d)* of feeding. (Courtesy Franz-Rainer Matuschka. From Matuschka FR, Spielman A: Risk of infection from and treatment of tick bite. *Lancet* 1993;342:529–30.)

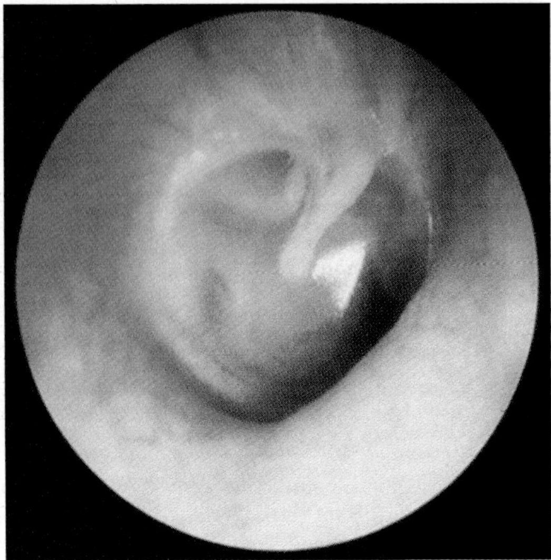

Plate 10A. Normal right tympanic membrane and middle ear.

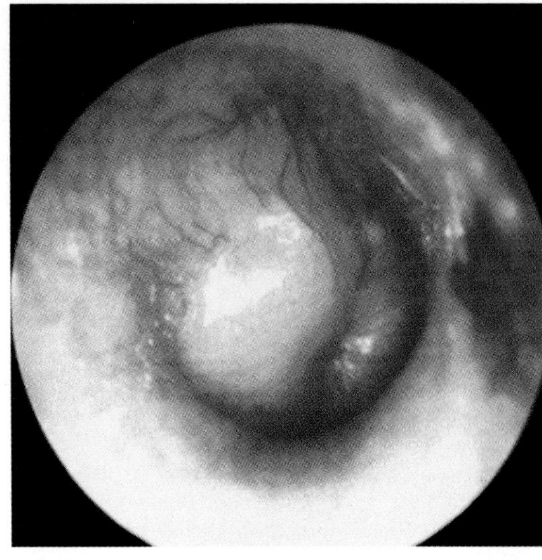

Plate 10B. Bulging right tympanic membrane in acute otitis media.

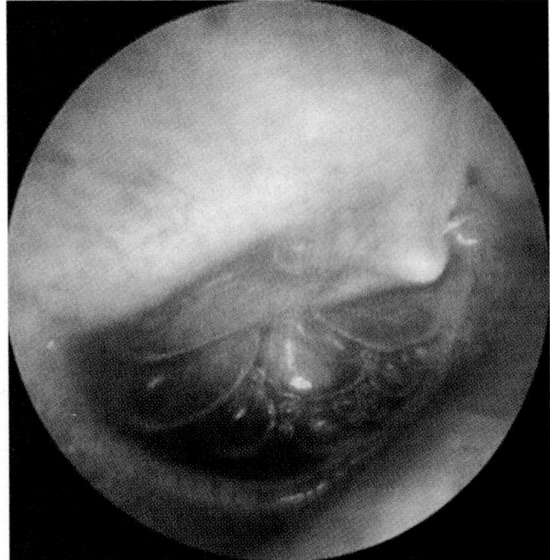

Plate 10C. Air-fluid level and bubbles visible through retracted, translucent right tympanic membrane in otitis media with effusion.

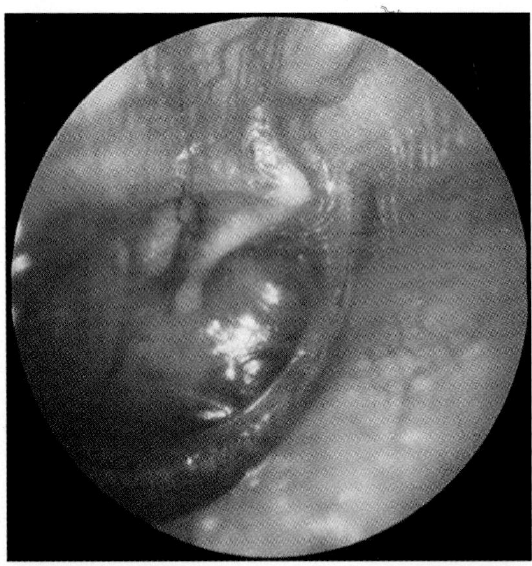

Plate 10D. Severely retracted, opaque right tympanic membrane in otitis media with effusion.

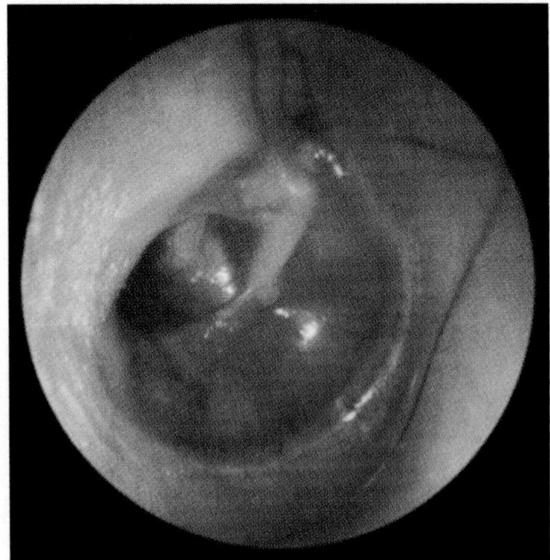

Plate 10E. Retraction pocket in the posterosuperior quadrant of right tympanic membrane in otitis media with effusion.

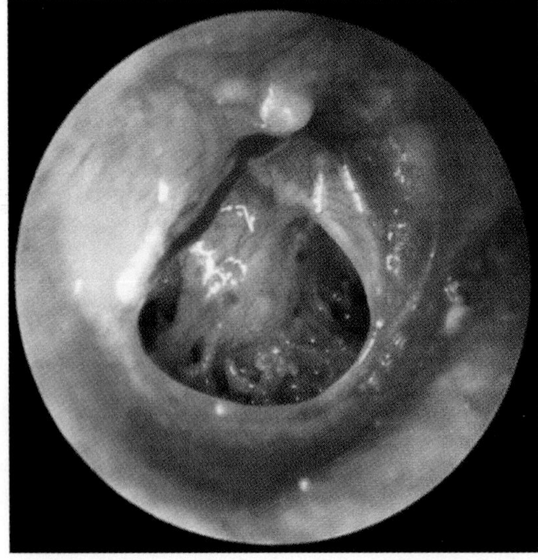

Plate 10F. Large "dry" central perforation of right tympanic membrane.

(Plates 10A to E from Bluestone CD, Klein JO: *Otitis Media in Infants and Children,* 3rd ed. Philadelphia, Saunders, 2001.)

Glossary of Abbreviations

AAP American Academy of Pediatrics
ACIP Advisory Committee on Immunization Practices
AIDS acquired immunodeficiency syndrome
ALC absolute lymphocyte count
ANC absolute neutrophil count
APACHE II Acute Physiology and Chronic Health Evaluation II
ARDS acute respiratory distress syndrome; adult respiratory distress syndrome
ATL adult T cell leukemia
BCG bacille Calmette-Guérin
BSA body surface area
BUN blood urea nitrogen
CBC complete blood cell count
CDC Centers for Disease Control and Prevention
CF complement fixation or complement-fixing
cfu colony-forming units
CMV cytomegalovirus
CMV-IG cytomegalovirus immune globulin
CNS central nervous system
CRP C-reactive protein
CSD cat-scratch disease
CSF cerebrospinal fluid
CSF colony stimulating factor
CT computed tomography
CTF Colorado tick fever
DIC disseminated intravascular coagulopathy
DNA deoxyribonucleic acid
EA early antigen
EA-D early antigen (diffuse)
EA-R early antigen (restricted)
EBNA Epstein-Barr virus nuclear antigen
EBV Epstein-Barr virus
ECG electrocardiogram
EEE Eastern equine encephalitis
EEG electroencephalogram
EIA enzyme immunoassay
EITB enzyme-linked immunotransfer blot, or Western blot
ELISA enzyme-linked immunosorbent assay (see EIA)
ERCP endoscopic retrograde cholangiopancreatography
ESR erythrocyte sedimentation rate
FDA United States Food and Drug Administration
FUO fever of unknown origin
GABHS group A β-hemolytic *Streptococcus*
G-CSF granulocyte colony stimulating factor
GI gastrointestinal
GM-CSF granulocyte-macrophage colony stimulating factor
gp glycoprotein
HAART highly active antiretroviral therapy (a combination HIV treatment regimen usually comprising two nucleoside reverse transcriptase inhibitors and a protease inhibitor)
HAM HTLV-I-associated myelopathy (also known as TSP)
HAV hepatitis A virus
HBeAg hepatitis B e antigen
HBIG hepatitis B immune globulin
HBsAg hepatitis B surface antigen
HBV hepatitis B virus
HCPS hantavirus cardiopulmonary syndrome
HCV hepatitis C virus
HDV hepatitis D virus
HEV hepatitis E virus
HGE human granulocytic ehrlichiosis
HGV hepatitis G virus
HHV6 human herpesvirus type 6
HHV7 human herpesvirus type 7
HHV8 human herpesvirus type 8
HIV human immunodeficiency virus
HLA human leukocyte antigen
HME human monocytic ehrlichiosis
hpf high-power field
HPV human papillomavirus(es)
HSV herpes simplex virus
HSV-1 herpes simplex virus type 1
HSV-2 herpes simplex virus type 2
HTLV-I human T-cell lymphotropic virus type I
HTLV-II human T-cell lymphotropic virus type II
HUS hemolytic uremic syndrome
ICAM-1 intercellular adhesion molecule-1
IFA immunofluorescence assay
IFN interferon (e.g., IFN-α, IFN-β, IFN-γ)
IG immune globulin
Ig immunoglobulin
IgA immunoglobulin A
IgD immunoglobulin D
IgE immunoglobulin E
IgG immunoglobulin G
IgM immunoglobulin M
IHA indirect hemagglutination assay
IL interleukin (e.g., IL-1, IL-2)
IPV inactivated poliovirus vaccine
IQ intelligence quotient
ISH in situ hybridization
IVIG intravenous immune globulin
kbp kilobasepair (or kilobasepairs)
kDa kilodalton
KOH potassium hydroxide
KS Kawasaki syndrome
LA latex agglutination
LCM lymphocytic choriomeningitis virus
LGV lymphogranuloma venereum
LPS lipopolysaccharide
LTB laryngotracheobronchitis
MAC *Mycobacterium avium* complex
MALT mucosa-associated lymphoid tissue
MBC minimum bactericidal concentration
MHC major histocompatibility complex

MIC minimum inhibitory concentration
MMR measles-mumps-rubella
MRI magnetic resonance imaging
mRNA messenger RNA
MRSA methicillin-resistant *Staphylococcus aureus*
MU million units
NEC necrotizing enterocolitis
NK cells natural killer cells
OPV oral poliovirus vaccine
PCP *Pneumocystis carinii* pneumonia
PCR polymerase chain reaction
PET positron emission tomography
pfu plaque-forming units
PML progressive multifocal leukoencephalopathy
PPD purified protein derivative (for tuberculin skin test)
PSAGN poststreptococcal acute glomerulonephritis
RIA radioimmunoassay
RID radioimmunodiffusion
RIG rabies immune globulin
RMSF Rocky Mountain spotted fever
RNA ribonucleic acid
RNC radionuclide cystography
RPR rapid plasma reagin (a nontreponemal serologic test for syphilis)
RSV respiratory syncytial virus
RSV-IG respiratory syncytial virus immune globulin
RT-PCR reverse transcriptase–polymerase chain reaction
SD standard deviation
SLE St. Louis encephalitis
SPA suprapubic percutaneous aspiration
STD sexually transmitted disease
TAT tetanus antitoxin
TIG tetanus immune globulin
TMP-SMZ trimethoprim-sulfamethoxazole
TNF tumor necrosis factor
TSP tropical spastic paralysis (also known as HAM)
TSST-1 toxic shock syndrome toxin-1
TTV TT virus
TU tuberculin unit
UTI urinary tract infection
VAHS virus-associated hemophagocytic syndrome
VAPP vaccine-associated paralytic poliomyelitis
VCA viral capsid antigen
VCUG voiding cystourethrography
VDRL Venereal Disease Research Laboratories (a nontreponemal serologic test for syphilis)
VEE Venezuelan equine encephalitis
VIG vaccinia immune globulin
VZIG varicella-zoster immune globulin
VZV varicella-zoster virus
WBC white blood cell
WEE Western equine encephalitis
WHO World Health Organization
XLP X-linked lymphoproliferative syndrome

CHAPTER 1

Microbial Virulence Factors

James K. Todd

The occurrence of most infectious diseases is influenced by an interrelationship of factors from the host, the microorganism, and the environment. The microorganism produces various virulence factors that allow it to adapt and cause disease in a susceptible host (Fig. 1–1). Transmission from the environmental reservoir to the host may occur by direct contact, by contact with vectors (e.g., arthropods), or by ingestion of food or water contaminated as a result of poor sanitation. Other factors (e.g., famine, injury, chemotherapy) that compromise the host may increase the risk of infection. The host may resist infection by any of several general and specific host defenses (e.g., phagocytes, antibodies, cellular immunity) and by external influences (i.e., anti-infective therapy, host defense–enhancing agents).

Microbes produce a wide variety of virulence factors that are species and often strain specific. Each organism, and frequently different strains of the same organism, may have a combination of factors that determine not only the propensity to cause disease but also the tissues affected (cell adhesion factors) and the type of disease (e.g., toxic, locally destructive). For every infectious disease, the interplay of host, environmental, and microorganism factors determines the nature and severity of infection.

PATHOGENESIS OF DISEASE

Epidemiologic factors define the reservoir of the microorganism, the mechanism of transmission within the population, and the subgroups of the population that are at increased risk (Chapter 3). After an individual is exposed to an organism, **colonization** may occur, permitting the growth and replication of the organism, usually on the skin or mucosal surface, without causing disease. A **commensal organism** that persists at the colonization site and does not cause disease may become established as part of the normal flora (Chapter 2). The organism may penetrate or evade the surface host defenses, gaining a portal of entry into the host and causing **disease.** An organism may be an **opportunistic pathogen** if altered host defenses are usually necessary to provide it the opportunity to cause infection. Other organisms possess virulence factors that may diminish the effect of the host defenses, giving the organism an opportunity to persist within the normal host or to spread farther and cause local or generalized tissue damage. These organisms are considered **primary pathogens** because they regularly cause disease in nonimmune hosts.

An **infectious disease** is any symptom or illness caused by a microorganism. A **contagious disease** represents an infectious disease that is effectively transmitted, usually by person-to-person spread. Not all persons have severe infections with classic symptoms. Depending on the host's genetic makeup and immune response, symptoms may be mild or even **subclinical** (i.e., inapparent) in some cases. The classic signs and symptoms of infection with a particular microorganism represent only the ''tip of the iceberg'' (Fig. 1–2). For every patient with overt infection, there are many others with mild or subclinical infections. A patient may be cured of the symptoms of infection or may remain colonized after recovery (**chronic carriers**). Persons who are actively infected or who remain carriers serve as a reservoir with the potential for transmitting the infection to others. Thus clinical cure does not necessarily equate with elimination of the organism. Some organisms (e.g., tuberculosis, hepatitis B, herpesviruses, retroviruses) may persist for the life of the patient, who, even though free of symptoms, may transmit the infection to others.

VIRULENCE FACTORS

The virulence factors of microorganisms determine their relative pathogenicity (Fig. 1–3). These factors include cell adhesion (attachment) factors, which permit attachment to particular cells; growth and protective factors, which play a role in protection of the microorganism from host defenses and antimicrobial agents; and toxins, which, if produced, may cause direct injury to the host. Microorganisms may possess more than one virulence factor. For example, *Neisseria meningitidis* is protected by its capsule from phagocytosis, and it also produces an endotoxin that commonly causes shock.

In addition, the host's own inflammatory response to the infection may mitigate symptoms or, in some cases, actually play a role in the pathogenesis of disease (e.g., rheumatic fever). Many toxins, mainly of *Staphylococcus* and *Streptococcus,* act as **superantigens** (see Fig. 5–8), which cause symptoms by release of immune cytokines (e.g., TNF, IL-1) that can cause capillary leakage resulting in shock. Thus the host's own inflammatory response to the infection may have deleterious effects that contribute to the nature and severity of disease.

Attachment Factors

Adherence is the initial contact of the microorganism with the target cells or tissues. **Adhesins** are cell adhesion factors expressed on the surface of the microorganism that bind to specific host cell receptors, or **ligands,** and mediate attachment to host tissues (Table 1–1). Cell adhesion factors also determine the **tropism** (i.e., preference) of the organism for particular tissues, thus determining the site of damage of the organism and disease symptoms. Viruses especially demonstrate selective tropisms.

Bacteria have **fimbriae** or **pili,** proteinaceous rodlike organelles on the surface that mediate attachment to host tissues. *Escherichia coli* typically have 100 to 1000 fimbriae per cell. Specific *E. coli* fimbriae, such as the *p*ili-*a*ssociated *p*yelonephritis (P, or Pap) fimbriae, mediate adherence to urinary tract epithelium, promoting colonization and infection.

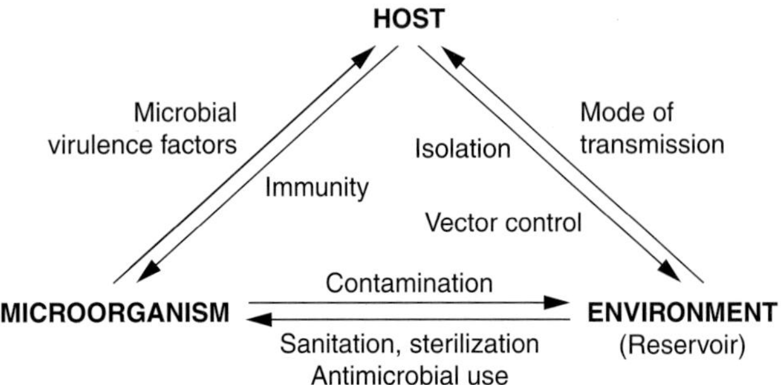

FIGURE 1–1. Interactions among host, microorganism, and environment in the pathogenesis of infectious diseases.

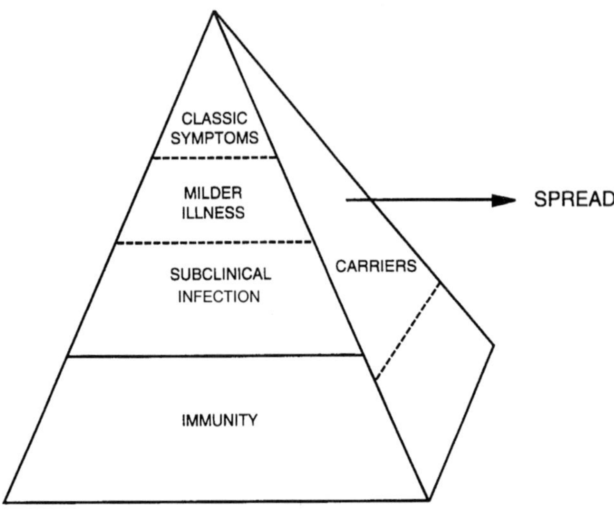

FIGURE 1–2. Manifestations of infectious disease in a population.

Growth and Protective Factors

Growth and protective factors protect the microorganism from host defenses and allow persistence and growth within the host (Table 1–2). These virulence factors are often essential to the pathogenesis of disease. Some factors interfere with the activity of immune globulin or host defense cells that would otherwise be effective in elimination of the microorganism. The extracellular slime produced by coagulase-negative staphylococci creates a thick glycocalyx that effectively cements the microorganism to indwelling catheters or other foreign body materials, allowing an otherwise commensal organism to survive and cause infection. Many bacteria produce proteases, lipases, and nucleases that break down host molecules to simple nutrients (amino acids, fatty acids, nucleotides) that can then be assimilated for the growth of the microorganism. Group A *Streptococcus* produces a fibrinolysin and hyaluronidase that catabolize fibrin and hyaluronic acid, thus permitting the spread of infection through soft tissue.

Intracellular Growth. All viruses and some bacteria replicate by intracellular growth, which protects them from extracellular host defenses (e.g., antibodies) and provides a vehicle for dissemination throughout the body. Antibodies previously produced by the host in response to vaccination (active immunization) or exogenous

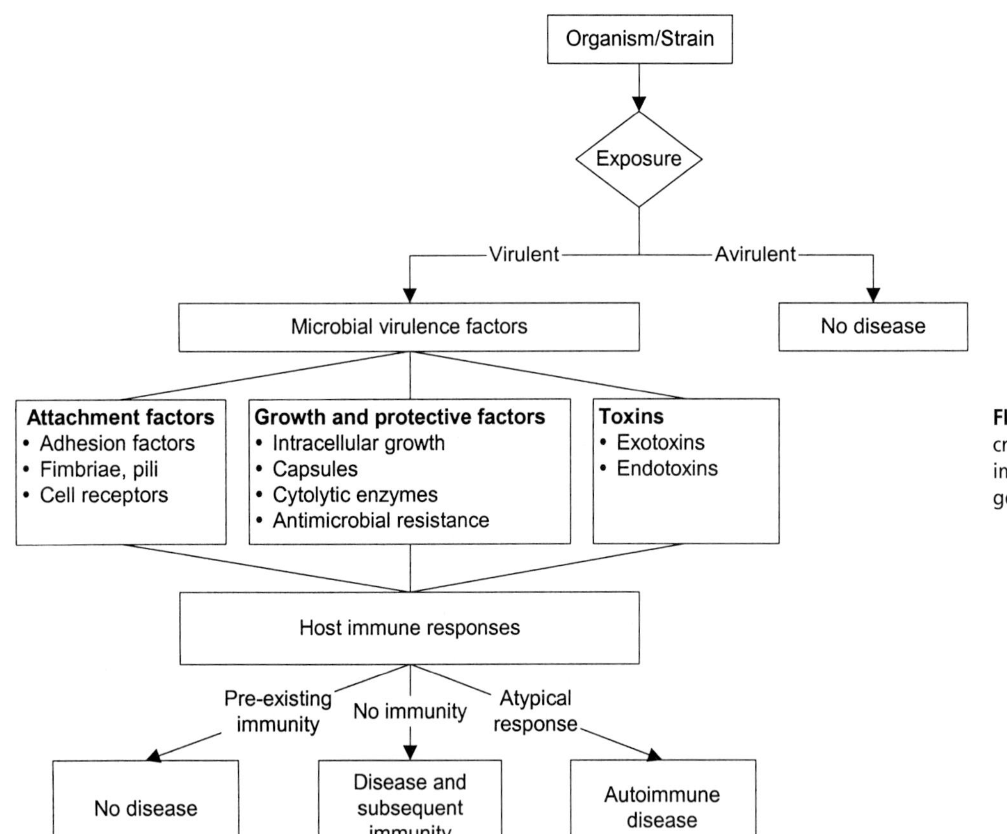

FIGURE 1–3. Interactions of microbial virulence factors and host immune responses in the pathogenesis of infectious diseases.

TABLE 1–1. Microbial Virulence Factors in Pathogenesis of Infection: Attachment Factors

Factor	Organism	Attachment Site	Disease
Pili (fimbriae)	*Escherichia coli*	Urothelium	Urinary tract infection
		Intestinal epithelium	Enteritis
	Vibrio cholerae	Intestinal epithelium	Cholera
	Neisseria gonorrhoeae	Urinary epithelium	Gonorrhea
Lipoteichoic acid	Group A *Streptococcus*	Pharyngeal cells	Pharyngitis
Hemagglutinin	Influenza virus	Respiratory epithelium	Influenza
	Bordetella pertussis	Respiratory epithelium	Pertussis
gp120	HIV	CD4 (on CD4 lymphocytes)	AIDS

antibodies administered soon after exposure (passive immunization) may neutralize free extracellular virus, but once inside cells, antibodies no longer affect viruses. Antibiotics that penetrate the cell poorly are less effective in the treatment of intracellular bacteria than indicated by in vitro susceptibility testing. Human bacterial pathogens that exist or replicate intracellularly include *Salmonella, Listeria, Legionella,* and *Mycobacterium.* Additional immune factors, such as cell lysis by killer macrophages, may be essential to free the intracellular organism from its protective environment and permit antibiotic therapy to be effective. Many protozoa (e.g., *Plasmodium, Babesia, Cryptosporidium, Toxoplasma, Leishmania*) are obligate intracellular pathogens.

Antimicrobial Resistance. Many bacterial organisms produce extracellular products that do not have a direct toxigenic effect but nonetheless play a role in the pathogenesis of disease. The β-lactamases produced by many organisms are excreted into the external environment and degrade the β-lactam ring of penicillins, thus inactivating the antibiotic and protecting the microorganism from its effects. Microorganisms produce many types of resistance factors, including extracellular enzymes and including factors that limit the permeability of the cell wall to antibiotics or alter antibiotic receptor sites. These resistance factors are often carried on plasmids or transposons that may be transmitted to other bacteria by recombination. Thus a resistance factor possessed by one organism may be transferred to another, which explains in part why the excessive use of antibiotics often provides an environment that selects for resistant strains.

Toxins

In addition to microbial factors that determine local invasion and pathogenesis of disease caused directly by growth and multiplication of organisms at the site of infection, many bacteria produce toxins that may freely diffuse throughout the host and cause damage at distant sites (Table 1–3). **Endotoxins,** which include components of the cell wall and intracellular toxins released only with lysis of the microorganism, mediate shock through complex interactions with host defense mechanisms. **Lipopolysaccharide,** an endotoxin that is an integral component of the gram-negative bacterial cell wall, is responsible for most of the toxic effects of gram-negative bacterial sepsis. The molecule is complex and consists of three distinct regions with unique pathogenic and antigenic properties: (1) the O-antigen polysaccharide, which is the major antigenic determinant of bacterial strains; (2) the core region, linking the O-antigen to the lipid A region; and (3) lipid A, which is the toxic moiety. Lipopolysaccharide interaction with the cell membrane of macrophages triggers release of TNF-α, IL-1, IL-6, and IL-8. **Exotoxins** are bacterial proteins that are secreted during growth of the microorganism and are toxic for target cells. For example, the diphtheria toxin produced by *Corynebacterium diphtheriae* is an exotoxin that causes local tissue damage both at the site of the

TABLE 1–2. Microbial Virulence Factors in Pathogenesis of Infection: Growth and Protective Factors

Factor	Organism	Effect
Capsule	*Streptococcus pneumoniae*	Blocks phagocytosis
	Haemophilus influenzae type b	
	Neisseria meningitidis	
Slime	Coagulase-negative staphylococci	Blocks phagocytosis
IgAse	*Neisseria gonorrhoeae*	Cleaves immunoglobulin
Protein A	*Staphylococcus aureus*	Interferes with activity of immunoglobulin
Cytolysins (hemolysins, leukocidins)	Group A *Streptococcus*	Destroys phagocytes and other cells
	S. aureus	
	Pseudomonas aeruginosa	
Fibrinolysins, hyaluronidase	Group A *Streptococcus*	Local spread of infection
Proteases, lipases, nucleases	Bacteria	Assimilation of extracellular nutrients
Intracellular growth	Some bacteria	Protects from host defenses
	All mycobacteria	
	Histoplasma capsulatum	
	All viruses	
	Some protozoa	
Antimicrobial resistance	Bacteria	Decreased antimicrobial effectiveness

TABLE 1–3. Clinical Effects of Bacterial Toxins

Clinical Effect or Disease	Organism and Toxin*	
	Exotoxins	Endotoxins
Shock	*Staphylococcus aureus* Toxic-shock syndrome toxin (TSST-1) Enterotoxins B, C Group A *Streptococcus* Pyrogenic exotoxins A, B, C	*Neisseria meningitidis* *Haemophilus influenzae* type b Other gram-negative organisms
Rash	*S. aureus* Exfoliatins A, B TSST-1 Group A *Streptococcus* Pyrogenic exotoxins A, B, C	
Gastritis	*Helicobacter pylori* Vacuolating cytotoxin (vacA)	
Vomiting	*S. aureus* Enterotoxins A, B, C_1, C_2, C_3, D, E, G	
Diarrhea	*Vibrio cholerae* Cholera toxin *Shigella dysenteriae* Shiga toxin (Stx) *Salmonella* Enterotoxin *Escherichia coli* Enterotoxins Heat-labile enterotoxin Heat-stable enterotoxin Cytotoxins Shiga-like toxins (Stx1, Stx2) *Yersinia* Enterotoxin *Campylobacter* Enterotoxin *Aeromonas* Enterotoxin *S. aureus* Enterotoxins A, B, C_1, C_2, C_3, D, E, G *Clostridium perfringens* Enterotoxin *Clostridium difficile* Enterotoxin (toxin A) Cytotoxin (toxin B) *Bacillus cereus* Enterotoxin	
Neuromuscular symptoms	*Clostridium botulinum* Botulinum toxins A, B, C_1, C_2, D, E, F, G *Clostridium tetani* Tetanus toxin *Corynebacterium diphtheriae* Diphtheria toxin	
Pertussis syndrome	*Bordetella pertussis* Pertussis toxin (and others)	
Anthrax	*Bacillus anthracis* Anthrax toxin	
Invasive *Pseudomonas* infections	*Pseudomonas aeruginosa* Exotoxins A, S, other cytotoxins	

*Exotoxins are commonly produced by both gram-positive and some gram-negative bacteria. Endotoxins are produced by gram-negative bacteria.

diphtheritic infection (e.g., a pharyngeal membrane) and at distant sites (e.g., myocarditis, neuritis) as it spreads through the bloodstream. Antibodies to toxoid vaccines are protective of the effects of toxemia.

Toxins may also be classified by their cellular tissue or mechanism of action. Certain strains of *Staphylococcus aureus* and other bacteria produce **enterotoxins,** which may be secreted into contaminated foods. When ingested, the preformed enterotoxin affects the vagal nerves of the gastrointestinal tract, causing vomiting and diarrhea—the typical result of picnic food poisoning. Other *S. aureus* strains produce **exfoliatins,** which diffuse from the site of actual infection (usually the nose) into the bloodstream and cause damage to the granular cell layer of the skin, resulting in the staphylococcal scalded skin syndrome. Other *S. aureus* strains produce **toxic shock syndrome toxin-1 (TSST-1)**, which can diffuse from a focal site of infection, often the vagina or an abscess, to cause shock mediated by the production of TNF and IL-1 by host macrophages. Group A *Streptococcus* produces **pyrogenic exotoxins** with similar effects, causing scarlet fever and a toxic shock–like syndrome. *Clostridium tetani* and *Clostridium botulinum* produce **neurotoxins** with effects on the neuromuscular junction, causing tetanus and botulism, respectively.

REVIEWS

Ades EW, Rest RF, Morse SA (editors): *Microbial Pathogenesis and Immune Response.* New York, New York Academy of Sciences, 1996: vol 2.

Ayoub EM, Cassell GH (editors): *Microbial Determinants of Virulence and Host Response.* Washington, DC, ASM Press, 1990.

Kado CI (editor): *Molecular Mechanisms of Bacterial Virulence.* Dordrecht, The Netherlands, Kluwer Academic Publishers, 1994.

Moss J, Tu AT, Vaughan M (editors): *Bacterial Toxins and Virulence Factors in Disease.* New York, Marcel Dekker, 1995.

Patrick S, Larkin MJ (editors): *Immunological and Molecular Aspects of Bacterial Virulence.* Chichester, NY, John Wiley & Sons, 1995.

Ron EZ, Rottem S (editors): *Microbial Surface Components and Toxins in Relation to Pathogenesis.* New York, Plenum Press, 1991.

Roth JA (editor): *Virulence Mechanisms of Bacterial Pathogens.* Washington, DC, ASM Press, 1995.

KEY ARTICLES

Arbuthnott JP, Poxton IR: Determinants of bacterial virulence. In Linton AH, Dick HM (editors): *Principles of Bacteriology, Virology, and Immunity.* Philadelphia, BC Decker, 1990.

Berkowitz FE: Bacterial exotoxins: How they work. *Pediatr Infect Dis J* 1989;8:42–7.

Cassell GH: Microbial surfaces: Determinants of virulence and host responsiveness. *Rev Infect Dis* 1998;10:S273–456.

Foxman B, Zhang L, Palin K, et al: Bacterial virulence characteristics of *Escherichia coli* isolates from first-time urinary tract infection. *J Infect Dis* 1995;171:1514–21.

Gotschlich EC: Thoughts on the evolution of strategies used by bacteria for evasion of host defenses. *Rev Infect Dis* 1983;5:S778–83.

Law D: Adhesion and its role in the virulence of enteropathogenic *Escherichia coli. Clin Microbiol Rev* 1994;7:152–73.

Quinn FD, Newman GW, King CH: In search of virulence factors of human bacterial disease. *Trends Microbiol* 1997;5:20–6.

Svanborg C, Godaly G: Bacterial virulence in urinary tract infection. *Infect Dis Clin North Am* 1997;11:513–29.

CHAPTER 2

Normal Microbial Flora

Robert S. Baltimore ▪ Hal B. Jenson

A relatively limited number of the thousands of bacteria, rickettsiae, viruses, parasites, and other pathogens that humans may contact cause the majority of infectious diseases. Various mechanisms are responsible for the disease potential of these organisms (Chapter 1). Most of the other nonpathogenic microorganisms are identified in various settings in the environment but are generally not isolated from human tissues.

However, certain species of microbes can be regularly isolated from the skin and mucosal surfaces of healthy persons. These **normal flora,** sometimes referred to as **indigenous flora,** include numerous species of bacteria. The normal flora live on the surface of epithelial tissues and do not appear to cause disease in their usual location. Recognition of normal flora in culture specimens is of practical importance because they are generally unlikely to be the source of illness in a patient, although some of these microorganisms may cause disease if they are transported to another location or if there are disturbances in ecologic relationships. Species that are normally found in or on the host but that cause no harm are termed **commensal organisms** to differentiate them from species with pathogenic potential.

Colonization versus Infection. **Colonization** is the state in which normal flora exist and multiply at a low rate and do not harm the host. Colonizing microorganisms do not invade tissue beyond the superficial layers of the epithelial-lined tissues that are exposed either to the external environment or generally beyond the internal exposed surfaces of the upper respiratory tract to the level of the glottis, the lower genitourinary tract, and the entire gastrointestinal tract. Such tissues include the ocular conjunctivae, nose, mouth, pharynx, and vagina. Some surfaces, such as the paranasal sinuses, are normally free of colonizing bacteria but may temporarily be contaminated by microorganisms.

Infection is the multiplication of microbes in normally sterile fluids or tissues, or the invasive proliferation of potentially harmful microorganisms. Infection induces an inflammatory and immune response in the immunocompetent host. In contrast, colonization does not lead to signs of inflammation, although a modest immune response may develop.

Microbiologic cultures do not differentiate between colonization and infection unless the tissue being sampled is normally sterile. Thus cultures of normally sterile fluids, such as blood, and of solid organs can be processed for growth and recovery of any microorganisms. Their presence is interpreted as apparent evidence of invasion and infection. Cultures of surfaces, fluids, or tissues that normally harbor colonizing microorganisms, such as the oropharynx, rectum, or vagina, should be specially processed to isolate organisms with a pathogenic potential from the vast array of normal flora present.

ROLE OF NORMAL FLORA IN PROTECTION AGAINST INFECTION

Many barriers, known collectively as host defenses, protect humans from infection. These defenses include **anatomic barriers** such as intact integument, nasal hair, sphincters at luminal orifices to prevent ascending infection, acidic gastric contents, ciliated respiratory epithelium with a mucociliary transport system that can physically move microorganisms, and the immune system (Chapter 5). Established colonization with numerous organisms of low virulence limits dominance of any one species and minimizes acquisition of exogenous, potentially pathogenic organisms. Other mechanisms by which indigenous flora afford protection include **bacterial interference** (competition for host nutrient sources), **colonization resistance** (nonspecific or specific blocking of cell-surface receptors or mucous blanket adhesions by other bacteria), and production of **bacteriocins** (bacterial products that are cytotoxic to other bacteria, usually a related species).

Both normal flora and pathogenic microbes appear to attach to human tissue. Specific binding occurs between specialized surface elements of the microorganisms (pili as well as other specific proteins and carbohydrates) and molecules on the skin and mucosal cellular surfaces. Some evidence exists that abundant normal bacterial and fungal flora may occupy most receptor molecules on mucosal cells, leaving very few receptor molecules available for the attachment of pathogens that may transiently enter the respiratory or gastrointestinal tract. Pathogens are therefore easily eliminated by mechanical means (e.g., washing, coughing, sneezing, intestinal peristalsis). Reduction of normal flora by the use of antibiotics or other measures, such as enemas, washing with disinfectants, and certain chemotherapies, permits new flora to attach more readily to the exposed receptor molecules on tissue surfaces. If these new flora have pathogenic potential, such as the ability to invade or to generate toxins, infection and subsequent illness are much more likely. Several familiar complications of antibiotic therapy, such as oral and vaginal candidiasis, which frequently accompanies treatment with broad-spectrum antimicrobial agents, and antibiotic-induced *Clostridium difficile*–associated diarrhea, are representative of this phenomenon. In the absence of antibiotic treatment, these offending species are normal flora commensals. Infection resulting from overgrowth of these organisms, typically *Candida,* is sometimes referred to as a **superinfection** or **suprainfection.**

In the hospital, elimination of pre-existing normal flora and acquisition of a new flora environment often result in colonization with microorganisms that are resistant to frequently used antimicrobial agents. This is the major mechanism for the spread of antibiotic-resistant flora in hospitals. These resistant organisms are selected and survive preferentially over the normal flora that are generally susceptible to commonly used antibiotics. These microbes are not more virulent or more likely to cause infection solely because of their antibiotic resistance, but they are usually more difficult to treat if they do cause infection.

OTHER BENEFITS OF NORMAL MICROBIAL FLORA

Normal flora are beneficial in many ways other than providing protection against infection. These organisms are probably responsible for normal stimulation of the immune system, especially in the infant; for metabolism of fatty acids in the skin; for digestion of foods in the gastrointestinal tract; for production of essential vitamins, such as vitamin K; and possibly for some degree of resistance to cancer.

NORMAL FLORA AS CAUSE OF INFECTION

Although colonizing microorganisms normally survive on skin and mucosal surfaces without harming the host, changes in the host may alter this relationship. The four most important events involved in the causation of infection by normal flora are (1) disruption of mucosal integrity by local inflammation, (2) obstruction of drainage of body secretions and excretions, (3) direct inoculation of organisms into deeper tissues by injury from a penetrating foreign body, and (4) movement of microorganisms across mucosal barriers by translocation.

Disruption of Mucosal Integrity. The skin and the mucosal epithelia of the respiratory, genitourinary, and gastrointestinal tracts are effective barriers to infection in the healthy person. Breakdown of these barriers may result in infection with normal flora. Inflammatory disorders of the skin, such as eczema or psoriasis, or skin injury, such as that seen with pressure (decubitus) ulcers or chickenpox lesions, may permit organisms from the skin surface access to deeper tissues. Bacterial species, such as *Staphylococcus aureus,* coagulase-negative staphylococci, and anaerobic diphtheroids, or fungi, such as *Candida albicans,* may become the agents of inflammation such as cellulitis. In the upper respiratory tract, inflammation caused by viral infections may allow normal oral bacterial flora to invade the tissues of the oropharynx. Anaerobic streptococci and even group A streptococci and *Haemophilus influenzae* may cause deep pharyngeal infections, potentially including bacteremia, in previously symptom-free carriers of these normal flora. Individuals with gastrointestinal inflammatory disorders such as Crohn's disease or infections caused by intestinal pathogens such as *Salmonella* may develop small ulcerations. These breaks allow normal gastrointestinal flora, such as enteric gram-negative aerobic bacilli or anaerobic bacteria, to gain access to the submucosal tissue and either cause local infection or enter the blood circulation.

Obstruction of Drainage. Mucous secretions, which are commonly contaminated with or contiguous to other surfaces colonized by normal flora, are part of the barrier to infection of many epithelial surfaces. Obstruction of normal drainage of secretions permits proliferation of normal flora and development of focal infection. Such infections are often polymicrobial, reflecting the polymicrobial nature of the normal flora, and may involve organisms of increased pathogenicity. Such microbes predominate as the actual infection develops. This scenario occurs in paranasal sinusitis with obstruction of the ostiomeatal complex, in otitis media with dysfunction of the eustachian tube, and in infections associated with obstruction of normally sterile excretions such as urine and bile.

Direct Inoculation. The introduction of organisms into deeper tissues by injury caused by a penetrating foreign body may result in a wide variety of infections from normal flora. Knife or bullet wounds or bite wounds through the skin or crossing mucosal barriers in the mouth or the gut may result in the inoculation of organisms from mucosal surfaces into deep tissues. Surgical wound infections, infections at the site of percutaneous insertion of intravascular catheters, and infections at the site of intramuscular injections may all be caused by species considered to be normal flora.

Translocation. **Translocation** is the process whereby intraluminal organisms in the intestine move across the mucosal barriers and lamina propria of the intestine into the deeper tissues. The organisms may reach the regional mesenteric lymph nodes and may subsequently spread to other tissues. This process appears to be important in the pathogenesis of infection associated with such gut processes as bowel obstruction, toxic megacolon, necrotizing enterocolitis, and neutropenic enteropathy (cecitis or typhlitis). Disorders that predispose to translocation include profound immunodeficiency, gastrointestinal ischemia, and alteration of the normal gut flora. In these circumstances, organisms of the normal flora in the intestinal contents may cause a range of infection, including transmural inflammation, focal infection limited to a segment of the intestine, mesenteric lymphadenitis, abscess, peritonitis, or sepsis. The cause of increased permeability for bacteria at the cellular level has not yet been established.

DEVELOPMENT OF NORMAL FLORA IN THE NEWBORN

During a normal vaginal delivery, the newborn departs the sterile environment and is exposed to the vaginal, skin, and enteric flora of the mother. These microorganisms rapidly colonize the infant. Organisms transmitted by the hands of caretakers and contaminated surfaces are also important. By the end of the first week of life, colonization of the upper respiratory tract, gastrointestinal tract, and skin with organisms typical of older humans has begun. In the gastrointestinal tract, development of anaerobic gram-negative bacillary flora lags, occurring between the first and the second weeks of life. This rapid colonization of previously sterile surfaces means that the infant is particularly susceptible to acquisition of **"abnormal" flora** if normal mechanisms are modified by antibiotic use, contact with contaminated animate and inanimate surfaces, and ingestion of fluids that contain microorganisms.

Feeding practices may also influence infant gastrointestinal colonization patterns. Although breast milk–fed infants acquire mostly *Lactobacillus* and *Bifidobacterium* in the first week of life, formula-fed infants have more *Escherichia coli* and other gram-negative bacilli and fewer *Bifidobacterium* organisms. Lactobacilli are an important part of the healthy neonatal flora and probably are responsible for much of the **colonization resistance.** Acquisition of lactobacilli is relatively deficient in infants who are born by cesarean delivery, are born preterm, spend a prolonged period in an Isolette, or receive antibiotics.

Acquisition of pharyngeal flora is also influenced by early events. Healthy infants generally have α-hemolytic streptococci as the predominant flora of the pharynx. Colonization of the pharynx with *E. coli* and other gram-negative aerobic species, probably originating from the gastrointestinal tract, is a common phenomenon in the young infant and may be transient or long term. Colonization with these bacterial species is more common in formula-fed than breast-fed infants in the first 6 months of life. These colonizing gram-negative bacteria are not associated with invasive infections in most healthy infants. Infants with protracted stays in newborn

TABLE 2–1. Predominant Microorganisms Indigenous to Various Locations of the Body (Normal Flora)

Commonly Present	Occasionally Present
Skin	
Bacteria	
Propionibacterium acnes	*Streptococcus*
Propionibacterium (other species)	*Peptococcus*
	Bacillus
Corynebacterium	*Mycobacterium*
Coagulase-negative staphylococci	Enterobacteriaceae
Staphylococcus aureus	*Escherichia coli*
Micrococcus	*Klebsiella*
	Proteus
	Enterobacter
	Pseudomonas
Fungi	
Malassezia furfur	*Candida*
	Mucor
Respiratory Tract	
Mouth and Throat	
Bacteria	
Streptococcus (α-hemolytic) (especially *S. mitis* and *S. salivarius*)	*Streptococcus pneumoniae*
	Enterococcus
	Neisseria meningitidis (nontypeable)
Micrococcus	Non–group A *Streptococcus*
Coagulase-negative staphylococci	Group A *Streptococcus*
*S. aureus**	Enterobacteriaceae
Peptostreptococcus	*E. coli*
Neisseria	*Klebsiella*
Haemophilus influenzae (nontypeable)	*Proteus*
Haemophilus parainfluenzae	*Enterobacter*
Moraxella catarrhalis	*Pseudomonas* (including *P. aeruginosa*)
Veillonella	*Eikenella corrodens*
Bacteroides (except *B. fragilis*)	*Capnocytophaga*
Fusobacterium	*Kingella*
Actinomyces	*Cardiobacterium hominis*
	Campylobacter sputorum
	Lactobacillus
	Corynebacterium
	Mycoplasma (including *M. pneumoniae*)
Spirochetes	
Treponema denticola	
Treponema refringens	
Fungi	
Candida albicans	Other *Candida*
Protozoa	
	Entamoeba gingivalis
	Trichomonas tenax
Nose	
Bacteria	
Coagulase-negative staphylococci	Enterobacteriaceae (in young children)
S. aureus	*E. coli*
Streptococcus (α-hemolytic)	*Klebsiella*
	Proteus
	Enterobacter
	Enterococcus (in young children)
	S. pneumoniae
	Group A *Streptococcus*
Paranasal Sinuses	
Usually sterile	
Trachea, Bronchi, Bronchioles, and Alveoli	
Usually sterile	
Gastrointestinal Tract	
Esophagus	
Contaminated with microorganisms from the mouth, pharynx, and ingested food	
Stomach	
Surviving microorganisms from the mouth, pharynx, and ingested food	
Hepatic Ducts, Gallbladder, Pancreatic Ducts, and Small Intestine (Except Lower Ileum)	
Usually sterile, or low numbers of anaerobic organisms	
Lower Ileum	
Bacteria†	
Gram-negative anaerobic	*S. aureus*
Lactobacillus	
Enterobacteriaceae	
E. coli	
Klebsiella	
Proteus	
Enterobacter	
Enterococcus	
Bacteroides	
Clostridium	
Mycobacterium	
Large Intestine and Feces	
Bacteria‡	
Gram-negative anaerobic	Group B *Streptococcus*
Bacteroides (including *B. fragilis*)	*Pseudomonas*
	Acinetobacter
Fusobacterium	*Alcaligenes faecalis*
Gram-positive anaerobic	Coagulase-negative staphylococci
Peptococcus	*S. aureus*
Peptostreptococcus	*Lactobacillus*
Enterobacteriaceae	*P. aeruginosa*
E. coli	*Campylobacter*
Klebsiella	*Corynebacterium*
Proteus	*Nontuberculous mycobacteria*
Enterobacter	Actinomycetes
Clostridium	*Treponema*
C. perfringens	
C. welchii	
Enterobacter	
Enterococcus	
Streptococcus	
Fusobacterium	
Flavobacterium	
Eubacterium	
Fungi	
	Yeasts (especially *Candida*)
	Filamentous fungi
Viruses	
	Adenoviruses (in children)
Protozoa	
	Entamoeba dispar
	Entamoeba moshkovskii
	Entamoeba coli
	Entamoeba hartmanni
	Endolimax nana
	Iodamoeba bütschlii
	Trichomonas hominis
	Chilomastix mesnili
Intestinal Flora	
Of Breast-Fed Infants	
Bifidobacterium	Enterobacteriaceae
	E. coli
	Klebsiella
	Proteus
	Enterobacter
	Enterococcus
Of Bottle-Fed Infants	
Lactobacillus acidophilus	*Enterococcus*
Gram-negative aerobes	
Clostridium	

TABLE 2–1. Predominant Microorganisms Indigenous to Various Locations of the Body (Normal Flora) *(Continued)*

Commonly Present	Occasionally Present
Genitourinary Tract	
Vagina (normal flora depends on age, glycogen content, pH, enzymes)	
Newborn period	
Usually sterile	
Neonatal period	
Bacteria	
Staphylococcus	
Corynebacterium	
Enterococcus	
Prepubertal period	
Bacteria	
Streptococcus (α- and γ-hemolytic)	
Corynebacterium	
Enterobacteriaceae	
E. coli	
Klebsiella	
Proteus	
Enterobacter	
Adult period	
Bacteria	
L. acidophilus	*Propionibacterium*
Coagulase-negative staphylococci	Group B *Streptococcus*
	Enterococcus
S. aureus	*Gardnerella vaginalis*
Streptococcus	*Acinetobacter*
Peptostreptococcus	*Mobiluncus*
Clostridium	Enterobacteriaceae
Corynebacterium	*E. coli*
	Klebsiella
	Proteus
	Enterobacter
	Neisseria
	Actinomycetes
	Mycoplasma
Fungi	
C. albicans	Other *Candida*
Pregnancy	
Increased coagulase-negative staphylococci, *Lactobacillus,* and yeasts	
Postmenopausal period	
Similar to prepubertal flora	
Cervix	
Usually sterile or harbors microorganisms similar to those in the upper vagina	
External Genitalia and Anterior Urethra	
Bacteria	
Coagulase-negative staphylococci	*Peptococcus*
Streptococcus	*Bacteroides*
Corynebacterium	*Fusobacterium*
S. aureus	Gram-negative anaerobic
Nontuberculous mycobacteria (uncircumcised males)	*Mycoplasma*
	Ureaplasma urealyticum
	Peptostreptococcus
	Enterococcus
	Enterobacteriaceae
	E. coli
	Klebsiella
	Proteus
	Enterobacter
Fungi	
C. albicans	

Commonly Present	Occasionally Present
Conjunctiva	
Bacteria	
Coagulase-negative staphylococci	*Streptococcus* (α-hemolytic)
S. aureus	Group A *Streptococcus*
Haemophilus aegypticus	*Streptococcus pneumoniae*
H. influenzae (nontypeable)	*Corynebacterium*
	Neisseria
	M. catarrhalis
	Enterobacteriaceae
	E. coli
	Klebsiella
	Proteus
	Enterobacter
Fungi	
	Malassezia furfur
Ear Canal	
Bacteria	
Coagulase-negative staphylococci	*S. pneumoniae*
Corynebacterium	*Bacillus*
Pseudomonas (including *P. aeruginosa*)	Enterobacteriaceae
	E. coli
	Klebsiella
	Proteus
	Enterobacter
Body Fluids	
Normal Voided Urine	
Bacteria	
(Usually sterile or harbors $<$1,000 cfu/mL)	
Coagulase-negative staphylococci	*Bacillus*
Corynebacterium	Nontuberculous mycobacteria
Streptococcus (α- and β-hemolytic)	
S. aureus	
Fungi	
C. albicans	
Smegma (Uncircumcised Males)	
Bacteria	
Mycobacterium smegmatis	Nontuberculous mycobacteria
Usually Sterile Body Fluids and Tissues	
Blood	
Cerebrospinal fluid	
Joint fluid	
Pleural fluid	
Pericardial fluid	
Peritoneal fluid	
Tissues without epithelial surfaces	

**S. aureus* and anaerobic cocci are rare in the edentulous mouth.

†10^{8-10} bacteria per gram; at least 95% of species are obligate anaerobes.

‡10^{11} bacteria per gram; at least 95% of species are obligate anaerobes.

intensive care units and who are treated with antibiotics frequently acquire other species as the predominant flora. Apparently, as in older persons, neonates are protected from transient colonization with potential pathogens by competition with normal flora.

NORMAL FLORA BY BODY SITE

The actual microorganisms colonizing a body site reflect a complex interaction between the microenvironment and the microorganism. At all body sites, including the skin, the majority of colonizing bacteria are anaerobic. However, their presence is not usually noted because they are generally avirulent and not involved in causing infection, and usual culture methods are often inadequate for optimal recovery.

The interpretation of cultures obtained from colonized sites must take into account the flora normally found at the site (Table 2–1). In addition, the method of obtaining the culture is important. For example, cultures of specimens from the lower respiratory tract, which is usually sterile, obtained through the oropharynx may be contaminated with the usual oropharyngeal organisms.

Perturbation of normal flora may permit colonization with unusual organisms that have the potential for pathogenic invasion. Infection does not necessarily follow. The interpretation of **surveillance cultures** (cultures of specimens from body sites, taken without a suspicion of infection) of mucosal-surface specimens from patients who are taking antimicrobial agents or in whom the normal flora is otherwise altered can be difficult. Surveillance cultures, which are most useful in the monitoring of the nosocomial spread of organisms and in the evaluation of a disease outbreak, are used to identify possible infecting organisms to guide empirical antimicrobial therapy if signs of infection develop. The diagnosis of an actual infection requires corroborating evidence. Surveillance cultures of samples from normally sterile sites (e.g., blood) without suspected infection are unnecessary. Under these circumstances a culture is more likely to show a false-positive result (i.e., to show a contaminant) than a true-positive result.

REVIEWS

Fonkalsrud EW, Krummel TM (editors): *Infections and Immunologic Disorders in Pediatric Surgery.* Philadelphia, WB Saunders, 1993.

Mackowiak PA: The normal microbial flora. *N Engl J Med* 1982;307:83–93.

KEY ARTICLES

Almuneef MS, Baltimore RS, Farrel PA, et al: Molecular typing demonstrating transmission of gram-negative rods in a neonatal intensive care unit in the absence of a recognized epidemic. *Clin Infect Dis* 2001;32:220–7.

Baley JE, Kliegman RM, Boxerbaum B, et al: Fungal colonization in the very low birth weight infant. *Pediatrics* 1986;78:225–32.

Baltimore RS, Duncan RL, Shapiro ED, et al: Epidemiology of pharyngeal colonization of infants with aerobic gram-negative rod bacteria. *J Clin Microbiol* 1989;27:91–5.

Barrie JD, Gallacher JB: The significance of *Escherichia coli* in the upper respiratory tract of children under 2 years of age. *Postgrad Med J* 1975;51:373–81.

Goldmann DA: Bacterial colonization and infection in the neonate. *Am J Med* 1981;70:417–22.

Hall MA, Cole CB, Smith SL, et al: Factors influencing the presence of faecal lactobacilli in early infancy. *Arch Dis Child* 1990;65:185–8.

Long SS, Swenson RM: Development of anaerobic fecal flora in healthy newborn infants. *J Pediatr* 1977;91:298–301.

Sprunt K, Leidy G, Redman W: Abnormal colonization of neonates in an intensive care unit: Means of identifying neonates at risk of infection. *Pediatr Res* 1978;12:998–1002.

Stark PL, Lee A: The microbial ecology of the large bowel of breast-fed and formula-fed infants during the first year of life. *J Med Microbiol* 1982;15:189–203.

CHAPTER 3

Epidemiology of Infectious Diseases

John C. Christenson

Certain environmental risk factors and exposures are necessary for the development of many infectious diseases. Exposures to contaminated fomites and environmental reservoirs such as food, water, and animals, as well as infected persons and vectors, place individuals at risk of infection. Humans interact with many sources of potential infection, and sound, systematic epidemiologic investigation is necessary to identify possible associations with infection (Fig. 3–1). **Epidemiology** is the science that helps determine the relationship between certain behaviors, acts, exposures, and risk factors and the acquisition of an infectious agent and later development of infection or disease. Without proper epidemiologic analysis, the development and proper implementation of preventive measures and immunizations would be almost impossible.

BASIC CONCEPTS OF EPIDEMIOLOGY

Epidemiology assists clinicians in determining the relationship of a certain behavior or exposure to an infection or disease. To provide this assistance, epidemiologists have various types of study designs available to them. The most commonly used study design is the **descriptive study** of the clinical features of medical conditions. These descriptions are used in further studies of the condition and in the process of identifying additional cases. Descriptive studies, because of their design, are generally retrospective and may be susceptible to observer bias. An **analytic study** involves the collection of data that are later analyzed with the intent of making an association between an event, exposure, or feature and an infection or disease. Analytic studies can be **retrospective** or **prospective.** A **case-control study** matches patients with certain diseases or infections with persons having similar demographic features (e.g., age, sex, presence of underlying conditions) to determine the relationship between events, exposures, or risk factors and the disease or infection being studied. Case-control studies are done in a retrospective manner once the features of the condition are known. In contrast, through the use of a **cohort study,** at-risk individuals can be observed in a prospective fashion, and in this manner the investigator can determine which exposures correlate with infection and disease. When planning an epidemiologic investigation with the intent of identifying a cause, one must carefully define the condition that is to be observed; the result is called the **case definition.**

Statistics as an Epidemiologic Tool

Once a clinical feature or association is suspected, the strength of association as it relates to the observed disease or infection is determined by statistical analyses including relative risk or odds ratio. A **two-by-two table** can be used to determine the association.

	Disease Present	*Disease Absent*
Exposure present	a	b
Exposure absent	c	d

$$\text{Relative ratio} = [a/(a + b)] \div [c/(c + d)]$$

$$\text{Odds ratio} = a/c \div b/d$$

The **relative risk (RR)** is defined as the ratio of the rate of illness or infection among exposed individuals to the rate of illness or infection among persons who were not exposed. These rates are usually determined by means of observational cohort studies. The **odds ratio (OR),** usually determined after completion of a case control study, provides an estimate of the RR of newly diagnosed cases of the disease or infection in relation to an exposure or possibly related event. If an RR or OR is greater than 1.0, there is a strong association between the exposure or risk and the disease or infection. If both are less than 1.0, then there is no observed relationship. In an examination of the relationship of an event, exposure, or potential risk factor to a disease or infection, the RR or OR is extremely important in determining the significance of this relationship.

Two epidemiologic concepts used frequently in clinical medicine are sensitivity and specificity. **Sensitivity** indicates how well a test or procedure predicts or identifies affected individuals among persons with the disease or infection. **Specificity** indicates how well the test or procedure identifies unaffected individuals among those individuals without the disease or infection. The higher the sensitivity and specificity, which are usually expressed as percentages, the better the test. A **two-by-two table** can be used to determine sensitivity and specificity.

	Disease Present	*Disease Absent*
Test positive	A	B
Test negative	C	D

$$\text{Sensitivity} = A/A + C$$

$$\text{Specificity} = D/B + D$$

Predictive values can better reflect how likely **(positive predictive value)** or unlikely **(negative predictive value)** it is that a test will identify a disease. The higher the predictive values, which are expressed as percentages, the better the test. These values are computed by using the following formulas.

$$\text{Positive predictive value} = A/A + B$$

$$\text{Negative predictive value} = C/C + D$$

Terminology That Defines Populations, Infections, and Disease Activity

Various terms are used to define at-risk or affected populations and disease outbreaks. **Incidence** refers to the number of new

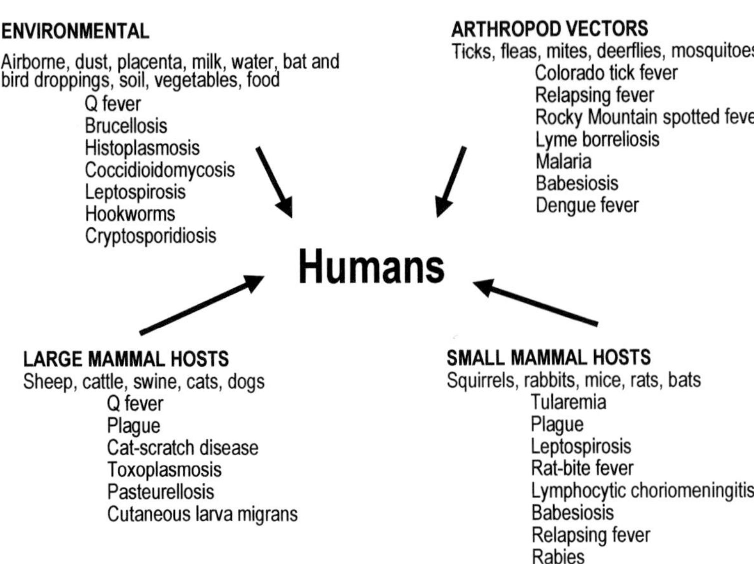

FIGURE 3–1. Interaction between humans and various environmental and zoonotic diseases.

infections per unit of population in a defined period. **Prevalence** indicates the presence of an infection, or number of cases per unit of population, at a given time of observation. **Seroprevalence** documents the presence of an infection per population unit at a given time based on the presence of organism-specific antibodies. Recognition of new infections or increased frequency of diseases during a short period or in a given location is important. This **clustering** of cases may be indicative of a common source outbreak. A **foodborne disease outbreak** consists of two or more cases of a similar illness resulting from the ingestion of a common food. A waterborne disease consists of two or more cases of a similar illness resulting from either ingestion of drinking water or exposure to water used for recreational purposes, with evidence that the water is the probable source of the illness. The requirement of two cases is waived for single cases of primary amebic meningoencephalitis and for chemical poisoning if supported by laboratory testing of the water. An infection or disease that is **endemic** occurs in a localized, confined region on a regular basis, with periods of increase and decrease. An **epidemic** refers to an increased incidence of disease in a defined population that is beyond the expected variation. A **pandemic** is an international epidemic. Continuous baseline surveillance is usually required to be able to identify an epidemic.

Zoonoses are infections that are transmitted in nature between vertebrate animals and humans. The terms **enzootic** and **epizootic** refer to concepts similar to endemic and epidemic but pertain to animal populations and are particularly important in an assessment of the risk of acquiring a zoonotic infection. Zoonoses are more likely to occur if humans venture into an area where an epizootic is present. Many zoonotic pathogens are maintained in nature by means of an **enzootic cycle,** in which mammalian hosts and arthropod vectors reinfect each other.

In an investigation the **index case** is usually the first identified case. During an epidemiologic investigation, **secondary cases** of disease or infection can be easily recognized with the assistance of an appropriate case definition or tests. In secondary cases the onset of disease occurs later than 24 hours after the appearance of the initial symptoms of the index case. The time of appearance of secondary cases may vary significantly depending on the incubation period of the organism. Secondary cases are clearly observed in individuals with close contact with the index case. The majority of infections represent **sporadic cases,** where there is no demonstrable epidemiologic link or association by person, place, time, or source to another case. On occasion, several individuals may develop signs or symptoms of the disease or evidence of infection within hours of identification of the index case; these represent **co-primary cases** that usually are caused by exposure to the same source of infection as the index case.

Attack rate is the number of new infections divided by the number of individuals exposed during a specific period. **Case-fatality rate** is the number of deaths due to infections or disease divided by the number of persons with the disease or infection. These rates are reported as percentages. **Mortality rate** is similar but refers to the ratio of individuals who have died in a certain period in a defined population. It is often expressed as a disease-specific rate.

Individuals or objects may be able to transmit infectious pathogens. Some persons may have **colonization** with an organism without evidence of disease or infection. These **carriers** may be responsible for the transmission of microorganisms. Microorganisms may colonize, multiply, and invade an individual, causing **infection** that may have signs and symptoms, or the infection may be ''silent''—a **subclinical infection.** What distinguishes colonization from infection is the host immune response, with microorganism-specific antibody production or cell-mediated immunity to the offending organism. The presence of signs and symptoms caused by the microorganism and the host's immune response reflect evidence of **disease,** or **illness.** After an infection, individuals may develop **immunity,** which may be cell mediated or humoral, against a microorganism that may provide **protective immunity** against all future infections or disease caused by that microorganism. Immunity may be strain or serotype specific. **Reservoirs** are humans, animals, or inanimate objects, or **fomites,** in an environment where microorganisms may survive or replicate and may serve as an agent of transmission of an infection. Animals such as rodents, cats, sheep, and prairie dogs are some of the important reservoirs in the environment and are responsible for many of the zoonotic diseases.

TRANSMISSION OF INFECTIOUS PATHOGENS

Multiple modes of transmission of infectious agents are apparent. Transmission may be direct or indirect. **Direct transmission** involves contact with a reservoir; for example, an infected individual may touch or may sneeze or cough on a susceptible person. **Indirect transmission** usually involves the presence of a **vector** such as food, water, blood, animal, or inanimate device that transfers an infective agent from one host to another. The term *vector* is often used to imply an arthropod intermediate. **Airborne diseases** such as tuberculosis, chickenpox, and measles are commonly transmitted through **small-particle aerosols,** which allow the infectious agent to be suspended in the environment for extended periods. Contact with **large-size droplets** results in transmission of other infectious agents, including respiratory viruses such as RSV. Contact with **contaminated body fluids or secretions** may place the recipient at risk of infection from **bloodborne** pathogens such as hepatitis B virus and HIV. Vectorborne transmission requires the presence of an invertebrate or arthropod vector to transmit an infectious agent and usually occurs through a bite or by contamination of food. Many of the zoonotic infections are acquired in this way.

In this era of air travel, persons incubating infections may travel while still symptom-free and within hours arrive in areas of the world where these infections do not usually occur. Clinicians in the nonendemic areas may fail to consider or recognize the disease, delaying the implementation of proper preventive measures and effective therapy, which may lead to local outbreaks as a consequence.

Nosocomial Transmission. **Nosocomial infections** signify infections that originate in the hospital but that are not present or incubating before admittance (Chapter 105). These infections usually occur in patients, but hospital personnel may also develop nosocomial infections. Many factors influence the nosocomial transmissibility of infectious agents. In hospitals, contaminated fomites such as stethoscopes, thermometers, or countertops are common sources of nosocomial pathogens. Most important, contaminated hands of health care workers are commonly associated with transmission of these pathogens. The likelihood of transmission depends on many factors such as the quantity of organisms in the vector or source, duration of vector exposure, and host susceptibility. Host susceptibility is a key factor that influences both the likelihood of a person's developing disease and the severity of the disease. For example, immunocompromised persons, persons with diabetes mellitus, achlorhydria, or gastric resection, and persons taking antacids may develop disease with a smaller inoculum of a bacterial pathogen than may be normally required to cause disease. Some organisms are more **virulent,** or **pathogenic,** than others, which is reflected in the inoculum required to cause infection, which varies significantly among organisms.

THE ENVIRONMENT AND INFECTION

Humans actively interact with nature's resources, plants, and other animals. Individuals are now spending considerably more time involved in outdoor activities as part of recreational or exploration activities. In addition, urbanization of rural areas, population growth, and overcrowding are increasing. Many modes of transmission exist for infections acquired in the outdoors, including ingestion, inhalation, skin or percutaneous contact, and direct contact with infected animals. Recreational activities such as hunting, hiking, camping, swimming in streams and ponds, and exploring caves are considered high-risk activities is relation to environmentally acquired and zoonotic infections.

Several common as well as some uncommon pathogens may be acquired from contact with contaminated soil and water (Table 3–1).

Soilborne Pathogens and Disease

Microorganisms contained in feces, urine, birth products, and carcasses of colonized or infected animals are the predominant soil contaminants that can lead to infection of humans, as well as other animals. Soil conditions that promote the growth of organisms, such as proper humidity, temperature, and the presence or absence of organic materials, are critical for the survival and transmission of certain infectious agents. For example, *Coccidioides immitis* is found in the superficial layers of the soil and is endemic to the semiarid regions of the southwestern United States, from California to Texas, where temperatures are high and humidity is low. Precipitation is predictable, with short but sometimes intense rainy seasons. Construction, archaeologic digs, and windstorms disturb the soil and allow the arthroconidia to become airborne and infect humans through inhalation. Examples of other soilborne fungi that cause disease include *Histoplasma capsulatum* and *Blastomyces dermatitidis,* which are both endemic to the eastern, southeastern, and central regions of the United States. Concentrated in the Ohio and Mississippi river basins, these organisms range throughout the midwestern states, as well as the Canadian provinces that border the Great Lakes. In addition, *H. capsulatum* is occasionally found in the extreme western United States. This fungus is spread through aerosol inhalation and contact with droppings of bats and birds.

Some infectious agents may survive in the soil even in the harshest conditions. *Coxiella burnetii,* the cause of Q fever, is resistant to many physical and chemical conditions. The sporelike forms of the organism may survive in the environment for months, even when the infected animal that contaminated the soil is no longer present. *C. burnetii* requires no animal or human host for its transmission.

Use of dust masks may prevent inhalation of infected dust particles when one is visiting arid areas. Dust masks should also be used when exploring caves, where large amounts of bat and bird droppings contaminate the soil, or when one is participating in archaeologic digs in the southwestern United States.

Waterborne Pathogens and Disease

Infected animals may be involved in contaminating water; for example, leptospiruric animals may urinate near streams or ponds. Contact with this water by other animals and humans may result in infection. Standing water of rivers and ponds contaminated by animal fecal material may serve as the mode of transmission of some zoonoses. Avoidance of contaminated areas, and especially avoidance of drinking unpurified water, is the preferred mode of prevention.

Infections by free-living amoebae living in water are uncommon but serious infections, including central nervous system infections caused by *Naegleria fowleri* (primary amebic meningoencephalitis) and *Acanthamoeba* (granulomatous amebic encephalitis). *Acanthamoeba* has been implicated in outbreaks of keratitis associated with the use of homemade saline products for contact lens users.

In the United States, there are approximately 10–15 waterborne-disease outbreaks annually (Fig. 3–2). Outbreaks are most common during the summer and fall months. The median outbreak size is approximately 10 persons per outbreak, but the range is from two to several hundred. Approximately 60% of outbreaks have an identifiable infectious cause, 10% are attributed to chemical

TABLE 3–1. Pathogens Associated with Soil and Water

Organism	Distribution
Organisms Frequently Found in Soil or Untreated Water Often without Direct Fecal Contamination	
Bacteria	
Aeromonas	Water
Bacillus anthracis (anthrax)	Soil
Chromobacterium violaceum	Water and soil
Clostridium botulinum	Soil
Clostridium tetani	Soil
Legionella pneumophila	Water
Plesiomonas	Water
Pseudomonas	Water and soil
Vibrio cholerae	Salt and brackish water
Vibrio vulnificus	Salt and brackish water
Yersinia	Water
Mycobacteria	
Mycobacterium marinum	Water
Fungi	
Blastomyces dermatitidis	Soil
Coccidioides immitis	Soil
Cryptococcus neoformans	Soil
Histoplasma capsulatum	Soil
Sporothrix schenckii	Soil
Viruses	
Adenoviruses	Water
Enteroviruses (including hepatitis A virus)	Water
Protozoa	
Cryptosporidium parvum	Water
Naegleria fowleri (primary amebic meningoencephalitis)	Water and soil
Acanthamoeba	Water and soil
Helminths	
Schistosoma	Fresh water
Organisms Frequently Found in Soil or Water Usually with Direct Fecal Contamination	
Bacteria	
Escherichia coli O157:H7	Water
Salmonella	Water
Shigella	Water
Spirochetes	
Leptospira	Water
Rickettsiae	
Coxiella burnetii (Q fever)	Soil
Protozoa	
Entamoeba histolytica	Water
Giardia lamblia	Water
Toxoplasma gondii	Soil
Helminths	
Hookworms (*Ancylostoma duodenale* and *Necator americanus*)	Soil
Ascaris lumbricoides	Soil
Strongyloides stercoralis	Soil
Toxocara canis	Soil
Trichuris trichiura	Soil

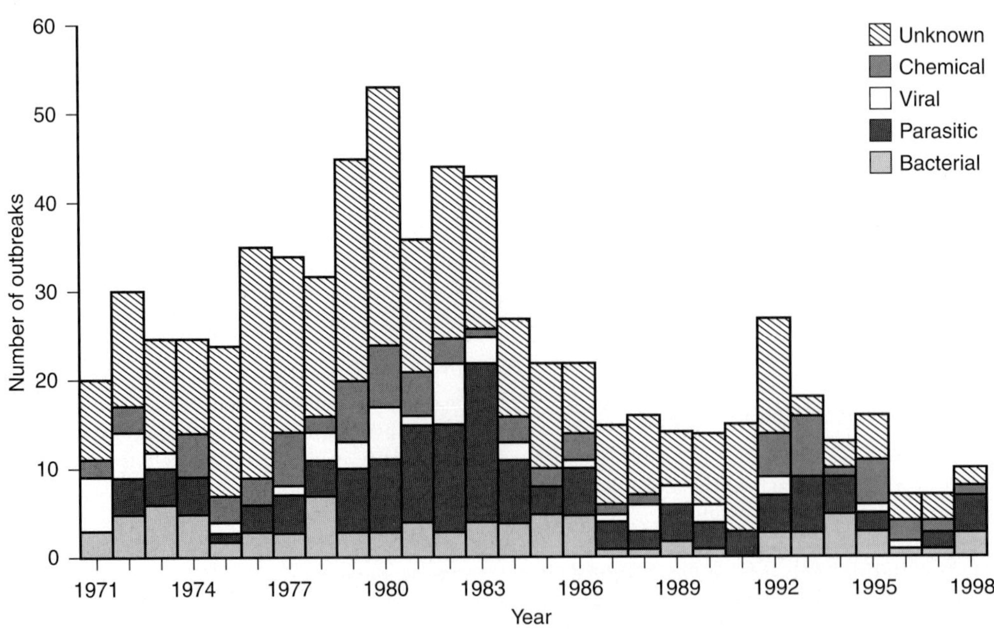

FIGURE 3–2. Number of waterborne-disease outbreaks associated with drinking water, by year and etiologic agent, United States, 1971–1998. (From Centers for Disease Control and Prevention: Surveillance for waterborne-disease outbreaks—United States, 1997–1998. *MMWR Morb Mortal Wkly Rep* 2000;49[SS-4]:1–21.)

poisoning, and 30% are of unknown cause. The most commonly identified infectious causes are the parasites *Cryptosporidium parvum,* which is the most common infectious cause, and *Giardia lamblia;* the bacteria *Escherichia coli* O157:H7 and *Shigella;* and Norwalk-like viruses. Uncommon infectious causes are *Legionella,* which causes pneumonia, and *Pseudomonas aeruginosa* and *Schistosoma,* which cause dermatitis. Approximately 50% of outbreaks are associated with community water systems, 30% with noncommunity water systems, and 25% with individual water systems. Only approximately 10% of all outbreaks are associated with surface water systems.

Swimming. Swimming in contaminated water or ingestion of such water, whether intentional or accidental, may also result in the spread of many infectious agents (Table 3–2). Many pathogens are spread by human fecal material in **swimming pools** and **hot baths.** Infants who are not toilet-trained should not be allowed to swim in public pools even if they are wearing diapers. Inadequate chlorination and improper maintenance of pH also increase the likelihood of propagation and spread of pathogens. Saunas and hot baths, and occasionally swimming pools, are associated with pustular folliculitis caused by *P. aeruginosa.* This infection may result from increased perspiration at higher temperatures and the increased numbers of bathers in a small space.

Swimming in streams and ponds, especially near farming areas, should be avoided. Swimming is not associated with the spread of the pathogens that cause sexually transmitted diseases. Women who swim in properly maintained public pools during pregnancy do not have an increased risk of intrauterine infections.

Foodborne Pathogens and Disease

The consumption of food products, whether animal or vegetable, that are grown or harvested in areas with contaminated soil or water or that are contaminated in storage or preparation may result in infection (Table 3–3). Use of fecal fertilizers or irrigation with contaminated water may contaminate foods. Vegetables and fruits that are not properly washed before consumption may result in enteric infections with *Salmonella* and *Listeria.* Outbreaks of enteric infections such as enterohemorrhagic *E. coli* O157:H7 and *Salmonella muenchen* infections may be related to changes in dietary preferences (sprouts, unpasteurized apple and orange juices). The consumption of raw or undercooked shellfish grown in polluted water or of meats from contaminated areas has been implicated in severe enteric infections with *Vibrio cholerae* and *E. coli* O157:H7. There is a wide range of minimum inoculum of enteric pathogens required to cause disease (Table 3–4).

TABLE 3–2. Infectious Agents Associated with Swimming

Freshwater Lakes and Rivers
Leptospira
Giardia lamblia
Cryptosporidium parvum
Naegleria fowleri (primary amebic meningoencephalitis)
Pseudomonas aeruginosa (otitis externa)
Fresh or Brackish Water
Austrobilharzia, Trichobilharzia, Ornithobilharzia (swimmer's itch)
Schistosoma (Africa, Asia, South America, Caribbean)
Streptococcus iniae
Mycobacterium marinum (and other mycobacteria)
Aeromonas hydrophila
Microbilharzia (swimmer's itch, clam-digger's itch)
Seawater
Vibrio cholerae
Vibrio vulnificus
Erysipelothrix rhusiopathiae
M. marinum
Swimming Pools and Sauna Baths
Enteric gram-negative bacilli, especially *Shigella*
Escherichia coli O157:H7
Pseudomonas aeruginosa (pustular folliculitis)
Adenovirus
Enteroviruses
Hepatitis A virus
Entamoeba histolytica
G. lamblia

Zoonotic and Vectorborne Pathogens and Disease

Zoonotic and vectorborne pathogens are important causes of human disease (Table 3–5), and many of them exhibit regional distribution and seasonal variation. The causative agent may not necessarily cause disease in nonhuman vertebrates. For some zoonotic organisms, humans may be a **dead-end host,** disrupting the life cycle of the organism. For other zoonotic species, humans may be a necessary part of the life cycle and may serve as either an **intermediate host** or a **definitive host.** Of the more than 150 different zoonotic diseases that have been described, *Borrelia burgdorferi,* the cause of Lyme disease, and a few other organisms account for most of the cases of vectorborne infections occurring in the United States (Fig. 3–3). Lyme disease accounts for approximately 90% of the reported cases of vectorborne infections in the United States (Chapter 29).

Enzootic foci of vectorborne illnesses require a favorable environment for the animal reservoir of the microbial pathogen as well as for the vector, which sometimes results in highly focal localization of the disease. Subtle environmental changes between different locales or states may account for significant differences in the incidence of a particular zoonosis in certain regions.

Reservoirs may include wild or domestic animals, and arthropods may be both vectors and reservoirs of disease. An infected animal may transmit a zoonotic pathogen directly to humans by close contact with oral or fecal secretions, by contact with the animal's coat, by animal bites or scratches, or by the consumption of contaminated flesh. Uncommon routes of inoculation may permit relatively innocuous animal pathogens to cause life-threatening human infection, such as B virus (herpesvirus simiae) infection from infected nonhuman primates. Zoonotic pathogens can also be transmitted to humans via an arthropod vector. In some instances the arthropod itself causes human disease; for example, *Sarcoptes scabiei* infestation is responsible for scabies.

The major vectors of zoonotic pathogens are fleas, flies, mosquitoes, and ticks. Fleas can transmit most rodentborne diseases. Blackflies may inject a poison into the skin with their bite, causing localized pain, numbness, and swelling that may persist for days. Horseflies and deerflies also give painful bites. Mosquitoes bite man and warm-blooded animals and are the principal vectors of the arboviral encephalitides, as well as of malaria, yellow fever, and dengue fever. Ticks can transmit many diseases (Table 3–6). *Dermacentor andersoni,* the wood tick, and *Dermacentor variabilis,* the dog tick, are probably the most common vectors of disease in the United States. These ticks are the vectors of RMSF and human ehrlichiosis. Another common vector, *Ixodes,* transmits *Babesia* and *B. burgdorferi,* the cause of Lyme disease.

The community-level risk of acquiring tickborne infections is a direct function of tick density, which in turn is causally related to the density of the reproductive host of the tick. The **transovarian transmission** rate of rickettsiae from female adult ticks to their

TABLE 3–3. Major Causes of Food-Borne Disease Outbreaks in the United States, 1993–1997*†

	Outbreaks		Cases		Deaths		
Etiologic Agent	No.	(%)	No.	(%)	No.	(%)	Common Food Sources
Bacterial							
Bacillus cereus	14	(0.5)	691	(0.8)	0	(0.0)	Fried rice, meats, vegetables
Brucella	1	(0.0)	19	(0.0)	0	(0.0)	Unpasteurized cow and goat milk, and cheese; blood sausages
Campylobacter	25	(0.9)	539	(0.6)	1	(3.4)	Poultry, raw milk, cheese
Clostridium botulinum	13	(0.5)	56	(0.1)	1	(3.4)	Vegetables, fruits, fish, honey
Clostridium perfringens	57	(2.1)	2,772	(3.2)	0	(0.0)	Beef, poultry, gravy, Mexican food
Escherichia coli (O157:H7)	84	(3.1)	3,260	(3.8)	8	(27.6)	Unpasteurized fruit juices, hamburgers, bean sprouts
Listeria monocytogenes	3	(0.1)	100	(0.1)	2	(6.9)	Unpasteurized milk and cheese products; poultry
Salmonella	357	(13.0)	32,610	(37.9)	13	(44.8)	Fruit, beef, poultry, eggs, dairy products, raw milk
Shigella	43	(1.6)	1,555	(1.8)	0	(0.0)	Egg salads, lettuce
Staphylococcus aureus	42	(1.5)	1,413	(1.6)	1	(3.4)	Ham, poultry, egg salads, pastries
Streptococcus, group A	1	(0.0)	122	(0.1)	0	(0.0)	
Streptococcus, other	1	(0.0)	6	(0.0)	0	(0.0)	
Vibrio cholerae	1	(0.0)	2	(0.0)	0	(0.0)	Shellfish
Vibrio parahaemolyticus	5	(0.2)	40	(0.0)	0	(0.0)	Shellfish, crabs
Yersinia enterocolitica	2	(0.1)	27	(0.0)	1	(3.4)	
Other bacterial	6	(0.2)	609	(0.7)	1	(3.4)	
Total bacterial	**655**	**(23.8)**	**43,821**	**(50.9)**	**28**	**(96.6)**	
Chemical							
Ciguatoxin	60	(2.2)	205	(0.2)	0	(0.0)	Barracuda, snapper, amberjack, grouper
Heavy metals	4	(0.1)	17	(0.0)	0	(0.0)	
Monosodium glutamate	1	(0.0)	2	(0.0)	0	(0.0)	
Mushroom poisoning	7	(0.3)	21	(0.0)	0	(0.0)	
Scombrotoxin	69	(2.5)	297	(0.3)	0	(0.0)	Tuna, mackerel, mahi-mahi
Shellfish	1	(0.0)	3	(0.0)	0	(0.0)	Shellfish
Other chemical	6	(0.2)	31	(0.0)	0	(0.0)	
Total chemical	**148**	**(5.4)**	**576**	**(0.7)**	**0**	**(0.0)**	
Parasitic							
Giardia lamblia	4	(0.1)	45	(0.1)	0	(0.0)	Raw vegetables
Trichinella spiralis	2	(0.1)	19	(0.0)	0	(0.0)	Contaminated pork; less frequently, contaminated horse meat, wild game
Other parasitic	13	(0.5)	2,261	(2.6)	0	(0.0)	
Total parasitic	**19**	**(0.7)**	**2,325**	**(2.7)**	**0**	**(0.0)**	
Viral							
Hepatitis A	23	(0.8)	729	(0.8)	0	(0.0)	Raw fruits and vegetables
Norwalk	9	(0.3)	1,233	(1.4)	0	(0.0)	Shellfish, salads
Other viral	24	(0.9)	2,104	(2.4)	0	(0.0)	
Total viral	**56**	**(2.0)**	**4,066**	**(4.7)**	**0**	**(0.0)**	
Confirmed Etiology	878	(31.9)	50,788	(59.0)	28	(96.6)	
Unknown Etiology	1,873	(68.1)	35,270	(41.0)	1	(3.4)	
Total 1993–1997	**2,751**	**(100.0)**	**86,058**	**(100.0)**	**29**	**(100.0)**	

*Includes Guam, Puerto Rico, and the U.S. Virgin Islands.
†Totals might vary by <1% from summed components because of rounding.
Adapted from Centers for Disease Control and Prevention: Surveillance for foodborne-disease outbreaks—United States, 1993–1997. *MMWR Morb Mortal Wkly Rep* 2000;49(SS-1):1–62.

TABLE 3–4. Inoculum of Enteric Pathogens Required to Cause Disease

Organism	Number of Organisms
Campylobacter	500
Cryptosporidium parvum	132
Entamoeba histolytica	10–100
Enterotoxigenic *Escherichia coli*	1,000,000–1,000,000,000
Giardia lamblia	10–25
Salmonella typhi	10,000–100,000,000
Nontyphoidal *Salmonella*	1,000–10,000,000,000
Shigella	10–100
Vibrio cholerae	1,000,000
Yersinia enterocolitica	1,000,000,000

offspring approximates 100%. These offspring are infected for life. In areas endemic for these tickborne diseases, 14,000 ticks are estimated to exist per acre of land. Fortunately, only 2–11% of these ticks harbor rickettsial organisms that may cause disease. The vast majority of ticks contain no rickettsial organisms, and a significant portion of these ticks are infected with nonpathogenic rickettsiae. The low incidence of pathogenic rickettsiae in some endemic regions may result from an interference phenomenon between nonpathogenic and pathogenic rickettsiae. For example, few cases of RMSF are reported on the eastern side of the Bitterroot River in Montana, whereas multiple cases of the disease are described on the western side.

The interaction of the vectors and their animal reservoirs, such as ground squirrels, rabbits, chipmunks, wood rats, meadow mice, weasels, and domestic pets (e.g., dogs and cats), ensures a constant source of pathogens in the environment. Infections in animal reservoirs are commonly inapparent. Humans, who are commonly accidental hosts in the cycle, are often exposed during recreational activities. Clinicians should suspect zoonotic infections in individuals returning from areas where the infectious disease is endemic, even when there is no history of known exposure to a vector or animal reservoir.

Tick Paralysis. Not all vectorborne diseases are infectious. For example, tick paralysis, or **tick toxicosis,** is a disease of animals that was first reported in North America in 1912. About 60 tick species can cause paralysis in animals, but only *D. andersoni* (the North American wood tick), *D. variabilis* (the common dog tick), and *Ixodes holocyclus* (the Australian marsupial tick) can affect humans. Tick paralysis is especially common among children in the spring and summer in the southeastern and northwestern United States and in British Columbia, Canada. Children are more frequently affected than adults, presumably because of their smaller body mass.

Tick paralysis results from a neurotoxin produced in the tick's salivary glands that either blocks the release of acetylcholine at the synapse or inhibits motor-stimulus conduction. Symptoms begin 2–7 days after the tick begins feeding, with symmetric weakness starting in the lower extremities and progressing as an ascending flaccid paralysis for several hours or days. Sensory function is usually spared, and the sensorium is clear. The CBC and CSF are normal. Nerve conduction velocity and compound muscle action potentials are decreased. The diagnosis is established by finding an engorged tick, which is usually embedded on the scalp. After the removal of the tick, symptoms generally resolve within several hours or days. If untreated, tick paralysis can be fatal, with a reported mortality rate of 12%.

Preventive Measures. Preventive measures are extremely important for persons visiting endemic or high-risk areas. Arthropod vectors are usually more active during the late spring and summer months because of the warm climate, and the incidence of zoonotic disease is highest between the months of June and September. Individuals should avoid grassy or marshy woodland areas during this time. The risk of mosquitoborne transmission is highest from dusk to dawn. Individuals should remain in screened areas at night and while sleeping, using indoor spray insecticides at sundown. Minimizing rodent burden and contact with rodents will minimize exposure to hantaviruses and to fleas that may transmit rodentborne disease such as plague (Table 3–7).

There are several preventive measures to minimize tick exposure and zoonoses (Table 3–8). It is especially important for persons at increased risk who are in endemic areas, such as asplenic individuals or those with HIV, to avoid habitats where ticks may be common.

Insect repellents should be applied to thin clothing and exposed areas of the skin, with repeated application as directed on the product insert. Most personal insect repellents contain **DEET** (*N, N*-diethyl-*m*-toluamide) and are available in aerosol and pump-spray products for treating clothing and skin and in liquid, cream, lotion, and stick products for precise skin application. There are no unreasonable adverse effects of DEET with normal recommended use. Repellents should be applied only to exposed skin and clothing, and not to cuts, wounds, irritated skin, eyes, mouth, or underclothing. They should not be applied to the hands of young children, who are prone to putting their hands in their mouths. Lower-concentration DEET products are appropriate for most situations where exposure to insects is minimal or for shorter exposure periods. Higher-concentration products provide increased efficacy and duration of protection and are particularly useful in highly infested areas. After a person returns indoors, the skin should be washed with soap and water. This is particularly important when repellents are used repeatedly in a single day or on consecutive days. Adverse reactions to DEET are exceptional but may include skin rash, toxic encephalopathy, and seizure.

Tick removal should be performed as soon as possible. After exposure to tick-infested sites, the body should be thoroughly examined while the person is showering; feeling for new bumps (ticks) may be facilitated by soap. To remove a tick, one should use blunt forceps or tweezers, grasping the tick as close to the skin as possible and steadily pulling the tick outward. Squeezing, twisting, or crushing the tick should be avoided because a tick's bloated abdomen can act like a syringe if squeezed. The application of heat and suffocation methods (e.g., using petrolatum jelly or nail polish) are of no benefit and may cause the tick to regurgitate into the bloodstream. Should the ''head'' stay in the skin, the site should be disinfected with alcohol or iodine. The mouth parts of the tick are not infectious and usually become encapsulated in a foreign-body reaction or eventually work themselves out of the site of the bite. Persons do not need to receive prophylactic antibiotics after each tick bite but should be alerted to signs and symptoms of disease.

Prophylactic antimicrobial therapy after a tick bite or exposure is not recommended because a majority of persons would be treated unnecessarily. A grace period exists for tick transmission of tickborne infections (Plate 9E). Infection appears to be most efficient after 30–36 hours of nymphal tick attachment for human granulocytic ehrlichiosis, after 36–48 hours for *B. burgdorferi,* and after 56–60 hours for *Babesia.* Active immunization for protection against zoonoses is available only for Lyme disease. Long-term antimicrobial prophylaxis to prevent zoonoses is not effective or cost-effective.

Text continued on page 22

TABLE 3–5. Epidemiology of Major Zoonotic and Vectorborne Infections

Disease	Causative Agent	Common Animal Reservoirs	Vectors/Modes of Transmission	Geographic Distribution
Bacterial Diseases				
Anthrax	*Bacillus anthracis*	Cattle, goats, sheep, swine, cats, wild animals	Aerosol inhalation of spores in hides and other animal by-products, direct contact	Worldwide; rare in United States
Bartonellosis (Oroya fever, verruga peruana)	*Bartonella bacilliformis*	Infected humans	Sandfly bite (*Phlebotomus verrucarum*)	Andes Mountains, Bolivia, Chile, Colombia, Ecuador, Peru
Brucellosis	*Brucella*	Cattle, sheep, goats, swine, horses, dogs	Aerosol inhalation, direct contact, ingestion of contaminated goat cheese and milk	Worldwide
Campylobacteriosis	*Campylobacter jejuni*	Rodents, dogs (puppies), cats, fowl (chicken), swine	Direct contact, ingestion of contaminated food or water	Worldwide
Cat-scratch disease	*Bartonella henselae*	Cats, dogs	Bites and scratches	Nationwide
Erysipeloid	*Erysipelothrix rhusiopathiae*	Sheep, swine, turkeys, ducks, fish	Direct contact	Worldwide
Listeriosis	*Listeria monocytogenes*	Cattle, fowl, goats, sheep	Ingestion of contaminated food, unpasteurized cheese and dairy products	Worldwide
Plague	*Yersinia pestis*	Wild and domestic rodents, cats, dogs	Direct contact, flea bite	New Mexico, Arizona, Utah, Colorado, California
Rat-bite fever (streptobacillary fever)	*Streptobacillus moniliformis*	Mice, rats, hamsters	Bites, ingestion of contaminated food or water	Japan, Asia; rare in United States
Salmonellosis	Nontyphoid *Salmonella*	Fowl, dogs, cats, reptiles, amphibians	Direct contact, ingestion of contaminated food or water	Worldwide
Tularemia	*Francisella tularensis*	Rabbits, squirrels, dogs, cats	Aerosol inhalation, direct contact, ingestion of contaminated meat, tick bite, deerfly bite	California, Utah, Arkansas, Oklahoma
Yersiniosis	*Yersinia enterocolitica, Yersinia pseudotuberculosis*	Rodents, cattle, goats, sheep, swine, fowl, dogs	Direct contact, ingestion of contaminated food or water	Worldwide
Whooping cough	*Bordetella bronchiseptica*	Cats, dogs, pigs, rabbits	Direct contact	Worldwide
Wound infection, bacteremia	*Pasteurella multocida, Capnocytophaga canimorsus*	Cats, dogs, rodents	Direct contact, bites and scratches	Worldwide
Mycobacterial Diseases				
Wound infection	*Mycobacterium marinum, Mycobacterium fortuitum, Mycobacterium kansasii*	Fish, aquarium	Direct contact, scratches	Worldwide
Spirochetal Diseases				
Leptospirosis	*Leptospira interrogans*	Dogs, rodents, livestock	Direct contact, contact with water or soil contaminated by urine of infected animals	Worldwide
Lyme disease	*Borrelia burgdorferi*	Deer, rodents	Tick bite (*Ixodes scapularis, Ixodes pacificus*)	Northeast, Midwest United States, California
Rat-bite fever (Haverhill fever)	*Spirillum minus*	Mice, rats, hamsters	Bites, ingestion of contaminated food or water	Japan, Asia, rare in United States

TABLE 3–5. Epidemiology of Major Zoonotic and Vectorborne Infections *(Continued)*

Disease	Causative Agent	Common Animal Reservoirs	Vectors/Modes of Transmission	Geographic Distribution
Spirochetal Diseases *(Continued)*				
Relapsing fever	*Borrelia*	Rodents, fleas	Louse bite, flea bite, transplacental transmission	Western and southern United States
Rickettsial Diseases				
Human granulocytic ehrlichiosis	Human granulocytic agent	Deer, rodents	Tick bite (*I. scapularis, I. pacificus*)	North-central and northeastern United States
Human monocytic ehrlichiosis	*Ehrlichia chaffeensis*	Dogs, ticks	Tick bite (*Amblyomma americanum*)	South-central and south Atlantic United States
Murine typhus	*Rickettsia typhi, Rickettsia felis*	Cats, rats, rodents	Flea bites	Southeastern and southern United States including Gulf Coast
Q fever	*Coxiella burnetii*	Sheep, goats, cattle, rabbits, parturient cats	Aerosol inhalation, direct contact, ingestion of contaminated milk	Nationwide
Rickettsialpox	*Rickettsia akari*	Common house mice	Mite bite	Urban areas in eastern United States, Korea, Russia, Africa
Rocky Mountain spotted fever	*Rickettsia rickettsii*	Dogs, small wild animals, rodents, ticks	Tick bite	Midwest and south Atlantic United States
Sennetsu fever	*Ehrlichia sennetsu*	Fish	Ingestion of raw fish	Japan
Chlamydial Diseases				
Psittacosis	*Chlamydia psittaci*	Birds	Aerosol inhalation	Worldwide
Fungal Diseases				
Cryptococcosis	*Cryptococcus neoformans*	Pigeons	Aerosol inhalation, contact with fecal material	Nationwide
Dermatophytoses	*Microsporum* *Trichophyton* *Epidermophyton*	Dogs, cats, rabbits	Direct contact, scratch	Worldwide
Histoplasmosis	*Histoplasma capsulatum*	Bats, birds	Aerosol inhalation, contact with fecal material	Mississippi and Ohio river valleys
Viral Diseases				
Colorado tick fever	Orbivirus	Rodents, ticks	Aerosol inhalation, tick bite, blood transfusion, ingestion of contaminated food	Rocky Mountains, Pacific Northwest, western Canada
Dengue fever	Dengue viruses (types 1–4)	Humans	Mosquito bite (*Aedes aegypti, Aedes albopictus*)	Tropical areas of the Caribbean, the Americas, and Asia
Hantavirus cardiopulmonary syndrome	Hantavirus	Rodents, mice, cats	Aerosol inhalation	Southwestern United States
Herpesvirus B infection	Herpesvirus B	Old World primates (rhesus, *Macaca cynomolgus*)	Animal bite	Africa, Asia (and primate centers worldwide)
Lymphocytic choriomeningitis	Lymphocytic choriomeningitis virus	Rodents, hamsters, mice	Aerosol inhalation, direct contact, bite	Worldwide
Rabies	Rabies virus	Dogs, skunks, bats, raccoons, foxes, cats	Bites and scratches	Worldwide
Vesicular stomatitis	Vesicular stomatitis virus	Horses, cattle, swine	Direct contact	The Americas
Protozoan Diseases				
African trypanosomiasis	*Trypanosoma brucei rhodesiense*	Wild and domestic animals	Insect bite (tsetse fly)	East Africa
	Trypanosoma brucei gambiense	Wild and domestic animals	Insect bite (tsetse fly)	West Africa

Table continued on following page

TABLE 3–5. Epidemiology of Major Zoonotic and Vectorborne Infections *(Continued)*

Disease	Causative Agent	Common Animal Reservoirs	Vectors/Modes of Transmission	Geographic Distribution
Protozoan Diseases *(Continued)*				
American trypanosomiasis (Chagas' disease)	*Trypanosoma cruzi*	Wild and domestic animals	Insect bite (reduviid bug); contact with fecal material of reduviid bug	South America, Central America, South Texas
Babesiosis	*Babesia*	Cattle, wild and domestic rodents	Tick bite (*I. scapularis*), blood transfusion	Worldwide
Leishmaniasis, mucocutaneous and cutaneous	*Leishmania*	Domestic and wild dogs	Sandfly bite	Tropics
Leishmaniasis, visceral	*Leishmania donovani* complex	Domestic and wild dogs	Sandfly bite	Tropics
Malaria	*Plasmodium*	Humans	Mosquito bite (*Anopheles*)	Usually imported to the United States, Southern California
Toxoplasmosis	*Toxoplasma gondii*	Cats, livestock	Ingestion of oocysts in fecally contaminated material or ingestion of tissue cysts in poorly cooked meat	Worldwide
Helminthic Diseases				
Anisakiasis	*Anisakis simplex*	Whales and dolphins	Ingestion of raw fish	Worldwide
Baylisascariasis (visceral larva migrans)	*Baylisascaris procyonis*	Raccoons	Ingestion of eggs contaminated with fecal material	Worldwide
Clonorchiasis	*Clonorchis sinensis*	Wild and domestic animals	Ingestion of metacercariae (raw fish)	Far East
Cutaneous larva migrans	*Ancylostoma braziliense*	Cats, dogs	Direct contact	Worldwide
Diphyllobothriasis	*Diphyllobothrium latum*	Wild and domestic animals	Ingestion of raw fish	North America, Europe
Dipylidiasis	*Dipylidium caninum*	Dogs, cats	Ingestion of infected fleas	Worldwide
Dracunculiasis	*Dracunculus medinensis*	Humans	*Cyclops* ingestion	Africa and Asia
Echinococcosis	*Echinococcus granulosus, Echinococcus multilocularis*	Dogs, carnivores, livestock (especially sheep)	Ingestion of eggs or food contaminated with fecal material	Worldwide
Fascioliasis	*Fasciola hepatica*	Wild and domestic animals	Ingestion of metacercariae (aquatic vegetation)	Worldwide
Filariasis	*Wuchereria bancrofti*	Humans	Mosquito bite	Tropics
	Brugia malayi	Wild and domestic animals	Mosquito bite	Asia
Loiasis	*Loa loa*	Primates	Tabanid fly bite (*Chrysops*)	Africa
Onchocerciasis	*Onchocerca volvulus*	Humans	Blackfly bite	Sub-Saharan Africa, Central and South America
Opisthorchiasis	*Opisthorchis viverrini*	Wild and domestic animals	Ingestion of metacercariae (raw fish)	Eastern Hemisphere
Paragonimiasis	*Paragonimus*	Wild and domestic animals	Ingestion of metacercariae (crustaceans)	Tropics
Schistosomiasis	*Schistosoma mansoni* *Schistosoma japonicum* *Schistosoma haematobium*	Wild and domestic animals	Cutaneous penetration of cercariae in water	Tropics
Taeniasis	*Taenia saginata* *Taenia solium*	Humans	Ingestion of raw beef (*T. saginata*) or raw pork (*T. solium*)	Worldwide
Toxocariasis (visceral larva migrans)	*Toxocara canis* *Toxocara cati*	Dogs Cats	Ingestion of eggs contaminated with fecal material	Worldwide
Trichinellosis	*Trichinella spiralis*	Wild and domestic animals	Ingestion of raw meat	Worldwide
Hymenolepiasis	*Hymenolepis nana*	Wild and domestic animals	Ingestion of eggs or food contaminated with fecal material	Worldwide
	Hymenolepis diminuta	Wild rodents	Ingestion of infected fleas or insects	Worldwide

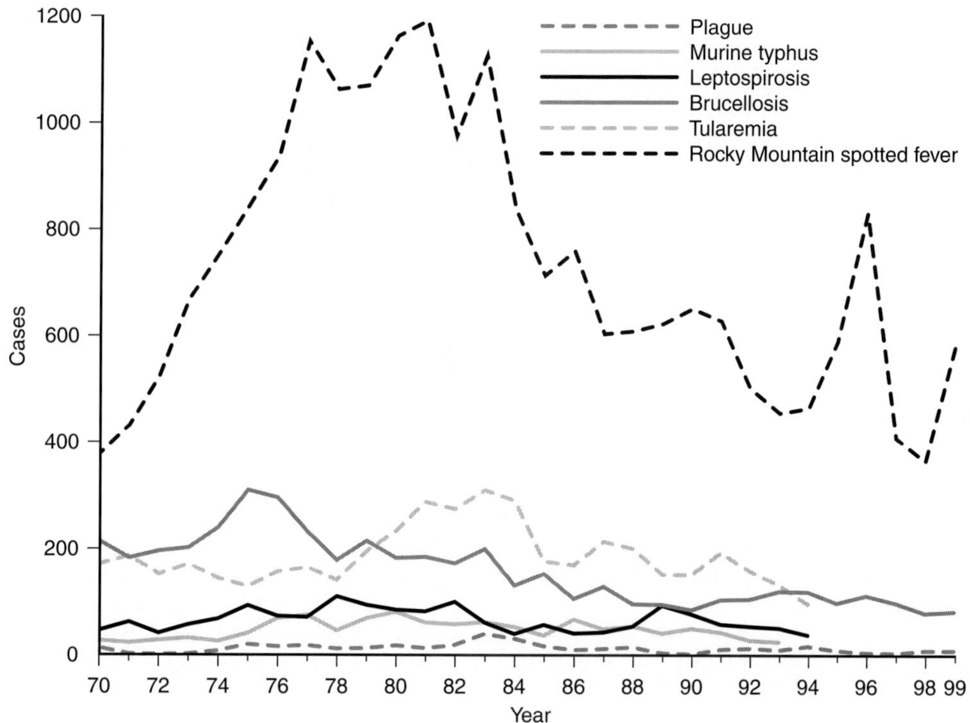

FIGURE 3–3. Number of reported cases of common zoonotic diseases other than Lyme disease in the United States, 1980–1999. See Figure 29–1 for Lyme disease. (Data from the Centers for Disease Control and Prevention.)

TABLE 3–6. Common Ticks Associated with Disease

Tick	Common Name	Associated Diseases*
Dermacentor andersoni	Rocky Mountain wood tick	Rocky Mountain spotted fever Colorado tick fever Tularemia
Dermacentor variabilis	American dog tick	Rocky Mountain spotted fever
Amblyomma americanum	Lone Star tick	Human monocytic ehrlichiosis Lyme disease–like illness (*Borrelia lonestari*)
Amblyomma maculatum	Gulf Coast tick	Human monocytic ehrlichiosis
Ixodes scapularis	Black-legged tick	Lyme disease Babesiosis Human granulocytic ehrlichiosis
Ixodes pacificus	Western black-legged tick	Lyme disease
Ornithodoros	Soft body ticks	Relapsing fever

**Dermacentor andersoni, Dermacentor variabilis,* and *Ixodes holocyclus* (the Australian marsupial tick) can cause tick paralysis in humans.

TABLE 3–7. Preventive Measures to Avoid Rodentborne Diseases (Hantaviruses, *Yersinia pestis*)

Eliminate rodent harborage
- Keep cooking, eating, and food storage areas clean
- Cover human food and animal feed
- Contain and elevate garbage
- Seal holes and cracks in dwellings to prevent entrance by rodents
- Clear brush and trash from around homes and outbuildings

Control rodent populations by maintaining snap traps or using rodenticides or both; in areas where plague occurs, control fleas with insecticides

Safely clean up rodent-infested areas
- Air out infested spaces before cleanup
- Spray areas of infestation and all excreta, nesting, and other materials with household disinfectant or 10% bleach solution; then clean up, seal in bags, and dispose of bags
- Avoid sweeping, vacuuming, or stirring dust until the area is thoroughly wet with disinfectant
- Wear rubber gloves; disinfect gloves before removal, and wash hands afterward
- In areas where plague occurs, spray insecticide on trapped rodents and nesting materials to prevent fleas from abandoning rodents to find new hosts

Avoid rodents when outdoors
- Do not disturb rodent droppings or camp or sleep near burrows or areas where trash is present
- Avoid feeding or handling rodents, even if they appear friendly

Adapted from Centers for Disease Control and Prevention: Update: Hantavirus pulmonary syndrome—United States, 1999. *MMWR Morb Mortal Wkly Rep* 1999:48:524.

TABLE 3–8. Preventive Measures to Avoid Tickborne Diseases

Avoid tick-infested habitats (e.g., thick scrub oak, briar, poison ivy sites) if possible
Avoid excretory products of wild animals
Wear shoes or boots, not sandals
Wear long-sleeved shirts and long trousers that cover the arms and legs, with trousers tucked into shoes or socks to prevent ticks from crawling under clothing
Wear light-colored clothing to facilitate detection of crawling ticks
Use insect repellants on skin (DEET) or on clothing (permethrin)
Conduct thorough inspection of the body and of pets after returning from the outdoors
Remove ticks promptly and carefully

For the deer tick–transmitted zoonoses, deer reduction has drastically diminished human risk. Host-seeking ticks may be killed by applications of acaricide to vegetation around yards or by targeted application with impregnated cotton, which mice carry back to their nests (Damminix). Deer ticks and Lone Star ticks are dependent on humid microclimates, and accordingly, vegetation management (brush cutting and removal, controlled burns) might prove useful.

Preventive occupational measures to minimize exposure are important for persons involved in farming, sheepherding, veterinary work, butchering, meatpacking, slaughterhouse work, and fowl processing.

REVIEWS

Bailar JC, Mosteller F (editors): *Medical Uses of Statistics,* 2nd ed. Boston, Massachusetts Medical Society, 1992.

Benenson AS (editor): *Control of Communicable Diseases in Man,* 16th ed. Washington, DC, American Public Health Association, 1995.

Hierholzer WJ: Principles of infectious disease epidemiology. In Mayhall CG (editor): *Hospital Epidemiology and Infection Control.* Baltimore, Williams & Wilkins, 1996.

Weber R: *Communicable Disease Epidemiology and Control.* London, CAB International, 1996.

Wiener HW, Vermund SH: Epidemiology in tropical medicine. In Guerrant RL, Walker DH, Weller PF (editors): *Tropical Infectious Diseases. Principles, Pathogens and Practice.* Philadelphia, Churchill Livingstone, 1999.

KEY ARTICLES

Centers for Disease Control and Prevention: Surveillance for foodborne-disease outbreaks—United States, 1993–1997. *MMWR Morb Mortal Wkly Rep* 2000;49(SS–1):1–62.

Centers for Disease Control and Prevention: Surveillance for waterborne-disease outbreaks—United States, 1997–1998. *MMWR Morb Mortal Wkly Rep* 2000;49(SS–4):1–35.

Chomel BB: Zoonoses of house pets other than dogs, cats, and birds. *Pediatr Infect Dis J* 1992;11:479–87.

Dworkin MS, Shoemaker PC, Anderson DE: Tick paralysis: 33 human cases in Washington State, 1946–1996. *Clin Infect Dis* 1999;29:1435–9.

Favero MS: Microbiologic indicators of health risks associated with swimming. *Am J Public Health* 1985;75:1051–4.

Felz MW, Smith CD, Swift TR: A six-year-old girl with tick paralysis. *N Engl J Med* 2000;342:90–4.

Fradin MS: Mosquitoes and mosquito repellents: A clinician's guide. *Ann Intern Med* 1998;128:931–40.

Goscienski PJ: Zoonoses. *Pediatr Infect Dis J* 1983;2:69–81.

Mead PS, Slutsker L, Dietz V, et al: Food-related illness and death in the United States. *Emerg Infect Dis* 1999;5:607–25.

Mills JN, Childs JE: Ecologic studies in rodent reservoirs: Their relevance for human health. *Emerg Infect Dis* 1998;4:529–37.

Raoult D, Roux V: The body louse as a vector of reemerging human diseases. *Clin Infect Dis* 1999;29:888–911.

CHAPTER 4

Infectious Agents and Oncogenesis

Hal B. Jenson

The epidemiology and course of many noninfectious human maladies suggest that infectious agents may play an etiologic role in the pathogenesis of these maladies. The environment has a principal role in causing sporadic cancers, and infectious agents, especially viruses, have been shown to contribute to a significant percentage of all human cancers worldwide. Viruses may contribute *directly* to oncogenesis by the effects of viral gene products as oncoproteins, such as transcriptional transactivators of host promoter sequences, or by the integration of viral genomes into host genomes, which can transactivate host proto-oncogenes. Viruses, bacteria, and parasites can contribute *indirectly* to oncogenesis by increased cellular proliferation of a target tissue or by persistent induction of an inflammatory response. Chronic inflammation and increased cell division increase the likelihood of mutagenesis. Another indirect means of carcinogenesis is modulation of the immune system, as with HIV infection, which permits the emergence and proliferation of tumor cells.

VIRUSES IN ONCOGENESIS

Several groups of viruses demonstrate in vitro cell-transforming properties and oncogenic potential, including the herpesviruses (HSV-1, HSV-2, CMV, EBV, VZV, HHV6, HHV7, and HHV8), the polyomaviruses (BK virus and JC virus), the adenoviruses (especially types 12 and 18), and the poxviruses (e.g., molluscum contagiosum virus). The strongest clinical association of infectious agents and tumorigenesis, on the basis of both epidemiologic and experimental data, exists for EBV, hepatitis B virus, hepatitis C virus, retroviruses, and papillomaviruses (Table 4–1). There is insufficient evidence for a causal link of HSV-1, HSV-2, CMV, HHV6, adenoviruses, or molluscum contagiosum virus with cancer.

Viruses contribute to approximately 15% of all cancers worldwide. Hepatocellular carcinoma, associated with hepatitis B virus and hepatitis C virus, and cancer of the cervix, associated with the human papillomaviruses, account for about 80% of virus-associated cancers. None of these viruses are capable of inducing cancer independently but require additional physical or chemical factors.

Most virus-associated tumors do not develop or manifest clinically during childhood or adolescence, which underscores the long clinically silent period between acquisition of infection and development of cancer. Yet the acquisition of these infections during childhood facilitates eventual malignant transformation, with the actual development and timing modulated by additional environmental influences. The recognized association of these infectious agents with cancer provides great potential for reducing the incidence of these cancers through the development of effective vaccines and immunization strategies in childhood, before exposure to and acquisition of these pathogens. The strategy to immunize against an infectious agent to reduce the incidence of cancer has already been successfully demonstrated for hepatitis B and hepatocellular carcinoma.

Epstein-Barr Virus

Epstein-Barr virus (EBV), a member of the Herpesviridae family, was the first virus demonstrated to contribute to human cancers. EBV causes several benign proliferations including infectious mononucleosis (Chapter 37) and, in persons with AIDS (Chapter 38), oral hairy leukoplakia and lymphoid interstitial pneumonitis. It is also associated with several lymphoid, epithelial, and soft tissue neoplasias (Table 4–1).

Nasopharyngeal Carcinoma. Nasopharyngeal carcinoma is a lymphoepithelioma that originates from epithelial cells of the posterior nasopharynx. It occurs sporadically in Western countries but is 10 times more common among persons from southern China, where it is the most common tumor among males. The pathogenesis of the tumor in China may be associated with genetic factors, such as the overrepresentation of certain HLA haplotypes (A2 Bsin2, Aw19, Bw46, and B17), and with volatile *N*-nitrosamines, ingested in smoked fish and perhaps inhaled from herbal extracts, which may stimulate B lymphocytes. Nasopharyngeal carcinoma is also endemic among whites in North Africa and among the Inuit in North America. The increased incidence persists even after emigration.

Malignant cells of undifferentiated nasopharyngeal carcinomas contain a high copy number of EBV episomes and express several EBV-encoded proteins. Patients with undifferentiated and partially differentiated, nonkeratinizing nasopharyngeal carcinoma have characteristic antibody patterns with high antibody titers to VCA, EA-D, viral DNase, and DNA polymerase that are both diagnostic and prognostic (Table 37–3). High levels of IgA antibody to VCA and EA can be detected in the asymptomatic period of tumor development and can be used to follow the efficacy of tumor therapy in persons with the undifferentiated form of the disease. In contrast, persons with the well-differentiated, keratinizing form of nasopharyngeal carcinoma have a low copy number of EBV genomes and have EBV serologic patterns similar to those of control populations.

Burkitt's Lymphoma. **Endemic (African) Burkitt's lymphoma** is the most common childhood cancer in equatorial East Africa and New Guinea (Table 4–2). These regions are characterized by holoendemic *Plasmodium falciparum* malaria and a high rate of EBV infection early in life. The constant malarial exposure operates as a B-lymphocyte mitogen that contributes to the polyclonal B-lymphocyte proliferation of EBV infection. It also impairs T-lymphocyte control of the EBV-infected B lymphocytes. Approximately 98% of persons with endemic (African) Burkitt's lymphoma harbor the EBV genome and express EBNA-1, compared with only 20% of persons with **nonendemic (sporadic or American) Burkitt's lymphoma**. Persons with Burkitt's lymphoma demonstrate unusually and characteristically high levels of EBV-specific antibody to VCA and to EA-R that correlate with the risk of tumor development (Table 37–3).

TABLE 4–1. Cancers Associated with Infectious Agents

Infectious Agent	Associated Cancers
Viruses	
Epstein-Barr virus	Burkitt's lymphoma Nasopharyngeal carcinoma Non-Hodgkin's lymphoma in immunocompromised persons Leiomyosarcoma in immunocompromised persons Hodgkin's disease (some forms) Palatine tonsil carcinoma (possible association) Primary central nervous system lymphoma (possible association)
Human herpesvirus type 8 (HHV8)	Kaposi's sarcoma Primary effusion lymphoma
Hepatitis B virus	Hepatocellular carcinoma
Hepatitis C virus	Hepatocellular carcinoma
Human papillomaviruses (Table 46–11)	Cutaneous and mucosal papillocarcinomas, including cervical carcinoma
HTLV-I	Adult T-cell leukemia (ATL) T-cell lymphoma
Polyomaviruses (JC, BK, and SV40)	Osteosarcoma Mesothelioma Brain tumors (ependymomas, glioblastomas, oligodendrogliomas)
Human immunodeficiency virus (HIV) (secondary to immunocompromise)	Non-Hodgkin's lymphoma (associated with EBV) Leiomyosarcoma (associated with EBV) Kaposi's sarcoma (associated with HHV8) Primary effusion lymphoma (associated with HHV8) Carcinomas of skin and cervix (associated with human papillomaviruses)
Bacteria	
Helicobacter pylori	Gastric adenocarcinoma Mucosa-associated lymphoid tissue (MALT) non-Hodgkin's lymphoma
Mycobacterium tuberculosis	Bronchogenic carcinoma
Fusobacterium nucleatum and *Treponema vincentii*	Squamous cell carcinoma arising from tropical phagedenic ulcer
Salmonella typhi and *Salmonella paratyphi*	Gallbladder cancer
Vibrio cholerae (possible association)	Immunoproliferative small intestinal disease
Trophermyma whippelii (possible association)	Small intestinal lymphoma
Chlamydiae	
Chlamydia trachomatis	Cervical carcinoma
Parasites	
Schistosoma haematobium	Squamous cell carcinoma of the urinary bladder
Schistosoma japonicum (possible association)	Colorectal carcinomas
Opisthorchis viverrini	Cholangiocarcinoma
Opisthorchis felineus	Cholangiocarcinoma
Clonorchis sinensis (possible association)	Cholangiocarcinoma
As Cofactors with Viruses	
Plasmodium falciparum	Burkitt's lymphoma (associated with EBV)
Strongyloides stercoralis	HTLV-associated leukemia (associated with HTLV-I)

TABLE 4–2. Comparison of Endemic and Nonendemic Burkitt's Lymphoma

Characteristic	Endemic (Classic or African)	Nonendemic (Sporadic or American)
Association with EBV	100%; usually EBV-2	15–25%; usually EBV-1
Chromosome breakpoints	Upstream of *c-myc*	Within *c-myc*
Occurrence	Africa: 8–10 cases per 100,000 population per year America: 4 cases per 100,000 children <15 yr of age	America: 0.2 per 100,000 children <15 yr of age
Common sites	Jaw, abdomen, orbit, paraspinal	Abdomen, bone marrow, lymph nodes, nasopharynx
Response to treatment	Good	Poor

Burkitt's lymphoma is a monoclonal proliferation. In all cases of Burkitt's lymphoma, whether with or without EBV, the c-*myc* proto-oncogene, located on chromosome 8, is invariably fused by nonrandom chromosomal translocation to the constant region of the immunoglobulin heavy chain locus on chromosome 14, t(8;14), the κ constant light chain locus on chromosome 2, t(2;8), or the λ constant light chain locus on chromosome 22, t(8;22). The gene on the chromosome involved in the translocation is deregulated and constitutively transcribed, possibly by virtue of the adjacent immunoglobulin locus. This results in an overproduction of a normal c-*myc* product that autosuppresses the c-*myc* allele on the nontranslocated chromosome.

The precise interaction of EBV-encoded proteins and c-*myc* deregulation and the contribution of EBV infection to the development of Burkitt's lymphoma is not yet defined. EBV likely plays a role as a nonessential cofactor in the development of Burkitt's lymphoma by promoting proliferation of the pre-B-cell population. This correspondingly increases the chances of a critical chromosomal translocation involving c-*myc*.

Hodgkin's Disease. Prospective studies have shown that EBV infection increases the risk of developing Hodgkin's disease by a factor of two to four. Persons with Hodgkin's disease consistently have elevated EBV antibody titers preceding the development of Hodgkin's disease. EBV is detectable in the Reed-Sternberg cells, the pathognomonic malignant cells of Hodgkin's tumors, in approximately 50% of the cases of Hodgkin's disease in developed countries and in up to 100% of the cases in developing countries. This geographic variation parallels the association of EBV with Burkitt's lymphoma. The **mixed cellularity** and **nodular sclerosing** histologic subtypes are most frequently positive for EBV (80% and 30%, respectively). The **lymphocyte-predominant** subtype is typically negative for EBV.

Lymphoproliferative Disease in Immunocompromised Persons. The most common EBV-associated tumor in the United States is lymphoproliferative disease, a non-Hodgkin's lymphoma associated with immunocompromise. Failure to control EBV replication can result from several different immunologic defects (Table 4–3). The prototype is the **X-linked lymphoproliferative (XLP) syndrome,** which has been described in 161 persons in 44 kindreds. About two thirds of persons with XLP syndrome die with fulminating and fatal infectious mononucleosis during the primary EBV infection. Survivors have hypogammaglobulinemia or B-cell lymphoma or both. About 85% of these persons die by 10 years of age. The XLP syndrome should be considered in any male patient with acute fatal primary EBV infection and in any kindred with a family history of hypogammaglobulinemia or with lymphoma in related males.

TABLE 4–3. Immunocompromised Conditions Predisposing to Epstein-Barr Virus–associated Lymphoma

Congenital Immunodeficiency
X-linked lymphoproliferative (XLP) syndrome
Common variable immunodeficiency
Ataxia-telangiectasia
Wiskott-Aldrich syndrome
Chediak-Higashi syndrome
Acquired Immunodeficiency
Acquired immunodeficiency syndrome (AIDS)
Immunocompromise associated with solid organ and bone marrow transplantation

Several other congenital immunodeficiency syndromes are also associated with an increased incidence of EBV-associated lymphomas. Lymphoproliferative syndromes arise from B lymphocytes and increase in incidence in parallel with the degree of immunocompromise. The B-cell tumors in immunocompromised persons may be focal or diffuse, and they may be polyclonal, oligoclonal, or monoclonal. Many of these tumors are probably polyclonal, but certain growth advantages favor the progression to oligoclonality or monoclonality.

In posttransplant recipients, who are severely immunocompromised, EBV infection may result in a self-limited infectious mononucleosis syndrome, fatal lymphoproliferation involving internal organs and progressing for 1 to 2 months, or extranodal non-Hodgkin's lymphoma. The incidence of malignant lymphoproliferation after transplantation is approximately 1% in adults; in children it is about 4%, presumably because of an increased incidence of primary EBV infection in seronegative children. Polyclonal posttransplant EBV-associated lymphoproliferative disease usually regresses when immunosuppressive therapy is decreased or discontinued, which indicates the importance of early immune control of EBV proliferation by cytotoxic T-cell responses. Cessation of immunosuppression with monoclonal posttransplant lymphoma, however, has no effect, an indication that the progression of the initial polyclonal lymphoproliferative response is followed by evolution to more aggressive tumors that are less inhibited by immune surveillance.

Immunodeficiency from HIV infection is associated with an approximately 300-fold risk of developing B-cell nonHodgkin's lymphoma. HIV-infected persons with lymphoma have increased numbers of EBV-infected circulating B lymphocytes and an increased EBV viral burden, in comparison with HIV-infected persons without cancer. EBV is detected in approximately 50% of these lymphomas. Improved antiretroviral therapy and longer survival among persons with AIDS may increase tumor incidence.

Primary **central nervous system lymphoma** is a relatively rare tumor that is typically found in persons with AIDS, organ transplant recipients, persons with congenital immunodeficiencies, and elderly individuals, especially men. EBV is detectable in the cells of the majority of central nervous system lymphomas, especially in persons with AIDS.

Other Tumors. EBV is associated with **leiomyosarcoma** in persons with AIDS or other immunocompromised persons, especially transplant recipients. EBV has been putatively associated with many other types of tumors on the basis of the detection of anti-EBV antibodies in serum or cerebrospinal fluid or because of the presence of EBV DNA or antigens in tissue samples. These tumors include lymphocyte lymphoma, angioimmunoblastic lymphadenopathy–like lymphoma, thymomas and thymic carcinomas derived from thymic epithelial cells, supraglottic laryngeal carcinomas, lymphoepithelial tumors of the respiratory tract and gastrointestinal tract, gastric adenocarcinoma, and leiomyosarcomas. The precise contribution of EBV to these various malignancies is not well defined.

Human Herpesvirus Type 8

Human herpesvirus type 8, also known as **Kaposi's sarcoma–associated herpesvirus,** appears to be necessary but not sufficient for the development of at least three types of tumors. **Kaposi's sarcoma** is a vascular spindle-cell disease occurring in approximately 15–25% of adults with AIDS. **Classic Kaposi's sarcoma,** occurring without HIV infection, is rare but is found in elderly Mediterranean and African men. HHV8 is detected in all clinical forms of Kaposi's sarcoma, including those associated with both HIV infection and classic Kaposi's sarcoma. HHV8 is also consistently found in a specific type of non-Hodgkin's lymphoma called **primary effusion lymphoma,** also known as body cavity–based lymphoma, which occurs in peritoneal, pleural, and pericardial spaces. Most cases of primary effusion lymphoma occur in HIV-infected persons, and the lymphoma cells are usually dually infected with both EBV and HHV8. HHV8 is also found in most cases of **multicentric Castleman's disease,** an atypical lymphoproliferative disorder that occurs in two variants, the hyaline-vascular variant and the plasma cell variant. Most HIV-infected persons with Castleman's disease, especially the plasma cell variant, harbor HHV8, in comparison with only approximately half of HIV-uninfected persons with multicentric Castleman's disease.

HHV8 has also been found in the dendritic cells of patients with **multiple myeloma,** a malignancy of B cells that represents the second most common hematologic malignancy in the United States. The results of serologic studies linking HHV8 to multiple myeloma remain controversial. HHV8 encodes a viral IL-6 homolog (vIL-6) that may stimulate exogenous B-cell populations in the bone-marrow microenvironment to proliferate nonspecifically.

Hepatitis B Virus

Hepatitis B infection (Chapter 78) may result in chronic carriage of HBsAg in approximately 5–10% of infected adults and 20% of infected children. Persistent proliferation of hepatocytes with chronic hepatitis B infection is associated with a 20- to 40-fold increased risk of **hepatocellular carcinoma.** Because approximately 200 million persons worldwide are chronic HBsAg carriers, hepatocellular carcinoma is one of the most common human cancers in the world, especially in the hepatitis B virus–endemic areas of Southeast Asia, China, Japan, sub-Saharan Africa, the Middle East, and the Mediterranean basin. Other noninfectious factors and conditions associated with the development of hepatocellular carcinoma include alcohol-induced cirrhosis, mycotoxins, petrochemicals, anabolic steroids, hemochromatosis, and α_1-antitrypsin deficiency.

Integrated hepatitis B virus DNA is found in hepatic tumors from all persons with HBsAg positivity and in 38% of those with antibody to HBsAg (anti-HBs). Although the precise mechanism for viral oncogenicity is unclear, it is likely that hepatitis B virus is integrated into the host genome at some time during persistent infection and precedes the appearance of malignant cells. The integration of viral DNA may modify expression of normal cellular proteins or may produce viral proteins such as the viral X gene, which acts as a transcriptional transactivator of host promoter sequences, including those associated with oncogene expression. Alternatively, integrated viral genomes can activate host protooncogenes. The oncogenic effect most likely operates indirectly or synergistically with the development of cirrhosis, a major cofactor for the development of hepatocellular carcinoma independent of hepatitis B virus infection, which is present in 60–90% of persons with hepatocellular carcinoma.

Hepatocellular carcinoma usually occurs in adults between 40 and 60 years of age, but in geographic areas where hepatitis B is endemic, it is more common in children and can occur as early as 3 years of age. Virtually all children with hepatocellular carcinoma are HBsAg-positive, and over 90% of their mothers are also HBsAg-positive, indicating the importance of perinatal hepatitis B virus transmission. Most of these children do not have HBeAg but do have antibody to HBeAg. The conversion from HBeAg positivity to anti-HBeAg positivity indicates a change from a viral-replicative to an integrated state, which appears to be an important antecedent in the development of the cancer. Although the majority of children with hepatocellular carcinoma do not have a clinical history of chronic liver disease, cirrhosis is usually present on liver biopsy.

Universal hepatitis B vaccination during childhood has already been shown to have a significant impact on decreasing the incidence of hepatitis B infection and the incidence of hepatocellular carcinoma in endemic areas.

Hepatitis C Virus

Infection with hepatitis C virus is the major risk factor for the development of hepatocellular carcinoma in the United States, where there are an estimated 3.5 million chronic carriers. The duration of hepatitic C infection and the degree of persistent hepatic injury are the major determinants in the development of hepatocellular carcinoma. Hepatitis C subtype 1b, which has been present in the United States the longest, causes 5–20% of cases of hepatitis C but is found in 90% of hepatocellular carcinomas associated with hepatitis C.

The mechanism by which chronic hepatitis C infection gives rise to hepatic tumors remains unknown. The hepatitis C virus genome is detected by PCR in both tumor and pericancerous cirrhotic liver tissue. However, hepatitis C virus is a positive-stranded RNA virus that does not replicate through a DNA intermediate and thus does not integrate into the host genome. Alcohol-related cirrhosis is present in the majority of cases of hepatocellular carcinoma associated with hepatitis C, which suggests that hepatitis C virus, similar to hepatitis B virus, may play an indirect role in carcinogenesis through the development of cirrhosis, rather than having a direct oncogenic effect.

Retroviruses

Retroviridae, the family of retroviruses, are widely distributed among vertebrate species and include three subfamilies: the Spumavirinae, Lentivirinae, and Oncovirinae. All RNA tumor viruses belong to this family, which are responsible for a variety of oncogenic diseases in humans and other animals. Not all retroviruses are oncogenic or even pathogenic, however. These viruses share many attributes of biology, transmission, and cellular specificity and yet demonstrate a diversity of clinical expression, which is largely a result of their different cell tropisms, potential for cytotoxicity, and direct and indirect roles in oncogenesis.

Retroviruses are positive-sense, single-stranded RNA viruses. They are distinguished by encoding RNA-dependent DNA polymerase and a ribonuclease collectively known as **reverse transcriptase,** which transcribes the viral single-stranded RNA into a DNA copy that integrates into the cell DNA genome at random sites to form the **provirus.** In any particular cell the retrovirus-cell relationship may develop along different paths. The virus may remain quiescent, in an inactive or latent state, and may not affect cellular function. The provirus is stable and is replicated and passed to progeny cells as part of the chromosomal genome. In a portion of infected cells, viral RNA is transcribed for production of structural proteins and enzymes for assembly of new infectious viral particles. The production of new virions may proceed without significant effect to the host cell, except that it is now continually producing new virions, or may take place rapidly, accompanied by cell death.

The **spumaviruses,** or foamy viruses (*spuma* means foam), are named because of the characteristic vacuolar multinuclear giant cells they induce in cultured cells. Several spumaviruses have been isolated from a variety of mammalian species, including humans, with up to 5% of persons in East Africa and the Pacific Islands being seropositive. An association of **human foamy virus** and subacute thyroiditis has been suggested, but these viruses have not been conclusively demonstrated as the cause of specific human or animal disease.

The **lentiviruses** include the cytopathic retroviruses associated with profound immunodeficiency, which include the retroviruses that cause AIDS in humans, **human immunodeficiency virus type 1 (HIV-1)** and **type 2 (HIV-2).** The **simian immunodeficiency virus (SIV)** causes simian AIDS, an AIDS-like illness in Old World monkeys. Infection with HIV is associated with a few types of tumors that develop as a result of cytolytic destruction of cell populations responsible for normal mechanisms of immune surveillance (e.g., CD4 cells) and other associated immune perturbations (Chapter 38). In children, non-Hodgkin's lymphomas, especially Burkitt's lymphoma, occur most frequently, followed by leiomyosarcomas. Other tumors include Kaposi's sarcoma, cervical dysplasia and squamous cell carcinomas, and possibly seminomas and testicular cancer. Viral cofactors are essential for the development of many of these tumors and include EBV for lymphoma and leiomyosarcoma, human papillomaviruses for carcinomas of the skin and cervix, and HHV8 for Kaposi's sarcoma and primary effusion lymphoma.

The **oncoviruses,** or RNA tumor viruses, constitute the largest subfamily of retroviruses and include **human T-cell leukemia/lymphoma (lymphotropic) virus type I (HTLV-I)** and **type II (HTLV-II).** A remarkably similar virus, designated simian T-cell lymphotropic virus (STLV), is ubiquitous in several species of Old World primates. Infection and seropositivity are lifelong. These transforming retroviruses contribute directly to the development of leukemia. The oncogenic retroviruses can transform the cell directly, leading to malignant growth.

Human T-cell Leukemia/Lymphoma Virus Type I. HTLV-I, discovered in 1980, is the cause of **adult T-cell leukemia (ATL;** also known as **adult T-cell leukemia/lymphoma [ATLL])** and **tropical spastic paresis (TSP;** also known as **chronic progressive myelopathy** or **HTLV-I-associated myelopathy [HAM]),** a progressive neurologic disease. HTLV-I is endemic in the southwestern portion of Japan, in the Caribbean basin, in Melanesia, in parts of Africa, and in Micronesia and New Guinea, where the seroprevalence in the general population is 3–20% and increases with advancing age. In older age groups the infection is more prevalent in women than in men. A high degree of familial clustering of infection exists in these endemic areas. There is no difference in antibody levels between patients with ATL and asymptomatic HTLV-I infection, in contrast to the higher antibody titers to EBV found in patients with Burkitt's lymphoma. Infection with *Strongyloides stercoralis* has been shown to be an independent risk factor for ATL in Jamaica.

The causal association of HTLV-I with ATL is based on the usual integration of the HTLV-I genome as a single copy in the ATL tumor cell; reproducible isolation of the virus from persons with ATL; a high titer of HTLV-I antibodies in 80–100% of persons with ATL; and overlapping geographic distribution of HTLV-I infection and ATL that is virtually identical. Individuals from areas endemic for HTLV-I remain at risk of having ATL even if they move to an area of low prevalence. The lifelong risk of ATL in endemic regions with HTLV-I infection early in childhood is approximately 2–4%. In Jamaica, up to half of non-Hodgkin's lymphoma cases are associated with perinatal HTLV-I acquisition and are not associated with acquisition of HTLV-I by transfusion or other means later in life.

Based on the volunteer blood donors, the combined seroprevalence rate of HTLV-I and -II in the United States is 0.016%. Most seropositive persons in the United States are born in endemic areas or report sexual contact with individuals from such areas. Intravenous drug abusers in the United States have a seroprevalence ranging from 7% to 49%. Transmission of HTLV-I occurs by sexual contact, by sharing of contaminated needles or other injection paraphernalia among injection drug users, by use of contaminated blood products, and perinatally from infected mother to child, either transplacentally or by breast-feeding. In endemic areas, transmission by breast-feeding is the major mode of spread, with approximately 25% of breast-fed infants born to HTLV-I seropositive mothers acquiring infection. Public health policy in endemic areas of Japan advises against breast-feeding by HTLV-I-seropositive mothers to curtail the incidence of ATL. Intrauterine transmission occurs much less frequently, and only 5% of children born to HTLV-I-infected mothers acquire infection if they are not breast-fed. The risk of male-to-female transmission by sexual contact is approximately 60% during a 10-year period, in comparison with a <1% risk of female-to-male transmission. In the United States, approximately 25–30% of sex partners of persons with seropositivity for HTLV-I or -II are also seropositive. Routine serologic screening of all blood for HTLV-I and -II was implemented in the United States in November 1988.

HTLV-I infects CD4 lymphocytes and is not associated with specific clinical manifestations at the time of primary acquisition. However, viral infection is implicated in the development of a spectrum of progressive lymphoproliferations ranging from subclinical lymphoproliferation, to chronic leukemia, to acute ATL. Chronic HTLV-I lymphoproliferative disease is manifested by low-grade lymphocytic proliferation with abnormal-appearing lymphocytes, with or without mild peripheral lymphadenopathy. ATL may remain suppressed for years before progressing to the acute form, which is manifested by hypercalcemia, lytic bone lesions, lymphadenopathy sparing the mediastinum, hepatomegaly and abnormal liver function, splenomegaly, and cutaneous lymphomas. Leukemia with polylobulated malignant circulating lymphocytes possessing mature T-cell markers, called flower cells, also occurs. ATL has an extremely long latent period, with a unimodal age distribution peaking at approximately 50 years of age. Conventional chemotherapy is not curative and relapses are common, with a median survival time of 11 months from diagnosis. There is no recognized chromosomal abnormality or oncogene associated with ATL.

Tropical spastic paraparesis is characterized by gradual onset and a slow progression of neurologic degeneration involving the corticospinal tracts and, to a lesser extent, the sensory system. Evidence of a causal role for HTLV-I is the appearance of HTLV-I DNA in the peripheral blood mononuclear cells of affected persons, the increased frequency of antibodies in case versus control subjects, detection of HTLV-I antibodies in the cerebrospinal fluid, and geographic epidemiology of TSP that parallels that of ATL. Not all persons with a diagnosis of TSP have antibodies to HTLV-I. Unlike ATL, TSP has an incubation period that may be as short as 3 years.

Human T-cell Leukemia/Lymphoma Virus Type II. HTLV-II was initially isolated from the tumor cells of a person with hairy cell leukemia, a rare lymphoproliferative disease characteristically of B-cell origin, and from cells of T-cell lymphoproliferation of another person with B-cell hairy cell leukemia. However, most persons with hairy cell leukemia do not harbor HTLV-II, and this virus has also been isolated from persons without evidence of malignancy. Rarely, HTLV-II has been isolated from persons with TSP-like neurologic illnesses or malignancies, but this virus has not been clearly identified as the cause of any specific disease.

HTLV-II shares approximately 65% nucleotide sequence homology with HTLV-I and is indistinguishable from HTLV-I when standard serologic assays are used. The licensed serologic tests use HTLV-I antigens and vary in their sensitivity to detect HTLV-II antibodies. Differentiation using the PCR method suggests that approximately half of patients with serologically diagnosed HTLV-I and -II infection are infected with HTLV-I and half with HTLV-II, which complicates the interpretation of early HTLV-I studies.

HTLV-II is prevalent among injecting drug users in the United States and Europe and may account for up to 90% of HTLV-I and -II seropositivity in these regions. HTLV-II is also endemic in Native Americans in Florida and New Mexico. HTLV-II is transmitted by sexual contact, sharing of blood-contaminated needles or other injection paraphernalia, and use of contaminated blood products. The virus has been found in human milk, although transmission by breast-feeding has not been documented.

Human Papillomaviruses

The human papillomaviruses (HPVs) are members of the family Papovaviridae, which includes 85 fully analyzed genotypes and more than 120 additional putative genotypes distinguished by both tissue specificity and malignant potential. These epitheliotropic viruses are found in many benign lesions and in squamous cell carcinomas of the skin and genital tract, especially malignancies of the uterine cervix (Table 46–11). They account for about 10% of cancers worldwide, including approximately 95% of cervical cancers. The high-risk types 16 and 18, which are associated with 50–60% and 10–20% of cervical cancers, respectively, interact with cellular factors in deregulating the normal growth of the cell. Low-risk types 6 and 11 probably depend on additional external influences. It is uncertain whether HPVs are a risk factor for the development of oral tumors and skin cancers. They may also have a role in the development of epithelial carcinomas of the bladder, esophagus, and lungs.

HPV causes permissive infection of basal epithelial cells but with a hyperplastic proliferation that results in vacuolization, or koilocytosis. The production of mature virions is restricted to terminally differentiated keratinocytes, causing acanthosis and hyperkeratosis. Once viral infection is established, HPV genomes persist in benign lesions as episomes. In malignant cells the virus is characteristically integrated into the cellular genome at the same location in the viral genome, at a break in the E1 and E2 open reading frames, but at random locations in the cellular genome. The site of integration into the cellular genome may be an important facet in the development of malignancy.

HPV infection of apparently normal cervical epithelium occurs, but the prevalence is unknown. HPV types 6 and 11 typically cause condyloma acuminatum, which is the most common viral sexually transmitted disease in the United States. These HPV types are rarely associated with malignant lesions and are considered to pose very low risk. Infection with HPV type 16, and to a lesser degree type 18, is associated with a higher risk of cervical cancer, vulvar cancer, penile cancer, and perianal and anal cancer. These HPV types have not been found in benign lesions.

Both oral-genital transmission of HPV and vertical transmission from infected mothers may occur. Between 20% and 30% of infants born to HPV-infected mothers may acquire HPV perinatally, apparently developing subclinical but possibly latent infection of foreskin and penile epithelium or nasopharyngeal epithelium or both.

Epidermodysplasia verruciformis, a rare autosomal recessive disorder, is associated with infection with many different HPV types. Beginning in young adulthood, tumors develop in approximately one third of the affected persons, primarily in papillomas in skin-exposed areas and characteristically associated with HPV-5 and to a lesser extent HPV-8. These tumors are examples of the cooperative effects of genetic, infectious, and environmental factors in oncogenesis.

Transcripts from two viral oncogenes, E6 and E7, are found in all HPV-positive cervical carcinomas. These HPV proteins from high-risk but not low-risk HPV types can immortalize human epithelial cells and can induce chromosomal instability, which may account for the somatic mutations seen in 15–20% of HPV-infected cancer cells. These oncoproteins can efficiently bind cellular tumor suppressors, including E7 binding of the retinoblastoma gene product (pRb) and E6 binding of p53, which subsequently promotes the degradation of p53. Such binding may inactivate these cellular proteins and eliminate the normal regulatory constraints of these tumor suppressors. In addition, the E6 and E7 oncoproteins activate cyclins A and E, which stimulates cell proliferation. Acting together, E6 and E7 immortalize keratinocytes in vitro, but an interval of several decades may intervene between HPV infection and the development of epithelial neoplasia in vivo. Additional influences must act on the cells in a stepwise transformation to a malignant state. However, the successful elimination of HPV infection appears to remove an important contributing factor in the development of these epithelial tumors.

Polyomaviruses

The polyomaviruses, also members of the Papovaviridae family, are small, nonenveloped, double-stranded circular DNA viruses. The two polyomaviruses that infect humans, JC virus and BK virus, share 75% genome homology. Both viruses are tropic for renal epithelium; JC virus also infects brain oligodendrocytes and is the etiologic agent of **progressive multifocal leukoencephalopathy (PML),** a fatal demyelinating disease (Chapter 55). The simian virus 40 (SV40) causes semipermissive infection of human fibroblasts. These viruses inactivate both the growth-arrest pathway dependent on retinoblastoma protein (pRb) and the p53-dependent apoptotic mechanism.

Polyomavirus sequences have been identified in several human tumors that occur in children, including osteosarcomas, mesotheliomas, and brain tumors (e.g., ependymomas, glioblastomas, oligodendrogliomas). The etiologic role of these viruses in human oncogenesis remains uncertain.

BACTERIA IN ONCOGENESIS

A few bacteria have been associated with certain malignancies on the basis of the pathophysiology of continuous inflammation and chronic proliferation of target tissue before the development of cancer (Table 4–1).

Helicobacter pylori

Helicobacter pylori, the most common cause of superficial gastritis and of gastric and duodenal ulcers, causes acute inflammation, as well as chronic inflammation that may persist for years (Chapter 75). After several decades the inflammation associated with *H. pylori* may progress to **chronic atrophic gastritis,** a recognized precursor condition for **adenocarcinoma of the stomach**. Several studies confirm the association of *H. pylori* infection with adenocarcinoma of the stomach, especially for adenocarcinomas of the distal portion of the stomach, with an odds ratio of 2.7 to 6. Genetic factors such as blood type and HLA type, host factors such as hypochlorhydria, and microbial virulence factors such as *cagA* virulence factor, may contribute to or modulate the development of gastric adenocarcinoma.

H. pylori is also associated epidemiologically with gastric lymphoma, the most common type of extranodal lymphoma. Persistent *H. pylori* infection contributes directly to localized oligoclonal or polyclonal proliferations of B cells in **mucosa-associated lymphoid tissue (MALT)** in the stomach, which predisposes the affected person to the development of non-Hodgkin's B-cell MALT lymphoma. The persistence and accumulation of MALT tumor cells may require continued *H. pylori* infection, suggesting an antigen-, superantigen-, or cytokine-driven proliferative response. Early gastric MALT lymphomas may regress with antibiotic treatment of *H. pylori* infection, suggesting that the identification and treatment of *H. pylori* are important elements in the prevention of both gastric lymphoma and gastric adenocarcinoma.

Mycobacterium tuberculosis

Mycobacterium tuberculosis can persist in a clinically dormant or smoldering state for decades, and bronchogenic carcinoma of the lung may occur up to 20 times more frequently in persons with tuberculosis than in persons matched for a comparable total of cigarette smoking. Carcinoma can cause reactivation of quiescent tuberculosis, and local tuberculous infection is associated with scar carcinoma. The historical association of tuberculosis with bronchogenic carcinoma has been significantly diminished by the prompt recognition and early treatment of tuberculous infection.

Salmonella typhi and *Salmonella paratyphi*

Chronic bacterial colonization of the gallbladder with *Salmonella typhi* and *Salmonella paratyphi* is associated with an increased risk of gallbladder cancer. This risk is additional to the risk posed by the presence of gallstones, which is an independent major risk factor for gallbladder cancer. Typhoid or paratyphoid fever without biliary colonization confers no increased risk.

CHLAMYDIA IN ONCOGENESIS

Serologic studies link *Chlamydia trachomatis* with a twofold to threefold increased risk for development of invasive squamous cell carcinoma of the uterine cervix, independent of the association with HPV. Increasing exposure to different *C. trachomatis* serotypes also increases risk of cervical carcinoma, especially to serotype G. The mechanisms of this association are not known.

PARASITES IN ONCOGENESIS

A few parasites have been associated with certain malignancies, also based on the pathophysiology of continuous inflammation and chronic proliferation of target tissue before the development of cancer (Table 4–1). Chronic *Schistosoma haematobium* infection causes chronic inflammation, fibrosis, and proliferation of the urinary bladder at the site of egg deposition, leading to squamous cell carcinoma of the bladder. *Schistosoma japonicum* infection is associated with colorectal cancer, but the evidence is less strong. *Schistosoma mansoni* has been inconsistently associated with cancers. Chronic biliary tract inflammation with *Opisthorchis viverrini, Opisthorchis felineus,* and possibly *Clonorchis sinensis* similarly predisposes the affected person to cholangiocarcinoma, although animal studies suggest that liver flukes cannot induce bile duct cancers in the absence of other factors.

The immunosuppressive effects of malaria appear to act as a cofactor that may predispose the affected person to EBV-associated Burkitt's lymphoma. Similarly, infection with *Strongyloides stercoralis* may result in a predisposition to HTLV-associated leukemia.

REVIEWS

Evans AS, Mueller NE: Viruses and cancer: Causal associations. *Ann Epidemiol* 1990;1:71–92.

Goedert JJ (editor): *Infectious Causes of Cancer: Targets for Intervention.* New Brunswick, NJ, Humana Press, 2000.

McCance DJ (editor): *Human Tumor Viruses.* Washington, DC, American Society for Microbiology, 1998.

Parsonnet J (editor): *Microbes and Malignancy. Infection as a Cause of Human Cancers.* Oxford, Oxford University Press, 1999.

Persing DH, Prendergast FG: Infection, immunity, and cancer. *Arch Pathol Lab Med* 1999;123:1015–22.

zur Hausen H: Viruses in human cancers. *Eur J Cancer* 1999;35: 1878–85.

KEY ARTICLES

Antilla T, Saikku P, Koskela P, et al: Serotypes of *Chlamydia trachomatis* and risk for development of cervical squamous cell carcinoma. *JAMA* 2001;285:47–51.

Antman K, Chang Y: Kaposi's sarcoma. *N Engl J Med* 2000;342: 1027–38.

Beasley RP, Hwang LY, Lin CC, et al: Hepatocellular carcinoma and hepatitis B virus. A prospective study of 22,707 men in Taiwan. *Lancet* 1981;2:1129–33.

Bergsagel DJ, Finegold MJ, Butel JS, et al: DNA sequences similar to those of simian virus 40 in ependymomas and choroid plexus tumors of childhood. *N Engl J Med* 1992;326:988–93.

Biggar RJ, Frisch M, Goedert JJ: Risk of cancer in children with AIDS. AIDS-Cancer Match Registry Study Group. *JAMA* 2000;284:205–9.

Centers for Disease Control and Prevention and the U.S.P.H.S. Working Group: Guidelines for counseling persons infected with human T-lymphotropic virus types I (HTLV-I) and type II (HTLV-II). *Ann Intern Med* 1993;118:448–54.

Chang KL, Flaris N, Hickey WF, et al: Brain lymphomas of immunocompetent and immunocompromised patients: Study of the association with Epstein-Barr virus. *Mod Pathol* 1993;6:427–32.

Franco EL: Viral etiology of cervical cancer: A critique of the evidence. *Rev Infect Dis* 1991;13:1195–206.

Gaffey MJ, Weiss LM: Association of Epstein-Barr virus with human neoplasia. *Pathol Ann* 1992;27:55–74.

Hjelle B: Human T-cell leukemia/lymphoma viruses. Life cycle, pathogenicity, epidemiology, and diagnosis. *Arch Pathol Lab Med* 1991;115:440–50.

Houghton M, Weiner A, Han J, et al: Molecular biology of the hepatitis C viruses: Implications for diagnosis, development and control of viral disease. *Hepatology* 1991;14:381–8.

Imrie C, Rowland M, Bourke B, et al: Is *Helicobacter pylori* infection in childhood a risk factor for gastric cancer? *Pediatrics* 2001;107:373–80.

Jenson HB, Leach CT, McClain KL, et al: Benign and malignant smooth muscle tumors containing Epstein-Barr virus in children with AIDS. *Leuk Lymphoma* 1997;27:303–14.

Koskela P, Anttila T, Bjørge T, et al: *Chlamydia trachomatis* infection as a risk factor for invasive cervical cancer. *Int J Cancer* 2000;85:35–9.

Lichtenstein P, Holm NV, Verkasalo PK, et al: Environmental and heritable factors in the causation of cancer—analysis of cohorts of twins from Sweden, Denmark, and Finland. *N Engl J Med* 2000;343:78-85.

Morrison EA: Natural history of cervical infection with human papillomaviruses. *Clin Infect Dis* 1994;18:172–80.

Parsonnet J, Hansen J, Rodriguez L, et al: *Helicobacter pylori* infection and gastric lymphoma. *N Engl J Med* 1994;320:1267–71.

Parsonnet J, Hansen J, Rodriguez L, et al: *Helicobacter pylori* infection and the risk of gastric carcinoma. *N Engl J Med* 1991;325:1127–31.

Paya CV, Fung JJ, Nalesnik MA, et al: Epstein-Barr virus–induced post-transplant lymphoproliferative disorders. ASTS/ASTP EBV-PTLD Task Force and The Mayo Clinic Organized International Consensus Development Meeting. *Transplantation* 1999;68:1517–25.

Reeves WC, Rawls WE, Brinton LA: Epidemiology of genital papillomavirus and cervical cancer. *Rev Infect Dis* 1989;11:426–39.

Schulz TF: Kaposi's sarcoma–associated herpesvirus (human herpesvirus-8). *J Gen Virol* 1998;79:1573–91.

Shijo H, Okazaki M, Koganemara F, et al: Influence of hepatitis B virus infection and age on mode of growth of hepatocellular carcinoma. *Cancer* 1991;67:2626–32.

Tsukuma H, Hiyama T, Tanaka S, et al: Risk factors for hepatocellular carcinoma among patients with chronic liver disease. *N Engl J Med* 1993;328:1797–801.

Vokes EE, Liebowtiz DN, Weichselbaum RR: Nasopharyngeal carcinoma. *Lancet* 1997;350:1087–91.

CHAPTER 5

Host Defenses Against Infection

Anthony J. Infante

BASIC PRINCIPLES OF THE IMMUNE SYSTEM

Many basic concepts of host resistance to infectious diseases were well established before the development of Pasteur's germ theory (1860–1880) and certainly before the existence of any detailed knowledge of the immune system. Collective human experience taught that there is an innate resistance to illness and that such resistance is more highly developed in certain individuals than others. Furthermore, there was a fairly sophisticated folk understanding that factors such as stress (''standing out in the rain'') and nutrition (''chicken soup'') play a role in modifying innate disease resistance.

In addition to innate, nonspecific resistance, there was also an understanding that there is a system of acquired, or adaptive, specific immunity and that, after significant exposure to or acquisition and subsequent recovery from certain specific illnesses, a state of lifelong protection from that illness, but not others, usually follows. These concepts of immunologic specificity and memory were put to use by Jenner (1796–1798) to immunize against smallpox, although still in an empirical way. In addition to the properties of specificity and memory, full appreciation of a third important attribute of the immune response, diversity, awaited the direct measurements of the early immunochemists. The work of Landsteiner and others (1900–1920) showed that the immune system is capable of responding to and differentiating among an almost limitless array of antigens, including novel organic chemical compounds never encountered in nature.

The solution of the dual problems of how immunologic specificity and diversity are generated has taken up the greater part of the second half of the twentieth century. Recent progress has also been made in determining the basis of immunologic memory. Now immunologists are turning increasingly to understanding the integration of the processes of innate and adaptive immunity, which appears to be critical for a regulated, protective immune response.

This chapter presents an overview of the cellular and molecular mechanisms responsible for innate and acquired immunity, including the properties of specificity, diversity, and memory, and other selected topics important to a contemporary understanding of host defenses against infections. The organization of the chapter is intentionally different from more formal textbooks of immunology and emphasizes, where possible, the sequential engagement of host defense mechanisms that might occur during an infection.

INNATE IMMUNITY

Innate immunity is the set of nonspecific protective mechanisms that does not require prior exposure to an antigen for full activity. Innate immune mechanisms exhibit a relatively low degree of antigen specificity and diversity and lack the property of antigen-specific memory (Table 5–1). An important advantage of innate immunity, however, is the ability to be rapidly and fully deployed without the extensive cellular differentiation and proliferation necessary for adaptive immunity. The protective mechanisms involved in innate immunity therefore provide an important first line of defense against infection, temporally as well as anatomically.

Barriers to Infection

The passive and active barrier functions of skin and mucous membranes are important and often overlooked elements of protection against infection. Breaches in these barriers, as well as alterations in the normal microbial flora, are major predisposing factors in susceptibility to infectious disease.

Skin and Mucous Membranes. Intact skin and mucous membranes play an important role in host resistance. The keratinized outer layer of skin provides an inert barrier to microorganisms, and the inner layers of the dermis contain cell types that provide both specific and nonspecific protection, including specialized macrophages called **Langerhans cells** and a subset of T lymphocytes known as **intraepithelial lymphocytes.** In addition to simple breaches in skin integrity (e.g., wounds, abrasions) that lead to increased susceptibility to infection, environmental factors, such as the potent immunosuppressive effect of ultraviolet-B irradiation on dermal T-cell immunity, are important. Burns and thermal injury not only cause destruction of the skin barrier but, when extensive, incite an intense inflammatory response that appears to suppress many macrophage and neutrophil functions, locally as well as systemically.

Mucous membranes likewise provide a combination of passive barrier and active protection. **Mucus** has a surprisingly complex biochemistry. The alteration in its viscosity in cystic fibrosis retards bacterial clearance and facilitates the pulmonary infections of cystic fibrosis. The normal beating action of **cilia** on certain epithelial cell types promotes the clearance of trapped microorganisms. Defects in ciliary motility are rare but instructive causes of increased susceptibility to infection. **Lysozyme,** an enzyme present in certain secretions, directly attacks bacterial cell walls. Secretory IgA is part of specific mucosal immunity.

Normal Microbial Flora. The normal indigenous microbial flora (Chapter 2) on skin and mucous membranes plays an important function in protecting the host from invasion of pathogens and is therefore a part of innate host defenses. Established colonization with numerous organisms of low virulence limits dominance of any one species and minimizes acquisition of exogenous pathogenic organisms. The mechanisms by which indigenous flora afford protection include competition for the host nutrient sources (**bacterial interference**); nonspecific or even specific blocking of cell-surface receptors or mucous blanket adhesions by other bacteria (**colonization resistance**); and the production of **bacteriocins,** bacterial products that are cytotoxic to other bacteria, usually of related species. The resident flora in the oropharynx and gastrointestinal

TABLE 5–1. Properties that Distinguish Mechanisms of Innate and Adaptive Immunity

Characteristic	Innate Immunity	Acquired Immunity
Specificity	Broad	Fine
Diversity	Limited	Extensive
Memory	No	Yes

tract also induces production of varying degrees of local and serum antibodies, called **natural antibodies,** that react with other bacteria, thereby inducing cross-reactive or cross-protective immunization. Reduction or disturbance of the normal flora, which accompanies antibiotic treatment, may result in diminished host resistance to certain pathogens.

Cellular and Soluble Components of Innate Immunity

Once an invading pathogen penetrates the first line of passive defenses, a series of more responsive elements come into play. The most important of these appear to be endothelial cells, granulocytes and macrophages, and the complement system (Fig. 5–1). Endothelial cells play an important role in focusing lymphocytes, macrophages, granulocytes, and other inflammatory cells to the site of infection. Granulocytes and macrophages have several key roles. First, they nonspecifically respond to and kill microorganisms, primarily bacteria, which limits the initial phase of pathogen replication. Macrophages then participate in a key phase of the host response, namely the activation of specific helper T lymphocytes. Finally, granulocytes and macrophages respond with increased bactericidal activity under the influence of products of activated T and B lymphocytes, including antibodies, certain interleukins, and IFN-γ. The **complement system** can be activated directly by microorganisms via the **alternative pathway** and by the action of specific antibodies in the **classical pathway.** In addition to direct action against microorganisms, complement components are also involved in the enhancement of granulocyte and macrophage antimicrobial function (Fig. 5–1).

A strategy used commonly by the cells and soluble factors of innate immunity is the recognition of fundamental biochemical differences between pathogenic microorganisms and host tissues. The major components that trigger nonspecific protective mechanisms are complex cell wall structures such as bacterial LPS and phosphorylcholine, fungal glycans (e.g., zymosan), and similar substances that do not occur on the surface of mammalian cells. The receptors involved in these types of recognition events have been termed **pattern receptors** to distinguish them from the highly specific receptors on lymphocytes. An example of such a pattern recognition system is the CD14 system for monocyte and macrophage LPS responsiveness. LPS binds to a serum protein, LPS-binding protein (LBP), which appears necessary for LPS transport. LPS is then transferred to CD14 on the surface of monocytes and macrophages. However, CD14 lacks an intracellular domain and does not appear capable of transmitting a signal to the cell interior. A member of the Toll-like receptor (TLR) family, TLR2, appears to associate with CD14 and to transmit the LPS signal to the cell interior.

Endothelial Cells. Skin and mucous membranes are a rich source of endothelial cells lining small blood vessels. These cells are highly responsive to injury, and they release several substances that are proinflammatory, causing the migration and activation of cells with antibacterial properties. Bacterial products, particularly LPS and the cytokines derived from local macrophages, especially IL-1 and TNF, activate endothelial cells to release additional cytokines and to up-regulate specific adhesion molecules on their cell surface. A newly recognized class of molecules that regulate leukocyte trafficking and migration in response to inflammation are the **chemokines** (chemoattractant cytokines). Two families of chemokines are currently recognized: the **CC family,** in which two cysteine (C) residues important for biologic activity are adjacent, and the **CXC family,** in which the cysteines are separated by another amino acid (X) (Table 5–2). Once cells are attracted to an inflammatory focus, adhesion molecule interactions come into play to keep them there (Table 5–3). Differential attraction and retention of leukocytes are based on the types of chemokine-receptor and adhesion molecule–ligand interactions that take place at the site of infection.

Granulocytes. Polymorphonuclear leukocytes, or granulocytes, consist of neutrophils, eosinophils, and basophils. A direct role for neutrophils in antibacterial immunity has long been accepted. Eosinophils and basophils have been well studied in terms of

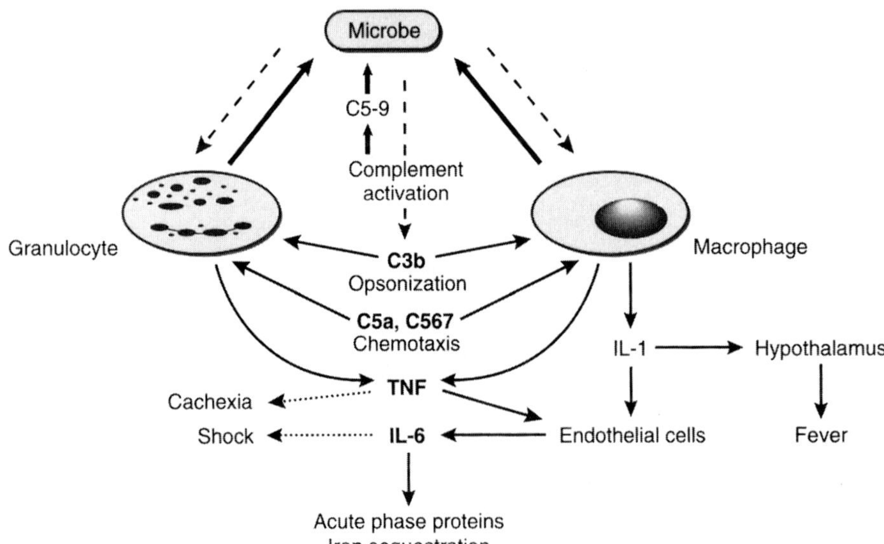

FIGURE 5–1. Integrated view of some important innate, nonspecific host responses to bacterial infection. Recognition of pathogenic components (*dashed lines*) initiates regulatory host interactions (*thin solid lines*) that results in beneficial host responses against the microbe (*dark solid lines*) but also include adverse effects (*dotted lines*).

TABLE 5–2. Some Important Human Chemokines, Their Receptors, and Cellular Specificity

Family	Receptor	Ligand(s)	Cells
CC	CCR1	RANTES, MIP-1α, MCP-2, -3	Eosinophils Monocytes
	CCR2	MCP-1, -2, -3, -4	Neutrophils Basophils Monocytes NK cells T lymphocytes B lymphocytes
	CCR3	Eotaxin RANTES, MCP-3, -4	Eosinophils Basophils NK cells
	CCR4	RANTES, MIP-1α, MCP-1	T lymphocytes
	CCR5*	RANTES, MIP-1α, -1β	Dendritic cells T lymphocytes
CXC	CXCR1	IL-8	Neutrophils
	CXCR2	IL-8, GRO-α, -β, -γ, NAP-2, ENA78, GCP-2	Neutrophils Basophils B lymphocytes
	CXCR3	IP-10, Mig	Eosinophils NK cells T lymphocytes
	CXCR4	SDF-1	Dendritic cells NK cells T lymphocytes B lymphocytes

*CCR5 is a cellular coreceptor with CD4 for HIV-1. The corresponding chemokines, RANTES, MIP-1α, and MIP-1β, block HIV-1 entry in vivo.
Adapted from Baggiolini M, DeWald B, Moser B: Human chemokines: An update. *Annu Rev Immunol* 1997;15:675–705.

their contributions to hypersensitivity disease, but their physiologic roles in host defense remain unclear. A role for eosinophils in protection against metazoan parasitic infections has been proposed on the basis of the observation of direct killing of certain parasites in vitro by eosinophils and by the protein products of eosinophilic granules. Basophils may serve as a fixed source of inflammatory mediators, particularly histamine and leukotriene B_4 (LTB_4), in various tissues.

Neutrophils can respond directly to bacterial components, a process that is mimicked in vitro by LPS and the synthetic peptide *N*-formyl-methionyl-leucyl-phenylalanine (N-FMLP), resulting in **chemotaxis,** which is the directed migration of inflammatory cells to the site of infection. Neutrophils are also attracted by products of host inflammatory reactions for which they have cell surface receptors, such as complement fragment C5a and the complex of C567, inflammatory lipid mediators such as platelet-activating factor (PAF) and LTB_4, and chemokines such as IL-8 (formerly neutrophil-activating factor). Complement and lipid mediators are most likely involved in initial neutrophil recruitment, with cytokines providing for a sustained response. The mobilization of granulocytes in response to bacterial infection includes an increase in bone marrow production above basal levels, resulting in the characteristic release of **bands,** or immature granulocytes, into the peripheral blood. This effect is mediated by activated T cells and specifically by the cytokines IL-6, IL-3, IL-4, and CSF.

Granulocytes and other leukocytes express receptors, such as L-selectin, for complex cell surface carbohydrates on the surface of endothelial cells. This causes a low affinity interaction (**primary adhesion**) that slows the granulocyte and allows it time to sense and respond to inflammatory signals emanating from infected tissues. This intravascular process can be mimicked in vitro by studying leukocytes under fluid-flow shear stress, and the cells can be seen to roll along endothelial cell monolayers (**leukocyte rolling**). When inflammatory signals are detected, granulocytes rapidly express cell surface molecules that mediate high-affinity adherence (**secondary adhesion**) to receptors on endothelial cells and transmigration through endothelial cells lining small blood vessels (**diapedesis**). An important family of adhesion molecules in this secondary adhesion step are the ***β_2*-integrins,** which are detected by antibodies against a shared subunit, CD18. The key ligand for CD18-bearing molecules on endothelial cells is intercellular adhesion molecule-1 (ICAM-1; Table 5–3).

On recruitment to the site of infection, granulocytes are activated to bactericidal activity, which is mediated by the products of specific granules. Killing may take place by the release of products into the extracellular environment and by bacterial phagocytosis and fusion of phagocytic vacuoles with lysosomal granules, creating **phagolysosomes,** inside the cell. Killing is mediated within the phagolysosome by both **oxygen-dependent** and **oxygen-independent** mechanisms. Activated neutrophils undergo a burst of oxygen consumption, which accompanies the production of several highly reactive antibacterial oxygen-containing moieties, including **superoxide** (O_2^-), hydrogen peroxide, hydroxyl radical, oxyhalides, and nitric oxide. These compounds are generated by a specific phagocytic oxidase (phox) enzyme complex and scavenged by other specific enzymes (e.g., superoxide dismutase) to prevent host tissue damage. Non-oxygen-dependent mechanisms include degradative enzymes such as lysozyme, phospholipases, elastase, collagenase, and a variety of proteases. The neutrophil is a potent antibacterial weapon; as a result, quantitative and qualitative neutrophil deficiencies are important causes of increased susceptibility to extracellular bacterial pathogens.

Mononuclear Phagocytes. Tissue macrophages are mononuclear phagocytes that develop from bone marrow–derived circulating monocytes. Resident macrophages take on recognizable phenotypic features depending on their location. Such specialized macrophages include **Kupffer cells** in the liver and **Langerhans cells** in the

TABLE 5–3. Adhesion and Other Cell Surface Molecules Involved in Immune and Inflammatory Responses

Receptor	Ligand	Function
Fcγ receptors: CD16, CD32, CD64	IgG Fc region	Opsonization, immune complex clearance
Complement receptors: CD11/18, CD21 (EBV receptor), CD35	C3 fragments	Opsonization
β_1 integrins: VLA-1, -2, -3, -4, -5, -6	Fibronectin, collagen, laminin	Leukocyte–extracellular matrix adhesion
β_2 (leukocyte) integrins: CD11a,b,c/CD18	ICAM-1, ICAM-2	Leukocyte–endothelial cell adhesion

skin. Macrophages at the site of infection may therefore include local residents and cells recruited from the circulation. Recruitment occurs in a fashion similar to that used by granulocytes.

Mononuclear phagocytes also share many important antibacterial mechanisms with granulocytes, which includes the ability to phagocytize and kill ingested bacteria using lysosomal enzymes and reactive oxygen species. Mononuclear phagocytes appear to require activation by products of concomitant specific immune reactions, particularly the T-cell product IFN-γ, to express maximal antimicrobial activity. Many organisms that are actively killed by IFN-γ-activated macrophages can persist and even proliferate inside resting macrophages. Activated macrophages are not themselves specific, having enhanced activity against unrelated pathogens. Mononuclear phagocytes are important in defense against intracellular pathogens such as *Mycobacterium, Salmonella, Listeria, Candida,* and *Histoplasma.* Persons who lack adequate T-cell function frequently are infected with these organisms and are therefore unable to generate fully activated macrophages.

Macrophages play an important role in initiating specific immune reactions through the process of antigen processing and presentation and are therefore an important bridge between innate and adaptive immunity. Small peptides are formed from the proteins of killed, ingested microorganisms by the activity of protease enzymes. These peptides are loaded onto newly synthesized MHC proteins that become expressed on the cell surface. It is in the form of peptide-MHC complexes that T lymphocytes recognize antigens and activate specific immune reactions. The antigen-presenting function of macrophages for T-cell activation is detailed later. T cell–macrophage communication is bidirectional. The expression of MHC molecules on macrophages is enhanced by T cell–derived IFN-γ. Macrophages are, conversely, an important source of IL-1, a potent costimulus of T-cell activation. In addition, IL-1 is an important stimulus of inflammatory responses, including fever and the acute-phase response.

Complement. Complement refers to a series of at least 20 distinct serum proteins that provide a number of important antibacterial activities (Table 5–4). The name refers to the ability of nonimmune serum to restore (complement) the antibacterial activity of immune serum that has been destroyed by heating. The mechanism involves the ability of heat-labile complement proteins to combine with heat-stable antibody molecules and to activate multiple antibacterial mechanisms. Similar to the activation of granulocytes and macrophages, the complement system can be activated specifically by antigen-antibody complexes (**classical pathway**) as well as nonspecifically (**alternative pathway**) (Fig. 5–2). Nonspecific activation appears to result from contact with certain bacterial surface components, including LPS and endotoxin. Sialic acid, an important component of mammalian cell surface glycoproteins, and specific membrane proteins such as decay-accelerating factor (DAF) appear to prevent complement activation by and damage of host cell surfaces during immune and inflammatory responses.

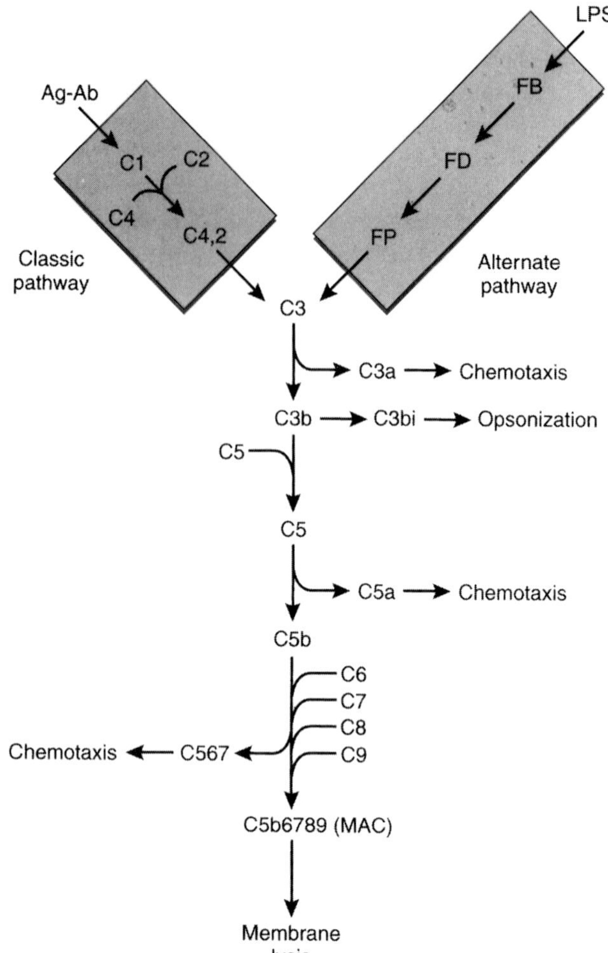

FIGURE 5–2. Pathways of complement activation. Boxes denote the classical pathway, activated by antigen-antibody (Ag-Ab) complexes, and the alternative pathway, triggered by lipopolysaccharide (*LPS*). The central role of C3 is apparent. Components with specific functions are noted. *MAC,* membrane attack complex.

TABLE 5–4. Important Complement Components and Products in Host Responses to Infection

Component	Activity
C3a, C5a	Mast cell degranulation, histamine release, smooth muscle contraction, chemotaxis
C3 fragments (C3b, C3bi)	Enhanced phagocytosis
Soluble C567 complex	Neutrophil chemotaxis
Membrane-bound complex of C5-9 (MAC)	Bacteriolysis

Initial, direct activation of C3, the most abundant complement protein, can occur by the action of LPS on enzymes of the alternative pathway. After initial activation a series of enzymatic reactions involving factors P, B, and D occurs that amplifies the system in a cascade-like fashion (Fig. 5–2). The result may be the production of additional C3b, C5a, and C5b67; the latter two are chemotactic for neutrophils. C3b can bind to numerous bacterial components by the creation of a covalent thioester linkage and can enhance phagocytosis of bacteria by polymorphonuclear leukocytes and macrophages, a process called **opsonization.** Recognition of C3b-coated bacteria by host cells is achieved by specific C3b receptors (CR1) on the host cell surface. Finally, physiologically active components are produced by proteolytic cleavage and macromolecular assembly and are capable of direct lysis of bacteria. The **membrane attack complex** (MAC), a macromolecular complex of C5, C6, C7, C8, and C9, produces a channel in biologic membranes, resulting in osmotic lysis. Figure 5–3 illustrates three mechanisms by which

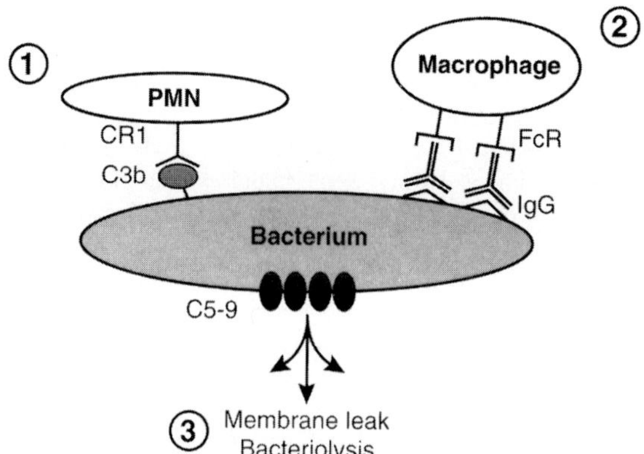

FIGURE 5–3. Multiple mechanisms involved in destruction of a pathogenic bacterium. *1,* Polymorphonuclear leukocytes (*PMN*) use complement receptor CR1 to recognize bacterium via C3b, formed through activation of the alternative pathway of complement (see Fig. 5–2). *2,* Macrophage uses receptor for Fc region of IgG (Fcγ R) to recognize bacterium coated with antibody IgG (antibody-dependent cellular cytotoxicity). *3,* Membrane attack complex, formed by either pathway of complement activation, inserts into the bacterial membrane, causing bacteriolysis.

pathogenic bacteria may be targeted for destruction. Evidence exists for antiviral activities of some complement components.

Metabolic Responses to Infection

A number of characteristic metabolic responses to infection occur that are not, strictly speaking, antimicrobial but that nevertheless assist the host defenses. The best studied of these responses are fever, the acute-phase reaction, and the sequestration of iron. Not all host metabolic responses are beneficial. Cachexia, resulting from the release of lipids from storage and protein breakdown for the release of energy stores (gluconeogenesis), may meet the short-term energy needs of the infected host but clearly has long-term deleterious consequences. Similarly, circulatory collapse and shock may be an extreme response initially designed to increase perfusion and speed the migration of inflammatory cells and mediators to the site of infection. Both of these nonspecific host responses are mediated by the soluble mediators TNF (cachexin) and IL-6 (Fig. 5–1), which are further enhanced and additionally regulated by T and B lymphocytes.

Fever. The association of fever and infection is an ancient observation. However, it is surprisingly difficult to find direct evidence for the beneficial effects of fever as a component of the host response. For example, the replication of many bacteria and viruses is directly sensitive to temperatures in the physiologic range. This has been used to explain the predilection of certain mycobacteria (e.g., *Mycobacterium leprae*) for infections of the distal extremities. It is unclear whether fever contributes in any meaningful way to the acceleration of beneficial host responses.

The ability of all kinds of pathogens (e.g., bacteria, viruses, parasites) to elicit fever, as well as the association of fever with noninfectious diseases such as rheumatologic and malignant conditions, has long indicated a final common pathway for fever as part of the host response. Recent evidence clearly implicates IL-1 and possibly TNF as leukocyte products that can directly induce fever in intact animals by causing a direct increase in prostaglandin synthesis in the hypothalamus. Bacterial cell wall products, including endotoxin, are potent inducers of IL-1, as are certain viral proteins and double-stranded RNA.

Acute-Phase Responses. The acute-phase response or reaction is actually a coordinated set of responses that occurs in many inflammatory conditions, including infections. The complete acute-phase response consists of fever, leukocytosis, thrombocytosis, adrenocorticotropic hormone (ACTH) and cortisol secretion, and a characteristic change in serum proteins (Chapter 10).

The acute-phase protein response is most readily detected by measuring an increased **erythrocyte sedimentation rate (ESR)** of erythrocytes, a response that was noted by the ancient Greeks. The increased ESR results from the alteration of the hemodynamic properties of the blood, which is caused by increased synthesis of **C-reactive protein (CRP),** serum amyloid A, haptoglobin, fibrinogen, and certain other α-globulins. CRP, named for its ability to bind pneumococcal group C polysaccharide, is the most prominent acute-phase protein in man. Whether this binding activity contributes significantly to general host defenses is unknown. Serum transferrin is decreased in the acute-phase response, and this change probably plays a role in iron sequestration. The coordinated expression of genes for many of these acute-phase proteins can be induced directly in liver by IL-6; IL-1 and TNF may also be involved. These mediators are secreted in coordinated fashion by endothelial cells, polymorphonuclear leukocytes, and macrophages.

Iron Sequestration. Iron is a vital trace nutrient for all living things because of its involvement in several key enzymatic reactions. In vitro bacterial growth is sensitive to iron concentration, and the competition for iron between the host and many bacterial species is intense. Bacteria use small molecules called **siderophores** to absorb and transport iron for their needs. Certain bacterial species produce **hemolysins,** which liberate iron from an important host source, erythrocytes.

As part of the acute-phase response to bacterial infection, the host sequesters iron in the reticuloendothelial system; the result can be measured as a decrease in serum transferrin, the major iron transporter. In addition, serum haptoglobin increases, presumably to scavenge iron released into the circulation. Multiple soluble factors, including IL-6, IL-1, TNF, and other factors involved in the acute-phase response, regulate iron sequestration. Although numerous case reports appear to document deleterious effects of acute iron administration or chronic iron overload on susceptibility to infection, this effect may be limited to certain bacterial species (e.g., *Yersinia*), and there is still some disagreement concerning the magnitude of the contribution of iron status to overall susceptibility to bacterial infection in the normal host.

INTERFACE BETWEEN INNATE AND ADAPTIVE IMMUNITY

Data accumulated in the past several years have facilitated an understanding of the links between innate and specific adaptive immunity. Mechanisms have been described that sense the result of the innate response to infection and fine-tune the adaptive response that follows so as to provide the right type of protection and to minimize the potential injury to the host that might result from an overzealous response. The dual roles of macrophages and complement in this process have been discussed. Recent research in this arena has also focused on the roles of dendritic cells, innate cytokine-producing cells, and NK cells. Specialized subsets of T lymphocytes that act in a somewhat similar fashion are described later.

Dendritic Cells. Dendritic cells are unique hematopoietic cells characterized by long finger-like projections (dendrites). Currently, two general types of dendritic cells are recognized. One type is derived from myeloid cell precursors, whereas the other appears to derive from lymphoid precursors, possibly T cells. Resting, or immature, dendritic cells are nonphagocytic, but actively pinocytic cells that synthesize and express large quantities of MHC class II molecules and actively transport them to the cell membrane. In this configuration, dendritic cells are poised to be active sampling centers for processing and presenting foreign antigens to CD4 T cells, the cells that drive the specific immune response. On a per-cell basis, dendritic cells appear to be the most efficient of all the antigen-presenting cells that can activate specific T cells, particularly naive T cells (those that have not previously recognized antigen). In addition to MHC molecules, they also express other molecules important for T-cell activation, especially members of the B7 family (CD80 and CD86).

After maturing under the guidance of cytokines, dendritic cells then enter a phase in which they no longer synthesize new MHC class II molecules. Instead, MHC molecules bearing antigenic peptides, derived during the earlier stage of active antigen processing, exist as long-lived complexes on the cell surface. Here dendritic cells appear to act as antigen depots for the later phases of the specific immune response, in particular the memory response.

Innate Cytokine-Producing Cells. An important transition, apparently made relatively early in an immune response, is that between a largely inflammatory response, involving cell-mediated effector functions, and a predominantly antibody-mediated response. These two responses are characterized by skewing of the cytokine secretion profiles of specific CD4 and CD8 T cells, with important physiologic consequences. A major determinant of the cytokine profile of the adaptive, specific response is the cytokine profile of the initiating, innate response. This realization has led to the search for antigen-nonspecific, innate cytokine-producing (ICP) cells that could prime the cytokine-secretion programs of antigen-specific CD4 and CD8 T cells. These cells are just beginning to be identified. Dendritic cells and macrophages are important ICP cells in skewing T-cell responses toward cell-mediated immunity by the production of IL-12. The ICP cells that point T-cell responses in the direction of antibody-mediated immunity by the secretion of IL-4 have yet to be definitively identified.

Natural Killer Cells. Another important cell that bridges both innate and acquired immunity is the NK cell. Operationally, NK cells were first described as cells with spontaneous cytotoxic activity that could lyse allogeneic tumor cells without previous priming. This is in contrast to conventional cytotoxic CD8 T cells, which require antigenic and cytokine stimulation before expressing cell-killing function. From a cell lineage standpoint, at least two types of NK cells are recognized. These are the CD56-bearing lineage of NK cells and the T cell lineage–derived NK cells. In addition to tumor immune responses, NK cells play an important role in certain viral and bacterial infections, particularly in limiting the initial spread of the infection. This is accomplished by direct killing and by secretion of cytokines, especially IFN-γ. NK cells have a unique arrangement of receptors and signaling. They spontaneously lyse cells that do not express MHC molecules; cells that do express MHC molecules engage NK cell receptors, called **killer inhibitory receptors (KIR),** that inhibit NK cell function. This mechanism is thought to be an important mechanism for eliminating virus-infected cells, many of which have low expression of MHC molecules as a result of the action of specific viral proteins.

ADAPTIVE IMMUNITY

Properties of T and B Lymphocytes

The nonspecific actions of the various cells and soluble mediators provide an important first line of defense against conventional bacteria. However, the spectrum or repertoire of the types of specificities that can distinguish between host and pathogen is limited. The cells that mediate adaptive, specific immunity are T and B lymphocytes. Identification and quantitation of T and B cells with immunofluorescence and flow cytometry are now routine in the research and clinical setting. Some important cell surface markers used in T- and B-cell identification are listed in Table 5–5.

In infectious diseases, antibody is usually found to be the primary specific host factor necessary for protection against or resolution of infection with encapsulated bacteria. The natural history of agammaglobulinemia in children demonstrates the requirement for antibody immunity in defense against pyogenic bacteria, especially gram-positive organisms. Although antibody-based protective mechanisms work well against extracellular pathogens, certain bacterial organisms (e.g., *Mycobacterium, Salmonella, Listeria*) evade protective mechanisms by adopting an intracellular lifestyle that includes residence in macrophages themselves. Viruses adopt an obligate intracellular localization, and for some viruses free viral particles are enveloped within host cell membranes. Fungi and parasites are also capable of relatively sophisticated active and passive means of evading host responses. As a result, the unique antigenic structures of intracellular bacteria, viruses, and fungi are made unavailable for direct recognition by antibodies, macrophages, neutrophils, and complement. The recognition mechanism of T cells is specially adapted to deal with these kinds of pathogens and is critical for adequate host defense.

The strategy of both T and B cells for providing the host with specificity and diversity is to generate an enormous number (estimated to be 10^{12}–10^{15}) of receptor molecules in an apparently random fashion and to express individual receptors on small numbers of cells, referred to as **clones,** which are derived from a single precursor. The random process of generating specificity and diversity might be expected to generate numerous receptors capable of recognizing not only foreign but also host components **(immunologic self),** and this expectation has been verified experimentally. The elimination of many self-reactive clones occurs while the lymphocytes are at an immature stage of development. Mature lymphocytes whose receptors display some threshold of affinity for a given antigen are expanded **(clonal selection).** The expanded population contains **effector cells,** which are activated and functional cells, and long-lived **memory cells** (Fig. 5–4). After the immune response is finished, the effector cells die and the memory cells survive.

TABLE 5–5. Additional Clinically Relevant Leukocyte Cell Surface Markers

Marker (Alternative Name)	Cell Type(s)
CD3	All mature T lymphocytes (T cells)
CD4	Helper T cells
CD5	T cells, B-cell subset
CD8	Cytotoxic T cells
CD14 (LPS receptor)	Macrophages, granulocytes
CD16 (FcγRIII)	Macrophages, granulocytes, NK cells
CD19	B cells
CD25 (IL-2 receptor)	Activated T cells
CD40	B cells
CD45 (LCA)	All lymphocytes
CD56 (NCAM)	T cells, NK cells
CD95 (Fas)	Activated lymphocytes
CD154 (CD40 ligand)	Activated T cells

LCA = leukocyte common antigen; *NCAM* = neural cell adhesion molecule.

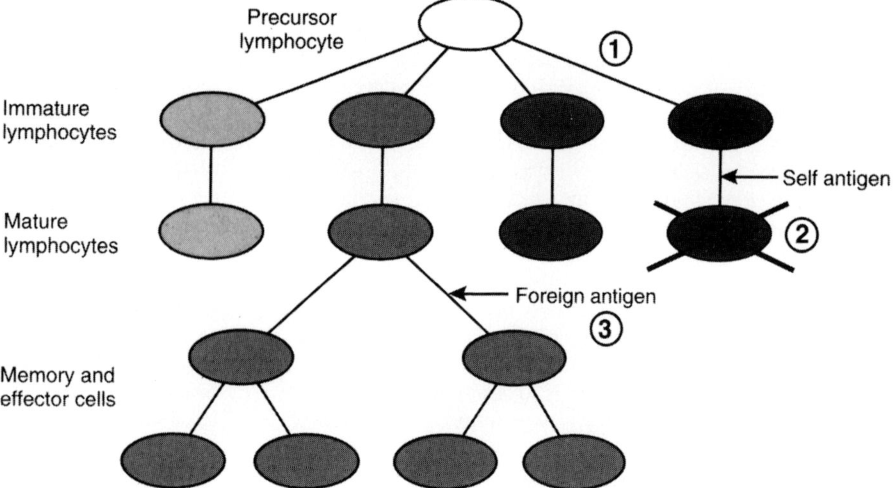

FIGURE 5–4. Receptor diversification and clonal selection in the development of the immune repertoire. The immune repertoire (spectrum of reactivity) of the adult animal is a function of (*1*) a random process of receptor diversification with unique receptors expressed on individual clones of cells, (*2*) mechanisms that eliminate self-reactive, receptor-bearing clones, and (*3*) expansion of useful clones by contact with antigens.

Both T and B lymphocytes participate in the generation of immunologic memory. Memory appears to have two components: clonal expansion and changes in activation requirements. Activated, antigen-specific lymphocytes proliferate and a certain number survive for long periods, providing an increased frequency of cells able to respond to secondary antigenic challenge. In addition, the surviving cells have a different phenotype: they are more easily triggered to activate their functional programs than are antigenically naive (virgin) T and B cells. There is currently no single cell surface marker or set of markers that reliably distinguishes recently activated lymphocytes from memory cells.

T Cell–Mediated Responses

Antigen-specific T cells recognize and respond to polypeptide fragments of bacterial, viral, or fungal proteins that have been derived from intracellular denaturation and proteolytic events collectively called **antigen processing.** These peptides are then bound to host MHC molecules and displayed on the surface of various cells for recognition by T cells **(antigen presentation).** These important steps are responsible for many of the critical regulatory aspects and genetic determinants of immune reactivity.

Major Histocompatibility Complex. The MHC, an evolutionarily conserved genetic region encoding a number of molecules of immunologic interest, plays a key role in the regulation of immune responses. MHC molecules are highly polymorphic within a population, and these polymorphisms control individual susceptibility and resistance to both infections and autoimmune diseases. As a by-product, they also make the major contribution to the ability of the immune system to accept or reject tissue allografts **(histocompatibility).** Human MHC products are called **HLA** (for human leukocyte antigen) molecules. The clinical manifestations of MHC polymorphisms are a direct result of their structure and function in antigen processing and presentation and in shaping the specificity repertoire of T lymphocytes.

The polymorphic MHC molecules of primary interest in immune recognition are the so-called class I and class II molecules (Fig. 5–5). The **MHC class I molecules** (human **HLA-A, -B,** and **-C**)

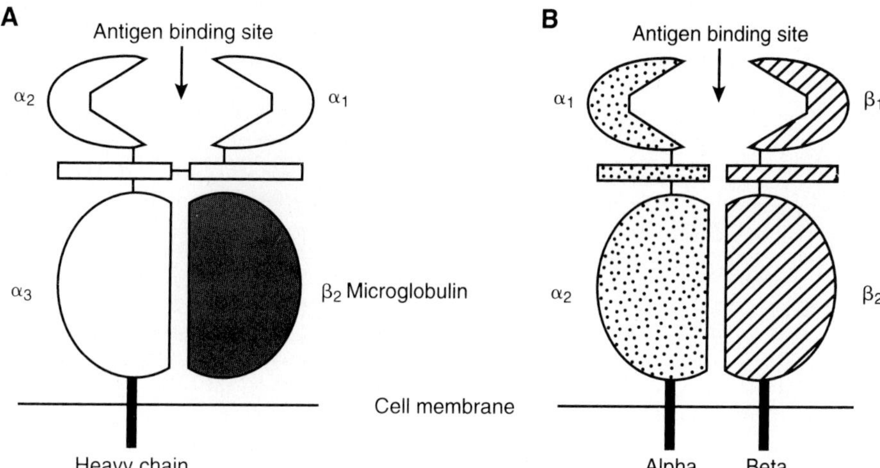

FIGURE 5–5. Structure of MHC molecules. MHC class I (**A**) and class II (**B**) molecules are shown schematically. Class I molecules (designated HLA-A, -B, and -C in man) are composed of a heavy chain (*unshaded*) noncovalently associated with β_2-microglobulin (*dark shading*). Class II molecules (HLA-DP, -DQ, and -DR in man) are composed of two chains, α (*stippled*) and β (*striped*), of approximately equal size and associated noncovalently. The class I heavy chain folds into compact "domains," α_1 and α_2 domains, which form an antigen-binding site. A similar binding site is made by the class II α_1 and β_1 domains. The binding site domains have a novel conformation, whereas the remaining domains (class I α_3 and β_2-microglobulin, and class II α_2 and β_2) resemble immunoglobulin domains.

consist of an MHC-encoded 45 kDa heavy chain and a noncovalently associated small subunit identical to the serum protein β_2-microglobulin. The membrane distal domains, which contain most of the polymorphisms between MHC molecules of different individuals, combine to form a unique binding site for the processed peptides derived from foreign antigens. This binding site is somewhat degenerate and able to bind numerous peptides that share only general motifs of structure, unlike the exact fit of many enzymes and their substrates, for example.

Nevertheless, the set of antigenic peptides capable of binding one MHC molecule is distinct from the set of peptides that binds another MHC molecule. This selectivity of MHC-peptide interaction underlies the association of certain polymorphisms (**HLA types**) with disease susceptibility. A postulated role of MHC polymorphism in immunity to infection is to ensure that at least some individuals in a population will be able to respond to and survive infection with a particular pathogen.

The **MHC class II molecules** (human **HLA-DR, -DP,** and **-DQ**) consist of two noncovalently linked polypeptides, α and β, of similar size, both of which are membrane inserted. Despite their differences in primary structure, MHC class I and II molecules assume a very similar three-dimensional structure.

An important difference between class I and II molecules is their tissue distribution. Whereas class I molecules are present on the surface of nearly all nucleated cells, class II molecules are restricted in their expression to B cells, macrophages, and dendritic cells. In response to cytokines, especially interferon-γ, class II molecules are also expressed on activated T cells and on other cells that are actively involved in an immune response, including the target organ cells in chronic autoimmune diseases. The restricted tissue distribution of class II molecules presumably reflects their participation in regulatory T-cell interactions rather than in effector functions.

Antigen Processing and Presentation. The classic **antigen-presenting cell (APC)** is the macrophage. The ability of macrophages to take up and destroy any number of classes of pathogenic organisms is well known. Purified macrophages that have processed antigen are clearly able to activate specific helper T cells effectively in the absence of other cell types. Recently it has been demonstrated that both dendritic cells and B cells, which are not able to engage in phagocytosis effectively, also possess the ability to process and present soluble protein antigens. An important common property of these APCs is the expression of class II molecules on their cell surface. It is likely that macrophages, B cells, and dendritic cells all function in vivo as APCs under certain circumstances. It is attractive to postulate that macrophages are of primary importance in the initiation of specific immune responses to bacteria, fungi, and protozoa, which they ingest and kill. Antigen-specific B cells may be important in secondary, or memory, responses by virtue of the expression of high-affinity receptors for soluble antigen in the form of membrane immunoglobulin. This cell surface antibody may act as a pump to concentrate the antigen inside the B cell, causing antigen-specific B cells to be effective APCs for T cells with the same antigen specificity. Dendritic cells may be potent APCs in specific anatomic locations (e.g., skin) that are macrophage poor. Dendritic cells are especially active with regard to processing and presenting soluble proteins, and they also appear to be important stimulators of graft rejection.

The antigen-processing pathways within the APCs are increasingly well understood (Fig. 5–6). Limited proteolysis is necessary for most exogenous protein antigens that are taken up into endocytic vesicles. For other antigens, simple unfolding of the protein is sufficient. At some point the endosomal degradative pathway of protein digestion intersects with the pathway of class II molecule synthesis. Peptides are loaded onto class II molecules, and the complexes are exported to the cell surface for recognition by T cells. Antigens synthesized within the cytoplasm (e.g., newly synthesized viral antigens) are processed by a different pathway, leading to presentation by class I molecules. This pathway appears to involve a large complex of cytoplasmic protease enzymes (**multiproteinase complex,** or **proteasome**) that degrades the antigen to peptides. Specialized transporter proteins translocate the peptides into the lumen of the endoplasmic reticulum, where they bind to newly synthesized class I molecules. The peptide–class I complexes then reach the cell surface.

Although the binding functions of class I and class II molecules are similar, the differences in antigen-processing pathways with which they are involved (exogenous vs endogenous) and the different tissue distributions are critical to determining which types of T cells are activated in response to infection. Conversely, inhibition of or interference with various aspects of antigen processing and presentation is a common escape mechanism in virus-infected cells or cancer cells. Some specific examples are given in Table 5–6.

T-Lymphocyte Recognition of MHC Bound Antigen. T lymphocytes bearing individually specific receptor molecules, known as T-cell receptors (TCRs), scan the environment for antigenic peptide-MHC complexes. TCRs are disulfide-linked heterodimeric structures that occur as two distinguishable types. TCRs composed of α and β chains are associated with most (>95%) peripheral T cells, including those in the blood, lymph nodes, and spleen. TCRs of a second type, composed of γ and δ subunit chains, appear on few recirculating T cells but are found on increased numbers of T cells at or near epithelial sites such as the skin and gastrointestinal tract. All four TCR chains are immunoglobulin-like in their overall structure and their pairing. The combinations of $\alpha\beta$ and $\gamma\delta$ TCRs are apparently exclusive.

Individual TCRs recognize specific MHC-peptide complexes as a unit, making contact with both peptide and MHC molecule amino acids (Fig. 5–7). Specific binding affinities of TCRs for peptide-MHC complexes are apparently weak and must be augmented by other ligand systems. TCR $\alpha\beta$–bearing cells with specificity for endogenous antigen bound to class I molecules coexpress a molecule called CD8. The ligand for CD8 is a nonpolymorphic region of the same class I molecule that binds the antigenic peptide for recognition by TCR $\alpha\beta$–bearing cells. Similarly, TCR $\alpha\beta$–bearing cells specific for exogenous antigen–MHC class II complexes coexpress the CD4 molecule. CD4 appears to corecognize a nonpolymorphic region of the class II molecule. As a result, TCR $\alpha\beta$–bearing cells can be separated into two functional subsets: CD4 MHC class II–restricted helper T cells and CD8 MHC class I–restricted cytotoxic T cells.

An alternative means of antigen and T-cell interaction has been described for a special class of viral and bacterial proteins, primarily exotoxins of *Staphylococcus aureus* and *Streptococcus,* including TSST-1. These extracellular proteins have been termed **superantigens** because they activate a larger and more diverse population of T cells than antigens that undergo the usual processing and presentation steps. Superantigens interact directly with MHC class II and cross-link it with the V_β region of the TCR (Fig. 5–7). This interaction occurs outside the antigen-binding groove area formed by the MHC class II molecule and the TCR. Individual superantigens typically activate 5–25% of total CD4 T cells, compared with about 1 in 10^5 for specific antigens recognized in the conventional manner. This type of recognition appears to be pathologic because it unleashes a **cytokine storm** that is responsible for the manifestations of toxic shock and related syndromes.

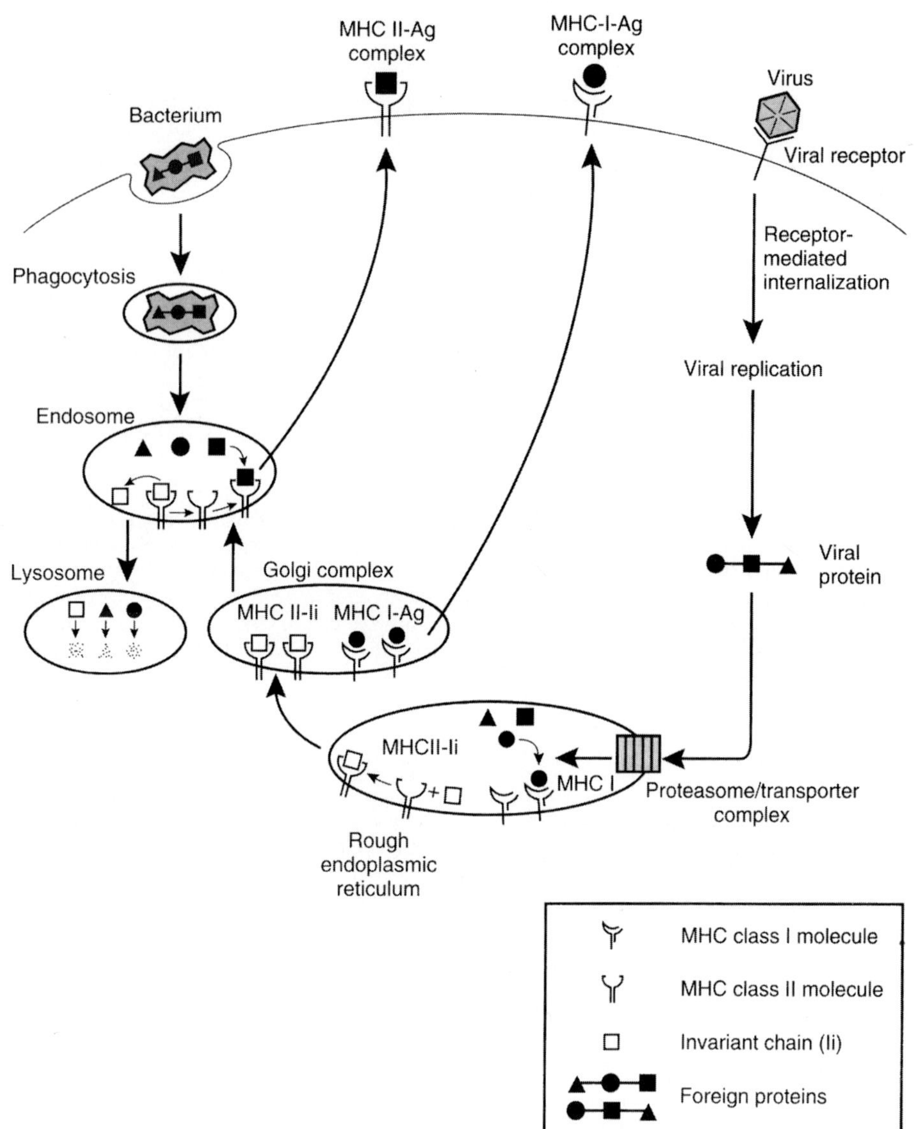

FIGURE 5–6. Antigen processing and presentation pathways for exogenous and extracellular antigens (e.g., derived from bacteria) compared with endogenous and intracellular antigens (e.g., derived from replicating viruses). Antigenic peptides (*dark triangles, circles,* and *boxes*) derived from enzymatic digestion of exogenous proteins in an endosomal compartment are loaded onto MHC class II molecules that have been prevented from acquiring endogenous peptides by invariant chain (*open boxes*). Alternatively, MHC class I molecules pick up endogenous peptides that have been transported into a Golgi compartment after proteolysis in the cytoplasm. In this way, MHC class I and class II molecules are able to specifically "sample" antigens derived from different sources and present them to CD4 and CD8 lymphocytes (Fig. 5–7).

TABLE 5–6. Specific Examples of Virus Inhibition of Antigen Processing and Presentation

Mechanism	Example(s)
Inhibition of MHC molecule biosynthesis	Adenovirus E1A
Enhanced degradation of MHC molecules	Cytomegalovirus US2 and 11
Inhibition of transporter of antigen presentation (TAP) function	Herpes simplex virus type 2 ICP47
Inhibition of T-cell costimulation	Epstein-Barr virus vIL-10

T-Cell Activation. T-cell $\alpha\beta$ and $\gamma\delta$ antigen–specific receptors are noncovalently linked to a complex of signaling molecules (at least five polypeptides) collectively termed CD3. Inositol phosphate turnover and a rise in intracellular free Ca^{2+} are important early events linked to the transmembrane signals. Subsequently a cascade of phosphorylation events, mediated by a series of protein kinases and their adapter molecules, occurs, leading eventually to the recruitment of transcription regulatory proteins and specific gene activation in the cell nucleus. CD4 and CD8 are also linked to specific intracellular signal-generating molecules, especially a lymphocyte-specific protein tyrosine kinase, $p56^{lck}$; CD45, a cell surface molecule with phosphatase activity, is also important.

Four other independent ligand-receptor systems also participate in T-cell activation after T cell–APC interaction. These systems are CD28:B7 (CD80 and CD86), LFA-1:ICAM-1, CD2:LFA-3, and CD5:CD72. Current understanding of the function of these so-

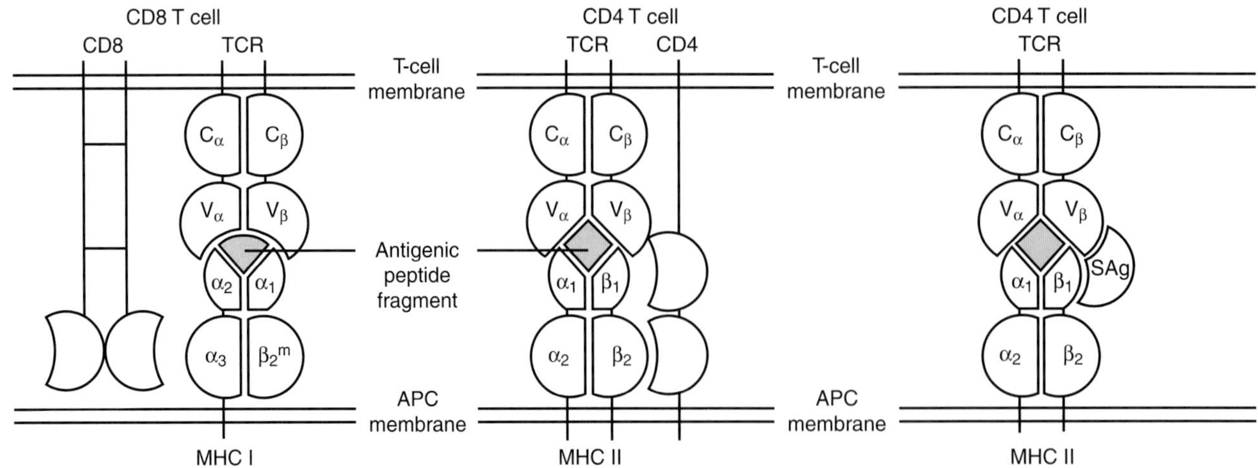

FIGURE 5–7. Schematic illustration of T-cell receptor (*TCR*) and accessory molecule involvement in recognition of peptide antigens bound to MHC molecules; class I and class II molecules (Fig. 5–5) are shown with peptide antigens (*dark shading*) filling their binding sites. Antigen-specific TCRs are composed of α and β chains. TCR variable (V_α, V_β) and constant (C_α, C_β) domains are labeled. T cells recognizing antigenic peptides bound to class I molecules express the accessory molecule CD8, which interacts with the class I molecule (*left panel*). Similarly, CD4 is an accessory molecule involved in recognition of class II–bound antigen (*middle panel*). The interactions of superantigens (*SAg*) with class II and TCR V_β domains occur outside the antigen-binding sites (*right panel*) without regard for MHC-bound peptide. Antigen-presenting cells (*APC*) include dendritic cells, macrophages, and B lymphocytes. β_2m, β_2-microglobulin.

called costimulating molecules is that they provide a "second signal" to T cells. The "first signal," recognition of antigen-MHC by the TCR, is necessary but not sufficient for T-cell activation. Furthermore, in many cases the recognition of the first signal without engagement of costimulatory molecules results in T cells' becoming functionally inactivated (anergic). This may be a fail-safe mechanism to prevent inappropriate or excessive T-cell activation.

Cytokine Secretion, T-Cell Subsets, and Effector Functions. An important set of gene activation events that occurs after T-cell activation involves secreted molecules called lymphokines and their cell surface receptors. **Lymphokines** (lymphocyte cytokines) are a diverse group of molecules that signal the proliferation and functional activation of lymphocytes and other cell types (Table 5–7). Antigen-induced lymphocyte proliferation is an important component of the host immune response that leads to amplification of function and the development of memory. IL-2 is the primary lymphokine that drives clonal expansion of T lymphocytes. Its major source is CD4 T cells. Thus a significant degree of clonal expansion is autocrine in nature.

TABLE 5–7. Some Important Lymphokines, Their Cellular Sources, and Principal Effects Related to Immune Responses to Infection

Name	Source	Effect
IL-1	Macrophages	T-cell activation
		Acute-phase response
IL-2	T cells (Th1)	T- and B-cell clonal expansion
IL-3	T cells	Stem cell, erythroid, and myeloid progenitor growth
IL-4	T cells (Th2)	IgE secretion
		T-, B-, and mast-cell growth
		Th2-cell differentiation
IL-5	T cells (Th2)	Eosinophil differentiation
		IgA secretion
IL-6	Macrophages	IgG secretion
		Acute-phase response
IL-7	Bone marrow stromal cells	T and B cell progenitor growth
IL-8	Macrophages, endothelial cells	Neutrophil chemotaxis
IL-10	T cells	Monocyte inhibition
		B cell activation
IL-12	Macrophages, dendritic cells	Th1 cell differentiation
IFN-γ	T cells (Th1)	IgG secretion
		Macrophage activation
TGF-β	T cells, monocytes	Inhibition of T-cell and monocyte activation
TNF-α	Macrophages	Acute-phase response

TGF = Transforming growth factor.

The importance of various subsets of T lymphocytes in the response to particular organisms has been well documented. The markers CD4 and CD8 define mutually exclusive, reciprocal subpopulations of mature, circulating T lymphocytes. The population of CD4 T cells contains mostly cells with executive functions such as macrophage-activating capability and antibody helper activity for B cells. The CD8 cell population contains the majority of cells with cytotoxic activity against virally infected cells and tumor targets. The critical role for CD8 T cells and their recognition of newly synthesized antigens of intracellular infectious organisms mediated by class I molecules is emphasized by the recognition of antigens that are not exposed on the surface of pathogenic organisms (e.g., viral nucleocapsid proteins). These antigens are nevertheless capable of stimulating strong T-cell immunity and in vivo protection against infection. CD8 cells therefore represent an important means of eliminating the cellular reservoirs of replication for intracellular pathogens.

An exciting recent development concerning the immunity of infection has been the finding that CD4 T cells can be subdivided on the basis of the secretion of lymphokines (Fig. 5–8). Probably as a result of the method of immunization or sensitization or both, totipotent CD4 cells capable of making many lymphokines generate two distinct T-helper subsets, Th1 and Th2. **Th1 cells** secrete IL-2 and IFN-γ and induce cell-mediated effector functions. The most important cytokine in polarizing T cells toward a Th1 phenotype is IL-12, which is secreted primarily by APCs, including dendritic cells and macrophages. **Th2 cells** secrete IL-4 and IL-5 and induce antibody-mediated effector functions. The primary influence polarizing T cells toward the Th2 phenotype is IL-4. The source of this early IL-4, which must be present before the Th2 cells can make IL-4, is still controversial.

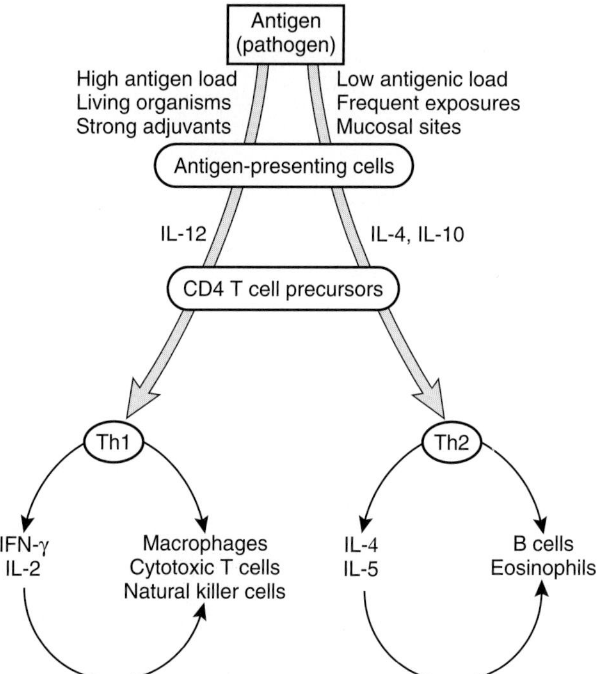

FIGURE 5–8. Simplified view of the polarization of T-cell responses into Th1 or Th2 phenotypes. Antigens presented under conditions (*A*) that induce IL-12 production (e.g., large quantities, living organisms, strong adjuvants) cause the differentiation of helper T-cell precursors into Th1 cells, which secrete IL-2 and IFN-γ. Th1 cells mediate cell-mediated effector functions by activating macrophages, cytotoxic T cells, and NK cells. In contrast, antigens presented under conditions (*B*) that induce IL-4 production (e.g., low quantities, frequent exposure, mucosal sites) cause the differentiation of helper T-cell precursors into Th2 cells, which secrete IL-4 and IL-5. Th2 cells mediate immunity to parasites and allergic disease by activating B cells (especially those that secrete IgE antibodies) and eosinophils. Cytokines secreted by Th1 and Th2 cells are counterregulatory (not shown), enhancing and maintaining polarization.

This compartmentalization of lymphokine secretion has significant physiologic relevance. Th1 cells play a critical role in delayed cutaneous hypersensitivity reactions (similar to tuberculosis skin test reactions), which are characterized by T-cell, macrophage, and monocyte infiltration. Th1-cell activation and the production of IL-2 and IFN-γ are key features in resistance to experimental *Trypanosoma cruzi* and *Schistosoma mansoni* infections in mice. Th1 responses are presumed to be important for intracellular bacterial and protozoan infections in humans.

Hypersensitive individuals have a significant Th2-cell response to allergens, those antigens that induce their symptoms. Th2-derived IL-4 is the primary lymphokine involved in the synthesis of IgE, the antibody responsible for triggering many allergic reactions. IL-4 also stimulates mast cell growth and activation, which are important in allergic disease. Th2 cells also make IL-5, a potent stimulator of eosinophil differentiation, further strengthening the connection between allergen-specific Th2 subset responses and hypersensitivity symptoms. Similar pathways also appear to be activated by helminthic infestation, in which IgE and eosinophil responses are notable. It is presently unclear whether the Th2 responses in these situations are primarily beneficial or harmful to the host.

Specialized T-Cell Subsets. The major subpopulations of T cells, in particular those found in the blood and peripheral lymphoid tissues (e.g., spleen, lymph nodes), have a high level of diversity in their receptors. However, certain T-cell subpopulations have uniform, stereotyped receptor structures and specificities for particular subspecies of antigens. For example, a recently discovered T-cell population has been described that uses a restricted subset of TCRs to recognize mycobacterial glycolipids presented by non-polymorphic MHC-like molecules of the CD1 family. This represents a highly conserved system of recognition, similar to the pattern recognition of innate immunity, using structures and cells that are characteristic of adaptive immunity. Other, similar specialized T-cell populations occur prominently in specific tissues, such as the skin and gastrointestinal tract, where initial contact with foreign antigens occurs. These T-cell populations are best considered as important intermediates in properties and function, bridging gaps between innate and adaptive immunity.

B Lymphocytes and Antibodies

B cells are lymphocytes that are capable of secreting antibody molecules. Mature B cells can be identified by the presence of immunoglobulin molecules or antibodies on the cell surface in the form of integral membrane proteins anchored by a short transmembrane tail. This form of immunoglobulin, usually IgM, serves as one of the triggers for B-cell activation and is identical in specificity to the antibody secreted when the activated B cell becomes a plasma cell. Membrane immunoglobulin is associated with additional non-polymorphic, signal transduction molecules, including Igα and Igβ, which form a B-cell receptor (BCR) complex analogous to the TCR-CD3 complex of T cells. Secreted antibody lacks the transmembrane tail, a result of alternative mRNA splicing. B-cell development is directly linked to the genetic events responsible for constructing antibody molecules. Pre-B cells, an important intermediate stage of B-cell development, are recognized by the presence of IgM heavy chains (μ chains) in the cytoplasm but not on the cell surface. Pre-B cells become B cells when immunoglobulin light chains are synthesized, resulting in the assembly of intact immunoglobulin molecules and their transport to the cell surface.

Several functionally important B-cell surface molecules are recognized. Class II molecules are critical for antigen-specific T cell–B cell interactions, which are required for antibody production to most antigens. A second key molecule in T cell–B cell interaction and B-cell activation is CD40. Engagement of CD40 on the B cell by CD154, an activation-induced molecule on helper T cells, is required for **antibody class switching,** the shift from making IgM to other antibody isotypes, particularly IgG. Activated B cells express receptors for certain cytokines that also regulate their ability to produce antibodies, including IL-2, IL-4, IL-5, IL-6, and IFN-γ.

General Structure of Antibodies. Antibody molecules are symmetric heterodimeric proteins consisting of two identical **heavy (H) chains** (50–70 kDa) and two identical **light (L) chains** (20–25 kDa) joined together by covalent disulfide bonds (Fig. 5–9). Each chain is composed of domains of 100–110 amino acids each, which fold into a characteristic three-dimensional structure of β-pleated sheets. Paired domains from opposing chains form strong noncovalent interactions, whereas the linear structure connecting adjacent domains of the same chain is somewhat flexible. This is especially true of the so-called **hinge region,** which has consequences for antibody function; changes in the hinge region account for divalent antigen binding and the ability to activate complement. The hinge region is susceptible to cleavage with proteases, including some specific bacterial enzymes that may act as virulence factors. Such cleavage results in the formation of fragments that retain antigen-binding properties **(Fab)** and other fragments that could be crystallized **(Fc).**

There are numerous differences in the first 100–110 amino acids (starting from the NH_2-terminus) of different human antibody light chains, with virtually complete conservation of sequence of the next 100–110 residues. This finding gave rise to the terms **variable (V)** and **constant (C)** regions and to two important hypotheses that have since been elegantly and thoroughly verified: the variable regions are the sites responsible for antigen-binding specificity; and the V and C regions are encoded by individual genes. The first hypothesis has been directly confirmed by x-ray crystallography of antigen-antibody complexes. The antigen-binding site consists of a series of loops that protrude from the edges of the variable domains. Both the H and L chains contribute such loops to the binding site. The amino acid sequences of these loops are even more variable than the remainder of the V region and are sometimes called **hypervariable regions.** They are also referred to as **complementarity determining regions (CDR),** referring to their antigen-binding function. The remainder of each V domain, consisting of seven protein strands that form two β-pleated sheets held together by a disulfide bond, is often called the

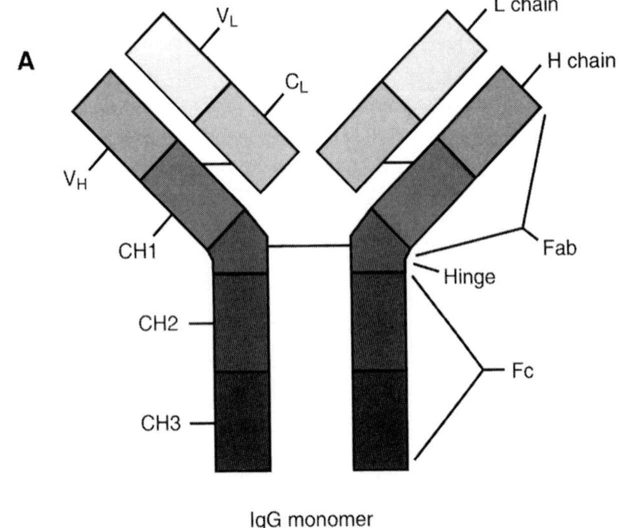

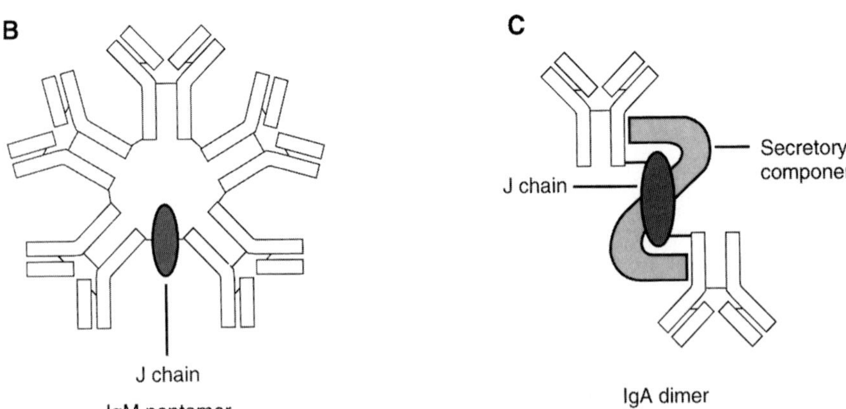

FIGURE 5–9. Schematic diagram of the major antibody classes: IgG **(A),** IgM **(B),** and IgA **(C).** Heavy *(H)* and light *(L)* chains, variable *(V)* and constant *(C)* domains, and Fab, hinge, and Fc portions are labeled for IgG. Additional features are shown for IgM (J chain) and IgA (J chain, secretory component) multimers.

framework. The three-dimensional structure of the antibody V regions explains the molecular basis of specificity, in which individual variation in amino acid composition, sequence, and orientation of the CDR loops contribute to the recognition of different antigens by individual antibodies. The C domains and the V regions have a similar structure, but the C domains lack the extended CDR loops that characterize the V region antigen-binding site.

Antibody Diversity. The vast number of specific antibodies and the peculiar structure of variable and conserved regions on the same protein chain presented a challenge for immunologists who wished to account for these properties at the genetic level. The explanation for these phenomena, given early on by several individuals, proved to be simple, elegant, heretical, and, ultimately, correct. What these investigators hypothesized was that two genes (one for V and one for C) could be combined to code for one polypeptide chain. This solved the dual problems of avoiding carrying millions of identical copies of C region information while at the same time providing a means for diversity-generating mechanisms to act on V regions independent of C regions. The two gene–one polypeptide hypothesis was later confirmed directly by recombinant DNA techniques.

Eventually it was found that the V regions themselves are formed from individual **gene segments,** or **minigenes.** For example, the germline organization of an immunoglobulin light chain locus (Fig. 5–10) consists of clusters of **V genes,** encoding about 90% of the V region ultimately found in the protein chain, that are found upstream of a smaller cluster of **J genes,** encoding the remaining 10% of the V region. The **C region gene** is located further downstream. Each V gene and each J gene is somewhat different from other members of the same cluster. About 150–200 light chain V genes and 4–6 J genes exist in mice, with somewhat more in humans. Separate and distinct V and J gene clusters exist for the two types of light chains, κ and λ. Diversity is produced by the combination of two mechanisms. First, an apparently random combination of V and J genes by DNA rearrangement occurs in maturing B cells. Second, the joining of V and J segments at their boundaries is not precise. Nuclease enzymes can remove nucleotides from the ends of the V and J gene segments, and terminal deoxynucleotide transferase (TdT) can add nucleotides that are not encoded in the germline DNA. These added nucleotides are referred to as the nontemplate, or **N segment,** and this mechanism for generating additional diversity has been labeled **N segment diversity.** These processes lead to tremendous increases in the diversity of the antibody produced. As a result, greater than 10^5 different light chains can be generated from fewer than 10^3 genes. The V gene encodes the CDR 1 and 2 loops, whereas the highly variable V-J junction contributes diversity to the hypervariable CDR 3 loop.

Antibody heavy chains are capable of even greater diversity. There are perhaps 1,000 heavy chain V gene segments. In addition to V and J segments, heavy chain V regions also include amino

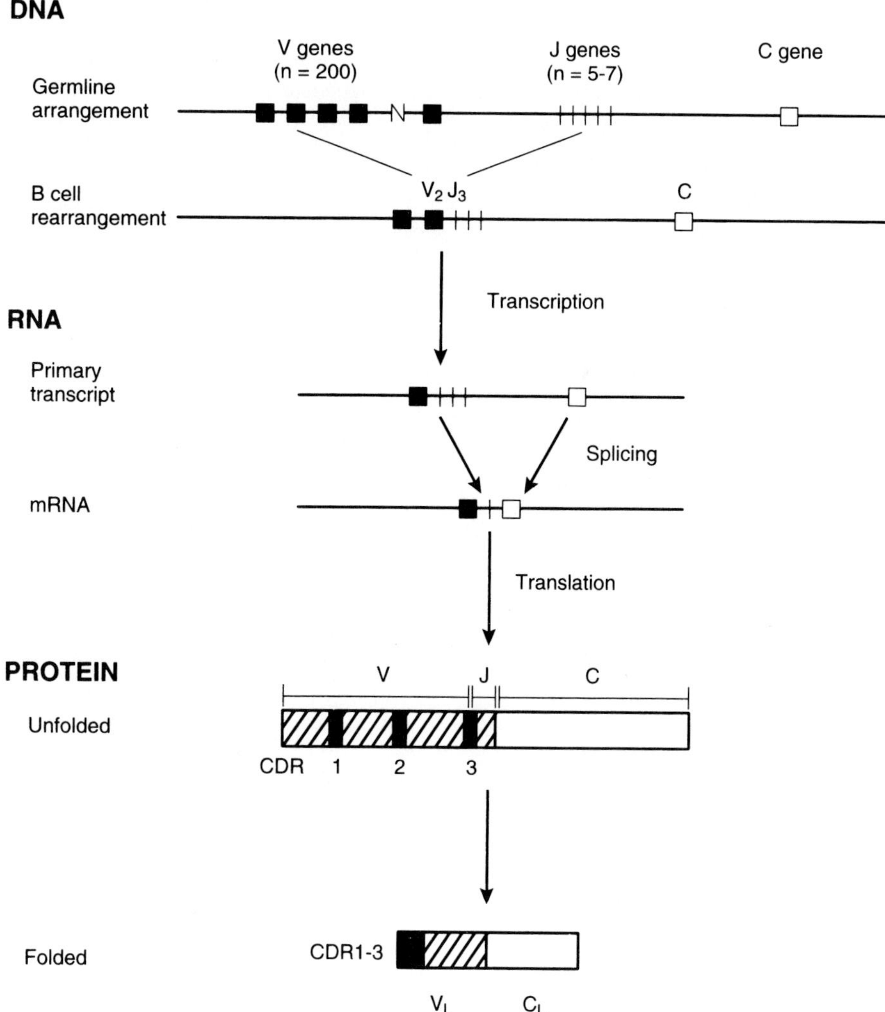

FIGURE 5–10. Correlation of genetic information and protein structural characteristics with antibody light chain function. Rearrangement of DNA coding for V and J gene segments forms a complete V region, which is then transcribed along with a C region gene and processed into mRNA. When translated into protein, the regions labeled CDR1 and CDR2 (contributed by the V gene segment) and the region labeled CDR3 (contributed by the V-J junction) are brought together by protein folding to form the antigen-combining site. The remaining V region structure forms a framework that holds the CDR loops in the proper orientation. The C region folds into a similar structure but without the extra loops. A similar process occurs for heavy chain, which then pairs with light chain to form an intact antibody (Fig. 5–9). CDR regions of the heavy chain complete the antigen-binding site.

acids encoded by **D (diversity) gene segments,** located between the V and J gene clusters. Thus two DNA rearrangements occur in heavy chain synthesis: D-to-J rearrangement occurs first, preceding V-to-DJ joining. The D segments provide for additional junctional diversity because nuclease and TdT activity can act at both the V-D and D-J junctions.

Therefore the number of possible heavy chain protein products is on the order of 1,000 times greater than for light chains (i.e., more than 10^8). If the pairing of heavy and light chains to form an intact antibody is relatively random, then a staggering 10^{13} or more individual antibody molecules can potentially be constructed from a relatively few (probably fewer than 10^4) germline encoded gene segments.

However, even this enormous degree of potential diversity of the antibody repertoire is apparently not enough to keep humans perfectly healthy. During an antibody response, the variable regions of heavy and light chains undergo point mutations **(somatic mutation)** that allow the selection of antibodies with significantly increased affinity for the offending pathogen. This process requires help from T lymphocytes participating in the response.

The antigen receptors of T lymphocytes are constructed from gene segments, similarly to the way that antibodies are constructed. Junctional diversity appears to be greater in TCRs than in immunoglobulins, particularly in β chains, because of the ways in which the D segments are used. However, TCRs do not appear to undergo somatic mutation. This possibility is reflected in the comparatively low affinity of TCRs for the corresponding antigen-MHC complexes. The failure of T cells to increase their affinity for antigen during the immune response **(affinity maturation)** is believed to be the result of pressure to avoid self-recognition and autoimmune disease. As a result of this limitation on TCR affinity, the T cells may have developed the additional ligand systems to yield sufficient total affinity for cellular activation, signaling, and function. The three-dimensional structure of several TCRs has recently been identified, and these TCRs show significant similarity, in their three-dimensional structure, to the Fab fragments of antibodies. It appears that the TCR makes contact with both the MHC molecule and the peptide fragment of antigen that forms the TCR ligand (Fig. 5–7).

Antibody Classes and Subclasses. Antibodies come in several different but related forms, designated **classes** and **subclasses** and sometimes known as **isotypes.** Different antibody classes and subclasses are the result of the usage of different constant region genes that differ in amino acid sequence. Two antibodies may share identical light chains and heavy chain V regions but are of different classes because they have different heavy chain C regions. Historically the finding of two such antibodies strongly supported the idea that multiple gene segments encode antibodies.

The five major classes of human antibodies are (in order of their appearance in ontogeny and phylogeny) IgM, IgD, IgG, IgA, and IgE. The heavy chains of these different antibody classes are 20–30% identical in amino acid sequence and highly homologous in overall structure. Four IgG subclasses (IgG1, IgG2, IgG3, and IgG4) and two IgA subclasses (IgA1 and IgA2) have been identified. The amino acid sequences of the heavy chain C regions of different subclasses within a class are more than 90% identical. The various C region differences endow the respective classes and subclasses with distinct biologic properties (Table 5–8). These properties have important clinical implications for antibody responses to infectious disease and for immune deficiencies.

IgM. IgM antibodies are formed early in the primary response to antigenic challenge. They are lower in affinity and broader in specificity than IgG antibodies, which follow in a T cell–dependent antigen response. Serum IgM antibodies are pentamers (Fig. 5–9), consisting of five 4-chain (H_2L_2) subunits linked together with a nonimmunoglobulin subunit called a **J chain** (not to be confused with the J gene segment). The overall binding avidity of the pentamer with more available binding sites partially makes up for the lower specific binding affinity of the individual IgM binding sites.

IgM antibodies are characteristic of T cell–independent B cell responses and are triggered by highly repetitive polymeric antigenic structures such as bacterial polysaccharides. Although these responses are clearly of protective value, they do not generate affinity maturation characteristic of IgG responses, nor do they generate memory. Recent evidence suggests that serum IgM may come predominantly from CD5 B cells.

IgD. IgD antibodies are present in the serum in vanishingly small amounts and probably serve no protective purpose there. IgD is usually found on the surface (sIgD) of B cells along with IgM (sIgM), both having identical specificity. The exact role of sIgD is unclear. It has been postulated that cells bearing sIgM alone differ in their signaling pathways from B cells bearing sIgM and sIgD. This may have some relevance to activation or tolerance in the B-cell compartment.

IgG. IgG is quantitatively and qualitatively an important component of host defenses. IgG is made late in the primary response and is briskly synthesized on secondary exposure to antigen. The switch from IgM to IgG production **(class switching)** in response to infection is heavily influenced by T cells through CD40 signaling and lymphokines. IgG responses to the high level of antibody secretion are marked by a continuous increase in affinity for the immunizing antigen **(affinity maturation),** which is the result of accumulation of point mutations in antibody V regions. As a consequence, T

TABLE 5–8. Biologic Properties of Antibody Classes and Subclasses

			IgG				IgA		
Property	**IgM**	**IgD**	**1**	**2**	**3**	**4**	**1**	**2**	**IgE**
Mean serum concentration (mg/dL)	150	<1	840	240	80	40	270	30	<0.01
Serum half-life (days)	5	2.8	23	23	9	23	7	7	2.3
Placental transfer	–	–	++	±	+	+	–	–	–
Complement fixation (classic pathway)	+	–	++	+	+	–	–	–	–
Cell binding									
Macrophages	–	–	++	±	++	±	–	–	+
Neutrophils	+	±	+	+	+	+	+	+	±
Mast cells	–	–	–	–	–	–	–	–	–
Presence in secretions	–	–	+	+	+	+	+	++	±

cell–dependent IgG responses are critical to the development of resistance to infection.

The four subclasses of human IgG have interesting differences in their ability to fix, or activate, complement and bind to effector cells, such as macrophages. In addition, a curious relationship between the type of antigen and the IgG subclass elicited can be found. Bacterial polysaccharides are excellent inducers of IgG2 and, to a lesser extent, IgG4 antibodies, whereas viral proteins and bacterial toxoids characteristically elicit IgG1 and IgG3 antibodies. The mechanism of this association is unknown but suggests some connection between antigen specificity (a V region function) and subclass (a C region property).

IgA. The primary interest in IgA stems from its abundance in mucosal secretions, although it is also found in the serum. Not only is IgA relatively more abundant than IgM and IgG in secretions, but the IgA is produced and secreted locally. In addition, B lymphocytes traffic between mucosal sites. For example, sensitization of IgA-bearing B cells in the gut results not only in local IgA production but in IgA secretion at additional mucosal sites (e.g., in breast milk).

IgA is usually isolated as J chain–containing dimers and tetramers (Fig. 5–9), particularly in secretions. In addition to the J-chain component, secretory IgA also includes a **secretory component (SC).** SC is produced by epithelial cells and acts as a cell surface receptor for IgA secreted by adjacent plasma cells. The IgA-SC complex is then vectorially transported to the luminal side of the epithelial cell and released into the secretions.

Two IgA subclasses exist, IgA1 and IgA2. Differences in the ratio of IgA1 to IgA2 in various fluids and differential sensitivities of the two IgA subclasses to certain bacterial proteolytic enzymes suggest distinctive roles for the two subclasses.

IgE. IgE antibodies are present in the sera of healthy individuals, with increased levels in hypersensitivity disease states and in parasitic infections. Production of IgE in response to antigen stimulation is highly dependent on T cells and IL-4. IgE is taken up by high-affinity receptors on mast cells and tissue basophils. Subsequent antigen exposure causes the rapid release of numerous mediators of inflammation, resulting in immediate hypersensitivity. The protective role of this response in parasitic disease and hypersensitivity is controversial. Physical expulsion of offending antigens from the respiratory and gastrointestinal tracts may be important.

Light Chains. Two light chain classes, **kappa** (κ) and **lambda** (λ), are found in all species examined thus far. Either light chain may be found in association with any heavy chain class or subclass antibody. The use of κ and λ chains differs widely among different species. Rodents (e.g., mice, rats) express κ chains on more than 90% of their antibodies, whereas cows and other ungulates produce mainly λ-bearing antibodies. Human antibodies fall within these extremes, with a $\kappa:\lambda$ ratio of about 2:1. The functional significance of these variations is unclear.

Antibody-Mediated Effects. Specific antibodies can trigger two important pathways, complement and antibody-dependent cellular cytotoxicity, leading to destruction or clearance of the offending antigen. In this way, antigen-specific responses augment nonspecific protective mechanisms.

IgM and IgG antibodies, with the exception of IgG4, can trigger **complement activation** (Fig. 5–2; Table 5–8). Aggregation of antibodies by binding to a multivalent antigen generates a binding site on the antibody Fc region for the complement component C1q. Antibody-C1q complexes then activate the classical complement cascade, resulting in the generation of chemotactic factors, opsonins and the membrane attack complex (MAC).

Non-antigen-specific cytotoxic cells participate in antigen-specific reactions mediated by specific antibodies through **antibody-dependent cellular cytotoxicity (ADCC)** (Fig. 5–3). Cells involved in ADCC include any cell with cytolytic capability that expresses receptors for the Fc region of antibodies (FcR). These include monocytes and NK cells. Antigen-specific cytotoxic T lymphocytes can also participate in ADCC, at least in vitro.

Regulation of Specific Immune Responses

Because immune system activation may be harmful or beneficial for the host, a number of mechanisms regulate the magnitude, duration, and localization of the immune responses. Some of these mechanisms are simple, such as antigen persistence and the limited half-life of activated cells or molecules. Others are more complex, such as the circuits and networks of interacting cells. It has been estimated that more than 70% of lymphocytes may have a regulatory rather than a direct protective function.

Selection of Lymphocyte Receptor Repertoire. If the development of immune receptors is random, production of self-reactive and potentially immunopathologic antibodies and T-cell receptors would be expected, and powerful mechanisms would be needed to limit the receptor repertoire of lymphocytes. Substantial evidence exists that self-reactive receptors are regularly generated and are subjected to a purging process. This evidence has had a significant impact on theories of autoimmunity. The current paradigm is that autoimmune receptors (antibody and TCR) are not abnormal receptors but that their expression is evidence of faulty or subverted regulatory mechanisms.

No specific exclusion of host peptides from MHC molecules for presentation to T cells is apparent. Thus antigen processing and presentation mechanisms do not appear to specifically discriminate host components and prevent recognition by T cells. Similarly, B-cell autoreactivity has been demonstrated in healthy individuals on several occasions. Low-level, low-affinity, naturally occurring IgM autoantibodies can be detected in normal serum, whereas most pathogenic autoantibodies are IgG antibodies that have variable region mutations reflecting T-cell help. Thus a considerable amount of B-cell autoreactivity appears to be tolerated in the healthy host. Through inappropriate activation and somatic mutation, however, the B-cell repertoire can form a substrate for pathologic autoantibodies.

T-cell autoreactivity appears to be stringently regulated at several levels. More than 95% of all T cells undergoing TCR gene rearrangement during development in the thymus die there by a specific programmed cell death mechanism known as apoptosis. Two distinct processes, positive and negative selection, that are mediated by different types of accessory cells in the thymus appear to be at work (Fig. 5–11). First, T cells are positively selected for recognition of antigen-MHC complexes present in the thymus. T cells whose TCR rearrangements result in some measurable affinity for selfantigen-MHC complexes are rescued from apoptosis. Second, T cells with high affinity for self-antigen-MHC complexes are negatively selected. The effect of these two selection processes is sufficient to eliminate most autoreactive T cells. In addition, postthymic T cells can also be **tolerized** in the peripheral (i.e., extrathymic) lymphoid tissue by exposure to self-antigen-MHC complexes on cells that lack costimulatory molecules (i.e., cells other than functional [''professional''] antigen-presenting cells). T cells also appear to lack an ability to introduce somatic mutations into TCR V regions. Thus, in contrast to B cells, T cells are unable to acquire autoreactivity somatically.

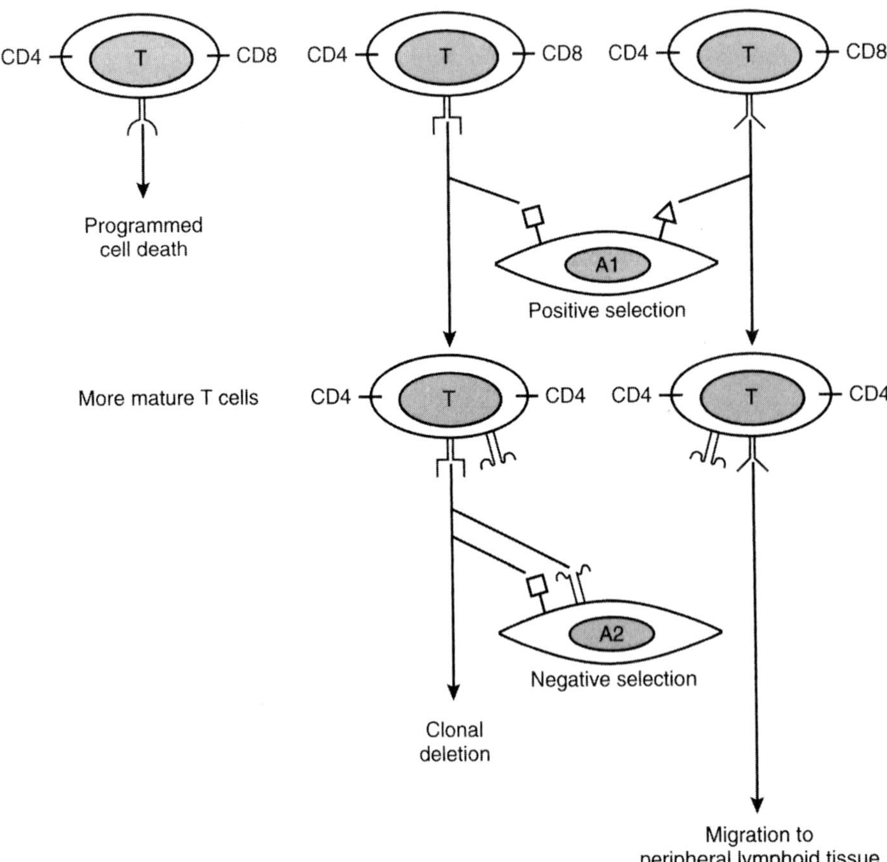

FIGURE 5–11. Positive and negative selection mechanisms act in the thymus to limit the T-cell receptor repertoire (illustrated for CD4 cells; an analogous process occurs to selected CD8 cells). Immature T cells expressing both CD4 and CD8 must encounter and bind to an MHC-bound "self"-antigen or, failing to do so, must die. Many T cells bearing irrelevant receptors fail to make this transition, called positive selection. Cells successfully engaging antigen in this step then express higher levels of receptor and become "single positive" for either CD4 (as shown) or CD8. These more mature T cells then must pass a second test. Those with high-affinity for self-antigen at this stage are deleted in a process called negative selection. The differing and somewhat contradictory requirements of positive and negative selection are shown here as being mediated by two different types of accessory cells (A1, A2) but are not well understood. As a result of this stringent selection process, few T cells escape from the thymus, in comparison with the large numbers that die in the thymus.

In summary, both B- and T-cell repertoires are constrained in their expression of specific receptors. T cells appear to have a more stringent set of requirements for repertoire development and expression. This may reflect their critical role in **self-nonself-discrimination,** which is critical in responding to pathogenic challenge while remaining unresponsive to autologous components.

Persistence of Antigen. It seems axiomatic that immune responses would subside after antigen is eliminated. The role of antigen persistence in the maintenance of immunologic memory arises because the phenotypic characteristics of activated and putative memory lymphocytes overlap to a considerable degree. It is possible that depots containing minute quantities of antigen may persist in long-lived antigen-presenting cells in the spleen and lymph nodes, constantly reinforcing immunologic memory. Mature dendritic cells, which contain a population of long-lived nonrecirculating MHC-peptide complexes on their cell surface, are candidates for long-lived memory-reinforcing, antigen-presenting cells.

Death of Activated Lymphocytes. Transient lymphadenopathy is the natural consequence of acute infection, which reflects the accumulation and then resolution of activated and expanded cells. During the later stages of activation, lymphocytes express the CD95 molecule, also called Fas or Apo-1. When CD95 is engaged by its ligand, FasL, which is found on the surface of other cells including other lymphocytes, CD95-expressing cells are triggered to undergo programmed cell death, or apoptosis. The CD95/Fas system appears to be a key regulator of lymphocyte homeostasis. Persons with CD95 mutations exhibit generalized, persistent, histologically benign lymphadenopathy. They also have elevated IgG levels and are prone to certain types of autoimmunity. The CD95/Fas pathway is one of several pathways by which accumulated cells of the immune system are eliminated on resolution of infections. Memory lymphocytes apparently find some way around these cell death pathways, but the mechanisms are currently obscure.

Regulatory T-Cell Circuits. The compartmentalization of T cells into various defined subsets has both regulatory and functional, protective effects. The interaction of counterregulating cells specific for the same antigen is said to define a **circuit.** Immune regulation is based on the secretion of lymphokines with counterbalancing properties (Fig. 5–8). The switch between lymphokines promoting cell-mediated (Th1) and those inducing antibody-mediated (Th2) effector functions may critically affect the outcome of an infectious process. The choice between these two pathways may be in part genetically determined and may also be affected by route and form of exposure or immunization.

Network Theories of Immune Regulation. The random process of immune receptor (antibody and TCR) generation results in the production of minute quantities of vast numbers of unique protein structures. Each new receptor is potentially capable of being recognized as a unique antigen (**idiotype**) by antibodies made against it (**anti-idiotype**). It has been proposed that such interactions are actually a predictable outcome of the system of immune receptor generation and may help regulate immune responses. Such a regulatory pathway of receptor-antireceptor (**idiotype-anti-idiotype**) interaction is termed an **idiotypic network.** Although the concept of regulation through idiotype networks remains controversial, idiotype-anti-idiotype interactions can produce useful probes to follow and manipulate specific immune reactions. It may provide a particularly useful immunization method for highly virulent or difficult-to-isolate viruses (Fig. 5–12).

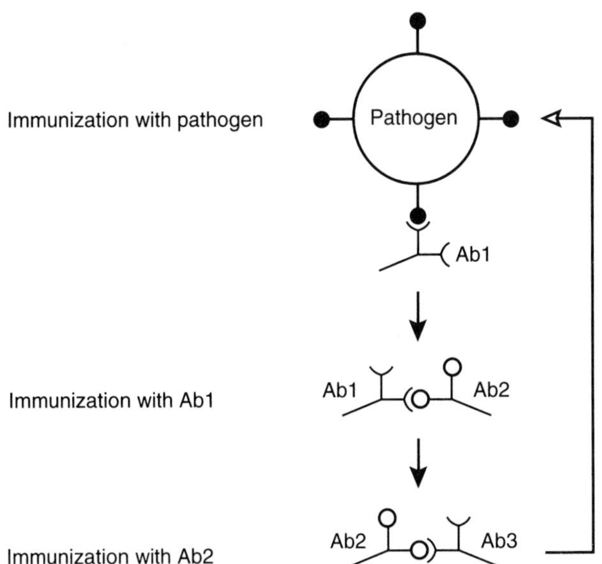

FIGURE 5–12. Practical application of idiotype-anti-idiotype principles for vaccine development. An antibody (*Ab1*) is produced against a pathogen. Ab1 is then used to produce a second antibody (*Ab2*) that specifically recognizes Ab1. Ab2 is likely to possess a structure that may mimic a pathogen protein structure that induced Ab1 and that also fits into the Ab1 binding site. If so, Ab2 can then be used for immunization to induce a third antibody (*Ab3*) similar to Ab1 and specific for the pathogen, which may protect against infection. In this way, a vaccine may be developed that does not require isolation of or exposure to the pathogen. This approach has now been successfully used in several viral infection models.

DEVELOPMENTAL ASPECTS AND PHYSIOLOGIC ALTERATIONS OF IMMUNITY

As a result of the adaptive nature of the immune system in response to a constantly changing antigenic environment, the immune system undergoes significant alterations during development and in times of stress. These alterations significantly affect susceptibility and resistance to infection.

Immunity in the Fetus and Neonate

The fetus and neonate occupy a special niche in terms of immunity and the external environment. The developing immune system must learn to tolerate host constituents while preparing to do battle with external pathogens. Given the random way in which the set of immune receptors (antibody and TCR) develops during the lifetime of a single individual, this requires a delicate balance. Likewise, given the significant role that prior antigenic exposure (''original antigenic sin'') and memory play in host defense, it is obvious that the fetal and neonatal immune system must not function in exactly the same way as the adult immune system. Rather than portraying the idea of an immunodeficiency of immaturity, however, the differences between fetal and adult immunity represent specific adaptations to different physiologic situations. The increased susceptibility of the newborn to infection is the price paid for these adaptations.

The Fetus as Allograft. The maternal immune system, which tolerates the embryo implanted in the uterus but can readily reject a skin or organ graft from an offspring, is fascinating. Current evidence suggests that the trophoblast does not express classic polymorphic HLA-A, -B, or -C transplantation antigens but, instead, displays a unique truncated, nonpolymorphic antigen called **HLA-G.** Although the lack of HLA-A, -B, and -C target antigens seems to be an obvious mechanism for avoiding rejection, the actual role of HLA-G is unclear. Studies suggest that the fetal tissue in contact with the maternal immune system is immunologically hypoantigenic. Evidence that active immune recognition may play a role in fetal survival also exists. In particular, animal strains with a high rate of fetal loss, as well as women with recurrent spontaneous abortion, may be induced to carry pregnancy to term after immunization with paternal cells. This suggests that specific T-cell recognition of alloantigens may be beneficial to fetal survival, at least in certain circumstances. Recent data do not appear to support theories of the uterus as an immunologically ''privileged'' site or of specific suppression of maternal immune responses against fetal antigens.

The Fetus as Host. Protective immune responses are present in the human fetus as early as the seventh week of gestation. Shortly after recognizable T cells can be detected, antibody responses of fetal origin to intrauterine infection can be detected by 12 weeks. Thus the fetal immune system is capable of significant immune reactivity fairly early in development (Table 5–9). Before this time, protection against infection must be provided exclusively by the mother. Replicating antigens (e.g., viruses) present before and during the time of immune repertoire development are capable of causing significant immune deviation. Such viruses may actually induce a state of **tolerance** in the developing immune system, resulting in prolonged viral replication and ongoing pathologic changes. Relatively innocuous viruses, such as rubella, may cause significant morbidity during this period.

TABLE 5–9. Development of Immunity in the Human Fetus

Week of Gestation	Event(s)
2–3	Stem-cell proliferation and differentiation
6	Primordial thymus develops; T cells detected in liver; MHC molecules detected
7	T cells in liver capable of mixed lymphocyte reaction
8	Lymphocytes appear in thymus
9	Maternal IgG detected in serum; B cells appear in liver
10	IgM synthesis detectable in spleen; thymocytes respond to mitogens (e.g., phytohemagglutinin)
11	Thymocytes can form E rosettes; B cells with surface Ig detectable in lymphoid tissue
12	Lymph nodes detectable
13	Peripheral T cells respond to phytohemagglutinin
14	Thymic cortex and medulla demarcated; peripheral T cells capable of cytotoxicity; B cells in blood reach adult normal levels

Further protection of the developing fetus is provided by maternal IgG acquired transplacentally beginning at 8–10 weeks and accelerating during the last trimester (Fig. 5–13). This placental transfer is active and specific for IgG. Low levels of antibodies against carbohydrate antigens in fetal and cord blood probably reflect the failure of the placenta to transfer IgM, rather than reflecting an antigen-specific or V region–specific mechanism. Although neonates of certain other species acquire serum antibody orally through milk, the human gut is impermeable to IgA and other antibody classes present in colostrum.

Despite the presence of adequate numbers of T and B cells, antigen-presenting cells, neutrophils, and adequate amounts of antibody and complement, the newborn is more susceptible to certain infections than at any other stage of life. The lymphocytes of newborns have a reduced ability to provide T-cell help for antibody production, in comparison with that of adults. This is accompanied by an increase in inhibitory activity. This alteration is apparently not antigen specific. Neonatal T cells also produce less IFN-γ than adult T cells. The best cellular marker of the altered T-cell activity in neonates is an increase in the percentage of CD4 T cells that also express CD45RA and, conversely, a decrease in the population of CD4 T cells that express CD29. Because CD45RA is sometimes considered a marker of virgin lymphocytes and CD29 a marker for memory cells, neonatal T-cell function may reflect the lack of antigenic experience of the fetal immune system. This is supported by evidence that in vitro activation of neonatal T cells by mitogens rapidly converts the cells to the CD29 phenotype, eliminates the inhibitory effect on antibody production, and up-regulates IFN-γ production.

Alterations in neonatal B-cell function are also specific. A subset of B cells bearing the CD5 marker, which is usually associated with T cells, is increased in neonates. This subset is notable for the production of polyreactive antibodies that often cross-react with self-antigens. Decreased responsiveness to carbohydrate antigens in

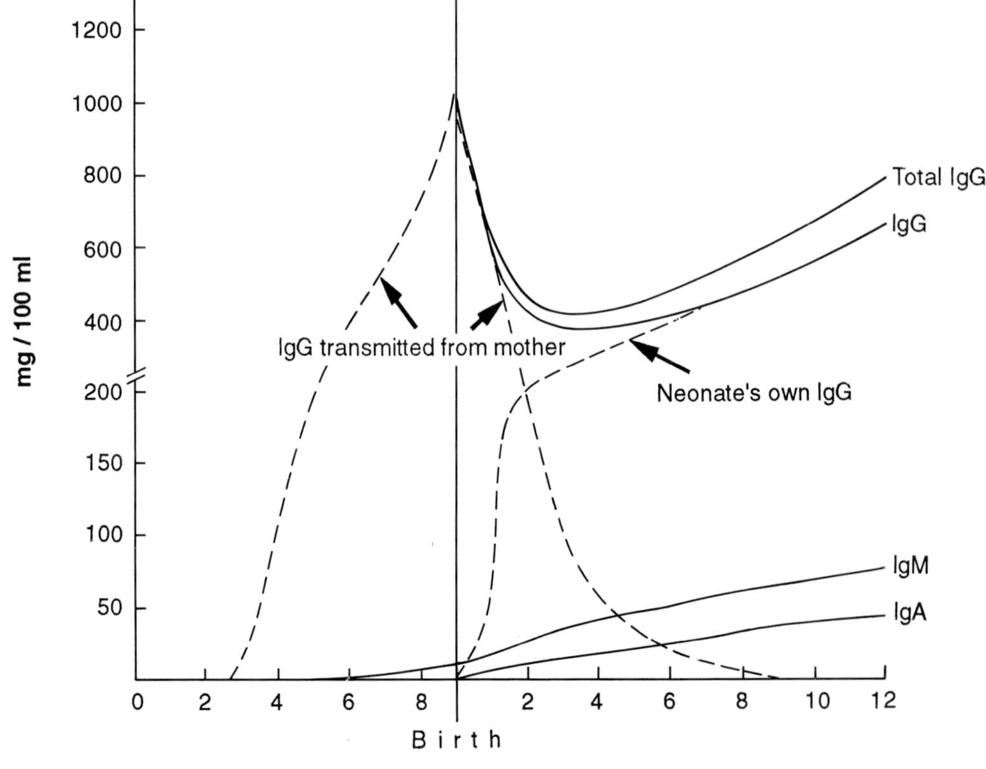

FIGURE 5–13. Serum Ig levels in fetuses and infants, reflecting the contribution of placental transfer of maternal IgG and the neonate's own antibody synthesis. (From Stiehm RE: Fetal defense mechanisms. *Am J Dis Child* 1975;129:438–43. Copyright 1975, American Medical Association.)

newborns and young infants is well known and clinically important. This response can be enhanced in vitro by the drug 8-thioguanine, an effect that appears to be mediated by enhancement of IL-6 production.

Neonatal T and B cells express a more limited set of V genes and have reduced N-segment diversity in their receptor molecules compared with adult T and B cells. Thus it is possible that newborns lack the full range of receptor diversity seen in adults. The functional significance of this interesting and specific finding remains to be explored.

The newborn also has quantitatively decreased activity of neutrophils, macrophages, and NK cells in comparison with adults. These differences are likely to be secondary to reduced IFN-γ production and reduced antibody and complement C3 production, because the deficits are reversible in vitro by IFN-γ and adult serum, respectively.

Why is the newborn saddled with these specific immune deficits? In one respect the reduced activity of T cells seems unavoidable. If memory T cells are more efficient than virgin T cells and if repeated antigenic exposure is needed to arm the immune system with enough memory cells, the neonate is simply an innocent bystander in the normal developmental program of immunity. Alternatively the decreased response to carbohydrate antigens and the failure to transport anticarbohydrate IgM across the placenta suggests a specific adaptation, perhaps related to allowing the acquisition of normal gut flora. Finally, the N-segment diversity and CD5 B-cell alterations appear to reflect a need to avoid autoreactivity during development. The human immune system matures rapidly, and most immune functions reach normal adult values by 2–3 years of age. The transition is gradual, probably reflecting the effect of progressive and continuous exposure to antigenic stimulation.

Physiologic Changes in Immune Responsiveness

Once the immune system has developed fully, immune reactivity remains intact for several decades in the absence of other factors. In later life a program of senescence emerges, with a gradual decrease in responsiveness. Occasionally, however, events may have a significant negative impact on immune reactivity, resulting in periods of increased susceptibility to infection. Although important observations have been made, much remains to be learned and understood concerning the mechanisms leading to decreased responsiveness and potential therapies to correct the immunocompromised state.

Malnutrition. Malnutrition, especially protein malnutrition, is probably the leading cause of immunosuppression on a global scale. Malnutrition directly causes immune hyporesponsiveness, which precedes clinically apparent infection. Moreover, although the number of episodes of infection is somewhat greater in malnourished than in healthy hosts, a substantial increase in the duration and severity of infectious illnesses occurs in malnourished persons. As in many other forms of stress and in aging, the primary target of most forms of malnutrition is the T lymphocyte.

Protein-calorie malnutrition is associated with decreased production of T cells, observed as decreased thymic size and decreased circulating levels of both CD4 and CD8 T cells. The functions of T cells, including specific antigen and mitogen responses, are decreased. As a result, T cell–dependent antibody responses are diminished, whereas intrinsic B-cell function appears to be preserved. Finally, there are decreased levels of complement components, particularly C3, in the serum of malnourished persons. Although much less common, specific micronutrient deficiencies are also associated with decreased function of various components of the immune system (Table 5–10). Specific micronutrient deficiencies, particularly of iron, zinc, and vitamin C, have been implicated in altered immune responses in elderly persons.

TABLE 5–10. Specific Micronutrient Deficiencies Associated with Decreased Immune Function

	Affected Cell			
Nutrient	**T Cell**	**B Cell**	**Macrophage**	**Neutrophil**
Vitamin A	+	+		
Vitamin B_6	+	+		
Vitamin C			+	+
Vitamin E	+	+		
Copper				+
Iron	+	+	+	+
Zinc	+	+		

Physical and Psychological Stress. Recent studies suggest that physical trauma and emotional stress can cause immunosuppression and increased susceptibility to infection and cancer. The mechanisms involved in these effects appear to be complicated and involve the interaction of inflammatory responses, endocrine effects, and neurotransmitters.

Physical stress in the form of severe trauma leads to persistent inflammatory responses mediated by nonspecific pathways. An important consequence of these pathways is the activation of macrophages and the suppression of T-cell function. Macrophage activation is reflected by increased production of IL-1 and TNF, decreased generation of nitrous and nitric oxides, and decreased antigen-presenting function. Suppression of T-cell function is measured as decreased skin test and mitogen reactivity. The end result is a transient state of immune unresponsiveness. These effects are probably compounded in most severe cases by a negative protein balance and other nutritional effects. A variety of specific and nonspecific immunologic and anti-inflammatory therapies, including pharmacologic and nutritional interventions, have been tried with some success to correct the immune abnormalities associated with severe trauma.

The observed immunosuppressive effects of significant psychological stress are probably mediated by the neuroendocrine system. Lymphocytes have specific receptors for a number of hormones and neurotransmitters. The administration of corticosteroids, catecholamines, and thyroid hormone has resulted in immune dysfunction in vivo and in vitro. In addition, psychological stress also targets T lymphocytes for decreased production and function. Observations include decreased size of the thymus and lymph nodes, decreased mitogen and antibody responses, and recurrences of latent infection with herpes simplex virus.

Aging. Although not strictly relevant to the pediatric population, the process of **immunosenescence** is informative regarding the developmental program of immunity and the regulation of immunologic reactivity and susceptibility to illness. Average values for measurements of T-cell immunity steadily decline after the sixth decade of life, although many persons maintain near normal reactivity. As a consequence, even after correction for the effects of age alone, decreased T-cell reactivity is associated with about a twofold increase in morbidity and mortality risk in otherwise healthy elderly persons. T cells are specifically targeted, and B cells and monocytes are relatively preserved. Decreased thymic production of mature T cells may play an important role. For example, elderly persons show decreased primary T-cell responses to newly encountered antigens while maintaining memory responses to recall antigens, reflecting the long life span of memory T cells. In addition to decreased production, there appear to be qualitative changes resulting in less efficient activation of T cells in elderly persons.

The mechanisms for the altered immune function in aging are unclear. They are probably multifactorial but may include the effects of nutrition. Proponents of the network theory of immune regulation suggest that immunosenescence in part reflects an intrinsic limitation on the development of new T- and B-cell receptors with time. According to this concept, the expression of each new receptor introduced into the network is dampened in time by interaction with those receptors already present. Support for this concept has been obtained from experimental animals. Whether perturbations of mechanisms involved in normal age-related changes in immune responses may prematurely lead to illness in children is entirely hypothetical at this time.

REVIEWS

Baggiolini M, DeWald B, Moser B: Human chemokines: An update. *Annu Rev Immunol* 1997;15:675–705.

Banchereau J, Steinman RM: Dendritic cells and the control of immunity. *Nature* 1998;392:245–52.

Butcher EC, Picker LJ: Lymphocyte homing and homeostasis. *Science* 1996;272:60–6.

Fearon DT, Locksley RM: The instructive role of innate immunity in the acquired immune response. *Science* 1996;272:50–3.

Fenton MJ, Golenbock DT: LPS-binding proteins and receptors. *J Leukocyte Biol* 1998;64:25–32.

Miller DM, Sedmak DD: Viral effects on antigen processing. *Curr Opin Immunol* 1999;11:94–9.

Morel PA, Oriss TB: Crossregulation between Th1 and Th2 cells. *Crit Rev Immunol* 1998;18:275–303.

Schelonka RL, Infante AJ: Neonatal immunology. *Semin Perinatol* 1998;22:2–14.

CHAPTER 6

Evaluation of Immune Function

Anthony J. Infante ▪ Naynesh Kamani

The incidence of primary immunodeficiency disorders is low, but recognition is important because some defects are lethal and early recognition can be lifesaving. In the evaluation of the person with "too many" common infections or an unusual infection, it is convenient to think in terms of the four principal arms of the host defense system: T cells, B cells (antibodies), phagocytic cells, and complement. A complete evaluation includes a thorough history including family history, physical examination, and laboratory screening directed at evaluating each of the four major components. Although it is generally believed that immunologists rely largely on laboratory testing, clinical acumen is as important in clinical immunology as in any other area of medicine. Numerous sophisticated probes of immune function are available, although an adequate laboratory screening can be done with a few simple tests. After the initial screening, however, persons thought to have a bona fide immunodeficiency disorder should be referred to a specialist.

CLINICAL EVALUATION OF IMMUNE FUNCTION

Recognizable Patterns of Illness. By applying principles of host defenses (Chapter 5), one can distinguish certain patterns of signs and symptoms indicative of a defect in T-cell, B-cell, phagocyte, or complement function (Table 6–1). These clues can guide the diagnostic evaluation and assist in planning therapy. A detailed family history with a pedigree can often yield clues to the diagnosis because many primary immunodeficiencies are inherited in an X-linked or autosomal recessive manner. In this respect, a family history of early death due to infection in the antibiotic era may be significant.

Infants with unusual or opportunistic infections, failure to thrive, and a variety of skin manifestations in the first few months of life characteristically have abnormalities of T-cell function. Although maternal antibody acquired transplacentally and the infant's own phagocytic cells and complement are sufficient to protect these infants from pyogenic bacteria, they are highly susceptible to viral, fungal, and protozoal illnesses. When antibody levels fall, which may occur more rapidly than in healthy infants because of failure of endogenous T-cell help as well as increased IgG catabolism, the infant also becomes susceptible to bacterial infection. Later in life, those patients who survive their childhood infections have lymphoid malignancies at an increased rate, as high as 10–30%.

Children who have serious bacterial infections later in the first year of life are likely to have B-cell defects. This timing coincides with the disappearance of maternal IgG from the infant's circulation (see Fig. 5–13). These children are often normal in height, weight, development, and activity. Malignancies in these children are rare compared with malignancies in children with T-cell disorders but may occur more often than in the general population.

Phagocytic cell defects may be seen first by the dermatologist or periodontist because skin and periodontal infections are common in these patients. As might be expected, culture-proven infection without the expected degree of inflammation is suggestive of phagocytic cell disorders.

Complement deficiency may be manifested in exactly the same way as B-cell deficiency, with serious pyogenic bacterial infections. Because complement is not transmitted across the placenta, complement deficiency may occur at any age. Curiously, many complement disorders have rheumatologic manifestations rather than resulting in recurrent infections.

Infection History. To make an appropriate referral for immunologic evaluation, the primary care physician must answer the basic question, How many infections are too many? The answer may be one infection if the infection is an unusual one, such as *Pneumocystis carinii* pneumonia, or many infections if episodes of otitis media are counted. Because immunodeficiency disorders, even in aggregate, are uncommon, only up to 1% of persons seen by primary physicians for frequent infections should be considered for further evaluation. Even among these persons, few will have an identifiable immunodeficiency, and many of those who do will have some additional feature that distinguishes them from similar cases.

A single episode of disease caused by an opportunistic organism, at any age, is suggestive of immunodeficiency. Symptomatic infection due to *P. carinii, Cryptosporidium, Toxoplasma, Aspergillus,* CMV, or atypical mycobacteria is moderately predictive of immunodeficiency, as is infection with *Candida,* VZV, or measles virus if the infection is severe. More than one serious infection with even a common bacterial pathogen should be suspected as an indication of an underlying immune defect, particularly if the infections occur in a young infant or within a short period. This possibility needs to be distinguished from recurrence due to inadequate treatment. Although patients with serious bacterial infections may also have recurrent otitis media and sinusitis, these latter two infections by themselves rarely lead to a diagnosis of immunodeficiency even when recurrences are frequent. Otherwise healthy infants and young children can have anywhere from 6 to 12 episodes of otitis media and upper respiratory tract and gastrointestinal infections annually (Table 6–2). Infants and toddlers attending daycare centers are likely to have more frequent respiratory and gastrointestinal tract infections.

The patient most commonly referred for immunologic evaluation is the young child with multiple episodes of otitis media, sinusitis, pharyngitis, and upper respiratory tract infections but without convincing evidence of pneumonia. Although such children may have serious immunodeficiency and may have escaped more serious illness by virtue of prompt recognition and treatment or by sheer chance, it is more likely that they have a problem other

TABLE 6–1. Clinical Manifestations of Immunodeficiency and Organisms Causing Associated Infections

Deficiency	Manifestations	Organisms Causing Infections
T cells	Persistent oral thrush	*Candida albicans*
	Chronic diarrhea	*Pneumocystis carinii*
	Skin rash	Atypical mycobacteria
	Failure to thrive	Cytomegalovirus
	Interstitial pneumonitis	
B cells	Recurrent otitis media	*Haemophilus influenzae* type b
	Sepsis	*Streptococcus pneumoniae*
	Meningitis	*Staphylococcus aureus*
	Suppurative arthritis	Echoviruses (chronic meningitis)
	Pneumonia	
	Sinusitis	
Phagocytic cells	Abscesses of soft tissue, skin, lungs, liver, and periodontium	*S. aureus*
	Mouth ulcers	*Serratia marcescens*
	Delayed separation of umbilical cord	*Klebsiella*
		Pseudomonas
		Candida
		Aspergillus
Complement	Recurrent otitis media	*S. aureus*
	Sepsis	*H. influenzae* type b
	Meningitis	*S. pneumoniae*
	Suppurative arthritis	*Neisseria meningitidis*
	Pneumonia	
	Sinusitis	
	Autoimmune disorders	

than immunodeficiency. The most common ''other'' problem, by far, is unrecognized hypersensitive upper airway disease manifested by hypersensitive rhinitis, sinusitis, otitis media resulting from mucosal edema and obstruction, and asthma. A careful history and selected laboratory studies usually reveal this disease. Many of the children with this disease have no clinical or laboratory evidence of either immunodeficiency or hypersensitivity.

Physical Examination. Certain primary immunodeficiency disorders are often first suspected on the basis of physical findings (Table 6–3). The primary care physician should not hesitate to involve subspecialists with expertise in the evaluation of these manifestations.

The physical examination of the person being evaluated for immunologic causes of recurrent infection focuses on three questions. First, does the person have other ongoing infections in addition to those that prompted the evaluation? Second, are there physical anomalies suggesting an anatomic basis for recurrent infection or suggesting a particular diagnosis? Third, are there physical findings of a normal or abnormal immune response? The initial physical examination of persons with recurrent infections should be comprehensive because infections and the associated immune responses can occur anywhere in the body. The majority of immunodeficiency

TABLE 6–2. Expected Episodes of Infection per Year in Healthy Children

Age	Acute Upper Respiratory Tract Infections	Acute Otitis Media (range)	Gastroenteritis
Birth to 1 yr	6–7	1 (0–6)	1–2
1–2 yr	8	1 (0–6)	2
In child care	11–13	1 (0–6)	3
3–5 yr	6–8	0–1 (0–6)	1–2
In child care	9	0–1 (0–6)	2
6–10 yr	5–6	<1	1–2
11–16 yr	4–5	<1	<1

TABLE 6–3. Characteristic Manifestations Associated with Primary Immunodeficiency Disorders

Signs and Symptoms	Syndrome
Eczema, bruising (thrombocytopenia with small platelets)	Wiskott-Aldrich syndrome
Hypocalcemia, cardiac anomalies	DiGeorge syndrome
Ataxia, ocular or cutaneous telangiectasias	Ataxia-telangiectasia
Skin abscesses, pneumatoceles	Hyper-IgE syndrome
Mild bleeding diathesis, partial oculocutaneous albinism, progressive peripheral neuropathy	Chédiak-Higashi syndrome
Recurrent, severe, or disseminated chickenpox or zoster	Common variable immunodeficiency
Delayed separation of umbilical cord (>21 days)	Phagocytic cell dysfunction

disorders are systemic diseases and therefore may be manifested at any anatomic location.

Acute or chronic otitis media, rhinitis, and sinusitis are frequent infections in persons with immunodeficiency but are also common in the general population. Thin, watery secretions may indicate hypersensitivity disease, whereas purulent drainage is more consistent with bacterial infection and suggests the possibility of immunodeficiency, particularly antibody deficiency. Similarly, the presence of nonproductive cough and wheezing suggests asthma, whereas sputum production, rales, and decreased breath sounds indicate possible bacterial pneumonia. Dyspnea, rales, and evidence of hypoxemia suggest interstitial lung disease and the possibility of T-lymphocyte defects. Radiologic evaluation is necessary to confirm the presence of paranasal sinus or lower respiratory tract disease.

Careful attention should be given to the lymph nodes, especially in the neck, axillae, and groin. Absent lymph nodes in the presence of local infection suggests cellular immune defects. Enlarged lymph nodes draining a site of infection but lacking characteristic warmth, erythema, and tenderness may indicate a functional neutrophil defect because mediators released from these cells are responsible for the signs of inflammation. Generalized lymphadenopathy may suggest the presence of HIV infection or an underlying lymphoproliferative disorder. Lymphoproliferative disorders may accompany primary immunodeficiency disorders at presentation or as late sequelae, or they may be the underlying cause of increased susceptibility to infection, such as Hodgkin's disease or chronic lymphocytic leukemia.

LABORATORY EVALUATION OF IMMUNE FUNCTION

Although relatively sophisticated immunologic testing is readily available through large national reference laboratories, routine screening of immune functions of most children with recurrent infections can usually be accomplished with a limited number of standard tests available locally. Additional testing can be reserved for children who have abnormal screening results. Children with characteristic opportunistic infections or syndromes should be studied with the more specific tests immediately. Clinical immunology consultation is usually advisable for the interpretation and correlation of results of the more sophisticated studies.

Interpretation of test results must be age specific and method specific, with the use of age-equivalent comparative normal values determined in equivalent assays. Despite the best efforts of even the most careful laboratories, many immunologic assays are subject to substantial and unavoidable biologic variation. Results that are unusual or that do not correlate with the clinical picture should be confirmed by repeated testing, preferably by using a reference laboratory. Similarly, it is usually advisable to defer immunologic studies until after recovery from serious acute infections. In particular, cellular immune function is dynamic and may appear abnormal during acute infection and convalescence, in comparison with values obtained in healthy control subjects.

Screening Studies

As with the history and physical examination, laboratory evaluation should be directed at probing the four major components of the immune system: T-cells, B cells, phagocytic cells, and complement. Each component should be tested quantitatively and qualitatively, which may require two separate tests for each component (Table 6–4). Similar clinical manifestations may be due to either absence or dysfunction of a particular component, as in many biochemically or cellularly determined diseases.

Most components of the immune system travel from their points of origin to sites of infection via the peripheral blood. The CBC, including differential count, platelet count, and the morphologic features of the erythrocytes, provides much information about the overall health of the ultimate leukocyte "factory," the bone marrow. Any cytopenia or persistent morphologic abnormality deserves further evaluation. Neutropenia is the most common phagocytic cell disorder. Serial neutrophil counts may be needed to confirm a diagnosis of cyclic neutropenia. Marked leukocytosis, often with a WBC count of more than 50,000/mm^3, is a common feature of leukocyte adhesion deficiency. Qualitative phagocytic cell defects that are reflected in abnormal morphologic features can be identified on the blood smear. Chédiak-Higashi syndrome is confirmed by the finding of "giant" granules in WBCs. An appropriate left shift during bacterial infection or lymphocytosis after viral infection is evidence of normal immune function.

TABLE 6–4. Screening Studies for Evaluation of Immune Function

Initial Screening Tests
CBC including differential WBC count, platelet count, peripheral smear
Delayed hypersensitivity skin test responses
Serum IgG, IgA, IgM, and IgE levels
Antibody titers to diphtheria, tetanus, *Streptococcus pneumoniae*
Serum complement activity (total hemolytic complement [CH_{50}])
Additional Screening Tests for Selected Patients
Lymphocyte subset analysis
Nitroblue tetrazolium test or flow cytometry
HIV antibody

T Cells. Lymphopenia is a cardinal sign of T-cell deficiency, since 60–80% of peripheral blood lymphocytes are T cells. The absolute lymphocyte count is insensitive to the absence of B cells. However, lymphopenia is not present in all cases of T-cell immunodeficiency, although these cases are revealed by functional assays. T-cell function can be measured in vivo by testing responses to previously encountered antigens. In children more than 1–2 years of age a reliable and inexpensive method is the assessment of delayed (at 48 hours) hypersensitivity skin test responses to intradermal antigens such as tetanus toxoid (1.5 Lf/mL), *Candida albicans* (1:100), or *Trichophyton* (1:30). The erythema and, most important, induration measured at the site of antigen deposition reflects antigen-specific T-lymphocyte and monocyte infiltration. A positive response, defined as a minimum of 5 mm induration, virtually ensures adequate T-cell and monocyte function. Unfortunately a negative response is less meaningful, since rates of sensitization to individual antigens in healthy subjects rarely exceed 60–70%. Negative responses also occur during immunosuppressive therapy, including therapy with corticosteroids. In children less than 1 year of age in whom T-cell deficiency is suspected, in vitro studies of T-cell function are required because many healthy children will not be adequately sensitized to the skin test antigens. Although chest x-ray evidence of a thymic shadow can be helpful, it should never preclude direct evaluation of T-cell number and function. Any person with an opportunistic infection or evidence of T-cell dysfunction should be tested for HIV infection.

B Cells. Measuring the serum levels of IgM, IgG, and IgA adequately screens for antibody deficiency. One, two, or all three major antibody classes may be deficient and may contribute to susceptibility to infection. As with all immunologic test results, it is imperative to compare results with age-adjusted normal values (Table 6–5). Results showing low levels should be repeated and reinforced by specific functional assays. The value of measuring IgG subclasses continues to be debated and is not as reliable as determination of total IgG. The routine measurement of serum IgA1 and IgA2 subclasses or of secretory IgA is not indicated. Serum IgE should be done to identify persons with the hyper-IgE syndrome or persons whose symptoms may be due to hypersensitivity. The classic serum protein electrophoresis does not contribute additional information to the evaluation for immunodeficiency.

Quantitative measurements of specific antibody titers to defined antigens are valuable studies in persons with borderline values for Ig class or subclass levels. Available tests measure antibodies to protein toxoids (diphtheria, tetanus) and polysaccharides (*Streptococcus pneumoniae*) to which the person has been exposed naturally or by immunization. A particularly definitive test is to measure antibody levels just before and 3–4 weeks after immunization with diphtheria-tetanus booster or the pneumococcal vaccine. A significant rise, defined as a fourfold or greater increase, in antibody levels indicates an adequate, integrated immune response. Responses to protein antigens correlate with the serum level of IgG1, whereas polysaccharide responses correlate with the serum level of IgG2. An important caveat is that most children less than 2 years of age are developmentally hyporesponsive to polysaccharide antigens.

Phagocytic Cells. Unfortunately, no readily available functional screening test for phagocytic cell defects currently exists. Specialized studies of adherence, chemotaxis, oxygen consumption, and bactericidal activity are labor intensive and require specially trained personnel. These tests are most commonly performed in connection with research studies. Assays of neutrophil oxidative function by tube or slide test using **nitroblue tetrazolium (NBT)** dye or by **flow cytometry** using dihydrorhodamine are sometimes available in larger hospital-based laboratories and will identify patients with and carriers of chronic granulomatous disease. Identification of persons with phagocyte dysfunction requires persistence and a high index of suspicion.

Complement. Serum complement analysis can be accomplished by measuring **total hemolytic complement (THC),** also called **CH_{50},** for the end point of the analysis. A defect in any of the components involved in the classic pathway of complement lysis, C1 through C9, will result in an abnormal value. A specific component deficiency can then be identified by using individual specialized assays. However, the most common cause of marginally low THC results is improper sample handling. Immediate analysis of a freshly drawn, chilled serum sample should be used to confirm an abnormal value. A low THC value will identify most complement deficiencies leading to increased susceptibility to infection.

Additional Studies

Persons with abnormal screening results or those with characteristic patterns of illness require further diagnostic study to define the exact nature of the defect. In most cases this entails the identification of a missing lymphocyte subpopulation or a functional defect at the cellular level. The cellular and molecular defects underlying several primary immunodeficiency disorders have been determined in recent years (Chapter 98).

T Cells. Immunophenotyping to quantify T cells, as well as B cells and NK cells, should be determined for persons in whom an obvious cause of recurrent or unusual infections cannot be readily identified. Relative and absolute numbers of lymphocyte subsets are determined by flow cytometry with the use of fluorescence-tagged monoclonal antibodies against CD (cluster of differentiation) cell surface molecules (Table 6–6). The sum of the percentages of **CD4 (T helper)** and **CD8 (T cytotoxic)** cells should generally equal the percentage of **CD3 (total T)** cells. There is a decline in each subset that parallels the overall decline in the total lymphocyte count during childhood, although the relative proportions of the subsets are maintained (Table 6–7). Probably the single most important value from this assessment of immune function is the absolute number of CD4 cells. As studies in AIDS have shown, there is an almost linear relationship between the number of CD4 cells and susceptibility to infection.

Further evaluation of T-cell disorders first involves confirmation of defective T-cell function by in vitro analysis. The most widely

TABLE 6–5. Normal Serum Immunoglobulin Levels by Age*†

				Total Ig	
Age	IgG	IgM	IgA	mg/dL	Percent of Adult Level
Newborn	1031 ± 200	11 ± 5	2 ± 3	1044 ± 201	67 ± 13
1–3 mo	430 ± 119	30 ± 11	21 ± 13	481 ± 127	31 ± 9
4–6 mo	427 ± 186	43 ± 17	28 ± 18	498 ± 204	32 ± 13
7–12 mo	661 ± 219	54 ± 23	37 ± 18	752 ± 242	48 ± 15
13–24 mo	762 ± 209	58 ± 23	50 ± 24	870 ± 258	56 ± 16
25–37 mo	892 ± 183	61 ± 19	71 ± 37	1024 ± 205	65 ± 14
3–5 yr	929 ± 228	56 ± 18	93 ± 27	1078 ± 245	69 ± 17
6–8 yr	923 ± 256	65 ± 25	124 ± 45	1112 ± 293	71 ± 20
9–11 yr	1124 ± 235	79 ± 23	131 ± 60	1334 ± 254	85 ± 17
12–16 yr	946 ± 124	59 ± 20	148 ± 63	1153 ± 169	74 ± 12
Adults	1158 ± 305	99 ± 27	200 ± 61	1457 ± 353	100 ± 24

*The values are in mg/dL except where noted and were derived from measurements made in 296 normal children and 30 adults. Levels were determined by the radial diffusion technique using specific rabbit antisera to human immunoglobulins.

†Mean ± SD.

Adapted from data in Stiehm ER, Fudenberg HH: Serum levels of immune globulins in health and disease: A survey. *Pediatrics* 1966;37:715–27.

TABLE 6–6. Clinically Useful Cell Surface Markers* for Lymphocyte Subset Analysis in Suspected Immunodeficiency

Total Lymphocytes	
CD45	Leukocyte common antigen (LCA)
T Cells	
CD3	T-cell receptor (TCR)–associated, "pan T cell" marker (CD4 plus CD8 cells should equal CD3 cells)
CD2, CD5	Pan T-cell markers not associated with TCR complex
CD4	T cells with predominant helper function
CD8	Cytotoxic and suppressor T cells
B Cells	
sIg	Surface immunoglobulin; defines mature B cells
CD19, CD20	B-cell markers not associated with sIg
HLA-DR	Also present on monocytes but not on T cells, unless activated
NK Cells	
CD16, CD56	NK cell markers (CD16 plus CD56 equals total NK cells)
Monocytes	
CD18	Lymphocyte function–associated antigen type 1 (absence defines a recognized phagocytic cell disorder [leukocyte adhesion deficiency])

*Using the cluster of differentiation (CD) system to codify cell surface markers.

available and reliable methods are measurements of cellular proliferation in response to mitogens and allogeneic cells. Peripheral blood lymphocytes proliferate in response to cell surface molecule cross-linking induced with plant lectins. Cellular proliferation is quantitated by uptake of radiolabeled precursors into newly synthesized DNA. Commonly used mitogens are **phytohemagglutinin, concanavalin A,** and **pokeweed mitogen.** Stimulation with unrelated allogeneic lymphocytes in a **mixed lymphocyte reaction (MLR)** also causes polyclonal lymphocyte activation and proliferation. Certain variant syndromes may show abnormalities of responsiveness to only one or two mitogens, or to mitogens but not MLR, or vice versa. It is important to analyze peripheral blood lymphocytes from at least one normal individual to serve as a positive control at the same time as the patient is being studied.

Studies of stimulated lymphocytes for in vitro lymphokine production may be helpful in persons with unexplained T-cell immunodeficiency. Analysis of cell surface molecules released into the circulation (e.g., CD8, IL-2 receptor) may be helpful in autoimmune diseases but does not contribute much to the evaluation of persons with recurrent infection.

B Cells. The analysis of screening studies for B-cell function, antibody titers, and antibody response to immunization is usually sufficient to determine the presence of significant deficiency. Classification of the three major antibody deficiency syndromes, X-linked agammaglobulinemia (XLA), X-linked hyper-IgM syndrome (XHIM), and common variable hypogammaglobulinemia (CVH), is assisted by cell surface marker analysis. Mature B cells bearing surface Ig are usually present in XHIM and CVH but absent in XLA. Direct stimulation of B cells in culture with pokeweed mitogen or EBV and subsequent measurement of antibody secretion may be helpful in understanding a person's defect but will not change the diagnosis or management.

TABLE 6–7. Normal Values for Lymphocyte Subpopulations by Age

Lymphocyte Subpopulations	Age Groups									
	Newborns	1 wk to 2 mo	2–5 mo	5–9 mo	9–15 mo	15–24 mo	2–5 yr	5–10 yr	10–16 yr	Adults
Lymphocytes (absolute count)*	4.8 (0.7–7.3)	6.7 (3.5–13.1)	5.9 (3.7–9.6)	6.0 (3.8–9.9)	5.5 (2.6–10.4)	5.6 (2.7–11.9)	3.3 (1.7–6.9)	2.8 (1.1–5.9)	2.2 (1.0–5.3)	1.8 (1.0–2.8)
CD19 B lymphocytes:										
Percent	12% (5–22%)	15% (4–26%)	24% (14–39%)	21% (13–35%)	25% (15–39%)	28% (17–41%)	24% (14–44%)	18% (10–31%)	16% (8–24%)	12% (6–19%)
Count*	0.6 (0.04–1.1)	1.0 (0.6–1.9)	1.3 (0.6–3.0)	1.3 (0.7–2.5)	1.4 (0.6–2.7)	1.3 (0.6–3.1)	0.8 (0.2–2.1)	0.5 (0.2–1.6)	0.3 (0.2–0.6)	0.2 (0.1–0.5)
CD3 T lymphocytes:										
Percent	62% (28–76%)	72% (60–85%)	63% (48–75%)	66% (50–77%)	65% (54–76%)	64% (39–73%)	64% (43–76%)	69% (55–78%)	67% (52–78%)	72% (55–83%)
Count*	2.8 (0.6–5.0)	4.6 (2.3–7.0)	3.6 (2.3–6.5)	3.8 (2.4–6.9)	3.4 (1.6–6.7)	3.5 (1.4–8.0)	2.3 (0.9–4.5)	1.9 (0.7–4.2)	1.5 (0.8–3.5)	1.2 (0.7–2.1)
CD4 T lymphocytes:										
Percent	41% (17–52%)	55% (41–68%)	45% (33–58%)	45% (33–58%)	44% (31–54%)	41% (25–50%)	37% (23–48%)	35% (27–53%)	39% (25–48%)	44% (28–57%)
Count*	1.9 (0.4–3.5)	3.5 (1.7–5.3)	2.5 (1.5–5.0)	2.8 (1.4–5.1)	2.3 (1.0–4.6)	2.2 (0.9–5.5)	1.3 (0.5–2.4)	1.0 (0.3–2.0)	0.8 (0.4–2.1)	0.7 (0.3–1.4)
CD8 T lymphocytes:										
Percent	24% (10–41%)	16% (9–23%)	17% (11–25%)	18% (13–26%)	18% (12–28%)	20% (11–32%)	24% (14–33%)	28% (19–34%)	23% (9–35%)	24% (10–39%)
Count*	1.1 (0.2–1.9)	1.0 (0.4–1.7)	1.0 (0.5–1.6)	1.1 (0.6–2.2)	1.1 (0.4–2.1)	1.2 (0.4–2.3)	0.8 (0.3–1.6)	0.8 (0.3–1.8)	0.4 (0.2–1.2)	0.4 (0.2–0.9)
CD4:CD8 ratio	1.8 (1.0–2.6)	3.8 (1.3–6.3)	2.7 (1.7–3.9)	2.5 (1.6–3.8)	2.4 (1.3–3.9)	1.9 (0.9–3.7)	1.6 (0.9–2.9)	1.2 (0.9–2.6)	1.7 (0.9–3.4)	1.9 (1.0–3.6)

*Absolute counts are in cells × 10^3/mm^3. Percentages are percent of total lymphocytes. Ranges (5th–95th percentile) are shown in parentheses.

Adapted from Comans-Bitter WM, de Groot R, van den Beemd R, et al: Immunophenotyping of blood lymphocytes in childhood. Reference values for lymphocyte subpopulations. *J Pediatr* 1997;130:388–93.

Phagocytic Cells. Specialized phagocytic cell studies, where available, will pinpoint qualitative defects. A useful panel includes tests that are sensitive to defects in adherence, chemotaxis, and production of reactive oxygen compounds used in killing microorganisms. Such studies are usually available only in research laboratories. Direct analysis of leukocyte expression of CD18 should be performed in the appropriate clinical setting to assess the possibility of leukocyte adhesion deficiency type 1. Similarly, the NBT dye test or flow cytometry using dihydrorhodamine should be used to assess for chronic granulomatous disease.

Complement. Specific complement defects are identified by immunochemical detection and functional assays of individual components. Functional analyses use the THC test and a standard panel of patient sera known to be deficient in a single component. The patient's serum sample is mixed with each known deficient serum and will fail to restore the activity of serum from patients with the same deficiency.

Ancillary Studies

Careful clinical and microbiologic documentation of infection and evaluation of sites of chronic or recurrent infection may be of value. Because a history of recurrent infection dictates the need for further evaluation, it is important to document that serious infections have, in fact, occurred. It is particularly helpful to distinguish viral from bacterial causes of recurrent, acute upper and lower respiratory tract infections. Recurrent bacterial infections are much more likely to indicate serious immune defects, usually B-cell disorders, whereas persistent interstitial lung disease due to viruses or *P. carinii* may indicate the presence of cell-mediated immune defects. In addition to cultures, which may need to be obtained by invasive methods, radiologic examination of the chest and sinuses aids in diagnosis and in the evaluation of treatment. Sinusitis, chronic bronchitis, and recurrent pneumonia are common consequences of antibody deficiency syndromes; chronic obstructive pulmonary disease is now a major cause of premature death in this group. Yearly pulmonary function studies are recommended for older children and adults with these immune disorders.

HLA typing should be performed on any patient with T-cell deficiency. Bone marrow transplantation (BMT) is indicated for all patients with severe T-cell deficiency disease. The availability of an HLA-matched sibling donor may tip the balance in favor of BMT in children with less severe deficiency because other available therapies are unable to restore T-cell function adequately. In addition to enabling the identification of potential donors for a BMT, HLA typing will help confirm the presence of HLA class I and class II antigens on patient lymphocytes. The absence of these important markers is a rare cause of one type of severe combined immunodeficiency, the ''bare lymphocyte'' syndrome.

REVIEWS

Noroski LM, Shearer WT: Screening for primary immunodeficiencies in the clinical immunology laboratory. *Clin Immunol Immunopathol* 1998;86:237–45.

Ochs HD, Smith CIE, Puck JM (editors): *Primary Immunodeficiency Diseases: A Molecular and Genetic Approach.* New York, Oxford University Press, 1999.

Stiehm ER (editor): *Immunologic Disorders in Infants and Children,* 4th ed. Philadelphia, WB Saunders, 1996.

KEY ARTICLES

Comans-Bitter WM, de Groot R, van den Beemd R, et al: Immunophenotyping of blood lymphocytes in childhood. References for lymphocyte subpopulations. *J Pediatr* 1997;130:388–93.

Wheeler GS, Streiner D: Evaluation of humoral responsiveness in children. *Pediatr Infect Dis J* 1992;11:304–10.

Yang K, Hill HR: Assessment of neutrophil function disorders: Practical and preventive interventions. *Pediatr Infect Dis J* 1994;13:906–19.

CHAPTER 7

Diagnostic Microbiology

Joseph M. Campos

For the clinician, the diagnostic microbiology laboratory is the essential link in defining the causes of bacterial, mycobacterial, and fungal infections. The types of specimens submitted for identification are generally the same for these three groups, although bacteria are the most commonly encountered organisms. Specimens for parasites (Chapter 8) and viruses (Chapter 9) require different collection and handling procedures.

Microbiologic diagnosis requires proficiency at examining microscopic smears and experience with specialized culture techniques. Although some laboratories continue to perform mycobacterial testing, many laboratories, especially those located in smaller or exclusively pediatric hospitals, refer testing to laboratories with more experience. Laboratories in the United States must observe the Occupational Safety and Health Administration (OSHA) requirements for early identification of individuals with suspected or confirmed tuberculosis and for protection of health care workers who may be exposed to aerosolized *Mycobacterium tuberculosis* in the course of performing workplace responsibilities.

CLASSIFICATION OF BACTERIA AND FUNGI

Microbiologists classify bacteria and fungi into groups to facilitate laboratory identification. Familiarity with this classification scheme can be useful to clinicians when they are communicating with the microbiology laboratory.

Classification of Bacteria

Proper classification requires knowledge of Gram-stain morphologic features, oxygen requirements, and catalase and oxidase test reactions (Table 7–1). Each of these characteristics is either instantly apparent or quickly established on detection of a culture positive for an organism.

Gram-Stain Morphologic Features. The **Gram stain** is a differential stain that divides the bacterial kingdom into two groups on the basis of cell wall structure. **Gram-positive bacteria** possess a thick, predominantly hydrophilic cell wall that resists the decolorizing effects of hydrophobic solvents like ethanol and acetone. **Gram-negative bacteria** have a much thinner cell wall surrounded by a hydrophobic **outer membrane (lipopolysaccharide layer)** that is readily dissolved by ethanol and acetone. Consequently the cell wall of gram-negative bacteria is more easily decolorized.

The **Gram-stain morphologic features** of bacteria consist of both the **Gram reaction** (gram positive or gram negative) and the shape (**coccus** or **bacillus**) of the organism. Additional description of the cellular arrangement (e.g., pairs, chains, clusters) may be helpful or misleading. Smears prepared from body fluids or broth cultures are more likely to accurately reflect the correct cellular arrangement than are smears prepared from colonies on a culture plate.

Atmospheric Oxygen Requirements. Bacteria can be divided into five categories according to their oxygen requirements: obligate aerobes, microaerophilic aerobes, facultative anaerobes, aerotolerant anaerobes, and obligate anaerobes (Table 7–2). **Obligate aerobes** (e.g., *Neisseria, Acinetobacter,* most *Pseudomonas* species) secure energy in the form of adenosine triphosphate solely from oxygen-dependent metabolic pathways (**aerobic respiration**). **Microaerophilic aerobes** (e.g., *Campylobacter, Helicobacter*) also require oxygen for energy generation but at concentrations below that present in the earth's atmosphere. Atmospheric levels of oxygen are poisonous for this group of bacteria. **Facultative anaerobes** (e.g., members of the Enterobacteriaceae family, *Staphylococcus*) obtain energy from either **oxygen-dependent** or **oxygen-independent (fermentative)** pathways. Because considerably higher quantities of energy per mole of substrate are produced by aerobic respiration than by fermentation, facultative anaerobes preferentially use oxygen-dependent metabolism when given the opportunity. **Aerotolerant anaerobes** (e.g., *Streptococcus, Enterococcus,* a few species of *Clostridium*) rely on fermentative pathways exclusively and are able to tolerate the toxic effects of atmospheric oxygen. **Obligate anaerobes** (e.g., *Bacteroides, Fusobacterium,* most species of *Clostridium*) also derive all of their energy from fermentation, but atmospheric levels of oxygen are either bacteriostatic or bactericidal.

Catalase and Oxidase Reactions. The enzyme **catalase** is one of a limited spectrum of enzymes responsible for eliminating intracellular peroxides, which are toxic by-products of oxidative metabolism. Catalase catalyzes the conversion of H_2O_2 to O_2 and H_2O. The **slide catalase test** requires less than 30 seconds to perform and is used to further subdivide gram-positive and gram-negative bacteria. The most frequent use for the test is to differentiate *Staphylococcus,* which is catalase positive, from *Streptococcus* and *Enterococcus,* which are catalase negative.

Cytochrome-*c* oxidase (aa_3) is another enzyme synthesized by certain bacteria that carry out oxidative metabolism. This enzyme, usually referred to as **oxidase,** is one of several capable of catalyzing the reduction of molecular oxygen to water, which is the final step of oxidative metabolism. The presence or absence of this enzyme is a key biochemical marker used in the initial identification of aerobic bacteria. Positive oxidase test results, which also require less than 30 seconds to obtain, are most often used for differentiation of *Neisseria, Moraxella, Pseudomonas,* and members of the Vibrionaceae family from oxidase-negative, gram-negative bacteria.

Classification of Actinomycetes

The actinomycetes consist of several genera of non-spore-forming gram-positive bacilli, many of which are capable of forming branching filaments (Table 7–3). Most genera are obligate aerobes

TABLE 7–1. Classification of Medically Important Human Bacteria

Obligate Aerobe
Gram-Negative Rods
Oxidase-positive species
- *Alcaligenes*
- *Bordetella*
- *Brucella* (except *B. ovis* and *B. neotomae*)
- CDC groups EF-4b, EO-2, IVc-2, M5, and M6
- *Flavobacterium*
- *Legionella* (some species)
- *Moraxella* (except *M. catarrhalis*)
- *Oligella*
- *Pseudomonas*

Oxidase-negative species
- *Acinetobacter*
- *Brucella ovis* and *Brucella neotomae*
- *Chryseomonas*
- *Flavimonas*
- *Francisella*
- *Legionella* (some species)
- *Xanthomonas*

Gram-Negative Cocci
Oxidase-positive species
- *M. catarrhalis*
- *Neisseria*

Gram-Positive Rods
Catalase-positive species
- *Actinomadura*
- *Bacillus* (some species)
- *Mycobacterium* (almost all strains)
- *Nocardia*
- *Nocardiopsis*
- *Streptomyces*

Catalase-negative species
- *Mycobacterium* (some isoniazid-resistant strains)

Gram-Positive Cocci
Catalase-positive species
- *Micrococcus*

Microaerophilic Aerobes
Gram-Negative Rods
Oxidase- and catalase-positive species
- *Campylobacter* (except *C. concisus, C. curvus, C. rectus,* and *C. sputorum*)

Facultative Anaerobes
Gram-Negative Rods
Oxidase-positive species
- *Actinobacillus* (some strains)
- *Aeromonas*
- *Cardiobacterium*
- CDC groups EF-4 and HB-5 (some strains)
- *Chromobacterium* (some strains)
- *Kingella*
- *Pasteurella*
- *Plesiomonas*
- *Vibrio*

Oxidase-negative species
- *Actinobacillus* (some strains)
- *Capnocytophaga*
- CDC group HB-5 (some strains)
- *Cedecea*
- *Citrobacter*
- *Edwardsiella*
- *Eikenella*
- *Enterobacter*
- *Escherichia*
- *Ewingella*
- *Haemophilus*
- *Hafnia*
- *Klebsiella*
- *Kluyvera*
- *Leclercia*
- *Leminorella*
- *Moellerella*
- *Morganella*
- *Pantoea*
- *Proteus*
- *Providencia*
- *Rahnella*
- *Salmonella*
- *Serratia*
- *Shigella*
- *Tatumella*
- *Trabulsiella*
- *Yersinia*
- *Yokenella*

Gram-Positive Rods
Catalase-positive species
- *Bacillus* (some species)
- *Corynebacterium*
- *Listeria*

Catalase-negative species
- *Arcanobacterium*
- *Erysipelothrix*

Gram-Positive Cocci
Catalase-positive species
- *Staphylococcus*
- *Stomatococcus*

Aerotolerant Anaerobes
Gram-Positive Rods
Catalase-positive species
- *Actinomyces viscosus*

Catalase-negative species
- *Actinomyces* (except *A. meyeri* and *A. viscosus*)
- *Clostridium histolyticum*
- *Clostridium tertium*
- *Lactobacillus* (most strains)

Gram-Positive Cocci
Catalase-negative species
- *Aerococcus*
- *Enterococcus*
- *Gemella*
- *Lactococcus*
- *Leuconostoc*
- *Pediococcus*
- *Streptococcus*

Obligate Anaerobe
Gram-Negative Rods
Catalase-positive species
- *Bacteroides* (some strains)
- *Bilophila*

Catalase-negative species
- *Bacteroides* (some strains)
- *Campylobacter concisus, C. curvus, C. rectus,* and *C. sputorum*
- *Fusobacterium*
- *Porphyromonas*
- *Prevotella*
- *Wolinella*

Gram-Negative Cocci
Catalase-positive species
- *Veillonella* (some strains)

Catalase-negative species
- *Acidaminococcus*
- *Megasphaera*
- *Veillonella* (some strains)

Gram-Positive Rods
Catalase-positive species
- *Propionibacterium*

Catalase-negative species
- *Actinomyces meyeri*
- *Bifidobacterium*
- *Clostridium*
- *Eubacterium*
- *Lactobacillus* (some strains)

Gram-Positive Cocci
Catalase-negative species
- *Peptococcus niger*
- *Peptostreptococcus* (most strains)

Catalase-positive species
- *Peptostreptococcus* (few strains)

TABLE 7–2. Oxygen Requirements of Bacteria

Organism Category	Mode of Energy Generation
Obligate aerobe	O_2-dependent aerobic respiration
Microaerophilic aerobe	O_2-dependent aerobic respiration
Facultative anaerobe	O_2-dependent aerobic respiration or O_2-independent anaerobic fermentation
Oxygen-tolerant anaerobe	O_2-independent anaerobic fermentation
Obligate anaerobe	O_2-independent anaerobic fermentation

TABLE 7–3. Classification of Medically Important Human Actinomycetes

Requires Oxygen for Growth
Partially Acid-Fast
- *Nocardia*
- *Rhodococcus* (some strains)

Not Acid-Fast
- *Actinomadura*
- *Nocardiopsis*
- *Rhodococcus* (some strains)
- *Streptomyces*

Grows Preferentially without Oxygen
Not Acid-Fast
- *Actinomyces*

(e.g., *Nocardia, Streptomyces, Actinomadura, Rhodococcus*). However, the genus *Actinomyces* contains obligately anaerobic and oxygen-tolerant anaerobic species only.

Classification of Mycobacteria

The clinically important mycobacteria have been classified by several schemes. One system divides the genus into two groups, the **tuberculous** or **typical mycobacteria** (e.g., *M. tuberculosis, M. bovis,* and *M. africanum*) and the **nontuberculous** or **atypical mycobacteria** (e.g., *M. kansasii, M. aviumintracellulare,* and *M. fortuitum*). The descriptive terms *typical* and *atypical* have since fallen into disfavor and are no longer recommended. The term ***Mycobacterium* other than *tuberculosis* (MOTT)** is currently preferred.

A second scheme, the **Runyon group classification** (Table 7–4), divides the species into several groups. The *M. tuberculosis* complex from the first scheme remains, but the MOTT group is further categorized into four Runyon groups: **photochromogens** (e.g., *M. kansasii, M. marinum*), which produce yellow-orange pigment only after exposure to bright light; **scotochromogens** (e.g., *M. scrofulaceum*), which produce pigment regardless of light exposure; **nonchromogens** (e.g., *M. avium-intracellulare*), which do not produce pigment under any circumstances; and **rapid growers** (e.g., *M. fortuitum, M. chelonei*), which form visible colonies on standard mycobacterial culture media in less than 7 days. *M. leprae,* the cause of Hansen's disease, is a MOTT that is not cultivable on artificial growth media and thus not classified by the Runyon scheme.

TABLE 7–4. Classification of Medically Important Human Mycobacteria (Runyon Group)

***Mycobacterium tuberculosis* Complex**
Niacin positive, nitrate reduction positive
M. tuberculosis
Niacin positive, nitrate reduction negative
M. bovis (rarely niacin positive)
Niacin negative, nitrate reduction negative
M. africanum
M. bovis (almost always niacin negative)
Photochromogens
Niacin positive, nitrate reduction negative
M. marinum (occasionally niacin positive)
M. simiae
Niacin negative, nitrate reduction positive
M. kansasii
Niacin negative, nitrate reduction negative
M. asiaticum
M. marinum (usually niacin negative)
Scotochromogens
Niacin negative, nitrate reduction positive
M. flavescens
M. szulgai
Niacin negative, nitrate reduction negative
M. gordonae
M. scrofulaceum
M. xenopi
Nonchromogens
Niacin negative, nitrate reduction positive
M. terrae
M. triviale
Niacin negative, nitrate reduction negative
M. avium-intracellulare
M. gastri
M. haemophilum
M. malmoense
Rapid Growers
Niacin positive, nitrate reduction positive
M. fortuitum (sometimes niacin positive)
Niacin positive, nitrate reduction negative
M. chelonei (sometimes niacin positive)
Niacin negative, nitrate reduction positive
M. fortuitum (sometimes niacin negative)
Niacin negative, nitrate reduction negative
M. chelonei (sometimes niacin negative)

Classification of Fungi

Fungi are eukaryotic organisms with cell walls containing chitin, cellulose, or both. The medically important fungi can be divided into two categories, yeasts and molds (Table 7–5). **Yeasts** are unicellular organisms that multiply asexually by formation of **buds,** or **blastoconidia.** Most yeasts are identified in the laboratory on the basis of microscopic morphologic features plus the results of biochemical tests. **Molds** are filamentous organisms that form **aerial hyphae** and multiply asexually by formation of **conidia** (e.g., microconidia, macroconidia, phialoconidia, annelloconidia, arthroconidia) or sporangiospores. Molds are identified by examination of the microscopic morphologic features of their reproductive, usually asexual, structures. Some yeasts and molds may exhibit sexual reproductive structures (e.g., asci and ascospores) when growing in the laboratory. **Conidia** are not surrounded by a membranous sac and can be formed individually, in chains, or in clusters directly from hyphae, pseudohyphae, or yeast cells or from the tips of hyphal stalks known as **conidiophores. Sporangiospores** are encased within a membranous sac, known as a **sporangium,** found at the end of a stalk known as a **sporangiophore.** Several of the pathogenic fungi can grow either as yeasts or molds and are known collectively as **dimorphic fungi.** Examples include *Histoplasma capsulatum, Blastomyces dermatitidis, Sporothrix schenckii,* and *Penicillium marneffei.*

SPECIMEN COLLECTION

The clinical utility of microbiology laboratory test results depends heavily on the quality of the specimens obtained and the manner in which they are transported to the laboratory. The site of specimen collection must be selected carefully to provide high yields of the infectious agent, its antigens, its nucleic acids, its toxins, or the antibodies produced by the host in response to its presence. Specimen collection must be conducted in a manner that ensures minimal contamination with commensal host flora. Specimen transport to the laboratory must occur under conditions that sustain the viability of infectious agents for culture and the integrity of their components or products for other assays (Table 7–6).

Body sites harboring large amounts of normal bacterial flora should be avoided if possible because of the likelihood of bacterial overgrowth of mycobacterial and fungal cultures. The conditions for transport of mycobacterial and fungal specimens to the laboratory in most instances are not as critical as they are for bacterial specimens because most mycobacteria and fungi survive adequately in specimens held at room or refrigerator temperature. Storage of specimens at room temperature for more than 60 minutes, however, does increase the probability of bacterial overgrowth.

Swab Specimens. Because of the ease of collection and transport, the temptation to obtain microbiology specimens on swabs is great. However, the yield from swab specimens, in most situations, is

TABLE 7–5. Classification of Medically Important Human Fungi

Yeasts	***Dimorphic Fungi***
Germ Tube Positive	*Blastomyces dermatitidis*
Candida albicans	*Coccidioides immitis*
Candida dubliniensis	*Histoplasma capsulatum*
Candida stellatoidea	*Paracoccidioides brasiliensis*
	Sporothrix schenckii
Germ Tube Negative	
Caffeic Acid Pigment Positive	***Opportunistic Fungi***
Cryptococcus neoformans	*Absidia*
Caffeic Acid Pigment Negative	*Acremonium*
Candida (not *C. albicans, C. stellatoidea,* or *C. dubliniensis*)	*Alternaria*
Cryptococcus (not *C. neoformans*)	*Aspergillus*
Rhodotorula	*Beauveria*
Saccharomyces	*Bipolaris*
Torulopsis	*Chrysosporium*
Trichosporon	*Cunninghamella*
Requires Exogenous Fatty Acids for Growth	*Curvularia*
Malassezia furfur	*Dreschlera*
	Fusarium
Molds	*Helminthosporium*
Dematiaceous Molds	*Mucor*
Cladosporium	*Paecilomyces*
Exophiala	*Penicillium*
Fonsecaea	*Rhizopus*
Phialophora	*Scedosporium*
Wangiella	*Scopulariopsis*
Dermatophytes	*Syncephalastrum*
Epidermophyton floccosum	*Verticillium*
Microsporum	
Trichophyton	

TABLE 7–6. Specimen Collection for Bacterial, Mycobacterial, and Fungal Testing

Specimen	Container	Other Considerations
Anaerobic Culture		
Aspirate, exudate	Anaerobic transport device, capped needleless syringe	Deliver to laboratory immediately
Rayon/Dacron swab	Anaerobic transport device	Deliver to laboratory immediately; preparation of smears requires separate swabs
Blood for Culture		
Bacteria (aerobic)	Aerobic blood culture bottle	0.5–10 mL blood recommended, depending on age and size of patient
Bacteria (anaerobic)	Anaerobic blood culture bottle	0.5–10 mL blood recommended, depending on age and size of patient (to be ordered only in situations in which anaerobic bacteremia is likely)
Mycobacteria	AFB blood culture bottle or Isolator 1.5 Microbial Tube	0.5–10 mL blood recommended, depending on age and size of patient
Fungi	Aerobic blood culture bottle or Isolator 1.5 Microbial Tube	0.5–10 mL blood recommended, depending on age and size of patient
Body Fluid for Culture		
CSF	Sterile, leakproof tube	Deliver to laboratory immediately; 2 mL for each culture type is optimal
Other body fluids	Sterile, leakproof tube	Deliver to laboratory immediately; 2 mL for each culture type is optimal
Body Fluid for Antigen Detection		
CSF	Sterile, leakproof tube	0.5 mL required; recommended for partially treated meningitis only
Other body fluids	Sterile, leakproof tube	Not available except under approved circumstances

TABLE 7–6. Specimen Collection for Bacterial, Mycobacterial, and Fungal Testing *(Continued)*

Specimen	Container	Other Considerations
Dermatophyte Culture		
Hair, skin, nails	Sterile, leakproof container	Hair: clip to within ½ inch of scalp, pluck remaining hair for culture; skin: cleanse with alcohol, culture scrapings from active edge of lesion; nail: cleanse with alcohol, scrape nail with sterile scalpel blade, discard initial scrapings, culture deeper scrapings
Respiratory Tract		
Throat (to identify group A *Streptococcus*)	Two rayon/Dacron swabs	One swab is for antigen detection; second swab should be used for culture or DNA probe if antigen detection result is negative
Throat (to exclude *Neisseria gonorrhoeae*)	Selective agar plate	Inoculate and streak agar with freshly collected specimen; deliver to laboratory immediately
Throat (to exclude *Corynebacterium diphtheriae*)	Rayon/Dacron swab	Notify laboratory to identify *C. diphtheriae*
Nasopharynx	Calcium alginate mini-tip swab (Regan-Lowe transport medium for *Bordetella pertussis*)	Notify laboratory to identify *Staphylococcus aureus* or *B. pertussis*
Tracheal aspirate	Sterile, leakproof container	Deliver to laboratory immediately
Sputum for bacteria	Sterile, leakproof container	Collect at least 2 mL from deep cough and deliver to laboratory immediately
Sputum for fungi or mycobacteria	Sterile, leakproof container	Collect at least 5 mL from deep cough and deliver to laboratory immediately
Chlamydia antigen detection (DFA)	Methanol-fixed smear	Nasopharyngeal aspirate preferred; nasopharyngeal smear acceptable
Chlamydia culture	Viral and chlamydial transport medium	Nasopharyngeal aspirate preferred
Stool		
Bacteria	Leakproof container, rayon/Dacron swab	Deliver to laboratory immediately
Ova and parasites	Leakproof container, formalin- and PVA-based preservative	Deliver to laboratory immediately if specimen is unpreserved stool; notify laboratory if *Cryptosporidium* is suspected
Clostridium difficile toxin	Leakproof container	Sample of 25 g stool required; deliver on ice to laboratory immediately
Clostridium botulinum toxin	Leakproof container	Sample of 25 g stool required; deliver on ice to laboratory immediately
Pinworm examination	Clear cellophane tape	Collect specimen in early morning, before defecation or bathing
Urine		
Clean-catch or catheterized specimen	Sterile, leakproof container	Deliver on ice to laboratory immediately
Suprapubic aspiration	Sterile, leakproof container, anaerobic transport device for anaerobic culture	Deliver on ice to laboratory immediately
Mycobacterial or fungal culture	Sterile, leakproof container	Deliver on ice to laboratory immediately; 10 mL of urine required
Genital Tract		
Neisseria gonorrhoeae culture	Selective agar plate	Inoculate and streak agar with freshly collected specimen; deliver to laboratory immediately
Routine culture	Rayon/Dacron swab, calcium alginate mini-tip swab	Preparation of smears requires separate swabs; Gram stain for *N. gonorrhoeae* performed on urethral swabs only
Chlamydia PCR	Roche Amplicor specimen transport medium	FDA-licensed for testing cervical, urethral, and urine specimens at present
Chlamydia culture	Viral and chlamydial transport medium	Cervical swabs only on postpubertal females; vaginal swabs acceptable for prepubertal females
Trichomonas wet preparation	Sterile, leakproof tube containing 1 mL saline solution	Collect fresh vaginal or urethral discharge specimens and deliver to laboratory immediately
Tissue/Bone		
Biopsy material	Sterile, leakproof container	Deliver to laboratory immediately

Table continued on following page

TABLE 7–6. Specimen Collection for Bacterial, Mycobacterial, and Fungal Testing *(Continued)*

Specimen	Container	Other Considerations
Ear		
Middle ear	Sterile, leakproof container	Tympanocentesis aspirate preferred
External ear	Rayon/Dacron swab	Preparation of multiple smears requires separate swabs
Eye		
Conjunctiva	Rayon/Dacron swab, calcium alginate mini-tip swab	Preparation of multiple smears requires separate swabs
Chlamydia antigen detection (DFA)	Methanol-fixed smear	Pus-free specimens yield best results
Chlamydia culture	Viral and chlamydial transport medium	Pus-free specimens yield best results
Wound/Abscess		
Aspirate or pus	Sterile, leakproof container, rayon/Dacron swab, anaerobic transport device for anaerobic culture	Preparation of smears requires separate swabs
Catheter Tip		
After withdrawal	Sterile, leakproof tube	Disinfect skin surrounding insertion site, remove catheter, and clip off distal 3 cm of tip aseptically into sterile tube
Serum		
Infectious disease serologic testing (Chapter 11)	Red-top tube	Collect at least 2 mL blood
Serum bactericidal titer	Red-top tube	Not available except under approved circumstances; collect at least 2 mL blood: trough specimen collected immediately before antimicrobial agent administration, and peak specimen collected 30 min (IV or IM) or 60 min (oral) after antimicrobial agent administration

AFB = acid-fact bacillus; DFA = direct fluorescent antibody; PVA = polyvinyl alcohol.

lower than that from corresponding aspirates, exudates, body fluids, or tissue specimens. This is especially true when a group of specimens are obtained by swab from the same site for multiple cultures. Many pathogenic fungi are found growing in tissue in the mold phase, and therefore pieces of tissue or biopsy material are the specimens of choice rather than specimens obtained by swab. Swabs should be reserved for collecting specimens that cannot be collected more effectively by other means. Sterile cotton, rayon, Dacron, and calcium alginate swabs on wooden, plastic, or flexible aluminum shafts are commercially available for specimen collection. However, some microorganisms are killed by exposure to the natural oils present in cotton fibers and wooden shafts. Accordingly, synthetic fiber swabs with plastic shafts are generally preferred for specimen collection.

Specimen-laden swabs should be inserted into or moistened with transport medium promptly. Liquid or semisolid transport medium (e.g., modified Stuart or Amies medium) is frequently included in the swab container and is intended to maintain the viability of microorganisms during transport. Pharyngeal swabs for collection of group A *Streptococcus* organisms are a notable exception because these bacteria survive equally well on dry or transport medium–saturated swabs. In fact, the yield of positive culture results is higher from dry pharyngeal swabs because of decreased numbers of surviving normal flora.

Specimens for Anaerobic Culture. Obligate anaerobes constitute the overwhelming majority of the microflora of the respiratory tract, gastrointestinal tract, and female genital tract. Even human skin is heavily colonized with anaerobes. Most microbiology laboratories deem requests for anaerobic culture of specimens collected from sites known to be colonized by anaerobic organisms as inappropriate and do not honor them. Laboratory work involved in anaerobic cultures is tedious, time-consuming, and expensive. Moreover, culture results cannot be interpreted with accuracy. The best interests of patients, physicians, and laboratories are served by ordering anaerobic cultures only on specimens collected carefully from appropriate sites.

Atmospheric oxygen results in intracellular accumulation of toxic metabolites (e.g., peroxides) in obligate anaerobes. Successful culture of anaerobes is contingent on their survival from specimen collection, inoculation, and anaerobic incubation. Many different transport devices that chemically remove oxygen from specimens are available to maintain the viability of obligately anaerobic bacteria and *Actinomyces.* Most microbiology laboratories reject specimens for anaerobic culture unless measures have been taken to ensure survival of anaerobic bacteria during transport.

Blood

Bacteremia in children differs from that in adults in four key respects (Table 7–7). First, the magnitude of the bacteremia (colony-forming units per milliliter) in children is higher, on average. Second, the quantity of blood that is usually submitted for culture is considerably less in children. Third, certain bacteria (e.g., *Streptococcus pneumoniae, Neisseria meningitidis, Salmonella*) are more frequent causes of bacteremia in children, whereas others

TABLE 7–7. Bacteremia in Children Compared with Adults

Magnitude of bacteremia tends to be higher in children.
Less blood is collected for culture in children.
Distribution of causative organisms is different in children.
Incidence of polymicrobial bacteremia is lower in children.

(e.g., obligate anaerobes) are more common in adults. Fourth, polymicrobial bacteremia is less common in children than in adults. These differences influence the choice of laboratory methods for detection of bacteremia in children.

Many laboratories furnish paired sets of blood culture bottles containing broth, one for aerobic and the other for anaerobic incubation. Some laboratories restrict the availability of anaerobic bottles because of the infrequency of anaerobic bacteremia in children. Blood is collected from patients and placed into bottles before transport. **Venting,** the purposeful introduction of oxygen into the aerobic bottle, should be performed by laboratory personnel only, once the bottles have reached the laboratory. Other collection methods for blood culture include the use of rubber-stoppered tubes containing sodium polyanetholesulfonate (SPS) as an anticoagulant and rubber-stoppered tubes containing a saponin-based lysis reagent plus SPS. When either of these tubes is used, laboratory personnel are responsible for inoculating specimens into broth or directly onto an agar medium.

The issues of when to collect, how much to collect, and how to collect specimens are important considerations in the collection of blood culture specimens. Although these variables have been investigated thoroughly in studies of adults, similar data from children are not as abundant. The following recommendations for the use of blood cultures in the management of children are generalized from published experience with both adults and children.

Timing of Blood Collection. The onset of fever and chills in a patient with intermittent bacteremia occurs approximately 1 hour after microbial invasion of the bloodstream. Therefore specimens harboring the highest numbers of bacteria are obtained immediately before or during a fever spike. Collection at other times yields specimens with lesser numbers because of eradication of bacteria from the bloodstream by the reticuloendothelial system. Culture of small volumes of blood containing low colony counts increases the likelihood of false-negative results.

In persons with constant fever and elevated WBC counts who have persistent bacteremia, cultures may be obtained at any time before administration of antimicrobial therapy. Blood culture specimens do not need to be obtained more frequently than once per day.

Technique for Collection of Blood. The importance of aseptic technique during blood culture collection cannot be overemphasized. Contamination of specimens with microorganisms from exogenous sources such as the patient's or phlebotomist's skin greatly confounds interpretation of culture results. A two-step disinfection process is recommended for preparation of skin for venipuncture (Table 7–8). First, oils and fatty substances that may be shielding microorganisms at the venipuncture site should be removed from the skin surface and pores by applying **70% isopropyl alcohol.** Second, the site should be treated with **providone-iodine** or **tincture of iodine** as skin disinfectants, which are allowed to remain on the skin for at least 30 seconds. Residual povidone-iodine can be removed before venipuncture with a second application of 70% isopropyl alcohol. Contact of the venipuncture site with nonsterile or nondisinfected objects, including the phlebotomist's gloved fingers, should be avoided. The rubber stoppers of specimen containers or blood culture bottles should be disinfected before the specimen is added.

TABLE 7–8. Preparation of Skin for Collection of Blood Culture Specimens

Application of 70% isopropyl alcohol to venipuncture site
Application of povidone-iodine or tincture of iodine to venipuncture site for 30 sec
Removal of povidone-iodine or tincture of iodine stain from skin with 70% alcohol (optional)

TABLE 7–9. Indications for Pediatric Anaerobic Blood Cultures

Signs and symptoms of abdominal infection
Sacral decubitus ulcers or cellulitis
Poor dentition, severe oral mucositis, or chronic sinusitis
Neutropenia or high-dose conticosteroid therapy
Sickle cell disease
Suspected bacteremia after human bite wounds or crushing trauma
Prolonged rupture of membranes or chorioamnionitis at birth

Adapted from Zaidi AKM, Knaut AL, Mirrett S, et al: Value of routine anaerobic blood cultures for pediatric patients. *J Pediatr* 1995;127:263–8.

The rate of contamination of blood culture specimens from children, which generally exceeds 3%, is invariably higher than that of specimens from adults. Because children with fever and elevated WBC counts often present with symptoms of rhinorrhea or diarrhea, their skin tends to be colonized with high counts of bacteria from the upper respiratory and gastrointestinal tracts. The sheer numbers of bacteria may render routine skin disinfection less effective than in adults. Another factor is the lack of cooperation by children approached for phlebotomy, which leads to inadequate skin disinfection.

Quantity of Blood Collected. Data on adults indicate that the probability of positive blood culture results rises proportionately with the quantity of blood collected. Current recommendations for adults call for culturing 20–30 mL of blood with inoculation in both aerobically and anaerobically incubated media. Collection of such a large amount from young children is not feasible. Fortunately, the higher magnitude of bacteremia in children allows satisfactory results when as little as 1–5 mL of blood is cultured. If <0.5 mL of blood can be collected, aerobically incubated media should be inoculated preferentially because anaerobic bacteremia in children is rare. Because of the rarity of anaerobic bacteremia in children, some laboratories elect not to inoculate anaerobically incubated media on a routine basis. Instead they commit the entire blood sample to aerobically incubated media unless anaerobic incubation is specifically requested, as it is for certain indications (Table 7–9).

Mycobacteria. Mycobacteremia occurs primarily in persons with AIDS. The main species involved (*M. avium-intracellulare, M. tuberculosis,* and *M. kansasii*) grow very slowly, and their detection requires 2–8 weeks of incubation by classic culture techniques. Newer techniques to shorten the time to detection or improve the sensitivity of mycobacterial blood culture (e.g., lysis centrifugation, radiometric broth culture, fluorometric broth culture, continuously monitored broth culture) have been developed and are in use in many laboratories.

Fungi. Several characteristics make detection of some fungi in blood more difficult than detection of bacteria. First, many fungi grow at rates considerably slower than bacteria, and cultures should be incubated for longer periods before results are considered negative. Most laboratories hold fungal blood cultures for 21 days or longer, compared with 5–7 days for routine bacterial blood cultures. Second, *Malassezia furfur,* an important cause of catheter-related fungemia in hospitalized neonates receiving lipid-containing hyperalimentation therapy, has a nutritional requirement for medium to long chain fatty acids that is not met by conventional blood culture media. Most laboratories supplement media with a source of these fatty acids (e.g., sterile olive oil) for growth of this yeast. Third, detection of molds (e.g., *Aspergillus*) in blood from persons with disseminated infection is hampered by the heterogeneous distribution of fungal elements in blood specimens and the undependable growth of molds in broth media. Collection of larger volumes of blood increases the likelihood that fungal hyphae will be present and will yield positive culture results. Inoculation of blood to solid media also improves the chances that molds will be detected because they are more easily recognized when growing on the surface of agar media. Recovery of most yeasts (e.g., *Candida* and *Cryptococcus*) from persons with fungemia is satisfactorily achieved by agitation of aerobically incubated routine bacterial blood culture specimens.

Body Fluids

Body fluids from closed cavities (e.g., CSF, pleural fluid, pericardial fluid, peritoneal fluid, and synovial fluid) should be collected in sterile, leakproof containers and transported to the laboratory promptly. If fluid collection is effected by a transcutaneous needle, the aseptic technique described for blood culture collection should be used.

Separate tubes for the hematology, clinical chemistry, and microbiology laboratories should be prepared if fluids are to be analyzed for cell count and differential, glucose level, and protein level, as well as Gram stain and culture. At least 1 mL of fluid should be placed in each tube. A fourth tube may be needed if additional tests, such as bacterial antigen testing or viral culture, are requested. When a mycobacterial or fungal infection is likely, the probability of recovering pathogens is maximized by submitting 5–10 mL of fluid to the microbiology laboratory for testing.

Mycobacteria. Body fluids harboring mycobacteria generally exhibit low colony counts, and therefore it is not unusual to encounter smear-negative but culture-positive specimens. The sensitivity of the culture itself can be seriously compromised when limited quantities of body fluids are submitted for analysis. Ideally, 5–10 mL of fluid should be collected to enable the laboratory to concentrate the specimen at least tenfold by centrifugation. Mycobacterial smears and cultures can then be prepared from the resuspended sediment, resulting in improved sensitivity.

Upper Respiratory Tract

Nasopharyngeal specimens for diagnosis of pneumonia caused by *Bordetella pertussis* and *Chlamydia trachomatis* should be collected with flexible, wire-shaft, mini-tip swabs composed of calcium alginate fibers. The child's head is titled backward and the swab is inserted into one of the nares until the tip reaches the posterior wall of the nasopharynx. The swab is gently rotated to scrape off ciliated epithelial cells and is then carefully withdrawn from the nose.

Pharyngeal specimens for culture of group A *Streptococcus, Arcanobacterium haemolyticum, Corynebacterium diphtheriae,* and *Neisseria gonorrhoeae* are collected by inserting rayon or Dacron swabs into the oral cavity so that the tip comes into contact with exudative, inflamed areas of the posterior pharynx and tonsils. Careful specimen collection, especially from young persons, is crucial. Carelessly collected specimens often amount to mere tongue- or saliva-soaked swabs. Such specimens, even when obtained from persons with bacterial pharyngitis, may yield negative results.

B. pertussis is exquisitely sensitive to toxic substances found in routine collection swabs, transport media, and growth media, and specimens should be placed in a protective transport medium such as **Regan-Lowe semisolid charcoal blood agar** or dilute **casamino acids broth** and transported immediately to the laboratory. These precautions are unnecessary for specimens submitted for *B. pertussis* antigen detection because viable organisms are not required.

Throat swabs for culture of *C. diphtheriae* should be sent to the laboratory promptly or placed on **Loeffler's medium** after collection for transport to the laboratory.

Lower Respiratory Tract

Laboratory diagnosis of bacterial lower respiratory tract infections in children is usually achieved by examining nasopharyngeal swabs, especially for viral agents (Chapter 9), and endotracheal aspirates. Such specimens inevitably are contaminated with upper respiratory tract flora whose presence can interfere with identification or be misleading in determining the cause of infection. Alternative, more invasive means of specimen collection that avoid contamination include bronchoalveolar lavage, by means of a suction apparatus protected from upper respiratory flora contamination during insertion, percutaneous needle aspiration, or open lung biopsy.

Mycobacteria. Laboratory diagnosis of tuberculosis in children is hampered by the difficulty in acquiring lower respiratory tract secretions. Unlike adolescents and adults, young children are unable to expectorate sputum on demand. Because young children swallow their sputum, gastric aspirate containing swallowed sputum has served successfully as an alternative specimen. Although mycobacteria are somewhat resistant to the deleterious effects of a low pH environment, long-term exposure does reduce their viability. Gastric aspirate (5–10 mL) should be delivered to the laboratory promptly and the pH titrated to neutrality if further delay in processing is unavoidable. The main disadvantage to the use of gastric aspirates is that the tap water acid-fast bacillus, *M. gordonae,* may be present in the stomach, and therefore positive results from acid-fast smears should be interpreted cautiously. Identification procedures for positive culture results should include provisions to exclude *M. gordonae.*

Fungi. The presence of certain fungi in the lower respiratory tract (e.g., *Histoplasma capsulatum, Blastomyces dermatitidis,* and *Coccidioides immitis*) is pathognomonic of infection. The culture of other fungi (e.g., *Candida* and *Aspergillus*) may reflect only the contamination of specimens with upper respiratory tract secretions.

Gastrointestinal Tract

Gastric and duodenal aspirates should be collected to minimize contamination with upper respiratory tract flora. If delay in specimen processing is anticipated, gastric acidity should be titrated to neutrality with sodium hydroxide or neutralized with a strong buffer to prevent killing of microorganisms during storage.

Gastric mucosal biopsy specimens for detection of *Helicobacter pylori* should be collected with the aid of direct visualization of the biopsy site by gastroscopy. Samples taken from the periphery of lesions provide the best chance of yielding pathogens.

Stool should be transported to the laboratory promptly after collection or placed into a suitable transport medium. Certain pathogens (e.g., *Shigella*) rapidly lose viability in stool because acidic waste products from bacterial fermentation accumulate and decrease the stool pH. A transport medium, such as buffered glycerolized saline solution, can be used to minimize loss of viability if specimens cannot be cultured immediately. *Campylobacter* organisms, unfortunately, do not tolerate buffered glycerolized saline solution well, and a different transport medium (e.g., Cary-Blair) is recommended. Stool is preferred over rectal swabs for diagnosis of enteritis, because swab specimens are often inadequately collected or improperly stored before testing. Macroscopic examination of stool allows identification of blood- or mucus-laden portions for further study. Such contents are likely to harbor pathogens at highest concentrations. Because young children cannot produce stool on demand, properly obtained rectal swab specimens are acceptable for detection of the agents of enteritis. Separate swabs should be submitted for each type of smear or culture requested.

Stool for toxin studies, such as *Clostridium botulinum* and *Clostridium difficile,* should be transported to the laboratory immediately or frozen to prevent loss of heat-labile toxin activity. Rectal swabs are not suitable for toxin detection studies.

Mycobacteria. Persons with AIDS who have disseminated *M. avium-intracellulare* infection may harbor large numbers of acid-fast bacilli in stool. Positive results on acid-fast-stained stool smears are easily obtained and may be the first laboratory indication of *M. avium-intracellulare* infection. Stool cultures for *Mycobacterium* should be discouraged because of the likelihood of bacterial overgrowth with normal bacterial flora.

Fungi. Fungal esophagitis is not uncommon among patients with defects of cellular immunity. The most frequent cause is *Candida albicans.* The source of infection is the colonized or infected upper respiratory tract or mouth. It may be difficult to distinguish colonization from infection by positive culture results alone, and diagnosis usually requires correlation of culture with direct examination. Overgrowth of *C. albicans* in the stool is common in patients receiving oral or systemic broad-spectrum antimicrobial agents, which may be reflected by overgrowth of stool cultures with *C. albicans.*

Urinary Tract

The optimal time to collect urine for evaluation of urinary tract infection is in the early morning during the day's first voiding. Pathogens generally are present in high numbers, and differentiation of clinically significant and insignificant bacteriuria is easiest. Specimens may be obtained by clean-catch collection, bladder catheterization, or suprapubic aspiration. Clean-catch and catheterized specimens require disinfection of the periurethral area before collection. Bagged specimens obtained by application of a sterile bag are not recommended because of frequent contamination despite attempts at disinfection. Clean-catch specimens should be collected in midstream to reduce contamination from periurethral flora. Despite these safeguards, clean-catch and catheterized specimens invariably are contaminated with small numbers of microorganisms, and measures must be taken during transport to the laboratory to minimize multiplication of contaminants. Refrigeration of urine after collection and transport on ice to the laboratory is an effective means of stabilizing colony counts. Transport of specimens on ice or the addition of boric acid as a urine preservative is indicated when long delays in specimen transport are anticipated. Agar-coated dipslides that are inoculated immediately after specimen collection are also helpful in circumventing the problems caused by delays in specimen delivery. Urine obtained by suprapubic aspiration or collected directly from the ureters is, in effect, a body fluid and should be transported in the manner described for body fluids.

Mycobacteria. Urine specimens for *M. tuberculosis* from persons with renal or miliary tuberculosis yield positive culture results in some cases. The recommended specimen is at least 10 mL of the first voided urine for the day. A clue to the existence of a mycobacterial urinary tract infection is the presence of sterile pyuria.

Genital Tract

A wide variety of commensal microorganisms inhabit the genital mucosa of males and females. Laboratory testing to identify causes of infection is facilitated when specimens contain minimal numbers of endogenous flora. Selection of suitable sites for specimen collection is crucial. In evaluations of female patients for gonococcal or chlamydial cervicitis, vaginal swabs and samples of vaginal discharge are inferior to direct sampling of the endocervical canal. Endocervical specimens should be collected after removing and discarding excess discharge with a swab. A second swab is inserted 1–2 cm into the cervical os, gently rotated, carefully removed to avoid contamination, and sent to the laboratory for testing. Concurrent sampling of the urethra and rectum further enhances the likelihood of pathogen detection.

Specimens for culture of *Neisseria gonorrhoeae* and *Chlamydia trachomatis* have unique collection and transport requirements. The viability of *N. gonorrhoeae* is rapidly reduced by abrupt changes in temperature and atmosphere, and therefore many laboratories furnish selective agar warmed to room temperature for inoculation immediately after specimen collection. Provision can also be made for placement of the culture plate in an atmosphere enriched with carbon dioxide during transport if immediate delivery to the laboratory is not possible. The survival of *C. trachomatis* en route to the laboratory is prolonged by placing specimens in a buffered transport medium, such as 2-sucrose phosphate broth.

Freshly expressed discharge or material from properly collected urethral swabs should be sent to the laboratory for diagnosis of infections in male patients with symptoms. A flexible-shaft minitip swab should be inserted 1–2 cm into the urethral orifice and gently rotated.

Syphilis can be diagnosed by dark-field microscopic examination of freshly collected transudate from a chancre of primary-stage infection or a condyloma latum of secondary-stage infection. Lesions should be gently abraded with dry gauze or a scalpel blade to express fluid. A drop of the fluid, with or without the addition of saline solution as a volume expander, is placed on a microscope slide, a coverslip is placed, and the specimen is examined under a microscope equipped with a dark-field condenser.

Fungi. *Candida,* especially *C. albicans,* is an important cause of vaginal infection in postpubertal females. Organisms may be detected microscopically or by culture. Because small numbers of yeasts may be present in healthy patients, large numbers of organisms accompanied by appropriate symptoms or vaginal pathology are indicative of infection. Special techniques are unnecessary for collection of vaginal specimens.

Soft Tissues

The optimum specimen for laboratory confirmation of skin and soft tissue infections is aspirated pus. If sufficient pus has not accumulated, whatever can be aspirated from the leading edge of the infection site should be sent to the laboratory for analysis. Simple direct aspiration of cellulitis yields bacteria in approximately 50% of cases, compared with injection of saline solution followed by aspiration, which yields bacteria in approximately 20% of cases. Swab collection of specimens from infected tissue is less desirable, albeit acceptable, although contamination of the specimens with adjacent skin flora must be avoided. Swabs for collection of specimens from open wounds are unsuitable because of contamination of tissue colonized with organisms not involved in infection.

The causes of burn wound infections are best ascertained by quantitative culture of affected tissue. Approximately 1 g of tissue from beneath the burn eschar should be removed and submitted to the laboratory (Chapter 49).

Mycobacteria. Certain mycobacteria (e.g., *M. marinum, M. ulcerans, M. haemophilum*) may cause cutaneous infections. Biopsy material is preferred over lesion swabs because the numbers of mycobacteria present may be low. These cutaneous mycobacteria, like the fungal dermatophytes, usually do not grow well at standard incubator temperatures (35–37°C) but can be cultured at 30–32°C with growth within 4–8 weeks.

Bone

Identifying the cause of bone and joint infections can be achieved by blood culture but is better determined by culture of needle or surgical aspiration of infected bone or by culture of joint fluid for joint infections. Aspirate or biopsy specimens should be placed in a sterile, leakproof container and immediately transported to the laboratory. Excessive drying is the primary concern during specimen transport and can be avoided by suspending biopsy specimens in small quantities of sterile, nonbacteriostatic saline solution.

Ear

Clinical circumstances sometimes dictate a need for laboratory confirmation or determination of the cause of middle ear infection. Tympanocentesis, aspiration of middle ear fluid, requires techniques that avoid contamination with organisms colonizing the external ear duct. Both the ear duct and the tympanic membrane should be disinfected with 70% isopropyl alcohol before the procedure (see Fig. 64–4).

Laboratory confirmation of otitis externa can be obtained by examining scrapings from the epidermal surface of the visibly inflamed ear duct. Scrapings must be collected in a manner that minimizes contamination with cutaneous flora present in the ear duct. Cerumen should be removed and discarded. A thin-tipped sterile swab is inserted into the ear duct and, without coming into contact with uninfected areas, used to absorb exudative material. The swab should be removed with equal care and sent to the laboratory for testing.

Eye

Specimens from persons with conjunctivitis should be obtained before application of preservative-containing topical medications. Fresh or dried exudate should be removed with a swab and discarded, which facilitates visualization of the conjunctiva. Ideal specimens consist of scrapings collected from the conjunctival membranes with a flexible-tip platinum spatula. Less desirable is collection of ocular discharge with a swab. Pus from infected eyelids should be collected on a premoistened swab.

Laboratory documentation of keratitis can be confirmed by examining corneal scrapings. Specimens should be collected with a platinum spatula by an experienced ophthalmologist. Swabs of infected corneal sites offer much poorer yields of microorganisms than corneal scrapings.

Intraocular fluid should be obtained by needle aspiration by an ophthalmologist. Fluid from both the anterior chamber and the vitreous cavity should be collected and placed in sterile tubes. Specimens must be delivered to the laboratory rapidly.

Infections Related to Use of Intravenous Catheters

Although exit site and tunnel infections are diagnosed on the basis of local signs of infection, catheter-related bacteremia is often difficult to prove without removal of the catheter and culture of the catheter tip. The use of **quantitative blood culture** by the **lysis direct plating method** or by direct inoculation of 0.5 mL of blood on an agar plate, to permit counting of colonies, can also be useful for identifying a catheter as the source of bacteremia. If the concentration of bacteria in blood obtained via the catheter is significantly (5–10 times) greater than that in blood obtained peripherally, a catheter-associated infection is likely.

If the catheter is removed, catheter-related infection should be documented by culture of the catheter tip. The distal tip should be cut with sterile scissors and sent in a sterile container to the laboratory for **semiquantitative culture** by the **roll plate method** and then also placed into broth. Other methods of processing catheter tips include sonication of the tip and culture in liquid medium. If the roll plate technique is used, growth of >15 colonies is considered significant and indicates catheter-associated infection. Fewer colonies likely represent contamination of the catheter as the catheter was removed.

Mycobacteria. *M. fortuitum* and *M. chelonei* are rapidly growing mycobacteria that have emerged as opportunistic causes of catheter-related infections. Because large numbers of these organisms may result in visible growth in agar or broth cultures after as few as 3 days of incubation, they may be misidentified as *Corynebacterium* species (diphtheroids).

Fungi. Many yeasts have been documented as causes of catheter-related sepsis, especially *Candida* and *M. furfur,* which is common in hospitalized neonates receiving lipid hyperalimentation.

SPECIMEN TRANSPORT AND INITIAL PROCESSING

The cardinal rule regarding transport of specimens is that specimens should be delivered to the laboratory in a manner that guarantees survival of pathogens, or their products, within a time frame that minimizes growth of nonpathogens present in the specimen.

If more than 1 mL of body fluid is submitted for Gram stain and culture, specimens should first be centrifuged at 1,500*g* for 15 minutes unless they are too viscous to allow sedimentation. After centrifugation, sediments should be resuspended in approximately 200 μL of supernatant and used for preparation of smears, wet mounts, and inoculation of cultures. The remainder of the supernatant should be retained for a short time for unanticipated tests. If ≤1 mL of body fluid is received, the advantages afforded by centrifugation are not sufficient to risk contamination or breakage of specimen tubes and loss of the specimen.

Many laboratories have obtained superior results with Gram stain smears prepared by **cytocentrifugation,** instead of drops of body fluid sediments allowed to air-dry on microscope slides. Cytocentrifugation is effective with specimen volumes <1 mL. The cytocentrifuge deposits all cellular elements, including microorganisms, onto a small area of the slide, effectively increasing the sensitivity of smear preparation.

Cerebrospinal Fluid. Guidelines as to which area should receive which tube of CSF vary from laboratory to laboratory (Table 7–10).

TABLE 7–10. Allocation of CSF Specimens to Various Laboratories

Tube 1:	Microbiology for bacterial antigen detection (if desired), viral culture (if desired), or storage for unanticipated tests
Tube 2:	Microbiology for Gram stain and culture
Tube 3:	Chemical analysis for glucose and total protein determinations
Tube 4:	Hematologic testing for cell count and differential count

In general, the first tube collected should not go to the hematology or clinical chemistry areas, because peripheral blood contamination markedly affects the cell and differential counts and the glucose and protein results, nor should the first tube go to the microbiology area for culture, because the initial fluid is most likely to be contaminated with skin flora.

Mycobacteria. Transport of specimens for mycobacterial testing carries the risk of exposure to infectious aerosols if a specimen harboring *M. tuberculosis* leaks or spills. Care should be taken to minimize the possibility of such an event. Initial processing of mycobacterial specimens, which poses risks to laboratory personnel, should be undertaken only within the confines of a certified biologic safety cabinet (class 2). Because the number of mycobacteria in specimens from infected patients may be very low, concentration of specimens by centrifugation is a common practice. **Centrifugation** may take place within a biologic safety cabinet or in the open laboratory if sealed rotor heads or centrifuge safety cups are used. Rotor heads or safety cups must be opened in a biologic safety cabinet. Liquid specimens >1 mL should be concentrated before testing. Centrifugation of specimens must be thorough for successful concentration of mycobacteria. Centrifugation at 3,000*g* for 30 minutes is necessary to sediment mycobacteria effectively. Viscous, tenacious specimens like sputum must be liquefied first if centrifugation is to have any value. Treatment with mucolytic agents such as *N*-acetyl-L-cysteine, trisodium phosphate, or dithiothreitol is generally helpful. If specimens are likely to contain high numbers of the host's endogenous flora, chemical decontamination of the specimen with sodium hydroxide, benzalkonium chloride, or oxalic acid is indicated. Aseptically collected body fluids do not need decontamination before cultures are inoculated.

Decontamination of waste contaminated with *M. tuberculosis* should take place within, or as near as possible, to the laboratory work area. Only methods known to destroy *M. tuberculosis* effectively (e.g., autoclaving, chemical disinfection, or incineration) should be used.

RAPID DIAGNOSTIC METHODS

Microscopic Evaluation for Bacteria

Light microscopy still plays an important role in the diagnosis of infections, despite significant advances in immunodiagnostic and nucleic acid probe–based assays for infectious agents. Microscopic examination of specimens frequently yields the earliest direct laboratory evidence of infection that can greatly influence clinical decision making during the initial stages of patient management. Because fungi form much larger structures than bacteria, microscopic detection of fungi is not difficult provided sufficient numbers of organisms are present in specimens.

Gram Stain. The most frequently requested microscopic examination is the Gram stain (Table 7–11). It was initially described more than a century ago and remains popular for two important reasons: stained bacteria are more readily seen than unstained bacteria, and bacteria are stained differently according to their cell wall structure. Knowledge of an organism's Gram reaction assists clinicians in selecting empirical antimicrobial therapy (Plates 1A, 1B, 1C).

Modifications of the procedure for counterstain-refractory bacteria, including *Campylobacter, Legionella,* and *Bartonella henselae,* have been described and generally involve use of dilute carbol-fuchsin to replace safranin. The decolorization step is the most critical step of the Gram stain procedure, during which either over- or under-decolorization may occur. Knowledge of the decolorization agent being used is essential because 95% ethanol is a much slower decolorizer than acetone. The most widely used decolorizer is a 1:1 mixture of 95% ethanol and acetone, which results in a moderate rate of decolorization. Staining of quality control smears known to contain both gram-positive and gram-negative bacteria confirms that proper technique is being used. Excessive heat fixation of the smear is another problem that may interfere with correct reading of bacterial and inflammatory cell morphologic features. Use of methanol fixation instead of heat fixation avoids the problem.

TABLE 7–11. Standard Gram Staining Procedure

Prepare thin smear of specimen, allow to air-dry, and fix with gentle heat or methanol.
Flood smear with crystal violet (gentian violet) for 10 sec. Rinse with tap water.
Flood smear with Gram's iodine for 10 sec. Rinse with tap water.
Briefly decolorize smear with 95% ethanol, acetone, or ethanol-acetone mixture until readily leachable crystal violet has disappeared (1–5 sec). Rinse with tap water.
Flood smear with safranin for 10 sec. Rinse with tap water. Gently blot dry or air-dry the smear.
Examine under conventional light microscope, using oil-immersion magnification (×1,000).

Correct understanding of Gram stain reports by clinicians requires familiarity with the laboratory's reporting format and nomenclature. Most laboratories report the quantity of microorganisms, inflammatory cells, erythrocytes, and epithelial cells observed. Further categorization of inflammatory cells as mononuclear or polymorphonuclear is feasible, but providing a precise differential count from a Gram-stained smear is not possible. Such information is better left to the hematology laboratory.

Observation of ≥1 bacteria per oil immersion field (×1,000) suggests that at least 100,000 cfu/mL of specimen are present. This relationship is especially helpful when smears of urine are examined.

Gram staining may also be used for detection of fungi and usually appear gram positive (Plate 2A). Fungi that do not stain well with crystal violet or safranin, the dyes used in the Gram stain, pose more of a problem. The hyphae of molds growing in tissue are excellent examples and may be detected by identifying areas of smears that are unstained and that morphologically resemble fungal hyphae.

Acridine Orange Stain. A disadvantage of Gram-stained smears is the difficulty in differentiating gram-negative bacteria from similarly stained cellular debris and protein strands found in some specimens. This problem is avoided if smears are stained with the fluorescent dye acridine orange, which intercalates within the double helix of prokaryotic and eukaryotic cellular DNA (Table 7–12). Examination of smears with ultraviolet light illumination reveals fluorescent orange microorganisms and human cells (Plate 1D).

Because of the high degree of contrast between stained microorganisms and unstained background material, the acridine orange method affords greater sensitivity than the Gram stain method. From 5- to 10-fold fewer organisms per milliliter of specimen are required to yield positive results on acridine orange smears. Although bacteria detected in acridine orange–stained smears cannot be classified as gram positive or negative, the same smears may be restained with Gram reagents to determine the Gram reaction of microorganisms detected.

TABLE 7–12. Acridine Orange Staining Procedure

Prepare thin smear of specimen, allow to air-dry, and fix with methanol.
Flood smear with 0.01% acridine orange (pH 4.0) for 60 sec. Rinse with tap water. Gently blot dry or air-dry the smear.
Examine under ultraviolet light microscope, using ×100–500 magnification.

Dark-Field Examination. Because most spirochetes are extremely thin, they are invisible under a conventional transmitted light microscope because there is insufficient contrast between the spirochetes and the background. Replacement of the standard microscope condenser with a dark-field condenser alters the microscope from one dependent on transmitted light to one dependent on reflected light. Thus spirochetes appear as bright objects against a black background, and the contrast is sufficient for resolution.

Even though dark-field examination is highly recommended for definitive diagnosis of primary and secondary syphilis, most laboratories offer the test infrequently. The reasons are that most laboratory microscopes today are not equipped with dark-field condensers, and chancres and condylomata lata of primary or secondary syphilis may be healed or too dry to yield positive results by the time they are sampled.

Dark-field examinations are performed by placing liquid specimens on microscope coverslips, adding small drops of sterile nonbacteriostatic saline solution to adhere coverslips to slides, and examining wet mounts immediately before the spirochetes lose their motility. *Treponema pallidum,* the agent of syphilis, appears as long, thin organisms exhibiting corkscrew-like motility (Fig. 7–1). The dark-field examination may also be used for detection of *Leptospira* and *Borrelia burgdorferi* in clinical specimens.

Acid-Fast Stains. All mycobacterial species exhibit some degree of acid fastness. **Acid fastness** refers to the resistance to decolorization of stained cell walls, even when the decolorization agent consists of a mixture of 95% ethanol and concentrated hydrochloride. *Nocardia* organisms are partially acid-fast; they resist decolorization by 2% H_2SO_4 but are usually decolorized by a mixture of 95% ethanol and concentrated hydrochloric acid. Almost all other actinomycetes are not acid-fast.

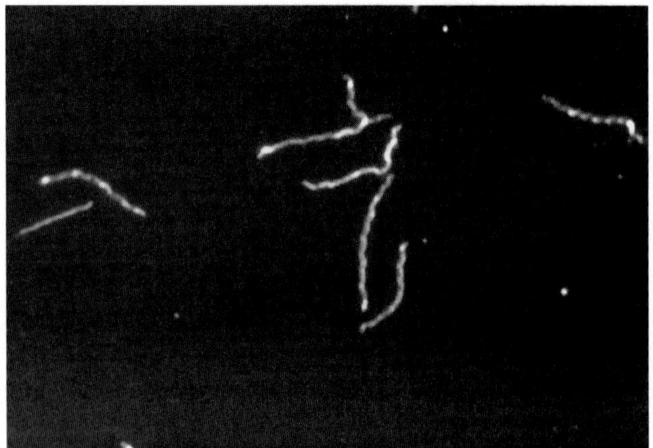

FIGURE 7–1. Dark-field examination of exudate from a primary chancre of syphilis. (From Pocket Picture Guide to Microbiology of Infectious Diseases, by D.K. Bannerjee, Mosby-Wolfe an imprint of Times Mirror International Publishers Ltd., UK, 1985.)

TABLE 7–13. Kinyoun Acid-Fast Staining Procedure

Prepare thin smear of specimen, allow to air-dry, and fix with heat at 80°C for 15 min.
Flood smear with Kinyoun carbol-fuchsin reagent for 5 min. Rinse with tap water.
Decolorize smear with acid-alcohol (95% ethanol and 3% hydrochloric acid) until no more stain leaves smear. Rinse with tap water.
Flood smear with 0.3% methylene blue (in H_2O) counterstain for 30 sec. Rinse with tap water. Gently blot dry or air-dry the smear.
Examine under conventional light microscope, using oil-immersion magnification (×1,000).

Several acid-fast staining methods are available. All are based on the same principles but differ from one another in the staining reagents and decolorizers used. The generic procedure calls for preparation of a thin smear of the specimen, followed by air drying and thorough heat fixation. The smear is then treated with a penetrative primary stain, decolorized with a strong mineral acid containing reagent, and counterstained (Plate 1F).

The **Ziehl-Neelsen** staining procedure requires heating the primary stain (carbol-fuchsin) to the point of steaming during the first step of the staining process. The decolorizer is a mixture of concentrated hydrochloric acid and 95% alcohol, and the counterstain is methylene blue.

The **Kinyoun** staining procedure differs from the Ziehl-Neelsen procedure in that heating of the primary stain (carbol-fuchsin) is not necessary (Table 7–13). Use of a more concentrated carbol-fuchsin reagent results in the penetration of the mycobacterial cell wall without the assistance of heat. Because the Kinyoun method is simpler, it has largely replaced the Ziehl-Neelsen method in most laboratories.

The **fluorochrome stain** is unique in that a microscope equipped for ultraviolet illumination or quartz-halogen illumination must be used. In either case the microscope must have appropriate excitation and barrier filters in place to enhance observation of fluorescence. Unlike the fluorescent immunoassays available for detection of a variety of microbial antigens, the fluorochrome staining method does not use fluorescent antibody conjugates (Table 7–14). The primary stain is a mixture of auramine O and rhodamine B dyes in a carbol-glycerol base. The hydrochloric acid–ethanol decolorizing agent of the fluorochrome procedure is not as strong as those used in the Ziehl-Neelsen and Kinyoun procedures. The counterstain, potassium permanganate, is used to quench background fluorescence. The primary advantage of the fluorochrome staining proce-

TABLE 7–14. Auramine-Rhodamine Fluorochrome Acid-Fast Staining Procedure

Prepare thin smear of specimen, allow to air-dry, and fix with heat at 80°C for 15 min.
Flood smear with auramine-rhodamine reagent for 15 minutes. Rinse with tap water.
Decolorize smear with acid-alcohol (70% ethanol and 0.5% hydrochloric acid) for 3 min. Rinse with tap water.
Flood smear with 0.5% potassium permanganate counterstain for 4 min. Rinse with tap water. Gently blot dry or air-dry the smear.
Examine under ultraviolet light microscope at ×100–500 magnification.

TABLE 7–15. Modified Kinyoun Acid-Fast Staining Procedure for *Nocardia*

Prepare thin smear of isolate, allow to air-dry, and fix with heat as for Gram stain.
Flood smear with Kinyoun carbol-fuchsin reagent for 5 min. Rinse with tap water.
Decolorize smear 5–10 sec with 0.5–1% sulfuric acid. Rinse with tap water.
Flood smear with 0.3% methylene blue (in water) counterstain for 30 sec. Rinse with tap water. Gently blot dry or air-dry the smear.
Examine under conventional light microscope, using oil-immersion magnification (×1,000).

dure is the greater sensitivity afforded by the sharp contrast between acid-fast organisms and the background (Plate 1G). Smears may be screened at lower magnification for more rapid examination of specimens.

The **modified acid-fast** staining procedures (e.g., **modified Kinyoun stain**) are the key to differentiating *Nocardia* from other aerobic actinomycetes (Table 7–15). Use of 0.5–1% H_2SO_4 or briefer exposure to the decolorizers used with the conventional Ziehl-Neelsen and Kinyoun procedures differentiates this staining procedure from the standard acid-fast staining procedure (Plate 1H).

India Ink Preparation. The india ink preparation is a technique for rapid, presumptive identification of *Cryptococcus neoformans* in body fluids by negative staining (Table 7–16). Microscopic examination of specimens with the organism reveals tiny carbon particles that are unable to penetrate the thick polysaccharide capsule of *C. neoformans,* creating the appearance of halo-surrounded organisms (Fig. 7–2). Care must be taken to avoid confusion with inflammatory cells, which may be surrounded by a thin halo. Encapsulated budding yeast cells should be seen before concluding that the india ink preparation result is positive. The india ink preparation usually shows a negative result when specimens contain fewer than 10,000/mL of *C. neoformans.* The particle agglutination assay for cryptococcal antigen is more sensitive and almost as rapid a test.

Potassium Hydroxide Preparation. Most fungi, when present in large numbers, can be detected reliably by Gram-stained smears of clinical specimens. Hair, skin, and nail scrapings from persons with dermatophyte infections, however, are not suitable for Gram staining. The use of 10–20% **potassium hydroxide (KOH)** can be used to clarify such specimens without altering the morphologic appearance of fungi (Table 7–17). Care must be taken, when one is examining skin scrapings, to avoid confusing fungal elements with cellular division planes (Fig. 7–3). The combination of dyes such as calcofluor white or indelible ink with 10–20% KOH sharpens the contrast between fungal elements and background material.

TABLE 7–16. India Ink Preparation

Place small drop of India ink next to drop of body fluid on microscope slide.
Place coverslip over both drops, causing drops to mix with each other.
Examine preparation under conventional light microscope at ×100–500 for presence of budding yeast cells surrounded by clear halo.

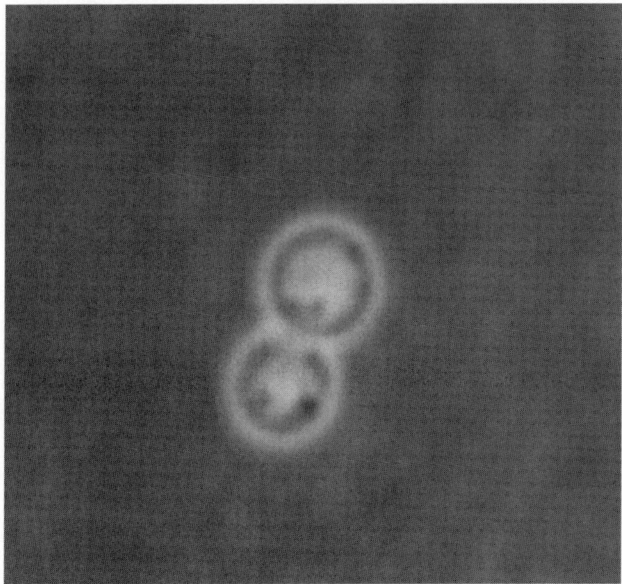

FIGURE 7–2. India ink preparation of cerebrospinal fluid containing *Cryptococcus neoformans.*

Calcofluor White Stain. Laundry detergent manufacturers discovered years ago that the addition of brighteners like **calcofluor white M2R** and **Tinopal CBS-X** to their products increased the "whiteness" of clothing. These fluorescent dyes, which bind efficiently to polysaccharides found in vegetable fibers, also bind to fungal cell walls. Smears are stained with these dyes for 1 minute and examined microscopically under ultraviolet illumination (Table 7–18). Fungal elements exhibit a bright whitish or bluish green fluorescence that stands out dramatically against an unstained background (Fig. 7–4).

Detection of Bacterial and Fungal Antigens

Immunoassays for direct detection of microbial antigens in specimens have enjoyed great popularity during the past three decades (Table 7–19). The primary appeal of these tests is the rapidity with which results can be made available, especially in comparison with classic culture methods. For persons with conditions such as group A streptococcal pharyngitis and certain of the sexually transmitted diseases, diagnosis and treatment may be achieved during a single visit. Same-visit therapy ensures treatment of noncompliant persons if single-dose therapy is available. Rapid diagnosis also facilitates prompt antimicrobial prophylaxis for contacts at risk of acquiring infection.

Some disadvantages are associated with antigen detection. First, the sensitivity or specificity of these assays is generally inferior to those of conventional, more time-consuming methods of direct visualization and culture. Antigen detection results may require confirmation by more sensitive or specific methods to exclude

TABLE 7–17. KOH Preparation

Place specimen into drop of 10–20% KOH on microscope slide.
Place coverslip on preparation and gently heat to just below boiling point.
After 5 min, examine preparation under conventional light microscope at ×100–500 for presence of fungal elements (usually hyphae).

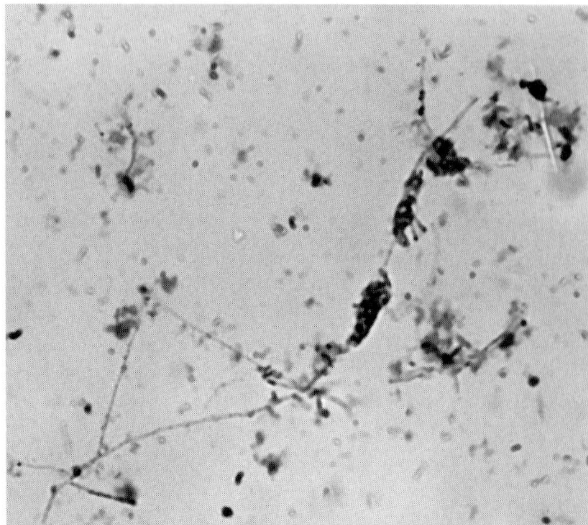

FIGURE 7–3. KOH preparation of skin scrapings containing a dermatophyte fungus.

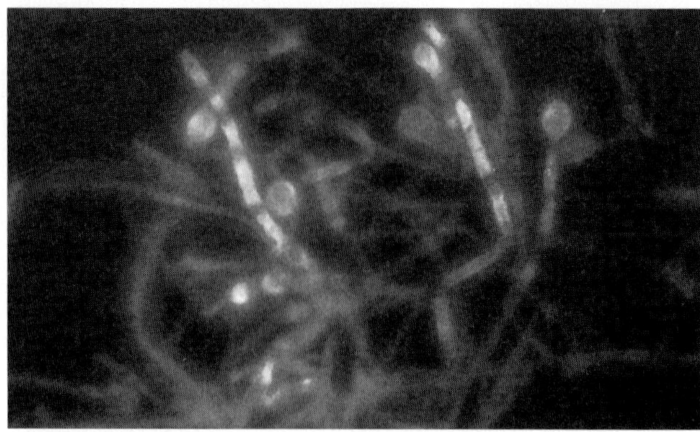

FIGURE 7–4. Calcofluor white–stained smear of skin scrapings containing *Candida albicans.* (From Tsieh Sun, American Society for Clinical Pathology.)

false-positive or false-negative results. Second, the cost of reagents for antigen detection assays is usually greater than that of the conventional tests. Cost is an important consideration, especially when large numbers of specimens need to be tested by both the rapid and confirmatory methods. Third, antigen detection results provide no guidance concerning the antimicrobial susceptibility of infectious agents. When an organism's antimicrobial susceptibility is unpredictable, specimens need to be cultured and isolates tested to obtain these results. Another significant disadvantage of the rapid antigen detection tests is the temptation to perform these tests on patients who would not otherwise have been tested by slower conventional methods. The relative convenience and ease of performance of these tests have encouraged their indiscriminate use, especially with assays configured in point-of-care of office laboratory testing formats. With inappropriate use, rapid antigen detection tests, in effect, become nothing more than screening tests, and positive results then require confirmation by more specific methods that entail extra costs and more time to complete.

Counterimmunoelectrophoresis. Counterimmunoelectrophoresis (CIE) tests were popular during the 1970s and early 1980s. Virtually all body fluids (CSF, serum, urine, synovial fluid, pleural fluid, pericardial fluid) are amenable to testing by CIE. Even sputa liquefied by treatment with disulfide bridge-breaking reagents like dithiothreitol or *N*-acetyl-L-cysteine can be tested. Antigens are detectable in the nanograms-per-milliliter range from *Haemophilus influenzae* type b, *Streptococcus pneumoniae, Neisseria meningitidis,* and group B *Streptococcus.*

The advantages of CIE are the rapidity of results and the potentially wide variety of specimens that could be tested. The disadvantages are the specialized electrophoresis equipment required for testing, lack of sensitivity compared to methods that were developed later, and inability of the standard assay to detect the capsular antigens of *S. pneumoniae* serotypes 7 and 14, two common pediatric serotypes. CIE is no longer widely used.

TABLE 7–18. Calcofluor White Staining Procedure

Flood specimen with drop of 0.1% calcofluor white M2R stain.
Place coverslip on mixture.
Examine slide under ultraviolet light–equipped microscope at ×100 magnification for presence of fluorescent fungal elements (usually hyphae).

Immunofluorescence. Microbiology laboratories commonly perform two types of immunofluorescence assays. **Direct immunofluorescence assay (DFA),** in which antibodies conjugated with a fluorescent dye react directly with antigens, is used only for antigen detection. **Indirect immunofluorescence assay (IFA),** in which antigens and antibodies initially react, followed by a second reaction with fluorescent dye conjugated antibodies directed against the immunoglobulin class of the first antibodies, is used for both antigen and antibody detection.

The advantages of immunofluorescence assays are the rapidity of results and the ability to assess the quality of the specimen while simultaneously identifying antigens. The disadvantages of these assays are the need for a microscope equipped with ultraviolet illumination, the inherent lack of sensitivity of assays that are read under a microscope, and the high level of skill required by microscopists to interpret results accurately.

Numerous immunofluorescence assays for detection of microbial antigens are in use today. Among the more common are those for *Chlamydia trachomatis, Legionella pneumophila, Bordetella pertussis, Giardia lamblia, Cryptosporidum parvum,* herpes simplex virus, varicella-zoster virus, cytomegalovirus, respiratory syncytial virus, influenza virus, parainfluenza virus, and adenovirus.

Latex Agglutination. The first easily performed assays for rapid detection of microbial antigens were based on latex agglutination (LA), a form of **particle agglutination** using latex beads. Many commercial kits are available for detection of groups A and B *Streptococcus, H. influenzae* type b, *S. pneumoniae* (multiple serotypes), *N. meningitidis* (multiple serogroups), *Escherichia coli* K1, *Cryptococcus neoformans,* and rotaviruses, among others. Specimens amenable to LA testing include urine and nonviscous body fluids and specimen extracts. Vicous specimens interfere with LA tests because of nonspecific clumping of latex particles.

TABLE 7–19. Methods for Rapid Detection of Bacterial and Fungal Antigens

Counterimmunoelectrophoresis
Direct or indirect immunofluorescence
Latex particle agglutination
Enzyme immunoassay
Immunochromatography
Optical immunoassay

Typical LA includes the use of two microscopic latex particle suspensions. The test latex is coated with antibodies directed against the antigen(s) being sought, and the other (control latex) is coated with nonspecific antibodies of the same immunoglobulin class used in the test latex. Positive results are indicated by agglutination of the test latex, but not the control latex, in less than 10 minutes. Assay sensitivities are superior to those of CIE and immunofluorescence.

Enzyme Immunoassay. Enzyme immunoassay (EIA), which produces colored reaction end points, became popular for detecting microbial antigens in the 1980s because of the difficulties some laboratories had in recognizing LA patterns consistently. Theoretically, EIA is at least an order of magnitude more sensitive than LA. The underlying principle of EIA involves attachment of antigen-capturing antibodies to a solid phase, such as a nitrocellulose membrane, a plastic dipstick, plastic beads, or the inner walls of a plastic tube or a microtiter tray well. The specimen is added, and after antigen binding by the capture antibodies, enzyme-conjugated detection antibodies are added. Substrate is then added to each reaction tube, and the newly formed capture antibody-antigen-detection antibody-conjugate complexes trigger conversion of colorless substrate to a colored end product that can be recognized with a spectrophotometer or in some cases with the unaided eye. EIA lends itself well to standardized, reproducible protocols that can be handled by automated or semiautomated instruments.

EIA can be configured to detect either antigens or antibodies. Antigen detection EIA tests currently available are numerous and include assays for groups A and B *Streptococcus, Chlamydia trachomatis, Neisseria gonorrhoeae, Helicobacter pylori, Campylobacter jejuni, Giardia lamblia, Cryptosporidium parvum,* HBsAg and HBeAg, rotavirus, respiratory syncytial virus, influenza virus, parainfluenza virus, adenovirus, herpes simplex virus, and human immunodeficiency virus-1.

Immunochromatography. One of the newer antigen detection assay types is immunochromatography, which is based on the reaction of a microbial antigen with antibodies conjugated to colored particles. The resultant immune complexes then flow (chromatograph) through the membrane to a reaction region coated with capture antibodies to the same microbial antigens. A positive signal is indicated by visible retention of the colored particles in the reaction region of the test device. The assay continues until the advancing front encounters a second set of capture antibodies directed against nonmicrobial components of the migrating particles. Assay completion is indicated by visible retention of the flowing particles in the quality control region of the test device. Antigen assays for detection of groups A and B *Streptococcus* are available in this format. Undoubtedly the list of antigen detection assays based on immunochromatography will increase with time. The chief advantage of the immunochromatographic method is its simplicity.

Optical Immunoassay. The newest antigen detection assay format is optical immunoassay (OIA), a name designated by the assay manufacturer. This technique depends on optically coated silicon wafers to which are attached capture antibodies directed against the microbial antigens of interest. Specimens are applied to the surface of the wafers and washed off, and the wafers are examined under bright light. The appearance of a purple reaction zone superimposed on a gold background is evidence of a positive reaction. OIA tests for detecting antigens of groups A and B *Streptococcus, C. trachomatis,* and influenza A and B viruses are commercially available. Similar to immunochromatography, the major advantages of OIA are the simplicity and rapidity of the assay, with results available in 5–21 minutes. Moreover, the OIA method appears able to detect smaller quantities of antigen than any of the other rapid antigen assays.

Detection of Bacterial Toxins

Many infectious microorganisms produce metabolic products that are toxic to the host. Toxins may be produced within the host at the site of infection, by organisms such as *Corynebacterium diphtheriae, Clostridium difficile, Clostridium tetani, Vibrio cholerae,* and *E. coli* O157:H7, or produced externally and then ingested by the host by organisms such as *Clostridium botulinum, Staphylococcus aureus,* and *Bacillus cereus.*

The biochemical bases of toxin action are diverse; they include inhibition of host cell protein synthesis by *C. diphtheriae* toxin and interference with acetylcholine release by *C. botulinum* toxin. Some internally produced toxins, such as toxin A of *C. difficile,* exert their effects locally at the site of toxin production, and others, such as tetanus toxin of *C. tetani,* act systemically. Some microbial toxins are cytotoxic and can be demonstrated by inoculation of specimens in cell cultures. For example, the toxins produced by hemorrhagic *E. coli* are readily demonstrable by inoculation of stool extracts to African green monkey kidney cells.

Clostridium difficile. *C. difficile* **cytotoxin (toxin B)** synthesis correlates highly with production of an **enterotoxin (toxin A)** that is responsible for enterocolitis. The toxin can be detected in stool extracts inoculated to one of several cell culture lines. Performance of the *C. difficile* cytotoxin assay requires bacteria-free stool extracts, appropriate cell culture lines, such as WI-38 human diploid lung fibroblasts, and *C. difficile, Clostridium sordellii,* or gas gangrene polyvalent antitoxin. Specimen extracts are added to individual cell culture tubes and incubated at 35°C, and the cells are examined microscopically for cytopathic effect after 4, 24, and 48 hours of incubation. A positive result is indicated by observing the cytopathic effect (e.g., rounding of the cells).

Several companies have developed commercial EIAs for *C. difficile* toxin A or toxin B or both. These assays are faster to perform and can be adapted to automated or semiautomated equipment. Even faster than the conventional EIA are a group of membrane-bound color end point immunoassays that detect *C. difficile* toxin A or *C. difficile* common antigen (glutamate dehydrogenase) in stool specimens. These assays appear to be less sensitive than EIA but provide results in as little as 15 minutes.

Positive results of *C. difficile* toxin A and toxin B assays in adults correlate highly with each other and with sigmoidoscopic evidence of *C. difficile*–associated enterocolitis. Similar results in children less than 1 year of age, however, must be interpreted carefully. Culture of stools from infants may be positive for both *C. difficile* and cytotoxin, even though the infants have no symptoms and there may be no histologic evidence of *C. difficile*–associated enterocolitis.

Clostridium botulinum. Only a handful of laboratories today maintain animal colonies necessary for detection of certain toxins, such as botulism toxins. Testing is usually referred to a centralized reference laboratory for confirmation of foodborne, wound, and infant botulism. All these tests require demonstration of neutralizable botulinum antitoxin in serum, stool, or gastric contents. The **suckling mouse assay** is still the assay method of choice.

Escherichia coli. Enterotoxigenic strains of *E. coli* are one of the major causes of traveler's diarrhea. The disease results from the action of two toxins of *E. coli,* **heat-labile (LT) enterotoxin** and **heat-stable (ST) enterotoxin,** on the mucosal epithelium of the small intestine. LT is similar in structure and activity to the cholera toxin of *Vibrio cholerae.* Biologic assays for the toxins include the **rabbit ileal loop assay** for LT and the **suckling mouse assay** for ST, but they are rarely performed in clinical laboratories. Immunoassays for both toxin types have been developed and are mostly available from reference laboratories.

Enterohemorrhagic *E. coli* organisms are the primary cause of hemorrhagic enterocolitis and hemolytic-uremic syndrome. Member strains of more than a dozen serotypes of *E. coli* have been shown to be capable of producing the **Shiga-like toxins (SLT I and II;** also known as **Vero toxin**) responsible for the disease, but most cases and outbreaks of infection in the United States have been associated with ***E. coli* serotype O157:H7.** SLT-1 is virtually identical to the **Shiga toxin** produced by *Shigella dysenteriae.* Both a biologic assay, the **Vero cell assay,** and several EIA tests have been developed for detection of SLT I and II. The latter assays are being performed by increasing numbers of hospital laboratories, particularly those in hospitals serving large numbers of pediatric patients.

CULTURE

Culture is still the definitive means for diagnosis of most infections. Liquid and solid growth media are available for cultivation of many bacteria and fungi. Cell culture lines for propogation of many viruses and chlamydiae are also available. Live animals may be inoculated to detect microorganisms not readily grown in vitro.

Types of Artificial Culture Media. Three categories of liquid and solid growth media are in common use: nonselective, selective, and differential (Table 7–20). **Nonselective media** are used most often and support the growth of a wide variety of microorganisms, usually at rapid growth rates. **Selective media** are intended to inhibit growth of all but a selected group of organisms. The growth-restrictive conditions may be due to the pH of the media (e.g., acidic pH of Sabouraud dextrose agar), the presence of growth-inhibitory chemicals in the media (e.g., high NaCl content of mannitol salt agar), or the presence of antimicrobial agents in the media (e.g., vancomycin, colistin, and nystatin in modified Thayer-Martin agar). **Differential media** reveal phenotypic characteristics of organisms that aid in their identification (e.g., determination of lactose-fermenting ability in MacConkey agar). Media frequently belong to more than one category (e.g., 5% sheep blood agar is both a nonselective and a differential medium; MacConkey agar is both a differential and a selective medium).

TABLE 7–20. Examples of Artificial Culture Media

Nonselective Media: Growth of Wide Variety of Microorganisms
5% Sheep blood agar
Chocolate agar
Mueller-Hinton broth/agar
Trypticase soy broth
Selective Media: Growth of Selected Groups of Microorganisms
Streptococcal selective agar (groups A and B *Streptococcus*)
Mannitol salt agar (*Staphylococcus*)
MacConkey agar (gram-negative bacilli)
Thayer-Martin agar (pathogenic *Neisseria*)
Differential Media: Differential Growth of Groups of Microorganisms
5% Sheep blood agar (α-, β-, and γ-hemolysis)
Mannitol salt agar (mannitol fermentation)
MacConkey agar (lactose fermentation)
Triple sugar iron agar (glucose, lactose, and sucrose fermentation, H_2S production, H_2 production)

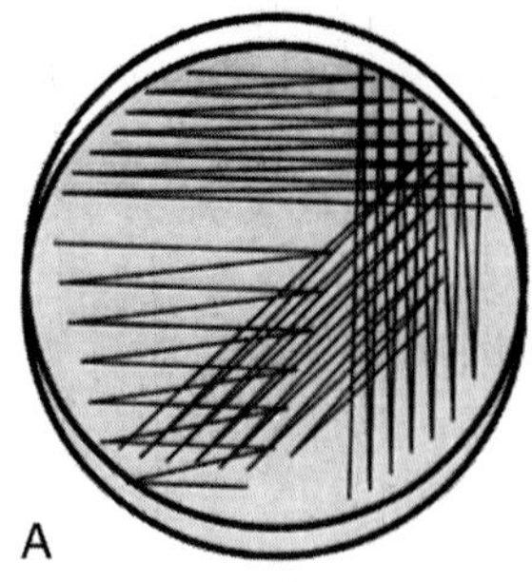

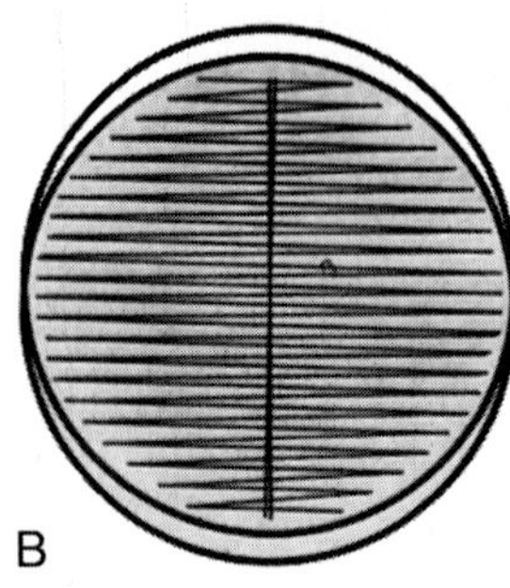

FIGURE 7–5. A, Four-quadrant streaking method for obtaining isolated colonies on agar culture media. **B,** Colony-count streaking method for obtaining estimates of the organism's viable count in clinical specimens.

The list of growth media from which to choose when one is inoculating bacterial cultures is almost endless. Most laboratories select their media according to the site of specimen collection unless detection of specific pathogens has been requested. The pathogens most likely to be recovered from specific body sites dictate the medium or combination of media that are inoculated. Thus the personnel collecting specimens must identify the source of the material sent to the laboratory and indicate whether unusual pathogens are suspected, so that suitable growth media are inoculated.

Most agar media are inoculated by using the **four-quadrant streaking method** (Fig. 7–5, *A*) to obtain well-isolated colonies. If quantitative results are desired (e.g., for urine cultures), the **colony-count streaking method** (Fig. 7–5, *B*) can be used. Agar media in tubes are inoculated by streaking the specimen onto the slanted agar surface, stabbing the inoculum into the agar itself, or both. Liquid culture media in tubes or bottles are inoculated by introducing the specimen directly into the broth.

The standard incubation temperature for bacterial cultures is 35–37°C. Other incubation temperatures are used when circumstances warrant (e.g., 42°C to culture *Campylobacter jejuni*). The incubation atmosphere for aerobic blood or chocolate agar cultures should be supplemented with 5–10% carbon dioxide. Growth of most aerobic bacteria is stimulated by additional carbon dioxide, and several important pathogens (e.g., *Neisseria gonorrhoeae*) may not grow without added carbon dioxide. Differential media that display color differences because of pH changes (e.g., MacConkey agar and mannitol salt agar) should be incubated in an unsupplemented atmosphere to prevent acidification of the media by added carbon dioxide. Reduced oxygen tension is necessary for growth of microaerophilic bacteria such as *C. jejuni.*

The incubation period varies with the group of pathogens being cultured. In general, agar media are held for 48–72 hours and enrichment broth media for 1–14 days. If slow-growing, fastidious pathogens are suspected in a specimen, the laboratory should extend the incubation time of cultures appropriately. The cost-effectiveness of inoculating enrichment broth media is dubious, and their use should be discouraged for most specimen types. The inclusion of a broth capable of growing *Propionibacterium acnes* from CSF collected from persons with central nervous system shunts is a notable exception.

Anaerobic Cultures. Anaerobic infections occur infrequently in children. Nonetheless, all microbiology laboratories must be prepared to process pediatric specimens for anaerobic culture. Specimens must not have been collected from body sites ordinarily colonized with anaerobes and must have been transported to the laboratory in a manner consistent with the survival of anaerobes. After these requirements have been met, it is the laboratory's responsibility to use culture methods that maximize detection of anaerobes.

Some laboratories **prereduce** their anaerobic culture media before use by overnight storage in an oxygen-free atmosphere. The purpose is to remove dissolved oxygen from the media and eliminate potentially lethal exposure of anaerobes to oxygen early in incubation.

Culture media should contain sufficient amounts of vitamin K and hemin to satisfy the growth requirements of fastidious *Prevotella* and *Porphyromonas.* Selective media containing kanamycin and vancomycin should be inoculated to promote recovery of *Bacteroides fragilis*–group organisms, which are likely to exhibit penicillin resistance and require alternative therapy. *B. fragilis*–group colonies can be difficult to detect otherwise, since positive cultures often are mixed with facultative anaerobes.

The pigmented members of *Prevotella* and *Porphyromonas,* another group that may be penicillin resistant, are best detected by growth on media containing **laked blood,** which are media with blood lysed by repeated freeze-thaw cycles. Young colonies on these media typically display brick red fluorescence under long-wave ultraviolet illumination, whereas older colonies exhibit visible black melanin pigment. A set of aerobically incubated media should be inoculated along with the anaerobically incubated media to permit side-by-side comparison of culture results from the same specimens. Facultative and oxygen-tolerant anaerobes should grow on both sets of media, whereas obligate anaerobes should grow only on the anaerobically incubated media. Anaerobic cultures should be incubated at 35–37°C. Because obligate anaerobes usually grow at slower rates than other bacteria, culture plates should be incubated for at least 5 days.

An anaerobic environment for incubation can be created in the laboratory in several ways. For example, either an air-tight, oxygen-free enclosure **(anaerobic glove box),** complete with a self-contained incubator, or a gas-tight container in which the original ambient atmosphere has been replaced with an oxygen-free gas mixture or in which the oxygen has been chemically removed can be used. Cultures do not have to be inoculated within an oxygen-free enclosure to obtain clinically relevant results. In fact, most laboratories that handle primarily pediatric specimens cannot justify the cost of an oxygen-free enclosure because of the low numbers of anaerobic cultures processed. After inoculation, however, culture media should be placed in an anaerobic environment immediately. Commercially available anaerobic jars and heat-sealable plastic bags are popular, cost-effective alternatives to anaerobic glove boxes for laboratories today.

Chlamydia. Chlamydiae are obligate intracellular parasites that are not able to grow on artificial culture media. Accordingly, cultures of chlamydiae must be inoculated to living cells, either monolayers of replicating cells derived from humans or other animals, or to an animal itself, such as an embryonated egg or infant mouse. Culture for *C. trachomatis* is becoming less frequently available from clinical microbiology laboratories. Most laboratories today prefer the antigen detection or nucleic acid probe method. *C. psittaci* and *C. pneumoniae* are difficult to grow in the laboratory, and diagnosis of infections is usually based on serologic testing. Specimens for *C. trachomatis* culture should be placed in *Chlamydia* transport medium (e.g., 2-sucrose phosphate) immediately after collection. In the laboratory, specimens are inoculated into a suitable cell culture line, such as cycloheximide-treated McCoy cell cultures, by centrifugation of specimens onto the cells. The shell vial culture format is ideal for *C. trachomatis.* After 48–72 hours of incubation at 35°C, cultures are examined for the presence of inclusion bodies by staining with Giemsa, iodine, or immunofluorescence reagents. Cell cultures with negative results after 72 hours of incubation can be blindly passed by processing them in a vortex mixer in the presence of glass beads and then reinoculating the supernatant into fresh cell cultures. The yield of positive culture results can be increased by as much as 10% by blind passage.

Mycoplasma. Mycoplasmas are the smallest free-living microorganisms known. Because they lack cell walls, they are exquisitely sensitive to osmotic changes in their environment. Three species in particular are currently considered to be human pathogens: *M. pneumoniae, M. hominis,* and *Ureaplasma urealyticum.* Culture media for mycoplasmas must be isotonic to protect them from lysis and nutritionally rich to meet their fastidious growth requirements. SP-4 glucose broth/agar and Shepard's 10B urea broth/A8 agar are recommended. They contain sodium chloride or glucose as osmotic stabilizers and horse serum, yeast extract, or fetal bovine serum as sources of necessary nutrients. Broth cultures should be incubated at 37°C in an ambient atmosphere, and agar cultures should be incubated at 37°C in an aerobic atmosphere containing 5% carbon dioxide.

Specimens for *M. pneumoniae* culture should be inoculated to SP-4 glucose broth or agar media or both. Broth cultures demonstrating color change should be subcultured to fresh broth and to agar media. Colonies displaying the "fried egg" morphologic picture typical of *M. pneumoniae* usually become evident after 8–15 days. Cultures negative for *M. pneumoniae* should be incubated for 28 days before being discarded.

U. urealyticum cultures should be inoculated into Shepard's 10B urea broth initially and examined twice daily for color changes indicative of urea splitting. Frequent examinations are important because survival of *Ureaplasma* in the alkaline environment created during their growth is short-lived. Broth undergoing color change should be subcultured immediately to agar media to confirm the presence of *U. urealyticum.* Broth cultures should be incubated for 7 days before being discarded as negative for the organism.

The same media used for *M. pneumoniae* or *U. urealyticum* cultures can also be used for *M. hominis* provided extra arginine is present. *M. hominis* grows somewhat slower than *U. urealyticum* in broth but more rapidly than *M. pneumoniae* on agar, with colonies becoming apparent after 2–5 days of incubation. Cultures negative for *M. hominis* should be held for 7 days before being discarded as negative for the organism.

Mycobacteria. Mycobacteria are obligate aerobes that differ from other bacteria in the acid fastness of their cell walls and, in most instances, their slow growth rate. Except for the Runyon group 4 species, clinically important mycobacteria form visible colonies on solid media only after 2–8 weeks of incubation. Because of the extended incubation periods required, precautions must be taken to avoid deterioration of media and overgrowth of cultures by other microorganisms. Solid media are frequently prepared in screw-capped tubes to prevent dehydration. Solid media in Petri plates must be sealed or stored in high-humidity environments to maintain their moisture content during incubation. The media themselves are highly selective for mycobacteria. This feature, combined with the use of one of the specimen-decontamination procedures described earlier, prevents most instances of culture overgrowth.

Several selective media for growth of mycobacteria are available (Table 7–21). Solid media include (1) opaque, inspissated, egg-based media (e.g., **Lowenstein-Jensen medium**) that contain no agar and (2) clear, agar-based media (e.g., **Middlebrook-Cohn 7H10 or 7H11 agar**) that should not be exposed to light because the formaldehyde that is generated could kill the mycobacteria.

TABLE 7–21. Commonly Used Mycobacterial Culture Media

Medium	Purpose
Lowenstein-Jensen medium	Primary culture for most mycobacteria
Middlebrook 7H10 or 7H11 agar	Primary culture for most mycobacteria
Middlebrook 7H9 broth	Primary culture for most mycobacteria from sterile body sites

The agar-based media tend to yield earlier positive results, but the egg-based media tend to furnish positive results more often. Media supplemented with blood or a chocolate-blood mixture is necessary to grow *M. haemophilum.* Laboratories that elect to use solid growth media should inoculate specimens into both types of media. Supplemental inoculation of broth media (e.g., **Dubos Tween albumin** or **7H9 broth**) may increase culture yields when specimens are processed from ordinarily sterile body sites.

Mycobacterial cultures should be incubated aerobically at 35–37°C in an atmosphere enriched with 5–10% carbon dioxide. Cutaneous lesion and bone aspirate cultures should include a second set of media incubated at 30–32°C to permit growth of *M. marinum, M. ulcerans,* and *M. haemophilum* because these species may not grow at higher temperatures. Cultures on solid media should be held for at least 8 weeks before a negative report is issued.

Use of carbon 14–labeled substrates in broth media for detection of mycobacterial growth has been successful in many laboratories. The principle is that growing mycobacteria release ^{14}C-labeled CO_2 as a metabolic by-product that can be detected radiometrically by sampling the gas in the headspace of the culture vessel. Although this method is laborious, experience has shown that it significantly reduces the time to detection of positive culture results compared with growth on solid media.

Recently, automated systems that continuously monitor for growth of mycobacteria in proprietary broth media have been introduced. Unlike the radiometric method described herein, these systems do not require manual transfer of cultures from an incubator to a reading instrument, nor are there radioisotopes in the culture media that may require specialized disposal. These systems monitor the liquid media for growth by detecting oxygen consumption or carbon dioxide production. Similar to the radiometric method, the automated systems shorten the time to detection of positive culture results. They also eliminate much of the laboratory staff time associated with use of manual culture methods.

Laboratories that grow mycobacterial cultures should at least be able to presumptively identify acid-fast isolates as members of the *M. tuberculosis* complex. The minimum steps in the process include demonstrating that isolates are acid-fast and determining whether isolates produce niacin from egg-based media and are capable of reducing NO_3 to NO_2. *M. tuberculosis* is capable of reducing both niacin and nitrate. Alternatively, laboratories may use commercially available DNA probes to identify an isolate as a member of the ***M. tuberculosis* complex,** composed of *M. tuberculosis, M. bovis,* and *M. africanum.*

Fungi. A large percentage of clinically significant fungal isolates are yeasts that grow equally well on bacterial or fungal culture media. Many clinically significant molds, particularly those which cause opportunistic infections in immunocompromised persons, grow rapidly on bacterial culture media. Fungal cultures are intended for yeasts or molds that might otherwise be overgrown by faster-growing bacteria on routine culture media. Fungal cultures also are incubated for longer periods and therefore allow detection of growth that might not be visibly evident at the end of the routine culture incubation period.

Bacterial growth on nonselective culture media can easily mask the presence of fungi. Selective fungal culture media inhibit the growth of bacteria either because of a low pH (e.g., **Sabouraud dextrose agar**) or because of the action of antimicrobial agents (e.g., chloramphenicol and gentamicin) added to the medium (Table 7–22). Accordingly, the yield of positive culture results from sites harboring bacterial flora is greater from selective fungal media than from nonselective culture media.

Other features that distinguish fungal from routine bacterial cultures are the incubation temperature and the duration of incubation. Many clinically important fungi do not grow at standard incubator temperatures (35–37°C) or form visible colonies within standard incubation periods (24–72 hours).

Routine fungal cultures should be inoculated into at least one medium lacking antimicrobial agents (e.g., Sabouraud dextrose agar). They should also be inoculated into another medium containing antibacterial agents (e.g., chloramphenicol and gentamicin) and an antifungal agent (e.g., cycloheximide). Cycloheximide prevents the growth of many environmental airborne fungi that occasionally contaminate fungal cultures. If a systemic dimorphic fungal infection is suspected (e.g., histoplasmosis, blastomycosis, or coccidioidomycosis), then a nutritionally enriched medium containing 5–10% sheep blood should be inoculated to obtain more rapid growth.

At least one of these culture media should support the growth of virtually all clinically significant fungi. Requests for culture of the few fungi that call for special media (e.g., media for *M. furfur* that require an exogenous source of medium chain to long chain fatty acids) require notification of the mycology laboratory. Another point to remember is that a few important fungal pathogens (e.g., *Cryptococcus neoformans, Scedosporium apiospermum*) cannot grow on cycloheximide-containing media. Thus at least one cycloheximide-free medium should be inoculated with each culture.

Cultures for body surface **dermatophyte** fungi should be incubated at 25–30°C for growth of fungi inhibited by temperatures of 35–37°C. A second set of cultures may be incubated at the higher temperature to hasten the growth of heat-tolerant fungi. Routine fungal cultures should be incubated for at least 3 weeks because many agents that cause dermatophytic, subcutaneous, or systemic infections may grow slowly. When only rapidly growing yeasts or molds are being sought, 5 days of incubation at 35–37°C is sufficient.

When cultures are positive for fungi, preliminary identification of isolates is accomplished by recognizing macroscopic and micro-

TABLE 7–22. Commonly Used Fungal Culture Media*

Medium	Purpose
Sabouraud dextrose agar	Primary culture for most fungi
Inhibitory mold agar	Primary culture for most fungi
Brain-heart infusion agar with added blood and antibiotics	Primary culture for accelerated growth of cycloheximide-resistant fungi
Corn meal agar	Secondary culture for induction of sporulation
Potato dextrose agar	Secondary culture for induction of sporulation

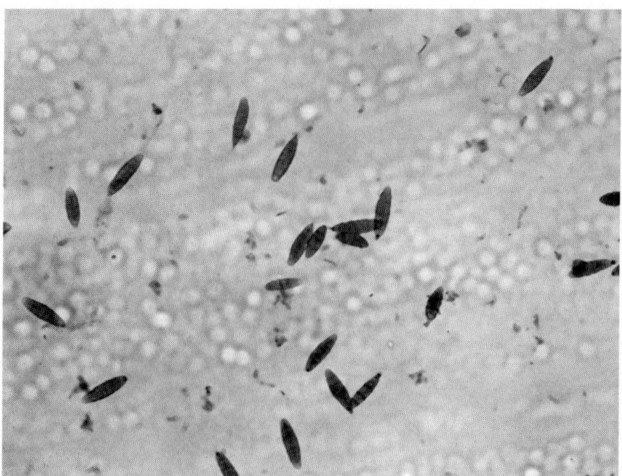

FIGURE 7–6. Macroconidia of *Microsporum canis.*

scopic morphologic features. Yeasts should be tested for production of germ tubes in serum or plasma after incubation at 35–37°C for 2–3 hours. Germ tubes are small-diameter, cylindrical, nonseptate appendages to yeast cells. Of the yeasts, only *Candida albicans, Candida stellatoidea,* and *Candida dubliniensis* produce germ tubes under the standard assay conditions. An alternative rapid test used by laboratories for presumptive identification of *C. albicans* is detection of both L-proline aminopeptidase and β-galactosaminidase enzymatic activities. This assay can be completed in 30 minutes and does not require skill at recognizing microscopic morphologic features. Definitive identification of commonly encountered yeasts requires microscopic examination for the morphologic features of hyphae, pseudohyphae and conidia, as well as assessment of biochemical test parameters (e.g., sugar assimilation and fermentation, urease and nitrate reduction tests). Filamentous fungi should be examined in lactophenol cotton blue wet mounts for characteristic conidial or sporangial structures (Fig. 7–6). Preparation of tease mounts from colonies grown on primary culture media may be unrewarding. In this case the laboratory should prepare coverslip slide cultures on starvation media such as potato dextrose or cornmeal agar.

ANTIMICROBIAL SUSCEPTIBILITY TESTING

Determination of the antimicrobial susceptibility of pathogenic microorganisms is one of the most important functions of the microbiology laboratory, especially in the case of microorganisms that do not have predictable susceptibility to antimicrobial agents. Results guide clinicians in selecting antimicrobial therapy. The selected regimen frequently replaces more expensive, empirically chosen, broad-spectrum antimicrobial agents that may cause undesirable side effects when administered for more than a few days.

Approved standards published by the **National Committee for Clinical Laboratory Standards (NCCLS)** exist only for testing rapidly growing aerobic bacteria, anaerobic bacteria, and yeasts. Several antimicrobial susceptibility methods for testing bacteria are in current use (Table 7–23). A method for testing *M. tuberculosis* has received tentative status, and methods for testing conidium-forming filamentous fungi and viruses have received proposed status. Methods for testing parasites and other infectious agents have not yet been standardized. The reproducibility of results from the same laboratory and the comparability of results from different laboratories for these microorganisms should not be assumed. Further, all antimicrobial susceptibility test results are obtained in an artificial laboratory environment that is very different from the host environment. It should not be assumed that laboratory results accurately predict clinical responses in patients.

Agar Diffusion. The agar diffusion test is still widely performed today. The advantages of this method over the others include a greater flexibility in selecting antimicrobial agents to test, the relative ease with which mixed cultures are detected, and the lower cost of test materials.

In the **Kirby-Bauer** version of the disk diffusion test, an exponentially growing broth culture or suspension prepared from overnight agar culture is used as an inoculum. The density of the inoculum is adjusted to match a McFarland 0.5 turbidity standard. Bacteria are inoculated with a saturated Dacron/rayon swab onto Mueller-Hinton agar plates, which may be supplemented with defibrinated sheep blood for growth of fastidious organisms. *Haemophilus* test medium (HTM) is used instead of Mueller-Hinton agar for testing *Haemophilus* species. Filter paper disks (maximum of 12 disks per 150 mm diameter plate) impregnated with standard quantities of antimicrobial agents are applied to the agar surface, and plates are incubated for 16–18 hours at 35°C in an ambient atmosphere. The use of a CO_2-enriched atmosphere is contraindicated because of the effects of an acidic medium pH on the activities of some antimicrobial agents, although carbon dioxide supplementation is permissible for bacteria that require it for growth.

Antimicrobial agents diffuse into the agar and quickly establish moving concentration gradients. Within the first few hours of incubation, the interactions between the changing concentrations of the antimicrobial agents and the increasing numbers of bacteria determine the diameters of the zones of growth inhibition that will form later around each disk. The zone diameters are measured and interpreted by using the NCCLS reference tables. The tables list breakpoints that assign zone diameters to susceptible (S), intermediately susceptible (I), and resistant (R) categories.

The disk diffusion method is intended for testing bacteria that grow rapidly on Mueller-Hinton agar. Virtually every factor that affects test results has been studied and addressed by the NCCLS standardized procedure. For certain fastidious bacteria (e.g., *Haemophilus, N. gonorrhoeae, Streptococcus*), deviations from the standardized procedure have been authorized by the NCCLS to enable testing.

The **E-Test** is a variant of the disk diffusion test that also provides quantitative MIC susceptibility results. Calibrated plastic strips coated with antimicrobial agent gradients are placed on the surface of inoculated agar media (maximum of six strips per 150 mm diameter plate). The point of intersection between the elliptical zone of growth inhibition and the calibrated strip establishes the antimicrobial agent's MIC. The E-Test has proved most useful for testing fastidious and anaerobic bacteria versus a limited number of antimicrobial agents.

TABLE 7–23. Antimicrobial Susceptibility Test Methods for Bacteria

- Broth dilution (MIC, MBC determination)
- Agar dilution (MIC determination)
- Agar diffusion (Kirby-Bauer disk diffusion, E test)
- Nonroutine tests
  - β-Lactamase assay
  - Anaerobic susceptibility testing
  - Antimicrobial agent synergy testing
  - Body fluid bactericidal activity determination

Broth Dilution. The reference method for antimicrobial susceptibility testing is the broth dilution method, which provides quantitative susceptibility results, is adaptable to measuring both inhibitory and bactericidal activities, and is suitable for miniaturization and automation. The latter feature has led to the development of instruments that furnish antimicrobial susceptibility data in as little as 4 hours.

The **minimum inhibitory concentration (MIC)** of an antimicrobial agent is the lowest concentration tested that inhibits visible growth of the microorganism. Knowledge of an antimicrobial agent's MIC, the routes of administration, and the levels of antimicrobial agents achievable at various body sites enables laboratories to categorize microorganisms as **susceptible (S), intermediately susceptible (I),** or **resistant (R).**

An antimicrobial agent's MIC can be determined according to NCCLS standardized procedures by several methods. One approach is to inoculate microorganism suspensions into tubes of growth media supplemented with stepwise increases of antimicrobial agent concentrations. The MIC can be determined similarly in a miniaturized format (e.g., within the wells of microtiter trays or within tiny chambers inside a clear plastic card). In either case, microorganism suspensions are prepared and matched to a turbidity standard. The final inoculum is prepared by diluting standard suspensions to yield final cell densities of 5×10^5 cfu/mL. Cultures are incubated for 16–20 hours at 35°C in an atmosphere appropriate for microorganism growth. MICs are determined by visual or photometric examination of the tubes, wells, or chambers for turbidity indicating microbial growth.

The **minimum bactericidal concentration (MBC)** of an antimicrobial agent is the lowest concentration tested that kills at least 99.9% of the original inoculum. Nonturbid tubes or wells from an MIC determination are subcultured to agar media to determine the number of viable microorganisms remaining after exposure to antimicrobial agents for 16–20 hours. If the number of survivors is ≤0.1% of the original inoculum, killing has occurred. Knowledge of antimicrobial MBCs is not routinely necessary to the selection of appropriate therapy for infections. Because the bactericidal properties of antimicrobial agents are predictable against most microorganisms, qualitative disk diffusion or quantitative MIC results are generally sufficient for the selection of successful therapy.

The bactericidal properties of some antimicrobial agents against staphylococci and streptococci are not always predictable because of the phenomenon known as antimicrobial **tolerance.** The physiologic basis of tolerance is greatly diminished autolytic enzyme activity in bacteria that have ceased cell wall synthesis. Autolytic enzyme activity is a normal component of *de novo* cell wall synthesis. Bacteria are usually killed by agents that inhibit cell wall synthesis, because excessive weakening of the existing cell wall is a result of continuing autolytic enzyme activity. If this activity is missing, the bacteria are not killed, even though cell wall synthesis has terminated.

The definition of tolerance for *Staphylococcus, Streptococcus,* and *Enterococcus* is an MBC:MIC ratio ≥32. With truly tolerant bacteria, the antimicrobial agent MIC is used to indicate susceptibility and the MBC is used to indicate the level of resistance. Although this concept is controversial, the clinical correlation between tolerance in the laboratory and therapeutic outcome has been close enough to convince many clinicians to alter their choice of antimicrobial therapy when tolerance has been reported.

Agar Dilution. The agar dilution method for determining an antimicrobial agent's MIC is particularly well suited to testing large groups of bacteria versus identical ranges of antimicrobial agent concentrations. An antimicrobial agent's MBC cannot be determined by agar dilution. According to the NCCLS standard agar dilution method, bacterial suspensions are prepared and matched to a turbidity standard. The suspensions are diluted to facilitate transfer of approximately 1×10^4 bacteria to agar media by means of a calibrated loop or a multitipped device like the Steers replicator. The inocula are approximately 1–2 μL to facilitate rapid absorption into the agar. Culture plates are incubated at 35°C for 16–20 hours in an aerobic atmosphere lacking added carbon dioxide. The MIC is the lowest antimicrobial concentration that inhibits visible growth on the agar surface; a barely visible haze of growth or the growth of a single colony is ignored.

Actinomycetes. Antimicrobial susceptibility testing of **actinomycetes** is not standardized and is rarely performed because of the relative lack of resistance of these microorganisms to first-line antimicrobial agents.

Mycobacteria. The reference susceptibility test method uses antimicrobial agents eluted from filter paper disks immersed in solid growth medium to yield uniform concentrations of each agent. After inoculation and suitable incubation, the number of colonies growing on antimicrobial agent–containing agar is compared with the number growing on a control agar that is free of antimicrobial agents. If the number of colonies on the treated agar is <1% of the number on the control agar, then the isolate is reported as susceptible. Colony numbers >1% of the control indicate resistance. More rapid methods for obtaining antimycobacterial susceptibility results, although not yet standardized by NCCLS, are increasing in popularity. They involve the use of the radiometric or nonradiometric broth culture monitoring systems. Isolates are inoculated into antimicrobial agent–containing broth media, and the rate of growth is compared with that in antimicrobial agent–free broth. Slower growth rates in antimicrobial agent–containing broth media indicate susceptibility, and similar growth rates suggest resistance.

Fungi. Although broth dilution, agar dilution, and disk diffusion procedures for fungal susceptibility testing have been described, only the broth dilution method has been designated by the NCCLS as a reference method for testing yeasts and filamentous fungi. The list of antifungal agents deemed suitable for testing is limited, however. Results with agents not on the list are not standardized and may not be accurate because of problems inherent with the test methods themselves.

Special Testing of Antimicrobial Agents

Occasionally, clinical circumstances warrant the performance of nonroutine tests involving antimicrobial agents. The laboratory's response to these situations depends on the complexity of the testing and the staffing and capability of the laboratory. Laboratories that are unable to perform such tests usually refer them to a regional or national reference laboratory for testing.

β-Lactamase Testing. The most common mechanism of resistance affecting the penicillins, cephalosporins, cephamycins, monobactams, and carbapenems is the production of one or more β-lactamases, which are enzymes that inactivate certain of these agents by hydrolyzing the β-lactam ring present in all of them (Fig. 7–3).

The β-lactamase test rapidly establishes whether isolates produce these enzymes. However, bacteria may be resistant to these agents by mechanisms other than β-lactamase production. Although positive results indicate bacterial resistance to the enzyme-labile agents in the group, negative results do not ensure susceptibility.

β-Lactamase tests are performed by exposing isolates to enzyme substrates for periods ranging between 10 seconds and 60 minutes (the time is dependent on the microorganism and the substrate). Three methods are in general use: the acidimetric method, the iodometric method, and the chromogenic cephalosporin method. The latter has emerged as the most satisfactory method and is in general use.

In the **chromogenic cephalosporin method,** nitrocefin and cefesone are chromogenic cephalosporins that are susceptible to the action of β-lactamases and that change color on hydrolysis of their β-lactam rings. These tests can be performed in liquid or on filter paper and involve exposing the test isolate to the buffered chromogenic substrate. After a suitable incubation period (up to 60 minutes for *Staphylococcus*), the substrate is examined for a color change. The method has been shown to produce accurate positive results with anaerobic gram-negative bacilli, *Enterococcus, Haemophilus, Moraxella catarrhalis, N. gonorrhoeae,* and *Staphylococcus.* Positive results indicate resistance to the penicillinase-labile penicillins, including ampicillin, amoxicillin, azlocillin, carbenicillin, mezlocillin, piperacillin, and ticarcillin.

Anaerobic Susceptibility Testing. Under most circumstances, β-lactamase testing of anaerobic gram-negative bacilli is all that is necessary to facilitate management of anaerobic infections with antimicrobial agents. However, laboratories located in regions that have had high rates of penicillin (not mediated by β-lactamase), cefoxitin, clindamycin, or metronidazole resistance in anaerobes should consider providing more comprehensive susceptibility data. The reference method for anaerobic susceptibility testing is based on the NCCLS agar dilution MIC method. Adaptations of the broth dilution and E-Test MIC methods for obtaining results from anaerobes have also been described but have not yet been standardized by the NCCLS. Periodic surveys of antimicrobial resistance in anaerobes are recommended to detect trends toward increasing resistance.

Antimicrobial Synergy Testing. Simultaneous administration of two or more antimicrobial agents results in additive, antagonistic, or synergistic effects in patients (Fig. 7–7). **Additive effects** are evident when the observed activity of a combination of antimicrobials approximates the sum of the activities exhibited by the agents individually. **Antagonistic effects** result when the activity of the combination is markedly less than the sum of the individual activities. **Synergistic effects** result when the activity of the combination is markedly greater than the sum of the individual activities. Clinicians usually rely on the published experience of investigators to predict the efficacy of antimicrobial combinations. On rare occasions, however, testing of antimicrobial combinations against patient isolates may be necessary to guide therapy with antimicrobial agents. Such testing is difficult, time-consuming, and expensive and should be reserved for situations in which results are truly necessary.

Synergy testing via the **checkerboard titration method** is usually performed in microtiter trays. MICs of two antimicrobial agents are determined individually and in combination by testing isolates versus stepwise concentrations of the agents alone and versus all possible concentration combinations of the agents together. Synergy is reported when the MIC of one or both agents is reduced at least a factor of 4 in the presence of subinhibitory concentrations of the other agent.

The **killing curve synergy test** method is performed in broth culture. The viability of organisms after exposure to antimicrobial agents alone is compared with that after exposure to the same antimicrobial agents in combination. Killing curves are constructed by plotting the log of the number of surviving bacteria in each culture with time. Synergy is reported when the number of survivors in the culture exposed to the antimicrobial agent combination is at least tenfold lower than that in the culture exposed to the most effective antimicrobial agent alone.

Determination of Bactericidal Activity in Body Fluid. Correlation between the bactericidal activity of sera and the clinical outcome of antimicrobial therapy exists for persons with endocarditis, osteomyelitis, bacteremia (in immunocompromised persons), and meningitis. The serum bactericidal test has not been shown to predict outcome in patients with other infections and therefore should not be ordered in those situations. Determination of body fluid bactericidal titers has been useful for documenting that systemically administered antimicrobial therapy has reached fluid-containing closed spaces (e.g., CSF in persons with a central nervous system shunt-associated infection). The test procedure has received tentative status from the NCCLS. **Serum bactericidal tests** should be performed on paired sera to yield the most useful clinical information. The first specimen (trough specimen) is collected just before administration of an antimicrobial agent dose, and the second specimen (peak specimen) 30–90 minutes after administration of the same dose (timing depends on the route of administration and the antimicrobial agent). Twofold dilutions using antimicrobial agent–free pooled human serum as a diluent are prepared serially. Because pooled human serum maintains the serum protein concentration constant in each tube, the effect of protein binding on antimicrobial agents is not variable from tube to tube. The organism inoculum is composed of a turbidity-standardized suspension of the patient's isolate and is added to each serum dilution tube and to a growth-control tube containing no serum (positive control).

The final cell density of organisms in each tube should approximate 5×10^5 cfu/mL. A viable count determination should be performed on the inoculum to determine actual cell density. Tubes are incubated at 35°C for 20 hours in an atmosphere consistent with the growth of the organism, agitated manually, and reincubated for 4 additional hours. Agitation of the tubes exposes organisms that may have avoided contact with antimicrobial agents by adhering to the walls of the tube. The serum inhibitory titer is calculated by determining the highest serum dilution that inhibits visible growth of the patient's organism. Tubes exhibiting no visible growth are subcultured (0.1 mL) to 5% sheep blood or chocolate agar and incubated for 24 hours. The number of colonies yielded from each subculture is counted and the serum bactericidal titer defined as the highest dilution of serum that kills at least 99.9% of the original inoculum.

In a correlation of test results with clinical outcomes in adults with endocarditis, peak serum bactericidal titers ≥1:64 and trough titers ≥1:32 predicted bacteriologic cure. Peak and trough titers as low as 1:8 usually predicted successful outcomes, but bacteriologic failures also occurred. Test results were not helpful in predicting bacteriologic failure.

In adults with acute osteomyelitis, peak serum bactericidal titers had no predictive value, but trough titers ≥1:2 predicted bacteriologic cure, and trough titers <1:2 predicted bacteriologic failure. Interpretation of test results differed in adults with chronic osteomyelitis. Peak serum bactericidal titers ≥1:16 and trough titers ≥1:4 predicted bacteriologic cure, and peak titers <1:16 and trough titers <1:4 predicted failure. These data suggest that adults with acute osteomyelitis should have trough serum bactericidal titers ≥1:2 and that those with chronic osteomyelitis should have trough serum bactericidal titers ≥1:4 throughout the course of therapy.

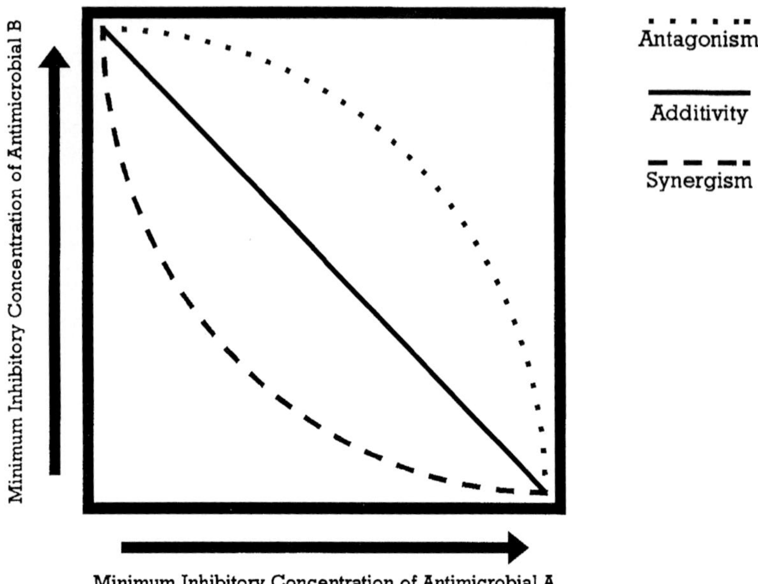

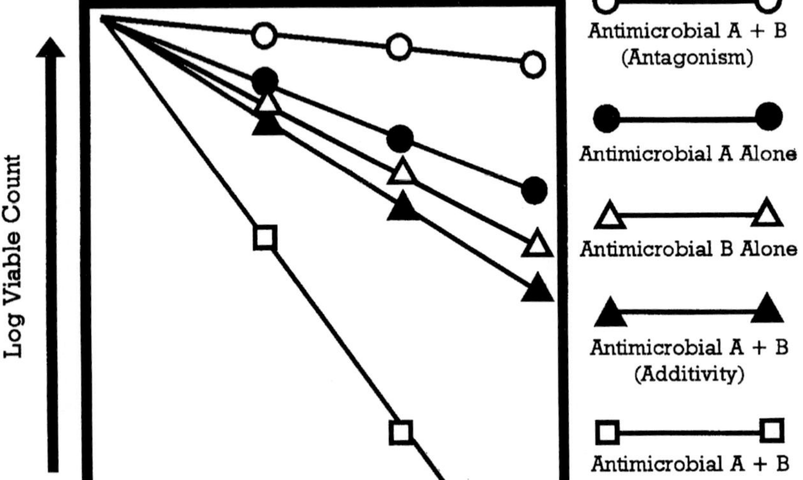

FIGURE 7–7. Graphic display of additive, antagonistic, and synergistic effects of simultaneous administration of two or more antimicrobial agents. *Top,* Isobolographic depiction. *Bottom,* Killing curve depiction.

For children with any infection and adults with infections other than those described herein, studies correlating serum bactericidal titers with clinical outcome have been less thorough. In general, peak titers ≥1:32 and trough titers ≥1:8 are considered satisfactory.

Measurement of Antimicrobial Agent Levels

Certain antimicrobial agents (e.g., aminoglycosides, vancomycin, chloramphenicol, 5-flucytosine) have narrow ratios of therapeutic to toxic levels. Additionally, these antimicrobial agents may rapidly accumulate to toxic concentrations in persons with renal or hepatic dysfunction. The blood levels of these antimicrobial agents should be monitored during therapy so that necessary dose adjustments can be made before patients are harmed. Serum levels for most of these agents can be monitored with rapid, very accurate instrument-assisted immunoassays.

Antimicrobial agents for which automated immunoassays do not exist can be measured with bioassays or by high-pressure liquid chromatography. For bioassays the most critical component is the assay organism, which must be susceptible to the agent being measured and yet resistant to other agents that may be present in clinical specimens. This is especially important if the other agents cannot be destroyed enzymatically or chemically beforehand. Bioassays are performed by adding assay organisms to molten agar that has cooled to 45–50°C and pouring the mixture into petri plates. After the agar has hardened, carefully measured volumes of patient sera are added to cylindrical wells cut into the agar or onto filter paper disks applied to the surface of the agar. A set of antimicrobial standards is tested at the same time. The plates are incubated at 35°C for as long as necessary to discern measurable zones of growth inhibition around the wells or filter paper disks.

The zone diameters for the antimicrobial standards are used to construct a linear regression equation or a linear standard curve on semilogarithmic graph paper. The antimicrobial concentrations in patient sera can be calculated by using the equation or extrapolating from the standard curve.

REVIEWS

Baron EJ, Finegold SM: *Diagnostic Microbiology,* 8th ed. St. Louis, Mosby, 1990.

Bruckner DA, Colonna P, Bearson BL: Nomenclature for aerobic and facultative bacteria. *Clin Infect Dis* 1999;29:713–23.

Garcia LS, Bruckner DA: *Diagnostic Medical Parasitology.* New York, Elsevier Science Publishing, 1988.

Howard BJ, Klaas J II, Rubin SJ, et al: *Clinical and Pathogenic Microbiology.* St. Louis, Mosby–Year Book, 1987.

Jousimies-Somer H, Summanen P: Microbiology terminology update: Clinically significant anaerobic gram-positive and gram-negative bacteria (excluding spirochetes. *Clin Infect Dis* 1999;29:724–7.

Larone D: *Medically Important Fungi,* 2nd ed. New York, Elsevier Science Publishing, 1987.

Markell EK, Voge M, John DT: *Medical Parasitology,* 7th ed. Philadelphia, WB Saunders, 1992.

McGinnis MR, Sigler L, Rinaldi MG: Some medically important fungi and their common synonyms and names of uncertain application. *Clin Infect Dis* 1999;29:728–30.

Murray PR, Baron EJ, Pfaller MA: *Manual of Clinical Microbiology,* 7th ed. Washington, DC, American Society for Microbiology Press, 1999.

Rippon JR: *Medical Mycology,* 3rd ed. Philadelphia, WB Saunders, 1988.

Summanen P, Baron EJ, Citron DM: *Wadsworth Anaerobic Bacteriology Manual,* 5th ed. Belmont, Calif, Star Publishing, 1993.

Woods GL, Gutierrez Y: *Diagnostic Pathology of Infectious Diseases.* Philadelphia, Lea & Febiger, 1993.

CHAPTER 8

Diagnostic Parasitology

Joseph M. Campos

Human parasites may inhabit the intestinal tract, genital tract, respiratory tract, circulatory system, central nervous system, and muscle tissue. Parasitic infections are usually confirmed by direct observation of the organism, which requires much skill to differentiate forms of closely related parasites, distinguish parasites from artifacts, and interpret specimens, such as stool, that have deteriorated. Laboratory diagnosis of parasitic infections usually involves macroscopic visualization of adult helminths or microscopic visualization of protozoa or helminth eggs and larvae. Reliable antigen-detection assays are also available for detection of some parasites. Cultures for parasites are rarely required or used. Histologic specimens are useful for identifying parasites that are causing tissue infections. Arthropods and arachnids are not truly parasitic, and infestations rarely require laboratory assistance.

CLASSIFICATION OF PARASITES

Parasites can be classified as **protozoa** and **helminths** (Table 8–1). The taxonomy of *Pneumocystis carinii* remains controversial. This organism shares many morphologic features with protozoa but has ribosomal RNA most closely resembling that of fungi.

SPECIMEN COLLECTION

Because culture of parasites is not usually required, specimen collection methods do not have to include maintenance of the viability of parasites.

Blood

Blood for examination for protozoa (e.g., *Plasmodium* and *Trypanosoma*) and helminths (e.g., microfilarial nematodes) should be collected in tubes containing ethylenediaminetetraacetic acid (EDTA) as an anticoagulant. The time of specimen collection should be noted so that results can be correlated with the patient's clinical status and fever pattern.

Central Nervous System

Laboratory detection of parasites in the central nervous system is difficult because organisms are few and because of the highly localized nature of the infectious process. For diagnosis of primary amebic meningoencephalitis or central nervous system trypanosomiasis, large quantities of CSF ($\geq$5 mL) should be sent to the laboratory to ensure that the specimen can be concentrated by centrifugation. Laboratory confirmation of neurocysticercosis, if necessary, is performed on aspirates from cystic lesions or biopsy specimens collected in the operating room.

Respiratory Tract

The ova of *Paragonimus westermani* are deposited in the lungs by adult female flukes and expelled from the body in coughed sputum. Thus microscopic examination of sputum is the laboratory test of choice for diagnosis of paragonimiasis. Larvae of *Ascaris lumbricoides, Ancylostoma duodenale, Necator americanus,* and *Strongyloides stercoralis* are transiently present in the lungs and may also be observed in sputum. Although removal is risky for the patient because of the possibility of spillage and anaphylaxis, the contents of echinococcal cysts may be examined to confirm the presence of *Echinococcus granulosus.*

Microscopic examination of bronchoalveolar lavage specimens has become the method of choice for diagnosis of *P. carinii* infection in immunocompromised persons. Specimen smears can be stained with one of several biologic stains (e.g., Giemsa, toluidine blue, methenamine silver) or fluorescent antibodies to highlight the presence of *P. carinii* cysts.

Gastrointestinal Tract

Stool is the specimen of choice for diagnosing most intestinal parasite infections. Watery or loose specimens are preferable and generate the highest yield of positive results. Specimens should be collected in a clean, leak-proof, capped container. Soiled diapers are discouraged as a source of specimens because of the possible negative impact of urine or diaper-associated chemicals on parasite morphologic features. Rectal swabs are not acceptable for ova and parasite examination.

Stool is especially subject to deterioration of parasitic morphologic features unless preventive measures are taken. Bacterial fermentation by stool flora, which occurs even at room temperature, results in production of large amounts of acidic waste products. As the stool pH decreases, the integrity of parasitic structures also decreases. The best preventive action is to place stool into a preservative (e.g., 5–10% formalin, merthiolate-iodine-formalin, sodium acetate–formalin, polyvinyl alcohol) that kills bacteria instantly and prevents further accumulation of acidic waste products. The next best option is to store stool at refrigerator temperature (4°C) to prevent further microbial growth and acid production.

The **cellophane tape preparation** is the method of choice for diagnosis of *Enterobius vermicularis* (pinworm) infection. Because *E. vermicularis* ova are deposited in the perianal folds by the nocturnally active gravid female worm, stool from an infected patient is unlikely to contain high numbers of ova. Instead, a segment of transparent cellophane adhesive tape is pressed against the patient's perianal region in the early morning before a bath or a bowel movement. The tape is applied to a microscope slide and examined microscopically under low power for *E. vermicularis* ova. Alternatively, a clear plastic paddle coated with adhesive can be used for specimen collection.

The **Enterotest (string test)** can be especially helpful for diagnosis of *Giardia* and *Strongyloides* infections. Patients are instructed to swallow a gelatin capsule attached to a thread that is

TABLE 8–1. Classification of Medically Important Human Parasites (Protozoa and Helminths)

PROTOZOA

Amebae (Intestinal)
Entamoeba histolytica
Blastocystis hominis

Flagellates (Intestinal)
Giardia lamblia
Dientamoeba fragilis

Ciliates (Intestinal)
Balantidium coli

Coccidia, Microsporidia (Intestinal)
Coccidia
Cryptosporidium parvum
Cyclospora cayetanensis
Isospora belli
Sarcocystis

Microsporidia
Enterocytozoon bieneusi
Encephalitozoon intestinalis

Sporozoa, Flagellates (Blood, Tissue)
Sporozoa (Malaria and Babesiosis)
Plasmodium vivax
Plasmodium ovale
Plasmodium malariae
Plasmodium falciparum
Babesia

Flagellates (Leishmanias, Trypanosomes)
Leishmania
Trypanosoma brucei gambiense
Trypanosoma brucei rhodesiense
Trypanosoma cruzi

Amebae, Flagellates (Other Body Sites)
Amebae
Naegleria fowleri
Acanthamoeba species
Balamuthia mandrillaris (Leptomyxid ameba)

Flagellates
Trichomonas vaginalis

Coccidia, Sporozoa (Other Body Sites)
Coccidia
Toxoplasma gondii
Sarcocystis "lindemanni"

Sporozoa
Pneumocystis carinii

HELMINTHS

Nematodes (Roundworms)
Intestinal
Ascaris lumbricoides
Enterobius vermicularis
Ancylostoma duodenale
Necator americanus
Strongyloides stercoralis
Trichuris trichiura

Tissue
Trichinella spiralis
Toxocara canis
Toxocara cati
Ancylostoma braziliense
Ancylostoma caninum
Dracunculus medinensis
Angiostrongylus cantonensis
Angiostrongylus costaricensis
Gnathostoma spinigerum
Anisakis species (larvae from saltwater fish)
Phocanema species (larvae from saltwater fish)
Contracaecum species (larvae from saltwater fish)

Blood and Tissues (Filarial Worms)
Wuchereria bancrofti
Brugia malayi
Brugia timori
Loa loa
Onchocerca volvulus
Dirofilaria immitis

Trematodes (Flukes)
Intestinal
Fasciolopsis buski
Echinostoma ilocanum
Heterophyes heterophyes
Metagonimus yokogawai

Liver/Lung
Clonorchis (Opisthorchis) sinensis
Opisthorchis viverrini
Fasciola hepatica
Paragonimus

Blood
Schistosoma mansoni
Schistosoma haematobium
Schistosoma japonicum
Schistosoma intercalatum
Schistosoma mekongi

Cestodes (Tapeworms)
Intestinal
Diphyllobothrium latum
Dipylidium caninum
Echinococcus granulosus
Echinococcus multilocularis
Hymenolepis nana
Hymenolepis diminuta
Taenia solium
Taenia saginata

metered out as the capsule passes through the esophagus and stomach and into the duodenal region of the small intestine. After the gelatin is digested from the thread, the end of the thread issuing from the patient's mouth is gently pulled until the entire length of thread has been removed from the gastrointestinal tract. The secretions adhering to the distal end of the thread are removed and examined microscopically for *Giardia* trophozoites and cysts and for *Strongyloides* larvae.

Genital Tract

Diagnosis of *Trichomonas vaginalis* infections can be performed by microscopic examination of vaginal or urethral discharge specimens suspended in a small volume of sterile nonbacteriostatic saline solution. Specimens should be promptly examined under the microscope while trophozoites are still motile. Their motility assists greatly in their detection because rapid movement helps identify their presence.

Tissue

Tissue and organ biopsy material from persons with suspected echinococcosis, trypanosomiasis, leishmaniasis, trichinosis, loaiasis, and onchocerciasis and aspirates from cutaneous ulcers and lymph nodes of persons with suspected trypanosomiasis, leishmaniasis, and toxoplasmosis must be delivered to the laboratory immediately after collection to prevent drying.

SPECIMEN TRANSPORT

The transport and initial processing of specimens for ova and parasite examination differ from those used with other specimens. Because examinations for parasites depend largely on recognition of characteristic structures under the microscope, preventing morphologic deterioration is more important than maintaining the viability of the parasites. Thus many specimens are placed promptly into preservatives that kill not only contaminating microorganisms but also the parasites themselves.

DIAGNOSIS OF PARASITIC INFECTIONS

Most parasitic infections are initially diagnosed or confirmed by microscopic examination. Appropriate training and a great deal of experience are the requisites for accurate examination. The most frequent mistake made by novice microscopists is not in recognizing that a parasite is indeed a parasite but, rather, in misidentifying a specimen artifact as a parasite. An atlas of photographs of common parasites should be available for quick reference. All microscopes used in the parasitology laboratory should be equipped with a properly calibrated ocular micrometer, which is a valuable tool for determining the size of suspect structures and for accurately distinguishing between parasites and artifacts.

Before microscopic examination, both preserved and unpreserved stools are usually extracted or concentrated or both. The original **formalin-ether procedure** has been supplanted by the **formalin–ethyl acetate concentration procedure** to avoid ether-related laboratory accidents. Hemo-De, a xylene substitute, is now replacing ethyl acetate in stool concentration protocols because it is even safer. The goal of the extraction procedures is to remove fatty material from stool and to concentrate what remains by centrifugation. Another concentration method used by some laboratories is the **zinc sulfate flotation technique.** In this technique, stool is added to a column of zinc sulfate solution adjusted to a specific gravity of 1.18. Ova and parasites float on the top of the solution because of their lower specific gravity. Wet mounts are prepared from the material present in the meniscus of the solution.

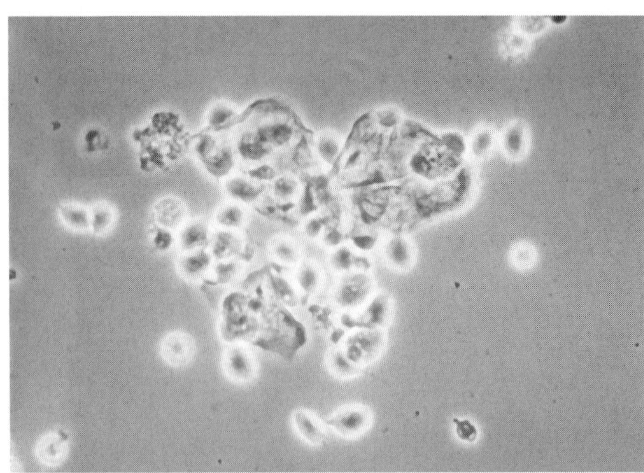

FIGURE 8–2. Direct specimen (saline wet preparation) of vaginal discharge containing *Trichomonas vaginalis* trophozoites.

Cellophane Tape Preparation. The sole purpose of this test is detection of the ova of *E. vermicularis.* The ova are recognized by their oval shape with one flattened side and the usual presence of larvae within the ova (Fig. 8–1). Occasional larvae that have emerged from ruptured ova may be seen.

Direct Specimen Wet Mount. Only when the number of parasites in specimens is high is the direct wet mount clinically useful. Wet mounts are moderately effective for diagnosis of vaginal trichomoniasis, with a sensitivity of approximately 50% compared to culture (Fig. 8–2). Heavy parasitic burdens in the gastrointestinal tract may be detected in unconcentrated wet mounts. In patients with more than one parasite, however, the organism present in smaller numbers may very well be missed. Thus, when a direct specimen wet mount is positive, the result is helpful, but a negative result does not exclude infection.

Concentrated Specimen Wet Mount. Stool specimens are extracted and concentrated before microscopic examination (Fig. 8–3). Wet mounts should be examined under low power (×100) initially to screen for helminth ova, followed by examination under high, dry magnification (×450) to screen for protozoa. Oil immersion magnification (×1,000) may be necessary for identification of certain protozoa.

Permanently Stained Smear. All stool specimens should also have a permanently stained smear prepared for examination for protozoa. Wheatley's trichrome stain is the choice of most laboratories, although the more difficult iron-hematoxylin stain is still favored by some (Fig. 8–4). Stained smears are examined under oil immersion magnification (×1,000) for protozoa.

Stained Smears for Pneumocystis carinii. A variety of staining methods have been developed for detection of *P. carinii* cysts and trophozoites in lower respiratory tract specimens. Perhaps the easiest to interpret are the **methenamine silver** and **toluidine blue** stains specific for cyst wall (Fig. 8–5). The **Giemsa stain** is the method of choice for visualizing *P. carinii* trophozoites but requires greater expertise to obtain accurate results. **Immunofluorescence** assays for *P. carinii* antigens have become popular in recent years. These assays feature relatively short staining times and facilitate screening smears rapidly at low magnification because of the heightened contrast between cysts and background material.

Modified Acid-Fast Stain. *Cryptosporidium* and *Isospora* are difficult to detect. *Cryptosporidium* is easily overlooked during routine ova and parasite examinations because its size and morphologic features resemble those of yeasts. Both *Cryptosporidium parvum*

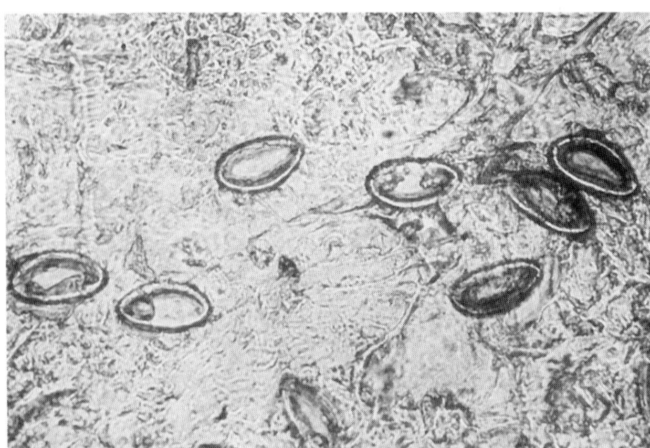

FIGURE 8–1. Cellophane tape preparation of *Enterobius vermicularis* (pinworm) ova.

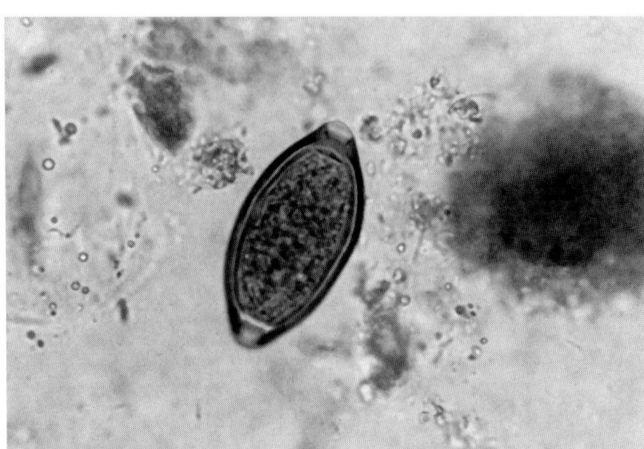

FIGURE 8–3. Concentrated wet mount preparation of stool containing *Trichuris trichiura* ova.

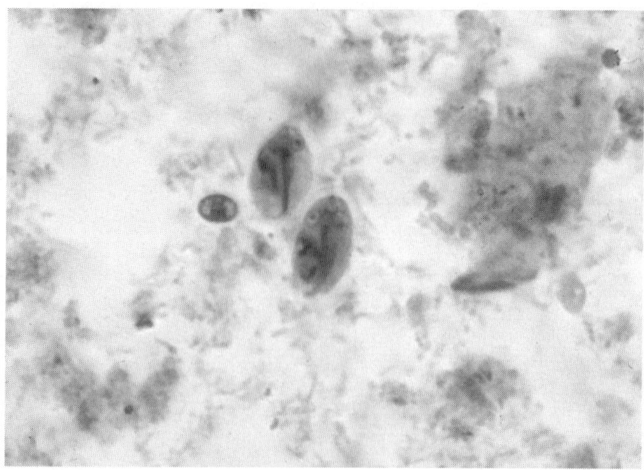

FIGURE 8–4. Trichrome-stained smear of stool containing *Entamoeba histolytica* trophozoites.

and *Isospora belli* oocysts are acid-fast when subjected to a modified staining protocol similar to that used for detection of *Nocardia* (Chapter 7). In the modified Kinyoun stain the carbol-fuchsin staining time is 5 minutes, the decolorization step is 5–10 seconds with 0.5–1% H_2SO_4, and the methylene blue counterstain is 30 seconds. Smears should be examined under oil immersion magnification (×1,000) for protozoa.

Giemsa and Wright Stains for Blood Parasites. Giemsa and Wright stains are effective for recognizing and identifying protozoa and helminths in blood smears. Both thick and thin blood smears, or films, should be prepared if blood parasites are suspected. A **thick smear** is prepared from two or three drops of blood spread over an area approximately 2 cm in diameter. The purpose of the thick smear is to screen larger volumes of blood so that light infections may be detected. The thick smear is not fixed before the staining process is begun. The Giemsa or Wright staining process lyses the unfixed erythrocytes and leukocytes in specimens, freeing intracellular parasites in the process. Extracellular parasites are not affected. Definitive identification of blood parasites seen in thick smears, however, is extremely difficult. The **thin smear** is prepared from a single drop of blood in the same manner as the differential count smear is prepared in the hematology laboratory. The smear should be fixed with methanol before being stained with Giemsa or Wright stain reagents. Intracellular parasites remain intracellular and display the morphologic features necessary for definitive identification. Stained smears should be examined under oil immersion magnification (×1,000). Careful attention to the details of an organism's morphologic characteristics is necessary to obtain accurate identification, which often requires comparison with a color atlas (Plates 2C and 2D).

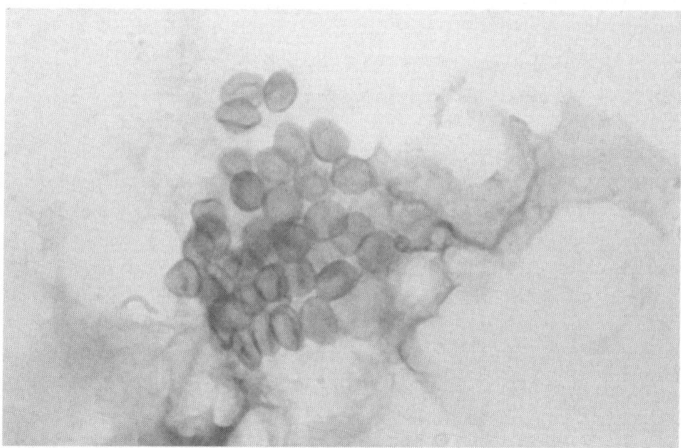

FIGURE 8–5. Toluidine blue–stained smear of bronchoalveolar lavage containing *Pneumocystis carinii* cysts. (From Tsieh Sun, American Society for Clinical Pathology.)

CULTURE

Culture is rarely required for laboratory diagnosis of parasitic infections, nor is it feasible for parasites with complicated life cycles that are difficult or impossible to mimic in the laboratory. Even for parasites that can be cultured in the laboratory, such as *Entamoeba histolytica, Trichomonas vaginalis,* and *Toxoplasma gondii,* the time required to obtain results is too long to furnish clinically useful information. Culture of *T. gondii* from placenta may be an adjunct for diagnosis of congenital toxoplasmosis. Cultures are grown in fibroblast cell lines and may show positive results within several days.

ANTIMICROBIAL SUSCEPTIBILITY TESTING

There are no routinely available methods for determining the susceptibility of parasites to drugs.

REVIEWS

Baron EJ, Finegold SM: *Diagnostic Microbiology,* 8th ed. St. Louis, CV Mosby, 1990.

Garcia LS: Classification of human parasites, vectors, and similar organisms. *Clin Infect Dis* 1999;29:734–6.

Garcia LS (editor): *Diagnostic Medical Parasitology,* 4th ed. Washington, DC, American Society for Microbiology Press, 2001.

Howard BJ, Klaas J II, Rubin SJ, et al: *Clinical and Pathogenic Microbiology.* St. Louis, CV Mosby, 1987.

Markell EK, Voge M, John DT: *Medical Parasitology.* Philadellphia, WB Saunders, 1986.

Murray PR, Baron EJ, Pfaller MA, et al: *Manual of Clinical Microbiology,* 7th ed. Washington, DC, American Society for Microbiology Press, 1999.

Woods GL, Gutierrez Y. *Diagnostic Pathology of Infectious Diseases.* Philadelphia, Lea & Febiger, 1993.

CHAPTER 9

Diagnostic Virology

Joseph M. Campos

Correct diagnosis of viral infections requires two-way communication between clinicians and laboratorians. In general, clinicians develop preliminary diagnoses based on clinical features, epidemiologic considerations, and specific organ involvement. These same criteria are used by laboratorians to determine the etiologic agents most likely involved. Viral diagnosis uses classic microscopy, antigen detection, nucleic acid detection, culture, and detection of antibodies. Because viruses may cause infections in some individuals without causing clinical disease, establishing causal relationships between viral detection and patient symptoms is not always possible.

Viruses are among the smallest agents known to cause human infection, ranging in diameter from 25 to 300 nm. They consist of **nucleic acid cores** surrounded by **protein coats (capsids),** which may or may not be surrounded by **lipid-containing envelopes.** Capsids are usually icosahedral or spherical in shape, but brick-shaped, bullet-shaped, and filamentous morphologic characteristics exist. Viral envelopes contain host cell lipids and proteins derived from the cell membranes of infected cells. Envelopes become part of viral particles when they are released from infected cells by a process known as **budding.** Viruses released by lysis of host cells are usually not enveloped.

Even smaller than viruses are disease-producing subviral particles known as **prions.** Several features distinguish prions from viruses. Prions exhibit multiple morphologic characteristics, whereas viruses tend to display consistent morphologic features. Prions are not immunogenic, whereas viruses almost always stimulate immune responses. Prions do not contain nucleic acids, whereas viruses possess nucleic acid genomes that function as templates for replication. Finally, prions consist of a single component of protein **(PrPSc)** encoded by a host chromosomal gene. Viruses are composed of nucleic acids and proteins. Prions are not detectable with routine laboratory tests.

CLASSIFICATION OF VIRUSES

More than 1,400 viruses have been assigned to approximately 60 families of viruses by the International Committee on Nomenclature of Viruses. At least 20 of the families contain members that cause human infection (Table 9–1). Viruses are broadly classified by their nucleic acid content as either **DNA viruses** or **RNA viruses** and are further divided by having **single-stranded nucleic acid** or **double-stranded nucleic acid.** Viruses can be further characterized by their ability to perform **reverse transcription.** The sense of the RNA in single-stranded RNA viruses is also incorporated into the classification scheme: **positive-stranded RNA** can be translated directly into protein, and **negative-stranded RNA** must first be replicated to create homologous positive strands that then serve as templates for protein synthesis.

SPECIMEN COLLECTION

Appropriate specimen collection based on the site of illness is essential to facilitate accurate virologic diagnosis (Table 9–2). The two primary goals of specimen transport are (1) to keep the material in specimens intact, viable, and infectious and (2) to prevent microbial overgrowth of specimens. Swab specimens, vesicular fluid, and small pieces of tissue should always be sent in **viral transport medium;** dry swabs are unacceptable because desiccation reduces virus viability. The main components of viral transport medium are veal infusion broth, bovine serum albumin, sodium bicarbonate ($NaHCO_3$), phenol red pH indicator, and antimicrobial agents to prevent bacterial and fungal growth. Screw-capped containers should be used to transport specimens to the laboratory. Normally sterile body fluids, such as CSF and bile, should not be diluted but should be transported in capped, sterile tubes. Blood should be collected and transported in tubes containing an anticoagulant.

To maximize culture yields, clinicians should collect specimens for viral isolation from patients as soon as possible after the onset of symptoms. Wire or plastic shaft swabs are suitable for specimen collection, although collection of cellular aspirates, body fluids, and tissues is strongly encouraged. Wooden shaft and cotton swabs should not be used because of the deleterious effects of plant-derived oils on viruses.

SPECIMEN TRANSPORT

From the moment specimens are collected, the quantity of infectious viruses present begins to decline. Temperature, time in transit, and the quantity of live viruses originally present are factors that influence the rate of viral survival in specimens. Specimens should be transported to the laboratory, preferably on wet ice, as soon as possible after collection. If transport delay is inevitable, specimens may be kept at 4°C for as long as 24 hours. For longer periods of transport, specimens should be frozen at −20°C or lower, although most viruses lose infectivity during the freezing and thawing process.

DIAGNOSIS OF VIRAL INFECTIONS

Viral isolation by culture, detection of viral antigens and nucleic acids, and serologic testing are the principal methods used in diagnostic virology. The specific tests performed depend on the suspected viral pathogens, the availability of tests for the suspected virus, the type of specimen to be tested, and the specific question, such as presence of virus, quantitation of virus, or determination of immunity (Table 9–3).

Conventional Cell Culture. After receipt by the laboratory, specimens are processed and inoculated to cell cultures growing in tubes

Text continued on page 89

TABLE 9–1. Classification of Medically Important Human Pathogenic Viruses

Family	Subfamily	Genus	Species
Double-Stranded DNA Viruses			
Adenoviridae		Mastadenovirus	Human adenoviruses 1–50
Herpesviridae	Alphaherpesvirinae	Simplexvirus	Human herpes virus 1 (herpes simplex virus type 1)
			Human herpes virus 2 (herpes simplex virus type 2)
			Cercopithecine herpesvirus 1 (monkey B virus)
		Varicellovirus	Human herpes virus 3 (varicella-zoster virus)
	Betaherpesvirinae	Cytomegalovirus	Human herpes virus 5 (human cytomegalovirus)
		Roseolovirus	Human herpesvirus 6
			Human herpesvirus 7
	Gammaherpesvirinae	Lymphocryptovirus	Human herpesvirus 4 (Epstein-Barr virus)
		Rhadinovirus	Human herpesvirus 8 (Kaposi's sarcoma–associated herpesvirus)
Papovaviridae		Papillomavirus	Human papillomaviruses 1–80
Polyomaviridae		Polyomavirus	BK virus
			JC virus
			SV40 (simian virus 40)
Poxviridae	Chordopoxvirinae	Molluscipoxvirus	Molluscum contagiosum virus
		Orthopoxvirus	Variola virus (smallpox)
			Vaccinia virus
		Parapoxvirus	Orf virus (contagious pustular dermatitis)
			Pseudocowpox virus (milker's nodule)
Double-Stranded DNA Viruses That Perform Reverse Transcription			
Hepadnaviridae		Orthohepadnavirus	Hepatitis B virus
Single-Stranded DNA Viruses			
Parvoviridae	Parvovirinae	Erythrovirus	Human parvovirus B19
Double-Stranded RNA Viruses			
Reoviridae		Coltivirus	Colorado tick fever virus
		Orbivirus	Orungo virus
			Kemerovo virus group
		Rotavirus	Human rotaviruses A, B, C (numerous subtypes)
Single-Stranded RNA Viruses That Perform Reverse Transcription			
Retroviridae		Deltaretrovirus	HTLV-I virus
			HTLV-II virus
		Lentivirus	HIV-1 virus
			HIV-2 virus
Single-Stranded RNA Viruses (Negative-Stranded)			
Arenaviridae		Arenavirus	Lassa fever virus
			Lymphocytic choriomeningitis virus
			Junin virus (Argentinian hemorrhagic fever)
			Machupo virus (Bolivian hemorrhagic fever)
Bunyaviridae		Bunyavirus	Bunyamwera virus
			California encephalitis virus
			La Crosse virus
			Viruses (>161) of other serogroups (mosquito-borne)
		Hantavirus (see Table 68–12)	Hantaan virus
			Dobrava virus
			Seoul virus
			Puumala virus
			Sin Nombre virus
			Black Creek Canal virus

Table continued on following page

TABLE 9–1. Classification of Medically Important Human Pathogenic Viruses *(Continued)*

Family	Subfamily	Genus	Species
Single-Stranded RNA Viruses (Negative-Stranded) *(Continued)*			
Bunyaviridae *(Continued)*		Nairovirus	Crimean-Congo hemorrhagic fever virus
			Viruses (>33) of other serogroups (tick-borne)
		Phlebovirus	Rift Valley fever virus
			Sandfly fever viruses
Filoviridae		Ebola-like viruses	Ebola virus (Zaire Ebola virus, Reston Ebola virus)
		Marburg-like viruses	Marburg virus
Orthomyxoviridae		Influenzavirus A	Influenza virus A
		Influenzavirus B	Influenza virus B
		Influenzavirus C	Influenza virus C
Paramyxoviridae	Paramyxovirinae	Morbillivirus	Measles virus
		Respirovirus	Parainfluenza viruses 1 and 3
		Rubulavirus	Mumps virus
			Parainfluenza viruses 2, 4A, 4B
	Pneumovirinae	Pneumovirus	Respiratory syncytial virus
Rhabdoviridae		Lyssavirus	Rabies virus
		Vesiculovirus	Vesicular stomatitis virus
Single-Stranded RNA Viruses (Positive-Stranded)			
Astroviridae		Astrovirus	Human astroviruses (8)
Caliciviridae		Calicivirus	Hepatitis E virus
			Human caliciviruses (including Norwalk, Hawaii, and Snow Mountain viruses)
Coronaviridae		Coronavirus	Human coronaviruses (2)
Flaviviridae		Flavivirus	Dengue viruses 1–4
			Japanese encephalitis virus
			Murray Valley encephalitis virus
			Powassan virus
			St. Louis encephalitis virus
			West Nile fever virus
			Yellow fever virus
		Hepacivirus	Hepatitis C virus
Picornaviridae		Enterovirus	Coxsackieviruses A 1–22, 24
			Coxsackieviruses B 1–6
			Echoviruses (30)
			Polioviruses 1–3
			Enteroviruses 68–71 (4)
		Parechovirus	Human parechovirus (formerly echovirus 22)
		Hepatovirus	Hepatitis A virus (formerly enterovirus 72)
		Rhinovirus	Human rhinoviruses (>115)
Togaviridae		Alphavirus	Chikungunya virus
			Eastern equine encephalitis virus
			Mayaro virus
			O'nyong-nyong virus
			Ross River virus
			Venezuelan equine encephalitis virus
			Western equine encephalitis virus
		Rubivirus	Rubella virus
Subviruses			
Prions (agents of spongiform encephalopathies)		Scrapie	Creutzfeldt-Jakob disease
			Gerstmann-Sträussler-Scheinker syndrome
			Kuru
			Bovine spongiform encephalopathy
Satellite viruses		Delta virus	Hepatitis delta (D) virus

TABLE 9–2. Specimen Collection for Virologic Testing

Body Site or Illness	Specimens for Direct Detection or Culture or Both	Serology
Body Site		
Upper respiratory tract	Nasopharyngeal aspirate	Paired sera
	Nose or throat wash, or both	
	Nose or throat swab, or both	
Lower respiratory tract	Bronchoalveolar lavage	Paired sera
	Lung biopsy	
Gastrointestinal tract	Stool or rectal swab[1]	None[2]
	Relevant organ biopsy	
Liver	Serum[3]	Single serum
	Liver biopsy	
Genital tract	Vesicle fluid, ulcer scraping for antigen detection	
	Urethral and endocervical swabs for culture	
Eye	Conjunctival scraping for antigen detection	Paired sera
	Conjunctival and corneal[4] swabs for culture	
	Throat swab	
Skin	Vesicle fluid, ulcer scraping and swab, crust, biopsy, stool, nose and throat swabs, urine	Paired sera
Illness		
Febrile illness	Nasopharyngeal aspirate	Paired sera
Nose and throat swabs		
Urine		
Stool[1]		
Anticoagulated blood		
Fever and lymphadenopathy (infectious mononucleosis)	Nasopharyngeal aspirate	Paired sera
	Nose and throat swabs	
Throat gargle[5]		
Urine		
Anticoagulated blood		
Meningitis, encephalitis	Cerebrospinal fluid	Paired sera
	Brain biopsy	Cerebrospinal fluid
	Corneal impression smear[6]	
	Stool[1]	
	Nose and throat swabs	
	Urine	
	Anticoagulated blood[7,8]	
	Serum[8]	
Myocarditis, pericarditis	Cardiac biopsy	Paired sera
	Pericardial fluid	
	Stool[1]	
	Nose and throat swabs	
Congenital and perinatal infections	Nasopharyngeal aspirate	Single serum from both mother and baby[9]
	Nose and throat swabs	
	Urine (for CMV)	
	Stool[1]	
	Cerebrospinal fluid	
	Vesicle fluid, ulcer scraping	

[1]Although rectal swabs rarely contain detectable levels of virus, they are an alternative when stool cannot be readily obtained.
[2]Serologic tests are not reliable for viruses that cause diarrhea.
[3]For detection of hepatitis A, B, and C antigens, or antibodies, or both.
[4]For corneal ulceration.
[5]For isolation of Epstein-Barr virus, gargle with 10 mL of RPMI-1640 medium.
[6]For detection of rabies virus antigen only.
[7]For detection of arboviruses.
[8]For viruses causing hemorrhagic fever (Filoviridae and Arenaviridae).
[9]Both are preferred, but cord blood specimens from newborns are satisfactory.

TABLE 9–3. Summary of Diagnostic Virology Methods for Specific Viruses

Virus	Test	Laboratory Time to Results
Adenovirus		
Serotypes 1–39, 42–47	Culture	3–21 days
Serotypes 1–39, 42–47	Antigen detection	1–4 hr
Serotypes 40–41	Antigen detection	2–4 hr
Arboviruses	Serology (IgG and IgM)	4 hr
Cytomegalovirus (CMV)	Culture	2–21 days
	Antigen detection (antigenemia)	4 hr
	Serology (IgG and IgM)	10 min to 4 hr
	Nucleic acid detection (qualitative and quantitative)	1–2 days
Enterovirus	Culture	2–21 days
	Nucleic acid detection (qualitative)	1–2 days
Epstein-Barr virus (EBV)	Serology (heterophile antibody)	10 min
	Serology (VCA-IgG, VCA-IgM, EA, EBNA)	4 hr
	Nucleic acid detection (qualitative and quantitative)	1–2 days
Hepatitis A virus	Serology (IgM, IgG/IgM)	4 hr
Hepatitis B virus	Antigen detection (HB_s, HB_e)	10 min to 4 hr
	Serology (HB_c IgM, HB_c, IgG/IgM, HB_s IgG, HB_e, IgG)	4 hr
	Nucleic acid detection (qualitative)	1–2 days
Hepatitis C virus	Serology (IgG)	4 hr
	Serology immunoblot (recombinant immunoblot assay [RIBA])	1–2 days
	Nucleic acid detection (qualitative and quantitative)	1–2 days
	Genotype	7 days
Hepatitis D virus	Serology (IgG)	4 hr
Herpes simplex viruses 1 and 2	Microscopy (Tzanck preparation)	30 min
	Culture	1–4 days
	Antigen detection	2–4 hr
	Serology (IgG, IgM)	4 hr
	Nucleic acid detection (qualitative)	1–2 days
HIV-1	Culture	6 wk
	Antigen detection (p24)	4 hr to 2 days
	Serology (IgG)	4 hr
	Serology by immunoblot	6 hr
	Nucleic acid detection (qualitative and quantitative)	4 hr to 2 days
	Genotype	7 days
	Phenotype	6 wk
HIV-2	Serology (IgG)	4 hr
	Serology by immunoblot	6 hr
HTLV-I/II	Serology (IgG)	4 hr
	Serology by immunoblot	6 hr
Human papillomaviruses	Nucleic acid detection (qualitative)	1–2 days
Influenza A and B viruses	Culture	3–21 days
	Antigen detection	30 min to 4 hr
Measles virus	Serology (IgG, IgM)	4 hr
Mumps virus	Serology (IgG, IgM)	4 hr
Parainfluenza 1–3 viruses	Culture	3–21 days
	Antigen detection	2–4 hr
Parvovirus B19	Serology (IgG, IgM)	4 hr
	Nucleic acid detection (qualitative)	1–2 days
Rabies virus	RT-PCR	
Respiratory syncytial virus (RSV)	Culture	3–21 days
	Antigen detection	30 min to 4 hr
Rotaviruses	Antigen detection	10 min to 4 hr
Rubella virus	Serology (IgG, IgM)	10 min to 4 hr
Varicella-zoster virus (VZV)	Microscopy (Tzanck preparation)	30 min
	Culture	4–10 days
	Antigen detection	4 hr
	Serology (IgG, IgM)	4 hr
	Nucleic acid detection (qualitative and quantitative)	1–2 days

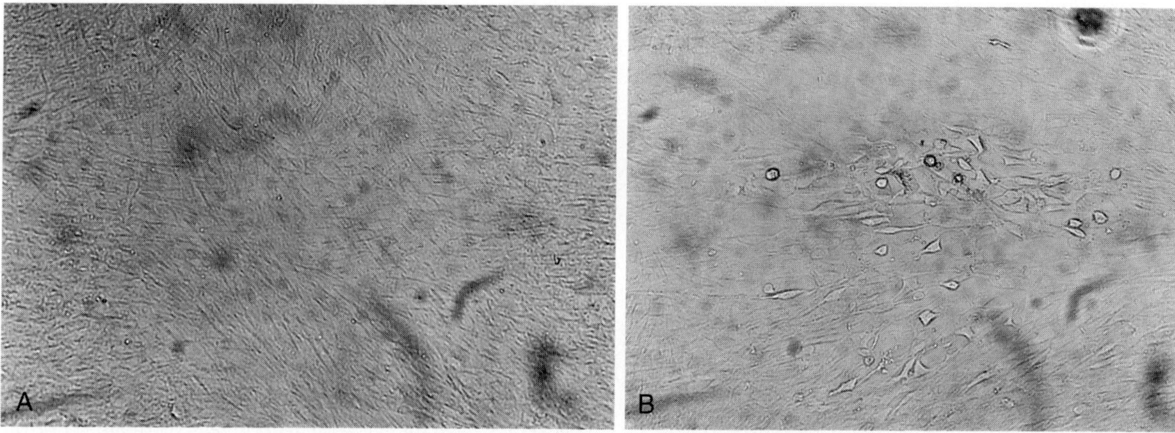

FIGURE 9–1. CPE induced by CMV isolate in human foreskin fibroblast monolayers. **A,** Uninfected cells. **B,** CMV-infected cells. Magnification: ×100.

or flasks. Cell lines for viral propagation may be **primary cells,** passaged once or twice, such as primary monkey kidney cells from rhesus monkeys; **diploid cells,** passaged 20–50 times, such as WI-38 and MRC-5 cells; or **continuous cells,** passaged an infinite number of times, such as HeLa and HEp-2 cells. Cell culture passage refers to continued growth of a cell line after transfer of a small number of cells to fresh culture medium.

The choice of cell lines depends on the viruses being sought. Human diploid fibroblasts (e.g., WI-38, human foreskin, or MRC-5 cells) are dependable for growth of HSV, CMV, and varicella-zoster virus; primary monkey kidney cells for enteroviruses and the respiratory viruses; and human continuous cell lines (e.g., HEp-2 or HeLa cells) for RSV and the respiratory adenoviruses. As a general rule, knowledge of the patient's clinical illness and origin of specimens aids virologists in deciding which cell lines to inoculate. If a specific virus is being sought, inoculation of one or two cell lines known to support growth of the suspected virus is recommended. If several viruses are possible, two or more cell lines capable of supporting growth of a variety of viruses should be inoculated.

Once cell cultures have been inoculated, they are incubated and examined microscopically for development of **cytopathic effect (CPE).** Typical CPE includes **increased refractility** and **rounding of cells, syncytium formation,** and the appearance of **plaques** in cell culture monolayers resulting from cellular lysis (Fig. 9–1). Other indicators of viral growth in the absence of visible CPE are the appearance of hemadsorbing regions in cell cultures, the presence of hemagglutinating activity in liquid growth media bathing cell cultures, the existence of stainable inclusion bodies, and the detection of viral antigens in cell cultures with immunofluorescence and immunoperoxidase staining. The time to develop CPE varies from 1–3 days for HSV to 2–21 days for CMV. Several important human viruses produce little, if any, visible CPE.

Some laboratories perform **blind passages** of apparently sterile cultures to increase the yield of positive results. Cell monolayers are disrupted by agitation in the presence of tiny glass beads and then used to inoculate fresh cell cultures. The second set of cultures are incubated and examined for CPE.

Some viruses of clinical importance are not cultivable or grow very poorly in conventional cell lines, such as coxsackie A viruses; hepatitis A, B, and C viruses; human parvovirus B19; human papillomaviruses; measles virus; arboviruses; and several gastrointestinal tract viruses including rotaviruses, coronaviruses, caliciviruses, astroviruses, and the enteric adenoviruses.

Shell Vial Culture. Detection of positive culture results can be accelerated for certain viruses with the shell vial culture technique, which has gained wide acceptance as a rapid method for detecting growth of CMV. Some laboratories have adapted the same technique for growth of RSV, influenza viruses, parainfluenza viruses, adenoviruses, HSV, and enteroviruses. Cell cultures growing on the surface of small coverslips are inoculated by centrifugation of specimens onto the coverslips. Coverslip cultures are housed in small shell vials containing liquid growth medium and incubated. After 1–5 days, cells are stained for expression of viral antigens by means of antibodies conjugated with a fluorescent dye. Visualization of nuclear or cytoplasmic fluorescence indicates that viral replication virus has occurred, confirming the presence of the virus (Fig. 9–2).

Antigen Detection. Antigen detection methods provide rapid results, usually within hours of receipt in the laboratory, and are especially useful for viruses that grow slowly or are labile, impairing recovery in culture. They permit greater flexibility in handling and transport of specimens. Methods in common use include

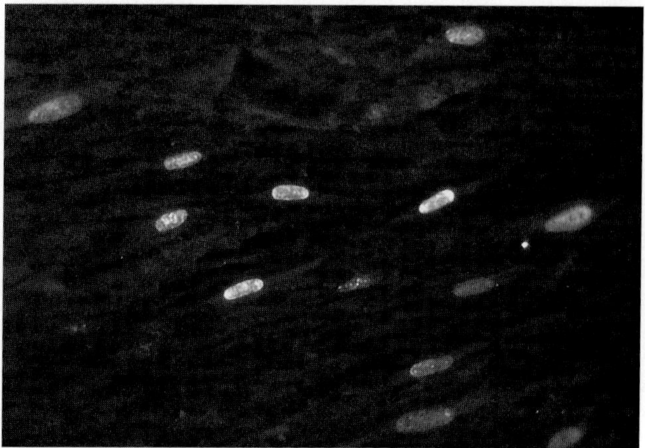

FIGURE 9–2 Shell vial assay for detection of CMV indirect immunofluorescence photomicrograph of human foreskin fibroblasts infected by the shell vial assay with a clinical specimen containing CMV and reacted with anti-CMV monoclonal antibodies. The presence of CMV is indicated by the appearance of typical strictly nuclear and bright fluorescence within infected cells. Magnification: ×250.

EIA, IFA, and particle agglutination (PA). Viruses for which EIA methods are popular include RSV, influenza A and B viruses, rotavirus, hepatitis B virus for HBsAg, and HIV-1. IFA is often used for detection of RSV, influenza A and B viruses, parainfluenza 1–3 viruses, adenovirus, HSV, and varicella-zoster virus antigens, as well as CMV antigenemia. PA has shown utility in the detection of rotavirus antigens. Antigen detection tests are not suitable for viruses with extensive antigenic heterogeneity, such as the enteroviruses and rhinoviruses.

Nucleic Acid Hybridization. Hybridization of viral nucleic acids with **probes,** or of small fragments of nucleic acids complementary to portions of the viral genome, for detection of DNA **(Southern blotting)** or RNA **(Northern blotting)** is a powerful tool for the detection and identification of viruses (Chapter 12). Techniques for amplification of target nucleic acid sequences, such as **PCR,** or for amplification of the signals generated once hybridization between probe and target has occurred, such as **probe amplification** or **signal amplification** assays, are extremely sensitive assays for diagnosis of infections. These assays have proved beneficial for diagnosing infections caused by viruses that are difficult or time-consuming to detect by other laboratory methods. Incorporation of reverse transcriptase in the PCR method, for **RT-PCR**, permits both detection and quantitation of viral RNA, such as quantitative assays for HIV-1 and hepatitis C virus that are used for diagnosis and also to monitor the response to antiviral therapy. Quantitative methods are being developed for other DNA and RNA viruses.

The extreme sensitivity of these assays requires caution in the interpretation of test results. For example, the lifelong latent infections of herpesviruses in host cells lead to frequent detection of herpesvirus DNA with target- or signal-amplified assays, indicating that the viral genome is present but not proving that active infection is ongoing. Assays that document the existence of short-lived messenger RNA or large numbers of target nucleic acid sequences in specimens provide much more convincing evidence of active herpesvirus infections.

Electron Microscopy. In laboratories with large virology workloads, a skilled workforce, and the necessary equipment, electron microscopy may still be used for detection of enteric viruses, particularly for rotavirus and caliciviruses. Stool suspensions are spotted on copper grids, negatively stained with phosphotungstic acid or uranyl acetate, and examined for virus particles. The size, shape, and structural characteristics of the particles are used for identification of the specific agents (Fig. 9–3).

Histopathologic Stains. The histologic stains that were used in the past for rapid diagnosis of viral infections largely have been supplanted by antigen detection tests. The **Tzanck preparation,** in which specimens are stained with Giemsa, Papanicolaou, or Wright reagents, can be used to demonstrate **multinucleated giant cells** and **ballooning cytoplasm** in specimens with HSV and varicella-zoster virus infections. Histologic stains can also highlight the enlarged cells with dense central inclusions, or **owl eyes,** characteristic of CMV infections.

Serology. Serologic diagnoses of recent viral infections (Chapter 11) can be established in three ways: (1) detection of specific IgM antibodies in sera collected during the acute phase of the illness, (2) demonstration of IgG seroconversion, from seronegative to seropositive status, or (3) documentation of a fourfold or greater change in IgG titer in specimen pairs obtained a minimum of 10–15 days, and preferably 3–4 weeks, after the initial specimen collected during the acute phase of the illness. It is highly desirable to test both sera simultaneously, 2–4 weeks apart.

IgM antibodies are usually the first immunoglobulins to appear, and they disappear within a few weeks to a few months after most primary viral infections. Detection of specific IgM antibodies can be helpful in diagnosing congenital infections caused by CMV, HSV, rubella, and parvovirus B19 and in recognizing infections caused by viruses that do not grow well in the laboratory, such as hepatitis A virus, hepatitis B virus, rubeola virus, and mumps virus. Caution is necessary in interpreting the results from patients with IgM antibodies directed against HSV, CMV, and varicella-zoster virus because some persons have low levels of detectable IgM antibodies long after primary infection.

IgG antibodies arise several weeks after the onset of infection and may persist at detectable levels for life. Thus the diagnostic value of a single IgG titer is limited during the acute phase of infection. Individual IgG titers are meaningful for evaluating the immune status of individuals and for determining the need for immunization against viral infections such as measles, mumps, rubella, and hepatitis B. Such measurements are also useful in assessing bone marrow and organ donors and recipients for evidence of latent infections with HSV, CMV, and varicella-zoster virus before transplantation.

ANTIVIRAL SUSCEPTIBILITY TESTING

The availability of increasing numbers of antiviral agents has prompted the emergence of strains resistant to these agents. Stan-

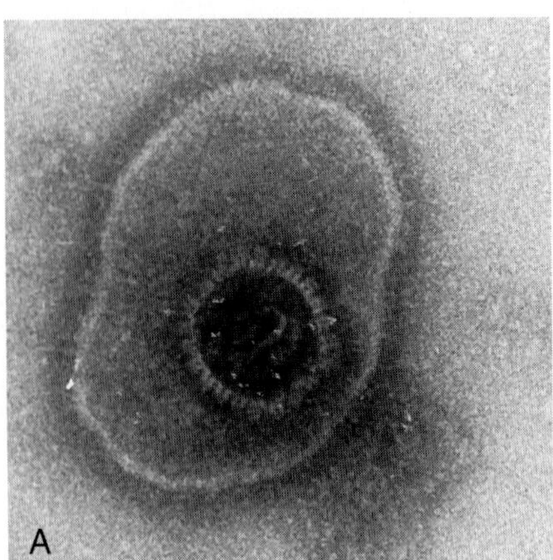

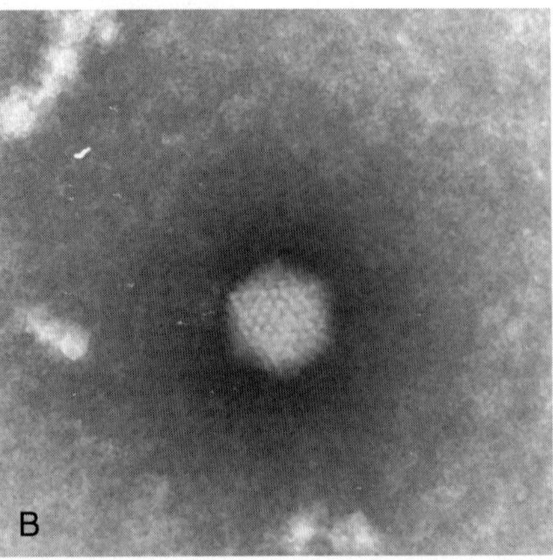

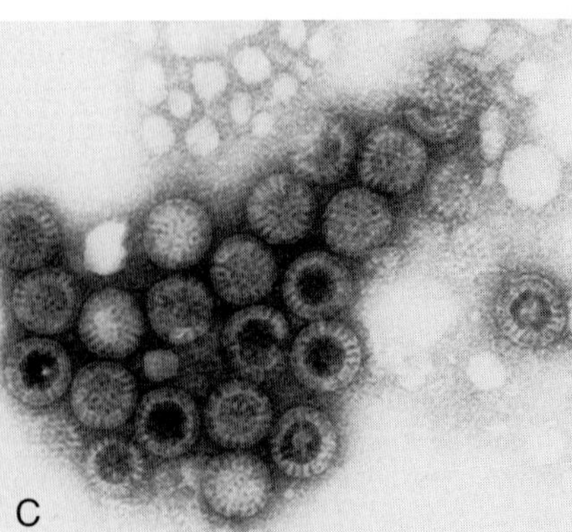

FIGURE 9–3. Electron micrographs showing characteristic morphologic features. **A,** Herpesvirus in vesicle fluid, showing the envelope nucleocapsid. **B,** Adenovirus particle in a urine specimen. **C,** Rotavirus particles in a stool specimen. Magnification: ×195,000.

dardized phenotypic methods for determining the susceptibility of isolates to antiviral agents are under development, and a plaque reduction assay for testing HSV is nearing approved status. Non-standardized phenotypic assays for determining the susceptibility of HIV-1 isolates to antiretroviral agents are also available, albeit extremely expensive. Genotypic assays involving nucleic acid sequencing of areas of the HIV-1 genome to detect mutations known to confer antiviral resistance are faster, less expensive alternatives. Antiviral susceptibility testing has also proved useful for persistent or worsening HSV or varicella-zoster virus infections in persons treated with acyclovir, for persistent or worsening CMV infections in immunocompromised persons treated with ganciclovir, and for patient-to-patient spread of influenza A virus in individuals receiving prophylaxis or treatment with antiviral drugs.

REVIEWS

Evans AS, Kaslow RA (editors): Viral infections of humans. In *Epidemiology and Control,* 4th ed. New York, Plenum, 1997.

Fields BN, Knipe DM, Chanock RM, et al (editors): *Fields' Virology,* 3rd ed. New York, Raven Press, 1996.

Greenberg SB, Krilov LR: *Laboratory Diagnosis of Viral Respiratory Disease. Cumitech 21.* Washington, DC, American Society for Microbiology, 1986, p 1–16.

Miller MJ: Viral taxonomy. *Clin Infect Dis* 1999;29:731–3.

Murray PR, Baron EJ, Pfaller MA, et al: *Manual of Clinical Microbiology,* 7th ed. Washington, DC, American Society for Microbiology Press, 1999.

Lennette EH, Lennette DA, Lennette ET (editors): *Diagnostic Procedures for Viral, Rickettsial, and Chlamydial Infections,* 7th ed. Washington, DC, American Public Health Association, 1996.

Sherlock CH, Brandt CJ, Middleton PJ, et al: *Laboratory Diagnosis of Viral Infections Producing Enteritis. Cumitech 26.* Washington, DC, American Society for Microbiology, 1989, p 1–12.

Specter SC, Hodinka RL, Young SA (editors): *Clinical Virology Manual,* 3rd ed. Washington, DC, American Society for Microbiology Press, 2000.

Storch GA: Diagnostic virology. *Clin Infect Dis* 2000;31:739–51.

Storch GA (editor): *Essentials of Diagnostic Virology.* New York, Churchill-Livingstone, 2000.

van Regenmortel MHV, Fauquet CM, Bishop DHI, et al (editors): *Virus Taxonomy. Seventh Report of the International Committee on Taxonomy of Viruses.* San Diego, Academic Press, 2000.

CHAPTER 10

Laboratory Evaluation of the Inflammatory Response

Robert S. Baltimore ▪ Hal B. Jenson

Some laboratory tests, such as a CBC and an ESR, are frequently ordered as part of the evaluation of patients with presumed infection but are not diagnostic of any particular infection. These tests reflect the hematologic response to inflammation by the total WBC count and the differential cell count, the production of proteins known as acute-phase reactants, and other metabolic changes in response to inflammation whether of an infectious or a noninfectious cause. These tests have a high degree of sensitivity for the presence of infection and inflammation, so normal values are sometimes used to support the clinical impression of the absence of serious infection. They have limited use as screening tests for infection, however, because they have wide ranges of normal values, especially in children, and require clinical correlation for correct interpretation. With some notable exceptions, their diagnostic specificity for any particular infection is extremely low.

Microbiologic diagnosis of a specific infection requires isolation of organisms, detection of antigens, or detection of antibodies developed in response to infection. However, characteristic changes of the leukocyte count and differential cell count may suggest certain infections, clarifying the need for additional, more specific tests, and in some circumstances may sufficiently confirm the clinical diagnosis to permit empiric management while awaiting results of definitive microbiologic tests. The changes in the WBC count and differential cell count and in acute-phase reactants are often useful in monitoring the person's response to treatment, and they also provide some assurance of the diagnosis as the values return to normal during the expected time interval.

NEUTROPHILS

Neutrophils normally constitute approximately 30–60% of the total leukocytes in the peripheral blood of children. The absolute number and percentage of the total WBC count are age dependent (Table 10–1). The initial cellular immunologic response to infection, especially in children, is usually a **leukocytosis,** an increase in the number of circulating leukocytes, with a neutrophilic response to both bacterial and viral agents. With most viral infections the initial neutrophilic response is transient and is quickly followed by a mononuclear response. In general, bacterial infections are associated with greater neutrophilia than are viral infections. Lymphocytes and monocytes are generally more numerous in established viral infections, although the consistency, as well as the height of this response, is less striking than that of neutrophilia with bacterial infections. Certain viral infections, such as infections with CMV and EBV, are frequently characterized by prominent lymphocytosis with relative neutropenia. However, the wide range of total and differential leukocyte counts seen with infections markedly compromises their diagnostic specificity and, to a lesser extent, their sensitivity. Without clinical correlation and relevance, the leukocyte count and the differential cell count are insufficient to confirm a specific diagnosis.

Neutrophilia

Neutrophil counts, which are normally 5,000–15,000/mm^3, as well as the percentage of neutrophils, which is normally 30–60%, in the blood of normal persons can vary considerably depending on many factors, including age (Table 10–1). **Neutrophilia** is a concentration of neutrophils in the blood that is above the normal number. Infections, and to a lesser extent other inflammatory disorders, stimulate the marrow to produce a larger number of leukocytes of the neutrophilic series. The degree of neutrophilia associated with infection depends on the cause, stage of illness, duration of infection, and systemic invasiveness, as well as on the immunocompetence of the host. A **leukemoid reaction** is defined as a total leukocyte count higher than 40,000/mm^3. A leukemoid marrow response is usually neutrophilic, but in certain circumstances other leukocyte types may predominate. A **shift to the left** is an increase in the numbers of circulating immature cells of the neutrophil series, including band forms, metamyelocytes, and myelocytes. Such an increase indicates the rapid release of cells from the bone marrow and is characteristically seen in the early stages of infection. A shift to the left is not the same as neutrophilia.

Neutrophilia is often used to identify the presence of infection, but caution must be taken because of the nonspecificity. The circulating neutrophilic blood elements are in equilibrium with the marginal compartment that consists of neutrophils sequestered in small blood vessels. Stress, vigorous exercise, or epinephrine injections may cause the marginated leukocytes to be mobilized into the circulation. This may be misinterpreted as a response to infection. Neutrophilia may also occur in certain noninfectious conditions, such as juvenile rheumatoid arthritis, especially when the inflammation is not under control; sickle cell disease; administration of corticosteroids; after splenectomy; in trisomy 21 syndrome in infancy; and in leukemic states.

Neutropenia

Neutropenia is a low concentration of circulating cells of the neutrophil series (mature plus immature cells). The **absolute neutrophil count (ANC)** is derived by adding the percentages of mature neutrophils and immature neutrophils (band forms, myelocytes, and metamyelocytes) in the peripheral blood and multiplying the total percentage by the total leukocyte count. Neutropenia is generally defined as an ANC of $<500/mm^3$ or sometimes of $<1,000/mm^3$. Neutropenia is generally not considered to be clinically significant until levels of $<1,000/mm^3$ are sustained.

Neutropenia can be caused by underproduction of neutrophil precursors in the bone marrow, a defect in neutrophil maturation, or an increased rate of cell destruction or consumption of neutrophils.

TABLE 10–1. Normal Leukocyte Counts*

	Total Leukocytes		Neutrophils†			Lymphocytes			Monocytes		Eosinophils	
Age	**Mean**	**Range**	**Mean**	**Range**	**%**	**Mean**	**Range**	**%**	**Mean**	**%**	**Mean**	**%**
Birth	—	—	4.0	2.0–6.0	—	4.2	2.0–7.3	—	0.6	—	0.1	—
12 hr	—	—	11.0	7.8–14.5	—	4.2	2.0–7.3	—	0.6	—	0.1	—
24 hr	—	—	9.0	7.0–12.0	—	4.2	2.0–7.3	—	0.6	—	0.1	—
1–4 wk	—	—	3.6	1.8–5.4	—	5.6	2.9–9.1	—	0.7	—	0.2	—
6 mo	11.9	6.0–17.5	3.8	1.0–8.5	32	7.3	4.0–13.5	61	0.6	5	0.3	3
1 yr	11.4	6.0–17.5	3.5	1.5–8.5	31	7.0	4.0–10.5	61	0.6	5	0.3	3
2 yr	10.6	6.0–17.0	3.5	1.5–8.5	33	6.3	3.0–9.5	59	0.5	5	0.3	3
4 yr	9.1	5.5–15.5	3.8	1.5–8.5	42	4.5	2.0–8.0	50	0.5	5	0.3	3
6 yr	8.5	5.0–14.5	4.3	1.5–8.0	51	3.5	1.5–7.0	42	0.4	5	0.2	3
8 yr	8.3	4.5–13.5	4.4	1.5–8.0	53	3.3	1.5–6.8	39	0.4	4	0.2	2
10 yr	8.1	4.5–13.5	4.4	1.8–8.0	54	3.1	1.5–6.5	38	0.4	4	0.2	2
16 yr	7.8	4.5–13.0	4.4	1.6–8.0	57	2.8	1.2–5.2	35	0.4	5	0.2	3
21 yr	7.4	4.5–11.0	4.4	1.8–7.7	59	2.5	1.0–4.8	34	0.3	4	0.2	3

*Numbers of leukocytes are thousands per cubic millimeter (or $\times 10^9$/L); ranges are estimates of 95% confidence intervals, and percentages refer to differential cell counts.
†Neutrophils include band cells at all ages and a small number of metamyelocytes and myelocytes in the first few days of life.
From Dallman PR: White blood cells. In Rudolph AM (editor): *Rudolph's Pediatrics,* 19th ed. Stanford, Conn, Appleton & Lange, 1996, p 1222.

Congenital disorders of the hematopoietic system may result in transient, chronic, or cyclic neutropenia (Chapter 98). Acquired neutropenia may result from microorganisms infecting the bone marrow space or leukocyte precursor cells, the hematologic toxicity of a large number of drugs, or immune-mediated leukocyte destruction caused by the development of cross-reacting antibody in response to infection or as a hypersensitive response to a drug.

Acute and usually transient decreased neutrophil production may result from the systemic effects of bacterial toxins or from viral infections of bone marrow cells. During acute infection the number of circulating neutrophils may decrease because of **margination,** the adherence of neutrophils to vascular endothelium. Acute leukopenia and neutropenia are often observed during the course of bacterial sepsis, with successful management of the underlying infection accompanied by restoration of leukocyte counts. Transient and usually mild neutropenia is characteristic of certain viral infections, such as hepatitis A and hepatitis B; infection with RSV, influenza A and B viruses, and poliomyelitis virus; measles, rubella, and roseola; VZV; and EBV infection. No specific additional care or management is required because the neutropenia usually resolves within several hours to several days.

Prolonged neutropenia resulting from anticancer therapy or from any other cause is associated with considerable risk of acquiring bacterial or fungal infections (Chapter 99). In general, the likelihood of infection increases as the neutropenia becomes more severe, with a substantial risk of prolonged duration of an ANC of $<100/mm^3$. The issue is complex, however, because neutropenia often exists in combination with other risks of infection that may be additive or synergistic.

Neonatal Neutrophil Counts. The leukocyte count rapidly changes in the first week of life (Fig. 10–1). For term infants the neutrophil count rises during the first hours of life, peaks at 12 hours (range, $8{,}000–14{,}400/mm^3$), and then gradually falls until 60 hours of life. The bounds of the normal range for the remainder of the first month of life remain constant in the range of $1{,}800–5{,}400/mm^3$. For very low birth weight neonates the normal range is greater.

A high proportion of neonates with bacterial infections have a higher than normal concentration of immature neutrophils in the blood and an elevated ratio of immature to total number of neutrophils (**I:T ratio**). In the normal neonate population, the maximum proportion of immature to total neutrophils can be as high as 0.16 in the first 24 hours of life but falls to 0.13 by 60 hours of life and remains steady with a maximum of 0.12 from 5 to 28 days of age.

Toxic Granulation and Döhle Bodies. The morphologic features of peripheral WBCs on Wright stain may demonstrate changes typically associated with bacterial infections but occasionally seen with viral infections. An increased size of neutrophil granules (**toxic granulation**) may be evident as younger neutrophils are released from the bone marrow in response to infection. **Döhle bodies** are pale blue inclusions in the peripheral cytoplasm of neutrophils. **Vacuolization** of the cytoplasm may also be seen. These morphologic changes are nonspecific for infection and may also be seen with trauma, burns, malignancy, and as a reaction to some drugs.

LYMPHOCYTES

Lymphocytes generally constitute 40–60% of the circulating leukocytes (Table 10–1). Through production of lymphokines, they are important in initiating, mediating, and modulating the immune response because of their unique role in immunologic memory and their ability to direct the activities of monocytes and granulocytes (Chapter 5). **Cell-mediated immunity,** or **cellular immunity,** refers to the lymphocytic cell response and is especially important in the control of the intracellular component of infections caused by some bacteria such as *Salmonella* and *Listeria,* mycobacteria, fungi such as *Candida* and *Histoplasma,* viruses, and protozoa such as *Leishmania.* Certain opportunistic infections are associated with specific defects of lymphocyte subsets.

Lymphocytosis

The normal lymphocyte count reaches a peak at 6–12 months of age and then declines throughout childhood until about 21 years of age, when the adult value is reached. **Lymphocytosis** is an unusually high concentration of lymphocytes in the peripheral blood and is characteristic of several infectious diseases. The **absolute lymphocyte count (ALC)** is derived by multiplying the percentage of lymphocytes in the peripheral blood by the total leukocyte count. During infancy, the ALC is normally more than twice

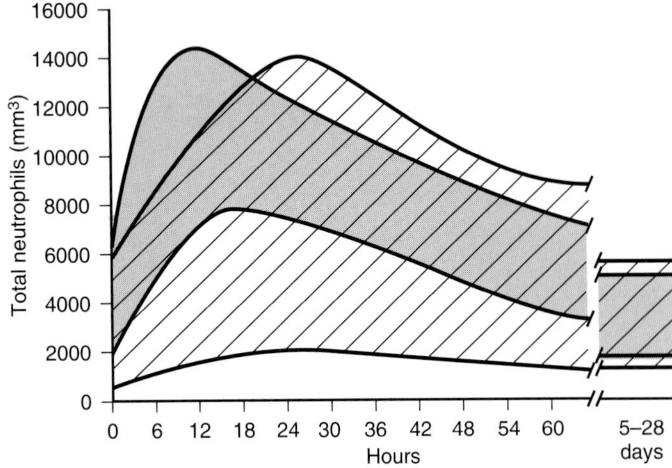

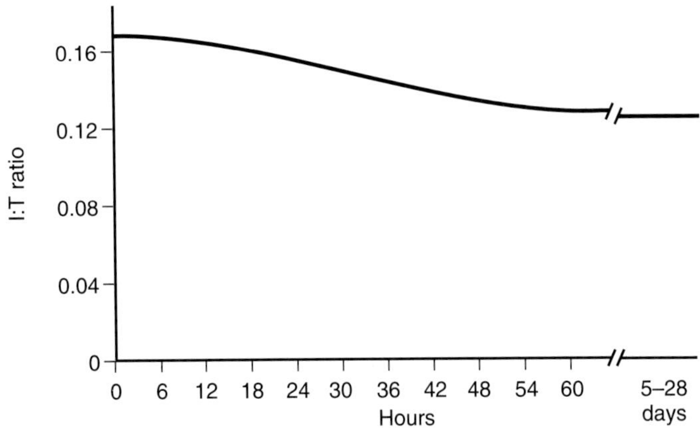

FIGURE 10–1. *Top:* Normal range of the total neutrophil count in term (*shaded*) and very low birth weight neonates (*hatched*). *Bottom:* Maximum proportion of the ratio of immature to total (I:T ratio) neutrophils in the neonate. (Data from Manroe BL, Weinberg AG, Rosenfeld CR, et al: The neonatal blood count in health and disease. I. Reference values for neutrophilic cells. *J Pediatr* 1979;95:89–98; and Muozinho A, Rosenfeld CR, Sánchez PJ, et al: Revised reference ranges for circulating neutrophils in very-low-birth-weight neonates. *Pediatrics* 1994;94:76–82.)

that in adulthood. Lymphocytosis may be characterized as **relative lymphocytosis** (>50% of the total WBCs) or **absolute lymphocytosis** (>4,500/mm^3).

Profound lymphocytosis classically is seen in pertussis, infectious mononucleosis caused by EBV, and the infectious lymphocytosis syndrome caused by an enterovirus. Lymphocytosis is also characteristic of infection with CMV, HSV-1 and HSV-2, HHV6 (roseola), *Toxoplasma gondii,* hepatitis B virus, rubella virus, adenovirus, and influenza B virus.

Pertussis. The principal agent of pertussis, *Bordetella pertussis,* produces **lymphocytosis-promoting factor (LPF),** which causes proliferation of both T and B lymphocytes. Lymphocytosis is present in approximately 75–85% of cases of pertussis, although the frequency is much lower in young infants. The total leukocyte count in pertussis may increase from 20,000/mm^3 to more than 50,000/mm^3, with the majority of the cells being mature lymphocytes. A leukocyte count greater than 40,000/mm^3 is considered to be a leukemoid reaction, which may indicate overwhelming pertussis infection or superinfection with another bacterial pathogen. Lymphocytosis also usually accompanies infection due to *Bordetella parapertussis,* which causes a milder syndrome of pertussis.

Atypical Lymphocytosis. **Atypical lymphocytes** are mature T lymphocytes that have been antigenically activated and that vary greatly in size and shape. In comparison with regular lymphocytes, atypical lymphocytes are larger and also have larger, eccentrically placed, indented, folded nuclei with a lower nucleus:cytoplasm ratio. The cytoplasm may appear vacuolated or foamy, with variable degrees of basophilia.

Although atypical lymphocytosis may be present in many of the infections that usually cause lymphocytosis, the highest levels of atypical lymphocytes are classically seen with EBV infection. The acute symptomatic phase of infectious mononucleosis is characterized by 20–30% atypical lymphocytes in the circulating leukocytes, although a wide range is seen. Other syndromes associated with atypical lymphocytosis include acquired CMV infection, toxoplasmosis, viral hepatitis, rubella, roseola, mumps, and some drug reactions.

Lymphopenia

Transient lymphopenia with rapid onset at the beginning of illness and lasting up to 24–48 hours has been described with many infections, including poliomyelitis virus, Coxsackievirus type A, rhinovirus, VZV, rubella, influenza virus, and Norwalk virus. The lymphopenia usually affects T cells, B cells, and null cells. This coincides with the accumulation of lymphocytes in tissues, which may be the major mechanism in the depletion of circulating lymphocytes that remain functionally intact.

CD4 Lymphocytopenia. The most common cause of CD4 (T4 or helper T cells) lymphocytopenia is HIV infection, and all persons with CD4 lymphocytopenia should be evaluated for HIV infection. Although transient low CD4 cell counts may occasionally be seen in apparently normal persons, persistently low counts are highly unusual. Table 6–7 lists the normal lymphocyte subsets for children and adults. Idiopathic CD4 lymphocytopenia in persons who are seronegative for HIV-1, HIV-2, HTLV-I, and HTLV-II is recognized, although it is rare. The natural history of this condition is unknown, although these persons do not demonstrate a progressive drop in CD4 lymphocyte counts with time, unlike persons with AIDS.

CD4:CD8 Ratio. The normal ratio of CD4 (T4 or helper cells) to CD8 (T8 or suppressor cells) T lymphocytes is 2:1. Diminution or even reversal of this ratio to less than 1:1 may result from CD4 cell depletion, as occurs in HIV infection, or expansion of the CD8 cell population, which occasionally is seen transiently with primary CMV or EBV infection.

EOSINOPHILS

Eosinophils primarily are tissue-dwelling WBCs and are hundreds of times more abundant in tissues than in the blood. They survive longer than neutrophils, probably for weeks in tissues. The increased production of eosinophils in the bone marrow and their appearance in the peripheral blood depends on their stimulation by specific cytokines. At least three major cytokines—IL-5, which is the principal eosinophil growth factor, GM-CSF, and IL-3—have so far been implicated in eosinophilopoiesis. These cytokines act together in the terminal differentiation of eosinophils and activate them by altering their morphologic features and their metabolism. Activated eosinophils are endowed with certain unique effector functions, such as the capacity to destroy parasitic helminths by releasing **major basic protein,** lipid mediators such as leukotrienes, and other helminth-toxic molecules contained within eosinophilic granules.

Infectious diseases commonly associated with eosinophilia are those in which the offending pathogen stimulates immunocompetent cells to release eosinophilopoietic cytokines, which occurs most often when multicellular parasites invade tissues. Thus eosinophilia is characteristic of human helminthic infections when the larval stages of the parasite migrate through skin, connective tissue, and viscera (Table 10–2). High-grade eosinophilia (>30% eosinophils, or a total eosinophil count >3,000/mm^3) frequently occurs during the muscle-invasion phase of trichinellosis, the pulmonary phases of ascariasis and hookworm infection (eosinophilic pneumonia), and the hepatic and central nervous system phases of visceral larva migrans. Eosinophilia subsequently diminishes as the larvae enter into the intestinal tract to resume development (e.g., ascariasis) or if they are cut off from the host by encapsulation or cyst formation (e.g., cysticercosis, echinococcosis). In contrast, eosinophilia is seldom seen in helminthic infections caused by pinworms and adult tapeworms, in which little or no tissue invasion occurs because the parasites develop almost exclusively within the lumen of the gastrointestinal tract.

Occasionally, eosinophilia is associated with nonhelminthic infections (Table 10–3). Tissue invasion by fly larvae (myiasis) commonly elicits eosinophil production. Approximately 10% of patients with active tuberculosis have mild eosinophilia, and eosinophilia has been described in patients with lepromatous leprosy. Eosinophilia is not usually associated with invasive fungal infec-

TABLE 10–2. Association of Helminthic Infections with Eosinophilia

Commonly Associated with Eosinophilia
Nematode Infections
Angiostrongylosis
Anisakiasis
Ascariasis
Capillariasis
Filariasis (including tropical pulmonary eosinophilia)
Hookworm infection
Ocular larva migrans
Strongyloidiasis
Trichinellosis (trichinosis)
Trichuriasis
Visceral larva migrans
Trematode Infections
Clonorchiasis
Fascioliasis
Opisthorchiasis
Paragonimiasis
Schistosomiasis
Cestode Infections*
Cysticercosis
Echinococcosis
Not Associated with Eosinophilia
Nematode Infection
Enterobiasis (pinworms)
Cestode Infection
Adult tapeworm infections

*Eosinophilia with cysticercosis or echinococcosis tends to occur primarily with inflammation associated with parasite death or cyst rupture.

TABLE 10–3. Nonhelminthic Infectious Diseases Associated with Eosinophilia

Disease	Comments
Bacterial	
Tuberculosis (*Mycobacterium tuberculosis*)	Up to 10% of patients with active disease Eosinophilia more common in men than women
Lepromatous leprosy (*Mycobacterium leprae*)	
Group A *Streptococcus*	Usually with resolving scarlet fever
Syphilis (*Treponema pallidum*)	Rare cause of eosinophilic pleocytosis
Fungal	
Coccidioidomycosis (*Coccidioides immitis*)	Usually 2nd–3rd week of infection May coincide with erythema nodosum
Aspergillosis (*Aspergillus*)	Allergic, bronchopulmonary type
Protozoan	
Isosporiasis (*Isospora belli*)	
Dientamoeba fragilis	
Viral	
Human T-cell leukemia/lymphoma virus (HTLV-I)	In association with T-cell leukemia
Human immunodeficiency virus (HIV)	May be associated with skin eruptions
Arthropod	
Myiasis	Invasion of tissues by fly larvae

TABLE 10–4. Noninfectious Systemic Diseases Associated with Eosinophilia

Hypersensitivity disorders
  Asthma
  Food hypersensitivity
  Allergic rhinitis
  Urticaria
Rheumatic (collagen-vascular) diseases
Immunodeficiency disorders
  Hyper-IgE syndrome
  Wiskott-Aldrich syndrome
  Graft-versus-host disease
Pulmonary disorders
  Loeffler's syndrome
  Hypersensitivity pneumonias
Gastrointestinal disorders
  Inflammatory bowel disease
  Eosinophilic gastroenteritis
Malignant disorders
  Hodgkin's disease
  T-cell leukemia or lymphoma (probably HTLV-I associated)
  Eosinophilic leukemia
  Myeloproliferative disorders
Miscellaneous disorders
  Sarcoidosis
Hypersensitivity drug reactions (Table 10–5)

tions, with the exception of invasive coccidioidomycosis and allergic bronchopulmonary aspergillosis, which is a hypersensitivity response to inhalation of the spores of *Aspergillus fumigatus.* Parasitic infections caused by protozoa are not usually associated with eosinophilia except in the case of some coccidial infections such as toxoplasmosis or isosporiasis. Persons with toxoplasmosis occasionally can have an eosinophilic pleocytosis in association with central nervous system involvement.

Occasionally eosinophilia is a feature of some noninfectious systemic diseases (Table 10–4). The mechanism has been established for only a few diseases. For example, the pathognomonic cell of Hodgkin's disease, the Reed-Sternberg cell, produces IL-5, which probably accounts for the association of eosinophilia in the nodular sclerosis and the mixed cellularity forms of the disease. Presumably the increased IL-5 production occurs during the inflammatory processes associated with some other neoplasms and collagen-vascular diseases. The administration of certain drugs is a common reason for eosinophilia (Table 10–5). Antimicrobial agents, in particular, are frequently responsible. The eosinophilia can develop at any time during therapy but typically occurs after several days of therapy.

TABLE 10–5. Drugs Commonly Associated with Eosinophilia

Antimicrobial Agents
Penicillins
Sulfonamides
Cephalosporins
Ciprofloxacin
Rifampin
Nitrofurantoin
Isoniazid

Amino Acids
L-Tryptophan

Anti-inflammatory Agents
Aspirin (especially for patients with nasal polyposis)

Antihypertensive Agents
Hydralazine

Central Nervous System Agents
Phenothiazines
Methyldopa
Phenytoin
Chlorpropamide

Cardiac Agents
Quinidine

Heavy Metals
Nickel

Radiographic Agents
Myelography dye

NONSPECIFIC ACUTE-PHASE REACTANTS

Inflammation is the response of living tissue to sublethal injury. The entirety of the nonspecific metabolic and inflammatory response to infection, trauma, autoimmune disease, and some malignancies is referred to as the **acute-phase response.** This response occurs immediately with injury or insult and is mediated by the pyrogenic cytokines IL-1, IL-6, and TNF-α. The acute-phase response includes a myriad of metabolic and endocrinologic perturbations, as distinguished from specific and nonspecific immunologic responses to infection (Chapter 5). Inflammation is associated with a hypermetabolic state, accentuated by the presence of fever, with decreased use of fats and increased catabolism of protein leading to negative nitrogen balance. Serum levels of albumin, prealbumin, and transferrin are decreased. Serum iron and zinc levels decrease as a result of increased cell uptake, and the serum copper level rises because of increased hepatic production of ceruloplasmin.

Within hours of the onset of infection, especially during bacterial infections and also during chronic disease such as rheumatoid arthritis and certain cancers, the liver increases production of several normal plasma proteins such as ceruloplasmin and fibrinogen. In addition, the liver produces proteins such as **C-reactive protein (CRP)** and **serum amyloid A** protein, both of which are not normally detected in healthy individuals. These **acute-phase reactants** reach a peak concentration in 3–5 days and are identified as positive acute-phase proteins, in contradistinction to those proteins whose concentration decreases (Table 10–6). The precise beneficial role of CRP and many of the other acute-phase proteins in protection from disease is not known. Although an elevated ESR or CRP concentration is supportive evidence of underlying inflammation, a normal ESR or CRP level does not exclude the presence of a pathologic condition.

Erythrocyte Sedimentation Rate. The ESR constitutes an indirect means of quantifying rouleau formation, which results from the aggregation of red blood cells, which in turn reflects the concentration of several proteins, particularly fibrinogen. During rouleau formation, the apparent surface:volume ratio of erythrocytes decreases and the denser rouleaux overcome the buoyant forces of plasma and sink. Consequently anything that alters the tendency to form rouleaux can affect the ESR. Fibrinogen and IgM increase the ESR by accelerating rouleau formation; hypofibrinogenemia results in a lower ESR by slowing rouleau formation. The erythrocyte size and concentration directly affect the ESR test. Lower erythrocyte mass due to anemia increases the ESR, and polycythemia and abnormally shaped erythrocytes (e.g., sickle cells) can

TABLE 10–6. Elements of the Acute-Phase Response

Component	Change with Infection
Erythrocyte Sedimentation Rate (ESR)	Increased
Acute-Phase Proteins	
Positive Acute-Phase Proteins	Increased
C-reactive protein (CRP)	
Serum amyloid A	
α_1-Acid glycoprotein	
Fibrinogen	
α_1-Antitrypsin	
Haptoglobin	
Ceruloplasmin	
β_2-Macroglobulin	
Platelet-activating factor	
Components of complement	
IL-6	
IL-8	
Negative Acute-Phase Proteins	Decreased
Albumin	
Prealbumin	
Transferrin	
Retinol-binding protein	
Lipids and Lipoproteins	
Triglycerides	Increased
High-density lipoproteins (HDL)	Decreased
Low-density lipoproteins (LDL)	Decreased
Very low density lipoproteins (VLDL)	Increased
Minerals	
Iron	Decreased
Zinc	Decreased
Copper	Increased
Platelets	Increased

result in a lower ESR. The ESR is directly related to age and sex; younger persons and females tend to have higher normal ESR values.

The ESR may be measured by either the Westergren or the Wintrobe method. A normal **Westergren ESR** is 0–15 mm/hr at all ages. A normal **Wintrobe ESR** is 0–10 mm/hr for males and 0–20 mm/hr for females. Measurement of the ESR as part of routine screening in symptom-free persons is valueless because 4–8% of such persons have an elevated ESR. Persons with extreme, sustained elevation of the ESR are more likely to have an underlying disorder, which is usually determined on the basis of other findings on careful history taking and thorough physical examination. Although the ESR does not rise and fall as fast as the CRP level, the ESR is nevertheless useful as a prognostic marker for the resolution of certain infectious diseases during therapy (e.g., osteomyelitis).

C-Reactive Protein. CRP is a hepatic protein that is normally present in usually undetectably low levels in serum ($\leq$10 mg/L) and serous fluids. Levels increase several hundred times within 6–8 hours after the onset of infection or injury and peak approximately 48–72 hours later. CRP levels remain elevated for the entire duration of the inflammatory process and then decrease rapidly as the disease resolves. CRP has a short half-life, which means that levels rise and fall faster than the ESR, roughly in parallel with the severity of ongoing inflammation. It can be measured by a wide variety of methods, including the tube precipitin assay, CF, RIA, a latex test, RID, and nephelometry. Typically, mild inflammation but severe viral infections may be associated with serum CRP levels between 10 and 40 mg/L; significant active inflammation or bacterial infection with levels of 40–200 mg/L; and burns and serious bacterial infections with levels of 300 mg/L or more. With successful antimicrobial treatment of bacterial infections, CRP levels fall rapidly and can be used as a prognostic marker. In certain cases of chronic inflammation, little or no increase in the CRP concentration is observed.

In neonates, CRP levels above 10 mg/L have moderate specificity for infection. Sensitivity and specificity can be increased by obtaining repeated CRP levels in the first 2 days of life or by a combination of CRP levels with other measures of inflammation, such as the I:T ratio and IL-6, IL-8, and TNF-α levels. Negative CRP values may be useful in making the decision to discontinue antibiotic therapy in premature infants with a high risk of infection and negative culture results and in determining when to stop antibiotic treatment in proven infection.

COLD AGGLUTININS

Cold agglutinins are cold-reacting, autoimmune, antierythrocyte antibodies. They react with defined groups of erythrocyte antigens, most often with the I-i system and sometimes with the P system. The I and i antigens are glycolipids or glycoproteins found on the surface of erythrocytes, polymorphonuclear leukocytes, lymphocytes, monocytes and macrophages, and platelets. The I antigen is normally present in the erythrocytes of most adults, and a low concentration of anti-I IgM, also normally present in healthy individuals, causes erythrocytes to agglutinate in the cold. Its allelic i antigenicity is typically found in fetal and umbilical cord erythrocytes, although I antigenicity predominates from early infancy through adulthood even if the i antigens persist. Consequently a cold-active antibody that strongly agglutinates normal adult erythrocytes and fails to agglutinate cord blood cells in a comparable manner may be identified as the anti-I antibody.

A cold agglutinin test measures antibodies that can agglutinate human erythrocytes in the cold but not at 37°C (98.6°F). The test is performed by adding a human group O erythrocyte suspension to serial dilutions of the test serum and incubating the mixtures at 4°C. At the time of reading, samples demonstrating agglutination at 4°C are warmed to 37°C, which should release the antibodies if the agglutination was due to a cold-active antibody. The end point is the highest dilution of serum that agglutinates erythrocytes at 4°C and is reversible at 37°C. Dilutions at which no agglutination is observed are reported as negative.

The presence of cold agglutinins can be ascertained in a simple bedside test by placing 4 drops of whole blood in an equal volume of sodium citrate (e.g., a Vacutainer tube with a light blue stopper) and placing the mixture on crushed ice for 1–2 minutes. When the tube is held up to the light and rotated, agglutination is seen as cell clumping in the thin film of blood clinging to the tube. The clumping disappears when the tube is warmed in the hands and then returns with reincubation on ice. Although this test is not quantitative, it generally correlates with a cold agglutinin titer of 1:64.

Elevated titers of cold agglutinins may be obtained in association with many infectious diseases but are obtained most classically with *Mycoplasma pneumoniae* infection and, less often, with infectious mononucleosis caused by EBV. The antibodies are heterogeneous populations of IgM, with anti-I specificity in *M. pneumoniae* infection and anti-i specificity in the case of EBV infectious mononucleosis. Although low titers of cold agglutinins are relatively nonspecific for a specific infection, higher titers (>1:64) of cold agglutinins are more specific for infection with *M. pneumoniae.* Cold agglutinins develop acutely and are transient, with a short duration. They are sometimes accompanied by cold-dependent clinical symptoms, such as pallor or cyanosis of the extremities, and can occasionally cause hemolytic episodes.

ANEMIA

Some acute infections, especially viral infections, and infection with parvovirus B19 in particular (Chapter 26), may cause transient bone marrow aplasia or selective erythroid hypoplasia. Anemia is demonstrable by laboratory testing in one third to one half of otherwise healthy children with acute febrile illness and roughly correlates with the degree of inflammation indicated by the duration and height of fever and the degree of elevation of the ESR. On this basis, symptoms of anemia are unusual because of the long half-life of normal erythrocytes and are usually only seen in persons with an underlying hemolytic anemia or shortened erythrocyte life span (e.g., with sickle-cell anemia).

Prolonged bone marrow hypoplasia, usually affecting most or all bone marrow precursor lines, is characteristic of latent viral infection with HIV or CMV.

A mild immune hemolytic anemia mediated by cold agglutinins may be seen with infection by many organisms, most characteristically with *Mycoplasma.* Clostridial infections are classically associated with severe and dramatic hemolytic anemia resulting from production of hemolysins, although a similar anemia may result from sepsis caused by other bacterial organisms.

Intrauterine infection with *Treponema pallidum,* CMV, rubella, or *T. gondii* may result in anemia due to bone marrow suppression or hemolysis, even though anemia is an uncommon manifestation of infection acquired later in life in healthy persons. Iron deficiency anemia may also result from gastrointestinal blood loss associated with parasitic infections, especially hookworm.

REVIEWS

Saez-Llorens X, Lagrutta F: The acute phase host reaction during bacterial infection and its clinical impact in children. *Pediatr Infect Dis J* 1993;12:83–7.

Wilson ME (editor): *A World Guide to Infections: Disease, Distribution, Diagnosis.* New York, Oxford University Press, 1991.

Wilson ME, Weller PF: Eosinophilia. In Guerrant RL, Walker DH, Weller PF (editors): *Tropical Infectious Diseases. Principles, Pathogens and Practice.* Philadelphia, Churchill Livingstone, 1999.

KEY ARTICLES

Butterworth AE: Cell-mediated damage to helminths. *Adv Parasitol* 1984;23:143–235.

Ehl S, Gering B, Bartmann P, et al: C-reactive protein is a useful marker for guiding duration of antibiotic therapy in suspected neonatal bacterial infection. *Pediatrics* 1997;99:216–21.

Franz AR, Steinbach G, Kron M, et al: Reduction of unnecessary antibiotic therapy in newborn infants using interleukin-8 and C-reactive protein as markers of bacterial infections. *Pediatrics* 1999;104:447–53.

Gresser I, Lang DJ: Relationships between viruses and leucocytes. *Prog Med Virol* 1966;8:62–130.

Jansson LT, Kling S, Dallman PR: Anemia in children with acute infections seen in a primary care pediatric outpatient clinic. *Pediatr Infect Dis* 1986;5:424–7.

Manroe BL, Weinberg AG, Rosenfeld CR, et al: The neonatal blood count in health and disease. I. Reference values for neutrophilic cells. *J Pediatr* 1979;95:89–98.

Muozinho A, Rosenfeld CR, Sánchez PJ, et al: Revised reference ranges for circulating neutrophils in very-low-birth-weight neonates. *Pediatrics* 1994;94:76–82.

O'Brien RT, Santos JI, Glasgow L, et al: Pathophysiologic basis for anemia associated with *Haemophilus influenzae* meningitis: Preliminary observations. *J Pediatr* 1981;98:928–31.

Pourcyrous M, Bada HS, Korones SB, et al: Significance of serial C-reactive protein responses in neonatal infection and other disorders. *Pediatrics* 1993;92:431–5.

Smith DK, Neal JJ, Holmberg SD: Unexplained opportunistic infections and $CD4^+$ T-lymphocytopenia without HIV infection. An investigation of cases in the United States. The Centers for Disease Control Idiopathic $CD4^+$ T-lymphocytopenia Task Force. *N Engl J Med* 1993;328:373–9.

Weller PF: Cytokine regulation of eosinophil function. *Clin Immunol Immunopathol* 1992;62:S55–9.

CHAPTER

11

Serologic Diagnosis of Infectious Diseases

Joseph M. Campos ▪ Hal B. Jenson

Serologic methods play an important role in the laboratory diagnosis of many infectious diseases, especially when attempts to recover suspected pathogens by culture are unsuccessful, impractical, or unavailable. These methods may be applied either to detection of specific antibodies as immunologic evidence of infection or to detection of microbial antigens in clinical specimens, with or without culture. Because serologic diagnosis by antibody testing requires some degree of host humoral immune response, it may be of limited usefulness in immunocompromised persons and is confounded by exogenous immunoglobulin administration before specimen collection.

ANTIBODY DETECTION

The ideal serologic test is highly sensitive and specific, is easily performed, is reproducible, is able to identify recent infection, and yields results comparable to those of other methods. Unfortunately, the clinical utility of most serologic tests is limited by the immunogenicity of the pathogen, the vigor of the host immune response, and the serologic method employed. Sensitivity and specificity are usually inversely related. In some cases the results of highly sensitive serologic tests that are easily performed and relatively inexpensive are confirmed by highly specific tests that are technically more difficult and more expensive. Many tests are based on commercially available reagents or test kits that have variable or sometimes unknown sensitivity and specificity. Results often depend on the skill of the operator and may vary considerably from laboratory to laboratory. Of the five classes of immunoglobulin (IgG, IgM, IgA, IgD, and IgE), only IgG, IgM, and IgA are formed in response to infection. Most serologic assays detect both the IgG and IgM classes. A positive IgG antibody result merely indicates an intact immune response after exposure to that immunogen but does not necessarily indicate recent or even symptomatic infection. Definitive serologic evidence of a current or recent infection requires either the detection of antibodies that are present during the acute phase of the illness, such as specific IgM antibodies, or the demonstration of a significant rise or fall of antibody titer in serial serum samples. It is desirable to test both sera simultaneously to avoid interassay variability, which could affect the comparison of titers.

IgM Antibodies. IgM antibodies characteristically appear 7–10 days after infection, reach a peak level at 2–3 weeks, and decline for several weeks to undetectable levels. Because the presence of IgM antibodies generally indicates current or very recent infection, only one serum sample taken during the acute phase of illness is usually needed for diagnostic purposes. The intensity of the IgM response is variable, and a weak or absent response with some infections limits the diagnostic usefulness of the assay. Determination of specific IgM antibodies, however, is a well-established method for rapidly diagnosing many different infections, especially viral infections, provided that sera were obtained at a time when IgM antibodies should be detectable. Cross-reactions with related viruses and IgM responses observed with reactivation of some latent viral infections (e.g., those caused by herpesviruses) decrease the specificity of IgM testing.

A false-negative IgM finding may result if both IgG- and IgM-specific antibodies are present, as in newborn infants with congenital infections (maternal IgG and fetal IgM) or in any patient during the transition between the early IgM and the later IgG responses to infection. Because IgG has a greater avidity for antigens than IgM or may be present at much higher titers, competition for available binding sites on assay-provided antigens could generate false-negative IgM test results.

Rheumatoid factor is an immunoglobulin, usually of the IgM class, that has anti-IgG binding activity to the Fc portion of the IgG molecule. It may interfere with assays for IgM-specific antibodies, particularly in sera from infants who have produced antibodies directed against maternal IgG. The problem arises when organism-specific maternal IgG in the sera of noninfected infants reacts with antigens in an immunoassay. Rheumatoid factor in the same specimens can bind to these immune complexes, falsely mimicking the appearance of a positive IgM test result. The incidence of false-negative and false-positive IgM results can be reduced by separating the IgM and IgG fractions of sera before assay performance. Ion exchange chromatography with inexpensive, disposable minicolumns, sucrose gradient ultracentrifugation, affinity chromatography with protein A–coated Sepharose beads, and reaction of sera with precipitating goat antihuman-IgG antisera have all been used successfully for this purpose.

IgG Antibodies. IgG antibodies are produced shortly after the IgM response, reach their highest levels 2–3 weeks after infection, and may remain detectable for life. IgG production also exhibits an **anamnestic response** after reinfection—a rapid, heightened antibody response that is not seen with IgM production. Detection of organism-specific IgG in serum samples can be used to characterize individuals as **immune.** However, it may not be helpful in the diagnosis of current or recent infection because of the variably prolonged duration of IgG production after infection.

Serologic diagnosis of infection with IgG antibody testing requires demonstration of a change in the IgG titer by testing paired sera. The first serum (**"acute" specimen**) should be collected during the acute phase of the illness. The second serum (**convalescent specimen**) should be collected at least 10–15 days later and preferably 3–6 weeks later. Because the IgG immune response does not coincide directly with the onset of clinical symptoms for all infectious diseases, serologic diagnosis may be established by demonstrating either **seroconversion,** defined as the production of antibody in a previously **seronegative** person, or a fourfold or greater increase in specific IgG antibody titer. If specimen pairs are collected later in the course of disease, they may demonstrate falling titers, indicating that peak IgG antibody production was occurring when the acute specimens were obtained. Thus a fourfold or greater fall in titer may also be considered diagnostic of recent infection. Both specimens should be tested simultaneously with the same reagents if titer comparisons are to be meaningful. A twofold rise or fall in titer is not considered significant because this degree of change is within the methodologic limitations of serial dilution tesing.

As a result of the delay in obtaining convalescent-phase sera, the diagnosis of infections with IgG-specific assays is often retrospective, an obvious disadvantage in most clinical situations. However, results of these tests may be important if culture, antigen detection, and nucleic acid detection assays fail to provide a definitive diagnosis.

IgA Antibodies. IgA antibodies are formed in response to infections of cells with secretory activity (e.g., the cells lining the respiratory, gastrointestinal, and genitourinary tracts). **Secretory IgA** is released at the sites of infection, and **serum IgA** is found in the blood. Determination of IgA titers for diagnosis of infections is uncommon, and the necessary reagents are available for limited situations.

Antibody Analyses in Fluids Other Than Serum. Detection of antibodies in body fluids other than serum or plasma can indicate infection in the vicinity of the fluid reservoir. Such analyses are usually performed on CSF or aqueous ocular fluid. Interpretation of positive results can be complicated by breakdown of the barriers between the bloodstream and the fluid reservoir, permitting ingress of serum immunoglobulins. Use of the **CSF-IgG index** aids in results interpretation by comparing the ratio of CSF IgG and serum IgG to the ratio of CSF albumin and serum albumin. For example:

$$\frac{\text{CSF IgG}}{\text{Serum IgG}} \bigg/ \frac{\text{CSF albumin}}{\text{Serum albumin}}$$

The normal range for this index is 0.4–0.6. In general, values greater than 0.7 are significant and indicate local production of IgG in the central nervous system. The specificity of this type of analysis can be substantially increased by comparing organism-specific antibody levels in CSF and serum. The ratio of specific antibody titers is compared with the ratio of another serum component, such as albumin or total immunoglobulin. For example:

$$\frac{\text{Organism-specific CSF antibody}}{\text{Organism-specific serum antibody}} \bigg/ \frac{\text{CSF albumin or total IgG}}{\text{Serum albumin or total IgG}}$$

Local production of antibodies is suspected if the ratio for specific antibody is significantly higher than the ratio for the other serum component.

Serologic Analyses in Newborns and Infants. The transplacental transfer of maternal IgG antibodies to the fetus confounds serologic diagnosis of congenital infections. Because pentameric IgM molecules are too large to cross placental membranes, their presence in a newborn's blood helps diagnose in utero and prenatal infections, provided placental rupture did not occur before birth. The longevity of maternal IgG antibodies in the fetus traditionally was considered the first 6 months of life. More sensitive assay methods in use today, however, can detect maternal IgG for as long as 15 months. Accordingly, the clinical significance of positive IgG serologic findings in the first year of life must be interpreted with caution. Stable or rising IgG antibody titers during the first year of life indicate primary infection. Falling titers are uninterpretable until the child reaches 15 months of age, at which time any detectable antibody represents exposure to an infectious agent, including those that cause congenital infections.

Labeled-Antibody Techniques

The general principles underlying **enzyme immunoassay (EIA)** (also known as **enzyme-linked immunosorbent assay [ELISA]**), **radioimmunoassay (RIA), fluorescence immunoassay (FIA),** and **immunofluorescence assay (IFA)** are similar. With the use of assay-dependent interpretive criteria, specimens are reported as **negative (nonreactive)** or **positive (reactive),** sometimes indicating the highest dilution that yields positive results when tests are performed on serial specimen dilutions. The major difference between the assays is the anti-human antibody labeling mechanism. For EIA, the label is an enzyme, usually **horseradish peroxidase, *β*-galactosidase,** or **alkaline phosphatase,** and a colored signal is generated by adding the enzyme's substrate to the assay tube. For RIA, the label is a radioisotope. For FIA, the label is a chelated form of a rare earth metal, europium. For IFA, the label is a fluorescent dye such as **fluorescein isothiocyanate (FITC).**

Of these tests, EIA, RIA, and FIA are most adaptable to automation. The signal obtained with EIA is measured with a spectrophotometer, that of RIA with a gamma counter, and that of FIA with a time-resolved fluorometer. In contrast, IFA requires a fluorescence microscope and subjective interpretation by visual inspection. These tests require more experience and expertise and therefore are significantly more time consuming. In contrast to these disadvantages, IFA offers an advantage over the other immunoassays by permitting direct visualization and discrimination of a variety of immunofluorescent patterns at the cellular and subcellular levels, such as nuclear, perinuclear (or cytoplasmic), and homogeneous or heterogeneous distribution. IFA is used as a standard test to evaluate the performance of other types of assays, including EIA or RIA.

Both EIA and RIA are sensitive assays. Although RIA is still used, EIA has replaced it in many applications because of the hazards and expense associated with using radioactive material. Some enzyme substrates are carcinogenic, but EIA is nevertheless generally less hazardous than RIA. FIA is now as sensitive as EIA and RIA. Time-resolved FIA, which exhibits reduced nonspecific background fluorescence, is a promising version of this technology.

All these labeled-antibody techniques can be applied to various antibody detection assays, the most common of which are the indirect sandwich assay and the reverse IgM-class "capture" assay.

Indirect Sandwich Assay. The indirect sandwich assay is the most widely used antibody detection assay. *Indirect* refers to the use of anti-human anti-immunoglobulins produced in other species, which are then conjugated to a fluorescent dye or enzyme and used to detect antibody binding to a known antigen fixed to a solid-phase support. The test serum is incubated with the antigen, washed, reacted with the conjugated anti-human immunoglobulin, and washed again. For EIA, it is also incubated with the enzyme substrate (Fig. 11–1). The solid-phase support for EIA, RIA, or FIA may be the well of a microtiter plate or a bead, or, for IFA, a glass slide. The antigen preparation is generally a mixture of uninfected and infected cells, especially for IFA, and may also be a recombinant molecule or a synthetic peptide for EIA or RIA.

To measure IgM by indirect sandwich assay, IgG in the sample must be removed or neutralized to minimize false-negative results, and rheumatoid factor must be removed to minimize false-positive IgM test results.

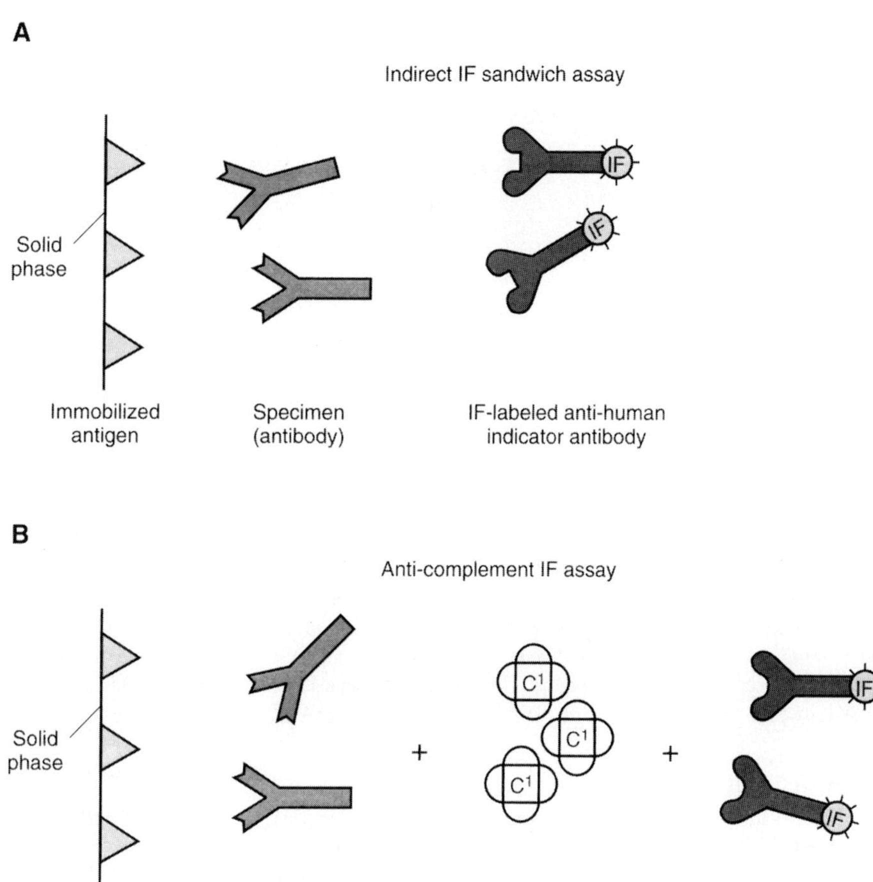

FIGURE 11–1. Immunofluorescence *(IF)* for antibody detection. **A,** Indirect sandwich assay. **B,** Anticomplement immunofluorescence assay (ACIF).

The indirect immunofluorescence sandwich assay has a few important variants: the **anticomplement immunofluorescence (ACIF) assay** and the **fluorescent antibody to varicella-zoster virus (VZV)–induced membrane antigen (FAMA) assay.** These tests are generally available only in reference laboratories. The ACIF test involves incubating the patient serum on the antigen slide, followed by the addition of human complement fixed to the cells in the presence of antibodies and then by the addition of FITC-conjugated anticomplement immunoglobulin (Fig. 11–1). The ACIF assay has several advantages compared with the indirect IFA, such as avoidance of nonspecific staining, which results from Fc receptors binding to human immunoglobulin nonspecifically, and brighter staining because of the amplifying effect of the complement system, since each IgG molecule can bind many complement molecules. However, more controls are necessary because of the addition of an extra step.

In the FAMA test, patient serum is incubated with a suspension of live, unfixed VZV-infected cells, after which a fluorescent anti-human immunoglobulin is added. Although the FAMA method is somewhat cumbersome, it is considered a standard test for the determination of VZV immune status because of its excellent sensitivity and specificity. The use of live cells, which preserves the native conformational structure of VZV antigens on the surface of infected cells, may explain the greater sensitivity of this assay.

Reverse Class "Capture" Assay. The reverse class "capture" assay has been traditionally used to detect antigen-specific IgM or IgA and avoids the problems of competitive interference and nonspecific reactivity found in indirect immunoassays (Fig. 11–2). The solid-phase support is coated with anti-IgM (or anti-IgA) antibody to "capture" and bind a representative sample of the IgM (or IgA) population present in the serum. After incubation of the serum sample and a washing step, antigen is then added. After a second washing step, bound antigen is detected by using a labeled anti-antigen antibody. This assay has proved to be both sensitive and specific.

For complete elimination of rheumatoid factor–IgM interference, which may occur with this type of assay, labeled $F(ab')_2$ fragments can be used as the indicator antibody. Rheumatoid factor binds only to the Fc portion of the IgG molecule, and therefore any rheumatoid factor present in the serum sample is not detected.

Competitive Inhibition Assay. Competitive inhibition has been applied mostly for RIA (Fig. 11–3) but can be used for EIA or FIA as well. This two-step procedure involves a first incubation of the test serum specimen with the solid-phase antigen. The immobilized antigen captures specific antibodies that are present in the sample. Then a predetermined amount of radiolabeled antibody directed against the same species antigens is added and binds to any remaining binding sites on the solid-phase antigen. Therefore in this assay format the radioactivity count measured is inversely proportional to the amount of specific antibody present in the specimen.

Direct Sandwich Assay. As in the indirect sandwich assay, the test serum is first applied to a solid-phase antigen. However, a soluble,

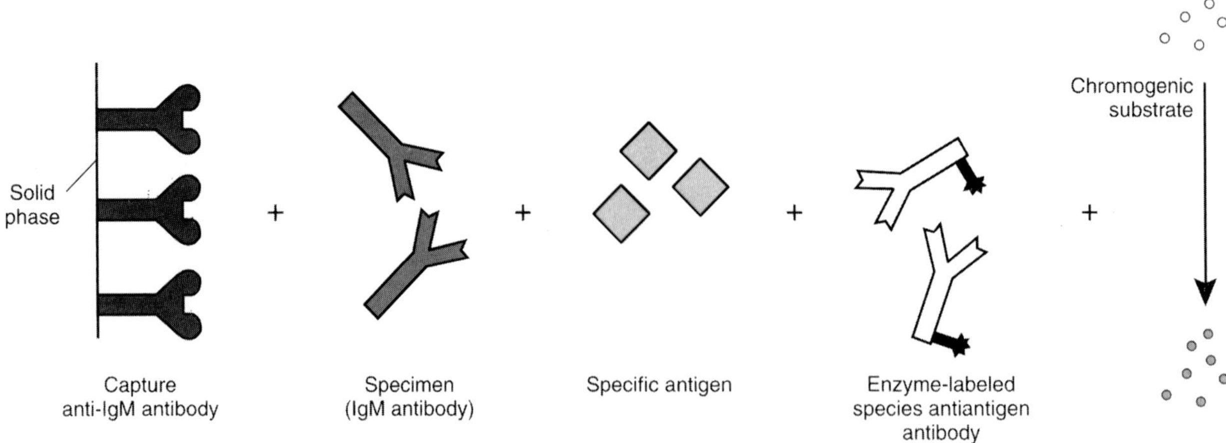

FIGURE 11–2. Principle of the reverse class "capture" enzyme immunoassay (EIA) for IgM antibody detection.

labeled antigen, instead of a labeled antihuman immunoglobulin, is then added to the mixture. Species-specific antibodies can therefore form immune complex bridges between soluble, labeled antigen and antigen coated on the solid phase. This format has been used mostly in RIA procedures but can be adapted to other types of assays.

Agglutination Assays

The agglutination assays for antibodies are very similar in principle to the particle agglutination assays for microbial antigens, with the obvious difference that the particles are coated with antigens instead of antibodies. **Passive agglutination** and **passive hemagglutination (HA)** allow identification and measurement of a specific antibody by agglutination to corresponding particulate, insoluble antigen. If the antigen is soluble, it can be adsorbed to the surface of inert particles, such as latex, bentonite, polystyrene, charcoal, or erythrocytes, for assay by particle agglutination. Microscopic latex particles, for **latex agglutination (LA),** are commonly used. Once coated or sensitized, these inert particles play a passive role as carrier molecules and react as if they themselves had the antigenic specificity of the coating antigen. For agglutination to occur, an antibody must be able to bridge the gap between particles so that at least one Fab portion is attached to a binding site on two antigenic particles. This results in generation of a lattice framework generally detectable by visual inspection. IgM molecules are generally better than IgG at forming such lattices. In the standard assay, serum dilutions are mixed with antigen-coated particles on a glass slide, placed on a mechanical rotator for 10 minutes, and examined macroscopically for visible particle agglutination. Despite the subjectivity of the interpretation of these tests, they have gained popularity because of ease of use, ability to be read visually without other equipment, and a high degree of sensitivity.

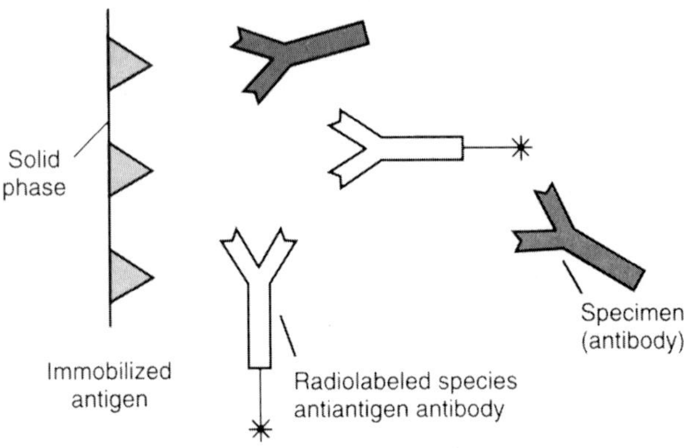

FIGURE 11–3. Competitive inhibition solid-phase radioimmunoassay (RIA) for antibody detection.

Particle Agglutination Inhibition. Most particle agglutination inhibition assays are based on the competition between antibody-coated particles and serum antibodies for a limited number of soluble antigen binding sites. Antigens that are complexed with serum antibodies are not available to react with antibody-coated particles, and particle agglutination is inhibited.

Complement Fixation

The **complement fixation (CF)** test involves competition between two antigen-antibody systems, representing the test and indicator systems that are incubated in sequence and are capable of complement activation. The CF test is based on antigen-antibody fixation of complement and consists of two stages. First, a known antigen and test serum are mixed with a predetermined amount of complement, usually from guinea pig serum. If specific antibody to the antigen is present, they react and form antigen-antibody immune complexes, and complement will be consumed, or "fixed." If antigen-antibody complexes do not form, the complement does not become attached and remains free in the mixture. Second, sheep erythrocytes sensitized, or coated, with specific antibodies (hemolysin) are added to the reaction mixture as the indicator. Because unfixed complement is a lytic agent, the absence of specific antibody from the test system results in the hemolysis of sensitized sheep erythrocytes. Therefore erythrocyte lysis signifies a negative result. Conversely, if an antigen-antibody reaction occurs in the first stage, no hemolysis will be observed because complement has already been fixed to the antigen-antibody complex. This positive result indicates the presence of specific antibody in the test serum.

The CF assay, despite its theoretical simplicity, is complicated and tedious and typically requires 2 days to complete. For reliable results, all reagents except for the unknown serum must be carefully titrated and used in precisely measured amounts. Both IgM and IgG are capable of fixing complement, but IgM is more efficient than IgG in this regard, at least theoretically. Although in many cases CF has been replaced with simpler techniques that are more direct, rapid, and sensitive, this assay remains important for the diagnosis of certain viral, rickettsial, and fungal infections. The CF test is generally performed only in reference laboratories.

Hemagglutination Inhibition and Neutralization Assay

The underlying mechanism for **hemagglutination inhibition (HI)** and for the neutralization assays is the same. The inhibitory effect of the type of antibody detected is directed against a specific biologic function of the antigen, in contrast to most other antibody assays that detect formation of immune complexes. Because both the HI and neutralization assays detect only antibodies to special functional sites on the infectious agent, these assays tend to be very specific. The presence of such antibodies at a predetermined titer correlates well with immunity to disease because these tests measure antibody that inhibits an essential biologic function of the microorganism. These antibodies do not necessarily predict immunity against reinfection, however.

Hemagglutination Inhibition Assay. The HI assay is based on the ability of certain viruses to hemagglutinate erythrocytes from specific animal sources under certain conditions. This aggregation occurs directly between specific antigens, the hemagglutinins, which are present on the surface of a virus, and receptors on the erythrocyte surface. If specific antibodies are mixed with known virus before the addition of erythrocytes, they will coat the hemagglutinins and prevent hemagglutination. This interaction is the basis of the HI test, which is relatively easy to perform. Test serum must be treated before performing the assay, however, because it frequently contains nonspecific viral inhibitors of hemagglutination or natural agglutinins of erythrocytes.

Neutralization Assay. **Neutralizing antibodies** prevent viral infection by blocking adherence of the virus to its target cells. Thus antibodies detected by the neutralization assay generally are considered protective. The efficacy of new vaccine preparations is frequently predicted by measuring neutralizing antibodies.

In the neutralization assay, incubation of virus with serum that contains neutralizing antibody prevents the virus from infecting a susceptible cell line and producing its characteristic cytopathic effect. Although the neutralization assay is one of the more sensitive, specific, and clinically relevant serologic tests available, it is cumbersome to perform. This assay is seldom used for routine diagnostic testing outside of research laboratories.

Precipitation Assays

Immunoprecipitation, or the precipitin reaction, involves the formation of complexes between soluble antibodies and antigens that become visible when their concentration is high enough to be insoluble.

The simplest method for detecting precipitation is the **tube precipitation** technique. This is performed by mixing soluble antigen and antibody (e.g., serum) in a test tube or capillary tube and observing the turbidity that results if specific reactants are present. Assays generally require overnight incubation, with visual flocculation serving as the end point. The tube precipitation method is relatively insensitive.

Immunodiffusion assays facilitate identification of specific bands of precipitation, increasing the diagnostic value of the test results. In this technique, precipitating immune complexes form after the diffusion of one or both of the reactants through a gel matrix such as agar or agarose. Diffusion may be passive or forced by an electric field in a process known as **electroimmunodiffusion.** Among the various passive immunodiffusion assays in use, the most important are the **Ouchterlony double-diffusion (DD) assay** and **radial immunodiffusion (RID).** In the DD assay, antigen and serum are allowed to diffuse toward each other through the gel matrix. If the serum contains specific antibody, a precipitin **line of identity** or partial identity develops at the junction of the advancing fronts. This line is characterized as indicating identity or partial identity by a comparison of its reactivity with that of a standard serum. The RID assay is used more often for detecting antigens than antibodies and involves incorporating the antibody into the gel and adding the antigen in a well punched into the gel. A ring of precipitation forms when optimal proportions of antigen and antibody are attained. Both DD and RID may require up to 48 hours before results are visible.

The major advantage of electroimmunodiffusion is that the time required for immune complex precipitation is significantly decreased. Of the available electroimmunodiffusion techniques, **counterimmunoelectrophoresis (CIE)** has been used most often. CIE is essentially a DD assay with electrical voltage applied across the gel to move negatively charged antigens and positively charged or uncharged antibodies toward each other. Uncharged antibodies migrate toward the negative pole by a phenomenon known as electroendosmosis (the flow of water toward the negative pole). Thus CIE requires that the buffer, pH, and voltage conditions selected result in negatively charged antigens and positively charged (or uncharged) antibodies. Because of the concentrating effects of the electrical field, CIE is 10–20 times more sensitive than the DD assay.

Immunoblotting

Immunoblotting, or **Western blotting,** is a powerful technique that allows direct visualization of antibody reactions with specific infectious-agent antigens (Fig. 11–4). A suspension of the infectious agent is disrupted with detergent or sonication, or both, to yield a solution of its antigenic components. The components are separated from one another according to size and electrical charge by electrophoresis through a rectangular two-dimensional polyacrylamide gel. The result is an array of the agent's component bands in the gel. The individual components are transferred electrophoretically in the third dimension from the gel to a rectangular immobilizing support membrane, such as nitrocellulose paper, causing formation of a replica of the gel's band pattern. Strips of the immobilizing support membrane are cut from the rectangular sheet so that each strip includes a portion of each of the agent's component bands. The strips are incubated first with test sera and then with a signal-generating antihuman immunoglobulin probe.

In a variation of the immunoblotting assay, pure antigens produced by recombinant DNA technology, rather than antigens harvested from infectious agent lysates, are used. This adaptation, known as a **recombinant immunoblot assay (RIBA),** has been used by many laboratories to confirm screening tests positive for hepatitis C virus.

The manner in which results of immunoblot and RIBA assays are visualized depends on the signal-generating probe used. If the probe was radiolabeled, the blot is placed in contact with x-ray film, for **autoradiography,** and then developed. The antigen bands that have been bound with the probe are evident on the x-ray film. Other signal-generating probes, such as enzyme-coupled antibodies and biotinylated antibodies that react with avidin–horseradish peroxidase, can also be used. Reactive antigen bands are revealed by the addition of a suitable chromogen (e.g., enzyme substrate), which deposits an insoluble precipitate directly onto the blot.

The interpretation of immunoblot results is qualitative and usually based on two criteria: (1) which band(s) are evident and (2) how intensely the bands are stained. Interpretation is subjective,

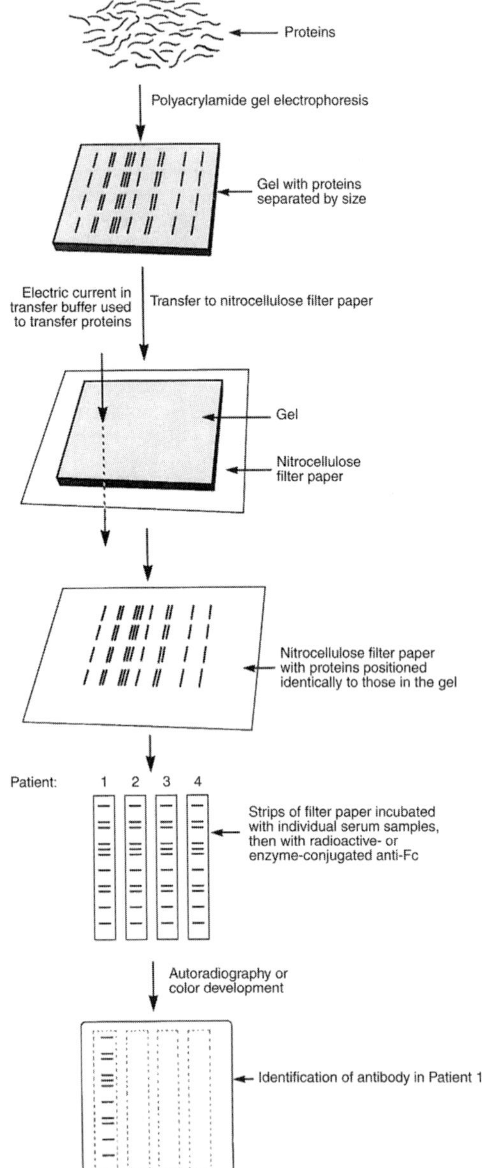

FIGURE 11–4. Immunoblotting (Western blotting) method for antibody detection. Proteins from a purified culture, or from a cell line harboring a virus, are harvested, denatured in a solution containing sodium dodecyl sulfate (SDS), and separated according to mass by using polyacrylamide gel electrophoresis. The separated proteins are transferred to a nitrocellulose filter paper by electrical current. As the filter is incubated with patients' serum, specific antibodies in the serum bind to the target proteins fixed on the filter paper. Antibodies bound to the filter paper are identified by incubating the filter with either radioactive or enzyme-conjugated anti-Fc, which are then detected by autoradiography or color development, respectively. (From Jenson HB: Retrovirus infections and the acquired immunodeficiency syndrome. *Adv Pediatr Infect Dis* 1990;5:113.)

and determining the significance of faint bands can be difficult. Immunoblot results are as sensitive as and more specific than those from conventional EIAs.

Radioimmunoprecipitation Assay

The **radioimmunoprecipitation assay (RIPA)** is an assay carried out in a liquid-phase system using purified or crude protein extracts as antigens. The infectious agent is grown in culture in the presence of radiolabeled amino acids that are incorporated during protein synthesis. The culture is then lysed, the lysate is incubated with patient serum, and the antigen-antibody complexes that form are precipitated. Radiolabeled proteins will be in the precipitate if the patient serum contains antibodies against the proteins. The precipitated material is chemically dissociated, and the labeled protein fraction is collected and applied to a gel for electrophoretic separation. After electrophoresis, the gel is exposed to x-ray film for autoradiography and the antigen bands containing radiolabeled antibodies are identified.

In general, RIPA is confined to research and reference laboratories because it is very labor intensive and requires the use of radioisotopes and live microorganisms. Both RIPA and immunoblotting are currently used as confirmatory tests for the serodiagnosis of HIV-1 infection. RIPA can help in resolving indeterminate patterns obtained by immunoblotting.

Antibody Test Panels

The majority of serologic tests, and those with the most clinical usefulness, detect antibodies directed against the infecting organism (Table 11–1). In contrast, tests that detect nonspecific, or cross-reacting, antibodies that are associated with a particular infection are usually less sensitive and almost always less specific. Two such tests, the nontreponemal antibody test for syphilis and the heterophile antibody test for infectious mononucleosis, still function as useful screening tests, however.

Febrile Agglutinin Tests. Febrile agglutinin tests are a panel of serologic tests originally intended to detect antibodies to bacteria such as *Salmonella* (Widal's reaction), *Francisella tularensis,* and *Brucella,* as well as certain of the rickettsiae (Weil-Felix test). The components of the febrile agglutinin panel, which vary from laboratory to laboratory, may include these and other serologic tests. These tests are nonspecific and insensitive. They are recommended neither as diagnostic tests nor as screening tests in the diagnostic study of patients with fever. More specific antibody, antigen, nucleic acid probe, or culture assays for these organisms should be ordered, rather than a febrile agglutinin panel.

TORCH Titers. The acronym TORCH is derived from the names of nonbacterial pathogens associated with neonatal infections: *Toxoplasma gondii, r*ubella virus, *c*ytomegalovirus, and *h*erpes simplex virus. However, this conceptual grouping is inappropriate because neonatal HSV infection is very different at presentation from these other intrauterine infections. In addition, the standard TORCH panel does not include important pathogens such as *Treponema pallidum,* HIV-1, and parvovirus. More important, interpretation of serum IgG results from specimens collected during the neonatal period must take into account possible interference from transplacentally acquired maternal antibodies. Thus the conventional TORCH titers should not be relied on for screening or obtaining specific diagnoses.

Antibody Tests for Bacteria

Group A Streptococcus. Group A *Streptococcus* infections usually are diagnosed by culture, antigen detection, or nucleic acid detection. However, serologic testing is clinically useful for documenting recent group A *Streptococcus* infection during the diagnosis of acute rheumatic fever or poststreptococcal glomerulonephritis (Chapter 40). The most commonly used streptococcal antibody tests are **antistreptolysin O (ASO), anti-deoxyribonuclease B (anti-DNase B),** and **antihyaluronidase** assays. When two or more streptococcal antibody tests are performed, increased titers are found within the first few months of onset in almost all persons with acute rheumatic fever, except for persons who also have late-onset carditis or isolated chorea.

The ASO test is an enzyme neutralization procedure. Dilutions of patient serum are mixed with a specific quantity of streptolysin O and then washed with human type O erythrocytes before examination for hemolysis. The ASO titer is the highest dilution of serum that completely prevents hemolysis of the erythrocytes. A diagnostic ASO titer is above the upper limit of normal of 120–160 Todd units for children 2–5 years of age, 240 Todd units for children 6–9 years of age, 320 Todd units for children 10–12 years of age, or ≥240 Todd units for other ages in a single specimen, or an increase in titer between acute and convalescent specimens of at least two dilutions. Because of the complicated dilution scheme used in performing the ASO test, a two-dilution rise in titer is not equivalent to a fourfold increase. ASO antibodies are present in approximately 85% of persons 2–4 weeks after group A *Streptococcus* pharyngitis. Streptolysin O is also produced by groups C and G *Streptococcus,* and the ASO test result may be positive in these infections also. The greatest value of the ASO test is serologic documentation of group A *Streptococcus* infection in acute rheumatic fever. The ASO test is not reliable for confirming antecedent group A *Streptococcus* skin infections complicated by acute poststreptococcal glomerulonephritis.

The anti-DNase B test, which uses substrate DNA, is also an enzyme neutralization assay. Depolymerized DNA is identified by the loss of alcohol precipitability or by a loss or change in color of a DNA-dye complex, such as DNA–methyl green. These antibodies are produced after both pharyngeal and skin group A *Streptococcus* infections. Thus this test is superior to the ASO test for confirmation of group A *Streptococcus* infection complicated by acute poststreptococcal glomerulonephritis. Anti-DNase B antibodies persist longer than ASO antibodies and can be used to document past group A *Streptococcus* infection in acute rheumatic fever when the ASO titer has fallen to normal levels. However, more convincing evidence of antecedent infection is the demonstration of at least a two-tube dilution or greater rise in titer between acute and convalescent sera. The upper limit of normal for anti-DNase B titers is 240–480 U for children 4–6 years of age and 480–800 U for children 7–12 years of age.

The antihyaluronidase test is an enzyme neutralization test that uses potassium hyaluronate. Hydrolysis of hyaluronate is recognized by failure of a clot to form on addition of 2N acetic acid. This test, like the anti-DNase B test, is an indicator of either pharyngeal or skin group A *Streptococcus* infection. A fourfold or greater rise in titer is considered positive. Because the anti-DNase B test is generally considered to be easier to read, the antihyaluronidase test is often used as a third-line test.

The Streptozyme test is an indirect hemagglutination assay that simultaneously detects antibodies to five streptococcal antigens (streptolysin O, DNase B, streptokinase, hyaluronidase, and adenine dinucleotide glycohydrolase) coated on erythrocytes. Poor reproducibility between the Streptozyme test and conventional ASO and anti-DNase B titers appears to be due to poor standardization of the Streptozyme reagents. This test is not recommended as a screening test and cannot be used as evidence of preceding group A *Streptococcus* infection for the diagnosis of rheumatic fever or poststreptococcal glomerulonephritis.

Legionellosis. At one time the indirect IFA for *Legionella pneumophila* antibodies was the method of choice for diagnosing legionellosis, but this has been supplanted by assays for *Legionella* antigens in lower respiratory tract and urine specimens. In addition, selective media for recovery of slow-growing *Legionella* organisms from respiratory specimens harboring mixed flora are available. Serologic evidence of *L. pneumophila* infection requires at least a fourfold rise in titer between acute and convalescent sera, with the latter specimen showing a titer of ≥1:128. Alternatively, if paired sera are not available, a single titer of ≥1:256 is presumptive evidence of recent infection.

Helicobacter pylori. Both EIA and immunoblot methods have been developed to detect serum antibodies to *Helicobacter pylori.* Antibodies are generally present in affected individuals as well as in some symptom-free individuals. Antibodies persist at high stable titers in untreated individuals, and although the titer may fall with effective treatment of *H. pylori* gastritis, it usually persists for a prolonged period after therapy. The nonspecificity of current serologic tests for *H. pylori* limits their usefulness as either screening or confirmatory tests. Recently developed stool antigen assays for *H. pylori* are now commercially available. Early studies indicate that these assays are superior to the antibody assays for diagnosis of infection. The main disadvantage to the use of the antigen assays has been their high cost.

Salmonella. The **Widal test** refers to the subset of the febrile agglutinin panel for detection of antibodies to *Salmonella typhi* using killed *Salmonella* suspensions harboring **O (somatic) and H (flagellar) antigens.** In immunologically naive populations, the serologic response to *S. typhi* O and H antigens characteristically is minimal and may not reach titers indicative of infection. The frequency of cross-reactions with other species and bioserotypes of *Salmonella* in persons with previous *Salmonella* infection is high, typically demonstrating a rapid rise to high levels on reinfection. Properly processed cultures of blood, bone marrow, stool, and bile are much superior to the Widal test for diagnosis of typhoid fever or the carrier state.

Syphilis. Because *Treponema pallidum* cannot be cultivated on artificial growth media, serologic diagnosis and dark-field microscopy are the mainstays of microbiologic diagnosis. Serologic diagnosis is generally established by using a combination of two tests: the **nontreponemal antibody (reagin) test** for screening and for monitoring response to therapy and the **treponemal antibody test** for diagnosis confirmation. Nontreponemal antibodies are directed against lipid-containing antigens, known as **cardiolipins,** that are derived from damaged host cells or perhaps from the treponemes themselves. Treponemal antibodies are specifically directed against surface antigens of *T. pallidum.*

The two most commonly used nontreponemal antibody tests are the **Venereal Disease Research Laboratory (VDRL)** test and the **rapid plasma reagin (RPR)** card test, which is a simplified variation of the VDRL test. The VDRL test uses cardiolipin complexed with lecithin, which then coats cholesterol particles. This test must be read microscopically. The RPR test, most often used today, uses cardiolipin-coated charcoal particles on a cardboard slide. Results of both of these tests can be quantified by testing serial dilutions of serum. The titers rise with the appearance of clinical lesions and with increasing duration of infection. Because they fall with appropriate antisyphilis therapy, they can be used to follow response to treatment. These tests are sensitive and inexpensive but not specific, because many noninfectious inflammatory states may give positive results.

Confirmatory treponemal antibody tests used to verify the diagnosis of syphilis include the **fluorescent treponemal antibody test absorbed with nonpallidum treponemes (FTA-ABS, or FTA)** and the **microhemagglutination–*T. pallidum* test (MHA-TP).** For the FTA-ABS, which is an IFA, the serum is heat-inactivated and absorbed with **sorbent** before testing, which removes antibodies to commensal treponemes that could cause false-positive results. The MHA-TP is a hemagglutination test per-

TABLE 11–1. Microbes and Infections for Which Specific Antibody Tests Are Often Used for Laboratory Diagnosis

		Primary Role of Antibody Testing in Laboratory Diagnosis*		
Organism	**Disease**	**As a Principal Means**	**As an Adjunct to Other Laboratory Tests**	**Not Generally Used**
Bacteria				
Group A *Streptococcus*	Acute rheumatic fever		X	
(streptolysin O, DNase B,	Poststreptococcal glomerulonephritis		X	
others)	Focal and systemic infections			X
Staphylococcus aureus	Focal and systemic infections			X
Bordetella pertussis	Pertussis		X	
Legionella pneumophila	Legionnaires' disease		X	
Brucella	Brucellosis	X		
Francisella tularensis	Tularemia		X	
Yersinia pestis	Plague		X	
Salmonella typhi	Typhoid fever		X	
Nontyphoidal *Salmonella*	Salmonellosis			X
Helicobacter pylori	Gastritis		X	
Spirochetes				
Treponema pallidum	Syphilis	X		
Leptospira	Leptospirosis		X	
Borrelia burgdorferi	Lyme disease			
By EIA				X
By immunoblot		X		
Mycoplasma				
Mycoplasma pneumoniae	Pneumonia		X	
Rickettsia				
Rickettsia rickettsii	Rocky Mountain spotted fever	X		
Rickettsia typhi	Murine typhus	X		
Coxiella burnetii	Q fever	X		
Ehrlichia	Ehrlichiosis	X		
Chlamydia				
Chlamydia psittaci	Psittacosis	X		
Chlamydia pneumoniae	Pneumonia	X		
Fungi				
Candida albicans	Candidiasis		X	
Aspergillus	Aspergillosis		X	
Blastomyces	Blastomycosis		X	
Coccidioides immitis	Coccidioidomycosis		X	
Cryptococcus	Cryptococcosis		X	
Histoplasma capsulatum	Histoplasmosis		X	
Sporothrix schenkii	Sporotrichosis			X
Protozoa				
Plasmodium	Malaria			X
Babesia	Babesiosis		X	
Pneumocystis carinii	Pneumonia			X
Toxoplasma gondii	Toxoplasmosis	X		
Entamoeba histolytica	Amebiasis			
Intestinal infection				X
Extraintestinal infection			X	
Trypanosoma cruzi	Chagas' disease (American trypanosomiasis)		X	
Leishmania	Visceral leishmaniasis		X	
	Cutaneous leishmaniasis			X
Helminths				
Nematodes				
Toxocara canis, Toxocara cati	Toxocariasis			
	Visceral larva migrans	X		
	Ocular larva migrans		X	

TABLE 11–1. Microbes and Infections for Which Specific Antibody Tests Are Often Used for Laboratory Diagnosis *(Continued)*

		Primary Role of Antibody Testing in Laboratory Diagnosis*		
Organism	**Disease**	**As a Principal Means**	**As an Adjunct to Other Laboratory Tests**	**Not Generally Used**
Helminths *(Continued)*				
Nematodes *(Continued)*				
Baylisascaris procyonis	Visceral larva migrans			X
Wuchereria bancrofti	Filariasis		X	
Brugia malayi	Filariasis		X	
Onchocerca volvulus	Onchocerciasis		X	
Loa loa	Loiasis		X	
Trichinella spiralis	Trichinellosis		X	
Strongyloides stercoralis	Strongyloidiasis		X	
Trematodes				
Schistosoma	Schistosomiasis			X
Cestodes				
Taenia solium	Cysticercosis		X	
Echinococcus granulosus, Echinococcus multilocularis	Echinococcosis		X	
Viruses				
Adenoviruses	Respiratory and systemic infections		X	
Arenaviruses	Systemic infection; hemorrhagic fever	X		
Arboviruses	Encephalitis	X		
Cytomegalovirus	Systemic infections		X	
Enteroviruses (polioviruses, coxsackieviruses, echoviruses)	Encephalitis; cutaneous and systemic infections		X	
Epstein-Barr virus	Infectious mononucleosis	X		
Flaviviruses	Systemic infections, hemorrhagic fever	X		
Filoviruses	Systemic infections; hemorrhagic fever	X		
Hantavirus	Respiratory and systemic infections	X		
Hepatitis A virus	Hepatitis	X		
Hepatitis B virus	Hepatitis	X		
Hepatitis C virus	Hepatitis	X		
Hepatitis D virus	Hepatitis	X		
Hepatitis E virus	Hepatitis	X		
Herpes simplex virus types 1 and 2	Cutaneous and systemic infections		X	
Human herpesvirus types 6 and 7	Roseola infantum	X		
Human herpesvirus type 8	Kaposi's sarcoma, primary effusion lymphoma	X		
Human immunodeficiency virus	AIDS	X		
Human T-cell leukemia/lymphoma virus type I and type II	Adult T-cell leukemia (also known as adult T-cell leukemia/ lymphoma) and tropical spastic paraparesis (also known as chronic progressive myelopathy or HTLV-I–associated myelopathy)	X		
Influenza viruses	Pneumonia		X	
Measles virus	Measles	X		
Mumps virus	Mumps	X		
Parainfluenza viruses	Laryngotracheobronchitis		X	
Parvovirus B19	Erythema infectiosum	X		
Respiratory syncytial virus	Bronchiolitis			X
Rubella virus	Rubella	X		
Varicella-zoster virus	Chickenpox; zoster		X	

*All IgG serologic tests can be used to confirm past infection and existing immunity to the infectious agent in an individual patient, as well as in population-based seroepidemiologic surveys. All positive IgG serologic test results during the first several months of life may represent transplacentally acquired maternal antibodies.

formed in the wells of microtiter trays. Sheep erythrocytes that have been sensitized with *T. pallidum* are mixed with sorbent-treated serum. A positive result is signaled by hemagglutination of the sensitized erythrocytes without hemagglutination of the non-sensitized erythrocytes. The MHA-TP has replaced the FTA-ABS in most laboratories, although clinicians still sometimes refer to it as the FTA test. Treponemal antibody titers are specific but do not correlate with disease activity and are not quantitative.

A positive RPR or VDRL test result should be followed by a specific test for *T. pallidum* antibodies because a large number of situations can cause biologic false-positive nontreponemal antibody test results. False-positive results in serum have become less common since the introduction of purified **cardiolipin-lecithin-cholesterol antigen.** Nontreponemal antibodies become detectable 1–4 weeks after infection and remain elevated until antimicrobial therapy begins or, in some cases, when untreated persons enter the late phase of the infection. The nontreponemal antibody titer then begins to fall and is usually undetectable before the cessation of treatment.

The specific treponemal antibody titers are the first to rise after infection, and the antibodies remain detectable in most persons for life, even after cure. Antibodies detected by FTA-ABS appear slightly before antibodies detected by MHA-TP. Both FTA-ABS and MHA-TP are principally used to confirm positive nontreponemal antibody test results. Because treponemal antibody test results are reported only qualitatively, and because these titers are affected very little by antimicrobial therapy, repeating these tests is of no value in monitoring response to treatment.

Diagnosis of *T. pallidum* infection in the newborn can be problematic because of the presence of transplacentally acquired nontreponemal and treponemal maternal antibodies. Serum from the infant is preferred for both nontreponemal and confirmatory tests in the diagnosis of congenital syphilis because blood from the umbilical cord may produce both false-negative and false-positive results. Pregnancy itself rarely, if ever, gives a false-positive nontreponemal antibody result; *all* positive maternal serologic test results, regardless of the titer, necessitate thorough investigation for the possibility of congenital syphilis. Comparison of the maternal and infant quantitative nontreponemal antibody titers may indicate fetal infection if the titer of the infant is at least fourfold (i.e., a two-tube dilution) higher than the maternal titer. Serial nontreponemal antibody tests should be performed for the infant with a positive test result at birth. Increasing or stable titers indicate infection or inadequate therapy; decreasing titers or disappearance of antibody indicates transplacentally acquired antibody or adequate treatment. Only a nonquantitative VDRL test should be performed for testing of CSF. The VDRL test of CSF is highly specific but is relatively insensitive (22–69%) for neurosyphilis. Use of the RPR, MHA-TP, or FTA-ABS for testing of CSF is not recommended because these tests have not been standardized for this purpose and have a high incidence of false-positive results.

Lyme Disease. The causative agent of Lyme disease, *Borrelia burgdorferi,* is difficult to grow in culture. The diagnosis of Lyme disease is usually established on the basis of clinical presentation and supported by serologic evidence of infection. Many of the currently commercially available serologic tests for Lyme disease suffer from poor sensitivity and specificity. These tests cross-react with other spirochetal antibodies, including antibodies against *Borrelia recurrentis, T. pallidum,* and *Leptospira.* Because antibody levels remain elevated for years after infection, a positive serologic test result does not distinguish recent or active infection from past infection. In addition, interlaboratory and intralaboratory variability of test results has been a significant problem. Some research and reference laboratories are able to perform sensitive and specific antibody tests that combine detection of IgG and IgM antibodies by enzyme immunoassay and immunoblot. Only approximately 55% of serologic test results reported positive by general laboratories can be confirmed by these laboratories.

Antibody Tests for Mycoplasma

Infections caused by *Mycoplasma pneumoniae* and *Ureaplasma urealyticum* are best diagnosed by culture. Serologic tests for *M. pneumoniae* include the nonspecific test for cold agglutinins (Chapter 10). Although low titers of cold agglutinins are rather nonspecific for any particular infection, titers of 1:64 and especially ≥1:128 are more specific for infection with *M. pneumoniae.* Both enzyme immunoassays and complement fixation assays for *M. pneumoniae* antibodies are available. Enzyme immunoassays for *M. pneumoniae* IgM antibodies are effective for diagnosis of acute infections. A single complement fixation antibody titer ≥1:128, or a fourfold or greater rise in titer between acute and convalescent sera, is evidence of recent *M. pneumoniae* infection.

Antibody Tests for Rickettsia

The **Weil-Felix test,** sometimes incorporated into the febrile agglutinin panel, is based on cross-reaction of selected *Proteus vulgaris* and *Proteus mirabilis* strains (OX-19, OX-2, and OX-K) with the rickettsiae that cause Rocky Mountain spotted fever, murine typhus, and endemic typhus. The end point is the highest dilution of the patient's serum that results in bacterial agglutination. These tests are not specific; positive test results are also seen with *Proteus* urinary tract infections and with certain spirochetal infections. Specific serologic assays for rickettsial antibodies are available from state health departments and the CDC and are the preferred tests for laboratory diagnosis of these infections.

Antibody Tests for Fungi

Immunodiffusion methods have been used to demonstrate antibodies to several fungi, primarily *Aspergillus* and *Candida albicans.* The sensitivity and specificity of these tests vary considerably. In some instances these tests are diagnostic, and sometimes they are used as prognostic indicators and for evaluating the therapeutic response. In most cases the information from these tests is ancillary to other, more sensitive and specific tests.

These tests should not be used as screening tests because of the high rate of false-positive results. Unfortunately, these fungal infections frequently occur in immunocompromised persons who may be incapable of mounting an adequate or diagnostic antibody response. Negative fungal serologic test results for such persons should not be used to exclude the possibility of fungal infections.

Aspergillosis. The majority of persons with allergic bronchopulmonary aspergillosis or pulmonary aspergilloma have *Aspergillus* precipitins in their blood. Sera may be screened for genus-specific precipitins, and if the results are positive, then for species-specific precipitins. *A. fumigatus, A. flavus,* and *A. niger* cause more than 95% of *Aspergillus* infections. The complement fixation test for *Aspergillus* antibodies is not as sensitive as immunodiffusion.

Candidiasis. Immunodiffusion and LA assays for antibodies directed against **mannan,** a cell wall polysaccharide, and cytoplasmic protein antigens are usually used. The LA assay gives quantitative results and requires only a few minutes to perform. An LA titer of ≥1:8 is suggestive of invasive infection. Lower titers indicate early invasive infection, mucocutaneous infection, or colonization.

Blastomycosis. An EIA test for *Blastomyces dermatitidis* detects antibodies in >75% of infected persons. Immunodiffusion and CF, formerly the tests of choice for serodiagnosis of blastomycosis, give positive results in fewer than 30% and 10% of persons, respectively. All three tests demonstrate excellent specificity. An EIA titer of ≥1:32 in a single specimen or a fourfold or greater rise in titer between acute and convalescent sera is indicative of a recent or current *B. dermatitidis* infection. A single titer of 1:8 or 1:16 is suggestive of blastomycosis.

Coccidioidomycosis. Serologic tests using CF, immunodiffusion, tube precipitation, and LA are available for *Coccidioides immitis* and are useful for diagnosis and for following the course of infection. The quantitative CF and qualitative immunodiffusion assays use heat-labile factors in coccidioidin (a skin test antigen) as an antigen. Any positive CF antibody titer is presumptive evidence of infection, with titers of ≥1:32 suggesting disseminated infection. CF titers of ≤1:8 that are corroborated by positive immunodiffusion results indicate recent infection. The CF antibody titers, which rise with advancing infection and decline with successful therapy, can be used to monitor response to therapy. The quantitative tube precipitation and LA assays give positive results earlier in the course of infection than the CF and immunodiffusion assays. These tests both use heat-treated **coccidioidin** as an antigen. The precipitation assay may take as long as 5 days, whereas the LA assay may be performed in a few minutes. Compared with tube precipitation, the LA assay is more sensitive but less specific. Antibodies detected by both methods are usually undetectable within 6 months, regardless of the patient's condition.

Histoplasmosis. Immunodiffusion, CF, and LA are currently available to test for histoplasmosis. Unfortunately, one of the antigens used for these tests, **histoplasmin,** cross-reacts to varying degrees with antibodies directed against *Blastomyces, Coccidioides,* and *Paracoccidioides,* and therefore a positive result must be interpreted in the context of the patient's travel history and clinical findings. Moreover, because recent histoplasmin skin testing causes transiently elevated antibody titers, it is essential that patients be questioned about past skin tests.

The CF test may also be performed by using an intact yeast cell antigen suspension. Antibody titers in infected persons rise earlier and are generally higher with the yeast cell antigen than with histoplasmin. A CF titer of ≥1:32 or a fourfold or greater rise in titer between acute and convalescent sera is strong evidence of infection. A single titer of 1:8 or 1:16 is suggestive of histoplasmosis. The immunodiffusion test, when it gives a positive result, provides a qualitative indication of infection if precipitin bands in the sera form similar lines of identity in comparison with positive control specimens. The M band is the first to appear after infection and provides inferential evidence of a recent skin test or current or past infection. The H band, if it appears, strongly correlates with active infection.

Usually the LA test result is positive before the CF and immunodiffusion tests. This quantitative test is performed in tubes and requires approximately 24 hours. The antibodies detected by LA rise quickly after the onset of infection. A titer of ≥1:32 is indicative of recent infection, but false-positive results because of cross-reactive antibodies or a recent *Histoplasma* skin test are possible.

Antibody Tests for Parasites

Most parasites are not routinely cultured in microbiology laboratories. Infections are diagnosed by direct visualization of the agent itself or by detection of antibodies in patient specimens.

Amebiasis. The diagnosis of *Entamoeba histolytica* dysentery (Chapter 76) and especially extraintestinal infection (Chapter 79) is greatly facilitated by serologic testing. More than 85% of infected persons possess detectable serum antibodies. Symptom-free intestinal carriers of *E. histolytica* have much lower rates of seropositivity. Microscopic examination of stained stool smears or concentrated stool suspensions is the preferred method for documenting asymptomatic carriage.

The indirect HA assay, CIE, and indirect IFA are most often used to detect *E. histolytica* antibodies. The HA assay uses erythrocytes coated with *E. histolytica* antigens and can be quantitated. A single titer of ≥1:256 is strongly suggestive of extraintestinal amebiasis.

Toxoplasmosis. Past or present *Toxoplasma gondii* infections are almost always diagnosed serologically. Baseline screening during pregnancy is recommended for selected women in the United States (see Table 94–3). Infants showing signs of intrauterine infection should be tested for IgM-specific *T. gondii* antibodies. The assays most often used are the IFA, which uses smears of *T. gondii* trophozoites, and EIA, which uses *T. gondii* antigen. The **Sabin-Feldman dye exclusion assay,** once the reference method for detection of *T. gondii* IgG antibodies, is now rarely performed. An advantage of the IFA and EIA is that IgG- or IgM-specific antibodies can be assayed. An IFA IgG titer of ≥1:1024 in an adult suggests recent infection. Any detectable IgM in a neonate or an IgM titer of ≥1:64 in an adult is proof of recent infection, although the onset of toxoplasmosis cannot be determined precisely because IgM antibodies may be detected for weeks to several months and may persist for years in approximately 5% of persons.

Special serologic tests for diagnosis of toxoplasmosis are available from the Toxoplasma Research Laboratory (Research Institute, Palo Alto Medical Foundation, Palo Alto, CA; telephone 650-853-4828). An **IgM immunosorbent agglutination assay (ISAGA),** an adaptation of the direct agglutination test, appears to be more sensitive and more specific than other tests for IgM antibodies. The **AC/HS test,** used only in adults with both IgG and IgM antibodies, is a differential agglutination test using formalin-fixed tachyzoites **(AC antigen)** and acetone- or methanol-fixed tachyzoites **(HS antigen).** AC antigen is recognized by IgG antibodies produced early in infection, and therefore a single serum sample can be used to distinguish between acute and remote infection. Also available are EIA tests for IgA antibody, which is most useful in the diagnosis of congenital infection, and for IgE antibody, which is most useful in the diagnosis of acute infection in adults.

Cysticercosis. The diagnosis of human neurocysticercosis, caused by the larval form of *Taenia solium,* is usually accomplished by demonstrating *T. solium* antibodies rather than by brain biopsy. The most reliable serologic assays are the EIA and immunoblot. A diagnostic EIA or immunoblot titer for cysticercosis is ≥1:64. Another assay, based on indirect hemagglutination (HA), is usually performed in reference laboratories. An HA titer diagnostic for cysticercosis is ≥1:128. False-positive reactions occur commonly in persons with echinococcosis.

Echinococcosis. Serologic testing for *Echinococcus granulosus* provides adjunctive evidence of infection to support radiographic findings. The sensitivity and specificity of serologic tests vary widely, however. The EIA test, the preferred method, and the indirect HA test are performed in reference laboratories. A diagnostic HA titer for echinococcosis is ≥1:128. False-positive reactions occur commonly in the sera of persons with cysticercosis.

Toxocariasis. Detection of *Toxocara* antibodies is the most precise means of diagnosis of visceral and ocular larva migrans. An EIA using larval antigens obtained from embryonated *Toxocara* ova is the serologic test of choice. The diagnostic titers for visceral organ involvement or ocular involvement are ≥1:32 and ≥1:8, respectively.

Trichinellosis. The diagnosis of trichinellosis is usually suggested by the history and clinical findings and confirmed by positive *Trichinella spiralis* serologic findings. The EIA for IgG or IgM antibodies is the test of choice. A diagnostic titer for trichinellosis is >1:5 in a person with symptoms or a fourfold or greater rise between acute and convalescent specimens. The bentonite flocculation test is an older serologic assay using serial dilutions of sera mixed with a suspension of bentonite (clay) particles sensitized with *T. spiralis* larval antigens and examined for flocculation of the particles.

Antibody Tests for Viruses

Culture, antigen detection, and nucleic acid detection methods are generally preferred for diagnosis of viral infections. Serologic tests are useful for suspected congenital infection in neonates for which IgM-specific antibody assays are available, for suspected infection with a virus that is difficult or impossible to culture, for documentation of past infection, and for screening organ and blood donors before donation of tissues or blood for transplantation or transfusion. The herpesviruses (herpes simplex virus types 1 and 2, cytomegalovirus, varicella-zoster virus, Epstein-Barr virus, human herpesvirus 6) all have the property to maintain lifelong infection after primary infection, with continuing antigen exposure and ongoing humoral immune response. Therefore a single positive IgG test result for these viruses indicates only past infection and cannot be used to diagnose acute infection.

Herpes Simplex Viruses. Virtually all sera from adults contain detectable antibodies to one or both types of HSV. The currently available commercial antibody tests for HSV are very sensitive, but many cannot reliably distinguish between HSV-1 and HSV-2 antibodies, in part because of the high level of antigenic overlap between these two very homologous organisms. Glycoprotein G–based EIA tests have been shown to be both sensitive and specific when used for herpesvirus testing in adult populations (Ashley, 1998) and have been approved in the United States for use in persons ≥18 years of age; however, they have unexplained low specificity for testing among children and adolescents. Many research laboratories can differentiate HSV-1 from HSV-2 antibodies, but results of tests based on commercial reagents or test kits should be interpreted cautiously, as only positive or negative for HSV.

Cytomegalovirus. Many persons symptomatically infected with CMV, such as organ transplant recipients and persons with AIDS, are immunocompromised and may be incapable of mounting a serologic response to CMV, or they may have received exogenous immune globulin. These circumstances often limit the usefulness of serologic diagnosis of active CMV infection in these patients. Culture is the method of choice for diagnosis of CMV infection.

Both EIA and indirect IFA are commonly performed for CMV antibodies, and both tests may also be used to detect IgM-specific antibodies. More complex assays, such as CF, ACIF, and HA, are available from reference laboratories. Detection of IgM-specific antibodies is diagnostic of infection, either current or acquired in recent weeks, or of reactivation. Congenital CMV infection is best diagnosed by culture of CMV from the newborn during the first few days of life but may be supported by the presence of IgM-specific CMV antibodies in the newborn or by rising or stable levels of CMV antibodies in serial specimens from the infant for several months. The CMV status of potential organ donors and recipients is determined by testing single serum specimens for IgG and IgM antibodies. Because variation in IgG antibody levels is normally found, there is little diagnostic utility in determination of serial IgG antibody titers.

Varicella-Zoster Virus. The main rationale for assaying for VZV antibody titers is to determine the susceptibility of unvaccinated persons with a negative or uncertain history of varicella infection. Both LA and EIA are more sensitive than CF and are most often used. The LA test is rapid and inexpensive but is relatively insensitive. This is a potential advantage for screening because positive results indicate relatively high, and therefore likely protective, antibody titers. A negative LA test result does not necessarily indicate susceptibility but is often used to determine the need for vaccination. The FAMA test is still considered the standard for determination of VZV immune status because of its excellent sensitivity and specificity, but it is infrequently performed.

Serologic diagnosis of recent chickenpox is possible by detection of IgM antibodies or by demonstration of a fourfold or greater rise in CF or IgG antibody titers between acute- and convalescent-phase sera. High levels of antibody are found in patients with reactivated infection, or zoster, but a single IgG determination cannot be used to distinguish chickenpox, zoster, or quiescent latent infection.

Epstein-Barr Virus. Culture of EBV is difficult and may take several weeks. Furthermore, isolation of EBV from a patient's saliva or blood does not prove current infection. Both the heterophile antibody assay and the EBV-specific antibody assay are used for diagnosis of EBV-associated infectious mononucleosis. The **Paul-Bunnell heterophile antibody** associated with acute EBV-associated infectious mononucleosis agglutinates sheep and horse erythrocytes, among others. Beef red blood cells, but not guinea pig kidney cells, adsorb this antibody. The latter adsorption property differentiates this response from the response to other heterophile antibodies (e.g., Forssmann antibodies) found in persons with serum sickness and rheumatic diseases and in some healthy persons.

The **heterophile antibody test** can be performed as a rapid test on a microscope slide (Monospot test). The IgM antibodies detected are unrelated to those directed against specific EBV antigens. Children younger than 4 years have a lower heterophile response that may not be detectable, presumably because of the milder illness observed in this age group. There is no anamnestic response for this antibody. A titer of >1:40 in a person with symptoms is diagnostic of infectious mononucleosis.

EBV-specific antibodies are directed against EBV **viral capsid antigen (VCA),** with an IgM response early in infection and an IgG response that persists for life; **early antigen-diffuse (EA-D)** and **early antigen-restricted (EA-R)**, which appear at the time of infection in about 70% of individuals and diminish to low or undetectable levels 3–6 months after infection; and **Epstein-Barr nuclear antigen (EBNA),** which appear 2–6 months after infection and persist at low levels for life (Fig. 37–3). Immunofluorescent tests are available for all these antigens. A positive VCA-IgM antibody titer is diagnostic of current or very recent infection (Table 37–3). The presence of EBNA anti-body dates the initial infection to at least several months previously. After primary infection and acute illness, significant fluctuations in VCA-IgG antibody titer occur without recognized correlation to clinical status. The presence of EA antibody without EBNA antibody indicates recent infection or immunosuppression, but EA antibody may be detectable intermittently and at low levels in approximately 10% of healthy individuals with remote infection. EIA tests for VCA-IgM, VCA-IgG, EBNA-IgG, EA-IgM, and EA-IgG antibodies have become available. Their sensitivity and specificity vary considerably in comparison with those of IFA.

HTLV-I and HTLV-II. The presence of antibodies to human T-cell leukemia/lymphoma viruses, type I (HTLV-I) and type II (HTLV-II), is evidence of infection with one of these viruses (Chapters 4 and 56). Current EIA serologic screening tests, based on HTLV-I antigens, do not differentiate between these two viruses, and they vary in their sensitivity to detect antibodies to HTLV-II. Supplemental tests, such as the immunoblot and RIPA, are available but may not reliably differentiate HTLV-I from HTLV-II. When PCR is used to detect HTLV-I or HTLV-II infection in volunteer blood donors, approximately half of the infections are shown to be with HTLV-I and half with HTLV-II.

Persons seropositive for HTLV-I or HTLV-II should be counseled not to donate blood, semen, body organs, or other tissues; not to share drug needles or syringes; to refrain from breast-feeding; and to consider the use of latex condoms, especially for persons with multiple sex partners, for persons in a sexual relationship that is not mutually monogamous, and for persons in a monogamous relationship with a partner who is seronegative for HTLV-I or HTLV-II.

Other Viruses. Serologic methods are the mainstay of diagnosis of recent or acute infection by IgM detection and of the determination of immune status through IgG detection for measles (Chapter 23); mumps (Chapter 36); rubella (Chapter 24); parvovirus B19 (Chapter 26); hepatitis A, hepatitis B, and hepatitis C (Chapter 78); HIV (Chapter 38); and hantaviruses (Chapter 68).

ANTIGEN DETECTION

Culture of microorganisms can sometimes be difficult, may require several days to weeks, and requires survival of microorganisms during transit to the laboratory. Some microorganisms are extremely fastidious, not amenable to culture, or patients may be receiving therapy that may interfere with culture. For these reasons, direct antigen detection offers a useful alternative or adjunct to culture and a more rapid method for diagnosis of infection (Table 11–2). The presence of intact, viable, or infectious microorganisms in specimens is not a requirement for antigen detection. In fact, individual structural and nonstructural proteins of the agent usually constitute the targets of these assays. The clinical significance of detecting such antigens varies with the agent. Because antigen detection cannot differentiate between colonizing and infecting microorganisms, it is prudent to test specimens from sites that are normally free of the microorganisms in question. For immunofluorescence-based antigen detection assays, specimens must contain infected cells or intact microorganisms. Assays that do not involve visualization of agents or infected cells (e.g., enzyme immunoassay and particle agglutination) perform well with specimens containing soluble antigens.

Labeled-Antibody Techniques

Direct and indirect assays can be used for antigen detection (Fig. 11–5). In a direct assay, antigens react directly with labeled antibodies. In an indirect assay, antigens react first with an unlabeled antibody, followed by reaction of the resulting immune complex with a second labeled antibody. The second antibody is directed against the first antibody, rather than the antigen, and increases the sensitivity of the assay compared with that of the direct method. Unfortunately, with the increase in sensitivity comes a decrease in specificity and a longer assay procedure. The indirect approach is attractive in many situations because it is more sensitive and more convenient if several different antigens are being sought in the same specimen.

Direct or indirect sandwich ''capture'' assays are widely used for antigen detection (Fig. 11–6). With enzyme immunoassay used as an example, the solid phase (e.g., tube wall or plastic bead) is coated with monoclonal or polyclonal antibodies directed against the antigen in question. The specimen is incubated in the presence of the solid phase–attached antibody, and after the washing step, labeled (in a direct assay) or unlabeled (in an indirect assay) antibody to the antigen is added. This is followed, in the case of the indirect assay, by the addition of a labeled antibody directed against the previously added unlabeled antibody. These capture assays can be adapted to most signal-generating systems. As is true of all indirect approaches for antigen detection, the animal species used to produce the second antibody must be different from the one used to produce the capture antibody.

EIA and RIA tests to detect fungal antigens in serum, urine, and CSF are useful as diagnostic adjuncts to culture and for monitoring the response to therapy in complicated cases. Commercial EIA tests are available for *Candida* and *Coccidioides* but suffer from poor sensitivity and specificity and are not recommended. A specific RIA test for *Histoplasma* antigen with approximately 90% sensitivity in serum and up to 98% sensitivity in urine, is available only from the Histoplasmosis Reference Laboratory (Indianapolis, IN; telephone 800-447-8634).

Competitive inhibition has also been applied to antigen detection (Fig. 11–7). This two-step procedure involves an initial incubation of the specimens with a well-characterized preparation of radiolabeled anti-antigen antibodies. Then the mixture is added to a solid phase coated with antigen. If antigen is present in the sample, it initially binds the radiolabeled antibodies and prevents them from binding to the solid phase. Therefore, in this assay format, the radioactivity bound to the solid phase is inversely proportional to the amount of antigen present in the specimen.

Particle Agglutination Assays

In general, the techniques used for particle agglutination–based antigen detection assays are similar to those described earlier for antibody detection, except that the target in the specimen is an antigen instead of an antibody. Thus, compared with antibody detection, the techniques for antigen detection are correspondingly reversed. Particles are coated with antibodies instead of antigen. Particle agglutination assays are in use for detection of several bacterial, fungal, parasitic, and viral agents.

Particle agglutination methods for antigen detection have long enjoyed popularity because of the simplicity and short turnaround time of the assay procedures. They detect antigens in specimens by visible lattice formation between the particles used in the assay. The sensitivity of the particle agglutination tests is usually not as high as that of the solid-phase immunoassays. Furthermore, the interpretation of test results is subjective. Despite these caveats, particle agglutination is widely used because the tests are simple and rapid.

Particle agglutination assays have largely replaced counterimmunoelectrophoresis for the detection of *Haemophilus influenzae* type b, *Neisseria meningitidis, Streptococcus pneumoniae,* and group B *Streptococcus* capsular antigens in urine, blood, and CSF. In the setting of partially treated infections, this method is especially useful when results are positive, but it is not a substitute for properly

TABLE 11–2. Antigen Detection Tests

Infectious Agent	Test	Laboratory Time to Results
Bacteria		
Bordetella pertussis	Direct immunofluorescence	30 min
Campylobacter jejuni	Enzyme immunoassay	2 hr
Chlamydia trachomatis	Direct immunofluorescence Enzyme immunoassay Optical immunoassay	30–120 min
Clostridium difficile toxin	Cytotoxicity neutralization Enzyme immunoassay	30 min to 48 hr
Escherichia coli Shiga-like toxins	Enzyme immunoassay	2 hr
Helicobacter pylori	Enzyme immunoassay	2 hr
Legionella pneumophila	Enzyme immunoassay Radioimmunoassay	2–4 hr
Meningitis pathogens *Escherichia coli* K1 *Haemophilus influenzae* type b *Neisseria meningitidis* serogroups, A, B, C, D, W135, X, Y, Z Group B *Streptococcus* *Streptococcus pneumoniae*	Particle agglutination Counterimmunoelectrophoresis	20 min
Group A *Streptococcus*	Particle agglutination Enzyme immunoassay Optical immunoassay Immunochromatography	5–10 min
Fungi		
Cryptococcus neoformans	Particle agglutination	30 min
Pneumocystis carinii	Direct immunofluorescence	60 min
Parasites		
Cryptosporidium parvum	Enzyme immunoassay Direct immunofluorescence	2 hr
Entamoeba histolytica	Enzyme immunoassay	2 hr
Giardia lamblia	Enzyme immunoassay Direct immunofluorescence	30–120 min
Trichomonas vaginalis	Direct immunofluorescence	60 min
Viruses		
Adenovirus		
Serotypes 1–39, 42–47	Direct or indirect immunofluorescence	1–4 hr
Serotypes 40–41	Enzyme immunoassay	2–4 hr
Cytomegalovirus	Indirect immunofluorescence	4 hr
Hepatitis B virus	Enzyme immunoassay Radioimmunoassay	10 min to 4 hr
Herpes simplex virus	Direct immunofluorescence Enzyme immunoassay	2–4 hr
HIV-1 (p24)	Enzyme immunoassay	4 hr to 2 days
Influenza A and B viruses	Direct or indirect immunofluorescence	30 min to 4 hr
Parainfluenza viruses 1–3	Direct or indirect immunofluorescence	2–4 hr
Respiratory syncytial virus	Direct or indirect immunofluorescence	30 min to 4 hr
Rotavirus	Enzyme immunoassay Particle agglutination	10 min to 4 hr
Varicella-zoster virus	Direct immunofluorescence	4 hr

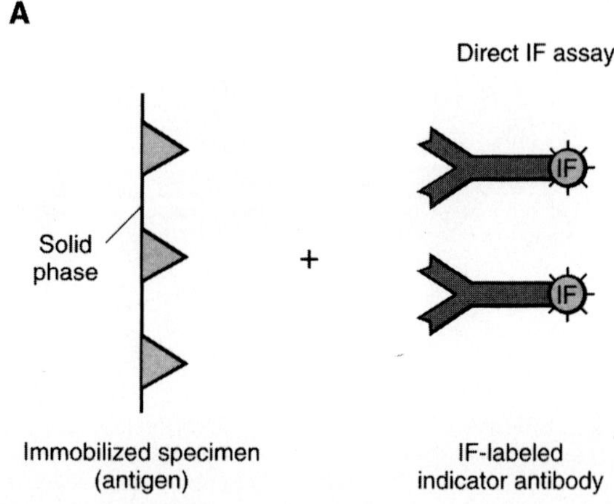

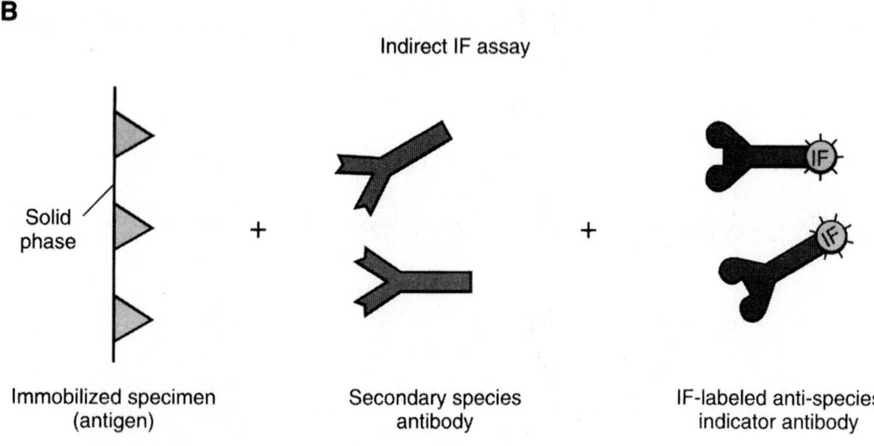

FIGURE 11–5. Principle of direct **(A)** and indirect **(B)** sandwich immunofluorescence *(IF)* assay for antigen detection.

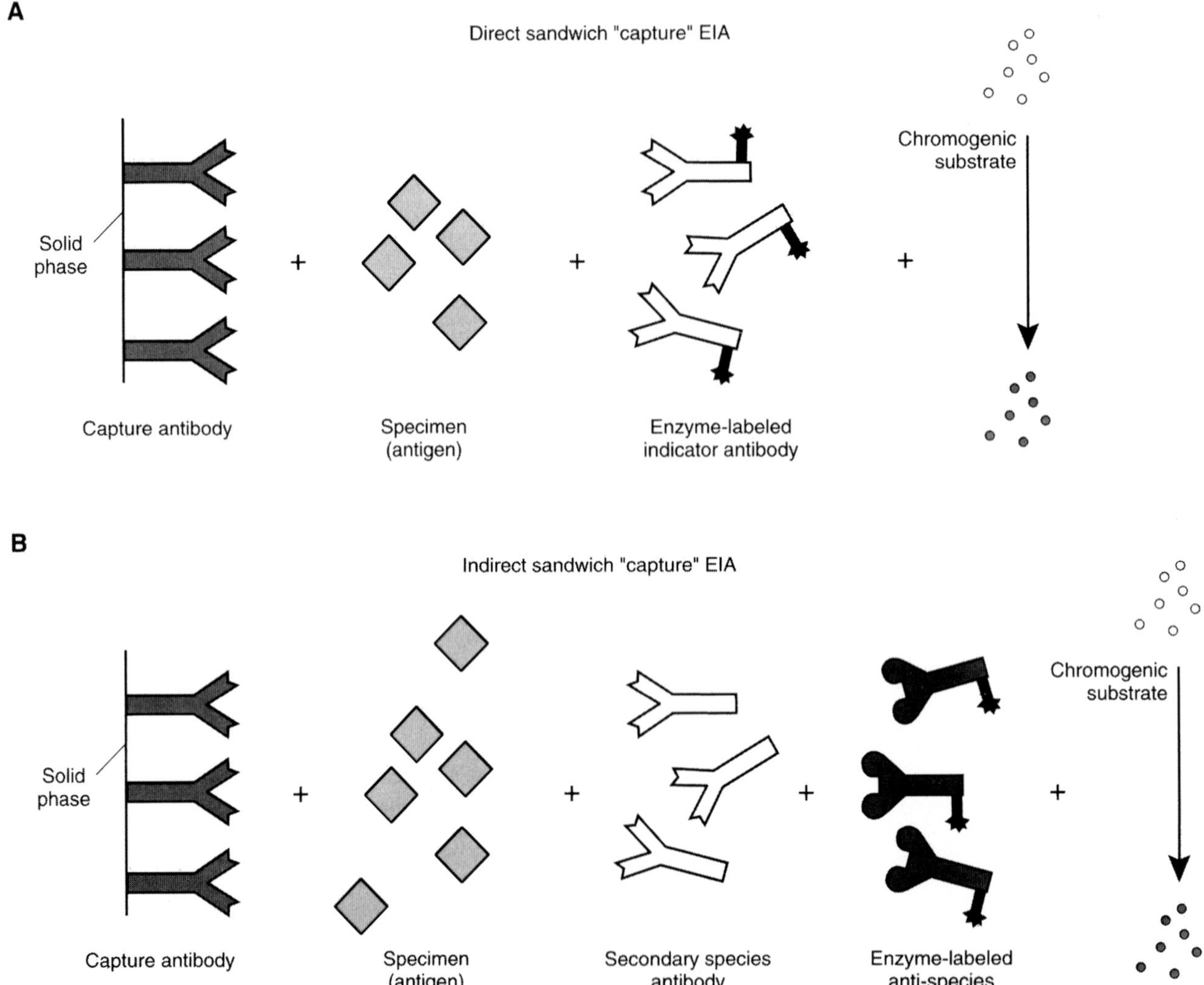

FIGURE 11–6. Principle of direct **(A)** and indirect **(B)** sandwich "capture" enzyme immunoassay *(EIA)* for antigen detection.

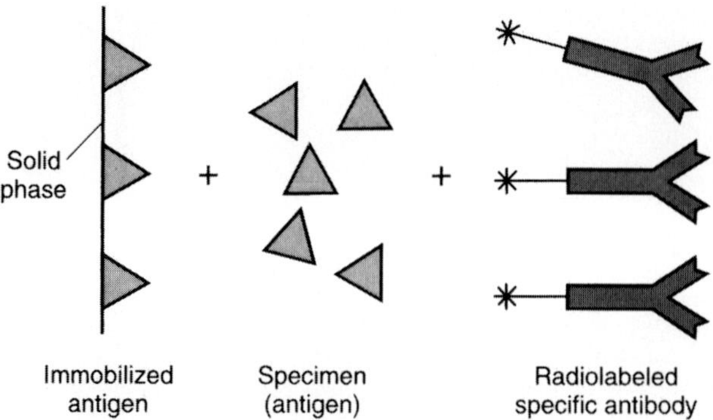

FIGURE 11–7. Competitive inhibition solid-phase radioimmunoassay (RIA) for antigen detection.

processed Gram stain and culture. Particle agglutination is also useful for detecting cryptococcal antigen in persons with serious *Cryptococcus neoformans* infections.

Immunoprecipitation Assays

The three immunodiffusion techniques described earlier for antibody detection, DD, RID, and CIE, although amenable to antigen detection, are rarely used for this purpose. DD is still used occasionally to detect fungal antigens associated with histoplasmosis, coccidioidomycosis, and aspergillosis. These assays are not especially reliable for these organisms and may be replaced by enzyme immunoassays as they are developed.

Toxin Neutralization Assay

Detection of cytotoxins associated with microorganisms can be demonstrated by neutralization of their cytotoxic effects with specific antisera. The cytoxicity assay for *Clostridium difficile* is an example in which stool extracts with and without *C. difficile* antitoxin are inoculated to growing cell cultures. If cytotoxicity is seen in the cells exposed to unneutralized stool extract, but not in the cells exposed to neutralized stool extract, then *C. difficile* toxin is present in the specimen.

REVIEWS

James K: Immunoserology of infectious diseases. *Clin Microbiol Rev* 1990;3:132–52.

Miller LE (editor): *Manual of Laboratory Immunology,* 2nd ed. Philadelphia, Lea & Febiger, 1991.

Murray PR, Baron EJ, Pfaller MA, et al: *Manual of Clinical Microbiology,* 7th ed. Washington, DC, American Society for Microbiology Press, 1999.

Rose NR, de Macario EC, Folds JD, et al: *Manual of Clinical Laboratory Immunology,* 5th ed. Washington, DC, American Society for Microbiology Press, 1997.

Steward M, Male D: Immunological techniques. In Roitt I, Brostoff J, Male D (editors): *Immunology,* 3rd ed. St. Louis, CV Mosby, 1993.

KEY ARTICLES

Andiman WA: Organism-specific antibody indices, the cerebrospinal fluid–immunoglobulin index and other tools: A clinician's guide to the etiologic diagnosis of central nervous system infection. *Pediatr Infect Dis J* 1991;10:490–5.

Ashley RL, Wu L, Pickering JW, et al: Premarket evaluation of a commercial glycoprotein G–based enzyme immunoassay for herpes simplex virus type-specific antibodies. *J Clin Microbiol* 1998;36:294–5.

Kaplan EL, Rothermel CD, Johnson DR: Antistreptolysin O and anti-deoxyribonuclease B titers: Normal values for children ages 2 to 12 in the United States. *Pediatrics* 1998;101:86–8.

Levine DP, Lauter CB, Lerner AM: Simultaneous serum and CSF antibodies in herpes simplex virus encephalitis. *JAMA* 1978;240:356–60.

CHAPTER 12

Diagnostic Pathology of Infectious Diseases

Claudia P. Molina ▪ Michael B. Smith ▪ A. Brian West

Although the majority of infections are diagnosed by culture or serologic investigations or by molecular studies of fluids or secretions, a small but important minority depends for diagnosis on morphologic or molecular studies of tissue samples. These studies usually are performed because of circumstances related to the sampling or to the pathogen. In both of these settings, morphologic studies are the first line of investigation. Sampling-related circumstances arise when a tissue specimen such as a biopsy or resection has been obtained for histologic evaluation and fixed in formalin in the usual manner, without submission of samples for culture; on histologic examination the tissue reaction is suggestive of an infectious process. Organism-related circumstances occur when a pathogen is suspected but cannot be easily cultured or is slow growing. The application of molecular techniques in clinical microbiology has allowed the detection of unculturable organisms (e.g., *Tropheryma whippleii,* hepatitis C virus [HCV]), identification of new agents (e.g., West Nile virus), characterization of previously unrecognized species (e.g., *Mycobacterium genavense*), screening of patient populations for panels of probable pathogens (e.g., otitis media, urethritis), monitoring of therapeutic responses (e.g., HIV or HCV viral burdens), and subtyping of microorganisms for prognostic purposes (e.g., HPV types 6 and 11 vs types 16 and 18; group A RSV vs group B RSV).

The detection of pathogens in histologic sections of tissue specimens has both advantages and limitations. Organisms can be localized to a site of injury, thereby implicating them in pathogenesis. Identification is frequently possible to a relatively precise level, and if not specific, the tentative identification can generally direct further investigations expeditiously. Conversely, identification is often not specific, and susceptibility to antimicrobial agents cannot be determined. A strength of histologic examination is that it embodies an enormous wealth of experience based on classic staining techniques, many a century old. Dramatic advances resulting from the introduction of immunohistochemistry and in situ hybridization during the last 25 years have greatly enhanced the power of this approach.

Critical to the diagnosis of an infection by these approaches is an adequate tissue sample from an active lesion that is properly fixed, coupled with a thorough clinical history. The starting point for detecting pathogens in tissues is characterization of the findings on the routinely prepared histologic or cytologic slide (Fig. 12–1). The clinician and pathologist must work together for the proper interpretation of pathologic findings. It is particularly important to know whether the patient has known or suspected immunodeficiency because the patient's immune status will influence the tissue reaction that is seen under the microscope and may significantly alter the interpretation of the differential diagnosis. History of travel and contact with animals may focus investigations on exotic infections or zoonotic diseases that would otherwise be less seriously considered.

HISTOLOGY AND CYTOLOGY

In histologic sections stained routinely with hematoxylin and eosin, and in routinely stained cytologic preparations, infections can be detected or suspected in three circumstances: when the organisms are visible, when there are distinctive cellular changes, and when there is a characteristic tissue reaction (Fig. 12–2).

Organisms Detected by Direct Visualization. Organisms that can be readily seen in tissues include metazoan parasites (*Dirofilaria* in the lung, cysticercosis in the brain, and *Enterobius* in the appendix), protozoa (*Entamoeba histolytica, Giardia lamblia,* and *Cryptosporidium parvum*), fungi (*Candida* and *Aspergillus*), and bacterial colonies such as those of gram-positive cocci and intestinal spirochetes, the sulfur granules of *Actinomyces,* and the occasional individual bacterium such as *Helicobacter pylori.*

Organisms Detected by Cellular Changes. Organisms that cause distinctive cellular changes fall into three groups according to their associated morphologic patterns (Table 12–1). The first group of organisms cause **cytopathic or cytoproliferative changes.** These changes, caused by a minority of viruses that can be readily recognized and may even be specific, include the presence of **multinucleated cells** (respiratory syncytial virus, herpesviruses, measles virus) and **viral inclusions,** which may be nuclear (herpes simplex viruses, varicella-zoster virus, adenoviruses), cytoplasmic (rabies virus, hepatitis B virus), or both (cytomegalovirus). The second group of organisms cause a **foam cell reaction** that is seen in histiocytes unable to stem the proliferation of intracellular cytoplasmic pathogens, which may be bacterial (*Mycobacterium avium, Mycobacterium leprae, Rhodococcus equi, T. whippleii*) or fungal (*Histoplasma capsulatum*). The third group of organisms cause **cytoplasmic granularity,** which is associated with non-foam-cell intracytoplasmic pathogens such as *Ehrlichia, Toxoplasma gondii, Leishmania, Isospora,* microsporidia, *Plasmodium,* and *Babesia.* These organisms tend to be smaller and require careful scrutiny and a high index of suspicion for detection, often using special stains.

Organisms Detected by Tissue Reactions. Organisms that cause characteristic tissue reactions constitute a large group of pathogens that may be difficult or impossible to see without the use of special staining techniques (Table 12–2). Instead, the nature of the tissue reaction suggests a differential diagnosis and thereby guides further investigations. A pattern of **tissue necrosis** with little inflammation suggests a toxin-driven process early in its development (*Clostridium difficile*), whereas an **exudative reaction** indicates including infection with pyogenic bacteria and certain fungi (*Candida* and *Aspergillus*). **Granulomatous reactions** are complex and are usually subdivided into **caseating, noncaseating, necrotiz-**

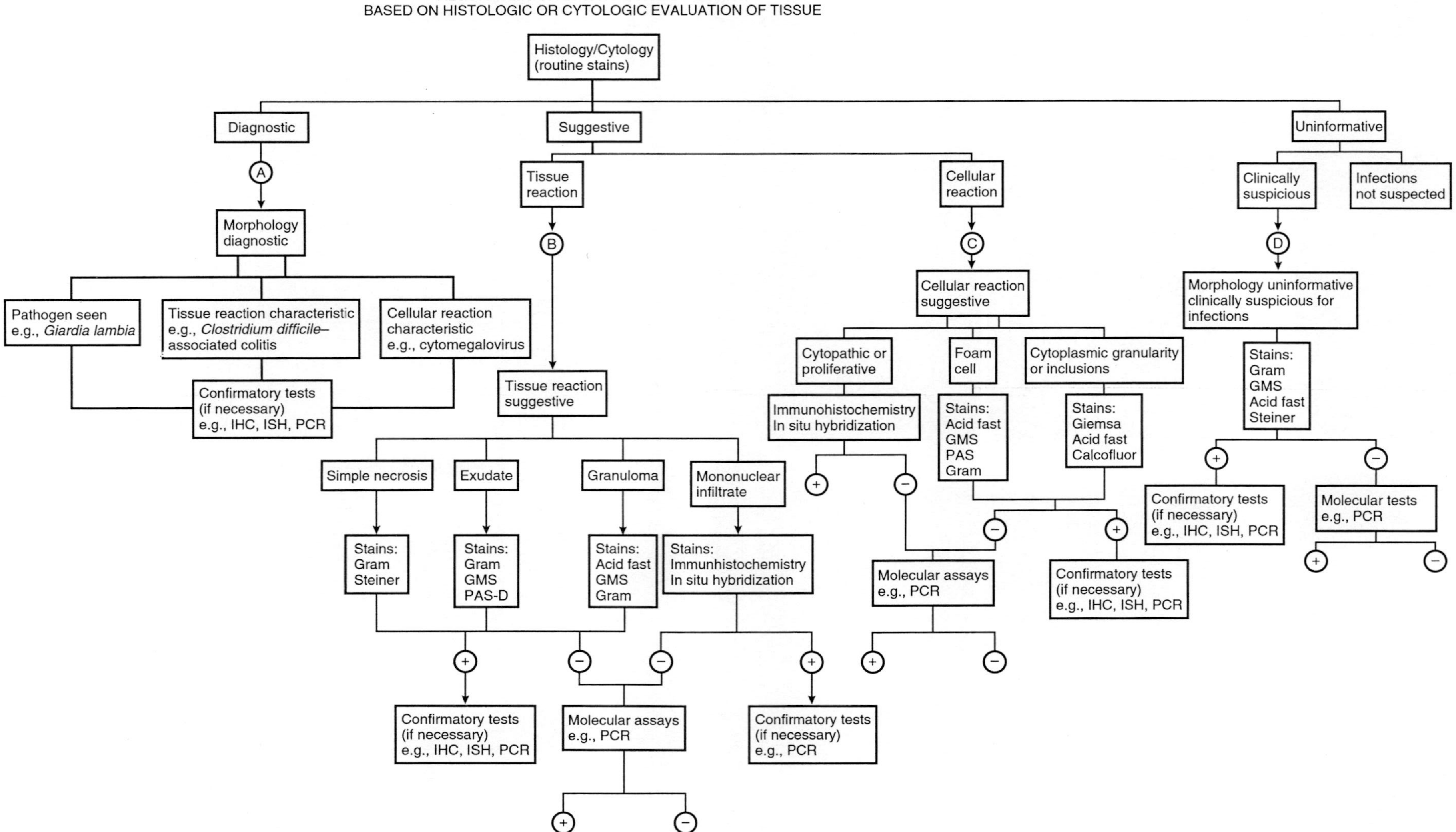

FIGURE 12–1. Algorithm for diagnosing infections in tissues by methods other than culture. GMS = Grocott-methenamine silver stain; PAS-D = periodic acid–Schiff–diastase; IHC = immunohistochemistry; ISH = in situ hybridization; PCR = polymerase chain reaction. The Steiner stain is a silver stain for bacteria; alternatively, the Warthin-Starry or Dieterle stain could be used.

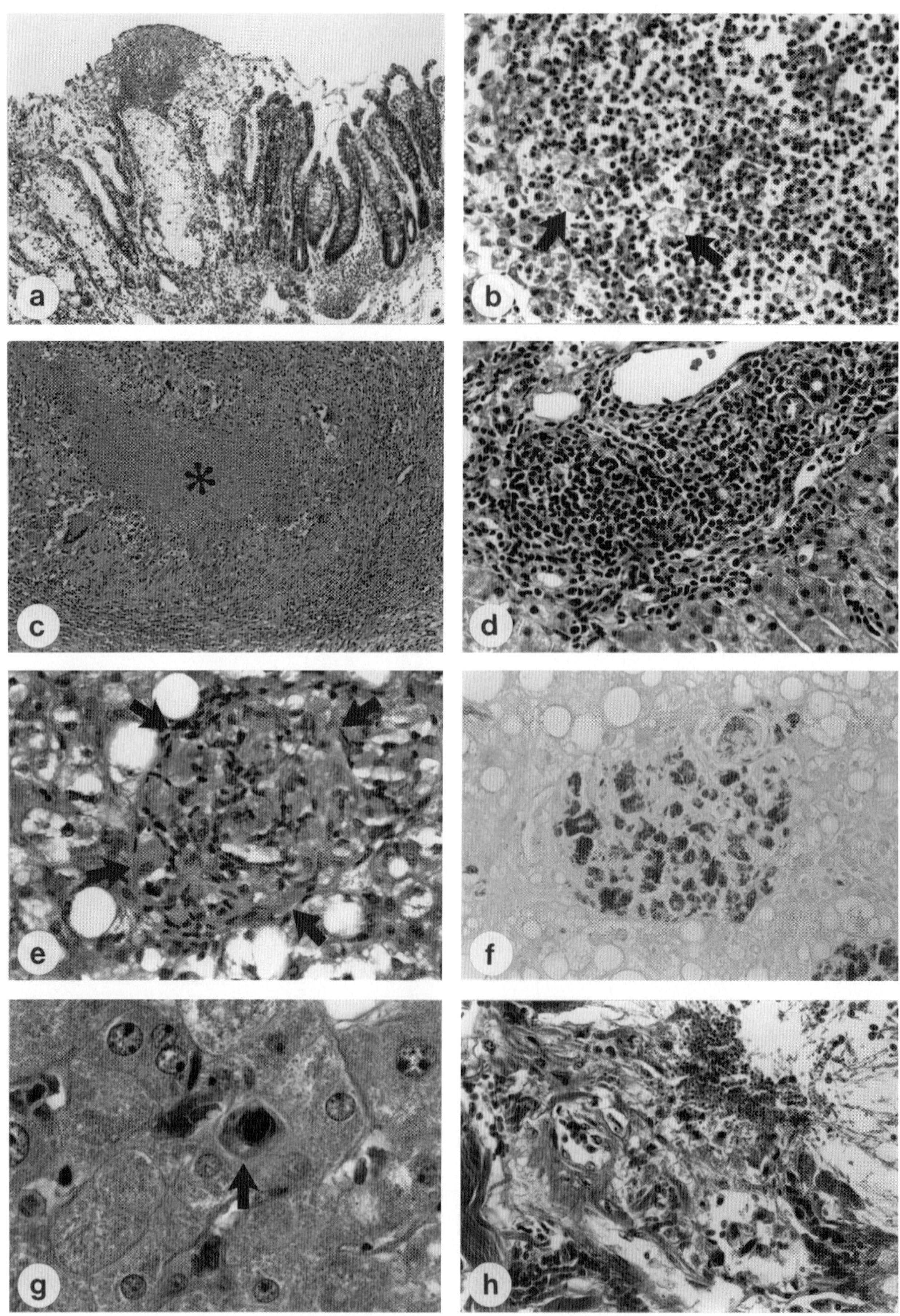

FIGURE 12–2. *See legend on opposite page*

TABLE 12–1. Pathogens Causing Distinctive Cellular Changes

Cytopathic or Cytoproliferative Reaction	Foam Cell Reaction
Adenoviruses	*Histoplasma capsulatum*
BK virus	*Mycobacterium avium* complex
Cytomegalovirus	*Mycobacterium leprae* (lepromatous form)
Hepatitis B virus	*Rhodococcus equi*
Herpes simplex viruses 1 and 2	*Tropheryma whippleii*
Human papillomaviruses	**Cytoplasmic Granularity**
JC virus	*Isospora*
Measles virus	*Leishmania*
Molluscum contagiosum virus	*Sarcocystis*
Parvovirus B19	*Septata intestinalis*
Rabies virus	*Toxoplasma gondii*
Respiratory syncytial virus	
Vaccinia virus	
Varicella-zoster virus	
Variola virus	

ing, and **fibrin ring** types, each with its own associated differential diagnosis (Table 12–2). An **interstitial mononuclear reaction** results from those organisms that cause a foam cell reaction, which often takes the form of aggregates of foamy histiocytes.

ELECTRON MICROSCOPY

Electron microscopy has a limited role to play in pathogen detection, in part because it is a poor tool for searching a large area of tissue for sparsely distributed organisms. It is of value in a few specific situations, such as screening fecal samples for viruses, determining viral morphologic features in cells showing viral injury, and distinguishing between different microsporidia.

IMMUNOHISTOCHEMISTRY

Fluorescence-tagged antibodies have been used for detection of pathogens by **immunofluorescence** in tissue sections in research for many years but are infrequently used in routine surgical pathology. The development in the last 25 years of **immunohistochemistry** using **immunoperoxidase** and **immunoalkaline phosphatase** methods for permanent sections, which includes methods for signal amplification and visualization with intensely colored chromogens, has greatly enhanced the capability for both detection and identification of pathogens in tissue sections (Plate 2H). Many highly specific antibodies are available, especially for viruses (Table 12–3).

IN SITU HYBRIDIZATION

In situ hybridization (ISH) combines molecular biologic and histochemical detection techniques to study gene expression in tissue sections and cytologic preparations (Fig. 12–3). The method involves a hybridization reaction between a labeled nucleotide probe and complementary target RNA or DNA sequences. The hybrids can be detected by histochemical chromogen development when

FIGURE 12–2. Characteristic tissue reactions (**a** to **d** and **h**) and cellular reactions (**e** to **g**). **a, Necrotizing reaction,** toxin induced, often with endothelial injury, edema, hemorrhage, and necrosis, with few neutrophils, as seen in infections by bacteria such as clostridia and the enterohemorrhagic *E. coli.* In this example of pseudomembranous colitis due to *C. difficile,* edema and red blood cell extravasation from damaged capillaries are seen in the deep mucosa and there is necrosis of the mucosal surface with exudation of fibrinomucoid material in the left half of the field. (H&E; ×75.) **b, Exudative reaction,** with neutrophil aggregation, edema, and abscess formation; commonly induced by extracellular pyogenic organisms such as staphylococci. Predominance of eosinophils is often seen in helminth infections. The photomicrograph shows a paraovarian abscess from a patient with pelvic inflammatory disease. In addition to neutrophils, which predominate, foamy macrophages are present (*arrows*), indicative of a prolonged process. (H&E; ×75.) **c, Granulomatous reaction.** Aggregates of epithelioid histiocytes, with or without necrosis, often form in response to intracellular bacteria and organisms with tough resistant cell walls, such as mycobacteria, fungi, and helminths. The illustration is of granulomatous peritonitis caused by *M. tuberculosis.* Epithelioid histiocytes form a palisade around a central area of necrosis (*asterisk*); multinucleate giant cells of histiocytic origin and small numbers of lymphocytes are present. (H&E; ×75.) **d, Interstitial mononuclear reaction.** Pure lymphoid infiltrates may be seen in viral or protozoal infections, as well as in mixed lymphoplasmacytic and histiocytic infiltrates in the late stage of any infection. The lymphoid infiltrate illustrated is mainly localized to the portal tract of this liver biopsy from a patient with chronic HCV infection. (H&E; ×75.) **e and f, Foam cell reaction.** In anergic hosts, intracellular pathogens may stimulate the aggregation of foamy rather than epithelioid macrophages, in which numerous organisms may be demonstrated (e.g., in infections with *Mycobacterium avium* complex). An example from a liver biopsy specimen of a patient with AIDS is shown in hematoxylin-eosin stain in **e** (*arrows*). The distended macrophages contrast markedly with the epithelioid histiocytes of *M. tuberculosis* granulomas in **c.** Acid-fast stain of an adjacent section (**f**) shows numerous mycobacteria forming dense clumps in the cytoplasm of each foam cell. (**e** and **f** ×275.) **g, Cytopathic or cytoproliferative reaction.** Nuclear and cytoplasmic inclusions and multinucleation are common effects of intracellular viral infections. Viruses also may stimulate hyperproliferation of infected cells. *Chlamydia* organisms cause cytoplasmic inclusions. In the example shown, CMV infection of one hepatocyte (*arrow*) has resulted in a huge nuclear inclusion. A few coarse granular cytoplasmic inclusions are present in the cytoplasm of this cell. (H&E; ×750.) **h, Null reaction.** The presence of pathogens in tissue in the absence of a host inflammatory reaction indicates that either the person is immunocompromised or the pathogens are evading the immune system. In the case illustrated, an immunocompromised transplant recipient shows no inflammatory response to intra-alveolar and invasive pulmonary candidiasis. (H&E; ×275.) (Adapted from von Lichtenberg F: *Pathology of Infectious Diseases.* New York, Raven, 1991.)

TABLE 12–2. Pathogens Causing Distinctive Tissue Reactions

Necrotizing Reaction with Little Inflammation	Mycobacteria
Toxin-Producing Organisms Including	*Nocardia*
Clostridium	*Sporothrix schenckii*
Enterohemorrhagic *Escherichia coli*	***Necrotizing Granulomas***
Vibrio vulnificus (early infection)	*Acanthamoeba*
Exudative Reaction	*Bartonella henselae*
Actinomycetes	*Blastomyces dermatitidis*
Aspergillus	*Chlamydia trachomatis*
Candida	*Chromoblastomycetes*
Pyogenic bacteria	*Francisella tularensis*
Zygomycetes	Nontuberculous mycobacteria
Granulomatous Reaction	*Paracoccidioides brasiliensis*
Noncaseating Granulomas	*Phaeohyphomycetes*
Brucella	*Sporothrix schenckii*
Dirofilaria immitis	*Yersinia enterocolitica*
Ehrlichia	*Yersinia pseudotuberculosis*
Histoplasma capsulatum	***Fibrin Ring Granulomas***
Mycobacteria	*Coxiella burnetii*
Schistosoma	Cytomegalovirus
Toxoplasma gondii	**Interstitial Mononuclear Reaction (Foam Cell)**
Caseating Granulomas	Coxsackieviruses
Aspergillus	*Cryptosporidium parvum*
Blastomyces dermatitidis	Hepatitis B and C viruses
Brucella	Lymphocytic choriomeningitis virus
Coccidioides immitis	Rabies virus
Cryptococcus neoformans	*Toxoplasma gondii*
Histoplasma capsulatum	*Treponema pallidum*

appropriately labeled probes are used. ISH localizes nucleotide sequences in the cell and visualizes portions of genome or message while preserving cell integrity within the heterogeneous tissue, permitting important anatomic interpretations. Many DNA probes are available for ISH identification of microorganisms including bacteria, fungi, and viruses (Table 12–4).

NUCLEIC ACID AMPLIFICATION METHODS

Nucleic acid amplification techniques increase the sensitivity of detection assays for nucleic acids and offer the possibility of automation and nonradioactive detection formats. There are three categories of amplification: (1) **target amplification** systems, which use PCR, transcription-mediated amplification, or strand displacement amplification; (2) **probe amplification** systems, which use Qβ replicase or thermostable DNA ligase for ligase chain reaction; and (3) **signal amplification** systems, which use compound probes or branched-probe technology to increase the signal in proportion to the amount of target in the reaction. Probe and signal amplification methods have been used primarily for research.

Polymerase Chain Reaction. PCR assays have been widely used for the detection of all types of microorganisms in tissues (Table 12–5), and numerous PCR-based kits are commercially available, including HIV type 1, HCV, cytomegalovirus, herpes simplex viruses, *Chlamydia trachomatis, Neisseria gonorrhoeae,* and *Mycobacterium tuberculosis.* The FDA has approved only a few PCR tests for use in clinical diagnosis.

The PCR assay occurs in three steps: melting or denaturing of double-stranded DNA at high temperatures to form two single-stranded fragments of DNA; cooling to allow annealing of oligonucleotide primers to complementary sequences of interest; and extension, in which *Taq* polymerase, a thermostable DNA polymerase from *Thermus aquaticus,* synthesizes DNA by extending the primers. The number of copies of the target DNA is geometrically amplified during 20–50 cycles, permitting detection of the target by electrophoresis followed by ethidium bromide staining, immunofluorescence detection, or a radioactive probe.

PCR assay is susceptible to interfering substances and to false-positive results. It must be performed with strict attention to avoiding contamination between samples, especially contamination of fresh, unamplified samples with amplified products from previous reactions. This is critical for the accurate diagnosis of infectious pathogens. Another drawback of PCR, if the assay result is positive, is that a culture of the infectious agent is not available for antimicrobial testing. Positive PCR results must be interpreted carefully because they may also be positive in the recovery phase of disease, when the infection is no longer contagious. Another drawback of PCR is that generally only one microorganism can be tested for at a time.

Several modifications of PCR technology have been developed. **Solution PCR,** the classic form of the procedure, offers substantially increased sensitivity over dot blotting, Southern blotting, or ISH. However, its utility may be restricted in certain situations because it detects only the presence of microbial DNA and does not localize the DNA to a specific cell or area of the tissue. **Reverse transcriptase–PCR (RT-PCR)** is used to amplify RNA targets. **Reverse transcriptase (RT)** is employed to synthesize a **complementary DNA (cDNA)** strand using RNA as the initial template, followed by PCR amplification. This is necessary in identifying specific mRNA and a wide array of RNA viral genomes, such as HIV and HCV. **Real-time PCR** provides information as the nucleic

TABLE 12–3. Infectious Agents Identified in Routinely Processed Tissues Using Monoclonal and Polyclonal Antibodies for Immunofluorescence or Immunohistochemistry

Bacteria	Viruses	Fungi
Actinomyces	Adenoviruses	*Absidia*
Afipia felis	Coronaviruses	*Aspergillus*
Bacillus anthracis	Coxsackie B viruses	*Blastomyces dermatitidis*
Bacteroides gingivalis	Cytomegalovirus	*Candida*
Bartonella	Dengue fever virus	*Coccidioides immitis*
Borrelia burgdorferi	Eastern equine encephalitis virus	*Cryptococcus neoformans*
Brucella	Ebola virus	*Fusarium*
Campylobacter	Echoviruses	*Histoplasma capsulatum*
Clostridium	Epstein-Barr virus	*Paracoccidioides brasiliensis*
Enterococcus	Hantaviruses	*Pneumocystis carinii*
Escherichia coli	Hepatitis A virus	*Pseudallescheria boydii*
Escherichia coli (O157:H7)	Hepatitis B virus	*Rhizomucor*
Gardnerella vaginalis	Hepatitis C virus	*Sporothrix schenckii*
Haemophilus ducreyi	Hepatitis D virus	*Trichosporon beigelii*
Haemophilus influenzae	Hepatitis E virus	**Protozoa**
Helicobacter pylori	Herpes simplex viruses 1 and 2	*Acanthamoeba*
Klebsiella	Human herpesvirus 6	*Cryptosporidium parvum*
Legionella pneumophila	Human herpesvirus 7	*Entamoeba histolytica*
Leptospira interrogans	Human herpesvirus 8	*Giardia lamblia*
Listeria monocytogenes	Human immunodeficiency virus	*Leishmania*
Mycobacterium	Human papillomaviruses	Microsporidia
Mycoplasma	Human T-lymphotropic virus type I	*Plasmodium falciparum*
Neisseria gonorrhoeae	Influenza viruses	*Toxoplasma gondii*
Pseudomonas aeruginosa	Lassa virus	*Trichomonas vaginalis*
Salmonella	Marburg virus	*Trypanosoma cruzi*
Shigella	Measles virus	**Others**
Staphylococcus	Parvovirus B19	*Chlamydia*
Streptococcus	Polioviruses	*Coxiella burnetii*
Treponema pallidum	Polyoma viruses (BK and JC)	*Ehrlichia chaffeensis*
Vibrio	Poxvirus	*Rickettsia*
Yersinia	Rabies virus	
	Respiratory syncytial virus	
	Rift Valley fever virus	
	Rotavirus	
	Varicella-zoster virus	
	Yellow fever virus	

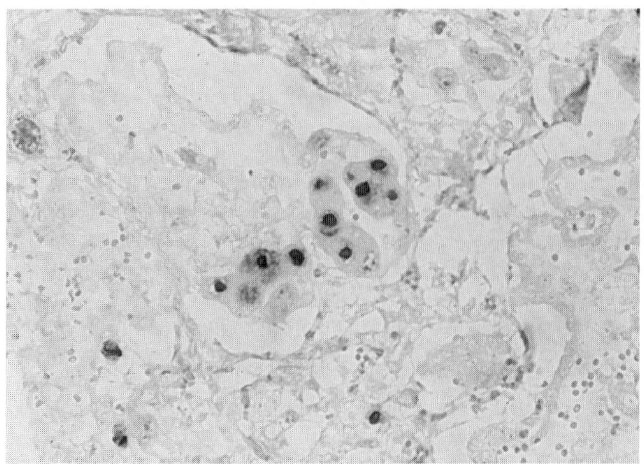

FIGURE 12–3. Cytomegalovirus-specific staining by in situ hybridization in a lung biopsy specimen. The presence of target DNA of CMV is indicated by dark inclusion-like deposits in infected cells. (×140.) *(Courtesy of Dr. Pierre Russo.)*

acid amplification process occurs that permits quantification determining the reaction cycle at which specific PCR products are first detected. This technique takes advantage of the 5′ to 3′ exonucleolytic activity of *Taq* polymerase, which cleaves a dually labeled (fluorescent dye and quencher), nonextendable hybridization probe during the extension phase of PCR and releases the fluorescent reporter dye from the probe. The relative increase in fluorescent dye emission is then measured with a special thermal cycler analyzer. **In situ PCR** is a technically much more difficult procedure that takes advantage of the extreme sensitivity of PCR while at the same time maintaining the integrity of the specimen to allow localization of the amplified DNA in histologic sections. **Nested PCR** was designed to overcome contamination of samples by using two sets of amplification primers. The target DNA is amplified by using one set of primers and is then reamplified with a second set of primers that are internal to the original set. This method requires that the tubes be opened during the amplification process for the addition of more reagents, and therefore it is impossible to ensure that there is no carryover of amplified DNA between the first and second rounds of amplification. **Multiplex PCR** was designed for amplification of more than one target sequence in a specimen at the same time. However, the assay often results in lower sensitivity.

TABLE 12–4. Infectious Agents Identified in Clinical Specimens Using DNA Probes for Hybridization Assays

Bacteria	Viruses	Fungi
*Campylobacter**†	Adenoviruses	*Aspergililus*
*Enterococcus**†	Coxsackie B viruses	*Blastomyces dermatitidis**†
Gardnerella vaginalis	Cytomegalovirus	*Candida*
*Haemophilus influenzae**†	Dengue fever virus	*Coccidioides immitis**†
Legionella pneumophila†	Ebola virus	*Cryptococcus neoformans*
*Listeria monocytogenes**†	Epstein-Barr virus	*Histoplasma capsulatum**†
*Mycobacterium**†	Hantaviruses	**Protozoa**
Mycoplasma	Hepatitis B virus	*Leishmania*
*Neisseria gonorrhoeae**†	Hepatitis C virus	*Plasmodium falciparum*
Rhodococcus equi	Herpes simplex viruses 1 and 2	*Trichomonas vaginalis*
*Staphylococcus**†	Human herpesvirus 6	**Other**
*Streptococcus**†	Human herpesvirus 7	*Chlamydia*
Ureaplasma urealyticum	Human herpesvirus 8	
	Human immunodeficiency virus	
	Human papillomaviruses	
	Human T-lymphotropic virus type I	
	Lassa virus	
	Marburg virus	
	Measles virus	
	Parvovirus B19	
	Polioviruses	
	Polyomaviruses (BK and JC)	
	Poxviruses	

*Nucleic acid probes currently approved by the FDA.
†Available for culture confirmation only.

Transcription-Mediated Amplification. The transcription-mediated amplification (TMA) assay is based on the isothermal amplification of either RNA or DNA; ribosomal RNA (rRNA) is often the preferred target because several thousand copies of rRNA are present in each cell. TMA uses two primers. The first primer contains a promoter sequence for RNA polymerase and a region complementary to the 16S rRNA target. After the primer anneals to the target, RT extends the primer to make a cDNA-RNA hybrid molecule. The RNA strand is removed from the hybrid molecule by ribonuclease H activity of RT. The single-stranded cDNA is available for the second primer, which is complementary to a portion of the cDNA. RT extends this primer, creating a double-stranded DNA molecule that contains a promoter for RNA polymerase, which generates multiple copies of rRNA. This rRNA is available for amplification with TMA, with billion-fold amplification achieved in less than 2 hours. The amplified RNA can be detected in a chemiluminescent assay by adding single-stranded, ester-labeled DNA. The Gen-Probe rRNA amplification system is a TMA assay that has been applied for detection of acid-fast bacilli in smear-positive specimens and for detection of *C. trachomatis* in urethral, cervical, and urine samples.

Qβ Replicase Amplification. The Qβ replicase amplification assay relies on the RNA-dependent RNA polymerase that originally was identified in the genomic RNA of a bacteriophage (Qβ bacteriophage). It is an enzyme that recognizes either the secondary structure of base-paired RNA from the Qβ genome or short probe inserts. After a given probe anneals to a target, the nonhybridized material can be removed and the probe is enzymatically replicated by Qβ replicase in vitro at colorimetrically detectable levels. This method is used to identify *C. trachomatis.*

Ligase Chain Reaction. The ligase chain reaction (LCR) assay is a type of probe amplification assay that uses two large fragments of DNA as primers that span the entire DNA target sequence. After hybridization to the target, the two primers are covalently linked by the enzyme ligase. After ligation the DNA is denatured and new probes are allowed to anneal. The use of this assay in clinical microbiology is limited to targets with stable nucleotide sequence, and it has been used for detection of *Listeria monocytogenes, M. tuberculosis, C. trachomatis,* and *N. gonorrhoeae.*

NEWER MOLECULAR METHODS

Molecular techniques have become an important part of a diagnostic laboratory's arsenal for infectious diseases. They tend to be more expensive than other diagnostic assays but generally offer a short turnaround time that facilitates earlier treatment and reduces the length of hospital stays. Improvements in instrumentation will make these assays easier, less expensive, and more widely available.

Laser Capture Microdissection. One of the constraints affecting molecular methods for detection of pathogens in tissue sections is the relatively minute amount of pathogen nucleic acid available to be targeted in a background that is a veritable ocean of potentially interfering host nucleic acid. Laser capture microdissection allows microdissection and capture of pieces of tissue from a histologic section (frozen or formalin-fixed, paraffin-embedded tissue) or cytology preparation that are precisely identified under the microscope and are as small as a single host cell, 7 μm in diameter. Thus the pathologist can greatly improve the signal:noise ratio of the molecular techniques by selecting pathogen-rich, host cell–poor samples for analysis.

The area of interest in the section is selected with an inverted microscope. Retrieval of selected cells is achieved by activation of a transparent transfer film (e.g., ethylene vinyl acetate) placed in contact with a tissue section, by a focused laser beam 30 or 60 μm in diameter. The precise area of film targeted by the laser bonds to the tissue beneath it, which is then lifted free of surrounding tissue, retaining its exact morphologic features. Once

TABLE 12–5. Infectious Agents Most Commonly Identified by PCR Assays

Bacteria	Viruses	Fungi
Actinomyces	Adenoviruses	*Aspergillus*
Afipia felis	Astroviruses	*Candida*
Alloiococcus otitidis	Coxsackie B viruses	*Coccidioides immitis*
Bartonella	Cytomegalovirus*	*Pneumocystis carinii*
Bordetella pertussis	Dengue fever virus	**Protozoa**
Borrelia burgdorferi	Eastern equine encephalitis virus	*Babesia*
Borrelia recurrentis	Ebola virus	*Cryptosporidium parvum*
Branhamella catarrhalis	Epstein-Barr virus*	*Cyclospora cayetanensis*
Brucella	Hantaviruses	*Entamoeba histolytica*
Campylobacter	Hepatitis B virus	*Leishmania*
Clostridium difficile	Hepatitis C virus*	Microsporidia
Corynebacterium diphtheriae	Hepatitis D virus	*Plasmodium*
Escherichia coli	Hepatitis E virus	*Toxoplasma gondii*
Escherichia coli (O157:H7)	Herpes simplex viruses 1 and 2	*Trichomonas vaginalis*
Francisella tularensis	Human herpesvirus 6	*Trypanosoma cruzi*
Haemophilus ducreyi	Human herpesvirus 7	**Others**
Haemophilus influenzae	Human herpesvirus 8	*Chlamydia*
Helicobacter pylori	Human immunodeficiency virus*	*Coxiella burnetii*
Kingella kingae	Human papillomaviruses	*Ehrlichia chaffeensis*
Legionella pneumophila	Human T-lymphotropic virus type I*	*Orientia tsutsugamushi*
Leptospira interrogans	Lassa virus	*Rickettsia*
Listeria monocytogenes	Marburg virus	
Mycobacterium	Parvovirus B19	
*Mycobacterium tuberculosis**	Polioviruses	
Mycoplasma	Polyomaviruses (BK and JC)	
*Neisseria gonorrhoeae**	Poxviruses	
Neisseria meningitidis	Rabies virus	
Nocardia	Rift Valley fever virus	
Pasteurella multocida	Rotavirus	
Salmonella	Toscana virus	
Shigella	Varicella-zoster virus	
Staphylococcus	West Nile virus	
Streptococcus	Yellow fever virus	
Treponema pallidum		
Tropheryma whippleii		
Vibrio		
Yersinia		

*PCR assays currently approved by the FDA.

captured, the DNA, RNA, or protein can be easily extracted from the isolated cells and analyzed by conventional PCR, RT-PCR, or polyacrylamide gel electrophoresis. Although still primarily a tool for research laboratories, applications of this method to infectious diseases range from research to diagnosis to monitoring of disease progression. It has important potential for detecting and identifying pathogens from tissue sites when additional samples are difficult or impossible to obtain.

DNA Microarrays. An important advance that has great potential for pathogen detection and identification in tissue extracts, although which as yet has not been widely applied, is DNA microarray technology, by which minute amounts of tissue nucleic acid can be screened against huge numbers of probes specific for known pathogens. DNA microarrays are tiny chips that can hold thousands of single-stranded DNA molecules with different specific sequences attached on a solid surface (e.g., glass). When a sample containing unknown sequences of single-stranded DNA is added to a chip, any sequences complementary to those found on the chip will hybridize to form double-stranded DNA. Duplex formation can be detected by fluorescence or by mass spectrometry. **Mass spectrometry** is a detector system that ionizes and separates molecules according to their atomic masses, resulting in a **mass spectrum** displaying different masses of charged molecules and their relative abundance. The instrument then identifies which area of the chip was able to bind the unknown DNA. Although this system is still a research tool, its advantages include a short turnaround time and ease of automation. In addition, the chips contain a regular array of DNA with a number of different sequences, allowing searching for, and detection of, many different microorganisms in the same assay.

MOLECULAR METHODS FOR SPECIFIC PATHOGENS

Bacteria. PCR is currently used in the typing of staphylococcal strains. Rapid nonradioactive DNA probes are currently available in culture confirmation tests for the detection of *Streptococcus pneumoniae,* group B *Streptococcus, Haemophilus influenzae,* and *Enterococcus.* A DNA probe assay is available for the rapid identification of *L. monocytogenes* and *Legionella* colonies on primary isolation plates. PCR methods are available for confirmation of virulent isolates, but as yet the procedures for direct diagnosis have not been fully developed.

Detection of *R. equi* in tissues by in situ hybridization by means of a biotinylated probe is available. The 16S rRNA gene of *T. whippleii* can be identified by PCR in intestinal and heart biopsy tissue, as well as in pleural effusion cells. A PCR-based direct detection system for *Corynebacterium diphtheriae* toxin is available and permits diagnosis from diphtheria membranes or biopsy tissue. *Borrelia burgdorferi* and *Borrelia recurrentis* can be identified by PCR in urine, serum, and CSF, a technique that may be helpful in the rapid diagnosis of infection at its early stages. Nasopharyngeal swabs or aspirates can be used for the detection of *Bordetella pertussis* by PCR, which has shown diagnostic potential. Simultaneous detection and discrimination of *Bordetella pertussis, Bordetella parapertussis,* and *Bordetella bronchiseptica* have also been reported.

Molecular tests have been developed for the presumptive diagnosis of gonococcal infections. A nucleic acid probe test (Gen-Probe) and an LCR test detect *N. gonorrhoeae* in urogenital and endocervical specimens. Concurrent infection with *C. trachomatis* is detected by PCR or TMA in clinical specimens, including urine. DNA hybridization techniques for *Mycoplasma* and *Ureaplasma urealyticum* are available by using 16S rRNA genes as targets. Molecular techniques for detection in clinical specimens are also available for these microorganisms but offer less value than cultures.

Multiplex PCR assays have been shown to be useful in the presumptive identification of four bacterial species that are causative agents of otitis media: *Branhamella catarrhalis, S. pneumoniae, H. influenzae,* and *Alloiococcus otitidis.* Similarly, simultaneous PCR detection of *Haemophilus ducreyi, Treponema pallidum,* and herpes simplex viruses directly from genital ulcers has been reported.

DNA probes exist for culture confirmation of *M. tuberculosis, M. avium, Mycobacterium intracellulare, Mycobacterium gordonae,* and *Mycobacterium kansasii.* Direct detection of toxigenic *Pasteurella multocida* by PCR has been reported in blood and CSF, as well as for culture confirmation. Cat-scratch disease and other *Bartonella* infections can be diagnosed by PCR amplification methods. PCR has also been used to demonstrate infection both by *Francisella tularensis* in skin lesions and by toxigenic and nontoxigenic strains of *C. difficile* in stools, but the methods are not commercially available. Isolate identification of *Actinomyces* and *Nocardia* by PCR techniques has been reported by reference laboratories. PCR assays are available for detection of *Leptospira* in serum, urine, and CSF.

PCR assays for the specific detection of *Escherichia coli* and *Shigella* and other enterobacteria are not commercially available; their use is limited to research purposes. A genus-specific probe for culture confirmation is available for *Campylobacter,* and PCR techniques for detection in stool samples are limited to research only. PCR is also available for detection of *H. pylori* in gastric tissue biopsies.

PCR tests for *Chlamydia pneumoniae, Chlamydia psittaci,* and *Coxiella burnetii* are available in research laboratories. Diagnosis of *Ehrlichia, Orientia tsutsugamushi, Rickettsia prowazekii, Rickettsia rickettsii,* and *Rickettsia typhi* infections by PCR amplification can be established by testing blood or plasma collected during acute infection; however, few reports have demonstrated detection of these organisms in frozen and paraffin-embedded tissues.

Fungi. PCR assays for the diagnosis of invasive disease by *Aspergillus* have been developed and tested in blood, sera, and lung tissue. Nucleic acid probes for the identification of dimorphic fungi in cultures are available for *H. capsulatum, Blastomyces dermatitidis,* and *Coccidioides immitis.*

Protozoa. PCR amplification tests for detection of *Pneumocystis carinii* in clinical specimens such as bronchloalveolar lavage and transbronchial biopsy specimens are available but offer little clinical utility. PCR assays are commercially available for detection of *Leishmania mexicana* and *Leishmania braziliensis* in skin lesions and of *Toxoplasma gondii* in clinical specimens including amniotic fluid. *Leishmania donovani* can be detected by PCR in blood and splenic aspirates. *Trichomonas vaginalis* can be detected in vaginal specimens by PCR. *Cryptosporidium parvum, Cyclospora cayetanensis,* and microsporidia can be identified by PCR in tissue biopsy and stool specimens, but the methods are available for research only. A DNA probe for the direct identification of *T. vaginalis* is available that allows the concomitant identification of *Candida* and pathogens associated with bacterial vaginosis.

Viruses. Nucleic acid amplification techniques are used for the detection and characterization of viruses when culture and serologic methods are difficult, extremely expensive, or unavailable, such as for detection of human papillomaviruses and parvovirus and to distinguish between HTLV-I and HTLV-II. In situ hybridization is used to detect polyomaviruses and papillomaviruses in tissues and to detect EBV in associated tumors. RT-PCR tests for HIV are used for early diagnosis and monitoring of treatment. Quantitative EBV PCR is used to monitor transplant recipients for development of posttransplantation EBV-associated lymphoproliferative disorders.

Multiplex PCR can be used for the detection and the typing and subtyping of influenza viruses in clinical specimens. The use of nested RT-PCR has been reported for prenatal and postnatal diagnosis of congenital rubella and for the detection of adenoviruses, caliciviruses, astroviruses, and rotaviruses in stool specimens. RT-PCR can be used for the definitive diagnosis of filovirus infections.

PCR methods for detecting and cloning hepatitis B virus DNA and HCV RNA have been developed. PCR for detection of HCV is useful when HCV serologic analysis shows indeterminate results and during monitoring of therapy for HCV infection. HCV genotypes can be determined by the use of RT-PCR. Analysis of liver tissue by PCR is useful for determination of hepatitis D virus in the presence of infection with hepatitis B virus.

PCR is the method of choice for diagnosis of central nervous system infection by enteroviruses, herpes simplex viruses, measles virus, and mumps virus. PCR is used to detect JC virus in CSF and blood. It can also be useful for diagnosis of primary central nervous system lymphoma caused by EBV. PCR is also used for the detection and quantification of cytomegalovirus in immunocompromised persons and in infants with congenital infection.

REVIEWS

Connor DH, Chandler FW, Schwartz DA, et al (editors): *Pathology of Infectious Diseases.* Stamford, Conn, Appleton & Lange, 1997.

Gutierrez Y (editor): *Diagnostic Pathology of Parasitic Infections with Clinical Correlations,* 2nd ed. New York, Oxford University Press, 2000.

Woods GL, Walker DH: Detection of infection or infectious agents by use of cytologic and histologic stains. *Clin Microbiol Rev* 1996;9:382–404.

Woods GL, Walker DH, Winn WC, et al (editors): *Infectious Disease Pathology: Clinical Cases.* Woburn, Mass, Butterworth-Heinemann, 1999.

KEY ARTICLES

Emmert-Buck MR, Bonner RF, Smith PD, et al: Laser capture microdissection. *Science* 1996;274:998–1001.

Fodor SP, Rava RP, Huang XC, et al: Multiplexed biochemical assays with biological chips. *Nature* 1993;364:555–6.

Jin L, Lloyd RV: In situ hybridization: Methods and applications. *J Clin Lab Anal* 1997;11:2–9.

Marshall A, Hodgson J: DNA chips: An array of possibilities. *Nat Biotechnol* 1998;16:27–31.

McHale RH, Stapleton PM, Bergquist PL: Rapid preparation of blood and tissue samples for polymerase chain reaction. *Biotechniques* 1991;10: 20–3.

Post JC, Ehrlich GD: The impact of the polymerase chain reaction in clinical medicine. *JAMA* 2000:283:1544–6.

Sandhu GS, Kline BC, Stockman L, et al: Molecular probes for diagnosis of fungal infections. *J Clin Microbiol* 1995;33:2913–9.

Tang YW, Procop GW, Persing DH: Molecular diagnostics of infectious diseases. *Clin Chem* 1997;43:2021–38.

Wagar EA: Direct hybridization and amplification applications for the diagnosis of infectious diseases. *J Clin Lab Anal* 1996;10:312–25.

Weiss JB: DNA probes and PCR for diagnosis of parasitic infections. *Clin Microbiol Rev* 1995;8:113–30.

Wetmur JG: DNA probes: Applications of the principles of nucleic acid hybridization. *Crit Rev Biochem Mol Biol* 1991;26:227–59.

CHAPTER 13

Diagnostic Imaging

Richard I. Markowitz

The goal of modern diagnostic imaging is to noninvasively depict organs and, by analysis of their appearance and relationships, derive useful diagnostic information. Plain film radiography has been enhanced and often superseded by modern cross-section imaging techniques. CT, MRI, and PET use computer technology to create images and differentiate tissues by using quantitative data generated by the interaction of tissues with different energy forms: conventional x-rays in CT or electromagnetic waves in MRI. These techniques allow physicians to view the body section by section, slice by slice, in planes and at angles hitherto unobtainable, even at autopsy.

Ultrasonography has been particularly successful as a noninvasive, nonirradiating, cross-sectional imaging technique suited to infants and children. Solid organs such as the kidneys, liver, and spleen are particularly well demonstrated by ultrasonography. High-resolution, real-time equipment and Doppler wave analysis, including color display, have made ultrasonography the major noninvasive modality for cardiovascular imaging. Ultrasound probes placed in body orifices permit transesophageal cardiac imaging, as well as high-resolution depiction of the male and female genitourinary tracts.

The diagnostic medical use of radionuclide scanning has expanded because of the wide choice of safe radioactive isotopes, which can be designed to have specific biologic activities. Computer analysis provides tomographic imaging that permits anatomic localization and increases sensitivity.

The ultimate usefulness of diagnostic imaging tests depends on two factors: (1) the innate sensitivity and specificity of each method in depicting or revealing the desired anatomic or physiologic information and (2) the skill, experience, and expertise of the diagnostic radiologist in interpreting the raw data to reach an accurate diagnostic conclusion. In some instances the pictures ''speak for themselves'' and the answers are fairly obvious even to the unsophisticated or untrained observer. In most cases, especially for infants and children, the correct information can be obtained only through the use of the latest state-of-the-art equipment, the experienced hands and minds of skilled technologists, and the trained eyes and minds of knowledgeable physicians. The fundamental difference between other diagnostic laboratory tests, which are quantitative, and most diagnostic imaging procedures, which are primarily pictorial and therefore qualitative, is the process of expert interpretation and consultation. Ideally, consultation with the radiologist should start before a test is performed, so that the necessary and appropriate diagnostic tests can be determined along with the order in which they should be performed. Several valid options, including the option of watching and waiting, are usually available.

Given all these options, the basic questions that a clinician should always ask include the following: Why am I ordering this test? What do I expect it will show? How will the results influence my thinking about the diagnosis? How will this information affect the treatment plan? Are there any alternative ways to acquire the same information with less radiation, morbidity, discomfort, time, or expense? Finally, will the information gleaned from this test be new, or will it duplicate information that I already have? Imaging of infants and children should always be directed toward answering a specific question. Rarely should these tests be used broadly to ''rule out disease,'' as is often the case in adult medicine. Identifying the goals and purposes of each test for each patient and consulting with the radiologist or imaging specialist when in doubt most often result in less expense and in faster, more specific, and more useful diagnostic information.

The expense and risk of a diagnostic procedure must be balanced carefully with the anticipated benefit. In a health care environment where increasingly sophisticated and specific diagnosis is possible and desired, gatekeepers who require verification and justification before authorization for payment are mandating limitations to the use of technology. As funding for health care becomes more restricted, technical resources must be used wisely and efficaciously. Although a given positive or negative imaging test might have great value to the treating physician, duplication of information and unnecessary or repetitive examinations should be avoided.

IMAGING METHODS

Technologic and anatomic considerations, as well as patient acceptability, local availability, expense, and accessibility, will direct the choice of the appropriate imaging modality (Table 13–1). There is often more than one acceptable approach to deriving the information necessary to arrive at the correct conclusion. Certain diagnostic imaging modalities are particularly well suited to imaging a specific organ or to answering a specific question that may be pertinent in the evaluation of pediatric infections (Table 13–2). Individual clinicians and radiologists often have favorite diagnostic approaches, and medical centers may have unique strengths and experience in certain areas. Ancillary issues may be determining factors such as the need for specially trained personnel for sedation of young children who will need to lie quietly for some tests or scans. As technology continues to evolve, continual re-evaluation of recommendations of diagnostic methods in the context of individual circumstances is necessary.

In the absence of localizing signs or symptoms, imaging of the entire body by multiple modalities is not productive. Money, time, and patient confidence can be lost if multiple tests are ordered indiscriminately without a specific question in mind.

Head and Neck

Brain. For the majority of focal or diffuse infections involving the central nervous system, the modalities of choice are CT, especially for bone detail, and MRI, especially for neurologic detail. Both require the patient to remain motionless for the duration of the scan procedure, which can range from 10 minutes to 1 hour. Scans of the neural axis to identify infection include contrast-enhanced CT (Fig. 13–1) and gadolinium-enhanced MRI (Fig. 13–2). In

TABLE 13–1. Use of Diagnostic Imaging Modalities for Pediatric Patients

Study	Usage	Ionizing Radiation	Use of Contrast	Expense	Operator Dependency*	Sedation Required†	Spatial Resolution‡	Contrast Resolution§
Plain film	Common	Minimal	No	Low	+ (T)	No	Excellent	Poor
Upper GI series; barium enema	Common	Moderate	Always	Moderate	++ (T and R)	No	Excellent	Good
VCUG	Common	Moderate	Always	Moderate	++ (T and R)	No	Excellent	Good
IV urography	Very low	Moderate	Always	Moderate	+ (T)	No	Excellent	Good
Ultrasonography	Common	No	No	High	++++ (T and R)	Sometimes	Good	Very good
Radionuclide scan	Common	Low	No	High	+++ (T)	Sometimes	Poor	None
CT	Common	Moderate	Often	High	++ (T)	Yes	Very good	Excellent
MRI	Moderate	No	Often	Very high	+++ (T and R)	Yes	Good	Best
Angiography	Low	High	Always	Very high	++++ (T and R)	Yes	Excellent	Very good

*The technologist (T) or radiologist (R).
†Sedation may be necessary, especially in the 1–4-year-old age group.
‡Spatial resolution is the ability to distinguish fine detail.
§Contrast resolution is the ability to distinguish different tissues by density.

general, CT is more readily available, less expensive, and easier to obtain than MRI, although the sensitivity of MRI, especially in the early detection of diffuse infections such as viral encephalitis, has made it increasingly attractive. Monitoring of sedated or comatose patients during scanning is essential, but it is more complicated in the MRI suite because of the prohibition and danger of ferromagnetic materials. Further developments in MRI technology have resulted in faster scanning, which is particularly important for pediatric patients.

Infection may involve the brain parenchyma itself (Figs. 13–3 and 13–4), the meningeal coverings (Fig. 13–2, *A*), and various real and potential intracranial spaces (Fig. 13–2, *B*). Intracranial fluid collections may develop in relation to necrosis of infected tissue (Fig. 13–5) or may be secondary to alteration of the normal CSF flow pattern caused by infection of the meninges. Inflamed but viable tissue may show enhancement after the injection of contrast material for CT, whereas dead or poorly perfused tissue is not enhanced (Figs. 13–3 and 13–4). Calcifications, which show very well on CT (Fig. 13–6), will appear as signal-free areas on MRI. Often these modalities are complementary, but because they demonstrate the same anatomic structures, the information provided may be redundant. The ability of MRI to depict and differentiate neural tissue and structure is particularly impressive and accounts for its great popularity despite high cost.

Ultrasonography of the brain of young infants through the anterior fontanel has been useful in identifying intracranial hemorrhage and hydrocephalus. It is an attractive method of examination because of the lack of radiation and the portability of the equipment,

TABLE 13–2. Use of Diagnostic Imaging Modalities for Anatomic Areas

Anatomic Area	Most Useful Imaging Modalities	Other Useful Imaging Modalities
Central nervous system	CT and MRI	
Neural structures	MRI (gadolinium enhanced)	CT (contrast enhanced)
Bony structures	CT	Plain film
Chest and airway		
Upper and middle respiratory tract	Plain film	Fluoroscopy, CT
Lower respiratory tract	Plain film	CT (contrast enhanced)
Heart	Plain film, echocardiography	MRI, magnetic resonance angiocardiography
Abdomen		
Mucosal lesions	Contrast studies (upper GI series, barium enema)	
Appendicitis	Plain film, CT	Ultrasonography, barium enema
Intestinal obstruction or perforation	Plain film	
Solid abdominal organs	Ultrasonography, CT	MRI
Genitourinary tract		
Anatomy	Ultrasonography, contrast studies of the bladder (VCUG) and kidneys (IV urogram)	CT
Renal scarring	Radionuclide scan (DMSA)	
Scrotum	High-resolution ultrasonography, color and power Doppler, radionuclide testicular scan	
Musculoskeletal system		
Bones and joints	Plain film, radionuclide scan, CT, MRI, ultrasonography	
Muscles and soft tissues	MRI, CT	

DMSA, dimercaptosuccinic acid.

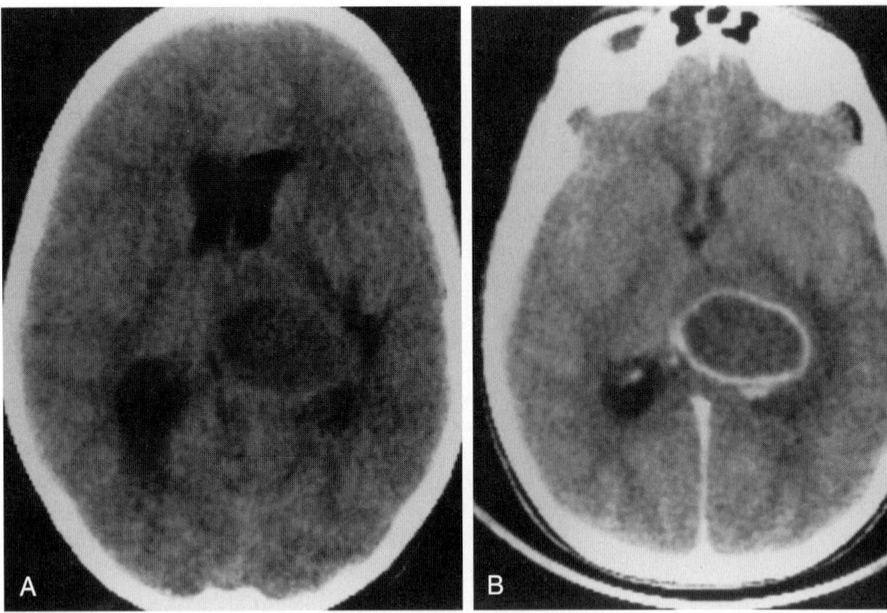

FIGURE 13–1. Brain abscess. **A,** Noncontrast transaxial CT demonstrates a focal area of low attenuation to the left of the midline, causing a mass effect. **B,** After intravenous injection of contrast medium, peripheral ring enhancement is observed. Low attenuation lateral to the lesion extending into the surrounding brain represents edema adjacent to the abscess.

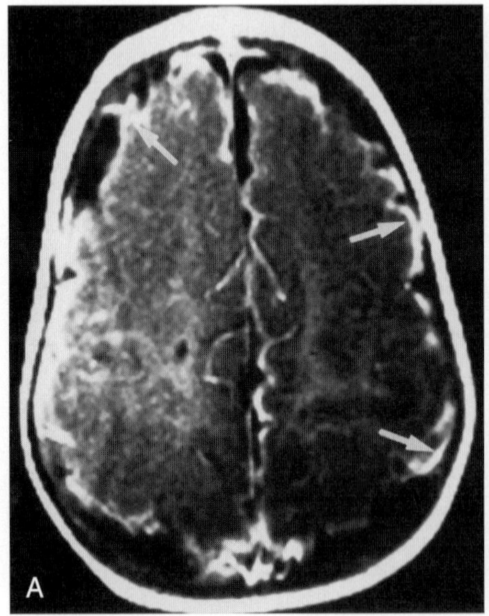

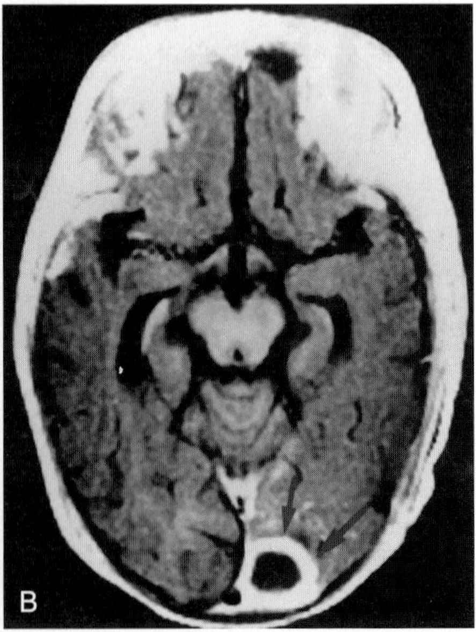

FIGURE 13–2. A, Meningitis caused by *Haemophilus influenzae* type b in a 4-month-old girl. Transaxial T1-weighted gadolinium-enhanced MRI at the level of the cerebral hemispheres shows enhancement of the pachymeninges (*arrows*) and small bilateral subdural effusions (peripheral low signal areas). **B,** Infected subdural collection after Hib meningitis. Transaxial T1-weighted gadolinium-enhanced MRI at the level of the midbrain shows a thick ring or rind of high signal intensity (*arrows*) surrounding an area of signal void between the two occipital lobes posteriorly and extending to the left.

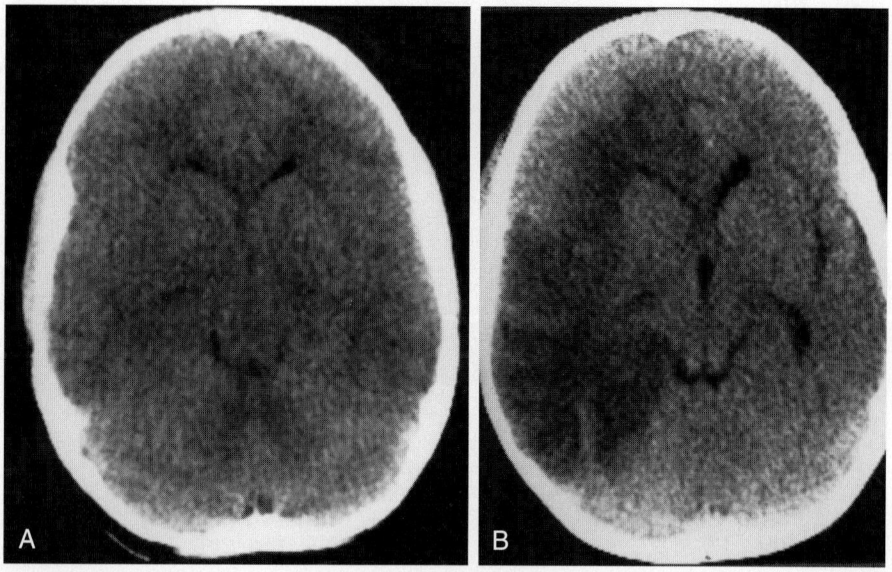

FIGURE 13–3. Herpes simplex virus encephalitis. **A,** Noncontrast transaxial CT shows slitlike ventricles and poor gray-white matter differentiation. **B,** Postcontrast CT reveals a large area of low density on the right, representing edema and poor perfusion.

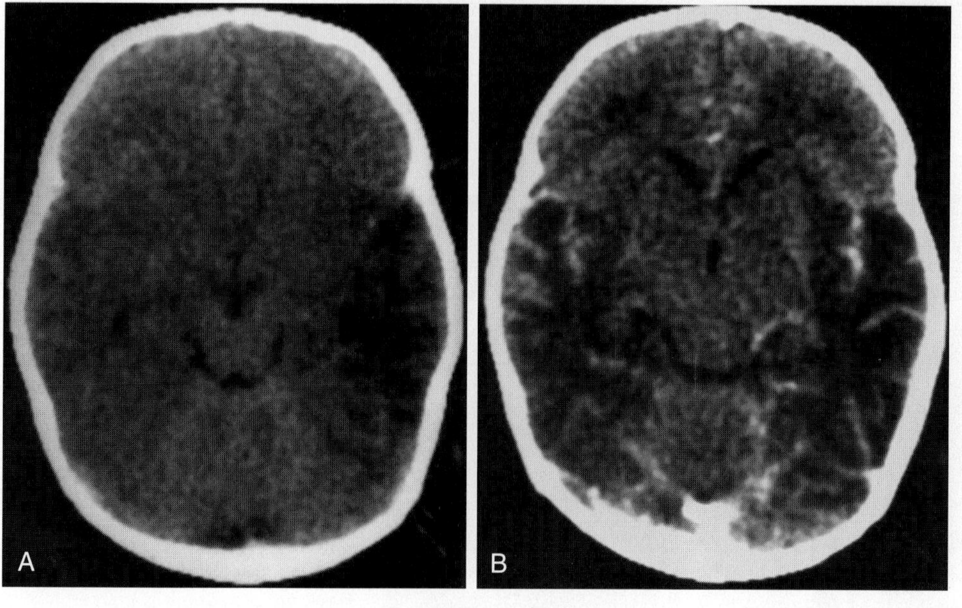

FIGURE 13–4. Neonatal herpes simplex virus encephalitis in a 3-week-old infant with drowsiness and poor feeding. **A,** Noncontrast CT of the brain shows bilateral, diffuse areas of low density that involve both parietotemporal lobes. **B,** Postcontrast CT shows bilateral gyral enhancement and accentuation of the hypodense cortex.

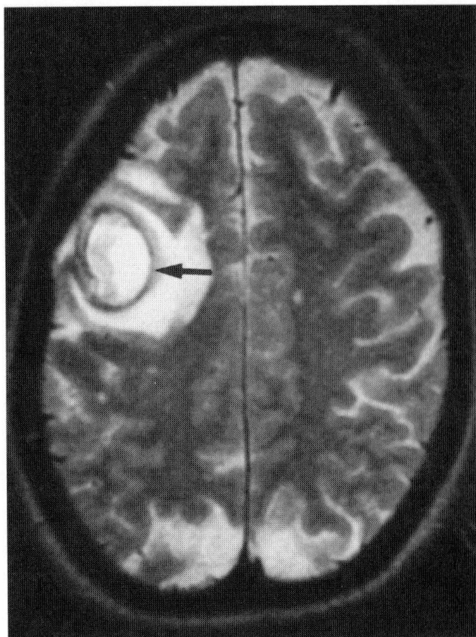

FIGURE 13–5. Brain abscess. Transaxial T2-weighted MRI shows a single round area of high signal intensity within the right cerebral hemisphere. The lesion has a thin wall of lower signal intensity (*arrow*) and is surrounded by high-signal edema extending into the brain, obliterating normal anatomic landmarks.

making routine bedside examination possible. Ultrasonography of the head is less sensitive than CT in depicting small, peripheral fluid collections and early cerebral ischemia and has no use in children whose anterior fontanel is closed. **Transcranial Doppler ultrasonography** is a technique used to evaluate cerebral blood flow, which may be useful among children with sickle cell anemia who have cerebrovascular complications, but it has no role in the evaluation of infection. Intracranial calcifications are readily detected by either ultrasonography or CT but appear as signal voids on MRI. Intraoperative ultrasonography can help neurosurgeons locate deep-seated fluid or pus collections within the brain that may not be apparent on the surface.

Skull. Except for infections of the bony cranium itself, plain film skull radiography has a limited role in the evaluation of intracranial infection. In utero infection with cytomegalovirus and *Toxoplasma gondii* may produce dystrophic calcification within the brain that can be detected on plain films (Fig. 13–7). Old calcified granulomas due to tuberculosis may also be evident. Usually, in these cases, CT is also performed and shows the calcifications in greater detail with finer anatomic localization (Figs. 95–6 and 95–8).

Paranasal Sinuses. The value of plain film examination of the paranasal sinuses remains controversial among radiologists and clinicians. Opacification of a sinus by fluid is frequently demonstrable radiographically, although the significance of the fluid is controversial. It has been conventional thought that an air-fluid level within a sinus on upright films correlates well with the presence of bacterial sinusitis. However, CT and MRI frequently show air-fluid levels within the sinuses of symptom-free patients. The common cold, allergic rhinitis, and crying in younger patients may be responsible for the accumulation of liquid mucus within these cavities. Similarly, mild mucosal thickening may be normal or related to allergy rather than to acute infection. Thus the diagnostic significance of abnormal findings on examination of the paranasal sinuses is debatable despite the popularity of conventional radiography. Conversely, normal paranasal sinus plain films appear to have significant negative predictive value for bacterial sinusitis.

In cases where complications of sinusitis, such as orbital cellulitis or epidural abscess are suspected, cross-sectional imaging with CT or MRI provides much more detailed and extensive information, making plain radiographs superfluous (Fig. 65–5). As in other anatomic areas, CT of the head and neck is better than MRI to evaluate bone detail, whereas MRI better delineates the neurologic components. Thus the anatomic detail provided by high-resolution, thin-cut CT of the sinuses, nasal passages, and mastoids provides otolaryngologists with the information necessary to plan surgery more intelligently and effectively.

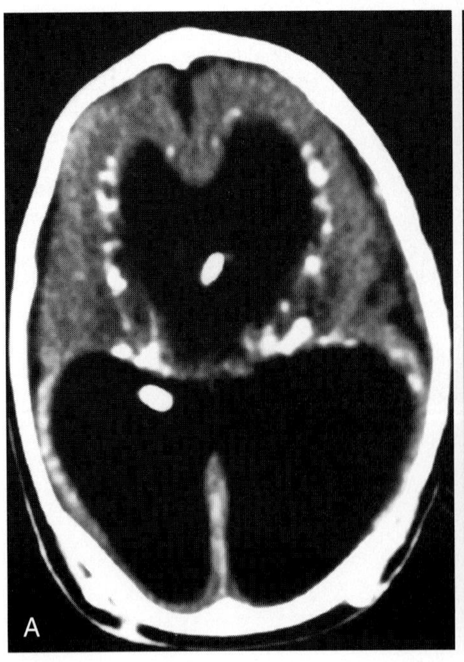

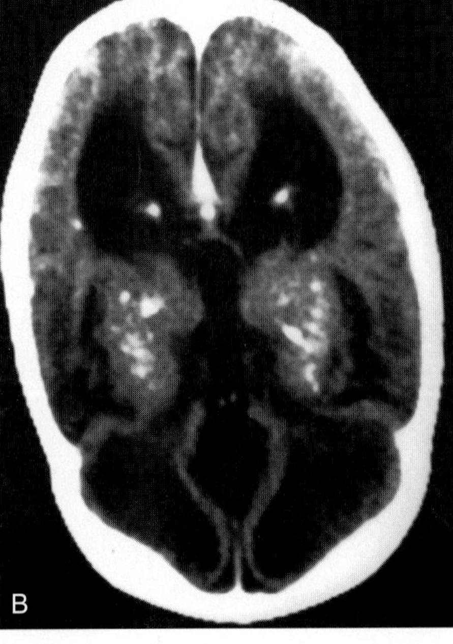

FIGURE 13–6. Congenital cytomegalovirus infection with hydrocephalus in a newborn. **A,** Transaxial CT shows marked cortical loss and multiple calcifications lining the enlarged ventricles. Segments of the shunt tube are seen within the ventricles. **B,** Transaxial CT shows heavy calcification within the basal ganglia. There is marked loss of brain tissue, especially in the occipital lobes.

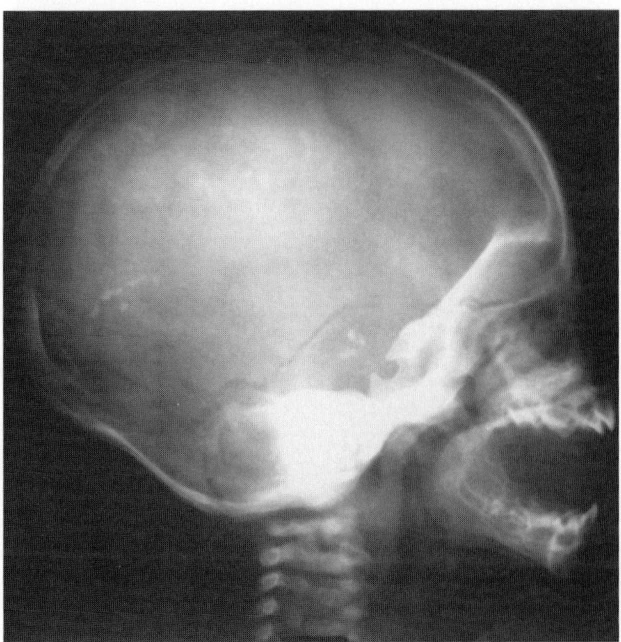

FIGURE 13–7. Lateral skull radiograph of a neonate, showing multiple coarse calcifications scattered throughout the brain in a periventricular distribution. Congenital toxoplasmosis or cytomegalovirus infection would be most likely.

Spinal Column. The spinal column can be imaged well by either CT or MRI. The need for positive-contrast myelography has greatly diminished as MRI has become the primary imaging modality for the spinal cord and the adjacent soft tissues.

Airway and Chest

Conventional radiographic examination of the chest remains the most widely used diagnostic imaging test in children and adults for primary evaluation of the airway, lungs, and overall heart size.

Upper and Middle Respiratory Tract. Plain films of the upper and middle airway are readily available and can be obtained rapidly to identify tonsillar hypertrophy (Fig. 13–8), retropharyngeal abscess (Fig. 59–2), peritonsillar abscess (Fig. 59–3), croup (Figs. 66–3 and 66–4), and epiglottitis (Fig. 66–4). Fluoroscopy and CT are occasionally used to supplement these studies.

Lower Respiratory Tract. The clinical and radiologic assessment of infection of the lower respiratory tract is an everyday event in the practice of most physicians. Findings range from minimal and subtle to overwhelming and obvious. When the clinical diagnosis is clear, radiographic confirmation may add little new information and may not necessarily affect the treatment plan or outcome. However, when there is some doubt or uncertainty in the clinician's mind, the results of the chest x-ray examination may influence the clinician's treatment decisions considerably.

Common radiologic findings of lower chest infection in infants include diffuse hyperinflation, as seen in viral bronchiolitis, or scattered perihilar, peribronchial thickening radiating from the central portions of the lung, indicating bronchopneumonia (Fig. 13–9). This pattern is not pathognomonic for a particular organism. However, when the patient's age and clinical presentation are taken into account, specific infections among the variety of viral and bacterial pathogens may be suspected. Lobar infiltration of normally aerated lung having fluid density can indicate pulmonary consolidation (Figs. 13–10 and 13–11), which is most often due to bacterial infection, usually pneumococcal pneumonia (Fig. 13-12). This is particularly common when the pattern of involvement is unilobar and the patient is otherwise healthy, with a normal immune system. Pleural effusion, either reactive or suppurative, may accompany bacterial infection (Fig. 13–13). Contrast-enhanced CT is helpful in the evaluation and management of cases of community-acquired lobar pneumonia complicated by large pleural effusion, focal necrosis, abscess, or empyema.

Overwhelming pulmonary infection, especially in the immunocompromised person, can lead to diffuse airspace consolidation (Fig. 13–14). *Pneumocystis carinii* and cytomegalovirus are commonly responsible, especially in T cell–deficient persons.

High-resolution CT has an important role in early detection of pulmonary infection in immunocompromised persons, especially in those with fungal disease (Figs. 13–15 and 13–16). The use of CT to stage the disease and to follow persons with tuberculosis has been helpful as an adjunct to plain radiographs (Fig. 35–13). The use of bronchography to diagnose and stage bronchiectasis has been supplanted by CT.

Primary tuberculosis is not uncommon in children, although secondary, or reactivation, pulmonary tuberculosis is unusual. Primary pulmonary infection and its associated immunologic response can appear as an area of peripheral or subpleural consolidation anywhere within the lung. Unilateral hilar lymphadenopathy (Fig. 13–17) may be part of the immunologic reaction. Extensive lymphadenopathy may cause atelectasis, especially of the right middle lobe (Fig. 13–18). The initial infiltrate may be absent or so small as to be overlooked at the time of diagnosis. With time and treatment the site of initial infection and the involved lymph nodes may calcify, producing calcified granulomas (Fig. 13-17). When infection is more virulent or the affected person less immunocompetent to fight the disease, infection may spread via endobronchial or hematogenous routes, the latter appearing as miliary disease (Fig. 35–12). The radiographic appearance may range from multiple areas of lobar consolidation or

Text continued on page 136

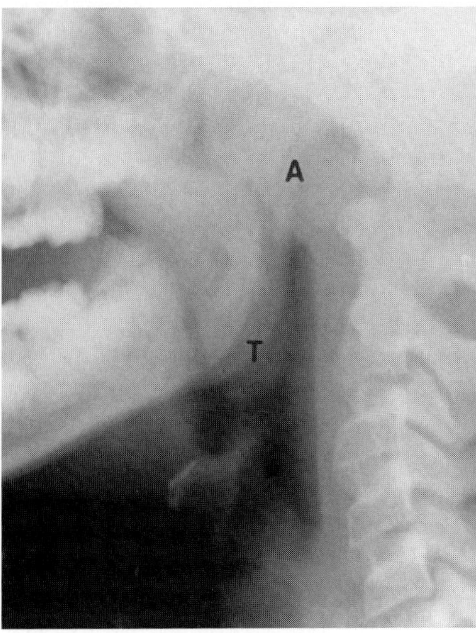

FIGURE 13–8. Enlarged tonsils and adenoids resulting from infectious mononucleosis. Lateral view of the soft tissues of the neck reveals marked enlargement of the tonsils (*T*) and adenoids (*A*), causing narrowing of the airway.

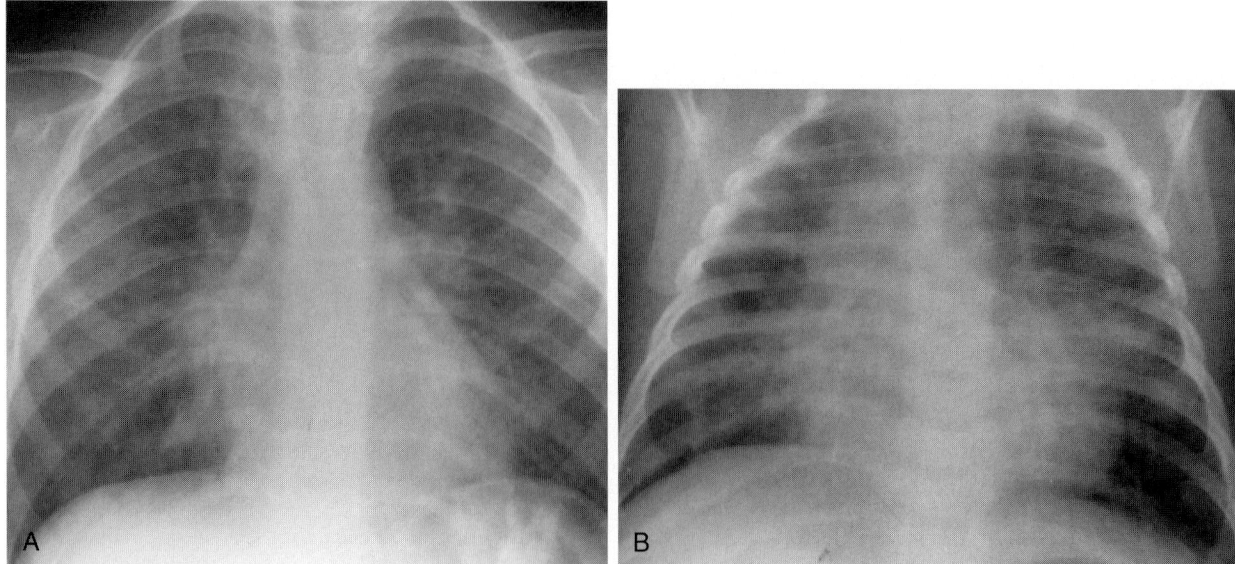

FIGURE 13–9. A, Diffuse viral bronchopneumonia in a 12-year-old boy with cough, fever, and wheezing. Frontal chest radiograph shows bilateral, perihilar, peribronchial thickening and shaggy infiltrate. Focal airspace disease representing consolidation or atelectasis is present in the medial portion of the right upper lobe. The findings are typical of bronchopneumonia. **B,** Pertussis pneumonia in a 2-month-old boy with fever and cough. Frontal chest radiograph shows bilateral patchy areas of infiltrate radiating from the hilar regions. There are scattered areas of focal consolidation as well as overall hyperinflation. This pattern of severe bronchopneumonia is typical but not specific for pertussis.

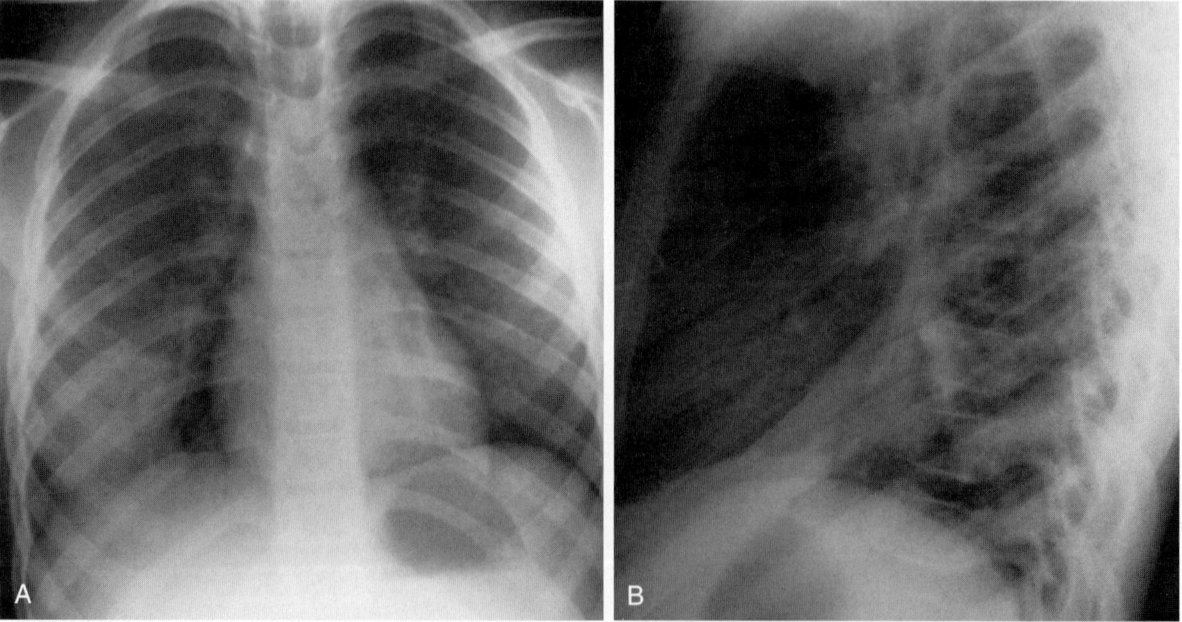

FIGURE 13–10. Segmental bacterial pneumonia of the anterior segment of the right lower lobe in a 7-year-old boy with chills, fever, and malaise. **A,** Frontal chest radiograph shows ill-defined airspace opacity in the right lower lobe. **B,** Lateral radiograph shows sharp demarcation of the consolidation by the major fissure anteriorly, although the remaining portions of the right lower lobe are clear.

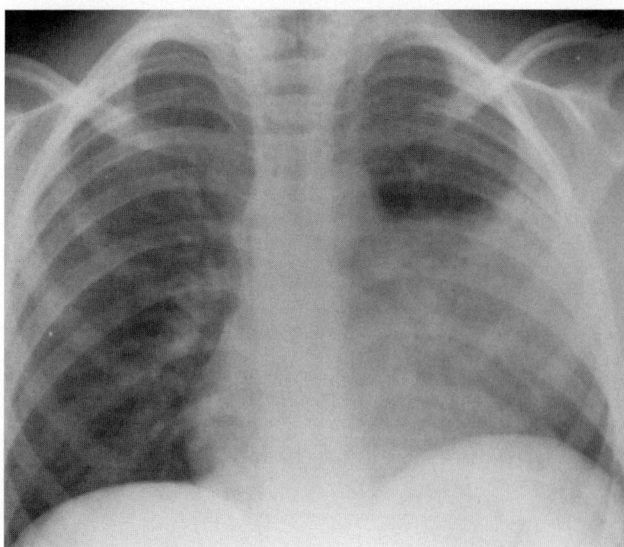

FIGURE 13–11. Acute lobar pneumonia of the lingula in a 6-year-old child with high fever, cough, and chest pain. Frontal chest radiograph demonstrates airspace consolidation, which obliterates the silhouette of the heart border on the left. The left hemidiaphragm is mildly elevated as a result of splinting.

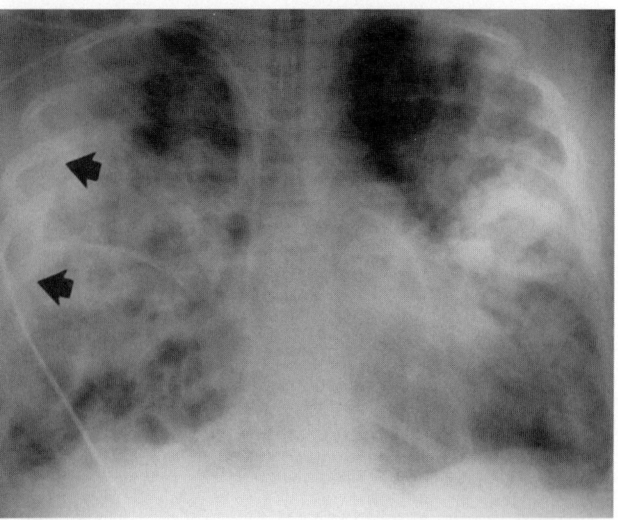

FIGURE 13–13. Diffuse necrotizing pneumonia caused by *Pseudomonas aeruginosa* in a15-year-old girl with respiratory failure and circulatory collapse. Supine frontal chest radiograph shows extensive, bilateral pulmonary infiltrates with scattered bleblike lucencies suggesting multifocal necrosis. There is a pleural effusion on the right (*arrows*).

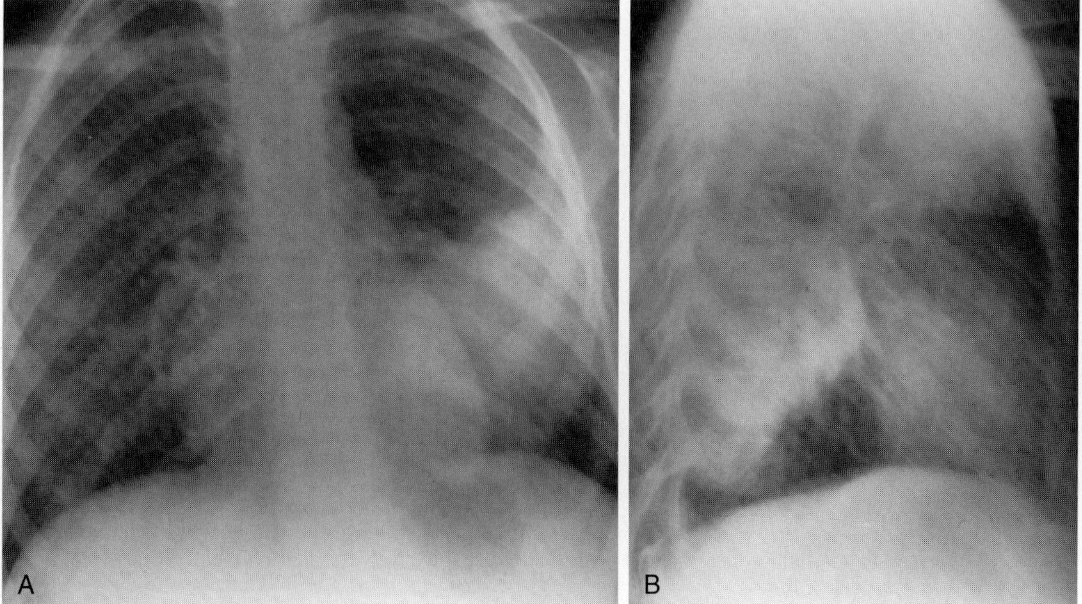

FIGURE 13–12. "Round pneumonia" of the left lower lobe, caused by pneumococcal infection in a 10-year-old boy with high fever, cough, and chest pain. **A,** Frontal chest radiograph shows a large, round density simulating a mass on the left, partially overlapping the cardiac shadow. **B,** Lateral radiograph shows that this mass is actually consolidation in the left lower lobe that appears round on the frontal projection.

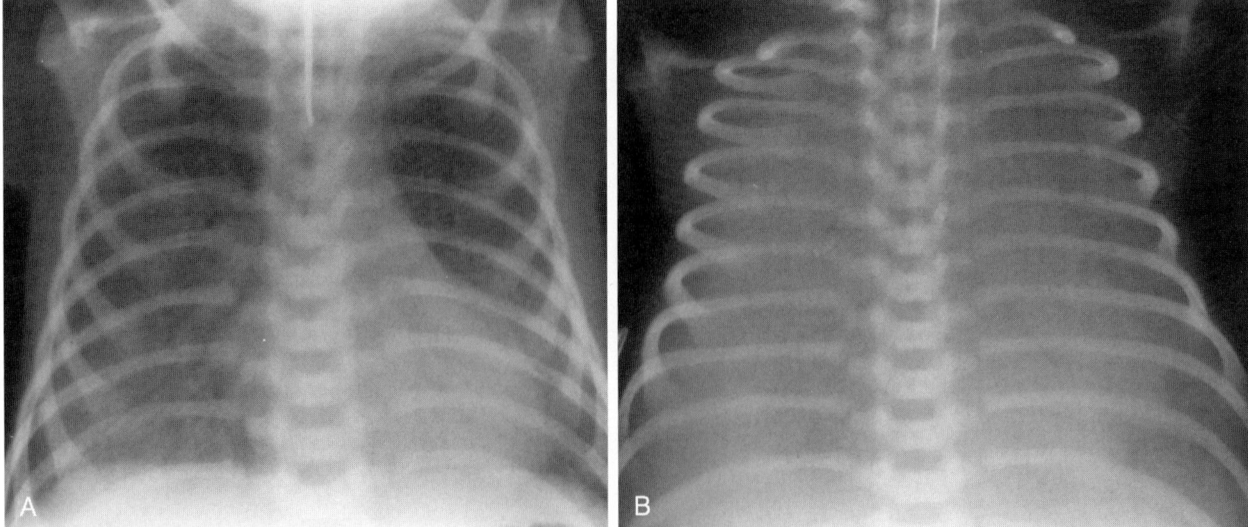

FIGURE 13–14. Diffuse viral pneumonia caused by herpes simplex virus in a neonate who was initially well at birth but had tachypnea at 48 hours of life. **A,** Diffuse pattern of fine, almost sandlike infiltrate involving both lungs is similar radiographically to moderate hyaline membrane disease. **B,** Twenty-four hours later, progression to complete consolidation and opacification of the lungs has occurred. The child died shortly thereafter. This rapid progression implies overwhelming infection and may be seen in association with group B *Streptococcus,* HSV, and other neonatal pathogens.

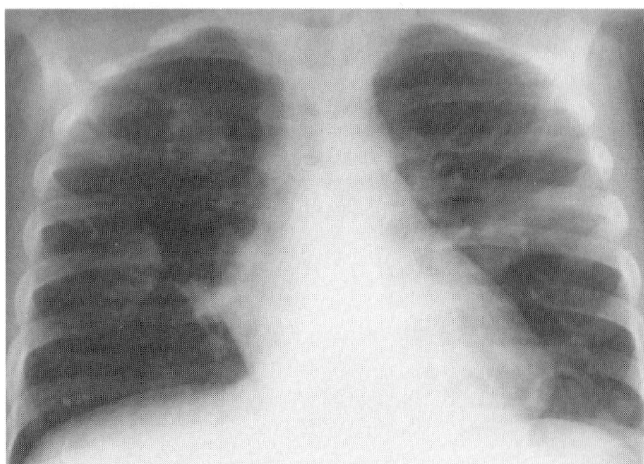

FIGURE 13–15. Fungal pneumonia caused by *Aspergillus* in an immunocompromised patient with persistent fever. Frontal chest radiograph shows faint, bilateral, patchy pulmonary infiltrates, as well as left lower lobe consolidation. The early stage of this type of infection is often subtle on plain films but may be easily demonstrated on CT.

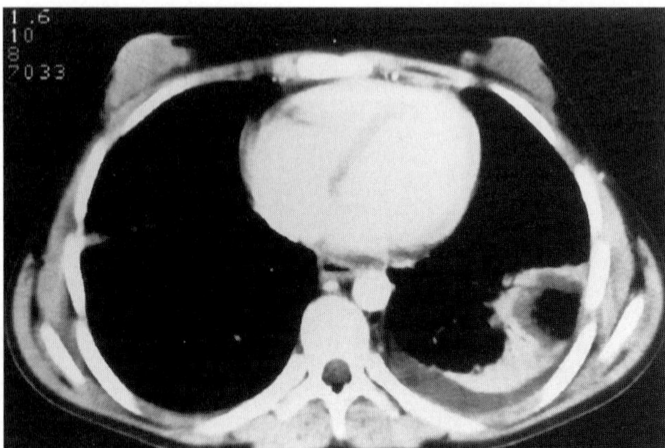

FIGURE 13–16. Necrotizing pneumonia caused by *Mucor* in a 12-year-old diabetic girl. Infection of the paranasal sinuses was the source. Contrast-enhanced CT of the chest shows brightly enhancing consolidation in the periphery of the left lower lobe. A gray zone of nonenhancing, nonperfused lung tissue surrounds a central round air collection, representing lung necrosis. A small, posterior pleural effusion is also present. Necrotizing pneumonia is typical of mucormycosis because of the underlying vasculitis and focal thrombosis that *Mucor* causes.

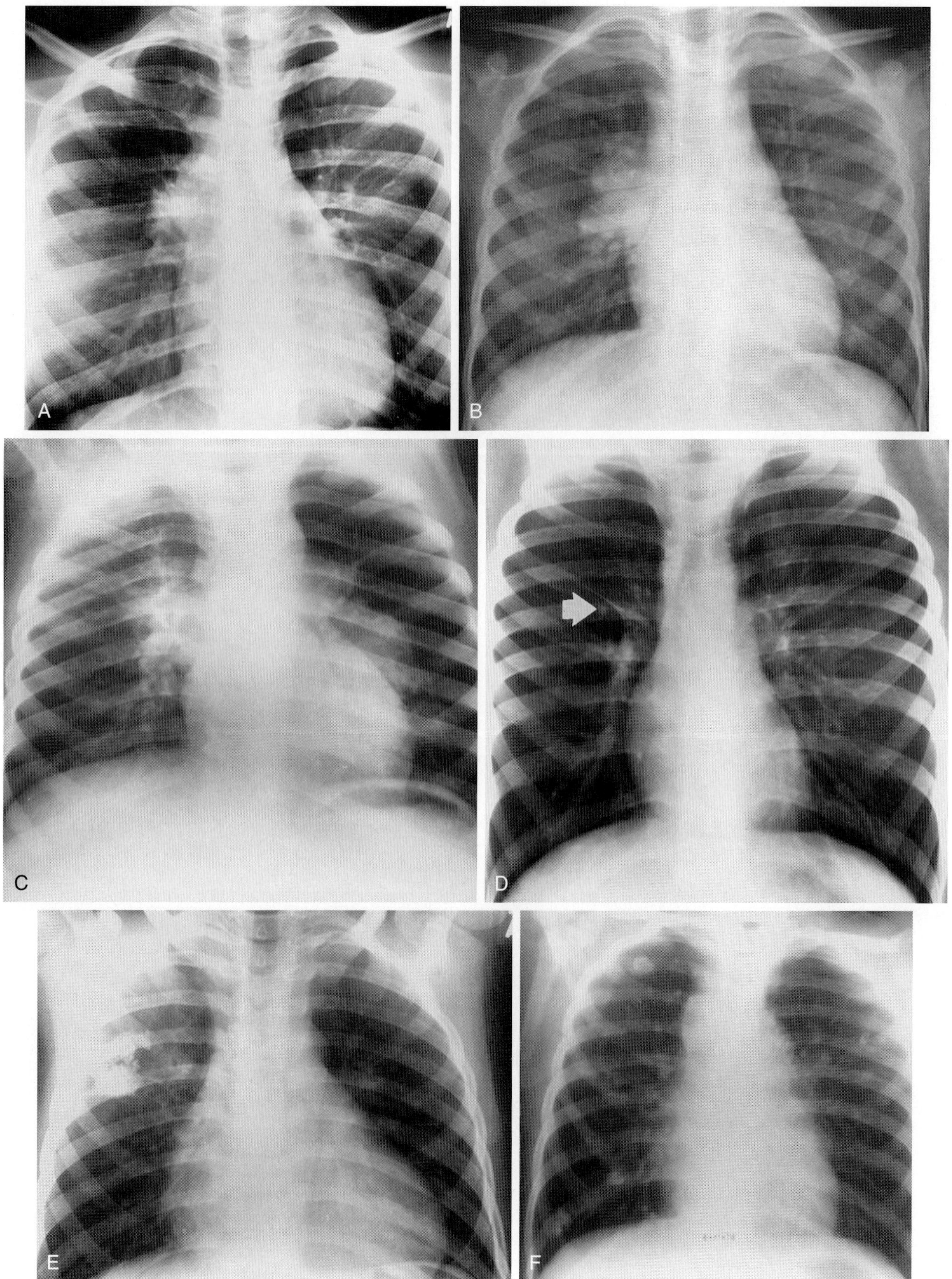

FIGURE 13–17. Primary pulmonary tuberculosis. **A** to **C,** Lymphadenopathy resulting from primary tuberculosis in three different children. **D** to **F,** Examples of calcified granulomas due to "healed" or inactive tuberculosis in three other children. **A,** Unilateral right hilar lymphadenopathy. **B,** Extensive right hilar and right paratracheal lymphadenopathy with localized bronchoconstriction. **C,** Bilateral hilar lymphadenopathy with left lower lobe pulmonary infiltrate. **D,** Single calcified granuloma (*arrow*) located below the minor fissure on the right. **E,** Unusual cluster of calcifications in the right upper lobe. **F,** Multiple pulmonary and nodal calcifications resulting from previous widespread pulmonary tuberculosis. (From Agrons GA, Markowitz RI, Kramer SS: Pulmonary tuberculosis in children. *Semin Roentgenol* 1993;28:2.)

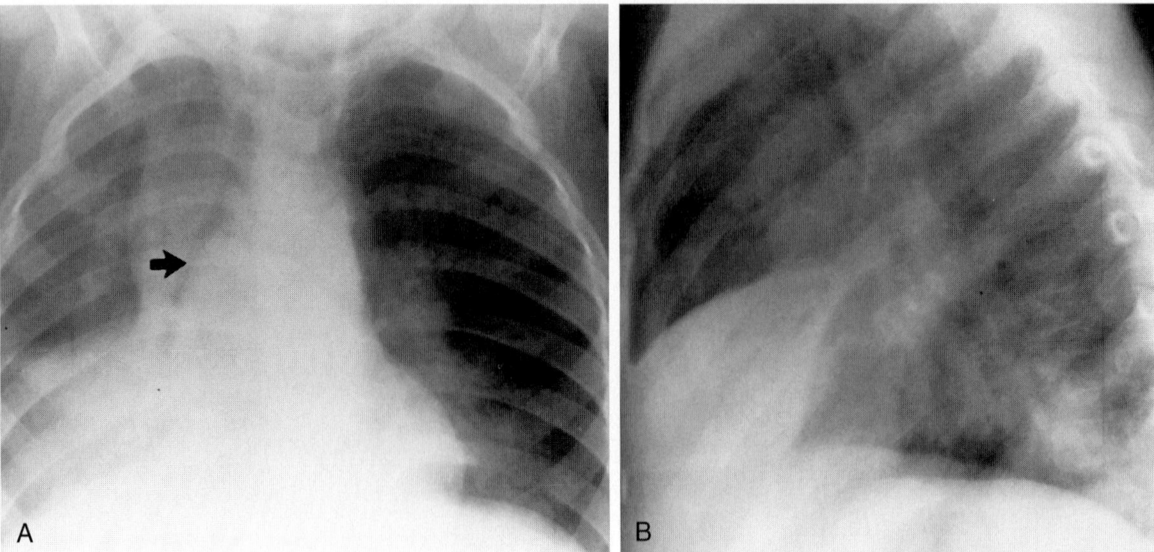

FIGURE 13–18. Primary tuberculosis with right middle lobe atelectasis resulting from lymph node compression of the bronchus intermedius in a 2-year-old boy with cough, wheezing, and a history of family exposure to pulmonary tuberculosis. **A,** Frontal chest radiograph shows consolidation and volume loss of the right middle lobe. Marked right hilar, paratracheal, and subcarinal lymphadenopathy is present, as well as severe narrowing of the bronchus intermedius (*arrow*). **B,** Lateral projection reveals the wedge-shaped, collapsed right middle lobe, as well as air space infiltrate in the lower lobe.

atelectasis to a disseminated pattern of widespread interstitial nodular disease. The radiographic appearance can be similar to that of varicella pneumonia, lymphocytic interstitial pneumonitis of AIDS (Fig. 13–19), or even metastatic disease, particularly thyroid malignancy. A high index of suspicion should be maintained for tuberculosis, especially when pulmonary infiltrates persist despite adequate treatment of the usual causative agents, and for unexplained mediastinal lymphadenopathy. Histoplasmosis, which has a more regional geographic distribution, can have radiographic findings similar to those of tuberculosis (Figs. 13–20 and 13–21).

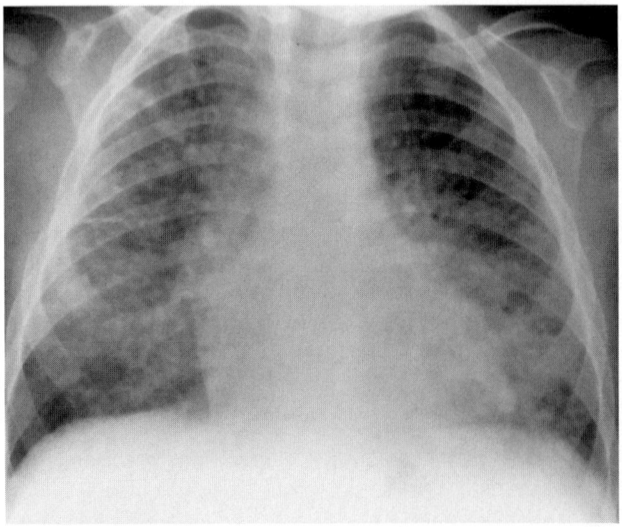

Heart

Conventional radiography of the chest is useful for evaluation of overall heart size and pulmonary status in cases of acute cardiac and pericardial infection. Echocardiography is invaluable for noninvasive delineation of heart valves and detection of lesions of endo-

FIGURE 13–19. Lymphocytic interstitial pneumonitis (LIP) in an 18-month-old-child with AIDS and mild tachypnea. Frontal chest radiograph shows an extensive and widespread pattern of multiple pulmonary nodules and mild mediastinal lymphadenopathy typical of LIP seen in infants and children with AIDS. This pattern is similar radiographically to that of varicella pneumonia, miliary tuberculosis, and metastatic disease, particularly thyroid carcinoma. The cause of LIP is unknown, although it may represent a hyperimmune reaction to Epstein-Barr virus. LIP responds to corticosteroid therapy but tends to rebound when therapy is discontinued.

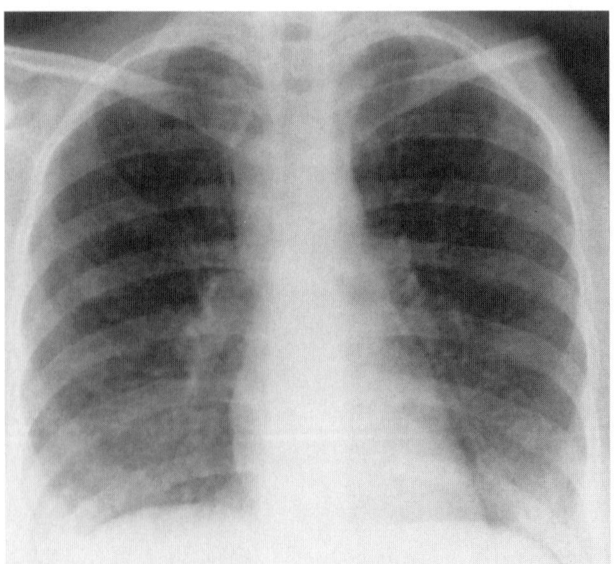

FIGURE 13–20. Histoplasmosis in a 14-year-old girl previously treated for leukemia. Frontal chest radiograph shows a widespread reticulonodular pattern of interstitial lung disease. Mild widening of the superior mediastinum represents lymphadenopathy.

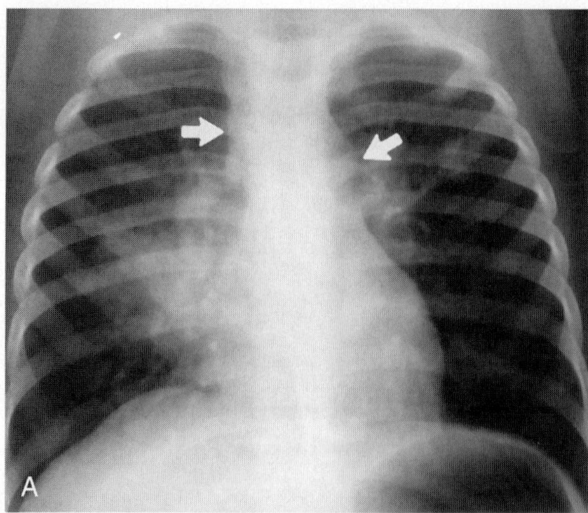

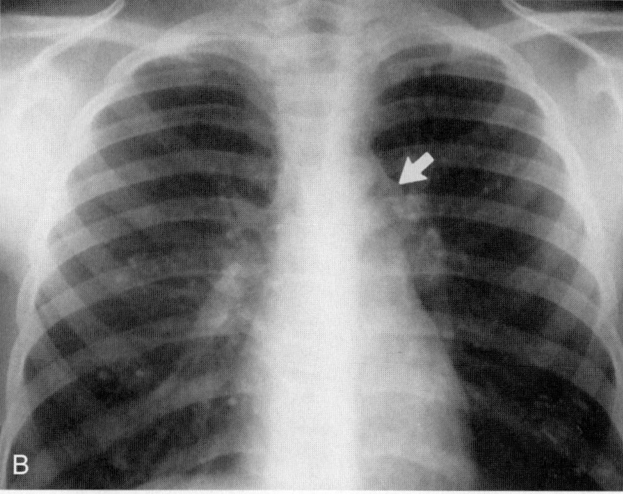

FIGURE 13–21. Histoplasmosis. **A,** Frontal chest radiograph during the acute phase shows a perihilar infiltrate extending into the right middle lobe, with bilateral hilar and paratracheal lymphadenopathy (*arrows*). **B,** Chest radiograph several years later shows complete resolution of the infiltrates. Scattered small calcifications persist within the lungs, with an enlarged left hilar lymph node (*arrow*).

carditis (Plate 8D) and is also especially good for detection of pericardial fluid. MRI can be used in special cases in which the usefulness of echocardiography is limited, such as after valve replacement, in calcified conduit, and in obesity. Mycotic aneurysms may also be evaluated with magnetic resonance angiography.

Abdomen

Gastrointestinal Tract. Diagnostic imaging of the gastrointestinal tract begins with contrast delineation of the mucosal outline (Fig. 13–22) or, alternatively, with direct endoscopic inspection, which is more expensive, is associated with greater morbidity, and requires sedation and skilled pediatric endoscopists.

Viral gastroenteritis does not require diagnostic imaging unless prolonged or changing symptoms, especially in the infant and young child, suggest the possibility of intussusception. Bacterial infections of the gut, especially the colon, may produce spasm and mucosal disruption that can be demonstrated by contrast enema. The radiologic findings of edema, mucosal ulceration, and spasm are not specific for any infection and can also be seen in noninfectious colitis. Changes in the bowel adjacent to an intra-abdominal inflammatory mass, such as an appendiceal abscess, may mimic the changes seen in infectious diarrhea and should not be mistaken for the primary abnormality (Fig. 13–23).

Appendix. The appropriate use of imaging in the diagnosis of acute appendicitis remains controversial. Conventional plain films of the abdomen are frequently normal or show nonspecific findings and may not be helpful. Although there is a good correlation between the presence of a calcified appendicolith and acute disease (Fig. 13–24), the finding of an appendicolith in a symptom-free person raises the question of whether such a person needs surgery. In the past, barium enema was used for the evaluation of suspected appendicitis, but ultrasonography and CT are now the diagnostic modalities of choice (Fig. 13–25). A false-negative result on ultrasonographic examination may be obtained because of the inability of the sonographer to perform deep compression or obtain adequate images, especially in obese individuals. CT, with or without oral or rectal contrast medium, is less operator dependent but uses ionizing radiation. Diagnostic imaging is helpful only when the clinical diagnosis is inconclusive. Patients with clinically obvious appendicitis need prompt surgical management, not additional radiologic evaluation.

Solid Abdominal Organs. Cross-sectional imaging with ultrasonography, CT, or MRI is the best way to image infections of the kidneys, liver, spleen, and retroperitoneum. The usefulness of MRI is limited because of long scan times, although new technical advances and the use of sedation have improved diagnostic quality.

CT is widely available, although strict attention to technique, including immobilization, is important (Fig. 13–26). Both oral and

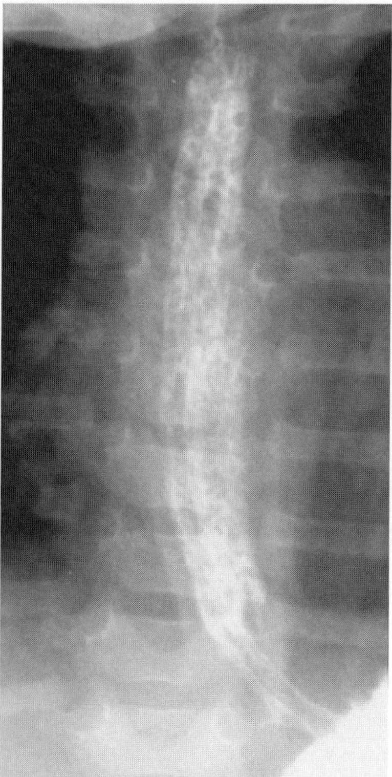

FIGURE 13–22. Fungal esophagitis caused by *Candida albicans* in a 9-month-old boy with failure to thrive. Barium esophagram shows diffuse mucosal irregularity.

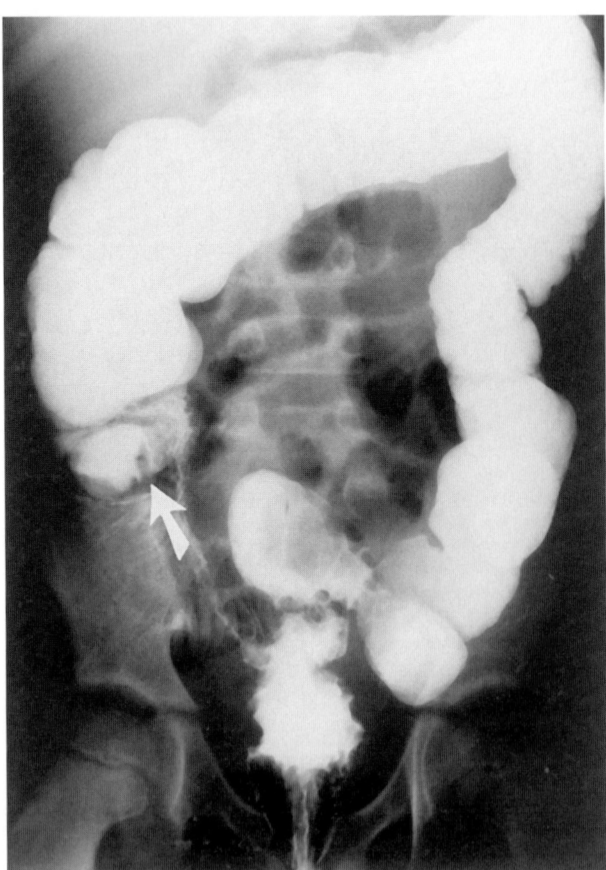

FIGURE 13–23. Acute appendicitis in a 5-year-old girl with fever, diarrhea, and abdominal pain. Barium enema demonstrates "sawtooth" irregularity of the rectosigmoid colon and spasm of the cecum. A filling defect at the base of the cecum (*arrow*) is noted, with nonfilling of the appendix. At surgery the appendix had perforated, causing generalized inflammation of the adjacent pelvic organs but no discrete abscess.

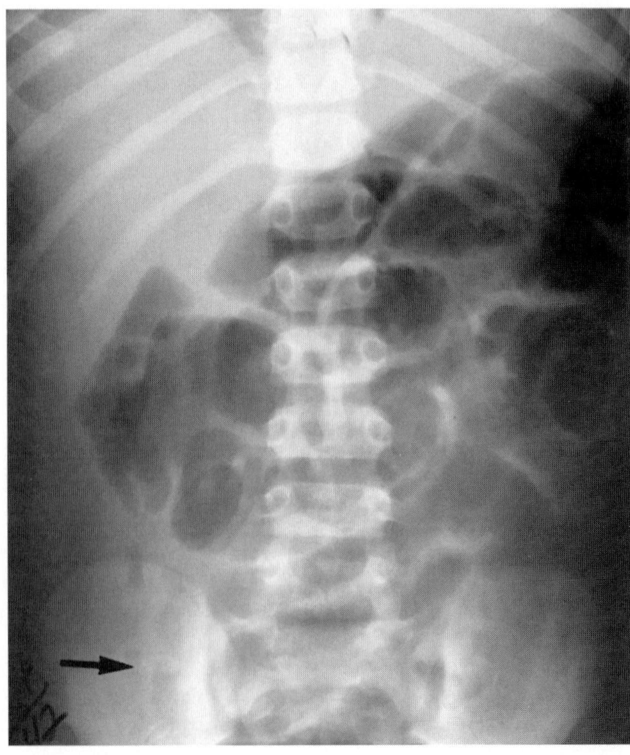

FIGURE 13–24. Acute appendicitis. Abdominal radiograph shows dilated small bowel loops consistent with ileus. A faint ovoid calcification (*arrow*) in the right lower quadrant represents an appendicolith in the inflamed appendix.

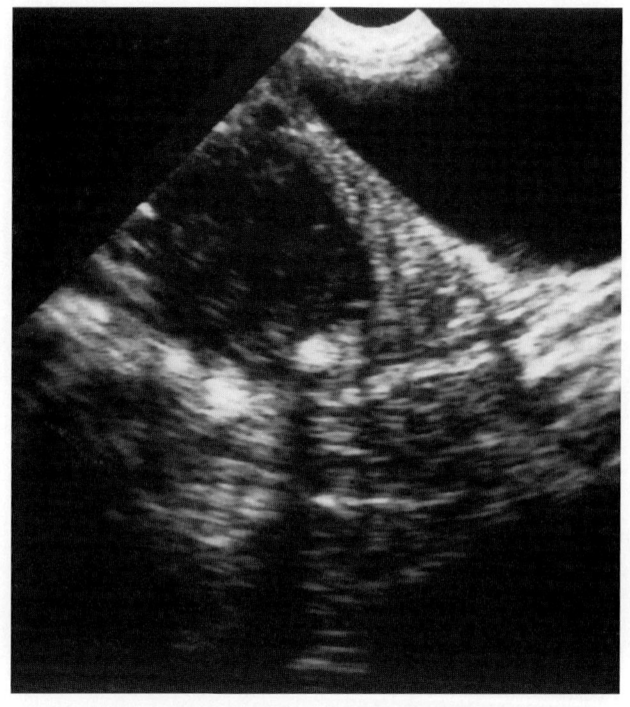

FIGURE 13–25. Appendiceal abscess with fecalith in a 9-year-old boy with abdominal pain and low-grade fever. Sonogram of right lower quadrant shows complex, hypoechoic, round mass with a single, highly echogenic stone at the bottom that represents the calcified appendicolith within the abscess.

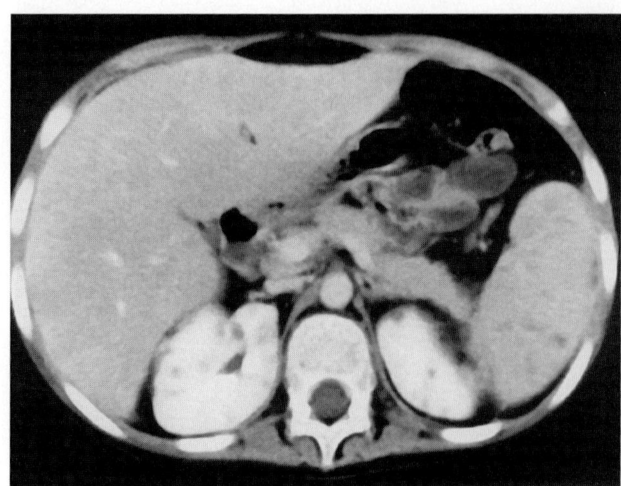

FIGURE 13–26. Disseminated fungal infection caused by *Candida albicans* in an 11-year-old girl with acute lymphocytic leukemia. Contrast-enhanced CT of upper abdomen shows multiple small foci of low attenuation throughout the kidneys and spleen in association with systemic candidiasis. The liver is not involved.

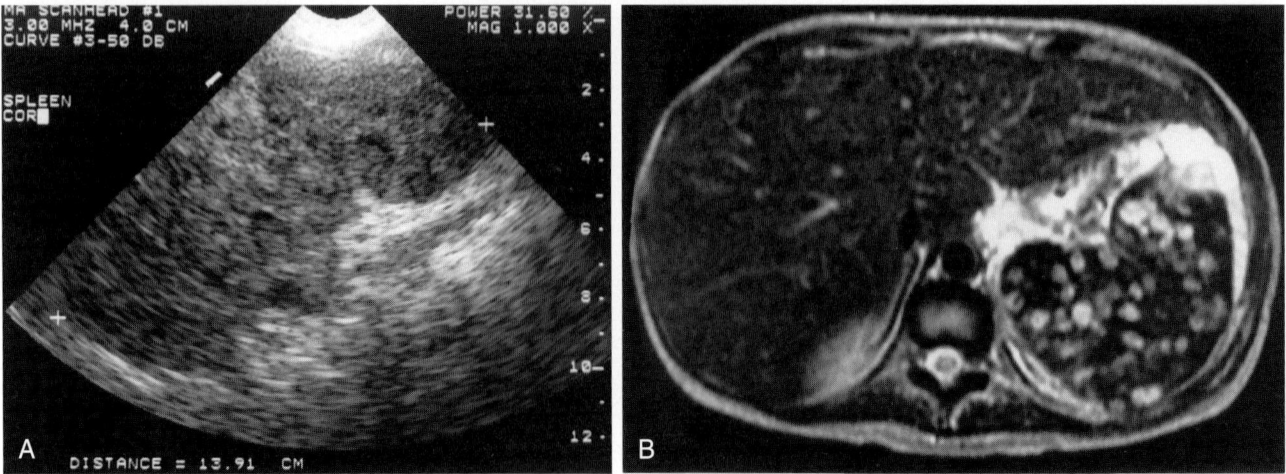

FIGURE 13–27. Fungal infection of spleen caused by *Candida albicans* in a 17-year-old immunocompromised girl with fever and anemia. **A,** Sagittal sonogram of spleen shows diffuse enlargement with inhomogeneity of spleen texture. **B,** Transaxial T1-weighted MRI of abdomen shows multiple foci of high-signal intensity within the enlarged spleen that represent multiple fungal lesions.

intravenous contrast are recommended. It is important to fill the entire bowel with contrast medium before scanning because unopacified bowel may be mistaken for an inflammatory or neoplastic mass. Motion artifact can be a serious problem, which is the reason that sedation is often advised.

Ultrasonography of the pediatric abdomen is an attractive diagnostic option because of the avoidance of radiation and contrast administration (Fig. 13–27). Sedation is sometimes necessary in younger and less cooperative persons to ensure an adequate examination. In general, complete ultrasonographic examination of the abdomen takes considerably longer than a CT examination, and its usefulness is limited by the presence of overlying bowel gas. Obese or uncooperative persons are more difficult to image and often require another imaging approach. The portability of ultrasound equipment is an advantage for patients in the intensive care unit, who cannot be easily transported.

Abscess drainage by an interventional radiologist with CT or ultrasonographic guidance is routinely performed in pediatric patients. It can obviate the need for immediate surgery in those for whom the risk associated with general anesthesia in high; in selected patients, this procedure can provide definitive treatment.

Genitourinary Tract

Ultrasonography, VCUG, and intravenous urography or pyelography are the most common radiologic methods used in the evaluation of urinary tract infections in children. The pertinent issues include evaluation for any underlying anatomic abnormality, such as a bladder outlet obstruction or malformation that predisposes the child to infection; the presence and severity of vesicoureteral reflux; the symmetry of size and shape of both kidneys; chronic parenchymal loss or scarring; and acute renal abscess or acute focal pyelonephritis. Different modalities are used to address these issues. CT or radionuclide studies may be helpful in clarifying abnormalities detected on the primary screening examinations (Fig. 13–28). Radionuclide technetium 99m dimercaptosuccinic acid renal scans can delineate scars from previous pyelonephritis.

Acute inflammatory conditions of the scrotum, including epididymitis and orchitis, must be distinguished from testicular torsion and infarction. High-resolution ultrasonography with color and power Doppler is useful in these situations. Radionuclide testicular scanning may show diminished flow in cases of torsion, whereas the blood flow may be increased in inflammatory conditions.

Ultrasonography is useful in diagnosing complications of pelvic inflammatory disease such as tubo-ovarian abscess (Fig. 13–29) and in excluding other causes of pelvic pain such as acute appendici-

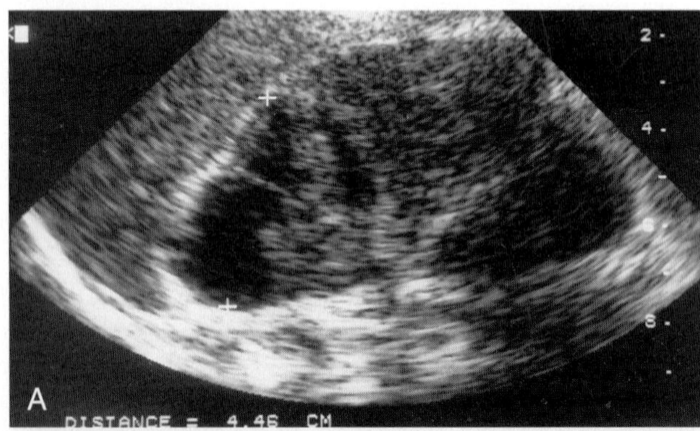

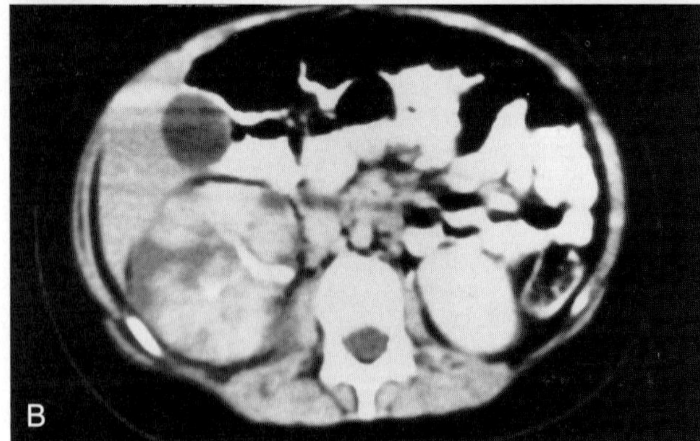

FIGURE 13–28. Acute bacterial focal nephritis in a 10-year-old girl with high fever, back pain, and pyuria. **A,** Sagittal sonogram of right kidney shows focal swelling of the upper pole with diminished echo texture simulating a renal mass. **B,** Contrast-enhanced abdominal CT confirms swelling of the right kidney with irregular segments of diminished perfusion (low attenuation) resulting from focal bacterial infection.

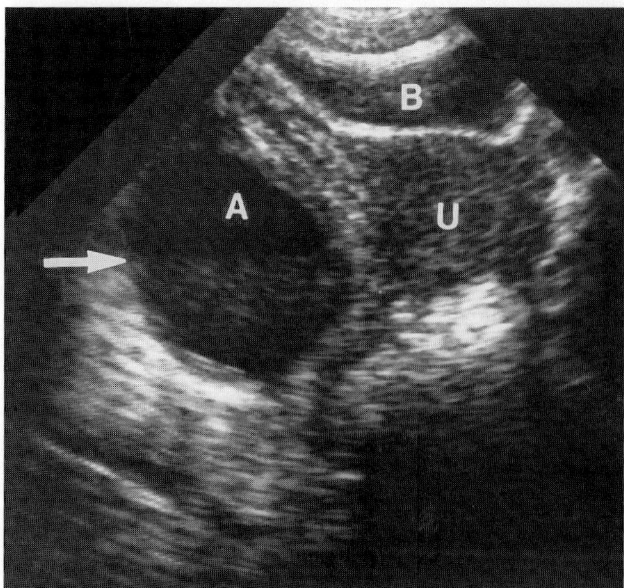

FIGURE 13–29. Pelvic inflammatory disease with tubo-ovarian abscess. Transverse pelvic sonogram shows a large, round fluid-filled abscess (*A*) replacing the normal right adnexa. There is a faint fluid-debris level within the abscess (*arrow*). Posterior to the bladder (*B*), the uterus (*U*) is mildly edematous.

tis or ovarian cyst. Percutaneous drainage of such abscesses recalcitrant to medical management can be performed under ultrasonographic or CT guidance.

Musculoskeletal System

Plain films are usually the first diagnostic modality employed in the study of the pediatric skeleton because of the high calcium content of bone. Radiographs provide excellent contrast, spatial resolution, and fine bone detail. Plain films also show soft tissue swelling and obliteration of normal deep fascial planes in children with serious infections, but these findings are often not definitive.

Radionuclide studies are helpful in the diagnosis of osteomyelitis. Because destruction of bone takes 10–14 days to identify on plain film (Fig. 13–30), other methods of early detection are required. Radionuclide bone scans have the advantage of being extremely sensitive to alterations in normal bone physiology. These changes, although not specific, may be detectable fairly early in the course of the disease (Fig. 13–31). Although the double-phase (early scanning during the flow phase and delayed scanning several hours later, during the static phase) bone scanning with technetium-99m diphosphonate remains the technique of choice for the detection of osteomyelitis, other agents and methods are useful. These include the tagging of white blood cells with gallium 67 and indium 111 (Fig. 13–32). Because traumatized bone may also concentrate radionuclide to a variable degree, scan findings should be interpreted in light of the clinical situation. A brief phase of diminished radionuclide uptake may occur early in the course of acute osteomyelitis, probably as a result of transiently diminished blood flow, which then progresses to a prolonged phase of increased uptake. If scans are performed during the time of transition from the "cold" to the "hot" phase, a false-negative result may be obtained. Scan technique is important in children with open epiphyses and growing bones. Meticulous positioning and immobilization and high-resolution "pinhole" camera views are necessary to reveal subtle differences between the two sides of the body.

CT can also demonstrate fine detail and help localize and characterize abnormalities that alter the calcified bone trabeculae. CT is also useful for demonstrating abscess or other anatomic alterations within muscle. MRI more readily demonstrates diseases that primarily affect the marrow or noncalcified components of bone. This is particularly true for osteomyelitis, which, although frequently destroying calcified bone, usually begins as an infection within the marrow (Fig. 13–31). Joint effusions and soft tissue abscesses are also well demonstrated by MRI, which is now the primary imaging modality for osteomyelitis.

High-resolution ultrasonography is used less frequently to detect subperiosteal changes of osteomyelitis but is especially helpful in guiding needle aspiration of fluid collections and joint effusions (Fig. 13–33).

The diagnosis of chronic osteomyelitis is more readily apparent on conventional radiographs (Fig. 13–34). Periosteal reaction, focal bone destruction, and reactive sclerosis occur in varying degrees depending on the aggressiveness of the lesion and the immune reaction to the infection. Occasionally, neoplasms such as Ewing's sarcoma and neuroblastoma, both of which are small, round cell tumors, can mimic the appearance and behavior of chronic osteomyelitis.

Congenital syphilis affects the metaphyses and diaphyses, which show periosteal new bone formation (Fig. 13–35). Congenital cytomegalovirus and rubella cause demineralization of the metaphyses, resulting in linear striations known as celery stalking (Fig. 95–7).

Text continued on page 146

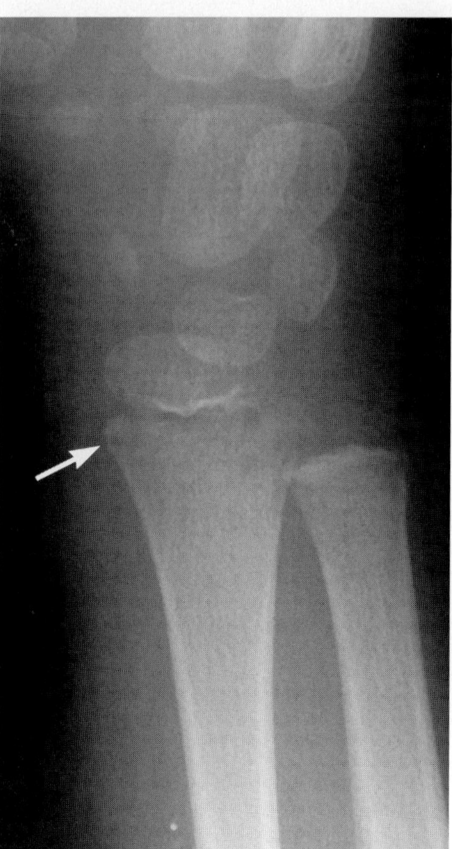

FIGURE 13–30. Acute osteomyelitis of the distal radius in a 7-year-old boy with a swollen, painful wrist. Oblique radiograph shows mild soft tissue swelling. Subtle, poorly demarcated demineralization is present at the metaphysis, indicative of early bone resorption (*arrow*) and early osteomyelitis.

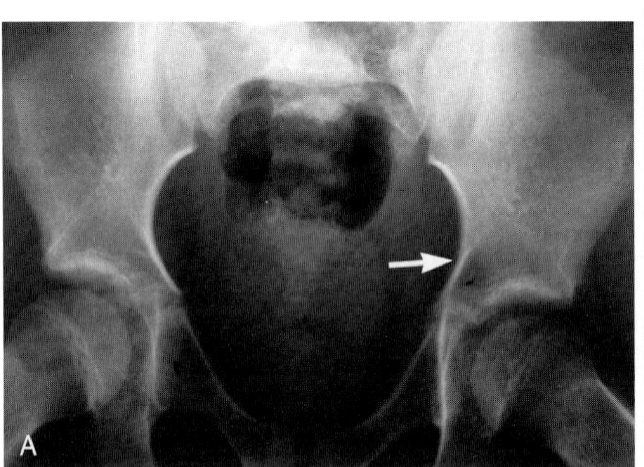

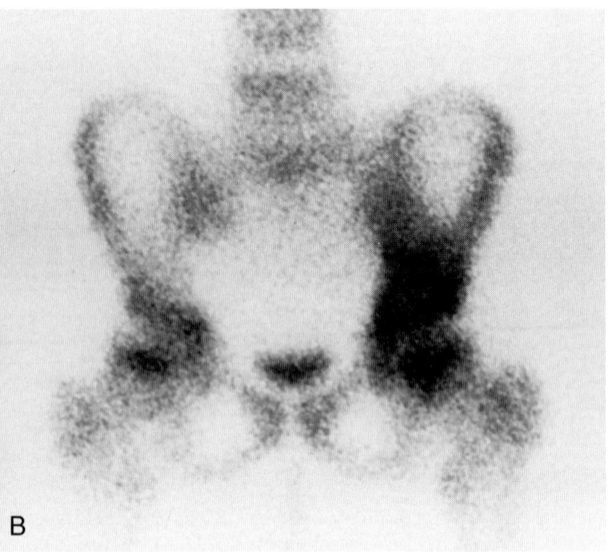

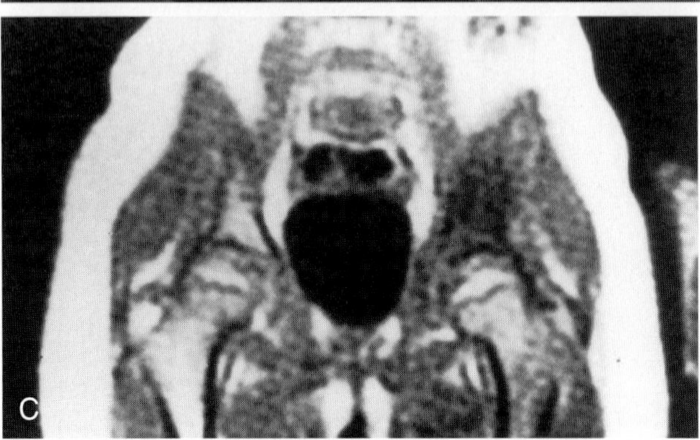

FIGURE 13–31. Osteomyelitis of the pelvis in a 12-year-old girl (a ballet dancer) with pain in the left hip of 1–2 weeks' duration. **A,** Frontal radiograph of pelvis shows mild demineralization of the acetabular portion of the left iliac bone adjacent to the triradiate cartilage. There is subtle periosteal reaction (*arrow*). **B,** Technetium 99m bone scan shows increased uptake by the left iliac bone and femoral head. **C,** Coronal T1-weighted MRI shows decreased signal from the marrow of the left iliac bone, compared with the bright signal from the normal fatty marrow on the right. The femoral head is normal, and there is no joint effusion. Needle aspiration of the iliac bone yielded *Staphylococcus aureus.*

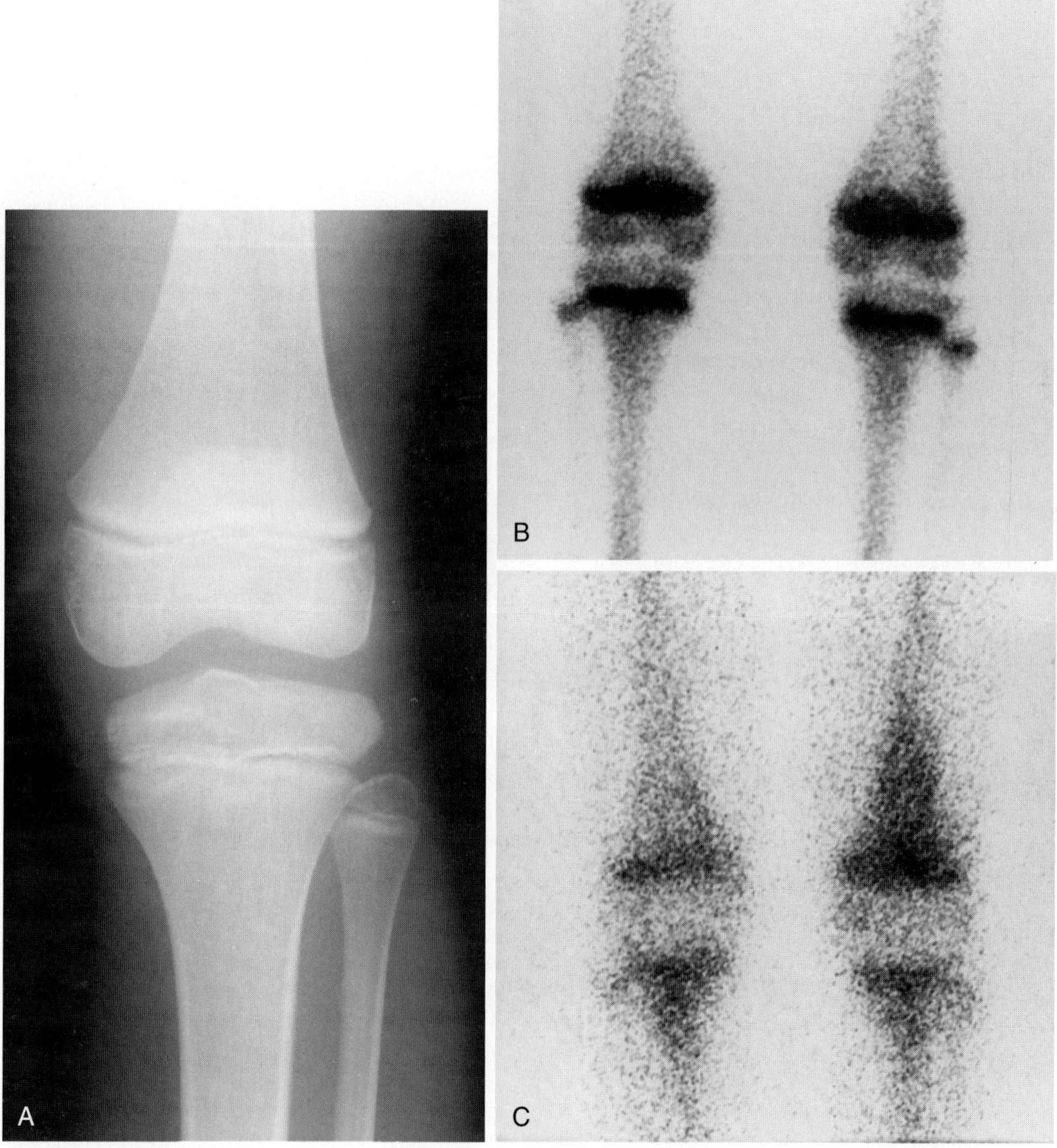

FIGURE 13–32. Osteomyelitis of the distal femur in a 12-year-old girl with pain in the left knee. **A,** Frontal radiograph of the left knee is normal. **B,** Technetium 99m bone scan performed shortly after the x-ray film was obtained is normal. **C,** Indium 111 white blood cell scan performed 2 days later shows increased uptake in the distal femoral metaphysis, consistent with osteomyelitis. (Courtesy of Gerald A. Mandell.)

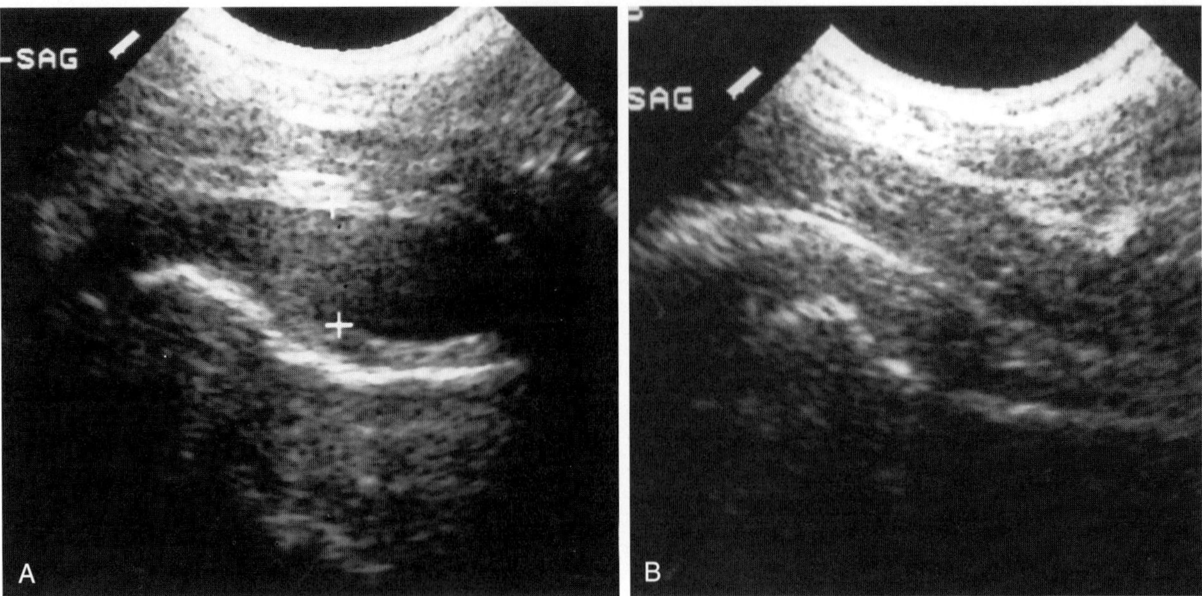

FIGURE 13–33. Hip joint effusion in a 4-year-old girl with pain and refusal to walk for 1 week. **A,** Anterior sagittal sonogram of right hip shows ovoid bulging of thickened joint capsule due to fluid. The *curved white line* at the bottom is the anterior surface of the femur. **B,** Similar view of normal left side for comparison.

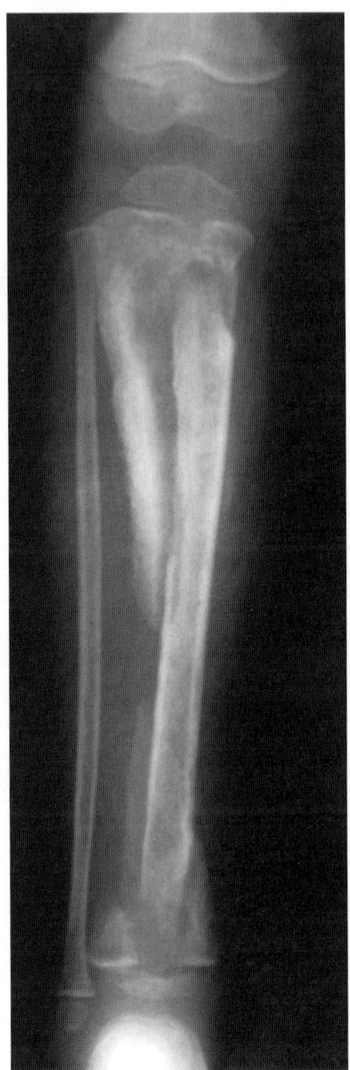

FIGURE 13–34. Chronic osteomyelitis of the tibia in a 4-year-old child with long-standing leg pain and swelling. Frontal radiograph shows extensive destruction and reactive sclerosis of the tibia. The dense central bone fragment represents the dead sequestrum. The surrounding partially reconstituted bone is the involucrum.

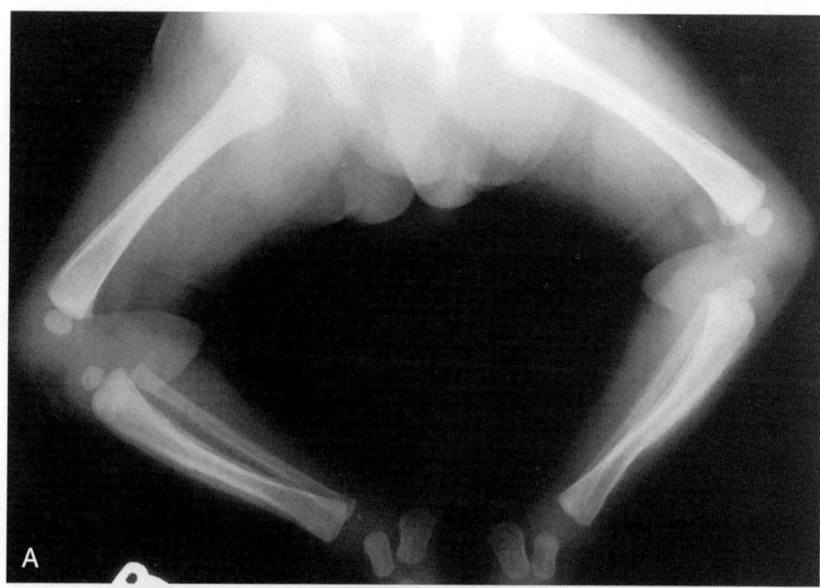

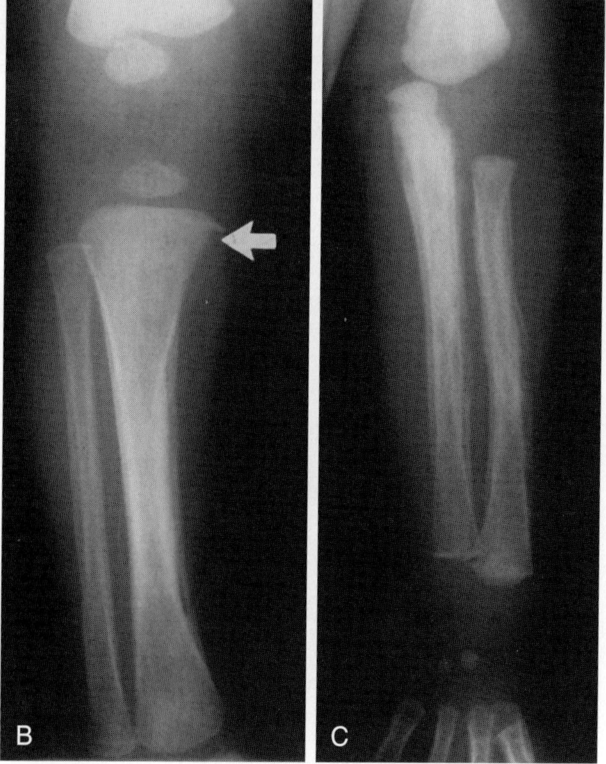

FIGURE 13–35. Term infant with congenital syphilis. **A,** Lateral view of both lower extremities reveals periosteal reaction of the long bones. **B,** Frontal view of the right tibia and fibula shows early destructive changes at the proximal tibial metaphysis (*arrow*) and diffuse periostitis. **C,** Similar periosteal and sclerotic changes involve the radius and ulna.

INTERPRETATION OF DIAGNOSTIC IMAGING STUDIES

Cross-sectional imaging usually entails a large number of individual images that must be viewed and mentally integrated. Despite the urging of concerned clinicians to take just a "quick peek" at a study, it does the patient a disservice if the examination is not interpreted completely and methodically. Comparison with prior examinations and other imaging studies may be critical and may greatly modify or even reverse a preliminary interpretation. The comparison and correlation of imaging findings often require additional time and effort. If a diagnostic imaging test is worth obtaining, all the images must be studied thoroughly and thoughtfully to fully appreciate their diagnostic significance. Multimodality imaging redundantly demonstrating the same pathologic change is useless without the knowledge and skill necessary to recognize and understand the information displayed.

A reasonable approach to diagnostic image interpretation is based on a thorough knowledge of anatomy, physiology, and pathology. The age, sex, and history of the patient, as well as geographic considerations and laboratory findings, should be considered before the final diagnosis is established. Experienced radiologists usually need relatively few imaging studies to determine the correct diagnosis. Despite great achievements in technology, the start of a diagnostic search still begins with the patient, whose history and physical findings should always be the primary impetus for the diagnostic study. The phrase "clinical correlation is advised" may be a cliché, but it has merit.

REVIEWS

Kirks DR, Griscom NT (editors): *Practical Pediatric Imaging,* 3rd ed. Philadelphia, Lippincott-Raven, 1998.

Silverman FN, Kuhn JP (editors): *Caffey's Pediatric X-ray Diagnosis,* 9th ed. St Louis, Mosby, 1993.

Swischuk LE (editor): *Imaging of the Newborn, Infant and Young Child,* 3rd ed. Baltimore, Williams & Wilkins, 1989.

KEY ARTICLES

Bova JG, Villalobos LB: Utilization review of simultaneously ordered multiple radiologic tests for the same symptom. *Am J Med Qual* 1998; 13:81–4.

Bramson RT, Meyer TL, Silbiger ML, et al: The futility of the chest radiograph in the febrile infant without respiratory symptoms. *Pediatrics* 1993;92:524–6.

Davies HD, Wang EE, Manson D, et al: Reliability of the chest radiograph in the diagnosis of lower respiratory infections in young children. *Pediatr Infect Dis J* 1996;15:600–4.

Dick PT, Feldman W: Routine diagnostic imaging for childhood urinary tract infections: A systematic overview. *J Pediatr* 1996;128:15–22.

Gylys-Morin VM: MR imaging of pediatric musculoskeletal inflammatory and infectious disorders. *Magn Reson Imaging Clin N Am* 1998;6: 537–59.

Kramer MS, Roberts-Brauer R, Williams RL: Bias and "overcall" in interpreting chest radiographs in young febrile children. *Pediatrics* 1992;90:11–3.

O'Marcaigh AS, Jacobson RM: Estimating the predictive value of a diagnostic test. How to prevent misleading or confusing results. *Clin Pediatr* 1993;32:485–91.

Rosenquist CJ: Pitfalls in the use of diagnostic tests. *Clin Radiol* 1989; 40:448–50.

Scally PM: Decision making in diagnostic radiology. *Australas Radiol* 1993;37:336–41.

CHAPTER 14

Anti-infective Therapy

Michael D. Reed ▪ Jeffrey L. Blumer

Anti-infective therapy has a history that dates back several thousand years. However, until the microbiologic basis for infectious diseases was established in the nineteenth century, this therapy was essentially empirical. The discovery of the antibacterial activity of aminoazo dyes, which led to the introduction of the sulfonamide antibiotics in the 1930s, revolutionized the practice of medicine. For the first time, infectious diseases could be specifically and effectively treated with agents that were relatively nontoxic to the patient.

The demonstration in 1933 in both Europe and the United States of the clinical efficacy of the sulfonamide Prontosil, the prodrug that is metabolized to sulfanilamide in children, heralded the birth of the ''golden age'' of antibiotics. This clinical triumph catalyzed a concerted search for new drugs to treat systemic infections. This search soon resulted in the ability of Florey, Chain, and their associates, in 1941, to capitalize on the discovery of penicillin by Fleming in 1929. During the next 3 decades, virtually all classes of agents used in current clinical practice were either isolated or synthesized.

Today antibiotics are responsible for more than $2 billion in annual health care costs. More than 30% of hospitalized patients in the United States receive at least one antimicrobial agent. Anti-infectives remain among the most common drugs prescribed on any outpatient basis throughout the world.

GENERAL PRINCIPLES OF ANTI-INFECTIVE THERAPY

Antimicrobial Therapeutics

The widespread use of anti-infective agents in medicine today is a testimony to their efficacy and safety. As such, these agents appear to fulfill the most basic precepts of chemotherapy—they are drugs that injure the invading organism without injuring the host. In fact, this principle of **selective toxicity** has been fundamental to the development of anti-infective agents from the earliest days of their clinical applications.

Selectivity is believed to exist when an agent influences the function of one type of living cell without affecting other types, even when these cells are close neighbors. Antibiotics are selective agents that are produced either by a microorganism or, in modern terms, by total or partial chemical synthesis. These substances have the capacity, in dilute concentrations, to inhibit the growth of other microorganisms (i.e., bacteriostatic) or to kill them (i.e., bactericidal).

The selectivity of antimicrobial agents can be divided into three categories on the basis of physical characteristics (Table 14–1). Some agents are selective because they capitalize on biochemical differences between the host and the infecting pathogen. For example, the sulfonamides inhibit the enzyme dihydrofolate reductase, which is essential to bacteria but not important to mammals because the latter can absorb folate from their diet. Bacteria lack the permease required for folate uptake and therefore must synthesize folate in situ. Other antibiotics are selective because they target structural differences between host cells and the infecting bacteria. For example, the β-lactam antibiotics inhibit the synthesis of bacterial cell walls, which are structures essential to bacterial survival but are not present on mammalian cells. Last, drugs such as griseofulvin manifest their selective toxicity by selectively accumulating in cells infected with certain microorganisms. As a result, the wide variety of anti-infective agents available today have a finite number of mechanisms through which they exert their antimicrobial effects (Table 14–2).

Matching an infecting organism's susceptibility to a list of the antibiotics to which it is susceptible does not always result in optimal treatment. The reasons that underlie the failure of this strategy represent the essence of the science of anti-infective therapeutics (Fig. 14–1). **Therapeutics** is the discipline within pharmacology that deals with the use of drugs in the prevention or treatment of disease. Although matching isolates with a list of antibiotics that are active in vitro may result in treatment choices that are, in the strictest sense, pharmacodynamically correct, they may be therapeutically misguided. The pharmacodynamic decision is based almost entirely on the susceptibility of a particular pathogen to the toxic effects of the drug under fairly rigid laboratory conditions. In contrast, the therapeutic approach considers characteristics of the host, the pathogen, and their individual and shared environments, as well as the physicochemical properties of the drugs available that fulfill the pharmacologic criteria for potential effectiveness. It is only within the past decade that the true importance of a therapeutic approach rather than simply a pharmacodynamic one has become apparent. Essential to this realization are several key questions regarding anti-infective therapy that must be addressed before drug is ever administered to a patient (Table 14–3). Unfortunately, definitive answers to these questions are lacking in most situations. Finding the answers represents one of the real challenges to anti-infective research for the next decade.

Determinants of Effective Therapy

Essential to the practice of anti-infective therapeutics is an understanding of the elements of effective therapy. From a pharmacologic perspective, there are basically three key determinants of effective therapy (Fig. 14–2). In a given clinical situation, if a drug can be identified that has favorable characteristics in each of these areas, it will, by definition, provide effective therapy.

Pharmacodynamics is the discipline within pharmacology that relates drug administration to drug concentration-effect relationships. In other words, it deals with the drugs' mechanisms of action and safety profiles. There is probably no other area of medicine in which the pharmacodynamic aspects of therapy are understood as well as in infectious diseases. In the context of clinical medicine, the pharmacodynamic effects of anti-infective drugs are assessed through the determination of anti-infective drug susceptibility in vitro.

TABLE 14–1. Physical Basis for Antimicrobial Selectivity

Comparative Biochemistry
Capitalizes on difference in macromolecular synthetic processes or intermediary metabolism between the host and the infecting agent (e.g., sulfonamides, quinolones)

Comparative Cytology
Capitalizes on differences in overall cell structure or composition of subcellular organelles between the host and the infecting agent, such as the presence of cell walls in bacteria in contrast to mammalian cells (e.g., β-lactams) and the differences in structure of bacterial ribosomes from mammalian ribosomes (e.g., aminoglycosides, macrolides)

Drug Accumulation
Capitalizes on pharmacokinetic differences between the host and infecting agent (e.g., griseofulvin, tetracyclines)

A number of procedures are available for testing the susceptibility of various microorganisms to anti-infective drugs. These procedures have been established best for bacteria and less so for fungi; they are poorly developed for other infectious agents. The susceptibility of bacteria to the toxic effects of various antibiotics is usually tested with the Kirby-Bauer disk technique or by broth dilution. In the former procedure a zone of growth inhibition that corresponds to a drug concentration associated with clinical effectiveness is measured. In the latter test the bacteria are inoculated into nutrient broth containing serial dilutions of the drug being tested. The greatest dilution associated with the inhibition of bacterial growth is termed the **minimum inhibitory concentration (MIC).** If further dilution can be achieved without a recurrence of bacterial growth, then this dilution is also the **minimum bactericidal concentration (MBC)** for the drug. If bacterial growth does recur, then the MBC is at a higher dilution.

MIC and MBC values provide some indication of the potency of the antibiotic with regard to the infecting bacterial pathogen. As such, these values reflect pharmacodynamic correlates of antibiotic effectiveness. Nevertheless, they must be interpreted with some caution. MIC values are determined under a very strict and standard set of laboratory conditions that may not readily reflect the clinical situation (e.g., a constant drug concentration for a prolonged period, lack of protein [albumin], standardized bacterial colony count). In addition, the values cannot be interpreted without additional information; potency is not synonymous with efficacy. For example, if two drugs have **MIC_{90}** values (antibiotic concentration that will inhibit growth of 90% of strains tested) for *Staplylococcus aureus* of 0.1 μg/mL and 1 μg/mL, respectively, it is tempting to consider the first drug to be superior. However, if the concentrations of the two drugs at the site of infection are 0.15 μg/mL and 100 μg/mL, respectively, the second agent may turn out to be more effective for pharmacokinetic reasons.

With the increasing understanding of the clinical limitations of the MIC and MBC, it has become clear that optimal antibiotic dosing requires an integration of a drug's pharmacokinetic profile with its in vitro pharmacodynamic correlates. This integration accounts for both the individual antibiotic's cellular mechanism of action and the time course of drug within the body. Considering the dose regimens used clinically, it is intuitive that the drug's disposition characteristics would be of paramount importance to the overall safety and efficacy of the prescribed medical therapy. Intensive animal research and evolving human research have been successful in determining the primary **pharmacokinetic (PK) and pharmacodynamic (PD)** parameters that correlate best with the efficacy of certain antibiotics. For many drugs and the β-lactams in particular, the therapeutic efficacy is highly dependent on the time that the free drug concentration exceeds the pathogen MIC. Thus the drugs with this PK-PD correlate are referred to as time-dependent antimicrobials. In contrast, certain other antibiotics (e.g., aminoglycosides, quinolones) have antibacterial efficacy that is dependent on the magnitude at which the antibiotic concentration exceeds the pathogen MIC, not on duration. These later drugs are termed concentration-dependent antimicrobials. An understanding of which antibiotic's therapeutic efficacy best correlates with the time above the MIC (time-dependent agents) or with the magnitude of drug concentration above the MIC (concentration-dependent antibiotics) gives the clinician the ability to determine the optimal antibiotic dosing regimen for the specific pathogen infecting an individual patient. For concentration-dependent agents, the ratio of the **peak drug concentration,** or **C_{max},** or **area under the drug concentration (AUC)** time curve to the pathogen MIC has been determined to best reflect the magnitude of concentration above a target MIC. This understanding of antimicrobial PK-PD interrelationships has permitted the development of contemporary dosing regimens such as once-daily dosing with aminoglycosides.

The PK-PD correlates for selected antibiotics are shown in Table 14–4. The target PK-PD parameter value for optimal efficacy of penicillin antibiotics is maintenance of the free drug concentration above the MIC for ≥40% of the dosing interval and about

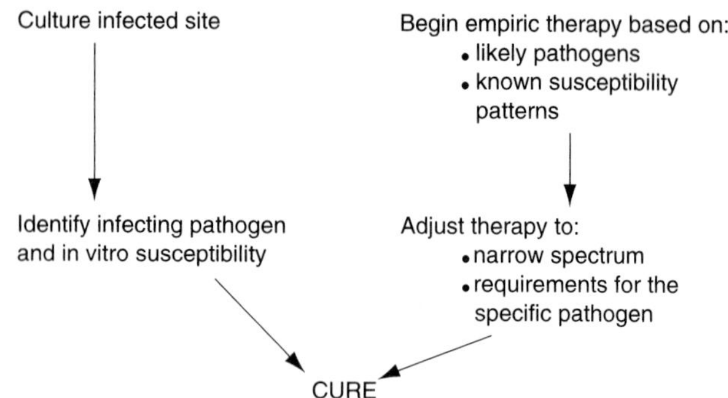

FIGURE 14–1. Expectations in anti-infective therapeutics.

TABLE 14–2. Mechanisms of Anti-infective Action

Inhibitors of cell wall synthesis
Inhibitors of protein synthesis
Antimetabolites
Altered membrane permeability
DNA gyrase inhibitor

TABLE 14–3. Fundamental Questions in Anti-infective Therapeutics

What is the optimal anti-infective drug for the treatment of *this* infectious process in *this* person?
What is the proper dose of this drug for the treatment of this infectious process in this person?
What is the most appropriate route of administration for this drug to this person?
What is the necessary duration of therapy for this infectious process in this person with the selected anti-infective agent?

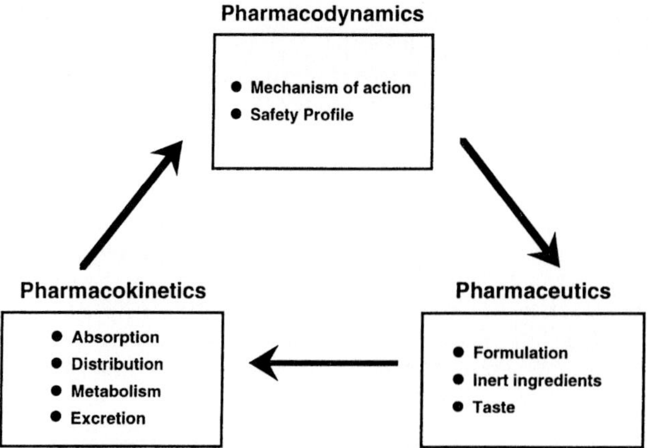

FIGURE 14–2. Determinants of effective therapy.

≥50% of the dosing interval for cephalosporins. With respect to the concentration-dependent antibiotics, such as the aminoglycosides and quinolones, either the C_{max}:MIC ratio or the AUC:MIC ratio must be used. The C_{max} for aminoglycosides and quinolones should be ≥8–10 times the MIC. For quinolones the AUC:MIC ratio should be ≥35 for gram-positive pathogens and ≥100 (to 125) for gram-negative pathogens, which best correlates with therapeutic efficacy. With increasing experience, our understanding of the optimal correlate values continues to expand. It is likely that with further research the true PK-PD parameter value for each antibiotic class will be refined and will likely be specific for specific pathogens at sites of infection.

Pharmacodynamics also deals with the safety profiles of the various anti-infective agents, as well as their mechanisms of action. Drug toxicity has posed little difficulty in treating pediatric patients with anti-infective agents, although some dramatic examples of adverse drug effects have occurred in infants and children. Because most of the drugs used were either synthesized or adapted with the principle of selective toxicity as a guiding premise, very few significant side effects have been reported. When adverse reactions occur, understanding their existence and having a monitoring plan that is likely to identify problems at an early stage are essential.

Pharmaceutics deals with the drug formulation that is actually administered to the patient. With intravenous drugs, this may simply relate to the type of salt or counter ion used. For oral preparations it is important to know whether the drug is a tablet, capsule, liquid, suspension, or elixir. When one is treating infants and children, there are additional considerations. First, the taste of the liquid preparations used may be an important determinant of compliance with therapy, and therefore the inactive ingredients in many liquid preparations may be of some concern. These ingredients are not regulated and may be changed by the manufacturer without notice. This possibility often becomes of particular importance with generic substitutions for brand name products. Second, some of the sugars, preservatives, and dyes may cause serious and even life-threatening reactions in sensitive persons.

Pharmacokinetics is the final determinant of effective therapy. This aspect of pharmacology relates drug administration to the concentration-time profile that the drug achieves in body fluids. To a large extent this profile is determined by what the body does to the drug rather than what the drug does to the body. It quantitatively describes the processes of drug absorption, distribution, metabolism, and excretion.

Pharmacokinetics can be bewildering to most clinicians, but certain aspects must be understood so that anti-infective therapy can be prescribed on a rational basis. It is essential to understand the central role of pharmacokinetics as a determinant of anti-infective efficacy. Because it is known that a given agent is effective against an isolated microorganism or likely pathogen before drug administration (pharmacodynamics) and that the formulation is safe and appropriate for the patient before drug administration (pharmaceutics), then almost any deviation from the expected therapeutic effect must have a pharmacokinetic basis. Generally these problems involve issues of drug distribution or drug elimination.

The aspect of pharmacokinetics familiar to most clinicians is the **elimination half-life ($t_{1/2\beta}$):** the period required for the concentration of drug in the biologic fluid to drop to half of its previously measured value. This parameter is clinically important because it can be related directly to the frequency of drug administration. Thus, in general, the longer the $t_{1/2\beta}$, the less frequently a drug must be administered.

In addition, the pharmacokinetic characteristics of a drug are those that may be altered in the face of disease or may be affected by drug-drug interactions. The need to adjust anti-infective dosing in the case of hepatic or renal functional impairment is determined by the effect that these disease states have on drug distribution, metabolism, and excretion. The pharmacologic basis of most drug-drug interactions is also related to alterations in drug distribution and metabolism.

Integration of these pharmacodynamic, pharmaceutic, and pharmacokinetic considerations should allow the description of the ideal anti-infective agent (Table 14–5). Such an approach results in a

TABLE 14–4. Pharmacokinetic-Pharmacodynamic Efficacy: Correlates for Selected Antibiotics

Concentration-Dependent Agents (C_{max}:MIC or AUC:MIC)	Time-Dependent Agents (Time Above MIC)
Aminoglycosides	Penicillins
Quinolones	Cephalosporins
Azithromycin	Carbapenems
Tetracyclines	Monobactams
Vancomycin	Macrolides
Ketolides	Clindamycin
Streptogramins	Oxazolidinones

C_{max} = peak plasma/serum drug concentration; AUC = area under the plasma/serum drug concentration-time curve; MIC = minimum inhibitory concentration.

TABLE 14–5. Ideal Anti-infective Agent

- Selective and effective in its anti-infective activity
- Capable of tissue penetration in concentrations that exceed by severalfold the minimum bactericidal concentration (MBC) of potential bacterial pathogens
- Bactericidal rather than bacteriostatic
- High affinity for site of action
- Resistant to inactivation by bacterial enzymes, tissue fluids, or products of inflammation
- Must not readily stimulate bacterial resistance
- Orally active
- Long elimination half-life
- Devoid of drug-drug interactions
- Absence of major organ system toxic effects
- Absence of developmental or behavioral toxic effects

rational selection among a variety of therapeutic choices (Fig. 14–3).

Selection of an Appropriate Anti-infective Agent

Most therapy for infectious diseases is initiated on an empirical basis. A commitment to rational anti-infective therapeutics requires a thorough knowledge of the pathogens likely to be responsible for a given infectious process and an understanding of the spectrum of coverage of the available anti-infective drugs (Table 14–6). In the selection of an anti-infective agent for empirical therapy, a number of factors related to the patient, microbiologic factors, and drug factors must be considered (Table 14–7).

Patient-related factors are the most numerous and complex determinants of drug selection for an infectious problem. Space does not permit an in-depth discussion of these issues. It is clear, however, that because the pathogens likely to be responsible for a given disease (e.g., pneumonia) vary with age, the presence of an underlying disease (e.g., cancer), and the status of the patient's hepatic or renal function, these factors must all be considered before prescribing empirical anti-infective therapy. Similarly, a history of allergic reactions to certain types of drugs or long-term immunosuppressive therapy weighs heavily in therapeutic decision making.

The microbiologic factors that must be considered in prescribing empirical therapy are fairly straightforward but no less important. Although knowledge of what pathogens are likely to be involved in a given infectious process is vital, knowledge of the anti-infective susceptibility patterns of these pathogens in the hospital or community in which the infection occurs is equally essential. Some wide geographic differences in anti-infective susceptibility patterns must be considered in prescribing empirical anti-infective therapy. For example, in a community with a high incidence of β-lactamase-producing *Haemophilus influenzae,* amoxicillin may not be a prudent choice for the empirical treatment of respiratory tract infections.

A number of drug-related issues must also be considered when one is prescribing anti-infective therapy. It is obvious that the intrinsic anti-infective activity of an agent is an important consideration in empirical drug therapy, but if the agent cannot reach the site of infection because of its physicochemical properties, it cannot provide effective therapy. Thus the pharmacokinetic characteristics of a drug may be an overriding consideration. Recognition of these issues allows the development of effective strategies for empirical anti-infective treatment (Table 14–8).

Concepts in Combination Anti-infective Therapy

Most infections in infants and children can be treated with a single anti-infective agent. The problem with this approach is that most anti-infective therapy is begun on an empirical basis until the results of culture and susceptibility testing are available. Combination therapy has therefore become extremely common in pediatric practice to ensure that the patient has adequate anti-infective coverage.

Three types of responses can be demonstrated in vitro when anti-infective agents are combined: additivity, synergism, and antagonism. These observations have spawned a widespread clinical practice of combination therapy. A number of reasons have been used to justify such treatment, including (1) prevention of the emergence of resistant organisms, (2) treatment of polymicrobial infections, (3) the need to start therapy in neutropenic, immunocom-

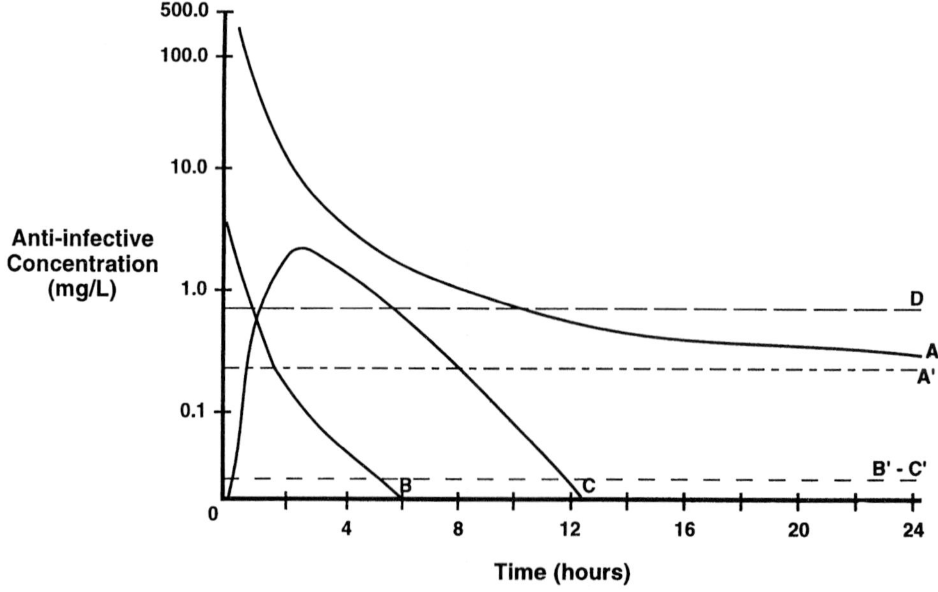

FIGURE 14–3. Integration of anti-infective pharmacodynamics and pharmacotherapeutics. The figure depicts the concentrations of three anti-infective agents, *A, B,* and *C,* at the site of infection, with time, after a single dose. Drugs *A* and *B* are administered intravenously, whereas drug *C* is the oral formulation of drug *B.* The *horizontal dashed lines* intersect with the *y*-axis at an anti-infective concentration equal to the MIC_{90} for an infecting bacterial pathogen. *Lines A'* and *B'-C'* represent one bacterial pathogen and intercept the *y*-axis at the MIC_{90} for drug *A* and drug *B/C,* respectively. *Line D* represents a second pathogen that has the same MIC_{90} for both drug *A* and drug *B/C.*

The figure shows that drug *B/C* is more potent than drug *A* in inhibiting the growth of the first pathogen, as depicted by the lower *y*-axis intercept for *line B'-C'* than for *line A.* However, the duration of the drug's effectiveness in inhibiting bacterial growth at the site of infection is far shorter for drug *B/C* than for drug *A.* To achieve the same duration of effective concentration at the site of infection, one must give drug *B/C* in multiple doses. Thus drug *A* may be a more rational choice than drug *B/C* for the first pathogen.

For the pathogen with the MIC_{90} depicted by *horizontal dashed line D,* the two drugs are equipotent. The graph indicates that both drugs need to be given in multiple doses for a 24-hour period to maintain effective anti-infective concentrations at the site of infection. Again, drug *A* may be a more rational therapeutic choice because of the less frequent dosing requirement.

TABLE 14–6. Generic and Trade Names of Anti-infective Agents*

Generic Name	Trade Name
Antibiotic Drugs	
Penicillins	
Natural penicillins	
Benzathine penicillin G	Bicillin Long-Acting
Penicillin G	Pentid, Pfizerpen
Penicillin G procaine	Crysticillin A.S., Wycillin
Penicillin V (phenoxymethyl penicillin)	Penapar-VK, Pen-Vee-K, V-Cillin K, Veetids
Penicillinase-resistant penicillins	
Cloxacillin	Cloxapen, Tegopen
Dicloxacillin	Dynapen, Pathocil
Nafcillin	Nafcil, Unipen
Oxacillin	Bactocill, Prostaphilin
Aminopenicillins	
Amoxicillin	Amoxil, Larotid, Polymox, Trimox, Wymox
Amoxicillin + clavulanate	Augmentin
Ampicillin	Amcill, Omnipen, Penbriten, Polycillin, Totacillin
Ampicillin + probenecid	Polycillin-PRB
Ampicillin + sulbactam	Unasyn
Bacampicillin	Spectrobid
Extended-spectrum penicillins	
Azlocillin	Azlin
Carbenicillin	Geopen, Pyopen
Carbenicillin indanyl sodium	Geocillin
Mezlocillin	Mezlin
Piperacillin	Pipracil
Piperacillin + tazobactam	Zosyn
Ticarcillin	Ticar
Ticarcillin + clavulanate	Timentin
Cephalosporins	
First generation	
Cefadroxil	Duricef, Ultracef
Cefazolin	Ancef, Kefzol
Cephalexin	Keflex, Keftab
Cephalothin	Keflin
Cephapirin	Cefadyl
Cephradine	Anspor, Velosef
Second generation	
Cefamandole	Mandol
Cefonicid	Monocid
Ceforanide	Precef
Cefprozil	Cefzil
Cefuroxime	Kefurox, Zinacef
Cefuroxime axetil	Ceftin
Carbacephem	
Loracarbef	Lorabid
Cephamycins	
Cefaclor	Ceclor
Cefotetan	Cefotan
Cefoxitin	Mefoxin
Third generation	
Cefdinir	Omnicef
Cefixime	Suprax
Cefoperazone	Cefobid
Cefotaxime	Claforan
Cefpodoxime proxetil	Vantin
Ceftazidime	Ceptaz, Fortaz, Tazicef, Tazidime
Ceftibuten	Cedax
Ceftizoxime	Cefizox
***Cephalosporins** (Continued)*	
Ceftriaxone	Rocephin
Fourth generation	
Cefepime	Maxipime
β-Lactamase Inhibitor Combinations	
Amoxicillin + clavulanate	Augmentin
Ampicillin + sulbactam	Unasyn
Piperacillin + tazobactam	Zosyn
Ticarcillin + clavulanate	Timentin
Penicillin Adjuvant	
Probenecid	Benemid
Monobactam	
Aztreonam	Azactam
Carbapenems	
Imipenem + cilastatin	Primaxin
Meropenem	Merrem
Aminoglycosides	
Amikacin	Amikin
Gentamicin	Garamycin
Kanamycin	Kantrex
Neomycin	Mycifradin
Netilmicin	Netromycin
Streptomycin	
Tobramycin	Nebcin, Tobrex
Glycopeptides	
Teicoplanin	Investigation in United States
Vancomycin	Vancocin, Vancoled
Streptogramin	
Quinupristin + dalfopristin	Synercid
Oxazolidinone	
Linezolid	Zyvox
Macrolides/Azalides	
Azithromycin	Zithromax
Clarithromycin	Biaxin
Dirithromycin	Dynabac
Erythromycin	E-mycin, Eryc, Erypar, Ery-Tab
Erythromycin estolate	Ilosone
Erythromycin ethylsuccinate	E.E.S., EryPed
Erythromycin ethylsuccinate + sulfisoxazole	Eryzole, Pediazole
Erythromycin gluceptate	Ilotycin
Erythromycin lactobionate	Erythrocin
Troleandomycin	Tao
Tetracyclines	
Chlortetracycline	Aureomycin
Demeclocycline	Declomycin
Doxycycline	Doryx, Doxychel, Vibramycin, Vibra-Tabs
Minocycline	Minocin
Oxytetracycline	Terramycin, Urobiotic
Tetracycline hydrochloride	Achromycin, Panmycin, Robitet, Sumycin
Quinolones	
Cinoxacin	Cinobac
Ciprofloxacin	Cipro
Enoxacin	Penetrex
Fleroxacin	Megalone
Gatifloxacin	Tequin
Levofloxacin	Levaquin
Lomefloxacin	Maxaquin

Table continued on following page

TABLE 14–6. Generic and Trade Names of Anti-infective Agents* *(Continued)*

Generic Name	Trade Name
Quinolones *(Continued)*	
Moxifloxacin	Avelox
Nalidixic acid	NegGram, Wintomylon
Norfloxacin	Noroxin
Ofloxacin	Floxin
Sparfloxacin	Zagam
Lincosamides	
Clindamycin	Cleocin
Lincomycin	Lincocin
Sulfonamides	
Mafenide	Sulfamylon
Silver sulfadiazine	Silvadene
Sulfacetamide*	AK-Sulf, Bleph-10, Cetamide, Sulamyd, Sulf-10
Sulfadiazine	Microsulfon
Sulfadoxine + pyrimethamine	Fansidar
Sulfamethizole	Thiosulfil
Sulfamethoxazole	Gantanol, Urobak
Sulfisoxazole	Gantrisin
Polymyxins	
Colistimethate	Coly-Mycin M
Colistin (polymyxin E)	Coly-Mycin S
Polymyxin B	Aerosporin
Miscellaneous Antibiotics	
Chloramphenicol	Chloromycetin
Erythromycin + sulfisoxazole	Pediazole
Furazolidone	Furoxone
Metronidazole	Flagyl, Protostat
Mupirocin (topical)	Bactroban
Nitrofurantoin	Furadantin, Macrodantin
Novobiocin	Albamycin
Spectinomycin	Trobicin
Trimethoprim	Proloprim, Trimpex
Trimethoprim-sulfamethoxazole (TMP-SMZ; cotrimoxazole)	Bactrim, Cotrim, Septra, Sulfatrim
Antimycobacterial Drugs	
Aminosalicylic acid	Paser
Clofazimine	Lamprene
Cycloserine	Seromycin
Dapsone	Avlosulfon
Ethambutol	Myambutol
Ethionamide	Trecator-SC
Isoniazid	Laniazid, Nydrazid
Pyrazinamide	
Rifabutin	Mycobutin
Rifampin	Rifadin, Rimactane
Streptomycin	
Combinations	
Isoniazid + rifampin	Rifamate
Isoniazid + rifampin + pyrazinamide	Rifater
Antifungal Drugs	
Amphotericin B	Fungizone
Liposomal amphotericin B	AmBisome
Amphotericin B colloidal dispersion (ABCD)	Amphotec
Amphotericin B lipid complex (ABLC)	Abelcet
Butoconazole	Gynazole-1
Caspofungin	Cancidas
Clotrimazole	Mycelex, Lotrimin, Gyne-Lotrimin
Antifungal Drugs *(Continued)*	Diflucan
Fluconazole	
Flucytosine	Ancobon
Griseofulvin	Fulvicin P/G, Fulvicin U/F, Gris-PEG, Grisactin
Itraconazole	Sporanox
Ketoconazole	Nizoral
Miconazole	Micatin, Monistat
Nystatin	Mycostatin, Nilstat
Terconazole	Terazol
Tioconazole	Vagistat-1
Tolnaftate	Aftate, NP-27, Tinactin
Antiviral Drugs	
Acyclovir	Zovirax
Amantadine	Symadine, Symmetrel
Cidofovir	Vistide
Famciclovir	Famvir
Foscarnet	Foscavir
Ganciclovir	Cytovene
Idoxuridine	Herplex, Stoxil
Ribavirin	Virazole
Rimantadine	Flumadine
Trifluridine	Viroptic
Valacyclovir	Valtrex
Vidarabine	Vira-A
Monoclonal Antibody	
Palivizumab	Synagis
Antiretroviral Drugs	
Nucleoside Reverse Transcriptase Inhibitors (NRTIs)	
Abacavir	Ziagen
Didanosine (ddI)	Videx
Lamivudine (3TC)	Epivir
Stavudine (d4T)	Zerit
Zalcitabine (ddC)	Hivid
Zidovudine (ZDV, AZT)	Retrovir
Combinations	
Zidovudine + lamivudine	Combivir
Nonnucleoside Reverse Transcriptase Inhibitors (NNRTIs)	
Delavirdine	Rescriptor
Efavirenz	Sustiva
Nevirapine	Viramune
Protease Inhibitors (PIs)	
Amprenavir	Agenerase
Indinavir	Crixivan
Nelfinavir	Viracept
Ritonavir	Norvir
Saquinavir	Fortovase, Fortovase Softgel
Combinations	
Lopinavir + ritonavir	Kaletra
Antiparasitic Drugs	
Antiprotozoal Drugs	
Atovaquone	Mepron
Atovaquone + proguanil	Malarone
Furazolidone	Furoxone
Iodoquinol	Yodoxin
Metronidazole	Flagyl, Protostat
Paromomycin	Humatin
Pentamidine aerosol	NebuPent
Pentamidine isethionate	Pentam 300
Trimethoprim-sulfamethoxazole (TMP-SMZ; Cotrimoxazole)	Bactrim, Cotrim, Septra, Sulfatrim

TABLE 14–6. Generic and Trade Names of Anti-infective Agents* *(Continued)*

Generic Name	Trade Name	Generic Name	Trade Name
Anthelmintic Drugs		***Antimalarial Drugs***	
Albendazole	Albenza	Chloroquine	Aralen
Diethylcarbamazine	Hetrazan	Hydroxychloroquine	Plaquenil
Mebendazole	Vermox	Mefloquine	Lariam
Niclosamide	Niclocide, Yomesan	Primaquine phosphate	
Niridazole	Ambilhar	Pyrimethamine	Daraprim
Oxamniquine	Vansil	Quinacrine	Atabrine
Piperazine citrate		Quinidine gluconate	
Praziquantel	Biltricide	Quinine sulfate	
Pyrantel pamoate	Antiminth	Sulfadoxine + pyrimethamine	Fansidar
Quinacrine	Atabrine		
Thiabendazole	Mintezol		

*See Table 63–2 for topical otologic antibiotics and Table 89–4 for topical ophthalmologic antibiotics.

TABLE 14–7. Considerations in the Selection of an Anti-infective Agent

Patient Factors	Microbiologic Factors
Age	Likely bacterial pathogens
Genetic factors	Anti-infective susceptibility patterns
Pregnancy	Prior antimicrobial therapy
Concurrent disease	**Drug Factors**
Allergy	Intrinsic anti-infective activity
Central nervous system disorders	Pharmaceutical properties
Hepatic function	Protein binding
Renal function	Tissue penetration
Indigenous microbial flora	Elimination half-life
Host defense mechanisms	Mode of elimination
Family and social setting	Safety profile

promised, and critically ill patients while one is awaiting culture results, (4) the use of lower doses of component agents to decrease drug toxicity, and (5) the possibility of synergy. Unfortunately, convincing clinical support for the use of combination anti-infective therapy is minimal with the exception of the documented benefit of older antibiotics used to provide empirical therapy for febrile patients with neutropenia and in other, carefully selected cases (e.g., the clinician may use penicillin plus an aminoglycoside to treat enterococcal endocarditis).

In contrast, in a number of examples of clinical antagonism with various anti-infective combinations, the combination therapy resulted in excess mortality. In 1951 an experience with treating pneumococcal meningitis in children with penicillin G, in comparison with the combination of penicillin G and chlortetracycline, was reported. The mortality in the two groups of patients were 21% and 79%, respectively. With the availability of a number of very broad spectrum agents today, it is not at all clear that combination therapy plays a role at all. In pediatric practice only a few indications for its use are well documented (Table 14–9).

TABLE 14–8. Strategies for Empirical Anti-infective Prescribing

- Identify likely pathogens
- Use locally generated anti-infective susceptibility data
- Consider spectra of activity of available agents
- Consider physicochemical barriers to drug distribution in the context of site of infection
- Be aware of patient factors that may mitigate drug choices

In addition to the extemporaneous combinations discussed herein, two fixed-combination anti-infectives are now widely used in pediatric practice: trimethoprim-sulfamethoxazole and erythromycin-sulfisoxazole. The former is a rational fixed combination that capitalizes on the sequential inhibition of bacterial folate synthesis to transform two bacteriostatic agents into a bactericidal combination. This combination drug is an effective second-line agent for a variety of moderate to severe infections in infants and children. The latter is a fixed combination that is labeled only for acute otitis media. With increases in antibiotic resistance of respiratory pathogens, it has very little to recommend it.

Monitoring Anti-infective Therapy

Before prescribing or administering any anti-infective agent, the clinician should have clear expectations concerning the effectiveness and safety of the drug for the person being treated. Thus a prospective plan for therapeutic monitoring must be in place. The clinician must to able to expect the resolution of signs and symptoms and negative culture results within a reasonable time while drug therapy continues. With respect to safety, the adverse effect profile for the drug to be used must be understood. A regimen for detecting these effects at a time when they are of minimal severity or are reversible also must be in place. Thus, for drugs known to cause end-organ dysfunction, serial monitoring of serum parameters reflecting the functioning of these target organs may be necessary. In some cases, monitoring may need to be performed by parents or by the patients themselves. In such cases, patient and family education concerning the effects of various drugs may be essential.

The concept of therapeutic drug monitoring is often considered synonymously with serum concentration monitoring. In fact, this type of monitoring is available for very few anti-infective agents. Moreover, even for drugs such as the aminoglycosides, chloramphenicol, and vancomycin, where the technology is readily available, the true clinical importance of such monitoring is debatable (see the section on aminoglycosides).

ANTIBACTERIAL DRUGS

β-LACTAM AGENTS

The β-lactam agents are among the most useful of the antimicrobial agents available to the clinician who cares for children. In general,

TABLE 14–9. Suggested Indications for Combination Anti-infective Therapy in Infants and Children

Indication	Drug Combination	Monotherapy Alternative
Premature infant with suspected sepsis where coagulase-negative staphylococci may be a pathogen	Vancomycin plus either cefotaxime or aminoglycoside	None
Newborn to 3-month-old infant with suspected sepsis where *Listeria monocytogenes* or *Enterococcus* may be a pathogen	Ampicillin plus cefotaxime	Ampicillin-sulbactam, piperacillin-tazobactam, imipenem, meropenem
Intra-abdominal sepsis	Aminoglycoside plus clindamycin with or without ampicillin	Ampicillin-sulbactam, piperacillin-tazobactam, imipenem, meropenem
Enterococcal endocarditis	Penicillin or ampicillin plus aminoglycoside	None
Febrile person with neutropenia	Ceftazidime or cefepime plus aminoglycoside with or without vancomycin*	Ceftazidime, imipenem, meropenem, piperacillin-tazobactam
Bacterial meningitis with penicillin-resistant *Streptococcus pneumoniae*	Vancomycin plus ceftriaxone	Meropenem

*In immunocompromised persons, no difference in clinical outcome has been reported when vancomycin has been added after the isolation of coagulase-negative staphylococci, in comparison with its empirical use.

these agents are bactericidal for susceptible pathogens and have an excellent safety record. As a result, these agents are often the drugs of first choice for treatment of infections caused by susceptible organisms. They are among the most useful antimicrobials for empirical therapy for both hospital- and community-acquired infections.

β-Lactam antimicrobial agents include the penicillins, cephalosporins, carbapenems, and monobactams (Table 14–6). These agents all have a **β-lactam ring** with variable rings and side chains. When bacteria develop resistance to β-lactam antibiotics, it is most often a result of their ability to elaborate a β-lactamase enzyme that is able to cleave the β-lactam ring.

The ring structure is the defining characteristic of the β-lactam agents. For example, the penicillins contain a thiazolidine ring attached to the β-lactam ring, the cephalosporins contain a dihydrothiazine ring attached to the β-lactam ring, and the monobactams have all side chains directly linked to the β-lactam ring. The nature of the side chains added to the ring structure is responsible for both the antibacterial spectrum of this compound and its pharmacokinetic properties.

Spectrum of Activity. Despite widespread clinical use for more than 5 decades, the precise mechanism(s) responsible for the bactericidal effect of the β-lactam class of antibiotics is unknown. It is probable that these drugs bind a group of proteins associated with bacterial cell wall synthesis referred to as **penicillin-binding proteins (PBPs).** These proteins vary in size, amount present, and specific enzymatic activity from one species of bacteria to another. PBPs serve many different functions for bacteria. For example, in *Escherichia coli,* PBP-1 is responsible for cell elongation and PBP-2 has a role in the cell cycle, whereas PBP-3 catalyzes a carboxypeptidase reaction that is necessary for cell division. Different classes of β-lactams may bind to different PBPs in specific bacteria, causing different cellular effects (e.g., cell elongation vs cell lysis). The interactions between β-lactam and PBPs may also stimulate the release of bacterial autolysins, causing cell death. Alterations in PBP configuration have been identified as an important cause of bacterial resistance to β-lactam antibiotics; examples of such bacteria are **methicillin-resistant *S. aureus* (MRSA)** and penicillin intermediate and resistant *Streptococcus pneumoniae.*

The antibacterial spectrum of the penicillins depends on their class (Table 14–10). The **natural penicillins,** penicillin G and penicillin V, are primarily effective against gram-positive bacteria, with the notable exception of the enterococci. In addition, certain anaerobic bacteria and important gram-negative cocci, including *Neisseria gonorrhoeae* and *Neisseria meningitidis,* are treated effectively. The **aminopenicillins** (e.g., amoxicillin) possess an expanded spectrum of activity, retaining the spectrum of the natural penicillins with added activity against *Enterococcus* and, importantly, gram-negative pathogens (e.g., *E. coli, Proteus mirabilis, Salmonella*). Like the natural penicillins, aminopenicillins are also susceptible to inactivation by bacterial β-lactamases. Subsequently the emergence of *Pseudomonas aeruginosa* as an important hospital-acquired pathogen stimulated the development of penicillins with antipseudomonal activity (e.g., ticarcillin, piperacillin).

The ability of certain bacteria to elaborate **β-lactamases** (i.e., **penicillinase**) that cleave the β-lactam bond, rendering the penicillin antibacterially inactive, fostered the development of the penicillinase-resistant penicillins (e.g., nafcillin) and the β-lactamase inhibitors (e.g., clavulanate). The penicillinase-resistant, antistaphylococcal penicillins retain much of the activity of the penicillins, although they are highly active against penicillinase-producing *S. aureus* and are ineffective against gram-negative cocci. The addition of a β-lactamase inhibitor with an aminopenicillin (e.g., amoxicillin-clavulanate) enhances the antibacterial spectrum of activity of amoxicillin to encompass many β-lactamase–positive pathogens, including penicillin-resistant *S. aureus, H. influenzae,* and *Bacteroides fragilis.* The addition of a β-lactamase inhibitor with an antipseudomonal penicillin (e.g., piperacillin-tazobactam) enhances the drug's spectrum of activity in a manner similar to that observed with amoxicillin.

Clinical Indications. This era is one of transition with respect to the clinical use of the penicillins. Although pediatricians have always been partial to the penicillins, the continued emergence of pathogen resistance combined with the increasing availability of a wide variety of cephalosporins with equivalent efficacy, a more favorable safety profile, and superior pharmacokinetics continues to challenge the supremacy of the penicillins.

Penicillin is still effective in the treatment of infections caused by group A *Streptococcus* and most infections due to *S. pneumon-*

TABLE 14–10. Comparative in Vitro Susceptibility of Selected Pathogens to Penicillin Antibiotics

	Minimum Inhibitory Concentrations (MIC_{50}) (mg/L)						
Organism	**Penicillin G**	**Penicillin V**	**Ampicillin, Amoxicillin**	**Oxacillin, Cloxacillin, Dicloxacillin,**	**Nafcillin**	**Carbenicillin, Ticarcillin**	**Azlocillin, Mezlocillin, Piperacillin**
Cocci							
Streptococcus pneumoniae	0.01	0.02	0.02	0.04	0.02	0.4	0.02
Group A *Streptococcus*	0.005	0.01	0.02	0.04	0.02	0.2	0.02
Group B *Streptococcus*	0.005	0.01	0.02	0.06	0.02	0.2	0.15
Viridans streptococci	0.01	0.01	0.05	0.1	0.06	0.2	0.12
Enterococcus faecalis	3.0	6.0	1.5	>25	>25	50	1.5
Staphylococcus aureus							
Penicillinase-negative	0.02	0.02	0.05	0.3	0.25	1.2	0.8
Penicillinase-positive	R	R	R	0.4	0.25	R	R
Coagulase-negative staphylococci	0.02	0.02	0.05	0.2	0.2	0.8	1.6
Neisseria gonorrhoeae	0.01	0.1	0.03	R	R	0.3	0.05
Neisseria meningitidis	0.05	0.25	0.05	R	R	0.1	0.05
Selected Bacilli and Anaerobes							
Clostridium perfringens	0.5		0.05	0.5		0.3	0.05
Corynebacterium diphtheriae	0.1		0.02	0.1		0.2	1.0
Listeria monocytogenes	0.5		0.5	R		4	0.5
Haemophilus influenzae							
β-Lactamase-negative	0.8		0.5	R		0.5	0.1
β-Lactamase-positive	R		R	R		R	R
Prevotella melaninogenica	0.5		0.5	R		0.5	0.5
Fusobacterium nucleatum	0.5		0.1	R		0.5	0.5
Bacteroides fragilis	R		R	R		R	32
*Moraxella catarrhalis**	R		R	R		R	R
Enterobacteriaceae and Pseudomonas							
Escherichia coli	R		3	R		6	8
Proteus mirabilis	R		3	R		1.5	1
Klebsiella	R		R	R		R	16
Enterobacter	R		R	R		R	16
Citrobacter diversus	R		R	R		12	8
Citrobacter freundii	R		R	R		12	32
Serratia	R		R	R		R	32
Salmonella	R		1.5	R		3	4
Shigella	R		1.5	R		3	8
Proteus vulgaris	R		R	R		12	16
Providencia	R		R	R		12	8
Morganella	R		R	R		25	8
Acinetobacter	R		R	R		25	32
Pseudomonas aeruginosa	R		R	R		R	16
Pseudomonas (other species)	R		R	R		R	R

R = resistant.
*Virtually all are β-lactamase producers.

iae. Unfortunately, the increasing resistance of *S. pneumoniae* to penicillin in most regions of the United States and around the world necessitates the use of alternative drugs as first-line agents against this common pathogen. Amoxicillin remains the drug of choice for acute otitis media. If the infection is suspected or known to be caused by β-lactamase-producing pathogens, the combination drug amoxicillin-clavulanate should be prescribed. In persons with suspected or known infections caused by penicillin-resistant strains of *S. pneumoniae,* high doses of amoxicillin (80–90 mg/kg/day), ceftriaxone, vancomycin, or meropenem are necessary for effective therapy.

Penicillins remain the drug of choice for prophylaxis against rheumatic carditis and against infections in persons with sickle cell disease. As a result of the changing susceptibility pattern of many pathogens, penicillin-β-lactamase inhibitor combinations have become the preferred agents for empirical therapy for infections involving the upper respiratory tract, skin, and soft tissue and in critically ill persons.

Metabolism and Disposition. The penicillins vary markedly in their disposition characteristics, both from drug to drug and with patient age (Table 14–11). With the notable exceptions of penicillin V and amoxicillin, these drugs are not well absorbed from the gastrointestinal tract. Thus, for most serious infections, the penicillins are administered parenterally. Protein binding varies markedly from a low of approximately 17% with ampicillin and amoxicillin to more than 95% with cloxacillin and dicloxacillin. Few of these drugs undergo any significant metabolism, although some agents, including nafcillin, cloxacillin, dicloxacillin, ampicillin, carbenicillin, ticarcillin, mezlocillin, and piperacillin, display significant he-

TABLE 14–11. Pharmacokinetic Characteristics of Penicillins

				$t_{1/2\beta}$ (hr)		
Drug	**Bioavailability**	**Protein Binding (%)**	**Metabolism (%)**	**Neonate (at 0–30 Days)**	**Infant and Child**	**Adult**
Penicillin G	20–30	65	10–30	1.5–3	0.5–1.2	0.5–0.75
Penicillin V	60–70	80	10–30			
Methicillin*	—†	40	20–30	1.5–3	0.8–1.2	0.5–0.8
Oxacillin	30–60	90–95	70	1.5–2	0.9–1.2	0.4–0.7
Cloxacillin	50	90–98	50	—	0.6–0.8	0.5–0.6
Dicloxacillin	40–75	96	30	—	0.8–1	0.6–0.8
Nafcillin	Poor	90	70–90	2.2–6	0.75–2	0.5–1.5
Ampicillin	30–50	15–25	10	2–8	0.75–1.8	0.5–1
Amoxicillin	80	20	20	2–4	1–2	0.5–1
Carbenicillin	30–40‡	50	10–20	3–6	0.8–1.8	1–1.5
Ticarcillin	—†	45–65	10	2–6	0.8–1.5	1–1.5
Azlocillin	—†	30	10	2.5–4	1–2	1–1.2
Mezlocillin	—†	30	5–10	2.5–4	0.5–1	0.5–0.75
Piperacillin	—†	22	5–10	2.5–4	0.5–1	0.5–0.75

*No longer available; shown for comparison only.
†Poor, clinically insignificant oral bioavailability.
‡Indanyl salt for oral administration only.

patic elimination. Most excretion is via the kidney, by processes of both filtration and tubular secretion.

Virtually all of the parenteral penicillins penetrate into the cerebrospinal fluid when meningeal inflammation is present, usually in concentrations adequate to treat meningitis. In the absence of inflammation, and with an intact blood-brain barrier, little penetration occurs.

Because the elimination of the penicillins is mainly renal, significant developmental changes occur in $t_{1/2\beta}$ during the first year of life (Table 14–11). In addition, disease-associated alterations in renal function necessitate dosing modifications.

Available Formulations for Penicillins. Available formulations are outlined in Table 14–12.

Recommended Dosing and Dosing Strategies. Ongoing changes in microbial susceptibility have long resulted in an increase in the dose of penicillin G used for most of its indications. For the other drugs, the doses are fairly standard but do vary somewhat with the age of the child (Table 14–13).

Adverse Effects. One of the reasons for the sustained popularity of the penicillin antibiotics in pediatric practice has been their safety profile. Adverse events, which can be extremely varied in their presentation, occur very rarely (Table 14–14). Little information is available concerning the mechanisms that account for most of the reported events. Among the hematologic effects, the alterations in platelet function are related to the binding of carbenicillin and ticarcillin (much less with piperacillin) to the adenosine diphosphate binding site, thus preventing normal aggregation.

The clinical syndrome of interstitial nephritis associated with penicillin therapy includes fever, a macular rash, eosinophilia, proteinuria, eosinophiluria, and hematuria. Progression from nonoliguric renal failure to anuria may occur. Renal function usually returns to normal with discontinuation of the drug's use. This reaction is rare but was most commonly reported with methicillin.

The hypokalemia seen with the antipseudomonal and extended-spectrum penicillins is related to the large doses of drug used clinically. In these instances the penicillin represents a nonreabsorbable anion that is presented to the distal renal tubules. The result is altered hydrogen ion excretion and secondary potassium ion loss.

The major toxic effects associated with the penicillins are allergic reactions, which range from IgE-mediated anaphylaxis to delayed-hypersensitivity reactions, including contact dermatitis. The mechanisms responsible for these allergic reactions relate to the ability of the penicillins to act as haptens and combine with proteins. The most important antigenic component of the penicillins is the penicilloyl determinant produced by the opening of the β-lactam ring, which permits amide linkage to proteins. Other breakdown products include the penicillanic acid derivatives that form in solution at high temperature or low pH. A number of minor determinants, including benzyl penicillin itself, can also act as sensitizing agents or can elicit major allergic reactions themselves.

Anaphylactic reactions to penicillin are estimated to occur in 0.01–0.05% of persons receiving this class of compounds. Approximately 10% of these reactions will be life threatening and 1% of reactions may be fatal. With the availability of a wide variety of antibiotics today, it is seldom necessary to expose penicillin-allergic or sensitized persons to the inciting drug. Fortunately, children with atopic dermatitis and allergic rhinitis do not appear to be at greater risk of having penicillin-allergic reactions. Even children who have had life-threatening reactions to a penicillin in the past may receive the drug without incident when a protracted period between exposures has occurred. It is often possible to substitute other β-lactam agents, such as extended-spectrum cephalosporins, monobactams, or carbapenems, for a penicillin with minimal risk of cross-reactivity. Nevertheless, re-exposure to a penicillin may sometimes be required, or concern associated with exposure of the patient to a β-lactam antibiotic may be considerable. In these circumstances a trial of desensitization may be prudent (Table 14–15).

Drug Interactions. Few drug-drug interactions of clinical significance with the penicillins have been reported (Table 14–16). The interaction with probenecid, a drug that competes with the penicillins for renal tubular secretion, is the only one of note. The

TABLE 14–12. Available Formulations of Penicillin Antibiotics

Antibiotic	Oral Formulation		Parenteral Formulation*
	Dosage Form	Amount	
Penicillin V	Suspension	125 and 250 mg/5 mL	None available
	Tablet	125, 250, and 500 mg	
Methicillin	No longer available		No longer available
Oxacillin	Suspension	250 mg/5 mL	Yes
	Capsule	250 and 500 mg	
Cloxacillin	Suspension	125 mg/5 mL	None available
	Capsule	250 and 500 mg	
Dicloxacillin	Suspension	6.25 mg/5 mL	None available
	Capsule	125, 250, and 500 mg	
Nafcillin	Suspension	250 mg/5 mL	Yes
	Capsule	250 mg	
	Tablet	500 mg	
Ampicillin	Suspension	125, 250, and 500 mg/5 mL	Yes
	Oral drops	100 mg/mL	
	Capsule	250 and 500 mg/5 mL	
Amoxicillin	Suspension	125 and 250 mg/5 mL	None available
	Oral drops	50 mg/mL	
	Capsule	250 and 500 mg	
	Tablet, chewable	125 and 250 mg	
Carbenicillin	Tablet	382 mg	None available in USA
Ticarcillin	None available		Yes
Azlocillin	None available		Yes
Mezlocillin	None available		Yes
Piperacillin	None available		Yes
Ampicillin-sulbactam	None available		Yes
Amoxicillin-clavulanate	Suspension	125, 200, 250, 400 mg/5 mL	None available in USA
	Tablet	250, 500, 875 mg	
	Tablet, chewable	125, 200, 250, 400 mg	
Ticarcillin-clavulanate	None available		Yes
Piperacillin-tazobactam	None available		Yes

*Antibiotics are available as sterile powder for reconstitution before intramuscular or intravenous administration. Standard recommended dilutions are available from the manufacturers in their respective package inserts. Clinically relevant, concentrated solutions should be obtained from the hospital pharmacy.

penicillin-probenecid interaction is used clinically to prolong the $t_{1/2\beta}$ of penicillin or ampicillin in the treatment of certain sexually transmitted diseases.

Obviously the potential exists for penicillin to interact with any drug that shares the renal organic anion secretory system as part of its elimination pathway. Because of the overall decrease in penicillin use in infants and children, these reactions are not likely to be important.

The antipseudomonal penicillins and to some extent the extended-spectrum penicillins have been shown to interact in solution with aminoglycosides, causing degradation of the aminoglycosides. This interaction occurs when the two agents are mixed in the same infusion solution for administration or in vivo in the face of renal failure. The aminoglycosides vary in their susceptibility to breakdown, with gentamicin ≥ tobramycin > amikacin ≥ netilmicin. It is recommended that these drugs should not be mixed in solution and that their administration should be temporally separated by 30–60 minutes.

Several recent cases of drug-drug interactions involving nafcillin and both cyclosporine and warfarin have also been reported. Until the clinical significance of these interactions is better defined, these combinations should be avoided. Patients who must receive these combinations must be carefully monitored.

THE CEPHALOSPORINS

The increasing emergence of bacterial resistance to available antibiotics and the need for broad-spectrum agents stimulated the search and ultimate discovery of the cephalosporin class of antibiotics. Isolated from a fungus found in the sewage dumping into the sea near Cagliari, Sardinia, the cephalosporin nucleus has spawned the development of more than 80 analogs (Table 14–17). These cephalosporins are now among the most prescribed of all anti-infective agents in the world.

Spectrum of Activity. As with the penicillins, the precise mechanism of action of the cephalosporins is unknown, although they appear to work via the same receptor complex. Cephalosporins bind to and inactivate PBPs, which, as discussed previously, are enzymes that are responsible for the synthesis of the bacterial cell wall and that include transpeptidases, carboxypeptidases, and endopeptidases.

The antibacterial activity of the various cephalosporins depends largely on their generation of origin. Unlike the natural penicillins, the **first-generation cephalosporins** are active against both gram-positive and gram-negative bacteria (Table 14–18), as well as being acid stable and resistant to β-lactamase hydrolysis. The activity of

TABLE 14–13. Penicillin Dosing Recommendations

Drug	Route	Age/Weight	Daily Dose*	Frequency	Sodium Content
Penicillin G (benzylpenicillin)	IM, IV	At ≤2,000 g	50,000 U/kg/day†	q12hr	
		(meningitis)	100,000 U/kg/day	q12hr	
		At >2,000 g	75,000–100,000 U/kg/day	q8hr	
		(meningitis)	150,000 U/kg/day	q8hr	
		Infant/child	100,000–250,000 U/kg/day	q4–6hr	
	IM, IV	Adult	2–24 million U/day	q4–6hr	2.8 mEq Na/g: 2.7 mEq K/g
Penicillin V	PO	Infant/child	15–30 mg/kg/day	q6–8hr	
	PO	Adult	1–2 g/day	q6–8hr	
Oxacillin	IM, IV	At ≤2,000 g			
		Age ≤7 days	50 mg/kg/day	q12hr	
		Age >7 days	100 mg/kg/day	q8hr	
		At >2,000 g			
		Age ≤7 days	75 mg/kg/day	q8hr	
		Age >7 days	150 mg/kg/day	q6–8hr	
	IM, IV, PO	Infant/child	50–200 mg/kg/day	q4–6hr	
	IM, IV	Adult	2–12 g/day	q4–6hr	
	PO		2–6 g/day	q4–6hr	2.8 mEq Na/g
Cloxacillin	PO	Infant/child	50–100 mg/kg/day	q6hr	Capsule: 0.6 mEq/250 mg
	PO	Adult	1–2 g/day	q6hr	Suspension: 0.48 mEq/5 mL
Dicloxacillin	PO	Infant/child	12.5–100 mg/kg/day	q6hr	Capsule: 0.65 mEq
	PO	Adult	0.5–2 g/day	q6hr	Suspension: 2.9 mEq/5 mL
Nafcillin	IM, IV	At ≤2,000 g			
		Age ≤7 days	50 mg/kg/day	q12hr	
		Age >7 days	75 mg/kg/day	q6hr	
		At >2,000 g			
		Age ≤7 days	50 mg/kg/day	q8hr	
		Age >7 days	75 mg/kg/day	q6hr	
	IM, IV	Infant/child	50–400 mg/kg/day	q4–6hr	
	PO		75–100 mg/kg/day	q4–6hr	
	IV	Adult	3–12 g/day	q4–6hr	
	IM		2–3 g/day	q4–6hr	2.9 mEq/g
Ampicillin	IM, IV	At ≤2,000 g			
		Age ≤7 days	50 mg/kg/day	q12hr	
		(meningitis)	100 mg/kg/day	q12hr	
		Age >7 days	75–100 mg/kg/day	q8hr	
		(meningitis)	150 mg/kg/day	q8hr	
		At ≥2,000 g			
		Age ≤7 days	75–100 mg/kg/day	q8hr	
		(meningitis)	150 mg/kg/day	q8hr	
		Age >7 days	75–100 mg/kg/day	q6hr	
		(meningitis)	200 mg/kg/day	q4–6hr	
	IM, IV	Infant/child	100–300 mg/kg/day	q4–6hr	
	PO		50–100 mg/kg/day	q4–6hr	
	IM, IV	Adult	8–12 g/day	q4–6hr	
	PO		1–2 g/day	q6hr	Injection: 3 mEq/g; suspension: 0.4 mEq/5 mL (250 mg)
Amoxicillin	PO	Infant/child‡	20–50 mg/kg/day	q8hr	
	PO	Adult	0.75–1.5 g/day	q8hr	
Carbenicillin	IM, IV	At ≤2,000 g			
		Age ≤7 days	225 mg/kg/day	q8hr	
		Age >7 days	400 mg/kg/day	q6hr	
		At ≥2,000 g			
		Age ≤7 days	300 mg/kg/day	q6hr	
		Age >7 days	400 mg/kg/day	q6hr	
	IM, IV	Infant/child	400–600 mg/kg/day	q4–6hr	
	PO		30–50 mg/kg/day	q6hr	
	IM, IV	Adult	18–36 g/day	q4–6hr	4.7–6.5 mEq/g

TABLE 14–13. Penicillin Dosing Recommendations *(Continued)*

Drug	Route	Age/Weight	Daily Dose*	Frequency	Sodium Content
Ticarcillin	IM, IV	At ≤2,000 g			
		Age ≤7 days	150 mg/kg/day	q12hr	
		Age >7 days	225 mg/kg/day	q8hr	
		At >2,000 g			
		Age ≤7 days	225 mg/kg/day	q8hr	
		Age >7 days	300 mg/kg/day	q6–8hr	
	IM, IV	Infant/child	200–300 mg/kg/day	q4–6hr	
	IM, IV	Adult	12–24 g/day	q4–6hr	5.2–6.5 mEq/g
Azlocillin	IM, IV	Infant/child	300–450 mg/kg/day	q4–6hr	
	IM, IV	Adult	12–24 g/day	q4–6hr	2.2 mEq/g
Mezlocillin	IM, IV	Age ≤7 days	150 mg/kg/day	q12hr	
		Age >7 days	225 mg/kg/day	q8hr	
	IM, IV	Infant/child	200–300 mg/kg/day	q4–6hr	
	IM, IV	Adult	12–24 g/day	q4–6hr	1.8 mEq/g
Piperacillin	IM, IV	Neonate	100 mg/kg/day	q12hr	
	IM, IV	Infant/child	200–300 mg/kg/day	q4–6hr	
	IM, IV	Adult	12–24 g/day	q4–6hr	1.85 mEq/g
Amoxicillin-clavulanate	PO	Infant/child	45–90 mg/kg/day	q8–12hr	
Ticarcillin-clavulanate	IM, IV	Infant/child	200–300 mg/kg/day	q4–6hr	
		Adult	12–18 g/day	q4–6hr	
Piperacillin-tazobactam	IM, IV	Infant/child	240 mg/kg/day	q4–6hr	
		Adult	12–18 g/day	q4–6hr	

*Dose provided as usual dosage range for age as total for 24 hours. Doses are higher for patients with cystic fibrosis (see Table 67–3).
†For potassium penicillin G, 1 mg = 1,595 U; for sodium penicillin G, 1 mg = 1,667 U.
‡Uncomplicated gonorrhea (<2 yr of age): 50 mg/kg + probenecid 25 mg/kg. Infective endocarditis prophylaxis: 50 mg/kg + probenecid 25 mg/kg 1 hr before procedure.

these agents against gram-negative rods is somewhat variable. Thus the first-generation cephalosporins require careful monitoring when used in this setting.

The **second-generation cephalosporins** were synthesized in order to broaden coverage against respiratory pathogens and to provide additional, more reliable gram-negative activity. With the advent of these agents, the cephalosporins truly began to make inroads into pediatric practice. In many respects these drugs proved that they could provide ideal empirical coverage for community-acquired infections in infants and children >3 months of age. They provided therapeutic activity against *S. pneumoniae,* group A *Streptococcus, H. influenzae,* and *Moraxella catarrhalis,* which cause respiratory tract infections, whether or not the latter two organisms were β-lactamase producers. In addition, they offered reliable activity against *S. aureus* in the treatment of skin and skin-structure infections and against *E. coli* in the treatment of urinary tract infections.

However, the history of the use of second-generation cephalosporins in pediatrics is somewhat marred. None of the orally active agents achieve sufficient concentrations in the central nervous system to treat or prevent bacterial meningitis. Furthermore, several reports of the development of bacterial meningitis in children during treatment with cefamandole, the first parenteral second-generation cephalosporin available in the United States, reflected the lack of adequate penetration of the central nervous system by earlier analogs. Finally, although cefuroxime, the quintessential second-generation cephalosporin, was shown to be safe and effective in treating bacterial meningitis, concerns related to delayed cerebrospinal fluid sterilization have limited its use for this indication.

At about the same time the second-generation cephalosporins were being developed, the **cephamycin** group of antibiotics was isolated from certain streptococcal species. The cephamycins contain a methyoxy group at the 7-position of the β-lactam ring. These drugs include cefaclor, which has in vitro activity similar to that of second-generation cephalosporins, and the drugs cefoxitin and cefotetan, which are generally less potent than the second-generation cephalosporins against respiratory pathogens but have clinically significant anaerobic activity.

In the mid-1970s and early 1980s, the search for antibiotics with a broader spectrum resulted in the synthesis of a group of parenteral **third- and then fourth-generation cephalosporins.** These have become among the most widely used drugs for the empirical treatment of infants and children with moderate to severe infections. A large part of the increased gram-negative activity results from the addition of an aminothiazole moiety to the amide group at the 7-position of the β-lactam ring. In addition to the enhanced gram-negative potency, all of these advanced-generation cephalosporins achieve concentrations in the central nervous system that are adequate to treat bacterial meningitis. In fact, ceftazidime is also efficacious in treating meningitis caused by *P. aeruginosa.*

Unfortunately, with the increased gram-negative spectrum and potency, third-generation cephalosporins have less gram-positive potency than first-generation drugs. Nevertheless, they are clinically effective in treating most infections caused by susceptible gram-positive organisms.

More recently, two additional advances in cephalosporin therapy have occurred. First, several orally effective agents with the anti-infective activity of third-generation cephalosporins have become available for clinical use. These include cefixime, cefpodoxime proxetil, and ceftibuten. It is important to remember that neither cefixime nor ceftibuten has any clinically useful antistaphylococcal activity. Cefpodoxime may not have adequate antistaphylococcal activity other than in superficial skin infections.

Second, the first **fourth-generation cephalosporin,** cefepime, was developed. This drug has excellent potency against both gram-

TABLE 14–14. Adverse Reactions to Penicillins

Type of Reaction	Comment
Allergic	
Anaphylaxis	Occurs most frequently with penicillin G
Hemolytic anemia	
Serum sickness	
Contact dermatitis	Occurs with ampicillin
Electrolytic	
Sodium overload	Usually related to anti-*Pseudomonas* penicillins at higher doses
Hypokalemia	
Gastrointestinal	
Diarrhea	
Enterocolitis	
Hematologic	
Hemolytic anemia	
Neutropenia	
Platelet dysfunction	Related to inhibition of ADP-dependent aggregation by the carboxypenicillins (carbenicillin and ticarcillin)
Hepatic	
Elevated adenosine triphosphate	Occurs more commonly with penicillins, showing significant hepatic elimination
Neurologic	
Seizures	Usually with overdose or associated with drug accumulation in renal failure
Renal	
Interstitial nephritis	Most common with methicillin
Hemorrhagic cystitis	
Idiopathic	
Rash	Ampicillin-amoxicillin causes rash in persons with infectious mononucleosis
Fever	
Late-onset urticaria	

positive and gram-negative organisms, with a broad spectrum of activity but with limited activity against *P. aeruginosa.* It also retains activity against many organisms resistant to ceftazidime.

Clinical Indications. The cephalosporins have assumed an important role in pediatric therapy. Because of their favorable pharmacodynamic, pharmaceutic, and pharmacokinetic properties, these drugs are rapidly replacing the penicillins as the drugs of choice for the treatment of infections in infants and children. It is important to remember that there are a number of organisms for which they do not have reliable activity (Table 14–19).

In the outpatient setting where amoxicillin remains the drug of choice for treating respiratory and urinary tract infections, the second- and third-generation cephalosporins offer more reliable coverage with less frequent dosing and more palatable preparations. Therefore compliance with therapy is more likely to result. With infections of the skin and skin structures, the oral second-generation (not third-generation) cephalosporins offer less frequent dosing, greater palatability, and efficacy comparable to that of the antistaphylococcal penicillins.

The cephalosporins have truly become the drugs of choice for the empirical treatment of infants and children with moderate to severe infections. In the newborn period, the use of ampicillin plus

TABLE 14–15. Penicillin Desensitization

The affected person must be admitted to a critical care area. A secure intravenous line is placed. In the presence of professionals trained and prepared to treat acute anaphylaxis, desensitization can be achieved by either of the following protocols:

Cutaneous Protocol

Give 5 U crystalline penicillin G, injected intracutaneously into lower forearm.

At 60–90 minute intervals, 10, 100, and 1,000 U are given intracutaneously.

This is followed by 10,000 U and then 50,000 U SC.

Penicillin is given IV at the same dose, and the dosage is increased until the therapeutic dose is reached.

or

Oral Protocol

Give 100 U penicillin V elixir PO.

Oral dose is doubled and given every 15 minutes until about 1,300,000 U is given.

Penicillin IV is then begun.

No prior therapy with hydrocortisone or diphenhydramine is given. Mild cutaneous reactions are allowed to resolve spontaneously or may be treated with diphenhydramine 25 mg given intravenously. These protocols may be used with other β-lactam antibiotics. Treatment should begin with 1/10,000 of the therapeutic dose and increase incrementally (e.g., 1/10,000, 1/5,000, 1/1,000, 1/100, 1/10, 1/5) until a full therapeutic dose is given.

cefotaxime has become a frequently used regimen for the treatment of infants with suspected sepsis or meningitis. After the first month of life, ceftriaxone, cefotaxime, and in some cases cefuroxime have become standard therapeutic agents for use in children with serious infections after admission to the hospital. In critically ill children, those with fever and neutropenia, and those with nosocomially acquired infections in the intensive care unit, cefepime is becoming a standard agent for empirical therapy. The choice of cefepime as initial therapy continues to expand markedly as bacterial resistance to ceftazidime rapidly increases in some hospitals.

Finally, the use of ceftriaxone on an outpatient basis in pediatric patients is increasing, with the majority of the drug administered as single intramuscular doses to young children who have fever without a known source. The drug is also sometimes used as single-dose therapy for acute otitis media. Ceftriaxone has truly become a pediatric workhorse.

TABLE 14–16. Clinically Relevant Drug-Drug Interactions: Penicillins

Drug	Action/Reaction
Probenecid*	Inhibits renal tubular secretion and systemic accumulation of penicillins
Aminoglycosides	Antipseudomonal penicillins are inactivated when admixed in same solution with aminoglycosides; depends on time, temperature, and pH of solution (e.g., IV, dialysis solution). The order of susceptibility to breakdown is as follows: gentamicin ≥ tobramycin ≥ amikacin ≥ netilmicin.

*Used clinically in the treatment of certain infections (e.g., certain sexually transmitted diseases).

TABLE 14–17. Comparative in Vitro Susceptibility of Selected Pathogens to Cephalosporin Antibiotics

	Minimum Inhibitory Concentrations (MIC_{90}) (mg/L)								
Organism	**Cephalexin, Cefadroxil, Cefazolin**	**Cefprozil, Loracarbef**	**Cefamandole, Cefuroxime**	**Cefaclor**	**Cefoxitin, Cefotetan**	**Cefixime, Ceftibuten, Cefpodoxime**	**Cefotaxime, Ceftizoxime, Ceftriaxone**	**Ceftazidime**	**Cefepime**
Cocci									
Streptococcus pneumoniae	4	1	0.25	1	4	<0.5	0.5	2	0.5
Group A *Streptococcus*	0.5	0.25	0.125	0.25	2	0.25	0.25	0.5	0.5
Group B *Streptococcus*		0.5	0.125	2		0.25	0.07	0.05	0.07
Viridans streptococci	6	4	0.5	R	2	R	0.5	4	>0.05
Enterococcus faecalis	R	R	R	R	R	R	R	R	R
Staphylococcus aureus									
Penicillinase-negative	16	2	0.5	4	4				
Penicillinase-positive	R	8	1	16	4	4*	4	8	16
Staphylococcus epidermidis	R	R	R	R	R	4*	R	R	R
Neisseria gonorrhoeae[†]									
β-Lactamase–positive	4		2	2	0.25	<0.25	1	0.5	0.25
Neisseria meningitidis	4		0.5		1–2		0.25	0.5	0.25
Selected Bacilli and Anaerobes									
Clostridium perfringens	R		0.5		8		4	0.1	0.1
Corynebacterium diphtheriae									
Listeria monocytogenes	R	R	R	R	R	R	R	R	R
Haemophilus influenzae									
β-Lactamase–negative	R	0.5	1	8	2	<0.25			
β-Lactamase–positive	R	0.5	2	8	8	<0.25	0.25	0.25	0.25
Prevotella melaninogenica	R	R	8	R	1–2	R	2		
Fusobacterium nucleatum					4				
Bacteriodes fragilis	R	R	R	R	4	R	R	R	R
Moraxella catarrhalis									
β-Lactamase–negative	R	1	1	1		<0.25			
β-Lactamase–positive	R	2	2	2	<0.25	0.5	0.5	0.25	0.5
Enterobacteriaceae and *Pseudomonas*									
Escherichia coli	16–32	2–8	2	16–32	2	1	0.25	0.25	0.25
Proteus mirabilis	16–32	4	2	8	4	0.5	0.25	0.25	0.25
Klesbsiella	16–32	8–32	4	16–32	8	0.5	0.25	0.5	0.25
Enterobacter[‡]	R	R	8–16	R	R	R	1–2	0.5	0.25
Citrobacter diversus	16	4		8			0.5	4	0.5
Citrobacter freundii						R		4	R
Serratia	R	R	R	R	R	R	R	R	0.5
Salmonella	R	R	2	R	4	0.5	1	0.5	0.25
Shigella	R	16	4	32	8	1	1	0.5	0.25
Proteus vulgaris	R	R	R	R	8	2	0.5	0.25	0.25
Providencia	R	R	16	R	4	1	0.5	1	0.5
Morganella	R		4	R	8	R	2	2	1
Acinetobacter	R			R				8	
Pseudomonas aeruginosa	R	R	R	R	R	R	R	16	32
Pseudomonas (other species)	R	R	R	R	R	R	R	8	16

R = resistant.
*Cefixime resistant.
†Includes β-lactamase–positive strains.
‡Many *Enterobacter* species are resistant to third-generation cephalosporins.

TABLE 14–18. Available Formulations of Cephalosporin Antibiotics

Drug	Oral Formulation		Parenteral Formulation*
	Dosage Form	Amount	
First Generation			
Cefadroxil	Suspension	125, 250, and 500 mg/5 mL	None
	Capsules	500 mg	
	Tablets	1 g	
Cefazolin	None available		Yes
Cephalexin	Suspension	125 and 250 mg/5 mL	None
	Oral drops	100 mg/mL	
	Capsules	250 and 500 mg	
	Tablets	250 and 500 mg	
Second Generation			
Cefamandole	None available		Yes*
Cefprozil	Suspension	125 and 250 mg/5 mL	None
	Tablets	250 and 500 mg	
Cefuroxime (axetil salt orally)	Tablets	125, 360, and 500 mg	Yes*
Loracarbef	Suspension	100 and 200 mg/5 mL	None
	Capsules	200 mg	
Cephamycins			
Cefaclor	Suspension	125, 187, 250, and 375 mg/5 mL	Yes
	Capsules	250 and 500 mg	
Cefotetan	None available		Yes
Cefoxitin	None available		Yes
Third Generation			
Cefixime	Suspension	100 mg/5 mL	None
	Tablets	200 and 400 mg	
Cefoperazone	None available		Yes
Cefotaxime	None available		Yes
Cefpodoxime	Suspension	50 and 100 mg/5 mL	None
	Tablets	100 and 200 mg	
Ceftazidime	None available		Yes
Ceftibuten	Suspension	90 mg/5 mL	
	Capsules	400 mg	
Ceftizoxime	None available		Yes
Ceftriaxone	None available		Yes
Fourth Generation			
Cefepime	None available		Yes

*Antibiotics are available as sterile powder for reconstitution before intramuscular or intravenous administration. Standard recommended dilutions are available from the manufacturers in their respective package inserts. Clinically relevant, concentrated solutions should be obtained from the hospital pharmacy.

TABLE 14–19. Organisms for Which Cephalosporins Lack Reliable Activity

Streptococcus pneumoniae (penicillin-resistant)
Staphylococcus aureus (methicillin-resistant)
Coagulase-negative staphylococci
Enterococcus faecalis
Listeria monocytogenes
Legionella pneumophila
Clostridium difficile
Stenotrophomonas maltophilia
Campylobacter jejuni
Pasteurella multocida

Metabolism and Disposition. The cephalosporins vary markedly in biodisposition, both from drug to drug and with patient age (Table 14–20). Oral first- and second-generation cephalosporins are generally well absorbed from the gastrointestinal tract. The oral third-generation cephalosporins show poor to moderate bioavailability but do achieve adequate systemic concentrations to treat infections of the upper and lower respiratory tract and the urinary tract.

Cephalosporins demonstrate varying degrees of protein binding, ranging from approximately 10% for cephalexin to 90% for cefoperazone. A third-generation cephalosporin, ceftriaxone, displays rather unique protein binding characteristics. The drug has a long $t_{1/2\beta}$ because it is highly protein bound. In addition, this binding shows saturation when the drug is administered in its usual therapeutic doses. Therefore, when ceftriaxone is administered as a single daily dose, an initial bolus of free drug is distributed rapidly to tissues as a result of the saturation of the protein binding sites, followed by a continual release of active drug from bound reservoirs for more than 24 hours. Administration of the total daily ceftriaxone

TABLE 14–20. Pharmacokinetic Characteristics of Cephalosporins

Drug	Bioavailability (%)	Protein Binding (%)	Metabolism (%)	$t_{1/2\beta}$ (hr) Neonate (0–30 Days)	$t_{1/2\beta}$ (hr) Infant/Child*	$t_{1/2\beta}$ (hr) Adult
First Generation						
Cefadroxil	90–95	5–10	5–10	—	1.3–1.7	1.4
Cefazolin	—	75–85	5–10	—	1.3–2.2	1.5–2
Cephalexin	90	6–10	5–10	3–5	0.75–1.5	0.9
Second Generation						
Cefaclor	90–95	25	5–20	NA	0.6–1	0.5–1
Cefamandole	—	70–75	5–10	1–2	1	0.5–1.5
Cefprozil	95	36	40	—	—	1.3
Cefuroxime	35–52	33–50	10–20	4–6	1–1.5	1–2
Loracarbef†	90	25	<5	NA	—	1
Cephamycins						
Cefotetan	—	88	<10	NA	NA	2.8–4.6
Cefoxitin	—	65–80	5–10	NA	NA	0.7–1.1
Third Generation						
Cefixime	30–50	65–70	60	3	—	2.4–4
Cefoperazone	—	90–93	70–85	6–12	1.5–2.5	1.6–2
Cefotaxime	—	13–38	20–30	2–6	0.9–1.2	1–1.5
Cefpodoxime	50	20–33	<5	NA	2.5–3	2.1–2.8
Ceftazidime	—	15–20	5–10	2.2–5	1.3–2	1.4–2
Ceftibuten‡	≅70‡	60–64	<10	—	1.9–2.5	2.4–2.8
Ceftizoxime	—	28–31	5–10	5–7	1.2–2.5	1.4–1.9
Ceftriaxone	—	25–98	40–60	9–16	4–8	5–9
Moxalactam§	—	50	5–10	4.5–7	1.5–2	1.5–2.5
Fourth Generation						
Cefepime	—	19	10–20	NA	1.5–1.7	1.7–2.0

NA = reliable published data not available.
*Transition from child to adult varies with the drug under consideration.
†First carbacephem antibiotic.
‡Preliminary bioavailability data; bioavailability decreases as individual doses increase >400 mg.
§No longer available; shown for comparison only.

dose as a single total dose (i.e., every 24 hours) achieves much higher active free-drug concentrations than are achieved if the same dose is administered in a divided, twice-daily regimen.

Of the four generations of cephalosporins, only the drugs in the third and fourth generations penetrate into the central nervous system reliably enough so that they can be used to treat bacterial meningitis. Among the second-generation drugs, cefuroxime has also been demonstrated to be effective in treating bacterial meningitis. It is not recommended for this indication, however, because of several reports of delayed cerebrospinal fluid sterilization in children who otherwise did well clinically. In every case the extent of penetration was directly related to the degree of inflammation.

Few of the cephalosporins undergo any significant metabolism. Those in the third generation do have sufficient biliary excretion to make them useful in the treatment of hepatobiliary infections. Most excretion, however, is renal and is confined to filtration. Few of the cephalosporins undergo tubular secretion.

Because the elimination of the cephalosporins is mainly renal, significant developmental changes occur in $t_{1/2\beta}$ during the first year of life (see Table 14–20). Disease-associated alterations in renal function necessitate dosing modifications. In addition, because of the high degree of protein binding of ceftriaxone and related concerns about bilirubin displacement, this drug is not recommended for the treatment of infants in the first month of life. The true significance of this potential displacement reaction is unknown.

Available Formulations. Parenteral cephalosporins are available in the United States in the form of a dry powder that can be reconstituted for injection as needed. Orally administered cephalosporins are available in a variety of dosage forms (see Table 14–18). The tablets and capsules have a fairly long shelf life, and the liquid formulations are stable with refrigeration for 2 weeks. Some of the newer liquid preparations such as cefixime and loracarbef do not require refrigeration and are therefore easy to transport with children going to daycare, to school, or on trips. In general, the suspensions are better tasting than the liquid penicillin preparations. Some cephalosporin suspensions, such as cefixime, cefaclor, cephalexin, cefprozil, and loracarbef, are considered palatable.

Recommended Dosing and Dosing Strategies. Most of the parenteral cephalosporins require two or three doses per day to maintain plasma concentrations in excess of the MIC values for susceptible pathogens (Table 14–21). However, ceftriaxone should be administered once a day.

The oral cephalosporin preparations vary greatly in required dosing frequency. Cefadroxil, a first-generation drug, and all three of the third-generation drugs can probably be administered as a single daily dose for most indications. One important aspect of oral cephalosporin dosing is strict adherence to dosing guidelines. In the past, most oral antibiotic dosing was based on that universally standard measuring device, the teaspoon. With the second- and

TABLE 14–21. Cephalosporin Dosing Recommendations

Drug	Route	Age/Weight	Daily Dose*	Frequency
First Generation				
Cefadroxil	PO	Infant/child	30 mg/kg/day	q12–24hr
	PO	Adult	1–2 g/day	q12–24hr
Cefazolin	IM, IV	Age ≤7 days	40 mg/kg/day	q12hr
		Age >7 days		
		At ≤2,000 g	40 mg/kg/day	q12hr
		At >2,000 g	60 mg/kg/day	q8hr
	IM, IV	Infant/child	50–100 mg/kg/day	q8hr
	IM, IV	Adult	1.5–8 g/day	q6–8hr
Cephalexin	PO	Infant/child	25–100 mg/kg/day	q4–8hr
	PO	Adult	1–4 g/day	q4–8hr
Second Generation				
Cefamandole	IM, IV	Infant/child	50–100 mg/kg/day	q4–6hr
	IM, IV	Adult	1.5–6 g/day	q4–8hr
Cefadroxil	PO	Infant/child	30 mg/kg/day	q12hr
	PO	Adult	0.5–1 g/day	q12–24hr
Cefuroxime	IM, IV	Infant/child	75–200 mg/kg/day	q8hr
	IM, IV	Adult	2.25–4.5 g/day	q8hr
	PO	Infant/child	0.125–0.5 g/day	q12hr
	PO	Adult	0.25–1.0 g/day	q12–24hr
Loracarbef	PO	Infant/child	15–30 mg/kg/day	q12hr
	PO	Adult	400–800 mg/day	q12hr
Cephamycins				
Cefaclor	PO	Infant/child	20–40 mg/kg/day	q8hr
	PO	Adult	0.75–1.5 g/day	q8hr
Cefotetan	IM, IV	Infant/child	40–60 mg/kg/day	q8–12hr
	IM, IV	Adult	2–6 g/day	q12hr
Cefoxitin	IM, IV	Infant/child	40–60 mg/kg/day	q8–12hr
	IM, IV	Adult	2–6 g/day	q12hr
Third Generation				
Cefixime	PO	Infant/child	8 mg/kg/day	q12–24hr
	PO	Adult	400 mg/day	q12–24hr
Cefoperazone	IM, IV	Infant/child	100–150 mg/kg/day	q8–12hr
	IM, IV	Adult	3–12 g/day	q8–12hr
Cefotaxime	IM, IV	Age ≤7 days	100 mg/kg/day	q12hr
		Age >7 days	150 mg/kg/day	q8hr
	IM, IV	Infant/child	100–200 mg/kg/day	q6–8hr
		Meningitis	200–300 mg/kg/day	q6–8hr
	IM, IV	Adult	3–12 g/day	q6–8hr
Cefpodoxime	PO	Infant/child	10 mg/kg/day	q12hr
	PO	Adult	200–400 mg/day	q12hr
Ceftazidime	IM, IV	At ≤2,000 g		
		Age ≤7 days	60–100 mg/kg/day	q12hr
		Age >7 days	90–100 mg/kg/day	q8hr
		At >2,000 g	100–150 mg/kg/day	q8hr
	IM, IV	Infant/child	100–150 mg/kg/day	q8hr
	IM, IV	Adult	2–6 g/day	q8–12hr
Ceftibuten	PO	Infant/child	9 mg/kg	q24hr
	PO	Adult	200–400 mg/day	q24hr
Ceftizoxime	IM, IV	Infant/child	90–200 mg/kg/day	q6–8hr
	IM, IV	Adult	3–6 g/day	q8–12hr
Ceftriaxone†	IM, IV	Age ≤7 days	50 mg/kg/day	q24hr
		Age >7 days	50–75 mg/kg/day	q24hr
	IM, IV	Infant/child	50–75 mg/kg/day	q12–24hr
		Meningitis	100 mg/kg/day	q12hr
	IM, IV	Adult	1–2 g/day	q24hr
Moxalactam‡	IM, IV	Age ≤7 days	100 mg/kg/day	q12hr
		Age >7 days	100–150 mg/kg/day	q8hr
	IM, IV	Infant/child	100–150 mg/kg/day	q8hr
	IM, IV	Adult	2–6 g/day	q8–12hr
Fourth Generation				
Cefepime	IM, IV	Infant/child	100–150 mg/kg/day	q8–12hr
			1–2 g/day	q8–12hr

*Dose provided as usual dosage range for age as total for 24 hours.
†For neonatal gonococcal prophylaxis: 25–50 mg/kg (maximum dose: 125 mg).
‡No longer available; shown for comparison only.

third-generation oral drugs, the administration of doses that are a bit too high (e.g., 9 mg/kg instead of 8 mg/kg) can result in a marked increase in the incidence of gastrointestinal side effects. Underdosing, particularly with the oral third-generation drugs that have only modest bioavailability, may result in therapeutic failure.

Adverse Effects. The cephalosporins are the safest class of antibiotics and perhaps the safest group of drugs available in medicine today. For this reason they have enjoyed an ever-increasing popularity. Adverse effects of cephalosporins occur in ≤7% of persons receiving the drugs, and apparently the incidence is even less frequent in infants and children.

The most common adverse effects associated with cephalosporins are gastrointestinal in nature and are usually limited to nausea, bloating, and diarrhea. They can be eliminated in large part with strict adherence to dosing recommendations.

Allergic reactions also occur but are not as common as those seen with the penicillins. The acyl side chains appear to participate as antigenic determinants in addition to metabolites of the core structure. The cross-reactivity of cephalosporins with penicillins in persons with documented penicillin allergy is largely unknown. The risk is considered to be somewhat higher than in the general population. When cephalosporins were given to persons in whom penicillin allergy was documented by skin testing, only 1 person in 99 developed a clinically significant reaction.

A significant incidence of serum sickness reaction has been associated with the use of the drug cefaclor. Risk factors include age <10 years and two or more courses of treatment with the drug. This reaction appears to be a problem unique to cefaclor and may be related to its instability in solution.

Other rare adverse reactions that have been associated with cephalosporins include positive Coombs' reactions, bone marrow suppression, thrombocytosis, acute tubular necrosis, and mild aminotransferase elevations. Ceftriaxone has been associated with the formation of biliary sludge in the gallbladder. In some critically ill patients, this may lead to the signs and symptoms of cholecystitis. The incidence of this effect is low.

Finally, the cephalosporins that contain the thiomethyltetrazole ring (e.g., cefamandole, cefonicid, cefoperazone, cefotetan, moxalactam) have been implicated in two interesting and unusual reactions rarely seen in children. First, patients receiving these drugs display alcohol intolerance similar to that seen with disulfiram. Second, hypoprothrombinemia may occur, especially with moxalactam. Some experts recommend the coadministration of vitamin K with these parenteral third-generation cephalosporins.

Drug Interactions. Few drug-drug interactions of any significance have been reported with the cephalosporins. Probenecid will decrease the renal clearance of cefixime, leading to systemic accumulation of this cephalosporin. Ceftriaxone has been implicated in several drug displacement interactions involving warfarin and phenytoin, but these are poorly documented. Overall, drug interactions are not a problem with the cephalosporins.

A MONOBACTAM: AZTREONAM

Aztreonam is the first monocyclic β-lactam antibiotic referred to as a monobactam.

Spectrum of Activity. Aztreonam, like other β-lactam antibiotics, is bactericidal against susceptible bacteria. Aztreonam interferes with bacterial cell wall synthesis in a manner similar to that of other β-lactam antibiotics; the drug binds to PBP 3. The spectrum of antibacterial activity for aztreonam is narrow and limited to aerobic gram-negative bacteria (Table 14–22). Gram-positive bacteria are generally resistant to this drug. In terms of activity, it resembles the aminoglycoside antibiotics. Synergy with aztreonam has been described for combinations including aminoglycosides and extended-spectrum cephalosporins.

TABLE 14–22. Representative in Vitro Susceptibility to Aztreonam for Selected Bacteria

	Aztreonam Concentration (mg/L)	
Pathogen	**MIC_{50}**	**MIC_{90}**
Escherichia coli	<0.1–0.25	0.2–0.5
Klebsiella	<0.1–0.125	0.2–0.5
Enterobacter	0.1–0.5	4–64
Serratia	0.1–1	0.4–2
Proteus mirabilis	<0.1–0.125	0.1–0.125
Proteus, indole-positive	<0.1–0.125	<0.1–1.56
Providencia stuartii	<0.01	<0.01
Citrobacter freundii	0.2	0.7
Pseudomonas aeruginosa	3.12–16	8–16
Haemophilus influenzae		
β-Lactamase–negative	<0.1	<0.1
β-Lactamase–positive	<0.1	<0.1
Yersinia enterocolitica	0.5	14
Acinetobacter calcoaceticus	16	4
Neisseria meningitidis	<0.06	<0.06
Neisseria gonorrhoeae	<0.1	0.2

Clinical Indications. Aztreonam is not considered first-line therapy for any infections in pediatric patients. Nevertheless, it may play a role in situations in which an aminoglycoside antibiotic is indicated and the patient has problems related to impaired renal function or is concurrently receiving other potentially nephrotoxic agents (e.g., amphotericin B, cisplatin). Aztreonam is a suitable alternative to aminoglycosides in these situations for two reasons: (1) the antimicrobial spectrum of activity of aztreonam is essentially identical to that of the aminoglycosides, and (2) the drug is stable in the face of degradation by β-lactamases and is associated with no nephrotoxicity.

Metabolism and Disposition. Aztreonam is poorly absorbed into the systemic circulation after oral dosing. After intramuscular (100% bioavailable) or intravenous administration, the drug is well distributed into most body fluids and tissues including the cerebrospinal fluid of patients with bacterial meningitis, where it reaches effective antibacterial concentrations. Approximately 30–50% of the drug is bound to plasma protein. Aztreonam is eliminated from the body by both hepatic and renal mechanisms. Approximately 70% of an administered dose is excreted unchanged in the urine by a combination of glomerular filtration and renal tubular secretion. Aztreonam pharmacokinetics in older infants and children appears to be similar to that described in adults. Volume of distribution (Vd) values range from 0.18 to 0.25 L/kg, and the $t_{1/2\beta}$ is approximately 1.6–2 hours. Disposition characteristics appear to be different in neonates and in persons with cystic fibrosis.

Recommended Dosing and Dosing Strategies. Dosing recommendations for aztreonam in children and adults is shown in Table 14–23. Aztreonam may be infused intravenously for 3–5 minutes or may be administered as an infusion for 20–30 minutes. Because of the extent to which the drug is eliminated from the body by the

TABLE 14–23. Aztreonam Parenteral Dosing Recommendations*

Neonates
Postnatal: age ≤7 days
Weight ≤2,000 g: 60 mg/kg/day divided q12hr
Weight >2,000 g: 90 mg/kg/day divided q8hr
Postnatal: age >7 days
Weight ≤2,000 g: 90 mg/kg/day divided q8hr
Weight >2,000 g: 120 mg/kg/day divided q6hr

Children >1 Mo of Age
General use: 90–120 mg/kg/day divided q6–8hr
Cystic fibrosis: 50 mg/kg/dose q6–8hr (i.e., up to 200 mg/kg/day); max 6–8 g/day

Adults
Urinary tract infection: 500–1,000 mg q8–12hr
Moderately severe systemic infections: 1–2 g q8–12hr
Severe systemic or life-threatening infections (especially caused by *Pseudomonas aeruginosa*): 2 g q6–8hr; max 8 g/day
Dosage adjustment in renal impairment
CrCl 10–30 mL/min: reduce dose 50%; administer at usual interval
CrCl <10 mL/min: reduce dose by 75%; administer at usual interval

CrCl = creatinine clearance.
Doses may be administered by the intramuscular or intravenous route.

kidneys, dose adjustments are necessary for neonates and for persons with compromised renal function.

Hemodialysis effectively removes approximately 30–50% of the drug, which suggests the need for supplemental redosing after hemodialysis. Only small amounts of the drug, approximately 10% of a dose, are removed by peritoneal dialysis.

Adverse Effects. Adverse effects associated with aztreonam use are similar to those described after the administration of other penicillin and cephalosporin antibiotics. Local injection site reactions appear to be the most commonly reported adverse drug effect, followed by rash, diarrhea, nausea, and vomiting. Overall, the incidence of adverse effects associated with aztreonam appears to approximate 7%. The drug is weakly immunogenic and does not appear to precipitate allergic reactions in persons allergic to penicillin. Nevertheless, aztreonam should be used cautiously in persons allergic to penicillin (allergic to β-lactam). The first dose should be administered under close physician supervision to confirm a lack of cross-allergenicity.

Drug Interactions. Probenecid, a competitive inhibitor of renal tubular secretion, may decrease aztreonam tubular secretion by 50%. Nevertheless, interaction with this drug does not appear to reduce aztreonam total body elimination or to alter plasma drug concentrations to any appreciable extent. This lack of probenecid effect most likely reflects the limited dependence of overall aztreonam body clearance on renal tubular secretion. Solutions for intravenous administration are incompatible and should not be mixed with metronidazole or nafcillin.

CARBAPENEM ANTIBIOTICS: IMIPENEM AND MEROPENEM

Spectrum of Activity. Carbapenems possess a broad spectrum of antibacterial activity against aerobic and anaerobic gram-positive and gram-negative pathogens. Imipenem, the prototype carbapenem, binds to all of the PBPs but possesses greatest affinity for PBPs 1 and 2. All the drugs in this group are highly resistant to degradation by both plasmid and chromosomally mediated β-lactamases. Despite this resistance, the carbapenems appear to be effective inducers of bacterial β-lactamases. This may limit their overall clinical utility, particularly when used as monotherapy. Comparative in vitro activity for the two commercially available carbapenems, imipenem and meropenem, is shown in Table 14–24.

Clinical Indications. The carbapenems are very broad spectrum agents that provide rational and effective empirical antimicrobial coverage in most clinical situations. Although they have been demonstrated to be safe and effective in pediatric patients with community-acquired respiratory tract infections, skin and soft tissue infections, uncomplicated urinary tract infections, and intra-abdominal infections, the real strength of these agents is in the

TABLE 14–24. Comparative in Vitro Susceptibility of Selected Pathogens to Imipenem and Meropenem

		Minimum Inhibitory Concentration Range	
Pathogen	No.	Imipenem (mg/L)	Meropenem (mg/L)
Staphylococcus aureus	94	0.016–0.5	0.03–2
Streptococcus pneumoniae	30	≤0.008–0.06	≤0.008–0.13
Enterococcus faecalis	22	0.5–8	1–8
Haemophilus influenzae	48	≤0.008–4	≤0.008–0.25
Moraxella catarrhalis	13	0.03–0.25	≤0.008–0.06
Neisseria meningitidis	23	0.06–0.13	≤0.008–0.03
Escherichia coli	41	≤0.008–0.05	≤0.008–0.6
Klebsiella pneumoniae	9	0.13–2	≤0.008–0.03
Enterobacter cloacae	70	≤0.008–2	≤0.008–0.5
Enterobacter aerogenes	16	≤0.008–2	≤0.008–1
Serratia marcescens	59	0.5–4	≤0.008–0.13
Proteus mirabilis	19	0.13–2	≤0.016–0.06
Morganella morganii	20	0.5–2	≤0.016–0.13
Pseudomonas aeruginosa	124	0.13–16	0.03–8
Bacteroides fragilis	56	≤0.06–0.5	≤0.06–2
Clostridium difficile	12	2–4	1–2

No. = number of strains tested.

treatment of serious infections in hospitalized persons. They offer a therapeutic alternative for the treatment of gram-negative sepsis in immunocompromised persons, of nosocomial infections in critically ill children, of bacterial meningitis, and of conditions in which therapy with other broad-spectrum antibiotics or antibiotic combinations has failed. Meropenem is an effective antibiotic for the treatment of infections caused by penicillin-resistant, cephalosporin-resistant *S. pneumoniae,* including meningitis.

The mechanism of action of carbapenems varies somewhat from that of the penicillins or cephalosporin in that they have somewhat different penicillin-binding protein targets from those primarily inhibited by these other β-lactam agents. For this reason, it is recommended that these agents not be used as first-line drugs. Instead, they should be reserved for the settings in which other agents have failed or the infecting pathogens are susceptible to no other drugs.

Metabolism and Disposition. Imipenem and meropenem are not absorbed after oral administration and are available only for parenteral administration. Like other β-lactam antibiotics, these drugs are well distributed in most body fluids and tissues, including the central nervous system in persons with meningitis. Approximately 20% of imipenem and meropenem is bound to plasma proteins.

Both drugs are excreted by the kidney, primarily by glomerular filtration and with only small amounts undergoing tubular secretion. Unlike meropenem, imipenem is efficiently degraded by a proximal tubular brush-border enzyme, dehydropeptidase I. From 6% to 38% of an administered imipenem dose is recovered in the urine as active drug. As a result, urinary concentrations may be ineffective in treating serious urinary tract infections. Thus for clinical use imipenem is administered along with a competitive inhibitor of dehydropeptidase I, cilastatin. Cilastatin possesses no inherent antibacterial activity but prevents the destruction of the imipenem penem ring. It is coadministered in a 1:1 ratio with imipenem and is handled by the body in a pharmacokinetically similar way. Meropenem is resistant to degradation by the dehydropeptidase enzyme.

The imipenem $t_{1/2\beta}$ range is 1.5–3 hours in neonates, 1–1.4 hours in infants and children, and 0.8–1.3 hours in adults with normal renal function. The meropenem $t_{1/2\beta}$ range is 1.1–1.4 hours in infants and children and 0.8–1.2 hours in adults.

Recommended Dosing and Dosing Strategies. The recommended dosing for imipenem-cilastatin and meropenem in children and adults is shown in Table 14–25. Considering the dependence of these drugs on renal function for elimination, doses should be reduced in persons with moderate to severe renal disease. A simple means of dosage adjustment involves the reduction of individual doses in proportion to the reduction in glomerular filtration based on creatinine clearance.

Adverse Effects. The adverse effect profile of carbapenems is similar to that of other β-lactam antibiotics. The most common adverse effects associated with carbapenems include gastrointestinal complaints (nausea, vomiting, and diarrhea), skin rash, and the rare occurrence of a reversible neutropenia. Slowing the rate of intravenous infusion may reduce the occurrence of nausea and vomiting. Seizures have been reported in some persons with reduced renal function who are receiving high-dose therapy. Persons with an underlying seizure disorder should take carbapenems with caution.

Drug Interactions. Probenecid may decrease the renal elimination of carbapenem antibiotics.

TABLE 14–25. Carbapenem Dosing Recommendations

Imipenem*
Neonates
  <1,200 g: 20 mg/kg/day once daily IV
  >1,200 g: 40 mg/kg/day divided q12hr IV
  >2,000 g: 40–60 mg/kg/day divided q8–12hr IV
Infants and children: 40–60 mg/kg/day divided q6–8hr IV
Adults: 1–4 g/day divided q6–8hr IV
Renal disease
  CrCl <50 mL/min: reduce dose by 50% q6–8hr
  CrCl 20–50 mL/min: reduce dose by 60% q8–12hr
  CrCl <20 mL/min: reduce dose by 75% q12hr

Meropenem
Neonates: 40 mg/kg/day divided q12hr† IV
Infants and children: 60 mg/kg/day divided q8hr IV
  Meningitis: 120 mg/kg/day divided q8hr IV (max 6 g/day)
Adults: 1.5–3 g/day divided q8hr IV
  Meningitis: 6 g/day divided q8hr IV
Renal disease
  CrCl <50 mL/min: reduce dose by 50% q6–8hr
  CrCl 20–50 mL/min: reduce dose by 60% q8–12hr
  CrCl <20 mL/min: reduce dose by 75% q12hr

CrCl = creatinine clearance.
*Dosing recommendations for imipenem-cilastatin based on imipenem component.
†Preliminary dosing recommendation.

THE AMINOGLYCOSIDE ANTIBIOTICS

The aminoglycoside antibiotics represent one of the most important classes of antimicrobial agents available for the treatment of bacterial infections. Before their introduction into clinical medicine in 1944, the number of antibiotics effective against gram-negative organisms was limited. Since their introduction, scientists and clinicians have attempted to replace these agents with newer, more effective, and safer antibiotics with only limited success. The extended-spectrum cephalosporins, monobactams, and carbapenems were claimed to be replacements for the aminoglycosides and were predicted to reduce the clinical need for this group of antibiotics substantially. Such assertions are no longer made, and the aminoglycosides remain important components of the therapeutic armamentarium.

The discovery of streptomycin launched 4 decades of investigative endeavors that yielded neomycin, kanamycin, gentamicin, tobramycin, and the newer analogs amikacin and netilmicin. Early recognition of the frequent incidence of serious adverse effects associated with systemic neomycin therapy (e.g., ototoxicity and nephrotoxicity) limited the use of neomycin to topical applications. In 1972 a semisynthetic derivative of kanamycin, amikacin, was introduced in the first attempt to design an aminoglycoside that was resistant to inactivation by bacterial enzymes known to metabolize aminoglycosides. A number of semisynthetic derivatives (e.g., netilmicin) have since been constructed in efforts to increase the spectrum of antibacterial activity, enhance the resistance to degradation by bacterial inactivating enzymes, and reduce the ototoxic and nephrotoxic potential.

Spectrum of Activity. The aminoglycoside antibiotics inhibit bacterial protein synthesis by binding primarily to the 30S ribosomal subunit. Some agents, including gentamicin, kanamycin, and tobramycin, bind to multiple sites on both ribosomal subunits. These drugs appear to bind irreversibly to specific proteins, thus inhibiting cellular initiation of protein synthesis. As a consequence, the aminoglycosides are rapidly bactericidal against most aerobic gram-negative bacilli. Cellular uptake of an aminoglycoside by susceptible bacteria is an oxygen-dependent active transport process, which makes anaerobic bacteria universally resistant.

Comparison of in vitro antibacterial activity of selected aminoglycoside antibiotics is shown in Table 14–26. Gentamicin, tobramycin, and amikacin possess no clinically useful activity against *Mycobacterium tuberculosis.* Although variable in vitro antibacterial activity is often observed for aminoglycosides against *H. influenzae, Mycoplasma,* and gram-positive bacteria, their therapeutic usefulness in infections caused by these pathogens is limited. Aminoglycosides may exhibit synergistic activity with other antimicrobial agents against *Staphylococcus, Streptococcus,* and *Enterococcus.*

Bacterial resistance to newer aminoglycoside antibiotics is uncommon despite their extensive clinical use. The reasons for this less-than-expected rate of resistance is unclear but may reflect a positive consequence of the rapid bactericidal action of these agents. This causes a prolonged postantibiotic effect that may delay or prevent the development of resistance. In contrast, shifts in patterns of susceptibility to aminoglycosides are often observed from year to year and from region to region, depending on the major agent used and the duration of its predominant or exclusive use. Nevertheless, these differences in antibacterial susceptibility are usually of minor clinical importance.

Bacterial enzymes capable of inactivating aminoglycosides by acetylation, adenylation, or phosphorylation are the most common mechanisms of bacterial resistance to an aminoglycoside. These inactivating enzymes are transferred as plasmids with individual agents that differ in their susceptibility to enzymatic degradation. Amikacin is the most stable drug, tobramycin is intermediate, and gentamicin is the least stable in regard to the effects of these inactivating enzymes.

Clinical Indications. The aminoglycosides are used predominantly to treat serious infections caused by gram-negative bacilli, especially those caused by more resistant organisms such as *Pseudomonas.* For empirical therapy it is important to know the aminoglycoside susceptibility pattern of organisms in a given community. For example, in some hospital nurseries, gentamicin can be used in empirical therapy for possible sepsis in newborns, but in other nurseries resistance to gentamicin is significant and amikacin should be selected.

Continuing use of aminoglycosides along with β-lactam antibiotics is common practice in treating severe infections or highly resistant organisms. This practice is based on the premise that combination therapy for infection with gram-negative bacilli usually provides synergy and theoretically a better outcome. Clinical evidence for this finding is best for infections caused by *P. aeruginosa.* In immunocompromised persons who are infected with this organism, data clearly show better survival and cure rates in those treated with an aminoglycoside and an antipseudomonal penicillin. This additive, or synergistic, effect of the aminoglycoside–β-lactam combination is less pronounced for the newer third- and fourth-generation cephalosporins. Another argument for two-drug therapy is the possibility that resistance induction is less likely to occur when an aminoglycoside is used with the β-lactam agent. Evidence exists to both support and refute this contention.

An aminoglycoside and ampicillin are used most frequently in pediatrics as empirical therapy for sepsis in newborns. More recently a combination of ampicillin and cefotaxime has also been employed. The presence of meningitis with gram-positive organisms, most likely group B *Streptococcus,* might make the older regimen of ampicillin and aminoglycoside preferable. The presence of gram-negative rods favors the use of the third-generation cephalosporin with or without the aminoglycoside, but the development of resistance to cephalosporins has been documented when this combination is used empirically for a large proportion of the infants. Final treatment should be guided by the pathogen isolated and by its antimicrobial susceptibility pattern.

Because the aminoglycosides do not cross the blood-brain barrier well, concentrations in the central nervous system are low and variable. Therefore the aminoglycosides should not be used as single agents to treat meningitis. In the past, gram-negative bacillary meningitis was treated with aminoglycosides because they were often the only active agents available. The drugs were administered via the intrathecal route to be most effective. This route was not uncommon in the newborn nursery in persons with *E. coli* and *Klebsiella* meningitis. Such treatment is rarely indicated now, except in the setting of ventriculoperitoneal shunt–related infections where an intraventricular reservoir is in place. The expanded spectrum–generation cephalosporins (e.g., cefotaxime) are responsible for an improved outcome in gram-negative meningitis, and their availability has virtually eliminated the need for intrathecal administration of aminoglycoside antibiotics. Occasionally a very resistant organism does require two-drug therapy, and an aminoglycoside is then selected for intrathecal therapy. It is important in intrathecal or intraventricular aminoglycoside therapy that a preservative-free preparation be employed. Moreover, the intraventricular route of aminoglycoside administration may be associated with increased morbidity or mortality particularly in persons with a large central nervous system bacterial burden. The very high local aminoglycoside concentration resulting from central drug administration may precipitate rapid bacterial cell lysis, stimulating an acute, profound systemic inflammatory response.

Aminoglycosides are also indicated in the treatment of enterococcal infections. Although not susceptible to the aminoglycosides alone, *Streptococcus* and *Enterococcus* are killed synergistically when an aminoglycoside is added to penicillin or ampicillin. This result correlates with improved clinical outcome. In serious infections such as endocarditis, the specific isolate should be tested in vitro for high-level aminoglycoside resistance as an indicator of the likelihood that synergy will occur. Increasingly, however, *Enterococcus* is becoming resistant both to β-lactams and to the synergistic effects of the aminoglycosides, resulting in the increasing use of vancomycin.

The synergy between aminoglycosides and β-lactams is useful in the treatment of penicillin-susceptible *Streptococcus* and *Enterococcus.* In the treatment of endocarditis caused by viridans streptococci, the addition of an aminoglycoside decreases failure rates

TABLE 14–26. Comparative in Vitro Antibacterial Activity of Aminoglycoside Antibiotics

	Antibiotic		
Pathogen	**Gentamicin/ Netilmicin**	**Tobramycin**	**Amikacin**
Escherichia coli	1–1.5	1–1.5	4
Klebsiella pneumoniae	0.5–1	0.5–1	2–4
Proteus mirabilis	1.5–2	1.5–2	8
Morganella morganii	2–4	1–2	4–8
Proteus vulgaris	2–4	2–4	8–16
Pseudomonas aeruginosa	1–2	0.5–1	2–4
Enterobacter aerogenes	0.5–1	0.5–1	2–4
Serratia marcescens	1–2	2–4	4–8
Providencia stuartii	2–4	2–4	8

and can shorten the course of therapy from 4 weeks to 2 weeks. In complicated cases a usual 4-week course of penicillin is often given with an aminoglycoside during the first 2 weeks. Unfortunately, because of the increasing resistance of *Enterococcus* to the aminoglycosides and their combinations (50% or greater), alternative therapies are necessary with increasing frequency. Synergy with penicillin or ampicillin is also cited as the reason for initially treating group B *Streptococcus* infections in newborns with aminoglycosides. Because of the incidence of relapse and the seriousness of these infections, many clinicians recommend continuing the drug combination in newborns with group B *Streptococcus* sepsis or meningitis until their condition has stabilized and they have completed the course with high-dose penicillin or ampicillin therapy alone.

Aminoglycosides are also synergistic with nafcillin or oxacillin against staphylococcal isolates. In endocarditis caused by *S. aureus*, more rapid clearing of the bloodstream has been demonstrated with combination therapy, but an improved clinical outcome has not clearly been established. Unlike with enterococcus, synergy should be assumed only if the organism is susceptible to the aminoglycoside in vitro. Coagulase-negative staphylococci can also be treated synergistically if the organisms are susceptible to one of the aminoglycosides. In ventriculoperitoneal shunt infections the addition of an intraventricular aminoglycoside may speed clearing of infection when the drug is added to parenteral therapy alone. Gentamicin is available in a preservative-free form for this use.

In children as in adults with sepsis syndrome, gram-negative pathogens should be suspected, and aminoglycosides are usually one of the antimicrobial agents first used on an emergent basis. Because *S. aureus* and group A *Streptococcus* can also produce this syndrome, the aminoglycoside should be given with a drug that has excellent gram-positive activity, such as vancomycin.

Metabolism and Disposition. After oral administration the aminoglycoside antibiotics are poorly absorbed into systemic circulation. Thus, for the treatment of systemic infections, these drugs must be administered either intramuscularly or intravenously. Aminoglycosides, particularly neomycin or gentamicin, may be administered orally as part of bowel sterilization–flora suppression therapy, thus capitalizing on their poor oral bioavailability. These drugs are not metabolized by the body and are excreted completely unchanged by the kidney via glomerular filtration. Hepatic disease does not interfere with the body elimination of aminoglycosides, whereas renal dysfunction directly influences the aminoglycoside body clearance.

Recommended Dosing and Dosing Strategies. For the treatment of systemic infections, aminoglycoside antibiotics can be administered intravenously by bolus injection, by intermittent intravenous infusion for 30–60 minutes, or by continuous 24-hour intravenous infusion. Previous dosing regimens for aminoglycoside antibiotics were based on the pharmacokinetic profiles (e.g., $t_{1/2\beta}$ and total body clearance) of each of the individual agents, in combination with a desire to achieve a predetermined target peak and trough drug concentration in the blood. However, these traditional dosage regimens did not capitalize on these drugs' clear concentration-dependent pharmacodynamic characteristics. On the basis of these PK criteria, gentamicin, tobramycin, and netilmicin were most often administered in three equally divided daily doses, or every 8 hours (Table 14–27), whereas amikacin and kanamycin are most often administered in two equally divided doses, or every 12 hours (Table 14–28).

The recognition that the antibacterial efficacy of the aminoglycoside antibiotics correlates best with the magnitude by which the drug concentration exceeds the pathogen's MIC (i.e., concentration-dependent antibacterial activity), reflected by such parameters as the ratio of peak drug concentration to MIC or by the ratio of the area under the drug concentration-time curve to MIC, has resulted in a re-evaluation of how these drugs are administered. For maximal antibacterial efficacy of a ''concentration-dependent'' drug such as an aminoglycoside, these drugs are best administered as a single daily dose rather than as divided daily doses. The single larger dose achieves maximal concentrations relative to pathogen MIC and thus improved bacterial killing. The traditional aminoglycoside dosing strategies have undergone considerable critique, and once-daily dosing of an aminoglycoside is increasingly common for adult patients (Table 14–29).

What permits the total-dose, once-daily dosing regimen is the overall safety profile of these agents. Although serious adverse effects are associated with the use of this class of antibiotics, these effects are not related to specific serum drug concentrations. Thus the routine monitoring of serum aminoglycoside serum concentrations with conventional divided daily dosing or with total-dose, once-daily dosing is not necessary.

TABLE 14–27. Dosing Guidelines for Gentamicin, Tobramycin, and Netilmicin

Age	Normal Renal Function*	Mild Impairment† (CrCl >50 mL/min)	Moderate Impairment† (CrCl 10–50 mL/min)	Severe Impairment† (CrCl <10 mL/min)	Hemodialysis
Preterm neonates (<1 kg)	3.5 mg/kg q24hr IV	3.5 mg/kg q24–36hr IV	3.5 mg/kg q36–48hr IV	3.5 mg/kg q48–72hr IV	NA
Preterm neonates (≥1 kg) and term neonates	5 mg/kg/day divided q12hr IV	2.5 mg/kg q12–18hr IV	2.5 mg/kg q18–36hr IV	2.5 mg/kg q36–72hr IV	NA
Infants, children, and adolescents‡	7.5 mg/kg/day divided q8–24hr IV or IM	1.9–2.5 mg/kg q8–12hr IV or IM	1.25–2.5 mg/kg q12–24hr IV or IM	0.6–2.5 mg/kg q24–48hr IV or IM	1.25–1.75 mg/kg IV after dialysis
Adults‡	3–5 mg/kg/day divided q8–24hr IV or IM	0.75–1 mg/kg q8–12hr IV or IM	0.5–1 mg/kg q12–24hr IV or IM	0.25–1 mg/kg q24–48hr IV or IM	0.5–0.7 mg/kg IV after dialysis

CrCl = creatinine clearance; NA = data not available.

*Aminoglycosides may be administered intravenously (for 20–30 minutes) or intramuscularly. The intravenous route is preferable, especially in newborns.

†Alternatively, aminoglycoside dosing in persons with varying degrees of renal function may be guided by serum drug concentration monitoring.

‡Total daily dose administered once daily (i.e., q24hr) should be initiated in infants, children, and adults with normal renal function (see Table 14–29 and text for complete discussion).

TABLE 14–28. Dosing Guidelines for Amikacin

Age	Dosing*
Preterm neonates	
Postnatal age ≤7 days	
At 1,200–2,000 g	7.5 mg/kg q12–18hr IV
At >2000 g	10 mg/kg q12hr IV
Postnatal age >7 days	
At 1,200–2,000 g	7.5 mg/kg divided q8–12hr IV
At >2,000 g	10 mg/kg divided q18hr IV
Infants, children, and adolescents†	15–30 mg/kg/day divided q8–12hr IV or IM
Adults†	15 mg/kg/day divided q8–12hr IV or IM
Renal disease	Adjust dose on basis of serum amikacin concentrations
Hemodialysis or peritoneal dialysis	Depending on renal impairment, provide 50–100% supplemental dose after dialysis

*Total daily dose administered once daily (i.e., q24hr) should be initiated in infants, children, and adults with normal renal function (see Table 14–29 and text for complete discussion).

†Aminoglycosides may be administered intravenously (for 20–30 minutes) or intramuscularly. The intravenous route is preferable, especially in newborns.

The monitoring of serum drug concentrations has often been suggested as an objective means of directing aminoglycoside dosing for maximal efficacy and safety. The traditionally targeted therapeutic peak and trough serum concentrations for aminoglycoside antibiotics are shown in Table 14–30. Peak concentrations are usually obtained 30 minutes after completion of a 30-minute intravenous infusion, immediately on completion of a 60-minute infusion, or 60 minutes after an intramuscular injection. These recommendations accommodate the early, rapid distribution period for aminoglycosides, permitting a more accurate quantitation of the postdistribution peak serum drug concentration. Trough concentrations are obtained at the end of the dosing interval, just before the next dose.

Unfortunately, wide acceptance of a target aminoglycoside serum concentration occurred in the absence of any clear relationship between the purported serum aminoglycoside concentration and either efficacy or safety. Nevertheless, these data do demonstrate that with routine weight- and age-based dosing achievable, aminoglycoside concentrations are efficacious and have limited toxicity. Thus the routine monitoring of serum aminoglycoside concentrations is no longer recommended. In selected clinical scenarios, monitoring may still be warranted (Table 14–31).

Considering the close relationship between aminoglycoside clearance and the glomerular filtration rate, some investigators use either the gentamicin or the tobramycin clearance rate as an estimate

TABLE 14–29. Once-Daily Dosing of Aminoglycoside Antibiotics

Gentamicin, Tobramycin, and Netilmicin
Infants and children: 5–7.5 mg/kg/day
Adults: 3–5 mg/kg/day
Children with cystic fibrosis: 10–20 mg/kg/day

Amikacin
Infants, children, and adults: 25–30 mg/kg/day

TABLE 14–30. Traditional Target Therapeutic Serum Aminoglycoside Concentrations

	Target Range (mg/L)	
Drug	Peak*	Trough*
Amikacin	25–40	2–10
Gentamicin	6–12	0.5–2
Netilmicin	6–12	0.5–2
Tobramycin	6–12	0.5–2

*See text for proper timing of peak and trough samples.

of the patient's creatinine clearance. Furthermore, because the primary route of aminoglycoside body elimination is the kidney, numerous dosing rules and nomograms have been published to direct initial doses of these drugs. The substantial variation observed between individuals in aminoglycoside disposition, particularly during the neonatal period and in persons with cystic fibrosis, however, reduces the clinical utility of these rules in pediatric practice. These dosing rules are recommended only as general guidelines. All doses should be modified as needed on the basis of individual requirements as indicated by predetermined objective end points.

Adverse Effects. The most commonly recognized and feared adverse effects associated with aminoglycoside administration are drug-induced ototoxicity and nephrotoxicity. All these agents have the potential to induce reversible or irreversible vestibular, cochlear, or renal toxicity. The true incidence of these important adverse effects is unknown, and their reported frequency most often depends on the variable definitions and methods used by the clinical investigators. More important, the incidence of these adverse effects in pediatrics is unknown. The majority of reports of these effects are from studies performed in adults, with no particular stratification to the younger ages.

In adults, the incidence of ototoxicity has been estimated to range anywhere from 2% to 25% and to differ depending on the population studied, the method used to determine function in cranial nerve VIII, and the specific aminoglycoside administered. Overall, it appears that the incidence of ototoxicity with the use of newer agents (e.g., gentamicin, tobramycin, amikacin, netilmicin, sisomicin) approximates 2%. The incidence of transient effects on vestibu-

TABLE 14–31. Indications for Monitoring Serum Aminoglycoside Concentrations

General Indications
Uncertain clinical response
Atypical body constituency (e.g., obesity, expanded extracellular fluid volume, low birth weight)

Specific Indications
Renal impairment
Rapidly changing renal function
Hemodialysis
Chronic ambulatory peritoneal dialysis
Prematurity
Burns
Cystic fibrosis
Therapeutic failure
Signs of nephrotoxicity
Signs of ototoxicity

lar or auditory function is most likely higher. The incidence in children as compared with that in adults is unknown.

Animal and human studies have demonstrated aminoglycoside accumulation in the perilymph and endolymph of the inner ear. Preliminary data suggest that aminoglycosides may alter the activity of the sodium-potassium pump, causing a change in electrical potential and osmotic pressure within the endolymph. Early toxicity usually involves outer hair cells of the organ of Corti, which affects high-pitched (high-frequency) sound outside the general range of conversational hearing. Further hearing impairment results from the progressive destruction of vestibular or cochlear sensory hair cells, which are very sensitive to aminoglycosides. The extent of permanent hearing loss depends on the number of permanently altered or destroyed sensory hair cells. Ototoxicity may occur more frequently in cases where high serum aminoglycoside concentrations persist for prolonged periods. Prolonged peak serum aminoglycoside concentrations delay back-diffusion of drug from the inner ear to the blood, possibly increasing the likelihood of ototoxicity. To date, no range of serum aminoglycoside concentrations or duration of exposure has been specifically correlated with the development of ototoxicity.

Clinically the monitoring of patients for the development or presence of aminoglycoside-induced ototoxicity is difficult. Initial decreases in hearing most often involve hearing outside the normal conversational range and are thus not perceived by patients. The clinical utility and cost-effectiveness of routine audiometry testing remain questionable. Early symptoms of cochlear toxicity include a high-pitched tinnitus, which is often accompanied by a feeling of fullness. The tinnitus may persist for several days to weeks after the drug has been stopped. Nausea, vomiting, and vertigo are often the first signs suggestive of vestibular toxicity. Symptoms of acute labyrinthitis, including vertigo in the upright position in association with difficulty in sitting or standing, may worsen. If these symptoms are allowed to persist, patients may have symptoms consistent with more chronic labyrinthitis. In severe cases, recovery from vestibular toxicity may take as long as 12–18 months, with many persons having some degree of residual damage.

Aminoglycoside-associated nephrotoxicity has been reported to occur in approximately 8–26% of patients who receive these drugs. The mechanism responsible for this nephrotoxicity is unclear, but it appears to result from proximal tubular necrosis, which causes subsequent compromise in glomerular function. The use of any aminoglycoside may result in a decrease in renal function. All aminoglycosides are selectively and avidly concentrated in renal cortical cells, although the degree and extent to which these agents are concentrated by proximal tubular cells are variable. This characteristic of differential renal cortical uptake has led some investigators to suggest the possible existence of a connection between the nephrotoxic potential of a specific aminoglycoside and its concentration in tubular cells. Although animal studies have suggested the occurrence of such relationships, no clinical evidence is available to support such relationships in humans.

Aminoglycoside-associated nephrotoxicity usually occurs after a minimum of 5 days of therapy. Early signs of toxicity with tubular involvement are most often observed as abnormalities in urinalysis findings, including proteinuria, an increased number of hyaline and cellular casts, and the loss of concentrating ability (decreasing specific gravity). Although many investigators have described acute increases in the urinary concentrations of certain proximal tubular cell enzymes and β_2-microglobulin, these laboratory tests appear too sensitive to be of any real clinical value in identifying which persons will develop drug-induced renal toxicity. If the process proceeds, tubular toxicity will compromise glomerular filtration, as reflected by increases in blood urea nitrogen and serum creatinine concentrations. Nonoliguric renal failure eventually occurs.

Fortunately the majority of cases of nephrotoxicity are reversible, reflecting the regenerative capacity of the primary cellular target. The true incidence of aminoglycoside-associated nephrotoxicity in unknown. As with the reported data describing aminoglycoside-associated ototoxicity, the incidence of this adverse effect is very much dependent on the definitions and methods used by the various clinical investigators. Data on children are lacking.

Allergic reactions, including rash, fever, and eosinophilia, are uncommon and occur in approximately 1–3% of persons who receive aminoglycosides.

Neuromuscular blockade associated with or induced by aminoglycosides is an uncommon adverse reaction. It leads to weakness in the skeletal muscles and may precipitate respiratory depression. The exact mechanism responsible for this adverse effect is unknown, but it may be a result of competitive antagonism of acetylcholine activity at the neuromuscular junction, both prejunctionally by inhibition of transmitter release and postsynaptically by a decrease in postsynaptic sensitivity to the neurotransmitter. Early epidemiologic evaluations indicate that neomycin is most likely to cause this adverse effect: neomycin > kanamycin > amikacin > gentamicin = tobramycin. Persons at particular risk of having aminoglycoside-induced neuromuscular blockade include those with myasthenia gravis, severe hypocalcemia, or infantile botulism or those who have recently received neuromuscular blocking agents. This adverse effect has been most commonly reported after intrapleural or intraperitoneal instillation of an aminoglycoside, but it has also been found in persons receiving aminoglycoside antibiotics via any route of administration. Intravenous infusion of a calcium salt (e.g., calcium chloride) successfully antagonizes this adverse drug effect.

Drug Interactions. Clinically significant drug-drug interactions with aminoglycoside antibiotics are rare. The most commonly implicated compounds involve those which possess some inherent propensity to induce ototoxicity or nephrotoxicity. Drugs frequently believed to interact with aminoglycoside antibiotics, resulting in clinically important effects, are shown in Table 14–32. The coadministration of an aminoglycoside with a loop diuretic has been suggested to enhance the ototoxic potential of both these agents.

TABLE 14–32. Drug Interactions with Aminoglycoside Antibiotics

Interacting Drug(s) or Drug Class	Nature of Interaction
Amphotericin B	Additive nephrotoxicity
Cephalothin-cephaloridine	Enhanced nephrotoxicity and ototoxicity
Cisplatin	Additive nephrotoxicity
Indomethacin	Reduced renal clearance
Loop diuretics*†	Enhanced ototoxicity
Neuromuscular blocking agents	Enhanced neuromuscular blockade, especially in low birth weight infants
Penicillins, especially carbenicillin-ticarcillin	Physiochemical interaction in vivo or in vitro reducing aminoglycoside activity
Vancomycin†	Enhanced nephrotoxicity

*Bumetanide, ethacrynic acid, furosemide.
†Rarely of clinical significance (see text for discussion).

Although potentiation of ototoxic effects with this drug combination has been observed in animals, its clinical relevance in humans, particularly with furosemide, is suspect. Similarly it is logical to assume an additive or synergistic renal toxic effect when known nephrotoxins (e.g., amphotericin B, cisplatin) are coadministered with aminoglycosides. Accurate discrimination of such effects in humans is difficult. Nevertheless, persons receiving multiple drugs known to affect renal function adversely should be monitored closely for evidence of renal damage. If such damage occurs, appropriate dose or drug selection adjustments should be made.

THE GLYCOPEPTIDES, STREPTOGRAMINS, AND OXAZOLIDINONES

Gram-positive bacterial pathogens remain one of the most common causes of infections arising in pediatric patients. Furthermore, the number of serious infections caused by methicillin-resistant *S. aureus* and penicillin-resistant *S. pneumoniae* are increasing at an alarming rate. For decades the prototypical glycopeptide vancomycin possessed potent in vitro activity against a broad spectrum of clinically important pathogens. Unfortunately, gram-positive pathogens have developed a host of mechanisms to evade antibacterial activity, including the emergence of glycopeptide-resistant *Enterococcus*, particularly *E. faecium*. As a result, investigators have worked diligently to identify effective alternatives to vancomycin, leading to the discovery of the streptogramin and oxazolidinone class of antibiotics.

Mechanism and Spectrum of Activity. The glycopeptides (vancomycin and teicoplanin), like the β-lactam antibiotics, inhibit cell wall formation of susceptible bacteria by prohibiting peptidoglycan synthesis. These drugs complex with the terminal amino acyl-D-alanyl-D-alanine portion of bacterial cell wall building blocks, which inhibits the peptidoglycan polymerase and the transpeptidation reactions. In contrast, the streptogramin (quinupristin-dalfopristin) and oxazolidinone (linezolid) antibiotics are protein synthesis inhibitors.

Vancomycin resistance, particularly among *Enterococcus* species, is occurring at an alarming rate. The VanA phenotype is encoded by a gene located on a plasmid that is easily transferable by means of conjugation to other enterococci and renders the pathogen resistant to both vancomycin and teicoplanin. The VanB phenotype is also transferable, coding resistance to vancomycin but not to teicoplanin. Moreover, in the laboratory *S. aureus* can receive and express enterococcal-resistant genes, conferring cross-species resistance. This ability heightens the concern regarding the widespread staphylococcal resistance to vancomycin.

Quinupristin and dalfopristin are two different, naturally occurring compounds administered in combination at a 30:70 ratio in a commercially available product called Synercid. Quinupristin and dalfopristin sequentially bind to different sites on the 50S ribosome subunit, which results in a stable ternary drug–ribosome complex that prevents newly synthesized peptide chains from extruding from this complex. Bacterial resistance to streptogramins can develop through decreased ribosomal binding by either drug component or through efflux mechanisms.

An oxazolidinone, linezolid (and eperezolid), inhibits protein synthesis by inhibiting the initiation complex at the 30S ribosome subunit. This binding interacts with a translational component involved in mRNA binding during the initiation of translation. As a result of this unique mechanism of action for the oxazolidinones, no cross resistance with currently available antimicrobials has been identified. To date, a mechanism for bacterial resistance to oxazolidinones has not been defined.

Comparative in vitro antibacterial activity of these agents is shown in Table 14–33.

Clinical Indications. Vancomycin is indicated for the treatment of infections caused by methicillin-resistant *S. aureus* and coagulase-negative staphylococci. This drug may also be used as an alternative to β-lactam therapy in the treatment of streptococcal and staphylococcal infections in penicillin-allergic children. It is also indicated as oral therapy in infants and children with antibiotic-associated colitis caused by *Clostridium difficile.*

The use of vancomycin as part of an empirical antibiotic regimen in the treatment of febrile, immunocompromised, or critically ill persons remains controversial. Although it is clear that gram-positive organisms account for an increasing number of infections in this patient population, the empirical use of vancomycin, as contrasted with adding it after infection with a susceptible organism is established, appears to have no benefit.

The clinical position of the streptogramin and oxazolidinone classes of antibiotics is evolving. The clinical utility of quinupristin-dalfopristin and linezolid appears to be in the treatment of persons with suspected or documented infections caused by vancomycin-resistant *E. faecium* and possibly glycopeptide-intermediate-resistant *S. aureus* (GISA; strains of *S. aureus* with vancomycin MICs of 8–16 μg/mL). Both drug classes have been shown to be effective in the treatment of gram-positive pneumonia and of skin and skin-structure infections.

Metabolism and Disposition. The glycopeptide antibiotics are not absorbed after oral administration. The oral use of glycopeptides in the treatment of *C. difficile* antibiotic-associated pseudomembranous colitis exploits this pharmacokinetic characteristic. Comparison of the pharmacokinetic characteristics of vancomycin relative to a patient's age's is shown in Table 14–34. Far fewer data are available on the pharmacokinetics of teicoplanin or on the streptogramins or oxazolidinones in pediatrics. Comparative disposition characteristics for these later drugs in adults are shown in Table 14–35.

Recommended Dosing and Dosing Strategies. Usual dosing recommendations for vancomycin are outlined in Table 14–36, teicoplanin dosing suggestions are shown in Table 14–37, and those for linezolid and quinupristin-dalfopristin in Table 14–38. For the treatment of systemic infection, vancomycin and teicoplanin are administered intravenously. Because vancomycin is very irritating, intramuscular injection should be avoided. Vancomycin should be diluted in a large volume (minimum dilution: 5 mg/mL) and administered as a controlled 1–2 hour infusion because of its irritant properties. Although vancomycin can be infused intravenously for 30 minutes without incident, rapid infusions (<60 minutes) are often complicated by "red man" syndrome (see Adverse Effects). In contrast, teicoplanin appears to be much less irritating than vancomycin and may be administered by intravenous bolus injection, intravenous infusion, or intramuscular injection. Better than 90% bioavailability is achieved by the latter route.

The use of intraventricular or intrathecal vancomycin to augment systemic administration in the treatment of persons with meningitis or infected central nervous system shunts and reservoirs is controversial. Intraventricular doses have ranged from 5 to 20 mg administered daily, with close monitoring of vancomycin concentrations in the cerebrospinal fluid. Current practice suggests targeting trough cerebrospinal fluid vancomycin concentrations at values of <10 mg/L.

Serum Drug Concentration Monitoring. For decades the monitoring of serum peak and trough vancomycin concentrations has been

TABLE 14–33. Comparative in Vitro Activity of Glycopeptide, Streptogramin, and Oxazolidinone Antibiotics

	Reported Range of MIC_{90} Values (mg/L)			
	Glycopeptide			
Organism	Vancomycin	Teicoplanin	Quinupristin-Dalfopristin	Linezolid
Staphylococci				
S. aureus				
Penicillin-sensitive	0.78–1	0.2–1		
Penicillin-resistant	1–3.12	1–3.12		
Methicillin-sensitive	0.78–1	0.39–1	1	2–4
Methicillin-resistant	0.5–3.12	0.2–3.12	2	0.5–4
Coagulase-negative staphylococci				
Methicillin-sensitive			0.5	2
S. epidermidis	2	0.25–2		
Methicillin-resistant			1	1–2
S. epidermidis	2–3.1	0.25–12.5		
S. hominis		0.5		
S. haemolyticus	4	1–32		
S. saprophyticus	1.56	0.78–1.56		
Streptococci				
Group A *Streptococcus*	0.5–0.78	0.03–0.25	0.5	
*S. pneumoniae**	≤0.25–0.78	0.12–0.2	1	0.5–1
Group B *Streptococcus*	0.5–1	0.12–0.4		
S. bovis	1	0.4–0.5		
S. milleri	1	0.03		
S. mitis	0.5	0.015		
S. sanguis	0.5	0.015		
Viridans group	1	0.1–1	2	
Group C *Streptococcus*	0.5	0.1–0.25		
Group F *Streptococcus*	1	0.5		
Group G *Streptococcus*	0.5	0.5		
Enterococcus	3.1–4	0.2–1.6		
E. faecalis	1–4	≤0.024–3.1	8	1–4
Vancomycin-resistant	R		14	2–4
E. faecium	0.5–2		2	2–4
Vancomycin-resistant	R		1	2–4

advocated. Peak concentrations are most often obtained either immediately after a 1- or 2-hour intravenous infusion or 30–60 minutes after completion of a 1-hour infusion, as some investigators suggest. Trough concentrations are obtained immediately before the next dose. Recommended serum vancomycin concentrations are 25–35 mg/L (peak) and 5–10 mg/L (trough). The data supporting routine monitoring of vancomycin concentrations are very limited, particularly in pediatric patients, as with aminoglycoside antibiotics. Such routine monitoring can no longer be recommended in children. Data support the monitoring of vancomycin serum concentrations only in those who are not responding to usual doses, those with compromised renal function, and those undergoing dialysis procedures. Currently there are no guidelines for therapeutic drug monitoring during teicoplanin, quinupristin-dalfopristin, or linezolid therapy.

Adverse Effects

Vancomycin. A large number of adverse effects have been associated with vancomycin administration, most of which have been attributed to impurities in earlier pharmaceutical formulations. Newer, purer formulations are claimed to be associated with a markedly reduced incidence of associated adverse effects.

The most common adverse effects associated with vancomycin and teicoplanin are outlined in Table 14–39. An early incidence of drug-induced thrombophlebitis, fever, and chills in as many as 50% of persons treated with the drug in the 1950s decreased mark-

TABLE 14–34. Pharmacokinetics of Vancomycin Relative to Age

Pharmacokinetic Parameter	Premature Neonate	Infant	Child	Adult
$t_{1/2\beta}$ (hr)	7–10	5–6	2–4	1.5–4
Vd_{ss} (L/kg)	0.5–0.7	0.5	0.3–0.5	0.5–1
Cl (mL/min/kg)	0.6–0.7	0.8–1.5	1–2	1.2–2

$t_{1/2\beta}$ = elimination half-life; Vd_{ss} = steady-state volume of distribution; Cl = body clearance (values will change depending on renal function).

TABLE 14–35. Comparative Pharmacokinetics of Glycopeptide, Streptogramin, and Oxazolidinone Antibiotics

Pharmacokinetics Parameter	Teicoplanin*	Quinupristin†	Dalfopristin	Linezolid‡
C_{max} (mg/L)		2.5–3§	7–9§	18‖
%Protein bound	90	55–78	11–26	31
$t_{1/2\beta}$ (hr)	45–70	1	0.75	3
Vd (L/kg)				
Cl (mL/min)		0.8§	0.9¶	100–200
F (%)				100
Metabolism	3%	Extensive	Extensive	Liver/renal

C_{max} = maximum concentration; $t_{1/2\beta}$ = elimination half-life; Vd = volume of distribution; Cl = body clearance; *F* = bioavailability.
*Teicoplanin available for intravenous and intramuscular administration only.
†Quinupristin-dalfopristin available as a combination product for intravenous administration only.
‡Linezolid available for intravenous and oral administration.
§Intravenous dose: 7.5 mg/kg.
‖Oral dose: 625 mg.
¶Values in liters per kilogram per hour.

TABLE 14–36. Vancomycin Dosing Recommendations

Premature Infants (<36 Wk Postconceptional Age)
Dose: 20 mg/kg/day divided q12hr

Neonates
Postnatal age ≤7 days
Body weight <1,200 g: 15 mg/kg/day q24hr 1,200–2,000 g: 20 mg/kg/day divided q12hr
Body weight >2,000 g: 30 mg/kg/day divided q12hr
Postnatal age >7 days
Body weight <1,200 g: 15 mg/kg/day q24hr
Body weight ≥1,200 g: 30 mg/kg/day divided q8hr

Infants Aged >1 Mo and Children
Dose: 45–60 mg/kg/day divided q6–8hr

Infants Aged >1 Mo and Children with Staphylococcal Central Nervous System Infection
Dose: 60 mg/kg/day divided q6–8hr

Adults
Normal renal function: 0.5 g q6hr or 1 g q12hr
Dosing interval in renal impairment
CrCl >90 mL/min: administer q6hr
CrCl 70–89 mL/min: administer q8hr
CrCl 46–69 mL/min: administer q12hr
CrCl 30–45 mL/min: administer q18hr
CrCl 15–29 mL/min: administer q24hr

Dialysis
Intermittent hemofiltration or peritoneal dialysis: no dose adjustment necessary
Continuous hemofiltration or peritoneal dialysis: no dose adjustment necessary

Intrathecal Administration*
Neonates: 5–10 mg/day
Children: 5–20 mg/day
Adults: 20 mg/day

Oral Administration
Children: 10–50 mg/kg/day divided q6–8hr; max 2 g/day
Adults: 0.5–2 g/day divided q6–8hr

CrCl = creatinine clearance.
*Monitor vancomycin concentration in cerebrospinal fluid to guide dosing (see text for details).

TABLE 14–37. Suggested Teicoplanin Dosing Recommendations

Children (Age 3–12 Yr)*
Dose: 10 mg/kg q12hr for 3 doses, followed by 6–10 mg/kg once daily

Adults†
Dose: 400 mg on day 1, followed by 200–400 mg once daily

Renal Disease
Dose adjustments as necessary

These dosing recommendations are preliminary; higher doses, administered more frequently, may be required for seriously ill persons.
*Seriously ill children may require 12 mg/kg/day.
†Seriously ill adults may require 6–12 mg/kg every 12 hours for 1–2 days, followed by 6 mg/kg once daily.

TABLE 14–38. Linezolid and Quinupristin-Dalfopristin Dosing Recommendations

Linezolid
Children: 10 mg/kg q8–12hr*
Adults: 600 mg q12hr IV or PO

Available Forms
Tablets: 400 mg, 600 mg
Oral suspension: 100 mg/5 mL
Intravenous injection: infuse IV for 30–120 min

Quinupristin-Dalfopristin
Children: 7.5 mg/kg q8–12hr*
Adults: 7.5 mg/kg q8–12hr
Dialysis: no dose adjustment necessary for peritoneal dialysis or hemodialysis

Available Forms
Intravenous injection: infuse in saline-free solutions for 60 min

*Suggested pediatric dosing (pediatric doses under investigation).

TABLE 14–39. Common Adverse Effects Associated with Vancomycin, Teicoplanin, Quinupristin-Dalfopristin, and Linezolid

Vancomycin	**Quinupristin-Dalfopristin**
Phlebitis (~10%)	Phlebitis (30–75%)
"Red man" ("red neck") syndrome	Increased conjugated bilirubin (?)
Nephrotoxicity (?)	Arthralgia (6%)
Ototoxicity (?)	Myalgias (8.5%)
Neutropenia (<2%)	**Linezolid**
Teicoplanin	Gastrointestinal disturbances (diarrhea 8.3%)
Injection site intolerance (~3%)	Headache (6.5%)
Hypersensitivity reaction (~5%)	Increase in liver and renal function tests (?)
Nephrotoxicity (?)	Neutropenia (may be severe)
Ototoxicity (?)	
Neutropenia (?)	

Numbers in parentheses represent approximate incidence.

edly to less than 10% in the 1980s. These percentages may decrease even further with the use of purer formulations.

The ''red man'' or ''red neck'' syndrome, which is characterized by flushing, pruritus, tachycardia, and an erythematous rash involving the face, neck, upper trunk, back, and arms, is associated with the rapid intravenous administration of vancomycin. This syndrome has not been reported after teicoplanin administration. The ''red man'' syndrome is most likely a result of vancomycin-induced histamine release. Pretreatment with antihistamines (e.g., diphenhydramine) or slowing the infusion rate to less than 7.5–15 mg/min or both will reduce the frequency and severity of this reaction.

Ototoxicity and nephrotoxicity have long been attributed to vancomycin therapy. Nevertheless, the true incidence of these important adverse effects is low. Only casual relationships, at best, are likely between vancomycin administration, resultant serum vancomycin concentrations, and auditory or renal toxicity. Current estimates suggest that the incidence of vancomycin-associated ototoxicity and nephrotoxicity approximates 2% and 5%, respectively, and that the occurrence of these adverse effects may depend on the presence of other confounding variables such as concurrent administration of known ototoxic drugs (e.g., aminoglycosides, cisplatin, diuretics), patient age, and severity of disease.

A reversible neutropenia with the use of vancomycin has been described with increasing frequency and may depend on dose and duration of therapy (administration for >14 days).

Teicoplanin. The lack of a clinically available formulation of teicoplanin limits a critical assessment of the overall safety profile. With the exception of the absence of the ''red man'' syndrome, preliminary safety data on teicoplanin suggest a profile similar to that seen with vancomycin.

Quinupristin-Dalfopristin and Linezolid. The occurrence of adverse effects associated with quinupristin-dalfopristin administration appears high. In clinical trials, approximately 63% of persons receiving the drug had at least one adverse event. The most common adverse effects associated with quinupristin-dalfopristin are shown in Table 14–39. When administered via a peripheral intravenous line, quinupristin-dalfopristin appears to be very irritating, resulting in the drug-associated, venous-related events described in 35–75% of persons receiving at least one infusion. The drug combination may also be associated with a high incidence of myalgias and arthralgias. The mechanism of this drug-induced reaction is unknown and is reversible on discontinuation of use. In some persons this reaction resolves when the dosing interval is increased to 12 hours or with the administration of analgesics or both.

TABLE 14–40. Possible Drug Interactions with Vancomycin, Quinupristin-Dalfopristin, and Linezolid

Vancomycin (Teicoplanin)
Possible additive ototoxicity and nephrotoxicity with other agents (e.g., loop diuretics, aminoglycosides, amphotericin B, cisplatin)
Quinupristin-Dalfopristin (Synercid)
Cytochrome P-450 3A4 (CYP-450 3A4) inhibitor blocks metabolism of carbamazepine, cyclosporine, corticosteroids, benzodiazepine, cisapride, and terfenadine
Linezolid
Reversible, nonselective inhibitor of monoamine oxidase; may intensify effects of sympathomimetic and serotonergic drugs (e.g., epinephrine, dopamine)

Linezolid appears to be relatively well tolerated after either oral or intravenous administration (see Table 14–39). However, the drug is a reversible, nonselective inhibitor of monoamine oxidase and therefore has the potential to augment both endogenously and exogenously administered sympathomimetic and serotonergic drugs. More experience is needed to assess the clinical relevance of these possible adverse effects and interactions. Recently a warning about severe neutropenia associated with this drug has been given.

Possible drug interactions with these classes of antimicrobial agents are shown in Table 14–40. As already discussed, the possibility of linezolid-induced interactions resulting from its ability to inhibit monamine oxidase activity requires continued evaluation.

MACROLIDE AND AZALIDE ANTIBIOTICS

The macrolide antibiotics represent a group of drugs that have been used extensively in pediatric practice. This class of drugs, first reported in 1952, was referred to as ''macrolides'' because the large macrocyclic ring structure is the primary nucleus of each of these agents. Although the immense clinical utility of erythromycin spawned the development of a large number of related analogs, only a few are actually used in clinical practice. Macrolide antibiotics and the subclass azalide antibiotics of current clinical interest are shown in Table 14–41 and comparative in vitro antibacterial activity in Table 14–42.

For more than 3 decades, erythromycin has been the primary macrolide in use. The drug and its many different salt formulations (see Table 14–41) are commonly used in the treatment of infections of the upper and lower respiratory tract, particularly in persons who are intolerant of or allergic to penicillins. Numerous attempts to modify the basic nucleus to enhance clinical effectiveness and reduce the incidence of distressing erythromycin-associated adverse gastrointestinal effects have been met with limited success until recently. The one identifiable end product of these investigations was the development of a large number of different pharmaceutical formulations of erythromycin. Many of these formulations are used clinically today, although the newer ones resulted in no significant decrease in the occurrence of adverse gastrointestinal effects. In contrast, the macrolide clarithromycin and the azalide azithromycin have a broader spectrum of activity than does erythro-

TABLE 14–41. Macrolide and Azalide Antibiotics

Azithromycin
Clarithromycin
Erythromycin
Enteric-coated pellets
Enteric-coated particles
Enteric-coated tablets
Base, ethylsuccinate, and estolate salts
Ointment
Troleandomycin

The azalide antibiotics are a subclass of the macrolide class of antibiotics.

mycin (see Table 14–42), and yet they cause fewer adverse gastrointestinal effects.

Mechanism of Action. The macrolide and azalide antibiotics competitively bind to the 50S ribosomal subunit, thus antagonizing bacterial RNA-dependent protein synthesis. This binding interferes with translocation of transfer RNA and formation of peptide bonds. The binding site on the 50S ribosome subunit appears to be the same target site used by other antibiotics, most notably chloramphenicol and clindamycin. This similarity in the site of antibacterial action of these different drug classes may result in antibacterial antagonism after coadministration to the same person. A comparison of the in vitro activity of selected macrolide antibiotics and the azalide azithromycin against important pathogens is shown in Table 14–42.

Bacterial resistance to the macrolide and azalide antibiotics involves alteration of the ribosomal target site, thus reducing or preventing drug binding. This alteration in binding results from bacteria that have acquired the ability to methylate macrolide-specific ribosomal target sites. All macrolide antibiotics are inducers of methylase activity. Bacterial resistance to erythromycin implies cross-resistance to other macrolides regardless of their ring structure (i.e., 14-membered clarithromycin, 15-membered azithromycin). Permeability mutations have also been reported.

Metabolism and Disposition. After oral administration the macrolide and azalide antibiotics are only moderately well absorbed. The bioavailability of erythromycin is dependent on the formulation. Among the preparations frequently prescribed for children, ethylsuccinate is the most erratic in its absorption. Comparison of the pharmacokinetics of erythromycin, clarithromycin, and azithromycin is shown in Table 14–43.

Once in the bloodstream, the macrolide and azalide agents are widely distributed throughout the body. Serum protein binding is modest and variable. Moreover, in contrast to the β-lactam and aminoglycoside antibiotics, significant amounts of these drugs are found in the intracellular fluid space, as contrasted with the extracellular space. In fact, for azithromycin, more than 95% of the drug in the body is in the intracellular space.

All three of the currently available macrolide and azalide drugs—erythromycin, clarithromycin, and azithromycin—undergo extensive hepatic metabolism. In the case of clarithromycin, the 14-hydroxy metabolite, which accumulates in the circulation to concentrations that exceed those of the parent drug, is also

TABLE 14–42. Comparative in Vitro Activity of Selected Macrolide and Azalide Antibiotics

	Erythromycin		Clarithromycin		14-Hydroxy-clarithromycin		Azithromycin	
Organism	**MIC_{50}**	**MIC_{90}**	**MIC_{50}**	**MIC_{90}**	**MIC_{50}**	**MIC_{90}**	**MIC_{50}**	**MIC_{90}**
Gram-Positive Aerobes								
Methicillin-sensitive *Staphylococcus aureus*	0.12–0.5	>128	0.06–0.25	>128	0.12	>128	0.12–1	>128
Coagulase-negative staphylococci	8–32	>128	4	>128	4	>128	16	>128
Group A *Streptococcus*	<0.03–0.12	0.03–4	0.012–0.03	0.012–2	0.015	0.03	0.12–1	0.12–4
Streptococcus pneumoniae	0.03–0.12	0.03–1	0.015–0.06	0.015–0.5	0.008	0.015	0.06–0.5	0.12–2
Group B *Streptococcus*	<0.03–0.12	<0.03–0.25	<0.03–0.12	<0.03–0.25	0.06	0.06	0.12–0.5	0.12–0.5
Erythromycin-sensitive *Enterococcus*	1–2	4	0.5–1	2			8	16
Erythromycin-resistant *Enterococcus*	>32		>32				>32	
Listeria monocytogenes	0.25–0.5	0.5–2	0.12–0.25	0.12–2	0.5	0.5	1–2	2–4
Gram-Negative Aerobes								
Moraxella catarrhalis	0.12–0.5	0.25–2	0.06–0.12	0.25–1	0.06	0.12	<0.015–0.12	0.03–0.12
Neisseria gonorrhoeae	0.12–0.5	0.25–2	0.125–0.25	0.25–2	0.25	0.5	<0.025–0.12	0.05–0.25
Legionella pneumophila	0.5–1	1–2	0.12–0.25	0.25	0.25	0.5	0.5	2
Haemophilus influenzae	1–8	4–32	1–8	2–16	2	4	0.25–4	0.5–4
Campylobacter	0.5–2	1–4	0.5–2	1–8			0.25	0.5
Helicobacter pylori	0.12	0.25	0.03	0.03	0.06	0.06	0.25	0.25
Anaerobes								
Bacteroides fragilis	2–8	4–32	1–2	2–8	1	1	2–3.12	2–6.25
Bacteroides (other species)	0.25–4	4–64+	0.25–4	2–64	0.12	1	0.25	1
Clostridium perfringens	1	1	0.25–0.5	0.5–2	0.5	0.5	0.25–0.78	0.25–0.78
Propionibacterium acnes	<0.03	<0.03	<0.03	0.25	0.03	0.06	<0.004	0.03
Anaerobic gram-positive cocci	<0.12–2	2–32+	0.25–2	4–32+	1	4	0.25–1	2–4
Chlamydia								
Chlamydia trachomatis	0.06–1	0.06–2	0.004–0.062	0.008–0.125			0.031–0.063	

MIC_{50} and MIC_{90} = minimum inhibitory concentrations for 50% and 90% of tested pathogens, respectively (in milligrams per liter).

TABLE 14–43. Single-Dose Pharmacokinetics of Selected Macrolide and Azalide Antibiotics in Adults

Parameter	Erythromycin Base	Clarithromycin	Azithromycin	14-Hydroxyclarithromycin
C_{max} (μg/mL)*	0.3–1.9	2.1	0.4	0.6–1
t_{max} (hr)	4	1.8	2.3	1.8
$t_{1/2\beta}$ (hr)	2	4.3	35–40	5.5–7.2
Vd (L/kg)	0.64	NA	23	60
AUC (μg hr/mL)	14.2	11.8 (AUC_{0-12})	2.36 (AUC_{0-24})	35
F (%)	—†	55	37	NA
Protein binding (%)	65–90	65–70	7–50	NA
Urine recovery	5–10%	18%	12%	NA

C_{max} = maximum serum drug concentrations; t_{max} = time after dose to reach C_{max}; $t_{1/2\beta}$ = elimination half-life; Vd = volume of distribution; AUC = area under the serum concentration–time curve after a 500 mg oral dose; F = bioavailability; NA = not available.
*For 500 mg dose.
†Dependent on formulation.

antimicrobially active (see Table 14–42). In general, less than 20% of these drugs is excreted in the urine as parent compound.

These rather unusual disposition characteristics have important clinical consequences. The relatively modest absorption and large volume of distribution result in rather low serum and extracellular fluid concentrations. Thus, although all macrolide and azalide agents are potent in vitro against a wide range of bacterial pathogens, they are not always clinically effective against these same organisms (e.g., *H. influenzae*) because of the low concentrations achieved in the blood and extracellular fluid. In contrast, their high intracellular concentrations enhance their effectiveness against intracellular pathogens such as *Mycoplasma, Chlamydia,* and *Legionella.* The clinical indications for the macrolide and azalide antibiotics in pediatrics are outlined in Table 14–44.

Available Formulations. A large number of different salt and ester formulations of erythromycin are available for clinical use (Table 14–45). Delayed-release erythromycin formulations include oral capsules containing enteric-coated pellets (e.g., Eryc); tablets containing enteric-coated particles (e.g., PCE Dispertab); enteric-coated tablets; film-coated tablets; ethylsuccinate drops, granules, suspension, and chewable tablets; and estolate salt as capsules, tablets, and suspension. The stearate and ethylsuccinate forms remain susceptible to gastric acid inactivation, whereas the estolate salt is much more resistant to acid inactivation. As mentioned earlier, true differences among these various salt (ester) forms and drug absorption, patient tolerance, and clinical efficacy appear minimal.

Erythromycin is available for intravenous administration as either a gluceptate or lactobionate salt. These formulations are usually diluted in either dextrose or saline solution to concentrations that do not exceed 5 mg/mL and administered intermittently for 20–60 minutes.

TABLE 14–44. Clinical Indications for Macrolide and Azalide Antibiotics in Pediatrics

- Alternative to β-lactams for streptococcal pharyngitis
- Alternative for persons allergic to β-lactam antibiotics
- New analogs (clarithromycin and azithromycin) for infections caused by *Haemophilus influenzae* (typeable and nontypeable) and in the treatment of acute otitis media
- Infections caused by *Mycoplasma pneumoniae* and *Legionella*
- Infections caused by *Chlamydia* and *Ureaplasma*
- Ophthalmic infections (newborn gonococcal ophthalmitis prophylaxis)

Recommended Dosing and Dosing Strategies. Erythromycin dosing recommendations relative to age and chemical formulation are outlined in Table 14–45. Newer analogs, which have a longer $t_{1/2\beta}$, are given much less frequently than erythromycin. Although these drugs are extensively metabolized by the liver, dosage adjustments do not appear necessary unless the patient has severe hepatic insufficiency. However, significant renal function impairment may necessitate dosage adjustment as a result of metabolite accumulation. Data defining specific dose reduction recommendations for macrolide use in persons with hepatic or renal disease are lacking. In persons with severe hepatic or renal insufficiency, it is recommended that the clinician either make a slight dose reduction (25% of daily dose) or maintain a normal dose but prolong the dosing interval. Dialysis techniques would not be expected to remove much macrolide from the body, considering the degree of protein binding, extensive tissue distribution, extensive hepatic metabolism, and biliary excretion of these drugs.

Adverse Effects. Overall, the safety profiles for erythromycin and its various salt formulations and analogs are excellent. The incidence of serious debilitating adverse effects with the use of these drugs is low. The most common adverse effect associated with erythromycin use is gastrointestinal discomfort. Nausea, vomiting, severe abdominal cramping, and epigastric distress have all been reported in varying frequencies with the use of erythromycin. Such problems are the most common reason that patients discontinue therapy.

For decades, most clinicians have suggested administering erythromycin with food to reduce the degree and extent of associated gastrointestinal discomfort. Erythromycin appears to mimic the effects of the gastrointestinal polypeptide motilin, which stimulates interdigestive (between meals) but not postprandial intestinal motility. Drug administration after a meal takes full advantage of the ameliorative effect of food on the promotilin activity of erythromycin.

Another approach to altering the incidence and severity of this important adverse drug reaction involved modifications of salt formulations of erythromycin. However, erythromycin-associated gastrointestinal distress occurs with all salt formulations. This discomfort can be so severe that many patients discontinue their therapy and refuse subsequent courses of erythromycin. Drug-induced gastrointestinal distress does not appear to be a common problem

TABLE 14–45. Dosing Guidelines for Macrolide and Azalide Antibiotics

Erythromycin
Neonates
- Postnatal age ≤7 days: 20 mg/kg/day divided q12hr PO
- Postnatal age >7 days:
  - Weight ≤1,200 g: 20 mg/kg/day divided q12hr PO
  - Weight >1,200 g: 30 mg/kg/day divided q8hr PO
- Prophylaxis of neonatal gonococcal or *Chlamydia* conjunctivitis: apply ointment into each conjunctival sac once

Infants and children
- Base and ethylsuccinate: 40 mg/kg/day divided q6hr PO
- Estolate: 30–50 mg/kg/day divided q8–12hr PO
- Stearate: 20–40 mg/kg/day divided q6hr PO
- Infusion*: 20–40 mg/kg/day (max 4 g/day) divided q6hr IV

Adults
- Estolate, stearate, or base: 250–500 mg q6hr PO
- Ethylsuccinate: 400 mg q6hr PO
- Infusion: 1–2 g/day divided q6hr IV or as continuous infusion for 24 hr

Clarithromycin
Children: 15 mg/kg/day divided q12hr PO
Adults: 250–500 mg q12hr PO

Azithromycin
Children: 10 mg/kg on day 1, followed by 5 mg/kg once daily for 4 days PO
Adults: 500 mg on day 1, followed by 250 mg once daily for 4 days PO; *or* 250 to 500 mg once daily IV†

*Infuse intravenously for 60 minutes.
†Infuse intravenously 30–60 minutes.

with two newer analogs, clarithromycin and azithromycin, which suggests a potential clinical advantage of these drugs over earlier erythromycin preparations.

More serious adverse effects associated with erythromycin administration include hepatic, otic, and cardiac toxicity. Erythromycin-induced hepatotoxicity was once believed to be a direct result of the salt formulation used, with the estolate salt most often deemed the hepatotoxin. However, all forms of erythromycin, including the base formulation, have been associated with this adverse effect. In addition, the clinical course of erythromycin-associated hepatotoxicity is strongly suggestive of a hypersensitivity reaction. Signs and symptoms are usually manifested after 2–3 weeks of erythromycin therapy in persons who have never before received the drug, whereas symptoms may occur within 1–2 days in persons who have taken erythromycin in the recent past. The incidence of this hypersensitivity reaction is unknown but is estimated to be approximately 0.1% in children and 0.25% in adults who receive the drug. Any person who develops severe nausea and epigastric distress that mimics acute cholecystitis, with or without an elevated body temperature, increased liver enzyme values, and peripheral eosinophilia in the blood should be evaluated for this reaction.

Erythromycin-associated ototoxicity and cardiotoxicity appear to be most frequent after parenteral administration, often after higher doses are administered. These clinical findings, combined with the near lack of association with oral administration, suggests that a relationship may exist between the occurrence of these adverse effects and the very high blood concentrations of parent drug achieved with parenteral administration. Bilateral sensorineural hearing loss, usually in the range of 30–80 decibels, has been reported and occurs most commonly in elderly persons (i.e., after the fifth decade of life). Complete normalization of hearing deficits occurs promptly after the drug is discontinued.

In contrast, erythromycin-associated cardiotoxicity represents a serious, life-threatening adverse effect that has been described in both children and adults. Like erythromycin-associated ototoxicity, the mechanism of cardiotoxicity is unknown, but it is unlikely to result from the lactobionate salt, considering the safety of lactobionate as a key component of organ transplant preservation fluids. Prolongation of the QT interval and ventricular tachydysrhythmias are the most common cardiac abnormalities reported. Dysrhythmias associated with intravenous erythromycin lactobionate therapy are similar to those observed in persons receiving quinidine or in persons with prolonged QT syndrome. Clinical findings are essentially the same as those in persons with QT interval prolongation, frequent premature ventricular contractions, or torsades de pointes. Thus the treatment of this adverse effect includes discontinuation of erythromycin and magnesium administration. Adverse otic and cardiac effects do not appear to be associated with intravenous azithromycin administration.

Drug Interactions. A number of important drug-drug interactions have reportedly occurred in persons receiving macrolide antibiotics. Drugs that result in clinically important drug interactions with macrolides are shown in Table 14–46. One of the earliest drug interactions described with macrolides involved the so-called steroid-sparing effect attributed to troleandomycin. This therapeutic drug interaction was often used by the pharmaceutical manufacturer as a promotional tool to encourage the use of this drug in persons with airway diseases, particularly if they were receiving corticosteroid therapy.

The macrolide antibiotics appear to interfere competitively with the hepatic metabolism of drugs that are metabolized by the cytochrome P-450 3A4 isoenzyme system. Coadministration of a macrolide antibiotic usually results in the accumulation of the long-term medication, often leading to adverse drug effects. Numerous cases of serious theophylline, cisapride, terfenadine, and carbamazepine intoxication have been reported after a macrolide has been added to the drug regimen of a person receiving one of these other medications. In contrast, no metabolic-based drug-drug interactions have been reported for the azalides.

TABLE 14–46. Drug Interactions with Macrolide and Azalide Antibiotics

Macrolides (Erythromycin and Clarithromycin)*
Carbamazepine
Cisapride
Corticosteroids
Cyclosporine
Digoxin
Terfenadine
Theophylline
Warfarin
Azalides (Azithromycin)
No metabolic-based drug-drug interactions with azalides

*Coadministration of erythromycin and clarithromycin decreases their body clearance, leading to accumulation and toxic effects (see text for discussion).

CHLORAMPHENICOL

Spectrum of Activity. Chloramphenicol was one of the first truly broad-spectrum antibiotics. The drug inhibits bacterial protein synthesis by binding to the 50S subunit of the ribosome. Unlike some of the other protein synthesis inhibitors, chloramphenicol is considered a bacteriostatic rather than a bactericidal drug. However, bactericidal activity can be demonstrated at clinically achievable concentrations against *S. pneumoniae, H. influenzae,* and meningococcus. Chloramphenicol possesses a broad spectrum of activity, including activity against most gram-positive and gram-negative aerobic and anaerobic bacteria, *Rickettsia, Chlamydia,* certain *Mycoplasma* species, and the molluscous phase of *Schistosoma.* Representative in vitro antibacterial activity is shown in Table 14–47.

Clinical Indications. Historically, chloramphenicol has enjoyed a position of prominence in the treatment of children with serious infections, including bacterial meningitis. With the availability of the newer broad-spectrum parenteral cephalosporins, this prominence has diminished markedly. It is now possible to achieve the same degree of clinical activity with a much lower risk of serious toxic effects, reflecting the rare use of this antibiotic today.

Metabolism and Disposition. The extent to which chloramphenicol is absorbed into the systemic circulation depends on which pharmaceutical formulation is administered. Chloramphenicol is one of the rare drugs for which the extent of drug absorption into the systemic circulation, or bioavailability, is greater when the drug is administered orally as a capsule than when either the oral suspension or the intravenous formulation is used. The reason for this unusual feature is that the oral solution and parenteral formulations are inactive ester forms of chloramphenicol (palmitate and succinate esters, respectively) that require ester cleavage to liberate active drug. The palmitate ester is split by pancreatic lipase, whereas the succinate ester is cleaved by nonspecific plasma and hepatic esterases. This process has a tremendous effect on the amount of active drug that reaches the blood and is distributed within the body.

Immaturity of plasma esterase activity is frequently observed in neonates and other young infants, necessitating the monitoring of both serum chloramphenicol and serum chloramphenicol succinate concentrations to assess the infant's ability to cleave the ester adequately, whereas persons with pancreatic disease (e.g., cystic fibrosis) may not have sufficient pancreatic lipase to cleave the palmitate ester.

Once liberated, active chloramphenicol is widely distributed throughout the body, including the central nervous system. This extensive distribution pattern is independent of the presence of inflammation. Approximately 60% of the drug is bound to plasma proteins. The majority of chloramphenicol in the body is rapidly conjugated to glucuronic acid in the healthy, mature liver and excreted from the body in the urine. Only 5–10% of the administered dose is excreted as unchanged chloramphenicol in the urine. The $t_{1/2\beta}$ of chloramphenicol varies with age and the maturity of the hepatic drug-metabolizing system (>24 hours in premature and newborn infants; ≥12 hours during the first 2 weeks of life; and 1.5–3.5 hours in older infants, children, and adults). This age-related maturation in renal function is reflected in the age-based dosing recommendations for chloramphenicol in pediatrics (Table 14–48).

TABLE 14–47. Pathogens Usually Susceptible in Vitro to Chloramphenicol

Gram-Positive Bacteria	Anaerobes
Staphylococcus aureus	*Bacteroides*
Coagulase-negative staphylococci	*Bacteroides fragilis*
Streptococcus pneumoniae	*Clostridium perfringens*
Group D *Streptococcus*	*Fusobacterium*
*Enterococcus**	*Peptococcus*
Listeria monocytogenes	*Peptostreptococcus*
Gram-Negative Bacteria	**Others**
Escherichia coli	*Rickettsia*
Haemophilus influenzae	*Chlamydia*
Klebsiella pneumoniae	*Mycoplasma*
Neisseria gonorrhoeae	
Neisseria meningitidis	
Salmonella	

*Variable in vitro susceptibility.

TABLE 14–48. Chloramphenicol Dosing Recommendations*

Neonates
Postnatal age ≤7 days: 25 mg/kg once daily IV
Postnatal age >7 days
≤2,000 g: 25 mg/kg once daily IV
>2,000 g: 50 mg/kg/day divided q12hr IV
Meningitis
Infants (>30 day, ≤8–10 mo): 60–75 mg/kg/day divided q6–8hr PO or IV
Children: 75–100 mg/kg/day divided q6hr PO or IV
Other Infections
Infants and children: 50–75 mg/kg/day divided q6hr PO or IV; max 4 g/day
Adults: 50 mg/kg/day divided q6hr PO or IV; max 4 g/day
Children and Adults
Ophthalmic: apply 1–2 drops or small amount of ointment q3–6hr; increase interval between applications after 48 hr
Topical: apply to affected area tid or qid
Dialysis
Hemodialysis/hemofiltration: effectively removes chloramphenicol and supplemental doses needed
Peritoneal: no dose adjustment needed
Liver disease: dosing should be avoided; if needed, dose carefully, titrating to effect and serum concentrations

*Bioavailability of the oral suspension is variable.

Available Formulations. Chloramphenicol is available as an oral capsule containing 250 mg of chloramphenicol base; a chloramphenicol palmitate suspension, with each 5 mL equivalent to 150 mg of chloramphenicol; a sodium succinate ester for intravenous administration; topical formulations for use on the skin; and ophthalmic suspensions and ointment containing 1% chloramphenicol. In many countries outside the United States, various concentrations of chloramphenicol may be found in nonprescription, over-the-counter antidiarrheal medications.

Serum Drug Concentration Monitoring. The tremendous interpatient and intrapatient variation in chloramphenicol disposition, particularly in infants and children with maturing hepatic, pancreatic, and plasma esterase activity, and the temporal relationship between drug toxicity and serum concentrations exceeding 25 mg/L have all fostered the routine practice of monitoring chloramphenicol serum concentrations. It is important to recognize that the recommended serum chloramphenicol concentrations were not derived from systematic, controlled comparative studies but rather from inferences gleaned by comparing patient toxicity data and in vitro susceptibility data. Despite these limitations, most authorities recommend that peak serum chloramphenicol concentrations be maintained at ≤25 mg/L and that trough concentrations be maintained between 5 and 10 mg/L. Peak serum concentrations are most often obtained 1 hour after completion of the intravenous infusion and 2 hours after oral administration, whereas trough concentrations are obtained just before the next dose of the drug.

Routine measurement of chloramphenicol or chloramphenicol succinate concentrations does not appear to be necessary in older persons with normal renal and hepatic function. In contrast, serum chloramphenicol concentrations should be measured in persons with immature or compromised hepatic function, those who do not appear to be responding appropriately to therapy, and those with immature or compromised renal function who are receiving chloramphenicol succinate. Determination of the chloramphenicol succinate concentration should be considered in persons with unexpectedly low serum chloramphenicol concentrations, particularly in young infants.

Adverse Effects. Adverse effects associated with chloramphenicol administration are unusual. On rare occasions, treatment with this drug is associated with nausea, vomiting, stomatitis, optic neuritis, or allergic hypersensitivity reactions. However, chloramphenicol administration can result in serious and life-threatening drug-induced toxicity. The most serious adverse effects include chloramphenicol-associated bone marrow suppression, aplastic anemia, and gray syndrome.

The most common hematopoietic toxicity of chloramphenicol is a dose-related, reversible anemia, thrombocytopenia, or leukopenia. These adverse effects appear to occur more commonly when serum chloramphenicol concentrations persistently exceed 25 mg/L. Such high levels serve as the foundation for monitoring serum concentrations. Reversible forms of bone marrow toxicity can be observed in nearly all persons receiving therapeutic doses of chloramphenicol for >5 days. Chloramphenicol is a competitive antagonist of the enzyme heme synthetase, which is responsible for coupling heme with protoporphyrin in hemoglobin. Inhibition of this enzyme causes a decrease in red cell iron uptake, with a consequent increase in circulating serum iron and a depression of erythropoiesis, manifested by a reticulocytopenia. A simultaneous increase in the erythroid:myeloid ratio with vacuolization of precursors of the bone marrow occurs. With continued administration for >10 days, mild anemia, thrombocytopenia, or neutropenia can be observed. These hematologic effects are reversible after the chloramphenicol dose is reduced or the drug therapy is discontinued.

TABLE 14–49. Drug Interactions with Chloramphenicol

Chloramphenicol interferes with body elimination
Barbiturates
Iron
Phenytoin
Sulfonylurea hypoglycemics
Warfarin
Drug stimulates chloramphenicol body clearance
Barbiturates
Rifampin

The most feared and notorious of chloramphenicol-associated adverse effects is irreversible bone marrow aplasia. Several epidemiologic studies suggest that the incidence of marrow aplasia approximates 1 in 24,000 to 1 in 200,000 individuals treated with the antibiotic. No variables have yet been identified as important risk factors predisposing an individual to the development of this adverse effect. Chloramphenicol-induced aplastic anemia is not related to dose or duration of therapy and has been reported to occur after a single dose and even after ophthalmic use. Whether this serious reaction occurs only after oral chloramphenicol administration, as a result of the production of a marrow toxic metabolite by gut flora, or after parenteral and topical use of the drug, is controversial. The true relationship between route of administration and development of irreversible bone marrow aplasia is unknown. Because the clinical need for chloramphenicol is decreasing, a resolution to this debate is unlikely.

Gray syndrome is another serious side effect of chloramphenicol. This syndrome was first described in 1958, when large numbers of neonates receiving parenteral chloramphenicol developed a characteristic pattern of symptoms that frequently resulted in death. Infants typically received high doses of chloramphenicol (100 to >300 mg/kg/day) for several days. Usually within 4–5 days, they began to vomit. Abdominal distention, greenish diarrhea, anorexia, and respiratory distress gave way to profound hypotension and a characteristic ashen gray color. Shock followed. The mechanism of this reaction is unknown but appears to be associated with high serum concentrations of chloramphenicol (>50 mg/L), underscoring the importance of serum chloramphenicol monitoring in neonates, infants, and any persons with compromised hepatic function. Possible drug-drug interactions involving chloramphenicol are outlined in Table 14–49.

THE TETRACYCLINES

Introduced soon after the discovery of penicillin and sulfonamide, the tetracycline class of antibiotics was once commonly used for the treatment of a wide variety of systemic and topical infections. Unacceptable adverse effects, including the permanent discoloration of teeth, has limited the use of these drugs in children. Increasing bacterial resistance to tetracyclines and the availability of safer, more effective antibiotics has dramatically reduced the clinical utility of these drugs to the treatment of only a few infectious diseases.

Spectrum of Activity. The tetracyclines were the first class of drugs that possessed a broad spectrum of antimicrobial activity that includes gram-positive and gram-negative bacteria, *Mycoplasma pneumoniae,* Rickettsiaceae, and *Chlamydia* (both *C. trachomatis* and *C. psittaci*). Representative comparative inhibitory activities for selected tetracycline analogs are shown in Table 14–50.

Tetracyclines inhibit bacterial protein synthesis by binding the 30S ribosomal subunit. This reversible ribosomal binding by tetra-

TABLE 14–50. Representative in Vitro Activity for Selected Tetracyclines

Pathogen	Minimum Inhibitory Concentration (mg/L)		
	Tetracycline	Doxycycline	Minocycline
Gram-Positive Bacteria			
Staphylococcus aureus	3.1	1.6	0.78
Group A *Streptococcus*	0.78	0.39	0.39
Streptococcus pneumoniae	0.8	0.2	0.2
Viridans streptococci	3.1	0.39	0.39
Enterococcus faecalis	>100	50	100
Gram-Negative Bacteria			
Escherichia coli	12.5	12.5	6.3
Enterobacter	25	25	12.5
Klebsiella	50	50	25
Serratia	200	50	25
Proteus mirabilis	>100	>100	>100
Neisseria gonorrhoeae	0.78	0.38	0.39
Neisseria meningitidis	0.8	1.6	1.6
Haemophilus influenzae	1.6	1.6	1.6
Legionella pneumophila	5.2	1.0	0.43
Mycoplasma and Chlamydia			
Mycoplasma pneumoniae	1.6	1.6	1.6
Ureaplasma urealyticum	0.4	0.1	0.13
Chlamydia	0.6	0.06	0.02

cyclines appears to inhibit aminoacyl tRNA binding on the mRNA-ribosome complex, thus preventing the addition of amino acids to the growing peptide chain. At very high concentrations, as encountered in overdoses in persons with renal disease, tetracyclines may interfere with mammalian protein synthesis. This interference is reflected by increases in blood urea nitrogen concentrations.

Bacterial resistance to tetracyclines may be natural or acquired. Natural resistance is usually mediated by decreased permeability of the bacterial cell membrane to tetracycline, thus preventing drug access to the binding sites on the ribosome. Acquired resistance is usually an inducible, plasmid-mediated resistance. Plasmid-mediated resistance to various tetracycline analogs, as well as to other antibiotic drugs including the aminoglycosides, chloramphenicol, or the sulfonamides, can be transferred across bacterial species.

Clinical Indications. The clinical indications for tetracycline antibiotics continue to decrease as the number of susceptible bacteria declines and the availability of safer, more effective bactericidal agents increases. Moreover, important adverse effects, including photosensitivity and staining of teeth, have resulted in admonitions regarding their use in children. At present, these drugs are recommended for only two indications in children. They remain primary therapeutic agents for the treatment of Rocky Mountain spotted fever and for the treatment of nongonococcal pelvic inflammatory disease and urethritis in adolescents. Tetracyclines may also be used to treat older children and adolescents with mycoplasmal disease or *Legionella.* The clinical value of systemic tetracycline administration as adjunctive treatment for acne vulgaris remains unclear.

Metabolism and Disposition. The pharmacokinetic characteristics of selected tetracycline derivatives are shown in Table 14–51. These data should be used as representative values; very limited data concerning the pharmacokinetics of tetracycline are available for pediatric patients. The tetracyclines are widely distributed to most body fluids and tissues, including ascitic fluid; bronchial secretions; sputum; and pleural, synovial, prostatic, and seminal fluids. The tetracyclines diffuse poorly into the central nervous system in the absence of inflammation. Although they diffuse well into breast milk, the bioavailability to the infant is most likely very low because of the complex formation with milk. Doxycycline and minocycline appear to distribute to body fluids and tissues to a greater extent than other tetracycline analogs because of their greater degree of lipid solubility.

Demeclocycline, oxytetracycline, and tetracycline do not appear to be metabolized and are eliminated unchanged in the urine. In contrast, doxycycline and minocycline are primarily eliminated from the body by nonrenal routes, most likely the bile. All tetracycline derivatives are excreted into the gastrointestinal tract, bound (complexed) to fecal material, and excreted from the body. Very little tetracycline is removed during hemodialysis or peritoneal dialysis.

Recommended Dosing and Dosing Strategies. Pediatric and adult dosing recommendations for selected tetracycline analogs are presented in Table 14–52. With few exceptions the American Academy of Pediatrics recommends that tetracyclines be used only in children 9 years of age or older because of tetracycline-associated retardation in skeletal development and associated enamel hypoplasia and permanent discoloration of the teeth.

Parenteral administration of tetracycline agents should be used only when oral administration is not possible. Intramuscular administration is associated with local pain at the injection site and is often less bioavailable than the oral form. In persons with renal disease, dosing reductions are necessary for most tetracyclines, including tetracycline and demeclocycline. Insufficient data are

TABLE 14–51. Pharmacokinetic Characteristics of Selected Tetracycline Antibiotics

Drug	Oral Bioavailability (%)	Effect*			Protein Binding (%)	Half-Life (hr)	Urinary Excretion (%)
		Food	Ca^{++}	Fe^{++}			
Tetracycline HCl	60–80	++	++	++	30–60	6–12	60
Demeclocycline	50–80	+	++	++	75–90	10–17	40
Doxycycline	90–100	±	+	++	80–85	15–25	40
Minocycline	90–100	±	+	++	80–90	11–25	10–15

Data derived primarily from adult subjects.
*± = <20%; + = 20–30%; ++ = >30% effect on drug bioavailability.

TABLE 14–52. Dosing Recommendations for Selected Tetracycline Antibiotics

Tetracycline Hydrochloride
Children
Oral: 25–50 mg/kg/day divided q6hr; max 3 g/day
Ophthalmic suspension: 1–2 drops 2–4 times daily; ointment: instill q2–12hr
IM route*: 15–25 mg/kg/day divided q8–12hr
Adults
Oral: 250–500 mg q6–12hr
Ophthalmic suspension: 1–2 drops 2–4 times daily; ointment: instill q2–12hr
IM route*: 250–300 mg/day divided q8–12hr

Available Forms
Suspension: 125 mg/5 mL
Capsules: 100 mg, 250 mg, 500 mg
Tablets: 250 mg, 500 mg

Demeclocycline
Children: 8–12 mg/kg/day divided q6–12hr
Adults: 150 mg qid or 300 mg bid
Uncomplicated gonorrhea: 600 mg initially; then 300 mg q12hr for 4 days (3 g total)
SIADH: 900–1,200 mg/day *or* 13–15 mg/kg/day divided q6–8hr initially; then decrease to 0.6–0.9 g/day

Available Forms
Capsule: 150 mg
Tablets: 150 mg, 300 mg

Doxycycline
Children: 2–5 mg/kg/day in 1–2 divided doses; max 200 mg/day
Adults: 100–200 mg/day in 1–2 divided doses

Available Forms
Suspension: 25 mg/5 mL, 50 mg/5 mL
Capsules: 50 mg, 100 mg
Delayed-release capsule: 100 mg
Tablet: 100 mg
Intravenous infusion: 100 mg, 200 mg/vial

Minocycline
Children >8 yr of age: 4 mg/kg on day 1, followed by 2 mg/kg/day thereafter divided q12hr
Adults: 200 mg initially, followed by 100 mg q12hr

Available Forms
Suspension: 50 mg/5 mL
Capsules: 50 mg, 100 mg
Tablets: 50 mg, 100 mg
Intravenous infusion: 100 mg/vial

SIADH = syndrome of inappropriate secretion of antidiuretic hormone.
*The intramuscular route for tetracycline administration is associated with severe local pain and should be avoided whenever possible.

available to determine whether similar dosing adjustments are needed for minocycline. In contrast, no dosage adjustment is necessary for doxycycline, which should be considered the preferred tetracycline for use in persons with compromised renal function.

A large number of adverse effects have been associated with the clinical use of tetracycline analogs. The more common and important adverse effects associated with these drugs are outlined in Table 14–53.

Drug Interactions. Tetracyclines readily chelate divalent and trivalent cations that are contained in oral antacids and vitamin preparations. Concurrent oral administration of tetracyclines with compounds containing these agents can result in complex formation, which markedly reduces oral bioavailability. This effect with calcium, aluminum, magnesium, and iron varies depending on the specific tetracycline analog. The impact of this interaction on the bioavailability of selected tetracycline analogs is shown in Table 14–54. Similarly, many antidiarrheal preparations that contain kaolin, pectin, or bismuth subsalicylate may also impair the oral absorption of these drugs. When any of these agents must be administered to persons receiving tetracyclines, the tetracycline should be administered 1–2 hours before or after administration of these other medications.

Tetracyclines may enhance the hypoprothrombinemic effect of oral anticoagulants (e.g., warfarin) by their suppressant effect on vitamin K–producing gastrointestinal flora. Drugs that stimulate hepatic drug–metabolizing enzymes, including carbamazepine, phenobarbital, phenytoin, and rifampin, have been reported to enhance the rate of elimination of tetracyclines. The use of tetracycline in a person receiving methoxyflurane anesthesia may result in fatal hepatotoxicity by an as-yet-undefined mechanism.

TABLE 14–53. Tetracycline-Associated Adverse Effects

Skeletal and Dental
Retardation of skeletal development in utero and in infants
Discoloration of permanent teeth (in children <9 yr of age)

Gastrointestinal
Nausea; vomiting; diarrhea; anorexia; flatus; epigastric burning; rare tablet-associated esophagitis; oral candidiasis; rare pseudomembranous colitis

Dermatologic
Photosensitivity (primarily demeclocycline)
Nail discoloration
Skin rash (rare)

Renal
Prerenal azotemia (rare)
Reversible Fanconi's syndrome (see text)

Gynecologic
Impaired fertility (minocycline?)

Local
Thrombophlebitis common with intravenous administration
Intramuscular administration painful

TABLE 14–54. Potential Drug Interactions with Tetracyclines

Chelation of Tetracycline Antibiotic and Decreased Intestinal Absorption
Di-trivalent cations (aluminum, calcium, magnesium, zinc)
Iron
Drug products
Kaolin, bismuth-containing products

Decreased Clinical Effect
Digoxin
Oral contraceptives
Warfarin

TRIMETHOPRIM-SULFAMETHOXAZOLE

The sulfonamides are broad-spectrum bacteriostatic agents that have been used extensively for the treatment of a wide variety of systemic infections for more than 5 decades. The increasing bacterial resistance to sulfonamide drugs has stimulated research to identify companion antibiotics that when combined with sulfonamides enhance, either additively or synergistically, the overall antibacterial activity of each component. The fixed-dose combination of two bacteriostatic agents, trimethoprim and sulfamethoxazole, was designed to combine two agents with similar pharmacokinetic characteristics in a 1:5 ratio (TMP:SMZ).

Spectrum of Activity. Trimethoprim and sulfamethoxazole, when administered in combination, demonstrate additive or synergistic antibacterial activity against a number of clinically important pathogens. Although the two components are bacteriostatic, the combination is bactericidal. Pathogens usually susceptible in vitro to TMP-SMZ are listed in Table 14–55.

Clinical Indications. A large number of antibiotics with antibacterial activity similar to that of TMP-SMZ are available. Thus the use of this antibiotic drug combination is limited to only a few clinical indications. TMP-SMZ is often used for the prophylaxis and treatment of urinary tract infections caused by gram-negative pathogens, for the treatment of acute and chronic bronchitis, and for infections caused by *Nocardia.* It remains the primary therapeutic agent for the prophylaxis and treatment of *Pneumocystis carinii* pneumonia and is a second-line drug for the treatment of acute otitis media.

Metabolism and Disposition. Trimethoprim and sulfamethoxazole are both well absorbed from the gastrointestinal tract after oral administration. Once absorbed into the systemic circulation, these drugs are widely distributed into most body fluids and tissues, including the central nervous system. In the absence of inflammation, TMP-SMZ concentrations in the cerebrospinal fluid approximate 50% of the drug concentration in plasma. Approximately 45–70% of TMP-SMZ is bound to plasma protein. Both components are metabolized in the liver; trimethoprim is metabolized to oxide and hydroxylated metabolites, whereas sulfamethoxazole is primarily *N*-acetylated and conjugated with glucuronide. Parent drug and metabolites are excreted from the body in the urine; approximately 80% of the trimethoprim and 30% of the sulfamethoxazole is excreted in the urine as unchanged drug, necessitating dosage adjustments in persons with significant renal function impairment. Peak plasma trimethoprim concentrations of approximately 1–2 mg/L and sulfamethoxazole concentrations of approximately 40–60 mg/L are usually observed within 1–3 hours of oral dosing.

TABLE 14–55. Pathogens Usually Susceptible in Vitro to Trimethoprim-Sulfamethoxazole

Gram-Positive Organisms
*Staphylococcus aureus**
*Streptococcus pneumoniae**
Nocardia

Gram-Negative Organisms
Escherichia coli
Klebsiella pneumoniae
Citrobacter freundii
Proteus
Salmonella typhi
Neisseria meningitidis
Yersinia
Aeromonas
Stenotrophomonas maltophilia
*Haemophilus influenzae**
*Moraxella catarrhalis**

Protozoa
Pneumocystis carinii

TMP-SMZ is administered in a 1:5 trimethoprim:sulfamethoxazole ratio.
*Pathogens demonstrate variable in vitro susceptibility.

Recommended Dosing and Dosing Strategies. TMP-SMZ dosing recommendations in children and adults and the available formulations are shown in Table 14–56. Clinical dosing calculations, in milligrams per kilogram of body weight, for TMP-SMZ are based on the trimethoprim component.

Adverse Effects. Adverse effects associated with TMP-SMZ administration include reactions involving either trimethoprim or sulfamethoxazole. The extent to which each component is responsible for a particular reaction is unknown. With few exceptions, the types and overall incidence of adverse effects of TMP-SMZ appear similar to those observed with sulfonamides alone. Nausea, vomiting, anorexia, and skin reactions, including rash and urticaria, are the most common adverse effects associated with TMP-SMZ administration.

An unusually high incidence of adverse effects of TMP-SMZ has been reported in persons with AIDS. A diffuse maculopapular and erythematous skin rash, fever, leukopenia, thrombocytopenia, and increased serum concentrations of hepatic aminotransferases have been described in up to 80% of persons with AIDS who receive this drug combination. These adverse effects most often recur after rechallenge with TMP-SMZ, although some persons have been successfully desensitized. The reason for this increased incidence of toxic effects in such persons is unknown. Moreover, the incidence is higher in white persons than in black persons.

TABLE 14–56. Dosing Recommendations for Trimethoprim with or without Sulfamethoxazole

Children >2 Mo
Mild to moderate infections: 6–12 mg TMP/kg/day divided q12hr
Serious infections (e.g., *Pneumocystis carinii*): 15–20 mg TMP/kg/day divided q6hr
Prophylaxis
- UTI prophylaxis: 2 mg TMP/kg once daily
- *P. carinii* prophylaxis: 5–10 mg TMP/kg/day divided q12hr 3 days/wk; dose should not exceed 320 mg TMP and 1,600 mg SMZ 3 days/wk (see Table 68–14)

Adults
UTI, chronic bronchitis: 1 double-strength tablet q12hr for 10–14 days*

Dialysis
Hemodialysis: single-dose supplementation required
Peritoneal: no dose needed

Available Formulations
- Oral suspension: 40 mg TMP with 200 mg SMZ/mL
- Oral tablets: 80 mg TMP with 400 mg SMZ per tablet
- Double-strength tablets: 160 mg TMP with 800 mg SMZ per tablet
- Parenteral: 16 mg TMP with 80 mg SMZ/mL

Dose calculations based on the trimethoprim component.
*In persons with renal impairment the dose or frequency may need to be adjusted. If creatinine clearance is 15–30 mL/min, reduce dose by 50%.

TABLE 14–57. Potential Drug Interactions with Trimethoprim-Sulfamethoxazole

Cyclosporine
Methotrexate
Phenytoin
Oral anticoagulants (e.g., warfarin)
Oral hypoglycemics (e.g., tolbutamide)

Interactions are unpredictable.

Skin reactions, including exfoliative dermatitis and Stevens-Johnson syndrome, have been reported with the use of sulfonamides alone, as well as with the use of TMP-SMZ. Less severe skin rashes are often generalized, maculopapular, erythematous, and pruritic in nature and most often occur within 10–14 days of the start of therapy. Hematologic toxicity with anemia, leukopenia, neutropenia, and thrombocytopenia has rarely been described in persons receiving TMP-SMZ. These possible toxic effects may reflect trimethoprim antagonism of mammalian folate metabolism in folate-deficient persons, including malnourished persons and those receiving additional bone marrow suppressant medications. When necessary, folic acid or folinic acid (leucovorin) may be administered along with TMP-SMZ without affecting antibacterial activity. Sulfonamides do not interfere with mammalian folate metabolism; mammalian cells require preformed folic acid and are incapable of synthesizing it. In contrast, the cell wall of sulfonamide-susceptible bacteria is impermeable to preformed folic acid. These organisms must synthesize it from *p*-aminobenzoic acid.

Considerable controversy continues to surround the use of sulfonamide-containing drugs in newborn infants, and concern persists about the possibility of drug-induced displacement of bilirubin and the development of kernicterus. Although elevations in the unbound (free) concentration of bilirubin only partially explains the propensity of sick neonates to develop kernicterus, it is clear that these increased bilirubin concentrations are a major predisposing factor. The sulfonamides and sulfonamide-containing drugs have been implicated as potent competitors for bilirubin binding sites on albumin. They are presumed to cause displacement of bilirubin, thus increasing free, circulating concentrations. Despite the decades of debate regarding possible sulfonamide-bilirubin displacement reactions, only very limited data on a small number of sulfonamide derivatives are available. In fact, sulfonamides display a highly variable ability to displace bilirubin from albumin binding sites. Sulfisoxazole clearly competes for albumin binding, whereas sulfadiazine and sulfanilamide appear to displace little or no bilirubin.

In addition, some questions have been raised regarding the role of the propylene glycol present in the early parenteral formulations used in the infants who developed kernicterus after receiving sulfisoxazole. Propylene glycol is a potent displacer of bilirubin. Published data to establish the safety or toxicity of sulfamethoxazole or of sulfamethoxazole combined with trimethoprim in the newborn are insufficient. Although case reports described the safe and efficacious use of this drug combination in neonates for selected infections (e.g., *Nocardia* infections), TMP-SMZ should be administered to neonates with caution and close monitoring. TMP-SMZ manufacturers recommend that the drug not be used in persons younger than 2 months.

Many possible drug interactions have been associated with sulfonamide administration (Table 14–57).

QUINOLONES

The quinolone agents are not yet labeled by the FDA for use in persons 18 years of age or younger because of cartilage toxicity seen during preclinical testing in beagle puppies. Despite these findings in animals, no age-specific skeletal-muscle or other related adverse effects have been defined for the quinolone class of antibiotics in humans. Thus the use of these drugs in pediatrics is increasing, and soon, age-specific dosing recommendations and FDA labeling for use in pediatrics will be available for many compounds. Nalidixic acid is the precursor to the increasing number of newer quinolone derivatives available for clinical use. The new quinolone derivatives are potent antibiotics that possess a broad spectrum of in vitro antibacterial activity. Moreover, newer analogs have been effective in the treatment of infections caused by difficult-to-treat gram-negative and multidrug-resistant pathogens. This highly desirable spectrum of antibacterial activity combined with excellent clinical efficacy after oral dosing continues to foster immense interest in this class of compounds.

Spectrum of Activity. The newer quinolone derivatives possess a broad spectrum of antibacterial activity. Comparative in vitro activity against important pathogens for selected quinolone derivatives is shown in Table 14–58. Quinolones inhibit DNA topoisomerase, often referred to as DNA gyrase, which is necessary for bacterial DNA replication and for some aspects of transcription and repair. This antagonism of DNA gyrase activity prohibits adenosine triphosphate–dependent DNA supercoiling, thus promoting breakage of the DNA strand. Although mammalian cells contain a DNA gyrase (i.e., type II) similar to the one found in bacteria, quinolones do not appear to interact with this enzyme at the concentrations achieved after routine dosing. This potential lack of interaction with mammalian cells may also reflect functional differences between bacterial and mammalian activity of DNA gyrase.

Bacterial resistance to quinolones is most likely a result of mutations that alter quinolone binding to DNA gyrase. Bacterial resistance is more often a chromosome-mediated rather than a plasmid-mediated process. When it occurs, it usually confers cross-resistance to other quinolones. In contrast, cross-resistance does not usually occur between quinolone and other antibiotic drug classes (e.g., β-lactams, aminoglycosides). The development of resistance by previously susceptible bacteria during quinolone therapy continues to complicate therapy and can restrict the use of these drugs.

Metabolism and Disposition. Comparison of important pharmacokinetic parameters for selected quinolone antibiotics derived from adults is shown in Table 14–59. With the exception of gatifloxacin and levofloxacin, the newer quinolones are primarily metabolized by the liver and do not require dose adjustments in persons with mild to moderate renal functional impairment (adjust only if creatinine clearance <30 mL/min). In contrast, dosage adjustments may be necessary in patients with liver disease. No systematic data that describe the influence of age on quinolone pharmacokinetic profiles are available.

Clinical Indications. Potential clinical uses of quinolone in pediatrics are outlined in Table 14–60 and dosing recommendations in Table 14–61.

Adverse Effects. Adverse effects associated with the clinical use of quinolone antibiotics are usually mild and transient in nature. Nausea, abdominal distress, headache, and dizziness appear to be the most common adverse effects associated with quinolone use in adults. Less common adverse effects have included photosensitivity reactions with skin rashes and central nervous system manifestations including depression, hallucinations, and seizures.

The most important quinolone-associated adverse effect for pediatrics is the possibility of drug-induced arthropathy. Preliminary

TABLE 14–58. Susceptibility of Common Bacterial Pathogens to Selected Quinolone Antibiotics

	Minimum Inhibitory Concentration$_{50/90}$ (mg/L)			
Organism	**Ciprofloxacin**	**Gatifloxacin**	**Levofloxacin**	**Moxifloxacin**
Gram-Negative Aerobes				
Escherichia coli	0.016/8	0.03/4	0.03/8	0.16/8
Klebsiella pneumoniae	0.06/8	0.06/4	0.13/16	0.13/8
Enterobacter cloacae	0.016/0.03	0.03/0.06	0.016/0.06	0.03/0.08
Serratia marcescens	0.13/9	0.25/4	0.25/8	0.25/8
Shigella	0.008	0.016	0.016	0.016/0.03
Salmonella	0.016	0.03/0.06	0.03	0.06/0.13
Proteus mirabilis	0.016/0.06	0.13/0.25	0.03/0.25	0.06/0.25
Proteus vulgaris	0.06	0.25	0.13	0.25/0.5
Morganella morganii	0.03	0.25	0.06	0.13
Haemophilus influenzae	0.016	0.016	0.06	0.06
Neisseria gonorrhoeae	0.016	0.016	0.008	0.03
Pseudomonas aeruginosa	0.5/8	4/32	2/32	4/32
Gram-Negative Anaerobes				
Bacteroides fragilis	8/8	0.5/1	2/2	1/2
Bacteroides (other species)	8/16	0.5/2	2/4	0.5/4
Gram-Positive Aerobes				
Staphylococcus aureus				
Methicillin-sensitive	0.5	0.13	0.25	0.06
Methicillin-resistant	1/32	0.13/16	0.5/16	0.06/4
Staphylococcus epidermidis	1	0.25	1	0.13
Streptococcus pneumoniae				
Penicillin-susceptible	1/4	0.25/1	1/2	0.25/1
Penicillin-resistant	1/2	0.25/0.5	1/2	0.25
Group A *Streptococcus*	1/1	0.25	0.5	0.25
Streptococcus	1/2	0.5	1	0.5
Enterococcus faecalis	1/4	0.5/2	1/2	0.25/1
Enterococcus faecium	4/16	2/4	2/8	1/4
Listeria	1	0.5	2	0.5

toxicity studies in animals described destructive lesions of cartilage. Subsequent evaluations and clinical experience, however, suggest an absence of quinolone-induced arthropathy in humans and provide the scientific foundation to undertake controlled clinical trials of quinolones in pediatrics. Two of the newer quinolones (i.e., gatifloxacin and levofloxacin) are undergoing active clinical investigation targeting labeling by the FDA for use in pediatric patients. The success of these research programs emanates from the lack of quinolone-associated and age-associated skeletal toxicities.

Of particular concern with quinolone agents has been their propensity to interfere with cardiac conduction. In particular, certain analogs can interfere with relaxation of the ventricles, leading to a prolongation of the QT or corrected-QT (QTc) interval on the electrocardiogram. Drugs that may prolong the QTc include class I (e.g., quinidine) and class III (e.g., sotalol) antiarrhythmic drugs, erythromycin, cisapride, and tricyclic antidepressants. This prolongation of ventricular relaxation, reflected by prolongation of the QTc interval, appears to be due to a drug's ability to bind to the *HERG* (human ether-a-go-go–related gene), which regulates the outward rectifier potassium current in cardiac muscle. The greatest risk of QTc prolongation occurs with sparfloxacin and grepafloxacin, with much less effect occurring with ciprofloxacin, moxifloxacin, levofloxacin, or gatifloxacin.

Drug Interactions. A number of potentially important drug-drug interactions have been reported with various quinolone antibiotics (Table 14–62). Concomitant administration of quinolones with divalent and trivalent cation-containing antacids (e.g., aluminum, calcium, magnesium), sucralfate (aluminum salt of sulfated disaccharide), and iron substantially reduces the oral absorption of quino-

TABLE 14–59. Comparative Pharmacokinetic Profiles for Selected Quinolone Antibiotics in Adults

Drug	Oral Dose (mg)	F (%)	C_{max} (mg/L)	t_{max} (hr)	$t_{1/2\beta}$ (hr)	AUC (mg · hr/L)	Metabolized (%)
Ciprofloxacin	750	70	3.3	1.25	4.2	35.2	35
Gatifloxacin	400	96	3.4	1.5	8.4	32.4	<1
Levofloxacin	500	90	5.2	1.5	7.4	61.1	5
Moxifloxacin	400	85	2.5	NA	13.1	26.9	10
Sparfloxacin	200	40–60	0.6	4	3.8	16.4	40

F = drug bioavailability; C_{max} = maximal plasma drug concentration at t_{max}; t_{max} = time after dosing to reach C_{max}; $t_{1/2\beta}$ = elimination half-life; AUC = area under plasma drug concentration–time curve.

TABLE 14–60. Potential Clinical Indications for Quinolones in Pediatric Practice

Predisposing Factors or Underlying Conditions	Infectious Disease	Pathogen(s)	Comments
Cystic fibrosis	Bronchopulmonary exacerbation	*Pseudomonas aeruginosa* *Staphylococcus aureus*	May replace parenteral antipseudomonal combination therapy; duration 1–3 mo
Urologic abnormality	Upper urinary tract infection	*P. aeruginosa* *Escherichia coli*	Duration 2–3 wk
Subacute form or atypical location	Osteomyelitis	*P. aeruginosa*	Duration 6–8 wk
Central nervous system	Shunt-related infection	Coagulase-negative staphylococci *S. aureus*	Initially plus intraventricular therapy with another agent; duration 3–4 wk
	Bacterial meningitis	*Enterobacter* *P. aeruginosa*	
Developing country	Endemic or epidemic shigellosis	*Shigella flexneri* *Shigella boydii* *Shigella dysenteriae*	
Nasopharyngeal carrier state	Prevention of meningitis	*Neisseria meningitidis* *Haemophilus influenzae* type b	
Immunocompromised person who is intolerant to or has not responded to therapy with β-lactam antibiotics	Sepsis	Enterobacteriaceae	
Acute otitis media		*H. influenzae* *Streptococcus pneumoniae* (penicillin resistant)	
Pneumonia		Atypical pneumonia Drug-resistant pathogens	

TABLE 14–61. Quinolone Dosing Recommendations

Nalidixic Acid
Children: 55 mg/kg/day divided q6–8hr
 UTI prophylaxis: 30–35 mg/kg/day divided q6–8hr
Adults: 1 g qid
 UTI prophylaxis: 500 mg qid

Available Forms
Oral suspension: 250 mg/5 mL
Tablets: 250 mg, 500 mg, 1,000 mg

Ciprofloxacin*
Children: 20–30 mg/kg/day divided in 2–3 doses (max 1.5 g/day)
 UTI prophylaxis: 30–35 mg/kg/day divided q6–8hr
Adults: 250–750 mg q12hr
 Modify dose interval in persons with creatinine clearance <30 mL/min; administer dose q8–24hr

Available Forms
Tablets: 100 mg, 250 mg, 500 mg, 750 mg
Oral suspension: 250 mg/5 mL, 500 mg/5 mL
Injection: 10 and 20 mg/mL for infusion for 30–60 min

Levofloxacin†
Children: 20–30 mg/kg/day divided q12hr PO/IV
Adults: 250–500 mg q24hr PO/IV

Available Forms
Tablets: 500 mg, 750 mg
Injection: 5 and 25 mg/mL infuse for 60 min

*Intravenous dose approximates 80% of oral dose.
†Preliminary dosing recommendation.

lone antibiotics. This decreased absorption most likely results from chelation of the quinolone by these cations, thus forming a poorly soluble complex. Similarly the presence of food in the stomach (from meals or tube feedings) may delay the rate and overall extent of quinolone absorption. As a result of these interactions, quinolones should not be coadministered with oral antacids, multivitamin-iron formulations, or sucralfate whenever possible. If one of these agents must be prescribed along with quinolone, the time between administration of the two drugs should be as long as possible (>3–4 hours). Until more data are available, a similar quinolone dosing strategy should be used with persons receiving tube feedings.

Quinolone antibiotics are effective inhibitors of hepatic cytochrome P-450 monooxygenases. The exact cytochrome P-450 iso-

TABLE 14–62. Quinolone-Based Drug-Drug Interactions

	Quinolone			
Compound	Ciprofloxacin	Gatifloxacin	Levofloxacin	Moxifloxacin
Antacids*	Yes	Yes	Yes	Yes
Iron	Yes	Yes	Yes	Yes
Calcium	Yes	?	Yes	Yes
Cimetidine	Yes	?	?	?
Sucralfate	Yes	?	Yes	?
Theophylline	Yes	No	No	No

? = questionable and unlikely to occur, but patients should be monitored for possible variable effect.
*Intestinal complexion decreasing bioavailability (calcium, magnesium, and aluminium ions). Administer quinolone 1 hour before or 2 hours after administration of a divalent or trivalent cation containing antacids.

enzymes involved and the extent to which parent compounds and metabolites inhibit this enzyme activity are unclear. Until these pathways are described more definitively, it remains difficult to predict which agents will show altered clearance when various quinolones are administered simultaneously. For example, both ciprofloxacin and enoxacin markedly interfere with the metabolism of theophylline and caffeine, whereas gatifloxacin, levofloxacin, and moxifloxacin may have no or only slight influence on the elimination of these two compounds. All persons receiving theophylline and a quinolone antibiotic should be checked closely for the development of theophylline toxicity. Clinical symptoms or serum theophylline concentrations, or both, should be monitored. Quinolones may also alter the metabolism of warfarin by means of a stereoselective mechanism that decreases the elimination of the less active R-enantomer. Close monitoring of prothrombin times for persons receiving ciprofloxacin and warfarin is necessary.

THE LINCOSAMIDES: LINCOMYCIN AND CLINDAMYCIN

Lincomycin was the first lincosamide isolated from a strain of *Streptomyces lincolnensis* in the early 1950s. Recognition of potent in vitro activity of lincosamides against gram-positive pathogens and clinical use of these drugs as possible alternatives to β-lactams fostered their early clinical development.

Spectrum of Activity. The lincosamides inhibit bacterial protein synthesis by binding to the 50S subunit of the ribosome. With few important exceptions, their spectrum of antibacterial activity is similar to that of erythromycin. These drugs are effective against most anaerobic bacteria, although most strains of *Bacteroides* are resistant to lincomycin and highly sensitive to clindamycin. Comparative in vitro activity of lincomycin and clindamycin against selected pathogens is shown in Table 14–63, and in vitro activity of clindamycin against anaerobes in shown in Table 14–64.

TABLE 14–63. Comparative in Vitro Activity of Lincomycin and Clindamycin Against Selected Pathogens

Pathogen	Representative Minimum Inhibitory Concentrations (mg/L)*	
	Lincomycin	Clindamycin
Gram-Positive Bacteria		
Staphylococcus aureus	1.6	0.1
Group A *Streptococcus*	0.04	0.04
Streptococcus pneumoniae	0.2	0.01
Viridans streptococci	0.04	0.02
Enterococcus faecalis	R	R
Gram-Negative Bacteria		
Escherichia coli	R	R
Neisseria gonorrhoeae	R	3.1
Neisseria meningitidis	R	R
Haemophilus influenzae	R	R
Anaerobic, Gram-Negative Bacteria		
Bacteroides fragilis	R	4
Prevotella melaninogenica	0.4	0.2
Fusobacterium	4	2
Anaerobic, Spore-Forming Bacilli		
Clostridium perfringens	8	4
Clostridium (other species)	8	4

R = resistant.
*MIC for 90% of strains.

Metabolism and Disposition. Lincomycin and clindamycin are both absorbed from the gastrointestinal tract after oral dosing. The bioavailability of lincomycin is 20–35%, and for clindamycin it exceeds 80%. These drugs are distributed to most body fluids and tissues; clindamycin is approximately 50 times more lipid soluble than lincomycin and is more extensively distributed. Despite this degree of lipid solubility, neither of these agents penetrates well into the central nervous system. Protein binding for clindamycin approximates 60–90%; for lincomycin, it approximates 70–80%.

The lincosamides are extensively metabolized by the liver before excretion by the kidney. Less than 10% of lincomycin or clindamycin is excreted unchanged in the urine. The metabolic rate of lincomycin is poorly understood. In contrast, clindamycin is metabolized by the liver to two primary active metabolites: *N*-demethylclindamycin, which is three times more active than the parent drug, and clindamycin sulfoxide, which is seven times less active than the parent drug.

Assessment of lincosamide pharmacokinetic data is difficult because most studies use bioassay techniques to quantitate biologic fluid samples, and these techniques cannot discriminate between parent drug and active metabolites. The importance of these renally eliminated metabolites to the development of drug toxicity is also unknown. Reported $t_{1/2\beta}$ values for clindamycin range from 2 to 4 hours in infants and children and from 0.8 to 5 hours in adults. Available pharmacokinetic data for lincomycin are insufficient.

Recommended Dosing and Dosing Strategies. Usual dosing recommendations for clindamycin are shown in Table 14–65. Pharmacologic and clinical data for lincomycin are insufficient to provide pediatric dosing guidelines; preliminary pediatric lincomycin dosing guidelines are given in Table 14–65.

Adverse Effects. The most common adverse effect associated with lincosamide administration is diarrhea. Although the incidence of diarrhea may be less with clindamycin than lincomycin, the use of either of these drugs is associated with the development of pseudomembranous colitis. The severity of the diarrhea is highly variable and can range from a mild, self-limiting process to a fatal condition. Death most often results from profound dehydration and shock. The occurrence of this serious adverse effect does not appear to be related to the dose or duration of lincosamide therapy but appears to result from *C. difficile* toxin elaborated from lincosamide-resistant *C. difficile* present in the gastrointestinal tract. Other, less common adverse effects associated with the use of these antibiotics include skin rash and thrombophlebitis.

Drug Interactions. Coadministration of a lincosamide with kaolin- and pectin-containing products should be avoided to prevent decreased or delayed lincosamide absorption.

METRONIDAZOLE

Metronidazole, the first drug available for the treatment of *Trichomonas vaginalis* infections, was synthesized by Rhone-Poulenc Pharmaceuticals in 1957. Systematic chemical modification of a 2-nitroimidazole compound, azomycin, elaborated from a *Streptomyces* isolated by Japanese researchers in 1953, yielded metronidazole. Subsequent studies in animals and humans demonstrated the effectiveness of this drug for amebiasis and for infections caused by *Giardia lamblia.* Today metronidazole is probably best known for its potent and broad activity against anaerobic bacteria.

TABLE 14–64. Comparative in Vitro Activity of Selected Antibiotics Against Anaerobic Bacteria

Pathogen (No.)	Minimum Inhibitory Concentration (mg/L)*			
	Metronidazole	Cefoxitin	Clindamycin	Piperacillin + Tazobactam
Bacteroides fragilis (32)	2	32	2	16
Bacteroides (23)	1	32	4	16
Fusobacterium (10)	<0.5	4	0.125	8
Clostridium difficile (13)	0.25	>64	>32	16
Clostridium perfringens (10)	8	4	2	<0.5
Clostridium (15)	4	64	8	8

*MIC for 90% of strains.
Data from Venezia RA, Yocum DM, Robbiano EM, et al: Comparative in vitro activities of a new quinolone, WIN 57273, and piperacillin plus tazobactam against anaerobic bacteria. *Antimicrob Agents Chemother* 1990;34:1858–61.

Recognition of the effectiveness of metronidazole for anaerobic infections was serendipitous and first described in 1962. The clinical observation that metronidazole effectively treated acute ulcerative gingivitis in a person who was taking the drug for trichomonal vaginitis led to studies that identified the antianaerobic activity of the drug. Subsequent investigations clearly demonstrated the potent, broad-spectrum activity of metronidazole against anaerobic bacteria.

However, concerns about the drug's possible carcinogenic and teratogenic potential limited its use to short-term therapy for amebiasis and for infections caused by *Trichomonas* and *Giardia.* The lack of substantive human data describing any real link between metronidazole and carcinogenic or teratogenic effects after more than 35 years of clinical use has fostered renewed interest in the use of this drug in treating systemic infections.

TABLE 14–65. Clindamycin and Lincomycin Dosing Recommendations

Clindamycin
Postnatal age <7 days
  ≤2,000 g: 10 mg/kg/day divided q12hr
  >2,000 g: 15 mg/kg/day divided q8hr
Postnatal age >7 days
  <1,200 g: 10 mg/kg/day divided q12hr
  1,200–2,000 g: 15 mg/kg/day divided q8hr
  >2,000 g: 20 mg/kg/day divided q6–8hr
Infants and children
  Oral: 10–30 mg/kg/day divided q6–8hr
  IV, IM: 25–40 mg/kg/day divided q6–8hr
Children and adults
  Topical: apply liberally twice daily
Adults
  Oral: 150–450 mg/dose q6–8hr (max 1.8 g/day)
  IV, IM: 1.2–1.8 g/day divided q6–12hr (max 4.8 g/day)
Available forms
  Oral capsules: 75 mg, 150 mg, 300 mg
  Oral suspension: 75 mg/5 mL
  Injection: 150 mg/mL (IM/IV); infuse for 60 min
  Vaginal cream
  Topical gel, lotion, solution

Lincomycin*
Children
  Oral: 30–60 mg/kg/day divided q6–8hr
  IM: 10 mg/kg q12–24hr
Adults
  Oral: 500 mg divided q6–8hr
  IM: 600 mg q12–24hr
Available forms
  Oral capsules: 250 mg, 500 mg
  Injection: 300 mg/mL (IM/IV) infuse IV for 60 min

*Doses are initial suggestions because insufficient data are available to make pediatric dose recommendations.

Spectrum of Activity. The mechanism of action of nitroimidazoles, from which metronidazole is derived, remains to be elucidated. In metronidazole, the nitro group appears to accept electrons from electron transport proteins, and these chemically reactive reduced forms of the drug produce cytotoxic compounds that accumulate and cause cell death. More recent studies have identified disruption of the helical structure of DNA and strand breakage by reduced metronidazole; this leads to cell death. Representative comparative in vitro activity of metronidazole is shown in Table 14–64.

Clinical Indications. Metronidazole is indicated for the treatment of anaerobic bacterial infections, including infections involving the central nervous system and brain abscess, trichomoniasis, amebiasis, and giardiasis.

Metabolism and Disposition. The disposition profile for metronidazole in both children and adults is poorly described. The tremendous variability observed in drug disposition, combined with a lack of uniformity in analytic methods used to analyze metronidazole concentrations in biologic fluids, limits the usefulness of available data. Many early studies used bioassay techniques that do not differentiate between the activity of the parent compound, metronidazole, and any of its active metabolites.

After oral administration, metronidazole appears to be completely absorbed. Peak serum concentrations are usually observed within 1–3 hours of administration. Serum metronidazole concentrations after rectal administration (bioavailability: 60–80%) and vaginal suppository administration (bioavailability: 20–30%) are much more variable and are often accompanied by a prolonged absorption phase. These suppository routes for metronidazole administration cannot be relied on for treatment of systemic infection.

Metronidazole distributes well into most body tissues and fluids, including the central nervous system, and protein binding approximates 10%. The drug is extensively metabolized by the liver to two primary hydroxylated acetic acid metabolites and other glucuronide and sulfated conjugates. The hydroxylated metabolite retains 60–80% of the bioactivity of the parent compound and accumulates in the blood after routine metronidazole dosing. Only about 20% of a total metronidazole dose is excreted unchanged as parent compound in the urine.

Less information is available on pediatric patients. In older infants, children, and adults, the metronidazole $t_{1/2\beta}$ and hydroxymetronidazole metabolite $t_{1/2\beta}$ are 6–12 hours and 9.5–20 hours,

TABLE 14–66. Metronidazole Dosing Recommendations

Neonates
Postnatal age <7 days
1,200–2,000 g: 7.5 mg/kg q24hr
>2,000 g: 7.5 mg/kg q12hr
Postnatal age >7 days
1,200–2,000 g: 7.5 mg/kg q12hr
>2,000 g: 15 mg/kg q12hr
Infants and Children
Amebiasis: 12–17 mg/kg q8hr
Other parasitic infections: 4–7.5 mg/kg q6hr
Anaerobic infections: 7.5 mg/kg q6hr
Adults
Amebiasis: 500–750 mg q8hr
Other parasitic infections: 250 mg q8hr
Anaerobic infections: 7.5 mg/kg q6hr, max 4 g/24-hr
Patients with Severe Liver Disease
Empirically decrease to one third to one half of normal daily dose; monitor daily for desired effect
Dialysis
Hemodialysis: dose supplementation
Available forms
Oral tablets: 250 mg, 500 mg
Injection: 5 mg/mL (avoid aluminum-containing equipment); neutralize infusion with bicarbonate (infuse for 60 min)

respectively. In premature and newborn infants and in persons with severe liver disease, metronidazole metabolism is markedly reduced and $t_{1/2\beta}$ values exceeding 24 hours have been described. Decreased total body clearance and drug accumulation are expected in premature and term infants during the first few months of life because of the immaturity of hepatic clearance mechanisms. The hydroxy metabolite has been detected in all preterm infants >35 weeks of age but in only two infants born at <35 weeks' gestation, although both mothers received betamethasone. Metronidazole doses must be adjusted to account for the maturation of hepatic and renal excretory pathways. Dosing recommendations are outlined in Table 14–66.

Adverse Effects. The types and severity of adverse effects that have been described after usual, routine metronidazole dosing are most often mild and self-limiting (Table 14–67). Mild nausea, abdominal cramping accompanied (rarely) by vomiting, headache, drowsiness, skin rashes, and an unpleasant metallic taste in the mouth have all been reported after oral metronidazole was received. More severe gastrointestinal effects, including prolonged anorexia, nausea, and vomiting, are usually associated with large single doses (>75 mg/kg/dose), as in radiosensitization, or with high-dose therapy (>180 mg/kg/day). Pseudomembranous colitis has been directly linked to oral metronidazole use in at least three patients, with only one case report of a metronidazole-resistant strain of *C. difficile.* Ironically the drug has been used successfully to treat many patients with antibiotic-associated pseudomembranous colitis (pediatric dose: 5 mg/kg administered every 6 hours for 10–14 days).

Neurotoxicity, including paresthesias, peripheral neuropathies, confusion, hallucinations, and seizures, have been described with metronidazole. These adverse effects appear to occur most commonly in persons who are receiving large doses for prolonged periods (>2 weeks). However, one case report describes a person who developed mental status changes after receiving metronidazole, 1 g every 12 hours for only 72 hours. Full recovery from these neurologic effects appears to occur after dose reduction or discontinuation of metronidazole therapy. An ''Antabuse type'' (disulfiram type) of reaction characterized by flushing, diaphoresis, throbbing headache, hyperventilation, tachycardia, confusion, and, in some persons, a toxic psychosis can occur when metronidazole is coadministered with alcohol. Like disulfiram, metronidazole most likely inhibits hepatic alcohol dehydrogenase, leading to acetaldehyde accumulation and the associated unpleasant effects.

Concerns regarding potential carcinogenic or teratogenic effects of metronidazole have severely limited the use of this drug to short courses, primarily in nonpregnant adults. The mutagenic potential of metronidazole and some urinary metabolites has been described in some bacteria and when bacterial test systems were used. A possible carcinogenic effect of high-dose metronidazole therapy was described in one preliminary rodent study, although other investigators have not been able to reproduce earlier findings. The relationship of these data from bacteria and rodents to humans is unknown. Numerous epidemiologic surveys have been unable to identify any link between metronidazole use and these effects in humans.

TABLE 14–67. Metronidazole-Associated Adverse Effects*

Nausea, vomiting, diarrhea
Metallic taste in mouth
Neutropenia (transient; rare: 2–4%)
Paresthesias, confusion, hallucinations
Disulfiram-like reaction
Carcinogenic, teratogenic potential (possible)

*See text for detailed descriptions.

TABLE 14–68. Potential Drug Interactions with Metronidazole

Cimetidine*
Ethanol (disulfiram-like reaction)
Lithium*
Phenobarbital†
Phenytoin*
Rifampin†

*Metronidazole decreases drug's body clearance (accumulation).
†Increases metronidazole metabolism.

Drug Interactions. A number of possible drug-drug interactions have been reported in persons receiving metronidazole, although the true clinical significance of most of these studies is questionable. A list of drugs that have been reported to result in drug interactions with metronidazole is shown in Table 14–68.

MUPIROCIN

Mupirocin, which was first isolated in 1971, is a fermentation product of *Pseudomonas fluorescens.* This drug is useful only for topical administration because of its rapid in vivo metabolism to antibacterially inactive metabolites (Table 14–69).

Spectrum of Activity. Mupirocin is active against a broad spectrum of gram-positive bacteria, including most strains of methicillin-sensitive and methicillin-resistant *Staphylococcus, Streptococcus* (but not *Enterococcus*), and *Listeria monocytogenes.* Some gram-negative bacteria, including *Moraxella catarrhalis* and most species

TABLE 14–69. Mupirocin

Drug Administration	Comment
Dosing	Topical application as needed 3–5 times daily (includes intranasal topical use for *Staphylococcus aureus* carriage)
Clinical indications	Impetigo, folliculitis; furunculosis, minor wounds, burns and ulcers; IV catheter exit site
Adverse effects	Rare, related to topical application
Drug interactions	None
Available forms	Ointment 2% (polyethylene glycol base)

of *Neisseria* and *Haemophilus,* are susceptible in vitro to mupirocin. The drug reversibly binds to the isoleucyl-tRNA synthetase of susceptible bacteria, preventing isoleucine incorporation and thereby inhibiting cellular protein synthesis.

Clinical Indications. Mupirocin is used topically for treatment of superficial skin infections such as impetigo. It is also administered intranasally to eradicate nasal carriage of *S. aureus,* such as in infection control programs to eliminate nosocomial transmission of methicillin-resistant strains of *S. aureus.*

Metabolism and Disposition. Mupirocin is well absorbed after oral administration but is rapidly and extensively metabolized to the antibacterially inactive metabolite monic acid. Thus the drug is of clinical value only when administered topically. When administered topically to intact skin, only small amounts of mupirocin appear to be absorbed into the systemic circulation. An increased amount of drug is absorbed when it is applied to traumatized or diseased skin. Nevertheless, the portion of drug that is not metabolized within the various layers of the skin (approximately 5–30%) is rapidly metabolized by the liver to monic acid.

ANTIFUNGAL DRUGS

AMPHOTERICIN B

Amphotericin B is considered by most physicians to be the "gold standard" for assessing the efficacy of systemic antifungal drugs. It is the agent to which all new antifungal drugs must be compared before clinical acceptance. A member of the polyene group of antifungal drugs (e.g., nystatin), amphotericin B was isolated from *Streptomyces nodosus,* which was discovered in the Orinoco River valley in Venezuela in 1953. Amphotericin B is an amphoteric compound (hence its name) that forms soluble salts in basic or acidic media. It remains the most effective antifungal agent in the therapeutic armamentarium. Recent advances in the formulation of amphotericin B with lipid complexes and liposomal delivery systems are promising approaches to enhanced efficacy and reduced toxicity.

Spectrum of Activity. The polyene antifungal agents bind to the membrane sterol ergosterol, resulting in increased membrane permeability and leakage of cellular contents, which culminates in cell death. Amphotericin B possesses a broad spectrum of activity against many fungal species but has no clinically important activity against bacteria, rickettsiae, *Chlamydia,* or viruses.

Comparison of fungal pathogen susceptibility to amphotericin B and other important antifungal drugs is shown in Table 14–70.

Metabolism and Disposition. Amphotericin B is poorly absorbed after oral administration and is irritating to tissue, thus precluding intramuscular administration. For the treatment of systemic infections, the drug is administered by slow intravenous infusion, usually for 4–6 hours. Little is understood about the disposition profile of amphotericin B in the body, although the drug has been used clinically for many years. Once in the systemic circulation, amphotericin B binds avidly to serum proteins (>95%), primarily to cholesterol moieties of β-lipoproteins. Amphotericin B also distributes to many organs and body fluids to varying degrees, but the actual sites and overall extent of drug distribution are poorly defined.

Studies attempting to quantitate drug in the cerebrospinal fluid have usually reported low and extremely variable concentrations, which suggests poor central nervous system penetration. However, amphotericin B monotherapy can be effective treatment for fungal meningitis, particularly when adequate doses have been administered for a sufficient period. Some clinicians have advocated supplemental intraventricular administration of amphotericin B in severely ill persons with central nervous system fungal infections.

Approximately 3% of amphotericin B is excreted in the urine unchanged in a 24-hour period. Detectable concentrations in urine have been described for as many as 27–35 days after discontinuation of therapy. The bile appears to be another important route of amphotericin B elimination from the body. Amphotericin B dosing recommendations have been derived largely from clinical experience. Dosing recommendations for amphotericin B and liposomal amphotericin B are shown in Table 14–71. General guidelines for the administration of amphotericin B are outlined Table 14–72.

Adverse Effects. For many years amphotericin B has gained a reputation as an exceedingly toxic drug (Table 14–73). For this reason, most clinicians avoid prescribing it until a diagnosis of a serious, systemic fungal infection has been made on the basis of blood or biopsy culture. The complexity of the biodisposition of amphotericin B, along with its slow distribution into tissues, would support the idea that an earlier initiation of therapy might result in greater clinical success. However, virtually every person who receives amphotericin B has some form of drug-induced adverse effect. Most of these effects are mild, but some may be life-threatening.

Nephrotoxicity is the most feared and most common adverse effect associated with amphotericin B administration. Up to 80% of adults who receive amphotericin B have some form of drug-associated reduction in renal function.

Administration of amphotericin B is associated with a decrease in renal blood flow and glomerular filtration, as well as impairment of proximal and distal tubular reabsorption of electrolytes, most notably potassium and magnesium. In nearly every adult who receives therapeutic doses of the drug, the glomerular filtration rate (GFR) drops initially by approximately 40% and stabilizes to between 20% and 60% of its normal value during prolonged therapy. This reduction in GFR is accompanied by increases in serum creatinine and blood urea nitrogen levels. After discontinuation of therapy, renal function usually returns to pretreatment values. This normalization process can take as long as weeks to months in some persons. However, similar effects on GFR have not been reported in infants and children, and the impact of amphotericin B therapy on renal function in pediatric patients is largely unknown. The incidence of renal problems in these persons appears to be lower than in adults.

TABLE 14–70. Comparative Susceptibility of Fungi to Important Antifungal Drugs

Antifungal Drug	Clinically Useful Activity Spectrum	Less Susceptible Fungi	Commonly Resistant Fungi
Amphotericin B	*Aspergillus* *Blastomyces dermatitidis* *Candida* *Coccidioides immitis* *Cryptococcus neoformans* *Histoplasma capsulatum* Zygomycetes	*Fusarium* *Candida lusitaniae*	*Aspergillus terreus* *Pseudallescheria boydii* (*Scedosporium apiospermum* is the asexual form)
5-Flucytosine (5-FC)	*Candida* *C. neoformans*		Other fungal pathogens
Fluconazole	*Candida* Dermatophytes *C. immitis* *C. neoformans*	*Blastomyces* *Candida glabrata* *Candida krusei* *Candida parapsilosis* *H. capsulatum*	*Aspergillus* Zygomycetes
Itraconazole, voriconazole, posiconazole*	*Aspergillus* *B. dermatitidis* *Candida* *C. immitis* *C. neoformans* Dermatophytes *H. capsulatum*	Fluconazole-resistant *Candida*	
Caspofungin	*Aspergillus* *Candida* *C. immitis* *H. capsulatum* *B. dermatitidis* *Pneumocystis carinii*		*Cryptococcus* *Fusarium* Zygomycetes

*Voriconazole and posiconazole have activity against *Fusarium* and *Pseudallescheria boydii.*

If nephrotoxicity is observed, alternate-day amphotericin B dosing with the usual (approximately 0.75 mg/kg) or twice-usual (approximately 1.5 mg/kg) doses has been suggested by some clinicians to afford better patient tolerance and retard the rate at which renal toxicity occurs. The actual benefit of alternate-day amphotericin B dosing is unclear, but such dosing may allow therapy in persons with marked renal toxicity to continue. In either case, single amphotericin B doses should not exceed 1.5 mg/kg in any 24-hour period. Irreversible renal toxicity resulting from amphotericin B therapy alone is extremely rare but has been reported when total doses have exceeded 4–5 g or after severe acute overdoses.

TABLE 14–71. Dose Recommendations for Amphotericin B

Colloidal suspension product: fungizone
- Neonates, infants, children, and adults: 0.5–1 mg/kg once daily, infused for 4–6 hr IV

Lipid-based formulation: liposomal amphotericin B (AmBisome); amphotericin B colloidal dispersion (ABCD; Amphotec); amphotericin B lipid complex (ABLC; Abelcet)
- Neonates, infants, children, and adults: 3–5 mg/kg once daily infused for 30 min IV
- Dialysis: no dose adjustment necessary
- Available forms: Lyophilized powder for injection preferably infused via a large vein in a dextrose-containing solution (do not filter any amphotericin B formulations); also available for topical application as a 3% cream, ointment, or lotion and 100 mg/mL suspension

*Serum concentrations monitoring may aid in avoiding bone marrow suppression (serum concentrate <100 mg/L).

No specific therapy to prevent or reverse amphotericin B–associated nephrotoxicity has been identified. A number of different strategies have been advocated with varying degrees of success. The most promising therapy to date appears to be the supplemental administration of sodium, often referred to as sodium loading or salt loading. Although controlled studies assessing the benefit of sodium supplementation are lacking, preliminary investigations and clinical experience have demonstrated success in preventing or reversing amphotericin B–associated nephrotoxicity. The mechanism of this renal protective effect of sodium is unknown. Nevertheless, it is currently recommended that persons receiving amphotericin B who are considered to be at risk of having nephrotoxicity receive supplemental sodium (1 mEq/kg/day) just before each daily dose of amphotericin B unless additional sodium is contraindicated. Routine clinical and laboratory monitoring of fluid and electrolyte balance is required for all persons receiving supplemental sodium. The substitution of a lipid-based amphotericin B product in persons with decreasing renal function induced by administration of the original colloidal suspension formulation will often reverse the observed decrease in GFR. For this reason, many centers are initiating amphotericin B therapy with a lipid-based complex (e.g., ABLC or liposomal) in persons predisposed to a marked amphotericin B–induced decrease in GFR. However, the high cost of the lipid formulations makes their routine use impractical. The importance of close monitoring of serum (urinary) electrolyte concentrations, including potassium and magnesium, in persons receiving amphotericin B cannot be overemphasized. Hypokalemia and hypomagnesemia, which can be profound, are common after just a few weeks of amphotericin B administration.

Shaking chills (rigors) and fevers frequently occur during the intravenous infusion of amphotericin B. The mechanism responsi-

TABLE 14–72. General Guidelines for the Administration of Amphotericin B

Administer a test dose (0.1 mg/kg children; 1 mg adult) either by mixing in 25–50 mL dextrose 5% in water or a 1 mg aliquot of the initial daily dose, infused for 20–30 min
If person has a reaction to the test dose or develops cardiopulmonary impairment, cautiously try a second test dose of 50–100 μg
If tolerated, prepare the drug in a concentration of 0.1 mg/mL of 5% dextrose water; do not use 0.9% sodium chloride solution, which may cause the drug to precipitate
Institute therapy with 0.25 mg/kg administered for 2–6 hr
Adjust dosage to patient tolerance
Increase daily dose gradually on subsequent days to a maximum of 0.5–0.6 mg/kg in most cases, not to exceed 1–1.5 mg/kg/day
Administer total daily dose by slow intravenous infusion (for 4–6 hr)
Lipid-based formulation may be infused for 30–60 min
Duration of treatment for most deep-seated mycoses is usually 6–12 wk; in severe or recalcitrant infections, the daily dose may range up to 1 mg/kg for many months (alternatively, dose escalation of a lipid-based formulation (8+ mg/kg/day) may be employed
If person is critically ill or immunocompromised, the first dose of 0.25 mg/kg can be given 2–4 hr after test dose; the next 2 or 3 doses can be given at 8-hr intervals, not exceeding a total of 0.6 mg/kg for 24 hr; monitor renal function closely
Amphotericin B can be given on alternate days by doubling daily dose up to a maximum of 1.5 mg/kg/dose; switching to lipid-based formulation in these patients would be optimal
Total daily dose should never exceed 1.5 mg/kg
Consider concomitant sodium administration (sodium or salt loading), 1 mEq/kg/day, routinely when using conventional colloidal suspension formulation

ble for these reactions is unknown, but they may result from amphotericin B–induced stimulation of prostaglandin synthesis, specifically prostaglandin E. Numerous therapies have been suggested to abate these uncomfortable side effects. Pretreatment with meperidine (0.5–1 mg/kg/dose), but not other opioids, approximately 10–30 minutes before amphotericin B administration is effective in ameliorating the associated shaking chills. In severe cases the meperidine dose can be repeated in the middle of the infusion if it is tolerated by the patient. More recent preliminary studies suggest that pretreatment with an NSAID (e.g., ibuprofen, 10 mg/kg) may also be effective, but the data are insufficient to recommend this alternative. The addition of hydrocortisone (25–100 mg) to amphotericin B infusion solutions has also been suggested to help reduce the febrile reactions associated with amphotericin B. The benefit of concurrent hydrocortisone administration has not been demonstrated in controlled clinical trials, however.

In addition, thrombophlebitis is reported frequently in persons receiving amphotericin B through peripheral veins. The addition of heparin (0.5–1 U/mL) to the infusion solution is often advocated as a means to minimize the incidence and severity of this reaction, although the use of heparin is unsubstantiated. Whenever possible, amphotericin B should be administered through a central venous catheter, and infusate concentrations should not exceed 0.1 mg/mL.

TABLE 14–73. Adverse Effects and Drug-Drug Interactions Associated with Amphotericin B

Adverse Effects
Hypokalemia, hypomagnesemia
Nephrotoxicity*
Fever and chills*
Nausea, vomiting, diarrhea
Thrombophlebitis
Bone marrow suppression (rare)
Peripheral neuropathy (intrathecal dosing)

Drug-Drug Interactions
Additive or synergistic nephrotoxic effects when coadministered with other nephrotoxins: aminoglycosides, cisplatin, cyclosporine, tacrolimus

*Incidence remarkably decreased with lipid-based formulations.

Many persons receiving amphotericin B are found to be anemic. The anemia, which usually occurs weeks into therapy, is normochromic and normocytic. It is usually mild and reverses without specific therapy after discontinuation of amphotericin B therapy. This possible drug reaction may be a result of inhibition of erythrocyte or erythropoietin production, or it may be a secondary effect of the amphotericin B–associated renal disease. Severely ill, debilitated persons may require intermittent transfusions to maintain an adequate hematocrit value. Leukopenia and thrombocytopenia have also been only rarely observed in persons receiving amphotericin B.

FLUCYTOSINE

Flucytosine (5-fluorocytosine [5-FC]) is a fluorinated pyrimidine synthesized in 1957 as part of a search for new drugs effective in the treatment of leukemia. The drug's antileukemic activity was limited, but flucytosine was later found to be effective therapy in the murine model of *Candida* sepsis. The drug enters the cell wall of yeasts by means of the permease system responsible for the normal cellular transfer of natural cytosine. Once inside the yeast cell, flucytosine is rapidly deaminated by cytosine deaminase to the antimetabolite 5-fluorouracil and incorporated into fungal RNA, thus inhibiting cell growth. Depending on its intracellular concentration, flucytosine can promote a fungistatic or a fungicidal effect. Amphotericin B may act synergistically with flucytosine against some fungi, most notably *Candida, Aspergillus,* and *Cryptococcus neoformans,* by altering the plasma membrane and increasing intracellular flucytosine concentrations.

Flucytosine possesses no inherent antibacterial activity. Primary resistance and the development of resistance by fungi during therapy have been major limitations to the clinical use of this drug as monotherapy for fungal infections. The mechanisms of resistance include fungal cell loss of deaminase activity, overproduction of pyrimidines, and loss of permease activity. Preliminary data suggest that a more rapid emergence of fungal resistance to flucytosine may be observed when lower doses (e.g., 100 mg/kg/day) rather than higher doses (e.g., 150 mg/kg/day) are used. Rapid development of resistance and possibly synergy underscores the primary clinical use of coadministration with amphotericin B.

Metabolism and Disposition. Flucytosine is rapidly and almost completely absorbed into systemic circulation following oral administration. The oral bioavailability range is 75–90% or higher. The rate and extent of flucytosine absorption have been reported to be delayed and reduced in patients with severely impaired renal function. Peak serum concentrations are usually observed 1–2 hours after an oral dose. The drug is well distributed in most body fluids and tissues, including the central nervous system. Approximately 3–5% of the drug is bound to plasma proteins.

The majority of flucytosine (85–95%) is excreted unchanged in the urine by means of glomerular filtration. Thus the elimination half-life ($t_{1/2\beta}$) of flucytosine is dependent on renal function. As expected, the drug's $t_{1/2\beta}$ is prolonged in premature and newborn infants with immature renal function and in patients with compromised renal function. In individuals with normal renal function, $t_{1/2\beta}$ usually ranges from 2.5 to 6 hours. In neonates the $t_{1/2\beta}$ range is reported to be 4–34 hours, and in adult patients with creatinine clearance values less than 10 mL/min the $t_{1/2\beta}$ exceeds 100 hours.

The usual dose of flucytosine in older infants, children, and adults is 100–150 mg/kg/day administered in four equal doses. Dosing should be modified proportionately in patients with compromised or immature renal function. Preliminary experience with premature and newborn infants has revealed highly variable flucytosine disposition characteristics and suggests an initial flucytosine dose of 50–100 mg/kg administered once daily. Both peritoneal dialysis and hemodialysis remove varying amounts of flucytosine; therefore supplemental dosing should be guided by the patient's clinical response to therapy, severity of underlying disease, and serial measurements of serum flucytosine levels. In the United States flucytosine is available as 250 mg or 500 mg capsules. These may be reformulated into a liquid or syrup for oral administration.

Adverse Effects. Aside from bone marrow suppression, adverse effects associated with flucytosine therapy appear to be unusual (Table 14–74). When they do occur, reactions are mild, especially in children. Gastrointestinal intolerance, including nausea and vomiting, has been reported to occur in up to 6% of patients receiving the drug. Rare cases of gastric mucosal necrosis and perforation have been reported.

The most significant adverse effect associated with flucytosine therapy is reversibly bone marrow suppression. Leukopenia or thrombocytopenia occurs in as many as 30% of patients and is more common in patients with compromised renal function. The myelosuppressive effects of flucytosine are most likely a result of the drug's in vivo conversion to 5-fluorouracil and represent the most common reason for discontinuing the drug. Marrow-suppressive effects are often observed after 10–26 days of therapy and appear to correlate well with high serum flucytosine concentrations. Maintenance of serum flucytosine concentrations below 100 mg/L is generally well tolerated by most patients. To avoid marrow-suppressive effects, serum flucytosine concentrations should be monitored in patients with compromised or fluctuating renal function and in those undergoing dialysis, including hemofiltration.

TABLE 14–74. Adverse Effects and Drug-Drug Interactions Associated with Flucytosine

Adverse Effects
Dose-related bone marrow suppression* (doses >150 mg/kg/day or decreased renal function)
Gastrointestinal intolerance (~6%)
Gastric mucosal necrosis or perforation (rare)
Drug-Drug Interactions
Additive or synergistic adverse effect when coadministered with other drugs known to suppress bone marrow function

*Leukopenia or thrombocytopenia unusual when serum flucytosine concentration is maintained at <100 mg/L.

Drug Interactions. The coadministration of oral antacids and aluminum or magnesium salts delays the rate but not the overall extent of flucytosine absorption. When coadministered with other drugs known to suppress bone marrow function, flucytosine may enhance associated bone marrow suppression.

FLUCONAZOLE AND INTRACONAZOLE

Fluconazole is the first in a series of new triazole antifungal agents and the most widely studied in pediatrics. The growing number of azole compounds reflects the continuing search for alternative antifungal drugs that are more effective and less toxic than the "gold standard," amphotericin B.

Spectrum of Activity. Ergosterol, the primary membrane sterol of fungal cells, is necessary for the formation of a competent cell wall. The azole antifungal drugs, including the imidazoles (e.g., miconazole, ketoconazole) and the triazoles (e.g., fluconazole, itraconazole), inhibit the C-14 demethylation of lanosterol, the primary precursor of ergosterol. The accumulation of ergosterol precursors causes disruptive changes in the permeability of the fungal cell membrane, inhibiting cell growth or causing cell death. Lanosterol demethylation is a cytochrome P-450-dependent process. The imidazole drugs appear less selective than triazole compounds in their inhibition of cytochrome P-450 enzyme activity, which may explain their greater propensity for interfering with the metabolism of other drugs metabolized by hepatic cytochrome P-450 enzymes. This mechanism of antifungal action of the imidazole drugs is different from that observed with amphotericin B, which binds to fungal cell ergosterol and promotes pore formation and cell leakage. Pathogenic fungi usually responsive to triazoles are listed in Table 14–70.

Metabolism and Disposition. Fluconazole is well absorbed after oral administration. Comparison of the disposition characteristics of fluconazole, itraconazole, and voriconazole is shown in Table 14–75. Current dosing recommendations are shown in Table 14–76 and important azole-induced adverse effects in Table 14–77.

TABLE 14–75. Comparative Pharmacokinetics of Selected Azole Antifungal Drugs in Adults

Parameter	Fluconazole	Itraconazole	Voriconazole
Oral bioavailability (%)	>90	50*	>90
T_{max} (hr)	1–2	1.5–4	1–2
Protein binding (%)	<15	>90	65
Vd (L/kg)	0.7–0.8	10.7	2
Primary route of elimination	Renal	Hepatic	Hepatic
Unchanged drug in urine (% of dose)	80	<1	<5
$t_{1/2\beta}$ (hr)	25–30†	20–40	6
Hemodialysis	Yes	No	?

T_{max} = time to peak serum drug concentration; Vd = volume of distribution; $t_{1/2\beta}$ = elimination half-life.

*Capsule formulation ~100% bioavailable when administered immediately after a meal ~40% with food; syrup formulation best administered on an empty stomach.

†Fluconazole $t_{1/2\beta}$ relative to age: premature infant ~70 hours; 12-day-old neonates ~40–50 hours; 9–13 months of age 20–25 hours; 5–15 years of age 15–18 hours.

TABLE 14–76. Dosing Recommendations for Selected Azole Antifungal Drugs

Fluconazole
Neonates <14 days of age: 3–12 mg/kg q72hr IV/PO
Children: 6–12 mg/kg once daily IV/PO
Adults: 200–800 mg once daily IV/PO

Available Forms
Oral tablets: 50 mg, 100 mg, 150 mg, 200 mg
Oral suspension: 10 mg/mL, 40 mg/mL
Injection: 2 mg/mL for slow IV infusion over 1–2 hr (≤200 mg/hr)

Itraconazole
Neonates: 5 mg/kg once daily or divided bid IV/PO
Children: 5 mg/kg once daily or divided bid IV/PO
Adults: 200 mg once daily or divided bid IV/PO

Available Forms
Oral capsule: 100 mg
Oral syrup: 10 mg/mL

Voriconazole*
Children: 6 mg/kg load; 4–6 mg/kg q12hr PO
Adults: 200 mg q12hr

*Investigational doses are preliminary suggestions.

Drug Interactions. Because fluconazole and other triazoles possess a high affinity for fungal cytochrome P-450 enzymes, it inhibits C-14 demethylase activity mediated by these enzymes, which leads to diminished ergosterol synthesis. The affinity of triazoles for mammalian cytochrome P-450 isoenzymes appears to be much less. Nevertheless, numerous metabolism-based drug-drug interactions have been reported with the use of triazole antifungal drugs (Table 14–78), primarily because of the ability of these drugs to interfere with the drug-metabolizing cytochrome P-450 enzymes. Although the affinity by individual triazole compounds for mammalian cytochrome P-450 varies, insufficient data are available to define specific cytochrome P-450 isoenzymes (other than CYP 3A4). Thus, until further data are available, caution should be employed whenever a cytochrome P-450 substrate (particularly 3A4) is coadministered with a triazole antifungal drug in the same person (Table 14–78).

ECHINOCANDINS

The echinocandins are a new class of antifungal drugs with tremendous promise. Caspofungin is the first analog approved for use in humans, to be followed by micafungin. These agents inhibit the synthesis of (1,3)-β-glucan, which is a glucose polymer essential for the structural integrity of fungal cell walls. This inhibition leads to structural damage of the cell wall of susceptible fungi, ultimately leading to cell lysis. In vitro susceptibility testing has demonstrated potent activity against *Candida, Aspergillus, Histoplasma capsulatum, Blastomyces dermatitidis,* and *P. carinii* (see Table 14–70). *Cryptococcus neoformans* and members of the Mucorales order are resistant to the echinocandins, reflecting the small amount of (1,3)-β-glucan synthase present in the cell wall of these later fungal pathogens. Most important, preliminary clinical efficacy trials of these agents reveal a high cure rate in the treatment of superficial and systemic infections caused by susceptible fungi (Table 14–70), particularly infections caused by *Candida.* Moreover, these drugs appear to possess a high therapeutic index with only mild adverse effects. To date, pediatric experience with echinocandins is limited. Clearly the results of clinical trials in both children and adults are needed to better define the role of these agents in clinical practice.

TABLE 14–78. Azole-Associated Drug-Drug Interactions

Azoles block the body clearance of the following drugs: benzodiazepine, astemizole, cisapride, cyclosporine, corticosteroids, digoxin, 3-hydroxy-3-methylglutaryl–coenzyme-A (HMG-CoA) reductase inhibitors, oral contraceptives, sulfonylureas, warfarin.
Enzyme inducers can stimulate metabolism of azoles: carbamazepine, phenobarbital, phenytoin, rifampin, rifabutin.
Gastric alkalizers reduce absorption of itraconazole and butoconazole*: antacids, cimetidine, didanosine, famotidine, lansoprazole, nizatidine, omeprazole, pantoprazole, ranitidine.
Metabolic-based interactions: fluconazole, itraconazole, and ketoconazole interfere with cytochrome P-450 drug–metabolizing enzymes (primarily cytochrome P-450 3A4). The magnitude of interaction is dependent on the affinity of the specific azole for the specific cytochrome P-450 isozyme, which varies among different azole compounds.

*Itraconazole and butoconazole require gastric acidity for oral absorption.

GRISEOFULVIN

Griseofulvin is effective in vitro against nearly all strains of *Trichophyton,* including *T. rubrum, T. tonsurans, T. mentagrophytes, T. verrucosum, T. megninii, T. gallinae,* and *T. schoenleinii.* The drug also demonstrates in vitro activity against *Epidermophyton floccosum* and species of *Microsporum,* including *M. audouinii, M. canis,* and *M. gypseum.* Griseofulvin is ineffective against other fungi.

TABLE 14–77. Important Adverse Effects of the Two Primary Azole Antifungal Drugs Used in Pediatrics

	Itraconazole	Fluconazole
Gastrointestinal tract	Nausea, vomiting (<10%)	Nausea (2%), vomiting (<5%), diarrhea (2%)
Skin and appendages	Pruritus, rash	Rash (~1.8%), possibly exfoliative
Hepatobiliary system	Elevations of aminotransferase values (<5%); hepatitis (rare)	Elevations of aminotransferase values (<7%); hepatitis (rare)
Endocrine system	Syndrome of mineralocorticoid excess; pedal edema; decreased testosterone synthesis (all rare)	Hypercholesterolemia Hypertriglyceridemia
Nervous system	Headache, dizziness, fatigue	Headache 1.9%, seizures

An investigational azole, voriconazole, may cause a transient visual disturbance (~25–30%), which tends to occur most often early in therapy with intravenous administration.

The antifungal activity of griseofulvin most likely results from its ability to disrupt the mitotic spindle structure of susceptible fungi. This antimitotic activity, which appears to involve a mechanism different from that of colchicine, causes cell arrest during metaphase. Deposition of griseofulvin in keratin precursor cells inhibits fungal invasion.

Griseofulvin remains the drug of choice for the treatment of dermatophyte infections, including tinea corporis (face and trunk), tinea capitis (scalp, eyebrows, and eyelashes), tinea cruris (groin, perineal and perianal areas), tinea pedis (feet), tinea barbae (beard and mustache), and tinea unguium (nails). This recommendation is based largely on the long history of the drug's clinical use, rather than on any thorough understanding of its clinical pharmacology in children.

Metabolism and Disposition. The oral bioavailability of griseofulvin is highly variable, often unpredictable, and extremely dependent on the pharmaceutical formulation administered. Approximately 25–75% of an oral dose of the microsize formulation (referring to drug particle size) is absorbed into the systemic circulation. The ultramicrosize formulation is the preferred formulation because nearly all of an administered dose is absorbed and the overall rate and extent of drug absorption are more consistent and predictable. Absorption of the microsize formulation is enhanced when the drug is coadministered with a meal high in fat content. Although this drug-food interaction is often discussed, the potential benefit to the patient is limited.

Once absorbed, griseofulvin is concentrated in skin, hair, nails, liver, fat, and skeletal muscle. The drug is deposited into keratin precursor cells with a high affinity for diseased tissue, which makes new keratin resistant to fungal invasion. Griseofulvin does not eradicate fungus that has infected the outer keratin layers of the hair, skin, or nails. Instead, the drug promotes cure through the natural shedding of fungus-infected keratin cells and replacement by sterile, griseofulvin-rich keratin cells. Thus the duration of griseofulvin therapy is directed by the time needed for normal desquamation—approximately 4–6 weeks for fungal infections of the skin or hair. In contrast, infections of the nails take longer; for example, toenail infections may require more than 1 year of continuous griseofulvin treatment.

Griseofulvin is metabolized in the liver to inactive metabolites that are excreted from the body in the urine. Less than 1% of the absorbed dose is excreted as parent griseofulvin in the urine. The $t_{1/2\beta}$ of griseofulvin has been reported to range between 9 and 22 hours.

Usual griseofulvin dosing recommendations are shown in Table 14–79. Dosage adjustment is unnecessary for persons with renal insufficiency, but the dose may need to be reduced or therapy discontinued in persons with moderate to severe hepatic functional impairment.

Adverse Effects. Adverse effects associated with griseofulvin administration are unusual and, when they occur, appear to be mild (see Table 14–79). Headache, which usually occurs during the first few weeks of therapy and resolves with continued therapy, appears to be the most common adverse effect of the drug. Gastrointestinal upset (nausea, vomiting), skin rashes, irritability, and mental confusion have been reported. Rare adverse effects include albuminuria and cylindruria, with no evidence of renal insufficiency, photosensitivity, or leukopenia. Griseofulvin interferes with porphyrin metabolism without clinical effect in healthy persons, but in persons with porphyria the drug may precipitate an acute exacerbation of the disease.

TABLE 14–79. Griseofulvin Dosing Recommendations, Adverse Effects, and Drug Interactions

Children
Microsize: 10–20 mg/kg/day in single or divided doses
Ultramicrosize: 5–10 mg/kg once daily or divided bid

Adults
Microsize: 500–1,000 mg once daily or divided bid
Ultramicrosize
- 330–375 mg/day in single or divided doses
- Doses up to 750 mg/day for infections more difficult to eradicate, such as tinea unguium (onychomycosis)

Adverse Effects
Headache, dizziness, nausea, vomiting
Albuminuria, cylindruria (rare)
Photosensitivity

Drug Interactions
Phenobarbital, rifampin, warfarin, alcohol

Available Forms
Microsize
- Oral capsules: 250 mg
- Oral suspension: 125 mg/5 mL
- Oral tablets: 250 mg, 500 mg

Ultramicrosize: Oral tablets: 125 mg, 165 mg, 250 mg, 330 mg

Drug Interactions. Griseofulvin reportedly stimulates the hepatic metabolism of warfarin and oral contraceptive steroids, thus reducing their pharmacodynamic effect (Table 14–79). Phenobarbital has been reported to result in lower griseofulvin serum concentrations. The mechanism of this possible phenobarbital-griseofulvin drug interaction is unclear and may be due to enhanced griseofulvin metabolism or decreased gastrointestinal absorption caused by phenobarbital.

KETOCONAZOLE AND MICONAZOLE

Ketoconazole is a synthetic imidazole antifungal drug that is very similar in pharmacology and antifungal activity to miconazole. The primary difference between these drugs is the relative clinical effectiveness of ketoconazole after oral administration. Ketoconazole is not available for parenteral administration. Moreover, with the availability of fluconazole and the newer, more advanced generation of triazoles (e.g., voriconazole, pozaconazole) and echinocandins, systemic ketoconazole is rarely used, particularly in children. Miconazole, also a synthetic imidazole antifungal agent, is used primarily as topical treatment for superficial fungal infections.

Metabolism and Disposition. Ketoconazole is rapidly absorbed after oral administration. The extent of this absorption is variable, however, and it may be decreased by the presence of food because it depends on low gastric pH. An acidic environment enhances ketoconazole dissolution to the hydrochloride salt, thus increasing systemic absorption. Concomitant administration of medications that increase gastric pH (e.g., antacids, histamine 2–receptor antagonists [cimetidine, ranitidine]) may decrease the rate and extent of ketoconazole absorption.

Approximately 84–99% of the drug is bound to plasma proteins. Only limited data concerning the distribution characteristics of ketoconazole are available. The drug has been detected in many body fluids, including urine, saliva, sweat, cerumen, and synovial fluid. Cerebrospinal fluid concentrations appear low and highly variable relative to plasma concentrations. The drug is partially metabolized in the liver to multiple inactive metabolites. Less than 20% of an administered dose is excreted unchanged in the urine.

Adverse Effects. The most common adverse effect associated with ketoconazole is gastrointestinal upset, including nausea and vomiting. These symptoms have been reported to resolve spontaneously, with no changes in drug dosing. Ketoconazole is a competitive inhibitor of testosterone, and at daily doses consistently exceeding 400 mg, males often have tender gynecomastia and decreased libido. These effects appear reversible on discontinuation of therapy.

Abnormalities in liver function test results, primarily transient asymptomatic elevations in hepatic serum aminotransferases, can also occur at any time during ketoconazole therapy. These elevations appear to return to normal despite continued ketoconazole administration and do not appear to signal more severe hepatotoxicity.

Drug Interactions. The concomitant administration of ketoconazole may decrease the hepatic metabolism of cyclosporine, corticosteroids, and possibly warfarin. Rifampin may stimulate the metabolism of ketoconazole.

NYSTATIN

Nystatin is a polyene antifungal drug originally isolated in 1950 for *Streptomyces noursei.* Until recently nystatin has been too toxic for systemic administration and has been used only as a topical agent. A systemically administered liposomal formulation is undergoing clinical investigation. The results of these clinical investigations and the role of liposomal nystatin in clinical practice have yet to be defined.

Nystatin possesses a broad spectrum of antifungal activity against yeast and yeastlike fungi. Susceptible microorganisms include species of *Candida, Aspergillus, Trichophyton, Microsporum, Histoplasma,* and *Coccidioides.* Nystatin binds to cell membrane sterols of susceptible fungi, thus disrupting the integrity of the fungal cell membrane. These characteristics and its broad spectrum of antifungal activity underscores the renewed interest in formulating a safe, systemically administered nystatin formulation.

Nystatin is most commonly used in the treatment of mild, superficial candidal infections, such as oral thrush, and as a prophylactic agent in critically ill and immunocompromised persons. Swabbing the oropharynx or instilling the drug by means of nasogastric tube or swallowing may prevent nosocomial fungal disease in such patients.

Metabolism and Disposition. Nystatin is poorly absorbed from the skin and the gastrointestinal tract. The drug is available as a suspension or cream for topical administration and as tablets for vaginal and oral use. One milligram of nystatin is equivalent to 3,500 units of nystatin.

Adverse Effects. Virtually no adverse effects are associated with the topical administration of nystatin. No drug interactions involving topical nystatin have been identified.

ANTIVIRAL DRUGS

ACYCLOVIR, FAMCICLOVIR, AND GANCICLOVIR

Acyclovir, an acyclic purine nucleoside of guanine, is relatively nontoxic and is effective against herpesviruses. During trials it was discovered that the drug identifies adenosine analogs capable of competing with adenosine deaminase activity for possible use as immunosuppressants.

Famciclovir is a synthetic, acyclic purine nucleoside analog of guanine possessing no inherent antiviral activity. The drug is an orally administered prodrug that is metabolized within the intestinal wall and liver, liberating antivirally active penciclovir. Penciclovir is structurally related to ganciclovir with pharmacologic activity related to acyclovir. Like acyclovir and ganciclovir, penciclovir is converted intracellularly to the active triphosphate moiety.

Ganciclovir is structurally and pharmacologically similar to acyclovir. The structural modifications in ganciclovir give the compound substantially greater antiviral activity against CMV, with less selectivity for viral DNA in comparison with acyclovir.

Spectrum of Activity. Considerable controversy persists regarding determination of antiviral drug susceptibility patterns in vitro and the appropriate way to report this activity. Nevertheless, in vitro and animal data suggest that these three antiviral drugs possess marked activity against human herpesviruses (HSV-1 and HSV-2), with less effectiveness against varicella-zoster virus (VZV). Acyclovir and ganciclovir appear to inhibit replicating Epstein-Barr virus (EBV) but have no effect on latent cellular infection. Adenoviruses and RNA viruses, including rhinovirus, measles virus, respiratory syncytial virus, and influenza virus, are usually resistant to these drugs.

Overall, ganciclovir is a more potent antiviral drug than acyclovir. Acyclovir possesses no clinically useful activity against CMV, but ganciclovir is very active in vitro against this virus and is used primarily for the treatment of serious CMV infections. In vitro studies show that ganciclovir is approximately 100 times more potent against CMV than acyclovir.

The role of penciclovir in clinical practice remains to be elucidated, particularly in pediatrics, for which few data exist. Most important, optimal dosing recommendations for these drugs have not been defined, which severely limits the use of oral famciclovir, a highly bioavailable agent. The excellent bioavailability of famciclovir with oral dosing favors its use in pediatrics when appropriate dosing recommendations become available.

Once inside cells infected with herpesvirus, acyclovir is converted to acyclovir monophosphate by herpes-induced deoxynucleoside kinase, which is also referred to as thymidine kinase. Intracellular acyclovir monophosphate is further phosphorylated to acyclovir triphosphate, which accumulates and inhibits herpesvirus DNA polymerase activity. Resistance by herpesviruses can be demonstrated in vitro and in animals. The primary mechanism of resistance appears to be cell mutation, which leads to the lack of herpes deoxynucleoside kinase activity necessary for the initial phosphorylation step in the initiation of drug activity.

Similarly, ganciclovir and penciclovir are phosphorylated intracellularly to the triphosphate moiety and competitively inhibit the incorporation of deoxyguanosine triphosphate into DNA. Ganciclovir triphosphate also interferes with viral DNA polymerase selectivity.

Metabolism and Disposition. Acyclovir is poorly absorbed after oral administration. The bioavailability of acyclovir is inversely proportional to the dose administered. As much as 15% is absorbed by oral doses of 100 mg, whereas only approximately 5% is absorbed at oral doses of 600 mg. Although the bioavailability is poor, serum acyclovir concentrations after repeated oral dosing in adults (200–600 mg per dose administered every 4 hours) may be adequate to treat most HSV infections. The drug is poorly absorbed after topical administration. No preparation is available for intramuscular administration.

Acyclovir is well distributed to most body fluids, tissues, and organs of the body, including the heart, lung, liver, kidney, saliva, zoster vesicular fluid, and central nervous system. Drug concentrations in cerebrospinal fluid approach 50% of simultaneously determined serum concentrations. Approximately 15% of the drug is bound to plasma proteins. The majority of acyclovir (>85% of the dose) is eliminated via the kidney after it is absorbed. The drug is excreted primarily by glomerular filtration, although some of the drug most likely undergoes active tubular secretion. Normal doses must therefore be modified in persons with reduced renal function; they can be adjusted in direct proportion to the reduction in creatinine clearance.

Ganciclovir has a disposition profile similar to that of acyclovir. Ganciclovir is poorly absorbed after oral administration, and the amount of orally administered drug absorbed is inversely related to the dose administered. An oral preparation has recently been approved for the treatment of CMV retinitis. The drug is well distributed to most body fluids, tissues, and organs, including the central nervous system. Approximately 1–2% of ganciclovir is bound to plasma proteins. Nearly 100% of the administered drug is excreted unmetabolized in the urine, and dosage adjustments are necessary in persons with reduced renal function. As with acyclovir, ganciclovir doses should be adjusted in proportion to reductions in creatinine clearance.

In contrast to acyclovir and ganciclovir, famciclovir is well absorbed after oral administration. Approximately 70–85% of oral dose is absorbed as penciclovir. Once the penciclovir is absorbed into the systemic circulation, its disposition characteristics is nearly identical to those of acyclovir and ganciclovir. The drug is well distributed in the body, with <20% bound to plasma proteins. Penciclovir is eliminated from the body primarily via the kidney (~70%), and the remainder is eliminated in the feces.

Dosing recommendations for acyclovir and ganciclovir are shown in Table 14–80. No pediatric dosing recommendations exist for famciclovir, which is available as 125 mg, 250 mg, and 500 mg tablets.

Adverse Effects. Adverse effects directly attributable to acyclovir, ganciclovir, or penciclovir administration are uncommon. Irritation at the site of intravenous infusion appears to be the most common adverse effect associated with the administration of these drugs. This irritation may be a result of the high pH of the intravenous formulation (e.g., pH 10–11.6).

Transient, reversible reductions in glomerular function have been reported with acyclovir. These reactions usually occur after rapid intravenous administration, thus supporting the current recommendations for 1-hour intravenous infusions. Acyclovir is poorly soluble, and after rapid intravenous infusion, high peak concentrations may result in drug crystallization within renal collecting tubules. Dehydration may lead to the development of acyclovir renal crystals, particularly in persons receiving moderate to high doses. Acyclovir renal crystallization appears reversible when the rate of intravenous infusion is slowed (for at least 1 hour) and adequate hydration is maintained. Although alterations in serum creatinine and blood urea nitrogen concentrations have also been described in some persons receiving acyclovir (<2% of patients), the relationship between these changes and ganciclovir use, versus the effect of concomitant use of known nephrotoxins (e.g., cyclosporine, amphotericin B), is unknown.

Seizures have rarely been reported in persons receiving these drugs. Adverse hematologic effects (e.g., neutropenia, thrombocytopenia) may occur in as many as 20–40% of persons receiving ganciclovir and are reversible on discontinuation of therapy. The actual contribution of ganciclovir versus the contribution of the underlying disease to the development of these effects is difficult to discriminate in many of these cases.

Drug Interactions. Probenecid, a competitive inhibitor of renal organic acid secretion, can decrease the renal tubular secretion of acyclovir. Administration of probenecid in combination with acyclovir can prolong the acyclovir $t_{1/2\beta}$ by as much as 30%. A similar drug interaction may also occur with ganciclovir. Concomitant administration of zidovudine may enhance the adverse hematologic effects observed with acyclovir and ganciclovir.

Generalized seizures have been reported in persons receiving concomitant ganciclovir and imipenem-cilastatin therapy, although the true nature of this possible interaction is unclear. Thus, until more definitive information is available regarding the possible drug-drug interaction between ganciclovir and imipenem-cilastatin, this drug combination should be used cautiously or avoided.

FOSCARNET

Foscarnet (phosphonoformic acid), an organic analog of inorganic pyrophosphate, is useful in the treatment of infections caused by herpesviruses.

Spectrum of Activity. Foscarnet has been shown in vitro to inhibit replication of all known herpesviruses, including CMV, HSV-1 and HSV-2, HHV6, EBV, and VZV. In addition, foscarnet appears to selectively inhibit pyrophosphate binding on virus-specific DNA polymerases and reverse transcriptases. Unlike many other antiviral drugs, foscarnet does not require in vivo activation (e.g., phosphorylation) by cellular kinases and is therefore active against thymidine kinase–deficient mutants. Foscarnet is indicated for the treatment of CMV retinitis. Therapy is initiated with a higher dose induction regimen, followed by a lower dose. Once-daily administration is used for maintenance therapy. Because foscarnet therapy is not a cure for CMV retinitis in the immunocompromised person, lifelong administration of the drug may be required.

Metabolism and Disposition. Foscarnet is administered by intravenous infusion only. The exact metabolic fate is unknown. The drug appears to be distributed throughout most of the body. Foscarnet binds avidly to developing tooth enamel and bone. Penetration into the cerebrospinal fluid has been reported as variable in the small number of subjects studied and may depend on the degree of inflammation. Approximately 14–17% of foscarnet is bound to plasma protein.

Foscarnet does not appear to undergo appreciable metabolism within the body. Between 80% and 90% of the dose is excreted unchanged as parent foscarnet in the urine. The exact nature of the renal excretion of foscarnet is unknown, but it appears to undergo glomerular filtration with tubular secretion and probably some tubular reabsorption. Some studies have demonstrated a direct relationship between foscarnet body clearance and measures of glomerular filtration (i.e., creatinine clearance). The direct proportion has been used to adjust doses in persons with compromised renal function. In adults, foscarnet $t_{1/2\beta}$ is 3–4.5 hours in persons with normal renal function and is prolonged in persons with renal dysfunction. Current foscarnet dosing recommendations and available forms are shown in Table 14–81.

Adverse Effects. Foscarnet administration appears to be associated with a large number of varied and often serious adverse effects

TABLE 14–80. Acyclovir and Ganciclovir Dosing Recommendations

Acyclovir

Neonates

Neonatal HSV infection: encephalitis, mucocutaneous infection, disseminated infection

30–60 mg/kg/day (or 1,500 mg/m²/day) divided q8hr IV for 2–3 wk*

Premature infants (≤34 wk gestation)

20–40 mg/kg/day divided q12hr IV for 2–3 wk*

Children and Adults

HSV encephalitis or disseminated infection

Children ≤12 yr: 60 mg/kg/day divided q8hr IV for 2–3 wk

Adolescents ≥12 yr and adults: 30 mg/kg/day divided q8hr IV for 2–3 wk

Mucocutaneous (orolabial or genital) HSV infection (see Table 85–7)

Severe disease: 15–20 mg/kg/day (or 750 mg/m²/day) divided q8hr IV for 5–10 days

Mild disease: 200 mg q4hr while awake (5 times/day) PO

Prophylaxis: 200 mg tid or qid (or 400 mg bid) PO

Varicella (chickenpox) in immunocompetent persons

Children: 40–80 mg/kg/day (max 800 mg/dose) divided qid PO for 5 days

Adults: 600–800 mg 5 times/day PO for 7–10 days or 1,000 mg q6hr PO for 5 days

Disseminated zoster in immunocompetent persons: chickenpox and localized and disseminated zoster in immunocompromised persons

Severe disease

Children <12 yr: 60 mg/kg/day (or 1,500 mg/m²/day) divided q8hr IV for 5–10 days

Adolescents ≥12 yr and adults: 30 mg/kg/day divided q8hr IV for 5–10 days

Mild disease

Children: 250–600 mg/m² 4–5 times/day PO for 7–10 days

Adults: 600–800 mg 5 times/day PO for 7–10 days or 1,000 mg q6hr PO for 5 days

Prophylaxis in bone marrow recipients

Autologous transplant recipients who are HSV seropositive: 250 mg/m² q12hr IV

Persons with clinical symptoms of herpes simplex: 150 mg/m² q8hr IV

Autologous transplant recipients who are CMV seropositive: 500 mg/m² q8hr IV

Persons with clinical symptoms of CMV infection: ganciclovir should be used in place of acyclovir

Prophylaxis of varicella or zoster in adults with HIV

400 mg 5 times/day PO

Suggested Dose Adjustments for Persons >6 Mo with Renal Impairment

Intravenous administration

CrCl 25–50 mL/min: administer usual dose q12hr

CrCl 10–25 mL/min: administer usual dose q24hr

CrCl <10 mL/min: decrease usual dose 50% and administer usual dose q24hr

Oral administration

200 mg 5 times/day

CrCl <10 mL/min: administer usual dose q12hr mg 5 times/day

800 mg 5 times/day

CrCl 10–25 mL/min: administer usual dose q8hr

CrCl <10 mL/min: administer usual dose q12hr

Available Forms

Capsule: 200 mg

Tablets: 400 mg, 800 mg

Oral suspension: 200 mg/5 mL

Intravenous injection: 50 mg/mL

Topical ointment: 5%

Ganciclovir

Retinitis in Children (Age >3 Mo) and Adults

Induction therapy: 10 mg/kg/day for 1–2 hr divided q12hr IV for 14–21 days, followed by maintenance therapy

Maintenance therapy: 5 mg/kg once daily for 7 days/wk *or* 6 mg/kg once daily for 5 days/wk

CMV Prophylaxis in Transplant Recipients

Initially 10 mg/kg/day divided q12hr for 7–14 days, followed by 5 mg/kg once daily 7 days/wk *or* 6 mg/kg once daily 5 days/wk

Other CMV Infections

Induction therapy: 10 mg/kg/day divided q8–12hr for 14–21 days, followed by maintenance therapy

Maintenance therapy: 5 mg/kg once daily for 7 days/wk *or* 6 mg/kg once daily for 5 days/wk

Suggested Dose Adjustments for Persons >6 Mo of Age with Renal Impairment (IV Induction Doses)

CrCl 50–70 mL/min: 2.5 mg/kg q12hr

CrCl 25–49 mL/min: 2.5 mg/kg q24hr

CrCl 10–24 mL/min: 1.25 mg/kg q24hr

CrCl <10 mL/min: 1.25 mg/kg 3 times/wk

Available Forms

Oral capsules: 250 mg, 500 mg

Intravitreal implant: 4.5 mg (released for 5–8 mo)

Intravenous injection: 50 mg/mL

CrCl = creatinine clearance.

*Acyclovir doses of 45–60 mg/kg/day are not approved by the FDA for neonates and have not been shown to be superior in clinical studies, but they are recommended by many experts for neonatal HSV disease in term newborns.

TABLE 14–81. Foscarnet Dosing Recommendations

CMV Retinitis
Adolescents and adults
Induction therapy: 180 mg/kg/day divided q8hr for 14–21 days
Maintenance therapy: 90–120 mg/kg once daily as a single infusion

Acyclovir-Resistant HSV Infection
Therapy: 120 mg/kg/day divided q8–12hr until lesions heal (usual maximum duration: 3 wk)

Available Form
Intravenous injection: 24 mg/ml

Dosage Adjustment for Renal Dysfunction

CREATININE CLEARANCE (mL/min/kg)	INDUCTION DOSAGE FOR HSV (in mg/kg): EQUIVALENT TO 40 mg/kg q12hr	INDUCTION DOSAGE FOR HSV (in mg/kg): EQUIVALENT TO 40 mg/kg q8hr	INDUCTION DOSAGE FOR CMV (in mg/kg): EQUIVALENT TO 60 mg/kg q8hr	INDUCTION DOSAGE FOR CMV (in mg/kg): EQUIVALENT TO 90 mg/kg q12hr
>1.4	40 q12hr	40 q8hr	60 q8hr	90 q12hr
>1–1.4	30 q12hr	30 q8hr	45 q8hr	70 q12hr
>0.8–1	20 q12hr	35 q12hr	50 q12hr	50 q12hr
>0.6–0.8	35 q24hr	25 q12hr	40 q12hr	80 q24hr
>0.5–0.6	25 q24hr	40 q24hr	60 q24hr	60 q24hr
>0.4–0.5	20 q24hr	35 q24hr	50 q24hr	50 q24hr
<0.4	Not recommended	Not recommended	Not recommended	Not recommended

(Table 14–82). Important adverse effects include anemia (sometimes severe enough to require transfusion), granulocytopenia, leukopenia, alterations in renal function, and systemic electrolyte abnormalities. Foscarnet effectively chelates divalent cations such as calcium and magnesium, and prolonged administration may lead to clinically significant reductions in body stores of these important minerals. Persons receiving this drug should have blood values of these cations monitored routinely to avoid deficiency abnormalities. Furthermore, foscarnet must not be administered in any intravenous fluids or as a piggyback with fluids containing calcium or magnesium (e.g., parenteral nutrition solutions, lactated Ringer's solution).

The mechanism of foscarnet-associated nephrotoxicity is unknown, but nephrotoxicity appears in as many as 33% of adults who receive the drug. Drug-induced renal toxicity is manifested as a decrease in the measured creatinine clearance and a rise in the serum creatinine concentration. This effect appears to be reversible once therapy has been discontinued. Although foscarnet-associated alterations in renal function may be observed at any time during therapy, toxicity appears to occur most frequently after the second week of induction therapy with the higher dose. Persons with underlying compromised renal function or drug-induced changes in renal function should receive the drug only if absolutely necessary. Foscarnet doses may be modified as outlined in Table 14–81 or may be altered in direct proportion to changes in the measured creatinine clearance. Furthermore, the hydration status of these persons must also be carefully monitored to maintain or promote

TABLE 14–82. Adverse Effects Associated with Foscarnet

Nephrotoxicity (usually reversible)
Electrolyte imbalance (calcium and magnesium ions)
Neurotoxicity (paresthesias, seizures)
Development of tooth enamel*
Anemia
Granulocytopenia, leukopenia
Headache
Nausea and vomiting

*Animal studies reveal greatest effect in young, growing animals, suggesting an adverse effect on children younger than 9 years.

urinary ''dilution'' of the drug in an attempt to prevent adverse irritant effects of foscarnet on the genitourinary epithelium.

The association of foscarnet with delayed or otherwise abnormal tooth enamel is important to pediatricians. Studies performed in mice and rats have demonstrated an adverse drug effect on developing enamel; this effect was most prominent in young, developing animals. The drug deposits in both enamel and bone in the developing human and the consequences of this deposition are not known.

Drug Interactions. The potential for foscarnet to enhance, either adaptively or synergistically, the adverse effects associated with other nephrotoxic or hematopoietic drugs must be considered when the drug is used in combination with these agents. Examples include the nephrotoxic drugs (e.g., cisplatin, amphotericin B, aminoglycosides), myelotoxic drugs (e.g., zidovudine), and drugs that may augment calcium or magnesium excretion (e.g., diuretics, pentamidine). The combination of foscarnet and pentamidine has been associated with severe hypocalcemia.

VIDARABINE

Vidarabine, also known as **adenosine arabinoside (Ara-A),** is a purine nucleoside analog that was first synthesized in the late 1950s as part of a search for new anticancer medications. The drug's antiviral activity was recognized in the mid-1960s.

Vidarabine is a virostatic drug that possesses a broad spectrum of antiviral activity. The drug appears to be of limited clinical utility and useful only for infections caused by herpes simplex and varicella-zoster viruses. This difference between in vitro and in vivo activity is most likely the result of rapid metabolism and logistic limitations associated with administration of the drug. Vidarabine selectively inhibits viral DNA synthesis by a mechanism that is not yet fully elucidated. Newer drugs such as acyclovir have supplanted the use of vidarabine.

Metabolism and Distribution. Vidarabine is poorly absorbed after oral, intramuscular, or subcutaneous administration. After intravenous administration, this drug is rapidly deaminated by red cell adenosine deaminase to its primary metabolite, a hypoxanthine derivative, arabinosyl hypoxanthine (Ara-HX), which is excreted in the urine. The majority of the antiviral activity of vidarabine in vivo is attributed to this metabolite, which is approximately 30 times less active than the parent compound. In addition, vidarabine most likely also undergoes phosphorylation to various phosphate nucleosides, including a triphosphate derivative, with presumed antiviral activity.

Both vidarabine and arabinosyl hypoxanthine (Ara-HX) appear to be widely distributed to most body fluids and tissues, including the central nervous system. Approximately 20–30% of the vidarabine and <3% of Ara-HX are bound to plasma protein. The reported $t_{1/2\beta}$ for vidarabine approximates 1.5 hours in adults with normal renal function; for Ara-HX this value is 3.3 hours. Preliminary data on infants and children suggest $t_{1/2\beta}$ values of 2.5–3 hours in infants and approximately 2.7 hours in children.

Serum concentrations and elimination characteristics of vidarabine in term infants are reported to be similar to those in older children and adults. Such similarity in disposition profiles across such an age range most likely reflects the rapid deamination of the drug in vivo. Approximately 3% of the administered dose is excreted in the urine as vidarabine and >50% as Ara-HX. Vidarabine dosing recommendations and available forms are shown in Table 14–83.

Adverse Effects. Adverse effects associated with vidarabine administration are usually mild and reversible on discontinuation of therapy. As mentioned earlier, poor drug solubility requires that large volumes of fluid be coadministered with the drug. This may be difficult or contraindicated in neonates and in persons with compromised renal function. Approximately 15% of treated persons have adverse gastrointestinal effects such as anorexia, nausea, vomiting, and diarrhea. Numerous neurotoxic reactions have been reported, including tremors, myoclonus, hallucinations, confusion, psychosis, and seizures, but the true incidence of these effects and their relationship to vidarabine administration is difficult to ascertain because of the known occurrence of these manifestations in persons with encephalitis. Nevertheless, case reports suggest possible neurotoxic effects directly attributable to vidarabine administration, and treated persons should be monitored for the possible occurrence of these effects. In addition, mild and reversible reductions in hemoglobin, hematocrit, and leukocyte and platelet counts have been described.

Drug Interactions. Allopurinol, a competitive inhibitor of xanthine oxidase, may interfere with the metabolism of Ara-HX, thus leading to the accumulation of this metabolite in the body and to possible vidarabine-related adverse effects. Until additional data are available for assessing the true nature of this possible interaction, the two drugs should be coadministered to the same patient cautiously.

TABLE 14–83. Vidarabine Dosing Recommendations

Age Categories
Neonates: 15–30 mg/kg for 18–24 hr IV*
Children and adults: 10–15 mg/kg for 12–24 hr IV*

Keratoconjunctivitis
Topical application ~5 times/day until complete epithelialization and then twice daily for an additional 7 days

Available Forms
IV injection: 200 mg/mL
Ophthalmic ointment 3%

*Drug administered by continuous intravenous infusion. Dose adjustments may be advisable in persons with renal disease; the vidarabine dose should be reduced in proportion to the decrease in creatinine clearance.

RIBAVIRIN

Ribavirin, a nucleoside analog, was first synthesized in 1970 as part of a search for a universally effective antiviral drug. This drug appears to have some therapeutic activity against several respiratory viruses. The exact role of ribavirin in clinical medicine remains controversial.

Ribavirin is a ribose-containing triazole ring that is structurally similar to natural nucleosides, most notably guanosine. Intracellular ribavirin is phosphorylated to a 5′-phosphate derivative, which is responsible for the observed antiviral activity. The precise mechanism by which ribavirin exerts its antiviral effect is unknown. Ribavirin may be of clinical value in the treatment of severe lower respiratory tract viral infections with influenza A and B viruses and RSV. The primary use of ribavirin is in the treatment of RSV pneumonia in severely ill patients with debilitating underlying diseases, including immunodeficiency, bronchopulmonary dysplasia, prematurity, and congenital heart disease, and in persons receiving immunosuppressive drug therapy.

Metabolism and Disposition. Only limited data describing the disposition of ribavirin in humans are available. The drug is rapidly absorbed after oral and aerosol administration. Preliminary pharmacokinetic data in children with HIV infection suggest approximately 40% bioavailability after oral administration. After aerosol administration, the highest ribavirin concentrations are observed in the lungs and erythrocytes. The drug appears to be distributed slowly into the central nervous system after long-term administration. Ribavirin is metabolized, most likely by the liver, to deribosylated ribavirin, which appears to retain the same antiviral activity as the parent compound. Approximately 40% of an administered dose is excreted in the urine as unmetabolized parent ribavirin.

Available Formulations. In North America, ribavirin is available only as a sterile lyophilized powder for aerosol administration. After reconstitution, this preservative-free solution is colorless, odorless, and tasteless, with a pH of 5.0–6.9.

Recommended Dosing and Dosing Strategies. Ribavirin is administered as an aerosol delivered by a small-particle aerosol generator (SPAG). The aerosol may be administered into an infant oxygen hood, face mask, or oxygen tent, or with caution, through an endotracheal tube. Aerosolized ribavirin administration after intubation may interfere with the function of mechanical ventilator equipment because of drug precipitation within the ventilatory apparatus and endotracheal tube. The currently recommended aerosol drug concentration is 20 mg/mL in the drug reservoir of the SPAG unit. The drug is administered as a continuous aerosolization for 18–20 hours. Shorter daily exposures and higher doses have been tried with no apparent change in outcome.

Adverse Effects. Clinical use of ribavirin has been associated with few clinically important adverse effects. Reversible anemia, most likely due to hemolysis, and suppression of mature erythrocyte release from bone marrow have been described. Anemia has not been reported in children receiving aerosolized ribavirin.

Bronchospasm may result from the aerosolization of ribavirin, but it is unclear whether the bronchospasm occurs because of the drug or the underlying respiratory lung disease.

Controversy persists regarding the possible teratogenic potential of ribavirin and the possible risks to pregnant health care workers who are exposed to ribavirin in the ambient environment. Most authorities suggest that pregnant health care workers avoid environmental exposure to ribavirin. The most common ribavirin-associated adverse effects seen in health care workers include eye irritation, particularly in workers wearing contact lenses, headache, and less frequently, nasal and throat irritation. Until the potential risks associated with environmental ribavirin exposure are better defined, it is advisable to administer ribavirin aerosol only within a confined, well-demarcated space with limited contact by patient visitors and health care personnel. Individuals who are pregnant or lactating should avoid contact with ribavirin.

Drug Interactions. No drug interactions have been described with ribavirin. Ribavirin may antagonize the antiviral activity of zidovudine.

AMANTADINE AND RIMANTADINE

Amantadine (*l*-adamantanamine) was synthesized in 1941, but the drug's virostatic activity was not appreciated until the early 1960s. Although amantadine has been available for more than 30 years, several factors have limited its use. First, amantadine is effective against influenza A viruses, and the clinical recognition of influenza A infection is difficult. Rapid antigen and antibody detection techniques are relatively new. Second, the clinical efficacy of amantadine has been questioned, and the frequency of adverse effects has been problematic. Rimantadine, an analog of amantadine, has been used extensively outside the United States for chemoprophylaxis against influenza infection. Renewed clinical interest in both these drugs has arisen from the many positive reports of their clinical efficacy. Their true clinical efficacy remains to be determined.

The antiviral activities of amantadine and rimantadine are similar. Both drugs possess antiviral activity against influenza A viruses and, in some culture systems, against parainfluenza viruses types 2 and 3 and some strains of respiratory syncytial virus. Because of the tremendous variability in the susceptibility of influenza A strains tested against amantadine and rimantadine, defining a true clinical role for these drugs is complicated. The mechanism of action against influenza viruses and other viruses is unknown. Amantadine and rimantadine dosing recommendations and available forms are outlined in Table 14–84.

TABLE 14–84. Amantadine and Rimantadine Dosing Recommendations

Age Categories
At 1–9 yr*: 5 mg/kg (max 150 mg) once daily or divided bid PO
At 10–13 yr*: 5 mg/kg (max 200 mg) once daily or divided bid PO
At 14–64 yr*: 200 mg divided bid PO
At ≥65 yr: 100 mg once daily PO

Duration
Treatment
Continue for 24–48 hr after disappearance of signs and symptoms
Prophylaxis
Continue for at least 10 days

Dosage Adjustments for Renal Impairment
Amantadine
CrCl 30–50 mL/min: usual daily dose on day 1; half of usual daily dose each day thereafter
CrCl 15–29 mL/min: usual daily dose on day 1; half of usual daily dose every other day thereafter
CrCl <15 mL/min: usual daily dose once every 7 days
Rimantadine
CrCl <10 mL/min: half of usual daily dose

Dosage Adjustments for Hepatic Impairment
Amantadine: no dosage reduction is necessary
Rimantadine: half of usual dose with severe hepatic dysfunction

Available Forms
Amantadine: oral capsule, 100 mg; oral syrup, 50 mg/5 mL
Rimantadine: oral tablet, 100 mg; oral syrup, 50 mg/5 mL

CrCl = creatinine clearance.
*Amantadine is approved for prophylaxis and treatment in children ≥1 year of age and adults. Rimantadine is approved for prophylaxis in children ≥1 year of age and adults, and for treatment in adults ≥18 years of age.

Metabolism and Distribution. Published data describing amantadine disposition in children are limited; the majority of the available pharmacokinetic data have been obtained from studies of adults. Amantadine appears to be well absorbed from the gastrointestinal tract with oral administration, with peak blood concentrations observed between 1 and 4 hours after drug administration. The drug appears to be extensively distributed throughout the body, achieving high concentrations in the lungs, heart, and brain. The large distribution volume of amantadine indicates extensive tissue binding by the drug and may partially explain the low blood concentrations achieved with long-term dosing. The drug is not metabolized, and the entire dose is excreted unchanged in the urine by both glomerular filtration and tubular secretion.

Amantadine dosing must be adjusted for changes in renal function and should be decreased in proportion to the reduction in the glomerular filtration rate. The average amantadine $t_{1/2\beta}$ is 24 hours. Because the drug is not removed by peritoneal dialysis or hemodialysis, no dosage adjustment is necessary after these procedures.

Even fewer published data concerning the disposition of rimantadine in either children or adults are available. Preliminary pharmacokinetic evaluations suggest a rapid rate of absorption, extensive tissue distribution, and $t_{1/2\beta}$ values averaging 28 hours in young adults and 25 hours in children, similar to those observed with amantadine. Unlike amantadine, rimantadine undergoes metabolism to *ortho-*, *para-*, and *meta-*hydroxylated metabolites. The nature and extent of rimantadine metabolism have not been elucidated.

Adverse Effects. Numerous bothersome and clinically important adverse effects are associated with amantadine therapy. The common occurrence of these adverse effects has been one of the primary factors limiting the clinical use of amantadine. Common adverse effects are listed in Table 14–85. In adults, daily amantadine doses of 200 mg, in comparison with higher daily doses of 300 mg, appear to be associated with only minor adverse effects. Effects on the nervous system appear to be the most prominent and include nervousness, insomnia, difficulty in concentration, confusion, and hallucinations. The occurrence of adverse effects, particularly those involving the central nervous system, is more frequent in persons with decreased renal function and in elderly persons. This finding underscores the importance of dosage adjustment in accordance with renal function.

The adverse effect profile for rimantadine appears to be identical to that of amantadine, although the frequency and severity of adverse effects may be less. In comparative studies of adults using identical doses, amantadine was associated with a greater incidence of adverse effects. The reason for this difference is unknown. Preliminary data suggest that when serum concentrations are com-

TABLE 14–85. Adverse Effects Associated with Amantadine and Rimantadine

Central Nervous System Symptoms
Headache
Nervousness, anxiety
Difficulty in concentration, slurred speech
Light-headedness, insomnia
Dizziness, tremor
Depression, confusion, hallucinations
Seizures
Other Effects
Rashes
Postural hypotension
Leukopenia

Majority of data were obtained in adult studies. Incidence of adverse effects increases in persons with impaired renal (amantadine) or hepatic (rimantadine) function without dosage adjustments.

parable, amantadine and rimantadine cause the same number and severity of adverse reactions. The greater in vitro potency combined with equal or slightly better clinical effectiveness and enhanced patient tolerance of rimantadine may explain the renewed interest in the clinical use of this drug.

Drug Interactions. No specific drug-drug interactions have been reported with either amantadine or rimantadine. The concurrent administration of antihistamine or anticholinergic drugs should be avoided, however, considering the frequent occurrence of anticholinergic effects associated with the use of amantadine or rimantadine.

The coadministration of rimantadine (but not amantadine) with acetaminophen or aspirin may result in a decreased peak rimantadine plasma concentration and a decreased amount of rimantadine absorbed into the systemic circulation, each by ~10%. Coadministration of cimetidine may decrease the rimantadine body clearance, suggesting the need for rimantadine dose reduction with concurrent administration with cimetidine.

OSELTAMIVIR AND ZANAMIVIR

Oseltamivir and zanamivir are the first of a new class of neuraminidase inhibitors developed for use in the prophylaxis or treatment of influenza caused by influenza viruses A and B. The influenza virus contains two surface glycoproteins, hemagglutinin and neuraminidase, which interact with viral receptors that contain neuraminic acid. Hemagglutinin binds to cellular receptors, initiates virus penetration, and promotes fusion of viral and cellular membranes. Neuraminidase is a tetramer in which the active site is highly conserved among all influenza A and B strains. Normally, neuraminidase destroys receptors recognized by hemagglutinin, allowing the virus to penetrate secretions and allowing viral replication and viral release from the cell surface. Inhibiting the action of neuraminidase by a neuraminidase inhibitor thus prevents infection by inhibiting the release of newly formed virus from the surface of infected cells and preventing viral spread across respiratory tract mucosal lining. Both of these agents are potent and specific inhibitors of influenza neuraminidase.

Metabolism and Distribution. Oseltamivir phosphate is the orally available ethyl ester prodrug of oseltamivir carboxylate, the active moiety. Once administered, the ethyl ester is rapidly metabolized to active oseltamivir carboxylate, which is approximately 80% bioavailable after oral administration. The drug's $t_{1/2\beta}$ is 6–10 hours. In contrast, zanamivir is poorly bioavailable with oral administration (~5%), underscoring the drug's clinical availability as an aerosol preparation. After aerosol administration, zanamivir concentrations in sputum are high, exceeding those necessary for neuraminidase inhibition for 6–12 hours. Plasma zanamivir concentrations are very low after aerosol administration. The sustained concentrations achieved in the respiratory tract with both drugs foster their twice-daily dosing for treatment and once-daily dosing for prophylaxis. The primary route of elimination of either drug is the kidney. However, because little drug reaches the systemic circulation after the use of zanamivir aerosol, no dosage adjustment is necessary in persons with poor renal function. In contrast, persons with creatinine clearance rates <30 mL/min who are treated with oseltamivir should receive a dose once daily rather than twice daily. Hemodialysis does not appear to remove oseltamivir, so no dosage adjustment is needed for the dialysis session over the appropriate reduction in dose because of poor renal function. Dosing recommendations and associated adverse effects for these agents are shown in Table 14–86.

TABLE 14–86. Oseltamivir and Zanamivir Dosing Recommendations and Adverse Effects

Oseltamivir*
Treatment (≥1 yr of age)
≤15 kg: 30 mg bid for 5 days
>15–23 kg: 45 mg bid for 5 days
>23–40 kg: 60 mg bid for 5 days
>40 kg: 75 mg bid for 5 days
Prophylaxis (≥13 yr of age)
75 mg once daily for at least 7 days
Zanamivir†
Treatment (≥7 yr of age)
2 inhalations via inhaler (10 mg) bid for 5 days
Prophylaxis
Not approved
Adverse Effects
Nausea, vomiting, diarrhea, headache, dizziness (rare)
Zanamivir: may precipitate bronchospasm; use with caution in persons with asthma or chronic obstructive pulmonary disease; have albuterol inhaler available.

*Oseltamivir is approved for treatment in children ≥1 year of age and adults, and for prophylaxis in persons ≥13 years of age.
†Zanamivir is approved for treatment in children ≥7 years of age and adults. Zanamivir is not approved for prophylaxis.

ANTIRETROVIRAL DRUGS

Advances in the discovery of new antiretroviral drugs and methods of achieving the optimal combination administration for maximal anti-HIV replication have revolutionized the treatment of AIDS. The various manifestations of HIV infection and disease and contemporary treatment recommendations are outlined in Chapter 38. Classes of antiretroviral drugs include nucleoside reverse transcriptase inhibitors, nonnucleoside reverse transcriptase inhibitors, and protease inhibitors (Table 14–87). Antiretroviral drugs have numerous clinically important drug-drug interactions (Table 14–88).

TABLE 14–87. Dose Guidelines, Adverse Effects, and Available Forms for Antiretroviral (HIV) Therapy

Drug	Dose Guidelines				Major Adverse Effects	Food Effect	Available Forms
	Neonate	Infant/Child	Adult	Dose Interval			
Nucleoside Reverse Transcriptase Inhibitors							
Abacavir (ABC)	—	8 mg/kg	300 mg	q12hr	Nausea, vomiting, headache, fever, rash, fatigue	No	Oral solution: 20 mg/mL Tablet: 300 mg
Didanosine (ddI)	50 mg/m^2	90–150 mg/m^2	200 mg	q12hr	Diarrhea, abdominal pain, nausea, vomiting, peripheral neuropathy, electrolyte imbalance	Yes (need buffering for best absorption)	Oral solution: 10 mg/mL Chewable tablets with buffers: 25, 50, 100, and 150 mg
Lamivudine (3TC)	2 mg/kg	4 mg/kg	150 mg	q12hr	Headache, nausea, diarrhea, rash, abdominal pain, pancreatitis, peripheral neuropathy	No	Oral solution: 10 mg/mL Tablet: 150 mg
Stavudine (d4T)	—	1 mg/kg	40 mg	q12hr	Headache, gastroesophageal distress, rash, peripheral neuropathy (rare), pancreatitis (rare)	No	Oral solution, 1 mg/mL Capsules: 15, 20, 30, 40 mg
Zalcitabine (ddC)	—	0.005–0.01 mg/kg	0.75 mg	q8hr	Headache, gastrointestinal upset, peripheral neuropathy, oral ulcers, pancreatitis, liver dysfunction	Yes	Oral syrup: 0.1 mg/mL Tablets: 0.375, 0.75 mg
Zidovudine (ZDV)	2 mg/kg q6hr 1.5 mg/kg q6hr	90–180 mg/m^2 q6–8hr PO 120 mg/m^2 q6hr IV	200 mg	q12hr	Hematologic toxic effects, headache, myopathy (unusual)	No	
Nonnucleoside Reverse Transcriptase Inhibitors							
Delavirdine			400 mg	q8hr	Headache, fatigue, gastrointestinal distress, rash (may be severe)	No	Tablet: 100 mg
Efavirenz		Body weight adjusted: 10 to <15 kg: 200 mg 15 to <20 kg: 250 mg 20 to <25 kg: 300 mg 25 to <32.5 kg: 350 mg 32.5 to <40 kg: 400 mg	600 mg	qd	Rash, somnolence, confusion, teratogenic in primates	No increased absorption with high-fat meal	Capsules: 50, 100, 200 mg
Nevirapine	Investigational	120–200 mg/m^2*	200 mg	q12hr	Rash (Stevens-Johnson syndrome), sedation, headache, diarrhea	No	Oral suspension: 10 mg/mL Tablets: 200 mg

Table continued on following page

TABLE 14–87. Dose Guidelines, Adverse Effects, and Available Forms for Antiretroviral (HIV) Therapy *(Continued)*

	Dose Guidelines						
Drug	**Neonate**	**Infant/Child**	**Adult**	**Dose Interval**	**Major Adverse Effects**	**Food Effect**	**Available Forms**
Protease Inhibitors							
Amprenavir		Oral solution: 22.5 mg/kg q12hr *or* 17 mg/kg q8hr Capsule: 20 mg/kg q12hr *or* 15 mg/kg q8hr	1,200 mg	q12hr	Nausea, vomiting, diarrhea, perineal paresthesias, severe rash (Stevens Johnson syndrome)	No; caution: oral solution contains propylene glycol	Oral solution: 15 mg/mL Capsules: 50, 150 mg
Indinavir	—†	500 mg/m^2	800 mg	q8hr	Nausea, gastrointestinal distress, headache, metallic taste, nephrolithiasis	Yes	Capsules: 200, 400 mg
Nelfinavir	40 mg/kg q12hr	30 mg/kg	750 mg	q8hr	Diarrhea, gastrointestinal distress, rash	Best administered with food	Oral powder for suspension: 50 mg/1 g scoop Tablet: 250 mg
Ritonavir		350–500 mg/m^2	600 mg	q12hr	Nausea, vomiting, diarrhea, headaches, circumpolar paresthesias	Best administered with food	Oral solution: 80 mg/mL Capsule: 100 mg
Saquinavir			600 mg	q8hr	Diarrhea, gastrointestinal distress, nausea, headache, rash, bleeding in persons with hemophilia	Best administered within 2 hr of a full meal	Hard or soft-gel capsules: 200 mg

*Initiate therapy with 120 mg/m^2 daily for 14 days; then increase as tolerated.

†Hyperbilirubinemia is an associated adverse effect, which limits use of indinavir in neonates.

TABLE 14–88. Drug Interactions of Antiretroviral Medications

Inhibitors	Drug Interactions
Nucleoside Reverse Transcriptase Inhibitors	
Abacavir	Ethanol may decrease abacavir body clearance
Didanosine	Didanosine decreases absorption of ketoconazole, itraconazole, tetracyclines, quinolones (e.g., ciprofloxacin); separate drug administration by 2 hr
Lamivudine	Lamivudine clearance decreased by TMP-SMZ
Stavudine	Drugs that decrease renal function will lead to a decrease in stavudine clearance
Zalcitabine	Amphotericin, foscarnet, aminoglycoside can decrease zalcitabine clearance; antacids can decrease zalcitabine absorption
Zidovudine	Enhanced marrow suppression with TMP-SMZ, acyclovir, ganciclovir, and others; zidovudine clearance decreased by probenecid, atovaquone, fluconazole, valproic acid, cimetidine; zidovudine clearance increased by rifampin, rifabutin, carbamazepine, phenobarbital, phenytoin (with or without effects)
Nonnucleoside Reverse Transcriptase Inhibitors	
Delavirdine	Delavirdine decreases body clearance of astemizole, terfenadine, cisapride, benzodiazepines, calcium-channel antagonists (e.g., nifedipine), warfarin, ketoconazole, fluconazole, fluoxetine; delavirdine clearance increased by rifampin, rifabutin, phenytoin, carbamazepine, phenobarbital; antacids (liquid antacids) and H_2 receptor antagonists may decrease delavirdine absorption
Efavirenz	Efavirenz can decrease clearance of astemizole, terfenadine, cisapride, benzodiazepines, ergot alkaloids, warfarin, oral contraceptives; enzyme inducers (e.g., rifampin, carbamazepine, phenobarbital) may increase efavirenz clearance; possibility of protein-displacement drug-drug interaction with efavirenz has been raised but is not documented
Nevirapine	Nevirapine (induces CYP 3A4) can increase clearance of many drugs: oral contraceptives, benzodiazepine, digoxin, phenytoin, calcium-channel antagonists
Protease Inhibitors	
Amprenavir	Amprenavir (inhibits CYP 3A4) decreases clearance of astemizole, terfenadine, cisapride, benzodiazepine, calcium-channel blockers, sildenafil; amprenavir clearance increased by rifampin, rifabutin, carbamazepine, phenytoin, phenobarbital
Indinavir	Indinavir (metabolized by CYP 3A4) decreases clearance of astemizole, terfenadine, cisapride, ergot alkaloids, and benzodiazepine; indinavir clearance decreased by ketoconazole and itraconazole
Nelfinavir	Nelfinavir (partially metabolized by CYP 3A4) decreases clearance of astemizole, terfenadine, cisapride, benzodiazepine, ergot alkaloids, and quinidine; nelfinavir clearance increased by rifampin and probably other inducers (e.g., carbamazepine)
Ritonavir	Ritonavir (metabolized by CYP 3A4) may decrease clearance of astemizole, terfenadine, calcium/ channel antagonists, benzodiazepines, cisapride, digoxin (variable); ritonavir increases metabolism of theophylline and estradiol; ritonavir clearance increased by carbamazepine, rifampin, phenobarbital, phenytoin, corticosteroids
Saquinavir	Saquinavir (metabolized by CYP 3A4) may decrease clearance of astemizole, terfenadine, calcium-channel antagonists, benzodiazepines, cisapride, digoxin (variable); saquinavir clearance increased by carbamazepine, rifampin, phenobarbital, phenytoin, corticosteroids

CYP = cytochrome P-450.
+/− =.

ANTIMYCOBACTERIAL DRUGS

A resurgence in the incidence of infections caused by mycobacteria has occurred during the past decade(Chapter 35). Comparative pharmacokinetic characteristics of drugs used in the treatment of mycobacterial infections are shown in Table 14–89, dosing recommendations and available forms in Table 14–90, important adverse effects associated with their use in Table 14–91, and clinically important drug-drug interactions in Table 14–92.

ETHAMBUTOL

Ethambutol was discovered in 1961 at Lederle Research Laboratories during a search for synthetic compounds with effective antitubercular activity. This tuberculostatic drug is commonly used in combination with other agents in the treatment of tuberculosis. Ethambutol is infrequently used in children before the age of 5 years, primarily because of the drug's potential for ocular toxicity.

Metabolism and Disposition. Ethambutol is well absorbed (75–80%) after oral administration. Coadministration with food does not appear to alter gastrointestinal drug absorption. Only limited data describing the distribution characteristics of ethambutol are available. On the basis of the clinical efficacy of ethambutol, it presumably achieves therapeutic concentrations in vital tissues and organs. Therapeutic concentrations have been described in the cerebrospinal fluid of persons with tuberculosis meningitis, but ethambutol does not appear to enter the spinal fluid in persons with normal meninges. Approximately 80% of the administered dose is excreted in the urine as unmetabolized ethambutol, and 10–15% is metabolized to either an aldehyde or a dicarboxylic acid derivative, both of which are microbiologically inactive. Hepatic insufficiency does not appear to alter ethambutol disposition, whereas

TABLE 14–89. Comparative Pharmacokinetics of Primary Antimycobacterial Drugs

Parameter	Ethambutol	Isoniazid	Rifampin
Bioavailability (%)	75–80	~100	~100
Cerebrospinal fluid penetration	Yes	Yes	Yes
Metabolism	Partial (~15%)	Extensive (~70%)	Primarily feces (~30% urine)
$t_{1/2\beta}$ (hr)	2–4	1.5–4	3–4
Protein binding (%)	20–30	10–15	80
Dialyzable (%)	5–20	50–100	Negligible

$t_{1/2\beta}$ = elimination half-life.

proportional dosage adjustments are necessary in the presence of renal insufficiency (see Table 14–90). Ethambutol dosing recommendations and available forms are shown in Table 14–90.

Adverse Effects. Overall, ethambutol is a well-tolerated drug when used in usual therapeutic doses (i.e., 15 mg/kg/day). Ethambutol-associated adverse reactions include diminished visual acuity, rash, fever, gastrointestinal upset, malaise, headache, mental confusion, disorientation, and joint pain (see Table 14–91). Ethambutol may decrease urinary excretion of uric acid, increasing serum urate concentrations by as much as 50%.

The most important adverse effect associated with ethambutol administration is a retrobulbar neuritis that results in decreased visual acuity and red-green color blindness. This ocular effect, which may be unilateral or bilateral, is dose related. The incidence of this adverse effect has been estimated to occur in persons receiving ethambutol doses of 50, 25, and 15 mg/kg/day at percentages of 15%, 5%, and <1%, respectively. This ocular toxicity is most often reversible after discontinuation of ethambutol therapy, although color blindness may persist for some time. Continued drug administration after the onset of symptoms may result in optic atrophy with irreversible impairment of vision. Because of the difficulties inherent in visual acuity testing of young children, this complication of ethambutol therapy limits the usefulness of the drug in children less than 5 years of age.

ISONIAZID

Isoniazid (INH), the hydrazine of isonicotinic acid, was discovered independently in 1952 at both Squibb and Roche Research Laboratories. Despite the long-term and widespread use of isoniazid, it remains one of the most important antituberculosis drugs available today. Most authorities agree that all persons with disease caused by isoniazid-susceptible strains of *M. tuberculosis* should receive this drug.

Metabolism and Distribution. Isoniazid is well absorbed after oral administration. Intramuscular administration produces serum isoniazid concentrations comparable to those measured after oral drug administration (see Table 14–89). Isoniazid is well distributed to most body fluids and tissues, including the central nervous system. The majority of an isoniazid dose (approximately 75–95%) is excreted as urinary metabolites within 24 hours of administration. The primary route for isoniazid metabolism is through acetylation by the enzyme *N*-acetyltransferase. The resulting acetylisoniazid undergoes further hydrolysis to yield isonicotinic acid and acetylhydrazine. The rate of acetylation is genetically controlled, and patients may be subdivided phenotypically into two district populations: slow and rapid acetylators. Obviously the rate of acetylation markedly influences isoniazid $t_{1/2\beta}$, total body clearance, and resulting serum drug concentrations. The acetylator phenotype may be an important determinant of drug efficacy when used in once-weekly dosing regimens, and it is a major determinant of the susceptibility to some of the side effects of the drug. Dosing recommendations and available forms of isoniazid are shown in Table 14–90.

Adverse Effects. Overall, isoniazid is associated with a low order of toxicity, particularly in children receiving <20 mg/kg/day (see Table 14–91). The associated peripheral neuropathy, which is more likely to occur in slow acetylators, is responsive to pyridoxine administration; malnourished persons should receive pyridoxine supplementation. Moreover, the American Academy of Pediatrics recommends that children with low milk and low meat consumption receive concomitant pyridoxine therapy. Concurrent pyridoxine administration prevents or reverses pyridoxine deficiency without affecting the antimycobacterial activity or serum concentration of isoniazid.

The most serious, potentially life-threatening adverse reaction associated with isoniazid is drug-induced hepatitis. This form of hepatitis is clinically, biochemically, and histologically similar to viral hepatitis. The exact mechanism responsible for this reaction is unknown; age appears to be the most important determinant of risk. Isoniazid-associated hepatic damage is rare in persons <20 years of age, and it occurs in approximately 2.3% of persons aged >50 years. It is found more frequently in persons of Japanese or Chinese origin. Almost all individuals of Chinese descent are rapid acetylators.

Drug Interactions. Isoniazid competitively inhibits the metabolism of carbamazepine and phenytoin, leading to accumulation and toxicity (see Table 14–92). Carbamazepine and phenytoin dosing may require downward adjustments when these drugs are coadministered with isoniazid. Serum anticonvulsant concentrations should be monitored closely in persons who are also taking isoniazid.

Concurrent antacid administration decreases the oral absorption of isoniazid. The antimycobacterial agent should be administered 1 hour before or 2 hours after antacid administration.

RIFAMPIN

The rifamycins are a group of complex macrocyclic antibiotics that were first isolated from *Streptomyces mediterranei* in Italy in the early 1960s. Unlike isoniazid and ethambutol, rifampin is active against many non-mycobacterial organisms. Rifampin is a potent bactericidal and tuberculocidal agent.

Metabolism and Distribution. Rifampin is well absorbed after oral administration (see Table 14–89). Peak plasma concentrations usually occur within 2–4 hours of a dose. The coadministration of *p*-aminosalicylic acid may delay the absorption of rifampin, resulting in blunted peak concentrations. Because food may de-

TABLE 14–90. Dosing Recommendations for the Primary Antimycobacterial Drugs

Ethambutol
Children
  Dosing: 15–25 mg/kg once daily
Adolescents and adults
  Dosing: 15 mg/kg once daily; may increase to 25 mg/kg/day if organism is isoniazid resistant during first 1–2 mo; max 2.5 g/day
Dose adjustment for persons with renal impairment
  CrCl 10–15 mL/min: administer q24–36hr
  CrCl <10 mL/min: administer q48hr or reduce daily dose
Available forms
  Oral tablets: 100 mg, 400 mg

Isoniazid
Children*
  Daily treatment: 10–15 mg/kg (max 300 mg) once daily†
  Twice-weekly treatment‡: 20–30 mg/kg (max 900 mg) twice weekly under supervision
  Prophylaxis: 10 mg/kg (max 300 mg) once daily
Adults
  Daily treatment: 5–10 mg/kg (max 300 mg) once daily†
  Twice weekly treatment‡: 15 mg/kg (max 900 mg) twice weekly under supervision
  Prophylaxis: 300 mg once daily
Available forms
  Oral tablets: 100 mg, 300 mg
  Oral syrup: 50 mg/5 mL
  Oral combinations
    Oral capsules: 300 mg rifampin and 150 mg isoniazid
    Oral tablets: 120 mg rifampin, 50 mg isoniazid, and 300 mg pyrazinamide
  Injection: 100 mg/mL

Rifampin (Oral)
Children
  Daily treatment: 10–20 mg/kg/day divided q12–24hr
  Twice-weekly treatment: 10–20 mg/kg (max 600 mg) twice weekly under supervision
Adults
  Daily treatment: 10 mg/kg (max 600 mg) once daily
  Twice-weekly treatment: 10 mg/kg (max 600 mg) twice weekly under supervision
Neisseria meningitidis prophylaxis (see Table 16–4)
  Neonates (age <1 mo): 10 mg/kg/day divided q12hr PO for 2 days
  Infants and children: 20 mg/kg/day divided q12hr PO for 2 days
  Adults: 600 mg q12hr PO for 2 days
Haemophilus influenzae type b prophylaxis (see Table 16–5)
  Infants and children: 20 mg/kg once daily PO for 4 days
  Adults: 600 mg once daily PO for 4 days
Nasal carriers of *Staphylococcus aureus*
  Adults: 600 mg once daily PO for 5–10 days (in combination with other antibiotics)
Available forms
  Oral capsules: 150 mg, 300 mg
  Oral combinations
    Oral capsules: 300 mg rifampin and 150 mg isoniazid
    Oral tablets: 120 mg rifampin, 50 mg isoniazid, and 300 mg pyrazinamide
  Injection: 60 mg/mL

CrCl = creatinine clearance.
*Supplemental pyridoxine is not necessary routinely but is recommended for breast-feeding infants, for children and adolescents with pre-existing nutritional deficiencies or diets low in meat and milk, and for women during pregnancy.
†Oral and intramuscular doses are identical.
‡The American Thoracic Society and the Centers for Disease Control and Prevention currently recommend twice-weekly directly observed therapy as a part of a short-course regimen that follows 1–2 months of daily treatment of uncomplicated pulmonary tuberculosis in the compliant person (Chapter 35).

crease the overall amount of rifampin absorbed, the drug should be administered before meals whenever possible.

Once absorbed, the drug is distributed throughout most body fluids and tissues, including the central nervous system. Rifampin is rapidly eliminated in the bile, undergoing enterohepatic circulation and progressive deacetylation in the liver. The deacetylated metabolite retains most if not all of the antibacterial activity of the parent compound. Rifampin is a potent inducer of hepatic drug-metabolizing enzymes; the $t_{1/2\beta}$ of rifampin is progressively shortened by approximately 40% during the first 14 days of uninterrupted therapy. Rifampin dosing recommendations are shown in Table 14–90.

TABLE 14–91. Important Adverse Effects Associated with Antimycobacterial Drugs

Ethambutol
Dose-related (>20 mg/kg/day) retrobulbar neuritis leading to decreased visual acuity and red-green color blindness.

Isonizid*
Nausea, vomiting, diarrhea
Hypersensitivity reactions including rash and fever
Hematologic: leukopenia, thrombocytopenia, anemia
Acne
Seizures, primarily after overdose or in persons with underlying seizure disorder
Pyridoxine responsive peripheral neuropathy
Hepatitis (rare)

Rifampin†
Rash (1–5%) including rare "red man" syndrome
Hepatitis (<1%)
Nausea, vomiting, diarrhea (~1%)
Influenza-like syndrome (fever, chills, myalgias)

*Adverse reactions are uncommon in children with daily doses <20 mg/kg/day.
†Most common with higher doses (e.g., adult dose exceeding 1,200 mg/day).

Adverse Effects. The incidence of adverse reactions to rifampin approximates 4% overall when the drug is used in usual therapeutic dosing schedules (see Table 14–91). This incidence increases when daily doses exceed 1,200 mg, which may occur when the drug is used as part of an intermittent treatment schedule for tuberculosis. The most common adverse effects associated with therapeutic doses are skin rash, fever, nausea, and vomiting. A cutaneous syndrome including flushing or itching of the skin, with or without a rash (usually involving the face and scalp), has been described early in the course of rifampin therapy. Other rare hypersensitivity reactions include hemolysis, thrombocytopenia, interstitial nephritis, and acute renal failure. An influenza-like syndrome characterized by fever, chills, and myalgias has been described in as many as 20% of persons receiving high-dose rifampin therapy (e.g., >1,200 mg/day in adults).

Liver disease has also been described in persons receiving rifampin. Rifampin-associated hepatitis occurs rarely in persons with normal hepatic function. Chronic alcoholism, underlying liver disease, or advanced age appears to predispose persons to the development of this potentially fatal adverse reaction. Hepatotoxic reactions to rifampin, when it is administered alone or in combination with isoniazid, are rare in children. Again, these reactions may be associated with excessive rifampin doses. Considerable controversy has surrounded a possible hepatotoxic interaction from combination isoniazid and rifampin therapy.

TABLE 14–92. Drug-Drug Interactions with Selected Antimycobacterial Drugs

Ethambutol
Absorption based
Aluminum-containing compounds may decrease ethambutol bioavailability.

Isoniazid
Absorption based
Aluminum-containing compounds may decrease isoniazid bioavailability.
Metabolism based
Isoniazid may interfere with metabolism of carbamazepine, cyclosporine, and phenytoin, leading to accumulation.
Other
Chronic ethanol may increase isoniazid-associated hepatitis.

Rifampin
Metabolism based
Rifampin is a highly effective stimulator of cytochrome P-450 drug-metabolizing enzymes and can increase the metabolism of many drugs, including acetaminophen, benzodiazepines, oral contraceptives, carbamazepine, cyclosporine, calcium-channel antagonists, phenytoin, theophylline.*

*Most likely also applies to rifabutin.

Drug Interactions. Rifampin has been shown to interfere with the metabolism of a number of substances and drugs (see Table 14–92). The majority of these drug-drug interactions result from the ability of rifampin to stimulate hepatic drug metabolism. Rifampin competes with and thus reduces biliary excretion of bilirubin, sulfobromophthalein, and certain cholecystography contrast media.

ANTIPARASITIC DRUGS

ANTIPROTOZOAL DRUGS

PENTAMIDINE

Pentamidine is an aromatic diamidine with antiprotozoal activity, particularly against *P. carinii.* This drug was first discovered more than 50 years ago as part of a concerted effort to identify effective antiprotozoal drugs, but its use was soon abandoned in favor of other drugs with less associated toxicity. A continued need for effective antiprotozoal and anti-*Pneumocystis* drugs, combined with the need for a better understanding of the drug-related adverse effects and the identification of an alternative route of administration, stimulated a resurgence in the development and clinical use of pentamidine.

Mechanism and Spectrum of Activity. Despite decades of clinical use, the mechanism of action of the diamidines is unknown. Several mechanisms have been proposed, but their relative individual or combined actions on protozoa and fungi are unknown. In fact, the mechanism may differ with the genus of the organism. Overall, the majority of in vitro studies involving a variety of susceptible species have demonstrated a relatively consistent inhibition of protein and nucleic acid synthesis by pentamidine. The effect of the inhibition of glucose metabolism by pentamidine on the drug's anti-infective activity is unknown. Such interference clearly influences the drug's adverse effect profile in humans, however.

Metabolism and Disposition. Only limited pharmacokinetic studies have been performed to evaluate the biodisposition of pentamidine. The vast majority of these limited data were derived from adults. Bioavailability after oral pentamidine administration is unknown, but it is believed to be poor, according to early studies demonstrating low bioavailability of stilbamidine, the prototype diamidine compound. Apparently no direct oral bioavailability studies have been performed and published for pentamidine itself. After intramuscular administration the drug appears to be well absorbed, achieving plasma pentamidine concentrations approaching 50% of

TABLE 14–93. Pentamidine Dosing Recommendations

***Pneumocystis carinii* Infection**
Treatment: 4 mg/kg once daily IV (preferred)* or IM for 14–21 days
Prophylaxis: 4 mg/kg q2–4wk IV or IM *or* inhalation of aerosolized pentamidine 300 mg via Respirgard II nebulizer once monthly

Trypanosomiasis
Treatment: 4 mg/kg once daily IV or IM for 10 days

Visceral Leishmaniasis
Treatment: 2–4 mg/kg once daily or every 2 days for 15 doses

Available Forms
Inhalation: 300 mg (as isethionate salt)
Powder for injection: 300 mg

*Intravenous infusion for at least 1 hour.

those observed after an intravenous infusion. In contrast, only small amounts of the drug are absorbed into the systemic circulation after aerosol administration.

The distribution of pentamidine after parenteral administration is unknown. The majority of tissue distribution data have been derived at autopsy from adults with AIDS. The drug appears to bind avidly to tissues and plasma proteins. Studies have demonstrated pentamidine in tissues up to 1 year after the last dose of drug. The highest concentrations of pentamidine have been described in the liver, kidneys, adrenals, spleen, lungs, and pancreas. After aerosol administration, the majority of the drug is found in the bronchoalveolar fluid at concentrations greatly exceeding those achieved with intravenous or intramuscular pentamidine administration.

The discrepancy in achievable pulmonary and systemic pentamidine concentrations between the two routes of administration is the basis for the preference for the aerosol route in the treatment of pulmonary infections. However, it is important to recognize that the actual amount of pentamidine deposition and the pulmonary distribution after aerosol administration depend on a number of important clinical factors central to all drugs administered via the aerosol route. Such factors include particle size, breathing pattern, ventilation (breaths per minute), extent of pulmonary disease, and associated regional ventilation and patient position. The ineffectiveness of pentamidine for the treatment of trypanosomal infections involving the central nervous system has been used as evidence of poor drug penetration into the central nervous system.

Pentamidine does not appear to undergo any appreciable metabolism and is primarily eliminated from the body in the urine. The $t_{1/2\beta}$ of pentamidine has been reported to range between 6 and 9 hours in adults. Similar values are observed in children. The effect of renal impairment on pentamidine elimination has not been studied adequately. Recommended doses for pentamidine administered via a variety of routes are outlined in Table 14–93.

Adverse Effects. As expected, the incidence of pentamidine-associated adverse effects depends on the dose and route of drug administration. The most common adverse effects observed with parenteral pentamidine include nephrotoxicity (in approximately 25% of patients), hypotension, cardiac dysrhythmias (often associated with rapid intravenous administration), sterile abscess formation, pain, erythema or tenderness at the site of deep intramuscular injection (in approximately 10% of patients), and hypoglycemia, which usually occurs after 5–7 days of therapy (in approximately 5–10% of patients). Pentamidine-associated nephrotoxicity most often develops gradually after the second week of therapy and is usually reversible on discontinuation of therapy. The observed nephrotoxicity is manifested as elevations in serum creatinine and blood urea nitrogen concentrations. Hypotension, when it occurs, may be due to rapid intravenous infusion, which emphasizes the administration recommendations that call for a slow infusion for 1–2 hours. Nevertheless, severe pentamidine-associated hypotension has been reported to occur during a slow drug infusion and to persist for hours afterward. The mechanisms underlying these renal and cardiovascular effects are unknown. Last, pentamidine-associated hypoglycemia can be profound (blood glucose concentration <25 g/dL) and prolonged. Blood glucose levels should be routinely monitored in persons receiving parenteral pentamidine.

The most common adverse effects associated with pentamidine aerosol are cough and bronchospasm; the relationship of these effects to the drug or to the extent of the underlying disease remains to be determined. Some studies have noted a decreased ability of investigators to obtain bronchoalveolar fluid or sputum for diagnostic tests from persons receiving pentamidine by aerosol. The possibility of a pentamidine-related drying effect on pulmonary secretions requires further investigation.

Drug Interactions. No specific drug interactions involving pentamidine have yet been reported. The possibility of additive or synergistic nephrotoxic effects should be considered whenever pentamidine is administered to a person who is receiving other known nephrotoxins such as aminoglycosides, amphotericin B, cisplatin, and possibly vancomycin.

ANTHELMINTIC DRUGS

MEBENDAZOLE, THIABENDAZOLE, AND ALBENDAZOLE

Mebendazole, thiabendazole, and albendazole are synthetic benzimidazole derivatives that possess a broad spectrum of activity against a wide range of helminths (worms) that infest humans (Table 14–94).

Mechanism and Spectrum of Action. Mebendazole and most likely albendazole appear to inhibit the uptake of glucose and other low-molecular weight nutrients by susceptible helminths. This inhibi-

TABLE 14–94. Helminths Usually Susceptible to Mebendazole, Thiabendazole, and Albendazole

Ancylostoma duodenale (hookworm)
Angiostrongylus cantonensis
Ascaris lumbricoides (roundworm)
Capillaria philippinensis (Philippine threadworm)
Enterobius vermicularis (pinworm)
Gnathostoma spinigerum
Hymenolepis nana (dwarf tapeworm)
Mansonella perstans
Necator americanus (hookworm)
Onchocerca volvulus
Strongyloides stercoralis (threadworm)*
Taenia saginata (beef tapeworm)
Taenia solium (pork tapeworm)
Trichinella spiralis (pork worm)
Trichuris trichiura (whipworm)

*Thiabendazole is preferred for *S. stercoralis*.

tion appears to be selective and irreversible for these compounds, causing degeneration of cytoplasmic microtubules in intestinal and tegmental cells of intestinal helminths. None of these agents appears to interfere with cellular functions of mammalian cells.

Thiabendazole appears to inhibit the fumarate reductase enzyme specific to helminths. In animal studies, thiabendazole has also been shown to exhibit anti-inflammatory, antipyretic, and analgesic effects.

Clinical Indications. Mebendazole, thiabendazole, and albendazole are indicated for the treatment of intestinal worm infestations including mixed helminth infestations. Mebendazole is effective for the majority of intestinal helminth infestations; thiabendazole may be the drug of choice for the treatment of *Strongyloides stercoralis* infestations. Mebendazole appears to be the anthelmintic of choice for persons with any degree of renal or hepatic disease, because of the degree of thiabendazole systemic absorption.

Metabolism and Distribution. Mebendazole and albendazole are poorly and erratically absorbed after oral administration; the estimated bioavailability approximates 2–10% of the orally administered dose. This low systemic bioavailability is most likely a combined result of poor drug absorption from the gastrointestinal tract and a rapid first-pass metabolism. Once absorbed, approximately 95% of mebendazole in blood is bound to plasma proteins. The drug $t_{1/2\beta}$ has been reported to range between 2.8 and 10 hours in both children and adults. Mebendazole is extensively metabolized in the liver, and <2–10% of the administered dose is excreted unchanged in the urine. In contrast, albendazole is rapidly metabolized in the liver to the active sulfoxide metabolite. The drug $t_{1/2\beta}$ of albendazole sulfoxide is approximately 8.5 hours.

Thiabendazole is rapidly and nearly completely absorbed from the gastrointestinal tract into the systemic circulation. Distribution characteristics of thiabendazole have not been described. Once absorbed, the drug is rapidly metabolized in the liver by means of hydroxylation. Mebendazole and thiabendazole dosing recommendations and available forms are outlined in Table 14–95.

Adverse Effects. Both mebendazole therapy and thiabendazole therapy are usually well tolerated and rarely are associated with adverse effects. When adverse effects do occur, they are most common after high-dose therapy. Transient abdominal pain with or without diarrhea has been reported in a few persons receiving the drug. Other rarely reported mebendazole- or thiabendazole-associated adverse effects include nausea, vomiting, headache, alopecia, skin rash, flushing, and abnormalities in the results of serum laboratory tests of liver and kidney function. A reversible myelosuppression manifested as neutropenia or thrombocytopenia has been reported in a small number of persons receiving prolonged, high-dose mebendazole therapy (e.g., for treatment of hydatid disease). Preliminary experience with albendazole suggests adverse effects similar to those of mebendazole.

Drug Interactions. Limited data suggest that the anticonvulsants carbamazepine and phenytoin may increase the hepatic metabolism of mebendazole, thiabendazole, and albendazole. Interference with the anthelmintic effect of mebendazole and albendazole is limited, at best, however, especially because the anthelmintic effect of mebendazole is due to local nonabsorbed drug concentrations. In contrast, possible drug-drug interactions including other agents (e.g., rifampin, phenobarbital) may be of clinical significance in persons receiving either drug for the treatment of extraintestinal infections. Thiabendazole may interfere with the hepatic metabolism of theophylline, and persons receiving this drug combination should be closely monitored.

TABLE 14–95. Albendazole, Mebendazole, and Thiabendazole Dosing Recommendations

Albendazole

Hydatid disease
- ≥60 kg: 400 mg bid with meals for 3 cycles of 28 days each, 14 days apart
- <60 kg: 15 mg/kg/day divided bid (max 800 mg/day) with meals for 3 cycles of 28 days each, 14 days apart

Neurocysticercosis
- ≥60 kg: 400 mg bid for 8–30 days
- <60 kg: 15 mg/kg/day divided bid (max 800 mg/day) for 8–30 days

Mebendazole (Children and Adults)

Pinworms: 100 mg once; may need to repeat after 2 wk

Whipworms, roundworms, hookworms: 100 mg bid for 3 consecutive days; may need to repeat course after 3–4 wk

Capillariasis: 200 mg bid for 20 days

Thiabendazole (Children and Adults)

50 mg/kg/day divided bid (max 3 g/day)
- Strongyloidiases: for 2 consecutive days (≥5 days for disseminated disease)
- Cutaneous larva migrans: for 2–5 consecutive days*
- Visceral larva migrans: for 5–7 consecutive days
- Trichinosis: for 2–4 consecutive days

Angiostrongyliasis: 50–75 mg/kg/day divided into 2–3 equal doses (q8hr or q12hr) for 3 days

Dracunculiasis: 50–75 mg/kg/day divided into 2 equal doses divided every 12 hours for 3 days

Available Forms

Albendazole: 200 mg tablets

Mebendazole: 100 mg chewable tablet

Thiabendazole
- Chewable tablet: 500 mg
- Suspension: 500 mg/5 mL

*Preliminary data suggesting efficacy with an extemporaneous topical ointment (10% thiabendazole suspension in white petrolatum) applied to lesions 4–6 times/day.

PRAZIQUANTEL

Praziquantel, which was discovered in 1972, is a synthetic heterocyclic anthelmintic agent. It is effective in the treatment of a wide range of cestode (tapeworm) and trematode infections in both animals and humans. Praziquantel is active against all *Schistosoma* species pathogenic to humans. Other trematodes and cestodes effectively eradicated by praziquantel are listed in Table 14–96.

The anthelmintic activity of praziquantel is most likely a result of two distinct actions of the drug on the helminth (worm). Praziquantel is rapidly and reversibly taken up by the helminth. At low concentrations the drug increased muscle activity, thus leading to spastic paralysis and causing the worm to lose attachment to host tissues. At higher concentrations, which are easily achieved with routine therapeutic dosing, the drug causes vacuolization and vesiculation of the integument of susceptible parasites. The molecular basis of these effects is unknown.

Clinical Indications. Praziquantel is used in the treatment of schistosomiasis, clonorchiasis, opisthorchiasis, other trematode infections (e.g., with intestinal flukes), and cestodiasis. Praziquantel is

TABLE 14–96. Anthelmintic Activity of Praziquantel

Trematodes
Schistosoma: All species pathogenic to humans
Liver flukes
Clonorchis sinensis
Opisthorchis viverrini
Fasciola hepatica
Lung flukes
Paragonimus uterobilateralis
Paragonimus westermani
Paragonimus kellicotti
Intestinal flukes
Metagonimus yokogawai
Nanophyetus salmincola
Fasciolopsis buski
Heterophyes heterophyes

Cestodes
Diphyllobothrium latum (fish tapeworm)
Dipylidium caninum (dog and cat tapeworm)
Hymenolepis nana (dwarf tapeworm)
Taenia saginata (beef tapeworm)
Taenia solium (pork tapeworm)
Cysticercus cellulosae (larval stage of *T. solium*)

rapidly absorbed after oral administration. Peak concentrations in blood are usually observed within 1–2 hours. The drug is rapidly and extensively metabolized by the liver to many hydroxylated and conjugated metabolites. The $t_{1/2\beta}$ of praziquantel approximates 0.8–1.5 hours in adults. Only traces ($<$0.1%) of parent drug are excreted unchanged in the urine. Praziquantel dosing recommendations and available forms are outlined in Table 14–97.

Adverse Effects. When administered in recommended doses for 1–2 days, praziquantel is usually well tolerated and is associated with only mild adverse effects, the most common of which appear to involve the nervous system and the gastrointestinal tract. Adverse central nervous system reactions have included dizziness, headache, and malaise. As a result, persons who drive an automobile or operate motorized machinery should be cautioned that praziquantel may temporarily interfere with their ability to operate these machines on the day of administration and for 1 day afterward. Common gastrointestinal effects primarily involve abdominal discomfort with or without accompanying nausea or diarrhea. These adverse effects, which are usually transient and mild, occur more frequently with higher praziquantel doses.

TABLE 14–97. Praziquantel Dosing Recommendations

Trematodes
Schistosoma: 20 mg/kg/day divided q8hr or q12hr PO for one 24-hr period
Flukes
Liver, intestine: 75 mg/kg/day divided q8hr PO for 1 day
Lung: 75 mg/kg/day divided q8hr PO for 2 days
Nanophyetus salmincola: 60 mg/kg/day divided q8hr PO for 1 day

Cestodes
*Cysticercus**: 50 mg/kg/day divided q8hr PO for 15 days
Tapeworms: 5–10 mg/kg as a single dose PO

Available Form
Tablet: 600 mg

*For cysticercosis, adjunctive therapy with dexamethasone should be given to persons with numerous cysts and in those with neurologic or intracranial hypertension. For neurocysticercosis, dexamethasone therapy should be started before praziquantel administration (Chapter 44).

Drug Interactions. Limited data assessing clinically important drug interactions with praziquantel are available. Carbamazepine, phenytoin, and rifampin may increase the metabolism of praziquantel, whereas cimetidine may decrease praziquantel metabolism.

PYRANTEL PAMOATE

Pyrantel pamoate was first used as a broad-spectrum anthelmintic agent in veterinary medicine. The drug's efficacy and lack of associated adverse effects prompted study and subsequent use in humans. In the United States, pyrantel pamoate is available as an over-the-counter medication.

Spectrum of Activity. Pyrantel pamoate is effective in the treatment of intestinal infestations involving *Enterobius vermicularis* (pinworm), *Ascaris lumbricoides* (roundworm), *Ancylostoma duodenale* (hookworm), *Necator americanus* (hookworm), and *Trichostrongylus orientalis* (hairworm).

Pyrantel pamoate is a depolarizing neuromuscular blocking agent that promotes release of acetylcholine and inhibition of acetylcholine-esterase in susceptible helminths, thus leading to prolonged (over)stimulation of ganglionic (nicotinic) receptors. These combined effects result in spastic paralysis of the worm. The drug is poorly absorbed from the gastrointestinal tract after oral administration. The majority of the administered dose is excreted in the feces; only a small proportion, approximately 7%, is excreted in the urine.

Recommended Dosing and Dosing Strategies. In the treatment of roundworm or pinworm, single-dose pyrantel 11 mg/kg (1 g maximum single dose) is administered to both children and adults. The dose may be repeated 2 weeks later to ensure complete eradication of pinworm infestations. For the treatment of hookworm infestations, 11 mg/kg (1 g maximum) is administered once daily for 3 consecutive days. Pyrantel pamoate is available as a suspension formulation containing 250 mg pyrantel per 5 mL and 62.5 mg (of pyrantel) tablets.

Adverse Effects. Adverse effects occur rarely after oral administration of pyrantel pamoate. Reported adverse effects of the drug have included nausea, vomiting, anorexia, abdominal cramps, diarrhea, headache, dizziness, drowsiness, and skin rash. Very rarely, pyrantel pamoate administration may be associated with transient, reversible elevations in values obtained from serum laboratory tests of liver function. Because the mechanism of anthelmintic action of piperazine is antagonistic to that of pyrantel, these two medications should not be administered concomitantly.

ANTIMALARIAL DRUGS

CHLOROQUINE

Chloroquine, a semisynthetic 4-aminoquinolone, is used primarily for the treatment of malaria. Today, the existence of many chloroquine-resistant and multidrug-resistant strains of *Plasmodium* has reduced the clinical usefulness of this prototypical compound for the treatment of malaria. Nevertheless, the drug remains the treatment of choice for uncomplicated or mild to moderate malaria caused by *P. vivax, P. ovale, P. malariae*, and sensitive strains of *P. falciparum*. In addition to antiprotozoal activity, the drug has limited usefulness as a second-line agent in the treatment of rheumatoid arthritis, discoid lupus erythematosus, porphyria cutanea tarda, solar urticaria, and polymorphous light eruption.

Spectrum of Activity. Chloroquine, like hydroxychloroquine, is active against the asexual erythrocytic forms of most strains of *P. vivax, P. ovale,* and *P. malariae.* However, the number of chloroquine-resistant strains of *P. falciparum,* the species that accounts for >85% of all cases of malaria, continues to increase in most geographic regions of the world. The mechanism of this plasmodial resistance to chloroquine is unknown. Preliminary studies indicate that resistant plasmodia fail to concentrate the drug within the digestive vacuoles of the parasite. It is also possible that drug-resistant organisms develop alternate pathways to utilize erythrocyte hemoglobin.

Unfortunately, chloroquine-resistant strains of *P. falciparum* are often resistant to quinine and combination regimens of antimalarial agents, including pyrimethamine and sulfadoxine or quinine and tetracycline. This increasing incidence of drug resistance underscores the need to identify newer compounds with improved safety profiles that are effective against plasmodia by means of various mechanisms. Chloroquine has no activity against exoerythrocytic tissue stages of plasmodium.

Clinical Indications. Chloroquine is used primarily for the treatment of acute malaria or as prophylaxis for malaria-exposed individuals.

Metabolism and Disposition. Chloroquine, a chiral compound, is administered as a 50:50 mixture of R and S chloroquine. The drug is well absorbed from the gastrointestinal tract after oral drug administration; bioavailability approximates 90% or greater. One study performed in adult volunteers suggests improvement in chloroquine bioavailability when the drug is taken with a meal, in comparison with dosing on an empty stomach. Patients should be instructed to take their dose of drug just before or just after a meal, as desired. Chloroquine is also well absorbed after subcutaneous or intramuscular administration, achieving plasma concentrations similar to those observed after intravenous administration.

Once absorbed, chloroquine is extensively distributed within most body fluids and tissue; the estimated volume of distribution ranges from 116 to 285 L/kg (mean: 240 L/kg) and reflects the extensive sequestration of the drug in body fluids and tissue. Chloroquine is concentrated in the liver, spleen, kidney, and lung (at approximately 200–700 times plasma concentration) and, to a lesser extent, in the brain and the spinal cord (at approximately 10–30 times plasma concentration). The drug also binds to melanin-containing cells in the eyes and skin and is concentrated in the erythrocytes. In addition, chloroquine crosses the placenta, and the drug and its desethyl metabolite can be found in small concentrations in human milk. Approximately 50–65% of the drug is bound to plasma proteins

About 50% of the absorbed chloroquine undergoes hepatic biotransformation to a number of metabolites. The primary chloroquine metabolite, monodesethylchloroquine, retains antimalarial activity and reaches plasma concentrations approaching 20–35% of parent chloroquine. Chloroquine and its metabolites are slowly excreted from the body via the kidney. Approximately 50% of unchanged chloroquine and 25% of monodesethylchloroquine are excreted in the urine. Accurate determination of the $t_{1/2\beta}$ for chloroquine has been difficult as a result of the drug's extensive tissue sequestration and subsequent slow redistribution after discontinuation of administration. Estimates of the chloroquine $t_{1/2\beta}$ are 70–125 hours or more. Chloroquine dosing strategies that include a loading dose have been designed to account for the extensive degree of tissue sequestration while limiting the incidence of drug-related adverse effects.

Assessment of the pharmacokinetics of individual chloroquine enantiomers has been performed in a small group of adults and reveals divergent pharmacokinetic behavior. No data describing any stereoselectivity of chloroquine activity or toxicity exist, and thus the clinical significance, if any, of these data is unknown. Oral chloroquine dosing schedules and available forms are shown in Table 14–98. The intramuscular route of chloroquine administration should be used only when oral therapy is not feasible.

Adverse Effects. When used for malaria prophylaxis, chloroquine is relatively free of adverse effects. When used orally in the treatment of malaria, adverse effects are uncommon but may include mild gastrointestinal upset, pruritus, mild and transient headache, and rarely, visual disturbances. These visual disturbances, which are often manifested as blurred vision or difficulty in focusing, occur most often after long-term administration. They may be associated with the extensive deposition of chloroquine in the eye.

The majority of adverse effects associated with chloroquine administration appear to be dose related and to occur most often when the drug is administered parenterally rather than orally. The discrepancy in the incidence of adverse effects between parenteral and oral chloroquine administration appears to result from the rapid attainment of high plasma drug concentrations that occur after parenteral, but not oral, administration. Chloroquine is a vasodilator, and serious, sometimes fatal cardiovascular toxicity (e.g., severe hypotension) has occurred after parenteral drug administration.

TABLE 14–98. Oral Chloroquine Dosing Recommendations

Treatment of Acute Attack of Malaria: Chloroquine Dose (mg base)*		
	Pediatric	*Adult*
Dose 1 (immediately)	10 mg/kg	600 mg
Dose 2 (6 hr after dose 1)	5 mg/kg	300 mg
Dose 3 (18 hr after dose 2)	5 mg/kg	300 mg
Dose 4 (24 hr after dose 3)	5 mg/kg	300 mg

Suppression or Prophylaxis of Malaria
Children: 5 mg base/kg once weekly (max 300 mg)
Adults: 300 mg
Prophylaxis is administered on the same day each week. Initiate therapy ~1–2 wk before exposure and continue weekly until 4 wk after departing endemic area

Treatment of Extraintestinal Amebiasis
Children: 10 mg base/kg once daily (max 300 mg) for 2–3 wk
Adults: 600 mg base once daily for 2 days, followed by 300 mg once daily for 2–3 wk

Available Forms
Tablets: 250 mg (as phosphate salt) equals 150 mg base *or* 500 mg (phosphate salt) equivalent to 300 mg base
Injection: Phosphate salt equivalent to 40 mg base per 5 mL

Chloroquine therapy assumes malaria caused by chloroquine-susceptible *Plasmodium.*
*Doses are presented as chloroquine base, not salt, formulation (see text for dose equivalents). Intramuscular dosing may be used when oral not feasible: 5 mg/kg base (max 200 mg) repeated in 6 hours for max 10 mg base/kg in a 24-hour period. (Adult intramuscular dosing: 200 mg q6hr.)

Drug Interactions. No clinically significant chloroquine drug-drug interactions have been described. It is possible that the concomitant administration of chloroquine with phenylbutazone or gold salts may be associated with an increased incidence of cutaneous reactions. Chloroquine at antimalarial doses may interfere with concurrent intradermal human diploid cell rabies vaccination.

QUININE

Literary descriptions of quinine date back as far as 1639, when books described the use of compounds obtained from the cinchona tree for the treatment of malaria. Quinine is the primary alkaloid isolated from bark obtained from this tree, which has also been described as the "fever" tree. By 1820, quinine and cinchonine were isolated from bark extract; even today, quinine is still obtained from natural sources. Quinine is the levorotatory isomer of quinidine and possesses cardiovascular effects qualitatively similar to those of quinidine.

Spectrum of Activity. Like chloroquine, quinine is a blood schizonticidal drug active against the asexual erythrocytic forms of most strains of *P. falciparum, P. vivax, P. ovale,* and *P. malariae.* Plasmodial resistance to quinine has been reported, and cross-resistance to chloroquine-resistant strains has been observed. The mechanism of antimalarial activity or plasmodial resistance is unknown.

Clinical Indications. Quinine is indicated for malaria prophylaxis or in the treatment of the acute disease. The drug is much less effective and more toxic than chloroquine. It is most often reserved for use in persons who have malaria caused by chloroquine-resistant strains or who cannot tolerate other antimalarial drugs. In addition, quinine is the drug of choice for cerebral malaria.

Metabolism and Disposition. Quinine is rapidly and nearly completely absorbed from the upper portion of the small intestine after oral administration. Limited data indicate that the drug is well absorbed even in the presence of diarrhea. Plasma quinine concentrations after oral administration have been reported to be only 10–20% less than those observed after intravenous infusion. Once absorbed into systemic circulation, the drug is well distributed to most body fluids and tissues, including the central nervous system. Quinine crosses the placenta and is distributed to human milk. The apparent volume of distribution of quinine, which is lower in persons with malaria than in uninfected individuals, averages approximately 1.9 L/kg in adults and 0.8 L/kg in children. Approximately 70% of quinine is bound to plasma proteins.

Quinine is extensively metabolized in the liver primarily via hydroxylation pathways. After oral administration, only 5–10% of a dose is excreted unchanged in the urine, and the remainder is excreted as less active metabolites. The quinine $t_{1/2\beta}$ has been reported to range from 8 to 21 hours in adults who are acutely ill with malaria, compared with 7–12 hours in convalescing persons. Corresponding $t_{1/2\beta}$ values in children 1–12 years of age with acute disease are 11–12 hours, in comparison with 6 hours in convalescing persons. The reasons for these differences in quinine pharmacokinetics—the contracted volume of distribution, increased $t_{1/2\beta}$, and a corresponding decrease in body clearance during the acute phase of the infection—are unknown but appear to be of no clinical significance. Quinine dosing recommendations and available forms are shown in Table 14–99.

TABLE 14–99. Dosing Recommendations for Quinine

Chloroquine Resistant Malaria
Children: 30 mg/kg/day (max 2 g/day) divided q8hr for 3–7 days in conjunction with another agent
Adults: 650 mg q8hr for 3–7 days in conjunction with another agent

Babesiosis
Children: 25 mg/kg/day (max dose 650 mg) divided q8hr for 7 days
Adults: 650 mg q6–8hr for 7 days

Available Forms
Capsules (sulfate salt): 65 mg, 200 mg, 300 mg, 325 mg
Tablets (sulfate salt): 162.5 mg, 260 mg

Adverse Effects. The adverse effects profile for quinine is highly variable; the majority of associated adverse effects are bothersome and self-limiting. With prolonged quinine administration or after a single large acute overdose, a typical dose-related cluster of symptoms, termed cinchonism, has been described. In mild cases, cinchonism is usually manifested as ringing in the ears, headache, nausea, and vomiting. If quinine dosing continues or an overdose is given, symptoms intensify, with progressive deterioration, including respiratory depression, hypotension, and cardiac conduction disturbances. Quinidine-like effects on the heart have been described in persons receiving appropriate quinine doses, but they occur most often after parenteral rather than oral administration. These effects may reflect the higher initial plasma drug concentrations obtained with intravenous dosing, and they underscore current intravenous dose recommendations for slow, intermittent infusions for 2–4 hours.

Other quinine-associated adverse effects include hypersensitivity reactions (e.g., cutaneous flushing, pruritus, skin rash), visual disturbances, and hypoglycemia. The drug may precipitate hemolysis and is contraindicated in persons with glucose-6-phosphate dehydrogenase deficiency. Persons with hypersensitivity to quinine should not receive the drug and should be counseled to avoid products that contain quinine, such as tonic water and certain cold preparations.

Drug Interactions. Quinine, like quinidine, may competitively decrease the renal clearance of digoxin or digitoxin, leading to increased plasma concentrations of these cardiac glycosides and resultant toxicity. Furthermore, because quinine possesses cardiac effects qualitatively similar to those of its isomer, quinidine, it should be administered with caution to persons who have underlying cardiac disease or who are taking drugs that suppress cardiac conduction and prolong the refractory period. Similarly, quinine and mefloquine should not be used concomitantly because associated adverse cardiac effects may be additive. Cimetidine, but not ranitidine, has been reported to decrease the body clearance and prolong the $t_{1/2\beta}$ of quinine. Quinine may potentiate the neuromuscular blocking effects of anesthetics, specifically pancuronium, succinylcholine, and tubocurarine. Last, quinine may depress the hepatic synthesis of vitamin K, which could enhance the activity of oral anticoagulants (e.g., warfarin).

REVIEWS

Butler DR, Kuhn RJ, Chandler MH: Pharmacokinetics of anti-infective agents in paediatric patients. *Clin Pharmacokinet* 1994;26:374–95.
Gregg CR: Drug interactions and anti-infective therapies. *Am J Med* 1999;106:227–37.

Henry NK, Hoecker JL, Rhodes KH: Antimicrobial therapy for infants and children: Guidelines for the inpatient and outpatient practice of pediatric infectious diseases. *Mayo Clin Proc* 2000;75:86–97.

Levison ME: Pharmacodynamics of antibacterial drugs. *Infect Dis Clin North Am* 2000;14:281–91.

San Joaquin VH, Stull TL: Antibacterial agents in pediatrics. *Infect Dis Clin North Am* 2000;14: 341–55.

Temple ME, Nahata MC: Pharmacotherapy of acute sinusitis in children. *Am J Health Syst Pharm* 2000;57:663–8.

KEY ARTICLES

Antifungal Drugs

Amichai B, Grunwald MH: Adverse drug reactions of the new oral antifungal agents—terbinafine, fluconazole and itraconazole. *Int J Dermatol* 1998;37:410–5.

Bennett ML, Fleischer AB, Loveless JW, et al: Oral griseofulvin remains the treatment of choice for tinea capitis in children. *Pediatr Dermatol* 2000;17:304–9.

Patel R: Antifungal agents. Part 1. Amphotericin B preparations and flucytosine. *Mayo Clin Proc* 1998;73:1205–25.

Richardson MD, Kokki MH: Antifungal therapy in ''bone marrow failure.'' *Br J Haematol* 1998;200:619–28.

Suarez S, Friedlander SF: Antifungal therapy in children: An update. *Pediatr Ann* 1998;27:177–84.

Antibacterial Drugs

Alpuche-Aranda CM: Beta-lactamase production and the role of ampicillin/sulbactam. *Pediatr Infect Dis J* 1998;17:S8–11; discussion S20–1.

Alvarez-Elcoro S, Enzler MJ: The macrolides: Erythromycin, clarithromycin, and azithromycin. *Mayo Clin Proc* 1999;74:613–34.

Bhatt-Mehta V, Schumacher RE, Faix RG, et al: Lack of vancomycin-associated nephrotoxicity in newborn infants: A case-control study. *Pediatrics* 1999;103:E48.

Bucher HC, Griffith L, Guyatt GH, et al: Meta-analysis of prophylactic treatments against *Pneumocystis carinii* pneumonia and toxoplasma encephalitis in HIV-infected patients. *J Acquir Immune Defic Syndr Hum Retrovirol* 1997;15:104–14.

Burkhardt JE, Walterspiel JN, Schaad UB: Quinolone arthropathy in animals versus children. *Clin Infect Dis* 1997;25;1196–204.

De Moor RA, Egberts AC, Schroder CH: Ceftriaxone-associated nephrolithiasis and biliary pseudolithiasis. *Eur J Pediatr* 1999;158:975–7.

Fisman DN, Kaye KM: Once-daily dosing of aminoglycoside antibiotics. *Infect Dis Clin North Am* 2000;14:475–87.

Groll AH, Muller FM, Piscitelli SC, et al: Lipid formulations of amphotericin B: Clinical perspectives for the management of invasive fungal infections in children with cancer. *Klin Padiatr* 1998;210:264–73.

Hampel B, Hullmann R, Schmidt H: Ciprofloxacin in pediatrics: Worldwide clinical experience based on compassionate use—safety report. *Pediatr Infect Dis J* 1997;16:127–9; discussion 160–2.

Mofenson LM: Rifabutin. *Pediatr Infect Dis J* 1998;17:71–2.

Mustafa MM, Pappo A, Cash J, et al: Aerosolized pentamidine for the prevention of *Pneumocystis carinii* pneumonia in children with cancer intolerant or allergic to trimethoprim/sulfamethoxazole [see Comments]. *J Clin Oncol* 1994;1:258–61.

Norrby SR, Gildon KM: Safety profile of meropenem: A review of nearly 5,000 patients treated with meropenem. *Scand J Infect Dis* 1999; 31:3–10.

Norrby SR: Carbapenems in serious infections: A risk-benefit assessment. *Drug Saf* 2000;22:191–4.

Reed MD, Blumer JL: Azithromycin: A critical review of the first azilide antibiotic and its role in pediatric practice. *Pediatr Infect Dis J* 1997;16:1069–83.

Reed MD: A reassessment of ticarcillin/clavulanic acid dose recommendations for infants, children and adults. *Pediatr Infect Dis J* 1998; 17:1195–9.

Robinson RF, Nahata MC: A comparative review of conventional and lipid formulations of amphotericin B. *J Clin Pharm Ther* 1999;24:249–57.

Rodvold KA, Everett JA, Pryka RD, et al: Pharmacokinetics and administration regimens of vancomycin in neonates, infants and children. *Clin Pharmacokinet* 1997;33:32–51.

Shapiro LE, Knowles SR, Shear NH: Comparative safety of tetracycline, minocycline and doxycycline. *Arch Dermatol* 1997;133:1224–30.

Siber GR, Gorham CC, Ericson JF, et al: Pharmacokinetics of intravenous trimethoprim-sulfamethoxazole in children and adults with normal and impaired renal function. *Rev Infect Dis* 1982;4:566–78.

Somech R, Arav-Boger R, Assia A, et al: Complications of minocycline therapy for acne vulgaris: Case reports and review of the literature. *Pediatr Dermatol* 1999;16:469–72.

Weinthal J, Frost JD, Briones G, et al: Successful *Pneumocystis carinii* pneumonia prophylaxis using aerosolized pentamidine in children with acute leukemia [see Comments]. *J Clin Oncol* 1994;12:136–40.

Wispelwey B, Pearson RD: Pentamidine: A review. *Infect Control Hosp Epidemiol* 1991;12:375–82.

Antimycobacterial Drugs

Donald PR: Preventing tuberculosis in childhood. *Indian J Pediatr* 2000;67:383–5.

Douglas JG, McLeod MJ: Pharmacokinetic factors in the modern drug treatment of tuberculosis. *Clin Pharmacokinet* 1999;37:127–46.

Graham SM, Daley HM, Banerjee A, et al: Ethambutol in tuberculosis: Time to reconsider? *Arch Dis Child* 1998;79:274–8.

Lazarus A, Sanders J: Management of tuberculosis. Choosing an effective regimen and ensuring compliance. *Postgrad Med* 2000;108:71–4, 77–9, 83–4.

McMaster P, Isaacs D: Critical review of evidence for short course therapy for tuberculous adenitis in children. *Pediatr Infect Dis J* 2000;19:401–4.

Mitchison DA: The role of individual drugs in the chemotherapy of tuberculosis. *Int J Tuberc Lung Dis* 2000;4:796–806.

Nobert E, Chernick V: Tuberculosis. 5. Pediatric disease. *CMAJ* 1999;160:1479–82.

Roos KL: *Mycobacterium tuberculosis* meningitis and other etiologies of the aseptic meningitis syndrome. *Semin Neurol* 2000;20:329–35.

Singh M, Jayanthi S, Kumar L: Drug-resistant tuberculosis. *Indian J Pediatr* 2000;67:S41–6.

Stowe CD, Jacobs RF: Treatment of tuberculous infection and disease in children: The North American perspective. *Paediatr Drugs* 1999; 1:299–312.

Swaminathan S: Treatment of tuberculosis. *Indian J Pediatr* 2000; 67:S14–20.

Telenti A, Iseman M: Drug-resistant tuberculosis: What do we do now? *Drugs* 2000;59:171–9.

Van Scoy RE, Wilkowske CJ: Antimycobacterial therapy. *Mayo Clin Proc* 1999;74:1038–48.

Yew WW: Therapeutic drug monitoring in antituberculosis chemotherapy. *Ther Drug Monit* 1998;20:469–72.

Antiviral Drugs

Anonymous: Antiretroviral therapy and medical management of pediatric HIV infection and 1997 USPHS/IDSA Report on the Prevention of Opportunistic Infections in Persons Infected with Human Immunodeficiency Virus. *Pediatrics* 1998;102:999–1085.

Balfour HH: Drug therapy: Antiviral drugs. *N Engl J Med* 1999; 340:1255–68.

Couch RB: Drug therapy: Prevention and treatment of influenza. *N Engl J Med* 2000;343:1778–87.

Crumpacker CS: Drug therapy: Ganciclovir. *N Engl J Med* 1996;335:721–9.

Englund JA, Fletcher CV, Balfour HH Jr: Acyclovir therapy in neonates. *J Pediatr* 1991;119:129–35.

Farley J, Vink P: Pediatric antiretroviral therapy from research to practice. *Pediatr AIDS HIV Infect* 1996;7:9–13.

Francavilla R, Mieli-Vergani G: Treatment of hepatitis C virus infection in children. *Can J Gastroenterol* 2000;14:41B–44B.

McDonald CK, Kuritzkes DR: Human immunodeficiency virus type 1 protease inhibitors. *Arch Intern Med* 1997;157:951–9.

McKinney RE Jr: Combination antiretroviral therapy. *Pediatr Infect Dis J* 1998;17:515–6.

Moscona A: Management of respiratory syncytial virus infections in the immunocompromised child. *Pediatr Infect Dis J* 2000;19:253–4.

Oram RJ, Herold BC: Antiviral agents for herpes viruses. *Pediatr Infect Dis J* 1998;17:652–3.

U.S. Public Health Service and Infectious Diseases Society of America: 1999 USPHS/IDSA guidelines for the prevention of opportunistic infections in persons infected with human immunodeficiency virus: U.S. Public Health Services (USPHS) and Infectious Diseases Society of America (IDSA). *MMWR Morb Mortal Wkly Rep* 1999;48(RR-10):1–66.

Zerr DM, Frenkel LM: Advances in antiviral therapy. *Curr Opin Pediatr* 1999;11:21–7.

Zoulim F, Trepo C: Drug therapy for chronic hepatitis B: Antiviral efficacy and influence of hepatitis B virus polymerase mutations on the outcome of therapy. *J Hepatol* 1998;29:151–68.

Antiparasitic Drugs

Cowden J, Hotez P: Mebendazole and albendazole treatment of geohelminth infections in children and pregnant women. *Pediatr Infect Dis J* 2000;19:659–60.

Davidson RN: Practical guide for the treatment of leishmaniasis. *Drugs* 1998;56:1009–18.

Dickson R, Awasthi S, Demellweek C, et al: Antihelmintic drugs for treating worms in children: Effects on growth and cognitive performance. *Cochrane Database Syst Rev* 2000;CD000371.

Geerts S, Gryseels B: Drug resistance in human helminths: Current situation and lessons from livestock. *Clin Microbiol Rev* 2000;13:207–22.

Hay RJ: Therapeutic potential of terbinafine in subcutaneous and systemic mycoses. *Br J Dermatol* 1999;141:36–40.

Lamp KC, Freeman CD, Klutman NE, et al: Pharmacokinetics and pharmacodynamics of the nitroimidazole antimicrobials. *Clin Phamacokinet* 1999;36:353–73.

Macreadie I, Ginsburg H, Sirawaraporn W, et al: Antimalarial drug development and new targets. *Parasitol Today* 2000;16:438–44.

Mumcuoglu KY: Prevention and treatment of head lice in children. *Paediatr Drugs* 1999;1:211–8.

Newton P, White N: Malaria: New developments in treatment and prevention. *Annu Rev Med* 1999;50:179–92.

Sangster NC, Gill J: Pharmacology of antihelmintic resistance. *Parasitol Today* 1999;15:141–6.

Stephenson I, Wiselka M: Drug treatment of tropical parasitic infections: Recent achievements and developments. *Drugs* 2000;60:985–95.

Warhurst DC: Drug resistance in *Plasmodium falciparum* malaria. *Infection* 1999;27:S55–8.

White NJ: Drug resistance in malaria. *Br Med Bull* 1998;54:703–15.

Zaat JO, Mank TH, Assendelft WJ: Drugs for treating giardiasis. *Cochrane Database Syst Rev* 2000;(2):CD000217.

CHAPTER 15

Immunotherapy and Immunomodulation

Gerald W. Fischer

The host immune response to invading microbes is a complex interaction that involves both cellular and humoral factors contributing to nonspecific immune enhancement and inflammation and to specific responses targeted to a specific pathogen (Chapter 5). In general, the host immune response is beneficial. However, a vigorous immunologic response may also result in enhanced tissue destruction, such as respiratory distress syndrome, or in physiologic instability, such as septic shock induced by TNF. **Immunotherapy** encompasses active immunization (Chapter 17) but is often used to refer to the use of immune components such as immune globulins (passive immunization), antitoxins, leukocyte transfusions, and immunopotentiators and immunosuppressants, alone or in combination, to enhance immunity or modulate unwanted physiologic responses and tissue destruction (Table 15–1).

IMMUNE GLOBULINS

IGs from humans and antisera derived from animals have been available for many years for prevention or treatment of infections. High-titer specific IG preparations are prepared from donors identified by screening or after immunization, and newer products are engineered monoclonal antibodies.

Many standard human IG preparations are currently available (Table 15–2). IG, previously known as immune serum globulin or gamma globulin, was used for many years as replacement therapy for patients with Ig deficiency but was limited by the necessity of intramuscular administration. The increased availability of **intravenous immune globulin (IVIG)** affords the ability to infuse large quantities of IgG rapidly with minimal discomfort. Animal-derived antitoxins and antisera such as TAT and RIG are generally not used in the United States unless specific human IG preparations are not available, as is the case for the treatment of botulism and respiratory diphtheria.

Standard IG and standard IVIG are derived from pooled human plasma (Fig. 15–1). Specific antibodies representative of the population providing the plasma may vary according to the infection and immunization experience of the donors. All IVIG products available in the United States contain functional IgG capable of neutralizing viruses, promoting phagocytosis of bacteria, and enhancing or modulating a variety of other immunologic responses, although titers to individual bacteria and viruses may vary. These large IG pools generally contain some antibodies to the majority of common human pathogens. When IVIG is targeted for prevention or treatment of specific viral, bacterial, and immunologic diseases, it is sometimes necessary to ensure that the appropriate antibodies are present to provide effective therapy. Because the levels of specific antibodies are not ensured and cannot easily be assayed, standard IG and IVIG preparations are not formally approved for such uses.

Preparations of IG have had an exceedingly good safety record. The plasma fractionation process is virucidal and partitions most virions that may be present in donor plasma to non-IgG fractions. Additional virucidal processing steps, such as heating or treatment with solvent-detergent, have been added recently to several preparation methods to enhance safety and should further minimize transmission of infectious agents by these products. All donors of blood products in the United States are screened for several viral infections including hepatitis B, hepatitis C, HIV, and HTLV-I and HTLV-II infections. Antibodies to hepatitis B, present in many donors, may further minimize transmission of remaining hepatitis B virus. Rare cases of hepatitis B and hepatitis C (non-A, non-B hepatitis) were traced to IG administration before wider incorporation of heating or solvent-detergent treatment. Transmission of HIV by IG products has not been documented. Although the accumulated data indicate that IVIG is exceedingly safe, physicians should never consider blood- and plasma-derived products to be totally without risk.

Immune Globulin Therapy

IG is a sterile preparation that is provided as a 16.5% (165 mg/mL) protein solution for intramuscular administration only. Intravenous administration may induce severe systemic reactions and anaphylaxis. Although 95% or more of the preparation is IgG, trace

TABLE 15–1. Components of Nonspecific (Innate) and Specific (Adaptive) Immunity That Can Be Modulated by Immunotherapy

Immune Component	Function
Nonspecific (Innate) Immunity	
Neutrophils and macrophages	Ingest and destroy microorganisms
Cytokines	Enhance immunity and inflammation
Interferons	Inhibit viruses; induce effector proteins and cytokines
Antibody Fc binding	Regulatory function; modulate phagocytosis
Specific (Adaptive) Immunity	
Opsonic antibody	Facilitate phagocytosis
Bactericidal antibody	Destroy bacteria
Antitoxin	Neutralize bacterial toxins
Virus neutralizing antibody	Destroy virus
Antibody-dependent cell-mediated cytotoxicity (ADCC)	Facilitate cell-mediated elimination of virus infected cells

TABLE 15–2. Immune Globulin Preparations and Antitoxins Available in the United States

Immunobiologic	Trade Name (and Manufacturer)	Type	Indication(s)
Botulinum antitoxin	Aventis Pasteur (distributed by the CDC)	Specific equine antibodies	Treatment of botulism (Chapter 56)
Cytomegalovirus immune globulin (CMV-IG)	CytoGam (MedImmune)	Pooled human antibodies from persons with high antibody titers to CMV	Prophylaxis for bone marrow and kidney transplant recipients (Chapter 100)
Diptheria antitoxin	Aventis Pasteur (distributed by CDC)	Specific equine antibodies	Treatment of respiratory diphtheria (Chapter 58)
Immune globulin (IG)	Gammar-P.I.M. (Centeon)	Pooled human antibodies	Measles postexposure prophylaxis (Chapter 23) Hepatitis A pre-exposure and postexposure prophylaxis (Chapter 78)
Intravenous immune globulin (IVIG)	See Table 15–3	Pooled human antibodies	Replacement therapy for antibody deficiency disorders (Chapter 98) Hypogammaglobulinemia in chronic lymphocytic leukemia Kawasaki syndrome (Chapter 39) Immune thrombocytopenic purpura
Hepatitis B immune globulin (HBIG)	H-BIG (North American Biologicals) BayHep B (Bayer Biological)	Specific human antibodies	Hepatitis B postexposure prophylaxis (Chapter 78)
Rabies immune globulin (RIG)*	Imogam Rabies Immune Globulin (Aventis Pasteur) Bayrab (Bayer Biological)	Specific human antibodies	Rabies postexposure management of persons not previously immunized with rabies vaccine (Chapter 50)
Respiratory syncytial virus immune globulin (RSV-IG)	RespiGam (MedImmune)	Pooled human antibodies from individuals with high neutralizing antibody titers to RSV	Prophylaxis of pneumonia caused by respiratory syncytial virus in infants born prematurely or with bronchopulmonary dysplasia (Chapter 67)
Respiratory syncytial virus monoclonal antibody (palivizumab)	Synagis (MedImmune)	Specific RSV monoclonal antibody	Prophylaxis of pneumonia caused by respiratory syncytial virus in infants born prematurely or with bronchopulmonary dysplasia (Chapter 67)
Tetanus immune globulin (TIG)	Baytet (Bayer Biological)	Specific human antibodies	Tetanus treatment (Chapter 56) Postexposure prophylaxis of persons not adequately immunized with tetanus toxoid (Chapter 48)
Vaccinia immune globulin (VIG)	Hyland Therapeutics (distributed by CDC)	Specific human antibodies	Treatment of eczema vaccinatum, vaccinia necrosum, and ocular vaccinia
Varicella zoster immune globulin (VZIG)	VZIG (American Red Cross)	Specific human antibodies	Postexposure prophylaxis of susceptible immunocompromised persons, certain susceptible pregnant women, and perinatally exposed newborn infants (Chapter 27)

*As much as possible of the full dose of RIG is infiltrated into and around the wound(s), and any remaining volume is administered intramuscularly at an anatomic site distant from rabies vaccine.

amounts of IgA and IgM are also present. There are three indications for IG use: (1) replacement therapy for antibody deficiency disorders, (2) hepatitis A pre-exposure and postexposure prophylaxis, and (3) measles postexposure prophylaxis.

The volume required for effective prophylaxis complicates treatment with IG. Generally, not more than 5 mL should be given at any single intramuscular injection site (1–3 mL for young children), and the total IG volume at all sites should not exceed 20 mL. Injections should be given into a large area of muscle mass. Serum IgG levels peak in approximately 48–72 hours and persist for 3–4 weeks. Live-virus vaccination is not recommended within 5 months after IG administration (6 months if 0.5 mL/kg was administered) because of interference of the passive antibodies with viral replication and development of immunity (Table 17–4).

Immunodeficiency. IG is not generally used for antibody replacement therapy for antibody deficiency disorders because IVIG provides higher serum IgG levels with less discomfort.

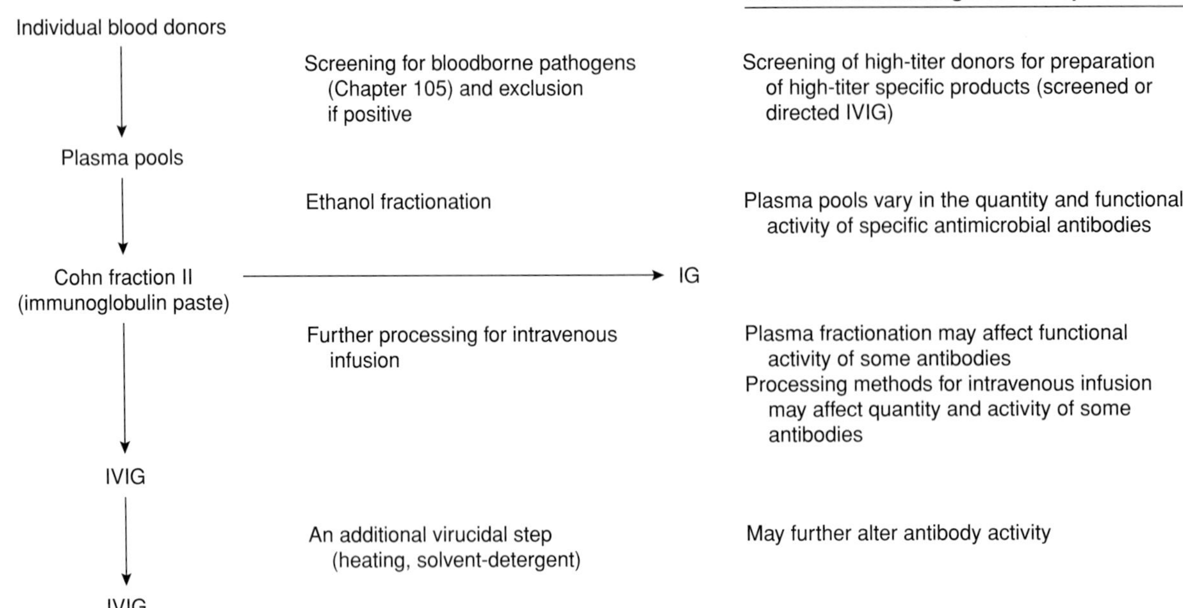

FIGURE 15–1. General steps for preparation from plasma of immune globulin for intramuscular administration, and intravenous immune globulin.

Hepatitis A. Hepatitis A vaccination is preferred to IG administration for pre-exposure hepatitis A prophylaxis, but IG is used for children less than 2 years of age or if protection is required within 14 days (Chapter 78). The pre-exposure prophylaxis regimen for hepatitis A, with IG used for nonimmune travelers, is 0.02 mL/kg, or 0.06 mL/kg every 5 months if the duration of a visit to a developing country exceeds 3 months. An IG dosage of 0.02 mL/kg is still commonly used for hepatitis A postexposure prophylaxis and should be given as soon as possible after exposure, but within 14 days (Chapter 78).

Measles. Measles postexposure prophylaxis is rarely indicated, but IG given within 6 days of exposure to measles in a household or hospital setting can prevent or modify disease in individuals for whom postexposure vaccination is not recommended (Chapter 23). Persons at high risk include infants less than 12 months of age; immunocompromised persons regardless of the previous vaccination status, including those with symptomatic HIV infection; and possibly susceptible pregnant women because of the risk of fetal death. Maternally derived antibodies should provide protection to the infant younger than 6 months. Infants between 6 and 12 months of age should receive postexposure prophylaxis within 72 hours with measles vaccination and concurrent IG. If the exposure occurred more than 72 hours but less than 6 days previously, IG may be given alone to modify the course of the disease. For immunocompetent persons exposed to measles, a single dose of IG, 0.25 mL/kg (maximum, 15 mL), is administered as soon after exposure as possible. For immunocompromised persons exposed to measles, a single dose of IG, 0.5 mL/kg (maximum, 15 mL), is used. Administration of IG is not needed in persons, including HIV-infected persons, receiving IVIG, 100–400 mg/kg, at regular intervals if the last dose was administered within 3 weeks of the exposure to measles. Administration of IVIG, 100–400 mg/kg, for postexposure measles prevention may be as effective as IG, but no data are available.

Intravenous Immune Globulin Therapy

Many standard IVIG products are now licensed for use in the United States (Table 15–3). These products are produced by different processes from plasma pooled from as many as 50,000 donors. Plasma fractionation and processing may alter the IgG characteristics by inducing IgG aggregation, fragmenting the antibodies, or adding heterologous proteins. Thus all plasma pools may not be similar. In addition, each lot may have its own characteristics, particularly in reference to pathogen-specific antibody titers. Recent studies have shown lot-to-lot variation in antibody titers to both bacterial and viral pathogens, in addition to differences resulting from the preparation procedure.

IVIG initially should be given by slow infusion, usually for several hours, with an initial infusion rate of 0.5 mL/kg/hr for 30 minutes, gradually increased at subsequent 15–30 minute intervals to a maximum of 2–4 mL/kg/hr. The person receiving the infusion should be observed for acute reactions during IVIG administration. Some persons have local discomfort at the infusion site or become flushed and light-headed. Slowing or stopping the infusion for 15–30 minutes usually alleviates the reaction and permits resumption of IVIG administration. The vasomotor reactions tend to occur early in the course of infusion and are generally related to the infusion rate. Hypotension is uncommon and rarely severe enough to warrant complete discontinuation of therapy. Anaphylaxis is rare but may be fatal. Renal toxic effects, reported in persons with underlying kidney disease who are receiving large doses of IVIG, may be related to substances in the IG preparation other than IgG. Renal function should be monitored in persons with known kidney disease. Congestive heart failure has been documented in sick persons, especially if higher IVIG doses are used, as in persons with Kawasaki syndrome who are given a single 2 g/kg dose. Although this therapy can be generally managed without difficulty, persons with underlying heart disease should be carefully monitored during IVIG administration.

Immunodeficiency. Administration of IVIG has been a major advance in the treatment of primary immunodeficiency diseases. Using larger doses in persons with immunodeficiency has routinely produced higher serum antibody levels and appears to be beneficial. At doses of 150 mg/kg, serum IgG levels reach approximately 400 mg/dL, and with doses of 400 mg/kg, serum IgG levels approach normal levels. Although it seems apparent that the higher serum levels of IgG are important, it is not known whether it is necessary to reach normal serum IgG concentrations.

To establish an optimal regimen, the clinician should monitor serum IgG levels regularly during administration of the first two IVIG doses. The serum IgG level increases approximately 200–250 mg/dL for each 100 mg/kg dose of IgG infused. Because the half-life of infused IgG is about 28 days (it may be less in neonates), trough levels should be obtained 3–4 weeks after infusion. The goal is to determine an IVIG dose and cycle of administration that maintains serum IgG levels of at least 350 mg/dL throughout the postinfusion period.

Many children with AIDS have dysregulation of immunoglobulin and low titers of antibody to specific pathogens, and IVIG administration has been used to prevent life-threatening bacterial infections in these children. Currently the use of IVIG is not standard therapy for all HIV-infected children but may benefit selected HIV-infected children with recurrent bacterial infections (Chapter 38). There is no evidence that IVIG alters the progression of HIV infection.

Prophylaxis of Neonatal Infections. After birth the immunoglobulin level in the infant begins to fall, and relative hypogammaglobulinemia may persist for several months. Because most maternally derived IgG crosses the placenta in the last 4–6 weeks of pregnancy, premature infants are generally born with a deficiency of IgG. Young infants, and especially premature neonates, are susceptible to encapsulated bacteria that require opsonic antibody for efficient phagocytosis and killing, including group B *Streptococcus, Escherichia coli, Haemophilus influenzae* type b, and *Staphylococcus.*

IVIG therapy in neonates has been shown to be exceedingly safe in several clinical trials involving more than 5,000 babies. The published studies that have evaluated IVIG prophylaxis have not clearly established the role of IVIG in preventing early-onset or late-onset neonatal infections. One reason may be the variability of specific antibacterial antibodies in different IVIG preparations and lots used in these studies. Of the three larger masked, placebo-controlled trials, one study showed benefit and two studies demonstrated no difference between IVIG and placebo for prophylaxis of neonatal sepsis. Meta-analysis of 12 studies of IVIG prophylaxis in 4,933 evaluable babies found that IVIG administered prophylactically to premature low birth weight newborns is of minimal but demonstrable benefit in preventing sepsis. The diversity of neonatal infections and the variability in IVIG preparations and lots confound the current studies. Because of the minimal benefit that has been demonstrated and the relatively large population that would require treatment, IVIG administration cannot be considered standard for prevention of neonatal infections. Staphylococci are now the leading cause of neonatal late-onset sepsis, and specific IVIG therapy for infection with staphylococci or other neonatal pathogens may be required to ensure uniform efficacy. Until specific preparations are available, premature neonates with recurrent infections may benefit from therapy with IVIG, 500 mg/kg per dose, every 2–3 weeks as prophylaxis, because serum IgG levels are often low in these babies.

Treatment of Neonatal Infections. IVIG has also been studied as an adjunct to appropriate antibiotic therapy for treatment of neonatal sepsis. In addition to enhancing opsonization, IVIG increases and maintains peripheral blood neutrophils in newborns with sepsis. Thus, by both preventing neutropenia and enhancing bacterial opsonization, antibodies may provide a valuable adjunct to antibiotic therapy. Several studies have shown a twofold to fourfold increased risk of death in babies with sepsis who did not receive IVIG in addition to antibiotic therapy. Meta-analysis of three studies of

TABLE 15–3. Standard Intravenous Immune Globulin (IVIG) Preparations Available in the United States

Manufacturer	Trade Name	Plasma Source	Preparation	Form	Formulation
Alpha Therapeutic	Venoglobulin-S	Paid and volunteer	PEG fractionation, DEAE Sephadex treatment, solvent-detergent treatment	Solution	5% and 10% IgG with 5% sorbitol
American Red Cross	Polygam S/D	Volunteer only	DEAE Sephadex treatment, solvent-detergent treatment	Lyophilized powder	5% IgG with 2% glucose, 0.2% PEG, 0.3% albumin
Aventis Pasteur	Panglobulin	Volunteer only	Acid (pH 4.0) with traces of pepsin	Lyophilized powder	10% IgG with 4% glucose, 0.4% PEG, 0.6% albumin 3%, 6%, 9%, and 12% IgG with 10% sucrose
Baxter Centeon	Gammar-P.I.V.	Paid and volunteer	Ultrafiltration, pasteurization	Lyophilized powder	5% IgG with 5% sucrose, 3% albumin
	Gammagard S/D	Paid and volunteer	DEAE Sephadex treatment, solvent-detergent treatment	Lyophilized powder	5% IgG with 2% glucose, 0.2% PEG, 0.3% albumin 10% IgG with 4% glucose, 0.4% PEG, 0.6% albumin
Bayer	Gamimune N	Paid and volunteer	Ultrafiltration, acid (pH 4.25) in final product	Solution	5% IgG with 10% maltose 10% IgG with glycine 0.16–0.24 mol/L
Immuno (distributed by Baxter)	Iveegam	Paid and volunteer	Immobilized trypsin, sequential PEG preparation	Lyophilized powder	5% IgG with 5% glucose
Novartis	Sandoglobulin	Volunteer only	Acid (pH 4.0) with traces of pepsin	Lyophilized powder	3%, 6%, 9%, and 12% IgG with 10% sucrose

PEG = polyethylene glycol; DEAE = diethylaminoethyl.

110 babies with neonatal sepsis showed a significantly decreased mortality rate when IVIG was given with standard antibiotics and supportive care, with a short-term mortality rate that was nearly sixfold higher in neonates not given IVIG.

Newborns with sepsis, especially small preterm babies (<1000 g) or those with neutropenia, may benefit from a 500 mg/kg dose of IVIG in addition to antibiotics. A second dose of IVIG may be given in 24 hours if the WBC count has not risen into the normal range. The total dose should not exceed 1,000 mg/dL because very high doses of IVIG may inhibit the killing of bacteria by antibiotics.

Specific Immune Globulin Preparations

Specific immune serum globulin preparations, commonly referred to as hyperimmune globulins, are prepared from the plasma of donors with high titers of the desired antibody, either naturally acquired **(screened or directed IVIG)** or induced by immunization. Several products with high antibody titers to specific pathogens have been available for many years to prevent, modify, or treat a variety of infections (Table 15–2).

Hepatitis B Immune Globulin. HBIG is used to prevent hepatitis B infection (Chapter 78) and should be given as soon as possible after hepatitis B exposure in conjunction with hepatitis B vaccine. HBIG with hepatitis B vaccine should also be given within 12 hours of birth to the infant born to a woman with HBsAg positivity.

Varicella-Zoster Immune Globulin. VZIG can prevent or modify the course of chickenpox in immunocompromised persons (Chapter 27). Individuals exposed to varicella who are considered at risk of having complications if infected should receive VZIG within 96 hours of exposure. VZIG is not effective after the illness is manifested.

Rabies Immune Globulin. RIG should be given in conjunction with rabies vaccine to individuals receiving postexposure rabies prophylaxis, with the exception of the preimmunized person with a documented serum antirabies antibody titer who should receive vaccine (two doses) alone (Chapter 50). Both RIG and rabies vaccine should be given as soon as possible after exposure. As much as possible of the full dose of RIG is infiltrated into and around the wound(s), and any remaining volume is administered intramuscularly at an anatomical site distant from rabies vaccine.

Tetanus Immune Globulin. TIG is used to treat tetanus (Chapter 56), with part of the dose infiltrated around the wound and part given intramuscularly. The TIG available in the United States is not licensed for intravenous or intrathecal use. If TIG is not available, equine **tetanus antitoxin (TAT)** should be used after appropriate testing for sensitivity and, if necessary, desensitization. Part of the antitoxin should be given intravenously. IVIG, 500–1,000 mg/kg, may contain sufficient antibodies to tetanus and may be used to treat tetanus if TIG is not available.

Cytomegalovirus Immune Globulin. CMV is an important pathogen in immunocompromised persons. CMV-IG is highly efficacious in the prevention and treatment of CMV infections in kidney and bone marrow transplant recipients and significantly reduces the incidence and mortality rate of CMV disease, especially interstitial pneumonia. Although standard IVIG may prevent CMV infections in such patients, specific CMV-IG ensures high titers of CMV-specific antibody, appears to have equal or better efficacy, and can be administered less frequently and at lower doses.

Prophylaxis is indicated for CMV-seronegative organ transplant recipients, with the first dose within 72 hours after transplantation. The recommended regimen for kidney transplant recipients is CMV-IG, 150 mg/kg, followed by 100 mg/kg at 2, 4, 6, and 8 weeks and by 50 mg/kg at 12 and 16 weeks. For other solid organ transplant recipients, the recommended regimen is CMV-IG, 150 mg/kg initially and at 2, 4, 6, and 8 weeks and 100 mg/kg at 12 and 16 weeks.

CMV-IG is also used to treat CMV pneumonia in transplant recipients (Chapter 100). Although either CMV-IG or ganciclovir used alone results in less than 20% survival, combination therapy using both IG and ganciclovir leads to 50–70% survival.

Respiratory Syncytial Virus Immune Globulin and Palivizumab. Two products currently available for the prevention of RSV lower respiratory tract infection are palivizumab, a neutralizing IgG monoclonal antibody directed against the RSV fusion protein, and **RSV-IG,** a polyclonal hyperimmune IG preparation. The products are indicated for the prevention of RSV infection in high-risk infants and children (Chapter 67) and are given monthly from the beginning of the RSV season (October to December) until the end of the RSV season (March to May). Palivizumab, 15 mg/kg IM, is preferred to RSV-IG, 750 mg/kg IV, because it is delivered in small fluid volume, can be administered intramuscularly, and does not interfere with live virus immunizations. RSV-IG may provide additional protection against other viral infections and may be preferable for persons with immunodeficiency who require routine IVIG in addition to RSV prophylaxis.

Immune Globulin Therapy for Other Viral Infections. Other viruses may ultimately be amenable to immunotherapy. Adenoviruses can cause a progressive pneumonia that can be particularly severe in some immunocompromised persons. No controlled trials are available, but IVIG has been used successfully in some patients. Enteroviruses, such as echovirus 11, can cause overwhelming illness in neonates and young infants. IG therapy has been shown to be capable of interrupting epidemics and may also be therapeutic. Persons with immunodeficiency and meningoencephalitis caused by echovirus have also responded to IVIG therapy. Direct instillation of IG into the ventricles has been used to attain sufficient antibody activity in the central nervous system of some patients. Testing preparations to identify a lot with a high titer of antibodies against these viruses will probably be required to ensure reliable therapy.

ANTITOXINS

Antitoxins are solutions of antibodies derived from the serum of animals immunized with a specific antigen, such as botulinum toxin, diphtheria toxin, and tetanus toxin. Botulinum antitoxin is used for treatment of food-borne botulism in infants (Chapter 56), and diphtheria antitoxin is used for the treatment of respiratory diphtheria (Chapter 58). TAT is used in the treatment of tetanus only if TIG is not available (Chapter 56). Human RIG has supplanted the use of equine products for rabies immunoprophylaxis (Chapter 50).

The products available in the United States are generally derived from the serum of horses. The serum globulin fraction of these products is concentrated by using ammonium sulfate. Some, but not all, products are also subjected to an enzyme digestion process in an attempt to decrease reactions to foreign proteins.

IG products prepared from animal sera pose a special risk to the recipient, and therefore their use should be strictly limited to certain indications when human antibody is not available. Specific antitoxins may be the only form of passive antibody available for prophylaxis or therapy for some conditions such as botulism and diphtheria.

TABLE 15–4. Desensitization Schedule for Animal Antisera

Dose Number*	Route of Administration†	Dilution of Serum in Normal Saline Solution	Dosage
1	IV or ID	1:1,000	0.1
2	IV or ID	1:1,000	0.3
3	IV or SC	1:1,000	0.6
4	IV or SC	1:100	0.1
5	IV or SC	1:100	0.3
6	IV or SC	1:100	0.6
7	IV or SC	1:10	0.1
8	IV or SC	1:10	0.3
9	IV or SC	1:10	0.6
10	IV or SC	Undiluted	0.1
11	IV or SC	Undiluted	0.2
12	IV or IM	Undiluted	0.6
13	IV or IM	Undiluted	1

*Administer at 15-minute intervals.
†ID = intradermal; IM = intramuscular; IV = intravenous; SC = subcutaneous. (If IV route is used, it should be used for all dilutions. Do not interchange IV with ID, SC, or IM. However, ID, SC, and IM routes change at the indicated doses.)

Before any animal serum is injected, it is critical to elicit a careful history of reactions such as asthma, hay fever, or urticaria to previous injections of animal serums. Persons with a history of asthma, allergic rhinitis, or other allergic symptoms may be dangerously sensitive to the corresponding serum and should be given animal serum only with the utmost caution.

Testing and Desensitization. Reactions that may be due to injection of animal serum include anaphylaxis, acute febrile reactions, serum sickness, arthritis, glomerulonephritis, neuritis, myocarditis, and Guillain-Barré syndrome. Testing for possible allergic reaction is necessary before administration of animal serum to any patient. Testing and desensitization should be performed only under controlled conditions by trained personnel familiar with the treatment of anaphylaxis, and the appropriate equipment and drugs (e.g., aqueous epinephrine, 0.3 mL of a 1:1,000 dilution) must be available within immediate reach.

Using the **scratch test,** apply one drop of a 1:100 dilution of the serum in normal saline solution to the site of a superficial scratch, prick, or puncture on the volar aspect of the forearm. A positive test result is a wheal with surrounding erythema at least 3 mm larger than the reaction to a control normal-saline-solution scratch, prick, or puncture test, read at 15–20 minutes. If the scratch test result is negative, an **intradermal test** is performed. In persons with a history of hypersensitivity, especially to animal extracts or serums, a 0.02 mL dose (enough to raise a small intradermal wheal) of serum diluted 1:1,000 in normal saline solution is administered. In persons with a negative history and negative scratch test result, a 0.02 mL dose of serum diluted 1:100 in normal saline solution is used. Antihistamines and decongestants may block the scratch and intradermal hypersensitive skin test reaction, and testing should not be done for at least 12 and preferably 24 hours after administration of these drugs.

The scratch test appears to be the safest and should always precede the intradermal test, which has resulted in fatalities from anaphylaxis. Positive test results indicate the probability of sensitivity, but a negative skin test result is not an absolute guarantee that an individual will not have a severe reaction. Therefore animal sera should be administered with caution even to persons whose test results are negative.

Patients with a positive scratch or intradermal test result or with a history of anaphylaxis after previous administration, should be referred to an allergist for desensitization (Table 15–4). No single desensitization schedule may be appropriate for all patients. Although escalating intravenous doses are preferable, the intradermal-subcutaneous-intramuscular route may also be used. The intravenous route is considered safest because it offers the best control if a reaction develops. If the intravenous route is used, it should be maintained throughout the desensitization. During desensitization an oral or intramuscular antihistamine may be used with or without intravenously administered hydrocortisone or methylprednisolone. Epinephrine should be administered immediately if signs of anaphylaxis are observed. Administration of sera as part of a desensitization procedure must be continuous because protection from desensitization is lost once administration is interrupted.

WHITE BLOOD CELL TRANSFUSIONS

Neutrophils play an important role in immunity to bacterial and fungal infections. Early clinical trials suggested some benefit from WBC transfusions in children with neutropenia caused by cancer chemotherapy. Neonates often deplete bone marrow neutrophil reserves, and survival after neonatal sepsis is improved if the transfused WBCs are collected by flow cytocentrifugation but not if they are collected from buffy coat preparations. WBC transfusions have also been used to treat fungal infections in persons with neutropenia. Several factors have diminished the appeal of WBC transfusions to treat persons with sepsis: (1) limited availability of suitable donors, (2) the necessary rapid processing of cells after harvesting, and (3) the need for immediate and around-the-clock availability. For WBC transfusions to be regularly used, physicians must have cells available whenever they are needed. In addition, in the absence of opsonic antibody, WBC transfusions may not promote enhanced microbial clearance.

CORTICOSTEROIDS

Corticosteroids have been used for many years as adjunctive therapy for a wide variety of infectious diseases because they exert a profound effect on inflammation, affecting many organ systems, and are immunosuppressive, affecting both humoral and cellular immunity. The immunosuppressive effects are most evident if prednisone, >0.3 mg/kg/day (or the equivalent), is used. When doses exceed 1 mg/kg/day for several weeks, susceptibility to a wide variety of infections is also increased. Short-term corticosteroid use (<5 days) has minimal impact on the predisposition to infections.

Because of the potential complications of corticosteroid use, the risk:benefit ratio should be weighed carefully. For some infectious conditions there is clear evidence to support corticosteroid use, whereas in others there are few objective data and only clinical experience. There are also some infectious diseases for which steroids should not be used (Table 15–5).

CYTOKINES

Rapid advances in the understanding and availability of cytokines such as interferons and colony-stimulating factors have made them suitable for innovative approaches to immunotherapy, although in some cases their adverse effects may limit their usefulness.

Interferons

IFNs are a family of proteins that comprise an integral part of the natural host defenses against microbial invasion and malignant cell

TABLE 15–5. Overview of Recommendations for the Use of Corticosteroids in Treatment of Infections

Infection	Recommendation*	Infection	Recommendation*
Use According to Organ System		**Use for Generalized Infections**	
Central Nervous System		Gram-negative sepsis associated with shock (routine)	E
Bacterial meningitis (routine)	C	Toxic shock syndrome (routine)	C
Infants and children with meningitis due to *Haemophilus influenzae* type b (selective)	B	Typhoid fever (routine)	C
Brain abscess (routine)	D	Critically ill patients in shock (selective)	A
Elevated intracranial pressure (selective)	C	Tetanus (routine)	B
Facial nerve paralysis in Lyme disease (routine)	D	Tuberculosis	
Neurocysticercosis (routine)	C	Pericarditis (selective)	A
Therapy with praziquantel (selective)	C	Meningitis (selective)	B
Cerebral malaria (routine)	E	Debilitated patients (severe constitutional symptoms, severe hypoxia, pleurisy, peritonitis selective)	C
Respiratory Tract		Herpes zoster (routine)	E
Pneumocystis carinii pneumonia (selective for hypoxia in early illness)	A	Older patients with postherpetic neuralgia (selective)	C
Chronic bronchitis (routine)	C	Bone marrow effects associated with viral infection (routine)	C
Viral bronchitis (routine)	E	Epstein-Barr virus infection (routine)	D
Acute laryngotracheobronchitis (croup) (selective for severe illness requiring hospitalization)	B	Impending airway obstruction (selective)	B
Acute epiglottitis (routine)	C	Hepatitis, pericarditis, myocarditis encephalitis (selective)	C
Allergic bronchopulmonary aspergillosis (routine)	B	Hemorrhagic fever with renal syndrome (routine)	E
Cardiac		Trichinosis (routine)	C
Viral pericarditis (routine)	C	Kawasaki syndrome (routine)	D
Viral myocarditis (routine)	C	Miscellaneous therapeutic uses	
Liver, Gastrointestinal Tract, Abdomen		To reduce fever associated with infection	C
Acute viral hepatitis (routine)	E	To minimize reactions to certain antimicrobial agents	C
Chronic hepatitis with hepatitis B virus (routine)	E		
Therapy with interferon alfa-2b (selective)	C		
Chronic hepatitis with non-A, non-B hepatitis (routine)	D		
Oral/hypopharyngeal/esophageal ulcers in HIV-infected patients (routine)	C		
Eye and Ear			
Infective endophthalmitis (routine)	C		
Eye manifestations of other infections (routine)	C		
Chronic effusion after otitis media (routine)	B		

*A, strong evidence for use; B, moderate evidence for use; C, poor evidence for or against use; D, moderate evidence against use; E, good evidence against use.
From McGowan JE Jr, Chesney PJ. Crossley KB, et al: Guidelines for the use of systemic glucocorticosteroids in the management of selected infections. Working Group on Steroid Use, Antimicrobial Agents Committee, Infectious Diseases Society of America. *J Infect Dis* 1992;165:1–13.

proliferation. There are three distinct IFN groups: IFN-α, IFN-β, and IFN-γ. There are at least 17 IFN-α genes but only one IFN-β and one IFN-γ gene. IFNs are produced by a variety of cells (Table 15–6) and function as intracellular signaling proteins. In a complex interaction with cytokines (IL-I and IL-2) and the cellular immune system, IFNs comprise a powerful immunologic defense. For example, IFN acts on virus-susceptible cells through specific receptors to alter intracellular protein synthesis. By induction or repression of cellular protein synthesis, viral activity is suppressed as different parts of the virus replication cycle are impaired. In addition, IFN enhances specific antibody formation and activates macrophages. IFNs are now being used to treat a wide variety of infectious and noninfectious diseases (Table 15–7).

The major side effects of IFNs are fever, headaches, chills, and local reaction at the site of injection.

Hepatitis B. Approximately one third of persons with chronic hepatitis B respond to 4–6 months of treatment with IFN-α (5–10

TABLE 15–6. Types of Interferons

Interferon	Types	Source
IFN-α	Many	Macrophages/monocytes Dendritic cells B lymphocytes
IFN-β	One	Fibroblasts Epithelial cells Macrophages
IFN-γ	One	T lymphocytes NK cells

MU daily) with normalization of liver function and loss of serum viral replication markers (HBeAg and DNA polymerase). Another 15% of initial nonresponders may clear HBsAg up to 1 year after completing the IFN-α treatment and thus cease to be carriers. The response of children with chronic hepatitis B to IFN-α therapy has been more variable and may be related to a variety of factors including mode of viral acquisition. In children, IFN-α doses of <10 MU/m^2 appear to be well tolerated.

Hepatitis C. Approximately 40–50% of persons with chronic hepatitis C may respond to 6 months of therapy with IFN-α (1–3 MU per dose, 3 times a week). A significant percentage of persons have relapse.

Human Papillomaviruses. IFN-α has been used to treat condylomata acuminata, plantar warts, and laryngeal papillomatosis. Intralesional administration of IFN-α for refractory condylomata acuminata (1 MU per lesion weekly for 3 weeks) is effective in up to 60% of patients. HIV-infected persons have a significantly poorer response. Plantar warts are less responsive to IFN-α therapy.

Laryngeal papillomatosis is caused by human papillomavirus transmitted during delivery to the newborn from maternal condylomata acuminata. Infection of the vocal cords may result in severely debilitating multiple papillomas that impair breathing and speech and may be life-threatening. Recurrence is common after laser surgery. However, laser surgery followed by repeated injections of IFN-α three times each week for up to 13 months has induced long-term remissions.

The long-term response of persons given systemic IFN-α therapy for juvenile laryngeal papillomatosis has been variable. Although a short-term decrease in lesion size may occur, the persistence of virus in the lesion may lead to resurgence after treatment is completed. Laser therapy alone may have an equal long-term benefit.

Chronic Granulomatous Disease. Persons with chronic granulomatous disease have recurrent serious infections with bacteria and fungi. Antibiotic prophylaxis provides some success. However, IFN-γ (50 μg/m^2 SC 3 times a week) produces a two-thirds reduction in serious infections that require hospitalization. There was a general overall improvement in all patient groups, but children <10 years of age demonstrated the greatest benefit. Side effects were generally mild and alleviated by symptomatic treatment.

Colony-Stimulating Factors

The isolation, production, and licensure of **CSF** for use in humans to promote WBC production has been a great scientific and medical achievement. Currently, CSF therapy is used primarily in immunocompromised persons and in persons with dysfunctional myelopoiesis to increase the number of neutrophils and monocytes. **GM-CSF** and **G-CSF** are available commercially. Although CSF treatment has potential applications in many settings, such as congenital and acquired neutropenia and HIV infection, most studies to date report the use of CSF in the prevention of neutropenia and infections

TABLE 15–7. Cytokines for Infectious Disease Indications

Cytokine	Trade Name (and Manufacturer)	Source	Indications	Chapter Where Information Can Be Found
Interferon				
α	Roferon-A, Injection (Roche)	Recombinant from *Escherichia coli*	Hepatitis C	78
α	Intron-A, Injection (Schering)	Recombinant from *E. coli*	Hepatitis B and C, condylomata acuminata	78
α	Alferon N, Injection (Interferon Sciences)	Human leukocyte derived	Condylomata acuminata	85
α	Avonex (Biogen)	Recombinant from mammalian cells	Multiple sclerosis	
α	Infergen, Injection (Amgen)	Recombinant from *E. coli*	Hepatitis C	78
β	Betaseron, SC Injection (Berlex)	Recombinant from *E. coli*	Hepatitis C	78
γ	Actimmune, SC injection (Genentech)	Recombinant from *E. coli*	Chronic granulomatous disease	98
Colony-Stimulating Factors				
GM-CSF	Leukine (Immunex)	Recombinant from yeast (*Saccharomyces cerevisiae*)	Reduce duration of neutropenia in immunocompromised persons; enhance neutrophil numbers during infection if low	99
G-CSF	Neupogen (Amgen)	Recombinant from *E. coli*	Same as GM-CSF	99

in patients receiving cancer chemotherapy. GM-CSF and G-CSF are currently licensed for use in bone marrow transplant recipients to enhance recovery of WBCs. The use of CSFs has reduced the duration of neutropenia and has also reduced the incidence and severity of infections in persons with cancer and in bone marrow transplant recipients. However, indications for CSF therapy for specific infections have not been identified.

GM-CSF and G-CSF can cause a number of side effects, including fever, anorexia, malaise, arthralgia, bone pain, elevated liver enzymes, and capillary leak syndrome.

Neonatal Infections. Because both GM-CSF and G-CSF have been shown to induce proliferation of myeloid precursors, to increase the release of cells from the bone marrow, and to enhance functional activity of mature neutrophils, it seems plausible that they would be beneficial for treating neonatal sepsis. However, clinical trials have not shown a clear benefit for GM-CSF or G-CSF in treating neonatal sepsis.

REVIEWS

Baron S, Tyring SK, Fleischmann WR Jr, et al: The interferons. Mechanisms of action and clinical applications. *JAMA* 1991;266:1375–83.

Dale DC: Potential role of colony-stimulating factors in the prevention and treatment of infectious diseases. *Clin Infect Dis* 1994;18: S2180–8.

Dwyer JM: Manipulating the immune system with immune globulin. *N Engl J Med* 1992;326:107–16.

Fischer GW: Immunoglobulin therapy in older infants and children. *Infect Dis Clin North Am* 1992;6:97–116.

The IMpact-RSV Study Group: Palivizumab, a humanized respiratory syncytial virus monoclonal antibody, reduces hospitalization from respiratory syncytial virus infection in high-risk infants. *Pediatrics* 1998; 102:531–7.

The International Chronic Granulomatous Disease Cooperative Study Group: A controlled trial of interferon gamma to prevent infection in chronic granulomatous disease. *N Engl J Med* 1991;324:509–16.

Lau AS, Lehman D, Geertsma FR, et al: Biology and therapeutic uses of myeloid hematopoietic growth factors and interferons. *Pediatr Infect Dis J* 1996;15:563–75.

Liles WC, Van Voorhis WC: Review: Nomenclature and biologic significance of cytokines involved in inflammation and the host immune response. *J Infect Dis* 1995;172:1573–80.

Nossal GJ: Current concepts: Immunology. The basic components of the immune system. *N Engl J Med* 1987;316:1320–5.

Ratko TA, Burnett DA, Foulke GE, et al: Recommendations for off-label use of intravenously administered immunoglobulin preparations. University Hospital Consortium Expert Panel for Off-Label Use of Polyvalent Intravenously Administered Immunoglobulin Preparations. *JAMA* 1995;273: 1865–70.

KEY ARTICLES

American Society of Hospital Pharmacists Commission on Therapeutics: ASHP therapeutic guidelines for intravenous immune globulin. *Clin Pharm* 1992;11:117–36.

Baker CJ, Melish ME, Hall RT, et al: Intravenous immune globulin for the prevention of nosocomial infection in low-birth-weight neonates. The Multicenter Group for the Study of Immune Globulin in Neonates. *N Engl J Med* 1992;327:213–9.

Christensen RD, Brown MS, Hall DC, et al: Effect on neutrophil kinetics and serum opsonic capacity of intravenous administration of immune globulin to neonates with clinical signs of early-onset sepsis. *J Pediatr* 1991;118:606–14.

Fanaroff AA, Korones SB, Wright LL, et al: A controlled trial of intravenous immune globulin to reduce nosocomial infections in very-low-birth-weight infants. National Institute of Child Health and Human Development Neonatal Research Network. *N Engl J Med* 1994;330:1107–13.

Givner LB: Human immunoglobulins for intravenous use: Comparison of available preparations for group B streptococcal antibody levels, opsonic activity and efficacy in animal models. *Pediatrics* 1990;86:955–62.

Groothuis JR, Simoes EA, Levin MJ, et al: Prophylactic administration of respiratory syncytial virus immune globulin to high-risk infants and young children. The Respiratory Syncytial Virus Immune Globulin Study Group. *N Engl J Med* 1993;329:1524–30.

Hemming VG, Rodriguez W, Kim HW, et al: Intravenous immunoglobulin treatment of respiratory syncytial virus infections in infants and young children. *Antimicrob Agents Chemother* 1987;31:1882–6.

Jenson HB, Pollock BH: Meta-analysis of the effectiveness of intravenous immune globulin for prevention and treatment of neonatal sepsis. *Pediatrics* 1997;99(2):E2.

Johnson S, Oliver C, Prince GA, et al: Development of humanized monoclonal antibody (MEDI-493) with potent in vitro and in vivo activity against respiratory syncytial virus. *J Infect Dis* 1997;176:1215–24.

Kim KS: High-dose intravenous immune globulin impairs antibacterial activity of antibiotics. *J Allergy Clin Immunol* 1989;84:579–86.

McGowan JE Jr, Chesney PJ, Crossley KB, et al: Guidelines for the use of systemic glucocorticosteroids in the management of selected infections. Working Group on Steroid Use, Antimicrobial Agents Committee, Infectious Diseases Society of America. *J Infect Dis* 1992;165:1–13.

The PREVENT Study Group: Reduction of respiratory syncytial virus hospitalization among premature infants and infants with bronchopulmonary dysplasia using respiratory syncytial virus immune globulin prophylaxis. *Pediatrics* 1997;99:93–9.

Rodriguez WJ, Gruber WC, Groothuis JR, et al: Respiratory syncytial virus immune globulin treatment of RSV lower respiratory tract infection in previously healthy children. *Pediatrics* 1997;100:937–42.

Snydman DR, Werner BG, Heinze-Lacey B, et al: Use of cytomegalovirus immune globulin to prevent cytomegalovirus disease in renal-transplant recipients. *N Engl J Med* 1987;317:1049–54.

Subramanian KN, Weisman LE, Rhodes T, et al: Safety, tolerance and pharmacokinetics of a humanized monoclonal antibody to respiratory syncytial virus in premature infants and infants with bronchopulmonary dysplasia. MEDI-493 Study Group. *Pediatr Infect Dis J* 1998;17:110–5.

Weisman LE, Stoll BJ, Kueser TJ, et al: Intravenous immune globulin prophylaxis of late-onset sepsis in premature neonates. *J Pediatr* 1994;125:922–30.

Weisman LE, Stoll BJ, Kueser TJ, et al: Intravenous immune globulin therapy for early-onset sepsis in premature neonates. *J Pediatr* 1992;121:434–43.

CHAPTER 16

Prophylaxis of Infectious Diseases

Robert S. Baltimore

The prophylaxis of infectious diseases, which encompasses many different clinical situations, uses a few distinct approaches singly or in combination directed against many, but not all, infectious agents. The goal of prophylaxis is to reduce the incidence of illness and risk to susceptible individuals who are placed at increased risk as contacts of an **index case,** the sentinel infection that identifies the presence of the organism. The index case may be a **confirmed case** (e.g., culture of the organism, positive PCR test result) or a **presumptive case** (e.g., positive Gram stain, positive antigen test result in the setting of a compatible clinical illness). Prophylaxis for susceptible individuals after exposure to infection may include **chemoprophylaxis** with antibiotics, **passive immunoprophylaxis** with immune globulin (Chapter 15), or **active immunoprophylaxis** by vaccination (Chapter 17). The appropriateness of prophylaxis for many infectious agents is limited by the availability of antimicrobial agents, specific immune globulin products, or vaccines that are effective in the limited time frame available to protect the exposed susceptible person. Vaccines for diphtheria, pertussis, tetanus, measles, mumps, hepatitis B, varicella, meningococcus, and rabies are used not only to prevent disease by pre-exposure vaccination but also for postexposure prophylaxis.

Prophylaxis can be used to prevent (1) the acquisition of organisms not already part of the individual's own flora, (2) the development of invasive infection by usually nonpathogenic organisms that are already part of the individual's own flora, or (3) clinical manifestations of infection in an individual who may already be contaminated with pathogens that may cause symptoms if no treatment is given (Table 16–1). The third category is actually **anticipatory therapy** and not prophylaxis, because it is believed that infection is already present but is still at the stage preceding overt clinical manifestations or physical findings. Prophylaxis is not effective at halting disease in persons who already are in the early stages of invasive disease, however. Anticipatory therapy is included here for contrast with true prophylaxis because occasionally confusion arises as to the logic of preventing of certain diseases. Table 16–2 summarizes prophylactic regimens and anticipatory therapies generally regarded as efficacious in children.

Prophylaxis can also be categorized as primary or secondary. **Primary prophylaxis** is used to prevent infection before a first occurrence. **Secondary prophylaxis** is to prevent recurrence of infection after a first episode, such as is indicated to prevent group A streptococcal infection in those who have had rheumatic fever.

Neisseria meningitidis

One of the most emotionally difficult situations for physicians is dealing with families or the community after a serious case of invasive infection caused by *Neisseria meningitidis.* Although the majority of these situations arise after an index case of sepsis or meningitis, decisions regarding chemoprophylaxis should be the same for all invasive *N. meningitidis* infections because they all may be associated with the spread of serious infections to susceptible contacts in the community.

Susceptible persons at risk of having meningococcal infection are those who lack bactericidal antibody and who have had prolonged close contact with the index case during the incubation period of infection. The decision as to which individuals require prophylaxis is based on experience and estimation of risk, which is dependent on the closeness of contact (Table 16–3). Indirect contact, such as contact with high-risk contacts, does not indicate increased risk. The incidence of secondary cases of meningococcal infection among household contacts is two or three cases per 1,000 individuals, more than 300 times greater than the attack rate in the general population. The rate is higher for children less than 5 years of age because these children have a lower prevalence of protective antibody. Other persons who have been shown to be at significantly greater risk than the general community are those in enclosed populations such as the military, retarded individuals in group homes, or similar groups. In other situations the intimacy and duration of contact are important practically to determine whether a specific individual's contact with an index case is sufficiently close to warrant prophylaxis. A practical criterion for prophylaxis is for persons who have frequently slept, eaten in, or otherwise resided in the same dwelling as the index patient. Chemoprophylaxis is often extended to daycare center attendees, although data showing efficacy in such situations are lacking. Medical personnel who perform the usual medical duties are not considered to be at exceptional risk and do not require prophylaxis unless they have had direct exposure to oral or respiratory secretions of the index

TABLE 16–1. Categories of Antimicrobial Prophylaxis

Category 1: Prevention of acquisition of an exogenous organism that is not normally part of the human flora
Example: Malaria prophylaxis

Category 2: Prevention of organisms naturally present (e.g., commensal organisms) or transiently colonizing one area of the body from gaining access to a normally sterile site
Example: Prevention of ascending urinary tract infections in which the responsible bacteria typically originate from the resident fecal or vaginal flora

Category 3: Prevention of organisms already present or presumed to be present from causing disease (anticipatory therapy)
Examples:
a. Administration of isoniazid to healthy persons with positive tuberculin skin-test results
b. Administration of antibiotics for penetrating abdominal wounds

Adapted from Hirschmann JV, Inui TS: Antimicrobial prophylaxis: A critique of recent trials. *Rev Infect Dis* 1980;2:1–23.

TABLE 16–2. Summary of Prophylactic Regimens and Anticipatory Therapy Generally Regarded as Efficacious for Children

Disease	Prophylaxis Category (Table 16–1)	Prophylactic Agent(s)	Chapter Where Information Can Be Found
Anti-infective Prophylaxis			
Animal bites (postexposure)	3	Amoxicillin-clavulanate	50
Chlamydia trachomatis, urogenital or neonatal exposure	1, 3	Tetracycline, erythromycin, azithromycin	68, 85
Cholera (*Vibrio cholerae*)	1, 3	Tetracycline, doxycycline, TMP-SMZ	76
Diphtheria (*Corynebacterium diphtheriae*)	2	Penicillin, erythromycin, vaccine	17, 58
Endocarditis, for individuals with structural heart defects undergoing procedures	2	Amoxicillin, others	71
Fever and neutropenia (with malignancy or transplantation)	2, 3		99, 100
Bacterial infections		Broad-spectrum antibiotics	
Fungal infections		Antifungal agents	
Haemophilus influenzae type b	2	Rifampin	16 (Table 16–5)
Human immunodeficiency virus (HIV-1)	1	Antiretroviral agents	38
Influenza A viruses	1	Amantadine, rimantadine, oseltamivir	68 (Table 68–11)
Influenza B viruses	1	Oseltamivir	68 (Table 68–11)
Lyme disease	1	Doxycycline	29
Malaria (*Plasmodium*)	1	Chloroquine, others	32
Meningococcal infections (*Neisseria meningitidis*)	2	Rifampin, sulfadiazine, ceftriaxone, ciprofloxacin	16 (Table 16–4)
Mycobacterium avium-intracellulare complex (MAC; in patients with AIDS)	2	Azithromycin, clarithromycin, rifabutin	38
Neonatal omphalitis (*Staphylococcus aureus*)	2	Triple dye to umbilical stump	96
Neonatal sepsis (group B *Streptococcus*)	3	Penicillin or ampicillin administered to the mother	94
Ophthalmia neonatorum (*Neisseria gonorrhoeae*)	3	Topical silver nitrate, erythromycin, tetracycline	89
Otitis media (recurrent)	2	Amoxicillin, sulfisoxazole	64
Pertussis (*Bordetella pertussis*)	2	Erythromycin, vaccine	17, 67
Plague (*Yersinia pestis*)	1	Tetracycline, sulfonamide	34
Pneumocystis carinii pneumonia (primary and secondary prevention in immunocompromised persons)	2	TMP-SMZ, aerosolized pentamidine, others	68 (Table 68–14)
Rheumatic fever (group A streptococcal pharyngitis, secondary prevention)	1	Penicillin, sulfadiazine	40
Streptococcus pneumoniae, with anatomic and functional asplenia	1, 2	Penicillin	101
Syphilis (*Treponema pallidum*)	1, 3	Penicillin	85
Transplant recipients			100
Herpes simplex virus infection	2, 3	Acyclovir	
Tuberculosis (primary and secondary prevention)	1, 3	BCG vaccine, isoniazid	35
Urinary tract infections (recurrent)	2	TMP-SMZ, others	82 (Table 82–4)
Varicella-zoster virus (chickenpox)	1, 3	Acyclovir, vaccine	17, 27
Immunoprophylaxis			
Hepatitis A	1, 3	Immune globulin	15, 78
Hepatitis B	1, 3	Hepatitis B immune globulin, vaccine	15, 17, 78
Measles	1, 3	Immune globulin, vaccine	15, 17, 23
Rabies	3	Rabies immune globulin, vaccine	15, 17, 50
Respiratory syncytial virus	1	Anti-RSV monoclonal antibody, RSV-IG	15, 67
Tetanus (*Clostridium tetani*)	1, 3	Antitoxin, tetanus immune globulin, vaccine	15, 17, 48
Varicella-zoster virus (disseminated infection in immunocompromised persons)	3	Varicella-zoster immune globulin	15, 27, 99
Transplant recipients			
Bacterial infections	1	Intravenous immune globulin	15, 100
Fungal infections	1, 3	Fluconazole	15, 100
Cytomegalovirus	1, 3	Cytomegalovirus immune globulin	15, 100

TABLE 16–3. Disease Risk for Contacts of Index Cases of *Neisseria meningitidis* Infection*

High-Risk Factors (Chemoprophylaxis Recommended)
Household contacts, especially young children
Child care or nursery school contact in previous 7 days
Direct exposure to the index patient's secretions through kissing or sharing of toothbrushes or eating utensils
Mouth-to-mouth resuscitation or unprotected contact during endotracheal intubation within 7 days before onset of illness
Frequently sleeps or eats in the same dwelling as the index patient

Low-Risk Factors (Chemoprophylaxis Not Recommended)
Casual contact with no history or direct exposure to the index patient's oral secretions (e.g., school or work mate indirect contact)
Indirect contact (i.e., the only contact is with a high-risk contact, with no direct contact with the index patient)
Medical personnel without direct exposure to the patient's oral secretions

Outbreak or Cluster
Chemoprophylaxis for persons other than those at high risk should be given only after consultation with local and state public health authorities

*Nasopharyngeal aspirate or throat swab cultures are not useful in determining risk.
Adapted from American Academy of Pediatrics Committee on Infectious Diseases and Canadian Paediatric Society Infectious Diseases and Immunization Committee: Meningococcal disease prevention and control strategies for practice-based physicians. *Pediatrics* 1996;97:404–11.

patient. Medical or laboratory personnel who are parenterally exposed to organisms in a laboratory accident require parenteral treatment.

Persons who have had any contact with a case must be closely observed. Only 1–2% of cases of meningococcemia occur among family members of persons with a confirmed case, and therefore chemoprophylaxis will not prevent the majority of cases. Contacts who become ill and are thought to have meningococcal disease, regardless of whether they received prophylaxis, require parenteral treatment. Continuation of treatment is based on the results of cultures of specimens taken before antimicrobial therapy was begun.

Rifampin is recommended for prophylaxis in children and adolescents and is 72–90% effective (Table 16–4). Rifampin may stain soft contact lenses and may affect metabolism of oral contraceptives, anticoagulant, and seizure medications. Ciprofloxacin may be used in persons 18 years of age or older and is 90–95% effective. Ceftriaxone may be used but must be given intramuscularly; it is 97% effective. Sulfadiazine may be used only if the isolate from the index case is known to be susceptible to sulfa compounds, or it may be used for outbreak control of an epidemic caused by a sulfa-susceptible strain. Drugs such as penicillin and ampicillin, which are effective in treating invasive meningococcal infections, do not achieve sufficiently high salivary levels to kill the organisms in the pharynx and are therefore ineffective for prophylaxis.

Throat cultures are not used for deciding who is to receive prophylaxis because the cultures take too long to process, do not identify individuals who are at risk because of lack of antibody, and do not distinguish between individuals carrying nonvirulent *Neisseria* strains and those carrying a strain similar to the index-case strain unless special, time-consuming serogrouping tests are performed. No tests for the determination of protective antibodies are commercially available.

Vaccination for postexposure prophylaxis is part of outbreak control when there is more than one related case caused by any of serogroups A, C, Y, or W135, which are included in quadrivalent vaccine (Chapter 17). This vaccine is also used for travelers to highly endemic areas (Chapter 104). Recently there has been increased concern regarding meningococcal disease in college students, with data showing that freshmen living in dormitories are at increased risk. College students and their parents should be given information about meningitis and the advantages of vaccination, and meningococcal vaccination should be offered. Some colleges and states are recommending or even requiring meningococcal vaccine for all matriculating freshmen.

Haemophilus influenzae Type b

For many years, contacts of cases of *H. influenzae* type b infection were not believed to be at sufficiently high risk to make chemoprophylaxis worthwhile, but several epidemiologic investigations showed the risk in families to be two or three cases per 1,000 individuals, similar to the risk for contacts of *N. meningitidis* infection. It was then determined that rifampin eliminated throat carriage and reduced the incidence of infection in household contacts. Studies in daycare centers before the development of conjugate *H.*

TABLE 16–4. Chemoprophylaxis Regimens for Contacts of Persons with *Neisseria meningitidis* Infection

Drug	Age at Contact	Dosage
Recommended Regimen		
Rifampin	Adult	600 mg q12hr PO × 2 days
	1 mo to 12 yr	10 mg/kg (max 600 mg q12hr PO × 2 days
	≤1 mo	5 mg/kg q12hr PO × 2 days
Alternative Regimens		
Ceftriaxone	>12 yr	250 mg as a single injection
	≤12 yr	125 mg as a single injection
Ciprofloxacin*	Adult ≥18 yr (nonpregnant)	500 mg orally as a single dose
Only if Organism Is Known to Be Susceptible to Sulfadiazine†		
Sulfadiazine (orally)*	Adults	1 g q12hr PO × 2 days
	1–12 yr	500 mg q12hr PO × 2 days
	<1 yr	500 mg q24hr PO × 2 days

*Quinolones are contraindicated for pregnant and lactating women and for children and adolescents younger than 18 years.
†If the strain is known to be susceptible to sulfonamides.

influenzae type b vaccines have shown that the risk of having secondary infections is relatively high for children younger than 4 years.

As with *N. meningitidis,* decisions regarding *H. influenzae* type b chemoprophylaxis should be the same for all invasive infections in the index patient because apparently they all may be associated with spread to susceptible contacts in the community. Susceptible individuals at risk are those who lack bactericidal antibody and have had prolonged close contact with an index case during the incubation period of infection. Because lack of bactericidal antibody is uncommon in persons older than 5 years, secondary cases almost always involve unimmunized children younger than 5 years. Bactericidal antibody may not prevent nasopharyngeal acquisition and carriage, however. Thus the strategy for *H. influenzae* type b prophylaxis is to prescribe chemoprophylaxis (Table 16–5) only when contacts include one or more children younger than 48 months who are not fully immunized, defined as having received at least one dose of *H. influenzae* type b conjugate vaccine at 15 months of age or older, or two doses between 12 and 14 months of age, or a two- or three-dose series when younger than 12 months with a booster dose at 12 months of age or older. If the household contacts include an immunocompromised child, regardless of age, then prophylaxis is given regardless of immunization status of the child because of the possibility that the immunization may not have been effective. When *H. influenzae* type b prophylaxis is indicated, all household members are given prophylaxis so that older children and adults do not serve as reservoirs for transmission of the organism to the younger children after prophylaxis is completed. In addition, index patients treated with parenteral antibiotics may still harbor *H. influenzae* type b in the pharynx because the drugs used for treatment do not achieve a sufficiently high salivary concentration to eradicate pharyngeal *H. influenzae* type b. Therefore the index patient should be treated with rifampin in the 4 days immediately preceding hospital discharge as part of the prophylactic strategy.

Chemoprophylaxis for *H. influenzae* type b infection is not effective at halting disease in those who are in the early stages of invasive disease. Exposed persons who are already ill should be treated empirically for infection. Throat cultures are not used for deciding who is to receive prophylaxis because they take too long to process and do not identify individuals at risk. No tests for protective antibodies are commercially available.

Since 1990 there has been almost universal immunization of infants in the United States with conjugate vaccines against *H. influenzae* type b. Because of the high efficacy of conjugate vaccines, children who are healthy and have been fully immunized are at minimal risk of having *H. influenzae* type b disease even if exposed directly to an index case of invasive disease. Household contacts do not require rifampin prophylaxis when all contacts are older than 4 years or when contacts younger than 4 years are fully immunized. Rifampin prophylaxis is indicated for all household contacts if there is a contact younger than 1 year, regardless of the vaccination status of that infant, or if the contact is a child younger than 4 years who is immunocompromised, because the previous vaccination may have been ineffective.

TABLE 16–5. Chemoprophylaxis Regimens for High-Risk Contacts of Index Patients with Invasive *Haemophilus influenzae* Type b Infection*

Drug	Age at Contact	Dosage
Recommended Regimen		
Rifampin (PO)	Adult	600 mg q24hr × 4 days
	1 mo to 12 yr	20 mg/kg (max 600 mg) q24hr × 4 days
	<1 mo	10 mg/kg q24hr × 4 days

*Unvaccinated or incompletely vaccinated children should receive one dose of vaccine and should be scheduled to complete the age-specific *H. influenzae* type b immunization schedule (Chapter 17).

Results of efficacy studies of prophylaxis in daycare centers have been inconclusive. Immunization of all children who attend daycare is the best measure against *H. influenzae* type b disease. At present, chemoprophylaxis in a daycare center with an index case may still be considered as for household settings, but supervising physicians should consider each situation on an individual basis. Prophylaxis is deemed reasonable only when administered to all attendees and workers. Chemoprophylaxis is recommended in a daycare center when a second case of invasive *H. influenzae* type b infection occurs within a short time of the index case.

Because vaccination for *H. influenzae* type b is now routine in the United States, unvaccinated, exposed, susceptible individuals should be vaccinated as appropriate for age (Chapter 17). This measure is not part of outbreak control or prophylaxis per se.

ANTIBIOTIC PROPHYLAXIS FOR PEDIATRIC SURGERY

A considerable amount of antibiotic use in pediatrics, as well as for adults, involves surgical prophylaxis. Studies of the efficacy of surgical prophylaxis as it applies specifically to infants and children are limited, and therefore most recommendations are extrapolations of recommendations for adults.

Surgical procedures may be classified on the basis of the risk of wound infection (see Table 105–7). **Clean procedures,** which do not involve a break in aseptic technique and incision through sterile tissues, have a low wound infection rate of about 1–2%. **Clean-contaminated procedures** that involve incision through a hollow organ and potential spillage or gross spillage of contaminated fluids have a 7–15% expected wound infection rate. **Contaminated procedures, or "dirty" surgery,** involving a ruptured or penetrated hollow viscus or contaminated wounds, may have a wound infection rate of 40% or more.

The benefits of a short course of surgical prophylaxis have been demonstrated mostly for procedures with intermediate infection rates. Clean procedures have such a low infection rate that it is difficult to demonstrate the value of antibiotic prophylaxis. Perioperative prophylaxis is usually given for clean procedures involving insertion of prosthetic material such as orthopedic appliances, pacemakers, and indwelling catheters. Dirty surgery requires antimicrobial therapy for several days that is more correctly considered empirical treatment and not just perioperative prophylaxis.

Clinical human studies and experimental animal research have demonstrated that antibiotics are effective in preventing surgical infection if the tissues are saturated with antibiotic from the time of incision until the end of the procedure. Antibiotic use substantially before or after the procedure has no demonstrable value. Most studies have shown that a dosing regimen with the first dose given approximately 30 minutes before the procedure (definitely <2 hours beforehand) and another given during the procedure if the operating time is long (>4 hours) is all that is required. Some regimens include one or two doses after the procedure, but doses given more than 24–48 hours after the procedure are unnecessary. Many hospitals have an automatic stop order 24 hours after the first dose to discourage such use.

Most recommendations for surgical prophylaxis include the use of cephalosporins. The first-generation cephalosporins, such as cephalothin or cefazolin, are active against normal skin flora,

TABLE 16–6. Common Surgical Procedures for Which Perioperative Prophylactic Antibiotics Are Recommended

Surgical Procedure	Likely Pathogens	Recommended Antibiotics and Dosage (IV Unless Stated Otherwise)*†
Clean Surgery		
Cardiac Surgery		
Prosthetic valve, coronary artery bypass, other open heart surgery, pacemaker or defibrillator implant	Coagulase-negative staphylococci *Staphylococcus aureus* *Corynebacterium* Enteric gram-negative bacilli	Cefazolin *or* cefuroxime 12.5–20 mg/kg (max 1–2 g) *or* Vancomycin 10–15 mg/kg (max 1 g)‡
Thoracic, Noncardiac Surgery	*S. aureus* Coagulase-negative staphylococci *Streptococcus* Enteric gram-negative bacilli	Cefazolin *or* cefuroxime 12.5–20 mg/kg (max 1–2 g) *or* Vancomycin 10–15 mg/kg (max 1 g)‡
Vascular Surgery		
Arterial surgery involving a prosthesis, the abdominal aorta, a groin incision; lower extremity amputation for ischemia	*S. aureus* Coagulase-negative staphylococci Enteric gram-negative bacilli	Cefazolin 12.5–20 mg/kg (max 1–2 g) *or* Vancomycin 10–15 mg/kg (max 1 g)‡
Neurosurgery		
Craniotomy	*S. aureus* Coagulase-negative staphylococci	Cefazolin 12.5–20 mg/kg (max 1–2 g) *or* Vancomycin 10–15 mg/kg (max 1 g)‡
Orthopedic Surgery		
Total joint replacement, internal fixation of fractures	*S. aureus* Coagulase-negative staphylococci	Cefazolin 12.5–20 mg/kg (max 1–2 g) *or* Vancomycin 10–15 mg/kg (max 1 g)‡
Ophthalmic Surgery	Coagulase-negative staphylococci *S. aureus* *Streptococcus* Enteric gram-negative bacilli *Pseudomonas*	Gentamicin, tobramycin, ciprofloxacin, ofloxacin, or neomycin-gramicidin-polymyxin B as multiple drops topically for 2–24 hr *and* Cefazolin 100 mg subconjunctivally
Clean-Contaminated Surgery		
Head and Neck Surgery		
Incisions through oral or pharyngeal mucosa	Oral anaerobes Enteric gram-negative bacilli *S. aureus*	Clindamycin 10 mg/kg (max 600–900 mg) *and* Gentamicin 1.5 mg/kg
Gastrointestinal Surgery		
Esophageal, gastroduodenal (for high risk only: morbid obesity, esophageal obstruction, decreased gastric acidity, or decreased gastrointestinal motility)	Enteric gram-negative bacilli Gram-positive cocci	Cefazolin 12.5–20 mg/kg (max 1–2 g)
Biliary tract (for high risk only: age >70 yr, acute cholecystitis, nonfunctioning gallbladder, obstructive jaundice, or common duct stones)	Enteric gram-negative bacilli *Enterococcus* *Clostridium*	Cefazolin 12.5–20 mg/kg (max 1–2 g)
Colorectal surgery	Enteric gram-negative bacilli Anaerobes *Enterococcus*	Children IV: cefoxitin 20–40 mg/kg (max 1 g) PO: See text Adults IV: cefoxitin 20–40 mg/kg (max 1 g) *or* cefotetan 1 g *or* Cefazolin 12.5–20 mg/kg (max 1–2 g) *and* metronidazole (500 mg) PO: After appropriate diet and catharsis, neomycin 1 g *and* erythromycin base 1 g at 1 PM, 2 PM, and 11 PM on day before 8 AM operation
Appendectomy, nonperforated	Enteric gram-negative bacilli Anaerobes *Enterococcus*	Cefoxitin 20–40 mg/kg (max 1 g) *or* Cefotetan 1 g (adults)

Table continued on following page

TABLE 16–6. Common Surgical Procedures for Which Perioperative Prophylactic Antibiotics Are Recommended *(Continued)*

Surgical Procedure	Likely Pathogens	Recommended Antibiotics and Dosage (IV Unless Stated Otherwise)*†
Clean-Contaminated Surgery *(Continued)*		
Genitourinary Surgery		
(for high risk only: urine culture positive or unavailable, preoperative catheter, transrectal prostatic biopsy)	Enteric gram-negative bacilli *Enterococcus*	Children: Amoxicillin-clavulanate Amoxicillin 25 mg/kg PO (max 500 mg) *or* Piperacillin-tazobactam Piperacillin 50 mg/kg (max 6 g) *or* As directed by urine culture results Adults: Ciprofloxacin 500 mg PO *or* Ciprofloxacin 400 mg IV *or* As directed by urine culture results
Gynecologic and Obstetric Surgery		
Vaginal or abdominal hysterectomy	Enteric gram-negative bacilli Anaerobes Group B *Streptococcus* *Enterococcus*	Cefazolin 12.5–20 mg/kg (max 1–2 g) *or* Cefoxitin 20–40 mg/kg (max 1 g) *or* Cefotetan 1 g (adults)
Cesarean section (for high risk only: active labor or premature rupture of membranes)	Same as for hysterectomy	Cefazolin 1 g after cord is clamped
Abortion	Same as for hysterectomy	*First trimester* (for high risk only: previous pelvic inflammatory disease, previous gonorrhea, or multiple sex partners): aqueous penicillin G 2 MU *or* doxycycline 100 mg 1 hr before abortion PO *and* 200 mg 30 min afterward PO *Second trimester:* cefazolin 1 g
Contaminated, or "Dirty," Surgery‡		
Ruptured Viscus	Enteric gram-negative bacilli Anaerobes *Enterococcus* Nosocomial pathogens with ruptured viscus in postoperative setting	Cefoxitin 20–40 mg/kg (max 1 g) q6hr *or* Cefotetan 1 g (adults) q12hr *with or without* gentamicin 1.5 mg/kg q8hr *or* Clindamycin 10 mg/kg (max 600 mg) q6hr *and* gentamicin 1.5 mg/kg q8hr
Traumatic Wound	*S. aureus* Group A *Streptococcus* *Clostridium*	Cefazolin 12.5–20 mg/kg (max 1–2 g)

*Parenteral prophylactic antimicrobials can be given as a single intravenous dose approximately 30 minutes before the procedure. For prolonged operations, additional intraoperative doses should be given every 4–8 hours for the duration of the procedure. Recommended doses are approximate, because no standard dosing has been established for some uses of surgical prophylaxis in pediatrics.
†Vancomycin is used in hospitals in which methicillin-resistant *S. aureus* and coagulase-negative staphylococci are frequent causes of postoperative wound infection and for patients who are hypersensitive to penicillins or cephalosporins. Vancomycin should be infused for a period of at least 1 hour.
‡For contaminated, or "dirty," surgery, therapy should be continued for about 5 days.
Modified for use in pediatrics from Antimicrobial prophylaxis in surgery. *Med Lett Drugs Ther* 1999;41:75–9.

especially *Staphylococcus aureus* and coagulase-negative staphylococci that are commonly associated with wound infections. Extended-spectrum cephalosporins, which have greater activity against many gram-negative bacilli, are generally no better for surgical prophylaxis than the first-generation agents but cost substantially more and are more likely to disturb the patient's own protective gastrointestinal flora. Some pediatric surgeons prefer a combination of ampicillin and gentamicin to first-generation cephalosporins for surgical prophylaxis in the neonate and young infant because the spectrum of activity is more appropriate for the organisms that cause neonatal sepsis.

Table 16–6 lists the recommended surgical prophylaxis for common surgical procedures in children and adolescents. Because many procedures in pediatric surgery are performed in low volume or only in a few centers, comprehensive guidelines for surgical prophylaxis are lacking. In such cases, surgeons use a regimen that is an extrapolation from similar but higher-volume procedures. Recommendations may vary from center to center.

In addition to the use of parenteral antibiotics for surgical procedures, bowel antisepsis is often used for elective colorectal surgery. This involves an appropriate diet, the use of cathartics for 36–48 hours before surgery, and the use of oral antibiotics such as neomycin (50 mg/kg/day; maximum, 1 g per dose) and erythromycin base (50 mg/kg/day; maximum, 1 g per dose) in three divided doses (at 1 PM, 2 PM, and 11 PM on the day before an 8 AM operation). Sometimes a combination of oral and parenteral antibiotics is used, although it is unclear whether this is more effective than either alone. Cefoxitin is generally recommended for adults, but a first-generation cephalosporin plus metronidazole should be effective for children. Other acceptable regimens for gastrointestinal surgery include broader antibiotic coverage with piperacillin-tazobactam, an aminoglycoside, and metronidazole, either with or without oral antibiotics.

REVIEWS

Antimicrobial prophylaxis in surgery. *Med Lett Drugs Ther* 1999;41: 75–9.

Shapiro ED: Prophylaxis for bacterial meningitis. *Med Clin North Am* 1985;69:269–80.

KEY ARTICLES

American Academy of Pediatrics Committee on Infectious Diseases: Meningococcal disease prevention and control strategies for practice-based physicians. *Pediatrics* 1996;97:404–12.

American Academy of Pediatrics Committee on Infectious Diseases and Committee on Drugs and Section on Surgery: Antimicrobial prophylaxis in pediatric surgical patients. *Pediatrics* 1984;74:437–9.

Azizkhan RG: Appropriate use of antibiotics in infants and children with infections. In Fonkalsruid EW, Krummel TM (editors): *Infections and Immunologic Disorders in Pediatric Surgery*. Philadelphia, WB Saunders, 1993.

Centers for Disease Control and Prevention: Control and prevention of meningococcal disease: Recommendations of the Advisory Committee on Immunization Practices (ACIP). *MMWR Morb Mortal Wkly Rep* 1997;46(RR–11):1–10.

Centers for Disease Control and Prevention: Control and prevention of serogroup C meningococcal disease: Evaluation and management of suspected outbreaks. Recommendations of the Advisory Committee on Immunization Practices (ACIP). *MMWR Morb Mortal Wkly Rep* 1997;46(RR–5):13–21.

Classen DC, Evans RS, Pestotnik SL, et al: The timing of prophylactic administration of antibiotics and the risk of surgical-wound infection. *N Engl J Med* 1992;326:281–6.

Ehrenkranz NJ: Antimicrobial prophylaxis in surgery: Mechanisms, misconceptions and mischief. *Infect Control Hosp Epidemiol* 1993;14: 99–106.

Kaiser AB: Antimicrobial prophylaxis in surgery. *N Engl J Med* 1986; 315:1129–38.

Mangram AJ, Horan TC, Pearson ML, et al: Hospital Infection Control Practices Advisory Committee: Guideline for prevention of surgical site infection, 1999. *Infect Control Hosp Epidemiol* 1999;20:250–78.

Nichols RL, Smith JW, Garcia RY, et al: Current practices of preoperative bowel preparation among North American colorectal surgeons. *Clin Infect Dis* 1997;24:609–19.

Schwartz B, Al-Tobaiqi A, Al-Ruwais A, et al: Comparative efficacy of ceftriaxone and rifampicin in eradicating pharyngeal carriage of group A *Neisseria meningitidis*. *Lancet* 1988;1:1239–42.

CHAPTER 17

Immunizations

Colin D. Marchant ▪ Mary Lou Kumar

Active immunization has dramatically reduced the incidence of many infectious diseases that were once common. Advances in biomedical science continue to yield new vaccines for previously unpreventable diseases and improved vaccines for many controllable diseases. Recommendations for vaccine use continue to evolve, and clinicians are urged to keep abreast of new directives formulated by (1) the American Academy of Pediatrics (AAP), (2) the Advisory Committee on Immunization Practices (ACIP) of the United States Public Health Service, (3) the American Academy of Family Physicians, and (4) the National Advisory Committee on Immunization (NACI) of Canada. The AAP publishes recommendations in the Report of the Committee on Infectious Diseases, with updated recommendations appearing periodically in the journal *Pediatrics.* Both publications are available from the AAP at 141 Northwest Point Blvd, PO Box 927, Elk Grove Village, IL 60009-0927. The ACIP recommendations are published periodically by the Centers for Disease Control and Prevention (CDC) in *Morbidity and Mortality Weekly Report,* which is available at www.cdc.gov/mmwr or by print subscription from The Massachusetts Medical Society, Boston, Mass. The NACI directives are published by Health and Welfare Canada in the Canadian Immunization Guide, with periodic updates in the Canada Communicable Disease Report. These are available from Canada Communication Group—Publishing, Ottawa, Ontario, Canada K1A OS9. Clinicians in other countries should consult health authorities in their home countries. Persons administering vaccines should also be thoroughly familiar with the product circular of the particular vaccines they are administering.

GENERAL CONSIDERATIONS

Clinicians should be familiar with active immunization in five distinct situations: (1) universal immunization of healthy infants and children, (2) immunization of persons who are compromised immunologically, physiologically, or anatomically, (3) immunization of persons who live or work in settings where their risk of exposure to vaccine-preventable diseases is increased, (4) immunization of persons who have been exposed to a particular disease, and (5) immunization of travelers to areas where the risks of particular diseases are increased.

Routine Immunization of Infants and Children

Universal immunization of healthy infants and children against diphtheria, tetanus, pertussis, poliomyelitis, hepatitis B, and measles is recommended worldwide. In the United States and many other developed countries, universal immunization for *Haemophilus influenzae* type b, *Streptococcus pneumoniae,* hepatitis B, mumps, rubella, and varicella is also part of standard pediatric practice, whereas hepatitis A is recommended for high-risk groups and populations (Table 17–1). In developing countries, prevention of tuberculosis with bacille Calmette-Guérin (BCG) vaccine is recommended for all newborn infants (Table 17–2), and yellow fever vaccine is recommended in countries with substantial risk of this disease, primarily for 33 countries in Africa.

All states require immunization of children entering grade school and licensed daycare; immunization also may be required for upper grades and college entry. The CDC publishes an annual survey of current school and college immunization requirements in the State Immunization Requirements for School Attendance, available from the National Immunization Program, Mailstop E-52, CDC, Atlanta, GA 30333 (www.cdc.gov/nip).

Delayed, Interrupted, and Unknown Immunization Status

When routine immunizations are not initiated in early infancy or are interrupted and resumed later in childhood, some modifications of the routine immunization schedule are made to achieve immunization as quickly as possible (Table 17–3). With increasing age, fewer immunizations for *H. influenzae* type b, *S. pneumoniae,* pertussis, diphtheria, tetanus, and polio may be required to achieve protective immunity. However, persons immunized after their thirteenth birthday require two doses of varicella vaccine for adequate protection. For all vaccines, if the immunization schedule has been interrupted, the doses that have already been given need not be repeated. However, if immunization status is unknown, the child should be considered unimmunized and an appropriate series of immunizations for age should be given.

Informed Consent

Vaccines should be administered only after informed consent has been obtained from the parent, guardian, and, in some cases, the vaccine recipient. In the United States, informed consent should be in writing and should include an explanation of the disease to be prevented, the benefits and risks of immunization, and the adverse events that parents should look for after immunization. The National Childhood Vaccine Injury Act of 1986 requires detailed notification of parents as to the risks of immunization. Every time a public or private health care provider in the United States administers a particular vaccine (i.e., diphtheria, tetanus, pertussis, poliomyelitis, measles, mumps, rubella, *H. influenzae* type b, hepatitis A, hepatitis B, pneumococcus, and varicella), the provider is required to provide a legal representative of any child (or any other adult individual receiving a vaccine) with a copy of the vaccine information statement prepared by the CDC. No other materials are acceptable for these vaccines. In addition to the names of the vaccinee and parent, the date, site of immunization, dose, manufacturer, vaccine lot number, name of the person who administered the vaccine, and place where the vaccine was administered should be recorded. This information is important if an untoward reaction occurs after immunization. Health care providers are not required

TABLE 17–1. Recommended Routine Childhood Immunization Schedule, United States, 2001

Vaccine	Age[1]											
	Birth	1 mo	2 mo	4 mo	6 mo	12 mo	15 mo	18 mo	24 mo	4–6 yr	11–12 yr	14–18 yr
Hepatitis B[2]	Hep B No. 1											
		Hep B No. 2			Hep B No. 3						(Hep B)	
Diphtheria and tetanus toxoids and pertussis[3]			DTaP	DTaP	DTaP		DTaP			DTaP	Td	
Haemophilus influenzae type b[4]			Hib	Hib	Hib	Hib						
Inactivated polio[5]			IPV	IPV	IPV					IPV		
Pneumococcal conjugate[6]			PCV	PCV	PCV	PCV						
Measles-mumps-rubella[7]						MMR				MMR	(MMR)	
Varicella[8]						Var					(Var)	
Hepatitis A[9]									Hep A in selected areas			

▭ Range of recommended ages for vaccination.

⬭ Vaccines to be given if previously recommended doses were missed or were given earlier than the recommended minimum age.

▒ Recommended in selected states or regions or both.

Approved by the Advisory Committee on Immunization Practices (ACIP), the American Academy of Pediatrics (AAP), and the American Academy of Family Physicians (AAFP).

Adapted from Centers for Disease Control and Prevention: Recommended childhood immunization schedule—United States, 2001. *MMWR Morb Mortal Wkly Rep* 2001;50:7–10, 19.

[1]This schedule indicates the recommended ages for routine administration of currently licensed childhood vaccines for children through 18 years of age. Licensed combination vaccines may be used whenever any components of the combination are indicated and the vaccine's other components are not contraindicated. Providers should consult the manufacturer's package inserts for detailed recommendations.

[2]**Infants born to hepatitis B surface antigen (HBsAg)-negative mothers** should receive the first dose of hepatitis B vaccine (Hep B) by age 2 months. The second dose should be administered at least 1 month after the first dose. The third dose should be administered at least 4 months after the first dose and at least 2 months after the second dose, but not before age 6 months. **Infants born to HBsAg-positive mothers** should receive Hep B and 0.5 mL hepatitis B immune globulin (HBIG) within 12 hours of birth at separate sites. The second dose is recommended at age 1–2 months and the third dose at age 6 months. **Infants born to mothers whose HBsAg status is unknown** should receive Hep B within 12 hours of birth. Maternal blood should be drawn at delivery to determine the mother's HBsAg status; if the HBsAg test result is positive, the infant should receive HBIG as soon as possible (no later than age 1 week). **All children and adolescents (through age 18 years)** who have not been immunized against hepatitis B should begin the series during any visit. Providers should make special efforts to immunize children who were born in or whose parents were born in areas of the world where hepatitis B virus infection is moderately or highly endemic.

[3]The fourth dose of diphtheria and tetanus toxoids and acellular pertussis vaccine (DTaP) may be administered as early as age 12 months, provided 6 months has elapsed since the third dose and the child is unlikely to return at age 15–18 months. Tetanus and diphtheria toxoids (Td) is recommended at age 11–12 years if at least 5 years has elapsed since the last dose of diphtheria and tetanus toxoids and pertussis vaccine (DTP), DTaP, or diphtheria and tetanus toxoids (DT). Subsequent routine Td boosters are recommended every 10 years.

[4]Three *Haemophilus influenzae* type b (Hib) conjugate vaccines are licensed for infant use. If Hib conjugate vaccine (PRP-OMP) (PedvaxHIB or ComVax [Merck]) is administered at ages 2 and 4 months, a dose at age 6 months is not required. Because clinical studies in infants have demonstrated that using some combination products may induce a lower immune response to the Hib vaccine component, DTaP/Hib combination products should not be used for primary immunization in infants at ages 2, 4, or 6 months unless approved by the Food and Drug Administration for these ages.

[5]An all-inactivated poliovirus vaccine (IPV) schedule is recommended for routine childhood polio vaccination in the United States. All children should receive four doses of IPV at age 2 months, at age 4 months, between ages 6 and 18 months, and between ages 4 and 6 years. Oral poliovirus vaccine should be used only in selected circumstances.

[6]The heptavalent pneumococcal conjugate vaccine (PCV) is recommended for all children aged 2–23 months. It is also recommended for certain children age 24–59 months.

[7]The second dose of measles, mumps, and rubella vaccine (MMR) is recommended routinely at age 4–6 years but may be administered during any visit, provided at least 4 weeks has elapsed since receipt of the first dose and that both doses are administered beginning at or after age 12 months. Those who previously have not received the second dose should complete the schedule no later than the routine visit to a health-care provider at age 11–12 years.

[8]Varicella vaccine (Var) is recommended at any visit on or after the first birthday for susceptible children (i.e., those who lack a reliable history of chickenpox [as judged by a health-care provider] and who have not been immunized). Susceptible persons aged ≥13 years should receive two doses given at least 4 weeks apart.

[9]Hepatitis A vaccine (Hep A) is recommended for use in selected states and/or regions and for certain high-risk groups.

Updated information about the immunization schedule is available on the National Immunization Program World-Wide Web site, http://www.cdc.gov/nip, or by telephone (800)232-2522 (English) or (800)232-0233 (Spanish).

TABLE 17–2. Expanded Program on Immunization of the World Health Organization: Recommended Immunization Schedule

	Vaccine and Dose Number					
Age	BCG	OPV	HBV*	DTP	Measles Vaccine	Tetanus Toxoid
Birth	No. 1	No. 1	No. 1			
6 wk		No. 2	No. 2	No. 1		
10 wk		No. 3		No. 2		
14 wk		No. 4		No. 3		
9 mo			No. 3		No. 1	
Women of childbearing age						≥2 doses

*HBV is recommended for all children in countries with a prevalence of hepatitis B antigenemia of 2% or more.

to obtain the signature of the vaccinee, parent, or other legal representative to acknowledge receipt of the vaccine information statement.

Site and Route of Administration

Most vaccines are administered by intramuscular or subcutaneous injection. A few should be administered by intradermal injection. The route of administration of each vaccine should be as recommended in the manufacturer's product information. The preferred sites for intramuscular and subcutaneous administration are the anterolateral aspect of the thigh in infants and the deltoid region in children and adults. The buttocks should not be used for the following reasons: (1) the vaccine is often injected into fatty tissue rather than muscle; (2) there is some risk of damage to the sciatic nerve; and (3) immune response is diminished when some vaccines, such as hepatitis B, are administered into the buttocks. The volar aspect of the forearm is preferred for intradermal injection of vaccines such as BCG. For optimal immune response, care must be taken not to administer intradermal preparations subcutaneously.

The needle length for intramuscular administration of vaccines into the anterolateral aspect of the thigh of infants is $\frac{7}{8}$ inch or longer. Use of shorter needles may result in injection into fatty tissues rather than muscle.

Simultaneous Administration of Vaccines

In general, multiple vaccines can be administered at separate sites without diminishing the immune response, although data are not complete for all vaccine combinations. Diphtheria and tetanus toxoids and acellular pertussis (DTaP) vaccine, measles-mumps-rubella (MMR) vaccine, *H. influenzae* type b conjugate vaccine (HbCV), hepatitis B vaccine (HBV), and either oral polio vaccine (OPV) or inactivated polio vaccine (IPV) may be administered simultaneously without impairing the immune response. Vaccines that are not already premixed should not be administered in the same syringe or at the same site. For other vaccines, it is preferable, for simultaneous administration, to inject each into a separate limb. If a single limb must be used for immunization, then the anterolateral aspect of the thigh is the preferred site and injections should be placed several centimeters apart so that local reactions do not overlap.

A notable exception to simultaneous administration involves the cholera and yellow fever vaccines, where simultaneous administration results in diminished immune response to both antigens. Optimally, there should be ≥3 weeks between these immunizations. Successive doses of OPV should be separated by ≥6 weeks to avoid serotype-specific interference with the immune response.

Use of Blood Products and Immune Responses to Immunization

Immune globulin preparations, including hyperimmune preparations to tetanus and hepatitis B, may be administered simultaneously with the corresponding vaccines by using separate injection sites without interfering with the immune response to active immunization. Rabies immune globulin given at twice the recommended dose can diminish the immune response to inactivated rabies vaccine, although not at the recommended dose (20 IU/kg). Immune globulin does not interfere with the immune response to oral polio, oral typhoid, yellow fever, and cholera vaccines.

Immune globulin administration can diminish the immune response to measles and rubella vaccines and possibly to mumps and varicella vaccines. If live parenteral viral vaccines are administered 2 weeks or more before immune globulin administration, then there should be no interference because viral replication will have occurred and an adequate immune response is expected.

On the basis of serologic studies and the expected half-life of passively administered immune globulin, suggested intervals between the use of immune globulin preparations and live measles vaccine vary from as little as 3 months to as long as 11 months, depending on the dose of immune globulin administered (Table 17–4). Transfusion with blood products other than immune globulin preparations may also inhibit immune responses to live measles vaccine. If measles immunization is given after immune globulin or other blood products within these intervals, measles immunization should be repeated after the recommended interval, or, alternatively, antibody testing after the interval should be performed to document immunity to measles.

Adverse Reactions

Clinical, scientific, and legal viewpoints on adverse reactions to immunization present conflicting perspectives. A few general statements can be made. Nonspecific symptoms, including fever, irritability, lethargy, and crying, are common during the ages when infants usually receive immunizations and occur somewhat more frequently after immunization but are self-limited. Local reactions at the injection site may occur with any vaccine but are more common after administration of whole cell pertussis vaccine and parenteral typhoid vaccine. Most of these reactions are transient, but sterile abscesses sometimes occur with killed vaccines.

Anecdotal reports of illnesses of all kinds that have begun after an immunization are numerous. A list of potential reactions can usually be found in the manufacturer's product circulars; these are given for the purpose of limiting the manufacturer's liability. Most of these reactions have not been causally related to the vaccine. However, some rare adverse reactions are clinically distinctive (e.g., paralytic polio from OPV, severe hypersensitivity reactions such as urticaria or anaphylaxis); therefore causal inference is reasonable. Controlled studies, especially rigorous controlled studies that demonstrate that vaccines cause other serious adverse events, are few. In the United States, the National Childhood Vaccine Injury Act of 1986 requires that health care providers report adverse events after immunization (Table 17–5).

Contraindications

General contraindications to vaccination include (1) hypersensitivity to the vaccine or its components, as manifested by urticaria, shock, wheezing, or evidence of airway obstruction; (2) immunocompromised states or pregnancy (for administration of live virus vaccines); (3) undefined illnesses, including febrile and neurologic

TABLE 17–3. Immunization Schedules for Children Whose Immunizations Have Been Delayed*

HBV	DTaP	Hib	IPV	PCV	MMR	Var
Age at First Immunization: <6 mo						
Two doses 1 mo apart; dose No. 3 given 4–12 mo later	Three doses 4–8 wk apart; dose No. 4 at 15–18 mo of age; dose No. 5 at 4–6 yr of age	Three doses of HbOC or PRP-T 2 mo apart and dose No. 4 at age 12–15 mo; or 2 doses of PRP-OMP 2 mo apart and dose No. 3 at age 12–15 mo	Two doses 2 mo apart; dose No. 3 at 15–18 mo; dose No. 4 at 4–6 yr	Three doses 4–8 wk apart; dose No. 4 at 12–15 mo of age	Dose No. 1 at 12–15 mo of age; dose No. 2 at age 4–6 yr	At 12–18 mo
Age at First Immunization: 7–11 mo						
Two doses 1 mo apart; dose No. 3 given 4–12 mo later	Three doses 2 mo apart; dose No. 4 given 6–12 mo later; dose No. 5 at 4–6 yr	Two doses of HbOC, PRP-T, or PRP-OMP 2 mo apart; dose No. 3 (HbOC, PRP-T, PRP-OMP, or PRP-D) at 12–15 mo (≥8 wk after dose No. 2)	Two doses 2 mo apart; dose No. 3 given 6–12 mo later; dose No. 4 at 4–6 yr	Two doses 4–8 wk apart; dose No. 3 at 12–15 mo of age (≥8 wk after dose No. 2)	Dose No. 1 at 12–15 mo of age; dose No. 2 at age 4–6 yr	At 12–18 mo
Age at First Immunization: 12–14 mo						
Two doses 1 mo apart; dose No. 3 given 4–12 mo later	Three doses 2 mo apart; dose No. 4 given 6–12 mo later; dose No. 5 at 4–6 yr only if dose No. 4 was given before fourth birthday	Two doses of HbOC, PRP-T, PRP-OMP, or PRP-D 2 mo apart	Two doses 2 mo apart; dose No. 3 given 6–12 mo later; dose No. 4 at 4–6 yr	Two doses ≥8 wk apart	Dose No. 1 at 15 mo of age; dose No. 2 at age 4–6 yr	Immunize at first contact
Age at First Immunization: 15–59 mo						
Two doses 1 mo apart; dose No. 3 given 4–12 mo later	Three doses 2 mo apart; dose No. 4 given 6–12 mo later; dose No. 5 at 4–6 yr only if dose No. 4 was given before fourth birthday	One dose of any conjugate vaccine; high-risk children should be immunized with 2 doses of any conjugate vaccine ≥8 wk apart	Two doses 2 mo apart; dose No. 3 give 6–12 mo later; a fourth dose at age 4–6 yr if dose No. 3 was given before fourth birthday	At 15–23 mo 2 doses ≥8 wk apart; ≥24 mo routine immunization not recommended, but high-risk children should be immunized with 2 doses ≥8 wk apart	Dose No. 1 at first contact; dose No. 2 at age 4–6 yr (≤4 wk after first dose)	Immunize at first contact
Age at First Immunization: 5–6 yr						
Two doses 1 mo apart; dose No. 3 given 4–12 mo later	Three doses 2 mo apart; dose No. 4 given 6–12 mo later *Note:* After seventh birthday, Td should be substituted for DTaP	Routine immunization not indicated; high-risk children should be immunized with 2 doses of any conjugate vaccine ≥8 wk apart	Two doses 2 mo apart; dose No. 3 given 6–12 mo later	Routine immunization not recommended	Dose No. 1 at first contact; dose No. 2 given ≥1 mo later (by 11–12 yr of age)	Immunize at first contact

Table continued on following page

TABLE 17–3. Immunization Schedules for Children Whose Immunizations Have Been Delayed* *(Continued)*

HBV	DTaP	Hib	IPV	PCV	MMR	Var
Age at First Immunization: After Seventh Birthday						
Two doses 1 mo apart; dose No. 3 given 4–12 mo later	Two doses Td given 2 mo apart; dose No. 3 given 6–12 mo later; booster doses at 10-yr intervals	Routine immunization not indicated; high-risk children should be immunized with 2 doses of any conjugate vaccine 1–2 mo apart	Two doses 2 mo apart; dose No. 3 given 6–12 mo later	Routine immunization not recommended	Dose No. 1 at first contact; dose No. 2 given ≥1 mo later (by 11–12 yr)	Immunize at first contact (2 doses 4–8 wk apart for persons ≥13 yr)

*For interrupted immunizations, previously administered doses should be counted as completed doses and immunizations resumed according to recommendations for current age. Assume that individuals of unknown immunization status are unimmunized and immunize according to current age.

conditions in which administration of vaccine may produce confusion in the diagnosis or in monitoring the therapeutic response; and (4) prior severe reactions that might be related to the vaccine when the benefits of further immunization do not outweigh the perceived risks of a further reaction. Components that may be responsible for hypersensitivity include traces of egg or egg antigens, thimerosal (added as a preservative), antibiotics (neomycin and streptomycin), or components of the infectious agent itself. Hypersensitivity reactions to vaccines and vaccine components must be evaluated carefully. Current preparations of measles and mumps vaccines do not contain significant amounts of egg cross-reacting proteins and may be given without skin testing to children with egg allergy. Influenza and yellow fever vaccines contain egg proteins, and a history of anaphylactic-like reactions to eggs is a contraindication to immunization with these vaccines, except under controlled circumstances. Protocols are available for testing and immunizing persons with a history of egg allergy with influenza and yellow fever vaccines, but use of these protocols is rarely necessary. A history of anaphylactic reactions to neomycin is a contraindication to MMR immunization. Local delayed hypersensi-

TABLE 17–4. Recommended Intervals Between Administration of Immune Globulin Preparations or Blood Products and Vaccination with Preparations Containing Live Measles Virus

Indication	Product, Dose, and Route	Equivalent mg IgG/kg	Suggested Interval Before Measles Vaccination (mo)
Immunoprophylaxis			
Tetanus prophylaxis	TIG 250 units IM	10 mg IgG/kg	3
Hepatitis A prophylaxis			
Contact prophylaxis	ISG 0.02 mL/kg IM	3.3 mg IgG/kg	3
International travel	ISG 0.06 mL/kg IM	10 mg IgG/kg	3
Hepatitis B prophylaxis	HBIG 0.06 mL/kg IM	10 mg IgG/kg	3
Rabies prophylaxis	RIG 20 IU/kg IM	22 mg IgG/kg	4
Varicella prophylaxis	VZIG 125 units/10 kg (maximum: 625 units) IM	20–40 mg IgG/kg	5
Measles prophylaxis			
Normal contact	ISG 0.25 mL/kg IM	40 mg IgG/kg	5
Immunocompromised contact	ISG 0/50 mL/kg IM	80 mg IgG/kg	6
Immune Globulin Replacement Therapy	IVIG 300–400 mg/kg	300–400 mg IgG/kg	8
Treatment of:			
Immune thrombocytopenic purpura	IVIG 400 mg/kg	400 mg IgG/kg	8
	IVIG 1,000 mg/kg	1,000 mg IgG/kg	10
Kawasaki syndrome	IVIG 2 g/kg	2,000 mg IgG/kg	11
Blood Transfusion			
Red blood cells, washed	10 mL/kg IV	Negligible	0
Red blood cells, adenine–saline solution added	10 mL/kg IV	10 mg IgG/kg	3
Red blood cells, packed	10 mL/kg IV	60 mg IgG/kg	6
Whole blood	10 mL/kg IV	80–100 mg IgG/kg	6
Platelets	10 mL/kg IV	160 mg IgG/kg	7
Plasma	10 mL/kg IV	160 mg IgG/kg	7

Adapted from Centers for Disease Control and Prevention: General recommendations on immunization: Recommendations of the Advisory Committee on Immunization Practices (ACIP). *MMWR Morb Mortal Wkly Rep* 1994;43(RR-1):1–38.

TABLE 17–5. Reportable Events Following Vaccination

Vaccine/Toxoid	Event	Interval from Vaccination
Tetanus in any combination; DTaP, DTP, DTP-Hib, DT, Td, TT	Anaphylaxis or anaphylactic shock	7 days
	Brachial neuritis	28 days
	Any sequela (including death) of above events	No limit
	Events described in manufacturer's package insert as contraindications to additional doses of vaccine*	See package insert
Pertussis in any combination; DTaP, DTP, DTP-HIB, P	Anaphylaxis or anaphylactic shock	7 days
	Encephalopathy (or encephalitis)	7 days
	Any sequela (including death) of above events	No limit
	Events described in manufacturer's package insert as contraindications to additional doses of vaccine*	See package insert
Measles, mumps and rubella in any combination; MMR, MR, R	Anaphylaxis or anaphylactic shock	7 days
	Encephalopathy (or encephalitis)	15 days
	Any sequela (including death) of above events	No limit
	Events described in manufacturer's package insert as contraindications to additional doses of vaccine*	See package insert
Rubella in any combination; MMR, MR, R	Chronic arthritis	42 days
	Any sequela (including death) of above events	No limit
	Events described in manufacturer's package insert as contraindications to additional doses of vaccine*	See package insert
Measles in any combination; MMR, MR, M	Thrombocytopenic purpura	30 days
	Vaccine-strain measles viral infection in an immunocompromised recipient	6 mo
	Any sequela (including death) of above events	No limit
	Events described in manufacturer's package insert as contraindications to additional doses of vaccine*	See package insert
Oral Polio (OPV)	Paralytic polio	
	In a nonimmunocompromised recipient	30 days
	In an immunocompromised recipient	6 mo
	In a vaccine-associated community case	No limit
	Vaccine-strain polio viral infection	
	In a nonimmunocompromised recipient	30 days
	In an immunocompromised recipient	6 mo
	In a vaccine-associated community case	No limit
	Any sequela (including death) of above events	No limit
	Events described in manufacturer's package insert as contraindications to additional doses of vaccine*	See package insert
Inactivated Polio (IPV)	Anaphylaxis or anaphylactic shock	7 days
	Any sequela (including death) of above events	No limit
	Events described in manufacturer's package insert as contraindications to additional doses of vaccine*	See package insert
Hepatitis B	Anaphylaxis or anaphylactic shock	7 days
	Any sequela (including death) of above events	No limit
	Events described in manufacturer's package insert as contraindications to additional doses of vaccine*	See package insert
Haemophilus influenzae type b	Early-onset *H. influenzae* disease	7 days
	Any sequela (including death) of the above events	No limit
	Events described in manufacturer's package insert as contraindications to additional doses of vaccine*	See package insert
Rotavirus†	Events described in manufacturer's package insert as contraindications to additional doses of vaccine*	See package insert
Varicella	Events described in manufacturer's package insert as contraindications to additional doses of vaccine*	See package insert
New vaccines	No conditions specified	See package insert

*The Reportable Events Table reflects what is reportable by law (42U.S.C. 300aa-25) to the Vaccine Adverse Event Reporting System (VAERS) including conditions found in the manufacturer's package insert. In addition, individuals are encouraged to report ANY clinically significant or unexpected events (even if you are not certain the vaccine caused the event) for ANY vaccine, whether or not it is listed on the Reportable Events Table.

†Rotavirus vaccine was withdrawn from the United States in 1999.

tivity reactions to neomycin and thimerosal are not indicative of anaphylactic reactions and are not contraindications to immunization with vaccines that contain these substances.

Contraindications to immunization are not necessarily absolute. The risks of live viral vaccines in immunocompromised persons may be outweighed by the risks of disease, and some live viral vaccines are recommended if risks of disease are high. Acute diseases may subside or stabilize so that immunizations can be resumed. The risk of disease in an epidemic situation may make further immunization advisable despite a history of reactions. Contraindications to specific vaccines are considered in the following sections discussing the individual vaccines. In addition to the previously mentioned recommendations concerning contraindications, there are a number of myths and misconceptions about contraindications. Mild to moderate infectious illness with or without low-grade fever, exposure to infectious diseases, and antimicrobial therapy for infectious illnesses are not contraindications to immunization. However, some experts believe that febrile children should not be immunized, so as to avoid confusion in the interpretation of signs and symptoms that may be caused either by the vaccines administered or by an evolving infectious illness. Children with a family history of seizure disorders, of sudden infant death syndrome, or of adverse reactions to vaccines other than those related to immunodeficiency should be immunized. Histories of allergies other than to specific components of a particular vaccine should not influence decisions to immunize. The presence of a pregnant woman in the infant's household is not a reason not to immunize. Breast-feeding is not a contraindication to immunization with any vaccine. Most reactions to diphtheria-tetanus-pertussis (DTP) vaccination are not contraindications to further use of DTP.

Vaccine Injury Compensation Program

Widespread public belief that whole-cell pertussis vaccine causes encephalopathy and permanent neurologic sequelae resulted in the cessation of immunization programs in some Western countries and many lawsuits in the United States. In recent years, critical review of the evidence that pertussis vaccine causes neurologic impairment has led to the conclusion that pertussis vaccine rarely if ever causes brain damage; the damage is too rare to be apparent in the largest epidemiologic studies. Nevertheless, the pressures of litigation and the potential for adverse impact on vaccine supply and development led to passage of the **National Childhood Vaccine Injury Act of 1986.** This act provides for compensation of persons who have specific injury after administration of vaccines for tetanus, pertussis, measles, mumps, rubella, polio, hepatitis B, *H. influenzae* type b, and varicella (Table 17–5). Claims are reviewed by a panel of experts, and acceptance of compensation by the injured party is linked to a waiver of further litigation for the injury. The law also mandates that informed consent be obtained before immunization and that adverse events be reported to the **Vaccine Adverse Event Reporting System (VAERS)** of the United States Department of Health and Human Services (telephone: 800-822-7967) (Table 17–5). Further limitation of the injuries that are eligible for compensation and the continuation of the vaccine injury compensation act itself are subject to ongoing action by the United States Congress. Physicians must seek updates on the current status of the Vaccine Injury Compensation Program (www.fda.gov/cber/vaers/vaers.htm).

Immunization of Compromised Persons

Compromised persons are susceptible to the same illnesses as healthy infants and children, and in some cases either the risk of infection or the severity of disease is increased. Immunodeficient and immunocompromised persons are often also at risk of serious infection if live vaccines are administered. Data on the efficacy of immunization of compromised persons are limited, however. General guidelines for the immunization of immunologically, physiologically, and anatomically compromised persons are outlined in Table 17–6.

Immunization of Special Groups

Pregnant Women. There is a theoretic risk to immunization with any vaccine during the period of organogenesis, the first trimester of pregnancy. Thus it is wise to avoid immunization during this time. Because of the potential for infection of the fetus, live viral vaccines such as MMR and varicella are generally contraindicated in women who expect to become pregnant in the following 3 months and throughout pregnancy. Vaccine strains of mumps and rubella viruses, but not of measles virus, are known to infect placental tissues. Despite placental infection, no cases of symptomatic congenital rubella syndrome due to rubella vaccine have been reported, and as yet no harmful effects of the MMR vaccine on the fetus have been documented. Thus the inadvertent administration of live viral vaccines is not an indication for termination of pregnancy. Oral polio and yellow fever vaccines can be given to pregnant women if risk of exposure is substantial and unavoidable. Inactivated viral and bacterial vaccines are not known to produce harmful fetal effects. Tetanus toxoid is efficacious and widely used in the third trimester in developing countries to prevent tetanus neonatorum by transplacental transfer of antitoxin antibody to the fetus. Women who have not received tetanus-diphtheria toxoid (Td) in the 10 years before pregnancy should receive a Td immunization. Hepatitis B, influenza, pneumococcal, and rabies vaccines are recommended for pregnant women at risk of having these diseases. Meningococcal, plague, and inactivated typhoid vaccine should be administered if the risk of disease is substantial. Live oral typhoid vaccine is not indicated in pregnancy.

Preterm Infants. Premature infants are capable of immune responses to vaccines and should be immunized according to their postnatal chronologic age with vaccine dosages recommended for term infants. Hepatitis B immunization may be initiated at birth; administration of hepatitis B vaccine and hepatitis B immune globulin immediately after birth is particularly important for infants of HBsAg-positive mothers. During hospitalization, OPV should be avoided because of possible transmission in the nursery to others for whom it may be contraindicated, but IPV, DTP, and HbCV should be administered. At hospital discharge, additional immunizations should be given as indicated and not be delayed. Infants with bronchopulmonary dysplasia, other pulmonary disease, or hemodynamically significant cardiac disease should also receive influenza vaccine at 6 months of age or older.

Children in Residential Institutions. Residential institutions are settings in which the risk of disease transmission is increased. All recommended childhood vaccines should be current for age unless contraindications are substantial. Individuals who did not receive hepatitis B vaccine as part of routine immunizations in infancy should be immunized with hepatitis B vaccine, because the risk of transmission is increased in residential settings. Influenza may also spread rapidly in institutional settings, and some residents may be physiologically compromised. Annual, timely influenza immunization programs are recommended for all residential institutions with children.

Adolescents and College Students. Individuals in these groups are less likely to receive appropriate immunizations than are infants and young children, in part because public clinics for immunization

TABLE 17–6. Immunization of Compromised Persons

Condition	Vaccine Contraindications	Vaccine Indications	Additional Considerations
Congenital immunodeficiency	*T-cell disorders:* all live bacterial and viral vaccines including MMR and OPV. *B-cell disorders:* live bacterial vaccines and OPV (i.e., MMR can be considered). *Phagocyte disorders:* live bacterial vaccines. *Complement disorders:* none. OPV should **not** be given to persons living in the same household.	Inactivated vaccines, including DTP, IPV, HbCV, PCV, and HBV, are indicated. After age 2 yr, additional doses of PCV may be required if fewer than 4 doses were administered before age 2 yrs. Pneumococcal polysaccharide vaccine should be given after age 2 yrs and after immunization with PCV is complete, and then repeated 3–5 yr later. Influenza and meningococcal vaccines may be indicated.	Immune response to vaccines may be inadequate.
Immunosuppressive therapy	Live viral vaccines, including MMR and OPV, during periods of immunosuppression. OPV should **not** be given to persons living in the same household.	Inactivated vaccines, including DTP, IPV, HbCV, PCV, and HBV, are indicated. After age 2 yr, additional doses of PCV may be required if fewer than 4 doses were administered before age 2 yr. Pneumococcal polysaccharide vaccine should be given after age 2 yr and after immunization with PCV is complete, and then repeated 3–5 yr later. Influenza immunization should be given annually. Varicella vaccine and MMR vaccine should be administered at least 3 mo after chemotherapy.	Immunization during chemotherapy or radiation therapy should be avoided because the immune response to immunization may be inadequate. Influenza vaccine should be administered at least 3–4 wk after chemotherapy when neutrophil and lymphocyte counts are higher than 100 mm^3. Live virus vaccines should not be administered for at least 3 mo after chemotherapy.
Corticosteroid therapy	May give live viral vaccines to previously healthy persons if corticosteroid therapy is of brief duration (less than 2 wk with moderate doses; *or* on alternate days in moderate doses of short-acting corticosteroids; *or* topically, via respiratory tract; *or* instilled at local sites (e.g., intra-articularly). Otherwise, guidelines for receiving immunosuppressive therapy should be applied.		Persons receiving the equivalent of 2 mg/kg or a total of 20 mg of prednisone per day for 2 wk or longer should be considered immunocompromised. Live virus vaccines should not be administered for at least 3 mo after therapy has been discontinued.
Hodgkin's disease	Live viral vaccines, including MMR and OPV, during periods of immunosuppression. OPV should **not** be given to persons living in the same household.	Inactivated vaccines, including DTP, IPV, HbCV, PCV, HBV. The HbCV vaccine is given according to age or as a single dose if splenectomy is performed after 15 mo of age. After age 2 yr, additional doses of PCV may be required if fewer than 4 doses were administered before age 2 yr. Pneumococcal polysaccharide vaccine should be given after age 2 yr and after immunization with PCV is complete, and then repeated 3–5 yr later.	If possible, immunize 2 wk before splenectomy or start of chemotherapy. Live viral vaccines should not be given until at least 3 mo after completion of chemotherapy.

Table continued on following page

TABLE 17–6. Immunization of Compromised Persons *(Continued)*

Condition	Vaccine Contraindications	Vaccine Indications	Additional Considerations
Solid organ transplants	Live viral vaccines. Data on immunization after transplantation are limited. OPV should **not** be given to persons living in the same household.	All routine immunizations, including MMR vaccination before transplantation if possible. Pneumococcal polysaccharide vaccine should be given after age 2 yr and repeated 3–5 yr later. Influenza vaccine should also be given.	Measles serologic testing is helpful to guide decisions for active immunization before transplantation. Response to immunization after transplantation is unknown, but patients probably respond poorly during high-dose immunosuppression.
Bone marrow transplants	Live viral vaccines (except MMR—see vaccine indications in column to the right). OPV should **not** be given to persons living in the same household.	Routine immunization schedule at 12, 14, and 24 mo after BMT and should include 3 doses of DTaP or DT, or Td (depending on age and contraindications), IPV, HbCV, and HBV, provided there is no GHVD. MMR vaccine is given 2 yr after transplantation if person does not have chronic GVHD and is not receiving long-term immunosuppressive therapy. Two doses of pneumococcal polysaccharide vaccine should be given 1 yr apart, if age >2 yr (there is no specific recommendation at this time for PCV). Influenza vaccines should be given annually beginning 12–24 mo after transplantation. Household members and health care workers in close contact with BMT patients should be appropriately immunized with MMR, varicella, polio, hepatitis A, and influenza (annually) vaccines.	The decision to immunize may be based on serology.
Human immunodeficiency virus infection	OPV, BCG if tuberculosis risk is low, as in the United States. OPV should **not** be given to persons living in the same household.	Routine immunizations with DTP, IPV, HBV, HbCV, PCV, MMR (unless CDC category 3 or severe immunosuppression; see Tables 38–2 and 38–3), and varicella (2 doses 3 mo apart if CD4 percent >25%). After age 2 yr, additional doses of PCV may be required if fewer than 4 doses were administered before age 2 yr. Pneumococcal polysaccharide vaccine should be given at ≥2 yr of age and after immunization with PCV is complete and is then repeated 3–5 yr later. Influenza split virus vaccine should be given annually, beginning after age 6 mo.	Immune responses may not be adequate for protection. If person is receiving immune globulin IV, consider administering MMR 2 wk before the next dose, and repeat MMR immunization at the recommended interval after immune globulin therapy.
Asplenia, sickle cell disease, or thalassemia	None	Routine immunizations with DTP, IPV, HBV, PCV, and MMR. HbCV should be given according to age or as a single dose if splenectomy was performed after 15 mo of age. After age 2 yr, additional doses of PCV may be required if fewer than 4 doses were administered before age 2 yr.	If possible, immunization should be initiated 2 wk before splenectomy. Antimicrobial chemoprophylaxis is also recommended for prevention of invasive bacterial infections (see Table 101–2).

TABLE 17–6. Immunization of Compromised Persons *(Continued)*

Condition	Vaccine Contraindications	Vaccine Indications	Additional Considerations
Asplenia, sickle cell disease, or thalassemia *(Continued)*		Pneumococcal polysaccharide vaccine should be given after age 2 yr and after immunization with PCV is complete, and then repeated 3–5 yr later. Meningococcal vaccine with serogroups A, C, Y, and W-135 can be given after age 2 yrs.	
Cardiorespiratory disease, diabetes mellitus, or chronic renal or metabolic disease	None	Routine immunizations with DTP, IPV, HBV, HbCV, PCV, and MMR. After age 2 yr, additional doses of PCV may be required if fewer than 4 doses were administered before age 2 yr. Pneumococcal polysaccharide vaccine should be given after age 2 yr and after immunization with PCV is complete, and then repeated 3–5 yr later. Influenza vaccine can be given annually and pneumococcal vaccine after age 2 yr. ***Note:*** Persons with renal failure require immunization with increased doses of HBV.	
Nephrotic syndrome, cerebrospinal fluid leak	None	Routine immunizations with DTP, IPV, HBV, HbCV, PCV, and MMR. After age 2 yr, additional doses of PCV may be requiired if fewer than 4 doses were administered before age 2 yr. Pneumococcal polysaccharide vaccine should be given after age 2 yr and after immunization with PCV is complete, and then repeated 3–5 yr later.	
Long-term aspirin therapy	None	Influenza vaccine should be given annually.	

BMT = bone marrow transplantation; GVHD = graft-versus-host disease.

of these age groups rarely exist. Immunization records for these individuals should be sought and reviewed to determine whether appropriate immunizations, including Td boosters, two prior doses of MMR, hepatitis B, and varicella vaccines, and age-appropriate polio immunizations have been administered. The American College Health Association (ACHA) recommends these vaccinations as a prematriculation requirement. Additionally, the ACHA and many colleges and universities recommend meningococcal vaccine before matriculation, especially for freshmen living in dormitories.

Health Care Workers. For protection of both themselves and others, health care workers should have immunity to measles, rubella, hepatitis B, and influenza. Those born on or after January 1, 1957, should have proof of physician-documented measles, should have serologic evidence of measles immunity, or should have received two doses of measles vaccine. Women who may become pregnant and persons in contact with pregnant women (i.e., those in pediatric and obstetric care settings) should be immune to rubella, as demonstrated by proof of rubella vaccine immunization or serologic test results. All health care workers should receive three doses of hepatitis B vaccine. Influenza poses an increased risk to many children encountered by health care workers. Infants younger than 6 months of age are at risk but should not be immunized. Health care workers, particularly those who care for young infants, should be offered annual, timely influenza immunization.

Immunization After Exposure to Disease

When an individual has contact with a known case of a particular disease or has otherwise been exposed or is presumed to have been exposed (e.g., bites or wounds), active immunization may prevent or modify disease (Table 17–7). In addition, antimicrobial chemoprophylaxis and passive immunization with immunoglobulin preparations are often indicated. For some vaccine-preventable diseases, including meningococcal disease due to serogroups A, C, Y, and

TABLE 17–7. Immunization After Disease Exposure

Disease	Exposure	Vaccine Use	Additional Measures
Diphtheria	Household contact	Younger than 7 yr: DTaP or DT; 7 yr or older: Td for persons: (1) unimmunized, (2) underimmunized for age, (3) unknown immunizations status, and (4) no diphtheria booster in last 5 yr.	Antimicrobial prophylaxis with erythromycin (40–50 mg/kg/day for 7 days PO; max 2 g/day; or benzathine penicillin G 600,000–1,200,000 U IM).
Measles	Household, school, workplace, or other exposure	Immunization with measles vaccine or MMR vaccine within 72 hr of exposure is preferred to passive immunoprophylaxis for all persons without documented, age-appropriate measles immunization. This also applies to infants 6–14 mo of age who would normally not yet have received measles vaccine.	Immune globulin (0.25 mL/kg IM; 0.5 mL/kg for immunocompromised persons; max dose: 15 mL) may be given instead of vaccine. Immune globulin is particularly useful for young infants, immunocompromised persons, and those exposed more than 3 but less than 6 days previously. If measles immunization is incomplete, measles vaccine should be given at the appropriate interval after immune globulin administration (Table 17–4).
Hepatitis B	Infant born to HBsAg-positive mother or mother of unknown HBsAg status.	Immunization with 3 doses of HBV at recommended doses and schedule (Table 17–12).	Mothers of unknown HBsAg status should be tested immediately. All infants born to HBsAg-positive mothers should also receive hepatitis B immune globulin (0.5 mL IM) within 12 hr of birth.
	Infant younger than 12 mo of age and primary caregiver has acute hepatitis B; household contact with acute hepatitis B and unknown exposure; sexual exposure to acute hepatitis B; inadvertent percutaneous or mucosal exposure to carrier or acute case of hepatitis B	Immunization with 3 doses of HBV at recommended doses and schedule if not previously immunized.	Hepatitis B immune globulin (0.6 mL/kg IM) if infant younger than 12 mo of age or if exposed person is unimmunized or inadequately immunized.
	Continuing household exposure or sexual exposure to a chronic HBsAg carrier.	Immunization with 3 doses of HBV at recommended doses and schedule.	None.
Mumps	Household, institutional	Known to be safe but not proved effective for prevention during mumps incubation. Consider for persons who are (1) unimmunized and were born after 1957 or (2) seronegative and born before 1957.	None.
Pertussis	Household, other close contact, daycare	If younger than 7 yr, give DTaP if persons are (1) unimmunized, (2) have had 2 or fewer doses of DTaP but none within the last 6 mo, or (3) have had 4 doses of DTaP but none within the last 3 yr and are less than 6 yr of age.	Erythromycin prophylaxis (40–50 mg/kg/day; max 3 g/day in 4 divided doses for 14 days) for all household and close contacts. Shorter courses of 7–10 days have also been reported to be effective.
Tetanus	Wounds, bites (see Table 47–5)	Younger than 7 years: DTaP or DT if 7 years or older: Td for persons who are (1) unimmunized, (2) underimmunized for age, (3) of unknown immunization status, and (4) have not had a tetanus booster in the last 10 yr (clean, minor wounds).	Tetanus immune globulin (250–500 U IM) for contaminated wounds, puncture wounds, or devitalized tissue for persons not known with certainty to have had 3 prior tetanus immunizations.

TABLE 17–7. Immunization After Disease Exposure *(Continued)*

Disease	Exposure	Vaccine Use	Additional Measures
Rabies	Animal bites or saliva from an animal with proven rabies or with significant risk of having rabies. Consultation with local public health authorities for risk assessment is strongly recommended.	If unimmunized: 5 doses of human diploid rabies vaccine or rabies vaccine absorbed on days 0, 3, 7, 14, and 28. Previously immunized persons: 2 doses on days 0 and 3.	Rabies immune globulin (RIG) (20 IU/kg, if possible, half of the dose injected into the wound site and the other half given IM in separate sterile syringe). RIG should be given within 7 days of exposure to all persons with significant exposure who are unimmunized and to those previously immunized if vaccine is not available.
Tuberculosis	Repeated exposure to isoniazid and rifampin-resistant strains of *Mycobacterium tuberculosis* or tuberculin-negative infants and children with repeated household exposure to a persistent inadequately treated case of sputum-positive tuberculosis.	Bacille Calmette-Guérin (BCG)	Appropriate antituberculosis chemotherapy (Chapter 35)

W-135 and including invasive *H. influenzae* type b infection, antimicrobial chemoprophylaxis rather than immunization is recommended (Chapter 16), in part because of the short incubation period of these diseases. In many other diseases, exposure cannot be identified in time for active immunization to be effective.

Immunization Before International Travel

Travel to foreign countries may entail the same risk of vaccine-preventable disease as at home, increased risk of these same diseases, or risk of diseases not encountered in the home country. Immunizations should be current for age whenever possible. Immunization for specific diseases should also be considered for travel to endemic areas (Table 17–8). For up-to-date details regarding travel to specific countries, physicians should consult the most recent edition of *Health Information for International Travel,* which is published by the CDC and available at the CDC website (www.cdc.gov/travel/yellowbook.pdf) or from the Public Health Foundation (telephone: 877-252-1200). The CDC also maintains the **International Travelers' Hotline** for up-to-date information (telephone: 404-3132-4559) and at the CDC website (www.cdc.gov/travel). Immunization should not be a substitute for other measures, including, but not limited to, avoidance of water or food that may be contaminated, prevention of sexually transmitted diseases, prevention or avoidance of bites by disease-transmitting insects, and avoidance of close contact with wild and domestic animals. (See Chapter 104 for recommendations for travelers.)

BACTERIAL VACCINES

Bacille Calmette-Guérin Vaccine (Tuberculosis)

Although the incidence of disease due to *Mycobacterium tuberculosis* has been comparatively low in developed countries, it is a major cause of morbidity and death worldwide. Isolates with resistance to multiple chemotherapeutic agents have appeared. Primary control of tuberculosis in the United States and many other countries has relied on detection of active cases and contacts and appropriate antituberculosis therapy rather than on immunization.

BCG vaccine is an attenuated live vaccine that was developed between 1910 and 1921 by serial passage of *Mycobacterium bovis* in animals. BCG has been found to protect children against disseminated tuberculosis and tuberculous meningitis, but evidence for the efficacy of BCG in the prevention of pulmonary tuberculosis is conflicting. The mechanisms underlying protection have not been defined, and no serologic methods for determining immune status are available. Cutaneous hypersensitivity is often induced by BCG but rarely exceeds 10 mm of induration, does not predict protection against disease, and typically wanes 10 years after BCG administration. Development of a papule or ulceration at the site of inoculation is believed to indicate immune response to BCG.

Standards for vaccine manufacture from seed BCG strains have been established by the World Health Organization (WHO). The exact efficacy of various licensed preparations in humans is not known, however, because mutations may occur with serial passage of the organism in culture and there is no laboratory correlate for efficacy. In the United States, BCG vaccines produced by two manufacturers are licensed: Organon Teknika Inc., Durham, N.C., and Connaught Laboratories, Willowdale, Ontario. BCG is administered intradermally, on the volar aspect of the forearm, by means of a sterile multiple-puncture disk.

The WHO Expanded Program on Immunization recommends universal immunization of newborn infants with a single dose of BCG in developing countries (Table 17–9). In the United States, BCG vaccine is recommended for persons with extended close contact with an active case of tuberculosis who cannot take isoniazid chemoprophylaxis and for persons with extended close contact with an active case of tuberculosis caused by isoniazid- or rifampin-resistant organisms. BCG is also recommended for health care workers at high risk of drug-resistant tuberculosis when other preventive or control methods are not effective. In persons 2 months of age and older, BCG should be administered only to those with the indications noted herein who have had a negative tuberculin skin test result. Whenever chemotherapy with isoniazid and other agents is feasible, chemotherapy is preferred because of its proven efficacy and because there is some uncertainty concerning the effectiveness of BCG. Reimmunization with BCG is not indicated.

Adverse effects of BCG, which occur in 1–10% of cases, include prolonged ulceration at the site of injection, regional lymphadenopathy, and lupus vulgaris. Osteomyelitis or disseminated infection

TABLE 17–8. Immunization for International Travel

Vaccine	Vaccine Use	Areas of Disease Risk
DTaP/Td	Immunizations should be current for age	Worldwide
HbCV	Immunizations should be current for age	Worldwide
IPV (OPV)	If younger than 18 years of age, all those unimmunized or partially immunized or those with unknown immunizations should have immunizations updated to include a total of at least 3 doses of IPV (can be given at 6-wk intervals). An unimmunized child who cannot be fully immunized before travel should receive a single dose of OPV. Persons 18 years of age or older who have received a primary series of IPV or OPV should receive a booster dose of IPV before travel to areas with endemic polio.	Worldwide, but risk may be higher in developing countries
Hepatitis A	Travelers to, or persons relocating to, areas of high endemicity.	All areas of the world *except:* Canada and the United States, Northern and Western Europe, Australia, New Zealand, and Japan
Hepatitis B	High-risk groups (e.g., health care workers) should complete recommended immunizations before travel to moderate or high prevalence areas even for short periods. Short-term travelers to high prevalence areas who expect to be exposed to blood, to have sexual contact, or to live in close quarters with local residents should also be immunized. Prolonged stay (e.g., 6 mo or longer) in high prevalence area warrants immunization.	Worldwide, but high prevalence exists in East Asia, Southeast Asia, Middle East, Africa, Amazon basin, South America, and in Eskimo and Inuit populations of the United States, Canada, and Greenland. Low prevalence is found in North America, temperate South America, Northern and Western Europe, Australia, and New Zealand. In all other areas, prevalence is intermediate.
Measles	Immunizations should be current for age. If 6–11 months of age monovalent should be given; if 12–14 months of age, MMR should be given. Persons born after 1957 should consider having a second dose of measles vaccine before international travel.	Worldwide
Cholera	Current vaccine has limited efficacy and is not recommended. Cholera risk to travelers is low if only cooked food and boiled water are consumed. Proof of cholera immunization may be required for travel to certain countries.	Tropical areas of Asia, Africa, and recently South America. Cholera is rare elsewhere.
Japanese B encephalitis	Travel to rural areas in warm and rainy seasons or to an endemic area for longer than a few weeks warrants immunization. The vaccine is now licensed in the United States and is available in most countries with endemic disease. Primary series of 3 immunizations with inactivated viral vaccine.	Japan (now rare), Korea, China, Southeast Asia, Indian subcontinent
Meningococcus	Travel to endemic regions or countries with outbreaks caused by vaccine serogroups A, C, Y, and W-135 warrants immunization. A single dose of capsular polysaccharide vaccine should be given ≥2 yr of age.	Endemic in sub-Saharan Africa during rainy season, December through June. Epidemics may occur in other countries; CDC may issue advisories.
Rabies	Occupational risk of animal contact in any country with rabies, high risk of contact with dogs in high prevalence countries, prolonged stay (e.g., more than 30 days) in high prevalence countries warrant immunization.	Almost worldwide. Highest risk in countries with rabid dogs: Central America, northern countries of South America, Indian subcontinent, and Southeast Asia. Rabid dogs also occur in other Asian and South American countries and in Africa.
Typhoid	For persons age 6 yr or older a primary series of either oral or parenteral vaccine should be given for travel to endemic areas where contact with contaminated food and water is anticipated (e.g., rural areas, small towns and villages, nontourist facilities). Children aged 2–6 yr should receive the Vi capsular polysaccharide vaccine.	Rare in developed countries but prevalent in many area of Asia, Africa, and Central and South America.
Yellow fever	Travel to endemic areas, even brief visits to urban areas, warrant immunization. An International Certificate of Vaccination may be required for travel to or from endemic countries. The single dose should be given for those 9 mo of age and older.	Tropical South America and Africa.

TABLE 17–8. Immunization for International Travel *(Continued)*

Vaccine	Vaccine Use	Areas of Disease Risk
Yellow fever *(Continued)*	There is a risk of vaccine-induced encephalitis. The vaccine should be given to infants 6–8 mo of age only if they are traveling to an area with an ongoing epidemic, should be given to infants 4–5 mo of age only in exceptional circumstances, and should never be given to infants younger than 4 mo of age.	
Varicella	Travelers who have not had varicella nor received varicella vaccine should consider receiving varicella vaccine before travel.	Worldwide

TABLE 17–9. Bacterial Vaccines and Their Indications

Vaccine	Indications
Anthrax	Laboratory personnel who work with *Bacillus anthracis*
	Handling of imported, potentially contaminated animal products (e.g., hides, hair)
Bacille Calmette-Guérin (BCG)	Routine immunization of newborn infants in developing countries
	Persons with repeated or extended exposure to isoniazid- and rifampin-resistant strains of *Mycobacterium tuberculosis*
	Persons with extended close contact with an active case of tuberculosis who cannot take isoniazid chemoprophylaxis
	Tuberculin-negative infants and children with two indications above
	Health care workers at high risk of drug-resistant tuberculosis where other preventive or control measures are not effective
Cholera	Travel to an endemic area; efficacy of vaccine is limited and therefore vaccination not recommended
	May be required for travel to certain countries
Diphtheria (DTaP, DTP, DT, Td)	Routine immunization of all infants beginning at 2 mo of age (not needed after age 6 yr)
	Persons with sickle cell disease, anatomic or functional asplenia, Hodgkin's disease
Meningococcal	Sickle cell disease, anatomic or functional asplenia, deficiency of terminal complement components
	Military recruits
	College-bound students, particularly those who will live in dormitories, should be informed about risks of meningococcal disease and offered option of immunization
	Travel to an area with increased risk of diseases (e.g., sub-Saharan Africa)
Pertussis: DTaP (or DTP)	Routine immunization of infants beginning at 2 mo of age and extending through age 6 yr
	After exposure to pertussis, primary DTaP series brought up-to-date if not current and age under 7 yr
Pneumococcal conjugate vaccine	Routine immunization of infants between 2 mo and 2 yr of age
	High risk of pneumococcal disease in children aged 24 to 59 mo: sickle cell disease, asplenia, congenital immunodeficiencies, immunosuppressive therapy, chronic cardiac disease, chronic pulmonary disease, chronic renal insufficiency, nephrotic syndrome, diabetes mellitus, cerebrospinal fluid leaks
	Moderate risk of pneumococcal disease: children aged 25 to 35 mo, children 36 to 59 mo of age who attend out-of-home day care, children 36 to 59 mo of age who are of Native American or African American descent
Pneumococcal polysaccharide	High risk of pneumococcal disease in children aged 24 to 59 mo: sickle cell disease, asplenia, congenital immunodeficiencies, immunosuppressive therapy, chronic cardiac disease, chronic pulmonary disease, chronic renal insufficiency, nephrotic syndrome, diabetes mellitus, cerebrospinal fluid leaks
Plague	Regular contact with potentially infected rodents or their fleas (e.g., biologists, laboratory workers)
	Travel to an area where plague occurs and there are rat infestations
Tetanus (DTaP, DTP, DT, Td)	Routine immunization of infants beginning at 2 mo of age (DTP) and extending through adult life (Td)
	Wound prophylaxis
Typhoid	Travel to endemic areas (e.g., Africa, Asia, and South and Central America if exposure to contaminated food or water is likely)
	Persistent household contact with a *Salmonella typhi* carrier
	Persons with repeated laboratory exposure to *S. typhi*
Tularemia	Occupational exposure to infected animal and insect (e.g., biologists, laboratory workers)

is found very rarely, typically occurring in immunocompromised persons. BCG is contraindicated in persons with proven or suspected cellular or combined immunocompromise and in persons receiving immunosuppressive therapy, including systemic corticosteroid therapy, because of the risk of disseminated infection. BCG is also contraindicated in infants and children with HIV infection in the United States, where the risk of tuberculosis is low, again because of the risk of disseminated BCG infection. The WHO recommends BCG immunization despite HIV infection in countries with substantial tuberculosis risk, however. BCG should not be used during pregnancy or in persons with burns.

Cholera Vaccine

Vibrio cholerae secretes a potent toxin that causes cholera. A phenol-killed whole-cell cholera vaccine has been in use for decades but has limited efficacy that lasts only 3–6 months. Reimmunization is required every 6 months. Killed whole-cell vaccines, with or without the purified B subunit of cholera toxins, have been evaluated in field trials, but efficacy was only approximately 50%. Two doses of cholera vaccine 1–4 weeks apart are administered intramuscularly or subcutaneously at doses that vary with age: 0.2 mL for children from 6 months to 4 years of age, 0.3 mL for children 5–10 years of age, and 0.5 mL for all individuals beyond age 10 years. Cholera vaccine is not recommended for infants younger than 6 months.

Cholera vaccine is not recommended before travel to endemic areas because the risk of cholera in travelers is very low, the vaccines efficacy is low, and cholera can be prevented by avoidance of potentially contaminated food and water. However, for travel to or between certain countries, immigration officials require a single dose of cholera vaccine. Immunization with cholera vaccine may interfere with the immune response to yellow fever vaccine, so these vaccines should be administered at least 3 weeks apart. Oral cholera vaccines have been developed and administered in field trials, but none has been licensed.

Diphtheria Toxoid

Diphtheria is caused by *Corynebacterium diphtheriae,* which produces a potent exotoxin that causes cell damage by inhibition of protein synthesis. Diphtheria toxin enters the circulation and causes organ damage at distant sites, particularly myocarditis and toxic peripheral neuritis. The severe complications of diphtheria can be prevented or ameliorated by circulating toxin-neutralizing antibodies, but antibodies have no effect once the toxin has entered the cell. Diphtheria toxoid induces neutralizing antibodies (antitoxin). Levels of at least 0.01 U/mL are generally regarded as protective.

Widespread universal immunization with formalin-inactivated diphtheria toxoid has resulted in a marked decline in the incidence of disease in Western countries. From 1980 to 2000, fewer than five cases of respiratory tract diphtheria were reported annually in the United States. Ninety-seven percent of schoolchildren in the United States have protective titers from primary immunization, and this is believed to be the reason that diphtheria is such a rare disease. Immunization does not, however, prevent nasopharyngeal acquisition or person-to-person transmission of *C. diphtheriae.* Antitoxin antibody is demonstrable in only some individuals after recovery from respiratory tract diphtheria, so immunization with diphtheria toxoid is recommended. Cutaneous diphtheria is more likely to induce immunity.

Formalin-inactivated diphtheria toxoid is combined with tetanus toxoid (DT and Td) with or without **whole-cell or acellular pertussis vaccine (DTP or DTaP).** These preparations are adsorbed on aluminum phosphate or aluminum hydroxide, and thimerosal is added as a preservative. The amount of diphtheria toxoid in pediatric preparations, measured in flocculation units (Lf), is between 10 and 20 Lf but varies among manufacturers. Vaccines containing diphtheria toxoid are indicated for routine immunization of infants and children, followed by booster immunizations throughout adult life at 10-year intervals. Diphtheria toxoid should also be given to those exposed to diphtheria and to those who recover from diphtheria. Preparations for adult use (Td) contain no more than 2 Lf of diphtheria toxoid, a dose that provides adequate immunogenicity without increasing the frequency of adverse reactions, in comparison with tetanus toxoid alone. Adverse reactions include local pain at the injection site and mild systemic symptoms. Reactions observed during the early development of diphtheria toxoid were markedly reduced by purification of diphtheria toxin and reduction in dosage.

Haemophilus influenzae Type b Vaccines

H. influenzae type b was the leading cause of bacterial meningitis in infants and children before the introduction of *H. influenzae* type b vaccine. The capsular polysaccharide of *H. influenzae* type b is a major virulence factor, enabling the organism to evade phagocytosis. A vaccine composed of purified capsular polysaccharide was licensed in 1985 for use in children ≥2 years of age. This vaccine induced a thymic-independent immune response characterized by no T-cell recruitment, which resulted in poor immune responses in young infants and little or no booster response. Because this vaccine was unable to protect young infants who are at the highest risk of *H. influenzae* type b disease, the polysaccharide has been covalently linked, or conjugated, to protein carriers. These ***H. influenzae*** **type b conjugate vaccines (HbCV)** induce thymic-dependent immune responses with recruitment of T cells. Immune responses to these vaccines are of greater magnitude than for the polysaccharide vaccine and demonstrate booster responses with subsequent doses. Some antibody response to the carrier protein is detectable but is not protective and does not substitute for vaccination against the organism from which the carrier is derived. The success of conjugate *H. influenzae* type b vaccines has prompted the rapid development of conjugate vaccines against *S. pneumoniae* and also for *N. meningitidis.*

Since licensure and implementation of routine HbCV immunization of infants beginning at 2 months of age, the decline in the incidence of meningitis and other invasive *H. influenzae* type b diseases has been dramatic. In addition, these conjugate vaccines reduce the rate of nasopharyngeal carriage of *H. influenzae* type b. Hence they may reduce the spread of the organism to susceptible contacts. The serum antibody concentration, as measured by radioimmunoassay, that provides long-term protection after immunization is estimated to be 1 μg/mL. A concentration of 0.15 μg/mL is believed to be adequate to provide protection against immediate infection. Immunization with HbCV does not protect against *H. influenzae* encapsulated strains other than type b or against unencapsulated strains.

Three *H. influenzae* type b protein conjugate vaccines are licensed in the United States. A fourth vaccine, *H. influenzae* type b diphtheria toxoid conjugate vaccine (PRP-D [polyribosylribitol phosphate with diphtheria vaccine]), was less immunogenic in young children. It was licensed only for the booster dose and not for primary immunization of infants. This vaccine is no longer produced.

H. influenzae type b–diphtheria CRM_{197} (HbOC [cross reacting membrane protein conjugate vaccine]) is composed of oligosaccharide units of type b saccharide linked to a mutant diphtheria protein. HbOC, manufactured by Wyeth Lederle Vaccines as HibTITER, is formulated to contain 10 μg of purified *H. influenzae* type b polysaccharide and approximately 25 μg of CRM_{197} protein. HbOC is administered as a 0.5 mL dose by intramuscular injection and is approved for use in a four-dose schedule at 2, 4, 6, and 15 months of age. Few infants have an immune response after the first dose, but the majority have a clear response after the second dose. After two doses, protective efficacy has been virtually 100% in a clinical trial. HbOC should not be used for immunization against diphtheria.

H. influenzae type b–meningococcal protein conjugate vaccine (PRP-OMP [polyribosylribitol phosphate–outer membrane protein]) is composed of capsular polysaccharide linked to an outer membrane protein of *Neisseria meningitidis* serogroup B. PRP-OMP, manufactured by Merck as PedvaxHIB, is a lyophilized vaccine that, when reconstituted with aluminum hydroxide diluent, contains 25 μg of polysaccharide and 250 μg meningococcal outer membrane protein complex. PRP-OMP is administered by intramuscular injection in a three-dose schedule at 2, 4, and 12 months of age. PRP-OMP induces an immune response in the majority of infants when a single dose is administered at 2 months of age. After a second dose at age 4 months, most of the remaining infants mount an immune response. Unlike other conjugate vaccines, a marked booster response is not seen after the second dose. When the third dose is administrated at 12 months of age, a booster response occurs. The significance of these differences has not been elucidated. Since most infants develop an antibody response to PRP-OMP after the first dose, this vaccine is preferred for immunization of high risk populations where disease onset is often in the first few months of life, such as Alaskan natives groups. Whether immune responses to the meningococcal outer membrane component provide protection against meningococcal infection is not known.

H. influenzae type b–tetanus toxoid conjugate vaccine (PRP-T) is manufactured by Aventis Pasteur and is distributed by Aventis Pasteur (ActHIB) and by GlaxoSmithKline (OmniHIB). The vaccine contains 10 μg PRP and 24 μg tetanus toxoid in 0.5 mL and may be used to immunize infants beginning at 2 months of age. It may also be combined in the same syringe with Aventis Pasteur DTaP vaccine (Tripedia) in infants 15–18 months of age. A first dose administered at 2 months of age induces an immune response in most infants, and almost all infants show a substantial response after the second dose at 4 months of age.

H. influenzae type b conjugate vaccines are recommended for universal immunization of infants beginning at 2 months of age. Because the immune response to *H. influenzae* type b conjugate vaccines is greater with increasing age, fewer doses of vaccine are required when immunization is initiated at older ages. After 15 months of age, a single dose of any of the three licensed vaccines is adequate. Although HbCVs from different manufacturers induce different patterns of immune response in infants, the vaccines should be considered interchangeable. Moreover, if primary immunization is initiated with PRP-OMP, a second dose of PRP-OMP is preferable to complete the primary series, but any conjugate vaccine would be suitable for a booster dose at 12–15 months of age. If more than one type of HbCV is used for primary immunization of infants or if the type is unknown, three doses should be given during infancy, followed by a booster dose at 12–15 months of age.

Children younger than 2 years of age who develop invasive *H. influenzae* disease should receive age-appropriate immunization with HbCV because natural disease does not reliably induce immunity in infants and young children. Adverse reactions to this vaccine are limited to moderate systemic symptoms and mild reactions at the injection site. HbCV should not be used for prevention after exposure in households or daycare centers because it is not known to be effective after exposure. Chemoprophylaxis with rifampin is recommended for prevention in these settings (Chapter 36).

Lyme Disease Vaccine

Lyme disease is caused by the tickborne spirochete *Borrelia burgdorferi.* A vaccine consisting of recombinant outer surface protein A (rOspA) induces antibodies directed against the **OspA** lipoprotein, which is expressed by the spirochete primarily while it is in the tick and less so when the spirochete has infected humans. The effectiveness of the vaccine appears to depend on antibody entering the tick while the tick is ingesting a blood meal. Thus an adequate concentration of anti-OspA antibody is thought to be important for protection, and an amnestic human response presumably has no role in protection.

The vaccine is approximately 80% effective for the prevention of Lyme disease. It is licensed for persons 15–70 years of age and may be licensed for children in the future. Two doses of vaccine are given 1–2 months apart, followed by a third (booster) dose after 6 months. Whether additional doses are required to boost antibody concentrations in subsequent years for persons at continued risk of having Lyme disease has not been established.

Vaccine against Lyme disease should be considered for persons ≥15 years of age who live in or travel to areas where Lyme disease is endemic and who will be at high or moderate risk of tick exposure in the course of work or recreational activities in tick-infested habitats. However, precise quantification of risk is not possible, and the cost-effectiveness of immunization against Lyme disease has not been established. It is not clear that vaccination against Lyme disease is better than taking precautions to avoid tick bites or receiving timely treatment of Lyme disease when it occurs. The vaccine should not be a substitute for personal precautions to avoid tick bites, nor should it be given to persons who are at low risk or to those who do not live in or expect to travel to endemic areas. Immunization of persons with a history of Lyme disease should be considered for those at continued risk, but persons with treatment-resistant chronic arthritis should not receive the vaccine because of possible increased immune reactivity to rOspA. Vaccine against Lyme disease should not be given to pregnant women because safety has not been established. The manufacturer, GlaxoSmithKline (800-366-8900, ext. 5231), has established a vaccine pregnancy registry for monitoring the effects of the vaccine in cases in which it was inadvertently administered during pregnancy.

Meningococcal Vaccine

Meningococcal disease, caused by *N. meningitidis,* is endemic worldwide, with peak incidence of endemic disease in infants in the first year of life or, during epidemics, in school-age children and adolescents. Persons with deficiencies of the terminal complement components or asplenia appear to be at increased risk of having meningococcal disease. Nine serogroups, based on capsular polysaccharide composition (A, B, C, D, X, Y, Z, 29-E, and W-135), cause disease in humans. Serogroups C, B, and Y have been responsible for outbreaks in recent years, and these three serogroups plus W-135 have been responsible for most sporadic cases in the United States. Serogroup A of *N. meningitidis,* which is rare in the United States, causes epidemic disease in other countries. During the 1990s there was an increase in the proportion of meningococcal disease caused by serogroups C and Y in the United States. It also became apparent that adults 18–20 years of age have an increased incidence of meningococcal disease in the United States and that college students living in dormitories are at increased risk. Other risk factors include low socioeconomic status, crowding, bar patronage, exposure to tobacco smoke, and prior upper respiratory tract infection.

Group A meningococcal polysaccharide induces an immune response in very few 3-month-old infants; 85% of 1-year-old children demonstrate seroconversion. A second dose induces an anamnestic response even in those initially immunized at 3 months of age. In field trials, protective efficacy of group A meningococcal polysaccharide vaccine ranged between 85% and 100% in children more than 1 year of age and in adults. In another study, efficacy was 89% during the first year after immunization but declined to 62% by the end of the third year in children 3 months to 16 years of age. In children younger than 4 years of age, efficacy was 10% after 3 years. Group B meningococcal polysaccharide is not immunogenic in humans, presumably because of immunologic tolerance. The group B meningococcal polysaccharide has sialic acid oligosaccharide linkages that are also found in fetal and neonatal nervous tissue. Immune responses to group C meningococcal polysaccharide vaccine are poor in infants younger than 2 years, decline more rapidly than those induced by group A meningococcal vaccine, and do not boost with a second dose. In field trials, group C meningococcal vaccine was 90% efficacious in adults and 75% protective in children 25–36 months of age, but the vaccine failed to protect infants 6–24 months of age. Polysaccharides of serogroups Y and W-135 meningococcus are immunogenic in adults and in children 2 years of age and older, but efficacy data are not available.

Meningococcal polysaccharide-protein conjugate vaccines to serogroups A, C, Y, and W-135 have been developed and demonstrate improved immunogenicity in infants. A meningococcal serogroup C polysaccharide-protein conjugate vaccine has been licensed and used in Great Britain, resulting in a marked decline in serogroup C meningococcal disease. Meningococcal protein conjugate vaccines have not yet been licensed in the United States. Vaccines for serogroup B meningococcal disease, composed of protein antigens, have been used to control outbreaks in Scandinavia and South America but are not licensed in the United States.

The meningococcal vaccine currently licensed in the United States is quadrivalent vaccine manufactured by Connaught and contains 50 μg of each of serogroups A, C, Y, and W-135 polysaccharides per dose. A 0.5 mL dose is administered subcutaneously. Adverse reactions consist of mild local reactions at the injection site, and up to 2% of children have fever.

Meningococcal vaccine is indicated in persons aged 2 years and older with sickle cell disease, anatomic or functional asplenia, deficiency of terminal complement components, or Hodgkin's disease. Military recruits routinely receive meningococcal vaccine. Travel to endemic areas with increased risk of disease, such as sub-Saharan Africa during the dry season, September through June, and epidemics caused by one of the four serogroups are additional indications. It is also recommended that students bound for college and their parents, particularly if the student will live in a dormitory, should be informed of the increased risk of meningococcal disease associated with attending college and should be offered the option of receiving meningococcal vaccine before college entry. Meningococcal vaccine does not prevent nasopharyngeal colonization with *N. meningitidis.* Under epidemic conditions, meningococcal vaccine may be given to household contacts as an adjunct to, but not a substitute for, chemoprophylaxis, because an antibody to immunization may take 7–14 days to develop and many secondary cases occur during this period. Second attacks of meningococcal disease with the same serogroup are rare, and immunization after recovery from disease has not been recommended. The duration of immunity after immunization is not known but has been estimated from serologic studies to be as short as 3 years in young children and as long as 10 years in adults. Revaccination after 3–5 years should be considered if the person is still at risk.

Pertussis Vaccine

Pertussis is caused by *Bordetella pertussis,* which attaches to the epithelium of the upper respiratory tract and produces several extracellular toxins (Table 67–8) that disrupt cilia, inhibit local host defenses, and have toxic effects on cells at distant sites. **Pertussis toxin** is believed to be responsible for effects at distant sites and for the prolonged coughing characteristic of pertussis. Clinical disease probably confers long-lasting immunity against severe disease but not against milder coughing illnesses, and the antigen specificities of antibodies responsible for protection have not been fully defined.

Whole-cell vaccines consisting of inactivated whole *B. pertussis* bacteria have been used for universal immunization of infants since the 1940s and are used in many countries. Whole-cell pertussis vaccines greatly reduced pertussis morbidity and mortality but frequently caused marked adverse effects. Acellular pertussis vaccines, composed of purified pertussis antigens, were developed, in part to improve the safety of pertussis vaccines, and are now the preferred vaccines for prevention of pertussis in the United States and many other countries. These vaccines contain purified, inactivated pertussis toxin and may also contain up to four additional protein antigens. Pertussis toxin is an extracellular protein toxin that is believed to produce many of the clinical manifestations of whooping cough. Filamentous hemagglutinin (FHA) is a protein that mediates attachment of *B. pertussis* to respiratory epithelium. Three surface proteins, pertactin, fimbriae 2, and fimbriae 3, are immunogenic surface proteins of uncertain pathogenic role. All five antigens (pertussis toxin, FHA, pertactin, fimbriae 2, and fimbriae 3) induce protection against *B. pertussis* infection in animals when given separately. In humans, pertussis toxoid is the principal protective antigen and is 70–75% efficacious for prevention of clinical whooping cough. The addition of FHA improves efficacy slightly. Because clinical trials of pertussis vaccine were not designed to determine systematically whether each additional antigen provided additional protection, the merits of each additional antigen are not known. Vaccines with three to five antigens achieve efficacy of 85% for protection against clinical pertussis, and all acellular pertussis vaccines achieve protection in the same range as that achieved by whole-cell pertussis vaccines.

Four acellular pertussis vaccines have been licensed in the United States, but two (ACEL-Imune and Certiva) have been withdrawn for commercial reasons. Tripedia (Aventis Pasteur) is a two-antigen vaccine composed of 23.4 μg each of formalin-inactivated pertussis toxoid and FHA; it is manufactured by the Research Foundation for Microbial Diseases of Osaka University (Biken), Japan, and is combined with diphtheria and tetanus toxoids. The vaccine does not contain pertactin or fimbriae. After a 3-year follow-up, a two-dose regimen of Biken-type vaccine in Swedish infants was shown to be 77% efficacious against all culture-confirmed pertussis and 92% against pertussis with cough lasting 30 days or longer. ActHIB (PRP-T) reconstituted with Tripedia is licensed for the fourth dose of pertussis vaccination. Infanrix (GlaxoSmithKline) is a three-antigen acellular pertussis vaccine composed of purified pertussis toxoid, FHA, and pertactin and combined with diphtheria and tetanus toxoids. This vaccine was 85% efficacious in a field trial for prevention of clinical pertussis.

Acellular pertussis vaccines combined with diphtheria and tetanus toxoids (DTaP vaccines) are indicated for universal immunization beginning at 2 months of age. A primary series of three doses is recommended at approximately 2, 4, and 6 months of age, followed by booster doses at 15–18 months of age and a fifth dose at 4–6 years of age. If there is a community pertussis outbreak, immunization may be initiated as early as 6 weeks of age and doses can be given every 4 weeks. Pertussis immunization after 7 years of age is not recommended; however, immunity wanes after 5–10 years, leaving many adolescents and adults susceptible to pertussis. Nevertheless, to date there has been no recommendation for immunization of adults and adolescents with acellular pertussis vaccines.

Anecdotal reports suggest that immunization after disease exposure may be of benefit. Household or other close contacts should have immunization with pertussis vaccine initiated or brought up-to-date according to recommended schedules. Children less than 7 years of age who have received three previous DTP or DTaP immunizations, with the last dose administered more than 6 months before exposure, should receive a booster dose. Those younger than 7 years who have received four previous DTP or DTaP immunizations, with the last dose administered more than 3 years earlier, should also receive a booster immunization. However, postexposure immunization should not be the sole preventive measure. Chemoprophylaxis with erythromycin or another appropriate antibiotic is indicated for all close contacts after disease exposure regardless of immunization status.

Acellular pertussis vaccines cause fewer adverse effects than whole-cell pertussis vaccines. Local reactions include pain, tenderness, redness, swelling, and induration at the injection site, and more uncommon reactions include swelling of the entire limb after the fourth or fifth dose of vaccine and, rarely, sterile abscess. Local reactions resolve spontaneously without sequelae. Common systemic reactions include anorexia, vomiting, lethargy, irritability, and low-grade fevers that also resolve spontaneously. Allergic reactions, such as urticaria, unless they appear immediately, do not carry a risk of anaphylaxis and are not a contraindication to subsequent immunization. The risk of anaphylaxis after administration of DTaP vaccine is remote. Of the more severe adverse effects associated with whole-cell pertussis vaccines, high fever (40.5°C or greater), prolonged crying, and hypotonic-hyporesponsive episodes have been observed after administration of DTaP vaccines but appear to be rare effects. Similarly, febrile convulsions are also less frequent. Acellular pertussis vaccines have not been causally associated with permanent neurologic deficits.

Despite the safety of acellular pertussis (and DTaP) vaccines, many of the contraindications and precautions that evolved with whole-cell DTP vaccines persist. Immediate anaphylaxis is a contraindication to any further immunization with any of the antigens in DTaP vaccines. Encephalopathy occurring within 7 days of DTaP vaccine is a contraindication to further immunization with pertussis vaccine. Precautions include febrile or afebrile seizures within 3 days; persistent, inconsolable crying for 3 hours or more within 2 days; collapse or shocklike state within 2 days; and unexplained fever with temperature greater than or equal to 40.5°C (104.9°F) within 2 days. Although the risks of subsequent immunization are unknown after these events, whenever any of these precautionary events occur, the decision not to immunize with pertussis vaccine must be weighed against the risk of pertussis disease.

Another concern is that immunization with DTaP vaccines in infants and children with neurologic disorders will result in the vaccines' being blamed as the cause of these disorders. In general, children with unstable or evolving neurologic conditions and those in whom the diagnosis is uncertain should have pertussis immunization deferred until the condition becomes stable or the diagnosis becomes established. However, children with stable neurologic conditions, including those with controlled seizure disorders, should be immunized. A family history of seizures is not a contraindication to pertussis immunization. When children with a history of seizures are immunized, administration of acetaminophen for fever control is recommended. If pertussis immunization is deferred during the first year of life, the use of diphtheria and tetanus toxoids can also be deferred because the risk of these diseases is extremely low in the first year of life in the United States. However, in the second year of life, if pertussis vaccination must still be deferred, then immunization with diphtheria-tetanus toxoids (DT) should be undertaken.

Pneumococcal Vaccines

Pneumococcal disease, caused by *Streptococcus pneumoniae,* is the predominant cause of otitis media and bacteremia in infants and young children and is also a common cause of pneumonia, sinusitis, and meningitis in all age groups. Certain individuals have increased mortality rates for bacteremic pneumococcal infection, including children with congenital immunodeficiencies, sickle cell disease, asplenia, splenic dysfunction, or AIDS and children receiving immunosuppressive therapy for cancer or after organ transplantation. Children with diabetes, cyanotic heart disease, congestive heart failure, chronic pulmonary disease, and renal insufficiency are also believed to be at increased risk for developing systemic pneumococcal infections. Children with nephrotic syndrome are particularly susceptible to pneumococcal peritonitis. Children with communications between the subarachnoid space and the respiratory tract, such as those with basal skull fractures, are at risk of having recurrent pneumococcal meningitis. Certain other groups are at moderate risk, including children 24–35 months of age, children 36–59 months of age who attend out-of-home daycare, and children who are of Native American or African American descent.

A polysaccharide capsule enables *S. pneumoniae* to avoid phagocytosis and intracellular killing. There are more than 90 capsular serotypes, but types 14, 6, 18, 19, 23, 4, 9, 7, 1, and 3 are responsible for most disease in children. Phagocytosis of pneumococci opsonized with type-specific anticapsular antibody is an important defense mechanism against systemic pneumococcal infection. The risk of pneumococcal disease is highest during the month after acquisition of a new serotype, but prolonged carriage does not increase the risk of disease.

Polysaccharide Pneumococcal Vaccines. Pneumococcal vaccines composed of purified capsular polysaccharides induce type-specific immunity, but like other polysaccharide vaccines, they often fail to induce immune responses in infants and children younger than 2 years of age. Some serotypes (e.g., type 3) induce immune responses in infants, whereas other types (e.g., types 14 and 19) induce immune responses in children older than 2 years. In contrast, type 6 is poorly immunogenic even in children. The currently licensed polysaccharide vaccines are composed of 23 separate capsular polysaccharides, which account for serotypes causing more than 95% of cases of bacteremia and meningitis and 85% of cases of otitis media in children. Pneumococcal vaccine has been shown to reduce pneumococcal bacteremia in children with sickle cell disease and asplenia. In adults, vaccine efficacy for invasive disease is approximately 50% but is lower with advanced age and with immunocompromise. Pneumococcal polysaccharide vaccine does not prevent colonization of the nasopharynx and thus does not affect transmission of the organism. Merck and Lederle each manufacture a 23-valent pneumococcal polysaccharide vaccine containing 25 μg of each polysaccharide per milliliter of vaccine. Pneumococcal vaccines may be administered either intramuscularly or subcutaneously. Adverse reactions are limited to mild transient local reactions at the injection site. Systemic symptoms, except occasional low-grade fever, are rare. Early studies of revaccination with pneumococcal vaccine suggested that the incidence of local reactions increased with the second immunization, but subsequent studies show that most persons can be reimmunized safely. Pneumococcal vaccine is not indicated for immunization of children younger than 2 years. In children older than 2 years, pneumococcal polysaccharide vaccine is recommended only for high-risk patients previously immunized with pneumococcal conjugate vaccine to increase protection against the additional pneumococcal serotypes in the polysaccharide vaccine.

Pneumococcal Conjugate Vaccines. In 2000, pneumococcal polysaccharide/oligosaccharide–diphtheria CRM_{197} conjugate vaccine (Prevnar) containing the capsular polysaccharides of the seven most common pneumococcal serotypes was licensed in the United States for prevention of invasive pneumococcal disease. This vaccine contains 4 μg of type 6B polysaccharide; 2 μg of each of types 4, 9V, 14, 19F, and 23F polysaccharides; and 2 μg of type 18C oligosaccharide, all conjugated to diphtheria protein CRM_{197}. This vaccine was 90% efficacious for the prevention of pneumococcal bacteremia in children and decreased the incidence of radiologically confirmed pneumonia by one third. The efficacy of the vaccine against acute otitis media caused by vaccine serotypes was approximately 60%, but an increase of 30% of acute otitis media episodes caused by nonvaccine serotypes resulted in an overall reduction of only 30% for all episodes of pneumococcal acute otitis media. The overall reduction of clinical episodes of all acute otitis media episodes was less than 10%, but there was a larger effect on recurrent acute otitis media, resulting in a 25% reduction in the use of tympanostomy tube insertion among vaccinees. Pneumococcal conjugate vaccine (PCV) reduces nasopharyngeal colonization by *S. pneumoniae* vaccine strains by approximately 50%. Immunization of children in daycare centers with PCV reduces transmission of pneumococci to their siblings at home. Pneumococcal–diphtheria CRM_{197} conjugate vaccines containing capsular antigens of 9 and 11 pneumococcal serotypes are under development and are expected to be licensed in the near future.

PCVs using other protein carriers are also being developed. Polysaccharides conjugated with tetanus and diphtheria toxoids have been shown to be safe and immunogenic and to reduce nasopharyngeal carriage of *S. pneumoniae.* A seven-valent PCV containing pneumococcal polysaccharides conjugated to an outer membrane protein of *N. meningitidis* has been shown to be safe and immunogenic and to reduce pneumococcal acute otitis media by 30%, an effect similar to that of the licensed diphtheria CRM_{197} conjugate. To date, the diphtheria CRM_{197} protein conjugate vaccine is the only PCV licensed in the United States. Four doses of PCV are recommended for universal immunization of healthy infants beginning as early as 6 weeks of age (Table 17–1). Infants immunized between 6 and 23 months of age should receive a reduced number of doses (Table 17–3).

Infants 24–59 months and older who are at high risk of pneumococcal disease, including those with sickle cell disease, asplenia, primary immunodeficiency, HIV infection, and immunosuppressive therapy, should complete PCV immunization before age 2 years; after age 2 years they should receive a dose of pneumococcal polysaccharide vaccine to expand serotype coverage. Children who have received four doses of PCV should be given a dose of 23-valent polysaccharide vaccine at least 6–8 weeks after the last dose of PCV. Children who have received 1–3 doses of PCV before 24 months of age should be given a single additional dose of PCV at least 6–8 weeks after the last dose of PCV, followed by a dose of polysaccharide vaccine at least 6–8 weeks later. An additional dose of polysaccharide vaccine should be given no earlier than 3–5 years after the initial dose of polysaccharide vaccine. Children 24–59 months of age who have received only a single previous dose of prior polysaccharide vaccine should receive two doses of PCV at an interval of 6–8 weeks. PCV immunization should be started no earlier than 6–8 weeks after the last dose of polysaccharide vaccine, and an additional dose of polysaccharide vaccine is recommended 3–5 years later. High-risk children 24–59 months of age who have received no previous doses of either polysaccharide vaccine or PCV should receive two doses of PCV given at an interval of 6–8 weeks, followed by a single dose of polysaccharide vaccine at least 6–8 weeks after the last dose of PCV and by an additional dose of polysaccharide vaccine 3–5 years after the previous dose.

Children 24–59 months of age at moderate risk of pneumococcal disease include those who receive out-of-home childcare and Native American and African American children. Additional factors that may be considered are crowding, homelessness, exposure to household tobacco smoke, history of recurrent otitis media, and tympanostomy tube placement in the previous year. If not previously immunized in the first 2 years of life, these children should be considered for either PCV or polysaccharide vaccine. However, some children may not have adequate immune responses to some of the serotypes in the polysaccharide vaccine, so PCV may be preferred. Furthermore, some groups such as Native Americans should receive a dose of PCV followed 6–8 weeks later by the polysaccharide vaccine.

Tetanus Toxoid

Tetanus is a severe neuromuscular disease caused by **tetanospasmin,** commonly called **tetanus toxin** and produced by *Clostridium tetani.* Tetanus rarely, if ever, induces protective antibody, but the disease can be prevented or ameliorated by tetanus toxin neutralizing antibodies of either human or animal origin. Active immunization with formalin-inactivated tetanus toxoid induces such antibodies. An antitoxin antibody concentration of 0.01 IU/mL is considered protective, but this level is not absolute. With universal immunization using tetanus toxoid, tetanus has become rare, with fewer than 50 cases reported annually in the United States. In developing countries, immunization of women of childbearing age with at least two doses of tetanus toxoid, either before pregnancy or during the third trimester of pregnancy, reduces the mortality from tetanus neonatorum.

Tetanus toxoid is prepared by formalin inactivation of purified tetanus toxin. The toxoid is formulated as a monovalent preparation or combined with diphtheria toxoid (DT and Td) or with both diphtheria toxoid and pertussis vaccine (DTP and DTaP). Most preparations contain 4–5 Lf of tetanus toxoid and are adsorbed on aluminum phosphate or aluminum hydroxide. Thimerosal is added as a preservative. Monovalent tetanus toxoid may be either in fluid (4–10 Lf) or in adsorbed form. Adsorbed vaccine induces protective antibody levels after three doses, whereas four doses of fluid vaccine are required to induce a comparable immune response. Adsorbed toxoid must be administered intramuscularly, but fluid toxoid may also be given subcutaneously.

Tetanus toxoid is among the most immunogenic vaccines. Antibody responses are induced even in newborn infants. Vaccines containing tetanus toxoid are indicated for universal immunization beginning at 2 months of age and extending throughout adult life (Tables 17–1, 17–2, and 17–3). Intervals of 1 month between primary immunizations are adequate for achieving a protective response. After primary immunization, booster doses of tetanus and diphtheria toxoids for adult use (Td) are recommended at 10-year intervals to maintain adequate levels of neutralizing antibody.

Tetanus toxoid vaccines should also be given for presumed exposure to tetanus, that is, to those individuals with possibly contaminated wounds (Table 17–7). Td, rather than tetanus toxoid alone, should be given because most people also benefit from booster immunization with diphtheria toxoid. For those with contaminated wounds, puncture wounds, and those with devitalized tissue who are not known with certainty to have had at least three previous doses of tetanus toxoid, tetanus immune globulin administered at a separate site is also indicated (Chapter 48). Tetanus immune globulin and other immune globulins do not interfere with the active immune response to tetanus toxoid.

The most common adverse reactions to immunization with tetanus toxoid are local pain and swelling at the injection site. These reactions are more frequent with successive doses of tetanus toxoid. Use of the combined preparation, Td, is associated with no more than a minimal increase in local reactions compared with the use of tetanus toxoid alone. Persons who have severe local reactions to tetanus toxoid often have elevated levels of circulating antitoxin antibody. These persons should not receive further doses of tetanus toxoid without monitoring of serum antitoxin levels. Some persons have fever and mild systemic symptoms after administration of tetanus toxoid, but these reactions are usually transient. Immediate hypersensitivity reactions such as anaphylaxis are extremely rare. Peripheral neuropathy that occurs a few hours to several weeks after administration of tetanus toxoid is rare and seems to be mediated by formation of immune complexes. Immediate severe hypersensitivity reactions and neurologic events after immunization with tetanus toxoid are contraindications to further administration.

Typhoid Vaccines

Typhoid is an acute illness caused by ingestion of food or water contaminated with *Salmonella typhi.* Immunity to *S. typhi* is complex and appears to include local secretory immunity in the gut to prevent mucosal invasion, circulating antibody to limit bloodborne dissemination, and cellular immunity directed against intracellular organisms. Natural infection induces partial immunity that may be overcome by ingestion of a large number of organisms. Multiple factors contribute to the virulence of *S. typhi,* including Vi polysaccharide capsule, O lipo-oligosaccharide, and H flagellar antigens. The Vi polysaccharide and O lipo-oligosaccharide appear to enable *S. typhi* to survive intracellularly. Typhoid is endemic in most developing countries, and in the United States most cases occur in persons who have traveled to other countries.

Since the first parenteral vaccine was developed in 1896 by inactivating whole *S. typhi* with heat and adding phenol as a preservative, a variety of typhoid vaccines have been made. No vaccine provides completely satisfactory protection. Three different types of typhoid vaccines have been licensed in the United States: (1) an oral live-attenuated vaccine, (2) a parenteral inactivated (heat-phenol) vaccine, and (3) a parenteral capsular polysaccharide vaccine. A fourth vaccine, an acetone-inactivated parenteral vaccine, is currently available only to the armed forces. No prospective comparative trials have been conducted, but the efficacy of each vaccine has been demonstrated in field trials.

Either parenteral or oral typhoid vaccine is indicated for immunization of travelers to developing countries, particularly countries in Asia, Africa, and Latin America with endemic typhoid, when prolonged exposure to potentially contaminated water or food is expected. However, immunization is not a substitute for consumption of purified water and foods that have been prepared properly, because vaccines are not 100% effective and the vaccine's protection may be overwhelmed by large inocula of *S. typhi.* Immunization is also indicated for persons with intimate exposure (e.g., household contact) to a documented *S. typhi* carrier and for laboratory technicians with repeated exposure to *S. typhi.* Routine immunization of schoolchildren with typhoid vaccine is also practiced in some countries with substantial typhoid risk. Typhoid vaccine is not indicated for prevention of secondary cases in common-source outbreaks or after natural disasters, including floods. Routine vaccination of sewage sanitation workers is not indicated in the United States but may be implemented in typhoid-endemic areas.

The licensed vaccines vary by contraindications, adverse reactions, lower age limits for use among children, and the time required for primary vaccination. Oral live typhoid vaccine should not be given to persons with immunodeficiencies, including HIV infection, or to persons taking antibiotics at the time of administration. Either of the parenteral typhoid vaccines is contraindicated only in persons with a history of severe local or systemic reactions after a previous dose. There are no data on safety or efficacy of oral or parenteral vaccines during pregnancy. The parenteral heat-phenol-inactivated vaccine is not generally recommended because it causes substantially more reactions and is no more effective than the oral live attenuated or parenteral purified polysaccharide vaccine. The lower age limits for use in children are 6 years for the oral vaccine, 6 months for the heat-phenol inactivated vaccine, and 2 years for the purified polysaccharide vaccine. Primary vaccination requires 1 week for oral vaccine, 4 weeks for the heat-phenol-inactivated vaccine, and a single injection for the purified polysaccharide vaccine.

It is not known whether simultaneous immunization with both parenteral and oral vaccines induces satisfactory immunity, and such use is not recommended. No information is available on the use of one vaccine as a booster after primary immunization with another, different vaccine. For persons previously vaccinated with heat-phenol-inactivated vaccine with continued or repeated exposure to *S. typhi,* vaccination with a primary series of oral typhoid vaccine or purified polysaccharide vaccine is reasonable.

Oral Live-Attenuated Typhoid Vaccine. Oral live-attenuated typhoid vaccine (Vivotif Berna, manufactured by the Swiss Serum and Vaccine Institute) is prepared from the Ty21a strain of *S. typhi* and must be refrigerated (not frozen). The Ty21a strain is deficient in the enzyme uridine diphosphate–galactose 4-epimerase. Accumulation of galactose metabolites in Ty21a eventually results in bacteriolysis, which accounts for the safety of the oral vaccine. The mechanism by which the Ty21a vaccine induces protection is not known. This vaccine induces some intestinal secretory antibody response but only modest concentrations of circulating antibody, in comparison with parenteral vaccines. It also elicits a cell-mediated immune response directed largely at the O antigen. Vaccine organisms are shed transiently in the stool of vaccinees, although secondary transmission has not been documented.

Three doses of oral live-attenuated typhoid vaccine administered on alternate days reduces infection by 33–67% during a follow-up period of 3–5 years. A four-dose regimen may be better than either three- or two-dose regimens, but because trials did not include a placebo group, precise efficacy results cannot be determined. Weekly and triweekly dosing regimens are less effective than alternate-day dosing. The efficacy of this vaccine has not been studied in children younger than 5 years, and the safety has not been tested in children younger than 1 year. A liquid formulation of Ty21a is more effective, but only enteric-coated capsules are available in the United States.

The recommended regimen consists of an enteric-coated capsule, containing 2–6 × 109 viable *S. typhi* Ty21a, and 5–50 × 109 nonviable *S. typhi* Tv21a on alternate days, for four doses. Each capsule should be taken on an empty stomach with a cool liquid no warmer than 37°C (98.6°F) approximately 1 hour before a meal. The vaccine is not recommended for children younger than 6 years. Oral live typhoid vaccine should not be given to persons with immunodeficiencies including HIV infection or to persons taking antibiotics (including antimalarial prophylaxis) within 24 hours before oral typhoid vaccine administration. Oral typhoid vaccine may be given to persons receiving parenteral immune globulin products. There are no data on the immunogenicity of oral typhoid vaccine administered concurrently with viral vaccines; if typhoid vaccination is warranted, it should not be delayed because of simultaneous administration of viral vaccines. The duration of immunity has not yet been established, but immunity has been documented for at least 5 years. A booster dose of one capsule is recommended every 5 years for persons with continued or repeated exposure to *S. typhi.*

Adverse reactions are no more common in vaccine recipients than in those who have received a placebo, and they are substantially fewer than in recipients of either of the parenteral vaccines.

Heat-Phenol-Inactivated Typhoid Vaccine. The heat-phenol-inactivated typhoid vaccine manufactured by Wyeth-Ayerst is a whole-cell *S. typhi* vaccine and must be refrigerated. The efficacy of the primary series of two doses in reduction of cases is 51–77%. The efficacy of the acetone-inactivated parenteral vaccine, available only to the armed forces, in reducing cases is 75–94%. Clinical efficacy correlates with the induction of agglutinating antibodies to flagellar H antigen, but clinical protection cannot be predicted from an individual's antibody titer. Modest agglutinin responses to Vi and O antigens are also elicited by this vaccine.

Primary vaccination for persons 10 years of age or older consists of two 0.5 mL subcutaneous injections, each containing approximately 5×10^8 killed bacteria, administered at least 4 weeks apart. Children 6 months to 10 years of age are given two doses of 0.25 mL. The vaccine is not recommended for children younger than 6 months. If time constraints do not permit the use of two doses at least 4 weeks apart, an alternative but less effective schedule of three doses given at weekly intervals has been used. Intradermal administration using doses of 0.1 mL produces antibody responses almost as high as subcutaneous administration produces and is associated with fewer local and systemic reactions, but this has not been evaluated in efficacy trials. A booster dose given either subcutaneously (0.25 mL for children 6 months to 10 years of age or 0.5 mL for persons 10 years of age or older) or intradermally (0. 1 mL regardless of age) every 3 years is sufficient for persons with continued or repeated exposure to *S. typhi.*

Adverse reactions in recipients of heat-phenol-inactivated whole-cell vaccine include fever (7–24%), headache (9–10%), and severe local pain or swelling (3–35%). Reactions result in absences from school or work in 21–23% of vaccinees. Severe reactions, including hypotension and shock, have been reported sporadically.

Vi Capsular Polysaccharide Vaccine. The parenteral Vi capsular polysaccharide vaccine (Typhim Vi, manufactured by Pasteur-Mérieux-Connaught, is composed of purified Vi antigen. A single 25 μg injection produces seroconversion in 93% of adults. Field trials have demonstrated a 74% reduction of cases at 20 months, a 61% reduction of cases at 1 year, a 52% reduction of cases at 2 years, and a 50% reduction of cases at 3 years. The efficacy of this vaccine has not been studied in persons from areas without endemic disease who travel to areas with endemic typhoid or in children younger than 5 years. It has not been tested in children younger than 1 year.

The vaccine is administered as a single intramuscular injection of 0.5 mL containing 25 μg of purified polysaccharide. It is not recommended for children younger than 2 years of age. A booster of 0.5 mL intramuscularly is recommended every 2 years for persons with continued or repeated exposure to *S. typhi.*

Adverse reactions in recipients of purified polysaccharide vaccine are few and include fever (0–1%) or headache (1–3%), and erythema or induration (7%). Reactions are significantly less frequent than with heat-phenol inactivated vaccine probably because the purified polysaccharide vaccine contains negligible amounts of lipopolysaccharide.

VIRAL VACCINES

Hepatitis A Vaccine

Two monovalent hepatitis A vaccines are currently available in the United States (Havrix [GlaxoSmithKline] and Vaqta [Merck]). Both vaccines are formalin-inactivated viruses propagated in human fibroblasts with the addition of aluminum hydroxide adjuvant. Havrix was licensed in 1995, followed by Vaqta in 1996. Both vaccines are currently licensed for children ≥2 years of age. In addition, a bivalent hepatitis A and hepatitis B vaccine (Twinrix [GlaxoSmithKline]) was approved in 2001 for persons ≥18 years of age. The approved schedule is a three-dose regimen (0, 1, and 6 months). This vaccine is intended for adults not previously immunized against hepatitis A and hepatitis B who are at risk for exposure to both hepatitis viruses.

Efficacy of hepatitis A vaccines is excellent in adults and children. Virtually 100% of children and young adults develop protective levels of antibody within 2 weeks after the first dose, with anamnestic responses and a further increase in titer after the second dose. As with hepatitis B, vaccine is less immunogenic in adults >40 years of age, and protective levels may not be achieved until after the booster dose.

The level of antibody considered protective was defined as a titer equal or greater than that level achieved by protective passive immunization. The level of antibody to hepatitis A virus (HAV) after a single dose of vaccine is generally higher than the level produced by administration of intramuscularly administered immune globulin, although lower than the titer after natural infection. Postvaccine anti-HAV, although protective, may be below the level detected by commercially available anti-HAV assays.

In the United States, hepatitis A vaccine is currently recommended for anyone ≥2 years of age at increased risk of hepatitis A, including children living in counties or states where rates of hepatitis A are ≥20 cases per 100,000 population, or approximately twice the national average (Table 17–10). These 11 states include Alaska, Arizona, California, Idaho, Nevada, New Mexico, Oklahoma, Oregon, South Dakota, Utah, and Washington. Children living in areas where rates of hepatitis A are greater than the national average but lower than twice the national average should be considered for routine vaccination. These six states include Arkansas, Colorado, Missouri, Montana, Texas, and Wyoming. The recommended dose for hepatitis A vaccination differs for children and adults (Table 17–11). All susceptible persons traveling to or working in countries that have high or intermediate hepatitis A endemicity should be immunized, including travelers to most regions of the world except Canada, Western Europe, Scandinavia, Japan, Australia, and New Zealand. Other target groups include children ≥2 years of age living in defined communities within the United States with high endemic rates or periodic outbreaks of hepatitis A, such as Native Americans and Inuits; persons with chronic liver disease, including hepatitis C; recipients of blood- or plasma-derived products; persons with an occupational risk of exposure; men who have sex with men; and injection drug users.

From a public health perspective, universal hepatitis A immunization is necessary to significantly impact the overall incidence of

TABLE 17–10. Viral Vaccines and Their Indications

Vaccine	Indications
Influenza	Adults at increased risk of influenza-related complications, including all persons ≥50 yr of age, adults with chronic pulmonary or cardiovascular disease, and adults with chronic diseases requiring medical follow-up or hospitalization during the preceding year; women who will be in the second or third trimester of pregnancy during the influenza season; children ≥6 mo of age with chronic pulmonary disease (moderate to severe asthma, bronchopulmonary dysplasia, cystic fibrosis) or hemodynamically significant cardiac disease; children ≥6 mo of age with sickle cell disease or other hemoglobinopathies; children ≥6 mo of age receiving immunosuppressive therapy; children ≥6 mo of age with chronic disease (diabetes, chronic renal and metabolic disease, symptomatic HIV infection) or on long-term aspirin therapy (rheumatoid arthritis or Kawasaki syndrome); and close contacts of any of the groups named above, including physicians, nurses, and other health care personnel in both hospital and outpatient facilities, employees of nursing homes and long-term care facilities, providers of home care, and household members
Hepatitis A	Travelers to, or persons relocating to, areas of high endemicity; children (≥2 yr of age) living in communities with high endemic rates and/or periodic outbreaks of hepatitis A (including Native Alaskans and Native Americans); persons engaging in high-risk sexual activity such as men who have sex with men and users of illicit injectable drugs; staff of institutions for developmentally disabled persons and in child daycare centers; and laboratory workers who handle live hepatitis A virus.
Hepatitis B	Routine immunization for all infants; children at high risk of early childhood HBV infection (Alaskan Native and Asian–Pacific Islander children) and children born to first-generation immigrants from HBV-endemic areas); all adolescents not previously immunized; members of households of adoptees who are HBsAg-positive; international travelers to areas in which HBV infection is endemic; persons undergoing hemodialysis; persons with bleeding disorders who receive clotting factor concentrates; inmates of juvenile detention and other correctional facilities; sexually active heterosexual persons with more than one sex partner during the previous 6 months or who have a sexually transmitted disease; sexually active men who have sex with men; and injection drug users
Japanese encephalitis	Travel to an endemic area with anticipated stay of ≥30 days
Measles-mumps-rubella (MMR)	Routine immunization of children at 12–15 mo of age with a second dose at either 4–6 yr or 11–12 yr (before entry to elementary or middle school); any person born after 1957 who has not been immunized or has no serologic evidence of immunity
Polio—inactivated (IPV)	Routine immunization of all infants beginning at 2 mo of age (Until the recommended all-IPV schedule is fully implemented, 4 doses of any combination of IPV and OPV are considered a complete immunization series.)
Polio—oral (OPV)	Unimmunized or partially immunized children at risk of exposure to poliovirus within 4 wk; children or adults at future risk of exposure to poliomyelitis who had received ≥1 dose of OPV or IPV; adults at risk of exposure to poliomyelitis within 4 wk who are unimmunized; adults at risk of exposure to poliomyelitis within 4 wk who are unimmunized; adults at risk of exposure to poliomyelitis within 4 wk who have had a partial or complete series with IPV
Rabies	Before exposure: persons at high risk of exposure to rabies (e.g., veterinarians, travelers with a prolonged stay [≥30 days] in endemic areas, animal handlers, spelunkers) After exposure: persons sustaining animal bites with potential for transmission of rabies, including bites by wild animals (e.g., skunks, raccoons, bats) and certain bites by domestic animals (see text)
Yellow fever	Travelers to areas of endemic infection (tropical Africa and areas of Central and South America); International Certificate of Vaccination may be required
Varicella-zoster	Routine immunization of children 12–18 mo of age; children aged 19 mo to 12 yr without a history of chickenpox; adolescents ≥13 yr of age and adults with susceptibility to infection

HAV infection. Recent reports of widespread multistate outbreaks of foodborne hepatitis A infection highlight the potential for hepatitis A to occur in individuals not targeted for vaccine by the present high-risk strategy. Further study of the vaccine's immunogenicity and efficacy in children <2 years of age is required before consideration can be given to universal immunization.

Hepatitis B Vaccine

The first hepatitis B vaccine was licensed in 1981. This unique vaccine consisted of hepatitis B surface antigen (HBsAg) purified from plasma of chronic hepatitis B virus carriers. The highly purified 22 nm HBsAg particles were potent immunogens and elicited protective anti-HBs. Improved molecular understanding of HBV, its genome, and its viral gene products, coupled with concerns about the use of a plasma-derived vaccine, led to the development of yeast-derived HBV recombinant vaccine in 1986. The vaccine is produced by insertion of a plasmid containing the HBsAg gene in *Saccharomyces cerevisiae* (baker's yeast). The resulting 17–25 nm particles are immunologically equivalent to HBsAg of human origin. The efficacy of the yeast-derived vaccine was demonstrated in infants of HBsAg-positive mothers who were also positive for hepatitis B e antigen (HBeAg). In the United States,

TABLE 17–11. Recommended Doses and Schedules for Monovalent Hepatitis A Vaccines

Age (years)	Dose	Volume (mL)	Doses	Schedule
Havrix (GlaxoSmithKline)				
2–18 yr	720 EL.U.	0.5	2	Initial and 6–12 mo later
≥19 yr	1,440 EL.U.	1	2	Initial and 6–18 mo later
Vaqta (Merck)				
2–18 yr	25 U	0.5	2	Initial and 6–12 mo later
≥19 yr	50 U	1	2	Initial and 6 mo later

EL.U. = enzyme-linked immunosorbent assay units.

yeast-derived vaccine quickly replaced the plasma-derived vaccine. The plasma-derived hepatitis B vaccine is no longer produced in the United States, although a small stock is maintained for the rare individuals with known allergy to baker's yeast.

Two yeast-derived monovalent vaccines are licensed in the United States: Recombivax HB (Merck) and Engerix-B (GlaxoSmithKline). Three doses of either hepatitis B vaccine, given in one of the recommended schedules, results in a protective antibody response (anti-HBs ≥10 mIU/mL) in more than 95% of infants, children, and adolescents. Although there have been a few reports of hepatitis B infection in vaccinated individuals despite protective levels of anti-HBs, these vaccine failures are rare. It has been hypothesized that these infections may be the result of mutations in the viral genome **(escape mutants),** which affect critical epitopes involved in binding of anti-HBs to surface antigen.

A bivalent hepatitis A and hepatitis B vaccine (Twinrix [GlaxoSmithKline]) has been available in Europe since 1997 and was approved in the United States in 2001 for persons ≥18 years of age. The approved schedule is a three-dose regimen (0, 1, and 6 months). This vaccine is intended for adults not previously immunized against hepatitis A and hepatitis B who are at risk for exposure to both hepatitis viruses.

With the availability and more widespread acceptance of yeast-derived HBV vaccine, indications for hepatitis B immunization expanded in the 1990s. Universal immunization is required for eventual elimination of the transmission of HBV. Accordingly, hepatitis B vaccine has been recommended by the ACIP since 1991 for all infants in the United States and, since 1997, for all unvaccinated children from birth to age 18 years. In 1999 a two-dose schedule for adolescents aged 11–15 years was approved; in these children, two 10 μg/1 mL doses of Recombivax HB, with the second dose given 4–6 months after the first dose, provides immunity comparable to that provided by three 5 μg doses, with the second and third doses given 1 and 6 months, respectively, after the first dose. Additionally, hepatitis B immunization continues to be recommended for all persons at increased risk of hepatitis B infection (Table 17–10).

Pediatricians need to be aware of differences in hepatitis B vaccine recommendations for infants of HBsAg-positive versus HBsAg-negative mothers. Infants of HBsAg-positive mothers require HBIG, as well as the first vaccine dose, within the first 12 hours of life. The subsequent two vaccine doses should be administered at 1 month and 6 months of age. When immunizing infants of HBsAg-negative mothers, the vaccine schedule can be more flexible, with administration of three doses of vaccine before 18 months of age (Table 17–12). Production of the 2.5 μg/mL doses of Recombivax-B previously used for infants of HBsAg-negative mothers and children less than 11 years of age, was discontinued in 1998, simplifying the immunization schedule for children. Immunization of infants of HBsAg-negative mothers immediately after birth was temporarily halted in 1999 because of concerns regarding possible exposure to thimerosal. With the expanded availability of thimerosal preservative–free hepatitis B vaccine, immunization of term infants in the immediate newborn period has resumed.

Experience with health care providers has revealed the importance of age at the time of immunization; seroconversion rates are lower in vaccinees ≥40 years of age. In addition, intramuscular administration must occur, and the vaccine should be injected in the deltoid, not gluteal, muscle to aid inadvertent deposition in adipose tissue.

At present there is no recommendation for a hepatitis B vaccine booster. Follow-up studies show a decline in antibody titer that is not unexpected with time. However, protection against hepatitis B persists even in individuals who no longer have detectable antibody. Further long-term studies are necessary to determine whether a booster will ultimately be required to maintain lifelong immunity. For selected high-risk individuals, a booster dose may be given if the anti-HBs level is less than 10 mIU/mL.

Influenza Vaccine

Influenza viruses present unique challenges because of their potential for year-to-year antigenic variation. Minor antigenic variation, or **drift,** and major antigenic changes, or **shift,** occur in the viral hemagglutinin and neuraminidase glycoproteins. Influenza A viruses in particular undergo constant antigenic change. Strategies for immunization to prevent influenza must address the inherent instability of the virus, as well as the fact that the only licensed influenza vaccines at present are inactivated and do not provide long-lasting protection. Cold-adapted nasally administered influenza vaccines have demonstrated efficiency against both influenza A and B but are not yet licensed.

Inactivated influenza vaccines are usually prepared as trivalent preparations containing two influenza A subtypes and an influenza B strain. Although methods of preparation vary, all vaccine manufacturers use the same virus strains. Influenza vaccine is reformulated every year; the decision concerning inclusion of new strains is based principally on the influenza viruses in circulation during the preceding winter.

Production of vaccine viruses is accomplished with high-yield reassortant viruses cultivated in chick embryo allantoic sacs. These reassortants allow a virus known to replicate to high titer (high-yield donor virus) to combine genetically with a virus of the desired

TABLE 17–12. Two Regimens for Timing of Hepatitis B Immunization of Infants of HBsAg-Negative Mothers

Regimen	Age
Recommended	
Dose 1	Birth
Dose 2	1–2 mo
Dose 3	6–18 mo
Alternate	
Dose 1	1–2 mo
Dose 2	4 mo
Dose 3	9–18 mo

antigenic phenotype. The use of such reassortants shortens the time needed to produce the desired influenza strains.

Several problems in the distribution of influenza vaccine in recent years highlight the potential pitfalls of a vaccine program reliant on yearly immunization. An influenza strain with potential for epidemic infection but not included in the vaccine may appear. For example, the trivalent vaccine for 1986–1987 contained A/Chile/83(H1N1), A/Mississippi/1/85(H3N2), and B/Ann Arbor/1/86. A new H1N1 strain, A/Taiwan/1/86, began to circulate widely in the fall of 1986. Anticipating possible epidemic spread of this new strain, monovalent A/Taiwan vaccine was prepared by December 1986. Considerable additional effort and expense were required to manufacture, distribute, and administer the new H1N1 vaccine.

Another problem occurred in 1991–1992, when influenza A virus began to circulate early in the fall. Because yearly influenza immunization programs were targeted primarily for late October and November, many eligible potential vaccine recipients had not yet been immunized when the influenza epidemic peaked. The optimal time for influenza immunization is from October through mid-November, although any time from September through the end of the influenza season is appropriate. Protection conferred by influenza vaccine generally begins 1–2 weeks after administration. If influenza viruses are already circulating in the community at the time vaccine is administered, consideration should be given to administration of anti-influenzal chemoprophylaxis to prevent infection in the immediate postvaccination period.

Inactivated influenza vaccines are available as either whole-virus or ''split'' preparations. Whole-virus vaccines have been available for many years and are purified by zonal gradient centrifugation or chromatography. Such vaccines are generally more immunogenic than the more highly purified subunit, or ''split,'' vaccines, but reactogenicity is also enhanced. Because of the occurrence of adverse effects in children immunized with whole virus vaccines, the more highly purified split vaccines should be used in this age group. These vaccines are prepared by treatment of whole virus with organic solvents or detergents. Regardless of whether the purification involves treatment with ether or a detergent such as sodium dodecyl sulfate, the immunogenicity and reactogenicity are similar. In children under the age of 9 years who are receiving vaccine for the first time, two doses given 1 month apart are recommended. Influenza vaccine is not recommended for infants <6 months of age (Table 17–13).

Yearly influenza vaccine is now recommended for all adults older than 50 years. Additionally, annual immunization is recommended for other individuals at risk of having influenza complications (Table 17–10). Adverse reactions to the vaccine, which are diminished in recipients of the split vaccine, may include fever and pain at the site of injection. Although concern about a possible relationship between Guillain-Barré syndrome and influenza vaccine has existed since the ''swine flu'' vaccine experience in 1976, there has subsequently been no evidence of neurologic disease in influenza vaccine recipients. Influenza vaccine may occasionally produce a false-positive enzyme immunoassay result for HIV and hepatitis C antibody. These false-positive results appear to be temporary, but their exact duration is unknown.

TABLE 17–13. Dosage Regimen for Influenza Virus Vaccination

Age Group	Type of Vaccine	Dosage (mL)	Number of Doses
6–35 mo	Split virus only	0.25	Initial series: 2; 1 dose annually thereafter
3–8 yr	Split virus only	0.5	Initial series: 2; 1 dose annually thereafter
9–12 yr	Split virus only	0.5	1 (initially and annually)
>12 yr	Whole or split virus	0.5	1 (initially and annually)

Japanese Encephalitis Vaccine

Japanese encephalitis is a mosquitoborne infection caused by a flavivirus antigenically related to other encephalitic flaviviruses, such as St. Louis and Murray Valley encephalitis viruses and West Nile virus. The arthropod vector is the *Culex* mosquito, a common species in rural Asia. An inactivated vaccine has been licensed in Japan since 1954. In the United States the vaccine was available through the CDC from 1983 to 1987 and licensed in 1992. It consists of formalin-inactivated infected mouse brains, extensively purified and free of myelin basic protein, and is recommended for persons who plan to reside for longer than 1 month in areas where Japanese encephalitis occurs. The vaccine is not recommended for travelers to Asia if visits are short and chiefly to urban areas.

The vaccine's efficacy, evaluated in a two-dose trial in Thailand, was approximately 90%. The level of antibody required for protection has been defined in animal challenge experiments as a neutralizing antibody titer greater than 1:10. In the United States a three-dose schedule at days 0, 7, and 30 is recommended. Alternatively, a regimen at 0, 7, and 14 days can be used, although postvaccination antibody titers are lower with the abbreviated schedule. Local reactions occur in approximately 20% of vaccinees; systemic adverse effects (e.g., fever, headache, malaise, myalgia, rash) are seen in approximately 10% of vaccinees. Since 1989, postvaccination hypersensitivity reactions, including urticaria, angioedema, and respiratory distress, have also been noted. A specific vaccine component responsible for these newly described allergic reactions has not been identified.

Measles Vaccine

Measles vaccine development proceeded rapidly after tissue culture identification of the virus in 1954. Two vaccines were introduced in 1963, an inactivated and an attenuated live vaccine. Administration of the attenuated vaccine, Edmonston B, was frequently associated with symptoms of mild measles, necessitating concomitant administration of immune serum globulin (ISG). Although the use of ISG diminished the vaccine's reactogenicity, immunogenicity was also diminished. Neither of the early measles vaccines proved satisfactory for long-term use.

Two additional attenuated live vaccines derived from the Edmonston strain were licensed in 1965 and 1968. Both vaccines were available in the United States until 1976. Since 1976, only the **Moraten strain** vaccine (Attenuvax [Merck]) has been marketed in the United States. Most measles vaccine is administered as a trivalent preparation, MMR, which is combined with vaccine strains of mumps and rubella. The vaccine has dramatically reduced the incidence of measles in the United States, although measles virus is still capable of epidemic spread, as demonstrated by widespread outbreaks during 1989–1991.

The immunogenicity of measles vaccine presently in use is excellent, with seroconversion in approximately 95% of vaccine recipients. Seroconversion may be decreased after administration of immune globulin and other blood products; specific intervals between administration of any blood product and measles vaccine are based on the amount of immune globulin used (Table 17–4). The addition of a vaccine stabilizer in 1979 appears to have decreased the number of primary vaccine failures (seroconversion failures) that may occur if the vaccine is improperly stored. At present, the manufacturer recommends storage of the vaccine at 2–8°C (36–46°F) before reconstitution. Once reconstituted, vaccine should be protected from sunlight and kept for no longer than 8 hours at 2–8°C. Proper handling of the vaccine is required to maintain the infectivity necessary to achieve successful immunization with this attenuated virus.

Primary vaccine failures due to interfering maternal antibody, in addition to those that result from improper handling of the vaccine, are well documented. In the United States, such failures are avoided by administering vaccine to infants at 12–15 months of age, by which time transplacentally acquired maternal antibody is no longer present. Before 1994, administration of vaccine at ≥15 months was advised, to allow for disappearance of maternal antibody that may interfere with vaccine response. At present, however, the majority of women of childbearing age have vaccine-induced immunity and neonates have lower antibody titers that decline rapidly, leaving infants susceptible to measles at an earlier age. Accordingly, the recommended age for measles vaccine was decreased from 15 months to 12–15 months of age.

In addition to primary vaccine failures, secondary vaccine failures (loss of immunity with time) may also occur. Although some investigations have indicated a trend toward a higher attack rate with increasing time since immunization, most studies indicate that protection is long-standing. A two-dose vaccine schedule has been recommended since 1989. A second dose of vaccine (as MMR vaccine) can be administered at either 4–6 years or 11–12 years of age, but the period from 4 to 6 years of age is recommended. Regardless of the timing of the second dose, the two-dose schedule enhances immunity, reflected by the low incidence of measles in the 1990s.

Adverse reactions to measles vaccine are generally mild. Fever (temperature >39.4°C) occurs in 5–15% of the vaccinees during the second week after immunization; rash may occur in 3–5% of vaccinees. Vaccine reactions in adults are similar to those in young children, although subjective complaints are often increased. Contraindications to measles vaccine are infrequent; egg allergy is no longer considered a contraindication. Rarely a hypersensitivity reaction from other vaccine components (gelatin or neomycin) may occur. Although live attenuated vaccines are generally contraindicated in individuals who are immunocompromised by underlying disease or immunosuppressant medication, measles vaccine may be given to children and adults with HIV infection unless CD4 cell counts are low.

Mumps Vaccine

The mumps vaccine was licensed in 1967, four years after licensure of live measles vaccine and 2 years before licensure of rubella vaccine. Before 1967 a formalin-inactivated mumps vaccine was available but never widely used because immunity was not long-lasting. The attenuation of the **Jeryl Lynn strain** by M. R. Hilleman provided a vaccine that has stood the test of time and remains in use today in the United States. Elsewhere in the world, other attenuated mumps vaccines have been developed, including Leningrad and Urabe AM9. Neither has the track record of safety, immunogenicity, and efficacy achieved by the Jeryl Lynn vaccine.

In the United States, mumps vaccine is available as a monovalent vaccine or combined with rubella, but it is usually administered with measles and rubella as trivalent MMR vaccine. The number of cases of mumps declined sharply after the introduction of mumps vaccine in 1967, even though the vaccine was not widely used until 1971, when it was combined with measles and rubella. Mumps virus has continued to circulate, and the number of reported cases increased from 2,982 in 1985 to 12,848 in 1987. The reported incidence of mumps infection in 1986 was 14-fold higher in the 15 states without a mandatory grade K–12 requirement. Since 1987 the number of cases per year has further diminished. The two-dose MMR vaccine schedule in place since 1989 has enhanced protection from this highly contagious virus.

Adverse reactions are uncommon. Egg allergy is no longer considered a vaccine contraindication. Low-grade fever, parotitis, rash, pruritus, and purpura occur in fewer than 1% of vaccine recipients. Central nervous system complications from Jeryl Lynn vaccine are extremely rare, and the incidence of these complications is no higher than the background rate of acute-onset neurologic diseases in the general population. Higher rates of central nervous system disease, however, have been noted in recipients of Leningrad and Urabe AM9 strain vaccines.

Polio

Polioviruses are RNA viruses in the Picornaviridae family. Like the other enteroviruses in this family, polioviruses are hardy viruses that survive the pH extremes of the gastrointestinal tract and transit readily from person to person by the fecal-oral route. Cultivation of type 2 virus in the late 1940s provided the breakthrough for development of highly effective polio vaccines.

Both the inactivated polio vaccine (IPV) and the oral polio vaccine (OPV) have played important roles in the control of the disease. In 1988 WHO set a target to globally eradicate polio by the year 2000. Based on successes in the Americas, WHO defined four principle strategies for global polio eradication: (1) 90% vaccine coverage in all countries; (2) national immunization days during which all children <5 years of age, regardless of immunization status, receive two doses of OPV spaced approximately 1 month apart; (3) surveillance for acute flaccid paralysis (AFP); and (4) "mopping up" immunizations (house to house) in high-risk areas identified through AFP disease surveillance. Although continued availability of OPV is critical for global immunization, the vaccine strategy in the United States has undergone modification from reliance on OPV from 1962 until 1997, to a sequential IPV/OPV schedule ("2 shots/2 drops") from 1997 through 1999, and finally, in January 2000, to universal immunization with four doses of IPV. Until the recommended all-IPV schedule is fully implemented, four doses of any combination of IPV and OPV is considered a complete immunization series.

Inactivated Polio Vaccine. Introduction of IPV in the United States in 1955 resulted in a dramatic reduction in the number of cases of paralytic polio. The inactivated vaccine was developed as a trivalent product because all three polio serotypes possess neurovirulence and because immunity to polioviruses is type specific. All three serotypes are inactivated with formalin without altering antigenic sites critical for the development of protective immune responses.

Adaptations of the original methods of IPV preparation, including use of human diploid cell lines and microcarrier systems to increase the yield of virus, resulted in production of an enhanced-potency vaccine (eIPV), which is more immunogenic than the original IPV. Licensed for use in the United States in 1988, eIPV is administered by intramuscular injection as a primary series at 2, 4, and 6–15 months of age, with a supplemental dose before school entry at 4–6 years.

Oral Polio Vaccine. Introduction of IPV in 1955 dramatically reduced the number of cases of paralytic polio in the United States, but polioviruses continued to circulate. Orally administered live attenuated vaccine offered the theoretical advantages of enhanced mucosal immunity and the practical advantages of ease of administration and lower cost. OPV was licensed in the United States in 1962 and was quickly embraced as the preferred polio vaccine. Trivalent OPV, licensed in 1964 to replace the three original monovalent vaccines, is now the only formulation distributed (Table

17–1). The vaccine contains 8×10^5, 1×10^5, and 8×10^5 median tissue culture infective doses of types 1, 2, and 3, respectively, administered in a volume of 0.5 mL. Because type 2 poliovirus replicates more efficiently in the gastrointestinal tract than types 1 and 3, a lower titer of type 2 vaccine is required.

As with other live attenuated vaccines, "cold chain" problems may interfere with the vaccine's infectivity. The U.S. manufacturer (Lederle) adds sorbitol as a stabilizer. The vaccine must still be shipped and stored at temperatures below freezing. A number of WHO-approved manufacturers of OPV add magnesium chloride as a thermal stabilizer, avoiding loss of vaccine potency when the vaccine is used in countries where vaccine storage at low temperatures cannot be guaranteed.

Immunologically, OPV comes close to being the perfect vaccine; both humoral and secretory immune responses mimic the responses to wild-type poliovirus infection. The mucosal immunity achieved from oral administration of the vaccine offers protection not just from disease but from infection. Eradication of wild-type polioviruses in the United States can be attributed in part to the presence of mucosal immunity in OPV recipients. An additional benefit is derived from the fecal excretion of polio vaccine viruses in recent vaccinees. Studies in both the United States and Japan indicate that person-to-person spread of vaccine viruses contributes to boosting of antibody titers.

With time, two drawbacks to OPV emerged. First, the occurrence of reversion from an attenuated to a neurovirulent strain is well documented. The mutation rate is highest in the brief period of intestinal replication that follows soon after vaccine administration. Such vaccine-associated mutations and reversions account for most of the rare polio cases in the United States. Second, 10–15% of reported cases of **vaccine-associated paralytic poliomyelitis (VAPP)** occur in immunocompromised OPV recipients or immunocompromised family contacts of OPV recipients. The occurrence of these cases was not evident when wild-type polioviruses were still in circulation because vaccine-associated cases are so rare (approximately six cases per year). During the past decade, identification of VAPP prompted review of the country's polio vaccine strategy and recommendations to shift to universal vaccination with eIPV. Since January 2000, eIPV has been recommended for all doses in the primary series as well as for the supplementary dose given at 4–6 years of age. Use of oral vaccine, if available, is limited to (1) unvaccinated children who will be traveling in <4 weeks to areas where polio is endemic, (2) children of parents who do not accept the recommended number of vaccine injections, and (3) persons vaccinated during mass vaccination campaigns to control outbreaks of paralytic polio. Children of parents who do not accept the recommended number of vaccine injections (second category) may receive OPV only for the third or fourth dose or both. In this situation, health care providers should administer OPV only after discussing the risk of VAPP with parents or other caregivers.

Rabies Vaccine

The pioneering efforts of Pasteur and others culminated in the first use of rabies vaccine in 1885. Fortunately, the treatment offered to Joseph Meister after he sustained multiple bites from a rabid dog was successful and immunization efforts continued to move slowly forward. Early rabies vaccines consisted of air-dried suspensions of virus-infected tissue from spinal cords of infected animals. Although no studies exist to document the early vaccine's immunogenicity or reactogenicity, its efficacy was attested by survival of at least some of the vaccinees.

During the next 70 years, little progress was made in the development of a vaccine against this RNA virus from the rhabdovirus family. In the early 1900s, vaccine preparation was modified by the addition of phenol to inactivate the virus more completely. By 1956, vaccine was prepared from infected suckling mouse brains. This preparation was free of myelin and the incidence of adverse neurologic effects was decreased. The development of methods to cultivate virus in vitro allowed preparation of vaccine in embryonated duck eggs. Duck embryo vaccine was introduced in the 1960s and proved safer than vaccine of nervous system origin. However, immunogenicity was diminished. Daily inoculations were required, given initially in conjunction with rabies immune globulin (RIG). Despite daily inoculation, immunity after completion of the vaccine series was not always achieved.

Further efforts to develop a safe, more effective vaccine culminated in the development of the human diploid cell vaccine (HDCV). The vaccine is effective even when given with RIG. Vaccine efficacy was demonstrated in a field trial in Iran. Since licensure in 1976, HDCV is the most frequently administered rabies vaccine for both pre-exposure and postexposure immunization. In the United States, it is estimated that approximately 100,000 doses are used each year, of which approximately 85% are given after exposure. A newer rabies vaccine, prepared from purified chick embryo cells (PCEC), is also now available.

The pre-exposure administration schedule for the United States is at 0, 7, and 28 days; some countries recommend vaccination only at 0 and 28 days. After exposure, a five-dose schedule is recommended (days 0, 3, 7, 14, and 28); the first dose is given in conjunction with RIG. The HDCV vaccine can be given by intradermal or intramuscular injection; PCEC is given only intramuscularly. Intradermal administration of HDCV requires only 0.1 mL, as opposed to 1 mL for intramuscular administration of HDCV and PCEC. Antibody titers are lower after intradermal administration, however. Although pre-exposure immunization with intradermal rabies vaccine may be less costly than intramuscular immunizations, decreased immunogenicity is a concern and intradermal administration is not recommended in the United States. In developing countries the immune response appears to be affected by the concomitant administration of chloroquine for antimalarial chemoprophylaxis.

The currently licensed rabies vaccines have an excellent safety record. The most frequent adverse reaction is local pain at the site of injection. The rate of neurologic abnormalities after HDCV administration is extremely low (1:150,000). Although this is higher than the background rate of neurologic abnormalities in the overall population, the reduction in adverse neurologic effects achieved by use of HDCV is significant. With vaccines containing neural tissue, neurologic abnormalities occurred in approximately 1:2,000 to 1:8,000 of recipients.

Although decisions about postexposure rabies immunoprophylaxis must be individualized, a few general principles should be kept in mind. First, the species of the biting animal is important. Bats and raccoons are major reservoirs of rabies in many parts of the United States. Rabies has also been identified in other wild animal species, including fox, skunks, and groundhogs. Second, the risk of rabies should be determined. Information regarding the risk of rabies in particular geographic areas can usually be obtained from local health departments. The risk of transmission of rabies must be weighed against the inconvenience and cost of postexposure immunoprophylaxis.

With bites from domestic animals, observation of the biting animal for a 10-day quarantine is extremely helpful. Dogs and cats with rabies virus in saliva will develop evidence of disease within this period. For wild animals, information regarding periods of transmissibility is incomplete and pathologic examination of brain tissue is required to exclude rabies.

After a bite by a domestic animal, additional information is required, including the animal's immunization history. If this information is available, the decision to administer rabies immunoprophylaxis often rests on whether the bite was provoked or unprovoked. If the bite was provoked and there has been no rabies in the area, immunoprophylaxis is not usually required.

Rotavirus Vaccine

After discovery of human rotavirus in 1973, early natural history studies revealed that immunity after wild-type rotavirus infection is incomplete, with recurrent infections following primary infection. Pre-existing immunity, however, modifies disease, and recurrent infections are mild or asymptomatic. Efficacy of rotavirus vaccine, therefore, needs to be judged by the vaccine's success in prevention of severe dehydrating rotavirus diarrheal disease, not prevention of rotavirus infection.

Rhesus monkey rotavirus produces an attenuated infection in humans and protects against human rotavirus serotype 3. To provide protection against the other three important human serotypes, three rhesus-human rotavirus reassortants were produced, each of which contained a gene from human serotypes 1, 2, and 4. The rhesus rotavirus was combined with the three rhesus-human reassortants in an oral quadrivalent vaccine (RRV-TV). In clinical trials RRV-TV prevented severe rotavirus gastroenteritis in 69–91% of vaccine recipients. On the basis of vaccine efficacy trials in infants immunized at 2, 4, and 6 months of age, RRV-TV was approved in August 1998. Common prelicensure adverse effects were limited to low-grade fever and decreased appetite and irritability, which clustered 3–4 days after administration of the first vaccine dose. After FDA approval, RRV-TV was quickly incorporated into recommended immunization schedules for infants beginning at 2 months of age. However, postmarketing surveillance within the first year of distribution revealed a temporal association between intussusception and recent administration of rotavirus vaccine. The vaccine was voluntarily withdrawn from the market in 1999.

This experience demonstrates the tremendous value of postmarketing surveillance. Prelicensure vaccine studies had noted only 5 cases of intussusception among approximately 10,000 vaccine recipients. Post-marketing surveillance, through the Vaccine Adverse Event Reporting System as well as several postlicensure surveillance studies, during the first post-licensure year, when an estimated 1.5 million doses of vaccine were distributed, revealed a 21.7 fold increased risk of intussusception 3–14 days after the first dose of RRV-TV. There was also a smaller increase in the risk of intussusception after the second dose of the vaccine. An estimated one case of intussusception attributable to the vaccine occurred for every 4,670–9,474 infants vaccinated. Ongoing trials of other investigational rotavirus reassortant viruses continue in an effort to develop a safe and effective vaccine to prevent severe dehydrating rotavirus infections.

Rubella Vaccine

Rubella virus was first isolated in tissue culture in 1962. The occurrence of a rubella epidemic a few years later provided impetus for vaccine development. During the 1964–1965 rubella epidemic in the United States, an estimated 12,000,000 cases of rubella occurred, with intrauterine infection in approximately 30,000 infants. The need to prevent congenital rubella hastened vaccine development, and several attenuated strains were licensed in 1969.

Since introduction of the vaccine, the number of cases of rubella has sharply declined. Congenital rubella has been almost eliminated; no more than 10–50 cases per year occur in the United States at present. In the first 10 years after vaccine licensure, several different vaccine strains were used, including HPV-77 (grown in duck embryo cultures), HPV-77 (grown in dog kidney culture), and Cendehill (grown in rabbit kidney). The RA27/3 strain, licensed in 1979, had enhanced immunogenicity and reduced reactogenicity and quickly replaced the earlier strains. The RA27/3 strain, grown in human diploid cells, is the only rubella vaccine in use in the United States. The vaccine is usually administered with measles and mumps as trivalent MMR vaccine. RA27/3 rubella vaccine is also available as a bivalent vaccine combined with measles.

MMR vaccine contains 1,000 pfu of RA27/3 virus; the vaccine's immunogenicity is excellent and immune responses occur with doses as low as 3 pfu. RA27/3 is remarkably stable. At 4°C (39°F) vaccine potency is maintained for years, and at room temperature viability is present as long as 3 months.

The immune response after use of RA27/3 vaccine is qualitatively similar to the immune response after wild-type infection, and virtually 100% of vaccinees demonstrate humoral immune responses. Additionally, secretory IgA antibodies can be found in nasopharyngeal secretions. Quantitatively, as expected after administration of an attenuated virus, immune response is less than after wild-type infection. Protection achieved by the vaccine appears to be long lasting. Primary vaccine failure is rare, and secondary vaccine failure has not been described. Nevertheless, routine administration of a second dose of MMR, as presently recommended in the United States at ages 4–6 years or at 11–12 years of age (4–6 years preferred), further enhances rubella immunity.

The most important vaccine adverse effect is arthritis or arthralgia. One compelling reason for the shift from the earlier vaccine strains to RA27/3 was that joint symptoms were decreased in RA27/3 vaccinees in comparison with recipients of the HPV-77 and Cendehill strains. In children immunized with RA27/3, joint symptoms are unusual. Transient arthralgia may occur in as many as 10–25% of adult vaccinees. This age-related difference reflects the age-related variation in joint symptoms noted after natural rubella infection. Although RA27/3 can to be given to rubella-seronegative adults (primarily women identified as seronegative by prenatal serologic findings), diminished reactogenicity in children is a compelling reason to immunize routinely in childhood.

Vaccinia (Smallpox) Vaccine

Vaccinia (smallpox) vaccine is highly effective as an immunizing agent to prevent smallpox, which is caused by **variola virus.** Vaccinia vaccine contributed significantly to the global eradication of smallpox. The last naturally occurring case occurred in Somalia in 1977, and in May 1980 the World Health Assembly certified that the world was free of naturally occurring smallpox. Because of the decreasing worldwide incidence of smallpox, recommendations for routine smallpox vaccination in the United States were rescinded in 1971. Routine smallpox vaccination of health care workers was discontinued in 1976, and vaccination of all military personnel was discontinued in 1990.

In 1980 the Advisory Committee on Immunization Practices (ACIP) of the CDC recommended the use of vaccinia vaccine to protect laboratory workers from possible infection while working with nonvariola orthopoxviruses (e.g., vaccinia and monkeypox). In 1984 these recommendations were expanded to include persons working in animal-care areas where studies with orthopoxviruses are being conducted. In addition, revaccination was recommended every 3 years. In 1991 the ACIP further expanded the recommendations to include health care persons involved in clinical trials using recombinant vaccinia virus vaccines and increased the recommended interval for revaccination for all persons to every 10 years.

Vaccinia vaccine should not be used therapeutically for any reason. There is no evidence to support value in treating or preventing recurrent herpes simplex, papillomavirus, or other virus infections. Severe complications, including death, have been reported from such misuse.

If a bioterrorist release of smallpox (variola) virus occurs, the CDC has recommended **postrelease vaccination** for the following groups: persons who were exposed to the initial release of the virus; persons who had face-to-face, household, or close-proximity contact (<6.5 feet or 2 meters) with a confirmed or suspected smallpox patient at any time from the onset of the patient's fever until all scabs have separated; personnel involved in the direct medical or public health evaluation, care, or transportation of confirmed or suspected smallpox patients; laboratory personnel involved in the collection or processing of clinical specimens from confirmed or suspected smallpox patients; and other persons who have an increased likelihood of contact with infectious materials from a smallpox patient (e.g., personnel responsible for medical waste disposal, linen disposal or disinfection, and room disinfection in a facility where smallpox patients are present).

The CDC is the only source of vaccinia vaccine that is currently licensed in the United States. Vaccinia vaccine does not contain smallpox (variola) virus. The vaccine has previously been prepared from calf lymph using a vaccinia seed virus, but a reformulated vaccine produced using sterile cell-culture techniques is being developed. The vaccine is a lyophilized, live-virus preparation of infectious vaccinia virus that is administered by **multiple-puncture technique** using a sterilized **bifurcated needle.** The needle is inserted into the vaccine vial, resulting in a droplet of recommended dosage adhering to the prongs of the needle. With the needle perpendicular to the skin over the deltoid region, 15 punctures are rapidly made with strokes of sufficient force to result in a trace of blood appearing after 15–20 seconds. Any remaining vaccine is wiped off with dry sterile gauze, which is disposed of in a biohazard waste container. A **major (or primary) reaction** is defined as a vesicular or pustular lesion of palpable induration surrounding a central crust or an ulcer, which usually forms 7–11 days after vaccination. By the end of the third week the scab falls off, leaving a permanent scar that is initially pink in color but eventually becomes flesh colored. Recently immunized health care workers preferably should avoid contact with unimmunized patients, especially immunocompromised persons, until the scab has separated from the skin at the vaccination site. Alternatively, the site should be kept covered with a semipermeable polyurethane dressing (e.g., Opsite), which should be changed daily, and hands should be washed thoroughly, especially after changing the bandage.

Varicella-Zoster Virus Vaccine

Vaccine development for herpesviruses, including VZV, has proceeded cautiously. A live attenuated VZV vaccine (Varivax [Merck]) was licensed in the United States in 1995. The vaccine was first developed in Japan in the 1970s with attenuation of a viral isolate from a child with chickenpox by multiple passages in human embryonic lung fibroblasts, guinea pig embryo cells, and human fibroblasts. Vaccine preparations consist of approximately 1,500–5,000 pfu per dose. Markers for attenuated vaccine virus are available, including vaccine-specific DNA restriction endonuclease patterns. The vaccine's thermolability necessitates careful handling; the lyophilized vaccine must be stored at −15°C to preserve infectivity, and once reconstituted it must be used within 30 minutes.

Varicella vaccine is recommended for routine immunization of all children at 12–18 months of age. Children 19 months through 12 years of age without a history of chickenpox should also be immunized. The dose for children from 12 months to 13 years of age is a single 0.5 mL subcutaneous injection. Adolescents ≥13 years and adults who have not had varicella should be immunized with two 0.5 mL doses given 4–8 weeks apart. Serologic testing to determine varicella immune status before immunization is not necessary. Postvaccination testing is not recommended because commercially available serologic tests may fail to detect vaccine-induced antibody.

Varicella vaccine reactions in healthy children and adults are mild. Rashes occur in approximately 5% of children, typically 7–10 days after immunization. These rashes may consist of erythema at the injection site or mild varicelliform eruptions with scattered lesions distant from the site. Lesions may be attenuated, without progression beyond the early maculopapular stage. A few may become vesiculated and may progress as typical varicella lesions. Low-grade fever may accompany the rash. Fever (temperature ≥38°C [100°F]) has been reported in approximately 10% of adolescent and adult vaccinees.

Varicella vaccine should not be routinely given to children with proven or suspected cell-mediated or T-lymphocyte immunodeficiency. In particular, children in three distinct groups require individualized decisions. Children with acute lymphocytic leukemia who have been in continuous remission for at least 1 year, with lymphocyte counts greater than 0.7×10^9/L and platelet counts greater than 100×10^9/L, may be candidates for varicella vaccine. Immunization decisions for such children should be discussed with an infectious diseases or hematology-oncology specialist. Children with HIV infection must also be considered individually. In children with a CD4 lymphocyte percentage of ≥25% (CDC class 1), benefits of vaccine may outweigh risks. Such children should be observed closely and seen immediately if they develop postimmunization varicella rashes. Because of the possible decrease in immune response, two doses of vaccine are recommended with a 3-month interval between doses. Children receiving or recently treated with high doses of corticosteroids (2 mg/kg/day for ≥14 days) should not receive varicella vaccine. After discontinuation of steroid therapy, vaccine may be administered when a 1-month interval has elapsed. Children with asthma who are using inhaled corticosteroids also require special consideration. Administration of low doses of inhaled corticosteroids usually should not result in systemic immunocompromise, but consultation with an immunologist or infectious diseases specialist may be desirable if there is concern about possible immunocompromise.

Varicella vaccine should not be given to pregnant women because the possible effects of the live attenuated virus on fetal development are uncertain. The vaccine manufacturer, in collaboration with the CDC, has established a Varivax Pregnancy Registry (800-989-8999) to monitor maternal and fetal outcomes when varicella vaccine is inadvertently given within 3 months before or during pregnancy.

Vaccine efficacy in healthy children is 85–100%. Some children who respond to the vaccine with seroconversion nonetheless develop infection when exposed to wild-type virus. These illnesses are usually mild, with low-grade or no fever (''breakthrough'' infections). Skin lesions are usually sparse and frequently attenuated, although some proceed through the typical varicella vesiculation. Breakthrough infections result in an anamnestic boost of VZV antibody, with development of antibody titers that approximate natural infection. When followed for 8–20 years, immunized children maintained stable antibody titers. To date, there is no evidence that breakthrough infections increase with time.

Varicella vaccine may be given simultaneously with MMR, but separate syringes and injection sites should be used. Studies are in progress to determine whether varicella vaccine can be combined with MMR (MMR-V) as a single injection. MMR-V vaccine would be an ideal way to accomplish universal varicella immunization. Proper handling of combined vaccine would be critical because of the thermolability of varicella vaccine.

Yellow Fever Vaccine

Vaccination against yellow fever is recommended for travelers to those parts of the world where yellow fever is endemic, including central Africa (latitudes +15 to −15 degrees) and parts of Latin America. The requirement of an International Certificate of Vaccination against Yellow Fever depends on the occurrence of infection within specific countries or regions, so travelers to endemic areas should obtain up-to-date information on requirements. If an International Certificate of Vaccination is required, the certificate must be signed and stamped at an official WHO-designated vaccine center.

The vaccine in use throughout the world is a live attenuated strain, designated 17D, that originally was isolated from an African patient in 1927. The cumbersome and time-consuming passages of the original viral strain to develop the attenuated 17D virus attest to the tenacity of the early medical virologists. Because of concerns about reversion of 17D to a more virulent strain, current regulations require that all vaccine be manufactured from virus that is no more than one passage from a seed lot that has passed all safety tests. At least 17 countries, including the United States, produce yellow fever vaccine.

The successful control of yellow fever in many epidemics attests to the vaccine's efficacy. Several of the studies on vaccine efficacy were extremely large, including one involving more than 59,000 subjects in Brazil. Protective immunity from yellow fever after a single dose of subcutaneously administered vaccine appears to be lifelong.

Overall, approximately 2–5% of vaccinees report adverse effects, including headaches, myalgia, and low-grade fever. Hypersensitivity reactions to the vaccine, which contains some egg protein, are rare (<1:1,000,000 vaccinees). Central nervous system symptoms from 17D vaccine are rare, but the vaccine is not recommended for infants younger than 4 months because of concern about this possible complication.

Increased levels of interferon have been documented in vaccine recipients. The presence of interferon may explain the diminished response seen when yellow fever vaccine is administered in conjunction with another vaccine such as cholera. Although data on concurrent use of yellow fever vaccine with other vaccines are incomplete, it is recommended that administration of yellow fever and cholera vaccines be separated by at least a 3-week interval.

REVIEWS

Ad Hoc Working Group for the Development of Standards for Pediatric Immunization Practices: Standards for pediatric immunization practices. *JAMA* 1993;269:1817–22.

Centers for Disease Control and Prevention: General recommendations on immunization. Recommendations of the Advisory Committee on Immunization Practices (ACIP). *MMWR Morb Mortal Wkly Rep* 1994;43(RR-1):1–38.

Centers for Disease Control and Prevention: Update: Vaccine side effects, adverse reactions, contraindications and precautions. Recommendations of the Advisory Committee on Immunization Practices. *MMWR Morb Mortal Wkly Rep* 1996;45(RR-12):1–35.

Gardner P, Eickhoff T, Poland GA, et al: Adult immunizations. *Ann Intern Med* 1996;124:35–40.

Gershon AA, Gardner P, Peter G, et al: Quality standards for immunization. Guidelines from the Infectious Diseases Society of America. *Clin Infect Dis* 1997;25:782–6.

Minister of Supply and Services Canada: Canadian Immunization Guide, 5th ed. National Health and Welfare, 1998.

Plotkin SA, Orenstein WA (editors): *Vaccines,* 3rd ed. Philadelphia, WB Saunders, 1999.

KEY ARTICLES

American Academy of Pediatrics: Combination vaccines for childhood immunization. Recommendations of the Advisory Committee on Immunization Practices (ACIP), the American Academy of Pediatrics (AAP), and the American Academy of Family Physicians (AAFP). *Pediatrics* 1999;103:1064–8.

American Academy of Pediatrics, Committee on Infectious Diseases: Universal hepatitis B immunization. *Pediatrics* 1992;89:795–800. [Published erratum: *Pediatrics* 1992;90:715.]

American Academy of Pediatrics, Committee on Infectious Diseases: *Haemophilus influenzae* type b vaccines: Recommendations for immunization with recently and previously licensed vaccines. *Pediatrics* 1993;92:480–8.

American Academy of Pediatrics, Committee on Infectious Diseases: Recommended timing of routine measles immunization for children who have recently received immune globulin preparations. *Pediatrics* 1994;93:682–5.

American Academy of Pediatrics, Committee on Infectious Diseases: Update on timing of hepatitis B vaccination for premature infants and for children with lapsed immunization. *Pediatrics* 1994;94:403–4.

American Academy of Pediatrics, Committee on Infectious Diseases: Recommendations for the use of live attenuated varicella vaccine. *Pediatrics* 1995;95:791–6. [Published erratum: *Pediatrics* 1995;96(1 Pt 1):preceding 151 and following 171.]

American Academy of Pediatrics, Committee on Practice and Ambulatory Medicine: Recommendations for preventive pediatric health care. *Pediatrics* 1995;96:373–4.

American Academy of Pediatrics, Committee on Infectious Diseases: The relationship between pertussis vaccine and central nervous system sequelae: Continuing assessment. *Pediatrics* 1996;97:279–81.

American Academy of Pediatrics, Committee on Infectious Diseases: Meningococcal disease prevention and control strategies for practice-based physicians. *Pediatrics* 1996;97:404–12.

American Academy of Pediatrics, Committee on Infectious Diseases: Prevention of hepatitis A infections: Guidelines for the use of hepatitis vaccine and immune globulin. *Pediatrics* 1996;98:1207–15.

American Academy of Pediatrics, Committee on Infectious Diseases: Acellular pertussis vaccine: Recommendations for use as the initial series in infants and children. *Pediatrics* 1997;99:282–8.

American Academy of Pediatrics, Committee on Infectious Diseases: Immunization of adolescents: Recommendations of the Advisory Committee on Immunization Practices, the American Academy of Pediatrics, the American Academy of Family Physicians, and the American Medical Association. *Pediatrics* 1997;99:479–88.

American Academy of Pediatrics, Committee on Infectious Diseases: Age of routine administration of the second dose of measles-mumps-rubella vaccine. *Pediatrics* 1998;101:129–33.

American Academy of Pediatrics, Committee on Infectious Diseases: Poliomyelitis prevention: Revised recommendations for use of inactivated and live oral poliovirus vaccine. *Pediatrics* 1999;103:171–2.

American Academy of Pediatrics, Committee on Infectious Diseases: Possible association of intussusception with rotavirus vaccination. *Pediatrics* 1999;104:575.

American Academy of Pediatrics, Overturf GD, Committee on Infectious Diseases: Technical Report: Prevention of pneumococcal infections, including the use of pneumococcal conjugate and polysaccharide vaccines and antibiotic prophylaxis. *Pediatrics* 2000;106:267–76.

American Academy of Pediatrics, Committee on Infectious Diseases: Policy Statement: Recommendations for the prevention of pneumococcal infections, including the use of pneumococcal conjugate vaccine (Prevnar), pneumococcal polysaccharide vaccine, and antibiotic prophylaxis. *Pediatrics* 2000;106:362–6.

American Academy of Pediatrics, Committee on Infectious Diseases: Meningococcal disease prevention and control strategies for practice-based physicians. [Addendum: Recommendations for college students.] *Pediatrics* 2000;106:1500–4.

Bisgard KM, Kao A, Leake J, et al: *Haemophilus influenzae* invasive disease in the United States, 1994–1995: Near disappearance of a vaccine-preventable childhood disease. *Emerg Infect Dis* 1998;4:229–37.

Braun MM, Terracciano G, Salive ME, et al: Report of a US Public Health Service Workshop on hypotonic-hyporesponsive episode (HHE) after pertussis immunization. *Pediatrics* 1998;102:E52.

Centers for Disease Control: National childhood vaccine injury act: Requirements for permanent vaccination records and for reporting of selected events after vaccination. *MMWR Morb Mortal Wkly Rep* 1988;37: 197–200.

Centers for Disease Control: Cholera vaccine. Recommendations of the Advisory Committee on Immunization Practices (ACIP). *MMWR Morb Mortal Wkly Rep* 1988;37:617–24.

Centers for Disease Control and Prevention: Yellow fever vaccine. Recommendations of the Advisory Committee on Immunization Practices (ACIP). *MMWR Morb Mortal Wkly Rep* 1990:39(RR-6):1–6.

Centers for Disease Control and Prevention: Recommendations for preventing transmission of human immunodeficiency virus and hepatitis B virus to patients during exposure-prone invasive procedures. *MMWR Morb Mortal Wkly Rep* 1991;40(RR-8):1–8.

Centers for Disease Control and Prevention: Diphtheria, tetanus, and pertussis. Recommendations for vaccine use and other preventive measures. Recommendations of the Immunization Practices Advisory Committee (ACIP). *MMWR Morb Mortal Wkly Rep* 1991;40(RR-10):1–28.

Centers for Disease Control and Prevention: Inactivated Japanese encephalitis virus vaccine. Recommendations of the Immunization Practices Advisory Committee (ACIP). *MMWR Morb Mortal Wkly Rep* 1993;42 (RR-1):1–15.

Centers for Disease Control and Prevention: Recommendations of the Advisory Committee on Immunization Practices (ACIP). Use of vaccines and immune globulins in persons with altered immunocompetence. *MMWR Morb Mortal Wkly Rep* 1993;42(RR-4):1–18.

Centers for Disease Control and Prevention: Typhoid immunization. Recommendations of the Advisory Committee on Immunization Practices (ACIP). *MMWR Morb Mortal Wkly Rep* 1994;43(RR-14):1–7.

Centers for Disease Control and Prevention: Update: Recommendations to prevent hepatitis B virus transmission. *MMWR Morb Mortal Wkly Rep* 1995;44:574–5.

Centers for Disease Control and Prevention: The role of BCG vaccine in the prevention and control of tuberculosis in the United States. A joint statement by the Advisory Council for the Elimination of Tuberculosis and the Advisory Committee on Immunization Practices. *MMWR Morb Mortal Wkly Rep* 1996;45(RR-4):1–18.

Centers for Disease Control and Prevention: Prevention of varicella. Recommendations of the Advisory Committee on Immunization Practices (ACIP). *MMWR Morb Mortal Wkly Rep* 1996;45(RR-11):1–36.

Centers for Disease Control and Prevention: Immunization of adolescents. Recommendations of the Advisory Committee on Immunization Practices, the American Academy of Pediatrics, the American Academy of Family Practice, and the American Medical Association. *MMWR Morb Mortal Wkly Rep* 1996;45(RR-13):1–16.

Centers for Disease Control and Prevention: FDA approval for infants of a *Haemophilus influenzae* type b conjugate and hepatitis B (recombinant) combined vaccine. *MMWR Morb Mortal Wkly Rep* 1997;46:107–9.

Centers for Disease Control and Prevention: Control and prevention of serogroup C meningococcal disease: Evaluation and management of suspected outbreaks. Recommendations of the Advisory Committee on Immunization Practices (ACIP). *MMWR Morb Mortal Wkly Rep* 1997;46(RR-5):13–21.

Centers for Disease Control and Prevention: Pertussis vaccination: Use of acellular pertussis vaccines among infants and young children. Recommendations of the Immunization Practices Advisory Committee (ACIP). *MMWR Morb Mortal Wkly Rep* 1997;46(RR-7):1–25.

Centers for Disease Control and Prevention: Prevention of pneumococcal disease. Recommendations of the Advisory Committee on Immunization Practices. *MMWR Morb Mortal Wkly Rep* 1997;46(RR-8):1–24.

Centers for Disease Control and Prevention: Immunization of health-care workers. Recommendations of the Advisory Committee on Immunization Practices (ACIP) and the Hospital Infection Control Practices Advisory Committee (HICPAC). *MMWR Morb Mortal Wkly Rep* 1997;46(RR-18):1–42.

Centers for Disease Control and Prevention: National, state and urban area vaccination coverage levels among children aged 19–35 months—United States, 1997. *MMWR Morb Mortal Wkly Rep* 1998;47:547–54.

Centers for Disease Control and Prevention: Measles, mumps, and rubella—vaccine use and strategies for elimination of measles, rubella, and congenital rubella syndrome and control of mumps. Recommendations of the Advisory Committee on Immunization Practices (ACIP). *MMWR Morb Mortal Wkly Rep* 1998;47(RR-8):1–57.

Centers for Disease Control and Prevention: Recommendations of the Advisory Committee on Immunization Practices: Revised recommendations for routine poliomyelitis vaccination. *MMWR Morb Mortal Wkly Rep* 1999;48:590.

Centers for Disease Control and Prevention: Withdrawal of rotavirus vaccine recommendation. *MMWR Morb Mortal Wkly Rep* 1999;48:1007.

Centers for Disease Control and Prevention: Human rabies prevention—United States, 1999. Recommendations of the Advisory Committee on Immunization Practices (ACIP). *MMWR Morb Mortal Wkly Rep* 1999;48(RR-1):1–21.

Centers for Disease Control and Prevention: Combination vaccines for childhood immunization. Recommendations of the Advisory Committee on Immunization Practices (ACIP), the American Academy of Pediatrics (AAP), and the American Academy of Family Physicians (AAFP). *MMWR Morb Mortal Wkly Rep* 1999;48(RR-5):1–15.

Centers for Disease Control and Prevention: Prevention of varicella. Recommendations of the Advisory Committee on Immunization Practices. *MMWR Morb Mortal Wkly Rep* 1999;48(RR-6):1–5.

Centers for Disease Control and Prevention: Recommendations for the use of Lyme disease vaccine. Recommendations of the Advisory Committee on Immunization Practices (ACIP). *MMWR Morb Mortal Wkly Rep* 1999;48(RR-7):1–25.

Centers for Disease Control and Prevention: Prevention of hepatitis A through active or passive immunization: Recommendations of the Advisory Committee on Immunization Practices (ACIP). *MMWR Morb Mortal Wkly Rep* 1999;48(RR-12):1–37.

Centers for Disease Control and Prevention: Poliomyelitis prevention in the United States. Updated recommendations of the Advisory Committee on Immunization Practices (ACIP). *MMWR Morb Mortal Wkly Rep* 2000;49(RR-5):1–22.

Centers for Disease Control and Prevention: Prevention and control of meningococcal disease: Recommendations of the Advisory Committee on Immunization Practices (ACIP). *MMWR Morb Mortal Wkly Rep* 2000;49(RR-7):1–10.

Centers for Disease Control and Prevention: Preventing pneumococcal disease among infants and young children: Recommendations of the Advisory Committee on Immunization Practices (ACIP). *MMWR Morb Mortal Wkly Rep* 2000;49(RR-9):1–35.

Centers for Disease Control and Prevention: Use of anthrax vaccine in the United States. Recommendations of the Advisory Committee on Infectious Practices (ACIP). *MMWR Morb Mortal Wkly Rep* 2000; 49(RR-15):1–20.

Centers for Disease Control and Prevention: Vaccinia (smallpox) vaccine. Recommendations of the Advisory Committee on Immunization Practices (ACIP), 2001. *MMWR Morb Mortal Wkly Rep* 2001;50(RR-10):1–25.

Centers for Disease Control and Prevention: Prevention and control of influenza: Recommendations of the Advisory Committee on Immunization Practices (ACIP). *MMWR Morb Mortal Wkly Rep* 2001; 50(RR-4):1–44.

Engels EA, Falagas ME, Lau J, et al: Typhoid fever vaccines: A meta-analysis of studies on efficacy and toxicity. *BMJ* 1998;316:110–6.

Evans G: National Childhood Vaccine Injury Act: Revision of the vaccine injury table. *Pediatrics* 1996;98:1179–81.

Feikin DR, Lezotte DC, Hamman RF, et al: Individual and community risks of measles and pertussis associated with personal exemptions to immunization. *JAMA* 2000;284:3145–50.

Henning KJ, White MH, Sepkowitz KA, et al: A national survey of immunization practices following allogeneic bone marrow transplantation. *JAMA* 1997;277:1148–51.

James JM, Zeiger RS, Lester MR, et al: Safe administration of influenza vaccine to patients with egg allergy. *J Pediatr* 1998;133:624–8.

Lavi S, Zimmerman B, Koren G, et al: Administration of measles, mumps, and rubella virus vaccine (live) to egg-allergic children. *JAMA* 1990;263:269–71.

Murphy TV, Gargiullo PM, Massoudi MS, et al: Intussusception among infants given an oral rotavirus vaccine. *N Engl J Med* 2001;344:564–72.

Singleton JA, Lloyd JC, Mootrey GT, et al: An overview of the vaccine adverse event reporting system (VAERS) as a surveillance system. *Vaccine* 1999;17:2908–17.

CHAPTER 18

Approach to the Child with Fever

Paul L. McCarthy

Fever is the response of warm-blooded animals to various inciting agents such as viruses or pathogenic bacteria. The febrile response is carefully regulated by a central temperature control mechanism located in the preoptic region of the hypothalamus. In response to a stimulus, polymorphonuclear leukocytes and other phagocytic cells of the reticuloendothelial system derived from the bone marrow release endogenous **pyrogen,** a cytokine that acts on the thermoregulatory center through the mediation of prostaglandins. Usually the **thermoregulatory center** is set at approximately 37°C (98.6°F). During a febrile response, however, the thermoregulatory center is set to maintain a higher level of body temperature. The center maintains this elevated temperature by increased heat production, especially through increased muscle activity such as shivering; increased heat conservation, especially through peripheral vasoconstriction; decreased sweating; and behavioral measures such as covering with blankets in response to chills even though the body temperature is elevated.

The thermoregulatory center during febrile episodes has an upper physiologic limit of 41.1°C (106°F). Temperatures beyond this limit should be considered potentially harmful to the host because of the possibility of damage to the central nervous system. There are conflicting data as to the value of an elevated temperature, from 37.8°C to 41°C (100–105.8°F), for the preservation of the host. Some types of microorganisms (e.g., treponemes) are destroyed, whereas others, such as selected strains of *Streptococcus pneumoniae,* grow poorly at higher temperatures. One form of treatment for syphilis in the preantibiotic era was to induce fever. Other studies have documented enhancement of certain immune responses if elevated temperature is present. In some cold-blooded animals, elevated body temperature is achieved by moving to an area of higher ambient temperature, which increases survival during bacteremic episodes. However, studies using animal models have shown that survival is poorer during episodes of gram-negative sepsis when the body temperature is elevated. Deterioration of selected immune responses when the temperature is greater than 40°C (104°F) has been documented. Thus the value of fever for host preservation during infectious episodes continues to be the subject of debate. Most of the studies that address this issue have been performed in vitro or in animals, and their applicability to humans is unclear.

It is certain that fever places increased metabolic demands on the host. High temperatures exaggerate the pulmonary vasoconstriction induced by hypoxemia. The patient who is febrile often has tachycardia and is uncomfortable and irritable; assessment for an underlying serious illness is therefore difficult. Finally, there is a strong correlation between the height of fever and the occurrence of febrile seizures in children at temperatures of 40–41.1°C (104–106°F).

FEBRILE ILLNESSES IN CHILDREN

Most acute febrile illnesses in children are caused by viral infections. As a practical matter, one of the most important challenges in the diagnostic evaluation of children with fever is differentiating those with serious illnesses from those with self-limited viral infections. The cause and risk of serious illness among children with acute febrile illnesses vary greatly depending on age. In the first 2 months of life, infants are more susceptible to sepsis and meningitis caused by gram-negative organisms and group B *Streptococcus.* Urinary tract infections in young male infants are more likely to be associated with underlying anatomic abnormalities of the urinary tract than in older children.

Children 3–36 months of age have five or six acute episodes of infection per year, with a decrease in frequency with increasing age (see Table 6–2). Thus fever in young children is a common problem confronting physicians. In addition, compared with older children, those 3–36 months of age more often have serious infections such as bacteremia, meningitis, and cellulitis associated with bacteremia. Approximately 50% of children with fever due to infection have a diagnosis of a viral syndrome such as an upper respiratory tract infection or viral gastroenteritis, and approximately 30% have otitis media. The incidence of serious infectious illnesses in young, febrile children varies with the patient population, from approximately 9% in children coming to an emergency center (Table 18–1), which includes referrals from other sites, to 1–3% in a cohort of children in a primary care setting (Table 18–2).

As children mature beyond 36 months of age, they acquire infection and develop immunity to the common bacterial pathogens. *Neisseria meningitidis* becomes the leading cause of bacterial meningitis. Pharyngitis caused by group A *Streptococcus* is a common bacterial infection. *S. pneumoniae* continues to be the most common

TABLE 18–1. Serious Illnesses During 996 Episodes of Acute Infectious Illness in Febrile Children Younger than 36 Months in an Emergency Center

Diagnosis	No.	%
Bacterial meningitis	9	0.9
Aseptic meningitis	12	1.2
Pneumonia	30	3.0
Bacteremia	10	1.0
Focal soft tissue infection	10	1.0
Urinary tract infection	8	0.8
Bacterial diarrhea	1	0.1
Abnormal electrolyte or blood gas values	9	0.9
Total	89	8.9

TABLE 18–2. Serious Illness During 1,221 Episodes of Acute Infectious Illnesses in 369 Children Followed Up for the First 32 Months of Life in Primary Care Settings

Diagnosis	Primary Care Center (761 Visits) No.	%	Private Practice (460 Visits) No.	%
Bacterial meningitis	0	0	0	0
Aseptic meningitis	1	0.14	0	0
Pneumonia	9	1.27	1	0.19
Bacteremia	2	0.28	2	0.39
Focal soft tissue infection	1	0.14	1	0.19
Urinary tract infection	2	0.28	1	0.19
Bacterial diarrhea	5	0.71	0	0
Abnormal electrolyte or blood gas values	3	0.42	0	0
TOTALS	23	3.24	5	0.96

cause of bacterial pneumonia, and *Mycoplasma pneumoniae* assumes increasing importance as a cause of pulmonary infiltrates in children after 5 years of age.

DIAGNOSIS

The determination of fever is based on data obtained with rectal thermometers. Oral thermometry is generally acceptable for older children and adults, but recorded temperatures usually are as much as 0.56°C (1°F) lower than rectal temperatures. Other methods of thermometry, including determination of the cutaneous, aural, or axillary temperatures, are unreliable.

The diagnostic approach to acute episodes of fever in children up to 36 months of age encompasses many of the complexities of the pediatric clinical evaluation. The common serious illnesses in febrile children represent a diagnostic challenge in these children. Serious infections such as occult pneumococcal bacteremia (Chapter 19), meningitis, and urinary tract infection are often manifested as only an upper respiratory tract infection or as only nonspecific findings such as fever, irritability, decreased feeding, and mild gastrointestinal symptoms, without localizing signs. An optimal chest examination in young children is often difficult because of noncooperation and the higher normal respiratory rate.

The diagnostic challenge in evaluating children with acute infectious illnesses is the identification of patients with serious illnesses by observation, careful history and physical examination, assessment of age and temperature risk factors, and the judicious use of laboratory tests. As the child matures, additional historical information can be obtained directly from the child.

Observation

Because young children with fever may have serious illnesses and because these serious illnesses may not be manifested in typical findings suggestive of disease (e.g., children with meningitis may not have nuchal rigidity), experienced pediatricians use **observational assessment** as a key part of the diagnostic process (McCarthy et al, 1980, 1981, 1982a). The two key elements of the observational assessment performed before the history and physical examination are "looking at the observer" and "looking around the room." Normal eye appearance or behavior may be described as "shiny," "bright," and "looks at observer," whereas descriptions that indicate severe impairment include "glassy" and "stares vacantly into space." These descriptions of eye function and appearance are a reflection of what pediatricians mean by the term **alertness.**

Other observations frequently used by pediatricians include a variety of descriptions of normal motor ability, such as "sitting," "moving arms and legs on table or lap," and "sitting without support," whereas severe impairment may be indicated by "no movement in mother's arms" and "lies limply on table." Many common observations describe characteristics that are usually referred to as playfulness, such as "vocalizing spontaneously," "playing with objects," "reaching for objects," "smiling," and "crying with noxious stimuli," or, if the child is impaired, as **"irritability."**

Another common observation is the response of a crying child to being held by the parent. For example, a normal response is "stops crying when held by the parent," whereas severe impairment is indicated by "continual crying despite being held and comforted." These descriptions are more precise than the commonly used term **consolability.**

Traditionally it has been believed that as pediatricians are forming judgments of the degree of illness by observation, they are assessing physical findings such as petechiae, bulging fontanel, or nasal flaring. Certainly these variables are crucial, but the studies showed that a majority of observations concern the child's response to stimuli. In variables relating to eye appearance or function, for example, stimulus-response data about the eyes (e.g. "looks at pen being offered") were noted much more often than organic data about the eyes (e.g., sunken, red, glassy). The more experienced pediatricians relied more heavily on stimulus-response data than did the physicians with less experience.

Thus the judgment of degree of illness by observation is based largely on the assessment of the interaction between the child and the environment. The extent of the interaction is often immediately apparent. For example, the child smiles at the observer and reaches for the proffered pen, and at other times the child cries and clings to the mother. After choosing a position of comfort for the child, usually on the parent's lap, the experienced examiner uses the stimuli in an attempt to elicit normal responses from the child. To orchestrate this interaction, pediatricians must be developmentalists and must be familiar with age-appropriate responses. Observation of febrile children is a complex process including both developmental skills and clinical skills. Pediatricians must assess the child's responses to multiple stimuli and must also be alert to clinical clues such as sunken eyes, cyanosis, and grunting.

Acute Illness Observation Scales. Six items, four of which concern response to stimuli, have been identified as the key predictors of serious illness in febrile children. These items compose the **Acute Illness Observation Scales (AIOS),** with the best possible score of 6 and the worst possible score of 30 (Table 18–3). Studies (McCarthy et al, 1982a) found that nearly two of three children with acute illnesses had AIOS scores ≤10 (i.e., they appear well), and fewer than 3% of these children had serious illnesses. However, children who appeared severely ill, with an AIOS score of ≥16, were relatively uncommon, but the chance of serious illness was high (92%). Approximately one in four children appeared moderately ill as defined by an AIOS score of 11–15, with a chance of serious illness that was high (26%). The occurrence of serious illness in febrile children who appeared moderately or severely ill, as defined by an AIOS score >10, was 13 times greater than the occurrence in children who appeared well (AIOS score ≤10).

History and Physical Examination

In a study (McCarthy et al, 1987) of the relationship between data gathered by observation and the results of the history and physical

TABLE 18–3. Acute Illness Observation Scales (AIOS)

Observation Element	1 (Normal)	3 (Moderate Impairment)	5 (Severe Impairment)
Quality of cry	Strong with normal tone *or* content and not crying	Whimpering *or* sobbing	Weak *or* moaning *or* high pitched
Reaction to parent stimulation	Cries briefly then stops *or* content and not crying	Cries off and on	Continual cry *or* hardly responds
State variation	Stays awake if awake *or* wakes up quickly if asleep and stimulated	Eyes close briefly then awakens *or* awakes with prolonged stimulation	Falls asleep *or* will not rouse
Color	Pink	Pale extremities *or* acrocyanosis	Pale *or* cyanotic *or* mottled *or* ashen
Hydration	Skin and eyes normal *and* mucous membranes moist	Skin and eyes normal *and* mouth slightly dry	Skin doughy or tented *and* dry mucous membranes *or* sunken eyes *or* both
Response (talk, smile) to social overtures	Smiles (*or* alerts if ≤2 mo of age)	Brief smile (*or* alerts briefly if ≤2 mo of age)	No smile, face dull and expressionless (*or* no alerting if ≤2 mo of age)

From McCarthy PL, Sharpe MR, Spiesel SZ, et al: Observation scores to identify serious illness in febrile children. *Pediatrics* 1982;70:802–9.

examination, ill appearance, a history of symptoms indicative of serious illness, and signs on physical examination suggestive of serious illness were of equal efficacy in detecting serious illnesses in 36 of 350 children. The history and physical examination, when combined, detected approximately 78% (28/36) of children with serious illnesses, but a combination of observation, history, and physical examination had the highest sensitivity, 86% (31/36). Abnormalities of the pulmonary and central nervous systems represented the majority of abnormal signs and symptoms and also had the strongest correlation with serious illness. This is not surprising, because many of the serious infectious illnesses in children involve these systems.

In a study (Alario et al, 1987) of observation, history, and physical examination in diagnosing pneumonia in children, observation of respiratory status (e.g., respiratory rate and work of breathing) was a critical clue. When physicians were consistent in believing that pneumonia was present or absent throughout the phases of observation, history, and physical examination, then a radiograph of the chest added new information in only 1 of 10 patients. Moreover, the roentgenogram of the chest changed the plan of management in only 6% of patients when the diagnostic impression was consistent.

Most studies of clinical judgment in pediatricians who see febrile children reach similar conclusions. When experienced physicians carefully perform the clinical evaluations, including observation, history, and physical examination, the great majority of serious illnesses, probably at least 90%, can be detected.

Age and Temperature Risks

Children younger than 3 months of age are at increased risk of having sepsis and meningitis caused by group B *Streptococcus* and gram-negative organisms, and these conditions may be difficult to diagnose by history and physical examination alone. There is also an association between temperature and serious illnesses. As fever increases, so does the occurrence of bacteremia. The incidence of bacteremia in young children is 7% when the temperature is 40°C (104°F) or above, 13% when the temperature is 40.6–41.1°C (105–105.9°F), and 26% when the temperature is 41.1°C (106°F) or more. In addition, there is a 10% occurrence of bacterial meningitis at temperatures of 41.1°C (106°F) and above (McCarthy and Dolan, 1976).

Laboratory Tests

Screening laboratory studies may be helpful in identifying the febrile child at increased risk of having the common serious infectious illnesses. In a study (Kuppermann et al, 1998) of 6579 children 3–36 months of age with fever (≥39°C [102.2°F]), including 164 children with pneumococcal bacteremia, an ANC of ≥10,000/mm^3 versus <10,000/mm^3 was associated with a 7.8% versus a 0.8% occurrence, respectively, of pneumococcal bacteremia. WBC counts of ≥15,000/mm^3 versus <15,000/mm^3 were associated with a 6% versus a 0.7% occurrence, respectively, of bacteremia. Higher temperatures indicated greater risk of bacteremia, with an odds ratio of 1.77 for bacteremia for each 1°C (1.8°F) increase in temperature. The risk of any serious illness in febrile children is approximately twice as great if the WBC count is ≥15,000/mm^3 or the ESR is ≥30 mm/hr than if neither of these elevations is present. Although screening laboratory tests are far from perfect in detecting serious illnesses in febrile children, they indicate an increased risk.

Screening studies may be most useful in combination with clinical evaluation. In a study (Baker et al, 1993) of 747 infants 29–56 days of age with fever, of the 287 infants who appeared well as determined by the AIOS without a recognized bacterial infection on physical examination and who had a peripheral WBC count <15,000/mm^3, a CSF leukocyte count <8/mm^3, a negative CSF Gram stain, and a urine spun specimen with leukocytes <10/hpf and few or no bacteria, only 1 (0.4%) infant had a serious bacterial infection. Of the remaining 460 infants with abnormalities on clinical evaluation or screening laboratory tests, 64 (14%) had serious bacterial illnesses.

Diagnostic Approach

The basis of the recommended diagnostic approach is a carefully performed observation period followed by the history and physical examination. Appreciation of age and temperature risks is also important. If the child appears well, has no indication of serious illness according to the findings of the history or physical examination, and has no age or temperature risk factors, then no laboratory evaluation is indicated. This profile typifies the majority of febrile children. Focal bacterial infections, such as otitis media, in well-appearing children should be treated with appropriate antibiotics without laboratory evaluation.

Alternatively, if the child appears ill or if abnormalities are present on history or physical examination, then laboratory studies appropriate for those findings are indicated. For example, the child with grunting and nasal flaring should have, at least, a chest roentgenogram. In the child with an acute onset of frequent watery stools flecked with blood, the presence of an enteric pathogen should be presumed until proved otherwise, and a stool culture should be performed. Often the presence of risk factors may indicate the direction in which the laboratory evaluation should proceed. For example, the infant younger than 3 months who appears ill without other findings should be tested for sepsis and should be admitted for intravenous administration of antibiotics. The irritable child with a temperature of 41.1°C (106°F) but no other findings is at high risk of having central nervous system disease, and the evaluation should include at least a lumbar puncture and blood culture.

The greatest controversy concerns how to proceed in those situations in which the clinical impression, after observation, history, and physical examination, indicates no serious illness even though age and temperature risk factors are present. Although assessment by clinical examination of the risk of sepsis and meningitis in infants younger than 3 months is fairly accurate, most physicians recommend that such children have a sepsis evaluation (Baker et al, 1993). Infants 30 days of age or younger should be admitted to the hospital for intravenous administration of antibiotics while awaiting culture results. Children 31–89 days of age often are admitted to the hospital for observation, but recent studies indicate that they may be followed up at home if results of the clinical evaluation and screening laboratory tests are noncontributory. If infants are followed up as outpatients, careful observation at home must be ensured. Some physicians have recommended administering ceftriaxone to febrile infants 31–89 days of age who are sent home, but this recommendation is not universally accepted (Baraff et al, 1993).

A blood culture may be considered for children 3–36 months of age without a focus of bacterial infection and with higher temperatures (≥39°C [102.2°F]) (Kuppermann et al, 1998). Blood cultures may be obtained from all such children initially or after laboratory screening with a finger-stick CBC, with cultures only for those children with an elevated WBC count (≥15,000/mm^3) or ANC (≥10,000/mm^3). Urine cultures should be considered for children in this age group who have fever without an identifiable source. This is especially important in young girls, in whom the occurrence of urinary tract infections is common. Urinalysis with microscopic examination may indicate an increased risk of urinary tract infection, but the urine culture is the definitive test.

ANTIPYRETIC THERAPY

Antipyresis is warranted when fever places undue stress on a physiologically compromised child (e.g., a child with pulmonary or cardiac disease) and is mandatory if the body temperature rises beyond the physiologic limit (41.1°C [106°F]). The necessity of antipyresis is less clear in the febrile child who is fussy and uncomfortable. However, increasing the child's comfort by reducing the fever is the reason most frequently given for antipyresis. In addition, the child's increased comfort with antipyresis can be a diagnostic aid to the physician in that the child may become more playful and interactive, which is good evidence against meningitis but not good evidence against occult bacteremia (Chapter 19).

The current mainstay of antipyretic therapy is **acetaminophen.** Acetaminophen is an antiprostaglandin that normalizes the thermoregulatory center's set point by interfering with the action of prostaglandins. Acetaminophen is well absorbed in the gastrointestinal tract, reaches peak levels in 1–2 hours, and has an effect that lasts 4–6 hours. It is not a gastrointestinal irritant, as are the nonsteroidal anti-inflammatory drugs (NSAIDs), and has not been associated with Reye's syndrome, which precludes the use of aspirin as an antipyretic agent in children. The acetaminophen dose for children is approximately 10–15 mg/kg orally every 4 hours, with a maximum adult dose of 640 mg (10 grains) every 4 hours (Table 18–4). No more than 5 doses should be given within a 24-hour period.

Ibuprofen and other NSAIDs are also useful for the treatment of fever. Similar to aspirin, these drugs are gastrointestinal irritants and affect the normal functioning of platelets. Ibuprofen generally is used as an alternative to acetaminophen in children 6 months of age or older who do not achieve satisfactory antipyresis with acetaminophen. The ibuprofen dose for children is 5–10 mg/kg orally every 6–8 hours and is adjusted on the basis of the initial temperature (Table 18–4). The effect on fever reduction in the first hour is the same with either acetaminophen or ibuprofen at 5 or 10 mg/kg, although the duration of the antipyretic effect of ibuprofen at the higher dose is generally 1–2 hours longer.

The efficiency of external cooling during acute febrile episodes has long been a subject of debate, but there appears to be no advantage to the use of antipyretics plus external cooling versus the use of antipyretics alone. When the temperature is elevated during an acute infectious illness and temperature reduction is desired, it is essential to reset the thermoregulatory center with antiprostaglandins. Otherwise, the body continues to produce and conserve heat even with external cooling. If external cooling is applied, it should be in the form of water at body temperature. As the water evaporates, calories are expended as the heat of evaporation. The use of cold water is not necessary unless the fever is extreme. The use of isopropyl alcohol as a method of external cooling should be discouraged because the alcohol may be absorbed. Sponging with tepid water should be reserved for those few patients in whom higher grades of fever (39.4–41.1°C [103–106°F]) do not respond to antipyretics and when the physician deems temperature reduction important.

Hospitalization or Outpatient Follow-up

Children with life-threatening infections should be admitted to the hospital for appropriate definitive treatment and supportive care. The majority of children with fever who are otherwise well and do not have life-threatening infections do not necessarily warrant admission. In many instances the immediate decision for inpatient observation versus outpatient follow-up depends on the answers to specific questions of parental adherence: Do the parents seem to be good observers of their child's condition? If the child's condition deteriorates, can the parents readily return to the hospital? Do the parents have transportation? Is there a telephone in the home? Can follow-up be ensured? When the answers to such questions are affirmative, nonthreatening but serious infections can be managed on an outpatient basis.

Physicians may choose to follow the child up as an outpatient either by telephone communication or by repeated examination, which is important for several reasons. First, additional encounters can be used to educate and support parents and to provide advice about management of symptoms in the future. Second, follow-up can be a useful part of the diagnostic process because a diagnosis that may not be apparent at the time of initial evaluation may become obvious on repeated examination; for example, the rash of roseola may not be apparent until the third or fourth day of illness. Third, follow-up documents the course of a more serious illness, such as pneumonia, during outpatient management. Such serious illnesses have a potential for clinical worsening, which mandates the monitoring of the child's progress.

TABLE 18–4. Use of Acetaminophen and Ibuprofen for Control of Fever in Children

Age	Weight (kilograms approximate)	Acetaminophen* (10–15 mg/kg per dose q4hr†)	Ibuprofen‡ Temperature ≤39.1°C (102.5°F) (5 mg/kg per dose q6–8hr)	Ibuprofen‡ Temperature >39.1°C (102.5°F) (10 mg/kg per dose q6–8hr)
0–3 mo	6–11 lb (2.5–5.4 kg)	40	—	—
4–5 mo	12 lb (5.5–5.9 kg)	80	—	—
6–11 mo	13–17 lb (6–7.9 kg)	80	25	50
12–23 mo	18–23 lb (8–10.9 kg)	120	50	100
2–3 yr	24–35 lb (11–15.9 kg)	160	75	150
4–5 yr	36–47 lb (16–21.9 kg)	240	100	200
6–8 yr	48–59 lb (22–26.9 kg)	320	125	250
9–10 yr	60–71 lb (27–31.9 kg)	400	150	300
11–12 yr	72–95 lb (32–43.9 kg)	480	200	400
Adult	≥96 lb (≥44 kg)	650	200	400

*Common dosage forms: infants' concentrated drops, 80 mg/0.8 mL (1 dropperful); children's suspension liquid, 160 mg/5 mL; children's chewable tablets, 80 mg; junior chewable tablets, 160 mg; junior-strength caplets, 160 mg; regular-strength tablets and caplets, 325 mg; extra-strength tablets, caplets, gelcaps, and geltabs, 500 mg.

†Not to exceed 5 doses in 24 hours.

‡Common dosage forms: oral drops, 40 mg/mL; suspension, 100 mg/5 mL; chewable tablets, 50 and 100 mg; adult tablets and caplets, 100, 200, 400, 600, and 800 mg.

REVIEWS

Alario AJ, McCarthy PL, Markowitz R, et al: Usefulness of chest radiographs in children with acute lower respiratory tract disease. *J Pediatr* 1987;111:187–93.

Baker MD, Bell LM, Avner JR: Outpatient management without antibiotics of fever in selected infants. *N Engl J Med* 1993;329:1437–41.

McCarthy PL, Jekel JF, Stashwick CA, et al: Further definition of history and observation variables in assessing febrile children. *Pediatrics* 1981;67:687–93.

McCarthy PL, Lembo RM, Fink HD, et al: Observation, history, and physical examination in diagnosis of serious illnesses in febrile children less than or equal to 24 months. *J Pediatr* 1987;110:26–30.

McCarthy PL, Sharpe MR, Spiesel SZ, et al: Observation scales to identify serious illness in febrile children. *Pediatrics* 1982a;70:802–9.

KEY ARTICLES

Baraff LJ, Bass JW, Fleisher GR, et al: Practice guideline for the management of infants and children 0 to 36 months of age with fever without source. Agency for Health Care Policy and Research. *Ann Emerg Med* 1993;22:1198–210.

Hoberman A, Wald ER, Reynolds EA, et al: Is urine culture necessary to rule out urinary tract infection in young febrile children? *Pediatr Infect Dis J* 1996;15:304–9.

Kauffman RE, Sawyer LA, Scheinbaum ML: Antipyretic efficacy of ibuprofen vs acetaminophen. *Am J Dis Child* 1992;146:622–5.

Kuppermann N, Fleisher GR, Jaffe DM: Predictors of occult pneumococcal bacteremia in young febrile children. *Ann Emerg Med* 1998;31:679–87.

McCarthy PL: Acute infectious illness in children. *Compr Ther* 1988;14:51–7.

McCarthy PL, Dolan TF Jr: Hyperpyrexia in children. Eight-year emergency room experience. *Am J Dis Child* 1976;130:849–51.

McCarthy PL, Cicchetti DV, Stashwick CA, et al: Diagnostic styles of attending pediatricians, residents, and nurses in evaluating febrile children. *Clin Pediatr* 1982b;21:534–7.

McCarthy PL, Jekel JF, Dolan TF Jr: Temperature greater than or equal to 40°C in children less than 24 months of age: A prospective study. *Pediatrics* 1977;59:663–8.

McCarthy PL, Jekel JF, Stashwick CA, et al: History and observation variables in assessing febrile children. *Pediatrics* 1980;65:1090–5.

McCarthy PL, Sznajderman SD, Lustman-Findling K, et al: Mothers' clinical judgment: A randomized trial of the Acute Illness Observation Scales. *J Pediatr* 1990;116:200–6.

Plaisance KL, Mackowiak PA: Antipyretic therapy. Physiologic rationale, diagnostic implications, and clinical consequences. *Arch Intern Med* 2000;160:449–56.

Samson JH, Apthorp J, Finley A: Febrile seizures and purulent meningitis. *JAMA* 1969;210:1918–9.

Wilson JT, Brown RD, Kearns GL, et al: Single-dose, placebo-controlled comparative study of ibuprofen and acetaminophen antipyresis in children. *J Pediatr* 1991;119:803–11.

CHAPTER 19

Fever and Occult Bacteremia in Infants and Young Children

M. Douglas Baker ▪ Paul L. McCarthy

The management of pediatric patients with fever in the absence of an apparent focus of infection presents problems unique to infants and young children. Research in this area has resulted in recommended approaches that minimize the chances of failing to recognize serious underlying infections while also minimizing unnecessary antibiotic use and hospitalization for those children who appear to be at low risk. There are two groups of children with special considerations: febrile children through 36 months of age, who are at risk of having bacteremia without a focus or evidence of sepsis (occult bacteremia), and younger febrile infants (<8 weeks of age), who may have bacteremia but also may have other foci of infection without apparent localizing signs or symptoms.

CHILDREN OLDER THAN 8 WEEKS OF AGE

EPIDEMIOLOGY

Bacteremia in febrile children, most notably in those up to 36 months of age, may be associated with focal soft tissue infections, such as buccal cellulitis, but often is also seen with apparently less serious clinical illnesses, such as viral upper respiratory tract infections or otitis media. **Ambulatory bacteremia,** or **occult bacteremia,** refers to bacteremia in those febrile children up to 36 months of age who have no focal soft tissue infections and who are not perceived as sufficiently ill to require hospitalization when seen initially but who subsequently have bacterial pathogens isolated in blood cultures.

Early studies performed at several medical centers documented that some young children with fever who are seen as outpatients do in fact have occult bacteremia. A study (McCarthy, 1988) of 996 consecutively enrolled children <36 months of age with temperatures of at least 38.3°C (101°F) documented occult bacteremia in 1% (10/996) of these children. Not all children had blood cultures, however. The occurrence of bacteremia increases as criteria for obtaining blood culture specimens, such as the degree of fever, are used that reflect the risk factors for bacterial bloodstream invasion. A study (Jaffe et al, 1987) of 955 children <36 months of age with temperatures of ≥39°C (≥102.2°F) and blood cultures for all children found that 2.8% (27/955) had bacteremia. During a period of approximately 1 year, a study (McCarthy et al, 1977) of 334 consecutive children <24 months of age with temperatures ≥40°C (≥104°F) evaluated in the emergency department at Yale–New Haven Hospital found that in 7.3% (24/329) of the children, blood cultures revealed bacteremia.

PATHOGENESIS

Bacteremia in outpatient children may occur either with or without an apparent focus of infection. Children may have fever and bacteremia associated with focal infections such as meningitis, buccal or periorbital cellulitis, epiglottitis, septic arthritis, osteomyelitis, pneumonia, bacterial enteritis, or urinary tract infection. A review (Alario et al, 1989) of 12 years of blood culture results obtained for outpatients found that 66% (318/482) of children with positive blood culture results were hospitalized immediately, most often presumably because of focal soft tissue complications. Only 34% (164/482) of children with bacteremia had so-called occult bacteremia. Many studies have demonstrated that the most common clinical syndromes without serious focal soft tissue involvement that are associated with bacteremia in outpatients are upper respiratory tract infections, influenza-like illnesses, fever with no associated findings, and otitis media. Children with diarrhea and fever may have *Salmonella* isolated from the blood. Other bacteria reported rarely to cause occult bacteremia are *Staphylococcus aureus,* group B *Streptococcus* (Garcia Pena et al, 1998), *Moraxella catarrhalis, Escherichia coli, Yersinia enterocolitica,* and *Enterobacter.* Bacteremia with group A *Streptococcus* has been associated with chickenpox, in some instances without evidence of a focal infection such as cellulitis or osteomyelitis (Doctor et al, 1995).

When bacteremia occurs with a seemingly less serious illness and without focal soft tissue infection, the organism isolated most often is *Streptococcus pneumoniae* (Table 19–1). This may change in the future because of the effectiveness of the conjugate pneumococcal vaccine approved in 2000.

SYMPTOMS AND CLINICAL MANIFESTATIONS

Several parameters are useful in predicting which febrile children without focal soft tissue infection at the initial visit do in fact have bacteremia. One of these parameters is the child's initial appearance. In a prospective study (Bass et al, 1993) of 519 children 3–36 months of age with either a temperature ≥40°C (≥104°F) or with a temperature ≥39.5°C (≥103°F) and a WBC count ≥15,000/mm^3, the child's appearance was assessed by scoring irritability, consolability, and social smile. The best total score for appearance was 3 and the worst was 10. As appearance worsened, the occurrence of bacteremia increased; at a clinical appearance score of 3, the occurrence of bacteremia was 8.5%, whereas if the score was 8 or greater, the occurrence of bacteremia was 19.7%. Another study (Baker et al, 1989) used the Acute Illness Observation Scales (AIOS) (Chapter 18) to assess the appearance of 154 children for whom blood cultures were to

TABLE 19–1. Organisms Isolated from Blood in Outpatient Children with Bacteremia (without Severe Focal Soft Tissue Infection)

Organism	Alario et al (1989) (n = 164)	Jaffe and Fleisher (1991) (n = 27)	Fleisher et al (1994) (n = 192)
Streptococcus pneumoniae	130	23	164
Haemophilus influenzae type b	29	2	9
Neisseria meningitidis	5	0	2
Salmonella	0	2	7
Others	0	0	10

Data from: Alario AJ, Nelson EW, Shapiro ED: Blood cultures in the management of febrile outpatients later found to have bacteremia. *J Pediatr* 1989;115:195-9; Jaffe DM, Fleisher GR: Temperature and total white blood cell count as indicators of bacteremia. *Pediatrics* 1991;87:670-4; and Fleisher GR, Rosenberg N, Vinci R, et al: Intramuscular versus oral antibiotic therapy for the prevention of meningitis and other bacterial sequelae in young, febrile children at risk for occult bacteremia. *J Pediatr* 1994;124:504-12.

be obtained, including 4 children with meningitis (Table 19–2). All children were then given antipyresis with acetaminophen, and AIOS scoring was repeated 1–2 hours later. Febrile children with bacteremia appeared more ill initially than children who did not have bacteremia but less ill than children with fever and severe focal bacterial infections such as meningitis. With antipyresis the appearance of children with bacteremia improved similarly to that of febrile children without bacteremia; hence the febrile child's appearance before antipyresis is critical in predicting bacteremia. Children with bacterial meningitis looked *more ill* 2 hours after antipyresis than they did initially.

These studies indicate that the occurrence of bacteremia is greater in ill-appearing children. Bacteremia, however, may occur in children who do not appear ill. In a study (Teach and Fleisher, 1995) that excluded ill-appearing children among 6,611 children 3–36 months of age with a temperature ≥39°C (≥102.2°F) and a nonfocal illness or uncomplicated otitis media, bacteremia was found in 2.9% (192/6,611) of the children. Neither the *change in appearance* after antipyresis nor the *response of fever* to antipyresis has been shown to be a predictor of bacteremia or to differentiate bacterial from nonbacterial infections (Baker et al, 1987, 1989) (Table 19–2).

Although a change in temperature in response to antipyresis does not predict bacteremia, several studies have demonstrated that the height of the initial fever is associated with bacteremia. As many as 7.3% of children up to age 24 months with a temperature ≥40°C (≥104°F) have bacteremia (McCarthy et al, 1977). However, the sensitivity of this degree of fever for all cases of bacteremia is only 52%; 48% of children with bacteremia have lesser fever (Jaffe and Fleisher, 1991). Hence additional screening studies have been sought to identify factors that predict bacteremia. A WBC count ≥15,000/mm^3 detects bacteremia in only approximately two thirds of children, although 23% of febrile children with temperatures ≥39°C (≥102.2°F) and a WBC count ≥15,000/mm^3 would be falsely identified as having bacteremia. Some experts (Jaffe and Fleisher, 1991) argue for a lower cutoff point of the WBC count to predict bacteremia in the hope of improving the sensitivity of diagnosis. At a WBC count of 10,000/mm^3, 92% of children with temperatures ≥39°C (≥102.2°F) and bacteremia will be identified. However, 57% of children with temperatures ≥39°C (≥102.2°F) and a WBC count ≥10,000/mm^3 will be falsely identified as having bacteremia. Nevertheless, some experts believe that a WBC count ≥10,000/mm^3 is the best compromise between sensitivity and false-positive rates in children with temperatures ≥39°C (≥102.2°F).

A study (Kuppermann et al, 1998) of 6,579 outpatient children 3–36 months of age with temperatures ≥39°C (≥102.2°F) who were previously enrolled in a study of occult bacteremia (Fleisher et al, 1994) specifically addressed the issue of prediction of occult pneumococcal bacteremia. The proportion of patients with occult bacteremia due to *S. pneumoniae* has increased since the vaccine against *Haemophilus influenzae* type b has been used. Occult pneumococcal bacteremia was seen in 2.5% (164/6,579) of the children who had blood cultures. For the total study sample, an ANC ≥10,000/mm^3 versus <10,000/mm^3 was associated with a 7.8% versus 0.8% occurrence of bacteremia; and a WBC count ≥15,000/mm^3 versus <15,000/mm^3 was associated with a 6% versus 0.7% occurrence of bacteremia. The authors favored the use of the ANC. Each 1°C increase in temperature was associated with an increased odds ratio of 1.77 favoring bacteremia. These data led the authors to characterize the following risk groups: (1) children 2–3 years of age with a temperature <39.5°C (<103.1°F) have a 1.1% risk of bacteremia; (2) children 2–3 years of age with a temperature

TABLE 19–2. Bacteremia and Response to Antipyresis

Factor	Bacteremic (n = 15)	Not Bacteremic (n = 135)	Meningitis (n = 4)
Clinical Appearance			
Initial appearance (mean AIOS score ± SD)	11.3 ± 3.5*	9.3 ± 2.9*	17.5 ± 4.7*
Appearance after antipyresis (mean AIOS score ± SD)	7.5 ± 1.4	7.7 ± 2.2	19.5 ± 5.9‡
Mean change in AIOS score	−3.8†	−1.6†	+2.0†
Temperature			
Initial temperature (mean ± SD)	40.1°C ± 0.5°C	40.4°C ± 0.4°C	
Temperature after antipyresis (mean ± SD)	38.5°C ± 0.6°C	38.4°C ± 0.6°C	
Mean change in temperature	−1.7°C§	−1.6°C§	

*p < .001 for mean AIOS score of all three groups.
†p < .05 for mean change in AIOS score among all three groups.
‡p < .05 for mean AIOS score between meningitis and other two groups.
§Not significant.
Adapted from Baker RC, Tiller T, Bausher JC, et al: Severity of disease correlated with fever reduction in febrile infants. *Pediatrics* 1989;83:1016–9.

≥39.5°C (≥103.1°F), and children 3–24 months of age with a temperature ≥39°C (≥102.2°F) have a 2.6% risk of bacteremia; and (3) children from group 2 with an ANC ≥10,000/mm^3 have an 8.3% risk of bacteremia.

Because the height of fever, WBC count, and clinical appearance have limitations as predictors of the presence of bacteria in the blood, recent studies have investigated the utility of more advanced technologies such as the PCR test to identify children with occult bacteremia. A study (Isaacman et al, 1998) reported PCR testing of 444 febrile outpatient children 3–36 months of age. The sensitivity of the PCR test for the 21 blood cultures that were positive for *S. pneumoniae* was 57%; 206 patients with a negative blood culture result had positive PCR text result. Thus PCR testing is not at this time sufficiently accurate to be used to identify children with occult bacteremia in an outpatient setting.

TREATMENT, COMPLICATIONS, AND PROGNOSIS

Expectant Antibiotic Therapy for Presumptive Bacteremia. The advisability of administering antibiotics while awaiting the results of the blood culture depends on the likelihood of subsequent focal soft tissue complications or persisting bacteremia and the efficacy of antibiotics in preventing such complications. Several studies have reported on focal complications and persisting bacteremia in children followed up as outpatients whose initial blood culture results were positive. A study (Alario et al, 1989) of 164 outpatient children with bacteremia found that 12% (20/164) of the cases were complicated by focal soft tissue involvement, including meningitis (n = 8), osteomyelitis (n = 2), and septic arthritis (n = 1), or with persisting bacteremia (n = 9) at follow-up. Of these 20 children with complications, 45% (9/20) returned to the hospital because the parents noted focal complications before being called back because of positive blood culture results. Of the remaining 11 children who returned after being called back because of positive blood culture results, 20% (4/20) had meningitis and 35% (7/20) had persisting bacteremia without other complications. This underlines the potential advantage of earlier intervention in an attempt to prevent complications in children who have had blood cultures and are followed up as outpatients; the mode of intervention is expectant antibiotic therapy.

The rate of complications of outpatient bacteremia correlates with the causal organism (Table 19–3). *S. pneumoniae* is less frequently associated with focal complications or persisting bacteremia than *H. influenzae* type b or *Neisseria meningitidis*. A study (Forman and Murphy, 1991) of 60 children with *H. influenzae* type b bacteremia followed up as outpatients found that 42% (25/60) developed invasive infections.

TABLE 19–3. Bacteremia and Complications by Organism

Organism	Proportion with Complications
Streptococcus pneumoniae	8/130 (6%)
Haemophilus influenzae type b	9/29 (31%)
Neisseria meningitidis	3/5 (60%)

Adapted from Alario AJ, Nelson EW, Shapiro ED: Blood cultures in the management of febrile outpatients later found to have bacteremia. *J Pediatr* 1989;115:195–9.

TABLE 19–4. Complications Associated with Bacteremia and Effect of Treatment with Oral Amoxicillin

Morbidity	Placebo (8/448)	Oral Amoxicillin (19/507)
Children with Major Complications		
Streptococcus pneumoniae	Persisting bacteremia (1)	Periorbital cellulitis (1)
Haemophilus influenzae type b	None	None
Salmonella	None	Persisting bacteremia (1)
Children with Minor Complications		
S. pneumoniae	Persisting fever (2) Otitis media (1)	Persisting fever (2) Otitis media (2)
H. influenzae type b	None	None
Salmonella	None	Enteritis (1)
Well without Complications		
S. pneumoniae	3	11
H. influenzae type b	1	1
Salmonella	0	0

Adapted from Jaffe DM, Tanz RR, Davis AT, et al: Antibiotic administration to treat possible occult bacteremia in febrile children. *N Engl J Med* 1987;317:1175–80.

Hence, if the efficacy of expectant antibiotics for presumptive bacteremia is being considered, use of an antibiotic effective against *H. influenzae* type b is warranted, although *S. pneumoniae* causes most instances of outpatient bacteremia. Now that the incidence of *H. influenzae* type b infections has dramatically fallen and a similar reduction in *S. pneumoniae* infections is likely to follow because of conjugate vaccines, these recommendations will require re-evaluation.

Several retrospective studies have found that the expectant use of antibiotics affects the occurrence of focal complications (Harper, 1995). In a rigorous prospective study (Jaffe et al, 1987), 995 children 3–36 months of age with temperatures ≥39°C (≥102.2°F) and no focal infections but who warranted antibiotic usage were randomly assigned to treatment with oral amoxicillin (507 children) or placebo (448 children). No differences in major morbidity between antibiotic and placebo groups occurred (Table 19–4). The numbers of children with major morbidity, however, were small, and the power of the study was insufficient to definitively assess the effect of antibiotics. The study did demonstrate that children with bacteremia who were given antibiotics became afebrile more quickly than those who were not given antibiotics.

Two studies (Kramer et al, 1989; Lieu et al, 1991) used decision analysis methods and compared several approaches to febrile children seen as outpatients. The data allowed a comparison between the two studies vis-à-vis the outcomes of hospitalizations and the number of major infections if a "blood culture" or a "no blood culture" strategy was used. In addition, data in one study (Lieu et al, 1991) permits a comparison of these two strategies with a third strategy, "blood culture for all and treat" (Table 19–5). These data indicate that obtaining blood cultures prevents two major infections per 1,000 patients (six vs four episodes of infection). In addition, the expectant use of antibiotics for all patients

TABLE 19–5. Comparison of Theoretical Outcomes of Bacteremia in Young Children Versus Initial Management

	Kramer (1989)		Lieu (1991)		
Outcome	Blood Culture for All	No Blood Culture	Blood Culture for All	No Blood Culture	Blood Culture for All and Treat
Patients	1000	1000	1000	1000	1000
Blood cultures performed	1000	0	1000	0	1000
Hospitalizations	24	6	14	6	8
Major infections	4	6	4	6	3

Adapted from Kramer MS, Lane DA, Mills EL: Should blood cultures be obtained in the evaluation of young febrile children without evident focus of infection? A decision analysis of diagnostic management strategies. *Pediatrics* 1989;84:18–27; and Lieu TA, Schwartz JS, Jaffe DM, et al: Strategies for diagnosis and treatment of children at risk for occult bacteremia: Clinical effectiveness and cost effectiveness. *J Pediatr* 1991;118:21–9.

who have blood cultures prevents one major infection per 1,000 patients, in comparison with blood culturing alone (four vs three episodes of infection).

Given the small number of major infections that are prevented by expectant use of antibiotics, it is not surprising that a study (Jaffe et al, 1987) of 955 children was unable to document a difference between placebo- and amoxicillin-treated groups. Another, much larger study (Fleisher et al, 1994) using two different methods of antibiotic intervention for potentially bacteremic febrile children enrolled 6,733 children between the ages of 3 and 36 months with temperatures ≥39°C (≥102.2°F) into a randomized trial of ceftriaxone (50 mg/kg as a single intramuscular dose) versus oral amoxicillin (20 mg/kg/dose every 8 hours for six doses). Bacteremia was documented in 2.8% (192/6,733) of these children: 164 with *S. pneumoniae,* 9 with *H. influenzae* type b, 7 with *Salmonella,* 2 with *N. meningitidis,* and 10 with other organisms. Of the 192 cases of bacteremia, 101 were in children randomly assigned to ceftriaxone therapy and 91 were in children treated with amoxicillin. Although the development of definite new focal bacterial infections differed significantly in the ceftriaxone- versus the amoxicillin-treated groups (0/101 vs 5/91, respectively), the development of definite or probable new focal bacterial infections did not differ significantly (3/101 vs 6/91, respectively). Additionally, four children treated with ceftriaxone were categorized as "unclassified," and yet on subsequent visits they had evidence of meningitis (n = 2), periorbital cellulitis (n = 1), or sinusitis (n = 1). If these four children are included in the comparison of the ceftriaxone- versus the amoxicillin-treated groups, the occurrence of focal complications is even more similar (7/101 vs 6/91, respectively).

Information from studies such as these led to an expert panel formulating guidelines for assessing and treating potential bacteremia in febrile children 3–36 months of age (Baraff et al, 1993). These guidelines call for a WBC count if the temperature is ≥39°C (≥102.2°F) and a blood culture for all such children, or for a blood culture only if the WBC count is ≥15,000/mm^3, followed by treatment with intramuscular ceftriaxone. Another option, according to this panel, is to treat all children with temperatures ≥39°C (≥102.2°F). These recommendations for therapy are highly controversial. Some experts (Kramer and Shapiro, 1997) have argued against obtaining CBCs and blood cultures for children in these risk groups, citing the poor predictive value of the WBC count, the cost of such an approach, patient discomfort associated with this testing, and associated unnecessary hospitalizations. They also argue against the use of expectant therapy with antibiotics while awaiting blood culture results because of the lack of data that clearly show their efficacy for prevention of complications, the side effects that could occur, and the likely emergence of resistant organisms.

These controversies and the lack of agreement among researchers are reflected in pediatric practice. In a recent survey (Wittler et al, 1998) of 175 pediatricians, when faced with the case of a child requiring blood culture and empiric antibiotics for potential occult bacteremia according to the guidelines of Baraff et al (1993), only 35% would start a blood culture and only 22% would treat empirically. It is our opinion that blood cultures are reasonable for children with higher grades of fever, such as temperatures ≥39°C (≥102.2°F). Many pediatricians may choose to follow such children without the use of blood cultures; if the follow-up is assiduous and communication is excellent between the family and the primary caregiver, then such an approach is reasonable. If blood cultures are obtained, the use of expectant antibiotics while one is awaiting blood culture results—given the results of studies, the ongoing controversy about this issue, and the impact on the development and spread of antimicrobial resistance—cannot be recommended as a routine practice.

Follow-up of Patients with Bacteremia. Approximately 3–5% of febrile children 3–36 months of age who have a blood culture will have positive results and will require re-evaluation. If findings indicate a focal soft tissue infection at re-evaluation, then repeated blood cultures, laboratory studies appropriate for the specific findings, and admission to the hospital for intravenous antibiotic therapy are warranted. Often, however, at the time of the return visit, evaluation is not straightforward because these children do not have a readily apparent focal complication. In these circumstances the child's clinical appearance and temperature and the specific organism identified in the blood culture are critical factors for clinical decision making.

A study (Bratton et al, 1977) of 97 episodes of unsuspected bacteremia with *S. pneumoniae* found that 55% (53/97) of the children had improved at follow-up, were afebrile and alert, and had no new focus of infection. All these children did well, and all who had repeated blood cultures (n = 40) had negative results. Of those who had not improved, 4 had meningitis, and in 13 of the 37 who had repeated blood cultures the bacteremia persisted. Hence, if a child with unsuspected *S. pneumoniae* bacteremia has clinically improved, a repeated blood culture is warranted, but the chance of focal complications or persisting bacteremia is small. The practice of using antibiotics while awaiting the result of the second culture is a reasonable approach but has not been studied rigorously. Children who have improved may be followed up as outpatients. Children with occult *S. pneumoniae* bacteremia who have not improved should have a full sepsis evaluation, including cerebrospinal fluid analysis and culture, with admission to the hospital for intravenous antibiotics pending laboratory and culture results. For *S. pneumoniae* bacteremia without meningitis, either cefotaxime (50–180 mg/kg/day q8hr IV) or ceftriaxone (50–75 mg/kg/day divided q12hr IV) provides empirical treatment until penicillin susceptibility is known. The total duration of treatment for children without a focus of infection who respond to antibiotics is 7–10 days. Children with *S. pneumoniae* bacteremia and meningitis should also receive vancomycin until antimicrobial susceptibilities are known (Chapter 52).

All children with occult *N. meningitidis* bacteremia should have a full sepsis evaluation, including cerebrospinal fluid analysis and culture and admission to the hospital for intravenous antibiotics. The poor outcome for many patients with unsuspected meningococcemia who are followed up as outpatients warrants this aggressive approach (Dashefsky et al, 1983; Wang et al, 2000). Penicillin G (200,000 U/kg/day divided q4hr IV; maximum, 24 MU/day) for 7 days provides treatment of meningococcal bacteremia.

Children with occult *H. influenzae* type b bacteremia represent a more complicated issue. A study (Forman and Murphy, 1991) found that by using a combination of ill appearance and the presence or absence of fever, a physician could predict not only focal soft tissue complications but also the results of cultures of normally sterile body fluids, including blood, obtained at the repeated evaluation (Table 19–6). These results indicate that the child who has a blood culture positive for *H. influenzae* type b at the initial visit and who is afebrile, well appearing, and without evidence of focal complications at follow-up has a small risk of ongoing invasive disease or of persisting bacteremia. The child who does not appear well or who continues to be febrile, however, should have a full sepsis evaluation, including CSF analysis and culture and admission to the hospital for intravenous antibiotics. Either cefotaxime (50–180 mg/kg/day divided q8hr IV) or ceftriaxone (50–75 mg/kg/day divided q12hr IV) provides empirical treatment until ampicillin susceptibility is known. The total duration of treatment for children who respond to antibiotics without a focus of infection is 7–10 days. The healthy-appearing, afebrile child with normal examination findings on follow-up should have a repeated blood culture and may continue to be followed up closely as an outpatient. The use of antibiotics in this circumstance has not been studied. It seems reasonable, however, to use intramuscular ceftriaxone daily for two doses until the repeated cultures are proved negative.

In summary, recent work has produced data that are useful in making clinical decisions regarding febrile children with bacteremia in an outpatient setting. Management strategies are evolving quickly. Certain key issues, such as the expectant use of antibiotics, continue to be the subject of debate.

TABLE 19–6. Complications Associated with *Haemophilus influenzae* Type b Bacteremia

Appearance	Total	Focal Soft Tissue Infection	Number with Positive Repeated Cultures of Blood or Body Fluids
Ill, with or without fever	25	20	14
Well and febrile	8	3	1
Well and afebrile	27	2*	0

*Pneumonia.

Adapted from Forman PM, Murphy TV: Reevaluation of the ambulatory pediatric patient whose blood culture is positive for *Haemophilus influenzae* type b. *J Pediatr* 1991;118:503–8.

INFANTS YOUNGER THAN 8 WEEKS OF AGE

The evaluation and management of fever in infants <8 weeks of age are somewhat different from those in older preschool children. Although the exact epidemiology of febrile illnesses in young infants is unclear, a large study (Baker and Bell, 1999) conducted in the emergency department of an urban pediatric referral center found the incidence of bacterial disease to be approximately 10% in febrile infants 1–2 months of age and approximately 13% in febrile infants <1 month of age. The bacterial diseases most commonly reported in this age group are urinary tract infections, which account for approximately one third of the total. However, bacterial gastroenteritis, bacteremia, meningitis, cellulitis, and other bacterial diseases are also seen with regularity. Although older reports of bacteremia in febrile infants suggested that observed incidences varied inversely according to age in weeks, more recent data indicate that the rate of bacteremia is between 2% and 3% in all febrile infants <8 weeks of age.

The reason for the relatively high overall rate of bacterial disease in this age group is not entirely clear. However, it is likely to be at least partly related to the immature immunologic function demonstrated in younger infants and to the increased susceptibility to certain bacterial pathogens, including *Listeria monocytogenes,* group B *Streptococcus,* and gram-negative enteric organisms.

TABLE 19–7. Protocols for Selection of Febrile Infants 1–3 Months of Age at Low Risk of Infection

Clinical Parameter	Baskin et al (1992)	Baker et al (1993)
Entry Criteria		
Age	28–89 days	29–56 days
Temperature	≥38°C	≥38.2°C*
Indicators of Low Risk of Infection		
AIOS score	—†	<10
WBC count	<20,000/mm³	<15,000/mm³
Band:neutrophil ratio	Not used	<0.2
Cerebrospinal fluid	No bacteria on Gram stain <10 WBC/mm³	No bacteria on Gram stain <8 WBC/mm³
Urinalysis	<10 WBC/hpf	<10 WBC/hpf
Chest x-ray film	Normal	Normal
Management		
Antibiotics prescribed for low-risk infants	Yes	No

*Temperature criteria changed to ≥38°C in a follow-up study (Baker et al, 1999).

†Acute Illness Observation Scales (AIOS) score was obtained but was not part of study entry criteria.

Adapted from Baskin MN, O'Rourke EJ, Fleisher GR: Outpatient treatment of febrile infants 28 to 89 days of age with intramuscular administration of ceftriaxone. *J Pediatr* 1992;120:22–7; and Baker MD, Bell LM, Avner JR: Outpatient management without antibiotics of fever in selected infants. *N Engl J Med* 1993;329:1437–41.

An important factor that distinguishes very young infants from older infants is the inconsistency of physical findings in the former with serious infection. The ability of a child to engage in interpretable social interaction with an adult is age related and inconsistent, if not absent, in infants <8 weeks of age. Although clinical scoring systems have been developed to help identify infants and toddlers at low risk of having bacterial disease (McCarthy et al, 1982), they have not been found to be reliable when applied to infants <8 weeks of age. In children of this age, a well appearance does not reliably ensure absence of bacterial disease.

These observations have influenced the practice of primary care physicians. Surveys indicate that most pediatricians, family practitioners, and emergency medicine physicians prefer to hospitalize febrile infants <8 weeks of age, including giving empirical antibiotic therapy.

Early studies of fever in infants showed that individual laboratory or clinical parameters, such as the CBC or the ESR, were not highly predictive of the presence of bacterial disease, thereby lending support to empirical hospitalization and administration of antibiotics. However, subsequent research has shown that for carefully selected infants, outpatient management can also be safe and effective. Of the studies that have tested screening tools to identify infants expected to be at low risk of having bacterial disease, two have used prospective, consecutive cohort designs. These studies were conducted in urban referral centers located in Boston (Baskin et al, 1992) and Philadelphia (Baker et al, 1993). From the entire reported population of young infants with fever, based on results of full evaluations for bacterial disease, each group of investigators identified subsets expected to be at minimal risk of having bacterial disease as the source of fever (Table 19–7). The specific components of the screening tools differed, which likely accounted for the failure of the Boston screen to predict the presence of bacterial disease in 5% of infants expected to be at minimal risk of having bacterial disease. The stricter Philadelphia screening criteria have consistently and accurately identified infants with fever due to nonbacterial diseases. Neither of these two screening tools has been prospectively tested in infants <1 month of age. Subsequent retrospective application of the Philadelphia and Boston screening tools to febrile infants <1 month of age have shown that 15–25% of these young infants with proven bacterial disease would have

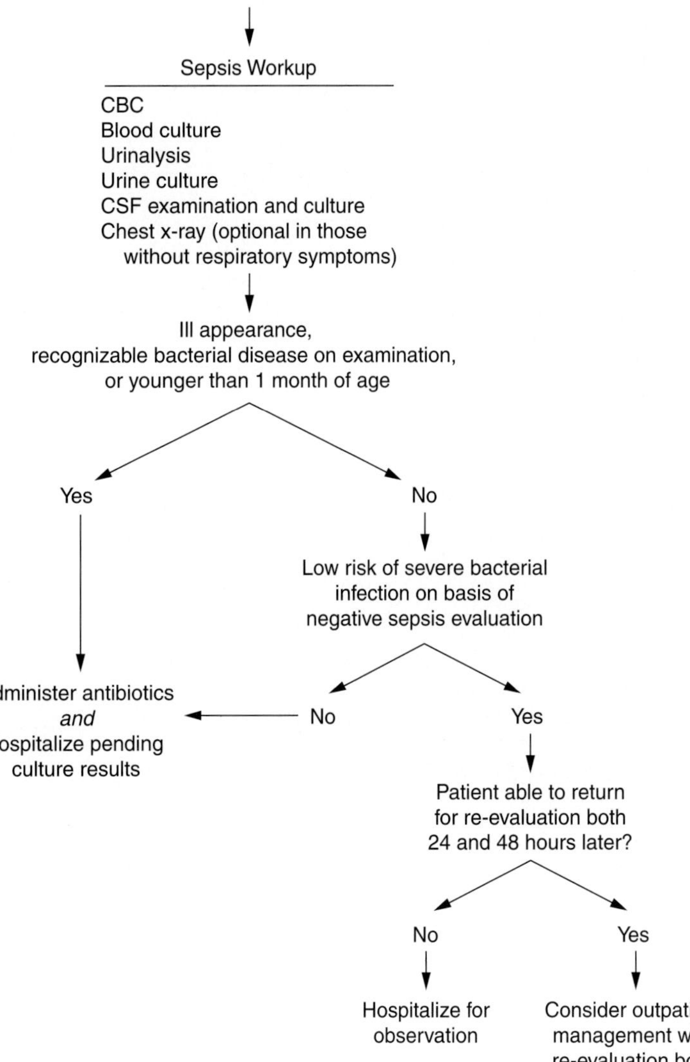

FIGURE 19–1. Algorithm for management of fever in infants <8 weeks of age.

been wrongly identified as being at low risk of having bacterial disease (Baker and Bell, 1999; Kadish et al, 1998).

The validity of some individual components of the infant fever screen has been challenged. Several investigators have concluded that the chest radiograph can be omitted from the evaluation of fever in infants who demonstrate no other signs or symptoms of respiratory disease. However, in several reports a substantial number of febrile infants with positive findings on chest radiography had no respiratory signs and symptoms. It is likely that many of those infants did not have bacterial pneumonia, despite their positive radiographic findings. This issue remains controversial.

Recommended Management

At present it seems prudent to approach fever in very young infants from an aggressive point of view (Fig. 19–1). Infants <8 weeks of age with measured rectal temperatures ≥38°C (≥100.4°F) should have a comprehensive evaluation including CBC, blood culture, urinalysis, urine culture, CSF analysis and culture, and a chest radiograph unless there are no respiratory signs or symptoms. Those with diarrhea should also have a stool culture, a test for the presence of fecal blood, and microscopic evaluation for fecal leukocytes. Those who are <4 weeks of age should be hospitalized and antibiotics administered empirically until bacterial cultures are proved negative. In the absence of meningitis or another focus of infection, either cefotaxime (50–180 mg/kg/day divided q8hr IV) or ceftriaxone (50–75 mg/kg/day divided q12hr IV) provides empirical treatment for *S. pneumoniae, H. influenzae* type b, *N. meningitidis, Salmonella,* and urinary tract pathogens. Ampicillin (200–300 mg/kg/day divided q6hr IV) should be added if *L. monocytogenes* or *Enterococcus* is suspected. The total duration of treatment for infants who have bacteremia without a focus of infection and who respond to antibiotics is 7–10 days. Antibiotic therapy can be discontinued at 48–72 hours if the infant appears well and results of the blood and other cultures are negative.

Infants between 4 and 8 weeks of age, if well appearing and otherwise found to be at low risk of having bacterial disease according to the Philadelphia criteria, can be managed as outpatients without antibiotics. Those who are not at low risk should be admitted to the hospital and antibiotics administered empirically until bacterial culture results are proved negative.

REVIEWS

Alario AJ, Nelson EW, Shapiro ED: Blood cultures in the management of febrile outpatients later found to have bacteremia. *J Pediatr* 1989; 115:195–9.

Baker RC, Tiller T, Bausher JC, et al: Severity of disease correlated with fever reduction in febrile infants. *Pediatrics* 1989;83:1016–9.

Baraff LJ, Bass JW, Fleisher GR, et al: Practice guideline for the management of infants and children 0 to 36 months of age with fever without source. Agency for Health Care Policy and Research. *Ann Emerg Med* 1993;22:1198–210.

Bratton L, Teele DW, Klein JO: Outcome of unsuspected pneumococcemia in children not initially admitted to the hospital. *J Pediatr* 1977;90:703–6.

Fleisher GR, Rosenberg N, Vinci R, et al: Intramuscular versus oral antibiotic therapy for the prevention of meningitis and other bacterial sequelae in young, febrile children at risk for occult bacteremia. *J Pediatr* 1994;124:504–12.

Jaffe DM, Tanz RR, Davis AT, et al: Antibiotic administration to treat possible occult bacteremia in febrile children. *N Engl J Med* 1987;317: 1175–80.

Kramer MS, Shapiro ED: Management of the young febrile child: A commentary on recent practice guidelines. *Pediatrics* 1997;100:128–34.

KEY ARTICLES

Baker MD, Fosarelli PD, Carpenter RO: Childhood fever: Correlation of diagnosis with temperature response to acetaminophen. *Pediatrics* 1987;80:315–8.

Baker MD, Bell LM, Avner JR: Outpatient management without antibiotics of fever in selected infants. *N Engl J Med* 1993;329:1437–41.

Baker MD, Bell LM: Unpredictability of serious bacterial illness in febrile infants from birth to 1 month of age. *Arch Pediatr Adolesc Med* 1999; 153:508–11.

Baker MD, Bell LM, Avner JR: The efficacy of routine outpatient management without antibiotics or fever in selected infants. *Pediatrics* 1999; 103:627–31.

Baskin MN, O'Rourke EJ, Fleisher GR: Outpatient treatment of febrile infants 28 to 89 days of age with intramuscular administration of ceftriaxone. *J Pediatr* 1992;120:22–7.

Bass JW, Steele RW, Wittler RR, et al: Antimicrobial treatment of occult bacteremia: A multicenter cooperative study. *Pediatr Infect Dis J* 1993; 12:466–73.

Dashefsky B, Teele DW, Klein JO: Unsuspected meningococcemia. *J Pediatr* 1983;102:69–72.

Doctor A, Harper MB, Fleisher GR: Group A beta-hemolytic streptococcal bacteremia: Historical overview, changing incidence, and recent association with varicella. *Pediatrics* 1995;96:428–33.

Forman PM, Murphy TV: Reevaluation of the ambulatory pediatric patient whose blood culture is positive for *Haemophilus influenzae* type b. *J Pediatr* 1991;118:503–8.

Garcia Pena BM, Harper MB, Fleisher GR: Occult bacteremia with group B streptococci in an outpatient setting. *Pediatrics* 1998;102:67–72.

Harper MB, Bachur R, Fleisher GR: Effect of antibiotic therapy on the outcome of outpatients with unsuspected bacteremia. *Pediatr Infect Dis J* 1995;14:760–7.

Isaacman DJ, Zhang Y, Reynolds EA, et al: Accuracy of a polymerase chain reaction based assay for detection of pneumococcal bacteremia in children. *Pediatrics* 1998;101:813–6.

Jaffe DM, Fleisher GR: Temperature and total white blood cell count as indicators of bacteremia. *Pediatrics* 1991;87:670–4.

Kadish JA, Bolte RB, Tobey J, et al: Applying outpatient protocols in febrile infants 1–29 days of age: Can the threshold be lowered [abstract]? Presented at the 38th Annual Meeting of the Ambulatory Pediatric Association, New Orleans, May 4, 1998.

Kramer MS, Lane DA, Mills EL: Should blood cultures be obtained in the evaluation of young febrile children without evident focus of infection? A decision analysis of diagnostic management strategies. *Pediatrics* 1989;84:18–27.

Kuppermann N, Fleisher GR, Jaffe DM: Predictors of occult pneumococcal bacteremia in young febrile children. *Ann Emerg Med* 1998;31:679–87.

Lieu TA, Schwartz JS, Jaffe DM, et al: Strategies for diagnosis and treatment of children at risk for occult bacteremia: Clinical effectiveness and cost-effectiveness. *J Pediatr* 1991;118:21–9.

McCarthy PL, Jekel JF, Dolan TF Jr: Temperature greater than or equal to 40°C in children less than 24 months of age: A prospective study. *Pediatrics* 1977;59:663–8.

McCarthy PL, Sharpe MR, Spiesel SZ, et al: Observation scales to identify serious illness in febrile children. *Pediatrics* 1982;70:802–9.

McCarthy PL: Acute infectious illness in children. *Compr Ther* 1988;14:51–7.

Teach SJ, Fleisher GR: Efficacy of an observation scale of detecting bacteremia in febrile children three to thirty-six months of age, treated as outpatients. Occult Bacteremia Study Group. *J Pediatr* 1995;126: 877–81.

Wang VJ, Malley R, Fleisher GR, et al: Antibiotic treatment of children with unsuspected meningococcal disease. *Arch Pediatr Adolesc Med* 2000;154:556–60.

Wittler RR, Cain KK, Bass JW: A survey about management of febrile children without source by primary care physicians. *Pediatr Infect Dis J* 1998;17:271–7.

CHAPTER 20

Fever of Unknown Origin

Paul L. McCarthy

Fever of unknown origin (FUO) is a diagnostic challenge to the pediatrician. The number of potential causes is great, and so is the array of laboratory tests that may be considered. The elements of clinical evaluation—history, physical examination, and observation—are the most critical in any diagnostic approach, after which appropriate laboratory studies may be ordered. The goal of the evaluation is to diagnose the cause accurately while minimizing trauma to the child as well as anxiety and cost for the family.

The normal body temperature of an adult is generally considered to be 37°C (98.6°F), although normal temperatures for an individual may vary from the average. The upper limit of normal temperature is 37.7°C (99.9°F), and the mean temperatures vary with the time of day, being lowest at 6 AM and highest at 4–6 PM, with a range of variability at these times of 0.5°C (0.9°F). Most clinicians agree that fever is present if the temperature is ≥38°C (≥100.4°F). Fever may be manifested in several patterns, including **sustained (continued or continuous) fever,** with no or little variation of not more than 0.556–0.834°C (1–1.5°F) each day and not returning to normal during any 24-hour period; **remittent fever** with diurnal variation of ≥1.11°C (≥2°F) and not falling to a normal level during any 24-hour period; **septic fever** with wide fluctuations, as with pyogenic infections; **hectic fever,** with daily recurring fever and with profound sweating, chills, and flushed countenance; **quotidian fever,** with daily fever (e.g., at 4–6 PM), as with *Plasmodium falciparum* infection and juvenile rheumatoid arthritis (JRA); **double-quotidian fever,** occurring twice a day, as with visceral leishmaniasis; **tertian fever,** occurring every third day, as with *Plasmodium vivax* or *Plasmodium ovale* malaria; **quartan fever,** occurring every fourth day, as with *Plasmodium malariae* malaria; **intermittent fever,** with small gaps of time without fever on most days, as with cholangitis (**Charcot's fever**); and **recurrent or relapsing fever,** with fever of any underlying fever pattern but with gaps of several days between long episodes of fever, as with Hodgkin's disease (**Pel-Ebstein fever**) or brucellosis.

The duration of fever qualifies an illness to be considered an FUO. However, the definition of duration differed in the major studies of FUO in children. FUO in children has been defined as temperatures ≥38.5°C (≥101.3°F) on more than four occasions for at least 2 weeks (Pizzo et al, 1975); fever for ≥3 weeks with an undiagnosed cause despite an evaluation as an outpatient, or fever for ≥1 week with an undiagnosed cause despite an evaluation as an inpatient (McClung, 1972; Lohr and Hendley, 1977); and temperatures ≥38°C (≥100.4°F) at least twice a week for 3 weeks (Steele, 1991). Fever associated with uncomplicated minor viral infections rarely lasts beyond 5 days. A practical criterion is that when a child has been febrile for more than 10 days and no cause is apparent, it is reasonable to consider the illness an FUO and to undertake the necessary evaluation. Fever of fewer than 10 days' duration with no identified caused is often referred to as **fever without localizing signs.**

ETIOLOGY

A vast number of diagnoses have been reported in children with FUO, although the cause is more likely to be an atypical presentation of a common disorder rather than the typical presentation of a rare disorder. Three major diagnostic categories—infection, collagen vascular disease, and malignancy—comprise one half to three fourths of cases of FUO (Table 20–1). In each of the four major studies of FUO in children, the major diagnostic category was infection, predominantly urinary tract infection, pneumonia, tonsillitis, sinusitis, and meningitis. Most infectious illnesses causing FUO do not represent rare or unusual diagnoses, but clinicians considering an infectious cause of an FUO should maintain a broad, searching perspective (Table 20–2). Certain infections, such as intra-abdominal bacterial infections, are currently less frequent causes of FUO than has previously been reported. Acute rheumatic fever and systemic lupus erythematosus are now comparatively rare causes of FUO, and Kawasaki syndrome has become a frequent cause of FUO, especially in younger children. Infectious causes are more common in younger children, whereas collagen vascular diseases, especially JRA, assume greater importance in children ≥6 years of age. Most malignancies associated with FUO in children are leukemias or lymphomas. A significant proportion of FUO cases in children and adults have no etiologic diagnosis.

DIAGNOSIS

It is of critical importance in the diagnostic evaluation of FUO to establish that the child does, in fact, have a fever. The technique of temperature taking may be incorrect (e.g., the mercury in the thermometer may not be shaken down before use). Temperatures of 37.7°C (99.9°F) may be considered by parents to be abnormal and reported as fever. Factitious fever may result from caregivers who seek secondary gain and report inaccurate temperature data. One study (Dinarello, 1978) of more than 400 patients reported to have FUO found that 18% actually did not have fever, but either the technique of temperature taking or the interpretation of temperatures was erroneous (12%), or the fever was factitious (6%). Hence the laboratory evaluation for FUO was averted in nearly one in five patients by reviewing the methods by which temperatures were taken and ascertaining that, in fact, elevated temperatures were documented.

Factitious fever, or fever that is produced intentionally by the patient (**Munchausen syndrome**) or the parent of a child (**Munchausen syndrome by proxy**), is an important consideration in the evaluation of FUO. It is usually the child's mother who fabricates the illness; she typically has had previous extensive exposure to the health care system and interacts well with medical personnel. Frequently she has experienced abuse or rejection in her own childhood and has a symbiotic relationship with the child. The

TABLE 20–1. Etiology of Fever of Unknown Origin in Children and Adults

	Children					Adults	
		Pizzo et al (1975)					
Etiology	McClung (1972) (n = 99)	Age <6 yr (n = 52)	Age >6 yr (n = 48)	Lohr and Hendley (1977) (n = 54)	Steele et al (1991) (n = 109)	Petersdorf and Beeson (1961) (n = 100)	Knockaert et al (1992) (n = 199)
Infection	29%	65%	38%	33%	20%	36%	23%
Bacterial or fungal	28%	38%	25%	30%	11%	36%	18%
Viral	1%	27%	13%	4%	9%	—	5%
Collagen vascular disease	11%	8%	35%	20%	8%	13%	21%
Juvenile rheumatoid arthritis	6%	6%	15%	13%	3%	—	3%
Systemic lupus erythematosus	3%	—	6%	—	2%	5%	1%
Rheumatic fever	—	—	—	2%	1%	6%	—
Other	2%	2%	15%	6%	3%	2%	18%
Malignancy	8%	8%	4%	13%	2%	19%	7%
Leukemia, lymphoma	4%	6%	2%	11%	2%	8%	3%
Sarcoma	4%	2%	2%	2%	—	2%	4%
Other	—	—	—	—	—	9%	—
Miscellaneous	10%	13%	4%	11%	2%	22%	20%
Factitious (Munchausen syndrome, or Munchausen syndrome by proxy [for children])		—	—	4%	1%	3%	4%
No etiologic diagnosis	41%	6%	19%	19%	67%	7%	26%

Data from Knockaert DC, Vanneste LJ, Vanneste SB, et al: Fever of unknown origin in the 1980s. An update of the diagnostic spectrum. *Arch Intern Med* 1992;152:51–5; Lohr JA, Hendley JO: Prolonged fever of unknown origin. A record of experiences with 54 childhood patients. *Clin Pediatr* 1977;16:768–73; McClung HJ: Prolonged fever of unknown origin in children. *Am J Dis Child* 1972;124:544–50; Petersdorf RG, Beeson PB: Fever of unexplained origin. Report on 100 cases. *Medicine* 1961;40:1–30; Pizzo PA, Lovejoy FH Jr, Smith DH: Prolonged fever in children: Review of 100 cases. *Pediatrics* 1975;55: 468–73; and Steele RW, Jones SM, Lowe BA, et al: Usefulness of scanning procedures for diagnosis of fever of unknown origin in children. *J Pediatr* 1991;119:526–30.

child's illness ensures attention and support in a medical environment. The bland, inappropriate affect of the caregiver despite the reported history of prolonged fever is often a key to recognizing that the ''fever'' is factitious, and careful temperature taking by medical staff will usually provide documentation.

The most important components in arriving at a diagnosis in a child with FUO are a carefully taken history and a carefully performed physical examination. Important aspects of the patient's history that may provide clues for further investigation of possible infectious diseases include contact with individuals who are ill; contact with animals, arthropods, or insects; travel; ingestion of contaminated food or water; ingestion of game meat, raw meat, or raw fish; pica; immunizations; hospitalizations, surgeries, and other treatments of medical illnesses; transfusions of blood or blood products; medications; and genetic and ethnic background. The most useful physical findings are skin findings, joint findings, heart murmurs, and hepatosplenomegaly.

In one study (Lohr and Hendley, 1977) of FUO in children, for the 44 of 54 patients with an FUO whose cause was established, there were 77 sources of information leading to a confirmation of the diagnosis. Of the 77 sources, 59 (77%) did not involve sophisticated diagnostic imaging or invasive procedures. The most useful sources of information were history (8 patients); physical examination (8 patients); observation of the clinical course (18 patients); and routine laboratory studies (25 patients) including a CBC, sickle cell preparation, hemoglobin electrophoresis, urinalysis, CSF analysis, bacterial cultures, serologic tests, blood chemistry tests, and radiographs.

There is a high yield of routine studies directed toward the diagnoses most commonly seen in childhood FUO. Invasive radiologic or surgical procedures (e.g., laparotomy) and biopsies (e.g., lymph node, liver) should be performed only if the child continues to have symptoms and no diagnosis has been established. The yield from biopsies and laparotomy in children is much less than in adults. Biopsy of the liver or lymph nodes should be reserved for those cases with specific findings (e.g., hepatitis, lymphadenopathy) or if a specific entity is suspected that requires histopathologic examination of tissue.

Laboratory Evaluation

Screening tests including WBC and differential cell counts, platelet count, ESR, and urinalysis should always be obtained. Careful examination of the blood smear is necessary in the evaluation of hematologic malignancies, abnormalities of the white blood cells, and malaria. In one series (McClung et al, 1972), in four of five children with FUO and leukemia there were abnormalities in the CBC. Anemia and an elevated ESR indicate an active inflammatory process, whereas an ESR <10 mm/hr most often indicates a minor or viral illness. Bacterial cultures of urine, blood, throat secretions, cerebrospinal fluid, and stool are important for diagnosing common serious bacterial infections that can cause an FUO. A PPD skin test for tuberculosis, along with *Candida,* mumps, or *Trichophyton* controls, should be performed. Serologic testing for specific bacterial, viral, and fungal infections is best guided by the history and physical examination.

Evaluation for collagen vascular disease should be part of the initial laboratory evaluation. Tests for antinuclear antibody, rheumatoid factor, quantitative immunoglobulins, and a serum complement profile (C3, C4, and total hemolytic complement [THC, also known as CH_{50}]) should be performed.

TABLE 20–2. Infectious Causes of Fever of Unknown Origin in Children

Systemic	
Septicemia	2
Malaria (*Plasmodium*)	1
Respiratory	
Tracheobronchitis, pneumonia	11
Pharyngitis, tonsillitis, peritonsillar abscess	7
Sinusitis	6
Chronic streptococcosis	5
Chronic otitis media	1
Tuberculosis (*Mycobacterium tuberculosis*)	1
Histoplasmosis (*Histoplasma*)	1
Central Nervous System	
Bacterial meningitis	8
Viral meningoencephalitis	3
Tuberculous meningitis (*M. tuberculosis*)	1
Gastrointestinal	
Bacterial enteritis	4
Pyogenic liver abscess	1
Cardiovascular	
Infective endocarditis	5
Renal	
Urinary tract infection, pyelonephritis	15
Musculoskeletal	
Osteomyelitis	4
Other	
Viral syndrome	19
Infectious mononucleosis (EBV)	12
Tuberculosis, other (*M. tuberculosis*)	4
Cat-scratch disease (*Bartonella henselae*)	3
Lyme disease (*Borrelia burgdorferi*)	2
Brucellosis	1
Psittacosis (*Chlamydia psittaci*)	1
Tick-borne typhus (*Rickettsia conorii*)	1
Generalized herpes simplex virus infection	1
Total	120

Combined data on 362 children in four studies of FUO in children: Lohr JA, Hendley JO: Prolonged fever of unknown origin. A record of experiences with 54 childhood patients. *Clin Pediatr* 1977;16:768–73; McClung HJ: Prolonged fever of unknown origin in children. *Am J Dis Child* 1972;124:544–50; Pizzo PA, Lovejoy FH Jr, Smith DH: Prolonged fever in children: Review of 100 cases. *Pediatrics* 1975;55:468–73; and Steele RW, Jones SM, Lowe BA, et al: Usefulness of scanning procedures for diagnosis of fever of unknown origin in children. *J Pediatr* 1991;119:526–30.

Bone marrow aspirates are important for diagnosing malignancies, as well as infections, especially in immunocompromised persons. A study (Hayani et al, 1990) of 414 episodes of FUO in children in whom bone marrow examination was part of the diagnostic evaluation showed its usefulness in detecting malignancy (28 children), hemophagocytic syndrome (3 children), histiocytosis (2 children), and infections (15 children) including bacterial (4 children), *Mycobacterium avium-intracellulare complex* (4 children), and fungal (3 children).

Diagnostic Imaging

Chest radiographs should be obtained routinely in the evaluation of FUO. Other diagnostic imaging studies are often informative but rarely lead to an unsuspected diagnosis, and therefore they should not be used as screening tests. Useful imaging studies may include abdominal ultrasonography and contrast (barium) examination of the upper and lower gastrointestinal tracts, which are especially useful in evaluating for regional enteritis. Abdominal CT or MRI should be performed before consideration is given to more invasive procedures such as laparotomy. The use of CT and MRI has virtually eliminated the need for exploratory surgery in patients with FUO.

MANAGEMENT

Children who do not appear severely ill and do not have specific findings to suggest a cause of FUO may be followed up as outpatients. Screening laboratory tests may be obtained. If doubt exists about the presence of fever, techniques of temperature taking should be reviewed with the parents and values recorded at home for several days. If the clinical suspicion is strong that the child has no underlying illness on the basis of observation, history, and physical examination, then laboratory evaluation may be delayed until the results of temperature values recorded at home for several days are reviewed.

Empirical antimicrobial therapy should generally be avoided for patients with no specific clues to a possible cause and no identifiable cause of FUO. Therapy may further obscure the diagnosis and provide a false sense of security in an infectious etiology. There is a possible role for selective use of an empirical trial of a nonsteroidal anti-inflammatory agent for patients in whom a collagen vascular disease is suspected. A rapid favorable response alleviates symptoms and provides additional evidence for a disorder that may become more apparent with time.

Inpatient evaluation of FUO is warranted if the clinical impression is that the child has a significant illness (e.g., the child is pale and listless), if necessary to document the fever pattern, or for repeated physical examinations (e.g., a quotidian fever patten with simultaneous observation of a fleeting salmon-color rash suggests JRA). Children should be admitted to the hospital for documentation of fever if there is any concern that the methods of temperature recording by caregivers are inaccurate or that the fever is factitious.

REVIEWS

Dinarello CA, Wolff SM: Pathogenesis of fever in man. *N Engl J Med* 1978;298:607–12.

Mackowiak PA (editor): *Fever: Basic Mechanisms and Management,* 2nd ed. New York, Raven Press, 1997.

McClung HJ: Prolonged fever of unknown origin in children. *Am J Dis Child* 1972;124:544–50.

Petersdorf RG, Beeson PB: Fever of unexplained origin. Report on 100 cases. *Medicine* 1961;40:1–30.

Pizzo PA, Lovejoy FH Jr, Smith DH: Prolonged fever in children: Review of 100 cases. *Pediatrics* 1975;55:468–73.

KEY ARTICLES

Buonomo C, Treves ST: Gallium scanning in children with fever of unknown origin. *Pediatr Radiol* 1993;23:307–10.

Forsyth BWC: Munchausen syndrome by proxy. In Lewis M (editor): *Child and Adolescent Psychiatry: A Comprehensive Textbook.* Baltimore, Williams & Wilkins, 1991.

Hayani A, Mahoney DH, Fernbach DJ: Role of the bone marrow examination in the child with prolonged fever. *J Pediatr* 1990;116:919–20.

Knockaert DC, Vanneste LJ, Vanneste SB, et al: Fever of unknown origin in the 1980s. An update of the diagnostic spectrum. *Arch Intern Med* 1992;152:51–5.

Lohr JA, Hendley JO: Prolonged fever of unknown origin. A record of experiences with 54 childhood patients. *Clin Pediatr* 1977;16:768–73.
Mackowiak PA, Wasserman SS, Levine MM: A critical appraisal of 98.6 degrees F, the upper limit of the normal body temperature, and other legacies of Carl Reinhold August Wunderlich. *JAMA* 1992;268:1578–80.
McCarthy PL: Fever. *Pediatr Rev* 1998;19:401–7.
Miller LC, Sisson BA, Tucker LB, et al: Prolonged fevers of unknown origin in children: Patterns of presentation and outcome. *J Pediatr* 1996; 12:419–23.
Steele RW, Jones SM, Lowe BA, et al: Usefulness of scanning procedures for diagnosis of fever of unknown origin in children. *J Pediatr* 1991;119:526–30.

CHAPTER 21

Bacteremia, Sepsis, and Septic Shock

Marc H. Lebel ▪ Bruce Tapiero

Bacteremia and *sepsis* both refer to the invasion of the bloodstream by a bacterial pathogen. **Bacteremia** is defined as a positive blood culture result. It may be transient and low grade (occurring during the course of dental or surgical procedures) and not associated with focal disease other than fever (primary occult bacteremia). Persistent bacteremia may represent a serious extension of an invasive bacterial infection (secondary bacteremia with focal infection). The child with bacteremia usually appears only mildly ill.

Sepsis is the systemic response to an infection manifested by hyperthermia (temperatures >38°C [100.4°F]) or hypothermia (temperatures <36°C [96.8°F]), tachycardia (heart rate >160/min in infants; >150/min in children), and tachypnea (respiratory rate >60/min in infants; >50/min in children). This systemic response can also be elicited by a variety of noninfectious causes. The clinical manifestations are similar and are mediated by the production of endogenous factors such as cytokines and other inflammatory mediators.

Children with septicemia and signs of central nervous system dysfunction (irritability, lethargy), cardiovascular impairment (cyanosis, poor perfusion), and DIC (petechiae, ecchymosis) are readily recognized as **"toxic appearing"** or **"septic."** This condition may progress to septic shock and eventually to death. An identified focus of infection, immunosuppression, or predisposing risk factor such as an intravascular device is often, but not always, present. A sepsis syndrome may occur in the absence of documented bacteremia that clinically cannot be differentiated from septic shock. This syndrome may result from endotoxemia; severe, localized gram-negative bacterial infection; slow-growing bacterial organisms; or rickettsial or viral infection.

Septic shock is defined as sepsis with hypotension (systolic blood pressure in infants: <65 mm Hg; in children: <75 mm Hg [or below the fifth percentile for age]) despite adequate fluid resuscitation in the presence of perfusion abnormalities. The resulting tissue ischemia leads to cell dysfunction and eventually cell death if hypoperfusion is prolonged.

In 1992 the American College of Chest Physicians and the Society of Critical Care Medicine developed consensus definitions of sepsis and organ failure in adult patients (Table 21–1). Although these definitions were not developed for pediatric patients, they are used to clarify the different syndromes, facilitate precise descriptions of patients for comparison between different institutions, and decrease the confusion that can exist in the interpretation of clinical trials.

ETIOLOGY

Bacteremia. The incidence and causes of bacteremia and sepsis vary according to age (Table 21–2). With the dramatic decline of the incidence of *Haemophilus influenzae* type b infections, *Streptococcus pneumoniae* now accounts for more than 85% of cases of bacteremia. New conjugate vaccines against *S. pneumoniae* should contribute to the overall decrease in the incidence of pneumococcal bacteremia in the first years of life. More recently, *Kingella kingae* has emerged as an important etiologic agent of invasive infections in young children, either as bacteremia alone or as endocarditis or osteoarticular infections.

Sepsis. The spectrum of etiologic agents of **overwhelming sepsis** changes with age and predisposing condition. In the newborn period the most common agents are group B *Streptococcus* and *Escherichia coli,* but fulminant sepsis has also been reported with *Listeria monocytogenes,* Enterobacteriaceae (e.g., *Enterobacter, Klebsiella*), *Staphylococcus aureus,* coagulase-negative staphylococci, and *Enterococcus* (Chapter 95). Yeast infections (e.g., with *Candida albicans* and other *Candida* species) and viral infections (e.g., with herpes simplex viruses, enteroviruses) can produce a clinical picture indistinguishable from that of fulminant bacterial neonatal sepsis.

The organism usually associated with fulminant sepsis in children beyond 8 weeks of age is *Neisseria meningitidis.* Meningococcemia is the prototype of fulminant pediatric infection without a primary focus of infection and leading to death in a matter of hours from the time of onset of symptoms. Approximately 3000 cases of meningococcemia occur annually in the United States. Of all cases of meningococcemia, 10–20% may be classified as fulminant, typically beginning with lethargy and a petechial rash and progressing rapidly to hypotension, shock, purpura, and DIC.

Other common but less frequent bacterial causes of sepsis in children include group A *Streptococcus, S. pneumoniae* (pneumococcus), and *H. influenzae* type b. *S. pneumoniae* is the most common cause of occult bacteremia in infants and young children, but the frequency of accompanying sepsis is far less than for *N. meningitidis* (Chapter 19). *H. influenzae* type b has historically been an important pathogen of sepsis in children, but universal immunization during infancy with conjugate *H. influenzae* type b vaccine has dramatically decreased the incidence of infections caused by this organism in countries that have adopted this vaccine. Other bacteria, such as *S. aureus, Pseudomonas aeruginosa,* and other enteric gram-negative bacilli, can also cause a similar picture of overwhelming sepsis but are uncommon in immunocompetent individuals without a risk factor such as an indwelling intravascular catheter.

In children with an immunologic defect, including functional or anatomic asplenia, encapsulated bacteria (*N. meningitidis, H. influenzae* type b, and *S. pneumoniae*) are the most common causes of overwhelming sepsis. *P. aeruginosa* and other gram-negative bacilli are also important pathogens in these patients.

Septic Shock. Many pathogens (bacteria, viruses, parasites, fungi, rickettsiae) can cause a sepsis syndrome and septic shock. The microbiologic causes vary according to the age of the patient, immune status, and other predisposing risk factors. Most of the

TABLE 21–1. Consensus Definitions for Sepsis and Organ Failure in Adults (American College of Chest Physicians and Society of Critical Care Medicine)

- ***Infection:*** microbial phenomenon characterized by an inflammatory response to the presence of microorganisms or the invasion of normally sterile host tissue by those organisms.
- ***Bacteremia:*** the presence of viable bacteria in the blood.
- ***Systemic inflammatory response syndrome:*** the systemic inflammatory response to a variety of severe clinical insults. The response is manifested by two or more of the following conditions:
  - Temperature >38°C (100.4°F) or <36°C (96.8°F)
  - Heart rate >90 beats/min
  - Respiratory rate >20 breaths/min or $Paco_2$ <32 mm Hg
  - WBC count >12,000/mm^3, <4,000/mm^3, or >10% immature (band) forms
- ***Sepsis:*** the systemic response to infection. This systemic response is manifested by two or more of the following conditions as a result of infection:
  - Temperature >38°C (100.4°F) or <36°C (96.8°F)
  - Heart rate >90 beats/min
  - Respiratory rate >20 breaths/min or $Paco_2$ <32 mm Hg
  - WBC count >12,000/mm^3, <4,000/mm^3, or >10% immature (band) forms
- ***Severe sepsis:*** sepsis associated with organ dysfunction, hypoperfusion, or hypotension. Hypoperfusion and perfusion abnormalities may include, but are not limited to, lactic acidosis, oliguria, or an acute alteration in mental status.
- ***Septic shock:*** sepsis with hypotension despite adequate fluid resuscitation, along with the presence of perfusion abnormalities that may include, but are not limited to, lactic acidosis, oliguria, or an acute alteration in mental status. Persons who are receiving inotropic or vasopressor agents may not be hypotensive at the time that perfusion abnormalities are measured.
- ***Hypotension:*** a systolic blood pressure of <90 mm Hg or a reduction of >40 mm Hg from baseline in the absence of other causes of hypotension.
- ***Multiple organ dysfunction syndrome:*** presence of altered organ function in an acutely ill patient to the extent that homeostasis cannot be maintained without intervention.

Reproduced with permission from American College of Chest Physicians/Society of Critical Care Medicine Consensus Conference: Definitions for sepsis and organ failure and guidelines for the use of innovative therapies in sepsis. *Crit Care Med* 1992;20:864–74. © Williams & Wilkins, 1992.

TABLE 21–2. Infectious Causes of Bacteremia and Sepsis in Otherwise Healthy Children, by Age Group

Neonatal Period	**Age 3–24 Mo**
Group B *Streptococcus*	*S. pneumoniae*
Escherichia coli	*N. meningitidis*
Other enteric gram-negative bacilli	*H. influenzae* type b
Listeria monocytogenes	***Rare:***
Coagulase-negative staphylococci	Group A *Streptococcus*
Rare:	*S. aureus*
Staphylococcus aureus	*Salmonella*
Salmonella	*Shigella*
Pseudomonas aeruginosa	**Age 2–5 Yr**
Age 1–3 Mo	*S. pneumoniae*
Haemophilus influenzae type b	*N. meningitidis*
Streptococcus pneumoniae	*H. influenzae* type b
Group B *Streptococcus*	***Rare:***
E. coli	Group A *Streptococcus*
Rare:	*Pseudomonas*
L. monocytogenes	Other gram-negative bacilli
Neisseria meningitidis	**Age ≥5 Yr**
Salmonella	*S. aureus*
	S. pneumoniae
	N. meningitidis
	Group A *Streptococcus*
	Rare:
	Other gram-negative bacilli
	Neisseria gonorrhoeae

pathogens causing bacteremia (Table 21–2) can eventually lead to septic shock, depending on the host and underlying condition.

Gram-negative enteric organisms are the most common pathogens involved in septic shock. One study (Jacobs, 1990) of septic shock in infants and children without predisposing risk factors reported that *H. influenzae* type b caused 41% of episodes, and *N. meningitidis* caused 18% (Table 21–3). Immunization against *H. influenzae* type b beginning at 2 months of age has caused a

TABLE 21–3. Septic Shock: Etiology and Mortality Rate for 143 Infants and Children

Pathogen	Total Episodes of Septic Shock (%)	Mortality (%)
Haemophilus influenzae type b	41	1.7
Neisseria meningitidis	18	11.5
Streptococcus pneumoniae	11	6.3
Group B *Streptococcus*	6	12.5
Staphylococcus aureus	5	28.6
Gram-negative enteric bacilli	5	0
Apparent meningococcemia	2	100
Pseudomonas aeruginosa	1	100
Other organisms	11*	6.3
TOTAL	**100**	**9.8**

*Includes eight cases of polymicrobial sepsis: *Listeria monocytogenes* (n = 2), *Proteus mirabilis* (n = 2), *Enterobacter sakazakii* (n = 1), *Staphylococcus epidermidis* (n = 1), *Enterococcus* (n = 1), and viridans streptococci (n = 1).

Adapted from Jacobs RF, Sowell MK, Moss MM, et al: Septic shock in children: Bacterial etiologies and temporal relationships. *Pediatr Infect Dis J* 1990;9:196–200. (Persons with malignancy, burn, or primary immunodeficiency were excluded from the analysis.)

sharp decline in the incidence of *Haemophilus* disease in North America, and other pathogens are now more likely to be encountered in children with septic shock.

Gram-positive organisms are also potential pathogens. *S. aureus* and group A *Streptococcus* can cause septic shock or toxic shock syndrome (Chapter 22). Infrequently, coagulase-negative staphylococci or *Enterococcus faecalis* causes a septic syndrome. Fungal infections caused by *C. albicans* can result in septic shock indistinguishable to the one caused by a gram-negative enteric pathogen. In the newborn period, perinatally acquired enterovirus and herpes simplex virus can cause multiorgan dysfunction and shock state (Chapter 97). In the older patient, adenoviral infections can cause a similar illness. Hantavirus infection has been associated with multiorgan failure, shock, and death (Chapter 68). Rocky Mountain spotted fever in the United States and Brazilian purpuric fever (caused by *Haemophilus aegyptius*) in South American can produce a meningococcemia-like illness (Chapter 30). Parasites such as *Plasmodium falciparum* can also induce septic shock (Chapter 32). Despite appropriate cultures, no pathogen is identified in up to 40% of patients with septic shock.

EPIDEMIOLOGY

Bacteremia and Sepsis. There are many predisposing risk factors for bacteremia in children (Table 21–4). The risk of bacteremia and sepsis is inversely related to advancing age. In the neonatal period the incidence of sepsis varies from 1 to 10 per 1,000 live births (average: 2–3 per 1,000). Premature infants have the highest incidence. In children younger than 3 months with fever, 15% have serious bacterial infection and 5% have bacteremia.

In children 6–24 months of age with fever but without localizing signs of infection at presentation, the incidence of bacteremia has decreased from 5% to 9% in the period before the availability of *H. influenzae* type b vaccines, to 1.6% after universal vaccination with *H. influenzae* type b conjugate vaccines (Lee, 1998). When there are signs of upper respiratory tract involvement, the reported incidence of bacteremia is 0.2%. The likelihood of bacteremia and sepsis in children 3–24 months of age is proportional to the degree of temperature elevation: bacteremia was found to be the cause of fever in 4% of infants with temperatures of 38.9–39.4°C (102–103°F), in 8% of those with temperatures of 40–41°C (104–105.8°F), and in 25% of those with temperatures above 41°C (105.8°F).

TABLE 21–4. Predisposing Risk Factors for Bacteremia in Infants and Children

- Agammaglobulinemia
- Acquired immunodeficiency syndrome (AIDS)
- Asplenia (anatomic or functional)
- Chemotherapy
- Complement and properdin deficiency
- Congenital heart disease
- Extensive burns
- Foreign body material
- Instrumentation of respiratory, gastrointestinal, or genitourinary tract
- Intractable diarrhea of infancy
- Intravascular or invasive monitoring device
- Malignancy (leukemia, lymphoma, or solid malignancy)
- Multiple trauma
- Neutropenia
- Prematurity
- Sickle cell disease
- Surgery
- Transplantation
- Urinary tract malformation

Bacteremia in young children without focal signs of infection has been termed occult bacteremia because the child does not appear to be critically ill (septic) despite the presence of bacteria in the bloodstream (Chapter 19).

After 2 years of age, bacteremia without an identifiable focus of infection is rare; the incidence of bacteremia will therefore depend on the type of associated infection.

Fulminant Sepsis. At the other end of the spectrum of disease severity, overwhelming, or severe, sepsis represents a group of life-threatening infections. The clinical evolution is one of a rapidly progressive sepsis syndrome, with multiorgan involvement that leads to death if not treated promptly and aggressively. There is often a predisposing factor such as prematurity, neutropenia, or functional asplenia, but fulminant sepsis can also occur in the otherwise healthy person. Sepsis may therefore be primary (with no localized source), or it may be secondary to a localized infection.

Septic Shock. The incidence of septic shock has increased in the adult population in the past few decades. In the United States it is estimated that 200,000 episodes of septic shock occur annually, with more than 100,000 deaths from this disease. This is the consequence of extensive use of invasive monitoring, more aggressive therapies such as chemotherapy and corticosteroids, and an increase in the number of organ transplantations.

It is difficult to determine precisely the incidence of septic shock in children because different levels of acute illnesses are treated at each reporting institution. Burned patients, organ transplant recipients, and immunocompromised patients may be treated at regional hospitals. Sepsis and septic shock are the ninth leading cause of death in children aged 1–4 years; the annual mortality rate is 0.5 per 100,000 population. In persons with bacteremia the incidence of septic shock, by infective organism, is 15% with *Enterobacter,* 14% with *E. coli,* 12% with *N. meningitidis,* 12% with *Enterococcus,* 10% with *H. influenzae* type b, and 3.5% with *Klebsiella pneumoniae.* The majority of infections caused by Enterobacteriaceae are nosocomially acquired.

Bacteremia with Focal Infection. Secondary bacteremia may accompany virtually any focal infection or focal mucosal invasion. In the otherwise healthy person, community-acquired sepsis is often the manifestation of an extension of focal tissue infection (Table 21–5). Secondary bacteremia itself may result in secondary metastatic foci of infection.

Bacteremia with the Use of Intravascular Devices. Bacteremia frequently complicates the use of peripheral and especially central indwelling catheters (Chapter 106).

Bacteremia and Sepsis in the Immunocompromised Person. Certain inherited or acquired disorders are associated either with higher-than-expected rates of infectious complications by organisms that produce no significant disease in most healthy individuals or with particularly severe manifestations of bacterial disease (Table 21–6). An opportunistic infection must be anticipated as a distinct possibility in every person with a transient derangement of host resistance. Hospitalization and prompt antibiotic therapy before a pathogen is identified are usually needed.

In a series (Aledo, 1998) of 140 episodes of septicemia in persons hospitalized on a pediatric hematology-oncology service,

TABLE 21–5. Pathogens of Sepsis According to Type of Infection

Type of Infection	Possible Pathogens
Buccal and periorbital cellulitis	*Staphylococcus aureus* *Haemophilus influenzae* type b *Streptococcus pneumoniae*
Endocarditis	Viridans streptococci *S. aureus* Coagulase-negative staphylococci *Enterococcus* *S. pneumoniae* *Kingella kingae*
Epiglottitis	*H. influenzae* type b *S. pneumoniae* Group A *Streptococcus*
Gastroenteritis	*Salmonella* *Escherichia coli* *Campylobacter jejuni* *Yersinia enterocolitica*
Meningitis	*S. pneumoniae* *Neisseria meningitidis* *H. influenzae* type b
Osteomyelitis or suppurative arthritis	*S. aureus* Group A *Streptococcus* *S. pneumoniae* *H. influenzae* type b *K. kingae*
Pericarditis	*S. aureus* *H. influenzae* type b *S. pneumoniae* *N. meningitidis*
Pneumonia	*S. pneumoniae* Group A *Streptococcus* *H. influenzae* type b *S. aureus*
Skin and wound infection	*S. aureus* Group A *Streptococcus* Coagulase-negative staphylococci
Urinary tract infection	*E. coli* *Proteus* *Enterobacter* *Klebsiella* *Enterococcus faecalis*

septic shock developed in 19% of children with positive blood culture results. Gram-negative bacteria were the major cause of septic shock, although they caused fewer infections than gram-positive pathogens did.

Children with Anatomic Defects. Children with congenital and acquired heart disease are at increased risk of having acute or subacute endocarditis, with the damaged tissues serving as a point of origin of infection. Obstructive lesions of the urinary tract, alone or in association with urinary catheters, significantly increase the risk of invasive infection. In addition to common gram-negative enteric bacteria, highly resistant organisms such as *P. aeruginosa, Serratia marcescens,* and *Acinetobacter* are also isolated. In children with short gut syndrome or other chronic gastrointestinal disorders, gram-negative enteric bacilli and enterococci can cause transient bacteremia or sepsis.

After surgery, invasive bacterial infection may occur because of disruption of the skin and mucosal membranes, use of urinary or intravenous devices, malnutrition, and possible placement in an intensive care environment. When fever develops in a child postoperatively, one must consider skin flora (*S. aureus,* coagulase-negative staphylococci, group A *Streptococcus,* and other streptococci), enteric gram-negative bacilli, and normal flora at the surgery site as potential agents of postsurgical sepsis.

TABLE 21–6. Pathogens Associated with Bacteremia in Immunocompromised Persons

Predisposing Factors	Pathogens Isolated Most Frequently
Acquired immunodeficiency syndrome (AIDS)	*Streptococcus pneumoniae* *Haemophilus influenzae* type b *Salmonella*
Asplenia/sickle cell disease	*S. pneumoniae* *H. influenzae* type b *Salmonella*
Burns	*Pseudomonas aeruginosa* *Staphylococcus aureus* Group A *Streptococcus*
Complement/properdin deficiency	*Neisseria meningitidis*
Malignancy/ transplantation	Coagulase-negative staphylococci *S. aureus* *P. aeruginosa* *Klebsiella* Viridans streptococci

Burns. Thermal injury is a serious problem at any age. Opportunistic infections account for approximately half of all burn-associated fatalities in children. In addition to the destruction of the normal skin and mucosal barriers, which allows skin bacteria and environmental contaminants a portal of entry, several immunologic perturbations have been described in burn patients: neutrophil dysfunction, abnormal response to antigens, delayed rejection of homografts, and diminished uptake of particles by the reticuloendothelial system. Despite the use of antibiotics, the rate of sepsis in burn patients has been stable for the past 25 years. Group A *Streptococcus* was the major pathogen at one time, but *S. aureus* (including methicillin-resistant strains) and gram-negative organisms (especially *P. aeruginosa*) should now be considered in the management of burns in children (Chapter 49).

Splenic Absence or Dysfunction. The major cause of splenic dysfunction is surgical removal, but congenital asplenia also occurs. Children who have undergone splenectomy for any reason and those whose splenic function is impaired by disease, such as sickle cell disease, are at significantly increased risk of having fatal septicemia (Chapter 101).

The risk of infection is increased for all individuals after splenectomy, but the susceptibility is influenced in large part by the underlying condition for which the spleen was removed. The risk of infection is 1% for children with posttraumatic splenectomy, 2% for those with idiopathic thrombocytic purpura, 10% for those with Hodgkin's disease, and 10–25% for those with thalassemia.

In many cases the infection is overwhelming and is typically caused by encapsulated organisms such as *S. pneumoniae, H. influenzae* type b, and *N. meningitidis.* Rarely do *Staphylococcus,*

Salmonella, P. aeruginosa, and *Klebsiella* cause septicemia. Fulminant sepsis caused by *Capnocytophaga canimorsus* (formerly CDC group DF-2) in persons who have undergone splenectomy after a dog bite is a well-known association.

Sickle Cell Disease and Related Hemoglobinopathies. Infection is the most frequent cause of death in children with sickle cell disease. The rate of septicemia in young patients with sickle cell disease has been estimated to be 400 times higher for those infected with *S. pneumoniae* and four times higher for those infected with *H. influenzae* type b than for immunocompetent persons. *Salmonella,* which invades the bloodstream through infarcted bowel wall, and *N. meningitidis* are also found in greater proportion in these patients. Sepsis is not only more frequent but also much more dramatic; overwhelming sepsis is common. Defective splenic filtering function because of increased trapping of abnormally shaped red blood cells and because of the diminished opsonization capacity of encapsulated organisms explains the increased incidence of severe sepsis in persons with sickle cell disease (Chapter 101).

Inherited Disorders of Immunity. Young patients with primary immunodeficiency are at increased risk of having invasive bacterial infection and sepsis (Chapter 98). Deficiencies of the terminal components of complement (C6, C7, C8, and C9) are associated with a markedly increased risk of serious infection with *N. meningitidis.*

Acquired Disorders of Immunity. The most important risk factors associated with bacteremia in patients with cancer are the depth and duration of granulocytopenia (Chapter 99). Other risk factors include oral mucositis, necrotizing enteropathy, and rectal fissures. Lymphoproliferative disorders (leukemia, lymphoma) appear to be an additional risk factor. In a study of fever and neutropenia in children with cancer, bacteremia was found in 58% of children with leukemia and in 35% of those with solid tumors.

Any infectious agent can produce disease in children with malignancy, but certain pathogens are more commonly seen. Septicemia in children with acute lymphocytic leukemia is most often caused by gram-negative organisms. Persistent fever is usually caused by fungi in children with leukemia in relapse and by gram-positive organisms in those with chronic lymphocytic leukemia. Bacteremia develops in 10–20% of those with febrile neutropenic cancer. The common sources of bacteremia include the lungs (25%), perianal cellulitis (10%), gastrointestinal tract (5%), and indwelling intravascular devices (0.6–1.3%). The most common etiologic agents isolated from pediatric cancer patients with bacteremia include, in equal distribution, gram-negative bacilli *(E. coli, Klebsiella, P. aeruginosa, Serratia)* and gram-positive organisms (coagulase-negative staphylococci, *S. aureus,* viridans streptococci, *Corynebacterium jeikeium, Bacillus*). The incidence of pneumococcal and *H. influenzae* type b bacteremia does not seem to be increased in children with cancer. Bacteremia or fungemia can occur while children are receiving antibiotic therapy.

Infectious complications are responsible for significant morbidity and mortality rates among children receiving organ transplantation and associated immunosuppressive therapy (Chapter 100). These complications are a threat to both the patient's life and the survival of the transplant tissue. The incidence of infections and the microorganisms involved depend on both the organ being transplanted (e.g., kidney, liver, heart, bone marrow) and the immunosuppressive agents used. Septicemia after organ transplantation tends to occur in the first month after transplantation, when the immunotherapy is more suppressive and risk factors for nosocomial infections are present (e.g., intubation, indwelling catheter, broad-spectrum antibiotics). Organisms responsible for bacteremia are the same as in malignancy.

PATHOGENESIS

For highly virulent encapsulated bacteria the initial stage in the pathogenesis of bacteremia is exposure to a bacterial pathogen, with subsequent nasopharyngeal colonization. Exposure to a carrier plays a major role in the rate of nasopharyngeal colonization. Specimens taken from 1- to 2-year-old children in daycare centers revealed that up to 50% of children are colonized with *S. pneumoniae* at the same time and that 15–20% are carriers of *H. influenzae* type b. During epidemics the rate of carriage of *N. meningitidis* among household contacts can be as high as 38%.

The encapsulated structure of *S. pneumoniae, H. influenzae* type b, and *N. meningitidis* explains the virulence of these bacteria. These organisms are capable of invading beyond the mucosal barrier into the bloodstream for reasons that are poorly understood. A concurrent viral infection may increase the likelihood of bacteremia in colonized individuals by disrupting the mucosal barrier. Infections with influenza virus types A and B have been associated with subsequent meningococcal sepsis and with pneumococcal bacteremia.

The factors that determine which children become colonized, which colonized children then have bacteremia, and which children with bacteremia either improve without treatment or go on to sepsis have not been totally defined. Host factors are certainly of major importance. Bactericidal antibodies in the serum have been shown to protect against meningococcal disease. The increased incidence of bacteremia in 3- to 24-month-old children may partly be the result of maturational immunodeficiency in the production of opsonic IgG antibodies to polysaccharide present on the encapsulated bacteria.

In immunocompromised persons, chemotherapy-induced mucositis and herpes simplex stomatitis often precede sepsis caused by gram-negative organisms or viridans streptococci. *S. aureus* and group A *Streptococcus* are common inhabitants of the normal skin flora. Any skin wound or foreign material within the skin makes the individual more susceptible to invasive infections by these agents through the portal of entry. There appears to be a continuum of disease, starting with colonization and progressing through bacteremia, that may have one of three outcomes: spontaneous resolution, sepsis, or focal infection. The gastrointestinal tract can be the source of infection by translocation of bacteria through the gut in infants and immunocompromised persons. Upper urinary tract infection with or without congenital malformation may be the primary focus of *E. coli* (or other gram-negative) sepsis.

Sepsis represents a failure of the host immune response to restrict the invading microorganisms, leading to an activation of the complement system and the coagulation system and the release of cytokines and prostaglandins. Profound multisystemic perturbations result.

Septic Shock. A variety of infectious and noninfectious causes can produce a sepsis syndrome. However, in septic shock the process begins with an infection. The pathogens may invade the bloodstream or release various toxic products in the blood. These two pathways activate the production of endogenous mediators that are responsible for severe pathophysiologic alterations that are seen in septic shock (Fig. 21–1).

One of the most potent endogenous mediators released in septic shock is TNF-α. This potent cytokine can induce a sepsis syndrome in experimental animals. TNF is secreted in response to endotoxin (lipopolysaccharide) of gram-negative bacteria and to teichoic acid of gram-positive pathogens, as well as to protozoa and viruses.

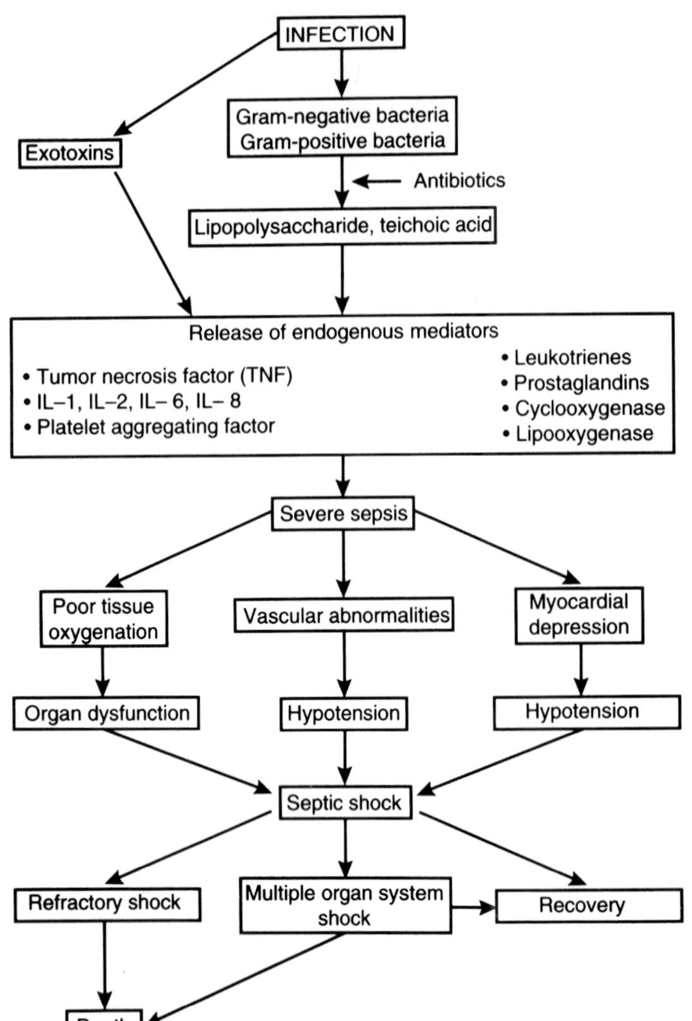

FIGURE 21–1. Pathogenesis of septic shock.

Elevated TNF concentrations have been found in severe infections in humans. Other mediators are also released that can cause profound physiologic effects on the heart, vasculature, and other organs.

Endotoxins are complex molecules of the outer cell wall of gram-negative bacteria. The **lipid A** portion, which is the best-conserved region of gram-negative endotoxin, is also its most active and toxic component. Increase of free endotoxin has been well documented in gram-negative infections after administration of bactericidal antibiotics. Injection of purified endotoxin has been shown to initiate the inflammatory cascade leading to septic shock.

The host possesses many systems for protection during endotoxemia. The reticuloendothelial system and anti-endotoxin antibodies are able to remove small quantities of circulating endotoxin. In the serum, there is a lipopolysaccharide-binding protein that can bind to the lipid A portion, thus enhancing opsonization of endotoxin and increasing the production of TNF by macrophages. The receptor for the lipopolysaccharide-lipopolysaccharide-binding protein complex is the CD14 receptor on the macrophage. When the concentration of lipopolysaccharide exceeds a critical level, an inflammatory response is initiated. The importance of this response will vary according to the extent of the production of endotoxins and according to the host's regulatory systems.

Products of gram-positive cell wall, including **peptidoglycan** and **lipoteichoic acid,** are biologically potent and can induce the production of the same cytokines involved in the pathogenesis of gram-negative bacillary septic shock. In a rat model of septic shock, peptidoglycan and lipoteichoic acid were shown to act synergistically to cause shock and multiple organ failure.

Once TNF is released, there is secondary secretion of mediators such as IL-1, IL-6, and IL-8; IFN-γ; platelet-activating factor (PAF); prostaglandins; and leukotrienes. The process continues with activation of neutrophils, endothelial cell synthesis of acute-phase reactants, and onset of coagulation activation. Endotoxin also activates the complement cascade with decreased concentrations of C3 in persons with septic shock.

IL-1 and TNF alter numerous physiologic functions of various organs and induce severe myocardial depression, hypotension, and increased endothelial permeability. IL-1 also induces the production of cytokines (IL-6, IL-8, TNF) and shock. IL-2 can act directly to cause hypotension and shock. Plasma levels of IL-6 correlate with mortality rates. Other mediators (PAF, leukotrienes, prostaglandins) increase the capillary leak syndrome and worsen tissue damage.

Nitric oxide is a potent vasodilator and is considered the primary regulator of vasomotor tone. Sepsis cascade induces the production of nitric oxide by endothelial cells and macrophages. Nitric oxide then diffuses into vascular smooth muscle cells, leading to muscle relaxation. Myocardial depression occurs in humans during the course of septic shock. The exact cause of this dysfunction is unknown, but it may result from the direct or indirect effects of some circulating myocardial depressant substance or from global myocardial ischemia caused by reduced coronary artery blood flow. Nitric oxide also influences myocardial function and likely is one of the final mediators that act as a myocardial depressant substance.

Many vascular abnormalities have been reported in persons with septic shock. Systemic vascular resistance is low with maldistribution of blood flow. Because inflammatory mediators can be released locally, local vasoconstriction or vasodilation, with accumulation of inflammatory cells, could occur. Most important, the peripheral use of oxygen and other nutrients is decreased. Eventually tissue hypoperfusion and anoxia result in multiple organ dysfunction.

SYMPTOMS AND CLINICAL MANIFESTATIONS

Children with sepsis appear "toxic," with multisystem clinical manifestations that include chills, gastrointestinal and neurologic complaints, and abnormal vital signs (Table 21–7). Fever is the single most common chief complaint made to physicians who evaluate children with suspected bacteremia or sepsis; however, sepsis can occur without fever, especially in neonates. Age and general appearance are of primary importance. The response to acetaminophen is not a clinically useful indicator to differentiate the causes of febrile illness in children; it cannot be used to distinguish children who have bacteremia from those who do not. The duration of fever before evaluation is also a poor indicator of the presence of bacteremia.

An observational scale (McCarthy, 1982) based on clinical observations (see Table 18–3) is used to correlate the overall appearance of the child with the presence of serious bacterial infection, usually bacteremia or sepsis. More than 90% of patients with a score of 16 or greater have a serious illness, compared with fewer than 3% when the score is 10 or less. The scale may be difficult to interpret in infants less than 6 weeks of age, however, because of the difficulty of assessing their response to social overtures.

In children more than 36 months of age, bacteremia without focus of infection is uncommon, and serious bacterial illness is recognized on the basis of clinical observation. In this age group, daycare and family contacts are important in the evaluation of children with suspected sepsis: more than one third of infants with *Salmonella* or *Shigella* infections have a family member infected with the same organism. It is important to provide prophylaxis to prevent secondary spread of invasive infections for contacts exposed to *H. influenzae* type b or *N. meningitidis.*

Knowledge of a specific immunologic impairment in febrile children may allow for accurate prediction of an invading pathogen. However, because the signs of infection (inflammation, tenderness) may be minimal and the rate of metastatic spread is high, thorough evaluation and examination of febrile, immunocompromised children for a possible focus of bacteremia is important. Unfortunately, more than 50% of persons with bacteremia and granulocytopenia lack specific physical findings. Blood pressure, capillary refill, peripheral perfusion, and pulse rate are essential for rapid assessment of cardiovascular integrity. Capillary refill time longer than 2 seconds, and cool, mottled extremities indicate insufficient circulation. Normal mental status and urine production are also indicators of the adequacy of circulation.

In newborns, jaundice can be seen in gram-negative sepsis and herpes simplex infections. Herpes simplex virus should always be considered in a neonate with symptoms of sepsis. Liver failure and multisystem involvement have been noted in both herpes simplex and enteroviral infections.

Fulminant Neisseria meningitidis Sepsis. Fulminant meningococcemia, sometimes known as **Waterhouse-Friderichsen syndrome,** represents a hyperacute form of meningococcemia, with nonspecific initial symptoms such as upper respiratory tract complaints, fever (>40°C [104°F] in 60% of cases), arthralgias, and myalgias. A macular, petechial, or purpuric rash is universally present (Plate 5D). Vomiting and diarrhea occasionally occur. Meningitis is variable. A profound and often irreversible state of shock, with DIC, capillary leak syndrome, and primary myocardial failure, is usually part of the terminal event of this devastating illness. The pathogenesis of the cardiovascular collapse seems to be a primary response to the endotoxin.

Fulminant Haemophilus influenzae Type b Sepsis. There are no epidemiologic, clinical, or laboratory clues by which to distinguish the etiologic diagnosis in a patient with fever, shock, petechiae, or purpura at presentation. Until the bacteriologic diagnosis is confirmed, the initial antibiotic therapy must be directed against *N. meningitidis, S. pneumoniae,* and *H. influenzae* type b. Deaths from *H. influenzae* type b–related overwhelming sepsis are also caused by intractable shock with progressive cardiac dysfunction. Adrenal hemorrhage occurs frequently in *Haemophilus* fulminant sepsis.

Septic Shock. Septic shock can be divided into two stages, early and late (Table 21–8). In early or hyperdynamic shock, the person presents with tachycardia, tachypnea, high fever or hypothermia, good capillary refill with warm extremities, and bounding pulses. However, signs of tissue hypoperfusion, such as alteration in mental status, weakness, abdominal cramps, or decreased urine output, may develop. Decreased central venous pressure and increased cardiac output, with decreased peripheral vascular resistance, also occur during the first stage. If treated aggressively, many persons will not progress to the second stage.

TABLE 21–7. Possible Clinical Signs and Symptoms in Persons with Sepsis

Cardiovascular	**Renal**
Hypotension	Oliguria
Poor perfusion	**Respiratory**
Tachycardia	Apnea
Gastrointestinal	Cyanosis
Diarrhea	Grunting
Metabolic	Hypoxia
Fever	Tachypnea
Hypoglycemia	**Dermatologic**
Hypothermia	Ecthyma gangrenosum
Metabolic acidosis	Jaundice
Rigors	Mottling
Neurologic	Petechiae
Confusion	Purpura
Decreased tone	Vasculitis
Irritability	
Lethargy	
Poor feeding	

TABLE 21–8. Clinical Stages of Septic Shock

Early (Warm) Septic Shock	Late (Cold) Septic Shock
Fever	Fever or hypothermia
Tachycardia	Tachycardia
Tachypnea	Tachypnea
Bounding pulses	Poor pulses
Altered mental status	Altered mental status
Widened pulse pressure	Narrowed pulse pressure
Increased capillary refill	Decreased capillary refill
Warm extremities	Cold extremities
Normal or decreased urine output	Decreased urine output
Normal or increased systolic blood pressure	Decreased systolic blood pressure
Increased, normal, or decreased cardiac output	Decreased cardiac output

In late septic shock, patients present with more manifestations of inadequate tissue perfusion, such as weak pulse, cold and moist skin, and cyanosis. Decreased central venous pressure, reduced cardiac output with lower blood pressure, and decreased urine output also occur. Peripheral vascular resistance can be either increased or decreased. Reduced tissue perfusion and oxygenation may lead to cellular death and multiorgan failure. Fulminant meningococcemia is a striking example of the process.

Physical Examination Findings

The initial clinical impression of a febrile child is important in the evaluation and future management of suspected sepsis. The **Acute Illness Observation Scale (AIOS)** (see Table 18–3) is a helpful tool in identifying children with serious illness. Vital signs, mental status, and peripheral perfusion should be evaluated routinely in febrile children. Assessment of the cardiovascular and respiratory function is essential to differentiate patients with bacteremia from those with septic shock (Table 21–8).

The presence of **fever and petechiae,** with or without localizing signs, places a person, independent of age, in a high-risk group for life-threatening bacterial infection, especially if the appearance is ''toxic'' (Table 21–9). Up to 10% of these persons have serious bacterial infection, meningococcal sepsis, or meningitis. Petechial and especially purpuric lesions should suggest the possibility of meningococcal or *Haemophilus* sepsis. Many patients with fulminant meningococcemia develop peripheral gangrene with disseminated intravascular coagulation and thrombosis of small vessels. Cardiac dysfunction occurs with a decrease in myocardial contractility. **Ecthyma gangrenosum** is associated with *P. aeruginosa* sepsis.

TABLE 21–9. Infectious Causes of Fever and Petechial Rash

Bacteria	**Viruses**
Neisseria meningitidis	Enteroviruses
Haemophilus influenzae type b	Rubella
Neisseria gonorrhoeae	Cytomegalovirus
Streptococcus pneumoniae	Epstein-Barr virus
Group A *Streptococcus*	Arboviruses
Yersinia pestis	Colorado tick fever
Streptobacillus moniliformis	**Other Causes**
Rickettsiae	*Mycoplasma pneumoniae*
Rocky Mountain spotted fever	

The presence of a cystic gingival mass in a febrile infant with fever should alert the clinician to the distinct possibility of concomitant pneumococcal bacteremia. This is almost the only pathognomonic finding of *S. pneumoniae* bacteremia. No other such physical findings have been related to occult bacteremia caused by other microorganisms.

In patients with septic shock, physicians should search carefully for primary foci of infection. Meningeal signs, the presence of rales on chest auscultation, abdominal tenderness, or redness over a catheter site may provide important clues as to the source of sepsis or to the extension of infection. Patients with sepsis or septic shock can develop multiple organ system dysfunction, which is defined by the presence of altered organ function in an acutely ill person to such an extent that homeostasis cannot be maintained without intervention.

DIAGNOSIS

Persons with septicemia are readily recognized as appearing ''toxic'' or ''septic'' in the presence of central nervous system dysfunction (irritability, lethargy), cardiovascular impairment (cyanosis, poor perfusion), and DIC (petechiae, ecchymosis).

The diagnosis of septic shock is made on the clinical presentation of sepsis: hyperthermia (temperatures >38°C [100.4°F]) or hypothermia (temperatures <36°C [96.8°F]), tachycardia (heart rate: infants, >160/min; children, >150/min), and tachypnea (respiratory rate: infants, >60/min; children, >50/min). Septic shock may be associated with hypotension (systolic blood pressure: infants, <65 mm Hg; children, <75 mm Hg [or below the fifth percentile for age]) and perfusion abnormalities despite adequate fluid resuscitation in persons who presumably are infected.

Differential Diagnosis

Children with many illnesses can present with a clinical picture similar to that of bacterial sepsis, and such diseases should be included in the differential diagnosis of this condition (Table 21–10). However, the most common cause of sepsis syndrome is overwhelming bacterial infection. Sepsis has been reported in association with several viruses (herpes simplex virus, adenoviruses, influenza viruses, parainfluenza viruses, hantaviruses). Rickettsial (Rocky Mountain spotted fever, ehrlichiosis), spirochetal (congenital syphilis), or protozoal (malarial) infections can also present with a sepsis-like picture.

Other noninfectious conditions may mimic septic shock (Table 21–10). Among these, cardiogenic shock is important to consider and rule out. Congestive heart failure may be the presentation of infants with coarctation of the aorta, hypoplastic left heart syndrome, anomalous coronary arteries, or supraventricular tachycardia. These patients may present with tachycardia, tachypnea, cyanosis, and poor peripheral perfusion. Early recognition is essential because management is drastically different from that of septic shock. Persons with hypovolemic shock resulting from severe dehydration during the course of another infectious process may appear to have sepsis, and several metabolic conditions, such as inborn errors of the urea cycle, may result in a sepsis-like presentation.

Laboratory Evaluation

A battery of blood tests can be considered in the initial evaluation of the child with suspected sepsis. None of these individual tests is sufficiently sensitive to predict bacteremia or invasive bacterial infections, but combined interpretation of those laboratory studies and the initial clinical impression of the physician help in the subsequent decision-making process.

The elevation of the total leukocyte count and the risk of bacteremia are linearly correlated. Febrile individuals with a WBC count

TABLE 21–10. Differential Diagnosis of Sepsis and Septic Shock

Infection	Gastrointestinal	Cardiopulmonary
Bacterial sepsis	Volvulus	Congenital heart disease
Meningitis	Intussusception	Paroxysmal atrial tachycardia
Viral infection	Gastroenteritis with dehydration	Myocarditis
Rickettsial infection	Fulminant hepatitis	Pericarditis
Protozoal infection	Peritonitis	Pulmonary embolism
Toxin-mediated reaction (toxic shock syndrome, staphylococcal scalded-skin syndrome)	**Other Conditions**	**Neurologic**
Metabolic/Endocrine	Vaccine reaction	Child abuse (intracranial bleeding)
Hypoglycemia	Anaphylaxis	Infant botulism
Congenital adrenal hyperplasia	Hemolytic-uremic syndrome	Guillain-Barré syndrome
Diabetes mellitus	Kawasaki syndrome	**Hematologic**
Diabetes insipidus	Reye's syndrome	Leukemia; lymphoma
Inborn errors of metabolism	Intoxication; drug abuse	Severe anemia
	Erythema multiforme	Methemoglobinemia
		Splenic sequestration crisis

of >15,000/mm^3 have a risk of bacteremia three times greater than those with counts <15,000/mm^3. Unfortunately the predictive value of this test is only 14%, which means that 86% of children with a WBC count >15,000/mm^3 do not have bacteremia. Alterations in the cellular distribution of the polymorphonuclear cells (elevated neutrophil count [>15,000/mm^3] and elevated band count [>500/mm^3]), often described as a **shift to the left,** suggest bacterial infection. Leukopenia (WBC count <5,000/mm^3), especially in the presence of neutropenia (neutrophil count <1,000/mm^3), is often observed late in the course of sepsis and could be a sign of imminent shock. **Neutrophil vacuolation, toxic granulation,** and **Döhle bodies** have also been observed in children with serious bacterial infections, but the relative value of those tests as accurate indicators of bacteremia remains to be clarified (Chapter 10).

Serum CRP, ESR, plasma fibronectin, elastase-α_1-proteinase inhibitor have all been shown to be of predictive value when studied in febrile patients. However, the addition of information provided by these tests does not seem to influence the decision-making process in the initial evaluation of children with serious bacterial infections (Chapter 10).

Laboratory evaluation of children with sepsis should also include tests that provide information about the systemic repercussion of the infection and any other clinical conditions that require specific management. Thrombocytopenia may occur as an isolated phenomenon or in the course of DIC. Prolongation of prothrombin time and partial thromboplastin time and the presence of fibrin split products or D-dimers and fragmented red blood cells are consistent with DIC. In the early phase of sepsis, arterial blood gas values show a mixed respiratory alkalosis and metabolic acidosis, but as the septic state progresses, metabolic acidosis, due to the accumulation of lactic acid (reflecting poor tissue perfusion), and respiratory decompensation, with or without adult respiratory distress syndrome (ARDS), may occur.

Among the other biologic perturbations, hypocalcemia, hypoglycemia or hyperglycemia, elevated aminotransferase values, and elevated blood urea nitrogen and serum creatinine concentrations are frequently noted.

Septic Shock. Many laboratory abnormalities found during the course of septic shock represent the effects of the shock state and hypoxia at the cellular level on the various organs (Table 21–11). Tests should be repeated frequently in persons in an unstable condition because the results are important for the patient management. The CBC may demonstrate thrombocytopenia with signs of intravascular hemolysis on the blood smear. Abnormal coagulation findings with the presence of fibrin split products are good indicators of DIC.

Arterial serum lactate concentration is a good reflection of tissue oxygenation and has good prognostic value in septic shock. In a recent study (Duke, 1997), serum lactate concentration discriminated survivors from those who died at 12 or 24 hours after admission but not at 48 hours. Electrolyte abnormalities (hyponatremia, hypocalcemia) can occur because of shock or renal insufficiency. They may also occur as a result of the massive fluid administration required for resuscitation. Hyperglycemia with secondary osmotic diuresis is seen with the use of inotropic agents such as epinephrine.

Decreased serum concentrations of proteins C and S have been associated with hereditary purpura fulminans. These episodes usually occur in infancy; levels of proteins C and S can be determined in these patients. In survivors of meningococcal infections, CH_{50} activity can be measured to detect terminal complement deficiencies. Such patients should be given meningococcal vaccine.

TABLE 21–11. Laboratory Abnormalities That Can Be Seen in Septic Shock

Hematologic
Anemia
Leukocytosis
Immature neutrophils (bands)
Thrombocytopenia (platelet count <100,000/mm^3)
Coagulation
Prolonged prothrombin time
Prolonged partial thromboplastin time
Presence of fibrin split products or D-dimers
Metabolic
Hyponatremia
Hypocalcemia (total and ionized)
Hyperglycemia or hypoglycemia
Hypoproteinemia
Hypoalbuminemia
Elevated serum lactate concentration
Hyperbilirubinemia
Elevated serum alanine and aspartate aminotransferases
Elevated creatinine phosphokinase
Renal
Abnormal urinary sediment
Azotemia (elevated blood urea nitrogen concentration)
Elevated serum creatinine concentration

Microbiologic Evaluation

Appropriate cultures of both blood and urine and any potentially infected site should be obtained. In overwhelming sepsis the demonstration of organisms from blood smear or buffy coat smear can confirm the clinical suspicion of septicemia and invasive infectious diseases. Antigen detection tests for rapid diagnosis of the infecting organism can be done in specimens from blood, urine, and cerebrospinal fluid.

Blood Cultures. Bacteremia can be diagnosed specifically only by appropriate blood cultures. Timing of blood collection is important for recovery of pathogens. Chills, sudden onset of fever, and hypotension are indications of bacteremia, and their occurrence presents the optimal time for obtaining blood cultures.

The ideal volume of blood is 10–15 mL in adults, 5–10 mL in older children, and a minimum of 1 mL in neonates. One study (Isaacman, 1996) showed that increasing the volume of blood inoculated into blood culture bottles improves the timely detection of bacteremia. Patients with an indwelling catheter should have blood drawn from the central line and from a peripheral vein. In case of multilumen intravenous devices, ideally, blood should be obtained through each lumen.

Two blood samples from two different sites of venipuncture are optimal for culturing. It has been shown that 91% of all bacteremic episodes are detectable by the first blood culture and that more than 99% of all episodes are identified by the first two blood cultures. The second set of blood cultures not only increases the yield of detection but also may help to differentiate true-positive blood culture results from the presence of skin flora contaminants. For possible catheter-associated infection, blood from the catheter site and additional peripheral blood should be cultured (Chapter 106).

Blood culture samples should be inoculated aerobically. If the suspected source of infection is the abdomen or if an anaerobic infection is suspected, anaerobic cultures should be obtained as well. False-negative blood culture results are found when persons are taking antibiotics. Blood culture results may be positive if the dilutional effect of the culture broth reduces the antibiotic concentrations below the minimal inhibitory concentration of the bacteremic pathogen. Use of blood culture bottles with resins to absorb antibiotics may enhance recovery (Chapter 7).

For quantification of organisms present and for increased recovery of intracellular organisms, the pediatric Isolator bottle is particularly useful. In this technique, 1.5 mL of the patient's blood is placed in a tube containing saponin, a rapid lysing agent of white and red blood cells. Then the blood is directly plated onto an agar medium (Chapter 7).

Without previous antimicrobial therapy, most pyogenic bacteria will show growth within 3 days of incubation. With the BACTEC system, the presence of viable bacteria is detected by CO_2 production, and most true instances of bacteremia will be detected within 12–48 hours of inoculation.

Lumbar Puncture. When meningitis is suspected, the clinician should perform a lumbar puncture for cerebrospinal fluid examination and culture. Lumbar puncture is specifically indicated for febrile children younger than 2 months of age, ill-appearing children of all ages, and patients with meningeal signs, petechial rash, and irritability. Lumbar puncture should not be withheld by fear of inducing meningitis in children with bacteremia. However, lumbar puncture should be postponed in children with signs of increased intracranial pressure (e.g., cranial nerve palsy, papilledema), focal neurologic findings, or other signs suggestive of an intracranial mass, until completion of CT or MRI scans. Cerebrospinal fluid examination also should be postponed in patients with hemodynamic or respiratory instability and in those with bleeding disorders or severe thrombocytopenia until these conditions are corrected. In these situations, empiric antimicrobial therapy should include coverage for meningitis until the diagnosis can be excluded by cerebrospinal fluid examination after the contraindication to lumbar puncture has resolved.

Other Cultures. Urine culture should be obtained, especially when there is no obvious clinical source of infection. The rate of urinary tract infection in febrile infants has been estimated up to 4%, and when an underlying congenital urinary tract anomaly exists, the percentage may be even higher. Specimens collected by urethral catheterization are of higher predictive value than bagged urine specimens, which are contaminated with skin or fecal flora in about 10–20% of cultures. Bladder aspiration, if not contraindicated, is the best means to obtain a reliable urine specimen in children younger than 6 months.

Organisms can also be found by Gram stain and culture of a purpuric skin lesion, especially in cases of suspected meningococcemia or gonococcemia. Cultures of stool specimens, abscesses, joint aspirate, endotracheal aspirate, or specimens from normally sterile body sites are obtained as clinically indicated. Cultures of specimens from body surfaces and from orifices such as the throat, nose, external auditory canal, and rectum have been useless in the identification of pathogens causing sepsis.

Rapid Diagnostic Tests. Many laboratory procedures are also available for the rapid identification of specific microorganisms within various body fluids. Countercurrent immunoelectrophoresis, EIA, or latex particle agglutination (Chapter 11) can detect the presence of polysaccharide antigens elaborated by *N. meningitidis, S. pneumoniae, H. influenzae* type b, and group B *Streptococcus.* These different techniques can be applied on virtually any fluid obtained from the patient: CSF, urine, serum, joint fluid, and pleural and pericardial fluid. Among the advantages of these tests are the possibility of a specific diagnosis within a matter of hours and an outcome that is not altered by the previous use of antibiotics. The results can provide useful information regarding the need for isolation procedures and antibiotic prophylaxis (*H. influenzae* type b, *N. meningitidis*). However, these techniques lack sensitivity (false-negative results because of inability to detect group B *N. meningitidis*) and specificity (false-positive results because of cross-reactivity in antigens of *H. influenzae, S. pneumoniae, N. meningitidis,* and *E. coli* K1). These tests should be used only in conjunction with, but not instead of, classic microbiologic culture methods. PCR to detect bacterial or fungal DNA in blood samples holds great promise for rapid diagnosis of pathogens in bacteremia and sepsis.

Diagnostic Imaging

Significant pulmonary infection is rarely found in febrile young infants who have a normal respiratory rate or normal auscultatory findings. A chest radiograph is necessary when pneumonia, ARDS, or pulmonary edema is suspected or in the child who has sepsis or appears ill but has no focus of infection. The radiograph may disclose an occult focus of infection (pleural, parenchymal, or pericardial) as well as unsuspected cardiac disease, which may be responsible for the critical condition of the child.

Other imaging studies, such as abdominal ultrasonography, CT, MRI, echocardiography, or nuclear medicine scans, are usually performed after the initial evaluation, depending on the clinical and laboratory findings, to determine the focus of infection and the cause of bacteremia or sepsis.

TREATMENT

The decision to admit febrile children to the hospital for parenteral antibiotic therapy for suspected bacteremia or sepsis is based initially on clinical evaluation. As a rule of thumb, children who appear ill, with signs of toxic effects or septic shock, should be admitted regardless of their age. Other indications for admitting children with suspected sepsis include high risk of severe infection (immunocompromise, central venous catheter [Fig. 21–2], asplenia, sickle cell disease, congenital heart disease), age less than 30–60 days, and parents who are too anxious or unreliable to be alert to changes in the general appearance of their child. Serious bacterial infections, such as those causing meningitis, osteomyelitis, suppurative arthritis, and severe pneumonia, also call for hospitalization.

The approach to well-appearing infants and young children at risk of having occult bacteremia is described in Chapter 19. Regardless of whether they have been treated with antibiotics, such children need to be re-evaluated as soon as the results of blood cultures are known, if their general status changes, or if focal infection develops. Multiple organ system failure should be carefully evaluated in persons with sepsis. Criteria for each system involved are delineated in Table 21–12.

The main objective in the management of children hospitalized with suspected sepsis is to prevent serious complications such as septic shock and death. For ill-appearing children hospitalized with suspected sepsis, the likely offending organisms dictate the initial choice of antibiotics. This primarily depends on the patient's age, the existence of any condition leading to impaired immune function, and the presence of a focal site of infection (Table 21–13). Local patterns of antibiotic resistance by common infective organisms should also be considered when one is selecting the initial antibiotic regimen. Many other alternative regimens can be used.

Definitive treatment should be tailored according to the susceptibility of the pathogen involved. The ultimate duration of treatment is based on the type of infection treated, on the offending pathogen and its susceptibility, on bacteriologic cure (negative results on subsequent blood cultures), and on the clinical response (temperature resolution, improved general condition). Some infections can be treated in the convalescent stages by orally administered antibiotics.

Initial Antimicrobial Therapy for Septic Shock

Antimicrobial treatment is instituted with parenterally administered antibiotics (Table 21–13). The initial antimicrobial therapy depends on the person's age, the presence or absence of a focal site of infection, and on whether the person is immunocompromised. The local pattern of antibiotic resistance, such as the presence of methicillin-resistant *S. aureus* and the in vitro susceptibility of gram-negative enteric bacilli, is important to consider when one is making a choice of initial empirical therapy for septic shock.

Multiresistant bacteria are expected if septic shock is developing while antibiotic therapy is being given. Fungal infections are also important to consider; *Candida* species can also produce septic shock. Amphotericin B therapy should be started promptly if fungal infection is suspected in the person with neutropenia who has septic shock at presentation.

In persons with septic shock, renal function can be altered and can even progress to complete renal failure because of decreased blood flow to the kidney and because of endotoxemia. In cases of

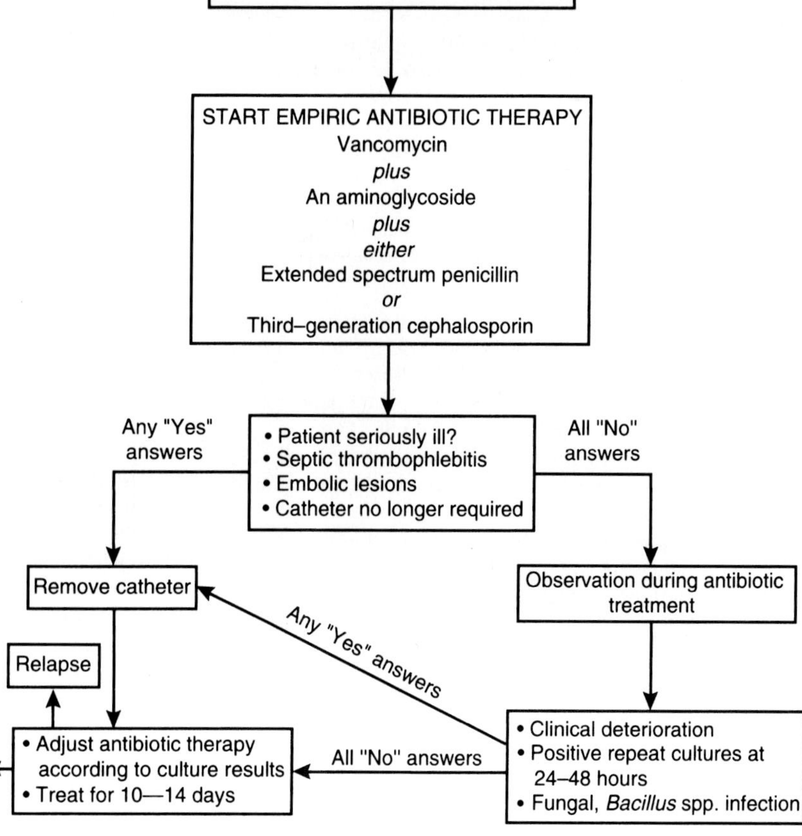

FIGURE 21–2. Approach to the management of catheter-related infection.

TABLE 21–12. Clinical and Laboratory Criteria for Failure of Specific Organ Systems

Cardiovascular
MAP <40 mm Hg (<12 mo of age)
MAP <50 mm Hg (≥12 mo of age)
HR <50 beats/min (<12 mo of age)
HR <40 beats/min (≥12 mo of age)
Cardiac arrest
Continuous vasoactive drug infusion for hemodynamic support

Respiratory
RR >90/min (<12 mo of age)
RR >70/min (≥12 mo of age)
Pa_{O_2} <40 mm Hg (in absence of cyanotic heart disease)
Pa_{CO_2} >65 mm Hg
Pa_{O_2}/F_{IO_2} <250 mm Hg
Mechanical ventilation (>24 hr if postoperative)
Tracheal intubation for airway obstruction or acute respiratory failure

Neurologic
Glasgow coma scale <5
Fixed, dilated pupils
Persistent (>20 min) intracranial pressure >20 mm Hg or requiring therapeutic intervention

Hematologic
Hemoglobin concentration <5 g/dL
WBC count <3,000/mm³
Platelet count <20,000/mm³
Disseminated intravascular coagulopathy (PT >20 sec or aPTT >60 sec in presence of positive FSP assay result)

Renal
Blood urea nitrogen concentration >100 mg/dL
Serum creatinine concentration >2 mg/dL
Dialysis

Gastrointestinal
Blood transfusion >20 mL/kg in 24 hr because of gastrointestinal hemorrhage (endoscopic confirmation optional)
Total bilirubin >5 mg/dL and AST or LDH more than twice normal value (without evidence of hemolysis)
Hepatic encephalopathy

AST = aspartate aminotransferase; FSP = fibrin split products; HR = heart rate; LDH = lactic dehydrogenase; MAP = mean arterial pressure; PT = prothrombin time; aPTT = activated partial thromboplastin time; RR = respiratory rate.
Reproduced with permission from Wilkinson JD, Pollack MM, Glass NL, et al: Mortality associated with multiple organ system failure and sepsis in pediatric intensive care unit. *J Pediatr* 1987;111:324–8.

renal failure, antibiotic therapy, particularly with aminoglycosides and vancomycin, should be adjusted and drug levels should be monitored (Chapter 14).

Definitive treatment should be tailored according to the susceptibility of the pathogen involved. The ultimate duration of treatment is based on the type of infection treated, the offending pathogen and its susceptibility, the bacteriologic cure (negative results on subsequent blood cultures), and the clinical response (temperature resolution, improved general condition).

Supportive Therapy for Septic Shock

The management of septic shock syndrome has many goals, including stabilization of the patient, removal of potentially infected foreign bodies or drainage of the abscesses, and treatment of the associated conditions. Children with septic shock, with or without respiratory insufficiency or multiorgan system failure, should be managed in a pediatric intensive care unit.

Initially, correction of hypovolemic shock is carried out by fluid resuscitation to achieve adequate tissue perfusion (Table 21–14). Large volumes of fluids and electrolytes are required because of the capillary leak syndrome and severe intravascular volume depletion. Some patients have protracted shock unresponsive to fluid therapy and require the use of inotropic agents (Table 21–15) such as dopamine and dobutamine. Invasive monitoring of cardiovascular function and urine output are necessary as well. This is important because the loss of vascular tone and the capillary leak syndrome can take many days to be corrected. Invasive monitoring helps determine the need for further fluid replacement and appropriate use of inotropic agents.

The introduction of more potent antimicrobial agents such as third-generation cephalosporins or carbapenems has not been associated with a significant reduction in the mortality and morbidity associated with septic shock. Microbial products in sepsis initiate an intense inflammatory response. Bactericidal antibiotics that lyse the bacteria may initially worsen the inflammatory cascade by liberating more endotoxin, which in turn induces the liberation of TNF-α, IL-1, and other inflammatory mediators. Besides early recognition and prompt treatment of septic shock, other therapies are needed to improve the survival rate of these patients.

Corticosteroids. High doses of methylprednisolone have been used widely in therapy for septic shock after early reports of efficacy. Early corticosteroid therapy before macrophage activation by endotoxins reduces the production of all cytokines and inhibits complement activation, histamine secretion by C3a and C5a, and endorphin release. However, carefully conducted clinical trials in the 1980s failed to demonstrate a beneficial effect of corticosteroid administration in adults with septic shock. The late mortality was increased in the corticosteroid group compared with the placebo group. Large corticosteroid doses were used in these studies and could account in part for the increased mortality. At present, there is a consensus that corticosteroids should not be used routinely in persons with septic shock. However, replacement doses should be given to persons with purpura fulminans thought to have adrenal insufficiency.

Naloxone. Endorphins are natural opiates that are liberated during the course of septic shock. In experimental studies they have been shown to cause hypotension. Naloxone, an opiate antagonist, could stabilize cellular membranes and prevent their dysfunction. Variable results have been reported with the use of naloxone in the treatment of septic shock in humans, however. Decreased mortality rates have never been described with the use of naloxone, and this drug is not recommended in the treatment of septic shock.

Ibuprofen. In a study (Bernard, 1997) of persons with sepsis, treatment with ibuprofen reduced levels of prostacyclin and thromboxane and decreased fever, tachycardia, oxygen consumption, and lactic acidosis but did not prevent the development of shock or the acute respiratory distress syndrome and did not improve survival rates.

Antibodies to Lipopolysaccharide. Endotoxins (lipopolysaccharides) of gram-negative bacteria play a major role in the activation of the inflammatory cascade of septic shock. Antibodies to the core region and the lipid A structure of lipopolysaccharides have been produced in an effort to offer passive protection by reactive antibodies that can neutralize the effects of the endotoxins.

TABLE 21–13. Initial Empiric Antimicrobial Therapy for Bacteremia and Septic Shock

Clinical Situation	Antibiotic	Duration*
No Identified Focus of Infection		
Newborn	Ampicillin *plus* An aminoglycoside	
Age 1 day to 1 mo	Ampicillin *plus* Cefotaxime *with or without* Nafcillin *or* oxacillin† *or* vancomycin	
Age 1–3 mo	Ampicillin *plus* Cefotaxime	
Age ≥3 mo	Third-generation cephalosporin *with or without* Nafcillin *or* oxacillin	
Identified Focus of Infection		
Meningitis	Cefotaxime *or* ceftriaxone *plus* Vancomycin	7–10 days
Pneumonia	Cefuroxime *plus* a macrolide	10 days
Endocarditis	Nafcillin *or* oxacillin *plus* An aminoglycoside *with or without* Penicillin G	4–6 wk
Catheter-associated		
Immunocompetent persons	Vancomycin *or* oxacillin *or* nafcillin *plus* Cefotaxime *or* ceftriaxone *or* ceftazidime	10–14 days
Identified Focus of Infection *(Continued)*		
Catheter-associated *(Continued)*		
Immunocompromised persons	Vancomycin *plus* Piperacillin-tazobactam *or* ticarcillin-clavulanate *plus* An aminoglycoside *or* Vancomycin *plus* ceftazidime	Variable
Gastrointestinal infection	TMP-SMZ *or* Third-generation cephalosporin	5–14 days
Intra-abdominal infection	Metronidazole *plus* Gentamicin *plus* Piperacillin-tazobactam *or* ampicillin	5–14 days
Urinary tract infection	Ampicillin *or* mezlocillin *plus* An aminoglycoside	10–14 days
Osteomyelitis or suppurative arthritis	Cefuroxime *or* nafcillin *plus* Third-generation cephalosporin	3–6 wk
Neutropenia	Piperacillin-tazobactam *or* ticarcillin-clavulanate *plus* An aminoglycoside *or* ceftazidime *plus* Vancomycin	Variable

*The duration of intravenous administration of antibiotics should be individualized on the basis of the identified focus of infection, clinical picture, and laboratory results. Selected persons may complete their treatment with orally administered antibiotics.

†Vancomycin may be substituted depending on the prevalence of oxacillin- or nafcillin-resistant *Staphylococcus*.

Suggested Dosages for Patients with Normal Renal Function

ANTIBIOTIC	INTRAVENOUS DOSAGE	MAXIMUM DAILY DOSE
Amikacin	15–22.5 mg/kg/day divided q8–12hr	15 mg/kg
Ampicillin	100–300 mg/kg/day divided q6hr	12 g
Cefotaxime	100–300 mg/kg/day divided q6–8hr	12 g
Ceftazidime	100–150 mg/kg/day divided q8hr	6 g
Ceftriaxone	50–100 mg/kg/day divided q12–24hr	4 g
Cefuroxime	100–150 mg/kg/day divided q8hr	4.5 g
TMP-SMZ	8–20 mg TMP/kg/day with 40–100 mg SMZ/kg/day divided q6–12hr	1.2 g TMP/6 g SMZ
Gentamicin	5–7.5 mg/kg/day divided q8hr	Adults: 5 mg/kg
Metronidazole	30 mg/kg/day divided q6–8hr	30 mg/kg
Mezlocillin	200–300 mg/kg/day divided q4–6hr	18 g
Nafcillin	150–200 mg/kg/day divided q6hr	9 g
Oxacillin	150–200 mg/kg/day divided q6hr	12 g
Piperacillin-tazobactam	Piperacillin 200–300 mg/kg/day divided q4–6hr	18 g
Ticarcillin-clavulanate	Ticarcillin 200–300 mg/kg/day divided q4–6hr	18 g
Tobramycin	5–7.5 mg/kg/day divided q8hr	Adults: 5 mg/kg
Vancomycin	40–60 mg/kg/day divided q6hr	2 g

Suggested Dosages for Neonates (use lower dose and longer dosing interval for neonates younger than 7 days of age)*

ANTIBIOTIC	INTRAVENOUS DOSAGE
Ampicillin	150–200 mg/kg/day divided q6–12hr
Cefotaxime	100–200 mg/kg/day divided q8–12hr
Gentamicin	5–7.5 mg/kg/day divided q8–12hr
Nafcillin	75–100 mg/kg/day divided q6–8hr
Vancomycin	30–45 mg/kg/day divided q8–12hr

*See Chapter 14 and Table 96–4.

TABLE 21–14. Supportive Therapy and Monitoring of Septic Shock

Apply basic principles of resuscitation: Airway
Breathing
Circulation
Oxygen administration (FIO_2: 0.4–1.0)
Early intubation and mechanical ventilation if necessary
Fluid resuscitation and hemodynamic stabilization
- Rapid boluses (20–30 mL/kg) of crystalloid solution; repeated as necessary (up to 60 mL/kg)
- If no response, administer colloid solution (5–10 mL/kg)
- Inotropic agents (dopamine, dobutamine, epinephrine) if no response to fluid resuscitation

Removal of catheters present at time of onset of shock; removal of other infected foreign bodies
Drainage of abscesses
Hydrocortisone, 25 mg/m²/dose every 6 hr (if purpura fulminans is present)
Therapy for multiorgan system failure (as needed)
- Acid-base status abnormalities
- Acute renal failure
- Adrenal insufficiency
- Adult respiratory distress syndrome
- Cardiac arrhythmias
- Cerebral edema
- Disseminated intravascular coagulation
- Electrolyte abnormalities or hypoglycemia
- Myocardial dysfunction

Continuous monitoring
- Heart rate
- Respiratory rate
- Arterial blood pressure
- Oxygen saturation
- Electrocardiographic findings
- Urine output
- Central venous pressure

Intermittent monitoring (as required)
- Temperature
- Glasgow coma scale
- Pulmonary capillary wedge pressure
- Cardiac index
- Blood gases and acid-base status
- CBC and platelet count
- Coagulation studies and fibrin split products
- Serum electrolyte values
- Serum glucose concentration
- Blood urea nitrogen and serum creatinine concentrations
- Total and ionized serum calcium
- Serum hepatic alanine and aspartate aminotransferases
- Total protein and albumin concentrations
- Serum lactate concentration

In experimental animal models, antibodies against the lipid A portion confer protection against gram-negative infection. Clinical trials using polyclonal (antiserum to *E. coli* J5 mutant strain) and monoclonal (E5 murine monoclonal IgM antibody, HA-1A human monoclonal antibody) antibodies to endotoxin have been performed in humans. The results of these studies have been variable, and some studies have been criticized for lack of information regarding the severity of sepsis at enrollment. Multiple organ failure and death were decreased in some subgroups of patients. E5 antibody appears to be helpful for persons with gram-negative infections who are not in shock, whether or not they have bacteremia. HA-1A is beneficial in cases of gram-negative bacteremia with or without shock but does not alter the course of nonbacteremic gram-negative infections. Antiendotoxin monoclonal antibodies are not licensed in the United States.

TABLE 21–15. Pharmacologic Agents Useful in the Treatment of Hemodynamic Abnormalities Associated with Septic Shock

Drug	Dose (μg/kg/min)	Effect on Receptors
Dopamine*	0–4	Dopaminergic
	4–10	β1, β2
	10–25	α, β1, β2
Dobutamine†	1.0–20	β1, (weak β2, α)
Epinephrine*‡	0.01–0.05	β2, β1
	0.05–1.0	β1, β2, α
Norepinephrine	0.01–1.0	α, β1
Phenylephrine	0.3–5.0	α
Nitroprusside	0.1–8.0	Decreased vascular resistance
Isoproterenol	0.05–1.0	β1, β2

*Effect variable according to dose.
†May widen pulse pressure at doses >10 μg/kg/min.
‡Increasing α effect with increasing dose.

Anti-Tumor Necrosis Factor Antibodies. TNF, an endogenous pyrogen, can stimulate the release of IL-1, IL-6, and PAF. It also promotes the metabolism of arachidonic acid. In the experimental model, anti-TNF antibodies improved some of the clinical manifestation of septic shock. In a large-scale trial of murine monoclonal TNF antibody conducted in adults, there was a modest beneficial effect in persons with septic shock but possible deleterious effects in those without shock.

Other Cytokine Therapies. IL-1–receptor antagonists, soluble receptors for TNF, lipid A analogs, nitric oxide inhibitors, endotoxin receptor antagonists, and other drugs are being developed for use in the treatment of sepsis and septic shock. Combination therapy with two or more drugs may be required to achieve significant clinical benefit in the majority of patients with septic shock. In experimental animal models of sepsis, antibodies against IL-1 and a receptor antagonist to IL-1 (IL-1ra) decreased hemodynamic alterations and improved outcome. In a study (Fisher et al, 1994) of IL-1ra in adults with sepsis and septic shock, treatment with IL-1ra did not improve the survival rate. In a study (Dhainaut, 1998) of 609 patients with severe sepsis, treatment with PAF receptor antagonist (PAFra) failed to demonstrate a significant benefit.

Activated Protein C. Drotrecogin alfa, or recombinant human activated protein C, has antithrombotic, antiinflammatory, and profibrinolytic properties and has been shown to produce a dose-dependent reduction in the levels of inflammatory markers. A study (Bernard et al, 2001) of 1,690 patients randomized to receive either drotrecogin alfa activated or placebo showed that treatment with drotrecogin alfa was associated with a reduction in the relative risk of death of 19.4% (95% confidence interval, 6.6–30.5%) and absolute reduction in the risk of death at 128 days of 6.1% ($p = .005$). However, the incidence of bleeding was higher in the group receiving drotrecogin alfa activated than in those receiving placebo (3.5% vs. 2%, $p = .06$). When available, activated protein C should be considered for adult patients with evidence of end-organ dysfunction associated with shock, acidosis, oliguria, or hypoxemia. It should not be given to persons with clinical signs of mild-to-moderate sepsis without evidence of end organ injury. Studies are needed to define the role of activated protein C in children.

Exchange Transfusion, Plasmapheresis, and Hemoperfusion. Mechanical removal of circulating mediators of inflammation and toxins has been used in a small number of persons. According to reports on dogs with gram-negative bacteremia, removal of all circulating mediators may do more harm than good. This procedure is not easy to perform in a person with septic shock and is not recommended on a routine basis.

Granulocyte Transfusions. WBC transfusion can be considered in severely ill neutropenic patients with persistent bacteremia or septic shock. Their efficacy is debatable, and the decision to use this mode of therapy should be individualized for each potential patient (Chapter 15). The efficacy of colony-stimulating factors such as G-CSF or GM-CSF has not been evaluated in persons with septic shock.

Intravenous Immunoglobulins. A meta-analysis (Jenson et al, 1997) of neonates with sepsis and proven bacteremia showed that the use of IVIG was associated with a sixfold decrease in fatality rate. A single IVIG dose of 500–750 mg/kg should be strongly considered in neonates with microbiologically proved sepsis. The use of IVIG beyond the neonatal age group has not been shown to be of benefit in the treatment of sepsis.

COMPLICATIONS AND PROGNOSIS

Regardless of the use of antibiotics, children with bacteremia may have one of three outcomes: self-limited disease, focal infection, or progression to sepsis and eventually septic shock. In a retrospective study (Bryan et al, 1984) of 713 episodes of bacteremia, the mortality rate of 7.6% was directly related to the age of the patient and the underlying condition. Death was a more frequent event in the youngest age groups. Mortality was 11% in neonates (0–30 days), 7% in infants (1–12 months), and 3% in younger children (1–2 years) and older children (3–16 years). No deaths occurred as a result of bacteremia from urinary tract infection, osteomyelitis, suppurative arthritis, or infected central venous line. Conversely, meningitis, pneumonia, and intra-abdominal infections were associated with 11% of the fatal bacteremias.

In another series (Wilkinson et al, 1987), persons with bacteremia and compromised defenses (related to cancer or nephrotic syndrome) or with underlying diseases (congenital heart disease, malnutrition) had a mortality rate of 26%. This was significantly greater than the 6% mortality for immunocompetent persons with bacteremia. Host susceptibility, particularly young or old age and underlying medical conditions, is the major determinant of the outcome from bacteremia. Polymicrobial gram-negative bacteremia has also been associated with increased mortality.

The risk of focal complications of persisting bacteremia is also related to the virulence of the offending organism. In a review (Shapiro, 1986) of 310 cases of occult bacteremia, the species causing bacteremia was significantly associated with the risk of developing subsequent meningitis in the 1.8% of individuals with occult bacteremia who developed meningitis. This risk was 15 times higher (13%) with *H. influenzae* type b occult bacteremia and 81 times higher with *N. meningitidis* (56%).

In unrecognized pneumococcal bacteremia, the illness is generally self-limited, with a mild clinical picture and spontaneous resolution in 40% of the cases. However, sequelae of occult pneumococcal bacteremia may develop. Meningitis occurs in 1–2% of cases and focal infections (pneumonia, osteoarticular infections) in 5% of cases. Approximately one quarter of untreated patients still have bacteremia at a visit 24–72 hours after the initial evaluation. In a study (Teach, 1998) of 178 immunocompetent children 3–36 months of age with pneumococcal bacteremia, the incidence of focal infection was significantly higher in children with pneumococcus counts >10 cfu/mL in the blood than in those with ≤10 cfu/mL (30.4% vs 12.9%, $p = .04$), regardless of the other clinical and laboratory characteristics.

The outcome of unsuspected *H. influenzae* type b bacteremia is associated with a higher risk of focal and serious infections: only 5% of the children have a transient, self-limited illness. Most often, they become sicker within hours and develop localizing signs of infections. In a study (Korones, 1992) of 69 patients with *H. influenzae* type b bacteremia who were managed as outpatients (40% were treated with antibiotics), approximately half of the children were either febrile or had a clinical focus of infection at a follow-up visit at 24–72 hours: meningitis (24%), pneumonia (7%), cellulitis (7%), epiglottitis (4%), and suppurative arthritis (4%) were the most common secondary infections. Of the remaining half who were afebrile and well appearing at follow-up, three children had persistent bacteremia and another five later developed focal infections. Therefore children with *H. influenzae* type b bacteremia are at high risk of having subsequent focal infection, regardless of whether they received antibiotics, and should be systematically recalled and carefully re-evaluated.

Many prognostic factors have been identified to predict an unfavorable outcome of *N. meningitidis* sepsis (Table 21–16). The **Glasgow Meningococcal Septicemia Prognostic Score** has been validated in a series of 100 children with meningococcemia (Table 21–17). No scoring system is able to predict survival or death for every single person, but these scoring systems are useful estimates of what could be the patient's outcome. A score >10 predicts death in 88%, and a score >8 predicts death in 73%. More recently the **Rotterdam prognostic scoring system** (Kornelisse, 1997), based on four laboratory features (serum CRP level, serum potassium level, base excess, and platelet count), has been shown to have good predictive value for death and survival (71% and 90%, respectively). With this scoring system, outcome was predicted correctly in 86% of patients. Other prognostic indicators have been associated with a poor outcome: hypothermia, seizures or shock on presentation, total peripheral leukocyte count <5,000/mm^3, platelet count <100,000/mm^3, the development of purpura fulminans, meningococcal serotype C, presence of circulating endotoxin, and high levels of circulating cytokines TNF-α, IL-1, and IFN-γ.

Febrile children with sickle cell disease are at increased risk of bacteremia when they have one or more of the following risk factors: hypotension, poor perfusion, temperature >40°C (104°F); WBC count <5,000/mm^3 or >30,000/mm^3; platelet count

TABLE 21–16. Unfavorable Prognostic Risk Factors in Meningococcal Infections

Presence of ≥3 factors prognosticates mortality rate of >85%
Presence of 0–2 factors prognosticates mortality rate of <10%

- Presence of petechiae for <12 hours before admission
- Presence of shock (systolic blood pressure ≤70 mm Hg)
- Absence of meningitis (WBC count ≤20/mm^3 in CSF)
- Normal or low peripheral WBC count (≤10,000/mm^3 in blood)
- Normal or low ESR (<10 mm/hr)

Adapted from Stiehm ER, Damrosch DS: Factors in the prognosis of meningococcal infection. Review of 63 cases with emphasis on recognition and management of the severely ill patient. *J Pediatr* 1966;68:457–67.

TABLE 21–17. Glasgow Meningococcal Septicemia Prognostic Score

Parameter	Points
Systolic blood pressure <75 mm Hg, age <4 yr	3
or	
Systolic blood pressure <85 mm Hg, age >4 yr	
Skin-rectal temperature difference >3°C	3
Modified coma scale score <8	3
or	
Deterioration of ≥3 points in 1 hr	
Deterioration in hour before scoring	2
Absence of meningism	2
Extending purpuric rash or widespread ecchymosis	1
Base deficit (capillary or arterial) >8.0	1
MAXIMUM SCORE	15

Adapted from Thompson APJ, Sill JA, Hart CA: Validation of the Glasgow Meningococcal Septicemia Prognostic Score: A 10-year retrospective survey. *Crit Care Med* 1991;19:26–30.

<100,000/mm^3; presence of pulmonary infiltrates on chest roentgenogram; history of pneumococcal sepsis; or complications of sickle cell disease such as a hemoglobin level <5 g/dL, dehydration, or severe pain. In one study (Wilimas, 1993), 6 of 70 persons (7 of 86 febrile episodes) with one of these risk factors had sepsis. These are useful guidelines of the need for hospitalization in this subgroup of patients.

The development of multiorgan system failure should be closely monitored and appropriately managed. Children develop ARDS more frequently than adults and may require ventilatory support. Renal insufficiency with secondary metabolic acidosis, hypocalcemia, and hyperphosphatemia may require dialysis for correction of metabolic and electrolyte abnormalities.

The mortality rate for septic shock varies from 40% to 60% in adults and is approximately 10% in immunocompetent children. This percentage can be higher (up to 40%) depending on the underlying disease and predisposing factors that lead to septic shock. It also depends on the early recognition of sepsis and the institution of appropriate therapy. The prognosis is worse if septic shock is recognized in the later stages. A scoring system may be used to predict the outcome in meningococcemia (Tables 21–16 and 21–17). The death rate is higher in neutropenic patients with *P. aeruginosa* or *C. albicans* septic shock, as well as in those with fulminant meningococcemia (Table 21–3).

When multiorgan dysfunction is present, the incidence of death is much higher, approaching 50%, and increases directly with an increasing number of failed systems. Survival also depends on whether the shock state can be reversed, whether tissues can be well perfused and oxygenated, and whether the focus of infection can be eradicated.

PREVENTION

Early detection of bacteremia and prompt recognition and initiation of therapy are key factors in preventing the progression from bacteremia to sepsis to septic shock. A high index of suspicion is needed, particularly in the neutropenic or immunocompromised person. In the critically ill child, good infection control measures (especially good hand-washing techniques) help decrease the incidence of nosocomially acquired infections. All invasive monitoring devices should be removed as soon as they are no longer required. Unexplained febrile episodes should be carefully evaluated.

For patients with anatomic or functional asplenia (sickle cell disease, splenectomy), chemoprophylaxis with penicillin V has reduced the risk of severe pneumococcal infections by 84% in comparison with placebo-treated infants (Chapter 101). In persons with leukemia, prophylaxis with TMP-SMZ decreases the incidence of *P. carinii* pneumonia (Chapters 68 and 99). Routine administration of other absorbable oral antibiotics to prevent bacterial disease is not recommended because it may predispose the patient to fungal or bacterial superinfection.

For patients with symptomatic HIV infection, monthly administration of IVIG has decreased the incidence of severe bacterial infections, particularly with encapsulated agents (Chapter 38). However, routine use of IVIG is not advised for other immunocompromised persons because this mode of preventive therapy has not been clearly shown to reduce the incidence of bacterial infection.

Immunization remains the mainstay of prevention for invasive bacterial disease. Since the introduction of routine vaccination with conjugated *H. influenzae* type b vaccines at 2 months of age, the rate of invasive disease caused by this organism has dramatically decreased. Routine immunization with conjugated pneumococcal vaccine is now recommended for infants and may have a similar effect. Routine use of meningococcal vaccine is not presently recommended, although it is likely that in the future conjugate vaccines against the meningococcus will be part of the strategy for prevention of this infection.

REVIEWS

Bone RC, Grodzin CJ, Balk RA: Sepsis: A new hypothesis for pathogenesis of the disease process. *Chest* 1997;112:235–43.

Dellinger RP: Current therapy for sepsis. *Infect Dis Clin North Am* 1999;13:495–509.

Hack CE, Aarden LA, Thijs LG: Role of cytokines in sepsis. *Adv Immunol* 1997;66:101–95.

Opal SM, Cross AS: Clinical trials for severe sepsis: Past failures and future hopes. *Infect Dis Clin North Am* 1999;13:285–97.

Parrillo JE: Pathogenic mechanisms of septic shock. *N Engl J Med* 1993;328:1471–7.

Rangel-Frausto MS, Pittet D, Costigan M, et al: The natural history of the systemic inflammatory response (SIRS): A prospective study. *JAMA* 1995;273:117–23.

Sáez-Llorens X, McCracken GH Jr: Sepsis syndrome and septic shock in pediatrics. Current concepts of terminology, pathophysiology and management. *J Pediatr* 1993;123:497–508.

Shapiro ED: Bacteremia in the febrile child. *Adv Pediatr Infect Dis* 1986;1:19–35.

Shenep JL: Septic shock. *Adv Pediatr Infect Dis* 1996;12:209–41.

Sriskandan S, Cohen J: Gram-positive sepsis: Mechanisms and differences from gram-negative sepsis. *Infect Dis Clin North Am* 1999;13:397–412.

Symeonides S, Balk RA: Nitric oxide in the pathogenesis of sepsis. *Infect Dis Clin North Am* 1999;13:449–63.

Van der Poll T, van Deventer SJ: Cytokines and anticytokines in the pathogenesis of sepsis. *Infect Dis Clin North Am* 1999;13:413–26.

KEY ARTICLES

Aledo A, Heller G, Ren L, et al: Septicemia and septic shock in pediatric patients: 140 consecutive cases on a pediatric hematology-oncology service. *J Pediatr Hematol Oncol* 1998;20:215–21.

Bernard GR, Vincent JL, Laterre PF, et al: Efficacy and safety of recombinant human activated protein C for severe sepsis. *N Engl J Med* 2001;344:759–62.

Bernard GR, Wheeler AP, Russell JA, et al: The effects of ibuprofen on the physiology and survival of patients with sepsis. The Ibuprofen in Sepsis Study Group. *N Engl J Med* 1997;27:912–8.

Bonadio WA: Evaluation and management of serious bacterial infections in the febrile young infant. *Pediatr Infect Dis J* 1990;9:905–12.

Bone RC, Fisher CJ Jr, Clemmer TP, et al: A controlled clinical trial of high dose methylprednisolone in the treatment of severe sepsis and septic shock. *N Engl J Med.* 1987;317:653–8.

Bryan CS, Reynolds KL, Derrick CW Jr: Patterns of bacteremia in pediatric practice: Factors affecting mortality rates. *Pediatr Infect Dis* 1984; 3:312.

Carcillo JA, Pollack MM, Ruttimann UE, et al: Sequential physiologic interactions in pediatric cardiogenic and septic shock. *Crit Care Med* 1989;17:12–6.

Carcillo JA, Davis AL, Zaritzky A: Role of early fluid resuscitation in pediatric septic shock. *JAMA* 1991;266:1242–5.

Cursons RT, Jeyetajah E, Sleight JW: The use of polymerase chain reaction to detect septicemia in critically ill patients. *Crit Care Med* 1999; 27:937–40.

Das I, Gray J: Enterococcal bacteremia in children: A review of seventy-five episodes in a pediatric hospital. *Pediatr Infect Dis J* 1998;17:1154–8.

Dhainaut JF, Tenaillon A, Hemmer M, et al: Confirmatory platelet-activating factor receptor antagonist trial in patients with severe gram-negative bacterial sepsis: A phase III, randomized, double-blind, placebo-controlled, multicenter trial. BN 52021 Sepsis Investigator Group. *Crit Care Med* 1998;26:1963–71.

Duke TD, Butt W, South M: Predictors of mortality and multiple organ failure in children with sepsis. *Intensive Care Med* 1997;23:684–92.

Fisher CJ Jr, Dhainaut JF, Opal SM, et al: Recombinant human interleukin 1 receptor antagonist in the treatment of patients with sepsis syndrome. Results from a randomized, double-blind, placebo-controlled trial. Phase III rhIL-1ra Sepsis Syndrome Study Group. *JAMA* 1994;271: 1836–43.

Greenes DS, Harper MB: Low risk of bacteremia in febrile children with recognizable viral syndromes. *Pediatr Infect Dis J* 1999;18:258–61.

Isaacman DJ, Karasic RB, Reynolds EA, et al: Effect of number of blood cultures and volume of blood on detection of bacteremia in children. *J Pediatr* 1996;128:190–5.

Jacobs RF, Sowell MK, Moss MM, et al: Septic shock in children: Bacterial etiologies and temporal relationships. *Pediatr Infect Dis J* 1990; 9:196–200.

Jenson HB, Pollock BH: Meta-analysis of the effectiveness of intravenous immune globulin for prevention and treatment of neonatal sepsis. *Pediatrics* 1997;99(2):E2.

Kornelisse RF, Hazelzet JA, Hop WC, et al: Meningococcal septic shock in children: Clinical and laboratory features, outcome, and development of a prognostic score. *Clin Infect Dis* 1997;25:640–6.

Korones DN, Marshall GS, Shapiro ED: Outcome of children with occult bacteremia caused by *Haemophilus influenzae* type b. *Pediatr Infect Dis J* 1992;11:516–20.

Lee GM, Harper MB: Risk of bacteremia for febrile young children in the post–*Haemophilus influenzae* type b era. *Arch Pediatr Adolesc Med* 1998;152:624–8.

Leibovici L, Drucker M, Konigsberger H, et al: Septic shock in bacteremic patients: Risk factors, features and prognosis. *Scand J Infect Dis* 1997;29:71–5.

Levi M, ten Cate H, van der Poll T, et al: Pathogenesis of disseminated intravascular coagulation in sepsis. *JAMA* 1993;270:975–9.

Levy I, Leibovici L, Drucker M, et al: A prospective study of gram-negative bacteremia in children. *Pediatr Infect Dis* 1996;15:117–22.

Mandl KD, Stack AM, Fleischer GR: Incidence of bacteremia in infants and children with fever and petechiae. *J Pediatr* 1997;131:398–404.

McCarthy PL, Sharpe MR, Spiesel SZ, et al: Observation scales to identify serious illness in febrile children. *Pediatrics* 1982;70:802–9.

Mok Q, Butt W: The outcome of children admitted to intensive care with meningococcal septicaemia. *Intensive Care Med* 1996;22:259–63.

Quartin AA, Schein RM, Kett DH, et al: Magnitude and duration of the effect of sepsis on survival. Department of Veterans Affairs Systemic Sepsis Cooperative Studies Group. *JAMA* 1997;277:1058–63.

Rosenstein NE, Perkins BA, Stephens DS, et al: The changing epidemiology of meningococcal disease in the United States, 1992–1996. *J Infect Dis* 1999;180:1894–901.

Shenep JL, Flynn P: Infections associated with long-term intravascular and cerebrospinal fluid shunt catheters. *Adv Pediatr Infect Dis* 1986;1: 145–62.

Smith-Elekes S, Weinstein MP: Blood cultures. *Infect Dis Clin North Am* 1993;7:221–34.

Teach SJ, Fleischer GR: Duration of fever and its relationship to bacteremia in febrile outpatients three to 36 months old. The Occult Bacteremia Study Group. *Pediatr Emerg Care* 1997;13:317–9.

Teach SJ, Dryja DM, Tristram D: Pneumococcal bacteremia and focal infection in young children. *Clin Pediatr* 1998;37:531–5.

Wilimas JA, Flynn PM, Harris S, et al: A randomized study of outpatient treatment with ceftriaxone for selected febrile children with sickle cell disease. *N Engl J Med* 1993;329:472–6.

Wilkinson JD, Pollack MM, Glass NL, et al: Mortality associated with multiple organ system failure and sepsis in pediatric intensive care unit. *J Pediatr* 1987;111:324–8.

Yagupsky P, Dagan R: *Kingella kingae:* An emerging cause of invasive infections in young children. *Clin Infect Dis* 1997;24:860–6.

Ziegler EJ, Fisher CJ Jr, Sprung CL, et al: Treatment of gram-negative bacteremia and septic shock with HA-1A human monoclonal antibody against endotoxin: A randomized, double-blind, placebo-controlled trial. The HA-1A Sepsis Study Group. *N Engl J Med* 1991;324:429–36.

CHAPTER 22

Toxic Shock Syndrome

Bruce Tapiero ▪ Marc H. Lebel

Toxic shock syndrome is an acute febrile illness with a diffuse, desquamating, erythematous eruption and generalized mucositis. There may be a prodrome of myalgia, malaise, headache, vomiting, and diarrhea. This condition can progress rapidly to hypotension and multiorgan system dysfunction.

Toxic shock syndrome gained great notoriety in the medical and lay literature in the early 1980s when the association between the disease, menstruation, and tampon use was recognized. Most of the cases in the early 1980s occurred in women (95%) and began during menstruation (90%), leading to the misconception among many physicians that toxic shock syndrome occurred only in association with tampon use. Nonmenstrual toxic shock syndrome has been reported with increasing frequency in children and men as well as women. It is important to appreciate the diversity of clinical situations in which toxic shock syndrome can occur, because this life-threatening condition necessitates early recognition and aggressive management.

ETIOLOGY

In 1978 Todd and colleagues originally described the disorder in 7 children 8–17 years of age. Five of these patients were colonized with phage group 1 *Staphylococcus aureus,* producing a toxin now known as **toxic shock syndrome toxin-1 (TSST-1).** Toxic shock syndrome is probably not a new entity, however, and cases of what is believed to have been toxic shock syndrome have been reported in the medical literature as **staphylococcal scarlet fever,** since at least 1927.

The association between toxic shock syndrome and *S. aureus* has been firmly established. Although isolation of *S. aureus* from the vagina or another site is not one of the diagnostic criteria of toxic shock syndrome, it is possible to isolate *S. aureus* in most cases of toxic shock syndrome before antimicrobial therapy is initiated. Vaginal isolation rates as high as 98% have been described in appropriately cultured menses-associated toxic shock syndrome, compared with the carriage rate in healthy control subjects of 8–10%. In persons with toxic shock syndrome associated with focal infections, *S. aureus* is typically the only organism found in the lesion.

Streptococcal Toxic Shock Syndrome. In the 1980s there was a resurgence of severe and even fatal acute group A *Streptococcus* infections, with the first description (Cone, 1987) of a toxic shock–like syndrome caused by group A *Streptococcus (Streptococcus pyogenes).* This syndrome is associated with soft-tissue infections that are complicated by hypotension and multiorgan failure. When this disease is associated with necrotizing fasciitis, the news media have labeled it as "flesh-eating disease."

EPIDEMIOLOGY

Carriage rates of *S. aureus* are 15–30% on the skin, 30–40% in the nasopharynx, and 5–15% in the vagina. The corresponding carriage rates for TSST-1-producing *S. aureus* are 5–15% for the nasopharynx and 1–5% for the vagina. The carriage of *S. aureus* with the potential of causing toxic shock syndrome is relatively high in comparison with the low incidence of toxic shock syndrome.

The incidence of toxic shock syndrome in the early 1980s ranged from 6 to 14 cases per 100,000 menstruating women. The last multistate active surveillance program, performed in 1986–1987, found the incidence of menstrual toxic shock syndrome to be 1 case per 100,000 women 15–44 years of age. For the past several years, the number of reported cases of toxic shock syndrome has decreased significantly (Fig. 22–1). In 2000 only 125 cases of toxic shock syndrome were reported. The majority of reported cases occur among white women 15–49 years of age, although the syndrome can occur in healthy subjects of any age and either sex.

A reduction in diagnosis and reporting, rather than an actual decrease in incidence, may have occurred as a result of diminished attention in the medical literature, changes in public awareness, possible changes in the accuracy of state surveillance, and fewer cases that fulfill the complete case definition because of earlier diagnosis and treatment.

Menses-Related Toxic Shock Syndrome. The mean age of patients with confirmed menses-associated toxic shock syndrome is 23 years, with a range of 11–61 years and 97% of cases in white females. One third of cases occur in teenagers 15–19 years of age, with 99% being tampon users; 1% of cases occurred with the exclusive use of napkins or mini pads. The relationship between toxic shock syndrome and menstruation led to the rapid association of toxic shock syndrome with the use of vaginal tampons. A number of case-control studies pointed to a particular high-absorbency brand of tampon (Rely), which was made of polyester foam impregnated with carboxymethylcellulose nodules. The manufacturer withdrew this tampon from the market in 1980. A decrease in the absorbency of tampons and changes in their chemical composition were temporally associated with a decrease in the incidence of toxic shock syndrome, but other factors may have contributed to the decline. Furthermore, because of public awareness, it is possible that fewer women use tampons regularly.

Nonmenstrual Toxic Shock Syndrome. In 1998, nonmenstrual toxic shock syndrome accounted for 59% of all the cases identified by active surveillance. Toxic shock syndrome is rare in prepubertal children of both sexes. The average age of persons with nonmenstrual toxic shock syndrome is 27 years, but the syndrome has been reported in newborn infants and in persons older than 80 years. The male:female ratio and the racial distribution of persons with nonmenstrual toxic shock syndrome closely resemble their distribution in the general population.

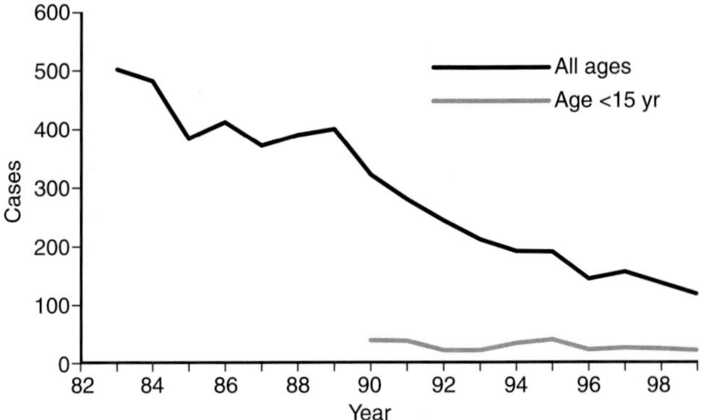

FIGURE 22–1. Reported cases of toxic shock syndrome by quarter in the United States, 1982–1999. (Data from the Centers for Disease Control and Prevention.)

Toxic shock syndrome has occurred with various staphylococcal infections, including surgical wound infection, abscess, osteomyelitis, lymphadenitis, and pneumonia. A variety of cutaneous and subcutaneous infections, such as impetigo, cellulitis, and infections associated with abrasions, burns, bites, insulin pump infusion sites, and ear piercing, have also been described. Sinusitis and nasal packing after otolaryngologic procedures account for many cases. Nonmenstrual toxic shock syndrome has also been associated with the use of the contraceptive sponge and contraceptive diaphragm, vaginal delivery, and therapeutic abortion. Risk factors for nonmenstrual cases have not been studied in a systematic fashion, but association with influenza A and B infections and bacterial tracheitis has been suggested. These infections alter the mucociliary clearance and disrupt the integrity of the mucosa in areas often colonized by *S. aureus,* which may result in a predisposition to toxic shock syndrome.

Streptococcal Toxic Shock Syndrome. Severe invasive infections caused by group A *Streptococcus* are not a reportable disease in all states in the United States. The incidence rate from population-based active surveillance studies of severe group A *Streptococcus* infections is 1.5–7 cases per 100,000 persons, with approximately 10,000 cases occurring nationwide each year. Streptococcal toxic shock syndrome accounted for only 6% of toxic shock syndrome among individuals younger than 10 years, compared with 21% among those older than 60 years.

Varicella infection is a major risk factor for invasive group A streptococcal infections among children. The risk of streptococcal toxic shock syndrome among children younger than 10 years with varicella is 39-fold higher within 2 weeks of illness onset (Davies, 1996).

Many other factors increase susceptibility to severe group A streptococcal infection and to the development of streptococcal toxic shock syndrome, including diabetes mellitus, chronic cardiac or pulmonary disease, HIV infection, intravenous drug use, and alcoholism. However, no predisposing factors are identified in at least 35% of cases. Several reports have suggested a relationship between the use of nonsteroidal anti-inflammatory drugs and necrotizing fasciitis attributable to group A streptococci. However, there have been no adequately controlled studies to confirm this association.

PATHOGENESIS

Staphylococcal Toxic Shock Syndrome. Toxic shock syndrome is the consequence of the pathogenic effects of several staphylococcal products, acting alone or together. Endogenous mediators released by the host in response to such toxins also have an effect. Bacterial endotoxin may play a complicating role.

Experimental studies demonstrate that toxic shock syndrome–associated *S. aureus* strains can cause a similar illness in rabbits. In addition, it has been found that persons receiving antistaphylococcal antibiotics, at least those with menses-associated cases, have a lower recurrence rate. In the rabbit model of toxic shock syndrome, TSST-1-producing strains cause a toxic shock–like illness. The biologic effects of TSST-1 are numerous, including reticuloendothelial system blockade; suppression of immunoglobulin synthesis; enhancement of delayed hypersensitivity reactions; activity as a **superantigen** (nonspecific polyclonal T-lymphocyte proliferation without regard to the antigenic specificity of the T-cell and macrophage activation [see Fig. 5–7]); induction of high fever; release of IL-1, TNF, and other lymphokines and monokines; and enhancement of host susceptibility to lethal shock by endotoxin. The other staphylococcal enterotoxins possibly associated with toxic shock syndrome can also act as superantigens to stimulate T cells with secondary release of lymphokines and monokines.

Investigations to define the factors in the vagina that promote TSST-1 production by staphylococcal strains while tampons are worn during menstruation show no evidence that microbial growth occurs within tampons, although such growth is possible. No association has been found between toxic shock syndrome and the frequency of changing tampons. Among a number of proposed theories, the potential role of magnesium has generated controversy. TSST-1 production in vitro is maximal in the presence of low concentrations of magnesium. Other studies have demonstrated that certain local conditions (e.g., aerobic environment, neutral pH, 6% CO_2, high protein levels, and low glucose content) could provide a rich environment for *S. aureus* growth and TSST-1 production, irrespective of any influence of the tampon. The relationship of tampon composition to the development and expression of the disease continues to be an area of active investigation.

The prevalence of antibodies against TSST-1 is 70% at age 10 years, 88% at age 20 years, and more than 95% in the general adult population. By contrast, pre-existing antibody titers to TSST-1 are absent or low in almost all cases of toxic shock syndrome. The increase in antibody against TSST-1 during recovery of nonmenstrual cases and the failure of antibody formation or the development of low antibody titers in recurrent menstrual cases are also strong evidence that TSST-1 plays a central role in the pathogenic mechanism of toxic shock syndrome. Approximately 90% of *S. aureus* bacteria isolated from the vagina in menstrual toxic shock syndrome produce TSST-1. No person with an anti-TSST-1 antibody titer of at least 1:100 who is infected with TSST-1-producing *S. aureus* has developed toxic shock syndrome.

However, between 30% and 60% of isolates of *S. aureus* associated with nonmenstrual toxic shock syndrome do not produce TSST-1. Furthermore, TSST-1-producing strains have also been isolated from children without anti-TSST-1 antibody who do not develop toxic shock syndrome. Thus TSST-1 is not the only toxin associated with toxic shock syndrome. Evidence in support of other staphylococcal enterotoxins (A, B, C_1, C_2, C_3, D, E, and G) as alternative toxic shock syndrome toxins in the appropriate clinical setting is increasing.

The toxic shock syndrome strain of *S. aureus* is more likely to make one or more enterotoxins than are strains in other clinical settings. This is particularly true for TSST-1-negative toxic shock syndrome–associated strains that almost always produce staphylococcal enterotoxin B. Paired sera from persons with TSST-1-negative toxic shock syndrome have demonstrated a rise in antibody titer to enterotoxins. In vitro studies have shown that the enterotoxins share several biologic activities with TSST-1, including induction of IL-1 by monocytes and immunoregulatory activities. Finally, several of the enterotoxins in laboratory animals can lead to a clinical picture that is indistinguishable from the toxic shock syndrome caused by TSST-1.

The most striking aspect of the pathophysiology of toxic shock syndrome is the rapid onset of hypotension, resulting in tissue ischemia and multisystem organ failure. The hypotension appears to have two causes: (1) a nonhydrostatic leakage of fluid from the vascular to the interstitial space, which leads to an extensive, generalized, nonpitting edema (particularly after fluid resuscitation), and (2) a decrease in vasomotor tone with pooling of blood in the peripheral vasculature. The capillary leakage and loss of vascular tone are probably mediated by *S. aureus* toxins or by toxin-induced mediators such as IL-1, TNF, and other endogenous mediators of septic shock.

These dramatic hemodynamic changes cause a decline in intravascular volume, central venous pressure, and eventually systemic blood pressure, resulting in poor tissue perfusion. The multiorgan involvement associated with the full clinical syndrome probably results from a combination of the direct effects of toxin or inflammatory mediators and the hemodynamic changes (Fig. 22–2). Multisystem organ dysfunction occurs more frequently in the presence of shock and poor tissue perfusion.

The migration of polymorphonuclear leukocytes is inhibited by TNF, which may explain the absence of a purulent response in surgical wound infections caused by TSST-1-producing *S. aureus.*

Streptococcal Toxic Shock Syndrome. The M-1 and M-3 serotypes of group A *Streptococcus* are associated with invasive disease but also are frequently associated with streptococcal toxic shock syndrome. The majority of these strains produce **streptococcal pyrogenic exotoxin A (SPEA);** only 15% of other isolates of streptococci produce exotoxin A. This exotoxin shares sequence homology with staphylococcal enterotoxins B and C_1 but not with TSST-1. Like TSST-1, exotoxin A is very active biologically and can induce high fever, enhance host susceptibility to lethal endotoxin shock, and act as a superantigen, resulting in T-cell proliferation without regard to the antigenic specificity of the T cell (see Fig. 5–7). Again, stimulation of the T cell by superantigens induces massive release of lymphokines and monokines with secondary multisystem illness. Streptococcal pyrogenic exotoxins B and C may also contribute to the pathogenesis of the disease.

Other streptococcal factors, such as streptolysin O, peptidoglycan, and lipoteichoic acid may also contribute to the pathogenesis of the toxic shock syndrome because those substances can induce production of TNF and IL-1β by human mononuclear cells, and they appear to function synergistically with exotoxin A.

A higher rate of invasive group A *Streptococcus* infection and streptococcal toxic shock syndrome has been linked with the appearance of a new dominant streptococcal serotype in the population. If prevalence of immunity to this new type is low, there will be an increase in the number of invasive infections. A higher rate of serious infection correlates with a lack of protective antibodies to the M protein and a low capacity of serum to neutralize the biologic activity of the toxins. There is no invasive strain. The same organism can produce necrotizing fasciitis, toxic shock, impetigo, or pharyngitis. It is the interactions between the microbial virulence factors (e.g., SPEA, M proteins) and an immune or nonimmune host that determines the epidemiology, clinical manifestations, and outcome of infection.

Once invasion of mucosal or epithelial barriers by group A *Streptococcus* occurs in a host without specific antibody to M protein, tissue invasion and possibly bacteremia will occur. If the invading strains also produce pyrogenic exotoxins A or B, toxic shock syndrome will develop in patients lacking specific antibody to pyrogenic exotoxin produced by the infecting strain.

In a reported case (Schlievert et al, 1993b) of group B *Streptococcus* toxic shock–like syndrome, the strain did not produce

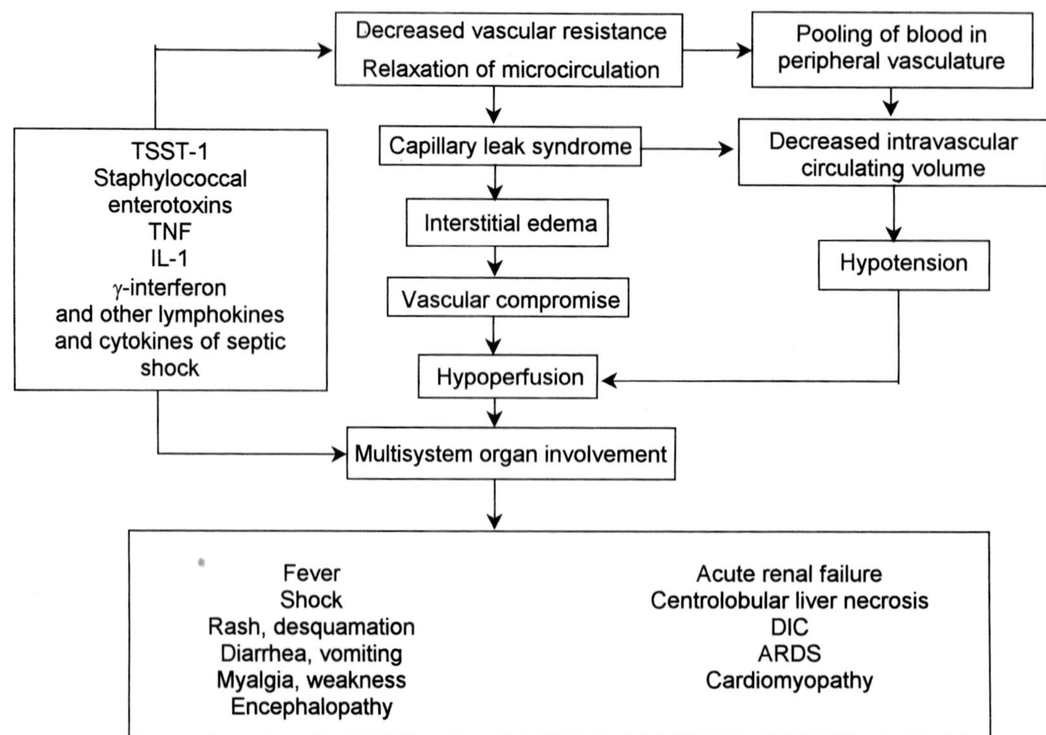

FIGURE 22–2. Sequence of events leading to multiorgan involvement in toxic shock syndrome.

TSST-1, staphylococcal enterotoxins, or streptococcal scarlet fever toxins but was producing a new pyrogenic toxin capable of causing toxic shock–like syndrome in animals. In three other persons with similar illnesses caused by group B *Streptococcus,* the bacterial strains were found to produce a toxin with similar properties capable of causing toxic shock–like illness.

SYMPTOMS AND CLINICAL MANIFESTATIONS

The clinical presentations of menstrual and nonmenstrual toxic shock syndrome are generally similar (Fig. 22–3). The syndrome most commonly occurs in women of reproductive age during the menstrual period or, occasionally, 1–2 days afterward. Nonmenstrual cases can occur in association with a wide variety of staphylococcal infections. When toxic shock syndrome is due to a surgical wound infection, it occurs most commonly 48 hours after surgery. The presentation is often shorter after nasal surgery; the nasal area is frequently colonized with *S. aureus.*

Illness due to toxic shock syndrome may be relatively mild or rapidly fatal. Typically the onset of the disease is abrupt, with high fever, myalgias, headaches, dizziness, diarrhea, and vomiting (Table 22–1). A diffuse sunburnlike erythroderma that blanches on pressure appears, and the eruption may resemble a scarlatiniform rash. It sometimes occurs initially over the trunk but inevitably spreads to the arms and legs. The erythema is most marked on the palms and soles. The rash may be petechial, but it is rarely purpuric.

Additional manifestations in the first 24–48 hours may include severe watery diarrhea, decreased urine output, peripheral cyanosis, and edema. Hypotension, oliguria, tachycardia, tachypnea, and a profound state of shock that can be refractory to fluid resuscitation rapidly develop. Intense conjunctival hyperemia and scleral involvement are frequent. Diffuse abdominal tenderness with no signs of peritonitis may be present. Many persons have neurologic symptoms such as confusion, hallucinations, and somnolence.

TABLE 22–1. Clinical Manifestations of Toxic Shock Syndrome

Symptoms	
Myalgia	96%
Vomiting	90%
Diarrhea	88%
Headaches	78%
Sore throat	75%
Clinical Signs	
Hypotension or orthostatic hypotension	100%*
Diffuse or palmar erythrodermia	100%*
Desquamation	100%*
Temperature	
≥38.9°C (102°F)	100%*
≥40°C (104°F)	87%
Oropharyngeal hyperemia	75%
Conjunctival hyperemia	71%
Neurologic abnormalities	58%
Vaginal hyperemia	35%
Vaginal discharge	27%
Rigors	25%

*Required by case definition.

Data from Tofte RW, Williams DN: Clinical and laboratory manifestations of toxic shock syndrome. *Ann Intern Med* 1982;96:843–7; Davis JP, Osterholm MT, Helms CM, et al: Tri-state toxic shock syndrome study. II. Clinical and laboratory findings. *J Infect Dis* 1982;145:441–8; Shands KN, Schmid GP, Dan BB, et al: Toxic-shock syndrome in menstruating women. Association with tampon use and *Staphylococcus aureus* and clinical features in 52 cases. *N Engl J Med* 1980;303:1436–42.

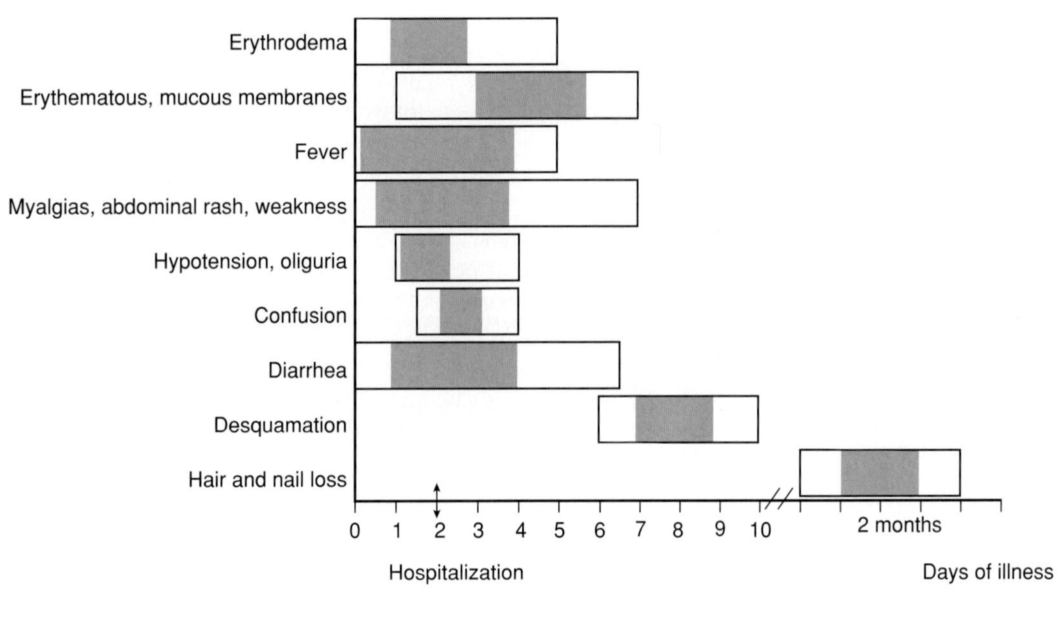

FIGURE 22–3. Profile of the typical clinical course of toxic shock syndrome.

Coma and increased intracranial pressure occurs in the most severe cases. The fever, headache, and diarrhea generally subside within the first week of the illness.

Depending on the severity of illness and shock, multisystem organ failure occurs to a variable extent. Acute renal failure, adult respiratory distress syndrome (ARDS), cardiac dysfunction and dysrhythmias, and DIC can be potentially fatal complications that require specialized care.

Progressively, patients can develop erythema of the mucous membranes with secondary ulcerations and eventually a late maculopapular eruption. The characteristic desquamation appears 1–3 weeks after initial presentation and can be extensive (Plate 6A). It is most often located on the fingers, palms, toes, and soles. The desquamation cleavage plane is at subepidermal level. Reversible nail and hair loss (telogen effluvium) is a tardive event.

In nonmenstrual toxic shock syndrome, it may be difficult to identify the source of infection because many toxic shock syndrome–associated staphylococci are nonpyrogenic. Focal signs of infection at the surgical wound site could be minimal or absent. It is important to examine the site carefully for a subcutaneous abscess and to obtain culture specimens from an apparently clean wound in the clinical setting of toxic shock syndrome.

Persons with AIDS can have multiple recurrences or a recalcitrant erythematous desquamating syndrome, which is actually an unrelenting toxic shock syndrome that can often result in death.

Streptococcal Toxic Shock Syndrome. The initial clinical presentation of severe invasive group A streptococcal infection is often nonspecific, and physicians should have a high index of suspicion regarding this rapidly evolving syndrome. Clues suggesting streptococcal toxic shock syndrome can include "flu like" symptoms such as myalgia, chills, and fever, but the pain is often more localized and severe than the generalized myalgia seen in influenza. Another common finding at presentation is local evidence of an abrasion, cut, or contusion at a body site, reflecting the entry point of group A *Streptococcus.*

In one study (Stevens, 1989) the clinical presentation of streptococcal toxic shock syndrome included severe pain in the involved extremity (85%), temperature greater than 38°C (100.4°F) (70%), localized swelling and redness (65%), confusion (55%), and tachycardia (25%). No subjects had rashes typical of scarlet fever. The incidence of complications was high: shock was present in 95% of patients (either at admission or within 4 hours), renal impairment in 85%, septicemia in 60%, and ARDS in 55%. The mortality rate was 30%.

DIAGNOSIS

The toxic shock syndrome case definition established by the CDC is based on the presence of six major diagnostic criteria (Table 22–2). There are no readily available laboratory tests to confirm the diagnosis of toxic shock syndrome. Some persons may not initially meet the diagnostic criteria, and therefore a high index of suspicion is required. Isolation of *S. aureus* from an infected site or isolation of *S. aureus* from the vagina and the presence of a tampon are strong evidence for a presumptive diagnosis in persons with atypical or milder forms of disease. However, isolation of the bacterium from a mucous membrane in the setting of nonmenstrual toxic shock syndrome is only suggestive of the diagnosis, even if the strain produces TSST-1, because some symptom-free persons are carriers. A presumptive diagnosis can be established retrospectively, with a significant increase in titers of anti-TSST-1 antibodies in paired sera in a patient with a compatible clinical presentation.

Streptococcal Toxic Shock Syndrome. In 1993 the Working Group on Severe Streptococcal Infections proposed a case definition for

TABLE 22–2. Toxic Shock Syndrome Case Definition

- **Fever:** temperature ≥38.9°C (102°F)
- **Rash:** diffuse macular erythroderma
- **Desquamation:** 1–2 weeks after onset of illness, particularly palms and soles
- **Hypotension:** systolic blood pressure ≤90 mm Hg for adults or less than 5th percentile for age for children and adolescents younger than 16 years of age; decrease in diastolic blood pressure ≥15 mm Hg with a change from lying to sitting position; orthostatic syncope or orthostatic dizziness
- **Multisystem involvement** of three or more of the following:
  - –Gastrointestinal: vomiting or diarrhea at onset of illness
  - –Muscular: severe myalgia or creatine phosphokinase at least twice the upper limit of normal for laboratory
  - –Mucous membranes: vaginal, oropharyngeal, or conjunctival hyperemia
  - –Renal: blood urea nitrogen or serum creatinine at least twice the upper limit of normal for laboratory or urinary sediment with pyuria (≥5 leukocytes per high-power field) in the absence of urinary tract infection
  - –Hepatic: total bilirubin, serum alanine aminotransferase (ALT), aspartate aminotransferase (AST) at least twice the upper limit of normal for laboratory
  - –Hematologic: platelet count ≤100,000/mm^3
  - –Central nervous system: disorientation or alterations in consciousness without focal neurologic signs when fever and hypotension are absent
- **Negative results** on the following tests, if obtained:
  - –Blood, throat, and cerebrospinal fluid cultures (blood culture may be positive for *Staphylococcus aureus*)
  - –Rise in antibody titers to Rocky Mountain spotted fever, leptospirosis, or measles

Case Classification

Probable: a case with five of the six clinical findings described above

Confirmed: a case with all six of the clinical findings described above, including desquamation, unless the patient dies before desquamation could occur.

From Centers for Disease Control and Prevention: Case definition for public health surveillance. *MMWR Morb Mortal Wkly Rep* 1990;39(RR-13):38.

TABLE 22–3. Proposed Case Definition for the Streptococcal Toxic Shock Syndrome*

I. Isolation of group A *Streptococcus*
  A. From a normally sterile site (e.g., blood; cerebrospinal, pleural, or peritoneal fluid; tissue biopsy; surgical wound)
  B. From a nonsterile site (e.g., throat, sputum, vagina, superficial skin lesion)
II. Clinical signs of severity
  A. Hypotension: systolic blood pressure ≤90 mm Hg in adults or less than 5th percentile for age for children and adolescents younger than 16 years
  and
  B. Two or more of the following signs:
    1. Renal impairment: creatinine ≥2 mg/dL (≥177 μmol/L) for adults or greater than or equal to twice the upper limit of normal for age. In patients with pre-existing renal disease, at least a twofold elevation over the baseline level.
    2. Coagulopathy: platelet count ≤100,000/mm^3 (≤100 × 10^9/L) or disseminated intravascular coagulation defined by prolonged clotting times, low fibrinogen level, and the presence of fibrin degradation products.
    3. Liver involvement: alanine aminotransferase (ALT), aspartate aminotransferase (AST), or total bilirubin levels greater than or equal to twice the upper limit of normal for age. In patients with pre-existing liver disease, at least a twofold elevation over the baseline level.
    4. Adult respiratory distress syndrome (ARDS), defined by acute onset of pulmonary diffuse infiltrates and hypoxemia in the absence of cardiac failure, or evidence of diffuse capillary leak manifested by acute onset of generalized edema, or pleural or peritoneal effusions with hypoalbuminemia.
    5. A generalized erythematous macular rash that may desquamate.
    6. Soft-tissue necrosis, including necrotizing fasciitis or myositis, or gangrene.

Case Classification
Probable: an illness fulfilling criteria IB and II (A and B), if no other cause of the illness is identified
Confirmed: an illness fulfilling criteria IA and II (A and B)

From The Working Group on Severe Streptococcal Infections. Defining the group A streptococcal toxic shock syndrome. Rationale and consensus definition. *JAMA* 1993;269:390–1. © 1993, American Medical Association.

the streptococcal toxic shock syndrome (Table 22–3). In this definition the occurrence of shock and multiorgan failure early in the course of infection characterizes streptococcal toxic shock syndrome, which is different from other types of invasive streptococcal diseases. Blood cultures and appropriate cultures of samples from any potentially infected site should be grown.

Differential Diagnosis

The differential diagnosis (Table 22–4) depends in part on the clinical presentation and its most noticeable features. In infants and young children with a febrile exanthematous illness, staphylococcal scalded skin syndrome, scarlet fever, and Kawasaki syndrome are often considered. Persons with these diseases rarely, if ever, develop hypotension. In staphylococcal scalded skin syndrome, extensive superficial desquamation and **Nikolsky's sign** often occur; shock and multisystem involvement are atypical. In scarlet fever the skin has a sandpaper-like texture, and Pastia's lines are apparent in the deep creases, particularly in the antecubital fossae. Children with Kawasaki syndrome generally develop thrombocytosis, not thrombocytopenia, they do not have hypotension unless myocardial infarction has occurred, and they rarely have multisystem organ failure.

TABLE 22–4. Differential Diagnosis of Toxic Shock Syndrome

- Drug reaction
- Kawasaki syndrome
- Leptospirosis
- Measles (typical and atypical)
- Meningococcemia
- Rocky Mountain spotted fever
- Streptococcal and staphylococcal scarlet fever
- Staphylococcal or gram-negative bacillary bacteremia
- Staphylococcal scalded skin syndrome
- Stevens-Johnson syndrome
- Toxic epidermal necrolysis
- Viral or toxin-mediated gastroenteritis
- Viral syndromes with exanthems

Depending on history of exposure, measles, leptospirosis, and Rocky Mountain spotted fever are other possible diagnoses. Target skin lesions, together with oral, anal, and conjunctival inflammation and drug exposure, suggest Stevens-Johnson syndrome. Although fever and hypotension are prominent in meningococcemia or bacterial sepsis, secretory diarrhea is almost always absent.

Laboratory Evaluation

Because of the multisystem involvement, the laboratory evaluation should include a CBC, urinalysis, and measurement of blood urea nitrogen, creatinine, liver enzymes, total bilirubin, creatine phosphokinase, serum electrolytes, and calcium (Table 22–5). Hypoproteinemia is present in most cases. Leukocytosis, thrombocytopenia, and azotemia are present in approximately 50% of patients. Any abnormal laboratory test results return to normal in the majority of patients by 7–10 days after onset of disease.

Electrocardiographic abnormalities are often nonspecific, but cardiac dysrhythmias may occur. The chest radiograph either may be normal or may demonstrate pulmonary edema or ARDS.

Microbiologic Evaluation

Appropriate cultures of samples from any potentially infected sites, including vaginal, blood, and cerebrospinal fluid cultures, should be obtained if clinically indicated. Bacteremia is rare, but frequently *S. aureus* can be isolated from one or more superficial sites. The strain can be sent to a reference laboratory to confirm the production of TSST-1. Paired sera can also be tested to identify a significant

TABLE 22–5. Laboratory Findings in Toxic Shock Syndrome

Finding	%
Hypoproteinemia	95%
Hypoalbuminemia	90%
Abnormal urinary sediment white blood cells (≥5/hpf; red blood cells ≥2/hpf)	69%
Elevated serum creatinine level (≥2 times upper limit of normal)	60%
Azotemia (≥2 times upper limit of normal)	55%
Hyperbilirubinemia (≥2 times upper limit of normal)	54%
Platelet count <100,000/mm³	50%
Hypocalcemia (serum calcium ≤7.5 mg/dL)	50%
Elevated creatinine phosphokinase level (≥2 times upper limit of normal)	49%
Leukocytosis (white blood cells ≥15,000/mm³)	48%
Elevated hepatic enzymes (≥2 times upper limit of normal)	47%
Hyponatremia	47%
Immature leukocytes (≥50%)	39%

Data from Davis JP, Osterholm MT, Helms CM, et al: Tri-state toxic shock syndrome study. II. Clinical and laboratory findings. *J Infect Dis* 1982; 145:441–8; Shands KN, Schmid GP, Dan BB, et al: Toxic-shock syndrome in menstruating women. Association with tampon use and *Staphylococcus aureus* and clinical features in 52 cases. *N Engl J Med* 1980;303:1436–42; Chesney PJ, Davis JP, Purdy WK, et al: Clinical manifestations of toxic shock syndrome. *JAMA* 1981;246:741–8.

rise in anti-TSST-1 titers. These tests (production of TSST-1 and serologic tests) are not performed on a routine basis and are available only in specialized research laboratories.

TREATMENT

The management of toxic shock syndrome has many goals, including stabilization of the patient, removal of potentially infected foreign bodies or drainage of abscesses, eradication of the primary focus of infection or colonization with toxin-producing staphylococci, and treatment of associated complications. Children in preshock or shock or with respiratory insufficiency or multiorgan system failure should be managed in a pediatric intensive care unit.

In menstrual toxic shock syndrome, gynecologic examination and removal of the tampon or the sponge is necessary. **Iodine vaginal douches** may help remove any preformed toxin. In nonmenstrual toxic shock syndrome, searches for potential sites of *S. aureus* infection, including sites of recent surgery, should be performed carefully. Abscesses should be drained and all foreign materials removed.

Initially, hypovolemic shock is corrected by fluid resuscitation to achieve adequate tissue perfusion (Table 22–6). Large volumes of fluids and electrolytes are required because of the severe capillary leakage and intravascular volume depletion. In certain persons who have protracted shock unresponsive to fluid therapy, the use of inotropic agents such as dopamine and dobutamine is necessary, as is monitoring of cardiovascular function and urine output. The loss of vascular tone and the capillary leak syndrome can take many days to abate, and monitoring helps determine the need for further fluid replacement and use of inotropic agents. Multiorgan system failure should be monitored and treated appropriately.

Specific treatment is instituted with a parenterally administered penicillinase-resistant β-lactam antibiotic such as nafcillin or oxacillin (Table 22–6). Treatment with vancomycin is indicated only when a person is considered to be at higher than usual risk of infection with MRSA or when there is a history of anaphylaxis to penicillin.

TABLE 22–6. Therapy and Monitoring of Staphylococcal Toxic Shock Syndrome

Fluid resuscitation and hemodynamic stabilization
- Boluses of crystalloid solution, 20–30 mL/kg; repeated as necessary
- Inotropic agents (dopamine, dobutamine, norepinephrine)

Removal of tampon or other infected foreign bodies

Drainage of abscesses

Intravenous antibiotic therapy:
- Oxacillin (150 mg/kg/day divided q6hr; maximum of 8–10 g/day) *or*
- Nafcillin (150 mg/kg/day divided q6hr; maximum of 8–10 g/day)

  and
- Clindamycin (25–40 mg/kg/day divided q6–8hr; maximum 2.7 g/day)

For penicillin-hypersensitive patients, alternative treatment is:
- Vancomycin (40 mg/kg/day divided q6hr; maximum 2 g/day)

Intravenous immunoglobulin (as needed):
- IVIG (400 mg/kg in a single dose)

Supportive therapy (as needed):
- Adult respiratory distress syndrome (ARDS)
- Electrolytes abnormalities
- Acid-base status abnormalities
- Myocardial dysfunction
- Cardiac dysrhythmias
- Acute renal failure
- Disseminated intravascular coagulation
- Cerebral edema

Continuous or intermittent monitoring (as needed):
- Heart rate
- Respiratory rate
- Arterial blood pressure
- Electrocardiogram
- Urine output
- Central venous pressure
- Pulmonary capillary wedge pressure
- Cardiac index
- Blood gases
- Serum electrolytes, calcium, serum creatinine, liver enzymes, coagulation studies
- Acid-base status

Laboratory studies suggest that antibiotics that inhibit protein synthesis, such as clindamycin, almost completely block production of TSST-1 by toxigenic strains of *S. aureus*. Experimental data suggest also that subinhibitory concentrations of β-lactam antibiotics actually may increase TSST-1 production by *S. aureus*. Although clinical studies are lacking, these results suggest a potential beneficial effect of adding clindamycin to a β-lactam drug when therapy for toxic shock syndrome is given.

Therapy should be continued for 14 days. There is no evidence that antibiotic therapy alters the course of the toxin-mediated disease unless an associated bacteremia exists. However, antistaphylococcal therapy seems to decrease the incidence of recurrence of toxic shock syndrome.

All commercially available preparations of immune globulin have high levels of antibody to TSST-1. In the rabbit model, IVIG decreases mortality rates when administrated up to 29 hours after inoculation of TSST-1-positive *S. aureus*. There are no clinical studies in humans to evaluate efficacy. Therefore IVIG should not be administered routinely to persons with toxic shock syndrome but should be reserved for those who did not respond or could not tolerate conventional therapies, including aggressive fluid administration, use of antibiotics, and surgical drainage. The dose most often used is 400 mg/kg, given as a single dose for several hours.

A retrospective study (Todd, 1984) suggested that early corticosteroid therapy reduces the severity of illness and duration of fever, although there was no difference in mortality. Corticosteroids appear to decrease toxin production by *S. aureus* in vitro. Because of a lack of clinical studies of the use of corticosteroids in toxic shock syndrome, they should be reserved for persons with serious illness refractory to treatment with fluid resuscitation, antibiotics, and IVIG. Replacement doses of corticosteroids should be given to persons thought to have adrenal insufficiency.

Streptococcal Toxic Shock Syndrome. The same therapeutic principles of fluid resuscitation and hemodynamic stabilization apply to both streptococcal and staphylococcal toxic shock syndrome.

Despite the universal susceptibility of group A *Streptococcus* to all β-lactam antibiotics, the outcome among children who have streptococcal toxic shock syndrome remains poor, with reported fatality rates exceeding 50%. Clinical failures may occur because of the **Eagle or inoculum effect,** which refers to reduced efficacy of penicillin and other cell wall–acting agents when group A *Streptococcus* is present in high concentrations. When the bacterial load is high, these bacteria reach a stationary phase and critical penicillin-binding proteins are not expressed, which is responsible for the decreased activity of penicillin in both human and experimental cases of severe streptococcal infection.

There is growing evidence that clindamycin may be the preferred drug for treating streptococcal toxic shock. The greater efficacy of clindamycin is multifactorial. Clindamycin is not affected by the bacterial growth cycle, it inhibits protein synthesis and hence toxin production, it appears to enhance phagocytosis of group A *Streptococcus,* and it may have an immunomodulatory effect by decreasing the production of TNF by lipopolysaccharide-stimulated monocytes. In a mouse model of group A *Streptococcus* myositis, the survival rate for mice treated with clindamycin was superior to that for mice treated with penicillin. A trend toward decreased mortality with the use of clindamycin was shown in a study (Kaul, 1997) of group A *Streptococcus* necrotizing fasciitis. Although resistance of group A *Streptococcus* to clindamycin has been reported, it remains less than 5% in the United States and Canada. The possibility of resistance to clindamycin dictates that it should not be used alone as therapy for severe group A *Streptococcus* infections. These data support the use of clindamycin (40 mg/kg/day, given intravenously in divided doses every 6–8 hours) in conjunction with high doses of penicillin G (200,000–300,000 U/kg/day, given intravenously in divided doses every 4 hours) as antimicrobial therapy for severe invasive group A streptococcal infections.

Adjunctive use of IVIG has been reported to be beneficial in the management of streptococcal toxic shock syndrome by its neutralizing activity against the toxins and cytokines released as a consequence of the streptococcal toxins. Dosages of 400 mg/kg/day for up to 5 days and a single dose of 1–2 g/kg have both been shown, in retrospective case-control studies, to increase superantigen-neutralizing activity and decrease the mortality rate.

Anecdotal reports suggest that hyperbaric oxygen is useful as adjunctive therapy for necrotizing fasciitis resulting from anaerobic and mixed bacterial agents. No controlled study of the use of hyperbaric oxygen has been performed for group A *Streptococcus* fasciitis, and therefore it should be considered experimental.

Prompt surgical exploration for diagnosis and extensive débridement can be lifesaving. MRI and CT are useful diagnostic tools that help define the extent of soft tissue involvement, although their use should not delay surgical exploration in a case of suspected fasciitis.

COMPLICATIONS

The case fatality rate of toxic shock syndrome is about 1–2%, with most fatalities occurring when there has been a long period of hypotension before initiation of therapy, which increases the likelihood of serious end-organ damage. The development of multiorgan system failure should be closely monitored and appropriately managed. Children develop ARDS more frequently than adults and may require ventilatory support. Renal insufficiency with secondary metabolic acidosis, hypocalcemia, and hypophosphatemia may require dialysis and correction of the metabolic and electrolyte abnormalities.

PROGNOSIS

In recent years, with earlier diagnosis and aggressive management, the case fatality rate has dropped to less than 3%. The mortality rate is higher in men, approximately 9–17%. When the syndrome occurs in children as a complication of influenza or influenza-like illness, the mortality can be greater than 50%. Persons with AIDS and toxic shock syndrome have a prolonged course with a worse prognosis.

The mortality rate for streptococcal toxic shock syndrome in the pediatric population is 5–10%, compared with a mortality rate of 30–80% for severe invasive group A *Streptococcus* infections in adults.

Sequelae are uncommon but may include vocal cord paralysis, chronic renal failure, muscle weakness, paresthesia, arthralgia, protracted myalgia, carpal tunnel syndrome, and amenorrhea. A pruritic, total body, maculopapular rash of late onset, at 9–13 days after onset of disease, has been reported in more than 50% of patients. It should not be confused with antibiotic allergy. Reversible hair and nail loss can occur 4–16 weeks after toxic shock syndrome.

Neuropsychologic sequelae have been reported at 2–12 months after recovery. Symptoms include concentration difficulties, headache, recent memory loss, and dysfunction of cognitive ability. Many of these patients were found to have electroencephalographic abnormalities. The exact pathogenesis or significance of these findings is uncertain.

Recurrence. In the early 1980s up to 34% of women with menstrual toxic shock syndrome had one or more confirmed or probable recurrent episodes (Table 22–7). In approximately 50% of patients the recurrence is classified as confirmed. Some persons may have more than one recurrent episode, which is generally less severe than the initial recurrence. This could be a result of absent or delayed production of antibodies. The use of antistaphylococcal antibiotics during the initial episode and discontinuation of tampon use are associated with a decreased risk of recurrent disease. Recurrence after nonmenstrual toxic shock syndrome is rare, with the exception of persons with AIDS.

PREVENTION

Toxic shock syndrome is not a contagious disease, but drainage and secretion precautions are recommended for the duration of

TABLE 22–7. Criteria for Confirmed or Probable Recurrence of Toxic Shock Syndrome

Confirmed Recurrence
Temperature: ≥38.9°C (102°F)
Rash: diffuse erythroderma
Hypotension: systolic blood pressure of ≤90 mm Hg for adults or <5th percentile for age for children and adolescent younger than 16 years, decrease in diastolic blood pressure of ≥15 mm Hg with a change from lying to sitting position; orthostatic syncope; or orthostatic dizziness
Mucous membranes hyperemia or myalgia
History of vomiting or diarrhea at the onset of illness
Desquamation

Probable Recurrence
Two of the first five criteria for a confirmed recurrence plus desquamation *plus* association with the menstrual period, *or*
Three of the first five criteria for a confirmed recurrence *without* desquamation but *with* association with the menstrual period

Modified from Davis JP, Osterholm MT, Helms CM, et al: Tri-state toxic shock syndrome study. II. Clinical and laboratory findings. *J Infect Dis* 1982;145:441–8.

illness. Discontinuation of tampon use is recommended for women with menses-associated toxic shock syndrome.

Prevention of Invasive Group A Streptococcal Disease. Opportunities for prevention are limited. Primary prevention of some sporadic community-acquired infections may be possible by reducing risk factors. Routine immunization against varicella should decrease the risk of invasive group A streptococcal invasive infections.

Some experts (Davies, 1996) recommend the use of antibiotic prophylaxis for persons who have been in close contact with persons who have severe invasive group A *Streptococcus* infection. This recommendation is based on the rate of invasive streptococcal infection in household members, which is 200 times that in the general population. However, no data are available about the effectiveness of any prophylaxis regimen for severe invasive group A streptococcal infections, and a working group on the prevention of cases among household contacts of persons with invasive group A streptococcal infections concluded that no definite recommendations can be made at this time.

REVIEWS

Ahmed S, Ayoub EM: Severe, invasive group A streptococcal disease and toxic shock. *Pediatr Ann* 1998;27:287–92.

American Academy of Pediatrics, Committee on Infectious Diseases: Severe invasive streptococcal infections: A subject review. *Pediatrics* 1998; 101:136–40.

Chesney PJ: Clinical aspects and spectrum of illness of toxic shock syndrome: Overview. *Rev Infect Dis* 1989;11:S1–7.

Davies HD: Invasive group A streptococcal infections in children. *Adv Pediatr Infect Dis* 1999;14:129–45.

Resnick SD: Toxic shock syndrome: Recent developments in pathogenesis. *J Pediatr* 1990;116:321–8.

Stevens DL: Invasive group A streptococcus infections. *Clin Infect Dis* 1992;14:2–11.

Stevens DL: Streptococcal toxic shock syndrome: Spectrum of disease, pathogenesis, and new concepts in treatment. *Emerg Infect Dis* 1995;1: 69–78.

Stevens DL: The flesh-eating bacterium: What's next? *J Infect Dis* 1999; 179:S366–74.

KEY ARTICLES

Barry W, Hudgens L, Donta ST, et al: Intravenous immunoglobulin therapy for toxic shock syndrome. *JAMA* 1992;267:3315–6.

Broome CV: Epidemiology of toxic shock syndrome in the United States: Overview. *Rev Infect Dis* 1989;11:S14–21.

Centers for Disease Control: Case definitions for public health surveillance. *MMWR Morb Mortal Wkly Rep* 1990;39(RR–13):38.

Chesney PJ, Davis JP, Purdy WK, et al: Clinical manifestations of toxic shock syndrome. *JAMA* 1981;246:741–8.

Chesney PJ, Crass BA, Polyak MB, et al: Toxic shock syndrome: Management and long-term sequelae. *Ann Intern Med* 1982;96:892–4.

Cone LA, Woodard DR, Schlievert PM, et al: Clinical and bacteriologic observations of a toxic shock–like syndrome due to *Streptococcus pyogenes. N Engl J Med* 1987;31:146–9.

Cone LA, Woodard DR, Byrd RG, et al: A recalcitrant, erythematous, desquamating disorder associated with toxin-producing staphylococci in patients with AIDS. *J Infect Dis* 1992;165:638–43.

Davies HD, McGeer A, Schwartz B, et al: Invasive group A streptococcal infections in Ontario, Canada. Ontario Group A Streptococcal Study Group. *N Engl J Med* 1996;335:547–54.

Forni AL, Kaplan EL, Schlievert PM, et al: Clinical and microbiologic characteristics of severe group A streptococcus infections and streptococcal toxic shock syndrome. *Clin Infect Dis* 1995;21:333–40.

Hoge CW, Schwartz B, Talkington DF, et al: The changing epidemiology of invasive group A streptococcal infections and the emergence of streptococcal toxic shock–like syndrome. A retrospective population-based study. *JAMA* 1993;269:384–9.

Jacobson JA, Kasworm EM, Reiser RF, et al: Low incidence of toxic shock syndrome in children with staphylococcal infections. *Am J Med Sci* 1987;294:403–7.

Kaul R, McGeer A, Norrby-Teglund A, et al: Intravenous immunoglobulin therapy for streptococcal toxic shock syndrome—A comparative observational study. The Canadian Streptococcal Study Group. *Clin Infect Dis* 1999;28:800–7.

Kaul R, McGeer A, Low DE, et al: Population-based surveillance for group A streptococcal necrotizing fasciitis: Clinical features, prognostic indicators, and microbiologic analysis of seventy-seven cases. *Am J Med* 1997;103:18–24.

MacDonald KL, Osterholm MT, Hedberg CW, et al: Toxic shock syndrome. A newly recognized complication of influenza and influenzalike illness. *JAMA* 1987;257:1053–8.

Norrby-Teglund A, et al: Relation between low capacity of human sera to inhibit streptococcal mitogens and serious manifestation of disease. *J Infect Dis* 1994;170:585–91.

Norrby-Teglund A, Basma H, Andersson J, et al: Varying titers of neutralizing antibodies to streptococcal superantigens in different preparations of normal polyspecific immunoglobulin G: Implications for therapeutic efficacy. *Clin Infect Dis* 1998;26:631–8.

Perez CM, Kubak BM, Cryer HG, et al: Adjunctive treatment of streptococcal toxic shock syndrome using intravenous immunoglobulin: Case report and review. *Am J Med* 1997;102:11–3.

Rosene KA, Copass MK, Kastner LS, et al: Persistent neuropsychological sequelae of toxic shock syndrome. *Ann Intern Med* 1982;96:865–70.

Schlievert PM: Role of superantigens in human disease. *J Infect Dis* 1993a; 167:997–1002.

Schlievert PM, Gocke JE, Deringer JR: Group B streptococcal toxic shock–like syndrome: Report of a case and purification of an associated pyrogenic toxin. *Clin Infect Dis* 1993b;17:26–31.

Stevens DL, Gibbons AE, Bergstrom R, et al: The Eagle effect revisited: Efficacy of clindamycin, erythromycin and penicillin in the treatment of streptococcal myositis. *J Infect Dis* 1988;158:23–8.

Stevens DL, Tanner MH, Winship J, et al: Severe group A streptococcal infections associated with toxic shock–like syndrome and scarlet fever toxin A. *N Engl J Med* 1989;321:1–7.

Stevens DL: Rationale for the use of intravenous gammaglobulin in the treatment of streptococcal toxic shock syndrome. *Clin Infect Dis* 1998; 26:639–41.

Todd JK, Fishauf M, Kapral F, et al: Toxic-shock syndrome associated with phage-group-I staphylococci. *Lancet* 1978;2:1116–8.

Todd JK, Ressman M, Caston SA, et al: Corticosteroid therapy for patients with toxic shock syndrome. *JAMA* 1984;252:3399–402.

Working Group on Severe Streptococcal Infections: Defining the group A streptococcal toxic shock syndrome: Rationale and consensus definitions. *JAMA* 1993;269:390–1.

Working Group on Prevention of Invasive Group A Streptococcal Infections. Prevention of invasive group A streptococcal disease among household contacts of case-patients: Is prophylaxis warranted. *JAMA* 1998; 279:1206–10.

CHAPTER 23

Measles

Charles T. Leach ▪ Hal B. Jenson

Measles, also known as **rubeola,** is a systemic respiratory illness characterized primarily by fever, cough, coryza, conjunctivitis, rash, and a distinctive enanthem. Measles is a potentially severe illness recognized since antiquity and caused by a virus that remains an important worldwide pathogen. In the United States, indigenous measles appears to have been eliminated as a result of an effective immunization program and aggressive surveillance.

Subacute sclerosing panencephalitis (SSPE), a rare but uniformly fatal form of degenerative encephalitis, develops an average of 8–10 years after a typical case of measles. SSPE is considered a slow encephalitis caused by measles virus.

ETIOLOGY

Measles is caused by **measles virus,** a single-stranded RNA virus of one antigenic type in the Paramyxoviridae family.

Transmission. Measles is spread primarily by large droplets from the upper respiratory tract and typically requires close contact between infected and uninfected persons. However, measles can also be spread by aerosolization. Persons with measles are considered contagious from 1 day before symptoms (about 5 days before onset of rash) to 4 days after appearance of the rash. The virus is not shed from cutaneous lesions. Humans are the only known natural hosts; measles virus has no animal reservoir and no insect vector. There is no recognized carrier state in humans.

EPIDEMIOLOGY

In the 1940s and 1950s, before the development of an effective vaccine, 150,000 to 900,000 measles cases were reported annually to the CDC (Fig. 23–1). The incidence was probably underreported, and it is likely that the actual attack rate approximated the annual birth cohort. Measles is a highly contagious disease and has a high attack rate among susceptible persons, which results in epidemics every 2–3 years in unvaccinated populations. The disease occurs throughout the year, but a distinct increase occurs between January and April. Measles occurs at equal rates in both males and females.

The first measles vaccine was licensed in 1963, and a dramatic fall in the number of reported measles cases ensued. However, between 1984 and 1990 an increase in measles cases occurred. After implementation of a new, two-dose measles vaccine requirement in 1989, the incidence of measles resumed its downward trend between 1991 and 1999. In 1999, only 100 cases of measles were reported in the United States, tying 1998 for the lowest ever recorded. The majority of cases in 1999 (66%) were epidemiologically or virologically linked to cases of measles from other countries with less stringent measles vaccine requirements. Of 11 measles outbreaks in the United States in 1999, seven were epidemiologically linked to an imported case. Most international visitors and United States residents with measles had received no measles vaccine. Although the primary vaccine failure rate has remained at 5% or less, outbreaks among small groups of susceptible persons have continued because of the high transmissibility of the disease.

PATHOGENESIS

Cellular receptors for measles virus are located on the upper respiratory tract epithelium, principally on the nasal mucosa. The virus replicates locally within upper respiratory tract epithelium and associated lymphoid tissue and is then disseminated via the bloodstream during a brief, low-titer, primary viremia to distant body sites including skin, respiratory tract, kidneys, intestinal tract, nervous system, and lymphoid tissue. Within these tissues the virus replicates in endothelial cells, epithelial cells, and monocytes. Finally, secondary viremia occurs and prodromal symptoms of measles soon follow. Viremia continues for 2–4 days and then rapidly clears coincident with the development of specific immunity. The characteristic rash follows. Virus can be recovered from the urine for several more days.

The most important characteristic of measles virus infection is the presence of large, multinucleated giant cells throughout reticuloendothelial tissues **(Warthin-Finkeldey cells)** and respiratory epithelia during prodromal and exanthematous stages of illness. These unusual cells are the result of cell fusion and contain microtubular structures resembling those seen within cells infected with measles virus in vitro. These giant cells typically measure 100 μm in diameter and contain up to 100 small or multilobulated nuclei with intranuclear and cytoplasmic inclusions (Fig. 23–2). Virus can be identified within the cells by electron microscopy.

Rash. The typical measles skin rash is characterized by vascular congestion, edema, and perivascular infiltrates of mononuclear cells. Viral antigens can be found in the epidermal layer. Hemorrhagic rashes, such as those seen in atypical measles, reveal extravasation of blood into the interstitial space. **Koplik's spots** resemble skin lesions histologically, although the amount of focal necrosis of the basal epithelium is usually larger and more endothelial proliferation is present. Giant cells and measles virus are not found in the mucous membrane lesions, although the virus may be seen around blood vessels and in capillary endothelial cells.

Pneumonia. Pulmonary involvement is frequent in uncomplicated cases of measles and reveals typical findings of a viral pneumonia with a predominantly monocytic response, including peribronchiolitis and variable interstitial inflammation. The lining of the respiratory tract, such as the laryngeal, tracheal, and bronchial mucosa, also shows changes as epithelial giant cells are formed and are frequently sloughed in the sputum along with macrophages and cellular debris. Severe measles pneumonia demonstrates an interstitial pattern and a picture similar to that of adult respiratory distress syndrome, with interstitial fibrosis and **bronchiolitis obliterans.**

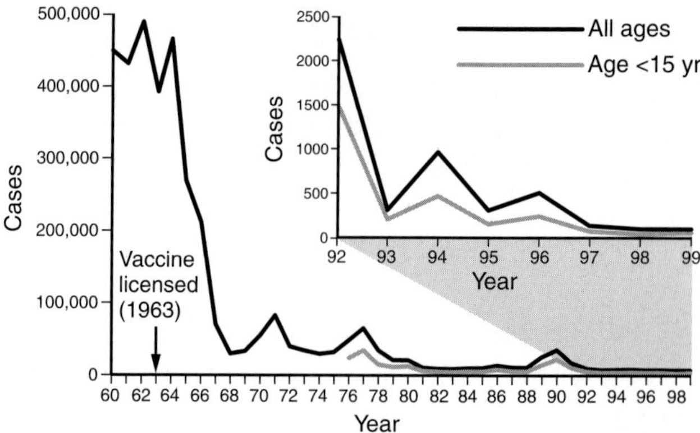

FIGURE 23–1. Reported cases (in thousands) of measles (rubeola) by year in the United States from 1950 to 1999. (Data from the Centers for Disease Control and Prevention, Atlanta, GA.)

Severe measles pneumonia may occur with increased frequency in immunocompromised children. It is characterized by the formation of giant cells, alveolar cell proliferation, and squamous metaplasia of bronchiolar epithelium, with prolonged excretion of giant cells and virus from the respiratory tract. Bronchopneumonia caused by bacterial infection, with findings of alveolar exudate, is a common complication of measles.

Encephalitis. Most cases of measles encephalitis in otherwise healthy persons have findings in common with other postinfectious encephalitides, including demyelination, gliosis, and a perivascular mononuclear cell infiltrate. Fat-laden macrophages may also be found near the blood vessels. In the majority of cases of measles encephalitis in immunocompromised persons, and in some cases in otherwise healthy persons, viral inclusions and viral antigens are present within the central nervous system, indicating invasion by measles virus.

Immune Suppression. Measles is associated with substantial cell-mediated immune suppression, probably accounting for the relatively high rate of secondary bacterial infections. This is demonstrated in vivo by diminished delayed-type hypersensitivity skin test reactivity. In addition, there is in vitro inhibition of lymphocyte proliferation, abnormal lymphokine production, and decreased natural killer cell activity. Recently, deficient production of IL-12, a critical immunoregulatory molecule, was demonstrated in monocytes exposed to measles virus. This may explain many of the immunologic abnormalities associated with measles.

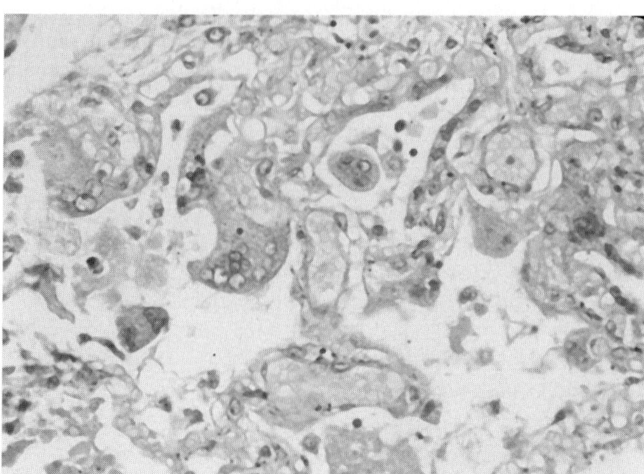

FIGURE 23–2. Giant cell pneumonia in a child with fatal measles infection. Multinucleated cells in the alveoli, containing acidophilic inclusion bodies. (Hematoxylin-eosin stain.)

SYMPTOMS AND CLINICAL MANIFESTATIONS

Incubation Period. The incubation period for measles is typically 8–12 days from exposure to the onset of symptoms. Longer incubation periods (up to 21 days) may be observed in partially immune persons and some adults.

Common Symptoms

Measles infection can be divided into four phases (Fig. 23–3): (1) the incubation phase, (2) the prodromal (catarrhal) phase, (3) the exanthematous (rash) phase, and (4) the recovery phase. The classic symptoms (Table 23–1) occur during the exanthematous phase.

Incubation Phase. No symptoms are evident during this precatarrhal phase.

Prodromal Phase. The prodromal phase of measles is defined by the onset of the first symptoms and is coincident with the highest level of measles viremia. The onset of the prodrome is usually a gradual phenomenon, with the most prominent symptoms being fever, cough, coryza, and conjunctivitis. Fever is frequently the first symptom noticed by the parent. The temperature usually rises steadily during the prodrome, with maximal temperatures in the range of 39.4°C (103°F) to 40°C (104°F) being reached by the time of the rash onset. In some cases the fever may remit for 1 or 2 days during the prodromal stage only to recur once the rash has appeared. The temperature reaches its maximum at the height of the exanthem and then usually falls rather rapidly. Development of fever during the later stages of illness or the lack of temperature lysis with the appearance of the rash suggests possible secondary bacterial infection.

Upper respiratory tract symptoms are prominent during the prodromal stage. Coryza develops with a profuse watery discharge from the nose, along with nasal congestion and sneezing. A pronounced cough, which sometimes resembles croup, is typically hoarse, dry, and hacking. The older child may complain of some tightening in the chest. Mild to moderate pharyngeal irritation also occurs.

Affliction of the eyes, another hallmark of measles, is characterized primarily by lacrimation, pain, and photophobia. Eye pain may be severe and is often likened to having sand in the eyes. Puffiness of the lower eyelids may also be noted. Other symptoms frequently observed during the prodromal period include malaise, myalgia, irritability, fretfulness, anorexia, headache, abdominal pain, constipation, and dry mouth and throat.

Exanthematous Phase. An average of 2–4 days usually elapses between the onset of symptoms and the first appearance of the measles rash; this period may occasionally be longer. Symptoms that occurred during the prodromal phase usually worsen with the onset of the rash but then begin to decrease in severity by the second day of the rash. Diarrhea may develop during the exanthematous phase.

Recovery Phase. After 4–5 days the rash begins to subside in order of appearance. The rash becomes brownish and is no longer brightly

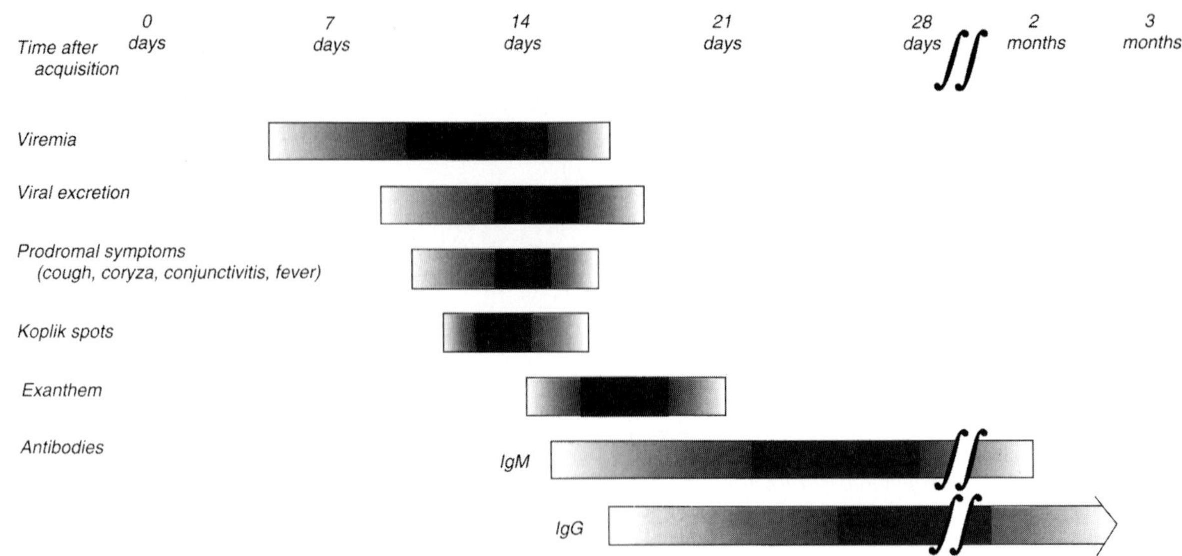

FIGURE 23–3. Profile of the typical clinical course of measles.

colored. Subsequently, a fine (branlike) desquamation of skin develops, which is most notable in the facial area. Desquamation of large flakes of skin is very uncommon. As the rash fades, constitutional and catarrhal symptoms continue to improve. By 10–14 days after the development of the rash, the child is usually back to a normal level of activity.

Physical Examination Findings

During the prodromal stage, typical physical findings include fever, dry cough, nasal congestion with clear rhinorrhea, conjunctivitis with photophobia, pharyngitis, anterior cervical lymphadenopathy, and crackles in the chest on auscultation. These findings may vary from person to person and may be attributed to the common cold.

Exanthem. The measles rash, which is maculopapular and not pruritic, usually first appears as irregular macules on the upper forehead or behind the ears and on the neck (Plate 3A). Within 24 hours the entire face, head, and neck are affected. Within 2–4 days the rash extends caudally to the chest, back, and extremities and includes the palms and soles; it becomes confluent on the cheeks. Lesions are palpable and frequently have a velvety texture. Single lesions may appear round, oval, or even irregular in shape. The lesions are initially sparse and punctate in appearance, but later they become larger and may coalesce to form plaques, especially on the upper portion of the body. Most lesions reach a diameter of 2–3 mm at maturity, after 24–36 hours. Early lesions easily blanch with pressure, although some petechiae may be seen. The rash is initially dark red, but the coloration subsequently becomes slightly purplish. When lesions become more mature, especially those on the face, pressure yields a yellowish or brownish hue. Skin unaffected with lesions is typically slightly edematous and may be slightly red. The term **morbilliform** is used to describe a measles-like rash.

TABLE 23–1. Clinical Manifestations of Measles

Prodrome
Fever, usually a temperature of 38.5°C (101°F)
Malaise
Measles
Fever, usually a temperature of 38.5°C (101°F)
Conjunctivitis
Photophobia
Cough
Coryza
Koplik's spots
Rash 3–4 days after onset of symptoms, spreads from face to extremities within 3–4 days
Convalescence
Rash fades in sequence of appearance within 3–4 days
Considered noncontagious by day 4 of rash

Enanthem. Measles can most easily be distinguished from other viral rash diseases by the presence of **Koplik's spots,** which are minute lesions on the oral mucosa that are pathognomonic for measles (Plate 3B). These tiny (1 mm) blue-white lesions occurring on a bright red, granular-appearing background first develop during the prodromal period, typically 1–2 days before the skin eruption, and are therefore reliable clinical markers for the diagnosis of measles. Initially a few discrete lesions develop on the buccal mucosa opposite the first lower molars. They increase in number rapidly for 24 hours and may spread to cover the buccal and perhaps some of the labial mucosa, becoming confluent in some areas. They are not found on the palate or in the posterior pharynx. These lesions should not be confused with other entities such as Fordyce's aphthae (common in adults and adolescents but lacking the bright red background) or aphthous ulcers (larger, painful ulcerative lesions present in much lower numbers). Koplik's spots begin to fade as the exanthem appears and usually disappear by the second day of the rash. However, the diffuse granular background of redness on the buccal mucosa can usually still be observed despite the absence of the tiny, discrete lesions. Koplik's spots in the mouth resemble rash lesions on the skin histologically.

Uncommon Symptoms

Modified Measles. Modified measles is a term commonly used to describe mild cases of measles occurring in persons with partial and inadequate protection against measles. Modified disease occurs after exposure to wild measles virus and may be a result of many different circumstances, including vaccination or natural measles infection at an early age (typically before 12 months of age, when levels of transplacentally acquired measles antibodies are not fully protective but may interfere with a normal immune response), administration of serum IG with measles vaccine (as practiced in the 1960s to reduce side effects of early vaccines), concomitant administration of IG with vaccine after measles exposure (e.g., during outbreaks of measles), or insufficient vaccine virus replication (e.g., vaccination with improperly stored vaccine). Recurrent measles infection with modified illness may rarely occur, typically in persons who have previously received postexposure prophylaxis with IG, which resulted in the development of partial immunity.

Children with modified illness may have subclinical illness with infection diagnosed only by serologic testing. Those with symptomatic modified measles have a shorter prodromal phase with minimal symptoms. Koplik's spots are infrequently observed and, if seen, are more transient than those found in typical cases of measles. Although the rash follows its usual progression, it does not become confluent. Modified measles may easily be confused with other exanthematous illnesses.

Atypical Measles. Reports of these unusual and severe cases of measles first appeared in 1965, with hundreds of similar cases subsequently reported. Atypical measles occurs almost exclusively in recipients of killed measles virus vaccine who later come in contact with natural (wild-type) measles virus. Recent experimental animal data suggest that the pathogenesis of the disease involves an anamnestic nonprotective antibody response leading to IgG immune complex deposition, complement activation, and abnormal cytokine production stimulating eosinophilia and high IgE levels. The killed vaccine was available in the United States between 1963 and 1967, and as many as 1 million persons may have received it. At present, these recipients are adults in the third or fourth decade of life. Vaccination with current live attenuated measles vaccine provides protection against atypical measles.

Like classic measles, atypical measles includes high fever and prominent cough; coryza and conjunctivitis are less common. The onset of atypical measles is usually abrupt and distinguished by severe headache; severe abdominal pain, often with vomiting; myalgias; pneumonia with pleural effusion; and an exanthem that is very different from the typical measles rash. The rash is variable, but typically it first appears on the peripheral extremities, especially the palms, wrists, soles, and ankles. The lesions then progress in a centripetal (cephalad) direction, eventually affecting the proximal extremities, trunk, and occasionally the face. In some persons the rash does not move significantly from the peripheral extremities. The lesions are maculopapular in the initial stages but normally become vesicular; eventually they may become purpuric or hemorrhagic. Koplik's spots rarely appear. Milder disease has been observed in the few cases of atypical measles in recipients of live measles vaccine.

The majority of patients with atypical measles have radiographic evidence of pneumonia, usually with segmental or lobar involvement that is frequently associated with pleural effusion and prominent hilar lymphadenopathy. Pulmonary infiltrates, which may coalesce into nodular densities, persist for years and can be mistaken for other disorders. Individuals with atypical measles are not generally considered to be infectious because measles virus can rarely be cultured from them.

Measles in Immunocompromised Persons. Compromised immunity, especially cell-mediated immunity, poses an increased risk of severe and frequently fatal disease after exposure to the measles virus. The diagnosis of measles is frequently delayed in immunocompromised persons because many of them do not exhibit the usual clinical findings associated with the disease. For example, prodromal symptoms may not be present, the rash may be mild, atypical, or absent, and Koplik's spots may not be observed. Prolonged excretion of measles virus within the respiratory tract and the development of severe complications such as giant cell pneumonia and encephalitis are frequent in immunocompromised children with measles. Although some immunocompromised children may have mild or even subclinical measles infection, measles in immunocompromised persons has a high overall mortality rate.

DIAGNOSIS

The diagnosis of measles is based primarily on clinical presentation and physical examination findings. Specific laboratory testing should also be performed for confirmation of this reportable disease.

Differential Diagnosis

The differential diagnosis includes many other exanthematous illnesses (Table 23–2). There is usually little difficulty in establishing a presumptive diagnosis of measles in a nonimmunized person with typical clinical findings, especially with a history of exposure. Most difficulty arises in the differentiation of the cutaneous and oral lesions of measles (especially modified measles) from those of rubella and scarlet fever (Table 23–3). A key finding in measles is the presence of Koplik's spots on the buccal mucosa. However, modified forms of illness cause greater difficulty in diagnosis because of the generally milder nature and the usual absence of Koplik's spots. Lymphadenopathy is not a regular occurrence in measles and, when present, does not occur in the same pattern as in rubella, where there is prominent involvement of the suboccipital, postauricular, and posterior cervical nodes.

Atypical Measles. Although atypical measles has a characteristic rash that should not be confused with the exanthem of typical measles, differentiation of atypical measles from other illnesses may be more difficult. The illness that most closely mimics atypical measles is RMSF, because the character and progression of the

TABLE 23–2. Differential Diagnosis of the Rash of Measles

Classic Measles
Rubella
Scarlet fever
Erythema infectiosum (fifth disease)
Enterovirus infection
Adenovirus infection
Roseola
Infectious mononucleosis
Mycoplasma pneumoniae infection
Kawasaki syndrome
Drug eruptions
Atypical Measles
Rocky Mountain spotted fever
Meningococcal infection
Rubella
Primary varicella
M. pneumoniae infection
Enterovirus infection
Bacterial or viral pneumonia
Henoch-Schönlein purpura
Drug eruptions

TABLE 23–3. Differentiation of the Skin Lesions of Measles, Rubella, and Scarlet Fever

	Measles	Rubella	Scarlet Fever
Color	Reddish-brown	Pink	Reddish
Distribution			
Initial appearance	Face and neck	Face and neck	Flexor surfaces; neck, axillary, inguinal, and popliteal skinfolds
Progression	Face, neck, trunk, and proximal extremities in 2–3 days	Face, neck, trunk, and extremities in 1–2 days	Generalized in 1 day; circumoral sparing
Confluent lesions	On face, neck, and upper trunk	Uncommon	Generalized in 1 day
Fades	By 5–6 days	By 3 days	Within several days
Desquamation	Mild hyperpigmentation with branny desquamation over upper trunk	Uncommon	Desquamation involving hands and feet
Oral lesions	Koplik's spots	Forchheimer's sign (petechiae on soft palate) in 20%	Strawberry tongue and circumoral pallor

rash are similar for both illnesses and because headache occurs frequently in both. Historical information useful in differentiating atypical measles from RMSF includes vaccination with killed measles vaccine, age of the patient, season of the year, tick exposure, chest radiograph findings, coagulation abnormalities, and the local incidence of measles. Any patient suspected of having RMSF should be treated presumptively.

Laboratory Evaluation

Routine laboratory evaluation is seldom necessary for evaluation of typical measles. During the prodrome and exanthem, mild neutropenia with absolute lymphopenia is usually observed, followed by a leukocytosis during the resolution phase. Mild elevations in aminotransferases, indicating hepatocellular injury, may occur during the course of measles, especially in adults, but they are rarely associated with clinical symptoms and resolve spontaneously. Cases of atypical measles usually display leukopenia early in their course, followed by eosinophilia. Approximately 30% of persons with measles develop cerebrospinal fluid pleocytosis. The urinalysis generally shows no abnormalities.

Microbiologic Evaluation

Specific microbiologic evaluation to confirm the diagnosis should be sought for all presumed cases of measles in the United States. This has become increasingly important because fewer practicing physicians are experienced in making a presumptive diagnosis based on clinical findings. The diagnosis can be confirmed by demonstrating one or more of the following: the presence of measles virus in any of several body fluid samples; a fourfold or greater increase in anti-measles IgG antibodies in acute and convalescent sera; or the presence of anti-measles IgM antibodies in serum. Serologic diagnosis is usually sufficient. Presumptive cases of measles should be reported promptly to the local health department, before laboratory confirmation is available.

Viral Culture. Culture of measles virus may not be generally available. Suitable sites and samples for culture of measles virus include blood (leukocytes), throat, nasopharynx, conjunctivae, urine, and, in unusual cases, cerebrospinal fluid or tissue. Samples should be collected as early as possible during the exanthematous period because virus concentrations begin to diminish during this phase. Nasopharyngeal samples are probably the best specimens. Samples from the upper respiratory tract should be collected by aspiration or by use of a sterile cotton-tipped swab, immediately placed in a vial containing appropriate medium with protein and antibiotics, and then transported to the laboratory. If transportation is delayed, specimens may be temporarily stored at 4°C.

Measles virus can be grown in several different cell lines, including primary human and simian kidney cells, EBV-immortalized B95-8 lymphocyte cells, and human umbilical cord cells. Typical multinucleated syncytial giant cells usually appear by 7–10 days after inoculation. Because other viruses may also form giant cells, the presence of measles virus within these cells must be confirmed by hemadsorption of infected cells to simian (but not nonsimian) red blood cells or by immunofluorescent methods.

Measles virus may also be detected directly from clinical specimens, such as nasopharyngeal swabs or urine. Cytologic examination of appropriately processed specimens from measles cases reveals giant cells and intranuclear inclusions (Fig. 23–2). A more specific approach involves immunohistochemical methods in which monoclonal or polyclonal anti-measles serum is used.

Serologic Diagnosis. The hemagglutination inhibition test has been the standard method used for measuring measles antibodies. Other suitable methods include complement fixation, neutralization, immunofluorescence, radioimmunoassay, and enzyme immunoassay. A fourfold or greater rise in the titer of measles IgG antibodies, measured in acute and convalescent serum samples drawn at least 10 days apart, confirms the diagnosis. Persons with atypical measles frequently develop extremely high titers of measles antibodies.

A positive measles IgM antibody test in a single serum sample can more rapidly confirm the diagnosis of measles. IgM antibodies are present within 1–2 days after the onset of the exanthem, reach a peak approximately 10 days later, and disappear within 1–2 months. A laboratory with expertise in measuring measles IgM antibodies should be used because false-positive and false-negative test results may be obtained. A capture enzyme immunoassay appears to be the most specific measles IgM test available.

Diagnostic Imaging. Diagnostic imaging is rarely indicated for the typical child with measles. However, imaging may be necessary for persons with measles whose cases have unusual features or complications. Bacterial bronchopneumonia is an important complication of measles. However, chest radiographs do not readily distinguish bacterial superinfection from pneumonia resulting from measles, which typically demonstrates interstitial, perihilar, and

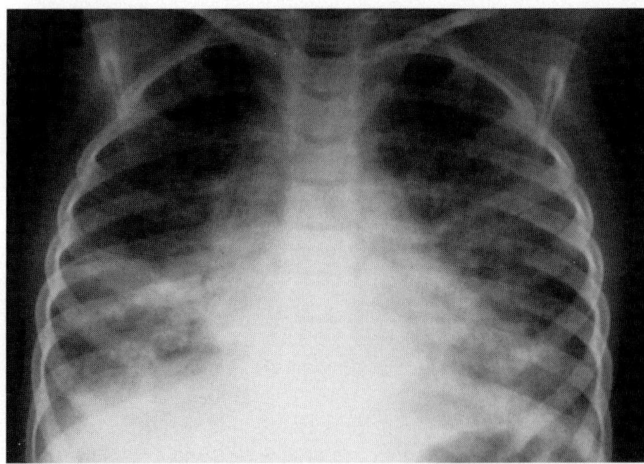

FIGURE 23–4. Measles pneumonia in a 5-year-old boy with leukemia. The frontal chest radiograph shows a diffuse interstitial infiltrate in the upper lung zones that becomes more nodular and coalesces in the lower lung zones to areas of frank consolidation. The perihilar regions are also involved, thus obscuring any lymphadenopathy that might be present.

lower lobe infiltrates (Fig. 23–4). Up to 50% of otherwise healthy children with uncomplicated measles have infiltrates on radiography of the chest.

Individuals with atypical measles (primarily adults) invariably develop high fever and severe cough. Chest radiographs of these patients frequently reveal focal infiltrates, either segmental or lobar, and sometimes persistent nodular densities.

Cases of measles encephalitis may require imaging of the central nervous system by CT or MRI for evaluation. The CT usually shows no abnormalities in measles encephalitis. Central nervous system imaging of SSPE is nonspecific and generally reveals atrophy and gray and white matter lesions. MRI is superior to CT for imaging of white matter and the basal ganglia in SSPE.

TREATMENT

Definitive Treatment

Specific antiviral therapy has not been convincingly shown to affect measles morbidity or mortality rates among children in the United States, despite in vitro susceptibility to several drugs and anecdotal reports of efficacy. Ribavirin therapy may be considered in cases of severe measles in immunocompromised children. However, such a decision should be made in consultation with an infectious disease specialist. Numerous antiviral compounds have been studied with little success in reversing the course of SSPE.

Vitamin A. Measles and other acute illnesses may induce a decrease in serum prealbumin and retinol-binding protein, precipitating acute vitamin A deficiency in marginally nourished children with little or no hepatic reserves of vitamin A. Measles in the presence of hypovitaminosis A, defined as a serum vitamin A level less than 10 μg/dL, is associated with lower levels of measles-specific antibody and increased measles morbidity and mortality. Although vitamin A deficiency is not acknowledged to be a significant problem in the United States, low serum levels of vitamin A have been found in both indigent and well-nourished children with measles. Information in developed countries regarding the association between low vitamin A levels and measles morbidity and mortality is incomplete.

In developing countries, vitamin A supplementation appears to improve morbidity and mortality among children with low vitamin A levels who develop severe measles, especially children younger than 2 years. Information about the need for additional vitamins in infants younger than 6 months is limited, however. The World Health Organization and the United Nations International Children's Emergency Fund (UNICEF) recommend vitamin A supplementation for children residing in regions where vitamin A deficiency is a recognized problem and the mortality rate for measles is 1% or greater. In the United States, the AAP recommends vitamin A supplementation for certain children older than 6 months who have measles and who are not already receiving supplemental vitamin A (Table 23–4).

A single dose of vitamin A (100,000 IU for infants 6 months to 1 year of age; 200,000 IU for older children) is administered at the time of diagnosis. The higher dose may be associated with headache and vomiting for a few hours. The dose is repeated 24 hours later and again at 4 weeks for children with ophthalmic symptoms or signs of hypovitaminosis A. No toxic effects have been reported at these dosages, although pseudotumor cerebri, with nausea, vomiting, headache, and a bulging fontanel in infants, and with abnormal liver function, may occur in association with acute vitamin A poisoning after cumulative intake usually of more than 1 million IU for 2–3 weeks. Vitamin A is teratogenic at therapeutic dosages and should not be administered to pregnant women.

Supportive Treatment

The mainstay of therapy for measles in children is supportive. Children should receive adequate bed rest in a room with subdued lighting. Oral nutrition should be maintained if possible. Acetaminophen or ibuprofen may be used for fever reduction and pain control. Over-the-counter medications for upper respiratory tract and ophthalmic symptoms are probably of no benefit. Clinicians must be alert for the emergence of bacterial superinfection during

TABLE 23–4. Vitamin A Supplementation for Patients with Measles

Vitamin A Supplementation Should Be Considered for:

Children 6 mo to 2 yr of age hospitalized for measles and its complications

Children older than 6 mo with measles *and* any one of the following:

- Immunodeficiency (primary or acquired, including immunosuppressive therapy)
- Ophthalmic signs of vitamin A deficiency
  - Night blindness
  - Bitot's spots (grayish white spots on the bulbar conjunctiva adjacent to the cornea)
  - Evidence of xerophthalmia
- Impaired intestinal absorption
- Moderate to severe malnutrition
- Recent immigration from an area of increased mortality due to measles

Administration

Children aged 6–11 mo: single dose of 100,000 IU PO

Children aged ≥12 mo: single dose of 200,000 IU PO

Children with ophthalmic evidence of vitamin A deficiency should be given additional doses the next day and at 4 wk.

Adapted from the American Academy of Pediatrics, Committee on Infectious Diseases: Vitamin A treatment of measles. *Pediatrics* 1993;91:1014–5.

the course of measles, especially in young infants, and treat accordingly.

COMPLICATIONS

The most frequent complications of measles in immunocompetent persons are diarrhea, bacterial otitis media, bacterial lower respiratory tract infections, and central nervous system disease. Measles infection of respiratory tract epithelium results in loss of normal local defenses, leading to otitis media, bacterial tracheitis, and bronchopneumonia. Other complications, including thrombocytopenia, hepatitis, tonsillitis, nephritis, ulcerative keratitis, iritis, panophthalmitis, peritonitis, appendicitis, myocarditis, pericardial effusion, pericarditis, and Stevens-Johnson syndrome, occur but are uncommon. In immunocompromised persons, pneumonia or encephalitis or both usually complicate measles.

Diarrhea. Diarrhea occurs in approximately 10% of persons with measles. Gastrointestinal illness usually occurs after the exanthem has appeared and lasts only a few days. The diarrhea is mild and usually does not require intravenous fluids.

Otitis Media. Otitis media is a frequent complication, occurring in approximately 5–15% of reported measles cases. Symptoms are usually delayed until the second week of illness, after the rash has faded, but may occur with the onset of the rash. Appropriate treatment with an antimicrobial agent is indicated.

Laryngotracheitis. Laryngotracheitis (**measles croup**) is a potentially severe and important complication of measles worldwide that occurs infrequently in the United States and other developed countries (approximately 5–20% of pediatric cases). Laryngotracheitis occurs more commonly with measles in infants, presumably because of their smaller airway. The most common finding at presentation is mild inspiratory stridor with no respiratory distress; some children develop more severe symptoms, however. Generally, children with measles croup should be admitted to the hospital, given supportive care (fluids and cool-mist oxygen), and observed for signs of worsening respiratory disease.

Bacterial Tracheitis. Bacterial tracheitis, although less common than measles croup, is a more severe complication and may occur in any age group. Illness may develop a few days after the exanthem appears or may not appear until more than 7 days after the onset of the rash. Children with bacterial tracheitis frequently present with severe upper airway distress and may require early intubation. Persons with suspected tracheitis should be hospitalized immediately. Consultation with an otorhinolaryngologist or pulmonologist should be sought, and prompt bronchoscopy or laryngoscopy should be performed to visualize the upper respiratory tract and obtain samples for bacterial cultures. Once specimens have been obtained, intravenous antibiotic treatment should be initiated. Because the most common organisms isolated from patients with measles and bacterial tracheitis are *Staphylococcus aureus* and *Streptococcus,* a penicillinase-resistant penicillin, such as nafcillin or oxacillin, or a first-generation cephalosporin, such as cefazolin, should be administered empirically, pending final culture and sensitivity results of the tracheal samples. Radiography of the chest should be performed because bronchopneumonia occurs frequently in persons with bacterial tracheitis.

Pneumonia. Children with measles commonly have radiographic evidence of pulmonary involvement characterized by interstitial, perihilar, and lower lobe infiltrates (Fig. 23–4). The development of pulmonary involvement early in the illness suggests that the virus itself is responsible. Measles pneumonia in immunocompetent persons is seldom severe but may progress to **bronchiolitis obliterans** and death, especially in infants. Corticosteroids have been reported to be beneficial in some patients with bronchiolitis obliterans and may be useful in selected patients.

Bacterial superinfection leading to **bronchopneumonia** is a serious complication that is associated with the majority of deaths occurring with measles. This condition typically develops when the exanthem is fading, and it is usually heralded by a recrudescent fever and worsening pulmonary status. The white blood cell count is frequently elevated, and a shift to more immature forms is apparent. The chest radiograph reveals interstitial or multilobar infiltrates.

Persons with bronchopneumonia should be hospitalized. A blood culture should be obtained in all cases, and a sputum culture may be obtained for older children and adolescents. Empirical antibiotic therapy should be initiated, including coverage for the most common etiologic agents (*S. aureus, Haemophilus influenzae* type b, group A *Streptococcus, Streptococcus pneumoniae*). An extended-spectrum cephalosporin such as cefuroxime or cefotaxime is appropriate empirical antibacterial therapy.

Persons with impaired immunity, especially cell-mediated immunity, exposed to measles frequently contract **giant cell (Hecht's) pneumonia,** a severe and usually fatal measles virus infection of the pulmonary parenchyma, often without a rash. It may develop during the acute measles illness but is frequently delayed for weeks or months. Fever, upper respiratory tract symptoms, and nonproductive cough are usually present. The cough worsens, and respiratory distress soon develops. The chest radiograph can show nodular, lobar, or interstitial infiltrates. The diagnosis is usually established when typical multinucleated giant cells are identified from lung tissue obtained by either an open lung biopsy or an autopsy (Fig. 23–2). Giant cell pneumonia has a high mortality rate. Favorable indicators for survival include resolution of giant cell shedding within the respiratory tract and development of specific measles antibodies.

Encephalitis. Encephalitis, which occurs in approximately 1–2 of every 1,000 cases of measles, is a dreaded complication because of its high morbidity and mortality. Measles-associated encephalitis encompasses a wide spectrum of disease entities, each form with distinctive characteristics of risk factors, incubation period, pathologic findings, and outcome.

Encephalitis may develop at any time from the prodrome phase until many years after a typical measles infection. Cases occurring within days of the measles illness are usually grouped under the broad name of acute measles encephalitis. Some cases show evidence of direct viral invasion of brain tissue and are characterized by inflammatory changes, intranuclear inclusion bodies, and frequent isolation of measles virus from cerebrospinal fluid or brain tissue. However, most cases of measles encephalitis resemble a classic postinfectious encephalitic process with prominent perivascular demyelination and no evidence of direct central nervous system invasion.

Acute measles encephalitis with inclusion bodies cannot be clinically distinguished from postinfectious measles encephalitis. The condition of persons with acute measles encephalitis usually deteriorates rapidly, and fever and signs of meningeal irritation develop. Seizures and focal neurologic signs may occur as the disease progresses. The onset of coma follows. The acute illness generally lasts a few days to weeks.

Immunocompromised children may contract measles encephalitis with central nervous system inclusion bodies but typically display a longer incubation period (1–7 months after acute measles infection) than immunocompetent children. This is sometimes referred to as subacute measles encephalitis, immunosuppressive measles encephalitis, measles inclusion body encephalitis, progressive measles encephalitis, or acute measles encephalitis of the delayed type. Most young persons with this type of encephalitis have acute lymphocytic leukemia. Encephalitis in immunocompromised persons carries a high mortality rate: most patients die within 4 months of diagnosis, although some are ill for several months. Illness is characterized by refractory seizures and altered mental status. Approximately one third of patients have epilepsia partialis continua, a condition characterized by seizures with unilateral, focal, persistent twitching. Diagnosis is based primarily on histologic findings of inclusions in brain biopsy specimens. Giant cell pneumonia occurs simultaneously in some children.

Subacute Sclerosing Panencephalitis. SSPE is a slow encephalitis that occurs in approximately 1 in every 1 million cases of measles. It evolves in an insidious fashion for months to years as a result of a persistent central nervous system infection with measles virus. Persons with SSPE are not contagious. The first stage affects intellectual and behavioral functions; subsequent stages affect motor abilities. Seizures, coma, and death result in a few years. SSPE is characterized by a diffuse lymphocytic infiltration of the brain and perivascular infiltration. Intranuclear inclusion bodies are seen within several types of cells. A characteristic EEG pattern (suppression burst) is present in most cases and often precedes the development of seizures. Serum measles antibody titers are characteristically extremely high; high levels also occur in cerebrospinal fluid.

The majority of SSPE cases occur after natural measles infection. Although SSPE has occurred in vaccinated persons with no history of measles, it is unclear whether the disease was caused by the vaccine viral strain or by unrecognized infection with wild-type measles virus. Evidence of an increased risk of SSPE after live measles booster vaccination in individuals who have previously had natural measles infection or who have received killed or live measles vaccine is nonexistent. Currently, indigenous cases of SSPE are rarely seen in developed countries, presumably because of the widespread use of measles vaccine.

Measles During Pregnancy. Most information regarding measles during pregnancy is based on outbreaks that occurred in Greenland between 1951 and 1962. These data and other studies have clearly shown that maternal measles is associated with a high fetal mortality rate if disease is acquired within the first 3 months of gestation. Approximately one third of women with first-trimester measles had spontaneous abortion, in comparison with fewer than 5% of those who acquired infection in later trimesters. The rate of stillbirths is also higher in women with measles during the first 3 months (10%), in comparison with those with measles in the second or third trimester (3%). Gestational measles may result in a higher rate of premature birth and a higher mortality rate during early infancy, but conclusive studies have not been performed. Unlike rubella, measles does not appear to cause a characteristic syndrome or congenital abnormalities in infants born live to mothers who have had gestational measles.

PROGNOSIS

The case-fatality rate for measles in the United States has averaged 0.1% in cases reported to the CDC in recent years, with the majority of deaths in infants with bronchopneumonia. A history of vaccination exists in 10% or fewer of the fatal cases. Higher mortality rates have been observed among immunocompromised persons, children younger than 5 years, and persons older than 19 years. The mortality rate among children with complications of diarrhea, otitis media, or measles croup is negligible. Bacterial tracheitis associated with measles has caused death.

Death from measles in adolescents and adults is usually associated with encephalitis. SSPE leads to death in virtually all cases. Other forms of measles encephalitis in immunocompetent persons are associated with a mortality rate of approximately 15%, with 20–30% of survivors having serious neurologic sequelae. Approximately 60–90% of patients with measles and underlying malignancy who develop pneumonia or encephalitis die, and survivors are invariably severely impaired. Measles in HIV-infected children carries a mortality rate of 30–50%, with most deaths associated with pneumonitis.

PREVENTION

Vaccination. The primary method of measles prevention in the United States is vaccination. Both a live-attenuated vaccine (Edmonston B strain) and a killed vaccine (formalin inactivated) first became available in 1963. A subsequent dramatic reduction in the number of measles cases followed (Fig. 23–1). Since that time, many changes in the type of vaccine and the age at vaccination administration have been recommended. The original vaccines were eventually discontinued (the killed vaccine in 1967; the Edmonston B live vaccine in 1975) after two improved live vaccines with fewer side effects were developed. Currently the sole measles vaccine in use in the United States, first licensed in 1968, is derived from the Moraten (''more attenuated'' strain of Edmonston B) strain of measles virus. Precautions, contraindications, and adverse effects of this live vaccine are discussed in detail in Chapter 17.

The measles vaccine is effective: more than 98% of persons receiving one dose develop an antibody response and long-term protection against the disease. Primary vaccine failure (i.e., the lack of an adequate protective immune response after immunization) is probably the major reason for susceptibility to measles after a single immunization, although waning immunity (i.e., diminishing antibody levels with time) may account for some loss of protection. Most cases of primary vaccine failure occur as a result of interference by transplacentally acquired antibodies when measles vaccine is given at too young an age (i.e., before 12 months of age). Other potential causes of primary vaccine failure include interference by antibodies from administered immunoglobulin preparations, mishandling of vaccine that leads to inactivation of the attenuated virus, inhibition of viral replication within the vaccine recipient by interferon or other substances, and unknown genetic factors.

Because antibody levels are significantly lower in vaccine recipients than in those with natural measles infection, infants born to women with vaccine-induced immunity have lower levels of passively acquired maternal antibody and increased susceptibility to measles at younger ages. This has prompted lowering of the recommended age for initial measles vaccination from 15 months to 12–15 months. In the future, when virtually all women of childbearing age will have vaccine-induced immunity, it may be prudent to lower the recommended age for initial vaccination further.

Routine immunization should be with the MMR vaccine at 12–15 months of age, with the second dose of MMR administered at 4–6 years of age. The two-dose series induces protective levels of antibodies in more than 99% of recipients. It is assumed that receipt of the second measles vaccination significantly reduces the number of persons (~5%) who do not respond to the first vaccination (i.e., primary vaccine failure).

For children who live in high-risk areas for measles, the initial MMR vaccination should be at 12 months of age. Such areas include counties with more than 5 cases of measles among preschool-aged children during each of the last 5 years, counties with a recent outbreak among unvaccinated preschool-aged children, and counties with large inner city populations. There is no evidence to indicate that persons already immune to measles, either from natural infection or previous vaccination, are at increased risk of having adverse reactions from the measles vaccine booster immunization.

Entrants to colleges and other educational institutions beyond high school and medical personnel with direct patient contact should have proof of immunity to measles. Adequate proof is a history of physician-diagnosed measles, serologic evidence of immunity to measles, birth before 1957, or dated documentation of two measles vaccinations administered on or after the first birthday. Adolescents and adults with no history of measles immunization should receive a dose on matriculation or employment, followed by a second dose 1 or more months later.

Certain groups of immunocompromised children should not receive measles or other live-virus vaccines because of poor antibody response and the risk of severe complications. However, HIV-infected children without severe immunosuppression and without evidence of measles immunity may receive measles vaccine. Children with cancer in remission who have not received chemotherapy in the previous 3 months, and children who have previously received immunosuppressive doses of corticosteroids (equivalent to 2 mg/kg/day, or 20 mg/day) for 14 days or longer but who have not received therapy in the previous month, may also receive measles vaccination. Studies have shown that such children have no more vaccine-related complications than immunocompetent children. All healthy members of families with an immunocompromised child for whom the measles vaccine is contraindicated should be fully immunized against measles. There is no evidence of spread of the viral vaccine strain from the vaccinee to other persons.

Postexposure Prophylaxis. Susceptible household or hospital contacts should receive postexposure prophylaxis (Table 23–5). This is especially important for persons at high risk of complications, including children younger than 12 months and immunocompromised children. Pregnant women are of concern because of the increased risk of fetal death with measles, especially during the first trimester.

TABLE 23–5. Postexposure Measles Prophylaxis for Susceptible Individuals

Susceptible Individual	Measles Vaccine (Given within 72 hr)	IG (Given within 6 days)
Age 0–5 mo		
Mother is immune	No	No
Mother is not immune	No	0.25 mL/kg (max 15 mL)
Age 6–11 mo	Yes	0.25 mL/kg if measles vaccine is not administered
Age ≥12 mo	Yes	No
Pregnant women	No	0.25 mL/kg (max 15 mL)
Immunocompromised person (including with symptomatic HIV infection)	No	0.5 mL/kg (max 15 mL)

Measles vaccine alone, given within 72 hours of exposure, can provide protection and is preferred for measles postexposure prophylaxis for persons 12 months of age or older. Vaccination should induce immunity if natural infection does not result. Live-virus vaccination is not recommended for immunocompromised persons or for pregnant women. For such individuals, standard IG given as soon as possible but within 6 days of exposure can prevent symptoms, prolong the incubation period, or modify the clinical illness. Infants are of special concern because of the inhibitory effect of transplacental antibodies on vaccination used alone as postexposure prophylaxis. Transplacental maternally derived antibodies generally protect infants younger than 6 months. Infants between 6 and 12 months of age should be vaccinated within 72 hours of exposure. If the exposure occurred more than 72 hours but less than 6 days previously, IG may be given alone to ameliorate the course of the disease. If a mother develops measles, all unvaccinated children in the household, regardless of age, should be vaccinated if they have no evidence of immunity.

For exposed persons for whom measles vaccine is contraindicated or not given within 72 hours, IG given within 6 days can provide protection. Infants and pregnant women should receive a single dose of IG, 0.25 mL/kg (maximum dose 15 mL). Immunocompromised persons should receive a single dose of IG, 0.5 mL/kg (maximum dose 15 mL). The IG should be given as soon as possible after exposure. Administration of IG is not needed in persons, including HIV-infected persons, receiving at least 100 mg/kg of IVIG at regular intervals if the last dose was administered within 3 weeks of the exposure to measles. All nonimmune persons exposed to measles that receive IG and do not develop measles or modified measles should later receive MMR vaccine. Depending on the specific immunobiologic agent and dose given, measles vaccination is not recommended within 5 months after IG administration (6 months if 0.5 mL/kg was administered) or 8 months after IVIG administration (if a dose of 300–400 mg/kg was administered) because of interference of the passive antibodies with viral replication and development of immunity (Table 17–4).

Outbreak Control. Important components of outbreak control include lowering the age at first vaccination to 6 months during preschool outbreaks; revaccination of all persons who have no evidence of measles immunity in institutional outbreaks; and revaccination and elimination of contact between susceptible exposed personnel and patients during outbreaks in medical facilities. Mass revaccination of entire populations is not necessary. IG should not be used to control measles outbreaks.

A measles outbreak in the United States is defined as a single case of confirmed measles. Administration of measles vaccine to susceptible individuals during the early course of an epidemic is beneficial, and therefore control measures should be initiated promptly, before confirmatory laboratory test results are obtained. Local public health officials should be enlisted to inform the medical community of a measles outbreak and to implement appropriate public health measures.

During an outbreak in preschool-age children, the age for initial measles vaccination should be lowered to 6 months in the outbreak population if cases are occurring in children younger than 12 months. Maternally derived antibodies should provide protection to the infant younger than 6 months. The combination MMR vaccine may be used if the monovalent measles vaccine is not readily available. Children initially vaccinated with measles or MMR vaccine before the first birthday should be revaccinated with MMR at 12–15 months of age and before school entry.

Outbreaks in institutions (e.g., daycare centers, schools, and colleges) should be managed by revaccination of all students, their siblings, and school personnel born on or after January 1, 1957, who do not have documentation of immunity to measles. To control outbreaks in daycare centers and schools, nonimmunized students should be excluded until vaccinated. Students may be readmitted immediately after vaccination. Nonimmunized persons who remain unvaccinated for medical, religious, or other reasons should be excluded from school until at least 21 days after the onset of rash in the last individual with measles.

Management of measles outbreaks in medical facilities should include revaccination of all medical workers born on or after January 1, 1957, who have direct patient contact and who do not have proof of immunity to measles. Vaccination may also be considered for workers born before 1957. Susceptible medical personnel who have been directly exposed to measles should be relieved from direct patient contact from day 5 to day 21 after exposure (regardless of whether they received measles vaccine or IG) or, if they become ill, for 4 days after the rash develops.

Hospital Isolation. Respiratory isolation of hospitalized persons is recommended for 4 days after the onset of rash. Immunocompromised persons should remain in isolation for the entire duration of their illness because of prolonged excretion of virus from the respiratory tract.

International Travel. Because measles remains endemic in much of the world, vaccination against measles should be performed for all international travelers born after January 1, 1957, who do not have documented immunity to measles or who have not received two doses of vaccine. Infants 6–11 months of age should receive a dose of monovalent measles vaccine before departure.

REVIEWS

Atkinson WL, Kaplan JM, Clover R: Measles: Virology, epidemiology, disease, and prevention. *Am J Prev Med* 1994;10:22–30.

Cherry JD: Viral exanthems. *Dis Mon* 1982;28:1–56.

Corlett WT: Rubeola. In *A Treatise on the Acute Infectious Exanthemata.* Philadelphia, FA Davis, 1901.

Van Rooyen CE, Rhodes AJ: Measles (morbilli). In *Virus Diseases of Man.* New York, Thomas Nelson, 1948.

KEY ARTICLES

American Academy of Pediatrics, Committee on Infectious Diseases: Vitamin A treatment of measles. *Pediatrics* 1993;91:1014–5.

Barkin RM: Measles mortality. Analysis of the primary cause of death. *Am J Dis Child* 1975;129:307–9.

Centers for Disease Control and Prevention: Measles, mumps, and rubella—vaccine use and strategies for elimination of measles, rubella, and congenital rubella syndrome and control of mumps: Recommendations of the Advisory Committee on Immunization Practices (ACIP). *MMWR Morb Mortal Wkly Rep* 1998;47(RR-8):1–57.

Centers for Disease Control and Prevention: Measles—United States, 1999. *MMWR Morb Mortal Wkly Rep* 2000;49:557–60.

Cherry JD, Feigin RD, Shackelford PG, et al: A clinical and serologic study of 103 children with measles vaccine failure. *J Pediatr* 1973;82:802–8.

Davidkin I, Valle M, Peltola H, et al: Etiology of measles- and rubella-like illnesses in measles-, mumps-, and rubella-vaccinated children. *J Infect Dis* 1998;178:1567–70.

Dunn RA: Subacute sclerosing panencephalitis. *Pediatr Infect Dis J* 1991;10:68–72.

Hussey GD, Klein M: A randomized, controlled trial of vitamin A in children with severe measles. *N Engl J Med* 1990;323:160–4.

Jespersen CS, Littauer J, Sagild U: Measles as a cause of fetal defects. A retrospective study of ten measles epidemics in Greenland. *Acta Paediatr Scand* 1977;66:367–72.

Kaplan LJ, Daum RS, Smaron M, et al: Severe measles in immunocompromised patients. *JAMA* 1992;267:1237–41.

Karp CL, Wysocka M, Wahl LM, et al: Mechanism of suppression of cell-mediated immunity by measles virus. *Science* 1996;273:228–31.

Kipps A, Dick G, Moodie JW: Measles and the central nervous system. *Lancet* 1983;2:1406–10.

Manning SC, Ridenour B, Brown OE, et al: Measles: An epidemic of upper airway obstruction. *Otolaryngol Head Neck Surg* 1991;105:415–8.

Markowitz LE, Albrecht P, Orenstein WA, et al: Persistence of measles antibody after revaccination. *J Infect Dis* 1992;166:205–8.

Markowitz LE, Albrecht P, Rhodes P, et al: Changing levels of measles antibody titers in women and children in the United States: Impact on response to vaccination. *Pediatrics* 1996;97:53–8.

Martin DB, Weiner LB, Nieburg PI, et al: Atypical measles in adolescents and young adults. *Ann Intern Med* 1979;90:877–81.

Mustafa MM, Weitman SD, Winick NJ, et al: Subacute measles encephalitis in the young immunocompromised host: Report of two cases diagnosed by polymerase chain reaction and treated with ribavirin and review of the literature. *Clin Infect Dis* 1993;16:654–60.

Quiambao BP, Gatchalian SR, Halonen P, et al: Coinfection is common in measles-associated pneumonia. *Pediatr Infect Dis J* 1998;17:89–93.

CHAPTER 24

Rubella

Charles T. Leach ▪ Hal B. Jenson

Rubella is a febrile exanthematous disease that is mild or inapparent in most children and adults. Rubella was first described by German physicians, leading to use of the term **German measles** in the English-language medical literature. Rubella is also known as **3-day measles** because of the characteristic duration of the rash. Rubella is a Latin diminutive meaning "little red."

Historically, rubella has been an important cause of epidemics that frequently have been confused with measles, but both diseases are now uncommon. The primary importance of rubella vaccination is the prevention of the potentially severe consequences of congenital infection (Chapter 95).

ETIOLOGY

Rubella is caused by **rubella virus,** a single-stranded RNA virus in the Togaviridae family. There is only one type of rubella virus.

Transmission. Rubella is a moderately contagious virus that is transmitted through direct person-to-person contact or by contaminated respiratory secretions. Rubella virus can be isolated from the blood and upper respiratory tract secretions during the week before the cutaneous eruption. Viremia ceases within 1–2 days after the appearance of the rash, but virus continues to be shed in the nasopharynx and throat from 7 days before to up to 14 days after the rash. No carrier state for rubella is recognized in humans, who are the only known natural hosts. There is no animal reservoir and no insect vector.

EPIDEMIOLOGY

Rubella typically has the highest incidence during the spring months but may be seen throughout the year. It occurs equally in both males and females. Before the introduction of rubella vaccine, epidemics of rubella occurred every 6–9 years and the majority of cases involved school-aged children (Fig. 24–1). Routine childhood vaccination has significantly altered the age distribution for rubella cases, and only 20% of cases now occur in persons less than 15 years of age. Hispanics have accounted for a large proportion of recent cases.

The 128 cases of rubella reported for 1995 is the lowest number ever reported and a greater than 99% decrease from the 45,000–58,000 cases reported annually in 1966–1971. In the United States, however, outbreaks of rubella in non-vaccinated groups continue to occur in adults in workplaces, prisons, colleges, and health care centers, with a total of 271 cases reported in 1999.

More than 20,000 infants had congenital rubella infection as a result of the last epidemic in the United States, in 1964–1965. Rubella vaccination has significantly reduced the incidence of congenital rubella syndrome, which has remained stable at 4–11 cases annually (Chapter 95).

PATHOGENESIS

Virus receptors exist in the respiratory epithelium, and after local replication a silent primary viremia occurs with systemic spread. Further replication occurs in the skin and lymph nodes and is followed by a secondary viremia and development of the typical clinical symptoms. Specific immunity develops as clinical manifestations of the disease resolve.

The pathogenesis of the rubella exanthem is not well understood. The virus can be found in both affected and unaffected areas of the skin, and thus the presence of virus alone does not appear to be the sole explanation for cutaneous lesions. Immunologic processes are likely to be important. When examined histologically, skin lesions show a mild, nonspecific perivascular lymphocytic infiltrate in the dermis.

SYMPTOMS AND CLINICAL MANIFESTATIONS

Incubation Period. The incubation for rubella is generally 16–18 days, with a range of 14–21 days (Fig. 24–2).

Common Symptoms

Symptoms of postnatal rubella infection in children are variable and generally mild. An estimated 25–50% of cases are asymptomatic. The principal manifestations of symptomatic disease are low-grade fever, lymphadenopathy, and rash (Table 24–1; Fig. 24–2).

The rubella prodrome is classically characterized by cervical lymphadenopathy, which appears the day before the onset of the rash. The suboccipital, postauricular, and posterior cervical lymph nodes are most commonly affected. The nodes are frequently tender and may cause a slightly stiff neck. Constitutional symptoms, such as malaise and anorexia, are not marked and temperatures rarely exceed 38.5°C (101.3°F). Conjunctivitis is minimal and is not usually associated with significant photophobia. Headache and eye pain are rare in children but may be distressing in older patients. Adults may also complain of a mild throat irritation and cough. Other upper respiratory tract symptoms are typically absent.

Exanthem. After a relatively short prodromal period of 12–24 hours (rarely longer than 2 days), the exanthem appears and any prodromal symptoms resolve rapidly. In children the rash is frequently the first sign of illness and is commonly noticed on awakening. The classic rubella exanthem is generalized and maculopapular (Plate 3C). It begins on the face and scalp and subsequently progresses in an orderly manner to the neck, trunk, and upper and lower extremities. Palms and soles may be involved to a lesser degree. It generally takes only 1–2 days for lesions to extend to the lower extremities. As the exanthem moves centrifugally, earlier lesions fade rather rapidly; facial and scalp lesions may therefore fade before the legs become involved, and lesions on the upper body

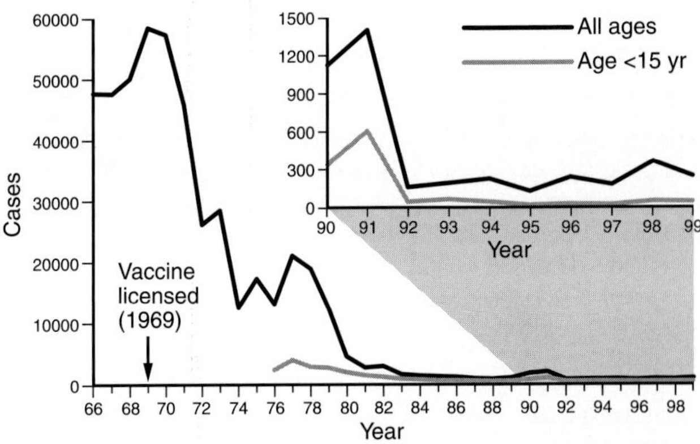

FIGURE 24–1. Reported cases of rubella in the United States by year, 1966–1999. Rubella vaccine was licensed in 1969. (Data from the Centers for Disease Control and Prevention.)

TABLE 24–1. Clinical Manifestations of Rubella

Low-grade fever	50–75%
Malaise (mild)	50–75%
Anorexia (mild)	50–75%
Lymphadenopathy (generalized or suboccipital, postauricular, or posterior cervical)	50–75%
Rash	50–75%
Forschheimer's spots	20%
Headache	
Children	Uncommon
Adults	Occasional
Polyarthralgia or polyarthritis	
Children	Uncommon
Adults	60%
Thrombocytopenia	Rare
Encephalitis	Rare

may not be visible by the time the child is first examined. The rash disappears within 2–3 days. It is commonly pruritic in adults but not in children.

Physical Examination Findings

Persons with rubella may seek medical attention shortly after the onset of the rash, at a time when the prodromal manifestations are resolving and significant findings on examination are few. A low-grade fever may be present. Conjunctivitis is minimal and involves predominantly the bulbar conjunctivae with no purulence. An enanthem known as **Forschheimer's spots** develops in approximately 20% of patients with rubella and is characterized by tiny, discrete 1–2 mm reddish spots on the soft palate and uvula. These lesions are transitory, appearing on the first day of the exanthem and lasting less than 24 hours. This enanthem is nonspecific: similar lesions may be seen with other infections. The posterior pharynx may be slightly injected, but there is no exudate. Generalized tender, nonfluctuant lymphadenopathy is present, and the posterior cervical, suboccipital, and postauricular nodes are most consistently involved.

Exanthem. Although somewhat variable, the classic rubella rash (Plate 3C) begins as discrete, tiny faint macules on the head. It progresses to the arms and legs as older lesions mature and become maculopapular. The color of rubella lesions is pale rose or pink, which contrasts with the darker coloration seen in measles and scarlet fever. A circumscribed areola surrounds the central portion of the lesion. Lesions usually are fairly discrete, with intervening unaffected skin, and are frequently elongated or irregularly round. Occasional areas of coalescence may develop, especially over the lower back and buttocks; however, a tendency to form large, crescentic areas of confluence or plaques, as often occurs in measles, is not apparent. Lesions blanch completely with pressure.

The rash subsides relatively quickly, and it may fade from the face on the second day. No evidence of skin involvement is noted after complete resolution within 2–4 days. Fine desquamation occasionally occurs as the rash subsides in areas of skin more intensely affected with the rash and in areas protected from frictional forces.

DIAGNOSIS

There is no single clinical finding pathognomonic for rubella. Instead, the presumptive clinical diagnosis of rubella is based on a collection of findings in an unvaccinated host. Suggestive findings include a mild illness with absent or minimal prodromal symptoms, a low-grade fever, and cervical lymphadenopathy immediately preceding a rash that begins on the face and rapidly evolves to include

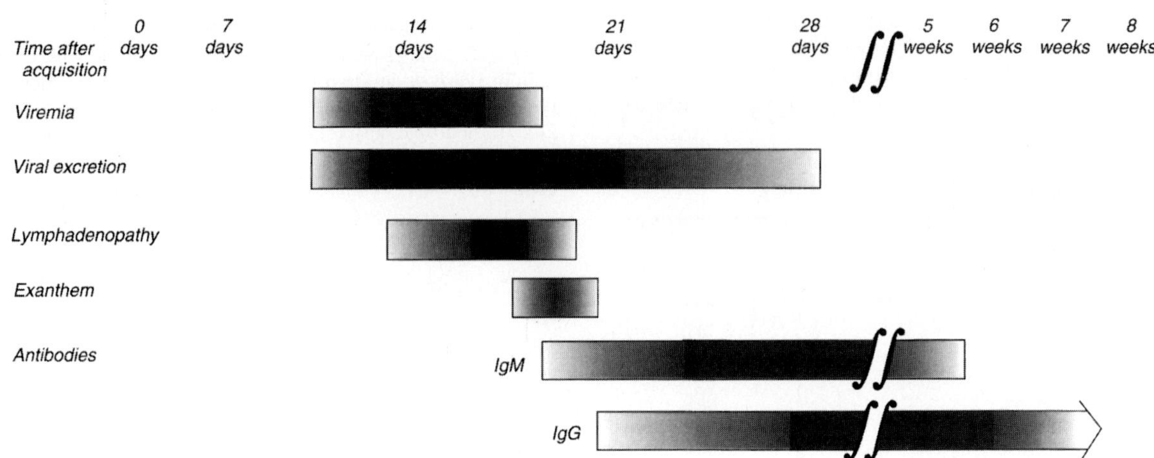

FIGURE 24–2. Profile of the typical clinical course of rubella.

the trunk and extremities before disappearing on the third day. Because rubella is mild, with variable clinical manifestations, clinical criteria are insufficient for establishing a diagnosis, and specific microbiologic testing is necessary for confirmation.

Although postnatal rubella is typically mild, congenital rubella may be severe. Therefore, in the attempt to identify cases and prevent further spread to pregnant women, every effort should be made to determine a specific diagnosis for all illnesses resembling rubella.

Differential Diagnosis

Because the rash of rubella is not easily discernible, rubella may be easily confused with several other acute febrile illnesses characterized by an exanthem (Table 24–2). Other viruses, including parvovirus B19, enterovirus, adenovirus, and HHV6, frequently cause measles- or rubella-like illnesses in MMR-vaccinated children.

Most difficulty arises in the differentiation of rubella from measles (especially modified measles) and scarlet fever (Table 23–2). Rubella has a short prodrome with characteristically mild or absent symptoms, in contrast to the symptomatic prodrome of measles, which lasts for several days and is characterized by fever, cough, coryza, and conjunctivitis. Scarlet fever begins abruptly with high fever, headache, and sore throat. The most notable aspects of the rash of rubella are the initial presence on the face and neck, lighter coloration of lesions, lack of confluence, rapid evolution, and rarely significant desquamation. Unlike measles, rubella has no pathognomonic oral lesions, although some patients have a nonspecific finding of petechiae on the soft palate (Forschheimer's spots). Scarlet fever is associated with the typical pharyngeal erythema and exudate of streptococcal pharyngitis.

Children with infectious mononucleosis may have a light-colored rash in addition to the typical fever and cervical lymphadenopathy. However, the fever is usually of longer duration than rubella, and the rash seldom affects the face. Erythema infectiosum begins as an intense rash on the face, especially the cheeks, which becomes prominent on the extensor surfaces of the extremities before spreading to the trunk. The rash is polymorphous and persists for a week or longer. Roseola usually occurs during infancy, with the exanthem occurring after lysis of fever. Many adenoviral and enteroviral infections are characterized by the presence of a maculopapular exanthem, but in contrast to rubella the duration of the rash is typically longer than 1–2 days.

Although the pattern of lymphadenopathy in rubella is characteristic, it is not pathognomonic. When present, lymphadenopathy in measles is more generalized and lacks prominence of the suboccipital and postauricular nodes. Scarlet fever primarily causes anterior cervical lymphadenopathy, and infectious mononucleosis is typically associated with generalized lymphadenopathy and hepatosplenomegaly. Lymphadenopathy is not a prominent feature of erythema infectiosum, roseola, or enteroviral infections.

TABLE 24–2. Differential Diagnosis of Rubella

Measles
Modified measles
Scarlet fever (group A *Streptococcus*)
Erythema infectiosum (parvovirus B19)
Enteroviruses
Adenoviruses
Roseola (HHV6)
Infectious mononucleosis
Mycoplasma pneumoniae
Kawasaki syndrome
Drug reaction

Laboratory Evaluation

Routine laboratory findings in cases of rubella are nonspecific and generally do not aid in diagnosis. Leukopenia with relative neutropenia and an elevated ESR are commonly observed. Plasma cells or Türk cells (developing plasma cells) may be seen in the peripheral smear. Thrombocytopenia occurs occasionally, although it is seldom associated with purpura. Liver enzymes are occasionally slightly elevated, but clinical manifestations are rare.

Microbiologic Evaluation

Serologic Testing. Serologic testing is the primary means of confirming the diagnosis of rubella. Demonstration of a fourfold or greater increase in specific IgG antibodies in paired acute and convalescent sera is diagnostic of infection. Acute-phase serum should be drawn within 7 days of the rash and convalescent-phase serum at least 10 days later. Paired sera should be tested simultaneously by the same laboratory method in the same laboratory. If testing of only a single serum is possible, specific IgM antibodies should be measured. Serum for IgM testing should be obtained within 1–2 weeks but not more than 4–5 weeks after rash onset.

Viral Culture. Rubella virus can be isolated from infected persons, but testing is expensive, time-consuming, and not routinely available. A specimen obtained by throat or nasopharyngeal swab is the most useful specimen for culture because virus persists in the upper respiratory tract for up to 2 weeks after the rash. During acute infection, rubella virus may also be cultured from blood, urine, feces, lymph nodes, skin, conjunctivae, cervix, CSF, and synovial fluid.

Other Methods. Other methods of identifying rubella virus, including electron microscopy, antigen detection (in tissues), and nucleic acid hybridization, may be used in selected cases, but these tests are currently available only in research settings.

Diagnostic Imaging

Imaging studies are not necessary for typical and uncomplicated cases of rubella but may be used to exclude other diagnoses. Rarely, persons with persistent arthritis attributable to rubella may require radiographs of affected joints to exclude other causes. MRI or CT of the head may be useful in the evaluation of persons with rubella encephalitis.

Pathologic Findings

Pathologic information is derived mostly from brain tissue obtained from rare fatal cases of rubella complicated by central nervous system disease. Histologically, these tissues show mononuclear perivascular infiltration, petechial hemorrhages, and variable degrees of neuronal destruction. Unlike other postinfectious encephalitides, perivascular demyelinization is uncommon. Rarely has rubella virus been identified in tissues.

TREATMENT

No specific therapy for rubella is available, although some antiviral agents inhibit growth of rubella virus in vitro. The efficacy of corticosteroids for rubella encephalitis is unproved. Routine supportive care includes adequate hydration and nutrition, with acetaminophen or ibuprofen administration for fever or pain relief.

COMPLICATIONS

Complications of rubella are uncommon or rare in children. The three most important complications are joint manifestations, thrombocytopenic purpura, and neurologic disease. The risk and severity of complications are not related to the degree of rubella illness.

Joint Manifestations. Although joint manifestations are less common in children and men, young women frequently have transient polyarthralgias or arthritis associated with rubella. The onset is usually within the first week of the exanthem. Multiple joints are typically affected, most often the joints in the fingers, knees, wrists, elbows, and ankles. Complete resolution characteristically occurs within 1–4 weeks, although rare cases of chronic arthritis have developed. The pathogenic basis for chronic joint symptoms may involve a cell-mediated response to persistent rubella antigen within the joint. A multidisciplinary team including a rheumatologist should manage persons with rubella who have chronic joint manifestations persisting beyond 1 month.

Thrombocytopenic Purpura. Thrombocytopenic purpura occurs in both children and adults with rubella at an overall rate of approximately 1 in 3,000 cases. Purpura usually develops within the first week after the rash appears and invariably is associated with thrombocytopenia, which probably results from anti-platelet antibodies. Thrombocytopenia and increased capillary wall fragility are responsible for the purpuric lesions. Complete recovery usually occurs within 2–8 weeks, but deaths have been reported as a result of this complication. Treatment with IVIG may be advisable but has not been studied. Optimal management includes consultation with a hematologist.

Neurologic Disease. Encephalitis and encephalopathy account for more than 90% of the neurologic complications of rubella but occur rarely, at a rate of 1 in 6,000 cases. Symptoms of central nervous system disease typically develop 2–5 days after appearance of rash, although rare cases have occurred either before or 2–3 weeks after the rash. Low-grade fever, sleepiness, headache, emesis, and seizures are the most common initial symptoms. The CSF usually displays a mild pleocytosis (5–100 cells/mm^3) with mononuclear cell predominance, a normal glucose concentration, and a normal to mildly elevated total protein concentration. The EEG shows abnormalities in all cases but is nonspecific, revealing generalized slowing and dysrhythmia. The severity of rubella encephalitis varies, with an overall mortality rate of 0–30%. In most fatal cases, progression to coma occurs rapidly. Most survivors recover without sequelae within 1–3 weeks. All cases of rubella with neurologic complications require consultation with a neurologist, and most persons will require hospitalization in an intensive care setting.

Less common neurologic complications include myelitis, peripheral polyneuritis, Guillain-Barré syndrome, and a rare progressive panencephalitis that more commonly follows cases of congenital rubella.

Other Complications. Pericarditis and myocarditis have been reported but are extremely rare.

Congenital Rubella Syndrome. Rubella infection during pregnancy may result in infection of the fetus, potentially resulting in a myriad of congenital symptoms in the newborn, including intrauterine growth retardation, cataracts, deafness, and atrial and ventricular septal defects (Chapter 95).

PROGNOSIS

The prognosis for persons acquiring rubella postnatally is excellent. The overall mortality rate is approximately 1 in 30,000 cases, with the majority of deaths in persons with encephalitis. Primary infection confers lifelong immunity.

PREVENTION

Vaccination. Live attenuated rubella vaccine was first introduced in the United States in 1969 (Chapter 17). The only current vaccine strain, RA27/3, was first licensed in 1979 and is available alone or in combination with measles vaccine or with mumps vaccine, although the combination MMR vaccine is the preferred immunizing agent for most children and adults. Whether administered alone or in combination, rubella vaccine elicits specific rubella antibodies in 99% of recipients and provides more than 90% protection. Immunity has been documented for more than 15 years and probably lasts a lifetime. Rare cases of primary infection in vaccinees have been reported.

Although receipt of only one dose of rubella vaccine is sufficient for proof of immunity, primary vaccination is recommended as the combination MMR vaccine at 12–15 months of age, with a second dose (also as MMR vaccine) recommended at 4–6 years of age. Children 11–12 years of age who have not received a second dose of MMR vaccine should be given the vaccine at that time. There is no evidence indicating an increased risk of adverse effects after rubella vaccination of immune versus nonimmune persons; therefore serologic testing before revaccination is not necessary.

The rubella component of MMR vaccine is rarely associated with adverse effects in children but in postpubertal females does cause arthralgias in 25% of vaccinees and acute arthritis-like symptoms in 10% of vaccinees. These symptoms typically develop 1–3 weeks after vaccination, last 1–3 days, and rarely recur. There is no causal association between rubella vaccine and chronic arthropathy.

All pregnant women should have prenatal serologic testing to determine their immune status to rubella, and all susceptible women should be vaccinated after delivery and before hospital discharge, provided no contraindications exist. Breastfeeding is not a contraindication to postpartum rubella immunization; vaccine virus has been transmitted by breastfeeding to infants, but the infants have remained asymptomatic. Opportunities to immunize susceptible women of childbearing age should also be sought during any other contact with health care providers. Documentation of immunity (by either serologic testing, confirmation of vaccination at ≥12 months of age, or birth before 1957) should be a prerequisite for employment of persons who will come in contact with patients in a medical setting. However, women who could become pregnant should not be considered immune to rubella solely on the basis of birth before 1957. In addition, it is recommended that workplaces employing women of childbearing age require all employees, and that colleges and universities require all entrants, to provide documented laboratory proof of immunity or receipt of vaccine before employment or enrollment.

Outbreak Control. The primary objective of rubella outbreak control is to reduce exposure of susceptible women in the childbearing age group to infected persons. This requires good communication between public health officials and the medical community. General management of rubella outbreaks includes identification of susceptible persons, prompt vaccination or exclusion of susceptible individuals, and careful monitoring to identify new cases and alter management when necessary. Although laboratory confirmation is necessary for all cases of rubella, it is important to institute control measures immediately, before verification. Children attending school or daycare who develop rubella should be excluded for 7 days after the onset of the rash, because the virus may be shed for several days.

Nonpregnant Contacts of Rubella Cases. The immune status of all persons exposed to a confirmed case of rubella should be determined. For nonpregnant persons, sufficient proof of immunity includes previous laboratory-confirmed rubella, documented receipt of one dose of rubella vaccine at ≥12 months of age, or birth before 1957. Susceptible nonpregnant persons may be offered rubella vaccine. Although there is no definite evidence that postexposure immunization prevents infection, vaccination is recommended because it is not harmful to persons incubating rubella and it protects the recipient from any future rubella exposure if the current exposure is not sufficient to transmit infection. If persons refuse vaccination or if contraindications to vaccination exist, they should be excluded from work or school for the entire incubation period (21 days after the last exposure to a case). Prophylaxis with IG is not recommended for nonpregnant contacts of rubella cases.

Pregnant Contacts of Rubella Cases. If a pregnant woman comes in contact with a confirmed case of rubella, immunity should be determined serologically in a prompt manner with a sensitive test. Immune women should be given reassurance. Susceptible pregnant women exposed to rubella should not receive vaccine because of the theoretical risk of transmission of vaccine-type virus to the fetus. Susceptible women should have repeated serologic testing performed 3 weeks after exposure and, if results are still negative, again 3 weeks later unless they are given IG prophylaxis, which precludes interpretation of subsequent serologic tests. Each follow-up specimen should be tested simultaneously with the previous specimen(s). A culture of a specimen from the nasopharynx should be performed if symptoms and signs of rubella develop. If all sera are negative for rubella antibodies, infection has not occurred. If seroconversion is detected at 3–6 weeks after exposure, the woman should be informed that she has been infected with rubella and counseled regarding the risk of transmission to the fetus and resulting anomalies.

Administration of IG may prevent or ameliorate symptoms of rubella if accomplished immediately after exposure. However, maternal infection and transmission to the fetus can still occur and has been documented in infants born to mothers given IG shortly after rubella exposure and despite the absence of maternal symptoms. For the susceptible pregnant woman who is exposed to rubella and for whom elective termination of pregnancy is an option, and when timing permits repeated serologic testing to document seroconversion while elective abortion is possible, IG administration is not recommended. The rationale for withholding IG is that it may provide an unjustified sense of security, and it precludes positive serologic diagnosis as the basis for termination of pregnancy. However, for the susceptible pregnant woman for whom elective abortion is not an option, or if exposure occurs later in gestation, IG should be administered in a dose of 0.55 mL/kg. IVIG may be preferable but has not been studied.

Hospitalization. Hospitalized infants with postnatal rubella should remain in respiratory isolation for 7 days after the onset of the rash. Approximately 10–20% of infants with congenital rubella may excrete virus from the respiratory tract at 6 months of age. Excretion of virus in respiratory secretions and urine may continue for up to 1 year or occasionally longer. These hospitalized infants should be in respiratory isolation, and standard precautions should be provided unless viral cultures of respiratory tract secretions show negative results. All health care workers caring for hospitalized infants with postnatal rubella infection or congenital rubella syndrome should have documented immunity to rubella.

International Travel. Rubella is both endemic and epidemic in many parts of the world. Therefore all international travelers without documented laboratory proof of immunity or receipt of vaccine should be vaccinated before departure. This is especially important for women of childbearing age.

REVIEWS

Atkinson IE: Rubella (Rötheln). *Am J Med Sci* 1887;93:17–34.

Centers for Disease Control and Prevention: Measles, mumps, and rubella—vaccine use and strategies for elimination of measles, rubella, and congenital rubella syndrome and control of mumps: Recommendations of the Advisory Committee on Immunization Practices (ACIP). *MMWR Morb Mortal Wkly Rep* 1998;47 (RR-8):1–57.

Cherry JD: Viral exanthems. *Dis Mon* 1982;28:1–56.

Corlett WT: Rubella. In *A Treatise on the Acute Infectious Exanthemata.* Philadelphia, FA Davis, 1901.

Horstmann DM: Problems in measles and rubella. *Dis Mon* 1978; 24:1–52.

Wesselhoeft C: Rubella (German measles). *N Engl J Med* 1947; 236:943–50, 978–88.

KEY ARTICLES

Bayer WL, Sherman FE, Michaels RH, et al: Purpura in congenital and acquired rubella. *N Engl J Med* 1965;273:1362–6.

Best JM, O'Shea S: Rubella virus. In Schmidt NJ, Emmons RW (editors): *Diagnostic Procedures for Viral, Rickettsial and Chlamydial Infections.* Washington, DC, American Public Health Association, 1989.

Centers for Disease Control and Prevention: Measles, rubella, and congenital rubella syndrome—United States and Mexico, 1997–1999. *MMWR Morb Mortal Wkly Rep* 2000;49:1048–50, 1059.

Davidkin I, Valle M, Peltola H, et al: Etiology of measles- and rubella-like illnesses in measles, mumps, and rubella–vaccinated children. *J Infect Dis* 1998;178:1567–70.

Dwyer DE, Hueston L, Field PR, et al: Acute encephalitis complicating rubella virus infection. *Pediatr Infect Dis J* 1992;11:238–40.

Heggie AD: Pathogenesis of the rubella exanthem: Distribution of rubella virus in the skin during rubella with and without rash. *J Infect Dis* 1978;137:74–7.

Smith CA, Petty RE, Tingle AJ: Rubella virus and arthritis. *Rheum Dis Clin North Am* 1987;13:265–74.

Urquhart GE, Crawford RJ, Wallace J: Trial of high-titre human rubella immunoglobulin. *BMJ* 1978:2:1331–2.

Walker JM, Nahmias AJ: Neurologic sequelae of rubella infection. *Clin Pediatr* 1966;5:699–702.

CHAPTER 25

Roseola

Charles T. Leach ▪ Hal B. Jenson

Roseola, also known as **roseola infantum, exanthem subitum,** and **sixth disease,** was first defined as a distinct disease at the turn of the 20th century. Roseola is a benign febrile, exanthematous illness that occurs almost exclusively during infancy. Children with roseola display a characteristic progression of illness that is seldom confused with other diseases.

ETIOLOGY

Studies performed in the late 1980s established **human herpesvirus 6 (HHV6)** as the principal cause of roseola. HHV6 has two viral subtypes, type A and type B. HHV6 type B is the principal cause of roseola. No disease has been consistently associated with HHV6 type A. **Human herpesvirus 7 (HHV7)** appears to cause 10–30% of cases of roseola. Subtypes have not been described for HHV7. HHV6 and HHV7 are double-stranded DNA viruses of the Betaherpesvirinae subfamily, along with cytomegalovirus, of the Herpesviridae.

Transmission. HHV6 and HHV7, like all herpesviruses, establish lifelong infections in the host after the primary infection. Most adults periodically excrete these viruses in saliva and are probably important sources of transmission of the viruses to infants. Both viruses are also shed at low rates in the female genital tract. Transmission from bone marrow and solid organ donors has been described. There is no evidence that infection is spread by breast milk or blood transfusion. Humans are the only known natural hosts. There is no animal reservoir and no insect vector.

EPIDEMIOLOGY

Roseola is the most common exanthem of infancy. Transplacental antibody protects most infants until 6 months of age, and susceptibility to infection increases as maternally derived antibody levels decline. By 12 months of age approximately 60–90% of children have developed antibodies to HHV6, and essentially all children are seropositive by 2–3 years of age. Infection with HHV7 occurs at a slightly later age. The incidence of clinically apparent disease is 10–15% during the first year of life and 30–35% during the first 3 years of life. The peak age for roseola is 6–15 months of age; more than 95% of cases occur in children younger than 3 years of age. These data indicate that a majority of children infected with HHV6 and HHV7 are asymptomatically infected or do not develop a distinct illness recognizable as roseola.

There are no sex or race differences in the epidemiology of roseola. Roseola occurs throughout the year, although some studies suggest a higher incidence during spring and fall months. Unlike some other childhood exanthems, a history of exposure to another child with roseola is extremely rare, and outbreaks are uncommon.

PATHOGENESIS

The basis for the unique pattern of rash after resolution of fever is intriguing but largely unexplored. There is no information about the pathogenesis of the exanthem. Most studies indicate that the causative agent is acquired from symptom-free healthy persons and enters the host through the oral, nasal, or conjunctival mucosa. After initial viral replication at an unknown site, viremia presumably occurs, as indicated by fever. The virus may establish a persistent silent or latent infection in salivary glands and within peripheral blood mononuclear cells after acute infection. Lifelong infection in apparently healthy individuals is associated with chronic, periodic shedding of virus in oral secretions.

SYMPTOMS AND CLINICAL MANIFESTATIONS

Incubation Period. The incubation period is generally 10 days, with a range of 5–15 days.

Common Symptoms

Primary HHV6 infection in the majority of healthy children is asymptomatic or has symptoms that are not recognizable as roseola. In one study of febrile children less than 3 years of age, only 17% with primary HHV6 infection had a rash. Children with classic roseola follow an almost unique progression of high fever without focal findings, followed by rash that is rarely confused with other childhood exanthems (Fig. 25–1). Roseola caused by HHV6 and HHV7 is clinically indistinguishable, although HHV6-associated roseola typically occurs in younger infants.

Prodrome. The first indication of illness is usually fever, which is characteristically abrupt in onset, relatively high, and sustained. In striking contrast to the high fever, most children are alert and behave normally, continuing with their usual play and daily activities. A small proportion of affected infants may become irritable and anorexic. Infrequent complaints include abdominal pain, vomiting, diarrhea, rhinorrhea, and sore throat. Febrile seizures may occur during this stage. Coryza, conjunctivitis, or cough is not significant in roseola. Fever continues for 3–5 days and then usually resolves rather rapidly, although sometimes the fever may gradually abate within 24–36 hours.

Exanthem. In classic cases a rash appears within 24 hours of fever resolution. In many cases the rash develops while the fever is rapidly resolving. The rash typically fades after 1–3 days, although some children have an evanescent rash lasting only a few hours.

Physical Examination Findings

Physical examination of patients during the febrile, pre-eruptive phase is usually unrewarding. Mild occipital or cervical lymphade-

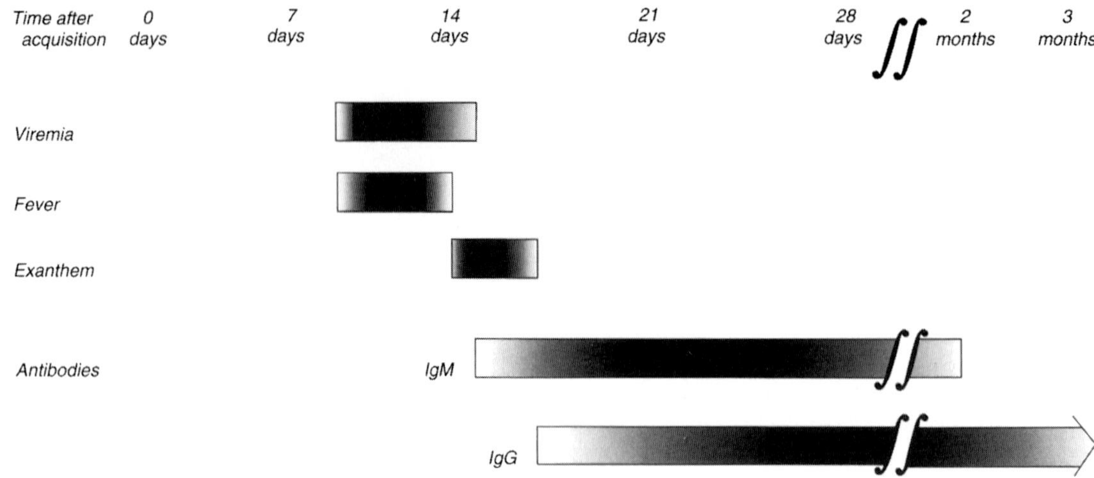

FIGURE 25–1. Profile of the typical clinical course of roseola (roseola infantum, or exanthem subitum).

nopathy have been inconsistently noted. Signs of mild upper respiratory tract infection, such as mild pharyngeal inflammation, erythematous papules on the soft palate, mild rhinorrhea, and minimal conjunctival redness may be observed. Some children may have slight palpebral edema. However, these physical findings have no distinct relationship to roseola and may simply reflect a concomitant viral upper respiratory tract infection. Fever associated with roseola usually ranges between 38.3°C (101°F) and 41.1°C (106°F), with an average maximum daily temperature of 39.4°C (103°F).

Exanthem. The rash of roseola is rose colored, as the name implies (Plate 3E). Although fairly distinctive, the rash may be confused with exanthems resulting from measles, rubella, or erythema infectiosum. It begins as discrete, small (2–5 mm), slightly raised pink lesions on the trunk and usually spreads to the neck, face, and proximal extremities. The lesions usually remain distinct but occasionally may become almost confluent and may blanch with pressure. The rash is not normally pruritic and does not develop vesicles, pustules, or desquamation.

Uncommon Manifestations

Roseola-like Illness. Variations in the usual presentation of roseola are frequently labeled **roseola-like illnesses.** Childhood illnesses with simultaneous high fever and rash cannot be labeled classic roseola and yet may resemble roseola in all other aspects, such as the characteristic appearance of the rash and an absence of significant toxic effects. It is not clear whether such illnesses represent infections with other agents, such as the enteroviruses, or encompass a spectrum of illnesses due to HHV6 and HHV7.

Neurologic Disease. Because most HHV6 and HHV7 infections occur in infants and young children, and because of the characteristically high fever associated with roseola, **febrile seizures** are the most common neurologic manifestation associated with roseola, occurring in 5–10% of cases. HHV6 infection is the underlying cause of approximately one third of febrile seizures, which may be the first manifestation of roseola. Compared with other causes of febrile seizures, HHV6-associated febrile seizures may develop at younger ages and are more likely to be atypical, although it is unclear whether there is a higher risk of recurrent seizures. Although HHV6 DNA has been identified by PCR in the CSF of patients with roseola complicated by febrile seizures, it is unlikely that the virus directly infects neurons. Rarely, encephalitis or meningoencephalitis may occur in either an immunodeficient or an immunocompetent person. Symptoms typically develop during the acute febrile period.

Other Manifestations. Thrombocytopenic purpura, characterized by the development of petechiae during the febrile, pre-eruptive stage, and rare cases of hepatitis and HHV6-associated hemophagocytosis have been reported. Prolonged bone marrow suppression has been attributed to HHV6 in some bone marrow transplant recipients. There may be a higher rate of progressive HIV disease in infants with HHV6 infection; similar studies in adults have not shown this relationship.

There is insufficient evidence to link HHV6 with interstitial pneumonitis, multiple sclerosis, heterophile-negative infectious mononucleosis, chronic fatigue syndrome (Chapter 41), lymphoproliferative disease, or malignancy.

Immunocompromised Persons. HHV6 infections after bone marrow or solid organ transplantation may be manifested as fever without specific findings.

Intrauterine Infection. Although 1–2% of umbilical cord blood specimens contain HHV6 DNA by PCR, suggesting intrauterine transmission, no congenital abnormalities or congenital syndrome has been described. Intrauterine HHV7 infection has not been documented.

DIAGNOSIS

The most important purpose for establishing the diagnosis of roseola is to differentiate this generally mild illness from other potentially more serious childhood rash illnesses. The diagnosis of roseola should be made on the basis of age, history, and clinical findings and seldom necessitates further laboratory investigation. Specific and rapid microbiologic tests for HHV6 may become available in the future.

Differential Diagnosis

Children with roseola may be at either of two different stages of the illness at presentation: during the febrile period, before the onset of the rash, and after the rash has appeared. Many illnesses may be easily confused with roseola during the pre-eruptive stage. However, the pattern of high fever without significant physical findings, rather rapid defervescence, and a subsequent rash are unique to roseola. Nevertheless, some cases may not display all these characteristics and may mimic other illnesses.

Drug Eruptions. Perhaps the most common condition that resembles roseola in populations immunized against rubella and measles is drug hypersensitivity reaction. Empirical administration of an antibiotic during the first few days of a febrile illness, followed by development of a drug eruption and coincidental resolution of the fever, may simulate the characteristic clinical pattern of roseola. A drug eruption may be distinguished by its morbilliform nature, pruritus, and resolution after discontinuation of the offending drug.

Rubella. Children with rubella invariably have a prodromal period, whereas no distinct prodrome develops in children with roseola. Suboccipital, postauricular, and posterior cervical lymphadenopathy occurs in the majority of children with rubella, but lymphadenopathy is an inconsistent finding in roseola. Rubella usually causes only low-grade fever that is coincident with the exanthem. In contrast, children with roseola characteristically have high fevers that resolve before the exanthem develops. The rash of rubella is usually more generalized, with greater coalescence than that seen with roseola. Furthermore a history of recent exposure is frequently elicited from individuals with rubella. Most important, persons vaccinated with rubella vaccine rarely develop rubella.

Measles. At the height of the fever, children with measles develop a morbilliform exanthem that is associated with cough, coryza, conjunctivitis, and Koplik's spots on the buccal mucosa in the early stages of disease.

Scarlet Fever. The features of scarlet fever that distinguish it from roseola are its rarity in infants, the simultaneous presence of fever and rash, the presence of pharyngitis, and the discrete, small cutaneous lesions with a sandpapery texture.

Laboratory Evaluation

Children with roseola typically develop a mild neutropenia and relative lymphocytosis coincident with the exanthem. Neutrophilia, lymphopenia, and normal WBC counts may be observed. Urinalysis and CSF findings are usually normal. Most persons with encephalitis have pleocytosis (30–200 cells/mm^3) with mononuclear cell predominance, elevated protein concentration, and normal glucose concentration.

Microbiologic Evaluation

Acute infection with HHV6 may be confirmed by viral culture, antibody testing, PCR, or other techniques.

Viral Culture. Traditional HHV6 and HHV7 viral culture uses fresh umbilical cord blood cells, requires 1–3 weeks, and is available only in research laboratories. A rapid shell vial culture for HHV6 requires 3–4 days and is available commercially.

Serologic Testing. Serologic testing for an IgM response may be useful for documenting acute infection. However, few laboratories offer this test, and false-positive results occur. Seroconversion or a fourfold or greater rise of specific IgG antibodies in sera drawn 2–3 weeks apart also confirms the diagnosis.

Other Methods. HHV6 and HHV7 can be identified in biologic specimens by PCR testing. The presence of viral DNA in noncellular specimens (e.g., serum, plasma, CSF) is clinically relevant because it indicates active viral replication. Identification of viral DNA in cellular material (e.g., peripheral blood mononuclear cells) does not necessarily indicate active infection because latent virus exists in these cells.

Other potentially useful diagnostic tests for HHV6 include antigen tests of serum and, for tissues, immunohistochemistry and in situ hybridization.

Diagnostic Imaging

Imaging studies are not necessary for the typical child with roseola. No pulmonary symptoms are associated with roseola, and the chest radiograph usually shows no abnormalities. In unusual cases of roseola complicated by encephalitis, CT or MRI of the head is warranted for complete evaluation.

TREATMENT

Definitive Treatment. HHV6 and HHV7 are inhibited in vitro by ganciclovir, cidofovir, and foscarnet at levels that are achievable in serum. However, these drugs have significant toxicity and their clinical efficacy for roseola has not been evaluated. They are unlikely to prevent development of latent viral infection. No specific therapy may ever be indicated for the otherwise healthy child with roseola because the illness almost invariably resolves without sequelae. However, future studies may address the role of specific antiviral therapy in unusual cases of roseola, such as roseola in children with significant neurologic complications, and in other forms of HHV6 and HHV7 infection associated with significant morbidity, such as infection in immunocompromised persons.

Supportive Therapy. Children in the febrile, pre-eruptive phase of roseola are usually otherwise comfortable and require little supportive therapy except administration of antipyretic agents. This is especially important for children who are fussy or uncomfortable or who have a history of febrile seizures or underlying neurologic problems that may predispose them to seizures. Maintenance of adequate fluid balance is important in all children with symptoms. Referral to a specialist should be considered in those rare circumstances in which unusual manifestations or complications develop, such as encephalitis or thrombocytopenic purpura.

COMPLICATIONS

Complications after roseola are uncommon and usually involve the central nervous system. Transient hemiparesis, lasting days to weeks, has been reported in several patients. Rarely, permanent sequelae, including mental retardation or hemiparesis, which may be attributable to brain anoxia during prolonged febrile seizures, have been reported.

PROGNOSIS

The prognosis for most children with roseola is excellent, with no sequelae. Few deaths directly attributable to HHV6 infection in infants and older children have occurred in children with roseola complicated by encephalitis, hepatitis, virus-associated hemophagocytosis syndrome, or multisystem involvement.

PREVENTION

Although roseola is a common illness, little information on which to base guidelines for prevention of secondary cases of infection is available. Whereas outbreaks of classic roseola are uncommon, occurrences of roseola-like illnesses have been associated with many different viruses, most commonly enteroviruses. It is likely that immunocompetent, healthy adults latently infected with HHV6 or HHV7 transmit the virus to susceptible infants and children via saliva. Until proper studies have been performed, no additional recommendations for prevention beyond good hand-washing technique can be made. If roseola caused by HHV6 is similar to other viral illnesses, the period of communicability is probably greatest during the period of high fever immediately preceding the appearance of the rash.

REVIEWS

Barenberg LH, Greenspan L: Exanthem subitum (roseola infantum). *Am J Dis Child* 1939;58:983–93.

Berenberg W, Wright S, Janeway CA: Roseola infantum (exanthem subitum). *N Engl J Med* 1949;241:253–9.

Braun DK, Dominguez G, Pellett PE: Human herpesvirus 6. *Clin Microbiol Rev* 1997;10:521–67.

Breese BB Jr: Roseola infantum (exanthem subitum). *N Y State J Med* 1941;41:1854–9.

Juretic M: Exanthema subitum. A review of 243 cases. *Helv Paediatr Acta* 1963;18:80–95.

Kimberlin DW: Human herpesviruses 6 and 7: Identification of newly recognized viral pathogens and their association with human disease. *Pediatr Infect Dis J* 1998;17:59–67.

KEY ARTICLES

Asano Y, Nakashima T, Yoshikawa T, et al: Severity of human herpesvirus-6 viremia and clinical findings in infants with exanthem subitum. *J Pediatr* 1991;118:891–5.

Asano Y, Yoshikawa T, Suga S, et al: Clinical features of infants with primary human herpesvirus 6 infection (exanthem subitum, roseola infantum). *Pediatrics* 1994;93:104–8.

Burnstine RC, Paine RS: Residual encephalopathy following roseola infantum. *Am J Dis Child* 1959;98:144–52.

Caserta MT, Hall CB, Schnabel K, et al: Primary human herpesvirus 7 infection: A comparison of human herpesvirus 7 and human herpesvirus 6 infections in children. *J Pediatr* 1998;133:386–9.

Cherry JD: Viral exanthems. *Curr Probl Pediatr* 1983;13:1–44.

Hall CB, Long CE, Schnabel KC, et al: Human herpesvirus-6 infection in children. A prospective study of complications and reactivation. *N Engl J Med* 1994;331:432–8.

Kositanont U, Wasi C, Wanprapar N, et al: Primary infection of human herpesvirus 6 in children with vertical infection of human immunodeficiency virus type 1. *J Infect Dis* 1999;180:50–5.

Leach CT, Newton ER, McParlin S, et al: Human herpesvirus 6 infection of the female genital tract. *J Infect Dis* 1994;169:1281–3.

Okada K, Ueda K, Kusuhara K, et al: Exanthema subitum and human herpesvirus 6 infection: Clinical observations in fifty-seven cases. *Pediatr Infect Dis J* 1993;12:204–8.

Pruksananonda P, Hall CB, Insel RA, et al: Primary human herpesvirus 6 infection in young children. *N Engl J Med* 1992;326:1445–50.

Suga S, Yoshikawa T, Asano Y, et al: Clinical and virological analyses of 21 infants with exanthem subitum (roseola infantum) and central nervous system complications. *Ann Neurol* 1993;33:597–603.

Suga S, Yoshikawa T, Nagai T, et al: Clinical features and virological findings in children with primary human herpesvirus 7 infection. *Pediatrics* 1997;99(3):E4.

Suga S, Suzuki K, Ihira M, et al: Clinical characteristics of febrile convulsions during primary HHV-6 infection. *Arch Dis Child* 2000:82;62–6.

Tanaka K, Kondo T, Torigoe S, et al: Human herpesvirus 7: Another causal agent for roseola (exanthem subitum). *J Pediatr* 1994;125:1–5.

Yamanishi K, Okuno T, Shiraki K, et al: Identification of human herpesvirus-6 as a causal agent for exanthem subitum. *Lancet* 1988;1:1065–7.

CHAPTER 26

Erythema Infectiosum (Fifth Disease)

Charles T. Leach ▪ Hal B. Jenson

The illness now known as **erythema infectiosum** was first described in Europe in the 1800s. The synonym "**fifth disease**" was derived from its description as the fifth childhood exanthem (Table 26–1). Erythema infectiosum is a mild, self-limiting malady in children that is characterized by fever and a distinctive rash. More severe manifestations can occur in persons with underlying chronic hemolytic anemia and in immunocompromised persons. Infection during pregnancy may cause hydrops fetalis, leading to spontaneous abortion and stillbirth (Chapter 95).

ETIOLOGY

Erythema infectiosum is caused by human parvovirus, sometimes referred to as **parvovirus B19** (B19), a single-stranded DNA virus with 5,500 base pairs in the family Parvoviridae. The designation *B19* refers to the laboratory number used to identify the first clinical isolate.

Transmission. Erythema infectiosum is highly contagious during the preexanthematous phase. Droplets from the respiratory tract spread most disease, although transmission through transfusion of contaminated blood products can occur. The rate of secondary spread to susceptible household contacts is as high as 50%, and during school outbreaks, 10–60% of children develop erythema infectiosum. Adults acquire B19 infection primarily through contact with children in the home, at school, or in daycare facilities. Most infected persons recall no contact with ill subjects because children with erythema infectiosum typically have mild or absent symptoms and are no longer infectious by the time the rash appears. However, the period of contagion is prolonged in persons who develop transient aplastic crises and in immunocompromised persons with pure red cell aplasia. There is no sex predilection for erythema infectiosum in childhood. B19 is the only parvovirus pathogenic for humans, although there are other pathogenic parvoviruses that infect animals.

EPIDEMIOLOGY

B19 predominantly infects school-aged children. B19 seroprevalence is only 2–9% in children less than 5 years of age but increases to 15–35% in older children (5–18 years of age) and 30–60% in adults. In the Northern Hemisphere, children frequently acquire B19 during the school months; such episodes typically last until May or June. B19 infections also take place sporadically throughout the year. Epidemics occur an average of every 6 years and last approximately 3 years.

PATHOGENESIS

B19 is tropic for rapidly dividing erythroid precursors in the bone marrow (Fig. 26–1). Erythrocyte P antigen, a surface glycolipid present on erythroid cells from most individuals, is the cellular receptor for B19. The virus infects, replicates, and destroys these cells, resulting in erythroid aplasia and anemia. B19 viral receptors have also been found on endothelial cells, placental tissues, and fetal heart and liver. Infection of these cells probably mediates the rash of erythema infectiosum, transplacental transmission, and fetal manifestations. Although B19 cannot replicate in granulocytic or megakaryocytic cell lines in vitro, it may abortively infect these cells in vivo and cause self-limited neutropenia and thrombocytopenia.

B19-associated anemia is usually subclinical in healthy persons. However, in children with underlying chronic anemia or shortened erythrocyte lifespan, such as sickle cell anemia, B19-induced erythroid aplasia usually causes a transient aplastic crisis. Immunocompromised children, including HIV-infected children, may be unable to clear the virus and may develop pure red cell aplasia as a result.

After infection of upper respiratory tract mucosa, viremia begins approximately 5 days later and peaks at 9 days. Reticulocytopenia and systemic symptoms develop during this initial viremic phase. The virus is simultaneously present in upper respiratory tract secretions. From 1 to 5 days after cessation of viremia, coincident with a specific humoral immune response, rash and joint manifestations may develop. Immunity generally persists for life, although in rare cases second episodes of B19 infection may develop.

The exanthem associated with erythema infectiosum is generally attributed to immunologic mechanisms because it develops at a time when viremia has ceased and neutralizing antibodies have appeared. Joint manifestations, which occur predominantly in adults, are also probably immune related.

Congenital B19 infection is acquired through placental transfer of virus with subsequent infection of fetal erythroid cells, leading to heart failure (manifested by hydrops fetalis) and death (Chapter 95).

SYMPTOMS AND CLINICAL MANIFESTATIONS

Incubation Period. The incubation period is typically 4–14 days and rarely may be as long as 21 days.

Common Symptoms

The clinical manifestations of B19 infection (Fig. 26–2) can occur at two different time points: during the viremic, erythroid infection phase (prodromal symptoms or anemia) and during the subsequent immunologic response to infection (exanthem or joint manifestations or both). One fifth of B19 infections in children are asymptomatic or subclinical.

Prodromal symptoms occur in 20–60% of cases of erythema infectiosum, but because manifestations are so mild, few children come for medical care during this phase. Symptoms of headache, low-grade fever, chills, malaise, sore throat, and coryza typically

TABLE 26–1. Classic Childhood Exanthems

Classic Order	Exanthem	Etiology
First disease	Rubeola (measles)	Rubeola virus
Second disease	Scarlet fever	Group A *Streptococcus*
Third disease	Rubella (German measles)	Rubella virus
Fourth disease	Filatov-Dukes disease*	
Fifth disease	Erythema infectiosum	Parvovirus B19
Sixth disease	Roseola infantum (exanthem subitum)	Human herpesvirus 6 (HHV6)

*A variant of scarlet fever caused by toxin-producing *Staphylococcus.*

develop several days before the exanthem appears. These manifestations coincide with viremia and resolve within a few days. In patients with prodromal symptoms, a symptom-free interval of 1–7 days usually precedes the exanthem.

Erythema infectiosum is associated with a classic exanthem that can be divided into three stages. A facial rash that produces an intense rose-red color on the cheeks with circumoral sparing is usually noted first and is often referred to as a ''**slapped cheek**'' appearance (Plate 4A). This rash lasts 1–4 days and subsequently fades. A less prominent rash typically occurs simultaneously or within 1 or 2 days on other parts of the body, especially the chest and proximal extremities, and defines the second stage (Plate 4B). The body rash is classically maculopapular and may be mildly pruritic. It rarely affects the palmar and plantar surfaces. Within a week the rash fades and appears more reticular or lacelike. The third stage is characterized by an evanescent rash that also involves the chest and proximal extremities but recurs and recedes in response to various stimuli. This stage typically lasts a few weeks but can persist for several months.

Arthritis. Although children infrequently (<10%) develop arthritis after B19 infection, in comparison with adults (60%), arthritis is the most common complication of erythema infectiosum. It typically appears at the time of the rash and is probably mediated by immune complexes. Most adults and children with B19-associated chronic arthritis are female. Approximately half of children with arthritis have polyarticular disease and half develop pauciarticular disease. Large joints, especially the knees, are affected more frequently than small joints. Symptoms usually resolve within 4 months but may persist for more than 1 year, with some patients fulfilling criteria for juvenile rheumatoid arthritis. B19-associated arthritis does not cause erosive arthritis. Children with persistent joint symptoms associated with erythema infectiosum should be referred to a pediatric rheumatologist.

Physical Examination Findings

Children with erythema infectiosum are seldom seen by a clinician during the prodromal phase, because symptoms are uniformly mild or absent. A low-grade fever (temperature 37.8–38.3°C [100–101°F]) and mild pharyngeal injection without exudate may be present. No consistent enanthem has been noted in cases of erythema infectiosum. Occasionally, clear rhinorrhea, mild conjunctivitis, and cough are observed. Lymphadenopathy may be present but is not usually prominent. There are no features during this phase of illness that distinguish B19 infection from other upper respiratory tract infections.

Exanthem. The first exanthematous phase of erythema infectiosum typically begins on the face but may develop concomitantly on other areas of the body. The facial rash does not develop in 20% of children. The facial rash is unique, beginning as red maculopapules on the cheeks that rapidly coalesce and develop into an intensely red symmetric exanthem on both cheeks (Plate 4A). The rash usually affects the nasal bridge, causing a butterfly distribution, but spares the nasolabial and chin areas, leaving circumoral pallor. The rash is warm and edematous with fairly sharp borders, is not tender, and is seldom pruritic. The facial rash fades within 4 days and does not desquamate.

The second-stage exanthem on body and extremities typically emerges 1–2 days after the facial rash, although these rashes may occur simultaneously. The most commonly affected sites are the extremities, especially the extensor surfaces, and the buttocks; the trunk and neck are less frequently involved, and the palms and

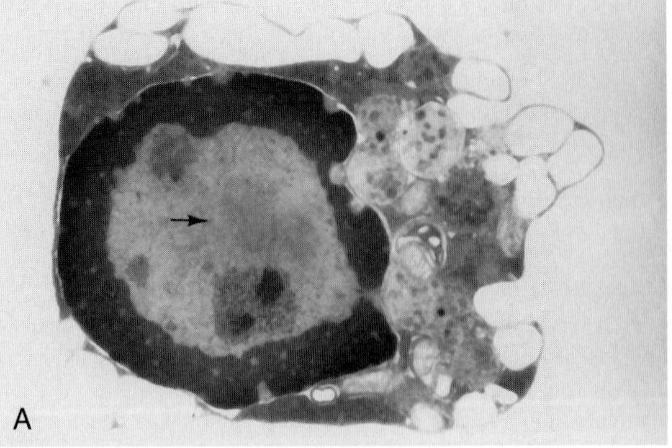

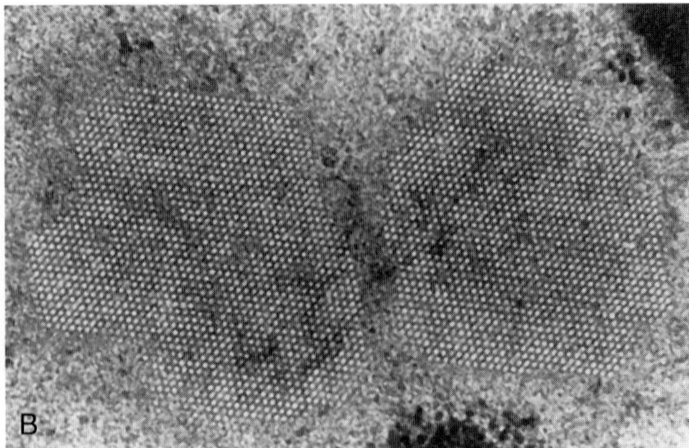

FIGURE 26–1. A, Electron microscopy of parvovirus B19–infected erythroid precursor cell, showing marginated chromatin and nuclear inclusions (*arrow*). Magnification: ×17,010. **B,** Electron microscopy of nuclear inclusions (**A,** *arrow*) consisting of a lattice or crystalline arrays of virions. Magnification: ×108,864. (From Sosa CE, Mahony JB, Luinstra KE, et al: Replication and cytopathology of human parvovirus B19 in human umbilical cord blood erythroid progenitor cells. *J Med Virol* 1992;36:125–30. Copyright © 1992 Wiley-Liss. Reprinted by permission of Wiley-Liss, a subsidiary of John Wiley and Sons, Inc.)

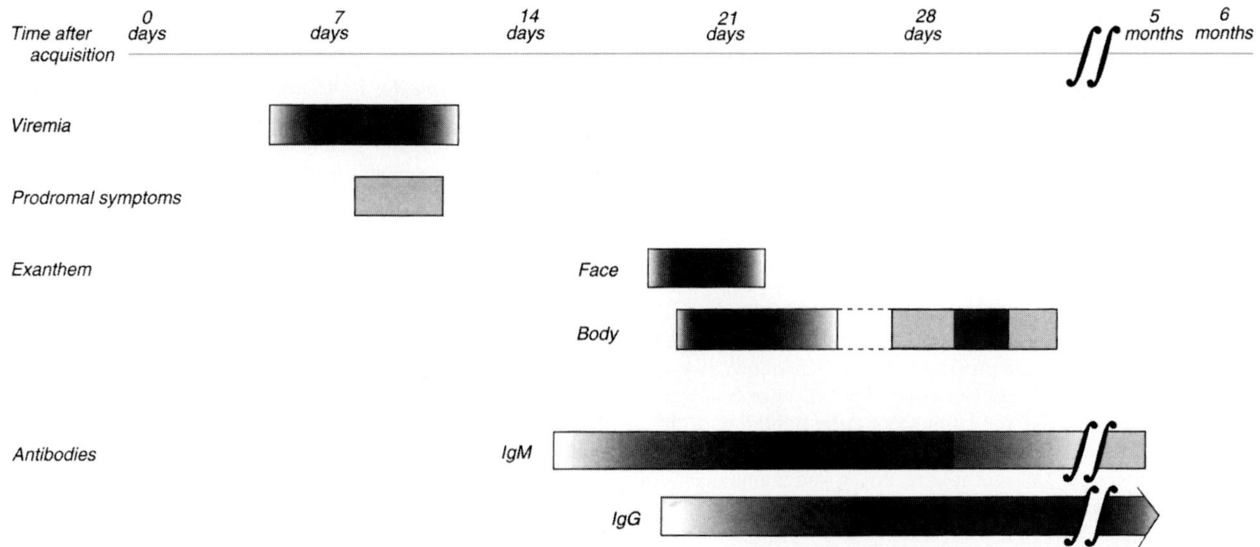

FIGURE 26–2. Profile of the typical clinical course of parvovirus B19 infection (erythema infectiosum or fifth disease).

soles are rarely affected. The body exanthem is less intense than the facial exanthem and first appears as fine, discrete red maculopapules that eventually enlarge and develop a violaceous hue. The central portions of the lesions gradually fade, leaving a distinctive rash that has been described as reticulated, lattice-like or lacelike (Plate 4B). The reticulated rash is the most common feature of erythema infectiosum. Pruritus is infrequent but can be prominent. Desquamation is rare.

In most children the exanthem gradually fades in approximately 7 days but may recur and recede in response to various stimuli. This evanescent feature of the exanthem is distinctive. Various triggers for recrudescence have been reported, including sunlight, environmental temperature changes, baths, exercise, and emotional stress. These episodes typically continue for 2–3 weeks but may recur for several months.

Recent cases of papular-purpuric **gloves and socks syndrome** have been associated with acute B19 infection. Petechial, urticarial, and vesicular rashes occur uncommonly in association with acute B19 infection.

Uncommon Symptoms

Unusual manifestations may develop in two general groups of children with B19 infection: children with an increased erythroid production requirement because of a shortened erythrocyte lifespan who develop a transient aplastic crisis, and children with immunodeficiency who acquire a persistent B19 infection that causes pure red cell aplasia. These children do not commonly display the typical manifestations of erythema infectiosum.

Transient Aplastic Crisis. Children with a variety of hematologic disorders characterized by ineffective erythroid production, increased erythroid hemolysis, or ongoing blood loss are at risk of having a symptomatic transient aplastic crisis after exposure to B19. Transient aplastic crises most often occur in children with chronic hemolytic anemias such as sickle cell anemia, thalassemia, hereditary spherocytosis, glucose-6-phosphate dehydrogenase deficiency, pyruvate kinase deficiency, and hereditary elliptocytosis. The crisis may be the first indication of a previously undiagnosed hematologic disorder. The crisis occurs only once, with initial B19 infection.

B19 infection is the most common cause of transient aplastic crisis among children in recognized risk groups. Most children with B19-induced transient aplastic crisis have multiple symptoms, including fever, lethargy, malaise, pallor, headache, gastrointestinal symptoms, and possibly respiratory complaints. The reticulocyte count is extremely low or zero, and the hemoglobin level is lower than usual for the patient. Transient neutropenia and thrombocytopenia also commonly occur. Transfusions are frequently required. Illness in most persons is self-limited, with recovery of reticulocytes by 1–2 weeks and return of peripheral blood counts to their preillness values by 3–4 weeks. Although rare fatalities have occurred from circulatory collapse or congestive heart failure, appropriate supportive therapy should result in recovery.

Signs identified on physical examination of children with transient aplastic crisis, such as pallor, tachypnea, tachycardia, and a gallop rhythm, are generally attributable to exacerbation of the anemia. Low-grade fever is frequently present. Uncommonly, an exanthem occurs at the onset of anemia, but it is rare for these children to display the typical rash of erythema infectiosum.

Pure Red Cell Aplasia. Susceptible immunodeficient persons can have a persistent B19 infection, with severe anemia resulting from pure red cell aplasia. Persons at risk include children with congenital immunodeficiencies, HIV-infected children, persons with cancer who are receiving chemotherapy, and recipients of bone marrow or solid organ transplants. Because of an absent or ineffective humoral immune response, B19 infection persists and continual viral replication occurs in the bone marrow. Although some persons may develop IgM or IgG antibodies (or both) against B19, these antibodies are ineffective in neutralizing the virus.

No consistent prodrome is identifiable, and a rash is uncommon. Virologic diagnosis requires demonstration of viral DNA in the blood or bone marrow or demonstration of giant pronormoblasts in the bone marrow. Hematologic abnormalities, including neutropenia and thrombocytopenia, may persist for months to years. Immunoglobulin administration may help resolve the anemia.

Physical findings of immunocompromised persons with B19-associated pure red cell aplasia are variable but seldom resemble erythema infectiosum, and they may include only low-grade fever, a nonspecific rash, and coryza. After administration of immunoglobulin, a maculopapular rash and joint manifestations, presumably mediated by immune complexes, may develop.

DIAGNOSIS

The diagnosis of erythema infectiosum in the healthy school-aged child is established on the basis of the clinical findings of a typical facial rash with absent or mild prodromal symptoms, followed by a reticulated body rash that waxes and wanes. Specific microbiologic testing should be reserved for immunocompetent children with an erythema infectiosum–like exanthem not occurring during an outbreak, children with transient aplastic crises, and immunocompromised persons with pure red cell aplasia.

Differential Diagnosis

Although erythema infectiosum is simple to diagnose during a community outbreak, distinguishing this disease from other disorders during other periods is more difficult. Illnesses most frequently confused with erythema infectiosum include rubella, measles, scarlet fever, enteroviral infections, systemic lupus erythematosus (SLE), and drug reactions. Epidemiologic aspects of infection such as seasonality, age, exposure history, incubation period, vaccination history, and history of other common rash-associated illnesses may be as important as clinical signs and symptoms in making a diagnosis.

Although the typically mild rubella prodrome is similar to erythema infectiosum, rubella is associated with prominent preauricular, postauricular, and suboccipital lymphadenopathy not observed in erythema infectiosum. Further, the rubella rash does not spare the circumoral area, is of short duration, and does not recur. Classic measles, with its prominent prodromal symptoms, pathognomonic enanthem, and typical rash, is seldom confused with erythema infectiosum. Rubella and measles are becoming increasingly rare in the United States as a result of effective immunization measures.

Scarlet fever may occasionally be confused with erythema infectiosum, principally because of the similar circumoral sparing of the facial rash. However, other features of scarlet fever, such as high fever, prominent pharyngeal findings, and characteristics of the rash (e.g., roughness of the skin) should clarify the diagnosis.

Nonpolio enteroviruses frequently cause various types of rashes during the summer and fall months but rarely cause erythema infectiosum–like facial rashes and do not cause recrudescent, reticulated rashes. However, as with erythema infectiosum, prodromal symptoms are absent or mild.

The exanthem typically associated with SLE occurs in a malar (butterfly) distribution and persists much longer than the facial rash of erythema infectiosum. However, other characteristics of the rash are dissimilar to erythema infectiosum. In addition, children with SLE usually have other SLE-associated manifestations such as renal disease, arthritis, or central nervous system symptoms.

Drug rashes occasionally mimic erythema infectiosum. A history of having received a medication, the presence of urticaria, and the lack of reticulation or recrudescence differentiate drug rashes from erythema infectiosum.

Transient Aplastic Crisis. Although B19 infection is the most common cause of transient aplastic crisis, other possible causes include bacterial infections (e.g., with *Salmonella* and *Streptococcus pneumoniae*), other viral infections (e.g., influenza, infection with Epstein-Barr virus), and drugs (e.g., chloramphenicol).

Pure Red Cell Aplasia. B19 is the most common cause of pure red cell aplasia in persons with compromised immunity, but other possible causes include Diamond-Blackfan anemia, drugs (e.g., zidovudine), autoimmune disease, malignancy, and other infections.

Laboratory Evaluation

Studies in healthy adult volunteers during the viremic phase of B19 infection reveal that many laboratory abnormalities occur, including reticulocytopenia lasting 7–10 days, mild anemia, thrombocytopenia, lymphopenia, and neutropenia. However, most otherwise healthy children present at the time of the rash, when viremia has already cleared. Laboratory results are usually normal by this time, but occasionally children have lymphocytosis, leukopenia, leukocytosis, thrombocytopenia, or mild eosinophilia.

Persons with transient aplastic crisis have reticulocytopenia and anemia, with the anemia generally proportional to the severity of the underlying hemolytic anemia. Other hematologic abnormalities, such as neutropenia, lymphocytosis and eosinophilia, may be seen, as in healthy children with erythema infectiosum. Immunocompromised children with pure red cell aplasia have anemia, reticulocytopenia, and varying degrees of abnormalities of other hematologic elements. Some children, especially organ transplant recipients, may develop pancytopenia.

Microbiologic Evaluation

Viral Culture. B19 virus does not grow on standard, commercially available cell lines, precluding this method of diagnostic testing.

Serologic Diagnosis. In children with normal humoral immunity, the best method for laboratory confirmation of acute B19 infection is the serum IgM antibody test, usually performed by RIA or EIA. IgM antibodies first appear during the prodromal, viremic phase of illness and persist for 1–2 months. Detection of B19-specific IgG antibodies is useful for determining past infection and immunity. IgG antibodies are detectable a few days after IgM antibodies and persist for years.

Serologic testing in immunocompromised persons may be problematic because they usually do not develop B19-specific IgM or IgG antibodies. Therefore, in these population groups, direct methods of detecting B19 virus or DNA are usually necessary. PCR, especially for persons with lower levels of detectable virus (e.g., those who have received immune globulin), and dot-blot hybridization are commonly used for direct detection of B19 DNA in serum. A less common method of detecting virus is B19 antigen detection in serum. Occasionally, children with transient aplastic crisis may be seen too early in the course of the disease, such as during the first few days of hospitalization, to allow detection of B19 IgM antibodies, and a direct method must be used to confirm the diagnosis.

Bone Marrow. Examination of the bone marrow may be required for immunocompromised persons with pure red cell aplasia. This reveals destruction of the erythroid series and the pathognomonic presence of giant pronormoblasts (Fig. 26–3). By electron microscopy, B19-infected cells display marginated chromatin and lattice-like nuclear inclusions (Fig. 26–1).

Diagnostic Imaging

Imaging studies usually are not necessary in children with B19-associated arthritis. Radiography has most often revealed only small

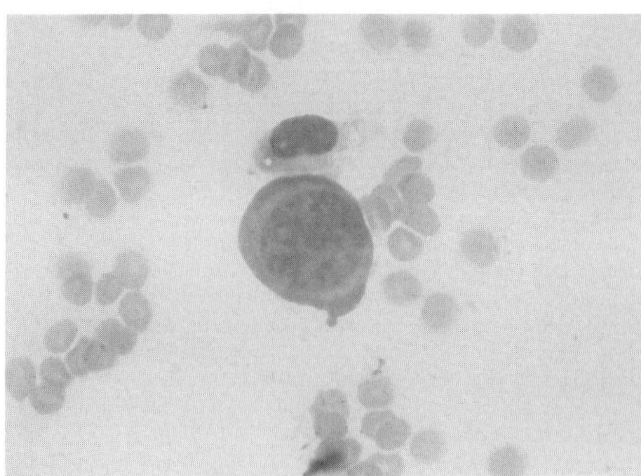

FIGURE 26–3. Wright-Giemsa stain demonstrating a giant pronormoblast from a bone marrow aspirate of a patient with parvovirus B19 infection. (From Krause JR, Penchansky L, Knisely AS: Morphological diagnosis of parvovirus B19 infection. A cytopathic effect easily recognized in air-dried, formalin-fixed bone marrow smears stained with hematoxylin-eosin or Wright-Giemsa. *Arch Pathol Lab Med* 1992;116:178–80. Copyright 1992, American Medical Association.)

joint effusions, and ultrasonography has demonstrated soft tissue swelling and synovial thickening.

TREATMENT

Definitive Treatment

No specific antiviral therapy is available for B19 infections. Although comparative trials have not been performed, administration of IVIG usually terminates B19-associated anemia in immunodeficient persons with persistent infection. Because approximately 50% of adults have IgG antibody, commercially available immune globulin preparations generally contain high levels of B19-specific antibodies. The IVIG dose is 400 mg/kg, administered intravenously daily for 5 days. Many persons develop immune complex–related symptoms, such as rash or arthritis, after IVIG treatments. Some persons, especially those with AIDS, may require further doses of IVIG, particularly if relapses occur.

Supportive Therapy

Discomfort associated with fever and pain associated with arthralgias are treated with acetaminophen or ibuprofen. A nonsteroidal anti-inflammatory agent such as ibuprofen is recommended for B19-associated arthritis. Other supportive measures for children with erythema infectiosum are rarely necessary. Children with transient aplastic crisis usually require hospitalization for intravenous fluid administration and transfusion. B19-associated pure red cell aplasia in immunocompetent children may necessitate repeated blood and platelet transfusions.

COMPLICATIONS

Complications are extremely rare in children with erythema infectiosum. Reported complications have included encephalitis, encephalopathy, aseptic meningitis, paresthesias, brachial plexus neuropathy, myocarditis, hepatitis, aplastic anemia, idiopathic thrombocytopenic purpura, transient erythroblastopenia of childhood, hemophagocytic syndrome, and systemic vasculitis. Because parvovirus B19 is not teratogenic, abortion because of possible malformation is not a consideration (Chapter 94).

PROGNOSIS

Erythema infectiosum in a healthy child is a benign exanthematous systemic viral infection. Only two reported fatalities have occurred in persons with transient aplastic crisis: one death from circulatory collapse and the other from heart failure.

PREVENTION

Preventive measures should focus on three high-risk groups of susceptible subjects: children with chronic hemolytic disorders, children with immunodeficiency, and pregnant women. The greatest risk to pregnant women is from children, including those in the household and, for daycare workers and teachers, those encountered on the job especially children 5–7 years of age. Effective measures for control of B19 infection in homes, daycare centers, and schools are limited. Because children are generally not infectious by the time the rash is present, the exclusion of affected children from school is not reasonable. Good hand-washing technique and prompt disposal of facial tissues are practical measures that should help reduce transmission.

Although B19 may be transmitted through transfusion of contaminated blood products, screening of blood for B19 is not routinely performed because of the moderately high seroprevalence of B19, the low incidence of transfusion-related infection, and the relatively minor severity of illness.

Vaccination. A B19 vaccine is not currently available. However, a recently developed B19 recombinant vaccine stimulates good antibody responses in laboratory animals, and phase 1 testing in humans is under way. If the vaccine proves to be safe and effective in preventing B19 infection, administration could be considered for susceptible members of high-risk groups.

Outbreak Control. When an outbreak of erythema infectiosum is identified, workers with children and parents of children should be informed of the risk of acquiring B19 infection and the consequences of such infection for persons in high-risk groups. Individuals may choose to avoid the workplace or school during the erythema infectiosum outbreak. Prolonged periods of avoidance would be necessary, however, because outbreaks typically last several months. Routine exclusion of children or adults in high-risk groups is not recommended. Avoidance does not eliminate the risk of acquiring B19 infection because workers are likely to have been exposed to infected schoolchildren, and children at home may transmit infection. The decision to avoid school or daycare facilities should be made only after careful discussion with local public health officials, private physicians, school or workplace administrators, and families. In selected cases, susceptibility to B19 may be determined by B19 IgG testing.

Hospital Isolation. In the rare instances in which otherwise healthy persons with erythema infectiosum are hospitalized, no special isolation precautions are necessary. Children are no longer considered contagious by the time the exanthem appears. However, children with transient aplastic crisis and immunodeficient children with B19-associated pure red cell aplasia are considered infectious and should remain in respiratory and contact isolation for the duration of their hospitalization. Nosocomial transmission of B19 has occurred; source patients were children with B19-associated transient aplastic crisis who were not isolated initially. A B19-infected person with transient aplastic crisis or pure red cell aplasia may share a room with another person with B19 infection as long as other contagious conditions are not present simultaneously. If possible, pregnant health care workers should avoid contact with children with transient aplastic crisis or B19-associated pure red cell aplasia.

REVIEWS

Anderson LJ: Role of parvovirus B19 in human disease. *Pediatr Infect Dis J* 1987;6:711–8.

Anderson LJ: Human parvoviruses. *J Infect Dis* 1990;161:603–8.

Balfour HH Jr: Erythema infectiosum (fifth disease). Clinical review and description of 91 cases seen in an epidemic. *Clin Pediatr* 1969;8: 721–7.

Brown KE, Young NS: Parvovirus B19 in human disease. *Annu Rev Med* 1997;48:59–67.

Shaw HLK: Erythema infectiosum. *Am J Med Sci* 1905;129:16–22.

Young NS: Parvovirus infection and its treatment. *Clin Exp Immunol* 1996;104:26–30.

KEY ARTICLES

Adler SP, Manganello AA, Koch WC, et al: Risk of human parvovirus B19 infections among school and hospital employees during endemic periods. *J Infect Dis* 1993;168:361–8.

Ager EA, Chin TD, Poland JD: Epidemic erythema infectiosum. *N Engl J Med* 1966;275:1326–31.

Anderson MJ, Higgins PG, Davis LR, et al: Experimental parvoviral infection in humans. *J Infect Dis* 1985;152:257–65.

Bansal GP, Hatfield JA, Dunn FE, et al: Candidate recombinant vaccine for human B19 parvovirus. *J Infect Dis* 1993;167:1034–44.

Bell LM, Naides SJ, Stoffman P, et al: Human parvovirus B19 infection among hospital staff members after contact with infected patients. *N Engl J Med* 1989;321:485–91.

Brown KE, Anderson SM, Young NS: Erythrocyte P antigen: Cellular receptor for B19 parvovirus. *Science* 1993;262:114–7.

Centers for Disease Control: Risks associated with human parvovirus B19 infection. *MMWR Morb Mortal Wkly Rep* 1989;38:81–97.

Cherry JD: Contemporary infectious exanthems. *Clin Infect Dis* 1993; 16:199–205.

Erdman DD, Usher MJ, Tsou C, et al: Human parvovirus B19 specific IgG, IgA, and IgM antibodies and DNA in serum specimens from persons with erythema infectiosum. *J Med Virol* 1991;35:110–5.

Gillespie SM, Cartter ML, Asch S, et al: Occupational risk of human parvovirus B19 infection for school and day-care personnel during an outbreak of erythema infectiosum. *JAMA* 1990;263:2061–5.

Koch WC, Massey G, Russell CE, et al: Manifestations and treatment of human parvovirus B19 infection in immunocompromised patients. *J Pediatr* 1990;116:355–9.

Nocton JJ, Miller LC, Tucker LB, et al: Human parvovirus B19–associated arthritis in children. *J Pediatr* 1993;122:186–90.

Pass RF: Day-care centers and the spread of cytomegalovirus and parvovirus B19. *Pediatr Ann* 1991;20:419–26.

Rao SP, Miller ST, Cohen BJ, et al: Transient aplastic crisis in patients with sickle cell disease–B19 parvovirus studies during a 7-year period. *Am J Dis Child* 1992;146:1328–30.

Smith PT, Landry ML, Carey H, et al: Papular-purpuric gloves and socks syndrome associated with acute parvovirus B19 infection: Case report and review. *Clin Infect Dis* 1998;27:164–8.

CHAPTER 27

Chickenpox and Zoster

Hal B. Jenson ▪ Charles T. Leach

Varicella-zoster virus (VZV) causes two distinct clinical entities from which it derives its name. Until the mid-1900s a separate herpesvirus was thought to cause zoster, previously known as **herpes zoster,** but this was shown to be the same virus that causes varicella. **Varicella,** commonly known as **chickenpox,** is the acute and generally benign illness resulting from primary infection with VZV. It is a highly contagious febrile illness characterized by a generalized, pruritic vesicular rash that was historically confused with smallpox. VZV establishes latency after primary infection that persists for the lifetime of the individual but usually does not lead to further illness. **Zoster,** which is commonly known as **shingles,** results from reactivation of latent VZV. In immunocompromised persons, primary VZV infection may be especially severe, and zoster may become disseminated with visceral involvement. With the availability of an effective vaccine, chickenpox is no longer an inevitable disease of childhood.

ETIOLOGY

VZV is a member of the Herpesviridae, a family with large, double-stranded DNA viral genomes, icosahedral capsid symmetry, and a surrounding envelope derived from nuclear membrane. Only enveloped virions are infectious. The envelope is sensitive to drying and detergents, which may account for the extremely labile nature of VZV.

Transmission. Even among viruses, VZV is remarkable for the high level of communicability among susceptible individuals, with a secondary attack rate in susceptible siblings of more than 90%. Spread occurs by direct person-to-person contact and by airborne droplets. Spread by aerosolization and airflow has been documented, especially with outbreaks. Fomites are apparently not important. Persons with varicella are most contagious 1–2 days before and shortly after the onset of rash, although contagiousness persists until all lesions are crusted. Transmission of virus from zoster lesions in immunocompetent persons is uncommon. Humans are the only host, and there is no animal vector.

EPIDEMIOLOGY

Chickenpox occurs throughout the year with consistent annual peaks from March through May in temperate climates. The temporal distribution of cases in colder climates shows earlier onset and longer seasonal duration. Before varicella vaccine, more than 3 million cases of chickenpox occurred annually in the United States, distributed equally between the sexes, with more than 9,000 hospitalizations. More than 90% of cases occur in children 1–14 years of age. Approximately 90% of individuals older than 15 years, even those without recollection of chickenpox during childhood, have antibody to VZV.

Zoster results from reactivation of latent infection and occurs without seasonality or sex prediction. Only 5% of cases occur in children younger than 15 years of age, with steadily increasing incidence with advancing age, putatively associated with waning immunity. The overall incidence of zoster (215 cases per 100,000 person-years) results in a cumulative lifetime incidence of approximately 10–20%, with 75% of cases occurring after 45 years of age. Recurrences are rare and are commonly associated with underlying illness, such as HIV infection. Zoster has been described in children born to mothers who had chickenpox during pregnancy, which reflects reactivation of latent VZV that was acquired in utero.

PATHOGENESIS

VZV is acquired by direct contact or by respiratory spread and infects epithelial cells of the respiratory tract, with cell-to-cell spread. The virus is spread systemically through the bloodstream by infected mononuclear leukocytes. Infection of the epithelial cells of the corium and dermis results in the characteristic cutaneous **pocks.** As the vesicles evolve, the clear fluid becomes cloudy from degenerating cells and infiltrating neutrophils. The vesicle may rupture, especially with excoriation, or the fluid may be resorbed.

VZV establishes lifelong latent infection in the cells of the dorsal root ganglia, usually without producing further clinical symptoms. Reactivation, which usually occurs in the setting of waning immunity or exogenous immunosuppression, and retroaxonal migration of virus leads to localized cutaneous eruption and pain in the distribution of the associated dermatomes, which results in zoster. Involvement of the anterior horn cells is associated with excruciating pain and may result in motor paralysis similar to that of poliomyelitis. No specific factors are recognized as responsible for the reactivation of latent VZV and the development of zoster. Children who have chickenpox before 1 year of age may not develop complete cell-mediated immunity and appear to be more prone to zoster during childhood. Significant genomic diversity exists among clinical isolates of VZV, but researchers have identified no genomic differences, including changes of virus isolates from the same person at the time of primary infection and at the time of zoster, that account for the variable clinical expression.

SYMPTOMS AND CLINICAL MANIFESTATIONS

Incubation Period. The incubation period is classically 14–16 days, although secondary cases may be seen from as soon as 10 days to as long as 20 days after exposure. In immunocompromised persons the incubation period may be shorter, or it may be longer if VZIG postexposure prophylaxis is given.

Common Symptoms

Chickenpox. A wide range of clinical severity of infection exists in immunocompetent hosts, although asymptomatic primary infection is uncommon. Primary VZV infection typically develops as

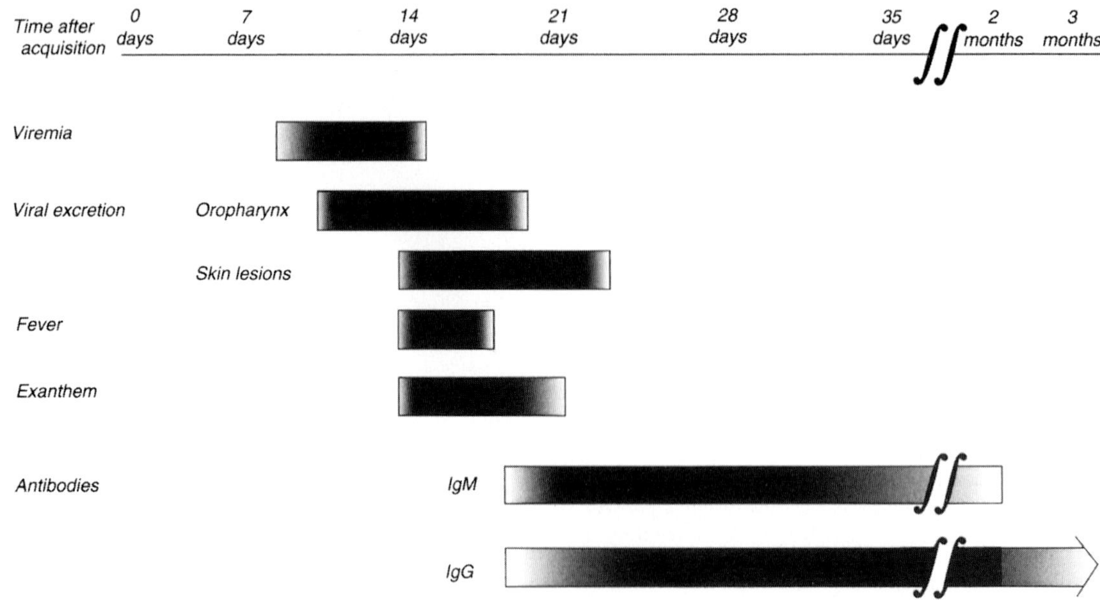

FIGURE 27–1. Profile of the typical clinical course of primary varicella (chickenpox).

a mild, pruritic vesicular rash, with mild to moderate fever paralleling the onset and severity of the rash (Fig. 27–1). The cutaneous lesions (Plate 4C) generally begin on the face, scalp, or trunk and spread centripetally to other areas of the body. The highest concentration of lesions occurs centrally over the trunk and proximal portions of the extremities. Occasionally a few lesions may be found on the mucous membranes of the mouth and conjunctivae and in the vagina and rectum. The vesicular rash is intensely pruritic. Lesions break out in successive crops for a 2–4 day period, with a total of approximately 300–500 lesions. Maximum daily temperature may range from slightly above normal to 40°C (104°F). Constitutional symptoms of malaise, anorexia, and lassitude accompany the fever but are generally mild. There are no associated symptoms of upper respiratory tract infection.

Secondary cases of chickenpox occurring in the same household typically are more symptomatic, with significantly more lesions, higher fever, and greater discomfort. This probably reflects the higher inoculum from closer and more prolonged contact of household members with the index case, in comparison with contact with playmates or schoolmates.

Modified Varicella-Like Syndrome. Breakthrough varicella occurring after varicella vaccination is significantly less severe than natural VZV infection. The rash is predominantly maculopapular, with only 30–50 lesions. Fever is usually absent or mild.

Progressive Varicella. In immunocompromised persons, especially those with hematologic malignancies, the symptoms may be significantly more intense, especially if untreated early in the course (Plate 4D). In approximately 25–50% of immunocompromised persons the fever is higher and more sustained; the rash continues to erupt for 1–2 weeks, usually with a much greater number of lesions; the cutaneous lesions show deeper involvement and more frequently have a hemorrhagic base, sometimes called **hemorrhagic varicella;** and symptomatic visceral involvement such as varicella pneumonia, meningoencephalitis, and hepatitis is more likely. The incidence of pneumonia is approximately 20%. Patients with leukemia with untreated primary VZV infection have an approximately 10% mortality rate.

Zoster. Zoster begins as a localized area of erythematous, maculopapular lesions that rapidly evolves and progresses into grouped, vesicular lesions typically involving from one to three sensory dermatomes, usually on the trunk (Fig. 27–2). A prodrome of fever, malaise, headache, and local pain or dysesthesia may occur 1–4 days before the onset of cutaneous lesions. New lesions continue to appear within the affected area for 3–5 days. Lesions typically last for 10–15 days. Zoster in children is usually only mildly painful. Conversely, in adults the pain of **acute neuritis** in the affected dermatomes is characteristically intense and constant. **Postherpetic neuralgia** is pain persisting longer than 1 month. There is usually no intervening period without pain, although postherpetic neuralgia can recur after pain-free intervals of various lengths of time. Fever and other systemic manifestations are typically absent.

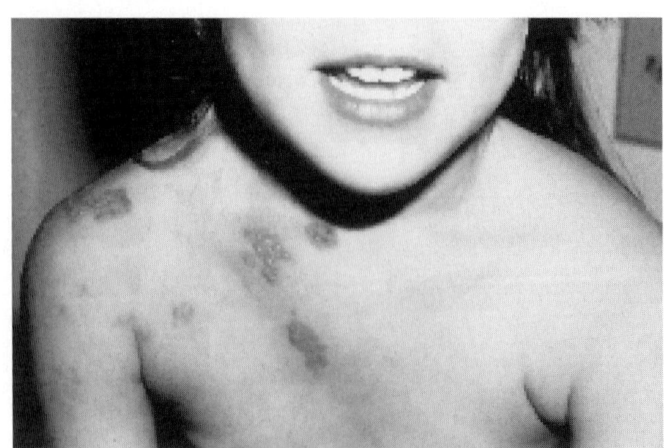

FIGURE 27–2. Zoster in a dermatomal distribution.

Disseminated Zoster. Disseminated zoster occurs almost exclusively in immunocompromised persons, with manifestations proportionate to the degree of cellular immune impairment. Development of localized zoster lesions is followed 4–11 days later by the generalized appearance of large numbers of vesicular lesions (Plate 4D). In untreated persons, sustained formation of new lesions continues for up to 2 weeks, with a prolonged interval to crusting. Approximately 5–25% of immunocompromised persons with zoster will develop cutaneous dissemination, and approximately 50% of these persons also have visceral involvement with varicella pneumonia, meningoencephalitis, and hepatitis. The mortality rate in untreated cases is approximately 33%, but with antiviral therapy it is less than 5%.

Physical Examination Findings

Chickenpox. The characteristic eruption begins as erythematous macules and rapidly progresses within hours to superficial, round vesicles on an erythematous base (Plate 4C). An evanescent generalized erythema may precede the vesicular rash. The majority of lesions are small, <5 mm in diameter, although some advanced lesions are more than twice as large (10–12 mm). The lesions continue to evolve for 1–2 days, with central umbilication of the vesicle, pustulation, sometimes spontaneous or traumatic disruption of the vesicle with drainage of turbid fluid, and finally maturation to a crusted ulceration. The surrounding erythema fades as the lesions crust and dry. Occasionally there may be a small amount of hemorrhage into the vesicopustules.

The rash is generalized but concentrated centrally and involves primarily the trunk and proximal extremities. The hallmark of the vesicular rash of chickenpox is its appearance in successive crops for 2–4 days, with lesions at all stages of development (macules, vesicles, pustules, crusting scabs) present at the same time in the same area. Lesions may be more heavily concentrated in areas of pre-existing dermal injury, such as with diaper dermatitis or sunburn. Generalized lymphadenopathy may occasionally be present, and regional lymphadenopathy may occur if there is secondary bacterial infection of lesions.

New lesion formation usually stops by 4 days, with crusting of all lesions by 6 days. The eschar typically remains for 1–2 weeks. When it falls off, it leaves pink, fresh skin with a slight depression that gradually resolves for 3–6 weeks with no residual scar formation. Excoriations may affect the appearance of the lesions. Scarring may develop from lesions that become secondarily infected or if eschars are removed prematurely.

Zoster. The grouped, vesicular lesions of zoster typically coalesce on an erythematous base and are distributed between one and three sensory dermatomes (Fig. 27–2). Lesions are unilateral and characteristically end abruptly at the midline, limited to the neural distribution. The vesicles may coalesce into bullous lesions. Occasionally a few solitary, isolated lesions on the contralateral side may be seen; they usually represent local rather than blood-borne spread of virus and are not indicative of disseminated disease. New lesions may continue to appear for 10–15 days. The affected area may not return to normal for 3–4 weeks.

Zoster in the distribution of the trigeminal nerve accounts for approximately 15% of zoster in adults (Fig. 27–3). Involvement of the maxillary or mandibular branch of the trigeminal nerve may result in lesions of the palate, tongue, or floor of the mouth. **Ramsay Hunt syndrome** is caused by zoster of the geniculate ganglion and results in a severe ipsilateral facial palsy, loss of taste in the anterior two thirds of the tongue, and cutaneous lesions involving the external auditory meatus. **Zoster ophthalmicus** is caused by involvement of the ophthalmic branch of the trigeminal nerve and results in well-demarcated zosteriform lesions over the forehead and eyelid. Lesions involving the retina may cause acute retinal necrosis and retinal detachment with a significant risk of blindness. Persons with zoster ophthalmicus may benefit from early antiviral and anti-inflammatory treatment to attempt to prevent loss of vision.

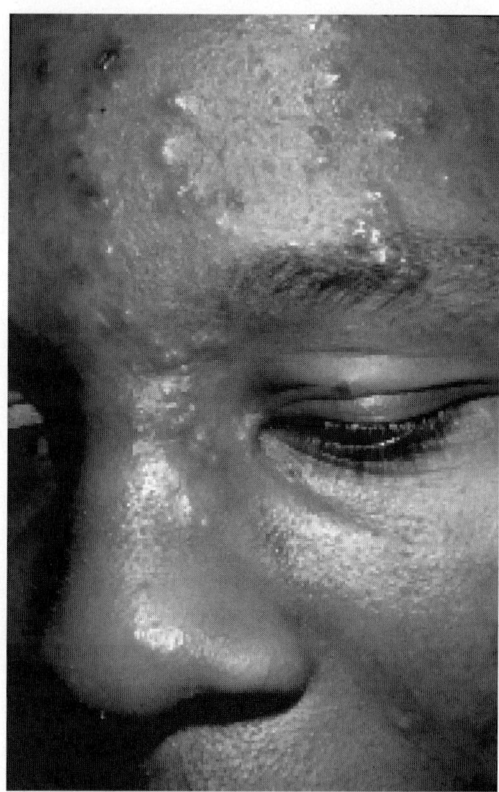

FIGURE 27–3. Zoster in the distribution of the trigeminal nerve (fifth cranial nerve).

Unusual Presentations

Bullous Varicella. Bullae occurring simultaneously with typical varicella vesicles are a result of secondary bacterial infection of varicelliform lesions with exfoliative toxigenic *Staphylococcus aureus.* Oral treatment with an antistaphylococcal agent such as a first-generation cephalosporin (e.g., cephalexin) or dicloxacillin is usually adequate.

Infection During Pregnancy and Fetal Infection. Pregnant women may be at increased risk of having varicella pneumonia, although the data are inconclusive. Infection of the fetus from the maternal viremia associated with chickenpox during the first trimester results in **congenital varicella embryopathy** in approximately 2% of cases (Chapter 94).

Perinatal Infection. Primary maternal VZV infection at the time of delivery, with onset of rash from 5 days before delivery to within 2 days after delivery, has an approximately 50% risk of severe systemic infection in the newborn. Neonatal infection is acquired by transplacental transmission associated with maternal viremia. Perinatal varicella is frequently complicated by visceral involvement, especially pneumonia, with a mortality rate in untreated newborns of approximately 25%. Maternal infection during this narrow window of time leads to the unique circumstances of transplacental transmission of a high burden of virus, and delivery of the newborn before development of the maternal humoral response and transmission of specific antibody to protect the fetus. Infants born to mothers with the onset of chickenpox rash from 5 days before delivery to within 2 days after delivery should receive VZIG postexposure prophylaxis.

Maternal infection that occurs more than 2 days after delivery represents a risk of horizontal transmission to the infant and is associated with neonatal illness approximately 2 weeks later but no increased risk of complications.

HIV Infection. Children with asymptomatic HIV infection generally tolerate primary VZV infection well. With progression of HIV infection to AIDS, chickenpox may have more severe cutaneous involvement and zoster may develop into chronic and recurrent zoster. Persons with AIDS should be considered immunocompromised for the purpose of treatment decisions regarding VZV infection.

DIAGNOSIS

The diagnosis of chickenpox, which is straightforward after known exposure or in the midst of a seasonal epidemic, is generally based on the distinctive characteristics of the rash. Laboratory testing for confirmation is usually not necessary.

Differential Diagnosis

In atypical cases or early in the course with few lesions, the rash may be confused with many other conditions (Table 27–1). The lesions of impetigo are characteristically located around the nares or mouth, are not associated with fever, and demonstrate gram-positive bacteria on Gram stain. The lesions of scabies may be localized or generalized but typically involve the hands and extremities predominantly; they are not as vesicular as chickenpox.

Historically the major differential diagnoses included smallpox and disseminated vaccinia. The eradication of smallpox and the discontinuation of smallpox vaccination have made the diagnosis of chickenpox less complicated.

Hand-Foot-and-Mouth Disease. This systemic febrile infection caused by coxsackievirus A is characterized by discrete, small, very tender vesicular lesions on the fingers, palms, and soles and in the oral cavity. The small number of lesions, their painful rather than pruritic nature, and the distal distribution differentiates this condition from chickenpox. The vesicles do not pustulate and crust.

Eczema Herpeticum. Eczema herpeticum, or **Kaposi's varicelliform eruption,** is a localized, vesicular eruption caused by herpes simplex virus. The eruption develops on skin with disruption of local cutaneous defenses, which results in a more aggressive, though localized, area of skin involvement. The classic underlying condition is eczema or atopic dermatitis, although trauma, burns, diaper dermatitis, or other cutaneous injury may permit more invasive skin infection by herpes simplex virus.

TABLE 27–1. Differential Diagnosis of Chickenpox

Impetigo
Insect bites
Scabies
Hand-foot-and-mouth disease
Disseminated herpes simplex virus infection
Eczema herpeticum
Rickettsialpox
Eczema vaccinatum
Generalized vaccinia
(Smallpox; no longer present)

Rickettsialpox. Rickettsialpox, caused by *Rickettsia akari,* is a zoonotic disease transmitted from mice to man by the bite of an infected mite. The resulting 5–30 mm papule at the original site of inoculation is followed by a febrile illness 7–10 days later (Chapter 34). The generalized papulovesicular rash of rickettsialpox appears within 2–3 days after the onset of fever with chills, rigor, headache, myalgia, and backache.

Smallpox. Smallpox, or **variola,** is caused by a poxvirus of the Orthopoxvirus genus. Smallpox is an important disease historically and through the late 1960s still caused 10–15 million cases annually in more than 30 countries. The last endemic case occurred in Somalia in 1977, although two laboratory-acquired cases occurred in 1978 in Birmingham, United Kingdom. Smallpox was declared eradicated by the World Health Organization on May 8, 1980. Today, virus stocks are kept only at the CDC in Atlanta and at the State Research Centre of Virology and Biotechnology in Novosibirsk, Russia. The successful global eradication of this disease is a unique accomplishment.

Smallpox is relatively noncontagious and requires close contact for spread by respiratory droplet. It is clinically characterized by an incubation period of 12 days (range, 7–17 days) and a prodromal period of 2–4 days of high fever, malaise, and prostration, followed by a rash that progresses for 7–14 days from macules to vesicles to crusting (Fig. 27–4). Unlike chickenpox, the lesions of smallpox are distributed centrifugally, affect primarily the distal limbs, and include the palms and soles. Pocks in any regional area are in the same stage of development. They are deeply embedded in the dermis and leave scars on healing. **Variola major,** or classic smallpox, had a case-fatality rate of 20% or more, with a mortality rate of almost 100% if associated with hemorrhagic lesions. **Variola minor,** caused by a less virulent strain, had a mortality rate of less than 1%. **Varioloid** was a mild illness that occurred in individuals immunized with smallpox who had pre-existing partial immunity.

Another Orthopoxvirus, **vaccinia,** is morphologically indistinguishable from smallpox virus, shares common antigens, and has been used for vaccination against smallpox. Cutaneous complications immediately after smallpox vaccination with vaccinia may resemble VZV lesions, with a localized vaccinial eruption in persons with eczema **(eczema vaccinatum)**, generalized vaccinia with vaccinial lesions appearing at sites distant from the inoculation, or progressive vaccinia in persons with underlying immunodeficiencies, leading to death in approximately 33% of persons.

Monkeypox. Monkeypox virus, another Orthopoxvirus, causes a vesicular illness in monkeys throughout Africa. Rare cases have occurred in humans after direct contact with infected monkeys. The resulting vesicular disease is similar to variola but is not generally communicable to other humans.

Laboratory Evaluation

The WBC count classically shows a leukocytosis with a predominance of neutrophils, although the degree varies. Asymptomatic thrombocytopenia resulting from transient viral depression of platelet formation may occur. Up to 75% of patients have mild to moderate elevation of hepatic aminotransferase values, which is sometimes accompanied by vomiting but no other specific evidence of Reye's syndrome (Chapter 55). Persons with varicella encephali-

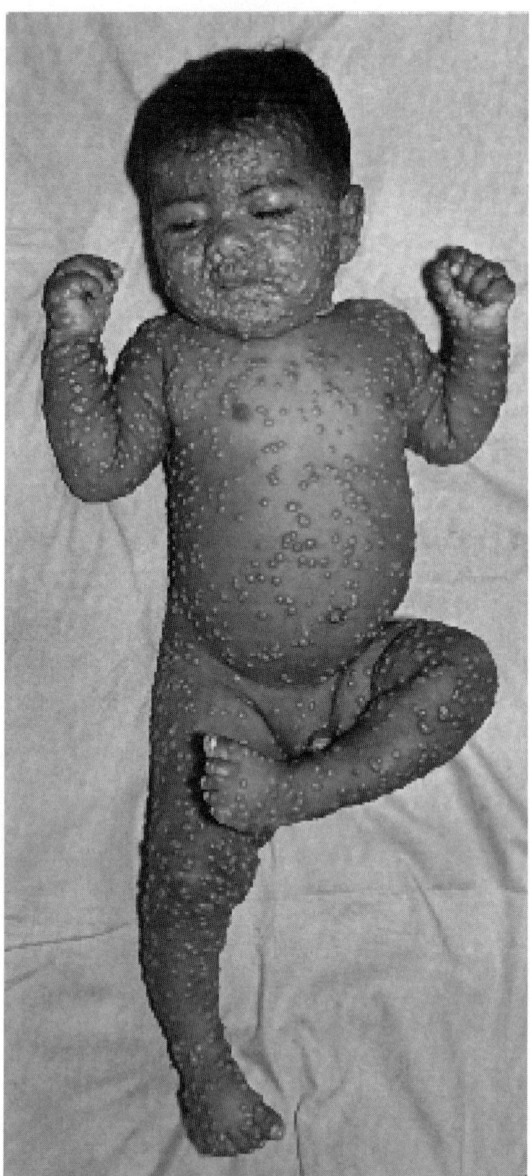

FIGURE 27–4. Lesions of variola major (smallpox) about 7 days after the onset of rash. (Courtesy World Health Organization.)

tis will have a modest, predominantly lymphocytic pleocytosis with an elevated protein value and normal cerebrospinal fluid glucose values. Many patients with zoster, especially that involving the cranial nerves, have mild pleocytosis even without specific central nervous system symptoms. The cerebrospinal fluid WBC count and protein level cannot be used alone to diagnose meningoencephalitis caused by VZV.

Microbiologic Evaluation

The diagnosis may be confirmed by direct examination or viral culture of vesicle fluid and by serologic testing. Immunofluorescence testing of the cellular debris or the roof of a vesicle provides rapid and accurate identification of VZV. Immunofluorescence tests have supplanted the less sensitive and less specific histopathologic smears such as the **Tzanck smear** for syncytial giant cells.

Viral Culture. Virus may be cultured from the blood immediately before and during the early vesicular stage and is easily cultured from vesicular lesions. The best material for viral isolation is the roof of a vesicular lesion. Although culture is not routinely necessary, it should be performed to confirm the diagnosis in immunocompromised persons with either localized or systemic involvement. This is especially important to distinguish disseminated infection caused by either VZV or herpes simplex virus. Viral culture of VZV usually requires 7–10 days. Virus also may be cultured from skin lesions of zoster, from peripheral blood mononuclear cells of persons with progressive varicella or of immunocompetent persons immediately before the onset of rash, and from the cerebrospinal fluid of persons with meningoencephalitis. Although transmission of VZV presumably occurs via respiratory spread, the virus cannot be isolated from the upper respiratory tract.

Serologic Testing. Antibodies to VZV are detectable by several methods, including the **fluorescent antibody to membrane antigen (FAMA) test,** immune adherence hemagglutination, enzyme-linked immunosorbent assay, and particle agglutination. Serologic diagnosis is established by seroconversion or by demonstration of at least a fourfold rise in antibody titer between acute- and convalescent-phase sera. The complement fixation test is inexpensive and may be used for diagnosis of acute infection. However, this test is not reliable for determination of immunity because antibodies detected by this method wane after acute infection, frequently yielding false-negative results.

Diagnostic Imaging

Radiographs of the chest are indicated for persons with chickenpox who have acute respiratory symptoms. In a prospective study (Weber, 1965), 16% of young men with chickenpox had radiographic abnormalities on chest radiography, although only 4% had a nonproductive cough and only 2% had dyspnea. Asymptomatic pulmonary involvement appears to occur frequently in adults with primary VZV infection.

TREATMENT

Both acyclovir and vidarabine have in vitro and in vivo efficacy against VZV, although acyclovir is generally preferred because it is less toxic, requires less additional fluid administration for intravenous administration, and is available in an oral formulation. The value of acyclovir for treatment of uncomplicated chickenpox in immunocompetent children is dubious, but early therapy is mandatory for immunocompromised persons to minimize dissemination and the associated complications (Table 27–2). Therapy for immunocompetent persons is recommended for zoster to minimize development of postherpetic neuralgia and is mandatory for disseminated zoster infection. Valacyclovir and famciclovir are preferred for treatment of zoster in adults.

Definitive Treatment

Chickenpox. Oral administration of acyclovir to immunocompetent persons with primary VZV infection within 24 hours of the onset of rash results in an approximately 15–30% reduction in the severity of cutaneous lesions (the number and duration of lesions, and the period of formation of new lesions) and a 1-day decrease in the duration and magnitude of fever and constitutional symptoms. Treatment has not been shown to decrease the severity of pruritus, rate of complications, spread of infection, or absence from school. The routine oral administration of acyclovir is not recommended in otherwise healthy children because of the marginal therapeutic benefit, the lack of difference in complications, and the cost of acyclovir treatment. Furthermore, the possible development

TABLE 27–2. Treatment of Varicella-Zoster Infections

Patient Group	Treatment: Recommended	Treatment: Alternative
Immunocompetent Persons		
Uncomplicated chickenpox in healthy children	Not routinely recommended	Acyclovir 20 mg/kg/dose (max: 800 mg) qid PO for 5 days
Uncomplicated chickenpox in selected persons Nonpregnant individuals ≥13 yr of age Children ≥12 mo of age: With a chronic cutaneous disorder With a chronic pulmonary disorder Receiving short-course, intermittent, or aerosolized corticosteroids Receiving long-term salicylate therapy as second cases in household contacts	***Children*** Acyclovir 20 mg/kg/dose (max: 800 mg) qid PO for 5 days ***Adolescents and Adults*** Famciclovir 500 mg tid PO for 7–10 days *or* Valacyclovir 1 g tid PO for 7–10 days	 ***Adolescents and Adults*** Acyclovir 800 mg PO 5 times a day for 5 days
Uncomplicated zoster	***Children*** Acyclovir 20 mg/kg/dose (max: 800 mg) PO 5 times a day for 5–7 days ***Adolescents and Adults*** Famciclovir 500 mg tid PO for 7–10 days *or* Valacyclovir 1 g tid PO for 7–10 days *And,* for relatively healthy persons ≥50 yr of age with moderate to severe pain at presention: Corticosteroids orally (adult regimen: prednisone, 60 mg for 7 days, 30 mg for 7 days, and 15 mg for 7 days)	 ***Adolescents and Adults*** Acyclovir 800 mg PO 5 times a day for 7–10 days
Varicella pneumonia Disseminated zoster Ophthalmic zoster	***Children*** Acyclovir 10–20 mg/kg/dose q8hr IV for 7–10 days ***Adolescents and Adults*** Acyclovir 10 mg/kg/dose q8hr IV for 7–10 days	***Children, Adolescents, and Adults*** Vidarabine 10 mg/kg/dose qd IV for 7–10 days
Immunocompromised Persons		
Chickenpox, or localized or disseminated zoster*	***Children*** Acyclovir 10–20 mg/kg/dose q8hr IV for 7–10 days ***Adolescents and Adults*** Acyclovir 10 mg/kg/dose q8hr IV for 7–10 days	
Acyclovir-Resistant VZV	Foscarnet 40 mg/kg/dose q8hr IV for 10 days	

*Oral therapy may be considered for selected immunocompromised persons with mild disease perceived to be at lower risk of severe varicella.

of virus resistance with widespread use of antiviral agents is a concern.

For selected persons who are not otherwise immunocompromised and are at increased risk, but not at high risk, of having severe chickenpox, oral acyclovir should be considered if it can be given within 24 hours after the onset of rash (Table 27–2). The decision to treat should be based on an informed discussion with the patient and the family, with emphasis on the modest clinical benefit and the continued risk of complications. Persons at increased risk of having severe chickenpox who might benefit from antiviral treatment include previously healthy nonpregnant individuals 13 years of age or older, children 12 months of age or older with a chronic cutaneous or pulmonary disorder, and persons receiving short-course or intermittent oral corticosteroids or aerosolized corticosteroids. If possible, corticosteroid use should be discontinued on recognized exposure to varicella. Children receiving long-term salicylate therapy who are at risk of developing Reye's syndrome may also benefit from oral acyclovir therapy. The use of oral acyclovir for uncomplicated infection in immunocompetent persons is not recommended during pregnancy or in children less than 12 months of age because there are insufficient data regarding the safety and efficacy of acyclovir in these groups. Treatment of second cases in household contacts of the index case is recommended because the population at risk is easily defined, the rate of transmission is very high among siblings and transmission is essentially unavoidable, the timing of illness (if it develops) can be anticipated because the incubation period is regular, and parents can be attuned to the symptoms so that oral therapy can be started early in the illness.

Unfortunately, selective administration of acyclovir for unusually severe but otherwise uncomplicated cases of chickenpox in immunocompetent persons is impractical. By the time the severity of illness is manifested, the disease is well established and the administration of acyclovir has an inconsequential mollifying effect on symptoms.

Zoster. Antiviral treatment of zoster is indicated to hasten the return to usual activity levels and of zoster ophthalmicus to mitigate loss of vision (Table 27–2). The principal complication of zoster is the often-debilitating pain, especially in adults, in association with acute neuritis and postherpetic neuralgia. Antiviral treatment accelerates cutaneous healing, hastens the resolution of acute neuritis, and reduces the risk of postherpetic neuralgia. Oral famciclovir, which is the prodrug of the active metabolite penciclovir, and valacyclovir, which is the L-valyl ester prodrug of acyclovir, have much greater bioavailability than acyclovir and are recommended for treatment of zoster in adults. Pediatric formulations of famciclovir and valacyclovir are not available. Acyclovir is recommended for children and is an alternative therapy for adults. The necessity of concomitant oral corticosteroids for zoster remains controversial, but this therapy is recommended for relatively healthy persons more than 50 years of age with moderate or severe pain at presentation. No studies of concomitant corticosteroids for zoster have been performed in children.

Immunocompromised Persons. Congenital or acquired immune defects (including HIV infection), hematogenous cancer or anticancer chemotherapy, or bone marrow or solid organ transplantation predisposes a person to more severe infection with primary VZV infection and to dissemination with zoster, including visceral involvement and death. To a lesser degree the use of corticosteroids, particularly with daily high doses (1–2 mg/kg/day), also increases the risk of severe infection. Immunocompromised persons who receive VZIG prophylaxis may still have a mild form of disease.

Immunocompromised persons who did not receive VZIG prophylaxis should be treated with intravenous acyclovir as soon as VZV infection is recognized. Oral therapy may be considered for selected immunocompromised persons with mild disease who are perceived to be at a lower risk of having severe varicella, such as HIV-infected persons with normal CD4 T-lymphocyte counts and persons who received VZIG immediately after exposure. When started early, antiviral therapy slows new lesion formation, decreases the time to healing, and significantly decreases the likelihood of visceral involvement. Immunocompromised persons may also require supportive treatment for pneumonia or encephalitis and should be managed in a center with adequate pediatric intensive care support.

Supportive Treatment

Chickenpox. Pruritus is the primary complaint of most children with chickenpox. Symptomatic local treatment includes the application of a drying antipruritic lotion such as calamine lotion, which can be used either alone or with 0.25% menthol, which serves as a local anesthetic and external analgesic. Bathing in colloidal oatmeal (Aveeno) may relieve pruritus. Lotion with phenol should not be used by pregnant women or for children younger than 6 months of age. Oral lesions may be treated with cool compresses with tap water or Burow's solution for 10 minutes 3–4 times a day. Cleansing mouthwashes with benzalkonium chloride (Zephiran) 1:1000 or with tetracycline suspension (250 mg/60 mL water) clean and soothe the mouth and help prevent secondary bacterial infection. Vulvovaginitis and perineal lesions should be managed by sitz baths in tepid water with or without colloidal oatmeal (Aveeno). Treatment with oral antihistamines (e.g., diphenhydramine hydrochloride) may be useful in more severely symptomatic cases, especially before bedtime, but may cause unwanted drowsiness at other times.

Fingernails of young children should be trimmed to minimize excoriation and reduce the likelihood of secondary bacterial infection. Lesions should be carefully cleansed with water and patted dry. Prophylactic therapy with antibiotics to prevent secondary bacterial infections of skin lesions is not warranted.

Acetaminophen should be used for control of fever. Because of the increased risk of Reye's syndrome with salicylate use during chickenpox, patients with chickenpox or zoster should not receive salicylates. Adequate intake of oral fluids should be encouraged.

Zoster. Burow's solution dressings are soothing and cleansing for lesions of zoster. Pain associated with zoster, either from the acute neuritis or postherpetic neuralgia, should be managed with appropriate analgesics. Acetaminophen should be used initially, followed by stronger agents if necessary, titrated according to their efficacy and adverse effects.

Postherpetic neuralgia refers to the characteristically intense, sometimes incapacitating, pain in the affected dermatomes that persists longer than 1 month after the resolution of cutaneous zoster lesions. It is uncommon in children but occurs with increasing frequency and is of longer duration with advancing age (Fig. 27–5). Approximately 67% of persons with postherpetic neuralgia are more than 30 years of age. The neuralgia has an inflammatory component; weekly intrathecal injections of methylprednisolone for up to 4 weeks is an effective treatment for intractable postherpetic neuralgia. There is no evidence of the efficacy of antiviral drugs in the treatment of postherpetic neuralgia.

Typically the pain is debilitating, which necessitates aggressive pain management. Numerous symptomatic treatment regimens have been suggested for severe cases of postherpetic neuralgia, but no single drug or treatment has emerged as clearly superior. In many cases such therapy may have to be continued for months. Oxycodone, gabapentin, several tricyclic antidepressants, and topical lidocaine patches have each demonstrated efficacy in the treatment of postherpetic neuralgia. A commonly used regimen recommended for initial management of severe cases in adults is a combination of a tricyclic antidepressant (amitriptyline 75–100 mg/day orally) and a substituted phenothiazine (perphenazine 4 mg 3 or 4 times per day orally; fluphenazine 1 mg 3 or 4 times per day orally; or thioridazine 25 mg 4 times per day orally). Capsaicin cream applied topically 3 or 4 times a day may also be useful. Severe cases may require treatment in conjunction with a dermatologist or pain management specialist experienced with postherpetic neuralgia.

COMPLICATIONS

Except for superficial secondary bacterial infection of cutaneous lesions, complications of chickenpox are uncommon in immunocompetent persons. Most complications are related to secondary bacterial infections of the skin or lower respiratory tract or to VZV infection of internal organs, leading to pneumonia, meningoencephalitis, or hepatitis (Table 27–3). Chickenpox is a systemic infection and is occasionally associated with nephritis, myocarditis, arthritis, myositis, uveitis, orchitis, and idiopathic thrombocytopenic pur-

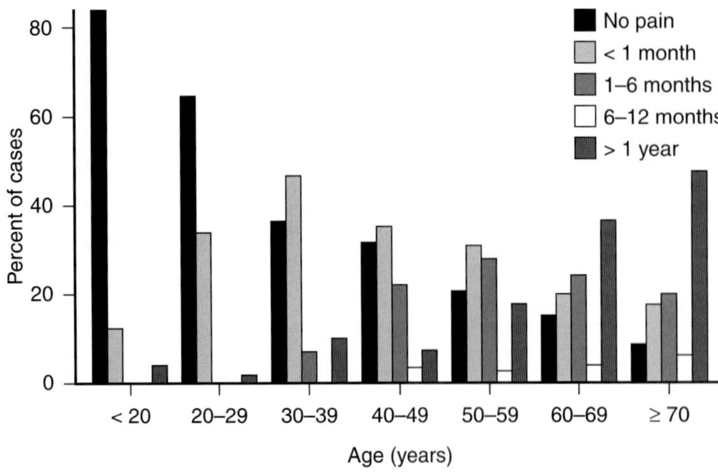

FIGURE 27–5. Age distribution and duration of postherpetic neuralgia in 916 patients with zoster. (Data from de Moragas JM, Kierland RR: The outcome of patients with herpes zoster. *Arch Dermatol* 1957;75:193.)

pura. Adults have complication rates 10–20 times that of children and account for more than half of deaths (Table 27–4). Successfully avoiding both the disease during childhood and vaccination incurs a continued risk of primary infection through adulthood, with the attendant increased risk of more severe complications.

Secondary Bacterial Infection. The disruption of the cutaneous barrier and the excoriation accompanying the pruritus commonly result in secondary bacterial infection of the skin lesions and cellulitis. This is the most common complication of chickenpox in children. The classic bacterium causing secondary bacterial infections associated with VZV infection is group A *Streptococcus,* although *Staphylococcus* is also frequently present. Secondary bacterial infection is suggested by fever (temperature >39°C [102.2°F]) more than 3 days after the onset of rash, increased fever, or recrudescence of fever. Bacteremia and distant foci of bacterial infection may occur, especially in immunocompromised persons. Topical antibiotic therapy with mupirocin may be used for local treatment of isolated secondarily infected lesions. Systemic treatment with an oral first-generation cephalosporin (e.g., cephalexin) or dicloxacillin is indicated for cellulitis or widespread bacterial infection, especially for involvement around the eyes, mouth, ear ducts, or perineum that precludes topical treatment.

TABLE 27–3. Complications of Chickenpox

Acute
Secondary bacterial infection of skin and soft tissues
Pneumonia
Bacteremia
Acute cerebellar ataxia
Meningitis
Encephalitis
Hepatitis
Reye's syndrome
Late
Guillain-Barré syndrome
Zoster, with:
Postherpetic neuralgia
Meningitis
Encephalitis
Keratitis
Retinitis
Pneumonitis

Pneumonia. Varicella pneumonia is uncommon in healthy children but is the most frequent serious complication of varicella in adults and immunocompromised persons. It occurs in 0.3–1.8% of healthy adults and in 42–47% of smokers with primary varicella. Pregnant women may be at increased risk, although the data are inconclusive. Varicella pneumonia usually occurs during the period of late cutaneous involvement and is clinically evident by tachypnea, dyspnea, cough, and sometimes pleuritic chest pain and hemoptysis. The chest radiograph shows bilateral involvement with a diffuse, variable amount of reticulonodular or interstitial infiltrate with a prominent peribronchial distribution (Fig. 27–6). The course of varicella pneumonia is extremely variable. It may resolve without significant respiratory distress or may progress to include severe pneumonia, pulmonary edema, and pleural effusion. Prompt initiation of acyclovir is associated with reduction of fever and tachypnea and with improvement in oxygenation.

Acute Cerebellar Ataxia. Acute cerebellar ataxia occurs in approximately 1 in 4,000 cases of chickenpox. It typically occurs toward the end of the first week after the onset of rash, but it may occur up to 21 days later and is manifested by fever, vomiting, and nuchal rigidity, with cerebellar signs of ataxia, vertigo, tremor, and nystagmus. The cerebrospinal fluid usually demonstrates a lymphocytic pleocytosis with elevated protein and normal glucose levels. The cerebellar symptoms are self-limited and resolve completely in 2–4 weeks.

Aseptic Meningitis and Encephalitis. Central nervous system involvement with chickenpox is usually manifested as acute cerebellar ataxia, although cerebral and cerebellar involvement may occur either alone or in combination. Clinical meningoencephalitis

TABLE 27–4. Estimated Risk of Varicella-Associated Complications in Adults and Children*

Complication	Adults	Children
Encephalitis	15/100,000	1.7/100,000
Reye's syndrome	Not reported	3.2/100,000
Hospitalization	18/1,000	1.7/1,000
Death	50/100,000	2.0/100,000

*From Plotkin SA, Friedman HM, Starr SE, et al: Vaccines against viruses of the herpes group. In Root RK, Warren KS, Griffiss JM, et al (editors): *Immunization.* New York, Churchill Livingstone, 1988, pp 65–92.

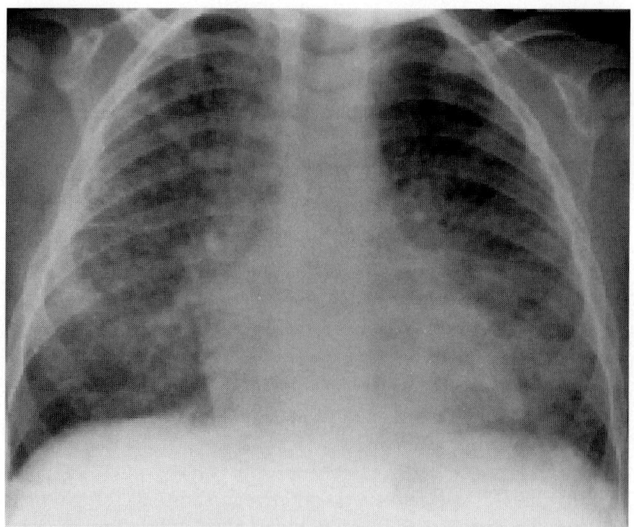

FIGURE 27–6. Varicella pneumonia in 3-year-old boy recovering from acute lymphocytic leukemia. A frontal chest radiograph shows extensive infiltration of both lungs with multiple nodular densities that sometimes overlap and coalesce. This pattern is typical of, but not exclusive for, varicella pneumonia. When healed, these lesions may leave small calcifications scattered throughout the lungs.

occurs in fewer than 0.1% of cases of varicella, and neither the incidence nor the severity correlates with the intensity of other symptoms. Symptoms of encephalitis, with fever, altered sensorium, seizures, and vomiting, usually develop toward the end of the first week after the onset of rash, although they occasionally appear simultaneously. The duration of symptoms is generally at least 2 weeks. The mortality rate for varicella encephalitis is 5–20%, with neurologic sequelae in approximately 15% of survivors.

Transverse myelitis, optic neuritis, and peripheral neuritis may occur during acute VZV infection. Guillain-Barré syndrome has also been reported.

Hepatitis. Subclinical hepatic involvement, detectable only by elevated hepatic aminotransferase levels, is frequently present during uncomplicated chickenpox. Vomiting suggests varicella hepatitis. More severe symptoms are uncommon but are seen with increased frequency in immunocompromised persons.

Reye's Syndrome. In persons with chickenpox and other viral infections, the higher risk of Reye's syndrome increases with salicylate administration during the viral illness. Therefore aspirin use is contraindicated in persons with chickenpox.

PROGNOSIS

Chickenpox. Primary varicella is generally a benign and uncomplicated illness. Lesions of chickenpox left to resolve spontaneously usually heal without scarring. Lesions complicated by secondary bacterial infection or premature removal of the eschar may leave a small scar. Historically, approximately 100 deaths related to varicella occurred each year in the United States before the introduction of the varicella vaccine. Less than 5% of varicella cases occur among persons older than 20 years of age, but this group accounts for 55% of varicella-related deaths. The mortality rate for untreated VZV infection among persons with hematogenous cancer is 7–14% among children and approaches 50% among adults. Although only 0.1% of VZV infections occur in immunocompromised persons, they account for 25% of fatalities.

Primary infection confers lifelong immunity, but asymptomatic reinfection may occur and has been documented, especially in adults with household VZV exposure. Symptomatic reinfection in immunocompetent persons is distinctly rare but may be more likely in immunocompromised persons.

Zoster. Zoster is usually a self-limited illness that resolves without complications even without specific antiviral treatment, especially in children. Advancing age and severity of pain at presentation and at 1 month are significant predictors of prolonged pain. The incidence and duration of postherpetic neuralgia is reduced with antiviral treatment of zoster. Scarring of affected areas is common in zoster because of deeper skin involvement.

PREVENTION

There is no indication for empirical prophylactic treatment with acyclovir of susceptible individuals after casual or even close contact with an index case. Persons receiving short, intermittent, or aerosolized corticosteroids should discontinue their use, if possible, after known exposure to varicella.

Vaccination. An attenuated live viral vaccine using the **Oka strain** of VZV was licensed in 1995. The vaccine is 85% effective in preventing disease and is 97% effective in preventing moderately severe and severe disease. The vaccine strain persists in vivo and appears to reactivate as antibody titers decline, with absent or only mild symptoms, and provides an immunologic boost that may extend the duration of immunity. Routine immunization is recommended for all children at 12–18 months of age and for children 19 months of age to the 13th birthday without a history of chickenpox. Susceptible persons ≥13 years of age at high risk of exposure or transmission should also be immunized. These include persons who live or work in environments where transmission is likely, such as teachers of young children, child-care employees, and residents and staff in institutional settings; persons who live or work in environments where transmission can occur, such as college students, inmates and staff of correctional institutions, and military personnel; adolescents and adults living in households with children; and international travelers. Serologic testing may be used to identify susceptible adolescents and adults, if desired. Varicella vaccination is recommended for all susceptible health care workers and for outbreak control of VZV in child-care facilities, schools, and institutions.

The dosage regimen for children 12 months to 12 years is a single 0.5 mL intramuscular injection; for persons ≥13 years of age the dosage is two 0.5 mL doses given 4–8 weeks apart. The age-specific incidence of zoster appears to be lower among children immunized with varicella vaccine than among children with natural infection. Studies of varicella immunization of older adults are in progress to evaluate the potential benefit of vaccination to decrease the incidence of zoster in persons who had chickenpox as children.

Persons with cellular immunodeficiencies, including blood dyscrasias, leukemia, lymphomas of any type, and malignant neoplasms affecting the bone marrow or lymphatic systems, should not be given varicella vaccination. The manufacturer provides free vaccine to any physician through an investigational protocol for use in persons with acute lymphocytic leukemia who meet certain criteria.

Persons with only humoral immunodeficiency should be immunized. Because HIV-infected children are at increased risk of morbidity from chickenpox and zoster, varicella vaccination should be considered for children with asymptomatic or mildly asymptomatic HIV infection in CDC class N1 or A1, with age-specific CD4 T-lymphocyte percentages of ≥25%. These children should receive two doses of varicella vaccine 3 months apart and should be encouraged to return for evaluation of any postvaccination varicella-like rash.

Isolation of Patients with Chickenpox. Immunocompetent persons are most contagious during the 1–2 days immediately preceding the onset of rash and for as long as 5 days later, coincident with the development and resolution of vesicular lesions. Crusting of lesions is considered an indication of resolution and diminished contagiousness. Immunocompetent persons with uncomplicated chickenpox should remain at home and excluded from school and other group settings until all lesions are crusted and no new lesions are appearing. This is usually about the sixth day after the onset of rash but may occur earlier in mild cases. Immunocompromised persons and others with prolonged illness should remain at home until all lesions are crusted.

Quarantine of persons with chickenpox and their contacts is not routine because the period of highest communicability is immediately preceding the onset of rash. Significant exposure has already occurred before diagnosis. Efforts to isolate siblings and household contacts are ineffective and are not recommended.

Isolation of Patients with Zoster. Although virus can be cultured from zoster lesions, the viral burden is typically low. Persons with zoster do not excrete virus in respiratory secretions. If the cutaneous lesions can be covered, they pose no risk even to susceptible individuals, and therefore persons with zoster may return to their school or usual daytime activities with adequate dressings covering the lesions. Persons with lesions that cannot be covered, either because of uncooperativeness or because of the anatomic location of the lesion, should be excluded until the lesions have crusted. All individuals who touch zoster lesions should wash their hands thoroughly.

Postexposure Prophylaxis

Postexposure prophylaxis is warranted for susceptible persons on the basis of the likelihood of susceptibility, the probability of transmission from the index case, and the probability of severe illness or complications if infection develops (Table 27–5). Children younger than 13 years without a history of chickenpox or vaccination are considered susceptible. Nonimmunized adolescents ≥13 years of age and adults are considered to be immune unless serologic testing demonstrates susceptibility. Most healthy adults with a negative or uncertain history of chickenpox have a high probability of having protective immunity. Serologic testing of immunocompetent older adolescents and adults can be performed if the results can be obtained within 72 hours from the time of exposure. Persons who routinely receive IVIG (100–400 mg/kg) are considered protected and do not require additional prophylaxis if IVIG was administered within 3 weeks, or within 2 weeks with HIV infection.

Immunocompetent Persons. Postexposure vaccination with varicella vaccine is effective in preventing illness or modifying severity in immunocompetent persons if administered within 72 hours, and possibly up to 120 hours, of exposure, and it is recommended for susceptible persons after exposure. There is no evidence that vaccination during the incubation or prodromal phase of chickenpox increases the risk of vaccine-associated adverse events. If exposure does not cause infection, the vaccination provides protection against subsequent exposure.

Acyclovir chemoprophylaxis is not routinely recommended, but chemoprophylaxis for healthy adult contacts with acyclovir beginning at 7–9 days after exposure may be used if vaccination is contraindicated or after late presentations. Chemoprophylaxis

TABLE 27–5. Postexposure Prophylaxis to Varicella-Zoster Virus

Varicella Immunization

Immunocompetent healthy persons ≥12 mo of age, within 72 (possibly 120) hr of exposure (as soon as possible)

VZIG (as soon as possible, but must be administered within 96 hr of exposure)

Newborn infants of mothers with onset of chickenpox from within 5 days before delivery to within 48 hr after delivery

Susceptible persons, defined as

- Immunocompromised persons (including HIV infection) without a history of chickenpox
- Susceptible pregnant women
- Hospitalized premature infants (≥28 wk gestational age) whose mothers lack a reliable history of chickenpox or serologic evidence of immunity
- Hospitalized premature infants (<28 wk gestational age, or ≤1,000 g birth weight), regardless of maternal history of chickenpox or serologic status
- With significant exposure to VZV, defined as
  - Household contact (residing in the same household)
  - Playmate contact (face-to-face contact of ≥1 hr*)
  - Hospital contact with chickenpox
    - In the same 2- to 4-bed room
    - Adjacent beds in a large ward
    - Face-to-face contact (≥1 hr*) with an infectious staff member
    - Visit by a person deemed infectious
  - Hospital contact with zoster
    - Close contact (e.g., touching or hugging) with a person deemed contagious

*Some experts suggest face-to-face contact of ≥5 minutes as constituting significant exposure for postexposure prophylaxis.

decreases the incidence and severity of the rash and fever, but seroconversion is variable and the protection afforded and the duration of immunity resulting from such subclinical infection are unknown.

Immunocompromised Persons. The use of VZIG is recommended for immunocompromised persons for postexposure prophylaxis. It may either prevent or ameliorate symptomatic illness and is thought to provide protection for 3 weeks. Modified infection after VZIG prophylaxis may not result in development of protective immunity, especially in immunocompromised persons, and these individuals should be considered as continuing to remain at risk with subsequent VZV exposure. VZIG can be given to healthy but susceptible adults for postexposure prophylaxis, but its use is not routinely recommended.

VZIG contains 10–18% globulin and is available in vials of 125 units in a volume of approximately 1.25 mL. It is administered as a single intramuscular injection in a dose of 125 units (the minimum dose) for each 10 kg increment of body weight, to a maximum dose of 625 units (i.e., 5 vials). VZIG should be administered as soon as possible after exposure but within 96 hours. IVIG is an alternative for persons with bleeding diatheses who cannot receive intramuscular injections.

Newborns. Newborns whose mothers develop chickenpox from 5 days before delivery to within 2 days after delivery may become infected by transplacental transmission associated with maternal viremia (Chapter 97). Administration of VZIG to mothers within 5 days of delivery is unlikely to result in protective levels of antibody in the fetus, so administration of VZIG directly to newborns immediately after birth is necessary. Newborns should be given 125 units of VZIG immediately after delivery or as soon as the maternal rash is recognized. Normal term infants whose mothers develop the rash of primary varicella 2 or more days postnatally or who are otherwise exposed to chickenpox or zoster do not have a higher risk of severe primary disease or complications than older children. Therefore VZIG is not indicated for these cases. Premature or low-birth-weight infants who have reached mature weight and who have been discharged from the hospital also do not require postexposure prophylaxis with VZIG.

Hospitalized Patients. Because of the highly contagious nature of VZV, hospitalization of patients with chickenpox should be carefully considered. If hospitalization is indicated, infected patients should not be located near immunocompromised persons. Hospitalization in an adolescent or adult unit, where the other patients are likely to be immune, may be preferable. Strict respiratory isolation in a negative pressure room for at least 5 days after the onset of rash, or until the vesicular lesions are crusting, is necessary.

Susceptible inpatients inadvertently exposed to VZV should preferably be discharged from the hospital before 10 days after the onset of rash in the index patient. If this is not possible, these inpatients should remain in strict isolation during days 8–21 after exposure. Hospitalized persons receiving VZIG should be isolated until 28 days after exposure.

Immunocompetent persons hospitalized with localized zoster do not require isolation beyond standard precautions; wound precautions are used in handling open lesions. Immunocompetent persons with disseminated zoster, and immunocompromised persons with zoster may shed the virus through the respiratory tract. These patients should remain in respiratory isolation in a negative pressure room until all cutaneous lesions are crusted.

Hospitalized infants born at or before 28 weeks of gestational age or with birth weights less than 1,000 g who are exposed to VZV in the hospital should receive 125 units of VZIG as soon as possible after exposure. Premature infants born after 28 weeks of gestation who are exposed to VZV and whose mothers have not had chickenpox should also receive 125 units of VZIG as soon as possible after exposure. Postexposure prophylaxis with VZIG is not necessary for preterm infants who have been discharged from the hospital because they have reached mature weight.

Medical Personnel. Health care workers exposed to VZV who have negative or unknown histories of previous varicella infection should have serologic testing performed as soon as possible. If immunity is demonstrated, workers may continue with their usual activities. Seronegative personnel should be furloughed or excused from patient care during days 8–21 after exposure. Susceptible health care workers should receive varicella immunization.

REVIEWS

Preblud SR, Orenstein WR, Bart KJ: Varicella: Clinical manifestations, epidemiology and health impact in children. *Pediatr Infect Dis* 1984;3: 505–9.

Preblud SR: Varicella: Complications and costs. *Pediatrics* 1986;78: 728–35.

Strauss SE, Ostrove JM, Inchauspe G, et al: NIH Conference. Varicella-zoster virus infections. Biology, natural history, treatment, and prevention. *Ann Intern Med* 1988;108:221–37.

KEY ARTICLES

American Academy of Pediatrics Committee on Infectious Diseases: The use of oral acyclovir in otherwise healthy children with varicella. *Pediatrics* 1993;91:674–6.

Asano Y, Itakura N, Kajita Y, et al: Severity of viremia and clinical findings in children with varicella. *J Infect Dis* 1990;161:1095–8.

Balfour HH Jr, Rotbart HA, Feldman S, et al: Acyclovir treatment of varicella in otherwise healthy adolescents. The Collaborative Acyclovir Varicella Study Group. *J Pediatr* 1992;120:627–33.

Centers for Disease Control and Prevention: Prevention of varicella. Recommendations of the Advisory Committee on Immunization Practices (ACIP). *MMWR Morb Mortal Wkly Rep* 1996;45:1–36.

Centers for Disease Control and Prevention: Varicella-related deaths among adults—United States, 1997. *MMWR Morb Mortal Wkly Rep* 1997; 46:409–12.

Centers for Disease Control and Prevention: Prevention of varicella. Update recommendations of the Advisory Committee on Immunization Practices (ACIP). *MMWR Morb Mortal Wkly Rep* 1999;48:1–5.

Choo PW, Donahue JG, Manson JE, et al: The epidemiology of varicella and its complications. *J Infect Dis* 1995;172:706–12.

Donahue JG, Choo PW, Manson JE, et al: The incidence of herpes zoster. *Arch Intern Med* 1995;155:1605–9.

Dunkle LM, Arvin AM, Whitley RJ, et al: A controlled trial of acyclovir for chickenpox in normal children. *N Engl J Med* 1991;325:1539–44.

Gershon AA, Steinberg SP, Gelb L: Clinical reinfection with varicella-zoster virus. *J Infect Dis* 1984;149:137–42.

Gershon AA, Mervish N, LaRussa P, et al: Varicella-zoster virus infection in children with underlying human immunodeficiency virus infection. *J Infect Dis* 1997;176:1496–500.

Gilden DH, Kleinschmidt-DeMasters BK, LaGuardia JJ, et al: Neurologic complications of the reactivation of varicella-zoster virus. *N Engl J Med* 2000;342:635–45.

Jackson JL, Gibbons R, Meyer G, et al: The effect of treating herpes zoster with oral acyclovir in preventing postherpetic neuralgia. A meta-analysis. *Arch Intern Med* 1997;157:909–12.

Krause PR, Klinman DM: Varicella vaccination: Evidence for frequent reactivation of the vaccine strain in healthy children. *Nat Med* 2000;6:451–4.

Laupland KB, Davies HD, Low DE, et al: Invasive group A streptococcal disease in children and association with varicella-zoster virus infection. Ontario Group A Streptococcal Study Group. *Pediatrics* 2000; 105:E60.

Lichtenstein PK, Heubi JE, Daughtery LL, et al: Grade I Reye's syndrome. A frequent cause of vomiting and liver dysfunction after varicella and upper-respiratory-tract infection. *N Engl J Med* 1983;309:133–9.

Lieu TA, Cochi SL, Black SB, et al: Cost-effectiveness of a routine varicella vaccination program for US children. *JAMA* 1994;271:75–81.

Lin F, Hadler JL: Epidemiology of primary varicella and herpes zoster hospitalizations: The pre-varicella vaccine era. *J Infect Dis* 2000; 181:1897–905.

Locksley RM, Flournoy N, Sullivan KM, et al: Infection with varicella-zoster virus after marrow transplantation. *J Infect Dis* 1985;152:1172–81.

Paryani SG, Arvin AM: Intrauterine infection with varicella-zoster virus after maternal varicella. *N Engl J Med* 1986;314:1542–6.

Petursson G, Helgason S, Gudmundsson S, et al: Herpes zoster in children and adolescents. *Pediatr Infect Dis J* 1998;17:905–8.

Potgieter PD, Hammond JM: Intensive care management of varicella pneumonia. *Respir Med* 1997;91:207–12.

Radetsky M: Smallpox: A history of its rise and fall. *Pediatr Infect Dis J* 1999;18:85–93.

Salzman MB, Garcia C: Postexposure varicella vaccination in siblings of children with active varicella. *Pediatr Infect Dis J* 1998;17:256–7.

Shepp DH, Dandliker PS, Meyers JD: Treatment of varicella-zoster virus infection in severely immunocompromised patients. A randomized comparison of acyclovir and vidarabine. *N Engl J Med* 1986;314:208–12.

Vázquez M, LaRussa PS, Gershon AA, et al: The effectiveness of the varicella vaccine in clinical practice. *N Engl J Med* 2001;344:955–60.

Weber DM, Pellecchia JA: Varicella pneumonia: Study of prevalence in adult men. *JAMA* 1965;192:228–9.

Whitley RJ, Weiss H, Gnann JW Jr, et al: Acyclovir with and without prednisone for the treatment of herpes zoster. A randomized, placebo-controlled trial. *Ann Intern Med* 1996;125:376–83.

Whitley RJ, Weiss HL, Soong SJ, et al: Herpes zoster: Risk categories for persistent pain. *J Infect Dis* 1999;179:9–15.

Wood MJ, Johnson RW, McKendrick MW, et al: A randomized trial of acyclovir for 7 days or 21 days with and without prednisolone for treatment of acute herpes zoster. *N Engl J Med* 1994;330:896–900.

CHAPTER 28

Cat-Scratch Disease

Kenneth M. Zangwill

Although the first clinical report of cat-scratch disease (CSD) appeared in the medical literature in 1950, which described a child seen in France in 1931, only in the last 10 years has the etiologic agent been identified and its broad spectrum of clinical disease appreciated.

ETIOLOGY

Bartonella henselae, Bartonella quintana, and *Bartonella clarridgeiae* have been linked to CSD, with *B. henselae* most commonly identified (Table 28–1). *Bartonella* organisms are small, curved, pleomorphic gram-negative bacilli with twitching motility and relatively fastidious growth characteristics. *B. henselae* was presumptively identified as the cause of CSD in 1992 when, using a serologic test to detect antibody against this organism, investigators noted that 36 (88%) of 41 sera from persons with clinical CSD showed positivity, compared with only 6% from healthy control subjects. Further reports of *Bartonella* DNA detected by PCR and identified by culture of clinical specimens from patients with presumed CSD and reports of the detection of *Bartonella* nucleic acid sequences in CSD skin test antigens solidified the etiologic role of these organisms.

Afipia felis was isolated in 1988 and putatively identified as a cause of CSD, but it rarely causes CSD, if at all.

Transmission. It appears that a different arthropod vector may transmit each pathogenic *Bartonella* species among the animal reservoir. Epidemiologic and PCR studies reveal that the cat flea, *Ctenocephalides felis,* can harbor *B. henselae* and may be the major vector for transmission among cats. There is a higher prevalence of *B. henselae* antibodies in the warmer, more humid climates that favor cat fleas, and cats bacteremic with *B. henselae* are more likely than nonbacteremic cats to be infested with fleas. In addition, an experimental kitten model has confirmed that fleas can transmit *B. henselae* to previously nonbacteremic, antibody-negative kittens, all of which developed high-level *B. henselae* bacteremia.

The mode of transmission to humans involves close contact with an infected cat, frequently with a few or sometimes numerous minor and apparently inconsequential cat bites and scratches that are sometimes recalled only in retrospect. Kittens appear more likely to harbor organisms and to facilitate transmission to humans.

In contrast to *B. henselae, B. quintana* is transmitted by the human body louse, *Pediculus humanus,* and *B. bacilliformis* is transmitted by the sandfly. *Bartonella* species have also been identified in ticks and lice.

EPIDEMIOLOGY

CSD has been reported worldwide. In the United States, large case-series and population-based surveillance studies suggest that CSD is most common in the pediatric population, with children 5–10 years of age at greatest risk (approximately 10 cases per 100,000 population per year). In addition, more than 40% of cases of CSD occur in persons >20 years of age, with an overall incidence of 3–4 per 100,000 population. Familial and geographic clusters have been reported rarely. Incidence peaks in the late fall and winter months, with some geographic variability, resulting in >2,000 hospitalizations annually in the United States. Lymph node biopsy for CSD patients accounts for >15% of all such procedures from September through January among children 5–14 years of age in the United States.

Cats and kittens appear to be the most important reservoirs of *Bartonella,* and this may be species dependent. Large case series and case-control evaluations have shown that being scratched, bitten, or licked by a cat (especially a kitten) is the most important risk factor for disease. Up to 15% of persons with CSD, however, do not report contact with cats or kittens, and person-to-person transmission has not been documented. Cats implicated in cases of CSD are more likely to have antibody against *B. henselae* than control cats. Other studies have shown a seroprevalence of 10–100% of anti-*Bartonella* antibody among community cats in the United States, with the highest rates found in areas of greatest humidity and warmth, as well as in France, Austria, Australia, Japan, the Netherlands, and Great Britain. Feline bacteremia among community cats is common, 10–41%, and has been shown to persist for up to a year. Younger cats and stray cats are more likely to be infected with *Bartonella* than older or domesticated cats. An immune response or bacteremia has also been detected in several other species, including coyotes, rodents, deer, and rarely in dogs. Several studies in the United States have shown that the seroprevalence of anti-*Bartonella* antibodies in humans is <4%. Higher rates are found in intravenous drug–using adults, veterinarians, and cat owners.

PATHOGENESIS

Lymph node pathology among persons with CSD is not specific to this infection and includes patchy, necrotic, granulomatous changes with microabscess formation and variable infiltration of leukocytes. Isolated nodal disease may occasionally spread into contiguous tissues, suppurate, and rupture with subsequent fistula formation. The histologic appearance of **bacillary angiomatosis,** which occurs predominantly in severely immunocompromised persons, however, typically reveals proliferation of small blood vessels with large, ''plump'' cuboidal endothelial cells with intermixed leukocyte infiltration and focal necrosis without granulomas, similar to that seen with bartonellosis, a febrile systemic illness caused by *B. bacilliformis* that is endemic to the Andean region of South America.

The pathogenetic mechanism of *Bartonella* infections, especially CSD, is unknown. It is likely that direct microbial invasion precipitates the pathologic changes described herein, but it has also

TABLE 28–1. Human Diseases Associated with *Bartonella*

Clinical Syndrome	*Bartonella* Species	Selected Clinical Details	At-Risk Populations
Cat-scratch disease (CSD)	*B. henselae** *B. quintana*† *B. clarridgeiae*	Solitary or regional lymphadenopathy, prolonged febrile illness; infrequently Parinaud's oculoglandular syndrome, encephalopathy or encephalitis, osteolytic bone lesions, granulomatous hepatitis, optic neuritis and chorioretinitis	Persons with contacts with cats, especially kittens
Bacillary angiomatosis, bacillary peliosis	*B. henselae* *B. quintana*†	Few to hundreds of cutaneous vascular nodules and exophytic lesions, bone, central nervous system, liver and spleen peliosis	Immunocompromised persons, especially HIV-infected persons
Trench fever	*B. quintana*†	Systemic febrile illness for 3–6 days that may cycle for several days or weeks with prolonged or relapsing fevers	Louse-infected areas (endemic in Poland, Eastern Europe, North Africa, and Russia)
Bartonellosis (Carrión's disease)	*B. bacilliformis*‡	Febrile hemolytic anemia (Oroya fever), followed 2–14 weeks later by vascular wartlike nodules (verruca peruana)	Endemic in Peru, Ecuador, and Colombia
Bacteremia	*B. quintana*† *B. henselae* *B. visonii*	Bacteremia may be prolonged despite therapy	Louse-infected areas, homeless persons
Endocarditis	*B. quintana*† *B. henselae* *B. elizabethae* *B. risonii*	A cause of "culture negative" endocarditis, usually left-sided	HIV-infected persons, alcoholism, homeless persons
Neurologic disorders	*B. henselae*	Aseptic meningitis, cranial and peripheral nerve dysfunction, acute psychiatric complex	HIV-infected persons

**B. henselae* is transmitted between cats by the cat flea *(Ctenocephalides felis).*
†*B. quintana* is transmitted by the human body louse *(Pediculus humanus).*
‡*B. bacilliformis* is transmitted by the sandfly *(Phlebotomus verrucarum).*

been postulated that certain late manifestations of CSD disease such as encephalopathy may result from a delayed hypersensitivity or immune complex–mediated response to the organism. Persons with CSD clearly have demonstrable anti-*Bartonella* antibody and develop specific cellular immunity. Adherence of *Bartonella* to cell surfaces may be facilitated by pili with internalization of bacteria by actin-dependent bacterial aggregation. Several clinical findings also suggest that *Bartonella* may persist intracellularly: (1) persistent bacteremia has been noted in humans and cats; (2) isolation is facilitated by lysis-centrifugation, which disrupts cellular membranes; (3) persons with bacillary angiomatosis may have clinical relapse; and (4) better clinical response has been noted with antimicrobial agents that penetrate intracellularly. *B. bacilliformis* has been shown to induce endothelial cell proliferation, possibly through an angiogenic factor, and to synthesize an extracellular protein that can deform red blood cells. This pathogenic feature is unique to *Bartonella.* Given the varied clinical presentations, response to therapy, and histopathologic findings in diseases due to *Bartonella,* pathogenesis likely varies with species, serotypes within species, changes in the virulence of a particular species with time, or modification by the immune status of the host.

SYMPTOMS AND CLINICAL MANIFESTATIONS

After an incubation period of up to 3 weeks, a wheal or papule or both develop at the inoculation site, although this is usually not present on physical examination because affected persons generally seek medical attention as a result of unresolving lymphadenopathy that does not appear until 1–4 weeks later. The most common sites of lymphadenopathy are the axillary, anterior cervical, and inguinal regions. Lymphadenopathy has also been reported in unusual locations, such as the epitrochlear, posterior auricular, and supraclavicular regions, reflecting the site of initial inoculation. Intervening lymphangitis does not occur. Up to 20% of persons will report lymphadenopathy at more than one site. Nodes are generally not tender, and overlying skin changes are minimal. Suppuration may occur and can result in fistula formation. Constitutional symptoms such as fever, headache, malaise, and anorexia accompany lymphadenopathy in approximately 50–80% of cases. Rarely, skin changes, including erythema nodosum, purpura, and transient nonspecific rashes, have been associated with CSD. In most cases the clinical illness resolves spontaneously, but lymphadenopathy may persist for weeks to months.

In addition to solitary or regional lymphadenopathy with fever, many atypical manifestations, which are now recognized because of the availability of diagnostic serologic testing, account for 5–25% of all cases of CSD. Central nervous system disease most commonly presents as encephalopathy, with associated seizures in 40–50% of patients. The onset is usually from a few days to 2 months after the development of lymphadenopathy. An abnormal EEG is present in the majority of patients, and mild cerebrospinal fluid lymphocytic pleocytosis is present in approximately one third of patients. Complete and rapid recovery is the rule, but severe disease with sequelae may occur. Status epilepticus, cranial and peripheral nerve pareses, and intracranial masses have also been reported. Ophthalmic disease usually presents as **Parinaud's oculoglandular syndrome,** which is characterized by bulbar conjunctivitis, preauricular lymphadenopathy, and conjunctival granuloma developing at the site of putative conjunctival or facial inoculation. Neuroretinitis, with a **macular star** or **stellate retinopathy** pattern, has also been described (Fig. 28–1, Plate 9D). Nearly 50 children have been described with hepatitis or splenitis, usually accompanied by prolonged fever, gait disturbance, abdominal pain, arthral-

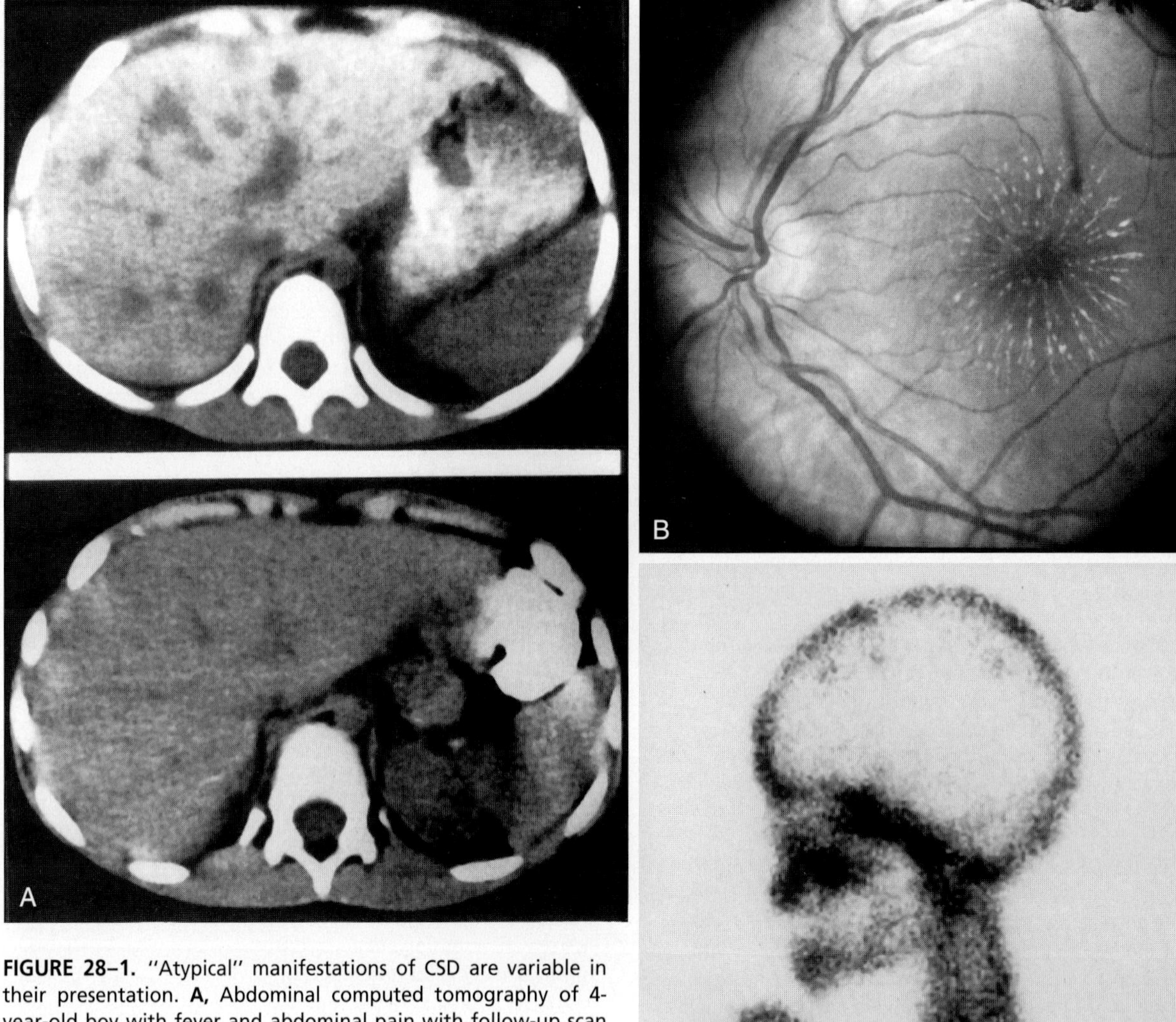

FIGURE 28–1. "Atypical" manifestations of CSD are variable in their presentation. **A,** Abdominal computed tomography of 4-year-old boy with fever and abdominal pain with follow-up scan obtained 2 months later. No antimicrobial therapy was given. **B,** Macular star in 11-year-old girl with 4 weeks of blurred vision. Improvement was noted after therapy with trimethoprim-sulfamethoxazole. **C,** Osteolytic lesions of the skull of 7-year-old boy, noted on bone scan. (From Zangwill KM: *Bartonella* infections. *Semin Pediatr Infect Dis* 1997;8:57–63.)

gias, and pleomorphic rashes. On CT there are usually multiple hypodense lesions of the liver or spleen or both (Fig. 28–1). Several patients have been described as having CSD osteomyelitis with osteolytic bone lesions (Fig. 28–1). Pulmonary disease has been described, usually with parenchymal disease and pleural effusion. Recurrent CSD has been described in only two persons, both adults.

Unusual Presentations

In addition to CSD and its varied manifestations, *Bartonella* organisms have been linked to several other syndromes. **Bacillary angiomatosis** is a vasoproliferative disease characterized by numerous brown to violaceous or colorless vascular tumors of the skin and subcutaneous tissues, which may number from a few to several hundred and vary in size from a few millimeters to several centimeters; the tumors occur primarily in adults in the later stages of AIDS, in persons with cancer, and in transplant recipients. **Bacillary peliosis** is a similar vasoproliferative disease that affects the liver (when it may be called **peliosis hepatis**), the spleen, and sometimes the lymph nodes and bone marrow of immunocompromised persons, primarily adults in the terminal stages of AIDS. Other unusual presentations include a febrile bacteremic syndrome with persistent or relapsing fever; endocarditis, usually among persons with various underlying chronic illnesses; several different central nervous system syndromes; bartonellosis; and trench fever (Table 28–1). It is clear that CSD, currently accepted as the most common manifestation of *Bartonella* infection, is merely a part of a broad range of illnesses caused by this organism. With increased use of diagnostic tests and further study of the epidemiology of these illnesses, the clinical spectrum of *Bartonella* infection has expanded and likely will continue to do so.

DIAGNOSIS

The diagnosis of CSD is usually suspected on the basis of the clinical presentation with regional, subacute lymphadenopathy and constitutional symptoms in persons with recent direct contact with a cat or kitten and is confirmed with a serologic test.

Differential Diagnosis

The most common alternative diagnoses to the unilateral subacute or chronic lymphadenopathy of CSD are suppurative lymphadenitis, neoplasm, and mycobacterial disease. Other important considerations include Kawasaki syndrome, infectious mononucleosis, toxoplasmosis, tularemia, brucellosis, dimorphic fungal infections, and noninfectious causes including structural abnormalities (e.g., hygroma, branchial cleft cyst) and collagen vascular diseases.

Microbiologic Evaluation

Bartonella can be identified in blood or tissue samples by special staining and bacterial culture. Organisms are best seen with silver staining methods using **Warthin-Starry** or **Steiner** stains. The Gram stain is usually unrevealing. Because *Bartonella* species are relatively fastidious organisms, culture techniques should be used that maximize recovery, including use of the lysis-centrifugation technique and a selective medium that contains hemin, followed by growth in a hypercapnic atmosphere for a minimum of 10 days. The organism grows slowly and may take 10–40 days. PCR is a highly sensitive and specific diagnostic tool for etiologic identification, including distinguishing between different species of *Bartonella,* but it is not readily available. With culture or PCR, *Bartonella* has been detected in several tissues from persons with CSD, including the site of skin inoculation, lymph nodes, bone, eye, conjunctivae, paraspinal lesions, liver, and spleen. Among persons with bacillary angiomatosis, *Bartonella* organisms have been identified in nearly every organ system including the brain.

Serologic Testing. The first serologic test, developed by the CDC, is an indirect immunofluorescence assay that is 70–85% sensitive and 90–95% specific for the diagnosis of CSD. Similar results have been noted among persons with bacillary angiomatosis. Among persons with CSD, antibody titers usually peak at 4–6 weeks after the development of lymphadenopathy and persist for 4–5 months thereafter, but some individuals exhibit variable antibody responses. Currently, most commercial diagnostic laboratories offer an enzyme immunoassay–based serologic test with comparable sensitivity and specificity, although there is some variability noted among different geographic regions. Currently, serologic testing does not reliably distinguish different species of *Bartonella.* Other techniques are being evaluated as tools for rapid species-specific identification but are not readily available.

Skin Test. The CSD antigen skin test **(Hanger-Rose test),** originally developed in 1946, used a nonstandardized preparation of aspirated pus from suppurative lymph nodes of patients with apparent CSD. It was available in limited quantities and was used by some physicians to confirm the diagnosis, but it should not be used because of the potential for transmission of infectious agents.

TREATMENT

The majority of cases of CSD resolve in 1–2 months without any antimicrobial therapy. Warm compresses have not been shown to enhance resolution of lymphadenopathy but may be helpful for symptomatic relief. Although *Bartonella* organisms appear to be susceptible to several antimicrobial agents when tested in vitro, such results do not reliably predict the clinical response to therapy. Anecdotal evidence and retrospective series suggest that for persons with CSD, some clinical response may be achieved with TMP-SMZ, rifampin, gentamicin, and, for adults, ciprofloxacin. One randomized trial (Bass et al, 1998) of 29 patients suggested that azithromycin might decrease lymph node size, as monitored by ultrasonography 30 days after therapy was initiated, compared with control subjects who received placebo. The clinical relevance of this finding is unclear because there was no significant effect on the eventual resolution of the lymphadenopathy. Antimicrobial therapy should be considered for patients with (1) lymphadenopathy that does not resolve within a reasonable period, such as longer than 6–8 weeks; (2) lymphadenopathy associated with significant morbidity, such as pain, limitation of movement, or persistence of debilitating constitutional symptoms; (3) severe systemic disease including encephalopathy, osteomyelitis, and neuroretinitis; or (4) an underlying medical disorder complicated by severe CSD. Proposed treatment regimens for bacteremia and endocarditis include various combinations of gentamicin plus ceftriaxone, erythromycin or another macrolide, and a quinolone. Most reported cases of *Bartonella* endocarditis have required surgical removal of the vegetation in addition to antibiotic therapy for cure.

Aspiration of inflamed, nonsuppurative lymph nodes in persons with CSD should be performed only to exclude other, more serious diagnoses or if superinfection is suspected. If such a procedure is performed, either fine needle aspiration or excisional biopsy should be performed; incision and drainage procedures may promote the development of fistulas. Suppuration may develop, which may require drainage or even excision. Ultrasonography is often useful in identifying suppuration that requires drainage.

Bacillary Angiomatosis and Bacillary Peliosis. Bacillary angiomatosis usually responds to treatment with macrolides or tetracyclines. Uncomplicated cutaneous disease in HIV-infected patients requires treatment with erythromycin, erythromycin plus rifampin, or doxycycline, usually for at least 6–8 weeks of therapy. Severe or invasive disease may require a minimum of 4–6 months of therapy and sometimes requires lifetime suppressive therapy. The activity of azithromycin and clarithromycin appears to be superior to the activity of erythromycin.

COMPLICATIONS

Encephalitis, encephalopathy, osteolytic bone lesions, granulomatous hepatitis, and optic neuritis and chorioretinitis may develop during the course of CSD. There are no controlled trials regarding the benefit of therapy in preventing or treating these uncommon manifestations.

PROGNOSIS

The majority of cases of CSD, including atypical cases, resolve completely in 1–2 months even without any antimicrobial therapy. No deaths have been directly attributable to CSD.

PREVENTION

The only specific recommendation for prevention is attentiveness toward avoidance of scratches and bites from cats and kittens. No data exist to support the usefulness of antimicrobial prophylaxis for persons after cat contact or for the implicated cat itself or the usefulness of aggressive flea eradication measures. Removal of the cat from the household or declawing is probably unnecessarily draconian. Mass vaccination of cats may be of value in the future.

REVIEWS

Anderson BE, Neuman MA: *Bartonella* spp. as emerging human pathogens. *Clin Microbiol Rev* 1997;10:203–19.

Bass JW, Vincent JM, Person DA: The expanding spectrum of *Bartonella* infections. I. Bartonellosis and trench fever. *Pediatr Infect Dis J* 1997; 16:2–10.

Bass JW, Vincent JM, Person DA: The expanding spectrum of *Bartonella* infections. II. Cat-scratch disease. *Pediatr Infect Dis J* 1997;16:163–79.

Breischwerdt EB, Kordick DL: *Bartonella* infection in animals: Carriership, reservoir potential, pathogenicity, and zoonotic potential for human infection. *Clin Microbiol Rev* 2000;13:428–38.

Carithers HA: Cat-scratch disease: Notes on its history. *Am J Dis Child* 1970;119:200–3.

Carithers HA: Cat scratch disease: An overview based on a study of 1200 patients. *Am J Dis Child* 1985;139:1124–33.

Carithers HA, Margileth AM: Cat-scratch disease: Acute encephalopathy and other neurologic manifestations. *Am J Dis Child* 1991;145:98–101.

Garcia-Caceres U, Garcia FU: Bartonellosis. An immunodepressive disease and the life of Daniel Alcides Carrión. *Am J Clin Pathol* 1991;95:S58–66.

Koehler JE, Tappero JW: Bacillary angiomatosis and bacillary peliosis and patients infected with human immunodeficiency virus. *Clin Infect Dis* 1993;17:612–24.

Margileth AM, Wear DJ, English CK: Systemic cat scratch disease: Report of 23 patients with prolonged or recurrent severe bacterial infection. *J Infect Dis* 1987;155:390–402.

Margileth AM, Baehren DF: Chest-wall abscess due to cat scratch disease (CSD) in an adult with antibodies to *Bartonella clarridgeiae:* Case report and review of the thoracopulmonary manifestations of CSD. *Clin Infect Dis* 1998;27:353–7.

KEY ARTICLES

Anderson B, Sims K, Regnery R, et al: Detection of *Rochalimaea henselae*–DNA in specimens from cat scratch disease patients by PCR. *J Clin Microbiol* 1994;32:942–8.

Arisoy ES, Correa AG, Wagner ML, et al: Hepatosplenic cat-scratch disease in children: Selected clinical features and treatment. *Clin Infect Dis* 1999;28:778–84.

Bass JW, Freitas BC, Freitas AD, et al: Prospective randomized double-blind placebo-controlled evaluation of azithromycin for treatment of cat-scratch disease. *Pediatr Infect Dis J* 1998;17:447–52.

Bergmans AMC, Peeters MF, Schellekens JFP, et al: Pitfalls and fallacies of cat scratch disease serology: Evaluation of *Bartonella henselae*–based indirect fluorescence assay and enzyme-linked immunoassay. *J Clin Microbiol* 1997;35:1931–7.

Chomel BB, Abbott RC, Kasten RW, et al: *Bartonella henselae* prevalence in domestic cats in California: Risk factors and association between bacteremia and antibody titer. *J Clin Microbiol* 1995;33:2445–50.

Chomel BB, Kasten RW, Floyd-Hawkins K, et al: Experimental transmission of *Bartonella henselae* by the cat flea. *J Clin Microbiol* 1996;34: 1952–6.

Dalton MJ, Robinson LE, Cooper J, et al: Use of *Bartonella* antigens for serologic diagnosis of cat scratch disease at a national referral center. *Arch Intern Med* 1995;155:1670–6.

Dunn MW, Berkowitz FE, Miller JJ, et al: Hepatosplenic cat-scratch disease and abdominal pain. *Pediatr Infect Dis J* 1997;16:269–72.

Giladi M, Avidor B, Kletter Y, et al: Cat scratch disease: The rare role of *Afipia felis*. *J Clin Microbiol* 1998;36:2499–502.

Hamilton DH, Zangwill KM, Hadler JL, et al: Cat-scratch disease—Connecticut, 1992–1993. *J Infect Dis* 1995;172:570–3.

Hopkins KL, Simoneaux SF, Patrick LE, et al: Imaging manifestations of cat-scratch disease. *Am J Roentgenol* 1996;166:435–8.

Jacobs RF, Schutze G: *Bartonella henselae* as a cause of prolonged fever and fever of unknown origin in children. *Clin Infect Dis* 1998;26:80–4.

Jameson P, Greene C, Regnery R, et al: Prevalence of *Bartonella henselae* antibodies in pet cats throughout regions of North America. *J Infect Dis* 1995;172:1145–9.

Koehler JE, Glaser CA, Tappero JW: *Rochalimaea henselae* infection: A new zoonosis with the domestic cat as reservoir. *JAMA* 1994;271:531–5.

Malatack JJ, Jaffe R: Granulomatous hepatitis in three children due to cat-scratch disease without peripheral adenopathy. An unrecognized cause of fever of unknown origin. *Am J Dis Child* 1993;147:949–53.

Margelith AM: Antibiotic therapy for cat scratch disease: Clinical study of therapeutic outcome in 268 patients and a review of the literature. *Pediatr Infect Dis J* 1992;11:474–8.

Ormerod LD, Dailey JP: Ocular manifestations of cat scratch disease. *Curr Opin Ophthalmol* 1999;10:209–16.

Regnery RL, Olson JG, Perkins BA, et al: Serological response to "*Rochalimaea henselae*" antigen in suspected cat-scratch disease. *Lancet* 1992; 339:1443–5.

Zangwill KM, Hamilton DH, Perkins BA, et al: Cat scratch disease in Connecticut: Epidemiology, risk factors and evaluation of a new diagnostic test. *N Engl J Med* 1993;329:8–13.

CHAPTER 29

Lyme Disease

Eugene D. Shapiro

Lyme disease **(Lyme borreliosis)** is the most common vector-borne disease in the United States. A cluster of children with unexplained arthritis in Lyme, Connecticut, was reported by one of their parents in the mid-1970s. Investigation of this "epidemic" of arthritis led to the description of "Lyme" arthritis in 1977 and ultimately to the discovery of its bacterial cause. Both the reported incidence of the disease and its geographic range have increased dramatically in recent years. Perhaps even more striking has been the attendant increase in publicity about the illness in the lay press, which at times has been accompanied by near hysteria about both risks and perceived complications of Lyme disease. This publicity, combined with a high frequency of misdiagnoses in persons with symptoms from other causes, has resulted in a degree of anxiety about Lyme disease—among both patients and physicians—that is out of proportion to the actual morbidity that it causes.

ETIOLOGY

Lyme disease is caused by the spirochete *Borrelia burgdorferi,* a fastidious, microaerophilic bacterium that replicates very slowly and requires special media to grow in the laboratory. Like other spirochetes, *B. burgdorferi* is a cylindrical organism, the cell membrane of which is covered by flagella and by a loosely associated outer membrane. The three major outer-surface proteins, **OspA, OspB,** and **OspC,** which are highly-charged basic proteins with molecular weights of about 31, 34, and 23 kDa, respectively, as well as the 41 kDa flagellar protein, are important targets of the immune response of humans. There are differences in the molecular structure of proteins from different strains of *B. burgdorferi.* Indeed, differences in the frequency of certain clinical manifestations of Lyme disease in Europe and in the United States (e.g., the greater frequency of meningopolyneuritis in Europeans) have been attributed to these biologic differences in the organism.

A Lyme disease–like illness caused by *Borrelia lonestari* that is limited to erythema migrans without progression to chronic disease has been reported in the Midwest United States.

Transmission. *B. burgdorferi* is transmitted by ticks of the *Ixodid* genus, which in the United States are primarily *Ixodes scapularis* (previously known as *Ixodes dammini*), the **deer tick** (Fig. 31–2; Plate 9E) and, less frequently, *Ixodes pacificus,* the **Western black-legged tick** in the Pacific states.

Several factors influence the risk of transmission of *B. burgdorferi* from ticks to humans. The proportion of infected ticks varies greatly both by geographic area and by the stage of the tick in its life cycle (Fig. 33–1). *I. scapularis* feeds on small mammals such as the **white-footed mouse** *(Peromyscus leucopus)* that are competent reservoirs for *B. burgdorferi.* In endemic areas the rates of infection of *I. scapularis* ticks are approximately 2% for larvae, 15–30% for nymphs, and 30–50% for adults. Infection rates of ticks as high as 60–90% have been reported in selected areas. By contrast, *I. pacificus* often feeds on lizards, which are not a competent reservoir of *B. burgdorferi.* Consequently only 1–3% of these ticks, even in the nymphal and adult stages, are infected with *B. burgdorferi.*

The risk of transmission of *B. burgdorferi* from infected deer ticks is also related to the duration of feeding. It takes hours for the mouthparts of ticks to implant fully in the host and much longer (i.e., days) for the tick to become fully engorged (Plate 9E). Experiments with animals have shown that nymphal-stage ticks must feed for 36–48 hours and adult ticks must feed for 48–72 hours before the risk of transmission of *B. burgdorferi* from infected ticks becomes substantial. The duration of time that a tick has fed can be estimated from indices of engorgement derived from experiments with animals. These indices indicate that approximately 75% of persons who recognize that they have been bitten by a deer tick remove the tick less than 48 hours after it has begun to feed.

The majority of persons who develop Lyme disease do not recall a tick bite. Unrecognized tick bites probably are associated with greater risk of transmission because unrecognized ticks may feed longer. A recognized tick bite is an indication that the person is at risk and should not be assumed to be the only exposure.

EPIDEMIOLOGY

Persons with increased occupational, recreational, or residential exposure to tick-infested woodlands and fields (the preferred habitat of ticks) in endemic areas are at increased risk of acquiring Lyme disease. Lyme disease occurs most commonly in areas where deer ticks are abundant and where the prevalence of *B. burgdorferi* in these ticks is high (20–50% of ticks). In the United States these areas include southern New England, southeastern New York, New Jersey, eastern Pennsylvania, eastern Maryland, Delaware, and parts of Wisconsin and Minnesota. There were 16,801 cases of Lyme disease reported to the CDC in 1998 (Fig. 29–1). More than 75% of the reported cases occurred in a small number (<70) of counties in endemic areas (Fig. 29–2). Lyme disease occurs in the Pacific states but is uncommon because few *I. pacificus* ticks are infected with the organism. To date, there have been no culture-confirmed cases of Lyme disease in persons whose only known exposure was in the south-central or southeastern United States.

Lyme disease occurs throughout the world. Cases have been reported throughout Europe, but most cases occur in the Scandinavian countries and in central Europe, especially Germany, Austria, and Switzerland.

The age distribution of Lyme disease is bimodal, with the highest reported incidence in children 5–9 years of age and adults 45–54 years of age. Approximately 52% of cases occur in males. Most cases have onset from June to August, although cases are reported to occur in all months of the year.

The incidence of Lyme disease varies tremendously from region to region and even within local areas. Information about the true incidence of the disease is complicated by reliance, in most in-

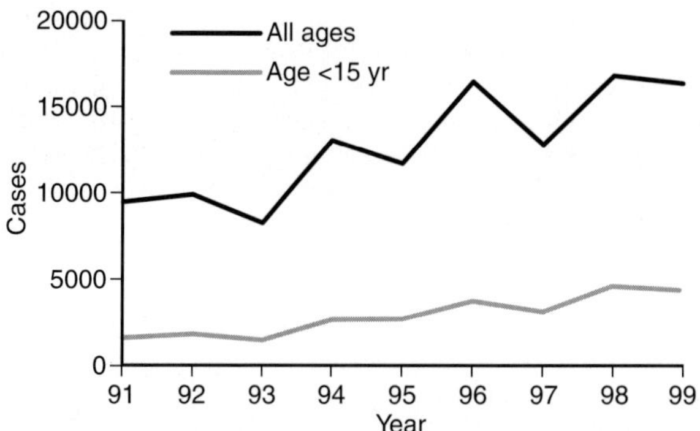

FIGURE 29–1. Reported cases (in thousands) of Lyme disease by year in the United States from 1991 to 1999. (Data from the Centers for Disease Control and Prevention.)

stances, on passive reporting of cases and by the high frequency of misdiagnosis. Furthermore, studies have indicated that as many as 50% of patients who have serologic evidence of recent infection with *B. burgdorferi* may be free of symptoms.

PATHOGENESIS

B. burgdorferi is transmitted when the organism is inoculated by an infected tick into the blood vessels of the skin of its host and then begins to multiply locally. The inflammation results in a **single erythema migrans** rash in approximately two thirds of persons with symptomatic disease. Days to weeks later the spirochete may disseminate, via either the bloodstream or the lymphatic vessels, to many other sites, including the skin (almost 25% of patients develop **multiple erythema migrans**), eye, synovial tissue, the central nervous system, and the heart. *B. burgdorferi* has been isolated from the blood or from tissue at all stages of the illness, but the small number of organisms that are present and the fastidious nature of in vitro growth make recovery of the spirochete difficult except for experienced laboratories. The spirochete has a preference for cell surfaces and adheres to a wide variety of different types of cells, which may explain why it is able to cause clinical manifestations in such a broad array of organ systems. Because the organism may persist in tissues for prolonged periods, symptoms may appear late in the course of infection.

It is likely that relatively few organisms actually invade the host, but mediators of inflammation such as IL-1 and other lymphokines amplify the inflammatory response and lead to much of the tissue damage and to symptoms of Lyme disease. Despite antimicrobial treatment, a very small subset of patients have refractory symptoms, such as recurrent Lyme arthritis, which may have an immunogenetic basis. There is substantial evidence that persons with the DR2, DR3, and DR4 HLA allotypes may have a genetic predisposition to the development of chronic, recurrent Lyme arthritis long after the bacteria have been killed.

SYMPTOMS AND CLINICAL MANIFESTATIONS

The clinical manifestations of Lyme disease generally are divided into two stages: **early Lyme disease** and **late Lyme disease.** Early Lyme disease often is further subdivided into **early localized dis-**

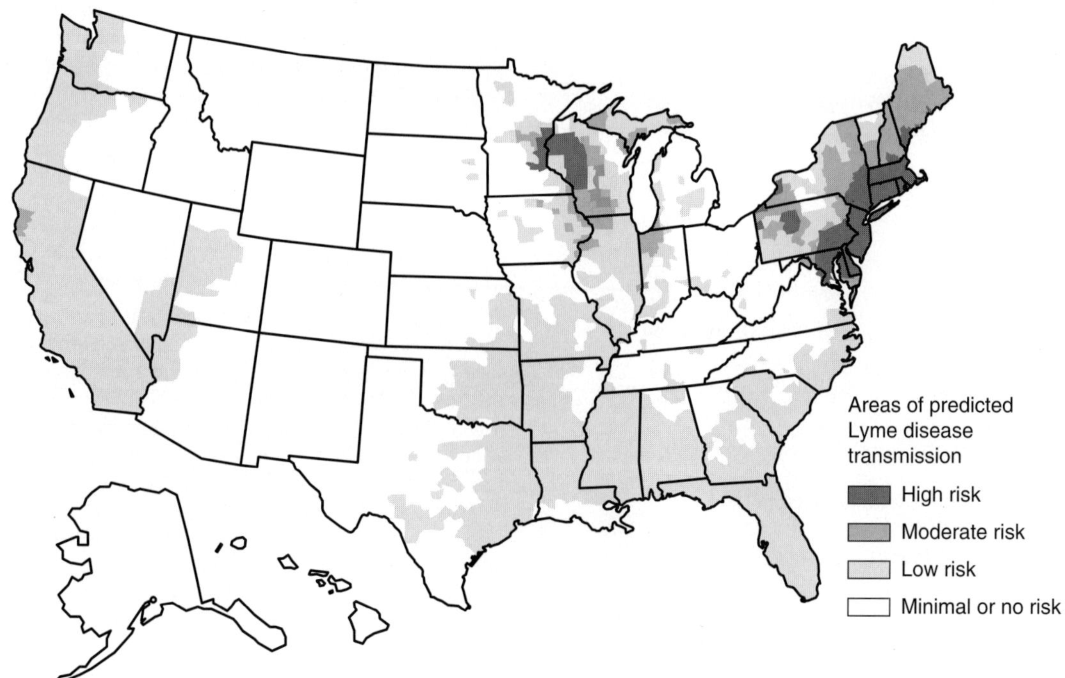

FIGURE 29–2. Approximate risk of Lyme disease in the United States. High-risk counties are where *I. scapularis* or *I. pacificus* is established, are where prevalence is predicted to be high, and are those in the top 10th percentile of counties reporting human cases during 1994–1997. Moderate-risk counties are where *I. scapularis* or *I. pacificus* is established and where prevalence is predicted to be high. Low-risk counties are where *I. scapularis* is established but prevalence is predicted to be low, or where *I. scapularis* is reported but not established, or where *I. pacificus* either is established or has been reported. Minimal- or no-risk counties are where neither *I. scapularis* nor *I. pacificus* is established or has been reported. The true risk might change from year to year. (From Centers for Disease Control and Prevention: Recommendations for the use of Lyme disease vaccine. Recommendations of the Advisory Committee on Immunization Practices. *MMWR Morb Mortal Wkly Rep* 1999:48[RR–7]:21.)

ease and **early disseminated disease** (Table 29–1). In the largest prospective study of children with Lyme disease that has been reported (a community-based study of 201 children with Lyme disease in Connecticut), the initial manifestations of Lyme disease were single erythema migrans (66%), multiple erythema migrans (23%), arthritis (7%), seventh-nerve palsy (3%), aseptic meningitis (1%), and carditis (0.5%). Erythema migrans was more likely to occur on either the head or neck in younger children and on the extremities in older children, a finding similar to that recently reported from Europe. Only about one third of the children with a single erythema migrans rash had serologic test results positive for *B. burgdorferi* at the time of presentation, whereas almost 90% of the children with multiple erythema migrans were seropositive. More than one fourth of the children had early disseminated Lyme disease when they were seen by a physician, and 89% had either single or multiple erythema migrans.

Early Localized Disease. The skin is the initial target organ for infection by *B. burgdorferi.* The first clinical manifestation is the typical annular rash, **erythema migrans.** It usually occurs 7–14 days after the tick bite, although the onset of the rash has been reported as few as 3 days and as many as 4 weeks later. The rash may be uniformly erythematous or it may appear as a target lesion with variable degrees of central clearing (Plate 6B). Occasionally there may be vesicular or necrotic areas in the center of the rash. The rash may be itchy, painful, or asymptomatic, and it may or may not be accompanied by systemic symptoms such as fever, myalgia, headache, and malaise. If the person is not treated, the rash gradually expands (hence the term *migrans*), sometimes to more than a foot in diameter. Without treatment the rash will remain for at least 1–2 weeks and usually for even longer. Approximately two thirds of children with Lyme disease will have single erythema migrans.

TABLE 29–1. Clinical Manifestations of Lyme Disease in Children

Early Localized Disease*
Erythema migrans (single)
Myalgia
Fatigue
Headache
Fever
Lymphadenopathy (regional)
Arthralgia
Early Disseminated Disease*
Erythema migrans (multiple)
Lymphadenopathy (regional or generalized)
Conjunctivitis
Cranial neuritis (especially facial palsy)
Aseptic meningitis
Carditis (usually manifests as heart block)
Radiculoneuritis
Fever
Headache
Myalgia
Arthralgia
Fatigue
Late Disease
Arthritis

*Nonspecific symptoms (e.g., headache, myalgia, arthralgia, fatigue) virtually always accompany the specific manifestations of Lyme disease (e.g., erythema migrans).

Early Disseminated Disease. A substantial proportion (approximately 25%) of children in the United States who are acutely infected with *B. burgdorferi* develop multiple erythema migrans lesions, a manifestation of early disseminated disease, which occurs approximately 3–10 weeks after the initial infection. The secondary skin lesions, which may develop several days or even weeks after the first lesion, are smaller than the primary lesion. Fever and myalgia usually accompany the secondary lesions. Patients may also complain of headache, neck pain, and malaise. Conjunctivitis and regional lymphadenopathy also may develop. Occasionally when the erythema migrans rash resolves, new evanescent lesions, which usually are small (1–3 cm), erythematous, annular lesions, may come and go for a period of several weeks. These lesions may appear at different sites, but generally they do not expand.

At this stage of the illness, aseptic meningitis may occur, although it is rare (about 1% of all patients). The DNA of *B. burgdorferi* has been detected in the cerebrospinal fluid of patients at this stage of the illness. Focal neurologic manifestations, specifically cranial neuropathies, also may occur at this stage. **Seventh-nerve palsy** (facial palsy) is relatively common and affects approximately 3% of children with Lyme disease. It may be the presenting as well as the only manifestation of Lyme disease. The palsy usually lasts for 2–8 weeks before it completely resolves, with or without treatment. Rarely, the palsy may resolve only partially or not at all. **Bannwarth's syndrome (meningopolyneuritis)** has been reported more commonly as a manifestation of Lyme disease in Europe. Encephalitis, with or without focal neurologic signs, occasionally occurs.

Late Disease. The classic manifestation of late Lyme disease is arthritis, which occurs in about 7% of children with Lyme disease. Arthralgia, a common, nonspecific symptom that frequently is present both among persons with early Lyme disease and among persons who do not have Lyme disease, should be differentiated from synovitis (e.g., manifest as an effusion), which is the hallmark of late Lyme disease. The arthritis occurs weeks to months after the initial infection. The large joints are primarily involved, especially the knees, which are affected in more than 90% of cases. Although the affected joint is swollen and tender, the patient usually does not have the exquisite pain that is typical of suppurative arthritis due to highly pathogenic, pyogenic organisms. Usually the joint swelling resolves within 1–2 weeks, although it may last for several weeks before recurring, often in other joints. Although large joints are most commonly involved, any joint, including small joints, may be affected. If untreated, the episodes of arthritis often increase in duration, sometimes lasting for months. However, even in persons who are untreated and who have had many recurrences of arthritis, the disease will usually resolve eventually. Most persons with Lyme arthritis will not have a history of erythema migrans because those with the rash usually are treated with antimicrobial agents and do not develop late manifestations of disease.

Late manifestations of Lyme disease of the central nervous system, sometimes termed tertiary **neuroborreliosis,** rarely have been reported in children. In adults, chronic demyelinating encephalitis, polyneuritis, and impairment of memory have been attributed to Lyme disease, although there is controversy about the frequency with which such late manifestations occur, especially among persons who have been treated. Other, rare manifestations of late Lyme disease include **acrodermatitis chronica atrophicans,** which is a chronic, atrophic sclerotic lesion of the skin, and *Borrelia* **lymphocytoma,** which is a localized, subcutaneous nodular lesion that usually occurs in either the earlobe or the breast.

Congenital Lyme Disease. Because clinical syndromes caused by congenital infection have been recognized with other spirochetal infections such as syphilis, there has been concern about the possible transmission of *B. burgdorferi* from an infected pregnant woman to her unborn fetus. Although case reports have been published in which *B. burgdorferi* has been identified from several abortuses and from a few live-born children with congenital anomalies, the placentas and abortuses, as well as tissues from affected children, did not show histologic evidence of inflammation. In addition, no consistent pattern of congenital malformations (as would be expected in a "syndrome" due to congenital infection) has been identified. In two small longitudinal studies of pregnant women with Lyme disease that were conducted by the CDC, the adverse outcomes that occurred could not be attributed to infection with *B. burgdorferi*. Furthermore, serosurveys conducted in endemic areas found no difference in the prevalence of congenital malformations among the offspring of women with serum antibodies against *B. burgdorferi* and the offspring of those without such antibodies.

Thus there is no definitive evidence that *B. burgdorferi* causes congenital disease, although the existence of such a syndrome also has not been excluded. There is no neurologic disorder that is attributed to congenital Lyme disease. Transmission of Lyme disease through breast-feeding has never been documented.

DIAGNOSIS

The diagnosis of Lyme disease, especially in the absence of the characteristic rash, may be difficult because the other clinical manifestations of Lyme disease are not specific and because the diagnosis generally is established by serologic testing. Even the diagnosis of erythema migrans sometimes may be difficult because the rash initially may be confused with nummular eczema, granuloma annulare, an insect bite, ringworm, or cellulitis (Table 29–2). However, the relatively rapid expansion of erythema migrans helps to distinguish it from these other conditions. A rash resembling erythema migrans has been associated with bites by *Amblyomma americanum,* the Lone Star tick, but is apparently not the result of *B. burgdorferi* infection. *A. americanum* is primarily found in the south-central and southeastern United States and is not a competent vector for *B. burgdorferi.*

Laboratory Evaluation

Routine laboratory tests rarely are helpful in diagnosing Lyme disease because the associated abnormalities also are nonspecific. The peripheral WBC count may be either normal or elevated. The ESR usually is elevated. The WBC count in joint fluid of persons with Lyme arthritis may range from 25,000 to 125,000/mm^3, often with a preponderance of polymorphonuclear cells. When the central nervous system is involved, there usually is a mild pleocytosis with a lymphocytic predominance.

Microbiologic Evaluation

Because the sensitivity of culture for *B. burgdorferi* is poor and it is necessary for patients to undergo an invasive procedure such as a biopsy or a lumbar puncture to obtain appropriate tissue or fluid for culture, such tests are indicated only in rare circumstances. Likewise, diagnostic tests, including PCR, that are based on the identification of antigens of *B. burgdorferi* have not been shown to be sufficiently accurate to be clinically useful under nonexperimental conditions, although preliminary studies in research laboratories suggest that PCR is very promising. Consequently the confirmation of Lyme disease by the laboratory usually rests on the demonstration of antibodies to *B. burgdorferi* in the patient's serum.

Serologic Diagnosis. It is well documented that the sensitivity and specificity of antibody tests for Lyme disease vary substantially.

TABLE 29–2. Differential Diagnosis of Lyme Disease

Stage of Disease and Clinical Manifestations	Differential Diagnoses
Early Localized Disease	
Erythema migrans (single)	Tinea corporis (ringworm) Nummular eczema Spider or insect bite Granuloma annulare
Early Disseminated Disease	
Erythema migrans (multiple)	Erythema multiforme Urticaria (hives)
Influenza-like symptoms	Viral or other bacterial infections
Seventh-nerve palsy (Bell's palsy)	Idiopathic Bell's palsy Tumor of the central nervous system
Carditis	Viral infections
Meningitis	Viral meningoencephalitis Parameningeal infections
Radiculoneuritis	Reflex sympathetic dystrophy
Late Disease	
Arthritis	Suppurative arthritis Juvenile rheumatoid arthritis Henoch-Schönlein purpura Serum sickness Collagen vascular disease
Encephalopathy	Degenerative neurologic illnesses Viral encephalitis Depression

The accuracy and reproducibility of prepackaged commercial kits are much poorer than those of tests performed by reference laboratories that maintain tight quality control and regularly prepare the materials that are used in the test. The use of Western immunoblots improves the specificity of serologic testing for Lyme disease. Official recommendations from the Second National Conference on Serologic Diagnosis of Lyme Disease (CDC, 1995) and from the CDC are that clinicians use a two-step procedure when ordering antibody tests for Lyme disease: first, a sensitive screening test, either an ELISA or IFA, and then, if results are positive or equivocal, an immunoblot to confirm the screening test result. If the ELISA or the IFA result is negative, an immunoblot is not necessary. The ELISA provides a quantitative estimate of the concentration of antibodies against *B. burgdorferi,* and the immunoblot provides information about the specificity of the antibodies. Most authorities require the presence of antibodies against at least either two or three (for IgM) or five (for IgG) proteins of *B. burgdorferi* (at least one of which is one of the more specific, low-molecular-weight outer-surface proteins) for the immunoblot result to be considered positive. Antibody tests are not useful for the diagnosis of early localized Lyme disease, because only a minority of persons with single erythema migrans will have a positive test result.

The predictive value of antibody tests (even of very accurate tests) is highly dependent on the prevalence of the infection among persons who are tested. Antibody tests for Lyme disease should *not* be used as screening tests for persons at low risk of infection. Unfortunately, because many lay persons as well as many physicians have the erroneous impression that chronic, nonspecific symptoms alone (e.g., headache, fatigue, or arthralgia) may be manifestations of Lyme disease, parents of a child with only nonspecific symptoms frequently demand that the child be tested for Lyme disease (and some physicians routinely order tests for Lyme disease for such children). Lyme disease will be the cause of the nonspecific symptoms in few such children (if any). However, because the specificity of even excellent antibody tests for Lyme disease rarely exceeds 90–95%, some of the tests in children without specific signs or symptoms of Lyme disease will give positive results; most of these (>95%) will be false-positive. Nevertheless, an erroneous diagnosis of Lyme disease, based on the results of these tests, frequently is made, and such children often are treated unnecessarily with antimicrobial agents.

Even though a person with symptoms has a serologic test positive for antibodies to *B. burgdorferi,* it is possible that Lyme disease may not be the cause of that person's symptoms. In addition to the possibility that the positive test result is falsely positive (a common occurrence), the person may have been infected with *B. burgdorferi* previously and the symptoms may be unrelated to the previous infection. Once serum antibodies to *B. burgdorferi* develop, they may persist for many years despite adequate treatment and clinical cure of the disease. In addition, because a substantial proportion of persons who become infected with *B. burgdorferi* never develop symptoms, in endemic areas there will be a background rate of seropositivity among those who have never had clinically apparent Lyme disease. When persons with previous Lyme disease (whether asymptomatic and untreated or clinically apparent and adequately treated) develop any symptoms and are tested for antibodies against *B. burgdorferi,* their symptoms may erroneously be attributed to active Lyme disease because of the positive serologic finding. Physicians should not routinely order antibody tests for Lyme disease for persons who have not been in endemic areas or for persons with only nonspecific symptoms.

TREATMENT

Recommendations for the treatment of children with Lyme disease (Table 29–3) have been extrapolated from studies of adults, because no clinical trials of treatment have been conducted among children. Children less than 8 years of age should not be treated with doxycycline for Lyme disease because it may cause permanent discoloration of their teeth. Although recent data suggest that discoloration is unlikely with a short course of doxycycline therapy, cefuroxime is effective and is approved for the treatment of Lyme disease. Preliminary results of treatment with azithromycin have been disappointing. There is little need for use of newer agents because the results of standard therapy with amoxicillin or doxycycline have been so good.

Symptoms such as fatigue, arthralgia, and myalgia sometimes persist for some time after completion of a course of treatment for Lyme disease. These nonspecific symptoms, which may accompany or follow more specific symptoms and signs of Lyme disease but almost never are the sole presenting manifestations of Lyme disease, usually resolve within a period of weeks. There is little evidence that such symptoms are related to persistence of *B. burgdorferi,* and there is no evidence that repeated courses of antimicrobials speed the resolution of such symptoms. Because antibodies against *B. burgdorferi* persist even after successful treatment of symptoms, there is no reason routinely to obtain follow-up tests of antibody concentrations against *B. burgdorferi.*

PROGNOSIS

There is a widespread misconception that Lyme disease is difficult to treat successfully and that chronic recurrences are common. In fact, the prognosis in children treated for Lyme disease is excellent. The most common reason for apparent failure of treatment is misdiagnosis (i.e., the person actually does not have Lyme disease). In a review of 65 children who were treated for erythema migrans, at follow-up at a mean of more than 3 years later, all the children were well and none had developed symptoms of late Lyme disease. In a larger, prospective follow-up study of 201 children with newly diagnosed Lyme disease (most had either early localized or early disseminated disease), at follow-up at a mean of 2½ years later, all the children were clinically cured.

The long-term prognosis for persons treated for late Lyme disease also is excellent. Recurrences of arthritis are rare, and most children who are treated for Lyme arthritis are permanently cured. Indeed, long-term follow-up of children with a diagnosis of Lyme disease before its cause was recognized (most of whom either were not treated with antimicrobials or were treated years after the onset of symptoms) indicated that the arthritis eventually resolved (after multiple recurrences) even in children who were never treated. One group of investigators performed neuropsychologic tests on

TABLE 29–3. Antimicrobial Treatment of Lyme Disease

Early Disease

Erythema Migrans and Disseminated Early Disease without Focal Findings, Facial Nerve Palsy (or Other Cranial Nerve Palsy), or First- or Second-Degree Heart Block

Doxycycline, 100 mg bid PO for 14–21 days (do not use in children <8 yr of age), or amoxicillin, 50 mg/kg/day divided tid (max: 500 mg/dose) PO for 14–21 days; alternatively, for those who cannot take either doxycycline or amoxicillin, use cefuroxime, 30 mg/kg/day (max: 500 mg/dose) divided bid PO for 14–21 days

Carditis with Third-Degree Heart Block

Treat as for late neurologic disease

Meningitis

Treat as for late neurologic disease

Late Disease

Neurologic Disease*

Ceftriaxone, 75–100 mg/kg/day in a single dose (max: 2 g) IV or IM for 14–28 days; or penicillin G, 200,000–400,000 U/kg/day (max: 18–24 MU/day) divided q4h IV for 14–21 days

Arthritis

Initial treatment, same as for erythema migrans except that treatment should be for 28 days; for symptoms that fail to resolve after 2 mo or for a recurrence, then either a repeated oral regimen or treatment as for late neurologic disease

*For isolated palsy of the facial nerve or other cranial nerves, treat as for erythema migrans.

children with Lyme disease up to 4 years after they were treated and found no evidence of any long-term sequelae of the infection. Other investigators who are conducting a community-based study of long-term outcome in persons with Lyme disease have also found no evidence of impairment of normal functioning in children 4–11 years after a diagnosis of Lyme disease.

PREVENTION

In endemic areas it is common for children to be bitten by deer ticks. Such bites often engender tremendous anxiety. However, the overall risk of acquiring Lyme disease is low (approximately 1–2%) even in areas in which Lyme disease is endemic. Furthermore, treatment of the infection, if it develops, is highly effective. In hyperendemic regions, prophylaxis of adults with doxycycline 200 mg as a single dose within 72 hours of a nymphal tick bite is effective in preventing Lyme disease but is not routinely recommended.

Testing to determine whether a tick is infected, such as PCR analysis, is not useful clinically, although it may provide important epidemiologic information; the predictive value, for infection of humans, of either a positive or a negative PCR result is unknown. The test result may be positive even if only very few organisms are present. Furthermore, the test provides no information about either the size of the inoculum delivered to the human host or the duration of feeding, both of which may be key determinants of the risk of transmission. In addition, false-positive and false-negative test results are common.

A more reasonable approach to preventing Lyme disease is to wear appropriate protective clothing (such as lightweight long pants) when entering tick-infested areas and to check for and remove ticks after spending time in such areas (Chapter 3). Insect repellants may provide temporary protection, but they may be absorbed from the skin, and if used frequently or in large doses, they may produce significant toxic effects, especially in children.

Vaccine. Vaccines that use recombinant OspA protein have been shown to be safe and efficacious in randomized clinical trials in persons ≥15 years of age. The vaccine, which is administered at 0, 1, and 12 months, has an efficacy of about 50% during the first year after 2 doses and 75% during the second year after the third (booster) dose. Because the spirochete expresses OspA in ticks and in later stages of human illness but not at the time of initial infection in human skin, the vaccine works because the tick ingests human blood during feeding before inoculating the spirochete into humans; antibody-dependent killing of *B. burgdorferi* occurs in the tick. Consequently, natural boosting of vaccine-induced immunity through exposure to the bacterium is not likely to occur, and additional booster doses of the vaccine may be necessary. Because the risk of Lyme disease in most populations is low and poor outcomes among persons with Lyme disease are rare, it is recommended that the vaccine be used selectively, not routinely, even in endemic areas, after discussion with each patient concerning risks and benefits. The vaccine is not currently licensed for children less than 15 years of age.

REVIEWS

Nadelman RB, Wormser GP: Lyme borreliosis. *Lancet* 1998;352:557–65.

Rahn DW, Malawista SE: Lyme disease: Recommendations for diagnosis and treatment. *Ann Intern Med* 1991;114:472–81.

Shapiro ED, Gerber MA: Lyme disease. *Clin Infect Dis* 2000;31:533–42.

Steere AC: Lyme disease. *N Engl J Med* 2001;345:115–25.

Wormser GP, Nadelman RB, Dattwyler RJ, et al: Practice guidelines for the treatment of Lyme disease. *Clin Infect Dis* 2000;31(Suppl 1):S1–14.

KEY ARTICLES

Adams WV, Rose CD, Eppes SC, et al: Cognitive effects of Lyme disease in children. *Pediatrics* 1994;94:185–9.

Centers for Disease Control and Prevention: Recommendations for test performance and interpretation from the Second National Conference on Serologic Diagnosis of Lyme Disease. *MMWR Morb Mortal Wkly Rep* 1995;44:590–1.

Centers for Disease Control and Prevention: Recommendations for the use of Lyme disease vaccine. Recommendations of the Advisory Committee on Immunization Practices. *MMWR Morb Mortal Wkly Rep* 1999:48(RR–7):1–25.

Centers for Disease Control and Prevention: Surveillance for Lyme disease—United States, 1992–1998. *MMWR Morb Mortal Wkly Rep* 2000;49(SS–3):1–11.

Dattwyler RJ, Luft BJ, Kunkel MJ, et al: Ceftriaxone compared with doxycycline for the treatment of acute disseminated Lyme disease. *N Engl J Med* 1997;337:289–94.

des Vignes F, Piesman J, Heffernan R, et al: Effect of tick removal on transmission of *Borrelia burgdorferi* and *Ehrlichia phagocytophila* by *Ixodes scapularis* nymphs. *J Infect Dis* 2001;183:773–8.

Gerber MA, Shapiro ED, Burke GS, et al: Lyme disease in children in southeastern Connecticut. Pediatric Lyme Disease Study Group. *N Engl J Med* 1996;335:1270–4.

Gross DW, Forsthuber T, Tary-Lehmann M, et al: Identification of LFA-1 as a candidate autoantigen in treatment-resistant Lyme arthritis. *Science* 1998;281:703–6.

Kalish RA, Kaplan RF, Taylor E, et al: Evaluation of study patients with Lyme disease, 10–20-year follow-up. *J Infect Dis* 2001;183:453–60.

Klempner MS, Hu LT, Evans J, et al: Two controlled trials of antibiotic treatment in patients with persistent symptoms and a history of Lyme disease. *N Engl J Med* 2001;345:85–92.

Nadelman RB, Nowakowski J, Fish D, et al: Prophylaxis with single-dose doxycycline for the prevention of Lyme disease after an *Ixodes scapularis* tick bite. *N Engl J Med* 2001;345:79–84.

Seltzer EG, Gerber MA, Cartter ML, et al: Long-term outcomes of persons with Lyme disease. *JAMA* 2000;283:609–16.

Seltzer EG, Shapiro ED: Misdiagnosis of Lyme disease: When not to order serologic tests. *Pediatr Infect Dis J* 1996;15:762–3.

Shapiro ED, Gerber MA, Holabird NB, et al: A controlled trial of antimicrobial prophylaxis for Lyme disease after deer-tick bites. *N Engl J Med* 1992;327:1769–73.

Sigal LH: Persisting complaints attributed to chronic Lyme disease: Possible mechanisms and implications for management. *Am J Med* 1994;96:365–74.

Sigal LH: The Lyme disease controversy. Social and financial costs of misdiagnosis and mismanagement. *Arch Intern Med* 1996;156:1493–500.

Sigal LH, Zahradnik JM, Lavin P, et al: A vaccine consisting of recombinant *Borrelia burgdorferi* outer-surface protein A to prevent Lyme disease. Recombinant Outer-Surface Protein A Lyme Disease Vaccine Study Consortium. *N Engl J Med* 1998;339:216–22.

Steere AC, Taylor E, McHugh GL, et al: The overdiagnosis of Lyme disease. *JAMA* 1993;269:1812–6.

Steere AC, Sikand VK, Meurice F, et al: Vaccination against Lyme disease with recombinant *Borrelia burgdorferi* outer-surface lipoprotein A with adjuvant. Lyme Disease Vaccine Study Group. *N Engl J Med* 1998;339:209–15.

Warshafsky S, Nowakowski J, Nadelman RB, et al: Efficacy of antibiotic prophylaxis for prevention of Lyme disease. *J Gen Intern Med* 1996;11:329–33.

CHAPTER 30

Rocky Mountain Spotted Fever

John C. Christenson

Rocky Mountain spotted fever (RMSF) is one of the most common vectorborne illnesses in the United States. The first documented cases of this disease were described in 1899 along the border of Idaho and Montana. Wilson and Chowning, in 1902, described in detail the geographic, seasonal distribution, age- and sex-specific incidence, mortality rate, clinical presentation, and pathology of the disease. Howard Ricketts subsequently identified a bacillus as the possible causative agent. In 1905, two physicians, McCalla and Brereton, began tick experiments in humans. In 1919, Wolbach described the etiologic agent of RMSF. The disease was finally linked to arthropod vectors in 1920.

ETIOLOGY

The causative agent of RMSF is *Rickettsia rickettsii,* a small, obligate gram-negative intracellular coccobacillary bacterium that is a member of the spotted fever group of the family Rickettsiae (Table 30–1).

Transmission. Ticks transmit rickettsiae to humans during the feeding process. *Dermacentor variabilis,* the dog tick, is the major vector in the United States. In the United States in areas where RMSF is highly endemic, 2–11% of ticks are infected with the organism. *Dermacentor andersoni,* the wood tick, is the major vector of the disease in the Rocky Mountain region. *Amblyomma americanum,* the Lone Star tick, is a vector for RMSF in the southwestern United States.

Ticks become infected by feeding on infected animals or through transovarian transmission or fertilization. Only adult ticks will feed on humans; larvae and nymphs feed on small animals.

EPIDEMIOLOGY

In 1998, 365 cases of suspected RMSF from 36 states were reported to the CDC. The majority of cases occurred in the South Atlantic region, with western extension through Tennessee and Oklahoma. The annual rate in the United States has been fairly stable over the past 8 years and is significantly less than the broad increase observed from the mid-1970s through the mid-1980s, which peaked in 1981 with 1,192 cases (see Fig. 3–2).

Most cases of RMSF in the United States occur during the months of May through October. The adult ticks usually feed on humans during late spring and summer months. In warmer regions, cases of RMSF can be observed during fall and early winter months. The age-specific incidence is highest in children 1–14 years of age, probably because of outdoor play and attraction to dogs. Only 60% of infected persons recall a tick bite.

PATHOGENESIS

R. rickettsii are in a dormant state in the salivary glands of ticks and undergo reactivation as ticks feed on fresh blood. Organisms are released from the salivary glands after the tick has been attached for at least 6–10 hours. The organisms may also be acquired from tick hemolymph if infected ticks are crushed and exposed to open skin lesions, as during tick removal. *R. rickettsii,* like other rickettsiae, migrate in the bloodstream and invade and proliferate within the endothelial cells of blood vessels, causing a focal, necrotizing vasculitis. This leads to thrombosis of small blood vessels with leakage of red blood cells and protein-rich fluid into surrounding tissues resulting in hypoalbuminemia, edema, hypovolemia, hypotension, and hypoperfusion of tissue. Vasculitis is responsible for findings in the skin, heart, lungs, kidneys, liver, and other organs.

SYMPTOMS AND CLINICAL MANIFESTATIONS

The incubation period for RMSF after a tick bite is 2–14 days, with an average of 7 days. The first 3 days of illness are characterized by fever and constitutional symptoms (Table 30–2). Older children and adults may complain of severe intractable headaches. Myalgias, especially of the calf or thigh muscles, are also common. Approximately 8–28% of patients may have hepatosplenomegaly and jaundice. The presence of periorbital edema and the degree of edema of the extremities correlate with the extent of vasculitis. The disease may last up to 3 weeks if untreated. No asymptomatic infection has been described.

Rash. From 75–96% of patients have a characteristic petechial rash (Plate 5C). This rash classically appears between days 3 and 5 of illness, appearing first on the feet and ankles, then on the wrists and hands, and within hours spreading centripetally to the trunk and head. The rash is present on the first day of symptoms in as many as 14% of patients and involves the palms and soles in approximately 50% of patients. The rash may start as a maculopapular exanthem and then evolve into a finely or grossly hemorrhagic, petechial rash.

In approximately 9–16% of laboratory-confirmed or probable cases there is no form of rash. Such "spotless" fever is more commonly seen in fatal cases, in African-Americans, and in older patients. A high index of suspicion is needed to detect these atypical cases because delays in recognition of the disease may result in a delay in treatment with increased mortality.

DIAGNOSIS

The diagnosis of RMSF is usually suspected on the basis of fever and petechial rash, especially when there is a history of a tick bite or possible tick exposure during outdoor activities between early spring and late summer in endemic regions. The diagnosis of RMSF should also be considered in cases of unexplained fever, macular or petechial rash, myalgias, electrolyte abnormalities, thrombocytopenia, or elevated hepatic transaminase levels. The absence of a

TABLE 30–1. Geographic Distribution of Major Human Rickettsioses

Disease	Organism	Geographic Area	Arthropod Vector	Vertebrate Host	Eschar
Spotted Fever Group					
Rocky Mountain spotted fever	*Rickettsia rickettsii*	Western hemisphere	Tick *(Dermacentor variabilis, D. andersoni, Amblyomma americanum, Ixodes)*	Wild rodents, dogs	No
Mediterranean spotted fever (Boutonneuse fever)	*R. conorii*	Mediterranean region, Africa, India	Tick *(Rhipicephalus sanguineus)*	Wild rodents, dogs	Yes
African tick-bite fever	*R. africae*	Southern Africa	Tick *(Amblyomma)*	Cattle	Yes
Queensland tick typhus	*R. australis*	Australia	Tick *(Ixodes)*	Wild rodents, marsupials	Yes
North Asian tick typhus	*R. sibirica*	Siberia, Mongolia	Tick *(Dermacentor)*	Wild rodents	Yes
Rickettsialpox	*R. akari*	Urban areas of eastern United States, former Soviet Union, Korea, Africa	Mite *(Allodermanyssus)*	Mouse	Yes
Typhus Group					
Epidemic typhus	*R. prowazekii*	South America, Asia, Africa	Body louse *(Pediculus humanus corporis)*	Humans, flying squirrels	No
Murine typhus	*R. typhi*	Worldwide	Flea *(Xenopsylla cheopis, Ctenocephalides felis)*	Small rodents	No
Scrub typhus	*R. tsutsugamushi*	South Pacific, Asia, Australia	Mite *(Leptotrombidium deliense)*	Wild rodents	Yes
***Ehrlichia* (Chapter 31)**					
Human monocytic ehrlichiosis	*Ehrlichia chaffeensis*	United States, Europe	Tick *(Amblyomma americanum)*	Deer	No
Human granulocytic ehrlichiosis	*Ehrlichia phagocytophila*-like organism	United States, Europe	Tick *(Ixodes scapularis)*	White-footed mouse, deer	No
Other Illness					
Q fever	*Coxiella burnetii*	Worldwide	Tick (animal-to-animal)	Cattle, sheep, goats (by inhalation of organism)	No

history of tick bite should not be misleading, because in approximately 10–20% of cases of RMSF there is no recognized tick exposure. Serologic assays are the most widely available and frequently used methods for confirming cases of RMSF, but these are often nonconfirmatory during the first 7–10 days of illness. Therapy for suspected RMSF should not be deferred pending laboratory confirmation.

Differential Diagnosis

The differential diagnosis of RMSF in the early stages includes not only several viral and bacterial infections but also some noninfectious conditions (Table 30–3). Meningococcemia is the disease that is most commonly confused with RMSF. Differentiation on the basis of clinical manifestations alone may be difficult, and empirical antimicrobial therapy covering both pathogens may be necessary initially. The exanthem of RMSF with its centripetal spread and petechial character should be easily distinguishable from those of measles and rubella.

Human ehrlichiosis (Chapter 31) shares many clinical symptoms as well as epidemiologic features with RMSF. Rash occurs in approximately 40% of cases of human monocytic ehrlichiosis but is rarely present with human granulocytic ehrlichiosis. The rash of ehrlichiosis is usually macular or maculopapular and distributed mainly on the trunk, but it may be petechial and distributed on the extremities as well, similar to the rash of RMSF.

Laboratory Evaluation

Approximately 50% of patients have thrombocytopenia (platelet count usually $<100{,}000/mm^3$). The majority of patients have a normal leukocyte count but with a neutrophilic predominance and often with a left shift. Anemia occurs in 30% of patients. Hyponatremia, which is observed in 20–88% of patients, is a common laboratory finding. Hepatic transaminase levels may be elevated.

Leukopenia and profound thrombocytopenia are more commonly seen in ehrlichiosis than in RMSF. Intracytoplasmic leukocyte inclusions, or **morulae,** are commonly observed in bone marrow mononuclear and polymorphonuclear cells of patients with acute ehrlichiosis (see Fig. 31-1). They are occasionally found in the peripheral blood with ehrlichiosis and are rarely seen in RMSF.

Microbiologic Evaluation

Serologic Diagnosis. Laboratory diagnosis can be established by specific serologic tests using one of the following assays: indirect IFA, LA, and EIA. A fourfold increase in antibody titers by any

TABLE 30–2. Symptoms and Signs of Rocky Mountain Spotted Fever

	Present During Illness	
Symptom or Sign	**Any Time (%)**	**First 3 Days (%)**
Fever		
37.7–38.8°C (100–102°F)	99	73
≥38.8°C (102°F)	90	63
Headache		
Mild or moderate	91	71
Severe	47	25
Rash		
Any	88	49
Maculopapular	82	46
Palms or soles	74	28
Petechial-hemorrhagic	49	13
Myalgias		
Mild or moderate	83	57
Severe	47	25
Triad of fever, rash, and history of tick exposure	67	3
Nausea, vomiting	60	38
Abdominal pain	52	30
Conjunctivitis	30	13
Lymphadenopathy	27	13
Stupor	26	6
Diarrhea	19	9
Edema	18	3
Ataxia	18	7
Meningismus	18	5
Splenomegaly	16	3
Hepatomegaly	12	2
Pneumonitis	12	2
Coma	9	1
Jaundice	9	2
Seizures	8	2
Shock	7	<1
Decreased hearing	7	1
Cardiac dysrhythmia	7	1
Myocarditis	5	0
Death	4	<1
Parotitis	4	<1
Orchitis (males)	1	0

Adapted from Helmick CG, Bernard KW, D'Angelo LJ: Rocky Mountain spotted fever: Clinical, laboratory, and epidemiological features in 262 cases. *J Infect Dis* 1984;150:480–6.

TABLE 30–3. Differential Diagnosis of Rocky Mountain Spotted Fever

Infectious
Meningococcemia *(Neisseria meningitidis)*
Gram-negative bacterial sepsis
Toxic shock syndrome
Leptospirosis
Secondary syphilis
Murine typhus *(Rickettsia typhi)*
Measles (rubeola)
Rubella
Enteroviral exanthem
Human ehrlichiosis

Noninfectious
Thrombotic thrombocytopenic purpura
Immune complex vasculitis
Drug reaction

TABLE 30–4. Antimicrobial Treatment for Rocky Mountain Spotted Fever

Recommended Therapy
Doxycycline 2–4 mg/kg/day (max adult dose, 200 mg/day) divided q12–24hr PO (may be administered IV initially) until patient is afebrile for 2–3 days. Usual course of therapy is 7–10 days.

Alternative Therapy
Chloramphenicol 50–75 mg/kg/day (max adult dose, 2–4 g/day) divided q6hr IV or PO until patient is afebrile for 2–3 days. Usual course of therapy is 7–10 days.

method is diagnostic. Early antimicrobial treatment may suppress the antibody response. A single titer of ≥1:64 with IFA or ≥1:128 with LA is also considered diagnostic of RMSF. All these tests are highly sensitive and specific. Antibodies in RMSF are usually detectable 7–10 days after onset of illness and fall to nondiagnostic levels by 2 months. The sensitivity and specificity of the *Proteus vulgaris* agglutination assays for strains OX-19 and OX-2 (**Weil-Felix test**) are so low that these tests should not be used for the diagnosis of RMSF.

Direct Detection. *R. rickettsii* can be identified in paraffin-embedded tissues by an immunohistochemical assay and in frozen tissue samples by an IFA assay. Immunohistochemical or immunofluorescent staining of a petechial lesion is highly specific, although the sensitivity of these methods decreases after the initiation of specific antimicrobial therapy. Organisms are often distributed sparsely through tissues, including skin, and there may be broad areas, even with petechial or ecchymotic lesions, with no demonstrable rickettsiae. These are the only currently available methods that can be used to confirm the diagnosis at the time of presentation, but they are available only through specialized research laboratories or the CDC.

Newer tests such as PCR are being developed and may be used for early diagnosis. Although highly specific, initial studies have demonstrated poor sensitivity.

Culture. Isolation of the organism can be achieved in cell culture but only in facilities with specialized laboratories.

Pathologic Findings

There are no histopathologic lesions that are pathognomonic for RMSF. Suggestive findings include multifocal lymphohistiocytic infiltrates in the interstitium of the kidneys, heart, and lung and in the hepatic portal triads. The brain may show multifocal glial nodules and arteriolar microinfarcts. Multifocal necroses, often containing rickettsial antigens, may be found in the adrenal cortices of persons dying of RMSF.

TREATMENT

The antimicrobial therapy of choice for RMSF is doxycycline for children older than 8 years of age, with chloramphenicol as an alternative (Table 30–4). The CDC and the AAP traditionally have recommended the use of chloramphenicol for children younger than 9 years of age because of the risk of permanent staining of developing teeth that may occur with the use of tetracyclines in this age group. However, several arguments support the use of tetracycline for the treatment of RMSF irrespective of age. The staining of teeth with the tetracyclines is related to dose. Tooth discoloration in children 5 years of age or younger who receive fewer than 6 courses of tetracycline therapy of approximately 6 days each is negligible. Some experts consider that the risk of discoloration is less when doxycycline is used. Chloramphenicol does have significant adverse effects. The risk of idiosyncratic aplastic anemia with chloramphenicol therapy is between 1 in 25,000 and 1 in 40,000 treated persons. Monitoring of serum chloramphenicol concentration is recommended to minimize the dose-related hematologic adverse effects of the drug. Ehrlichiosis sometimes mimics RMSF clinically, and whereas tetracyclines are highly effective for ehrlichiosis, *Ehrlichia* is usually resistant to chloramphenicol. However, if *Neisseria meningitidis* infection is considered in the differential diagnosis, chloramphenicol is the preferred agent for monotherapy. One study demonstrated a higher mortality in patients with RMSF who were treated with chloramphenicol than in those treated with tetracycline.

On the basis of in vitro susceptibility testing and animal studies, quinolones such as ciprofloxacin are active against *R. rickettsii.* Patients with Mediterranean spotted fever (MSF) have been successfully treated with quinolones. In a recent study, azithromycin was found to be equivalent to doxycycline for the treatment of MSF. Although additional information is needed concerning these newer agents for RMSF, they may be considered as alternatives for patients unable to receive doxycycline or chloramphenicol.

COMPLICATIONS

The pulmonary circulation is a major target of the infection. As a result of the severe vasculitis, pulmonary capillary leakage into the interstitial space and airspace frequently occurs, resulting in noncardiogenic pulmonary edema. This is manifested clinically by cough and respiratory distress with interstitial infiltrates on chest radiographs. Severe respiratory failure is observed in 12% of persons with RMSF. Adult respiratory distress syndrome has also been reported. The mortality rate is very high if mechanical ventilation is required.

Another target of the disease is the CNS, and signs of meningoencephalitis are commonly noted. This is clinically recognized in approximately 25–33% of persons with RMSF and may be manifested by confusion, stupor, delirium, ataxia, seizures, or coma. Approximately 33% of the persons with CNS involvement have severe neurologic dysfunction. Encephalitis associated with RMSF has a poor prognosis. The cerebrospinal fluid may have a mild pleocytosis (WBC count usually less than 200/mm^3) with a lymphocytic or polymorphonuclear predominance and a slightly elevated protein level. The glucose level is usually normal but is rarely depressed. Guillain-Barré syndrome has also been described with RMSF.

Severe cases of RMSF are characterized by profound vascular collapse, disseminated intravascular coagulopathy, and multiple organ failure. The prognosis under these circumstances is poor. Myocarditis as evidenced by abnormal electrocardiograms and arrhythmias is present in approximately 26% of patients. Acute renal failure may result from acute tubular necrosis. Severe peripheral vasculitis may result in skin necrosis and gangrene, requiring amputation.

Persons with glucose-6-phosphate dehydrogenase deficiency (G6PD) are at high risk of fulminant RMSF with increased mortality due to severe hemolysis.

PROGNOSIS

Without effective therapy, approximately 25% of patients with RMSF die. However, almost no patients die if antimicrobial therapy is initiated within a week of onset of symptoms. The overall case fatality rate is approximately 3.4%. For patients older than 20 years the mortality rate is 6.8%; for patients younger than 20 years it is 2.4%. Prognostic indicators for increased mortality are hepatomegaly, jaundice, stupor, marked neurologic dysfunction, inappropriate or delayed therapy, and renal failure. In one study a delay in therapy of more than 5 days after onset resulted in a mortality rate of 23%, whereas treatment within 5 days reduced the mortality rate to 6.5%. Delayed diagnosis and late treatment usually result from atypical initial symptoms and late appearance of rash. Therapy for suspected RMSF should not be postponed pending results of diagnostic tests.

PREVENTION

No effective vaccine is currently available for the prevention of RMSF. Preventive measures are extremely important for persons visiting endemic areas. Such measures include avoidance of tick-infested areas, thorough inspection after returning from the outdoors, wearing of protective clothing (long sleeves, long pants, shoes instead of sandals), use of insect repellants, and careful removal of ticks, if found (Chapter 3). Prophylactic antibiotics should not be given after a tick bite. Attention to preventive measures and to early signs and symptoms of disease with prompt evaluation is recommended.

REVIEWS

Hackstadt T: The biology of rickettsiae. *Infect Agents Dis* 1996;5:127–43.

La Scola B, Raoult D: Laboratory diagnosis of rickettsioses: Current approaches to diagnosis of old and new rickettsial diseases. *J Clin Microbiol* 1997;35:2715–27.

Raoult D, Roux V: Rickettsioses as paradigms of new or emerging infectious diseases. *Clin Microbiol Rev* 1997;10:694–719.

Thorner AR, Walker DH, Petri WA Jr: Rocky Mountain spotted fever. *Clin Infect Dis* 1998;27:1353–9.

KEY ARTICLES

Abramson JS, Givner LB: Should tetracycline be contraindicated for therapy of presumed Rocky Mountain spotted fever in children less than 9 years of age? *Pediatrics* 1990;86:123–4.

Archibald LK, Sexton DJ: Long-term sequelae of Rocky Mountain spotted fever. *Clin Infect Dis* 1995;20:1122–5.

Dalton MJ, Clarke MJ, Holman RC, et al: National surveillance for Rocky Mountain spotted fever, 1981–1992: Epidemiologic summary and evaluation of risk factors for fatal outcome. *Am J Trop Med Hyg* 1995;52: 405–13.

Helmick CG, Bernard KW, D'Angelo LJ: Rocky Mountain spotted fever: Clinical, laboratory, and epidemiological features in 262 cases. *J Infect Dis* 1984;150:480–6.

Kirkland KB, Wilkinson WE, Sexton DJ: Therapeutic delay and mortality in cases of Rocky Mountain spotted fever. *Clin Infect Dis* 1995;20: 1118–21.

Maxey EE: Some observations on the so-called spotted fever of Idaho. *Med Sentinel* 1899;7:348.

Meloni G, Meloni T: Azithromycin vs doxycycline for Mediterranean spotted fever. *Pediatr Infect Dis J* 1996;15:1042–4.

Paddock CD, Greer PW, Ferebee TL, et al: Hidden mortality attributable to Rocky Mountain spotted fever: Immunohistochemical detection of fatal, serologically unconfirmed disease. *J Infect Dis* 1999;179:1469–76.

Ricketts HT: Some aspects of Rocky Mountain spotted fever as shown by recent investigations. *Med Rec* 1909;76:843–55. (Reprinted in *Rev Infect Dis* 1991;13:1227–40.)

Rolain JM, Maurin M, Vestris G, et al: In vitro susceptibilities of 27 rickettsiae to 13 antimicrobials. *Antimicrob Agents Chemother* 1998; 42:1537–41.

Schutze GE: Prevention of tick infestation. *Semin Pediatr Infect Dis* 1994;5:157–60.

Wilson LB, Chowning WM: The so-called ''spotted fever'' of the Rocky Mountains. *JAMA* 1902;39:131–6.

Wolbach SB: Studies on Rocky Mountain spotted fever. *J Med Res* 1919;41:1–196.

CHAPTER 31

Human Ehrlichiosis

Sam R. Telford III ▪ Peter J. Krause

Human ehrlichiosis was first recognized in 1956 in Japan as **Sennetsu fever,** a mononucleosis-like syndrome with fever, lymphadenopathy, malaise, and anorexia. Two newly described human ehrlichioses caused by tick-transmitted rickettsiae have subsequently emerged in the United States (Table 31–1). These are similar illnesses with acute onset of fever accompanied by headache, malaise, myalgias, and rigors. Laboratory findings include leukopenia, thrombocytopenia, and elevated hepatic enzymes. Intraleukocytic clusters of bacteria (morulae) may be observed in peripheral blood smears. Symptoms generally resolve promptly with tetracycline therapy.

ETIOLOGY

Ehrlichia chaffeensis infects monocytes and is the causative agent of **human monocytic ehrlichiosis (HME)** (Fig. 31–1). The other *Ehrlichia* infects granulocytes and has yet to receive a specific name but is currently known as the **agent of human granulocytic ehrlichiosis (HGE), HGE agent,** *Ehrlichia phagocytophila* genogroup, or *Ehrlichia equi* (Fig. 31–1).

Transmission. Deer serve as the reservoir for *E. chaffeensis,* the cause of HME. The vector is the **Lone Star tick,** *Amblyomma americanum.* The prevalence of infection in host-seeking ticks appears to be minimal, approximately 1% for nymphs and adult ticks. Ticks at all three stages aggressively attack humans, but only nymphs and adults transmit infection.

The ecology of HGE is more comprehensively understood because the agent shares the same vector and reservoir as those of Lyme disease (Chapter 29) and babesiosis (Chapter 33). The natural cycle clearly depends on the interaction of *Ixodes scapularis* (previously known as *Ixodes dammini*), the **deer tick** (Fig. 31–2 and Plate 9E), and their main host, the **white-footed mouse** *(Peromyscus leucopus).* In northern California, *Ixodes pacificus,* the **western blacklegged tick,** serves as the vector of HGE. **White-tailed deer** *(Odocoileus virginianus)* serve as the host on which adult ticks most abundantly feed. Adult ticks feed during the fall and during the spring lay eggs that hatch synchronously in late July (Fig. 33–1). Larvae feed mainly during August and September, when they acquire ehrlichial infection. Unlike the agents of Lyme disease and babesiosis, that of HGE appears to behave more like an arbovirus in its ecology. A variety of reservoir hosts may contribute to the force of transmission, including mice, voles, chipmunks, deer, and sheep. In addition, reservoir infectivity appears to be transient, lasting only about 2 weeks. This is in sharp contrast to Lyme disease and babesiosis, whose reservoirs appear to be infective to the vector for their entire life. Larval ticks feed and overwinter and then molt to the nymphal stage during the spring. Nymphal ticks seek hosts during late April, May, June, and early July. The life cycle of the tick is completed when nymphs that have fed on a host molt to the adult stage in the fall. Thus, *I. scapularis* ticks develop from egg to egg over a span of at least 2 years. This permits cohorts of nymphal ticks to overlap, thereby buffering the population against years of host scarcity.

One case of HGE transmission by blood transfusion was described in a 75-year-old man in whom HGE developed 10 days after he was transfused with one unit of packed red blood cells from a blood donor who had both HGE and Lyme disease. Transplacental or perinatal transmission is not apparent in the reservoir rodents or in humans.

EPIDEMIOLOGY

Ehrlichiosis is not a nationally reportable disease, which limits accurate estimates of cumulative case numbers. At least 500 cases of HME, with 11 deaths, have been recorded. A similar number of HGE cases and case fatalities have been reported. Prospective studies of HME incidence in Oklahoma and Georgia suggest that it is as common as RMSF, occurring at the rate of approximately 5 cases per 100,000 population. Efforts to describe HGE incidence have been limited thus far to passive case detection. An early estimate of HGE incidence in a site of intense transmission was 58 cases per 100,000 population. The asymptomatic to symptomatic case ratio has not been described but is likely to be large.

Most HME infections occur in the late spring and summer. The Lone Star tick is distributed widely from New Jersey southward to Florida and westward through Oklahoma and Texas; therefore HME is found most commonly in the southeastern and south-central United States. Isolated populations of the Lone Star tick exist on Fire Island, New York, and in Narragansett Bay, Rhode Island.

The distribution of HGE closely parallels that of the deer tick vector. Most cases of HGE occur between April and September, with peak occurrence from May through July. Cases of HGE have been serologically confirmed in Minnesota, Wisconsin, New York, Maryland, Connecticut, Massachusetts, and Florida. Cases have been confirmed by PCR in Minnesota, Wisconsin, Maryland, Massachusetts, and Florida. Cases of HGE have been described from northern California, where the western black-legged tick *(I. pacificus)* serves as vector of equine granulocytic ehrlichiosis. The deer tick vector of HGE may be spreading southward along the Atlantic coast and may infest sites where Lone Star ticks are abundant. The relatively recent proliferation of deer, abandonment of farmland and subsequent succession to thick secondary vegetation, and increased use of coastal sites for human recreation or habitation have allowed deer ticks and Lone Star ticks to reach tremendous densities in certain areas. As a result the human ehrlichioses have emerged as a public health burden in much of the eastern United States.

PATHOGENESIS

Unlike *R. rickettsii,* the agent of RMSF (Chapter 30) that targets vascular sites, *Ehrlichia* infects phagocytic cells and may inhibit

TABLE 31–1. Major Pathogenic *Ehrlichia* Species

Organism	Major Target Cell	Host(s)	Disease(s)
Genogroup I			
E. chaffeensis	Monocytes and macrophages	Humans	Human monocytic ehrlichiosis
E. canis	Monocytes and macrophages	Dogs	Canine ehrlichiosis
Genogroup II			
Human granulocytic agent	Neutrophils	Humans, deer	Human granulocytic ehrlichiosis
E. equi	Neutrophils	Horses	Equine granulocytic ehrlichiosis
E. phagocytophila	Neutrophils	Sheep, cattle, deer	Tickborne fever
Genogroup III			
E. sennetsu	Monocytes and macrophages	Humans	Sennetsu fever
E. risticii	Monocytes and macrophages	Horses	Equine monocytic ehrlichiosis

their function. The profound leukopenia that is often associated with ehrlichiosis may render the host more susceptible to opportunistic pathogens. Many of the deaths due to ehrlichiosis appear to be associated with secondary bacterial or fungal infections.

SYMPTOMS AND CLINICAL MANIFESTATIONS

Incubation Period. The incubation period of HME and HGE appears to be 1–3 weeks, with a median of 11–12 days.

Common Symptoms

The spectrum of HME and HGE infection ranges from asymptomatic to fatal, but most affected persons experience an acute febrile illness lasting 1–2 weeks, which generally resolves spontaneously. Patients with either infection experience similar signs, symptoms, and clinical course (Table 31–2). Ehrlichiosis is characterized by fever, headache, chills, sweats, malaise, and myalgia. Patients may also experience arthralgia, nausea, vomiting, anorexia, weight loss, and, less frequently, confusion, prostration, vertigo, diarrhea, and cough. Rash occurs in approximately 40% of patients with HME but is rarely present with HGE. The rash may be macular, maculopapular, or petechial and involves the trunk and extremities. Meningitis and pneumonia are uncommon manifestations of ehrlichiosis.

Laboratory Findings

Laboratory features of ehrlichiosis include progressive reductions in circulating white blood cells and platelets. Anemia is frequently present. Bleeding is seldom noted, although DIC has been described. Slight elevations in hepatic and renal function tests, particularly aspartate aminotransferase and serum creatinine, as well as hyponatremia and hypoalbuminemia, may occur. These changes are presumably due to generalized vasculitis. The ESR is slightly elevated.

DIAGNOSIS

The interim case definition of the CDC for ehrlichiosis is ''undifferentiated fever'' and at least one of the following: (1) PCR-positive blood or tissue sample; (2) fourfold rise in antibody titer to the antigen of *E. equi* (testing paired serum samples with the convalescent sample taken at least 1 month after the acute sample); or (3) demonstration of the organism in blood smears or tissues.

Human ehrlichiosis is usually a presumptive clinical diagnosis. Failure to directly demonstrate the pathogen by microscopy, PCR,

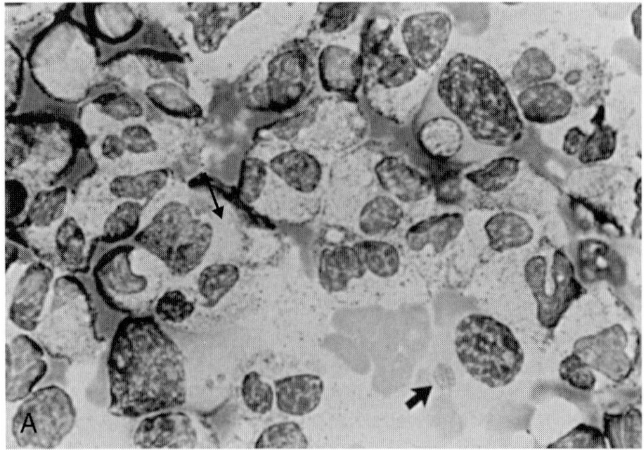

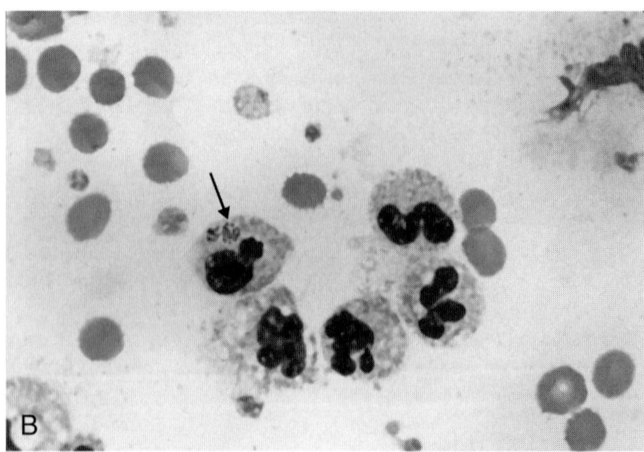

FIGURE 31–1. A, Morula *(arrow)* of *Ehrlichia chaffeensis* in the cytoplasm of a mononuclear leukocyte (probably a monocyte) in the peripheral blood smear of a patient with HME. **B** Morula *(arrow)* of the ehrlichial agent of HGE in the cytoplasm of a neutrophil from a patient with HGE. (Wright stain; ×1200). (**A** from Maeda K, Markowitz N, Hawley RC, et al: Human infection with *Ehrlichia canis,* a leukocytic Rickettsiaceae. *N Engl J Med* 1987;316:853–6. Copyright © 1987 Massachusetts Medical Society. All rights reserved.)

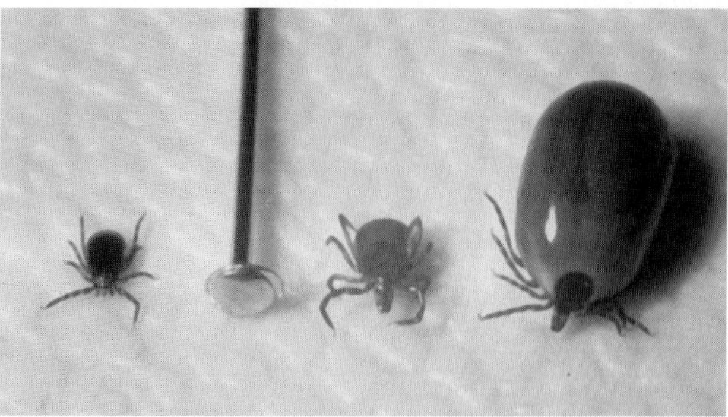

FIGURE 31–2. *Ixodes scapularis* (previously known as *Ixodes dammini*), which is the tick vector of HGE as well as Lyme disease and babesiosis. The ticks are an adult male, an adult female, and an engorged female. *Amblyomma americanum* is the tick vector of HME. (Courtesy of Mike Frigione.) (See also Plate 9E.)

cultivation, or subinoculation is common. The strategy for confirming the presumptive diagnosis thus rests upon seroconversion, as it does for all other rickettsial diseases.

Although it is not necessary to distinguish between the two American human ehrlichioses for patient management, assigning a specific identity to the etiologic agent is useful for epidemiologic purposes. All cases of ehrlichiosis should be reported to state health departments so that the public health burden of these emergent tickborne zoonoses may better be estimated.

Differential Diagnosis

The nonspecificity of signs and symptoms makes diagnosis dependent on a high index of suspicion by the physician and careful analysis of laboratory findings (Table 31–3). The differential diagnosis includes Lyme disease without erythema migrans (Chapter 29), babesiosis (Chapter 33), tularemia (Chapter 34), and RMSF (Chapter 30).

Microbiologic Evaluation

Direct Detection. Examination of a Giemsa- or Wright-stained thin blood smear for characteristic **morulae** (bacterial inclusions in leukocytes) establishes the diagnosis (Fig. 31–1), but failure to detect morulae within leukocytes is common. Thrombocytopenia and leukopenia, with elevated hepatic enzymes, should provide an incentive for prolonged scrutiny of multiple blood smears, perhaps taken at different times of the day. For both infections, buffy coat smears may facilitate microscopy. The leading edge of thin blood smears should be carefully examined because granulocytes tend to concentrate there. HME is extremely difficult to diagnose by microscopy because monocytes generally comprise <5% of all circulating leukocytes.

TABLE 31–2. Symptoms and Signs of Human Ehrlichiosis

Symptom or Sign*	Monocytic Ehrlichiosis (HME) (% of 156–211 cases)	Granulocytic Ehrlichiosis (HGE) (% of 12 cases)
Fever	97	100
Malaise	84	100
Headache	81	100
Myalgia	68	100
Rigors	61	100
Diaphoresis	53	91
Nausea	48	50
Vomiting	37	50
Cough	26	25
Arthralgias	41	25
Rash	36	8
Confusion	20	42

*At any time during the course of infection.

Adapted from Dumler JS, Bakken JS: Ehrlichial diseases of humans: Emerging tickborne infections. *Clin Infect Dis* 1995;20:1102–10.

TABLE 31–3. Laboratory Diagnosis of Human Ehrlichiosis

Routine Laboratory Tests
Leukopenia
Thrombocytopenia
Anemia
Elevated aspartate aminotransferase
Elevated creatinine

Microbiologic Evaluation
Identification of leukocyte morulae on blood smear
Isolation of causative agent in tissue culture
Amplification of *Ehrlichia* DNA using PCR
Detection of anti-*Ehrlichia* serum antibody

Molecular detection by PCR has been employed with some success, but it is performed as a research technique and is not generally available.

Culture. Direct cultivation of the agent of HGE from the patient by incubating whole blood with human promyelocytic (HL60) cells in vitro shows much promise for definitive diagnosis. The sensitivity of this procedure is unknown. Similarly, monolayers of canine histiocyte (DH82) cells may be used for cultivating the agent of HME. Mouse inoculation may serve as a confirmatory test for HGE, much as hamster inoculation is for babesiosis due to *Babesia microti.*

Serologic Testing. Acute samples should be stored and analyzed in parallel with the convalescent sample taken 1 month later. Multiple convalescent samples may be required to demonstrate seroconversion. Serology for ehrlichiosis is not yet standardized. IFAs for antibody use *E. equi* within horse neutrophils as a surrogate antigen or HL60 cells–cultivated HGE agent. The sensitivity and specificity of the indirect fluorescent antibody test have not been evaluated.

TREATMENT

Patients respond well to treatment with doxycycline or other tetracyclines for a minimum of 7 days. Defervescence is expected within 24–48 hours after the beginning of a regimen with oral doxycycline of 100 mg twice daily for adults or 3 mg/kg per day in two divided doses for children. The decision to use doxycycline in children under 8 years of age is difficult. Physicians must weigh the risks of not treating a possible life-threatening disease against the uncommon risk of permanent staining of teeth from the tetracycline. Rifampin has been suggested as an alternative for patients in whom tetracycline is contraindicated. Chloramphenicol, the second-line drug for treatment of RMSF, seems poorly effective against the agents of HME and HGE in vitro. Ciprofloxacin and other quinolones hold promise based on in vitro tests against the agent of HGE.

COMPLICATIONS

Persons with HME or HGE may require hospitalization. The case fatality rate is estimated to be 3–5%.

PROGNOSIS

Most persons with ehrlichiosis experience an acute febrile illness of 1–2 weeks' duration that spontaneously resolves. Chronic infections or sequelae have not yet been described, although weakness and fatigue appear to persist for as long as 1 month.

PREVENTION

No vaccine is available for the prevention of human ehrlichiosis. Preventive measures are extremely important for persons visiting endemic areas. Such measures include avoidance of tick-infested areas, thorough inspection after returning from the outdoors, wearing of protective clothing (long sleeves, long pants, shoes instead of sandals), use of insect repellents, and careful removal of ticks, if found (Chapter 3).

Prophylactic antibiotics should not be given after a tick bite. Attention to preventive measures and to early signs and symptoms of disease with prompt evaluation is recommended. A "grace period" exists for tick transmission of infection. Infection with HGE appears to be most efficient after 30–36 hours of nymphal tick attachment, as opposed to 36–48 hours for *Borrelia burgdorferi* and 56–60 hours for *Babesia.*

The community-level risk of acquiring ehrlichiosis is a direct function of tick density, which in turn is causally related to that of the reproductive host of the tick. For the zoonoses transmitted by the deer tick, deer reduction has served to drastically diminish human risk. Host-seeking ticks may be killed by applications of acaricide to vegetation around yards or by targeted application of Damminix via impregnated cotton, which mice carry back to their nests. Deer ticks and Lone Star ticks are dependent on humid microclimates, and therefore vegetation management (e.g., brush cutting and removal, controlled burns) might prove useful.

REVIEWS

Dumler JS, Bakken JS: Ehrlichial diseases of humans: Emerging tick-borne infections. *Clin Infect Dis* 1995;20:1102–10.

Edwards MS: Ehrlichiosis in children. *Semin Pediatr Infect Dis* 1994; 5:143–7.

KEY ARTICLES

Bakken JS, Krueth J, Wilson-Nordskog C, et al: Clinical and laboratory characteristics of human granulocytic ehrlichiosis. *JAMA* 1996;275: 199–205.

Bakken JS, Dumler JS, Chen SM, et al: Human granulocytic ehrlichiosis in the upper Midwest United States: A new species emerging? *JAMA* 1994;272:212–8.

Ewing SA, Dawson JE, Kocan AA, et al: Experimental transmission of *Ehrlichia chaffeensis* (Rickettsiales: Ehrlichieae) among white tailed deer by *Amblyomma americanum* (Acari: Ixodidae). *J Med Entomol* 1995;32:368–74.

Goodman JL, Nelson C, Vitale B, et al: Direct cultivation of the causative agent of human granulocytic ehrlichiosis. *N Engl J Med* 1996;334: 209–15.

Harkess JR, Ewing SA, Brumit T, et al: Ehrlichiosis in children. *Pediatrics* 1991;87:199–203.

Horowitz HW, Aguero-Rosenfeld ME, McKenna DF, et al: Clinical and laboratory spectrum of culture-proven human granulocytic ehrlichiosis: Comparison with culture-negative cases. *Clin Infect Dis* 1998;27:1314–7

Horowitz HW, Kilchevsky E, Haber S, et al: Perinatal transmission of the agent of human granulocytic ehrlichiosis. *N Engl J Med* 1998;339:375–8.

Lochary ME, Lockhart PB, Williams WT Jr: Doxycycline and staining of permanent teeth. *Pediatr Infect Dis J* 1998;17:429–31.

Maeda KN, Markowitz N, Hawley RC, et al: Human infection with *Ehrlichia canis,* a leukocytic rickettsia. *N Engl J Med* 1987;316:853–6.

Needham GR: Evaluation of five popular methods for tick removal. *Pediatrics* 1985;75:997–1002.

Ratnasamy N, Everett ED, Roland WE, et al: Central nervous system manifestations of human ehrlichiosis. *Clin Infect Dis* 1996;23:314–9.

Telford SR III, Dawson JE, Katavolos P, et al: Perpetuation of the agent of human granulocytic ehrlichiosis in a deer tick-rodent cycle. *Proc Natl Acad Sci USA* 1996;93:6209–14.

Telford SR III, Lepore TJ, Snow P, et al: Human granulocytic ehrlichiosis in Massachusetts. *Ann Intern Med* 1995;123:277–9.

Wilson ML, Telford SR III, Piesman J, et al: Reduced abundance of immature *Ixodes dammini* (Acari: Ixodidae) following elimination of deer. *J Med Entomol* 1988;25:224–8.

CHAPTER 32

Malaria

Peter J. Krause

Malaria is an acute and chronic illness characterized by paroxysms of fever, chills, sweats, fatigue, anemia, and splenomegaly. It has played a major role in human history, having arguably caused more harm to more people than any other infectious disease. Periodic fevers were mentioned in early Hindu and Chinese writings and were well described in ancient Greek and Roman texts. Malaria is of overwhelming importance in the developing world today, with an estimated 250 million cases and 1–2 million deaths each year. Malaria may be the leading infectious cause of death in the world, and most of these deaths occur in infants and young children.

ETIOLOGY

Malaria is caused by obligate intracellular protozoa of the genus *Plasmodium* and class Sporozoa, which also includes *Babesia, Cryptosporidium,* and *Toxoplasma gondii.* Malaria is caused by four species of *Plasmodium: P. falciparum, P. malariae, P. ovale,* and *P. vivax* (Table 32–1). *Plasmodium* species exist in a variety of forms and have a complex life cycle that enables them to survive in different cellular environments in the human host and in the mosquito vector. There are two major phases in the life cycle, an asexual phase (schizogony) in humans and a sexual phase (sporogony) in mosquitos (Fig. 32–1).

Schizogony, the asexual development of *Plasmodium* species in man, occurs in two sequential steps: the exoerythrocytic phase in hepatic cells and the erythrocytic phase in red blood cells. The **exoerythrocytic phase** begins with inoculation of **sporozoites** by a female *Anopheles* mosquito into the bloodstream. Within minutes the sporozoites enter the hepatocytes, where they develop and multiply asexually in multinucleated **exoerythrocytic schizonts.** After 1–2 weeks the hepatocytes rupture and release thousands of **merozoites** (10,000–30,000 merozoites per schizont) into the circulation. The tissue schizonts of *P. falciparum* and *P. malariae* rupture once, and none persist in the liver. There are two types of tissue schizonts for *P. ovale* and *P. vivax.* The primary type ruptures in 6–9 days, whereas a secondary type **(hypnozoite)** remains dormant in the liver cell for weeks, months, or as long as 5 years before releasing merozoites and thereby causing relapses.

The **erythrocytic phase** of *Plasmodium* asexual development begins when the merozoites from the liver penetrate erythrocytes. Once inside the erythrocyte, the parasite transforms into the **ring form,** which then enlarges to become a **trophozoite.** These latter two forms can be identified with Giemsa stain on blood smear, which is the primary means of confirming the diagnosis of malaria. The trophozoites multiply asexually as multinucleated **erythrocytic schizonts** to produce a number of small erthrocytic merozoites. Merozoites are released into the bloodstream when the erythrocyte membrane ruptures, which is associated with the production of fever. In patients with previous malaria who are partially immune, the merozoite release and accompanying febrile paroxysms are synchronous. Merozoite release occurs approximately every 48 hours for *P. ovale* and *P. vivax* and every 72 hours for *P. falciparum* and *P. malariae,* although *P. falciparum* infections are often asynchronous. In nonimmune patients, merozoite release is asynchronous, resulting in nonperiodic febrile episodes. Over time, some of the merozoites develop into female **(macrogamete)** and male **(microgamete) gametocytes.** It is the gametocytes that complete the *Plasmodium* life cycle when they are ingested during a blood meal by the female anopheline mosquito.

Sporogeny, the sexual phase of the *Plasmodium* life cycle, begins when gametocytes are ingested from man by the female mosquito during a blood meal. The male and female gametocytes fuse to form a **zygote** in the stomach cavity of the mosquito. The zygote matures into a motile **ookinete** that penetrates the outer wall of the stomach and transforms into an **oocyst.** In the oocyst, numerous haploid sporozoites subsequently form and burst out into the body cavity, enter the salivary gland, and are inoculated into a new host with the next blood meal.

Transmission. The parasites are transmitted to humans by female *Anopheles* mosquitoes. Malaria can also be transmitted through blood transfusion, through the use of contaminated needles, and from a pregnant woman to her fetus. The risk of blood transmission is small and is decreasing in the United States. Congenital malaria occurs when parasites are transmitted from the mother to the fetus via the placenta.

EPIDEMIOLOGY

Malaria is a worldwide problem, with transmission occurring in more than 100 countries with a combined population of more than 1.6 billion people. Malaria is the most important cause of fever and morbidity in the tropical world. The principal areas of transmission are sub-Saharan Africa, southern and southeast Asia, Mexico, Haiti, the Dominican Republic, Central and South America, Papua New Guinea, Vanuatu, and the Solomon Islands. Major cities in Asia and South America are nearly free of malaria; cities in Africa, India, and Pakistan are not (Fig. 32–2). There is generally less risk of malaria at altitudes above 4,500 feet. Regions that have successfully eliminated transmission of malaria include North America, western Europe, and the Caribbean, as well as Australia, Chile, Israel, Japan, Korea, Lebanon, and Taiwan. Hopes for worldwide eradication of malaria faded in the 1970s with the development of insecticide and drug resistance as well as administrative and political difficulties. The most accurate current information about areas in the world where malaria risk and drug resistance exist can be obtained from local and state health departments or the CDC.

In the United States more than half the states were endemic for malaria in 1882, with 14 states remaining endemic in 1912; endemic malaria had been eliminated by the 1950s (Fig. 32–3). Approxi-

TABLE 32–1. Important Characteristics of the Four *Plasmodium* Species of Human Malaria

Characteristic	*P. falciparum*	*P. vivax*	*P. ovale*	*P. malariae*
Exoerythrocytic cycle	5.5–7 days	6–8 days	9 days	12–16 days
Erythrocytic cycle	48 hr	42–48 hr	49–50 hr	72 hr
Prepatant period	9–10 days	11–13 days	10–14 days	15 days
Usual incubation period, and range	12 days (9–14 days)	13 days (12–17 days; may be as long as 6–12 mo)	17 days (16–18 days; may be longer)	28 days (18–40 days; may be longer)
Merozoites per hepatic schizont	30,000	10,000	15,000	2,000
Erythrocyte preference	Young erythrocytes but can infect all	Reticulocytes	Reticulocytes	Older erythrocytes
Usual parasite load (% erythrocytes infected)	1–5% (or greater)	1–2%	1–2%	1–2%
Secondary exoerythrocytic cycle (hypnozoites) and relapses	Absent	Present	Present	Absent
Duration of untreated infection	1–2 yr	1.5–4 yr (includes liver stage)	1.5–4 yr (includes liver stage)	3–50 yr
Severity of primary attack	Severe in nonimmune—A MEDICAL EMERGENCY—Failure to recognize and treat can lead to death	Mild to severe: Danger of splenic rupture, relapse related to persistence of latent exoerythrocytic forms	Mild: Danger of splenic rupture, relapse related to persistence of latent exoerythrocytic forms	Can be very chronic in subclinical and subpatent forms; can cause nephritis in children
Usual periodicity of febrile attacks	None	48 hr	48 hr	72 hr
Duration of febrile paroxysm	16–36 hr (may be longer)	8–12 hr	8–12 hr	8–10 hr

Adapted from Strickland GT: Malaria. In Strickland GT (editor): *Hunter's Tropical Medicine,* 7th ed. Philadelphia, WB Saunders, 1991, p. 589.

mately 1,000–2,000 imported cases are recognized annually in the United States, with most cases occurring in foreign civilians living in endemic areas who become infected and travel to the United States or in United States citizens who travel to endemic areas without taking appropriate chemoprophylactic drugs (Fig. 32–4).There is also a small number of transfusion-associated and congenital cases.

Between 1957 and 1994 the CDC identified 74 cases of malaria from 21 states. These were probably acquired by mosquitoborne transmission within the United States, with recent outbreaks of mosquitoborne malaria transmission in New Jersey, New York, and Texas. It is likely that untreated persons with malaria acquired in an endemic country traveled to the United States and infected indigenous *Anopheles* mosquitoes, which transmitted the disease to others. Anopheline mosquitoes capable of transmitting malaria currently exist in all 48 states of the continental United States, although under current conditions the average lifespan of anopheline mosquitoes in the United States is less than the duration of the sporogonic cycle in mosquitoes. Environmental changes (e.g., global warming), the spread of drug resistance, and increased air travel could lead to the re-emergence of malaria in the United States.

The geographic distribution of different malaria species is difficult to assess, but *P. falciparum* and *P. malariae* are found in most malarious areas. *P. falciparum* is the predominant species in Africa, Haiti, and New Guinea. *P. vivax* predominates in Bangladesh, Central America, India, Pakistan, and Sri Lanka. *P. vivax* and *P. falciparum* predominate in Southeast Asia, South America, and Oceania. *P. ovale,* the rarest species, is transmitted primarily in Africa.

PATHOGENESIS

Although current understanding of the pathogenesis of the clinical manifestations of malaria is incomplete, four important pathologic processes have been identified: fever, anemia, tissue anoxia resulting from cytoadherence of infected erythrocytes and impairment of local blood flow, and immunopathologic events. Malarial illness is manifest only during the erythrocytic cycle. Fever occurs when erythrocytes rupture and release merozoites into the circulation. The cause of fever is unclear, but it is thought to result from parasite- or tissue-derived pyrogens, especially tumor necrosis factor (TNF). Anemia is caused by hemolysis, sequestration of erythrocytes in the spleen and other organs, and bone marrow suppression. The cause of bone marrow suppression in patients with malaria is unclear, but it may be related to elevated levels of TNF. Cytoadherence of infected erythrocytes to vascular endothelium is thought to contribute to many of the clinical manifestations of severe *P. falciparum* malaria. Increased adherence of erythrocytes, as well as polymorphonuclear leukocytes and platelets, may lead to obstruction of blood flow and capillary damage with resultant vascular leakage of protein and fluid, followed by edema and tissue anoxia. The expression of several adherence molecules on infected erythrocytes (including thrombospondin, ICAM-1, and CD36) is thought to initiate adherence of infected erythrocytes to vascular endothelium in a variety of organs, including the brain, heart, lung, intestine, and kidney. Several immunopathologic events have been documented in patients with malaria; these include polyclonal activation resulting in both hypergammaglobulinemia and the formation of immune complexes; immunodepression, especially of T cell func-

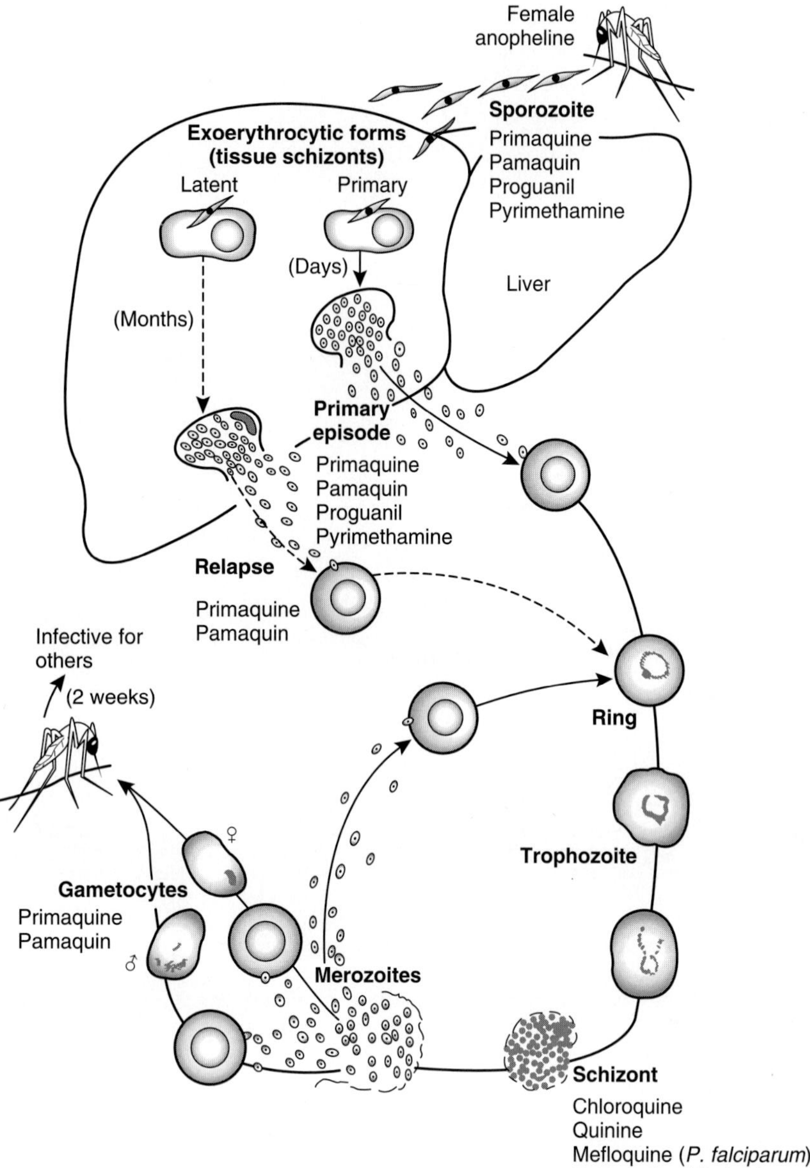

FIGURE 32–1. The life cycle of plasmodia in humans, including the sites of action of important antimalarial drugs. (Adapted from Wyler DJ: *Plasmodium* and *Babesia*. In Gorbach SL, Bartlett JG, Blacklow NR [editors]: *Infectious Diseases,* 2nd ed. Philadelphia, WB Saunders, 1998, p. 2407.)

tion; impairment of the phagocytic system in the spleen and liver; and release of cytokines such as TNF that may be responsible for much of the pathogenesis of the disease.

Immunity. The immune response to *Plasmodium* species infection is complex and not fully understood, especially for *P. malariae, P. ovale,* and *P. vivax.* In general, immunity following *Plasmodium* infection is incomplete, so that severe disease is averted but complete eradication or prevention of future infection is not achieved. In some cases, termed **premunition,** parasites circulate in small numbers for extended periods of time but are prevented from rapidly multiplying and causing severe illness. Prevention of **repeated episodes** of *Plasmodium* infection is not possible because the parasite has developed a number of immune-evasive strategies, such as intracellular replication, rapid antigenic variation, and alteration of the host immune system that includes partial immune suppression.

The human host response to *Plasmodium* infection includes natural immune mechanisms that prevent infection by other *Plasmodium* species, such as those of birds or rodents, as well as alterations in erythrocyte physiology that prevent or modify malarial infection. Examples of the latter include the following: erythrocytes lacking Duffy blood group antigen are resistant to *P. vivax* merozoite invasion; ovalocytes are resistant to penetration by *P. falciparum* merozoites; erythrocytes containing hemoglobin S (sickle cell anemia) resist malaria parasite growth; and erythrocytes containing hemoglobin F (fetal hemoglobin) resist *P. falciparum* growth.

The complex intracellular and extracellular life cycle of *Plasmodium* species elicits a broad range of acquired humoral responses. In general, extracellular *Plasmodium* organisms are targeted by humoral immune mechanisms, whereas intracellular organisms are targeted by cellular defenses, such as T lymphocytes, macrophages, polymorphonuclear leukocytes, and the spleen. *Plasmodium*-specific antibody blocks the invasion of erythrocytes by merozoites and acts as an opsonin during phagocytosis of the organisms. The spleen is thought to play a central role in limiting the number of circulating parasites because its removal can result in the exacerba-

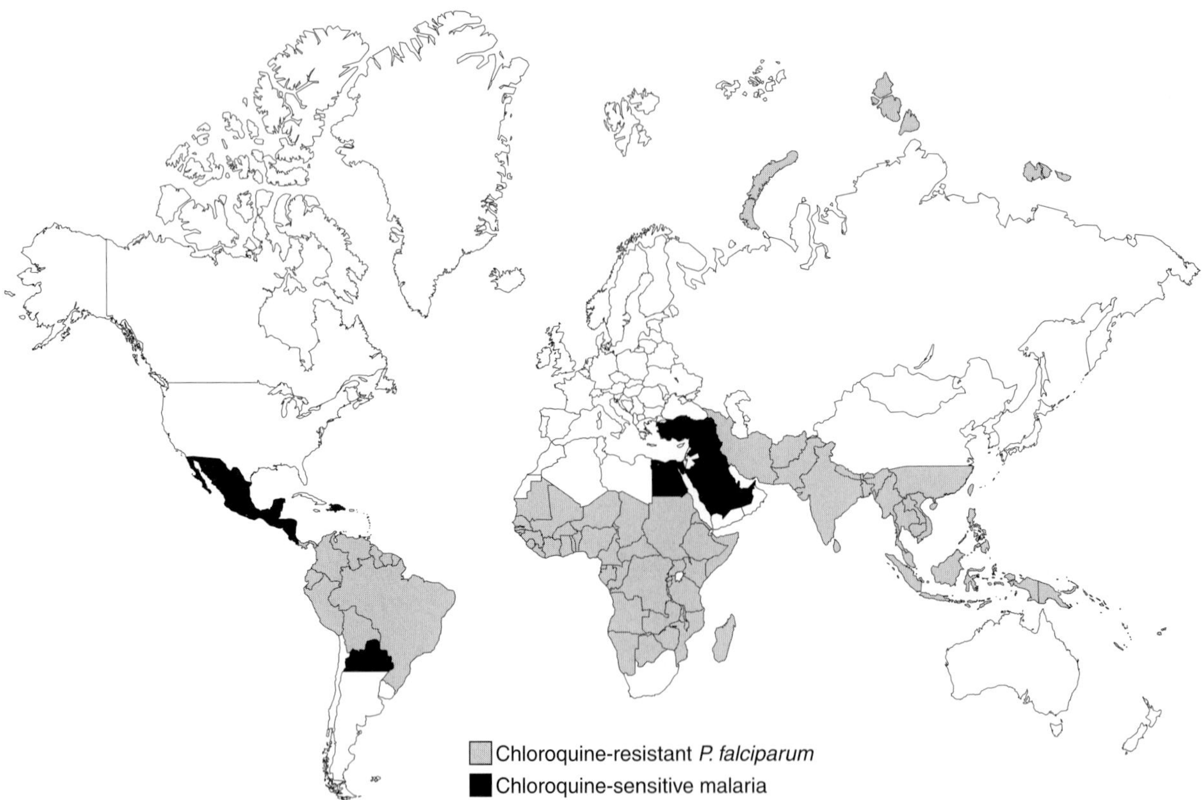

FIGURE 32–2. Worldwide distribution of malaria and chloroquine-resistant *Plasmodium falciparum* malaria, 1997. (From Centers for Disease Control and Prevention: Health Information for International Travel, 1999–2000.)

tion of disease in patients harboring a small number of organisms. In hyperendemic areas, newborns are resistant to acute malaria infection and rarely become ill with malaria, in part because of passive maternal antibody and high levels of fetal hemoglobin. The brunt of malarial morbidity and mortality in hyperendemic areas is borne by children from 3 months to 2–5 years of age who suffer yearly attacks of debilitating and potentially fatal disease. After this time, immunity is gradually acquired and severe illness with malaria is less common. Severe disease may occur, however, during pregnancy or after extended residence outside the endemic region. Interestingly, HIV-infected children and adults have not been found to have increased morbidity or mortality from *P. falciparum* malaria.

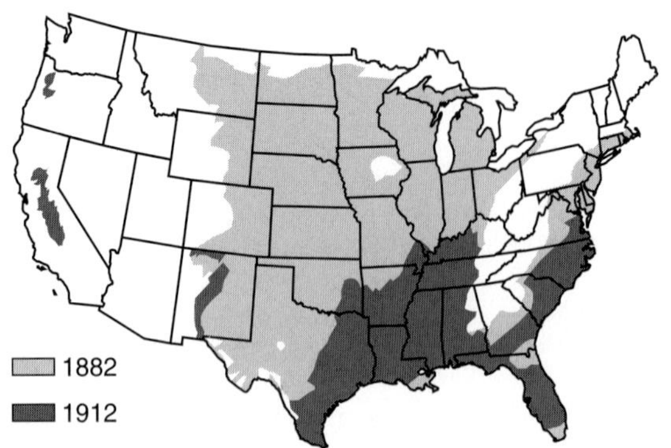

FIGURE 32–3. Areas of the United States where malaria was thought to be endemic in 1882 and 1912. (From Zucker JR: Changing patterns of autochthonous malaria transmission in the United States: A review of recent outbreaks. *Emerg Infect Dis* 1996;2:37–43.)

CLINICAL SYMPTOMS AND MANIFESTATIONS

The clinical manifestations of malaria range from asymptomatic infection to fulminant illness and death, depending on the virulence of the infecting malaria species and the host immune response.

Usual Presentation

The incubation period from the time of mosquito bite to the development of symptoms of malaria ranges from 6–30 days, depending on the *Plasmodium* species involved (Fig. 32–5). The incubation period can be prolonged in patients with partial immunity or incomplete chemoprophylaxis. A prodrome lasting 2–3 days may occur before parasites are detected in the blood, usually with symptoms of headache, fatigue, anorexia, myalgias, and slight fever and less frequently with pain in the chest, abdomen, or joints. The most characteristic clinical feature of malaria, which is seldom noted with other infectious diseases, is **febrile paroxysms** alternating with periods of fatigue but otherwise relative wellness. The classic symptoms of the febrile paroxysms of malaria include high fever, rigors, sweats, and headache. Myalgia, back pain, abdominal pain, nausea, vomiting, diarrhea, pallor, and jaundice may also occur. Paroxysms coincide with the rupture of schizonts that occur every 48 hours with *P. vivax* and *P. ovale* (**tertian periodicity**) and every 72 hours with *P. malariae* (**quartan periodicity**). Periodicity is less prominent with *P. falciparum* and mixed infections.

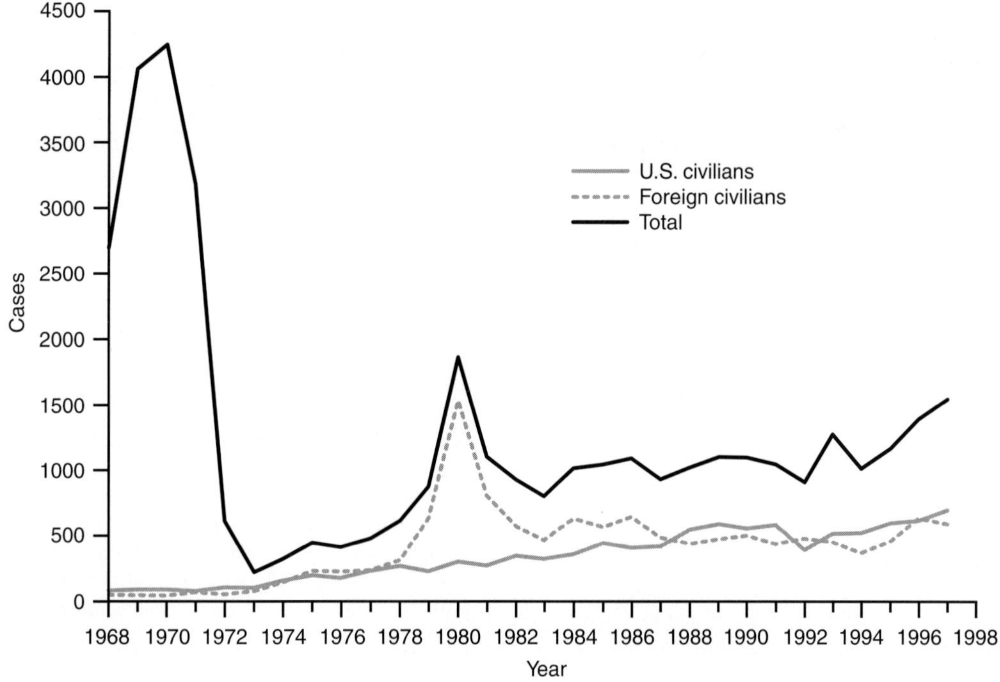

FIGURE 32–4. Number of malaria cases among United States and foreign civilians in the United States from 1968–1997. The increased number of cases for 1968–1972 reflects cases among U.S. military personnel during the Vietnam conflict and for 1980 reflects cases among immigrants from Southeast Asia after the Vietnam conflict. Total cases include those in which the nationality is unknown. (From Centers for Disease Control and Prevention, 2001).

Persons with primary infection, such as travelers from nonendemic regions, may also have irregular symptomatic episodes for 2–3 days before regular paroxysms begin. **Short-term relapse** describes the recurrence of symptoms after a primary attack that is due to the survival of erythrocyte forms in the bloodstream (Fig. 32–5). **Long-term relapse** describes the renewal of symptoms long after the primary attack, usually due to release of merozoites from an exoerythrocytic source in the liver. Long-term relapse occurs with *P. vivax* and *P. ovale* because of the persistence in the liver and with *P. malariae* because of persistence in the erythrocyte. A history of typical symptoms in a person more than a few weeks after return from an endemic area therefore indicates *P. vivax, P. ovale,* or *P. malariae* infection.

Clinical Manifestations in Children. Symptoms of malaria in children older than 2 months of age vary widely and range from low-grade fever and headache alone to temperature higher than 40°C (104°F) with headache, drowsiness, anorexia, thirst, nausea, vomiting, diarrhea, pallor, cyanosis, or hepatosplenomegaly. The most common presentation in children traveling to an endemic area consists of fever, anorexia, and vomiting with splenomegaly, anemia, thrombocytopenia, and a normal or low WBC count; classic

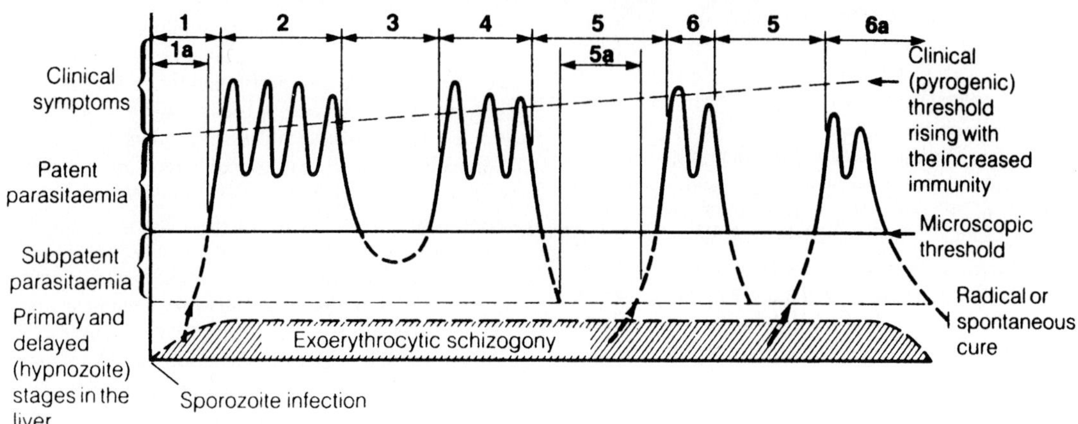

FIGURE 32–5. Phases of malaria infection showing short-term and long-term relapses. *1* = incubation period; *2* = primary attack composed of paroxysms; *3* = latent period (clinical latency); *4* = Short-term relapse; *5* = latent period; *5a* = parasitic latency; *6* = long-term relapse followed by parasitic relapse; *6a* = parasitic relapse. (From Manson-Bahr PEC, Bell DR: Malaria. In Manson-Bahr PEC, Bell DR [editors]: *Manson's Tropical Diseases,* 19th ed. Philadelphia, Bailliere Tindall, 1991, p. 14.)

malarial fever patterns are unusual. In endemic areas, it is estimated that infected mosquitoes bite children 50–150 times a year, with clinical illness that occurs once or twice a year although asymptomatic parasitemia occurs more frequently.

Congenital Malaria. Congenital malaria, acquired from the mother prenatally or perinatally, is a serious problem in tropical areas but is only occasionally reported in the United States. In endemic areas, congenital malaria is an important cause of abortions, miscarriages, stillbirths, premature births, intrauterine growth retardation, and neonatal deaths. The establishment of infection in utero is thought to be largely dependent on the immune status of the mother. Congenital malaria usually occurs in a nonimmune mother with *P. vivax* or *P. malariae* infection, although it can be observed with any of the human malaria species. Congenital malaria is more common in mothers who have acute attacks of malaria during pregnancy, with an estimated attack rate of 1–4%, compared with an estimated 0.3% rate in mothers with chronic, subclinical infections. The first sign or symptom most commonly occurs between 10 and 30 days of age but has been noted as early as 14 hours and as late as several months of age. Signs and symptoms of congenital infection include fever, restlessness, drowsiness, pallor, jaundice, poor feeding, vomiting, and diarrhea; cyanosis and hepatosplenomegaly in severe cases are also noted. Malaria is often severe during pregnancy and may have an adverse effect on the fetus because of maternal illness or placental infection, even in the absence of transmission from mother to child.

P. falciparum Malaria. The incubation period is usually 10–14 days but can be longer. *P. falciparum* malaria is the most severe form of malaria, with fatality rates of up to 25% in nonimmune adults and 31% in nonimmune infants if appropriate therapy is not instituted promptly. For this reason, the diagnosis of *P. falciparum* malaria constitutes a medical emergency. Unlike *P. ovale* and *P. vivax,* which primarily infect immature erythrocytes, and *P. malariae,* which infects only mature erythrocytes, *P. falciparum* infects both reticulocytes and mature erythrocytes. Relapses do not occur because there is no long-term liver or erythrocyte phase.

Malaria caused by *P. falciparum* is associated with intense parasitemia that can reach 60% or more, whereas malaria caused by *P. ovale, P. vivax,* and *P. malariae* usually results in parasitemias of less than 2%. *P. falciparum* malaria is most commonly associated with serious complications, such as cerebral malaria, renal failure, and blackwater fever. **Blackwater fever** is characterized by hemoglobinuria due to severe intravascular hemolysis, renal failure due to acute tubular necrosis, and a high mortality rate. Severe clinical manifestations of *P. falciparum* malaria include neurologic alterations, including coma, seizures, and upper motor neuron dysfunction; cardiac alterations, including decreased cardiac output; pulmonary alterations, including pulmonary edema and adult respiratory distress syndrome; renal alterations, including decreased renal function and acute renal failure; gastrointestinal alterations, including impaired liver function and small-bowel malabsorption; and biochemical and electrolyte alterations, including hyponatremia and hypoglycemia. Milder or asymptomatic infections occur in persons who are partially immune to *P. falciparum.*

P. vivax Malaria. The incubation period is 12–18 days but may be as long as 5–13 months. *P. vivax* malaria generally is less severe than *P. falciparum* malaria but may cause death due to ruptured spleen or in association with reticulocytosis following anemia. Relapse may occur if antihepatic malaria treatment is not given; it is common within 6 months after an acute attack but may occur as long as 4 years after initial infection.

P. malariae and P. ovale Malaria. The incubation period ranges from 18 days to many weeks, and long-term relapse has been observed 1½–4 years after an acute attack of *P. ovale* and 30–50 years after an acute attack of *P. malariae* malaria. *P. malariae* malaria is the mildest and most chronic of all malaria infections. Parasitemia is often low, which makes the diagnosis more problematic. Untreated *P. malariae* malaria can cause chronic ill health with anemia, recurrent fever, headache, malaise, fatigue, and sweats in addition to pronounced, acute febrile illness. *P. ovale* malaria is the least common type of malaria. It is clinically similar to *P. vivax* malaria and commonly is found in conjunction with *P. falciparum* malaria.

DIAGNOSIS

The most important aspect in the diagnosis of malaria in children is to consider the possibility of malaria in any child who has fever, chills, splenomegaly, anemia, or decreased level of consciousness and a history of recent travel or residence in an endemic area (Table 32–2). The diagnosis of malaria should be considered, regardless of the use of chemoprophylaxis. Certain criteria suggest *P. falciparum* malaria (Table 32–3). The differential diagnosis is broad and includes a number of infectious and noninfectious diseases (Table 32–4).

Microbiologic Evaluation

The diagnosis of malaria is established by identification of organisms on appropriately stained smears of peripheral blood (Fig. 32–6 and Plates 2C and 2D). In nonimmune persons, symptoms typically occur 1–2 days before parasites are detectable on blood smear. Although *P. falciparum* is most likely to be identified from blood during a febrile paroxysm, the timing of the smears is less important than their being obtained several times each day over a period of 3 successive days. It may be necessary to repeat the smears as often as every 4–6 hours each day to establish the diagnosis. Most patients with symptoms of malaria will have detectable parasites on thick blood smears during a 48-hour period. Both thick and thin blood smears should be examined. The concentration of erythrocytes on a **thick smear** is approximately 20–40 times greater than on a thin smear. Thick smears are used to quickly scan large numbers of erythrocytes. The thin smear allows for positive identification of the malaria species and determination of the percentage of infected erythrocytes, which is also useful in following the response to therapy.

It is important that the proper staining technique be used; Giemsa stain is better than Wright's stain or Leishman's stain. Identification and speciation are best performed by an experienced microscopist and checked against color plates of the various *Plasmodium* species and are most easily established by identification of gametocytes. Gametocytes of *P. falciparum* are banana-shaped (Plate 2D), whereas the gametocytes of the other *Plasmodium* are circular or ovoid (Fig. 32–6). Speciation of *Plasmodium* at other stages of the life cycle is possible but requires extensive experience. If malaria parasites are identified but no gametocytes are present for speciation, or if speciation is not possible, treatment for *P. falciparum* malaria is necessary. The available serologic tests use IFA, IHA, EIA, or immunoprecipitation but do not distinguish present from past infection. Serologic studies are used primarily for epidemiologic surveys and for screening of potential blood donors.

TREATMENT

Definitive Treatment

The development of resistance to antimalarial drugs in recent years, especially *P. falciparum,* has greatly complicated malaria therapy

TABLE 32–2. Diagnosis of Malaria

History
Common
Travel to an endemic area
Paroxysms of fever interspersed by periods of "wellness"
Less Common
Recent blood transfusion
Intravenous drug use
Symptoms
Common
Fever, chills, rigors
Headache
Less Common
Malaise, fatigue
Arthralgias
Chest, abdominal, and back pain
Nausea, vomiting
Decreased level of consciousness
Signs
Common
Fever
Pallor
Tachycardia, orthostatic hypotension
Less Common
Splenomegaly
Hepatomegaly
Jaundice
Rash (urticaria, petechiae)
Conjunctival suffusion
Flow murmur
Rales
Altered consciousness
Laboratory Findings
Common
Intraerythrocytic parasites
Anemia (normochromic, normocytic, hemolytic)
Leukopenia
Thrombocytopenia
Less Common
Elevated hepatic transaminases, bilirubin
Electrolyte alteration (especially hyponatremia)
Elevated BUN, creatinine
Hypoglycemia

and chemoprophylaxis. The process of *Plasmodium* drug resistance is ongoing, and physicians caring for patients with malaria or traveling to areas where malaria is endemic need to be aware of current information regarding malaria treatment and chemoprophylaxis. The best source for healthcare professionals for such information is the CDC Malaria Hotline, which is available 24 hours a day (telephone: 770-488-7788).

TABLE 32–3. Important Criteria Suggestive of *Plasmodium falciparum* Malaria

Ring forms are small with double chromatin dots
Erythrocytes infected with more than one parasite
Intense parasitemia (>2%)
Symptoms occurring less than 1 month after return from an endemic area

TABLE 32–4. Differential Diagnosis of Malaria

Viral Infections
Influenza
Poliomyelitis
Yellow fever
Prerash stage of many viral illnesses
Bacterial Infections
Tuberculosis
Brucellosis
Typhoid fever
Relapsing fever
Infective endocarditis
Parasitic Infections
Trypanosomiasis
Kala-azar
Amebic liver abscess
Other Conditions
Hepatitis
Gastroenteritis
Blood disorders

The pace of the evaluation and treatment of malaria depends on the suspected species of infecting organism (*P. falciparum* or other), the severity of the illness, and the immune status of the patient (immune or nonimmune). There are numerous antimalarial drugs available (Fig. 32–1 and Table 32–5). Chloroquine remains the primary antimalarial for treatment of non–*P. falciparum* malaria, even though rare cases of chloroquine-resistant *P. vivax* malaria have been described from Indonesia and New Guinea. Alternatives to chloroquine must be considered in the treatment of *P. falciparum* malaria. Empiric therapy for chloroquine-resistant *P. falciparum* malaria is also adequate for other forms of malaria. If definitive speciation cannot be established, treatment should consist of drugs effective against chloroquine-resistant *P. falciparum* malaria.

***P. falciparum* Malaria.** Any person who has fever without an obvious cause, who has left a *P. falciparum* endemic area within the incubation period of 9–14 days, and who is nonimmune should be considered to have a medical emergency. Thick and thin blood smears should immediately be obtained, and if they are positive, the patient should be hospitalized and therapy begun. If blood films are negative, they should be repeated every few hours; if the patient is severely ill, antimalarial therapy should be initiated without delay. The type of antimalarial drug used is determined in part by the severity of the illness and by the region where acquisition occurred. Resistance to chloroquine has been confirmed or is probable in all regions with *P. falciparum* malaria except Hispaniola, Central America north of Panama, and the Middle East (Fig. 32–2). Persons with *P. falciparum* malaria who are from an endemic area and are immune or semi-immune should be treated for chloroquine-resistant *P. falciparum* malaria.

Intravenous quinidine gluconate should be administered to patients with *P. falciparum* malaria who cannot retain oral fluids and medication because of vomiting; have neurologic dysfunction, pulmonary edema, or renal failure; have a peripheral asexual parasitemia that exceeds 5%; or have a peripheral asexual parasitemia of 1–4% with a severe attack and any doubt about chloroquine sensitivity. Intravenous treatment should be in an intensive care unit, with parenteral quinidine gluconate administered by slow intravenous infusion over 1–2 hours. Vital signs, hydration status,

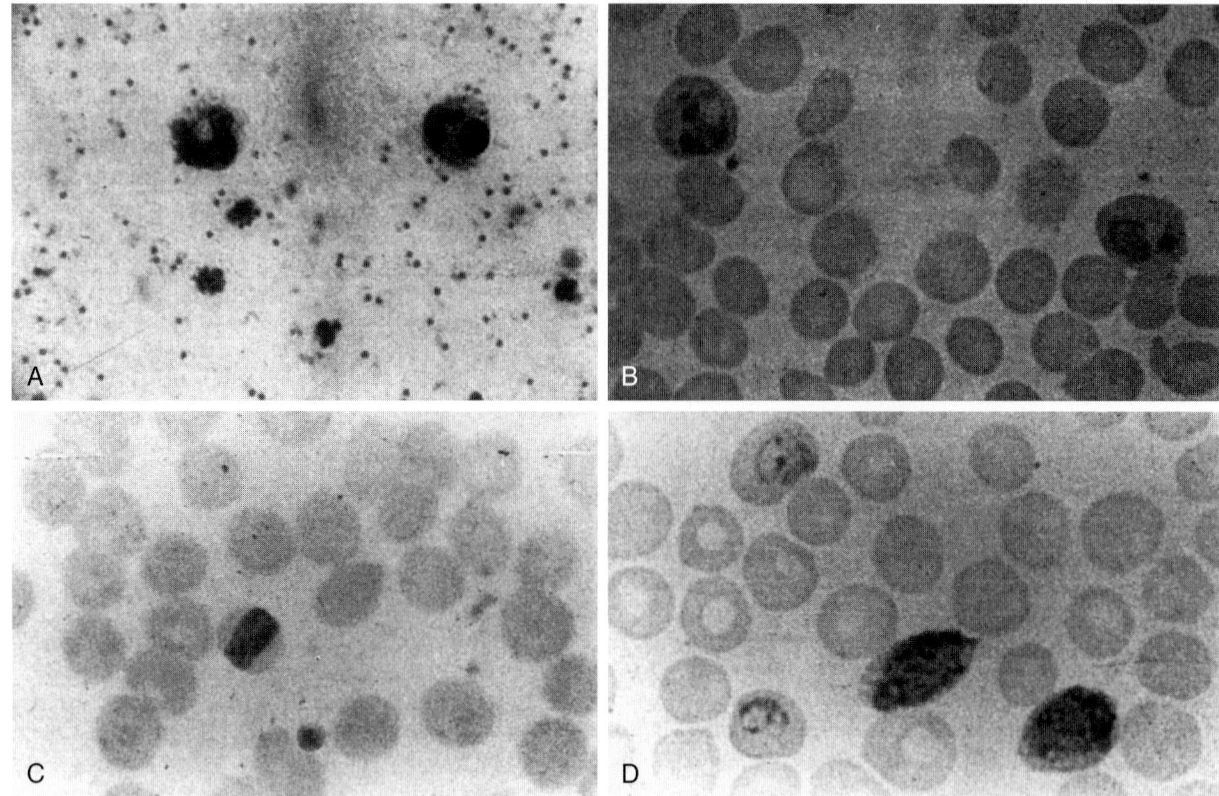

FIGURE 32–6. Morphology of plasmodia. **A,** Thick blood smear from a patient with heavy *P. falciparum* infection showing leukocytes, platelets, and numerous ring forms of the parasite. **B,** Thin blood smear from a patient with *P. vivax* infection showing ameboid trophozoites and Schüffner's dots in the enlarged erythrocytes. **C,** Thin blood smear from a patient with *P. malariae* infection showing a band-shaped trophozoite in the normal-sized erythrocyte. **D,** Thin blood smear from a patient with *P. ovale* infection showing two ameboid trophozoites in the enlarged stippled erythrocytes and two schizonts in oval (or elongated) erythrocytes. (From Strickland GT: Malaria. In Strickland GT [editor]: *Hunter's Tropical Medicine,* 7th ed. Orlando, Fla., WB Saunders, 1991, p. 594.)

blood glucose, and electrocardiographic status should be continuously monitored during the infusion. Indications for slowing the infusion rate include a plasma quinidine level >6 mg/L, QT interval >0.6 seconds, QRS widening beyond 25% of baseline, or development of significant hypotension. Parenteral therapy with quinidine to achieve blood levels of 3–6 mg/L should be continued until the parasitemia is less than 1%, which usually occurs within 48 hours, or until oral medication can be tolerated. Quinine sulfate is then given orally 3 times a day for a total of 3 days of combined quinidine/quinine therapy. Alternatively, tetracycline 4 times a day for 7 days or pyrimethamine-sulfadoxine (Fansidar) in one dose may subsequently be used to complete therapy. Tetracycline is usually avoided in children younger than 9 years of age and in pregnant women because of the risk of dental staining. Other adverse effects of tetracycline include gastrointestinal disturbances and photosensitivity. Pyrimethamine-sulfadoxine may cause gastrointestinal upset and skin reactions.

Patients with mild to moderate infection, a parasite count of <5%, and any doubt about chloroquine sensitivity should be given oral quinine sulfate 3 times a day for 3–7 days, with an additional antimalarial drug from one of the following: (1) a single dose of Fansidar on the last day of quinine administration; (2) doxycycline or tetracycline for 7 days; or (3) clindamycin for 5 days. Alternatives to these regimens include mefloquine given in 2 doses 12 hours apart, the combination of atovaquone and proguanil (Malarone) for 3 days, or atovaquone and doxycycline for 3 days. Important caveats are that the duration of quinine treatment should be for 7 consecutive days in persons who acquire *P. falciparum* in Thailand, and Fansidar should not be used in persons who acquire *P. falciparum* infections in Thailand, Myanmar (Burma), Cambodia, or the Amazon basin because of pyrimethamine-sulfadoxine resistance in these areas.

Patients with uncomplicated *P. falciparum* malaria acquired in areas without chloroquine resistance should be treated with oral chloroquine as for *P. vivax, P. ovale,* or *P. malariae* infections. Patients begun on chloroquine whose parasite count does not drop rapidly within 24–48 hours and whose blood smear results are not negative for the parasite after 4 days should be assumed to have a chloroquine-resistant organism and should be treated for chloroquine-resistant *P. falciparum* malaria.

P. vivax, P. ovale, and P. malariae Infection. Patients with *P. vivax, P. ovale,* or *P. malariae* infection should be given chloroquine phosphate orally. The clinical and blood smear responses to therapy should be monitored. Adverse effects of chloroquine include gastrointestinal irritation and vomiting. If vomiting precludes oral administration, chloroquine can be given by nasogastric tube or, in rare cases and with great care, by IM administration. Sudden death has been attributed to parenteral administration of chloroquine to children. Uncommon side effects of chloroquine include pruritus, headache, dizziness, blurred vision, acute psychoses, and exacerbation of psoriasis.

Patients with *P. vivax* or *P. ovale* malaria should be given primaquine once a day for 14 days to prevent relapse. Some strains

TABLE 32–5. Treatment of Malaria

Drug[1]	Adult Dosage	Pediatric Dosage
All *Plasmodium* Species Except Chloroquine-Resistant *P. falciparum*		
Oral Drug of Choice		
Chloroquine phosphate[2]	600 mg base (1 g) then 300 mg base (500 mg) 6 hr later, followed by 300 mg base (500 mg) at 24 and 48 hr	10 mg/kg base (max 600 mg) followed by 5 mg/kg base (max 300 mg) 6 hr later, and 5 mg/kg base daily (max 300 mg) at 24 and 48 hr
Parenteral Drug of Choice		
Quinidine gluconate[3]	10 mg/kg loading dose IV (max 600 mg) in normal saline solution slowly over 1–2 hr followed by a continuous infusion of 0.02 mg/kg/min until oral therapy can be started	Same as adult dose
Chloroquine-Resistant *Plasmodium falciparum*		
Oral Drug of Choice		
Quinine sulfate[4]	650 mg tid for 3–7 days	25 mg/kg/day (max 650 mg per dose) divided tid for 3–7 days
plus tetracycline[5]	250 mg qid for 7 days	25 mg/kg/day (max 250 mg per dose) divided qid for 7 days
Alternative Oral Regimens[6]		
Quinine sulfate *plus* pyrimethamine-sulfadoxine (Fansidar)[7]	Same as above Single dose of 3 tablets on the last day of quinine	Same as above <1 yr: single dose of 1/4 tablet1–3 yr: single dose of 1/2 tablet 4–8 yr: single dose of 1 tablet 9–14 yr: single dose of 2 tablets >14 yr: single dose of 3 tablets
or		
Mefloquine	Single dose of 1,250 mg	>15 kg: 25 mg/kg (max 1,250 mg) in a single dose
or		
Atovaquone *plus* proguanil (Malarone)[8]	2 tablets (500 mg atovaquone, 200 mg proguanil) bid for 3 days	11–20 kg: 1/2 tablet bid for 3 days 21–30 kg: 1 tablet bid for 3 days 31–40 kg: 1 1/2 tablets bid for 3 days >40 kg: 2 tablets bid for 3 days
Parenteral Drug of Choice		
Quinidine gluconate	Same as above	Same as above
Prevention of Relapses: *P. vivax* and *P. ovale* Only		
Primaquine phosphate[9] (after completion of chloroquine)	15 mg base (26.3 mg salt) once a day for 14 days or 45 mg base (79 mg salt) once a week for 8 weeks	0.3 mg/kg base (max 15 mg base [26.3 mg salt]) once a day for 14 days

[1] Review contraindications and adverse effects before use (see text).
[2] If chloroquine phosphate is not available, hydroxychloroquine sulfate is as effective (400 mg hydroxychloroquine sulfate is equivalent to 500 mg chloroquine phosphate).
[3] Quinine dihydrochloride is an alternative parenteral drug for treatment of non-chloroquine-resistant *Plasmodium* but is not available in the United States.
[4] Quinine sulfate should be given for 7 days for treatment of *P. falciparum* infections acquired in Thailand.
[5] Physicians must weigh the benefits of the tetracycline therapy against the possibility of dental staining in children younger than 9 years of age.
[6] Quinine sulfate *plus* clindamycin or halofantrine alone are other alternative oral regimens. There are limited data on efficacy of clindamycin for treatment of malaria in children. Quinine sulfate *plus* clindamycin is a treatment choice for pregnant women. Halofantrine is not available in the United States.
[7] Fansidar should be avoided for treatment of *P. falciparum* infections acquired in Thailand, Myanmar (Burma), Cambodia, or the Amazon basin because of Fansidar resistance in these areas.
[8] Available as a combination tablet (Malarone) containing atovaquone (250 mg) and proguanil (100 mg).
[9] Primaquine can cause hemolytic anemia in patients with glucose-6-dehydrogenase deficiency, which should be tested before administration. Primaquine should not be given during pregnancy.

may require two courses of primaquine. Primaquine can induce hemolytic anemia in persons with glucose-6-dehydrogenase (G6PD) deficiency, which should be evaluated before initiation of the drug. Primaquine should not be given during pregnancy. Patients with malaria of any type need to be monitored for possible recrudescence with repeat blood smears at the end of therapy because recrudescence may occur 90 or more days after therapy with low-grade resistant organisms. Mothers of children living in endemic areas should be encouraged to treat fever with an antimalarial drug. If such children are severely ill, they should be given the same therapy as nonimmune children.

Supportive Therapy

Supportive therapy for *P. falciparum* is important and may require blood transfusions to maintain the hematocrit above 20%; exchange transfusion in life-threatening malaria with parasitemia greater than 5%; supplemental oxygen or ventilatory support for pulmonary edema or cerebral malaria; careful intravenous rehydration for severe malaria, intravenous glucose for hypoglycemia, which may be severe and result in cerebral dysfunction; anticonvulsants for cerebral malaria with seizures; dialysis for renal failure; antibiotics for bacterial superinfection; and acetaminophen for fever. The value of anti-TNF antibody, deferoxamine, mannitol, prostacyclin, dextran, pentoxifylline, and acetylcysteine is unclear. Other therapeutic agents, including aspirin, hyperimmune serum, heparin, cyclosporine, and high-dose corticosteroids, either are of no value or are harmful.

COMPLICATIONS

Cerebral Malaria. Cerebral malaria is a complication of *P. falciparum* infection and a frequent (20–40%) cause of death, especially in children and nonimmune adults. Cerebral malaria rarely causes long-term sequelae if it is treated appropriately with prompt initiation of antimalarial therapy, fluid restriction, a single dose of intramuscular phenobarbital (3.5 mg/kg for children less than 60 kg) to reduce the possibility of seizures, and treatment of other potential complications such as hypoglycemia. Cerebral malaria usually develops after the patient has been ill for several days but may develop precipitously. As with other complications, cerebral malaria is more likely in patients with intense parasitemia (>5%). The symptoms range in severity but always include a decreased level of consciousness that may vary from severe headache to drowsiness, confusion, delirium, hallucinations, or coma. Physical findings may be normal or may include high fever (40–41.1°C [106–108°F]), seizures, muscular twitching, rhythmic movement of the head or extremities, contracted or unequal pupils, retinal hemorrhages, hemiplegia, absent or exaggerated deep tendon reflexes, and a positive Babinski sign. Lumbar puncture reveals increased intracranial pressure and CSF protein with minimal or no pleocytosis and normal glucose. There are no specific EEG findings with cerebral malaria.

Splenic Rupture. Splenic rupture is a rare complication that may occur with acute infection due to any malaria species. It can occur spontaneously but is usually the result of trauma, including overly vigorous palpation on physical examination. If causes severe internal hemorrhage and may result in death if removal of the spleen and blood transfusions are not performed in a timely manner.

Renal Failure and Blackwater Fever. A common complication of severe falciparum malaria is renal failure, which results from deposition of hemoglobin in renal tubules, decreased renal blood flow, and acute tubular necrosis. Blackwater fever is a clinical syndrome that consists of severe hemolysis and hemoglobinuria that contribute to renal failure. It is a rare complication that occurs when antibodies directed against parasite-laden erythrocytes and complement result in severe hemolytic anemia, hemoglobinuria, oliguria, and jaundice. Renal failure usually requires peritoneal dialysis or hemodialysis.

Pulmonary Edema. Pulmonary edema may occur several days after therapy has begun and is commonly associated with excessive intravenous fluids. It can develop rapidly and may be fatal. Care should be taken not to overhydrate patients with *P. falciparum* malaria.

Hypoglycemia. Hypoglycemia is more common in children, pregnant women, and patients receiving quinine therapy. A decreased level of consciousness may be confused with cerebral malaria. Hypoglycemia is associated with increased mortality and neurologic sequelae.

Thrombocytopenia. Thrombocytopenia is a common complication of *P. falciparum* and *P. vivax* malaria, with platelet counts as low as 10,000–20,000/mm^3.

Algid Malaria. A rare form of *P. falciparum* malaria, algid malaria occurs with overwhelming infection leading to hypotension and vascular collapse. Death may occur within a few hours.

PROGNOSIS

In children, asymptomatic parasitemia may last for weeks or months. It is associated with many undesirable outcomes, including anemia, splenomegaly, nephrotic syndrome, poor growth, and immunosuppression, and may contribute to increased risk of Burkitt's lymphoma. Death in infants and children may occur with any of the malarial species but is most frequent with complicated *P. falciparum* malaria. The likelihood of death is increased in children with pre-existing health problems, such as measles, intestinal parasites, schistosomiasis, anemia, and malnutrition. (Table 32–6).

PREVENTION

There are two components of malaria prevention: reduction of exposure to infected mosquitoes and chemoprophylaxis. Mosquito protection is needed because no chemoprophylactic or treatment regimen can guarantee protection in every instance because of the widespread development of resistant organisms.

Reducing Exposure to Malaria. Travelers to endemic areas should remain in well-screened areas from dusk to dawn, which is the period when the *Anopheles* mosquito usually feeds and when the risk of transmission is highest; spray pyrethrin or a similar insecticide indoors at sundown; and sleep under permethrin-treated mosquito netting if the bedroom is not air-conditioned or screened. Travelers should wear clothing that covers the arms and legs, with trousers tucked into shoes or boots, especially at night. The most

TABLE 32–6 Features Indicating a Poor Prognosis in Severe Malaria

Clinical Features
Impaired consciousness*
Repeated convulsions (>3 in 24 hr)
Respiratory distress (rapid, deep, labored breathing)
Substantial bleeding
Shock
Biochemical Features
Renal impairment (serum creatinine >3 mg/dL)†
Acidosis (plasma bicarbonate <15 mmol/L)
Jaundice (serum total bilirubin >2.5 mg/dL)†
Hyperlactatemia (venous lactate >45 mg/dL)
Hypoglycemia (blood glucose <40 mg/dL)
Elevated aminotransferase levels (>3 times normal)
Hematologic Features
Parasitemia (parasite count >500,000/mm^3 or mature trophozoite and shizont count >10,000/mm^3)‡
>5% neutrophils contain malaria pigment

*The prognosis correlates with the level of impaired consciousness.
†The combination of deep jaundice and renal failure is particularly grave.
‡Trophozoites are mature parasites in which pigment is visible under light microscopy.
Adapted from White NH: The treatment of malaria. *N Engl J Med* 1996;335:800-6.

TABLE 32–7. Chemoprophylaxis of Malaria

Regimen*†	Timing	Adult Dosage	Pediatric Dosage
Prophylaxis for Travel to Regions with Chloroquine-Sensitive Malaria			
Recommended Regimen			
Choroquine phosphate	1 wk before exposure and continuing weekly while in malarious area and for 4 wk after last exposure	300 mg base (500 mg salt) PO once a week	5 mg/kg base (8.3 mg/kg salt; max 300 mg base [500 mg salt]) PO once a week
Prophylaxis for Travel to Regions with Chloroquine-Resistant Malaria			
Recommended Regimen (All Areas Except the Thai-Cambodia and Thai-Myanmar [Burma] Border Areas)			
Mefloquine	1 wk before exposure and continuing weekly while in malarious area and for 4 wk after last exposure	228 mg base (250 mg salt) PO once a week	<5 kg: 4.6 mg/kg base (5 mg/kg salt) once a day 5–9 kg: 1/8 tablet once a week 10–19 kg: 1/4 tablet PO once a week 20–30 kg: 1/2 tablet PO once a week 31–45 kg: 3/4 tablet PO once a week >45 kg: 1 tablet PO once a week
Alternative Regimens‡			
Doxycycline (recommended for travelers to the Thai-Cambodia and Thai-Myanmar [Burma] border areas)	1–2 days before exposure and continuing daily while in malarious area and for 4 wk after last exposure	100 mg PO once a day	≥8 years: 2 mg/kg (maximum, 100 mg) PO once a day
or			
Atovaquone-proguanil (Malarone)	Same as above	1 adult tablet (250 mg atovaquone, 100 mg proguanil) PO once a day	11–20 kg: 1 pediatric tablet (62.5 mg atovaquone, 25 mg proguanil) PO once a day 21–30 kg: 2 pediatric tablets PO once a day 31–40 kg: 3 pediatric tablets PO once a day >40 kg: 4 pediatric tablets PO once a day
Presumptive Self-Treatment			
Pyrimethamine-sulfadoxine (Fansidar)	Self-treatment of febrile illness when medical care is not immediately available (within 24 hr); continue chemoprophylaxis regimen and *seek medical care immediately*	3 tablets (total of 75 mg pyrimethamine and 1,500 mg sulfadoxine) PO in one dose	<1 yr: ¼ tablet PO in one dose 1–3 yr (or 5–10 kg): ½ tablet PO in one dose 4–8 yr (or 11–20 kg): 1 tablet PO in one dose 9–14 yr (or 31–45 kg): 2 tablets PO in one dose >14 yr (or >45 kg): 3 tablets PO in one dose
or			
Atovaquone-proguanil (Malarone)	Same as above	4 tablets (total of 4,000 mg atovaquone and 1,600 mg proguanil) PO in one dose for 3 days	11–20 kg: 1 adult tablet PO in one dose for 3 days 21–30 kg: 2 adult tablets PO in one dose for 3 days 31–40 kg: 3 adult tablets PO in one dose for 3 days >40 kg: 4 adult tablets PO in one dose for 3 days
Individuals with Prolonged Exposure (e.g., Missionaries, Peace Corps Volunteers) from Areas Endemic for *P. vivax* and *P. ovale* (Almost All Areas Except Haiti) or with Intense *P. vivax* Exposure (e.g., Papua New Guinea)			
Primaquine	Daily during the last 2 weeks of chemoprophylaxis	30 mg base (52.6 mg salt) PO once a day for 14 days	0.5 mg/kg base (0.8 mg/kg salt; maximum, 15 mg base [26.3 mg salt]) PO once a day for 14 days

*Review contraindications and adverse effects before use (see text). No drug regimen guarantees protection against malaria. Travelers to countries with a risk of malaria should be advised to avoid mosquito bites by using personal protective measures (see text).

†In pregnancy, chloroquine and proguanil for prophylaxis have been used extensively and safely, but the safety of other chemoprophylactic regimens is uncertain. The Food and Drug Administration does not license mefloquine for use in pregnant women or in children who weigh less than 15 kg, but recent recommendations from the CDC allow the drug to be considered for use when travel to chloroquine-resistant *P. falciparum* areas cannot be avoided. Doxycycline and primaquine should not be used in pregnancy. Pyrimethamine-sulfadoxine should not be used in pregnant women at term or in infants younger than 2 months of age. Travel during pregnancy to chloroquine-resistant malarial areas should be discouraged.

‡Failures of prophylaxis with chloroquine and proguanil have been reported commonly. This regimen is only 40–60% effective and is no longer recommended.

effective mosquito repellents contain 20–35% **DEET** (N,N diethyl-m-toluamide) and are effective for about 4 hours. Children should not be taken outside from dusk to dawn, but if it is absolutely necessary for them to go outside, they should wear long-sleeved clothing and long pants, and DEET should be applied to exposed skin except for the eyes, mouth, and hands (because hands are often placed in the mouth). The repellent should then be washed off as soon as the children come back inside. Adverse reactions to DEET include skin rashes, toxic encephalopathy, and seizures. Even with these precautions, parents should seek professional medical care immediately if a child becomes ill while traveling in a malarious area.

Chemoprophylaxis. Chemoprophylaxis is necessary for all visitors to and residents of the tropics who have not lived there since infancy. Children of nonimmune women should have chemoprophylaxis from birth. Children of women from endemic areas have passive immunity until 3–6 months of age, after which they are increasingly likely to acquire malaria.

Chemoprophylaxis should be started 1–2 weeks before a person enters the endemic area except for doxycycline, which can be started 1–2 days before, and should continue for at least 4 weeks after the person leaves. In the few remaining areas of the world that are free of chloroquine-resistant malaria strains (e.g., the Dominican Republic, Haiti, Central America north of Panama, and the Middle East), chloroquine is given once per week on the same day of the week (Table 32–7). Chloroquine is distributed as 250 mg and 500 mg tablets in the United States and as a liquid in foreign countries, although it tastes bitter. The pharmacist should prepare powdered doses and place them in envelopes or gelatin capsules, which are easier to transport and which can be added to something sweet, such as chocolate syrup or jelly. Adverse effects are rare but include nausea and vomiting.

In areas where chloroquine-resistant *P. falciparum* exists, mefloquine is recommended for all ages except for travelers to the Thai-Cambodian and Thai-Myanmar (Burma) border areas, where mefloquine resistance is common and doxycycline is recommended. Pregnant women should be advised to postpone travel to a malaria-risk area until after parturition. If travel cannot be postponed, experience with chloroquine and limited experience with mefloquine suggest that they are safe to use during pregnancy, including the first trimester, whereas doxycycline and primaquine should not be used during pregnancy. Mefloquine is usually well tolerated, with the most common adverse effects being nausea and vomiting, but it is not recommended for persons with a known hypersensitivity to the drug, a history of epilepsy or severe psychiatric disorders, or cardiac conduction defects or who are taking β-blockers. Alternative chemoprophylaxis regimens are doxycycline, which is not approved for children <8 years of age, and atovaquone-proguanil (Malarone), although dosing is uncertain for children <11 kg (24 pounds). Doxycycline is equivalent to mefloquine for short-term prophylaxis but is not acceptable for long-term prophylaxis because of adverse effects associated with its long-term use. **Presumptive self-treatment** with pyrimethamine-sulfadoxine (Fansidar) or atovaquone-proguanil during travel is recommended for travelers with a febrile illness suspected to be malaria who cannot reach medical care within 24 hours. This is a temporary measure, and prompt professional medical care is imperative, especially for a febrile child. Atovaquone-proguanil is recommended for travelers to the Amazon River basin, Southeast Asia, and some countries in Africa because of sulfadoxine-pyrimethamine resistance. Mefloquine should not be used for self-treatment because of the frequency of serious adverse effects at treatment doses. There have been several reports of both melfoquine and pyrimethamine-sulfadoxine resistance.

Vaccine. Extensive efforts have been made to develop a malaria vaccine, but results to date have been disappointing.

REVIEWS

Bruce-Chwatt LJ: History of malaria from prehistory to eradication. In Wernsdorfer WH, McGregor I (editors): *Malaria: Principles and Practice of Malariology.* New York, Churchill Livingston, 1988.

Taylor TE, Strickland GT: Malaria. In Strickland GT (editor): *Hunter's Tropical Medicine,* 8th ed. Philadelphia, WB Saunders, 2000.

White NJ: Malaria. In Cook GC (editor): *Manson's Tropical Diseases,* 20th ed. Philadelphia, Bailliere Tindall, 1996.

Wyler DJ: Malaria: Overview and update. *Clin Infect Dis* 1993;16:449–56.

KEY ARTICLES

Campbell CC: Challenges facing antimalarial therapy in Africa. *J Infect Dis* 1991;163:1207–11.

Centers for Disease Control: Change of dosing regimen for malaria prophylaxis with mefloquine. *MMWR Morb Mortal Wkly Rep* 1991;40:72–3.

Centers for Disease Control: Mosquito-transmitted malaria—California and Florida, 1990. *MMWR Morb Mortal Wkly Rep* 1991;40:106–8.

Centers for Disease Control: Recommendations for the prevention of malaria among travelers. *MMWR Morb Mortal Wkly Rep* 1990;39:1–10.

Centers for Disease Control: Treatment with quinidine gluconate of persons with severe *Plasmodium falciparum* infection: Discontinuation of parenteral quinine from CDC Drug Service. *MMWR Morb Mortal Wkly Rep* 1991;40:21–3.

Centers for Disease Control and Prevention: Malaria surveillance—United States, 1997. *MMWR Morb Mortal Wkly Rep* 2001;50(SS–1):25–44.

Grau GE, Taylor TE, Molyneux ME, et al: Tumor necrosis factor and disease severity in children with falciparum malaria. *N Engl J Med* 1989;320:1586–91.

Hoffman SL, Nussenzweig V, Sadoff JC, et al: Progress toward malaria preerythrocytic vaccines. *Science* 1991;252:520–1.

Lobel HO, Miani M, Eng T, et al: Long-term malaria prophylaxis with weekly mefloquine. *Lancet* 1993;341:848–51.

Luzzatto L: Genetics of red cells and susceptibility to malaria. *Blood* 1979;54:961–76.

Lynk A, Gold R: Review of 40 children with imported malaria. *Pediatr Infect Dis J* 1989;8:745–50.

Miller KD, Greenberg AE, Campbell CC: Treatment of severe malaria in the United States with a continuous infusion of quinidine gluconate and exchange transfusion. *N Engl J Med* 1989;321:65–70.

Ockenhouse CF, Ho M, Tandon NN, et al: Molecular basis of sequestration in severe and uncomplicated *Plasmodium falciparum* malaria: Differential adhesion of infected erythrocytes to CD36 and ICAM-1. *J Infect Dis* 1991;164:163–9.

White NJ: The treatment of malaria. *N Engl J Med* 1996;335:800–6.

Wyler DJ: Immunology of malaria. In Wyler DJ (editor): *Modern Parasite Biology.* New York, WH Freeman, 1990.

Wyler DJ: Steroids are out in the treatment of cerebral malaria: What's next? *J Infect Dis* 1988;158:320–4.

Zucker JR: Changing patterns of autochthonous malaria transmission in the United States: A review of recent outbreaks. *Emerg Infect Dis* 1996;2:37–43.

CHAPTER 33

Babesiosis

Peter J. Krause

Babesiosis is a malaria-like, tickborne illness caused by intraerythrocytic protozoa. The disease is named after Victor Babes, the Hungarian microbiologist who discovered the causative microorganism. Although babesiosis has long been recognized as a clinically and economically important disease in livestock, the first human case was not described until 1957. Over the past 30 years the epidemiology of the disease has changed from a few isolated cases to the establishment of endemic areas in southern New England, New York, and the upper Midwest, and the disease has been reported from a wide geographic range in North America and Europe.

ETIOLOGY

There are more than 90 species in the genus *Babesia* that infect a variety of wild and domestic animals throughout the world. Most *Babesia* species are small (1–5 μm long) and pear shaped, round, or oval. Four *Babesia* species have been found to cause disease in humans: *Babesia microti*, WA-1, and MO-1 in North America and *Babesia divergens* in Europe.

Transmission. Human babesiosis is a zoonotic disease with transmission by a tick vector from an infected animal reservoir. In the northeastern United States, three animal species have been identified as important in the survival of *B. microti.* The **white-footed mouse** *(Peromyscus leucopus)* is the primary reservoir for *B. microti.* Approximately two thirds of mice in endemic areas are parasitemic. The primary vector for *B. microti* is *Ixodes scapularis* (previously known as *Ixodes dammini*), the **deer tick** (Fig. 29–1 and Plate 9E), which is the same tick that transmits *Borrelia burgdorferi,* the etiologic agent of Lyme disease (Chapter 29) and the agent of human granulocytic ehrlichiosis (Chapter 31). There are three active stages in the life cycle of *I. scapularis:* larva, nymph, and adult (Fig. 33–1). Nymphs are the primary vector for transmission of infection to humans. They feed in the late spring and summer and, if infected, transmit *B. microti* to rodents or man. Consequently, most human cases of babesiosis occur in the summer. The **white-tailed deer** *(Odocoileus virginianus)* is an important host of *I. scapularis* but is not a reservoir for *B. microti.* It is thought that the recent increase in the deer population has resulted in an increase in the number and distribution of *I. scapularis* and thus an increase in the incidence of human babesiosis, human granulocytic ehrlichiosis, and Lyme borreliosis. Rarely, babesiosis is acquired through blood transfusion. Transplacental-perinatal transmission of babesiosis has also been described.

EPIDEMIOLOGY

Most human cases of babesiosis have been reported from the coastal areas of southern New England and eastern Long Island and from Minnesota and Wisconsin, where the disease is endemic. Human babesiosis due to previously unreported species recently has been described in California and Washington State (WA-1) and in Missouri (MO-1). Human cases of *B. divergens* in Europe have been reported from Belgium, France, Great Britain, Ireland, Russia, and Yugoslavia.

Age is an important factor in the symptoms of babesial disease. Although published reports of pediatric babesiosis demonstrate that babesiosis may result in debilitating episodes of disease, the intensity of illness appears to be greater in persons older than 40 years of age. The majority of cases of babesiosis have been reported in adults 40–60 years old, although babesial infection is detected by serologic testing as commonly in children as in older adults in highly endemic areas. Babesiosis may be less likely to be considered by physicians caring for children than by those caring for adults because it is generally thought to be a geriatric rather than a pediatric disease. In addition, febrile illnesses in adults tend to be more aggressively evaluated, including evaluation for babesiosis, because febrile illness is less common in adults than in children. Additional work is needed to clarify the clinical spectrum of babesial illness in children as well as in adults.

PATHOGENESIS

Babesia species are intraerythrocytic protozoa. Extracellular forms are seen only in heavily parasitized cases. After adhesion and entry into the erythrocyte, the organism multiplies by asexual budding into two to four daughter cells or merozoites. Unlike *Plasmodium falciparum* merozoites, which are released from erythrocytes all at once (in synchrony), *Babesia* species are released at varying intervals. New erythrocytes are infected, and the cycle is repeated. The absence of synchrony decreases the possibility of sudden massive hemolysis and may explain why persons heavily parasitized with *Babesia* species are generally less ill than those parasitized with *P. falciparum.*

Alteration of the erythrocyte membrane and lysis caused by babesial infection of the erythrocyte is associated with many of the clinical manifestations and complications of babesiosis, including fever, hemolytic anemia, jaundice, hemoglobinemia, hemoglobinuria, and renal insufficiency. Ischemia and necrosis result from obstruction of blood vessels by parasitized erythrocytes, which may cause hepatomegaly and hepatic dysfunction, splenomegaly, and cerebral dysfunction. The spleen plays a critical role in protection against *Babesia* species. Most fatal cases of babesiosis in humans have occurred in persons who have undergone splenectomy, although asplenia does not always result in death or even in severe illness. The spleen is thought to protect against babesial infection by removing and phagocytizing parasites from infected erythrocytes and by the production of antibabesial antibody. Other host defense mechanisms that may help limit babesial infection

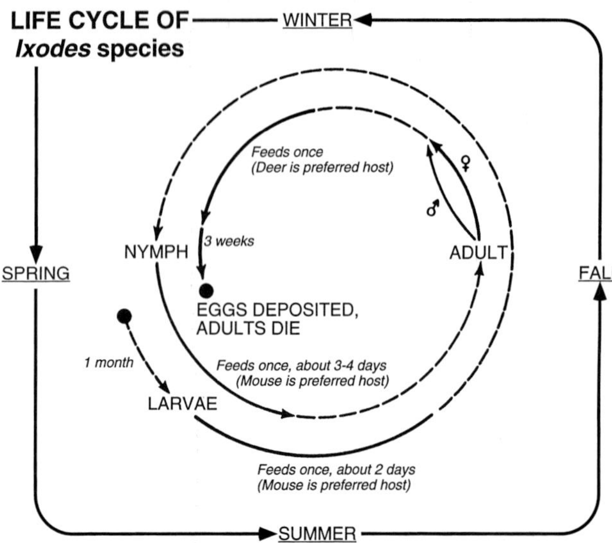

FIGURE 33–1. Life cycle of *Ixodes scapularis*, the arthropod vector for babesiosis, Lyme disease, and human granulocytic ehrlichiosis. (Adapted from Spielman A, Wilson ML, Levine JF, et al: Ecology of *Ixodes dammini*–borne human babesiosis and Lyme disease. *Annu Rev Entomol* 1985;30:439–60. With permission, from the *Annual Review of Entomology,* Volume 30 © 1985 by Annual Reviews www.AnnualReviews.org.)

include B and T lymphocytes, antibody, complement, a soluble nonantibody factor, macrophages and macrophage products such as tumor necrosis factor, and polymorphonuclear leukocytes.

SYMPTOMS AND CLINICAL MANIFESTATIONS

Incubation Period. In clinically apparent cases, symptoms of babesiosis begin after an incubation period of 1–6 weeks from the beginning of tick feeding.

Usual Symptoms

The clinical manifestations of babesiosis range from fulminating disease leading to (1) death or prolonged convalescence, (2) moderate to severe illness with symptoms that are similar to those of malaria, (3) nonspecific flulike illness, or (4) subclinical infection detected through retrospective serosurveys. Inapparent infection is the most common form of the disease according to data from several serosurveys in endemic areas. There is often no recollection of a tick bite, since the unengorged *I. scapularis* nymph is only about 2 mm long (Fig. 29–1 and Plate 9E).

Typical symptoms in moderate to severe infection include intermittent temperature spikes to as high as 40°C (104°F) and one or more of the following: chills, sweats, myalgias, arthralgias, fatigue, nausea, and vomiting (Table 33–1). Other less common clinical manifestations are emotional lability and depression, hyperesthesia, headache, sore throat, abdominal pain, conjunctival injection, photophobia, weight loss, and nonproductive cough. Rash seldom is noted with babesiosis. Erythema migrans occurring with babesiosis indicates concomitant Lyme disease. Coinfection with *B. microti* and *B. burgdorferi* may result in more severe acute illness than either infection alone and may possibly result in a higher incidence of long-term joint complications.

Physical Examination Findings

The findings on physical examination in patients with babesiosis generally are minimal, often consisting only of fever (Table 33–1).

TABLE 33–1. Clinical Manifestations of Babesiosis

Symptoms	Signs
Common	
Fever	Fever
Chills	Splenomegaly
Sweats	Hepatomegaly
Myalgia	
Arthralgia	
Fatigue	
Less Common	
Anorexia	Pharyngeal erythema
Nausea	Jaundice
Vomiting	Retinopathy
Headache	
Emotional lability	

Mild splenomegaly, hepatomegaly, or both are noted occasionally. Slight pharyngeal erythema, jaundice, and retinopathy with splinter hemorrhages and retinal infarcts have also been reported.

DIAGNOSIS

The diagnosis of babesiosis should be considered in patients who live or travel in endemic areas and who experience a flu-like illness. Laboratory findings reflect the invasion and subsequent lysis of erythrocytes by the parasite (Table 33–2). There is mild to moderately severe hemolytic anemia with an elevated reticulocyte count. The WBC count is normal to slightly decreased with a left shift. Thrombocytopenia is common. Tests show elevated liver function in about half of patients. Proteinuria and elevated BUN and creatinine levels may also occur.

Microbiologic Evaluation

Specific diagnosis of babesiosis is made by microscopic identification of the organism with Giemsa stains of thick or thin blood smears (Fig. 33–2). *Babesia* species are round, oval, or pear shaped and have a blue cytoplasm with a red chromatin. The ring form is most common and is similar to the rings of *P. falciparum* (Plate 2C). Multiple thick and thin blood smears should be examined because only a few erythrocytes are infected in the early stage of the illness, when most people seek medical attention. Maximum erythrocyte infection is approximately 10% in normal hosts but may be up to 85% in asplenic persons. Usually fewer than 1% of erythrocytes are parasitized early in the course of the illness, and therefore the laboratory investigation of possible babesiosis should include multiple examinations of blood smears.

Serologic testing, small animal inoculation, and PCR can be used to confirm babesial infection. Both IgG and IgM antibodies can be detected by indirect IFA. During the acute phase of the illness, titers usually exceed 1:1,024 but decline to 1:64 or less within 8–12 months. Thus a babesial antibody titer of 1:1,024 or

TABLE 33–2. Laboratory Tests for the Diagnosis of Babesiosis

Complete blood cell count, including platelet count
Giemsa stains of thick and thin blood smears
Acute and convalescent serology
Small-animal inoculation of blood
PCR of blood

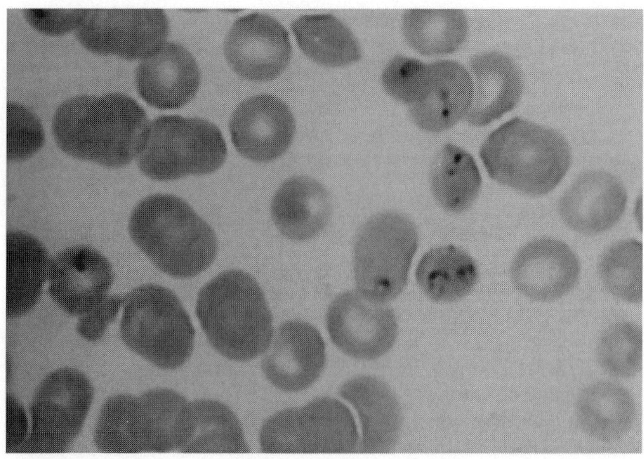

FIGURE 33–2. Ring forms of *Babesia microti* in human blood smear (×1000).

greater usually signifies active or recent infection. Although cross-reactions occur to different *Babesia* species and *Plasmodium* species with the IFA test, these titers are almost always low (1:16 or less). Where laboratory expertise exists, blood from the patient can be injected intravenously or intraperitoneally into small laboratory animals, such as hamsters or gerbils. If present in the patient's blood, *B. microti* usually appears in the blood of the inoculated animal within 2–4 weeks. PCR is also a sensitive and specific method for detection of *Babesia* DNA that should supplant the hamster inoculation test. Proper technique must be used to prevent false-positive results.

TREATMENT

The combination of clindamycin and quinine is the therapy of choice for babesiosis (Table 33–3), but it has not always been effective. Adverse effects occur in 50–70% of patients and include decreased hearing, tinnitus, vertigo, and diarrhea. Atovaquone and azithromycin have been used successfully for treatment of babesiosis in adults, with efficacy similar to that of clindamycin and quinine, but with reduction of adverse effects to about 15%. With both regimens, clearance of *B. microti* may be delayed and inconsistent and bloodborne parasites may persist for months. Pentamidine and TMP-SMZ have been used successfully to treat a case of *B. divergens* in France.

Exchange blood transfusion is an important therapeutic modality in patients with life-threatening babesial infections. Exchange transfusions can decrease the degree of parasitemia rapidly and remove toxic byproducts of babesial infection, but they should be used only in the most severe infections, as in patients with a high parasitemia (>5%) and coma, hypotension, congestive heart failure, pulmonary edema, or renal failure.

TABLE 33–3. Recommended Antibiotic Treatment for Babesiosis

Recommended Regimen	Alternative Regimen*
Clindamycin *plus* Quinine for 7–10 days	Atovaquone *plus* Azithromycin for 7–10 days
Severe Cases *plus* exchange transfusion	

*This regimen has been studied only in adults.

Recommended Dosages for Patients with Normal Renal Function

ANTIBIOTIC	DOSAGE	MAXIMUM DAILY DOSE
Atovaquone	40 mg/kg/day divided q12hr PO	1,500 mg
Azithromycin	10 mg/kg on day 1, then 5 mg/kg thereafter, once daily PO	500 mg day 1, then 250 mg thereafter
Clindamycin	20 mg/kg/day divided q8hr IM or IV	1,800 mg
Quinine	25 mg/kg/day divided q8hr PO	1,950 mg

COMPLICATIONS

A severe form of babesiosis that has been noted in some patients consists of fulminant illness lasting about a week and ending in death or a prolonged convalescence. Although more common in persons with *B. divergens* infection or prior splenectomy, severe babesiosis can occur in otherwise healthy persons who are infected with *B. microti*. In a retrospective study of 136 patients with *B. microti* infection from Long Island, New York, seven patients (5%) died. The patients with fatal illness ranged in age from 60 to 82 years, and only one was known to be immunocompromised. Signs and symptoms in severe cases include high fever, severe hemolytic anemia, hemoglobinemia and hemoglobinuria, jaundice, ecchymoses, petechiae, congestive heart failure, pulmonary edema, renal failure, adult respiratory distress syndrome, and coma.

PROGNOSIS

Clinically apparent illness usually lasts for a few weeks to several months, with prolonged recovery of up to 18 months. Parasitemia may continue even after the patient feels well, and it has been demonstrated in humans for as long as 27 months with subsequent relapse of illness. Although fatalities occur, complete recovery with or without specific antibabesial therapy is the rule.

PREVENTION

Prevention of babesiosis can be accomplished by avoiding areas in May through September where ticks, deer, and mice are known to thrive. It is especially important for those at increased risk in endemic areas, such as asplenic persons, to avoid tall grass and brush where ticks may abound. All those who travel in the foliage in endemic areas should wear clothing that covers the lower part of the body and is sprayed or impregnated with diethyltoluamide (DEET), dimethyl phthalate, or permethrin, in addition to searching for ticks on themselves and their pets. Ticks should be removed as soon as possible; the mouthparts should be grasped with tweezers without squeezing the body of the tick. Administration of prophylactic antibiotics after a tick bite to prevent babesiosis is not indicated. Attempts to reduce the tick, mouse, or deer populations in endemic areas are less effective. It has been recommended that prospective blood donors who reside in endemic areas and who present with a history of fever within the preceding 1 to 2 months be excluded from donating blood so as to prevent transfusion-related cases. Effective *Babesia bovis* and *Babesia bigemina* vaccines have been developed for use in cattle, but there is no effective *B. microti* vaccine.

REVIEWS

Dammin GJ: Babesiosis. In Weinstein L, Fields BN (editors): *Seminars in Infectious Disease.* New York, Stratton, 1978.

Spielman A, Wilson ML, Levine JF, et al: Ecology of *Ixodes dammini*-borne human babesiosis and Lyme disease. *Annu Rev Entomol* 1985; 30:439–60.

KEY ARTICLES

Centers for Disease Control: Clindamycin and quinine treatment for *Babesia microti* infections. *MMWR Morb Mortal Wkly Rep* 1983;32:65–72.

Dammin GJ, Spielman A, Benach JL, et al: The rising incidence of clinical *Babesia microti* infection. *Hum Pathol* 1981;12:398–400.

Esernio-Jenssen D, Scimeca PG, Benach JL, et al: Transplacental/perinatal babesiosis, *J Pediatr* 1987;110:570–2.

Healy GR, Ruebush TK II: Morphology of *Babesia microti* in human blood smears. *Am J Clin Pathol* 1980;73:107–9.

Herwaldt B, Persing DH, Precigout EA, et al: A fatal case of babesiosis in Missouri: Identification of another piroplasm that infects humans. *Ann Intern Med* 1996;124:643–50.

Krause PJ, Lepore T, Sikand VK, et al: Atovaquone and azithromycin for the treatment of babesiosis. *N Engl J Med* 2000;343:1454–8.

Krause PJ, Telford SR III, Ryan R, et al: Geographical and temporal distribution of babesial infection in Connecticut. *J Clin Microbiol* 1991; 29:1–4.

Krause PJ, Telford SR III, Pollack RJ, et al: Babesiosis: An underdiagnosed disease of children. *Pediatrics* 1992;89:1045–48.

Krause PJ, Telford SR III, Spielman A, et al: Concurrent Lyme disease and babesiosis: Evidence for increased severity and duration of illness. *JAMA* 1996;275:1657–60.

Krause PJ, Spielman A, Telford S III, et al: Persistent parasitemia after acute babesiosis. *N Engl J Med* 1998;339:160–5.

Mathewson HO, Anderson AE, Hazard GW: Self-limited babesiosis in a splenectomized child. *Pediatr Infect Dis* 1984;3:148–9.

Meldrum SC, Birkhead GS, White DJ, et al: Human babesiosis in New York State: An epidemiologic description of 136 cases. *Clin Infect Dis* 1992;15:1019–23.

Persing D, Mathiesen D, Marshall WF, et al: Detection of *Babesia microti* by polymerase chain reaction. *J Clin Microbiol* 1992;30:2097–103.

Rosner F, Zarrabi MH, Benach JL, et al: Babesiosis in splenectomized adults: Review of 22 reported cases. *Am J Med* 1984;76:696–701.

Ruebush TK II, Juranek DD, Chisholm ES, et al: Human babesiosis on Nantucket Island: Evidence for self-limited and subclinical infections. *N Engl J Med* 1977;297:825–7.

Scimeca PG, Weinblatt ME, Schonfeld G, et al: Babesiosis in two infants from Eastern Long Island, NY. *Am J Dis Child* 1986;140:971.

Steketee RW, Eckman MR, Burgess EC, et al: Babesiosis in Wisconsin: A new focus of disease transmission. *JAMA* 1985;253:2675–8.

Wittner M, Rowin KS, Tanowitz HB, et al: Successful chemotherapy of transfusion babesiosis. *Ann Intern Med* 1982;96:601–4.

CHAPTER 34

Other Zoonoses and Vectorborne Infections

John C. Christenson

More than 150 zoonotic infections causing a wide variety of human illnesses have been described. The possibility of environmental or zoonotic exposure to an infectious agent should always be considered in the evaluation for infection (Chapter 3). Lyme disease is the most common zoonosis in the United States (Chapter 29), followed by RMSF (Chapter 30) and human ehrlichiosis (Chapter 31). The relatively few other important zoonoses that are considered among the more common have a far lower incidence (<200 cases) per year in the United States (Fig. 3–3). These are characterized clinically by multisystem involvement but with nonspecific signs and symptoms (Table 34–1). Most other zoonoses are rarely diagnosed in the United States. The most important clue to an infection suspected of being zoonotic may be possible or known environmental exposure to the reservoir or vector, including living in an endemic area.

BRUCELLOSIS

Brucellosis, also known as **undulant fever** or **Malta fever,** is a worldwide infectious disease of mammals, including cattle, swine, dogs, sheep, goats, and occasionally humans. Brucellosis is an important endemic disease in many parts of the world, but it is mainly an occupational disease in the United States. Infection in children is reported infrequently.

ETIOLOGY

Brucellosis is caused by *Brucella,* which are small, aerobic nonmotile gram-negative coccobacilli. Infection is directly related to contact with animals that are infected or colonized with one of the four *Brucella* species known to cause human disease: *B. suis* in swine; *B. melitensis* in goats and sheep; *B. abortus* in cattle and bison; and *B. canis* in dogs, which is a rare cause of infection in humans.

Transmission. Humans may become infected by inhaling infected aerosol droplets, through direct skin contact, and through splash exposures to mucous membranes. Contact is likely in slaughterhouses, farms, laboratories, and during veterinary medicine activities. Udders, uteri, and testicles of infected cattle have large concentrations of bacteria. Consumption of unpasteurized milk products, such as raw milk and cheese, also contributes to transmission.

EPIDEMIOLOGY

The incidence of brucellosis in the United States has decreased in the past several decades (Fig. 3–3), with fewer than 100 cases reported annually. This decrease is most likely a result of the enforcement of governmental regulations within the meat and dairy industry, such as routine vaccination of animals or destruction of animals in whom brucellosis is identified. Spontaneous abortions and infertility may indicate *Brucella* infection in animals. Epidemic abortions among dogs, foxes, and coyotes suggest infection with *B. canis.* Exposure to aborted animal fetuses may place humans at risk. In the United States, brucellosis is endemic among the bison at Yellowstone National Park.

Many cases caused by the introduction and consumption of dairy products, such as cheese prepared from unpasteurized milk, continue to be reported in the United States. In addition, returning travelers may have consumed some of these products before reentry into the country and may present with signs of a febrile illness days after their arrival. *B. melitensis* infection usually reflects a recent visit to an endemic area, such as the Mediterranean or the Middle East, and consumption of unpasteurized milk products, especially goat cheese and milk. Occupational disease may occur in veterinarians and other persons who use the live-attenuated *B. abortus* strain 19 or *B. melitensis* strain Rev-1 vaccines for immunization of farm animals. The use of a newer vaccine containing a less virulent strain of *B. abortus,* RB51, may minimize this risk.

PATHOGENESIS

Brucella are intracellular pathogens that may survive within phagocytic cells, such as polymorphonuclear cells, for extended periods of time. The organisms tend to migrate to lymph node tissue and organs with reticuloendothelial systems, especially the liver and the spleen, where they continue to proliferate. The severity of the disease is dependent on the *Brucella* species involved: *B. melitensis* is associated with more severe disease; *B. abortus* tends to be milder and sporadic; and *B. suis* is more commonly associated with suppurative abscesses.

SYMPTOMS AND CLINICAL MANIFESTATIONS

The incubation period after exposure and acquisition ranges from 1 week to more than 30 days. The clinical features of brucellosis are nonspecific and may vary in severity from a mild febrile illness to a severe suppurative infection. Children frequently have a mild, self-limiting illness. More than 95% of patients report fever that is either persistent or spiking with daily defervescence, along with other generalized symptoms (Table 34–2).

Physical Examination Findings

Approximately 10–14% of patients have demonstrable splenomegaly and lymphadenopathy. Focal findings may be present in patients with suppurative abscesses.

TABLE 34–1. Differential Diagnosis of Major Zoonoses According to Clinical Syndromes

Syndrome / Exposure	Disease
Fever, Rash, and Multisystem Involvement	
History of tick bite or exposure, or during an endemic season, or exposure to domestic or wild animals	Rocky Mountain spotted fever Colorado tick fever Human ehrlichiosis Murine (or fleaborne) typhus
Exposure to fresh water (streams or ponds)	Leptospirosis
Musculoskeletal, central nervous system, cardiac involvement	Lyme disease
Biphasic Febrile Illness, Constitutional Symptoms (Headaches, Myalgias, Malaise)	
Occurrence in endemic regions or exposure to arthropod vectors	Colorado tick fever Dengue fever Relapsing fever
Exposure to rodents, hamsters, aseptic meningitis	Lymphocytic choriomeningitis
Arthralgias, regional lymphadenitis, maculopapular exanthem on extremities	Rat-bite fever
Fever, Mononucleosis-like Illness	
Consumption of unpasteurized milk products; occupational exposure	Brucellosis
Exposure to turtles, dogs, cats, poultry	Salmonellosis
Fever, Constitutional Symptoms (Chills, Sweats, Myalgias, Headaches), Exposure to Rodents	
Vesiculopapular exanthem, dark escharlike lesion, living in an urban dwelling	Rickettsialpox
Severe hemolytic anemia in an asplenic patient, occurrence in endemic regions	Babesiosis
Acute respiratory distress syndrome–like lung disease, fever, leukocytosis, thrombocytopenia, occurrence in endemic regions	Hantavirus cardiopulmonary syndrome
Atypical Pneumonia Unresponsive to Conventional Therapy	
Exposure to sheep, goats, cattle, parturient cats or dogs	Q fever
Exposure to skinned or dead animals, wild rabbits	Tularemia
Exposure to rodents, dead animals, with or without regional lymphadenitis	Plague Hantavirus cardiopulmonary syndrome
Exposure to wild imported birds	Psittacosis
Soft-Tissue Infections Secondary to Animal Bites	
Septicemia, asplenic patient	*Capnocytophaga canimorsus* (formerly DF-2)
Soft-tissue infection, cellulitis, septic arthritis, osteomyelitis: secondary to cat or dog bite or scratch	Pasteurellosis *(Pasteurella multocida)* Cat-scratch disease
Fever; Regional, Painful Lymphadenitis	
Occurrence in endemic regions	Tularemia Plague
Secondary to cat scratch	Cat-scratch disease
Contact with Rodents, Swine; Ingestion of Contaminated Food or Undercooked Pork Products	
Fever, diarrhea, abdominal pain	Yersiniosis caused by *Yersinia enterocolitica*
Fever, acute mesenteric lymphadenitis	Yersiniosis caused by *Yersinia pseudotuberculosis*
Fever, Leukocytosis, Eosinophilia, Hepatomegaly, Exposure to Dogs and Cats; Travel to the Tropics	
Visceral larva migrans *(Toxocara canis)*	
Unsteady Gait, Difficulty Standing, Paralysis, History of Tick Exposure	
Tick paralysis (tick toxicosis)	

DIAGNOSIS

Brucellosis can be categorized according to the duration of symptoms: **acute brucellosis** persists for <3 months, **subacute brucellosis** persists for 3–12 months, and **chronic brucellosis** persists for >12 months. The diagnosis of brucellosis is usually suspected from the clinical manifestations combined with a history of possible exposure and is confirmed by culture or serologic testing.

TABLE 34–2. Symptoms of Brucellosis

Symptoms	Signs
Fever	Hepatomegaly
Chills	Splenomegaly
Generalized weakness	Lymphadenopathy
Weight loss	**Laboratory Findings**
Myalgias	Anemia
Arthralgias	Elevated hepatic transaminases
Headache	

Differential Diagnosis

The febrile illness of brucellosis resembles the clinical presentation of other infectious diseases, such as infectious mononucleosis (caused by EBV, CMV, or *Toxoplasma gondii*), typhoid fever, tularemia, influenza, and miliary tuberculosis. *Brucella* sacroiliitis may resemble musculoskeletal infections by *Mycobacterium tuberculosis* or *Staphylococcus aureus.*

Laboratory Evaluation

A normal WBC count with a relative lymphocytosis is usually found, although leukopenia and thrombocytopenia occasionally can be present. Thrombocytopenia usually suggests hypersplenism or bone marrow aplasia secondary to granuloma formation within the bone marrow. A normocytic, normochromic anemia is present in more than one third of cases, and elevated serum liver enzymes are present in more than 50% of cases. Prolonged fever with hemophagocytosis has been described with brucellosis.

Microbiologic Evaluation

Brucellosis can be diagnosed by isolation of *Brucella* from the blood or from an infected site. The yield of blood cultures varies according to the duration of the infection; in acute illness, isolation of the organism from blood is achieved in 93% of cases, whereas in chronic disease, only 20% of patients have a positive culture. Routine blood cultures are capable of recovering the organism, but the conventional broth bottles need to be held for at least 2–4 weeks rather than the usual 7 days. When BACTEC is used, the organism will generally grow within 5 days.

Serologic Testing. Serologic diagnosis is also possible by detection of a fourfold increase in titers, or a single IgG titer of ≥1:160. The serum agglutination test is the one most often used. These antibodies may cross-react among species of *Brucella.* A specific antigen is needed for the detection of antibodies against *B. canis.* Although blocking IgG and IgA antibodies may cause false-negative tests, a positive IgM may be diagnostic. These false-negative results are caused by a **prozone phenomenon,** which may be eliminated by serial dilutions of sera; a 1:1,280 dilution is usually sufficient for the diagnosis under these circumstances. The regularly available *Brucella* antibody tests do not detect antibodies to *B. canis.* Specialized serologic testing is available from state health departments and the CDC.

A PCR assay with genus-specific primers has been found to be rapid, highly sensitive, and specific in research laboratories when compared with cultures and serologic tests. However, this PCR assay is not available in clinical laboratories.

TREATMENT

Antimicrobial therapy should always consist of combination therapy for a minimum of 4 weeks (Table 34–3). Because *Brucella* may survive for extended periods, some authorities suggest an even longer duration of therapy. More than 50% of relapses occur within 1 month of completing therapy. In studies with *B. melitensis,* treatment with combinations of rifampin plus gentamicin, doxycycline plus gentamicin, oxytetracycline plus gentamicin, doxycycline plus streptomycin, or TMP-SMZ plus gentamicin resulted in no relapses. When a tetracycline agent is selected, doxycycline is preferred because of its longer half-life. The use of TMP-SMZ alone resulted in a 30% relapse rate. Newer agents, such as ciprofloxacin or ofloxacin, are often effective in providing an excellent acute response but have a 27% relapse rate when used alone. Corticosteroids should be used to avoid a **Jarisch-Herxheimer reaction** (fever, rigors, hypotension, and prostration during the first hours of antimicrobial therapy).

TABLE 34–3. Recommended Antibiotic Therapy for Brucellosis

Children <9 yr
TMP-SMZ: TMP 10 mg/kg/day, SMZ 50 mg/kg/day (max 480 mg TMP/day, 2400 mg SMZ/day) divided q6hr IV *or* divided q12hr PO for 4–6 wk
plus
Rifampin 15–20 mg/kg/day (max 600–900 mg/day) in 1–2 daily divided doses PO for 4–6 wk

Children ≥9 yr
Doxycycline 4 mg/kg/day (max 200 mg/day) divided q12hr PO for 4–6 wk *or* tetracycline 30–40 mg/kg/day (max 2 g/day) divided 4 times a day PO for 4–6 wk
plus
Rifampin 15–20 mg/kg/day (max 600–900 mg/day) in 1–2 daily divided doses for 4–6 weeks

Severe Cases
Streptomycin 20 mg/kg/day (max 1 g/day) divided q12hr IM for 2 wk, *or* gentamicin 5 mg/kg/day divided q3hr IM for 7–14 days
plus
TMP-SMZ, *or* doxycycline, *or* tetracycline

COMPLICATIONS

Brucella has a tropism for the musculoskeletal system, and patients with brucellosis often complain of arthralgias as well as sciatica, bursitis, and tendonitis. Suppurative arthritis, spondylitis, and osteomyelitis are frequent, especially with *B. melitensis.* The sacroiliac joint is the most commonly involved; involvement tends to be unilateral and nondestructive and responds to antimicrobial therapy. Spinal joints may also be affected; 60% of these complications are localized in the lumbosacral region. These infections may spread to the vertebral bodies and surrounding tissues, causing irritation of the dorsal roots. Early surgical débridement may be useful.

Approximately one half of patients with brucellosis complain of neuropsychiatric symptoms, such as mental depression, nervousness, fatigue, insomnia, and inattention. The genitourinary tract in humans may be involved with orchitis, prostatitis, and epididymitis. Chronic pyelonephritis resembling renal tuberculosis has been described.

Manifestations of **neurobrucellosis,** which are rare, are variable and include meningitis, encephalitis, myelitis, radiculitis, neuritis, or any combination of these. Cerebrospinal fluid analysis demonstrates a lymphocytic pleocytosis of a few hundred cells, hypoglycorrhachia, and elevated protein. Nearly one third of patients have involvement of the cranial nerves, especially the sixth, seventh, and eighth. In *Brucella* meningitis, examination of the CSF for the presence of *Brucella* antibodies is commonly positive.

Brucella concentrates in tissues with high concentrations of reticuloendothelial function, such as the liver, the spleen, and the lymph nodes, and may cause a noncaseating granulomatous hepatitis. Bronchitis, pneumonia, pulmonary nodules, lung abscess, and hilar lymphadenopathy have been reported. An unusual presentation that occurs after skin contact with the organism is a hypersensitivity reaction with discrete, elevated, red papules that may subsequently progress to ulcer formation.

Infection during pregnancy may result in premature labor and congenital infection of the infant.

PROGNOSIS

Recurrent bacteremia is common after treatment with a single agent. Combination therapy is effective in reducing the number of relapses. Patients with focal disease are more likely to fail to respond to therapy. Prolonged treatment beyond 4 weeks may be necessary.

PREVENTION

The prevention of human brucellosis is based on the eradication of brucellosis from infected animals. Pasteurization of all milk products is essential for the control of brucellosis in children. Persons must avoid the consumption of unpasteurized dairy products. Avoidance of occupational hazards also minimizes infection. Bovine brucellosis has been greatly controlled in the United States by active immunization and serologic testing programs of cattle. Infected animals are usually destroyed.

No vaccine is currently available in the United States for use in humans.

TULAREMIA

ETIOLOGY

Tularemia was first recognized in 1911 as the cause of a plague-like illness of ground squirrels in Tulare County, California. McCoy and Chapin isolated a bacterium, which they named *Bacterium tularense,* as the causative agent. Pearse described the first reported human cases of ulceroglandular tularemia in 1911. From 1915–1917, three ophthalmologists in Cincinnati described the first human cases of bacteriologically confirmed tularemia. Francis, a physician in the United States Public Health Service, went to Utah in 1919 to investigate the cause of deerfly fever and isolated the organism from infected humans and from jackrabbits. It was soon realized that *B. tularense* was the cause of **market fever,** a common illness in persons who skinned and dressed wild rabbits. In recognition of Francis's contributions concerning the clinical, pathologic, and epidemiologic aspects of tularemia, the organism was renamed *Francisella tularensis. F. tularensis* is a small, strictly aerobic, gram-negative, nonmotile coccobacillus.

Transmission. More than 100 species of wild animals and 9 species of domestic animals are naturally infected with *F. tularensis* and may serve as a reservoir. *Dermacentor andersoni,* the common **wood tick,** is the most important vector for tularemia in the United States and feeds on snowshoe rabbits, horses, mountain goats, woodchucks, mountain rats, and ground squirrels. In the southern United States, *Amblyomma americanum,* the **Lone Star tick,** is the vector. *D. variabilis,* the **dog tick,** can also transmit the organism. Transovarian transmission allows the persistence of the organism in nature. Biting deerflies are common vectors in Utah, Nevada, and California. Bites by infected cats and squirrels have also resulted in infection.

EPIDEMIOLOGY

Infections occur after a tick or deerfly bite or when a person comes in contact with infected tissues or body fluids. Cases of tularemia are more common between May and September because of increased tick activity during this period. Rabbit hunting is a significant risk factor. Approximately 150–200 cases of tularemia are reported annually in the United States (Fig. 3–3), one half of which are reported from Arkansas, Oklahoma, Tennessee, Texas, and Missouri. High activity is also noted in Utah, Colorado, California, and Kansas. Nearly 21% of cases of tularemia occur in children younger than 14 years of age, and 36% of cases occur in persons younger than 24 years of age.

PATHOGENESIS

After entry through the skin or mucous membranes, the organism disseminates to many body tissues through the lymphatics and the blood. The organism may live intracellularly in the reticuloendothelial system for prolonged periods.

SYMPTOMS AND CLINICAL MANIFESTATIONS

The incubation period for tularemia is usually 3–10 days but may range up to 21 days. Various clinical syndromes of tularemia are observed in children (Table 34–4). **Ulceroglandular tularemia** is the most common form and accounts for 21–85% of cases. Regional lymphadenopathy proximal to the site of a tick or deerfly bite is typically present with a cutaneous ulcer, 0.3–0.4 cm in diameter, at the site of the inoculation. The ulcer may be present for several days, often persisting for ≥2 weeks after onset of symptoms. **Glandular tularemia,** which accounts for 3–20% of cases, has only regional lymphadenopathy. **Typhoidal tularemia,** which accounts for 5–30% of cases, presents as an acute febrile illness that may persist more than 2–3 weeks if untreated. Maculopapular to pustular exanthems, including pustules surrounding the site of the bite, are commonly observed. Patients with typhoidal tularemia may present with a sepsislike illness, with a mortality rate as high as 30–60%. **Pneumonic tularemia,** which accounts for 7–20% of cases, may be primary after inhalation of infected droplets or secondary to dissemination after untreated ulceroglandular or typhoidal disease. From 10–15% of cases of ulceroglandular tularemia disseminate and have pneumonic involvement, compared with 30–38% of the typhoidal form of disease with pneumonia. **Oropharyngeal tularemia,** which accounts for 0–12% of cases, occurs after the consumption of inadequately cooked meats. **Oculoglandular tularemia,** which accounts for 0–5% of cases, follows inoculation of the conjunctival sac. The eyelids become edematous, painful, and inflamed. Multiple, small, well-demarcated ulcers can be observed. The palpebral conjunctiva is most commonly involved.

TABLE 34–4. Symptoms of Tularemia

General Findings
Fever
Chills
Headache
Myalgia
Cough
Ulceroglandular Tularemia (21–85%)
Eschar or ulcer
Regional lymphadenopathy with a distal tick bite
Glandular Tularemia (3–20%)
Lymphadenopathy only
Typhoidal Tularemia (5–30%)
Abrupt onset of fever, chills, headaches, malaise, vomiting, photophobia
Hepatosplenomegaly
Pneumonia (7–20%)
Cough
Pulmonary infiltrates
Oropharyngeal Tularemia (0–12%)
Pseudomembranous pharyngitis
Cervical lymphadenopathy
Oculoglandular Tularemia (0–5%)
Unilateral painful, purulent conjunctivitis
Preauricular lymphadenopathy

DIAGNOSIS

The diagnosis of tularemia is usually suspected from the clinical manifestations combined with a history of possible exposure and is confirmed by culture or serologic testing.

Differential Diagnosis

Ulceroglandular tularemia may resemble bubonic plague, cat-scratch disease, rickettsialpox, sporotrichosis, and atypical mycobacterial lymphadenitis. Glandular tularemia may be confused with infectious mononucleosis. Pharyngeal tularemia is difficult to distinguish clinically from diphtheria. Typhoidal tularemia is the most difficult form to diagnose, and is commonly confused with typhoid fever, yersiniosis, and bacterial sepsis. In patients with meningitis, a primarily lymphocytic response is observed in the cerebrospinal fluid. Oculoglandular tularemia shares many clinical features with adenoviral pharyngoconjunctival fever and cat-scratch disease.

Microbiologic Evaluation

Ulcer scrapings, lymph node biopsies, sputum, and blood may be cultured. *F. tularensis* is a fastidious organism that usually requires a specialized medium for growth in the laboratory, generally either cystine glucose blood agar or modified charcoal-yeast extract. Modified Mueller-Hinton broth and chocolate agar supplemented with IsoVitale X will also support the growth of the organism. Methods such as the lysis-centrifugation or lysis-direct plating (Isolator) may be used, followed by inoculation on appropriate media. Atypical strains of *F. tularensis* that do not require enriched medium for growth have been isolated.

A PCR assay that appears to be as sensitive as blood culture for the diagnosis of tularemia has been developed. Material from ulcers can also be tested by PCR, with good sensitivity. However, this PCR test is still mainly a research tool and is not available in clinical laboratories.

Serologic Testing. The diagnosis of tularemia is most frequently confirmed by serologic testing. A fourfold increase in agglutinating antibody titers is diagnostic of tularemia, although a single titer of ≥1:160 suggests recent infection. These antibodies may cross-react with *Brucella* and other species of *Francisella.*

TREATMENT

Gentamicin and streptomycin, which are bacteriocidal for *F. tularensis,* are the antimicrobial agents of choice for tularemia (Table 34-5). Treatment is continued for 7–10 days, with at least 3 days of treatment after the patient becomes afebrile. Tetracycline and chloramphenicol are alternative agents but are bacteriostatic against *F. tularensis,* and clinical relapses occur in up to 50% of patients. Newer agents such as ceftriaxone, cefotaxime, and ceftazidime have in vitro activity against *F. tularensis,* although the in vitro MIC does not correlate with successful clinical outcome. Many treatment failures have been reported with ceftriaxone. Chloramphenicol, in combination with gentamicin, is recommended for the treatment of meningitis. However, gentamicin combined with doxycycline has been successfully used for meningitis. Quinolones have also been shown to be effective in the treatment of tularemia and can be used as an alternative treatment but are only approved for persons ≥18 years of age. Unfortunately, relapses with all regimens have been described.

TABLE 34–5. Recommended Antibiotic Therapy for Tularemia

Gentamicin 6 mg/kg/day divided q8hr IM or IV for 7–10 days
or
Streptomycin 30–40 mg/kg/day (max: 1 g/day) divided q12hr IM for 3 days, then reduced to 15 mg/kg/day for an additional 4 days
or
Ciprofloxacin* 15–20 mg/kg/day (max 1500 mg/day) divided q12hr PO for 7–10 days

*Ciprofloxacin and other quinolone antibiotics are contraindicated for pregnant and lactating women, children, and adolescents <18 years of age.

COMPLICATIONS

Complications secondary to tularemia are rare. Cases of pericarditis, meningitis, endocarditis, hepatitis, peritonitis, and osteomyelitis have been reported, primarily after typhoidal tularemia. In patients with no history of epidemiologic exposure the disease may go undiagnosed for extended periods of time, without receiving effective antibacterial therapy.

PROGNOSIS

Milder cases of tularemia in children may resolve spontaneously. Tularemia responds promptly to appropriate therapy, with defervescence and resolution of illness within several days and an overall mortality of <1%. The clinical response may appear delayed when nodes progress to suppuration.

PREVENTION

No effective natural control measures are available for tularemia. Important preventive measures are avoidance of endemic areas, use of protective clothing when outdoors (long sleeves, long pants, shoes instead of sandals), use of insect repellents, and careful removal of ticks if found (Table 3–8). Children should not play with or handle sick or dead rabbits, and wild rabbits should not become pets. Rubber gloves should be used for skinning rabbits or other potentially infected animals. Rabbit meat should be well cooked.

Many cases of laboratory-acquired disease have been described, and laboratory technicians should take precautions when attempting to isolate *F. tularensis.* If exposure occurs, such as splash injury or smelling of organisms on an agar plate, a 7-day course of doxycycline may be indicated, similar to postexposure prophylaxis for plague.

A live attenuated vaccine has been shown to reduce the incidence of typhoidal tularemia but did not significantly prevent ulceroglandular disease. This vaccine is recommended for those persons who anticipate frequent exposure to *F. tularensis* and may be available in the United States through the United States Armed Forces.

PLAGUE

Plague was responsible for some of the most devastating epidemics in history, including the death of nearly one third of Europe's population in the 14th century. The disease is endemic in the southwestern United States and in many parts of the world. Bubonic plague, a febrile painful lymphadenitis, is its most common clinical manifestation.

ETIOLOGY

Plague is caused by infection with the bacterium *Yersinia pestis,* a gram-negative, nonmotile, bipolar-staining pleomorphic coccobacillus that lives intracellularly.

Transmission. The natural reservoirs are rodents, such as rock squirrels, California ground squirrels, prairie dogs, and chipmunks. Fleas from infected animals may transmit the organism to humans, who serve as accidental hosts. Persons are commonly infected by flea bites or through skin lacerations or abrasions while skinning wild animals. Exposure to the carcasses of dead animals may also result in infection by means of contaminated aerosol droplets.

Domestic cats that are permitted to roam freely in endemic areas may feed on sick or dead plague-infected rodents or may be bitten by fleas and are at increased risk of infection and peridomestic transmission to humans. Increased peridomestic transmission is an important and probably underestimated source of infection in endemic states where suburbanization has increased the number of humans living near plague foci. Veterinarians are also at increased risk of exposure.

EPIDEMIOLOGY

Fewer than 500 cases of human plague have been reported in the past 50 years in the United States (Fig. 3–3). Approximately 90% of these cases were geographically confined to areas of New Mexico, Arizona, southern Colorado, and California. During this time, however, the number of states reporting disease has increased from 3 states during 1944–1953 to 13 states during 1984–1993, including several states previously considered to be free of this disease (Fig. 34–1). Plague was introduced into North America in San Francisco in 1900 and has migrated eastward in rodents and rodent-consuming carnivores to reach eastern Montana, western Nebraska, western North Dakota, and eastern Texas.

The majority of cases occur between May and September, with the highest number of cases occurring during July. Annual epizootic plague activity usually peaks during or immediately after years with cooler summer temperatures and rainfall above normal levels, resulting in increased populations of plague-susceptible rodent species. Most exposures occur at homesites.

PATHOGENESIS

Y. pestis enters the body through a bite or through the mucous membrane and migrates via the lymphatics to regional lymph nodes, where it is usually engulfed by phagocytic cells. The organism replicates in these cells, and further multiplication results in cell lysis and release of the bacilli, which disseminate to the lungs, eyes, meninges, joints, or skin. *Y. pestis* produces an endotoxin that may cause multisystem dysfunction and disseminated intravascular coagulation.

SYMPTOMS AND CLINICAL MANIFESTATIONS

Four clinical types of plague have been described: bubonic plague, septicemia, pneumonia, and meningitis. The most frequent presentation is **bubonic plague.** Initially there is a nonspecific febrile illness, and 2–7 days after exposure a **bubo,** a painful regional lymphadenitis with surrounding marked cellulitis, develops proximal to the flea bite or laceration. Buboes are most commonly observed in the groin and axillary area. **Septicemic plague** is most commonly observed as a progression of bubonic plague, especially when therapy is delayed. The septicemic type of plague mimics other sepsis syndromes. **Primary septicemic plague,** a rare entity that does not include regional lymphadenopathy, is fulminant and highly fatal if untreated. From 1980–1984, 18 cases of septicemic plague were described (Hull et al, 1987) in New Mexico, representing 25% of the total number of plague cases. Only 17% of the cases were in persons younger than 20 years of age; in contrast, 50% of the patients with bubonic plague were in this age group. Septicemic plague was more common in persons older than 40 years of age. Nausea, vomiting, diarrhea, and abdominal pain, probably secondary to mesenteric lymphadenitis, were more frequently reported in those patients with septicemic plague. Most of the recent cases of **pneumonic plague** have occurred as secondary pulmonary involvement in patients with septicemic plague. **Primary pneumonic plague,** which follows inhalation of infected droplets, occurs almost exclusively after contact with infected domestic cats and is usually a severe, fatal illness. Because of its potential for human-to-human transmission, pneumonic plague is a public health emergency. Meningitis has been reported in 5–50% of persons with bubonic or septicemic plague.

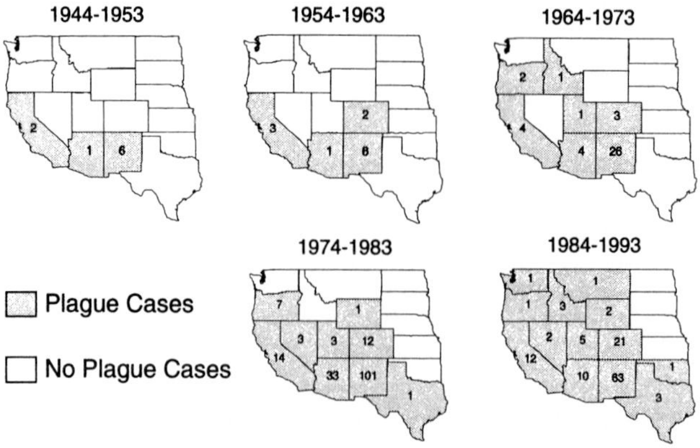

FIGURE 34–1. Number of human plague cases reported in the United States by state and decade, 1944–1993. (From Centers for Disease Control and Prevention: Human Plague—United States, 1993-1994. *MMWR Morb Mortal Wkly Rep* 1994;43:243.)

DIAGNOSIS

The diagnosis of plague is usually suspected from the clinical manifestations combined with a history of possible exposure and is confirmed by serologic testing. The diagnosis of plague meningitis can be confirmed by examination of the CSF, which usually reveals gram-negative coccobacillary organisms, pleocytosis with a predominance of polymorphonuclear cells, hypoglycorrhachia, and a high protein level.

Differential Diagnosis

Bubonic plague may resemble staphylococcal or streptococcal lymphadenitis, cat-scratch disease, and ulceroglandular tularemia. Septicemic plague may resemble other forms of sepsis. Pneumonic plague may have findings compatible with hantavirus cardiopulmonary syndrome, pneumococcal pneumonia, and pneumonic tularemia.

Microbiologic Evaluation

The diagnosis of plague is confirmed either by isolation of *Y. pestis* from blood, aspirates of the regional lymphadenopathy, or cutaneous lesions or by serologic testing. An indirect IFA assay can be used for examination of tissues. Visualization of gram-negative coccobacilli with **bipolar staining,** or a safety pin appearance, on Gram stain is characteristic. If plague is suspected, the clinical laboratory should be notified so that appropriate precautions can be taken in the handling of patient specimens.

Serologic Testing. Antibodies against *Y. pestis* can be detected with a hemagglutination inhibition assay. A fourfold rise in antibody titers to the F-1 antigen of *Y. pestis* confirms infection.

TREATMENT

If plague is suspected, empirical treatment should be initiated promptly before comfirmation of the diagnosis. Gentamicin and streptomycin are the drugs of choice (Table 34–6). Supportive care with intravenous fluids and vasopressive agents is extremely important for septicemic plague. Surgical drainage of buboes is usually not indicated, but if it is necessary, it should not be attempted until at least 24 hours after initiation of antimicrobial therapy because the drainage is highly contagious.

COMPLICATIONS

Septicemic plague most commonly occurs as a secondary entity in a patient with bubonic plague. Secondary pneumonia is a common complication. Plague meningitis is more likely with delayed diagnosis and hematogenous spread to the meninges. Complications during convalescence include polyarthritis, small lung abscesses, and delayed suppuration of buboes.

PROGNOSIS

Untreated plague has an estimated mortality exceeding 80%, but with appropriate antimicrobial therapy the majority of patients become afebrile within 3 days and recover. Most of the fatal cases of plague in the United States result from delays in seeking medical treatment and in establishing the correct diagnosis. Survival is more likely in persons who seek medical treatment early and are diagnosed and hospitalized early in the course, or who have an early onset of gastrointestinal symptoms. The mortality rate with septicemic plague is approximately 30% compared with approximately 10% with bubonic plague.

PREVENTION

Rodent surveillance and control is recommended for endemic areas (Table 3–7). Routine vaccination is not recommended for persons living in endemic areas, but the inactivated whole-cell vaccine should be given to those who are regularly exposed to potentially infected rodents and their fleas (Chapter 17). State public health authorities should be notified immediately of all suspected cases.

All patients with plague should be placed in strict respiratory isolation until pneumonia can be excluded or until they have received therapy for 48 hours. Patients with documented pneumonic plague should remain in respiratory isolation with droplet precautions until sputum cultures are negative. Persons exposed to pneumonic plague should receive antimicrobial prophylaxis with either doxycycline or TMP-SMZ for 7 days (Table 34–7). Patients with nonpneumonic plague require only standard precautions and not isolation. Bedding and the patient's residence should be disinfested of plague-infected animals.

TABLE 34–6. Recommended Antibiotic Therapy for Plague

Type of Infection	Recommended Regimen	Alternative Regimen
Plague without meningitis	Gentamicin* for 5–7 days *or* Streptomycin* for 5–7 days	Tetracycline for 10–14 days
Plague with meningitis	Chloramphenicol for 10 days	

*Serum concentrations of aminoglycosides should be monitored during therapy in persons with impaired renal function and in newborns.

Recommended Dosages for Patients with Normal Renal Function

ANTIBIOTIC	DOSAGE	MAXIMUM DAILY DOSE
Chloramphenicol	75–100 mg/kg/day divided q6hr IV or 75 mg/kg/day divided q6hr PO	4 g 3 g
Gentamicin	7.5 mg/kg/day divided q8hr IV or IM	Adults: 5 mg/kg
Streptomycin	30 mg/kg/day divided q12hr IM	1 g
Tetracycline	25–50 mg/kg/day divided q6hr IV	2–3 g

TABLE 34–7. Recommendations for Postexposure Prophylaxis for Persons Exposed* to *Yersinia pestis*

Children ≥2 mo
TMP-SMZ: TMP 8 mg/kg/day, SMZ 40 mg/kg/day divided q12hr PO for 7 days

Children ≥9 yr
TMP-SMZ: TMP 8 mg/kg/day SMZ 40 mg/kg/day divided q12hr PO for 7 days
or
Doxycycline 2–4 mg/kg/day divided q12hr PO for 7 days
or
Tetracycline 25–50 mg/kg/day divided q6hr PO for 7 days

Adults (≥18 yr)†
TMP-SMZ: TMP 320–640 mg, SMZ 1.6–3.2 g divided q12hr PO for 7 days
or
Doxycycline 100–200 mg divided q12hr PO for 7 days
or
Tetracycline 2 g/day divided q6hr PO for 7 days

*Exposure is defined as close exposure within 6.5 ft (2 m) to a person with pneumonic plague or exposure to *Y. pestis* in the laboratory.
†The use of tetracycline and doxycycline during pregnancy should be avoided.
Adapted from Centers for Disease Control and Prevention: Prevention of plague: Recommendations of the Advisory Committee on Immunization Practices [ACIP]. *MMWR Morb Mortal Wkly Rep* 1996;45(RR-14):1–15.

LEPTOSPIROSIS

Leptospirosis is a disease of wild and domestic animals. Humans are infected by contact with infected animals or their body fluids.

ETIOLOGY

Leptospirosis is caused by *Leptospira,* a motile, flexible, tightly coiled spirochete that is an obligate aerobe. Two species of this genetically diverse genus are recognized: *L. interrogans,* for the pathogenic leptospires, and *L. biflexa,* for the saprophytic members. More than 200 distinct serotypes of *L. interrogans* exist. Many serotypes share common agglutinogens and have been assembled into 23 serogroups; *icterohaemorrhagiae* and *canicola* are the most common in the United States. The serogroup *icterohaemorrhagiae* is thought to cause the most severe disease, although other strains are also known to cause serious disease in children. Leptospires survive in wet, mildly alkaline environments at temperatures of 82.4–89.60°F (28–32°C).

Transmission. Humans are dead-end hosts. Leptospires live for years in renal tubules of infected mammals, including rats, dogs, cattle, swine, raccoons, goats, and mice. Rats and dogs are the most important reservoir. Humans become infected by coming in contact with leptospiruric animals, contaminated soil, or bodies of infected water.

EPIDEMIOLOGY

Recent outbreaks have occurred among white-water rafters, triathletes, and swimmers. In many countries, outbreaks have followed heavy rains and flooding. High-risk occupations include the military, agricultural and aquacultural industries, meatpacking, animal husbandry, and veterinary medicine. Persons who work in rat-infested areas are also likely to become infected. For years, leptospirosis was believed to be a disease of rural areas, but in recent years urban and suburban predilection is becoming apparent. Urban rats have been found to be infected with *Leptospira,* and leptospirosis has been described in residents living in inner city neighborhoods in the United States. Approximately 50–200 cases were reported annually in the United States through 1994 (Fig. 3–3), but leptospirosis is no longer a reportable disease, so the precise incidence is unknown. In the United States, Hawaii has the highest number of cases.

PATHOGENESIS

Leptospires penetrate the skin or mucous membranes. They circulate in the blood and infect the endothelium of small blood vessels in target organs, such as renal tubules, liver, meninges, muscles, eyes, and placenta, resulting in localized ischemia. Endothelial damage may also lead to extravasation of fluids into surrounding tissues.

SYMPTOMS AND CLINICAL MANIFESTATIONS

After an incubation period of 1–2 weeks (range: 2–26 days), patients may experience a biphasic pattern illness consisting of an **initial leptospiremic phase** and a **secondary leptospiruric or immune phase** (Table 34–8). An asymptomatic period of 1–5 days may separate the two stages of the disease. The leptospiremic phase is characterized by profound myalgias, mainly of the lumbosacral areas, thighs, and calves, as well as conjunctival suffusion and prostration. During this first phase, which lasts 4–7 days, leptospires can be isolated from the blood and cerebrospinal fluid. A more severe illness consisting of an initial phase of fever accompanied by azotemia, jaundice, hemorrhage, anemia, mental status changes, and shock is the classic hepatorenal disease **Weil's disease,** which occurs in approximately 5–10% of cases. Signs of the onset of the leptospiruric phase are fever and headache in a presentation of aseptic meningitis that cannot be distinguished clinically from viral meningitis. Diarrhea has also been reported. The appearance of anti-leptospira agglutinating antibodies and the disappearance of the leptospires from the blood is characteristic of the immune phase, which may last 4–30 days or longer. During this stage leptospires can be isolated from the urine.

Atypical presentations of the disease have been described in children; these include acalculous cholecystitis (hydrops of the gallbladder), pancreatitis, uveitis, and abdominal causalgia, or a desquamating maculopapular skin rash with infarction of the distal extremities may be seen. An illness resembling adult respiratory distress syndrome and pulmonary hemorrhage have also been described with leptospirosis.

TABLE 34–8. Symptoms of the Biphasic Illness of Leptospirosis

Initial Leptospiremic Phase
Usually Asymptomatic
or
Abrupt Onset of Short Duration, Influenza-Like Illness
Fever
Headache
Chills
Profound myalgias
Arthralgias
Neck stiffness
Abdominal pain
Conjunctival suffusion
Nausea and vomiting
or
Icteric Leptospirosis or Weil's Disease (5–10% of cases)
Fever
Headache
Myalgias
Jaundice
Renal failure
Hypotension
Hemorrhage
Pulmonary hemorrhage
Secondary Leptospiruric Phase
Aseptic meningitis
Fever
Headache
Vomiting

DIAGNOSIS

The diagnosis of leptospirosis is usually suspected from the clinical manifestations combined with a history of possible exposure and is confirmed by serologic testing.

During the leptospiruric stage, patients may have mild proteinuria, pyuria, granular casts, and microscopic hematuria. Liver enzymes are usually normal. Thrombocytopenia is common, but platelet levels remain above 50,000/mm^3. CSF analysis demonstrates pleocytosis (cell count usually $<$500/mm^3) with normal or elevated protein levels but with normal glucose levels. There may be pulmonary findings on chest radiographs but minimal physical findings.

Differential Diagnosis

Anicteric leptospirosis may resemble influenza, malaria, dengue fever, Colorado tick fever, enteroviral meningitis, and infectious mononucleosis. If an exposure to rodents is evident, rat-bite fever may also be suspected. Weil's disease may resemble severe fulminant hepatitis, adenovirus infection, gram-negative sepsis, or hantavirus cardiopulmonary syndrome.

Microbiologic Evaluation

Leptospires can be isolated from blood and cerebrospinal fluid during the first week of illness; after this period, urine is the most likely source of positive cultures and dark-field examinations. Isolation can be achieved with the use of specialized media. Clinical specimens can also be injected intraperitoneally into laboratory animals, followed by examination under dark-field microscopy. A PCR assay appears to be an effective diagnostic tool in the early stages of the disease, including meningitis, but this is not available in clinical laboratories.

Serologic Testing. The diagnosis is usually confirmed by detection of a fourfold increase in specific antibodies. Several serologic tests are available. Although the microagglutination assay is highly sensitive and specific, it is technically difficult for general use because it requires live leptospires. The slide macroagglutination assay is a simple test but has an unacceptably high number of false-negative and false-positive results. More recently, an EIA with a sensitivity and specificity >90% has been used. A dipstick assay for detection of *Leptospira*-specific IgM antibodies has been found to be a simple and reliable method for serologic diagnosis, especially in field conditions away from laboratory facilities.

TREATMENT

Leptospirosis is self-limiting in >90% of untreated patients, although doxycycline given within 3 days of onset of illness is beneficial (Table 34–9). High-dose penicillin G is recommended for the treatment of CNS disease. Some patients may experience a **Jarisch-Herxheimer reaction** (fever, rigors, hypotension, and prostration during the first hours of antibiotic therapy). Supportive care is required for persons with dehydration, hypotension, hemorrhage, and renal failure. Some patients may require mechanical ventilation and hemodialysis.

COMPLICATIONS

Infections during pregnancy may lead to spontaneous abortions in the first trimester or may result in newborns with active disease. These complications are rare in the United States.

PROGNOSIS

Patients with mild disease almost always recover. Intensive supportive therapy may be necessary for those who are seriously ill. The mortality is high in Weil's syndrome, with renal failure the leading cause of death.

PREVENTION

The preferred preventive measure is the avoidance of potentially infected areas near streams and ponds. Swimming in these areas is considered risky. However, because vaccinated domestic animals and livestock may still excrete the organism in the urine, prevention of human infection may be difficult in many circumstances. Vaccination of animals, especially domestic dogs, prevents disease in the animals, but it does not stop renal infection and leptospiruria.

Doxycycline has also been shown to be effective as prophylaxis for persons working in highly endemic areas for short periods of time, such as military personnel on training exercises, or volunteers working in flooded areas. Long-term use of doxycycline for prophylactic purposes is not advised.

TABLE 34–9. Recommended Antibiotic Therapy for Leptospirosis

Mild Disease
Doxycycline 4 mg/kg/day (max 200 mg/day) divided q12hr PO for 7 days
Severely Ill Patients
High-dose penicillin G 300,000 U/kg/day (max 12–24 MU) divided q4hr IV for 7 days

RELAPSING FEVER

Relapsing fever, a common zoonotic disease in the western United States, involves mainly tickborne transmission.

ETIOLOGY

The spirochete *Borrelia hermsii* is the major cause of **tickborne relapsing fever** in the western United States, whereas *Borrelia dugesii* is the major cause of the disease in Mexico and Central America. Another species, *Borrelia recurrentis,* is transmitted by the louse *Pediculus humanus* and causes **louseborne relapsing fever.** This epidemic form is commonly associated with war, famine, floods, poor hygiene, overcrowding, and malnutrition and is not seen in the United States.

Transmission. *Borrelia* is transmitted by the soft-shell ticks of the genus *Ornithodoros,* which are parasites of rodents that live in dead trees, logs, woodpiles, burrows, and nests. They feed at night through a painless bite. The several species of *Ornithodoros* implicated in the transmission of the spirochete vary according to geographic areas: *O. turicata* in New Mexico, Texas, and Oklahoma; *O. parkeri* in Utah, Nevada, and Wyoming; and *O. hermsii* in Colorado, California, and British Columbia.

EPIDEMIOLOGY

The most recent outbreak of relapsing fever of clinical significance in the United States occurred in 1990 in Grand Canyon National Park. Rodent nests were found in the ceilings and below the floors of the cabins in which confirmed cases of relapsing fever were contracted. *O. hermsii* was found in these rodent nests. Sleeping in these infested cabins or sleeping near woodpiles correlated with infection. Similar outbreaks in 1973 and 1995 resulted in the infection of residents of multiple states and one foreign country. These outbreaks indicate the importance of obtaining a detailed epidemiologic history from persons with febrile illnesses, including a history of recent travel to endemic areas.

An increase in the number of cases of human disease is observed when rodent populations decrease because of rodent control programs or disease or because of the intrusion of humans into nesting areas of the ticks as a result of an increase in outdoor recreational activities. Cases of relapsing fever have been reported from throughout the United States and the U.S. Virgin Islands.

PATHOGENESIS

Borrelia organisms are introduced into the bloodstream via the bite of a tick or a louse. The spirochetes live in target organs, with spirochetemia during febrile episodes.

SYMPTOMS AND CLINICAL MANIFESTATIONS

The clinical manifestations of tickborne and louseborne relapsing fever are similar. The incubation period for relapsing fever is approximately 4–18 days (median: 6 days). A 2–3 mm pruritic eschar at the site of the tick or louse bite may be present. The initial phase of illness, which may last 3 days, is followed by an afebrile period of defervescence that may last approximately 3 days before relapsing into another febrile episode (Table 34–10). The afebrile stage may be variable in its occurrence and duration. Pa-

TABLE 34–10. Symptoms of Relapsing Fever

Abrupt Onset of the Following
Fever
Extreme fatigue
Chills and sweats
Headache
Myalgia
Arthralgia
Exanthem

tients may have one to six relapses of fever, with a mean of three episodes. Exanthems, which may be petechial, macular, maculopapular, or erythema multiforme–like, occur in nearly one third of patients. The duration of illness varies from 1–54 days, with a median of 18 days.

Neonatal Infection. Several cases of neonatal relapsing fever have been reported, implicating transplacental transmission of the organism. The mothers had nonspecific febrile illnesses, and the infants had severe disease with hepatosplenomegaly, coagulopathy, bleeding, hepatic dysfunction, profound jaundice, and evidence of CNS involvement with polymorphonuclear pleocytosis and elevated protein. The diagnosis was confirmed by observing the spirochetes in blood smears and occasionally in the CSF.

DIAGNOSIS

The diagnosis of relapsing fever is usually suspected from the clinical manifestations combined with history of possible exposure and is confirmed by examination of thick blood smears, which permits direct visualization of the spirochete. Acridine orange staining of blood smears (quantitative buffy coat method) may enhance sensitivity to 70%. Sensitivity may be increased to approximately 85% if combined with animal inoculation, although this is not available in most clinical laboratories.

Differential Diagnosis

Relapsing fever may resemble malaria, typhoid fever, leptospirosis, dengue fever, rat-bite fever, Colorado tick fever, rickettsialpox, and murine typhus.

TREATMENT

Tetracycline, erythromycin, chloramphenicol, and penicillin are effective in the treatment of relapsing fever (Table 34–11). A relapse rate of 20% has been reported with this disease, even with antimicrobial therapy. Corticosteroids should be used to avoid a **Jarisch-Herxheimer reaction** (fever, rigors, hypotension, and prostration during the first hours of antimicrobial therapy). An increased risk is associated with higher doses of the antimicrobial agents; the first dose should be lower than subsequent doses.

COMPLICATIONS

CNS involvement, usually consisting of a clinical appearance resembling aseptic meningitis, may occur in 8% of cases. CSF analysis demonstrates a lymphocytic pleocytosis with elevated protein. Iritis and iridocyclitis are found in 15% of patients. Bleeding may occur as petechial lesions, epistaxis, hemoptysis, or hematuria. Eye involvement may result in blindness. Myocarditis with arrhythmias, cerebral hemorrhages, and hepatic failure is usually associated with death.

TABLE 34–11. Recommended Antibiotic Therapy for Relapsing Fever

Type of Infection	Recommended Regimen
Afebrile	Erythromycin for 5 days
Febrile	Penicillin G *or* penicillin V, as a single dose followed by a 10-day course of doxycycline or erythromycin *with or without* Corticosteroids to avoid Jarisch-Herxheimer reaction

Recommended Dosages for Patients with Normal Renal Function

ANTIBIOTIC	DOSAGE	MAXIMUM DAILY DOSE
Doxycycline	4 mg/kg/day divided twice daily PO	200 mg
Erythromycin	40 mg/kg/day divided q6hr PO	2 g
Penicillin G	10,000 U/kg as a single dose IV	10,000 U/kg
Penicillin V	7.5 mg/kg as a single dose PO	7.5 mg/kg

PROGNOSIS

The prognosis depends on the extent of involvement. Fortunately, many milder cases may resolve spontaneously without therapy. Patients with multisystem involvement with failure are more likely to die. Physicians not familiar with the disease may not consider the diagnosis and may delay effective therapy.

PREVENTION

Avoidance of arthropod vectors and use of protective clothing are the best methods of prevention (Table 3–8). Rodent dwellings should be eradicated whenever possible. The use of insecticides may also reduce the likelihood of infection.

MURINE TYPHUS

Murine typhus, or **fleaborne typhus,** is found in all parts of the world. The primary natural reservoir is the rat. Active eradication programs and improvement in living standards have resulted in a decrease in the number of cases.

Louseborne typhus, or **epidemic typhus,** is caused by *Rickettsia prowazekii* and transmitted from person to person by the body louse *(Pediculus humanus corporis)*. It is a serious and sometimes fatal illness that is closely associated with devastation, war, and famine. It is found in areas of South America and Africa but is not endemic on the North American continent. **Brill-Zinsser disease** is the recrudescent form of epidemic typhus that occurs years after primary infection with *R. prowazekii* and is generally milder. This disease has been reported in the United States in immigrants from Eastern Europe.

ETIOLOGY

Rickettsia typhi, formerly known as *R. mooseri,* is a gram-negative intracellular bacillus that is the cause of murine typhus. It is endemic in the southern United States in the area around the Rio Grande Valley of south Texas, in the states bordering Mexico, and in the

Gulf Coast regions. *Rickettsia felis,* formerly known as ELB agent, is a newly recognized cause of fleaborne typhus.

Transmission. *R. typhi* is transmitted to humans by the rat flea, usually *Xenopsylla cheopis.* The important vector in Texas is the cat flea, *Ctenocephalides felis,* which infests cats, opossums, raccoons, and skunks. Cat flea vectors also appear to be responsible for the transmission of *R. felis.*

EPIDEMIOLOGY

In the mid-1940s, close to 5,000 cases were reported annually. With improved sanitation and reduction of the rat population, which is a reservoir, the number of cases has decreased considerably to only 25–50 cases annually through 1993 (Fig. 3–3). Murine typhus is no longer a reportable disease, so the precise incidence is unknown.

The majority of cases in the United States occur between April and August, with 80% of the cases occurring in south Texas. Approximately 40% of patients remember a flea exposure or bite. Other patients may recall exposure to infested animals. The median age of infected patients is approximately 50 years, with few cases reported in children.

Murine typhus is also endemic in many developing regions of Africa, Asia, Europe, Australia, and South America.

PATHOGENESIS

Like other rickettsial organisms, *R. typhi* invades the endothelium of blood vessels, causing a vasculitis, and may cause a multisystem disease mediated by the effect of cytokines.

SYMPTOMS AND CLINICAL MANIFESTATIONS

The presentation of murine typhus is similar to that of other rickettsial diseases (Table 34–12). From 48–79% of patients exhibit an exanthem, usually macular, papular, or maculopapular in appearance, including 6% with a petechial rash. The exanthem involves the trunk in the majority of patients and may affect the legs and arms. The rash appears on approximately the sixth day of illness.

Some patients may have abnormal chest radiographs with evidence of pulmonary edema, pleural effusions, and pneumonitis. From 5–45% of patients may have neurologic manifestations including coma, delirium, and stupor. These resolve rapidly as the fever decreases. The cerebrospinal fluid is usually normal, but a mild mononuclear pleocytosis with elevated protein and low glucose levels may be found.

DIAGNOSIS

The diagnosis of murine typhus is usually suspected from the clinical manifestations combined with a history of possible exposure and is confirmed by detection of *R. typhi*–specific antibodies. An indirect IFA or an EIA is the preferred method for serologic diagnosis. A fourfold increase in antibody titers or a single titer of ≥1:128 is diagnostic. Low antibody titers against *R. rickettsii* may indicate *R. typhi* infection. Immunohistochemical staining of skin lesions with the use of monoclonal antibodies may also be useful. A PCR assay is under development but is not available in clinical laboratories.

Many patients may present early in the course of the disease with leukopenia; evidence of a rebound leukocytosis appears later. Rarely, patients have a WBC count <3000/mm^3. Nearly 50% of patients have thrombocytopenia, and 73% have anemia. Approximately 90% of patients have abnormal liver enzymes. Hyponatremia and hypoalbuminemia are also common; these are believed to be a consequence of the increased capillary permeability secondary to the endothelial damage of blood vessels.

Differential Diagnosis

Murine typhus may resemble human ehrlichiosis, RMSF, meningococcemia, typhoidal tularemia, and dengue fever.

TREATMENT

Treatment with tetracycline results in a rapid resolution of symptoms only if given early in the course of the disease (Table 34–13). Treatment may prevent neurologic sequelae in those patients with CNS involvement.

COMPLICATIONS

Complications with murine typhus are infrequent. Coma, hallucinations, seizures, ataxia, renal insufficiency, and respiratory failure have been described most often. Retinal white dots have been reported as a complication of murine typhus. Disease severity is associated with older age, delayed diagnosis, thrombocytopenia, bleeding and coagulopathy, cardiac arrhythmias, hepatic and renal dysfunction, pulmonary compromise, CNS abnormalities, and previous therapy with sulfa agents.

PROGNOSIS

The disease tends to be mild in children. The prognosis of infected patients depends on the systems involved and pre-existing health. Complete recovery can usually be predicted in children treated with effective antimicrobial therapy. A case fatality rate of approximately 4% has been reported, which is similar to that of other rickettsial infections, especially RMSF.

PREVENTION

Combined efforts at rodent and opossum control and flea eradication are necessary to decrease the number of infections (Table 3–7).

TABLE 34–12. Symptoms of Murine Typhus

Fever
Headache
Chills
Myalgias
Nausea, vomiting, abdominal pain
Diarrhea
Exanthem

TABLE 34–13. Recommended Antibiotic Therapy for Murine Typhus

Doxycycline 2 mg/kg/day (max: 200 mg) as a single dose PO
or
Doxycycline 4–5 mg/kg/day (max: 200 mg/day) divided in 2 doses PO until afebrile for 2–3 days (usual duration: 5 days)

Q FEVER

Q fever, for **query fever,** is a rickettsial disease of worldwide distribution and differs from other such diseases in that it does not require an arthropod vector for transmission to humans.

ETIOLOGY

Coxiella burnetii, the causative agent of Q fever, is highly contagious. Inoculation with only one organism can cause infection. *C. burnetii* is highly resistant to various chemical and physical agents, which makes it extremely difficult to eradicate once it is established in a given area. It survives for long periods of time in the environment: in dust derived from animal milk, urine, feces, amniotic fluid, or placental membranes.

Transmission. Cattle, sheep, and goats are the primary animal reservoirs. Humans become infected by inhalation of contaminated dust or consumption of unpasteurized milk. The skinning of wild rabbits during the winter months is also associated with infection. Some anecdotal descriptions of infection in infants resulting from transplacental transmission and breast-feeding have been reported. More recently, parturient cats and dogs have been implicated as a source of Q fever in the northeastern United States and Nova Scotia. Amniotic fluid, placentas, mammary glands, and fetal membranes of infected animals have high concentrations of *C. burnetii,* which may become aerosolized during parturition. Infections in animals are usually subclinical. Apparently, ticks are responsible for the animal-to-animal transmission of the organism. The disease is not transmitted between humans.

EPIDEMIOLOGY

A high number of laboratory-related infections are reported from research laboratories that use sheep and goats and other potentially infected animals. The high infection rate results not only from handling of the animals but also from mere visiting of the facilities or passing through research areas.

PATHOGENESIS

Infection follows inhalation of contaminated dust or aerosols or ingestion of unpasteurized dairy products. *C. burnetii* is a strict intracellular pathogen that lives in the phagolysosomes of host cells.

SYMPTOMS AND CLINICAL MANIFESTATIONS

The incubation period for Q fever is 14–39 days (mean: 20 days). Commonly, Q fever is a chronic but self-limited illness (Table 34–14), eventually resulting in a complete recovery in several weeks in the majority of patients. The disease in children commonly presents as fever of unknown origin, pneumonia, and meningoencephalitis. In approximately 20% of children it may present as recurring episodes of fever that last 2–11 months. Fever is the only manifestation in approximately one third of patients. In contrast to other rickettsioses, there is no exanthem. Although commonly not observed, some patients may have an associated exanthem. Elevation of liver enzymes and jaundice is rare. Although pulmonary findings are scant on physical examination, many patients have radiographic evidence of pneumonia. Multiple, round, segmental opacities with atelectasis can be seen. In some regions of North America, Q fever is a common cause of **atypical pneumonia.**

TABLE 34–14. Symptoms of Q Fever

High fever, usually 40–40.6°C (104–105°F), or fever of unknown origin
Chills and sweats
Severe headaches
Fatigue
Retrobulbar pain
Myalgias
Hepatitis
Pneumonia
Meningoencephalitis

DIAGNOSIS

The diagnosis of Q fever is usually suspected from the clinical manifestations combined with a history of possible exposure and is confirmed by serologic testing.

Differential Diagnosis

Q fever pneumonia may resemble adenoviral pneumonia, influenza, hantavirus cardiopulmonary syndrome, or atypical pneumonia caused by *Mycoplasma pneumoniae, Chlamydia pneumoniae,* or *Legionella.* Q fever endocarditis should be considered as a cause of culture-negative endocarditis.

Microbiologic Evaluation

Routine microbiologic isolation in the laboratory should not be attempted because of the contagiousness of this organism. A minimum of Biosafety Level 3, which is not usually available in most clinical laboratories, is required.

Serologic Studies. Serologic diagnosis is the most appropriate diagnostic method. Two different assays can be used: CF and indirect IFA, which is preferred because of its higher sensitivity. Specific antibodies against *C. burnetii* generally peak between 4–8 weeks of illness. With CF, antibody levels are highest at 12 weeks. In 98% of infected patients, antibodies can be detected up to 1 year after infection. Nearly 90% of patients have a specific IgM detectable by the second week of the illness.

There is **antigenic phase variation** (phase I and II) demonstrated in the antibody response to *C. burnetii.* Not only are antibodies to these specific antigens useful for diagnosis, but they also help determine the stage of the disease and the prognosis after therapy. Antibodies against phase II antigens are observed during the acute, self-limited infection, whereas high levels of anti-phase-I antibodies suggest chronic Q fever. A phase II:phase I ratio (II:I ratio) >1 indicates primary Q fever; a ratio ≤ 1 is characteristic of Q fever endocarditis. A nested PCR of serum has been found to be highly sensitive in the diagnosis of acute Q fever pneumonia but is not available in clinical laboratories.

TREATMENT

The majority of acute infections caused by *C. burnetii* resolve spontaneously and require no antimicrobial therapy. Treatment is appropriate, however, because of the uncertainty of chronicity. Antibiotics that are clinically effective against *C. burnetii* include rifampin, TMP-SMZ, quinolones, and doxycycline. For the treatment of Q fever endocarditis a strict regimen of doxycycline and a quinolone for a minimum of 3 years is necessary.

COMPLICATIONS

Patients with underlying valvular cardiac disease, either congenital or prosthetic, are at risk of endocarditis, which may be difficult to eradicate. This disease entity evolves slowly in a subacute manner. It should be suspected in patients who have endocarditis, a suggestive epidemiologic medical history, and negative blood cultures and who fail to respond to antimicrobial therapy. Valve replacement is usually not indicated. Other complications consist of glomerulonephritis, pericarditis, myocarditis, hemophagocytosis, and infection during pregnancy.

PROGNOSIS

The majority of Q fever infections are self-limited. Pneumonia is rarely fatal, and when it occurs the patient usually has a pre-existing condition. Involvement of the heart may be difficult to eradicate and may result in worsening of the pre-existing heart disease. Vertebral osteomyelitis has also been reported.

PREVENTION

Prevention is an important aspect of the management of Q fever and should be targeted toward the workplace. Surveillance of researchers and animals through antibody titers should be implemented. Sheep should be confined to sheep facilities. Immunocompromised patients, pregnant women, or patients with valvular heart disease should not work in areas of high endemicity or with sheep. Persons at risk may also be vaccinated. Protection does not correlate with antibody titers; skin testing is a better predictor. A Q fever vaccine is available for high-risk persons in some countries, but in the United States it is used almost exclusively by the military.

RICKETTSIALPOX

Rickettsialpox, or **vesicular rickettsiosis,** was first recognized as a human disease in 1946 in the eastern United States. This condition has since been recognized as a cause of disease in the former Soviet Union, Korea, Africa, and Europe.

ETIOLOGY

Rickettsialpox is caused by *Rickettsia akari,* a small coccobacillus that is an intracellular organism. It is antigenically related to *R. rickettsii.* The rickettsial organism is transmitted by the mite of the common house mouse, *Mus musculus.* In Korea the vole appears to be the reservoir.

EPIDEMIOLOGY

Infections occur in large urban areas, mainly in large apartment dwellings infested with mice. Cases are now infrequently reported in the United States. A recent study (Comer et al, 1999) suggests that intravenous drug users in urban areas may be at increased risk of rickettsialpox. Exposures probably occur in mice-infested shooting galleries.

PATHOGENESIS

Following transmission via a mite bite, the rickettsial organisms disseminate to various target organs, such as the skin, lungs, and liver. As in other rickettsioses, *R. akari* replicates within endothelial cells of small blood vessels and results in vascular thrombosis and necrosis.

TABLE 34–15. Symptoms of Rickettsialpox

Symptoms
Fever
Malaise
Chills and sweats
Headaches
Myalgias
Decreased appetite
Dark escharlike lesion at site of inoculation
Papulovesicular exanthem

SYMPTOMS AND CLINICAL MANIFESTATIONS

The incubation period is usually 9–14 days (range: 9–21 days). The disease is a mild, nonfatal infection characterized by a painless, primary lesion at the site of the mite bite that begins as a firm red papule and vesiculates to an escharlike skin lesion covered with a black scab. There is regional lymphadenopathy. Fever and a generalized erythematous maculopapular exanthem develop and become papulovesicular in appearance within days. At this stage the illness may be confused with chickenpox. Symptoms of the disease usually last for about 1 week (Table 34–15).

DIAGNOSIS

The diagnosis of rickettsialpox is usually suspected from the clinical manifestations combined with a history of possible exposure and is confirmed by serologic testing. Because of the antigenic cross-reactivity, testing for antibodies to *R. rickettsii* using the indirect IF or CF assays can be used to confirm the diagnosis of rickettsialpox. *R. akari* can also be isolated from clotted human blood but only in specialized diagnostic and research facilities.

Differential Diagnosis

Rickettsialpox may resemble rat-bite fever, ulceroglandular tularemia, murine typhus, relapsing fever, and cat-scratch disease.

TREATMENT

Although most patients require no therapy, the use of doxycycline or chloramphenicol may shorten the duration of the disease (Table 34–16). Although tetracycline drugs generally are not recommended for children <9 years of age because of the risk of dental staining, a comparison of benefits versus the risk associated with the use of chloramphenicol may favor the use of doxycycline.

COMPLICATIONS AND PROGNOSIS

The illness is self-limited and usually mild, without complications. No fatal cases have been reported.

TABLE 34–16. Recommended Antibiotic Therapy for Rickettsialpox

Therapy
Doxycycline 4–5 mg/kg/day (max 200 mg/day) divided in 2 doses PO until afebrile for 2–3 days (usual duration: 5 days)
or
Chloramphenicol 50–75 mg/kg/day (max 4 g/day) divided q6hr IV or PO until afebrile for 2–3 days (usual duration: 5 days)

PREVENTION

Rodent control in large apartment dwellings is the most effective prevention measure (Table 3–7).

DENGUE FEVER

Dengue fever was first described in the Americas in 1780 as a large epidemic in Philadelphia. Epidemics, which have now become more frequent, occur almost every year. Severe forms of the disease are **dengue hemorrhagic fever (DHF)** and **dengue shock syndrome (DSS).**

ETIOLOGY

Dengue fever is caused by dengue virus, a flavivirus transmitted by the mosquito *Aedes aegypti.* Four serotypes, classified as DEN-1, DEN-2, DEN-3, and DEN-4, cause human disease. Multiple serotypes may circulate and cause disease in an endemic region at the same time. The dengue flaviviruses are known to be endemic in the Caribbean basin, which places parts of the United States at risk.

Transmission. This vector is prevalent in Southeast Asia, the Caribbean basin, Central and South America, and eastern and western tropical Africa. *A. aegypti* mosquitoes are present throughout the year in the southeastern and south central regions of the United States. *A. albopictus,* the vector of Asian dengue fever, is now also endemic in the eastern United States. The female mosquito, infected with the dengue virus for life, prefers to feed indoors and has a peak biting activity from 2–3 hours after daybreak to 3–4 hours before nightfall. The mosquitoes live and multiply in artificial water reservoirs, such as old tires, planters, gutters, animal-watering pans, buckets, and bromeliads around human habitats.

EPIDEMIOLOGY

The increase in international air travel has resulted in an influx of imported dengue fever cases into the United States. Approximately 150 suspected cases of imported dengue fever are reported annually. In 1995, 29 cases of indigenous transmission of dengue fever were confirmed in south Texas. In 1994, 23,693 cases of dengue fever–like illnesses were reported in the Commonwealth of Puerto Rico. In 1981, Cuba experienced an epidemic of DEN-2 with 116,243 hospitalized cases, and approximately 24,000 cases of DHF, with 158 deaths.

Some experts believe that the Americas are experiencing pandemics similar to those experienced by Southeast Asia 30 years ago. This increase in dengue fever activity is also associated with an increase in complications such as DHF and DSS. The increase in dengue fever cases in the Americas is most likely related to the failure to control *A. aegypti* populations, rapid dissemination of virus strains due to air travel, population growth with uncontrolled urbanization, and the ecologic factors that allow coexistence of multiple serotypes of dengue flaviviruses.

PATHOGENESIS

The vasculitis produced by the flaviviruses causes increased vascular permeability, resulting in the edema of surrounding tissues. These effects are commonly mediated by the deposition of immune complexes and other immunologic mediators. The more severe variants of dengue fever, DHS and DSS, are postulated to be related to immune enhancement resulting from previous infection with dengue virus. It is believed that this antibody-dependent enhancement increases replication of the virus in monocytes, resulting in the release of cytokines. Other experts have suggested that more virulent strains of the virus have been genetically selected in the environment.

SYMPTOMS AND CLINICAL MANIFESTATIONS

The incubation period of dengue fever is 3–15 days (mean: 5–8 days). The clinical manifestations of the disease (Table 34–17) are variable and range from an asymptomatic, subclinical infection in the majority of cases to a classic disease known as **breakbone fever** or **saddleback fever** pattern. The initial fever lasts approximately 3–7 days. A flushed face or a generalized transient, macular exanthem may be observed in the first 24–48 hours of the disease. An afebrile state abruptly follows, and intense sweating is noted. A secondary rise of fever may occur, and on the last day of fever a secondary morbilliform or maculopapular exanthem that lasts 1–5 days may occur. Itching of the palms and soles is classically associated with the exanthem. As the exanthem fades, petechiae may appear on the dorsum of feet, legs, hands, fingers, and oral cavity. Other common symptoms include severe headache, arthralgia, myalgia, nausea, and vomiting. Young children may have a cough, sore throat, and rhinitis. In some patients, CNS involvement, such as encephalitis, may develop.

DIAGNOSIS

The diagnosis of dengue fever is usually suspected from the clinical manifestations combined with history of possible exposure and is confirmed by either isolation of the virus or detection of virus-specific neutralizing antibodies. Leukopenia, granulocytopenia, thrombocytopenia, and hemoconcentration are also observed in patients with dengue fever and, if present, may suggest the diagnosis.

Differential Diagnosis

Persons with dengue fever may be confused with persons with influenza, malaria, murine typhus, relapsing fever, babesiosis, Colorado tick fever, and leptospirosis. The appearance of a petechial exanthem may suggest meningococcemia and RMSF.

Microbiologic Evaluation

Viral isolation usually requires the intrathoracic inoculation of the virus into mosquitoes. Although this method has a higher sensitivity than mosquito cell tissue cultures, it is performed only in specialized laboratories. If viral isolation is desired, serum or cerebrospinal fluid should be collected in the first week of illness, placed on dry

TABLE 34–17. Symptoms of Dengue Fever

Abrupt onset of high fever (usually 39.4–41.1°C [103–106°F])
Chills
Malaise
Frontal or retro-orbital headaches
Anorexia, nausea, and vomiting
Myalgias and arthralgias, lumbosacral pain
Generalized lymphadenopathy
Cutaneous hyperalgesia
Exanthem

ice, and transported to a specialized laboratory within 24 hours of collection. Serologic tests that use hemagglutination inhibition or EIA are available. A fourfold increase in antibody titers is diagnostic. Unfortunately, these antibodies may cross-react with various flaviviruses, including all serotypes of dengue virus. The detection of antibodies indicates only that the person was infected with a flavivirus in the last several weeks. A PCR assay has been found to be quite sensitive and specific in the diagnosis of dengue fever, and many laboratories in endemic regions have access to this technology. Immunohistochemical staining of infected tissues may also be useful. If necessary, specimens can be sent to the CDC Dengue Branch in Puerto Rico for assistance in confirming the diagnosis.

TREATMENT

No specific treatment is currently available for dengue fever. Proper fluid intake, bed rest, and antipyretic therapy are generally indicated and helpful. Acetaminophen is recommended for management of fever, thus avoiding the anticoagulant properties of aspirin. Aggressive supportive care may be necessary to correct the coagulopathy and shock observed with severe disease.

COMPLICATIONS

Most dengue infections result in relatively mild illness but may progress to DHF with bleeding diatheses and hemorrhagic complications, such as epistaxis, gingival bleeding, bleeding at venipuncture sites, large spontaneous ecchymoses, menorrhagia, and hematuria. Severe cases may manifest disseminated bleeding and gastrointestinal hemorrhage. DHF is usually observed in children younger than 15 years of age. Signs of circulatory failure or hemorrhagic manifestations usually appear 24 hours before or after patient defervescence. The criteria of the World Health Organization for DHF are fever, minor or major hemorrhagic manifestations, thrombocytopenia (platelets $\leq$100,000/mm^3), and objective evidence of **capillary leak syndrome** and increased capillary permeability, such as hemoconcentration (hematocrit increased by $\geq$20%), pleural effusion (by chest radiograph or other diagnostic imaging method), or hypoalbuminemia. A case of DSS must meet these criteria plus hypotension or narrow pulse pressure ($\leq$20 mm Hg). Approximately 20–30% of cases of DHF progress to DSS, which appears 2–5 days after the onset of a simple episode of dengue fever. Rapid clinical deterioration with cardiovascular collapse may ensue. It is believed that patients with dengue fever have a higher risk of DHF and DSS if they have been infected previously because of immune enhancement. Well-documented cases of DHF and DSS have occurred in patients with first time dengue infections, however. Most cases of DHF and DSS are reported in Southeast Asia. However, many cases have been reported in Central America and the Caribbean.

Although rare, vertical transmission of dengue fever has been reported.

PROGNOSIS

Convalescence from uncomplicated dengue fever is commonly characterized by profound bradycardia, marked asthenia, and psychomotor depression. However, complete recovery without sequelae eventually occurs. The mortality is 1–2% with DHF and 13–44% with DSS. Early diagnosis and aggressive fluid replacement therapy with good nursing care can reduce fatality rates to 1% or less. Administration of corticosteroids does not reduce the mortality in DSS.

Immunity is type-specific, and therefore it is possible to contract dengue fever four times. Previous infection may predispose to more serious illness upon subsequent infection with another serotype.

PREVENTION

The wearing of long pants, long sleeves, and shoes rather than sandals and the use of insecticides minimize the likelihood of infection in persons visiting endemic areas (Chapter 3). The implementation of vector control measures should reduce the vector population. Vector control should be continued even in years of low dengue activity.

Live attenuated dengue virus vaccines, which are currently serotype-specific, have been studied in humans with variable results. They are associated with mild adverse effects, such as fever and exanthems. Further studies are required to demonstrate safety and efficacy.

COLORADO TICK FEVER

Colorado tick fever (CTF) is the only human orbiviral disease in the United States. Early cases were confused with RMSF.

ETIOLOGY

CTF is an acute viral disease caused by an orbivirus of the genus *Coltivirus* in the Reoviridae family. This virus is maintained in nature by transmission among small mammals, principally rodents. It is transmitted by *Dermacentor andersoni,* the **wood tick.**

EPIDEMIOLOGY

Infections by this virus are frequently encountered in the western United States between April and August, with a peak during May and June. Approximately 115 cases were reported in Utah during 1960–1969, and 228 cases were reported in Colorado during 1973–1974. Since the disease is no longer a reportable disease, the current incidence is unknown. However, anecdotally, many cases are seen every summer in endemic areas.

SYMPTOMS AND CLINICAL MANIFESTATIONS

The incubation period is approximately 0–14 days (mean: 4–6 days). The classic presentation of this disease is a biphasic temperature pattern. The patient is initially febrile for 2–3 days, is afebrile for an equal period of time, and then is again febrile for another 2–3 days. This **saddleback fever** pattern resembles the same disease pattern observed with dengue fever. The patient then experiences the classic triad of fever, myalgias, and headaches, as well as other constitutional symptoms (Table 34–18). Approximately 5–12% of patients have an exanthem that may be either macular, maculopapular, or petechial. CNS involvement, usually a meningoencephalitis, has been documented, especially in children.

Approximately 90% of infected persons recall a tick exposure, and 52% are aware of a tick bite. This disease may be initially confused with RMSF, especially if the patient has an exanthem.

DIAGNOSIS

The diagnosis of CTF is usually suspected from the clinical manifestations of a biphasic febrile illness combined with a history of

TABLE 34–18. Symptoms of Colorado Tick Fever

Symptoms
Fever
Lethargy
Myalgias
Headaches
Abdominal pain and vomiting
Photophobia
Exanthem
Nuchal rigidity
Sore throat
Meningoencephalitis

possible exposure, such as recreational travel to an endemic area, and is confirmed by virus culture or serologic testing. During the second febrile episode, patients classically have leukopenia, WBC count usually between 2,000 and 3,000/mm^3, and neutropenia.

Several methods exist to confirm the diagnosis of CTF. The recommended method is culture of a ground blood clot from the infected person by intraperitoneal inoculation of laboratory mice for isolation of the virus. Neutralizing antibodies against the virus can also be detected. Approximately 90% of infected persons have a fourfold increase in specific neutralizing antibodies within 30 days with EIA and Western blot assays. Only one third of patients have detectable antibodies by day 10 of the illness. Preliminary work has demonstrated that PCR is a highly sensitive tool in the early diagnosis of CTF. Persistent viremia lasting >4 weeks is a common feature but does not appear to correlate with prolonged symptoms.

Differential Diagnosis

The diagnosis of CTF is frequently confused with that of human ehrlichiosis, RMSF, murine typhus, relapsing fever, and meningococcemia. If the patient recently has visited an endemic region, dengue fever should also be suspected.

TREATMENT

No effective therapy is available. The disease is self-limiting. Supportive care consisting of adequate fluid intake, bed rest, and antipyretic therapy is usually necessary.

COMPLICATIONS

Meningoencephalitis with lymphocytic pleocytosis (cells up to 500/mm^3) and elevation of CSF protein is commonly observed. Disseminated intravascular coagulation, pericarditis, myocarditis, atypical pneumonia, and gastrointestinal hemorrhage have been reported as unusual complications.

PROGNOSIS

Nearly 48% of affected patients have persistent symptoms of malaise and generalized weakness for longer than 3 weeks. The likelihood of prolonged symptoms correlates directly with age: 70% of patients >30 years of age have prolonged symptoms; 60% of patients <20 years of age have symptoms lasting longer than 1 week. The prognosis is good for the majority of patients. Resolution of symptoms is usually complete, even in patients with a prolonged convalescence.

PREVENTION

Avoidance of tick-infested areas and the use of protective clothing or insect repellents are the preferred modes of prevention (Table 3–8). Thorough inspection after returning from the outdoors is also important.

REVIEWS

Shapiro ED: Tick borne diseases. *Adv Pediatr Infect Dis* 1998;13:187–218.

Spach DH, Liles WC, Campbell GL, et al: Tick-borne diseases in the United States. *N Engl J Med* 1993;329:936–47.

Weinberg AN, Weber DJ (editors): Animal-associated human infections. *Infect Dis Clin North Am* 1991;5(1):1–175 and 1991;5(3):647–731.

Brucellosis

al-Eissa YA, al-Mofada SM: Congenital brucellosis. *Pediatr Infect Dis J* 1992;11:667–71.

Bannatyne RM, Jackson MC, Memish Z: Rapid diagnosis of *Brucella* bacteremia by using the BACTEC 9240 system. *J Clin Microbiol* 1997;35:2673–4.

Chheda S, Lopez SM, Sanderson EP: Congenital brucellosis in a premature infant. *Pediatr Infect Dis J* 1997;16:81–3.

Gottesman G, Vanunu D, Maayan MC, et al: Childhood brucellosis in Israel. *Pediatr Infect Dis J* 1996;15:610–5.

Lubani MM, Dudin KI, Sharda DC, et al: A multicenter therapeutic study of 1100 children with brucellosis. *Pediatr Infect Dis J* 1989;8:75–8.

McLean DR, Russell N, Khan MY: Neurobrucellosis: Clinical and therapeutic features. *Clin Infect Dis* 1992;15:582–90.

Queipo-Ortuno, MI, Morata P, Ocon P, et al: Rapid diagnosis of human brucellosis by peripheral-blood PCR assay. *J Clin Microbiol* 1997; 35:2927–30.

Street L Jr, Grant WW, Alva JD: Brucellosis in childhood. *Pediatrics* 1975;55:416–21.

Young EJ: An overview of human brucellosis. *Clin Infect Dis* 1995; 21:283–90.

Tularemia

Cross JT, Jacobs RF: Tularemia: Treatment failures with outpatient use of ceftriaxone. *Clin Infect Dis* 1993;17:976–80.

Francis E: Landmark article April 25, 1925: Tularemia. By Edward Francis. *JAMA* 1983;250:3216–24.

Fulop M, Leslie D, Titball R, et al: A rapid, highly sensitive method for the detection of *Franciscella tularensis* in clinical samples using the polymerase chain reaction. *Am J Trop Med Hyg* 1996;54:364–6.

Jacobs RF: Tularemia. *Adv Pediatr Infect Dis* 1996;12:55–69.

Johansson A, Berglund L, Gothefors L, et al: Ciprofloxacin for treatment of tularemia in children. *Pediatr Infect Dis J* 2000;19:449–53.

Rodgers BL, Duffield RP, Taylor T, et al: Tularemic meningitis. *Pediatr Infect Dis J* 1998;17:439–41.

Plague

Centers for Disease Control and Prevention: Prevention of plague. Recommendations of the Advisory Committee on Immunization Practices (ACIP). *MMWR Morb Mortal Wkly Rep* 1996;45(RR-14):1–15.

Craven RB, Barnes AM: Plague and tularemia. *Infect Dis Clin North Am* 1991;5:165–75.

Hull HF, Montes JM, Mann JM: Septicemic plague in New Mexico. *J Infect Dis* 1987;155:113–8.

Leptospirosis

Antony SJ: Leptospirosis—An emerging pathogen in travel medicine: A review of its clinical manifestations and management. *J Travel Med* 1996;3:113–18.

Farr RW: Leptospirosis. *Clin Infect Dis* 1995;21:1–8.

Takafuji ET, Kirkpatrick JW, Miller RN, et al: An efficacy trial of doxycycline chemoprophylaxis against leptospirosis. *N Engl J Med* 1984; 310:497–500.

Trevejo RT, Rigau-Perez JG, Ashford DA, et al: Epidemic leptospirosis associated with pulmonary hemorrhage—Nicaragua, 1995. *J Infect Dis* 1998;178:1457–63.

Vinetz JM, Glass GE, Flexner CE, et al: Sporadic urban leptospirosis. *Ann Intern Med* 1996;125:794–8.

Relapsing Fever

Centers for Disease Control and Prevention: Outbreak of relapsing fever—Grand Canyon National Park, Arizona, 1990. *MMWR* 1991;40:296–303.

Horton JM, Blaser MJ: The spectrum of relapsing fever in the Rocky Mountains. *Arch Intern Med* 1985;145:871–5.

Trevejo RT, Schriefer ME, Gage KL, et al: An interstate outbreak of tick-borne relapsing fever among vacationers at a Rocky Mountain cabin. *Am J Trop Med Hyg* 1998;58:743–7.

Yagupsky P, Moses S: Neonatal *Borrellia* species infection (relapsing fever). *Am J Dis Child* 1985;139:74–6.

Murine Typhus

Dumler JS, Taylor JP, Walker DH: Clinical and laboratory features of murine typhus in south Texas, 1980 through 1987. *JAMA* 1991;266:1365–70.

Fergie JE, Purcell K, Wanat D: Murine typhus in South Texas children. *Pediatr Infect Dis J* 2000;19:535–8.

Higgins JA, Radulovie S, Schriefer ME, et al: Rickettsia felis: A new species of pathogenic rickettsia isolated from cat fleas. *J Clin Microbiol* 1996;34:671–4.

Rauolt D, LaScola B, Enea M, et al: A flea-associated Rickettsia pathogenic for humans. *Emerg Infect Dis* 2001;7:73–81.

Whiteford SF, Taylor JP, Dumler JS: Clinical, laboratory, and epidemiologic features of murine typhus in 97 Texas children. *Arch Pediatr Adolesc Med* 2001;155:396–400.

Q Fever

Marrie TJ, Durant H, Williams JC, et al: Exposure to parturient cats: A risk factor of acquisition of Q fever in maritime Canada. *J Infect Dis* 1988;138:101–8.

Raoult D, Marrie T: Q fever. *Clin Infect Dis* 1995;20:489–96.

Richardus JH, Schaap GJ, Donkers A, et al: Q fever in infancy: A review of 18 cases. *Pediatr Infect Dis* 1985;4:369–73.

Ruiz-Contreras J, Gonzalez Montero R, Ramos Amador JT, et al: Q fever in children. *Am J Dis Child* 1993;147:300–2.

Rickettsialpox

Brettman LR, Lewin S, Holzman RS, et al: Rickettsialpox: Report of an outbreak and a contemporary review. *Medicine* 1981;60:363–72.

Comer JA, Tzianabos T, Flynn C, et al: Serologic evidence of rickettsialpox (*Rickettsia akari*) infection among intravenous drug users in inner-city Baltimore, Maryland. *Am J Trop Med Hyg* 1999;60:894–8.

Kass EM, Szaniawski WK, Levy H, et al: Rickettsialpox in a New York City hospital, 1980 to 1989. *N Engl J Med* 1994;331:1612–7.

Dengue Fever

Centers for Disease Control and Prevention: Dengue outbreak associated with multiple serotypes—Puerto Rico, 1998. *MMWR* 1998;47:952.

Dung NM, Day NP, Tam DT, et al: Fluid replacement in dengue shock syndrome: A randomized, double-blind comparison of four intravenous-fluid regimens. *Clin Infect Dis* 1999;29:787–94.

Gubler DJ: Dengue and dengue hemorrhagic fever. *Clin Microbiol Rev* 1998;11:480–96.

Kautner I, Robinson MJ, Kuhnle U: Dengue virus infection: Epidemiology, pathogenesis, clinical presentation, diagnosis, and prevention. *J Pediatr* 1997;131:516–24.

Malison MD, Waterman SH: Dengue fever in the United States: A report of a cluster of imported cases and review of the clinical, epidemiologic, and public health aspects of the disease. *JAMA* 1983;249:496–500.

Rigau-Perez JG, Gubler DJ, Vorndam AV, et al: Dengue: A literature review and case study of travelers from the United States, 1986-1994. *J Travel Med* 1997;4:65–7.

Vaughn DW, Green S, Kalayanarooj S, et al: Dengue viremia titer, antibody response pattern, and virus serotype correlate with disease severity. *J Infect Dis* 2000;181:2–9.

Colorado Tick Fever

Attoui H, Billoir F, Bruey JM, et al: Serologic and molecular diagnosis of Colorado tick fever viral infections. *Am J Trop Med Hyg* 1998;59:763–8.

Goodpasture HC, Poland JD, Francy DB, et al: Colorado tick fever: Clinical, epidemiologic, and laboratory aspects of 228 cases in Colorado in 1973–1974. *Ann Intern Med* 1978;88:303–10.

Johnson AJ, Karabatsos N, Lanciotti RS: Detection of Colorado tick fever virus by using reverse transcriptase PCR and application of the technique in laboratory diagnosis. *J Clin Microbiol* 1997;35:1203–8.

Spruance SL, Bailey A: Colorado tick fever: A review of 115 laboratory confirmed cases. *Arch Intern Med* 1973;131:288–93.

CHAPTER 35

Tuberculosis

Jeffrey R. Starke

Since about 1700, when John Bunyan coined the phrase "Captain of the Men of Death" to describe the impact of **consumption** on Europe, tuberculosis has been, and still is, the leading cause of morbidity and mortality worldwide from an infectious disease. Approximately one third of the world's population harbors *Mycobacterium tuberculosis* and is at risk of developing disease. From 1984 to 1992 the United States experienced a resurgence of tuberculosis. Potential reasons for this resurgence included (1) the epidemic of infection caused by HIV infection, which is a potent risk factor for the development of tuberculosis disease in an adult infected with the tubercle bacillus; (2) increases in other vulnerable populations, such as homeless, users of intravenous and other street drugs, alcoholics, and residents of correctional institutions; (3) increased immigration from countries with a high prevalence of tuberculosis, which enlarges the pool of infected persons in the United States; and (4) often inadequate public health service and access to health care, which hinders rapid diagnosis, early treatment, and completion of contact investigations. From 1992 to the present, tuberculosis case numbers have declined as adequate tuberculosis control measures have been reestablished in most areas of the United States.

Infection and Disease. The terminology used to describe various aspects of tuberculosis can be confusing, but it follows the pathophysiology of the disease. **Tuberculosis infection** describes the preclinical stage of infection with *M. tuberculosis,* sometimes termed **latent tuberculosis.** The tuberculin skin test is positive, but the chest radiograph is normal and no signs or symptoms of illness are evident. **Tuberculosis disease** occurs when clinical manifestations of pulmonary or extrapulmonary tuberculosis become apparent, either by clinical signs and symptoms or on chest radiographs. The term "tuberculosis" usually refers to the disease. The time interval between the initial tuberculosis infection and the onset of disease may be several weeks or many decades. In adults, the distinction between asymptomatic infection and clinical disease is usually clear. In young children, tuberculosis usually develops as an immediate complication of the primary infection, and the distinction between infection and disease may be less obvious. An infected child with any radiographic or clinical manifestations consistent with tuberculosis is usually considered to have tuberculosis disease, even if no symptoms are present.

Two major elements determine a person's risk of developing tuberculosis: the likelihood of exposure to an individual with infectious tuberculosis, which is primarily determined by the individual's environment, and the ability of the person's immune system to control the initial infection and keep it latent. An estimated 10–15 million persons in the United States have latent tuberculosis infection. Without treatment, disease will develop in 5–10% of immunologically normal adults with tuberculosis infection at some time during their lives. About one half of these adults experience disease within the first 3 years of infection. In children, the risk is greater; up to 40% of those less than 1 year of age with untreated tuberculosis infection develop radiographic evidence of disease, as do 20% of children aged 1–10 years and 15% of adolescents aged 11–15 years. Medical conditions or treatments that impair the cellular immune system further increase the likelihood that tuberculosis disease will develop in a person with latent infection.

ETIOLOGY

The agents of human tuberculosis—*M. tuberculosis, Mycobacterium bovis,* and *Mycobacterium africanum*—belong to the order Actinomycetales of the family Mycobacteriaceae. Disease from *M. africanum,* which is found in Africa and thought to be an intermediate between *M. tuberculosis* and *M. bovis,* is rare. The **tubercle bacilli** are non-spore-forming, nonmotile, pleomorphic, weakly gram-positive curved rods about 2–4 μm long. They may appear beaded or clumped in stained clinical specimens or culture media. They are obligate aerobes that grow in synthetic media containing glycerol as the carbon source and ammonium salts as the nitrogen source. These mycobacteria grow best at 37–41°C, produce niacin, and lack pigmentation. A lipid-rich cell wall accounts for resistance to the bactericidal actions of antibody and complement. A hallmark of all mycobacteria is **acid-fastness:** the capacity to form stable mycolate complexes with arylmethane dyes such as crystal violet, carbolfuchsin, auramine, and rhodamine. Once stained, they resist decoloration with ethanol and hydrochloric or other acids. The term **acid-fast bacilli** is practically synonymous with mycobacteria, although some organisms, such as *Nocardia,* are variably acid-fast.

Mycobacteria grow slowly, with a generation time of 12–24 hours. Isolation from clinical specimens on solid synthetic media usually takes 3–6 weeks, and drug-susceptibility testing requires an additional 4 weeks. However, growth can be detected in 1–3 weeks in selective liquid medium using radiolabeled nutrients, and drug susceptibilities can be determined in an additional 3–5 days.

Transmission. Transmission of *M. tuberculosis* is from person to person, usually by mucus **droplets** that become airborne when the ill individual coughs, sneezes, laughs, sighs, or even breathes. Infected droplets dry and become **droplet nuclei,** which may remain suspended in the air for hours, long after the infectious person has left the environment. Environmental factors, such as poor circulation of air, can enhance transmission. Only particles <10 μm in diameter can reach the alveoli and establish infection. Rarely, transmission occurs by direct contact with infected body fluids, such as urine and purulent sinus tract drainage, or with heavily infected fomites.

Several patient-related factors have been associated with an increased chance of transmission (Table 35–1). Of these, a positive acid-fast smear of the sputum is most closely correlated with infectivity. Extensive epidemiologic studies in orphanages, children's hospitals, and the community have shown that children with primary tuberculosis disease rarely, if ever, infect other children or

TABLE 35–1. Risk Factors for Transmission of Tuberculosis

A positive acid-fast smear of the sputum
Presence of a cavity or extensive infiltrate in the lung
Severe, forceful cough
Unwillingness or inability to cover a cough
A high volume or low viscosity of sputum
Forceful exhalation maneuvers, such as singing or shouting
Prolonged duration of respiratory symptoms
Inadequate chemotherapy, especially as a result of noncompliance or drug resistance

adults. Tubercle bacilli are relatively sparse in the endobronchial secretions of children with pulmonary tuberculosis, and a significant cough is usually lacking. When young children do cough, they rarely produce sputum and they lack the tussive force necessary to suspend infectious particles of the correct size.

Infectivity must be considered in several pediatric clinical situations. Older children and adolescents with reactivation forms of pulmonary tuberculosis, such as cavities or extensive infiltrates, should be considered potentially infectious to others. Although most children with pulmonary tuberculosis are not infectious, additional caution must be taken within the hospital setting to avoid infection of health care workers and other patients. Many experts place hospitalized children with suspected pulmonary tuberculosis in respiratory isolation initially if their parents or adult visitors have not been fully evaluated for tuberculosis. This isolation is actually directed more at high-risk adults than at the ill child.

Determining when a potentially infectious patient with pulmonary tuberculosis is no longer infectious is difficult. The decision must be based on improvement in symptoms, decreased number of acid-fast bacilli in the sputum smear, initial chest radiograph findings, and adherence to treatment. Previous studies of transmission to animals and retrospective epidemiology have indicated that most initially infectious patients become noninfectious within 2 weeks of starting effective treatment. Many patients become noninfectious within several days, but occasional adult patients remain infectious for weeks to months after beginning ultimately effective treatment. Several investigations have shown that the vast majority of close contacts are infected by the source case before diagnosis and treatment and that continued exposure to the source case after diagnosis leads to little or no incremental risk of infection.

EPIDEMIOLOGY

An estimated 8 million new cases of tuberculosis occur each year among adults, and 3 million deaths are attributed to the disease annually. In developing countries, 1.3 million new cases of the disease occur in children <15 years of age, and 450,000 children die each year of tuberculosis. The vast majority of children with tuberculosis infection and disease acquire *M. tuberculosis* from an adult with tuberculosis; understanding the epidemiology of tuberculosis in children requires a thorough knowledge of the epidemiology for adults.

Adults. Tuberculosis, the leading cause of death in the United States at the beginning of the twentieth century, decreased in incidence for several decades. Case rates began to fall during the first half of this century, long before the discovery of effective antituberculosis drugs, primarily as a result of improved living conditions and nutrition. From 1953 to 1984, the incidence of disease declined an average of about 6% per year. However, beginning in 1985, the downward trend was reversed for both adults and children (Fig. 35–1). In 1991, 26,283 cases were reported, an increase of 18% from 1985. The true incidence of tuberculosis is probably higher, because many cases are undiagnosed or unreported. Because of improvements in tuberculosis control in much of the United States, reported tuberculosis dropped to 17,531 cases in 1999.

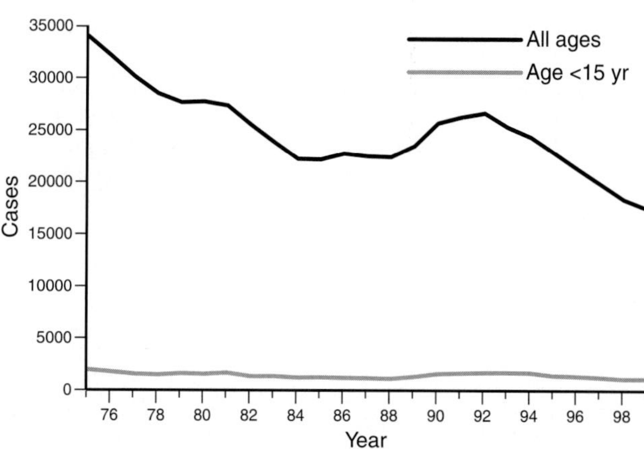

FIGURE 35–1. Reported cases (in thousands) of tuberculosis by year in the United States from 1975 to 1999. (Data from the CDC.)

Decades ago, when tuberculosis was more prevalent in the United States, the risk of exposure to an adult with infectious tuberculosis was high and fairly uniform across the population. This is currently true in many of the world's developing countries, where tuberculosis rates remain high. At present in North America, tuberculosis rates are highest in some fairly well-defined groups of high-risk persons (Table 35–2). Although tuberculosis case rates generally increase with age among the non-Hispanic white population, a strong trend toward increased case rates in young adults has developed, especially among minority populations. This trend is especially striking in urban areas. Cities with populations of more than 250,000 residents hold 18% of the United States population but account for more than 42% of tuberculosis cases. From 1985 to 1996 the median age of persons with tuberculosis dropped from 49 to 43 years, reversing a long-standing trend that had suggested that younger cohorts with fewer infected persons were replacing older, more heavily infected cohorts.

Among young adults in the United States, tuberculosis is predominantly a disease of racial and ethnic minorities, especially among African Americans, Hispanics, and Native Americans.

TABLE 35–2. High-Risk Groups for Tuberculosis in North America

Increased Risk of Becoming Infected
Foreign-born persons from high-prevalence countries
Residents of jails and prisons
Residents of nursing homes
Homeless persons
Users of illegal drugs
Poor and medically indigent persons
Health care workers who care for high-risk patients
Children exposed to adults in high-risk groups

Increased Risk of Developing Disease Once Infected
Coinfection with HIV and other immunocompromising diseases
Immunosuppressive therapies
Malnutrition
Age <4 years
Recent infection (within 2 years)

Some epidemiologic and immunologic evidence indicates that African Americans may be slightly more susceptible to tuberculosis infection than are non-Hispanic white persons. Genetic factors may partly control a person's susceptibility to tuberculosis infection and disease. In addition, extrinsic differences in socioeconomic status, nutrition, access to health care, and crowded living conditions undoubtedly contribute heavily to the increased tuberculosis case rates among minority groups.

Approximately 40% of persons with tuberculosis in the United States are foreign born. The number of tuberculosis cases in the United States is increasing among foreign-born persons from countries with a high prevalence of the disease. In 1995, the estimated tuberculosis case rate for foreign-born persons arriving in the United States was 13 times greater than the overall United States rate. Persons from six countries—Mexico, the Philippines, Vietnam, South Korea, Haiti, and China—accounted for about 65% of these cases. The majority of foreign-born persons in whom tuberculosis develops are identified within 5 years of immigration. Many of these cases could be prevented if high-risk persons were more effectively screened and treated for tuberculosis infection at or before immigration.

Certain settings harbor persons at high risk of acquisition and transmission of tuberculosis. The prevalence rates of tuberculosis infection and disease among adults in correctional institutions are often 10–20 times higher than in the general population because such persons are disproportionately poor and from minority racial and ethnic groups and therefore have a greater likelihood of being infected with HIV, and often they were infected during previous incarcerations. On release from these facilities, former inmates can unknowingly spread tuberculosis into the community. Tuberculosis case rates for elderly persons in nursing homes are often many times higher than among similar persons who live in other situations. Homeless persons, including those living in shelters, may have tuberculosis case rates 20–50 times higher than the general population. Migrant farm workers may have very high tuberculosis rates, and long-term treatment can be difficult to complete in this mobile population. Finally, health care settings where tuberculosis patients are cared for may promote transmission, especially if the physicians do not consider the diagnosis initially. For physicians, the time of greatest risk of acquiring tuberculosis infection appears to be during training in medical school and residency. The onset of tuberculosis disease often occurs years later, however.

The new factor that undoubtedly has had the greatest impact on the resurgence of tuberculosis has been the epidemic of HIV infection, which is the most potent risk factor yet identified for the development of clinical disease in adults with latent tuberculosis infection. In most locales that experienced increases in tuberculosis cases from 1985–1999 the demographic groups with the greatest tuberculosis morbidity also had large numbers of HIV-infected persons. In HIV-infected adults with a significant Mantoux tuberculin skin test reaction, tuberculosis disease develops at a rate of 5–10% per year, compared with the 5–10% lifetime risk in immunocompetent adults. Many HIV-infected adults with pulmonary tuberculosis are capable of spreading *M. tuberculosis* to contacts, especially if the organism is detected in sputum by acid-fast smear and a cavity or extensive infiltrate is present on a chest radiograph.

Children. Between 1953 and 1981, childhood tuberculosis rates in the United States declined about 6% per year. Between 1982 and 1988, the case rates remained relatively flat, but they began to increase in 1989 (Fig. 35–1). In 1993, 1,721 cases were reported in children <15 years of age, a 52% increase over 1988 cases. After improvements in tuberculosis control in the United States, the number of childhood tuberculosis cases dropped to 1,044 in 1999. About 60% of cases occur in infants and children <5 years of age. Children between the ages of 5 and 14 years, often called the "favored age," usually have the lowest rates of tuberculosis disease in any population. The gender ratio for tuberculosis in children is about 1:1, in contrast to adults, in whom there is male predominance.

Historically, tuberculosis case rates have been the highest between January and June in the Northern Hemisphere, possibly because of more extensive indoor contact with infectious adults during the colder months. The disease also is geographically focal in the United States, with seven states—California, Florida, Georgia, Illinois, New York, New Jersey, and Texas—accounting for 72% of reported cases among children <5 years of age. Disease rates are highest in cities with more than 250,000 residents.

Childhood tuberculosis case rates in the United States are strikingly higher among ethnic and racial minority groups and the foreign-born than in whites. Approximately 85% of cases occur among African American, Hispanic, Asian, and Native American children, which reflects the risk of transmission within the living conditions for these children. Although most of these children were born in the United States, from 1986 to 1990 the proportion of foreign-born children with tuberculosis rose from 13% to 16% for children <5 years of age, and from 40% to 49% among adolescents 15–19 years of age.

Most children are infected with *M. tuberculosis* in the home, but outbreaks of childhood tuberculosis centered in elementary and high schools, nursery schools, family day care homes, churches, school buses, and stores still occur. A high-risk adult working in the area has been the source of the outbreak in most cases.

The recent epidemic of HIV infection has had a profound effect on the epidemiology of tuberculosis among children as a result of two major mechanisms: HIV-infected adults with tuberculosis may transmit *M. tuberculosis* to children, some of whom will develop tuberculosis disease, and children with HIV infection may be at increased risk of progressing from tuberculosis infection to disease. Increased childhood tuberculosis case rates have been associated with a simultaneous increase among HIV-infected adults in the community. In general, HIV-infected children may be more likely to have contact with HIV-infected adults who are at high risk of tuberculosis. Tuberculosis is probably underdiagnosed among HIV-infected children for two reasons: the similarity of its clinical presentation to that of other opportunistic infections and AIDS-related conditions and the difficulty of confirming the diagnosis with positive cultures. Children with tuberculosis disease should have HIV serologic testing because the two infections are linked epidemiologically.

Although data on tuberculosis disease in children are readily available, data concerning tuberculosis infection without disease (i.e., a positive skin test only) are lacking. Tuberculosis infection is a reportable condition in only four states, and national surveys were discontinued in 1971. The most efficient method of finding children infected with *M. tuberculosis* is through contact investigations of adults with infectious pulmonary tuberculosis. On average, 30–50% of all household contacts of an index case have a reactive skin test.

In developing countries, tuberculosis infection rates among the young population average 20–50%. The prevalence is less than 1% for most U.S. children but reaches 2–9% in some urban school populations. The majority of infections occur among foreign-born students. Each tuberculosis infection in a young child is a sentinel health event representing transmission of *M. tuberculosis* within a community and a failure to control the disease. The recent upward trend in reported pediatric tuberculosis cases in the United States and the results from these skin test surveys in urban areas imply that the pool of infected children and young adults in the United States has grown.

PATHOGENESIS

The primary complex of tuberculosis consists of local disease at the portal of entry and the regional lymph nodes that drain the area of the primary focus. Tubercle bacilli within particles larger than 10 μm usually are caught by the mucociliary mechanisms of the bronchial tree and are expelled. Smaller particles are inhaled beyond these clearance mechanisms. However, primary infection may occur anywhere in the body. Ingestion of milk infected with bovine tuberculosis can lead to a gastrointestinal primary lesion. Infection of the skin or of a mucous membrane can occur through an abrasion, cut, or insect bite. The number of tubercle bacilli required to establish infection is unknown, but probably only several organisms are necessary.

The tubercle bacilli multiply initially within the alveoli and alveolar ducts. The initial accumulation of host immune cells in a previously uninfected person consists predominantly of polymorphonuclear leukocytes. Epithelioid cell proliferation and the appearance of **giant cells** with lymphocytic infiltration and **granuloma formation** occur later. Concurrently, some of the bacilli are ingested but not killed by macrophages, which carry them through lymphatics to the regional lymph nodes. When the primary lesion is in the lung, the hilar lymph nodes usually are involved, although an apical focus may drain into paratracheal nodes.

The incubation period after the tubercle bacilli enter the body to the development of cutaneous hypersensitivity is 2–12 weeks, most often 4–8 weeks. The onset of hypersensitivity may be accompanied by a febrile reaction that lasts 1–3 weeks. During this phase of intensified tissue reaction, the primary complex may become visible on chest radiographs. Animal studies suggest that a large infectious inoculum may be associated with a shorter incubation period, although this has never been proved in human beings. The primary focus grows larger but does not yet become encapsulated during this time. The inflammatory response becomes more intense as hypersensitivity develops, and the regional lymph nodes often enlarge. The parenchymal portion of the primary complex often heals completely by fibrosis or calcification after undergoing caseous necrosis and encapsulation. Occasionally, the parenchymal lesion continues to enlarge, resulting in focal pneumonitis and thickening of the overlying pleura. If caseation is intense, the center of the lesion liquefies, empties into the associated bronchus, and leaves a residual primary tuberculous cavity.

During the development of the parenchymal lesion and the accelerated caseation brought on by the development of hypersensitivity, tubercle bacilli from the primary complex spread via the bloodstream and lymphatics to many parts of the body. The areas most commonly seeded are the apices of the lungs, liver, spleen, meninges, peritoneum, lymph nodes, pleura, and bone. This dissemination involves either large numbers of bacilli, which leads to disseminated tuberculosis disease, or small numbers of bacilli that leave microscopic tuberculous foci scattered in various tissues. Initially these metastatic foci are clinically inapparent, but they are the origin of both extrapulmonary tuberculosis and reactivation pulmonary tuberculosis in some persons.

The tubercle foci in the regional lymph nodes develop some fibrosis and encapsulation, but healing is usually less complete than in the parenchymal lesions. Viable *M. tuberculosis* may persist for decades after calcification of the nodes. In most cases of primary tuberculosis infection, the lymph nodes remain normal in size and no thoracic complications develop. However, because of their location, hilar and paratracheal lymph nodes that become enlarged by the host's inflammatory reaction to the tubercle bacilli may encroach upon the regional bronchus. Partial obstruction caused by external compression may lead at first to hyperinflation in the distal lung segment. This compression occasionally causes complete obstruction of the bronchus, resulting in atelectasis of the lung segment. Inflamed caseous nodes attach to the bronchial wall and erode through it, leading to endobronchial tuberculosis or a fistulous tract. The extrusion of infected caseous material into the bronchus can transmit infection to the lung parenchyma, causing bronchial obstruction and atelectasis. The resultant lesion is a combination of pneumonia and atelectasis. The radiographic findings of this process have been referred to as "epituberculosis," "collapse-consolidation," and "segmental tuberculosis." Rarely, tuberculous intrathoracic lymph nodes invade adjacent structures, such as the pericardium or esophagus.

A fairly predictable timetable for primary tuberculosis infection and its complications in infants and children is apparent. Massive lymphohematogenous dissemination leading to miliary or disseminated disease occurs in only 0.5–2% of infected children, usually no later than 2–6 months after infection. Clinically significant lymph node or endobronchial tuberculosis usually appears within 3–9 months. Lesions of the bones and joints usually take at least a year to develop; renal lesions may be evident 5–25 years after infection. In general, complications of the primary infection occur within the first 2 years.

Tuberculosis disease that occurs more than a year after the primary infection is thought to be secondary to endogenous regrowth of persistent bacilli from the primary infection. In rare cases, exogenous reinfection may result in tuberculosis disease, but most cases of postprimary or reactivation tuberculosis are believed to be secondary to endogenous organisms. Reactivation tuberculosis is rare in infants and young children but is fairly common among adolescents and young adults. For unknown reasons, reactivation tuberculosis among adolescents affects girls twice as often as boys. The most common form of reactivation tuberculosis is an infiltrate or cavity in the apex of the lung, where oxygen tension is high and there is a heavy concentration of tubercle bacilli deposited during the primary subclinical dissemination of organisms. Dissemination during reactivation tuberculosis is rare among immunocompetent children.

The age of the child at acquisition of the primary tuberculosis infection seems to have a great effect on the occurrence of both primary and reactivation tuberculosis. Hilar lymphadenopathy and subsequent segmental disease complicating the primary infection occur most often in young children. Approximately 40% of children <1 year of age develop a radiographically significant lymphadenopathy or segmental lesion, compared with 24% of children 1–10 years of age and 16% of children 11–15 years of age. However, if young children do not have early complications, their risk of developing reactivation tuberculosis later in life appears to be low. Conversely, older children and adolescents rarely experience complications of the primary infection but have a much higher risk of developing reactivation pulmonary tuberculosis as adolescents or adults.

Pregnancy and the Newborn. True congenital tuberculosis is rare, with fewer than 300 cases reported. Congenital infection occurs by two mechanisms: by passage of *M. tuberculosis* via the placenta to the fetus or by fetal aspiration of contaminated amniotic fluid. The mothers of the infected infants frequently have tuberculosis pleural effusion, meningitis, or miliary disease during pregnancy or soon afterward. However, the diagnosis of tuberculosis in the newborn often leads to discovery of the mother's tuberculosis. The intensity of lymphohematogenous spread during pregnancy is one of the factors that determine whether congenital infection occurs. Primary infection in the mother just before or during pregnancy is more likely to lead to congenital infection than is latent infection. However, even massive involvement of the placenta with tuberculosis does not always give rise to congenital infection. Whether the fetus can be infected directly from the mother's bloodstream without a caseous tuberculous lesion forming first in the placenta is not clear. The tubercle bacilli first reach the fetal liver, where a primary focus may develop with associated involvement of the periportal lymph nodes. Organisms can pass through the liver into the main fetal circulation, leading to a primary focus in the lung. The bacilli in the lung usually remain dormant until after birth, when oxygenation and pulmonary circulation increase significantly.

Congenital tuberculosis may also occur by aspiration or ingestion of infected amniotic fluid if a caseous placental lesion ruptures directly into the amniotic cavity. This infection with tubercle bacilli is the most likely cause of congenital tuberculosis if multiple primary foci are present in the lung or gut and middle ear.

The most common route of infection for the neonate is undoubtedly postnatal acquisition of *M. tuberculosis* by airborne inoculation. The distinction between postnatal infection and true congenital infection is often impossible to establish on clinical grounds unless the placenta is available for inspection and culture. This determination is not of major importance to the infant, because the treatment regimens are the same. However, determining the true source and route of infection is vital for proper evaluation and treatment of the mother and other persons in the infant's environment.

Immunity

The exact immunologic mechanisms that characterize human resistance and reaction to *M. tuberculosis* remain undetermined. Conditions that adversely affect cell-mediated immunity, such as HIV infection, malignant disease, malnutrition, and the use of corticosteroids, predispose to the progression from tuberculosis infection to disease. Tuberculosis is associated with a vast antibody response, but these antibodies appear to play little role in host defense.

In the first several weeks after infection, tubercle bacilli undergo an initial period of uninhibited growth, either free in alveolar spaces or after ingestion by inactivated alveolar macrophages. Sulfatides in the cell wall of mycobacteria can prevent fusion of the phagosome with lysosomes within the macrophage, allowing organisms to escape the destructive effects of intracellular enzymes. Cell-mediated immunity starts to develop within 4–8 weeks of infection, about the time that tissue hypersensitivity begins. Initially, a small population of lymphocytes recognizes certain mycobacterial antigens after they have been processed and presented by macrophages. These lymphocytes proliferate and secrete lymphokines and other mediators, which attract other lymphocytes and macrophages to the areas where tubercle bacilli reside. The lymphokines also activate the macrophages, causing them to develop high concentrations of lytic enzymes that enhance their mycobacterial capacity. The activated macrophages release fibroblast-stimulating factor, resulting in collagen deposition and eventual fibrosis. A discrete subset of regulator lymphocytes, including both helper and suppressor cells, modulates the immune response. In most persons the development of specific cellular immunity prevents progression of tuberculosis infection, resulting in an asymptomatic primary infection.

While the population of activated lymphocytes expands, tissue hypersensitivity develops along with cell-mediated immunity. These two phenomena are similar but can be disassociated in animal models. Together they can be both beneficial and harmful to the host. They can destroy both tubercle bacilli and host tissue, leading to caseation and liquefaction, especially in the presence of large amounts of mycobacterial antigen. Tuberculosis may actually suppress the host's immune system in a variety of ways. A significant decrease in the number of helper lymphocytes commonly occurs, even in patients with clinically mild disease. Persons who are seriously ill with tuberculosis may lose their tissue hypersensitivity, leading to cutaneous **anergy** that may be global or specific for tuberculin.

SYMPTOMS AND CLINICAL MANIFESTATIONS

In the majority of children with tuberculosis infection, no signs or symptoms develop at any time. Occasionally the initiation of the infection is marked by several days of low-grade fever and mild cough. Rare patients experience a clinically significant disease with high fever, cough, malaise, and flulike symptoms that resolve within a week. Other children at the onset of tissue hypersensitivity experience a fever and mild systemic symptoms that resolve in 1–3 weeks.

The proportion of extrapulmonary tuberculosis cases has increased over the past two decades in the United States. About 15% of adult tuberculosis cases are extrapulmonary, and 25–30% of children with tuberculosis have an extrapulmonary presentation (Fig. 35–2).

Pulmonary Disease. The symptoms and physical signs of intrathoracic tuberculosis in children are usually surprisingly meager, considering the degree of radiographic changes often seen. The physical manifestations of disease tend to differ by age at onset. Young infants and adolescents are more likely to have significant signs or symptoms, whereas school-age children often have clinically silent disease (Table 35–3).

More than half of infants and children with radiographically moderate to severe pulmonary tuberculosis have no physical findings, and their diseases are discovered via contact tracing of an adult with tuberculosis. Infants are more likely to experience signs and symptoms, probably because of their small airway diameters relative to the parenchymal and lymph node changes in primary tuberculosis. Nonproductive cough and mild dyspnea are the most

Extrapulmonary Tuberculosis in Children

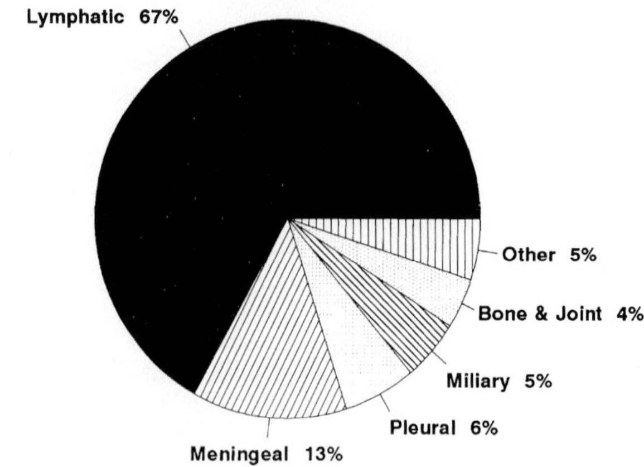

FIGURE 35–2. Distribution of tuberculosis cases by anatomic site among the 25% of cases of childhood tuberculosis that are extrapulmonary.

TABLE 35–3. Occurrence of Clinical Features of Pulmonary Tuberculosis in Infants, Children, and Adolescents

Clinical Feature	Occurrence		
	Infants	Children	Adolescents
Symptom			
Fever	Common	Uncommon	Common
Night sweats	Rare	Rare	Uncommon
Cough	Common	Common	Common
Productive cough	Rare	Rare	Common
Hemoptysis	Never	Rare	Rare
Dyspnea	Common	Rare	Rare
Sign			
Rales	Common	Uncommon	Rare
Wheezing (focal or diffuse)	Common	Uncommon	Uncommon
Fremitus	Rare	Rare	Uncommon
Dullness to percussion (pleural disease)	Rare	Rare	Uncommon
Decreased breath sounds (focal)	Common	Rare	Uncommon

common symptoms. Systemic complaints, such as fever, night sweats, anorexia, malaise, and decreased activity that is the equivalent of malaise, occur less often. Some infants have difficulty gaining weight or develop a failure-to-thrive presentation that often does not improve significantly until after several months of treatment.

Pulmonary signs are even less common. Some infants and young children with bronchial obstruction show signs of air trapping, such as localized wheezing or decreased breath sounds that may be accompanied by tachypnea or, rarely, frank respiratory distress. A two-headed stethoscope may reveal delayed exhalation of air on the affected side. Occasionally these nonspecific symptoms and signs are alleviated by antibiotics, suggesting that bacterial superinfection distal to the focus of tuberculous bronchial obstruction contributed to the clinical presentation of disease.

A rare but serious complication of primary tuberculosis in children occurs when the parenchymal focus enlarges and develops a large caseous center. The radiographic and clinical picture of progressive primary tuberculosis is similar to that of bronchopneumonia, with high fever, moderate to severe cough, night sweats, dullness to percussion, rales, and decreased breath sounds. Liquefaction in the center may result in formation of a thin-walled cavity, which may become a tension cavity as a result of a valvelike mechanism that allows air to enter but not escape. The enlarging focus may slough debris into adjacent bronchi, leading to intrapulmonary dissemination. Rupture of the cavity into the pleural space causes a bronchopleural fistula or pyopneumothorax; rupture into the pericardium causes acute pericarditis. Before the advent of antituberculosis chemotherapy, the mortality rate of progressive primary pulmonary tuberculosis was 30–50%. Currently, with effective treatment, the prognosis is excellent for full recovery.

Older children and adolescents, especially those with reactivation-type tuberculosis, are more likely to experience fever, anorexia, malaise, weight loss, night sweats, productive cough, chest pain, and hemoptysis than are children with primary pulmonary tuberculosis. However, findings on physical examination are usually minor or absent, even when cavities or large infiltrates are present. Most signs and symptoms improve within several weeks of starting effective treatment, although cough may last for several months. The most common sites for this type of tuberculosis are the original parenchymal focus, the regional lymph nodes, or the apical seedings **(Simon's foci)** established during the early bacillemia of the primary infection. This form of disease usually remains localized to the lungs because the presensitization of tissue to tuberculin evokes an immune response that prevents further lymphohematogenous spread.

Lymphohematogenous Disease. Tubercle bacilli are disseminated to distant sites in all cases of tuberculosis infection. Autopsy cultures of persons who died of other causes within days to weeks after infection with *M. tuberculosis* have grown the organisms from many tissues, most commonly liver, spleen, skin, and lung apices. The clinical picture produced by lymphohematogenous dissemination depends on the quantity of organisms released from the primary focus and the host's immune response.

Lymphohematogenous spread is usually asymptomatic. Patients rarely experience protracted hematogenous tuberculosis caused by the intermittent release of tubercle bacilli as a caseous focus erodes through the wall of a blood vessel in the lung. Although the clinical picture may be acute, more often it is indolent and prolonged, with spiking fevers accompanying the release of organisms into the bloodstream. Multiple organ involvement is common, leading to hepatomegaly, splenomegaly, and lymphadenitis in superficial or deep nodes or papulonecrotic tuberculids appearing in crops on the skin. Bones and joints or the kidneys may become involved. Meningitis, which occurs only late in the course of the disease, was often the cause of death in the prechemotherapy era. Early pulmonary involvement is surprisingly mild, but diffuse lung involvement becomes apparent if treatment is not given promptly. Culture confirmation can be difficult. Bone marrow or liver biopsy with appropriate stains and cultures may be necessary and should be performed if the diagnosis is considered and other tests are unrevealing. The tuberculin skin test is usually reactive.

Miliary Disease. The most common clinically significant form of disseminated tuberculosis is miliary disease, which occurs when massive numbers of tubercle bacilli are released into the bloodstream, causing disease in two or more organs. Miliary tuberculosis is usually an early complication of the primary infection. Although this form of disease is most common in infants and young children, it is also seen in older adults as a result of the breakdown of a previously healed or calcified pulmonary lesion that formed years earlier.

The clinical manifestations of miliary tuberculosis are protean and depend on the load of organisms that disseminate and where they lodge. Tissues have varying susceptibility to infection. Lesions are usually larger and more numerous in the lungs, spleen, liver, and bone marrow than in other organs. The distribution may be caused both by blood supply and by the numbers of reticuloendothelial cells and tissue phagocytes. This form of tuberculosis is most common in infants and malnourished or immunosuppressed patients, suggesting that host immune competency also plays a role.

The onset of clinical disease is sometimes explosive, with the patient becoming gravely ill in several days. More often the onset is insidious; the patient may not be able to pinpoint the time of initial symptoms accurately. Early systemic signs include malaise, anorexia, weight loss, and low-grade fever. At this time, abnormal physical signs are usually absent. Within several weeks hepatosplenomegaly and generalized lymphadenopathy develop in about one half of cases. About this time the fever becomes higher and more sustained, although the chest radiograph usually is normal and respiratory symptoms are few. Within several weeks the lungs become filled with tubercles, and dyspnea, cough, rales, or wheezing occur. As the pulmonary disease progresses, an alveolar air block syndrome may result in frank respiratory distress, hypoxia, and pneumothorax or pneumomediastinum. Signs or symptoms of meningitis or peritonitis are found in 20–40% of patients with advanced disease. Chronic or recurrent headache in a patient with miliary tuberculosis usually indicates the presence of meningitis, whereas the onset of abdominal pain or tenderness is a sign of tuberculous peritonitis. Cutaneous lesions, such as papulonecrotic tuberculids, nodules, or purpura, often appear in crops. Choroid tubercles occur in 13–87% of patients and are highly specific for miliary tuberculosis. The tuberculin skin test is nonreactive in up to 40% of patients.

Pleural Disease. Tuberculous pleural effusions, which can be local or general, usually originate in the discharge of bacilli into the pleural space from a subpleural pulmonary focus or caseated subpleural lymph nodes. Asymptomatic local pleural effusion is so frequent in primary tuberculosis that it is a component of the primary complex. Most large and clinically significant effusions occur months to years after the primary infection. Tuberculous pleural effusion is infrequent in children <6 years of age and rare in those <2 years of age. The effusions are usually unilateral but can be bilateral. They are virtually never associated with a segmental pulmonary lesion and are rare in miliary tuberculosis.

The clinical onset of tuberculous pleurisy is usually fairly sudden. It is characterized by low to high fever, shortness of breath, chest pain (especially on deep inspiration), dullness to percussion, and diminished breath sounds on the affected side. The presentation is similar to that of pyogenic pleurisy. The fever and other symptoms may last for several weeks after the start of antituberculosis chemotherapy. Although corticosteroids reduce the clinical symptoms, they have little effect on the ultimate outcome. The tuberculin skin test is positive in about 80% of cases. The prognosis is excellent; radiographic resolution takes months, however. Scoliosis rarely complicates recovery of a long-standing effusion.

Lymph Node Infection. Tuberculosis of the superficial lymph nodes, sometimes referred to as **scrofula,** is the most common form of extrapulmonary tuberculosis in children. Historically, drinking unpasteurized cow's milk laden with *M. bovis* usually caused scrofula. Through effective veterinary control, *M. bovis* has been virtually eliminated in North America. However, because of inadequate control measures, *M. bovis* disease persists in Mexico. Most current cases of scrofula caused by *M. tuberculosis* occur within 6–9 months of the initial infection, although some cases appear years later. The tonsillar, anterior cervical, and submandibular nodes become involved secondary to extension of a primary lesion of the upper lung fields or abdomen. Infected nodes in the inguinal, epitrochlear, or axillary regions, which are rare in children, result from regional lymphadenitis associated with tuberculosis of the skin or skeletal system.

In the early stages of infection, the lymph nodes usually enlarge gradually. The nodes are firm (but not hard), discrete, and nontender. The nodes often feel fixed to underlying tissue. Disease is most often unilateral, but bilateral involvement may occur because of crossover drainage patterns of lymphatic vessels in the chest and lower neck. As infection progresses multiple nodes are affected; this often results in a mass of matted nodes. Systemic signs and symptoms other than low-grade fever are usually absent. The tuberculin skin test is usually reactive. Although a primary pulmonary focus is virtually always present, it is visible radiographically in only 30–70% of cases. Pulmonary signs and symptoms are often lacking. The illness occasionally is more acute with rapid enlargement of nodes, high fever, tenderness, and fluctuance. The initial presentation is rarely a fluctuant mass with overlying cellulitis or skin discoloration.

If left untreated, the infection may resolve but more often progresses to caseation and necrosis of the lymph node. The capsule of the node breaks down, resulting in the spread of infection to adjacent nodes. The skin overlying the mass of nodes becomes thin, shiny, and erythematous. Rupture results in a draining sinus tract that may require surgical removal (Fig. 35–3).

Meningitis. Central nervous system tuberculosis is the most serious complication in children and is uniformly fatal without effective treatment. The brain stem is the most common focus, and cranial nerves III, VI, and VII are frequently involved. This condition usually arises from the formation of a metastatic caseous lesion in the cerebral cortex or meninges that develops during the occult lymphohematogenous dissemination of the primary infection. This lesion, called a **Rich focus,** increases in size and discharges small numbers of tubercle bacilli into the subarachnoid space. The resulting gelatinous exudate infiltrates the cortical or meningeal blood vessels, producing inflammation, obstruction, and subsequent infarction of cerebral cortex. This exudate interferes with the normal flow of cerebrospinal fluid in and out of the ventricular system at the level of the basal cisterns leading to a communicating hydrocephalus. The combination of vasculitis, infarction, cerebral edema, and hydrocephalus results in the severe damage that can occur gradually or rapidly. Profound abnormalities in electrolyte metabolism, especially hyponatremia, also contribute to the pathophysiology. The syndrome of inappropriate antidiuretic hormone secretion is common and may last for weeks. Other problems, such as salt wasting, make correction of the electrolyte disturbances difficult.

Tuberculous meningitis complicates about 0.3% of untreated primary infections. This condition is extremely rare in infants <4 months of age because pathologic events usually need this time to develop. It is most common in children between 6 months and 4 years of age. Because tuberculous meningitis is an early manifestation of the primary infection, occurring within 2–6 months after infection, the adult source case can usually be identified.

The clinical progression of tuberculous meningitis may be rapid or gradual. Rapid progression tends to occur more often in infants and young children who may experience symptoms for only several days before the onset of acute hydrocephalus, seizures, or cerebral

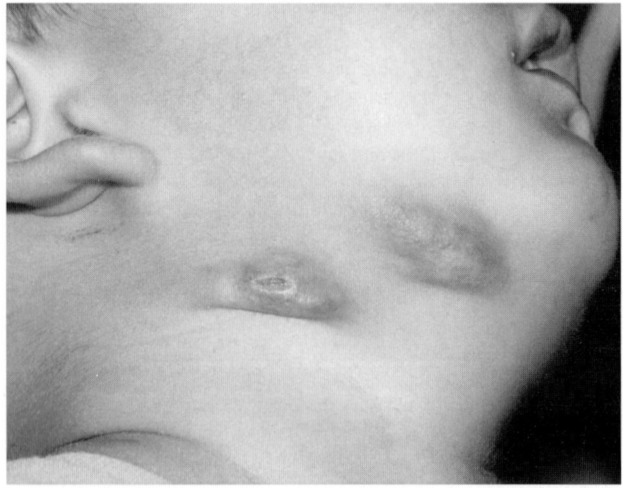

FIGURE 35–3. A draining sinus tract caused by tuberculosis of cervical lymph nodes in a child.

edema. More often, the signs and symptoms progress slowly over several weeks and can be divided into three stages. The first stage, which typically lasts 1–2 weeks, is characterized by nonspecific symptoms, such as fever, headache, irritability, drowsiness, and malaise. Focal neurologic signs are absent, but infants may experience a stagnation or loss of developmental milestones. The second stage begins more abruptly, and lethargy, nuchal rigidity, and Kernig's or Brudzinski's signs, seizures, hypertonia, vomiting, cranial nerve palsies, and other focal neurologic signs are apparent. The clinical picture usually correlates with the development of hydrocephalus, increased intracranial pressure, and vasculitis. Although some children have no evidence of meningeal irritation, they have signs of encephalitis, such as disorientation, abnormal movements, and speech impairment. The third stage is marked by coma, hemiplegia or paraplegia, hypertension, decerebrate posturing, deterioration in vital signs, and, eventually, death.

The prognosis of tuberculous meningitis correlates most closely with the clinical stage of illness at the time antituberculosis chemotherapy begins. The vast majority of patients in the first stage have an excellent outcome, whereas in the third stage most patients who survive have permanent disabilities, including blindness, deafness, paraplegia, diabetes insipidus, and mental retardation. The prognosis for young infants is also poor. It is imperative that antituberculosis treatment be considered for any child in whom basilar meningitis and hydrocephalus or evidence of vasculitis develops with no other apparent cause. Often the key to the diagnosis is identification of the adult source case.

Tuberculoma. Tuberculoma, a tumorlike mass resulting from the aggregation or enlargement of caseous tubercles, usually presents clinically as a brain tumor. Tuberculomas account for up to 40% of intracranial masses in some areas of the world, but they are rare in North America. They occur most often in children <10 years of age; they are usually singular but may be multiple. Lesions are most often supratentorial in adults, but in children they are often infratentorial, located at the base of the brain near the cerebellum. The most common symptoms are headache, fever, and convulsions. The tuberculin skin test is usually reactive, but the chest radiograph is usually unremarkable. Surgical excision may be necessary to distinguish tuberculoma from other brain tumors.

Since the advent of CT, the paradoxical development of tuberculomas in patients with tuberculous meningitis who are receiving ultimately effective chemotherapy has been recognized. The cause and nature of these tuberculomas are poorly understood. Their development is not a failure of drug treatment and does not necessitate a change in the therapeutic regimen. This phenomenon should be considered whenever a child with tuberculous meningitis deteriorates or develops focal neurologic findings while undergoing treatment. Corticosteroids may help alleviate the occasionally severe clinical signs and symptoms. It is unclear how long antituberculosis chemotherapy should be given when these lesions appear. The lesions may be very slow to resolve, persisting for months or even years.

Skeletal Infection. Skeletal tuberculosis usually results from lymphohematogenous seeding of tubercle bacilli during primary infection. Bone infection may also originate as a result of direct extension from a neighboring infected bone. The time interval between infection and clinical disease can be as short as 1 month in cases of tuberculous dactylitis or as much as 30 months or longer for tuberculosis of the hip. The infection usually begins in the metaphysis. Granulation tissue and caseation destroy bone both by direct infection and by pressure necrosis. Soft tissue abscess and extension of the infection through the epiphysis into the nearby joint often complicate the bone lesion. The infection becomes apparent clinically when joint involvement progresses.

Weight-bearing bones and joints are affected most commonly. Most cases of bone tuberculosis occur in the vertebrae, causing tuberculosis of the spine, also known as **Pott's disease.** Although any vertebral body can be involved, there is a predilection for the lower thoracic and upper lumbar vertebrae. Involvement of two or more vertebrae is common; such vertebrae are usually contiguous, but there may be skip areas between lesions. The infection is in the body of the vertebrae, leading to bony destruction and collapse. Tuberculous spondylitis usually progresses from initial narrowing of one or more disk spaces to collapse and wedging of the vertebral body with subsequent angulation of the spine (gibbus) or kyphosis. The infection may extend out from the bone, causing a paraspinal (Pott's), psoas, or retropharyngeal abscess.

The most frequent clinical signs and symptoms of tuberculous spondylitis in children are low-grade fever, irritability, and restlessness, especially at night, associated with back pain, usually without significant tenderness, and abnormal positioning and gait or refusal to walk. Spinal rigidity may be caused by profound muscle spasm. This condition often results from the patient's involuntary effort to immobilize the spine.

Other sites of skeletal tuberculosis, in approximate order of frequency, are the knee, hip, elbow, and ankle. The degree of involvement can range from joint effusion without bone destruction to frank destruction of bone and restriction of the joint caused by chronic fibrosis of the synovial membrane. These forms of tuberculosis, which usually evolve over months to years, most commonly cause mild pain, stiffness, limping, and restricted motion. The tuberculin skin test is reactive in 80–90% of cases. Culture of joint fluid or bone biopsy usually yields the organism. Tuberculosis should be considered in any child with a persistent bone or joint lesion.

Tuberculous dactylitis is a form of bone tuberculosis that is peculiar to infants. In affected children, distal endarteritis develops, followed by painless swelling and cystic bone lesions. Abscesses rarely occur. The tuberculin skin test is usually reactive.

Abdominal and Gastrointestinal Infection. Tuberculosis of the oral cavity or pharynx is very unusual. The most common lesion is a painless ulcer on the mucosa, palate, or tonsil with enlargement of the regional lymph node. Tuberculosis of the larynx causes chronic hoarseness and is often accompanied by upper lobe apical pulmonary disease and sputum production. Tuberculosis of the esophagus is rare in children but may be associated with a tracheoesophageal fistula in infants.

Tuberculous peritonitis occurs most often in young men but is uncommon in adolescents and rare in young children. Generalized peritonitis results from subclinical or miliary hematogenous dissemination. More localized peritonitis is caused by direct extension from an abdominal lymph node infection, an intestinal focus, or tuberculous salpingitis. Pain and tenderness are often mild initially. Rarely, the lymph nodes, omentum, and peritoneum become matted in children; they can be palpated as a "doughy," irregular, nontender mass. Ascites and low-grade fever commonly occur. The tuberculin skin test is usually reactive. The diagnosis can be confirmed by paracentesis with appropriate stains and cultures, but this procedure must be performed carefully to avoid entering bowel intertwined with the matted omentum.

Tuberculous enteritis can be caused by hematogenous dissemination or by swallowing tubercle bacilli discharged from the patient's own lungs or by drinking unpasteurized milk containing *M. bovis.* The jejunum and ileum near Peyer's patches and the appendix are the most common sites of involvement. Shallow ulcers that cause pain, diarrhea, or constipation and weight loss are the usual findings. Mesenteric adenitis usually complicates the infection. The nodes may cause intestinal obstruction or erode through the omentum to cause generalized peritonitis. The clinical presentation of tuberculous enteritis mimics many other conditions and should be suspected in any child with chronic gastrointestinal complaints and a reactive tuberculin skin test. Biopsy, stain, and culture of the lesions are often necessary to confirm the diagnosis.

Genitourinary Infection. Renal tuberculosis is rare in childhood because the incubation period is several years or more. Tubercle bacilli usually reach the kidney during lymphohematogenous dissemination. Before renal parenchymal disease develops, the organisms can be recovered from the urine in many cases of miliary tuberculosis and in some patients with primary pulmonary tuberculosis. In true renal tuberculosis, small caseous tubercles develop in the renal parenchyma and release *M. tuberculosis* into the tubules. A large mass may develop near the renal cortex and discharge large numbers of bacteria through a fistula into the renal pelvis. Infection then spreads locally to the ureters, prostate, or epididymis.

Renal tuberculosis is clinically silent in the early stages, with the only signs being sterile pyuria and microscopic hematuria. Dysuria, flank or abdominal pain, and gross hematuria develop as the disease progresses. Superinfection by other bacteria occurs frequently and may delay recognition of the underlying tuberculosis. Hydronephrosis or ureteral stricture may complicate the disease. Urine cultures for *M. tuberculosis* are positive in about 80–90% of cases; acid-fast stains of large volumes of urine sediment are positive less frequently. The tuberculin skin test is usually reactive.

Tuberculosis of the genital tract is uncommon in both boys and girls before puberty. This condition originates from lymphohematogenous spread, although it can arise from direct spread from the intestinal tract or bone. In adolescent girls, genital tract tuberculosis may develop during the primary infection. The fallopian tubes are most often involved (90–100% of cases), followed by the endometrium (50%), ovaries (25%), and cervix (5%). The usual symptoms are lower abdominal pain and dysmenorrhea or amenorrhea. Systemic manifestations are often absent, and the chest radiograph is normal in the majority of cases. Chronic infection leads to infertility.

Genital tuberculosis in adolescent boys causes epididymitis or orchitis, occurring as a nodular, painless swelling of the scrotum that is usually unilateral. Involvement of the glans penis is rare.

Other Sites of Infection. The most common form of cardiac tuberculosis is pericarditis, which arises by direct invasion or lymphatic drainage from subcarinal lymph nodes. The pericardial fluid is serofibrinous or slightly hemorrhagic early in the course of the disease. Presenting symptoms, including low-grade fever, malaise, and weight loss, are often nonspecific. Chest pain is unusual in children. A pericardial friction rub or distant heart sounds with pulsus paradoxus may be present. As infection progresses, fibrosis develops, leading to obliteration of the pericardial sac and constrictive pericarditis. The child may become extremely ill with respiratory distress and evidence of cardiac failure. Diagnosis usually requires pericardiocentesis with pericardial biopsy. Acid-fast stain of pericardial fluid is rarely positive, but cultures are positive in 30–70% of cases. In addition to antituberculosis chemotherapy, a partial or complete pericardiectomy may be required to relieve constrictive pericarditis.

Ocular tuberculosis is rare in children. This condition most often involves the conjunctiva or the cornea and usually occurs as a result of direct inoculation. Unilateral redness and lacrimation are associated with enlargement of the preauricular, submandibular, or cervical lymph nodes. Tuberculosis of the ciliary body or iris and tuberculous uveitis are exceedingly rare.

Tuberculosis of the middle ear results from a primary focus in neonates who aspirate infected amniotic fluid or from hematogenous dissemination in older children. The most common signs and symptoms are painless otorrhea, tinnitus, decreased hearing, facial paralysis, and a perforated tympanic membrane. Enlargement of lymph nodes in the preauricular or anterior cervical chains may accompany infection. Disease is almost exclusively unilateral. Diagnosis can be difficult for two reasons: stains and cultures are frequently negative, and histologic specimens of the affected tissue often show acute and chronic inflammation without granuloma formation.

Cutaneous tuberculosis was more common decades ago. It arises as an extension of disease from the primary complex, from hematogenous dissemination, or from hypersensitivity to the tubercle bacillus. Skin lesions associated with the primary complex can be caused by direct inoculation of the skin through an abrasion, cut, or insect bite. Regional lymphadenitis is striking, but systemic symptoms are usually lacking. The most common form of hypersensitivity lesion is erythema nodosum, which is characterized by large, painful, purple-brown, indurated nodules on the shins and forearms. **Scrofuloderma** occurs when a caseous lymph node ruptures to the outside, leaving an ulcer or a sinus tract. **Papulonecrotic tuberculids** are miliary lesions of the skin that appear most frequently on the face, trunk, and upper thighs. Their characteristic ''apple jelly'' center is best demonstrated by placing a glass slide over the lesions. **Tuberculosis verrucosa cutis** is a wartlike lesion, most common on the arms or legs, that may represent autoinoculation of tubercle bacilli in a person already sensitized to the organism (Fig. 35–4).

Congenital Infection. Symptoms of hematogenous congenital tuberculosis may be present at birth but more commonly begin by the second or third week of life. The most common signs and symptoms are the classic triad of respiratory distress, fever, and

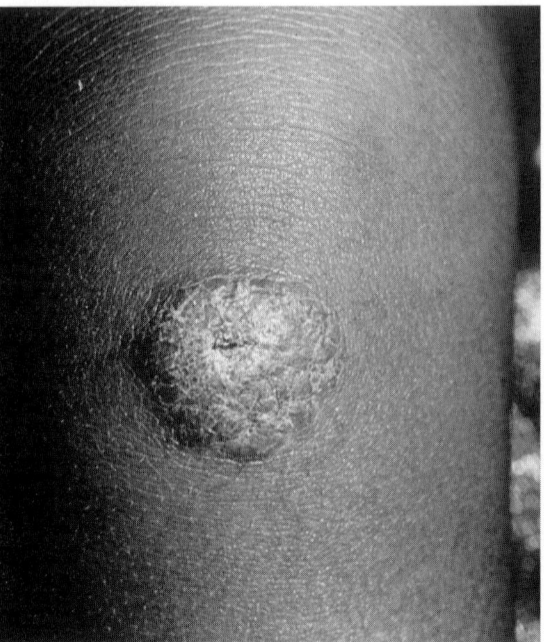

FIGURE 35–4. "Warty" tuberculosis (verrucosa cutis) below the knee of a child who also had pulmonary tuberculosis.

hepatic or splenic enlargement, which may be accompanied in order of frequency by poor feeding, lethargy or irritability, lymphadenopathy, abdominal distention, failure to thrive, ear drainage, and skin lesions. The clinical manifestations vary in relation to the site and size of the caseous lesions. Many infants have an abnormal chest radiograph, most often with a miliary pattern. In some infants with no pulmonary findings early in the course of the disease, profound radiographic and clinical abnormalities later develop. Hilar and mediastinal lymphadenopathy and parenchymal infiltrates are common.

The clinical presentation of congenital tuberculosis may be similar to that caused by bacterial sepsis and other congenital infections. Neonatal tuberculosis should be suspected in infants with signs and symptoms of bacterial or congenital infection whose response to antibiotic and supportive therapy is poor and whose evaluation for other infections is unrevealing.

The most important clue for rapid diagnosis of congenital tuberculosis is usually in the maternal or family history of tuberculosis. Frequently, the mother's disease is discovered after the neonate's tuberculosis is suspected. The tuberculin skin test in the infant is always negative initially but may become positive in 1–3 months. A positive acid-fast stain of an early morning gastric aspirate in a newborn usually indicates tuberculosis. Direct acid-fast stains on middle ear fluid, bone marrow, tracheal aspirates, or biopsy material (especially liver) can be useful and should be performed. The CSF should be examined and cultured, although the yield for isolating *M. tuberculosis* is low and less than 25% of affected infants have meningitis.

HIV-Infected Children. An increasing number of children with coexisting tuberculosis and HIV infection have been reported. The diagnosis of tuberculosis can be missed in an HIV-infected child because skin test reactivity may be absent, culture confirmation is difficult, and the clinical appearance of tuberculosis may be similar to that of other HIV-related infections. Tuberculosis in HIV-infected children appears similar clinically to that in immunocompetent children, but disease may be more severe and extrapulmonary manifestations are more common. Pulmonary symptoms accompanied by fever and weight loss are the usual presentation. There is an increased tendency toward progressive pulmonary disease with cavitation.

DIAGNOSIS

In many children, tuberculosis is discovered through contact investigations of adults who have infectious tuberculosis. In many cases, these children have asymptomatic disease that would have progressed or escaped detection if the contact tracing had not occurred. Some diagnoses are made after a symptomatic illness begins. A strong index of suspicion for tuberculosis is required to identify the cause of illness correctly because the signs and symptoms of most forms of the disease are similar to those of many other infections and conditions.

The diagnosis of disseminated or miliary tuberculosis is often difficult. For infants and children, discovery of an adult source case for the infection often leads to the correct diagnosis. Many young patients with tuberculosis present with fever of unknown origin and have few specific signs or symptoms. Up to 40% of infants and children have a negative tuberculin skin test initially, and most of these patients are globally anergic. Examinations of sputum, urine, or gastric contents may be unrevealing at first; biopsy of the liver or bone marrow may facilitate a more rapid diagnosis.

Confirming a presumptive diagnosis of tuberculous meningitis can be especially difficult if an adult index case cannot be found. The tuberculin skin test is negative in 30–50% of cases, and up to one half of children have a normal chest radiograph. Mycobacteria culture of gastric aspirates should be obtained from any child with suspected tuberculous meningitis. Treatment must often be empiric and based on a high index of suspicion.

The importance of the epidemiologic setting of the child in establishing the diagnosis of tuberculosis cannot be overemphasized. The child's relative risk of tuberculosis influences the interpretation of the skin test and chest radiograph.

Tuberculin Skin Test. A positive tuberculin skin test reaction is the hallmark of infection with *M. tuberculosis.* Within 8 years of his discovery of the tubercle bacillus in 1882, Koch found that subcutaneous injection of a broth culture filtrate of tubercle bacilli into a person with tuberculosis caused induration at the injection site. In 1939 Seibert developed a **purified protein derivative (PPD)** from tubercle bacilli in broth culture that became the standard, or **PPD-S.** Commercially produced PPD is standardized against the original lot of PPD-S. When tuberculin reactivity is caused by infection with *M. tuberculosis,* this test usually remains positive for the individual's lifetime. However, it returns to negative in a small number of persons who are treated with isoniazid soon after infection occurs.

Two techniques are used for tuberculin skin testing: **multiple puncture tests** and the **Mantoux test.** Multiple puncture tests were designed for mass screening, which is no longer performed. They should never be used in today's clinical practice.

The Mantoux tuberculin skin test technique uses the intradermal injection of 0.1 mL containing 5 tuberculin units (TU) of PPD stabilized with Tween 80. Technique must be precise and consistent. The results are interpreted as the transverse diameter of induration present after 48–72 hours (Fig. 35–5). Occasionally a significant reaction (interpreted as positive) will not be apparent until after 96 hours or more. Although experienced examiners usually

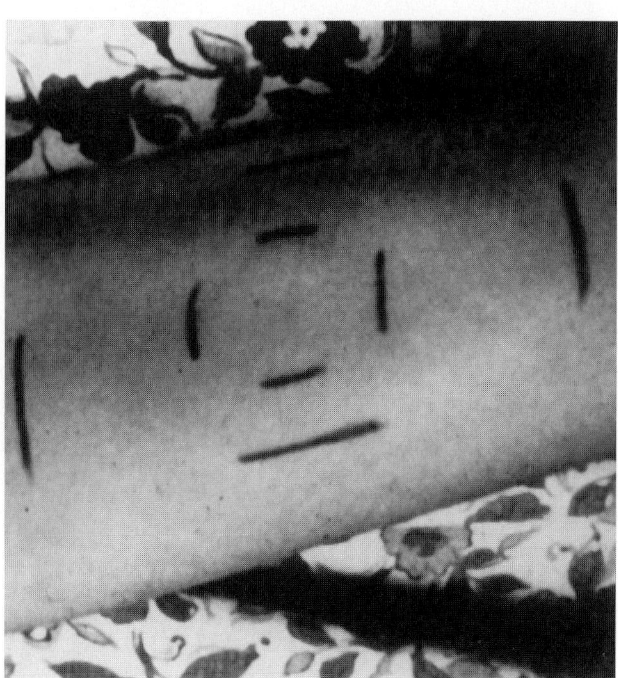

FIGURE 35–5. A positive Mantoux skin test for tuberculosis. The reaction consists of an inner zone of induration (inner marks) and an outer zone of edema and erythema (outer marks). Interpretation is based on the transverse diameter of induration after 48–72 hours.

agree on results, inexperienced observers, especially parents, frequently interpret and report results inaccurately.

A variety of host-related factors, such as very young age, malnutrition, immunosuppression by disease or drugs, viral infections (especially measles, varicella, and influenza), and overwhelming tuberculosis, can depress tuberculin reactivity in a child infected with *M. tuberculosis*. Corticosteroid therapy may decrease the reaction to tuberculin, but the effect is variable and may be limited to the first several months of steroid administration. However, tuberculin skin testing at the initiation of corticosteroid therapy is probably reliable. Approximately 10% of immunocompetent children with pulmonary tuberculosis do not react initially to 5 TU of PPD; most become reactive after several months of treatment, suggesting that the disease contributed to the anergy. Anergy may be global or specific to tuberculin; thus having positive control skin tests with a negative tuberculin test never rules out tuberculosis.

False-positive reactions to tuberculin can be caused by cross-sensitization to antigens of nontuberculous mycobacteria. These cross-reactions usually are transient over several months to years. They usually produce induration of less than 10 mm, although they occasionally reach 15 mm or more.

A history of prior BCG vaccination is never a contraindication to tuberculin testing. No reliable method distinguishes tuberculin reactions caused by BCG vaccination from those resulting from infection with *M. tuberculosis,* however. Many infants who receive BCG vaccine never have a tuberculin reaction. When a reaction does occur, the induration size is usually <10 mm, and the reaction wanes after several years. In general, a reactive area of ≥10 mm in a BCG-vaccinated child with risk factors for exposure to tuberculosis indicates infection with *M. tuberculosis* and necessitates further diagnostic evaluation and usually chemotherapy.

The interpretation of the Mantoux tuberculin reaction should be influenced by the purpose for which the test was given and the consequences of false classification. The appropriate size of induration indicating a positive test varies with related epidemiologic factors. For example, a person in a high-risk group for tuberculosis or with clinical signs or symptoms consistent with tuberculosis who has a mild reaction to a tuberculin test is more likely to be infected with *M. tuberculosis* than is a low-risk person with greater induration, who is probably demonstrating a false-positive result. For children, determination of whether there has been exposure to an adult with infectious tuberculosis is crucial.

Because there is always some overlap in reactions to the Mantoux test between groups of persons with and without tuberculosis infection, false-positive and false-negative results always occur. To minimize false results, reaction size limits for determining a positive result are established and patients are stratified by risk of infection (Table 35–4). For adults and children at high risk of having infection progress to disease, a reactive area of ≥5 mm is classified as a positive result. For other high-risk groups, including infants, a reactive area of ≥10 mm is considered positive. For all other low-risk persons, particularly in communities where the prevalence of tuberculosis is low, the cutoff point for a positive reaction may be raised to ≥15 mm. Classification of children by this scheme depends on the willingness and ability of the clinician to obtain a thorough history not only of the child but also of the adults who care for the child. To interpret the tuberculin skin test correctly, the physician must clearly understand tuberculosis case rates and characteristics within the community and the indication for tuberculin testing in the individual patient.

TABLE 35–4. Decision Rules for a "Positive" Mantoux Tuberculin Reaction

≥5 mm
Contacts to infectious cases
Abnormal chest radiograph or signs and symptoms
HIV-infected and other immunosuppressed patients
≥10 mm
Other high-risk individuals listed in Table 35–1
≥15 mm
Individuals with no risk factors

Bronchoscopy. Several excellent reported series of children with pulmonary tuberculosis in the 1940s through the 1960s used rigid-scope bronchoscopy to help define the pathophysiology and natural progression of the disease. At present, bronchoscopy plays a fairly minor role in the diagnosis and management of tuberculosis in children. Bronchoscopy cultures alone are not reliable; the culture yield from bronchoscopy for *M. tuberculosis* is usually lower than that for gastric aspirates. The greatest current use for flexible-scope bronchoscopy is to help diagnose tuberculosis initially when radiographic, skin test, and epidemiologic data are not clear or available. Bronchoscopy can also help exclude such diagnoses as foreign body aspiration and pyogenic infection. This procedure can establish the diagnosis of endobronchial tuberculosis with or without the presence of a fistulous tract. The information provided may help the clinician determine whether a course of corticosteroids is beneficial for the child, although this approach has not been subjected to adequate randomized clinical trials.

Laboratory Evaluation

Laboratory tests such as a CBC and cell differential count, ESR, urinalysis, and blood chemistries are usually normal in children with tuberculosis. Abnormalities in liver enzyme or function test findings may be indicative of hepatic involvement in miliary tuberculosis.

Pleural Fluid. Examination of pleural fluid and pleural membrane is vital to establish the diagnosis of tuberculous pleurisy. The pleural fluid is usually yellow and only occasionally tinged with blood. The chemistry results are indicative of a mild exudate: the specific gravity is 1.012–1.025, the protein level is usually 2–4 g/dL, and the glucose level may be low, although it is often in the low-normal range (20–40 mg/dL). Most typically, there are several hundred to several thousand WBC/mm^3 with an early predominance of polymorphonuclear cells followed by a high frequency of lymphocytes. Acid-fast smears of the fluid are rarely positive because of the relative paucity of organisms in the fluid. Cultures are positive in only 30–70% of cases. Biopsy of the pleura is more likely to yield a positive acid-fast stain or culture, and evidence of granuloma formation can be demonstrated. Some investigators have found assays for adenosine deaminase in the pleural fluid to be useful for distinguishing tuberculous from other plueral effusions, but this test is not generally available in North America.

Cerebrospinal Fluid. The most important laboratory test for the diagnosis of tuberculous meningitis is the examination and culture of the lumbar CSF. The CSF leukocyte count usually ranges from 10 to 500/mm^3 but occasionally is higher. Polymorphonuclear leukocytes may predominate initially, but in the large majority of cases, lymphocytes are predominant. The CSF glucose level is typically <40 mg/dL but is rarely <20 mg/dL. The protein level is elevated and may be markedly high (400–5,000 mg/dL) secondary to hydrocephalus and spinal block. Although the lumbar CSF is grossly abnormal, the ventricular CSF may have normal chemistries and cell counts because samples are obtained proximal to the site of the obstruction. The diagnosis of tuberculous meningitis can be missed if a ventricular CSF sample is the only one obtained. The success of microscopic examination of acid-fast stained CSF and mycobacterial culture is directly related to the amount of CSF sampled. Examinations or culture of <1 mL of CSF are unlikely to demonstrate *M. tuberculosis*. When 5–10 mL of lumbar CSF can be obtained, the acid-fast stain of the CSF sediment may be positive in up to 30% of cases, and the culture is positive in 70%.

Microbiologic Evaluation

The most important laboratory tests for the diagnosis and management of tuberculosis are the acid-fast stain and mycobacterial culture (Chapter 7). An estimated 10,000 organisms per milliliter are required for a positive smear; identification of a single organism on a slide is suspicious. The best culture specimen for pulmonary tuberculosis in a child is the early morning gastric aspirate obtained before the child has arisen and peristalsis has emptied the stomach of the pooled secretions that have been swallowed overnight. Unfortunately, even under optimal conditions, three gastric aspirates yield *M. tuberculosis* in fewer than 50% of cases; negative cultures never exclude the diagnosis of tuberculosis in a child. The yield from flexible bronchoscopy is less than from properly obtained gastric aspirates.

Fortunately, the need for culture confirmation is usually small. If the child has a positive tuberculin skin test, clinical or radiographic findings suggestive of tuberculosis, and previous contact with an adult source case, he or she should be treated for tuberculosis disease. The drug susceptibility test results from the source case's isolate can be used to determine the best therapeutic regimen. Cultures should be grown and susceptibility tests performed on specimens from a child with suspected tuberculosis when the source case is unknown or when the source case has a drug-resistant isolate. The yield from gastric aspirate acid-fast stains is much lower than for culture, but a markedly positive result from gastric fluid usually indicates pulmonary tuberculosis.

The serodiagnosis of tuberculosis has long been envisioned but, in practice, has been disappointing. A variety of whole cell and specific antigens have been studied, but none has been sufficiently successful to be considered for commercial application in North America. Detection of structural components of the cell wall of *M. tuberculosis* in patient specimens is another approach. Tuberculostearic acid, a mycolic acid that is almost unique to *M. tuberculosis,* has been found in the CSF and sputum of patients with tuberculosis. This fairly sensitive and highly specific test requires the use of gas chromatography and mass spectrometry with ion monitoring. It is available only from several research laboratories.

Nucleic Acid Amplification (PCR). The form of nucleic acid amplification studied in children with tuberculosis is PCR using the mycobacterial insertion element IS6110 as the DNA marker for *M. tuberculosis* complex organism (Chapter 12). Compared with a clinical diagnosis of pulmonary tuberculosis in children, the sensitivity of PCR has varied from 25–83% and specificity has varied from 80–100% in clinical trials. Some false-positive results occurred in children with disease caused by nontuberculous mycobacteria. The PCR test performed on gastric aspirate contents is positive in some children with recent tuberculosis infection and a normal chest radiograph, demonstrating the occasional arbitrariness of the distinction between tuberculosis infection and disease in children. The PCR may give suggestive results but has a limited role in evaluating children for tuberculosis. A negative PCR result does not eliminate tuberculosis as a diagnostic possibility, and a positive result does not represent absolute confirmation. PCR may help in evaluating children with significant pulmonary disease when the diagnosis of tuberculosis cannot be established on clinical and epidemiologic grounds. There have been published case reports of the use of PCR to diagnose extrapulmonary tuberculosis—meningitis using CSF, pleuritis using pleural fluid, and lymph node disease using tissues—but there have been no clinical trials.

Diagnostic Imaging

Because many cases of pulmonary tuberculosis in children are relatively silent clinically, radiography is a cornerstone for the diagnosis of disease. As expected, the radiographic findings mirror the pathophysiology of primary and reactivation disease.

The intial parenchymal inflammation that follows deposition of infected droplet nuclei in the alveoli of the lung usually is not visible radiographically. However, a localized, nonspecific infiltrate with an overlying pleural reaction may be seen. This lesion usually resolves within 1–2 weeks. All lobar segments of the lung are at equal risk of being the focus of infection. In 25% of cases two or more lobes of the lungs are involved, although disease usually occurs at only one site. Spread of infection to regional lymph nodes occurs early.

The hallmark of childhood pulmonary tuberculosis is the relatively large size and importance of the hilar lymphadenitis compared with the less significant size of the initial parenchymal focus, together historically referred to as **Ghon's complex** (with or without calcification of the lymph nodes). Because of the usual pattern of lymphatic circulation in the chest, a left-sided parenchymal focus often leads to bilateral hilar lymphadenopathy whereas a right-sided focus is associated only with right-sided adenitis. Hilar adenopathy is inevitably present with childhood tuberculosis, but it may not be detected on a plain radiograph when calcification is not present. Both calcified and noncalcified lymph nodes are detected by CT.

In most cases of tuberculosis infection, the mild parenchymal infiltrate and lymphadenitis resolve spontaneously, the chest radiograph remains normal, and the child has no symptoms. In some children, the hilar or mediastinal lymph nodes continue to enlarge, often best demonstrated in the lateral chest radiograph (Fig. 35–6). Partial bronchial obstruction caused by external compression from the enlarging nodes can cause air trapping, hyperinflation, and even lobar emphysema (Fig. 35–7). As the nodes attach to and infiltrate the bronchial wall, caesium fills the lumen, causing complete obstruction. This results in atelectasis that usually involves the lobar segment distal to the obstructed bronchial lumen. The resulting radiographic shadows are usually called collapse-consolidation or segmental lesions. These findings are similar to those caused by aspiration of a foreign body; in essence, the lymph node is acting as the foreign body. Segmental lesions are more common in infants than in older children, undoubtedly because of the smaller diameter of the infants' airways. Multiple segmental lesions in different lobes may be apparent simultaneously. Segmental atelectasis and hyperinflation lesions also occur together.

Other radiographic findings occur in some patients. Occasionally children have a picture of lobar pneumonia without impressive hilar lymphadenopathy. Newborns with congenital tuberculosis usually have extensive pulmonary disease (Fig. 35–8). In infants the radiographic appearance can be that of an exudative pneumonia with bowing of the fissure (Fig. 35–9). This appearance is similar to one caused by pyogenic pneumonia, particularly when caused by *Klebsiella pneumoniae.* Secondary bacterial infection may contribute to this appearance of tuberculosis. If the infection is progressively destructive, liquefaction of the lung parenchyma leads to formation of a thin-walled primary tuberculous cavity. Rarely, bullous lesions occur in the lungs and can cause pneumothorax. Enlargement of the subcarinal lymph nodes can cause compression of the esophagus and, rarely, a bronchoesophageal fistula. A sign of subcarinal tuberculosis is horizontal splaying of the mainstem bronchi.

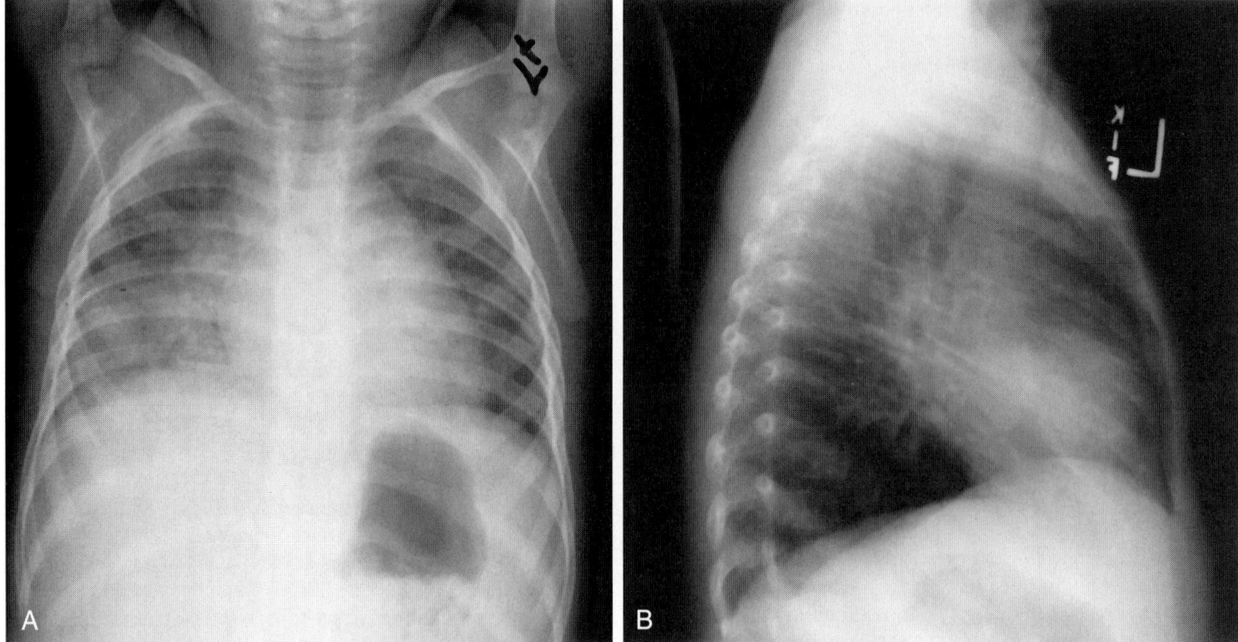

FIGURE 35–6. Pulmonary tuberculosis in a child. The posteroanterior view **(A)** shows a homogenous lesion, whereas the lateral view **(B)** shows more distinct hilar adenopathy and atelectasis.

Adolescents with pulmonary tuberculosis may develop segmental lesions with hilar lymphadenopathy or the apical infiltrates, with or without cavitation, that are typical of adult reactivation tuberculosis. Regional lymphadenitis is absent in this type of disease. Lordotic views or tomograms may be necessary to demonstrate small apical foci of disease.

The course of thoracic lymphadenopathy and bronchial obstruction can follow several paths if antituberculosis chemotherapy is not given. In many cases the segment or lobe re-expands and the radiographic abnormalities resolve completely. Of course, children still have infection with *M. tuberculosis* and are at high risk of reactivation tuberculosis in subsequent years. The calcified foci containing live organisms may break down later in life, leading to reactivation disease. In some cases, the segmental lesion resolves with residual calcification of the primary parenchymal focus or regional lymph nodes (Fig. 35–10). The calcification usually occurs in fine particles, creating a stippling effect. Calcification begins 6 months or more after infection. Finally, bronchial obstruction may cause scarring and progressive contraction of the lobe or segment, which is often associated with cylindrical bronchiectasis leading to chronic pyogenic infection. Complete radiographic and clinical resolution without calcification occurs in the vast majority of cases with early institution of adequate treatment for collapse-consolidation lesions.

Chest radiography is useful in the diagnosis of miliary and pleural tuberculosis. When first visible, the lesions of miliary tuberculosis are usually <2–3 mm in diameter (Fig. 35–11). As disease progresses, the smaller lesions coalesce to form larger lesions and sometimes extensive infiltrates. Hilar lymphadenopathy frequently accompanies the more diffuse milary lesions but is extremely rare with tuberculous pleurisy. Tuberculous pleural effusion may be localized or massive (Fig. 35–12). Often the radiographic picture is much more extensive than would be suggested by physical findings or symptoms. The effusion usually resolves completely over several months, although residual basilar scarring may be apparent.

Radiographic studies may aid greatly in the diagnosis of extrapulmonary tuberculosis in children. Plain radiographs, CT, and MRI of the tuberculous spine usually demonstrate collapse and destruction of the vertebral body with narrowing of the involved disk spaces (Fig. 35–13). Radiographic findings in bone and joint tuberculosis range from mild joint effusions and small lytic lesions to massive destruction of the bone (Fig. 35–14).

These studies also are useful in the diagnosis of tuberculosis of the CNS. CT or MRI of the brains of patients with tuberculous meningitis may be normal during early stages of the infection. As the disease progresses, basilar enhancement and communicating hydrocephalus with signs of cerebral edema or early focal ischemia are the most common findings. Tuberculomas usually appear as discrete lesions with a significant amount of surrounding edema (Fig. 35–15). Contrast enhancement is often impressive and may result in **ring enhancement** with a ringlike lesion. Angiographic studies show that, unlike many types of brain tumor, tuberculomas usually are avascular.

In children, with renal tuberculosis, intravenous pyelograms may reveal mass lesions, dilation of the proximal ureters, multiple small filling defects, and hydronephrosis if ureteral stricture is present (Fig. 35–16).

TREATMENT

Mycobacteria replicate slowly and can remain dormant in the body for prolonged periods. Tubercle bacilli can be killed only while replicating, and replication is most frequent among bacteria that are metabolically active. The treatment of tuberculosis is affected by the presence of naturally occurring drug-resistant organisms in large bacterial populations, even before chemotherapy is initiated. Although a population of bacilli as a whole may be considered drug susceptible, a subpopulation of drug-resistant organisms occurs at fairly predictable frequencies. The mean frequency for these drug-resistant organisms is about 10^{-6} but varies among drugs: for strep-

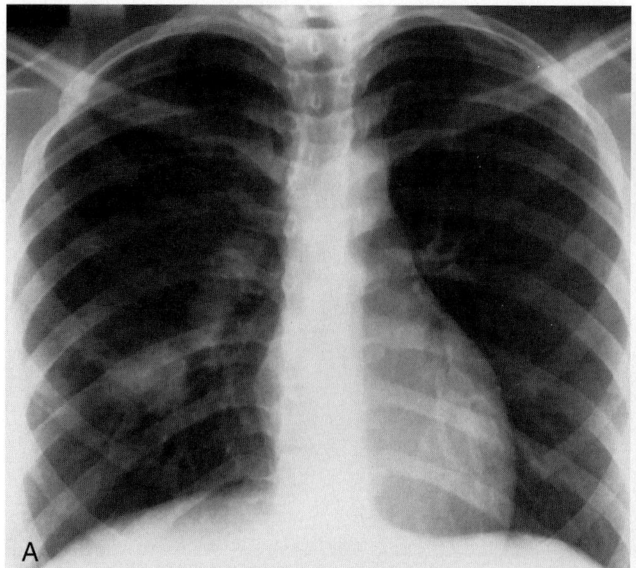

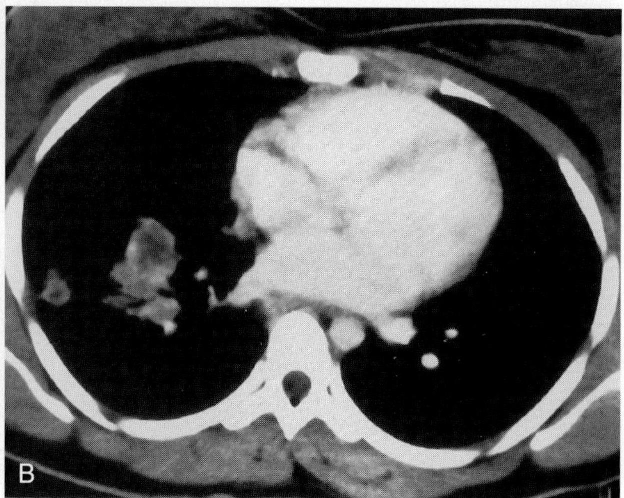

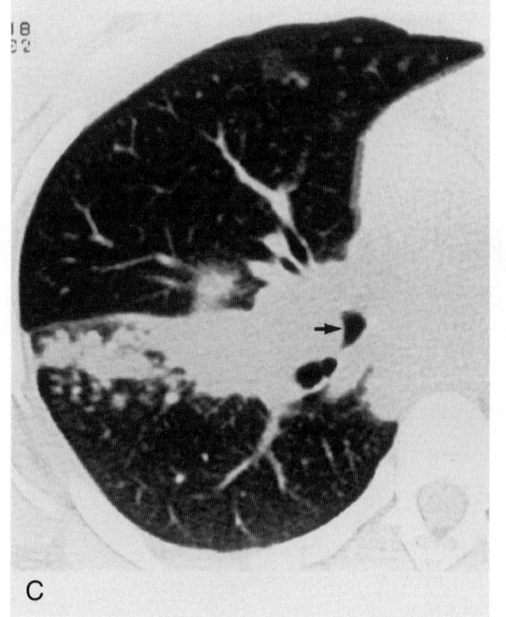

FIGURE 35–7. Primary tuberculosis in a 12-year-old symptom-free girl with a history of family exposure to tuberculosis. A frontal chest radiograph **(A)** shows a small parenchymal infiltrate in the right midlung with associated right hilar lymphadenopathy. A CT scan **(B)** with intravenous contrast shows low attenuation within the primary lesion as well as a smaller, more peripheral lesion. A thin-section, high-resolution CT scan **(C)** reveals endobronchial compression *(arrow)* by the adjacent enlarged lymph nodes, as well as the wide extent of pulmonary infiltration and its subpleural (minor fissure) location. (From Agrons G, Markowitz R, Kramer S: Pulmonary tuberculosis in children. *Semin Roentgenol* 1993;28: 158–72.)

tomycin, 10^{-5}; for isoniazid, 10^{-6}; and for rifampin, 10^{-7}. A cavity containing 10^{9} tubercle bacilli has thousands of drug-resistant organisms, whereas a closed caseous lesion with its much smaller population contains few, if any, resistant organisms.

These microbiologic characteristics of *M. tuberculosis* help explain why single antimicrobial drugs cannot cure cavitary tuberculosis. If a single drug is given to adults with cavitary tuberculosis, the vast majority of patients have a significant number of organisms resistant to that drug in several months. Fortunately, the occurrence of resistance to one drug is independent of resistance to any other drug. The chance that an organism is naturally resistant to two drugs is on the order of 10^{-11} to 10^{-13}. Because populations of this size rarely occur in patients, organisms naturally resistant to two drugs are essentially nonexistent.

The major biologic determinant of the success of antituberculosis therapy is the size of the bacterial population within the host. For patients with large populations of bacilli, such as adults with cavities or extensive infiltrates, many drug-resistant organisms are present initially and at least two antituberculosis drugs must be given. Conversely, for patients with tuberculosis infection but no disease, the bacterial population is small, drug-resistant organisms are rare or nonexistent, and a single drug such as isoniazid can be given. Children with primary pulmonary tuberculosis and patients with extrapulmonary tuberculosis have medium-sized populations in which significant numbers of drug-resistant organisms may or may not be present. In general, these patients are treated with at least two drugs.

Actions of Antituberculosis Drugs. The various antituberculosis drugs differ in their primary site of activity and their actions. Isoniazid and rifampin are bactericidal for *M. tuberculosis* and are effective against all populations of mycobacteria. Streptomycin and several other aminoglycosides are also bactericidal for tubercle bacilli. Pyrazinamide cannot be shown to be bactericidal in the

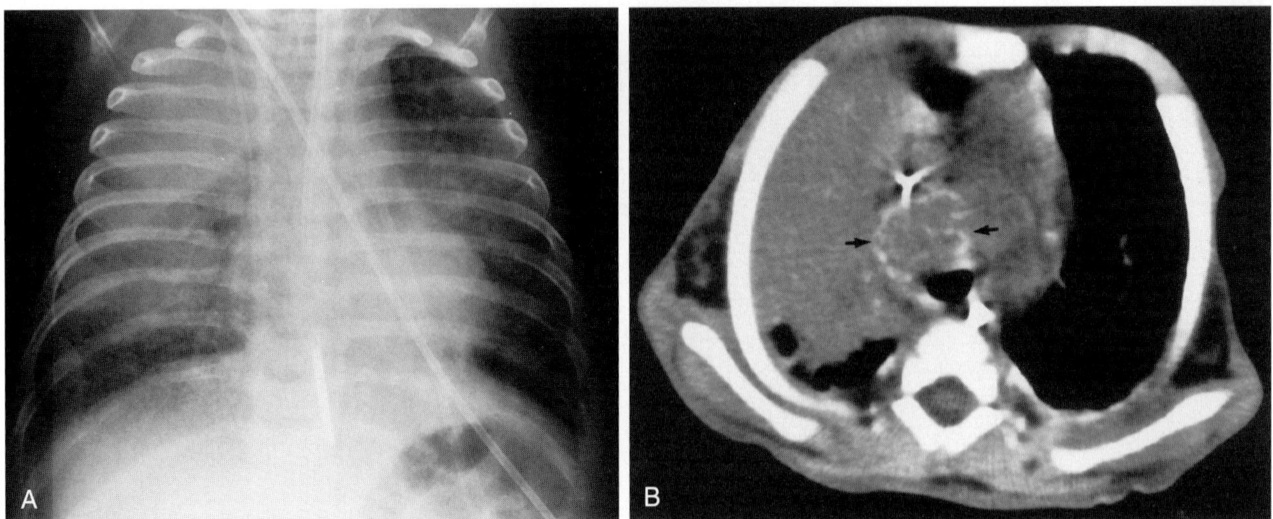

FIGURE 35–8. Congenital tuberculosis in a 6-week-old infant. A posteroanterior chest radiograph **(A)** reveals bilateral pulmonary infiltrates and complete opacification of the right upper lobe. A CT scan of the chest **(B)** shows the consolidation of the right lung and multiple small calcifications in the lymph nodes *(arrows)*. Dark areas in the subpleural posterior portion of the right upper lobe represent areas of frank necrosis. (From Agrons G, Markowitz R, Kramer S: Pulmonary tuberculosis in children. *Semin Roentgenol* 1993;28:158–72.)

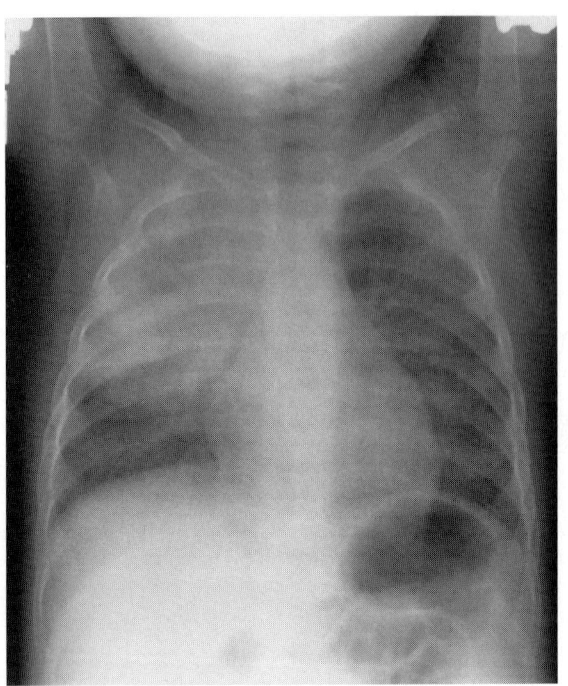

FIGURE 35–9. Pulmonary tuberculosis resulting in the appearance of an exudative pneumonia, with bowing of the horizontal fissure.

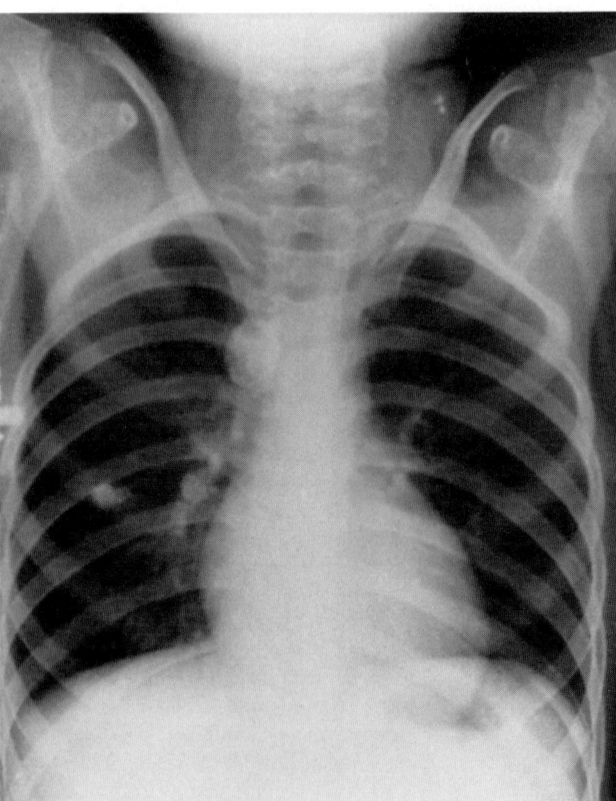

FIGURE 35–10. Calcified parenchymal lesion and mediastinal lymph nodes in a child with tuberculosis.

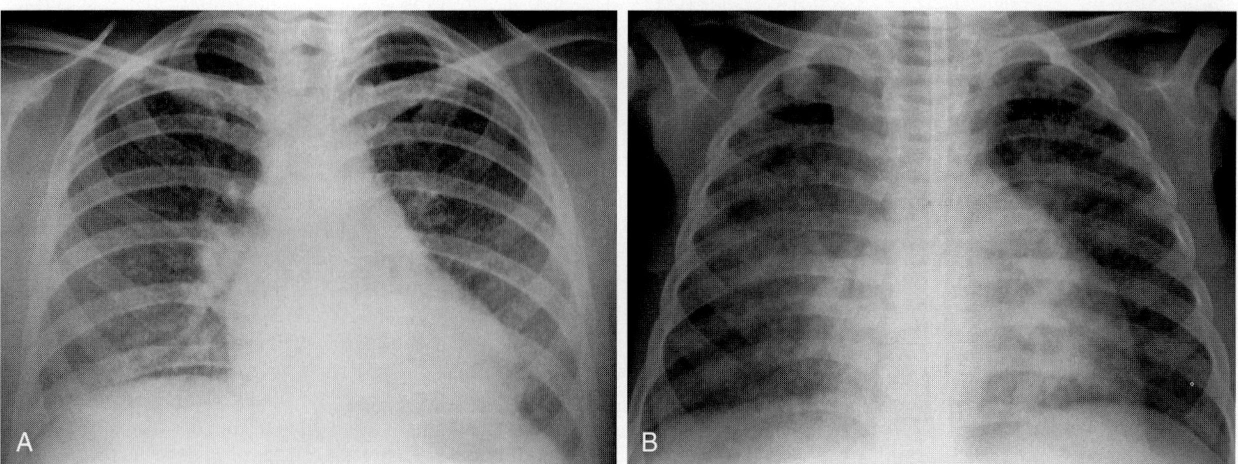

FIGURE 35–11. Miliary tuberculosis. **A,** Fine nodular pattern in a 2-year old child with fever and mild tachypnea. **B,** Coarse nodular pattern in a 1-year-old with moderate respiratory distress. The reticulonodular infiltrate tends to coalesce in the perihilar regions. The upper mediastinum is widened as a result of paratracheal lymphadenopathy. (From Agrens G, Markowitz R, Kramer S: Pulmonary tuberculosis in children. *Semin Roentgenol* 1993;28:158–72.)

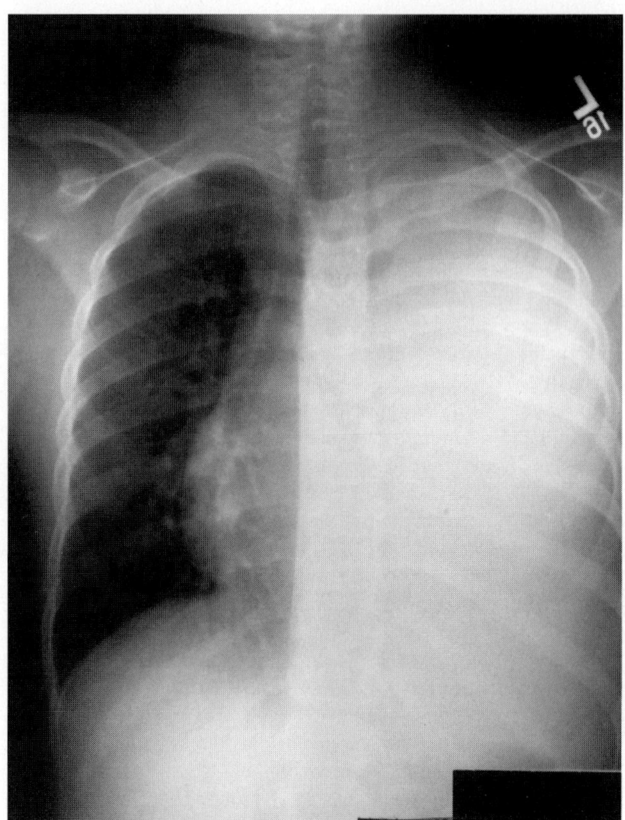

FIGURE 35–12. Massive tuberculous pleural effusion in an 8-year-old girl who was infected by a school janitor.

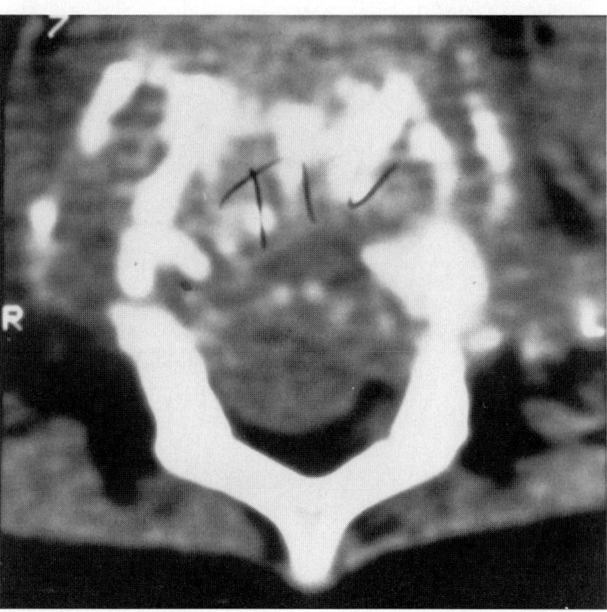

FIGURE 35–13. A CT scan of a child with tuberculosis of the spine, showing massive destruction of the twelfth thoracic vertebral body.

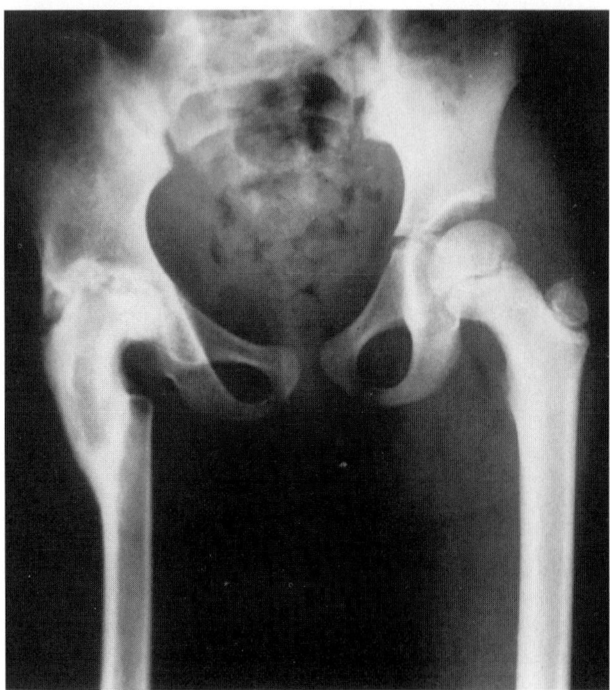

FIGURE 35–14. Tuberculosis of the hip and femur in a child.

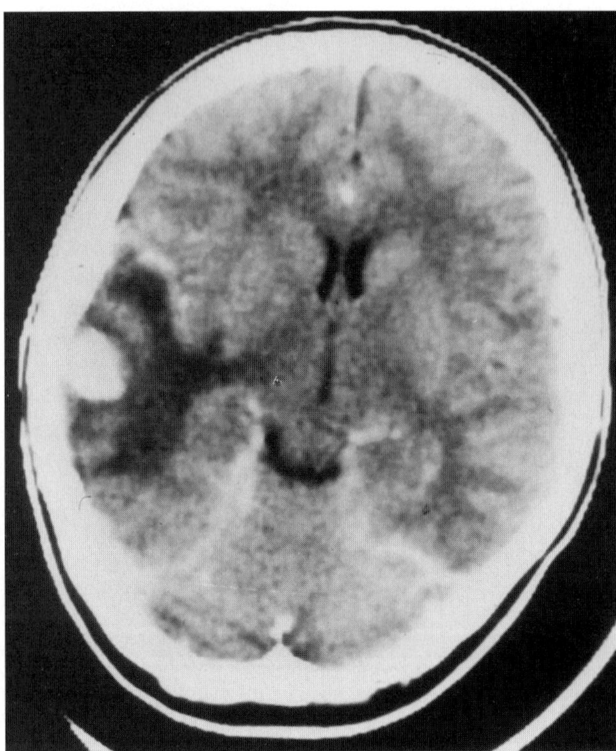

FIGURE 35–15. A CT scan of the brain of a 12-year-old Cambodian girl showing a large tuberculoma. A large area of edema surrounds the lesion.

laboratory but clearly contributes to the killing of *M. tuberculosis* in the patient. Other antituberculosis drugs, such as ethambutol at low doses (15 mg/kg/day), ethionamide, and cycloserine, are bacteriostatic for *M. tuberculosis*; ethambutol at 25 mg/kg/day has some bactericidal activity. The major purpose of bacteriostatic drugs is to prevent the emergence of resistance to the bactericidal drugs. Isoniazid and rifampin are also effective in preventing emergence of resistance to other drugs, but pyrazinamide has almost no similar activity.

The earliest treatment regimens for tuberculosis in adults and children combined the action of a bactericidal drug such as isoniazid with a bacteriostatic drug such as ethambutol. A small number of drug-susceptible organisms survived in spite of chemotherapy with these combinations, and 18–24 months of therapy was necessary to permit host defenses to eliminate persistent organisms. Even with this prolonged treatment, relapse rates were about 5–10%, mostly because of nonadherence with this long regimen.

The availability of rifampin and the ''rediscovery'' of pyrazinamide in the 1970s effected radical change in antituberculosis chemotherapy. Rifampin used with isoniazid has resulted in cure of almost 100% of patients with pulmonary tuberculosis in a period of only 9 months. Rifampin is important for treatment in children because it is particularly effective against mycobacteria in closed caseous lesions that are metabolically active in intermittent short spurts of only a few hours. When pyrazinamide is added to isoniazid and rifampin, a cure can be effected with only 6 months of treatment in almost 100% of patients with drug-susceptible tuberculosis.

Definitive Treatment

Historically, recommendations for treating children with tuberulosis have been extrapolated from clinical trials of adults with pulmonary tuberculosis. The trend over the last two decades has been to develop regimens that are increasingly intense and short. It is well established that a 9-month regimen of isoniazid and rifampin cures more than 98% of cases of drug-susceptible pulmonary tuberculosis in adults. After daily administration for the first 1–2 months, both drugs can then be given daily or twice weekly for the remaining 7–8 months with equivalent results and low rates of adverse reactions. Twice-weekly administration is supported by pharmacologic and animal model data and extensive clinic trials in adults and children. The addition of pyrazinamide at the beginning of the regimen reduces the duration of necessary treatment to 6 months. Therapy with isoniazid, rifampin, pyrazinamide, and streptomycin during the initial 2 months of treatment followed by isoniazid and rifampin in the remaining 4 months routinely yields cure rates of more than 98% with relapse rates below 4% in adults. If pyrazinamide is excluded from the initial phase of treatment, the rate of bacteriologic failure rises to 7–10%. However, the exclusion of streptomycin does not affect the cure or relapse rate appreciably.

Over the past two decades, a number of trials of antituberculosis therapy for children with drug-susceptible pulmonary tuberculosis have demonstrated that a 9-month regimen of isoniazid and rifampin is highly successful. As with adults, medication should be given daily at first but may be administered twice weekly during the final 7–8 months of treatment. The major drawbacks of this two-drug, 9-month regimen are the length of therapy, the need for good compliance, and the relative lack of protection against possible drug resistance. Several major studies of 6 months of therapy in children have reported using at least three drugs initially. Although the therapeutic regimens used in these various trials have been slightly different, the most common treatment involved 6 months of therapy with isoniazid and rifampin supplemented during the first 2 months with pyrazinamide. In general, the results from these trials in children have been very similar to those reported for

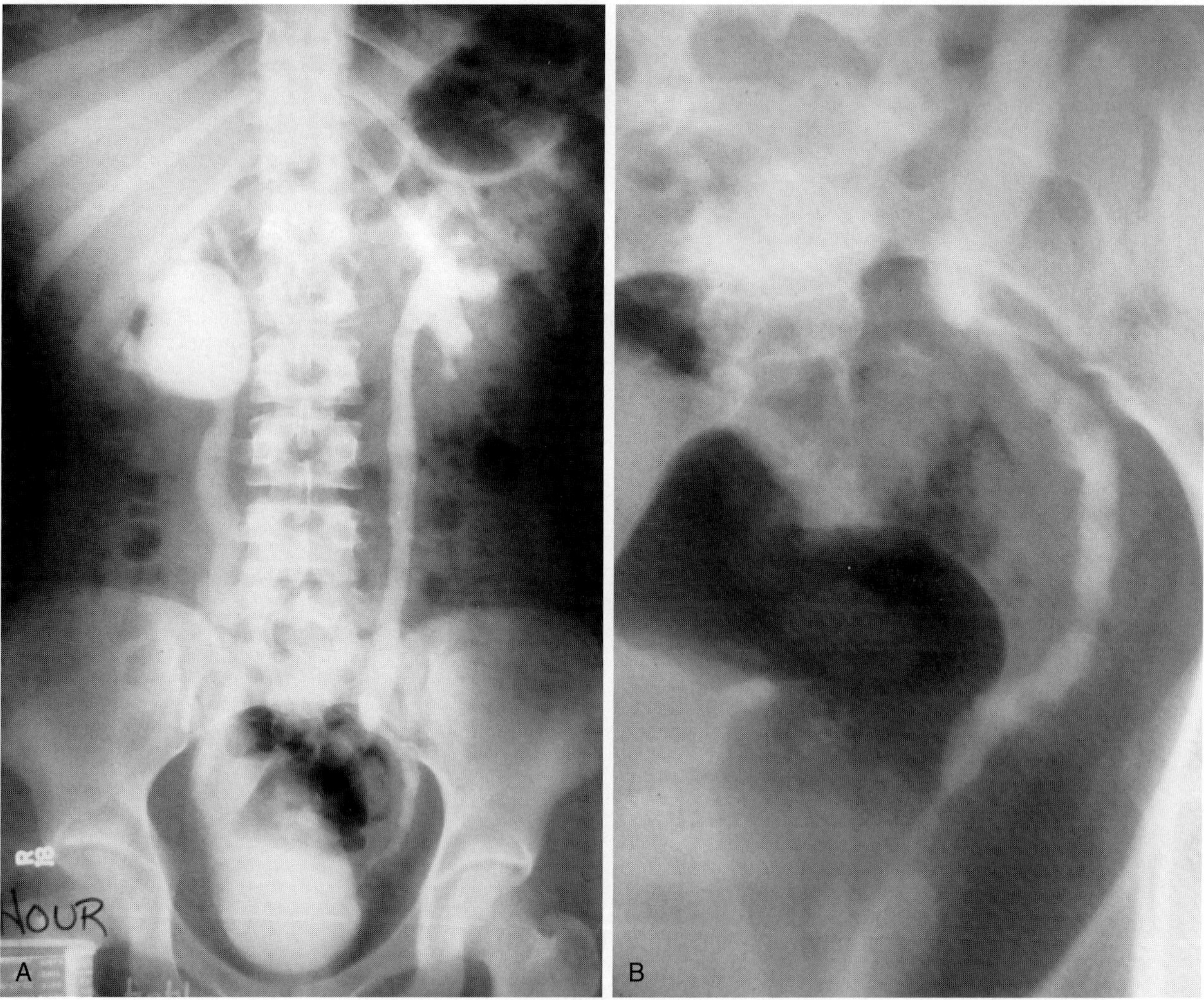

FIGURE 35–16. Renal tuberculosis in a 12-year-old girl. An intravenous pyelogram **(A)** reveals bilateral delayed excretion and mild hydroureteronephrosis. A detailed view of the left ureter **(B)** shows coarse irregularity of its wall reflecting small granulomatous foci. (Reprinted with permission from Elshihabi I, Brzowski A, Jenson H, et al: Renal tuberculosis in a child with hematuria. *Pediatr Infect Dis J* 1993;12:963–5.)

adults with pulmonary tuberculosis. Regimens that did not use streptomycin in the beginning of therapy were as successful as those that included it. Several trials demonstrated that direct observation of the administration of twice-weekly medications during the latter phase of therapy was as effective and safe as daily self-administration of medications. In all reported trials, the overall success rate was more than 95% for complete cure and 99% for significant improvement. The incidence of clinically significant adverse reactions was less than 2%.

On the basis of reported studies the AAP has endorsed a regimen of 6 months of isoniazid and rifampin supplemented during the first 2 months by pyrazinamide as standard therapy for intrathoracic tuberculosis in children (Table 35–5). Daily administration of medications for the first 2 weeks to 2 months is desirable, but after this period drugs can be given either daily by the family or twice weekly under direct observation of a health care provider. **Directly observed therapy** means that the health care worker is physically present when the medications are administered to the patient. A 9-month regimen using only isoniazid and rifampin is acceptable, although less desirable, only if the possibility of drug resistance to either isoniazid or rifampin is extremely low. For most areas of the United States and some areas of Canada, the incidence of drug resistance is high enough among the adult population that the three-drug, 6-month regimen is strongly preferred. Because this regimen requires administration of the drug for 50% less time than the 9-month regimen, adherence is improved.

Extrapulmonary Tuberculosis. Controlled clinical trials of treating various forms of extrapulmonary tuberculosis are virtually nonexistent. In many reports, extrapulmonary cases have been combined with pulmonary cases and often are not analyzed separately. Extrapulmonary tuberculosis is usually caused by fairly small numbers of mycobacteria because the large cavitary population in the lung is not present. Most non-life-threatening forms of extrapulmonary tuberculosis have responded well to a 9-month course of isoniazid and rifampin or a 6-month regimen using three or four drugs in the initial phase of treatment. In general, the treatment for these forms of extrapulmonary tuberculosis is the same as that for pulmonary tuberculosis. One exception may be bone and joint tuberculosis, which has been associated with a higher failure rate when 6-month chemotherapy is used, especially if surgical intervention has not been performed. Some experts recommend at least 9–12 months of effective chemotherapy for bone and joint tuberculosis (Table 35–5).

Tuberculous lymphadenitis responds well to antituberculosis chemotherapy, although involved nodes may remain enlarged for

TABLE 35–5. Recommended Treatment Regimens for Tuberculosis in Infants, Children, and Adolescents

Tuberculosis Infection/Disease	Regimens	Remarks
Asymptomatic infection (positive skin test, no disease)		At least 6 consecutive months of therapy with good adherence should be given.
Isoniazid-susceptible	9 months of isoniazid	
Isoniazid-resistant	6 months of rifampin	If daily therapy is not possible, twice-weekly therapy may be used for 9 months.
Pulmonary and hilar lymphadenopathy	6 months (standard regimen): 2 months of isoniazid, rifampin, and pyrazinamide daily, followed by 4 months of isoniazid and rifampin daily *or* 2 weeks to 2 months of isoniazid, rifampin, and pyrazinamide daily, followed by 4–5½ months of isoniazid and rifampin twice weekly, directly observed	If drug resistance is possible, an additional drug (ethambutol or streptomycin) should be added to the initial therapy until drug susceptibility is determined. Drugs can be given 2 or 3 times per week under direct observation in the initial phase if nonadherence is likely.
Meningitis, disseminated (miliary), and bone/joint	2 months of isoniazid, rifampin, pyrazinamide, and streptomycin daily, followed by 7–10 months of isoniazid and rifampin daily *or* 2 months of isoniazid, rifampin, pyrazinamide, and streptomycin daily, followed by 7–10 months of isoniazid and rifampin twice weekly, directly observed	Streptomycin used in initial therapy until drug susceptibility is known. For patients who may have acquired tuberculosis in geographic locales where resistance to streptomycin is common, capreomycin or kanamycin (15–30 mg/kg/day) may be used instead of streptomycin.
Extrapulmonary other than meningitis, disseminated (miliary), or bone/joint	Same as pulmonary disease	See pulmonary disease

Suggested Dosages for Patients with Normal Renal Function

DRUG	DAILY DOSE (mg/kg/dose)	TWICE WEEKLY DOSE (mg/kg/dose)	MAXIMUM DOSE
Isoniazid	10–15	20–30	Daily: 300 mg Twice weekly: 900 mg
Rifampin	10–20	10–20	600 mg
Pyrazinamide	20–40	40–60	2 g
Ethambutol	15–25	25–50	2.5 g
Streptomycin	20–40	20–40	1 g

months to years. Surgical removal alone is not adequate treatment, because the lymph node disease is only part of a systemic infection. However, surgical biopsy and culture may be necessary to distinguish tuberculous lymphadenitis from other entities, especially cat scratch disease or infection with nontuberculous mycobacteria. Excisional biopsy is preferred over incisional biopsy because of an increased risk of subsequent sinus tract formation or severe scarring with the incisional procedure.

Tuberculous meningitis usually has not been included in trials of extrapulmonary tuberculosis because of its serious nature and low incidence. As with other forms of extrapulmonary tuberculosis, the number of mycobacteria causing disease is usually small. Daily treatment with isoniazid and rifampin for 12 months is generally effective. Several recent reports have suggested that 6–9 months of therapy is effective if isoniazid, rifampin, and pyrazinamide are administered during the initial phase of treatment. At present, there probably are not sufficient data to recommend the 6-month treatment for most children with this form of tuberculosis. The official recommendation of the AAP for tuberculous meningitis is 12 months of therapy that includes at least isoniazid and rifampin and usually one or two other drugs in the initial phase of treatment. However, some experts believe that treatment for 6–9 months is adequate, especially if pyrazinamide is included in the initial treatment. Most experts add a fourth drug—usually streptomycin, ethambutol, ethionamide, or another aminoglycoside—at the beginning of therapy to protect against unsuspected initial drug resistance.

HIV-Infected Children. The optimal treatment of tuberculosis in HIV-infected children has not been established. Adults with tuberculosis who are seropositive for HIV usually can be treated successfully with standard regimens that include isoniazid, rifampin, and pyrazinamide. The duration of therapy should be a total of 9 months or 6 months after cultures of sputum become sterile, whichever is longer. Determining whether a pulmonary infiltrate in an HIV-infected child who has a positive tuberculin reaction or history of exposure to an adult with infectious tuberculosis is actually caused by *M. tuberculosis* is difficult. It is likely, as in immunocompetent children, that gastric aspirate or bronchoscopy cultures may be sterile even when tuberculosis disease is present. The radiographic appearance of other pulmonary complications of HIV infection in children, such as lymphoid interstitial pneumonitis, may be similar to that of tuberculosis. Treatment is usually empiric and based on epidemiologic and radiographic information. Therapy should be considered when tuberculosis cannot be excluded.

Most experts believe that HIV-infected children with drug-susceptible tuberculosis disease should receive isoniazid, rifampin, and pyrazinamide for 2 months followed by isoniazid and rifampin to complete a total treatment duration of 6–9 months. It is recommended that all children with tuberculosis disease be evaluated for HIV infection, because the two infections are epidemiologically linked.

Drug-Resistant M. tuberculosis. The incidence of drug-resistant tuberculosis appears to have increased in North America, particularly along the Mexican border and in large cities. In the entire United States, approximately 10% of isolates of *M. tuberculosis* are resistant to at least one drug. Many countries in Latin America and Asia routinely report drug resistance rates of 20–30%. There are two major types of drug resistance. **Primary resistance** occurs when a person is infected with *M. tuberculosis* that is already resistant to a particular drug. **Secondary resistance** occurs when drug-resistant organisms emerge as the dominant population during therapy. The major causes of secondary drug resistance are poor adherence with medication by the patient or inadequate management by the physician. Nonadherence with one drug is more likely to lead to secondary resistance than failure to take all drugs. Formulations that include multiple drugs in one capsule are designed to prevent selective resistance and should be used in the treatment of older children. Unfortunately, no practically usable multiple drug formulations are available for infants or small children.

Patterns of drug resistance among children tend to mirror those found among adults in the same population. Certain epidemiologic factors, such as being an immigrant from Asia or Latin America, homelessness, or a history of previous antituberculosis treatment, correlate with drug resistance in adults and their contacts.

Therapy for drug-resistant tuberculosis is successful only when at least two bactericidal drugs to which the infecting strain *M. tuberculosis* is susceptible are given. When a child has possible drug-resistant tuberculosis, at least three, and usually four or five, drugs should be administered initially until the susceptibility pattern is determined and a more specific regimen can be designed. The specific treatment plan must be individualized for each patient according to the results of susceptibility testing on the isolates from the child or the adult source case. Isoniazid-resistant tuberculosis disease in children usually can be treated successfully with rifampin, pyrazinamide, and ethambutol given for 9 months. Although primary resistance to pyrazinamide is rare, pyrazinamide is not effective in preventing the emergence of rifampin resistance during therapy when isoniazid resistance already exists. Therefore, the combination of isoniazid, rifampin, and pyrazinamide may not be adequate if initial isoniazid or rifampin resistance is present. A fourth drug—usually ethionamide, ethambutol, or streptomycin—should also be given initially. The CDC recommends that adults with suspected pulmonary tuberculosis who live in regions where the isoniazid resistance rate is ≥4% should routinely receive four antituberculosis drugs until the susceptibility pattern of their isolate is known. However, the bacterial burden in children with tuberculosis is much lower, and development of secondary resistance is rare. Because the volume of additional antituberculosis medications is large in a young child, most experts treat children with suspected tuberculosis with only isoniazid, rifampin, and pyrazinamide unless the source case is at risk of drug resistance, the child came from a country with high rates of drug resistance, or the child's tuberculosis is life threatening.

Several outbreaks of tuberculosis caused by strains of *M. tuberculosis* that have become resistant to isoniazid and rifampin with or without resistance to other drugs have been reported in hospitals in several North American cities. These strains are now referred to as **multidrug-resistant strains.** The outbreaks have affected primarily HIV-infected adults. Tuberculosis infection and disease have also occurred among hospital workers and other patients. Among the HIV-infected patients, the mortality rate associated with multidrug-resistant strains has been as high as 90%, and the time interval between initial infection and death has been as short as 4–6 weeks. Multidrug-resistant tuberculosis is extremely difficult to treat and requires combinations of up to five secondary drugs used for 18 months or longer. Multidrug-resistant tuberculosis has become more common in countries or regions with poor tuberculosis control practices. Nonimmunocompromised patients with multidrug-resistant tuberculosis respond much better to chemotherapy, but successful treatment requires 4–7 drugs for 12–24 months.

Corticosteroids. Corticosteroids are useful in the treatment of some children with tuberculosis, but only when administered with effective antituberculosis drugs. There is little evidence that one corticosteroid is better than another. The most commonly prescribed regimen is prednisone, 1–2 mg/kg/day for 4–6 weeks, with gradual tapering. Corticosteroids are beneficial when the host inflammatory reaction contributes significantly to tissue damage or impairment of organ function. There is convincing evidence that corticosteroids decrease mortality rates and long-term neurologic sequelae in some patients with tuberculous meningitis by reducing vasculitis, inflammation, and, ultimately, intracranial pressure. Lowering the intracranial pressure not only limits tissue damage but also probably favors the circulation of antituberculosis drugs through the brain and meninges. Short courses of corticosteroids may be effective for children with enlarged hilar lymph nodes that compress the tracheobronchial tree, causing respiratory distress, localized emphysema, or segmental pulmonary lesions. Several randomized clinical trials have shown that corticosteroids can help relieve symptoms and tamponade associated with acute tuberculous pericardial effusion. In patients with tuberculous pleural effusion and shift of the mediastinum and acute respiratory compromise, corticosteroids may cause dramatic improvement in symptoms; however, the long-term course of the disease is probably unaffected. Some children with severe miliary tuberculosis may have dramatic improvement with corticosteroids if the inflammatory reaction is so severe that alveolocapillary block is present.

Tuberculosis Infection Without Disease (Latent Infection). The treatment of children with asymptomatic tuberculosis infection to prevent the development of tuberculosis disease is an established practice. Such treatment has often been referred to as "preventive therapy" or "chemoprophylaxis." These terms are unfortunate because they imply that treatment is optional and not required therapy for an established infection. During the 1950s the U.S. Public Health Service conducted placebo-controlled trials of 1 year of daily isoniazid therapy in more than 125,000 subjects. These trials demonstrated a reduction of more than 90% in the incidence of subsequent tuberculosis disease in subjects with good adherence. The effectiveness of isoniazid therapy in children has approached 100% and has lasted for at least 30 years.

Isoniazid therapy for tuberculosis infection is clearly indicated for children with positive tuberculin skin test reactions who have no clinical or radiographic evidence of disease and also for persons of any age who demonstrate recent conversion of the tuberculin skin test reaction from negative to positive after exposure to an infectious person. Isoniazid therapy also should be started for children <4 years of age with negative tuberculin skin test reactions who have had recent exposure to an adult with contagious tuberculosis, including infants born to mothers who have tuberculosis disease. These children may already be infected with *M. tuberculosis* but have not yet developed delayed hypersensitivity. In small children and infants, significant tuberculosis disease may develop simultaneously with skin test reactivity, and illness may develop before the positive skin test reaction is recognized. For exposed children, tuberculin skin testing is usually repeated 3 months after contact with the adult source case has been interrupted. Broken contact is defined as either physical removal from the source case or effective chemotherapy that renders the source case noninfectious. If the repeat tuberculin skin test reaction is negative, isoniazid can be discontinued; if the reaction is positive, the child has tuberculosis infection and a full course of isoniazid therapy should be administered.

There is controversy concerning the optimal duration of isoniazid therapy for latent tuberculosis infection. Trials among infected adults in eastern Europe have shown that, although a 12-month program of isoniazid therapy is more effective than a 6-month treatment plan, the 6-month program is more cost-effective because of fewer toxic reactions to the drug and less need for monitoring patients for toxic effects. Relatively few comparable data for children are available. The AAP and the CDC currently recommend a 9-month period of isoniazid therapy for latent tuberculosis in children.

The optimal treatment for tuberculosis infection caused by drug-resistant strains of *M. tuberculosis* has not been established. For infections with strains that are resistant only to isoniazid, most experts recommend a 6- to 9-month course of rifampin. No data from controlled clinical trials support this practice, however. Similarly, no data are available concerning treatment of tuberculosis infection caused by organisms that are resistant to both isoniazid and rifampin. Some experts have recommended a combination of a fluoroquinolone, such as ofloxacin or ciprofloxacin, with pyrazinamide for 6–9 months. An alternative regimen is high-dose ethambutol (25 mg/kg/day) and pyrazinamide for a similar period of time. The efficacy and safety of these regimens in children are not established, and an expert in pediatric tuberculosis should be consulted for treatment of multidrug-resistant tuberculosis infection or disease in children.

Compliance (Adherence). Noncompliance, or nonadherence, is a major problem in tuberculosis control because of the long-term nature of treatment and the sometimes difficult social circumstances of the patients. As treatment regimens become shorter, adherence assumes an even greater importance. Suspected cases of tuberculosis must be reported to the local health department so it can compile accurate statistics, perform necessary contact investigations, and assist both patients and health care providers to overcome barriers to adherence with therapy. To adhere to treatment regimens, the patients and family must know what is expected of them through verbal and written instructions in the patient's main language. Postcard and telephone appointment reminders are helpful. Missed appointments should be followed up immediately by either the physician's office or the appropriate local health authority. Adherence with treatment is the responsibility of the clinician as well as of the patient and the family.

An assessment of potential nonadherence should be made at the initiation of therapy. Missed appointments should quickly be brought to the attention of the public health officials responsible for such matters. They may be able to support treatment by using various incentives or enablers, behavior modification, or, in extreme cases, confinement. Physicians should inquire about the color of urine of patients who are taking rifampin to be sure that the drug is being taken. Families can provide helpful information, such as reports of pill counts and medical knowledge, but these techniques are notoriously unreliable in proving adherence. If the physician suspects any chance of nonadherence with daily self-administered medications, directly observed therapy should be instituted with the help of the local health department. Responsible adults in the child's environment, such as grandparents, teachers, school nurses, or church workers, can often be used to help ensure that medication is properly given. Twice-weekly, directly observed therapy is extremely effective, and most experts consider it the standard of care for treating tuberculosis disease in children.

Following Up the Child With Tuberculosis. The physician and other health care workers must take an active role in the care of children with tuberculosis. Children receiving treatment should be followed up carefully to ensure adherence with therapy, monitor for toxic reactions to medications, and ensure that the tuberculosis is being adequately controlled. It is extremely important for the family that a single health care provider be identified as the primary caregiver. Nonadherence rates are significantly higher in clinical situations in which several physicians treat the same patients on a rotating basis, as frequently occurs in teaching hospitals with house staff clinics. In general, patients should be seen at monthly intervals and should be given enough medication at each visit to last until the next scheduled visit. The practice of dispensing several months of medications at one visit should be discouraged.

Anticipatory guidance with regard to the administration of antituberculosis medications to children is crucial. The physician should foresee difficulties that the family might have in introducing several new medications, often in very inconvenient dosage forms, to a young child. Until the family develops a workable dosing scheme, children may receive little medication in the first several weeks because of vomiting and difficult administration. Commercially available preparations of antituberculosis medications may be hard to give to small children. A liquid suspension of isoniazid is available, but its stability is variable and results in diarrhea and gastrointestinal upset in many children who take this preparation. Pharmacists can make rifampin into a stable suspension that is helpful for treating small children who cannot swallow capsules. This drug should be taken on an empty stomach if possible. Isoniazid and pyrazinamide pills can be crushed and given with small amounts of food.

The rates of adverse reactions to antituberculosis medications are sufficiently low in children that routine biochemical monitoring is not necessary. If there is any history of previous hepatitis or other chronic illness, it is advisable to obtain a baseline set of serum liver enzyme and serum uric acid levels. If the patient or family reports any symptoms that could be toxic reactions to antituberculosis medications, the child should have a complete physical examination, and serum hepatic enzymes and bilirubin should be measured. Serum liver enzyme elevations of two to three times the normal range are fairly common and do not necessitate discontinuation of medications if all other findings are normal. In addition, mild arthralgias or arthritis could be caused by pyrazinamide, but these problems are usually transient even when pyrazinamide is continued. Some patients taking pyrazinamide develop a troublesome pruritic morbilliform rash that is not allergic in nature. All children taking ethambutol should have regular monitoring of visual acuity and color discrimination.

Radiographic changes occur slowly with intrathoracic tuberculosis, and frequent chest radiograph monitoring is not necessary. A common practice is to obtain a chest radiograph at diagnosis and 1–2 months after the initiation of therapy to ensure that no unusual changes in radiographic appearance have occurred. If these radiographs are satisfactory, repeat chest radiographs are not necessary until the completion of 6 months of therapy. At this time, a normal chest radiograph is not required for discontinuation of treatment. The majority of children with significant intrathoracic lymphadenopathy have abnormal radiographic findings for 1–3 years, long after effective antituberculosis treatment has ceased. If improvement has occurred after 6 months of treatment, medications can be discontinued and the child can be followed up at intervals of 3–6 months with appropriate chest radiographs to document continued improvement in the radiographic appearance.

Supportive Therapy

In the prechemotherapy era, all the clinician was able to offer the child with tuberculosis was supportive care. With proper chemotherapy, such care plays a small role in the management of the child with tuberculosis. Activity does not need to be restricted unless the child develops respiratory embarassment or immobilization is necessary for treatment, as in some cases of vertebral tuberculosis. Adequate nutrition is important, although many small children who present with failure to thrive and tuberculosis do not begin to gain weight until several months after effective chemotherapy has been started.

Isoniazid can cause **pyridoxine (vitamin B_6) deficiency** by competitive inhibition. Although pyridoxine serum levels decline in children taking isoniazid, clinical symptoms are rare. The most common symptoms are paresthesias or numbness of the hands and feet. Routine administration of pyridoxine to children taking isoniazid is not necessary, but it should be given to breast-feeding infants, pregnant women, and children with meat- and milk-deficient diets. The usual dose is 25–50 mg orally per day.

PROGNOSIS

In general, the prognosis of tuberculosis in infants, children, and adolescents is excellent with early recognition and effective chemotherapy. In most children with pulmonary tuberculosis, the disease completely resolves and ultimately radiographic findings are normal. The prognosis for children with bone and joint tuberculosis and tuberculous meningitis depends directly on the stage of disease at the time antituberculosis medications are started. With extrapulmonary tuberculosis, the major problem is often delayed recognition of the cause of disease and delayed initiation of treatment.

PREVENTION

There are several major methods of preventing tuberculosis among children (Table 35–6). Primary methods prevent the initial tuberculosis infection and subsequent immunologic events, whereas secondary methods keep an established infection from progressing to disease. In the United States the public health system has relied primarily on secondary prevention with isoniazid chemotherapy.

TABLE 35–6. Major Methods of Tuberculosis Prevention

Primary Prevention
Interrupting transmission of infection
Case management: contact investigation
Environmental control: isolation, ultraviolet lights, and respirators
Vaccination: Bacille Calmette-Guérin (BCG)
Secondary Prevention
Chemotherapy for infection without disease (latent infection)

Interrupting Transmission. The highest priority of any tuberculosis control program should be case finding and treatment, which interrupt transmission of infection between close contacts. Infected close contacts can be identified and started on appropriate treatment in this manner. This system relies on effective and adequate public healtlh response and resources. Children, particularly young infants, should be given high priority during contact investigations because their risk of infection may be high and they are more likely to rapidly develop severe forms of tuberculosis. Mass screening of the general population for tuberculosis infection, an inefficient process, is generally discouraged. However, testing of known high-risk groups of adults or children should be encouraged only if effective mechanisms are in place to assure adequate evaluation and treatment of persons with positive test reactions.

Another important control measure for the prevention of tuberculosis involves the physical air around the source case. In the patients' usual surroundings, it is unlikely that this environmental factor can be controlled, but appropriate precautions must be taken in health care settings. Offices, clinics, and hospital rooms used by adults with possible tuberculosis should have adequate ventilation, with air exhausted to the outside. When air recirculation cannot be avoided, high-efficiency filtration or ultraviolet radiation of the air should be employed. Most established chest clinics already have these measures in place, but an increasing number of tuberculosis patients are cared for in other types of facilities. In general, children with tuberculosis are not infectious, and air quality control issues are less important for them. However, unless the adults accompanying the child have been thoroughly screened for infectious tuberculosis, they should be considered potentially contagious and appropriate air quality controls should be used.

Bacille Calmette-Guérin (BCG) Vaccination. The only available vaccine against tuberculosis is the bacille Calmette-Guérin (BCG), named for the two French investigators responsible for its development. The original vaccine organism was a strain of *M. bovis* attenuated by subculture every 3 weeks for 13 years. This strain was distributed to dozens of laboratories, each of which continued to subculture the organisms on different media under various conditions. The result has been production of many "daughter" BCG strains that differ widely in morphology, growth characteristics, sensitizing potency, and animal virulence.

The route of adminstration and the dosing schedule for BCG vaccine are important variables for determining vaccine efficacy. The preferred route of administration is intradermal injection with a syringe and needle because this is the only method that permits accurate measurement of an individual dose. Use of the intradermal route is relatively expensive, however, and in developing countries needles and syringes are reused, with the resulting danger of HIV and hepatitis virus transmission. A unit dose multipuncture technique, similar to that previously used for tuberculin skin testing, is the only technique available in the United States and many other parts of the world. There are no reported trials comparing various techniques of administration, although the complication rates generally are lower with multipuncture devices.

The BCG vaccines are extremely safe in immunocompetent hosts. Local ulceration and regional suppurative lymphadenitis occur in 0.1–1% of vaccinees. Local lesions do not suggest underlying host immune defects and appear not to affect the level of protection. They usually resolve spontaneously but occasionally require chemotherapy with either isoniazid or erythromycin. Rarely, surgical excision of a suppurative draining node is necessary, but this should be avoided if possible. Although osteomyelitis near the inoculation sites of BCG has been reported, this effect appears to be related to certain strains of the vaccine that are no longer in wide use.

Systemic complaints, such as fever, convulsions, loss of appetite, and irritability, are extraordinarily rare after BCG vaccination.

An accurate assessment of the efficacy of BCG vaccines throughout the world is extremely difficult. Recommended vaccine schedules vary widely in different countries. The official recommendation of the World Health Organization is a single dose administered during infancy. In the United Kingdom, a single dose is administered during adolescence. In many countries the first dose is given in infancy; then one or more additional vaccinations are given during childhood. In some countries repeat vaccination is universal; in others it is based either on tuberculin negativity or on the absence of a typical scar (Fig. 35–17). The optimal age for adminstration and schedule is completely unknown because adequate comparative trials have not been performed.

Although dozens of BCG trials on varying human populations have been reported, the most useful data have come from several controlled trials. The results of these studies were disparate; some demonstrated a great deal of protection from BCG, but others showed no efficacy at all. A variety of explanations for the different apparent responses to BCG vaccines in the major trials have been proposed, including methodologic and statistical variations among the populations, interactions with environmental mycobacteria that either enhance or decrease the protection afforded by BCG, different potencies among the various BCG vaccines, and genetic factors for BCG response within the study populations. BCG vaccination during infancy has little apparent effect on the ultimate incidence of tuberculosis among adults. However, many experts believe that BCG may be more effective in preventing tuberculosis among infants and young children than in the general population. Retrospective studies from Europe and Asia have yielded estimates of the protective effect of BCG in young children of 60–80%. The effect is particularly strong for tuberculous meningitis; the results are compatible with a protective effect of more than 70%.

In summary, BCG vaccination has worked well in some situations but poorly in others. BCG vaccination has had little effect on the ultimate control of tuberculosis throughout the world. It does not substantially influence the chain of transmission because those cases of contagious pulmonary tuberculosis in adults that can be prevented by BCG vaccination constitute a small fraction of the sources of infection in a population. Any protective effect created by BCG probably wanes over time. The best use of BCG appears to be for prevention of life-threatening forms of tuberculosis in infants and young children.

BCG vaccination has never been adopted as part of the strategy for the control of tuberculosis in the United States. However, it may contribute to tuberculosis control in narrowly selected population groups. BCG is recommended for tuberculin skin test–negative infants and children who are (1) at high risk of intimate and prolonged exposure to persistently untreated or ineffectively treated patients with infectious pulmonary tuberculosis and cannot be removed from the source of infection or placed on long-term preventive therapy and (2) continuously exposed to persons with tuberculosis who have bacilli that are resistant to isoniazid and rifampin. BCG is contraindicated in persons whose immunologic responses are impaired. Several studies in Africa have shown that BCG vaccine is tolerated well by infants with HIV infection. The only strain of BCG currently licensed in the United States is susceptible to isoniazid, although isoniazid-resistant strains are available in some countries. At present, isoniazid is not administered with BCG vaccination in the United States.

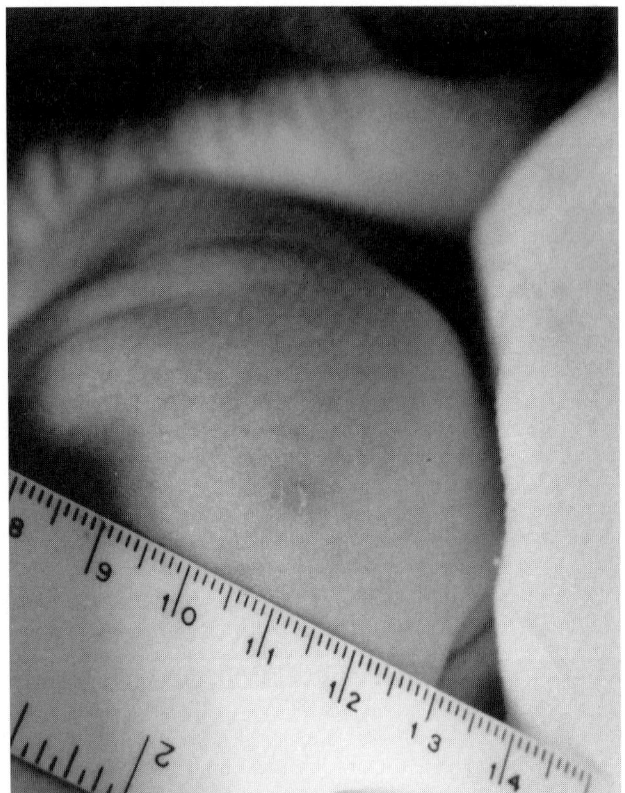

FIGURE 35–17. A scar resulting from vaccination with bacille Calmette-Guérin (BCG) on the deltoid region of an infant.

REVIEWS

American Thoracic Society: Targeted tuberculin testing and treatment of latent tuberculosis infection. *MMWR Morb Mortal Wkly Rep* 2000;49:1–51.

Raviglione MC, Snider DE Jr, Kochi A: Global epidemiology of tuberculosis: Morbidity and mortality of a worldwide epidemic. *JAMA* 1995;273:220–6.

Smith MH: Tuberculosis in children and adolescents. *Clin Chest Med* 1989;10:381–95.

Starke JR, Correa AG: Management of mycobacterial infection and disease in children. *Pediatr Infect Dis J* 1995;14:455–69.

Starke JR, Jacobs RF, Jereb J: Resurgence of tuberculosis in children. *J Pediatr* 1992;120:839–55.

Ussery XT, Valway SE, McKenna M, et al: Epidemiology of tuberculosis among children in the United States: 1985 to 1994. *Pediatr Infect Dis J* 1996;15:697–704.

KEY ARTICLES

American Academy of Pediatrics, Committee on Infectious Diseases: Update on tuberculosis skin testing of children. *Pediatrics* 1996;97:282–4.

Cantwell MF, Shehab ZM, Costello AM, et al: Brief report: Congenital tuberculosis. *N Engl J Med* 1994;330:1051–4.

Centers for Disease Control and Prevention: The role of BCG vaccine in the prevention and control of tuberculosis in the United States: A joint statement by the Advisory Council for the Elimination of Tuberculosis and the Advisory Committee on Immunization Practices. *MMWR Morb Mortal Wkly Rep* 1996;45:1–18.

Colditz GA, Brewer TF, Berkey CS, et al: Efficacy of BCG vaccine in the prevention of tuberculosis: Meta-analysis of the published literature. *JAMA* 1994;271:698–702.

Coovadia HM, Jeena P, Wilkinson D: Childhood human immunodeficiency virus and tuberculosis co-infections: Reconciling conflicting data. *Int J Tuberc Lung Dis* 1998;2:844–51.

Havlir DV, Barnes PF: Tuberculosis in patients with human immunodeficiency virus infection. *N Engl J Med* 1999;340:367–73.

Hsu KH: Thirty years after isoniazid: Its impact on tuberculosis in children and adolescents. *JAMA* 1984;251:1283–5.

Huebner RE, Schein MF, Bass JB Jr: The tuberculin skin test. *Clin Infect Dis* 1993;17:968–75.

Hussey G, Chisolm T, Kibel M: Miliary tuberculosis in children: A review of 94 cases. *Pediatr Infect Dis J* 1991;10:832–6.

Kendig EL Jr, Rodgers WL: Tuberculosis in the neonatal period. *Am Rev Tuberc Pulm Dis* 1958;77:418–22.

Lincoln EM, Davis PA, Bovornkitti S: Tuberculous pleurisy with effusion in children: A study of 202 children with particular reference to prognosis. *Am Rev Tuberc Pulm Dis* 1958;77:271–89.

Lincoln EM, Harris LC, Bovornkitti S, et al: Endobronchial tuberculosis in children: A study of 156 patients. *Am Rev Tuberc Pulm Dis* 1958;77:39–61.

Nemir RL, Cardona J, Vaziri F, et al: Prednisone as an adjunct in the chemotherapy of lymph node—bronchial tuberculosis in childhood: A double blind study. II. Further term observation. *Am Rev Respir Dis* 1967;95:402–10.

Nolan RJ Jr: Childhood tuberculosis in North Carolina: A study of the opportunities for intervention in the transmission of tuberculosis to children. *Am J Public Health* 1986;76:26–30.

Pablos-Mendez A, Raviglione MC, Laszlo A, et al: Global surveillance for antituberculosis drug resistance, 1994-1997. World Health Organization-International Union Against Tuberculosis and Lung Disease Working Group on Anti-Tuberculosis Drug Resistance Surveillance. *N Engl J Med* 1998;338:1641–9.

Starke JR, Taylor-Watts KT: Tuberculosis in the pediatric population of Houston, Texas. *Pediatrics* 1989;84:28–35.

Steiner P, Rao M: Drug-resistant tuberculosis in children. *Semin Pediatr Infect Dis* 1993;4:275–82.

Vallejo JG, Ong LT, Starke JR: Clinical features, diagnosis, and treatment of tuberculosis in infants. *Pediatrics* 1994;94:1–7.

Vallejo JG, Starke JR: Tuberculosis and pregnancy. *Clin Chest Med* 1992;13:693–707.

Waecker NJ Jr, Connor JD: Central nervous system tuberculosis in children: A review of 30 cases. *Pediatr Infect Dis J* 1990;9:539–43.

CHAPTER 36

Mumps

Hal B. Jenson ▪ Charles T. Leach

Mumps, historically known as **epidemic parotitis,** is an acute systemic febrile illness of variable severity affecting primarily glandular organs, most commonly the salivary glands. The term mumps is the plural of the dialectal verb "mump," which means "grimace," and describes the characteristic facial expression of persons with symptomatic parotitis.

ETIOLOGY

Mumps is caused by **mumps virus,** a single-stranded RNA virus in the Paramyxoviridae family, which also includes measles virus, parainfluenza viruses, and respiratory syncytial virus.

Transmission. Mumps virus is transmitted via oropharyngeal secretions by direct contact, droplet spread, or fomites. The disease is highly infectious via airborne transmission. Virus is present in saliva for up to 7 days before and for about 9 days after the first clinical symptoms of parotid involvement, with the highest levels shed immediately before and at the onset of parotitis. No carrier state for mumps is recognized in humans, who are the only known natural hosts. There is no animal reservoir and no insect vector.

EPIDEMIOLOGY

Mumps, which is endemic worldwide, was prevalent in the United States before introduction of the live virus vaccine in 1967 (Fig. 36–1). Closed populations were particularly susceptible to epidemics every 2–5 years. The peak incidence was during January to May, with a low level of background cases occurring throughout the year. The 387 cases of mumps reported for 1999 is the lowest number ever reported and a more than 99% decrease from the 152,209 cases reported in 1968, when mumps was first designated a reportable disease. In recent years approximately one half of cases have occured in children <15 years of age. Mumps is uncommon in infancy because of protective antibodies acquired transplacentally from the mother. At least 80–90% of persons >20 years of age are immune to mumps as determined by the presence of mumps-neutralizing antibodies.

PATHOGENESIS

After initial infection and proliferation within the salivary glands and the oral epithelium, a transient viremia occurs for 1–2 days with systemic spread of the virus. Mumps virus primarily infects glandular tissues, including the salivary glands, testicles and ovaries, occasionally the pancreas, and less frequently the CNS. In glandular tissue the virus causes inflammation and diffuse interstitial edema with perivascular lymphocytic infiltration. Polymorphonuclear cells and necrotic debris may accumulate, especially in the lumina of infected glands. Interstitial hemorrhage and focal areas of infarction are more common in orchitis as a result of development of intense edema within the constraints of a relatively inelastic tunica albuginea. Severe cases may result in testicular atrophy of the germinal epithelium with accompanying hyalinization and fibrosis. Mumps encephalitis may occur as either acute encephalitis with neurolysis or postinfectious encephalitis characterized by microglial reaction and demyelinization with sparing of the neurons. Specific immunity develops as clinical manifestations of the disease resolve.

SYMPTOMS AND CLINICAL MANIFESTATIONS

Incubation Period. The incubation period is generally 16–18 days, with a range of 12–25 days.

Common Symptoms

The majority of cases are mild. Up to one third of susceptible persons exposed to mumps virus become infected but do not have symptoms. Mumps is a systemic infection with the hallmark finding in symptomatic persons of parotitis (Table 36–1; Fig. 36–2). Epididymo-orchitis and meningitis are the most important of the less frequent manifestations.

Parotitis. After the onset of prodromal symptoms of low-grade fever, malaise, anorexia, abdominal pain, and headache, swelling and tenderness of the parotid glands develop within a day. The parotid swelling is usually first apparent in one gland, involves both glands in less than a day, and reaches a maximum size in 1–3 days. Parotid swelling involves only one gland in approximately one fourth of cases. Persons may complain of earache exacerbated by chewing or elicited by palpation of the gland. The fever usually subsides after 1–6 days and is followed by gradual resolution of the parotid swelling, which usually lasts for a total of about 6–10 days. The submaxillary salivary glands are also occasionally involved, and the sublingual salivary glands are least commonly affected. The incidence of salivary gland involvement is the same for both sexes.

Epididymo-Orchitis and Oophoritis. Epididymo-orchitis and oophoritis are rare in the prepubertal child. In postpubertal males the incidence of epididymo-orchitis with mumps is approximately 30%; this is the second most common specific manifestation of mumps infection in men. In contrast, the incidence of oophoritis with mumps in postpubertal females is approximately 5%. Gonadal involvement is manifest by gradual worsening of scrotal swelling and testicular pain, typically during the first week of parotitis, but is seen during the second week in one fourth of cases. Occasionally, gonadal involvement precedes parotitis or occurs as the only manifestation of mumps infection. Orchitis is usually unilateral; bilateral orchitis is seen in only one sixth of cases. Symptoms of testicular

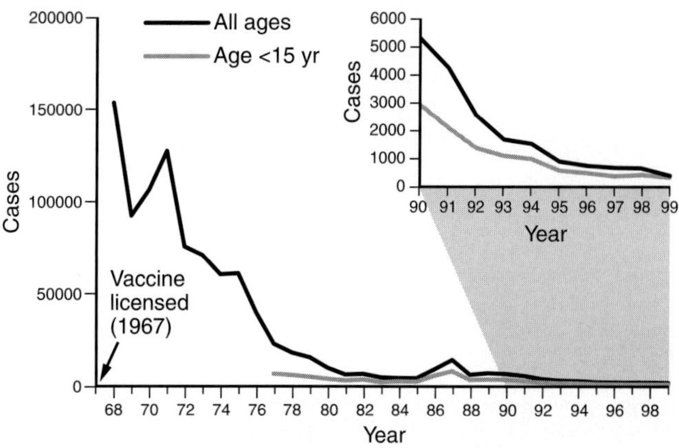

FIGURE 36–1. Reported cases of mumps in the United States by year from 1968–1999. Mumps vaccine was licensed in December 1967. (Data from the Centers for Disease Control and Prevention.)

TABLE 36–1. Frequency of Clinical Manifestations of Mumps

Fever	>90% of cases
Glandular Signs	
Parotitis	70%
Submandibular or sublingual sialadenitis, or both	10%
Epididymo-orchitis	
Prepubertal males	Rare
Postpubertal males	30%
Unilateral (25%)	
Bilateral (5%)	
Oophoritis	
Prepubertal females	Rare
Postpubertal females	5%
Mastitis	
Postpubertal females	30%
Pancreatitis	Uncommon
Neurologic Signs	
CSF abnormalities	60%
Meningitis	30%
Encephalitis	0.1%
Deafness	
Transient high-frequency hearing loss	4%
Permanent unilateral deafness	Rare
Cardiac Signs	
ECG changes	10%
Clinical myocarditis	Rare
Renal Signs	
Urinalysis abnormalities (microscopic hematuria and proteinuria)	60%
Clinical nephritis	Rare
Skeletal Signs	
Migratory polyarthralgia	
Adults	Occasional
Children	Rare

pain and lower abdominal pain, which generally subside within 5 days, may persist for weeks.

Meningitis and Encephalitis. Mumps meningitis is the most common CNS manifestation of mumps. Approximately two thirds of persons with mumps parotitis have pleocytosis, and about one third have signs and symptoms of aseptic meningitis, which is indistinguishable from other common causes. Meningitis usually appears within a few days after onset of parotid enlargement, although it may occur before parotitis develops or even in its absence. Meningeal symptoms include headache, nausea, vomiting, irritability, drowsiness, and neck stiffness. Mumps meningitis is generally benign, with complete recovery in 3–4 days.

Mumps encephalitis, an uncommon manifestation of mumps infection, may have permanent sequelae and is the principal complication associated with death from mumps. Although lethargy is frequently seen in uncomplicated mumps, profound changes in sensorium, depressed level of consciousness, vertigo, convulsions, psychosis, or hemiplegia with mumps infection suggest encephalitis. Coma is an unfavorable prognostic finding.

Physical Examination Findings

Salivary Glands. The parotid gland, the largest of the salivary glands, is roughly wedge shaped, with its base above and its apex behind the angle of the mandible. The gland is wedge shaped in the horizontal plane as well, with its base in the lateral position and its apex against the pharyngeal wall. The superior margin of the gland extends upward behind the temporomandibular joint into the posterior part of the mandibular fossa. The parotid gland is not normally palpable.

Parotid swelling with mumps is generally visibly apparent (Plate 3F), usually without overlying erythema, and is accompanied by tenderness to palpation. The enlargement obscures the angle of the mandible, unlike swelling associated with cervical lymphadenopathy. The submandibular salivary glands may also demonstrate tenderness to palpation if they are involved. The orifices of Stensen's and Wharton's ducts, which drain the parotid and submaxillary salivary glands, respectively, may appear reddened and edematous. Purulent discharge from the salivary glands is not characteristic of mumps.

Epididymo-Orchitis. Epididymitis is present in 85% of cases with orchitis and usually precedes testicular involvement. The infected testicle may be only slightly swollen or as much as four times normal size; it is also warm and tender, often with overlying erythema of the scrotum. During convalescence the affected testes may demonstrate a loss of turgor.

Meningitis and Encephalitis. CNS involvement with mumps may be designated as primary, with symptoms before or during the development of parotitis, or postinfectious, characterized by the appearance of symptoms 1–3 weeks after the onset of parotitis. Meningeal involvement is suggested by nuchal rigidity and positive Brudzinski's and Kernig's signs. Encephalitis is indicated by change in sensorium, impaired balance and ambulation, increased reflexes, and extensor plantar responses. Local weakness of the limbs with transient loss of tendon reflexes and subjective sensory loss may also occur.

Other Manifestations. Presternal edema (Fig. 36–3) develops in approximately 6% of persons with mumps. This is probably due to impaired lymphatic drainage from the anterosuperior part of the chest caused by enlarged submandibular salivary glands.

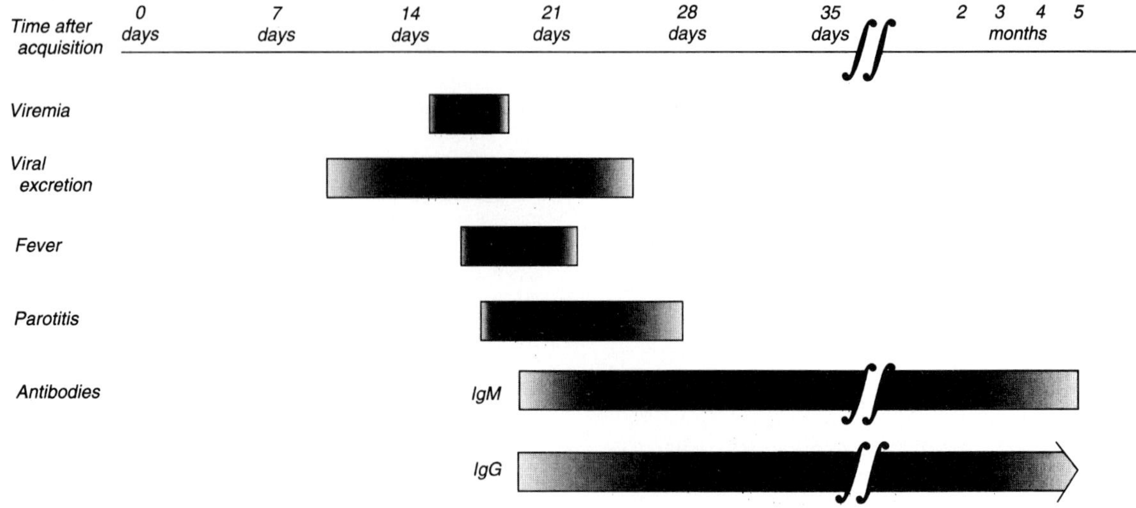

FIGURE 36–2. A profile of the typical clinical course of mumps.

Uncommon Symptoms

The clinical manifestations of mumps are generally more severe and more likely to include extrasalivary involvement in the postpubertal adolescent and adult than in the younger child. Mumps virus can infect the pancreas, kidneys, mammary glands, ovaries, heart, thyroid, joints, lungs, liver, and prostate (Table 36–1). Extrasalivary gland manifestations usually follow the onset of parotid swelling, although they can precede it or even occur as isolated findings in the absence of clinical parotitis.

Pancreatitis. Pancreatitis can result in severe epigastric pain and nausea accompanied by prostration and persistent emesis. Symptoms usually resolve completely in a few days, and affected persons require only supportive treatment.

Polyarthralgia and Polyarthritis. Migratory polyarthralgia, monoarticular arthritis, and even polyarticular arthritis are rarely seen in younger children but are occasionally seen in older persons with mumps infection. The duration of skeletal symptoms is quite variable, ranging from a few days to 3 months, with a median of about 2 weeks. The large joints are most commonly affected, especially the knees, ankles, shoulders, and wrists. The small joints (metacarpophalangeal and interphalangeal) as well as the temporomandibular joints are less commonly involved. The arthritis resolves with no residual joint damage, regardless of the duration or severity of symptoms.

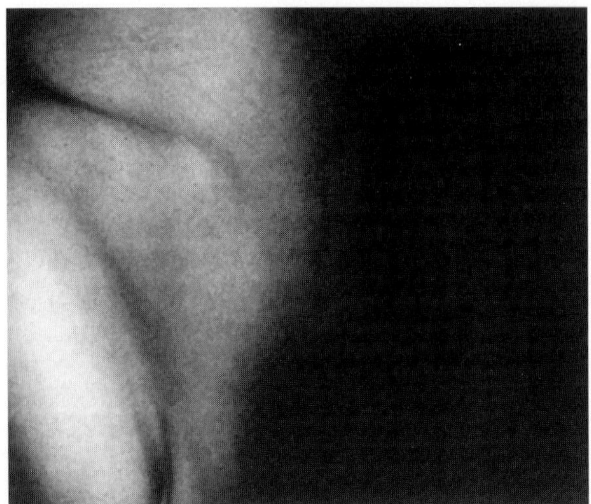

FIGURE 36–3. Presternal edema, which is due to obstructed lymph drainage, occurs in approximately 5% of cases of mumps. (Courtesy of Burtis B. Breese.)

Renal Involvement. Subclinical microscopic hematuria and proteinuria may occur with mumps. The virus can be isolated from urine in approximately three fourths of such cases during the first few days of illness.

Neonatal Infection. Infection with mumps virus during the neonatal period is uncommon because of the presence of protective maternal antibody. Mumps has been associated with respiratory symptoms in neonates.

DIAGNOSIS

The diagnosis of mumps is usually determined on the basis of fever and constitutional symptoms accompanied by parotid gland swelling, especially if symptoms develop 2–3 weeks after known exposure to mumps. Meningeal involvement is suggested by headache, nausea, vomiting, irritability, drowsiness, and neck stiffness.

Differential Diagnosis

Several viruses besides mumps virus are causally associated with acute parotitis (Table 36–2). Although additional symptoms or signs specific to each particular virus may accompany these infections, they can be conclusively differentiated from mumps only by viral culture, paired serologic testing, or both.

Acute suppurative parotitis or sialadenitis, usually caused by *Staphylococcus aureus,* is associated with high fever and unilateral symptoms involving a single salivary gland. Exquisite tenderness to palpation and purulent discharge from the associated salivary duct are characteristic (Chapter 62). Tumors, cysts, and obstruction of the salivary gland ducts as a result of stones (sialolithiasis) are almost always unilateral. Persistent, bilateral, usually asymptomatic parotid enlargement may be caused by drugs (e.g., phenylbutazone, thiouracil, iodides, and phenothiazines), metabolic disorders in-

TABLE 36–2. Differential Diagnosis of Parotid Swelling

Bilateral Parotid Swelling with Signs of Acute Inflammation	
Common	***Uncommon***
Mumps virus	Lymphocytic choriomeningitis virus
Parainfluenza virus type 3	Herpes simplex viruses
Coxsackieviruses	
Influenza virus A	
Unilateral Parotid Swelling with Signs of Acute Inflammation	
Mumps virus	
Acute suppurative parotitis or sialadenitis (usually caused by *Staphylococcus aureus*)	
Bilateral Parotid Swelling without Signs of Acute Inflammation	
HIV infection	
Diabetes mellitus	
Malnutrition	
Sjögren's syndrome	
Sarcoidosis (uveoparotid fever)	
Drug reaction	
Unilateral Parotid Swelling without Signs of Acute Inflammation	
Tumor	
Cyst	
Obstruction due to stones (sialolithiasis) or stricture	

cluding diabetes mellitus and malnutrition, autoimmune disorders (especially Sjögren's syndrome), and the lymphoid hyperplasia associated with HIV infection.

Cervical lymphadenitis is differentiated from parotitis by the characteristically well-defined borders of the enlarged lymph node as well as a location completely posterior and inferior to the ramus of the mandible. The borders of the parotid gland, especially along the anterior and inferior sides, are poorly defined in terms of surface anatomy. When the gland is enlarged, the ramus of the mandible is obscured.

Pyogenic or bacterial orchitis is usually unilateral and is caused by staphylococci, streptococci, or *Mycobacterium tuberculosis* (Chapter 83).

Laboratory Evaluation

In mumps infection the WBC and differential counts are generally normal to mildly elevated, with a lymphocytic predominance. The serum amylase level is elevated and may remain abnormal for 2–3 weeks, even in the absence of clinical salivary gland involvement. Mumps may also cause pancreatitis with resulting high serum amylase levels from the pancreas. The presence of pancreatitis with mumps can be confirmed by amylase isoenzyme analysis or demonstration of a concomitantly elevated serum pancreatic lipase. The EEG is normal in mumps meningitis but is abnormal in mumps meningoencephalitis.

Cerebrospinal Fluid. The CSF with mumps meningoencephalitis usually shows a cell count of 100–500 mm^3, occasionally reaches 1,000 mm^3, and rarely exceeds 2,000 mm^3. CSF protein is either normal or mildly elevated to approximately 50 mg/dL. The CSF glucose is generally normal, although values of less than 40 mg/dL have been reported. Hypoglycorrhachia, if present on initial evaluation, is usually present for only 3–4 days, although the pleocytosis may persist for up to 5 weeks. Mumps antibodies may also be detected in the CSF of persons with mumps meningitis or meningoencephalitis.

Microbiologic Evaluation

Viral Culture. Although isolation of mumps virus by culture definitively confirms the diagnosis, viral culture is usually unnecessary and is not a routine laboratory procedure. Mumps virus is difficult to recover from serum, reflecting the transient duration of viremia, which has been detected only rarely and typically is present for only 1–2 days during the very early phase of symptoms. Mumps virus can usually be isolated from saliva from 2–3 days before until 4–5 days after the onset of parotitis, from the CSF in persons with meningitis or meningoencephalitis during the first 3 days of meningeal symptoms, and from the urine in about 75% of persons during the first 2 weeks of illness (Fig. 36–2). Virus has also been isolated from breast milk and from testicular biopsy specimens.

Serologic Testing. The diagnosis of mumps infection is usually confirmed by demonstrating serologic conversion using complement fixation, hemagglutination inhibition, enzyme immunoassay, immunofluorescent assay, or neutralization tests in paired (acute and convalescent) sera tested simultaneously. The first serum sample should be obtained as soon as the infection is suspected, and the second serum sample 2–4 weeks later. A fourfold or higher rise in antibody titer is serologic evidence of mumps infection. The presence of IgG antibodies in a single serum sample is not diagnostic. Cross-reacting antibodies and technical limitations severely affect the reliability and clinical usefulness of IgM antibody test results. Antibodies to the mumps virus may cross-react with heterologous antibodies to the parainfluenza virus because these viruses share the same cell attachment site and viral epitopes.

Mumps antibodies may also be detected in CSF. Mumps meningitis may be confirmed by an elevated mumps CSF/serum antibody ratio using a serologic test that can be titered (Chapter 10).

Mumps Skin Test. The mumps skin test, which is sometimes used to demonstrate intact cell-mediated immunity, should not be used to determine immunity to mumps because it is unreliable for this purpose.

Diagnostic Imaging

Radiographic evaluation of painful joints or even joints with mumps arthritis is characteristically normal.

Pathologic Findings

Histologic study of involved glandular tissues reveals a diffuse interstitial infiltrate of lymphocytes and plasma cells with inflammatory edema, occasionally with focal necrosis. The ducts do not generally demonstrate accumulated secretions. CNS involvement is characterized by lymphocytic and plasma cell infiltrates within the meninges that do not extend appreciably into the cortical tissue. Polymorphonuclear leukocyte infiltration is rarely present in either glandular or CNS tissues.

TREATMENT

Definitive Treatment

No specific treatment is available for mumps infection. The efficacy of mumps immune globulin is unproved, and this product is no longer available or recommended.

Supportive Therapy

The management of mumps infection consists of symptomatic relief and supportive treatment. The principal symptoms of fever and pain associated with swelling of the salivary gland can be relieved by acetaminophen or ibuprofen. Application of warm or cold packs to the parotid gland according to the preference of the patient, may also be beneficial.

The treatment of orchitis is also symptomatic and consists of bed rest, scrotal support with a bridge constructed of adhesive tape between the upper thighs to support the inflamed testis, local cooling, and analgesics (acetaminophen, nonsteroidal anti-inflammatory drugs, or codeine or other narcotics) as needed. Most patients are treated initially with antibiotics because bacterial orchitis cannot be excluded at the initial presentation (Chapter 83). For intractable severe pain, an anesthetic block of 1% procaine hydrochloride may be helpful. There is no convincing evidence that corticosteroids or incision of the tunica albuginea will reduce pain or the incidence of subsequent atrophy, and neither of these is recommended. Most symptoms of mumps orchitis resolve in about 5 days, although in one fourth of cases the symptoms persist for >2 weeks.

COMPLICATIONS

Mumps orchitis engenders high levels of unnecessary anxiety in many men concerning possible testicular atrophy and sterility. Most men have unilateral testicular involvement that does not lead to sterility. Some degree of testicular atrophy is detectable months to years later, however, in about 50% of cases of mumps with testicular involvement. Even with severe unilateral atrophy, only a cosmetic imbalance results. Sterility from mumps is rare, even in cases of bilateral testicular involvement. Impotence is not a sequela of mumps.

Neurologic complications that are rarely associated with mumps include transverse myelitis, ascending polyradiculitis (Guillain-Barré syndrome), a poliomyelitis-like syndrome, facial nerve palsy, cerebellar ataxia, and aqueductal stenosis with resulting hydrocephalus. Transient, high-frequency hearing loss accompanies acute illness in 4% of cases but usually resolves. Permanent unilateral deafness occurs in only 1 in 20,000 cases of mumps.

Infection with mumps virus during the first trimester of pregnancy may be associated with a small risk of fetal death and low birth weight. A variety of congenital malformations have been reported with mumps infection during gestation, although incidence rates are not significantly higher than in the general population.

PROGNOSIS

Mumps is a self-limited, generally benign infection, even when extrasalivary complications such as meningitis occur. Pancreatitis, arthritis, and other symptoms of mumps infection generally resolve without sequelae. Mumps encephalitis is frequently associated with persistent EEG abnormalities, ataxia, and behavioral disturbances during convalescence; presentation with convulsions, altered level of consciousness, psychosis, or absence of salivary gland swelling are associated with an unfavorable prognosis. Recovery from mumps encephalitis is usually complete, although residual cranial nerve palsies involving the optic, facial, trigeminal, or oculomotor nerves occur rarely.

Mumps virus RNA has been detected in the myocardium of more than 70% of cases of **endocardial fibroelastosis,** indicating that this is a sequela of a viral myocarditis, perhaps associated with selection and persistence of defective virus mutants. Experimental infection of chick embryos, which demonstrates similar cardiac histopathologic traits, provides additional evidence. The dramatic decline of endocardial fibroelastosis in recent decades probably reflects universal mumps immunization. Mumps virus has also been suggested as a cause of juvenile diabetes mellitus on the basis of several case reports, although coincidental infection cannot be excluded.

Recurrence. Mumps virus does not persist after infection, with the possible exception of endocardial fibroelastosis. Any form of mumps infection, including subclinical infection, confers lifelong immunity. Symptomatic recurrent cases have been reported and have been suggested by serologic analyses, but the evidence is scarce and inconclusive.

PREVENTION

Persons born before 1957 are considered immune to mumps because of the high probability of natural infection and subsequent immunity.

Passive Protection. Standard immune globulin (IG) is ineffective in preventing secondary cases of mumps and is not recommended. A historical approach to passive protection was use of mumps immune globulin, which failed to reduce either the attack rate or the incidence of orchitis or meningoencephalitis. It is no longer available or recommended.

Vaccination. Live attenuated mumps vaccine was licensed in the United States in 1967 (Chapter 17). The only current vaccine strain, Jeryl Lynn, is available alone or in combination with measles or with rubella, although the combined measles, mumps, and rubella (MMR) vaccine is the preferred immunizing agent for most children and adults. Whether administered alone or in combination, mumps vaccine elicits protective immunity in more than 98% of vaccinees, although the levels of antibodies induced are lower than levels resulting from natural infection. Vaccine virus replicates in the parotid glands but is not detectable by culture in the oral secretions of vaccinees.

Although receipt of only one dose of mumps vaccine is sufficient for proof of immunity, primary vaccination is recommended as combined MMR vaccine at 12–15 months of age with a second dose (also as MMR) recommended at 4–6 years of age. Children 11–12 years of age who have not received a second dose of MMR should be given MMR at that time.

Outbreak Control. Epidemics among closed populations of immunized persons may occur. Proof of immunity is either a history of physician-diagnosed mumps, serologic evidence of mumps immunity, or dated documentation of mumps vaccination. To control outbreaks in day care centers and schools, unimmunized students should be excluded until vaccinated. Administration of mumps vaccine to susceptible persons during the early course of an epidemic is beneficial, and excluded students can be readmitted immediately after vaccination. Unimmunized persons who remain unvaccinated for medical, religious, or other reasons should be excluded from school until at least 26 days after the onset of parotitis in the last person with mumps. Local public health officials should be enlisted to inform the medical community of a mumps outbreak and to implement appropriate public health measures.

Hospital Isolation. To minimize spread to susceptible persons, it has traditionally been recommended that persons with mumps be isolated until the parotid swelling has subsided (9 days after the onset of parotid swelling). However, virus is present in saliva for several days before symptoms of parotitis are apparent, and thus spread to close contacts may already have occurred. Persons with inapparent infection are also contagious. Therefore, enforcement of strict isolation may be of little benefit. However, contact of acutely infected persons with persons with congenital or acquired immunodeficiency, including persons with cancer who are receiving immunosuppressive therapy, should be avoided. Respiratory isolation with standard precautions should be used for hospitalized persons with mumps.

REVIEWS

Beard CM, Benson RC Jr, Kelalis PP, et al: The incidence and outcome of mumps orchitis in Rochester, Minnesota, 1935 to 1974. *Mayo Clin Proc* 1977;52:3–7.

Centers for Disease Control and Prevention: Measles, mumps, and rubella—vaccine use and strategies for elimination of measles, rubella, and congenital rubella syndrome and control of mumps: Recommendations of the Advisory Committee on Immunization Practices (ACIP). *MMWR Morb Mortal Wkly Rep* 1998;47(RR-8):1–57.

Centers for Disease Control and Prevention: Mumps surveillance—United States, 1988–1993. *MMWR Morb Mortal Wkly Rep* 1995;44(SS-3):1–13.

McDonald JC, Moore DL, Quennec P: Clinical and epidemiologic features of mumps meningoencephalitis and possible vaccine-related disease. *Pediatr Infect Dis J* 1989;8:751–5.

KEY ARTICLES

Azimi PH, Cramblett HG, Haynes RE: Mumps meningoencephalitis in children. *JAMA* 1969;207:509–12.

Bang HO, Bang J: Involvement of the central nervous system in mumps. *Bull Hyg* 1944;19:503–4.

Brunell PA, Brickman A, O'Hare D, et al: Ineffectiveness of isolation of patients as a method of preventing the spread of mumps. *N Engl J Med* 1968;279:1357–61.

Casella R, Leibundgut B, Lehmann K, et al: Mumps orchitis: Report of a mini-epidemic. *J Urol* 1997;158:2158–61.

Candel S: Epididymitis in mumps, including orchitis: Further clinical studies and comments. *Ann Intern Med* 1951;34:20–36.

Gordon SC, Lauter CB: Mumps arthritis: A review of the literature. *Rev Infect Dis* 1984;6:338–44.

Hersh BS, Fine PE, Kent WK, et al: Mumps outbreak in a highly vaccinated population. *J Pediatr* 1991;119:187–93.

Johnstone JA, Ross CA, Dunn M: Meningitis and encephalitis associated with mumps infection. *Arch Dis Child* 1972;47:647–51.

Kameya S, Hayakawa T, Kameya A, et al: Clinical value of routine isoamylase analysis of hyperamylasemia. *Am J Gastroenterol* 1986;81:358–64.

Moroshima T, Miyazu M, Ozaki T, et al: Local immunity in mumps meningitis. *Am J Dis Child* 1980;134:1060–4.

Nagai T, Nakayama T: Mumps vaccine virus genome is present in throat swabs obtained from uncomplicated healthy recipients. *Vaccine* 2001; 19:1353–5.

Ni J, Bowles NE, Kim YH, et al: Viral infection of the myocardium in endocardial fibroelastosis: Molecular evidence for the role of mumps virus as an etiologic agent. *Circulation* 1997;95:133–9.

Koskiniemi M, Donner M, Pettay O: Clinical appearance and outcome in mumps encephalitis in children. *Acta Paediatr Scand* 1983;72:603–9.

Philip RN, Reinhard KR, Lackman DB: Observations on a mumps epidemic in a "virgin" population. *Am J Hyg* 1959;69:91–111.

Reman O, Freymuth F, Laloum D, et al: Neonatal respiratory distress due to mumps. *Arch Dis Child* 1986;61:80–1.

Utz JP, Houk VN, Alling DW: Clinical and laboratory studies of mumps. IV. Viruria and abnormal renal function. *N Engl J Med* 1964;270:1283–6.

Vuori M, Lahikainen EA, Peltonen T: Perceptive deafness in connection with mumps: A study of 298 servicemen suffering from mumps. *Acta Otolaryngol* 1962;55:231–6.

CHAPTER 37

Infectious Mononucleosis

Hal B. Jenson

Infectious mononucleosis defines a clinical syndrome characterized by systemic somatic complaints, primarily of fever, fatigue and malaise, lymphadenopathy, and sore throat. Originally described as **glandular fever** in the late nineteenth century, and still known by that name in Europe, this illness has been recognized as a distinct entity since 1921. The clustering of cases and the mononuclear lymphocytosis with atypical-appearing lymphocytes that accompanies the illness led to the name infectious mononucleosis.

ETIOLOGY

Infectious mononucleosis is classically caused by Epstein-Barr virus (EBV), a ubiquitous member of the Herpesviridae family. EBV is a relatively large, enveloped, double-stranded DNA virus that is composed of approximately 172,000 base pairs that encode about 100 gene products. After primary infection, EBV is maintained latently in multiple episomal copies in the cell nucleus and establishes lifelong infection in the host, which remains clinically silent or at least inapparent following the primary illness. The primary reservoir is **resting B lymphocytes.** During the **latent state** the viral episomes replicate with cellular DNA synthesis, only a limited number of viral genes are expressed, no virions are produced, and no clinical manifestations are evident. At least nine EBV-encoded proteins are expressed and are either necessary or responsible for latent maintenance of intracellular virus. Six of these proteins belong to a complex of nuclear neoantigens known as **EBV-determined nuclear antigens (EBNA),** the most prominent of which is **EBNA-1.** Three **latent membrane proteins** (**LMP-1, LMP-2A,** and **LMP-2B**) are detectable on the surfaces of latently infected EBV-transformed cells and are important in T-lymphocyte recognition of EBV-infected B lymphocytes. Under certain conditions in vitro (e.g., addition of carcinogenic chemicals) but poorly defined conditions in vivo, EBV in latently infected lymphocytes enters **lytic replication,** culminating in the release of mature virions and cell death. In contrast to the limited transcription of EBV genes during latency, active viral replication results in production of almost 100 polypeptides. Replicative proteins are classified according to their production relative to viral DNA synthesis; those that occur in the presence of inhibitors of viral DNA synthesis are termed **early antigens,** and those that appear only after viral DNA synthesis are termed **late antigens. Early antigens (EAs)** are a group of more than 20 proteins encoded over scattered regions of the EBV genome. A few of these are encompassed in two classes of EAs, defined on the basis of distribution in the cell and solubility in methanol and designated **diffuse (EA-D)** and **restricted (EA-R).** These and other early antigens are important in viral gene regulation and provide enzymatic activities needed for viral DNA replication. Late antigens include the **viral capsid antigens (VCAs),** a set of structural capsid proteins found in cells actively undergoing EBV replication. Infectious virions are intermittently shed from oropharyngeal and genital tract epithelial cells of infected but healthy persons. Viral replication or reactivation is asymptomatic and is not accompanied by recognizable clinical symptoms.

EBV-Negative Infectious Mononucleosis–like Illnesses. Approximately 10% of cases of infectious mononucleosis–like illness are not caused by EBV. In the majority of EBV-negative infectious mononucleosis–like illnesses the exact cause usually remains uncertain but is presumed to be another known infectious agent. Specific diagnosis is often not necessary because of the usually self-limited and uncomplicated clinical course of these diseases. Primary infections with CMV, *Toxoplasma gondii,* adenovirus, viral hepatitis, HIV, and possibly rubella virus have been identified as causative agents in some cases.

Transmission. Person-to-person spread of EBV is by oral transmission and respiratory spread of salivary secretions from infected persons. The efficiency of transmission is low and appears to require close contact; kissing and intimate family contact are most often implicated. Environmental sources and fomites do not seem to be important. The rate of transmission is highest for familial contact, but even then only about one third of susceptible family members contract EBV from index cases of infectious mononucleosis. EBV can be cultured from the oropharyngeal secretions of 75–100% of persons during the acute phase of infectious mononucleosis; EBV is shed sporadically in salivary secretions from 20–25% of seropositive healthy adults who have no symptoms. Transmission of EBV in blood or blood products is rarely recognized; most posttransfusion cases of infectious mononucleosis–like illness are attributable to CMV.

EPIDEMIOLOGY

EBV is distributed worldwide and infects up to 95% of the world's adult population. Significant relationships exist between age at primary EBV infection and both socioeconomic status and clinical symptoms (Fig. 37–1). In developing countries and in socioeconomically disadvantaged populations of industrialized countries, primary infection usually occurs during infancy and early childhood and is generally associated with no symptoms or only mild symptoms. Up to 95–100% of these children are seropositive by the age of 2–4 years. Among more affluent populations in industrialized countries early childhood infection is still most common, but about one third to one half of cases of infection occur during adolescence and early adulthood. Primary EBV infection in adolescents and young adults is manifest in approximately one half of the cases by the characteristic triad of fever, pharyngitis, and generalized lymphadenopathy. This symptom pattern is recognized clinically as the clinical syndrome of infectious mononucleosis. The clinical entity of EBV-associated infectious mononucleosis is most commonly observed among 15 to 24-year-old persons in higher socioeconomic groups in industrialized countries, despite the high inci-

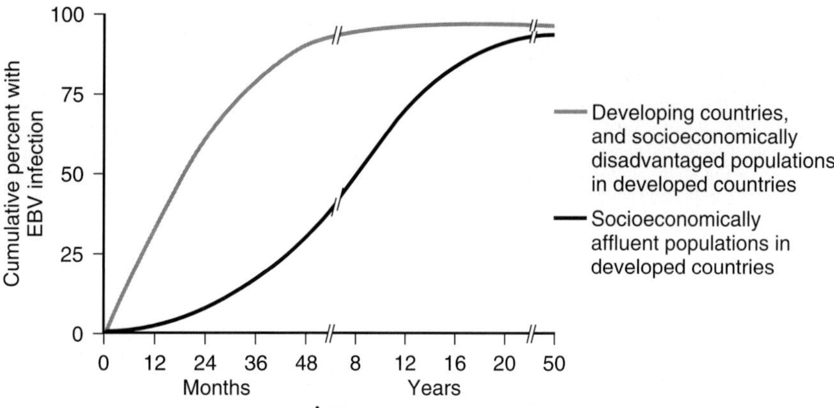

FIGURE 37–1. Age at acquisition of EBV infection in different populations.

dence of asymptomatic EBV infection among infants and young children (Fig. 37–2). The overall incidence of infectious mononucleosis is estimated to be 45 cases per 100,000 per year; in young adults the incidence rises to about 100 cases per 100,000 per year. True incidence rates are unknown because a specific diagnosis may not be made in all cases, and a nonspecific presentation may be attributed to other causes.

EBV shows no sex predilection, although the peak age-specific incidence for cases that occur outside childhood is approximately 18 years for males and 16 years for females. Primary infection is uncommon in women during the child-bearing years, and no real evidence of in utero or congenital infection resulting from the occasional cases of infectious mononucleosis that occur in women in this age group has been found. No seasonal variation has been noted. Outbreaks are distinctly uncommon compared with many other infectious diseases, although college and military populations experience a high incidence rate.

PATHOGENESIS

Via binding of the EBV gp340/220 glycoprotein, EBV infects cells expressing **complement receptor type 2 (CR2; CD21),** the receptor for the complement C3d component that is normally found on B lymphocytes and, to a lesser extent, on nonkeratinized and parakeratinized oral and cervical epithelial cells. The initial infection involves intracellular viral replication within oropharyngeal epithelial cells, cell lysis, and release of mature virus into oropharyngeal secretions. Patients may have fewer symptoms or may exhibit pharyngitis. Virions disseminate to contagious structures, such as the salivary glands, with eventual viremia and spread to mature B lymphocytes in the peripheral blood and other reticuloendothelial tissues. During the acute illness, EBV infects approximately 1% of circulating B lymphocytes. This progression to systemic infection occurs irrespective of oropharyngeal or systemic symptoms. The B lymphocytes infected during infectious mononucleosis include cells that produce all classes of immunoglobulin, although IgM is most common.

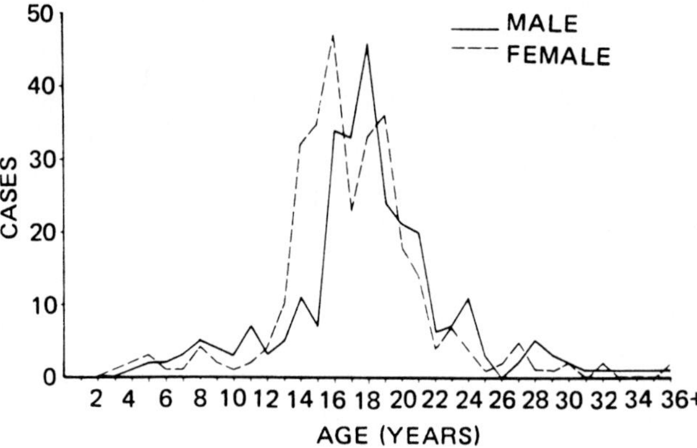

FIGURE 37–2. Cases of infectious mononucleosis by age and sex in metropolitan Atlanta, Georgia, in 1968. (From Heath CW Jr, Brodsky AL, Potolsky AL: Infectious mononucleosis in a general population. *Am J Epidemiol* 1972;95:46–52.)

The pharyngeal symptoms associated with classic EBV-associated infectious mononucleosis are caused by primary EBV infection of nasopharyngeal epithelium accompanied by hypertrophy and inflammation of pharyngeal lymphoid tissue. Infection of B lymphocytes and a mild polyclonal proliferation are quickly followed by an intense CD8 T-lymphocyte-mediated immunopathologic response that involves the liver, spleen, bone marrow, and brain. The circulating atypical lymphocytes that are characteristic of infectious mononucleosis are CD8 T lymphocytes that exhibit both suppressor and cytotoxic functions. This relative as well as absolute increase in CD8 lymphocytes results in a transient reversal of the normal 2:1 **CD4:CD8 T lymphocyte ratio.** Many of the clinical manifestations of infectious mononucleosis may be, at least in part, the result of the host immune response, which is effective in reducing the number of EBV-infected B lymphocytes to fewer than one per 10^6 lymphocytes, which are primarily resting B lymphocytes.

The entire lymphoreticular system is involved in infection. Lymph nodes throughout the body are affected, with moderate enlargement and increased numbers of active lymphoid follicles. Hepatocytes may demonstrate minimal swelling associated with lymphocytic and monocytic portal infiltration. The spleen is enlarged with hyperplasia of the red pulp, and the bone marrow is usually normocellular to mildly hypercellular.

In persons with AIDS, unregulated EBV replication in oropharyngeal epithelium may lead to the lesions of **oral hairy leukoplakia (OHL).** EBV replications in the lung may contribute to the development of **lymphocytic interstitial pneumonitis (LIP)** in children with AIDS (Chapter 38). Severe and even fatal systemic primary EBV infection has rarely occurred in persons who appear to be immunologically incapable of limiting the replication and dissemination of EBV-infected B cells. The **X-linked lymphoproliferative (XLP) syndrome,** also known as **Duncan's syndrome** after the first described kindred, is an X-linked genetic immunologic defect that permits overwhelming and sometimes fatal EBV infection. The defective gene product is known as **SAP** for **SLAM-associated protein.** SLAM is **signaling lymphocyte activate molecule,** which is upregulated on both T and B cells with infection. SAP inhibits the upregulation of SLAM, preventing uncontrolled lymphoproliferation of EBV infection in immunocompetent hosts. Males with XLP syndrome are healthy until they acquire primary EBV infection. It is possible to identify affected males of affected kindreds through genetic analysis before EBV infection develops. Unabated EBV replication may also be seen in Chédiak-Higashi syndrome.

EBV and Cancer. EBV has been intimately associated, though not necessarily causally associated, with Burkitt's lymphoma in Africa, nasopharyngeal carcinoma, Hodgkin's disease, and B cell lymphomas in organ transplant recipients and patients with immunodeficiency disorders, including AIDS. In normal hosts these cancers do not occur as manifestations of primary EBV infection (Chapter 4). Both Burkitt's lymphoma in Africa and nasopharyngeal carcinoma in southern Asia are remarkable for being highly endemic in regions with almost universal acquisition of EBV in early childhood decades before the tumors develop.

SYMPTOMS AND CLINICAL MANIFESTATIONS

The incubation period of EBV-associated infectious mononucleosis after exposure is approximately 2–6 weeks. The varied symptoms of primary EBV infection are modulated by age and immune response. Primary infection is symptomatic in one–half or more of older children and adults and is classically manifest as infectious mononucleosis. Primary EBV infection in infants and young children is usually asymptomatic, although the syndrome of infectious mononucleosis may be seen. The onset of symptoms may be abrupt or gradual.

Acute infectious mononucleosis caused by EBV is a clinically self-limited disease characterized by the cardinal manifestations of fever, fatigue and malaise, lymphadenopathy, and sore throat, with the signs of splenomegaly and hepatomegaly and several other generally mild, minor symptoms (Table 37–1). Symptoms typically develop slowly over several days and persist for a variable period, with gradual spontaneous resolution. The total duration of disease is usually 2–3 weeks.

Several features of EBV-associated infectious mononucleosis are apparent on physical examination. Lymphadenopathy is bilateral and diffuse. It is most prominent in the posterior cervical lymph chain, the anterior cervical and submandibular lymph nodes, and, less frequently, the axillary and inguinal lymph nodes. The nodes are freely mobile and mildly but not markedly tender to examination, with no other signs of inflammation. Splenomegaly is present in up to one half of patients, and hepatomegaly is found in up to 10% of patients; these appear during the acute phase with most other symptoms. Mild hepatic tenderness to percussion may occur, and jaundice is uncommon. Children younger than 4 years of age are more likely to have splenomegaly, hepatomegaly, rhinorrhea, and nonspecific skin rash. An erythematous pharynx, usually with enlarged tonsils that may have an exudate, is also found. Occasionally, a few petechiae at the junction of the hard and soft palate are evident. Various rashes, including macular, petechial, scarlatiniform, and urticarial eruptions, have been described in only approximately 5% of cases.

Ampicillin Rash. Primary viral infection with EBV or with CMV is associated with an unusual but nonspecific maculopapular, erythematous rash after administration of ampicillin (or amoxicillin). This vasculitic rash most likely results from ampicillin-antibody immune complexes resulting from polyclonal B-cell activation. This consistently occurs in adolescents and adults with infectious mononucleosis who are given ampicillin but resolves without specific measures. Since antimicrobial therapy is not necessary for infectious mononucleosis, the antibiotic should be discontinued. If antimicrobials are prescribed for a concomitant bacterial infection, an alternative to ampicillin should be used primarily for the disconcerting, though apparently not dangerous, appearance.

Neurologic Manifestations. Neurologic complications usually present at or shortly after the peak of other symptoms but occasionally may precede or alternatively follow resolution of classic symptoms. Headache is present in 50% of cases of infectious mononucleosis, with severe neurologic manifestations in up to 5% of cases. Meningoencephalitis is the most common severe neurologic manifestation and is characterized by altered consciousness, sometimes with combative behavior, with seizures occurring in approximately 30–40% of cases. Cerebrospinal fluid pleocytosis is seen in as many as 27% of cases, and diffuse slowing and occasional focal abnormalities on EEG are seen in as many as 23% of cases. Encephalitis may result in permanent sequelae in 40% of cases, but most neurologic symptoms resolve without sequelae in 1 week to 3 months. Both infectious and immunologic mechanisms may contribute to neurologic syndromes complicating infectious mononucleosis. EBV-specific antibodies have been detected in the CSF, and EBV genomic sequences have been detected in CSF and brains of persons with neurologic complications of infectious mononucleosis.

An **Alice-in-Wonderland syndrome** of **metamorphopsia,** which is the distortion of perception of sizes, shapes, and spatial relationships of objects, has been described, especially in children. Guillain-Barré syndrome, facial nerve palsy, optic neuritis, and transverse myelitis are rare components of infectious mononucleosis that usually occur when other symptoms are most severe, or shortly thereafter, but may precede or alternatively follow resolution of classic symptoms. The pathogenesis of these neurologic manifestations, which is largely unknown, may include either CNS infection or a postinfectious immune-mediated reaction. These neurologic manifestations typically resolve without sequelae.

Hematologic Manifestations. Autoimmune hemolytic anemia occurs in approximately 3% of cases of infectious mononucleosis, typically with onset during the first 2 weeks of illness and lasting for <1 month.

Mild thrombocytopenia with typical platelet counts of 100,000–150,000/mm^3 occurs in approximately 25–50% of patients during the second and third weeks of illness. Severe thrombocytopenia with platelet count <20,000/mm^3 occurs rarely. Both hypersplenism and antiplatelet antibodies may contribute to thrombocytopenia. Hemorrhagic manifestations are rare but have included purpura, epistaxis, gingival bleeding, hematuria, splenic hemorrhage with rupture, and, rarely, cerebral hemorrhage.

Mild, transient neutropenia to counts approximately 2,000–3,000/mm^3 occurs in 50–80% of cases of infectious mononucleosis, with a nadir during the third and fourth weeks of illness but occasionally persisting for as long as 8 weeks. An increased proportion of immature neutrophils (band forms) also occurs regularly but is short lived, with return to normal beginning by about 3 weeks. Severe neutropenia to counts <1,000/mm^3 and typically lasting only a few days to 1–2 weeks occurs in approximately 3% of cases. Neutropenia may result in part from production of antineutrophil antibodies as part of EBV-induced polyclonal B-cell activation.

TABLE 37–1. Clinical Manifestations and Complications of EBV Infectious Mononucleosis

Symptoms	
Common	
Fever and chills	90%
Sore throat	80
Fatigue and malaise	70
Headache	50
Anorexia	20
Myalgia	20
Abdominal discomfort or nausea	10
Uncommon	<5%
Cough	
Vomiting	
Arthralgias	
Signs	
Common	
Fever	90%
Lymphadenopathy	90
Pharyngitis	80
Splenomegaly	50
Hepatomegaly	10
Palatal enanthem (usually petechiae)	10
Periorbital edema	10
Rash	5
Uncommon	
Ampicillin rash	
Following administration of ampicillin or amoxicillin	95%
Following administration of other β-lactam antibiotics	40–60%
Neurologic manifestations	1–5%
Encephalitis or meningoencephalitis	
Altered consciousness	
Seizures	
Cerebellitis	
Cranial neuritis	
Optic neuritis	
Facial nerve (Bell's) palsy	
Sudden hearing loss	
Transverse myelitis	
Peripheral mononeuritis and polyneuritis	
Autonomic neuropathies	
Guillain-Barré syndrome	
Hemolytic anemia	3%
Jaundice	5%

Uncommon Complications	
Splenic rupture	Rare (<0.5%)
Airway obstruction	<5%
Hematologic complications	
Aplastic anemia	Rare
Agranulocytosis	Rare
Pancytopenia	Rare
Lower respiratory tract complications	Rare
Interstitial pneumonia	
Pleuritis	
Cardiac complications	Rare
Myocarditis	
Pericarditis	
Rhabdomyolysis	Rare
Psychological complications	Rare
Metamorphopsia (Alice-in-Wonderland syndrome)	
Depressive disorders	
Psychosis (visual, auditory, or gustatory hallucinations)	

Toxic granulation and **Döhle bodies** are almost always present in the first weeks of illness, with disappearance over several weeks. Granulocytopoiesis is not usually affected, although agranulocytosis has been reported with complete arrest at the promyelocyte stage.

Hepatitis. Lymphocytic infiltration of the liver and proliferation of Kupffer's cells lead to mild intrahepatic cholestasis but with maintenance of the lobular architecture and without necrosis. Mild, transient elevations in hepatic transaminase levels are common during the second to fourth weeks of illness, occurring in 50–80% of cases with levels that are usually up to 4 times normal, although the AST (SGOT) may reach 1,700 U/L and the ALT (SGPT) may reach 1,000 U/L. Coagulopathy is not seen. Hepatomegaly and hepatic tenderness are present in 10–15% of cases. Mild jaundice develops in approximately 5% of cases and may result from cholestasis as well as virus-induced hemolysis. Severe hepatitis may be complicated by ascites. Recovery is usually complete with only supportive care, although fatal hepatitis complicating infectious mononucleosis has been reported in rare cases.

X-linked Lymphoproliferative (XLP) Syndrome. XLP syndrome is a rare X-linked disorder that has been reported in 272 males in 80 kindreds. About two thirds of affected persons die with primary EBV infection, developing a fulminating and fatal infectious mononucleosis. The survivors develop either hypogammaglobulinemia, B cell lymphoma, or both, with a mortality approaching 85% by the age of 10 years. The XLP syndrome should be considered in any male patient with acute, fulminating, or fatal primary EBV infection and in any kindred with a family history of hypogammaglobulinemia or lymphoma in related males.

EBV in Transplant Recipients. In recipients of solid organ and bone marrow transplants, EBV infection may result in a self-limited infectious mononucleosis syndrome, fatal lymphoproliferation in internal organs progressing over a period of 1–2 months, or extranodal lymphoma. The incidence of malignant lymphoproliferations in transplant recipients is approximately 1% in adults and 4% in children, presumably reflecting an increased incidence of primary infection in seronegative children.

EBV Infection in Persons with AIDS. EBV infection is common during early childhood in children born to HIV-1-infected mothers, whether or not the children have HIV-1 infection. The cumulative EBV infection rate by the age of 3 years is approximately 80% for HIV-infected children and 85% for HIV-uninfected children. Children with rapidly progressive HIV-1 disease demonstrate more frequent EBV shedding. Neither acute nor persistently active EBV infection has a sustained effect on mean CD4 cell counts, percent CD4, IgG levels, HIV RNA levels, or lymphadenopathy, hepatomegaly, and splenomegaly.

LIP is an interstitial pneumonia in persons, primarily children, with AIDS and is characterized by peribronchial infiltration of cytotoxic T lymphocytes directed against alveolar epithelial cells. EBV has been isolated from the pulmonary secretions of many patients with LIP and demonstrated by in situ hybridization, although the causal link with EBV is not firmly established. Corticosteroid therapy is beneficial in both clinical and radiographic improvement (Chapter 38).

OHL is seen almost exclusively in persons with AIDS. The lesions appear as white, raised lesions measuring 5–30 mm with a corrugated, rough surface along the lateral margins of the tongue. EBV is found by in situ hybridization in the upper layers of the epithelium. If OHL is suspected on clinical grounds, the patient should be evaluated for HIV infection (Chapter 38).

DIAGNOSIS

A diagnosis of infectious mononucleosis implies primary infection with EBV. A presumptive diagnosis is based on the pattern of typical clinical symptoms in the setting of atypical lymphocytosis, but serologic tests confirm the cause. The diagnosis of an **infectious mononucleosis–like syndrome,** which is sometimes known as **heterophile-negative infectious mononucleosis,** implies an illness caused not by EBV but by one of a relatively small group of other infectious agents.

Differential Diagnosis

The spectrum of clinical manifestations of primary EBV infection is highly variable, and certain symptoms or signs may be more prominent in individual patients, especially in early stages of the disease. Infectious mononucleosis should be considered in the differential diagnosis of many conditions, even if only a portion of the classic symptoms or signs are present, however. The prominence of the nonspecific constitutional symptoms and the broad spectrum of severity of the individual symptoms often make diagnosis of nonclassic presentations on clinical grounds alone difficult. Focusing on one or two individual symptoms may mask the overall picture.

Those cases of infectious mononucleosis not caused by EBV but that have a recognized cause are most often caused by CMV, and less often by *Toxoplasma gondii,* HIV, viral hepatitis, and adenovirus. Heterophile-negative infectious mononucleosis in children younger than 4 years of age may actually be caused by EBV in approximately 50% of cases, compared with 5–10% in adults.

Acquired Cytomegalovirus Infection. CMV-associated infectious mononucleosis is manifested primarily by fever and malaise, characteristically with prominent splenomegaly. Sore throat or significant lymphadenopathy is usually present. Most patients demonstrate atypical lymphocytosis, negative heterophile antibody, mildly or moderately elevated hepatic transaminases, and evidence of subclinical hemolysis on serial specimens. CMV is the usual cause of infectious mononucleosis–like illnesses that follow blood transfusions. Positive IgM serologic tests for CMV and negative serologic tests for EBV confirm a presumptive clinical diagnosis of primary CMV infection. During the acute illness, CMV may be cultured from urine as well as from peripheral blood leukocytes.

Other Causes. Infectious mononucleosis–like illnesses may result from infection with other infectious agents. *T. gondii,* which causes toxoplasmosis, characteristically causes waxing and waning cervical lymphadenopathy with significant systemic symptoms (Chapter 51) and may also be accompanied by a low level of atypical lymphocytosis. Toxoplasmosis may be suspected on epidemiologic grounds if there is a history of close contact with a cat and confirmed by serologic diagnosis. Infection with hepatitis A virus or hepatitis B infection virus may also result in significant malaise, fever, and lymphadenopathy. Hepatic transaminase levels are markedly elevated at the time of initial presentation and are often accompanied by jaundice, unlike the mild elevations without jaundice that occur with infectious mononucleosis, usually during the second week of illness. Atypical lymphocytosis is less than with EBV-associated infectious mononucleosis. Although rubella typically presents with fever and lymphadenopathy, sometimes with a mild atypical lymphocytosis, the rash is usually diagnostic. Rubella can usually be excluded in persons with a history of previous disease or vaccination but may be evaluated by serologic testing. Even if EBV infection appears likely, HIV infection should be considered if any epidemiologic risk factors or other symptoms or signs of AIDS are present.

Although hepatosplenomegaly is not characteristic of streptococcal pharyngitis, the pharyngitis and cervical lymphadenopathy of group A *Streptococcus* pharyngitis may be indistinguishable from infectious mononucleosis. Testing for EBV heterophile antibody may be required in addition to a throat culture because up to 5% of persons with EBV-associated infectious mononucleosis have positive throat cultures for group A *Streptococcus.* Many of these persons are probably carriers of pharyngeal streptococci.

Laboratory Evaluation

The hallmark laboratory finding of infectious mononucleosis is the presence of **atypical lymphocytes,** usually between 10 and 30% of the total WBC count, which contributes to an absolute and relative lymphocytosis (Table 37–2). Atypical lymphocytes are not pathognomic for EBV infection, however, and may also be seen with a few other infections as well as with drug reactions (Chapter 10). The increase in circulating white blood cells in infectious mononucleosis is primarily a result of an increase in the number of CD8 T lymphocytes responding to EBV-infected B lymphocytes. The total WBC count is slightly elevated to 12,000–18,000/mm^3; monocytes and lymphocytes typically constitute 60–70% of the circulating white blood cells. A diminution or even a reversal of the normal 2:1 CD4/CD8 T lymphocyte ratio may also be apparent because of the intense proliferation of CD8 T lymphocytes. This finding, which is more noticeable in older persons, peaks during the second and third weeks of illness.

Transient neutropenia, both relative and absolute, may be seen during the first week of illness, especially in children. Thrombocytopenia is common and may result from an increased rate of platelet destruction resulting from autoimmune antiplatelet antibodies or from sequestration associated with hypersplenism. Thrombocyto-

TABLE 37–2. Laboratory Abnormalities of EBV Infectious Mononucleosis

Common	
Atypical lymphocytosis	80%
Reversal of CD4:CD8 T lymphocyte ratio	80%
Asymptomatic elevated hepatic transaminases	50–80%
Neutropenia	50–80% (early)
Severe neutropenia (neutrophil count <1,000/mm³)	<3%
Thrombocytopenia	25–50% (early)
Severe thrombocytopenia (platelet count <20,000/mm³)	Rare
Uncommon	
Autoimmune hemolytic anemia	<3%
Electrocardiograph (ECG) abnormalities (ST-T wave abnormalities)	Rare

penia with hemorrhages occurs in approximately 4% of cases. Autoimmune hemolytic anemia, usually associated with positive cold agglutinins, rarely appears during the second and third weeks of illness and usually resolves over 1–2 months.

Mild elevation of hepatic transaminases occurs in approximately 50% of otherwise uncomplicated cases, characteristically peaks during the second week of illness at 2–3 times normal levels, and gradually resolves in 3–4 weeks. Transient depression of delayed hypersensitivity, as determined by cutaneous anergy and in vitro lymphocyte proliferative responses to mitogens, has been reported during the acute phase of infectious mononucleosis.

Cerebrospinal Fluid. The CSF in patients with encephalitis or meningoencephalitis typically has a mononuclear cell count up to 200/mm³, a normal opening pressure, normal to mildly elevated protein concentration, and normal glucose concentration. Both atypical lymphocytes and low titers of EBV-specific antibodies have been reported in the CSF (Chapter 11).

Microbiologic Evaluation

The diagnosis of infectious mononucleosis caused by EBV is confirmed by serologic tests, either with the transient presence of heterophile antibodies or with the permanent emergence of EBV-specific antibodies (Fig. 37–3). Acute CMV-associated infectious mononucleosis may be diagnosed by testing for IgM antibodies to CMV.

Heterophile Antibody Test. **Heterophile antibodies** agglutinate cells from species different from those in the source serum. The heterophile antibodies in human serum associated with acute infectious mononucleosis, also known as **Paul-Bunnell antibodies,** agglutinate sheep and horse erythrocytes, among others, and are adsorbed by beef red blood cells but not by guinea pig kidney cells. The adsorption property distinguishes this response from other heterophile antibodies found in patients with serum sickness and rheumatic diseases and in some healthy persons with **Forssman antibodies.** Approximately 80% of children 4 years of age or older and 90% of adolescents and older patients with primary EBV infection have heterophile antibodies; children younger than 4 years of age have a lower heterophile response that may not be detectable. The antibody response usually peaks in the second and third weeks of illness and can usually be found for up to 6–9 months after resolution of symptoms (Fig. 37–3), especially in adults. Approximately 20% of patients have a positive heterophile test response for 18 months or longer; there is no anamnestic response. The titer does not correlate with the severity of illness. This is an IgM antibody and is unrelated to those antibodies directed to specific EBV antigens. Its role in the pathogenesis or recovery from EBV infection is not known.

The most widely used method for detection of Paul-Bunnell heterophile antibodies is the qualitative, rapid slide test, which is slightly more sensitive than the classic tube heterophile test. A test using horse erythrocytes is somewhat more sensitive than one using sheep erythrocytes and detects heterophile antibody in 90% of cases of EBV-associated infectious mononucleosis in adults but in only up to 50% of cases in children younger than 4 years of age. The false-positive rate is <10%. Erroneous interpretations by operators account for most of the false-positive results and some of the false-negative outcomes as well.

If the heterophile antibody test is negative and an EBV-associated disease is suspected, EBV-specific serologic testing is indicated to confirm the cause. This testing is also useful in evaluating a positive heterophile antibody test associated with clinical or

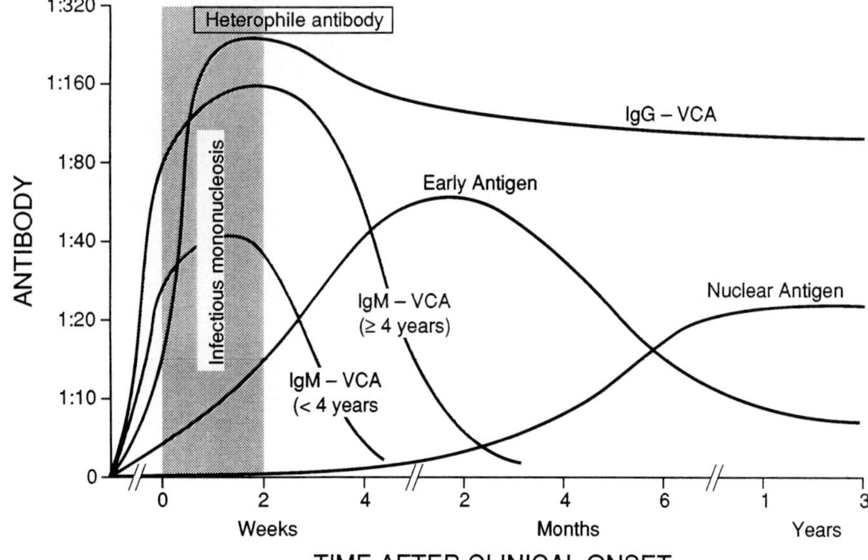

FIGURE 37–3. Schematic representation of the development of antibodies to various EBV antigens in patients with infectious mononucleosis. The titers are geometric mean values expressed as reciprocals of the serum dilution. The minimum titer tested for antibodies to VCA and EA is 1:10, and for nuclear antigen it is 1:2.5. The IgM response to VCA is divided because of the significant differences noted according to age of the patient. (From Jenson HB, Ench Y: Epstein-Barr virus. In Rose NR, de Macario EC, Folds JD, et al (editors): Manual of Clinical Laboratory Immunology, 6th ed. Washington, DC, American Society for Microbiology, 2001.)

laboratory findings uncharacteristic of infectious mononucleosis. Approximately 5–10% of cases of infectious mononucleosis–like illness are not caused by EBV and are not uniformly associated with a heterophile antibody response.

Specific EBV Antibody Tests. EBV-specific antigen-antibody testing is useful in determining susceptibility or immunity to primary EBV infection on an individual basis, especially in the evaluation of EBV infection in a heterophile antibody–negative, infectious mononucleosis–like episode. Several distinct EBV-associated antigen systems have been characterized (Table 37–3 and Fig. 37–3).

The EBNA, EA, and VCA antigen systems are the most useful for diagnostic purposes. The acute phase of infectious mononucleosis is characterized by rapid IgM and IgG antibody responses to VCA in all cases. The IgM response to VCA is transient and lasts approximately 1–3 months. The IgG response to VCA usually peaks during the acute illness, declines slightly over the next few weeks to months, and then remains at a relatively stable level for life. An IgG response to the EA complex is seen in most cases. Anti-EA antibodies are usually present for several months but may persist for several years after resolution of the acute infection. Anti-EBNA-1 antibodies, which typically appear much later, gradually emerge over several months following the onset of illness and last for life. Some immunocompromised patients with a poor clinical course demonstrate diminishing or undetectable levels of anti-EBNA-1 antibodies.

Some laboratories may offer tests for EBNA-2 antibodies in addition to tests for EBNA-1 antibodies. EBNA-2 antibodies, which are made in response to another latent EBV nuclear protein, are usually detectable at the onset of clinical symptoms and persist for at least 4 months. The EBNA-2 results do not contribute to information from the regular battery of tests, and thus these tests are not routinely performed. The EBNA-2 antibody titer gradually falls over the next few years, but the variable titer makes the result almost useless in dating the onset of infection.

The wide range of individual antibody responses can occasionally make interpretation of an individual antibody profile difficult (Table 37–3). The detection of IgM antibody to VCA is the most valuable and specific serologic test for the diagnosis of acute EBV infection, and it is generally sufficient to confirm an acute EBV infection. In almost all cases, the IgM-VCA antibody response can be detected for up to 4 months after clinical onset of the infectious mononucleosis, and in a few cases this period is even longer. The laboratory must take appropriate steps to remove rheumatoid factor, which may give a false-positive IgM-VCA result (Chapter 11). Antibody profiles that are not based on IgM-VCA are not as dependable for diagnosis of acute EBV infection. IgM antibody to CMV may be detected in serum of patients with EBV-associated infectious mononucleosis, but IgM antibody to EBV VCA does not appear to be detectable with CMV-induced, infectious mononucleosis–like episodes. High titers of IgG antibody to VCA do not by themselves necessarily indicate an acute EBV infection.

More than 80% of patients with infectious mononucleosis develop a transient antibody response to the EA-D component. In some adults, and especially in young children, however, this response may be directed mainly against the EA-R component.

The testing of a second, or convalescent, serum 4–6 weeks after clinical onset of disease is of minimal help in diagnosing acute EBV infection, because fewer than 10% of patients have a significant antibody titer rise over this interval.

A currently quiescent EBV infection is characterized by the concurrent presence of moderate but stable titers of IgG antibodies to VCA and EBNA and by the absence of IgM antibody to VCA. Antibodies to EA are usually absent, but may be intermittently present at low titers, predominantly to the EA-R component, in up to 10% of healthy persons.

High titers of IgG antibody to VCA and EA, considered to indicate enhanced EBV activity or reactivation, have been noted in persons with Burkitt's lymphoma, nasopharyngeal carcinoma, or immunosuppression or immunodeficient states (Chapter 4). The

TABLE 37–3. Correlation of Clinical Status and Virus and Antibody Pattern in EBV Infection

	Characteristic Response*					
	Heterophile Antibodies (Qualitative Test)	EBV-Specific Antibody				
Clinical Status		IgM-VCA	IgG-VCA	EA-D	EA-R	EBNA
Lower limit of detection	–	1:8†	1:10	1:10	1:10	1:2.5
Susceptible individual	–	<1:8	<1:10	<1:10	<1:10	<1:2.5
Acute primary infection: infectious mononucleosis	+	1:32 to 1:256	1:160 to 1:640	1:40 to 1:160	–‡	– to 1:2.5
Recent primary infection: infectious mononucleosis	+/–	– to 1:32	1:320 to 1:1280	1:40 to 1:60	–‡	1:5 to 1:10
Remote infection	–	–	1:40 to 1:160	–§	– to 1:40	1:10 to 1:40
Reactivation: immunosuppressed or immunocompromised patient	–	–	1:320 to 1:1280	–§	1:80 to 1:320	– to 1:160
Burkitt's lymphoma	–	–	1:320 to 1:1280	–§	1:80 to 1:320	1:10 to 1:80
Nasopharyngeal carcinoma	–	–	1:320 to 1:1280	1:40 to 1:160	–‖	1:20 to 1:160

*Individual responses outside the characteristic range may occur.

†1:10 may be the lowest dilution tested by some laboratories.

‡In young children and adults with asymptomatic seroconversion, the anti-EA response may be mainly to the EA-R component.

§A minority of individuals will have the anti-EA response mainly to the EA-D component.

‖A minority of individuals will have the anti-EA response mainly to the EA-R component.

Adapted from Jenson HB, Ench Y: Epstein-Barr virus. In Rose NR, de Mecario EC, Folds JD, et al (editors): Manual of Clinical Laboratory Immunology, 6th ed. Washington, DC, American Society for Microbiology, 2001.

antibody response to EA is directed principally to the EA-R component in patients with Burkitt's lymphoma and immunosuppression and to the EA-D component in patients with nasopharyngeal carcinoma. High levels of IgA antibody to VCA and EA are also found in persons with nasopharyngeal carcinoma, including the early occult or asymptomatic stages. In these patients, tumor activity and response to therapy may be monitored by serial IgA-VCA and IgA-EA determinations.

Virus Culture. EBV culture is performed by **transformation** of human umbilical cord lymphocytes into a nonmalignant, continuously growing, or **immortalized,** cell line. EBV cultures require 3–6 weeks. The EBV **transformation assay,** which is used primarily in research laboratories, is not usually recommended for evaluation of suspected infectious mononucleosis. The assay can semiquantitatively assess the level of infectious EBV by measuring induction of lymphoproliferation or activation of B cells to immunoglobulin production.

Transforming EBV can be cultured from the oropharyngeal secretions in approximately 75% of children during the acute phase of infectious mononucleosis. The rate of oropharyngeal viral excretion gradually decreases over a period of 18 months following acute infection, with asymptomatic and intermittent shedding of EBV in oropharyngeal secretions for life; at any given time, EBV can be sporadically isolated from saliva from approximately 20% of symptom-free seropositive healthy adults. The prevalence of oral shedding increases up to 50% in immunocompromised persons, such as transplant recipients or patients undergoing cancer chemotherapy.

Diagnostic Imaging

Radiographs are usually unnecessary in the evaluation of infectious mononucleosis. Enlarged pharyngeal tonsils may be observed on a lateral neck radiograph (see Fig. 13–9).

TREATMENT

Definitive Treatment

There is no effective specific treatment for EBV-associated infectious mononucleosis, which is usually a self-limited illness that lasts 2–3 weeks without sequelae. There have been five randomized clinical trials of treatment of infectious mononucleosis with acyclovir in a total of 339 patients; individually and by meta-analysis (Torre and Tambini, 1999), these trials show no statistically significant benefit or clinical effectiveness of acyclovir treatment. There is a significant reduction in the rate of oropharyngeal EBV shedding during 10 days of therapy but no difference in oropharyngeal shedding at 3 weeks. There is no evidence that antiviral therapy hastens resolution of symptoms or prevents development of complications of infectious mononucleosis. Small studies of various combinations of acyclovir, IVIG, and IFN-α may have limited effects on the duration of fever and a sense of well-being, although objective measures of improvement have not been demonstrated. The inhibitory effect on viral replication does not persist after discontinuation of therapy. Studies of small groups of patients with CMV-associated infectious mononucleosis have demonstrated a similar lack of efficacy of such treatments. Persons with fulminating disease believed to be caused by acute EBV infection, which is rare, and immunocompromised persons may benefit from acyclovir therapy. These patients should be managed in conjunction with an infectious diseases specialist.

Supportive Therapy

Rest and symptomatic therapy are the mainstays of management of infectious mononucleosis in immunocompetent persons. Acetaminophen should be used for fever. Blunt abdominal trauma may predispose to splenic rupture, which is rare, so it is customary and prudent to advise exclusion from contact sports and strenuous physical activities for the first 2–3 weeks of illness or if splenomegaly is present on physical examination, at least until the organomegaly is resolved. Although approximately 50% of patients with splenic rupture have a history of abdominal trauma, such recommendations have not been shown to reduce the incidence of splenic rupture.

Corticosteroids. The use of corticosteroids for complications of infectious mononucleosis has been advocated on the basis of anecdotal experience but has not been critically evaluated and remains controversial. Corticosteroids are unnecessary in mild, uncomplicated cases and should not be routinely administered to all persons with infectious mononucleosis. Indications include incipient upper airway obstruction, autoimmune hemolytic anemia or neutropenia, thrombocytopenia with hemorrhage, and meningoencephalitis and other neurologic complications. Intravenous dexamethasone (0.25 mg/kg every 6 hours) or methylprednisolone (1 mg/kg every 6 hours) or oral prednisone (40 mg daily) given for 1–3 days have been used with similar results of dramatic subjective improvement within 24 hours and objective improvement within 72 hours. Corticosteroid therapy may hasten resolution of complications in some, but not all, cases of infectious mononucleosis. Reluctance to use corticosteroids is based on the unknown long-term effects of using an immunomodulator for a virus that will establish intracellular latency and for which the normal immune response is usually quite effective in preventing progression as well as subsequent development of EBV-associated malignant diseases (Chapter 4). IVIG therapy may be as good or better for treatment of thrombocytopenia or hemolytic anemia associated with infectious mononucleosis, although this has not been critically evaluated. Both an infectious diseases specialist and a hematologist should be consulted about this complication.

COMPLICATIONS

The great majority of patients with infectious mononucleosis recover uneventfully without complications. Cumulative clinical experience coupled with biologic plausibility, and in some cases experimental data, supports the causal association of many manifestations and complications with EBV infectious mononucleosis (Table 37–1). Many of the complications of infectious mononucleosis were reported before the identification of EBV as the cause of infectious mononucleosis and therefore lack specific virologic confirmation. The sophistication of diagnostic testing has greatly improved over the past 30 years since many of these complications were first reported. The ability of EBV to maintain lifelong latency after primary infection with low levels of replication and viral shedding and enduring antigen exposure results in continued humoral immune response with long-standing and easily detectable levels of specific EBV antibodies, especially to viral capsid antigen and also to the early antigen complex. Variation in specific EBV antibody titers may be due to reactivation of latent virus, infection with heterologous virus with development of cross-reactive antibodies, selective stimulation of memory B cells by related antigens, or polyclonal B cell stimulation. These important differences from most other infectious agents in conjunction with the high prevalence of EBV infection have contributed to innumerable case reports (based on serologic test results alone) of EBV being erroneously implicated as a cause of a wide variety of complications. Although the associations of EBV with many of the putative complications are intriguing both individually and in toto, for many complications the small numbers of cases studied, the limitations of the methods and analyses employed, and in some instances reports of contradictory findings often result in inconclusive evidence to confirm a causal relationship to EBV.

Splenic Rupture. Subcapsular splenic hemorrhage and spontaneous rupture of the spleen are celebrated but rare complications of infectious mononucleosis, occurring in fewer than 0.5% of cases in adults. The rate in children is unknown but is likely much lower. The highest incidence is during the second and third weeks of illness. Splenic rupture is rarely fatal, although it is usually regarded as the most common peril associated with infectious mononucleosis. Abrupt or insidious onset of acute left upper quadrant abdominal pain, which may radiate to the left shoulder, suggests the possibility of splenic hemorrhage, especially if accompanied by shock. Although splenectomy traditionally has been advocated, numerous recent reports have documented favorable outcomes with nonoperative management for selected patients who meet certain criteria: (1) hemodynamic stability, (2) a normal level of consciousness, (3) age under 50 years, (4) transfusion requirements of less than 4 units of blood, (5) early resolution of splenic defects on imaging studies, and (6) rapid resolution of posttraumatic ileus. Conservative management may result in longer hospitalization and prolonged periods of limited physical activity with risk of recurrent hemorrhage.

Airway Obstruction. Significant upper airway obstruction results from palatal and nasopharyngeal tonsil hypertrophy and inflammatory edema of surrounding soft tissues. Airway obstruction with progressive symptoms occurs in fewer than 5% of all cases and is one of the most common indications for hospitalization of patients with infectious mononucleosis. Younger children appear to be at greater risk. Most cases can be managed with observation by pulse oximetry and treatment with head-of-bed elevation, intravenous hydration, humidified air, and systemic corticosteroids. Occasional cases require temporary nasopharyngeal stenting to bypass lymphoid hyperplasia and soft tissue edema. Severe airway obstruction that fails to respond to medical management should be relieved by tonsilloadenoidectomy followed by postoperative endotracheal intubation for 12–24 hours.

Aplastic Anemia. Aplastic anemia associated with infectious mononucleosis is a rare complication that presents approximately 3 weeks after the onset of illness, usually with recovery in 4–8 days. Some cases do require bone marrow transplantation.

Pneumonia. Pneumonia is an uncommon manifestation of infectious mononucleosis and is frequently the result of coinfection with bacterial, viral, or mycoplasmal pathogens. Bilateral interstitial infiltrates are most common, frequently with the presence of unilateral or bilateral pleural effusions. The pleural fluid typically has a leukocyte count of $<4,000/mm^3$ with a predominance of lymphocytes.

Cardiac Manifestations. Asymptomatic electrocardiographic changes are the most frequent cardiac abnormality, occurring in approximately 6% of cases during the first 3 weeks of illness, but these resolve without sequelae. Rarely, histiocytic and lymphocytic infiltration of the myocardium may result in myocarditis.

Rhabdomyolysis. Acute rhabdomyolysis and myoglobinuria have been reported rarely, and may be further complicated by nonoliguric renal failure.

Fulminant EBV Infection. Fulminant or fatal infectious mononucleosis in immunocompetent hosts is rare. Unusually severe immune responses during infectious mononucleosis may occur with exaggerated symptoms of persistent or intermittent fever, generalized lymphadenopathy, and hepatosplenomegaly with extremely high antibody titers and high viral burdens. Most cases of fatal infectious mononucleosis are the consequence of an apparently uncontrolled lymphoproliferative response to primary EBV infection and demonstrate **hemophagocytic lymphohistiocytosis.** EBV is considered to be the principal cause of severe cases of **virus-associated hemophagocytic syndrome (VAHS),** a hemophagocytic lymphohistiocytosis associated with a systemic viral infection of nonmalignant, generalized histiocytic proliferation with marked **hemophagocytosis,** which is phagocytosis by macrophages of erythrocytes, leukocytes, platelets, and their precursors in bone marrow and other tissues. Distinguishing VAHS and malignant histiocytosis is often difficult. EBV infection of T lymphocytes contributes to production of TNF-α and IFN-γ with excessive activation of monocytes that exhibit hemophagocytosis and produce high levels of IL-1, IL-6, and IL-18. Anti-TNF-α and anti-IFN-γ antibodies attenuate hemophagocytosis. Most patients with fatal infectious mononucleosis exhibit pathologic findings of VAHS. The fever, lymphadenopathy, and hepatosplenomegaly are further complicated by pulmonary infiltrates, rash, cytopenias, and hepatic dysfunction that can have a fulminant course, often leading to death. Treatment with etoposide, which reduces both monocyte and macrophage activity, and corticosteroids may be an effective therapy.

Psychological Complications. Visual hallucinations and acute psychotic reactions are reported occasionally, and auditory and gustatory hallucinations are reported rarely.

Both biologic and psychological determinants are important in the clinical expression of infectious mononucleosis in adolescents and adults. Transient psychological distress, somatization, and functional disability are common during acute infection, and depressive symptoms appear to occur more frequently with infectious mononucleosis than with other viral illnesses. Predictors of psychosocial distress at 2 months include both biologic factors (e.g., severity of symptoms during the first 2 weeks of illness, higher hepatic transaminase levels) and psychosocial factors (e.g., poorer social functioning in the month preceding diagnosis). Predictors of psychosocial distress at 6 months include an increase in the number of adverse life events over the previous 6-month period and a reduction of activities in the 2 weeks before illness. Infectious mononucleosis is not associated with prolonged depression or ''postviral'' depression, although major depressive disorders occur rarely.

Chronic Fatigue Syndrome. Prolonged convalescence after infectious mononucleosis usually indicates an underlying psychiatric disorder, a fatigue syndrome, or both. There is no basis for confirmation of the hypothesis that infection with EBV is the primary cause of the symptoms in the majority of cases of chronic fatigue syndrome (Chapter 41). The term ''chronic EBV infection'' is misleading because every person infected with EBV is infected for life. Reactivation of latent EBV during periods of immunosuppression is associated with T-cell lymphocytosis characteristic of primary infection and may contribute directly to lymphoma and other tumors in immunocompromised patients.

Intrauterine Infection. EBV is not believed to cause fetal anomalies or even fetal infection, in spite of symptomatic maternal infection during pregnancy. Concern about the potential teratogenic effect of nucleoside analogues such as acyclovir overrides any putative benefit regarding its use in pregnant women. The likelihood after either primary or reactivated EBV infection during pregnancy is there will be a normal outcome.

EBV and Cancer. EBV was the first virus shown to contribute to proliferative disorders in human beings; therefore it was the first virus to be identified as a human tumor virus. The first observation of EBV was in the cultured lymphoid cells of African Burkitt's lymphoma. Several types of lymphoid and epithelial neoplasia have been associated with EBV (see Table 4-1), most notably Burkitt's lymphoma, nasopharyngeal carcinoma, Hodgkin's disease, and B-cell lymphomas and leiomyosarcomas in patients with cancer, recipients of solid organ and bone marrow transplants, and persons with immunodeficiency disorders, including XLP syndrome and AIDS (Chapter 4). The precise etiologic role of EBV in the development of these tumors remains to be defined, however.

PROGNOSIS

The clinical course of most cases of infectious mononucleosis lasts up to 3 weeks, with maximal fever, lymphadenopathy, and sore throat occurring during the first 2 weeks of illness and then gradually resolving. The disease is much milder during the third week. The constitutional symptoms of malaise and fatigue may resolve more slowly, with convalescence continuing over several weeks to even months in otherwise unremarkable cases. Unusual persistence of fatigue for months to a few years after infection with EBV or influenza virus is well recognized, although a causal link is not firmly established and should not be inferred. Other signs of clinical depression are frequently evident in persons with persistent fatigue. Several studies of convalescence after acute systemic infection support the view that symptomatic recovery critically depends on the emotional state and attitude of the patient. A person with a propensity for depression is more likely to respond to acute infection with depression-like symptoms than a person who does not have such a vulnerability (Chapter 41).

Death associated with infectious mononucleosis is uncommon, although the disease has a historical reputation for mortality. Complications associated with death include meningoencephalitis, splenic rupture, secondary infection, fulminant hepatitis, airway obstruction, and heart block and cardiac dysrhythmia (Penman, 1970). Except for fulminating acute EBV infection in persons with the XLP syndrome and in immunocompromised patients, adequately documented fatal cases of infectious mononucleosis, even when they involve splenic rupture, are scarce. EBV-associated aplastic anemia is believed to have a good prognosis with supportive therapy during the acute stages.

After acute infection, EBV is shed intermittently and apparently asymptomatically in oropharyngeal secretions for life. The virus can be sporadically isolated from saliva in up to approximately 20% of symptom-free healthy, seropositive adults and in a lesser percentage of children. Immunodeficiency resulting from cancer or immunosuppressive therapy or AIDS is associated with oropharyngeal shedding of EBV in 50–75% of such patients.

Second attacks of infectious mononucleosis caused by EBV have not been documented, although similar symptoms may occur with infectious mononucleosis–like illnesses caused by other etiologic factors.

Prevention

EBV is ubiquitous. Because intimate contact is necessary for transmission, isolation of patients with infectious mononucleosis is unnecessary. It is practically impossible to prevent spread via oral secretions in children who share toys and other objects placed in their mouths. This is especially true in the case of adolescents and older persons who consciously engage in kissing, an activity that is highly effective in transmission. Because no substantive evidence of in utero or congenital infection exists, there is no indication for routine prenatal serologic testing.

Persons with infectious mononucleosis should not donate blood during acute illnesses or for at least 6 months afterward. Infection by transfusion of blood is possible but is uncommon because of the level of antibodies present in most donated blood, previous infection and antibodies in most recipients of blood products, and separation of the majority of white blood cells from erythrocytes and plasma. Most cases of posttransfusion infectious mononucleosis–like illness are caused by CMV. The risk of infection in neonates and immunocompromised hosts can be reduced by using seronegative donors or by appropriately preparing blood products to minimize the number of white blood cells and the corresponding cell-associated virus.

There is no vaccine against EBV, although numerous approaches are actively being pursued.

REVIEWS

Schlossberg D (editor): Infectious Mononucleosis. New York, Springer-Verlag, 1989.

Sumaya CV, Ench Y: Epstein-Barr virus infectious mononucleosis in children. I. Clinical and general laboratory findings. *Pediatrics* 1985;75:1003–10.

Sumaya CV, Ench Y: Epstein-Barr virus infectious mononucleosis in children. II. Heterophil antibody and viral-specific responses. *Pediatrics* 1985;75:1011–9.

Torre D, Tambini R: Acyclovir for treatment of infectious mononucleosis: A meta-analysis. *Scand J Infect Dis* 1999;31:543–7.

KEY ARTICLES

Alpert G, Fleisher GR: Complications of infection with Epstein-Barr virus during childhood: A study of children admitted to the hospital. *Pediatr Infect Dis* 1984;3:304–7.

Andiman WA: Epstein-Barr virus-associated syndromes: A critical reexamination. *Pediatr Infect Dis* 1984;3:198–203.

Asgari MM, Begos DG: Spontaneous splenic rupture in infectious mononucleosis: A review. *Yale J Biol Med* 1997;70:175–82.

Domachowske JB, Cunningham CK, Cummings DL, et al: Acute manifestations and neurologic sequelae of Epstein-Barr virus encephalitis in children. *Pediatr Infect Dis* J 1996;15:871–5.

Eshel GM, Evov A, Lahat E, et al: Alice in Wonderland syndrome, a manifestation of acute Epstein-Barr virus infection. *Pediatr Infect Dis* 1987;6:68.

Fleisher G, Bolognese R: Infectious mononucleosis during gestation: Report of three women and their infants studied prospectively. *Pediatr Infect Dis* J 1984;3:308–11.

Grierson H, Purtilo DT: Epstein-Barr virus infections in males with the X-linked lymphoproliferative syndrome. *Ann Intern Med* 1987;106:538–45.

Grose C, Henle W, Henle G, et al: Primary Epstein-Barr virus infections in acute neurologic diseases. *N Engl J Med* 1975;292:392–5.

Heath CW Jr, Brodsky AL, Potolsky AL: Infectious mononucleosis in a general population. *Am J Epidemiol* 1972;95:46–52.

Horwitz CA, Henle W, Henle G, et al: Clinical and laboratory evaluation of cytomegalovirus-induced mononucleosis in previously healthy individuals. Report of 82 cases. *Medicine (Baltimore)* 1986;65:124–34.

Imai S, Usui N, Sugiura M, et al: Epstein-Barr virus genomic sequences and specific antibodies in cerebrospinal fluid in children with neurologic complications of acute and reactivated EBV infections. *J Med Virol* 1993;40:278–84.

Imashuku S, Hibi S, Ohara T, et al: Effective control of Epstein-Barr virus-related hemophagocytic lymphohistiocytosis with immunochemotherapy. *Blood* 1999;93:1869–74.

Jenson H, McIntosh K, Pitt J, et al: Natural history of primary Epstein-Barr virus infection in children of mothers infected with human immunodeficiency virus type 1. *J Infect Dis* 1999;179:1395–404.

Katon W, Russo J, Ashley RL, et al: Infectious mononucleosis: Psychological symptoms during acute and subacute phases of illness. *Gen Hosp Psychiatry* 1999;21:21–9.

Lazarus KH, Baehner RL: Aplastic anemia complicating infectious mononucleosis: A case report and review of the literature. *Pediatrics* 1981; 67:907–10.

Okano M, Gross TG: Epstein-Barr virus-associated hemophagocytic syndrome and fatal infectious mononucleosis. *Am J Hematol* 1996;53: 111–5.

Penman HG: Fatal infectious mononucleosis: A critical review. *J Clin Pathol* 1970;23:765–71.

Pipp ML, Means ND, Sixbey JW, et al: Acute Epstein-Barr virus infection complicated by severe thrombocytopenia. *Clin Infect Dis* 1997;25:1237–9.

Reisman MD, Greco MA: Virus-associated hemophagocytic syndrome due to Epstein-Barr virus. *Hum Pathol* 1984;15:290–3.

Robinson JE, Brown N, Andiman W, et al: Diffuse polyclonal B-cell lymphoma during primary infection with Epstein-Barr virus. *N Engl J Med* 1980;302:1293–7.

Sayos J, Wu C, Morra M, et al: The X-linked lymphoproliferative-disease gene product SAP regulates signals induced through the co-receptor SLAM. *Nature* 1998;395:462–9.

Schnell RG, Dyck PJ, Bowie EJ, et al: Infectious mononucleosis: Neurologic and EEG findings. *Medicine (Baltimore)* 1966;45:51–63.

Seemayer TA, Gross TG, Egeler RM, et al: X-linked lymphoproliferative disease: Twenty-five years after the discovery. *Pediatr Res* 1995;38: 471–8.

Silverstein A, Steinberg G, Nathanson M: Nervous system involvement in infectious mononucleosis: The heralding and/or major manifestation. *Arch Neurol* 1972;26:353–8.

Sumaya CV, Ench Y: Epstein-Barr virus infections in families: The role of children with infectious mononucleosis. *J Infect Dis* 1986;154:842–50.

Torre D, Tambini R: Acyclovir for treatment of infectious mononucleosis: A meta-analysis. *Scand J Infect Dis* 1999;31:543–7.

Tynell E, Aurelius E, Brandell A, et al: Acyclovir and prednisolone treatment of acute infectious mononucleosis: A multicenter, double-blind, placebo-controlled study. *J Infect Dis* 1996;174:324–31.

Weigle KA, Sumaya CV, Montiel MM: Changes in T lymphocyte subsets during childhood Epstein-Barr virus infectious mononucleosis. *J Clin Immunol* 1983;3:151–5.

Wohl DL, Isaacson JE: Airway obstruction in children with infectious mononucleosis. *Ear Nose Throat J* 1995;74:630–8.

Wolfe JA, Rowe LD: Upper airway obstruction in infectious mononucleosis. *Ann Otol Rihinol Laryngol* 1980;89:430–3.

CHAPTER 38

Human Immunodeficiency Virus and Acquired Immunodeficiency Syndrome

Terence I. Doran ▪ Janet Squires

The first cases of **acquired immunodeficiency syndrome (AIDS)** in children were reported in 1983, two years after the syndrome was described in adults. Retrospectively, it has been recognized that there were a number of children born in the late 1970s to mothers infected with the **human immunodeficiency virus type 1 (HIV, or HIV-1),** the causative agent of AIDS. The 1990s brought changes in our understanding of HIV and significant advances in the treatment of persons with HIV disease and AIDS. New antiretroviral medications are being added to the treatment arsenal every year. AIDS deaths in the United States have decreased markedly in recent years. Treatment of pregnant HIV-infected women and their newborns has greatly decreased the number of vertically infected children in the United States and other developed countries. Physicians can readily monitor viral production and immune response, allowing better assessment of response to therapy and of disease progression.

Despite the remarkable successes, there continue to be significant problems. Antiretroviral medications have benefited a relatively limited population in the developed world while remaining entirely out of reach for 95% of the world's infected population because of costs. Resistance to antiretroviral medications is increasing. Treatment regimens are increasingly complex, beyond what many patients can manage. Globally an estimated 15,000 new infections occur daily, with little to impede the spread of disease. Education alone has not resulted in the behavioral changes that are necessary to curtail the spread of HIV. Vaccine development may be the best chance to control the spread of HIV. However, it is uncertain if or when a vaccine will ever be developed for widespread use.

ETIOLOGY

HIV-1 and HIV-2 are RNA retroviruses in the Lentivirinae subfamily of human retroviruses. HIV-1 is slightly more than 100 nm in diameter (Figs. 38–1 and 38–2) and is composed of two similar or identical strands of RNA, surrounded by core proteins and a lipid bilayer derived from the outer membrane of the host cell. Embedded in the membrane and extending outward are the 160 kDa glycoproteins (gp) that serve as the receptor binding molecules. The **gp160** molecules are composed of the **gp40** component, which spans the lipid bilayer, and the **gp120** molecule, which serves to bind HIV to cell receptors. The core of the virus within the bilayer comprises four proteins (**p24, p17, p9,** and **p7**) derived from a 53 kDa precursor by proteolytic cleavage by HIV-1 protease. The viral RNA is associated with molecules of a nucleic acid binding protein **(p9),** and reverse transcriptase (**p66** and **p51**), forming a complex surrounded by a cylinder of p24 protein molecules. The p17 protein molecules line the inner surface of the lipid bilayer around the viral core.

The genome of HIV-1, which is approximately 9,700 base pairs long, is similar to other human retroviruses in its basic structure (Fig. 38–1) and gene products (Table 38–1). Three major regions *(gag, env, pol)* encode structural proteins and viral enzymes. The ***gag* region** encodes the 53 kDa molecule that is cleaved into p24, p17, p9, and p7. The ***env* region** encodes the envelope glycoproteins gp40 and gp120, which together comprise gp160. The ***pol* region** encodes the **RNA-dependent DNA polymerase,** or **reverse transcriptase,** sometimes designated **p66** or **p51.** The *pol* region also carries information for an **integrase (endonuclease)** and a **protease.** The other HIV viral products generally serve as regulatory factors.

Human Immunodeficiency Virus Type 2. HIV-2, a somewhat distant cousin of HIV-1, is morphologically and genetically similar to HIV-1 and has a similar tropism for the CD4 molecules on the surfaces of lymphocytes and certain other cells. There are major antigenic differences between HIV-1 and HIV-2, with only 39% and 58% homology between *env* and *gag* proteins of the two viruses. HIV-2 is closer genetically to **simian immunodeficiency virus (SIV),** which causes an AIDS-like illness in macaques, than to HIV-1. The major differences are in the *env* and *gag* regions of the genome and in the presence of *vpx,* which is found in SIV and HIV-2 but not in HIV-1 (Table 38–1).

Retroviral Life Cycle. Our understanding of the life cycle of HIV continues to evolve. New information about host cell receptors, about the turnover of virions and the half-life of the virus inside and outside of various cells, and about the magnitude of viral production has revolutionized how HIV is viewed and treated.

The initial step in virus–host cell interaction is more complex than once believed. The CD4 molecule found predominantly on **T4 lymphocytes,** also known as **T-helper lymphocytes** or **CD4 lymphocytes,** is the primary receptor for HIV binding, which is mediated through the HIV gp120 portion of the gp160 molecule. HIV requires more than one receptor for binding and entrance into host cells.

It is likely that mucosal membrane exposure to HIV is followed by viral entry into **dendritic cells,** known as **Langerhans cells,** just below the mucosal surface. Langerhans cells have viral receptors and can be infected without being destroyed. After initial replication, regional spread to lymph nodes occurs, followed by replication there and in peripheral blood, at which time the initial evidence of disease is recognizable in some persons as the **acute retroviral syndrome.**

Evidence favors the macrophage as the first major cell target for HIV. In early infection, these macrophage-tropic viral particles attach via the gp120 protein to both the macrophage CD4 protein and another protein, **chemokine receptor 5 (CCR5).** Other recep-

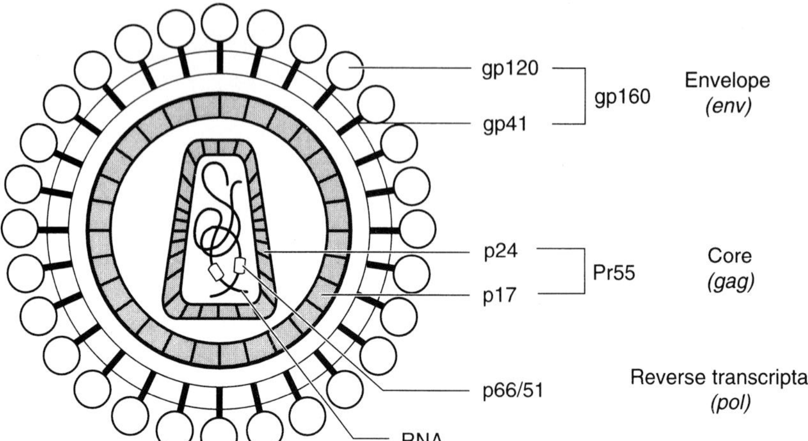

FIGURE 38–1. Structure of HIV. Numerous proteins are immunogenic and can be detected by the Western immunoblot test, although gp41 and p24 are the most prominent and reproducibly detectable.

tors **(CCR3** or **CCR2b)** are sometimes involved, although somewhat less effectively. In yet other cases the primary interaction is with the CD4 lymphocytes that have as a coreceptor the chemokine receptor **CXCR4.** The transmembrane portion of the gp160 molecule, gp40, is uncovered after gp120–CD4 binding and becomes involved with binding at an adjacent membrane site. A complex series of conformational changes follows, leading to viral insertion.

There is a subpopulation of persons of European ancestry who lack CCR5 co-receptors. Those persons who are homozygous for CCR5 proteins appear to be resistant to HIV infection. Those who are heterozygous for the deletion can become infected, but disease progression is delayed by several years.

When HIV attaches, a series of events occur, beginning with fusion of the viral membrane and the host cell membrane (Fig. 38–3). When HIV enters the target cell, the outer membrane and core proteins are removed and the two strands of viral RNA are transcribed by virally encoded reverse transcriptase into DNA. Virally encoded DNA is transported to the nucleus, where it is integrated into the target cell genome. This provirus remains integrated in a latent state indefinitely. Certain cofactors, such as other viruses, cytokines, and other factors, will trigger the proviral DNA to be translated back to viral RNA. Viral RNA serves two purposes. Some RNA is translated into a polyprotein, which is cleaved by viral protease into the individual structural and functional proteins that compose HIV. Viral RNA is packaged inside these new structural proteins and buds through the host cell membrane, into which newly produced viral envelope proteins (gp120 and gp40) are embedded.

HIV is well known for the rapidity with which it mutates. With time, macrophage-tropic viruses will become tropic for CD4 lymphocytes as well, and eventually the bulk of the virus particles become **T-tropic** and favor the CD4 T lymphocytes. This event appears to occur when the immune system begins to collapse and clinical disease accelerates.

EPIDEMIOLOGY

Worldwide Epidemic. A dramatic decline in AIDS cases and deaths has occurred in countries where the latest medical techniques and treatments are available. Unfortunately, 95% of HIV-infected people live in locations where even basic HIV testing is a luxury and antiretroviral therapy is unavailable. The World Health Organization (WHO) has estimated that since the beginning of the epidemic, 52 million persons in the world have become infected; of these, 19 million have died and 34 million were alive in 2000. In 1999 a total of 15,000 people became infected daily—approximately 5.4 million for the year.

Sub-Saharan Africa has accounted for 70% (34 million) of infected persons, of whom one third have died and 23.3 million are currently living with HIV. More than one fourth of the population of some countries is infected, with the highest rate occurring among young adults and increasingly among female adolescents. Hetero-

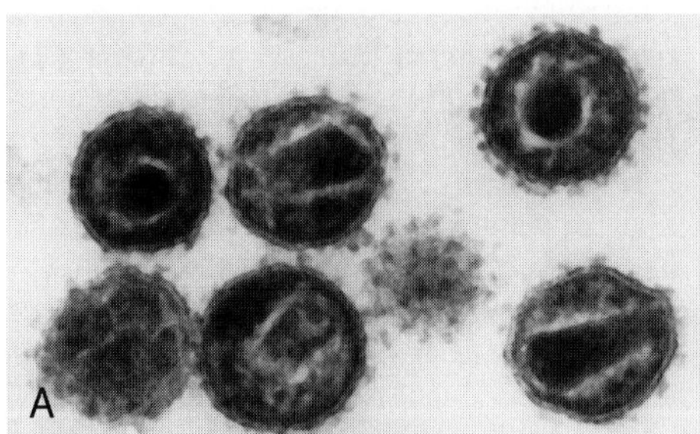

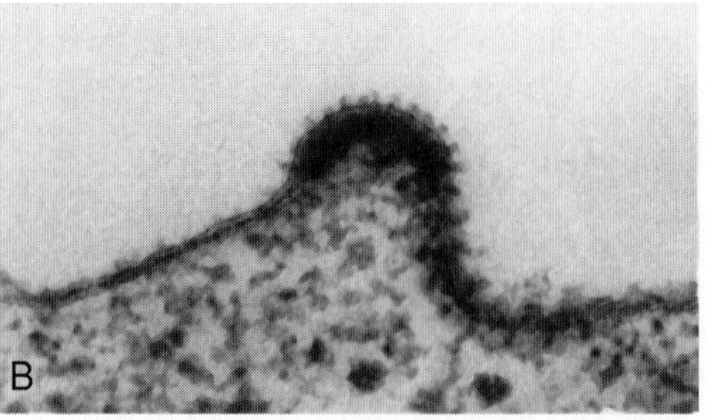

FIGURE 38–2. Transmission electron micrographs of HIV. **A,** The HIV virion is 100 nm in diameter and consists of a dense inner core and an outer lipid envelope. The two copies of genomic HIV RNA, reverse transcriptase, and other viral proteins are contained within the core, which is shaped like a truncated cone. Numerous glycoproteins project from the membrane surface ("knobs" on top of "spikes"). Magnification: ×200,000. **B,** Budding of a maturing HIV virion at the cell membrane. HIV envelope proteins combine with membrane lipids to form a maturing virion envelope as trial RNA and enzymes organize within the developing particle. Magnification: ×120,000. (Used with permission from Jenson HB: Retrovirus infections and the acquired immunodeficiency syndrome. *Adv Pediatr Infect Dis* 1990;5:99.)

TABLE 38–1. HIV Viral Genes, Gene Products, and Functions of Gene Products

Gene Name	Molecular Size	Gene Product Function	Comment
gag	$Pr55^{gag}$	Gag (structural capsid protein) precursor	
	p24	Core capsid antigen	Core internal structural proteins
	p17	Matrix antigen	
	p7, p6	Nuclear capsid protein (binds RNA; binds virus protein R)	
	p2		
	p1		
pol	$Pr170^{gag\text{-}pol}$	Pol (viral enzyme) precursor	
	p66/51	Reverse transcriptase (2 forms)	Transcription of viral RNA to DNA
	p31	Integrase (endonuclease)	
	p10	Protease	Cleaves viral precursor protein into individual proteins that form the viral capsid
env	gp160		
	gp120	Surface viral glycoprotein	Primary molecule binding HIV to CD4 molecule
	gp40	Transmembrane glycoprotein	Anchors gp120 to the viral surface; involved as secondary binding molecule
Regulatory			
tat	p14/p16	Transactivation protein	Transcriptional elongation; possibly involved with apoptosis
rev	p19	Rev protein	Transport of virally encoded RNA molecules from nucleus to cytoplasm
vif	p23	Viral infectivity factor	Involved in viral assembly near host cell membrane
vpr	p10–15	Virus protein R	Arrests cells in G_2 phase optimizing expression of viral genome
nef	p27	Negative regulator factor	Accelerates removal of CD4 from cell surface, promoting degradation
vpu	p16	Virus protein U	Binds to CD4 cellular receptor protein in endoplasmic reticulum (allows rapid degradation of CD4)
vpx	p14	(Found in HIV-2 and SIV)	Function is similar to *vpr* in HIV-1

sexual and vertical transmission are the predominant risk factors. Women have approximately 46% of the cases among adults, and in some countries women far exceed men in the rates of infection.

In the early 1990s a rapid increase in cases occurred in Thailand and other countries of Southeast Asia. Recently AIDS has surged in India, where 2–5 million people are estimated to be infected. The numbers will continue to rise dramatically unless significant medical, public health, and social changes occur. Heterosexual transmission accounts for three fourths of cases, with the remainder due to sharing of contaminated needles, use of contaminated blood products, and vertical transmission.

In South America, Central America, and the Caribbean, the HIV epidemic was well established in many countries in the early 1980s. WHO estimates that 1.4 million people in Latin America and 330,000 in the Caribbean countries are living with HIV infection.

HIV has had a variable impact in Europe. Western Europe has had a pattern similar to that seen in the United States, whereas Eastern Europe, which was largely spared in the first decade of the epidemic, has since had an increase in HIV cases. In Western Europe, more males than females were infected in the early years of the epidemic because of male-to-male sexual transmission. The population of Western Europe has had much of the same benefit from antiretroviral medications as people in the United States, including a sharp reduction in pediatric cases because of the use of zidovudine (ZDV) in pregnancy. In contrast, the spread in Eastern Europe has predominantly been among injection drug users and sex industry workers. New antiretroviral medications have largely been unavailable to this population.

United States. In 1996 AIDS deaths and the number of persons with HIV infection that progressed to AIDS declined for the first time. At the peak in 1995, a total of 49,897 persons died; the number declined to 21,437 in 1997. Through the end of 1999 a total of 733,374 Americans have been reported to have AIDS. Approximately 40,000 persons continue to become infected each year. As more persons become infected and fewer die of AIDS complications, the population of persons living with HIV disease grows each year. Approximately 650,000–900,000 persons are HIV infected in the United States, including those with AIDS.

Improved survival rates and outcome have not occurred uniformly across all racial and ethnic groups, genders, ages, and regions of the United States. Women now constitute 27% of new HIV cases, versus 16.3% of cumulative AIDS cases, indicating a recent proportional increase in new infections among women. From 1995 to 1996, AIDS cases decreased 8% among men but increased 1% among women, but this increase was much less than the 8% increase among women for the prior year. The largest decline in new AIDS cases has been among white (non-Hispanic) men, a group in which a 3% decline in new AIDS cases in 1995 was followed by a 13% decline in 1996. In 1996 the number of new AIDS cases in Hispanics declined for the first time, with a 5% decrease, but the number of new AIDS cases among African Americans remained constant.

HIV infection is concentrated in the largest metropolitan centers but has also decentralized into midsized metropolitan areas (50,000–500,000 population), small towns, and rural areas. One in six infections has been reported from the smaller towns and

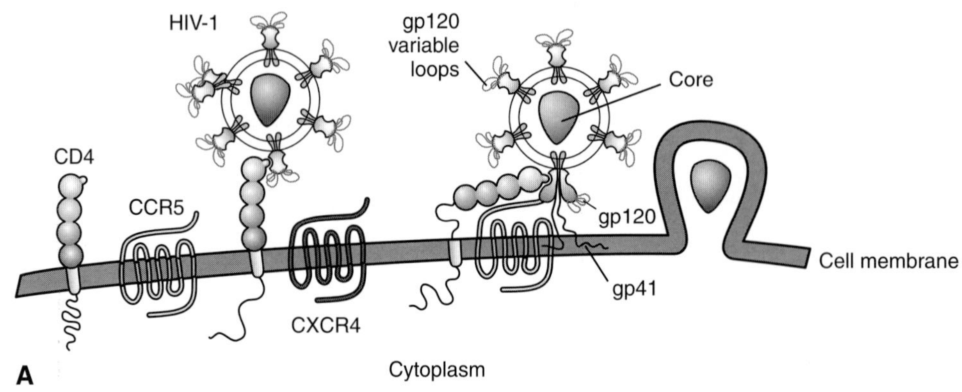

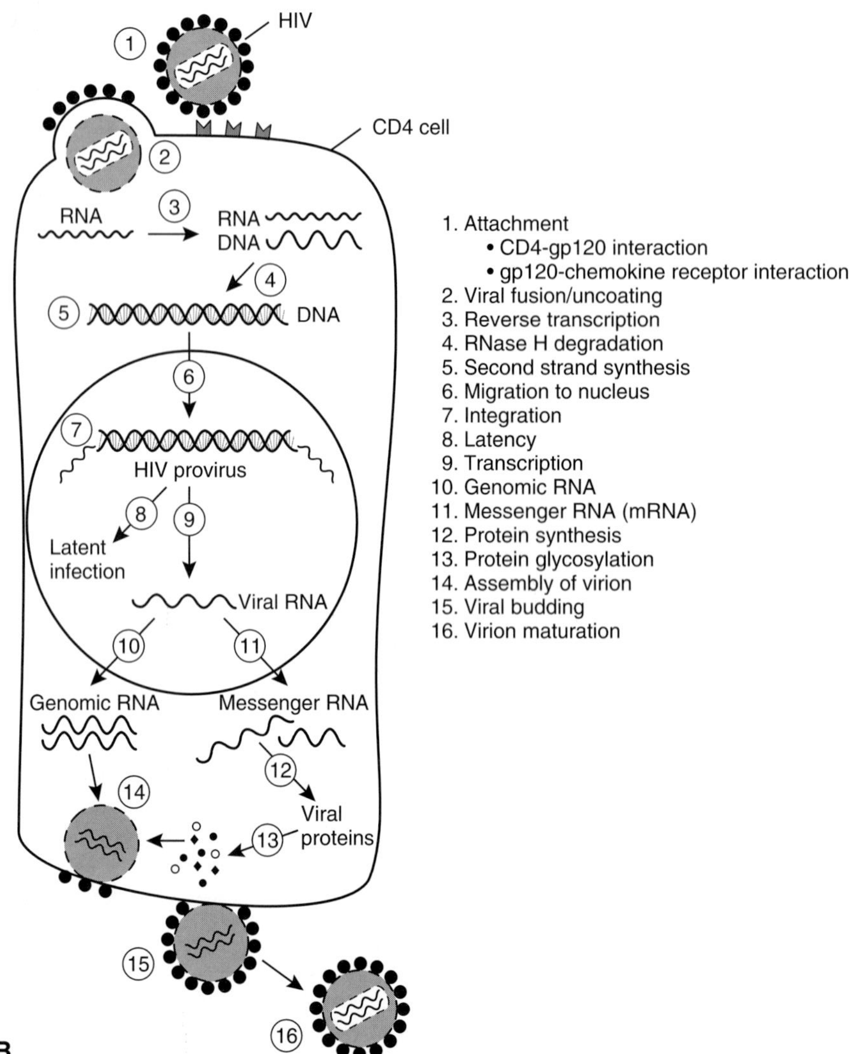

FIGURE 38–3. A, Viral attachment is mediated by attachment of the ligand gp120 with CD4 and a chemokine receptor, either CCR5 or CXCR4. CD4 is found primarily on helper T lymphocytes and also on macrophages and microglial, dendritic, and Langerhans cells. Fusion is mediated by gp41. **B,** The life cycle of HIV. After fusion and uncoating, reverse transcription of viral RNA begins, leading to double-stranded viral DNA. HIV integrase facilitates insertion of the viral DNA duplex into the host genome, giving rise to the HIV provirus. HIV is transcribed into regulatory, structural, and enzymatic proteins and also into new HIV RNA genomes. Viral proteins and RNA genomes combine into virions that bud from the host cell and reinitiate the cycle by infecting other cells.

rural areas. Every state and territory has reported cases of AIDS, although the disease remains relatively uncommon in the sparsely populated states of the West and the Upper Midwest. Nonetheless, many small towns and rural areas have HIV cases in both adults and children. The less populous areas are often ill equipped to deal with HIV and AIDS. These persons often live far from the specialized programs and support services that form the sophisticated AIDS infrastructure in many urban areas. It is common for people with HIV infection to receive their diagnosis in a large city and then to return to their hometowns as they become ill. Physicians with HIV expertise and the HIV infrastructure that is so commonly in place in urban areas are often lacking in rural areas, and patients fear discovery and stigmatization.

Women. More than 124,000 women have been reported to have AIDS in the United States, with many more having less advanced HIV disease. Cumulatively, 16.9% of adults with AIDS have been women. Between June 1998 and June 1999, women had 23.2% of new AIDS cases, compared with fewer than 7% of new cases in the mid-1980s. There has been marked improvement in early identification of HIV-infected women, especially those who are pregnant.

African Americans have accounted for 57% of cases among women and for 62.2% of the new AIDS cases reported from June 1998 to June 1999. Hispanic women have 20% of all cases, and white, non-Hispanic women have 21.7% of cases. The percentage of cases in minority women was already high in the early years of the epidemic and has continued to increase.

Approximately 85% of infected women are of childbearing age (15–44 years). Women are generally younger than men are when they become infected, often acquiring the disease as adolescents from older, more sexually experienced partners. However, they may not develop AIDS until adulthood.

Cumulatively, 42% of cases of AIDS in women were in injection drug users, whereas at least 40% of the women were infected through sexual transmission. The former group includes women who also had infected partners, so the actual mode of transmission is uncertain. Sexual transmission was the most common risk factor for women with AIDS diagnosed in 1999 (40%); injection drug users accounted for 27% of new cases. Risk factors are unknown or unreported for 32% of newly identified women with AIDS. Historically two thirds of women with unknown risk factors were later shown to have been infected sexually. Hence approximately 60% of new cases are the result of sexual transmission, a percentage that has steadily increased. For women with newly diagnosed HIV cases, a category that is variably reported, in 1999 38% of cases were sexually transmitted, 55% were a result of unknown exposure, and only 7% were a result of injection drug use. These figures emphasize the shift from the predomination of injection drug use as the primary risk factor to sexual transmission as the predominant risk in the most recent cases.

For new AIDS cases reported in 1999, 38% of African American women, 47% of Hispanic women, and 40% of white, non-Hispanic women were infected sexually; 25–36% had no identified risks, but most were likely infected by sexual transmission. More than 50% of women infected sexually have had partners whose risk factors remain unclear. It may be years after HIV infection before diagnosis, so the infecting partner may have been forgotten or may be unavailable.

Contaminated needles are responsible for more cases than might be apparent at first, because 16.3% of women infected sexually have had a partner who was an injection drug user. The percentage of cases among women directly infected through contaminated needles is declining, although many are infected sexually by partners who acquired the virus through this means. Directly or indirectly, drug injection has accounted for almost 58% of AIDS cases among women, although it accounted for only 38% of cases reported between June 1998 and June 1999.

Noninjection drug use also increases the risk of HIV acquisition. The use of **crack cocaine** is a well-known contributing risk factor for HIV, although its use declined sharply in the 1990s. It is common for crack cocaine–dependent women to resort to prostitution to obtain money or drugs. Consequently they are at increased risk of sexually transmitted diseases that can facilitate the spread of HIV.

Injection drug use contributes both medical and psychosocial complications, which affect the treatment of and prognosis for persons with HIV infection in these families. Failure to obtain prenatal care and a lack of adherence to medication regimens are common problems of drug users. Other substances, including alcohol, tend to lower inhibitions, which increases susceptibility to HIV infection by impairing judgment regarding partners, condom use, and other behaviors.

Children Younger than 13 Years. In the United States there has been a dramatic drop in AIDS cases among children less than 13 years of age. Infected children are living much longer than could have been anticipated a few years ago. This population of older children presents new medical, social, and psychological challenges. There has been an actual reduction in new pediatric HIV infections in recent years. In contrast, there is no slowing of new infections in adults and adolescents, although progression of HIV infection to AIDS and death is slowing.

The turning point for children was the 1994 **AIDS Clinical Trials Group (ACTG) 076 study,** which showed that the antiretroviral medication ZDV, when used by pregnant HIV-positive women and their offspring, decreased the risk of vertical transmission from 25.5% to 8% in comparison with a placebo control group. A subsequent United States Public Health Service Task Force recommendation urged HIV testing for all pregnant women. For those testing positive, it was recommended that treatment with ZDV should be offered. It is now estimated that 6,000–7,000 HIV-infected women deliver fewer than 500 infected infants annually in the United States, versus 1,500 before the ACTG 076 study. Although pediatric HIV infections are declining, the number of children who are exposed to HIV is increasing because of the rise in cases among women of childbearing age.

HIV infection in children is predominately due to transmission from infected women (91% of cumulative cases); contaminated blood products account for 7% (cumulative), although new cases are now rare. Five new cases were reported in 1999 (three children had hemophilia, and two had received blood products for other reasons), but they likely represent infection that occurred many years ago. A small percentage of cases results from sexual abuse of children by infected adults.

African American and Hispanic children account for 81.5% of all AIDS cases reported since 1982, a percentage that has continued to rise. White (non-Hispanic) children have accounted for 17.4% of all cases but only 12.9% of cases reported in 1999. More than one third of the children have mothers who are injection drug users, and many others have mothers who have used licit or illicit noninjection drugs and alcohol. Children may be exposed in utero to both HIV and drugs. These children are at significant risk of having developmental and physical problems.

Adolescents. Adolescents constitute a relatively small percentage of persons with AIDS. This fact is not indicative of the scope of the problem. It typically takes 10–11 years from the time of initial infection until HIV progresses to AIDS in an adolescent or adult. An estimated 20% of adults with AIDS were infected as adolescents. The mean age of infection declined from the mid-30s in the first years of the epidemic to the low 20s.

The proportion of female patients with AIDS is larger among the adolescent and young adult population than among older adults. In the 13- to 19-year-old group, 63.5% of new AIDS cases (1999) were in the female adolescents. This compares to 44% of cases in women in the 20- to 24-year-old group and 16% (cumulative) in women more than 25 years old. Many young adults likely acquired the virus as adolescents. Moreover, of the HIV cases reported in 1998, representing more recently acquired infection, percentages were even higher in females.

Adolescents often become infected through ''adult'' risk behaviors, including sexual transmission. Female adolescents and homosexual male adolescents frequently initiate sexual activity with partners who are years older and who have been sexually active for years. These older individuals often bring an increased risk of sexually transmitted diseases including HIV to the adolescent. Behaviors acquired in adolescence, including use or lack of use of barrier protection and birth control, high-risk sexual behaviors, substance use, and promiscuity, are often patterns that continue in adulthood. Through 1999, at least 52% of 13- to 19-year-old female adolescents with AIDS and 49% of 20- to 24-year-old women with AIDS had acquired the virus sexually, with 38% of 13- to 19-year-old male adolescents and 65% of 20- to 24-year-old men having been infected sexually by other males.

Among 13- to 19-year-old male adolescents with HIV infection, a cumulative 38% were infected by contaminated blood products. Only 4% of cumulative cases in the 20- to 24-year-old group were in this risk group. The majority of these were men with hemophilia. Among female patients with HIV infection, 7% of those 13–19 years of age and 2% of those 20–24 years of age were infected by contaminated blood. Before March 1985, blood products, including products containing coagulation factors, were responsible for a significant portion of HIV infections in young males, many of whom have subsequently developed AIDS. Up to 90% of people with factor VIII deficiency and 60% with factor IX deficiency may have become infected. Of males with AIDS cases newly reported in 1999, only 13% of those 13–19 years of age and 2% of those 20–24 years of age had HIV transmitted by contaminated blood. These persons acquired HIV before March 1985 and are just now progressing to AIDS. Cases attributable to blood products will continue to be increasingly uncommon in years to come because most such HIV infections have already progressed to AIDS.

Injection drug use as a risk factor is less common among adolescents than among adults. Cumulatively, 6% of 13- to 19-year-old male adolescents and 12% of 20- to 24-year-old men were injection drug users. For females, the percentages were 14% and 27%, respectively, for these age groups.

Many adolescents are unable to provide a risk factor for their infection. It is striking that 49% of female adolescents and 41% of male adolescents with newly reported cases of AIDS in 1999 were in the ''risk not reported or identified'' category. Among those 20–24 years of age, these figures are 22% and 39%, respectively. With time, at least two thirds of the cases are typically reclassified as being due to sexual transmission. Heterosexual transmission for females, and sex with other males for males, are clearly the predominant modes of HIV transmission.

Vertically infected children are increasingly surviving into the adolescent years. This outcome is attributable to advances in antiviral treatment and support services, and it presents new challenges to health service providers, parents and other caretakers, and the adolescents themselves. The difficulties of dealing with chronic illness, the need to adhere to complex medical regimens, neuropsychological factors, and adolescent issues such as sexuality and substance abuse are important issues for these persons.

Adolescents have different levels of risk acceptance and different needs for education about sexuality, sexual activity, and methods of prevention of pregnancy and disease and for information about substance use and abuse. Education needs to be tailored to the person's age, cultural beliefs, education, and presence or lack of risk factors.

Human Immunodeficiency Virus Type 2. In addition to HIV-1, which causes most AIDS cases worldwide, a related retrovirus (HIV-2) was discovered in West Africa in 1986. The transmission and epidemiology of HIV-1 and HIV-2 are similar, although HIV-2 cases have been largely limited to West Africa, with occasional cases reported in the Americas and Europe, primarily in persons who have traveled there from West Africa.

HIV-2 is less pathogenic than HIV-1, less readily transmitted sexually, and rarely, if ever, transmitted vertically from mother to child. Declines in CD4 lymphocyte counts are less dramatic and disease progression is slower. When first identified in 1986, HIV-2 was typically missed by serologic screening tests in up to 30% of cases. Separate, more sensitive assays, including EIA antibody screening assays and immunoblot confirmatory tests, that are specific for HIV-2 have been developed. Most commercial assays screen for both HIV-1 and HIV-2. Specific screening for HIV-2 outside of West Africa is largely unnecessary. The CDC recommends HIV-2 testing for persons from Central and Southern Africa, their sex partners or persons who may have been exposed to them through shared needles, persons who have received blood products in those countries, and the children of women at risk of having HIV-2 infection.

PATHOGENESIS

The understanding of the virology and the pathophysiology of HIV disease has progressed rapidly in recent years. An older theory of viral latency or near dormancy has been shown to be incorrect. In most infected persons, HIV is highly active, with viral replication and turnover occurring on an enormous scale beginning within a few weeks to months after the virus is acquired. A typical adult produces 10 billion viral particles daily, with half of the virus in circulation being cleared and replaced each day. The half-life of the virus is 1–2 days. In adults, approximately 2 billion CD4 lymphocytes are also produced daily. There are several subpopulations of HIV-infected CD4 lymphocytes with varying functions and life spans ranging from days to years. HIV can infect other CD4 cells, including monocytes and dendritic cells. Besides possible long-term survival inside certain cells, the human body has **sanctuary sites,** such as the central nervous system, where HIV remains largely free from attack by immune mechanisms and most antiretroviral agents. These sites potentially may serve to repopulate other sites after antiviral treatment.

Cellular Basis of HIV Infection. The availability of **viral load or viral burden** testing allows rapid feedback on the effectiveness of antiviral therapies and on prognostic information regarding disease progression. After an initial burst of viral production, the level of viral production achieves a fairly steady rate of production, the **set point,** in older children and adults (Fig. 38–4). A person with a high set point is more likely to progress rapidly in his or her disease than someone with a lower set point. This is a major determinant

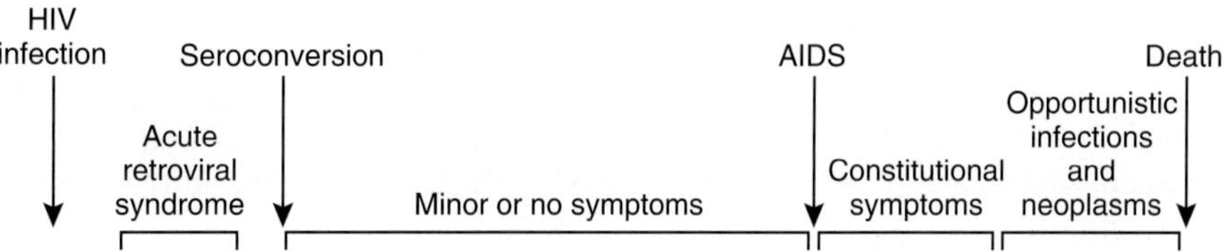

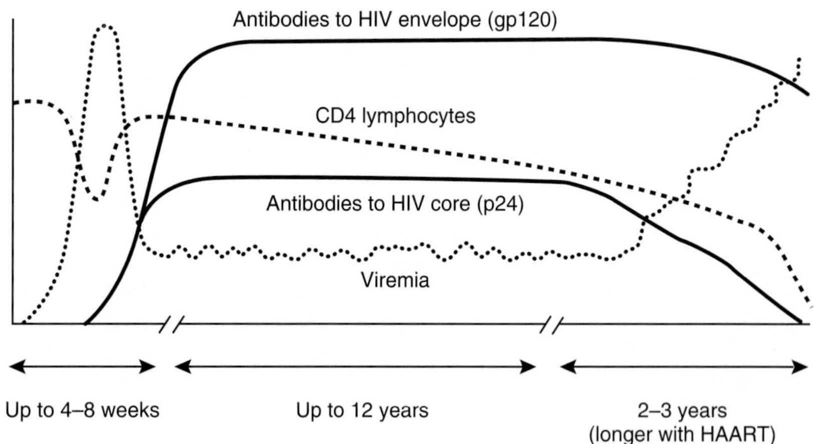

FIGURE 38–4. Characteristic pattern of detectable HIV viremia, p24 antigen, HIV antibody, and CD4 lymphocyte counts for HIV infection acquired during adolescence or adulthood. A clinically silent period follows the acute retroviral infection. Clinical AIDS typically takes many years to develop.

in the rate of disease progression to AIDS and ultimately to death. As HIV disease advances, destruction of CD4 lymphocytes impairs the immune response, which facilitates a wide spectrum of opportunistic infections and allows development of malignancies.

HIV is sometimes viewed as existing in several ''compartments'' of the body, including peripheral blood, tissues, and various subgroups of peripheral blood mononuclear cells. Production and turnover of virus varies by location. This has important implications for the development of medications and treatment protocols if there is to be a hope of viral eradication and cure. The half-life of free HIV is about 6 hours, with most HIV-infected peripheral blood mononuclear cells surviving for 1–2 days.

HIV is able to evade immune eradication by several methods. Integration of virally encoded genetic material into the cell genome is the major mechanism. Additionally, certain sanctuary sites are inaccessible or minimally accessible to currently available medications. For example, few currently available antiretroviral medications achieve significant levels in the central nervous system. This raises concerns about the ability to completely eradicate HIV, even if eradication could be achieved in the peripheral compartments. Current therapy is often able to suppress viral replication in the peripheral compartment to undetectable levels but has not been shown to eradicate HIV. Another concern is that if only low levels of antivirals are achieved in sanctuary sites, there is a potential for the virus to become resistant to those medications.

SYMPTOMS AND CLINICAL MANIFESTATIONS

Since the first descriptions of pediatric HIV disease in the early 1980s, both common and rare manifestations of HIV disease and AIDS in infants, children, and adolescents have been well described. In the first decade of the epidemic, emphasis was placed on identification of ''high risk'' women and infected children as evidenced by clinical signs and symptoms. Emphasis has shifted to identification, education, and treatment of HIV-infected women in order to decrease risk to their infants.

Classification of Children with HIV Disease and AIDS. In 1983 the CDC devised a surveillance case definition for AIDS for children <13 years of age, which was similar to the original AIDS classification scheme for adults, with minor differences for the few pediatric-specific illnesses known at that time. The most recent modification to the definition was developed in 1994. The current system, unlike the 1983 case definition, recognizes that HIV-infected children can be infected without manifesting symptoms, or they may manifest a range of symptoms from minor to advanced symptomatic disease (AIDS). It also recognizes that some HIV-positive children may be exposed but not infected.

Classification of HIV disease and AIDS in a child by this system requires knowledge of whether the child has been HIV exposed or is infected, of the immune status according to an age-specific CD4 lymphocyte count, and of the history of opportunistic infections or other clinical signs and symptoms of disease (Tables 38–2 through 38–4). Once classified, a child's case is never reclassified to a lower classification even if symptoms and immune status improve. The case is classified by the most advanced category that develops and may be reclassified only to a more advanced category as the immune status worsens or new clinical conditions occur.

HIV-seropositive children <18 months of age whose infection status is uncertain have the prefix *E* appended to the classification, indicating perinatal exposure. The classification EN1 indicates that in utero exposure occurred but that the child has no signs or symptoms of disease, has no history of illness attributable to HIV, and has a normal CD4 lymphocyte count for age. If the child proves to be infected, the *E* prefix is dropped and the case is reclassified consistent with the child's immune status and clinical history. With the widespread availability of better testing methods, the infection status of most children is known with near certainty by 4–6 months of age. Technically these children are still designated as having *E*

TABLE 38–2. Pediatric HIV Classification System

	Clinical Categories*†			
Immunologic Categories‡	N: No Signs or Symptoms	A: Mild Signs and Symptoms	B: Moderate Signs and Symptoms	C: Severe Signs and Symptoms
1. No evidence of immune suppression	N1	A1	B1	C1
2. Evidence of moderate suppression	N2	A2	B2	C2
3. Evidence of severe suppression	N3	A3	B3	C3

*Pending clarification of infection status of a perinatally HIV-exposed child, a letter *E* (for *E*xposed) is placed before the classification code (e.g., EN1).
†All category C conditions and one category B condition (lymphoid interstitial pneumonitis [LIP]) are AIDS-defining conditions and are reportable as AIDS.
‡Age-specific immunologic categories are defined in Table 38–3.

status until they lose maternal antibodies, at which time their status is reclassified as **seroreversion.**

For adolescents >13 years old and for adults, the same classification system is used and it is somewhat simpler than the system used for children. The CD4 lymphocyte categories are constant across the adolescent and adult populations and are identical to the categories used for children 6–12 years old (Table 38–3). For persons >13 years of age, there is no *N* category and no *E* designation.

Acute Retroviral Syndrome. The acute retroviral syndrome is associated with the initial burst of viral replication shortly after infection is transmitted (Fig. 38–4). This occurs in approximately 50% of adults within weeks or months of acquiring HIV. Acute retroviral syndrome is rare or is not obvious in infancy. The constellation of symptoms is somewhat reminiscent of infectious mononucleosis. Headaches, lymphadenopathy, generalized nonspecific rash, fever, aseptic meningitis, and other symptoms are common in adults with this syndrome. Night sweats, malaise, anorexia, weight loss, myalgias, and arthralgias may also occur. Less common symptoms include retro-orbital pain, photophobia, diarrhea, pharyngitis, depression, irritability, and mood changes. The period from HIV exposure to the onset of symptoms is typically 2–4 weeks, with a range of 5 days to 3 months. It is possible to culture the virus or perform a PCR assay for using blood lymphocytes, serum, or cerebrospinal fluid during this period. Often physicians and patients do not recognize the symptoms as being associated with HIV. Some patients will recall a severe influenza-like illness, which may represent acute retroviral syndrome and may give an approximate period at which the infection began.

Viral replication peaks at a high level during this time, and then the immune response controls the initial infection. Viral levels then drop to a baseline level, the set point, which is the ongoing level of viral production.

Progression of HIV Infection to AIDS. The relationship of HIV to AIDS is relatively straightforward (Fig. 38–4). AIDS represents the advanced stage of HIV disease. AIDS in adults or adolescents is defined by the presence of any category C conditions or by a CD4 lymphocyte count <200/mm^3. The category C conditions for adolescents differ from those for younger children (Table 38–4). Children <13 years of age are classified as having AIDS if they have ever had any category C conditions as defined for that age group (Tables 38–2 and 38–4) or lymphoid interstitial pneumonia (LIP), a category B disease. LIP is in category B rather than category C because it typically carries a somewhat better prognosis than the category C conditions. There is no CD4 lymphocyte level below which a child is considered to have AIDS. At the thirteenth birthday a child's status should be reclassified on the basis of the adult system.

When the term *AIDS* was first used, the cause of the disease was unknown and patients were diagnosed according to immunologic and clinical criteria. The term *HIV disease* was used later, after the cause of the disease was clarified. It was soon recognized that many infected people do not have symptoms of AIDS at the time of diagnosis and that signs and symptoms sometimes do not develop for years after diagnosis. Nonetheless, viral activity and damage to the immune system begin to occur at significant levels from the time of initial infection. The *HIV-AIDS* terminology is often confusing to patients and to the lay public. In casual usage, *HIV* and *AIDS* are sometimes incorrectly used as interchangeable terms.

HIV disease is a continuum, beginning with the acquisition of the virus, after which a transient period of mild to severe symptoms may occur. There is then generally an asymptomatic or minimally symptomatic period, which may persist for many years, although in some persons, especially infants, this period may last for only a few months. It is typically followed by the gradual onset of signs and symptoms, culminating in an AIDS-defining condition. In some cases the transition from an asymptomatic stage to AIDS is abrupt, with the sudden onset of severe diseases such as PCP, which ensues when cumulative damage to the immune system allows secondary complications. The median period between acquisition of HIV disease and AIDS is 10–11 years for untreated adults or adoles-

TABLE 38–3. Immunologic Categories Based on Age-Specific CD4 Lymphocyte Counts and Percentage of Total Lymphocytes*

	Age <12 Mo		Age 1–5 Yr		Age 6–12 Yr	
Immunologic Category*	Cells/mm^3	(%)	Cells/mm^3	(%)	Cells/mm^3	(%)
No evidence of suppression	≥1,500	(≥25)	≥1,000	(≥25)	≥500	(≥25)
Evidence of moderate suppression	750–1,499	(15–24)	500–999	(15–24)	200–499	(15–24)
Evidence of severe suppression	<750	(<15)	<500	(<15)	<200	(<15)

*Immunologic categories are used in conjunction with Table 38–2.

TABLE 38–4. Immunologic and Clinical Categories for Classification of Children with HIV Infection*

Category N: Not Symptomatic

Children who have no signs or symptoms considered to be the result of HIV infection or who have only one of the mild conditions listed in category A.

Category A: Mildly Symptomatic

Children with **2 or more** of the following conditions but none of the conditions listed in categories B and C:

- Lymphadenopathy (≥0.5 cm at ≥2 sites; bilateral = 1 site)
- Hepatomegaly
- Splenomegaly
- Dermatitis (seborrhea, atopic dermatitis)
- Parotitis
- Recurrent or persistent upper respiratory tract infection, sinusitis, or otitis media

Category B: Moderately Symptomatic

Children who have symptomatic conditions other than those listed for category A or C that are attributed to HIV infection, including but not limited to:

Secondary Infectious Diseases

Bacterial meningitis, pneumonia, or sepsis (single episode)
Candidiasis, oropharyngeal (thrush), persisting more than 2 mo in children >6 mo of age
Cytomegalovirus infection, with onset before 1 mo of age
Herpes simplex virus stomatitis, recurrent (>2 episodes within 1 yr); or bronchitis, pneumonitis, or esophagitis, with onset before 1 mo of age
Herpes zoster (shingles), ≥2 distinct episodes or involving >1 dermatome
Nocardiosis
Toxoplasmosis, with onset before 1 mo of age
Varicella, disseminated (complicated chickenpox)
Persistent fever (lasting >1 mo)

Secondary Cancer

Leiomyosarcoma

Other Diseases

Anemia (hemoglobin <8 g/dL), neutropenia (neutrophil count <1,000/mm³), or thrombocytopenia (platelet count <100,000/mm³) persisting ≥30 days
Cardiomyopathy
Diarrhea, recurrent or chronic
Hepatitis
Nephropathy
Lymphoid interstitial pneumonia or pulmonary lymphoid hyperplasia complex†

Category C: Severely Symptomatic†

Children who have any condition listed in the 1987 surveillance case definition for AIDS with the exception of lymphoid interstitial pneumonia **(see category B, above):**

Secondary Infectious Diseases

Serious bacterial infections, multiple or recurrent (i.e., any combination of ≥2 culture-confirmed infections within 2-y period) of the following types: septicemia, pneumonia, meningitis, bone or joint infection, or abscess of an internal organ or body cavity (excluding otitis media, superficial skin or mucosal abscesses, and indwelling catheter–related infections)
Candidiasis, esophageal or pulmonary (bronchi, trachea, lungs)

Category C: Severely Symptomatic* *(Continued)*

Secondary Infectious Diseases *(Continued)*

Coccidioidomycosis, disseminated (at site other than or in addition to lungs or cervical or hilar lymph nodes)
Cryptococcosis, extrapulmonary
Cryptosporidiosis or isosporiasis with diarrhea persisting >1 mo
Cytomegalovirus with onset of symptoms at ≥1 mo of age (at site other than liver, spleen, or lymph nodes)
Herpes simplex virus infection causing a mucocutaneous ulcer that persists >1 mo; or bronchitis, pneumonitis, or esophagitis for any duration affecting a child ≥1 mo of age
Histoplasmosis, disseminated (at a site other than or in addition to lungs or cervical hilar lymph nodes)
Mycobacterium tuberculosis, disseminated or extrapulmonary
Mycobacterium avium complex or *Mycobacterium kansasii,* disseminated (at a site other than or in addition to lungs, skin, or cervical or hilar lymph nodes)
Mycobacterium, other species or unidentified species, disseminated (at a site other than or in addition to lungs, skin, or cervical or hilar lymph nodes)
Pneumocystis carinii pneumonia
Progressive multifocal leukoencephalopathy (JC virus infection)
Salmonella (nontyphoidal) septicemia, recurrent
Toxoplasmosis of the brain with onset at ≥1 mo of age

Secondary Cancers

Kaposi's sarcoma
Lymphoma, primary, in brain
Lymphoma, small, noncleaved cell (Burkitt's), or immunoblastic or large cell lymphoma of B-cell or unknown immunologic phenotype

Other Diseases

Encephalopathy (≥1 of following progressive findings present for ≥2 mo in absence of a concurrent illness other than HIV infection that could explain the findings:

- Failure to attain or loss of developmental milestones or loss of intellectual ability, verified by standard scale or neuropsychologic tests
- Impaired brain growth or acquired microcephaly demonstrated by head circumference measurements or brain atrophy demonstrated by CT or MRI (serial imaging is required for children <2 yr of age)
- Acquired symmetric motor deficit manifested by ≥2 of the following: paresis, pathologic reflexes, ataxia, or gait disturbance

Wasting syndrome in absence of concurrent illness other than HIV infection that could explain the following findings:

- Persistent weight loss >10% of baseline, *or*
- Downward crossing of ≥2 of following percentile lines on weight-for-age chart (95th, 75th, 50th, 25th, 5th) in child ≥1 yr of age, *or*
- Less than 5th percentile on weight-for-height chart on 2 consecutive measurements ≥30 days apart, *plus* (1) chronic diarrhea (≥2 loose stools per day for ≥30 days), *or* (2) documented fever (for ≥30 days, intermittent or constant)

*Clinical and immunologic classifications are shown in Tables 38–2 and 38–3.
†All category C conditions and one category B condition (lymphoid interstitial pneumonia) are AIDS-defining conditions.

cents. In rare cases, AIDS ensues within months after the initial infection, and at the other extreme, some people have little progression of disease 15 years or longer after acquisition. With the trend to earlier diagnosis and treatment at the time of diagnosis, it is likely that the period will be significantly lengthened.

For infants and young children, the disease course is often more compressed, especially for vertically infected children. Children who manifest significant signs and symptoms or even AIDS within months or a few years of birth, sometimes within a few weeks of delivery, are known as **rapid progressors.** The **slow progressors,** a subgroup similar to adults in disease progression, often have a period of years with minimal or no symptoms before AIDS develops. The high level of virus production that occurs in infants compared with adults may be primarily responsible for the rapid progression of disease. Children infected through blood products typically have prolonged periods of 7–10 years without symptoms.

Factors Associated with Vertical HIV Transmission. Approximately 25% of infants born to HIV-infected mothers will become infected if no intervention occurs. Of those who are infected, an estimated one third appear to have become infected in utero and two thirds perinatally. Although rare in the United States, transmission through breast milk also occurs. As many as 50% of infected children manifest signs or symptoms in the first year of life. The group of rapid progressors was long believed to consist predominantly of those who were infected in utero, whereas the slow progressors were thought to be those infected perinatally. It appears that there is some overlap between these groups.

The most important determinant of disease progression is the infant's viral load. At 1 month of age this averages approximately 750,000 copies of virus per milliliter of blood in the rapid progressors. These children typically have detectable virus in the first few days of life, indicating in utero transmission and viral replication. In contrast, children who have no detectable virus in the first days of life but who later prove to be infected were apparently infected perinatally. Between 2 weeks and 2 months of age, most infected children not previously identified will develop detectable virus. This perinatally infected group will have a lower average viral load of approximately 300,000 copies per milliliter, which probably explains why these children are more likely to be slow progressors. Although the highest levels will occur among children infected in utero, the factors that determine when infection occurs and the magnitude of the viral load are not clear. Viral levels in infants and young children are usually manyfold higher than what is typical in adults. Moreover, adults will have a decline within a few weeks to a baseline set point, which represents a steady-state level of viral production and destruction. Infants have a slow decline in viral levels that may last 2–6 years before stabilizing.

Several factors are known to increase the risk of a newborn with an HIV-infected mother of acquiring HIV: breast-feeding; a high maternal viral load in pregnancy; prolonged labor; a mother who has advanced disease or who became infected while pregnant; and prematurity and low birth weight. Other factors such as maternal or fetal immune response and viral strain might also affect transmission. Some women and infants with multiple risk factors, such as high viral load and advanced disease, will nonetheless bear healthy children. Others with seemingly low risks will bear infected children.

Breast-feeding places an infant at increased risk of acquiring HIV. The risk of transmission solely through breast-feeding ranges from 8% to 18% for infants of women who were infected before beginning lactation. The risk is approximately doubled for infants of women who become infected while lactating. The duration of breast-feeding and the condition of the breast tissues, such as cracking of the nipples, increase the risk. What advice to give to infected women in regard to breast-feeding in developing countries where the HIV rates are tremendously high has been extensively debated. Formulas and clean water may be lacking in developing countries. Moreover, a woman may identify herself as being HIV infected by not breast-feeding and be ostracized.

Women who become HIV infected during pregnancy have an increased risk of delivering an infected infant. This is a difficult issue to study directly because people are often unaware when they became infected. It is likely that the increased risk occurs because there is a high level of virus production within a few weeks to months of acquiring HIV, which tapers off as the immune system responds and curtails viral reproduction.

Women with advanced disease (AIDS), including those with CD4 cell counts $<200/mm^3$, are more likely to have infected infants, probably resulting from rising viral loads in late-stage disease. Prolonged labor is associated with increased risk of many types of viral and bacterial infections including HIV, probably through ascending infection and prolonged exposure to blood and vaginal fluids containing the virus. Other factors such as prematurity and low birth weight have a somewhat lesser impact, although they are associated with an increased risk of infection as well.

Initial Clinical Presentation of Children with HIV and AIDS. Initial signs or symptoms of HIV infection can be acute and dramatic or gradual in onset and mundane in appearance (Table 38–5). Recurrent or difficult-to-eradicate oral candidiasis, generalized lymphadenopathy, splenomegaly, and hepatomegaly are common early signs of infection. In rare instances, children may be born already manifesting signs of disease, such as lymphadenopathy, hepatomegaly, or splenomegaly. Conditions that are common in the general pediatric population, including ear infections, upper respiratory tract infections, and pneumonia, occur more frequently in children with HIV than in other children.

AIDS-defining conditions are usually uncommon outside of the immunocompromised state, and these may also be the earliest indicators of disease. When unusual opportunistic diseases occur, an evaluation of the immune system including testing for HIV is indicated. Poor weight gain, lymphadenopathy, or recurrent oral candidiasis is sometimes actually present before the AIDS-defining presentation, but its significance may not be appreciated. Tuberculosis and Kaposi's sarcoma are common in adults with HIV but uncommon in children. Some occur when organisms that have been harbored in a quiescent state for years or decades become reactivated as the immune system becomes significantly damaged. *Pneumocystis carinii* pneumonia (PCP), cytomegalovirus (CMV) disease, and toxoplasmosis are common reactivation diseases in adults with AIDS. In children these conditions are often primary rather than reactivation diseases. Congenitally acquired CMV and toxoplasmosis are not AIDS-defining conditions (Table 38–4), but both are considered to be category B conditions. Nonetheless, HIV-infected children who are also born with congenital toxoplasmosis or CMV disease typically have a poor outcome.

Increasingly, HIV-exposed infants are identified at delivery because the mother is known before delivery to be infected. However, physicians should not assume that the mother has been tested. Some women assume that they must have been tested, even though they have not discussed testing with a physician and have not been given test results. A maternal history of HIV disease, sex with a high-risk partner, or sex with a partner with HIV disease, drug use, or multiple sexual partners is useful (Table 38–6), although a negative history does not rule out infection. Obtaining an accurate

TABLE 38–5. Common Presenting Symptoms and Signs of HIV Infection in Children

General Symptoms and Signs
Growth delay or failure to thrive
Weight loss
Recurrent fever
Generalized lymphadenopathy
Hepatomegaly
Splenomegaly

Neurologic Conditions
Progressive encephalopathy
Delayed development
Loss of developmental milestones
Acquired microcephaly
Hypertonicity and spasticity, especially of lower extremities

Pulmonary Conditions
Pneumocystis carinii pneumonia
Lymphoid interstitial pneumonitis (LIP)
Cytomegalovirus (CMV) pneumonia
Recurrent bacterial pneumonia

Oral Conditions
Thrush (chronic, recurrent, or difficult to eradicate)
Parotitis or enlarged salivary glands

Gastrointestinal Tract Conditions
Recurrent or chronic diarrhea

Hepatic Conditions
Hepatitis

Hematologic Conditions
Anemia
Leukopenia
Lymphopenia
Thrombocytopenia

Dermatologic Conditions
Atopic dermatitis
Seborrhea
Candida diaper dermatitis

Opportunistic Infections
Recurrent otitis media
Serious bacterial infections (pneumonia, sepsis, meningitis, osteomyelitis)
Tuberculosis
Mycobacterium avium complex infection
Candida esophagitis
Toxoplasmosis (>1 mo of age)
CMV, disseminated or organ specific
Disseminated herpes simplex virus infection
Pneumocystis carinii pneumonia

Other Conditions
Cardiomyopathy
Chronic or recurrent otitis media
Chronic rhinorrhea

Tumors
Lymphoma (non-Hodgkin's or primary central nervous system)
Leiomyosarcoma

history of risk factors may be difficult because many persons either are unaware that they have been exposed or deny risk factors. Heterosexual transmission is underappreciated as a risk factor. People are often unaware that they have had a partner who has engaged in risky behavior.

TABLE 38–6. Persons for Whom HIV Testing Is Recommended or Strongly Encouraged

Users of injectable drugs (particularly if associated with needle sharing)
Men who have had sexual intercourse (anal or oral) with other men since the mid-1970s
Persons (including those who have hemophilia) who received blood transfusions between 1976 and March 1985
Persons who have had multiple sex partners
Persons who have engaged in sex in exchange for money, drugs, or other favors
Persons who have engaged in sexual intercourse (vaginal, anal, or oral) with any persons in any of the above categories
Persons with other sexually transmitted diseases
Children born to adults or adolescents in any of the above categories
Children born to a known HIV-infected mother
Donors of organs, tissues, or fluids
Persons who have been subjected to unwanted sexual intercourse (vaginal, anal, or oral)
Persons who have had a significant exposure to blood or body fluid from an HIV-infected person, a high-risk person, or a person whose status cannot be determined
All pregnant women (testing is strongly encouraged)

DIAGNOSIS

Infants born to HIV-infected women acquire HIV antibodies passively from their mothers. Rare exceptions are infants born extremely early who have not yet acquired maternal antibodies and infants of women who were infected late in pregnancy and who underwent delivery before mounting an antibody response. Although virtually all infants of HIV-infected women are "HIV positive," only about one fourth are infected. In children, therefore, the term *HIV positive* does not equate to *HIV infected.* Maternal HIV antibodies typically persist for 9–12 months, with virtually 100% of uninfected infants losing antibodies by 18 months of age. It is desirable to identify infected children early, and improved diagnostic methods allow most children to be identified in the first weeks or months of life. Serial antibody testing is not an acceptable way to diagnose HIV infections in vertically infected children before 15–18 months of age.

The basic methods of HIV diagnosis in adults, adolescents, and older children (>18 months of age) has not changed significantly since serologic testing for HIV was introduced in 1985, except that the methods have become more refined and are increasingly sensitive and specific. In contrast, testing for children less than 18 months of age has evolved remarkably since that time. HIV testing is warranted if the medical and social histories indicate that the person is at risk.

Before laboratory testing, the patient or the parent or guardian of a minor child should be counseled. Counseling is usually a legal requirement and is a sound medical practice. Pretest counseling includes a discussion of HIV risk factors, an overview of HIV disease, the nature of the test, and the implications of test results. Permission should always be obtained for testing. Laws regarding an adolescent's legal right to grant permission for HIV testing and treatment vary by state and may differ from laws on other sexually transmitted diseases.

Pretest counseling and posttest counseling are as important as the serologic diagnosis itself because the diagnosis has such an emotional impact. Posttest counseling of a person with negative test results is another chance to educate about methods of prevention. A positive test result must be followed by counseling to discuss the need for further laboratory studies and therapeutic options, to provide psychological and social assistance as necessary, to plan for further testing of partners and children, and to discuss how to avoid transmission to others. Methods of risk reduction for children and sexual partners or needle-sharing partners should be discussed. For physicians with little HIV-related experience, local or regional centers or physicians providing care for infected persons should be contacted and a referral made. For physicians unfamiliar with such resources, local and state health departments or the nearest medical school should be able to provide assistance.

Laboratory Evaluation

Serologic Testing. Serologic testing for HIV-specific antibodies is the diagnostic gold standard for persons older than 15–18 months. The process begins with an EIA screening test, which has sensitivity and specificity >99%. The results are reported as positive (reactive) or negative (nonreactive). Typically the laboratory should repeat the EIA on the same serum sample if the initial test result is positive. The EIA result alone is not definitive evidence of HIV infection because false-positive results occur. A confirmatory test is always necessary to corroborate the result of a positive EIA result. Most laboratories use one of several commercially available immunoblot tests for confirmation (Chapter 11). Other methods such as radioimmunoprecipitation or immunofluorescence assays are occasionally used for confirmation.

Several organizations have developed minimum criteria for a positive result on an immunoblot test (Table 38–7). If a test result is positive by one set of criteria, it is usually but not always positive by the other criteria. The result is reported as positive (reactive) when at least two or three specific bands are present. Most infected individuals will have more than the minimum number. Many laboratories will report which bands are present. When no antibody-antigen bands are detected, the immunoblot result is reported as negative (nonreactive). A positive EIA finding followed by a negative immunoblot result is rare in a person who is truly infected. In some cases a test result is neither positive nor negative. These indeterminate tests do not meet the minimum requirements for a positive result (Table 38–7). They often have one or two bands, or they have bands that do not align with those present in the positive control. Under no circumstances should a person be told that he or she is HIV infected without a clearly positive confirmatory test result.

TABLE 38–7. Guidelines for Immunoblot Interpretation for HIV*

Organization	Minimum Requirements for a Positive Immunoblot Result
American Red Cross	≥1 band from each gene group (Table 38–1): *gag* (p55, p24, p17) *pol* (p66, p51, p31) *env* (gp160, gp120, gp41)
Association of State and Territorial Public Health Laboratory Directors/Centers for Disease Control and Prevention	Any 2 of: p24, gp41, or gp120/160
Consortium for Retrovirus Serology Standardization	p24 or p31 *and* either gp41 or gp120/160
DuPont	p24 and p31 *and* either gp41 or gp120/160

*Four standards exist defining a positive immunoblot result. In most, but not all cases, a positive immunoblot result by one standard is also positive by another.

Early in infection, before the onset of full antibody production, an indeterminate test result can be obtained. In such a case an infected person will always have a clearly positive immunoblot result within 6 months. Indeterminate results will sometimes be obtained with rheumatologic disorders, immunologic disorders, cancers, infections such as hepatitis, or in persons who have previously received blood products. In some cases there is not a good explanation for an indeterminate finding. A particularly difficult problem has been the situation in which a positive EIA result and an indeterminate immunoblot result are obtained in a pregnant woman. An increasing percentage of all HIV tests performed during pregnancy show false-positive results. The reason is that the emphasis has shifted from testing ''high risk'' women to testing all women. Hence the number of women with true positive results (infected women) is diluted by an increasing number of low-risk women for whom a positive test result has an increasing chance of being falsely positive.

For most pregnant women with indeterminate immunoblot results, a single band will be present, although occasionally two bands are seen. Rarely a test will meet the minimum requirement for a positive result in a person who is not infected. The physician should be especially vigilant when an immunoblot shows minimum positive criteria, especially if the presumably infected person has a subsequent undetectable viral load test and normal findings on immunologic studies.

Indeterminate immunoblot results require special handling, particularly when they are obtained during pregnancy. A person who has a positive EIA result and a negative or indeterminate immunoblot result should be counseled, reevaluated for risk factors, and told what can be done to clarify the results. In such cases a PCR test can rapidly help clarify the infection status. Another approach long recommended by the CDC is to repeat antibody testing 3 and 6 months after the indeterminate result. A person who is infected will have a positive immunoblot result in that time. A person whose test result becomes negative or who has a persistently indeterminate result for 6 months is not infected. Some people remain ''serofast,'' retaining the same pattern indefinitely.

Nonserologic Testing. Antibody tests are generally sufficient for older children and adults. Children of HIV-infected women will have passively acquired maternal antibodies, which can persist for as long as 18 months. It is possible to ascertain the infection status of most children by 4–6 months of life by using nonserologic methods.

The most widely used nonserologic HIV test method is the PCR assay, which has become the standard method for determining the HIV infection status of HIV-exposed children <18 months of age. The HIV **DNA PCR** method is preferred; it has a sensitivity and specificity of >99%. Recommendations from the American Academy of Pediatrics include HIV PCR testing at birth (within 48 hours), at 1–2 months of age, and at 4–6 months of age. Umbilical cord blood should not be used for HIV testing.

Approximately one third of infected infants will have a positive PCR test result in the first 48 hours of life. This has some prognostic significance because infants who were infected in utero are those who are likely to test positive in the first hours or days after birth and for whom the prognosis for progression to AIDS and long-term survival may be somewhat worse than for children infected perinatally.

Children who acquire the virus at or near the time of birth usually have negative PCR results in the first days after delivery, when viral titers are below detection level. About 40% of infected infants will have a positive HIV PCR test result within the first 2 days of life. By 2–4 weeks after delivery, 93–95% of infected infants will test positive. This includes children infected in utero and most of those infected perinatally. The final PCR test is usually performed between 4 and 6 months of age. Almost all of the infected but previously unidentified infants will have a diagnosis by 4–6 months. There are rare cases of infected children whose first positive PCR results are obtained beyond 6 months of age.

When an infant tests positive, a second confirmatory test should be performed as soon as possible. The confirmatory test might be a second PCR DNA, an HIV culture, or a viral load test. The latter has the advantage of both confirming the result and serving as a baseline before initiation of therapy. If all PCR results remain negative by 4–6 months of age, the infant has >99% chance of not being HIV infected. A negative antibody EIA result at 15–18 months of age is final confirmation that the child is not infected. Repeated HIV tests should be performed at any time in the first year of life if the child develops symptoms suggestive of HIV infection.

There is a trend to perform more tests earlier in life, for example, at 2 weeks of age, when there is an opportunity to provide antiretroviral therapy near the time of rapid viral replication. ZDV therapy has not decreased the sensitivity and predicted values of virologic assays. It is uncertain whether more potent antiretroviral combinations used in pregnancy might delay virologic diagnosis.

Diagnostic PCR tests are unnecessary beyond 15–18 months of age because antibody testing is adequate. One exception is a finding of positive EIA results but negative or indeterminate immunoblot results in a pregnant woman. Pregnancy is a time when an HIV-infected woman and her physician have to make critical decisions including implementation of ZDV therapy, the mode of delivery, and whether to breast-feed. A diagnosis has major emotional and social implications for the woman. A woman who has an indeterminate test result in the early months of pregnancy may elect to defer ZDV therapy while waiting for the PCR test result. A negative finding should give assurance that infection is unlikely and that ZDV need not be taken. An indeterminate test result obtained in the last days or hours before delivery may not allow time for PCR testing before delivery, and treatment decisions such as use of ZDV and cesarean delivery may have to be made without supportive data.

These individual decisions are based on risk factors, turnaround time for the test, and the woman's desires regarding treatment. There is no specific stage of therapy at which one approach or another is best, but the physician and patient must together make a decision regarding PCR testing and treatment when serologic test results are uncertain.

In addition to the DNA PCR method, **viral load or viral burden** test methods by HIV **RNA PCR** potentially may prove to be at least as sensitive as the DNA PCR method for early diagnosis. Three methods of viral load testing, with varying sensitivities, are in use.

The third nonserologic method that is available is viral culture. In contrast to PCR testing, which is widely available, few laboratories supply the laborious, time-consuming, and expensive viral culture. Culturing requires 1–4 weeks, compared with a few days for other methods. Because the sensitivity is the same as, or slightly less than, that of PCR testing, the predictive value of a negative test result is approximately the same as, or slightly less than, that of a DNA PCR test performed at the same age. A positive test result confirms infection.

Another method is the **p24 protein antigen test.** The p24 protein is a core viral protein that can be found free in serum and sometimes in the CSF of many infected persons. It was used as a marker of disease progression before the PCR methods became widely available. The original method of measuring p24 was recognized as very specific, but the test lacked sensitivity. As few as one half to one third of infected infants routinely tested positive by this method. In the early 1990s it was found that more p24 antigen was available than had generally been appreciated, but much of it was complexed with anti-p24 antibodies. A weak acid treatment liberates antigen from the complex before the assay is performed and increases yield to approximately 80% at the peak detection age of about 2 months. Although p24 antigen testing is widely available, inexpensive, and relatively simple to perform, it has been widely replaced by the PCR method.

TREATMENT

Treatment regimens for HIV-infected children and infants are complex and evolving (Table 38–8). Resources for updated information and treatment recommendations are provided in Table 38–9.

The HIV-Exposed Newborn. Most infants born to HIV-infected mothers do not have HIV infection. Nevertheless, these infants represent a uniquely vulnerable group, requiring many resources for appropriate care and follow-up.

Care for the infant begins with good prenatal care for the pregnant woman. With current medical practices the HIV perinatal transmission rate is 10% or less. An obstetrician who is knowledgeable about HIV disease is important to protect the mother's health and to provide therapies that minimize risks for the infant. Colleagues in obstetrics and pediatrics must collaborate before the birth to plan appropriate treatments during labor and therapy for the infant in the early hours of life.

The ACTG 076 study provided the basis for strong recommendations to use ZDV as a pharmacologic means of reducing perinatal HIV transmission. Treatment has three separate components: prepartum oral ZDV for the mother beginning at the fourteenth week of pregnancy, intravenous ZDV during labor, and oral ZDV for the infant for the first 6 weeks of life (Table 38–10). ZDV therapy should be offered to all pregnant women with a diagnosis of HIV infection during pregnancy. Multidrug regimens may be prescribed for the pregnant woman, consistent with current guidelines, which stress that all HIV-infected women should receive the most effective treatment regardless of pregnancy status. When possible, ZDV should be included in the treatment plan for the pregnant HIV-infected woman because it is the medicine best studied in terms of efficacy and safety for the infant. Data on partial implementation of the recommended three parts of ZDV therapy are incomplete. As a general rule, pediatricians should attempt to complete as much of the ACTG 076 protocol as possible.

The most common adverse effect described in infants receiving ZDV during the ACTG 076 study was a mild and transient anemia, which usually resolves without therapy. This condition is rarely of clinical significance unless there are other risk factors for anemia. No associations with congenital malformations or prematurity have been noted to date. Concerns about long-term effects of ZDV exposure for infants await follow-up studies. Other antiretroviral agents have not been as extensively studied as ZDV for pregnant women.

Long-term animal studies have shown that ZDV is associated with vaginal tumors in rodents and zalcitabine is associated with thymic lymphomas. There are no long-term human data on adults

TABLE 38–8. Recommended Treatment Regimens for Selected Opportunistic Infections in Children with HIV Infections

Organism	Children (≤13 Yr of Age)	Adolescents (>13 Yr of Age) and Adults
Bacteria		
Streptococcus pneumoniae *Haemophilus influenzae* type b *Shigella* *Campylobacter*	Antibiotics and duration of therapy are generally the same as for non-HIV-infected children with the same disease	Antibiotics and duration of therapy are generally the same as for non-HIV-infected adolescents and adults with the same disease
Nontypical *Salmonella*		
Enteritis	Cefpodoxime 10 mg/kg/day (max 400 mg) divided bid PO for 2–4 wk *or* TMP-SMZ 8–10 mg TMP/kg/day divided bid PO for 2–4 wk *or* Amoxicillin 50 mg/kg/day divided tid PO for 2–4 wk	Ciprofloxacin 500 mg bid PO for 2–4 wk *or* Ampicillin 8–12 g/day divided q6hr IV for 1–4 wk then amoxicillin 500 mg PO tid to complete 2–4 wk course
Bacteremia and invasive infections	Ceftriaxone 50–100 mg/kg/day divided q12–24hr IV for 2–4 wk *or* Cefotaxime 100–150 mg/kg/day divided q8hr IV for 2–4 wk	Ciprofloxacin 800 mg/day divided bid IV for 2–4 wk *or* Ceftriaxone 50–100 mg/kg/day divided q12–24hr IV for 2–4 wk *or* Cefotaxime 100–150 mg/kg/day divided q8hr IV for 2–4 wk
	Notes • Nontyphoidal enteritis in HIV-infected persons should be treated to decrease risk of invasive disease • Treatment of bacteremia and invasive infections in persons with HIV infection may need to be prolonged • Secondary prophylaxis for several months may be used	
Mycobacteria		
Mycobacterium tuberculosis		
Latent tuberculosis infection	Isoniazid 10–15 mg/kg (max 300 mg) once daily for 12 mo	Isoniazid 300 mg once daily for 12 mo
Pulmonary tuberculosis	Isoniazid 10–15 mg/kg (max 300 mg) once daily for 6–12 mo *plus* Rifampin 10–20 mg/kg (max 600 mg) once daily for 6–12 mo *plus* Pyrazinamide 15–30 mg/kg (max 2 g) once daily PO for 2 mo In areas with >4% isoniazid resistance or if resistance is suspected on the basis of culture result from a contact, one of the following should be added until drug susceptibility is determined: Streptomycin 20–40 mg/kg (max 1 g) once daily IM for 2 mo *or* Ethambutol 15–25 mg/kg (max 2.5 g) once daily PO for 2 mo	Isoniazid 5 mg/kg (max 300 mg) once daily for 6–9 mo *plus* Rifampin 10 mg/kg (max 600 mg) once daily for 6–9 mo *plus* Pyrazinamide 15–30 mg/kg (max 2 g) once daily PO for 2 mo In areas with >4% isoniazid resistance or if resistance is suspected on the basis of culture result from a contact, one of the following should be added until drug susceptibility is determined: Streptomycin 15 mg/kg (max 1 g) once daily IM for 2 mo *or* Ethambutol 15 mg/kg (max 2.5 g) once daily PO for 2 mo
Extrapulmonary or disseminated	Isoniazid, rifampin, pyrazinamide, and streptomycin (*or* ethambutol) for 2 mo *followed by* Isoniazid *plus* rifampin for 10 mo (total of 12 mo)	Isoniazid, rifampin, pyrazinamide, and streptomycin (*or* ethambutol) for 2 mo *followed by* Isoniazid *plus* rifampin for 10 mo (total of 12 mo)
	Notes • After 2 mo of daily therapy, therapy can be given 2–3 times/wk using directly observed therapy and higher doses (see Table 35–5) • Recommendations for treatment of pulmonary disease for HIV-infected children vary from 6 to 12 mo of total therapy • Rifampin-containing regimens are generally incompatible with protease inhibitors and non-nucleoside-reverse-transcriptase inhibitors; rifabutin may be substituted for rifampin, allowing protease inhibitors to be continued	

TABLE 38–8. Recommended Treatment Regimens for Selected Opportunistic Infections in Children with HIV Infections *(Continued)*

Organism	Children (≤13 Yr of Age)	Adolescents (>13 Yr of Age) and Adults
Mycobacteria *(Continued)*		
Mycobacterium tuberculosis (Continued)		
Extrapulmonary or disseminated *(Continued)*	• The potential for drug interactions is significant for persons treated for both HIV and tuberculosis • Pyridoxine 10 mg/kg/day PO is recommended to prevent neurologic adverse effects for persons with risk factors (pregnancy, breast-feeding infants, diabetes mellitus, uremia, alcoholism, malnourishment, some pre-existing seizure disorders) • Infectious disease consultation is recommended	
Mycobacterium avium-intracellulare complex (MAC)	Clarithromycin 30 mg/kg/day in 1–2 divided doses PO *plus* Ethambutol 15–20 mg/kg once daily PO *with or without* Rifabutin 5 mg/kg (max 300 mg) once daily PO *or* Ciprofloxacin 20–30 mg/kg once daily IV or PO *or* Amikacin 15–30 mg/kg/day (max 1.5 g/day) divided q8–12hr IV	Clarithromycin 500 mg bid PO *plus* Ethambutol 10–15 mg/kg once daily PO *with or without* Rifabutin 300 mg once daily PO *or* Ciprofloxacin 1–1.5 g divided bid PO *or* Amikacin 15–30 mg/kg/day (max 1.5 g/day) divided q8–12hr IV
	Notes • A minimum of 2 drugs is required for treatment of MAC; azithromycin 10 mg/kg (max 500 mg) once daily PO is sometimes substituted for clarithromycin • Regimens of 5–7 drugs have been used, although adverse effects and drug interactions are significant • Therapy is continued for life; treatment suppresses but does not cure MAC infection • Many medications used to treat MAC interact with antiretroviral drugs • Infectious disease consultation is recommended	
Coccidioides immitis		
Disseminated infection, diffuse pneumonia, meningitis	Amphotericin B 1 mg/kg/day IV (duration depends on clinical response) *or* Fluconazole 8–12 mg/kg/day (max 800 mg) PO ***Then Continue Lifelong Secondary Prophylaxis*** Fluconazole 3–6 mg/kg (max 400 mg) once daily PO	Amphotericin B 1 mg/kg/day IV (duration depends on clinical response) *or* Fluconazole 400–800 mg once daily PO *or* Itraconazole 400 mg divided bid PO ***Then Continue Lifelong Secondary Prophylaxis*** Fluconazole 400 mg once daily PO *or* Itraconazole 400 mg divided bid PO
	Notes • Fluconazole is preferred for meningitis • Intrathecal (intrareservoir) amphotericin B may be added for coccidioidomycosis meningitis that fails to respond to fluconazole • Infectious disease consultation is recommended	
Cryptococcus neoformans		
Meningitis	Amphotericin B 0.7–1 mg/kg once daily IV for 10–14 days *with or without* Flucytosine 50–150 mg/kg/day divided qid PO for 14 days ***Then Continue Lifelong Secondary Prophylaxis*** Fluconazole 6–12 mg/kg (max 400 mg) once daily or divided bid PO *or* Itraconazole 2–5 mg/kg (max 400 mg) once daily PO *or* Amphotericin B 0.5–1 mg/kg/day 1–3 times/wk IV	Amphotericin B 0.7–1 mg/kg once daily IV for 10–14 days *with or without* Flucytosine 50–150 mg/kg/day divided qid PO for 14 days *then* Fluconazole 400–800 mg/day divided bid PO ***Then Continue Lifelong Secondary Prophylaxis*** Fluconazole 200 mg once daily PO *or* Itraconazole 400 mg tablet *or* 200 mg suspension once daily PO *or* Amphotericin B 0.5–1 mg/kg/day 1–3 times/wk IV
Pulmonary, disseminated, or antigenemia	As for meningitis	Fluconazole 200 mg bid PO for 6–10 wk *or* Itraconazole 200 mg tablet *or* 100 mg suspension once daily PO for 6–10 wk

Table continued on following page

TABLE 38–8. Recommended Treatment Regimens for Selected Opportunistic Infections in Children with HIV Infections *(Continued)*

Organism	Children (≤13 Yr of Age)	Adolescents (>13 Yr of Age) and Adults
Mycobacteria *(Continued)*		
Cryptococcus neoformans (Continued)		
Pulmonary, disseminated, or antigenemia *(Continued)*		***Then Continue Lifelong Secondary Prophylaxis*** Fluconazole 200 mg once daily PO *or* Itraconazole 200 mg tablet *or* 100 mg suspension once daily PO *or* Amphotericin B 0.5–1 mg/kg/day 1–3 times/wk IV
Histoplasma capsulatum		
Pneumonia, disseminated infection	Amphotericin B 0.5–1 mg/kg/day IV (an equivalent dose of liposomal amphotericin B can be substituted for the deoxycholate salt of amphotericin B) IV (duration depends on clinical response, usually 7–14 days) *or* Itraconazole 5–12 mg/kg/day divided bid PO for 12 wk ***Then Continue Lifelong Secondary Prophylaxis*** Itraconazole 5–10 mg/kg/day (max 400 mg) once daily PO	Amphotericin B 0.5–1 mg/kg/day (an equivalent dose of liposomal amphotericin B can be substituted for the deoxycholate salt of amphotericin B) IV (duration depends on clinical response, usually 7–14 days) *or* Itraconazole 600 mg divided bid PO for 3 days, then 400 mg tablet divided bid PO *or* 200 mg suspension divided bid PO for 12 wk *or* Fluconazole 1600 mg once PO then 400–800 mg once daily PO for 12 wk ***Then Continue Lifelong Secondary Prophylaxis*** Itraconazole 400 mg divided bid PO *or* Amphotericin B 50 mg 1–2 times a week IV
Fungi		
Aspergillus		
Pneumonia, disseminated infection	Amphotericin B 1 mg/kg/day (an equivalent dose of liposomal amphotericin B can be substituted for the deoxycholate salt of amphotericin B) IV (duration depends on clinical response) ***Alternative Regimen*** Itraconazole 5–10 mg/kg/day divided bid PO	Amphotericin B 0.7–1.4 mg/kg/day (an equivalent dose of liposomal amphotericin B can be substituted for the deoxycholate salt of amphotericin B) IV (duration depends on clinical response) ***Alternative Regimen*** Itraconazole 600 mg divided bid PO for 3 days, then 400 mg tablet divided bid PO *or* 200 mg suspension divided bid PO for 12 wk
Candida		
Oral candidiasis (initial treatment until symptoms resolve, usually 10–14 days)	Nystatin 100,000–500,000 U qid PO (gargle or swish and swallow) *or* Clotrimazole 10 mg oral troches 3–5 times/day PO ***Alternative Regimens*** Fluconazole 3–6 mg/kg (max 100 mg) once daily PO *or* Ketoconazole 5–10 mg/kg once daily or divided bid PO *or* Amphotericin B 1 mL qid PO (gargle or swish and swallow) ***Then Maintenance Therapy as Needed*** Nystatin 100,000–500,000 U qid PO (gargle or swish and swallow) *or* Clotrimazole 10 mg oral troches 3–5 times/day PO *or* Fluconazole 3–6 mg/kg (max 100 mg) once daily PO	Clotrimazole 10 mg oral troches 3–5 times/day PO *or* Nystatin 500,000 U qid PO (gargle, or swish and swallow) ***Alternative Regimens*** Itraconazole 200 mg tablet or 100 mg suspension once daily PO *or* Fluconazole 100 mg once daily or divided bid PO *or* Amphotericin B 1–5 mL qid PO (gargle or swish and swallow) ***Then Maintenance Therapy as Needed*** Clotrimazole 10 mg oral troches 3–5 times/day PO *or* Nystatin 500,000 U qid PO (gargle or swish and swallow) *or* Fluconazole 100 mg once daily or 200 mg 3 times/wk PO

TABLE 38–8. Recommended Treatment Regimens for Selected Opportunistic Infections in Children with HIV Infections *(Continued)*

Organism	Children (≤13 Yr of Age)	Adolescents (>13 Yr of Age) and Adults
Fungi *(Continued)*		
Candida (Continued)		
Esophagitis (initial treatment until symptoms resolve, usually 2–3 wk)	Fluconazole 3–6 mg/kg (max 400 mg) 1–2 times/day *or* Amphotericin B 0.5–1 mg/kg once daily (an equivalent dose of liposomal amphotericin B can be substituted for the deoxycholate salt of amphotericin B) IV ***Then Maintenance Therapy as Needed*** Fluconazole 3–6 mg/kg (max 100 mg) once daily PO *or* Itraconazole 2–5 mg (max 100 mg suspension) once daily PO *or* Ketoconazole 200 mg once daily PO	Fluconazole 200 mg 1–2 times/day or 200 mg 3 times/wk PO *or* Itraconazole 200 mg tablet bid *or* 100 mg suspension once daily PO *or* Ketoconazole 200 mg once daily PO *or* Amphotericin B 0.5–1 mg/kg once daily (an equivalent dose of liposomal amphotericin B can be substituted for the deoxycholate salt of amphotericin B) IV (duration depends on clinical response) ***Then Maintenance Therapy as Needed*** Fluconazole 100 mg 1–2 times/day PO *or* Itraconazole 200 mg tablet bid *or* 100 mg suspension once daily PO *or* Ketoconazole 200 mg once daily PO
Parasites		
Pneumocystis carinii pneumonia	See Table 68–13 for treatment and Table 68–14 for primary and secondary prophylaxis	
Toxoplasma gondii		
Congenital infection	See Table 95–9	
Acquired encephalitis	Pyrimethamine 2 mg/kg/day PO loading dose for 2 days, then 15 mg/m²/day or 1 mg/kg/day (max 25 mg) once daily PO *plus* Sulfadiazine 100 mg/kg/day divided bid PO *plus* Leucovorin 5–10 mg 3 times/wk PO ***Then Continue Lifelong Secondary Prophylaxis*** Pyrimethamine 25–75 mg once daily PO *plus* Sulfadiazine 500–1,000 mg qid PO *plus* Leucovorin 10 mg 3 times/wk PO	Pyrimethamine 100–200 mg PO loading dose, then 25–75 mg once daily PO *plus* Sulfadiazine 4–8 mg once daily PO *plus* Leucovorin 10–25 mg once daily PO ***Then Continue Lifelong Secondary Prophylaxis*** Pyrimethamine 25–75 mg once daily PO *plus* Sulfadiazine 500–1,000 mg qid PO *plus* Leucovorin 10–25 mg once daily PO
	Notes • Consider adding prednisone 1 mg/kg/day divided bid PO for infants or persons with chorioretinitis, a high concentration of CSF protein (≥1,000 mg/dL), or systemic or generalized infection until improvement of chorioretinitis or resolution of elevated CSF protein • Infectious disease consultation is recommended	

or the offspring of women exposed during pregnancy. Several agents are associated with animal teratogenicity—most notably delavirdine, which has been associated with ventricular septal defects in animals and in several children. Didanosine, saquinavir, ritonavir, and nelfinavir are pregnancy category B drugs, meaning that animal studies have not revealed risk to the fetus. All others are category C medications, indicating incomplete data or that abnormalities were noted in animal studies. Reports from antiretroviral registries have generally not identified significant complications for infants exposed prenatally to antiretroviral drugs; the association with defects in some animal models and the lack of long-term data indicate the need for caution.

Multidrug regimens may be advantageous for both the mother and infant. While women should be considered for triple antiviral

TABLE 38–9. Sources for Updated HIV/AIDS Information

Internet Resources	
www.hivatis.org	HIV/AIDS Treatment Information Services Website (useful access to recent guidelines and recent data)
www.cdc.gov	National AIDS Clearinghouse Website
www.aap.org	American Academy of Pediatrics, HIV-Related Policies
www.pedhivaids.org	National Pediatric and Family HIV Resource Center
Hotlines for Health Care Providers	
800–448–0440	HIV/AIDS Treatment Information Service
800–362–0071	National Pediatric and Family HIV Resource Center for Texas and Oklahoma; AIDS Helpline for Health Professionals
800–933–3413	HIV Telephone Consultation Service at San Francisco General Hospital
888–448–4911	National Clinicians' Post-Exposure (e.g., needle stick) Prophylaxis Hotline
800–874–2572	National HIV Trials
Hotlines for the General Public	
800–342–2437	CDC National AIDS Hotline
800–344–7432	SIDA—Spanish Information Hotline (CDC)
800–822–7422	Project Inform (Info/Newsletter)
212–682–7440	AmFAR Quarterly Report on Drugs in Clinical Trials

therapy by the same criteria as other adults, and they should also be counseled about the potential, sometimes unknown risk for the fetus. An obstetrician experienced in the use of antiretroviral drugs or an infectious disease specialist who can advise the obstetrician should be consulted when multidrug therapy is used in pregnancy.

Additional measures to further reduce HIV perinatal transmission remain areas of research and interest and have worldwide implications for controlling the epidemic. Obstetric practices, such as washings of the birth canal during labor with antiviral agents, have been studied with mixed results. Several reports have shown that a cesarean delivery performed before the onset of labor decreases the risk of perinatal transmission. Peripartum use of single doses of oral medicines with prolonged viral suppression, such as nevirapine, has been reported to decrease rates of perinatal transmission in studies performed in other countries. However, these obstetric practices are not without complications or costs. There is growing concern that a short-term course of a nonnucleoside reverse transcriptase inhibitor such as nevirapine near delivery may result in subsequent maternal viral resistance to the entire class of similar medicines. Thus certain practices may be beneficial and worth the cost for selected groups of mothers, such as those with high viral loads caused by medical or compliance failures or those with HIV infection diagnosed late in pregnancy.

TABLE 38–10. Recommended Regimen to Prevent Perinatal HIV Transmission*

Mothers

During pregnancy: zidovudine 100 mg 5 times daily PO after wk 14 of pregnancy

During labor: zidovudine 2 mg/kg/hr loading dose IV, followed by 1 mg/kg/hr IV

Infants

At 8–12 hr of life: zidovudine 2 mg/kg q6hr and continued until 6 wk of age

*All three components are recommended, but treatment may be initiated with peripartum treatment or with treatment of the infant (beginning within 12 hours of life) even if previous therapy has not been administered. HIV-infected women should receive the most effective therapeutic treatment regardless of pregnancy status. When possible, ZDV should be included in the treatment plan for the pregnant HIV-infected woman, because it is the medicine best studied in terms of efficacy and safety for the infant.

Adherence by medical personnel to universal precautions is recommended for all deliveries; the precautions include the use of gowns, gloves, masks, and eye protection and the avoidance of mouth-suctioning devices. No special washings or isolation procedures are indicated for the HIV-exposed infant. HIV symptoms are almost never obvious in the newborn. If the infant has abnormal physical findings such as poor growth, microcephaly, lymphadenopathy, or hepatosplenomegaly, other causes should be considered. The mother's record should be reviewed for documentation of other maternal infections. If antepartum laboratory results are unavailable, tests of the infant for syphilis, toxoplasmosis, and CMV disease may be considered. A CBC may be helpful to assess the infant for conditions causing a predisposition to anemia, which could be exacerbated by the use of ZDV therapy.

ZDV should be given to the infant within the first 12 hours of life, at a dose of 2 mg/kg every 6 hours. If the child is not taking enteral feedings, ZDV can be provided through the intravenous route at the same dosage of 2 mg/kg/dose every 6 hours. Dosing adjustments for extreme prematurity are being evaluated. Ongoing studies of ZDV for infants born before 34 weeks' gestation use doses of 1.5 mg/kg every 12 hours from birth to 2 weeks and then increase the dose to 2 mg/kg every 8 hours. For critically ill premature infants, measurement of serum levels should be attempted. The ZDV dose may be adjusted to maintain a regimen of 2 mg/kg per dose if weight gain is significant.

HIV-exposed infants require attention to nutrition, growth and development, nurturing, and anticipatory guidance. Breast-feeding is contraindicated for HIV-infected mothers in the United States and other countries where suitable alternative sources of nutrition are available. Routine childhood immunizations should be provided. The live oral polio vaccine (OPV) should not be used in children born to HIV-infected mothers because HIV-infected household members may be at risk of acquiring the poliovirus. The administration of bacille Calmette-Guérin (BCG) vaccine to HIV-infected persons is contraindicated because of its potential to cause disseminated disease. Frequent health visits in the first year of life allow the health care provider to provide serial testing for HIV in the infant and to monitor for clinical signs of HIV infection, both of which are described earlier in this chapter. Typically the child is seen at 2 weeks, at 1 month, and at 1-month intervals until 6 months of age, followed by 3-month visits until final HIV testing at 15 months of age.

Recommendations for PCP prophylaxis for HIV-exposed infants are intended to protect infants who may be HIV infected during the period when diagnosis is uncertain. Prophylaxis may be started at 6–8 weeks and continued until serial HIV test results are negative, usually around age 4 months. TMP-SMZ is the prophylactic treatment of choice (see Table 68–14). The necessity of this recommendation has lessened as the rates of perinatal HIV transmission have fallen and the ability to make the diagnosis in the early months of life has improved.

There may be a tendency toward bacterial or other infectious illnesses in HIV-exposed infants, possibly because of suboptimal protection provided by transplacental maternal antibodies. Especially in the early months until HIV infection is excluded, fevers and respiratory illnesses must be evaluated for potential HIV-related conditions. Many HIV-infected women learn the diagnosis while being tested during pregnancy and have had little time to devote to their own issues and needs. Providing a single location for health care for multiple members of a family, including the infant, has been successful in some communities. In other settings the pediatric care team best uses the multiple infant health care visits as an opportunity to educate parents, to make referrals for social services, and to facilitate access to appropriate adult health care settings.

The HIV-Infected Child. Establishing the diagnosis of HIV infection in a child remains a sad and life-altering event. HIV disease is incurable and is associated with significant morbidity and mortality. However, the prognosis has improved dramatically in recent years. Families can be honestly counseled that early diagnosis of HIV infection allows the opportunity for intervention before clinical disease occurs. The long-term outlook is obviously unknown, but many children can look forward to years of reasonable health, albeit years filled with medicines and medical visits.

There has been a paradigm shift, from HIV infection as a fulminant disease culminating in early death to a chronic condition with an unpredictable outcome. This change results in a whole new set of challenges for the child and family and for the medical caregiver. In this time of rapid progress and change, it is impossible to present a discussion of treatment specifics that will not be outdated within months. Basic concepts of therapy are presented, again with the admonition that health care providers will need to continue to use the ever-expanding information resources to provide current information and care.

Definitive Treatment

In 1993 the first Working Group on Antiretroviral Therapy and Medical Management of HIV-infected Children was convened by the National Pediatric and Family HIV Resource Center. These specialists in the care of infants, children, and adolescents with HIV infection have produced and periodically update guidelines addressing the complex issues of treatment of pediatric HIV disease (Table 38–9). Certain principles of treatment have evolved that form the foundation for consideration of specific therapeutic options for HIV-infected children. Antiretroviral agents should be used in combination in the treatment of all HIV-infected children. Monotherapy is considered obsolete and should be avoided whenever possible. HIV can develop mutations that render the virus resistant to specific antiretroviral agents and that limit clinical usefulness of treatment. Adherence to multidrug regimens minimizes the development of resistance. Measures of virus load, specifically HIV RNA assays, should be used to assess the adequacy of medical therapies. The goal of treatment is suppression of HIV to below limits of detection or to levels as low as possible for as long as possible. Therapies for children require attention to dosages depending on age and size. Underdosing will foster the development of resistant HIV strains, whereas overdosing leads to problems related to drug toxicity. Drug formulations and dosing schedules for children remain a high priority in new therapy development. Information from clinical trials involving HIV-infected adults has generally been applicable to children. All therapies approved for HIV infection may be used for children when indicated. Ongoing research is needed to define safe and effective therapies for children. There are many barriers to the optimal use of antiretroviral medicines in children, including (1) lack of available and palatable liquid formulations, (2) complexity of medication schedules, (3) dependency on overwhelmed family members to provide medicine, (4) secrecy among caregivers, (5) potential drug interactions, and (6) adverse effects.

Initiation of Treatment. For all HIV-infected children with symptoms or other evidence of immunodeficiency, antiretroviral therapy is indicated regardless of age or the viral load. For the symptom-free child with normal immune system values, initiation of treatment may depend on individualized assessment of benefits and risks.

For newly diagnosed cases in infants, most experts recommend initiation of therapy as soon as a confirmed diagnosis is established. Data from recently infected adults have demonstrated that factors surrounding the early course of infection may influence the entire subsequent disease course. The rationale for early treatment during the primary infection of an infant is that aggressive, prompt therapy during early viral replication might preserve the child's immune function, decrease viral seeding, lower the viral set point, and result in improved clinical outcome. Clinical data proving the therapeutic benefit of aggressive early treatment in infants are not yet available. There are many pitfalls in dealing with HIV-infected infants, not the least of which are unknown optimal dosing and the concern that drug resistance may develop.

For children >12 months of age, most experts also recommend treatment whenever possible, although adherence to medical regimens is notoriously difficult in these young children. Some experts can support deferment of therapy in symptom-free children with normal immunity if there are concerns regarding adherence, safety, and long-term persistence of an antiviral effect. In this situation the use of the viral load assay as an indication to initiate treatment may be helpful. Although not absolute, current practical guidelines include the following: (1) treatment should be started in any child with HIV RNA levels of >100,000 copies/mL; (2) treatment should be strongly considered in a child with an HIV RNA level of 10,000–20,000 copies/mL; and (3) treatment should be offered to any child with a viral load that increases by fivefold before age 2 years or by threefold after age 2 years.

Combination Therapy. By the mid-1990s, studies were already showing the benefits of multidrug therapies over monotherapy. The introduction and success of protease inhibitor medicines in 1996 hastened the trend of using multiple antiretroviral agents in combination. The availability of different drugs with different actions ushered in the era of **highly active antiretroviral therapy (HAART),** usually meaning the use of three or more drugs including a protease inhibitor. It is also acceptable to use a combination regimen consisting of the triple nucleoside analog reverse transcriptase inhibitor (RTI) combination of zidovudine plus lamivudine plus abacavir for selected patients with viral loads <100,000 viral copies/mL. This combination is available as a single tablet (Trizivir), although no liquid combinations currently exist. One major advantage is reduction of the ''pill burden'' (to one tablet twice daily), which may have an advantage with poorly adherent populations, including adolescents. Substitution of a nonnucleoside RTI medication (nevirapine or efavirenz) is acceptable in selected situations. There is increasing experience with these non–protease inhibitor combinations, and specific guidelines for the use of various combinations will eventually be developed. Currently, physician experience and comfort with various combinations will determine when and how they are used. The somewhat fortuitous widespread availability of viral load measurement about the same time changed the whole focus of care to suppressing the viral load to below the limit of detection or as low as possible for as long as possible. Numerous subsequent studies have verified the justification of this treatment goal, because viral suppression has clearly been shown to correlate with improved levels of CD4 cells, a decrease in AIDS-associated complications, and improved health. Reduction of the mortality rate among HIV-infected children in the late 1990s, in comparison with prior periods, is attributable to the use of antiretroviral medications.

Numerous drugs acting at different stages in viral replication are available, including a few combination formulations (Table 38–11). Many antiretroviral drugs are associated with significant adverse effects and interactions (Table 38–12). Triple combination therapy is much more efficacious in the decreasing mortality rate than dual therapy, monotherapy, or especially no therapy (Table 38–13). The optimal regimens for primary therapy, intensification therapy, and salvage therapy in children and adolescents remain to be determined.

Nucleoside Analog Reverse Transcriptase Inhibitors. **Nucleoside reverse transcriptase inhibitors (NRTIs)** were historically the first general class of antiviral agents and remain the mainstay of treatment of HIV disease. They block viral replication by interfering with **reverse transcriptase (RT),** which causes a block of transcription of viral RNA into DNA. Drugs in this group include zidovudine (ZDV), didanosine (ddI), zalcitabine (ddC), stavudine (d4T), lamivudine (3TC), and abacavir (Table 38–11).

Nonnucleoside Analog Reverse Transcriptase Inhibitors. **Nonnucleoside RT inhibitors (NNRTIs)** also block RT, using a mechanism different from that of NRTI. Generally NNRTIs are capable of significant viral suppression, but a single virus mutation can confer resistance. Thus they are never used alone and typically should be only one part of regimens including three or more agents. Drugs in this group include nevirapine, delavirdine, and efavirenz (Table 38–11).

Protease Inhibitors. Protease inhibitors (PIs) interfere with viral protease, which cleaves polyprotein precursors during the final virion assembly stage of HIV replication. Resulting defective virions are incapable of infecting new cells. Once researchers identified the target protease enzyme, the development of PIs by several pharmaceutical firms was a triumph of science. The various drugs in this class act by the same mechanism but have widely different chemical structures with diverse side effects. The use of a PI with two or more other drugs defined the HAART regimens, which have revolutionized the management of HIV disease. With long-term use, undesirable side effects are being reported; they include disorders of triglyceride and cholesterol levels, a predilection to insulin resistance, and fat redistribution syndromes. Drugs in this group include indinavir, ritonavir, nelfinavir, saquinavir, amprenavir, and the combination formula of lopinavir-ritonavir (Table 38–11). Although lopinavir-ritonavir is a combination medication, the ritonavir is present only in low levels and is included to inhibit the cytochrome P-450 system, which impairs clearance of lopinavir and boosts its serum level above what could otherwise be achieved. Hence ritonavir is present in this case because of its pharmacologic property, not because of its antiretroviral activity.

Monitoring and Indications for Changing Antiretroviral Therapy. Children with HIV disease require frequent, often monthly, assessments in the first year of life. For older children who are clinically stable, the frequency of medical evaluations can be spaced between 1 and 3 months, depending on factors such as severity of symptoms, needs of the family, and accessibility to health care. Monitoring should be performed by clinicians familiar with the clinical symptoms of HIV disease and the signs and symptoms of toxic effects of the drugs.

Two HIV-specific laboratory tests important for routine monitoring are the **CD4 T-lymphocyte cell count and percentage** and the **quantitative HIV viral assay,** also referred to as **viral load.** Various commercially available assays can be used to measure the number of copies of plasma HIV RNA, and in clinical practice it is important to use the same assay to monitor an individual patient. These two HIV-specific laboratory tests are typically performed every 3–4 months in the clinically stable child. Transient intercurrent illnesses and some immunizations can affect both of these assays, so these tests should be performed when children are at their baseline health status. In both tests there is considerable variability with repeated testing of the same patient. Trends in changing laboratory CD4 cell counts or viral load values should result in only limited concern until a second confirmatory test is done, with a minimum of 1 week between assays.

There are three primary reasons to change antiretroviral therapy: (1) failure of the current regimen with evidence of disease progression clinically or worsening of laboratory values, (2) toxic effects or intolerance to current treatment, and (3) new data demonstrating that an alternative drug or regimen is superior to the current treatment. Treatment failure is not always easy to identify but is characterized by disease progression that can be seen clinically as growth failure, development of new diseases associated with immunodeficiency, or development or worsening of neurologic disease. Treatment failure as defined by deteriorating virologic measurements and immunologic markers may also warrant a change in therapy, but reliance on laboratory assays alone may not always be appropriate.

HIV RNA viral load measurement is the major measure for assessing adequacy of therapy and has been one of the great advances in recent years. In HIV-infected adults, it is now clearly established that prolonged periods of suppressed viral activity correlate with improved survival and health. Virologic treatment failure indicators include the following: (1) a $<$10-fold decrease from baseline HIV RNA levels after 12 weeks of therapy; (2) failure to achieve undetectable HIV RNA levels after 4–6 months of therapy, although undetectable levels are not achievable in every patient; (3) repeated detection of HIV RNA in children who had previously undetectable levels with therapy; and (4) persistent increase in HIV RNA levels after initiation of therapy ($>$5-fold for those $<$2 years of age; $>$3-fold for those $\geq$2 years of age). In children the interpretation of HIV RNA levels may be complicated. They are dramatically high in perinatally infected infants compared with typical adult values. There is marked overlap of HIV RNA levels in children who have and those who do not have rapid disease progression. The predictive value of a specific HIV RNA level in an individual child is only moderately good. Undetectable viral loads are not always achievable in children. Thus HIV RNA levels that denote virologic treatment failure are a relative indication for therapy change and must be used with appreciation for treatment options.

When a therapeutic failure occurs, it is reasonable to assume viral resistance. Ideally, the regimen would be changed to all new antiviral agents. Two rules are generally recommended: (1) never change only one drug at a time, and (2) never add a single drug to a failing regimen. However, there are only a limited number of treatment combination options available. When treatment appears inadequate, the first task is to evaluate whether the drug is failing or the family is failing to give the drug. Education, nonjudgmental monitoring, disclosure of HIV status to supporting community adults, and practical services such as home nursing visits and medically managed daycare may support adherence to medications for those families having difficulties. In selected cases, placement of gastrostomy tubes for medicine delivery in the very young child may be indicated. Knowledge of the family's ability to provide

TABLE 38–11. Antiretroviral Drugs for Treatment of HIV Infection

Antiretroviral Drug	Availability	Adults	Pediatric
NRTI			
Zidovudine (ZDV, AZT, Retrovir)	50 mg/5 mL 100 mg capsule 300 mg capsule	200 mg q8hr 300 mg q12hr	90–180 mg/m^2 q12hr to q8hr Neonate: 2 mg/kg q6hr for 6 wk
Lamivudine (3TC, Epivir)	10 mg/mL 150 mg tablet	150 mg q12hr PO	4 mg/kg q12hr PO
Zidovudine-lamivudine (ZDV/3TC, Combivir)	300 mg/150 mg tablet	One tablet q12hr PO	None
Didanosine (ddI, Videx)	10 mg/mL 25, 50, 100, 150 mg chewable tablet	35–49 kg: 125 mg q12hr 50–74 kg: 200 mg q12hr $\geq$75 kg: 300 mg q12hr	90–150 mg/m^2 q12hr
Stavudine (d4T, Zerit)	1 mg/mL 15, 20, 30, 40 mg capsule	$<$60 kg: 30 mg q12hr $\geq$60 kg: 40 mg q12hr	1 mg/kg q12hr
Zalcitabine (ddC, Hivid)	0.375 mg, 0.75 mg tablet	0.75 mg q8hr	0.01 mg/kg q8hr
Abacavir (Ziagen)	20 mg/mL 300 mg tablet	300 mg tablet	8 mg/kg q12hr
NNRTI			
Nevirapine (Viramune)	50 mg/5 mL 200 mg tablet	200 mg once daily for 14 days *then* 200 mg q12hr	120 mg/m^2 once daily PO for 14 days *then* 200 mg/m^2 q12hr PO
Efavirenz (Sustiva)	50, 100, 200 mg capsule	600 mg qd	10 to $<$15 kg: 200 mg 15 to $<$20 kg: 250 mg 20 to $<$25 kg: 300 mg 25 to $<$32.5 kg: 350 mg 32.5 to $<$40 kg: 400 mg $\geq$40 kg: 600 mg
Delavirdine (Rescriptor)	100 mg tablet	400 mg q8hr	Unknown
Protease Inhibitor			
Indinavir (Crixivan)	200 mg, 400 mg tablet	800 mg q8hr PO **without food**	350 mg/m^2 q8hr
Nelfinavir (Viracept)	50 mg/scoop powder 250 mg tablet	750 mg q8hr PO	25–30 mg/kg q8hr
Ritonavir (Norvir)	80 mg/mL 100 mg capsule	300 mg q12hr on day 1 400 mg q12hr on days 2, 3 500 mg q12hr on day 4 600 mg q12hr	400 mg/m^2 q12hr
Saquinavir (Fortovase softgel)	200 mg capsule	1,200 mg q8hr **with food**	Unknown
Saquinavir-ritonavir combination	200 mg capsule 100 mg capsule	400 mg q12hr 400 mg q12hr	Unknown
Amprenavir (Agenerase)	150 mg capsule	$\geq$13 yr *or* $\geq$50 kg: 1,200 mg q12hr	4–12 yr of age: 20 mg/kg q12hr *or* 15 mg/kg q8hr
Lopinavir-ritonavir (Kaletra)	400 mg/100 mg with 5 mL 133.3 mg/33.3 mg capsule	3 caps (or equivalent liquid) q12hr When concomitant therapy with efavirenz or nevirapine is used, dosing is as follows: 4 capsules (or equivalent liquid) q12hr	7 to $<$15 kg: (12 mg/3 mg)/kg q12hr 15 to $<$40 kg: (10 mg/2.5 mg)/kg q12hr $\geq$40 kg: adult dose When concomitant therapy with efavirenz or nevirapine is used, dosing is as follows: 7 to $<$15 kg: (13 mg/3.25 mg)/kg q12hr 15 to $<$50 kg: (11 mg/2.75 mg)/kg q12hr $\geq$50 kg: adult dose

NRTI = nucleoside reverse transcriptase inhibitors; NNRTI = nonnucleoside reverse transcriptase inhibitors.

TABLE 38–12. Characteristics of Antiretroviral Drugs: Major Toxic Effects, Interactions, and Special Instructions*

Antiretroviral Drug	Adverse Effects	Interactions	Instructions
Zidovudine (ZDV, AZT, Retrovir)	Main: anemia, neutropenia, headache Less: myopathy, myositis, liver toxic effects	Ganciclovir, interferon alfa, TMP-SMZ, acyclovir, atovaquone, methadone, probenecid, valproic acid, fluconazole, cimetidine, rifampin, rifabutin, clarithromycin, ribavirin, phenytoin	Should not be used with stavudine because of poor antiviral effect Typical doses are l60 mg/m² q8hr, or 180 mg/m² q12hr
Didanosine (ddl, Videx)	Main: gastrointestinal disturbance Less: pancreatitis (rare, serious, dose related), peripheral neuropathy (dose related), electrolyte disturbance, hyperuricemia, hepatitis, retinal depigmentation	Imidazoles, dapsone, tetracycline, quinolone, delavirdine	The didanosine formulation contains buffering agents or antacids Food decreases absorption; recommended on an empty stomach (1 hr before or 2 hr after meal) For oral solution: shake well and refrigerate; stable for 30 days Chewable tablets difficult for children; 2 tablets usually needed for adequate buffering effect
Lamivudine (3TC, Epivir)	Main: headache, fatigue, gastrointestinal disturbance, skin rash Less: pancreatitis, neuropathy, neutropenia, hepatitis	TMP-SMZ (rarely of significance)	
Stavudine (d4T, Zerit)	Main: headache, gastrointestinal disturbance, skin rashes Less: pancreatitis, peripheral neuropathy, hepatitis	Rarely of significance	Not for use with zidovudine
Zalcitabine (ddC, Hivid)	Main: headache, gastrointestinal disturbance, malaise Less: peripheral neuropathy, pancreatitis, hepatitis, oral and esophageal ulcers, skin rashes, marrow suppression	Cimetidine, amphotericin, foscarnet, aminoglycosides	Do not use with didanosine because of risk of neuropathy
Abacavir (GW1592, Ziagen)	Main: gastrointestinal disturbance, headache, fever, rash, anorexia, fatigue Less: diarrhea, pancreatitis, hepatitis, elevated triglycerides, elevated glucose, lactic acidosis		Not metabolized by hepatic cytochrome P-450 No interactions when used with zidovudine and lamivudine **Severe potentially fatal hypersensitivity reaction occurs in 5%,** characterized by fever, nausea, vomiting, diarrhea, and abdominal pain, with finding of skin rash, lymphadenopathy, and ulceration of mucous membranes; usually occurs in first 6 wk; main danger is in restarting because **hypotension and death have occurred on rechallenge**
Nevirapine (NVP, Viramune)	Main: skin rash (some severe and life-threatening, including Stevens-Johnson syndrome), sedation, headache, diarrhea, and nausea	Inducer of cytochrome P-450†	Interactions with protease inhibitors, with levels of indinavir and saquinavir decreased and ritonavir possibly decreased Given with initial 14-day lead-in period, then doubled Rash reaction usually develops in first 6 wk; nevirapine discontinued if rash severe or associated with fever or mucosal lesions

TABLE 38–12. Characteristics of Antiretroviral Drugs: Major Toxic Effects, Interactions, and Special Instructions* *(Continued)*

Antiretroviral Drug	Adverse Effects	Interactions	Instructions
Efavirenz (DMP-266, Sustiva)	Main: skin rash, central nervous system (somnolence, insomnia, confusion, abnormal thinking, impaired concentration, agitation, hallucinations, euphoria)	Mixed inducer-inhibitor of cytochrome P-450†	Complex interactions with protease inhibitors, leading to higher or lower concentrations Bedtime dosing recommended to improve tolerability of central nervous system effects High-fat meals may interfere
Delavirdine (DLV, Rescriptor)	Main: rash	Involves cytochrome P-450 enzyme system†	Dosage in pediatrics unknown
Indinavir (Crixivan)	Main: gastrointestinal disturbance, headache, metallic taste, dizziness, asymptomatic hyperbilirubinemia Less: nephrolithiasis, rare spontaneous bleeding (hemophilia), hyperglycemia, diabetes	Involves cytochrome P-450 enzyme system†	
Ritonavir (Norvir)	Main: gastrointestinal disturbance, asthenia, circumoral paresthesia, taste perversion, dizziness Less: spontaneous bleeding (hemophilia), hyperglycemia, diabetes	Involves cytochrome P-450 enzyme system†	Take with food; liquid may be mixed with various foods or liquids to minimize taste
Amprenavir (Agenerase)	Main: gastrointestinal disturbance, rash (may be severe), perioral tingling Less: spontaneous bleeding (hemophilia)	Involves cytochrome P-450 enzyme system† Contains propylene glycol, which is not adequately metabolized in children <4 yr of age, pregnant women, persons with hepatic or renal failure, and those treated with disulfiram or metronidazole; it is contraindicated in these groups	Take with or without food but not with fatty meals
Lopinavir-ritonavir (Kaletra)	Main: diarrhea, nausea, abdominal pain Less: spontaneous bleeding (hemophilia)	Involves cytochrome P-450 enzyme system† Dose must be increased when taken with NNRTI	Preferably take with food

*Hyperglycemia, new-onset diabetes mellitus, diabetic ketoacidosis, and exacerbation of pre-existing diabetes mellitus have been reported in persons receiving HAART. These metabolic derangements are strongly but not exclusively associated with protease inhibitors. Hypertriglyceridemia, hypercholesterolemia, and disturbances in fat distribution have been associated with all protease inhibitors, especially ritonavir.

†Drugs in the NNARTI group and the protease inhibitor group are metabolized by the liver and have effects on the cytochrome P-450 enzyme system. These agents will affect the metabolism of other drugs and each other. **Significant potential drug interactions are extensive** and vary by medication. Such drug interactions are outlined in detail in prescribing information for each medication. Other drugs that may exhibit aberrant metabolism from altered P-450 activity include the following: rifampin, rifabutin, sedative-hypnotics (e.g., triazolam, midazolam), oral anticoagulants (warfarin), digoxin, phenytoin, theophylline, antihistamines (astemizole, terfenadine), cisapride, clarithromycin, ergot alkaloid derivatives, oral contraceptives, St. John's wort, and many others. **This is not a complete list, and before beginning any antiretroviral medication, the complete list of prescribed, over-the-counter, and herbal medications or supplements should be reviewed.** Persons taking antiretroviral drugs should be instructed to avoid adding any medication or supplement without discussion with their physician first.

medicines consistently must be complete before one switches from one complex multidrug therapy to another.

Future Antiretroviral Therapy. In the near future, antiretroviral therapy is likely to concentrate on the availability of new antiviral agents and the search for better combinations of new and existing drugs. Desirable traits for new drugs include high potency with different mechanisms of antiviral activity and different resistance patterns. Medication adherence will be facilitated by easier and less frequent dosing, fewer dietary restrictions, fewer and less severe side effects and drug interactions, and less cost.

The use of HAART has reduced the amount of HIV in some persons to undetectable blood levels for prolonged periods, sometimes for several years. This success led to speculation that prolonged suppression might result in a "cure." Unfortunately, subsequent studies have consistently demonstrated that currently available drugs do not totally eradicate the virus and that small reservoirs of HIV remain in circulating blood cells. Searching for

TABLE 38–13. Recommendations for Combination Therapy

Recommended Regimens*		
Column A (One Choice)	**Column B (One Choice)**	**Regimens Not Recommended**
Zidovudine + Didanosine	Ritonavir	Zidovudine + Stavudine
Zidovudine + Lamivudine	Nelfinavir	Didanosine + Zalcitabine
Stavudine + Didanosine	Indinavir	Stavudine + Zalcitabine
Zidovudine + Zalcitabine	Saquinavir (softgel)	Lamivudine + Zalcitabine
Stavudine + Lamivudine	Ritonavir + Saquinavir (softgel)	Any monotherapy
Didanosine + Lamivudine	Efavirenz	
Zidovudine + Abacavir	Lopinavir-ritonavir	
Lamivudine + Abacavir		
Stavudine + Abacavir		
Didanosine + Abacavir		
Zidovudine + Lamivudine + Abacavir (omit column B choice)		

*Drugs not listed in order of preference.

the ''magic bullet'' involves creating more effective and less toxic medicines for even longer-term suppression of virus, immune system–enhancing modalities that reverse prior damage and maximize the body's curative powers, and novel strategies that actually purge residual virus from the body.

Supportive Therapy

Nutrition. Attention to appropriate nutrition is indicated for all children with HIV. Routine assessment of growth parameters at every medical visit and the charting of growth curves are essential. The failure-to-thrive condition is seen in young children with rapidly progressive disease. Anorexia and limited oral intake can result in nutritional deficiencies and inadequate growth. Oropharyngeal lesions, dental caries, gum disease, and intestinal disorders are common in older children. Pre-emptive education concerning nourishing diets and dental hygiene practices are important components of care. If inadequate growth is diagnosed, the first reaction should be an evaluation for adequacy of antiretroviral therapy. Dietary counseling may help the family provide optimal numbers of calories taken orally. Multivitamins should be used. Palatable supplements with high calorie and high protein content such as Pediasure or Ensure can be helpful. Dietary stimulants such as Periactin may be of limited value. For significant anorexia and growth failure, gastric feedings may be necessary. Gastrostomies must be surgically placed, but they provide long-term options for nutritional support and have the additional benefit of facilitating medicine intake. Education about food preparation and the avoidance of foods with a high risk of harboring an infectious organism such as *Salmonella* or *Giardia* are also indicated. Preliminary studies of the use of growth hormone and other growth enhancers are in progress.

Immunizations. Guidelines have been published by the American Academy of Pediatrics and the Advisory Committee on Immunization Practices of the CDC. Routine immunizations include diphtheria-pertussis-tetanus vaccine, IPV, *Haemophilus influenzae* type b vaccine, heptavalent pneumococcal conjugate vaccine, and hepatitis B vaccine, with the same schedule as for other children. OPV should not be used for HIV-infected children or any person requiring polio vaccine who lives in the same household because of the potential for transmission of poliovirus to persons with compromised immunity. Routine measles-mumps-rubella (MMR) immunization is recommended unless the child is classified as being in CDC category 3 or is severely immunocompromised (Tables 38–2 and 38–3), in which case MMR vaccine is avoided because of the theoretical risk of live virus vaccination. After known exposure to measles for all HIV-infected persons, immune globulin prophylaxis is indicated unless immune globulin has been administered within the previous 3 weeks. Varicella-zoster virus vaccine is recommended for selected children. Although this live virus was not recommended in the past, in 1999 the vaccine was recommended for consideration for those HIV-infected children who were generally healthy and had a CD4 cell percentage >25%. When used for HIV-infected children, the vaccine should be given in two doses 3 months apart. After known exposure to varicella for all HIV-infected persons without a reliable history of previous varicella or vaccination, VZIG administration is indicated within 72 hours if immune globulin has not been used within the previous 3 weeks.

Influenza vaccine should be provided for infants >6 months of age and repeated annually. BCG vaccine should be avoided for HIV-infected children in the United States. The WHO recommends BCG vaccination for symptom-free HIV-infected children in developing countries. Other live virus vaccines and the oral typhoid vaccine should be avoided in HIV-infected children.

Tuberculosis Screening. Annual tuberculosis testing is recommended for all HIV-infected and uninfected children who reside with HIV-infected individuals or adult members of other groups considered at high risk of having tuberculosis. Only the **Mantoux skin test** containing 5 TU of **purified protein derivative (PPD)** should be used. Skin test controls may be used to evaluate for anergy. The criterion for a positive PPD test result is a 5 mm induration for HIV-infected persons and for all children in close contact with a person with infectious tuberculosis.

Prevention of Opportunistic Infections. Much of the improvement in survival of HIV-infected persons in the 1990s was due to the improvement in management of opportunistic infections. Guidelines for prevention and treatment of selected opportunistic infections were most recently published in 1999 by a joint effort of the U.S. Public Health Service and the Infectious Diseases Society of America. Specific pediatric notes are included for each of the infectious agents.

Immune system deterioration is reflected in declining CD4 cell counts, which are often used to determine when prophylaxis should be initiated (Table 38–14). The advent of HAART has led to significant increases in CD4 cell counts in children with negligible levels before treatment. The extent of immunologic reconstitution after effective therapy is not yet fully understood. Clinical trials are under way to evaluate whether it is safe to discontinue prophylactic therapy in treated children in whom CD4 cell counts have increased to a level above which prophylaxis is normally begun. Specific

TABLE 38–14. Normal CD4 Cell Counts and CD4 Cell Counts at Which to Initiate Prophylaxis for *Pneumocystis carinii* Pneumonia, *Mycobacterium avium-intracellulare* Complex (MAC), and *Toxoplasma gondii* Infections

	Normal CD4 Cell Count per mm^3		CD4 Cell Count per mm^3 (or %) at Which Prophylaxis Is Initiated		
Age	Median	Lower Limit	PCP	MAC Infection	*Toxoplasma* Infection
1–11 mo	>3,000	1,500	All*	<750	—†
12–23 mo	2,600	1,000	750 (<15%)	<500	—†
24–71 mo	1,700	1,000	500 (<15%)	<75	—†
≥6 yr	1,000	500	200 (<15%)	<50	<100
Any age	NA	NA	Prior disease	Prior disease	Prior disease

NA = not applicable.
*All HIV-infected infants <1 year of age require prophylaxis. HIV-exposed infants may benefit from prophylaxis, starting at 6–8 weeks of age and continuing until HIV infection reasonably excluded.
†Guidelines not established for children but are assumed to be below the CD4 count at which PCP prophylaxis is initiated. Use of TMP-SMZ for PCP prophylaxis is also effective for *T. gondii* prophylaxis (Table 68–14).

recommendations are periodically updated and should be reviewed by caregivers (Table 38–15).

Pneumocystis carinii Pneumonia. PCP prophylaxis is indicated for all HIV-infected children <12 months of age who have had prior PCP, who have a CD4 cell percentage of less than 15%, or who have CD4 cell counts below certain critical levels (Table 38–14). For HIV-exposed infants, PCP prophylaxis is also currently recommended from the age of 6–8 weeks until the diagnosis of HIV can be reasonably excluded, usually at about 4 months. TMP-SMZ is the prophylactic treatment of choice (Table 68–14). It is typically better tolerated by children than by adults. Alternative regimens include dapsone and aerosolized pentamidine administered by the Respirgard nebulizer. Other agents and regimens may be effective in selected settings of patient intolerance, but data are incomplete.

Mycobacterium avium-intracellulare complex (MAC). MAC organisms are ubiquitous in the environment and pose risks to severely immunocompromised individuals. Thresholds for MAC prophylaxis are based on age and CD4 cell counts (Table 38–14). Recommended prophylaxis is with clarithromycin twice daily or azithromycin once weekly, with alternative rifabutin once daily or azithromycin once daily (Table 38–15). The use of prophylaxis for MAC has declined recently because of drug interactions with other drugs used in late-stage HIV disease, specifically the PIs. Assessment of the risks and benefits must be individualized.

Toxoplasma gondii. HIV-infected children beyond the age of 1 year should be tested for *Toxoplasma* IgG antibodies. Prophylaxis may be indicated in those with antibodies if the CD4 cell count falls to low levels (the levels for PCP prophylaxis are commonly used [Table 38–14]). The child with previous *Toxoplasma* antibody–negative status should be retested if the CD4 cell count falls to the level for initiation of PCP prophylaxis. Fortunately, TMP-SMZ, the first choice for PCP prophylaxis (Table 68–14), also provides prophylaxis against toxoplasmosis. For children who cannot tolerate TMP-SMZ, dapsone 2 mg/kg/day plus pyrimethamine 1 mg/kg/day plus leucovorin 5 mg twice weekly can be used for prophylaxis (Table 68–15). Families with HIV should receive education about the relation of *Toxoplasma* with cats.

Tuberculosis. Prophylaxis for tuberculosis is given to an HIV-infected person with a positive PPD skin test result (>5 mm for HIV-infected individuals) without evidence of active disease and with no prior antituberculosis treatment (Table 38–15). Similar treatment should also be considered for the child with skin-test negativity and close contact with an active case of tuberculosis, at least for several months until the skin tests can be repeated. First-line prophylaxis is isoniazid given once daily for 12 months. Directly observed therapy with isoniazid twice weekly is an alternative if needed to ensure adherence. For strains known to be INH resistant, rifampin 10–20 mg/kg (max 600 mg daily) is indicated.

Bacterial Respiratory Tract Infections. Infusions of IVIG 400 mg/kg per dose once monthly may be a benefit to selected HIV-infected children. This passive protection was first used in the 1980s, before effective antiretroviral therapies became available. A large placebo-controlled study showed decreases in the frequency of bacterial infections and hospitalizations for children with CD4 cell counts >200 cells/mm^3 and no benefit for children with late-stage AIDS. The overall assessment was that monthly treatments did not improve ultimate survival time but did improve the quality of life for those children who were not already very ill. Use of IVIG declined with increasing use of antiretroviral agents in children. These expensive treatments should be limited to selected HIV-infected children with demonstrated significant abnormalities of immunologic function and with a history of recurrent invasive bacterial infections. IVIG may not provide additional benefit to children treated with daily TMP-SMZ. Twice-daily penicillin may be used for prophylaxis against invasive pneumococcal infection. Conjugate vaccines for *H. influenzae* type b and pneumococcus are indicated.

Measles. Routine vaccines have been recommended if children are not severely immunocompromised. Immunoglobulin prophylaxis should be given for HIV-infected children exposed to measles, even if previously vaccinated.

Chickenpox and Zoster. Varicella vaccine should be considered for children with asymptomatic (N1) or minimally symptomatic (A1) HIV infection and CD4 lymphocyte percentages less than 25%. VZIG, one vial (250 U) per 10 kg body weight (max five vials), should be given within 96 hours of exposure to chickenpox or zoster if the child has an abnormal CD4 lymphocyte count or percentage for age and has not had prior varicella (Table 38–15). Selected children may benefit from acyclovir when it is used to prevent recurrent zoster. The optimal dose for this indication is unclear. Starting doses are 5 mg/kg twice daily, with an increase to 10–20 mg/kg three or four times daily if breakthrough occurs.

Herpes simplex Virus. Frequently recurring herpetic lesions may be controlled with the use of oral acyclovir at dosages used for chickenpox and zoster. Concerns regarding development of resistant strains mandate individualized treatment.

TABLE 38–15. Preventive Regimens for Major Opportunistic Infections in Children with HIV Infections

Organism	Indication	Preventive Regimens* First Choice	Alternatives
Strongly Recommended			
Pneumocystis carinii	See Table 38–14	See Table 68–14	See Table 68–14
Mycobacterium avium complex	See Table 38–14	Clarithromycin 7.5 mg/kg (max 500 mg) divided bid PO *or* Azithromycin 20 mg/kg (max 1,200 mg) once weekly PO	Children ≥6 yr: rifabutin 300 mg once daily PO Children <6 yr: rifabutin 5 mg/kg (max 300 mg) once daily PO Azithromycin 5 mg/kg (max 250 mg) once daily PO
Mycobacterium tuberculosis			
Isoniazid sensitive	Tuberculin skin test reaction ≥5 mm *or* Previous untreated positive tuberculin skin test reaction *or* Contact with case of active tuberculosis	Isoniazid 10–15 mg/kg once daily PO (or IM) for 12 mo *or* Isoniazid 20–30 mg/kg (max 900 mg) twice weekly PO for 12 mo	Rifampin 10–20 mg/kg (max 600 mg) once daily PO (or IV) for 12 mo
Isoniazid resistant	As above; high probability of exposure to isoniazid-resistant tuberculosis	Rifampin 10–20 mg/kg once daily PO (or IV) for 12 mo	Unclear
Multidrug (isoniazid, rifampin) resistant	As above; high probability of exposure to multidrug-resistant tuberculosis	Consult with public health authority or infectious disease specialist	None
Varicella-zoster virus	Significant exposure to varicella with no history of chickenpox or zoster	VZIG 1 vial (1.25 mL)/10 kg (max 5 vials) within 96 hr after exposure (ideally within 48 hr) IM	
Vaccine-preventable pathogens	HIV exposure/infection	Routine immunizations	
Generally Recommended			
Toxoplasma gondii	IgG antibody to *T. gondii* with severe immunosuppression; also based on CD4 cell count (Table 38–14)	TMP-SMZ: 150 mg TMP/m^2 bid PO†	Dapsone 2 mg/kg (*or* 15 mg/m^2) (max 25 mg) once daily PO *plus* Pyrimethamine 1 mg/kg once daily PO *plus* Leucovorin 5 mg once daily PO every 3 days
Not Recommended for Most Patients (Indicated Only in Special Circumstances)			
Invasive bacterial infections	Hypogammaglobulinemia	IVIG (400 mg/kg IV q4wk)	None
Candida	Severe immunosuppression	Nystatin (100,000 U/mL) 4–6 mL q6hr PO *or* Topical clotrimazole, 10 mg 5 times daily PO	None
Cryptococcus neoformans	Severe immunosuppression	Fluconazole 3–6 mg/kg once daily PO	Itraconazole 2–5 mg/kg once daily or divided bid
Histoplasma capsulatum	Severe immunosuppression (endemic geographic area)	Itraconazole 2–5 mg/kg once daily or divided bid PO	None

*Dose shown is **total daily dose** unless otherwise noted.
†Use of TMP-SMZ for PCP prophylaxis is also effective for *T. gondii* prophylaxis (Table 68–14).

Cytomegalovirus. Prophylaxis is not generally recommended unless prior end-organ disease has been diagnosed. There may be selected persons with extremely low CD4 lymphocyte counts who are seropositive for CMV and who could benefit from oral ganciclovir. Acyclovir is not effective in preventing CMV disease, and valacyclovir is not recommended.

Candida. Primary prophylaxis is not recommended, but for selected persons with recurring significant cutaneous or mucosal candidiasis, treatment may be helpful. For skin and scalp lesions, topical antifungal creams, Selsun lotion, and antiseborrheic shampoos should be tried first. For thrush, nystatin is rarely helpful. Half or whole clotrimazole 10 mg troches, which can be crushed and applied in the mouths of infants, can be used two to four times a day. For children with recurrent problems, fluconazole 3–6 mg/kg/day once daily or ketoconazole 5–10 mg/kg/day in 1 or 2 daily doses may be useful.

Adolescents

Adolescents span the gap between children and adults, with unique needs, problems, and approaches to treatment. The epidemiology was described previously, indicating the diverse experiences of children who are infected as adolescents, those with hemophilia-related HIV infection, and those who have reached adolescence after having acquired HIV vertically. Treatment for adolecents at Tanner stages I and II is as for the younger children, whereas adolescents at Tanner stage V are treated as for adults. Adolescents at Tanner stages III and IV receive individualized therapy and need to be monitored closely for evidence of drug benefit and adverse events.

Adherence to medications, isolation from peers and sometimes family because of the disease, lack of funding, low self-esteem, body image, and experimentation with substances and sex are all issues that need consideration when one is working with this population. Case management with psychological support services and other social support services, peer counseling, and support groups are often greater needs than the actual medical care. A physician who solely emphasizes medical issues is not likely to be successful with most HIV-infected adolescents. Family support is important but may not be forthcoming, particularly for men who have sex with men, injection drug users, and street children, who may be estranged from their families. There are few comprehensive adolescent HIV programs that are capable of providing the entire spectrum of services needed for success.

Psychosocial Support Services

Few women, children, adolescents, and families are prepared for the impact that HIV has on their lives. Many lack the necessary financial resources or lose them as illness ensues and employment is jeopardized. Social support networks normally provided by family and friends are often lacking, either because individuals with HIV are shunned or because the individuals do not disclose their illness. Many people have pre-existing psychological conditions or a history of substance abuse that makes adherence to clinical appointments and medication schedules difficult. This difficulty is compounded by situational depression, adverse effects of medications, and complications of the disease itself. Difficulty with housing, transportation, food, respite care, and childcare are always present. Seemingly intact, capable families with adequate finances, medical insurance, and social support often deteriorate with time in the face of HIV disease. These are the reasons that so much emphasis is placed on providing comprehensive programs that emphasize case management for individuals and families, rather than just medical models of care.

A physician working with an HIV-infected woman, child, or adolescent should strongly consider consulting a program where comprehensive care is provided. Many physicians working with HIV-positive children, women, and adolescents are willing to follow such patients jointly or to take over care, depending on the level of comfort of the referring physician.

COMPLICATIONS

HIV complications result from declining numbers of CD4 lymphocytes. The loss of immune system integrity allows viral, bacterial, fungal, and mycobacterial infections to occur. Noninfectious complications such as cancers, wasting, and HIV encephalopathy result from uncontrolled viral replication. Secondary disturbances include altered immunoglobulin production when the normal balance of T-helper and suppressor cells is disturbed and B cells are not regulated in the normal manner. Bacterial infections and viral infections occur as normal immunoglobulin responses are blunted.

The initial presentation of HIV in children often includes nonspecific and sometimes relatively unimpressive signs or symptoms. The acute retroviral syndrome so commonly described in adults is rare or is manifested more subtly in children. Lymphadenopathy is common and is often generalized in the first weeks or months of life. It may be transient or persistent and is often subtle. The lymph nodes are typically mobile, firm, and nontender. Hepatomegaly without evidence of hepatitis and splenomegaly are also frequent early signs of infection, as is oral candidiasis. In HIV-infected children, oral candidiasis may be persistent, severe, recurrent, or recalcitrant to treatment. These signs and symptoms alone do not portend a particularly poor prognosis. Nevertheless, any of these signs alone, especially when several of them exist together, may be indicative of HIV disease.

Neurologic Conditions

Encephalopathy. In children with HIV, progressive encephalopathy, the pediatric equivalent of AIDS dementia in adults, is a common complication of the disease. AIDS encephalopathy is an AIDS-defining condition for children. The frequency of HIV encephalopathy was once estimated to be 50–90%. More recent estimates have lowered this estimate considerably. As many as 10% of children have encephalopathy as the initial presentation of AIDS, and overall about 17% of children have had this condition reported as an AIDS-indicator condition. The true prevalence is difficult to determine because of variability in clinical presentation, the presence of psychosocial cofactors, and the lack of a specific test.

Exactly when the virus enters the central nervous system and why some children are affected while others are spared is not known; however, macrophages are believed to carry HIV into the central nervous system. The major cell affected by HIV in the central nervous system is the glial cell. Damage by HIV occurs through loss of support cells, rather than occurring directly to neurons.

Developmental slowing and failure to achieve developmental milestones are the hallmarks of encephalopathy. In more severe cases there is regression with loss of milestones. Acquired microcephaly accompanies encephalopathy in young children and may parallel or precede developmental delays. The older child may have loss of intellectual performance and declining school achievement. Changes in cognitive development, failure to achieve milestones or loss of milestones, acquired microcephaly, and onset of neurologic signs such as hyperreflexia or hypertonia should lead to the consideration of HIV encephalopathy in an infected child or of the possibility of HIV infection in a child whose status is unknown.

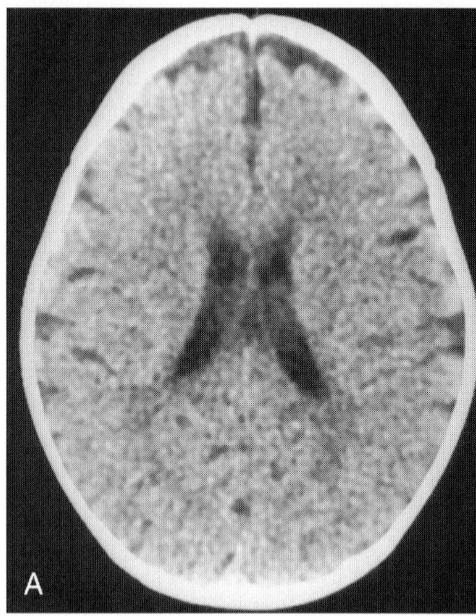

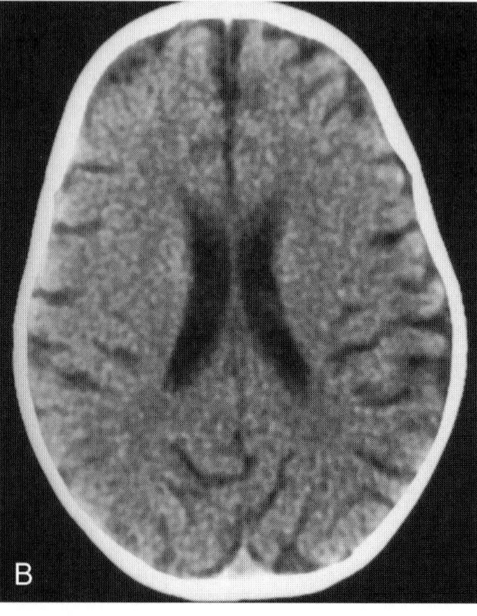

FIGURE 38–5. Progression of early HIV-associated encephalopathy demonstrated by CT. A CT scan at 8 months of age **(A)** in an infant with AIDS reveals essentially normal anatomy. A repeated CT scan at 10 months of age **(B)** shows generalized cortical atrophy with marked increase of the subarachnoid space and prominent sulci, dilated ventricles, and attenuation of white matter. This condition is accompanied by neurodevelopmental deterioration. (Used with permission from Jenson HB: Retrovirus infections and the acquired immunodeficiency syndrome. *Adv Pediatr Infect Dis* 1990;5:118.)

Other factors besides HIV encephalopathy that can impair cognition and development are common among children born to HIV-infected women. Drug or alcohol exposure in utero and congenital infections other than HIV infection, such as CMV infection or toxoplasmosis, are sometimes reported in HIV-infected children. Ongoing drug or alcohol use by parent or caretaker, depression in the parent or child, absence of the parent because of his or her own HIV disease, prolonged hospitalization of the child, and absence of the parent because of illness can limit stimulation and impair development. Malnutrition, poverty, and chaotic life frequently coexist with HIV and can contribute to developmental problems.

For the diagnosis of HIV encephalopathy to be considered as an AIDS-defining condition, the stringent criteria described in Table 38–4 must be met. Adherence to the guidelines allows children with non-HIV-related delays to be excluded. The progressive nature of the condition is emphasized, and static conditions such as cerebral palsy would be excluded.

Impaired brain growth with acquired microcephaly is the most common physical manifestation of HIV encephalopathy. Cerebral atrophy, the cause of the microcephaly, is the most common finding when central nervous system imaging is performed (Fig. 38–5). Basal ganglia calcifications are also common findings on CT scans (Fig. 38–6).

Other physical findings include progressive motor dysfunction, which is characterized by increased deep tendon reflexes, progressive weakness, and hypertonicity. Generalized weakness, progressive loss of fine-motor skills, gait ataxia, and spastic paraparesis or quadriparesis can occur. Children who functioned independently may deteriorate and lose most or all of their independent living skills.

HIV-infected children should undergo periodic developmental and neurologic testing by standard methods. A medical history should include information about in utero exposure to drugs and alcohol, in utero infections, perinatal history, and history of central nervous system infections. The physician might consider a baseline CT or MRI scan of the head. Physical examinations should include the head circumference measurement.

Assessment of the child's social environment is as important as the medical background. Nonprogressive (static) encephalopathy, which may be associated with prenatal or perinatal insults such as drugs, infections, or anoxia, should be evaluated. The static nature of such events can help to differentiate them from HIV encephalopathy.

Whether encephalopathy is HIV related or not, a thorough evaluation will allow the physician to recommend appropriate occupational, physical, and speech therapy or to address specialized medical needs by arranging for specialty care. Medical treatment of HIV encephalopathy has had limited success. Early clinical trials with ZDV showed promise in reversing or slowing encephalopathic changes in some children. The improvement was generally short lived, typically lasting a matter of months, with re-emergence of central nervous system manifestations possibly because of acquisition of viral resistance. There is some promise for the use of other combinations such as ZDV plus lamivudine (3TC) or ZDV plus didanosine. Optimism is guarded because central nervous system penetration by many antiretroviral agents is poor. The central nervous system is sometimes considered to be a sanctuary site where HIV is minimally affected by the profound declines in viral load

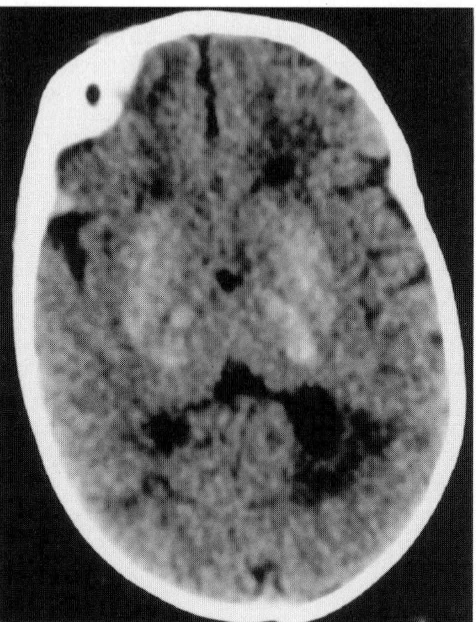

FIGURE 38–6. Advanced HIV encephalitis. A computed tomography scan of the brain shows advanced white matter involvement with bilateral basal ganglia calcifications caused by HIV infection.

occurring in the peripheral circulation and lymph nodes when combination therapy is used. Whether early, aggressive combination therapy will prevent HIV penetration of the central nervous system or prevent progression to encephalopathy has not yet been determined.

Secondary Infections and Tumors. Secondary central nervous system infections are somewhat less common in children than adults. Mass lesions, meningitis, and other infections of the central nervous system have clinical presentations that overlap with those of encephalopathy. The need for imaging studies and chemical, cellular, and culture evaluation of the CSF are based on the specific clinical findings. A CSF stain or culture and a brain biopsy can sometimes confirm specific infections, whereas imaging studies of the central nervous system may suggest but not confirm a diagnosis. The possibilities are numerous, and the clinician needs to consider common bacterial and viral agents as well as unusual fungal or parasitic infections.

Central nervous system toxoplasmosis is common in AIDS. A diagnosis of *Toxoplasma* encephalopathy is often based on *Toxoplasma* serologic findings indicating prior exposure and on the presence of one or more ring-enhancing lesions on CT scans of the brain. In older children and adults, toxoplasmosis is usually a reactivation disease—hence the presence of antibodies before the onset of symptoms. In newborns and infants it may represent primary disease. In selected cases it may be necessary to confirm the diagnosis by brain biopsy. The presence of characteristic lesions in a person who has fever, headache, reduced alertness, and focal deficits or seizures is adequate to initiate treatment for presumptive toxoplasmosis (Table 38–8).

Cryptococcus neoformans occasionally causes meningitis and central nervous system abscesses in children with severely compromised immune status. It is somewhat more insidious in onset than other forms of meningitis, typically taking days or weeks to evolve. Fever, headache, and nausea and vomiting are common. Most persons remain alert at the time of presentation, although there may be some malaise. Cranial nerve deficits, seizures, and stiff neck are less common, particularly early in the course. The diagnosis is established by positive results on a CSF latex cryptococcal antigen test, by the identification of organisms on an India ink preparation of spinal fluid, or by culture results. Treatment is with pyrimethamine and sulfadiazine and may require lifelong secondary prophylaxis (Table 38–8). Other infections that need to be considered include bacterial or viral meningitis, or encephalitis due to CMV, central nervous system tuberculosis, and myriad other organisms that can affect the immunocompromised host.

The most common primary central nervous system neoplasm is lymphoma. Infants are rarely affected, but the incidence of lymphoma increases with age and the degree of immunosuppression. Metastases from cancers other than in the central nervous system also occur, with lymphomas being the most common neoplasms. Multiple lesions suggest metastatic disease rather than a primary central nervous system tumor. Surgery, radiation, and chemotherapy have all been used with mixed success. The course is hampered by the impaired immune system and often by the poor general health status of persons who develop AIDS-related malignancies.

Pulmonary Conditions

Pneumocystis carinii Pneumonia. The lungs are frequent sites of HIV-related disease in adults and children. PCP was described in the initial reports of AIDS in 1981. Before the AIDS epidemic, PCP was primarily seen among immunocompromised persons such as those with cancer who were undergoing chemotherapy. Through 1998 PCP was the most common AIDS-defining condition in children (34% of cases). Early diagnosis of HIV infection and implementation of PCP prophylaxis has reduced the incidence of PCP. It remains the most common opportunistic infection among adults and children with AIDS, although rates are decreasing.

The peak incidence of PCP in children is 3–8 months of age, representing initial exposure to the organism. For many children it is the first manifestation of HIV disease and may be the first indication of HIV disease in a family. An estimated one half to three fourths of all children have been exposed to *Pneumocystis* by 3–4 years of age.

PCP may be manifested as a rapidly progressive respiratory deterioration or as a slow, insidious process with tachypnea, dyspnea, and fever. The presence of cough is variable. The lungs are often clear to auscultation. The chest radiograph typically reveals bilateral, diffuse interstitial infiltrates that may rapidly worsen within days to complete opacification (Fig. 38–7). Arterial blood gas analysis or pulse oximetry demonstrates the low oxygen saturation of hypoxemia, although hypercapnia may be absent. Hypoxemia may precede radiographic changes. Lactate dehydrogenase levels, although nonspecific, are frequently elevated to high levels.

Confirmation of PCP usually is best established by bronchoalveolar lavage (BAL) or occasionally by open lung biopsy. Lung biopsy is usually unnecessary and because of its invasiveness is used selectively. Sputum specimens will occasionally reveal the presence of *Pneumocystis* organisms, although sensitivity is low and only a positive result has significance. Children younger than 8 years are usually unable to cooperate enough or to generate a cough sufficient to produce a sputum sample. Methods used to stain tissue or BAL samples for *Pneumocystis* include the methenamine silver, toluidine blue, calcofluor white, and fluorescein-conjugated monoclonal antibody stains for the cyst wall. The Giemsa technique is the first choice for trophozoites but requires significant experience

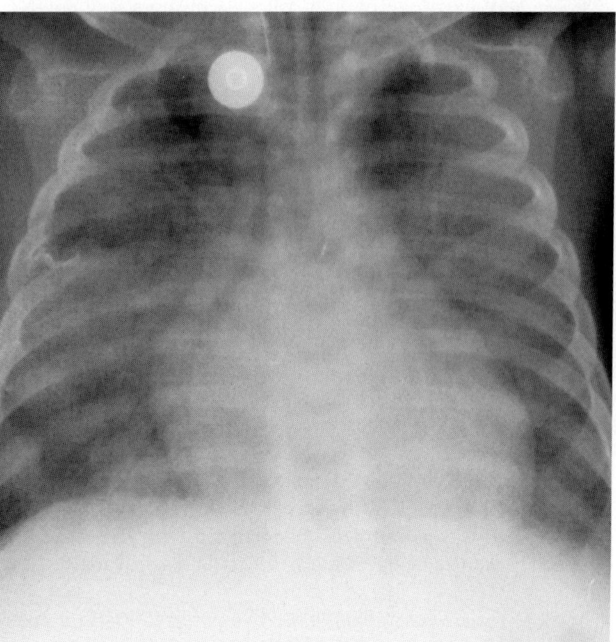

FIGURE 38–7. Chest radiograph of *Pneumocystis carinii* pneumonia (PCP) in a 6-month-old infant seropositive for HIV infection who developed severe tachypnea, dry cough, and progressive respiratory distress. The frontal chest radiograph shows the diffuse "ground glass–like" air space (alveolar) infiltration of the lungs typical of PCP. Sutures in the right lung are from a previous lung biopsy.

and skill. Fluorescent monoclonal antibodies are available in some laboratories.

Extrapulmonary *P. carinii* occurs in <1% of cases. It has occasionally been found in the central nervous system, retinas, lymph nodes, bone marrow, thyroid gland, spleen, or liver of persons with HIV. It was more common when inhaled pentamidine was occasionally used for PCP prophylaxis in adults. It generally prevented pulmonary disease, but the drug was confined to the lungs, occasionally allowing organisms to escape from the lungs via lymphatic or hematogenous routes. This is uncommon when systemic prophylaxis is used.

In a person for whom the physical findings, history, and radiographic evidence are supportive and in whom the CD4 lymphocyte level is in the severe range for age (Table 38–3), a presumptive diagnosis of PCP is reasonable and therapy should be initiated. The drug of choice remains intravenous or oral TMP-SMZ (20 mg TMP with 100 mg SMZ/kg/day) in four divided doses for 14–21 days, with 21 days for severe disease (Table 68–13). Therapy is usually initiated intravenously and, with improvement, completed by using oral TMP-SMZ. Intravenous pentamidine 4 mg/kg/day in a single daily infusion is often the alternative for persons who do not tolerate TMP-SMZ or who do not show improvement in 5–7 days. There is less experience in treating children with other agents such as dapsone (with or without trimethoprim) or atovaquone. Atovaquone is now available in suspension as well as capsule formulations but is not yet approved for use in children. Trimetrexate, a trimethoprim analog (dihydrofolate reductase inhibitor), is generally reserved for persons with severe or life-threatening intolerance of first-line therapeutic agents. These treatments should be used when other therapies fail or are not tolerated.

Corticosteroids are used as adjunctive therapy for moderate to severe PCP. A good indicator of severe disease is hypoxia, with Pao_2 <70 mm Hg. Methylprednisolone 2–4 mg/kg is given intravenously in four divided doses, usually for 5–14 days depending on response and severity of disease, followed by a tapering dose.

Prognosis for adults and adolescents with PCP has improved since the early days of the HIV epidemic as more aggressive treatment and new medications have become available. Survival is better in centers where there is the most experience with treatment of HIV infection and its complications. The percentage of infants with HIV who develop PCP has declined in recent years, but the mortality rate remains higher than for adults and older children.

The most important correlate of PCP risk is the age-specific CD4 lymphocyte count or percentage (Table 38–3). Adults and adolescents rarely develop PCP unless the CD4 lymphocyte count is $<200/mm^3$ (or <15%). Guidelines for testing children have been revised as new information has become available. Previous guidelines set a CD4 lymphocyte count of $\leq 1500/mm^3$ for children younger than 12 months. This was abandoned after reports describing children with PCP disease at higher CD4 levels. The guidelines issued in 1996 indicate that there is no clear CD4 lymphocyte level above which the child in the first year of life does not risk the development of PCP. Prophylaxis is begun for all HIV-exposed children at 4–6 weeks of age and continued until HIV disease is reasonably excluded, typically at 4–6 months of age (Table 68–14).

Lymphoid Interstitial Pneumonitis. **Lymphoid interstitial pneumonitis (LIP),** or **pulmonary lymphoid hyperplasia,** is the most common chronic lung disease in children with AIDS. It is uncommon in adults with AIDS or children with conditions other than AIDS. It was one of the original AIDS-defining conditions in children but is not an AIDS-defining condition in adults. LIP is unique in that it is the only category B, AIDS-defining condition (Table 38–4). This is due to the relatively mild nature of LIP compared with other category C, AIDS-defining conditions. Like the incidence of other opportunistic infections, that of LIP has declined in recent years. It occurs in approximately one fifth of infected children. This decline is probably due to the use of more intensive antiretroviral therapy in recent years. As many as 25–40% of children with AIDS were once reported to have LIP.

Although the pathogenesis of LIP is not completely understood, EBV antibodies are usually present in children with LIP, and EBV DNA has been demonstrated in biopsy specimens from children with LIP. An infiltration of the lungs by a pleomorphic mixture of lymphocytes, plasma cells, and immunoblasts with activation of T cells and an increased production of lymphokines, resulting in tissue damage, characterize LIP.

LIP differs from many other pulmonary complications found in children with AIDS in that it is chronic, often with few significant symptoms or signs. Patients may remain free of symptoms for years or may develop a chronic cough as the disease progresses. Generally there is no fever or tachypnea. Frequently there is coexisting enlargement of lymph nodes, liver, spleen, or salivary glands because of lymphocytic infiltrates similar to those seen in the lungs. There may be a gradual increase in symptoms, with chronic cough, wheezing, episodes of hypoxia, and development of digital clubbing. Right-sided heart failure occurs in some patients. Persons with LIP frequently develop secondary bacterial pneumonia but rarely develop PCP, possibly as a result of some protective effect of LIP in the lungs.

LIP is diagnosed by chest radiography, often in children with no clinical signs or symptoms. LIP has a characteristic radiographic appearance with a reticulonodular pattern and a lack of hilar lymphadenopathy (Fig. 38–8). The chest radiograph is fairly stable for months or years. Lung biopsy is rarely needed to confirm the diagnosis, although sometimes lung biopsies are performed to rule out other conditions and LIP is confirmed in the process. Histopathologic samples of biopsy tissues reveal germinal centers consisting of lymphocytes surrounded by plasma cells (Fig. 38–9). Other involved tissues have similar findings. Bronchoscopy with BAL has not proved to be necessary or especially useful in the diagnosis of LIP.

Antiretroviral therapy is probably in large part responsible for the decreased incidence of LIP. Decreased viral loads and improved immune status means that progression to LIP is less likely. There may be a direct therapeutic benefit of antiretroviral drugs as well.

Usually treatment for LIP is unnecessary early in the course of the disease. Therapy is indicated when a person has an acute exacerbation of symptoms, including tachypnea accompanied by a Pao_2 <65 mm Hg or significant worsening of radiographic findings. Some persons may respond to bronchodilators. For others, steroids are needed. Prednisone (or its equivalent) taken orally at 1–2 mg/kg daily for 2–4 weeks, with a gradual taper to 0.5 mg/kg every other day for several weeks, is typical. The duration of therapy should be determined by the clinical response. Oxygen therapy may be necessary for brief periods until Pao_2 levels become normal. Diuretics are sometimes helpful in persons with symptomatic LIP. Persons with clubbing and chronic hypoxemia (Pao_2 <85) may benefit from long-term steroid therapy. This regimen includes up to 3 months of daily therapy (prednisone 2 mg/kg/day), followed by slow tapering with long-term low-dose maintenance therapy (10–20 mg daily or every other day). Prognosis is generally good, although an increased incidence of bacterial infections and cor pulmonale can occur.

Bacterial Infections. Two documented invasive bacterial infections in a 2-year period constitute an AIDS-defining condition in children <13 years of age (Table 38–4). Invasive infections include sepsis, pneumonia, meningitis, bone and joint infections, and abscess of an internal organ. They do not include minor conditions such as

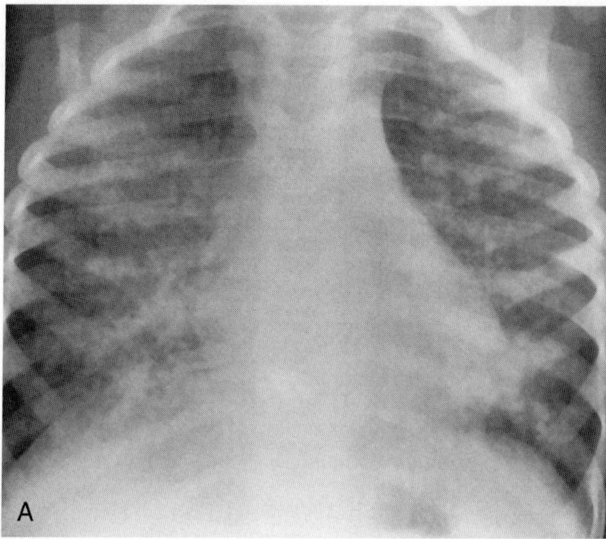

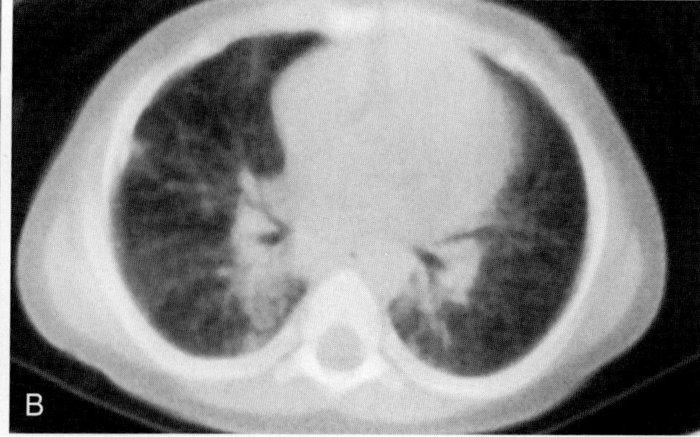

FIGURE 38–8. Lymphocytic interstitial pneumonitis in a relatively symptom-free 2-year-old boy seropositive for HIV infection. **A,** Frontal chest radiograph shows bilateral reticulonodular interstitial infiltrates scattered throughout both lungs in an uneven distribution. **B,** Computed tomography scan reveals bilateral hilar lymphadenopathy as well as the hazy interstitial infiltrates.

otitis media or infections occurring in the presence of a foreign body such as a catheter.

Bacterial pneumonia caused by *Streptococcus pneumoniae* or *H. influenzae* type b is frequent, although *H. influenzae* type b infections have been increasingly rare since the introduction of the conjugate *H. influenzae* type b vaccine in the early 1990s. Diagnosis is confirmed by blood culture or by culture and Gram stain of material obtained by bronchoscopy or from sputum samples. The emergence of penicillin-resistant *S. pneumoniae* in recent years has complicated treatment. It is prudent to begin empirical therapy with vancomycin plus cefotaxime or ceftriaxone. Antibiotic therapy is modified on the basis of antimicrobial susceptibility tests.

Tuberculosis. Tuberculosis has been reported in as many as 10% of adults with AIDS, and it is common in developing countries, where both diseases are common. It is not common in HIV-infected children in developed countries. Nevertheless, these children are at risk because of their immune impairment and because they often live in households with HIV-infected adults who are at risk of having tuberculosis. HIV-infected children are among those few children for whom annual PPD testing is recommended.

Cutaneous anergy complicates the diagnosis of tuberculosis in persons with HIV. Anergy worsens with declining CD4 lymphocyte levels. Any person with HIV is considered to be at risk of having tuberculosis. A history of exposure should be sought and a 5 TU PPD placed by using the Mantoux method. Other strengths (1 TU or 250 TU) are not recommended, and multiple puncture tests such as the tine test are unreliable and unacceptable. A cutaneous reaction with induration of ≥5 mm in response to a 5 TU skin test is considered a positive result in an HIV-infected person. A child with a positive skin test result should be evaluated for active disease by physical examination and chest radiography.

A negative PPD test result is inadequate to rule out tuberculosis in an HIV-infected child when there is a strong history of exposure,

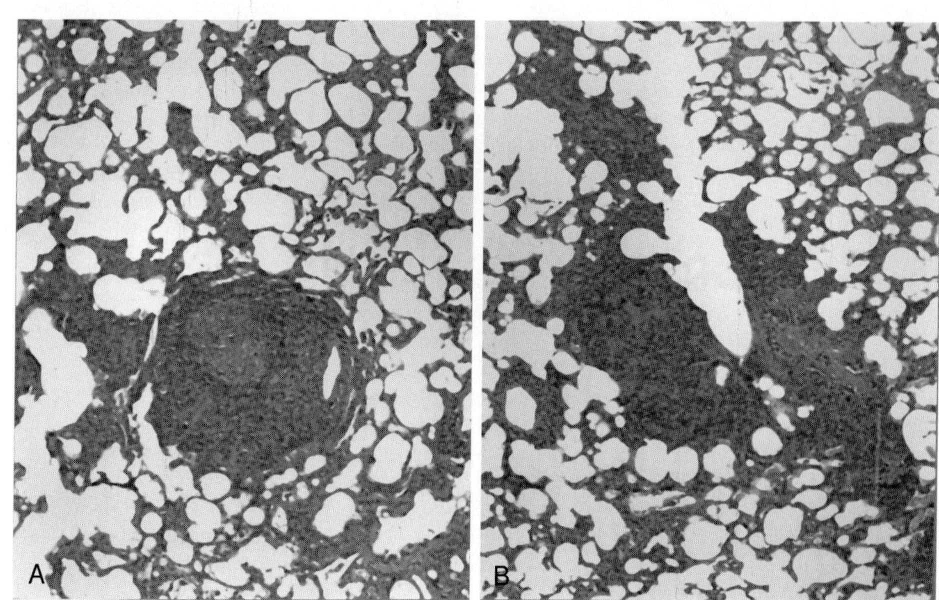

FIGURE 38–9. Microscopic pathologic changes in lymphoid interstitial pneumonitis in a child with AIDS. **A,** Diffuse pulmonary interstitital lymphoid infiltration, including development of a micronodular lymphoid follicle. Magnification: ×40. **B,** Peribronchiolar lymphoid interstitial infiltration. Magnification: ×40. (Used with permission from Jenson HB: Retrovirus infections and the acquired immunodeficiency syndrome. *Adv Pediatr Infect Dis* 1990;5:132.)

clinical evidence of disease consistent with tuberculosis, or advanced HIV disease with a low CD4 lymphocyte level. An HIV-infected child with pneumonia who responds poorly to standard antibiotic therapy or who has a positive PPD test result should be evaluated for tuberculosis by standard mycobacterial culture methods. An HIV-infected child with a family history or other significant exposure to tuberculosis should be evaluated by PPD testing. Even if the skin test result is negative, a symptom-free, HIV-infected child with a strong tuberculosis exposure history should be given isoniazid prophylaxis for 9–12 months. A positive skin test result should lead to more complete physical and radiographic evaluation and appropriate antimycobacterial therapy.

A child 8 years of age or older is usually able to produce adequate sputum samples. For younger children, gastric lavage samples from three consecutive first morning samples will sometimes yield mycobacteria from sputum that has been swallowed overnight. Three samples will yield organisms in fewer than 50% of cases. Alternatively, bronchoscopic samples may be needed. Nonpulmonary culture sources include CSF, urine, lymph nodes, bone, or pleural fluid from some persons with disseminated disease.

Treatment of tuberculosis in children with HIV depends on immune status, the site of infection, and potential or known resistance patterns of the organism. Treatment of pulmonary tuberculosis in a child with a normal or nearly normal immune system should include a minimum of three drugs for the first 2 months of therapy, followed by two drugs for 4 months to complete 6 months of therapy. A child with advanced AIDS should be treated for 9–12 months, although some specialists advocate a 6-month course of treatment for uncomplicated disease, as for persons with tuberculosis but not HIV infection. Extrapulmonary disease should be treated for 9–12 months.

Except in cases of known resistance or drug hypersensitivity, preferred therapy should include isoniazid 10–15 mg/kg (max 300 mg) in a daily single dose orally for the entire course. After 2 months of daily therapy, isoniazid may be given 20–30 mg/kg/day in a single dose twice weekly for the last 4 months of therapy. Rifampin is also included in all treatment protocols unless resistance or hypersensitivity is known to exist. It is given at 10–20 mg/kg (max 600 mg) in a single daily dose by mouth. After the initial 2 months of therapy, rifampin may be given twice weekly at the same daily dose.

In regimens requiring a third drug, pyrazinamide is usually included. It is given once daily for the first 2 months of the regimen in a dose of 20–40 mg/kg. When drug resistance is a concern, a four-drug regimen is used with the addition of streptomycin (20–40 mg/kg once daily given intramuscularly) or ethambutol (15–25 mg/kg in a single daily oral dose) for 2 months. Many pediatricians prefer streptomycin because ethambutol can cause optic neuritis and diminution of red-green color discrimination, which is difficult to monitor in young children. However, there is risk of ototoxicity with streptomycin, and it requires daily intramuscular injections.

For young children or adolescents who are being treated for tuberculosis and HIV disease simultaneously and who are receiving medications for prophylaxis against other opportunistic infections, the numbers of medications and potential drug interactions are daunting. In such cases it is strongly recommended that the physician work in conjunction with a pediatric infectious disease specialist. Suboptimal tuberculosis therapy would seriously jeopardize the possibility of eradicating the organism and is to be avoided.

Precautions are necessary for persons with HIV who usually will also be taking antiretroviral medications. Rifampin should generally not be administered to persons receiving PIs or NNRTIs. Rifampin, which is cleared through the cytochrome P-450 enzyme system of the liver, will reduce blood levels of some PIs. Conversely, rifampin levels will be increased especially by ritonavir and to a lesser degree by other PIs. The NNRTIs have variable effects on the cytochrome P-450 system. The other rifamycin drugs, rifabutin and rifapentine, are less potent cytochrome P-450 inducers than rifampin and are better tolerated than rifampin for persons taking both antiretroviral and tuberculosis medications. They should still be used with caution. The nucleoside analog medications are not metabolized by the cytochrome P-450 enzyme system.

Because of the numbers of medications and the chance of drug interactions, some specialists avoid PIs for the duration of tuberculosis treatment. Another approach is to drop rifampin after 2 months of therapy and continue with a combination such as isoniazid and ethambutol, allowing reintroduction of a PI. Rifabutin is sometimes used to treat or prevent MAC disease in persons with advanced AIDS and can be considered for use with a PI other than ritonavir, although it is not available as a pediatric formulation.

Fungal Infections. Invasive pulmonary fungal infections are occasionally seen in children with HIV. With patients surviving longer, fungal infections are more likely. Primary prevention is limited to avoidance of potential situations in which inhalation of fungal spores might occur. Because these spores are regionally or ubiquitously present environmental organisms, attempts at avoidance may be ineffective. Primary prevention of fungal infections by antifungal medications is generally not recommended because of the infrequency of infections, cost, potential drug interactions, and lack of data as to efficacy.

Coccidioidomycosis may occur in people who reside in or have a travel history to endemic areas of the southwestern United States. *Coccidioides immitis* infections in HIV-infected children appear to be rare. Diagnosis is often made serologically, by means of latex agglutination, enzyme immunoassay, complement fixation, and immunodiffusion. Skin tests do not correlate well with progression to disease and are not usually recommended. The most accurate diagnosis is made by determination of growth of the organism and by use of fungal stains of lung biopsy specimens. Material obtained by bronchiolar lavage may be cultured and subjected to special stains to reveal the characteristic spherules, providing an accurate diagnosis.

Two classes of antifungal agents are used for treatment. Mild to moderate infections including focal pneumonia can be treated with azoles, especially fluconazole or itraconazole. For the more severe infections such as diffuse reticulonodular pulmonary disease, which carries a 70% mortality rate, amphotericin B is used. The optimal duration of therapy is not well established. The duration of amphotericin B therapy for mild to moderate disease is typically several weeks, long enough for abnormalities of acute infection to resolve, whereas for more severe disease, primary treatment with amphotericin B extends for several months. After initial treatment, lifelong suppression with fluconazole or itraconazole is necessary. This approach has not been well studied in children, but extrapolation from adult data showing its efficacy is reasonable.

Histoplasmosis is common in the Ohio and Mississippi river valleys. It is often acquired by inhalation of spores of *Histoplasma capsulatum* from soil contaminated with bird droppings. Culture and fungal stains of sputum are the preferred methods of diagnosis. For disseminated disease, bone marrow or, blood cultures with the lysis centrifugation method or biopsy specimens of infected organs are potential sources of the organism. Fungal stains of biopsy tissues (Gomori's methenamine silver stain and others) will sometimes demonstrate intracellular budding yeast. Skin testing is not useful for diagnosis of acute pneumonia and is not recommended. Urinary

Histoplasma antigen testing by radioimmunoassay is a useful adjunct method of diagnosis and of following response to therapy. Although treatment is often unnecessary for uncomplicated primary disease in the healthy person, children with HIV should be treated with amphotericin B therapy for acute primary or disseminated disease. There is little experience with the treatment of histoplasmosis in HIV-infected children. Duration of therapy should be determined by clinical and laboratory evidence of response. Mild infections can be treated with itraconazole for 3 months, whereas moderate or severe disease should be treated with at least 2 weeks of intravenous amphotericin B therapy, followed by 10 weeks of itraconazole therapy. Lifelong suppressive therapy with itraconazole or fluconazole is necessary because of the high rate of relapse.

Cryptococcal infections in the healthy person are often subclinical, minimally symptomatic, or limited to pneumonia. They are less common in children with AIDS than in adults. Infection is initiated by inhalation of ubiquitous aerosols of contaminated soil. Immunocompromised persons are more likely to have dissemination from the lungs to other sites. Infection may evolve to fungemia or meningitis. Diagnosis is made by chest radiography and by culture and stains of sputum samples. Serum cryptococcal antigens can also be used for diagnosis and to monitor effectiveness of therapy. Blood and CSF samples should be sent for culture, India ink stain, and latex cryptococcal antigen. A CT scan of the head may be needed to assess the patient for central nervous system abscess.

Intravenous amphotericin B 0.5–0.7 mg/kg/day for 2–3 weeks (at least 6 weeks for meningitis) is recommended for treatment. The addition of flucytosine 50–150 mg/kg/day orally in four divided doses may improve response and often allows the lower amphotericin B dose (0.3 mg/kg/day) to be used. Fluconazole and itraconazole are sometimes used for primary treatment, although they have generally not been as effective as amphotericin B. Lifelong suppressive therapy is necessary to decrease the risk of relapse. Both itraconazole and fluconazole have been used, but in pediatric patients the experience with fluconazole (6 mg/kg/day orally in one dose) is greater. Amphotericin B at a dose of 0.5–1 mg/kg given intravenously once weekly is an alternative for suppressive therapy.

Aspergillus is an uncommon cause of pulmonary disease or disseminated disease in children with AIDS. Disease occurs in persons with severe immunosuppression, including a CD4 lymphocyte count <50 (or the equivalent in a younger child), severe and prolonged neutropenia, or long-term steroid use. The chest radiograph will sometimes reveal focal infiltrates, cavitation, or reticulnodular disease. In an adult or older child, diagnosis of *Aspergillus* is made by culture, 10% KOH treatment, or Gomori's methenamine–silver nitrate staining of sputum or bronchoalveolar lavage samples. In some children, including younger children who are unable to produce sputum, tissue diagnosis by lung biopsy may be needed. Treatment with amphotericin B (1–1.5 mg/kg/day) or liposomal amphotericin B (5 mg/kg/day) for 30 days or longer is recommended. If the immune system remains compromised, the outcome even with optimal therapy is generally poor.

Candida pulmonary disease is rare in children with HIV disease. Diagnosis must be confirmed by histologic evidence from lung tissue because sputum samples are frequently contaminated with oral *Candida.* Treatment should include amphotericin B or liposomal amphotericin B for 30 days or longer.

Viral Infections. Viral pneumonia is common in children with AIDS. Respiratory syncytial virus (RSV), adenovirus, influenza virus, and parainfluenza virus infections occur seasonally. HSV, CMV, or VZV pneumonia can occur in severely immunocompromised children. With some viruses the clinical course is similar to that of a healthy person, whereas others may cause severe, even fatal disease. RSV infections in infants are usually not very different from infections in uninfected children in terms of severity of disease, although viral shedding can last for weeks to 6 months (and occasionally longer). The diagnosis is made by rapid tests or culture of nasopharyngeal washings. HIV-infected infants may develop bronchiolitis that is similar in presentation to bronchiolitis in other infants. RSV pneumonia occasionally occurs in older children or adults.

Adenovirus may cause respiratory tract disease, gastroenteritis, hepatitis, meningoencephalitis, hemorrhagic cystitis, and conjunctivitis in persons with HIV. It is more likely to be disseminated in HIV disease. Mortality rates of 50% have been reported. In the respiratory tract, adenovirus can cause upper and lower respiratory tract infection, or there may be asymptomatic nasal carriage, diagnosed by culture of nasal washings. The diagnosis is sometimes made from cultures of urine or tissue biopsy specimens. Symptomatic and asymptomatic viremia can be diagnosed by culture of blood. Pneumonia occurring in severely immunocompromised persons typically has a poor outcome. No specific treatment is available.

The clinical presentation of influenza does not generally differ between HIV-infected and uninfected patients. There are a few reports of prolonged illness and prolonged shedding of virus. It can be diagnosed by culture of nasal washings, preferably within the first 3 days of illness, by serologic assay, or by several rapid tests of nasal washings. Prophylaxis and treatment of influenza is possible (see Table 68–11). Annual influenza immunization is recommended for persons with HIV infection.

Parainfluenza can cause upper respiratory tract infections, croup, bronchiolitis, and pneumonia in children with HIV. Severe or fatal infections may occur with severe immunocompromise or in persons who are coinfected with other organisms. Diagnosis is made by culture or rapid test methods using nasopharyngeal secretions. Viral shedding of parainfluenza is prolonged and has been reported for as long as a year. Aerosolized ribavirin has been used with modest success to treat parainfluenza infections in persons with severe combined immunodeficiency, but data on its use in persons with HIV are limited.

Measles virus pneumonia in HIV-infected persons has been reported, but measles is uncommon in the United States. Persons may be unaware that they have been exposed. Bronchial secretions or tissue from lung biopsy material may be needed to prove the diagnosis. Children with advanced HIV disease often lack the classic measles rash, delaying diagnosis. In such persons, measles pneumonia is often fatal. With a more intact immune system the rash is typical or slightly modified and the outcome is often similar to that in other children. Vitamin A supplementation has improved outcome in studies of measles-infected children from developing countries. These children are often malnourished and have low serum levels of vitamin A. Supplementation with vitamin A is recommended as adjunct therapy for children with measles. Children between 6 and 12 months of age are given 100,000 IU vitamin A at diagnosis, and older children are given 200,000 IU. Both aerosolized and intravenous ribavirin have been used with modest success to treat measles pneumonia and should be considered for HIV-infected children with measles.

Varicella pneumonia can occur with primary varicella disease or zoster in immunocompromised children, especially HIV-infected children with low CD4 lymphocyte counts. Viral dissemination to liver, lungs, and brain may occur with advanced HIV disease, often with a poor outcome. The clinical presentation of characteristic varicella lesions, accompanied by respiratory symptoms (dyspnea, hyperpnea, cough, pleuritic chest pain) and evidence of diffuse bilateral interstitial or reticulonodular infiltrates, is often enough to establish a presumptive diagnosis of varicella pneumonia. Culture of lesions and secretions from the respiratory tract to identify varicella can be used to confirm the diagnosis. Treatment should be initiated as soon as there is clinical suspicion of varicella disease. Acyclovir given intravenously at 500 mg/m^2 every 8 hours for 7–10 days is recommended for varicella pneumonia.

CMV may cause a variety of diseases including pneumonia in children with HIV. CMV pneumonia occurs in children with advanced disease. The prognosis is poor. The diagnosis is made difficult by the frequently widespread presence of CMV in body tissues and fluids (e.g., urine, blood, respiratory tract secretions) in persons who do not have invasive disease. Isolation of CMV from airway secretions is not adequate to establish it as the cause of lower respiratory tract disease. An example is the presence of CMV in some children who also have PCP who respond to PCP treatment alone, which indicates the commensal role of CMV. Tissue diagnosis demonstrating the presence of CMV in tissues is needed to establish it conclusively as the cause.

CMV pneumonia is usually treated with ganciclovir, and foscarnet is used for recalcitrant infections. Ganciclovir is available in several forms, including an intravenous formulation, an oral preparation that is poorly absorbed, and a slow-release intravitreal implant form for CMV retinitis. For CMV pneumonia, intravenous ganciclovir is given at 5 mg/kg/dose twice daily in an induction phase of 14–21 days. Daily maintenance with 5 mg/kg/day or 6 mg/kg for 5 days per week is lifelong maintenance after induction. The value of anti-CMV immune globulin in this situation is less clear.

Other viruses affecting the respiratory tract include rhinoviruses and coronaviruses. Clinical presentations typically do not differ significantly from what is seen in other children.

Cardiac Conditions

Cardiac abnormalities of structure and function have been described among HIV-infected children. Approximately 6–10% of children with HIV will develop clinically significant heart disease, especially congestive heart failure. Subclinical cardiac involvement may be much higher. Congenital heart disease is no more common than in uninfected children. Lymphocytic myocarditis with necrosis, lymphocytic pericarditis, dysrhythmias, disorders of contractility, and cardiomyopathy have been described. Direct HIV invasion of cardiac tissues has been documented but is often difficult to prove.

Other viral (EBV, CMV, coxsackievirus), fungal *(Candida, Aspergillus),* and parasitic *(Toxoplasma, Pneumocystis)* infections should be considered. Illicit drugs and occasionally medications, including antiretroviral medications, have been implicated in cardiac disease. Lymphomas can affect the heart. Persons with encephalopathy possibly develop cardiac disease as a result of autonomic neuropathy. Cardiomyopathy may occur as a secondary complication of pulmonary disease; for example, cor pulmonale may result from LIP.

Gastrointestinal Tract Conditions

The gastrointestinal tract is a frequent site of disease in children with HIV. Common infections, infections that are usually limited to immunocompromised persons, and noninfectious conditions are all part of the differential diagnosis when gastrointestinal tract disease occurs in children with HIV. Tissue biopsies or special culture techniques may be required to establish the cause.

Oral Disease. Oral candidiasis is often recurrent, may be severe in AIDS, and is sometimes slow to clear even with treatment. Several forms of oral candidiasis, including the classic white patches of pseudomembranous candidiasis, have been described. Thrush, angular cheilitis, erythematous candidiasis, and hyperplastic candidiasis are less common forms. The diagnosis can be made by the use of KOH-stained specimens, which display pseudohyphae or blastospores, by culture of scrapings, or by the testing of biopsy specimens. Oral candidiasis persisting >2 months in children >6 months of age is a clinical category B disease (Table 38–4).

Topical nystatin (100,000–500,000 U four times a day orally), clotrimazole troches (three to five times daily), or vaginal suppositories or creams used intraorally can all be considered for mild cases, although they require frequent dosing and responses may be slow or ineffective. Extensive or recalcitrant disease can be treated with a short course (typically 5 days) of fluconazole, itraconazole, or ketoconazole, with longer courses and repeated treatments as needed. Ketoconazole (5–10 mg/kg in one or two doses orally) is not approved for children less than 2 years of age and has potential for significant interactions with several antiretroviral medications. Fluconazole (5–6 mg/kg/day in one or two doses orally) for 5 days is generally well tolerated and has less potential for drug interactions than does ketoconazole. Itraconazole (5 mg/kg/day in one oral dose) for 5 days is effective and generally well tolerated. Repeated or prolonged treatment with azole antifungals may result in the development of resistant organisms, necessitating use of amphotericin B. When candidiasis recurs frequently, prophylaxis with nystatin or clotrimazole can be considered, but azole drugs (ketoconazole, itraconazole, fluconazole) are avoided, when possible, because of the propensity of *Candida* to develop resistance with prolonged use of these drugs.

HSV may cause occasional lesions or severe, prolonged, debilitating stomatitis. Acyclovir typically is given intravenously (500 mg/m^2 every 8 hours) for severe disease. To be effective, therapy should be started as soon as possible after lesions appear. Oral acyclovir (20 mg/kg every 6 hours) is an option for selected patients who have mild disease and who are able and willing to take oral medications. Famciclovir and valacyclovir are newer medications that allow less frequent dosing. They are effective but are not yet approved for children.

Aphthous ulcers are painful, shallow ulcerations that probably result from an autoimmune phenomenon and that frequently recur. These lesions can be both extensive and large in persons with HIV. They sometimes respond to oral dexamethasone elixir used once or twice daily as an oral rinse, or they may require systemic corticosteroids (prednisone). Some persons respond to cimetidine, viscous 2% lidocaine, or chlorhexidine. Periodontal disease, sometimes resulting from viral infections (EBV, CMV), is common.

Children with HIV are prone to **dental caries,** in part because of the large numbers of medications they ingest, many of which have a sucrose-based flavoring. Poor dental care and malnutrition compound the problem.

Oral hairy leukoplakia is more common among adults than children. It is a benign proliferation of EBV in oropharyngeal epithelial cells exclusive to people with HIV disease. The lesions found on the lateral margins and occasionally on the dorsum of the tongue or on the pharynx appear as white plaques with vertical folds. The diagnosis can be confused by *Candida* superinfection. Biopsy reveals epithelial hyperplasia with epithelial proliferations appearing as "hairs." EBV replication continues unimpaired by normal host defenses, with infection and reinfection of the basal and suprabasal epithelial cells. Some persons respond to oral acyclovir therapy. For persons who have a relapse, prolonged high-dose acyclovir therapy may be necessary. Other antiviral agents such as ganciclovir, foscarnet, famciclovir, valacyclovir, and cidofovir potentially may offer benefit, although the latter three are not approved for children.

The salivary glands (parotid, submaxillary, and submandibular) can become enlarged in children with HIV. The glands are typically firm, nontender or mildly tender, and without evidence of inflammation. Some persons develop xerostomia or secondary infections with acute pain, fever, and discharge from Stensen's duct. Typically, however, **parotitis** is a chronic process that may last for weeks or months. Like LIP, it represents a lymphocytic infiltration of the tissues, and the two conditions are often associated. It is unlikely to be confused with acute, severely painful parotitis, which may occur with infections caused by mumps virus, influenza virus, parainfluenza virus, or adenovirus. The typical HIV-associated parotitis does not require specific therapy. Acute, painful parotitis with discharge should be evaluated by culture of discharge and antibiotic therapy. If there is rapid enlargement, especially unilaterally, a biopsy may be necessary to rule out lymphoma, which has been reported in persons with HIV.

Esophagitis. *Candida* esophagitis can occur with immunocompromise. It is an AIDS-defining (category C classification) condition and the most common cause of esophagitis in the immunocompromised person. *C. albicans* is the most common causative species, although *C. parapsilosis, C. tropicalis,* and other species are occasional causes. HSV is the most common cause of esophagitis in the otherwise healthy person and is seen in HIV-infected children as well. CMV infection should also be considered in the differential diagnosis.

Persons with esophagitis have odynophagia, dysphagia, retrosternal pain, and decreased oral intake. The absence of contiguous disease (thrush, herpes stomatitis) in the mouth does not exclude disease in the esophagus. A barium swallow with an esophagogram is useful for confirming that esophagitis exists, but a negative test ressult does not rule out the diagnosis. Although this method may reveal the diagnosis, it does not confirm the cause. In selected cases, endoscopy and biopsy, with appropriate stains and cultures, may be needed to confirm the diagnosis.

Presumptive therapy based on symptoms may be initiated with oral fluconazole or ketoconazole or, for persons unable to swallow, with intravenous fluconazole. Failure to respond to presumptive therapy necessitates endoscopy to obtain biopsy samples. On confirmation of *Candida* esophagitis, an azole antifungal agent (as indicated for presumptive therapy) or intravenous amphotericin B should be used. Amphotericin B is used at a final dose of 0.75–1 mg/kg once daily. The newer lipid-complexed amphotericin B preparations can be considered in selected cases. Antiviral treatment with intravenous ganciclovir or foscarnet is indicated for proven CMV esophagitis, whereas intravenous acyclovir is the drug of choice for HSV esophagitis.

Bacterial Enteritis. The large and small intestines are the sites of numerous infectious and noninfectious complications of HIV. Fever, chills, abdominal cramps, and diarrhea are common, so history and physical examination alone will not establish the cause. Standard stool and blood cultures are a reasonable starting point because pathogens common in the general population are also common with HIV disease. Bacterial enteritis caused by nontyphoidal *Salmonella, Shigella,* and *Campylobacter* are even more prevalent in persons with HIV than in the general population, and the enteritis is more likely to be complicated by bacteremia, especially with *Salmonella.* Recurrent or severe infections are more likely to occur in HIV-infected persons. *Salmonella* enteritis may be associated with bloody diarrhea, and *Shigella* may involve the small bowel, causing watery diarrhea or, more commonly in the large bowel, causing severe bloody diarrhea.

Salmonella gastroenteritis in a person with HIV should be treated because the risk of invasive disease outweighs concerns about developing chronic carriage. Antibiotic choices include ampicillin, TMP-SMZ, cefotaxime, ceftriaxone, and quinolone antibiotics for 14 days. Quinolones are not approved for persons less than 18 years of age or for pregnant or lactating women.

For invasive *Salmonella* infection, including sepsis and meningitis, TMP-SMZ, ampicillin, chloramphenicol, and third-generation cephalosporins are used. The specific antibiotic, route of administration, and duration will depend on the organism's susceptibility, the site of infection, and the host. Long-term therapy is indicated, usually for 3–6 weeks depending on the patient and the type of infection.

Shigella infection is typically self-limited, and a short course (5 days) of the same antibiotics used for *Salmonella* infection is adequate to reduce the risk of spreading the organisms and may shorten the duration of symptoms. *Campylobacter* infection may be manifested as bacteremia or enteritis. Erythromycin, azithromycin, and quinolones are the antibiotics of choice. The latter are used in children after risks and benefits are weighed.

Mycobacteria. Atypical *Mycobacterium* infections, especially with MAC, are common causes of gastrointestinal disease in persons with AIDS. *M. chelonae, M. kansasii, M. marinum, M. scrofulaceum, M. fortuitum, M. abscessus,* and other species are occasionally implicated. Infections typically occur with CD4 lymphocyte counts $<100/mm^3$ in adults and older children and at somewhat higher counts in young children. There is an inverse correlation between the CD4 lymphocyte count and the risk of acquiring MAC disease. Multiple organ systems are affected and bacteremia is common. Weight loss, fever, anemia, night sweats, anorexia, abdominal pain, diarrhea, and hepatosplenomegaly are common manifestations of MAC disease. The respiratory tract may be affected, although generalized infections, often manifested by gastrointestinal symptoms, are more common. The gastrointestinal and respiratory tracts serve as portals of entry. These organisms are common in dust, soil, water, poultry, and milk products. The disease is uncommon in infants; it is more common in older, immunocompromised children and may occur in 30–50% of adults with advanced AIDS.

The diagnosis is often initially based on clinical assessment. Tissue specimens (from stool, bone marrow, blood, urine, or sputum) or liver or lung biopsy specimens may reveal acid-fast bacilli when appropriately stained. Sometimes they are only found by culture, which may require 4–6 weeks for growth. Recent improvements in diagnostic technology often allow earlier diagnosis than in the past.

Treatment is complex, requiring a minimum of 2 medications. Many physicians use three or more medications, although previous enthusiasm for regimens using five to seven drugs has faded. There is potential for drug interactions between antimycobacterial medications and antiretroviral medications, which are often used simultaneously. Between HIV treatment and MAC treatment, the number of medications prescribed often makes adherence beyond the capabilities of even dedicated persons, and many young children and their parents are not likely to be able to maintain the regimen. Difficult choices are sometimes necessary when one is treating such complications of HIV disease.

MAC treatment regimens should always include one macrolide antibiotic (clarithromycin or azithromycin). Clarithromycin is given at a dose of 15 mg/kg/day (max 500 mg) divided into two oral doses, whereas azithromycin is given at 10 mg/kg/day in one oral dose. Ethambutol (15–20 mg/kg [max 2.5 g] in one daily oral dose) is often the preferred second drug. Some experts also add rifabutin (5–10 mg/kg [max 300 mg] in one daily oral dose). Other choices include rifampin, clofazimine, amikacin, or ciprofloxacin. Typically it takes 4–6 weeks to achieve maximum benefit, but therapy is continued for the patient's lifetime. Although symptoms abate and bacterial loads can be reduced, mycobacteria are generally not eradicated. Survival after diagnosis of MAC disease is typically less than 1 year, although treatment generally improves quality of life and extends the duration of life as well.

Prevention of MAC infections is often possible. The CD4 lymphocyte values at which MAC prophylaxis should be initiated are shown in Table 38–14, and appropriate prophylactic medications are shown in Table 38–15. In addition, many persons filter drinking water, peel fruits and vegetables carefully, and avoid unpasteurized milk products to reduce exposure to atypical mycobacteria. Because no evidence strongly supports that these measures prevent MAC infections, whether to use them is a personal decision that each person should make.

Parasitic Infections. Parasites are common agents of disease in persons with HIV, and those who acquire some of them are considered to have AIDS-defining conditions. *Cryptosporidium parvum, Isospora belli,* and microsporidia are occasional causes of infection in otherwise healthy persons. Cryptosporidiosis among immunocompetent persons has been increasingly reported in recent years. *C. parvum* may cause frequent prolonged watery diarrhea, cramping pain, weight loss, and sometimes anorexia. It is generally confirmed by modified acid-fast stain of stool specimens or intestinal biopsy specimens. Paromomycin 25–35 mg/kg/day in two to four divided oral doses for 2–4 weeks and azithromycin may have limited efficacy.

I. belli causes foul-smelling, profusely watery, nonbloody diarrhea. It uncommonly affects children except in tropical climates and is rare or nonexistent in children with HIV in developed countries. It occasionally occurs in adults and adolescents with HIV. It is identified by modified acid-fast stains of stool specimens or intestinal biopsy specimens and is treated with a 10-day course of TMP-SMZ (TMP 10 mgkg/day and SMZ 50 mg/kg/day).

More than 700 species in at least six genera belong to the order Microsporida, which typically results in less severe gastrointestinal disease than *Cryptosporidium.* The organisms best associated with enteritis are *Enterocytozoon bieneusi* and *Septata intestinalis,* which may produce enteritis with voluminous watery diarrhea, cramping, and dehydration, but patients often are afebrile. Other microsporidia cause corneal infections, hepatitis, nephritis, or myositis in some adults with AIDS. Biopsy of intestinal tissues is usually necessary to prove that microsporidia are the cause of disease, although they sometimes can be detected in stool or in duodenal or jejunal aspirates. Special stains of biopsy tissues or light microscopic examination of stained, formalin-fixed, unconcentrated stool specimens may reveal the characteristic organism. Species identification is sometimes made by using fluorescein-tagged antibodies. Albendazole, metronidazole, and atovaquone will sometimes reduce symptoms, although they generally do not achieve eradication.

Prevention of *Cryptosporidium* infections requires close attention to numerous potential sources of exposure. Human and animal feces, surface water sources and products made from such sources (including ice), and raw oysters are known sources. Outbreaks associated with municipal water sources have occurred, and during an outbreak, water should be boiled or filtered with an appropriate filter, or alternative supplies should be obtained. Avoidance of contact with feces, including infants or animals with diarrhea, should be encouraged. There are no known control measures for microsporidia.

Strongyloides stercoralis, a helminth, is an occasional cause of infection in AIDS, as is *I. belli,* a protozoan, although both are uncommon, especially in the pediatric population. The former causes abdominal pain, weight loss, nausea and vomiting, and diarrhea after attachment to the mucosa of the small intestine, and if invasion occurs, it can cause eosinophilia, a papular rash, and pruritus. An urticarial perianal rash may occur, and bowel wall invasion may result in gram-negative septicemia. Identification is made by identification of larvae (rarely ova) in stool or duodenal fluid. Thiabendazole, ivermectin, and albendazole may be effective therapy.

Entamoeba histolytica causes ulcerations, bloody diarrhea, and abdominal pain in persons with AIDS. The biopsy may reveal the characteristic **flask-shaped mucosal lesions,** and biopsy specimens or fresh stools may yield the trophozoites or cysts. Serologic diagnosis can also be used. Treatment for older, nonpregnant persons is with metronidazole, 35–50 mg/kg/day (500–750 mg/dose for adults) given orally or intravenously, divided into three daily doses for 10 days. If extraintestinal disease occurs, metronidazole therapy is followed by iodoquinol, 40 mg/kg/day orally divided into three doses for 20 days. Paromomycin is the alternative choice. The safety of metronidazole, which is reserved for severe or life-threatening disease, has not been established for young children. Alternative therapies for asymptomatic carriers include iodoquinol, paromomycin, or diloxanide furoate (available from the CDC).

Cytomegalovirus. CMV can affect virtually every organ system, including the tissues of the gastrointestinal tract, where it may cause severe bloody diarrhea, abdominal pain, and weight loss when it affects the colon or profuse watery diarrhea when it affects the small bowel. Mucosal ulceration leading to perforation or toxic megacolon may occur.

Intestinal biopsy with tissue stains is generally necessary to prove that CMV is the cause of disease, because the organism is ubiquitous and culture of body fluids alone does not prove causation. A fourfold rise in CMV-specific antibodies offers presumptive diagnosis of infection but is not definitive and does not determine the site of disease. Quantitative PCR methods increasingly are used to follow the course of CMV disease, although interpretation of viral loads differs in various clinical situations and continues to evolve. Treatment with ganciclovir (5 mg/kg twice daily given intravenously) or foscarnet (40–60 mg/kg three times daily given intravenously) is variably successful, with decreased symptoms and weight gain. Recurrences are common, as for CMV infection at other sites, and lifelong suppressive therapy with the same agents should be considered. These medications are associated with significant toxic effects and frequent drug interactions. They should be used with appropriate caution.

A variety of other infectious agents, including rotavirus, adenovirus, *Giardia, Candida,* and various bacteria, as well as noninfectious causes that include medications and dietary factors, may cause gastrointestinal disease. Sometimes no cause is found, despite extensive diagnostic study, and the diagnosis is considered to be idiopathic disease with malabsorption and watery diarrhea.

Malignancies. The most common malignancies in children with HIV are lymphomas, with the most common site being the gastrointestinal tract. Leiomyosarcomas are the second most common tumors in HIV-infected children. Increasing numbers of children with lymphomas have achieved remission with aggressive regimens of chemotherapy and with adjunctive therapy. Treatment is complicated by the number of other medications taken for HIV, by complications of HIV, and by the pre-existing immunocompromised state of the children at the initiation of therapy.

Hepatic Complications

Hepatomegaly is common in children with HIV. Children with hepatomegaly, especially if the condition is accompanied by splenomegaly, lymphadenopathy, or failure to thrive, should be considered as candidates for an evaluation for HIV. Hepatitis resulting from infections or medications also occurs.

Hepatitis B and C virus infections are common in persons with hemophilia, transfusion recipients, intravenous drug users, gay men, and people with a history of multiple sexual partners, so HIV and hepatitis viruses often coexist. Infants born to women with hepatitis B are at high risk (60–90%) of not only acquiring the virus but of becoming chronically infected. Hepatitis C is much less commonly transmitted vertically. Because both are common in women infected with HIV, their children are at proportionally increased risk.

Hepatitis B and HIV each may increase viral levels of the other. Because the inflammation of hepatitis B disease results from an immune response, there is some evidence that inflammation is decreased in people with HIV because of immunocompromise. Some data do not support this possibility, although it appears that progression of AIDS in coinfected individuals is not worse. Viral carriage is prolonged.

Persons infected with both hepatitis C and HIV have more rapid progression of hepatitis and probably of HIV disease as well. Children born to coinfected mothers may be at somewhat higher risk of acquiring HIV. Treatment of both hepatitis B and hepatitis C is complicated, more so in HIV-coinfected persons who are receiving multiple, potentially hepatotoxic medications.

CMV frequently affects the liver or biliary tract of children with HIV. A urine culture positive for CMV does not verify that any particular complication, including hepatitis, is the result of CMV. Hepatic CMV infection causes a mixed hepatocellular and cholestatic pattern of disease. Confirmation of infection requires liver biopsy with demonstration of CMV by stains or in situ hybridization methods. Women with HIV are at increased risk of having active CMV infections with elevated viral levels, which places their children at increased risk of acquiring CMV and HIV. A few children have dual congenital acquisition of HIV and CMV, and these children typically have liver involvement. Treatment options for acute hepatic CMV infections include ganciclovir and foscarnet, after which long-term suppressive therapy with the same medications is necessary. Outcome is typically poor for such children.

HIV infection of the liver occurs. In the past it was associated with possible giant cell hepatitis, although often there are no specific characteristic changes. Reaching a diagnosis is not easy and requires elimination of other potential sources, liver biopsy with special stains of tissues, and possibly electron microscopy for verification. HIV hepatitis has been reported to be responsive to steroid therapy.

Cryptosporidium and microsporidia can affect the liver, often ascending via the common bile duct. Cholestatic or mixed liver disease may result. A variety of other organisms, including adenoviruses, *Candida, Coccidioides, Histoplasma,* MAC, and *M. tuberculosis,* may on occasion cause hepatic disease in children with HIV. Liver-specific laboratory tests are not helpful in differentiating these agents, and liver biopsy with appropriate stains or other organism-specific methods of identification are necessary.

Many HIV-specific medications used to treat HIV infections are hepatotoxic. When there is evidence of liver damage, these medications need to be considered as potential causes and their sequential elimination may be necessary to establish the cause of disease. By regularly monitoring aminotransferases, one may infer that a newly added medication is the cause of this complication if an increase occurs shortly after initiation of therapy. Empirical reduction in dosages of many of the antiretroviral medications should be considered in cases of hepatic failure. Data are limited and specific guidelines are frequently nonexistent.

Renal Conditions

Urinary tract infections and renal abscesses result from a patient's immunocompromised state. Additionally, several HIV-associated renal diseases may occur, including focal glomerulosclerosis, which occurs after infancy and generally leads to renal failure, mesangial hyperplasia, segmental necrotizing glomerulonephritis, and minimal change disease. Signs usually include proteinuria, sometimes with edema. Acidosis, hypernatremia, hematuria, hyperlipidemia, hypoalbuminemia, and hypoproteinemia may occur, depending on the specific condition. Corticosteroids have little impact on proteinemia, renal failure, or survival. Hemodialysis does not significantly improve survival. Supportive therapy includes increased dietary protein to replace renal losses and supplemental calcium plus phosphate binders to correct renally induced hypocalcemia and hyperphosphatemia. Antiretroviral medications, particularly some nucleoside analogs (zidovudine, didanosine, stavudine, zalcitabine, lamivudine) require dosage modifications for renal failure. Many of the drugs should be used with caution because data are limited.

Hematologic Conditions

Medications, secondary infections, malignancies, HIV-related renal disease, and HIV disease itself can cause disorders in any or all cell lines of the bone marrow. Malabsorption, malnutrition, and poor diet can result in deficiencies of protein, iron, or vitamins, which can also affect production of the formed elements of blood. Other disorders unrelated to HIV should also be considered as possible causes of hematologic abnormalities, including hemoglobinopathies, blood loss, toxic effects of lead, and other disorders.

Anemia. Anemia is the most common hematologic abnormality in HIV and is more common in advanced disease. Medications, including such antiretroviral drugs as zidovudine and some common antibiotics (TMP-SMZ) and antivirals (ganciclovir, acyclovir), can cause anemia. Additionally, an inadequate supply of protein, vitamins (folic acid, B_{12}), or iron due to inadequate diet, inadequate dietary intake, or malabsorption can cause anemia. Infections such as those with parvovirus B19 and HIV, neoplasias, and myelofibrosis can have a direct impact on bone marrow production of red cell precursors. Hereditary causes such as thalassemia and sickle cell disease should be considered. Relative erythropoietin (EPO) insufficiency is common. Hypersplenism and blood loss, whether occult or overt, should be considered as well.

An elevated mean corpuscular volume (MCV) or macrocytosis is common with ZDV treatment. The MCV often exceeds 100 fL and within several weeks may result in macrocytic anemia. It is not related to vitamin B_{12} or folic acid deficiency and generally improves with a decreased dose or cessation of ZDV treatment. Sometimes cessation of ZDV therapy for 1–4 weeks, followed by reintroduction at a lower dose (typically 30% lower), is adequate to improve outcome. Recombinant EPO therapy can be employed as another method of treatment and has become less commonly necessary in recent years because doses of ZDV have been reduced and treatment alternatives have become available. Other agents are less likely to cause anemia.

Normochromic, normocytic anemia is consistent with anemia of chronic disease or in some cases with ZDV therapy. In contrast, microcytic hypochromic anemia is more characteristic of iron deficiency anemia. Fragmented red blood cells are frequently seen with antibody-induced hemolytic anemia resulting from nonspecific hypergammaglobulinemia.

Bone marrow suppression caused by disseminated infections is common. Most infections result in suppression of all cell lines. The presumptive diagnosis may be established by using specific stains or cultures of marrow for fungi, viruses, bacteria, or parasites. The bone marrow should also be examined for lymphomas and other malignancies.

In some cases, no cause can be found for anemia, but antiretroviral treatment results in improvement. Presumably HIV itself is the causative agent of anemia in some of those cases. Treatment of anemia involves elimination of the cause if possible, treatment of the underlying causes if feasible, or treatment of the signs and symptoms when the other approaches are unsuccessful.

Leukopenia. Leukopenia is common in HIV and AIDS. Determining the cause of leukopenia can be complicated because potential causes are numerous. ZDV was once a major cause of leukopenia. In recent years, ZDV doses have been reduced and the use of ZDV has decreased in proportion to the availability of other medications. If ZDV is the suspected cause of leukopenia, its use can be discontinued until the white blood cell count has recovered. If leukopenia recurs, the medication may need to be permanently discontinued. An alternative course is to substitute another medication for ZDV. Medications including TMP-SMZ, ganciclovir, and acyclovir are sometimes implicated as causes of leukopenia. Eliminating these agents when feasible may result in improved white blood cell concentrations.

Bone marrow suppression by a variety of infectious causes or by malignancies can result in leukopenia. Pancytopenia is often more common than isolated leukopenia. HIV disease itself will frequently result in leukopenia, particularly lymphopenia. Injections of granulocyte colony–stimulating factor (G-CSF) can improve the white blood cell concentration, although daily or almost daily subcutaneous injections of G-CSF are necessary, resulting in significant expense and inconvenience.

Thrombocytopenia. Like anemia and leukopenia, thrombocytopenia is common in HIV. However, the most common cause of thrombocytopenia in HIV-infected children is immune thrombocytopenic purpura (ITP). As in non-HIV-related ITP, petechiae, easy bruising, low peripheral platelet counts, and normal numbers of megakaryocytes in the bone marrow are typical findings. The usual cause is hypergammaglobulinemia, resulting in nonspecific thrombocytopenia. ITP can be the initial presentation of HIV in children and should be considered in the differential diagnosis of ITP.

The evaluation and treatment of ITP in children with HIV is not significantly different from those in other children. Elimination of obvious potential causes should be performed when feasible. IVIG is usually the first choice for treatment. Doses as high as 2 g/kg given for 2–5 days have been successfully used in some persons, although success is sometimes transient. Repeated courses of IVIG therapy may be needed every 2–4 weeks to maintain the platelet count. Sometimes the effectiveness of therapy declines with time. If the initial course of therapy is unsuccessful, a bone marrow examination should be performed, in consultation with a hematologist, before the use of steroids. Other possible therapeutic approaches include high-dose, pulsed steroids and splenectomy in persons unresponsive to other therapies.

Medications, especially ganciclovir, suppression of bone marrow production by CMV or HIV itself, and infiltration of bone marrow with various infectious agents or malignancies may result in loss of platelet production. When marrow suppression is the cause, more than one cell line is usually involved.

Dermatologic Conditions

The skin is frequently a site of disease in children with HIV. Dermatologic conditions may be the first apparent manifestation of HIV disease. Many of the complications of HIV are expressed outwardly on the skin. Adverse effects of many therapeutic agents used for treatment of HIV are revealed on the skin.

Bacterial Infections. *Staphylococcus aureus* causes pustules, impetigo, abscesses, cellulitis, and ulcerations of skin. Standard cultures and stains of material from the infected site and blood cultures are used to confirm the diagnosis. Treatment ranges from mupirocin ointment for impetigo and minor skin infections, to a short course (7–10 days) of an oral antistaphylococcal antibiotic (dicloxacillin, first-generation cephalosporin, clindamycin), to intravenous antistaphylococcal antibiotics for widespread or systemic infections.

Pseudomonas aeruginosa can cause ecthyma gangrenosum, the cutaneous manifestation of serious underlying disease occurring in immunocompromised persons. Lesions occurring on skin and mucosal membranes rapidly progress from macules to nodules to black eschars. Patients are frequently ill appearing and have bacteremia. Blood cultures should be obtained before the start of intravenous antibiotic therapy with two anti-*Pseudomonas* drugs, including an extended-spectrum β-lactam and an aminoglycoside.

MAC disease can be manifested with ulcers, nodules, and macules—components of disseminated infection, usually occurring in the late stage of disease. Bacteria can be stained and cultured in specimens from multiple tissue sources, including blood, stool, bone marrow, and tissue biopsies. Appropriate therapy was described previously. Cure is generally not a realistic goal, although multidrug therapy can often control the organisms. Cutaneous lesions can occur with *Mycobacterium haemophilum,* and *M. marinum.*

Both *Bartonella henselae* and *Bartonella quintana* can cause **bacillary angiomatosis.** *B. henselae,* the agent of cat-scratch disease, is transmitted from the bites or scratches of a cat, usually a kitten, although some persons are unable to recall exposure to a cat. Cutaneous lesions appear as small, red papules. *B. quintana* is the louseborne cause of trench fever. Subcutaneous nodules caused by *B. quintana* are sometimes associated with lytic areas of cortical destruction of underlying bone. *Bartonella* can affect the liver, spleen, brain, lymph nodes, and lungs and may cause systemic signs and symptoms including weight loss or fever. Most disease caused by these organisms appears in persons with advanced disease. The diagnosis is typically established by biopsy, with appropriate stains including **Warthin-Starry stain.** Culture of these organisms is difficult. The treatment of choice is erythromycin given orally four times daily for 8 weeks or longer. Alternatives include other macrolide antibiotics or doxycycline.

Viral Infections. Infections by the herpes family of viruses are widespread in people with HIV, and cutaneous manifestations are common. HSV disease may be manifested on mucous membranes and may spread to perioral skin and beyond. Primary disease can be especially severe in children, and recurrences are fairly common. The diagnosis is made by clinical appearance, culture, and fluorescent immunocytologic assay of lesions. Treatment is with intravenous acyclovir, 750 mg/m^2/day divided every 8 hours for 5–14 days depending on severity and response. Oral acyclovir, 1,200 mg divided three times daily for 7–10 days, is used for mild cases.

Varicella virus may be manifested in several ways. Every effort should be made to have the person with HIV avoid varicella exposure, and VZIG given within 72 hours of exposure can abort or ameliorate the infection. Diagnosis is usually made on the basis of clinical appearance, although immunofluorescent antibody studies and culture may confirm diagnosis. Treatment is with acyclovir, 1,500 mg/m^2/day divided every 8 hours for 7–10 days or until all lesions are crusted. Oral acyclovir at 80 mg/kg (max 4 g) divided five times daily for the same duration is acceptable for mild disease. Disseminated disease is more common in immunocompromised persons, and physicians should be alert for pulmonary, hepatic, and central nervous system symptoms.

Zoster (shingles) is common in adults with or without AIDS and fairly common in children with AIDS. The diagnosis is usually based on the characteristic dermatomal distribution. Multidermatomal distribution and disseminated disease are less common and much more serious. The treatment is the same as for varicella.

A rare form of chronic varicella-zoster virus disease is seen in children and some adults with HIV and occasionally in other immunocompromised children. Lesions may persist or recur at some point after apparently healing. These lesions initially have the typical appearance of varicella, developing a hyperkeratotic, verrucous appearance with a heaped-up edge, often surrounding a central ulceration. Virus can persistently be isolated. Treatment may be effective initially; however, with time the response is usually poor. Prolonged treatment may result in the development of resistance to antiviral medications.

Kaposi's sarcoma is caused by human herpesvirus 8. HHV-8 is rare in children with HIV and is found less commonly in adults now than in the 1980s. It causes red or purple plaques or nodules on the skin and mucosa and in many internal organs. Biopsy and histologic studies are used to confirm the diagnosis, and a number of highly specialized treatments have been used.

Molluscum contagiosum, caused by a DNA poxvirus, causes 1–2 mm papules with a central umbilication (Chapter 46). These lesions may be larger and more numerous in children with AIDS. Treatment by curettage or liquid nitrogen therapy may temporarily improve appearance, but recurrence is common.

Fungal Infections. *Candida* infection in the form of mild to severe diaper dermatitis, with its characteristic red intertriginous distribution and satellite lesions, is common. Sometimes other areas of the body are infected. Nystatin diaper cream or ointment, 2% miconazole cream, or in severe cases perhaps oral (systemic) antifungal therapy can be used for treatment.

Tinea corporis or tinea capitis is similar in appearance in HIV-infected and uninfected children (Chapter 46). Skin scrapings for KOH preparation or dermatophyte culture can be used to confirm the diagnosis. Treatment is the same as for uninfected children, although the physician must be aware that some antifungal agents interact adversely with antiretroviral medications.

Occasionally other fungi will be manifested by cutaneous lesions. Most prevalent among them is *C. neoformans,* which can appear as papules or nodules. They vary with size, and the diagnosis is usually made by biopsy, with stains showing the characteristic organisms, or by culture of the specimen.

Drug Reactions. Cutaneous reactions caused by antiretroviral medications and other commonly used medications are common in adults and children with HIV (Table 38–12). Of special note is the severe, occasionally fatal hypersensitivity reaction reported with abacavir after about 2 weeks of treatment. If a hypersensitivity reaction has been proved or is likely, rechallenge with abacavir should be avoided. Efavirenz, an NNARTI, can produce a rash in one fourth of patients after about 2 weeks. Those with mild rash can continue the medication, and the rash typically will resolve within 2–4 weeks. If therapy is discontinued, patients can be considered for rechallenge, with caution. With a more severe bullous or desquamative rash, the medication should be discontinued. TMP-SMZ, commonly used for PCP prophylaxis, causes hypersensitivity reactions in about 16% of HIV-infected persons. The reactions range from mild maculopapular reactions to life-threatening Stevens-Johnson syndrome. Desensitization regimens can sometimes be used to allow reinstitution of prophylaxis or treatment of disease, should it recur. Alternative regimens should be considered.

Other Conditions. Scabies may present in the typical manner commonly seen in other children, or it may occur as the severe, matted form of **crusted scabies,** also known as **Norwegian scabies,** seen in severely immunocompromised children. The appearance ranges from generalized, papular discrete lesions that are intensely pruritic to crusted scabies that form hyperkeratotic, crusted, scaling plaques. Scrapings examined under the microscope can confirm diagnosis. Topical 5% permethrin cream applied for 8–14 hours and repeated in 7 days is often effective. For the severe, crusted form of scabies, ivermectin taken orally has been effective in adults and a small number of immunocompromised children. Limited experience suggests that ivermectin 0.2 mg/kg taken once orally or sometimes followed by a second dose after 7 days can be highly effective in eradication of crusted scabies.

Seborrheic dermatitis is common among infected infants and children. It may be the initial presenting sign of HIV infection, although it is not pathognomonic. The face, postauricular areas, and intertriginous folds in the diaper region are commonly affected. It may be seen as cradle cap in infants. Selenium-containing shampoos left on the affected areas for 10 minutes before washing are effective in controlling the symptoms in many children.

Atopic dermatitis is also more common in HIV-infected children. It occurs on the cheeks and extensor folds in infancy and is often red and pruritic. Treatment with moisturizing agents and judicious use of topical corticosteroids may help.

PROGNOSIS

Despite all the facets that are unknown or incompletely known, the prognosis appears to be better than ever for persons infected with HIV. The prognosis varies significantly among HIV populations, and it is difficult to predict survival accurately in individuals. The prognosis for children born to HIV-infected mothers has markedly improved because of antiretroviral prophylaxis and the use of planned cesarean deliveries. Such strategies have significantly decreased the number of HIV-infected children in developed countries but have had virtually no impact on the 95% of HIV-exposed children who live in developing countries.

The prognosis for children and adults infected with HIV appears to have been altered remarkably by the introduction of combination antiretroviral therapy. It has been only a few years since combination therapies have been introduced. Among adolescents and adults with an AIDS-defining opportunistic illness, median survival time has improved from 11 months in 1984 to 46 months for 1995 diagnoses. Too little time has passed for long-term evaluation of more recent treatments. However, these individuals can already be seen to be living better. There are fewer HIV-infected persons progressing to AIDS and fewer persons with AIDS who are dying from the disease than in past years.

No long-term studies are available regarding the durability of treatment for HIV infection. The significant short-term adverse effects of many medications and the lack of knowledge about long-term adverse effects are of concern. The large ''pill burden'' for adults or the ''liquid burden'' for children required to maintain viral suppression, the emergence of multidrug-resistant viruses, and the inability of many individuals to follow complex medication schedules for themselves and family members cause difficulty in maintaining the viral suppression needed for sustained benefit. For most of the infected population in developing countries, the benefits of antiviral medications remain out of reach.

In the past there was a significant correlation between a child's initial classification and the prognosis. It is not clear how early treatment might affect the prognostic value of the current classification scheme. Viral load testing has altered our understanding of the pathophysiology of disease and is a more sensitive correlate of disease progression than is the immune status. The person's viral load and the ability to suppress it to low levels appear to be the best correlates of short-term and presumably long-term survival. The CD4 lymphocyte count is also an important determinant of survival and prognosis, and some studies, particularly among adults, indicate that the combination of viral load and immune status together is the best laboratory indicators of prognosis.

HIV-infected children who survive into adolescence and perhaps eventually into adulthood will have to be monitored for psychological problems resulting from a lifelong chronic illness, from years of taking medications, and often from dealing with a secretive and unpopular illness. They often deal as well with the loss of one or more family members to HIV, dietary restrictions, and restricted social activities. HIV encephalopathy has been studied in young children, as has AIDS dementia in adults. It is not known whether long-term central nervous system infection might manifest differently in adolescents who were born infected and are reaching adulthood with their disease.

PREVENTION

Individuals can prevent HIV infection by eliminating risk behaviors such as injection drug use, unprotected sex, and sex with multiple partners. All blood is screened for HIV infection, with the risk of HIV transmission by contaminated blood estimated to be approximately 1 in 493,000 units (Chapter 105).

Vertical Transmission. Antiretroviral treatment of pregnant women and their offspring can prevent perinatal HIV transmission (see under Treatment).

Postexposure Prophylaxis. Recommendations to provide antiretroviral medicines to health care workers after significant occupational exposure to HIV have been issued by the CDC. A multicenter case-control study of health care workers after inadvertent needle-stick and other blood exposures showed a 79% reduction in the risk of acquiring HIV for workers who received postexposure prophylaxis.

Specifics of postexposure prophylaxis depend on the extent of the exposure and the potential HIV levels in the source (Table 105–30). Recommended prophylaxis for occupational HIV exposures for which there is a recognized transmission risk is with ZDV (600 mg/day: 300 mg twice daily orally, 200 mg three times a day orally, or 100 mg every 4 hours) and lamivudine (150 mg twice a day orally), both for 4 weeks (Table 105–31). Prophylaxis for occupational HIV exposures that pose an increased risk of transmission (e.g., large-bore hollow needle, deep puncture, visible blood on device or needle) is the basic regimen plus either indinavir (800 mg every 8 hours) or nelfinavir (750 mg three times a day), also for 4 weeks. The necessity of postexposure prophylaxis should be considered on an individual basis. Advice after the use of postexposure prophylaxis and the latest information is available through the National Clinicians' Post-Exposure Prophylaxis Hotline (telephone: 888-448-4911).

Prophylaxis may be considered after potential HIV exposure from sexual activity or injection drug use. The probability of HIV transmission by certain sexual acts is about the same magnitude as percutaneous occupational exposures. Rough estimates of probabilities for HIV transmission based on exposure include 0.3% after needle-stick injuries in health care workers, 0.1–0.3% after receptive anal sex, and 0.08–0.2% after receptive vaginal sex. For adults with recurring exposures, postexposure prophylaxis is controversial because of complications, costs, and concerns of drug resistance. Prophylaxis is increasingly offered to adults after a single potential exposure, such as a sexual assault event, although there is not yet any evidence that this measure is effective.

Presentation of children after proven or suspected sexual abuse often raises consideration for postexposure prophylaxis. Most child abusers are not HIV infected, most sexual acts do not transmit HIV, and most victims of child sexual abuse do not receive medical care soon after the event. However, there will be rare occasions when physicians caring for children who have been sexually assaulted should consider the extremely unlikely but devastating potential of HIV transmission. When indicated, two or three antiviral agents, as for occupational postexposure prophylaxis, should be used (Table 105–31). Postexposure prophylaxis is unlikely to have any effect if started beyond 36 hours after a sexual assault. Postexposure prophylaxis should be stopped if the perpetrator is identified and shown to be uninfected. There is no evidence that postexposure prophylaxis is effective in preventing HIV transmission after sexual exposure.

REVIEWS

Centers for Disease Control and Prevention: 1994 Revised classification system for HIV infection in children less than 13 years of age. *MMWR Morb Mortal Wkly Rep* 1994;43(RR-12):1–10.

Centers for Disease Control and Prevention: U.S. Public Health Service recommendations for human immunodeficiency virus counseling and voluntary testing for pregnant women. *MMWR Morb Mortal Wkly Rep* 1995;44(RR-7):1–15.

Centers for Disease Control and Prevention: Public Health Service Task Force recommendations for the use of antiretroviral drugs in pregnant women infected with HIV-1 for maternal health and for reducing perinatal HIV-1 transmission in the United States. *MMWR Morb Mortal Wkly Rep* 1998;47(RR-2):1–30.

Centers for Disease Control and Prevention: Guidelines for the use of antiretroviral agents in pediatric HIV infection. *MMWR Morb Mortal Wkly Rep* 1998;47(RR-4):1–43.

Centers for Disease Control and Prevention: Guidelines for the use of antiretroviral agents in HIV-infected adults and adolescents. *MMWR Morb Mortal Wkly Rep* 1998;47(RR-5):43–82.

Centers for Disease Control and Prevention: Management of possible sexual, injecting-drug-use, or other nonoccupational exposure to HIV, including considerations related to antiretroviral therapy. Public Health Service statement. *MMWR Morb Mortal Wkly Rep* 1998;47(RR-17):1–14.

Centers for Disease Control and Prevention: Guidelines for national human immunodeficiency virus case surveillance, including monitoring for human immunodeficiency virus infection and acquired immunodeficiency syndrome. *MMWR Morb Mortal Wkly Rep* 1999;48(RR-13):1–27.

Centers for Disease Control and Prevention: Surveillance for AIDS-defining opportunistic illnesses, 1992–1997. *MMWR Morb Mortal Wkly Rep* 1999;48(SS-2):1–22.

Centers for Disease Control and Prevention: Updated U.S. Public Health Service guidelines for the management of occupational exposures to HBV, HCV, and HIV and recommendations for postexposure prophylaxis. *MMWR Morb Mortal Wkly Rep* 2001;50(RR-11):1–42.

Committee on Pediatric AIDS: Evaluation and medical treatment of the HIV-exposed infant. *Pediatrics* 1997;99:909–17.

Dolin R, Masur H, Saag MS (editors): *AIDS Therapy.* Philadelphia, Churchill Livingstone, 1999.

National Pediatric and Family HIV Resource Center and National Center for Infectious Diseases, Centers for Disease Control and Prevention:

1995 Revised guidelines for prophylaxis against *Pneumocystis carinii* pneumonia for children infected with or perinatally exposed to human immunodeficiency virus. *MMWR Morb Mortal Wkly Rep* 1995; 44(RR-4):1–11.

Pizzo PA, Wilfert CM (editors): *Pediatric AIDS: The Challenge of HIV Infection in Infants, Children, and Adolescents,* 3rd ed. Baltimore, Williams & Wilkins, 1998.

U.S. Public Health Service (USPHS) and Infectious Diseases Society of America (IDSA): 1999 USPHS/IDSA guidelines for the prevention of opportunistic infections in persons infected with human immunodeficiency virus. *MMWR Morb Mortal Wkly Rep* 1999;48(RR-10):1–59.

Working Group on Antiretroviral Therapy and Medical Management of Infants, Children, and Adolescents with HIV Infection: Antiretroviral therapy and medical management of pediatric HIV infection. *Pediatrics* 1998;102:1005–56.

KEY ARTICLES

Aleixo LF, Goodenow MM, Sleasman JW: Zidovudine administered to women infected with human immunodeficiency virus type 1 and to their neonates reduces pediatric infection independent of an effect on levels of maternal virus. *J Pediatr* 1997;130:906–14.

American Academy of Pediatrics, Committee on Infectious Diseases and Committee on Pediatric AIDS: Measles immunization in HIV-infected children. *Pediatrics* 1999;103:1057–60.

American College of Obstetricians and Gynecologists: Joint statement of the American Academy of Pediatrics and the American College of Obstetricians and Gynecologists. *Pediatrics* 1999;104:128.

Andiman WA: Medical management of the pregnant woman infected with human immunodeficiency virus type 1 and her child. *Semin Perinatol* 1998;22:72–86.

Blanche S, Rouzioux C, Moscato ML, et al: A prospective study of infants born to women seropositive for human immunodeficiency virus type 1. HIV Infection in newborns. French Collaborative Study Group. *N Engl J Med* 1989;320:1643–8.

Bye MR: HIV in children. *Clin Chest Med* 1996;17:787–96.

Connor EM, Sperling RS, Gelber R, et al: Reduction of maternal-infant transmission of human immunodeficiency virus type 1 with zidovudine treatment. Pediatric AIDS Clinical Trials Group Protocol 076 Study Group. *N Engl J Med* 1994;331:1173–80.

Culnane M, Fowler M, Lee SS, et al: Lack of long-term effects of in utero exposure to zidovudine among uninfected children born to HIV-infected women. Pediatric AIDS Clinical Trials Group Protocol 219/076 Teams. *JAMA* 1999;281:151–7.

de Martino M, Tovo P-A, Balducci M, et al: Reduction in mortality with availability of antiretroviral therapy for children with perinatal HIV-1 infection. Italian Register for HIV Infection in Children and the Italian National AIDS Registry. *JAMA* 2000;284:190–7.

De Rossi A, Masiero S, Giaquinto C, et al: Dynamics of viral replication in infants with vertically acquired human immunodeficiency virus type 1 infection. *J Clin Invest* 1996;97:323–30.

Dunn DT, Newell ML, Ades AE, et al: Risk of human immunodeficiency virus type 1 transmission through breastfeeding. *Lancet* 1992;340:585–8.

Griffith BP, Booss J: Neurologic infections of the fetus and newborn. *Neurol Clin* 1994;12:541–64.

Guay LA, Musoke P, Fleming T, et al: Intrapartum and neonatal single-dose nevirapine compared with zidovudine for prevention of mother-to-child transmission of HIV-1 in Kampala, Uganda: HIVNET 012 randomised trial. *Lancet* 1999;354:795–802.

Johann-Liang R, Cervia JS, Noel GJ: Characteristics of human immunodeficiency virus-infected children at the time of death: An experience in the 1990s. *Pediatr Infect Dis J* 1997;16:1145–50.

Katz BZ, Berkman AB, Shapiro ED: Serologic evidence of active Epstein-Barr virus infection in Epstein-Barr virus associated lymphoproliferative disorders of children with acquired immunodeficiency syndrome. *J Pediatr* 1992;120:228–32.

Kind C, Rudin C, Siegrist CA, et al: Prevention of vertical HIV transmission: Additive protective effect of elective Cesarean section and zidovudine prophylaxis. Swiss Neonatal HIV Study Group. *AIDS* 1998;12:205–10.

Kline MW, Lewis DE, Hollinger FB, et al: A comparative study of human immunodeficiency virus culture, polymerase chain reaction and anti-human immunodeficiency virus immunoglobulin A antibody detection in the diagnosis during early infancy of vertically acquired immunodeficiency virus infection. *Pediatr Infect Dis J* 1994;13:90–4.

Lacaille F, Fournet JC, Blanche S: Clinical utility of liver biopsy in children with acquired immunodeficiency syndrome. *Pediatr Infect Dis J* 1999;18:143–7.

Lee LM, Karon JM, Selik R, et al: Survival after AIDS diagnosis in adolescents and adults during the treatment era, United States, 1984–1997. *JAMA* 2001;285:1308–15.

Lindegren ML, Byers RH Jr, Thomas P, et al: Trends in perinatal transmission of HIV/AIDS in the United States. *JAMA* 1999;282:531–8.

Lobato MN, Caldwell MB, Ng P, et al: Encephalopathy in children with perinatally acquired human immunodeficiency virus infection. Pediatric Spectrum of Disease Clinical Consortium. *J Pediatr* 1995;126:710–5.

Mandelbrot L, Le Chenadec J, Berrebi A, et al: Perinatal HIV-1 transmission: Interaction between zidovudine prophylaxis and mode of delivery in the French Perinatal Cohort. *JAMA* 1998;280:55–60.

Matheson PB, Abrams EJ, Thomas PA, et al: Efficacy of antenatal zidovudine in reducing perinatal transmission of human immunodeficiency virus type 1. The New York City Perinatal HIV Transmission Collaborative Study Group. *J Infect Dis* 1995;172:353–8.

Mayaux MJ, Burgard M, Teglas JP, et al: Neonatal characteristics in rapidly progressive perinatally acquired HIV-1 disease. The French Pediatric HIV Infection Study Group. *JAMA* 1996;275:606–10.

McIntosh K, Shevitz A, Zaknun D, et al: Age- and time-related changes in extracellular viral load in children vertically infected by human immunodeficiency virus. *Pediatr Infect Dis J* 1996;15:1087–91.

Miotti PG, Taha TE, Kumwenda NI, et al: HIV transmission through breastfeeding: A study in Malawi. *JAMA* 1999;282:744–9.

Mofenson LM, Yogev R, Korelitz J, et al: Characteristics of acute pneumonia in human immunodeficiency virus–infected children and association with long-term mortality risk. National Institute of Child Health and Human Development Intravenous Immunoglobulin Clinical Trial Study Group. *Pediatr Infect Dis J* 1998;17:872–80.

Nishanian P, Huskins KR, Stehn S, et al: A simple method for improved assay demonstrates that HIV p24 antigen is present as immune complexes in most sera from HIV-infected individuals. *J Infect Dis* 1990;162:21–8.

Owens DK, Holodniy M, McDonald TW, et al: A meta-analytic evaluation of the polymerase chain reaction for the diagnosis of HIV infection in infants. *JAMA* 1996;275:1342–8.

Shaffer N, Bulterys M, Simonds RJ: Short courses of zidovudine and perinatal transmission of HIV. *N Engl J Med* 1999;340:1042–3.

Shaffer N, Chuachoowong R, Mock PA, et al: Short-course zidovudine for perinatal HIV-1 transmission in Bangkok, Thailand: A randomised controlled trial. Bangkok Collaborative Perinatal HIV Transmission Study Group. *Lancet* 1999;353:773–80.

Shearer WT, Quinn TC, LaRussa P, et al: Viral load and disease progression in infants infected with human immunodeficiency virus type 1. Women and Infants Transmission Study Group. *N Engl J Med* 1997;336: 1337–42.

Simonds RJ, Lindegren ML, Thomas P, et al: Prophylaxis against *Pneumocystis carinii* pneumonia among children with perinatally acquired human immunodeficiency virus infection in the United States. *Pneumocystis carinii* Pneumonia Prophylaxis Evaluation Working Group. *N Engl J Med* 1995;332:786–90.

Simpson BJ, Shapiro ED, Andiman WA: Reduction in the risk of vertical transmission of HIV-1 associated with treatment of pregnant women with orally administered zidovudine alone. *J Acquir Immune Defic Syndr Hum Retrovirol* 1997;14:145–52.

Sleasman JW, Hemenway C, Klein AS, et al: Corticosteroids improve survival of children with AIDS and *Pneumocystis carinii* pneumonia. *Am J Dis Child* 1993;147:30–4.

Sperling RS, Shapiro DE, Coombs RW, et al: Maternal viral load, zidovudine treatment, and the risk of transmission of human immunodeficiency virus type 1 from mother to infant. Pediatric AIDS Clinical Trials Group Protocol 076 Study Group. *N Engl J Med* 1996;335:1621–9.

Srugo I, Israele V, Wittek AE, et al: Clinical manifestations of varicella-zoster virus infections in human immunodeficiency virus–infected children. *Am J Dis Child* 1993;147:742–5.

Steketee RW, Abrams EJ, Thea DM, et al: Early detection of perinatal human immunodeficiency virus (HIV) type 1 infection using HIV RNA amplification and detection. New York City Perinatal HIV Transmission Collaborative Study. *J Infect Dis* 1997;175:707–11.

Tardieu M, Le Chenadec J, Persoz A, et al: HIV-1-related encephalopathy in infants compared with children and adults. French Pediatric HIV Infection Study and the SEROCO Group. *Neurology* 2000; 54:1089–95.

The European Collaborative Study: Caesarean section and risk of vertical transmission of HIV-1 infection. *Lancet* 1994;343:1464–7.

The International Perinatal HIV Group: The mode of delivery and the risk of vertical transmission of human immunodeficiency virus type 1—a meta-analysis of 15 prospective cohort studies. The International Perinatal HIV Group. *N Engl J Med* 1999;340:977–87.

Thea DM, Lambert G, Weedon J, et al: Benefit of primary prophylaxis before 18 months of age in reducing the incidence of *Pneumocystis carinii* pneumonia and early death in a cohort of 112 human immunodeficiency virus–infected infants. New York City Perinatal HIV Transmission Collaborative Study Group. *Pediatrics* 1996;97:59–64.

Wade NA, Birkhead GS, Warren BL, et al: Abbreviated regimens of zidovudine prophylaxis and perinatal transmission of the human immunodeficiency virus. *N Engl J Med* 1998;339:1409–14.

Wiktor SZ, Ekpini E, Karon JM, et al: Short-course oral zidovudine for prevention of mother-to-child transmission of HIV-1 in Abidjan, Côte d'Ivoire: A randomised trial. *Lancet* 1999;353:781–5.

Working Group on Antiretroviral Therapy, National Pediatric HIV Resource Center: Antiretroviral therapy and medical management of the human immunodeficiency virus–infected child. *Pediatr Infect Dis J* 1993; 12:513–22.

CHAPTER 39

Kawasaki Syndrome

Anne H. Rowley ▪ Stanford T. Shulman

Kawasaki syndrome (KS) was first described in 1967 by Dr. Tomisaku Kawasaki in the Japanese-language medical literature. Kawasaki reported his experience with 50 children who manifested a distinctive clinical illness characterized by fever, rash, conjunctival injection, enanthem, redness and swelling of the hands and feet, and cervical lymphadenitis. KS was originally termed **mucocutaneous lymph node syndrome** and was believed to be a benign childhood illness. However, by late 1970 as many as 10 fatal cases of this illness had occurred in Japan, all in children under 2 years of age, usually when they appeared to be improving or recovered. In general, autopsy revealed complete occlusion of coronary artery aneurysms by thrombus, with resultant myocardial infarction.

The original English-language report by Kawasaki and coworkers in 1974 was followed in 1976 by that of Melish and coworkers, who described the same illness in 16 children in Hawaii. Melish had independently developed the same diagnostic criteria for KS in the early 1970s before learning of the Japanese reports of the illness. Echocardiography, which became available about 1979, has shown that approximately 20–25% of untreated patients with KS develop cardiovascular sequelae, with severity ranging from asymptomatic coronary artery ectasia or aneurysm formation to giant coronary artery aneurysms with the potential for rupture, thrombosis, myocardial infarction, and sudden death.

More than 150,000 cases of KS have been recognized in Japan through the end of 1998. KS now appears to have replaced acute rheumatic fever as the leading cause of acquired heart disease in children, both in the United States and elsewhere in the developed world.

ETIOLOGY

The etiology of KS remains unknown. Many striking clinical manifestations, such as the acute onset of a self-limited illness, and the epidemiologic characteristics of age distribution, seasonal peaks in winter and spring, and well-documented epidemics superimposed on an endemic incidence support an infectious cause. Conventional bacterial and viral cultures, as well as extensive serologic investigations, have failed to identify an infectious agent. Isolation of toxic shock syndrome toxin (TSST-1)–producing *Staphylococcus aureus* from KS patients more frequently than from controls has not been confirmed.

EPIDEMIOLOGY

KS is almost exclusively an illness of young children. Approximately 80% of the patients are less than 5 years of age, and only 2–3% of the cases occur after the age of 8 years. Occasional reports of acute KS in adults have been published, although in retrospect, many such early reports appear to have represented patients with toxic shock syndrome. However, documented cases of ischemic heart disease that appears to be the sequela of undiagnosed KS in childhood occur in teenagers and young adults. KS occurs worldwide and affects children of all races, with Asians (particularly Japanese and Koreans) at highest risk and white children apparently at lowest risk.

Because of striking racial differences in the incidence of KS, genetic factors have been investigated. Human leukocyte antigen (HLA) typing studies have yielded conflicting data but do not support an association of the disease with specific HLA types. In studies of immunoglobulin allotypes as possible genetic markers for KS, differences have been found between both white and Japanese patients with KS and appropriate race-matched controls with respect to allotypic frequencies. This suggests a genetic influence on an immune-mediated pathogenesis.

Little evidence of person-to-person spread of KS exists. However, a study (Fujita et al., 1989) of Japanese children with KS revealed that the risk that a second case will develop in a family within 1 year after onset of the first case was significantly higher (2.1%) than the risk for the general population of age-matched children (0.19%). In addition, 54% of the second cases developed within 10 days after the first case; the illness commonly appears on the same date in sets of twins who develop KS. These findings suggest that KS follows exposure to an infectious agent in genetically predisposed persons.

Japan. Epidemiologic studies in Japan have demonstrated no rural versus urban, geographic, or altitude-related differences in prevalence of KS. The number of cases increases in the late winter and spring. In Japan the peak age of patients with KS is 6–12 months; equal numbers of cases occur during the first and second years of life. Virtually every study has yielded a male-to-female ratio of approximately 1.5:1.

The incidence of KS in Japan increased from 1967 to the mid-1980s, apparently as a result of both improved recognition and an actual increase in incidence and has now plateaued at approximately 6,000 cases per year. The endemic annual incidence in Japan is about 105 cases per 100,000 children <5 years of age. Three nationwide epidemics of KS occurred in Japan in 1979, 1982, and late 1985 to early 1986. A wavelike spread of cases, which resembles that observed with known viral illnesses, has been noted during epidemics.

United States and Europe. The peak age of patients with KS is 8–24 months, greater than it is in Japan, with approximately 80% of cases in children <5 years of age. Cases peak in late winter and spring. Nationwide epidemics have not been observed. Clusters of cases have been reported from Hawaii (1978); Rochester, New York (1979); Finland (1981–1982); 10 areas of the United States between August 1984 and January 1985; Los Angeles (December 1985); and Denver (1997–1998). Investigations of these outbreaks showed that KS occurred most commonly in children of middle and upper socioeconomic status. National surveys have indicated that approximately 3,000–3,500 cases of KS occur annually in the United States.

The annual incidence in the United States is approximately 10 cases per 100,000 children <5 years of age, with the lowest incidence in white children, intermediate incidence in black children, and the highest incidence among children of Asian ethnicity, particularly Japanese and Korean. During outbreaks, the incidence may rise two- to tenfold. An association with exposure to recently shampooed carpets has been inconsistent in several studies of risk factors for KS. Another possible risk factor for KS is residence within 200 yards of a body of water, but this also has been an inconsistent finding.

TABLE 39–1. Associated Noncardiac Features of Kawasaki Syndrome

Extreme irritability, especially in infants
Arthralgia, arthritis
Aseptic meningitis
Hepatic dysfunction
Hydrops of the gallbladder
Diarrhea
Otitis media
Uveitis
Pneumonitis, mild; radiologically but not clinically apparent
Erythema and induration at site of BCG inoculation (rare in the United States, common in Japan)

PATHOGENESIS

In acute KS, inflammatory cells infiltrate the vascular wall, particularly of the coronary arteries. These cells include macrophages, monocytes, and lymphocytes, particularly CD8 T cells. Plasma cells, predominantly those producing IgA, also infiltrate the vascular wall in acute KS. The presence of IgA plasma cells in a nonmucosal, nonlymphoid site in the vascular wall is a new finding with important implications for the immunopathogenesis of KS. It suggests that the etiologic agent of KS enters via a mucosal portal of entry, antigen is processed in the gut or bronchus-associated lymphoid tissues, and B cells switch to IgA production and then enter the general circulation. IgA B cells then may enter the vascular tissue and terminally differentiate into plasma cells. An increase in IgA plasma cells in the respiratory tracts of children with acute KS, when compared with controls, is consistent with the hypothesis of a respiratory portal of entry of the pathogen. Other sites of IgA plasma cell infiltration in acute KS tissues include kidney and pancreas but not liver parenchyma or thyroid. Data indicate that the IgA produced in the vascular wall is oligoclonal, suggesting an antigen-driven immune response directed at epitopes of an etiologic agent.

Thus the epidemiologic features and clinical findings of KS suggest that this illness may be caused by an infectious agent that is likely to be entering the host via the respiratory route and may lead to a predominantly IgA immune-mediated syndrome in some genetically predisposed persons. Interest continues in a putative superantigen (Fig. 5–7) from an infectious agent as the cause of KS, but data at present are inconclusive.

SYMPTOMS AND CLINICAL MANIFESTATIONS

The course of KS can be divided into three clinical phases. The acute febrile phase, which usually lasts 7–14 days, is characterized by fever, conjunctival injection, mouth and lip changes, swelling and erythema of the hands and feet, rash, lymphadenopathy, aseptic meningitis, diarrhea, and hepatic dysfunction. In the subacute phase, which typically occurs from approximately day 10 to day 25 after the onset of illness, the fever, rash, and lymphadenopathy resolve, but irritability, anorexia, and conjunctival injection usually persist. Desquamation of the fingers and toes, arthritis and arthralgia, myocardial dysfunction, and thrombocytosis are seen during the subacute phase. The convalescent phase begins when all clinical signs of illness have disappeared and continues until the ESR returns to normal, usually 6–8 weeks after the onset of illness.

Occasionally a clinical rebound occurs with recurrence of fever and at least one other acute clinical sign, such as rash or conjunctival injection, after such signs have appeared to resolve. This occurs most often within a few days or weeks of onset of illness and is associated with an increased risk of coronary artery disease. KS has been reported to recur in 3% of Japanese and 1–2% of U.S. children with KS.

Several noncardiac manifestations may be present with acute KS (Table 39–1). Cardiac disease is the major complication of KS and occurs in about 20–25% of untreated patients.

Physical Examination Findings

Fever. Fever in the patient with KS is generally high (usually ≥40°C [104°F]), remittent, and prolonged. The duration of fever is usually 1–2 weeks in untreated patients, although it commonly resolves within 4–5 days after the administration of aspirin in doses of 50–100 mg/kg/day. Fever resolves much more promptly with intravenous immune globulin (IVIG) administration in addition to aspirin.

Conjunctival Injection. Nonsuppurative conjunctival injection, which is characteristic of KS, involves the bulbar conjunctivae much more severely than the palpebral or tarsal conjunctivae and is not generally associated with exudate. It usually begins shortly after the onset of fever and generally persists for 1–2 weeks in patients who are not treated with IVIG. Conjunctival injection may improve significantly almost immediately after IVIG treatment, although mild conjunctival injection may last for 1–2 additional weeks.

Oral Findings. Changes in the mouth are characterized by erythema; dryness, fissuring, peeling, and bleeding of the lips (Plate 5F); erythema of the oropharyngeal mucosa; strawberry tongue with diffuse erythema and prominent papillae (Fig. 39–1); and absence of oral or lingual ulcerations.

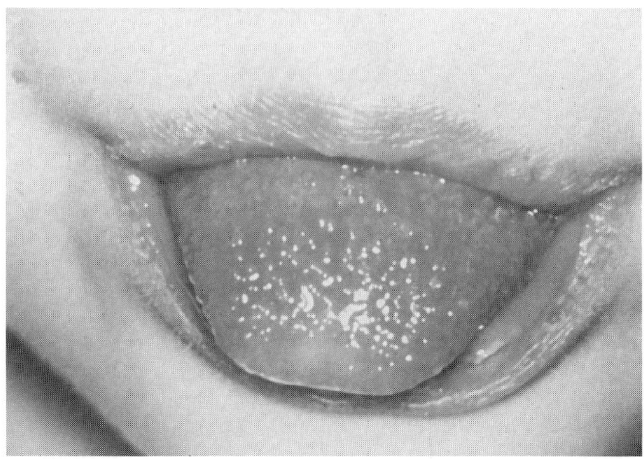

FIGURE 39–1. Strawberry tongue with prominent papillae in Kawasaki syndrome.

Peripheral Findings. The findings on the hands and feet are distinctive. Erythema of the palms and soles or firm induration of the hands and feet occurs. Induration may limit fine motor movements and be sufficiently painful to result in refusal to bear weight. **Desquamation** of the fingers and toes, which begins in the periungual region, may extend to involve the palms and soles as well (Fig. 39–2). The desquamation is not seen in the first week of illness but is characteristically noted 10–20 days after the onset of fever. Approximately 1–2 months after the illness begins, deep, transverse grooves across the nails **(Beau's lines)** may appear. These subsequently grow out with the nail, although occasionally some nails are shed.

Rash. The rash of KS, which usually appears within 5 days after onset of fever, may take many forms: an urticarial exanthem with large erythematous plaques; a morbilliform, maculopapular rash; an erythema multiforme-like rash with target lesions; a scarlatiniform erythroderma; or, rarely, a fine and micropustular rash (Plate 5E). Involvement of the trunk and extremities is usually extensive. Perineal accentuation may occur. Bullae and vesicles are not seen. Desquamation may occur in the perineal region during the acute phase.

Lymphadenopathy. Cervical lymphadenopathy occurs in 50–75% of patients with KS. At least one lymph node must be >1.5 cm in diameter to meet the diagnostic criteria. Affected lymph nodes, which may be unilateral or bilateral, are firm and somewhat tender. They may have overlying erythema but are nonfluctuant, do not yield pus when aspirated, and do not yield bacterial or viral growth when cultured by standard techniques.

The conjunctival injection, extremity changes, erythematous lips, and rash manifested by some patients are often overlooked in the face of severe cervical lymphadenitis. A study (Stamos et al., 1994) reported several patients, usually more than 3 years of age, in whom cervical lymphadenopathy was the most striking clinical symptom of KS, resulting in a delay in diagnosis. In patients with cervical lymphadenitis, particularly if it is not responding to antibiotic therapy, other clinical signs of KS should be sought.

Other Findings. Striking **irritability** of a much greater degree than that commonly observed in other febrile illnesses, particularly among younger patients, is typical in patients with KS. Infants, particularly those less than 6 months of age, quite frequently do not exhibit all the diagnostic signs of KS when they present with the illness, and a particularly high index of suspicion is necessary to establish the diagnosis in these children. Unfortunately, these younger infants with KS are at the highest risk of developing coronary artery abnormalities. Early diagnosis of acute KS and institution of appropriate therapy are particularly important in this age group.

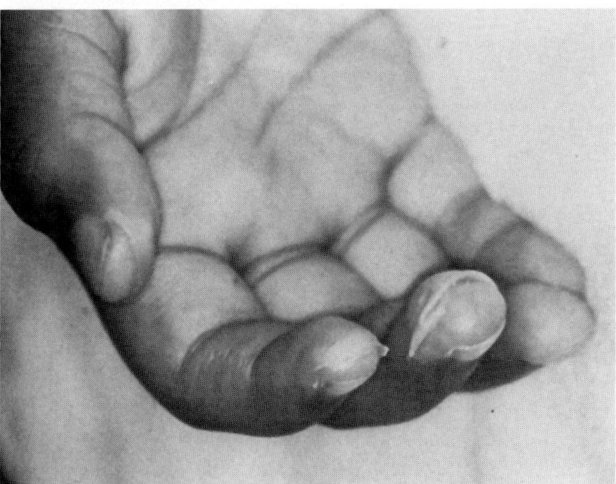

FIGURE 39–2. Periungual desquamation of the fingertips during the subacute stage of Kawasaki syndrome.

Associated features of KS include arthritis and arthralgia, which are seen in approximately 30% of patients not treated with IVIG and in about 10% of those who receive IVIG and aspirin. These patients are somewhat more likely to be older and to be girls. Onset of joint symptoms peaks around day 7 of illness, but such symptoms may develop as late as 3 weeks after onset of the disease. Polyarticular involvement is common, with knees and ankles most frequently involved. Synovial fluid WBC concentrations range from several thousand to more than 75,000/mm^3. Arthritis typically responds to nonsteroidal agents and persists up to 2 weeks. Patients with KS do not develop chronic arthritis.

Evidence of aseptic meningitis is found in at least one fourth of patients with KS who have lumbar puncture, with CSF WBC concentrations averaging 25–100/mm^3 with a lymphocytic predominance. The glucose and protein values are generally normal. Hepatic dysfunction with mild obstructive jaundice and mildly to moderately elevated levels of serum transaminases is seen occasionally. Acute, noncalculous distention of the gallbladder (hydrops of the gallbladder) commonly occurs in patients with KS, who present with a mass in the right upper quadrant or guarding in the first 2 weeks of illness. This resolves without surgical intervention.

Unusual Presentations

Atypical (or incomplete) KS, which refers to children who have fever and fewer than four other diagnostic criteria for KS, is recognized with increasing frequency and has been identified worldwide. It is characteristically seen in young infants, an age group in which the diagnosis of KS is particularly difficult. This form of illness may be more serious. Children with atypical presentations may develop severe coronary disease leading to myocardial infarction, aneurysm rupture, and sudden death. In general, atypical cases appear to have a laboratory profile similar to that of typical cases. Children with a prolonged febrile illness of unexplained cause who develop subsequent peripheral desquamation should be considered for echocardiography to identify any coronary abnormalities. Ultimately, accurate identification of all cases of KS will require identification of the etiologic agent and the development of a diagnostic test.

DIAGNOSIS

In the absence of a diagnostic test for KS, the diagnosis is established by the presence of fever and at least four of five other principal clinical criteria without other explanation for the illness (Table 39–2). Each of the diagnostic criteria is observed in about 90% of classic (or typical) cases with the exception of cervical lymphadenopathy, which is present in about 75% of cases.

Differential Diagnosis

The differential diagnosis of KS includes several infectious and noninfectious diseases (Table 39–3).

Laboratory Evaluation

Laboratory findings in patients with KS are nonspecific and nondiagnostic. However, certain findings are quite characteristic, including a moderate to marked leukocytosis with a predominance of neutrophils in the acute phase. Elevation of the ESR and other acute-phase reactants in the acute phase and persisting for 6–8

TABLE 39–2. Diagnostic Criteria for Kawasaki Syndrome

A. Fever of at least 5 days' duration*
B. Presence of *four* of the following *five* conditions:
   1. Bilateral conjunctival injection
   2. Changes of the mucosa of the oropharynx, including injected pharynx; injected or dry, fissured lips; strawberry tongue
   3. Changes of the peripheral extremities, such as edema or erythema of hands, feet, or both; desquamation, usually beginning periungually
   4. Rash, primarily truncal; polymorphous but nonvesicular
   5. Cervical lymphadenopathy
C. Illness not explained by other known disease process

*Many experts believe that in the presence of classic features of KS, the diagnosis can be made and treatment instituted by experienced persons before the fifth day of fever.

weeks is almost universal and can be very helpful in distinguishing KS from uncomplicated viral illnesses and drug reactions. A mild to moderate normochromic normocytic anemia is common, as are mild elevations of the transaminases. The platelet count, which is generally normal in the first week of illness, begins to rise in the second week, peaking at about 3 weeks at a mean count of 800,000/mm^3, although it may rise to as high as 2,000,000/mm^3. Antinuclear antibody and rheumatoid factor are not detectable. Sterile pyuria occurs in about 35% of patients and may be intermittent. Ultrasonography is useful in the evaluation of gallbladder hydrops.

Echocardiography

A baseline echocardiogram should be obtained at initial diagnosis, at 1–2 weeks, and at 6–8 weeks, even if the initial studies are unremarkable. Additional studies are unnecessary if all three echocardiograms are normal. Additional studies and cardiology consultation are needed if abnormalities are present on any of the three echocardiograms.

TREATMENT

Acute Phase. Therapy during the acute phase of illness is aimed at reducing inflammation in the myocardium and in the coronary artery wall (thus preventing coronary aneurysm formation) and preventing thrombosis by inhibiting platelet aggregation (Table 39–4). Discovery of the etiologic agent of KS will allow for more specific treatment.

Aspirin at high doses (80–100 mg/kg/day) is used to reduce inflammation in the acute phase of KS. Aspirin in combination with IVIG results in a more rapid anti-inflammatory effect than does aspirin alone. High-dose aspirin is usually reduced to low-dose aspirin (3–5 mg/kg/day) on day 14 of illness; this provides antithrombotic effects that are important in the subacute and convalescent phases of KS. Aspirin is discontinued after the ESR becomes normal and echocardiography at 6–8 weeks after the onset of illness detects no cardiac abnormalities. If the patient develops an illness suspected of being varicella or influenza, aspirin therapy may be interrupted to reduce the risk of Reye's syndrome. In patients at particularly high risk of myocardial infarction, the use of an alternative antiplatelet agent should be considered.

TABLE 39–3. Differential Diagnosis of Kawasaki Syndrome

Toxic shock syndrome
Scarlet fever
Leptospirosis
Rocky Mountain spotted fever
Measles
Stevens-Johnson syndrome
Drug reactions
Juvenile rheumatoid arthritis
Mercury poisoning

TABLE 39–4. Current Recommended Therapy for Kawasaki Syndrome

Acute Stage
- Aspirin, 80–100 mg/kg/day in 4 divided doses until about illness day 14
- Intravenous immune globulin, 2 g/kg as a single dose given over 12 hr

Convalescent Stage (after illness day 14 in afebrile patient)
- Aspirin, 3–5 mg/kg/day in single dose; discontinue 6–8 weeks after onset of illness after the ESR becomes normal and verifying by echocardiography that no coronary abnormalities are present

Chronic Therapy for Patients with Coronary Abnormalities
- Aspirin, 3–5 mg/kg/day in single dose; possible addition of dipyrimadole in selected patients deemed to be at high risk
- Some physicians use coumadin or heparin together with antiplatelet therapy in patients with particularly severe coronary findings or past evidence of coronary thrombosis

Acute Coronary Thrombosis
- Prompt fibrinolytic therapy with streptokinase, urokinase, or tissue plasminogen activator should be initiated at a tertiary care center under the supervision of a cardiologist

High-dose IVIG (2 g/kg administered as a 10- to 12-hour infusion) with aspirin is the treatment of choice for patients with KS and should be administered as soon as possible after diagnosis. This treatment has been shown to be effective when given within the first 10 days of illness, but optimally it should be administered as soon as possible. High-dose IVIG therapy with aspirin reduces the incidence of coronary artery abnormalities from 20–25% in patients treated with aspirin alone to 5% in patients who receive IVIG with aspirin. Treatment with both IVIG and aspirin not only reduces the prevalence of coronary disease but also results in significantly more rapid resolution of fever and normalization of acute-phase reactants and myocardial function when compared with treatment with aspirin alone. IVIG reduces the incidence of long-term coronary abnormalities and giant coronary artery aneurysms. In patients who develop coronary aneurysms despite IVIG, abnormalities appear more likely to resolve than in those who never receive this therapy. Doses of IVIG less than 2 g/kg appear to be less effective. The mechanism of action of IVIG in KS is unknown.

About 10% of patients with acute KS have persistent fever 3 days after completion of the IVIG infusion. In addition, some patients demonstrate initial defervescence but then develop recurrent fever after being afebrile for 24 hours or more. In both of these circumstances, referral to a center with substantial experience in the diagnosis and treatment of KS should be considered. Retreatment of these patients with a second dose of IVIG (2 g/kg) should be considered. Although the efficacy of IVIG after 10 days of illness has not been studied, IVIG should be strongly considered for a patient with KS who presents after 10 days of illness and is still febrile.

Although data from Japan from the 1970s and 1980s suggested that corticosteroids worsen coronary disease in KS when given as primary therapy, there has been renewed interest in the possible use of high-dose intravenous corticosteroid therapy in patients who do not respond to one or more infusions of IVIG. A study (Wright et al., 1996) reported that three of four patients with KS who had not responded to multiple doses of IVIG had resolution of fever after the administration of high-dose (30 mg/kg/day) intravenous methylprednisolone for 1–3 days. Further study is needed before corticosteroid therapy can be recommended. Consultation with a physician who has had considerable experience with the treatment of KS is recommended before corticosteroid therapy is offered.

The routine administration of live virus vaccines (MMR and varicella vaccines) should be delayed after IVIG treatment for KS (Table 17–20). Schedules for administration of other routine childhood vaccinations do not need to be interrupted.

Convalescent Phase. Patients with KS should undergo periodic physical examinations and CBC counts, determinations of ESR, and platelet counts until these values return to normal. Coronary aneurysms are likely to be first apparent 2–3 weeks after onset of illness. If the results of echocardiography are normal during the third week, the test can be repeated approximately 1–2 months later. If this third study also fails to demonstrate an abnormality and if the ESR and platelet count have returned to normal, aspirin can be discontinued. The development of aneurysms after 6 weeks of illness is extremely unusual unless clinical evidence of inflammation persists.

If the echocardiogram is abnormal during the subacute or convalescent stage of illness, aspirin is continued and echocardiography is repeated. Low-dose aspirin should be continued indefinitely even if aneurysms resolve, because data from intracoronary ultrasonographic studies demonstrate that a regressed aneurysm is not a normal blood vessel.

For patients with persistent small solitary aneurysms, long-term, low-dose aspirin should be administered. No restriction of physical activities is necessary for these patients and for those in whom coronary artery abnormalities have resolved. However, stress echocardiography should be considered for these patients, and coronary angiography may be indicated if stress testing, echocardiographic results, or clinical features suggest myocardial ischemia. If myocardial ischemia is suspected or proven, physical activities should be limited accordingly.

Patients with large or multiple coronary aneurysms without obstruction should receive long-term therapy with antiplatelet drugs (aspirin with or without dipyridamole). Some experts recommend additional anticoagulant therapy (heparin or warfarin). Activity restriction should be based on stress test results and degree of anticoagulation. Close cardiac follow-up, including yearly stress testing and angiography as indicated, is necessary. Thallium scintigraphy with exercise is useful in identifying patients with ischemia or old infarctions that did not exhibit ECG changes during exercise.

Patients with KS who develop obstructive changes in one or more coronary arteries present a difficult management problem. The obstruction may be the result of thrombosis or stenosis, or both, of the vessel secondary to intimal proliferation and fibrosis. Some patients with small thrombi can be managed with oral anticoagulant therapy alone. Intracoronary or intravenous thrombolytic therapy has been used with varying degrees of efficacy in selected patients with significant acute thrombosis. Experience with percutaneous transluminal coronary angioplasty to correct obstruction in KS is limited and has been complicated by intimal tears and neoaneurysm formation.

Coronary bypass has been used for obstructed coronary arteries. A review (Kitamura et al., 1994) of the Japanese multicenter experience of 170 patients with KS who underwent coronary bypass grafting from 1975–1990 found that two early and eight late deaths occurred; 141 of 170 patients (83%) were considered to have good operative results. The graft patency rate at 3 years or later was 46% for saphenous vein grafts and 77% for internal mammary or gastroepiploic artery grafts. Patency of saphenous vein grafts was particularly poor in patients younger than 8 years of age; such grafts should be avoided. Arterial grafts, such as those involving the internal thoracic and gastroepiploic arteries, grow in length and diameter as the patient grows.

COMPLICATIONS

KS was initially believed to be a benign childhood illness. Soon after Kawasaki's initial report, however, it became apparent that several children with KS died suddenly and unexpectedly, usually during the third or fourth week after onset of illness, when they appeared to be recovering. Death usually resulted from massive myocardial infarction secondary to coronary artery thrombosis in areas of previous coronary aneurysm or stenosis or occasionally from rupture of a giant coronary aneurysm.

Cardiac. Echocardiographic and angiocardiographic data have shown that approximately 20–25% of untreated patients with KS develop coronary artery abnormalities, including aneurysms. Although initial reports indicated a 1–2% fatality rate, more recent data from Japan document fatality rates as low as 0.08%. This is a consequence of improved therapy and recognition of milder cases.

Two-dimensional transthoracic echocardiography should be used routinely to detect and follow coronary artery changes in patients with KS. Angiography is reserved for selected patients with more severe echocardiographic abnormalities or ischemic features. Echocardiography detects more than 90% of aneurysms detected by angiography. Echocardiography gives a better view of the proximal portions of the coronary arteries than of the distal portions; aneurysms most often arise proximally.

The earliest cardiac complications occur within the first 10 days of illness and include myocarditis, occasionally with congestive failure manifested by severe tachycardia and gallop rhythm or rarely frank cardiogenic shock or arrhythmias; pericarditis with pericardial effusion; and mitral or aortic insufficiency. Electrocardiographic changes such as flattening and depression of the ST segment, flattening or inversion of the T wave, decreased voltage, and conduction disturbances such as heart block may be seen. Over the next 5 weeks, these findings generally resolve, but acute coronary arteritis during the first 2 weeks of illness may lead to the formation of coronary artery aneurysms.

Coronary dilatation is first detectable at a mean of 10 days after the onset of illness, and the peak frequency of coronary dilatation or aneurysms occurs within 4 weeks of onset. Ectasia of the coronary lumen may be seen earlier, but aneurysms usually form between the eighteenth and the twenty-fifth days. The development of new echocardiographic coronary abnormalities after 6 weeks is quite rare. Most deaths occur in the period from 2 to 12 weeks after the onset of illness. Death usually results from coronary thrombosis leading to myocardial infarction, from acute myocarditis, or, rarely, from rupture of a coronary aneurysm with resulting hemopericardium.

Aneurysmal changes of the coronary arteries may resolve or persist. The fate of coronary aneurysms in KS was well described by Kato et al. (1996). From 1 to 3 months after onset of KS, 25% of all patients with KS in this study had angiographic evidence of coronary aneurysms. Repeat angiography 1–2 years from onset in patients with abnormalities showed that about 50% of the aneurysms had resolved. Of those patients with persistent aneurysms, about 80% had aneurysms without stenosis and 20% had aneurysms with stenosis. Long-term follow-up 3–18 years after onset revealed that myocardial infarction occurred in 1.9% of all cases of KS, and 39% of patients with persistent aneurysms had stenosis. The fatality rate in these 598 cases diagnosed between 1973 and 1983 was 0.8%, and bypass surgery was performed in 1.2%. All episodes of myocardial infarction, all deaths, and all surgical bypasses in this long-term study occurred in patients who had coronary aneurysms with stenosis.

The availability of intracoronary ultrasonography has allowed assessment of coronary artery wall morphology in regressed aneurysms. These studies indicate that regressed aneurysms have a markedly thickened intima-media complex. Coronary reactivity to nitroglycerin in these vessels has been shown to be significantly lower than in normal vessels. Whether this predisposes to premature atherosclerosis is unclear.

Certain clinical factors appear to be predictive of increased risk of development of coronary artery disease and form the basis for several clinical scoring systems. Such scoring systems are not helpful in determining the need for therapies such as IVIG, because many features suggestive of a poorer prognosis are not early signs or symptoms, and many children with scores indicating low risk have developed significant cardiovascular disease. Therefore selective treatment with IVIG based on the presence of certain risk factors cannot be recommended. In addition, the presence or absence of risk factors should not preclude routine echocardiography for all patients with KS, including those with a lower than average predicted risk of developing aneurysms. Factors that are most strongly predictive of coronary disease include duration of fever for more than 16 days, recurrence of fever after an afebrile period of at least 48 hours, arrhythmias other than first-degree heart block, male sex, age less than 1 year, anemia, thrombocytopenia, hypoalbuminemia, and cardiomegaly. The prevalence of serious coronary abnormalities is particularly high among those <6 months of age.

Patients with giant coronary artery aneurysms, which are defined as having an internal diameter of at least 8 mm, are at greatest risk of developing coronary thrombosis, stenosis, and myocardial infarction. A study (Nakano et al., 1986) reported the clinical characteristics of 11 patients with KS who experienced myocardial infarction. Giant aneurysms were present in all 11 patients; most of these events occurred within several months of the onset of illness. Only 5 patients had clinical symptoms at the time of infarction, 2 of the 11 died, and 2 of the 9 survivors required continued digoxin therapy. Kato and colleagues (1986) reported that the usual clinical symptoms of myocardial infarction in KS were shock and vomiting; chest pain was not recognized unless the child was over 4 years of age. Infarctions were asymptomatic in 37% of the patients. Infarctions usually occurred within 1 year of acute KS, but 27% of the patients who developed this complication did so more than 1 year after onset. Myocardial infarction and sudden death resulting from coronary artery abnormalities have been reported in patients with a history of an illness consistent with KS or with no known history of previous illness. At least 13 patients have undergone cardiac transplantation because of severe sequelae of KS.

Valvular insufficiency in acute KS may rarely be severe enough to require valve replacement.

Other Complications. Sensorineural hearing loss is a rare complication of KS. Inflammation and resultant aneurysm formation in medium-sized muscular arteries throughout the body (excluding cerebral vessels) occur in 2.2% of patients with KS. Virtually all of these patients also have significant coronary involvement.

A rare but serious complication of KS is the development of severe peripheral ischemia with resultant gangrene. Approximately 20 cases of this complication, which appears to occur with equal frequency in boys and girls and predominantly in non-Asian children, have been reported exclusively in infants <7 months of age. Most of these patients also develop giant coronary artery aneurysms, the most severe form of coronary abnormality following KS, and also have evidence of peripheral arterial aneurysms, particularly axillary aneurysms. The pathogenesis of the peripheral ischemia is uncertain but may include severe arteritis of digital or other peripheral small arteries; arteriospasm of these small vessels, perhaps in association with severe vasculitis; thrombosis of these small vessels as a result of endothelial damage and stagnant blood flow; thrombosis of a more proximal arterial aneurysm (particularly axillary) with embolism distally; rarely, cardiogenic shock with poor peripheral perfusion; or a combination of several of these factors. Treatment has generally included anti-inflammatory therapy (salicylates and IVIG), vasodilator therapy (prostaglandin E_1 or sympathetic nerve block), and thrombolytic or anticoagulant therapy. Even with such treatment, the peripheral ischemia may result in autoamputation.

PROGNOSIS

The prognosis of KS is directly related to early treatment with IVIG and aspirin, careful serial cardiac evaluations (including echocardiography), and the development of complications (especially coronary aneurysms). Patients whose clinical symptoms have resolved and who have normal echocardiograms at 6–8 weeks have an excellent prognosis and are not considered to be at increased risk of subsequent disease.

Altered lipid metabolism occurs in acute KS, as it does in many infectious and inflammatory disorders. Whether long-term lipid abnormalities occur after KS is more controversial. At the present time, counseling of patients and parents should conform to standard recommendations on nutrition for children and adolescents (Dajani et al., 1994).

PREVENTION

Prevention of KS will not be possible until the etiologic agent and pathogenesis of the disorder are identified. No preventive measures are known.

REVIEWS

Mason WH, Takahashi M: Kawasaki syndrome. *Clin Infect Dis* 1999;28: 169–85.

Rowley AH, Shulman ST: Kawasaki syndrome. *Pediatr Clin North Am* 1999;46:313–29.

KEY ARTICLES

Barron KS, Shulman ST, Rowley AH, et al: Report of the National Institutes of Health Workshop on Kawasaki Disease. *J Rheumatol* 1999;26: 170–90.

Burns JC, Capparelli EV, Brown JA, et al: Intravenous gamma-globulin treatment and retreatment in Kawasaki disease. *Pediatr Infect Dis J* 1998;17:1144–8.

Checchia PA, Pahl E, Shaddy RE, et al: Cardiac transplantation for Kawasaki disease. *Pediatrics* 1997;100:695–9.

Council on Cardiovascular Disease in the Young: Diagnostic Guidelines for Kawasaki Disease. *Circulation* 2001;103:335–6.

Dajani AS, Taubert KA, Takahashi M, et al: Guidelines for long-term management of patients with Kawasaki disease: Report from the Committee on Rheumatic Fever, Endocarditis, and Kawasaki Disease, Council on Cardiovascular Disease in the Young, American Heart Association. *Circulation* 1994;89:916–22.

Fujita Y, Nakamura Y, Sakata K, et al: Kawasaki disease in families. *Pediatrics* 1989;84:666–9.

Han RK, Silverman ED, Newman A, et al: Management and outcome of persistent or recurrent fever after initial intravenous gamma globulin therapy in acute Kawasaki disease. *Arch Pediatr Adolesc Med* 2000; 154:694–9.

Kato H, Sugimura T, Akagi T, et al: Long-term consequences of Kawasaki disease: A 10- to 21-year follow-up study of 594 patients. *Circulation* 1996;94:1379–85.

Kato H, Ichinose E, Kawasaki T: Myocardial infarction in Kawasaki disease: Clinical analyses in 195 cases. *J Pediatr* 1986;108:923–7.

Kawasaki T, Kosaki F, Okawa S, et al: A new infantile acute febrile mucocutaneous lymph node syndrome (MLNS) prevailing in Japan. *Pediatrics* 1974;54:271–6.

Kitamura S, Kameda Y, Seki T, et al: Long-term outcome of myocardial revascularization in patients with Kawasaki coronary artery disease: A multicenter cooperative study. *J Thorac Cardiovasc Surg* 1994;107: 663–73.

Melish ME, Hicks RM, Larson EJ: Mucocutaneous lymph node syndrome in the United States. *Am J Dis Child* 1976;130:599–607.

Nakano H, Saito A, Ueda K, et al: Clinical characteristics of myocardial infarction following Kawasaki disease: Report of 11 cases. *J Pediatr* 1986;108:198–203.

Newburger JW, Takahashi M, Beiser AS, et al: A single intravenous infusion of gamma globulin as compared with four infusions in the treatment of acute Kawasaki syndrome. *N Engl J Med* 1991;324:1633–9.

Rosenfeld EA, Corydon KE, Shulman ST: Kawasaki disease in infants less than one year of age. *J Pediatr* 1995;126:524–9.

Rowley AH, Eckerley CA, Jack HM, et al: IgA plasma cells in vascular tissue of patients with Kawasaki disease. *J Immunol* 1997;159:5946–55.

Rowley AH, Gonzalez-Crussi F, Gidding SS, et al: Incomplete Kawasaki disease with coronary artery involvement. *J Pediatr* 1987;110:409–13.

Rowley AH, Shulman ST, Mask CA, et al: IgA plasma cell infiltration of proximal respiratory tract, pancreas, kidney, and coronary artery in acute Kawasaki disease. *J Infect Dis* 2000;182:1183–91.

Rowley AH, Shulman ST, Spike BT: Oligoclonal IgA response in the vascular wall in acute Kawasaki disease. *J Immunol* 2001;166:1334–43.

Shulman ST, Melish M, Inoue O, et al: Immunoglobulin allotypic markers in Kawasaki disease. *J Pediatr* 1993;122:84–6.

Stamos JK, Corydon K, Donaldson J, et al: Lymphadenitis as the dominant manifestation of Kawasaki disease. *Pediatrics* 1994;93:525–8.

Stockheim JA, Innocentini N, Shulman ST: Kawasaki disease in older children and adolescents. *J Pediatr* 2000;137:250–2.

Sugimura T, Kato H, Inoue O, et al: Intravascular ultrasound of coronary arteries in children: Assessment of the wall morphology and the lumen after Kawasaki disease. *Circulation* 1994;89:258–65.

Sundel RP, Newburger JW, McGill T, et al: Sensorineural hearing loss associated with Kawasaki disease. *J Pediatr* 1990;117:371–7.

Suzuki A, Yamagishi M, Kimura K, et al: Functional behavior and morphology of the coronary artery wall in patients with Kawasaki disease assessed by intravascular ultrasound. *J Am Coll Cardiol* 1996;27:291–6.

Tomita S, Chung K, Mas M, et al: Peripheral gangrene associated with Kawasaki disease *Clin Infect Dis* 1992;14:121–6.

Wright DA, Newburger JW, Baker A, et al: Treatment of immune globulin-resistant Kawasaki disease with pulsed doses of corticosteroids. *J Pediatr* 1996;128:146–9.

Yanagawa H, Nakamura Y, Ojima T, et al: Changes in epidemic patterns of Kawasaki disease in Japan. *Pediatr Infect Dis J* 1999;18:64–6.

CHAPTER 40

Rheumatic Fever and Poststreptococcal Glomerulonephritis

Michael A. Gerber

Rheumatic fever and poststreptococcal acute glomerulonephritis (PSAGN) are both well-recognized, nonsuppurative sequelae of infections with group A β-hemolytic *Streptococcus* (GABHS) that occur after an asymptomatic latent period. Both of these diseases are characterized by lesions remote from the site of the streptococcal infection. Although the pathogenic mechanisms of rheumatic fever and PSAGN are still poorly understood, these complications appear to be fundamentally different. Rheumatic fever and PSAGN differ in their clinical manifestations, epidemiology, and potential morbidity. In addition, PSAGN can occur after an infection with GABHS of either the skin or the upper respiratory tract, but rheumatic fever can occur only after an infection of the upper respiratory tract.

RHEUMATIC FEVER

Evidence to support the link between GABHS upper respiratory tract infections and acute rheumatic fever is considerable. As many as two thirds of patients with either an initial or a recurrent attack of rheumatic fever have had an upper respiratory tract infection several weeks before the rheumatic attack. Patients with acute rheumatic fever almost always have elevated or rising antibody titers to GABHS extracellular antigens, which indicate a recent acute infection with group A *Streptococcus*. In addition, antibody titers to these antigens are usually considerably higher than those seen in patients without rheumatic fever. The peak age and seasonal incidence of rheumatic fever also parallel those of GABHS infections. Outbreaks of streptococcal pharyngitis in closed communities, such as boarding schools or military camps, may be followed by outbreaks of acute rheumatic fever. Finally, antimicrobial therapy that eliminates GABHS from the upper respiratory tract or long-term, continuous antimicrobial prophylaxis that prevents GABHS pharyngitis also prevents initial attacks and recurrences, respectively, of acute rheumatic fever.

ETIOLOGY

GABHS, also known as *Streptococcus pyogenes,* is a common cause of infections of the upper respiratory tract (pharyngotonsillitis; Chapter 58) and the skin (impetigo or pyoderma; Chapter 46) in children. Streptococci, which are gram-positive, coccoid-shaped bacteria that tend to grow in chains, are broadly classified on the basis of their reactions on mammalian red blood cells. The zone of complete hemolysis that surrounds colonies grown on blood agar plates distinguishes β-hemolytic streptococci from α-hemolytic (green or partial hemolysis) and γ-hemolytic (nonhemolytic) species (Plate 1E). β-Hemolytic streptococci can be divided into groups on the basis of a group-specific polysaccharide (**Lancefield carbohydrate C**) located in the cell wall. More than 20 serologic groups have been identified, and they are designated by the letters A, B, C, and so on.

The **M protein,** a major component of the cell wall of the group A *Streptococcus,* is used to serotype strains of GABHS into more than 100 different M types. The M protein appears as roughened fimbriae, extending out from the cell wall, and is a virulence factor that helps the organism resist phagocytosis.

Humans are the only natural reservoir for GABHS. These highly communicable streptococci can cause disease in persons of any age who do not have type-specific immunity against the particular serotype involved. Disease in neonates is uncommon, however, probably because of maternally acquired antibodies. The incidence of upper respiratory tract infections is highest in young, school-age children.

Upper respiratory tract infections are most common in the northern regions of the United States, especially during the winter and early spring. GABHS is spread by airborne salivary droplets and nasal discharge; close proximity, as in a school or home, promotes transmission. Recent reports suggest that GABHS has the potential to be an important upper respiratory tract pathogen and to produce outbreaks of disease in daycare settings. Explosive outbreaks of streptococcal pharyngotonsillitis have also been caused by foods contaminated with group A *Streptococcus.*

EPIDEMIOLOGY

In some developing areas the annual incidence of rheumatic fever is currently as high as 280 per 100,000 population (Table 40–1). Worldwide, rheumatic heart disease remains the most common form of acquired heart disease in all age groups. In many developing countries, this disease accounts for as much as 50% of all cardiovascular disease and as many as 50% of all hospital admissions for this condition. However, striking differences are evident in the incidence of rheumatic heart disease among different ethnic groups in the same country; many of these differences appear to be related to differences in socioeconomic status.

In the early 1900s in the United States, rheumatic fever was the leading cause of death among children and adolescents and was the primary cause of heart disease in adults less than 40 years of age. As many as one fourth of the hospital beds nationwide were occupied by patients with rheumatic fever or its complications. Annual incidence rates of 100–200 per 100,000 population were common in the United States at that time. By the 1940s the annual incidence of rheumatic fever decreased to 50 per 100,000 population. Over the next four decades the decline in incidence accelerated rapidly, so that by the early 1980s the annual incidence in some areas of the United States was as low as 0.5 per 100,000 population.

TABLE 40–1. Incidence of Acute Rheumatic Fever

Location and Population Group	Time Period	Incidence (per 100,000)
Cyprus	1972	27–43
Iran	1972–74	80
Sri Lanka	1978	140
Sweden	1971–80	0.2
United States	1980	0.5
India	1984–95	44
Kuwait	1984–88	29
Turkey	1985–89	46
China	1986–95	20
Australia	1989–93	
Aboriginal		282
Nonaboriginal		3
Tunisia	1990	30
New Zealand	1995	
Maori		37
Non-Maori		9

This sharp decline in incidence has also been observed in other industrialized nations (Table 40–1).

The explanation for the dramatic decline in the incidence of rheumatic fever in the United States and other developed countries has never been clearly established. Improved socioeconomic conditions with better nutrition, hygiene, and access to medical care and less crowding could certainly have been contributing factors. Although the decrease in the incidence of rheumatic fever began before the antibiotic era, the use of antibiotics has also had a positive effect. Antibiotic therapy of GABHS pharyngitis has been important in preventing initial attacks and, particularly, recurrences of the disease. In addition, researchers have learned that different strains of GABHS vary in their ability to produce acute rheumatic fever. The decline in the incidence of rheumatic fever in this country can be attributed, at least in part, to a shift from **rheumatogenic strains** (M types 1, 3, 5, 6, and 18) to nonrheumatogenic strains in the prevalent GABHS.

A dramatic outbreak of acute rheumatic fever in the Salt Lake City area began in early 1985, with 198 cases reported by the end of 1989. Other focal outbreaks were reported between 1984 and 1988 from Columbus and Akron, Ohio; Pittsburgh; Nashville and Memphis, Tennessee; New York City; Kansas City, Missouri; Dallas; and among recruits at the San Diego Naval Training Center in California and at the Fort Leonard Wood Army Training Base in Missouri. A large proportion of the strains of GABHS associated with these outbreaks were very mucoid in appearance, a characteristic that had been epidemiologically associated with acute rheumatic fever. In addition, many of these strains belonged to the well-recognized rheumatogenic types. The appearance of rheumatogenic strains in selected communities was probably a major factor in these outbreaks of rheumatic fever. Evidence suggests that this resurgence of acute rheumatic fever was extremely focal and not nationwide. Although these outbreaks ceased within a few years, investigators in Salt Lake City have continued to report a markedly increased incidence of acute rheumatic fever in that area.

The precise risk of developing rheumatic fever after an untreated episode of GABHS pharyngitis is not known. During outbreaks of streptococcal pharyngitis in a military population in the 1950s, acute rheumatic fever developed in approximately 3% of untreated patients. Among schoolchildren in a nonepidemic setting in the 1960s, approximately 0.3% of the untreated patients eventually became ill with the disease. Rheumatic fever does not develop after GABHS infections at sites other than the upper respiratory tract or after non-group A *Streptococcus* infections.

Several host factors determine the risk of development of rheumatic fever in particular patients after an episode of GABHS pharyngitis. Children between 5 and 15 years of age are at greatest risk of GABHS pharyngitis; the incidence of both initial attacks and recurrences of rheumatic fever peaks in this population. Patients who have had one attack of rheumatic fever tend to have recurrences, and the clinical features of the recurrences tend to mimic those of the initial attack. In addition, a genetic predisposition to rheumatic fever appears to exist. Studies in twins have shown a higher concordance rate of rheumatic fever in monozygotic than in dizygotic twin pairs. Recent investigations have also demonstrated an association between the presence of specific HLA markers and a B-cell alloantigen (designated as D8/17) and susceptibility to rheumatic fever.

Historically, rheumatic fever has been associated with poverty, particularly in urban areas. Much of the decline in the incidence of rheumatic fever in industrialized countries during the preantibiotic era can probably be attributed to improvements in living conditions. Of the various manifestations of poverty, crowding, which contributes to the spread of GABHS infections, is the factor most closely associated with rheumatic fever. The significant decline in incidence of rheumatic fever in industrialized countries over the past four decades has been attributable in large measure to the greater availability of medical care and to the widespread use of antibiotics.

PATHOGENESIS

The pathogenic link between pharyngeal GABHS infection and the occurrence of acute rheumatic fever with organ and tissue involvement far removed from the upper respiratory tract is still not understood. One of the major obstacles to determining the pathogenesis of rheumatic fever has been the inability to establish an animal model. Several theories of the pathogenesis of rheumatic fever have been proposed, but currently only two are seriously considered—the cytotoxicity theory and the immunologic theory.

Proponents of the cytotoxicity theory have suggested that a streptococcal toxin may be involved in the pathogenesis of rheumatic fever. GABHS does produce several enzymes that are cytotoxic for mammalian cells. **Streptolysin O** is known to have a direct cardiotoxic effect on mammalian cells in tissue culture, and this enzyme is one of the most frequently considered as an active agent. However, one of the major problems with the cytotoxicity hypothesis is its inability to explain the latent period between the GABHS pharyngitis and the onset of acute rheumatic fever.

The concept of an abnormal host immunologic response to the GABHS is more widely accepted than the cytotoxicity theory. Most of the attention regarding this response has focused on the possibility of autoimmunity. Several GABHS antigens have been shown to cross-react immunologically with human tissue antigens. As a result of this antigenic mimicry in the course of the host's immune response to the GABHS, the host's antigens may be mistaken as foreign. A large number of cross-reactive GABHS antigens could potentially be involved in this proposed autoimmune process. Cross-reactivity between group A *Streptococcus* M protein and myocardial sarcolemma membranes and between group A *Streptococcus* carbohydrate and a structural glycoprotein of heart valves are two of the processes most likely to be involved. A potential initiating step is expression of anti–vascular cell adhesion molecule-1 (VCAM-1) on valvular endothelium of rheumatic valves, which facilitates extravasation of CD4 and CD8 lymphocytes through the activated endothelium into the valve.

SYMPTOMS AND CLINICAL MANIFESTATIONS

The episode of GABHS pharyngitis that precedes acute rheumatic fever ranges from subclinical to clinical. A subclinical episode can be recognized only retrospectively with a rise in the titers of streptococcal antibodies. When symptoms of acute pharyngitis are present, they usually resolve within 3–4 days even without antibiotic therapy. The patient then appears well before the onset of the major manifestations of acute rheumatic fever (Table 40–2); this interval is known as the latent period.

Latent Period. The length of the latent period, which can be measured only in rheumatic patients with a clear history of a sore throat, is variable. In the majority of patients, this period ranges between 1 and 3 weeks. The latent period of rheumatic fever is usually longer than that of PSAGN, which is about 10 days after an episode of GABHS pharyngitis. There is no evidence that the latent period is shortened during a recurrence of rheumatic fever.

Carditis. The most serious clinical manifestation of acute rheumatic fever is carditis, which is the only clinical feature of this disease that can be fatal during the acute stage of the illness or that can result in long-term sequelae. When rheumatic fever affects the heart, it usually involves the endocardium, myocardium, and pericardium to varying degrees. Clinically, rheumatic carditis is almost always associated with a murmur of valvulitis.

Arthritis. Arthritis, the most common major manifestation of acute rheumatic fever, occurs in approximately 75% of the patients. It appears early in the course of the disease and is almost always a migratory polyarthritis unless the clinical expression has been aborted by early administration of anti-inflammatory agents. The larger joints, particularly the knees, ankles, elbows, and wrists, are most frequently affected. Involvement of the small joints of the hands and feet is unusual and suggests another diagnosis.

Chorea. The chorea of acute rheumatic fever **(Sydenham's chorea, chorea minor, St. Vitus' dance)** indicates CNS involvement. Girls are affected with chorea twice as often as boys. The incidence of chorea among rheumatic patients, which has varied widely, appeared to be decreasing, but in one of the more recent outbreaks in the United States the incidence was 31%.

The latent period between the acute GABHS infection and the onset of chorea is, on the average, longer than the latent period for the other rheumatic manifestations, and usually ranges from 1–6 months. Consequently, chorea may either develop after other clinical signs of rheumatic fever or it may be the sole clinical manifestation of rheumatic disease. Patients with isolated chorea may have no evidence of an ongoing inflammation or an antecedent GABHS infection, which complicates the diagnosis of rheumatic fever. Because these patients are at risk of developing rheumatic heart disease and of experiencing recurrences of rheumatic fever, however, diagnosis is important.

Recently, it has been suggested that a group of neuropsychiatric disorders referred to as pediatric autoimmune neuropsychiatric disorders associated with *S. pyogenes* (PANDAS), which includes obsessive-compulsive disorder (OCD) and Tourette's syndrome (TS), are related to Sydenham's chorea. Although there is evidence supporting a link between OCD and TS and Sydenham's chorea, the concept that these neuropsychiatric disorders represent an extension of the spectrum of acute rheumatic fever remains unproved.

TABLE 40–2. Frequency of Major Manifestations in Recent Reports of Acute Rheumatic Fever in the United States

Condition	Frequency (%)
Carditis	58
Arthritis	75
Chorea	22
Erythema marginatum	4
Subcutaneous nodules	3

Subcutaneous Nodules. Subcutaneous nodules, which are a rare clinical manifestation of rheumatic fever, usually occur only in patients with carditis. These firm, painless nodules appear over the extensor surfaces of certain joints (e.g., elbows, knees, wrists), in the occipital region, or over the spinous processes of the thoracic or lumbar vertebrae.

Erythema Marginatum. Erythema marginatum is the only distinctive skin manifestation of rheumatic fever. This rare clinical manifestation usually occurs only in patients with carditis. Erythema marginatum generally occurs in the early stage of the rheumatic fever episode but often persists or recurs after all other manifestations of the disease have disappeared.

Physical Examination Findings

Cardiac Findings. The most commonly heard heart murmur during acute rheumatic fever is an apical systolic murmur of mitral regurgitation. This long, usually pansystolic, murmur of blowing quality and high pitch is best heard at the apex with transmission toward the left axilla. The intensity is variable and does not change substantially with phase of respiration or position.

Another murmur that is often heard in association with mitral regurgitation is an apical middiastolic murmur **(Carey Coombs murmur).** This low-pitched murmur is best heard through the bell portion of the stethoscope with the patient in the left lateral recumbent position and the breath held in expiration. It usually starts with the third heart sound, which is accentuated by mild mitral regurgitation, and ends before the first heart sound. The Carey Coombs murmur of acute rheumatic carditis must be differentiated from the rumbling, crescendo, apical presystolic murmur of established mitral stenosis that is often followed by an accentuated mitral first heart sound.

Less frequently heard is the high-pitched, blowing, decrescendo murmur of aortic regurgitation. This murmur begins immediately after the aortic component of the second heart sound and is best heard along the left sternal border after deep expiration with the patient leaning forward. It may be short, faint, difficult to hear, and occur only intermittently. Isolated aortic valve involvement without a murmur of mitral regurgitation is unusual in acute rheumatic carditis.

Myocarditis in the absence of valvulitis is not likely to be rheumatic in origin. If the myocardial involvement with rheumatic carditis is severe, clinical, radiographic, and echocardiographic evidence of congestive heart failure may be present.

Pericarditis, the least common finding in rheumatic carditis, is usually associated with severe pancarditis and is almost never seen as an isolated finding. Alternative causes of pericarditis should be sought in the absence of endocarditis and myocarditis.

Arthritis. Characteristically, rheumatic arthritis is associated with swelling, warmth, erythema, pain, and limitation of motion in two or more joints. The pain is usually severe, and patients may develop a pseudoparalysis secondary to guarding of the joint. The synovial fluid from affected joints has a WBC count of 10,000–100,000/mm^3, with predominantly neutrophils. It has a protein concentration of about 4 g/dL, a normal glucose level, and a good mucin clot. In untreated patients, findings in an individual joint usually persist for 1–5 days, and in most such patients the joint symptoms resolve completely within weeks. The response to salicylate therapy is characteristically dramatic. If treated patients have not substantially improved within 48 hours, the diagnosis of rheumatic arthritis should be questioned. The arthritis of rheumatic fever almost never produces permanent deformity of the affected joints.

Chorea. Chorea is characterized by purposeless, involuntary movements, emotional lability, lack of muscular coordination, and weakness. The movements are abrupt and can be suppressed by the patient's will, but for only a brief time. Although they disappear during sleep, they may occur at rest and interfere with voluntary activities. Stress, effort, and fatigue exacerbate the movements. All voluntary muscles may be involved, but the effect on the hands and face is usually the most striking. Facial grimacing or other inappropriate facial expressions are common. The emotional changes associated with chorea may present as outbursts of inappropriate behavior, including crying, frustration, and restlessness.

Choreic movements can be accentuated by having patients stretch their arms out in front of them, close their eyes, and stick out their tongues. They typically display undulating tongue movements with flexion of the wrists, hyperextension of the metacarpophalangeal joints, straightening of the fingers, and abduction of the thumb (''**spooning**'' or ''**dishing**'' of the hands). When patients are asked to raise their arms above their heads, they may also pronate one or both of their hands **(pronator sign).** Typically, the handwriting is sloppy and the speech is slurred. Choreic movements, which are generally more marked on one side of the body, are occasionally completely unilateral (hemichorea). The characteristic muscular weakness is best revealed by having the patient squeeze the examiner's hands. The resultant grip alternately increases and decreases in tension, producing the characteristic **''milking sign''** or **''relapsing grip.''**

Although the duration of the chorea is variable, the condition is self-limited, with eventual complete resolution of the symptoms. Improvement is usually seen within 1–2 weeks, but full recovery may take as long as 2–3 months. In some rare cases, symptoms may recur over a period of years, particularly in association with intercurrent illnesses.

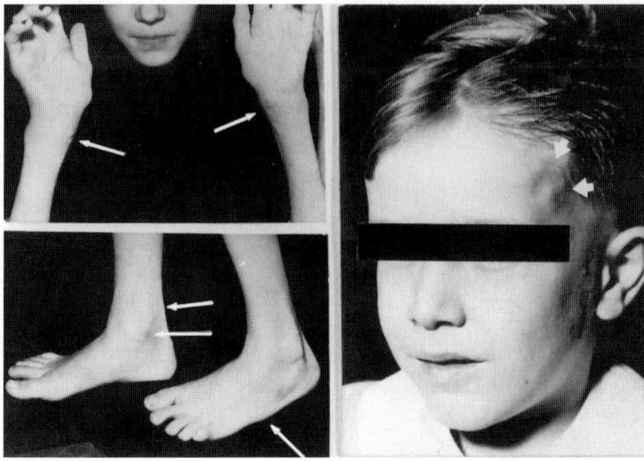

FIGURE 40–1. Subcutaneous nodules over bony prominences at different sites in three patients with acute rheumatic fever. (From Markowitz M, Gordis L: *Rheumatic Fever,* 2nd ed. Philadelphia, Saunders, 1972, p 73.)

Subcutaneous Nodules. Subcutaneous nodules, which are approximately round and vary from a few millimeters to as much as 2 cm in diameter (Fig. 40–1), usually first appear several weeks into the illness. The skin overlying the nodules moves freely and is not inflamed. The nodules typically disappear within 1–2 weeks but last no longer than 4 weeks.

Erythema Marginatum. The lesions begin as small, pink or red macules that may be slightly raised. Over time these lesions expand centrifugally, leading to areas with clear centers surrounded by distinct, pink, serpiginous, or circular margins. If the margins are circular, the rash is termed erythema annulare. The lesions are nonpruritic, nonindurated, blanch with pressure, and range in diameter from 1–3 cm. They are usually found on the trunk and sometimes on the proximal parts of the limbs but never on the face (Fig. 40–2). Erythema marginatum, which may be difficult to see in dark-skinned patients, may be accentuated by a hot bath or by the application of warm towels.

Nonspecific Manifestations. Other nonspecific clinical manifestations of rheumatic fever frequently occur, but because they are also often seen in numerous other diseases, their diagnostic value

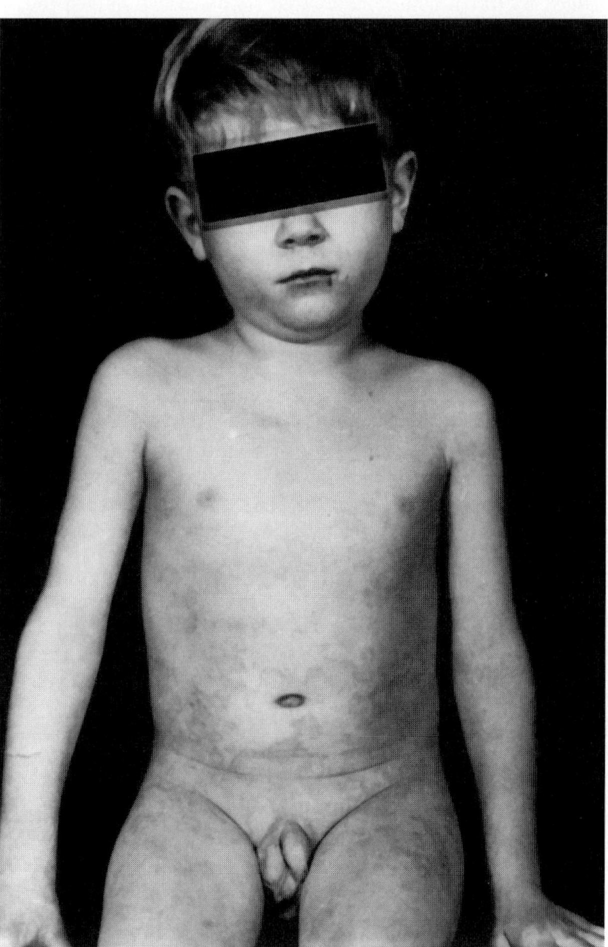

FIGURE 40–2. Erythema marginatum in an 8-year-old boy with acute rheumatic fever. (From Markowitz M, Gordis L: *Rheumatic Fever,* 2nd ed. Philadelphia, Saunders, 1972, p 75.)

is limited. Fever is almost always present at the onset of rheumatic arthritis, often occurs with isolated carditis, but is not usually apparent with isolated chorea. Arthralgia, which is pain in a joint without objective signs of inflammation, is another nonspecific clinical manifestation of rheumatic fever. The migratory arthralgia associated with rheumatic fever generally affects two or more large joints. Pain may be severe. Limitation of motion may result. Patients with rheumatic fever may also have abdominal pain. Anorexia, nausea, and vomiting also commonly occur, and severe epistaxis may be present.

DIAGNOSIS

Jones Criteria. No single sign, symptom, or laboratory test is pathognomonic or diagnostic of acute rheumatic fever. In 1944, Dr. T. Duckett Jones established a set of guidelines to aid in the diagnosis of the initial attack of acute rheumatic fever based on combinations of clinical and laboratory findings. Jones divided the clinical features of acute rheumatic fever into those that were most useful diagnostically **(major manifestations)** and those that were less characteristic **(minor manifestations).** The resulting scheme became known as the Jones criteria (Table 40–3). The presence of two major manifestations or one major and two minor manifestations indicates a high probability of acute rheumatic fever if supported by evidence of a preceding GABHS infection. Evidence of infection includes a recent episode of GABHS pharyngitis documented by throat culture or a rapid streptococcal antigen test, a positive throat culture for GABHS at the time of diagnosis of rheumatic fever, or positive streptococcal antibody titers. The Jones criteria were designed to establish the diagnosis of rheumatic fever during the acute stage of illness and not to measure rheumatic activity, diagnose inactive or chronic rheumatic heart disease, or predict the course or severity of the disease.

The diagnosis of rheumatic fever can be established in three clinical situations without strictly adhering to the Jones criteria. In each of these situations the diagnosis should remain presumptive, however, until other causes have been excluded. In some patients, chorea may be the only manifestation of rheumatic fever. Similarly, late-onset carditis may be the single characteristic feature of rheumatic fever in patients who come to medical attention months after the onset of the disease. In both of these cases, patients may have insufficient supporting historical, clinical, or laboratory findings to satisfy the Jones criteria. The third situation involves a recurrence of rheumatic fever, which can be diagnosed when only a single major manifestation is present in patients with a reliable history of rheumatic fever or established rheumatic heart disease if evidence of a preceding GABHS infection exists.

Differential Diagnosis

The differential diagnoses of rheumatic fever include many infectious as well as noninfectious illnesses (Table 40–4). The collagen vascular diseases must be considered in any child who presents with arthritis. In particular, rheumatoid arthritis must be distinguished from acute rheumatic fever. Children with rheumatoid arthritis tend to be younger and usually have less joint pain relative to their clinical findings. Spiking fevers, lymphadenopathy, and splenomegaly are evident. Response to salicylate therapy is much less dramatic with rheumatoid arthritis than with acute rheumatic fever.

When carditis is the sole major manifestation of acute rheumatic fever, viral myocarditis, viral pericarditis, and infective endocarditis must be considered. In general, the absence of a significant cardiac murmur excludes the diagnosis of acute rheumatic fever. Echocardiography can be very helpful in identifying functional murmurs and murmurs caused by congenital heart defects. Patients with infective endocarditis may present with both joint and cardiac manifestations. These patients can usually be distinguished from patients with acute rheumatic fever by positive blood cultures and the presence of associated findings (Chapter 71).

Microbiologic Evaluation

A throat culture or rapid streptococcal antigen test should be obtained from every patient in whom rheumatic fever is suspected. Only a minority of these patients have positive throat cultures at the time of presentation, however. Because the isolation or identification of GABHS from a throat swab cannot distinguish between an acute streptococcal infection and a streptococcal carrier,

TABLE 40–3. Guidelines for the Diagnosis of Initial Attack of Rheumatic Fever (Jones Criteria, Updated 1992)*

Major Manifestations*	Minor Manifestations	Supporting Evidence of Antecedent Group A Streptococcal Infection
Carditis Polyarthritis Chorea Erythema marginatum Subcutaneous nodules	Clinical features: Arthralgia Fever Laboratory features: Elevated acute phase reactants Erythrocyte sedimentation rate C-reactive protein Prolonged P-R interval	Positive throat culture or rapid streptococcal antigen test Elevated or rising streptococcal antibody titer

*The presence of two major or of one major and two minor manifestations indicates a high probability of acute rheumatic fever if supported by evidence of preceding group A streptococcal infection.

Reproduced with permission. Guidelines for the Diagnosis of Rheumatic Fever: Jones Criteria, Updated 1992. *JAMA* 1992;268:2069. Copyright American Heart Association.

TABLE 40–4. Differential Diagnosis of Acute Rheumatic Fever

Arthritis (Polyarticular)	Carditis	Chorea
Rheumatoid arthritis	Viral myocarditis	Huntington's chorea
Systemic lupus erythematosus	Viral pericarditis	Wilson's disease
Serum sickness	Infective endocarditis	Systemic lupus erythematosus
Sickle cell disease	Mitral valve prolapse	Cerebral palsy
Malignancies	Congenital heart disease	Tics
Gonococcal infection	Innocent murmurs	Hyperactivity
Reactive arthritis (e.g., *Shigella, Salmonella, Yersinia*)		

the best evidence of an antecedent streptococcal infection is a serologic response to GABHS. An elevated or preferably a rising streptococcal antibody titer can be used as serologic evidence of a recent GABHS infection. The most commonly used streptococcal antibody tests are the **antistreptolysin O (ASO), antideoxyribonuclease B (anti-DNase B),** and **antihyaluronidase** assays. ASO antibodies are present in approximately 85% of patients 2–4 weeks after streptococcal pharyngitis. When two or more different streptococcal antibody tests are performed, titers are increased within the first few months of onset in almost all cases of acute rheumatic fever, with the exception of cases of isolated chorea or late-onset carditis.

A rapid slide agglutination test for antibodies to GABHS extracellular enzymes (Streptozyme) exists but is not recommended. Because of poor standardization of reagents and poor reproducibility, it is not to be used as a definitive test for antecedent streptococcal infection.

Diagnostic Imaging

Echocardiography can be extremely helpful in confirming auscultatory evidence of valvulitis and in ruling out innocent murmurs, congenital lesions, or other acquired abnormalities. At present, however, echocardiographic evidence of valvular regurgitation without accompanying auscultatory findings is insufficient as the sole criterion for valvulitis in acute rheumatic fever. Although isolated myocarditis or pericarditis may be seen with rheumatic carditis, this presentation is extremely unusual in the absence of a murmur.

Pathologic Findings

Heart. The **Aschoff body,** the distinctive pathognomonic lesion of rheumatic fever, is an oval, perivascular aggregation of large cells with polymorphous nuclei and basophilic cytoplasm that are classically found in the heart, although similar lesions have been found in the joint synovium. The cells are arranged as a rosette around an avascular core of fibrinoid or necrotic protoplasm.

Myocardial damage predominates in patients who die early in the course of acute rheumatic fever. The myocardium is edematous, pale, flabby, and mildly hypertrophic, with some dilatation of the cardiac chambers. Endocardial involvement is also almost invariably present; tiny translucent nodules, or verrucae, occur along the edges of the valve. The atrial endocardium may be thickened, especially in the left atrium above the base of the posterior leaflet of the mitral valve, and a serofibrinous effusion may be present in the pericardial sac. Microscopically, diffuse swelling and degeneration of the collagen are apparent. Aschoff bodies or nodules that may persist long after any other evidence of active disease may be present.

In patients who die at a later stage of the initial attack or during an early recurrence of rheumatic fever, the valve leaflets are usually retracted, thickened, and deformed. The commissures may be fused, and the chordae tendineae may be retracted and fused.

Most patients who die of rheumatic fever do so many years after the initial attack, at a time when the heart is greatly enlarged from both dilatation and hypertrophy. The heart valves may be markedly deformed and calcified. Fibrin deposits in various stages of organization and fibrous replacement with thickening of the cusps and narrowing of the orifice contribute to valve deformation. Pericardial involvement, which may lead to calcification, is rarely constrictive. Although some Aschoff bodies may still be present, they are reduced to spindle-shaped or triangular scars.

Joints. In patients with rheumatic fever–associated arthritis, the articular and periarticular structures are swollen and edematous, but no erosion of the joint surfaces or pannus formation is evident. The exudate is turbid but not purulent.

Brain. In the few pathologic specimens that have been available from patients with Sydenham's chorea who have died of carditis, arteritis, cellular degeneration, and occasional emboli and infarction were present. These changes were scattered throughout the cortex, basal ganglia, substantia nigra, and cerebellum.

Subcutaneous Nodules. The structure of subcutaneous nodules resembles that of Aschoff bodies. These nodules contain a central zone of fibrinoid necrotic material surrounded by histiocytes and fibroblasts with none of the palisading or zoning seen in a rheumatoid nodule.

TREATMENT

Bed Rest. All patients with acute rheumatic fever should be placed on bed rest, preferably in a hospital, so they can be examined daily for evidence of carditis. If carditis is going to occur, it usually develops within 2–3 weeks of the onset of the illness. Patients with arthritis who have no evidence of carditis can be ambulant soon after the fever and signs of arthritis have subsided and after the acute-phase reactants (e.g., ESR, CRP) have begun to return to normal. Patients with carditis who have no apparent cardiomegaly or congestive heart failure should be confined to bed for 2 weeks and allowed up for meals and the bathroom over the following 2 weeks. Physical activities can then be increased gradually over the next month as long as the carditis shows no signs of progression. Patients with cardiomegaly should be on strict bed rest for 4–6 weeks and then gradually allowed to be ambulant over the following 4–6 weeks. If congestive heart failure is also present, bed rest should be continued until this condition is brought under control.

Antimicrobial Treatment. Once the diagnosis of acute rheumatic fever has been established, the patient should receive a course of penicillin (or erythromycin if allergic to penicillin) appropriate for the treatment of GABHS pharyngitis (Chapter 58). The purpose of this treatment is to eradicate any GABHS that may be present in the pharynx, even if the throat culture is negative. After this initial course of antibiotic therapy, the patient should be started on long-term antibiotic prophylaxis. Antibiotic therapy has no effect on the clinical manifestations of acute rheumatic fever, the duration of the episode, or the prognosis.

Anti-inflammatory Treatment. Anti-inflammatory agents (e.g., salicylates, corticosteroids) should be withheld if arthralgia or questionable arthritis is the only clinical reason for suspecting rheumatic fever. Premature treatment with one of these drugs may interfere with the development of migratory polyarthritis, thus obscuring the diagnosis of acute rheumatic fever. Acetaminophen can be used to control fever and pain while the patient is being observed for more definite signs of rheumatic fever or for evidence of another disease.

Patients with definite arthritis and those with carditis without cardiomegaly or congestive heart failure should be treated with aspirin (Table 40–5). Determination of the serum salicylate level is not necessary unless the arthritis does not respond or signs of salicylate toxicity (e.g., tinnitus, hyperventilation) develop. There is no evidence that nonsteroidal anti-inflammatory agents are more effective than aspirin.

Patients with cardiomegaly or congestive heart failure with carditis should receive corticosteroids (Table 40–5). The clinical impression is that severely ill patients with rheumatic carditis toler-

TABLE 40–5. Recommended Anti-inflammatory Agents for Acute Rheumatic Fever

Clinical Manifestation	Treatment
Arthralgia	No anti-inflammatory agents; analgesics only
Arthritis, carditis (mild)	Aspirin, 100 mg/kg/day in 4 divided doses for 3–5 days; then 75 mg/kg/day for 4 wk
Carditis (moderate or severe)	Prednisone, 2 mg/kg/day in 4 divided doses for 2–3 wk; then reduce by 5 mg/day every 2–3 days; at taper, begin aspirin, 75 mg/kg/day, for 6 wk

ate steroids better than aspirin and that congestive heart failure resulting from rheumatic carditis responds more rapidly to steroids than to aspirin.

Termination of the anti-inflammatory therapy may be followed by the reappearance of clinical manifestations or of laboratory abnormalities. These "rebounds" are best left untreated unless the clinical manifestations are severe, for which aspirin or corticosteroids should be reinstated.

Congestive Heart Failure. The congestive heart failure associated with rheumatic carditis can usually be controlled with bed rest and corticosteroids. If not, diuretics should be added first, followed by digitalis if necessary.

Surgical Treatment. For many years physicians believed that valvular surgery was contraindicated while the rheumatic inflammatory process was still active. In recent years, however, patients with life-threatening congestive heart failure who have not responded to medical management have been treated successfully with valve replacement.

Sydenham's Chorea. Children with chorea should be taken out of school and placed in a quiet environment, either at home or in the hospital. Bed rest is indicated in severe attacks, and care must be taken to prevent patients from injuring themselves. Because chorea often occurs as an isolated manifestation after the resolution of the acute phase of the disease, anti-inflammatory agents are usually not indicated. No well-controlled studies demonstrate the effectiveness of corticosteroids in treating chorea. Sedatives may be helpful early in the course of chorea; phenobarbital (16–32 mg every 6–8 hours) is the drug of choice. If phenobarbital is ineffective, then haloperidol (0.01–0.03 mg/kg/day in two divided doses) or chlorpromazine (0.5 mg/kg every 4–6 hours) should be given. The anticonvulsants valproate sodium and carbamazepine have also been used somewhat successfully to treat chorea. Patients with chorea, even in the absence of other manifestations, require long-term antibiotic prophylaxis.

COMPLICATIONS

Cardiac valvular disease secondary to rheumatic fever carries an increased risk of development of infective endocarditis during episodes of transient bacteremia. Therefore patients with these cardiac conditions require additional, short-term antibiotic prophylaxis before surgical or dental procedures that are associated with transient bacteremia. The antibiotic regimens used to prevent recurrences of acute rheumatic fever are inadequate for protection against infective endocarditis. The current recommendations of the American Heart Association regarding infective endocarditis prophylaxis should be followed (Chapter 71). The physician should also stress the importance of good dental hygiene in the prevention of infective endocarditis. Patients who have had rheumatic fever but have no evidence of residual valvular disease do not require endocarditis prophylaxis.

If the myocardial involvement with rheumatic carditis is severe, congestive heart failure may result. Patients with chronic rheumatic heart disease may develop atrial fibrillation, but this complication is much less common in children than it is in adults. Patients with chronic rheumatic heart disease are at risk of suffering recurrent episodes of bacterial or viral pneumonia.

PROGNOSIS

The prognosis for patients with rheumatic fever depends primarily on the clinical manifestations present at the time of the initial attack and the severity of the episode. In most of the older reports, the incidence of carditis during the initial attack is about 50%. In some of the more recent outbreaks, the incidence of carditis was considerably higher, perhaps because a less rigorous definition of carditis and the use of Doppler echocardiography to establish the diagnoses in the absence of physical findings increases the apparent sensitivity of diagnosis. Approximately 70% of the patients with carditis during the initial episode of acute rheumatic fever recover with no residual heart disease; the more severe the cardiac involvement at first, the greater the risk of residual heart disease. For example, patients who initially have marked cardiomegaly and congestive heart disease frequently have residual heart disease.

Patients with no carditis during the initial attack of acute rheumatic fever are unlikely to have carditis with recurrent attacks. In contrast, patients with carditis during the first attack are likely to have carditis with recurrent attacks; the risk of permanent heart damage increases with each recurrence. Approximately 20% of the patients who present with "pure" chorea who are not put on secondary prophylaxis develop rheumatic heart disease within 20 years.

Death during the initial attack of rheumatic fever is unusual. Approximately 75% of patients with acute rheumatic fever are well within 6 weeks of the onset of the attack, and fewer than 5% have symptoms, usually chorea or intractable carditis, beyond 6 months. In the absence of recurrent GABHS infections, rheumatic fever does not recur more than 8 weeks after the withdrawal of anti-inflammatory therapy. The joint manifestations of acute rheumatic fever resolve completely without sequelae; similarly, chorea resolves without any residual damage to the nervous system. The long-term sequelae of rheumatic fever are limited to the heart.

Before antibiotic prophylaxis was available, 75% of rheumatic patients had one or more recurrent attacks during their lifetime; these recurrences were a major source of morbidity and mortality. The risk of recurrent episodes is highest immediately after the initial attack and decreases with time.

PREVENTION

Prevention of both initial and recurrent episodes of acute rheumatic fever involves controlling GABHS infections of the upper respiratory tract. Prevention of initial attacks (primary prevention) depends on identification and eradication of the GABHS that produces episodes of acute pharyngitis. Persons who have already suffered an attack of acute rheumatic fever are particularly susceptible to recurrences of rheumatic fever with any subsequent GABHS upper respiratory tract infection, whether symptomatic or not. Such patients should receive continuous antibiotic therapy to prevent recurrences (secondary prevention).

Primary Prevention. Penicillin is the drug of choice for the treatment of GABHS pharyngitis except in patients who are allergic to this drug (Chapter 58). Erythromycin should be used for penicillin-allergic patients.

Secondary Prevention. Secondary prevention requires continuous antibiotic prophylaxis, which should begin as soon as the diagnosis of acute rheumatic fever has been made and immediately after the full therapeutic course of penicillin has been completed. Patients who have carditis with their initial episode of rheumatic fever are at a relatively high risk of having carditis with recurrences and of sustaining additional cardiac damage and should receive antibiotic prophylaxis well into adulthood and perhaps for life. Other patients with rheumatic fever have a relatively low risk of carditis with recurrences, and antibiotic treatment may be discontinued in these patients when they reach their early 20s and after a lapse of at least 5 years since the last episode of rheumatic fever. The decision to discontinue prophylactic antibiotics should be made only after careful consideration of potential risks and benefits and of epidemiologic factors such as the risk of exposure to GABHS infections.

The regimen of choice for secondary prevention is a single injection of 1.2 million units of benzathine penicillin G every 4 weeks (Table 40–6). In certain areas of the world where the incidence of rheumatic fever is particularly high, or in certain high-risk patients, use of benzathine penicillin G every 3 weeks may be necessary, as levels of penicillin may fall to marginally effective amounts after 3 weeks. Continuous oral antimicrobial prophylaxis can be used in compliant patients. Penicillin given twice daily and sulfadiazine given once daily are equally effective when used in such patients. For the exceptional patient who is allergic to both penicillin and sulfonamides, erythromycin may be given twice daily.

TABLE 40–6. Secondary Prevention of Rheumatic Fever (Prevention of Recurrent Attacks)

Agent	Dose	Route of Administration
Benzathine penicillin G	1,200,000 units q4wk*	Intramuscular
or		
Penicillin V	250 mg bid	Oral
or		
Sulfadiazine	0.5 g once daily for patients <45.4 kg (60 lb); 1 g once daily for patients >45.4 kg	Oral
For individuals allergic to penicillin and sulfadiazine: Erythromycin	250 mg bid	Oral

*In high-risk situations, administration every 3 weeks is justified and recommended.

From Dajani A, Taubert K, Ferrieri P, et al: Treatment of acute streptococcal pharyngitis and prevention of rheumatic fever: A statement for health professionals. Committee on Rheumatic Fever, Endocarditis, and Kawasaki Disease of the Council on Cardiovascular Disease in the Young, the American Heart Association. *Pediatrics* 1995;96:758–64.

Antistreptococcal Vaccines. Work on the development of an antistreptococcal vaccine has been ongoing for a number of years. The three major obstacles in the development of this vaccine are the multiplicity of GABHS serotypes, the risk of evoking cross-reactive antibodies, and difficulties in the development of a delivery system that would result in the production of both humoral and secretory antibodies. Recently, major advances have been made in the attempt to overcome these obstacles. A vaccine that could prevent GABHS upper respiratory tract infections and complications such as rheumatic fever appears to be much closer to being a reality than at any time in the past.

POSTSTREPTOCOCCAL GLOMERULONEPHRITIS

PSAGN can occur after an infection with GABHS of either the skin or the upper respiratory tract, in contrast to rheumatic fever, which can occur only after a GABHS infection of the upper respiratory tract.

ETIOLOGY

The characteristics of GABHS are described in the discussion of rheumatic fever. In contrast to upper respiratory tract infections, streptococcal skin infections occur most frequently during the summer in temperate climates. In warm climates such infections occur year-round. GABHS can be present on normal skin for at least a week before lesions are evident. Lesions do not usually appear on the skin in the absence of an abrasion or insect bite. The bacteria usually spread by cutaneous transmission, although skin serotypes may colonize the throat. Transmission is favored by both close proximity and poor hygiene.

EPIDEMIOLOGY

Although the actual incidence of PSAGN is difficult to determine because many of the cases are asymptomatic, it is by far the most common form of glomerulonephritis in children. The incidence of PSAGN in many industrialized countries has been steadily decreasing in the last several decades. Although PSAGN is most often a sporadic disease, it may also occur in epidemic forms. Sporadic disease associated with GABHS pharyngitis tends to occur in the winter and early spring, whereas sporadic disease associated with GABHS pyoderma tends to appear in the summer and early fall. The vast majority of sporadic cases of PSAGN are subclinical, and they usually come to medical attention only because of abnormally appearing urine. Only about 20% of the cases of epidemic PSAGN are subclinical.

PSAGN is primarily a disease of preschool- and school-age children. Approximately 60% of patients are between 2 and 12 years of age. Symptomatic PSAGN appears to affect boys predominantly. When both symptomatic and asymptomatic cases of PSAGN are included, however, the sex distribution of cases is nearly equal.

PSAGN can occur as a nonsuppurative complication of GABHS infections of either the upper respiratory tract or the skin. The asymptomatic latent period between an episode of GABHS pharyngitis and the appearance of PSAGN is approximately 10 days. The latent period after an episode of GABHS pyoderma is approximately 14–21 days. Second attacks of PSAGN are very uncommon, and acute rheumatic fever and PSAGN only very rarely occur simultaneously in the same patient.

Certain serotypes of GABHS that have been associated with PSAGN have been designated as **nephritogenic** strains. The nephritogenic strains associated with pharyngitis, which include M types 1, 4, 6, 12, and 25, are different from the nephritogenic strains associated with pyoderma, which include M types 49, 53, 55, 56, and 57. PSAGN appears to be less common after a GABHS infection of the skin than after a GABHS infection of the throat, but the overall attack rate after an infection at either site with a nephritogenic strain is approximately 15%.

PATHOGENESIS

Although the link between GABHS infections and PSAGN has been clearly established, the mechanism or mechanisms by which the renal injury is produced are as yet incompletely defined. The evidence that PSAGN results from the deposition of immune complexes in the kidney, however, is considerable. Whether the inciting antigen is a GABHS antigen or an autologous antigen that cross-reacts with streptococcal antibodies is not clear. How these immune complexes are formed is not known, although a number of theories have been proposed.

Recent investigations have identified several potential inciting antigens in the pathogenic mechanism that produces PSAGN. Evidence suggests that **endostreptosin** (also known as preabsorbing antigen), an intracellular antigen that is released when nephritogenic strains of GABHS are disrupted, may be the inciting antigen in PSAGN. **Nephritis strain-associated protein (NSAP),** an extracellular antigen of nephritogenic GABHS, is another potential candidate for this role. Finally, **vimentin,** an intermediate filament protein of glomerular mesangial cells, may cross-react with a portion of the M protein of nephritogenic GABHS. Therefore, vimentin may be involved in antigenic mimicry that induces an autoantibody response, which produces PSAGN.

SYMPTOMS AND CLINICAL MANIFESTATIONS

The clinical findings that usually bring patients with PSAGN to medical attention are edema and hematuria. The severity and distribution of the edema, which is typically first noticed in the periorbital area, varies among individual patients. The fact that most patients lose weight during recovery suggests that fluid retention with or without clinical edema commonly occurs. Approximately 30–50% of children with PSAGN have gross hematuria, which is typically described as "cola-colored," "smoky," or "rusty" urine. The gross hematuria may persist for as little as a few hours or for as long as 2 weeks.

Physical Examination Findings

Approximately 50–90% of children with PSAGN have hypertension. The hypertension is highly variable, but systolic pressures greater than 200 mm Hg and diastolic pressures greater than 120 mm Hg are not unusual. In a very small percentage of patients, the hypertension may be severe enough to cause hypertensive encephalopathy characterized by nausea, vomiting, headaches, seizures, or changes in the level of consciousness.

The majority of children with PSAGN also have evidence of circulatory congestion as a result of the expansion of the intracellular fluid volume. Dyspnea, orthopnea, cough, or audible pulmonary rales may be apparent, but congestive heart failure is unusual in a child with an otherwise normal cardiovascular system. Children with PSAGN, who may be pale, may have systemic symptoms such as lethargy, anorexia, fever, and abdominal pain, but seldom do they appear extremely ill. Occasionally, a child with PSAGN may present with a fulminant course, including severe oliguria and hypertensive encephalopathy (Table 40–7).

DIAGNOSIS

The diagnosis of PSAGN can usually be made on the basis of clinical and laboratory findings in children with serologic evidence of a recent GABHS infection. A renal biopsy is rarely indicated but should be considered if hypertension, hypocomplementemia, heavy proteinuria, or renal insufficiency persists. The histologic abnormalities identified in the renal biopsy specimen correlate with the clinical severity of the disease and with the long-term prognosis.

Differential Diagnosis

Other diseases that may have a presentation similar to PSAGN include a variety of primary renal diseases, such as nephrotic syndrome, Berger's disease, and familial nephritis, and a variety of multisystem diseases with renal involvement, such as Henoch-Schönlein purpura, SLE, and serum sickness. Other infectious diseases, such as infective endocarditis, bacterial sepsis, and hepatitis B, can be associated with acute glomerulonephritis and must be distinguished from PSAGN (Table 40–8).

Laboratory Evaluation

Virtually all children with PSAGN have microscopic hematuria, and 30–50% have gross hematuria. Most children with the disease also have proteinuria; approximately 30% have proteinuria in the nephrotic range, with more than 2 $g/m^2/24$ hours of protein loss. Affected children may also have pyuria or hyaline, granular, or red blood cell casts in their urine.

Depression of the total hemolytic complement activity and C3 levels are seen in almost all children during the initial 2 weeks of

TABLE 40–7. Signs and Symptoms of Poststreptococcal Acute Glomerulonephritis

Common Findings
Hematuria (microscopic or macroscopic)
Edema
Hypertension
Oliguria
Frequent Findings
Circulatory congestion
Pulmonary rales
Dyspnea
Orthopnea
Cough
Pallor
Variable Findings
Encephalopathy
Confusion
Headache
Somnolence
Convulsions
Systemic symptoms
Fever
Nausea
Anorexia
Abdominal pain
Uncommon Findings
Anuria and renal failure
Congestive heart failure

TABLE 40–8. Differential Diagnosis of Poststreptococcal Acute Glomerulonephritis

Nephrotic syndrome
Berger's disease
Familial nephritis
Henoch-Schönlein purpura
Systemic lupus erythematosus
Serum sickness
Infective endocarditis
Bacterial sepsis
Hepatitis B

PSAGN. About one third have modest elevations of their BUN and creatinine levels. Elevated levels of circulating immune complexes are seen in most patients during the first week of disease, and the quantity of immune complexes correlates with the severity of the PSAGN. Although an elevated erythrocyte sedimentation rate is common during the early stages of the disease, the height of the erythrocyte sedimentation rate does not correlate with the severity of the PSAGN. Urine output is often reduced; patients may produce concentrated urine with an acidic pH. With moderate to severe impairment of renal function, patients may develop metabolic acidosis, hyperkalemia, hyperchloremia, hyponatremia, hypoalbuminemia, or dilutional anemia.

The isolation of GABHS from a culture of the pharynx or skin can support the diagnosis of PSAGN. However, because the culture cannot distinguish between an acute streptococcal infection and a streptococcal carrier, the best evidence of an antecedent streptococcal infection is a serologic response to GABHS. With pharyngitis-associated PSAGN, 90–95% of the patients have an elevated ASO or antideoxyribonuclease B titer. With pyoderma-associated PSAGN, the ASO titer is not consistently elevated, but the antideoxyribonuclease B titer is elevated in 90–95% of these cases.

Pathologic Findings

Although renal biopsy is rarely indicated in patients with PSAGN, this procedure may be helpful in certain situations (see Diagnosis). The glomerular lesions of PSAGN may be either proliferative, exudative, or both; typically all of the glomeruli are diffusely involved in the process. The proliferative changes may involve the endothelial or epithelial cells of Bowman's capsule, and consequently crescent formation may occur. Although initially diffuse, the hypercellularity is usually confined to the mesangial cells as the acute stage of the PSAGN subsides. Electron microscopy reveals deposits consisting of IgG and C3, which are usually found in a subepithelial location during the first 3–6 weeks of the disease. These electron-dense deposits may also be found in the subendothelial, intramembranous, or mesangial regions. The glomerular basement membrane usually appears normal.

TREATMENT

Although antibiotic therapy does not affect the clinical course of PSAGN, it can eradicate the nephritogenic GABHS that may still be present and reduce the risk of transmitting these streptococci to others. Penicillin is the antibiotic of choice; erythromycin is the preferred agent for patients who are allergic to penicillin.

No therapies, including use of immunosuppressive agents, have been shown to accelerate the resolution of the renal lesions in PSAGN. Therefore, treatment consists primarily of palliative measures directed at the complications of the disease.

COMPLICATIONS

The hypertension sometimes found in children with PSAGN, which is occasionally severe, can be associated with encephalopathy. The circulatory congestion that may occur with this disease can also be severe; it can lead to congestive heart failure and pulmonary edema. Although oliguria is often seen in children with PSAGN, anuria and renal failure are unusual but can occur. The progression of acute PSAGN to chronic glomerulonephritis in children is extremely unusual.

PROGNOSIS

Overall, the prognosis for children with PSAGN is very favorable. More than 95% of children with the disease experience a spontaneous and complete resolution of symptoms, edema, and renal dysfunction; fewer than 5% have abnormal urinalyses 15 years after the acute episode. In 0.5–2% of hospitalized children with PSAGN, kidney damage is so severe that persistent or progressive renal failure develops.

PREVENTION

In contrast to acute rheumatic fever, which can be prevented with antibiotic therapy of the antecedent GABHS infection, evidence that PSAGN can be prevented once an infection with a nephritogenic strain of GABHS has occurred is lacking. Antibiotic treatment of patients with PSAGN who are still harboring the nephritogenic GABHS limits transmission to others, however. During outbreaks of nephritogenic GABHS infections, penicillin prophylaxis of children at risk may be beneficial. Because recurrences of PSAGN are very rare, long-term antibiotic prophylaxis after an episode of PSAGN is not indicated.

REVIEWS

da Silva NA, Pereira BA: Acute rheumatic fever: Still a challenge. *Rheum Dis Clin North Am* 1997;23:545–68.

Lewy JE, Salinas-Madrigal L, Herdson PB, et al: Clinico-pathologic correlations in acute poststreptococcal glomerulonephritis: A correlation between renal functions, morphologic damage and clinical course of 46 children with acute poststreptococcal glomerulonephritis. *Medicine (Baltimore)* 1971;50:453–501.

Markowitz M, Gordis L (editors): *Rheumatic Fever,* 2nd ed. Philadelphia, Saunders, 1972.

Simckes AM, Spitzer A: Poststreptococcal acute glomerulonephritis. *Pediatr Rev* 1995;16:278–9.

Stollerman GH (editor): *Rheumatic Fever and Streptococcal Infection.* Grune & Stratton, Orlando, Fla, 1975.

Stollerman GH: Nephritogenic and rheumatogenic group A streptococci. *J Infect Dis* 1969;120:258–63.

Stollerman GH: Rheumatic fever. *Lancet* 1997;349:935–42.

Tejani A, Ingulli E: Poststreptococcal glomerulonephritis: Current clinical and pathologic concepts. *Nephron* 1990;55:1–5.

Rheumatic Fever

Alban B, Epstein JA, Feinstein AR, et al: Rheumatic fever in childhood and adolescence. A long-term epidemiologic study of subsequent prophylaxis, streptococcal infections, and clinical sequelae. *Ann Intern Med* 1964;60(Suppl 5):1–129.

Albert DA, Harel L, Karrison T: The treatment of rheumatic carditis: A review and meta-analysis. *Medicine (Baltimore)* 1995;74:1–12.

Bisno AL: Group A streptococcal infections and acute rheumatic fever. *N Engl J Med* 1991;325:783–93.

Dajani A, Taubert K, Ferrieri P, et al: Treatment of acute streptococcal pharyngitis and prevention of rheumatic fever: A statement for health professionals. Committee on Rheumatic Fever, Endocarditis, and Kawasaki Disease of the Council on Cardiovascular Disease in the Young, the American Heart Association. *Pediatrics* 1995;96:758–64.

Denny FW, Wannamaker LW, Brink WR, et al: Landmark article May 13, 1950: Prevention of rheumatic fever. Treatment of the preceding streptococcic infection. *JAMA* 1985;254:534–7.

Gordis L: Effectiveness of comprehensive-care programs in preventing rheumatic fever. *N Engl J Med* 1973;289:331–5.

Gordis L, Lilienfield A, Rodriguez R: Studies in the epidemiology and preventability of rheumatic fever. I. Demographic factors and the incidence of acute attacks. *J Chronic Dis* 1969;21:645–54.

Kaplan EL, Johnson DR, Cleary PP: Group A streptococcal serotypes isolated from patients and sibling contacts during the resurgence of rheumatic fever in the United States in the mid-1980s. *J Infect Dis* 1989;159:101–3.

Kaplan MH, Meyeserian M: An immunological cross reaction between group A streptococcal cells and human heart tissue. *Lancet* 1962; 1:706–10.

Roberts S, Kosanke S, Dunn ST, et al: Pathogenic mechanisms in rheumatic carditis: Focus on valvular endothelium. *J Infect Dis* 2001;183:507–11.

Stollerman GH: The changing face of rheumatic fever in the 20th century. *J Med Microbiol* 1998;47:655–7.

Veasy LG, Weidmeier SE, Orsmond GS, et al: Resurgence of acute rheumatic fever in the intermountain area of the United States. *N Engl J Med* 1987;316:421–7.

Veasy LG, Hill HR: Immunologic and clinical correlations in rheumatic fever and rheumatic heart disease. *Pediatr Infect Dis J* 1997;16:400–7.

Veasy LG, Tani LY, Hill HR: Persistence of acute rheumatic fever in the intermountain area of the United States. *J Pediatr* 1994;124:9–16.

Poststreptococcal Glomerulonephritis

Anthony BF, Kaplan EL, Wannamaker LW, et al: Attack rates of acute nephritis after type 49 streptococcal infection of the skin and of the respiratory tract. *J Clin Invest* 1969;48:1697–704.

Bright R: Cases and observations illustrative of renal disease accompanied with the secretion of albuminous urine. *Guys Hosp Rep* 1836;1:338.

Clark G, White RH, Glasgow EF, et al: Poststreptococcal glomerulonephritis in children: Clinicopathological correlations and long-term prognosis. *Pediatr Nephrol* 1988;2:381–8.

Dodge WF, Spargo BH, Travis LB, et al: Poststreptococcal glomerulonephritis: A prospective study in children. *N Engl J Med* 1972;286:273–8.

Jordan SC, Lemire JM: Acute glomerulonephritis: Diagnosis and treatment. *Pediatr Clin North Am* 1982;29:857–73.

Rammelkamp CH Jr, Weaver RS: Acute glomerulonephritis—The significance of the variations in the incidence of the disease. *J Clin Invest* 1953;32:345–58.

Read SE, Zabriskie JB (editors): *Streptococcal Diseases and the Immune Response.* New York, Academic Press, 1980.

Stetson CA, Rammelkamp CH, Krause RM, et al: Epidemic acute nephritis: Studies on etiology, natural history and prevention. *Medicine* 1955; 34:431–50.

CHAPTER 41

Chronic Fatigue Syndrome

Hal B. Jenson

Numerous terms have been applied to the syndrome of easy fatigability in association with mild to debilitating somatic symptoms, including **chronic mononucleosis, chronic EBV infection, neurasthenia,** and **immune dysfunction syndrome.** It was formally defined in 1988 by the CDC as **chronic fatigue syndrome** because fatigue is the principal and invariable physical symptom, but it remains an enigma and a diagnostic dilemma. Chronic fatigue syndrome is neither a new disease nor the result of enhanced appreciation of previously unrecognized clinical illness. Descriptions of a similar illness are in Hippocrates' writings from approximately 400 B.C. Current understanding of chronic fatigue syndrome is derived largely from studies in adults and to a lesser extent in adolescents; very little information is available about this syndrome in young children.

ETIOLOGY

The cause of chronic fatigue syndrome is unknown. Chronic fatigue syndrome is an illness that is the subjective experience of symptoms representative of a variety of clinical conditions of organic, psychologic, and mixed causes. There is no conclusive evidence that this condition is a single disease with a single identifiable etiologic agent or even that there are characteristic physiologic abnormalities. Chronic fatigue syndrome is frequently purported to be associated with various infectious agents, however, and it shares various clinical manifestations with many recognized infectious illnesses.

EPIDEMIOLOGY

Chronic fatigue is a common presenting symptom of adolescents and adults; the incidence of chronic fatigue in children is unknown. Depending on demographic factors of age, sex, and ethnicity, the prevalence of chronic fatigue in adults in the United States is 0.3–0.6%. A community-based study (Jason, 1999) found the highest levels of chronic fatigue syndrome in women, minority groups, and persons with lower levels of education and occupational status. Women constitute approximately three fourths of patients who fit the current case definition. Prevalence rates vary significantly, but chronic fatigue syndrome is seen in all populations.

The majority of cases of chronic fatigue syndrome are sporadic and are not associated with secondary cases. More than 60 descriptions of clusters of cases have been reported, many in the 1950s, that gave rise to many eponyms derived from the geographic location or institution where the outbreak occurred. Most "epidemics" of chronic fatigue appear to have been the result of psychosocial phenomena, principally mass hysteria on the part of individuals or altered perception of disease in the community. There is no evidence of person-to-person, transplacental, or bloodborne transmission of chronic fatigue syndrome.

PATHOGENESIS

The pathogenesis of chronic fatigue syndrome is unknown. Numerous infectious agents associated with neuropsychiatric symptoms have been postulated to be the cause of the condition, but at present the contribution of recognized or possibly a new infectious agent is unsubstantiated.

Infectious Diseases. Many persons with a diagnosis of chronic fatigue syndrome correlate the onset with a viral-like illness as the inciting event, including infectious mononucleosis, influenza, chickenpox, or a nonspecific infection with symptoms of sore throat, fever, myalgia, or diarrhea. In many cases the clinical symptoms of depression, such as fatigue, lack of energy and interest, and inability to concentrate merge with or are intensified by the weakness normally found during convalescence from a systemic infectious disease. The result is chronic, sometimes disabling fatigue. Persistent fatigue after an otherwise uncomplicated primary infection is well recognized, especially with EBV and influenza virus. Symptoms of fatigue and exhaustion may last anywhere from a few months to a few years and may be accompanied by signs of depression. Similar but less frequent and dramatic postinfectious fatigue has been reported with cytomegalovirus infection, toxoplasmosis, hepatitis A, rubella, chickenpox, and even after adequately treated Lyme disease, brucellosis, and infections with group A *Streptococcus, Campylobacter jejuni, Escherichia coli* O157:H7, and *Mycoplasma pneumoniae.* Several studies of convalescence after acute infection demonstrate that symptomatic recovery is critically dependent on the emotional state and attitude of the individual. Persons with a propensity to become depressed are more likely to respond to acute infection with depression-like symptoms than individuals who do not have such a vulnerability.

Numerous reports have suggested various agents, including *Borrelia burgdorferi* (the cause of Lyme disease), overgrowth of *Candida,* EBV, HHV6, enteroviruses, or a new retrovirus, as the putative cause of chronic fatigue syndrome. Further careful investigations using strict epidemiologic criteria and enhanced laboratory methods have failed to confirm a causal relationship between chronic fatigue syndrome and these viruses or other infectious agents. At present, the hypothesis that infection with or replication of a known or new virus is the primary cause of the symptoms in the majority of cases of chronic fatigue syndrome has no firm basis.

It is frequently impossible to discern whether the isolation of an infectious agent, serologic evidence of infection, or any laboratory abnormality is evidence of a causal relationship to chronic fatigue, is the result of chronic fatigue syndrome, or is an epiphenomenon. Fatigue is a common symptom during and after many acute infections. Defining the etiologic role of any particular infectious agent is difficult; the infection could represent a benign secondary infection in minimally immunocompromised individuals. Alternatively, coinfection with more than one infectious agent may be necessary.

Immunologic Causes. Several modest, diverse, and sometimes conflicting immunologic abnormalities have been reported in persons with a diagnosis of chronic fatigue syndrome. These include hypogammaglobulinemia or hypergammaglobulinemia, immunoglobulin subclass deficiencies, the presence of antinuclear antibodies, elevated levels of circulating immune complexes, increased CD8 T-lymphocyte counts, T-lymphocyte dysfunction (both specific and nonspecific to EBV), qualitative defects in NK cell function, monocyte dysfunction, decreased in vitro lymphocyte proliferative responses to stimulation mitogens, impaired cell-mediated immune function as determined by delayed-type hypersensitivity skin testing, abnormalities in the ribonuclease L pathway in peripheral blood mononuclear cells, and high rates of skin test reactivity to common food or inhalant extracts. These alterations could represent primary immunologic defects or changes resulting from chronic infection or disease. Specific laboratory immune defects, occurring either in isolation or in a pattern, have not been identified. Furthermore, the magnitude of the abnormalities described is small compared with classic immune disorders, and the degree of immune aberrations does not appear to correlate with the severity of clinical symptoms. No opportunistic infections have been associated with chronic fatigue syndrome.

A complex relationship exists between the psyche and the immune system. In several studies, depression has been shown to affect cellular immune response. Therefore even abnormal in vitro immunologic findings may not be useful in differentiating organic from functional illness. The subtle perturbations of the immune system seen in persons with a diagnosis of chronic fatigue syndrome may be partially the cause of the somatic complaints or another manifestation of the primary process. This is unresolved at present.

Neuropsychiatric Causes. Approximately 80% of persons with chronic fatigue syndrome have psychological or neuropsychiatric difficulties among their principal complaints. Personality difficulty and disorder are increased in adolescents with chronic fatigue syndrome. Up to 25% of all patients meet the criteria for major (nonendogenous) depression at the time of initial diagnosis, and as many as 50% have a psychiatric diagnosis, usually major depression, associated with their somatic complaints. These somatic symptoms are not merely the result of an underlying psychological disorder. Depression and anxiety disorders may be an integral part of the primary disease process of chronic fatigue syndrome, a result of the fatigue and other symptoms, or some combination of the two.

TABLE 41–1. Frequency of Symptoms in Patients with Chronic Fatigue Syndrome

Symptom	Frequency (%)
Primary Somatic Complaints	
Fatigue	100
Myalgias	80–95
Postexertional malaise	70–80
Low-grade fever	40–95
Functional Disabilities	
Impaired memory or concentration	60–90
Sleeping during the day	40–90
Depression	70–85
Anxiety	50–75
Other Somatic Complaints	
Headache	40–90
Sore throat	50–75
Chest palpitations Muscle weakness Postexertional malaise Worsening of premenstrual symptoms Stiffness ("gelling phenomenon") Visual blurring Nocturia	50–60
Nausea Dizziness Arthralgias Tachycardia	40–50
Paresthesias Dry eyes Dry mouth Diarrhea Anorexia Cough Finger swelling Night sweats Painful or enlarged lymph nodes Rash	30–40

Adapted from Komaroff AL, Buchwald D: Symptoms and signs of chronic fatigue syndrome. *Rev Infect Dis* 1991;13:S8–11.

SYMPTOMS AND CLINICAL MANIFESTATIONS

The symptoms of chronic fatigue syndrome are protean, with a spectrum of gradation from subtle to debilitating. Although the perception of fatigue undoubtedly varies among individuals, fatigue as a symptom should not be dismissed as a minor ailment. Like pain, fatigue is a subjective symptom that can result in severe impairment and interference with work, school, and social activities. **Fatigue** is the increased discomfort and decreased efficiency to respond to stimulation, accompanied by the sensation that the skeletal muscles are unable to perform work, in contrast to **sleepiness,** which is the desire to close the eyes and increasingly relax in a position that supports the head while entering the sleep state.

Chronic fatigue syndrome is characterized by multiple somatic complaints of at least 6 months' to several years' duration, in association with impairment to <50% of the usual work or school schedule, activities of daily living, exercise tolerance, and interpersonal relationships (Table 41–1). Fatigue, the most consistent symptom, is generally manifested as lassitude, tiredness, weakness, intolerance to exertion with easy fatigability, significant sleeping during the day, and general malaise. Nocturnal sleeping patterns are usually unchanged and do not differ from those in unaffected individuals. The fatigue is usually accompanied by low-grade fever and myalgias. Emphasis on one particular symptom other than the constitutional symptoms of malaise and fatigability is somewhat uncommon and should prompt further investigation. Weight loss is infrequent. Symptoms of cognitive dysfunction are common and include confusion, difficulty in concentrating, impaired thinking, and forgetfulness. Adult patients often judge these as among the most debilitating symptoms.

The majority of patients correlate an abrupt onset of fatigue with an initial viral-like illness characterized by low-grade fever, sore throat, and cough. Less frequently the initial symptoms indicate gastrointestinal tract involvement with nausea and diarrhea. Persons with a diagnosis of chronic fatigue syndrome have been reported to have high rates of concomitant medical syndromes, including migraine headache, irritable bowel syndrome, or a history of depression, anxiety, or panic disorder. Many persons have signs and symptoms of depression on initial evaluation for chronic fatigue.

Familial rates of major depression are high in families of individuals with a diagnosis of chronic fatigue syndrome.

A history of food, inhalant, or drug allergy is reported by approximately two thirds of persons with chronic fatigue syndrome. Fatigue often accompanies the onset of allergic symptoms and in some cases may be the predominant symptom.

Symptoms in children appear to be similar to those in adolescents and adults. School absenteeism is a major problem. In a small retrospective study (Marshall et al, 1991) of 23 children with a median age of 14 years and a median duration of symptoms of 6 months, two thirds missed 2 or more weeks of school and one third required home tutoring.

Physical Examination Findings

A complete physical examination should be performed in the evaluation of chronic fatigue syndrome. Abnormal findings are conspicuously absent, however. Autonomic dysfunction and neurally mediated hypotension, shown by orthostatic intolerance with abnormal heart rate and blood pressure responses to tilt-table tests, have been reported in adolescents in whom chronic fatigue syndrome has been diagnosed. Physical examination findings diagnostic of an underlying condition are obtained only in approximately 2% of persons with chronic fatigue at presentation, but normal examination findings reassure both patients and physicians. Furthermore, a physical examination is essential to exclude physical causes of depression if a tentative diagnosis of major depression is being considered.

DIAGNOSIS

Chronic fatigue syndrome is a diagnostic subset of **chronic fatigue,** a broader category defined as unexplained fatigue of ≥6 months' duration, which in turn is a subset of **prolonged fatigue,** which is defined as fatigue lasting ≥1 month. The diagnosis of chronic fatigue syndrome is based on inclusionary and exclusionary criteria but remains a diagnosis of exclusion dominated by persistent or relapsing fatigue that is not due to ongoing exertion, is not relieved by rest, and results in a substantial reduction of previous levels of activity, accompanied by at least four specific symptoms for ≥6 months with no other identifiable cause (Fig. 41–1). There are no distinguishing demographic or clinical manifestations between chronic fatigue syndrome and **idiopathic chronic fatigue,** which is not associated with the other symptoms of chronic fatigue syndrome.

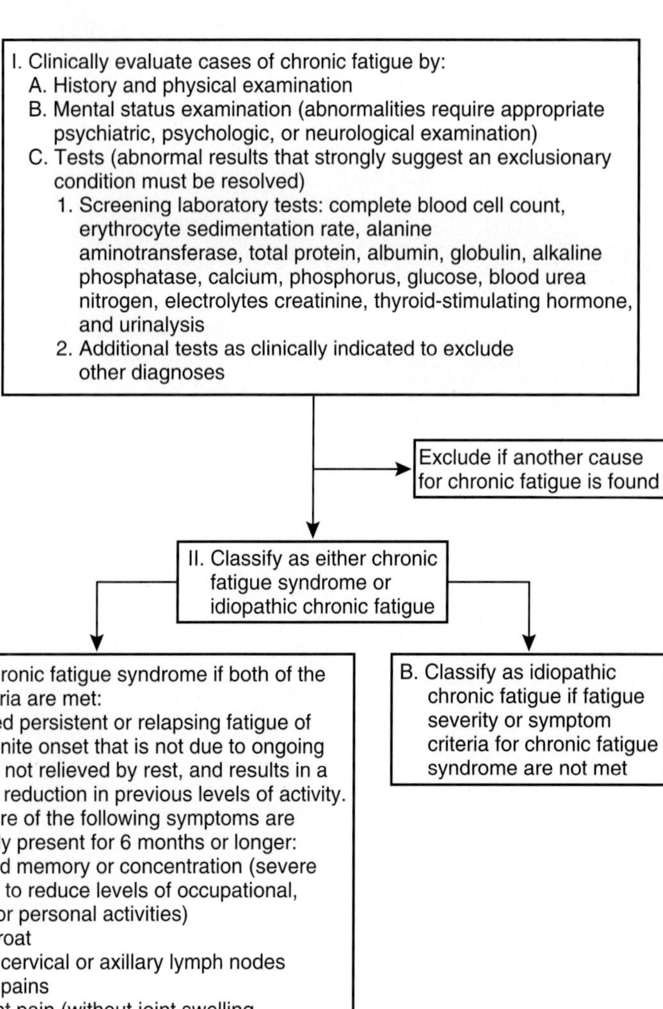

FIGURE 41–1. Clinical evaluation and classification of unexplained chronic fatigue. The case definition for chronic fatigue syndrome was proposed by the CDC in 1988 (Holmes et al, 1988) and refined and simplified in 1994 by an international working group. (Adapted from Fukuda K, Straus SE, Hickie I, et al: The chronic fatigue syndrome: A comprehensive approach to its definition and study. *Ann Intern Med* 1994;121: 953–9.)

The primary purpose of the diagnostic evaluation in persons with fatigue at presentation is to exclude other recognizable and potentially treatable conditions. The proposed criteria for chronic fatigue syndrome (Fig. 41–1) should not necessarily be strictly applied to individuals in clinical practice, but they do provide useful guidelines in the characterization of this symptom complex. Most persons, including children, who are referred to subspecialists for evaluation of chronic fatigue do not fulfill the diagnostic criteria for chronic fatigue syndrome. The diagnostic criteria do not differentiate persons with organic illness from those with similar symptoms arising from a primary affective disorder. One principal difference in these patient populations is the attribution of symptoms to physical rather than psychological causes in individuals who eventually have a diagnosis of chronic fatigue syndrome. When the history is elicited from a persons seen for evaluation of fatigue, it is often helpful to ask directly what the person thinks might be causing the symptoms and whether he or she has specific concerns or fears.

Chronic fatigue syndrome is difficult to diagnose in children, who have trouble describing their symptoms and articulating their concerns and who may not perceive themselves as being ill because they have no clear reference for normal health. As with any chronic illness in childhood, careful attention must be directed to the family dynamics to identify and resolve family problems or psychopathology that may be contributing to the child's perceptions of the symptoms. The diagnosis of chronic fatigue syndrome in a child should be entertained with a great deal of caution. Most patients, including children, with chronic fatigue syndrome attribute their symptoms to physical rather than psychological causes. Applying the label of chronic fatigue syndrome may delay the diagnosis of a treatable medical illness, avoid the detection of psychological problems or family dysfunction, and perpetuate inappropriate illness behaviors that may have a profound effect on the child's psychosocial development.

Differential Diagnosis

The diagnosis of chronic fatigue syndrome can be established only after recognized medical and psychiatric causes of fatigue, many of which are treatable, have been excluded (Table 41–2). These include any medical condition that may explain the presence of chronic fatigue, such as untreated hypothyroidism, sleep apnea and narcolepsy, an adverse effect of medication, and severe obesity. A previously diagnosed chronic medical condition, such as hepatitis B or hepatitis C, without documented resolution should be clarified. The diagnostic criteria for chronic fatigue syndrome closely parallel those for major depression. Although depression and other psychological symptoms may be manifestations of chronic fatigue syndrome, prior diagnoses of major depressive disorder with psychotic or melancholic features, bipolar affective disorders, schizophrenia of any subtype, delusional disorders of any subtype, dementias of any subtype, anorexia nervosa or bulimia nervosa, or alcohol or other substance abuse within 2 years before the onset of the chronic fatigue or at any time afterward are considered diagnostic exclusion criteria. Symptoms of other pre-existing medical conditions may also resemble chronic fatigue syndrome. Patients with fatigue resulting from underlying cardiopulmonary disease, malignancy, rheumatic disease, or neurologic disease rarely have isolated fatigue at presentation, however. Such organic illnesses are also considered exclusion criteria. The evaluation of chronic fatigue should not be confused with the evaluation of prolonged fever of unidentified origin (Chapter 20).

Fibromyalgia. Fibromyalgia **(fibrositis)** is a relatively common rheumatic condition characterized by unexplained widespread musculoskeletal pain in addition to multiple discrete painful point sites, or **trigger sites.** Fibromyalgia may occur in isolation or concomitantly with other rheumatic disorders. Although the symptoms of chronic fatigue syndrome are present in persons with fibromyalgia, the diagnostic criteria of fibromyalgia presented by the American College of Rheumatology require at least 3 months of widespread pain *plus* the presence of at least 11 of 18 specific trigger sites that are painful—not just tender—to digital palpation. These sites represent pain-associated irritations, are not truly inflammatory, and may be postinfectious phenomena. Fibromyalgia may represent a subset of persons with chronic fatigue syndrome having heightened musculoskeletal symptoms.

Laboratory Evaluation

Because the symptoms of chronic fatigue syndrome are diverse and the potential conditions that may lead to illness in particular individuals are numerous, some clinicians tend to pursue each possible diagnosis with a specific laboratory test. However, laboratory evaluation is helpful in only approximately 5% of cases of chronic fatigue syndrome. Discovery of an unsuspected organic illness by laboratory testing alone is very uncommon. Laboratory studies are aimed primarily not at diagnosing chronic fatigue syn-

TABLE 41–2. Differential Diagnosis of Chronic Fatigue Syndrome

Severe obesity (body mass index* ≥45)	Neuromuscular disease
Malignancy	Multiple sclerosis
Allergic disorders	Myasthenia gravis
Autoimmune disease	Endocrine disease
Chronic inflammatory disease	Hypothyroidism
Sarcoidosis	Adrenal insufficiency
Wegener's granulomatosis	Cushing's syndrome
Fibromyalgia	Diabetes mellitus
Postinfectious fatigue	Drug dependency or abuse
Lyme disease	Alcohol
Brucellosis	Psychotropic medications
Epstein-Barr virus infectious mononucleosis	Controlled-prescription medications
Acute cytomegalovirus infection	Illicit drugs
Influenza	Drug reaction
Acute toxoplasmosis	Environmental toxins
Chronic bacterial disease	Chemical
Occult abscess	Pesticide
Infective endocarditis	Heavy metal
Lyme disease	Chronic pulmonary, cardiac, gastrointestinal, hepatic, renal, or hematologic disease
Tuberculosis	Sleep disorders
Fungal disease	Sleep apnea
Histoplasmosis	Narcolepsy
Blastomycosis	Psychoses
Coccidioidomycosis	Psychotic depression
Chronic viral disease	Bipolar disorder
Chronic hepatitis B	Schizophrenia
Chronic hepatitis C	Nonpsychotic depression
HIV infection	Somatoform disorders
Parasitic disease	Generalized anxiety disorder
Toxoplasmosis	Panic disorder
Amebiasis	Pregnancy
Giardiasis	Postpartum symptoms
Systemic helminthic infection	

*Body mass index = (Weight in kilograms)/(Height in meters)^2.

drome but at excluding other treatable diseases with similar symptoms.

Although evaluation of each person should be individualized, screening laboratory studies should be limited to general tests that provide evidence of the absence of significant organic dysfunction (Fig. 41–1). Further tests should be directed toward excluding treatable diseases that may be suggested by specific symptoms or physical findings. In general, the greater the number of symptoms and the longer the duration of illness, the less extensive laboratory evaluation is required to exclude other organic disease.

Most patients with chronic fatigue syndrome show laboratory evidence of some type of immune dysfunction. However, because of the subtlety of the abnormalities, the extreme variability among individual patients, the normal longitudinal variability, and the lack of correlation with prognosis, these parameters are not routinely studied in the evaluation of chronic fatigue syndrome in an individual patient. No laboratory test or group of tests has been shown to correlate reliably with the severity of clinical symptoms or the likelihood of clinical improvement.

Microbiologic Evaluation

Extensive virologic or serologic studies in patients with chronic fatigue syndrome are not usually beneficial unless specifically indicated by the history, physical examination findings, or laboratory screening tests. Although some specific microbiologic tests have been suggested as part of the evaluation of chronic fatigue syndrome, close scrutiny has failed to demonstrate consistent differences between cases and controls that merit routine testing.

Diagnostic Imaging

Diagnostic imaging, including radionuclide imaging studies such as ^{67}Ga scans, ^{111}In scans, ^{99m}Tc bone scans, and liver-spleen scans, is not useful.

Psychologic Evaluation

Physicians often tend to evaluate symptoms by searching for physical or metabolic causes before considering psychiatric causes. Psychiatric factors are much more common in persons with chronic fatigue at presentation than in those with other illnesses, however. Evaluation of chronic fatigue should include psychologic evaluation for depression or anxiety disorders, which should precede exhaustive searches for organic causes. Sleep disorders and sleepiness may be distinguished from fatigue by polysomnography. Depression or other psychiatric conditions should be considered in periodic re-evaluations of patients with persistent fatigue and multiple somatic symptoms. The number of unexplained physical symptoms, the extent of disruption of activities of daily living, and the tendency to amplify symptoms all increase linearly in relation to the prevalence of current and past psychiatric diagnoses and lifetime depressive symptoms in patients with a diagnosis of chronic fatigue syndrome. Selection criteria that require multiple physical complaints, such as the current case definition, may in fact be selective for patients with the highest prevalence of lifetime psychiatric disorders.

TREATMENT

Development of definitive treatment for chronic fatigue syndrome awaits definition of the causes of the symptoms. No proven specific therapeutic agents for chronic fatigue syndrome are now available or are recommended. No data suggest relief of symptoms or cure of chronic fatigue by dietary or vitamin supplements. Treatment should involve emotional support, symptom relief, and minimizing of unnecessary and misleading diagnostic tests and unproved therapeutic trials. Psychologic or psychiatric intervention may be a principal component of supportive treatment.

Definitive Treatment

A variety of compassionate therapeutic approaches have been studied, including antibacterial, antifungal, antiviral, and anti-inflammatory agents; immunotherapies, including plasmapheresis; antidepressants; and opiates. However, none of these treatments is consistently beneficial in the management of persons with chronic fatigue syndrome. Randomized, double-blind, crossover studies using either acyclovir, chosen because of its ability to inhibit the replication of EBV both in vitro and in vivo, or nystatin, chosen because of the possible connection of chronic fatigue with *Candida,* failed to demonstrate any therapeutic effectiveness over placebo for the systemic or psychological symptoms. High-dose IVIG therapy has also failed to demonstrate reproducible clinical or psychological improvement. Strong placebo effects have been noted in most placebo-controlled trials. One randomized study (McKenzie et al, 1998) of low-dose hydrocortisone therapy showed mild symptomatic improvement, but the associated adrenal suppression argues against its use. Despite the increased frequency of neurally mediated hypotension, a study (Rowe et al, 2001) of treatment with fludrocortisone, which is often used to treat low blood pressure, did not demonstrate amelioration of symptoms of chronic fatigue syndrome. Patients and families should understand the limitations of conventional medical therapies.

At present, anti-infective or anti-inflammatory therapy or immunotherapy for chronic fatigue is not justified. Alternative therapies such as removal of dental fillings, elimination diets, or administration of megadoses of vitamins, essential fatty acids, or magnesium have not been adequately studied and may be dangerous, expensive, and exploitative. Because the diagnosis of chronic fatigue syndrome excludes many treatable clinical illnesses, no specific empirical medical therapy is currently recommended for patients with this diagnosis.

Supportive Therapy

The mainstay of management of chronic fatigue syndrome is comprehensive, supportive treatment centered around a combination of restoration of a normal sleep pattern, rehabilitation strategies including exercise, emotional sustenance for the patient and the family, and optimism. Rehabilitation strategies are most successful when they are initiated early in the illness, which can minimize some of the detrimental psychological consequences of chronic illness. Continuing psychological follow-up is especially important in pediatric cases. Family therapy can help patients, parents, and siblings deal with the debility by providing reassurance, improving self-esteem, and encouraging healthy discussion and help-seeking. This therapy may also allow for a better understanding into the possible initiating or contributing causes of symptoms and may possibly uncover potential remedies and solutions. Although the causes of chronic fatigue syndrome and the contribution of psychological factors are subjects of debate, the symptoms and the subsequent effects on the lives of affected individuals and their families are very real and should be addressed appropriately. In most instances, psychological or psychiatric intervention is a principal part of supportive therapy, but in some cases it is definitive treatment for depression or anxiety disorders. Unnecessary referral to medical specialists may only reinforce the patient's and family's perception that there is an underlying organic illness that needs to be detected.

Antihistamines may be helpful for alleviating difficulty in initiating or maintaining sleep. More severe symptoms of depression, anxiety, and sleep disorders may require low doses of tricyclic antidepressants or benzodiazepines. However, such therapies are rarely necessary and are not recommended, especially in children, unless clinically indicated by formal psychiatric evaluation as part of a comprehensive psychiatric management plan. Analgesics such as acetaminophen or ibuprofen should be used for headaches. Nonsteroidal anti-inflammatory drugs may be useful in the symptomatic relief of low-grade fever, myalgias, and arthralgias. Symptoms of light-headedness and postural syncope often abate with increased daily water and salt intake. In adolescents, corticosteroids or β-blockers can be effective. Fatigue is associated with reduced serotonin and may improve with **selective serotonin reuptake inhibitors (SSRIs)** such as fluoxetine or sertraline.

Patients with severe limitation of activity should be started on a schedule of gentle, carefully graded remobilization, determined by individual tolerance, to increase strength and resilience. Physical therapy beginning with 30 minutes of activity daily, divided into two periods and leading to a regular regimen of moderate exercise, can reduce fatigue and help restore a more active lifestyle. Complete bed rest and lack of exercise only perpetuate immobility and lead to deconditioning, whereas rapid remobilization, for whatever reason, may not be tolerated and may exacerbate symptoms. Return to school should be initiated gradually but systematically to resume normal attendance. Home tutoring may be an interim alternative. Patients and their families should clearly understand that no evidence shows that activity harms patients with chronic fatigue syndrome.

Continued empathy and support by the treating physician is important in maintaining a physician-patient relationship that is conducive to identification and resolution of both organic and psychological illness. Periodic medical re-evaluation approximately every 3 months is warranted for early detection of other identifiable causes of chronic fatigue, especially if new symptoms develop.

COMPLICATIONS

There are no long-term risks or increased rates of cancer, autoimmune disease, multiple sclerosis, opportunistic infections, or other complications. Development of unusual symptoms or findings should prompt re-evaluation or reconsideration of the original diagnosis of chronic fatigue syndrome.

PROGNOSIS

Chronic fatigue can persist for years with significant morbidity but no mortality. None of the diagnostic criteria for chronic fatigue syndrome and no laboratory tests appear to predict reliably the eventual clinical course, the rate of resolution of symptoms, or even the likelihood of clinical improvement. The clinical course of chronic fatigue syndrome is highly variable. About 20% of adults with a diagnosis of chronic fatigue syndrome return to their previous state of health for periods of at least 1 year without any specific medical intervention, although most adults never return to their preillness level of usual activity. Approximately 60% of adults report gradual but significant improvement in symptoms within 2–3 years without specific therapy, although some persons show no improvement or occasionally worsen. Patients who deal with stress by **somatization,** having physical rather than psychological symptoms, and who deny the modulating role of psychosocial factors have a less favorable prognosis. The eventual clinical course is unpredictable, and many of the adults remain functionally impaired for years. Children and adolescents with chronic fatigue appear to recover more readily, typically with an undulating course of gradual but substantial improvement, or complete resolution, in 80–100% of adolescents within 1–4 years after diagnosis. Personality disorder may be linked to poor outcome in adolescents with chronic fatigue syndrome.

Patients should be told that their symptoms will likely wax and wane. This contributes to the difficulty in evaluating the effectiveness of possible therapies, and patients should understand the need to consider cautiously the novel therapies that appear periodically in the lay press.

PREVENTION

Because the cause of chronic fatigue syndrome is unknown, there are no recognized preventive measures.

REVIEWS

Fukuda K, Strauss SE, Hickie I, et al: The chronic fatigue syndrome: A comprehensive approach to its definition and study. International Chronic Fatigue Syndrome Study Group. *Ann Intern Med* 1994;121:953–9.

Goodnick PJ, Klimas NG (editors): *Chronic Fatigue and Related Immune Deficiency Syndromes.* Washington, DC, American Psychiatric Press, 1993.

Holmes GP, Kaplan JE, Gantz NM, et al: Chronic fatigue syndrome: A working case definition. *Ann Intern Med* 1988;108:387–9.

Klonoff DC: Chronic fatigue syndrome. *Clin Infect Dis* 1992;15:812–23.

Levine PH (editor): Chronic fatigue syndrome: Current concepts. *Clin Infect Dis* 1994;18:S1.

Marshall GS: Report of a workshop on the epidemiology, natural history, and pathogenesis of chronic fatigue syndrome in adolescents. *J Pediatr* 1999;134:395–405.

Shafran SD: The chronic fatigue syndrome. *Am J Med* 1991;90:730–9.

Wessely S: Chronic fatigue syndrome: Summary of a report of a joint committee of the Royal Colleges of Physicians, Psychiatrists and General Practitioners. *J R Coll Physicians Lond* 1996;30:497–504.

KEY ARTICLES

Aaron LA, Burke MM, Buchwald D: Overlapping conditions among patients with chronic fatigue syndrome, fibromyalgia, and temporomandibular disorder. *Arch Intern Med* 2000;24;160:221–7.

Bell DS, Jordan K, Robinson M: Thirteen-year follow-up of children and adolescents with chronic fatigue syndrome. *Pediatrics* 2001;107:994–8.

Carter BD, Edwards JF, Kronenberger WG, et al: Case control study of chronic fatigue in pediatric patients. *Pediatrics* 1995;95:179–86.

Carter BD, Kronenberger WG, Edwards JF, et al: Psychological symptoms in chronic fatigue and juvenile rheumatoid arthritis. *Pediatrics* 1999; 103:975–9.

Garralda E, Rangel L, Levin M, et al: Psychiatric adjustment in adolescents with a history of chronic fatigue syndrome. *J Am Acad Child Adolesc Psychiatry* 1999;38:1515–21.

Gold D, Bowden R, Sixbey J, et al: Chronic fatigue. A prospective clinical and virologic study. *JAMA* 1990;264:48–53.

Hall GH, Hamilton WT, Round AP: Increased illness experience preceding chronic fatigue syndrome: A case control study. *J R Coll Physicians Lond* 1998;32:44–8.

Jason LA, Richman JA, Rademaker AW, et al: A community-based study of chronic fatigue syndrome. *Arch Intern Med* 1999;159:2129–37.

Jordan KM, Landis DA, Downey MC, et al: Chronic fatigue syndrome in children and adolescents: A review. *J Adolesc Health* 1998;22:4–18.

Katon W, Russo J: Chronic fatigue syndrome criteria. A critique of the requirement for multiple physical complaints. *Arch Intern Med* 1992; 152:1604–9.

Klimas NG, Salvato FR, Morgan R, et al: Immunologic abnormalities in chronic fatigue syndrome. *J Clin Microbiol* 1990;28:1403–10.

Krilov LR, Fisher M, Friedman SB, et al: Course and outcome of chronic fatigue in children and adolescents. *Pediatrics* 1998;102:360–6.

Kroenke K, Wood DR, Mangelsdorff AD, et al: Chronic fatigue in primary care. Prevalence, patient characteristics, and outcome. *JAMA* 1988; 260:929–34.

Kruesi MJ, Dale J, Straus SE: Psychiatric diagnoses in patients who have chronic fatigue syndrome. *J Clin Psychiatry* 1989;50:53–6.

Lloyd A, Hickie I, Wakefield D, et al: A double-blind, placebo-controlled trial of intravenous immunoglobulin therapy in patients with chronic fatigue syndrome. *Am J Med* 1990;89:561–8.

Manu P, Lane TJ, Matthews DA: The frequency of the chronic fatigue syndrome in patients with symptoms of persistent fatigue. *Ann Intern Med* 1988;109:554–6.

Marshall GS, Gesser RM, Yamanishi K, et al: Chronic fatigue syndrome in children: Clinical features, Epstein-Barr virus and human herpesvirus 6 serology and long-term follow-up. *Pediatr Infect Dis J* 1991;10:287–90.

McKenzie R, O'Fallon A, Dale J, et al: Low-dose hydrocortisone for treatment of chronic fatigue syndrome. A randomized controlled trial. *JAMA* 1998;280:1061–6.

Plioplys AV: Chronic fatigue syndrome should not be diagnosed in children. *Pediatrics* 1997;100:270–1.

Rangel L, Gerralda E, Levin M, et al: Personality in adolescents with chronic fatigue syndrome. *Eur Child Adolesc Psychiatry* 2000;9:39–45.

Rowe PC, Calkins H, DeBusk K, et al: Fludrocortisone acetate to treat neurally mediated hypotension in chronic fatigue syndrome: A randomized controlled trial. *JAMA* 2001;285:52–9.

Siegel DM, Janeway D, Baum J: Fibromyalgia syndrome in children and adolescents: Clinical features at presentation and status at follow-up. *Pediatrics* 1998;101:377–82

Smith MS, Mitchell J, Corey L, et al: Chronic fatigue in adolescents. *Pediatrics* 1991;88:195–202.

Stewart JM, Gewitz MH, Weldon A, et al: Orthostatic intolerance in adolescent chronic fatigue syndrome. *Pediatrics* 1999;103:116–21.

Straus SE, Dale JK, Wright R, et al: Allergy and the chronic fatigue syndrome. *J Allergy Clin Immunol* 1988;81:791–5.

Wessely S, Powell R: Fatigue syndromes: A comparison of chronic ''postviral'' fatigue with neuromuscular and affective disorders. *J Neurol Neurosurg Psychiatry* 1989;52:940–8.

Wilson A, Hickie I, Lloyd A, et al: Longitudinal study of outcome of chronic fatigue syndrome. *BMJ* 1994;308:756–9.

Wolfe F, Smythe HA, Yunus MB, et al: The American College of Rheumatology 1990 criteria for the classification of fibromyalgia. Report of the Multicenter Criteria Committee. *Arthritis Rheum* 1990;33:160–72.

CHAPTER 42

Nematode Infections

Peter J. Hotez

The parasitic nematodes, or **roundworms,** exert a devastating effect on childhood health and well-being. Ascariasis, hookworm infection, and trichuriasis rank one, two, and three, respectively, as the most prevalent identified communicable diseases among children in the developing world. Yet, because these helminth infections are not often associated with dramatic and acute symptoms their importance is often not appreciated. Young children who harbor parasitic nematodes have a wide range of systemic manifestations and unique clinical conditions that are not usually seen in adults, such as the swollen-belly syndrome of strongyloidiasis, the *Trichuris* dysentery syndrome with colitis, and infant ancylostomiasis (Table 42–1). Among children in developing countries, trichuriasis is the leading cause of inflammatory bowel disease, hookworm infection is a leading cause of childhood iron-deficiency anemia, and ascariasis and strongyloidiasis contribute significantly to childhood malnutrition. Each of these four nematode diseases directly impairs the growth and development of children.

HOOKWORM INFECTION

ETIOLOGY

The two major species of human hookworms, *Ancylostoma duodenale* and *Necator americanus,* cause different clinical syndromes in children. *A. duodenale,* which is larger, generally causes greater blood loss, can infect humans orally, and is more virulent than *N. americanus* (Table 42–2). In addition to the major anthropophilic hookworm *A. duodenale,* which causes classic hookworm infection, the genus *Ancylostoma* includes a less common zoonotic species, *A. ceylanicum,* found in India and Southeast Asia; *A. caninum,* the dog hookworm that has been implicated as a cause of eosinophilic enteritis in Queensland, Australia, and possibly the southern United States; and *A. braziliense,* the dog and cat hookworm. The larval stage of *A. braziliense* is the principal cause of **cutaneous larva migrans** (Chapter 46). *N. americanus,* the only representative of its genus, is also a major anthropophilic hookworm and causes classic hookworm infection.

The infective larval stages of the anthropophilic hookworms live in a developmentally arrested state in warm, damp soil. The emerging first-stage larva molts twice to become a nonfeeding, third-stage **filariform larva** (Fig. 42–1), which travels vertically in the soil as it migrates along films of moisture. The larvae infect humans either by penetrating through the skin (*A. duodenale* and *N. americanus*) or when they are ingested (only *A. duodenale*). Larvae entering the human host by skin penetration undergo extraintestinal migration through the venous circulation and lungs before they are swallowed, whereas orally ingested larvae may either undergo extraintestinal migration or remain in the gastrointestinal tract. Larvae returning to the small intestine undergo two molts to become adult, sexually mature male and female worms ranging in length from 5–13 mm. The buccal capsule of the adult *A. duodenale* hookworm has teeth, and the buccal capsule of *N. americanus* has cutting plates, to facilitate attachment to the mucosa and submucosa of the small intestine. Hookworms can remain in the intestine for 1–5 years, where they mate and produce eggs. Approximately 2 months is required for the larval stages of hookworms to undergo extraintestinal migration and develop into mature adults, although *A. duodenale* larvae may remain developmentally arrested for many months before resuming development in the intestine. Mature *A. duodenale* female worms produce about 30,000 eggs per day; daily egg production by *N. americanus* is less than 10,000 per day. The eggs are thin shelled and ovoid, measuring approximately 40 × 60 μm. Eggs that are deposited on soil with adequate moisture and shade will develop into first-stage larvae and hatch. During the ensuing several days, under appropriate conditions, the larvae will molt twice to the infective stage. Infective larvae are developmentally arrested and nonfeeding. They migrate vertically in the soil until they either infect a new host or exhaust their lipid metabolic reserves and die.

Because survival of the external stages depends on precise soil conditions, transmission of hookworm infection occurs primarily in children who live in rural or agricultural areas rather than urban areas. In endemic regions the number of hookworms that parasitize the intestine tends to increase in individuals during the first decade

TABLE 42–1. Major Pediatric Syndromes Caused by Parasitic Nematodes

Syndrome	Etiologic Agent	Transmission
Infant ancylostomiasis	*Ancylostoma duodenale*	Perinatal?
Hookworm iron deficiency	*A. duodenale*	Larval ingestion and penetration
	Necator americanus	Larval penetration
Trichuris dysentery	*Trichuris trichiura*	Egg ingestion
Trichuris colitis	*T. trichiura*	Egg ingestion
Neonatal ascariasis	*Ascaris lumbricoides*	Transplacental?
Swollen-belly syndrome	*Strongyloides fuelleborni*	Perinatal
Diarrhea, malabsorption ("celiac-like")	*Strongyloides stercoralis*	Larval penetration
Visceral larva migrans	*Toxocara* *Baylisascaris procyonis*	Egg ingestion
Cutaneous larva migrans	*Ancylostoma braziliense* (a zoonotic hookworm)	Larva penetration (and failure to migrate)

TABLE 42–2. Contrasts Between *Ancylostoma duodenale* and *Necator americanus*

Characteristic	*Ancylostoma duodenale*	*Necator americanus*
Geographic distribution	Worldwide in tropics; predominate in northern India, China, and northern Africa	Worldwide in tropics; predominate in Latin America, and sub-Saharan Africa
Size of adult female	10–13 mm	9–11 mm
Adult lifespan	1 yr	3–5 yr
Virulence for human	Greater	Lesser
Daily blood loss per worm (estimated)	0.26 mL	0.03 mL
Infects infants	Yes	No
Oral infectivity	Yes	No

of life and then either continues to increase throughout adulthood or reaches a plateau. Thus there is no clear evidence that humans acquire natural immunity to hookworms. Certain individuals appear to be especially prone to acquire large worm burdens, the basis of which is unknown. In parts of the world where *A. duodenale* infection occurs, clusters of hookworm cases have been reported in neonates and infants, which suggest that *A. duodenale* can be transmitted vertically via breast-feeding.

EPIDEMIOLOGY

Both major species of human hookworm are common in the underdeveloped nations of the tropics. Hookworm is still focally endemic in scattered rural areas of the southeastern United States, although it is no longer a major public health threat. *N. americanus* is the predominant species found in Latin America, but pockets of *A. duodenale* infection are also present. *A. duodenale* is highly prevalent in northern India and China, where infantile ancylostomiasis has been described, and is the predominant hookworm in Mediterranean countries.

PATHOGENESIS

Hookworm larvae infect humans either by penetrating the skin or, in the case of *A. duodenale,* by oral ingestion. Entry is facilitated by the release of parasite-derived hydrolytic enzymes, and the larvae release eicosanoids that elicit a vigorous host inflammatory response leading to a dermatitis known as **ground itch.** A similar syndrome known as **Wakana disease** can develop in the gastrointestinal tract.

Larvae that penetrate the skin enter the small venules and lymphatics, where they are routed to the right atrium, right ventricle, and pulmonary circulation before becoming trapped in the pulmonary capillaries. The larvae migrate through the lungs and are expectorated or swallowed. On entry into the gastrointestinal tract the larvae undergo two molts to become sexually mature, adult worms that live in the small intestine, where they attach to the mucosa with their cutting plates and suck a plug of intestinal mucosa into their buccal capsule. The ingested bolus of host tissue is degraded through the action of hydrolytic enzymes. Blood loss resulting from the action of parasite-derived anticoagulants occurs as capillaries in the lamina propria are ruptured within the tissue bolus. The development of hypochromic microcytic anemia from intestinal blood loss is highly dependent on the daily iron intake and iron reserves of the host. Certain individuals, especially growing children, are vulnerable to the effects of iron deficiency and have growth failure as well as attention deficit and intellectual impairment. Such impairment may occur by interfering with the development of dopaminergic receptors and the biosynthesis of iron-containing metalloenzymes that are essential for the turnover of endogenous neurotransmitters. Permanent deficits may result when iron deficiency occurs early in childhood.

Interruption of larval development has been described for *A. duodenale.* These larvae can remain developmentally arrested for months or possibly longer in body tissues such as muscle. The arrested or tissue-dwelling larvae have been postulated to migrate to the mammary glands during late pregnancy or parturition before transmission to neonates and infants through breast milk.

In addition to iron deficiency, plasma protein leakage from the intestine also occurs in association with blood loss and can result in hypoalbuminemia and protein malnutrition. Alterations in gastric motility, acidity, and absorption have also been described.

Cutaneous Larva Migrans. Cutaneous inflammation caused by migrating zoonotic hookworm larvae such as *A. braziliense* leads to **cutaneous larva migrans,** or **creeping eruption,** as the larvae fail to pass through the basement membrane of the epidermal-dermal junction but migrate laterally within the epidermis.

SYMPTOMS AND CLINICAL MANIFESTATIONS

Ground itch is an intensely pruritic, papular-vesicular dermatitis that develops at the cutaneous site of hookworm larval entry. This cutaneous inflammation is often exacerbated by scratching and excoriations that lead to secondary bacterial infection. Cough and dyspnea with wheezing occur in association with migration of larvae to the lung 1–2 weeks after skin invasion. Hookworm pneumonitis, however, is usually not severe. An immediate hypersensitivity-like syndrome known as **Wakana disease,** associated with the ingestion of large numbers of *A. duodenale* larvae, consists of nausea, vomiting, dyspnea, and eosinophilia.

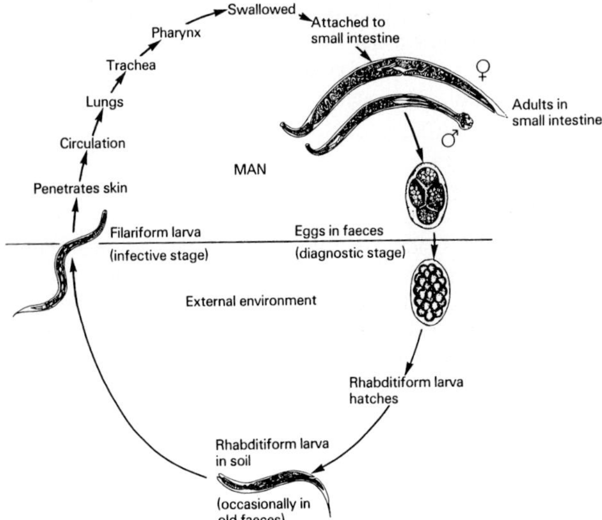

FIGURE 42–1. Life cycle of human hookworms *Ancylostoma duodenale* and *Necator americanus.* (From Zaman V: *Atlas of Medical Parasitology,* 2nd ed. Sidney, Adis Health Science Press, 1984.)

TABLE 42–3. Major Clinical Manifestations of Hookworm Disease

Cutaneous Larval Penetration
Ground itch
Cutaneous larval migrans (*Acylostoma braziliense*)
Gastrointestinal Larval Penetration
Wakana disease
Gastrointestinal Infection with Adult Worms
Iron-deficiency anemia
Physical growth retardation
Intellectual retardation
Chlorosis
Hypoproteinemia
Eosinophilia

The appearance of adult hookworms in the intestine can result in nonspecific gastrointestinal symptoms that precede the appearance of hookworm anemia, which develops approximately 10–20 weeks after initial exposure to infective larvae. Although light hookworm infections are often asymptomatic, heavy infections cause the symptoms of anemia, including dyspnea on exertion, palpitations, and fatigue (Table 42–3). Moderately and heavily infected children are described as being dull and apathetic, and they are often unable to concentrate on school lessons. Children in developing countries who are employed as day laborers must often stop working. In China a syndrome of infantile *A. duodenale* hookworm infection, with melena, diarrhea, anorexia, extremely low hemoglobin concentrations, and a high infant mortality, has been described.

Older children who are chronically infected with hookworms may exhibit delays in growth that are particularly apparent at the time of puberty. Similarly, chronic hookworm anemia may lead to impaired psychomotor, behavioral, and intellectual development. Many of these effects have been attributed directly to iron deficiency.

Physical Examination Findings

The physical signs of hookworm anemia include pale sclerae, koilonychia, and new cardiac murmurs. The skin can assume an unusual pale greenish yellow pallor known as **chlorosis.** In severe hookworm disease, the effects of protein-losing enteropathy can impart a kwashiorkor-like appearance with facial edema, potbelly, and sparse hair.

DIAGNOSIS

The diagnosis of syndromes caused by migrating larvae, including ground itch, cutaneous larva migrans (Fig. 46–26), and pneumonitis, is established by the clinical findings. Hookworm pneumonitis is similar to, but less severe than, other helminthic diseases that exhibit lung migrations, such as ascariasis, strongyloidiasis, and **tropical pulmonary eosinophilia,** a hypersensitivity syndrome associated with *Wuchereria bancrofti* and *Brugia malayi* microfilariae and microfilarial antigen in the lungs.

Laboratory Evaluation

Intestinal hookworm infection is usually diagnosed by identification of the characteristic eggs in the feces in the light microscope. Concentration techniques are usually not required to diagnose infections that are sufficiently heavy to cause clinically important disease. Many quantitative techniques are available that permit estimates of egg output. Ova of *A. duodenale* and *N. americanus* are very similar morphologically, and speciation usually requires raising and recovering infective larvae.

TREATMENT

Definitive Treatment

Several common anthelmintics for the eradication of adult hookworms from the human small intestine are available (Table 42–4). Although the benzimidazoles, including mebendazole and albendazole, are embryotoxic and teratogenic in laboratory animals and their safety has not been established in infants and young children, large-scale field trials indicate that they are well tolerated and safe. They are contraindicated in persons with blood dyscrasias, leukopenia, or liver disease. It is not known whether any of these agents eradicates extraintestinal, arrested *A. duodenale* larvae, which potentially can repopulate the gut or gain access to breast milk. High cure rates have been reported with mebendazole, but this drug is not well absorbed and is therefore ineffective for hookworm infection outside the gastrointestinal tract. Albendazole is also effective, usually as a single dose, although treatment for 3 consecutive days is often necessary to ensure complete removal of the adult worms. A metabolite of albendazole is absorbed and achieves anthelmintic therapeutic levels in tissues. Twice-yearly doses of benzimidazoles are currently being given to more than 1 million children in a study that will run for 3 years. In the pilot studies, no significant events were reported in more than 60,000 treated children.

Recent reports of drug failure with benzimidazoles have prompted concerns about possible emerging anthelmintic drug resistance among hookworms and other intestinal nematodes. This phenomenon has been well described among intestinal nematodes of livestock and results from selection of mutations in nematode tubulin, the target site for benzimidazoles. To date, the reports of drug failure have not been linked to bona fide anthelmintic drug

TABLE 42–4. Therapy for Hookworm Infection*

Ancylostoma duodenale* and *Necator americanus
Albendazole 400 mg PO as a single dose†
or
Mebendazole 100 mg bid PO for 3 days, or 500 mg PO once†
or
Pyrantel pamoate 11 mg/kg (maximum dose: 1 g) qd PO for 3 days
Cutaneous Larva Migrans (*Ancylostoma braziliense*)
Albendazole 400 mg qd PO for 3 days†
or
Ivermectin 200 μg/kg qd PO for 1 or 2 days
or
Thiabendazole topically (either the pediatric suspension or a mixture of 500 mg in 5 mg of petrolatum, applied to the affected area under occlusion several times a day, usually for several weeks)

Adapted from Drugs for parasitic infections. *Med Lett Drugs Ther* 2000; 42:1–11.

*Same dosages for children and adults.

†The benzimidazoles, including albendazole, mebendazole, and thiabendazole are embryotoxic and teratogenic in rodents. They are contraindicated in persons with blood dyscrasias, leukopenia, or liver disease.

resistance. As an alternative drug, pyrantel pamoate is available in suspension and has been reported to be effective against infant hookworm infection caused by *A. duodenale,* although multiple doses may be required. This drug is often formulated with oxantel pamoate, an agent that eradicates whipworm.

Supportive Therapy

Oral iron supplementation ameliorates the anemia seen in light to moderate hookworm infections. Many of the chronic effects of iron deficiency, such as intellectual and growth retardation, are reversible. However, permanent deficits from iron deficiency have been noted when the insult occurs during the first year of life. Life-threatening and hemodynamically significant hookworm anemia is an indication for transfusion and intensive monitoring.

COMPLICATIONS

The acute and chronic complications of hookworm anemia include detrimental effects on growth and development. Exacerbation of disease reportedly occurs with tropical sprue. In addition, fatalities from severe anemia have been described in association with infant ancylostomiasis. Long-standing hookworm infection may be associated with a higher incidence of secondary bacterial and viral infections, including measles pneumonia.

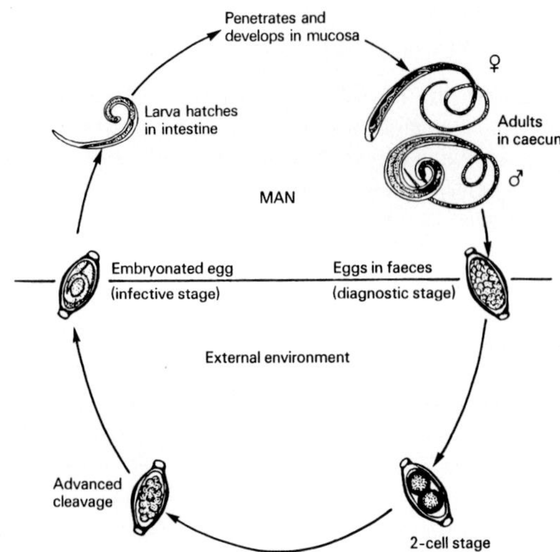

FIGURE 42–2. Life cycle of *Trichuris trichiuria.* (From Zaman V: *Atlas of Medical Parasitology,* 2nd ed. Sidney, Adis Health Science Press, 1984.)

PROGNOSIS

The prognosis of light to moderate hookworm infection after anthelmintic therapy is excellent. Long-term iron deficiency anemia, particularly in the clinical setting of kwashiorkor and marasmus, may lead to permanent intellectual and growth impairment.

PREVENTION

The combination of sanitary disposal of human feces and health education in association with chemotherapy often temporarily eradicates hookworm infection. These practices are not routinely implemented in developing countries, however, because of their expense and the high incidence of reinfection. Such control measures also do not eradicate populations of arrested larvae. The wearing of shoes does not prevent entry by larvae that enter the host by oral ingestion or penetrate the skin on areas other than the feet. Research directed toward defined vaccines is in progress.

TRICHURIASIS

ETIOLOGY

The life cycle of the **whipworm** *Trichuris trichiura* is less complex than the hookworm life cycle. Unembryonated eggs excreted in human feces can infect humans after approximately 2–4 weeks in moist, shaded soil. During this time an active second-stage larva develops within the characteristic bipolar-plugged egg, which is then ingested (Fig. 42–2).

EPIDEMIOLOGY

An estimated 800 million people have infection caused by *T. trichiura* throughout the world. Trichuriasis is less common in countries with temperate climates, but approximately 10% of the population of rural areas of the southeastern United States is infected. The prevalence of trichuriasis in children and adults is often similar, although the severity of the infection is greater in children because they acquire a greater number of worms. As a result of this greater worm burden, children later develop colitis and stunted growth. This increased childhood susceptibility may have an immunologic basis. As in hookworm infection, certain individuals appear to be predisposed to heavy *Trichuris* infections.

PATHOGENESIS

After ingestion of *T. trichiura* eggs by the host, the liberated second-stage larvae penetrate the mucosal epithelium of the cecum or colon and become intracellular. The larvae do not migrate outside the intestine to complete their development, but instead they mature within the cecal and colonic epithelium and create tunnels that enlarge to accommodate worm growth. This process is facilitated by the release of parasite pore-forming proteins. Eventually the thickened posterior portion of the worm ruptures the epithelial tunnel to protrude into the lumen, leaving the intracellular existence to the attenuated anterior end. In this way the adult whipworms disrupt the normal architecture of the colonic mucosa, which is further disrupted by the host inflammatory response. The worm measures approximately 40 mm in length. Egg deposition by maturing females begins 1–3 months after infection.

The clinical presentation of colitis accompanied with ulceration and bleeding that occurs in heavy infections has a striking resemblance to inflammatory bowel disease. Unlike inflammatory bowel disease, however, *Trichuris* colitis usually resolves completely after anthelmintic therapy. A syndrome similar to Crohn's disease is seen when heavy infections extend cephalad to the terminal ileum. The anemia of trichuriasis is probably not associated with direct blood-sucking behavior of the adult whipworm but, rather, is a combination of the anemia of chronic inflammation and leakage of erythrocytes from damaged and eroded capillaries in the mucosa. Gross hemorrhage can sometimes occur in association with dysentery, although the actual blood loss caused by each adult whipworm is usually much less than that caused by an adult hookworm.

SYMPTOMS AND CLINICAL MANIFESTATIONS

Light infections with *T. trichiura* are, for the most part, asymptomatic, although investigations concerning the possible long-term consequences, which may include malnutrition and growth retardation, are currently taking place. There is also evidence that *T. trichiura,* as well as other intestinal nematodes, may affect childhood cognitive and intellectual development. Two major syndromes, which overlap considerably, are associated with heavy *Trichuris* infections in childhood: dysentery and chronic colitis with growth retardation (Table 42–5).

Trichuris Dysentery. The hallmark of *Trichuris* dysentery, a generally acute condition associated with heavy trichuriasis, is diarrhea with blood and mucus. Infections heavy enough to extend to the rectum can produce tenesmus and rectorectal intussusception, resulting in rectal prolapse. Children with this condition are often emaciated and can develop a kwashiorkor-like appearance. Severe dysentery results in anemia.

Chronic Trichuris Colitis. Chronic *Trichuris* colitis has several extraintestinal manifestations that are similar to those caused by other forms of chronic inflammatory bowel disease. Malnutrition and growth retardation are prominent. Short stature has been directly correlated with the number of whipworms in the gut, with striking catch-up growth after expulsion with anthelmintics. Colitis-associated anemia and clubbing of the fingers, which are analogous to similar findings in Crohn's disease, are common features in this syndrome as well.

DIAGNOSIS

Trichuris dysentery can resemble other forms of bacterial and amebic dysentery, and chronic *Trichuris* colitis can be similar to other types of inflammatory bowel disease. The ESR is not elevated in trichuriasis. A specific diagnosis of trichuriasis is confirmed by demonstrating the presence of the characteristic bipolar plugged eggs in the feces. Concentration techniques may also be used.

TREATMENT

Definitive Treatment

Trichuriasis is often considered more refractory to treatment than ascariasis. Mebendazole is the recommended drug, and albendazole is an alternative (Table 42–6). As in hookworm infection, multiple dosage regimens are sometimes required, usually for 3 days. Oxantel pamoate is an effective alternative that is available in some countries, where it is formulated with pyrantel pamoate (effective against hookworms and other gastrointestinal nematodes) in a suspension suitable for pediatric use.

TABLE 42–5. Major Clinical Manifestations of Trichuriasis

Colitis (inflammatory bowel disease)
Physical growth retardation
Clubbing
Anemia of chronic disease
Dysentery
Intussusception

TABLE 42–6. Specific Chemotherapy for Trichuriasis*

Mebendazole 100 mg bid PO for 3 days, or 500 mg PO once†
Alternative: Albendazole 400 mg PO as a single dose†‡
or
Pyrantel pamoate and oxantel pamoate 10 mg/kg of each PO as a single dose§

Adapted from Drugs for parasitic infections. *Med Lett Drugs Ther* 2000; 42:1–11.

*Same dosages for children and adults.

†The benzimidazoles, including albendazole and mebendazole, are embryotoxic and teratogenic in rodents. They are contraindicated in persons with blood dyscrasias, leukopenia, or liver disease.

‡A single dose of albendazole may not be adequate. With heavy infections it may be necessary to extend therapy for 3 days.

§Oxantel pamoate is not generally available in the United States. It is formulated as a suspension of 50 mg pyrantel pamoate and 50 mg oxantel per milliliter, with a recommended single dose of 10 mg/kg of each constituent (Bundy and Cooper, 1989).

Supportive Therapy

Iron supplementation facilitates catch-up growth and ameliorates anemia. The symptoms of human trichuriasis frequently respond dramatically to specific anthelmintic therapy even in the absence of supportive treatment, however.

COMPLICATIONS

There is potential for rectal prolapse and secondary pyogenic bacterial invasion that leads to appendicitis and the extraintestinal manifestations similar to those encountered with inflammatory bowel disease.

PROGNOSIS

The prognosis for resolution of symptoms and catch-up growth after anthelmintic therapy is excellent.

PREVENTION

The prevention of trichuriasis, like other geohelminthic infections, requires public health measures directed at improved sanitation and health education. Some anthelmintics commonly used in conjunction with mass or targeted chemotherapy campaigns may have poor efficacy in the treatment of trichuriasis. Raw fruits and vegetables grown in endemic areas should be avoided, because *T. trichiura* eggs have been isolated from produce irrigated with sewage wastewater.

ASCARIASIS

ETIOLOGY

The infective stage of *Ascaris lumbricoides* is the mature larva-containing egg. It is broadly oval, has a thick shell with an outer mamillated covering, and measures approximately 40×60 μm. *Ascaris* eggs are hardier and more resistant to environmental stress than eggs of other human nematode species. Eggs are passed in the feces of infected individuals and mature in 5–10 days under favorable environmental conditions to become infective. After ingestion by the human host, larvae are released from the eggs and penetrate the intestinal wall before migrating to the lungs via the venous circulation. They then break through the pulmonary tissues into the alveolar spaces, ascend the bronchial tree and trachea, and are reswallowed. On arrival in the small intestine, the larvae develop into mature adult worms. Male worms measure 15–25 cm × 3 mm, and female worms measure 25–35 cm × 4 mm. Each female has a lifespan of 1–2 years, and the uterus can contain as many as 27 million eggs with the capacity for producing 200,000 eggs each day.

EPIDEMIOLOGY

Ascariasis, which is arguably the most prevalent helminthiasis of humans, affects more than 1 billion people worldwide. Young children are affected more frequently and tend to acquire higher worm burdens than adults. Ascariasis has a global distribution. In the United States, intestinal obstruction caused by *A. lumbricoides* occurs in children less than 6 years of age at a rate of 2 obstructions per 1,000 children per year.

Like hookworm infection and trichuriasis, the frequency distribution of the numbers of *Ascaris* worms per host is aggregated; thus a few individuals are predisposed to heavy worm burdens. The relatively high prevalence of ascariasis in temperate countries and in urban environments reflects the success of the infective stage of the parasite in surviving harsh environments.

PATHOGENESIS

After fully embryonated *Ascaris* eggs are swallowed, they enter the duodenum where the larvae emerge from their weakened shells to penetrate the intestinal mucosa (Fig. 42–3). After penetration, they then reach the mesenteric lymphatics or mesenteric portal venules en route to the right side of the heart and then to the lungs. Larvae leave the pulmonary circulation, enter the lung parenchyma, ascend the bronchioles, bronchi, and trachea, and are swallowed.

Minimal damage is produced by larval intestinal mucosa invasion, although some hepatic damage can occur when large numbers of larvae migrate through the portal hepatic venules. The lung sustains the greatest injury to migrating *Ascaris* larvae. In contrast to hookworms, these larvae cause both significant mechanical damage to the lungs, which results in pulmonary microhemorrhages, and pulmonary inflammation. The recruitment of neutrophils and eosinophils to the lung is followed by edema and exudation, which results in filling of the alveolar spaces. The pulmonary inflammation seen in ascariasis may occur in response to the release of the allergenic molting fluid by migrating larvae during ecdysis.

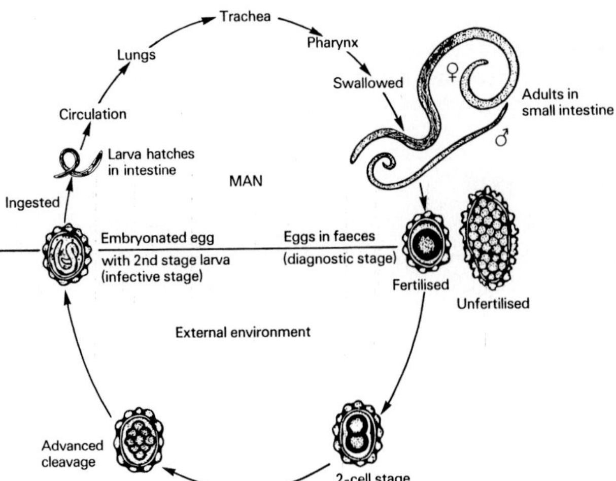

FIGURE 42–3. Life cycle of *Ascaris lumbricoides.* (From Zaman V: *Atlas of Medical Parasitology,* 2nd ed. Sidney, Adis Health Science Press, 1984.)

TABLE 42–7. Major Clinical Manifestations of Ascariasis

Löffler's syndrome
Nonproductive cough
Mild hemoptysis
Dyspnea
Wheezing
Eosinophilia
Abdominal discomfort
Malnutrition/malabsorption
Intestinal obstruction
Hepatobiliary disease

Once *Ascaris* larvae enter the small bowel, they develop into adults that may reach 20–35 cm in length. The adult worms can cause mechanical damage and obstruction by wandering into the biliary tree or by becoming entangled and matted in a bolus. In addition, the adults impair nutrition and cause malabsorption of proteins and fats, possibly because of villous atrophy. Vitamin A malabsorption may also occur. Infected animals and, presumably, humans may have lactase deficiency and impaired lactose digestion.

A syndrome of transplacentally acquired neonatal ascariasis has also been described. This syndrome may be more frequent than is commonly recognized. Infections with *Ascaris* and other intestinal nematodes during pregnancy may be associated with intrauterine growth restriction.

SYMPTOMS AND CLINICAL MANIFESTATIONS

The most common symptoms associated with the presence of adult *Ascaris* in the lumen of the small intestine are mild abdominal discomfort and intermittent acute epigastric pain (Table 42–7). Aside from the dramatic sequelae of hepatobiliary disease and acute intestinal obstruction caused by wandering adults, the greatest detrimental effect is on the nutritional status of the host. Moderate to heavy infections result in impaired digestion and malabsorption of dietary protein, fat, and vitamin A. Steatorrhea is a common feature in children with severe ascariasis. Even mild *Ascaris* infections contribute significantly to childhood malnutrition on a global scale.

DIAGNOSIS

The diagnosis of Löffler's syndrome caused by *Ascaris* pneumonitis is established by the presence of cough and wheezing, eosinophilia, infiltrates on chest radiographs, and the presence of eosinophils and Charcot-Leyden crystals on direct examination of the sputum. This syndrome can also be associated with strongyloidiasis, visceral larva migrans, tropical pulmonary eosinophilia, and, less commonly, hookworm infection.

When intestinal obstruction occurs in an endemic area, ascariasis should be considered. Intestinal ascariasis is diagnosed by direct examination of fecal films. Concentration methods are not usually required because a single adult female worm can produce an aver-

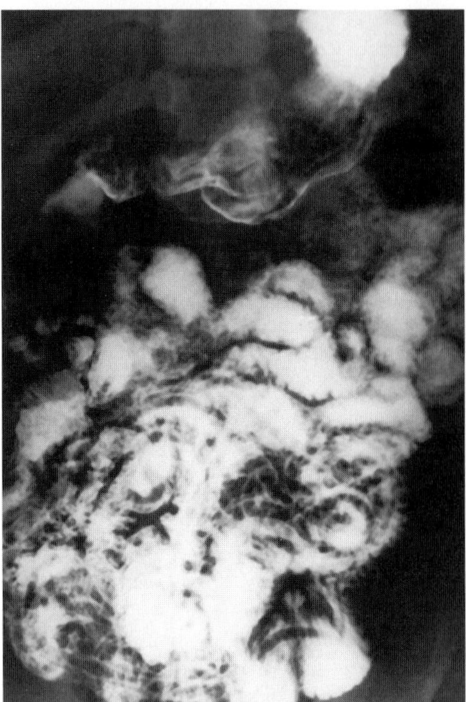

FIGURE 42–4. Intestinal ascariasis in a 4-year-old child with a history of malnutrition. A frontal supine abdominal radiograph from a small bowel examination shows barium-filling loops of small bowel in which long, smooth, filling defects (worms) are noted. Sometimes the worm ingests the barium, thus revealing a long; thin line within the worm that represents its own intestinal tract (not shown here).

age of 200,000 eggs per day. Occasionally roundworms in the gastrointestinal tract may be identified by radiographic contrast studies as an incidental finding (Fig. 42–4).

TREATMENT

Definitive Therapy

For most cases of intestinal ascariasis the recommended treatment is albendazole or mebendazole or, alternatively, pyrantel pamoate (Table 42–8). Where intestinal obstruction is imminent, some experts recommend using the older drug piperazine citrate, which paralyzes the worms and facilitates relaxation of the bolus. Piperazine and pyrantel pamoate are antagonistic and should not be used simultaneously.

TABLE 42–8. Therapy for Ascariasis*

Albendazole 400 mg PO as a single dose†
or
Mebendazole 100 mg bid PO for 3 days, or 500 mg orally once†
or
Pyrantel pamoate 11 mg/kg (maximum dose: 1 g) PO as a single dose‡

Adapted from Drugs for parasitic infections. *Med Lett Drugs Ther* 2000; 42:1–11.

*Same dosages for children and adults.

†The benzimidazoles, including albendazole and mebendazole, are embryotoxic and teratogenic in rodents. They are contraindicated in persons with blood dyscrasias, leukopenia, or liver disease.

‡For acute intestinal obstruction, piperazine citrate may be preferred because it paralyzes the adult worms. Piperazine is antagonistic to pyrantel pamoate.

Supportive Therapy

Intestinal obstruction as a complication of ascariasis requires appropriate supportive medical therapy and may necessitate surgical intervention. In the early stages of intestinal obstruction, blockage is often incomplete and can be managed conservatively with nasogastric suction, intravenous correction of fluid and electrolyte deficits, and anthelmintics. In some cases the administration of either mineral oil or the radiopague agent Gastrografin may relieve the obstruction. Surgery is warranted if the obstruction persists or if other complications develop.

COMPLICATIONS

The most dramatic complications of ascariasis occur when the adult worms migrate spontaneously or in response to irritants, including halogenated hydrocarbons such as tetrachloroethylene, which is sometimes used in poorer countries for treatment of hookworm infection. These complications frequently require surgical intervention.

Biliary Ascariasis. Adult *A. lumbricoides* may migrate into the biliary tree and cause hepatobiliary and pancreatic ascariasis, particularly in young children with heavy infections. The clinical presentation depends on the location of biliary invasion. Pancreatitis is seen when worms invade the pancreatic duct, cholecystitis is evident when worms enter the common bile duct and cause cystic duct obstruction, and cholangitis and hepatic abscess are seen when worms block the hepatic duct. Hepatobiliary ascariasis is difficult to diagnose by conventional imaging procedures (e.g., oral cholecystography or intravenous cholangiography) because the worms often move out of the ducts after producing biliary or pancreatic symptoms. Endoscopic retrograde cholangiopancreatography has been used in endemic areas both diagnostically and therapeutically. Ultrasonography is also helpful for diagnosis.

Acute Intestinal Obstruction. Acute small bowel obstruction and perforation are relatively common causes of surgical emergencies among young children who harbor large numbers of worms. These children often have abdominal distention and vomiting, sometimes with adult worms in the vomitus.

PROGNOSIS

Most cases of ascariasis resolve completely with anthelmintic therapy. The development of acute complications that require surgical intervention is often associated with severe morbidity and even death.

PREVENTION

The public health measures aimed at improved sanitation and health education are similar for both ascariasis and trichuriasis. However, a major difference in the biology and ecology of the parasite affecting control strategies is the higher resistance of *Ascaris* eggs to environmental stress.

TOXOCARIASIS AND BAYLISASCARIASIS (VISCERAL AND OCULAR LARVA MIGRANS)

ETIOLOGY

Visceral larva migrans (VLM) and ocular larva migrans (OLM) are zoonoses that occur when humans accidentally become the "dead end" aberrant host of a helminthic infection (Fig. 42–5). In temperate climates, and in the United States in particular, this situation develops when humans ingest the eggs of the canine ascarid *Toxocara canis* or, less commonly, the feline ascarid *Toxocara cati* or the raccoon ascarid *Baylisascaris procyonis* (Table 42–9). Adult ascarids are remarkably common in their definitive hosts. Almost all puppies are naturally infected with *T. canis;* nearly all juvenile raccoons contain *B. procyonis.* Infected animals, including pets, can shed millions of eggs per day that can survive for months in the soil.

EPIDEMIOLOGY

Small children are especially prone to acquire VLM from intimate contact with a family pet or from contaminated sandboxes or playgrounds. The overall seroprevalence of toxocariasis in the United States is reported to be 3%. However, this value may range up to 5% in the southeastern United States and is even higher among socioeconomically disadvantaged African American children. The major risk factors for acquiring VLM or OLM from *Toxocara* organisms appear to be a history of geophagia (pica) and exposure to a litter of puppies.

PATHOGENESIS

The extent of pathologic changes associated with VLM is proportional to the number of eggs ingested. Larvae that are liberated from eggs in the gastrointestinal tract invade the mucosa of the small intestine and migrate in human viscera. By so doing, they cause mechanical injury and immunopathologic damage by eliciting a delayed-type hypersensitivity response that includes eosinophils. Eosinophilic granule proteins such as **major basic protein** are released into the tissues and contribute to this damage. Many visceral organs, most commonly the liver, lung, heart, and brain, may be involved. Hepatitis, pneumonitis, myocarditis, and meningoencephalitis may result.

Ultimately the larvae are overcome by the host inflammatory response when they are consumed in an eosinophilic granuloma. Some larvae may survive for months or years by evading the host immune response through a process of antigen shedding that elicits granuloma formation. *B. procyonis* larvae develop considerably in humans and reach sizes as large as 2 mm, unlike *T. canis* larvae, which do not grow in the aberrant host. The larger size and the more aggressive somatic migratory behavior account for the greater virulence of *B. procyonis* larvae.

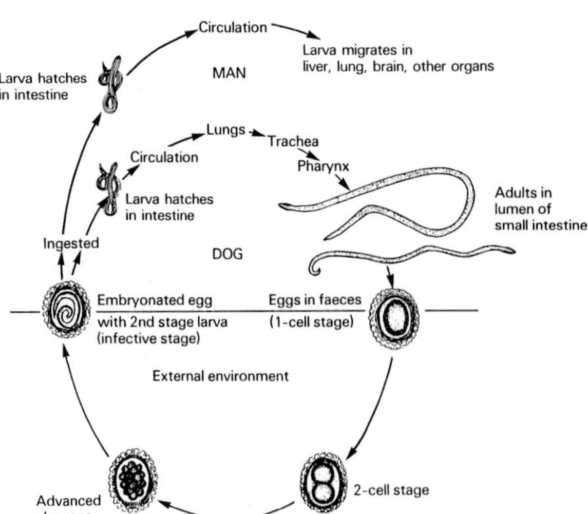

FIGURE 42–5. Life cycle of *Toxocara canis.* (From Zaman V: *Atlas of Medical Parasitology,* 2nd ed. Sidney, Adis Health Science Press, 1984.)

TABLE 42–9. Ascarids Commonly Associated with Visceral and Ocular Larva Migrans

Parasite	Definitive Host
Toxocara canis	Dogs
Toxocara cati	Cats
Baylisascaris procyonis	Raccoons
Lagochilascaris sprenti	Opossums

SYMPTOMS AND CLINICAL MANIFESTATIONS

Visceral Larva Migrans. The zoonotic ascarids can produce an asymptomatic infection, VLM, or OLM. The asymptomatic condition is the most common and is probably associated with only a few larvae outside the central nervous system. Asymptomatic patients may have a mild eosinophilia and do not often develop specific antibodies. A subset of patients may have only wheezing and asthma-like symptoms, leading to the suggestion, as yet unproved, that *T. canis* may be an environmental cause of asthma. The clinical presentation of VLM depends on the number of migrating larvae and whether the infection is primary or associated with repeat infection. The classic description involves a child who has fever, leukocytosis, eosinophilia, hepatomegaly, and pneumonitis with wheezing and hypergammaglobulinemia as part of the inflammatory response to repeated waves of migrating larvae (Table 42–10). VLM is usually diagnosed in very young children between 1 and 5 years of age. Larvae migrating during a primary infection may be better able to damage host viscera without being impeded by the host inflammatory response, and therefore they are more likely to reach the central nervous system. Children with central

TABLE 42–10. Major Clinical Manifestations of Visceral Larva Migrans

Eosinophilia
Pneumonitis (with wheezing)
Hepatomegaly
Leukocytosis
Fever
Hypergammaglobulinemia
Neuropsychiatric disturbances
Eosinophilic meningitis (with *Baylisascaris procyonis* infection)

nervous system involvement frequently have either neuropsychiatric disturbances or seizures. Seizures, when they occur, are typically generalized and tonic-clonic. A static encephalopathy from *T. canis* infection recently has been described. Severe eosinophilic meningitis has been attributed to *B. procyonis* infection.

Ocular Larva Migrans. In contrast to VLM, OLM typically occurs in older children, who often have isolated unilateral ocular signs and no systemic findings and symptoms. They often do not have eosinophilia or elevated antibody titers. Larvae probably enter the anterior vitreous of the eye from a peripheral branch of the retinal artery. After they gain access to the subretinal space, these larvae elicit granulomas in the posterior and peripheral poles that ''drag'' the retina. Unilateral vision loss and strabismus are common presenting features. A diffuse endophthalmitis may also occur.

TABLE 42–11. Therapy for Visceral Larva Migrans*†

Albendazole‡ 400 mg bid PO for 5 days
Alternative: Mebendazole‡§ 100–200 mg bid PO for 5 days

Adapted from Drugs for parasitic infections. *Med Lett Drugs Ther* 2000; 42:1–11.
*Same dosages for children and adults.
†The recommended treatment for both VLM and OLM is controversial. Diethylcarbamazine (6 mg/kg/day orally in 3 divided doses for 7–10 days) has also been shown to be effective. Corticosteroids and antihistamines may be useful adjuncts.
‡The benzimidazoles, including albendazole and mebendazole, are embryotoxic and teratogenic in rodents. They are contraindicated in persons with blood dyscrasias, leukopenia, or liver disease.
§Because mebendazole is poorly absorbed through the gastrointestinal tract, large doses are required to achieve therapeutic levels in the tissues; doses as large as 1–3 g/day have been used with some success.

DIAGNOSIS

Visceral Larva Migrans. The diagnosis of VLM is usually established by clinical symptoms. An EIA that measures serum antibody against excretory-secretory antigens from *T. canis* is available from the CDC. It has a high degree of sensitivity (78%) and specificity (92%) at a titer of more than 1:32. The sensitivity is somewhat lower for OLM and is probably related to lower larval worm burdens. The EIA measures antibodies that may arise from past exposure unrelated to the present illness; it does not reliably measure antibodies against *B. procyonis* and other zoonotic ascarid antigens and should not be used for this purpose. Some serum samples from patients with other nematode infections (e.g., ascariasis, filariasis, strongyloidiasis) may show reactivity and false-positive results. Patients with VLM often have elevated **anti-A or anti-B isohemagglutinin titers.**

Ocular Larva Migrans. OLM is generally diagnosed on the basis of characteristic migratory tracts and granulomas visualized on the retina, especially the posterior and peripheral pole, by ophthalmologic examination. Larvae are occasionally seen. Intraocular eosinophils have been reported on cytologic examination of the aqueous humor, and the detection of *T. canis* antigen in the aqueous and vitreous humors has also been described. OLM is often misdiagnosed as a retinoblastoma.

TREATMENT

Visceral Larva Migrans. The treatment of VLM is controversial (Table 42–11). Because a major component in the pathogenesis of VLM is the immunopathologic host response, exacerbation of symptoms by the administration of anthelmintics, with death and decay of the parasite, is a concern. Furthermore, the efficacy of anthelmintic treatment is questionable. Often with toxocaral VLM, the infection is self-limiting. Increasing experience with albendazole indicates that this anthelmintic is the treatment of choice, sometimes in combination with corticosteroids for severe symptoms or for central nervous system or eye involvement.

Ocular Larva Migrans. The treatment of OLM requires a combination of anthelmintic and corticosteroid therapy, in conjunction with ophthalmologic consultation and surgery (e.g., vitrectomy, membrane peeling) when appropriate. No drugs have been demonstrated to be effective, although albendazole, mebendazole, thiabendazole, levamisole, and ivermectin have been used. Corticosteroid therapy is considered helpful. Ocular baylisascariasis has been treated successfully with photocoagulation therapy to destroy intraretinal larvae.

COMPLICATIONS

VLM can involve the liver, lung, heart, and brain and can potentially result in several complications that require individualized management. Children with primary toxocariasis and central nervous system involvement may develop neuropsychiatric disturbances. *B. procyonis* infection can lead to much more severe central nervous system disease, including a fatal eosinophilic meningoencephalitis manifested by mental status changes, focal neurologic signs, and a cerebrospinal fluid pleocytosis with a high percentage of eosinophils.

PROGNOSIS

Toxocariasis usually has an excellent prognosis in children. *B. procyonis* infections have a higher probability of central nervous system involvement, which is associated with a poorer prognosis than toxocaral VLM. One study (Dinning, 1988) suggests that, with proper pharmacologic and surgical interventions, the visual prognosis of OLM may be better than previously believed.

PREVENTION

Prevention of VLM and OLM requires both the control and anthelmintic treatment of animal reservoirs, particularly dogs and cats, with a goal of reducing the number of infective eggs that contaminate playgrounds and sandboxes. Adequate prevention requires the cooperation of veterinarians, public health officials, and pet owners and breeders.

STRONGYLOIDIASIS

ETIOLOGY

Strongyloides stercoralis, one of only two major helminth species to replicate within the human host by **autoinfection** (the other being *Capillaria philippinensis*), is one of the most virulent helminths to infect humans. The life cycle of *S. stercoralis* is exceedingly complex because of several unique features of the parasite's biology (Fig. 42–6). This organism may be free-living in the soil for one or possibly more generations and may enter the **heterogonic cycle**

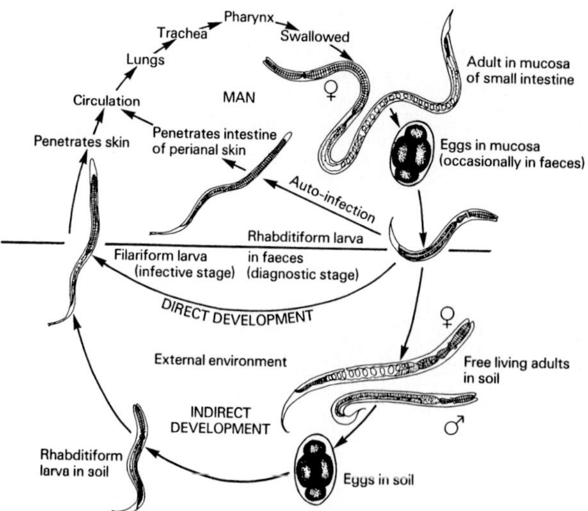

FIGURE 42–6. Life cycle of *Strongyloides stercoralis.* (From Zaman V: *Atlas of Medical Parasitology,* 2nd ed. Sidney, Adis Health Science Press, 1984.)

before undergoing the **homogonic cycle** in the host. In addition, larvae may reinvade the same host in an **autoinfective cycle,** which may lead to **hyperinfection** or **disseminated infection.**

A second form of strongyloidiasis, caused by *Strongyloides fuelleborni,* results in a fatal disease known locally as **swollen belly syndrome** in infants living in Papua, New Guinea. The prevalence of infection reaches 100% in 4-year-old children in some villages but drops precipitously in adults. This syndrome may occur as a result of perinatal transfer of larvae through breast milk.

EPIDEMIOLOGY

The overall prevalence of strongyloidiasis is probably underestimated because of the difficulties in establishing the diagnosis. Endemic foci of this disease occur in the southern United States, including Kentucky, eastern Tennessee, and North Carolina. Southeast Asian refugees have high rates of infection.

PATHOGENESIS

Humans usually become infected when the third-stage filariform larvae penetrate the skin. The *S. stercoralis* larvae follow a path of infection analogous to that of hookworm larvae as they enter venules and lymphatics, where they are swept by the circulation to the right side of the heart and to the lungs before being expectorated and swallowed. The parasite reaches adulthood in the small intestine, where it invades the mucosa and becomes lodged in the crypts. Generally only adult female worms are evident at this stage, suggesting that the parasite reproduces by parthenogenesis in the homogonic cycle. Eggs released by adult *S. stercoralis* in the intestinal mucosa hatch and release first-stage larvae, sometimes referred to as **rhabditiform larvae,** which migrate into the lumen and are passed with the feces.

Under certain conditions, as yet not well understood, first-stage larvae continue their development in the human host to become third-stage **filariform larvae** while still in the gastrointestinal tract. The filariform larvae reinvade the bowel wall and ultimately become parasitic adults. This autoinfection can lead to the accumulation of large worm burdens known as **hyperinfection syndrome.** Larvae may migrate to extraintestinal sites, including the lung and the central nervous system, to cause disseminated infection. The hallmark of moderate to severe strongyloidiasis in children is diarrhea associated with malabsorption, which occurs as a consequence of adult worms' invading the intestinal crypts and mucosa in association with a host inflammatory component of mononuclear cells and eosinophils. The villi become broad and blunted, similar to what is sometimes seen in tropical sprue. Villous blunting sometimes progresses, particularly during hyperinfection, to ulcerations, fibrosis, and thickening of the bowel wall. Parasites are encountered in all layers of the intestinal wall in persons with hyperinfection syndrome.

SYMPTOMS AND CLINICAL MANIFESTATIONS

A wide range of clinical syndromes, from asymptomatic infection to hyperinfection, is characteristic of strongyloidiasis (Table 42–12). Intermittent abdominal cramping accompanied with epigastric pain is often described. Young children develop a syndrome characterized by anorexia, vomiting, chronic diarrhea with fat malabsorption leading to steatorrhea, protein malabsorption resulting in hypoalbuminemia and peripheral edema, cachexia, and abdominal distention. The appearance of such children is "celiac-like." Deficiencies in vitamin B_{12} and folate may also occur. An exaggerated form of this clinical condition, known as **swollen belly syndrome,** has been described in young infants with *S. fuelleborni* infection. This syndrome has a high mortality rate and may occur as a result of perinatal transfer of larvae through breast milk. Growth restriction is also a prominent feature of the *Strongyloides*-associated malabsorption syndromes. Reversal of symptoms and dramatic catch-up growth has been described after anthelmintic therapy.

DIAGNOSIS

Diagnosis is based on the recovery of first-stage rhabditiform larvae from feces in persons with intestinal strongyloidiasis but is difficult because the female is much less fecund than other parasitic nematodes. As few as 50 progeny per day are released by each female adult, in contrast to at least 200,000 eggs per day produced by one female adult *Ascaris.* Furthermore, because the adult *S. stercoralis* releases progeny in a sporadic manner, the sampling error can be great. A number of concentration techniques are available to increase the likelihood of finding larvae. Alternatively, methods such as the **Baermann technique** have been developed for recovering larvae from larger quantities of feces. A sensitive **agar-plate method** can detect the tracts of larvae present in low numbers in feces, sputum, and other body fluids. Many different immunodiagnostic assays, including an EIA, are under investigation.

TABLE 42–12. Major Clinical Manifestations of Strongyloidiasis

Celiac-like syndrome/swollen belly syndrome
Diarrhea
Cachexia and anorexia
Abdominal distention
Protein and fat malabsorption
Physical growth retardation
Folate and vitamin B_{12} malabsorption
Autoinfection
Hyperinfection syndrome
Disseminated strongyloidiasis

TABLE 42–13. Therapy for Strongyloidiasis*

Ivermectin 200 μg/kg/day qd PO for 1–2 days†
Alternative: Thiabendazole 50 mg/kg/day PO divided in 2 doses (maximum dose 3 g/day) for 2 days‡

Adapted from Drugs for parasitic infections. *Med Lett Drugs Ther* 2000; 42:1–11.
*Same dosages for children and adults.
†In immunocompromised persons or in persons with hyperinfection syndrome or disseminated disease, it may be necessary to prolong or repeat therapy or use other agents.
‡This dose is likely to be toxic and may have to be decreased.

TREATMENT

Definitive Treatment

All infected individuals should be treated because of the potential for hyperinfection. Ivermectin is the drug of choice, and thiabendazole is an alternative (Table 42–13). For immunocompromised persons or persons with disseminated disease, it may be necessary to prolong the course for 5–14 days of therapy or to repeat the course. Demonstrating parasitologic cure conclusively may be difficult because of the inherent difficulties in identifying strongyloidiasis. Consecutive follow-up stool examinations should be performed several months after therapy.

Supportive Therapy

For hyperinfection syndrome, lifesaving supportive measures include respiratory and ventilatory support for pulmonary involvement, antimicrobial therapy for secondary gram-negative sepsis and meningitis, and tapering of the dosage of corticosteroids and other immunosuppressive drugs that predispose persons to hyperinfection.

COMPLICATIONS

Some persons with generalized inanition eventually develop the hyperinfection syndrome, in which larvae may disseminate to all tissues, including the central nervous system. Persons with cell-mediated immunosuppression from leukemia, lymphoma, high-dose corticosteroid therapy, transplantation-associated immunosuppression, or HIV or HTLV-I infection are particularly vulnerable to hyperinfection syndrome. Gram-negative sepsis and meningitis are common complications of hyperinfection syndrome as large numbers of larvae perforate the bowel and compromise the gastrointestinal endothelium. Overwhelming larval pulmonary invasion leads to fulminant pneumonia.

PROGNOSIS

Young children with malabsorption and growth failure often respond dramatically to anthelmintic therapy. Hyperinfection syndrome is difficult to treat and may require repeated courses of therapy. Mortality rates associated with the bacterial complications of hyperinfection syndrome are significant.

PREVENTION

Public health control methods used in the prevention of hookworm infection are often adequate to prevent strongyloidiasis. The filariform larvae of *S. stercoralis* are particularly active, and therefore clinical laboratory technicians should handle fecal samples cautiously. Diagnosis and treatment of children with strongyloidiasis who are undergoing immunosuppressive therapy generally require infectious diseases consultation.

ENTEROBIASIS (PINWORM)

ETIOLOGY

Human pinworm infection, caused by *Enterobius vermicularis,* is the most common helminthiasis in temperate climates, including the United States. This condition primarily affects children. In some elementary schools in the United States, up to 25% of children have pinworms. Transmission in daycare centers has also been described.

EPIDEMIOLOGY

Humans become infected with *E. vermicularis* when they ingest the embryonated eggs, which become infective shortly after being deposited by the gravid female worm. There are four routes of transmission: (1) direct, by finger contamination from anus to mouth, (2) indirect, by fomes contamination, (3) ingestion, by oral intake of airborne eggs, and (4) retroinfection, in which eggs hatch in the perianal area, giving rise to larvae that reenter the bowel and develop into adult worms.

PATHOGENESIS

Eggs containing the infective first-stage larvae are ingested and pass to the duodenum. The emerging larvae migrate to the jejunum and ileum, where they molt before the developing and adult stages of *E. vermicularis* reach the cecum. The adult worms produce minimal, if any, direct damage to the cecal or appendiceal mucosa, with only occasional development of minute ulcerations. In the absence of tissue injury, eosinophilia is not usually found. The gravid female leaves the cecum and migrates out of the rectum to deposit eggs, which elicit pruritus in the perianal area.

SYMPTOMS AND CLINICAL MANIFESTATIONS

Intense itching leading to **pruritus ani** is the hallmark of enterobiasis (Table 42–14). The syndrome is produced by wandering gravid female pinworms that provoke scratching of the irritated region, which causes excoriation and secondary bacterial infection. Vaginitis, sometimes accompanied by discharge, can also occur. In young

TABLE 42–14. Major Clinical Manifestations of Enterobiasis

Pruritus ani
Vaginitis
Neuropsychiatric disturbances
Insomnia
Restlessness and hyperactivity
Irritability
Anorexia
Nightmares
Teeth grinding

TABLE 42–15. Therapy for Enterobiasis (Pinworms)*

Albendazole 400 mg PO once, repeated in 2 wk†
or
Mebendazole 100 mg PO once, repeated in 2 wk†
or
Pyrantel pamoate 11 mg/kg (maximum: 1 g) PO once, repeated in 2 wk

Adapted from Drugs for parasitic infections. *Med Lett Drugs Ther* 2000; 42:1–11.
*Same dosages for children and adults.
†The benzimidazoles, including albendazole and mebendazole, are embryotoxic and teratogenic in rodents. They are contraindicated in persons with blood dyscrasias, leukopenia, or liver disease.

children, pruritus and vaginitis are often associated with a range of neuropsychiatric disturbances. Aberrant wandering by the adult pinworm in ectopic foci may produce more serious manifestations.

DIAGNOSIS

The diagnosis is established by recovering the eggs with transparent adhesive tape that is applied to the perianal skin and then placed on a microscope slide (Fig. 8–1). *E. vermicularis* eggs are not usually found in the feces. The best results are obtained by applying clear adhesive tape to the perianal skin in the morning as soon as the patient awakens and before a bath or bowel movement. False-negative results can be obtained, however, and the technique may have to be repeated several times before a diagnosis can be established. Occasionally, parents report discovering a worm in the perianal area. Laboratory evaluation distinguishes the pinworm from cestode proglottids.

TREATMENT

A single dose of albendazole, mebendazole, or pyrantel pamoate, with a repeated dose in 2 weeks, is usually adequate for treatment of most pinworm infections (Table 42–15). Because the commonly used anthelmintics are most effective against the adult stage, any eggs that are swallowed at the time the drug is given may ultimately develop into mature adults. Therefore therapy is repeated at 2 weeks, after the new adult worms have developed. Usually all members of the household must be treated. Most cases of apparent ''treatment failures'' are probably associated with reinfection rather than resistance to the anthelmintic. Although benzimidazole resistance has been reported for some nematodes of domestic animals, it has not yet been reported for *E. vermicularis.* At the time of treatment, laundering underwear, bedclothes, and towels in hot water is also prudent.

COMPLICATIONS

An association between pinworm infection and lower urinary tract infection (e.g., cystitis) has been reported. Urinary tract infection may occur after the introduction of bacteria into the urethra by migrating adult *E. vermicularis.* This pathogenesis may also explain some cases of enuresis. Gravid female pinworms have been reported to crawl into the uterus and fallopian tubes and cause salpingitis. Pinworms may also migrate into the appendix and result in appendicitis either by functioning as an obstruction-causing appendicolith, possibly in association with granuloma formation, or by introducing bacteria. Enterobiasis has been found in association with granulomas in a wide range of ectopic sites, including the peritoneum and the liver. Coinfections with an intestinal protozoan, *Dientamoeba fragilis,* have been described in children with pinworm. Concomitant *D. fragilis* infection should be suspected in children who harbor pinworms and have diarrhea or abdominal pain.

PROGNOSIS

The prognosis is excellent after anthelmintic therapy. Reinfection in the household or in school is extremely common, however, even after adequate drug treatment. Repeated therapy may be necessary.

PREVENTION

Good hand-washing technique and appropriate hygiene, especially in daycare and school settings, is important in the prevention of transmission. Laundering of underwear, bedclothes, and towels in hot water is sometimes helpful.

TRICHINELLOSIS (TRICHINOSIS)

ETIOLOGY

Trichinellosis, also known as **trichinosis,** is a parasitic zoonosis caused by 5 closely related members of the genus *Trichinella,* primarily *Trichinella spiralis* (Table 42–16).

EPIDEMIOLOGY

The infection is still a public health problem in North America because its most classic and common etiologic agent, *T. spiralis,* remains enzootic in domestic swine and some wild animals, including bears, in the continental United States. In the Arctic and sub-Arctic zones of Alaska and Canada, *Trichinella nativa* is enzootic in wildlife such as bears and walruses and is a significant pathogen among native Inuit. In the United States, the incidence of trichi-

TABLE 42–16. Members of the Genus *Trichinella*

	Pathogenicity in Humans	Distribution	Reservoirs	Resistance to Freezing
T. spiralis	High	Cosmopolitan	Hogs, rats	Low
T. nativa	High	Arctic	Bears, Canidae	High
T. nelsoni	Low	Africa	Hyenas, Felidae	Low
T. britovi	Moderate	Temperate zone	Canidae	Low
T. pseudospiralis	?	Cosmopolitan	Mammals, birds	Low

Modified from Murrell KD, Bruschi F: Clinical trichinellosis. *Prog Clin Parasitol* 1994;4:117–50.

nellosis has declined significantly, from an average of about 400 cases per year in the late 1940s to a current average of about 50 cases per year. The recent figure is probably an underestimate, because many cases go unreported. The downward trend has been attributed to a decrease in the amount of contaminated pork that is commercially purchased, which may reflect enactment of the Swine Health Protection Act, which prohibits the feeding of non-heat-treated garbage to swine.

Trichinella is found in virtually all warm-blooded animals. Contaminated commercial pork remains the most important source of trichinellosis and accounts for sporadic outbreaks. There is also some concern that sylvatic carnivore reservoirs may re-establish the disease in currently uninfected domestic swine populations. The largest number of cases occurs in the northeastern United States, although Alaska has the highest incidence of any one state. Most trichinellosis cases occur in young adults between 20 and 39 years of age. Certain ethnic groups are at particular risk of acquiring trichinellosis, including some Southeast Asian refugees, who have a preference for raw or lightly cooked pork, and Native Americans who live in Arctic and sub-Arctic areas. Outbreaks in Europe have been attributed to infected horsemeat. Several cases have resulted from consumption of wild game including bear, wild boar, walrus, and cougar. A history of ingestion of wild game, especially if not commercially prepared, is a risk factor for trichinellosis.

PATHOGENESIS

Humans acquire trichinellosis when they eat uncooked or undercooked meat infected with the encysted larvae of *Trichinella*. After encysting in the stomach, the larvae grow rapidly and molt in the small intestine. Like *Trichuris,* the adult worms have an intracellular phase in the cells that line the intestinal mucosa. After about 1 week, they produce larvae that disseminate via a hematogenous route and invade skeletal muscle and viscera, producing profound changes in the host cell's morphologic characteristics. Encysted larvae develop only in muscles, however. The **myogenic program** (i.e., the genes responsible for transcribing muscle cell–specific proteins such as myosin) is switched off in favor of a new program that permits the synthesis of host cell proteins essential for parasite survival. The morphologically altered cells, or **nurse cells,** are nourished by their own microvascular blood supplies, which presumably develop in response to angiogenic factors released by the parasite or infected cell.

The extent of infection is primarily related to the number of larvae that encyst in muscle, but considerable variation occurs depending on the species and type of muscle. Human invasion with 15 *T. spiralis* larvae per gram of diaphragmatic muscle can be fatal, whereas infections of more than 1,000 *Trichinella britovi* or *Trichinella nelsoni* larvae per gram are not lethal.

SYMPTOMS AND CLINICAL MANIFESTATIONS

The incubation period from the time of ingestion of *T. spiralis*–infected pork until the onset of symptoms is usually 5–15 days. The majority of infections are asymptomatic, but when clinical disease occurs, the course can be divided into an early phase and a late phase (Table 42–17). The **early phase** is intestinal and is associated with diarrhea, abdominal pain, and vomiting. In parts of the Canadian Arctic, possibly with *T. nativa* infection, the intestinal phase is exaggerated; prolonged diarrhea is a hallmark characteristic, and fever and muscle symptoms are absent.

TABLE 42–17. Major Clinical Manifestations of Trichinellosis

Early Phase (Intestinal)
Abdominal pain
Diarrhea
Vomiting
Acute Phase (Muscle)
Myalgias
Eosinophilia
Periorbital edema
Weakness
Fever

The **late phase** caused by *T. spiralis* begins approximately 1 week after infection and may last for several weeks. It is characterized by facial and periorbital edema, myalgias, muscle weakness, fever, and eosinophilia. Epidemiologically related infections from a single outbreak have been observed to be more severe in children. The second month of infection is associated with gradual resolution, although weakness and myalgias may continue.

DIAGNOSIS

A case of trichinellosis is defined by the CDC on the basis of either a *Trichinella*-positive muscle biopsy result or a serologic test positive for *Trichinella* in a person with compatible clinical symptoms. In an outbreak, at least one person must meet the first criterion, and the associated cases in persons who consumed the same meat product must have either a positive serologic test result or the clinical syndrome. Seroconversion typically occurs 3–5 weeks after infection. The most common associated laboratory findings include leukocytosis with eosinophilia, elevated immunoglobulin levels (particularly IgE), and elevated values for muscle enzymes (lactate dehydrogenase and creatine phosphokinase).

TREATMENT

Definitive Treatment

Because most anthelmintics are not well absorbed from the gastrointestinal tract, the larval stages can be difficult to eradicate (Table 42–18). Removal of the adult worms from the small intestine with either mebendazole or pyrantel pamoate may reduce the number of larvae that reach skeletal muscle via the hematogenous route. Mebendazole, which may reach therapeutic levels in tissues when given in high doses, has recently replaced thiabendazole, even though the latter drug is well absorbed. Albendazole may represent an appropriate alternative.

Supportive Therapy

Simultaneous administration of a corticosteroid such as prednisone (1–2 mg/kg/day) may prevent an exacerbation of symptoms associated with an immediate hypersensitivity response to the dying worms, described as a Jarisch-Herxheimer reaction. Corticosteroids may also be useful in ameliorating the inflammation resulting from life-threatening complications such as myocarditis or cerebritis. Corticosteroids should be used with caution, however, because of their immunosuppressive potential, especially in the absence of specific anthelmintic therapy. Nonsteroidal anti-inflammatory agents may help to alleviate myalgias.

TABLE 42–18. Therapy for Trichinellosis*

Corticosteroids for severe symptoms
plus
Mebendazole† 200–400 mg tid PO for 3 days, then 400–500 mg tid PO for 10 days
Alternative: Albendazole† 400 mg bid PO for 8–14 days

Adapted from Drugs for parasitic infections. *Med Lett Drugs Ther* 2000; 42:1–11.
*Same dosages for children and adults.
†The benzimidazoles, including albendazole and mebendazole, are embryotoxic and teratogenic in rodents. They are contraindicated in persons with blood dyscrasias, leukopenia, or liver disease.

COMPLICATIONS

Cardiovascular involvement occurs in about 20% of hospitalized cases. Electrocardiographic changes are frequently noted during this phase of trichinellosis. Myocarditis resulting from heart muscle invasion and neurotrichinellosis resulting from central nervous system invasion are serious complications that usually require adjunct corticosteroid therapy.

PROGNOSIS

The prognosis is generally good with treatment in the absence of cardiac or central nervous system involvement or underlying debilitation or immunosuppression.

PREVENTION

The overall prevalence of trichinellosis in commercial hogs in the United States has been estimated at 0.125%, although there are marked regional differences (e.g., 0.73% of hogs in New England have trichinellosis). Some states, such as Illinois, have instituted vigorous control programs to eliminate trichinellosis from hog populations, such as prohibiting feeding of garbage to swine. Enforcement of the Swine Health Protection Act at the state level, together with health education, may help to reduce trichinellosis.

Meat should be thoroughly cooked before eating to ensure that *Trichinella* organisms are killed. A temperature of 77°C (170°F) is above the thermal death point of the trichinae and is indicated by a change in color of the meat from pink or red to gray. Brine solutions and smoking processes used for preparing jerky may also kill the organisms; both temperature and total duration are important determinants of efficacy in these processes.

ANGIOSTRONGYLIASIS

ETIOLOGY AND EPIDEMIOLOGY

Abdominal angiostrongyliasis caused by *Angiostrongylus costaricensis* occurs from southern Mexico to Argentina and in Costa Rica. Humans are considered aberrant hosts because the parasite is unable to complete its life cycle, dying in the gastrointestinal tract. The majority of cases are in children, and two cases acquired in the United States have been described.

The most common infectious cause of **eosinophilic meningitis** in humans is inadvertent infection with *Angiostrongylus cantonensis,* the **rat lungworm,** which lives in the pulmonary arteries of the rat. *A. cantonensis* is enzootic in Southeast Asia, the South Pacific, Japan, and Taiwan. *A. cantonensis* is acquired by eating raw or undercooked freshwater snails, slugs, prawns, or crabs containing infectious third-stage larvae.

PATHOGENESIS AND CLINICAL MANIFESTATIONS

Abdominal angiostrongyliasis is acquired by the accidental ingestion of fruits and vegetables contaminated with infective larvae shed by slugs, which are the intermediate hosts. The adult worms, whose definitive hosts are usually black rats or cotton rats, reside in the mesenteric arteries near the cecum, where they elicit symptoms that can mimic acute appendicitis or symptomatic Meckel's diverticulum. This clinical syndrome is manifested by right lower quadrant pain, anorexia, vomiting, fever, and eosinophilia. The diagnosis is often established only after laparotomy.

Eosinophilic meningitis caused by *A. cantonensis,* sometimes accompanied with pulmonary infiltrates, results from helminthic spread after invasion into the pulmonary vessels. At presentation, persons with central nervous system involvement often have a headache, paresthesias, generalized weakness, and visual disturbances in association with an eosinophilic pleocytosis.

DIAGNOSIS AND TREATMENT

The diagnosis of abdominal angiostrongyliasis caused by *A. costaricensis* requires demonstration of the parasite or eggs in tissues. The worms usually localize to the mesenteric arteries of the ileocecal region. Diagnostic imaging may show bowel edema, but no forms of *A. costaricensis* are present in stool. Definitive treatment of abdominal angiostrongyliasis usually requires surgical resection, although adjunct anthelmintics may be beneficial. Mebendazole is currently recommended for treatment of *A. costaricensis* infections (Table 42–19). Although not yet studied extensively, albendazole may be preferable to mebendazole for treatment of *Angiostrongylus* infections.

The diagnosis of infection with *A. cantonensis* is established by a history of exposure and the presence of eosinophilic meningitis, with 15–90% eosinophils of greater than 100 cells/mm^3 in the CSF. The CSF protein level is elevated, and the glucose level is normal. The role of anthelmintics in the treatment of *A. cantonensis* eosinophilic meningitis is not clear (Table 42–19). Most persons recover spontaneously without treatment. Anthelmintics can provoke neurologic symptoms. Analgesics, corticosteroids, and careful removal of CSF at frequent intervals can relieve symptoms (Pien, 1999).

TABLE 42–19. Therapy for Angiostrongyliasis*

Angiostrongylus costaricensis (abdominal angiostrongyliasis)
Mebendazole† 200–400 mg tid PO for 10 days
Alternative: Thiabendazole† 75 mg/kg/day (maximum: 3 g/day) PO divided in 3 daily doses for 3 days
Angiostrongylus cantonensis (eosinophilic meningitis)
Mebendazole† 100 mg bid PO for 5 days

Adapted from Drugs for parasitic infections. *Med Lett Drugs Ther* 2000; 42:1–11.
*Same dosages for children and adults.
†The benzimidazoles, including albendazole, mebendazole, and thiabendazole, are embryotoxic and teratogenic in rodents. They are contraindicated in persons with blood dyscrasias, leukopenia, or liver disease.

FILARIASIS

ETIOLOGY AND EPIDEMIOLOGY

Wuchereria bancrofti and *Brugia malayi,* the major etiologic agents of human filariasis, including **elephantiasis,** are widely distributed in the tropics and cause enormous human morbidity. **Onchocerciasis,** or **river blindness,** caused by *Onchocerca volvulus,* is found in endemic foci primarily limited to West Africa, Central America, and northern parts of South America. Disease resulting from infection with these organisms usually becomes apparent only after many years of repeated exposure, and thus the dramatic clinical manifestations associated with these infections do not occur frequently in childhood.

PATHOGENESIS AND CLINICAL MANIFESTATIONS

Children living in endemic areas are often infected early in life through mosquito bites, and they frequently develop an asymptomatic microfilaremia. With repeated exposure, adolescents and young adults have one or more annual episodes of acute lymphangitis associated with systemic signs of a toxic reaction, including fever and rigors sometimes referred to as **filarial fever,** headache, malaise, and myalgias. Zoonotic *Brugia* infections (possibly from raccoon, rabbit, or cat animal reservoirs) that result in benign lymphadenopathy have been reported in the United States. Affected persons usually do not have circulating microfilariae. An immunodeficient infant with microfilaremia has been described.

Tropical pulmonary eosinophilia (TPE) is a hypersensitivity syndrome associated with microfilariae and microfilarial antigen in the lungs and manifested by cough and asthma with eosinophilia. TPE must be differentiated from other helminthiases with a lung migratory phase, such as ascariasis, hookworm infection, strongyloidiasis, and toxocariasis.

O. volvulus is acquired through the bite of black flies, of the genus *Simulium,* that breed along rivers and streams. Fly larvae remain in the subcutaneous tissues, where they ultimately become encased in a nodular **onchocercoma** before maturing. Microfilariae released from female adults often migrate to the eye, where they opacify and cause blindness as a late manifestation. Children living in endemic areas, especially Africa, however, typically have **onchodermatitis,** a pruritic skin rash composed of numerous discrete papules that contain microfilariae. Subcutaneous edema sometimes follows, leading to a characteristic **peau d'orange** appearance, which can become lichenified. In Central America, some children develop reddish purple lesions on the face that is sometimes referred to as **erisipela de la costa**.

DIAGNOSIS AND TREATMENT

The diagnosis of filariasis is traditionally established by identifying microfilariae in the blood. They appear in the peripheral circulation with a characteristic periodicity, the timing of which may vary for any given geographic location. New enzyme immunoassays for the detection of parasite antigen have been developed and may replace or supplement this time-honored diagnostic method. The microfilariae of *O. volvulus* are typically identified by examination of skin snips. In the case of West African onchocerciasis, the pelvic girdle, iliac crest, and back of the scapula have the highest yield, although one snip from each of six different sites should be obtained.

There is no ideal treatment for human filariasis that targets the adult worms, or macrofilariae. For treatment of lymphatic filariasis a standard course of oral diethylcarbamazine (DEC) for 12–14 days is still widely used (children: 1 mg/kg three times daily on days 1 and 2, 1–2 mg/kg three times daily on day 3, and 6 mg/kg/day divided in three daily doses on days 4–14; adults: 50 mg three times daily on days 1 and 2, 100 mg three times daily on day 3, and 6 mg/kg/day divided in three daily doses on days 4–14). A single dose of DEC (6 mg/kg) may be as macrofilaricidal as a multidose regimen against *W. bancrofti.* A single dose of ivermectin (200 μg/kg) is effective for treatment of microfilaremia but does not kill the adult worm. Neither DEC alone nor DEC in combination with ivermectin or albendazole has been shown to eliminate filarial antigenemia completely. Antihistamines or corticosteroids may be required to reduce the allergic response from disintegration of microfilariae after treatment of filarial infections.

For treatment of onchocerciasis, ivermectin (150 μg/kg once, repeated every 6–12 months until asymptomatic) will reduce microfilarial loads in the skin and subcutaneous tissues and may possibly reduce the likelihood of progression to ocular disease. Annual treatment with ivermectin can prevent blindness from ocular onchocerciasis.

KEY ARTICLES

Hookworm Infection

Biddulph J: Mebendazole and albendazole for infants. *Pediatr Infect Dis J* 1990;9:373.

Cowden J, Hotez P: Mebendazole and albendazole treatment of geohelminth infections in children and pregnant women. *Pediatr Infect Dis J* 2000;19:659–60.

De Clercq D, Sacko M, Behnke J, et al: Failure of mebendazole in treatment of human hookworm infections in the southern region of Mali. *Am J Trop Med Hyg* 1997;57:25–30.

Hotez PJ: Hookworm disease in children. *Pediatr Infect Dis J* 1989; 8:516–20.

Hotez PJ, Pritchard DI: Hookworm infection. *Sci Am* 1995;272:68–74.

Hotez PJ, Zheng F, Long-qi X, et al: Emerging and reemerging helminthiases and the public health of China. *Emerg Infect Dis* 1997;3: 303–10.

Prociv P, Croese J: Human eosinophilic enteritis caused by dog hookworm *Ancylostoma caninum. Lancet* 1990;335:1299–302.

Rossignol JF: Chemotherapy: Present status. In Schad GA, Warren KS (editors): *Hookworm Disease: Current Status and Future Directions.* Bristol, Penn, Taylor & Francis, 1990.

Schad GA, Banwell JG: Hookworms. In Warren KS, Mahmoud AAF (editors): *Tropical and Geographic Medicine.* New York, McGraw-Hill, 1984.

Trichuriasis

Bundy DA, Cooper ES: *Trichuris* and trichuriasis in humans. *Adv Parasitol* 1989;28:107–73.

Bundy DA, Cooper ES, Thompson DE, et al: Effect of age and initial infection intensity on the rate of reinfection with *Trichuris trichiura* after treatment. *Parsitology* 1988;97:469–76.

Cooper ES, Bundy DA, MacDonald TT, et al: Growth suppression in the *Trichuris* dysentery syndrome. *Eur J Clin Nutr* 1990;44:285–91.

MacDonald TT, Choy MM, Spencer J, et al: Histopathology and immunohistochemistry of the caecum in children with the *Trichuris* dysentery syndrome. *J Clin Pathol* 1991;44:194–9.

Nokes C, Grantham-McGregor SM, Sawyer AW, et al: Moderate to heavy infections of *Trichuris trichiura* affect cognitive function in Jamaican school children. *Parasitology* 1992;104:539–47.

Ascariasis

Chu WG, Chen PM, Huang CC, et al: Neonatal ascariasis. *J Pediatr* 1972;81:783–5.

Crompton DWT, Pawlowski ZS: Life history and development of *Ascaris lumbricoides* and the persistence of human ascariasis. In Crompton DWT, Nesheim MC, Pawlowski ZS (editors): *Ascariasis and Its Public Health Significance.* Bristol, Penn, Taylor & Francis, 1985.

Hall A: Intestinal parasitic worms and the growth of children. *Trans R Soc Trop Med Hyg* 1993;87:241–2.

Khuroo MS, Zargar SA, Mahajan R: Hepatobiliary and pancreatic ascariasis in India. *Lancet* 1990;335:1503–6.

Nesheim MC: Nutritional aspects of *Ascaris suum* and *A. lumbricoides* infections. In Crompton DWT, Nesheim MC, Pawlowski ZS (editors): *Ascariasis and Its Public Health Significance.* Bristol, Penn, Taylor & Francis, 1985.

Savioli L, Bundy D, Tomkins A: Intestinal parasitic infections: A soluble public health problem. *Trans R Soc Trop Med Hyg* 1992;86:353–4.

Villar J, Klebanoff M, Kestler E: The effect of fetal growth of protozoan and helminthic infection during pregnancy. *Obstet Gynecol* 1989;74:915–20.

Toxocariasis and Baylisascariasis (Visceral and Ocular Larva Migrans)

Bekhti A: Mebendazole in toxocariasis. *Ann Intern Med* 1984;100:463.

Dinning WJ, Gillespie SH, Cooling RJ, et al: Toxocariasis: A practical approach to management of ocular disease. *Eye* 1988;2:580–2.

Fortenberry JD, Kenney RD, Younger J: Visceral larva migrans producing static encephalopathy in an infant. *Pediatr Infect Dis J* 1991;10:403–6.

Fox AS, Kazacos KR, Gould NS, et al: Fatal eosinophilic meningoencephalitis and visceral larva migrans caused by the raccoon ascarid *Baylisascaris procyonis. N Engl J Med* 1985;312:1619–23.

Hotez PJ: Visceral and ocular larva migrans. *Semin Neurol* 1993;13:175–9.

Huff DS, Neafie RC, Binder MJ, et al: Case 4. The first fatal *Baylisascaris* infection in humans: An infant with eosinophilic meningoencephalitis. *Pediatr Pathol* 1984;2:345–52.

Kazacos KR, Boyce WM: *Baylisascaris* larva migrans. *J Am Vet Med Assoc* 1989;195:894–903.

Kazacos KR: Visceral and ocular larva migrans. *Semin Vet Med Surg (Small Anim)* 1991;6:227–35.

Marmor M, Glickman L, Shofer F, et al: *Toxocara canis* infection of children: Epidemiologic and neuropsychologic findings. *Am J Public Health* 1987;77:554–9.

Schantz PM: *Toxocara* larva migrans now. *Am J Trop Med Hyg* 1989; 41:21–34.

Sharghi N, Schantz PM, Caramico L, et al: Environmental exposure to *Toxocara* as a possible risk factor for asthma: A clinic-based case-control study. *Clin Infect Dis* 2001;32:E111–6.

Sturchler D, Schubarth P, Gualzata M, et al: Thiabendazole vs. albendazole in treatment of toxocariasis: A clinical trial. *Ann Trop Med Parasitol* 1989;83:473–8.

Strongyloidiasis

Arakaki T, Iwanaga M, Kinjo F, et al: Efficacy of agar-plate culture in detection of *Strongyloides stercoralis* infection. *J Parasitol* 1990;76: 425–8.

Ashford RW, Vince JD, Gratten MJ, et al: *Strongyloides* infection associated with acute infantile disease in Papua New Guinea. *Trans R Soc Trop Med Hyg* 1978;72:554.

Barnish G, Ashford RW: *Strongyloides* cf. *fuelleborni* and hookworm in Papua New Guinea: Patterns of infection within the community. *Trans R Soc Trop Med Hyg* 1989;83:684–8.

Burke JA: Strongyloidiasis in childhood. *Am J Dis Child* 1978;132: 1130–6.

Genta RM, Walzer PD: Strongyloidiasis. In Walzer PD, Genta RM (editors): *Parasitic Infections in the Compromised Host.* New York, Marcel Dekker, 1989.

Huchton P, Horn R: Strongyloidiasis. *J Pediatr* 1959;55:602–8.

Liu LX, Weller PF: Antiparasitic drugs. *N Engl J Med* 1996;334: 1178–84.

Naquira C, Jimenez G, Guerra JG, et al: Ivermectin for human strongyloidiasis and other intestinal helminths. *Am J Trop Med Hyg* 1989;40:304–9.

Schad GA, Aikens LM, Smith G: *Strongyloides stercoralis:* Is there a canonical migratory route through the host? *J Parasitol* 1989;75: 740–9.

Walzer PD, Milder JE, Banwell JG, et al: Epidemiologic features of *Strongyloides stercoralis* infection in an endemic area of the United States. *Am J Trop Med Hyg* 1982;31:313–9.

Enterobiasis (Pinworm)

Crawford FG, Vermund SH: Parasitic infections in day care centers. *Pediatr Infect Dis J* 1987;6:744–9.

Daly JJ, Baker GF: Pinworm granuloma of the liver. *Am J Trop Med Hyg* 1984;33:62–4.

Faust EC, Russell PF, Jung RC (editors): *Craig and Faust's Clinical Parasitology.* Philadelphia, Lea & Febiger, 1970.

Katz M: Parasitic infections. *J Pediatr* 1975;87:165–78.

Saffos RO, Rhatigan RM: Unilateral salpingitis due to *Enterobius vermicularis. Am J Clin Pathol* 1977;67:296–9.

Simon RD: Pinworm infestation and urinary tract infection in young girls. *Am J Dis Child* 1974;128:21–2.

Wagner ED, Eby WC: Pinworm prevalence in California elementary school children, and diagnostic methods. *Am J Trop Med Hyg* 1983;32:998–1001.

Weller TH, Sorenson CW: Enterobiasis: Its incidence and symptomatology in a group of 505 children. *N Engl J Med* 1941;224:143–6.

Trichinellosis (Trichinosis)

Bailey TM, Schantz PM: Trends in the incidence and transmission patterns of trichinosis in humans in the United States: Comparison of the periods 1975–1981 and 1982–1986. *Rev Infect Dis* 1990;12:5–11.

Landry SM, Kiser D, Overby T, et al: Trichinosis: Common source outbreak related to commercial pork. *South Med J* 1992;85:428–9.

MacLean JD, Viallet J, Law C, et al: Trichinosis in the Canadian Arctic: Report of five outbreaks and a new clinical syndrome. *J Infect Dis* 1989;160:513–20.

McAuley JB, Michelson MK, Schantz PM: *Trichinella* infection in travelers. *J Infect Dis* 1991;164:1013–6.

Murrell KD, Bruschi F: Clinical trichinellosis. *Prog Clin Parasitol* 1994; 4:117–50.

Schantz PM: Parasitic zoonoses in perspective. *Int J Parasitol* 1991;21: 161–70.

Stehr-Green JK, Schantz PM: Trichinosis in Southeast Asian refugees in the United States. *Am J Public Health* 1986;76:1238–9.

Angiostrongyliasis

Hsu WY, Chen JY, Chien CT, et al: Eosinophilic meningitis caused by *Angiostrongylus cantonensis. Pediatr Infect Dis J* 1990;9:443–5.

Hulbert TV, Larsen RA, Chandrasoma PT: Abdominal angiostrongyliasis mimicking acute appendicitis and Meckel's diverticulum: Report of a case in the United States and review. *Clin Infect Dis* 1992;14:836–40.

Koo J, Pien F, Kliks MM: *Angiostrongylus (Parastrongylus)* eosinophilic meningitis. *Rev Infect Dis* 1988;10:1155–62.

Pien FD, Pien BC: *Angiostrongylus cantonensis* eosinophilic meningitis. *Int J Infect Dis* 1999;3:161–3.

Shih SL, Hsu CH, Huang FY, et al: *Angiostrongylus cantonensis* infection in infants and young children. *Pediatr Infect Dis J* 1992;11:1064–6.

Filariasis

Baird JK, Alpert LI, Friedman R, et al: North American brugian filariasis: Report of nine infections of humans. *Am J Trop Med Hyg* 1986;35: 1205–9.

Burnham G: Onchocerciasis. *Lancet* 1998;351:1341–6.

Greene BM, Dukuly ZD, Munoz B, et al: A comparison of 6-, 12-, and 24-monthly dosing with ivermectin for treatment of onchocerciasis. *J Infect Dis* 1991;163:376–80.

Gutierrez Y, Petras RE: Brugia infection in Northern Ohio. *Am J Trop Med Hyg* 1982;31:1128–30.

McCarthy JS, Ottesen EA, Nutman TB: Onchocerciasis in endemic and nonendemic populations: Differences in clinical presentation and immunologic findings. *J Infect Dis* 1994;170:736–41.

Olness K, Francoisi RA, Johnson MM, et al: Loiasis in an expatriate American child: Diagnostic and treatment difficulties. *Pediatrics* 1987;80:943–6.

Simmons CF Jr, Winter HS, Berde C, et al: Zoonotic filariasis with lymphedema in an immunodeficient infant. *N Engl J Med* 1984;310:1243–5.

Whitworth JA, Maude GH, Downham MD: Clinical and parasitological responses after up to 6.5 years of ivermectin treatment for onchocerciasis. *Trop Med Int Health* 1996;1:786–93.

CHAPTER 43

Trematode Infections

Peter J. Hotez

Infections caused by the trematodes, or **flukes,** are significant causes of morbidity and growth retardation among children in developing countries and among refugees. With the exception of the schistosomes, all human trematodes are hermaphroditic; their life cycles are indirect, requiring one or more intermediate hosts. Of the major human trematodiases caused by hermaphroditic species (Table 43–1), schistosomiasis has tremendous global significance, is still endemic in many parts of South America and the Caribbean, and is frequently found in Latin American and Caribbean (including Puerto Rican) immigrants in the United States. A few autochthonous trematodiases occur in the United States, including zoonotic paragonimiasis caused by *Paragonimus kellicotti,* cercarial dermatitis from avian schistosomes, and rare cases of fascioliasis caused by *Fasciola hepatica.*

SCHISTOSOMIASIS

ETIOLOGY

The *Schistosoma* is a genus of flukes, or trematodes, that parasitize the bloodstream. The transmission of schistosomiasis requires a source of freshwater that is contaminated with human feces or urine that contains eggs, the presence of an appropriate snail species, and human contact with water.

EPIDEMIOLOGY

Schistosomiasis, also known as bilharziasis, is a major cause of liver and urinary tract disease among children in developing countries (Table 43–2). More than 200 million people, most of them children, are infected with schistosomes. *Schistosoma mansoni* is widespread in Africa and is the only human schistosome that is indigenous to the Western Hemisphere. Almost 10 million people in Brazil alone are infected, and the parasite is still a significant public health problem in Puerto Rico. *S. haematobium,* a cause of urinary tract disease, is also endemic in Africa, where dual infections with *S. mansoni* occur, as well as in the Middle East. *S. japonicum* is endemic in East Asia, particularly China and the Philippines. The *S. japonicum* complex includes *S. mekongi* in Southeast Asia. Schistosomiasis is a major problem among recent immigrants and refugees to the United States, particularly from the Caribbean and Southeast Asia. Almost half a million of these people in the United States may be infected. Animal reservoirs may have importance in some cases of human schistosomiasis. *S. japonicum* infects cattle and pigs and is considered a zoonosis. *S. mansoni* may infect some species of baboons and rodents.

Children appear to be particularly predisposed to heavy levels of infection with schistosomes and consequently have greater morbidity. Increased transmission from more frequent and repeated water contact is partly responsible, although one study (Butterworth, 1987) suggests that young children are predisposed to infection because of specific defects in host immune responses.

PATHOGENESIS

Humans become infected when they come into contact with freshwater containing free-swimming cercariae, which can survive for about 48 hours after leaving the snail (Fig. 43–1). Cercariae have a tail that allows them to actively penetrate skin. In response to host skin lipids the cercariae secrete hydrolytic enzymes and eicosanoids that facilitate entry. On host entry the cercariae lose their tails and undergo major morphologic and biochemical transformations to become schistosomula. The schistosomula migrate to the lungs. Ultimately the maturing adult worms gain access to the portal circulation of the liver in 1–3 weeks. There the worms reach sexual maturity and mate, the female living in the gynecophoric canal of the male (all other human trematodes are hermaphroditic). The mating pairs migrate to their final destination, which for *S. mansoni* and *S. japonicum* are the mesenteric veins and for *S. haematobium* is the vesicle plexus surrounding the bladder. After fertilization the female releases eggs having a characteristic spine that facilitates passage through the vessel wall into either the lumen of the intestine (for *S. japonicum* and *S. mansoni*) or the bladder (for *S. haematobium*), which allows for exit in the feces or urine, respectively. In freshwater the eggs hatch and release ciliated miracidia, which enter snail intermediate hosts. Here the intramolluscan stages develop to produce new cercariae.

Most of the pathology from human schistosomiasis occurs when the eggs do not exit the host but instead become entrapped in host tissues to form granulomas. Therefore an intact cell-mediated immune system is essential to initiate the immunopathology of schistosomiasis. In fact, recent evidence suggests that host tumor necrosis factor is recruited as a growth factor for the parasite. In schistosomiasis mansoni and japonica the eggs are typically either trapped in the intestinal wall or swept via the portal vein to the liver. Intestinal wall granuloma formation results in fibrosis while liver granuloma formation results in periportal fibrosis. The latter can progress to **Symmers' pipestem fibrosis** to cause portal hypertension and hepatosplenomegaly. Deposition of eggs in the bladder and ureters by *S. haematobium* causes granuloma formation in these tissues that may lead to an obstructive uropathy. It is believed that chronic inflammatory insults to the bladder resulting from *S. haematobium* egg deposition account for the unusually high rates of squamous cell carcinoma of the bladder seen in endemic areas.

Young and school-aged children are particularly vulnerable to the effects of chronic schistosomiasis, which includes both immunologic and nutritional components. Children acquire a selective immunodeficiency against the invading schistosomula through the production of blocking antibodies, which block the effector immune mechanisms against schistosomula. It has been postulated that

TABLE 43–1. Major Human Trematodiases (Other than Schistosomiasis) and Etiologic Agents

Disease/Etiology	Site of Pathology	Intermediate Host	Geographic Location	Treatment*
Clonorchiasis (Chinese Liver Fluke)				
Clonorchis sinensis	Bile duct Liver	Fish	East Asia, Hawaii	Praziquantel 75 mg/kg/day in 3 divided doses PO for 1 day *or* Albendazole 10 mg/kg PO for 7 days
Fascioliasis (Sheep Liver Fluke)				
Fasciola hepatica	Liver	Aquatic vegetation	Mideast, Africa, United States, United Kingdom	Triclabendazole 10 mg/kg PO once *or* Bithionol 30–50 mg/kg PO on alternate days for 10–15 doses
Fasciolopsiasis				
Fasciolopsis buski	Intestine	Aquatic vegetation	East Asia	Praziquantel 75 mg/kg/day in 3 divided doses PO for 1 day
Heterophyidiasis				
Heterophyes heterophyes	Intestine	Fish	East Asia	Praziquantel 75 mg/kg/day in 3 divided doses PO for 1 day
Metagonimiasis				
Metagonimus yokogawai	Intestine	Fish	East Asia	Praziquantel 75 mg/kg/day in 3 divided doses PO for 1 day
Metorchiasis (North American Liver Fluke)				
Metorchis conjunctus	Bile duct Liver	Fish	Latin America North America	Praziquantel 75 mg/kg/day in 3 divided doses PO for 1 day
Nanophyetiasis				
Nanophyetus salmincola		Salmon	United States (Washington)	Praziquantel 75 mg/kg/day in 3 divided doses PO for 1 day
Opisthorchiasis (Southeast Asian Liver Fluke)				
Opisthorchis viverrini	Bile duct Liver	Fish	Thailand	Praziquantel 75 mg/kg/day in 3 divided doses PO for 1 day
Paragonimiasis (Lung Fluke)				
Paragonimus pulmonalis	Lung	Crustacea	East Asia	Praziquantel 75 mg/kg/day in 3 divided
Paragonimus westermani	Lung	Crustacea	Asia	doses PO for 2 days
Paragonimus mexicana	Lung	Crustacea	Mexico	*or*
Paragonimus kellicotti	Lung	Crustacea	United States	Bithionol 30–50 mg/kg PO on
Paragonimus uterobilateralis	Lung	Crustacea	Africa	alternate days for 10–15 doses

*Treatment recommendations adapted from Drugs for parasitic infections. *Med Lett Drugs Ther* 2000;42:1–11.

TABLE 43–2. Etiologic Agents of Human Schistosomiasis

Etiologic Agent	Disease Syndrome	Geographic Location
Schistosoma mansoni	Intestinal, hepatic	South America, Caribbean, Africa, Middle East
Schistosoma japonicum	Intestinal, hepatic	Far East, especially China, Philippines, Japan
Schistosoma mekongi	Intestinal, hepatic	Southeast Asia (Laos, Thailand)
Schistosoma intercalatum	Intestinal, hepatic	Central Africa
*Schistosoma mattheei**	Intestinal, hepatic	Central Africa
Schistosoma haematobium	Urinary	Africa, Near and Middle East
*Schistosoma bovis**	Urinary	East and Central Africa

*Rare zoonosis.

blocking antibody production retards the development of immunity to the parasite until later, in adult life. As a result, schistosome worm burdens are often higher in children than adults. Heavy schistosome worm burdens in childhood adversely affect nutritional status and may be the mechanism by which schistosomes impair childhood growth.

SYMPTOMS AND CLINICAL MANIFESTATIONS

Many light schistosome infections are asymptomatic. Individuals harboring large numbers of *S. japonicum* and, to a lesser extent, *S. mansoni* frequently develop a syndrome associated with acute schistosomiasis called **Katayama fever.** It occurs with the onset of egg deposition approximately 2–8 weeks after entry by cercariae and is manifested as an acute onset of fever, chills, eosinophilia, and hepatosplenomegaly, often described as similar in clinical presentation to serum sickness. More commonly, children with intestinal schistosomiasis caused by *S. japonicum* and *S. mansoni* develop intermittent abdominal pain that is sometimes accompanied with bloody diarrhea (Table 43–3). The intestinal phase may be followed

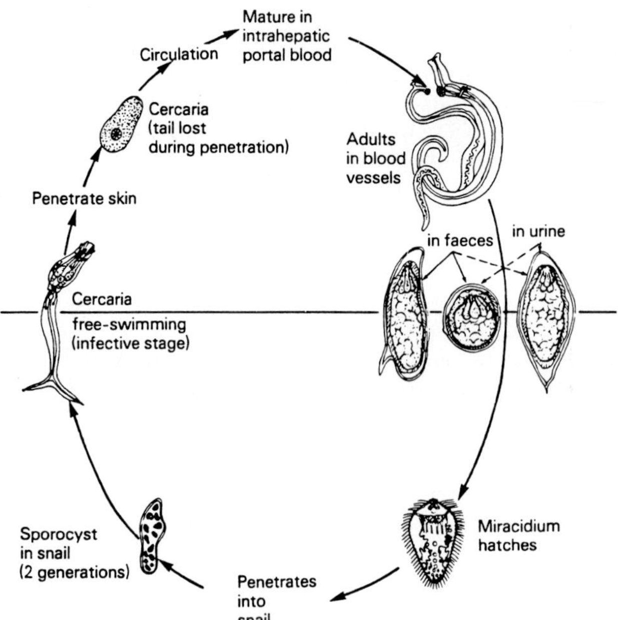

FIGURE 43–1. Life cycle of human schistosomes. (From Zaman V: *Atlas of Medical Parasitology,* 2nd ed. Sidney, Adis Health Science Press, 1984.)

by the appearance of signs of portal hypertension, including hepatosplenomegaly and ascites. There is tremendous variability in the clinical presentation, however. Some children develop only hepatic disease and others only intestinal symptoms, with the potential for numerous complications.

Children with *S. haematobium* infection may also be free of symptoms, but they commonly develop dysuria, hematuria, and increased frequency. Obstructive uropathies leading to hydronephrosis and hydroureter can develop in long-standing disease.

Schistosomes exert a strong negative effect on growth throughout childhood and adolescence. In a cross-sectional study (McGarvey, 1992) from the Philippines, infected male and female subjects were found to be significantly shorter and to have less limb muscle and subcutaneous adipose tissue than uninfected control subjects. Many of these deficits are reversible after anthelmintic chemotherapy.

Cercarial Dermatitis. In many parts of the world, including the United States (e.g., the Great Lakes area), humans can develop dermatitis (**"swimmer's itch"** or **"clam-digger's itch"**) after

TABLE 43–3. Major Clinical Manifestations of Schistosomiasis

Schistosoma japonicum* and *Schistosoma mansoni
Abdominal pain
Bloody diarrhea
Portal hypertension
Hepatosplenomegaly
Katayama fever (especially *S. japonicum*)
Schistosoma haematobium
Hematuria
Dysuria
Obstructive uropathy
Squamous cell bladder carcinoma (in late stages)

penetration by other mammalian schistosomes including *S. mattheei* and *S. douthitti* and also by cercariae of avian schistosomes including *Austrobilharzia, Trichobilharzia,* and *Ornithobilharzia,* which are associated with freshwater, and *Microbilharzia,* which is associated with seawater. Contact with freshwater or brackish water typically occurs during bathing. Cercarial dermatitis has an allergic or immunopathologic basis. The first exposure to zoonotic cercariae produces very mild symptoms. With repeated exposure a dermatitis comprising large papules, typically 3–5 mm, develops, accompanied by erythema and intense pruritus. The onset is often within 24 hours after exposure. The disease is self-limited, and cercariae seldom survive past the skin. Antihistamines help relieve the pruritus.

DIAGNOSIS

In the early stages of illness before the appearance of eggs in excreta, such as in Katayama fever, the diagnosis is predominantly based on clinical criteria. A definitive diagnosis of schistosomiasis requires an identification of eggs in either the feces or urine of an infected individual. Because adult female *S. mansoni* typically releases fewer than 300 eggs per day, a direct fecal smear is often insensitive. Stool examination by a Kato-Katz thick smear is an alternative. Studies in the Philippines, however, indicate that a single fecal examination using the **Kato-Katz smear** will miss 35% of lightly infected persons. Therefore multiple examinations may be required if there is a strong suspicion of clinical schistosomiasis. Serologic testing for adult worm specific antibody (by ELISA and immunoblot), available from the CDC, may offer additional and useful diagnostic data.

S. haematobium infection is diagnosed by examination of urine collected close to noon, when egg excretion is maximal. To obtain a semiquantitative estimate of intensity, 10 mL of urine is typically filtered through a membrane that is then examined. Eggs can also be identified by rectal biopsies in persons whose excreta have no eggs. Endoscopy and colonoscopy, cystoscopy, and liver function tests are useful adjuncts in the evaluation of intestinal, bladder, and liver disease.

TREATMENT

Praziquantel is the treatment of choice for human schistosomiasis when cost is not a consideration (Table 43–4). At $2 to $5 per dose required for antischistosomal therapy, however, treating large populations is too expensive for many developing countries. This is lamentable given studies that demonstrate a decrease in prevalence, incidence, and intensity of infections with regular population-based treatment programs in tropical developing countries. In some regions, oxamniquine is as effective as praziquantel in the treatment of *S. mansoni* infection, and metrifonate is as effective as praziquantel for the treatment of *S. haematobium* infection. Surgical intervention is sometimes required to treat portal hypertension.

COMPLICATIONS

In general, complications are more frequently reported from *S. japonicum* infections than *S. mansoni* infections because of the greater egg release and deposition by the former. Katayama fever in acute schistosomiasis japonica can be fatal, whereas it occurs less frequently with *S. mansoni* infection. Long-standing and severe portal hypertension in schistosomiasis japonica can lead to varices and hepatic encephalopathy, although usually enough liver parenchyma is preserved so that this is uncommon. *S. haematobium* may eventually cause obstructive uropathy leading to secondary

TABLE 43–4. Specific Chemotherapy for Schistosomiasis

Schistosome	Drug	Dosage
Schistosoma haematobium	Praziquantel	40 mg/kg/day in 2 divided doses PO for 1 day†
Schistosoma japonicum	Praziquantel	60 mg/kg/day in 3 divided doses PO for 1 day
Schistosoma mansoni	Praziquantel	40 mg/kg/day in 2 divided doses PO for 1 day
	Alternative: Oxamniquine*	Children: 20 mg/kg in 2 divided doses PO for 1 day; adults: 15 mg/kg PO once
Schistosoma mekongi	Praziquantel†	60 mg/kg/day in 3 divided doses PO for 1 day

*Dosages of oxamniquine may vary in a given geographic area because of strain differences. In East Africa the dose should be increased to 30 mg/kg/day, and in Egypt and South Africa, 30 mg/kg in 2 divided doses PO for 2 days. Some experts recommend 40–60 mg/kg in 2 divided doses PO for 2–3 days for all of Africa. Seizures and neuropsychiatric disturbances have been reported in some patients. Oxamniquine is contraindicated in pregnancy.

†Metrifonate is used in some countries where praziquantel is not available or is too expensive.

Adapted from Drugs for parasitic infections. *Med Lett Drugs Ther* 2000;42:1–11.

bacterial urinary tract infections and chronic renal failure. There is also an association with squamous cell carcinoma of the bladder. Pulmonary embolization leading to obstruction of pulmonary arterioles may cause pulmonary hypertension and cor pulmonale.

Egg deposition in the spinal cord can lead to transverse myelitis in all three forms of schistosomiasis. *S. japonicum* can be associated with cerebral involvement that results in focal granulomas in the cerebrum, leading to seizures or mass effect.

PROGNOSIS

Because life-threatening complications are relatively uncommon in endemic areas, the prognosis after anthelmintic chemotherapy is generally favorable. Although intestinal, liver, and bladder fibrosis is not reversible, anthelmintic chemotherapy will prevent its progression. Significant catch-up growth in response to anthelmintic chemotherapy has been observed for all three schistosomes. Improved physical fitness and appetite have also been noted after treatment of *S. haematobium* infection.

PREVENTION

Preventive measures include health education about the possible dangers of frequent contact with freshwater and the construction of latrines to discourage defecation and urination in freshwater. There has been a great effort to interrupt transmission by eliminating the intermediate snail host through the widespread use of molluscicides. In many cases, however, this approach has not been effective, and in a few cases it has been deleterious because of toxic effects in fish, rice crops, domestic animals, and humans. Mass, targeted chemotherapy with praziquantel has been suggested and in some cases implemented. There is an intense research effort to develop chemically defined vaccines against cercariae, schistosomula, or adult worms. Swimming in the ocean and in chlorinated freshwater pools is considered safe from trematodiases.

REVIEWS

Butterworth AE, Fulford AJ, Dunne DW, et al: Longitudinal studies on human schistosomiasis. *Philos Trans R Soc Lond B Biol Sci* 1988;321:495–511.

King CH, Mahmoud AA: Drugs five years later: Praziquantel. *Ann Intern Med* 1989;110:290–6.

Shuxian L, Guangchen S, Yuxin X, et al: Progress in the development of a vaccine against schistosomiasis in China. *Int J Infect Dis* 1998;2:176–80.

KEY ARTICLES

Bensted-Smith R, Anderson RM, Butterworth AE, et al: Evidence for predisposition of individual patients to reinfection with *Schistosoma mansoni* after treatment. *Trans R Soc Trop Med Hyg* 1987;81:651–4.

Boyce TG: Acute transverse myelitis in a 6-year-old girl with schistosomiasis. *Pediatr Infect Dis J* 1990;9:279–84.

Butterworth AE, Bensted-Smith R, Capron A, et al: Immunity in human schistosomiasis mansoni: Prevention by blocking antibodies of the expression of immunity in young children. *Parasitology* 1987;94:281–300.

Flavell DJ: Liver-fluke infection as an aetiological factor in bile-duct carcinoma of man. *Trans R Soc Trop Med Hyg* 1981;75:814–24.

Kammerer WS, Van Der Decker JD, Keith TB, et al: Clonorchiasis in New York City Chinese. *Trop Doct* 1977;7:105–6.

Latham MC, Stephenson LS, Kurz KM, et al: Metrifonate or praziquantel treatment improves physical fitness and appetite of Kenyan schoolboys with *Schistosoma haematobium* and hookworm infections. *Am J Trop Med Hyg* 1990;43:170–9.

Mariano EG, Borja SR, Vruno MJ: A human infection with *Paragonimus kellicotti* (lung fluke) in the United States. *Am J Clin Pathol* 1986;86:685–7.

McGarvey ST, Aligui G, Daniel BL, et al: Child growth and schistosomiasis japonica in northeastern Leyte, the Philippines: Cross-sectional results. *Am J Trop Med Hyg* 1992;46:571–81.

McGarvey ST, Aligui G, Graham KK, et al: Schistosomiasis japonica and childhood nutritional status in northeastern Leyte, the Philippines: A randomized trial of praziquantel versus placebo. *Am J Trop Med Hyg* 1996;54:498–502.

Olveda RM, Daniel BL, Ramirez BD, et al: Schistosomiasis japonica in the Philippines: The long-term impact of population-based chemotherapy on infection, transmission, and morbidity. *J Infect Dis* 1996;174:163–72.

Pachucki CT, Levandowski RA, Brown VA, et al: American paragonimiasis treated with praziquantel. *N Engl J Med* 1984;311:582–3.

Stephenson LS, Latham MC, Kurz KM, et al: Single dose metrifonate or praziquantel treatment in Kenyan children. II. Effects on growth in relation to *Schistosoma haematobium* and hookworm egg counts. *Am J Trop Med Hyg* 1989;41:445–53.

Tsang VC, Wilkins PP: Immunodiagnosis of schistosomiasis. Screen with FAST-ELISA and confirm with immunoblot. *Clin Lab Med* 1991;11:1029–39.

CHAPTER 44

Cestode Infections

Peter J. Hotez

The cestodes, or **tapeworms,** cause two major types of zoonotic disease syndromes depending on whether humans are the definitive or the accidental (''dead end''), intermediate host. When humans serve as definitive hosts, they develop infections with adult tapeworms that do not generally elicit severe disease. When humans serve as accidental, intermediate hosts for the larval cestode, serious morbidity and pathology can result. Cysticercosis and echinococcosis cause the greatest morbidity among the larval cestodiases and are a significant cause of death.

CYSTICERCOSIS

ETIOLOGY

Cysticercosis results from infection with the larval stages of the **pork tapeworm** *Taenia solium.* The cysticercus was formerly known as *Cysticercus cellulosae.* Humans acquire these larvae by ingesting eggs in the gravid segments, or **proglottids,** of adult tapeworms. Human cysticercosis is transmitted by fecal-oral contact through either heteroinfection from another individual, frequently a family member who harbors the adult pork tapeworm, or by autoinfection in the case of a person with adult *T. solium* (Fig. 44–1). Autoinfection probably occurs by transmission of eggs from anus to mouth, although researchers have suggested that eggs may also ascend to the duodenum and liberate oncospheres. Human cysticercosis is a biologic ''dead end'' for the organism, which does not develop into an adult tapeworm. Although cysticerci have been found in almost every organ of the body, cerebral cysticercosis leads to the most serious pathology.

EPIDEMIOLOGY

Cysticercosis, the most common helminth infection of the central nervous system, has a high prevalence in the developing countries of Latin America because pigs are raised in poor rural areas in close proximity to improperly disposed human feces and because large amounts of raw or uncooked pork are consumed. More than 90% of persons with cysticercosis in the United States were born in another country, usually Mexico or a Central American country. Cysticercosis has been increasingly recognized in U.S. cities with large Mexican and Central American populations, such as Los Angeles, and neurocysticercosis is now a leading cause of epilepsy among children living in Los Angeles County. Locally acquired cases have also been reported. However, epidemiologic investigations of many of these so-called autochthonous cases have revealed that they were acquired from index patients who still harbored the adult *T. solium* after emigrating from an endemic area. For example, an outbreak of neurocysticercosis among Orthodox Jews in New York City resulted from contact with domestic housekeepers who had recently emigrated from Latin American countries (Schantz, 1992).

PATHOGENESIS

After ingestion of the eggs of *T. solium,* an oncosphere is liberated in the duodenum, where it penetrates the intestinal mucosa, enters the mesenteric circulation, and spreads throughout the body. The muscles, subcutaneous tissues, eyes, and brain are most commonly involved. After approximately 2 months the oncospheres develop into cysticerci, each of which is a trilaminated structure that usually contains an invaginated scolex. In time they evoke a host inflammatory response involving lymphocytes, plasma cells, and eosinophils, which is greatest around dying and dead cysticerci. The response is highly variable, however, and some cysticerci live in the tissues for years, undisturbed by a histologically detectable host response. It has been suggested, partly because females develop a stronger response, that sex and human leukocyte antigen type may influence the degree of inflammation.

SYMPTOMS AND CLINICAL MANIFESTATIONS

Outside the central nervous system, even large numbers of cysticerci may not cause symptoms. In a study (Mitchell, 1988) among children admitted to the Children's Hospital of Los Angeles, the most common form of cerebral cysticercosis was a solitary inflamed parenchymal mass lesion with a number of characteristic radiographic CT findings (Fig. 44–2). Children with solitary lesions frequently have partial seizures that progress to generalized seizures. In contrast, children and adults who reside in endemic areas, such as Mexico and South Africa, are reported to have a higher proportion of complications, including elevated intracranial pressure, arachnoiditis, meningitis, encephalitis, and hydrocephalus. These differences may reflect the observation that children who immigrate to the United States leave sources of chronic re-exposure behind.

DIAGNOSIS

The diagnosis is suspected by clinical presentation and possible exposure and is confirmed by diagnostic imaging and serologic testing.

Laboratory Diagnosis

Limited diagnostic information can be obtained from the CSF of persons with neurocysticercosis. The CSF protein typically is elevated. A mild lymphocytic pleocytosis, with a mean cell count of $59/mm^3$, is present in approximately half of the cases, frequently with eosinophils. Lumbar puncture is contraindicated in those patients with elevated intracranial pressure.

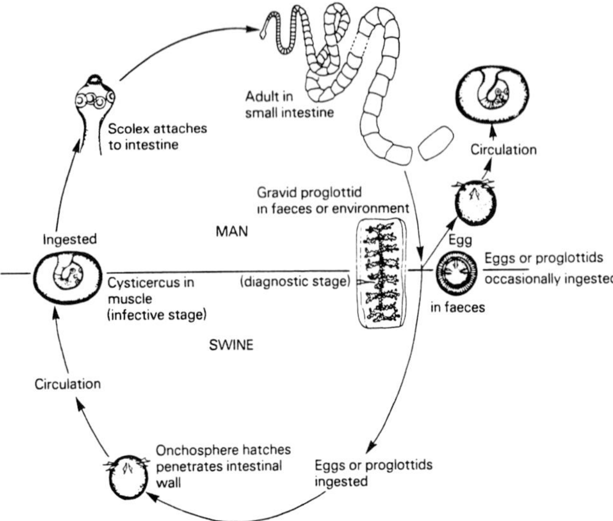

FIGURE 44–1. Life cycle of *Taenia solium* (formerly *Cysticercus cellulosae*). (From Zaman V: *Atlas of Medical Parasitology,* 2nd ed. Sidney, Adis Health Science Press, 1984.)

Serologic Testing. Although ELISA has been used traditionally to detect cysticercus antibodies in serum or CSF, it is being gradually replaced with an **enzyme-linked immunotransfer blot (EITB),** or **Western blot,** which has a high degree of sensitivity. The titers by EITB will decline in persons with fewer than two parenchymal cysts. Serum EITB may have a higher degree of sensitivity than CSF EITB and is therefore more commonly performed in specialized diagnostic laboratories, such as at the CDC. Persons with a single parenchymal cyst seen on diagnostic imaging but who have a negative serologic test result, pose a diagnostic dilemma that may be an indication for brain biopsy in areas of low endemicity.

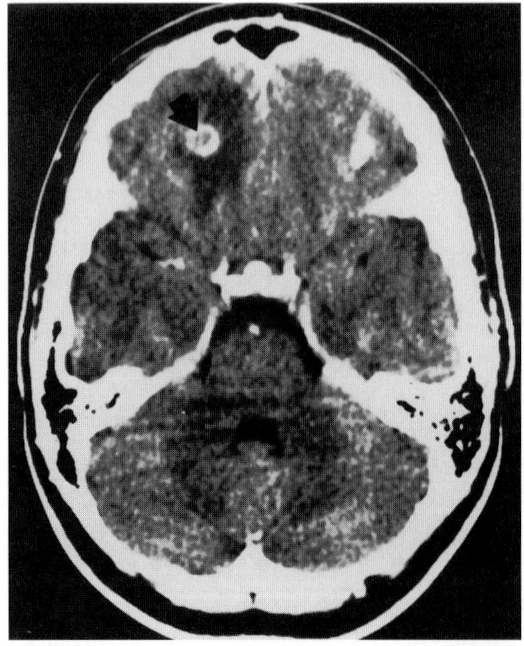

FIGURE 44–2. Contrast-enhanced CT scan showing an enhancing ring lesion from cysticercosis in the right orbital frontal region. The *arrow* indicates the cyst surrounded by edema. (From Mitchell WG, Crawford TO: Intraparenchymal cysticercosis in children: Diagnosis and treatment. *Pediatrics* 82:79;1988.)

Diagnostic Imaging

The diagnosis of neurocysticercosis is typically established by CT findings in an appropriate clinical setting. Common features of these mass lesions on CT scans (Table 44–1) include solitary distribution in most cases; demonstration of ring enhancement with contrast medium; typical size of 5–20 mm in diameter; location in the cortex or gray-white junction; and wide variability in the extent of secondary edema. Other, less common findings that are reported (del Brutto, 1988), particularly in endemic areas, include small calcifications or granulomas from old and destroyed cysts; hypodense lesions that do not demonstrate ring enhancement; and diffuse brain swelling with multiple nodular, ring-enhancing lesions **(cysticercosis encephalitis).**

MRI may be more sensitive than CT in the detection of small parenchymal cysticerci and for diagnosis of the brain edema that accompanies cysticercosis encephalitis. The presence of a hyperdense point within the cyst can suggest the presence of a pathognomonic parasite scolex. Intraventricular cysts may be isodense with CSF, and therefore the injection of a contrast medium may be required for identification.

TREATMENT

The initial therapy for neurocysticercosis should focus on alleviation of symptoms, including the use of anticonvulsant drugs if necessary. Treatment of uncomplicated neurocysticercosis with anthelmintics is controversial. Any cysticidal drug may cause irreparable damage if administered in the presence of ocular or spinal cysts, even when corticosteroids are also administered. An ophthalmologic examination should be performed before the start of anthelmintic therapy so that the presence of intraocular cysts can be excluded.

Definitive Treatment

A single enhancing lesion in children with neurocysticercosis in the United States may spontaneously resolve without the use of anthelmintics. Because ring enhancement is believed to be associated with inflammation around a dying or dead parasite, specific anthelmintic therapy may not be of benefit at this stage of disease. Similarly, there may not be benefit from anthelmintics for persons with CT scans that reveal only the calcifications associated with dead parasites. Randomized trials of anthelmintic therapy have not shown a benefit, but expectant observation for neurocysticercosis, especially in children, remains controversial, prompting some ex-

TABLE 44–1. Major Clinical Manifestations of Neurocysticercosis

"Simple": in Nonendemic Areas without Re-exposure
Solitary, 5–20 mm, ring-enhancing, parenchymal mass
Focal seizures
Secondary generalized seizures
"Complicated": in Endemic Areas with Re-exposure
Multiple cysts
Seizures
Increased intracranial pressure
Arachnoiditis
Meningitis
Encephalitis
Hydrocephalus

perts to recommend treatment for all children even with a single ring-enhancing lesion. Conversely, all persons with either multiple cysts or viable cysticerci without radiographic evidence of inflammation usually require specific anthelmintic therapy. In persons with associated seizures, marked remission or improvement usually occurs after administration of definitive anthelmintic therapy (Vasquez, 1992).

Two anthelmintics have been used for the treatment of neurocysticercosis: praziquantel and albendazole (Table 44–2). Albendazole is slightly more effective, leading to an 85–88% rate of disappearance of cystic lesions on CT scan, compared with 50–60% for praziquantel (Sotelo, 1990; Takaynagui, 1992). Anthelmintics are larvicidal and consequently hasten and exacerbate the inflammatory response and may increase intracranial pressure. Therefore anthelmintics are contraindicated and should be temporarily withheld from patients with severe cerebral edema from complicated neurocysticercosis until the accompanying swelling subsides. Corticosteroids and osmotic diuresis to reduce brain edema are important adjuncts in the treatment of complicated neurocysticercosis, especially in the presence of encephalitis, arachnoiditis, vasculitis, or cerebral edema. It is common practice to administer prednisone (1 mg/kg/day; maximum: 60 mg/day) or dexamethasone (0.1–0.3 mg/kg/day; maximum: 4–16 mg/day) 2–3 days before starting cysticidal therapy or on the second or third day of cysticidal therapy (Vasquez, 1992) and to continue during and until shortly after anthelmintic therapy is discontinued. Dexamethasone may lower plasma levels of praziquantel by as much as 50% but may raise the level of albendazole by 50%. Albendazole is commonly administered with a fatty snack to enhance intestinal absorption. In some centers, cimetidine (400 mg orally twice daily for adults) is administered to obtain higher serum levels of albendazole. The duration of anthelmintic therapy is also controversial, with recommendations from 8 days to several months; most recommendations are for 1 month.

TABLE 44–2. Therapy for Cysticercosis*

Albendazole 15 mg/kg/day (maximum dose: 800 mg) PO divided in 2 daily doses for 8–30 days; may be repeated as necessary†‡

or

Praziquantel 50–100 mg/kg/day PO divided in 3 daily doses for 30 days†

*Initial therapy for parenchymal disease with seizures should focus on asymptomatic treatment with anticonvulsant drugs. Treatment of parenchymal disease with albendazole and praziquantel is controversial, and randomized trials have not shown a benefit. Some experts recommend expectant observation for a single solitary mass lesion ("simple" neurocysticercosis). Corticosteroids (e.g., dexamethasone) should be given 2–3 days before anthelmintic therapy (*Med Lett Drugs Ther* 1990;32:23–35) or on the second or third day of anthelmintic therapy (Vasquez, 1992) and continued during and shortly after therapy. Corticosteroids can alter the pharmacokinetics of anthelmintic drugs, requiring adjustment of the dosage of either albendazole or praziquantel.

†Any cysticidal drug may cause irreparable damage when used to treat ocular or spinal cysts, even when corticosteroids are used (White, 2000). An ophthalmologic examination to exclude the presence of intraocular cysts should always be performed before anthelmintic treatment is started.

‡Prolonged courses of benzimidazoles require the monitoring of liver function and hematopoiesis. The benzimidazoles are embryotoxic and teratogenic in rodents and are contraindicated in persons with blood dyscrasias, leukopenia, and liver disease. Albendazole should be administered with a fatty meal to enhance absorption. Cimetidine can also be administered to increase serum albendazole levels.

Adapted from Drugs for parasitic infections. *Med Lett Drugs Ther* 2000;42:1–11.

Supportive Therapy

Seizures should be controlled with anticonvulsants alone. Their use may be tapered after the child is free of seizures for 1–2 years. Obstructive hydrocephalus requires surgical removal of the cyst or placement of a CSF shunt.

COMPLICATIONS

The complications of neurocysticercosis depend on the anatomic location of the lesions. Multiple lesions in the parenchyma may cause encephalitis with increased intracranial pressure. These persons should be treated with corticosteroids and osmotic diuretics before specific anthelmintic therapy. The presence of cysticerci in the subarachnoid space results in inflammatory occlusion of the foramina of Luschka and of Magendie, leading to hydrocephalus, which can also be caused by intraventricular neurocysticercosis. Affected persons often benefit from ventriculoperitoneal shunt placement, sometimes in association with surgical extirpation of clumps of cysticerci. Intraventricular cysts often require surgical removal. Tapeworm larvae in the sella may mimic pituitary tumors. Intraspinal neurocysticercosis may also occur. Heavy infections of cysticerci outside the central nervous system have been associated, rarely, with a pseudohypertrophic myopathy.

PROGNOSIS

The prognosis for a child with a solitary mass lesion is good, and approximately 60% of such children who are weaned from anticonvulsants remain free of seizures. The prognosis of complications from neurocysticercosis depends on the anatomic location and number of the lesions. In a study (Vasquez, 1992) with 3 years of follow-up of persons with neurocysticercosis, 54% who received definitive cysticidal therapy were seizure-free, in comparison with no seizure-free individuals in the untreated group.

PREVENTION

The refrigeration of pork infested with cysticerci at temperatures above 0°C does not affect parasite survival. In contrast, freezing of meat decreases the likelihood of survival. Storage of pork for 4 days at −5°C, 3 days at −15°C, or 1 day at −24°C kills most cysticerci.

ECHINOCOCCOSIS

ETIOLOGY

Human echinococcosis is a zoonosis caused by *Echinococcus* (Table 44–3). The helminths are acquired by the accidental ingestion of the eggs of *Echinococcus granulosus,* the **minute dog tapeworm,** passed in the feces of the definitive host, usually carnivores of the family Canidae such as dogs, wolves, coyotes, and jackals.

EPIDEMIOLOGY

E. granulosus infection is found worldwide and occurs wherever sheep, who serve as the natural intermediate host, graze. Human echinococcosis is associated with the practice of feeding sheep viscera to dogs. Hyperendemic foci occur in rural areas of Uruguay and Argentina. In the United States, echinococcosis is prevalent among American Indians in New Mexico, those of Basque descent

TABLE 44–3. Etiologic Agents of Human Echinococcosis

Etiologic Agent	Type of Cyst	Animal Reservoir	Distribution
Echinococcus granulosus	Unilocular	Sheep; dogs	Worldwide
Echinococcus granulosus var. *canadensis*	Unilocular	Caribou; moose; dogs	Arctic (sylvatic)
Echinococcus multilocularis	Alveolar	Voles; rodents; fox	Northern Hemisphere
Echinococcus vogeli	Polycystic	Pacas; bush dogs	South America, Central America
Echinococcus oligarthrus	Rare	Pacas; felids	South America, Central America

living in California, and the families of sheep ranchers in Utah. The Canadian Indian and Inuit populations of Canada are frequently infected with a less virulent, northern or sylvatic variant (sometimes designated *E. granulosus* var. *canadensis*) that is typically found in moose and caribou rather than sheep. *Echinococcus multilocularis,* which causes aggressive and fulminant alveolar hydatid disease in the Northern Hemisphere, is a zoonosis found in Arctic foxes that feed on rodents. Infections have been reported in Manitoba and Saskatchewan and in the North Central United States (North Dakota, South Dakota, Minnesota, Montana, Iowa, and Wyoming). Clinical manifestations seldom become apparent during childhood. Polycystic hydatid disease caused by *Echinococcus vogeli* is found in Central and South America.

PATHOGENESIS

After oral ingestion the activated oncospheres of *Echinococcus* are released in the gastrointestinal tract and penetrate the mucosa to enter the venous and lymphatic vessels (Fig. 44–3). Although the liver is the major site of hydatid cyst development, many oncospheres reach the lung and central nervous system. *E. granulosus* hydatid cysts form over a period of years, slowly increasing in size by 1–5 cm per year. Cyst growth is a three-step process: (1) metacestode growth, (2) asexual reproduction and budding to produce protoscolices, and (3) synthesis of a fluid-filled, laminated endocyst that is surrounded by connective tissue, known as the **ectocyst.** The so-called unilocular cyst is well tolerated until it enlarges to the point where it compresses on vital structures or causes pain. Between 50% and 70% of unilocular hydatid cysts are in the liver, and 20–30% are in the lung. Unilocular hydatid cysts from the sylvatic variant *E. granulosus* var. *canadensis* are usually found in the lung. Occasionally the cyst spontaneously ruptures and disseminates the protoscolices that form the nidus of secondary cysts. Cyst rupture can result in anaphylaxis.

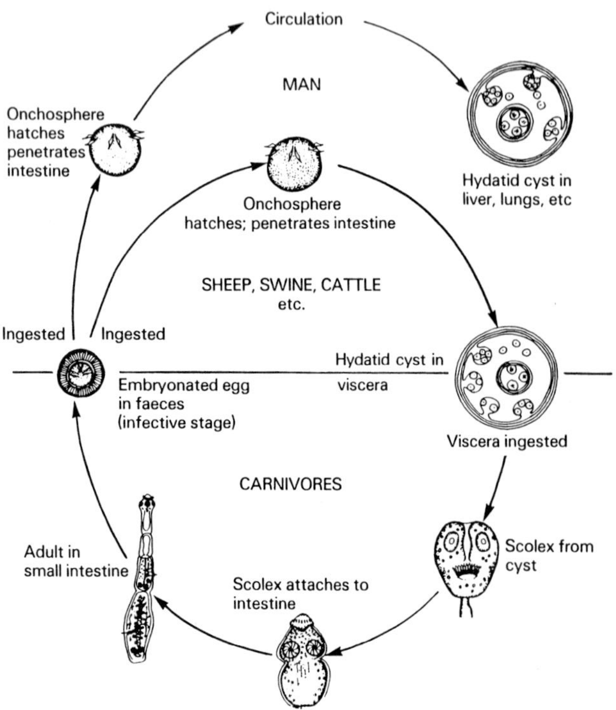

FIGURE 44–3. Life cycle of *Echinococcus granulosus.* (From Zaman V: *Atlas of Medical Parasitology,* 2nd ed. Sidney, Adis Health Science Press, 1984.)

Alveolar hydatid disease caused by *E. multilocularis* is much more aggressive than unilocular hydatid disease. The alveolar form proliferates indefinitely and causes progressive destruction of the liver parenchyma, leaving behind necrotic debris. Parasite entry into blood vessels facilitates metastasis to distant sites, including the brain.

SYMPTOMS AND CLINICAL MANIFESTATIONS

Unilocular hydatid cysts are slow growing, usually about 1 cm per year, and frequently cause no symptoms for years until they reach relatively large sizes. Consequently, echinococcosis is not usually diagnosed in childhood. Signs and symptoms of hepatic hydatid cysts include right upper quadrant pain and hepatic enlargement that is sometimes accompanied by a palpable mass (Table 44–4). Extension into the biliary tree can lead to obstructive jaundice and cholangitis. Unilocular cyst rupture or leakage is frequently associated with an immediate hypersensitivity syndrome with urticaria and pruritus. Severe anaphylaxis may occur. Persons with

TABLE 44–4. Major Clinical Manifestations of Echinococcosis

Unilocular Hydatid Cyst *(Echinococcus granulosus)*
Right upper quadrant mass
Right upper quadrant pain
Hepatomegaly
Obstructive jaundice
Immediate hypersensitivity reaction, anaphylaxis (cyst rupture)
Unilocular Hydatid Cyst *(Echinococcus granulosus* var. *canadensis)*
Asymptomatic lung mass
Cough, fever, hemoptysis
Urticaria (cyst rupture)
Alveolar Hydatid Disease *(Echinococcus multilocularis)*
Hepatomegaly
Jaundice
Hepatic failure
Multiple palpable abdominal masses
Central nervous system changes

intact pulmonary unilocular cysts often have no symptoms, but the rupture of pulmonary hydatid cysts is manifested by coughing, dyspnea, and hemoptysis.

Approximately one third of the cases of infection with the more benign sylvatic, or northern, variant of *Echinococcus* (*E. granulosus* var. *canadensis*) involve children. The majority of patients have single lung hydatid cysts that cause no symptoms and are often initially detected on chest radiographs obtained for tuberculosis screening. Rupture of these cysts causes comparatively few symptoms, including mild cough, fever, and slight hemoptysis. A few patients have urticaria but rarely manifest severe anaphylaxis.

Alveolar (multilocular) hydatid disease has an aggressive course that frequently leads to hepatic failure. Presenting clinical signs include hepatomegaly, jaundice, and multiple palpable abdominal masses.

DIAGNOSIS

Although epidemiologic history may offer important clues regarding diagnosis, hydatid cysts are often first identified radiographically. Serologic testing is useful as an adjunct for diagnosis. Alveolar hydatid disease frequently mimics hepatocellular carcinoma in its clinical presentation. Exploratory laparotomy delineates the extent of disease.

Laboratory Evaluation

Peripheral eosinophilia is usually not present. Mild elevation of hepatic enzymes may be present with hepatic hydatid cysts.

Microbiologic Evaluation

Protoscolices are sometimes recovered in the sputum of persons with pulmonary involvement, although this is inconsistent.

Serologic Testing. Serologic assays, usually based on EIA techniques, are useful adjuncts in the diagnosis of echinococcosis. The false-negative rate is high, however, particularly in persons with unruptured cysts. Persons with intact lung cysts induce the least antigenic stimulation, and nearly 50% of these persons are serologically nonreactive. Negative serologic findings are common in persons with *E. granulosus* var. *canadensis,* who typically have intact lung cysts at presentation. Detection of antibody to *Echinococcus* antigen 5 (arc 5) in serum confirms a positive EIA result. An EIA using purified *E. multilocularis* antigen is also available from the CDC. Approximately 5–10% of persons with cysticercosis are cross-reactive on serologic testing for echinococcosis. Use of Casoni's skin test with hydatid cyst fluid is not justified.

Diagnostic Imaging

Plain radiographs of the abdomen and lung are not specific. A radiograph of the chest may reveal an asymptomatic intrapulmonary mass (Fig. 44–4). The CT scan frequently reveals a mixture of hyperdensities and hypodensities with scattered calcifications. Demonstration of **internal septa** or **daughter cysts** by CT, MRI, or ultrasonography is pathognomonic for hydatid cysts. Such findings are present in approximately 50% of persons with unilocular liver cysts; daughter cysts are not seen in persons with northern, or sylvatic, unilocular cysts. Closed aspiration of hydatid cysts is contraindicated because it may result in rupture, leading to anaphylaxis or protoscolex dissemination.

TREATMENT

Until recently, surgical removal of cysts was the only therapeutic option and remains the treatment that has the best potential for immediate and complete cure. The benzimidazoles, especially albendazole, are effective in the treatment of hydatid disease, resulting in cyst regression or collapse, and are increasingly used to supplement or even supplant surgery (Table 44–5). Prolonged courses of therapy, for 60–90 days, are often required. Albendazole administered for one to three periods of 28 days, with drug-free intervals of 14 days, has been used with some success. Reversible toxic effects in the liver and bone marrow have been reported with

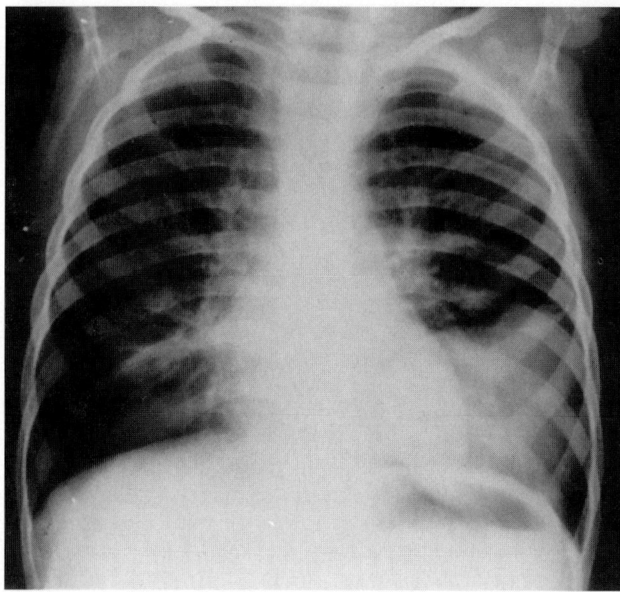

FIGURE 44–4. Echinococcal lung cyst in a 5-year-old boy with a history of asthma, low-grade fever, and eosinophilia. Frontal chest radiograph reveals a large, round, homogeneous mass within the left lower lobe. The mass is well demarcated with no surrounding Inflammatory reaction. In addition, there is bilateral central peribronchial thickening compatible with chronic reactive airway disease.

TABLE 44–5. Therapy for Echinococcosis

Unilocular Hydatid Cyst *(Echinococcus granulosus)*
Surgical resection*
plus
Albendazole 15 mg/kg/day (maximum: 800 mg/day) divided in 2 daily doses PO for 1–6 mo†
Unilocular Hydatid Cyst (*E. granulosus* var. *canadensis)*
Expectant observation
Alveolar Hydatid Disease (*Echinococcus multilocularis)*
Surgical resection is the only reliable means of treatment. Some reports suggest adjunct use of albendazole or mebendazole, which is controversial (Wen, 1994).
Albendazole 15 mg/kg/day (maximum: 800 mg/day) divided in 2 daily doses PO administered preoperatively and postoperatively†

*Praziquantel is useful preoperatively or in case of spillage during surgery. Percutaneous drainage with ultrasound guidance plus albendazole therapy has been effective for management of hepatitic cyst disease (Khuroo, 1997).

†Prolonged courses of benzimidazoles require monitoring of liver function and hematopoiesis. The benzimidazoles are embryotoxic and teratogenic in rodents and are contraindicated in persons with blood dyscrasias, leukopenia, and liver disease. Albendazole should be taken with a fatty meal to enhance absorption.

Adapted from Drugs for parasitic infections. *Med Lett Drugs Ther* 2000; 42:1–11.

prolonged treatment. Diagnostic imaging can be used to monitor therapeutic responses. The role of praziquantel in the therapy for echinococcosis is under evaluation.

Surgical treatment is still required for very large cysts and for cysts that cause biliary obstruction. Enucleation of the entire cyst, followed by the obliteration of the cavity (e.g., omentoplasty after hepatic cyst removal), is the treatment of choice. In one study (Tomkins, 1991), conservative surgical treatment was less effective in preventing recurrence than was a radical surgical procedure. Resections may be particularly important for alveolar echinococcal disease. Persons with alveolar disease may benefit from partial hepatectomy with adjunct anthelmintic therapy before and after surgery.

Complete removal of an intact cyst is not always possible. One successful resection technique involves circulating liquid nitrogen through a funnel attached to the cyst wall. The liquid nitrogen freezes the funnel to the edge of the cyst, allowing the contents to be evacuated. A common practice is percutaneous puncture of the cyst under sonographic guidance, aspiration of the cyst contents, and injection of protoscolicidal agents (e.g., 0.5% silver nitrate, hypertonic saline, solution, or formalin), followed by reaspiration of the cyst. This is known as **PAIR therapy.** Sclerosing cholangitis resulting from chemical leakage into the biliary tree is a major complication. Adjunct chemotherapy with albendazole may be beneficial, particularly in cases where spillage occurs.

Albendazole may also alter the natural history of alveolar hydatid disease. In Mongolian jirds, a type of rodent, with *E. multilocularis* infection, albendazole inhibits larval growth and protoscolex formation, decreases metastatic disease, and reduces mortality rates. Surgical resection of the entire larval mass, which frequently requires hepatic or pulmonary lobe resection, is the only therapy that has been proved effective.

Sylvatic unilocular hydatid disease caused by *E. granulosus* var. *canadensis* is usually mild and self-limited and therefore can be managed conservatively. Asymptomatic cysts and lesions that do not become secondarily infected or that grow rapidly may be followed up with periodic imaging studies.

COMPLICATIONS

Approximately 5–10% of unilocular cysts involve organs other than the liver or lungs. Central nervous system involvement is more common in children and is associated with elevated intracranial pressure and focal neurologic signs. Hydatid cysts in the kidney can lead to pain and hematuria, and those in the bone frequently cause pathologic fractures. Occasionally, cysts spontaneously rupture and disseminate the protoscolices that form the nidus of secondary cysts. Such rupture can result in anaphylaxis.

PROGNOSIS

The outcome of echinococcosis is variable and depends on the size, number, and anatomic location of the cysts and whether they have ruptured. The prognosis of sylvatic unilocular hydatid disease is generally excellent even in the absence of medical intervention.

Lesions of alveolar hydatid disease are frequently inoperable. Before albendazole and praziquantel became available, most persons with inoperable lesions died of their disease. It is not known how new developments in anthelmintic chemotherapy will alter the otherwise potentially grave prognosis of alveolar hydatid disease.

PREVENTION

Control measures for unilocular hydatid disease are directed against interrupting the transmission of *E. granulosus* from sheep and carnivore hosts. Such measures include the safe disposal of sheep viscera, mass chemotherapy in dogs, and health education. Eradication of human alveolar hydatid disease requires the avoidance of the definitive host, usually foxes, and the prevention of rodent consumption by pets. Chemically defined vaccines are being developed.

ADULT TAPEWORM INFECTIONS

Adult tapeworm infections may frequently interfere with human nutrition, but they are often asymptomatic and seldom life-threatening. Tapeworms share a number of common morphologic features, including a **scolex,** which is composed of either suckers or grooves that facilitate attachment to the intestinal wall, and a **strobila,** which is a chain of proglottids. The proglottids located close to the posterior end of the worm are usually gravid and consist of a uterus filled with eggs. Both the proglottids and the eggs have morphologic characteristics that allow for species identification based on stool examination.

DIPHYLLOBOTHRIASIS

Diphyllobothrium latum, the **fish tapeworm,** is found in many temperate climates. In the United States, endemic foci have been described in Minnesota and Michigan. In Canada, *Diphyllobothrium alascense,* a related parasite, has been described among the Inuit. *Diphyllobothrium* requires two intermediate hosts, a crustacean *(Cyclops)* and a freshwater fish. When humans ingest raw fish, they become the definitive host. Other fish-eating mammals may also serve as reservoirs.

The most striking clinical feature of infection with *D. latum* is the development of megaloblastic hematopoiesis and anemia caused by vitamin B_{12} deficiency. The pathogenesis of this deficiency has not been determined. Although host malabsorption and decreased intrinsic factor production contribute to this condition, there is some evidence that the deficiency occurs because of direct uptake by the worm. Praziquantel in a single dose of 25 mg/kg (more than that required for taeniasis) is the treatment of choice (Table 44–6).

DIPYLIDIASIS

Humans become infected with *Dipylidium caninum,* the **dog tapeworm,** when they accidentally ingest fleas *(Ctenocephalides)* containing cysticercoid larvae. Cysticercoids mature to adult tapeworms in 3–4 weeks. Most infections occur in young children,

TABLE 44–6. Therapy for Adult Tapeworm Infections

Taenia saginata	Praziquantel	5–10 mg/kg once PO*
Taenia solium		
Dipylidium caninum		
Diphyllobothrium latum		
Hymenolepis diminuta		
Hymenolepis nana†	Praziquantel	25 mg/kg once PO*

*A higher dose of praziquantel (25 mg/kg) may be required for treatment of *D. latum* infections.
†Because the larval stages of *H. nana* are also present in the human definitive host, praziquantel is considered the treatment of choice.
Adapted from Drugs for parasitic infections. *Med Lett Drugs Ther* 2000; 42:1–11.

frequently in infants. Children can remain free of symptoms, but often they develop diarrhea, anorexia, and abdominal pain. *D. caninum* infection is believed to be underreported. Often it is first seen by the children or their parents, who can observe actively motile proglottid segments that look like grains of rice in the stool. Commonly this observation is misinterpreted as a sign of pinworm infection. If possible, proglottid segments should be preserved in 5–10% formalin. Praziquantel is the treatment of choice (Table 44–6).

HYMENOLEPIASIS

Infection with *Hymenolepis nana* occurs in tropical and semitropical climates, including southern Europe. Infection with *Hymenolepis diminuta,* the **rat tapeworm,** has also been described in children. Humans are the only definitive host and become infected by fecal-oral transmission. Unlike many human tapeworm infections, *H. nana* has no absolute requirement for an intermediate host, although some species of beetles and fleas can serve this purpose. After ingestion the larva enters a villus to become a cysticercoid, which then continues to develop into an egg-producing adult. *H. nana* is one of the smallest tapeworms that infects humans. Infection with large numbers of adults can occur, however, and cause diarrhea, abdominal pain, anorexia, and nausea. Praziquantel is the drug of choice because it eliminates both the cysticercoids in the villi and the adults. Usually higher doses are required than those used for other tapeworm infections (Table 44–6).

TAENIASIS

Taenia saginata, the **beef tapeworm,** is found wherever undercooked or raw beef is consumed. The prevalence of this infection is particularly high in East Africa. Humans are the only definitive host. The eggs are passed within intact proglottids, which can migrate out of the anus and fall to the ground. Cattle, which are the major intermediate host, ingest the eggs that disperse from the proglottid segment. Oncospheres are liberated and penetrate the gastrointestinal tract to gain access to the circulation. In the muscles, they develop into cysticerci. When humans consume so-called ''measly'' beef, the cysticerci liberate a scolex that attaches to the intestinal wall. The adult tapeworm can reach 10 m in length.

Most infections are asymptomatic. When gastrointestinal symptoms occur, they are usually mild. Immediate hypersensitivity reactions accompanied with pruritus, urticaria, and asthma have been described. Praziquantel in a single dose is an effective treatment (Table 44–6).

Taenia solium, the **pork tapeworm,** is also found wherever undercooked or raw pork is consumed (Fig. 44–1). Like cysticercosis, the prevalence of this cestode in Mexico and other parts of Latin America is high. The life cycle and clinical manifestations of pork tapeworm infection are similar to those of *T. saginata.* Treatment is always recommended because of the possibility of autoinfection that may result in cysticercosis. Praziquantel is effective as a single oral dose (Table 44–6).

KEY ARTICLES

Cysticercosis

Baranwal AK, Singhi PD, Khandelwal N, et al: Albendazole therapy in children with focal seizures and single small enhancing computerized tomographic lesions: A randomized, placebo-controlled, double-blind trial. *Pediatr Infect Dis J* 1998;17:696–700.

Coyle CM, Wittner M, Tanowitz HB: Cysticercosis. In Guerrant RL, Walker DH, Weller PF (editors): *Tropical Infectious Diseases: Principles, Pathogens, and Practice.* Philadelphia, Churchill Livingstone, 1999.

del Brutto OH, Sotelo J: Neurocysticercosis: An update. *Rev Infect Dis* 1988;10:1075–87.

del Brutto OH, Zenteno MA, Salgada P, et al: MR imaging in cysticercotic encephalitis. *AJNR Am J Neuroradiol* 1989;10:S18–20.

del Brutto OH, Sotelo J: Albendazole therapy for subararchnoid and ventricular cysticercosis. Case report. *J Neurosurg* 1990;72:816–7.

Despommier DD: Tapeworm infection—the long and the short of it. *N Engl J Med* 1992;327:727–8.

Diaz JF, Verastegui M, Gilman RH, et al: Immunodiagnosis of human cysticercosis (*Taenia solium*): A field comparison of an antibody–enzyme-linked immunosorbent assay (ELISA), and antigen-ELISA, and an enzyme-linked immunoelectrotransfer blot (EITB) assay in Peru. The Cysticercosis Working Group in Peru (CWG). *Am J Trop Med Hyg* 1992;46:610–5.

Evans C, Garcia HH, Gilman RH, et al: Controversies in the management of cysticercosis. *Emerg Infect Dis* 1997;3:403–5.

Gottstein B: Molecular and immunological diagnosis of echinococcosis. *Clin Microbiol Rev* 1992;5:248–61.

Jung H, Hurtado M, Medina MT, et al: Dexamethasone increases plasma levels of albendazole. *J Neurol* 1990;237:279–80.

Mitchell WG, Snodgrass SR: Intraparenchymal cerebral cysticercosis in children: A benign prognosis. *Pediatr Neurol* 1985;1:151–6.

Mitchell WG, Crawford TO: Intraparenchymal cerebral cysticercosis in children: Diagnosis and treatment. *Pediatrics* 1988;82:76–82.

Morales NM, Agapejev S, Morales RR, et al: Clinical aspects of neurocysticercosis in children. *Pediatr Neurol* 2000;22:287–91.

Richards FO Jr, Schantz PM, Ruiz-Tiben E, et al: Cysticercosis in Los Angeles County. *JAMA* 1985;254:3444–8.

Schantz PM, Moore AC, Munoz JL, et al: Neurocysticercosis in an Orthodox Jewish community in New York City. *N Engl J Med* 1992;327:692–5.

Singhi P, Ray M, Singhi S, et al: Clinical spectrum of 500 children with neurocysticercosis and response to albendazole therapy. *J Child Neurol* 2000;15:207–13.

Sotelo J, Rosas N, Palencia G: Freezing of infested pork muscle kills cysticerci. *JAMA* 1986;256:893–4.

Sotelo J, del Brutto OH, Penagos P, et al: Comparison of therapeutic regimen of anticysticercal drugs for parenchymal brain cysticercosis. *J Neurol* 1990;237:69–72.

St. Geme JW III, Maldonado YA, Enzmann D, et al: Consensus: Diagnosis and management of neurocysticercosis in children. *Pediatr Infect Dis J* 1993;12:455–61.

Takaynagui OM, Jardim E: Therapy for neurocysticercosis. Comparison between albendazole and praziquantel. *Arch Neurol* 1992; 49:290–4.

Vazquez V, Sotelo J: The course of seizures after treatment for cerebral cysticercosis. *N Engl J Med* 1992;327:696–701.

White AC Jr: Neurocysticercosis: Updates on epidemiology, pathogenesis, diagnosis, and management. *Annu Rev Med* 2000;51:187–206.

Echinococcosis

Case Records of the Massachusetts General Hospital: Weekly clinicopathological exercises. Case 45–1987. A 16-year-old girl with hepatic and pulmonary masses after a sojourn in Bolivia. *N Engl J Med* 1987;317: 1209–18.

Filice C, Brunetti E: Echo-guided diagnosis and treatment of hepatic hydatid cysts. *Clin Infect Dis* 1997;25:169–71.

Finlay JC, Speert DP: Sylvatic hydatid disease in children: Case reports and review of endemic *Echinococcus granulosus* infection in Canada and Alaska. *Pediatr Infect Dis J* 1992;11:322–6.

Grunebaum M: Radiological manifestations of lung echinococcosis in children. *Pediatr Radiol* 1975;3:65–9.

Khuroo MS, Wani NA, Javid G, et al: Percutaneous drainage compared with surgery for hepatic hydatid cysts. *N Engl J Med* 1997;337: 881–7.

Lightowlers MW, Mitchell GF, Rickard MD: Cestodes. In Warren KS, Agabian N (editors): *Immunology and Molecular Biology of Parasitic Infections.* Cambridge, Mass, Blackwell Scientific, 1991.

Rowley AH, Shulman ST, Donaldson JS, et al: Albendazole treatment of recurrent echinococcosis. *Pediatr Infect Dis J* 1988;7:666–7.

Schantz PM, Brandt FH, Dickinson CM, et al: Effects of albendazole on *Echinococcus multilocularis* infection in the Mongolian jird. *J Infect Dis* 1990a;162:1403–7.

Schantz PM, Okelo GBA: Echinococcosis (hydatidosis). In Warren KS, Mahmoud AAF (editors): *Tropical and Geographical Medicine.* New York, McGraw-Hill, 1990b.

Tomkins RK: Management of echinococcal cysts of the liver. *Mayo Clin Proc* 1991;66:1281–2.

Wen H, Zou PF, Yang WG, et al: Albendazole chemotherapy for human cystic and alveolar echinococcosis in north-western China. *Trans R Soc Trop Med Hyg* 1994;88:340–3.

Adult Tapeworm Infections

Chappell CL, Enos JP, Penn HM: *Dipylidium caninum,* an underrecognized infection in infants and children. *Pediatr Infect Dis J* 1990;9:745–7.

Hamrick HJ, Bowdre JH, Church SM: Rat tapeworm (*Hymenolepis diminuta*) infection in a child. *Pediatr Infect Dis J* 1990;9:216–9.

CHAPTER 45

Cutaneous Signs of Systemic Infections

Kathryn Schwarzenberger ▪ Robert Sidbury

The skin is unique among organs in its visibility, and many infections in children have prominent cutaneous manifestations. The entire surface of the skin and mucous membranes can be easily examined. The morphology of a skin lesion reflects the underlying disease pathogenesis and, if properly interpreted, can narrow the diagnostic possibilities of a given disease. In some cases, the skin lesions are characteristic of a particular disease, and the diagnosis can be made on sight. Such lesions include the vesicular lesions of herpes infections or the red ''slapped cheeks'' of fifth disease. Other exanthems, however, are not specific and may suggest many different disease processes, including noninfectious causes. Diagnosis of skin lesions in the immunocompromised host can be particularly challenging, as common skin diseases may assume uncommon or unusual patterns. Accurate characterization of skin lesions provides a basis for clinical diagnosis and helps guide diagnostic procedures and initial therapy.

History. Despite the ready visibility of skin lesions, the history of a rash should always be considered when one is making a diagnosis. Skin lesions evolve over time, and it is important to characterize their presence as early or late in the course of the illness. Because certain exanthems have characteristic distribution patterns, details of where and how the lesions began and their change over time may provide important diagnostic information. The status of the child's general health preceding the illness and the prodromal symptoms must be established. History of the child's exposure to other persons, as at daycare or school, known exposure to persons with similar symptoms, travel, animal exposure, medications, and immunizations should be established. Knowledge of the child's immune status and factors that may predispose to certain illnesses should be determined. Trauma or skin conditions that result in open lesions predispose to infection. Sexual and menstrual history, including the use of tampons, is important in pursuing the diagnosis of sexually transmitted diseases and toxic shock syndrome. Other epidemiologic factors to be considered include the season of the year, geographic location, and the age of the child.

Physical Findings. Physical examination of the child must first determine whether the child is seriously ill. Assessment of vital signs, particularly the presence of fever or hypotension, is critical. A relative tachycardia should accompany fever, and its absence may be a clue to certain infectious diseases, including typhoid fever and *Mycoplasma* infections. The general physical examination should note the presence or absence of lymphadenopathy, hepatosplenomegaly, and joint abnormalities. The complete skin examination should include careful evaluation of the skin, oral and ocular mucous membranes, genital mucosa, nailbeds, and the hair and scalp. Although the hair is not frequently involved in acute infections, certain diseases can affect its growth or appearance, and the condition of the hair may indicate the general health of the child.

Accurate evaluation of the skin lesions is critical in establishing a correct diagnosis. Both the type of skin lesions and their distribution should be noted. Skin lesions associated with infections include the following:

Macules: Circumscribed, flat lesions of varied size and shape, distinguished from surrounding skin by color only. Macules may be erythematous, pigmented, or purpuric.

Papules: Raised, circumscribed elevations <1 cm in diameter that may be scaly, ulcerated, or may become pustular. An eruption of small papules mixed with erythematous macules is described as **maculopapular** or **morbilliform.**

Plaques: Papular lesions >1 cm in diameter.

Nodules: Large, palpable papules measuring $>0.5–1$ cm that are deep, extending into the dermis or subcutaneous tissues.

Wheals: Commonly called hives, wheals are evanescent, erythematous elevations of skin that may assume an annular or gyrate configuration.

Vesicles: Small fluid-filled epidermal lesions <1 cm in diameter.

Bullae: Larger fluid-filled lesions >1 cm in diameter, which may be flaccid or tense, reflecting their depth within the skin. Fluid is usually clear or straw-colored.

Pustules: Circumscribed elevations in the skin filled with pus, which may have an initial papular phase and are often surrounded by erythema.

Erosions: Shallow epidermal depressions with loss of the superficial epidermis.

Target lesions: Erythematous papules or plaques with a characteristic configuration consisting of a red to violaceous to dusky center surrounded by a raised, edematous, pale ring. The periphery is red, creating a targetlike impression.

Purpura: Lesions resulting from extravasation of red blood cells into the skin. Purpuric lesions include **petechiae,** which are small, red to purple macules measuring up to several millimeters, and **ecchymoses** which are larger, hemorrhagic macules. **Palpable purpura** is characteristic of leukocytoclastic vasculitis, which may occur in various conditions, including infection, collagen vascular disorders, serum sickness, and drug eruptions. Macular purpura suggests thrombocytopenia, coagulopathies, disseminated intravascular coagulation, trauma, and the benign pigmented purpuras.

More than one type of lesion may be present at a given time and may reflect evolution of the lesions of a particular infection. The location of a given skin lesion may affect its appearance. Vesicles on mucous membranes are usually short lived, and shallow erosions are more frequently seen. Crusts rarely develop in moist areas, as on mucosa or in skin folds. Lesions in thick-skinned areas, such as the palms and soles, may be particularly difficult to characterize as vesicles, and bullae may go unrecognized.

It is also important to recognize the configuration of skin lesions, as some infections have very distinctive patterns. Three common patterns include (1) grouped lesions, such as those of herpesvirus infections; (2) linear lesions, which may result from traumatic inoculation of an infection, such as warts or molluscum contagiosum; and (3) annular lesions, which are characteristic of Lyme disease, syphilis, and fungal infections. The patterns of distribution on the body of some infections, although not always fully understood, are sufficiently characteristic of some diseases that a differential diagnosis can be formed.

Skin lesions may appear different on individual skin colors. Erythema is often very subtle on darkly pigmented skin and may be missed by the untrained observer. Hyperpigmentation is a common response to inflammation in darkly pigmented skin, and that which appears red on lightly pigmented skin may appear dark brown or have a bluish or violet color on dark skin. Residual hyperpigmentation or hypopigmentation may persist in dark skin after inflammation has resolved.

ERYTHEMATOUS MACULAR RASHES

Several common pediatric infections are characterized by exanthems that consist primarily of macular erythema. These diseases include scarlet fever; staphylococcal scalded skin syndrome, staphylococcal toxic shock syndrome, and streptococcal toxic shock syndrome. These infections have in common the production of bacterial exotoxins that cause the systemic and cutaneous findings. Late desquamation is common to most of these diseases. The presence of localized or diffuse sunburnlike erythema should immediately suggest the possibility of a toxin-mediated bacterial infection (Table 45–1).

Scarlet Fever. Scarlet fever results from pharyngeal infection by group A *Streptococcus* that produces pyrogenic exotoxin. Systemic symptoms of fever, pharyngitis, nausea, vomiting, headache, and malaise are followed after several days by a diffuse erythema with a fine, rough, sandpaperlike texture (Plate 3D). The exanthem usually begins on the head and neck and spreads to the trunk and extremities. Erythema is often exaggerated in the antecubital and axillary skin folds as erythematous or petechial red lines known as **Pastia's lines.** Palms and soles are usually spared. The face is flushed with circumoral pallor, and the lips and oral mucous membranes are red. Petechiae may be present on the palate. Early in the illness, the papillae of the tongue hypertrophy and project through a thick, white coating, producing a **white strawberry tongue.** The coating subsequently sloughs, leaving a red, raw, denuded **red strawberry tongue** (Plate 3D). The pharynx is red, and a purulent exudate may be visible on the tonsils. Cervical lymphadenopathy is common.

The erythema begins to fade within 4–7 days, and affected areas of skin desquamate. This usually begins on the face and torso, where the skin sheds in superficial, fine scales. Skin on the hands and feet subsequently desquamate, often in large sheets. This pattern of desquamation suggests scarlet fever, but the exanthem of scarlet fever can resemble a viral exanthem or a drug reaction.

TABLE 45–1. Diseases With Macular Erythema

Disease	Characteristics	Distribution
Scarlet fever	Diffuse erythema with fine papules Sandpaper texture Erythema accentuated in skin folds (Pastia's lines) Mucosal erythema Desquamation follows	Neck, trunk, and extremities most involved
Staphylococcal scalded skin syndrome	Localized to diffuse erythema May blister Desquamation follows	Accentuated around mouth, eyes, axilla, neck, groin folds
Toxic shock syndrome	Diffuse, macular erythema Involves mucosa Desquamation occurs late	Generalized Prominent in flexures, palms, soles
Kawasaki syndrome	Diffuse, macular erythema Edema of the hands and feet Mucosal erythema Redness and fissuring of lips Desquamation follows	Trunk, proximal extremities, perineum

Staphylococcal Scalded Skin Syndrome. Staphylococcal scalded skin syndrome is caused by *Staphylococcus aureus* that produces **exfoliatin,** and occurs most frequently in young children, typically following an unrecognized infection. Early signs include conjunctivitis and a clear or purulent nasal discharge. Acute fever and irritability are followed by the onset of diffuse, tender **erythroderma.** Involved skin appears scalded or sunburned (Plate 6C). The redness is characteristically accentuated around the eyes, mouth, and in flexural areas (Figs. 45–1 and 45–2). **Pastia's lines** may develop in the flexures. Large, flaccid, superficial blisters develop in involved areas within 24–48 hours and slough, leaving moist, erythema-based erosions. Affected, intact-appearing skin can be easily denuded with firm rubbing **(Nikolsky's sign).** Superficial, often extensive desquamation of the skin follows as the erythema fades. Mucous membranes are not characteristically involved, but the lips may desquamate along with the perioral skin. The skin heals without scarring.

Staphylococcal scalded skin syndrome must be distinguished from Stevens-Johnson syndrome/toxic epidermal necrolysis (TEN), which usually occurs as a drug reaction. Erythema multiforme–like target lesions or the presence of significant mucosal involvement suggests the possibility of Stevens-Johnson syndrome/TEN. The depth of cutaneous involvement distinguishes staphylococcal

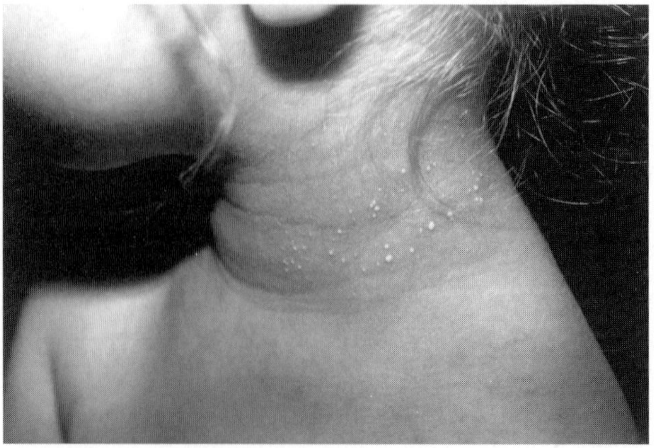

FIGURE 45–1. Staphylococcal scalded skin syndrome. Erythema in the neck folds with formation of small pustules.

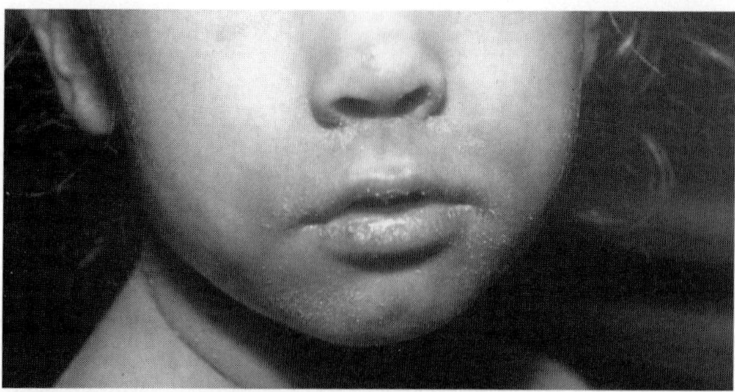

FIGURE 45–2. Staphylococcal scalded skin syndrome. Erythema and desquamation around the mouth. The pustule on the nose was the original site of *Staphylococcus aureus* infection.

scalded skin syndrome from Stevens-Johnson syndrome/TEN. The toxins responsible for staphylococcal scalded skin syndrome cleave the skin within the upper layers of the epidermis, causing superficial desquamation. In Stevens-Johnson syndrome/TEN, the skin separates between the epidermis and dermis and the entire epidermis is sloughed. Skin biopsy may be needed to clarify the depth of involvement. When rapid diagnosis is required, the skin should be examined by frozen section.

Toxic Shock Syndrome. Fever, hypotension, and an erythematous rash are the hallmarks of staphylococcal toxic shock syndrome, which is caused by *S. aureus* that produces TSST-1. It is uncommon in the pediatric population but must be considered whenever erythroderma is present in the setting of fever and multisystem illness. The exanthem of toxic shock syndrome consists of a sunburn-like erythema that may feel rough or resemble sandpaper in texture (Plate 6A). The rash is generalized but may be accentuated around an infected site. Palms and soles may be red, and there may be edema of the extremities. Mucous membranes are characteristically involved with intense conjunctival hyperemia, with a strawberry tongue. There may be mucosal erosions. Bullae are not characteristic of toxic shock syndrome. Generalized desquamation follows the acute illness in 1–3 weeks. Skin peels on the palms and soles in thick sheets. Patchy alopecia and shedding of the fingernails can occur as late sequelae but are unusual.

A similar clinical syndrome is caused by toxigenic group A *Streptococcus* and may be accompanied by bacteremia and a soft-tissue infection. The exanthem of toxic shock syndrome may resemble scarlet fever, which should not have associated hypotension or shock, and early staphylococcal scalded skin syndrome, which lacks hypotension and is characterized by subsequent formation of bullae. A skin biopsy cannot definitively confirm the diagnosis of toxic shock syndrome.

Kawasaki Syndrome. Kawasaki syndrome is a multisystem disease. It may have erythroderma (Plate 5E), but mucosal involvement is much more extensive than with toxic shock syndrome, usually with prominent redness and fissuring of the lips (Plate 5F). The skin lesions of Kawasaki syndrome are more varied than those of toxic shock syndrome, with papules, pustules, and urticarial and target lesions all having been reported.

MACULOPAPULAR RASHES

An erythematous, maculopapular exanthem is the rash most commonly associated with infectious diseases: it is usually caused by viruses but is also associated with various bacterial, rickettsial, and fungal infections (Table 45–2). The differential diagnosis of an erythematous, maculopapular eruption includes noninfectious causes, the most common of which is an allergic drug eruption. In the appropriate clinical setting, acute graft-versus-host disease and collagen-vascular diseases should also be considered in the differential diagnosis of a maculopapular eruption.

The history is important in distinguishing between these processes, as they are often indistinguishable by clinical and even histologic findings. Sometimes a nonspecific maculopapular eruption precedes the onset of lesions more characteristically associated with a specific disease. For example, a papular rash may occur early in the course of meningococcemia, preceding the more characteristic purpura. Similarly, the purpura of RMSF may begin with fine papules on the ankles and wrists. Papules may precede the onset of vesicles of varicella or herpes zoster.

A skin biopsy specimen from a maculopapular eruption may not provide a specific diagnosis. Many infectious rashes, particularly viral exanthems, have no specific histologic features that distinguish one from another. Bacterial or fungal organisms, however, may sometimes be identified in a skin biopsy specimen, and the skin can be easily submitted for cultures. A biopsy may help distinguish between infectious and noninfectious causes. The disease history, clinical appearance of the rash, and serologic test results may each be essential in establishing a diagnosis in specific cases.

Measles. The skin lesions of measles are preceded for 3–5 days by fever, cough, rhinitis, conjunctivitis, diarrhea, and vomiting. The exanthem, consisting initially of discrete red macules and papules, begins on the forehead or neck and spreads over several days to involve the face, trunk, and extremities (Plate 3A). The hands and feet are spared. The lesions coalesce into areas of confluent erythema, which persists for 4–7 days, then resolves with fine desquamation and mild hyperpigmentation.

Koplik's spots have long been considered pathognomonic of measles; however, similar mucosal lesions have been reported in association with parvovirus infections. These small, 1 mm, blue-white macules on an erythematous base are found on the oral mucosa during the prodromal phase of the illness (Plate 3B). They generally resolve before the exanthem erupts.

Atypical Measles. Atypical measles is preceded by a prodrome similar to that of measles. The exanthem develops 2–4 days after the onset of systemic symptoms and consists of erythematous macules and papules that begin on the hands and feet and spread over several days to involve the trunk and extremities. Petechiae, purpura, and vesicles may be present. Koplik's spots are unusual. The exanthem resolves within 7–10 days.

Rubella. The rash of rubella is usually preceded by no or only mild prodromal symptoms, although cervical and postauricular lymphadenopathy may be prominent. Multiple fine, discrete, red macules and papules erupt on the face and spread over 24 hours to involve the trunk and extremities. The oral mucosa may be erythematous, and there may be small, red-brown macules **(Forchheimer spots)** on the soft palate. The acute illness resolves within 2–3 days and may be followed by mild, superficial desquamation of the skin.

Roseola. **Roseola infantum,** or **exanthem subitum,** is caused by HHV6, or occasionally by HHV7. Roseola is distinguished by several days of high fever of up to 105°F (40.5°C) in a child who otherwise appears well, with abrupt onset of a rash at about the fourth day of illness as the fever resolves. The rash appears as

TABLE 45–2. Diseases With Maculopapular Rashes

Disease	Characteristics	Distribution
Measles	Generalized maculopapular rash. Blue-white macules on oral mucosa (Koplik's spots).	Starts on forehead, spreads to trunk and extremities.
Atypical measles	Generalized maculopapular rash. May become petechial or purpuric.	Initially on hands and feet, spreads to trunk and extremities.
Rubella	Generalized erythematous, maculopapular rash.	Starts on face, spreads to trunk and extremities.
Roseola infantum	Red to pink macules with surrounding pallor.	Trunk, buttocks, neck. May involve face and extremities.
Erythema infectiosum	Three-phase exanthem: facial erythema ("slapped cheeks"); followed by maculopapular rash; reticulated erythema. Erythema may recur.	Cheeks, trunk, extremities.
Epstein-Barr virus infection	Erythematous macular to maculopapular rash. May be hemorrhagic. Worsens with ampicillin.	Trunk, extremities.
Cytomegalovirus infection	Small erythematous macules and papules. May be petechial. Worsens with ampicillin	Face, trunk, extremities.
Echovirus	Numerous small macules and papules. Punched-out ulcers on palate, pharynx. May be exaggerated in sun-exposed skin.	Starts on face, spreads to trunk and extremities, palms and soles.
Viral hepatitis	Erythematous, maculopapular rash, urticaria, petechiae.	Trunk, extremities.
Gianotti-Crosti syndrome	Small, flat-topped, flesh-colored to red papules. Feels like lentils in skin.	Extremities, buttocks, face.
Salmonella enteric fever	Recurrent crops of blanchable small, pink papules.	Anterior chest, abdomen.
Syphilis	Vesicles, bullae, macules, papules, desquamation.	Acral areas, groin, face, mucosa.
Mycoplasma pneumoniae infection	Maculopapular, vesicular rash. Erythema multiforme.	Trunk, extremities.
Disseminated candidiasis	One to many red papules or nodules, which may become necrotic in center. Sunburnlike erythema in newborns.	Trunk, extremities.
Typhus	Erythematous macules. May become purpuric.	Starts on trunk, spreads to extremities; palms and soles spared.
Scrub typhus	Necrotic, erythematous papule at location of bite. Erythematous, maculopapular rash develops later.	Starts on trunk, spreads to extremities.

multiple pink, 2–3 mm macules and papules surrounded by a rim of pallor, which appear initially on the torso but may spread to the neck and extremities. Periorbital edema may be present. The exanthem lasts several days before resolving without desquamation or scarring.

Erythema Infectiousum (Fifth Disease). The exanthem of fifth disease characteristically begins on the face where erythema and edema give the cheeks a **slapped-cheek** appearance (Plate 4A). The degree of erythema is variable and can be quite subtle and also evanescent. Within several days of the onset of symptoms, an erythematous, macular eruption develops on the trunk, buttocks, and extremities. Lesions may coalesce to form a reticulated pattern (Plate 4B). Although the acute rash usually clears within 5–10 days, it may recur at irregular intervals during the succeeding few months. Recurrences may be precipitated by activities that induce vasodilation.

Epstein-Barr Virus Infections. Several cutaneous eruptions have been associated with EBV infection, although none are specific. A small percentage of children with acute mononucleosis will have a pruritic morbilliform eruption on the trunk and extremities during the first week of infection. Palatal petechiae may also be present. The most notable feature is the dramatic exacerbation that follows administration of ampicillin or another β-lactam antibiotic. The rash, thought to be immune complex–mediated, begins on the trunk 5–10 days after antibiotic administration is begun and spreads to involve the extremities. The palms and soles may be involved. Other symptoms of hypersensitivity reactions, such as arthralgia, edema, and gastrointestinal symptoms, may be associated. Development of the rash does not indicate an allergy to the antibiotic. A similar, nonspecific morbilliform eruption can occur with CMV infection, which can also worsen with the administration of β-lactam antibiotics. The presence of petechiae may suggest infection by EBV rather than CMV.

Papular acrodermatitis of childhood, or **Gianotti-Crosti syndrome,** has also been associated with primary EBV infection. This eruption, originally described in children with hepatitis B, occurs in young children and consists of numerous symmetrically distributed, flesh-colored to red papules on the face, buttocks, and extremities (Fig. 45–3). The trunk is usually spared. The firm lesions have been compared in shape and texture to lentils. The eruption is usually asymptomatic and resolves within 2–8 weeks without sequelae.

Viral Hepatitis. Although cutaneous manifestations other than jaundice are not prominent features of viral hepatitis, exanthems and other skin eruptions do accompany a small percentage of infections. Approximately 5% of patients with hepatitis A have an associated morbilliform eruption, which may be indistinguishable from rubella. Urticaria may occur early in the course of viral hepatitis and may be associated with a systemic serum sickness–

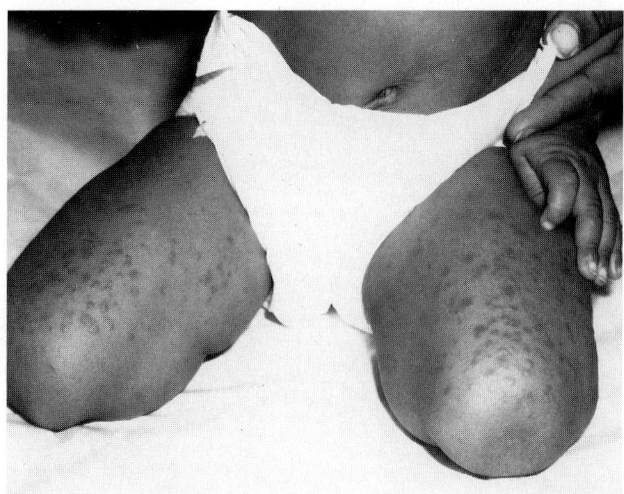

FIGURE 45–3. Gianotti-Crosti syndrome. Erythematous, lentil-like papules on the thighs.

like illness. Other nonspecific skin findings associated with viral hepatitis include papular acrodermatitis of childhood, or Gianotti-Crosti syndrome, leukocytoclastic vasculitis, erythema nodosum, lichen planus, erythema multiforme, and cryoglobulinemia.

Unilateral Laterothoracic Exanthem. The cause of this distinct exanthem has not yet been identified, although a viral origin seems likely, given the seasonal outbreaks and associated prodromal symptoms. Affected children have a mildly pruritic, morbilliform eruption consisting of 1 mm pink papules localized in a unilateral distribution, often in the flexures of the axilla or inguinal region. The rash spreads centrifugally during the first week, but it remains asymmetric with predominant involvement on the half of the body initially affected. The lesions persist for approximately 6 weeks and then resolve without sequelae. Young children around age 2 years are usually affected.

Other Viral Exanthems. Many other viral infections may be associated with exanthems. Their presentation and appearance are often too similar to permit easy distinction. In temperate climates, the nonpolio enteroviruses are the leading cause of "viral exanthems" in children during the summer and fall. These viruses include certain coxsackieviruses, enteroviruses, and echoviruses. Only some of these viruses cause syndromes with specific findings, such as herpangina or hand-foot-and-mouth syndrome, both caused by coxsackieviruses. Most other viral exanthems are much less distinctive.

Exanthems occur in association with at least half of the known echoviruses and are more common in children than in adults. Many varied forms have been described, including maculopapular, vesicular, and petechial eruptions. There is no close correlation between the virus type and the associated rash. Echovirus infection should be considered in a child with a fever and a maculopapular eruption that begins on the face and spreads to involve the trunk and extremities, including the palms and soles. Palatal petechiae or shallow mucosal ulcers may be found.

Adenoviruses are often associated with a diffuse, pink, maculopapular rash that spares the oral mucosa. Erythema multiforme and Stevens-Johnson syndrome have also been associated with adenoviruses. Respiratory syncytial virus may be associated with a generalized eruption consisting of poorly circumscribed red macules. The lesions begin during the acute phase of the infection and persist 3–5 days. Mumps is sometimes, but rarely, accompanied by a diffuse morbilliform eruption that lasts up to 10 days. Both Reovirus 2 and Colorado tick fever can produce morbilliform eruptions. The exanthem begins on the face with pink macules and papules that spread to the trunk and extremities. The rash of Colorado tick fever subsides as the fever wanes, but it may recur with subsequent episodes of fever. Rotavirus gastroenteritis may be accompanied by an erythematous, papular eruption that begins on the face and progresses to involve the trunk and extremities during its 4- to 7-day course.

Salmonella typhi (Typhoid Fever). Enteric fever, or typhoid fever, can be accompanied by a variety of skin lesions. The most characteristic are **rose spots,** which develop 7–10 days into the course of the illness. These small, pink, blanchable papules arise on the anterior chest in crops of spots that appear and resolve within several days. Lesions continue to develop over several weeks if untreated. Rose spots may occur with enteric fever caused by nontyphoidal *Salmonella.*

Syphilis. The cutaneous manifestations of congenital syphilis resemble those seen in adults with secondary syphilis. Lesions can take a variety of forms, including macules, papules, bullae, a maculopapular exanthem, and papulosquamous lesions. Maculopapular erythematous lesions resolve with scaly desquamation (Fig. 45–4). Copper-brown macules may be present on the palms and soles. Vesicobullous and eroded lesions, uncharacteristic of adult syphilis, may be present, especially over acral areas. Moist condyloma lata and mucous patches may be found on mucosal surfaces.

Primary acquired syphilis is characterized by a chancre. After a variable incubation period that averages 3 weeks, the chancre develops at the site of spirochete inoculation. Genital lesions are most common, although extragenital chancres in a variety of locations have been described. The classic chancre appears as a firm-based, nontender ulcer measuring up to 1 cm in diameter (see Plate 7A). Chancres in skin folds may develop a similar lesion on opposing skin **(kissing lesions).** Minimal erythema usually surrounds the ulcer. Extragenital chancres may have a different appearance, which complicates diagnosis.

A wide variety of skin lesions occur in secondary syphilis. Hyperpigmented macules on the palms and soles (**copper pennies**) are characteristic, as is a truncal eruption consisting of small pink or flesh-colored papules surrounded by a collarette of scale (see Plate 7B). Because of the long latency required for the development of tertiary syphilis, gummas are not likely to occur in the pediatric population.

Mycoplasma pneumoniae Infection. Skin manifestations occur in up to 10% of children with *M. pneumoniae* infection. Erythematous maculopapular or vesicular eruptions have been described, although none is distinctive for the infection. Boys are more frequently affected. The exanthem persists for 1–2 weeks. Erythema multiforme and Stevens-Johnson syndrome occur in a small number of patients with *Mycoplasma* infection that is usually less severe than Stevens-Johnson syndrome from other causes.

Candida Infection. Disseminated candidiasis occurs most frequently in the setting of immunosuppression from cancer, immunosuppressive therapy, corticosteroids, indwelling catheters, broad-spectrum antibiotics, long-term hospitalization, and prematurity. Skin lesions are found in a small percentage of patients with disseminated candidiasis and may occur more frequently with disseminated *Candida tropicalis* infection than with *C. albicans.* From one to several erythematous papules or small nodules usually arise on

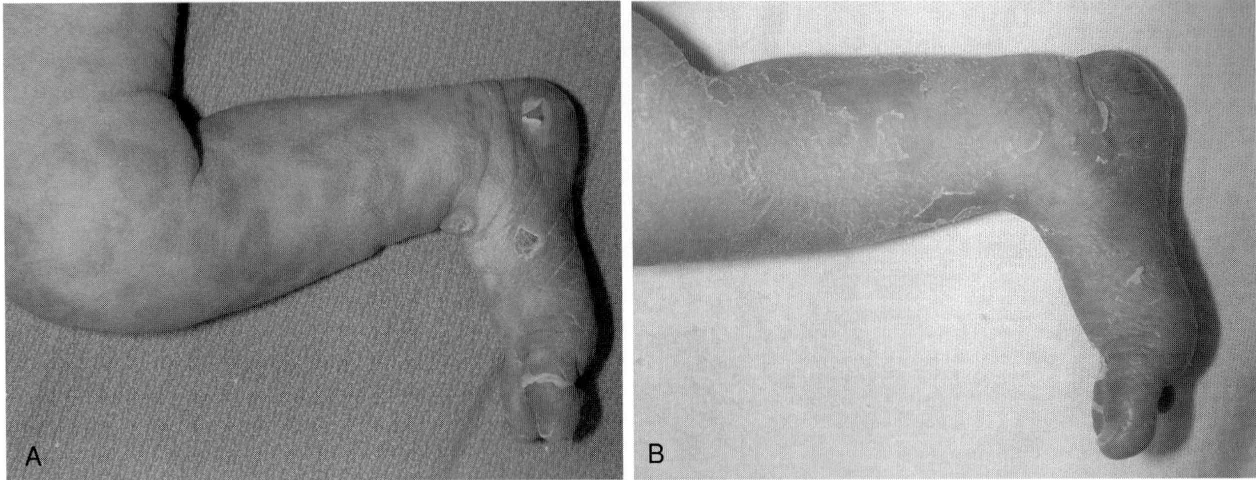

FIGURE 45–4. Congenital syphilis. **A,** At birth: Widespread, maculopapular, erythematous annular lesions with desquamation of the toes present at birth. **B,** Day 7: Resolving lesions with scaly desquamation that is especially prominent on the soles.

the trunk or extremities; the face is generally spared. Lesions may be hemorrhagic if there is thrombocytopenia. A diffuse, sunburnlike erythema may occur in low-birth-weight infants with disseminated candidiasis.

Typhus. Both epidemic and murine typhus have prominent cutaneous manifestations. Epidemic typhus, caused by *Rickettsia prowazekii,* begins with an acute onset of fever, chills, headache, myalgia, conjunctivitis, and photophobia. In most cases, after 3–7 days of illness, erythematous macules erupt on the trunk and spread to involve the extremities. The palms, soles, and face are usually spared. Lesions may become petechial or hemorrhagic, and acral gangrene may occur in severe cases. Murine typhus, caused by *R. typhi,* has clinical features similar to those of epidemic typhus but tends to be a milder illness, with rash in fewer than half of cases.

Scrub Typhus. Scrub typhus, caused by *Orientia tsutsugamushi,* presents after an incubation period of 1–3 weeks with the onset of fever, chills, headache, and myalgia. The **tache noire,** a vesicular papule or necrotic eschar with an erythematous rim, is found at the site of the infecting mite bite in approximately half of the cases. In approximately half of the cases an erythematous macular to papular eruption starts on the trunk and spreads to the extremities. The palms, soles, and face are usually spared.

TARGET LESIONS

Target lesions are distinct lesions that are the hallmark of erythema multiforme. The relationship of **erythema multiforme** and **Stevens-Johnson syndrome/toxic epidermal necrolysis (TEN)** has long been controversial, but these diseases can be logically divided into two categories based on etiology and clinical presentation: **erythema multiforme,** a relatively benign, recurrent condition associated with herpes simplex virus infection, and **Stevens-Johnson/TEN,** a potentially more serious condition usually caused by drugs (Table 45–3).

Erythema Multiforme. Erythema multiforme is a potentially recurrent condition characterized by target lesions and mucocutaneous erosions. Target lesions usually arise symmetrically on acral surfaces, including the hands, knees, elbows, and buttocks. Palms and soles, as well as the face, may be involved. The center of the lesion may blister and, in some cases, become hemorrhagic. In these circumstances, target lesions must be distinguished from autoimmune blistering diseases and Sweet's syndrome. Mucosal erosions or ulcers are frequently present, affecting primarily the lips, gingiva, and buccal mucosa. In some cases only the mucosa is affected. The degree of involvement varies greatly; some patients have only a few lesions, and others have more extensive involvement. Erythema multiforme rarely involves >10% of the body surface area. Lesions generally last 1–3 weeks before they heal without scarring.

Erythema multiforme has been clearly linked to herpes simplex virus infections. In many cases, erythema multiforme is triggered by an identifiable recurrence of herpes simplex, and it has been suggested that herpes simplex may be the only cause of recurrent benign erythema multiforme. However, in some cases, there is no clinically obvious herpes outbreak preceding the development of erythema multiforme, and the presence of herpes may be detected only by sensitive molecular techniques. Treatment of erythema multiforme with antiviral agents, both during the acute episodes and as suppressive therapy to prevent recurrences, has been successful in many cases. Other infections have been linked with erythema multiforme, including *Histoplasma capsulatum,* EBV, and coxsackievirus B5 infections, although the epidemiologic link with herpes simplex virus remains the strongest.

Stevens-Johnson Syndrome/TEN. Stevens-Johnson syndrome/TEN and erythema multiforme differ in their cause and clinical course. The two conditions are thought to represent spectrums of the same disease. Stevens-Johnson syndrome/TEN usually begins with acute onset of skin lesions ranging from a morbilliform or papular eruption to more widespread, tender erythroderma that lacks any characteristic distribution. Target lesions similar to those of erythema multiforme may be present, but they may be larger and more irregularly shaped, and they may progress rapidly to involve large areas of the body. Skin lesions may blister, and affected, intact-appearing skin can be easily denuded with firm rubbing **(Nikolsky's sign).** As the blistering progresses, affected skin sloughs in large sheets, leaving behind large denuded areas of skin. Full epidermal loss can be recognized by a loss of pigmentation in the denuded areas. This may be difficult to appreciate on lightly pigmented skin, but it is apparent on darker skin, where pigment loss reveals a moist, red dermis. Mucosal involvement is usual and may involve not only the mouth but also the conjunctiva and genital mucosa. The prognosis depends on the degree of involvement and the development of associated complications.

TABLE 45–3. Comparison of Erythema Multiforme and Stevens-Johnson Syndrome/Toxic Epidermal Necrolysis

	Erythema Multiforme	Stevens-Johnson Syndrome/Toxic Epidermal Necrolysis
Etiology	Herpes simplex virus infection	Drugs*
Course	Recurrent	Episodic
Typical lesions	Target lesions on acral surfaces Symmetrical distribution	Atypical target lesions, with confluent erythema, macules, and erosions
% BSA affected	Usually <10%	May be up to 100%
Nikolsky sign	Negative	Positive
Mucosal involvement	Frequently affects oral mucosa only	May have widespread mucosal involvement May heal with scarring and synechiae formation
Complications	Rare; pain can limit oral intake, resulting in dehydration	Multisystem involvement possible Sepsis frequent

*Classes of drugs frequently associated with Stevens-Johnson syndrome/TEN include antibiotics, especially sulfa drugs; anticonvulsants (e.g., phenytoin, carbamazepine, lamotrigine); nonsteroidal anti-inflammatory agents; and allopurinol.
Adapted from Fritsch PO, Ruiz-Maldonado R: Erythema multiforme. In Freedberg IM, Eisen AZ, Wolff K, et al (editors): *Dermatology in General Medicine,* 5th ed. New York, McGraw-Hill, 1999.

Children and infants can develop Stevens-Johnson syndrome/TEN, although adults are more frequently affected. Drugs are the leading cause of Stevens-Johnson syndrome/TEN. Frequent offenders include antibiotics, particularly sulfa drugs; anticonvulsant agents; nonsteroidal anti-inflammatory agents; and allopurinol. Severe reactions have occurred in HIV-infected persons treated with trimethoprim-sulfamethoxazole. Many other medications have anecdotally caused reactions.

Infectious causes of Stevens-Johnson syndrome/TEN are rare and are poorly documented. *Mycoplasma pneumoniae* is reported to cause Stevens-Johnson syndrome/TEN, although this association appears to be infrequent. It may ultimately be difficult to prove whether infections cause Stevens-Johnson syndrome/TEN.

PURPURA

The combination of fever and a petechial or purpuric skin eruption requires an immediate, thorough evaluation. Petechiae or purpura may be the manifestation of several life-threatening infections, including meningococcemia, bacterial sepsis with disseminated intravascular coagulopathy (DIC), infective endocarditis, or RMSF (Table 45–4). Purpura can also be caused by many noninfectious causes.

Purpura results from extravasation of red blood cells into the skin that can result from abnormal blood clotting, from inflammation, or from microvascular occlusion with subsequent ischemia. Purpura is distinguished from erythema by its resistance to compression. Erythematous skin blanches with pressure, whereas purpura remains red or purple. Careful examination of purpuric lesions should determine whether the purpura is palpable. Nonpalpable purpura is generally noninflammatory. Common causes of nonpalpable purpura include thrombocytopenia or defects in platelet function, which usually cause petechiae; coagulopathies, including DIC; trauma; and defects in blood vessels as occurs in sun-damaged skin or in persons who have received corticosteroids. **Palpable purpura** suggests associated inflammation and is considered to be the hallmark of **leukocytoclastic vasculitis.** Septic vasculitis is often palpable, as is most immune-mediated purpura.

Meningococcemia. Most persons with acute meningococcemia have skin lesions. Early in the illness, a viral type of exanthem may be present with a pink to red maculopapular eruption on the trunk, extremities, or both. This rash may be transient, and rarely it may be the only skin finding. Purpuric lesions develop in the majority of infected persons. The classic cutaneous exanthem consists of multiple, **palpable petechiae** on the proximal extremities and trunk. Lesions may develop central necrosis or may become bullous. In fulminant disease, the lesions coalesce into extensive ecchymoses. Acral areas are often prominently involved.

Children sometimes but rarely develop **chronic meningococcemia,** characterized by recurrent episodes of fever, arthralgias, myalgias, and skin lesions. The cutaneous lesions most frequently

TABLE 45–4. Diseases With Purpura

Disease	Characteristics	Distribution
Meningococcemia	Initial maculopapular rash followed by petechiae, widespread ecchymoses.	Trunk, proximal extremities.
Rocky Mountain spotted fever	Fine, blanchable macules and papules; progresses to petechial purpura.	Starts on wrists, ankles; progresses to involve trunk, proximal extremities.
Disseminated intravascular coagulation and purpura fulminans	Large symmetric ecchymoses.	Extremities, trunk.
Infective endocarditis	Petechiae, splinter hemorrhages, painful or painless macules on digits.	Chest, extremities, mucosa, digits.
Ecthyma gangrenosum	Erythematous nodule or plaque, enlarges with gray or violet center, becomes necrotic with central eschar.	Perineum, inguinal region, axilla.
Papular-purpuric gloves and socks	Pruritic papules that become purpuric.	Sharply demarcated on hands and feet.

consist of pink macules and papules that appear over joints in association with fever and joint pain. The lesions may be purpuric.

Rocky Mountain Spotted Fever. The cutaneous lesions of RMSF develop within several days of the onset of systemic symptoms. Small, blanchable, pink papules and macules characteristically begin on the wrists and ankles. Lesions progress to involve the trunk and extremities and may become petechial or purpuric. As many as 10% of persons with RMSF have no initial cutaneous lesions, and only a small percentage present with the triad of fever, petechial rash, and a history of a tick bite.

Disseminated Intravascular Coagulation (DIC) and Purpura Fulminans. DIC is a condition of widespread intravascular coagulation resulting from sudden activation of the coagulation cascade. Certain clotting factors are depleted faster than they can be replaced, ultimately causing a state of hypocoagulability. A variety of disorders, including infection, acidosis, hypoxemia, burns, leukemia, chemotherapy, venous hemangiomas, and snake bites, can trigger DIC. Homozygous and double heterozygous forms of **protein C deficiency** can cause neonatal thrombosis and purpura fulminans.

Purpura fulminans, a variant of DIC, can occur in children during or after an infection. A variety of infections, including meningococcemia, streptococcal infections, gram-negative bacterial sepsis, and varicella, may lead to purpura fulminans. Purpura fulminans develops rapidly with acute onset of fever, chills, and ecchymotic skin lesions. Acral areas are primarily involved. As a consequence of intravascular thrombosis, large areas of skin may blister and become necrotic. These affected areas may ulcerate or may ultimately progress to symmetric peripheral gangrene. Evidence of multisystem involvement is usually present, and the condition may progress to shock and death.

Infective Endocarditis. Skin lesions occur in up to 50% of cases of infective endocarditis. Most lesions result from small emboli or vasculitis, thus petechiae and purpura are the most common skin findings. Petechiae occur in successive crops during the course of endocarditis and are located on the chest, extremities, and mucosa, particularly the conjunctiva. **Splinter hemorrhages** occur in approximately 15% of patients.

Lesions considered to be specific for endocarditis include **Osler's nodes** and **Janeway lesions.** Osler's nodes occur in up to 15% of patients with endocarditis. They are small, painful red papules with a pale center that are usually located on the finger or toe pads or along the nailbed. Osler's nodes are caused by microemboli in the skin, which result in localized infarction. Janeway lesions, in contrast, are generally painless. These small erythematous or hemorrhagic macules on the palms or soles occur in a small minority of patients with endocarditis (Plate 8C).

Ecthyma Gangrenosum. Disseminated *Pseudomonas aeruginosa* infection is associated with a variety of cutaneous lesions, including cellulitis, papules, vesicles, and erythema multiforme–like lesions. The most characteristic cutaneous lesion is ecthyma gangrenosum, which results from disseminated infection that causes a localized septic vasculitis with subsequent infarction. The skin lesion is usually an erythematous papule or nodule with a central gunmetal gray color. Infection in the center may progress rapidly with development of a large eschar, or it may blister. Purpura and, ultimately, necrosis are common. Ecthyma gangrenosum frequently occurs in the perineum, inguinal region, and axilla.

Similar, rapidly progressive, necrotic lesions may occur with disseminated fungal infections with *Aspergillus* and the Zygomycetes. These organisms invade the deep blood vessel walls, causing infarction and subsequent cutaneous necrosis.

Ecthyma gangrenosum should be differentiated from **pyoderma gangrenosum,** a rapidly progressive, noninfectious process of cutaneous necrosis that is often associated with inflammatory bowel diseases and malignancy. Pyoderma gangrenosum begins with a small, tender nodule that rapidly enlarges. The center becomes dusky and violaceous and ulcerates with pus. A characteristic "rolled" border is seen at the edge of the ulcer, and there may be extensive undermining of the skin around the periphery of the ulcer. Pyoderma gangrenosum may be misdiagnosed as an infectious ulcer and is often subjected to aggressive débridement. Unfortunately, pyoderma gangrenosum exhibits pathergy, and surgery or trauma may actually precipitate or worsen the lesion. Pyoderma gangrenosum should be suspected in the setting of a rapidly progressive ulcer from which no bacterial or fungal organisms can be cultured.

Viral Infections. Some viral infections can cause petechial or purpuric eruptions. The cutaneous findings are rarely specific, and distinguishing the rash from that of a bacterial infection may be difficult. Petechial rashes have been associated with EBV, CMV, echovirus 9, coxsackievirus, atypical measles, varicella, and the viral hemorrhagic fevers.

Papular-purpuric gloves and socks is a unique eruption syndrome described in teenagers and young adults infected with parvovirus B19. Affected persons develop intensely pruritic, erythematous papules and edema of the hands and feet. There is sharp demarcation at the wrist and ankle. Lesions rapidly become purpuric after onset. Fever and oral erosions may be associated.

Palatal Petechiae. Petechiae are often seen on the soft palate but are not specific for any infection. They have been associated with congenital or acquired infections, including rubella, syphilis, toxoplasmosis, and infective endocarditis and infections caused by group A *Streptococcus,* EBV, CMV, herpes simplex viruses, and HIV. The presence of large areas of purpura on the mucosa should prompt evaluation of platelet number and function, as well as of coagulation status.

VESICULAR OR PUSTULAR ERUPTIONS

Fluid-filled cutaneous vesicles or pustules are characteristic of several common childhood infections (Table 45–5). Vesicles are frequently caused by viral infections, whereas pustules often reflect bacterial or fungal infections. This distinction is not absolute, as lesions of some infections begin as vesicles and evolve over time into pustules. This is common of herpes simplex virus infections. The history of the evolution of a given skin eruption may be invaluable in establishing a diagnosis.

Vesicles and pustules are, by definition, small. The presence of larger blisters or bullae may indicate an immune-mediated skin disease such as chronic bullous disease of childhood. Infectious exceptions include bullous impetigo and bullous tinea pedis. Blisters from both of these conditions can be large. The presence of numerous vesicles or pustules, especially if located on the palms or soles, may indicate a primary dermatologic condition such as dyshidrotic eczema or pustular psoriasis.

Although vesicles and pustules are characteristic of certain systemic infections, they can also result from superficial cutaneous infections. *S. aureus* infection of the skin or hair follicles often results in small pustules on an erythematous base. Both systemic and cutaneous candidiasis can cause from one to numerous cutaneous pustules. Dermatophyte infections frequently cause scaling of the skin, but vesicles or pustules are occasionally present.

TABLE 45–5. Diseases With Vesicles or Pustules

Disease	Characteristics	Distribution
Varicella (chickenpox)	Successive crops of small vesicles on erythematous base; become crusted.	Face, trunk.
Zoster	Grouped vesicles on an erythematous base; become crusted.	Over 1–3 sensory dermatomes, usually on the trunk.
Herpes simplex virus infection	Grouped to widespread vesicles on erythematous base may crust; ulcerate.	Lips, genitals; may disseminate.
Coxsackievirus infection	Painful, small vesicles on pharynx (herpangina).	Pharynx.
	Painful, small vesicles on pharynx, hands, and feet (hand, foot, and mouth disease).	Pharynx, hands, feet.
Gonococcemia	One to few dusky pustules on erythematous, papular base.	Acral areas, often overlying joints.

Varicella. The skin lesions of varicella, or **chickenpox,** begin on the face and rapidly spread to involve the trunk. The extremities are relatively spared, but there may be a few lesions on the palms or soles. Oral mucosa may be involved, but intact vesicles usually rupture, leaving behind only erythema-based erosions. The varicella lesion begins as a small rose-colored or red macule or papule. Within 24 hours, a small, thin-walled vesicle erupts on the surface. As the lesion matures, neutrophils fill the vesicle, creating a pustule. The pustule dries, becoming umbilicated and finally crusted. Most lesions heal without scarring. Lesions of varicella appear in successive crops throughout the course of the infection, and it is common to see lesions in all stages of development at one time. In rare cases, varicella becomes purpuric, and progression to purpura fulminans may occur.

Zoster. Zoster, commonly called **shingles,** results from reactivation of latent varicella-zoster virus and is uncommon in the pediatric age group. Severe pain or dysesthesia in the involved dermatome often precedes the cutaneous lesions of zoster. The localized area becomes red, and grouped vesicles erupt. The presence of vesicles may be obscured by severe edema. Lesions are most common on the trunk where they appear within the distribution of 1–3 sensory dermatomes. Any dermatome, however, can be affected. Zoster erupting in the sacral dermatomes may be confused with recurrent HSV infection. Vesicles become pustular with time and, in particularly severe cases, may be hemorrhagic. Zoster in children may be less painful than that in adults.

Herpes Simplex Virus Infections. A wide variety of vesicular or ulcerative skin lesions occur with herpes simplex virus, ranging from gingivostomatitis to widespread, disseminated infections. Disseminated disease or that occurring in immunocompromised patients may be particularly difficult to diagnose. Immunocompromised children, or those with an underlying eczematous skin disorder such as atopic dermatitis, are at risk of developing **eczema herpeticum,** which is widespread cutaneous dissemination of herpes simplex. Unlike the grouped vesicles of recurrent herpes simplex or zoster, these vesicles are often isolated but are spread over large areas. Abnormal skin, such as that affected by eczema, is usually involved, but normal skin can also be infected. Herpetic lesions on mucosal surfaces frequently have no intact vesicles and may appear only as punched-out, sharply demarcated ulcers.

Coxsackievirus Infections. Coxsackieviruses cause a variety of skin eruptions, many of which are nonspecific, morbilliform viral exanthems. Two syndromes, herpangina and hand-foot-and-mouth disease, have recognizable characteristics consisting primarily of vesicles.

Herpangina is caused by several coxsackieviruses and echoviruses. From one to many small, erythema-based painful vesicles erupt on the pharynx during the course of an illness associated with fever, headache, pharyngitis, dysphagia, and, rarely, a stiff neck. The lesions rupture, leaving a shallow, punched-out–appearing ulcer.

Similar pharyngeal vesicles or ulcers characterize **hand-foot-and-mouth disease** but are also accompanied by small, solitary, red to gray papulovesicles on the palms and soles (Fig. 45–5). Scattered lesions may be present on the dorsal parts of the hands and feet, and occasionally there may be a few vesicles on the buttocks or face.

Gonococcemia. Hematogenous dissemination of *Neisseria gonorrhoeae* occurs only in up to 3% of patients with gonorrhea. Pregnant women or those within 1 week of menses are at greatest risk. The most distinctive skin lesions of disseminated gonorrhea are seen in the acute **arthritis-dermatitis syndrome.** This syndrome, which may be misdiagnosed as disseminated meningococcemia, is characterized by recurrent episodes of arthritis, tenosynovitis, and skin lesions. Although a variety of skin lesions may be seen, the most characteristic is a tender, necrotic pustule with a grayish white center on an erythematous base (Fig. 45–6). These are most frequent on acral surfaces and, in contrast to lesions of meningococcemia, usually number fewer than 30. Skin lesions are uncommon in infants with disseminated gonorrhea.

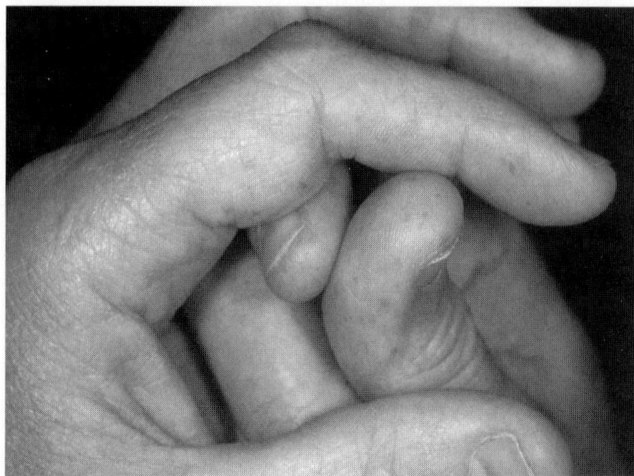

FIGURE 45–5. Hand-foot-and-mouth disease. Solitary, painful papulovesicles on the hands of a young adult.

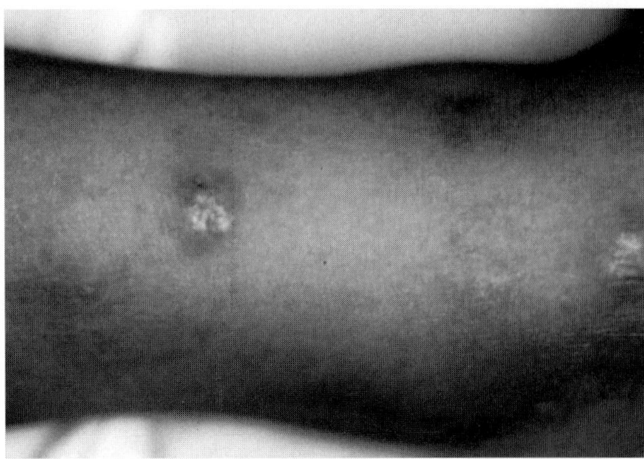

FIGURE 45–6. Disseminated gonococcemia. Small, necrotic papules on an extremity.

NODULES

Cutaneous nodules are, by definition, larger than papules. They result from inflammation deep in the dermis or subcutaneous tissues. Granulomatous reactions, such as that caused by mycobacterial or deep fungal infections, frequently produce nodules. Depending on the type of infection and the host immune response, nodules may remain intact or they may become suppurative or ulcerate (Fig. 45–7).

Careful examination of cutaneous nodules should note the presence or absence of warmth, erythema, fluctuance, tenderness, associated epidermal changes, and the pattern of distribution. Sporotrichoid spread, which is linear progression of infections along regional lymphatic vessels, is frequently seen in sporotrichosis and other fungal infections, atypical mycobacterial infections, cutaneous tuberculosis, nocardiosis, and CSD.

Cutaneous nodules may result from a variety of noninfectious causes, including inflammatory conditions, autoimmune diseases, and malignant diseases. A skin biopsy with appropriate cultures for mycobacteria and fungi may be required. In most cases, a deep incisional biopsy should be performed to ensure that the specimen is adequately sampled.

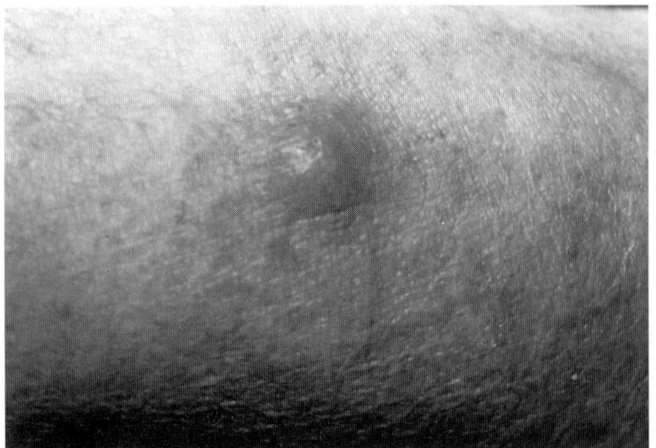

FIGURE 45–7. *Mycobacterium chelonae* cutaneous infection. Firm, erythematous nodule on a limb.

TABLE 45–6. Infectious Causes of Erythema Nodosum

Commonly Associated	Less Commonly Associated
Tuberculosis	*Mycoplasma pneumoniae*
Leprosy	Lymphogranuloma venereum
Streptococcal infections	Cat-scratch disease
Yersinia enterocolitica	Tularemia
Blastomycosis	Leptospirosis
Coccidioidomycosis	*Salmonella enteritidis*
Histoplasmosis	Hepatitis B
	Epstein-Barr virus
	Psittacosis
	Dermatophyte infections

Erythema Nodosum. Although not itself infectious, erythema nodosum is frequently a marker for certain underlying infections, and its presence should prompt appropriate evaluation (Table 45–6). Erythema nodosum is an inflammatory condition characterized by one or many tender, warm, nonsuppurative, erythematous nodules located primarily over the anterior shins. Other body sites are less frequently involved. The nodules arise spontaneously, persist for 3–6 weeks (without treatment), and heal without significant scarring. Postinflammatory hyperpigmentation may result in dark-skinned persons. They may be accompanied by arthritis or other systemic symptoms.

Erythema nodosum is a septal panniculitis, and a deep skin biopsy is needed to confirm the diagnosis. No infectious organisms have been identified within the nodules, which are thought to have an immunologic pathogenesis.

Sarcoidosis is a common cause of erythema nodosum. Tuberculosis and streptococcal infections are frequently associated infections. Erythema nodosum usually develops within 3 weeks of certain streptococcal infections. The occurrence may be episodic or, in some children, can become recurrent. Other mycobacterial infections, including leprosy, as well as deep fungal infections can also cause erythema nodosum. Less frequent infectious causes include *Mycoplasma pneumoniae,* tularemia, leptospirosis, *Salmonella enteritidis, Yersinia enterocolitica,* CSD, EBV, hepatitis B, and psittacosis. Drugs, particularly oral contraceptives and sulfonamides, are frequently implicated. Erythema nodosum can be associated with inflammatory bowel disease, certain malignant diseases, and Behçet's syndrome.

ALOPECIA

Hair loss in children has numerous possible causes, ranging from congenital abnormalities to nutritional deficiencies to behavioral problems. A complete and thorough evaluation of the hair shaft, scalp, body and facial hair, nails, and teeth should be performed. A biopsy of the scalp may be required to determine the cause of hair loss and may include evaluation of the hair shaft with light or electron microscopy.

Infectious causes of hair loss are relatively uncommon, with the exception of tinea capitis (Chapter 46). Any child with alopecia, either focal or diffuse, particularly when there is associated scale in the scalp, warrants evaluation for tinea capitis. Fungal culture is generally required to confirm the diagnosis.

Syphilis can also be associated with hair loss. Scalp hair loss does not accompany primary syphilis, unless the scalp is the site of the chancre. Patchy hair loss, often described as having a ''moth-eaten'' appearance, is seen in secondary syphilis, and there may be more diffuse hair loss resembling **telogen effluvium.** Biopsy of the scalp will reveal an inflammatory infiltrate with plasma cells, but the infecting organism is rarely identified.

Staphylococcus aureus may be isolated from certain inflammatory scalp conditions that cause alopecia, including **dissecting folliculitis** and **folliculitis decalvans.** It is unclear whether the process is primarily infectious, however. Antibiotics are often partially successful in treating these inflammatory conditions.

SKIN LESIONS ASSOCIATED WITH HIV INFECTION

Most children with HIV infection have some form of mucocutaneous disease during the course of their illness. In most cases, these are the common pediatric dermatoses but are more severe and less responsive to therapy than usual. The presentation may be atypical, particularly when infections become chronic, and the diagnosis may be more difficult to establish.

Mucocutaneous candidiasis, impetigo, herpes simplex, herpes zoster, and viral warts (papillomaviruses) are among the cutaneous infections that may be aggravated by underlying HIV-related immunocompromise. Children with HIV infection may have severe seborrheic dermatitis, and they are particularly likely to develop drug eruptions, especially with the sulfa component of trimethoprim-sulfamethoxazole. Kaposi's sarcoma is extremely unusual in children with AIDS.

REVIEWS

Cherry JD: Contemporary infectious exanthems. *Clin Infect Dis* 1993;16:199–205.

Frieden IJ, Resnick SD: Childhood exanthems: Old and new. *Pediatr Clin North Am* 1991;38:859–87.

Cohen B: Parvovirus B19: An expanding spectrum of disease. *Br Med J* 1995;311:1549–52.

Drago F, Rebora A: The new herpesviruses: Emerging pathogens of dermatological interest. *Arch Dermatol* 1999;135:71–5.

McCalmont C, Zanolli MD: Rickettsial diseases. *Dermatol Clin* 1989;7:591–601.

Prose NS, Resnick SD: Cutaneous manifestations of systemic infections in children. *Curr Probl Pediatr* 1991;21:92–113.

Schachner LA, Hansen RC (editors): *Pediatric Dermatology,* 2nd ed. Churchill Livingstone, 1995.

KEY ARTICLES

Baker RC, Seguin JH, Leslie N, et al: Fever and petechiae in children. *Pediatrics* 1989;84:1051–5.

Baley JE, Silverman RA: Systemic candidiasis: Cutaneous manifestations in low birth weight infants. *Pediatrics* 1988;82:211–5.

Bastiji-Garin S, Rzany B, Stern RS, et al: Clinical classification of cases of toxic epidermal necrolysis, Stevens-Johnson syndrome, and erythema multiforme. *Arch Dermatol* 1993;129:92–6.

Goodyear HM, Laidler PW, Price EH, et al: Acute infectious erythemas in children: A clinico-microbiological study. *Br J Dermatol* 1991;124:433–8.

Grossman ME, Silvers DN, Walther RR: Cutaneous manifestations of disseminated candidiasis. *J Am Acad Dermatol* 1980;2:111–6.

Halasz CL, Cormier D, Den M: Petechial glove and sock syndrome caused by parvovirus B19. *J Am Acad Dermatol* 1992;27:835–8.

Helmick CG, Bernard KW, D'Angelo LJ: Rocky Mountain spotted fever: Clinical, laboratory, and epidemiological features of 262 cases. *J Infect Dis* 1984;150:480–8.

Hook EW III, Holmes KK: Gonococcal infections. *Ann Intern Med* 1985;102:229–43.

Leibel RL, Fangman JJ, Ostrovsky MC: Chronic meningococcemia in childhood: Case report and review of the literature. *Am J Dis Child* 1974;127:94–8.

Levy M, Shear NH: *Mycoplasma pneumoniae* infections and Stevens-Johnson syndrome: Report of eight cases and review of the literature. *Clin Pediatr* 1991;30:42–9.

Marler RA, Neumann A: Neonatal purpura fulminans due to homozygous protein C or protein S deficiencies. *Semin Thromb Hemost* 1990;16:299–309.

Marzouk O, Thouson AP, Sills JA, et al: Features and outcome in meningococcal disease presenting with maculopapular rash. *Arch Dis Child* 1991;66:485–7.

Masi AT, Eisenstein BI: Disseminated gonococcal infection (DGI) and gonococcal arthritis (GCA): II. Clinical manifestations, diagnosis, complications, treatment, and prevention. *Semin Arthritis Rheum* 1981;10:173–97.

McCuaig CC, Russo P, Powell J, et al: Unilateral laterothoracic exanthem: A clinicopathologic study of forty-eight patients. *J Am Acad Dermatol* 1996;34:979–84.

Preblud SR, Orenstein WA, Bart KJ: Varicella: Clinical manifestations, epidemiology and health impact in children. *Pediatr Infect Dis* 1984;3:505–9.

Spicer TE, Rau JM: Purpura fulminans. *Am J Med* 1976;61:566–71.

Straka BF, Whitaker BL, Morrison SH, et al: Cutaneous manifestations of the acquired immunodeficiency syndrome in children. *J Am Acad Dermatol* 1988;18:1089–102.

Wong VK, Hitchcock W, Mason WH: Meningococcal infections in children: A review of 100 cases. *Pediatr Infect Dis J* 1989;8:224–7.

CHAPTER 46

Superficial Cutaneous Infections

Robert Sidbury ▪ Kathryn Schwarzenberger

The diagnosis and treatment of superficial cutaneous infections are a vital part of pediatric practice. Many diseases, such as impetigo, ringworm, warts, and head lice, are familiar to all physicians and are likely to be seen during the course of any day. Other cutaneous infections are much more rare and may be recognized only by the specialist. The epidemiology of some infections has changed in the past few decades, reflecting the effects of worldwide travel; today we see diseases in urban settings that were previously limited to rural areas. Many children today are immunocompromised, either by disease or by treatment, and many will develop cutaneous infections. Immunocompromised children are at risk of developing the same infections as any children; however, infections in these children may be more severe or persist longer than in immunocompetent children.

Most superficial cutaneous infections are relatively benign; others, however, such as eczema herpeticum, are potentially life threatening, and their recognition is necessary to ensure that appropriate therapy is promptly instituted. Some cutaneous infections, such as tinea capitis and scabies, are contagious, and early diagnosis and treatment may prevent spread to schoolmates and family members. Differentiation of cutaneous infections from other skin diseases requires a careful and thorough medical history and close attention to the morphology and location of the skin lesions. In some situations, additional information can be obtained from a Gram stain or potassium hydroxide preparation, culture of the skin, or a skin biopsy. In many cases, therapy will be initiated before the results of a culture or biopsy are available, and treatment must be based on the clinical diagnosis alone.

BACTERIAL INFECTIONS

IMPETIGO

ETIOLOGY

Impetigo, the most common cutaneous infection in children, is caused by *Staphylococcus aureus* and group A *Streptococcus.* Two clinical variants are recognized: **nonbullous impetigo,** also known as **crusted impetigo,** and **bullous impetigo.** Several decades ago, group A *Streptococcus* was considered to be the primary cause of nonbullous impetigo. More recently, *S. aureus* has been identified as the sole agent in up to 90% of cases of impetigo in industrialized countries. *S. aureus* and group A *Streptococcus* are cultured together in a smaller percentage of cases, and *Streptococcus* alone is identified in fewer than 10%. Group A *Streptococcus* remains a common cause of impetigo in developing countries. Bullous impetigo is caused by *S. aureus,* most often group II, phage type 71.

Transmission. Impetigo is very contagious. It is spread by direct person-to-person contact and by autoinoculation.

EPIDEMIOLOGY

Impetigo is primarily a disease of young children, although adolescents and adults may be affected. Heat, humidity, crowding, and poor hygiene are predisposing factors and may contribute to spread of the disease during epidemics. Impetigo occurs year-round in warm climates, and there is an increased incidence during the summer and fall in higher latitudes.

PATHOGENESIS

Intact skin is relatively resistant to bacterial invasion, and disruption of the skin integrity precedes infection. This may be from minor trauma, an insect bite, or a primary skin condition, such as atopic dermatitis. Nasal colonization with *S. aureus* serves as the source of infection in some cases. Bacterial invasion into the skin and hair follicle elicits a pyogenic response that results in the crusting that is characteristic of impetigo. Strains of *S. aureus* that cause bullous impetigo produce an **exfoliative toxin** that causes cleavage of the skin identical to that which occurs in staphylococcal scalded skin syndrome; in impetigo, however, the toxins remain localized and do not cause a systemic illness.

SYMPTOMS AND CLINICAL MANIFESTATIONS

Impetigo frequently arises on skin around the nose and mouth, possibly implicating the nose as the source of infection. The extremities and trunk can also be involved. A small erythematous papule or vesicle develops and then enlarges and ruptures and is rapidly covered with a characteristic honey-colored crust (Fig. 46–1). Removal of the crust reveals superficial erosion with a moist or oozing base. Although the base may be red, surrounding erythema is usually minimal. The lesions are generally nontender, but they may be pruritic. There may be regional lymphadenopathy, but systemic symptoms are unusual. Lesions usually heal without scarring.

Bullous impetigo may develop without evidence of antecedent skin trauma. The large, flaccid bulla easily ruptures, leaving a clean, shallow erosion that dries with a shiny, varnishlike surface. A collarette of scale may surround the erosion, but little crusting is present. Regional lymph nodes are usually not enlarged. Lesions heal without scarring (Table 46–1).

DIAGNOSIS

The diagnosis of impetigo is usually based on the characteristic clinical appearance. A bacterial culture confirms the diagnosis and allows for antibiotic susceptibility testing. Skin swabs should be obtained from early lesions from which the crust has been removed. Fluid from intact blisters may also be cultured. Serologic testing can be used in the diagnosis of group A *Streptococcus* impetigo but is most useful for retrospective diagnosis and is rarely used to establish the diagnosis of an acute infection. Unlike the antibody

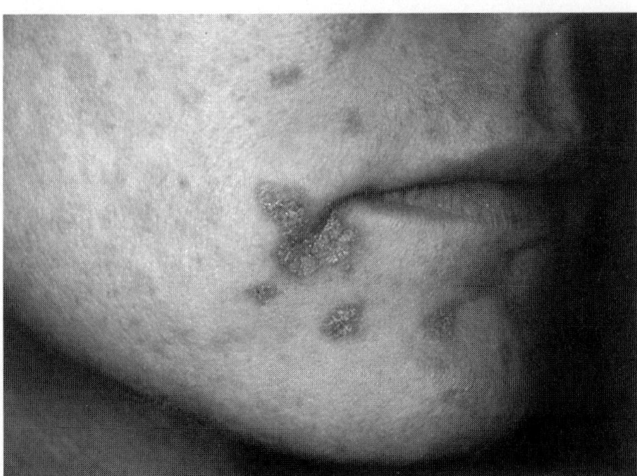

FIGURE 46–1. Impetigo. Typical honey-colored crusts grouped around the mouth.

response to group A *Streptococcus* pharyngitis, antistreptolysin-O antibody production is minimal or absent. The presence of antideoxyribonuclease B, however, correlates well with group A *Streptococcus* impetigo.

TREATMENT

The change in bacterial etiology from *Streptococcus* to primarily *Staphylococcus* has necessitated re-evaluation of the standard therapy for impetigo. Although penicillin was once effective, the predominance of β-lactamase-resistant *S. aureus* has made penicillin therapy inadequate in most cases. Penicillin should be used only if a culture identifies group A *Streptococcus* as the sole pathogen. Semisynthetic penicillins, first- or second-generation cephalosporins, and amoxicillin-clavulanate are all appropriate and effective treatments (Table 46–2). Staphylococcal resistance to erythromycin has become highly prevalent in some areas; however, studies have shown that the clinical response to macrolide therapy remains high despite in vitro resistance. Culture and antibiotic susceptibility testing should be performed in cases of treatment failure.

Topical therapy with mupirocin 2% ointment or cream may be appropriate for mild cases of impetigo and has been shown to be as effective as systemic erythromycin therapy. Topical therapy avoids the potential adverse effects of systemic medications, but its use may be limited in widespread disease, on areas of skin where it will be readily wiped off, or around the eyes or mouth. The cost of topical mupirocin therapy also may exceed that of some systemic medications.

COMPLICATIONS

Complications of impetigo are rare. If left untreated, impetigo may progress to ecthyma, in which infected areas enlarge into ulcerated nodules. Usually found on the lower extremities, these lesions require prolonged antibiotic therapy and may cause scarring. Staphylococcal scalded skin syndrome may result from exotoxin production by certain strains of *S. aureus* that cause bullous impetigo. Poststreptococcal glomerulonephritis can follow group A *Streptococcus* impetigo, as well as group A *Streptococcus* pharyngitis, but the incidence and severity of this complication appear to be decreasing in the United States. Nephritogenic strains of group A *Streptococcus* that cause impetigo include M types 49, 53, 55, 56, and 57. The role of antibiotics in preventing glomerulonephritis remains unclear, but prevention is unlikely when crusted lesions are already present. Because of the indolent nature of many cases of impetigo, glomerulonephritis may already be active at the time of initial presentation. Therapy leads to earlier clearing of skin lesions and helps prevent spread of the disease, which is especially important if the infection is caused by a nephritogenic strain. Acute rheumatic fever does not occur as a complication of impetigo caused by group A *Streptococcus,* but only as a complication of pharyngitis caused by group A *Streptococcus.*

PREVENTION

Good hygiene, especially good hand washing, and early antibiotic treatment may help limit spread within the community. Children with impetigo should remain out of school or daycare until 24 hours of antibiotic therapy has been completed. Close physical contact should be avoided while skin lesions are present.

FOLLICULITIS, FURUNCLES, AND CARBUNCLES

Common pyogenic skin infections in children include superficial folliculitis, furuncles, and carbuncles. All three conditions involve the hair follicle; the depth of infection determines the clinical lesion. Bacterial, fungal, and viral infections all can affect the follicle, as may a variety of noninfectious, inflammatory conditions, such as acne vulgaris.

ETIOLOGY

S. aureus is the usual pathogen in furuncles and carbuncles, and it can also cause a superficial folliculitis. Infrequently, gram-negative organisms, including *Escherichia coli, Proteus,* and *Pseudomonas aeruginosa,* are isolated. *P. aeruginosa* causes a distinctive follicu-

TABLE 46–1. Clinical Characteristics of Impetigo

	Nonbullous	Bullous
Etiology	*Staphylococcus aureus*, Group A *Streptococcus*	*Staphylococcus aureus* (usually group II, phage type 71)
Distribution	Face, extremities	Trunk, face, extremities
Clinical lesions	Pustules to "honey-colored" crusts on erythematous base	Flaccid bullae on erythematous base; ruptured lesions dry with shiny, "varnishlike" base
Associated signs and symptoms	Lesions asymptomatic to pruritic Regional lymph nodes occasionally enlarged Systemic signs rare	Lesions asymptomatic to pruritic Lymphadenopathy rare Systemic signs rare

TABLE 46–2. Antibiotic Treatment of Bacterial Skin Infections

Type of Infection	Antibiotic Regimen: Recommended Regimen	Antibiotic Regimen: Alternative Regimen
Topical treatment for folliculitis	Clindamycin 1% gel topically, applied 2 times daily for 7–10 days until lesions resolve	
Topical treatment for impetigo	Mupirocin 2% ointment or cream topically, applied 3 times daily for 7–10 days until lesions resolve	
Oral treatment for impetigo, folliculitis, furuncles, and carbuncles	Cephalexin *or* Cefadroxil *or* Dicloxacillin*	Amoxicillin-clavulanate *or* Cefuroxime axetil *or* Erythromycin
Cellulitis, erysipelas, erysipeloid, ecthyma gangrenosum	See Chapter 47, Table 47-1	
Lymphangitis (see Chapter 51)	See Chapter 51	

*The taste of dicloxacillin is objectionable to many children.

Recommended Dosages for Patients with Normal Renal Function

ANTIBIOTIC	DOSAGE (PO)	MAXIMUM DAILY DOSE
Amoxicillin-clavulanate	40–50 mg amoxicillin/kg/day divided 3 times a day	1.5 g
Cefadroxil	30 mg/kg/day divided 2 times a day	2 g
Cefuroxime axetil	30 mg/kg/day divided 2 times a day	1 g
Cephalexin	50–100 mg/kg/day divided 4 times a day	4 g
Dicloxacillin	25–50 mg/kg/day divided 4 times a day	2 g
Erythromycin	40 mg/kg/day divided 4 times a day	2 g

litis associated with the use of hot tubs or whirlpools. Anaerobic bacteria, including *Peptococcus, Peptostreptococcus, Lactobacillus,* and *Bacteroides,* as well as certain coagulase-negative staphylococci, have been implicated in the development of furuncles in the groin region.

EPIDEMIOLOGY AND PATHOGENESIS

Superficial folliculitis results from infection within the opening of the hair follicle. Areas frequently involved include the scalps of children and the faces of men who shave. Occlusion or other trauma predisposes the skin to the development of folliculitis. Superficial *P. aeruginosa* folliculitis is associated with the use of hot tubs or whirlpools.

A **furuncle,** or **boil,** is an inflammatory abscess arising deep within the hair follicle. A **carbuncle** results when several furuncles coalesce, producing a larger, deeper, nodular lesion. Furuncles develop in hair-bearing skin, frequently on the neck, trunk, axillae, and buttocks. Predisposing conditions include bacterial colonization of the skin or nares, occlusion, abnormalities of hair follicles, maceration, and high humidity. Furuncles occur more frequently during warm summer months. Recurrent furuncles may occur among family members. In children with immunodeficiencies that involve the skin, recurrent furuncles may develop. Chronic granulomatous disease, Chédiak-Higashi syndrome, hypocomplementemias, hypergammaglobulinemia E, and Wiskott-Aldrich syndrome all have been associated with recurrent furunculosis.

SYMPTOMS AND CLINICAL MANIFESTATIONS

The lesions of folliculitis consist of one to many small, dome-shaped fragile pustules or erythematous papules located within a hair follicle (Fig. 46–2). The underlying skin is red. Lesions are asymptomatic to slightly tender, and there is usually no associated fever.

P. aeruginosa folliculitis presents as pruritic papules, pustules, or deeper, purple-red nodules predominantly on areas of skin that had been covered by a swimsuit. The lesions develop 8–48 hours after exposure, usually without associated systemic symptoms, although lymphadenopathy, fever, and malaise have been reported.

A furuncle begins as a painful, red papule several millimeters in diameter, which increases in size over several days and evolves into a tender, violaceous nodule. The lesion may become fluctuant and exhibit a central pustule (Fig. 46–3). At this stage, the lesion may spontaneously drain with release of pus and resolution of pain. Carbuncles begin similarly, but they progress to involve several follicles, resulting in a large, painful nodule on which many pustules may be present. Most furuncles heal without scarring; however, because of their depth of involvement, carbuncles may leave irregular, depressed scars.

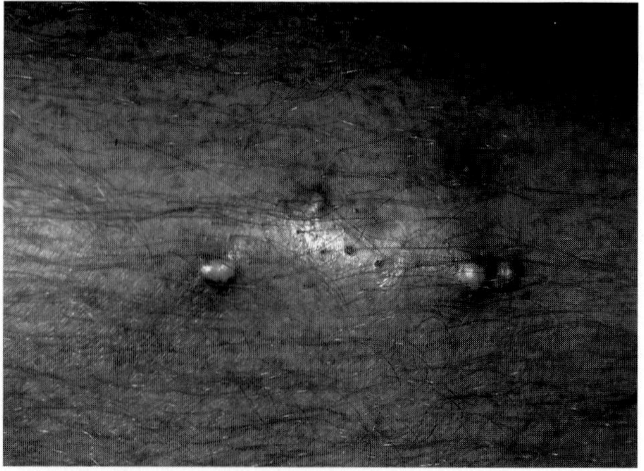

FIGURE 46–2. *Staphylococcus aureus* folliculitis. Small pustules on an erythematous base arising within neighboring hair follicles.

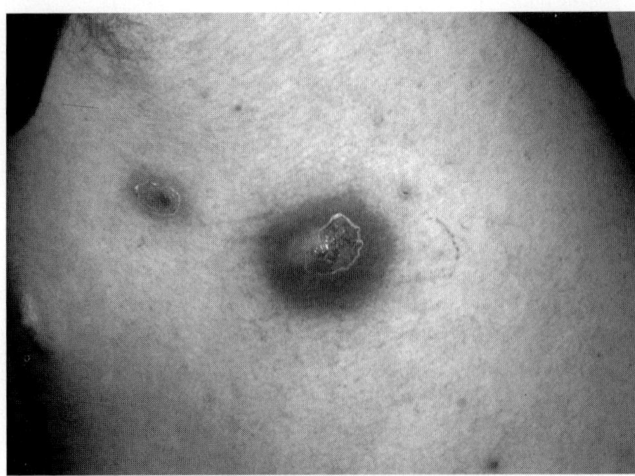

FIGURE 46–3. Furuncle. A large, tender, inflammatory nodule involving the superficial and deep layers of the skin. Pus is liberated on drainage.

Recurrent furunculosis is associated with skin or nasal carriage of phage group II strains of *S. aureus* in the patient or family members. Lesions typically recur several times a year but may resolve completely after several years. Treatment includes identification and eradication of the carrier state.

Recurrent furunculosis and carbuncles should be distinguished from **hidradenitis suppurativa,** a chronic, recurrent disease of the apocrine sweat glands in which, for unclear reasons, occlusion of the duct occurs. A suppurative infection develops in the occluded gland, producing tender, erythematous comedones, papules, and pustules. As the disease progresses, scarring and sinus tracts develop. Lesions are grouped in areas of skin where apocrine glands are distributed, particularly around the axilla, groin, and buttocks. The disease affects adults predominantly, but it can begin at or shortly before puberty. Severe, scarring acne, and dissecting folliculitis of the scalp may be associated.

Furuncles and carbuncles should be distinguished from fungal and viral infections, foreign body reactions, and even cutaneous malignant neoplasms. Persistent lesions warrant biopsy and culture.

DIAGNOSIS

The diagnosis of these superficial bacterial infections is usually made on the basis of clinical findings. A Gram stain of any drainage typically reveals polymorphonuclear leukocytes and gram-positive cocci consistent with *S. aureus,* the most common infecting organism.

TREATMENT

Folliculitis. Topical therapy with an antibacterial wash, such as chlorhexidine or an antibacterial lotion or solution, such as clindamycin 1%, applied twice a day for 7–10 days may be sufficient to clear a superficial infection. Oral antibiotics may be necessary in unresponsive or persistent cases, or when there is widespread involvement (Table 46–2). Folliculitis caused by *P. aeruginosa* is generally self-limited and resolves in 1–2 weeks without specific treatment. Because of the potential risk of dissemination, *P. aeruginosa* folliculitis in an immunocompromised patient should be treated aggressively with systemic antibiotic therapy that provides antipseudomonal coverage.

Furuncles and Carbuncles. Fluctuant lesions in most areas may be carefully incised and drained to hasten healing. Lesions in the external auditory canal, nares, and around the nose, however, should be treated with systemic antibiotics without attempting drainage because venous spread of infection from these areas may result in CNS infection or cavernous sinus thrombosis. Systemic antibiotics are also indicated for the treatment of lesions that have not responded to local care, for large or frequent lesions, with evidence of surrounding cellulitis, for immunocompromised patients, and in the presence of valvular heart disease because of the risk of infective endocarditis (Table 46–2).

PREVENTION

Prevention of recurrence requires correction of any conditions that predispose to furuncle formation. Occlusion should be avoided. When indicated, weight loss is recommended. Good hygiene, along with use of an antibacterial soap, may help decrease bacterial concentrations on the skin. Application of mupirocin 2% nasal ointment twice a day to the nares for 5–14 days may help eradicate staphylococcal carriage in patients with recurrent infections; however, recolonization occurs frequently.

ACNE VULGARIS

Acne vulgaris is a multifactorial skin disorder that predominantly affects adolescents, with up to 85% of teenagers experiencing some form of acne. Although acne is often dismissed as a benign disorder, the acute lesions and their potential lifelong scars may have considerable emotional impact on those who are affected.

ETIOLOGY

Although the cause of acne is multifactorial, proliferation of certain microbiologic agents, including *Propionibacterium acnes,* coagulase-negative staphylococci, and the yeast *Malassezia furfur* appear to be related to the development of lesions. *P. acnes* is an anaerobic gram-positive bacillus.

EPIDEMIOLOGY

Acne occurs worldwide with no apparent racial or ethnic predilection. It usually begins in the early teens, with a peak incidence at approximately 17 years of age. Most cases resolve by the late teens or early twenties, although persistence into adulthood is not uncommon. The incidence of acne is the same in both sexes, but boys may be more severely affected. Acne may also occur during early infancy.

PATHOGENESIS

Multiple factors are involved in the development of acne. These include abnormal follicular keratinization, sebum production, hormones, proliferation of *Propionibacterium acnes,* and inflammation. **Comedones** result from the abnormal proliferation and increased cohesion of keratinocytes lining the sebaceous follicle. The sebaceous gland, responding to androgens produced during puberty, hypertrophies and secretes excessive amounts of sebum that may contribute to comedone formation by providing a substrate for the proliferation of *P. acnes* at the base of the follicle. In the presence of sebum, *P. acnes* proliferates and elaborates products that attract neutrophils and may disrupt the integrity of the follicular epithelium. Neutrophils ingest the bacteria, releasing hydrolases that may further damage the follicle walls. The follicular contents rupture into the dermis, where further inflammation results in development of the pustule or cyst.

SYMPTOMS AND CLINICAL MANIFESTATIONS AND DIAGNOSIS

There is a wide spectrum of presentation of acne that is influenced by age (Table 46–3).

Neonatal Acne. Neonatal acne presents within the first 2–3 months of life and is thought to result from stimulation of the infant's sebaceous glands by maternal androgens. This benign condition resolves spontaneously.

Infantile Acne. Infantile acne develops after the first few months of life and is more common in boys. It usually resolves spontaneously within weeks to months but, rarely, may persist for as long as 5 years. Closed comedones, small papules, and pustules are characteristic. Therapy should be tailored to the type of lesions present. If comedones are prominent, topical tretinoin cream (0.025–0.05%) can be used with minimal irritation. If inflammation is present, 2.5-5% benzoyl peroxide cream or lotion, topical clindamycin 1% lotion, or topical erythromycin solution applied twice a day may be effective. Systemic erythromycin is the treatment of choice if moderate to severe inflammation is present.

TABLE 46–3. Clinical Spectrum of Acne

Type	Clinical Features
Neonatal acne	Present around birth Results from effects of maternal androgens Resolves spontaneously
Infantile acne	Onset 2–3 months of age Closed comedones, small papules, pustules on face Usually resolves within few months Rarely persists up to 5 years of age
Acne vulgaris	Onset in early to mid teens Mixture of open and closed comedones, inflammatory papules, pustules and cysts Face, back, and chest usual location May improve by late teens, twenties; may persist
Acne fulminans	Acute onset in adolescent boys Ulcerative, nodulocystic lesions on trunk and chest Associated fever, chills, arthralgia, bone lesions, weight loss Poor response to standard therapy; requires retinoids, systemic corticosteroids
Steroid-induced acne	Associated with use of topical or systemic corticosteroids Monomorphic papules, comedones May resolve with withdrawal of corticosteroids
Gram negative folliculitis	Usually occurs in patients receiving antibiotic therapy Pustules and inflammatory papules on face, around nose Responds to appropriate antibiotic therapy, retinoids

Acne may appear later in infancy and childhood. In the absence of other signs of hormonal excess, such as hirsutism, a complete endocrinologic evaluation is not indicated. Rarely, infants may develop nodulocystic acne, and systemic therapy with isotretinoin may be necessary to prevent scarring. Scarring rarely results from mild cases.

Adolescent Acne. Acne usually begins on the face and, particularly in boys, may involve the neck, back, and chest. A variety of lesions are characteristic of acne, and the different types are usually present simultaneously. **Comedones** are noninflammatory lesions that are seen early in the disease course and consist of small, white papules **(whiteheads)** or brownish-black, oily, follicular plugs **(blackheads).** Inflammatory lesions include erythematous papules, pustules, nodules, and cysts. These may cause scarring.

Acne Fulminans. Acne fulminans is a rare, disfiguring variant of acne seen almost exclusively in adolescent boys, and is characterized by the acute onset of ulcerating, nodulocystic lesions on the face, trunk, and chest in association with fever and leukocytosis. Myalgia, arthralgia, weight loss, and osteolytic bone lesions may be present. The cause of this condition is unknown, and the response to standard acne therapy is poor. Systemic corticosteroids and isotretinoin are often required to control this severe condition.

Steroid-Induced Acne. Use of systemic corticosteroids for as little as several weeks can induce an acneiform eruption suggestive of acne. Unlike those of acne vulgaris, the lesions tend to be monomorphic and are usually clustered on the trunk, shoulders, and upper arms. The face is usually less involved. Prolonged use of topical corticosteroids on the face can cause a similar eruption.

Gram-Negative Folliculitis. A folliculitis complication of antibiotic therapy should be considered in patients who develop new lesions that do not respond to previously effective systemic antibiotics. Superinfection by gram-negative organisms, including *Escherichia coli, Proteus mirabilis, Klebsiella,* and *Enterobacter* has been documented in acne patients who are receiving long-term antibacterial therapy. Diagnosis is confirmed with a culture obtained from an early pustule. The administration of systemic antibiotics according to culture results is indicated.

TREATMENT

Effective treatment of acne vulgaris should address the different causes and contributing factors of the disease. Individual therapy should be tailored to the specific clinical situation. Antibiotics, both topical and systemic, are frequently used and are particularly effective for the treatment of inflammatory skin lesions. Topical clindamycin and erythromycin are equally effective and may be adequate initial therapy for mild, inflammatory acne. Benzoyl peroxide, an organic peroxide available in strengths of 2.5–10%, is bactericidal for *P. acnes.* The combination of benzoyl peroxide and a topical antibiotic (clindamycin or erythromycin) produces a better response than either agent used alone. Systemic antibiotics should be considered when there is a significant inflammatory component, as evidenced by numerous deep papules or pustules, and they are particularly necessary when there are lesions on the chest or back. Oral tetracyclines are among the most effective antibiotics; it is likely that at least some of their efficacy results from a nonspecific, anti-inflammatory effect. Tetracycline is effective at a dose of 500 mg/day. Once control is established, maintenance doses may be reduced to as little as 250 mg/day. Tetracycline is contraindicated during pregnancy and should not be used in children under 9 years of age. Doxycycline, 100 mg/day, is also effective, and its once-a-day dosing may improve patient compliance. Dermatologists prescribe minocycline frequently, but recent reports of autoimmune hepatitis and lupuslike reactions from minocycline may necessitate re-evaluation of its use as first-line therapy. Alternative antibiotics include erythromycin and, rarely, ampicillin.

Retinoids are extremely effective in the treatment of comedonal and cystic acne. Tretinoin cream normalizes follicular keratinization and prevents the formation of comedones. It often works well as a single agent for treatment of comedonal acne, and it can be used in combination with topical or oral antibiotics. Adapalene gel, a derivative of naphthoic acid with retinoid and anti-inflammatory effects, is also available for the treatment of acne and may be less irritating than tretinoin for some patients.

Isotretinoin, an oral analog of vitamin A, is indicated for patients with severe, recalcitrant, nodulocystic acne. Its use is limited by numerous potential adverse effects, including serious teratogenicity. Patients receiving isotretinoin require careful selection, pretreatment counseling, and regular monitoring during therapy. Only physicians who are very familiar with its safety profile and use should use isotretinoin.

Some women develop acne flares in response to menstruation, which is often poorly controlled with standard therapies. Hormonal therapies with antiandrogenic effects, such as spironolactone and oral contraceptive pills, can be helpful. Spironolactone is effective at doses of 25–200 mg/day. Serum potassium levels and blood pressure must be monitored. Oral contraceptive agents with little to no androgenic effects, such as Ortho Tri-Cyclen, may also be effective.

Management of uncomplicated cases of adolescent acne by a pediatrician or primary care provider is appropriate; however, any patient who does not respond to conservative therapy or any person with scarring or nodulocystic acne should be referred to a dermatologist.

ERYTHRASMA

Erythrasma is a superficial infection of intertriginous skin caused by overgrowth of the gram-positive diphtheroid *Corynebacterium minutissimum.* Erythrasma occurs in all age groups, but it is uncommon in childhood. It occurs most frequently in warm, humid climates.

Erythrasma presents with sharply demarcated, reddish brown patches in intertriginous areas. Commonly involved sites include the groin, inframammary area, axilla, and gluteal crease. Fine scale may cover the surface of the lesions, which may be pruritic. A less common presentation, known as **tropical erythrasma,** produces widespread, annular lesions on the skin.

The diagnosis of erythrasma is confirmed by a Wood's light examination. The affected areas fluoresce with a characteristic coral red color, which helps distinguish erythrasma from tinea cruris and inverse psoriasis, which ordinarily do not fluoresce. Treatment with erythromycin (40 mg/kg/day orally divided every 6 hours) for 7 days is effective in most cases. Topical therapy with erythromycin 2% solution, clindamycin 2% solution, and imidazole antifungal agents also has been successful.

PITTED KERATOLYSIS

Pitted keratolysis is a superficial infection attributed to *Corynebacterium.* This asymptomatic foot condition occurs in all age groups and, like erythrasma, is seen most often in humid climates, particularly among those with chronically sweaty feet.

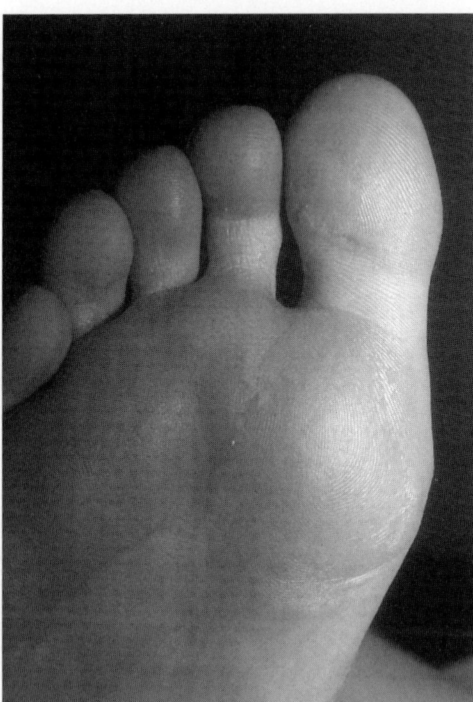

FIGURE 46–4. Pitted keratolysis. Multiple small, punctate erosions arising in areas of maceration on the plantar foot.

Pitted keratolysis presents with patterned, punched-out–appearing, 1–2 mm round to oval erosions on a background of maceration on the soles of the feet (Fig. 46–4). There is typically little to no erythema. The absence of scale helps distinguish it from tinea pedis. Treatment options include topical clindamycin 2% solution, erythromycin 2% solution, topical imidazole antifungal agents, or oral erythromycin.

BLISTERING DISTAL DACTYLITIS

Blistering distal dactylitis is a superficial infection of the distal fat pad of the finger, usually caused by group A *Streptococcus. Staphylococcus aureus* and group B *Streptococcus* also have been reported to cause dactylitis, but less commonly. Most cases of blistering distal dactylitis involve children. Clinically, the lesions consist of asymptomatic to tender superficial blisters on an erythematous base overlying the anterior fat pad of the finger (Fig. 46–5). Incision of the blister, which can measure up to 1 cm in diameter, usually yields a small amount of thin, white pus. A single digit is usually involved, although several fingers may be affected. There are usually no associated systemic symptoms or fever.

Blistering dactylitis must be distinguished from herpetic whitlow, staphylococcal bullous impetigo, primary bullous disorders, friction blisters, and thermal burns. Treatment consists of systemic antistreptococcal antibiotics. Penicillin V (25–50 mg/kg/day orally divided every 8 hours) or erythromycin (40 mg/kg/day orally divided every 6 hours) for 10 days is effective, as is a single dose of intramuscular benzathine penicillin G (600,000 units for children weighing less than 60 pounds; 1.2 million units for older children and adults). A Gram stain should be performed on the purulent drainage, and a Tzanck smear or viral culture should be obtained if

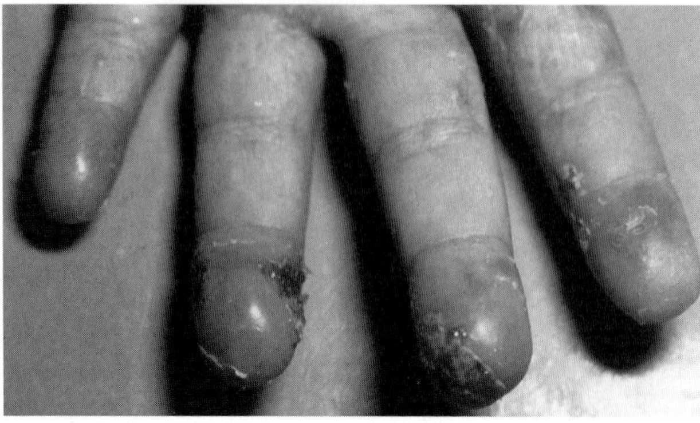

FIGURE 46–5. Blistering distal dactylitis. Blisters are present on the fat pads of the fingers.

herpetic whitlow is suspected. If a *S. aureus* infection is suspected, antimicrobial coverage should include a penicillinase-resistant penicillin, cephalosporin, or erythromycin. Incision and drainage is required when a large amount of pus is present. Compresses or warm soaks may help alleviate discomfort.

PERIANAL DERMATITIS

Perianal dermatitis, also called **perianal streptococcal disease,** is a distinct clinical entity characterized by well-demarcated, perianal erythema. Group A *Streptococcus* was originally identified as the cause of the condition, although *S. aureus* has also been cultured from similar clinical lesions. Affected children complain of anal pruritus and painful defecation. They may pass blood-streaked stools. Physical examination reveals well-marginated, flat, pink to beefy red perianal erythema extending as far as 2 cm from the anus (Fig. 46–6). Erythema may involve the vulva and vagina. Lesions may be tender, and they may fissure and bleed, particularly when chronic. Systemic symptoms and fever are unusual. Although overt pharyngitis is not usually present, group A *Streptococcus* can be isolated from the throat of many children with streptococcal perianal dermatitis. Impetigo is rarely associated. The presence of pustules on the buttock or perineum suggests a staphylococcal infection. Candidiasis can also cause satellite pustules.

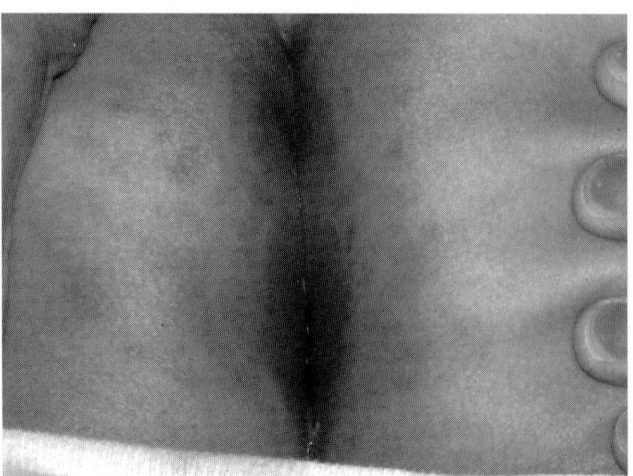

FIGURE 46–6. Perianal dermatitis (perianal streptococcal disease). Symmetrical, tender erythema around the anus of a child with a superficial group A *Streptococcus* infection.

The differential diagnosis includes inverse psoriasis, diaper dermatitis, candidiasis, pinworm infection, simple anal fissures, and irritant dermatitis. The diagnosis is suspected on clinical grounds and can be confirmed with a culture obtained by swabbing the affected area. The clinical laboratory should be notified that streptococci are suspected, as the perianal skin is usually heavily colonized with enteric flora.

Treatment is with systemic antibiotics. Penicillin V (25–50 mg/kg/day orally divided every 8 hours) or erythromycin (40 mg/kg/day orally divided every 6 hours) for 10 days is effective treatment of streptococcal infections. If *S. aureus* is suspected or cultured, dicloxacillin (12–25 mg/kg/day orally divided every 6 hours) or a first-generation cephalosporin (cephalexin 25–50 mg/kg/day orally divided every 6 hours) may be used.

DECUBITUS ULCERS

EPIDEMIOLOGY AND PATHOGENESIS

Decubitus ulcers, also known as **pressure sores,** can occur in any child who is bedridden or otherwise immobilized for a prolonged period of time. Ulcers develop as a consequence of local tissue ischemia that results when the tissue pressure exceeds the vascular perfusion pressure. This occurs most commonly at sites of bony prominence, and thus the sites most frequently involved in supine patients include the sacrum, the skin overlying the greater trochanters, and the heels. Friction, shearing forces, and local tissue trauma, such as maceration or excoriation, may contribute to the development of decubitus ulcers.

ETIOLOGY

The microbiology of decubitus ulcers in children, like that of adults, is polymicrobial. Both aerobic and anaerobic organisms have been cultured from ulcers, and several different organisms are usually recovered. The normal flora of the skin and organs surrounding the ulcer may influence the bacteria present in a given ulcer. Organisms commonly recovered from both children and adults include *S. aureus, Streptococcus faecalis,* gram-negative enteric bacteria, anaerobic gram-positive cocci, and *Bacteroides.*

SYMPTOMS AND CLINICAL MANIFESTATIONS AND DIAGNOSIS

Decubitus ulcers begin as an area of nonblanching erythema on intact skin. If pressure continues, the skin breaks down and ulcerates (Fig. 46–7). Ulcers may extend to involve the deep subcutaneous tissues, muscle, and bone. Necrotic tissue may be present in the ulcer and may become colonized or overtly infected with bacteria.

TREATMENT AND PROGNOSIS

The successful treatment of decubitus ulcers requires a reduction in the local tissue pressure. This can be accomplished by frequent turning and positioning and by the use of pressure-reducing devices, such as special mattresses, mattress overlays, or cushions. Specialized beds are available that maximize even weight redistribution, although the high cost of these beds makes their widespread use impractical.

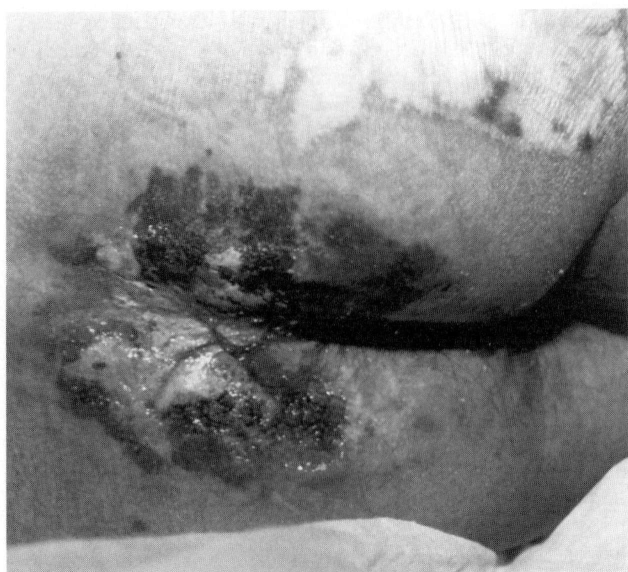

FIGURE 46–7. Decubitus ulcer.

Necrotic debris within the ulcer must be débrided, either surgically or mechanically. Healing within a clean or successfully débrided, relatively superficial ulcer can then be facilitated by the use of an occlusive dressing, such as hydrocolloid or semipermeable film dressing.

Ulcers involving deep subcutaneous tissues or muscle are best managed surgically, often requiring a tissue flap for healing. Antibiotics are indicated if there is evidence of cellulitis or overt wound infection. The antibiotic choice should be guided by a deep culture from the wound.

Decubitus ulcers are the cause of considerable morbidity among hospitalized and debilitated patients. Infectious complications include sepsis, osteomyelitis, and joint infections. Consultation with a specialist familiar with the care of ulcers, such as a dermatologist or plastic surgeon, is advisable.

ANTHRAX

ETIOLOGY

Anthrax is an acute bacterial infection by the organism *Bacillus anthracis,* a large, gram-positive rod that forms spores in culture and in the environment that remain viable for decades.

The organism is acquired by direct contact with or inhalation of spores from infected animals or animal byproducts or by ingestion of undercooked meat. Cutaneous lesions in humans contain infectious organisms, but person-to-person transmission by direct contact or respiratory spread is not recognized.

EPIDEMIOLOGY

Anthrax is a disease of wild and domestic animals; humans are incidental hosts. The areas of high prevalence in the world are the Near and Middle East and parts of South America and Europe. Most patients have had occupational or other exposure to infected animals or their products, including hides, hair, or carcasses of domesticated or wild animals. In the United States, cutaneous anthrax was not reported after 1992 until one case in North Dakota in 2000. Inhalation anthrax was last reported in 1976, and gastrointestinal anthrax has not been reported.

PATHOGENESIS

The organism secretes three proteins—protective antigen, lethal factor, and edema factor—that are collectively known as **anthrax toxin.** These proteins combine to produce two toxins: **edema toxin** and **lethal toxin.** Subcutaneous injection of edema factor produces edema and may contribute to the gelatinous nature of the exudate often present in the skin lesions, whereas intravenous injection of lethal toxin into experimental animals leads to death. Full virulence of *B. anthracis* also requires the presence of a poly-D-glutamic acid capsule. Production of the toxin and capsule is encoded by two large plasmids present in virulent strains.

SYMPTOMS AND CLINICAL MANIFESTATIONS

Infection with *B. anthracis* may take several forms. The most common form of anthrax is cutaneous disease, which accounts for more than 95% of reported cases in the United States. Other forms include a widespread pulmonary infection and a rare form of gastrointestinal disease. Sepsis and meningitis may complicate cutaneous, inhalation, or gastrointestinal diseases. Public awareness about anthrax has recently increased because of the potential use of anthrax spores as a biologic warfare agent. Aerosolization of spores results in pulmonary infection. There are no classic cutaneous findings associated with pulmonary anthrax.

Cutaneous anthrax begins when spores enter abraded or traumatized skin. Following a 2- to 5-day incubation period, a small, painless, erythematous papule develops at the site of inoculation. This enlarges rapidly, becoming edematous, gelatinous, and hemorrhagic. The center becomes necrotic, and a black eschar develops. Satellite pustules may surround the primary lesion. Despite extensive local involvement, the lesion is characteristically painless. Regional lymph nodes may be tender and enlarged, and there may be fever. Cutaneous anthrax infrequently disseminates, causing hypotension, tachycardia, and high fever.

Pulmonary anthrax, also known as **woolsorter's disease,** results from the inhalation of aerosolized spores that germinate in the lungs, producing an acute, necrotizing infection. Mild upper respiratory tract symptoms are followed within 2–4 days by respiratory distress with cyanosis that can progress to death.

Gastrointestinal anthrax is characterized by abdominal pain, vomiting, bloody diarrhea, and shock after the ingestion of spores.

DIAGNOSIS

The diagnosis of anthrax requires identification of the organism in the wound exudate or tissue. A Gram stain of the vesicle fluid or scrapings may reveal the large, gram-positive bacillus. The diagnosis is confirmed by isolation of the organism in culture. Serologic analysis provides retrospective diagnostic information.

TREATMENT

Parenteral high-dose penicillin G (300,000–400,000 U/kg/day) is the treatment of choice for cutaneous anthrax; it should be continued until the lesion has dried and the edema has resolved. Thereafter, oral penicillin G can be used to complete a 10- to 14-day course. Alternative drugs include tetracycline, erythromycin, and chloramphenicol. Débridement should be avoided because bacteremia may result.

COMPLICATIONS AND PROGNOSIS

Rapid defervescence and clinical improvement should follow appropriate treatment of cutaneous disease. The prognosis for persons with other forms of the disease, including pulmonary, gastrointestinal, and septicemic anthrax, is very poor. The disease may progress rapidly if not recognized and treated promptly.

PREVENTION

Prevention of anthrax is aimed at minimizing human exposure through animal vaccination and disease control. A human vaccine is available for persons at high risk of occupational exposure.

MYCOBACTERIAL INFECTIONS

LEPROSY

Leprosy, or **Hansen's disease,** is a chronic granulomatous disease caused by *Mycobacterium leprae.* Although the infection can involve many organ systems, it most commonly affects skin and nerves.

ETIOLOGY

M. leprae is a gram-positive, obligate intracellular, acid-fast bacillus that proliferates preferentially in cooler areas of the body. The organism has a variable generation time of up to 13 days, perhaps accounting for the long incubation period seen in human disease. In tissue sections, *M. leprae* is found either singly or in clumps of multiple bacilli called **globi.**

Transmission. Humans are the major host and reservoir of the leprosy bacillus. The upper respiratory tract is believed to be the most likely source of disease transmission because patients with multibacillary forms of the disease shed large numbers of bacilli in their nasal secretions. Bacilli are present in some skin lesions and have been identified in breast milk. There is also evidence of transplacental transmission.

Leprosy also occurs in three known animal species: the nine-banded armadillo (found wild in Louisiana and Texas), the chimpanzee, and the mangabey monkey. Disease transmission to humans is believed to be possible.

EPIDEMIOLOGY

Considerable progress has been made in the international fight against leprosy in the past 10–15 years. The WHO reported an estimated 1.2 million cases of leprosy in the world in 1997, a decrease from as many as 10–12 million cases in previous decades. Approximately 700,000 new cases were reported in 1997. This dramatic decrease in the prevalence of the disease has resulted from aggressive attempts to diagnose the disease in endemic countries and also reflects the successful adoption of effective treatment regimens involving multidrug therapy (MDT). More than 9 million patients were reported by the WHO to have been cured since 1985.

The highest concentrations of leprosy are found in Africa, India, Southeast Asia, South America, the Philippines, and on some South Pacific islands. India, Indonesia, and Myanmar account for 70% of all cases worldwide. Leprosy is relatively rare in the United States, where between 100 and 200 new cases are reported each year. An increase in cases seen in the 1980s was related to immigration of Indo-Chinese refugees, but the number has again stabilized (Fig. 46–8). Most cases of leprosy in the United States are imported, although the disease is indigenous in Louisiana, eastern Texas, and Hawaii.

About 20–30% of all reported cases of leprosy occur in children, most frequently during childhood and adolescence. Infants are rarely infected. Both sexes are equally affected. Racial, ethnic, and nutritional factors do not appear to affect disease susceptibility. However, genetic factors, including human leukocyte antigen (HLA) haplotypes, may influence susceptibility to infection and the subsequent expression of disease.

PATHOGENESIS

The clinical and histologic manifestations of leprosy are determined by the host immune responses to *M. leprae.* Varied levels of response to the organism result in a diverse spectrum of disease. Both humoral and cell-mediated immune responses are evoked in leprosy, but humoral immunity does not appear to be an important factor in disease resistance. Antibody titers to *M. leprae* antigens tend to correlate inversely with the intensity of the cell-mediated immune response.

Tuberculoid leprosy is characterized by a high level of cell-mediated immunity to *M. leprae* antigens. This may be functionally demonstrated by a positive response to the **lepromin test,** an intradermal skin test using a standardized, heat-killed suspension of *M. leprae.* The lepromin test is useful only in establishing the presence of an immune response to the organism. Because it is also positive in healthy persons sensitized to *M. leprae,* the lepromin test is not diagnostic. Histologically, the lesions of tuberculoid leprosy consist of dense, well-circumscribed, epithelioid cell granulomas within the dermis. A mantle of lymphocytes surrounds the granulomas, and **Langhans' giant cells** may also be associated. Acid-fast bacilli, if present, are few in number. The lymphocytes within the granuloma are predominantly of CD4 (T helper) phenotype, whereas CD8 (T suppressor) cells are present within the surrounding mantle. The CD4 : CD8 cell ratio is usually normal within the lesions and in the peripheral blood.

Lepromatous leprosy lies at the other end of the disease spectrum from tuberculoid leprosy and is characterized by a specific, cell-mediated immune unresponsiveness to *M. leprae.* The lepromin test is negative. In the absence of an adequate immune

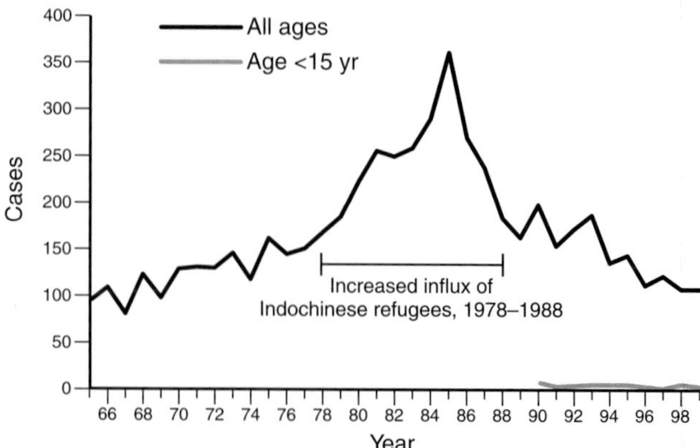

FIGURE 46–8. Reported cases of Hansen's disease by year in the United States from 1967–1999. (Data from Centers for Disease Control and Prevention.)

response, the bacillus proliferates diffusely and is seen easily in tissue sections and slit-skin smears. Histologically, lepromatous lesions consist of numerous foamy macrophages, which may nearly fill the dermis. Lymphocytes are scattered throughout the infiltrate, which is usually separated from the epidermis by a clear zone. Involved nerves have a thickened perineurium. CD8 cells predominate in lepromatous lesions with a reduced CD4 : CD8 ratio, usually 0.5–0.6. Although the total number of circulating peripheral blood lymphocytes may be reduced, the CD4 : CD8 ratio is usually normal. Moreover, patients with lepromatous leprosy generally have intact cell-mediated immunity against other antigens. The mechanisms of this specific anergy are incompletely understood and may involve the production of suppressor T cells. Other mechanisms, including genetic factors and clonal deletion of *M. leprae*–specific T cells, have been proposed. Macrophage dysfunction may also be involved.

SYMPTOMS AND CLINICAL MANIFESTATIONS

The clinical manifestations of leprosy encompass a wide range of findings that involve the skin, peripheral nerves, and mucous membranes (Table 46–4). Three cardinal signs of leprosy include cutaneous lesions, cutaneous anesthesia, and enlarged peripheral nerves.

Various classification systems have been used to describe leprosy. The system devised by Ridley and Jopling incorporates clinical, immunologic, and pathologic criteria to divide leprosy into five groups: tuberculoid, borderline-tuberculoid, borderline, borderline-lepromatous, and lepromatous. Indeterminate and pure neural forms of leprosy also are described. For purposes of treatment, the WHO divides leprosy into **paucibacillary** and **multibacillary** forms, depending on the absence or presence of acid-fast bacilli in a skin smear.

Indeterminate Leprosy. The incubation period for leprosy is prolonged, averaging 2–5 years. The earliest manifestations may include paresthesia and subtle changes in cutaneous sensation. **Indeterminate skin lesions** are subtle, consisting of poorly defined slightly hypopigmented to pink macules. Skin texture, hair, and sweating are preserved in these early lesions. A skin smear is usually negative. Indeterminate leprosy may heal spontaneously, remain stable, or progress to another form of leprosy.

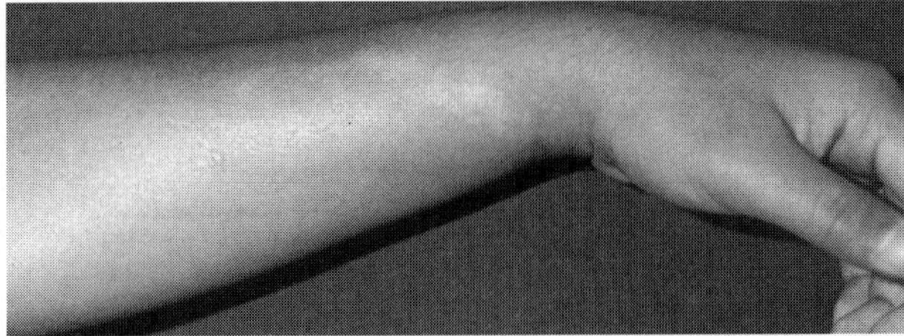

FIGURE 46–9. Tuberculoid leprosy. Subtle hypopigmented macules arising on the forearm of a child with leprosy. Involvement of the cutaneous nerves may render these areas insensate.

Tuberculoid Leprosy. Tuberculoid lesions evolve from indeterminate lesions or arise *de novo.* Lesions consist of single to multiple, well-defined, hypopigmented macules of any size distributed asymmetrically on the body (Fig. 46–9). A ring of papules may be present at the border of the lesion. These papules may spread centrifugally, leaving behind central atrophy.

Nerves are affected, with tactile and thermal sensation becoming impaired. Sweating is decreased, and hair loss may occur as follicles are infiltrated with inflammatory cells. Local cutaneous and peripheral nerves may be enlarged and palpable. Acid-fast bacilli are rarely demonstrable in skin smears.

Borderline Leprosy. Borderline leprosy encompasses a spectrum that includes features of both tuberculoid and lepromatous leprosy. It may have a wide range of manifestations. Borderline leprosy usually presents with more skin lesions than does the tuberculoid form. Lesions are usually larger and less well defined, and there may be satellite lesions at the border. Nodules may be present. Neural changes tend to be more severe than in tuberculoid leprosy and may cause deformities. Borderline leprosy is unstable and can evolve into either tuberculoid or lepromatous leprosy with time. Organisms may or may not be identifiable in tissue.

Lepromatous Leprosy. Anergy to *M. leprae* allows widespread proliferation of the bacillus, resulting in skin lesions ranging from

TABLE 46–4. The Clinical and Immunohistologic Spectrum of Leprosy

	Form of Leprosy		
Characteristic	**Tuberculoid**	**Borderline**	**Lepromatous**
Clinical features	One to several anesthetic macules or plaques distributed asymmetrically on the body Hair growth, sweating may be absent Peripheral nerves may be enlarged	Clinical lesions with features of either or both ends of the spectrum; usually several macules or plaques present. May be poorly circumscribed Neural changes more severe than in tuberculoid	Multiple, often widespread lesions with macules, papules, and nodules Skin may appear diffusely thickened. Leonine facies Neuropathy late, severe
Host immune response	High level of cell-mediated immunity to *M. leprae* Lepromin test positive	May see features of either form of leprosy	Specific, cell-mediated anergy to *M. leprae* Lepromin test negative
Histopathology	Well-circumscribed, epithelioid cell granulomas in dermis surrounded by lymphocytes Few bacilli present in skin		Numerous foamy macrophages in dermis with scattered lymphocytes Numerous bacilli present

diffuse, generalized skin thickening to widespread, generalized nodules called **lepromas.** Cooler parts of the body are preferentially involved. Early lesions may consist of subtly hypopigmented macules with no detectable sensory changes. Left untreated, lepromatous leprosy progresses to widely disseminated disease. Because of the weak immune response, damage to nerves progresses slowly but may ultimately occur as organisms infiltrate the nerves. Severe neuropathy can render the hands and feet insensitive, leading to deformities. For unknown reasons, lepromatous forms of leprosy occur infrequently in children.

A distinct form of lepromatous leprosy called **Lucio leprosy** occurs in some patients of Latin American ancestry. This highly anergic form of leprosy results in widely disseminated disease with neuropathy, skin changes, loss of body hair, and an obstructive vasculitis, which may infarct and ulcerate the skin.

Neuritic Leprosy. Involvement of peripheral nerves without cutaneous lesions can occur, but it does so infrequently. Patients may present with tender, palpable nerves and have associated anesthesia or paresthesia.

Acute Reactions. Acute inflammatory reactions may occur during the natural course or treatment of leprosy. Approximately 50% of all patients experience these episodes; however, these reactions occur less frequently in children than in adults. Two immunologically mediated reactions have been described: reversal reactions (type 1) and erythema nodosum leprosum (type 2).

Reversal reactions occur in patients with borderline or tuberculoid leprosy and represent a change in the degree of cell-mediated immunity. These reactions can be ''upgrading,'' reflecting an increased immune response, or ''downgrading,'' in which the immunity is decreased. **Upgrading reactions** result in pre-existing skin lesions becoming red and edematous and may be associated with neuritis. As upgrading reactions recur, the disease progresses toward the tuberculoid form. **Downgrading reactions** allow proliferation of the organism in the skin.

Erythema nodosum leprosum is thought to represent an Arthus type of hypersensitivity involving immune complexes. This reaction occurs most often in lepromatous leprosy and may occur before, during, or after antimycobacterial chemotherapy. Erythema nodosum leprosum is characterized by painful skin nodules, fever, malaise, anorexia, and wasting. Other organ systems can be involved, resulting in arthritis, adenitis, orchitis, and neuritis. A leukocytosis occurs in 85% of patients.

DIAGNOSIS

The diagnosis of leprosy should be suspected on clinical grounds, particularly in endemic areas or among immigrants from these regions. Tactile and thermal sensory testing should be performed on hypopigmented skin lesions. A **slit-skin smear** may be used to identify acid-fast bacilli in skin. In this procedure, involved skin is cleaned and pinched between the thumb and index finger of the left hand, and an incision measuring 5 mm in length by 2 mm in depth is made with a sterile scalpel. Blood is wiped away, and the base and sides of the incision are scraped at a right angle to the incision. The material obtained is smeared on a slide and stained for acid-fast bacilli by the Ziehl-Neelsen method. Smears also may be obtained from nasal mucosa.

The diagnosis of leprosy can also be established with a skin biopsy. A deep punch biopsy and special stains for acid-fast bacilli should be performed. The organism cannot be isolated in vitro.

TREATMENT

Four major drugs are used for the treatment of leprosy: dapsone and clofazimine, which are primarily mycobacteriostatic, and rifampin and the thioamides, which are mycobactericidal. Several other drugs, including ofloxacin, which is a fluoroquinolone, clarithromycin, which is a macrolide, and minocycline, also have bactericidal activity against *M. leprae.* Because drug resistance to one or more of the agents is common, combination therapy is recommended (Table 46–5). The recommended duration of treatment has been decreased on the basis of 1997 WHO recommendations. A single-dose treatment has been suggested for the treatment of single-skin-lesion paucibacillary leprosy. Treatment is provided on an outpatient basis.

Erythema Nodosum Leprosum. Therapy of erythema nodosum leprosum has been greatly enhanced by the availability of thalidomide. Approximately 90% of patients treated with thalidomide have a dramatic improvement. Thalidomide is usually started at adult doses of 100 mg nightly and can be increased up to 200 mg as needed. Doses in excess of 200 mg/day are usually not tolerated because of excessive sedation. Tumor necrosis factor-α (TNF-α) levels fall during thalidomide therapy, which is thought to contribute to clinical improvement. The greatest threat during reversal reactions is permanent nerve damage that can result from the destructive effects of the acute inflammatory response. If a rapid response to therapy is not seen, or if nerve tenderness does not improve with therapy, prednisone (0.5–1 mg/kg/day) should be added. An alternative therapy is clofazimine 200 mg/day.

COMPLICATIONS AND PROGNOSIS

Without treatment, the prognosis for persons with leprosy is poor. Some degree of irreversible nerve damage occurs in nearly all patients and can be severe, resulting in joint and extremity deformities. Secondary deformities, such as chronic skin ulcers and osteomyelitis, may follow neurologic impairment. Involvement of the motor nerves can produce paralysis. Acute reactions involving the eye may cause blindness. Secondary amyloidosis may complicate long-standing lepromatous leprosy and ultimately cause renal failure.

TABLE 46–5. Recommendations for Multidrug Therapy for Leprosy, World Health Organization, 1997

Multibacillary leprosy (lepromatous, borderline-lepromatous, and borderline forms)
- Rifampin 600 mg once a month (450 mg for children <35 kg)
- Dapsone 100 mg daily (1–2 mg/kg for children)
- Clofazimine 300 mg once a month and 50 mg daily
- Treatment duration 12 months

Paucibacillary leprosy (indeterminate, tuberculoid, and borderline tuberculoid forms)
- Rifampin 600 mg once a month (450 mg for children <35 kg)
- Dapsone 100 mg daily (1–2 mg/kg for children)
- Treatment duration 6 months

Single skin lesion paucibacillary leprosy
- Rifampin 600 mg
- Ofloxacin 400 mg
- Minocycline 100 mg

CUTANEOUS NONTUBERCULOUS MYCOBACTERIAL INFECTIONS

Cutaneous mycobacterial infections are caused by both tuberculous and nontuberculous mycobacteria. Although *Mycobacterium tuberculosis* remains the most common cause of mycobacterial skin infections worldwide, it rarely causes cutaneous disease in the United States.

ETIOLOGY

Many species of nontuberculous mycobacteria can cause skin and soft tissue infections (Table 46–6). *M. marinum* and *M. fortuitum*-complex organisms are most frequently reported. *M. marinum* is found worldwide as an opportunistic pathogen that affects marine animals and humans. It is classified in the Runyon Group I as an acid-fast, slow-growing photochromogen. *M. fortuitum* and *M. chelonae* are rapid-growing species classified in the Runyon group IV. Cutaneous infections by other atypical mycobacteria occur, but they are rare in children in the United States.

EPIDEMIOLOGY

M. marinum has been isolated from fresh and salt water, swimming pool walls, tropical fish tanks, well water, and infected marine animals. The organism enters the skin through a traumatic abrasion or cut and, after an incubation period averaging 3 weeks, causes clinical disease.

M. fortuitum and *M. chelonae* are important causes of nosocomial infection and have been associated with the use of indwelling venous and dialysis catheters, surgical implants, and coronary artery bypass operations.

SYMPTOMS AND CLINICAL MANIFESTATIONS

M. marinum produces a chronic, granulomatous infection commonly known as **swimming pool granuloma** or **fish tank granuloma.** Lesions are typically located on the extremities, elbows, or knees, where trauma may have occurred. A purple-red, asymptomatic to slightly tender papule develops and slowly enlarges. The surface may be verrucous or crusted and may ulcerate. The infection can spread along the regional lymphatic vessels, resulting in a linear distribution of lesions along the affected extremity. Rarely, cutaneous dissemination occurs. Associated systemic symptoms and lymphadenopathy are rare.

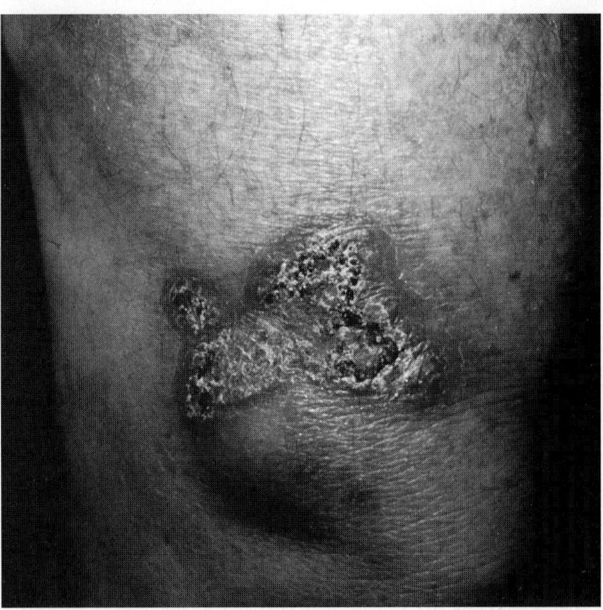

FIGURE 46–10. *Mycobacterium marinum.* Characteristic lesion on the knee.

M. fortuitum and *M. chelonae* cause localized, nodular, or suppurative lesions at the site of mycobacterial inoculation (Fig. 46–10). *M. kansasii* causes chronic granulomatous skin lesions. *M. ulcerans* infection, which is found predominantly in Africa and Australia, causes a chronic skin ulcer called **Buruli ulcer,** which is a painless nodule that enlarges, creating a large, necrotic ulcer.

DIAGNOSIS

The differential diagnosis of *M. marinum* infection includes mainly other mycobacterial infections and sporotrichosis. These may be

TABLE 46–6. Cutaneous Infections Caused by Nontuberculous (Atypical) Mycobacteria

Organism	Runyan Group	Disease Name	Distribution	Predisposing Factors	Clinical
M. marinum	Photochromogen (slow-growing)	Swimming pool granuloma, fish tank granuloma	Worldwide	Exposure to infected fresh or salt water, fish, fish tanks, pools	Single to multiple purple, pink papules that enlarge to nodules. May ulcerate
M. kansasii	Photochromogen (slow-growing)	None	Worldwide	Immunosuppression	Chronic, granulomatous skin nodule(s). Sporotrichoid spread may occur
M. fortuitum *M. chelonae*	Nonphotochromogen (rapid-growing)	None	Worldwide	Nosocomial exposure: inoculation, indwelling catheters, surgical implants	Nodules, cold abscesses at inoculation site
M. ulcerans	Nonchromogen (slow-growing)	Buruli ulcer	Africa, Australia, Latin America	None	Painless, subcutaneous nodule. Enlarges gradually, resulting in large ulcers

clinically indistinguishable. The history may suggest the diagnosis, but identification of the organism is needed for confirmation. Lesions should also be distinguished from foreign body granulomas, cutaneous leishmaniasis, deep fungal infections, primary cutaneous or metastatic malignant neoplasms, sarcoidosis, and chronic pyogenic infections.

Acid-fast bacilli may be identified in smears and culture of the wound exudate. In most cases the diagnosis is best established with a skin biopsy. Specimens should be evaluated by microscopic examination, including tissue stains for mycobacteria and fungi, and the tissue should be cultured. *M. marinum* grows well on Löwenstein-Jensen medium and develops a vivid yellow color when exposed to light. Growth requires 2–3 weeks and is optimal at temperatures of 30–33°C (86–91.4°F). To ensure that appropriate media and culture conditions are used, the laboratory should be notified if either *M. marinum* or *M. haemophilum* is suspected.

A high incidence of cross-reactivity between the mycobacterial antigens of different species renders skin testing nonspecific and insufficiently reliable for diagnosis.

TREATMENT

Left untreated, most *M. marinum* infections in an immunocompetent host resolve within several years, although scarring may result. Complications are rare; however, infections can extend locally into soft tissues or bone, causing arthritis, tenosynovitis, and osteomyelitis. Laryngeal granulomas have been reported.

Various treatment modalities for *M. marinum* infections have been used, including surgical excision of isolated nodules, electrodesiccation and curettage, local heat, radiation therapy, potassium iodide (SSKI), antibiotics, and antituberculous drugs. In vitro susceptibility testing should precede drug therapy, because resistance to standard antituberculous drugs, including isoniazid, para-amino salicylic acid, and streptomycin, is common. Successful treatment has been reported with antibiotics, including tetracycline, doxycycline, minocycline, rifampin, and cotrimoxazole. Prolonged therapy may be required.

Complications and dissemination of other atypical mycobacterial cutaneous infections are rare in an immunocompetent host. However, these complications have become serious problems for adults with AIDS. Cutaneous lesions may persist for several years in the absence of treatment. Therapeutic options are similar to those for *M. marinum* infection, although surgical excision of cutaneous lesions may be required for cure. If a catheter or prosthetic device is associated with atypical mycobacterial infection, it should be removed.

FUNGAL INFECTIONS

TINEA CAPITIS

ETIOLOGY

Tinea capitis results from infection of the scalp and hair shaft by keratophilic fungi of two genera, *Trichophyton* and *Microsporum. Microsporum audouinii* was once responsible for most cases of epidemic tinea capitis in the United States, but a dramatic shift in etiology occurred in the past several decades, and *Trichophyton tonsurans* now causes more than 90% of cases. *M. audouinii* and *Microsporum canis* are relatively rare causes of tinea capitis in the United States.

Transmission. The dermatophyte is transmitted by direct human contact in the case of anthropophilic fungi (e.g., *T. tonsurans* and *M. audouinii*) or between humans and animals when zoophilic fungi (e.g., *M. canis*) are involved. Dermatophytes also can be transmitted via fomites. Organisms have been recovered from a variety of objects, including combs and brushes, hats, furniture, and linens. *T. tonsurans* has been isolated from the scalps of symptom-free persons in endemic areas and from family members of infected persons. These persons may serve as asymptomatic carriers of the infection.

EPIDEMIOLOGY

Tinea capitis is the most common dermatophyte infection in children, with a higher incidence among urban African American and Hispanic children. Approximately 95% of cases occur in children and adolescents, predominantly in preadolescent children.

PATHOGENESIS

After inoculation of spores, the dermatophyte proliferates in the stratum corneum. Hyphae penetrate the surrounding hair follicles and infect the keratinized portion of the hair shaft. Actively growing, or anagen, hairs are preferentially invaded. Sporulation within the hair by endothrix organisms weakens the shaft, resulting in brittle hairs that break just above the surface of the scalp. The residual fragment of hair may be seen as a **"black dot."**

SYMPTOMS AND CLINICAL MANIFESTATIONS

The clinical presentation of tinea capitis caused by *Trichophyton* differs from that caused by *Microsporum* (Table 46–7). *M. audoui-*

TABLE 46–7. Clinical Spectrum of Tinea Capitis

	Organism	
Clinical Factor	***T. tonsurans***	***M. audouinii***
Incidence	Primary cause in U.S. in 1990s	Frequent cause in U.S. in early 1900s; now relatively rare
Clinical manifestations	"Black-dot" tinea capitis: diffuse scaling of scalp; short, broken hairs visible on scalp as "black dots"; mild inflammation to kerion formation	"Gray-patch" tinea capitis—annular patch of alopecia with fine scale, short, broken, gray-appearing hair fragments; mild inflammation to kerion formation
Wood's light examination	Negative	Positive
Resolution	Persistent course	Spontaneous resolution may occur at adolescence

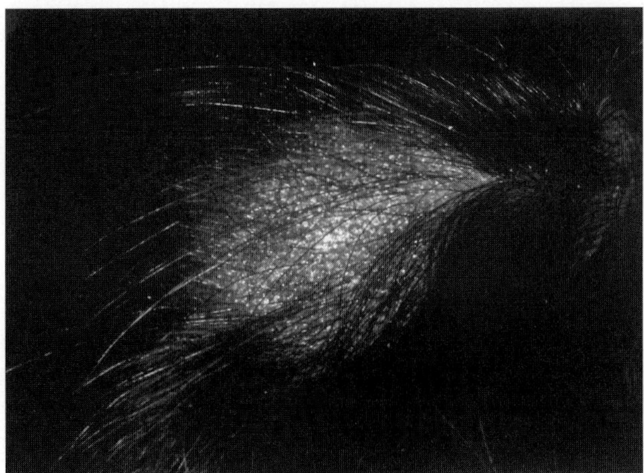

FIGURE 46–11. Black-dot tinea capitis. Infection of the hair follicles by *T. tonsurans* renders the hairs susceptible to breakage at the scalp level. This results in patches of alopecia with so-called "black dots" on the surface.

nii produces well-circumscribed, single patches of scaly alopecia that fluoresce when examined with a Wood's light. Tinea capitis due to *T. tonsurans* does not fluoresce. It may present in one of several patterns. **Black dot tinea,** in which there are many short, broken hairs on the scalp resulting from intrapilary sporulation, is common in *T. tonsurans* infections. Discrete scaly areas of hair loss are present (Fig. 46–11). Other children with *T. tonsurans* infections have only diffuse, fine scaling that may be difficult to detect unless the scalp is gently scratched. This form of tinea capitis, which may be itchy or asymptomatic, is easily confused with dandruff, seborrheic dermatitis, and atopic dermatitis. Diffuse hair loss may complicate long-standing infection.

In a few patients, a strong inflammatory response results in development of perifollicular pustules or a **kerion,** which is a boggy, tender, inflammatory mass (Fig. 46–12). A kerion results from an acute hypersensitivity reaction to the fungus and may be accompanied by fever, lymphadenopathy, and leukocytosis. Kerions may be misdiagnosed as cellulitis or impetigo. Secondary bacterial infection with skin pathogens, including *S. aureus,* can occur, however, and may require simultaneous treatment with systemic antibiotics. Because of the vigorous inflammatory reaction in a kerion, systemic corticosteroids and possibly antibiotic therapy may be required in addition to appropriate systemic antifungal therapy. Timely diagnosis and aggressive treatment of a kerion may prevent permanent scarring alopecia.

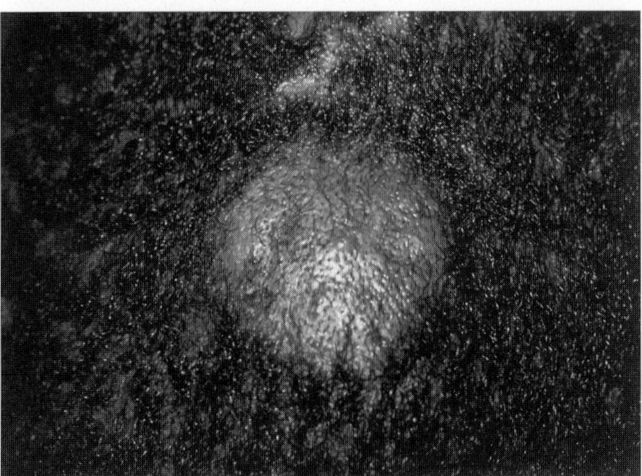

FIGURE 46–12. Kerion. Inflammatory scalp mass in tinea capitis.

Tinea capitis may be accompanied by a pruritic, papular eruption on the face, neck, and trunk known as an **id reaction,** which represents a hypersensitivity reaction to fungal allergens and may be mistaken for an allergic reaction to drug therapy. The rash resolves with treatment of the tinea. If symptomatic, an id reaction can be treated with topical corticosteroids.

DIAGNOSIS

Tinea capitis should be suspected in all children with scaling of the scalp or with hair loss. The diagnosis can often be confirmed by a **potassium hydroxide (KOH) examination** of infected hairs. Broken, **"black dot"** hairs should be obtained by gentle epilation, scraping with a scalpel blade, or wiping of the affected area with a moist piece of gauze. Hyphae may be identified within the hair shaft of hairs infected with *T. tonsurans. Microsporum* infection produces spores that surround the hair shaft. Because interpretation of a KOH preparation can be difficult, a negative result should not exclude infection. A fungal culture provides the definitive diagnosis and allows for identification of the infecting organism. Scalp scrapings, broken hairs, and plucked hairs can be cultured. Skin and pieces of infected hair may be collected by gently scraping the scalp with a sterile scalpel blade. The scrapings are then transferred to the culture medium. Similarly, a sterile toothbrush or cotton swab can be used to débride the scalp. The bristles should be pressed directly into the culture agar. Broken hairs can be carefully plucked and placed on the surface of the agar, with part of the hair implanted into the medium.

Specimens should be inoculated on **Sabouraud medium** with chloramphenicol and cycloheximide. **Dermatophyte test medium (DTM),** an alternative fungal culture medium, contains a phenol red indicator that turns red with dermatophyte growth. DTM is useful when a dermatophyte is suspected; however, growth of *Candida* or saprophytic fungi, which do not cause the indicator to change color, may go undiagnosed by the unskilled observer. Specimens should be incubated at room temperature, with the cap of the culture tube loosely applied. Dermatophyte growth can be slow, and cultures should be held at least 4 weeks before a negative result is determined.

TREATMENT

Systemic antifungal therapy is required for the treatment of tinea capitis (Table 46–8). Topical therapy alone is not effective. Griseofulvin, which is active against all species of *Trichophyton* and *Microsporum,* remains the drug of choice. Griseofulvin is primarily fungistatic, but it also may have fungicidal activity in actively metabolizing hyphae. **Microsize griseofulvin** is given in a dose of 20–25 mg/kg/day orally divided twice daily for 6–8 weeks. Absorption of the drug is maximized by administration with a fatty meal. Treatment failure may require retreatment with griseofulvin at maximal doses, or treatment with an ultramicrosize preparation. The dose of **ultramicrosize griseofulvin** is one half that of the microsize dose. Clinically significant adverse effects of griseofulvin are rare, and the routine monitoring of complete blood counts and liver function tests is not required in otherwise healthy children. Headaches and gastrointestinal upset are among the most frequent adverse effects.

Although griseofulvin remains the treatment of choice for uncomplicated tinea capitis, therapeutic failures are common and may be due to several factors. Underdosing is one of the most common

TABLE 46–8. Treatment of Tinea Capitis

Drug	Dosage/Form	Duration	Laboratory Evaluation
Griseofulvin	Microsize 20–25 mg/kg/day	6–8 wk	None routinely needed
	Ultramicrosize 10–15 mg/kg/day	6–8 wk	
Terbinafine*	Wt: <20 kg: 62.5 mg	2–4 wk	Consider baseline complete blood cell count and liver enzymes
	20–40 kg: 125 mg	2–4 wk	
	>40 kg: 250 mg	2–4 wk	
Itraconazole	Wt: <10 kg: 5mg/kg/day once daily	2–4 wk	Consider baseline complete blood cell count and liver enzymes. Repeat if therapy continued for longer than 4 weeks.
	10–20 kg: 100 mg every other day	2–4 wk	
	21–30 kg: 100 mg once daily	2–4 wk	
	31–40 kg: 100 mg once daily	2–4 wk	
	or		
	100 mg once daily alternating with 200 mg once daily	2–4 wk	
	41–50 kg: 100 mg once daily alternating with 200 mg once daily	2–4 wk	
	or		
	200 mg once daily	2–4 wk	
	>50 kg: 200 mg once daily	2–4 wk	

*Not effective for treatment of *M. canis* infection.
Adapted from Friedlander SF: Tinea capitis—past, present and future. *Curr Probl Dermatol* 2000;12:126.

reasons for treatment failure. Although many recommendations for microsize griseofulvin are for 10 mg/kg/day, in practice, doses of 20–25 mg/kg/day are required for efficacy. Treatment must be continued until there is resolution of clinical symptoms, but the 6- to 8-week course is difficult for many children to complete.

Although neither terbinafine nor itraconazole has yet been approved by the FDA for pediatric use, there is growing evidence to suggest that they are safe and efficacious for the treatment of tinea capitis in children. Itraconazole is primarily fungistatic, but it is lipophilic and has a high affinity for keratin, which results in the preferential accumulation of high tissue levels in the hair and nails. Like other azoles, itraconazole functions by inhibiting fungal cell wall synthesis through inhibition of cytochrome P450 enzymes. Because of this, there is potential for interactions with other drugs that use this metabolic pathway. Because of the presence of cyclodextrin in the oral solution of itraconazole, which has an unclear safety profile, some experts recommend against its use in children, favoring instead use of the capsule form. Terbinafine is an allylamine that has fungicidal properties in vitro through inhibition of fungal wall synthesis. It is also lipophilic and concentrates in hair and nails. Terbinafine has been used successfully in Europe since 1991 and appears to have fewer adverse effects and less potential for drug interactions than does itraconazole. The empiric use of terbinafine in the treatment of tinea capitis is limited, as it does not appear to be effective against *M. canis.* The safety profiles of both itraconazole and terbinafine are excellent; however, it is recommended that liver enzymes be checked at baseline and midway through the course of treatment. In addition to the daily dosing described, both terbinafine and itraconazole can be administered on an intermittent, pulsed-dose schedule. Because both drugs concentrate in the hair and nails, pulse dosing is effective and may reduce potential adverse effects. In addition, pulse dosing may be more cost-effective and may increase compliance.

Topical antifungal agents alone are not effective in the treatment of tinea capitis. Adjunctive use of selenium sulfide 2.5% shampoo daily for several weeks may help decrease spore shedding. Ketoconazole 2% shampoo is also available. Consideration should be given to evaluation and treatment of family members and close contacts.

COMPLICATIONS

Complications of tinea capitis are rare if the infection is recognized and treated. Most problems result from kerion formation, which may cause permanent scarring. Tinea from the scalp can spread to the surrounding skin, causing tinea corporis. Secondary bacterial infections may develop and require antibiotic treatment.

PROGNOSIS

Tinea capitis from *M. audouinii* has been reported to resolve spontaneously at puberty. Although spontaneous cures of *T. tonsurans* tinea have been reported, they appear to be rare. Indolent infection may persist for months to years if not treated. Treatment failures may actually represent reinfection.

PREVENTION

Early treatment is indicated to minimize spread of the disease. Hair articles, combs, and brushes should not be shared. No isolation is necessary, and infected children undergoing treatment may attend daycare and school. Shaving the hair and the use of stocking caps are of historical interest, but they are no longer recommended. An infected child should be reminded not to share brushes, combs, hats, or other articles that may come in contact with the scalp.

CUTANEOUS DERMATOPHYTE INFECTIONS

ETIOLOGY

Dermatophyte infections of glabrous, or non-hair-bearing, skin are caused by three genera: *Microsporum, Trichophyton,* and *Epidermophyton.* Because these three dermatophytes produce the same clinical signs and symptoms, tinea infections are classified by their anatomic region of involvement (Table 46–9).

TABLE 46–9. Causes of Superficial Dermatophyte Infections

Infection	Organism
Tinea corporis	*Microsporum canis* *Trichophyton rubrum* *Trichophyton mentagrophytes*
Tinea faciei	*M. canis* *Trichophyton verrucosum*
Tinea pedis and tinea manuum	
Interdigital	*T. rubrum* *T. mentagrophytes*
Moccasin-type	*T. rubrum*
Vesicular	*T. mentagrophytes* var. *interdigitale*
Tinea cruris	*T. rubrum* (*T. mentagrophytes* and *Epidermophyton floccosum* less commonly)
Tinea unguium (onychomycosis)	*T. rubrum* *E. floccosum*

Transmission. Dermatophytes are transmitted person-to-person, by contact with infected animals, and by fomites.

EPIDEMIOLOGY

Dermatophyte infections of glabrous skin occur worldwide but are more common in warm, humid regions. Tinea corporis, like tinea capitis, occurs frequently in children. Tinea infections of the hands, feet, and groin, however, are rare before adolescence.

SYMPTOMS AND CLINICAL MANIFESTATIONS AND DIAGNOSIS

Tinea Corporis. **Tinea corporis,** or **ringworm,** is most frequently caused by *M. canis, Trichophyton rubrum,* and *Trichophyton mentagrophytes.* If tinea capitis is associated, *T. tonsurans* may be found in both the hair and skin (Fig. 46–13). Tinea corporis usually presents with one or more well-circumscribed, erythematous, annular plaques. The lesion often starts as a small papule or plaque that expands outward; a raised ring of scale at the leading edge is characteristic. As the lesion grows, the central part of the plaque may clear. Pustules or vesicles may be present in the plaques. The lesions of tinea may be extensive in immunocompromised patients. Inappropriate treatment with high-potency topical corticosteroids may obscure the appearance, leading to large, multicentric lesions that may be difficult to diagnose if tinea is not suspected; this is sometimes referred to as **tinea incognito.** Tinea corporis must be distinguished from nummular eczema, psoriasis, atopic dermatitis, pityriasis rosea, and granuloma annulare. Because these can closely resemble tinea corporis, the diagnosis should be confirmed by KOH examination or culture.

Tinea Faciei. Tinea infections of the face occur in children of all ages, including infants. Sources of infection have included the mother's breast in a nursing child. *M. canis* and *Trichophyton verrucosum* are frequent pathogens, although any dermatophyte can be involved. Associated tinea capitis should be excluded whenever the face or neck is affected.

Tinea Pedis and Tinea Manuum. The organisms most frequently isolated from tinea infections of the hand and foot are *T. rubrum* and *T. mentagrophytes.* Tinea pedis is uncommon in young children, but it occurs with increasing frequency after puberty. Foot dermatitis in young children is more often caused by atopic dermatitis, juvenile plantar dermatosis, or allergic contact dermatitis. Confirmation with a KOH examination or fungal culture is recommended before treatment for tinea pedis.

Tinea pedis may be asymptomatic or pruritic. It has several different clinical forms, some of which may be present simultaneously. Intertriginous tinea pedis is most common and consists of scaling and erythema in the lateral toe web spaces. The skin may become macerated and fissured. Bacterial superinfection, particularly with gram-negative organisms, may follow.

Another form of tinea pedis, often caused by *T. rubrum,* is characterized by dry, hyperkeratotic, minimally erythematous scaling of the dorsal and lateral aspects of the feet. This is sometimes referred to as **moccasin-type tinea pedis** and may be associated with dermatophyte infection of one hand **("one hand, two feet").** Patients often confuse this type of tinea for dry skin.

The third, and least common, variant of tinea pedis is the vesicular type, usually caused by *T. mentagrophytes* var. *interdigitale.* Small vesicles are present on the instep or plantar surface of the foot and may be associated with scaling on the feet or between the toes. Larger bullae are unusual. The vesicles are often extremely pruritic.

Tinea Cruris. Tinea infections of the groin area are uncommon in young children, but they occur relatively frequently among adolescent boys. *T. rubrum* is the organism most commonly isolated, although *T. mentagrophytes* and *Epidermophyton floccosum* are occasionally found. Tinea cruris usually presents with symmetric, erythematous scaling on the upper, inner thighs and in the inguinal creases. The scaling is usually most prominent along the peripheral border. Dermatophyte infections spare the scrotum, and its involve-

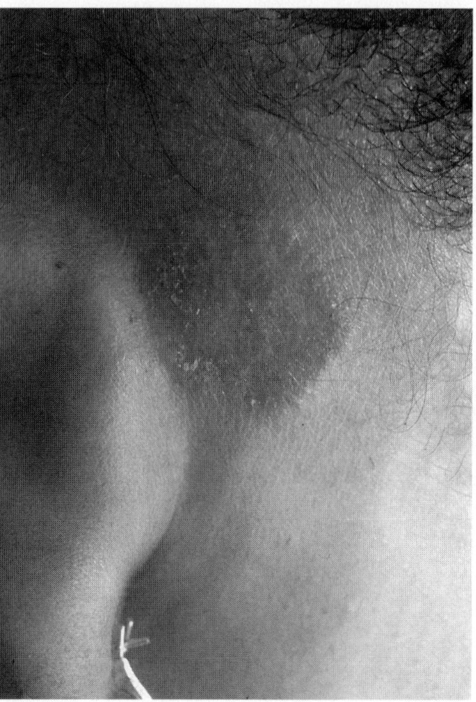

FIGURE 46–13. Tinea corporis. A typical lesion of tinea corporis, or ringworm. Lesions in this location, as well as on the face, may be associated with tinea capitis

ment suggests an alternative diagnosis, including candidiasis or inverse psoriasis. Tinea cruris should also be distinguished from erythrasma and, in infants, irritant dermatitis. Associated tinea pedis should be sought and treated if present. Chronic onychomycosis can serve as a reservoir for reinfection.

Tinea Unguium (Onychomycosis). Dermatophyte infections of the nail are uncommon in young children; the incidence increases after puberty, when tinea pedis becomes common. **Distal subungual onychomycosis,** characterized by thickening and yellowing of the distal aspect of the fingernail or toenail, is the most commonly observed pattern (Fig. 46–14). *T. rubrum* is most frequently isolated, and, occasionally *E. floccosum* is isolated. *Candida* species can infect the nail and may be associated with a **fungal paronychia.** Appropriate cultures should be obtained if this is considered, particularly among immunocompromised children. Nail abnormalities in children can be caused by psoriasis, lichen planus, several genetic conditions in which nail dystrophy is prominent including ''20 nail dystrophy,'' the ectodermal dysplasias, pachyonychia congenita, and dyskeratosis congenita. A thorough dermatologic examination is indicated for a child with abnormal nails.

TREATMENT

The suspected diagnosis of a superficial fungal infection should always be confirmed with a KOH examination or culture. Skin samples are obtained by carefully scraping the affected area with a glass slide, spatula, or a scalpel blade. Organisms are most likely to be found in the active, red, scaly border of the lesions or in vesicles or pustules. Examination of a large amount of scale improves the yield of positive results. Any topical medication or lotions on the skin should first be removed with an alcohol swab before the scrapings are obtained. When organisms are not demonstrated with a KOH examination, a culture should be performed if the clinical suspicion is high.

Superficial tinea infections limited to the skin respond well to topical therapy with any of several available antifungal creams or lotions (Table 46–10). Systemic therapy is rarely needed for simple skin infections. Onychomycosis usually requires systemic therapy and, because of the prolonged treatment course required with griseofulvin, its use is not recommended. Oral terbinafine and itraconazole are both effective, although their cost and potential toxicities must be considered. A topical antifungal lacquer has recently become available for the treatment of nail fungus.

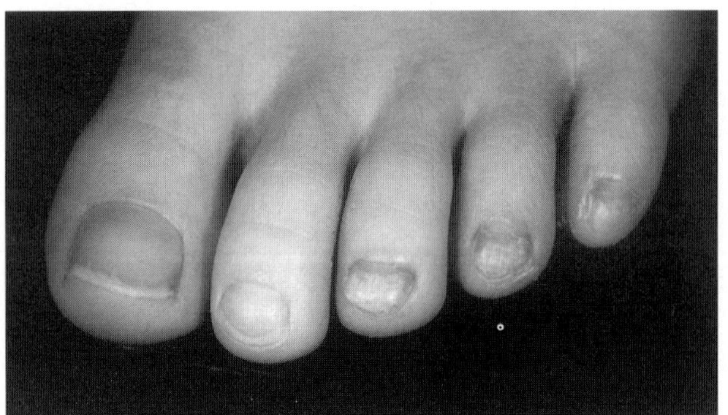

FIGURE 46–14. Onychomycosis (tinea unguium).

TINEA VERSICOLOR

Tinea versicolor, also known as **pityriasis versicolor,** is a common skin infection resulting from superficial invasion of the stratum corneum by the lipophilic yeast, *Malassezia furfur,* previously known as *Pityrosporum ovale* and *P. orbiculare.* This disease occurs most frequently in warm, moist climates and affects person of all ages. Affected persons usually complain of ''white spots'' on their skin. In some cultures, these are thought to be ''acid spots.'' Although pityriasis versicolor is benign and of primarily cosmetic consequence, *M. furfur* can cause nosocomial fungemia in premature infants.

Clinical lesions consist of one to multiple hypopigmented to brown macules located on the upper trunk, neck, and shoulders (Fig. 46–15). The lesions may be isolated, or they may coalesce into large patches that involve most of the trunk. Facial involvement is common in young children. Lesions are asymptomatic or may be mildly pruritic. Fine scale may be evident on the surface, which may be confirmed by gentle scratching.

Short hyphae and round spores **(''spaghetti and meatballs'')** can be identified in KOH preparations obtained from scaling areas and usually confirm the diagnosis. *M. furfur* can be cultured, but it requires a specialized medium with lipids to support its growth.

The differential diagnosis of tinea versicolor includes vitiligo, pityriasis alba, seborrheic dermatitis, tinea corporis, and postinflammatory hypopigmentation or hyperpigmentation. Treatment depends on the extent of involvement. Isolated lesions respond well to twice daily application of an antifungal cream, such as miconazole 2% cream, clotrimazole 1% cream, econazole nitrate 1% cream, or ketoconazole 2% cream. More widespread involvement can be treated with daily application of selenium sulfide 2.5% lotion, which is allowed to remain on the skin for 30 minutes daily for 7–10 days. Repeated monthly application may help prevent recurrences. Oral ketoconazole (400 mg taken about 1 hour before exercise or sweating once a week for 2 weeks) is also effective. Hypopigmentation may persist for weeks to months following successful therapy. Recurrences are common despite appropriate treatment.

CUTANEOUS AND ORAL CANDIDIASIS

Mucocutaneous *Candida* infections are common in young children. Most infections remain limited to the skin, nails, and mucous membranes; however, dissemination with systemic involvement can occur, especially in immunocompromised persons.

ETIOLOGY

Candida albicans causes up to 90% of human *Candida* infections. Less common pathogens include *C. tropicalis, C. parapsilosis, C. guilliermondii, C. pseudotropicalis, C. glabrata, C. krusei,* and *C. zelanoides. C. albicans* is an ovoid yeast measuring 3–6 μm in diameter. It reproduces asexually by budding, forming filamentous chains called pseudohyphae. Under certain circumstances, true septate mycelia may develop. A mixture of yeast and hyphae forms may be recovered from clinical lesions.

EPIDEMIOLOGY

C. albicans is a frequent saprophyte of human mucous membranes and the gastrointestinal tract. Approximately 6% of infants are

TABLE 46–10. Treatment of Tinea Infections of Skin and Nails

Disease	Therapy*	Duration	Monitoring for Adverse Effects
Tinea corporis, tinea pedis, tinea manuum, tinea cruris	Topical creams (OTC):		
	miconazole 2% bid	~2 wk†	Not required
	clotrimazole 1% bid	~2 wk	
	terbinafine 1% qd	1 wk	
	Topical creams (Rx):		
	econazole nitrate 1% qd	~2 wk	
	oxiconazole 1% qd	~2 wk	
	ketoconazole 2% qd	~2 wk	
	sulconazole 1% qd	~2 wk	
	naftifine 1% qd	~2 wk	
	butenafine 1% qd	1 wk	
	ciclopirox 1% bid	~2 wk	
Onychomycosis (always confirm with KOH prep or culture)	Definite pediatric dosages have not been established.		
	Adult doses:		
	terbinafine 250 mg once daily PO	12 wk	Check baseline complete blood cell count and liver enzymes
	or		
	itraconazole 200 mg once daily PO	12 wk	Repeat at 6 weeks for terbinafine, monthly for continuous itraconazole
	or		
	itraconazole 200 mg twice daily PO 1 wk of each month	3 mo	Not required for pulse dosing‡

*Some topical antifungal preparations are available in different vehicles, including creams, gels, sprays. Only the cream is referenced.
†Therapy for tinea pedis should be continued 1 week after clinical resolution.
‡Consider baseline liver enzymes before use of itraconazole.

colonized orally at birth, and the prevalence rises rapidly over the next few weeks of life. *C. albicans* may be part of the normal oral, gastrointestinal, and vaginal flora of healthy adolescents and adults. However, it is not considered part of the normal flora of adult skin. Colonization is more frequent among persons with chronic skin conditions, such as psoriasis and atopic dermatitis.

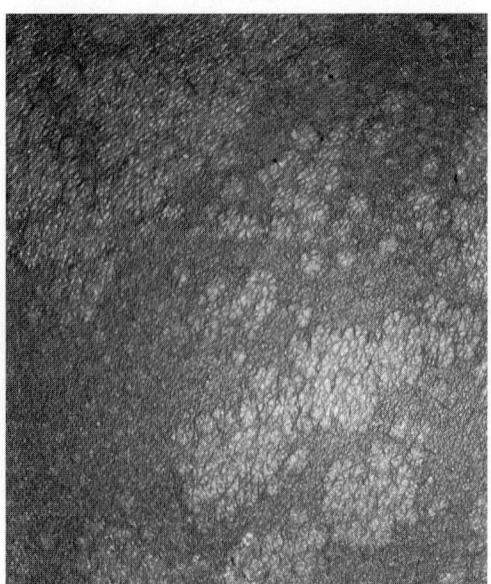

FIGURE 46–15. Tinea versicolor. Scaly, hyperpigmented lesions on the body.

Local factors, including warmth, humidity, occlusion, and maceration, predispose to candidiasis. Use of corticosteroids, oral contraceptives, or antibiotics and diabetes mellitus and immunosuppression are associated with an increased incidence of candidal infection. Most infections are of endogenous origin. Neonates may initially acquire *Candida* from the maternal vaginal tract. Transmission from the skin of health care workers, the mother, or other infants may contribute to colonization.

PATHOGENESIS

The mechanisms by which *Candida* produces disease are not completely understood. *Candida* exists in both yeast and mycelial forms; the yeast form appears to be necessary for colonization and may be active in hematogenous dissemination. Transformation to mycelial forms is associated with tissue invasion, although both forms are found in infected tissues. Successful colonization and subsequent infection initially require adherence of the yeast to host mucosal surfaces. This is mediated by mannoprotein constituents on the cell wall and may be affected by bacterial competition for adherence sites. Once attached, the yeast transforms into mycelial elements and can invade the epidermal barrier. Invasion appears to involve the production of keratolytic enzymes, phospholipases, or proteolytic enzymes by the fungus. *Candida* cell wall mannans activate the alternative pathway of the serum complement system, attracting polymorphonuclear leukocytes. These leukocytes aggregate, producing the microabscesses characteristic of cutaneous candidiasis. An increased rate of epidermal proliferation accompanies the local inflammation and may help confine the infection to the epithelium.

Host defense mechanisms against *Candida* infection are numerous and include both immune and nonimmune factors. The epithelial barrier functions as the first line of defense; an intact stratum corneum may prevent excessive colonization and infection. Local bacterial microflora compete for mucosal adherence sites and nutrients. Complement activation and subsequent inflammation, neutrophil migration, and killing complete the initial defense. Immune defenses against candidal infection consist primarily of cell-mediated processes, and their importance is evident in the increased incidence of candidiasis in patients with impaired cell-mediated immunity. Serum antibodies are not protective, and severe candidal infections are not characteristic of antibody-deficiency disorders.

SYMPTOMS AND CLINICAL MANIFESTATIONS AND DIAGNOSIS

Oral Candidiasis. Acute pseudomembranous candidiasis, or thrush, occurs in up to 5% of newborns. The infant's predisposition to infection probably results from inoculation with *Candida* before the normal bacterial flora is established. Oral thrush presents with discrete white, curdlike patches and plaques on the buccal mucosa, tongue, gingiva, and palate. The lesions are friable and, if forcibly removed, reveal an erythematous, denuded base. Erosions may be painful. **Perlèche,** or **angular cheilitis,** may accompany thrush and can result from repeated trauma, such as lip licking.

Oral candidiasis is usually a self-limited, benign infection that responds to local therapy. Resistance to therapy may indicate an underlying immunodeficiency, including primary immunodeficiencies and HIV infection. Thrush is very uncommon in older children and adolescents unless local factors predispose to infection or the immune system is compromised.

Congenital Candidiasis. Congenital candidiasis is a relatively rare disorder that results from ascending intrauterine infection by *C. albicans.* Although no maternal complications are associated, the umbilical cord and placental membrane may contain yellow papules and plaques consistent with *Candida* funisitis and chorioamnionitis. Skin lesions are present at birth, or arise soon thereafter, and consist of widespread, erythematous macules, papules, and pustules located on the trunk, face, and extremities. The palms and soles may be involved, but the oral mucosa and diaper area are initially spared. Congenital candidiasis is usually self-limited and responds to topical antifungal therapy. Infants at risk of complications are those of low birth weight or with respiratory distress.

Paronychia. *Candida* paronychia occurs most frequently in persons whose hands and fingers are frequently wet. In children, it may result from repeated trauma or sucking on fingers. An acute paronychia causes redness, swelling, and tenderness along the nail fold. A small abscess may develop, and there may be a purulent drainage. Chronic infection can cause dystrophic changes in the nail, such as ridging and fissuring, and the nail itself can become infected by *Candida.* Secondary bacterial infections may require antibiotic therapy.

Diaper Dermatitis. Inflammation of skin chronically occluded by diapers is a common problem that affects approximately 10% of children between birth and 2 years of age. Numerous factors are involved in the pathogenesis of diaper dermatitis. Whether the type of diaper used affects the incidence of diaper dermatitis is a subject of controversy. Several studies have suggested that the use of absorbent disposable diapers is associated with a lower incidence of irritation, whereas other studies produced conflicting results. It is clear that occlusion, such as that occurring under plastic diaper covers, predisposes the skin to maceration. Macerated skin is prone to injury and bacterial or candidal superinfection. Friction may injure the skin, particularly in areas of diaper contact or in skin folds. Urine and feces irritate the skin and may contribute to maceration. *C. albicans* is present in up to 70% of cases of diaper dermatitis and may serve as a primary or secondary pathogen.

Diaper dermatitis causes moist, symmetric red plaques within skin folds of occluded skin. The skin may be macerated and eroded, and there may be papules in the involved area. The presence of satellite pustules, small pustules with an erythematous base at or extending beyond the periphery of the erythema, suggests candidiasis. The diagnosis is confirmed by KOH preparation from skin scrapings. Yeast or pseudohyphae or both are found.

Several dermatologic conditions can mimic diaper dermatitis and should be considered in the differential diagnosis of diaper rashes that do not respond to conventional therapy. Psoriasis, seborrheic dermatitis, and Langerhans cell histiocytosis can present with an erythematous rash in the diaper area. Referral to a dermatologist should be considered for any child who does not respond to topical therapy after several weeks or whose rash recurs. The presence of other skin lesions may also warrant referral.

Chronic Mucocutaneous Candidiasis. Chronic mucocutaneous candidiasis is a group of syndromes characterized by recurrent and persistent *Candida* infections of the nails, skin, and mucous membranes. An underlying abnormality of cell-mediated immunity is present in most patients, and an endocrinopathy may also be present. Chronic mucocutaneous candidiasis usually presents within the first year of life with widespread, often disfiguring lesions of the skin, nails, and mucous membranes. Cutaneous lesions may be markedly hyperkeratotic (Fig. 46–16). Despite the extensive cutaneous involvement, systemic dissemination is rare. Lesions are resistant to topical therapy.

TREATMENT

Oral candidiasis in infants usually responds to treatment with nystatin suspension (100,000 U/mL) 100,000–400,000 U four times a day until symptoms are resolved. Alternatively, nystatin suppositories or clotrimazole troches (10 mg) can be inserted into a pacifier nipple, and the child can be allowed to suck on it. Older children and adults can be treated with clotrimazole troches or with nystatin. Fluconazole may be considered for severe cases, particularly with severe symptoms that inhibit eating and drinking. Oral or intravenous dosing of fluconazole for oropharyngeal or esophageal candidiasis is 6 mg/kg on the first day followed by 3 mg/kg/day until the course is completed, or for at least 2 weeks.

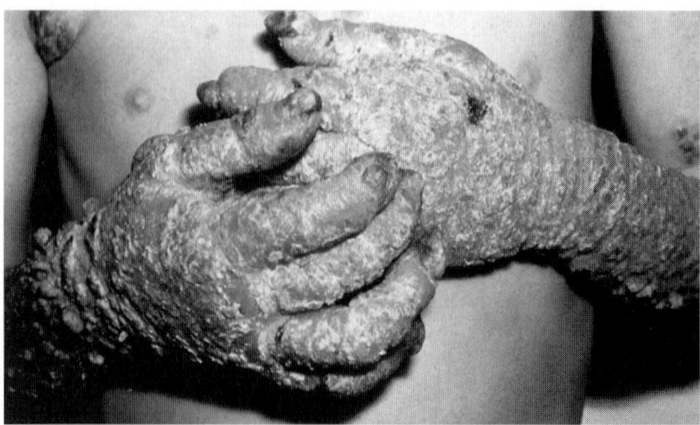

FIGURE 46–16. Chronic mucocutaneous candidiasis. Hyperkeratotic, verrucous lesions on the skin, with onychomycosis of nails.

Cutaneous candidiasis, including diaper dermatitis, paronychia, and congenital candidiasis, usually responds to treatment with topical antifungal agents, including nystatin and the imidazoles. Various imidazole creams are available, including miconazole 2% cream, econazole nitrate 1% cream, and clotrimazole 1% cream. Application twice daily is recommended. Associated oral involvement should also be treated. Chronic mucocutaneous candidiasis is resistant to topical therapy, but systemic treatment with an oral azole (ketoconazole, fluconazole, or itraconazole) may help clear the skin and mucosa. The nails are most recalcitrant to therapy and require a prolonged course. Amphotericin B is also effective but must be given intravenously.

Treatment of diaper dermatitis also requires keeping the involved area as dry as possible, which necessitates frequent diaper changes. The use of overlying plastic diaper covers or plastic-covered disposable diapers should be limited. The skin should be gently cleansed with a mild soap; excessive scrubbing or cleaning might increase irritation. Protective ointment, such as zinc oxide, may help prevent irritation; however, petrolatum may trap moisture in the skin, potentially increasing the risk of maceration. Irritant dermatitis may be treated with hydrocortisone 1% cream applied to the affected area twice daily until the dermatitis heals. If candidiasis is suspected or diagnosed, a topical antifungal cream should be added. Suitable preparations include miconazole 1% cream, econazole nitrate 2% cream, clotrimazole 1% cream, and nystatin. These should be applied to the affected area twice a day until the rash has cleared. Commercial preparations consisting of an antifungal agent combined with a topical corticosteroid are not recommended because the corticosteroid component may be too strong for use in the diaper area. If oral thrush is present, it should be treated with oral nystatin, 100,000–400,000 U four times a day.

SPOROTRICHOSIS

ETIOLOGY

Sporotrichosis is a chronic, granulomatous infection caused by the dimorphic fungus *Sporothrix schenckii.* High humidity and warm temperatures favor growth of the organism, which is present in soil and sphagnum moss and on plants and decaying vegetation.

Transmission. Cutaneous infection results from traumatic inoculation of the fungus. Adults are commonly affected on the upper extremities, and children frequently have lesions on the face. Inhalation or aspiration of spores may lead to pulmonary infection.

EPIDEMIOLOGY

S. schenckii is found worldwide. It is common in Central America, particularly Mexico, and in the United States along the Mississippi and Missouri River valleys.

SYMPTOMS AND CLINICAL MANIFESTATIONS

Cutaneous disease accounts for 75–80% of cases of sporotrichosis, but the organism can cause disseminated disease. Cutaneous sporotrichosis occurs in three clinical subtypes: lymphocutaneous, fixed cutaneous, and disseminated cutaneous disease. **Lymphocutaneous sporotrichosis** is the most common form of sporotrichosis. It classically presents as a painless, firm, pink, papule or pustule that rapidly enlarges to produce a violaceous, necrotic nodule. The infection spreads from the primary lesion along the draining lymphatic vessels, producing an ascending chain of subcutaneous nodules. These may suppurate and drain. Systemic signs and symptoms are unusual, and, unless the patient is immunocompromised, the disease remains limited to the skin, subcutaneous tissues, and lymphatic system. Untreated lesions may heal spontaneously, although scarring or sclerosis of the affected lymphatic system may result.

Fixed cutaneous sporotrichosis results from fungal replication at the site of inoculation but without spread to local lymphatic vessels. Deep inoculation may result in tenosynovitis.

Disseminated sporotrichosis is rare in children with intact cell-mediated immunity. It usually results from the hematogenous spread of pulmonary infection. Cutaneous disease rarely disseminates.

DIAGNOSIS

The diagnosis of sporotrichosis is best established with a fungal culture. *S. schenckii* grows well in several days on most routine fungal culture media. Suitable specimens for culture include exudate from draining lesions or aspirates from nonulcerated, subcutaneous nodules. If a skin biopsy is performed, the specimen should be submitted for both histologic examination and culture.

The differential diagnosis of sporotrichosis includes cutaneous mycobacterial infections, deep fungal infections, anthrax, cat-scratch disease, tularemia, and pyogenic bacterial infections.

The treatment of choice for localized cutaneous or lymphocutaneous sporotrichosis is oral itraconazole (100–200 mg orally once daily for 3–6 months). The alternative treatment with saturated solution of potassium iodide (SSKI; 1 g/mL), which is usually started as 5 drops in water or juice three times a day, gradually increasing to 10 drops a day for a young child, 20–40 drops three times a day for an adolescent, and up to a maximum of 40–50 drops three times a day for an adult, as tolerated. Treatment with SSKI is inexpensive, but it is problematic for many patients because of the difficult dosing regimen. Associated adverse effects of anorexia, nausea, a metallic taste, and rash contribute to poor patient compliance. SSKI is not effective for other forms of sporotrichosis.

A nonpharmacologic therapy is **hyperthermic treatment** in the forms of hot baths (45°C), hot compresses, or a hand-held heating device applied 40–60 minutes per day. This therapy may be appropriate for cutaneous or lymphocutaneous sporotrichosis in pregnant women or in patients who are intolerant of other therapies. It may be used as an adjunctive therapy for patients with osteoarticular sporotrichosis. Treatment is repeated daily for several months. Surgical excision may also be effective for localized disease.

Therapy with amphotericin B has not been as effective for systemic infections as for other systemic mycoses. The preferred treatment for subacute or chronic osteoarticular, pulmonary, or disseminated sporotrichosis is itraconazole 200 mg orally twice daily for 1–2 years. Amphotericin B is recommended for persons who are acutely ill with life-threatening illness or who have meningeal involvement. Amphotericin B is an alternative to itraconazole for other patients.

COMPLICATIONS

Sporotrichosis is usually localized with tissue involvement related to inoculation. Osteomyelitis, septic arthritis, and septic bursitis can be associated with overlying cutaneous infection and should be suspected if the penetrating trauma was deep. Hematologic dissemination and systemic sporotrichosis are rare in healthy persons but have been seen with increased frequency in immunocompromised persons or those with a history of alcohol abuse. The basis for the latter association is not known.

VIRAL INFECTIONS

HERPES SIMPLEX VIRUS

ETIOLOGY

Mucocutaneous herpes simplex virus (HSV) infection is a serious public health problem that affects both children and adults. The spectrum of disease caused by the two serotypes, designated HSV-1 and HSV-2, ranges from asymptomatic infection to disseminated fatal disease. A hallmark of HSV is its ability to establish lifelong latent infection from which it can reactivate.

Transmission. Infection results from contact of the virus, present either in lesions or in infectious secretions, with skin or mucosa. Sexual transmission and autoinoculation occur. Under certain conditions, the virus has been identified on fomites. However, no clear evidence of indirect transmission has been found.

EPIDEMIOLOGY

Herpes simplex viruses are found worldwide, and HSV infection is endemic in the United States. Seroepidemiologic studies of large United States populations show HSV-1 seroprevalence of 85–90% in some adult populations. HSV-1 is usually acquired during childhood; by the age of 5 years, up to 40% of children are seropositive. In contrast, HSV-2 infection is rare in childhood. Antibodies can be detected in fewer than 1% of children younger than 15 years of age. The incidence rises in the late teens and twenties to an estimated adult prevalence as high as 25%. The overall incidence of HSV-2 infection has risen in the past several decades. Poor correlation of clinical history with the presence of antibodies to both HSV subtypes suggests a high incidence of asymptomatic infection.

Recurrent disease occurs with both HSV-1 and HSV-2 infections. The site of infection influences recurrence rates. Genital infections recur more frequently and with a higher incidence than do oral infections. It is estimated that 33% of the adult population in the United States experiences recurrent herpes labialis infections.

Pregnant women with genital herpes, especially primary infections, at the time of delivery may transmit the infection to the newborn before or at the time of delivery.

PATHOGENESIS

Infection of epidermal cells results in cell lysis and death as the virus is released either extracellularly or directly into adjacent cells. Viral latency follows infection of local cutaneous neurons. The virus persists in a latent state in the sensory dorsal root ganglion, and cannot be eradicated by any known treatment. Reactivation can be triggered by stimuli, including trauma, fever, and exposure to ultraviolet light.

Both humoral and cellular defenses are involved in the immune response to HSV infection. The importance of cell-mediated immunity is reflected in the increased frequency and severity of infection experienced by patients with deficient cell-mediated immunity. Antibodies to HSV are formed during the initial infection; however, the presence of antibodies does not protect against recurrence. Moreover, no significant rise in antibody titer is seen during recurrent episodes. The presence of antibodies to either HSV subtype may lessen the risk and severity of subsequent infection by the heterologous virus; however, the antibodies do not provide complete protection against infection.

SYMPTOMS AND CLINICAL MANIFESTATIONS

In addition to skin infections, HSV can also cause herpes gingivostomatitis (Chapter 60), herpes labialis (Chapter 60), and genital herpes infections (Chapter 85).

Cutaneous Infections. Primary and recurrent HSV infections may occur at cutaneous sites other than the mouth and genital tract. The characteristic herpes skin lesions are grouped, 2–4 mm fluid-filled vesicles on an erythematous base (Fig. 46–17). Erythematous papules may precede the vesicles, and if there is significant edema, the vesicles may be difficult to identify. Removal of the vesicle roof with a scalpel blade typically reveals a small, sharply demarcated, ulcer with a ''punched-out'' appearance. Herpetic lesions may be painful, and they may be mistaken for cellulitis or other infectious processes. Within several days, the vesicles rupture, become crusted, and gradually heal. Some vesicles become pustular before crusting. Residual hyperpigmentation may persist, but clinically significant scarring is rare. Regional lymphadenopathy may accompany the skin lesions with primary HSV infection. Recurrences occur in roughly the same location and may be preceded by prodromal symptoms of tingling or burning.

Herpetic whitlow is a herpesvirus infection of the finger pulp (Fig. 46–18). Health care workers, including dentists, dental hygienists, and nurses with exposure to HSV-contaminated oral secretions, are at particularly high risk of contracting this form of infection. Children may inoculate their digits while sucking their thumbs or biting their nails.

Cutaneous herpesvirus infections can be spread during close physical contact. Disease spread among athletes during contact sports has been called **herpes gladiatorum.** The virus can be spread directly from active lesions on the skin or via contaminated oral secretions onto traumatized skin.

Eczema Herpeticum. Cutaneous HSV infection in patients with a compromised skin barrier can result in a widespread disseminated

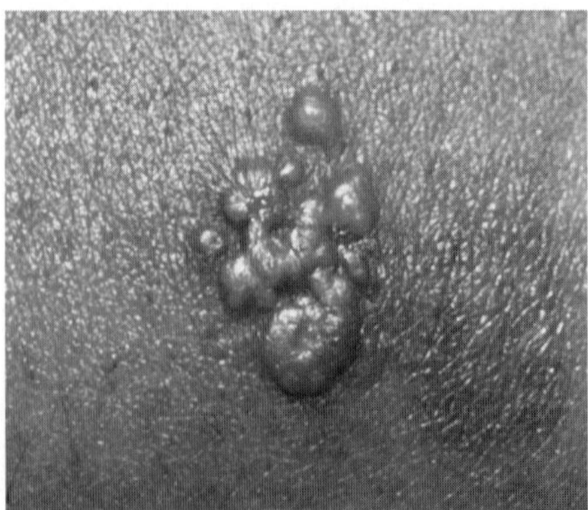

FIGURE 46–17. Recurrent cutaneous herpes simplex virus infection. Hyperpigmented macules around acute vesicles represent postinflammatory scarring from earlier lesions.

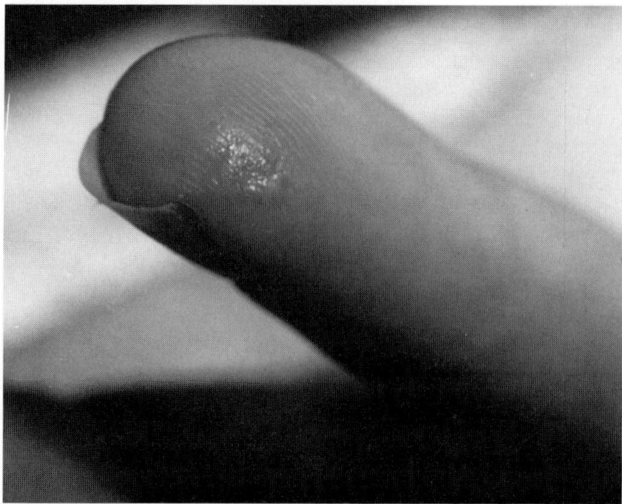

FIGURE 46–18. Herpetic whitlow. Painful herpetic vesicles involving distal fingertip.

infection called **eczema herpeticum,** or **Kaposi's varicelliform eruption.** Atopic dermatitis is the most common underlying disease. Disease results either from primary exposure to HSV or from recurrence of latent infection. Clinically, hundreds of herpetic vesicles may cover large areas of the body. Usually the infection spreads across otherwise abnormal skin; however, the vesicles can also arise on clinically normal skin (Fig. 46–19). Eczema herpeticum is clinically distinguished from herpes zoster by its random distribution, which may involve many dermatomes. In addition, lesions of eczema herpeticum are often isolated and are not grouped, as are the vesicles of herpes zoster. If untreated, lesions continue to erupt in successive crops over several weeks, often associated with fever and lymphadenopathy. There is a risk of secondary bacterial infection and systemic dissemination. Aggressive treatment with oral antiviral therapy is indicated. Similar eruptions have been described in association with vaccinia virus and coxsackievirus infections.

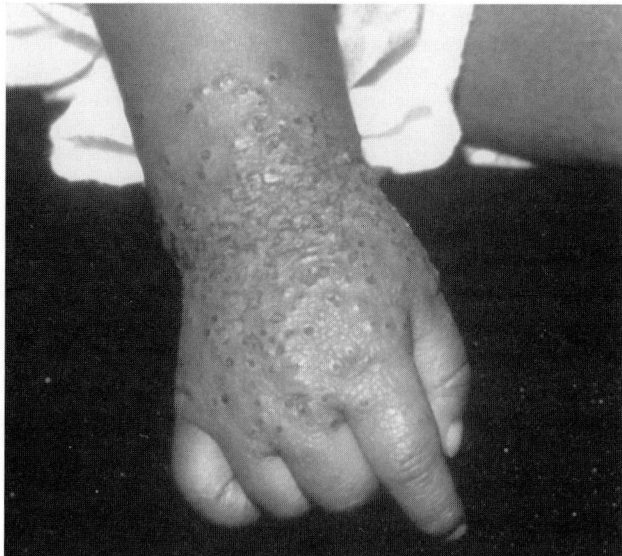

FIGURE 46–19. Eczema herpeticum. Multiple, widespread tender vesicles of HSV arising on the hand of a child with severe atopic dermatitis.

Herpes Simplex Infections in Immunocompromised Persons. HSV infections in immunocompromised persons tend to be more severe and prolonged than those in immunocompetent persons. Oral herpes infections may spread to cause pharyngitis, esophagitis, or pneumonitis. Viremia with visceral dissemination may occur during both primary and recurrent infections. Concurrent infections with other opportunistic pathogens such as *C. albicans* should be considered, particularly in cases resistant to therapy.

A chronic herpes simplex infection should be considered in the differential diagnosis of any nonhealing skin ulcer in an immunocompromised patient, particularly lesions around the mouth or genitals. Although the characteristic vesicles may have been present at the time of onset, as the lesion becomes chronic, skin ulceration is more common (Fig. 46–20). Ulcers may be large or small, and often one to many small, punctate ulcers persist. The diagnosis is difficult to establish with a Tzanck smear, and usually a culture or skin biopsy is needed. Prolonged antiviral therapy until the wounds have healed is necessary, with the duration determined by the clinical response.

DIAGNOSIS

In most cases, the diagnosis of herpes simplex infection can be established on the basis of clinical appearance. Direct immunofluorescence testing provides a rapid diagnosis of varicella-zoster virus infection. Immunofluorescence screening for HSV is also available at some institutions. However, the virus grows quickly in culture, and culture results are usually available within 24–48 hours. A viral culture remains the most sensitive and specific method of diagnosis of HSV infection. Positive cultures are obtained from up to 94% of vesicles, 87% of pustules, 70% of ulcers, and 27% of crusted lesions. Varicella-zoster virus can also be grown in culture, but it may require several days for isolation. Because varicella-zoster virus is highly cell-associated and extremely labile, the sensitivity of viral culture is relatively low.

Serologic tests may be helpful in the diagnosis of primary infection if seroconversion is documented. Elevated antibodies in-

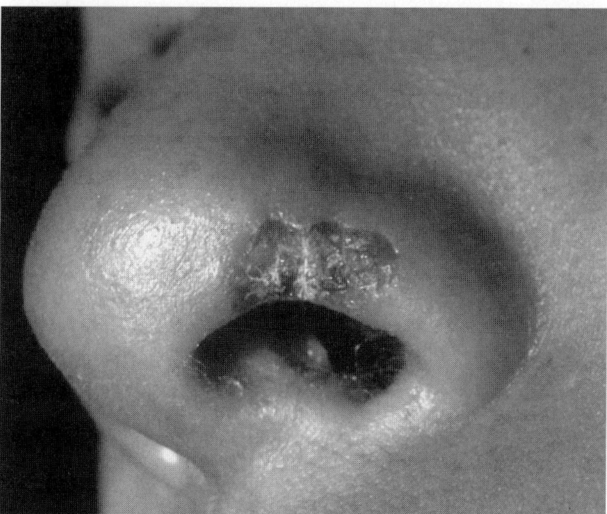

FIGURE 46–20. Herpes simplex in an immunosuppressed child. Autoinoculation of HSV from the finger of a child with HIV infection and herpetic whitlow resulted in this slowly healing ulcer.

dicate prior infection but are not helpful in the diagnosis of recurrent infections. Although commonly reported separately, commercial HSV antibody tests do not reliably distinguish between HSV-1 and HSV-2 antibodies.

The Tzanck smear provides cytologic confirmation when multinucleated giant cells can be identified (Fig. 46–21). This test is relatively easy and inexpensive to perform; however, proper interpretation requires experience. An early, intact vesicle is carefully swabbed with alcohol and unroofed with a No. 15 scalpel blade. The vesicle fluid is aspirated, the base and sides of the ulcer are gently scraped to obtain cellular material, and the sample is submitted for direct immunofluorescence studies and viral culture. The sensitivity of the Tzanck smear is highest when the sample is taken from an intact vesicle and decreases considerably when lesions have crusted or dried. A Tzanck smear cannot distinguish between HSV-1, HSV-2, and varicella-zoster infections. A skin biopsy may be performed when the diagnosis is unclear and may be necessary to establish the diagnosis of lesions in immunocompromised patients.

TREATMENT

Cutaneous herpesvirus infections are self-limited, and treatment is optional for uncomplicated infections in immunocompromised children. Treatment with topical or oral antiviral agents may shorten the duration of viral shedding and hasten the time to healing. Although its use in children has not been established, oral acyclovir or topical penciclovir 1% cream, applied to herpes labialis every 2 hours for 4 days, is used for oral herpetic gingivostomatitis (Table 60-3). Similar regimens could be used for localized cutaneous herpes infections in immunocompetent persons. Oral acyclovir, valacyclovir, and famciclovir are used for the treatment of primary and recurrent genital herpes (Chapter 85). Antiviral treatment does not, unfortunately, prevent development of latent infection or eradicate latent infection.

Eczema herpeticum often requires aggressive treatment in the hospital setting. Intravenous antiviral therapy should be continued until the patient is stabilized and no new lesions are seen. Oral or intravenous therapy should also be considered for children with chronic skin disorders that may predispose to the development of eczema herpeticum. Chronic infections should be treated until they heal.

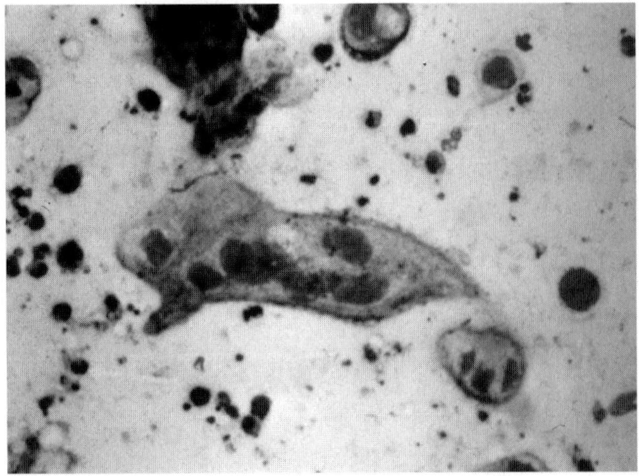

FIGURE 46–21. Tzanck preparation. Multinucleated giant cells that are consistent with a herpesvirus infection are present. Multinucleated giant cells are also seen with varicella-zoster virus (chickenpox).

COMPLICATIONS

Local or systemic dissemination can complicate herpes simplex infections. Herpes simplex keratitis is the most common cause of corneal blindness in the United States. Primary or recurrent HSV infection in children and adults may result in encephalitis, presumably by neurotropic spread of the virus through the olfactory bulb. Recurrent erythema multiforme has been clearly associated with HSV infection. Disseminated infection rarely occurs in immunocompetent children.

PROGNOSIS

HSV infections cause considerable morbidity in both immunocompetent and immunocompromised persons. The establishment of latency leaves infected patients at risk of lifelong recurrences. In some patients, however, the frequency of recurrence decreases with the duration of infection.

PREVENTION

Avoidance of exposure to the virus is at present the only certain preventive measure. Patients with oral or genital herpes should be reminded of the contagious nature of the disease and should avoid exposure to uninfected partners when active lesions are present. Patients should also be warned that, in some instances, HSV could be transmitted in the absence of apparent clinical lesions. Regular use of barrier contraceptive devices may provide some protection from genital transmission. Suppressive therapy with daily doses of acyclovir or other antiviral agents can also help limit outbreaks (Chapter 85).

HUMAN PAPILLOMAVIRUSES

ETIOLOGY

Human papillomaviruses (HPV) belong to the family Papovaviridae and cause a range of infection from asymptomatic, latent infection to squamous cell carcinoma. More than 80 HPV genotypes have been identified, although the actual number of types may exceed 200. Different types appear to have anatomic specificity and are linked with specific clinical findings (Table 46–11). Papillomaviruses are host-specific, and HPV infect only humans.

Transmission. HPV can be transmitted through direct person-to-person contact, including sexual contact, and by fomites. Warts may be transmitted to the genital area from other areas of the body, often by transmission on the hands of the patient, by autoinoculation, or by the caretaker. The number of infectious virion particles in a given wart varies by the type and age of the lesion; new lesions usually contain a greater number of infectious virions than do older lesions.

EPIDEMIOLOGY

Nongenital **warts** occur frequently in children and young adults, with an estimated incidence of 5–10%. The incidence may be higher among institutionalized children. Persons with a history of warts are likely to develop other lesions. Immunocompromised patients, particularly renal allograft recipients, and others with compromised cell-mediated immunity have a very high incidence of warts. Genital warts are a sexually transmitted infection (Chapter 85).

TABLE 46–11. Association of Common Human Papillomavirus (HPV) Types with Clinical Disease

Benign Proliferations	Malignant Proliferations
Type 1	
Deep plantar warts	
Types 1, 2, 4, 29	
Common and plantar warts	
Types 3, 10, 28	
Flat warts	
Types 26, 27, 49	
Common and flat warts in immunocompromised patients	
Types 5, 8, 9, 12, 14, 15, 17, 19–25, 36–38, 46, 47, 49, 50	
Flat warts and papillomas in patients with epidermodysplasla verruciformis	Skin carcinomas usually at sun-exposed sites in epidermodysplasia verruciformis patients
Types 6, 11 (16, 30, 42, 43, 44, 54 less often)	
Condyloma acuminatum	Verrucous carcinoma, Buschke-Löwenstein tumors
Types 16, 18 (31, 33, 35, 39, 45, 51, 52, 56, 59, 61 less often)	
Cervical, vulvar, penile, and perianal intraepithelial neoplasia	Cervical, vulvar, penile, perianal, and anal cancer

PATHOGENESIS

Minor skin trauma facilitates entrance of the virus into the skin. The incubation period varies from weeks to months. HPV infects the epidermis and stimulates hyperplasia, causing the characteristic verrucous lesions. Viral particles are detectable in the upper epidermis, at or above the granular layer. Two thirds of warts in healthy children resolve spontaneously within 2 years. Both humoral and cell-mediated immunity appear to be involved in wart regression.

SYMPTOMS AND CLINICAL MANIFESTATIONS

Common Warts (Verruca Vulgaris). Common warts are usually small, rough, hyperkeratotic papules, arranged singly or in groups (Fig. 46–22). They may be located on any skin surface but are most commonly found on the hands, fingers, and knees of children. Paring of the surface may expose **black dots** that are thrombosed capillaries. Warts distort dermatoglyphic lines, and periungual lesions may cause localized nail dystrophy. Most common warts are asymptomatic.

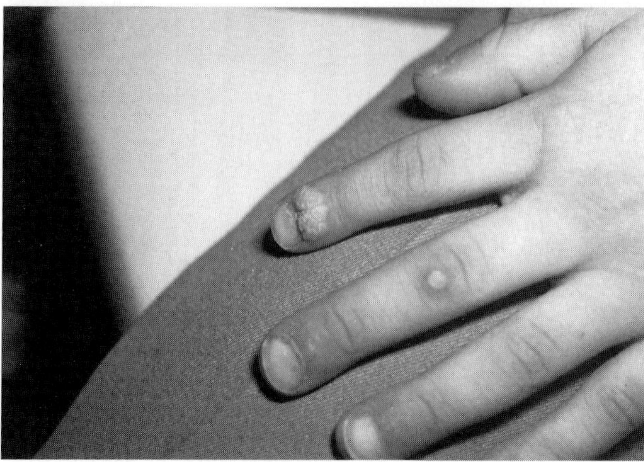

FIGURE 46–22. Common warts (verruca vulgaris).

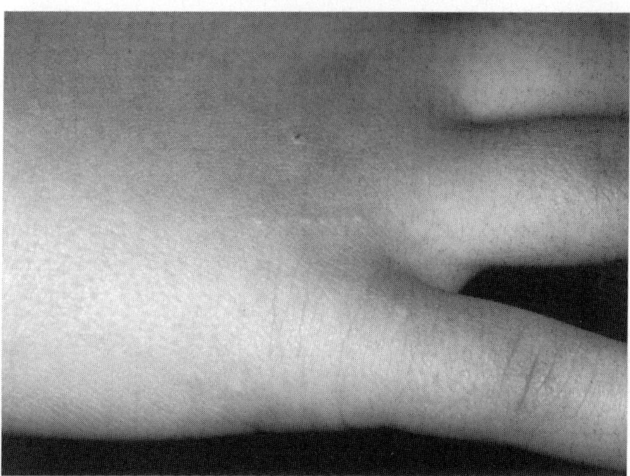

FIGURE 46–23. Flat warts (verruca plana). Subtle, flesh-colored papules in a linear distribution on the dorsum of the hand of a child. The distribution results from autoinoculation during trauma, such as scratching.

Plantar Warts. Plantar warts are commonly found on pressure sites of the foot, including the heel and metatarsal heads. Lesions are relatively flat, hyperkeratotic plaques that may be surrounded by a rim of thickened skin. Black dots are often present and, when found, help distinguish the lesions from corns and calluses. Multiple warts may coalesce into larger mosaic warts.

Flat Warts (Verruca Plana). Flat warts are smooth, slightly elevated papules that are clinically distinct from common warts. They are usually small, measuring less than 5 mm in diameter, with a color ranging from tan to pink. Flat warts are present most commonly on the face and extremities and may occur as multiple lesions (Fig. 46–23).

Filiform Warts. These long, slender projections are present most commonly on the face, around the eyelids, nares, and lips.

Anogenital Warts. Anogenital lesions may take several different forms. Large, hyperkeratotic, cauliflower-like lesions called **condylomata acuminata** usually occur in moist areas of the groin, such as around the labia and anus (Fig. 46–24). The lesions may become large and exophytic. Other lesions include sessile, verrucous papules found on the shaft of the penis and on the scrotum. The lesions generally remain smaller than the hyperkeratotic lesions.

Laryngeal Papillomas. Laryngeal or respiratory papillomas result from the acquisition of HPV at birth from maternal genital warts. The papillomas are extremely rare and usually are discovered during early childhood when the child develops an abnormal cry or a change in voice. They may extend to involve the trachea, bronchi, and lung parenchyma.

DIAGNOSIS

Most warts are diagnosed by their characteristic clinical appearance. Skin biopsy provides histologic confirmation when needed. HPV typing is not routinely performed.

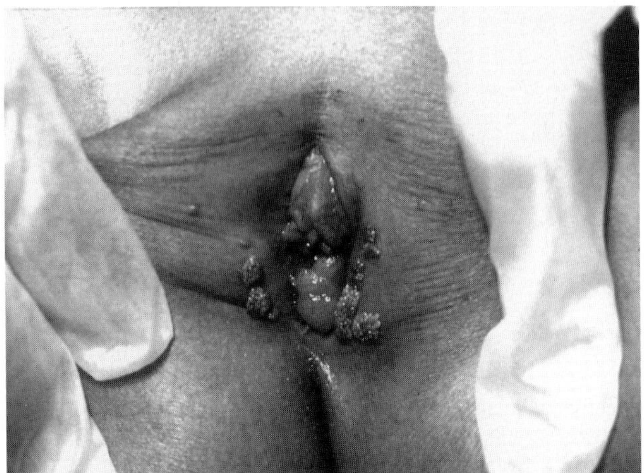

FIGURE 46–24. Perianal warts. Multiple verrucous papules arising around the anus in a victim of sexual child abuse.

TREATMENT

Because of the high rate of spontaneous resolution, treatment of warts should be designed to minimize the risk of scarring and trauma to the child. Common treatments for nongenital warts include cryotherapy and chemical destruction with topical salicylic acid or salicylic acid–lactic acid preparations. Application of topical agents for up to 6 weeks or longer may be necessary. Other acids, including trichloroacetic acid, have been used, as have pharmacologic agents, including podophyllin, cantharidin, topical retinoid acid, and 5-fluorouracil. Surgical removal of warts may be considered for lesions that are resistant to conservative therapy. Electrosurgery and carbon dioxide laser therapies are effective modalities. Periungual warts may be particularly difficult to eradicate, especially if the wart extends under the nail plate. Removal of the nail, followed by laser destruction of the wart, is often required to eliminate the wart. Because of the potential for permanent nail dystrophy, it is recommended that only experienced physicians perform this procedure.

Genital lesions are generally treated by cryotherapy, podophyllin, or a combination of the two. Purified podophyllotoxin is available for patient application. An immunomodulatory topical cream, imiquimod 5% cream, was recently approved for the treatment of genital warts in children and adults. Imiquimod induces local production of interferons and other cytokines that presumably enhance the cell-mediated immune response to papillomavirus-infected keratinocytes. The cream is applied three times a week to the affected areas until lesions resolve. Imiquimod cream is usually well tolerated and has few adverse effects other than occasional irritation. This is particularly important in the setting of child abuse, as aggressive, potentially painful interventions should be avoided in this vulnerable population. Laser surgery or excision may be needed to remove larger, exophytic lesions.

The pediatrician can initiate treatment of simple, common warts with topical preparations. Use of cryotherapy and electrocautery should be limited to physicians who are trained in their use. Immunocompromised children, as well as patients with lesions that do not respond to conservative measures, should be referred to a dermatologist for evaluation and treatment. Children with anogenital warts are best evaluated in a center with the resources to screen for child abuse.

Juvenile laryngeal papillomas causing airway or vocalization problems traditionally have been treated with laser surgery. Laser surgery used as a single modality usually requires repeated treatments, and recurrences are common. Repeated injections of IFN-α three times each week for up to 13 months have been used with some success. However, HPV persists in the lesions even after IFN-α therapy, and the ultimate response is variable.

Sexual Abuse. The presence of condylomata in children may serve as a marker of child abuse, but the presence of genital warts alone cannot be considered proof of sexual contact. Many genital warts in children contain HPV types that are usually isolated from nongenital warts. A complete evaluation should include a thorough history and, if possible, physical examination of all potential sources of wart exposure, including caretakers and siblings. Careful attention should be paid to the appropriateness of the child's response to both caretaker and physician during the office visit. The physical examination should include an evaluation for other signs of abuse, such as rectal or vaginal tears or scarring. Any findings suggestive of sexual abuse require the involvement of appropriate social service and law enforcement authorities.

COMPLICATIONS

Most warts are benign, transient infections that resolve without sequelae, either spontaneously or with therapy. Human papillomavirus infection has been associated with the development of various malignant neoplasms, including cervical carcinoma (related to HPV types 16 and 18), squamous cell carcinoma (particularly in immunocompromised patients), verrucous carcinoma, Bowen's disease, and certain carcinomas of the head and neck and gastrointestinal tract (Chapter 4).

MOLLUSCUM CONTAGIOSUM

ETIOLOGY

Molluscum contagiosum is a benign, papular skin infection common in children and young adults. It is caused by the molluscum contagiosum virus (MCV), a large DNA virus of the Poxviridae family. Three different MCV types (MCV I, II, and III) have been identified with the use of restriction endonuclease digestion techniques. Lesions caused by different subtypes are clinically indistinguishable. MCV III is uncommon.

Transmission. The virus can be spread by direct contact, autoinoculation, and possibly contact with fomites. Infectivity is generally low. Genital lesions can be sexually transmitted.

EPIDEMIOLOGY

Molluscum contagiosum occurs worldwide, with an annual incidence of 2–8%. Epidemiologic studies suggest that the incidence in the United States rose 11-fold between 1966 and 1983. Infection is most common in children and young adults; older adults are rarely infected. Immunocompromised persons are at risk of widespread lesions.

PATHOGENESIS

Viral replication occurs in the cytoplasm of epidermal keratinocytes. The epidermis hypertrophies, proliferating down into the dermis and extending upward to produce the clinical lesion. Infected cells contain characteristic eosinophilic, intracytoplasmic inclusion bodies called **Henderson-Paterson bodies.** Ultrastructural studies of lesions have identified viral particles in all layers of the epidermis.

SYMPTOMS AND CLINICAL MANIFESTATIONS

The incubation period varies from 2 weeks to 3 months. The site of infection varies among age groups. Children are most frequently infected on the face, trunk, and extremities, reflecting transmission of the virus by direct contact. Lesions may affect the eyelid or its margins. In adolescents, lesions are frequently found in the genital area and may be the result of sexual transmission. The characteristic skin lesion is a small, smooth, firm, flesh-colored to pink papule with **central umbilication** (Fig. 46–25). A **central core** can often be expressed. There are usually 1–20 papules present, which may be grouped or arranged in a linear array if they arise in a site of previous trauma. Isolated lesions usually measure 2–5 mm in diameter; however, giant mollusca measuring 10–15 mm may occur. Careful examination of these lesions will usually reveal multiple coalescing papules. Lesions are usually asymptomatic, but they may be pruritic or tender. Previously stable lesions may spontaneously become red and inflamed, representing the development of an immune response to the virus that typically heralds clearance of the lesion. The inflamed papules are frequently misdiagnosed and thought to be infected, leading to unnecessary treatment with antibiotics. In patients with impaired immunity or pre-existing skin diseases, such as atopic dermatitis, widespread lesions may develop.

DIAGNOSIS

The diagnosis of molluscum contagiosum is usually established on the basis of clinical appearance alone. The differential diagnosis includes common and flat warts, chickenpox, juvenile xanthogranuloma, adenoma sebaceum, syringomas, and trichoepitheliomas. Inflamed lesions may resemble folliculitis, furuncles, or cysts. Histologic evaluation of a skin biopsy specimen confirms the clinical diagnosis but is rarely necessary. Smears of the central core stained with Wright, Giemsa, or Gram stain demonstrate the characteristic inclusion bodies.

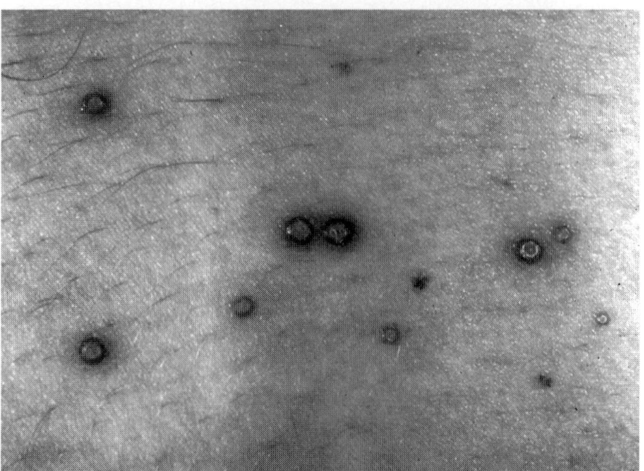

FIGURE 46–25. Molluscum contagiosum. Characteristic umbilicated papules.

TREATMENT

Molluscum contagiosum is usually a self-limited disease. Lesions left untreated in an immunocompetent person resolve spontaneously within several months to years. Treatment may lessen the incidence of autoinoculation and direct transmission to others. Immunocompromised persons and those with pre-existing skin diseases warrant more aggressive therapy. The age of the patient and site of the lesions should also be considered in the choice of therapy. In older patients with a limited number of lesions, sharp curettage with removal of the core is a reasonable choice. Pain can be minimized with topical application of anesthetic cream (2.5% lidocaine and 2.5% prilocaine) before treatment. In younger children or those with numerous lesions, topical 0.9% cantharidin is an effective, painless alternative. It is essential that the cantharidin be applied sparingly, and it must be washed off within 4 hours. Blistering may result. Occasionally, use of cantharidin is complicated by development of multiple molluscum lesions at the periphery of the blister. Some children tolerate cryotherapy with liquid nitrogen; application with a cotton-tipped applicator may minimize pain and trauma to uninvolved skin. Other treatment options include tretinoin cream or gel, podophyllin, salicylic acid-lactic acid preparations, and imiquimod cream.

COMPLICATIONS AND PROGNOSIS

Complications are rare, and most lesions resolve with time or treatment. Lesions on the eyelid margin shed virus and may produce a follicular conjunctional reaction and an irritating punctate keratitis, associated with light sensitivity. Treatment of periocular molluscum is potentially dangerous, and consultation with an ophthalmologist is strongly recommended. Patients with impaired systemic or cutaneous immunity may develop widespread lesions, although systemic spread of the virus has not been observed.

PARASITIC INFECTIONS

CUTANEOUS LARVA MIGRANS

Cutaneous larva migrans, also known as **creeping eruption,** is caused by the migration of nematode larvae within the skin. The most common pathogen in the United States is *Ancylostoma braziliense,* the dog and cat hookworm, and rarely *Ancylostoma caninum,* which is found only in dogs. This intensely pruritic eruption is found worldwide and is particularly common in warm, tropical regions. It is endemic to the southeastern and Gulf coasts of the United States.

Ova deposited in the feces of an infected animal mature into noninfectious, rhabditiform larvae, which, after feeding, molt into infectious, filiform larvae. These enter human skin on contact and migrate within the epidermis above the basal layer. Larvae migrate millimeters to centimeters a day, producing the characteristic **serpiginous tracts.**

Because of the source of contact, common areas of involvement include the dorsal feet, buttocks, hands, and knees. Skin between the toes may be infected. An erythematous, pruritic papule may be identified at the entry site, followed by development of serpiginous, red tracts or plaques (Fig. 46–26). Vesicles may develop along the tracts, and scratching may result in secondary impetiginization. Eosinophilia may be associated. Visceral dissemination can occur but is rare.

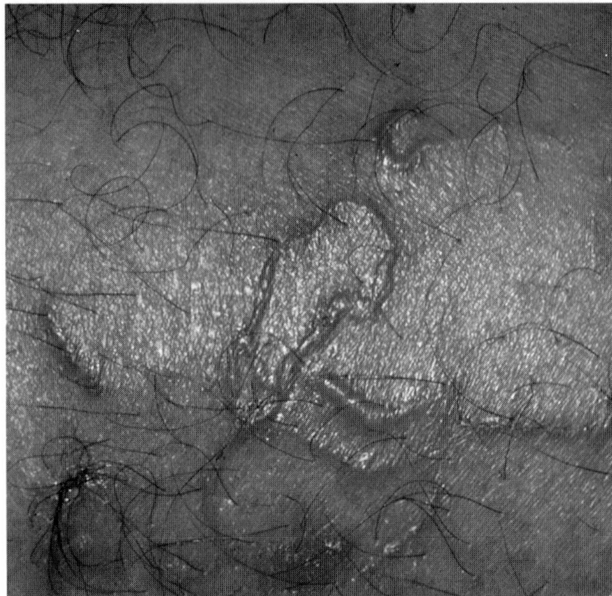

FIGURE 46–26. Cutaneous larva migrans (creeping eruption). Raised, red, pruritic serpiginous tracts in the skin caused by the migration of nematode larvae within the skin.

Cutaneous larva migrans is usually self-limited and resolves spontaneously within 1–3 months. Therapy is often necessary because of the intense pruritus. Effective treatment regimens include albendazole and ivermectin (Table 42-4).

CUTANEOUS LEISHMANIASIS

ETIOLOGY

Leishmaniasis is an infection caused by at least 12 different species of the genus *Leishmania,* which are intracellular parasitic flagellates. There are three clinical expressions of this infection: cutaneous, mucosal, and visceral leishmaniasis. The cutaneous form is the most common and the only form occurring in the United States. **Old World cutaneous leishmaniasis** is caused by *L. major, L. tropica,* and *L. aethiopica.* **New World cutaneous leishmaniasis** is caused by either *L. mexicana,* which is found in south Texas through Central America, or *L. brasiliensis.* **Visceral leishmaniasis** in the Old World is caused by *L. donovani,* and in the New World by *L. donovani chagasi,* which is found in Central and South America and rarely in Mexico. Cutaneous leishmaniasis is generally mild but may cause cosmetic disfigurement. Visceral leishmaniasis is associated with significant morbidity and mortality.

Transmission. Transmission may be either zoonotic (by rodents) or anthroponotic, with the common vector being the female sandfly (*Phlebotomus, Lutzomyia,* or *Psychodopygus*). Ingested amastigotes transform and multiply into the promastigote form and subsequently infect the sandfly bite wound. Once inoculated, promastigotes are engulfed by histiocytes and multiply. The promastigotes are released from the histiocytes to seed tissue and continue the life cycle.

EPIDEMIOLOGY

Descriptions of cutaneous leishmaniasis are found in the Old Testament, and throughout history this disease has had various names including Jericho boil, Delhi boil, Aleppo boil, and chiclero's ulcer. Cutaneous leishmaniasis is endemic in five continents, with an estimated annual incidence of 1–1.5 million cases. Although cutaneous leishmaniasis has been reported in more than 80 countries, 90% of all cases occur in Afghanistan, Iran, Saudi Arabia, Syria, Brazil, and Peru. In endemic areas, cutaneous leishmaniasis occurs most commonly in children, and many children in these areas demonstrate evidence of past infection. Cases of cutaneous leishmaniasis in the United States occur primarily in travelers or immigrants.

PATHOGENESIS AND CLINICAL MANIFESTATIONS

The clinical manifestations depend on the interplay of parasitic virulence and host defenses. Cutaneous leishmaniasis begins as an inflamed vesicopustule several weeks to months after a sandfly bite. The papule enlarges and crusts, often leaving a shallow ulcer with a sharp, indurated margin (Fig. 46–27). Lesions often heal within 2 weeks and leave a variable degree of scarring. More extensive cutaneous, nasal, and visceral involvement may occur, depending on the infecting species and the host immune response.

DIAGNOSIS

The development of one or several slowly progressive, nontender, nodular or ulcerative lesions combined with potential exposure in an endemic area suggests the possibility of cutaneous leishmaniasis. The differential diagnosis includes sporotrichosis, blastomycosis, cutaneous tuberculosis, cutaneous nontuberculous mycobacterial infections, leprosy, and ecthyma.

Examination of tissue from ulcerated skin lesions with Giemsa or Wright staining may reveal characteristic 2 to 4 μm oval bodies with a single nucleus and kinetoplast. Organisms can be grown from tissue biopsy in **Novy-MacNeal-Nicolle (NNN)** culture medium at 24°C in approximately two thirds of the cases. Serologic testing with the use of an ELISA assay has very high specificity and sensitivity. Skin biopsy is also characteristic, with granulomatous infiltration in the dermis and epidermis and, in advanced stages, showing dense infiltration by macrophages containing numerous amastigotes.

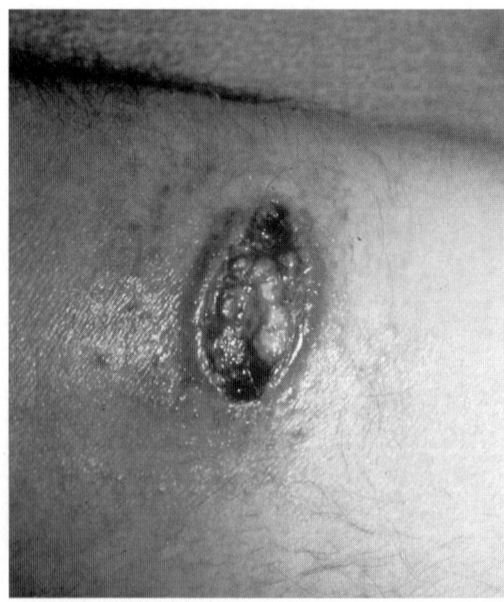

FIGURE 46–27. Cutaneous leishmaniasis. Shallow ulcer with a sharp, raised border on the extremities.

TREATMENT

Treatment should take into consideration host defenses, strain virulence, and the reality that many of these lesions will heal spontaneously. For limited cutaneous disease, physically destructive modalities, including liquid nitrogen cryotherapy, thermotherapy, electrocautery, and surgical excision, may be effective. Topical application of the aminoglycoside antibiotic paromomycin twice daily for 10–20 days can be curative. Topical antifungal agents have been used but do not appear to be effective. In cases in which spread beyond the skin is likely, because of either strain virulence or host immunosuppression, systemic therapy is warranted. Pentavalent antimony (20 mg/kg/day intravenously or intramuscularly for 20–28 days) is first-line therapy for cutaneous leishmaniasis with extensive spread or if there is facial involvement. Adverse effects include ECG changes, elevated transaminase levels, pancreatitis, and neuropathy. Alternative systemic agents include pentamidine, oral paromomycin, liposomal amphotericin B, allopurinol, azole antifungal agents, and dapsone. A new oral agent, miltefosine, a lecithin analog, appears promising.

COMPLICATIONS AND PROGNOSIS

Localized cutaneous leishmaniasis may result in significant hypopigmentation or hyperpigmentation and depressed, irregular scarring. New World cutaneous leishmaniasis, particularly that caused by *L. brasiliensis,* may cause ulcerative lesions of the nasopharynx and may spread in the skin via the lymphatic vessels. If there is nasal involvement (mucocutaneous leishmaniasis or espundia), significant mutilation of the mouth, palate, nose, and trachea can result, often leading to fatal sepsis. Prevention by avoidance of exposure to nocturnal sandflies and use of insect repellent can be helpful in controlling transmission. Community-based sandfly or host eradication programs have had some success. Vaccination of humans or domestic dogs may have a role in the future.

INFESTATIONS

MYIASIS

Myiasis is the infestation of mammalian tissues by the larvae, or maggots, of flies. Many species of flies are capable of causing the condition, and although animals are more frequently involved, humans can be affected after the appropriate exposure.

Myiasis occurs worldwide, but it is more common in tropical environments. The skin is the most frequently involved site, although any exposed organ can be affected, including the eye, nasopharynx, gastrointestinal tract, and urogenital tract. Two forms of cutaneous myiasis are recognized: wound myiasis and furuncular myiasis.

Wound myiasis in the United States is commonly caused by *Callitroga americana,* the screw worm fly. The common housefly, *Musca domestica,* is an infrequent, accidental parasite. Wound myiasis results when the fly, possibly attracted by blood or necrotic tissue, lays her eggs on the wound surface. The larvae hatch and feed on the necrotic debris. The maggots usually remain on the wound surface, and tissue invasion is rare; however, certain species can burrow into living tissue.

Treatment of wound myiasis involves application of 10–15% chloroform in vegetable oil to the ulcer for 30 minutes. The dead maggots can then be extracted. Successful use of ethyl chloride spray has also been reported.

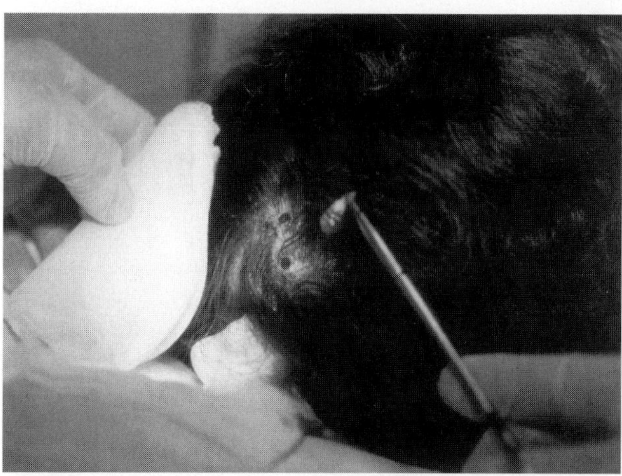

FIGURE 46–28. Furuncular myiasis. Surgical extraction of the larva from a pustule in the scalp.

Furuncular myiasis in the New World is frequently caused by the **human botfly,** *Dermatobia hominis.* The fly is common in parts of South and Central America, where cattle infestations are of serious economic importance. Cases found in the United States are usually imported. *D. hominis* is an obligate parasite that lays its eggs on the underside of another insect, such as a mosquito or tick. The larvae hatch and penetrate through the skin of the victim during feeding. Within several days, a red, raised, 2- to 4-mm papule develops at the site of penetration. A central pore, through which the larva breathes, may be visible in the center of the papule. The lesion may be tender or pruritic and may discharge pus or serum. If the lesion is not treated, the larva matures within 6–7 weeks, emerges, and drops off.

Treatment of furuncular myiasis usually involves surgical removal of the larva. Occlusion of the larval breathing tube by such substances as pork fat, beeswax, and chewing gum also has been used successfully to treat the infestation. As the larva is deprived of air, it emerges to the skin surface, from which it can be easily removed (Fig. 46–28). A thick coat of petrolatum might function similarly.

Complications of cutaneous myiasis are unusual. A secondary bacterial infection may develop in furuncular myiasis.

SCABIES

ETIOLOGY

Scabies is a common, often intensely pruritic dermatosis caused by the mite *Sarcoptes scabiei.* This infestation is estimated to affect at least 300 million people worldwide. Scabies can be complicated by secondary bacterial infections.

EPIDEMIOLOGY

Scabies occurs in all age groups and in both sexes. Transmission occurs through close personal contact with an infected person. Clustered outbreaks occur in hospitals and nursing homes and among families. The mite can survive off the human body for up to 34 hours, and fomite transmission is thought to be possible.

PATHOGENESIS

A gravid female mite burrows into the superficial epidermis, where she lays 2–3 eggs daily, leaving behind feces or **scybala.** This process continues for approximately 30 days. The eggs hatch, and the resultant larvae emerge to mature. An average of 10–20 mites is present on an immunocompetent patient at a given time. Patients who are immunocompromised or neurologically impaired may develop a severe form of the disease known as **Norwegian** or **crusted scabies** with infestation of up to 2 million live mites at one time.

The onset of clinical symptoms is delayed in primary infestations, as itching results from hypersensitivity to the mite or its byproducts. Allergic sensitization to the mite or mite products develops over several weeks, and, on subsequent infestation, symptoms begin within 24 hours.

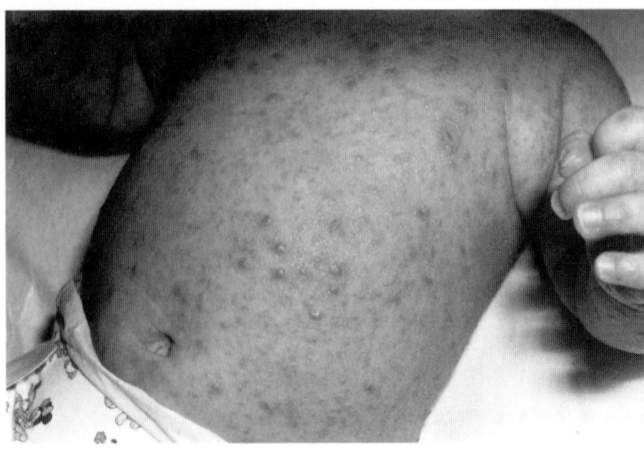

FIGURE 46–30. Scabies. Widespread infestation of an infant.

SYMPTOMS AND CLINICAL MANIFESTATIONS

Pruritus is the major symptom and may be more severe at night than during the day. Scabies is characterized by small, erythematous papules, pustules, and fine linear burrows that involve the finger webs (Fig. 46–29), the flexor aspect of the wrists, the elbows, the axillary folds, the waist, and the periumbilical skin. The penis, scrotum, and areola may be affected. Lesions in infants and young children often form vesicles or nodules and may involve the head and neck, diaper area, and axilla (Fig. 46–30). Palm and sole involvement is a distinctive feature of scabies infection during infancy.

If the infestation is untreated, the characteristic pattern of distribution may be lost, making the diagnosis more difficult to establish. Chronic lesions may become crusted or nodular. In crusted scabies, a thick, malodorous, scaly crust develops on affected areas, and the entire body may become red and scaly. Nail dystrophy may also be associated with scabies.

DIAGNOSIS

The diagnosis of scabies is confirmed by microscopic identification of the mite, eggs, larvae, and feces (Fig. 46–31). Multiple papules, vesicles, or burrows are carefully scraped with a No. 15 scalpel blade dipped in a drop of mineral oil. The oil helps collect the skin particles. The mite, eggs, or scybala should be evident on low-power microscopy. A skin biopsy is helpful in the diagnosis of atypical cases, particularly if lesions have become nodular.

TREATMENT

The safest and most effective treatment of scabies is permethrin 5% cream, which is applied overnight to the entire body. Treatment should be repeated in 1 week. Permethrin should not be used in infants younger than 2 months of age. Lindane 1% lotion is also effective, but rare reports of neurotoxicity have limited its use in young children. Crotamiton cream and precipitated sulfur (6% in petrolatum) are considerably less effective than the other agents. Precipitated sulfur is safe for use in young infants. It is applied nightly for 3 nights and washed off in 24 hours. Although not presently approved by the FDA for this use, the oral antiparasitic agent ivermectin (200 μg/kg orally as a single dose) has been used successfully for the treatment of scabies in both immunocompetent and immunocompromised persons.

Because the mite lives only a short time off the body, extensive fumigation of the home and furniture is not necessary. Clothing, towels, and bed linens should be laundered in hot water. In most cases, treatment of family members and close contacts is also indicated. Children with crusted scabies may require repeated treatments; the patient should be considered potentially infectious as long as any crusts persist.

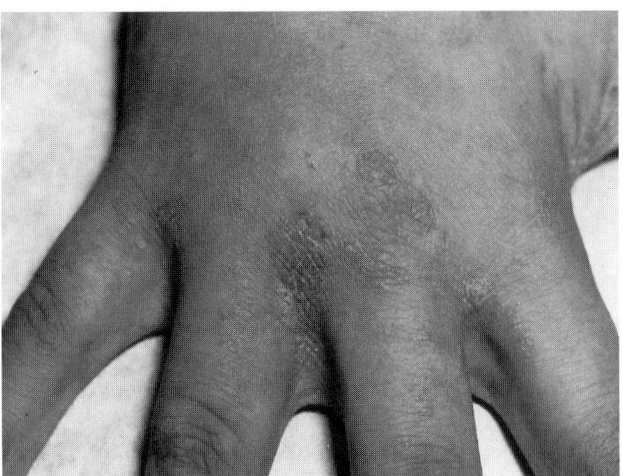

FIGURE 46–29. Scabies. Crusted and excoriated papules in the finger webs.

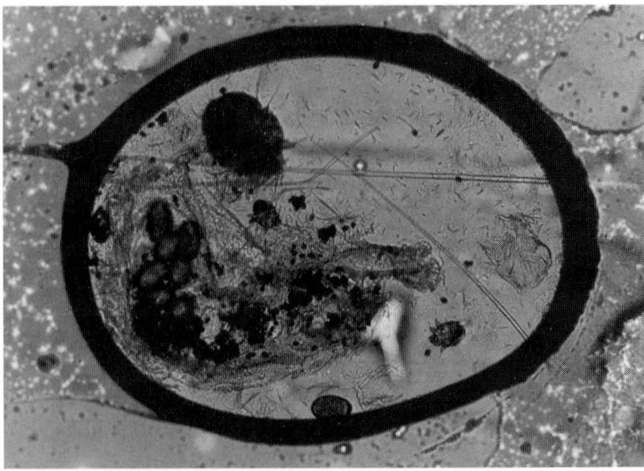

FIGURE 46–31. Scabies. Microscopic examination of superficial scraping reveals mite and eggs.

COMPLICATIONS

Pruritus may persist for several weeks or even months after successful therapy. This represents the prolonged hypersensitivity reaction and does not necessarily indicate treatment failure. Inadequate treatment or reinfestation should be suspected if new lesions develop after treatment, however. A secondary bacterial infection may complicate scabies, particularly the crusted variant, and should be treated with appropriate antibiotics.

OTHER MITE INFESTATIONS

Several specimens of mites other than *S. scabiei* are known to infest humans. These have been grouped into four categories: blood-sucking mites, including those of the families *Gamasidae* or *Dermanyssidae* (such as the chicken mite, house mouse mite, tropical fowl mite); the ''straw-itch'' or grain mites of the family Pyemotidae; pet or fur mites of the family Cheyletiellidae; and chiggers, larvae of the family Trombiculidae. The hair follicle mites, *Demodex folliculorum* and *D. brevis,* are present on the hair-bearing skin of many persons. These mites may be associated with several dermatoses, including folliculitis and **rosacea,** a cutaneous vascular disorder of adults that usually involves the cheeks and nose, producing flushing, papules, pustules, and telangectasia. Their possible role in the pathogenesis of this condition remains uncertain.

Clinical lesions from mite bites are caused by toxins produced by the mite or by allergic sensitivity to mite secretions. Unlike the scabies mite, these mites do not complete their life cycle on humans, so they are rarely identified on a patient.

Mite infestation should be considered in the differential diagnosis of an unexplained, pruritic, papular eruption. Lesions are usually small, up to several millimeters in diameter, and may have a central vesicle or hemorrhage. The distribution may provide clues to the diagnosis: chiggers tend to be distributed around the ankles and lower legs, whereas pet mites may be found on the face and arms where there was contact with the infested animal. A thorough history may identify possible exposure to mites.

Most mite infestations resolve spontaneously. A single application of lindane 1% lotion or permethrin cream 5% may hasten resolution. Clothing should be thoroughly washed, and carpets and upholstery may require cleaning if involved. Pets require treatment if infested.

The complications of mite infestation include secondary bacterial infections on excoriated skin. In addition, mites serve as vectors of several infectious diseases. *Liponyssoides sanguineus,* a blood-sucking parasite of the family Dermanyssidae, may transmit *Rickettsia akari,* the cause of rickettsialpox. Members of the Trombiculidae family can transmit *R. tsutsugamushi,* the etiologic agent in scrub typhus.

PEDICULOSIS (LICE)

ETIOLOGY

Three species of lice infest humans: *Pediculus humanus capitis,* the **head louse;** *Phthirus pubis,* the **pubic louse** or **crab;** and *P. humanus humanus* (also known as *P. humanus corporis*), the **body louse.** Pubic lice are transmitted sexually, and their presence in children may be a sign of child abuse. The body louse can function as a vector for several potentially serious infectious diseases.

The louse is a six-legged wingless insect (Fig. 46–32). Lice pierce the skin and suck blood, on which they live. A salivary substance enters the wound and may incite the associated dermatitis. Relatively few adult lice are present on the body at one time. Lice have a life span of 2–4 weeks and generally cannot survive being away from the host for more than 48 hours, although eggs of the body louse in clothing may survive for several days.

Transmission. Transmission results from person-to-person contact and is facilitated by the shared use of hairbrushes, clothing, and hair articles. Hair length does not influence infestation. The body louse persists in seams of clothing and bedding, from which it can be transmitted.

EPIDEMIOLOGY

The epidemiology of pediculosis differs considerably among the three types of infestation. **Pediculosis capitis,** or head lice, infestation occurs worldwide in all socioeconomic groups. Preschool and elementary school children are most frequently involved. It is less common among African Americans than among white or Hispanic persons.

Pediculosis pubis, pubic lice infestation, is more common among older adolescents and adults than among children. It is usually transmitted through sexual contact, and other sexually transmitted diseases may be associated. *Phthirus pubis* preferentially infests short-haired regions of the body and, in children, may involve the eyelashes. Transmission by fomites may occur.

Infestation by body lice, **pediculosis corporis,** is uncommon in the United States and generally affects indigent or vagrant populations with poor personal hygiene.

PATHOGENESIS

The head louse is the smallest of the three human lice (2–4 mm in length). It has a translucent, gray appearance and lives only in the hair or on the scalp. The female louse lays approximately 4 eggs per day in casings known as **nits.** In temperate climates, the eggs are deposited on the hair shaft near the scalp. The distance of the nit from the scalp provides an indication of the duration of infestation. Nits present on hair more than 1 cm from the scalp are usually older than 2 weeks and are unlikely to be viable.

The pubic louse has the appearance of a brown fleck on the skin. It may infest the eyelashes and eyebrows, as well as body and facial hair. Nits may be found on infested hairs.

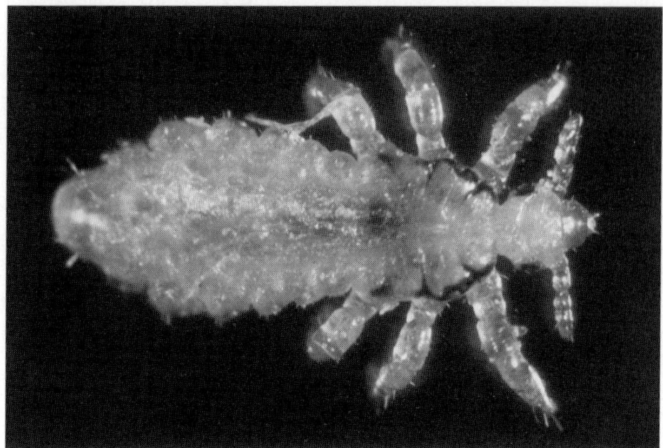

FIGURE 46–32. *Pediculosis humanus capitis,* the head louse. The adult louse is a wingless insect 2–4 mm in length with a translucent gray appearance.

The body louse is slightly larger than the head louse. It lives in the seams of undergarments and bedding and comes onto the body only to feed.

SYMPTOMS AND CLINICAL MANIFESTATIONS

Pediculosis capitis usually causes pruritus behind the ears or on the nape of the neck, although some children do not experience any symptoms. Some children may describe a crawling sensation in the scalp. Excoriations and crusting, with or without associated lymphadenopathy, may be present on the scalp.

Pediculosis pubis usually causes mild to severe pruritus in the groin area. Eyelash involvement in children may cause blepharitis with crusting, ulceration, scaling, and bleeding of the eyelid margin.

Pediculosis corporis causes pruritus that, because of repeated scratching, may result in lichenification of the skin or secondary bacterial infections.

DIAGNOSIS

The diagnosis of lice is usually suggested by symptoms of pruritus occurring simultaneously in several family members or, in the case of pediculosis pubis, in sexual partners.

Head lice are rarely found on the scalp, although nits are numerous and easily identified. These small, white shells are firmly attached to the hair close to the scalp; their identity can be confirmed by examination under the microscope.

Pubic lice or their nits may be found on visual examination and may be mistaken for a freckle. **Blue macules,** or **maculae ceruleae,** may be present in the thighs or buttocks.

Body lice are found in the patient's clothing. The skin bears marks of feeding, excoriation, and lichenification.

TREATMENT

Pediculosis capitis and pediculosis pubis can be treated successfully with permethrin 1% cream rinse, which is available without prescription. The hair should be washed with shampoo, after which the cream rinse is applied and allowed to remain for 10 minutes before it is rinsed off with water. Prophylactic use of permethrin is recommended for persons exposed to head lice epidemics in which at least 20% of the population of an institution is infested and for immediate members of the household of infested individuals. Casual use of permethrin, however, is strongly discouraged. Malathion 0.5% lotion applied for 8–12 hours is also effective for children 6 years of age and older, but the lotion is flammable; hair dryers and electric curlers must be avoided. Lindane 1% shampoo applied to the scalp for 4 minutes is also effective; however, misuse (e.g., ingestion or prolonged or repeated administration) can cause CNS toxicity. Lindane should not be used in infants, young children, pregnant or lactating women, or persons with seizures or other neurologic disorders. In cases of head lice resistant to other therapies, a single oral dose of ivermectin (200 μg/kg or 12 mg) may be considered.

Repeated treatment 7 days after initial therapy is recommended to kill any newly emerged nymphs. Children may return to school after their first treatment, however.

Nits should be mechanically removed with a fine-toothed comb. Wrapping the hair for 30–60 minutes in a towel soaked in an equal mixture of vinegar and water may facilitate mechanical removal.

Chemical pediculicides should never be applied to the eyelashes. Infestations in this location should be treated with repeated application of petrolatum 3–5 times daily for 7–10 days. Simultaneous treatment of other hairy portions of the body with a pediculocide is recommended.

In all cases, thorough cleaning of clothing and bed linens is necessary. Machine washing and drying with the use of hot cycles is advocated because high temperatures are lethal for both lice and eggs. Dry cleaning or storage of clothing in plastic bags for a minimum of 10 days is also effective. Combs and brushes should be disinfected with a pediculicide shampoo.

COMPLICATIONS

Complications of hair and pubic lice infestations are rare. Although the body louse can serve as a vector for infectious diseases, including *Rickettsia prowazekii* (epidemic typhus), *Bartonella quintana* (trench fever), and *Borrelia* (relapsing fever), infestations with lice represent more of a public health nuisance than a significant concern.

PROGNOSIS

Pediculicide treatment with appropriate disinfestation measures is highly effective. Reinfestation from untreated contacts or fomites, especially for pediculosis corporis, is more likely than primary treatment failure.

PREVENTION

Close contacts should be examined and treated if they are infested or if exposure warrants prophylactic treatment as described. Children sharing the same bed or personal articles (e.g., combs and brushes) should be treated simultaneously with the index patient. Children should be allowed to return to daycare or school the morning after treatment. Conservative ''no-nit'' policies in schools have not been shown to be effective in controlling head lice infestations.

REFERENCES

Impetigo

Baltimore RS: Treatment of impetigo: A review. *Pediatr Infect Dis* 1985; 4:597-601.

Barton LL, Friedman AD, Sharkey AM, et al: Impetigo contagiosa. III. Comparative efficacy of oral erythromycin and topical mupirocin. *Pediatr Dermatol* 1989;6:134–8.

Dagan R, Bar-David Y: Double-blind study comparing erythromycin and mupirocin for treatment of impetigo in children: Implications of a high prevalence of erythromycin-resistant *Staphylococcus aureus* strains. *Antimicrob Agents Chemother* 1992;36:287–90.

Dajani AS, Ferrieri P, Wannamaker LW: Natural history of impetigo. II. Etiologic agents and bacterial interactions. *J Clin Invest* 1972;51: 2863–71.

Ferrieri P, Dajani AS, Wannamaker LW, et al: Natural history of impetigo. 1. Site sequence of acquisition and familial patterns of spread of cutaneous streptococci. *J Clin Invest* 1972;51:2851–62.

Gisby J, Bryant J: Efficacy of a new cream formulation of mupirocin: Comparison with oral and topical agents in experimental skin infections. *Antimicrob Agents Chemother* 2000;44:255–60.

Melish ME: Staphylococci, streptococci and the skin: Review of impetigo and the staphylococcal scalded skin syndrome. *Semin Dermatol* 1982; 1:101–9.

Misko ML, Terracina JR, Diven DG: The frequency of erythromycin-resistant *Staphylococcus aureus* in impetiginized dermatoses. *Pediatr Dermatol* 1995;12:12–5.

Peter G, Smith AL: Group A streptococcal infections of the skin and pharynx (first of two parts). *N Engl J Med* 1977;297:311–7.

Folliculitis, Furuncles, and Carbuncles

Dahl MV: Strategies for the management of recurrent furunculosis. *South Med J* 1987;80:352–6.

Deobbeling BN, Breneman DL, Neu HC, et al: Elimination of *Staphylococcus aureus* nasal carriage in health care workers: Analysis of six clinical trials with calcium mupirocin ointment. The Mupirocin Collaborative Study Group. *Clin Infect Dis* 1993;17:466–74.

Hedstrom SA: Recurrent staphylococcal furunculosis. Bacteriological findings and epidemiology in 100 cases. *Scand J Infect Dis* 1981;13:115–9.

Hedstrom SA: Treatment and prevention of recurrent staphylococcal furunculosis: Clinical and bacteriological follow-up. *Scand J Infect Dis* 1985; 17:55–8.

Hoeger PH, Lenz W, Boutonnier A, et al: Staphylococcal skin colonization in children with atopic dermatitis: Prevalence, persistence and transmission of toxigenic and non-toxigenic strains. *J Infect Dis* 1992;165: 1064–8.

Rasmussen JE, Graves WH: *Pseudomonas aeruginosa,* hot tubs and skin infections. *Am J Dis Child* 1982;136:553–4.

Acne Vulgaris

Eady EA, Cove JH, Blake J, et al: Recalcitrant acne vulgaris: Clinical, biochemical and microbiological investigation of patients not responding to antibiotic treatment. *Br J Dermatol* 1988;118:415–23.

Goldstein B, Chalker DK, Lesher JL Jr: Acne fulminans. *South Med J* 1990;83:705–8.

Karvonen SL: Acne fulminans: Report of clinical findings and treatment of twenty-four patients. *J Am Acad Dermatol* 1993;28:572–9.

Leeming JP, Holland KT, Cuncliffe WI: The microbial colonization of inflamed acne vulgaris lesions. *Br J Dermatol* 1988;118:203–8.

Leyden JJ, Marples RR, Mills OH Jr, et al: Gram-negative folliculitis—A complication of antibiotic therapy in acne vulgaris. *Br J Dermatol* 1973; 88:533–8.

Pochi PE: The pathogenesis and treatment of acne. *Annu Rev Med* 1990;41:187–98.

Sawaya ME, Hordinsky MK: The antiandrogens. When and how they should be used. *Dermatol Clin* 1993;11:65–72.

Winston MH, Shalita AR: Acne vulgaris: Pathogenesis and treatment. *Pediatr Clin North Am* 1991;38:889–903.

Yonkosky DM, Pochi PE: Acne vulgaris in childhood: Pathogenesis and management. *Dermatol Clin* 1986;4:127–36.

Erythrasma

Cochran RJ, Rosen T, Landers T: Topical treatment for erythrasma. *Int J Dermatol* 1981;20:562–4.

Sarkany I, Taplin D, Blank H: The etiology and treatment of erythrasma. *J Invest Dermatol* 1961;37:283–90.

Pitted Keratolysis

Takama H, Tamada Y, Yano K, et al: Pitted keratolysis: Clinical manifestations in 53 cases. *Br J Dermatol* 1997;137:282–5.

Blistering Distal Dactylitis

Freiden IJ: Blistering dactylitis caused by group B streptococci. *Pediatr Dermatol* 1989;6:300–2.

McCray MK, Esterly NB: Blistering distal dactylitis. *J Am Acad Dermatol* 1981;5:592–4.

Schneider JA, Parlette HL: Blistering distal dactylitis: A manifestation of group A beta-hemolytic streptococcal infection. *Arch Dermatol* 1982; 118:879–80.

Woroszylski A, Duran C, Tamayo L, et al: Staphylococcal blistering dactyitis: Report of two patients. *Pediatr Dermatol* 1996;13:292–3.

Perianal Dermatitis

Kokx NP, Comstock JA, Facklam RR: Streptococcal perianal disease in children. *Pediatrics* 1987;80:659–63.

Krol AL: Perianal streptococcal dermatitis. *Pediatr Dermatol* 1990;7: 97–100.

Montemarano AD, James WD: *Staphylococcus aureus* as a cause of perianal dermatitis. *Pediatr Dermatol* 1993;10:259–62.

Rehder PA, Eliezer ET, Lane AT: Perianal cellulitis: Cutaneous group A streptococcal disease. *Arch Dermatol* 1988;124:702–4.

Spear RM, Rothbaum RJ, Keating JP, et al: Perianal streptococcal cellulitis. *J Pediatr* 1985;107:557–9.

Decubitus Ulcers

Berlowitz DR, Wilking SV: Risk factors for pressure sores: A comparison of cross-sectional and cohort-derived data. *J Am Geriatr Soc* 1989;37: 1043–50.

Brook I: Microbiological studies of decubitus ulcers in children. *J Pediatr Surg* 1991;26:207–9.

Woolsey RM, McGarry ID: The cause, prevention, and treatment of pressure sores. *Neurol Clin* 1991;9:797–808.

Anthrax

Brachman PS: Anthrax. *Ann N Y Acad Sci* 1970;174:577–82.

Burnett JW: Anthrax. *Cutis* 1991;48:113–4.

Dixon TC, Meselson M, Guillemin J, et al: Anthrax. *N Engl J Med* 1999; 341:815–26.

LaForce FM: Anthrax. *Clin Infect Dis* 1994;19:1009–13.

Manios S, Kavaliotis I: Anthrax in children: A long forgotten, potentially fatal infection. *Scand J Infect Dis* 1979;11:203–6.

Leprosy

Hastings RC, Gillis RP, Krahenbuhl JL, et al: Leprosy. *Clin Microbiol Rev* 1988;1:330–48.

Meyers WM: Leprosy. *Dermatol Clin* 1992;10:73–96.

Neill MA, Hightower AW, Broome CV: Leprosy in the United States, 1971-1981. *J Infect Dis* 1985;152:1064–9.

Sampaio EP, Sarno EN, Galilly R, et al: Thalidomide selectively inhibits tumor necrosis factor alpha production by stimulated human monocytes. *J Exp Med* 1991;173:699–703.

Cutaneous Nontuberculous Mycobacterial Infections

French AL, Benator DA, Gordon FM: Nontuberculous mycobacterial infections. *Med Clin North Am* 1997;81:361–79.

Grange JM, Noble WL, Yates MD, et al: Inoculation mycobacterioses. *Clin Exp Dermatol* 1988;13:211–20.

Huminer D, Pitlik SD, Block C, et al: Aquarium-borne *Mycobacterium marinum* skin infection: Report of a case and review of the literature. *Arch Dermatol* 1986;122:698–703.

Johnston JM, Izumi AK: Cutaneous *Mycobacterium marinum* infection (''swimming pool granuloma''). *Clin Dermatol* 1987;5:68–75.

O'Brien RJ: The epidemiology of nontuberculous mycobacterial disease. *Clin Chest Med* 1989;10:407–18.

Starke JR: Nontuberculosis mycobacterial infections in children. *Adv Pediatr Infect Dis* 1992;7:123–59.

Street ML, Umbert-Millet IJ, Roberts GD, et al: Nontuberculous mycobacterial infections of the skin: Report of fourteen cases and review of the literature. *J Am Acad Dermatol* 1991;24:208–15.

Wallace RJ Jr: The clinical presentation, diagnosis, and therapy of cutaneous and pulmonary infections due to the rapidly growing mycobacteria, *M. fortuitum* and *M. chelonae. Clin Chest Med* 1989;10:419–29.

Tinea Capitis

Aly R: Ecology, epidemiology and diagnosis of tinea capitis. *Pediatr Infect Dis J* 1999;18:180–5.

Caputo RV: Fungal infections in children. *Dermatol Clin* 1986;4:137–49.

Dragos V, Lunder M: Lack of efficacy of 6-week treatment with oral terbinafine for tinea capitis due to *Microsporum canis* in children. *Pediatr Dermatol* 1997;14:46–8.

Esterly NB: Fungal infections in children. *Pediatr Rev* 1981;3:41–9.

Freidlander SF: The evolving role of itraconazole, fluconazole and terbinafine in the treatment of tinea capitis. *Pediatr Infect Dis J* 1999; 18:205–10.

Gupta AK, Hofstader SL, Adam P, et al: Tinea capitis: An overview with emphasis on management. *Pediatr Dermatol* 1999;16:171–89.

Jacobs AH, O'Connell BM: Tinea in tiny tots. *Am J Dis Child* 1986; 140:1034–8.

Kearse HL, Miller OF: Tinea pedis in prepubertal children: Does it occur? *J Am Acad Dermatol* 1988;19:619–22.

Krowchuk DP, Lucky AW, Primmer SL, et al: Current status of the identification and management of tinea capitis. *Pediatrics* 1983;72:625–31.

McBride A, Cohen BA: Tinea pedis in children. *Am J Dis Child* 1992; 146:844–7.

Philpot CM, Shuttleworth D: Dermatophyte onychomycosis in children. *Clin Exp Dermatol* 1989;14:203–5.

Prevost E: The rise and fall of fluorescent tinea capitis. *Pediatr Dermatol* 1983;1:127–33.

Raimer SS, Petrusick TW: Superficial fungal infections in children. *Dermatol Clin* 1984;2:57–65.

Solomon LM: Special symposia: Tinea capitis: Current concepts. *Pediatr Dermatol* 1985;2:224–37.

Tack DA, Fleischer A Jr, McMichael A, et al: The epidemic of tinea capitis disproportionately affects school-aged African Americans. *Pediatr Dermatol* 1999;16:75.

Tanz RR, Hebert AA, Esterly NB: Treating tinea capitis: Should ketoconazole replace griseofulvin? *J Pediatr* 1988;112:987–91.

Weston JA, Hawkins K, Weston WL: Foot dermatitis in children. *Pediatrics* 1983;72:824–7.

Wilmington M, Aly R, Frieden IJ: *Trichophyton tonsurans* tinea capitis in the San Francisco Bay area: Increased infection demonstrated in a 20-year survey of fungal infections from 1974 to 1994. *J Med Vet Mycol* 1996;34:285–7.

Tinea Versicolor

Hebert A: Tinea versicolor. *Dermatol Clin* 1984;2:29–43.

Cutaneous and Oral Candidiasis

Butler KM, Baker CJ: Candida: An increasingly important pathogen in the nursery. *Pediatr Clin North Am* 1988;35:543–63.

Chapel TA, Gagliardi C, Nichols W: Congenital cutaneous candidiasis. *J Am Acad Dermatol* 1982;6:926–8.

Epstein JB, Truelove EL, Izutzu KT: Oral candidiasis: Pathogenesis and host defense. *Rev Infect Dis* 1984;6:96–106.

Hebert AA, Esterly NB: Bacterial and candidal cutaneous infections in the neonate. *Dermatol Clin* 1986;4:3–21.

Jordan WE, Lawson KD, Berg RW, et al: Diaper dermatitis: Frequency and severity among a general infant population. *Pediatr Dermatol* 1986;3:198–207.

Jorizzo JL: The spectrum of mucosal and cutaneous candidiasis. *Dermatol Clin* 1984;2:19–27.

Kirkpatrick CH: Chronic mucocutaneous candidiasis. *J Am Acad Dermatol* 1994;31:S14–7.

Kozinn PJ, Taschdjian CL, Dragutsky D, et al: Cutaneous candidiasis in early infancy and childhood. *Pediatrics* 1957;20:827–34.

Leyden JJ: Diaper dermatitis. *Dermatol Clin* 1986;4:23–8.

Ray TL: Oral candidiasis. *Dermatol Clin* 1987;5:651–62.

Singalavanija S, Frieden IJ: Diaper dermatitis. *Pediatr Rev* 1995;16:142–7.

Sporotrichosis

Belknap BS: Sporotrichosis. *Dermatol Clin* 1989;7:193–202.

Calhoun DL, Waskin H, White MP, et al: Treatment of systemic sporotrichosis with ketoconazole. *Rev Infect Dis* 1991;13:47–51.

Kauffman CA: Sporotrichosis: State of the art clinical article. *Clin Infect Dis* 1999;29:231–7.

Restrepo A, Robledo J, Gomez I, et al: Itraconazole therapy in lymphangitic and cutaneous sporotrichosis. *Arch Dermatol* 1986;122:413–7.

Smith PW, Loomis GW, Luckasen JL, et al: Disseminated cutaneous sporotrichosis: Three illustrative cases. *Arch Dermatol* 1981;117:143–4.

Winn RE: Systemic fungal infections: Diagnosis and treatment. I. Sporotrichosis. *Infect Dis Clin North Am* 1988;2:899–911.

Winn RE: A contemporary view of sporotrichosis. *Curr Top Med Mycol* 1995;6:73–94.

Herpes Simplex Virus

Bork K, Brauninger W: Increasing incidence of eczema herpeticum: Analysis of seventy-five cases. *J Am Acad Dermatol* 1988;19:1024–9.

Corey L: First-episode, recurrent, and asymptomatic herpes simplex infections. *J Am Acad Dermatol* 1988;18:169–72.

Corey L, Spear PG: Infections with herpes simplex viruses (1). *N Engl J Med* 1986;314:686–91.

Johnson RE, Nahmias AJ, Magder LS, et al: A seroepidemiologic survey of the prevalence of herpes simplex virus type 2 infection in the United States. *N Engl J Med* 1989;321:7–12.

Lafferty WE, Coombs RW, Benedetti J, et al: Recurrences after oral and genital herpes simplex virus infection: Influence of site of infection and viral type. *N Engl J Med* 1987;316:1444–9.

Novelli VM, Atherton DJ, Marshall WC: Eczema herpeticum: Clinical and laboratory features. *Clin Pediatr* 1988;27:231–3.

Schmitt DL, Johnson DW, Henderson FW: Herpes simplex type 1 infections in a group day care. *Pediatr Infect Dis J* 1991;10:729–34.

Spruance SL, Stewart JL, Rowe NH, et al: Treatment of recurrent herpes simplex labialis with oral acyclovir. *J Infect Dis* 1990;161:185–90.

Spruance SL, Rea TL, Thoming C, et al: Penciclovir cream for the treatment of herpes simplex labialis: A randomized, multicenter, double-blind, placebo-controlled trial. Topical Penciclovir Collaborative Study Group. *JAMA* 1997;277:1374–9.

Strauss SE, Rooney JF, Sever JL, et al: NIH Conference. Herpes simplex virus infection: Biology, treatment, and prevention. *Ann Intern Med* 1985;103:404–19.

Young TB, Rimm EB, D'Alessio DJ: Cross-sectional study of recurrent herpes labialis: Prevalence and risk factors. *Am J Epidemiol* 1988;127: 612–25.

Human Papillomaviruses

Baker GE, Tyring SK: Therapeutic approaches to papillomavirus infections. *Dermatol Clin* 1997;15:331–40.

Beutner KR: Human papillomavirus infection. *J Am Acad Dermatol* 1989; 20:114–23.

Beutner KR, Becker TM, Stone KM: Epidemiology of human papillomavirus infections. *Dermatol Clin* 1991;9:211–8.

Boyd AS: Condylomata acuminata in the pediatric population. *Am J Dis Child* 1990;144:817–24.

Cobb MW: Human papillomavirus infection. *J Am Acad Dermatol* 1990; 22:547–66.

Davis AJ, Emans SJ: Human papilloma virus infection in the pediatric and adolescent patient. *J Pediatr* 1989;115:1–9.

deVilliers EM: Papillomavirus and HPV typing. *Clin Dermatol* 1997;15: 199–206.

deVilliers EM: Importance of human papillomavirus DNA typing in the diagnosis of anogenital warts in children. *Arch Dermatol* 1995;131: 366–7.

Goldfarb MT, Gupta AK, Gupta MA, et al: Office therapy for human papillomavirus infection in nongenital sites. *Dermatol Clin* 1991;9: 287–96.

Highet AS: Viral warts. *Semin Dermatol* 1988;7:53–7.

Karabulut AA, Sahin S, Eksioglu M: Is cimetidine effective for nongenital warts: A double-blind, placebo-controlled study. *Arch Dermatol* 1997; 133:533–4.

Kraus SJ, Stone KM: Management of genital infection caused by human papillomavirus. *Rev Infect Dis* 1990;12:S620–32.

Massing AM, Epstein WL: Natural history of warts: A two-year study. *Arch Dermatol* 1963;87:306–10.

Melton JL, Rasmussen JE: Clinical manifestations of human papillomavirus infection in nongenital sites. *Dermatol Clin* 1991;9:219–33.

Obalek S, Jablonska S, Orth G: Anogenital warts in children. *Clin Dermatol* 1997;15:369–76.

Obalek S, Misiewicz J, Jablonska S, et al: Childhood condyloma acuminatum: Association with genital and cutaneous human papillomaviruses. *Pediatr Dermatol* 1993;10:101–6.

Obalek S, Jablonska S, Favre M, et al: Condylomata acuminata in children: Frequent association with human papillomaviruses responsible for cutaneous warts. *J Am Acad Dermatol* 1990;23:205–13.

Rock B, Naghashfar Z, Burnett N, et al: Genital tract papillomavirus infection in children. *Arch Dermatol* 1986;122:1129–32.

Molluscum Contagiosum

Becker TM, Blount JH, Douglas J, et al: Trends in molluscum contagiosum in the United States, 1966-1983. *Sex Transm Dis* 1986;13:88–92.

Brown ST, Nalley JF, Kraus SJ: Molluscum contagiosum. *Sex Transm Dis* 1981;8:227–34.

Porter CD, Archard LC: Characterisation by restriction mapping of three subtypes of molluscum contagiosum virus. *J Med Virol* 1992;38:1–6.

Cutaneous Larva Migrans

Caumes E, Carriere J, Datry A, et al: A randomized trial of ivermectin versus albendazole for the treatment of cutaneous larva migrans. *Am J Trop Med Hyg* 1993;49:641–4.

Herbener D, Borak J: Cutaneous larva migrans in northern climates. *Am J Emerg Med* 1988;6:462–4.

Hotez PJ: Hookworm disease in children. *Pediatr Infect Dis J* 1989;8: 516–20.

Jelinek T, Maiwald H, Nothdurft HD, et al: Cutaneous larva migrans in travelers: Synopsis of histories, symptoms, and treatment of 98 patients. *Clin Infect Dis* 1994;19:1062–6.

Kurgansky D, Burnett JW: Creeping eruption. *Cutis* 1990;45:399–400.

Cutaneous Leishmaniasis

El-On J, Halevy S, Grunwald MH, et al: Topical treatment of Old World cutaneous leishmaniasis caused by *Leishmania major:* A double-blind control study. *J Am Acad Dermatol* 1992;27:227–31.

Evans TG: Leishmaniasis. *Infect Dis Clin North Am* 1993;7:527–46.

Grimaldi G Jr, Tech RB: Leishmaniasis of the New World: Current concepts and implications for future research. *Clin Microbiol Rev* 1993;6:230–50.

Myiasis

Baird JK, Baird CR, Sabrosky CW: North American cuterebrid myiasis: Report of seventeen new infections of human beings and review of the disease. *J Am Acad Dermatol* 1989;21:763–72.

Elgart ML: Flies and myiasis. *Dermatol Clin* 1990;8:237–44.

Scabies, Other Mite Infestations, and Pediculosis (Lice)

Blankenship ML: Mite dermatitis other than scabies. *Dermatol Clin* 1990;8:265–75.

Burns DA: The treatment of human ectoparasite infection. *Br J Dermatol* 1991;125:89–93.

Elgart ML: Pediculosis. *Dermatol Clin* 1990;8:219–28.

Elgart ML: Scabies. *Dermatol Clin* 1990;8:253–63.

Gillis D, Slepon R, Karsenty E, et al: Seasonality and long-term trends of pediculosis capitis and pubis in a young adult population. *Arch Dermatol* 1990;126:638–41.

Green MS: Epidemiology of scabies. *Epidemiol Rev* 1989;11:126–50.

Hogan DJ, Schachner L, Tanglertsampan C: Diagnosis and treatment of childhood scabies and pediculosis. *Pediatr Clin North Am* 1991;38: 941–57.

Meinking TL, Taplin D: Safety of permethrin vs lindane for the treatment of scabies. *Arch Dermatol* 1996;132:959–62.

Meinking TL, Taplin D, Hermida JL, et al: The treatment of scabies with ivermectin. *N Engl J Med* 1995;333:26–30.

Meinking TL, Taplin D: Advances in pediculosis, scabies, and other mite infestations. *Adv Dermatol* 1990;5:131–50.

Mumcuoglu KY, Klaus S, Kafka D, et al: Clinical observations related to head lice infestation. *J Am Acad Dermatol* 1991;25:248–51.

Paller AS: Scabies in infants and small children. *Semin Dermatol* 1993; 12:3–8.

Schachner LA: Treatment resistant head lice: Alternative therapeutic approaches. *Pediatr Dermatol* 1997;14:409–10.

Schultz MW, Gomez M, Hansen RC, et al: Comparative study of 5% permethrin cream and 1% lindane lotion for the treatment of scabies. *Arch Dermatol* 1990;126:167–70.

Sterling GB, Janniger CK, Kihiczak G: Neonatal scabies. *Cutis* 1990;45: 229–31.

Taplin D, Meinking TL, Chen JA, et al: Comparison of crotamiton 10% cream (Eurax) and permethrin 5% cream (Elimite) for the treatment of scabies in children. *Pediatr Dermatol* 1990;7:67–73.

Taplin D, Meinking TL, Castillero PM, et al: Permethrin 1% creme rinse for the treatment of *Pediculus humanus* var *capitis* infestation. *Pediatr Dermatol* 1986;3:344–8.

CHAPTER 47

Cellulitis

John S. Bradley

Cellulitis results from inflammation of the epidermis, dermis, and adjacent subcutaneous tissue. It is typically characterized by redness, swelling, and pain. The clinical manifestations and extent of inflammation depend on the virulence of the bacterial pathogen and its mechanisms of tissue invasion and destruction, the mechanism of inoculation, and the type and vigor of the host response. This response is determined in part by age-specific immune function. Many microbiologic and clinical differences distinguish cellulitis of the extremities from cellulitis of the head and neck.

CELLULITIS OF THE EXTREMITIES AND TRUNK

ETIOLOGY

Staphylococcus aureus and group A *Streptococcus* are the predominant pathogens of cellulitis of the extremities at all ages. The spectrum of skin and soft tissue infections caused by these organisms ranges from impetigo (Chapter 46) to severe, rapidly progressive, invasive infections with bacteremia and sepsis.

Several other bacteria occasionally cause cellulitis. Certain organisms in soil and water, such as *Pseudomonas aeruginosa, Aeromonas hydrophila, Plesiomonas, Vibrio* (especially *V. vulnificus*), and *Pseudomonas pseudomallei,* can invade the skin through even minor breaks. In immunocompromised persons, cellulitis of the extremities can be caused by less pathogenic organisms and is also associated with more severe local tissue destruction, such as **ecthyma gangrenosum,** which is caused by *P. aeruginosa* or occasionally *Aspergillus* and often is associated with marked systemic toxic effects.

EPIDEMIOLOGY

The median age of children with cellulitis of the extremities is 5 years, somewhat older than the median age for facial cellulitis of 3 years. The affected age groups and the distribution of infections on the extremities are similar to those of skin abrasions and insect bites, which provide a point of entry for organisms. Chronic skin disorders, such as eczema, that facilitate access of organisms to the dermis may predispose a person to impetigo and cellulitis.

PATHOGENESIS

Colonization of the skin with these organisms usually precedes infection. Abrasions, cuts and scratches, insect bites, other cutaneous lesions (e.g., chickenpox, eczema), and penetrating trauma (e.g., animal or human bites) with direct inoculation usually facilitate inoculation. Cutaneous infection such as impetigo may remain superficial or may invade deeper tissues. Both *S. aureus* and group A *Streptococcus* elaborate growth and spreading factors that allow the organisms to evade host phagocytosis and to damage tissue locally, promoting local spread of organisms. Organisms may also spread through the lymphatics, resulting in erysipelas, or through deeper fascial planes, resulting in fasciitis (Chapter 48). Regional lymph nodes are often enlarged in children with chronic skin infections and occasionally become acutely infected (Chapter 51). The nodes may undergo suppurative necrosis with subsequent spread of organisms to the adjacent soft tissues. Neutrophils are essential in eradicating infections caused by *S. aureus* and group A *Streptococcus,* and thus impaired host neutrophil chemotaxis, phagocytosis, or intracellular killing of bacteria is associated with an increased risk of having these infections (Chapter 6).

SYMPTOMS AND CLINICAL MANIFESTATIONS

Tenderness, erythema, and swelling occur at the point of entry of organisms into the skin, with progressive local symptoms as infection spreads to adjacent areas. The central area of the cellulitis may suppurate, particularly with staphylococcal infection, resulting in an abscess. Regional lymphadenopathy or lymphadenitis is common. Fever is usually low grade, and the child generally does not appear toxic.

Erysipelas is a unique form of cellulitis caused by group A *Streptococcus.* It is characterized by a bright red, indurative, extremely tender, rapidly progressive area of cellulitis that may advance at a rate of several millimeters per hour (Plate 8A). Lesions usually occur on the extremities in children but may also occur on the face or trunk. The advancing margin of erysipelas is sharply demarcated and slightly raised and indurated, as opposed to the more diffuse, deeper swelling of other forms of cellulitis. Small, 1–2 mm bullae filled with clear or purulent fluid may develop several hours after erysipelas has been present. Higher fever and greater clinical toxicity are more frequent than in other forms of cellulitis.

Erysipeloid is an unusual cutaneous infection caused by *Erysipelothrix rhusiopathiae,* a gram-positive bacillus frequently isolated from poultry, fish, and animals. Erysipeloid shares some characteristics with erysipelas but has central clearing of the lesion, a much slower progression of erythema, and minimal systemic toxicity. Although the disease is believed to be mainly an occupational hazard for butchers and fishermen, cases have been reported in children with no obvious source of infection.

Ecthyma is usually caused by group A *Streptococcus* and frequently complicates impetigo. Initially it is characterized by increased edema and erythema, which is also characteristic of impetigo, followed by local invasion of subcutaneous tissues rather than remaining superficial. A rim of erythematous induration may develop around an eschar, which, if removed, reveals a shallow ulcer. **Ecthyma gangrenosum** is a particularly serious infection that occurs in immunocompromised persons. It results from hematogenous spread of septic emboli to the skin and is caused by *P. aeruginosa* or occasionally *Aspergillus* or other gram-negative organisms. The lesions are initially round, purple macules that undergo central necrosis to become deep, punched-out ulcers up to 2–3 cm in diameter with a dark necrotic base, raised red edges, and sometimes a yellowish green exudate. It is usually accompanied by high fever, myalgia, and exquisite local tenderness.

Rarely, certain fungi (e.g., *Coccidioides, Cryptococcus, Histoplasma,* and *Sporothrix*) and nontuberculous mycobacteria (e.g., *Mycobacterium marinum*) cause locally invasive disease with clinical findings consistent with mild cellulitis surrounding the inoculation site of the pathogen.

DIAGNOSIS

The diagnosis of facial cellulitis is usually established by the clinical manifestations and physical findings.

Differential Diagnosis

Lymphangitis is a soft tissue infection usually caused by group A *Streptococcus* (Chapter 51). A macular, blanching, tender red streak may develop proximal to the initial site of inoculation in the cutaneous tissue and extend for several centimeters along the lymphatic drainage of the lesion (Plate 8B). The margin may advance rapidly, as in erysipelas, although in lymphangitis the erythema is neither indurative nor raised. This relatively localized lymphatic spread of group A *Streptococcus* may occur without the development of either overt cellulitis or erysipelas. Initially, no fever or bacteremia is present, but if untreated, the infection frequently progresses to bacteremia accompanied by systemic signs of infection.

Laboratory Evaluation

The WBC count is usually elevated in cellulitis, particularly with erysipelas. Ecthyma gangrenosum is often associated with neutropenia resulting from cancer therapy or other immunosuppression.

Microbiologic Evaluation

Cultures of tissues and blood from immunocompetent persons with uncomplicated cellulitis and without unusual exposure to soil, freshwater, or saltwater are generally unnecessary before the initiation of empirical antibiotic therapy for presumed staphylococcal and streptococcal cellulitis. Cultures to identify the pathogen and determine antimicrobial susceptibilities are indicated for serious infections, for toxic appearance or signs of shock, in immunocompromised persons, with development or progression of inflammation during antibiotic therapy, or after unusual exposures, such as exposure to soil, freshwater, saltwater, or animal feces or products. Persons with infection in the deep tissue spaces may require surgical intervention to obtain the appropriate microbiologic samples, particularly if the infection is not responding to therapy.

Tissue Culture. Cultures or even a biopsy for bacterial and fungal stains of the involved area may be helpful for immunocompromised persons with cellulitis that may be caused by unusual bacteria or fungi, or for cellulitis that does not respond to empirical therapy, which suggests that the pathogen is resistant to the antibiotics.

Results comparing recovery of an organism by aspiration from the point of maximal inflammation and by aspiration from the leading edge are conflicting. Cultures from both sites may be desirable and are helpful in establishing the microbiologic cause in up to 60% of infections. One study (Traylor, 1998) found that simple direct aspiration of an area of cellulitis yields bacteria in approximately 50% of cases, compared to injection of saline solution followed by aspiration, which yields bacteria in approximately 20% of cases. The reason may be that the core material cut during simple aspiration is not subsequently ejected. A tissue aspirate of cellulitis is obtained for culture by preparing the site with povidone and isopropyl alcohol and then attaching a 21- to 23-gauge needle to a 5 mL syringe for aspiration of the involved area. Negative pressure is applied as the needle enters the skin and is advanced into the subcutaneous tissues to the area of maximum inflammation. Usually only a drop or two of serosanguineous fluid returns into the syringe, which should then be transported directly to the laboratory for Gram stain and culture.

Blood Culture. Blood cultures may be helpful, but results are positive in <5% of uncomplicated staphylococcal or streptococcal cellulitis. Cellulitis without an associated break in the skin as a portal of entry indicates the possibility of bacteremic spread or direct extension of underlying infection and therefore suggests the need for further evaluation before the start of empirical treatment. Bacteremia with group A *Streptococcus* is believed to be more common in children with erysipelas than with other forms of cellulitis. Bacteremia is common in immunocompromised persons with ecthyma gangrenosum.

Diagnostic Imaging

Extensive edema and tenderness with severe cellulitis of the extremities may preclude an accurate examination to determine the extent of infection. In these situations, CT or MRI allows for identification of deep abscesses and fasciitis that may require surgical débridement.

TREATMENT

Empirical therapy for moderate to severe cellulitis of the extremities of immunocompetent persons should consist of a β-lactam antibiotic that has excellent activity against both *S. aureus* and group A *Streptococcus,* such as cefazolin, nafcillin, or oxacillin (Table 47–1). In cases of severe infection, gentamicin may be added to the β-lactam antibiotic to increase bactericidal activity. For persons with hypersensitivity to β-lactam antibiotics, clindamycin and vancomycin are alternative agents.

Oral therapy is appropriate for mild cellulitis and for infections that have shown a rapid response to initial intravenous therapy. For children, cephalexin suspension is preferred over dicloxacillin suspension because of the rather bitter, metallic taste of dicloxacillin. Oral clindamycin suspension also may be used to treat staphylococcal or streptococcal infections and is preferred in persons with hypersensitivity to β-lactam antibiotics. Macrolides are not recommended for oral therapy because of the increasing rate of resistance of group A *Streptococcus.* Despite a higher MIC for group A *Streptococcus,* amoxicillin is preferable to penicillin V for oral therapy because of greater absorption and because palatability results in better adherence. Antibiotic treatment should continue until fever has resolved and signs of local inflammation are absent for several days—usually 7–14 days.

For erysipelas or lymphangitis, hospitalization and initial parenteral antibiotic therapy are recommended because of the greater risk of bacteremia and the possibility of the development of secondary sites of infection. Intravenous penicillin G is the preferred therapy for these streptococcal infections, although antistaphylococcal antimicrobial agents (e.g., cefazolin or nafcillin) may be administered empirically pending culture results. For erysipeloid, intravenous penicillin G is the treatment of choice.

TABLE 47–1. Antibiotic Therapy for Cellulitis of the Extremities and Trunk

	Antibiotic Regimen			
	Parenteral and Empiric Therapy		Oral and Convalescent Therapy	
Type of Infection	Recommended Regimen	Alternative Regimen	Recommended Regimen	Alternative Regimen
Cellulitis	Cefazolin *or* nafcillin *or* oxacillin	Clindamycin *or* vancomycin*	Group A *Streptococcus* Amoxicillin	Penicillin V *or* clindamycin *or* a macrolide
			Empirical or culture-negative Cephalexin *or* dicloxacillin	Clindamycin *or* a macrolide
Erysipelas	Penicillin G	Cefazolin *or* nafcillin *or* oxacillin	Penicillin V	Amoxicillin *or* a macrolide
Erysipeloid	Penicillin G		Penicillin V	
Ecthyma gangrenosum	Ceftazidime *plus* Vancomycin *with or without* an aminoglycoside*	Piperacillin-tazobactam *or* ticarcillin-clavulanate *or* ceftazidime *or* cefepime *plus* Vancomycin *with or without* an aminoglycoside*	Oral therapy is not recommended	
Lymphangitis (see Chapter 51)				

*Serum concentrations of vancomycin and aminoglycosides should be monitored during therapy in persons with impaired renal function and in newborns.

Recommended Dosages for Patients with Normal Renal Function

ANTIBIOTIC	DOSAGE	MAXIMUM DAILY DOSE
Parenteral Therapy (IV)		
Amikacin	15–20 mg/kg/day divided q8–12hr	(Same)
Cefazolin	100 mg/kg/day divided q8hr	3–6 g
Cefepime	100–150 mg/kg/day divided q8–12hr	6 g
Ceftazidime	150 mg/kg/day divided q8hr	6 g
Clindamycin	40 mg/kg/day divided q8hr	2.7 g
Gentamycin	7.5 mg/kg/day divided q8hr	5 mg/kg (adults)
Nafcillin	150 mg/kg/day divided q6hr	9 g
Oxacillin	150–200 mg/kg/day divided q6hr	12 g
Penicillin G	200,000–250,000 U/kg/day divided q4hr	18–24 MU
Piperacillin-tazobactam	Piperacillin 200–300 mg/kg/day divided q6hr	18 g
Ticarcillin-clavulanate	Ticarcillin 200–300 mg/kg/day divided q6hr	18 g
Tobramycin	7.5 mg/kg/day divided q8hr	5 mg/kg (adults)
Vancomycin	45–60 mg/kg/day divided q6hr	2 g

ANTIBIOTIC	DOSAGE	MAXIMUM DAILY DOSE
Oral and Covalescent Therapy		
Amoxicillin	40–50 mg/kg/day divided 3 times daily	1.5 g
Azithromycin	10 mg/kg on day 1, then 5 mg/kg once daily	500 mg on day 1, then 250 mg/day
Cephalexin	50–100 mg/kg/day divided 4 times daily	4 g
Clarithromycin	15 mg/kg/day divided 2 times daily	1 g
Clindamycin	10–20 mg/kg/day divided 4 times daily	1.2 g
Dicloxacillin	25–50 mg/kg/day divided 4 times daily	2 g
Erythromycin	40 mg/kg/day divided 4 times daily	2 g
Penicillin V	50 mg/kg/day divided 4 times daily	2 g

For immunocompromised persons, particularly if neutropenia is present, antibiotics highly active against both *S. aureus* and *P. aeruginosa* must be used pending culture results. Appropriate antibiotic combinations include ceftazidime, cefepime, or piperacillin-tazobactam, plus an aminoglycoside, as well as nafcillin, oxacillin, or vancomycin; meropenem may be used as single-agent therapy. The empirical antibiotic regimen should be adjusted after the organism has been isolated and the susceptibilities are known. Bacteremia caused by *P. aeruginosa* should be treated with a regimen that includes an active β-lactam antibiotic (e.g., ceftazidime, cefepime, piperacillin-tazobactam, or meropenem), usually in combination with an aminoglycoside.

Surgical débridement is important to hasten the resolution of cutaneous abscesses or suppurative regional lymph nodes. Cultures may continue to be positive for *Staphylococcus* or *Streptococcus* for several days, despite appropriate antibiotic therapy, if abscesses are not adequately drained. Drains may be required if all areas of suspected abscess formation cannot be easily reached and débrided, to allow for continuing drainage of smaller abscesses that may be peripheral to a central lesion.

COMPLICATIONS

Bacteremia may occur with either staphylococcal or streptococcal infections. Generally, the more ''toxic'' the patient's condition, the more likely that bacteremia is present. A notable exception is the systemic toxicity seen in toxic shock syndrome (Chapter 22), which is mediated by exotoxins. Bacteremia may lead to secondary sites of infection. Infection can also spread by direct extension to the deep muscle groups, causing fasciitis (Chapter 48).

PROGNOSIS

Most children who receive early, appropriate antimicrobial therapy, and drainage if necessary, recover completely from their acute cellulitis. Superficial or deep scars may develop as sequelae of necrotizing infections. Immune-mediated sequelae such as acute glomerulonephritis may occur after streptococcal infections of the skin or the upper respiratory tract, even if treated with appropriate antibiotics (Chapter 42).

PREVENTION

Good hygiene, including meticulous care of cuts and abrasions, can minimize the likelihood of developing cellulitis. Prophylactic antibiotics are not indicated for clean, superficial wounds, but early institution of antibiotic therapy, if fever and local signs of infection develop, may prevent progression and more invasive disease.

CELLULITIS OF THE HEAD AND NECK

Facial cellulitis is a bacterial infection of the soft tissues of the face that may occur with any trauma that disrupts the integrity of the skin, including abrasions, cuts or scratches, insect bites, other cutaneous lesions (e.g., chickenpox, impetigo), or penetrating trauma (e.g., animal or human bites). Infection may also reach the soft tissues of the face through the oral mucosa as a result of dental abscesses or intraoral trauma-related infections caused by oral flora. **Preseptal cellulitis,** or **periorbital cellulitis,** involves the soft tissues anterior to the orbit and the orbital septum (Fig. 47–1), both above and below the eye. **Buccal cellulitis** is caused by infection in the soft tissues overlying the buccinator muscle in the cheek.

ETIOLOGY

Organisms causing facial cellulitis are a direct reflection of the organisms on the skin or oral mucous membranes, those of the object penetrating the skin, or a combination of both. *S. aureus* and group A *Streptococcus* are the major pathogens in all age groups, especially if associated with a break in the skin or cervical lymphadenopathy. Preseptal and buccal cellulitis caused by *Streptococcus pneumoniae* or *Haemophilus influenzae* type b is associated with bacteremia in approximately 70% of cases. Facial cellulitis associated with dental infections is caused by oral flora, including microaerophilic *Streptococcus,* usually β-hemolytic, in 30%; by anaerobic cocci, including *Peptostreptococcus* and *Veillonella,* in 20–50%; by gram-negative anaerobic or facultative bacilli, including *Prevotella, Porphyromonas,* and *Fusobacterium,* in 20–50%; by staphylococci in 15%; by *Eikenella corrodens* in 15%; and by *Bacteroides fragilis* in 5–10%.

EPIDEMIOLOGY

Facial cellulitis occurs frequently in children, with a median age of 3 years. Cellulitis caused by spread of infection from regional lymph nodes of the neck, most commonly the anterior and superior

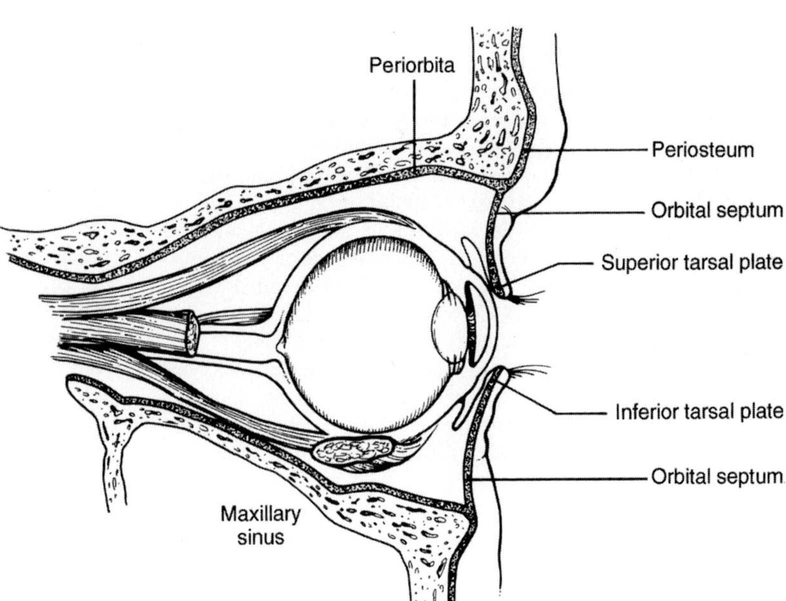

FIGURE 47–1. Preseptal cellulitis involves the soft tissues anterior to the orbital septum both superior to and inferior to the eye.

cervical nodes and less frequently the posterior cervical and preauricular nodes, is occasionally seen in children 6–24 months of age.

Preseptal and buccal cellulitis caused by *H. influenzae* type b and *S. pneumoniae* occurs primarily among children 6–24 months of age. Before widespread immunization against *H. influenzae* type b, this organism was responsible for approximately 60% of all cases of preseptal cellulitis, with most cases occurring in children younger than 2 years. Cellulitis caused by *H. influenzae* type b is rare in immunized children. *S. aureus,* group A *Streptococcus,* and *S. pneumoniae* now account for the great majority of the cases of preseptal cellulitis in children. Pneumococcal cellulitis occurs almost exclusively in children younger than 4 years but represents <5% of all bacteremia-associated pneumococcal disease. Several other organisms that colonize the skin, including coagulase-negative staphylococci and *Corynebacterium,* are occasionally cultured from samples obtained from children with preseptal cellulitis, although these organisms most likely represent skin contaminants.

PATHOGENESIS

The pathogenesis of head and neck cellulitis varies depending on the organisms causing the infection. If a portal of entry through the skin is identified, *S. aureus* or group A *Streptococcus* is the cause in >80% of cases. Multiple factors facilitate tissue invasion by *S. aureus* and group A *Streptococcus.* Encapsulation of *S. aureus* confers protection from opsonins. Extracellularly excreted enzymes such as fibrinolysin and hyaluronidase facilitate tissue necrosis and spread of organisms. Exotoxins, including staphylococcal toxic shock syndrome toxin (TSST-1) and streptococcal pyrogenic exotoxins A, B, and C, can potentially lead to multiple organ system failure such as toxic shock syndrome (Chapter 22).

Many tissues invaded by *S. aureus* or group A *Streptococcus* ultimately undergo some degree of tissue necrosis, with inflammation histologically characterized by a brisk polymorphonuclear leukocyte response and microabscess formation. These small abscesses may coalesce to form a clinically apparent abscess, which then may drain spontaneously through fistulas to either cutaneous or mucosal surfaces.

Preseptal and buccal cellulitis usually result from inoculation of soft tissues secondary to bacteremia, especially with *S. pneumoniae* or *H. influenzae* type b, but also by direct invasion of the buccal mucosa from organisms colonizing the mucosa and by secondary spread of organisms from an ipsilateral infected middle ear to buccal soft tissue through the lymphatics that supply both regions.

Cellulitis associated with suppuration of regional lymph nodes is also most commonly caused by *S. aureus* or group A *Streptococcus.* Bacteria enter regional nodes through the lymphatic drainage from the skin or through the oropharynx. Subsequent lymphadenitis and suppuration of the node may lead to spread of organisms into the surrounding soft tissues of the face or neck and development of cellulitis. On occasion, the originally involved node may be predisposed to infection because the normal architecture of the node is distorted by a previous or current indolent infection by other pathogens, such as nontuberculous mycobacteria or fungi.

Cellulitis of the head and neck may also be caused by infections originating in the oropharynx. Dental infections of the maxillary alveolar ridge may erode the bone, inoculating overlying soft tissues of the face. Dental infections of teeth in the mandible, after intraoral trauma, or peritonsillar abscesses may lead to cellulitis of the sublingual space, retropharyngeal space, and other deep soft tissues of the neck (Chapter 59).

Pott's puffy tumor is swelling of the soft tissues of the forehead that results from a communication between the frontal sinus and the medullary cavity of the frontal bone, in which the sinus is situated. Bacteria causing frontal sinusitis may be transported to the frontal bone, causing osteomyelitis, with subsequent erosion through the outer table of the bone and the development of a subperiosteal abscess. This abscess and the inflammation in the adjacent soft tissues produce the characteristic clinical findings of Pott's puffy tumor.

SYMPTOMS AND CLINICAL MANIFESTATIONS

The development of preseptal or facial cellulitis caused by *S. aureus* or group A *Streptococcus* in older children is relatively slow, occurring over several hours to a few days, with gradually increased swelling, erythema, and tenderness. Affected children do not have systemic toxicity and usually have little or no fever. On palpation, however, the central erythematous area is usually tender. A break in the skin, which served as the portal of entry for infection, is frequently seen.

The clinical presentation of preseptal cellulitis caused by *S. pneumoniae* and *H. influenzae* type b is usually acute and dramatic, as opposed to the relatively more indolent and slowly progressive cellulitis caused by *S. aureus* or group A *Streptococcus.* Many of the systemic symptoms of clinical toxicity, including moderate to high fever, irritability, and acute decrease in appetite and activity, may be attributed to the bacteremia that frequently accompanies cellulitis caused by *S. pneumoniae* and *H. influenzae* type b. Periorbital swelling and erythema develop quickly, within a few hours, and are associated with marked tenderness to palpation (Plate 7E). The edema is usually boggy but may be indurated centrally. Although a violaceous hue has been thought to indicate *H. influenzae* type b infection, it is not specific because it may reflect only the characteristics of the depth of infection and the degree of inflammation present at the time of the initial examination.

Buccal cellulitis is also frequently associated with bacteremia, with systemic toxicity similar to that occurring in preseptal cellulitis. An acute, tender, erythematous, indurated, unilateral swelling of the cheek occurs for a few hours, accompanied by a moderate to high fever and irritability (Plate 7F). A break in the skin is usually not seen with either preseptal or buccal cellulitis caused by *S. pneumoniae* or *H. influenzae* type b.

Facial cellulitis resulting from intraoral trauma or dental abscess may be slowly or rapidly progressive, depending on the location of the infection and on the bacteria involved. Cellulitis associated with dental infections usually is manifested by gradual swelling of the face for a few days and is associated with mild tenderness and mild overlying erythema. Indurative, woody edema of tissues is not usually seen. In sharp contrast, Ludwig's angina is characterized by dramatic, rapidly progressive, indurative, painful cellulitis of the tissues of the sublingual and submandibular spaces and may occur after intraoral trauma or in association with poor dentition. In addition to indurative edema, crepitus caused by gas-forming anaerobic organisms may occasionally be present. Suppuration is not usually present initially but may subsequently develop. Children are usually febrile and appear toxic. Difficulty in swallowing is a frequent complaint. Difficulty in speaking indicates involvement of the subglottic area and suggests involvement of the tissues surrounding the airway, which may then progress to airway obstruction.

Cellulitis resulting from regional lymphadenitis is usually suggested by a history of swelling and tenderness of a lymph node. Occasionally the diffuse swelling in the soft tissues overlying the node that occurs after suppuration of the node is so great that the node or cluster of nodes may no longer be able to be distinguished

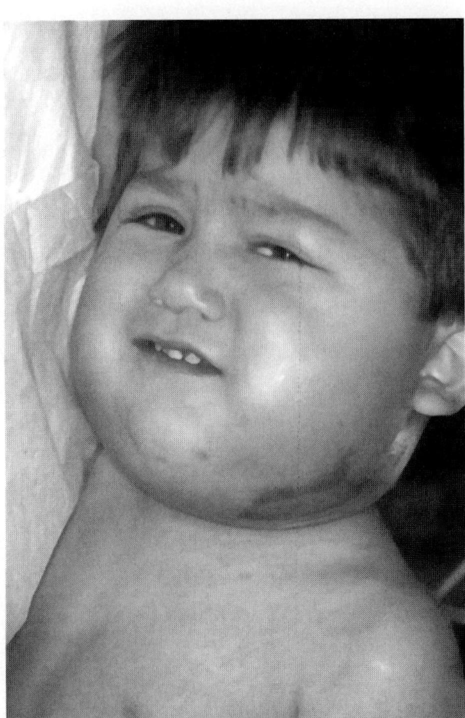

FIGURE 47–2. Two-year-old boy with cellulitis of the submandibular soft tissues complicating group A streptococcal pharyngitis and bilateral cervical lymphadenitis. A tissue aspirate from the center of maximal inflammation was positive on Gram stain for gram-positive cocci in chains and positive by culture for group A *Streptococcus.*

by palpation (Fig. 47–2). The secondary cellulitis may also progress to abscess formation, with fluctuation in the center of the cellulitis.

Symptoms of frontal sinusitis, such as headache, fever, persistent cough, congestion, and rhinorrhea, are usually present for several days to weeks before the onset of Pott's puffy tumor. Trauma also may result in a predisposition to this infection. Although swelling, redness, and tenderness are all usually present, tenderness with minimal swelling may be the only physical finding.

Ludwig's angina, a distinct clinical syndrome originally described as gangrenous induration of the connective tissues of the neck, primarily involves the sublingual and submandibular spaces. Normal oral aerobic and anaerobic flora, including *Bacteroides,* is responsible for most infections. Group A *Streptococcus* and *S. aureus* have also been occasionally isolated. *P. aeruginosa* and *Candida albicans* occasionally cause cellulitis in children with underlying immunodeficiency.

Pott's puffy tumor, an infection of the soft tissues overlying the frontal bone, is characterized by boggy swelling and tenderness of the forehead, with minimal erythema, and results from direct extension of frontal sinusitis through the frontal bone. It has been reported in children as young as 6 years, but is most often diagnosed in adolescents older than 12 years, after the frontal sinuses are developed. The causative organisms are those responsible for sinusitis, including aerobic and anaerobic respiratory tract flora, predominantly α-hemolytic streptococci, with *S. aureus* and *Bacteroides* each isolated in approximately 20% of reported cases.

DIAGNOSIS

The diagnosis of facial cellulitis is usually established by the clinical manifestations and physical findings.

Laboratory Evaluation

The WBC count is usually more elevated in preseptal and buccal cellulitis caused by *S. pneumoniae* and *H. influenzae* type b than in cellulitis caused by *S. aureus* and group A *Streptococcus,* with mean WBC counts of approximately 18,000/mm^3 and 13,000/mm^3, respectively. WBC counts are also generally elevated in children with dental abscesses, Ludwig's angina, and regional lymphadenitis.

Any child with preseptal or buccal cellulitis who appears toxic at the time of the initial examination, particularly those younger than 1 year, should have a lumbar puncture. Meningitis as a complication occurs in approximately 1% of bacteremic *S. pneumoniae* infections and 10% of bacteremic *H. influenzae* type b infections.

Microbiologic Evaluation

Cultures of facial cellulitis are not always necessary but may be performed using techniques as for other sites of cellulitis. Aspiration of fluctuant lymph nodes may be invaluable in children with facial cellulitis caused by regional lymphadenitis (Chapter 51). In facial swelling related to dental abscess, tissue aspirates usually are not helpful because the site of infection is deep and may be well localized adjacent to the root of the involved tooth. Drainage material should be cultured at the time of tooth extraction.

Blood Culture. Children with preseptal or buccal cellulitis may have bacteremia, and a blood culture may be helpful for confirming the cause of the infection. The appearance of facial cellulitis without a break in the skin as a portal of entry suggests the possibility of bacteremic spread or direct extension of underlying infection and the need for further evaluation.

Diagnostic Imaging

CT or MRI is important in the assessment of preseptal cellulitis with any degree of proptosis, ophthalmoplegia, chemosis, or diplopia, to exclude orbital involvement (Fig. 47–3). Nontender swelling of the preseptal tissues accompanied by erythema, which may appear clinically similar to preseptal cellulitis, occurs in children with ethmoid sinusitis when the venous drainage of the periorbital tissues by the ophthalmic vein is impaired by inflammatory edema. CT or MRI can identify ethmoid sinusitis and differentiate this cause of periorbital swelling from preseptal cellulitis. CT or MRI can also identify frontal sinus involvement in Pott's puffy tumor, as well as epidural abscess, another potential complication of sinusitis.

Ultrasonography is useful in the evaluation of regional cervical lymphadenopathy to identify abscess formation and to determine whether surgical drainage is necessary. With extensive soft-tissue swelling of the face and neck, as in Ludwig's angina (Chapter 61), CT or MRI can delineate areas of abscess formation within areas of inflammatory edema that should be considered for surgical drainage.

TREATMENT

The choice of empirical antibiotic therapy for facial cellulitis is dependent on many factors (Table 47–2). For children younger than 4 years, especially those not immunized against *H. influenzae* type b or with no identified portal of entry in the skin, therapy for preseptal and buccal cellulitis requires antibiotics active against *H. influenzae* type b and *S. pneumoniae,* as well as against *S. aureus* and group A *Streptococcus.* Ceftriaxone and cefotaxime are highly active against *S. pneumoniae* and *H. influenzae* type b, but neither is highly active against *S. aureus.* Cefuroxime is less active against *H. influenzae* type b than either ceftriaxone or cefotaxime, particu-

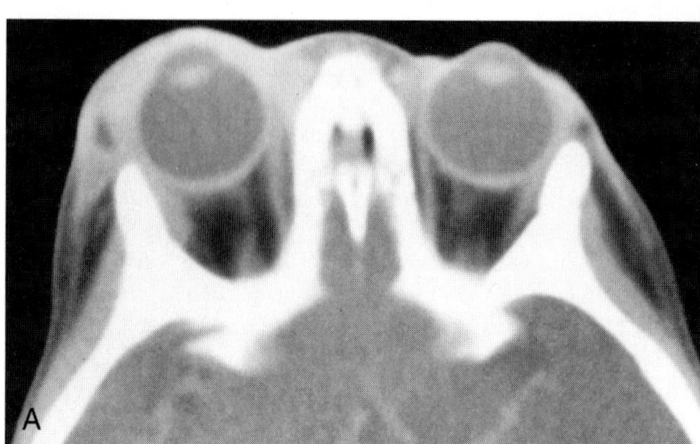

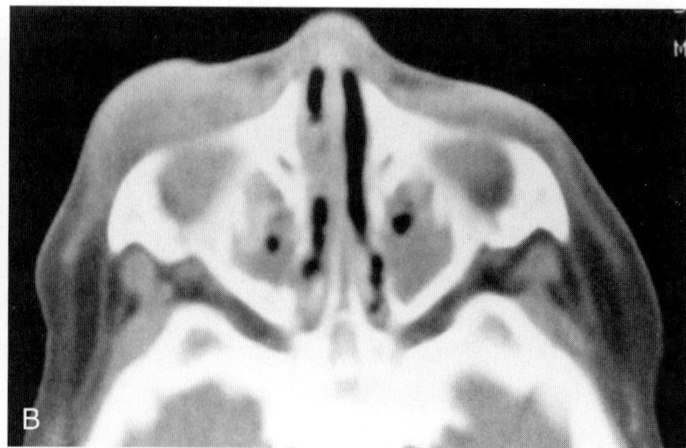

FIGURE 47–3. CT of preseptal cellulitis and sinusitis. **A,** Transaxial CT section through the orbits demonstrates superficial soft-tissue swelling external to the right orbit. Mild thickening of the lateral muscle cone is present, but there is no evidence of an intraorbital abscess. **B,** Transaxial CT section through the sinuses shows extensive fluid accumulation within both maxillary sinuses and mucus in the nasal airway just to the right of midline. Soft-tissue edema is present superficially over the right maxilla.

larly against β-lactamase-producing strains, and is less active against *S. aureus* than either cefazolin or nafcillin. However, cefuroxime as a single antibiotic represents an acceptable choice in most cases of preseptal cellulitis. For preseptal cellulitis confirmed as caused by *H. influenzae* type b, ceftriaxone or cefotaxime should be used because they have better CNS penetration than cefuroxime.

For children older than 4 years fully immunized against *H. influenzae* type b or with a portal of entry in the skin, either cefazolin or nafcillin should be used for empirical therapy because of the greater likelihood of infection caused by *S. aureus*. Facial infections caused by *S. aureus* or group A *Streptococcus* may progress to abscesses that require surgical incision and drainage, even when appropriate antibiotics have been administered.

Facial cellulitis associated with dental infections usually requires only penicillin G, or clindamycin as an alternative, because of the predominance of anaerobes and gram-positive oral flora causing these infections (Chapter 61). Extraction of the infected tooth is usually required for persons with facial cellulitis associated with dental abscesses. Ludwig's angina is associated with a greater potential for complications, and therapy with cefotaxime plus clindamycin, penicillin G plus metronidazole, or meropenem is recommended (Chapter 61). CT and MRI are helpful for defining abscess formation with Ludwig's angina and the need for surgical management. Infections characterized only by inflammatory edema can be managed medically rather than surgically. Immunocompromised children may require empirical therapy against *P. aeruginosa* with ceftazidime or cefepime.

Empirical antibiotic therapy for cellulitis associated with regional lymphadenitis should include antibiotics that are highly active against *S. aureus* and group A *Streptococcus,* such as cefazolin or nafcillin, with clindamycin or vancomycin as alternatives. For particularly severe, deep infections caused by *S. aureus,* some experts recommend adding either an aminoglycoside such as gentamicin because of the synergy against *S. aureus* or rifampin because of the increased tissue penetration, although improved outcomes after the use of these regimens have not been shown. CT, MRI, and ultrasonography are often helpful in defining the presence of tissue abscesses that may require surgical drainage. Facial cellulitis associated with cervical lymphadenitis that does not respond to empirical antibiotic therapy suggests the possibility of lymphadenitis with nontuberculous mycobacteria (Chapter 51).

Empirical treatment of Pott's puffy tumor should include antibiotics active against both *S. aureus* and respiratory flora, because sinusitis is the underlying infection. Cefazolin, nafcillin, or clindamycin should be used in combination with either ceftriaxone or cefotaxime. Sinus drainage may be required to prevent further complications of the infection such as epidural abscess and vascular thrombosis.

COMPLICATIONS

Most complications of facial cellulitis caused by *H. influenzae* type b and *S. pneumoniae* are a result of bacteremia rather than local extension, with meningitis occurring in 10% and 1% of children with bacteremia, respectively. Other sites including lung, pericardium, bones, and joints may also become secondarily infected from bacteremia. Because of the presence of the orbital septum, preseptal cellulitis rarely progresses to cause orbital cellulitis (Chapter 65; Fig. 47–1). Suspected involvement of the orbit requires CT or MRI and ophthalmologic consultation.

Edema with Ludwig's angina may progress rapidly with extensive soft-tissue swelling of the submandibular space that compromises the airway in the supraglottic or subglottic region. A tracheostomy may be required to maintain the airway.

PROGNOSIS

Most patients with facial or preseptal cellulitis recover fully with appropriate antimicrobial therapy. Recurrence is unexpected unless there is an underlying cause, such as poor dentition.

PREVENTION

Childhood immunization with *H. influenzae* conjugate vaccine has markedly reduced the incidence of infections caused by this organism, including facial cellulitis. Childhood immunization with *S. pneumoniae* conjugate vaccine may similarly reduce the incidence of facial cellulitis caused by this organism. Prophylactic antibiotics are not indicated for clean, superficial facial wounds, but early institution of antibiotic therapy if fever and local signs of infection develop may prevent progression and more invasive disease. Good dental hygiene and dental care minimize the development of facial cellulitis associated with dental infections.

TABLE 47–2. Antibiotic Therapy for Cellulitis of the Face and Neck

	Antibiotic Regimen			
	Parenteral Therapy		Oral and Convalescent Therapy	
Type of Cellulitis	Recommended Regimen	Alternative Regimen	Recommended Regimen	Alternative Regimen
Preseptal or buccal cellulitis:				
Point of entry identified and immunized against *Haemophilus influenzae* type b	Cefazolin *or* nafcillin *or* oxacillin	Cefuroxime *or* clindamycin *or* vancomycin	Cephalexin *or* dicloxacillin	Clindamycin
No point of entry identified or not immunized against *H. influenzae* type b	Ceftriaxone *or* cefotaxime	Cefuroxime	β-Lactamase-negative *H. influenzae* type b *or Streptococcus pneumoniae*	
			Amoxicillin	Amoxicillin-clavulanate
			β-Lactamase-positive *H. influenzae* type b *or* culture negative	
			Cefuroxime axetil *or* cefprozil *or* cefpodoxime *or* cefdinir	
Dental-associated facial cellulitis (see Chapter 61)	Penicillin G	Clindamycin *or* Metronidazole *plus* cefazolin *or* nafcillin *or* oxacillin	Clindamycin *or* amoxicillin-clavulanate	Penicillin V
Pott's puffy tumor	Ceftriaxone *or* cefotaxime	Cefuroxime *or* ampicillin-sulbactam	Cefuroxime axetil *or* cefprozil *or* cefpodoxime *or* cefdinir	Amoxicillin-clavulanate

*Serum concentrations of vancomycin and aminoglycosides should be monitored during therapy in persons with impaired renal function and in newborns.

Recommended Dosages for Patients with Normal Renal Function

ANTIBIOTIC	DOSAGE	MAXIMUM DAILY DOSE
Parenteral Therapy (IV)		
Cefazolin	100 mg/kg/day divided q8hr	3–6 g
Cefotaxime	150 mg/kg/day divided q8hr	6 g
Ceftriaxone	50 mg/kg/day divided q24hr	1 g
Clindamycin	40 mg/kg/day divided q8hr	2.7 g
Metronidazole	30 mg/kg/day divided q6hr	2.7 g
Nafcillin	150 mg/kg/day divided q6hr	9 g
Oxacillin	150–200 mg/kg/day divided q6hr	12 g
Penicillin G	200,000–250,000 U/kg/day divided q4hr	18–24 MU
Vancomycin	45–60 mg/kg/day divided q6hr	2 g

ANTIBIOTIC	DOSAGE	MAXIMUM DAILY DOSE
Oral and Convalescent Therapy		
Amoxicillin-clavulanate	Amoxicillin 40 mg/kg/day divided tid	1.5 g
Cefdinir	14 mg/kg/day divided bid	600 mg
Cefpodoxime	10 mg/kg/day divided bid	400 mg
Cefprozil	15 mg/kg/day divided bid	1 g
Cefuroxime axetil	30 mg/kg/day divided bid	1 g
Cephalexin	50–100 mg/kg/day divided qid	4 g
Clindamycin	10–20 mg/kg/day divided qid	1.2 g
Dicloxacillin	50–100 mg/kg/day divided qid	4 g
Pencillin V	50 mg/kg/day divided qid	2 g

REVIEWS

Blumer JL, Lemon E, O'Horo J, et al: Changing therapy for skin and soft tissue infections in children: Have we come full circle? *Pediatr Infect Dis J* 1987;6:117–22.

Powell KR: Orbital and periorbital cellulitis. *Pediatr Rev* 1995;16:163–7.

KEY ARTICLES

Donahue SP, Schwartz G: Preseptal and orbital cellulitis in childhood. A changing microbiologic spectrum. *Ophthalmology* 1998;105:1902–5.

Feder HM Jr, Cates KL, Cementina AM: Pott puffy tumor: A serious occult infection. *Pediatrics* 1987;79:625–9.

Fergie JE, Patrick CC, Lott L, et al: *Pseudomonas aeruginosa* cellulitis and ecthyma gangrenosum in immunocompromised children. *Pediatr Infect Dis J* 1991;10:496–500.

Fleisher G, Ludwig S, Campos J: Cellulitis: Bacterial etiology, clinical features, and laboratory findings. *J Pediatr* 1980;97:591–3.

Gross SJ, Nieburg PI: Ludwig angina in childhood. *Am J Dis Child* 1977;131:291–2.

Loyer EM, DuBrow RA, David CL, et al: Imaging of superficial soft-tissue infections: Sonographic findings in cases of cellulitis and abscess. *AJR Am J Roentgenol* 1996;166:149–52.

Nagy M, Pizzuto M, Backstrom J, et al: Deep neck infections in children: A new approach to diagnosis and treatment. *Laryngoscope* 1997; 107:1627–34.

Sadow KB, Chamberlain JM: Blood cultures in the evaluation of children with cellulitis. *Pediatrics* 1998;101(3):E4.

Traylor KK, Todd JK: Needle aspirate culture method in soft issue infections: Injection of saline vs. direct aspiration. *Pediatr Infect Dis J* 1998;17:840–1.

Uzcategui N, Warman R, Smith A, et al: Clinical practice guidelines for the management of orbital cellulitis. *J Pediatr Ophthalmol Strabismus* 1998;35:73–9.

CHAPTER 48

Wound and Deep-Tissue Infections

John S. Bradley

Broadly defined, wounds occur when the integrity of the skin or mucous membrane is breached as a result of either a traumatic injury or surgery. Once the normal cutaneous and mucosal barriers to bacterial invasion are no longer intact, infection of the epidermis and dermis, known as **cellulitis,** may result (Chapter 47), or it may progress to involve the deeper levels of connective tissue and fascial planes, when it is known as **necrotizing fasciitis,** and ultimately to the underlying muscle, when it is known as **myonecrosis.** Several clinical entities closely resembling or identical to necrotizing fasciitis have been described in the medical literature: **dry gangrene, streptococcal gangrene, synergistic necrotizing cellulitis, Fournier's gangrene** or necrotizing fasciitis of the perineum, **gangrenous erysipelas,** and **varicella gangrenosa.** These are variants of a destructive, usually rapidly progressive deep tissue infection, which involves the skin, subcutaneous tissue, and fascia but not the underlying muscle. Neonatal **omphalitis** is a form of necrotizing fasciitis. The deepest necrotizing infection, **clostridial myonecrosis** or **gas gangrene,** is distinguished from necrotizing fasciitis by involvement of muscle in addition to the fascia. The morbidity and mortality rates for these infections are considerable. Fortunately, myonecrosis is rare in children.

Infections may occur after such trivial injury to the skin as minor abrasions, insect bites, or varicella infection or after more extensive injury from accidental trauma, human or animal bites (Chapter 50), or surgery. As with all infections the severity and course of wound-related infections are the result of multiple interrelated factors including the type and extent of trauma, the organisms involved, and the host response. These infections may all be life threatening, and all require the physician to recognize the earliest signs of deep tissue involvement. Immediate hospitalization and aggressive surgical and medical therapy are essential to minimize tissue destruction and death.

ETIOLOGY

The organisms involved usually reflect the location of the tissue that is infected (Table 48–1), with skin flora being the predominant cause of infection on the extremities and trunk, mixed aerobic and anaerobic gastrointestinal flora responsible for infections of the perineum, and mixed aerobic and anaerobic respiratory flora causing deep tissue infections of the head and neck. Organisms infecting children after cutaneous injuries are generally skin or environment flora inoculated into traumatic wounds, leading to signs and symptoms characteristic of each organism. The organisms causing the infection clearly reflect the material contaminating the wound.

Surgery on an unruptured abdominal viscus is classified as **clean-contaminated surgery** in which there is no spillage of gastrointestinal contents into the peritoneal cavity or surgical incision. Surgery involving a ruptured viscus is classified as **dirty surgery** because at the time of surgery, microorganisms from the gastrointestinal tract have gained access into the abdominal cavity, which is then always treated as though it is infected. The majority of abdominal postsurgical infections result from leakage of the normal intestinal flora into the peritoneal cavity and the abdominal incision site.

Pediatric cases of necrotizing fasciitis historically have most often been caused by group A *Streptococcus* after varicella, although nonstreptococcal cases associated with trauma and surgery continue to be reported. A mixture of aerobes and anaerobes is present in 70–80% of trauma-related necrotizing fasciitis. Anaerobic streptococci are frequently associated with either enteric gram-negative organisms or *Staphylococcus aureus.* In soil-contaminated wounds, *Clostridium* has been documented as playing a role in necrotizing fasciitis without deeper muscle involvement.

Myonecrosis. Clostridial organisms are the most common pathogens causing myonecrosis, with *Clostridium perfringens* responsible for approximately 80% of cases. Other clostridial organisms, including *C. septicum* and *C. novyi,* have been associated with tissue destruction far less often than *C. perfringens. C. septicum* is a relatively aerotolerant anaerobe that is a reported cause of spontaneous, nontraumatic gas gangrene and is capable of bacteremic spread from the intestinal tract to establish a focal tissue infection without apparent antecedent trauma. Bacteremia is usually associated with intestinal tract abnormalities such as colon cancer, diverticulitis, necrotizing enterocolitis and bowel infarction. Approximately 90% of persons with *C. septicum* bacteremia have colon cancer, often occult.

Nonclostridial myonecrosis results from synergistic infection with multiple organisms other than *Clostridium.* In one study (Darke et al, 1977) of adults, 15% of persons with clinically diagnosed gas gangrene were infected with organisms other than *Clostridium.* Most of the organisms responsible for necrotizing fasciitis may also cause myonecrosis. These organisms include anaerobic streptococci or anaerobes in combination with either *S. aureus,* group A *Streptococcus,* or enteric gram-negative bacilli.

Neonatal Necrotizing Fasciitis. Necrotizing fasciitis in neonates most commonly occurs as a complication of omphalitis, which is a polymicrobial infection usually caused by skin or stool flora. In 75% of cases, both aerobes and anaerobes can be recovered from cultures. Aerobes include *S. aureus,* group A *Streptococcus,* group B *Streptococcus,* gram-negative enteric bacilli (*Escherichia coli, Klebsiella pneumoniae, Enterobacter,* and *Proteus*), *Enterococcus,* and viridans streptococci, and anaerobes include *Bacteroides fragilis* and *Clostridium.*

Soil- and Water-Associated Infections. Gram-negative enteric bacilli are the organisms most frequently isolated from infected soil-contaminated wounds. Approximately 40% are infected with enteric gram-negative bacilli (*Enterobacter, E. coli, Klebsiella, Citrobacter, Proteus,* and *Morganella*), 23% with environmental

TABLE 48–1. Deep Invasive Bacterial Soft-Tissue Infections

	Infection		
	Cellulitis	Necrotizing Fascilitis	Myonecrosis
	Anaerobic streptococcal cellulitis Nonclostridial crepitant cellulitis	Dry gangrene Streptococcal gangrene Fournier's gangrene	Necrotizing myositis Gas gangrene Clostridial myonecrosis
Soft-Tissue Layers Involved			
Dermis	Primary site of infection	Primary site of infection	Secondarily involved
Subcutaneous	Primary site of infection	Primary site of infection	Secondarily involved
Fascia	Not involved	Primary site of infection	Primary site of infection
Muscle	Not involved	Not involved	Primary site of infection
Systemic toxic effects	Mild to moderate	Moderate to severe	Severe
Mortality (%)	<5%	25–50%	50–90%
Causative Organisms			
Staphylococcus aureus	Common	Common	Uncommon
Group A *Streptococcus*	Common	Common	Uncommon
Enteric gram-negative bacilli	Rare	Uncommon	Rare
Anaerobic streptococci	Rare	Uncommon	Rare
Clostridium	Rare	Uncommon	Rare
Pseudomonas aeruginosa	Uncommon	Uncommon	Common
Bacteroides	Rare	Common	Common

gram-negative bacilli (*Acinetobacter* and *Pseudomonas*), 19% with *Enterococcus,* and 8% with anaerobes. *Aspergillus* infection after trauma tends to present in the second week after injury. Fungal infections may be underreported because of the limited culture techniques used in some studies,

Spores of *Clostridium tetani* are common in soil, and the anaerobic conditions that often develop in traumatic wounds are optimal for germination of spores and production of toxin by vegetative organisms. The risk of tetanus as a result of infection with *C. tetani* in a well-débrided and well-cleansed wound is low, especially because of the high level of immunization (Chapter 56). **Neonatal tetanus,** resulting from infection at the umbilical stump, is rarely seen in developed countries with appropriate antiseptic care of the umbilicus after birth.

Among the freshwater organisms, *Pseudomonas, Aeromonas,* and *Plesiomonas* have been documented as causing fasciitis. Saltwater organisms responsible for serious invasive infection in the United States include *Vibrio* species, especially *Vibrio vulnificus,* which occurs naturally in the warm estuaries of the Gulf of Mexico. Wounds contaminated by water containing these organisms may become infected after relatively minor cutaneous trauma. In addition to wound infections, *V. vulnificus* can cause septicemia in immunocompromised persons (Chapter 100). Nontuberculous mycobacteria, primarily *Mycobacterium marinum,* may cause a chronic cutaneous infection in immunocompetent persons after exposure to freshwater and saltwater, swimming pools, tropical-fish tanks, well water, or infected marine animals (Chapter 46).

EPIDEMIOLOGY

The most serious of the deep tissue infections, which may follow trauma but may also arise spontaneously, are necrotizing fasciitis and myonecrosis. Myonecrosis is very uncommon in children. Deep tissue infections may be less common in children than in adults, which may reflect fewer serious injuries among children, fewer underlying disease states associated with these syndromes (e.g., peripheral vascular disease, diabetes mellitus, carcinoma), or underreporting of infections. Since reporting of invasive streptococcal infections, including necrotizing fasciitis, became mandatory in certain counties in California in 1994, the documented incidence of these infections in children has been relatively constant at approximately 4 cases per 100,000 children per year.

Historically, war has been responsible for the greatest number of life-threatening, wound-related infections. Injury-related infections in civilian populations were not given extensive consideration until the second half of the 20th century. Currently, motor vehicle accidents are responsible for the majority of serious trauma-related infections in nonmilitary populations. One of the few categories of pediatric injuries investigated for posttraumatic risk of infection is the category of **farm injuries.** Injuries that break the skin and are associated with gross contamination of the wound with soil are those most likely to lead to infection. In one study (Brennan, 1990) 72% of injuries involving the long bones of the extremities associated with a deep laceration had complicating infections, compared with 29% of minor avulsions or finger amputations and only 5% of abrasions or crush injuries in which the skin did not require suturing.

Several factors appear to increase the incidence of postoperative wound infections, including length of hospitalization before surgery, penetrating trauma and contaminated wounds, emergent surgery, duration of surgery >2 hours, repeated surgical procedures, and surgery in neonates. Perioperative antibiotic prophylaxis can decrease the risk of postoperative infection (Table 16–6). The anterior abdominal wall is the site most often infected postoperatively, usually after appendectomy or other surgery on the bowel. The risk of developing a wound infection after appendectomy without rupture (clean-contaminated surgery) is approximately 10% in patients without perioperative antibiotic prophylaxis. However, the infection rate after appendectomy for a gangrenous or perforated appendix (dirty surgery) rises to about 35%.

Neonatal Necrotizing Fasciitis. In a review (Hsieh, 1999) of 69 neonates, necrotizing fasciitis was most often associated with an abdominal wall site of infection, occurring as a complication of **omphalitis** in more than 80% of cases. Mammary gland infection, balanitis, fetal scalp monitoring, and postoperative complications, including those occurring after circumcision, account for the predisposing factors in the remaining 20% of cases. The male-to-female ratio is 1:1, with onset at a mean of 1 week of age. The incidence of omphalitis is not easily determined because of the difficulty in clinically differentiating **funisitis,** a superficial cellulitis around the umbilicus, from deeper infections that involve the subcutaneous tissue, fascia, and muscle. No specific immunologic factors have been associated with neonatal necrotizing fasciitis.

PATHOGENESIS

Trauma or surgery results in damage to tissue, and infection may or may not arise in damaged tissues that are inoculated with bacteria. Several factors determine the ultimate progression of inoculation to the development of infection. Classification of the different deep soft-tissue infectious disease syndromes is based on the tissue layers involved in the infection. Although there is some overlap in these syndromes, the distinction allows for an analysis of the microbiology, pathogenesis, and treatment of the different syndromes. The layers of tissue can be divided into (1) the epidermis and dermis, containing subcutaneous fat and connective tissue, (2) deep fascia, and (3) underlying muscle (Table 48–1).

Involvement of only the more superficial layers of the epidermis and dermis leads to cellulitis, commonly caused by *S. aureus* and group A *Streptococcus* (Chapter 47). Gram-negative organisms, anaerobic streptococci, and clostridia only rarely cause superficial disease, but may lead to infection known as **anaerobic streptococcal cellulitis** or **nonclostridial crepitant cellulitis,** which is often injury related.

Necrotizing Fasciitis. For infections that involve the underlying fascia, necrotizing fasciitis has become the global name for this set of clinically similar infections. **Streptococcal gangrene** and **Fournier's gangrene** are two examples of necrotizing fasciitis that usually result in the destruction of the subcutaneous tissue and fascia but spare the deeper muscle. When muscle is involved in the destructive infectious process itself, the clinical entity is known variously as **myonecrosis, gas gangrene, clostridial myonecrosis,** or **necrotizing bacterial myositis,** depending on the microbiologic findings and the clinical features of the infection. Omphalitis in a neonate may involve the subcutaneous tissue, the fascia or, in extensive disease, the muscles of the abdominal wall.

The pathogenesis of necrotizing soft-tissue infections is a direct result of the production of factors by a single organism or by multiple organisms that lead directly to cell death, enzymatic destruction of supporting connective tissue, and evasion or destruction of host humoral and cellular responses to the infecting organisms. It is well known that group A *Streptococcus, S. aureus,* and *Clostridium* are able to invade and proliferate in necrotic tissue, to elaborate extracellular enzymes and toxins that can damage tissue and facilitate invasion through soft tissue planes, and to limit host defenses. These organisms are capable of causing extensive tissue damage when present as the sole infecting organism. Other organisms, including anaerobic streptococci such as *Peptostreptococcus,* gram-negative bacilli, and *Bacteroides* species other than *B. fragilis,* when present as the sole pathogen, usually do not produce such a rapidly destructive infection, but when present in combination with other bacteria, they can cause infection characterized by greater virulence with apparent pathogenic synergy. The multiple bacterial factors involved in the production of a synergistic soft-tissue infection have not been well defined. The pathologic changes in histologic specimens of necrotizing fasciitis include necrosis of the superficial fascia, polymorphonuclear leukocyte infiltration of the deep dermis and fascia, fibrinous thrombosis of arterioles and venules, and the absence of muscle involvement.

Of particular concern is the role of **nonsteroidal anti-inflammatory drugs (NSAIDs)** such as ibuprofen in streptococcal necrotizing fasciitis. In retrospective analyses a statistically significant association of these agents with the development of necrotizing fasciitis in children with varicella has been documented. At this time it has not been determined whether NSAIDs are causative or merely associated with use in the child with severe pain, who is more likely to have ongoing tissue destruction. In vitro, NSAIDs inhibit local inflammatory responses and may possibly play a role in allowing these organisms to evade host defenses.

Myonecrosis. Myonecrosis, or gas gangrene, represents the deepest level of infection, involving both fascia and muscle, and usually depends on conditions that facilitate the growth of anaerobic organisms (Table 48–2). These conditions include tissue devitalized by the injury; tissue with poor blood flow; tissue into which bleeding with hematoma formation has occurred; tissue that contains foreign material; and tissue in which an infection by aerobic bacteria, such as staphylococci or streptococci, has already developed. In mixed infections with both facultative aerobes and anaerobes, it is postulated that the aerobic organisms are responsible for using tissue oxygen, thereby reducing further the **redox potential** in tissues that may have been inoculated by *Clostridium* and other anaerobic bacteria.

Clostridium is capable of producing a large array of toxins. The most common is **α toxin,** which is present in all clostridial organisms, is a lecithinase that is destructive to cell membranes and is capable of altering capillary permeability. *C. perfringens* may produce several other toxins including **hyaluronidase, collagenase, hemolysin, lipase, protease,** and **deoxyribonuclease.** These biologically active toxins produced in the anaerobic environment of necrotic tissue allow for the rapid spread of organisms through tissue planes. More necrotic tissue is thus produced, allowing greater growth of organisms and increasing elaboration of toxins. Because of progressive deep-tissue destruction and subsequent systemic spread of toxins, *C. perfringens* infections, if untreated, are often fatal.

Soil- and Water-Associated Infections. Wound infections due to clostridial species other than *C. perfringens* do not routinely result in extensive tissue necrosis, but they may be life-threatening because of the systemic effects of absorbed toxins. Tetanus is perhaps the best known of these infections (Chapter 56). The spores of *Clostridium tetani* may germinate in devitalized tissue, leading to the production of **tetanospasmin,** a neurotoxin that may cause dramatic, intense skeletal muscle spasms in unimmunized persons. In immunized persons, however, the toxin is neutralized by circulating antibody produced in response to injected tetanus toxoid. Less commonly associated with wound infections is *Clostridium botulinum.* Spores of this organism are frequently present in soil and may contaminate a wound that breaks the skin. Germination of spores and vegetative growth in an anaerobic environment allow for production and absorption of toxin, resulting in the clinical syndrome of botulism indistinguishable from that associated with foodborne disease (Chapter 56).

Cutaneous diphtheria is essentially no longer seen in the United States because of the high level of immunization in the general

TABLE 48–2. Conditions That Favor Anaerobic Wound Infection

Devitalized tissue
Poor blood flow
Hematoma
Foreign material
Pyogenic infection

population. *Corynebacterium diphtheriae* organisms may be inoculated into a wound from the pharynx or the skin of another person who either is infected or is a carrier. **Diphtheria toxin** is elaborated only by certain strains of *C. diphtheriae* with lysogenic phage infection. The toxin is locally active, causing tissue necrosis and producing sharp peripheral wound margins and a purulent membranous base. Toxin may be systemically absorbed from an infected wound, leading to multiple organ effects, including myocarditis and neuritis, although to a much lesser degree than in children with pharyngeal diphtheria.

Trauma-associated infections caused by *V. vulnificus* are first characterized by erythema and swelling at the site of injury, followed by rapid progression of the infection to involve deeper fascial planes with the development of bullae and ultimately necrosis of the skin and subcutaneous tissues. Necrotizing fasciitis and myonecrosis have been reported with this organism, with local invasion of blood vessels noted in the histopathologic examination of surgical specimens.

Aeromonas, better known for causing diarrhea (Chapter 76), can also cause deep tissue infections. *Aeromonas* produces at least two different hemolysins, proteinases, and a leukocidin, all of which may participate in the pathogenesis of the infection. These infections generally develop within 1–2 days after exposure and rapidly progress to cellulitis, necrotizing fasciitis, and myositis. The infected tissue may be foul smelling, and abscess formation is occasionally present.

Cutaneous nontuberculous mycobacterial infection caused by inoculation of *M. marinum* into traumatized skin is usually associated with an indolent infection that may last several months (Chapter 46).

Frostbite. Frostbite, which most commonly affects the fingers, toes, nose, and ears, is associated with a variable degree of damage to the epidermis, dermis, and on occasion the subcutaneous tissue, fascia, muscle, and bone. Vascular damage results in extensive extravasation of fluid into the soft tissues. Local symptoms resulting from damage to the tissue depend on the degree of injury, but in milder frostbite rewarming is usually associated with erythema, considerable edema, and blister formation as vascular reperfusion occurs. Cutaneous infection may occur either in viable tissues after rewarming or in necrotic, devitalized tissue. Secondary infection of injured tissue usually leads to new clinical findings of tissue inflammation within hours or days after reperfusion. Systemic symptoms of infection frequently develop simultaneously with new local findings, facilitating differentiation of frostbite-mediated tissue damage from infection.

SYMPTOMS AND CLINICAL MANIFESTATIONS

Cellulitis complicating an injury shares many of the clinical characteristics of cellulitis due to *S. aureus,* group A *Streptococcus,* and mixed-organism infections (Chapter 46). The tissue layers involved (epidermis, dermis, or subcutaneous tissue) become inflamed as the inoculated bacteria multiply. In the span of hours to a few days after bacterial inoculation, the wound, which frequently shows some signs of inflammation from the tissue injury already present, exhibits increasing edema, erythema, pain, and discharge. Systemic symptoms of fever, myalgias, and headache may accompany the development of local findings in the wound and may be particularly prominent when bacteremia develops as a complication of wound infection or in infection with bacteria (e.g., *S. aureus,* group A *Streptococcus, Clostridium*) that elaborate extremely potent toxins capable of being absorbed from the wound. Lymphangitis associated with wound infections is most often caused by group A *Streptococcus* (Chapter 51).

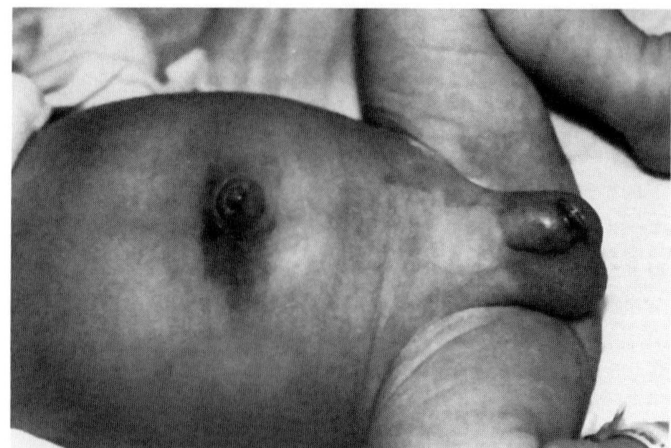

FIGURE 48–1. Abdominal wall in 3-week-old infant with omphalitis (necrotizing fasciitis). Minimal early cutaneous changes and marked edema are present in this infant, whose infection was confirmed at surgery.

Necrotizing Fasciitis. The infection initially resembles cellulitis originating at a site of trauma, at a varicella lesion or other tissue injury, or at the umbilical stump in neonates with omphalitis (Fig. 48–1). On occasion the infection spreads from deeper tissues, as is the case in necrotizing fasciitis related to colon cancer in adults. Erythema, tenderness, and edema may develop as early as 1–3 days or as late as 2 weeks after the initial trauma, depending on the organisms involved. The area of edema and tenderness spreads and is not sharply marginated, although the overlying skin may not show any dramatic changes early in the infection (Fig. 48–2). Blisters and bullae appear, and necrosis of the fascia produces thin, watery pus. The skin may become gangrenous and may slough. Crepitation may develop at this time. A higher fever and a toxic state develop as the infection progresses.

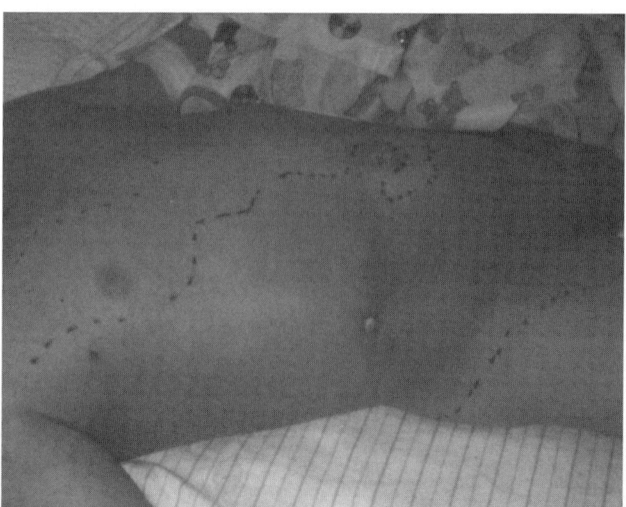

FIGURE 48–2. Group A streptococcal necrotizing fasciitis resulting from varicella, immediately before radical débridement in a 6-year-old boy. Note the prominent focal changes at sites of varicella lesions and the diffuse, edematous, dusky changes in the lateral abdominal wall, marked preoperatively.

When explored during an operation, the subcutaneous tissue planes offer no resistance to the spreading forceps because the substance of this tissue has become necrotic. The overlying skin, having lost its blood supply relatively late in the infection, also begins to show signs of necrosis. A thin, serosanguineous discharge may be noted from the trauma-induced or surgical wound, which previously may have been assessed as clean and well healed.

The clinical condition is often toxic, as though bacteremic, although blood cultures are usually sterile. Signs and symptoms of endotoxic shock may develop, with decreased myocardial contractility, adult respiratory distress syndrome, oliguria, and extensive extravasation of intravascular fluid. The mortality rate for this advanced infection is high. Marked soft-tissue edema in the area of infection and surrounding tissues may persist for up to 3–5 days despite appropriate surgical and medical management.

Fournier's gangrene usually begins with perineal pain and is rapidly progressive. The clinical condition may appear relatively nontoxic initially. The painful, inflamed, swollen tissue becomes gangrenous, and the disease spreads to the perineum, buttocks, groin, penis, and anterior abdominal wall.

Myonecrosis. Myonecrosis also is a life-threatening infection (Table 48–3). Myonecrosis involves the trunk more often in children than in adults, but the extremities may also be involved. Omphalitis that has progressed beyond involvement of the subcutaneous tissues and fascial planes to include the abdominal musculature is another example of myonecrosis.

About 1–9 days (most often 4–7 days) after an injury, pain and irritability out of proportion to the degree of local findings suddenly develop at the site of injury—or at the umbilical stump in the case of omphalitis. Rapid development of edema at the site of the wound and simultaneous progression of pain in the context of fever are the hallmark of infection in the deep tissue spaces. Mild erythema or a pale or dusky color of the skin surrounding the wound or umbilical stump may occur initially as the destructive process is localized deep to the dermis, resulting in minimal findings superficially at the onset of the infection. As the infection progresses and thrombi form in the vessels that supply the dermis, the superficial skin becomes progressively more dusky and necrotic. Crepitation may be noted early in the infection in up to 60% of adults with myonecrosis with either a clostridial or a nonclostridial cause. Infections associated with gas formation tend to occur earlier after trauma and tend to be more severe than those without gas formation. Large bullae may appear at the site of the wound. Depending on the organisms involved, these bullae contain a foul- or sweet-smelling, yellowish or brownish, thin discharge. With progressive local tissue edema and the development of systemic edema from movement of fluid out of the intravascular compartment, tachycardia develops at a level more pronounced than is easily explained by the child's fever.

Within several hours, systemic toxicity becomes marked. Altered mental status, progressive shock that is difficult to treat, acidosis, and coagulopathy develop. Deep tissue infections may be particularly fulminant in immunocompromised persons. Newborn infants with omphalitis that progresses to necrotizing fasciitis and myonecrosis frequently develop multiple organ system failure and die.

TABLE 48–3. Symptoms and Signs of Myonecrosis

Acute onset of severe pain out of proportion to degree of local findings at site of trauma or surgery
Extensive rapidly progressive edema around the wound
Mild erythema or dusky blue skin surrounding the wound, with later findings that may or may not include crepitus or the development of large bullae
Progressive tachycardia in the absence of high fever
Progressive clinical systemic toxic effects
Gram stain of wound exudate, showing either rare, large gram-positive bacilli (*Clostridium*) with scant polymorphonuclear neutrophils or rare polymorphonuclear neutrophils only
Progressive shock, with acidosis

DIAGNOSIS

Wounds exhibit inflammation from the tissue destruction produced at the time of injury. The inflammatory response increases during the first several hours after injury, depending on the location, type, and extent of injury. Tissue inflammation present during the first 12–24 hours after the injury is usually not a result of infection. However, after this relatively short time interval, bacteria introduced into the wound may proliferate in devitalized tissue, leading to a clear change in the degree and character of the local symptoms and a change in the characteristics of the wound discharge. In addition, systemic symptoms of infection such as fever may develop in response to systemic absorption of bacterial products.

The diagnosis of necrotizing fasciitis and myonecrosis is established on clinical findings. In the early stages of infection it may be difficult to distinguish cellulitis, necrotizing fasciitis, and myonecrosis. However, with aerobic cellulitis, wound pain and edema are less severe and systemic toxicity is usually absent.

These infections should be suspected in the context of the rapidly progressive clinical symptoms, particularly with soft-tissue crepitation, which occurs in approximately 10% of persons with these infections. For clinical findings consistent with a rapidly progressive soft-tissue infection, surgical evaluation, with wound biopsy, is mandatory for confirming the diagnosis and is an important component of therapy. The structural integrity of the subcutaneous and fascial tissues should be assessed when the wound is explored. If no resistance to forceps is noted in subcutaneous tissue and fascia, the surgeon is required to extend the original incision until normal, healthy, nonnecrotic areas are encountered. Examination of the deep fascia and muscle layer is mandatory in the differentiation between necrotizing fasciitis and myonecrosis. With visualization of the muscle beneath infected fascia, identification of obviously necrotic muscle confirms the diagnosis of myonecrosis. On occasion, however, even if it appears normal, the muscle may not bleed when cut or contract when cauterized. These findings also indicate muscle necrosis and mandate radical débridement.

A **frozen section** at the time of initial surgical exploration is valuable in identifying necrotizing fasciitis, indicating the need for aggressive débridement, which might not be performed otherwise. Both aerobic and anaerobic cultures are essential in assessing the full range of bacteria involved and their antibiotic susceptibilities.

Laboratory Evaluation

Laboratory evidence of infection includes an elevated WBC count that typically shows a dramatic increase in the number of circulating immature neutrophils. Advanced infection may be associated with progressive signs of metabolic acidosis and DIC, with thrombocytopenia, prolonged prothrombin time and partial thromboplastin time, and decreasing fibrinogen levels. If there is extensive tissue necrosis, hypocalcemia may occur because of saponification after necrosis of subcutaneous fat.

Microbiologic Evaluation

Microbiologic evaluation of the wound is essential in confirming the diagnosis and guiding antibiotic management. A Gram-stained smear of necrotic tissue gives clues to the diagnosis. The finding of large ''boxcar'' gram-positive bacilli is characteristic of infection with *Clostridium.* Multiple gram-positive cocci mixed with gram-negative bacilli suggest a nonclostridial bacterial cause.

Anaerobic and aerobic culture specimens should be obtained from both the central portion and the advancing edge of maximal inflammation of the infection for the best yield of organisms. Specimens for anaerobic culture should be processed as quickly as possible. Aerobic and anaerobic blood cultures are needed because of the propensity of organisms in deep tissue infections to disseminate.

Diagnostic Imaging

Plain radiographs of the extremities, or a cross-table lateral abdominal radiograph if the trunk is involved, may be helpful in confirming the clinical suspicion of crepitation by demonstrating gas in the subcutaneous tissues. This finding is present in approximately 40–80% of persons with necrotizing fasciitis and myonecrosis. Organisms other than *Clostridium,* including enteric gram-negative bacilli, also may be responsible for soft-tissue gas. Ultrasonography, CT, and particularly MRI have been shown to be more sensitive imaging procedures than standard radiography in assessing deep tissue necrosis present in necrotizing fasciitis or myonecrosis. These studies may help define the extent of disease, but performing them should not delay surgical débridement in rapidly progressive disease.

TREATMENT

The treatment of necrotizing fasciitis and myonecrosis as deep tissue infections requires an aggressive combination of surgical and medical management. First and foremost is the need for extensive surgical débridement of all involved areas down to healthy tissue with good blood flow. This procedure defines the extent of disease and provides for removal of nonviable necrotic tissue. Extensive débridement of all involved layers of tissue, from the dermis and the subcutaneous tissues through to muscle, is associated with optimal survival of the patient (Fig. 48–3). Even after adequate débridement, signs and symptoms of progressive infection may occur with increasing edema and erythema, presumably caused by tissue-bound toxins. Repeated daily surgical exploration may be required for necrotic tissue if clinical signs of progressive disease are present. If no devitalized tissue is found after successive operative evaluations of new tissue edema, the tissue changes can be attributed to toxins formed and released before therapy.

Definitive Treatment

Empirical antibiotic therapy for deep tissue infections may be accomplished with one of several combinations of antibiotics (Table 48–4). Clindamycin and either cefotaxime or ceftriaxone provide activity against *Clostridium* and anaerobic streptococci, as well as *S. aureus,* group A *Streptococcus,* and gram-negative enteric bacilli. Antibiotic regimens incorporating ceftazidime and an aminoglycoside provide activity against *P. aeruginosa,* a more common pathogen in environmental trauma-related infections and infections in immunocompromised children.

For invasive toxin-mediated infection caused by group A *Streptococcus,* retrospective data analysis suggests that clindamycin therapy is associated more often with a favorable outcome than is therapy with β-lactam antibiotics. Two theoretical explanations may support this observation. Toxin production by streptococcal organisms is inhibited more rapidly after exposure to clindamycin, a protein synthesis inhibitor, than after use of β-lactam antibiotics. In addition, penicillins are less active against a large inoculum of organisms approaching a stationary phase of growth **(Eagle effect)** than is clindamycin. In vitro studies have not documented antagonism between clindamycin and penicillin for the vast majority of

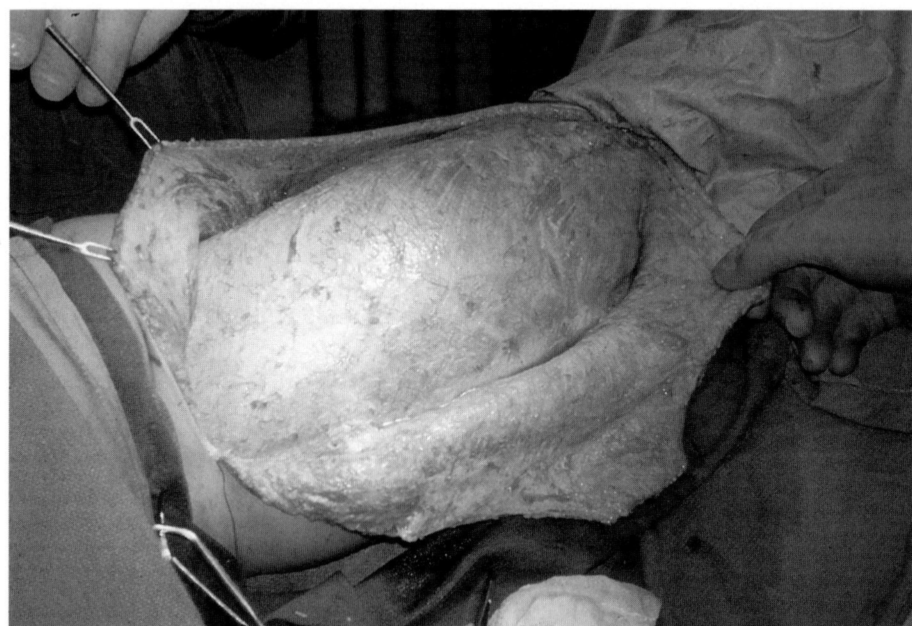

FIGURE 48–3. Extensive débridement of the lateral abdominal and chest wall subcutaneous and fascial tissues of the child shown at the preoperative stage in Figure 48–2. Devitalized tissue demonstrated typical surgery-related pathology with loss of tissue integrity.

TABLE 48–4. Antibiotic Therapy for Necrotizing Fasciitis and Myonecrosis*

Etiologic Agent	Recommended Therapy	Alternative Therapy
Empirical Antibiotic Therapy	Clindamycin *plus* cefotaxime *or* ceftriaxone *or* cefepime *with or without* an aminoglycoside†	Penicillin G *plus* nafcillin *or* oxacillin *plus* cefotaxime *or* ceftriaxone *or* an aminoglycoside† *or* Metronidazole *plus* vancomycin† *plus* cefotaxime *or* ceftriaxone *or* Meropenem *or* imipenem
Definitive Antibiotic Therapy		
Clostridium, anaerobic streptococci	Penicillin G	Clindamycin *or* metronidazole
Group A *Streptococcus*	Clindamycin *or* penicillin G	
Staphylococcus aureus		
Methicillin sensitive	Cefazolin	Nafcillin *or* oxacillin *or* clindamycin
Methicillin resistant	Vancomycin†	
Gram-negative enteric bacilli	Cefotaxime or ceftriaxone *plus* an aminoglycoside†	Ticarcillin-clavulanate *or* piperacillin-tazobactam *plus* an aminoglycoside† *or* Cefepime *or* Meropenem *or* imipenem
Pseudomonas aeruginosa	Ceftazidime *or* ticarcillin-clavulanate *plus* an aminoglycoside†	Meropenem *or* imipenem *with or without* an aminoglycoside†

*Aggressive surgical débridement of all involved tissue layers is essential.
†Serum concentrations of vancomycin and aminoglycosides should be monitored during therapy.

Suggested Dosages for Patients with Normal Renal Function

ANTIBIOTIC	INTRAVENOUS DOSAGE	MAXIMUM DAILY DOSE
Amikacin	15–20 mg/kg/day divided q8–12hr	15 mg/kg
Cefazolin	100 mg/kg/day divided q8hr	3–6 g
Cefepime*	150 mg/kg/day divided q8hr	6 g
Cefotaxime*	200 mg/kg/day IV divided q6hr	12 g
Ceftazidime*	150 mg/kg/day divided q8hr	6 g
Ceftriaxone*	100 mg/kg/day divided q12hr	2–4 g
	or 80 mg/kg/day (maximum 24 g) q24hr	2–4 g
Clindamycin	40 mg/kg/day divided q8hr	2.7 g
Gentamicin	7.5 mg/kg/day divided q8hr	Adults: 5 mg/kg
Imipenem	100 mg/kg/day divided q6hr	2 g
Meropenem*	120 mg/kg/day divided q8hr	3 g
Metronidazole	30 mg/kg/day divided q6hr	4 g
Nafcillin	150 mg/kg/day divided q6hr	9 g
Oxacillin	150–200 mg/kg/day divided q6hr	12 g
Penicillin G	250,000–400,000 U/kg/day divided q4hr	20–24 MU
Piperacillin*	200–300 mg/kg/day divided q6hr	18 g
Ticarcillin-clavulanate	Ticarcillin 200–300 mg/kg/day divided q6hr	18 g
Tobramycin	7.5 mg/kg/day divided q8hr	Adults: 5 mg/kg
Vancomycin	45–60 mg/kg/day divided q6hr	2 g

*Maximum doses as used for meningitis.

strains, supporting the common practice of combination therapy for presumed streptococcal necrotizing fasciitis with both clindamycin and penicillin.

Definitive antibiotic therapy is guided by culture and susceptibility testing (Table 48–4). Initial broad-spectrum therapy can be refined, particularly if a single organism is isolated. If culture results indicate infection caused by a gram-negative bacillus that is capable of being induced to produce chromosomal β-lactamase, such as *Enterobacter, Serratia, Citrobacter,* or *Pseudomonas,* an aminoglycoside should be used in addition to the third-generation cephalosporin to minimize the emergence of β-lactamase-producing organisms. Alternative β-lactam antibiotics that are relatively stable to these β-lactamases and are acceptable as monotherapy are cefepime, a fourth-generation cephalosporin, meropenem, and imipenem. Strains of *Klebsiella* and *E. coli* may harbor extended-spectrum β-lactamases active against the third-generation cephalosporins, requiring treatment with cefepime, meropenem, or imipenem.

For necrotizing fasciitis, a similar broad-spectrum empirical approach to therapy is required until culture results are obtained. If streptococci and anaerobes, excluding β-lactamase-positive *Bacteroides,* are the only organisms isolated, penicillin G or clindamycin may be used as a single agent.

Empirical antimicrobial treatment of Fournier's gangrene, usually caused by mixed aerobic and anaerobic enteric flora, is similar to that of omphalitis. Activity is required against enteric bacilli, *Bacteroides,* and gram-positive cocci including *S. aureus.*

For newborns with omphalitis, extensive surgical débridement is essential. Antibiotics are important adjunctive therapy. Broad-spectrum combination therapy, active against gram-positive cocci such as *S. aureus,* against enteric gram-negative bacilli, and against anaerobes, including β-lactamase-producing *Bacteroides,* is critical. Prospective comparative antibiotic treatment studies to determine optimal therapy have not been performed. Combinations that provide the required antibacterial activity are (1) cefotaxime plus clindamycin and (2) metronidazole plus nafcillin plus gentamicin. Culture results allow the antibiotic coverage to be focused more appropriately.

Empirical antimicrobial therapy of water-associated wound infections should include broad-spectrum coverage, including activity against *Pseudomonas,* such as a third-generation cephalosporin (e.g., ceftazidime) or an antipseudomonal penicillin plus an aminoglycoside. Surgical débridement is frequently necessary, at which time cultures of deep tissues can be obtained. Most strains of *Pseudomonas, Aeromonas,* and *Plesiomonas* are resistant to ampicillin and first-generation cephalosporins.

The medical treatment of wounds caused by *V. vulnificus* is controversial. Most experts recommend tetracycline or doxycycline as the treatment of choice. For children more than 8 years of age and for younger children and infants with overwhelming disease, tetracycline should be used, administered intravenously if the patient is too ill to tolerate oral therapy. Alternative therapies that are less well studied include high-dose penicillin G therapy, the use of aminoglycosides, and therapy with third-generation cephalosporins such as ceftazidime, cefotaxime, or ceftriaxone. The benefits of tetracycline therapy must be weighed against the minimal risk of dental staining in younger persons.

Hyperbaric Oxygen Therapy. The role of hyperbaric oxygen in the treatment of anaerobic necrotizing fasciitis, myonecrosis, and other anaerobic and mixed infections is controversial. Although not beneficial against anaerobic organisms in all tissue locations of infection, hyperbaric oxygen therapy may have some role in managing clostridial disease, particularly disease involving the extremities.

Hyperbaric oxygen therapy is delivered in specialized referral centers. In the treatment chambers, tissue levels of oxygen are maximized by having the patient breathe 100% oxygen under 2–3 atmospheres of pressure. No prospective, randomized evaluation of hyperbaric oxygen therapy for infection has been performed. Experts reporting retrospective data have found either no substantial benefit or rapid demarcation of devitalized areas on the extremities, allowing débridement or amputation of these areas, in contrast to other areas that still have perfusion. Delivery of high concentrations of oxygen to marginally perfused tissues may well have a detrimental effect on the growth of *Clostridium* and most anaerobes. However, the oxygen has no effect on preformed clostridial α toxin, which explains the progression of clinical findings after days into therapy despite negative culture results. Some centers reported a reduced mortality in the era of hyperbaric oxygen therapy, whereas other centers not using hyperbaric oxygen reported similar lower mortality during the same period. The populations treated are difficult to compare because of differences in time to diagnosis, extent of disease, and underlying conditions. All reported experience is also skewed toward older adults. Some experts believe that the sharper demarcation of viable versus nonviable tissue in the extremities allows for more conservative débridement of necrotic tissue, thereby sparing some persons limb amputation. Surgical therapy, however, has the highest priority, and transport to a facility with oxygen therapy capabilities should not replace radical emergent surgical débridement if deemed necessary after initial evaluation.

Tetanus Prophylaxis. Tetanus immunization status should be assessed with any wound involving damaged deep tissue or anaerobic conditions. With clean minor wounds, children with three or more tetanus immunizations, the most recent immunization having been given within 10 years before the injury, need no further immunization (Table 48–5). Tetanus immune globulin (TIG) is not indicated for clean minor wounds.

For deep wounds contaminated with soil or for wounds likely to be associated with anaerobic conditions, such as puncture wounds, no immunization is needed if three or more tetanus immunizations have been given, with the most recent immunization or booster within 5 years of the time of injury. The use of TIG is not indicated for children who are fully immunized. For children whose history of immunization is uncertain or for children who have not completed the initial course of three injections, tetanus immunization is recommended. Children with clean, minor wounds should be given prophylaxis with diphtheria and adsorbed tetanus toxoids with pertussis vaccine (DTaP) if younger than 7 years or prophylaxis with tetanus and diphtheria toxoids (Td) if 7 years of age or older. For the deep wounds contaminated with soil or with anaerobic conditions, such as puncture wounds, when immunization status is uncertain, TIG is recommended in a single dose of 250–500 U given intramuscularly, in addition to tetanus immunization.

COMPLICATIONS

Complications include extensive local tissue destruction and necrosis, abscess formation, peritonitis, sepsis, septic emboli, DIC, and death. Persons with myonecrosis and extensive muscle necrosis who recover frequently have a long-term disability and require rehabilitation. Reconstruction of muscle and fascial layers, as well as skin grafting, is usually required. The prolonged hospitalization usually required is associated with a high risk of nosocomial infection.

PROGNOSIS

The outcome of necrotizing fasciitis and myonecrosis depends greatly on prompt recognition and early and aggressive surgical exploration and débridement, along with broad-spectrum parenteral antimicrobial therapy. Even with appropriate surgical and antibiotic therapy, progressive local edema may take 3–5 days to begin to resolve, forcing the clinician to question the adequacy of therapy. Slow recovery is the rule, with extensive soft-tissue damage requiring several weeks to heal.

The mortality rate for necrotizing fasciitis has ranged in recent reports from 12.5% to 73%, even with appropriate, aggressive management. In children with Fournier's gangrene the mortality rate is approximately 9%. The mortality for myonecrosis is reported to be 7–95%, although several factors have been shown to affect survival. The extent of the infection, the location of the infection (extremity infections having a lower mortality than infections of the torso), the number of hours that symptoms lasted before treatment was sought, the surgical expertise and management of dé-

TABLE 48–5. Guide to Tetanus Prophylaxis in Wound Management

History of Tetanus Immunization (Doses)*	Clean Minor Wounds†		All Other Wounds‡	
	Td	TIG§	Td	TIG§
Uncertain or fewer than three	Yes	No	Yes	Yes
Three or more‖	No¶	No	No#	No

*Usually, tetanus toxoid as adsorbed toxoid. Although licensed, fluid tetanus toxoid is rarely used.
†Td = adult-type tetanus and diphtheria toxoids. If the patient is younger than 7 years, diphtheria and tetanus toxoids (DT) or diphtheria and tetanus toxoids with pertussis vaccine (DTaP) are given.
‡Including but not limited to wounds contaminated with dirt, feces, soil, or saliva; puncture wounds; avulsions; and wounds resulting from missiles, crushing, burns, and frostbite.
§Equine tetanus antitoxin should be used if TIG (tetanus immune globulin) is not available.
‖If only three doses of fluid toxoid have been received, a fourth dose of toxoid, preferable an adsorbed toxoid, should be given. Although licensed, fluid tetanus toxoid is rarely used.
¶Yes, if more than 10 years since the last dose.
#Yes, if more than 5 years since the last dose.
Used with permission of the American Academy of Pediatrics Committee on Infectious Diseases. Copyright, 2000. Tetanus. In Pickering LK (editor): *2000 Red Book: Report of the Committee on Infectious Diseases,* 25th ed. Elk Grove Village, Ill, The Academy, 2000, p. 566.

bridement, and the quality of intensive care of the critically ill child with multiple organ system failure all have been identified as important prognostic factors. A dramatically lower mortality among persons operated on within 12 hours of the onset of symptoms has been reported than among persons whose surgical treatment was delayed.

PREVENTION

The prevention of injuries will clearly decrease the number of injury-related wound infections. Surgical wound infections can be minimized by following current guidelines for sterile surgical technique and perioperative antibiotic prophylaxis (Table 16–6). Tetanus immunization is an effective method of preventing morbidity and death from *C. tetani* wound colonization and infection. Similarly, immunization against diphtheria has led to the virtual elimination of cutaneous diphtheria as a complication of wounds.

REVIEWS

American Academy of Pediatrics Committee on Infectious Diseases: Severe invasive group A streptococcus infections: A subject review. *Pediatrics* 1998;101:136–40.

Antimicrobial prophylaxis in surgery: *Med Lett Drugs Ther* 1999;41:75–9.

Barton LL, Jeck DT, Vaidya VU: Necrotizing fasciitis in children: Report of two cases and review of the literature. *Arch Pediatr Adolesc Med* 1996;150:105–8.

Fildes J, Bannon MP, Barrett J: Soft-tissue infections after trauma. *Surg Clin North Am* 1991;71:371–84.

Hsieh WS, Yang PH, Chao HC, et al: Neonatal necrotizing fasciitis: A report of three cases and review of the literature. *Pediatrics* 1999;103:e53.

KEY ARTICLES

Brennan SR, Rhodes KH, Peterson HA: Infection after farm machine–related injuries in children and adolescents. *Am J Dis Child* 1990; 144:710–3.

Brook I: Aerobic and anaerobic microbiology of necrotizing fasciitis in children. *Pediatr Dermatol* 1996;13:281–4.

Brook I: Microbiology of necrotizing fasciitis associated with omphalitis in the newborn infant. *J Perinatol* 1998a;18:28–30.

Brook I, Frazier EH: Aerobic and anaerobic microbiology of infection after trauma. *Am J Emerg Med* 1998b;16:585–91.

Choo PW, Donahue JG, Platt R: Ibuprofen and skin and soft tissue superinfections in children with varicella. *Ann Epidemiol* 1997;7:440–5.

Classen DC, Evans RS, Pestotnik SL, et al: The timing of prophylactic administration of antibiotics and the risk of surgical-wound infection. *N Engl J Med* 1992:326:281–6.

Darke SG, King AM, Slack WK: Gas gangrene and related infection: Classification, clinical features and aetiology, management and mortality: A report of 88 cases. *Br J Surg* 1977;64:104–12.

Farrell LD, Karl SR, Davis PK, et al: Postoperative necrotizing fasciitis in children. *Pediatrics* 1988;82:874–9.

Gettleman LK, Shetty AK, Prober CG: Posttraumatic invasive *Aspergillus fumigatus* wound infection. *Pediatr Infect Dis J* 1999;18:745–7.

Lally KP, Atkinson JB, Woolley MM, et al: Necrotizing fasciitis. A serious sequela of omphalitis in the newborn. *Ann Surg* 1984;199:101–3.

Schmid MR, Kossmann T, Duewell S: Differentiation of necrotizing fasciitis and cellulitis using MR imaging. *AJR Am J Roentgenol* 1998; 170:615–20.

Stamenkovic I, Lew PD: Early recognition of potentially fatal necrotizing fasciitis. The use of frozen-section biopsy. *N Engl J Med* 1984; 310:1689–93.

Zerr DM, Alexander ER, Duchin JS, et al: A case-control study of necrotizing fasciitis during primary varicella. *Pediatrics* 1999;103:783–90.

Zimbelman J, Palmer A, Todd J: Improved outcome of clindamycin compared with beta-lactam antibiotic treatment for invasive *Streptococcus pyogenes* infection. *Pediatr Infect Dis J* 1999;18:1096–100.

CHAPTER 49

Burn Wound Infections

John S. Bradley

Burns result from exposure to thermal, electrical, chemical, or radiation energy and represent an important cause of morbidity and death in children. In addition to cardiovascular instability and respiratory tract damage, infection also plays a major role in both morbidity and death from burns, with up to 20% of all burn deaths directly attributable to bacterial infection. Many factors contribute to susceptibility of burns to infection, including loss of the skin as a barrier to bacterial and fungal invasion, which is the most important factor, and also suppressed immune responses of persons with burns. Awareness of the increased susceptibility of children with burns to infection, knowledge of the microbiologic features of burns with appropriate use of topical and systemic antibiotics, and aggressive surgical management have led to improved outcomes for children with serious burns.

ETIOLOGY

A variety of bacteria are responsible for burn wound infections. The specific causative organisms vary from center to center, and also from year to year within each center. Isolation policies and prophylactic and empirical use of antibiotics, both intravenous and topical, differ among institutions and alter the colonizing flora that may ultimately cause infection.

Burn wounds quickly become colonized with *Staphylococcus* and other gram-positive cocci, which may progress to infection during the initial 1–2 weeks of hospitalization. Colonization of burn wounds in children also reflects the area of the child's body adjacent to the wound. For example, gastrointestinal flora, both aerobic and anaerobic, tends to colonize burns in the perianal area, and oral flora tends to colonize burn wounds on the face.

The most common gram-positive organism infecting burns is *Staphylococcus aureus,* especially burns of <20% of the BSA. *S. aureus* accounts for up to 50% of all invasive burn wound infections in some institutions. More extensive burn wounds are likely to be infected with *Pseudomonas aeruginosa,* which is the most common gram-negative organism infecting burns, as well as with enteric gram-negative bacilli (e.g., *Escherichia coli, Klebsiella, Enterobacter, Serratia*). These organisms begin to colonize the burn after the first week of hospitalization and continue to play a prominent role in colonization and infection throughout hospitalization (Table 49–1). Antibiotic-resistant nosocomial organisms often colonize and subsequently infect burns after the first few weeks of hospitalization, the result of selection from use of systemic and topical antibiotics that inhibit the more susceptible normal flora.

The rate of infection with *Candida* is low during the first few weeks of hospitalization but increases to a constant 5–10% of all documented infections during the later hospital course. Even though the rate of bacterial infection has decreased in many centers during the past 2 decades, the rate of fungal infection has not diminished. In some centers, *Aspergillus* now causes infection at a greater rate than *Candida.* The Zygomycetes fungi (e.g., *Mucor, Rhizopus*) have also become clinically significant pathogens in persons with burn wounds, perhaps in part as a result of improved long-term survival of those with extensive burns treated with aggressive antibiotic therapy and surgery.

Cutaneous infection of burns with HSV and VZV can occur with primary infection or with reactivation of latent infection. CMV also appears to reactivate in persons with burns and may cause systemic symptoms. The incidence of herpesvirus infections in persons with burns has not been studied prospectively. Respiratory viruses, particularly adenoviruses, have also been documented as a cause of fever in children with burns.

EPIDEMIOLOGY

Approximately 500,000 children seek medical attention each year for burns, resulting in approximately 25,000 hospitalizations and 1,500 deaths. House fires are the cause of 80–90% of deaths from burns in children. Scald burns from hot bathwater and other hot liquids are common in all pediatric age groups, particularly children younger than 4 years of age, who have approximately eight times more scald burns than flame burns.

The temporal distribution of invasive bacterial disease during hospitalization with burns is bimodal, with the first peak occurring during the second and third weeks of hospitalization, usually caused by *S. aureus,* and the second peak occurring after 4 weeks of hospitalization, usually cased by gram-negative bacilli. The proportion of deaths attributed to infectious complications of burns is probably at least 20%, but reported rates in adults vary considerably, from 1.6% to 75%.

Cutaneous HSV infection complicating burn wounds occurs most commonly in children younger than 10 years with significant burns, typically involving the head and neck. Both HSV and VZV infections of burns can occur as nosocomial infections.

PATHOGENESIS

Thermal injury to tissue from an energy source is the initial insult in a burned child. The severity of the injury depends on the type, strength, and duration of exposure to the source of energy. Deeper and more extensive burn injuries are associated with a greater mortality rate. Although there is considerable variability at different burn centers, burns covering ≥60% BSA are associated with at least a 50% mortality rate. Necrotic, devascularized burned tissue acts as a focus for the growth of pathogens. A burn eschar forms in areas of partial- and full-thickness skin damage and acts as a barrier that promotes the proliferation of bacteria and fungi present at the interface of viable and necrotic tissues (Fig. 49–1). As organisms continue to grow in necrotic tissue, invasion of viable tissue inevitably occurs, leading to burn wound infection and bacteremia. Histologic evidence from biopsy samples confirms both proliferation of organisms in viable tissue and invasion into blood

TABLE 49–1. Microorganisms Isolated from Blood, Burn Wound, and Lung Infections in Burn Victims*

	Source (%)		
Isolate	Blood	Burn	Lung
Pseudomonas aeruginosa	30	40	30
Staphylococcus aureus	20	20	5
Gram-negative enteric bacilli	15	10	15
Fungi and yeast	5	15	20
Others	30	15	30

*Numbers represent averages: documented differences exist between institutions, and organisms isolated vary with duration of hospitalization, percentage of BSA burn, and use of topical antibiotics. Physicians must be guided by culture results, including serial punch biopsy cultures of burn wounds for each patient.

vessels and lymphatics. Early surgical excision and grafting have dramatically decreased the infectious complications of third-degree and serious second-degree burns during the past 2 decades. These trends are particularly evident in burns of <20–40% BSA.

Instrumentation is an important risk factor for infection in critically ill persons with burns. Central venous catheters, endotracheal tubes, and urinary bladder catheters all breach the normal cutaneous and mucosal barriers to bacterial and fungal invasion. Abnormalities of the normal skin barrier associated with the burn may add to the risk of vascular catheter–associated infection.

Immunologic Perturbations. Clinically significant humoral and cellular immunologic abnormalities described in adults with burns are likely to be present in children. The extent of immunologic abnormalities is directly proportional to the extent of the burn injury, with the most profound abnormalities in patients with burns of >30% BSA. Immunoglobulin levels are transiently depressed with a nadir 2–5 days after the burn. During this time, extravasation of intravascular fluid into burned, necrotic tissues, as well as into healthy tissues as the result of capillary leak from systemic inflammation, is maximal. Complement levels also decrease transiently during the first week after the burn. Nonspecific complement activation by burned tissue may lead to nonspecific activation of polymorphonuclear leukocytes. Low levels of circulating complement may also lead to a depression in specific organism-directed chemotaxis by polymorphonuclear leukocytes. Levels of fibronectin, a nonspecific opsonin, are also decreased after burn injury. Polymorphonuclear leukocytes initially have diminished chemotaxis, which improves substantially by the end of the second week. In addition, polymorphonuclear leukocytes demonstrate decreased intracellular bactericidal activity against *S. aureus* in an in vitro assay system.

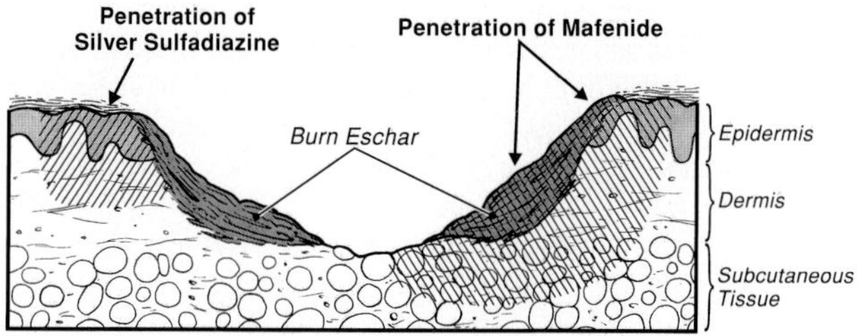

FIGURE 49–1. Cross section of a full-thickness burn demonstrates burn eschar extending through the dermis into the subcutaneous fat. Bacteria, which initially colonize the surface of the burn, may proliferate in necrotic tissue, reaching concentrations of more than 10^5 bacteria per gram of tissue, a concentration associated with a high risk of invasive disease. Also shown is the depth of penetration into burn tissue of two topical antibiotics, silver sulfadiazine and mafenide acetate.

Lymphocyte function defects lead to anergy to skin test antigens, which may be clinically associated with delayed skin graft rejection. Lymphocytes from persons with burns show decreased nonspecific mitogen responses, most likely because of the presence of unspecified circulating inhibitory factors that impair cellular responses. Increased CD8:CD4 cell ratios reflect increased numbers of circulating CD8 lymphocytes. In persons with burns, cellular responses to new antigens may be depressed because of inappropriate antigen-processing interactions between macrophages and T cells.

SYMPTOMS AND CLINICAL MANIFESTATIONS

Distinguishing infected burns from uninfected burns is frequently difficult. Symptoms and signs usually associated with infection, such as fever, wound exudates, and elevated WBC count, are more frequently a reaction to necrotic, burned tissue than to infection. Infants with extensive scald burns may have high, spiking fevers in the absence of infection, especially during the first few weeks of hospitalization, which complicates evaluation for infection. Changes in clinical examination with time are as important as any single facet of the examination.

Complete burn wound examinations at the time of dressing changes are essential, with particular attention to any changes in the appearance of the wound. Focal tissue changes at the site of the burn may occur with bacterial invasion of tissues and vessels surrounding the wound. An increase in pain at the wound site with an increased production of exudate about the wound, particularly a greenish exudate characteristic of *P. aeruginosa,* suggests a developing burn wound infection. Increasing necrosis at the periphery of the wound in areas previously believed to be viable may suggest invasive infection. Premature sloughing of the graft or focal areas where the graft will not ''take'' may be an indication of infection. Areas of graft with suspected infection should be excised and specimens from the wound cultured and then examined carefully for signs of infection.

S. aureus tends to cause focal suppurative disease with abscesses of burn wounds and occasionally of deeper adjacent tissues, but usually without sepsis. In contrast, *P. aeruginosa* tends to cause rapidly progressive cellulitis with early vessel invasion and bacteremia. *Candida* infection tends to be more indolent and focal, although it has been associated with a high mortality (10%).

Burn wound sepsis refers to clinical deterioration associated with clinical signs and symptoms of sepsis, although bacteremia or fungemia may not be present. The symptoms of burn wound sepsis (Table 49–2) occur as a result of systemic absorption of

TABLE 49–2. Signs and Symptoms of Burn Wound Sepsis

Fever or hypothermia
Increasing pain
Tachycardia
Increased oxygen requirement
Altered mental status
Eschar changes
Increased rate of exudate deposition in wound
Greenish discoloration of wound (*Pseudomonas aeruginosa*)
Increasing necrosis on periphery of burn wound
Early sloughing of xenograft, allograft, or autograft

inflammatory bacterial products and host cell production of cytokines such as TNF and IL-1 in response to necrotic tissue or localized bacterial infection. Local or systemic bacterial infection may cause either hyperthermia or hypothermia. Shock may develop, leading to tachycardia and altered mental status. Capillary leak syndrome may develop as a result of sepsis and may be initially noted by an increasing oxygen requirement due to increased levels of pulmonary interstitial fluid, rather than by peripheral edema.

Reactivation of HSV, VZV, and CMV can cause persistent fever, which may be difficult to differentiate clinically from fever and burn wound infection caused by bacterial pathogens. Single or grouped vesicles or ulcers on cutaneous or mucosal surfaces suggest HSV and VZV infections. CMV infection may be associated only with fever or occasionally with pneumonia or hepatitis. Respiratory and enteric viral pathogens responsible for community and nosocomial infections (e.g., rotavirus, RSV) can also cause intercurrent infections in children with burns.

DIAGNOSIS

Evaluation of burn wounds for infection is particularly difficult because fever is common with burns, the wound exudate is frequently profuse, and colonization of wounds with bacteria is universal. The most important aids in diagnosing burn wound infection are quantitative culture and histologic evaluation of the wound. The evaluation of burn wound sepsis involves evaluation of all areas of the burn for focal infection, in addition to evaluation for systemic spread of infection.

HSV and VZV infections usually cause cutaneous lesions and are identified by detection of specific viral antigens in lesions or by viral culture. CMV infection is more difficult to diagnose than HSV and VZV infections because of the absence of cutaneous lesions. CMV infection is identified by culture of urine or peripheral leukocytes or by testing plasma for CMV antigen or by PCR.

Nosocomial infections must also be considered in the evaluation of fever. Viral cultures and viral antigen testing may be indicated for children with high fever and respiratory or gastrointestinal symptoms suggestive of intercurrent viral infections, especially children with persisting symptoms whose surveillance culture results do not indicate invasive bacterial or fungal infection.

Laboratory Evaluation

Standard laboratory tests for infection, such as the WBC count or determination of the ESR, are rarely helpful. Widespread inflammation from necrotic tissue and repeated débridement may contribute to nonspecific elevation of these test results.

Microbiologic Evaluation

Skin Biopsy and Culture. An increased density of bacterial pathogens in burn wound tissue is associated with the likelihood of invasive infection. A density of $>10^5$ organisms per gram of tissue is frequently used to signify invasive disease. Biopsy samples of tissue, down to and including normal tissue, should be obtained from representative areas of the burn wound. The biopsy specimen is then divided and a portion submitted to the microbiology laboratory for weighing and quantitative culturing for aerobic and anaerobic bacteria. Another portion is submitted to the pathology laboratory to search for histologic evidence of bacteria or fungi invading viable tissue and vessels. In the original study (Pruitt and McManus, 1984), 96% of biopsy samples with $<10^5$ organisms per gram of tissue had no histologic evidence of infection, whereas 36% of biopsy specimens yielding $\geq 10^5$ organisms per gram of tissue had histologic evidence of invasive infection. The frequency of biopsy sampling from burn patients varies from institution to institution, with most performing routine biopsies two or three times per week, depending on the clinical status of the patient. Routine prospective monitoring by biopsy not only quantitates the density of organisms present in the burn wound but also provides the identity and antimicrobial susceptibilities of colonizing organisms.

Diagnostic Imaging

Persistent fever may indicate an abscess deep to the burn area that may not be clinically obvious. In particular, electrical burns may cause necrosis of deep tissue, which may become infected and require surgical drainage. CT or MRI may be used to identify and define deep tissue abscesses.

TREATMENT

Treatment of infected burn wounds includes both surgical management and antibiotic treatment. Improved outcomes have resulted from advances in both areas. A team approach involving the surgeon, the pediatrician, and the infectious disease specialist is usually required for optimal treatment of children with severe burns.

The status of tetanus immunization and the risk of tetanus should be assessed at the time of initial evaluation of burned children.

Definitive Treatment

Surgery. Surgical management with early burn eschar excision and wound closure, particularly of burn wounds of <30% BSA, has been widely accepted. In general, repeated tangential excision of burn wounds starts during the first week after the injury and continues every few days until the necrotic tissue has been removed, leaving behind healthy tissue with good perfusion. The wound may then be closed by graft material or biologic membrane. Surgical criteria for the type and extent of excision are based on the extent and location of the burn and the establishment of limits of blood loss during the operation. Although excision of burn eschar is clearly associated with an improved outcome, surgical complications have been reported. Transient bacteremia caused by organisms present in the burn eschar occurs during 15–50% of operative procedures. On occasion the bacteremia may persist and become clinically evident with sepsis. Although many burn centers use parenteral antibiotic therapy prophylactically at the time of excision of burn eschar, recent data suggesting lower rates of bacteremia, particularly for burns involving <40% BSA, support excision and cleansing without prophylactic therapy.

Maximal burn wound healing occurs if a moist membrane covers the open wound, forming a physiologic barrier to infection that allows for optimal wound healing and regeneration of tissue below the membrane. Many of the immunologic abnormalities present in persons with severe burns quickly resolve after the necrotic tissue has been excised and the wound has been closed. Various materials have been successfully used after débridement to close burn wounds, including xenografts (usually porcine), allografts, and ultimately autografts. Biologic synthetic membranes and techniques to propagate autologous fibroblasts in vitro to form autograft material are currently under investigation. Superficial abscesses may develop beneath graft material without being clinically apparent, requiring removal of graft material to examine underlying tissue.

Antibiotic Treatment. Antibiotic therapy for burn wounds includes both topical and systemic antibiotics. Infectious complications of severe burns have decreased substantially since the advent of prophylactic topical antibiotic therapy in burn wound management (Table 49–3), which is used primarily to decrease or prevent burn wound colonization and subsequent infection. Treatment of a burn wound infection still most often depends on administration of

TABLE 49–3. Topical Antibiotic Therapy

Type	Advantages	Disadvantages
Silver sulfadiazine (Silvadene)	Broad-spectrum bacterial activity Wound kept moist Not painful with application	Poor eschar penetration Transient reversible neutropenia Bacterial resistance
Mafenide acetate (Sulfamylon)	Broad-spectrum bacterial activity Excellent eschar penetration Wound kept moist	Painful on application Metabolic acidosis with widespread application Bacterial resistance Allergic reactions
Povidone-iodine (Betadine)	Broad-spectrum bacterial and fungal activity Good eschar penetration	Painful on application Wound surface dries easily Systemic absorption of iodine

systemic antibiotics, although mafenide acetate penetrates the burn eschar adequately to treat localized infection (Fig. 49–1).

The use of any antibiotic, topical or systemic, has profound effects on the colonizing flora. Although susceptible organisms may be inhibited by topical antibiotic therapy, they are seldom eradicated from burn wound surfaces. In this environment, antibiotic-resistant organisms have a selective advantage and may proliferate in burn wounds and subsequently cause infection. Decisions about antibiotic therapy must therefore be made carefully because the consequences of inappropriate or indiscriminate therapy can be disastrous for both the individual patient and the other patients in the burn unit.

Prophylactic intravenous penicillin, once believed to be effective in preventing infection, has not been shown in recent studies to be of substantial benefit in preventing burn wound infections. The use of systemic antibiotics in burn patients should be reserved for actual treatment of a suspected or documented infection. However, most children with serious burns are treated with intravenous antibiotic therapy soon after admission to the burn unit because many signs and symptoms of infection, present solely because of the tremendous inflammation caused by the burn, cannot be distinguished from infection.

Early burn wound infections are most frequently caused by *S. aureus,* and therefore empirical antibiotic therapy for suspected burn wound infections during the first week is with a first-generation cephalosporin or antistaphylococcal penicillin (Table 49–4). In situations of life-threatening sepsis a greenish wound exudate suggestive of *P. aeruginosa,* or a Gram stain indicating colonization or infection with a gram-negative bacillus, the use of an antibiotic such as a third-generation cephalosporin active against gram-negative organisms including *P. aeruginosa* is indicated. The possibility of methicillin-resistant *S. aureus* in life-threatening infection may be empirically treated by the addition of vancomycin. Other potential sites of infection (e.g., lung, upper respiratory tract, urinary tract) must also be considered in selecting an antibiotic regimen.

After the first week of hospitalization, nosocomial infections with hospital-acquired organisms, especially gram-negative bacilli, must be strongly considered. Because each burn unit has endogenous nosocomial bacterial flora that may vary with respect to both the types of organisms and the susceptibility patterns, knowledge of recently isolated pathogens is essential. Culture results from all persons with burns should be monitored to identify unusually resistant organisms and to assess the effectiveness of infection control procedures in the unit. This facilitates early identification of changes in organisms present in the unit and in antibiotic susceptibilities and of the need for stricter infection control practices to prevent spread of resistant organisms. Knowledge of the local prevalence of penicillin-, cephalosporin-, and aminoglycoside-resistant organisms, which are commonly found in many hospitals, is required to permit a knowledgeable choice of empirical therapy for suspected burn wound infections. Empirical therapy usually includes an antipseudomonas β-lactam antibiotic (e.g., ceftazidime, piperacillin), usually in combination with an aminoglycoside. This provides synergy to retard the development of β-lactam resistance, particularly in organisms with inducible β-lactamases such as *P. aeruginosa, Enterobacter,* and *Serratia.* Plasmid-mediated resistance to gentamicin and tobramycin may require the use of alternative aminoglycosides such as amikacin. Gram-negative bacilli resistant to penicillins, cephalosporins, and aminoglycosides may require the use of a carbapenem (e.g., meropenem or imipenem-cilastatin) or a quinolone (e.g., ciprofloxacin, levofloxacin, moxifloxacin, or gatifloxacin). Many burn units are also colonized with methicillin-resistant *S. aureus,* necessitating the addition of vancomycin for suspected *S. aureus* infection. Definitive antibiotic therapy is based on the results of cultures and susceptibility testing. A treatment course of 10–14 days is usually sufficient for most burn wound infections, assuming that the wound is adequately débrided and finally closed. Prolonged antibiotic therapy invites colonization by resistant bacteria as well as by yeast and fungi.

Antifungal Treatment. Fungal colonization with subsequent infection occurs after the first few weeks of hospitalization. Empirical therapy with amphotericin B (1 mg/kg/day administered for 3–4 hours intravenously) or one of its lipid-based formulations may be necessary for suspected infection that does not respond to antibiotic therapy or if cultures show growth of fungi. The newer parenteral azole antifungal agents such as fluconazole and itraconazole demonstrate substantially fewer organ toxic effects, although adequate studies in pediatric burn patients have not yet been reported.

Antiviral Treatment. Primary infection or reactivation of HSV and VZV, causing cutaneous disease or systemic symptoms, is treated with acyclovir (30 mg/kg/day divided every 8 hours intravenously) and usually requires 10–14 days of therapy. Surgery for wounds complicated by HSV or VZV infection should be deferred if possible until the viral infection is controlled. Ganciclovir is used to treat CMV infection, which responds more slowly to treatment than HSV and VZV infections. Antiviral therapy may need to be prolonged until the burn wound shows significant healing, which may parallel the return of normal immune function.

Supportive Therapy

Use of IVIG has been suggested as an appropriate therapy for persons with severe burns to reverse some of the documented humoral immunologic abnormalities. Theoretically, passively acquired opsonizing antibody to the infecting organisms should benefit the host. Intramuscular IG has not been shown to be of consistent benefit in reducing infection, but IVIG has been shown to be of benefit in experimental animals. Convincing data on efficacy in humans are currently unavailable. One unexpected difficulty in treating burns is the exceedingly short half-life of IVIG in these patients, which is as short as 2 days, compared with 3 weeks in healthy children and adults.

TABLE 49–4. Antibiotic Treatment for Bacterial Burn Wound Infections

Diagnosis or Etiologic Agent*	Recommended Regimen	Alternative Regimen
First Week After Burn		
Local infection	Cefazolin	Nafcillin *or* oxacillin
Life-threatening infection, greenish wound exudate, or gram-negative bacilli on Gram stain	Vancomycin *plus* ceftazidime *with or without* an aminoglycoside	Vancomycin *plus* piperacillin-tazobactam *with or without* an aminoglycoside
After First Week	Ceftazidime *or* ceftriaxone *or* piperacillin-tazobactam *plus* an aminoglycoside *with or without* vancomycin	Meropenem *or* cefepime *with or without* an aminoglycoside *with or without* vancomycin
Gram-Positive Cocci†		
Staphylococcus aureus		
Methicillin sensitive	Cefazolin	Nafcillin *or* oxacillin
Methicillin resistant	Vancomycin	Linezolid
Enterococcus		
Vancomycin sensitive	Ampicillin *with* an aminoglycoside *or* vancomycin	Linezolid
Vancomycin resistant	Linezolid	Quinupristin-dalfopristin
Group A *Streptococcus,* viridans streptococci	Cefazolin	Nafcillin *or* oxacillin
Gram-Negative Bacilli†		
Pseudomonas aeruginosa	Ceftazidime *or* piperacillin-tazobactam *plus* an aminoglycoside	Meropenem *or* cefepime *with or without* an aminoglycoside
Escherichia coli, Klebsiella, Enterobacter, Serratia	Cefotaxime *or* ceftriaxone *or* piperacillin-tazobactam *plus* an aminoglycoside	Meropenem *or* cefepime *with or without* an aminoglycoside
Fungi		
Candida albicans	Amphotericin B	Fluconazole

*Of the most frequently isolated organisms from punch biopsy cultures.
†Use susceptibility results from culture results.

Recommended Dosages for Persons with Normal Renal Function

ANTIBIOTIC	INTRAVENOUS DOSAGE	MAXIMUM DAILY DOSE	ANTIBIOTIC	INTRAVENOUS DOSAGE	MAXIMUM DAILY DOSE
Amikacin	15–20 mg/kg/day divided q8–12hr	(Same)	Gentamicin	7.5 mg/kg/day divided q8hr	5 mg/kg (adult dose)
Ampicillin	100–200 mg/kg/day divided q6hr	10–12 g	Meropenem	60–120 mg/kg/day divided q8hr	3 g
Cefazolin	100 mg/kg/day divided q8hr	3–6 g	Nafcillin	150 mg/kg/day divided q6hr	9 g
Cefepime	100–150 mg/kg/day divided q8–12hr	6 g	Oxacillin	150–200 mg/kg/day divided q6hr	12 g
Cefotaxime	200 mg/kg/day IV divided q6hr	12 g	Piperacillin-tazobactam	200–300 mg/kg/day divided q6hr	18 g
Ceftazidime	150 mg/kg/day divided q8hr	6 g	Tobramycin	7.5 mg/kg/day divided q8hr	5 mg/kg (adult dose)
Ceftriaxone	100 mg/kg/day divided q12hr *or* 80 mg/kg/day q24hr	2–4 g	Vancomycin	45–60 mg/kg/day divided q6hr	2 g

The pharmacokinetics of all systemically administered drugs have been shown to be altered considerably in persons with burns because of several simultaneously occurring events: increased metabolic rate, increased tissue distribution, increased glomerular filtration rate, and loss of drugs (including IG) by diffusion into the burn eschar. Doses of antibiotics usually need to be higher than doses used in persons without burns. Doses of potentially nephrotoxic drugs such as aminoglycosides or vancomycin need to be individualized by monitoring serum concentrations closely.

COMPLICATIONS

Necrotic tissue provides an ideal anaerobic environment for germination of the spores of *Clostridium tetani* with the production of tetanus toxin by the vegetative organisms. Cases of clinical tetanus in nonimmunized burned infants have been reported. For children who are not fully immunized, the appropriate immunization with diphtheria and adsorbed tetanus toxoids and pertussis vaccine (DTaP) or with tetanus and diphtheria toxoids (Td) should be administered. Children with extensive or full-thickness burns who are fully immunized but whose last tetanus booster was given more than 5 years previously should receive a booster Td.

Burn wound infections may lead to other foci of infection including pneumonia, catheter-associated infection, septic thrombophlebitis, infective endocarditis, sinusitis, urinary tract infection, and otitis media. Nosocomial pneumonia acquired during intubation may be caused by *Streptococcus pneumoniae,* by the person's own flora, or by hospital-acquired pathogens, especially *P. aeruginosa,* enteric gram-negative bacilli, and *S. aureus.* An indwelling nasogastric or nasojejunal tube is a risk factor for sinusitis, which may be diagnosed by CT and, if fevers persist despite empirical antibiotic therapy, by sinus aspiration. Almost all critically burned children have central venous catheters placed early in the hospital course to maximize nutritional support. Catheter-related sepsis is a common problem, particularly with extensive burns if a catheter must be placed through burned areas of skin or with extended hospitalization. Septic thrombophlebitis and endocarditis may occur as complications of catheter-related sepsis. Organisms responsible for catheter-related infections are usually the same as those colonizing the burn. Indwelling bladder catheters are often used to monitor urine output and may also be a focus of nosocomial infections, although meticulous catheter care and maintenance of a closed system may prevent infection. Nonspecific findings of fever may be the only clue to a catheter-related infection.

PROGNOSIS

Cardiovascular instability from extensive tissue damage, with increased vascular permeability, and respiratory tract inflammation from smoke inhalation are major contributors to the mortality, which is directly proportional to the extent of the burn injury. As many as 20% of all burn deaths are the direct result of bacterial infections. The two population groups at highest risk of dying from burn wound infections are the very young and the very old, with persons 20–30 years of age having the lowest mortality for burns covering an equivalent percentage of BSA. Both the mortality and the length of hospital stay for burn patients have decreased substantially in the past 2 decades, attributable in part to the decrease in infectious complications of burns. With aggressive surgical management to decrease the reservoir of necrotic burn tissue and routine microbial surveillance to assess the density of burn wound colonization and susceptibility patterns of pathogens, complications from burn wound sepsis have been minimized. However, as children with more serious and extensive burns survive, the chance of burn wound sepsis or nosocomial infection with organisms resistant to multiple antibiotics increases, providing a challenge in anti-infective management.

PREVENTION

Broad-spectrum topical antibiotic agents (Table 49–3) are used in initial empirical therapy for severe burns soon after children with symptoms are admitted to the burn unit, because many of the signs and symptoms of infection are present solely as a result of the tremendous inflammation caused by the burn. Sterile technique during dressing changes, surgical procedures, and physical therapy is important in minimizing colonization with hospital flora, which could include organisms resistant to multiple antibiotics. In general, systemic antimicrobial therapy has not been shown in prospective studies to be of benefit when used as prophylaxis and should be reserved for the actual treatment of a suspected or documented infection.

REVIEWS

Monafo WW, West MA: Current treatment recommendations for topical burn therapy. *Drugs* 1990;40:364–73.

Pruitt BA, McManus AT: Opportunistic infections in severely burned patients. Am J Med 1984;76(3A):146.

Pruitt BA Jr, McManus AT, Kim SH, et al: Burn wound infections: Current status. *World J Surg* 1998;22:135–45.

KEY ARTICLES

Becker WK, Cioffi WG Jr, McManus AT, et al: Fungal burn wound infection. A 10-year experience. *Arch Surg* 1991;126:44–8.

Bowser-Wallace BH, Graves DB, Caldwell FT: An epidemiological profile and trend analysis of wound flora in burned children: 7 years' experience. *Burns Incl Therm Inj* 1984;11:16–25.

Brook I, Randolph JG: Aerobic and anaerobic bacterial flora of burns in children. *J Trauma* 1981;21:313–8.

Deitch EA: The management of burns. *N Engl J Med* 1990;323:1249–53.

Finkelstein JL, Schwartz SB, Madden MR, et al: Pediatric burns. An overview. *Pediatr Clin North Am* 1992;39:1145–63.

Fukunishi K, Takahashi H, Kitagishi H, et al: Epidemiology of childhood burns in the Critical Care Medical Center of Kinki University Hospital in Osaka, Japan. *Burns* 26:2000;465–9.

Garrelts JC, Peterie JD: Altered vancomycin dose vs. serum concentration relationship in burn patients. *Clin Pharmacol Ther* 1988;44:9–13.

Linnemann CC Jr, MacMillan BG: Viral infections in pediatric burn patients. *Am J Dis Child* 1981;135:750–3.

Loirat P, Rohan J, Baillet A, et al: Increased glomerular filtration rate in patients with major burns and its effect on the pharmacokinetics of tobramycin. *N Engl J Med* 1978;299:915–9.

McGill SN, Cartotto RC: Herpes simplex virus infection in a paediatric burn patient: Case report and review. *Burns* 2000;26:194–9.

McManus AT, Kim SH, McManus WF, et al: Comparison of quantitative microbiology and histopathology in divided burn-wound biopsy specimens. *Arch Surg* 1987;122:74–6.

Mozingo DW, McManus AT, Kim SH, et al: Incidence of bacteremia after burn wound manipulation in the early postburn period. *J Trauma* 1997;42:1006–11.

Ou LF, Lee SY, Chen YC, et al: Use of Biobrane in pediatric scald burns—experience in 106 children. *Burns* 1998;24:49–53.

CHAPTER 50

Bite-Wound Infections

John S. Bradley

A **bite** is defined as a wound or puncture made by the teeth or other mouthparts of a living organism. Animal bites and human bites have different infectious disease implications.

ETIOLOGY

When the integrity of the skin is violated by the bite injury, bacterial pathogens from both the skin of the victim and the oral cavity of the biting animal or human can produce clinical infection. Viral pathogens may also be transmitted by either animal or human bites, causing systemic infection without an obvious local wound infection.

Animal Bites. The organisms isolated from infected animal bite wounds usually represent the skin flora of the victim and the oral flora of the animal. One study (Brook, 1987) of infected dog and cat bites showed a median of 2.8 aerobes and 1.8 anaerobes per infected bite, and another study (Talan et al, 1999) showed a median of 5 isolates per culture, reflecting the polymicrobial nature of oral flora. *Pasteurella, Staphylococcus,* and *Streptococcus* predominate in infected wounds (Table 50–1). *Bartonella henselae,* the cause of cat-scratch disease, can also be transmitted by cat bites or scratches, especially from young kittens (Chapter 28).

Bites by rodents may lead not only to local wound infections but also to systemic disease caused by the organisms responsible for **rat-bite fever,** *Streptobacillus moniliformis* and *Spirillum minus.* (**Haverhill fever** refers to *S. moniliformis* infection that occurs after ingestion of contaminated milk.) Bites by Old World monkeys can transmit **B virus,** a simian herpesvirus that is enzootic among rhesus and cynomolgus monkeys and that was named for the patient from whom it originally was isolated. It is also known as Herpesvirus simiae and formally is designated Cercopithecine herpesvirus 1.

Human Bites. The organisms responsible for infection by human bites are primarily oral flora, including *Streptococcus, Eikenella corrodens, Haemophilus,* and *Bacteroides,* as well as skin flora (Table 50–1). Although most of the oral flora cultured from human bite wounds are not highly pathogenic, they can cause a wide spectrum of severity of infection, from indolent to fulminant when inoculated directly into subcutaneous tissues.

As with certain zoonoses, human diseases spread primarily by other routes may on occasion be transmitted by bites. Syphilis, tuberculosis, and infection with actinomycetes have been reported after human bites. Viral infections may be transmitted by human bites, including hepatitis B virus, hepatitis C virus, HSV, and HIV.

EPIDEMIOLOGY

Animal Bites. It has been estimated by the CDC that approximately 3.73 million animal bites occur in the United States each year from dogs alone, with 757,000 requiring medical attention. Animal bites are responsible for up to 1% of all emergency health care visits, with dog bites representing up to 90% of all animal bites evaluated in this setting. In one study (Weiss, 1998) the median age of those who sought such emergency care was 15 years of age, with the highest incidence of bites occurring in boys 5–9 years of age (60.7 per 10,000 boys 5–9 years of age). Most emergency health care visits for animal bites occur during the summer months in the afternoon and evening hours, presumably reflecting the time of maximal contact between children and pets. Approximately half of animal bites occur on the hands and one fourth on the forearm or arm. Most of the animal bites to children are caused by animals known to the children, either their own pets or those of a neighbor, rather than by wild or stray animals. Children younger than 4 years are particularly likely to be bitten by the family dog, with 90% of these injuries actually occurring in the home.

Between 5% and 60% of all bite wounds are complicated by infection. Approximately 50% of cat bites, 16% of human bites, and 4% of dog bites will become infected, even with optimal initial wound management. Among children hospitalized for dog bite injuries, two thirds of the wounds are complicated by infection. Infections from bites by pets such as mice or rats are much less common, accounting for only 2.5% of all animal bite-wound infections. Bites by wild animals, farm animals, and reptiles have been anecdotally complicated by infection, but accurate incidence data are not available. Rat bites primarily affected children ≤5 years of age, with the majority of bites inflicted on the face and hands and occurring in the bedroom between midnight and 8 AM. The incidence of rat-bite fever after a rodent bite is unknown, but the disease has been noted to occur after up to 10% of rodent bites of such severity that they are brought to medical attention. Most B virus infections in humans occur in adult animal handlers in medical research facilities.

Human Bites. Human bites occur with regularity among children 2–4 years of age. Bite wounds occur more frequently among boys by a ratio of 2:1 until 13 years of age, when girls are bitten at a higher rate than boys. Human bites are responsible for approximately 1 in 600 emergency department visits, with the highest number of emergency health care visits during the summer and early fall. Although most bites occur during fights between children, predominantly with injury to the fingers, forearms, and cheeks, bites during play are not uncommon in young children. As children grow to adolescence, bites occur during other activities, such as during sporting contests and during lovemaking, as has also been docu-

TABLE 50–1. Infections Transmitted by Bites

Common Pathogens Causing Bite-Wound Infections

Animal Bite Wounds	
Organism	***Average Incidence in Infected Bites (%)****
Staphylococcus aureus	40
Pasteurella multocida	40
Streptococci	40
Corynebacterium	20
Coagulase-negative staphylococci	20
Aerobic enteric gram-negative bacilli	15
Anaerobic streptococci	40
Bacteroides	20
Human Bite Wounds	
Organism	***Average Incidence in Infected Bites (%)****
Streptococci	50
S. aureus	45
Corynebacterium	25
Eikenella corrodens	15
Haemophilus	15
Bacteroides	60
Anaerobic streptococci	50

Less Common Pathogens Causing Bite-Wound Infections

Animal Bite Wounds
Bartonella henselae (cat-scratch bacillus)
Fusobacterium
Pseudomonas
Clostridium tetani
Capnocytophaga canimorsus
Herpesvirus simiae (herpes B virus)

Human Bite Wounds
Actinomycetes
Fusobacterium
Herpes simplex virus

Systemic Infections Transmitted by Bites

Animal Bite Wounds	
Organism	***Disease***
B. henselae	Cat-scratch disease
Francisella tularensis	Tularemia
Yersinia pestis	Plague
Streptobacillus moniliformis	Rat-bite fever (streptobacillary)
Spirillum minus	Rat-bite fever (spirillary)
Rabies virus	Rabies
Herpesvirus simiae (herpes B virus)	Encephalitis
Human Bite Wounds	
Organism	***Disease***
Treponema pallidum	Syphilis
Mycobacterium tuberculosis	Tuberculosis
Hepatitis B virus	Hepatitis
Hepatitis C virus	Hepatitis
Human immunodeficiency virus	Acquired immunodeficiency syndrome (AIDS)

*Percentages add up to more than 100% because of the polymicrobial nature of bite-wound infections.

mented in adults. Another adult type of injury, the **clenched-fist injury,** occurs after a fistfight or after an accidental sports injury, with the opponent's tooth inoculating the deeper tissue planes and tendon sheaths of the hand with oral bacteria, leading to a rapidly progressive and potentially destructive infection.

PATHOGENESIS

Injuries from animal bites reflect the anatomy of the teeth and the strength of the jaws of the biting animal. Dog bites tend to cause lacerations, with crush and avulsion injuries as a function of the large, broad, sharp teeth and powerful jaws. Bites by cats, mice, rats, and snakes tend to cause puncture wounds because of the characteristic sharp, elongated needle-like teeth. In one study (Talan, 1999), 85% of cat bites were punctures, 3% were lacerations, and 12% a combination of the two, in comparison with dog bites, in which 60% were punctures, 10% were lacerations, and 30% were a combination. Human bites more closely resemble dog bites than cat bites, with abrasions and lacerations being more common than punctures. Bacteremia occurs rarely after an animal or human bite wound in an immunocompetent person.

The severity of bacterial bite-wound infections depends on several factors: (1) the oral flora of the person or animal inoculating the wound, (2) the anatomic location and structures damaged by the bite, (3) the organisms contaminating the wound from the environment or the skin, and (4) the time elapsed after the bite and before the wound is brought to medical attention. Rabies presents a unique situation as a complication of a bite, because the infection itself is extremely uncommon, the incubation period may last up to 1 year, and the consequences of the infection can be fatal.

Animal Bites. Most infections develop at the site of the bite wound and adjacent tissue. Puncture wounds tend to seal quickly, producing an environment that facilitates growth of anaerobic organisms. With any bite, but particularly with cat bites, the teeth may penetrate not only the skin but also underlying structures such as joints, bones, tendons, or tendon sheaths, allowing for inoculation of organisms into deeper tissue spaces. Puncture wounds may appear innocuous immediately after the injury, but infection often develops in the deeply inoculated tissues within a few hours and may not be recognized. Once infection develops, if it is not appropriately managed, it can spread along deep tissue spaces and lead to abscess formation.

Snakebite wounds appear to have a higher rate of infection by enteric gram-negative bacilli than mammalian bites. This finding is thought to reflect the manner in which a snake swallows its prey headfirst, with the animal's fecal flora subsequently colonizing the snake's mouth. Snake venom itself is sterile, although extensive necrosis of tissue may occur after snakebite, providing an optimal environment for growth of inoculated organisms. Gram-positive skin flora are also frequently isolated from snakebite-wound infections.

Risk factors for infection after a dog bite, which can be extrapolated to other bite wounds, include (1) bites to the hand, which are twice as likely to become infected as bites to the arm or leg; (2) delay of more than 24 hours in seeking treatment of the bite; and (3) bite victims more than 50 years of age. One retrospective study (Callahan, 1978) found that children less than 4 years of age had a decreased risk of infection.

Although the evaluation of a bite is usually focused on the degree of local injury and the presence of local infection, some systemic bacterial and viral infections may be transmitted by relatively innocuous animal bites (Table 50–1). These include streptobacillary rat-bite fever caused by *S. moniliformis,* cat-scratch disease caused by *B. henselae,* tularemia caused by *Francisella tularensis,* and plague caused by *Yersinia pestis,* although plague is usually spread by respiratory and enteric routes. Systemic viral infections transmitted by animal bites include rabies and B virus (Herpesvirus simiae) infections.

Human Bites. Although human bites tend to be more superficial than animal bites and are as easily irrigated and débrided as dog bites, the infection rate is greater. Presumably this is a result of the large numbers of aerobic and anaerobic organisms inoculated into the wound, because human saliva contains up to 10^8 organisms per milliliter.

With a clenched-fist injury, the deeper tissue spaces of the hand are inoculated at the time of injury. The tooth causes injuries ranging from a small laceration to more extensive soft-tissue, tendon, joint, and bone injuries. Organisms inoculated through a laceration may extend down through the skin over the metacarpophalangeal joint, through the thin synovial capsule, and into the joint itself. When the injured person opens the fist, the extensor tendon of the finger retracts proximally, carrying the inoculated oral flora into the tendon sheath and simultaneously sealing off the wound. This process produces conditions optimal for the development of an anaerobic infection, which can be devastating and can lead to long-term disability of the hand.

SYMPTOMS AND CLINICAL MANIFESTATIONS

Animal Bites. The clinical features of infection depend on the character and extent of the wound, the anatomic location of the injury, and the organisms responsible for the infection (Fig. 50–1). Characteristically, *Pasteurella* infections become symptomatic during the first 24 hours after the injury; symptoms include erythema, swelling, tenderness, and drainage at the site of the bite wound. Infections due to *Pasteurella* most often remain localized to the inoculated wound, but direct extension to surrounding tissues may occur, leading to lymphangitis and regional lymphadenopathy, and bacteremia may occur with metastatic foci including osteomyelitis, arthritis, tenosynovitis, sepsis, meningitis, brain abscess, pneumonia, and endocarditis. Wounds that appear infected more than 24 hours after an injury are more likely to be infected with *Staphylococcus* or *Streptococcus,* among other oral flora. A careful search for sites of infection deeper than the obviously inoculated skin is important, especially in puncture wounds inflicted by cats, in which the sharp teeth may inoculate underlying bones, joints, or tendons.

Infection caused by *B. henselae,* the cause of cat-scratch disease (Chapter 28), may result in the formation of a small 5–10 mm papule at the site of the bite and in the more characteristic suppurative regional lymphadenopathy. In addition to the local infection, systemic disease such as osteomyelitis, encephalitis, pneumonia, hepatitis, and fever of unknown origin has also been reported.

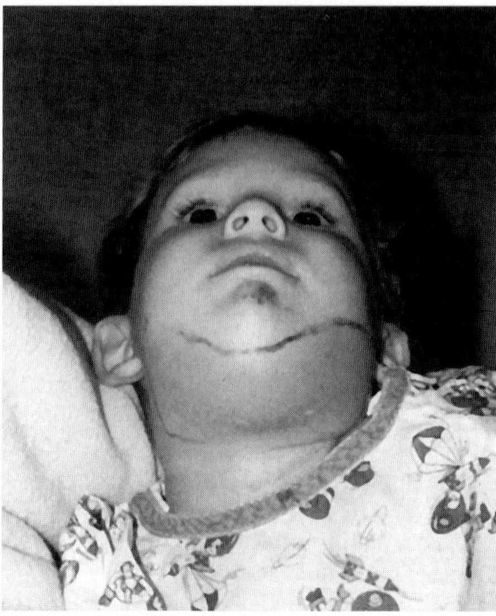

FIGURE 50–1. A 3-year-old boy with cellulitis that developed 24 hours after a puncture type of dog-bite wound of the chin, after a provoked attack from a neighbors pet.

Infections with *B. henselae* may also occur after a cat licks a superficial wound, presumably inoculating organisms directly into the tissue.

Rat-bite fever is a clinical syndrome caused by one of two different organisms, both normal oral flora of the rodent and each producing a slightly different clinical syndrome. *S. moniliformis* is a gram-negative bacillus that may cause infection within 12 hours to 10 days after a bite. Although the bite may be associated with initial local inflammation, healing often occurs before the onset of systemic symptoms. Irregularly spiking fevers with chills may occur for up to 3 weeks after the onset of symptoms. An associated morbilliform or petechial rash occurs in 75–95% of cases. The rash has a generalized distribution but is most prominent on the extremities, including the palms and soles. Arthralgia and arthritis, usually involving more than one joint, occur in up to 97% of cases; the knees, ankles, elbows, and shoulders are most often involved. If the infection is untreated, joint symptoms will occur, slowly resolve, and then spontaneously recur in 56–73% of cases. Endocarditis, pneumonia, myocarditis, hepatitis, pericarditis, and neonatal sepsis have been reported as complications.

Rat-bite fever caused by *S. minus* has an incubation of 7–21 days, with clinical disease that is generally milder than with *S. moniliformis.* Although some healing occurs at the site of inoculation, some ulceration or eschar is usually still present when systemic symptoms develop. A maculopapular rash occurs in 75% of infections. Arthritis is uncommon (2%), as are endocarditis and nephritis.

Herpes B virus infection manifests clinically in Old World macaque primates in a manner similar to infection with HSV in humans, with reactivation of latent virus producing infectious oral secretions in a symptom-free animal. For the person who is bitten, the virus may produce a vesicular rash at the site of the bite. However, a high rate of associated complications occurs with ascending paresthesias and numbness of the involved extremity, ascending flaccid paralysis, and subsequent development of encephalitis with fever, lethargy, and confusion. A mortality of 70% has been associated with infections in humans.

Human Bites. Approximately three fourths of human bite wounds in children are superficial abrasions in which the integrity of the epidermis is not completely broken. These wounds have a far lower rate of infection than puncture and laceration wounds. Parents tend to bring children to medical attention rather quickly after a human bite; 70–80% of children with bites present for medical care within 12 hours of the injury. Signs of inflammation are present within 12 hours in many cases, with rapid progression seen within 24–48 hours of the bite, particularly if the wound is neglected.

DIAGNOSIS

The diagnosis of a wound infection in the context of the history of a bite with increasing inflammation at the site of inoculation is usually straightforward. Localized infection is characterized by swelling, erythema, and tenderness with progressive inflammation involving adjacent tissues, with or without the formation of an abscess. Systemic signs of infection are not usually present. In one study (Feder et al, 1987) only one third of persons with infected bite wounds had fever at the time of hospitalization. Laboratory tests such as a CBC and ESR are not particularly helpful in diagnosing infection. In the same study (Feder et al, 1987), only 10% of persons hospitalized with bite-wound infections had an elevated WBC count, and only 23% had an elevated ESR.

Cultures from bite lesions obtained within a few hours of the bite have yielded a vast array of organisms. Only a few of the organisms cultured, however, may ultimately be responsible for an infection; therefore most experts believe that routine cultures of bite lesions without signs of infection are not indicated. For wounds that appear infected, both aerobic and anaerobic cultures should be performed. Blood cultures should be considered as well, although the yield of positive results is only about 5%. Because *S. moniliformis* is inhibited by an anticoagulant added to most commercial blood culture media, the microbiology laboratory must be made aware of this suspected pathogen for optimal recovery.

A careful search for deeper sites of infection must be undertaken for puncture wounds or deep lacerations. Examination of bones for point tenderness and an assessment of range of motion of joints adjacent to a bite should be performed. Physical findings of soft tissue, bone, or joint inflammation may occur up to 1–2 weeks after the injury. If physical findings suggest osteomyelitis or septic arthritis, a radionuclide scan may help identify the infection. Aspiration of clinically involved joints is indicated to confirm the diagnosis and obtain material for culture. For deeper infections in which an adequate examination is not possible, surgical exploration may be warranted. Biopsies of bone, regional lymph nodes, or soft tissue, with special stains for bacterial, fungal, or viral pathogens, may be helpful in the diagnosis. This is particularly important for infections possibly caused by *B. henselae* because routine bacterial media do not support growth of this organism.

Serologic testing is helpful to confirm cat-scratch disease. Serologic tests for the agents of rat-bite fever are not available. An examination of a blood smear for spirochetes may lead to the diagnosis of rat-bite fever due to *S. minus.*

For infections presenting 5–7 days after a bite, fungal cultures should be obtained in addition to bacterial cultures. Viral cultures for HSV infection should be obtained if this pathogen is suspected on the basis of a history of exposure or a physical examination suggesting characteristic vesicles.

TREATMENT

Local Care. Although many areas of surgical and medical treatment of animal and human bites are controversial, one facet of care is universal: the need for adequate cleansing and débridement. Aggressive wound management of dog-bite wounds is associated with a dramatic decrease in the infection rate, from 60% to 5%. Cleansing of the wound with high-pressure irrigation using a few hundred milliliters of normal saline solution is usually effective. Removal of devitalized tissue is also important to prevent a nidus of infection for inoculated organisms. The low rate of infection from properly managed dog-bite lacerations is equivalent to the infection rate of all nonbite lacerations.

Puncture wounds are difficult to débride. The wound should be irrigated if possible, but if tissue edema increases during the irrigation process, the possibility of spreading infection through tissue planes exists and aggressive irrigation may be contraindicated. Surgically opening a puncture wound to allow for irrigation will cause increased tissue damage and is not recommended unless signs of infection are already present. Suturing of puncture wounds is usually not indicated.

For adequately débrided dog-bite wounds, primary closure can be accomplished without increasing the risk of infection. However, for extensive wounds in which devitalized tissue may remain, primary closure is not recommended. Re-evaluation within 24–48 hours of the wounds should occur for additional débridement, possibly with delayed primary closure if no signs of infection are present.

Human bite wounds, given the high risk of infection, are generally not sutured but are cleaned, débrided, and loosely dressed. Serious human bite wounds of the head and neck or the hand usually require hospitalization and surgical consultation for optimal wound management. Human bites of the head and neck are best managed by delayed closure and late reconstruction to achieve an optimal cosmetic result. Bites to the hand, particularly clenched-fist injuries, may need surgical exploration to determine the extent of the injury. Surgical intervention also allows for optimal débridement of all inoculated tissue spaces, which should decrease the risk of infection.

Antimicrobial Therapy for Infected Wounds. For wounds that appear infected at the time of initial assessment, whether as the result of an animal bite or a human bite, antibiotic therapy should be started after a Gram stain and aerobic and anaerobic cultures have been obtained. Persons with signs of systemic toxic effects or a rapidly progressing infection should be hospitalized for parenteral antibiotic therapy and surgical consultation. For infected animal or human bites in which local signs of infection are minimal and evidence of systemic toxicity is absent, oral antibiotic therapy may be used if adequate wound débridement can be accomplished and there is good compliance. However, if there are doubts regarding the adherence to an oral antibiotic regimen or a return for follow-up examination, the patient should be hospitalized and a clear response to parenteral antibiotic therapy demonstrated before outpatient oral therapy is begun.

Few antibiotics offer optimal coverage for all potential pathogens (Table 50–2). Penicillin, the drug of choice for *Pasteurella multocida,* has minimal activity against most strains of *Staphylococcus aureus.* However, nafcillin, dicloxacillin, cefazolin, and cephalexin, which are some of the most active drugs against *S. aureus,* have little activity against most strains of *Pasteurella.* Oral amoxicillin-clavulanate offers the best coverage for the majority of pathogens found in wound infections and is considered by most experts to be the drug of choice for infected wounds in outpatients (Table 50–3). Selected second- and third-generation oral or parenteral cephalosporins may provide an alternative based on in vitro susceptibility testing. Cefuroxime axetil and cefpodoxime have moderate activity against strains of *S. aureus* in addition to having much better activity against *Pasteurella* than most other oral cephalosporins. For persons with hypersensitivity to β-lactam antibiotics, macrolides may be used as an alternative. Azithromycin has better activity against *Pasteurella* than erythromycin, in addition to providing activity against most anaerobes and skin flora. Other antibiotics that may be considered for persons with a hypersensitivity to β-lactam drugs include tetracycline, chloramphenicol, and TMP-SMZ. Quinolones such as levofloxacin, moxifloxacin, and gatifloxacin have excellent in vitro activity against aerobic and anaerobic bite-wound pathogens, including *Pasteurella,* and may represent an option for the adolescent and adult, although little clinical data are available to support these in vitro observations.

For intravenous treatment a combination of penicillin G and an antistaphylococcal agent (nafcillin or cefazolin) provides optimal coverage. Parenteral β-lactam–β-lactamase inhibitor combinations such as ampicillin-sulbactam demonstrate excellent in vitro activity against the majority of bite-wound pathogens, including *Pasteurella.* Alternatives include second-generation cephalosporins (cefoxitin, cefuroxime) and third-generation cephalosporins (ceftriaxone, cefotaxime), but there is minimal evidence to support their use. Although various aerobic gram-negative bacilli, such as *Pseudomonas, Enterobacter,* or β-lactamase-positive *Bacteroides* may be resistant to antibiotic therapy directed at *S. aureus* and *Pasteurella,* these organisms are not sufficiently prevalent in bite-wound infections to necessitate specific empirical therapy. Gram-stain and culture results should direct subsequent antibiotic therapy.

For persons with a history of a rodent bite and systemic symptoms consistent with rat-bite fever, parenteral therapy should include penicillin G, which is active against both of the organisms responsible for rat-bite fever. For uncomplicated rat-bite fever (fever, rash, arthralgia), oral penicillin or tetracycline may be effective therapy. Parenteral therapy should be used for complicated rat-bite fever involving the lung or heart. Other antibiotics that show in vitro activity against *S. moniliformis* include cephalosporins and vancomycin. Erythromycin has variable activity against *S. moniliformis.*

Infections after bite wounds from snakes are not common unless tissue destruction from a fasciotomy or envenomation occurs. Cefazolin has been used for empirical treatment of hospitalized patients

TABLE 50–2. Antibiotic Susceptibilities of Common Bite-Wound Pathogens

	Organism			
Antibiotic	***Staphylococcus aureus***	***Pasteurella multocida***	**Streptococci**	***Eikenella corrodens***
Oral				
Amoxicillin	0	+++	+++	++
Penicillin V	0	+++	+++	+++
Dicloxacillin	+++	0	+++	0
Amoxicillin-clavulanate	++	+++	+++	+++
Cephalexin	+++	++	+++	0
Cefuroxime	++	+++	+++	++
Erythromycin	++	0	+++	0
Tetracycline	++	+++	+++	+++
Parenteral				
Penicillin G	0	+++	+++	+++
Nafcillin	+++	0	+++	0
Ampicillin-sulbactam	++	+++	+++	+++
Ticarcillin-clavulanate	++	+++	+++	+++
Cefazolin	+++	++	+++	+
Ceftriaxone or cefotaxime	++	+++	+++	+++

0 = no activity; + = minimal activity against some isolates; ++ = moderate activity; +++ = good to excellent activity.

TABLE 50–3. Empiric Therapy for Infected Bite Wounds (Dog, Cat, Human)

Route	Recommended Therapy	Alternative Therapy
Parenteral Therapy	Penicillin G *plus* Cefazolin *or* nafcillin *or* oxacillin	Cefuroxime *or* Cefotaxime *or* ceftriaxone *or* ceftazidime *with or without* Cefazolin *or* nafcillin *or* oxacillin
Oral Therapy	Amoxicillin-clavulanate	Cefuroxime axetil *or* Penicillin V *plus* Cephalexin *or* dicloxacillin

No significant prospective comparative trials for clinical and microbiologic efficacy have been performed. These recommendations are based on in vitro susceptibilities and anecdotal reports.

Suggested Dosages for Patients with Normal Renal Function

ANTIBIOTIC	INTRAVENOUS DOSAGE	MAXIMUM DAILY DOSE
Parenteral Therapy		
Ampicillin-sulbactam	200 mg/kg/day divided by q6hr	8g
Cefazolin	100 mg/kg/day divided q8hr	3–6 g
Cefotaxime	150 mg/kg/day divided q8hr	12 g
Cefoxitin	80–160 mg/kg/q6hr	8 g
Ceftazidime	150 mg/kg/day divided q8hr	6 g
Ceftriaxone	50 mg/kg q24hr	2–4 g
Cefuroxime	150 mg/kg/day divided q8hr	4.5 g
Nafcillin	150 mg/kg/day divided q4–6hr	9 g
Oxacillin	150–200 mg/kg/day divided q4–6hr	12 g
Parenteral Therapy (Continued)		
Penicillin G	200,000–250,000 U/kg/day divided q4hr	18–25 MU
Ticarcillin-clavulanate	200–300 mg/kg/day divided q6hr	8 g
Oral Therapy		
Amoxicillin-clavulanate	50 mg/kg/day divided tid	1.5 g
Cefuroxime axetil	30 mg/kg/day divided bid	1 g
Cephalexin	25–50 mg/kg/day divided qid	2 g
Dicloxacillin	12–25 mg/kg/day divided qid	2 g
Penicillin V	50 mg/kg/day divided qid	2 g

with venomous snakebites. With the extensive inflammation caused by venom-related tissue destruction, infection is not easy to recognize in the initial 24–48 hours after the bite. Cefazolin is active against skin flora and many of the gram-negative organisms isolated from infected bites. Other antibiotics or antibiotic combinations with activity against *S. aureus* and enteric gram-negative bacilli should also be effective.

COMPLICATIONS

Baseline serologic tests for hepatitis B virus, hepatitis C virus, or HIV should be performed if any of these viruses could possibly have been transmitted, in conjunction with appropriate postexposure prophylaxis for hepatitis B (see Table 78–10) and HIV (see Table 105–31). There is no means of postexposure prophylaxis for hepatitis C, although close monitoring is recommended (Chapter 105).

Tetanus. Although the risk of tetanus from a well-débrided and cleansed wound is low, the possibility of inoculating spores of *Clostridium tetani* into a bite wound does exist. Of particular concern are wounds that are sutured closed and puncture wounds, in which anaerobic conditions may exist, allowing germination of *Clostridium* spores and production of toxin by vegetative bacteria, leading to clinical disease. The tetanus immunization status should be assessed for any bite wound that breaks the skin. A superficial, minor wound that can be cleansed requires no further therapy to prevent tetanus if the patient is fully immunized. A deep wound, particularly a wound contaminated with dirt, may require tetanus immunization, tetanus immune globulin, or both, depending on the characteristics of the wound and the immunization status (see Table 48–5).

Rabies. A decision about the need for rabies immune globulin (RIG) therapy and active immunization must be made as soon as possible. Rabies presents a clinical dilemma to physicians treating animal bites, particularly if the animal is wild or the bite of a domestic animal appears unprovoked. Each year in the United States between 16,000 and 39,000 persons receive postexposure rabies prophylaxis. Between 1980 and 1997, only two cases of human rabies attributable to bites from dogs indigenous to the United States occurred; during the same period, 12 cases attributable to dogs from outside the United States occurred. Although rabies is endemic in certain wild animal populations, rabies in domestic animals has been uncommon. Most rabid domestic animals have been reported along the United States–Mexico border. Local health departments will be aware of rabies activity in both wild and domestic animal populations and need to be consulted to assess the risk of infection after a bite. In one study (Moore, 2000), 59% of owned dogs were up-to-date on rabies vaccinations, in comparison with 41% of owned cats.

Since 1980, 21 (58%) of the 36 cases of human rabies in the United States have been associated with insectivorous bats, reversing a historical pattern of rabies primarily transmitted by dogs. However, in only one or two of these cases was a clear history of a bite elicited, although in the majority of cases a nonbite contact with bats was recognized. Recent changes in the recommendations address the low risk of rabies exposure in cases in which a bat is found in a room with a person who might be unaware of the bat or unable to relate that a bite or direct contact with a bat has occurred, such as a mentally disabled or intoxicated person, a sleeping child, or an unattended young infant. These persons are now considered candidates for postexposure prophylaxis.

Any healthy-appearing domestic dog, cat, or ferret responsible for an apparently unprovoked bite should be captured and observed for 10 days by a veterinarian without immediate treatment of the victim. In this way the signs of rabies may be noted in the animal at the earliest possible time. Symptoms appear in most animals within only 3 days of virus shedding. If the signs appear, a rapid diagnosis of rabies virus infection can be established by examination of the brain tissue of the animal, and the bitten person can be treated. Captured wild animals should be killed without a period of observation. If the biting animal is not captured, particularly if it is a wild animal of a species known to harbor the virus in the region, rabies should be assumed to be present, and the victim should be given both passive and active protection from rabies. The wild animals that most frequently transmit rabies in the United States are skunks, foxes, raccoons, and bats (see Fig. 55–2).

Because the virus is present in animal saliva, a break in the skin from a bite or exposure to animal saliva on abraded skin or a mucous membrane may lead to infection. The incubation period may last from days to weeks depending on the severity and the anatomic location of the bite (Chapter 55).

Immediate and thorough washing of wounds and scratches with soap and water is indicated in all bites in which rabies exposure is suspected. For persons believed to be at risk of rabies after exposure, the following treatment guidelines apply. First, RIG in a dosage of 20 IU/kg should be given, with the full dose of RIG infiltrated subcutaneously into the area around the wound if possible. Any remaining RIG that cannot be infiltrated into the wound should be given as an intramuscular injection. Second, inactivated rabies vaccine should be initiated at the same time that RIG prophylaxis is given. Currently approved rabies vaccines include the human diploid cell rabies vaccine (HDCV), rabies vaccine adsorbed, and purified chick embryo cell vaccine. The vaccines should be administered intramuscularly in a volume of 1 mL as soon as possible after the risk of exposure has been determined to be high, with additional vaccine doses on days 3, 7, 14, and 28. All three vaccines are thought to be equally safe and effective. The deltoid muscle is the preferable site of injection in older children, but the outer aspect of the thigh may be used in younger infants. Although approved for pre-exposure vaccination, intradermal HDCV is not recommended for postexposure prophylaxis.

B Virus (Herpesvirus simiae). Exposure to the bite or to the infectious secretions of a macaque monkey requires immediate evaluation for possible exposure to B virus. Guidelines have been developed to assess the risk of exposure based on assessments of infection in the monkey and on the type and severity of the exposure; immediate consultation with an expert in B virus infections is necessary. Immediate and thorough cleansing of the wound is important, as are culture and serologic assessment of the animal for active B virus infection. For high-risk exposures, intravenous acyclovir is recommended; for moderate-risk exposures, acyclovir is administered orally for 2 weeks. Close clinical and serologic follow-up is important after the bite. Aggressive treatment with intravenous acyclovir for the person with symptomatic infection is important to minimize the progression of neurologic symptoms in the bitten extremity and the development of encephalitis. After intravenous acyclovir, long-term suppressive therapy with continuous oral acyclovir for at least 5–7 years is recommended to prevent latent virus from reactivating with subsequent neurologic disease. The optimal duration of acyclovir therapy is unknown.

Immunocompromised Persons. Immunocompromised persons have an increased risk of progression of disease both locally and systemically after a bite. In addition to the more common wound pathogens, less invasive bacteria may also cause disease. *Capnocytophaga canimorsus* is a gram-negative bacillus that is part of the normal oral flora in the dog and is of low virulence in immunocompetent persons. In immunocompromised persons, including persons with asplenia, this organism can cause necrotizing cellulitis at the site of inoculation, as well as sepsis, disseminated intravascular coagulation, pneumonia, meningitis, arthritis, and endocarditis.

PREVENTION

The most controversial area in the management of bites is antibiotic prophylaxis. Well-controlled, prospective, double-blind studies of dog, cat, or human bite wounds of similar severity and anatomic location, with standardized surgical management and evaluation of infection, have not been performed. Some of the first reports of penicillin prophylaxis suggested that the rate of infection of hand wounds by animal bites dropped from as high as 70% to 10% with prophylaxis, although the numbers of patients enrolled was not sufficient to achieve statistical significance. Other studies of dog-bite wounds have indicated that wound management and not antibiotic prophylaxis is the most important factor in preventing infection. In a recent meta-analysis (Cummings, 1994) of eight studies on antibiotic prophylaxis of dog-bite wounds, prophylaxis was associated with a significant decrease in wound infections, in addition to the benefits of prompt evaluation and aggressive wound care. In serious human bites a prospective study (Zubowicz, 1991) of adults suggested that antibiotics given either orally or intravenously decreased the rate of infection. However, two retrospective studies (Baker et al, 1987; Schweich et al, 1985) suggest that oral antibiotics have no clinically significant impact on the subsequent development of infection following human bites of children. A notable finding was that even appropriate oral antibiotic prophylaxis was occasionally associated with treatment failure, as demonstrated by the development of an infection caused by organisms susceptible to the antibiotic.

Despite the lack of consistent data, however, most experts continue to recommend antibiotics after human bites because of the high rate of infection. Animal or human bites to the hand or face may cause considerable morbidity; these wounds, even if not infected at the time of presentation, should be considered for antibiotic prophylaxis. Puncture wounds and those wounds neglected for more than 24 hours are also at high risk of infection (Table 50–4) and should also be considered for prophylactic treatment. Antibiotic choices for prophylaxis should logically correspond to those used for treatment of developed infections, with amoxicillin-clavulanate representing the most widely recommended oral therapy.

TABLE 50–4. High-Risk Factors for Bite-Wound Infection

Hand, foot, or face bite wounds (animal or human)
Puncture wounds, including cat bites
Human bite wound
Delay in seeking therapy (>24 hr)

REVIEWS

Goldstein EJ: Current concepts on animal bites: Bacteriology and therapy. *Curr Clin Top Infect Dis* 1999;19:99–111.

Marcy SM: Infections due to dog and cat bites. *Pediatr Infect Dis* 1982;1:351–6.

Trott A: Care of mammalian bites. *Pediatr Infect Dis J* 1987;6:8–10.

KEY ARTICLES

Aghababian RV, Conte JE Jr: Mammalian bite wounds. *Ann Emerg Med* 1980;9:79–83.

Baker MD, Moore SE: Human bites in children. A six-year experience. *Am J Dis Child* 1987;141:1285–90.

Basadre JO, Parry SW: Indications for surgical debridement in 125 human bites to the hand. *Arch Surg* 1991;126:65–7.

Boenning DA, Fleisher GR, Campos JM: Dog bites in children: Epidemiology, microbiology, and penicillin prophylactic therapy. *Am J Emerg Med* 1983;1:17–21.

Brook I: Microbiology of human and animal bite wounds in children. *Pediatr Infect Dis J* 1987;6:29–32.

Callaham ML: Treatment of common dog bites: Infection risk factors. *J Am Coll Emerg Physicians* 1978;7:83–7.

Centers for Disease Control and Prevention: Human rabies prevention—United States, 1999. Recommendations of the Advisory Committee on Immunization Practices (ACIP). *MMWR Morb Mortal Wkly Rep* 1999; 48:1–21.

Cummings P: Antibiotics to prevent infection in patients with dog bite wounds: A meta-analysis of randomized trials. *Ann Emerg Med* 1994; 23:535–40.

Elenbaas RM, McNabney WK, Robinson WA: Evaluation of prophylactic oxacillin in cat bite wounds. *Ann Emerg Med* 1984;13:155–7.

Feder HM, Shanley JD, Barbera JA: Review of 59 patients hospitalized with animal bites. *Pediatr Infect Dis J* 1987;6:24–8.

Fleisher GR: The management of bite wounds. *N Engl J Med* 1999; 340:138–40.

Hirschhorn RB, Hodge RR: Identification of risk factors in rat bite incidents involving humans. *Pediatrics* 1999;104:e35.

Holmes GP, Chapman LE, Stewart JA, et al: Guidelines for the prevention and treatment of B-virus infections in exposed persons. The B virus Working Group. *Clin Infect Dis* 1995;20:421–39.

Krebs JW, Smith JS, Rupprecht CE, et al: Rabies surveillance in the United States during 1998. *J Am Vet Med Assoc* 1999;215:1786–98. (Published erratum appears in *J Am Vet Med Assoc* 2000;216:1223.)

Leung AK, Robson WL: Human bites in children. *Pediatr Emerg Care* 1992;8:255–7.

Moore DA, Sischo WM, Hunter A, et al: Animal bite epidemiology and surveillance for rabies postexposure prophylaxis. *J Am Vet Med Assoc* 2000;217:190–4.

Noah DL, Drenzek CL, Smith JS, et al: Epidemiology of human rabies in the United States, 1980–1996. *Ann Intern Med* 1998;128:922–30.

Schweich P, Fleisher G: Human bites in children. *Pediatr Emerg Care* 1985;1:51–3.

Shirley LR, Ross SA: Risk of transmission of human immunodeficiency virus by bite of an infected toddler. *J Pediatr* 1989;114:425–7.

Stucker FJ, Shaw GY, Boyd S, et al: Management of animal and human bites in the head and neck. *Arch Otolaryngol Head Neck Surg* 1990; 116:789–93.

Talan DA, Citron DM, Abrahamian FM, et al: Bacteriologic analysis of infected dog and cat bites. Emergency Medicine Animal Bite Infection Study Group. *N Engl J Med* 1999;340:85–92.

Weiss HB, Friedman DI, Coben JH: Incidence of dog bite injuries treated in emergency departments. *JAMA* 1998;279:51–3.

Zubowicz VN, Gravier M: Management of early human bites of the hand: A prospective randomized study. *Plast Reconstr Surg* 1991;88:111–4.

CHAPTER 51

Lymphadenopathy, Lymphadenitis, and Lymphangitis

Toni Darville ▪ Richard F. Jacobs

Lymphadenopathy is defined literally as disease of the lymph nodes but is used interchangeably with lymph node enlargement. Enlargement of the lymph nodes occurs in response to a wide variety of infectious, inflammatory, and neoplastic processes. It is most helpful to divide the approach to lymphadenopathy into generalized lymphadenopathy with enlargement of two or more noncontiguous lymph node regions, regional lymphadenopathy involving only one lymph node group, and lymphadenitis. The upper limit of normal lymph node size is 10 mm in diameter in most anatomic sites, with the exceptions of 15 mm for inguinal nodes, 5 mm for epitrochlear nodes, and 2 mm for supraclavicular nodes, which are usually undetectable.

Lymph nodes are well-defined structures surrounded by a fibrous capsule perforated at various points by afferent lymphatic vessels, which drain specific regions of the body. Lymph empties into a nodal sinus subjacent to the capsule, filters through the lymphoid tissue, and terminates at the hilus, where the efferent lymphatics emerge. The cortex, or periphery of a node, contains spherical aggregates of lymphoid cells composed primarily of B lymphocytes. T lymphocytes are found primarily in the area between these follicles and in the deep cortex of the node. The medullary cords occupying the central portion of the node contain mostly plasma cells, and it is there that antibody is made.

Lymph nodes are extremely labile structures. Even though lymph nodes are not normally palpable in the neonate, a considerable amount of lymphoid tissue is present at birth. This intrinsic lymphoid tissue steadily enlarges until puberty, when it undergoes progressive atrophy throughout life. Lymph nodes are most prominently palpable in children 4–8 years of age. Lymph nodes are strategically located in groups, and they filter particulate antigens from the lymphatic drainage of well-defined anatomic areas. On antigenic stimulation, lymphocyte or lymphoblast proliferation usually occurs. This results in a greatly increased number of lymphocytes within the node and consequent nodal enlargement. If the antigen is cleared, antigenic stimulation ceases and the nodal enlargement is transient. **Chronic lymphadenopathy** results if the antigen persists, as in the case of intracellular parasites capable of prolonged survival. Lymphoid hyperplasia with resulting lymphadenopathy can also occur in the absence of antigenic stimulation, as with hyperthyroidism and lymphomas. Histiocytic hyperplasia occurs in the histiocytoses, some lipid storage diseases, some forms of Hodgkin's disease, and in the benign condition sinus histiocytosis. Lymphadenopathy results from invasion of nodes with malignant cells of leukemias or metastatic tumors.

Lymphadenitis is acute or chronic inflammation of lymph nodes. Acute lymphadenitis results when bacteria and toxins from a site of acute inflammation are carried via lymph to regional nodes. Not only does intranodal lymphocytic and histiocytic proliferation occur, but also extrinsic polymorphonuclear leukocytes invade the node. These nodes become enlarged because of cellular infiltration and edema. Distention of the nodal capsule results in tenderness. Chronic lymphadenitis can occur with a variety of chronic infections; those caused by organisms that represent B-cell antigens induce follicular hyperplasia, and microorganisms that stimulate T cells induce paracortical lymphoid hyperplasia. Both of these processes result in chronically enlarged nodes. Characteristically, these lymph nodes are not tender because they are not under increased pressure.

Regional Lymphadenopathy. Regional lymphadenopathy can be further subdivided on the basis of the various anatomic groups of lymph nodes strategically located throughout the body. Major regional lymph node groups have anatomic designations: occipital, preauricular, submaxillary and submental, cervical, supraclavicular, mediastinal, axillary, epitrochlear, inguinal, iliac, abdominal, and pelvic. Individual groups of nodes become enlarged most often because of the presence of an infectious or inflammatory process proximal to the node(s).

Occipital nodes drain the posterior portion of the scalp and are frequently enlarged when inflammatory conditions such as pediculosis capitis, tinea capitis, or seborrheic dermatitis are present. Rubella may cause isolated enlargement of the occipital nodes.

Preauricular nodes drain the lateral portion of the eyelids, conjunctivae, skin of the cheek, and temporal region of the scalp. The **oculoglandular syndrome of Parinaud** consists of conjunctival pathologic changes associated with ipsilateral preauricular lymphadenopathy. Trachoma, caused by *Chlamydia trachomatis,* is the most common cause of this syndrome worldwide. Although uncommon in the United States, trachoma may still be found on some American Indian reservations and in the Mexican American population of the Southwest. *Chlamydia* is also responsible for neonatal inclusion conjunctivitis (blennorrhea), which occurs 1–2 weeks after birth. The presence of preauricular lymphadenopathy may help to differentiate chlamydial from gonococcal ophthalmitis, which it closely resembles. Adenovirus infections may cause pharyngoconjunctival fever, characterized by sore throat, follicular conjunctivitis, fever, and enlarged preauricular nodes or anterior cervical nodes or both. Other causes of the oculoglandular syndrome include tularemia, listeriosis, cat-scratch disease, tuberculosis, syphilis, HSV infection, and sporotrichosis.

Submaxillary, submental, and cervical nodes are commonly enlarged and are grouped under the term *cervical lymphadenopathy.* Supraclavicular nodes drain the entire upper body, including the abdomen. The left supraclavicular node may be enlarged because of intra-abdominal pathologic changes resulting from its relation to the thoracic duct. The right supraclavicular node drains areas of the lung and mediastinum and may become enlarged in instances of thoracic disease.

Mediastinal nodes receive lymph drainage from the thoracic viscera and therefore may become enlarged in pulmonary disease states. Chronic pulmonary diseases cause mediastinal lymphadenopathy, in contrast to the rare occurrence in acute bacterial or viral infections. Coccidioidomycosis and histoplasmosis can cause bilateral hilar lymphadenopathy. Sarcoidosis commonly has bilateral hilar lymphadenopathy as a clinical finding, and the paratracheal nodes are also frequently involved. Tuberculosis usually causes unilateral hilar lymphadenopathy that is four times more frequently found on the right side, but bilateral involvement mimicking sarcoidosis has been reported. Calcification is typical of tuberculosis, histoplasmosis, and coccidioidomycosis, and it also occurs in sarcoidosis. Childhood lymphomas result in bilateral hilar lymphadenopathy; these nodes do not calcify.

Axillary nodes drain the hand, arm, chest wall, upper and lateral abdominal wall, and part of the breast. The most common cause of axillary lymphadenopathy is inflammation or infection of the upper extremity. However, if the axillary nodes enlarge rapidly without an infectious focus, then malignancy must be considered.

Epitrochlear nodes receive lymphatic drainage from the middle, ring, and little fingers and from the medial portion of the hand and forearm. Lymphadenopathy of epitrochlear nodes is most often because of a primary pyoderma or secondarily infected skin lesions. *Staphylococcus aureus* and group A *Streptococcus* are implicated most often. Chronically enlarged bilateral epitrochlear nodes can be found in secondary syphilis.

Iliac nodes drain the lower abdominal wall and portions of the genitalia, urethra, and bladder and receive afferents from the superficial and deep inguinal nodes. These are located along the external and common iliac arteries in the anterior retroperitoneal space and can be detected by deep palpation over the inguinal ligament. Acute iliac adenitis may develop from infection of the lower extremities, lower abdominal wall, perineum, or the urinary tract, or rarely it may result from hematogenous infection. After infection develops, it breaks through fascial compartments, allowing for abscess formation in the space between the posterior peritoneum and the psoas and iliac fascia. An unexplained limp may be the initial symptom; the acute onset of fever may not occur for days or weeks. Hip and back pain become prominent, and patients will lie in bed with the thigh flexed and abducted. Extension of the thigh is very painful. Examination at this point suggests the diagnoses of suppurative arthritis or osteomyelitis. No limitation of hip motion except for extension may help to distinguish this condition from true hip disease. Only after some days or weeks does lower abdominal pain develop, and the person becomes acutely ill with high fever and leukocytosis. When the symptoms are on the right side, the diagnosis of retrocecal appendicitis with abscess may be suggested, but the lack of nausea and vomiting and the antecedent limp may help with differentiation. Abdominal CT scanning can be helpful in making the diagnosis. An abscess abutting the psoas and iliac muscles will be delineated. *S. aureus* is by far the most common infectious agent, followed in frequency by group A *Streptococcus*.

Abdominal and pelvic nodes drain the lower extremities and all the pelvic and abdominal organs. Any inflammatory condition of the bowel may lead to their enlargement. Any disorder that causes generalized lymphadenopathy will also result in abdominal lymphadenopathy. Symptoms of abdominal node enlargement may include abdominal pain, backache, constipation, urinary frequency, jaundice, and intestinal obstruction. About half of all childhood lymphomas involve abdominal nodes. This nodal enlargement may lead to ascites from portal vein compression or to edema of the lower abdominal wall and lower extremities from iliac vein obstruction.

Lymphocutaneous syndromes are characterized by regional lymphadenitis associated with a characteristic skin lesion at the site of inoculation. Agents implicated include *Francisella tularensis, Bartonella henselae* (cat-scratch disease), *Nocardia, Bacillus anthracis, Yersinia pestis* (plague), cutaneous diphtheria, sporotrichosis, histoplasmosis, coccidioidomycosis, *Pasteurella multocida* (dog or cat bite), and *Spirillum minus* and *Streptobacillus moniliformis* (rat-bite fever).

Lymphangitis is an inflammation of subcutaneous lymphatic channels that usually presents as an acute bacterial infection.

GENERALIZED LYMPHADENOPATHY

Generalized lymphadenopathy is defined as enlargement of two or more noncontiguous lymph node regions. Hepatosplenomegaly often accompanies generalized lymphadenopathy.

ETIOLOGY

Generalized lymphadenopathy is frequently a manifestation of disseminated infection and includes bacterial, fungal, and protozoal causes (Table 51–1).

EPIDEMIOLOGY

Lymphatic tissues are at the peak of their development during the early school years, and the nodal response to a variety of stimuli is rapid and often prolific in this age group, in comparison with responses in adults. Infections are the most common causes of enlarged lymph nodes. Viral infections are more likely to cause generalized enlargement than any other type of infection. Disorders causing generalized lymphadenopathy usually are associated with other findings in the history, physical examination, and laboratory data that make a diagnosis relatively easy.

TABLE 51–1. Infectious Causes of Generalized Lymphadenopathy

Viral
Rubella
Rubeola
Epstein-Barr virus
Cytomegalovirus
Human immunodeficiency virus
Hepatitis viruses A through E
Varicella
Adenovirus
Bacterial
Septicemia
Endocarditis
Brucellosis
Secondary syphilis
Tuberculosis
Leptospirosis
Fungal
Coccidioidomycosis
Histoplasmosis
Protozoal
Toxoplasmosis

PATHOGENESIS

Systemic viral infection is the most common cause of generalized lymphadenopathy in children. After initial acquisition of viruses by the oral or respiratory route, infection occurs in the pharynx and within 1 day spreads to the regional lymph nodes, where antigenic stimulation leads to lymphoid hyperplasia and lymphadenopathy. On about the third day, **minor viremia,** or **primary viremia,** occurs, involving many secondary organs. Viral multiplication in these sites coincides with the onset of clinical symptoms. A major viremia then occurs during the period of secondary organ infection, usually lasting from days 3–7 of infection. It is during this period of **major viremia,** or **secondary viremia,** that antigenic stimulation in multiple lymph node groups results in generalized lymphadenopathy. Cessation of viremia and resolution of clinical symptoms occurs with the host immune response.

In contrast to viral infections, which are frequently associated with generalized lymphadenopathy, it is a rare development in bacterial infections. Bacterial infections with bacteremia may occasionally result in generalized lymphadenopathy. In these diseases, the immune response to the bacterial organism, as well as direct infection of the node with subsequent invasion by polymorphonuclear leukocytes, leads to nodal enlargement.

SYMPTOMS AND CLINICAL MANIFESTATIONS

Viral infections usually produce soft and only minimally tender nodes. Other symptoms are specific for the particular virus involved and are helpful in establishing a specific diagnosis. Disseminated bacterial infection may produce nodes that are painful, warm, tender, and red. These nodes usually remain discrete and may suppurate or drain spontaneously. When infections due to fungal and parasitic agents cause lymphadenopathy, it is most often of a subacute or chronic nature, and the nodes are granulomatous and mildly tender.

Viral illnesses that cause exanthems are often associated with lymphadenopathy. Measles causes hyperplasia of all lymphoid tissue, with the lymph nodes at the angle of the jaw and in the posterior cervical region most commonly involved. Mesenteric lymphadenopathy may result in abdominal pain, and appendiceal mucosa involvement may obliterate the lumen and cause symptoms of appendicitis. Rubella is classically associated with tender posterior auricular, suboccipital, and posterior cervical lymphadenopathy that develops at least 24 hours before the onset of the rash and may remain for a week or more. No other disease causes such tender enlargement of these nodes as rubella. Other exanthematous viral illnesses that may present with generalized lymphadenopathy include varicella and adenovirus infections.

Infectious Mononucleosis. Mononucleosis syndromes frequently have generalized lymphadenopathy as a prominent clinical sign. Other findings include fever, sore throat, malaise, and fatigue. EBV causes 85–95% of mononucleosis syndromes, with CMV, *Toxoplasma gondii,* adenoviruses, rubella, the hepatitis viruses, and, in more recent years, the HIV as occasional causes. Tender, enlarged cervical nodes are the hallmark of infectious mononucleosis caused by EBV. The posterior cervical nodes are most often enlarged, but other groups are also affected. Individual nodes are freely movable, are not spontaneously painful, and are only mildly tender to palpation. Hepatomegaly can be found in 10–15% of patients, and splenomegaly in about half.

CMV is the most frequent cause of heterophile-negative mononucleosis and is clinically difficult to distinguish from EBV-induced mononucleosis. CMV more frequently follows transfusion of blood products and more frequently has fever as the only symptom, with few other findings. Pharyngitis, especially with a membranous exudate, is much more characteristic of EBV than CMV mononucleosis. Splenomegaly may be slightly more prominent with CMV-induced disease, whereas atypical lymphocytosis is usually less intense than with EBV infection.

Acquired *T. gondii* infection may give rise to an infectious mononucleosis-like illness, although 80–90% of persons who become infected with this parasite do not develop any symptoms. When clinical findings occur, the most common presentation is asymptomatic cervical lymphadenopathy, but any or all lymph node groups may be enlarged. The nodes are usually discrete and nontender, rarely more than 3 cm in diameter, and do not suppurate. Lymphadenopathy may wax and wane for months, persisting in some unusual cases beyond 1 year. The clinical course is benign and self-limited in immunocompetent persons. A history of eating undercooked meat or of exposure to cats or kittens can often be elicited.

Hepatitis viruses may also cause mononucleosis-type symptoms, especially those of hepatitis B. Infectious mononucleosis accompanied by jaundice is more likely to represent viral hepatitis. Aminotransferase levels rise more slowly with EBV and CMV infection and are usually lower than with viral hepatitis.

Acute HIV infection in adolescents and adults is associated with a mononucleosis-like illness consisting of fever, malaise, myalgias, headache, sore throat, diarrhea, and maculopapular rash, accompanied by lymphadenopathy in 50% of patients. After other acute symptoms have resolved, the lymphadenopathy may remain as **persistent generalized lymphadenopathy (PGL),** involving at least several extrainguinal sites, of at least 3 months' duration. The nodes are distributed symmetrically and are discrete and nontender, and suppuration does not occur. Regression of the lymphadenopathy may occur after 8–19 months in some persons. However, opportunistic infections or neoplastic disease can develop in some persons after regression. The diagnosis of HIV infection can be confirmed by serologic testing. Most persons with PGL require no invasive evaluation.

Children with perinatally acquired HIV often have generalized lymphadenopathy at presentation, together with other nonspecific findings that may include failure to thrive, fever, hepatosplenomegaly, persistent oral candidiasis, and recurrent or chronic diarrhea. These findings, in addition to the history of a mother at risk of HIV infection, should prompt an evaluation.

Bacterial Infections. Bacterial infections causing generalized lymphadenopathy are uncommon. Bacterial sepsis or septic emboli associated with infective endocarditis may rarely result in generalized lymphadenopathy.

Marked lymphadenopathy is a common finding in persons with primary immunodeficiency, such as persons with chronic granulomatous disease. In most cases the nodes eventually become purulent and spontaneously drain. Hepatosplenomegaly is common, with hepatic or perihepatic abscesses frequently reported. All these findings reflect the accumulation of infecting microorganisms within phagocytic cells deficient in microbiologic killing ability.

Dissemination of *Treponema pallidum* organisms in secondary syphilis may result in various constitutional symptoms and signs including fever, sore throat, headache, rash, and generalized painless lymphadenopathy. These nodes seldom become extensively enlarged but may remain palpable for months. Enlargement of the epitrochlear lymph nodes is a unique finding that should prompt consideration of secondary syphilis. Diagnosis is most easily made by serologic methods.

Lymphohematogenous dissemination of tubercle bacilli in miliary tuberculosis results in hepatosplenomegaly and generalized lymphadenopathy in about half of these persons. Dissemination may develop as an early complication of primary infection, before the development of tuberculin hypersensitivity, or as a result of hematogenous spread from a clinically silent lesion that formed years earlier. A history of tuberculosis is unusual, and symptoms and signs including fever, malaise, weight loss, and weakness are nonspecific. As many as one fourth to one third of persons with disseminated tuberculosis will have negative tuberculin skin test results. For most of these persons there is a clear history of contact with a household case of tuberculosis. A miliary infiltrate on a chest roentgenogram is reported in 92% of infants and children and in 93–97% of adults with disseminated tuberculosis infection. This disease carries a 14–21% mortality, with death most often attributed to a delay in diagnosis and treatment, which emphasizes the need for vigorous diagnostic measures. Lymph node biopsy and culture can be diagnostic and can be pursued promptly when lymphadenopathy is present.

Generalized lymphadenopathy occurs with brucellosis and leptospirosis, in association with other clinical symptoms specific for these diseases. Occupational or environmental exposure to animals is an important clue to the diagnosis.

Fungal Infections. Fungal infections rarely lead to generalized lymphadenopathy, even with disseminated disease. *Coccidioides immitis* infection results from inhalation of airborne spores and produces symptomatic respiratory disease in 40% of patients. Hilar nodes may be prominent, also suggesting a diagnosis of sarcoid. Disseminated disease with generalized lymphadenopathy, meningitis, bony lesions, and abscesses does occur in about 0.5% of patients. Dissemination and fatal disease seems to occur more often in very young children, immunocompromised persons, and persons of dark-skinned races. The endemic areas of coccidioidomycosis are confined to the Western Hemisphere and in the United States include the desert Southwest. Histoplasmosis, another fungal disease that produces respiratory symptoms and hilar lymphadenopathy, may become disseminated in infants and immunocompromised persons. Generalized lymphadenopathy, hepatosplenomegaly, fever, endocarditis, pericarditis, meningitis, and bone marrow invasion may develop. Although this infection occurs worldwide, it is most common in the Ohio and Mississippi River Valleys of the United States. In both of these disease conditions the diagnosis can be suspected by clinical presentation and serologic testing and confirmed by the isolation and identification of organisms from infected secretions of lymph node or lung.

Physical Examination Findings

Physical examination should include the exact location and detailed measurements of the size and number of involved nodes, the shape of the nodes, and the character of the nodes, including consistency, mobility, tenderness, warmth, fluctuance, firmness, and adherence to adjacent structures. Other pertinent physical findings, such as hepatosplenomegaly and skin lesions, are also important.

DIAGNOSIS

Although lymphadenopathy, whether generalized or localized, is a frequently encountered childhood problem, determining its cause can frequently be somewhat difficult. The evaluation of generalized lymphadenopathy begins with a careful history and detailed physical examination, with laboratory tests as indicated (Fig. 51–1). The history should include the duration of lymphadenopathy, the presence and duration of any associated systemic symptoms or signs, exposure to animals or contact with persons infected with tuberculosis, sex history, travel history, preceding trauma, current medications (especially phenytoin), food and ingestion history (especially of undercooked meat or unpasteurized dairy products), medical and surgical history, and family history. A history of trauma or of other infections in the region drained by the involved nodes should be elicited. Findings in the history or physical examination or epidemiologic characteristics that suggest a specific or uncommon diagnosis should prompt the performance of additional or more specific laboratory testing.

Measurements of the involved nodes and notations of any changes in nodal characteristics or of the appearance of any new systemic symptoms should be recorded carefully at every office visit. Failure of the node or nodes to diminish in size or persistence of symptoms is an indication for further diagnostic study and consideration for excisional biopsy.

Differential Diagnosis

There are many noninfectious causes of generalized lymphadenopathy (Table 51–2). Autoimmune disorders and hypersensitivity states may be associated with generalized lymphadenopathy. Children with systemic-onset juvenile rheumatoid arthritis often have lymphadenopathy and splenomegaly, together with high-spiking fever, usually in combination with a rheumatoid rash. Seventy percent of persons with active systemic lupus erythematosus have lymphadenopathy, which is generalized in 34%. Serum sickness is an immune hypersensitivity reaction occurring after exposure to foreign proteins, often drugs; it is characterized by urticaria, edema, fever, polyarthralgia, and generalized lymphadenopathy. Autoimmune hemolytic anemia has been associated with greatly enlarged nontender lymph nodes during episodes of hemolysis. Lymphadenopathy associated with phenytoin and other antiepileptic drug administration has been well documented. Other drugs that have been implicated include allopurinol, isoniazid, antithyroid medications, and pyrimethamine.

Lymph nodes enlarged because of malignant disease are usually nontender and are not associated with overlying erythema. The nodes may feel rubbery or hard, and groups of nodes may become matted together with others or may become surrounded by relatively normal reactive nodes. More than 90% of children with Hodgkin's disease have a painless, enlarged node or nodes in the cervical or supraclavicular regions at presentation. The size of the lymph node may have fluctuated for several months. Systemic symptoms of fever, anorexia, nausea, night sweats, or weight loss may be present in up to one third of these patients.

Non-Hodgkin's lymphomas of childhood and adolescence are a heterogeneous group of lymphoid malignancies. In contrast to Hodgkin's disease, localization of lymphoma is unusual, and most persons have evidence of generalized disease at presentation, although symptoms resulting from involvement of specific lymphoid organs are common. Various lymph nodes, including those of the pharynx in Waldeyer's ring, Peyer's patches of the ileum, and other organs including the thymus, pelvic organs, the liver, and the spleen, may be involved. Enlargement is rapid, with time of onset of symptoms to diagnosis being relatively brief.

Generalized lymphadenopathy has been reported in 70% of children with acute lymphoblastic leukemia and in 30% of children with acute nonlymphoblastic leukemia; however, this is usually an incidental finding and not the presenting complaint. In metastatic neuroblastoma the left supraclavicular node, involved because of extension upward in the thoracic duct as a result of primary disease in the abdomen, may be the initial clinical finding. Occasionally neuroblastoma will present with generalized lymphadenopathy.

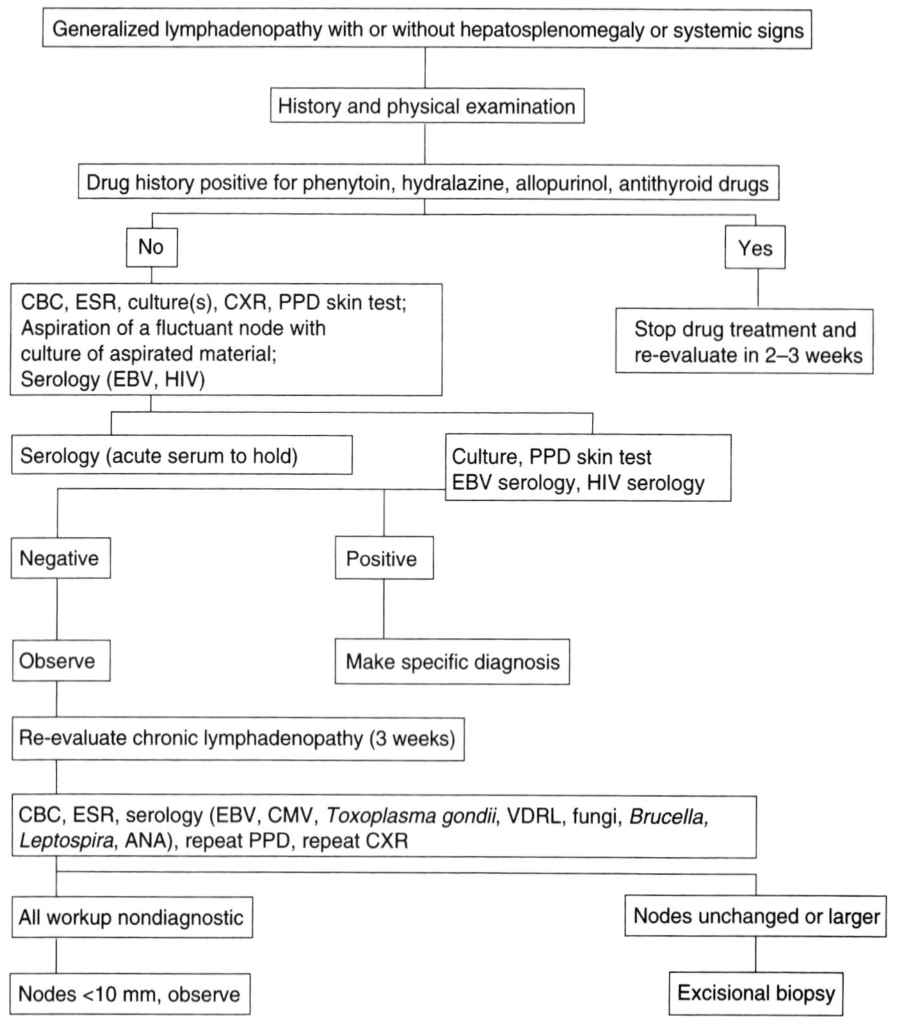

FIGURE 51–1. Evaluation of a child with generalized lymphadenopathy. CBC = complete blood cell count; ESR = erythrocyte sedimentation rate; CXR = chest radiograph; PPD = purified protein derivative; HIV = human immunodeficiency virus; EBV = Epstein-Barr virus; CMV = cytomegalovirus; VDRL = Venereal Disease Research Laboratories; ANA = antinuclear antibody.

The histiocytic disorders are a group of diseases that have as their main feature the infiltration of tissues by histiocytic cells. They may present with local, multifocal, or disseminated disease. In the disseminated form, generalized lymphadenopathy and massive hepatosplenomegaly are seen in addition to seborrheic rash, marrow failure, chronic otorrhea, and bony lesions.

Storage diseases are rare causes of lymphadenopathy. In Niemann-Pick and Gaucher's diseases, lipid-laden macrophages accumulate in the lymph nodes, liver, and spleen, resulting in detectable enlargement. The primary manifestation of these diseases is neurologic deterioration.

The endocrinologic disorders of hyperthyroidism and adrenal insufficiency are sometimes associated with nonspecific lymphoid hyperplasia.

Almost all patients with sarcoidosis exhibit either generalized or hilar lymphadenopathy. Bilateral cervical nodes, when enlarged, are firm, rubbery, and discrete with little tendency to coalesce. Other symptoms include fatigue, cough, fever, dyspnea, and weight loss.

Laboratory Evaluation

Initial laboratory evaluation includes a CBC and ESR. In cases in which a specific diagnosis is not readily apparent from the initial history and physical examination, acute titers for EBV and HIV infections and for syphilis can be obtained if indicated. It is advisable to obtain an extra blood specimen to hold for acute titers for future serologic diagnosis of coccidioidomycosis, histoplasmosis, brucellosis, and leptospirosis. Other specific tests, such as a radiograph of the chest and a tuberculin skin test, should be suggested by findings in the history and physical examination.

Microbiologic Evaluation

Needle aspiration of a fluctuant node may be performed either at the initial office visit or at follow-up visits. All aspirated material should be examined by Gram and acid-fast stains and cultured for aerobic and anaerobic bacteria, mycobacteria, and fungi.

In some cases neither needle aspiration, serologic studies, skin tests, nor a therapeutic trial of antimicrobial therapy is sufficient to confirm the cause of the infection or to exclude a more serious cause of the lymph node enlargement. In such circumstances, excisional biopsy for histologic examination and culture should be performed if there is no decrease in the size of the node within 4–8 weeks of follow-up. Children with supraclavicular lymphadenopathy and children with persistent fever or weight loss for which a specific diagnosis is not readily available should undergo early biopsy. Consistency, tenderness, and unilaterality are not helpful for discriminating the cause of lymphadenopathy in children and should be disregarded as considerations for the need for biopsy.

When the decision is made to biopsy an enlarged node, the surgeon should remove the largest, firmest palpable node available. In general, biopsy of cervical or supraclavicular nodes is preferable

TABLE 51–2. Noninfectious Causes of Generalized Lymphadenopathy

Autoimmune Disorders
Juvenile rheumatoid arthritis
Systemic lupus erythematosus
Autoimmune hemolytic anemia

Hypersensitivity States
Serum sickness
Drug reactions

Neoplasms
Hodgkin's disease
Non-Hodgkin's lymphoma
Metastatic to the lymph nodes
  Acute stem-cell leukemias
  Neuroblastoma
Histiocytoses

Storage Diseases
Niemann-Pick disease
Gaucher's disease

Endocrine Disorders
Hyperthyroidism
Adrenal insufficiency

Other Disorders
Chronic granulomatous disease
Acquired immunodeficiency syndrome
Chronic pseudolymphomatous lymphadenopathy
Sarcoidosis

to biopsy of inguinal nodes when other considerations are the same. More than one node should be removed if possible. Lymph nodes must be meticulously handled during the procedure, because the interpretation of the biopsy specimen often depends primarily on cellular characteristics. In addition to histopathologic examination, Gram and acid-fast stains and aerobic, anaerobic, acid-fast, and fungal cultures should be obtained.

TREATMENT

The treatment of generalized lymphadenopathy will depend on the specific etiologic diagnosis. Most of the infectious causes are viral diseases for which there is no specific treatment.

COMPLICATIONS

The cost and morbidity of lymph node biopsies should be considered. The morbidity of excisional biopsy is generally limited to minor wound infections at the operative site. Excisional biopsy can usually be performed in a day surgery center without the need for overnight hospitalization; for older children local anesthesia often suffices. The cost can be justified if a delay in the diagnosis of a treatable disease is minimized by biopsy.

PROGNOSIS

A review (Knight and Reiner, 1983) of 239 children with peripheral lymphadenopathy who underwent peripheral lymph node biopsy found 31 (13%) to have neoplastic disease. In this series, findings in the history and physical examination that were more often associated with serious diseases (e.g., cancer, histiocytosis, or infection with *Mycobacterium tuberculosis*) were supraclavicular lymphadenopathy, persistent fever or weight loss, and fixation of the node to the skin and deep tissues. Generalized lymphadenopathy in this series was most often due to benign reactive hyperplasia. The demonstration of nondiagnostic hyperplasia usually suggests benign antigenic stimulation, such as viral infection. However, 17–25% of children with nondiagnostic node biopsy specimens will develop severe lymphoreticular disease, including lymphoma and tuberculosis. This emphasizes the need for close follow-up of these persons.

INGUINAL LYMPHADENOPATHY AND LYMPHADENITIS

Inguinal and femoral lymphadenopathy may be asymptomatic, and inguinal nodes ≤15 mm in diameter are regularly palpable in virtually all children. However, when nodes in this region become inflamed, they may produce noticeable pain, stiffness, or swelling in the groin. Inguinal nodes drain the lower extremities, the scrotum and penis in the male, the distal part of the urethra in both sexes, the lower part of the anal canal, and the skin of the lower abdomen, perineum, and gluteal region. Isolated inguinofemoral lymphadenopathy usually results from infection, inflammation, or neoplasm involving one of its drainage areas.

ETIOLOGY

Infection is the most common cause of inguinal lymphadenopathy. The organisms causing inguinal lymphadenitis can be divided into those of nonvenereal origin and those associated with sexually transmitted diseases. As with regional lymphadenitis of other lymph node groups, *S. aureus* and group A *Streptococcus* are the most common causes of the presence of skin or soft tissue infections distal to the nodes. Inguinal lymphadenopathy in postpubertal adolescents and adults and in instances of sexual abuse of children results from sexually transmitted organisms including *Neisseria gonorrhoeae, T. pallidum,* HSV, *Haemophilus ducreyi,* and *C. trachomatis* (Chapter 85).

EPIDEMIOLOGY

Skin infections associated with insect bites on the lower extremities or with diaper dermatitis in infants are readily overlooked causes of *S. aureus* and group A *Streptococcus* inguinal lymphadenitis. Inguinal lymphadenopathy may also occur in response to the inoculation of organisms by traumatic injury to the lower extremities.

Cat-scratch disease, which most often affects children and young adults, is caused by the inoculation of *B. henselae* by the scratch or bite of a domestic cat and may result in isolated inguinal or femoral node involvement when the inoculation site is on the lower extremities.

Bubonic plague results from the bite of rodent fleas infected with *Y. pestis.* Humans also rarely become infected by the direct handling of infected animal tissues or by ingestion of contaminated animal tissues. Although plague occurs worldwide, most of the human cases are reported from the developing countries of Asia and Africa. In the United States it occurs in the Southwest during the summer and fall, when people are outdoors and come into contact with rodents and their fleas, with 60% of cases in persons less than 20 years of age.

Ulceroglandular tularemia may involve the inguinal nodes as a result of infected arthropod bites on the lower extremities. *F.*

tularensis is most often transmitted to humans by infected ticks, but infection may also commonly occur after contact with tissues or body fluids of infected wild mammals (e.g., rabbits, squirrels, beavers, deer). Less commonly, the disease is transmitted by animal bites (e.g., cat, coyote, squirrel). Infection may also occur by ingestion of infected, inadequately cooked meat or by exposure to contaminated water via the conjunctiva, the oropharynx, or the skin. Although the disease occurs in all 50 states, the majority of cases are reported from Arkansas, Tennessee, Texas, Oklahoma, and Missouri. In the past few decades the incidence has peaked in the spring and summer, suggesting that vectorborne tularemia is becoming the most common form of disease.

Sexually Transmitted Diseases. Inguinal lymphadenopathy in sexually active persons is more often due to sexually transmitted diseases. These diseases are rarely seen in prepubertal children, and when they are, they raise suspicions of sexual abuse.

Although gonorrhea is a common sexually transmitted disease, inguinal lymphadenopathy resulting from this infection is uncommon. Similarly, lymphadenopathy appears rarely to accompany cases of nongonococcal urethritis. In contrast, inguinal lymphadenopathy occurs in 50–70% of cases of primary syphilis and in 80% of cases of primary genital herpes. Inguinal lymphadenopathy is also reported in 20% of men and 30% of women with recurrent genital herpes. The vast majority of cases occur in persons 15–30 years of age. Markers associated with increased risk of these venereal diseases include nonwhite ethnicity, lower socioeconomic status, less education, urban residence, and unmarried status.

Chancroid, which is caused by *H. ducreyi,* a small, pleomorphic, gram-negative bacillus, is frequently associated with tender inguinal buboes. This infection is worldwide in distribution and is typically associated with low socioeconomic status and poor hygienic conditions. Only 10% of the reported cases are in women. Major outbreaks of infection have recently been reported in California.

Lymphogranuloma venereum (LGV), caused by the LGV biovars of *C. trachomatis,* is uncommon in the United States, with fewer than 1,000 cases reported each year. Cases in children have been rarely recognized, with only approximately 20 cases in children reported since 1935. Most of these children are girls 3–12 years of age. Also notable is the apparent occurrence of LGV in other adult family members of those infected with LGV, especially the mothers of the infected girls. Although the disease is usually acquired in childhood as a result of genital contact by sexual assault, infection may be transmitted by handling of contaminated fomites. LGV occurs worldwide and is endemic in Asia, Africa, and South America. In the United States, LGV has been reported three times as frequently in men as in women, with the highest occurrence in persons of low socioeconomic status living in the Southeast, in men who have sex with men, and in persons returning from endemic regions outside the United States. Humans are the sole natural host.

Granuloma inguinale, caused by *Calymmatobacterium granulomatis,* is common in the tropics, but fewer than 100 cases are reported in the United States each year. It is seen more frequently in nonwhite persons. It is rare in prepubertal children, but it can be transmitted to children by contaminated fomites. The disease is only mildly contagious, and repeated exposure is apparently necessary for infection to occur. Although this sexually transmitted disease does not truly involve the lymph nodes, the granulomatous lesions that it produces in the groin area are often confused with lymphadenopathy.

PATHOGENESIS

The inguinofemoral nodes serve as filters trapping the various microbes infecting the lower extremities and the genital region, resulting in inguinofemoral lymphadenopathy. Depending on the nature of the infecting organism, host defenses, and antimicrobial therapy, the process may or may not progress to abscess formation.

In prepubertal children, in whom the most common cause of inguinal lymphadenopathy is infection with *S. aureus* or group A *Streptococcus,* infection is presumed to enter the inguinal and femoral lymphatics from the skin of the lower abdominal wall, from the perineal or gluteal regions, or from the lower extremities. The primary focus can be undetectable. Pyodermas of the skin, repeated minor infections of the feet, insect bites, and diaper dermatitis are all possible mechanisms whereby pyogenic organisms gain access to the inguinofemoral nodes.

Zoonotic infections result in inguinal lymphadenopathy by the inoculation of organisms via arthropod bites, animal bites or scratches, or contact of damaged skin with contaminated animal tissues. Many of these cause lymphocutaneous syndromes, in which a characteristic skin lesion is associated with regional lymphadenopathy.

SYMPTOMS AND CLINICAL MANIFESTATIONS

Inguinal lymphadenitis caused by *S. aureus* and group A *Streptococcus* produces a relatively acute enlargement of the affected nodes. Inguinal lymphadenopathy due to pyogenic infections is usually unilateral, and the nodes characteristically are exquisitely tender, firm, red, and warm. Systemic symptoms are usually minimal unless cellulitis, metastatic foci of infection, or bacteremia is present. If treatment is delayed or the infection does not respond to antibiotics, the nodes are likely to suppurate and require drainage.

Cat-scratch disease involves the inguinal nodes in 10–25% of persons, although the most frequent site of involvement is the axillary nodes (Chapter 28).

Bubonic plague is manifested most commonly as isolated, painful, inguinal or femoral lymphadenopathy. During an incubation period of 2–8 days after the bite of an infected flea, bacteria proliferate in the regional lymph nodes. Only rarely is a papular or pustular lesion at the site of the insect bite evident at the onset of clinical illness. Affected persons typically develop the sudden onset of fever, chills, weakness, and headache, accompanied by intense pain in the region of the involved node. Swelling evolves in this area, which is so exquisitely tender that patients will avoid any movement of the involved area. The buboes of persons with plague may vary from 1–10 cm and are firm and nonfluctuant. The overlying skin is warm, and edema surrounds the involved nodes. Plague is virtually unique for the suddenness of onset of the fever and bubo and for the fulminant clinical course, which can produce death as quickly as 2–4 days after the onset of symptoms.

Tularemia that results from exposure to infected animals (e.g., rabbits, squirrels, deer) most often involves the upper extremity, but tickborne infections frequently produce inguinal lymphadenopathy, which is observed in 20–50% of adult cases. Approximately 2 days after the onset of fever and systemic symptoms, tender lymphadenopathy develops. Within 24 hours the portal of entry may become evident when a painful, swollen papule appears distal to the involved nodes. The tick prefers warm, moist areas, and the initial lesion is often found on the scrotum or penis or in the groin. This papule ruptures, leaving an ulcerated lesion **(ulceroglandular tularemia),** which in untreated cases can persist for months. Rarely the lesion may be subtle or absent **(glandular tularemia).** Involved nodes are enlarged and tender, and the skin overlying the nodes is frequently inflamed. These nodes may suppurate and drain in about half of the cases.

Brucellosis and infectious mononucleosis are diseases that may rarely be causes of inguinal lymphadenopathy, usually in association with generalized lymphadenopathy. **Nontuberculous mycobacteria,** also known as **atypical mycobacteria,** and *M. tuberculosis* infections can rarely cause isolated inguinal lymphadenopathy, but these infections more often produce cervical lymphadenopathy.

Sexually Transmitted Diseases. Gonococcal and nongonococcal urethritis may occasionally produce bilateral or unilateral inguinal lymphadenopathy. With either infection, the nodes are usually discrete and are not fixed to the overlying skin.

Primary genital herpes is commonly associated with tender, nonsuppurative inguinal lymphadenopathy, which is frequently bilateral. There is likely to be a prodromal period of fever and malaise, often accompanied by vulvar paresthesia and burning, before the onset of the primary vesicles characteristic of this infection. Occasionally the lymphadenopathy actually precedes the appearance of skin lesions. The lymphadenopathy is described as lasting 1–2 weeks in persons with primary disease. Although lymphadenopathy is occasionally seen in episodes of recurrent disease, it is usually of shorter duration.

Primary syphilis results in relatively painless and usually bilateral inguinal lymphadenopathy **(satellite bubo)** in 50–70% of cases. Nodes usually become enlarged about 7 days after the appearance of the chancre. The chancre may frequently be missed in women because it is frequently situated on the cervix or vaginal wall. The examiner usually palpates a chain of nodes rather than a single node, and these nodes are firm, discrete, nonsuppurative, painless, and freely movable. The overlying skin is not inflamed. Constitutional symptoms are usually absent. Generalized lymphadenopathy occurs in secondary syphilis.

Chancroid is usually accompanied by painful inguinal lymphadenopathy. The incubation period is usually 3–7 days but may be longer. The first sign of infection is a small, hyperemic macule that progresses to become a papule, then a pustule, and finally a small, painful ulcer. The primary lesion may be on the vulva, the vaginal mucosa, or the cervix but is usually on one of the labia minora. Multiplication by autoinoculation creates a number of small ulcers, which coalesce to form an eroded area. This area is covered with a gray base laden with organisms. The lymphadenopathy of chancroid develops about 1 week after the primary lesion appears and is present while the ulcer is still active. The chancroidal bubo is typically unilateral, markedly painful, and composed of fused inguinal nodes, which may suppurate and drain.

The primary genital lesion of LGV is usually transient and asymptomatic. The initial manifestation of the disease is usually the characteristic inguinal bubo, occurring 1–4 weeks after sexual exposure to LGV biovars of *C. trachomatis.* The lymphadenopathy is most often unilateral. Initially the node is tender, discrete, and movable, but subsequently the inflammatory process involves multiple nodes in the area. Chills, fever, and constitutional symptoms are common at this stage. If left untreated, within a matter of weeks the inguinal nodes and subcutaneous tissues become a brawny mass adherent to the indurated, purplish red overlying skin. The inguinal nodes increase in size and form abscesses. Unless they are aspirated, the buboes rupture and form multiple fistulous tracts. A central lengthwise linear depression, the **groove sign** of LGV, is produced by involvement of nodes above and below the inguinal ligament. If LGV is left untreated, periadenitis causes progressive vascular and lymphatic obstruction. These pathologic processes, together with increased connective tissue proliferation, result in induration and hypertrophy of the vulvar and perineal skin and subcutaneous tissues. Eventually the inguinal, vulvar, perineal, and anal areas are the site of deep, shaggy, granulomatous ulcerations with rectal and colonic strictures and massive fibrosis of the deep pelvic lymphatics and connective tissues. LGV proctitis is manifested as tenesmus, hematochezia, purulent rectal discharge, and abdominal pain.

Donovanosis (granuloma inguinale) is a sexually transmitted chronic disease characterized by granulomatous lesions in the groin that may be confused with true lymphadenopathy. The disease is caused by *C. granulomatis,* an encapsulated bacillus that forms intracytoplasmic inclusions in large mononuclear cells that are pathognomonic of the disease (Donovan's bodies). Granuloma inguinale has a long incubation period of 3–4 months, allowing for low detection rates in sexual partners. The initial lesion is a small, relatively painless vesicle or reddish nodule most often found on the prepuce or glans penis in the man and on the labia in the woman. The early lesion becomes a small, soft mass of red granulation tissue, which progresses to ulceration. This progresses slowly, often coalescing with adjacent lesions or forming new lesions by autoinoculation. The patient has no systemic symptoms, and the perineal lesions are relatively painless early in the disease. Later, the ulcerative process may extend to the anus and urethra, making defecation and urination difficult. If left untreated, the ulcerative area continues to enlarge and its margins become thickened by an edging of granulation tissue. Lymphedema and scarring make walking and sitting difficult. Occasionally the lymphatics are involved, but the frequently seen **suppurating bubo** of the groin is in fact a subcutaneous granuloma **(pseudobubo).** Hematogenous dissemination occasionally occurs and is more frequent in women, particularly in those with the primary lesion on the cervix. When this occurs, disease may involve the bones, joints, and liver. Systemic disease causes severe toxemia, associated with prolonged spiking fever, progressive anemia, and weight loss. A diagnosis of granuloma inguinale is established by the microscopic identification of Donovan's bodies in tissue taken from a lesion.

Physical Examination Findings

Physical examination should include exact location and detailed measurement of the size and number of involved nodes, their shape, and their character, including consistency, mobility, tenderness, warmth, fluctuance, firmness, and adherence to adjacent structures. Other pertinent physical findings, such as hepatosplenomegaly and skin lesions, are also important.

Specific findings on physical examination of the involved nodes can help in the determination of the infectious agent. Inguinal nodes that are bilateral suggest venereal infection. Firm nodes accompany most acute inflammatory processes and are of little diagnostic significance. Nodes may become fluctuant when the infectious process goes untreated. Fluctuant nodes are characteristic of *S. aureus* and group A *Streptococcus* infections, plague, and LGV, are found in half of the cases of tularemia, and are rare in syphilis and genital herpes. The sign of the groove suggests LGV but has been reported with suppurative bacterial lymphadenitis and with lymphomatous involvement of the inguinal nodes. Redness of the overlying skin is typical of lymphadenitis with *S. aureus,* group A *Streptococcus,* tularemia, and chancroid. A purplish hue to the overlying skin has been reported with lymphadenopathy due to the LGV biovars of *C. trachomatis.*

DIAGNOSIS

Persons with regional inguinal lymphadenopathy can be approached similarly to persons with generalized lymphadenopathy. Differences in the diagnostic study will be due to the likelihood of specific disease states, causing enlargement of nodes in a specific region of the body. Evaluation begins with a careful history and detailed physical examination, with laboratory tests as indicated

(Fig. 51–1). The history should include the duration of the lymphadenopathy, the presence and duration of any associated systemic symptoms or signs, exposure to animals or contact with persons infected with tuberculosis, sex history, travel history, preceding trauma, current medications (especially phenytoin), food and ingestion history (especially of undercooked meat or unpasteurized dairy products,) medical and surgical history, and family history. A history of trauma or other infections in the region drained by the involved nodes should be elicited. Findings in the history or physical examination or epidemiologic characteristics that suggest a specific or uncommon diagnosis should prompt the performance of additional or more specific laboratory testing.

Once it is determined that an inguinal mass is truly an enlarged lymph node, the aim of the evaluation is to identify infection of the external or internal genitalia or of the lower extremities and to determine whether other lymph node groups are involved. In persons who are sexually active, the evaluation will obviously be much different from that in a prepubertal child.

Historical information can be extremely helpful in establishing the diagnosis. An outdoor occupation may place a person at risk of tularemia or plague. Chancroid, granuloma inguinale, and LGV are all rare in the United States; a history of travel to areas in which these diseases are endemic is important. Plague is extremely rare in patients who have not lived or passed through the southwestern United States or Southeast Asia.

The duration of lymphadenopathy can help to narrow the differential diagnosis. Most infections produce a relatively acute enlargement of the affected nodes, but cat-scratch disease and malignancy are more often relatively chronic. Gradually increasing indolent lymphadenopathy may accompany repeated minor injuries to the lower extremities. A history of pain or tenderness is consistent with many acute infections but is characteristic of cat-scratch disease, tularemia, gonorrhea, genital herpes, chancroid, and infection with pyogenic cocci. Tenderness is unusual in nodes involved with syphilis, lymphoma, or other malignancies. A history of trauma may suggest specific cat-scratch disease or tickborne tularemia. In persons with suspected lymphadenopathy of venereal origin, a history of prior genital lesions should be sought. An indolent, indurated, relatively painless genital ulcer that heals spontaneously is suggestive of syphilis. A history of a painless papule or ulcer of the external genitalia that has disappeared is consistent with LGV, but the majority of these lesions go completely unnoticed. A history of purulent genital discharge suggests gonococcal urethritis or cervicitis. A history of prior sexually transmitted disease increases the probability of a genital infection.

Differential Diagnosis

Several conditions mimic inguinal lymphadenopathy. Abscesses of the skin or soft tissue overlying the groin area may produce a tender mass easily confused with inguinal lymphadenopathy. The mass will be fixed to the overlying skin, and the examiner may be able to press his or her fingers behind the mass to establish its separation from the inguinal or femoral lymphatic chains. This picture will be confused further if such an infection leads to true local lymphadenopathy. An intra-abdominal abscess such as a psoas abscess may occasionally dissect into the inguinal canal. Inguinal and femoral hernias are common masses in the groin, but their softness and variation with respiration serve as clues to the diagnosis. An inguinal hematoma or aneurysm, ectopic testes, ectopic spleens, and inguinal endometriosis can also be confused with enlarged inguinal nodes. Ultrasonography or computed tomography may help to distinguish these conditions from true lymphadenopathy.

Malignancy arising in the genital tract or lower extremities or an unknown primary tumor may metastasize to the inguinal nodes. This is somewhat more common in elderly persons. Lymphadenopathy due to neoplasm is usually nontender.

Microbiologic Evaluation

Laboratory investigation should be guided by findings in the history and physical examination. In persons with acute unilateral adenitis associated with skin or soft tissue infection of the lower extremities, a trial of antibiotics with activity against *S. aureus* and group A *Streptococcus* can be instituted before extensive laboratory evaluation. A clinical response should be noted in 36–48 hours. If this response is not seen, further diagnostic investigation should be undertaken.

Tularemia is diagnosed on the basis of clinical manifestations, a thorough history of possible exposure, and results of serial antibody tests. There are no absolute pathognomonic clinical features of tularemia. Agglutinating antibodies are usually detectable by the second week of illness but occasionally do not appear until 4–6 weeks. A titer of 1:160 or greater is presumptive evidence of infection, but confirmation of the diagnosis depends on a rising titer. Gram-stained smears of material from these patients do not usually reveal the organism. There is no danger in collecting these specimens, however, and examination of direct smears can exclude other possible causes. Specimens should not be cultured for *F. tularensis* in the common hospital laboratory because of danger to laboratory personnel but should be sent to a laboratory with appropriate facilities and expertise.

Serologic tests for brucellosis and infectious mononucleosis are available. Diagnosis of nontuberculous mycobacterial infection and of *M. tuberculosis* infection requires culture of these organisms from aspirated material or excised nodes.

Lymphadenopathy associated with gonococcal and nongonococcal urethritis or cervicitis is diagnosed by appropriate stains and cultures of urethral or cervical discharge.

Syphilis is most easily diagnosed with serologic tests. Results of these tests are almost always positive for a person with inguinal lymphadenopathy, and a nonreactive treponema-specific antibody test essentially rules out syphilis.

The diagnosis of genital herpes can usually be established clinically but may be confirmed with viral culture. Detection of HSV in direct smears of open lesions, although less sensitive than culture, may allow for a rapid, specific diagnosis.

Chancroid may occasionally be diagnosed on the basis of a Gram-stained smear from an ulcerated lesion. The finding of short gram-negative rods, sometimes in a parallel array resembling a school of fish, is highly suggestive of the diagnosis. The edge of an ulcerated lesion is the best site for obtaining material. Fluid from the edge of the lesion can be cultured for *H. ducreyi*. However, this organism is extremely fastidious, and the laboratory should be notified that this organism is suspected.

A diagnosis of LGV is considered whenever a patient has tender, enlarged inguinal nodes or an ulcerative or granulomatous lesion of the perineal region. An acutely painful, unilateral inguinal lymphadenopathy is particularly suspicious. The diagnosis is confirmed by identification of *C. trachomatis,* LGV serovars, in cultures of material from a bubo, from an ulcer, or from the rectum, cervix, or urethra. Unfortunately, bubo aspirates are positive for the organism in only about 30% of the suspected cases. Serologic complement fixation tests with chlamydial antigen will show a high ($>$1:32) or rising titer in 95% of the persons with LGV.

Aspiration. Before the advent of effective antimicrobial therapy, needle aspiration of enlarged nodes was frequently complicated by sinus tract formation, but this complication is now rare. Needle aspiration findings may reveal the etiologic agent if other diagnostic measures have failed and the person has not responded to empirical antimicrobial therapy. The certainty that a mass is an inguinal lymph node is important because the procedure is contraindicated with inguinal hernia or aneurysm. Ultrasonography may help to resolve these questions. The largest, most fluctuant node having the most direct access is the best target. The overlying skin should be cleansed and anesthetized. A sterile 18-gauge needle attached to a 10 mL syringe should be used to evacuate thickened pus if present. The node should be entered from an area of healthy skin. If no purulent material is obtained on aspiration, the syringe may be disconnected from the needle and replaced with another containing a small amount of nonbacteriostatic saline solution, which is injected into the node and then aspirated. After aspiration, the air should be evacuated from the syringe and needle, and the needle immediately capped. The specimen should be delivered to the microbiology laboratory promptly. In general, surgical incision and drainage of the nodes should be avoided. Pus from fluctuant nodes should be examined by Gram stain and then cultured. Wayson or Wright's stain should be performed if bubonic plague is suspected. If the presence of nontuberculous mycobacteria or *M. tuberculosis* is a consideration, acid-fast staining should also be done. The aspirate should be cultured, as indicated, for *S. aureus,* group A *Streptococcus, N. gonorrhoeae,* and *H. ducreyi.* Material recovered from nonfluctuant nodes should be examined by dark-field microscopy if available. A good specimen contains about 10 lymphocytes per oil-immersion field and reveals spirochetes in about 95% of cases of syphilis. These specimens should be handled with extreme care because many of the possible etiologic organisms are contagious.

Biopsy. Eventually, **excisional biopsy** may be necessary to establish a diagnosis. Few pathologic features are differentially diagnostic in acute infection. Noncaseating granulomas are frequently seen with gonorrhea, syphilis, and LGV. Langerhans-type giant cells are not specific for mycobacterial infection because they may also be seen in syphilis and LGV. Fibrosis of the capsule and pericapsular tissues with phlebitis or endarteritis is highly suggestive of syphilis. The combination of follicular hyperplasia, granulomas with giant cells, and microabscesses in the same specimen is highly suggestive of cat-scratch disease.

TREATMENT

If a specific diagnosis can be established initially, the person should be treated with the most effective and least toxic antimicrobial agent available for that specific disease. In persons with acute pyogenic lymphadenitis suspected to be caused by *S. aureus* or group A *Streptococcus,* empirical therapy may be instituted before aspiration or other diagnostic evaluation. Penicillinase-resistant penicillins or first-generation cephalosporins with good antistaphylococcal coverage can be used. In persons allergic to β-lactam antibiotics a macrolide or clindamycin can be given. If a clinical response to antibiotics is not seen within 36–48 hours, further diagnostic evaluation should be performed, including needle aspiration of the involved node for stains and cultures. Subsequent therapy should be based on the results of these tests. Persons who are systemically ill should be hospitalized and antimicrobial therapy instituted promptly. Persons who have more indolent, slowly progressive inguinal lymphadenopathy may await the results of laboratory investigations (Table 51–3).

If Gram stain of the lymph node aspirate suggests an organism other than *S. aureus* or group A *Streptococcus,* treatment should be directed at the most likely organism until culture results are known. Final bacteriologic identification and the results of antimicrobial susceptibility tests should guide the ultimate antimicrobial therapy for unusual infections such as cat-scratch disease (Chapter 28), tularemia (Chapter 34), plague (Chapter 34), and rat-bite fever (Chapter 50).

Inguinal lymphadenopathy associated with sexually transmitted infections, including gonorrhea, syphilis, chancroid, LGV, genital herpes, and granuloma inguinale, is treated as for other forms of these infections (Chapter 85). Initial therapy with ceftriaxone, 250 mg intramuscularly, or cefotaxime, 500 mg intramuscularly, followed by erythromycin, 500 mg orally 4 times a day for 14 days, will adequately treat gonorrhea, including penicillinase-producing strains, most cases of syphilis, nongonococcal urethritis, chancroid, LGV, and staphylococcal and streptococcal infections. Close follow-up is necessary in these patients while results of cultures and other laboratory investigations are pending. Once an accurate diagnosis is made, more specific therapy may be instituted (Chapter 85).

COMPLICATIONS AND PROGNOSIS

The prognosis for nonvenereal inguinal lymphadenitis caused by *S. aureus* and group A *Streptococcus* is extremely good because of the availability of effective antimicrobial therapy. Even with nodes that become fluctuant, appropriate drainage combined with antimicrobial therapy is effective, with only rare complications or relapses.

Unfortunately, persons who develop inguinal lymphadenitis associated with venereal disease frequently become reinfected with the same or different sexually transmitted organisms in ensuing years because of the continued presence of high-risk behaviors. Although most of the sexually transmitted diseases respond well to specific antimicrobial therapy, repeated infection is not uncommon (Chapter 85). In the case of LGV, repeated infection or prolonged infection without appropriate treatment can lead to vascular and lymphatic obstruction of the lower extremities and perineal region.

PREVENTION

Appropriate medical therapy for infections of the lower extremities should reduce the incidence of inguinal lymphadenitis due to *S. aureus* and group A *Streptococcus.* Prevention of the zoonotic infections of plague and tularemia include vector control and public education pertaining to the epidemiology of these diseases (Chapter 34), as well as personal protective measures against tickborne and rodentborne infections (Chapter 3). The prevention of the sexually transmitted diseases causing inguinal lymphadenopathy involves public education and the identification and proper treatment of infected persons, both with and without symptoms (Chapter 85).

CERVICAL LYMPHADENOPATHY AND LYMPHADENITIS

Cervical node enlargement is characterized by inflammation of one or more lymph nodes of the neck and is the most frequently encountered childhood lymphadenopathy. Cervical lymph nodes are considered enlarged if they are greater than 10 mm in diameter. Causes of cervical lymphadenopathy include among others infection, neoplasm, and histiocytoses. Nonlymphoid cervical masses may also mimic lymphadenopathy in this region.

The **superficial cervical lymph nodes** lie on top of the sternocleidomastoid muscle and include the **anterior group,** which lie along the anterior jugular vein, and the **posterior group,** which are found in the **posterior triangle** along the course of the external

TABLE 51–3. Sources of Inguinal Lymphadenitis, Node Characteristics, and Recommended Treatment

Primary Disease or Cause	Node Characteristics	Treatment*
Nonvenereal Origin		
Staphylococcus aureus or group A *Streptococcus*	Acute onset; unilateral tender, red, warm, indurated node	Penicillinase-resistant penicillins, first-generation cephalosporins
Bartonella henselae (cat-scratch disease)	Associated skin papule distal to node; unilateral warm, red, indurated node	No specific antimicrobial therapy; aspiration if fluctuant; azithromycin may speed resolution (Chapter 28)
Yersinia pestis (plague)	Acute onset; systemic symptoms common with fulminant clinical course; intensely painful, firm, nonfluctuant node	Streptomycin, doxycycline, chloramphenicol (Chapter 34)
Francisella tularensis (tularemia)	Associated painful skin papule from tick bite; unilateral tender, red, warm node	Gentamicin, tetracycline, chloramphenicol (Chapter 34)
Sexually Transmitted Organisms		
Neisseria gonorrhoeae and nongonococcal urethritis	Only occasional, discrete, minimal tenderness	Ceftriaxone or cefotaxime, followed by doxycycline or erythromycin (Table 85–2)
Treponema pallidum (syphilis)	Painless bilateral chain of nodes	Benzathine penicillin G, doxycycline, erythromycin (Table 85–6)
Herpes simplex virus	Tender, nonsuppurative, frequently bilateral	Acyclovir, famciclovir, valacyclovir (Table 85–7)
Haemophilus ducreyi (chancroid)	Associated painful genital ulcer; unilateral markedly painful nodes	Erythromycin, azithromycin, ciprofloxacin (Table 85–8)
Chlamydia trachomatis, LGV biovars (lymphogranuloma venereum)	Tender, multiple nodes, unilateral, progress to abscesses with fistulous tracts; constitutional symptoms frequent; if untreated, progressive vascular and lymphatic obstruction develops	Doxycycline, erythromycin sulfisoxazole, (Table 85–4)

jugular vein (Fig. 51–2). These receive afferents from the superficial tissues of the neck, mastoid, superficial parotid (preauricular) nodes, and submaxillary glands. Their efferents terminate in the upper deep cervical nodes. The **submental lymph nodes,** located between the digastric muscles of the chin, receive superficial and deep drainage from the anterior part of the tongue, the lower lip, and the chin. The **mastoid lymph nodes,** located near the mastoid process of the temporal bone, drain the parietal scalp and the inner surface of the pinna. The **occipital lymph nodes** lie at the base of the occiput and receive afferents from the occipital scalp and superficial portions of the upper posterior part of the neck. The submental, mastoid, and occipital nodes all send efferents to the deep cervical nodes. The **deep cervical lymph nodes** lie deep to the sternocleidomastoid muscle along the whole length of the internal jugular vein and are divided into upper and lower groups. One member of the upper group, the **jugulodigastric gland,** or **tonsillar node,** drains the palatine tonsil and frequently becomes enlarged in persons with tonsillitis or with tuberculous infection originating from the tonsils. The lower deep cervical lymph nodes receive drainage from the larynx, trachea, thyroid gland, and esophagus. The **submandibular lymph nodes** lie adjacent to the submandibular salivary gland, where they receive superficial drainage from the lower lip, the vestibule of the nose, the cheeks, the medial parts of the eyelids, and the forehead. They also receive deep drainage from the posterior part of the mouth, gums, teeth, and tongue, as well as from superficial and submental lymph nodes. It

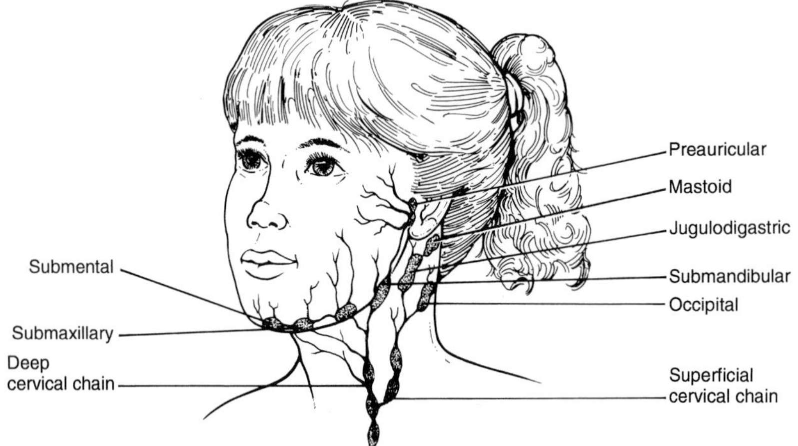

FIGURE 51–2. Lymphatic drainage and lymph nodes involved in patients with cervical lymphadenitis.

is not surprising that these nodes, together with the deep cervical nodes, are affected in the majority of cases of cervical lymphadenitis in young children. The lymphatic flow follows the venous flow and empties into the subclavian veins.

ETIOLOGY

Infection is by far the most common cause of cervical lymphadenopathy in the pediatric age group. The most common causes of cervical node enlargement in children are reactive hyperplasia due to an infectious stimulus in the head and neck region, and infection of the node itself. Injury or invasion most frequently occurs proximal to the involved lymph node or nodes, which then become secondarily infected by drainage from afferent lymphatics. Cervical lymphadenitis most commonly is associated with a systemic viral illness and resolves in a few days to 2 weeks.

Acute suppurative lymphadenitis is usually caused by only a few bacterial species, with symptoms developing rapidly within a few days. The likelihood that a given organism is responsible varies with the age of the child. In neonates, *S. aureus* and group B *Streptococcus* are the most common pathogens. *S. aureus* infection is most common in older infants. In children, acute bacterial cervical lymphadenitis is equally likely to be caused by *S. aureus* or group A *Streptococcus.* Dental infections caused by aerobic and anaerobic bacteria associated with dental caries and periodontal disease may be accompanied by cervical lymphadenopathy (Chapter 61). In older children and adolescents, EBV infection is a relatively common cause of posterior cervical lymphadenitis (Chapter 37).

Subacute or chronic lymphadenitis that progresses gradually for 2 or more weeks, although occasionally due to *S. aureus,* is caused most commonly by nontuberculous mycobacteria, *B. henselae* (Chapter 28), or *T. gondii* and infrequently by EBV or CMV. Infection and reactive hyperplasia in response to infection continue to be the most common causes of lymphadenopathy in children with a duration of 3 weeks or longer. Among children in the United States, 70–95% of mycobacterial cervical lymphadenitis is caused by nontuberculous mycobacteria, commonly *Mycobacterium avium-intracellulare* complex. Other nontuberculous mycobacteria that are common causes of cervical lymphadenitis include *M. kansasii, M. fortuitum,* and *M. haemophilum. M. haemophilum* causes infection of the perihilar or cervical lymph nodes. There are reports of immunologically normal children having cervical and perihilar lymphadenitis caused by *M. haemophilum,* but all reported cases in adults have been in immunocompromised persons.

EPIDEMIOLOGY

The epidemiology of cervical adenitis is that of the causative infectious agents. Most commonly cervical adenitis occurs as part of a lymphoreticular response to a systemic viral illness. The mode of spread for most viral cases of cervical lymphadenitis and for bacterial infections with group A *Streptococcus* and *M. tuberculosis* is by dropletborne transmission via the respiratory route. Except in newborns, in whom male dominance has been reported in cases of group B *Streptococcus* lymphadenitis, infectious lymphadenitis displays no sexual or seasonal predilection.

Subacute granulomatous lymphadenitis due to mycobacteria displays distinct epidemiologic characteristics (Table 51–4). Cervical lymphadenopathy caused by nontuberculous mycobacteria occurs more often in white persons, in contrast with that caused by *M. tuberculosis,* which occurs more often in African Americans and Hispanics. Children with lymphadenitis due to nontuberculous mycobacteria are characteristically 1–4 years of age and live in suburban or rural communities with no history of contact with tuberculosis. Nontuberculous mycobacteria, or atypical or "environmental" mycobacteria, are widely distributed in soil, water, and cold-blooded animals, and in general they are of relatively low pathogenicity in warm-blooded animals. Human infection probably arises from inhalation of aerosols. Human-to-human spread has never been proved.

Scrofula caused by *M. tuberculosis,* formerly a common disease in children and young adults, has become much less frequent but is still occasionally seen in older adults who many years earlier immigrated to this country from endemic areas or who live in rural areas in this country. In this setting the disease represents reactivation of prior cervical node tuberculosis, acquired either by ingestion of milk infected with *Mycobacterium bovis* (**bovine tuberculosis**) or by lymphohematogenous spread of infection from an initial pulmonary focus of *M. tuberculosis* to this group of lymph nodes. Tuberculous lymphadenitis is occasionally reported in children in this country, usually in older children and adolescents.

PATHOGENESIS

Although cervical lymphadenitis is a common entity in pediatric practice, its pathophysiology is not completely understood. Bacteria gain access to the cervical lymph nodes through the lymphatics from the upper respiratory tract, anterior nares, mouth, or skin of the head or neck. The common occurrence of group A *Streptococcus* lymphadenitis in infants and children less than 3 years of age, in contrast to the infrequency with which streptococcal pharyngitis is observed in this age group, indicates the importance of the interaction between the host and a specific microorganism. Periodontal disease and dental caries predispose children to the development of cervical lymphadenitis and usually involve mouth anaerobic bacteria (Chapter 61). Certain infections are characterized by direct inoculation of the skin proximal to cervical lymph nodes with such organisms as *S. aureus, B. henselae, F. tularensis,* and *Nocardia.*

SYMPTOMS AND CLINICAL MANIFESTATIONS

Cervical lymphadenopathy caused by infection can be categorized on the basis of clinical findings as either acute or subacute and chronic. Cervical lymphadenitis of acute onset may be further categorized as either bilateral or unilateral. In most situations acute bilateral cervical lymphadenitis is either part of the lymphoreticular response to a systemic infection or a localized reaction to acute pharyngitis. Lymph nodes are usually small and rubbery and may or may not be tender. There is little or no redness or warmth of the overlying skin. The presence of distinguishing clinical features such as gingivostomatitis (HSV), herpangina (coxsackievirus or echovirus), or rash (rubella or rubeola) may help establish a cause.

Acute unilateral pyogenic cervical lymphadenitis is caused by *S. aureus* or group A *Streptococcus* in 53–89% of cases. The male-to-female ratio is equal, and 70–80% of cases occur in children 1–4 years of age. Systemic symptoms are usually minimal or absent unless associated with cellulitis, metastatic foci of infection, or bacteremia. Clinically there is little that helps to differentiate streptococcal from staphylococcal infections, although staphylococcal infections tend to have a longer duration of symptoms and a greater likelihood of suppuration at presentation. There are no significant differences in the incidence of associated otitis media, nasal discharge, pharyngitis, skin lesions, conjunctivitis, or the size and site of lymph node involvement. Submandibular involvement is the most frequent, followed by upper cervical and then submental. Involved nodes are usually 2–6 cm in diameter, and one fourth to

TABLE 51–4. Differentiation of *Mycobacterium tuberculosis* and Nontuberculous Mycobacterial Cervical Lymphadenitis

Factor	*M. tuberculosis*	Nontuberculous Mycobacterial
Age	All ages (most >5 yr)	1–4 yr
Race	Predominantly African American and Hispanic	Predominantly white
Exposure to tuberculosis	Present	Absent
Chest roentgenograms	Abnormal (20–70%)	Normal (97%)
Residence	Urban	Rural
PPD >15 mm of induration*	Usual	Uncommon
Bilateral involvement	Not uncommon	Rare
Response to antimycobacterial drugs	Yes	Partial

*PPD refers to 5 tuberculin unit (5 TU) intracutaneous skin test.

one third become fluctuant. Of those nodes that become fluctuant, 86% will become suppurative within 2 weeks of enlargement. Tenderness is moderate to intense and is often accompanied by erythema and warmth of the overlying skin.

Cervical lymphadenitis in the newborn is most often caused by *S. aureus,* with clinical features similar to those in older infants and children. In recent years, group B *Streptococcus* has been described as the cause of a ''cellulitis-adenitis'' syndrome in infancy. Infants with this condition differ from those with staphylococcal adenitis in that they are younger, between 3 and 7 weeks of age, are more often male, and have a greater incidence of systemic symptoms including irritability, fever, and poor feeding. Bacteremia occurs in almost all these infants, and rarely CSF cultures have shown positive results. Appropriate intravenous antibiotic therapy effects rapid resolution.

Cervical lymphadenitis may also be part of the **streptococcosis** syndrome of infancy caused by group A *Streptococcus.* These infants have coryza, a low-grade fever, nasal discharge with excoriation and crusting around the nares, vomiting, and anorexia. Within a few days of onset, cervical lymph node enlargement occurs. Without treatment, these nodes may suppurate after several weeks, but this is uncommon if appropriate therapy is given early in the course of the illness.

Lymphocutaneous syndromes are conditions in which regional lymphadenitis is associated with a characteristic skin lesion at the site of inoculation. Such lesions are associated with cervical lymphadenitis when the inoculation site occurs in the head or neck region. A history or presence of tick bites on the head or neck suggests ulceroglandular tularemia as a possible cause of acute cervical lymphadenitis (Fig. 51–3). Cat-scratch disease is a relatively common cause of subacute or chronic cervical lymphadenopathy in children and also represents a lymphocutaneous syndrome (Chapter 28).

A common cause of childhood chronic cervical lymphadenitis, especially in certain regions of the United States, is nontuberculous mycobacterial infection (Table 51–4). The signs and symptoms of lymphadenitis due to nontuberculous or tuberculous mycobacteria are virtually identical. Nontuberculous lymphadenitis is located more consistently in the anterior cervical region (82–93%), typically high in the neck close to the mandible, whereas tuberculous lymphadenitis may be observed in posterior cervical, axillary, and inguinal regions in 40% of cases. A substantial proportion of persons with tuberculous lymphadenitis will have hilar lymphadenopathy or generalized lymphadenopathy or both. In both disease states the nodes are usually relatively painless and rather firm initially, but in time they gradually soften, then rupture, and drain. Enlargement is initially rapid and then plateaus after 2 weeks. The local reaction is circumscribed, and although the skin overlying the node may develop a pinkish discoloration, it is not warm to the touch. Systemic illness is minimal or absent (Fig. 51–4).

Compared with nontuberculous mycobacterial lymphadenitis, cervical lymphadenitis caused by *M. tuberculosis* is more likely to occur in children more than 5 years of age, who are more likely to have bilateral node enlargement (10% of cases), a history of exposure to tuberculosis, and an abnormality noted on a chest roentgenogram (20–70%). Mantoux skin testing, or the PPD skin test, is a helpful discriminator because the diameter of the reaction to the standard tuberculin skin test with 5 tuberculin units of human PPD usually exceeds 15 mm with cervical lymphadenitis caused by *M. tuberculosis,* whereas reactions ranging from 5 to 15 mm are common with nontuberculous mycobacteria. In one study (Margileth et al, 1984) the reaction to the standard tuberculin skin test was positive at greater than 15 mm in 85% of persons determined to have tuberculous adenitis on an initial test and in 100% on retest. In this same study, 83% of persons with nontuberculous adenitis had skin test reactions of 5–15 mm, and 17% had negative reactions. In disease due to *M. haemophilum* the lymphadenopathy is usually cervical but may also involve perihilar nodes. With perihilar lymphadenitis, the symptoms and signs may be indistinguishable from those of primary tuberculosis. In addition, Mantoux testing may lead to further confusion because it may yield results >10 mm.

Acquired toxoplasmosis may also cause chronic posterior cervical lymphadenitis. Most patients are free of symptoms, but in

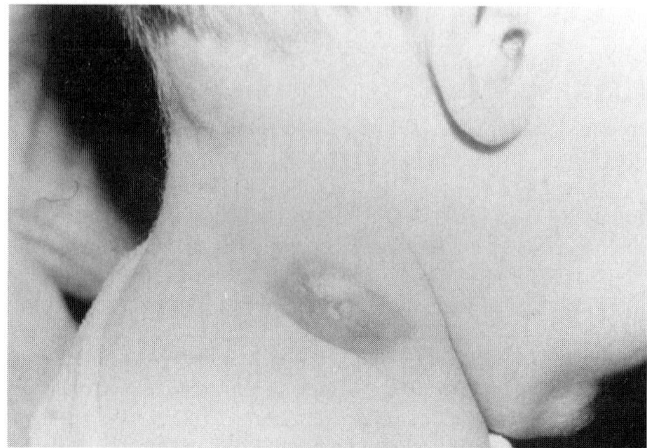

FIGURE 51–3. A 5-year-old boy with fever and unilateral inflammation of occipital and posterior cervical nodes of 3 days' duration. An ulcerated lesion from an antecedent tick bite was found on the posterior aspect of the scalp. Streptomycin injections resulted in complete resolution of fever and lymphadenitis.

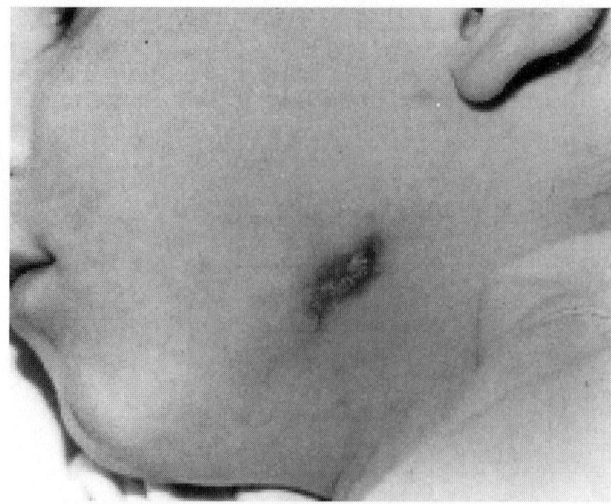

FIGURE 51–4. A 4-year-old boy who had unilateral nontender enlargement of the lymph nodes of 4 weeks' duration without other symptoms. Spontaneous drainage had been present for several days. Tuberculin skin testing resulted in a 9-mm induration; an excisional biopsy acid-fast stain was positive, and cultures grew *Mycobacterium avium* complex.

approximately 10% of cases of acquired toxoplasmosis, lymphadenopathy and fatigue occur without fever. In about half of the cases, toxoplasmosis is manifested by a single enlarged node in the posterior cervical area that is nontender and that fluctuates in size. A history of eating undercooked meat or of contact with cats or cat litter is usually elicited. Other causes of chronic posterior cervical or occipital lymphadenopathy that are easily recognizable on physical examination include tinea capitis, seborrhea of the scalp, and head lice.

Physical Examination Findings

Physical examination should include the exact location and a detailed measurement of the size and number of involved nodes, their shape, and their character, including consistency, mobility, tenderness, warmth, fluctuance, firmness, and adherence to adjacent structures. Bimanual examination with one finger in the mouth is extremely helpful when one is examining nodes in the cheek or mandibular areas. Ultrasonographic examination may be extremely useful in establishing whether the mass is cystic or solid or contains areas of fluctuance. The physical examination should also include the presence or absence of dental disease, oropharyngeal or skin lesions, ocular disease, other nodal enlargement, and any other signs of systemic illness such as hepatosplenomegaly and skin lesions.

DIAGNOSIS

The evaluation of cervical lymphadenopathy begins with a careful history and detailed physical examination, with laboratory tests as indicated (Fig. 51–5). The history should include the duration of lymphadenopathy, which is characterized as acute or subacute and chronic; the presence and duration of any associated systemic symptoms or signs; exposure to animals or contact with persons infected with tuberculosis; travel history; preceding trauma; current medications, especially phenytoin; food and ingestion history, especially of undercooked meat or unpasteurized dairy products; medical and surgical history; and family history. A history of trauma or of other infections in the region drained by the involved nodes should be elicited. Findings in the history, physical examination, or epidemiologic characteristics that suggest a specific or uncommon diagnosis should prompt the performance of additional or more specific laboratory testing. Findings in the history, physical examination, or epidemiologic circumstances that suggest a specific cause of the lymphadenitis should prompt the performance of specific diagnostic tests early in the presentation.

Differential Diagnosis

The noninfectious causes of cervical lymphadenopathy are often associated with generalized lymphadenopathy. Congenital and acquired cysts, pilomatricomas that are believed to be hamartomas of hair follicle origin, and benign neoplasms (e.g., lipoma, neurofibroma, lymphangioma) account for the majority of noninflammatory neck lesions in children and adolescents.

A study (Knight et al, 1983) of 775 superficial lumps excised in children and adolescents less than 17 years of age found neoplasm in 11, or 1.4%. At the same institution, malignancy was found in 24 (13%) of 182 enlarged cervical nodes in children referred for excisional biopsy. Malignant lymph nodes are usually painless, not inflamed, and firm in consistency. Most malignant conditions that produce cervical lymphadenopathy are chronic in nature. Nodes located in the posterior triangle are more often due to malignancy than those located in the anterior triangle. The cause of malignant cervical nodes varies with the age of the child. During the first 6 years of life, neuroblastoma and leukemia are the most common causes. In children more than 6 years of age, Hodgkin's disease is the most common cause, followed by non-Hodgkin's lymphoma. Thyroid tumors are the third most frequent neck malignancy in the pediatric age group and, in contrast to the others, may present as an isolated cervical mass without associated systemic symptoms. Rhabdomyosarcoma, which is the most common solid tumor of the head and neck region in children 1–6 years of age, may present with enlarging cervical lymphadenopathy and chronic serosanguineous nasal discharge.

Histiocytic causes of cervical lymphadenopathy include **sinus histiocytosis** with massive lymphadenopathy and other histiocytoses. Sinus histiocytosis with massive lymphadenopathy is a benign form of histiocytosis of unknown origin, usually occurring in African Americans, that is associated with massive, painless lymphadenopathy, usually in the cervical area; however, other regions are also involved in three fourths of affected persons. Rarely, extranodal sites such as the orbit may be involved. Lymphadenopathy may persist for months or years and then gradually resolve.

Kawasaki syndrome, originally called mucocutaneous lymph node syndrome, has an inconsistent clinical finding of unilateral cervical lymphadenopathy in 50–82% of cases, typically larger than 1.5 cm in diameter. The enlarged node is firm, minimally tender, or red and nonsuppurative. It usually rapidly subsides at the time of defervescence, although some persons have had persistent cervical lymphadenopathy for more than 3 weeks (Chapter 39).

The **periodic fever, aphthous stomatitis, pharyngitis, cervical adenitis syndrome (PFAPA syndrome),** characterized by periodic fevers associated with aphthous stomatitis, pharyngitis, and cervical lymphadenitis, has been described. Symptoms are cyclic, occurring at 4–6 week intervals. The PFAPA syndrome persists for years, but complications have not been reported. Results of immunologic studies, including neutrophil function and number, are reported as normal, and cultures have been negative for bacteria and viruses. The cause of this syndrome is unknown. Systemic corticosteroids usually are helpful (Chapter 58).

At the initial examination there may be some uncertainty as to whether the mass actually represents an enlarged node. The most common neck masses of congenital origin are thyroglossal duct cyst, branchial cleft cyst, and cystic hygroma. Each has a character-

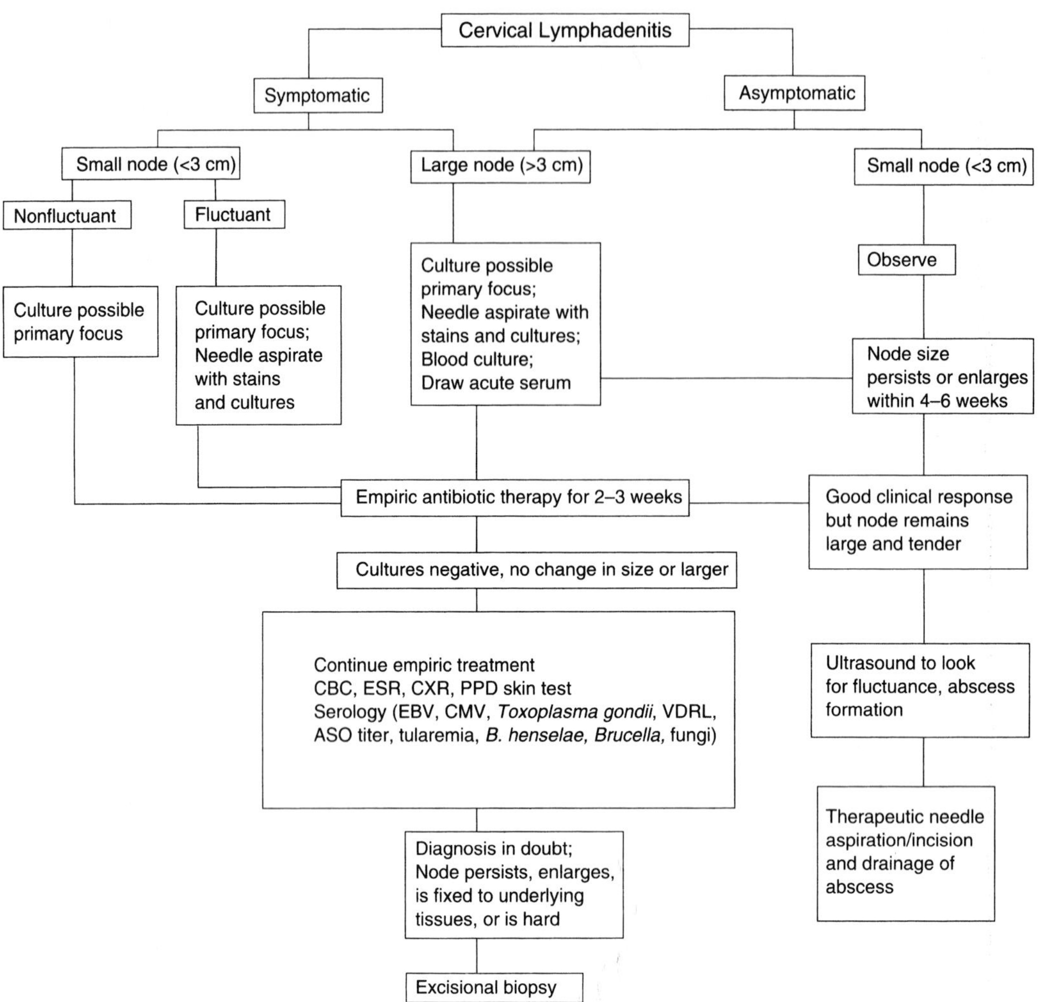

FIGURE 51–5. Diagnostic evaluation of a child with cervical lymphadenitis. ASO = anti-streptolysin titer; CXR = chest radiography; CBC = complete blood cell count; CMV = cytomegalovirus; EBV = Epstein-Barr virus; ESR = erythrocyte sedimentation rate; HIV = human immunodeficiency virus; PPD = purified protein derivative; VDRL = Venereal Disease Research Laboratories.

istic location. **Thyroglossal duct cysts** are the most common of the midline masses found in the neck and are usually located at the level of the hyoid in the midline or lateral to the midline. They retract with protrusion of the tongue or move with swallowing and may have an associated fistula. When these cysts become infected, they resemble suppurative nodes. Other midline masses include epidermoid cysts, lipomas, thyroid tumors, and the rare midline lymph node. **Branchial cleft cysts** are located at the anterior border of the sternocleidomastoid muscle. They usually arise from the second branchial cleft and manifest themselves as skin dimples. They, too, may become secondarily infected, leading to diagnostic confusion. A careful examination should detect a sinus tract. **Cystic hygromas,** considerably less common than thyroglossal duct or branchial cleft cysts, arise from the lymphatics and are most commonly found posterior to the sternocleidomastoid muscle in the supraclavicular fossa. Cystic hygromas compress, transilluminate, and enlarge with straining.

Hemangiomas are similar to cystic hygromas but have a red or bluish tinge. Sternocleidomastoid tumors are transient, hard, spindle-shaped fibromas found in the sternocleidomastoid muscle of young infants. These tumors may look and feel like adenitis of a deep jugular node. Other lesions to be considered include neurofibromas, which are often associated with café au lait spots, dermoid cysts, which are found in the midline and do not transilluminate, and teratomas, which may show calcifications on radiographs. Mumps sialadenitis and dental abscesses are often mistaken for massive enlargement of a tonsillar or submandibular node. Careful observation, serial examinations, and appropriate laboratory studies (e.g., a serum amylase test to rule out parotitis, dental films for periapical abscess) help to exclude these conditions. Biopsy is often required to determine the cause of tumors of the head and neck region.

Laboratory Evaluation

If the diagnosis remains uncertain and empirical therapy fails to elicit a response, findings in the history and physical examination should guide further diagnostic study, which may include CBC, ESR, chest roentgenogram, antistreptolysin O titer, and serologic tests for syphilis, toxoplasmosis, CMV and EBV infection, tularemia, *Brucella* infection, histoplasmosis, and coccidioidomycosis. Intradermal skin testing for tuberculosis should be performed with the standard (5 TU) Mantoux test. Skin test reactions of >10–15 mm strongly suggest infection with *M. tuberculosis,* whereas smaller reactions are more indicative of a nontuberculous mycobacterial infection. Intradermal testing with nontuberculous mycobacterial antigens is not commercially available.

Microbiologic Evaluation

Cultures of infected skin lesions and tonsillar exudates should also be performed, although isolation of group A *Streptococcus* from either of these foci does not confirm the cause of the streptococcal lymphadenitis. A blood culture specimen should be obtained from children with systemic signs and symptoms suggestive of bacteremia. A blood specimen from a person with a large cervical node can be held for acute-phase serologic titers if it is needed later.

Aspiration. Further evaluation is indicated for cervical lymph nodes >3 cm in diameter, fluctuant nodes, or nodes associated with moderate fever and systemic symptoms. If lymphoma is suspected, biopsy should be performed. An etiologic agent can be recovered by needle aspiration of the affected node in 60–88% of cases. Only inflamed nodes should be aspirated, but these need not be fluctuant. The procedure is safe and relatively easy to perform and, when properly performed, is not associated with serious complications. Concerns about the possible formation of a persistent draining skin sinus after aspiration of a node infected with mycobacteria are not a contraindication because this is uncommon and could be cured by excision once the diagnosis is established. The largest, most fluctuant node having the most direct access is the best target. The overlying skin should be cleansed and anesthetized. A sterile 18-gauge needle attached to a 10 mL syringe should be used to evacuate thickened pus if present. The node should be entered from an area of healthy skin. If no purulent material is obtained on aspiration, the syringe may be disconnected from the needle and replaced with another containing a small amount of nonbacteriostatic saline solution, which is injected into the node and then aspirated. After aspiration, the air should be evacuated from the syringe and needle, and the needle should immediately be capped. The specimen should be delivered to the microbiology laboratory promptly. Pus from fluctuant cervical nodes should be examined by Gram stain or acid-fast stain and cultured for aerobic and anaerobic bacteria and mycobacteria. *M. haemophilum* has specific culture requirements for optimal growth, including an iron- or blood-enriched medium and a low temperature. When specific culture requirements are not provided, the organism may not be identified. If the node remains enlarged and tender, ultrasonography can reveal the presence of pus reaccumulation, and the need for repeated aspiration or for incision and drainage.

Biopsy. If laboratory tests, skin tests, and aspiration fail to yield a diagnosis and the lymphadenopathy persists, enlarges, becomes fixed to underlying tissues, or becomes hard, an excisional biopsy should be performed. The entire node should be excised if possible because this approach is curative for nontuberculous mycobacterial infection. Biopsy material should be submitted for Gram, acid-fast, Giemsa, periodic acid–Schiff, Warthin-Starry silver (for cat-scratch disease), and methenamine silver stains. Cultures for aerobic and anaerobic bacteria, mycobacteria, and fungi should be performed.

Histopathologic assessment of all excised nodes should be performed. Examination of lymph nodes infected with a variety of mycobacterial species reveals a broad spectrum of possible inflammatory responses. Both acute and chronic inflammatory responses have been observed. Acute suppuration, nonnecrotic epithelioid tubercles, and caseation may occur alone or in combination in the same lymph node. These different pathologic features reflect the degree of immunologic reactivity or tissue hypersensitivity and the local concentration of antigen. Careful studies have failed to detect gross or microscopic abnormalities that might permit differentiation of one mycobacterial infection from another. Therefore, because initial pathology reports of excised tissue will indicate only the presence of acid-fast bacilli or granulomatous changes compatible with mycobacterial infection, a specific diagnosis will depend on culture results. Older children more frequently have negative results on culture of lymph node aspirates and therefore are more often candidates for excisional lymph node biopsy. These are also the persons more likely to have lymphomas. Thus it is important that the node be removed carefully, without disruption of the cellular characteristics.

TREATMENT

Most cases of cervical lymphadenitis in children require very little diagnostic study and no specific therapy. Persons with several nodes that are only slightly enlarged and minimally tender, in association with few inflammatory signs, require only observation. Most such lymph nodes usually regress within 2–3 weeks. Should one or more lymph nodes continue to enlarge, with increasing tenderness and signs of inflammation, the need for diagnostic evaluation before the start of therapy depends on the age of the person, the associated findings, the size and location of the nodes, and the severity of the acute systemic symptoms. Neonates with lymphadenitis require a complete sepsis evaluation in addition to needle aspiration of the involved nodes. Older infants and children with localized cervical lymphadenitis will often respond to empirical antibiotic therapy for *S. aureus* and group A *Streptococcus* with a decline in fever and symptoms; thus there is often no need for any evaluation beyond a careful history and physical examination to exclude other possible causes. This is especially true if the inflamed node is <3 cm in diameter and nonfluctuant and if systemic symptoms are absent or mild. The patient should be examined carefully for evidence of a primary focus such as pharyngitis, conjunctivitis, otitis media, skin infection, or dental abscess. If one of these conditions is found, appropriate microbiologic stains and cultures should be obtained and appropriate treatment given.

The specific treatment of cervical lymphadenopathy depends on the underlying cause. Because almost all cases in infants and children are associated with an infectious agent, therapy should be guided by Gram and acid-fast stains and, ultimately, by culture and antimicrobial susceptibility testing of aspirated material from the involved node. However, when a child has minimal systemic symptoms and findings typical of acute bacterial lymphadenitis, empirical antibiotic therapy is appropriate without the prior performance of a needle aspiration. Close follow-up is a necessity in this situation because the absence of a clinical response within 36–48 hours of the start of therapy is an indication for this diagnostic procedure.

The most common etiologic agents of acute suppurative cervical lymphadenitis are *S. aureus* and group A *Streptococcus,* and empirical treatment should include antibiotics with activity against both of these organisms. Parenteral therapy is beneficial in persons who have marked lymph node enlargement, moderate to severe systemic symptoms, and associated cellulitis. Oxacillin, 150–200 mg/kg/day, or nafcillin, 150 mg/kg/day, is recommended, or, especially for persons with hypersensitivity to penicillins, cefazolin, 100 mg/kg/day. For persons with hypersensitivity to β-lactams, vancomycin, 40 mg/kg/day, is appropriate. Clindamycin, 30 mg/kg/day, for parenteral or oral use has good antistaphylococcal activity and good anaerobic coverage. Treatment of cervical lymphadenitis associated with dental infections should include an antibiotic regimen with good anaerobic coverage (Chapter 61).

For bacteriologically proved group A *Streptococcus* lymphadenitis, penicillin G, 50,000 U/kg/day, or penicillin V, 50 mg/kg/day, is recommended. Erythromycin ethyl succinate, 40 mg/kg/day, or cephalexin, 25–50 mg/kg/day, is appropriate for children with hypersensitivity to penicillins. The average duration of therapy is 10 days unless abscess formation occurs. In this situation, incision and drainage are indicated, and antibiotics should be administered for 5–7 days after resolution of the acute process.

Clinical improvement evidenced by a decline in fever and other systemic symptoms, together with a decrease in inflammation and tenderness of the involved node, should be observed within 36–48 hours of the start of therapy. If such a response does not occur, needle aspiration should be performed. The size of the involved nodes may not change for many days, with regression often requiring 4–6 weeks. On initial presentation and at subsequent follow-up visits, careful measurements should be taken and recorded to allow for objective evidence of lymph node evolution during therapy. Once signs of acute inflammation have resolved, continued antimicrobial therapy is of little value because penetration of antibiotics through the fibrous capsule of the node is poor. Persistence of significant enlargement beyond 6–8 weeks indicates the need for further diagnostic evaluation and consideration of excisional biopsy.

If a Gram stain of the lymph node aspirate suggests an organism other than *S. aureus* or group A *Streptococcus,* treatment should be directed at the most likely etiologic organism until culture results are known. Final bacteriologic identification and antimicrobial susceptibility tests should guide the ultimate antimicrobial therapy for unusual infections such as cat-scratch disease (Chapter 28), tularemia (Chapter 34), plague (Chapter 34), and rat-bite fever (Chapter 50).

Cervical lymphadenitis caused by some nontuberculous mycobacteria may respond to antituberculosis drugs, but the treatment of choice is surgical excision (Table 51–5). To direct chemotherapy, one must determine the nontuberculous *Mycobacterium* species causing infection (Table 51–5). Specific species, including *M. kansasii, M. marinum, M. xenopi, M. gordonae, M. malmoense,* and *M. szulgai,* and some strains of the *M. avium* complex and *M. haemophilum,* are susceptible to some antituberculosis drugs. Treatment of the rapidly growing mycobacteria and of most strains of the *M. avium* complex requires other antibiotics. Multiple drug therapy is used for essentially all infections other than some *M. marinum* skin infections because of the propensity of mycobacteria to develop resistance to single drugs. When chemotherapy is being considered, it is essential that adequate drug susceptibility information be obtained from a qualified laboratory. Drug susceptibility testing should be performed on all isolates believed to be clinically significant. Most experts recommend total removal of all visibly infected nodes, deep as well as superficial. When this is impossible or when it would result in considerable cosmetic problems, thorough curettage has been found to be effective in selected patients, and a few patients have been reported to respond to antibiotic therapy. Surgical excision remains an important element of therapy.

The treatment of cervical lymphadenitis caused by *M. haemophilum* should also be surgical removal. In persons with perihilar nodes caused by this organism, full excision may not be possible, so long-term chemotherapy based on in vitro susceptibility testing may be used.

Recommended therapy for lymphadenitis caused by *M. tuberculosis* is the same as that for pulmonary disease caused by this organism (Chapter 35). Response to antituberculosis therapy is typical, with marked regression of lymph nodes being evident within 3 months. However, nodes may remain palpable for months because of the fibrous scarring that occurs as part of the healing process. Surgery is indicated only for diagnostic purposes; draining sinuses that may occur spontaneously or as a result of incision and drainage resolve readily with medical treatment.

TABLE 51–5. Agents Most Commonly Used for Nontuberculous Mycobacterial Infections

Organism	Drug
Mycobacterium avium complex (disseminated)	Amikacin, ciprofloxacin, clarithromycin, azithromycin, clofazimine, ethambutol, rifampin, rifabutin
M. kansasii	Ethambutol, isoniazid, rifampin, streptomycin
M. marinum	Doxycycline, ethambutol, rifampin, TMP-SMZ
M. fortuitum, *M. chelonae,* *M. abscessus*	Amikacin, cefoxitin, ciprofloxacin, erythromycin, TMP-SMZ, clarithromycin, azithromycin

COMPLICATIONS AND PROGNOSIS

The majority of acute infections caused by *S. aureus* and group A *Streptococcus* respond to treatment with a minimal likelihood of complications. Most of the other uncommon bacterial causes have an excellent prognosis with specific treatment. Delay in diagnosis and treatment can obviously prolong the clinical course and may even result in complications or sequelae such as abscess formation, cellulitis, and bacteremia. Except for abscess formation, these complications are rare. The complication of abscess formation can be readily cured with incision and drainage in conjunction with appropriate antimicrobials.

Subacute and chronic cervical lymphadenitis caused by nontuberculous mycobacteria has an excellent prognosis. With prompt surgical excision of cervical lymphadenitis caused by nontuberculous mycobacteria, cure can be expected in approximately 97% of cases. Infection with *M. tuberculosis* also has an excellent prognosis with treatment of antituberculosis drugs.

PREVENTION

Appropriate treatment of predisposing conditions, such as dental disease, streptococcal pharyngitis, otitis media, impetigo, and other infections involving the face and scalp, should decrease the incidence of pyogenic cervical lymphadenitis. The incidence of subacute lymphadenitis caused by *M. tuberculosis* should be decreased by minimizing exposure of infants and children to active tuberculosis. In addition, avoidance of cat feces can help prevent acquired toxoplasmosis.

LYMPHANGITIS

Lymphangitis is an inflammation of the lymphatic channels, usually in the subcutaneous tissues. It occurs either as an acute process of bacterial origin or as a chronic process of fungal, mycobacterial, or filarial origin.

ETIOLOGY

Acute lymphangitis develops when an infection, commonly on an extremity, rapidly spreads along lymphatic channels and is most often caused by group A *Streptococcus.* **Chronic granulomatous lymphangitis** is an indolent process in which infection, frequently introduced by minor trauma to the skin or subcutaneous tissues, extends proximally along the course of regional lymphatics, slowly producing multiple subcutaneous nodules. The fungus *Sporothrix schenckii* is the most common cause of chronic lymphangitis in the United States. Other infectious agents occasionally producing chronic lymphangitis in this country include *M. marinum, Nocardia brasiliensis,* and rarely *M. kansasii* and *Nocardia asteroides.* Rare filarial causes that are seen only in immigrants from endemic areas include *Wuchereria bancrofti* and *Brugia malayi.*

EPIDEMIOLOGY

Streptococcal lymphangitis may occur in areas of tissue damage due to trauma, operative wounds, or stasis ulceration. This may or may not be associated with frank cellulitis. Although group A *Streptococcus* is frequently a normal inhabitant of the skin, these organisms can be transmitted by person-to-person spread.

Chronic lymphangitis due to *S. schenckii* most often arises as a result of contact with thorny plants, such as roses or sphagnum moss, that implant the dimorphic fungus in the subcutaneous tissues of the host. Most patients with this disease are previously healthy adults <30 years old with occupations involving exposure to plant products.

M. marinum, an atypical mycobacterium that grows best at 25–32°C and is found in swimming pools and aquariums, may cause cutaneous disease in persons who have had contact with these sources.

PATHOGENESIS

A break in skin integrity may allow invasion of pathogenic organisms into the subcutaneous tissues and hence into the lymphatics. When such an infection is not contained locally but spreads along lymphatic channels, lymphangitis results. Group A *Streptococcus* is the most common cause of acute lymphangitis. These organisms possess many virulent properties, such as the ability to release toxic and digestive enzymes that allow them to spread rapidly up the lymphatic vessels, inducing a pyogenic inflammatory process. Chronic lymphangitis results from the inoculation of less virulent organisms into the skin, such as *S. schenckii,* which produce granulomatous inflammation.

SYMPTOMS AND CLINICAL MANIFESTATIONS

Acute lymphangitis is rapidly progressive, often with systemic manifestations. It is characterized by the appearance of red linear streaks extending from the initial site of infection to the draining regional lymph nodes, which are often enlarged and tender. Systemic symptoms, including chills, fever, malaise, and headache, are prominent, and the process may be accompanied by bacteremia. Peripheral edema of the involved extremity often occurs. The time from initial lesion to lymphangitis to complicating bacteremia may be as little as 24–48 hours.

Unlike acute lymphangitis, chronic granulomatous lymphangitis is an indolent process associated with little pain or systemic symptoms. Sporotrichosis is most commonly the underlying disease. Cutaneous sporotrichosis begins at the site of inoculation, where a small, red, painless papule arises, enlarges slowly, becomes violaceous, and intermittently discharges a small amount of serosanguineous exudate. During the next several weeks, similar nodules form proximally along the lymphatic channel. Ulceration may occur. Despite infection of the lymphatics, the lymph nodes are frequently not infected. Isolation of *S. schenckii* from nodes is uncommon. Fortunately this infection most often remains confined to the subcutaneous tissues and, when untreated, may wax and wane for several months or years. The proximal extension of these lesions, often with skip areas, is distinctive but may be mimicked by lesions of *M. marinum, N. brasiliensis,* or, rarely, *M. kansasii* or *N. asteroides.*

Less common manifestations of infection with *S. schenckii* involve extracutaneous sites. Ocular sporotrichosis results from traumatic inoculation of the conjunctiva or cornea. Osteoarticular sporotrichosis, which comprises about 80% of the extracutaneous cases, produces an indolent arthritis, usually without signs of cutaneous disease or other organ involvement. Pulmonary sporotrichosis is rare and usually presents as a single chronic cavitary lesion in an upper lobe.

DIAGNOSIS

The combination of a peripheral infection or traumatic lesion and the acute onset of fever with a proximal red linear streak directed toward regional lymph nodes is clinically diagnostic of acute lymphangitis. Thrombophlebitis may produce linear areas of tender erythema, but the absence of an initiating lesion and of tender regional nodes is helpful in distinguishing it from lymphangitis. The etiologic agent often can be identified on Gram-stained smears and cultures of specimens obtained from the initial lesion. Blood cultures are often positive for group A *Streptococcus.*

Sporotrichosis is considered when chronic lymphangitis presents in combination with a history of the patient's working among plants, timbers, or soil. Culture of pus or of a skin biopsy specimen is the preferred method of diagnosis. Identification by histopathologic section is less precise because of variability in the shape and size of yeastlike cells.

If sporotrichoid *M. marinum* infection is suspected, the diagnosis should be confirmed by demonstration of acid-fast bacilli and by culture of the organism at 30°C on an appropriate medium.

TREATMENT

Penicillin is the treatment of choice of acute lymphangitis. In a mildly ill patient, therapy with penicillin V may be instituted. For more severe disease, penicillin G should be given intravenously. For persons with hypersensitivity to penicillins, a first-generation cephalosporin should be used. For persons with hypersensitivity to β-lactams, clindamycin or a macrolide can be used.

The treatment of choice for localized cutaneous or lymphocutaneous sporotrichosis is oral itraconazole (Chapter 46). Alternative treatments include saturated solution of potassium iodide and **hyperthermic treatment** in the form of hot baths (45°C), hot compresses, or a hand-held heating device applied 40–60 minutes per day.

Localized sporotrichoid lesions caused by *M. marinum* may be treated by surgical excision. Chemotherapy is reserved for the more extensive infections due to this organism (Table 51–5). Specific antimicrobial therapy should be chosen on the basis of susceptibility data because this species is often resistant to the most commonly used antimycobacterial drugs.

COMPLICATIONS

Complications of acute lymphangitis include group A *Streptococcus* bacteremia, and hematogenously disseminated infection. In persons with conditions that predispose them to repeated episodes of lymphangitis, such as lower extremity edema and stasis ulceration, especially if associated at times with congestive heart failure, lymphatic obstruction often occurs on healing and results in persistent lymphedema.

PROGNOSIS

Acute lymphangitis responds rapidly to antibiotic therapy. There are no sequelae if infection remains localized to the lymphatics.

Cutaneous sporotrichosis responds well to therapy, and the prognosis is good. Extracutaneous sporotrichosis is more difficult to eradicate and necessitates the use of systemic antifungal treatment.

The prognosis of sporotrichoid lesions caused by *M. marinum* is good because most of these infections are localized and can be cured with local excision.

PREVENTION

The prevention of acute lymphangitis involves the prompt and vigorous treatment of predisposing skin conditions. Prompt diagnosis and the rapid institution of specific antimicrobials can reduce the potential complications associated with bacteremia. Wearing protective skin covering when in contact with mulch, hay, timbers, and other plant products can reduce the risk for sporotrichosis.

REVIEWS

Bedros AA, Mann JP: Lymphadenopathy in children. *Adv Pediatr* 1981; 28:341–76.

Kelly CS, Kelly RE Jr: Lymphadenopathy in children. *Pediatr Clin North Am* 1998;45:875–88.

Lake AM, Oski FA: Peripheral lymphadenopathy in childhood. Ten-year experience with excisional biopsy. *Am J Dis Child* 1978;132:357–9.

Scobie WG: Acute suppurative adenitis in children: A review of 964 cases. *Scot Med J* 1969;14:352–4.

Sisson BA, Glick L: Genital ulceration as a presenting manifestation of infectious mononucleosis. *J Pediatr Adolesc Gynecol* 1998;11:185–7.

Zuelzer WW, Kaplan J: The child with lymphadenopathy. *Semin Hematol* 1975;12:323–34.

Generalized Lymphadenopathy

Arisoy ES, Correa AG, Wagner ML, et al: Hepatosplenic cat-scratch disease in children: Selected clinical features and treatment. *Clin Infect Dis* 1999;28:778–84.

Canale VC, Smith CH: Chronic lymphadenopathy simulating malignant lymphoma. *J Pediatr* 1967;70:891–9.

Enderlin G, Morales L, Jacobs RF, et al: Streptomycin and alternative agents for the treatment of tularemia: Review of the literature. *Clin Infect Dis* 1994;19:42–7.

Jacobs RF: Tularemia. *Adv Pediatr Infect Dis* 1996;12:55–69.

Jacobs RF, Condrey YM, Yamauchi T: Tularemia in adults and children: A changing presentation. *Pediatrics* 1985;76:818–22.

Kendig EL Jr: The clinical picture of sarcoidosis in children. *Pediatrics* 1974;54:289–92.

Knight PJ, Mulne AF, Vassy LE: When is lymph node biopsy indicated in children with enlarged peripheral nodes? *Pediatrics* 1982;69:391–6.

Knight PJ, Reiner CB: Superficial lumps in children: What, when, and why? *Pediatrics* 1983;72:147–53.

Inguinal Lymphadenopathy and Lymphadenitis

Akers WA: Tender inguinal lymph nodes and gonococcal urethritis. *Milit Med* 1972;137:107–8.

Corey L, Adams HG, Brown ZA, et al: Genital herpes simplex virus infections: Clinical manifestations, course and complications. *Ann Intern Med* 1983;98:958–72.

D'Costa LJ, Bowmer I, Nsanze H, et al: Advances in the diagnosis and management of chancroid. *Sex Transm Dis* 1986;3:189–91.

Drusin LM: Syphilis: Clinical manifestations, diagnosis and treatment. *Urol Clin North Am* 1984;11:121–30.

Goens JL, Schwartz RA, De Wolf K: Mucocutaneous manifestations of chancroid, lymphogranuloma venereum and granuloma inguinale. *Am Fam Physician* 1994;49:415–8, 423–5.

Hart G: *Chancroid, Donovanosis, Lymphogranuloma venereum.* Atlanta, U.S. Department of Health, Education, and Welfare, 1974.

Kaufman AF, Boyce JM, Martone WJ: From the Centers for Disease Control. Trends in human plague in the United States. *J Infect Dis* 1980;141:522–4.

Maull KI, Sachatello CR: Retroperitoneal iliac fossa abscess. A complication of suppurative iliac lymphadenitis. *Am J Surg* 1974;127:270–4.

Thorsteinsson SB: Lymphogranuloma venereum: Review of clinical manifestations, epidemiology, diagnosis and treatment. *Scand J Infect Dis* 1982;32:127–31.

Cervical Lymphadenopathy and Lymphadenitis

Baker CJ: Group B streptococcal cellulitis-adenitis in infants. *Am J Dis Child* 1982;136:631–3.

Barton LL, Feigin RD: Childhood cervical lymphadenitis: A reappraisal. *J Pediatr* 1974;84:846–52.

Benson-Mitchell R, Buchanan G: Cervical lymphadenopathy secondary to atypical mycobacteria in children. *J Laryngol Otol* 1996;110:48–51.

Brook I: Aerobic and anaerobic bacteriology of cervical adenitis in children. *Clin Pediatr (Phila)* 1980;19:693–6.

Feder HM Jr, Bialecki CA: Periodic fever associated with aphthous stomatitis, pharyngitis and cervical adenitis. *Pediatr Infect Dis J* 1989;8:186–7.

Hazra R, Robson CD, Perez-Atayde AR, et al: Lymphadenitis due to nontuberculous mycobacteria in children: Presentation and response to therapy. *Clin Infect Dis* 1999;28:123–9.

Knight PJ, Mulne AF, Vassy LE: When is lymph node biopsy indicated in children with enlarged peripheral nodes? *Pediatrics* 1982;69:391–6.

Knight PJ, Reiner CB: Superficial lumps in children: What, when, and why? *Pediatrics* 1983;72:147–53.

Lai KK, Stottmeier KD, Sherman IH, et al: Mycobacterial cervical lymphadenopathy: Relation of etiologic agents to age. *JAMA* 1984;251:1286–8.

Lampe RM, Baker CJ, Septimus EJ, et al: Cervicofacial nocardiosis in children. *J Pediatr* 1981;99:593–5.

Marcy SM: Infections of lymph nodes of the head and neck. *Pediatr Infect Dis* 1983;2:397–405.

Margileth AM, Chandra R, Altman RP: Chronic lymphadenopathy due to mycobacterial infection: Clinical features, diagnosis, histopathology and management. *Am J Dis Child* 1984;138:917–22.

Peters TR, Edwards KM: Cervical lymphadenopathy and adenitis. *Pediatr Rev* 2000;21:339–405.

Powell KE, Meador MP, Farer LS: Recent trends in tuberculosis in children. *JAMA* 1984;251:1289–92.

Ramadan HH, Wax MK, Boyd CB: Fine-needle aspiration of head and neck masses in children. *Am J Otolaryngol* 1997;18:400–4.

Rosai J, Dorfman RF: Sinus histiocytosis with massive lymphadenopathy: A pseudolymphomatous benign disorder. Analysis of 34 cases. *Cancer* 1972;30:1174–88.

Schaad UB, Votteler TP, McCracken GH Jr, et al: Management of atypical mycobacterial lymphadenitis in childhood: A review based on 380 cases. *J Pediatr* 1979;95:356–60.

Thomaidis T, Anastassea-Vlachou K, Mandalenaki-Lambrou C, et al: Chronic lymphoglandular enlargement and toxoplasmosis in children. *Arch Dis Child* 1977;52:403–7.

Ying M, Ahuja A, Metreweli C: Diagnostic accuracy of sonographic criteria for evaluation of cervical lymphadenopathy. *J Ultrasound Med* 1998; 17:437–45.

Lymphangitis

Craliana J, Conti-Diaz IA: Healing effects of heat and rubefacient on nine cases of sporotrichosis. *Sabouraudia* 1963;3:64.

Crout JE, Brewer NS, Tompkins RB: Sporotrichosis arthritis: Clinical features in seven patients. *Ann Intern Med* 1977;86:294–7.

Duran RJ, Coventry MB, Weed LA, et al: Sporotrichosis: A report of twenty-three cases in the upper extremity. *J Bone Joint Surg* 1957;39(A):1330.

Kauffman CA: Sporotrichosis. *Clin Infect Dis* 1999;29:231–7.

Orr ER, Riley HD Jr: Sporotrichosis in childhood: Report of ten cases. *J Pediatr* 1971;78:951–7.

Pluss JL, Opal SM: Pulmonary sporotrichosis: Review of treatment and outcome. *Medicine* (*Baltimore*) 1986;65:143–53.

Restrepo A, Robledo J, Gomez I, et al: Itraconazole therapy in lymphangitic and cutaneous sporotrichosis. *Arch Dermatol* 1986;122:413–7.

Sanders WJ, Wolinsky E: In vitro susceptibility of *Mycobacterium marinum* to eight antimicrobial agents. *Antimicrob Agents Chemother* 1980; 18:529–31.

CHAPTER 52

Meningitis

Ram Yogev

Meningitis can be classified on the basis of the duration of symptoms before the disease is recognized (acute, subacute, and chronic) or by the causative organism (bacterial, viral, fungal). A wide variety of microorganisms can cause infection of the meninges. Most bacteria cause an acute onset of signs and symptoms, but some bacteria cause a slower onset (subacute) and still fewer bacteria cause a very gradual onset of symptoms (chronic).

Viral infection of the meninges, usually referred to as **aseptic meningitis,** is the most common cause of meningitis and commonly presents with a less acute onset of signs and symptoms than does bacterial infection. However, with better culture techniques it has become clear that the term *aseptic* is not synonymous with *viral* because other etiologic agents, such as *Mycobacterium tuberculosis, Borrelia burgdorferi, Mycoplasma,* and fungi, can cause moderate CSF pleocytosis in which no bacteria grow on routine culture. In addition, autoimmune diseases and malignant neoplasms can present as aseptic meningitis. Thus the term *aseptic* should be used with caution and then only to suggest that bacteria of common causes were not isolated from the CSF.

If the duration of symptoms is longer than 1 week, the term **subacute meningitis** is used. Subacute meningitis is usually caused by slow-growing bacteria such as *M. tuberculosis* or by fungi such as *Cryptococcus neoformans.* If the duration of symptoms is several months or longer, the term **chronic meningitis** is used. Syphilitic and coccidioidal meningitides represent such infections. The meningitis syndrome can occur with many other entities, such as posttraumatic meningitis, eosinophilic meningitis, Mollaret's meningitis, and CNS shunt infections.

ETIOLOGY

Bacterial Meningitis. Virtually any organism can cause meningitis, but a relatively small number of organisms cause most cases (Table 52–1). A variety of predisposing factors, such as age, race, immune status, and specific environmental conditions, contribute to increased susceptibility to a given organism. The most common organisms causing meningitis are *Streptococcus pneumoniae* and *Neisseria meningitidis.* After the introduction of *Haemophilus influenzae* type b conjugate vaccine in 1988, there was a greater than 99% decline in invasive disease caused by *H. influenzae* type b, including meningitis. Thus by 1995 the overall incidence of bacterial meningitis declined by 87% in children 1 month to 5 years of age. In children less than 2 years of age, *S. pneumoniae* is the etiologic agent in almost half of the cases, and *N. meningitidis* is the cause of almost one third. In children older than 2 years, *N. meningitidis* is responsible for more than 60% of the cases, and *S. pneumoniae* is the cause of only 30%. *N. meningitidis* invasive disease is more common in young children than in adults, with an attack rate that is 16-fold higher, or 8 cases per 100,000 children. The most common isolate is *N. meningitidis* serogroup C, which causes 45% of the cases. A small number of cases of *H. influenzae* type b meningitis occur, mainly in young children who did not receive at least two doses of the conjugate vaccine.

Several risk factors predispose persons to bacterial meningitis (Table 52–2). Persons with IgG or complement deficiencies and congenital or functional asplenia have an increased risk of meningitis from *S. pneumoniae* or *H. influenzae* type b regardless of their age. Certain environmental situations such as household or dormitory contact increase the incidence of *N. meningitidis* infection. In contrast, coagulase-negative staphylococci and *Staphylococcus aureus* are the most common causes of meningitis associated with CNS shunts. *S. pneumoniae* and group A *Streptococcus* are the most common causes of posttraumatic meningitis. Communication between the skin and the subarachnoid space, which occurs in congenital midline defects of the skull or lumbosacral area, predispose children to *S. aureus* or *Escherichia coli* meningitis.

Neonatal Meningitis. Group B *Streptococcus, E. coli,* and *Listeria monocytogenes* are the most common causes of bacterial meningitis in infants younger than 1 month. Other gram-negative bacilli, such as *Enterobacter, Klebsiella,* and *Pseudomonas,* can be acquired nosocomially; they cause severe meningitis, with a mortality of

TABLE 52–1. Bacterial Causes of Meningitis

Age	Common	Uncommon	Rare
0–2 mo	Group B *Streptococcus* *Escherichia coli* *Listeria monocytogenes* *Klebsiella* *Enterobacter*	*Staphylococcus aureus* Coagulase-negative staphylococci *Salmonella* *Pseudomonas aeruginosa*	*Streptococcus pneumoniae* Group A *Streptococcus* *Citrobacter diversus* *Haemophilus influenzae* types a through f and nontypeable *Enterococcus faecalis*
≥2 mo	*S. pneumoniae* *Neisseria meningitidis*	Group A *Streptococcus* Gram-negative bacilli	*L. monocytogenes* *S. aureus* *H. influenzae* type b

almost 50%. Meningitis due to *Citrobacter diversus* and *Citrobacter freundii,* which may occur as sporadic cases or an epidemic, is commonly associated with multiple brain abscesses. *S. aureus* and coagulase-negative staphylococci are also important causes of nosocomial infections in newborns, especially premature newborns.

Viral Meningitis. Acute viral meningitis is common, although in most patients the specific viral agent is not identified. Many viruses cause acute meningitis, but only a few are responsible for most cases (Table 52–3). From 70% to 85% of all acute viral meningitides are caused by enteroviruses, especially coxsackieviruses, with most of the cases occurring in young children. Transmission is from person to person by the fecal-oral and possibly the respiratory routes. From 5% to 7% of acute viral meningitides are caused by arboviruses, which are transmitted by various arthropod vectors. St. Louis encephalitis virus is the most common cause of arboviral meningitis. Adenovirus is an uncommon cause of meningitis, but the symptoms and signs are usually more severe than those of enteroviral meningitis. HSV-2 rarely causes meningitis during or soon after genital infection. Mumps meningitis, although rare in developed countries, is common in regions where the vaccine is not available. HIV is rarely associated with meningitis.

Aseptic Meningitis. In addition to viral causes, many other disorders can cause signs and symptoms of acute meningitis, with the CSF showing moderate pleocytosis containing lymphocytes primarily. These disorders are grouped as ''aseptic meningitis'' syndrome (Table 52–4). Early bacterial infections and partially treated

TABLE 52–2. Risk Factors for Bacterial Meningitis

Predisposing Factor	Common	Uncommon
IgG deficiency	*Streptococcus pneumoniae* *Haemophilus influenzae* type b	*Neisseria meningitidis* *Staphylococcus*
Complement deficiency	*N. meningitidis* *S. pneumoniae*	*H. influenzae* type b
Congenital or functional asplenia	*S. pneumoniae* *Salmonella*	*H. influenzae* type b
Household or daycare center contact	*N. meningitidis* *S. pneumoniae*	*Staphylococcus aureus* *Escherichia coli*
Head injury	Group A *Streptococcus* *N. meningitidis*	*Klebsiella pneumoniae* *H. influenzae* *E. coli*
Central nervous system shunt	Coagulase-negative staphylococci *S. aureus*	*Pseudomonas aeruginosa* *Propionibacterium acnes*
Dermal fistula	*S. aureus* *E. coli*	

TABLE 52–3. Viral Causes of Meningitis

Virus	Common	Uncommon	Rare
Enteroviruses*	+		
Arboviruses	+		
Adenovirus		+	
Herpes simplex virus type 2		+	
Mumps		+	
Human immunodeficiency virus		+	
Herpes simplex virus type 1			+
Varicella-zoster virus			+
Influenza			+
Parainfluenza			+
Epstein-Barr virus			+
Measles			+
Cytomegalovirus			+
Lymphocytic choriomeningitis			+
Rotavirus			+

*Cause 70–85% of all known cases of acute viral meningitis.

TABLE 52–4. Causes of Aseptic Meningitis

Duration of Symptoms	Cause	Frequency	
		Common	Uncommon
Acute (days)	Viral	+	
	Partially treated bacterial meningitis	+	
	Parameningeal infections	+	
	Early bacterial meningitis		+
	Brucella		+
	Mycoplasma		+
	Rocky Mountain spotted fever		+
	Kawasaki syndrome		+
	Chemical		+
	Intracranial hemorrhage		+
	Neurosurgical procedure		+
	Drugs		+
	Eosinophilic meningitis		+
	Mollaret's meningitis		+
	Naegleria fowleri (primary amebic meningoencephalitis)		+
Subacute (wk)	Tuberculosis	+	
	Lyme disease	+	
	Malignant neoplasia	+	
	Mycoplasma		+
	Leptospirosis		+
	Cat-scratch disease		+
	Candida		+
	Cryptococcosis		+
	Toxoplasma gondii		+
	Acanthamoeba (granulomatous encephalitis)		+
	Behçet's syndrome		+
	Heavy-metal poisoning		+
	Autoimmune diseases		+
	Sarcoidosis		+
Chronic (mo)	Tuberculosis	+	
	Neurosyphilis	+	
	Brucella		+
	Cryptococcosis		+
	Coccidioidomycosis		+
	Candida		+
	Paracoccidioidomycosis		+
	Histoplasmosis		+
	Autoimmune disease		+

meningitis should always be considered and excluded, because a delay in providing therapy may affect the outcome severely. Unrecognized early bacterial infection can occur in neonates infected with group B *Streptococcus* and *L. monocytogenes* and in children infected with *S. pneumoniae.* At presentation, persons who receive oral antibiotics may have a longer duration of symptoms and CSF findings indistinguishable from those of viral meningitis. The clinical findings, age, and some laboratory findings may be helpful in differentiating these patients from those with aseptic meningitis due to other infectious agents.

Parameningeal infections such as vertebral osteomyelitis, ethmoid or sphenoid sinusitis, epidural or subdural abscess, venous sinus thrombosis, and mastoiditis can cause meningeal irritation simulating aseptic meningitis. Tuberculous meningitis can also be seen as aseptic meningitis at presentation; early recognition of this disease will prevent severe neurologic sequelae. *Mycoplasma pneumoniae* rarely causes aseptic meningitis after respiratory infection with this organism. In newborns, other members of the Mycoplasmataceae family, such as *Ureaplasma urealyticum* and *Mycoplasma hominis,* rarely cause aseptic meningitis. *Brucella, Borrelia burgdorferi* (Lyme disease), *Borrelia recurrentis* (relapsing fever), *Bartonella henselae* (cat-scratch disease), and *Leptospira* may invade the meninges to cause aseptic meningitis. Infection due to rickettsiae such as *Rickettsia rickettsii* (Rocky Mountain spotted fever) commonly presents with meningitis. The rash that accompanies these cases of meningitis serves as an important diagnostic clue. Irritation of the meninges by injection of various materials, such as myelography, antibiotics, and anticancer medications, or by neurosurgical procedures, especially subtentorial operations, can cause aseptic meningitis. Certain drugs, such as azathioprine, nonsteroidal anti-inflammatory agents, and carbamazepine, and certain antibiotics, such as sulfa-containing compounds, are rarely associated with acute aseptic meningitis. Kawasaki syndrome rarely causes aseptic meningitis, usually as a minor component of the other manifestations.

Eosinophilic Meningitis. Eosinophilic meningitis is a rare form of acute meningitis and is usually caused by invasion of the meninges by parasites (Table 52–5). *Angiostrongylus cantonensis,* the rat lungworm, is a common cause in Southeast Asia. In the United States, eosinophilic meningitis is rare; when it occurs, malignant neoplasia and tuberculous meningitis should be considered before the exotic parasites.

TABLE 52–5. Etiologic Agents Associated with Eosinophilic Meningitis

Type	Agent
Parasites	*Angiostrongylus cantonensis*
	Taenia solium
	Paragonimus westermani
	Echinococcus
	Schistosoma
	Trichinella spiralis
	Toxocara canis
	Toxoplasma gondii
Bacterial	*Treponema pallidum*
	Mycobacterium tuberculosis
Viral	Lymphocytic choriomeningitis virus
	Rabies vaccination
Fungal	Coccidioidomycosis
Drugs	Ibuprofen
Malignant neoplasia	Lymphoma
Other	Foreign bodies
	Hypereosinophilic syndrome
	Demyelinating diseases

TABLE 52–6. Causes of Recurrent Meningitis

- Mollaret's meningitis
- Head trauma
- Congenital anatomic defect
  - Cribriform plate defect
  - Epidermoid cyst
  - Dermal fistula
  - Meningomyelocele
- Immunodeficiency
  - Human immunodeficiency virus
  - Hypogammaglobulinemia
  - Complement deficiency
  - Leukemia, lymphoma
  - Drug induced
  - Ibuprofen
  - Sulfa
  - Quinolones

Recurrent Meningitis. There are many causes of recurrent meningitis (Table 52–6). **Mollaret's meningitis** is a rare form of acute meningitis characterized by recurrent benign episodes of meningeal signs and symptoms. The CSF findings resemble viral meningitis, but the CSF contains endothelial-like cells known as **Mollaret cells.** HSV-1 and EBV have been implicated as the etiologic agents. Each episode of meningitis resolves spontaneously within several days. Skull fractures and congenital anatomic defects are the most common causes. Radioisotope studies and exploratory surgery are helpful in detecting these causes. If meningococci are recovered during recurrent episodes, serum complement or IgG deficiency should be considered. Drug-induced recurrent meningitis may occur with the use of antibiotics (e.g., penicillin, ciprofloxacin, sulfa-containing drugs, isoniazid), nonsteroidal anti-inflammatory drugs (e.g., ibuprofen), and intravenous immunoglobulin.

Primary Amebic Meningoencephalitis. Amebic meningitis is a rare cause of acute meningitis. *Naegleria fowleri* is the principal pathogen of acute and usually fatal **primary amebic meningoencephalitis (PAM).** Other amebic causes include *Acanthamoeba, Balamuthia mandrillaris,* and *Leptomyxa. Acanthamoeba* and *Leptomyxa* also cause **granulomatous amebic encephalitis,** which is also usually fatal.

N. fowleri has been recovered from water reservoirs and soil in temperate areas. Typically, patients with PAM will have a history of swimming in freshwater reservoirs 1–2 weeks before the onset of the disease. The clinical presentation of PAM is indistinguishable from that of other causes of acute meningitis. High fever, photophobia, headache, and vomiting accompanied by abnormal smell and taste sensations will progress to irritability, confusion, stupor, and coma within several days. The disease rarely presents itself subacutely with a low-grade fever, headache, and focal signs that imitate a brain abscess or a tumor. CSF examination is not helpful in the differential diagnosis unless PAM is suspected and a warm specimen of CSF is carefully examined for moving amebas. The CSF shows predominance of neutrophils in acute cases, but predominance of mononuclear cells is seen in subacute cases. Because PAM is rare, most cases are diagnosed only post mortem.

Subacute Meningitis. The most common cause of subacute meningitis is tuberculosis. Although it can present as an acute episode, most patients have a more indolent course of nonspecific symptoms such as anorexia, nausea, vomiting, and behavior changes. *M. tuberculosis* is by far the major cause of tuberculous meningitis, but rarely *Mycobacterium bovis* and, in immunocompromised hosts, other atypical mycobacteria, such as *Mycobacterium avium-intracellulare,* and *Mycobacterium kansasii,* can cause meningitis. *B. burgdorferi* transmitted by a tick bite (Lyme disease) is another cause of subacute meningitis that is relatively common in certain geographic regions of the United States. Approximately 4 weeks from the onset of symptoms, meningitis may occur. In some patients, meningitis may be the first manifestation of Lyme disease. Leptospirosis can also cause subacute meningitis and, as with *Borrelia,* the meningitis usually appears in the second stage of the disease (the immune phase), when antibodies against the leptospires develop and an inflammatory response is initiated. The severity of the meningitis does not correlate with the severity of clinical manifestations that occur in the first stage of the disease.

Subacute meningitis is a rare complication of cat-scratch disease. Some fungi, such as *Cryptococcus* and *Candida,* are increasingly recognized as causing subacute meningitis, especially in an immunocompromised person. Toxoplasmosis should be suspected as a cause of subacute meningitis in immunocompromised persons with vague, indolent neurologic symptoms. Noninfectious causes of subacute meningitis include malignancies such as leukemia and CNS tumors and autoimmune diseases such as lupus erythematosus, rheumatoid arthritis, and Behçet's syndrome (recurrent genital ulcers, aphthous stomatitis, and ocular inflammation). Sarcoidosis, a granulomatous disease of unknown origin, very rarely causes subacute meningitis. Heavy metal poisoning, such as lead poisoning, which usually causes encephalopathy, may sometimes present with symptoms suggestive of subacute meningitis and CSF findings indistinguishable from those of meningitis.

Chronic Meningitis. When symptoms and signs of meningeal irritation are present for several weeks or months without improvement, chronic meningitis should be considered. There are many causes of chronic meningitis (Table 52–4). Indolent tuberculous meningitis may be a diagnostic challenge because it may be the first manifestation of tuberculosis. Although approximately 50% of persons with tuberculous meningitis have miliary tuberculosis that is evident on chest radiographs, in many persons the primary focus cannot be identified. **Neurosyphilis** is another example of chronic meningitis. In 10–20% of untreated infants with congenital syphilis, CNS symptoms and signs develop after a long latent period. The CSF of infants with asymptomatic congenital syphilis in the first months of life is often abnormal, suggesting a chronic disease course. *Brucella* meningitis usually presents as acute meningitis, but a more indolent course of meningoencephalitis that occurs 2 months to 2 years after the initial systemic disease has been reported. Persons with agammaglobulinemia are particularly prone to develop prolonged enteroviral infection of the CNS. The most common cause is an echovirus. Many fungal infections can have a chronic presentation. *Cryptococcus neoformans* and *Candida* are both etiologic agents of subacute meningitis that sometimes present with a more gradual disease course consistent with chronic meningitis. *Coccidioides immitis* infection, which is usually confined to the lung and hilar lymph nodes, may disseminate to other organs; rarely, chronic meningitis may be the only manifestation of this infection. *Histoplasma capsulatum* is another fungus that rarely causes chronic meningitis. Autoimmune diseases such as lupus erythematosus and juvenile rheumatoid arthritis may rarely progress to chronic meningitis.

EPIDEMIOLOGY

Bacterial Meningitis. The true incidence of bacterial meningitis is difficult to state because many cases go unreported. The incidence of bacterial meningitis is highest among children younger than 1 year. An extremely high incidence is found among American Indians, Alaskan Natives, and Aboriginal Australians, suggesting that genetic factors play a role in susceptibility. Although racial differences in the overall incidence of bacterial meningitis are reported, with an incidence 2–4 times greater among black and Hispanic populations than among European American populations, evidence supports socioeconomic differences rather than genetic predisposition as the major contributing factor.

Other risk factors for meningitis include acquired or congenital deficiencies of host immunity, such as IgG or complement deficiency, and splenectomy or congenital asplenia. Persons with hemoglobinopathies such as sickle cell disease, who eventually develop functional asplenia, have an increased risk of bacterial meningitis. Environmental conditions such as crowding, as in some households, daycare centers, and college and military dormitories, increase the risk of airborne transmission of bacteria from person to person and lead to secondary cases and even epidemics. A CSF leak resulting from congenital anomalies or skull fracture increases the risk of meningitis, especially that caused by *S. pneumoniae.*

Neonatal Meningitis. Group B *Streptococcus* infection of newborns can present itself as **early onset,** which usually occurs in the first day of life but can occur in the first week of life, and **late onset,** which occurs weeks after birth and rarely presents during the second week of life. Although there is some overlap between these two entities, the differences in the presenting signs and symptoms and the outcome make the separation practical (Table 52–7).

TABLE 52–7. Early-Onset and Late-Onset Neonatal Bacterial Infections

Factor Analyzed	Early Onset	Late Onset
Age (days)	<7	>7
Pathogens		
Group B *Streptococcus*	Common	Common
Escherichia coli	Common	Uncommon
Listeria monocytogenes	Uncommon	Common
Obstetric Complications (%)	50	10
Detection of Bacteria		
Blood	Common	Uncommon
Cerebrospinal fluid	Uncommon	Common
Urine, throat, or rectum	Common	Uncommon
Signs and Symptoms (%)		
Hyperthermia	50	65
Hypothermia	15	<5
Respiratory distress	35	20
Apnea	25	10
Anorexia and vomiting	30	50
Lethargy	25	50
Irritability	15	30
Diarrhea	10	20
Jaundice	40	30
Seizures	<5	40
Bulging fontanelle	—	25
Nuchal rigidity	—	15
Mortality (%)	15–20	5–10

The most common manifestations of early-onset disease are those of respiratory insufficiency and cardiovascular collapse. Meningitis is not common with early-onset disease but, in contrast, is a common manifestation of late-onset disease, and it should be considered in any neonate with fever, poor appetite, and lethargy. The risk of the disease among African American neonates is 35 times that among white neonates. Prematurity and young age of the mother (<20 years of age) are other risk factors for newborns. Although more than 5% of newborns born to a colonized mother acquire the organism in the birth canal, only a small percentage of those who became colonized (2–3%) eventually have invasive disease. If the newborn is colonized at multiple sites, the chance of developing invasive disease increases.

E. coli is the second most common cause of neonatal meningitis. Organisms with the capsular antigen K1, one of almost 80 different capsular antigens, are especially associated with neonatal meningitis. The **K1 antigen** is an important factor in the invasiveness of the bacteria and in the severity of the infection. Like group B *Streptococcus, E. coli* can be acquired by newborns during the birth process because both species of bacteria may be present in the birth canal. In addition, because *E. coli* K1 antigen is often prevalent in nursery personnel, postnatal transmission to newborns and subsequent development of meningitis may occur. For both group B *Streptococcus* and *E. coli,* low birth weight inversely affects the rate of meningitis—the smaller the newborn, the higher the incidence of meningitis. Other risk factors include immediate postpartum fever in the mother, resuscitation of the newborn at birth, and prolonged (longer than 24 hours) premature rupture of the membranes. The incidence of *E. coli* meningitis increases severalfold among newborns who receive parenteral iron. In addition, galactosemia is a risk factor for *E. coli* sepsis and meningitis.

Approximately 5% of neonatal meningitis is caused by *L. monocytogenes,* and its incidence seems to be increasing. Newborns acquire *L. monocytogenes* from the mother's intestinal tract during delivery. Consumption of contaminated food such as dairy products or prepared meats may be responsible for the acquisition of the bacteria by a pregnant mother. *L. monocytogenes* serotypes 4b and 2a are the most frequent causes of *L. monocytogenes* meningitis. Similar to group B *Streptococcus* infections, *L. monocytogenes* infections can present in two forms: as early-onset sepsis, which usually represents in utero infection manifested as sepsis after delivery, usually in a premature newborn, and as late-onset disease, which is manifested as meningitis 2 weeks or longer after birth.

The increased survival rate among very small premature newborns because of improved resuscitation and maintenance techniques has caused an increase in nosocomial infections with enteric gram-negative bacilli and staphylococci. Approximately 5% of all neonatal cases of meningitis are due to staphylococci. The risk factors for these pathogens are the immature immune system of prematurity and the use of vascular catheters, which allow staphylococci, which are present on the skin, access to the bloodstream and from there to the meninges.

Viral Meningitis. The enteroviruses cause meningitis during the summer and fall in temperate climates and year-round in tropical climates. These infections are more prevalent in low socioeconomic groups, among young children, in immunocompromised persons, and possibly among athletes. The incubation period is 3–6 days, but fecal excretion and transmission are continuous for several weeks. The prevalence of arboviral meningitis is determined by the geographic distribution and seasonal activity of the arthropod vector. In the United States most arboviral infections occur during the summer and fall. The incubation periods vary from agent to agent, with a range of 4–21 days.

Tuberculous Meningitis. The epidemiology of tuberculous meningitis reflects that of tuberculosis (Chapter 35). Children are usually infected by adults, especially in socioeconomically deprived situations. Tuberculous meningitis occurs in 0.5% of primary tuberculous infections and is most common among children 6 months to 6 years of age. The incubation period is 2–6 months, and miliary tuberculosis can be identified in 50% of patients.

Syphilitic Meningitis. The rate of syphilis, and subsequently congenital syphilis, has decreased in the past decade. It persists in socioeconomically deprived populations with poor prenatal care, particularly in residents of urban centers, in adolescents, and among prostitutes and women infected with HIV.

Fungal Meningitis. Fungal meningitis usually occurs in immunocompromised persons. The impaired immunity allows fungi with low pathogenicity to invade the meninges and cause an infection (Table 52–8). Frequent use of broad-spectrum antibiotics facilitates the process by killing sensitive bacteria and allowing the colonized fungus in the gastrointestinal tract or the skin (e.g., *Candida*) to multiply and reach the bloodstream. Other risk factors are exposure to environmental sources (e.g., *Aspergillus* during construction or from ventilation systems), intravenous or other catheters, extension of local infection (e.g., oral thrush or esophageal candidiasis), and underlying immunocompromising diseases and therapies. Fungal meningitis can occur in the absence of any predisposing factors but usually occurs in endemic areas. For example, about 0.1% of healthy people with primary infections with *C. immitis* after

TABLE 52–8. Risk Factors for Fungal Meningitis

Risk Factor	Organism	Frequency
Endemic area	*Coccidioides*	Uncommon
	Histoplasma	Uncommon
	Blastomyces	Uncommon
Immunocompromised host	*Paracoccidioides*	Uncommon
Neonate	*Candida*	Common
Malignant neoplasia	*Candida*	Common
	Aspergillus	Uncommon
	Histoplasma	Uncommon
Organ transplant	*Cryptococcus*	Common
	Aspergillus	Uncommon
AIDS	*Cryptococcus*	Common
	Histoplasma	Uncommon
	Coccidioides	Uncommon
Severe combined immunodeficiency	*Candida*	Uncommon
	Cryptococcus	Uncommon
Chronic granulomatous disease	*Aspergillus*	Common
Neutropenia	*Candida*	Common
	Aspergillus	Uncommon
Corticosteroids	*Candida*	Common
	Cryptococcus	Uncommon
	Coccidioides	Uncommon
Diabetes mellitus	Zygomycetes	Uncommon
Antibiotics	*Candida*	Common
Hyperalimentation	*Candida*	Common
Intravenous catheter	*Candida*	Common
Pregnancy	*Coccidioides*	Uncommon*

*Although rare, this infection is more common in this population than in others.

inhalation in an endemic area eventually develop meningitis, usually several months after the primary infection.

PATHOGENESIS

Bacterial Meningitis. Meningitis caused by encapsulated bacteria usually begins with respiratory colonization of the potentially pathogenic agent (Figure 52–1). Specific virulence factors are important in the establishment of a carrier state. Bacteria must adhere to epithelial cells for colonization to occur. Bacterial capsules seem to be an important factor for adhesion in gram-positive bacteria such as group B *Streptococcus* and *S. pneumoniae,* whereas **pili** increase the ability of gram-negative bacteria such as *N. meningitidis, H. influenzae,* and *E. coli* to become attached. Respiratory viral infections facilitate the colonization and local invasion of bacteria by damaging the respiratory epithelial cells, thereby adversely affecting the protective host mechanisms such as macrophage function and neutrophil chemotaxis. It is estimated that 5–10% of healthy adults and children are nasopharyngeal carriers of *N. meningitidis,* and 25–50% of young children are colonized with *S. pneumoniae.* Daycare attendance increases the rates of colonization and particularly the percentage of penicillin-resistant strains.

The exact mechanism by which bacteria invade from the surface of the epithelial cells into the bloodstream is unknown. Some bacteria (e.g., *N. meningitidis, S. pneumoniae*) produce IgA protease, which cleaves IgA, the principal immunoglobulin of the mucosal surface that facilitates bacterial invasion through the mucosa. Several observations suggest that the bacterial capsule is an important factor for invasion. For example, of the 84 serotypes of *S. pneumoniae,* fewer than 20 serotypes cause almost all of the cases of bacteremia and meningitis.

In addition to the capsule, other surface components of bacteria, such as **outer membrane proteins** and **lipopolysaccharides,** appear to play a role in bacterial virulence and ability to invade the mucosa. The transport of bacteria across the mucosa appears to occur by different mechanisms for different species. It is speculated that *H. influenzae* invades the mucosal cells by a process involving the microfilaments and microtubules and is then transported to the blood through the lymphatics. *N. meningitidis* is transported within a phagocytic vacuole. The exact transport mechanism of *S. pneumoniae* remains unknown, but the bacterium gains access to the blood via the lymphatics.

Once bacteria have entered the bloodstream, the progression to sustained bacteremia or the abortion of the invasion depends on intact host defense mechanisms such as opsonization, type-specific antibodies, and complement, as well as the presence or absence of a bacterial capsule that inhibits phagocytosis, complement activation, and opsonization.

Specific antibodies against the capsular polysaccharides of the invading bacteria are acquired with age. Multiple mechanisms have been suggested for the poor humoral response in young infants. Delay in maturation of the specific immunity is probably the main reason. This delay accounts for the increased prevalence of pneumococcal and meningococcal infections in young children. Clearance of intravascular microorganisms occurs mainly in the liver

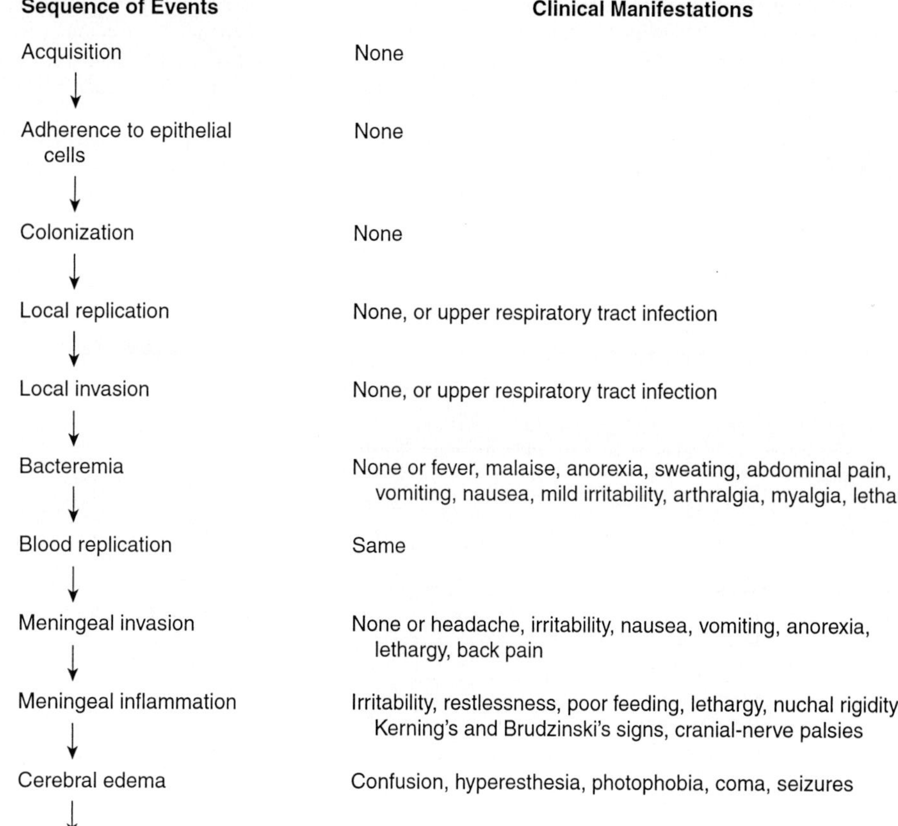

FIGURE 52–1. Pathogenesis of bacterial meningitis and clinical manifestations.

and spleen and requires complement activation and opsonization. This requirement may explain the increased incidence of pneumococcal and meningococcal infections in persons without a functioning spleen or with an impaired complement system. The clinical manifestations of bacteremia may be vague and nonspecific (Fig. 52–1). In some persons, bacteremia may be asymptomatic. In most persons, nonspecific symptoms such as fever, malaise, poor appetite, myalgia, and mild irritability are present.

Bacteria survive in the blood because the capsule effectively resists complement activity and phagocytosis. Sustained bacteremia is achieved by efficient and rapid intravascular replication *(H. influenzae, N. meningitidis)* or replication at an extravascular focus *(S. pneumoniae)*. The magnitude of the bacteremia is also an important factor in the pathogenesis of meningitis. In an animal model of meningitis, it was shown that almost all animals with bacteremia and counts of $>10^4$/mL developed meningitis, whereas only 25% of animals with bacteria counts $<10^4$/mL developed meningitis. This observation of the effects of higher and lower levels of bacteria may explain why meningitis does not occur in all cases of *S. pneumoniae* bacteremia.

Bacteria gain access to the meninges though the choroid plexus. The low concentration of complement components and immunoglobulins in normal CSF facilitates prompt access of bacteria to the leptomeninges and rapid replication, causing meningitis. Inflammation of the meninges usually causes headache, nausea, vomiting, irritability, lethargy, and fever (Fig. 52–1). Although the bacteria are usually confined to the subarachnoid space, the intimate contact of this space with the brain parenchyma may explain the involvement of the brain in meningitis. Inflammation of sensory nerves produces hyperesthesia, photophobia, nuchal rigidity, and Kernig and Brudzinski signs. In addition, mental changes ranging from confusion to coma, seizures, and transient or permanent focal neurologic signs occur with more severe involvement of the brain.

The specific pathophysiologic changes that cause brain damage are the result of bacterial products and the host inflammatory response (Fig. 52–2). The **endotoxin** of gram-negative bacteria is probably the first inducer of the inflammatory response. In gram-positive bacteria the **peptidoglycans,** especially those containing **teichoic acids,** are the inducers of the inflammatory response. The intense inflammatory reaction starts with the release of cytokines from the macrophages, monocytes, and other cells, such as vascular endothelial cells, astrocytes, and microglial cells. The primary mediators of the inflammatory response are **tumor necrosis factor (TNF)** and **interleukin 1 (IL-1).** Other cytokines involved in the host inflammatory response include **plasma-activating factor (PAF), macrophage inflammatory proteins (MIP-1 and MIP-2),** and **prostaglandins.** PAF recruits and activates neutrophils and monocytes and, by direct action on vascular smooth muscle, causes vasoconstriction and vasodilation. In addition, it causes changes in the vascular endothelial cells that lead to increased vascular permeability and edema formation. MIP-1 and MIP-2 induce chemotaxis and the oxidative burst in neutrophils. They also elicit brain edema by increasing the permeability of the blood-brain barrier. Prostaglandins such as prostaglandin E_2 play a role in cytotoxic edema of the gray matter and, to a lesser extent, in the development of vasogenic edema of the white matter.

TNF and IL-1 play a major role in the host response to gram-negative bacteria. They induce an influx of neutrophils and low molecular weight serum proteins into the CSF. They also cause increased vascular permeability by inducing morphologic changes in the endothelial cells and neurologic damage by direct toxic effects on oligodendrocytes. The proteins of the complement system, such as C5a, that reach the CSF produce intense chemotactic activity, which further increases the influx of neutrophils. The ability of neutrophils to eliminate bacteria from the CSF is limited because of low concentrations of specific antibodies and complement components in the CSF, resulting in suboptimal opsonization. However, the increased number of activated neutrophils in the CSF may potentiate brain cell damage. Thus it appears that limiting the number of neutrophils in the CSF during meningitis may be beneficial. In contrast to gram-negative bacteria, PAF seems to play a prominent role in inducing the inflammatory response in gram-positive bacterial infections. These differences in the initiation of the host response may have implications for our understanding of the subtly different clinical manifestations of bacterial meningitis. Studies of animal models of meningitis suggest that the addition of dexamethasone before or immediately after the initiation of antibiotic therapy reduces the inflammatory response. Dexameth-

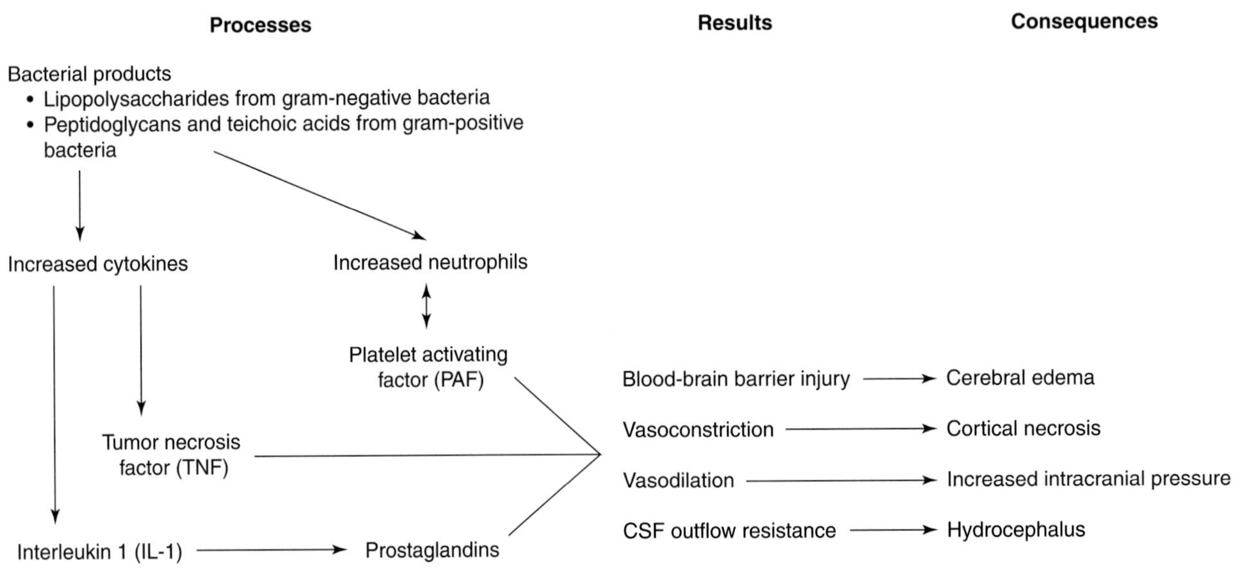

FIGURE 52–2. Pathophysiologic mechanisms of meningitis.

asone inhibits the production of TNF and IL-1 and thus reduces the inflammatory changes in the CSF. These observations led to the suggestion that the addition of dexamethasone to antibiotic therapy may be beneficial to persons with bacterial meningitis. In addition, removal or neutralization of endotoxin, TNF, IL-1, or PAF by specific antibodies in the animal model of meningitis reduced the inflammatory response, which suggested that attenuation of the inflammatory response might reduce the severity of meningitis and its neurologic sequelae. Thus antiendotoxin or anticytokine therapies, or their combination, will likely play a major role in the future in improving the outcome of bacterial meningitis.

Increased intracranial pressure is common in bacterial meningitis. It is the result of increased fluid leakage through the blood-brain barrier, interstitial cerebral edema from metabolic abnormalities of the brain cells, and abnormal cerebral blood flow and fluid collection in the subdural space. Increased intracranial pressure presents clinically as severe headaches, irritability, bulging fontanelle, and rarely as papilledema. Cerebral edema decreases cerebral blood flow and increases venous obstruction and stasis, which may cause focal ischemia, thrombosis of cortical veins, or cortical necrosis. These changes present as focal neurologic signs, and such findings suggest a poor outcome. The purulent material in the subarachnoid space may interfere with the flow of CSF, causing hydrocephalus. In addition, subdural fluid collection may also cause enlargement of the head. The clinical symptoms are vomiting, seizures, persistent fever despite appropriate antibiotic therapy, and bulging fontanelle. A severe complication of increased intracranial pressure is transtentorial herniation of the brain. This rare complication, which occurs in $<2\%$ of children with increased intracranial pressure, presents with sudden worsening of respiratory and hemodynamic measurements, sluggish pupillary reaction, and deterioration in the level of consciousness.

Viral Meningitis. Most viruses reach the meninges by the hematogenous route. After replication at the site of entry, which is usually the gastrointestinal tract or the respiratory tract, or in the regional lymph nodes, a transient primary viremia that is asymptomatic spreads the virus to the reticuloendothelial system, including the liver, spleen, and lymph nodes. If virus replication is not terminated in these organs, a more persistent secondary viremia occurs; it is manifested by nonspecific signs and symptoms that include fever, malaise, myalgia, nausea, vomiting, poor appetite, and mild irritability. Specific receptors in the CNS probably play an important role in the attachment of the virus to the meninges and in entry into the CSF. It is presumed that passive viral transport across the blood-brain barrier contributes to the establishment of viral meningitis. The inflammatory host response to viral meningitis is not well studied because of the generally benign nature of the disease. The involvement of cytokines in the host response is limited; TNF and IL-1 are not detected or are present at very low concentrations, which may explain the milder clinical manifestations of this disease. The severity of the clinical manifestations depends on the extent of viral replication in the CNS and on the progression of the infection into the brain. Once the virus is no longer confined to the meninges and brain involvement occurs, resulting in **meningoencephalitis,** more serious manifestations occur. These include disorientation, severe changes in consciousness, seizures, behavioral and speech disturbances, focal nerve paralysis, and hemiparesis. Demyelination may follow destruction of oligodendroglia cells, which results in more permanent neurologic sequelae.

SYMPTOMS AND CLINICAL MANIFESTATIONS

In the presence of the specific signs and symptoms of meningitis, such as bulging fontanelle, stiff neck, and seizures, it is relatively easy to consider the disease. Unfortunately, in many cases of meningitis the clinical manifestations are nonspecific (Table 52–9). It is not possible to differentiate the common bacterial causes of meningitis in children (Table 52–10). This is particularly true for newborns and young infants, who may have only fever, lethargy, and poor feeding. It is especially reasonable to perform a lumbar puncture for CSF analysis in an attempt to diagnose meningitis in young children: if the history or the clinical manifestations raise a doubt about the putative cause of the disease; if a febrile person develops an unexplained alteration in mentation or level of alertness and consciousness; or if the severity of the clinical manifestations cannot be explained by the apparent clinical findings (e.g., the person appears sicker than should be suggested by the diagnosis of otitis media). Thus, if a physician is considering the need for a lumbar puncture, it should be performed. Lumbar puncture for CSF analysis identifies the presence of meningitis and is the key to distinguishing the type of meningitis.

Infants and Children. An insidious onset is common for viral meningitis and in younger infants with bacterial meningitis. The symptoms usually start with a nonspecific febrile illness, such as an upper respiratory tract infection that progresses to poor feeding, nausea, and vomiting. Listlessness, lethargy, and sleepiness may develop for several days. In this setting it is difficult to consider meningitis, particularly early, especially if another infection such as otitis media, pharyngitis, or an upper respiratory tract infection is diagnosed and if oral antibiotics are administered. Extrameningeal infections are common with meningitis, and all patients with infections should have close follow-up to identify the development of more specific signs and symptoms of meningitis. In infants and children who are old enough to report their symptoms, the most common complaints are headache, neck pain, and nausea. Confusion, photophobia or other visual abnormalities, and hyperesthesia also may be noted.

Another presentation pattern of meningitis in children is an acute and fulminant condition with manifestations of sepsis developing rapidly, usually within a few hours. This progressive form is associated with the rapid development of fever, loss of appetite, nausea, and vomiting, which are the result of increased intracranial pressure. Seizures are common, and the level of consciousness progressively deteriorates from lethargy and irritability to somnolence, obtundation, and coma. Nuchal rigidity and bulging fontanelle (when the fontanelle is open) are common. The rapid development of brain edema in these children may lead to transtentorial herniation and death. This fulminant presentation is relatively uncommon and occurs primarily with bacterial meningitis. Even immediate initiation of appropriate antibiotic therapy may not affect the outcome in these persons.

Fewer than 1% of children with bacterial meningitis have no classic signs and symptoms of meningitis, but they do have unexplained fever associated with behavioral changes or a few petechial skin lesions. Although petechiae are usually associated with *N. meningitidis* infections, they also occur with *S. pneumoniae* and many viral infections. The quality of the child's cry, skin color and perfusion, level of consciousness, hydration, and reaction to parents or social stimuli are helpful observational tools in assessing the possibility of meningitis. In addition, the peripheral WBC count may be helpful because in many persons with bacterial meningitis the WBC count is greater than 15,000/mm^3, with a predominance

TABLE 52–9. Signs and Symptoms of Meningitis

Signs and Symptoms	Neonates	Infants	Children
Signs			
Fever	Common	Common	Common
Seizures	Common	Less common	Less common
Diarrhea	Less common	Uncommon	Rare
Abdominal distention	Less common	Uncommon	Rare
Jaundice	Less common	Rare	Rare
Respiratory distress	Less common	Rare	Rare
Shock	Less common	Uncommon	Uncommon
Nuchal rigidity	Uncommon	Less common	Common
Kerning's or Brudzinski's sign	Uncommon	Less common	Common
Opisthotonos	Uncommon	Less common	Common
Bulging fontanelle	Uncommon	Less common	NA
Ataxia	Rare	Uncommon	Uncommon
Symptoms			
Vomiting	Common	Common	Less common
Anorexia (poor feeding)	Common	Common	Less common
Lethargy	Common	Common	Common
Irritability	Less common	Common	Less common
Nausea	Unknown	Common	Common
Headache	Unknown	Less common	Common
Neck pain	Unknown	Less common	Common
Confusion	Unknown	Less common	Less common
Photophobia	Unknown	Less common	Less common
Hyperesthesia	Unknown	Less common	Less common

Common = >50% of cases; less common = 10–50% of cases; uncommon = 1–10% of cases; rare = <1% of cases; NA = not applicable.

of immature neutrophils. In fulminant bacterial meningitis the peripheral WBC count is usually low, and as a result the WBC count in the CSF may also be low, resembling that of aseptic meningitis. The poor clinical condition of the patient should serve as a clue in differentiating fulminant bacterial meningitis from viral meningitis.

Neonatal Meningitis. In neonates the signs and symptoms of meningitis, including bacterial meningitis, may be subtle (Table 52–9). Fever is probably the most common sign but unfortunately is also common with many other noninfectious diseases in newborns. Dehydration, hematoma, medications such as atropine, anoxia and kernicterus that damage the thermoregulatory mechanisms, and external modification of the newborn's temperature by thermoregulated incubators are a few examples of such causes. Approximately one third of newborns with meningitis have no fever, or hypothermia. Gastrointestinal signs and symptoms such as regurgitation, vomiting, diarrhea, and abdominal distention appear in half of newborns with meningitis. Respiratory distress, manifested as tachypnea, grunting, flaring of the alae nasi, retractions, or apnea, is present in one third of patients. These findings also may be caused by many other conditions, such as aspiration pneumonia, cardiovascular disease, dehydration, metabolic disease (e.g., acidosis), and respiratory distress syndrome. Lethargy is probably the most common manifestation of CNS dysfunction in newborns, whereas irritability is less common, noted in approximately one third of affected newborns. Lethargy or irritability is also a sign of hypoglycemia of the newborn, narcotic withdrawal, congenital heart disease, hypoxia, and genetic disorders such as dysautonomia, which should be included in the differential diagnosis.

Approximately 40% of newborns with meningitis have seizures, but subtle focal seizures may be present although undocumented in another 20–40%. Focal signs, in order of frequency, include hemiparesis, paresis of eye movements, and cranial nerve palsies. Seizures are twice as common in newborns as in older children with meningitis, especially in the presence of other risk factors such as hypoxia, hypoglycemia, hypocalcemia, intracranial hemorrhage, kernicterus, congenital malformations, and a narcotic-addicted mother.

TABLE 52–10. Differences in Clinical Manifestations of Bacterial Meningitis

Manifestation	*Haemophilus influenzae* type b	*Streptococcus pneumoniae*
Prodrome	Protracted or fulminant	Usually not rapid
Irritability	Common	Less common
Shock, disseminated intravascular coagulopathy (%)	10	<3
Obtunded, semicomatose (%)	10	25
Focal neurologic signs (%)	15	35
Hearing loss (%)	5–20	30–45
Mortality (%)	3–5	7–10

Physical Examination Findings

Nuchal rigidity, or **stiff neck,** is an important sign of meningitis in older children but is relatively rare in newborns, occurring in only 10–15% of newborns with meningitis. Nuchal rigidity may also occur in persons with pharyngitis, pneumonia, rheumatoid arthritis, trauma to the neck muscles, retropharyngeal abscess, and tetanus. Sudden neck flexion that causes flexion of the knees **(Brud-**

zinski's sign) and the inability to completely extend the leg when the thigh is flexed on the abdomen **(Kernig's sign)** are also common in older children but are rare in newborns. The same observation is true for **opisthotonos.**

Because newborns have open sutures, the skull can respond to brain edema with an increase in head size and thus reduce the intensity of the increased intracranial pressure. As a result a **bulging fontanelle** is uncommon in term newborns (occurring in 15–20% with meningitis) and rare in premature infants. This sign is present in one third of infants with meningitis who still have an open fontanelle. Ataxia, a rare sign of meningitis, is not seen in newborns and young infants.

DIAGNOSIS

The nonspecific signs and symptoms that often occur early in the course of meningitis require careful observation and examination of the patient. The level of consciousness, mental status, reaction to parents or social stimuli, quality of the child's cry, and skin color, hydration, and perfusion are helpful observational tools in assessing the possibility of meningitis, which should be considered if any of these observations show abnormalities. In addition, meningitis should always be suspected if the severity of the clinical manifestations cannot be explained by the physical examination findings. Neuroimaging with CT and MRI contributes little to the diagnosis of acute meningitis and should be performed only if signs of increased intracranial pressure or focal neurologic deficits are found.

Differential Diagnosis

Many disorders may show signs and symptoms of meningeal irritation and increased intracranial pressure imitating meningitis, including infectious causes (i.e., bacterial, viral, fungal, protozoal) and noninfectious causes (e.g., hemorrhage, tumors, collagen vascular disease). Differentiation of these disorders in most instances is relatively simple because the history, physical examination, and CSF examination usually give a clear indication of the appropriate diagnosis. In some situations, additional tests such as immunologic and radiographic studies may help in the differential diagnosis. Unfortunately, in a few cases the diagnosis must be deferred because none of the available tests is helpful in differentiating among similar disorders.

Other conditions may suggest the possibility of meningitis. Seizures may be associated with meningitis, encephalitis, and intracranial abscess, or they can be the sequelae of brain edema, cerebral infarction, or vasculitis. Young infants and children may have a febrile seizure, or a seizure may occur in a person with an underlying seizure disorder and a lowered seizure threshold to fever. Most **febrile seizures** occur in children between 6 months and 4 years of age, with the highest incidence being in the second year of life. Febrile seizures are usually brief in duration, usually less than several minutes, are generalized rather than focal, and occur without other signs or symptoms to suggest CNS infection. They usually occur soon after a rapid increase in temperature, characteristically at the beginning of an otherwise uncomplicated infectious illness such as otitis media or an upper respiratory tract infection. If a child has had a fever for more than 24 hours without a seizure, it is unlikely that a seizure occurring after this period is due to fever. The condition is also more common in children with a family history of febrile seizures. Most children have only one episode of febrile seizures, with the exception of children with cerebral palsy, epilepsy, or other underlying neurologic disorders. In children with these disorders, multiple episodes (including some occurring in the absence of fever) may more appropriately be called **seizures with fever.** In some instances a violent seizure may lead to peripheral leukocytosis and fever. Thus the documentation of fever before a seizure is helpful in deciding whether it is a febrile seizure.

Common metabolic disorders that cause seizure can be evaluated by checking the serum electrolyte, glucose, urea, and calcium levels. An EEG is also indicated in complex cases. The best information can be obtained when the test is done 7–10 days after the episode because diffuse slow waves may be found if the EEG is done immediately after the seizure. The need for a lumbar puncture depends on the history and the physical examination findings. A lumbar puncture should be performed if the child is younger than 6 months, when febrile seizures are rare, if the physical examination is inconclusive, or if the child has had the fever for longer than 24 hours, with no sudden increase in temperature occurring before the seizure. If there is doubt whether the child has had a febrile seizure or a seizure due to an acute CNS infection, examination of the CSF is urgently indicated.

LABORATORY EVALUATION

Lumbar Puncture. If meningitis is deemed likely on the basis of history and clinical presentation, a lumbar puncture should be performed immediately to obtain CSF for examination. There are few contraindications to lumbar puncture. In mild to moderate increased intracranial pressure, which is relatively common in bacterial meningitis, a lumbar puncture should be done as soon as possible because the benefits of performing it outweigh the minimal risks of herniation, especially in young infants if the fontanelles are open. Before a lumber puncture is done, the optic fundi should be examined to exclude papilledema. Although this finding is rare in children with meningitis, if papilledema is found, a neuroimaging study, such as CT, should be performed before the lumber puncture. If severe increased intracranial pressure is suspected because of dilated, nonreactive pupils, abnormal ocular mobility suggesting sixth nerve palsy, bradycardia, hypertension, or stupor, the lumbar puncture should be postponed until CT is performed. A few focal CNS infections, such as a brain abscess, subdural empyema, or epidural abscess, may present with clinical signs and symptoms indistinguishable from those of meningitis. Because brain herniation may occur after lumbar puncture if any one of these conditions, each of which is rare in children, is present, the procedure should be delayed until CT is performed. In emergency situations a cisternal puncture may be performed. Alternatively a lumbar puncture can be performed safely, even if increased intracranial pressure is present, by first giving an intravenous bolus of mannitol. Then, 20–30 minutes after administration of the bolus, a small (22-gauge) needle is used to collect up to 1 mL of CSF, which is sufficient for the diagnosis of meningitis.

Other conditions, such as Reye's syndrome or herpes simplex encephalitis, which may result in severe brain edema without papilledema, extensive intracranial bleeding, or obstructive hydrocephalus, may require a delay in performing a lumbar puncture. Persons whose condition is clinically unstable because of hypotension and shock may require empirical therapy for sepsis and meningitis, with postponement of the lumbar puncture until the procedure can safely be tolerated.

Lumbar puncture is a relatively safe procedure with few complications. Using a needle without a stylet may cause fragments of skin to be implanted directly into the subarachnoid space, resulting in **intraspinal epidermoid tumors.** Another controversial complication relates to reports that performing lumbar puncture on infants younger than 1 year who have bacteremia may lead to meningitis. Although such an association has been reported in a few infants, it is possible that the bacteremia was already advanced, with a high concentration of bacteria in the blood, and that their ill appearance was the result of early meningitis before the CSF reflected diagnostic changes. Thus a normal CSF profile at the time of lumbar puncture does not completely exclude the possibility that meningeal infection is present in its early stages, before the inflammatory response is reflected in the CSF. In addition, the importance of lumbar puncture in excluding meningitis in a febrile child who does not have a focus of infection outweighs the very small risk of seeding bacteria into the CSF during the procedure. If there is evidence of local infection (e.g., overlying cellulitis) at the site of a proposed lumbar puncture, the subarachnoid space should be entered at a different place, such as by cisternal puncture performed by a skilled specialist. Persons with severe blood clotting problems (e.g., hemophilia, anticoagulant therapy, or thrombocytopenia [platelet count <20,000/mm^3]) may have bleeding after the lumbar puncture. The blood may then collect in the subdural space, rarely causing compression of the spinal cord and neurologic damage. In a young infant, flexing of the neck while lying in a lateral position for a lumber puncture can cause respiratory deterioration; therefore the sitting position is preferred to avoid this complication.

Traumatic lumbar puncture occurs in 15–20% of children, and the percentage is even higher among newborns. It seems plausible that if the ratio of WBCs/mm^3 to RBCs/mm^3 in the CSF exceeds the ratio in the peripheral blood, then pleocytosis could be identified. Therefore, by calculating the number of WBCs contributed by the contaminating blood (the predicted count), one would be able to determine whether the CSF WBC count (the observed count) represents actual pleocytosis of the CSF. However, multiple studies have demonstrated that such a calculation is usually inaccurate in children. Only about 20% of the predicted number of WBCs have been found in the CSF, and therefore mild pleocytosis, especially with viral or early bacterial meningitis, may escape recognition. Patients who have had a traumatic lumbar puncture must therefore be followed closely, and if the possibility of bacterial meningitis cannot be otherwise excluded, empirical antibiotic therapy should be started until the CSF culture result is reported to be negative. Although traumatic lumbar punctures are relatively common, the possibility of subarachnoid hemorrhage from child abuse or trauma should be considered. Normal CSF is colorless, whereas the CSF of patients with hemorrhage has **xanthochromia,** or a yellow pigmentation, from the breakdown of RBCs. The CSF should be centrifuged as soon as possible after the lumbar puncture, at least within 2 hours, and if the supernatant is clear, the lumbar puncture was traumatic. A hemorrhage should be suspected if the supernatant is xanthochromic. **Crenation** of RBCs in the CSF occurs too quickly for differentiation of a traumatic lumbar puncture from bleeding from other causes.

The collected CSF should always be examined for total WBC count (quantifying the percentage of neutrophils and mononuclear cells), RBC count, protein level, glucose level, and the presence of bacteria by Gram stain and culture. Additional tests include acid-fast stain and mycobacterial culture if tuberculosis is suspected, fungal stains and culture if fungal infection is suspected, and PCR for viruses and viral culture if viral infection is suspected. There are fewer WBCs and a higher level of glucose in normal ventricular fluid than in the CSF obtained by lumbar puncture.

White Blood Cells. Normal CSF does not contain more than 5 WBCs/mm^3 (Table 52–11). In very young children the total WBC count in normal CSF is increased and inversely related to age. Thus the upper limit of normal for the total WBC count in the CSF of term newborns at birth is 30 cells/mm^3, for premature newborns at birth 32 cells/mm^3, and for newborns 4–8 weeks of age 25 cells/mm^3. By 6–8 weeks of age the total WBC count in the CSF decreases to 10/mm^3 and then slowly decreases to 5/mm^3. The differential count for normal CSF of premature and term newborns has up to 60% polymorphonuclear cells. Usually the differential count of normal CSF in infants shows fewer than 1% polymorphonuclear cells. Only 5% of children older than 6 weeks with normal CSF have a polymorphonuclear cell count of 1–3/mm^3. CSF cell counts should be performed soon after collection. If the procedure is delayed by more than an hour, the number of neutrophils may decrease because of lysis and adherence of WBCs to the walls of the tube.

The causes of pleocytosis are numerous (Table 52–12). Bacterial meningitis is almost always associated with marked CSF pleocytosis, cell counts usually from 1,000/mm^3 to sometimes greater than 10,000/mm^3. Usually *N. meningitidis* and *H. influenzae* infections cause more severe pleocytosis than infection with *S. pneumoniae.* It is relatively uncommon (<2% of cases) to identify bacterial meningitis without CSF pleocytosis in older children. In contrast, nearly 10–15% of neonates with bacterial meningitis may have a normal WBC count in the CSF, reflecting the wider range of normal CSF WBC counts in neonates. The differential cell count for bacterial meningitis classically shows a predominance of polymorphonuclear cells, usually greater than 85%. The cellular response in most cases of acute viral meningitis is a predominance of monocular cells. However, the early cellular response in viral meningitis may have a predominance of polymorphonuclear cells. In that event it is difficult to differentiate early viral or early bacterial meningitis from partially treated bacterial meningitis.

The predominance of polymorphonuclear cells and a reduced glucose concentration in the CSF is important for differentiating bacterial and viral meningitis. It has been shown that when these two factors are considered in relation to the age of the child and the season of the year, they can serve as excellent predictors of whether the meningitis is bacterial or viral. If the interpretation of the predominance of neutrophils in the CSF on initial evaluation is still questionable, a repeated lumbar puncture 4–6 hours after the first lumbar puncture typically shows the shift to lymphocyte predominance characteristic of viral meningitis.

TABLE 52–11. Limits of Normal Values for Cerebrospinal Fluid Parameters*

Parameter	Premature†	Term†	Infant/Child	Adolescent/Adult
WBC count (/mm^3)	32	30	10	5
Neutrophils (%)	60	60	10	20
Mononuclear (%)	40	40	90	80
Glucose (mg/dL)	25	35	40	40
Protein (mg/dL)	150	150	55	55

*Upper limits for WBC count and protein level; lower limit for glucose level.
†Until 1 month of age.

TABLE 52–12. Differential Diagnosis of Cerebrospinal Fluid Pleocytosis and Hypoglycorrhachia

	Predominantly Polymorphonuclear		Predominantly Mononuclear	
	Normal Glucose Level	Reduced Glucose Level	Normal Glucose Level	Reduced Glucose Level
Common	Bacterial meningitis Early viral meningitis Partially treated bacterial meningitis	Bacterial meningitis Partially treated bacterial meningitis	Viral meningitis Partially treated bacterial meningitis Parameningeal infection Lead encephalopathy	Viral meningitis Partially treated bacterial meningitis
Less common	Viral encephalitis Early tuberculous meningitis Early fungal meningitis Parameningeal infection Acute hemorrhagic encephalitis	Viral meningoencephalitis Ventricular empyema Ruptured subdural abscess Ruptured brain abscess	*Mycoplasma* meningitis Lyme disease Infectious mononucleosis Early tuberculosis Brain abscess Rocky Mountain spotted fever Chemical meningitis Leukemia Syphilis	Tuberculous meningitis Fungal meningitis Leukemia
Rare		Amebic meningitis Subarachnoid hemorrhage	Cat-scratch disease Sarcoidosis Leptospirosis Behçet's syndrome	Toxoplasmosis Sarcoidosis Cysticercosis

Glucose. The glucose level in normal CSF of premature and term newborns can be as low as 25 mg/dL and 35 mg/dL, respectively (Table 52–11). Glucose is an important indicator of severe brain involvement because a decrease in its concentration suggests decreased glucose transport across the blood-brain barrier and increased glycogenolysis. A decreased CSF glucose concentration of 19–30 mg/dL (**hypoglycorrhachia**) is found in most cases of bacterial meningitis but is also found in many other diseases (Table 52–12). In approximately 75% of cases the CSF glucose level returns to normal within 48 hours of adequate antibiotic therapy. This is important if the differential diagnosis is between bacterial meningitis and a more chronic infection such as tuberculosis, in which the decreased CSF glucose level persists.

Protein. The normal CSF protein level is 25–40 mg/dL (Table 52–11) but is altered in many diseases (Table 52–13). The amount of protein in the normal ventricular fluid is 50% of its concentration in the CSF. In newborns the level is higher and usually ranges from 20 to 170 mg/dL. The CSF protein level increases in most cases of bacterial meningitis to 100–500 mg/dL. Normal CSF protein values are occasionally seen in bacterial meningitis and other CNS diseases, whereas in 10–15% of cases, protein levels of 1,000 mg/dL or higher are found, which indicates the sometimes questionable usefulness of measuring the CSF protein level. In viral meningitis the protein level usually ranges from 50 to 150 mg/dL. Although a consistent CSF protein level >150 mg/dL argues against a viral cause, the protein concentration is the least specific of the CSF measurements. Tuberculous and fungal meningitis, subdural brain abscess, encephalitis, and brain tumors can cause moderate elevation of CSF protein, usually 200–1,000 mg/dL. Guillain-Barré syndrome and spinal subarachnoid block are usually associated with high protein levels, >1,000 mg/dL, although such levels can also be the result of tuberculous or fungal meningitis.

Stains. The **Gram stain** is valuable in rapidly determining the pathogen of bacterial meningitis. Most cases of pediatric bacterial meningitis due to *N. meningitidis, S. pneumoniae,* and *H. influenzae* type b have a positive Gram stain (Table 52–14). In contrast, fewer than 50% of meningitis cases due to *L. monocytogenes* have a positive Gram stain. The sensitivity of the Gram stain in diagnosing the pathogen depends on the number of bacteria present in the CSF and the skills of the observer. If the number of bacteria is lower than 10^3–10^4/mL, as may occur in early bacterial meningitis or in

TABLE 52–13. Cerebrospinal Fluid Protein Levels in Various Diseases

Mildly Elevated (50–200 mg/dL)
Viral meningitis
Bacterial meningitis
Tuberculous meningitis
Fungal meningitis
Brain abscess
Epidural abscess
Subdural empyema
Syphilis
Encephalitis
Subdural hematoma
Collagen vascular disease
Tumors
Moderately Elevated (200–1,000 mg/dL)
Bacterial meningitis
Tuberculous meningitis
Fungal meningitis
Brain abscess (especially if ruptured)
Subdural abscess
Encephalitis
Tumors
Markedly Elevated (>1,000 mg/dL)
Bacterial meningitis
Tuberculous meningitis
Fungal meningitis
Guillain-Barré syndrome
Spinal subarachnoid block

TABLE 52–14. Rapid Antigen Tests of Cerebrospinal Fluid for Meningitis

Test	Sensitivity (%)	Specificity* (%)
Bacterial		
Gram Stain		
Streptococcus pneumoniae	95	100
Neisseria meningitidis	95	100
Haemophilus influenzae type b	75	100
Latex Agglutination		
S. pneumoniae	75	≥95
N. meningitidis	75	≥95
H. influenzae type b	95	≥95
Fungal		
India ink	≤50	≥95
Cryptococcal latex agglutination	90	≥95
Cryptococcal enzyme immunoassay	100	≥95

*The specificity of latex agglutination tests for bacterial antigens in urine is approximately 75% compared with cerebrospinal fluid.

partially treated meningitis, the Gram stain is positive in only 25–50% of cases. When the number of bacteria exceeds 10^5/mL, which is the usual number of bacteria in most cases of bacterial meningitis, the smear is positive in 75–95% of cases. A Gram stain can show false-positive results if bacterial contamination is present in the collecting tubes, slides, or reagents used for the procedure. In addition, the results can be misinterpreted: *S. pneumoniae* can be mistaken for *N. meningitis, L. monocytogenes* for diphtheroids, and *S. aureus* for *Streptococcus.*

An **acid-fast stain** is an important test if there is suspicion of tuberculosis. When a large volume of CSF (10–20 mL) is centrifuged, the sensitivity of the acid-fast stain increases to 40%. However, with the small volume of 1–2 mL of CSF usually available from pediatric patients, the sensitivity is only approximately 10%. The **latex agglutination** and **EIA tests for *Cryptococcus*** are sensitive for identifying cryptococcal meningitis; an **India ink** examination of CSF may also be used but is less sensitive (Table 52–14). **Silver stain** as well as Gram stain may be used to detect fungi such as *Candida, Coccidioides,* or *Blastomycosis.* Unfortunately the yield of these techniques is low, probably because the number of organisms in the CSF is low.

Antigen Detection Tests. The **particle agglutination test** provides a rapid and accurate method of detecting bacterial antigens in the CSF and is useful in diagnosing meningitis due to *S. pneumoniae, N. meningitidis* (except serogroup B), *H. influenzae* type b, and group B *Streptococcus.* Antigen detection test results are positive in 75–95% of cases of bacterial meningitis due to these organisms. However, not all persons in whom meningitis is suspected need a particle agglutination test. Only CSF specimens with negative results on Gram stain should be tested routinely by particle agglutination. Particle agglutination may be especially helpful in suspected and partially treated bacterial meningitis with negative culture results. Bacterial antigens are also found in the urine of many persons with meningitis, and therefore both urine and CSF should be tested. The specificity of the urine test is 75%, in comparison with the specificity of the CSF test.

Cultures. The CSF should always be cultured with appropriate media (i.e., blood, chocolate agar, and broth) even if the CSF appears to be normal. Blood cultures should be part of the routine tests because they may show the cause of the condition. For persons previously treated with antibiotics, diluting the CSF 1:100 and 1:10,000 may increase bacterial recovery by separating the antibiotic from the CSF. If a person has received penicillin or other penicillinase-susceptible antibiotics, the addition of penicillinase to the media may increase the chance of recovering the bacteria. Anaerobic cultures should be considered for immunocompromised persons and for persons with dermal sinuses, recurrent meningitis, or postsurgical or posttraumatic meningitis.

When tuberculous or fungal meningitis is suspected, the appropriate culture media should be used. The yield of mycobacterial cultures is only 50–75%, and multiple cultures of large volumes of CSF (10–20 mL) may be required. The same may be true of fungal meningitis. Only 70% of persons with cryptococcal meningitis have a positive culture result after the first lumbar puncture, but 90% have a positive result after multiple lumbar punctures.

Viral cultures are usually disappointing, with a yield of less than 25%. Enteroviral meningitis may also be confirmed by isolating virus from stool and pharyngeal secretions from patients with compatible clinical findings. Because there is no specific antiviral therapy that can significantly shorten the course of viral meningitis, the major value of viral cultures is epidemiologic. Viral cultures should also be obtained if HSV encephalitis is included in the differential diagnosis (Chapter 55).

Polymerase Chain Reaction. PCR testing of CSF requires small amounts of clinical material and is rapid, sensitive, and specific. The PCR test is becoming more widely available for enteroviruses and also for HSV (Chapter 55), although there are currently no commercially available tests. PCR testing for enteroviruses has been thoroughly studied and is superior to viral culture for the diagnosis of many enterovirus infections, particularly enteroviral meningitis. The use of PCR for the diagnosis of enteroviral meningitis provides prompt results, usually within 24–48 hours, which can reduce unnecessary diagnostic and therapeutic interventions, reduce antibiotic use, shorten hospital stays, and decrease costs.

Other Tests. Many other tests that may help in the diagnosis of meningitis are available. The level of lactic acid in the CSF is more often elevated in bacterial meningitis, >35 mg/dL, than in viral meningitis. Noninfectious conditions such as cerebral ischemia, recurrent seizures, and subarachnoid hemorrhage may produce similar elevations of lactic acid. Thus the CSF lactic acid may add to the differential diagnosis, although its specificity is too low for diagnosis.

The use of acute-phase reactants such as **CRP** has been suggested to differentiate bacterial and viral meningitis. CRP levels greater than 100 ng/mL suggest bacterial meningitis. If the CRP test result is negative, bacterial meningitis can be excluded with almost 100% certainty. It appears that these tests add little to the currently available tests and that their predictive value in equivocal cases still needs to be evaluated. A low CSF chloride level was previously associated with tuberculous meningitis, but it has been shown that this reflects the low serum chloride levels often seen in bacterial and viral meningitis and therefore the test is not useful for differentiating the cause of the meningitis.

Although a thorough investigation of the CSF specimen is traditionally performed and the dictum "the more, the better" is the rule, it appears that an abbreviated CSF evaluation in a previously healthy child is safe and cost-effective in excluding the possibility of bacterial meningitis. If the CSF of a child with suspected meningitis who has not previously received antibiotics, is not immunosuppressed, has not had a neurosurgical procedure, and is not having seizures contains fewer than 6 nucleated blood cells per cubic millimeter, the probability of bacterial meningitis is less than 2%. Thus for young infants who have fever but no clinical manifestations of bacterial meningitis and for whom the CSF evaluation is performed solely to exclude bacterial meningitis, the CSF should be analyzed only for nucleated cells. If the absolute number of cells is $\leq 5/\text{mm}^3$, only the CSF culture should be obtained. In contrast, if the number of nucleated cells is $\geq 6/\text{mm}^3$, then other diagnostic tests are needed to exclude bacterial meningitis.

Unusual Presentations

Partially Treated Bacterial Meningitis. Children treated with oral antibiotics before meningitis is diagnosed have a longer duration of symptoms. Yet, because oral antibiotics given before the lumbar puncture do not alter the CSF findings substantially, the diagnosis of bacterial meningitis can still be established. There is a tendency for pretreatment with oral antibiotics to decrease the total number of WBCs, the percentage of polymorphonuclear leukocytes, the CSF protein concentration, and the percentage of positive Gram stain or culture results, but the differences are minor. Therefore, if (1) a child has no clinically significant neurologic signs or symptoms such as seizures, focal neurologic signs, or severe alteration of consciousness, (2) the CSF glucose level is not grossly abnormal, and (3) the WBC count in the CSF is $<500/\text{mm}^3$ and predominantly mononuclear, intravenous antibiotic therepy can be discontinued 72 hours after it is begun if the blood and CSF culture results are negative and the patient's condition has improved clinically. For an older child who has received oral antibiotics and has CSF findings suggestive of viral meningitis, intravenous antibiotic therapy should not be started and the child should be observed closely. If no spontaneous improvement is noted in 12 hours, the CSF should be re-examined. If the clinical features suggest bacterial meningitis even when the CSF culture result is negative, which can happen in partially treated cases, a complete course of intravenous antibiotic therapy is recommended. Although a full course of intravenous therapy is usually recommended for persons with evidence of bacterial meningitis who seem to respond to oral antibiotics in such a way that their CSF findings are modified to imitate those of viral meningitis and who have a negative CSF culture result, 72–96 hours of continued intravenous antibiotic therapy is probably sufficient for full recovery.

Diagnostic Imaging

CT and MRI should not be routinely performed for persons with evidence of meningitis. When there is evidence of increased intracranial pressure, the CT or MRI is helpful in deciding whether "to tap or not to tap." If meningitis is present, loss of sulci is noted on CT or MRI and the inflamed meninges show enhancement with contrast (Fig. 13–2). Hydrocephalus resulting from CSF flow obstruction can be seen, as well as arterial or venous infarction.

TREATMENT

Prompt treatment of bacterial meningitis is essential for prevention of additional damage to the brain. The initial antimicrobial therapy should be tailored according to the age of the patient, the expected pathogens, and their known susceptibility to the antibiotic (Table 52–15).

Definitive Treatment

The choice of an antibiotic for treatment of meningitis depends on the ability of the drug to penetrate into the CSF and to achieve a sufficiently high bactericidal concentration. Multiple factors influence antibiotic penetration. The inflammatory response to the offending pathogen enhances the passive diffusion of the antibiotic through the blood-brain barrier. The penetration declines as the meningeal inflammation subsides during recovery or treatment with steroids and is one of the theoretical contraindications to using steroids for persons with meningitis. Because the currently available third-generation cephalosporins achieve high bactericidal titers in the CSF, the minor reduction in their penetration into the CSF caused by corticosteroids does not substantially affect their bactericidal activity. Highly lipophilic substances such as chloramphenicol, isoniazid, and rifampin enter the CSF more readily through the lipid layers of the blood-brain barrier than do nonlipophilic drugs such as the cephalosporins and aminoglycosides. The penetration of vancomycin into the CSF is erratic. In addition, the coadministration of corticosteroids with vancomycin to an animal model of meningitis significantly reduced the CSF concentrations of vancomycin. These data suggest that although vancomycin may achieve adequate levels in the CSF to eradicate most *S. pneumoniae* isolates, in a few persons the concentrations may not be sufficient. Therefore vancomycin should not be used alone if the drug is given with corticosteroids.

The host immune response in the CNS is limited, and phagocytosis of encapsulated bacteria is inefficient. Therefore antibiotics are the main mechanism to fight the CNS invader, but the delivery of antibodies and complement is restricted by the blood-brain barrier. Antibiotics must not only reach the CNS but also achieve a sufficiently high concentration to kill the bacteria constantly. Studies using animals have shown that the antibiotic concentration in the CSF must be at least 10–20 times higher than the amount needed to kill the bacteria in vitro (i.e., the minimum bactericidal concentration [MBC]). The reason for recommending the third-generation cephalosporins as the drugs of choice for the initial therapy for presumed bacterial meningitis is recent changes in bacterial susceptibility to antibiotics. The prevalence of *S. pneumoniae* strains that are relatively resistant or highly resistant to penicillins and cephalosporins is increasing. Cefotaxime or ceftriaxone appears to be effective if the in vitro susceptibility of the isolated *S. pneumoniae* to these antibiotics is $<0.5\ \mu\text{g/mL}$. Unfortunately, recent reports suggest that these agents may not be effective in eradicating the

TABLE 52–15. Initial Antimicrobial Therapy by Age for Presumed Bacterial Meningitis

Age	Drug of Choice*	Alternative Drug*
Newborns (0–28 days)	Cefotaxime or ceftriaxone,† plus ampicillin with or without gentamicin	Gentamicin plus ampicillin; ceftazidime plus ampicillin
Infants and toddlers (1 mo to 4 yr)	Ceftriaxone‡ or cefotaxime and vancomycin§	Cefotaxime or ceftriaxone and rifampin
Children and adolescents (5–13 yr) and adults	Ceftriaxone or cefotaxime and vancomycin§	Ampicillin plus chloramphenicol

*For dosage see Table 52–16.
†Not for newborns younger than 1 week with hyperbilirubinemia because of the possibility of bilirubin displacement from albumin.
‡For patients 4–6 weeks of age the addition of ampicillin in areas where *Listeria monocytogenes* is prevalent is recommended.
§Vancomycin should be discontinued as soon as possible if the isolate is *Streptococcus pneumoniae* susceptible to penicillin or cefotaxime (or ceftriaxone).

bacteria in some cases of meningitis. Reported failures occurred when the CSF *S. pneumoniae* isolate had a cefotaxime or ceftriaxone MIC ≥2 μg/mL. Therefore, if the CSF isolate is not sensitive to penicillin and the MIC to cefotaxime or ceftriaxone or both is ≥0.5 μ/mL, vancomycin (or chloramphenicol) should be the drug of choice if the strain is susceptible in vitro. Currently there are *S. pneumoniae* strains resistant to chloramphenicol, but there are as yet no *S. pneumoniae* strains resistant to vancomycin. With the increased use of vancomycin, development of resistance is almost inevitable. In areas where penicillin-resistant *S. pneumoniae* is prevalent, vancomycin in combination with ceftriaxone or cefotaxime is recommended as the initial empirical management for children older than 3 months with suspected bacterial meningitis. This combination should be continued until the etiologic agent is defined and the susceptibility results are available.

Once the etiologic agent is defined by particle agglutination or culture and its susceptibility to antibiotics is determined, a specific single drug or combination of drugs should be chosen (Table 52–16). Penicillin G should be used for susceptible strains of *S. pneumoniae*. If the *S. pneumoniae* isolate is relatively resistant to penicillin (MIC between 0.1 and 1 μg/mL, or no inhibition of bacterial growth around a 1 μg oxacillin disk), ceftriaxone or cefotaxime is recommended if the isolate is susceptible (MIC <0.5 μg/mL). Ceftriaxone may be preferred because of its convenience of administration. The drug can be given once daily (80 mg/kg, not to exceed 3 g), and if the intravenous route is inaccessible, an intramuscular injection at the same dosage is as effective as the intravenous therapy. If the isolate is intermediately resistant (MIC 0.5–1 μg/mL) or resistant (MIC ≥2 μg/mL) to the extended-spectrum cephalosporin, vancomycin or chloramphenicol is the antibiotic of choice. Failures with vancomycin alone have been reported with both penicillin-sensitive and penicillin-resistant pneumococcal meningitis. This may be attributed to the variability in CSF penetration of this antibiotic. Therefore the combination of vancomycin and ceftriaxone is recommended. Other options include the addition of rifampin to vancomycin or treatment with meropenem.

N. meningitidis can be treated effectively with intravenous penicillin G or ampicillin. Although a few reports have suggested that *N. meningitidis* can be resistant to penicillin, the clinical significance of this observation is not yet clear. Ceftriaxone or cefotaxime is an excellent alternative, or, as in the case of *S. pneumoniae,* they may be used as the drug of choice. Meropenem is another alternative, and chloramphenicol can be used in areas where penicillin-resistant strains have appeared or if the person has β-lactam hypersensitivity. Another advantage of chloramphenicol is the ability to treat meningitis with oral antibiotics. In persons without circulatory collapse, as in clinical sepsis, oral administration of chloramphenicol achieves therapeutic levels in the CSF. The oral dose (75 mg/kg/day divided every 6 hours) can be used either after several days of intravenous administration or when intravenous access is impossible. It is advisable to monitor the chloramphenicol blood level if oral therapy continues for more than 3 days. A peak serum level of 15–25 μg/mL (2–3 hours after the dose) is recommended.

Meningitis due to *H. influenzae* type b should be treated with ceftriaxone or cefotaxime. The once-daily dosage regimen of ceftriaxone permits persons with an uncomplicated course to complete therapy at home. The prevalence of ampicillin-resistant strains (>40%) in many regions of the United States and the increased resistance to chloramphenicol worldwide suggest that the traditional combination of ampicillin and chloramphenicol should be used only if the third-generation cephalosporins are unavailable.

If the duration of therapy depends on eradication of bacteria from the CSF, it seems logical to shorten the course of therapy because the newer antibiotics (e.g., the third-generation cephalosporins) eliminate bacteria more rapidly from the CSF. It is recommended that *S. pneumoniae* meningitis be treated for 10–14 days, *N. meningitidis* for 5–7 days, and *H. influenzae* for 7–10 days.

Neonatal Meningitis. In newborns with group B *Streptococcus* meningitis, the traditional combination of ampicillin and either gentamicin or amikacin is still considered to be the combination of choice. These drugs have demonstrated synergy in vitro against group B *Streptococcus.* Although parenteral penicillin G alone (400,000–500,000 U/kg/day every 6–8 hours) or ampicillin (300 mg/kg/day every 6–8 hours) is also considered to be a drug of choice, the more rapid killing of the bacteria by the ampicillin-aminoglycoside combination points toward preference for the combination. Cefotaxime has been shown to be effective for the treatment of group B *Streptococcus* infections and therefore should be considered as a drug of choice because it is easier to administer. Ceftriaxone should not be used in newborns younger than 7 days because of the possibility of increasing levels of free bilirubin in the serum by displacing it from albumin. In older newborns, ceftriaxone, given once daily, is probably as effective as cefotaxime, but experience with it is limited. Vancomycin or chloramphenicol is an alternative drug for patients with β-lactam hypersensitivity. Experience with the use of these drugs is limited in neonates, and adverse effects unique to this age group, such as circulatory collapse and the gray baby syndrome, should be considered when the drugs are used.

L. monocytogenes is highly susceptible to ampicillin, which is the drug of choice. None of the third-generation cephalosporins is active against this organism, and thus they should never be used for definitive treatment or alone for empirical treatment of neonatal meningitis. Infants allergic to penicillin have been treated successfully with intravenous TMP-SMZ. Because sulfonamides may displace bilirubin from albumin and therefore increase the risk of toxic CNS effects of bilirubin in icteric newborns, the combination should not be used in the first week of life or in infants with hyperbilirubinemia.

E. coli is the most common gram-negative bacterium that causes neonatal meningitis in the United States. The drug of choice is cefotaxime because it does not interfere with bilirubin binding to albumin. Because the aminoglycosides are inferior to the third-generation cephalosporins, their use is associated with a lower cure rate and thus they are rarely indicated. Many experts recommend the combination of cefotaxime with either gentamicin or amikacin. Meropenem has been used successfully in persons with gram-negative bacterial meningitis whose treatment with third-generation cephalosporins failed, but experience with this drug is limited. In the rare occurrence of *Pseudomonas* meningitis, ceftazidime (150–225 mg/kg/day divided every 8 or 12 hours; the lower dose and longer interval should be used for newborns <7 days) is the drug of choice. If the CSF culture result remains positive, the addition of an aminoglycoside should be considered. The use of aztreonam and the quinolones should be reserved for the very rare occurrence of a multiply resistant gram-negative infection. The experience with these compounds in neonates is limited, and their routine use is not recommended.

For neonatal meningitis with its higher tendency toward recurrence, a longer course of therapy is recommended. Group B *Streptococcus* and *L. monocytogenes* meningitis should be treated for 14 days, and gram-negative bacterial meningitis therapy should be extended to 21 days.

Other Causes of Meningitis. Many other bacteria can rarely cause meningitis (Table 52–16). The specific therapy for tuberculous meningitis is discussed in Chapter 35. There is no proven therapy

TABLE 52–16. Recommended Antibiotic Therapy for Meningitis According to the Etiologic Agent

Etiologic Agent	Recommended Therapy	Alternative Therapy
Bacteria		
Streptococcus pneumoniae		
Penicillin susceptible (MIC ≤0.06 μg/mL)	Penicillin G	Ampicillin *or* Cefotaxime (or ceftriaxone) *or* Meropenem *or* Chloramphenicol
Penicillin resistant (intermediate [MIC 0.1–1 μg/mL] or absolute [MIC ≥2 μg/mL]) and cefotaxime susceptible (MIC ≤0.5 μg/mL)	Cefotaxime *or* Ceftriaxone	Vancomycin *or* Chloramphenicol *or* Meropenem
Penicillin resistant (intermediate [MIC 0.1–1 μg/mL] or absolute [MIC ≥2 μg/mL]) and cefotaxime resistant (intermediate [MIC 1 μg/mL] or absolute [MIC ≥2 μg/mL])	Vancomycin with cefotaxime *or* Ceftriaxone *or* Chloramphenicol	Vancomycin plus rifampin with or without cefotaxime (or ceftriaxone) *or* Meropenem*
Neisseria meningitidis	Penicillin G	Ampicillin *or* Cefotaxime (or ceftriaxone) *or* Meropenem *or* Chloramphenicol (for penicillin-resistant strains)
Haemophilus influenzae type b	Cefotaxime *or* Ceftriaxone	Ampicillin (if susceptible) *or* Meropenem *or* Chloramphenicol
Group B *Streptococcus*	Penicillin G *or* Ampicillin plus an aminoglycoside *or* Cefotaxime	Ceftriaxone *or* Vancomycin *or* Chloramphenicol
Listeria monocytogenes	Ampicillin with or without an aminoglycoside	Vancomycin plus an aminoglycoside or TMP-SMZ
Escherichia coli, Klebsiella, Enterobacter	Cefotaxime or ceftriaxone	Aminoglycoside (e.g., gentamicin, amikacin) *or* Meropenem or a quinolone
Salmonella	Cefotaxime or ceftriaxone	Ampicillin (if susceptible) *or* Chloramphenicol *or* TMP-SMZ
Staphylococcus aureus, coagulase-negative staphylococci		
Methicillin susceptible	Nafcillin or oxacillin	Vancomycin
Methicillin resistant	Vancomycin	Vancomycin plus rifampin
Group A *Streptococcus*	Penicillin G	Ampicillin
Enterococcus faecalis	Ampicillin plus an aminoglycoside	Vancomycin plus an aminoglycoside
Pseudomonas	Ceftazidime with or without an aminoglycoside	Ticarcillin (or piperacillin) plus an aminoglycoside
Fungi		
Candida	Amphotericin B with or without flucytosine	
Histoplasma capsulatum	Amphotericin B	
Cryptococcus neoformans	Amphotericin B with or without flucytosine	

*Should be used cautiously.

Table continued on following page

TABLE 52–16. Recommended Antibiotic Therapy for Meningitis According to the Etiologic Agent *(Continued)*

Etiologic Agent	Recommended Therapy	Alternative Therapy
Ameba		
Naegleria fowleri	Amphotericin B plus intrathecal amphotericin B (0.1 mg) plus rifampin	

Suggested Dosages for Persons with Normal Renal Function

DRUG	DOSAGE	MAXIMUM DAILY DOSE	DRUG	DOSAGE	MAXIMUM DAILY DOSE
Amikacin	22.5 mg/kg/day divided q8–12hr IV	750–900 mg	Meropenem	120 mg/kg/day divided q8hr IV	6 g
Ampicillin	200–400 mg/kg/day divided q6hr IV	12 g	Nafcillin	150–200 mg/kg/day divided q6hr IV	9 g
Cefotaxime*	200–300 mg/kg/day divided q6hr IV	12 g	Oxacillin	150–200 mg/kg/day divided q6hr IV	12 g
Ceftriaxone	100 mg/kg/day divided q12hr IV or IM or 80 mg/kg/day divided q24hr IV or IM	3–4 g 3–4 g	Penicillin G	250,000–500,000 U/kg/day divided q6hr IV	20–24 MU
Chloramphenicol	75–100 mg/kg/day divided q6hr IV or 75 mg/kg/day divided q6hr PO	2–4 g 2–4 g	Rifampin	20 mg/kg/day divided q12hr IV	600 mg
TMP-SMZ	15 mg/kg/day (as trimethoprim) divided q8hr IV	1.2 g (as trimethoprim)	Tobramycin	7.5 mg/kg/day divided q8hr IV	250–300 mg
Gentamicin	7.5 mg/kg/day divided q8hr IV	250–300 mg	Vancomycin	45–60 mg/kg/day divided q6hr IV	2 g

Suggested Dosages for Neonates*
(Use lower dose and longer dosing interval for neonates younger than 7 days of age; see Chapter 14 and Table 96–4)

DRUG	DOSAGE	DRUG	DOSAGE
Amikacin	15–22.5 mg/kg/day divided q8–12hr IV	TMP-SMZ	10 mg/kg/day (as trimethoprim) divided q8–12hr IV
Ampicillin	150–200 mg/kg/day divided q6–12hr IV	Gentamicin	5–7.5 mg/kg/day divided q8–12hr IV
Cefotaxime	100–200 mg/kg/day divided q8–12hr IV	Penicillin G	150,000–300,000 U/kg/day divided q6–8hr IV
Ceftriaxone	50–100 mg/kg/day q24hr IV (do not use in neonates younger than 7 days of age)	Vancomycin	30–45 mg/kg/day divided q8–12hr IV
Chloramphenicol	25–50 mg/kg/day divided q12–24hr IV		

Suggested Dosages of Antifungal Agents

	DOSAGE		DOSAGE
Amphotericin B	1 mg/kg once daily for 3–4hr IV	Flucytosine	150 mg/kg/day divided q6hr PO

*Cefotaxime 300 mg/kg/day is recommended when used for emipirical therapy (until identification and susceptibilities are known) and for cefotaxime-resistant (intermediate or absolute) *S. pneumoniae.* Cefotaxime 200–225 mg/kg/day is adequate for susceptible organisms.

for amebic meningoencephalitis, but one person was successfully treated with intravenous and intrathecal amphotericin B and miconazole, plus rifampin. For *Candida* meningitis, amphotericin B is the drug of choice. The addition of flucytosine appears to be reasonable because the two drugs have synergistic activity, and several reports have documented a good cure rate. *Histoplasma* meningitis has a better cure rate if amphotericin B is given at a dosage of 1 mg/kg once daily than if a lower dosage (0.25–0.5 mg/kg once daily) is given. Results of fluconazole therapy for *Histoplasma* meningitis in adults are not encouraging. In addition, itraconazole should not be used for *Histoplasma* meningitis because the drug penetrates the CSF poorly. For cryptococcal meningitis the combination of amphotericin and flucytosine is recommended. The relapse rate is proportional to the severity of the immunosuppression of the affected person. Among HIV-infected persons the relapse rate exceeds 50%; in other persons the relapse rate is less than 25%. Fluconazole (4–6 mg/kg once daily) is the drug of choice for maintenance therapy to prevent relapses. Fluconazole is inferior to amphotericin B as primary therapy for cryptococcal meningitis. It has a higher failure rate than amphotericin, and thus it should not be used for primary treatment but only for suppression and prevention. Coccidioidal meningitis responds best to amphotericin B. Recent studies suggest that the oral administration of fluconazole may be successful in suppressing the infection.

Supportive Therapy

Persons with bacterial meningitis are usually hospitalized. Those with mild viral disease can be treated as outpatients at the physician's discretion. The temperature, blood pressure, pulse rate, respiratory rate, and neurologic status should be monitored periodically. More frequent monitoring is required for persons with severe disease, beginning soon after hospitalization. Initially, oral feeding should be avoided to prevent vomiting and aspiration and to allow careful assessment for inappropriate antidiuretic hormone (ADH) secretion. The **syndrome of inappropriate ADH (SIADH) secretion** is found in more than 75% of persons with bacterial meningitis but is rare in other causes of meningitis. Retention of fluid in excess of salts may occur, and thus body weight and serum sodium concentration should be carefully monitored in the first 24–48 hours of treatment while the patient receives intravenous fluids (750–1,000 mL/m^2/day). When the serum sodium concentration is 136 mEq/L or greater, fluid restriction can be discontinued. In persons with dehydration, fluid restriction should be avoided, but close monitoring of the serum sodium concentration allows careful reassessment of fluid and electrolyte balance.

Corticosteroids. Prompt antibiotic therapy for bacterial meningitis results in release of cytokines that augment the inflammatory response and amplify the damage to the brain tissue. Several studies in children with *H. influenzae* type b meningitis have shown that dexamethasone (0.6 mg/kg/day divided every 6 hours for 2–4 days) reduces the likelihood of neurologic complications, primarily hearing loss. Thus the American Academy of Pediatrics Committee on Infectious Diseases recommended dexamethasone for the treatment of *H. influenzae* type b meningitis. Because the efficacy of dexamethasone in children with pneumococcal or meningococcal meningitis has not been demonstrated satisfactorily, expert opinion is divided. Several multicenter prospective studies from the United States and Europe concluded that dexamethasone did not improve hearing status or neurologic or developmental outcome when compared with placebo. In addition, a recent meta-analysis (McIntyre et al, 1997) of 10 studies that included children with pneumococcal meningitis did not find any significant benefit from therapy with dexamethasone in regard to hearing loss or neurologic deficit. The differences in the inflammatory response to infection caused by gram-negative bacteria (e.g., *H. influenzae* type b) and gram-positive bacteria (e.g., *S. pneumoniae*) may be the reason for the different effects of dexamethasone on the outcome of these infections. Another concern about using dexamethasone is that the drug may diminish penetration of antibiotics into the CSF, an especially important consideration when treating penicillin-resistant *S. pneumoniae* meningitis with vancomycin. Thus the routine use of dexamethasone as adjunctive therapy for all bacterial meningitis seems to be unjustified; the drug should be used only if there is strong evidence that *H. influenzae* type b is the etiologic agent in a child who did not receive at least two doses of a conjugated *H. influenzae* type b vaccine. Because *H. influenzae* type b meningitis is a rare disease in the United States, and because the routine use of dexamethasone in the treatment of other causes of meningitis has not yet been shown to be efficacious, it seems reasonable not to use the drug.

Anticonvulsants. Persons with seizures should be given appropriate anticonvulsants. Phenobarbital (5–10 mg/kg/per dose repeated at 20-minute intervals until seizures are controlled or a total dose of 40 mg/kg is reached) administered intravenously is the most commonly used drug. Lorazepam (0.05 mg/kg intravenously) is an anticonvulsant with a rapid onset of action that can be used acutely for terminating seizure activity. Phenytoin (15–20 mg/kg), a long-acting anticonvulsant, is effective in controlling seizures without affecting the level of consciousness and can be used for termination of seizures or for maintenance. The combination of phenobarbital and phenytoin controls seizures in most children. If seizure activity resolves after the first 48 hours and the neurologic examination findings are normal at discharge, anticonvulsants can be discontinued. An EEG is indicated only if the seizures continue for longer than 3 days or if they are focal.

Increased Intracranial Pressure. Persons with increased intracranial pressure should have the head of the bed elevated to 30 degrees. If signs of cerebral herniation are noted, the patient should undergo intubation and mechanical hyperventilation to decrease the $PaCO_2$, which causes cerebral vasoconstriction. Hyperventilation may be effective for only 24–36 hours, after which it should be discontinued. Mannitol (0.25–1 g/kg infused for 10–30 minutes) may be helpful in reducing brain edema. If the first dose has no effect, further intravenous boluses can be given. The benefit of corticosteroids for edema with bacterial meningitis is controversial. Because corticosteroids have been proved effective in reducing edema around brain tumors, dexamethasone (10 mg/m^2/day divided every 6 hours) is recommended. The disadvantage of corticosteroids is that they reduce the concentration of antibiotics in the CSF by reducing the inflammatory response. Therefore, if corticosteroid therapy is used, it should be discontinued after 2–4 days. Pentobarbital in a high dose (loading dose of 20–30 mg/kg, followed by a maintenance dose of 1 mg/kg/hr) was found to be useful when treatment with hyperventilation and mannitol failed.

COMPLICATIONS

Fever During Antimicrobial Therapy. Fever usually resolves within days after appropriate antimicrobial therapy. Approximately 75% of persons with *S. pneumoniae* or *N. meningitidis* become afebrile by day 4 of treatment, and 90% are afebrile by day 6. In contrast, persons with *H. influenzae* meningitis have a longer duration of fever, with only 75% afebrile by day 6 and 90% afebrile by day 10. Thus **prolonged fever** (more than 10 days) is relatively common in *H. influenzae* meningitis (10–15% of cases) and less common in *S. pneumoniae* and *N. meningitidis* meningitides (6–9% of cases). **Secondary fever,** defined as recurrence of fever after an afebrile period of at least 24 hours, occurs in approximately 25% of affected persons. Although recrudescence of the infection must be considered for persons with a prolonged or secondary fever, this complication is rare, occurring in $<1\%$ of patients. The most likely causes of fever are CNS complications, such as subdural effusion or empyema, drug fever, or another focus of infection, such as pneumonia or arthritis (Table 52–17). Sterile subdural effusion seems to be a common cause of prolonged fever or secondary fever. Another focus of infection is a common cause of prolonged fever (almost a third of the patients) but is uncommon (3% of patients) in secondary fever. In contrast, nosocomial infections, such as urinary tract infections, upper respiratory tract infections, and phlebitis, are common in secondary fever (30% of patients) but relatively uncommon ($<10\%$ of patients) in prolonged fever. Drug fever is a common cause of prolonged fever (20% of patients) but an uncommon cause of secondary fever (5% of patients). For many persons the cause of fever remains unknown (15% of persons with prolonged fever and 30–40% of persons with secondary fever). Thus for a person with meningitis who has an abnormal fever pattern, if the physical examination and laboratory studies (e.g., CT scan of the head, urinalysis, complete blood cell count and differential cell count, chest radiographs) do not reveal evidence of an untreated infection and the person appears well, careful observation is necessary and the option to change or discontinue antibiotic therapy should be considered. If no cause of the fever is found and the child still has a fever more than 48 hours after a change in or discontinuation of antibiotic therapy, any change in the child's appearance such as irritability or development of persistent neurologic signs necessitates a repeated lumbar puncture. If the CSF has a substantial proportion of polymorphonuclear cells and a low glucose level, renewed efforts to rule out the possibility of persistent infection in the CNS are prudent. Corticosteroids tend

TABLE 52–17. Causes of Fever in Infants and Children Treated for Bacterial Meningitis

Cause	Prolonged Fever	Secondary Fever
Unknown	Common	Very common
Subdural	Common	Common
Another focus (e.g., pneumonia, arthritis)	Common	Rare
Drug fever	Common	Rare
Empyema	Rare	Rare
Nosocomial infection	Rare	Common
Phlebitis	Rare	Rare

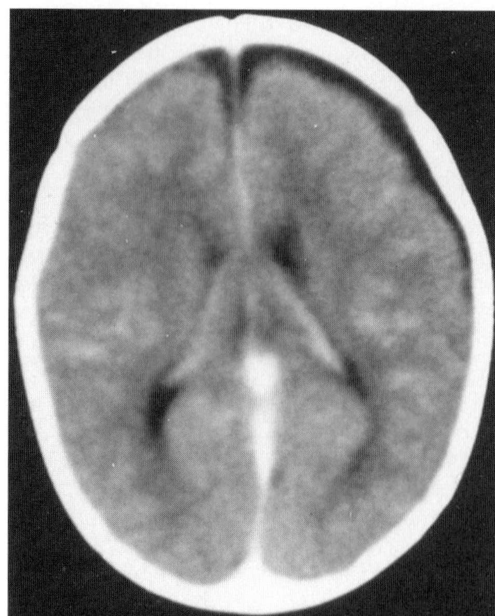

FIGURE 52–3. Subdural effusion after meningitis. Eight-month-old infant with recent *H. influenzae* type b meningitis. Contrast-enhanced CT of the head shows asymmetric subdural effusions, left greater than right, along the frontoparietal region. Note the lack of any enhancement of the adjacent brain tissue. (Courtesy of Alison S. Smith.)

to shorten the febrile period. In persons receiving the drug for 2–4 days as adjunct therapy, the fever may recur when the drug therapy is discontinued. The recurrence does not represent a secondary fever but a temporarily suppressed prolonged fever.

Neither the duration of the fever nor its pattern adversely affects whether neurologic abnormalities are noted at the time of discharge.

Subdural Empyema or Effusion. Local extension of bacterial infection to produce subdural empyema (or a brain abscess) is a rare complication (Chapter 54). If CT or MRI documents extension to the subdural space, a subdural tap should be performed and the person should be examined for other sites of infection (e.g., endocarditis).

In contrast to subdural empyema, sterile subdural effusions are a frequent complication of bacterial meningitis, occurring in 30–40% of patients. Young age (<1 year) and rapid onset of disease are associated with a higher incidence of subdural effusion. Most effusions are detected during the first 5–7 days of the disease. Persons with effusion are more likely to have seizures or other neurologic abnormalities at presentation, but there is no increase in developmental delay or neurologic abnormalities in comparison with persons without effusion. CT or ultrasonography through an open anterior fontanel may be helpful in confirming the presence of effusions (Figure 52–3). Most of these effusions resolve slowly within weeks to months of the acute episode, without any intervention. Subdural paracentesis is necessary only if symptoms of increased intracranial pressure are present or if the effusions are believed to contribute to focal neurologic symptoms or seizures.

PROGNOSIS

The survival rate for bacterial meningitis has increased with the appropriate use of antimicrobial agents and supportive therapy. However, several factors are believed to contribute to the long-term sequelae of the disease, although the importance of some of these factors is controversial. The specific cause (bacterial or viral), the age of the patient (newborn or child), the concentration of the bacteria in the initial CSF specimen (>10^7 cfu/mL), the concentrations of cytokines in the blood or the CSF, the time from initiation of therapy to sterilization of the CSF, the presence of focal neurologic findings at admission suggesting involvement of brain parenchyma, the occurrence of seizures during the acute phase, and a low ratio of glucose in the CSF to glucose in the blood are some of the factors that indicate the risk of sequelae.

Many neurologic abnormalities detected soon after the acute illness resolve slowly over the course of weeks to months after treatment. Approximately 33% of survivors have neurologic abnormalities at the time of discharge, but only 11% have neurologic deficits 5 years later. Thus close follow-up for an extended period is recommended to evaluate the outcome for individual patients. The family should not be discouraged about the ultimate outcome.

Bacterial Meningitis. The mortality for bacterial meningitis in children is estimated to be 3–10%; the rate is higher for neonatal meningitis. In the United States the mortality due to *S. pneumoniae* meningitis is 7–10%. The mortality for *N. meningitidis* is 5% and is higher if accompanied by fulminant meningococcal septicemia (Table 21–18). The mortality rate for *H. influenzae* type b meningitis is only about 3% in the United States but is 20% in developing countries. This discrepancy is mainly due to differences in access to care, although malnutrition probably also plays an important role. The mortality for neonatal group B *Streptococcus* meningitis is 8–20%, depending on gestational age, and for neonatal *E. coli* meningitis it is 25–30%.

Approximately 60–70% of survivors are considered to be healthy. **Sensorineural hearing loss** is one of the most common sequelae of bacterial meningitis. It occurs in 30–40% of persons with *S. pneumoniae* meningitis, 10–15% of persons with *H. influenzae* meningitis, and 5% of persons with *N. meningitidis* meningitis. The hearing loss usually occurs early in the course of the infection and only occasionally improves. Persons with severe disease, seizures, prolonged fever, and low CSF glucose levels at the time of admission have a higher incidence of hearing loss. The incidence of hearing loss can be reduced in persons with *H. influenzae* type b meningitis if dexamethasone is given before or with the first dose of antibiotic. A similar effect has not been demonstrated in persons with pneumococcal or meningococcal meningitis. Because hearing loss is relatively common in persons with bacterial meningitis, audiometric evaluation should be performed before discharge, and if results are abnormal, repeated tests are recommended.

Ataxia is often associated with severe hearing loss, probably because of concomitant involvement of the auditory and vestibular systems in the inner ear. In most children the balance disturbances resolve within several months.

Controversy exists about the frequency of minimal brain dysfunction and speech and language delays in this population. Although some studies have suggested that the mean IQ of children who had meningitis is considerably lower than that of children serving as control subjects, other studies have demonstrated a much better outcome. A recent study (Grimwood, 1995) examining the outcome of bacterial meningitis in school-age survivors found that 27% of them had abnormal neurologic and audiometric findings that adversely affect their learning ability, academic performance, and behavior. Although many of these children had neurologic complications during or after meningitis, a proportion of them seem to be normal. Therefore all survivors of bacterial meningitis should be carefully followed up for learning disabilities. Academic performance after minor brain injury can remain normal in some of these children if academic support is available at school and at home to compensate for the subtle deficits in learning and performance efficiency. Most of the older studies about outcome were performed largely with children recovering from *H. influenzae* meningitis, and it is not clear whether these results can be applied directly to persons recovering from *S. pneumoniae* meningitis or *N. meningitidis* meningitis, currently the most common types of bacterial meningitis.

Among children without evidence of cerebral injury, the incidence of late-onset seizures (or epilepsy) is low. Thus, if a child has normal findings on neurologic examination soon after the acute illness, the likelihood that seizures will develop is negligible. In contrast, children with persistent neurologic abnormalities are at greater risk of having a seizure disorder within 5 years of the acute illness. Although seizures during the acute illness statistically are associated with the development of late-onset seizures and neurologic sequelae, most children with seizures during the acute illness recover completely without any sequelae.

Severe neurologic sequelae such as hemiplegia, quadriplegia, hyperactivity, and mental retardation are the result of severe damage to the brain parenchyma and are found in fewer than 5% of children recovering from bacterial meningitis. The frequency of these sequelae is higher after meningitis during the neonatal period. Hydrocephalus is an uncommon complication of childhood meningitis, but it occurs more frequently after neonatal meningitis. In most cases the complication develops insidiously within weeks to months, and a careful follow-up is recommended. Blindness is a very rare complication; it may result from optic neuritis or occipital cortical damage. In many cases the patient recovers with time.

Viral Meningitis. A large prospective study (Rorabaugh et al, 1993) of infants younger than 2 years with aseptic meningitis, in whom a viral cause was suggested, revealed that although 9% of infants with aseptic meningitis had acute CNS complications such as a complex seizure, increased intracranial pressure, and coma, most patients improved quickly and had no long-term sequelae. In addition, the long-term prognosis for infants with acute neurologic complications appeared to be as favorable as the prognosis for infants without these complications. Considerably more acute complications were noted in infants older than 3 months than in younger infants. The outcome of viral meningitis is most favorable, although neurologic, behavioral, and psychological evaluations should be part of the follow-up to identify early the few patients who will benefit from more intensive interventions.

PREVENTION

Contacts. Prophylactic therapy for all intimate contacts of persons with *N. meningitidis* infection is recommended (Chapter 16). A practical criterion for prophylaxis is for individuals who have frequently slept, eaten in, or otherwise resided in the same dwelling as the index case, which include household members; daycare contacts; military recruits; college students, boarding school students, and persons using other dormitory housing; and medical personnel performing mouth-to-mouth resuscitation (Table 16–3). Rifampin or ceftriaxone is usually used for prophylaxis (Table 16–4). Schoolroom classmates and medical personnel performing routine care usually do not need chemoprophylaxis.

The risk of secondary disease with *H. influenzae* in household contacts younger than 4 years is low (0.5–1%). Prophylaxis is recommended to all household contacts if one of the contacts is a child less than 4 years of age with incomplete *H. influenzae* type b immunization (Chapter 16). Rifampin is used for prophylaxis (Table 16–5). Chemoprophylaxis for attendees of a daycare center with one case of *H. influenzae* invasive disease is not recommended.

The prevention of viral meningitis is difficult. Particular attention to hand washing and personal hygiene reduces the transmission of enteroviruses. The development of vaccines against specific viruses will be an effective measure in reducing the rate of meningitis, as was shown by the poliomyelitis and mumps vaccines. For reduction of arboviral meningitis, effective methods to control the insect vectors are needed.

The prevention of fungal meningitis depends on the etiologic agent. *Candida* colonization may be minimized by judicious and sparing use of broad-spectrum antibiotics for as short a time as possible, as well as by meticulous care of intravascular catheters. For persons with neutropenia, prophylactic therapy with oral antifungal drugs may prevent the colonization and spread of *Candida.* For prevention of *Aspergillus* meningitis, the sources of this fungus (e.g., air-conditioner filters and construction projects) should be carefully monitored. It is almost impossible to prevent cryptococcal or coccidioidal meningitis in immunocompromised persons. Because these fungi are acquired by inhalation and are not transmitted from person to person, there are no effective means to prevent their spread.

Vaccination. Vaccines have been proved to be the most effective measure in preventing bacterial meningitis. Immunization of infants with conjugate vaccines of *H. influenzae* type b (Chapter 17) has been followed by a dramatic decrease in meningitis caused by this organism. The seven-valent conjugate pneumococcal vaccine is also effective in preventing invasive pneumococcal disease, including meningitis, in infants less than 2 years of age (Chapter 17).

Several vaccines to prevent *N. meningitidis* infection are available, including the monovalent A or C, the bivalent A/C, and the quadrivalent A/C/Y/W-135. There is no effective vaccine against meningococcal serogroup B. The response to the meningococcal vaccines is different at different ages. Although the current vaccine against serogroup A is protective in infants as young as 3 months, the current vaccine against serogroup C is protective only in children older than 2 years. Field trials of an investigational conjugate meningococcal C vaccine suggest that it may be protective in infants younger than 2 years, but it is not currently available in the United States.

Recently there has been increased concern regarding meningococcal disease in college students, with data showing that freshmen living in dormitories are at increased risk. College students and their parents should be informed about risks of meningitis and the advantages of vaccination, and meningococcal vaccination should be offered. Some colleges and states are recommending or even requiring meningococcal vaccination for all matriculating freshmen.

REVIEWS

Dawson KG, Emerson JC, Burns JL: Fifteen years of experience with bacterial meningitis. *Pediatr Infect Dis J* 1999;18:816–22.

Kaplan SL: Adjuvant therapy in meningitis. *Adv Pediatr Infect Dis* 1995;10:167–86.

McIntyre PB, Berkey CS, King SM, et al: Dexamethasone as adjunctive therapy in bacterial meningitis. A meta-analysis of randomized clinical trials since 1988. *JAMA* 1997;278:925–31.

Pfister HW, Fontana A, Täuber MG, et al: Mechanisms of brain injury in bacterial meningitis: Workshop summary. *Clin Infect Dis* 1994; 19:463–79.

Quagliarello VJ, Scheld WM: Treatment of bacterial meningitis. *N Engl J Med* 1997;336:708–16.

Riedo FX, Plikaytis BD, Broome CV: Epidemiology and prevention of meningococcal disease. *Pediatr Infect Dis J* 1995;14:643–57.

Tuomanen EI: The biology of pneumococcal infection. *Pediatr Res* 1997;42:253–8.

KEY ARTICLES

Ahmed A: A critical evaluation of vancomycin for treatment of bacterial meningitis. *Pediatr Infect Dis J* 1997a;16:895–903.

Ahmed A, Brito F, Goto C, et al: Clinical utility of the polymerase chain reaction for diagnosis of enteroviral meningitis in infancy. *J Pediatr* 1997b;131:393–7.

Arditi M, Ables L, Yogev R: Cerebrospinal fluid endotoxin levels in children with *H. influenzae* meningitis before and after administration of intravenous ceftriaxone. *J Infect Dis* 1989;160:1005–11.

Arditi M, Mason EO Jr, Bradley JS, et al: Three-year multicenter surveillance of pneumococcal meningitis in children: Clinical characteristics, and outcome related to penicillin susceptibility and dexamethasone use. *Pediatrics* 1998;102:1087–97.

Ashwal S, Perkin RM, Thompson JR, et al: Bacterial meningitis in children: Current concepts of neurologic management. *Adv Pediatr* 1993; 40:185–215.

Barquet N, Domingo P, Cayla JA, et al: Prognostic factors in meningococcal disease: Development of a bedside predictive model and scoring system. Barcelona Meningococcal Disease Surveillance Group. *JAMA* 1997; 278:491–6.

Berlin LE, Rorabaugh ML, Heldrich F, et al: Aspeptic meningitis in infants <2 years of age: Diagnosis and etiology. *J Infect Dis* 1993;168:888–92.

Booy R, Kroll JS: Bacterial meningitis and meningococcal infection. *Curr Opin Pediatr* 1998;10:13–8.

Doit C, Barre J, Cohen R, et al: Bacterial activity against intermediately cephalosporin-resistant *Streptococcus pneumoniae* in cerebrospinal fluid of children with bacterial meningitis treated with high doses of cefotaxime and vancomycin. *Antimicrob Agents Chemother* 1997;41:2050–2.

Fiore AE, Moroney JF, Farley MM, et al: Clinical outcomes of meningitis caused by *Streptococcus pneumoniae* in the era of antibiotic resistance. *Clin Infect Dis* 2000;30:71–7.

Franco SM, Cornelius VE, Andrews BF: Long-term outcome of neonatal meningitis. *Am J Dis Child* 1992;146:567–71.

François M, Laccourreye L, Huy ET, et al: Hearing impairment in infants after meningitis: Detection by transient evoked otoacoustic emissions. *J Pediatr* 1997;130:712–7.

Friedland IR, Klugman KP: Cerebrospinal fluid bactericidal activity against cephalosporin-resistant *Streptococcus pneumoniae* in children with meningitis treated with high-dosage cefotaxime. *Antimicrob Agents Chemother* 1997;41:1888–91.

Green SM, Rothrock SG, Clem KJ, et al: Can seizures be the sole manifestation of meningitis in febrile children? *Pediatrics* 1993;92:527–34.

Grimwood K, Anderson VA, Bond L, et al: Adverse outcomes of bacterial meningitis in school-age survivors. *Pediatrics* 1995;95:646–56.

Hamilton MS, Jackson MA, Abel D: Clinical utility of polymerase chain reaction testing for enteroviral meningitis. *Pediatr Infect Dis J* 1999; 18:533–8.

Joffé A, McCormick M, DeAngelis C: Which children with febrile seizures need lumbar puncture? A decision analysis approach. *Am J Dis Child* 1983;137:1153–6.

John CC: Treatment failure with use of a third-generation cephalosporin for penicillin-resistant pneumococcal meningitis: Case report and review. *Clin Infect Dis* 1994;18:188–93.

Kilpi T, Anttila M, Kallio MJ, et al: Length of prediagnostic history related to the course and sequelae of childhood bacterial meningitis. *Pediatr Infect Dis J* 1993;12:184–8.

Klugman KP, Dagan R: Randomized comparison of meropenem with cefotaxime for treatment of bacterial meningitis. Meropenem Meningitis Study Group. *Antimicrob Agents Chemother* 1995;39:1140–6.

Kornelisse RF, Westerbeek CM, Spoor AB, et al: Pneumococcal meningitis in children: Prognostic indicators and outcome. *Clin Infect Dis* 1995; 21:1390–7.

Ma P, Visvesvara GS, Martinez AJ, et al: *Naegleria* and *Acanthamoeba* infections: Review. *Rev Infect Dis* 1990;12:490–513.

Marshall GS, Hauck MA, Buck G, et al: Potential cost savings through rapid diagnosis of enteroviral meningitis. *Pediatr Infect Dis J* 1997;16:1086–7.

McKinney RE Jr, Katz SL, Wilfert CM: Chronic enteroviral meningoencephalitis in agammaglobulinemic patients. *Rev Infect Dis* 1987; 9:334–56.

Nava JM, Bella F, Garau J, et al: Predictive factors for invasive disease due to pencillin-resistant *Streptococcus pneumoniae:* A population-based study. *Clin Infect Dis* 1994;19:884–90.

Pomeroy SL, Holmes SJ, Dodge PR, et al: Seizures and other neurologic sequelae of bacterial meningitis in children. *N Engl J Med* 1990; 323:1651–7.

Prober CG: The role of steroids in the management of children with bacterial meningitis. *Pediatrics* 1995;95:29–31.

Radetsky M: Duration of symptoms and outcome in bacterial meningitis: An analysis of causation and the implications of a delay in diagnosis. *Pediatr Infect Dis J* 1992;11:694–8.

Rodewald LE, Woodkin KA, Szilagyi PG, et al: Relevance of common tests of cerebrospinal fluid in screening for bacterial meningitis. *J Pediatr* 1991;119:363–9.

Rorabaugh ML, Berlin LE, Heldrich F, et al: Aseptic meningitis in infants younger than 2 years of age: Acute illness and neurologic complications. *Pediatrics* 1993;92:206–11.

Rothrock SG, Harper MB, Green SM, et al: Do oral antibiotics prevent meningitis and serious bacterial infections in children with *Streptococcus pneumoniae* occult bacteremia? A meta-analysis. *Pediatrics* 1997; 99:438–44.

Schuchat A, Robinson K, Wenger JD, et al: Bacterial meningitis in the United States in 1995. Active Surveillance Team. *N Engl J Med* 1997;337:970–6.

Sharief MK, Ciardi M, Thompson EJ: Blood-brain barrier damage in patients with bacterial meningitis: Association with tumor necrosis factor-alpha but not interleukin-1 beta. *J Infect Dis* 1992;166:350–8.

Singhi SC, Singhi PD, Srinivas B, et al: Fluid restriction does not improve the outcome of acute meningitis. *Pediatr Infect Dis J* 1995;14:495–503.

Snedeker JD, Kaplan SL, Dodge PR, et al: Subdural effusion and its relationship with neurologic sequelae of bacterial meningitis in infancy: A prospective study. *Pediatrics* 1990;86:163–70.

Spellerberg B, Prasad S, Cabellos C, et al: Penetration of the blood-brain barrier: Enhancement of drug delivery and imaging by bacterial glycopeptides. *J Exp Med* 1995;182:1037–43.

Unhanand M, Mustafa MM, McCracken GH Jr, et al: Gram-negative enteric bacillary meningitis: A twenty-one-year experience. *J Pediatr* 1993; 122:15–21.

Waler JA, Rathore MH: Outpatient management of pediatric bacterial meningitis. *Pediatr Infect Dis J* 1995;14:89–92.

CHAPTER 53

Central Nervous System Shunt-Related Infections

Ram Yogev

Hydrocephalus is commonly seen in persons with anatomic abnormalities such as meningomyelocele and Chiari malformations and in premature newborns with intraventricular hemorrhage. Other causes include intracranial infections (e.g., congenital cytomegalovirus infection, congenital toxoplasmosis infection, bacterial meningitis), central nervous system malignancies, benign tumors (e.g., cysts), and intraventricular bleeding after head trauma. The most common procedure to divert CSF fluid for symptomatic hydrocephalus is insertion of a shunt. The standard shunt system has three components: a proximal ventricular catheter, a unidirectional flow valve, and a distal catheter, which is usually inserted into the peritoneal cavity to create a **ventriculoperitoneal shunt (VP shunt),** into the right atrium to create a **ventriculoatrial shunt (VA shunt),** or, less frequently, into the pleural cavity or the gallbladder. CSF shunts are prone to complications, with a 10-year failure rate of more than 50%, mainly because of obstruction or overdrainage (from siphoning).

ETIOLOGY

Gram-positive bacteria, especially *Staphylococcus,* are the most common cause of infections involving shunts. Coagulase-negative staphylococci (e.g., *S. epidermidis, S. capitis,* and *S. hominis*) are isolated in 40–70% of cases. *Staphylococcus aureus,* the second most common gram-positive bacterial cause, is isolated in 10–40% of cases. Other gram-positive organisms that cause these infections include other group C *Streptococcus* strains, group A *Streptococcus, Enterococcus, Propionibacterium,* and *Corynebacterium* (diphtheroids). Poor culture techniques (e.g., failure to use anaerobic culture media; incubation for less than 5–7 days) may lead to underreporting of *Propionibacterium* and *Corynebacterium* infections involving shunts.

Gram-negative bacteria (e.g., *Escherichia coli, Klebsiella,* and *Proteus*) cause 5–25% of shunt-related infections. *Pseudomonas* and *Acinetobacter* are reported much less commonly. The infections caused by gram-negative bacteria are more common in patients with myelomeningocele and in patients in whom the distal end of the VP shunt was inserted into the peritoneal cavity by a percutaneous trocar, which may result in inadvertent perforation of the intestinal tract.

Many other microorganisms, such as *Streptococcus pneumoniae, Neisseria meningitidis, Haemophilus influenzae, Pasteurella multocida,* and fungi, have been reported but are uncommon causes of shunt-related infections.

EPIDEMIOLOGY

The reported incidence of shunt-related infections varies considerably and ranges from <1% to 40%. Almost two thirds of the central nervous system infections occur within 1 month of placement of the shunt, and 90% of infections are manifested within 6 months. The incidence of these infections is significantly higher in infants in the first 6 months of life than in older children, and it is even higher in newborns with intraventricular hemorrhage treated with a shunt in the first week of life. The reasons for the increased incidence of infections involving shunts in very young children are not completely understood, but suggested mechanisms have included delayed wound healing, higher skin density of bacteria that are more resistant to antibiotics and more adherent to the shunt than in older children, longer duration of hospitalization, and increased exposure to antibiotics just before the shunt is placed.

There is no significant difference between the incidence of infections involving VP shunts and that involving VA shunts, but lower infection rates are found with lumboperitoneal and cholecystic shunts. Increased infection risk exists for shunts placed after removal of a previous contaminated shunt, probably because of incomplete bacterial eradication. Several other factors have been reported to affect the incidence of infection, including the cause of the hydrocephalus, the neurosurgeon's experience, the duration of surgery, the number of people in the operating room, and the operative technique (e.g., use of prophylactic antibiotics, method of skin preparation, open surgery to insert the abdominal catheter vs direct puncture of the abdominal wall with a trocar).

PATHOGENESIS

Central nervous system shunts become contaminated at the time of surgery, by hematogenous spread, or by extension of infection that contaminates the distal end and spreads in a retrograde manner through the catheter. Most infections are a result of contamination at the time of surgery, as evidenced by the occurrence of almost two thirds of infections within 1 month of surgery, and skin flora are the predominant causative organisms. Coagulase-negative staphylococci are particularly important causes of shunt-related infection, which is due to the production of an **exopolysaccharide slime,** or **glycocalyx,** that facilitates binding to the foreign body and protects the organism from host defenses by inhibiting neutrophil phagocytosis. Slime production increases the likelihood of shunt obstruction and reduces antibiotic penetration, which predisposes the patient to treatment failure when antibiotics alone are used.

Skin flora are the most common organisms associated with infections involving shunts, but VA shunts are more susceptible to contamination with organisms associated with bacteremia, and VP shunts are more prone to contamination from intestinal organisms. There may be no specific abdominal symptoms or only abdominal pain associated with distal VP shunt-related infections. Rarely the catheter tip of a VP shunt may erode or even puncture a viscus.

SYMPTOMS AND CLINICAL MANIFESTATIONS

Most persons with shunt-related infection present with nonspecific signs and symptoms, such as mild to moderate fever, malaise, irritability, nausea and vomiting, vague abdominal pain, and headache. Few persons have the classic signs and symptoms of central nervous system inflammation, such as stiff neck, bulging fontanelle (in infants), change of mental status, cranial nerve palsies, and papilledema. In some persons the **shunt tract** may be infected, with evidence of cellulitis or dehiscence of the surgical wounds (e.g., of the head; of the abdomen, as with a VP shunt) or tenderness, edema, and erythema along the tract itself. The type of shunt may also affect the presentation of the infection. For example, infections involving VP shunts may present with symptoms and signs confined only to the abdominal cavity, such as abdominal pain, tenderness with or without guarding, intestinal obstruction, or an abdominal mass (i.e., **pseudocyst**). Infections involving VA shunts may present with signs and symptoms of bacteremia, sepsis, or rarely endocarditis or as immune-complex disease manifested clinically as arthritis, skin rash, or nephritis **(shunt nephritis).**

DIAGNOSIS

In most cases the major difficulty in diagnosing shunt-related infections is the nonspecific and insidious onset of associated signs and symptoms. Therefore any person with a central nervous system shunt who develops fever without an obvious source should be evaluated for such an infection. A higher index of suspicion is needed for persons who develop fever within 3–6 months after shunt placement.

Because the clinical features of an infection involving a shunt are often nonspecific, appropriate laboratory tests are essential. Tapping the shunt or sampling fluid in direct contact with the shunt is the only specific diagnostic test available. Culturing of the shunt wound, blood, or CSF obtained by lumbar puncture often is not revealing or misleading. Although bacteremia is often present in persons with VA shunts and may help identify the cause of the infection, blood culture results are usually negative for persons with all other types of shunts. Blood culture results showing coagulase-negative staphylococci are difficult to interpret because these organisms are the most common contaminants of blood cultures. Evaluation and culture of lumbar CSF obtained by a lumbar puncture are often not informative because there is often no communication between the lumbar space and the ventricular fluid and shunt.

The fluid obtained from the direct tap of the shunt reservoir or the ventricular system should be tested for differential cell count, glucose concentration, Gram stain, and culture. Shunt fluid pleocytosis with a predominance of polymorphonuclear cells indicates a shunt-related infection, although in some cases a normal cell count (<10 WBCs/mm^3) may be obtained. Other cells such as mononuclear cells or eosinophils may predominate during an infection. **CSF eosinophilia** can also occur with allergy to the shunt material (e.g., silicone) or to the materials used for sterilization (e.g., ethylene oxide), or it can occur with intraventricular administration of antibiotics (e.g., vancomycin). A low glucose level suggests an infection, but in many shunt-related infections the level is within the normal range. The protein concentration is commonly measured, but it is of limited use in determining the presence or absence of infection. High protein levels are found in many persons with shunt malfunction but without infection, and normal protein levels have been reported in many persons with shunt-related infections.

If the cell count reveals a high number of red blood cells, the interpretation of the CSF WBC count should be done cautiously because bleeding may have stimulated an inflammatory response, with an increased number of WBCs resulting from blood spilled into the CSF without any infection. A positive Gram stain with an increased CSF WBC count or a reduced glucose level is helpful for preliminary identification of the pathogen (i.e., gram-positive or gram-negative bacterium) and for choosing empirical antibiotic therapy. Caution should be exercised in interpreting a positive Gram stain when the CSF has a normal glucose level and WBC count. Such findings may be due to contamination of the CSF sample, the stains used for the procedure, or the slide on which the sample was placed. A negative Gram stain does not exclude an infection, and one should wait for the culture results. Ventricular fluid should always be cultured both anaerobically and aerobically. In some cases the culture result is positive even though other CSF parameters are normal. The possibility of contamination of the CSF specimen or colonization of an uninfected shunt should be considered. Some anaerobic bacteria (e.g., *Propionibacterium*) or cultures from persons who received prior antibiotics require a longer time to grow, and therefore the laboratory should be asked to observe these cultures longer (5–7 days).

Blood or CSF C-reactive protein may be helpful in the diagnosis of shunt-related infection. In patients with VA shunts, measurement of serum antistaphylococcal antibodies or C3 and C4 components of the complement system has been suggested but any benefits remain unproved.

TREATMENT

The published literature suggests five different approaches regarding therapy for infection involving a shunt:

1. Use of systemic antibiotics alone, or with intraventricular antibiotics and without replacement of the shunt
2. Removal of the shunt and immediate insertion of a new shunt, with the use of systemic or intraventricular antibiotics or both
3. Removal of the shunt, administration of systemic or intraventricular antibiotics or both, and insertion of an **extraventricular device (EVD)** to monitor the response to the antibiotic therapy, with a new shunt inserted only when the ventricular system has become sterile
4. Removal of the shunt, followed by a stereotactic third ventriculostomy and systemic antibiotic therapy
5. Externalization of only the distal (e.g., peritoneal) portion of the catheter, with the use of systemic or intraventricular antibiotics or both

The lack of large prospective, randomized studies makes it difficult to decide the optimal approach.

Use of antibiotics alone without surgery is justified by the need to maintain CSF drainage to prevent increased intracranial pressure and avoid costly operations and lengthy hospital stays. The low success rate and the higher mortality rate of this approach suggest that it should be rarely used. Only in cases of shunt placement associated with purulent meningitis due to *S. pneumoniae, N. meningitidis,* or *H. influenzae* type b does the use of systemic antibiotics alone, without removal of the shunt, appear to be an acceptable option.

Immediate replacement of the shunt with a new shunt, in combination with antibiotic therapy, has a higher rate of success than the use of antibiotics alone, but it is less effective than removal of the shunt accompanied by the insertion of an EVD and the administration of antibiotics. In addition, the inability to monitor ventricular fluid and the time to sterilization results in a longer period of systemic antibiotic therapy, up to 4–8 weeks, which may lead to increased iatrogenic infections and increased costs.

Internal shunting by third ventriculostomy, with avoidance of a prosthetic device, is effective in managing noncommunicating hydrocephalus and refractory shunt-related infections. Shunt independence for extended periods may be possible in many persons without myelomeningocele. The disadvantages of this technique include increased morbidity (e.g., hypothalamic injury, subarachnoid hemorrhage), technical difficulty in younger children, and, if a stereotactic technique is used, increased costs and limited availability of the necessary equipment.

When it is suspected that only the distal portion of the shunt is contaminated (e.g., pseudocyst, appendicitis, erythema or swelling along the shunt tract, surgical wound infection), externalization of only the distal end of the shunt, in combination with antibiotic therapy, is favored by some neurosurgeons. The advantages of this technique include ready access to the CSF for frequent sampling, diversion of the CSF and shunt from an infected area to avoid ascending infection, and maintenance of CSF flow to prevent increased intracranial pressure. The disadvantage is that colonization or early contamination of the proximal portion of the shunt may be obscured by antibiotic treatment, and the infection may become active after discontinuation of therapy and reinsertion of the distal portion of the shunt.

The most widely accepted management of shunt-related infections is removal of the entire shunt, insertion of an EVD to control intracranial pressure and to provide access to CSF for monitoring the infection and administration of parenteral antibiotics and, if necessary, intraventricular antibiotics. After successful antibiotic therapy, the EVD is removed and a new shunt is placed. The treatment success rate with this approach is high, with more rapid clearance of infection and a shorter duration of antibiotic therapy.

Antibiotic Treatment. The choice of antibiotic depends on local patterns of antimicrobial susceptibility and the ability of the antibiotic to penetrate the blood-brain barrier. In most areas, local resistance of *Staphylococcus* to semisynthetic penicillins (e.g., nafcillin, oxacillin) is greater than 10–15%, and therefore vancomycin should be used as initial empirical therapy during the wait for culture results and antibiotic susceptibilities. Vancomycin therapy should be discontinued as soon as the infecting organism is known to be susceptible to the semisynthetic penicillins, which will reduce the likelihood that the organism will develop resistance to vancomycin. None of the first-generation cephalosporins (e.g., cephalothin, cefazolin, or cephapirin) should be used for shunt-related infections, even if in vitro data suggest that the isolate is susceptible, because they penetrate the blood-brain barrier poorly.

The choice of initial antibiotic therapy before the CSF culture results are known is determined by the patient's clinical condition and the CSF findings (Fig. 53–1). Persons with coagulase-negative staphylococcal shunt-related infections usually have only mild symptoms, whereas persons with *S. aureus* or gram-negative bacterial infections are more seriously ill. The CSF Gram stain can be helpful in preliminary identification of the bacteria. If the Gram stain shows gram-positive bacteria (e.g., *Staphylococcus*), vancomycin is the drug of choice. If the Gram stain shows gram-negative bacteria, the drug of choice is cefotaxime or ceftriaxone. Treatment with an aminoglycoside is associated with a less favorable outcome because of poorer penetration into the CSF. If the Gram stain is negative, the CSF WBC count and the glucose level are determined. If either is abnormal and the person is not severely ill, vancomycin alone should be given because the likelihood of a gram-negative infection is low. In contrast, if the person is severely ill, the combination of vancomycin and cefotaxime (or ceftriaxone) provides coverage of gram-negative bacteria as well. In well-appearing persons with normal CSF parameters and without other signs of infection (e.g., peritonitis, wound infection, shunt tract infection), antibiotic therapy can be withheld until CSF culture results are known. If other signs of infection are present, antibiotic therapy is tailored according to the site of infection, with vancomycin used for persons with skin involvement, and the combination of clindamycin, which is active against gram-positive bacteria and anaerobic bacteria, and cefotaxime (or ceftriaxone) can be used for febrile persons with abdominal symptoms.

The antibiotic dosage and the dosing interval (Table 53–1) should be optimal (i.e., **meningeal schedule**) to achieve a CSF level above the in vitro minimum inhibitory concentration of the organism. Eradication of the bacteria occurs more consistently if the CSF drug level is at least 10 times higher than the MIC of the organism. Therefore, if the CSF is not sterile after 2–3 days of antibiotic treatment, measurement of the ventricular fluid bactericidal titer should be considered. For determination of the bactericidal titer, 1 mL of CSF at the expected peak antibiotic level (i.e., 2–3 hours after the antibiotic is given intravenously) is serially diluted with culture medium to produce dilutions of 1:2, 1:4, 1:8, and 1:16, and an equal volume of medium with 10^5 colonies of the organism per milliliter is added to each dilution to yield final CSF dilutions of 1:4, 1:8, 1:16, and 1:32. After 24 hours of incubation, the tubes are observed for turbidity, reflecting growth of bacteria. If no turbidity is present at the 1:4 and 1:8 dilutions, the achieved CSF level of the antibiotic is probably sufficient and the continued growth of bacteria from the CSF may be due to colonization of the EVD or contamination. Alternatively, if turbidity is present at a 1:8 dilution, the CSF level of the antibiotic may not be sufficient and the addition of another antibiotic or a change to a different antibiotic is warranted. In vitro susceptibility results, including results of synergism studies, should be used to determine the optimal antibiotic regimen.

The duration of treatment is empirical and depends on the etiologic agent, the CSF findings at presentation, and the time to sterilization. If the CSF parameters are normal but the culture yields coagulase-negative staphylococci, the duration of therapy depends on the time to sterilization. For example, if the only culture with a positive result is an intraoperative CSF or shunt culture of a specimen taken at the time of shunt removal, therapy is necessary only for 72–96 hours. Alternatively, if subsequent postoperative CSF culture results are also positive, therapy should continue until negative CSF culture results are achieved for 7 days. If the CSF parameters are abnormal and the only culture with a positive result is an intraoperative CSF or shunt culture, therapy should continue for 7 days. If subsequent CSF samples show abnormal CSF findings and positive culture results, therapy should be extended until negative CSF culture results are achieved for 10 days.

A longer duration of antibiotic therapy is recommended with other bacteria (e.g., *S. aureus,* gram-negative bacteria). If the CSF findings are normal and the only culture with a positive result is an intraoperative CSF or shunt culture, treatment should continue until negative CSF culture results are achieved for 7 days. In all other situations, therapy should continue until negative CSF culture results are achieved for 10 days.

Persistent positive CSF culture results after shunt removal despite appropriate antibiotic therapy indicate the possible need for EVD replacement. If CSF culture results continue to be positive, the addition of intraventricular antibiotic treatment should be considered.

Reshunting should occur immediately at the end of treatment. Abnormal CSF findings such as low glucose levels or mildly elevated cell counts or elevated protein levels at the end of antibiotic

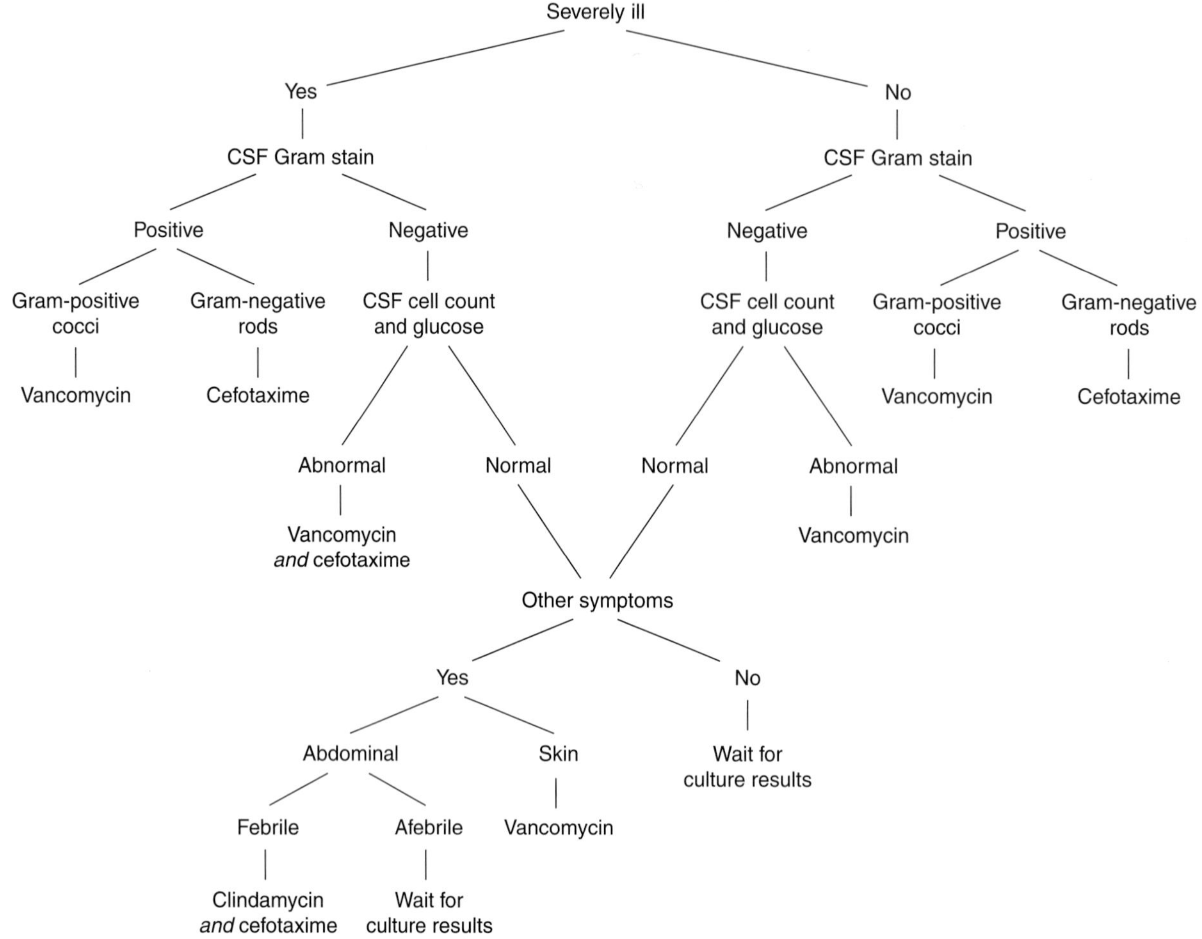

FIGURE 53–1. Empirical management of CNS infection involving a shunt. This algorithm should not be used for suspected infection in neonates or immunocompromised persons because they often present with less severe clinical symptoms and less CSF inflammatory response.

therapy should not delay reshunting. There is no benefit in prolonged hospitalization for observation after completion of antibiotic therapy for signs of relapse of the infection. Treated persons should have close follow-up as outpatients.

Intraventricular Antibiotic Treatment. Some experts recommend direct instillation of antibiotics into the ventricular system; caution should be used because of potential neurotoxic effects. The suggested dosages for intraventricular treatment have been determined empirically from use in a small number of patients (Table 53–1). In addition, preservative-containing antibiotic preparations should be checked for appropriateness for intraventricular instillation. If intraventricular antibiotics are used, they should be administered once or twice daily, and, if possible, the EVD should be closed for 30–60 minutes after drug administration. If the EVD cannot be closed and the amount of CSF drainage exceeds 7–10 mL/hr, the frequency of antibiotic instillation should be increased. Pleocytosis and eosinophilia may occur in persons receiving intraventricular vancomycin or gentamicin.

If the ventricular fluid culture continues to show positive results despite changes in systemic antibiotic therapy and replacement of the EVD, intraventricular treatment should be considered. Because of the potential neurotoxicity of the empirically recommended antibiotic doses and the unpredictability of the CSF antibiotic levels, irrigation of the ventricular system with a known concentration of an antibiotic solution is preferred. The insertion of two EVDs is required for a continuous flow of the solution. The concentration of the antibiotic in the solution should equal the highest safe plasma level when the drug is given intravenously. For example, for treating a person with susceptible gram-negative bacteria, amikacin at a concentration of 30 mg/L in saline solution, yielding a concentration of 30 μg/mL, is recommended. Gentamicin at a concentration of 10–12 mg/L (with a special intrathecal preparation) is an acceptable alternative when the MIC of gentamicin for the isolate is <1 μg/mL. The antibiotic solution is administered through one EVD at a rate of 10–20 mL/hr, and the second EVD is left open to drain the fluid and to remove debris and pus from the ventricles. Intraventricular antibiotics are continued until sterility of the drained fluid is achieved, with the duration of systemic antibiotics as previously described.

COMPLICATIONS

Infections involving shunts increase the morbidity and mortality for central nervous system shunts. The mortality in persons with shunt-related infections is double the mortality of patients with shunts who do not have a shunt-related infection; they also have three times as many shunt-related operations, which contribute to increased morbidity and costs. Even when the initial infection was successfully treated, a secondary infection or colonization of the

TABLE 53–1. Recommended Intravenous and Intraventricular Antibiotic Doses for Central Nervous System Infections Involving Shunts

Antibiotic	Intravenous Dose	Intraventricular Dose (Once or Twice a Day)
Oxacillin	200–300 mg/kg/day divided q6–8hr	—
Nafcillin	200 mg/kg/day divided q6–8hr	50 mg/day
Vancomycin	60 mg/kg/day divided q6–8hr	5 mg/day
Gentamicin	7.5 mg/kg/day divided q8hr	1–4 mg/day
Amikacin	22.5 mg/kg/day divided q8hr	2–15 mg/day
Tobramycin	7.5 mg/kg/day divided q8hr	1–4 mg/day
Cefotaxime	200 mg/kg/day divided q6hr	—
Ceftriaxone	100 mg/kg/day divided q12hr	—
Ceftazidime	200 mg/kg/day divided q8hr	—
Chloramphenicol	100 mg/kg/day divided q6hr	25 mg/day
Penicillin G	400,000 U/kg/day divided q6hr	—
Ampicillin	200–400 mg/kg/day divided q6hr	25–50 mg/day
Metronidazole	30 mg/kg/day divided q8hr	—
Amphotericin B	1 mg/kg/day q24hr	0.1–0.5 mg/day

EVD occurred in 3–5% of cases. The risk of secondary infection is minimized by using a sterile closed drainage system that is carefully maintained; in addition, injections into the system are avoided and only trained personnel are allowed to drain CSF samples from the system. The continuous external drainage of CSF also causes loss of electrolytes and fluids. Therefore the routine assessment of serum electrolytes once or twice weekly is recommended, and the total daily amount of fluid lost as drained CSF should be replaced.

PROGNOSIS

With appropriate combination medical and surgical therapy, the mortality rate for infections involving shunts is low. Incomplete initial therapy for a first episode increases the risk of a second episode. Long-term morbidity after a shunt-related infection includes seizures, psychomotor retardation, and cognitive deficiency. A study (McLone et al, 1982) showed that the IQ scores of children who had an infection involving a shunt were significantly lower (mean IQ = 72) than those of children with a shunt but without infection (mean IQ = 95).

PREVENTION

The temporal proximity of most shunt-related infections to the time of the shunting procedure suggests that greater attention to the area adjacent to the shunt during surgery may reduce shunt colonization and subsequent infection. Therefore bactericidal shampoos (e.g., chlorhexidine) should be used to reduce bacterial density of the scalp before surgery. Only essential personnel should be present during the operation, and the skin should be cleaned with a fat solvent, followed by preparation with soap and an antibiotic solution, with attention to avoiding contact between the shunt and the skin. A detailed perioperative protocol (Choux et al, 1992) reduced the infection rate from more than 7% to less than 1%.

Surgical Prophylaxis. Several studies have examined the effect of prophylactic antibiotics on the reduction of the infection rate. Major variations in study design and the small number of subjects in each study preclude definitive conclusions. Meta-analyses of well-designed studies suggest that the use of prophylactic antibiotics is associated with significant reduction in the incidence of infections if the baseline infection rate involving shunts is greater than 10%. If the baseline infection rate is lower than 10%, prophylactic antibiotics are not recommended. The choice of antibiotics should be based on the local antibiotic susceptibility patterns of the pathogens commonly causing infections involving shunts in that area. If used, prophylaxis preferably should be started 1–2 hours before surgery, to allow higher levels of drug in the skin tissues. The duration of prophylaxis should not exceed 6–8 hours postoperatively.

REVIEW ARTICLES

Hanekom W, Yogev R: Cerebrospinal fluid shunt infections. *Pediatr Infect Dis* 1996;11:29–54.

Schoenbaum SC, Gardner P, Shillito J: Infections of cerebrospinal fluid shunts: Epidemiology, clinical manifestations, and therapy. *J Infect Dis* 1975;131:543–52.

KEY ARTICLES

Choux M, Genitori L, Lang D, et al: Shunt implantation: Reducing the incidence of shunt infection. *J Neurosurg* 1992;77:875–80.

Cotton MF, Hartzenberg B, Donald PR, et al: Ventriculoperitoneal shunt infections in children. A 6-year study. *S Afr Med J* 1991;79:139–42.

Di Rocco C, Marchese E, Velardi F: A survey of the first complication of newly implanted CSF shunt devices for the treatment of nontumoral hydrocephalus. Cooperative survey of the 1991–1992 Educational Committee of the ISPN. *Childs Nerv Syst* 1994;10:321–7.

Grabb PA, Albright AL: Intraventricular vancomycin-induced cerebrospinal fluid eosinophilia: Report of two patients. *Neurosurgery* 1992;30:630–4.

James HE, Walsh JW, Wilson HD, et al: Prospective randomized study of therapy in cerebrospinal fluid shunt infection. *Neurosurgery* 1980; 7:459–63.

Jimenez DF, Keating R, Goodrich JT: Silicone allergy in ventriculoperitoneal shunts. *Childs Nerv Syst* 1994;10:59–63.

Jones RF, Stening WA, Kwok BC, et al: Third ventriculostomy for shunt infections in children. *Neurosurgery* 1993;32:855–9.

Kontny U, Höfling B, Gutjahr P, et al: CSF shunt infections in children. *Infection* 1993;21:89–92.

Luer MS, Hatton J: Vancomycin administration into the cerebrospinal fluid: A review. *Ann Pharmacother* 1993;27:912–21.

McLone DG, Czyzewski D, Raimondi AJ, et al: Central nervous system infections as a limiting factor in the intelligence of children with myelomeningocele. *Pediatrics* 1982;70:338–42.

Piatt JH Jr: Cerebrospinal fluid shunt failure: Late is different from early. *Pediatr Neurosurg* 1995;23:133–9.

Pople IK, Bayston R, Hayward RD: Infection of cerebrospinal fluid shunts in infants: A study of etiological factors. *J Neurosurg* 1992;77:29–36.

Rodgers J, Bayston R: Characterisation of the IgG response to cell proteins of coagulase-negative staphylococci in hydrocephalus shunt infections. *Eur J Pediatr Surg* 1992;2:22–9.

Stamos JK, Kaufman BA, Yogev R: Ventriculoperitoneal shunt infections with gram-negative bacteria. *Neurosurgery* 1993;33:858–62.

Tung H, Raffel C, McComb JG: Ventricular cerebrospinal fluid eosinophilia in children with ventriculoperitoneal shunts. *J Neurosurg* 1991; 75:541–4.

Vinchon M, Vallee L, Prin L, et al: Cerebro-spinal fluid eosinophilia in shunt infections. *Neuropediatrics* 1992;23:235–40.

Walters BC: Cerebrospinal fluid shunt infection. *Neurosurg Clin North Am* 1992;3:387–401.

Wyatt RJ, Walsh JW, Holland NH: Shunt nephritis. Role of the complement system in its pathogenesis and management. *J Neurosurg* 1981; 55:99–107.

Yogev R: Cerebrospinal fluid shunt infections: A personal view. *Pediatr Infect Dis* 1985;4:113–8.

CHAPTER 54

Brain and Parameningeal Abscesses

Sheral S. Patel ▪ John R. Schreiber

One of the most feared complications of common upper respiratory tract infections in children is a brain or parameningeal abscess. These infections are defined by their anatomic location. A **brain abscess** begins as an area of cerebritis that develops into an encapsulated area of pus. A **subdural empyema** is located between the cranial dura and the arachnoid membrane, whereas a **cranial epidural abscess** is located between the dura and the skull. A high index of suspicion is necessary to recognize intracranial infections because signs and symptoms are often nonspecific and can range from fever and headache to focal neurologic defects and seizures. A **spinal epidural abscess** is defined as purulent material outside the dura within the spinal canal. Spinal epidural abscesses are usually a result of bacteremia and can present with fever and back pain or even paralysis. Prompt neurosurgical intervention and antimicrobial therapy are critical for the management of brain and parameningeal abscesses, as well as spinal epidural abscesses.

BRAIN ABSCESS

A brain abscess begins as a localized area of **cerebritis** that develops into a collection of pus surrounded by a capsule. Before the introduction of antibiotics such as penicillin and chloramphenicol, brain abscesses were usually fatal. Advances in the past 30 years have greatly facilitated the early diagnosis and management of brain abscesses. These advances include the advent of CT, stereotactic brain biopsy and aspiration, better anaerobic culture techniques, and newer antibiotics. Close cooperation among the infectious diseases specialist, the neurosurgeon, and the primary care physician is needed for optimal patient care.

ETIOLOGY

A mixed bacterial population is usually isolated from brain abscesses complicating chronic otitis media, sinusitis, and mastoiditis, including anaerobes such as *Streptococcus milleri,* viridans or microaerophilic streptococci, *Bacteroides fragilis,* and other *Bacteroides* species (Table 54–1). Other organisms infrequently isolated from brain abscesses include gram-negative bacilli, *Proteus,* Enterobacteriaceae, *Pseudomonas aeruginosa,* and *Staphylococcus aureus. Streptococcus pneumoniae* is a rare cause of brain abscess but is associated with infections from contiguous structures and rarely is isolated after meningitis. Abscesses associated with dental infections are caused by a greater variety of organisms, including *Actinomyces* and *Fusobacterium.*

Immunocompromised persons can develop brain abscesses from fungi or *Nocardia* as a result of direct extension from sinuses or from hematogenous spread. *Nocardia* can present as an isolated central nervous system lesion or as part of a disseminated infection associated with pulmonary or cutaneous disease. *Aspergillus* is the most common fungal cause of brain abscesses and is associated with rapid progression and high mortality.

Mycobacterium tuberculosis is a rare cause of brain abscesses but should be considered in the differential diagnosis in areas where tuberculosis is endemic or in persons with disseminated disease. Forms of central nervous system tuberculosis include tuberculomas and tuberculous brain abscesses (Chapter 35). A **tuberculoma** is an area of dense granulation tissue that contains epithelioid and giant cells; it is not a true abscess. A **tuberculous brain abscess** is a focal collection of pus containing acid-fast bacilli surrounded by vascular granulation tissue forming a dense capsule.

Frequent causes of parasitic brain lesions include toxoplasmosis and neurocysticercosis. *Toxoplasma gondii* is the most common cause of parasitic brain abscesses in persons with AIDS. **Neurocysticercosis,** a central nervous system infection caused by the larval form of *Taenia solium* (Chapter 44), is characterized by a cystic or calcified lesion seen on CT or MRI.

EPIDEMIOLOGY

Brain abscesses can occur at any age. Approximately one fourth of all brain abscesses occur in children less than 15 years of age, with most occurring from 4–7 years of age. The ratio of males to females is about 2:1. The most common predisposing factor is a contiguous infection such as chronic otitis media, mastoiditis, and sinusitis. Other risk factors include use of corticosteroids, cranial trauma (including surgery), and cyanotic congenital heart disease. Penetrating orbital trauma from pencils or wooden toys is a frequently unrecognized cause of brain abscesses in children. In these cases the external wound over the eye will heal rapidly and the serious nature of the wound is overlooked. A less common predisposing factor is bacteremia associated with a distant focus of infection such as pneumonia.

The epidemiology of brain abscesses in children is changing. The incidence of brain abscesses in organ transplant recipients and other immunocompromised persons is rising as this population increases. At the same time, the widespread use of antimicrobial therapy for otitis media and pharyngitis has led to a decrease in the incidence of otogenic temporal lobe and cerebellar abscesses. As more children have early surgical correction of their cardiac anomalies, the incidence of brain abscesses in this population has also decreased. Brain abscesses in children less than 2 years of age are uncommon and are usually caused by gram-negative organisms as a complication of meningitis. Frontal lobe abscesses as a complication of frontal sinusitis most frequently occur in adolescent boys.

PATHOGENESIS

Animal models have been used to describe four stages in the development of brain abscesses, providing the basis for establishing

TABLE 54–1. Culture Results of Brain Abscess and Subdural Empyema

Bacteria	Brain Abscess	Subdural Empyema	Extradural Abscess
Anaerobes	37	42	1
Streptococci	33	54	3
Staphylococci	30	15	4
Proteus vulgaris	10	1	0
Streptococcus pneumoniae	7	0	0
Escherichia coli	4	0	0
Haemophilus aphrophilus	2	1	0
Haemophilus influenzae	1	0	0
Klebsiella pneumoniae	1	1	0
Unknown	20	19	0
Total number of cultures	145	133	8

Adapted from Yogev R: Suppurative intracranial complications of upper respiratory tract infections. *Pediatr Infect Dis J* 1987;6:324–7.

the timing and nature of surgical intervention. The first stage is **early cerebritis,** with focal areas of inflammation and edema occurring 1–3 days after direct inoculation of the organism into the brain parenchyma. Expansion of cerebritis and the beginning of a necrotic central focus is noted in **late cerebritis,** during days 4–9. The **early capsule stage** occurs on days 10–14 and is characterized by the establishment of a ring-enhancing capsule of well-vascularized tissue associated with an early appearance of gliosis and fibrosis. Finally, during the **late capsule stage,** a well-formed capsule develops as the abscess is walled off.

The brain has an abundant blood supply and an impermeable blood-brain barrier, making it relatively resistant to bacterial infections. The four primary settings in which brain abscesses occur are direct spread from a contiguous source, as a complication of meningitis, with hematogenous spread from a distant site of infection, and after cranial trauma or craniotomy (Table 54–2).

In children, parameningeal foci such as otic, sinus, or mastoid infections are the most common predisposing factors for brain abscesses. Valveless emissary veins drain these areas and permit either direct or retrograde flow into the venous systems of the

TABLE 54–2. Predisposing Conditions for Intracranial Abscesses and Empyema

	Patients (%)		
Primary Site	Brain Abscess (107 Patients)	Subdural Empyema (67 Patients)	Extradural Abscess (14 Patients)
Middle ear infection	24	21	29
Sinus infection	13	48	57
Cyanotic heart disease	12	0	0
Cerebral trauma	10	1	0
Lung infection	7	3	0
After neurosurgery	6	6	0
Meningitis	6	15	0
Unknown	22	6	14

Adapted from Yogev R: Suppurative intracranial complications of upper respiratory tract infections. *Pediatr Infect Dis J* 1987;6:324–7.

brain, leading to vascular spread of sinus infection (Fig. 54–1). Direct extension through the bone can also occur. Abscesses that arise from sinus or mastoid infections are usually single and are found in the temporal or frontal lobe. **Cerebellar abscesses** are typically associated with chronic otitis media and mastoiditis. Dental abscesses are a rare cause of brain abscesses in infants and children.

The most common pathogens causing neonatal meningitis, including group B streptococci and *Escherichia coli,* are rare causes of brain abscesses in neonates. In contrast, neonatal meningitis or septicemia caused by *Proteus* or *Citrobacter diversus* is associated with a high risk (up to 40%) of brain abscess. These abscesses are often multiple and are found in periventricular locations. Other facultative gram-negative organisms associated with neonatal brain abscesses include *Serratia marcescens* and *Enterobacter* species.

Persons with ventriculoperitoneal shunts may develop brain abscesses caused by *S. aureus,* coagulase-negative staphylococci, gram-negative enteric bacilli, and *P. aeruginosa.*

Bacteremia and hematogenous spread of infection from a remote location can occur, particularly in children with cyanotic congenital heart disease. In these children the **right-to-left shunt** bypasses the filtering mechanism of the pulmonary system and leads to an increased risk of brain abscess. In addition, decreased arterial oxygenation can result in an elevated hematocrit, with increased blood viscosity causing focal areas of ischemia that serve as a nidus for infection in the brain. The most common organisms isolated in this setting include viridans and microaerophilic streptococci, anaerobic streptococci, and, occasionally, *Haemophilus* species. Brain abscesses associated with right-to-left shunting are rare in children less than 2 years of age, which suggests that another factor such as microinfarcts preceding bacteremia are important as a nidus.

Brain abscesses are an uncommon complication of open skull fracture, penetrating brain trauma, or craniotomy. There can be a significant delay from the time of injury until the abscess is recognized. After head trauma, *S. aureus* is the most common organism

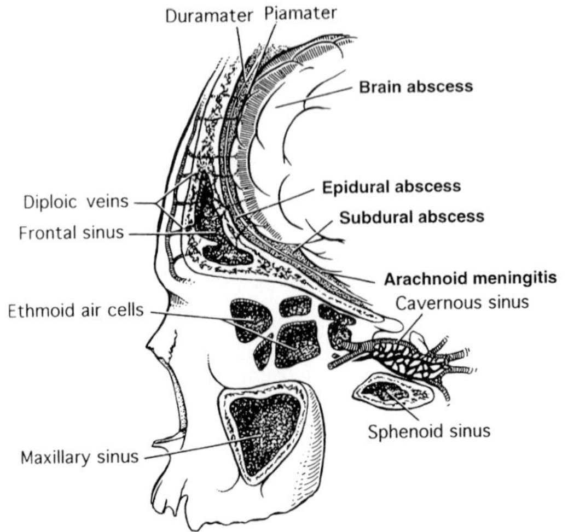

FIGURE 54–1. Major anatomic routes for intracranial extension of infection. Intracranial infection (brain abscess, subdural abscess, epidural abscess, and meningitis) may result from direct spread of a contiguous infection (e.g., osteomyelitis, sinusitis) or spread of organisms by the vascular supply, especially through the cavernous sinus. (From Chow AW: Life threatening infections of the head and neck. *Clin Infect Dis* 1992;14:991–1002. copyright 1992, The University of Chicago Press.)

isolated. If the wound is contaminated with soil, then infection with *Clostridium* species and facultative gram-negative organisms is also possible. *Nocardia* is an uncommon etiologic agent of brain abscesses associated with penetrating head trauma.

SYMPTOMS AND CLINICAL MANIFESTATIONS

The classic triad of headache, fever, and focal neurologic deficit is an uncommon presentation of brain abscess, especially in children. The size and location of the abscess, the virulence of the infecting organism, and the presence of underlying systemic conditions can influence the clinical presentation of a brain abscess. A high index of suspicion is essential because the symptoms and signs are often nonspecific. A dull, aching, and poorly localized headache is the most common presenting symptom (Table 54–3). The interval between the onset of the first symptom and the time of diagnosis averages about 1 month. The development of high fever in a patient with a chronic infection such as chronic sinusitis or chronic otitis media may be a clue to a developing brain abscess. Acute worsening of a pre-existing headache accompanied by onset of severe meningismus may reflect **rupture of the brain abscess** into the ventricular space.

Depending on the abscess location, neurologic findings such as seizures, changes in mental status, and focal neurologic deficits can occur. Papilledema is less common, and immediate neurosurgical evaluation is needed if papilledema is found on physical examination. Cerebellar abscesses often are manifested by nausea, vomiting, and headache rather than classic cerebellar findings. Brainstem abscesses usually extend longitudinally along fiber tracts in the brainstem, rather than expanding transversely, thus making a well-defined brainstem syndrome unlikely.

Neonates and immunocompromised persons are less likely to have the classic triad of fever, headache, and neurologic deficits at presentation. The initial symptoms and signs of a brain abscess in neonates include seizures, respiratory compromise, vomiting, poor feeding, and increasing head circumference. Immunocompromised persons may have a poor inflammatory response and usually present with overt neurologic findings such as seizures and stroke.

TABLE 54–3. Symptoms and Signs of Intracranial Abscess and Empyema

	Patients (%)		
	Brain Abscess	Subdural Empyema	Extradural Abscess
Headache	81	74	100
Fever	44	86	82
Vomiting	50	62	30
Altered consciousness	54	79	50
Seizures	39	52	20
Papilledema	35	42	0
Dilated pupils	5	27	0
Ocular palsy	5	28	0
Hemiparesis or hemiplegia	20	68	15
Stiff neck	48	53	16

Adapted from Yogev R: Suppurative intracranial complications of upper respiratory tract infections. *Pediatr Infect Dis J* 1987;6:324–7.

DIAGNOSIS

Differential Diagnosis

The differential diagnosis of a brain abscess includes any disease process that results in an expanding intracranial mass lesion (Table 54–4). Because of the nonspecific nature of the presentation of brain abscess, both infectious and noninfectious causes must be considered (Fig. 54–2). These causes include meningitis, subdural abscess, cranial epidural abscess, solid tumor, lymphoma, intracerebral hemorrhage, cerebral infarction, and migraine headaches.

Laboratory Evaluation

There are no pathognomonic laboratory data for brain abscesses. An elevated WBC count and an elevated ESR are common. One or more of the causative pathogens are occasionally isolated from blood cultures. Review of past hospitalizations may reveal previous bacteremia or infections. The electroencephalogram usually shows nonspecific focal changes localizing the abscess.

Lumbar puncture should not be performed if a brain abscess is suspected, because there is a significant risk of **brainstem herniation.** This risk far outweighs the benefits of any laboratory values obtained. Cerebrospinal fluid findings, including cell count and protein concentration, are usually abnormal, but culture results are negative unless the abscess has ruptured. The best opportunity to establish the microbiologic diagnosis is at the time of surgery.

Microbiologic Evaluation

Prompt transport, including the use of anaerobic transport media, and cultures of abscess aspirate obtained at the time of surgery are crucial to the recovery of the infecting organism. Specimens for Gram stain and aerobic and anaerobic cultures should be obtained at the time of surgical drainage, regardless of prior antibiotic treatment. Gram stains can help guide empirical antimicrobial therapy before culture results are known. Acid-fast and fungal stains and cultures for mycobacteria, fastidious slow-growing organisms such as *Actinomyces* and *Nocardia,* and fungi should be obtained for immunocompromised persons or those with a history of exposure to tuberculosis. Blood, otic, sinus, or mastoid cultures can reliably predict the microbiology of the brain abscess and should be sent for Gram stain and for aerobic and anaerobic cultures.

Diagnostic Imaging

The advent of CT and MRI has greatly facilitated earlier diagnosis and precise localization of brain abscesses. CT scan with contrast material shows the classic ring-enhancing lesion associated with a mature brain abscess (Fig. 54–3). In cases of suspected cerebritis, a delayed CT scan 30–60 minutes after contrast material is given will show focal areas of edema characterized by filling in of the

TABLE 54–4. Differential Diagnosis of Brain Abscess

Infectious	Noninfectious
Subdural abscess	Brain tumor (primary or metastatic)
Cranial epidural abscess	Lymphoma
Bacterial meningitis	Intracerebral hemorrhage
Viral meningitis	Cerebral infarction
Encephalitis	Venous sinus thrombosis
Tuberculomas	Migraine headache
Cysticercosis	
Toxoplasmosis	
Cryptococcosis	

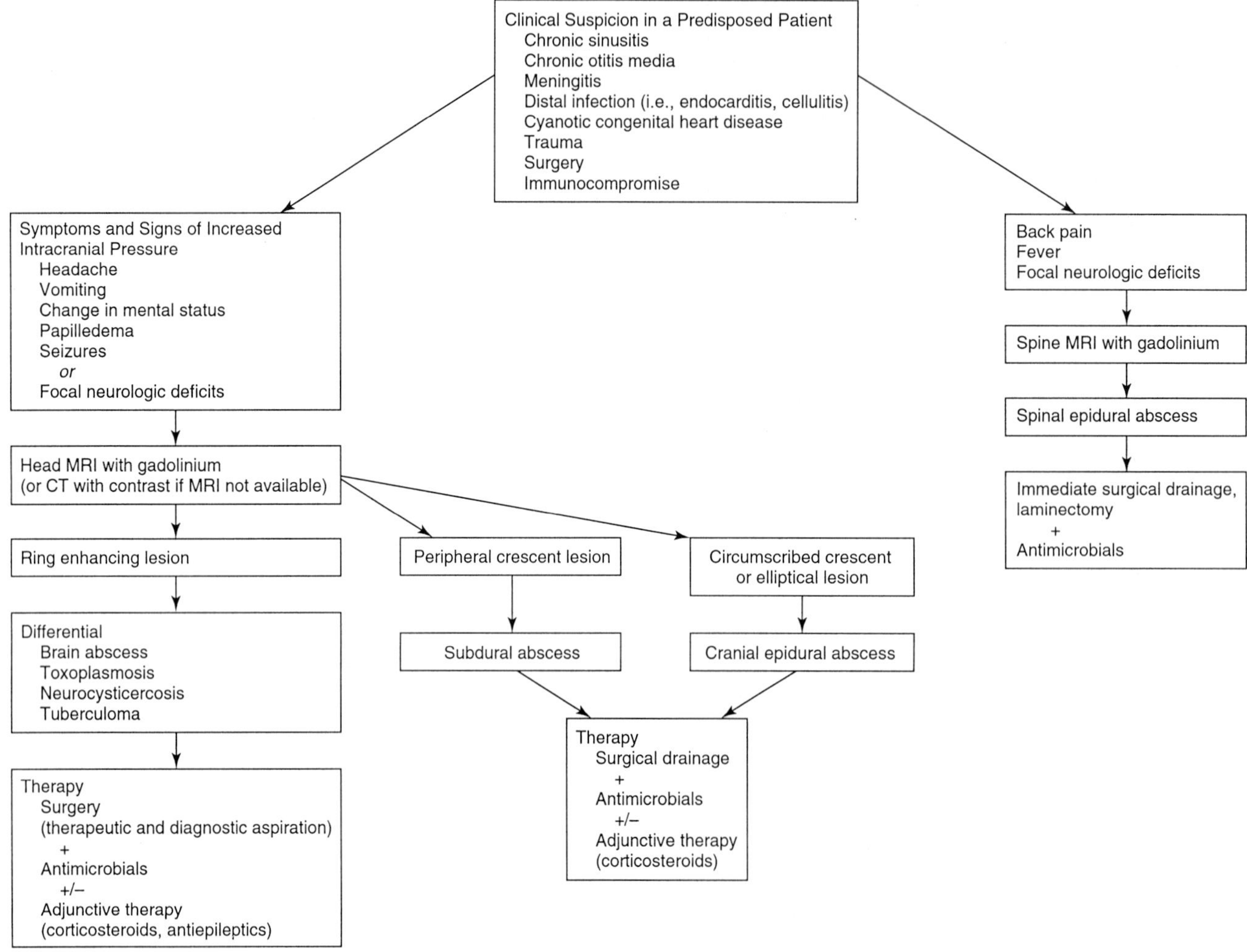

FIGURE 54–2. Management algorithm for brain and parameningeal abscesses.

central hypointense area by contrast material, which indicates that a central necrotic area has not yet developed. Serial weekly or biweekly CT or MRI aids in monitoring the response to treatment and in timing repeated surgery, if needed.

MRI is superior to CT for soft tissue resolution and evaluation of the posterior fossa. Brain abscesses will appear hypointense on T1-weighted sequences, showing ring enhancement after intravenous administration of gadolinium (Fig. 54–4). A hyperintense area of pus surrounded by a well-defined capsule and surrounding edema will be evident on T2-weighted sequences of a mature brain abscess.

CT or MRI is less likely to show enhancement and surrounding edema in immunocompromised persons. It can also be difficult to differentiate between metastatic brain abscesses and metastatic brain tumors. Brain abscesses tend to occur at watershed regions between vascular distributions and to appear as lesions with hypodense centers with peripheral enhancement, whereas tumors usually have irregular borders and diffuse enhancement.

Other radiographic modalities such as arteriography, radionuclide scans, and ventriculography are not optimal for diagnosing brain abscesses but can be helpful in diagnosing other processes such as aneurysms and arteriovenous malformations.

TREATMENT

Cornerstones of the management of brain abscesses include empirical antibiotic therapy, surgery, and serial imaging. Empirical antibiotic therapy can be initiated on the basis of history, the presumptive source of infection, and Gram stain of purulent material, if available. CT or MRI provides rapid and precise localization of brain lesions that require surgical intervention. Stereotactic needle aspiration provides both therapeutic drainage and a diagnostic specimen for culture and special studies. Serial imaging is helpful in an evaluation of the response to therapy and the need for further surgery.

Antimicrobial Therapy. Empirical antimicrobial therapy should be started in all patients having a presumptive diagnosis of a brain abscess. Preoperative therapy should not significantly reduce the isolation rate of organisms from the abscess at the time of surgery. Empirical antibiotic therapy is guided by the possible pathogens causing the abscess and by the penetrability of antibiotics into brain tissue and the abscess cavity (Table 54–5). Once culture results are known, the spectrum of antibiotic coverage can be narrowed.

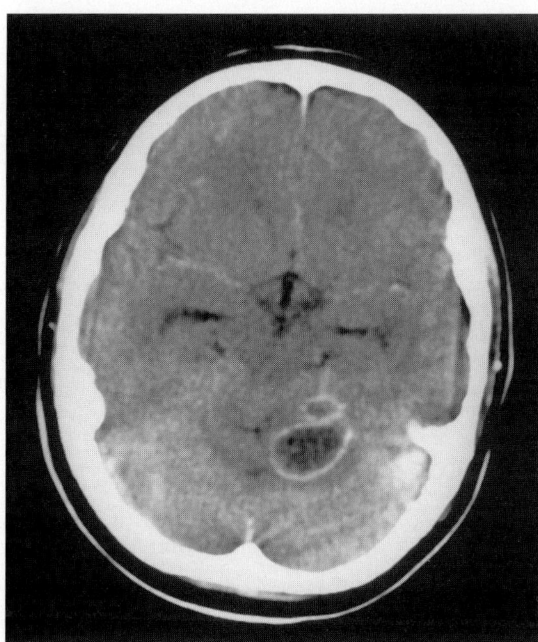

FIGURE 54–3. Ring-enhancing lesion consistent with a left cerebellar abscess seen on CT scan with contrast medium in a 10-year-old boy as a complication of chronic otitis media and mastoiditis.

Penicillin G is bactericidal against some of the common etiologic organisms, including many *Streptococcus* species and anaerobes other than *B. fragilis*. Despite a relatively poor central nervous system penetration, penicillin G has measurable therapeutic concentrations within the purulent material of brain abscesses. Minimum inhibitory concentrations for sensitive pathogens are exceeded in the abscess cavity with high doses.

Although limited data are available on the use of semisynthetic penicillins such as nafcillin, they have been successfully used to treat brain abscesses caused by *S. aureus*. First-generation cephalosporins have poor central nervous system penetration and are generally not recommended. Vancomycin has been used to treat brain abscesses despite its poor central nervous system penetration but has been reserved for situations in which antimicrobial resistance to drugs with better penetration is suspected. Vancomycin is effective against *S. aureus* including MRSA, coagulase-negative *Staphylococcus,* penicillin- and cephalosporin-resistant *S. pneumoniae,* aerobic and anaerobic *Streptococcus,* and *Clostridium.*

Third-generation cephalosporins such as ceftriaxone and cefotaxime are frequently used in empirical treatment of brain abscesses because they are bactericidal and because they achieve adequate minimum inhibitory concentrations in CSF and brain abscesses for a variety of pathogens. Cefotaxime and ceftriaxone are active against gram-negative bacilli, *S. pneumoniae,* and *Haemophilus influenzae.* Ceftazidime and cefepime have less gram-positive coverage but better activity against *Pseudomonas* species. Because gram-negative organisms such as *Citrobacter* and *Proteus* are frequent pathogens in neonatal brain abscesses, the combination of cephalosporins (especially cefotaxime) and aminoglycosides plays a major role in the treatment of brain abscesses in neonates. Monotherapy with β-lactams such as ampicillin is inadequate empirical therapy for brain abscesses because of its limited spectrum and the frequent resistance found in *E. coli* and *Proteus.* The combination of ampicillin and sulbactam has shown therapeutic success in a small series of patients, but data on the penetration of the sulbactam component into the brain abscess cavity are limited.

Metronidazole has good oral absorption and excellent CSF and brain abscess cavity penetration. It is bactericidal against strict anaerobes such as obligate gram-negative anaerobic bacilli, *Clostridium, Peptostreptococcus,* and *Peptococcus.*

Carbapenem antibiotics such as imipenem and meropenem have been used successfully in the treatment of both cerebral pyogenic brain abscesses and nocardiosis. Meropenem is associated with a lower incidence of seizures than imipenem. It has been used successfully in the treatment of bacterial meningitis and may be used in the treatment of brain abscesses caused by more resistant pathogens such as penicillin-resistant *S. pneumoniae* and β-lactam–resistant gram-negative bacilli.

Other classes of antibiotics have occasionally been used in the treatment of brain abscesses. Trimethoprim-sulfamethoxazole has good central nervous system penetration and covers many aerobic gram-positive and gram-negative organisms. Quinolones also have good central nervous system penetration and provide excellent activity against gram-negative facultative anaerobes such as Enterobacteriaceae and *Pseudomonas.* Because of the theoretical effects on developing cartilage, quinolones must be used with caution in young children.

Chloramphenicol has been used in the past because its antimicrobial spectrum includes anaerobes, *S. pneumoniae,* viridans streptococci, and *H. influenzae.* It also has excellent oral absorption and excellent central nervous system penetration. Chloramphenicol has fallen out of favor as first-line treatment of brain abscesses because of its lack of bactericidal activity for certain organisms, association with idiosyncratic aplastic anemia, and increasing bacterial resistance.

Antibiotics including bacitracin and gentamicin have been instilled into the abscess cavity after aspiration, but this approach is not recommended because efficacy and potential toxic effects have not been evaluated. Seizures can occur if the instilled antibiotics diffuse rapidly into the surrounding brain parenchyma.

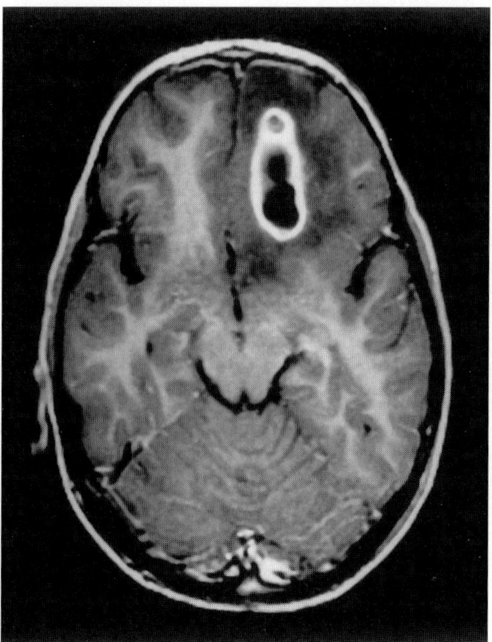

FIGURE 54–4. Classic ring-enhancing lesion and surrounding edema seen on MRI with gadolinium in an 8-year-old boy with a mature left frontal brain abscess as a complication of sinusitis.

TABLE 54–5. Recommended Empirical Antimicrobial Therapy for Brain Abscess

Source of Abscess	Site of Abscess	Microbial Flora	Empirical Antimicrobial Therapy
Paranasal sinus	Frontal lobe	Aerobic streptococci (usually *Streptococcus milleri* group) Anaerobic streptococci *Haemophilus* *Bacteroides* (non-*fragilis*)	Cefotaxime *or* ceftriaxone *plus* Metronidazole *plus* Vancomycin *or* penicillin G
Otogenic infection	Temporal lobe, cerebellum	*Streptococcus* Enterobacteriaceae *Bacteroides* species (including *B. fragilis*) *Pseudomonas aeruginosa*	Cefepime *or* ceftazidime *plus* Metronidazole *plus* Vancomycin *or* penicillin G
Metastatic spread	Multiple cerebral lesions common, especially in middle cerebral artery distribution, but any lobe can be involved	Depends on source: Endocarditis *Staphylococcus aureus* Viridans streptococci Urinary tract Enterobacteriaceae *Pseudomonas* Intra-abdominal *Streptococcus* Enterobacteriaceae Anaerobes Lung abscess *Streptococcus* *Actinomyces* *Fusobacterium*	Cefotaxime *or* ceftriaxone *plus* Metronidazole *plus* Vancomycin *or* nafcillin *or* oxacillin
Penetrating trauma	Depends on site of wound	*S. aureus* *Clostridium* Enterobacteriaceae *Pasteurella multocida*	Cefotaxime *or* ceftriaxone *plus* Vancomycin *or* nafcillin *or* oxacillin
Postoperative		Coagulase-negative staphylococci *S. aureus* Enterobacteriaceae *P. aeruginosa*	Cefepime *or* ceftazidime *plus* Vancomycin

Adapted from Mathisen GE, Johnson JP: Brain Abscess. *Clin Infect Dis* 1997;25:763–9.

Suggested Dosages for Persons with Normal Renal Function

ANTIBIOTIC	DOSAGE	MAXIMUM DAILY DOSE	ANTIBIOTIC	DOSAGE	MAXIMUM DAILY DOSE
Cefepime	100–150 mg/kg/day divided q8–12hr IV	4–6 g	Nafcillin	150–200 mg/kg/day divided q6hr IV	12 g
Cefotaxime	200–300 mg/kg/day divided q6–8hr IV	12 g	Oxacillin	150–200 mg/kg/day divided q6hr IV	12 g
Ceftriaxone	100 mg/kg/day divided q12–24hr IV or IM	3–4 g	Penicillin G	300,000–500,000 U/kg/day divided q6hr IV	24 MU
Ceftazidime	150 mg/kg/day divided q8hr IV	6 g	Vancomycin	60 mg/kg/day divided q6hr IV	2 g
Metronidazole	30 mg/kg/day divided q6hr IV	30 mg/kg (adults)			

Fungal brain abscesses most commonly occur in immunocompromised persons and should be managed aggressively with open craniotomy, surgical débridement, and antifungal chemotherapy. *Aspergillus* is one of the most common causes of fungal brain abscesses. Amphotericin B is the treatment of choice, and in vitro synergy studies suggest that amphotericin B in combination with flucytosine or rifampin may be more effective than amphotericin B alone. Mucormycosis should also be treated with amphotericin B. In vitro studies have shown the combination of amphotericin B and rifampin also to be effective for *Mucor,* but the clinical benefit of combination therapy is unproved. Candidiasis can present with diffuse microabscesses too small to be seen on CT or MRI. Treatment should be with amphotericin B and flucytosine. The addition of flucytosine is useful against susceptible *Candida* species because it has better central nervous system penetration than amphotericin B. Soil fungi such as *Blastomyces, Histoplasma,* and *Coccidioides* may be resistant to amphotericin B, and azole therapy (i.e., fluconazole or itraconazole) may be necessary for amphotericin B–resistant organisms.

Tuberculous brain abscesses require prolonged antituberculosis therapy after initial needle aspiration. Because tuberculous brain abscesses are so uncommon, no randomized treatment studies are available. Optimal therapy requires the use of multiple drugs to which the organism is susceptible and should be continued for at least 1 year (Chapter 35). Open craniotomy and excision should be avoided.

The treatment of choice for brain abscesses caused by *Nocardia* is sulfadiazine in combination with craniotomy and complete excision. The combination of trimethoprim and sulfamethoxazole is also effective against *Nocardia.* A prolonged course of oral antibiotics for more than 1 year is often required to prevent recurrence of *Nocardia* infection.

Parasitic brain lesions caused by toxoplasmosis and neurocysticercosis require different therapy. Persons with AIDS who have lesions consistent with toxoplasmosis on imaging can initially be treated with pyrimethamine and sulfadiazine or pyrimethamine and clindamycin without needle aspiration (Chapter 38). Persons who do not respond to empirical antimicrobial therapy for toxoplasmosis should have diagnostic needle aspiration. Persons with cysticercosis caused by *T. solium* should be treated with albendazole (Table 44–2).

Surgery. Prompt surgical drainage can lead to identification of the responsible organism and can simplify the antibiotic regimen needed. There is no alternative to surgical drainage except during the early phases of cerebritis or in persons with small, deeply situated abscesses. Even in cases of multiple abscesses, the largest and most superficial lesion should be aspirated for a microbiologic diagnosis and to reduce the intracranial mass effect. **Stereotactic biopsy** is a minimally invasive closed surgical drainage procedure that can be performed with CT guidance. Risks of hemorrhage or other complications are low. A frame is attached to the patient's head to localize the abscess with 1–2 mm accuracy. It is particularly useful in obtaining material from deeper critical regions. In neonates, certain brain abscesses can be tapped through the anterior fontanelle with guidance by real-time ultrasonography.

Both **excision** and **needle aspiration** are equally effective in the management of bacterial brain abscesses. Craniotomy and excision can be reserved for persons who have not responded to treatment after needle aspiration and drainage, persons with multiloculated abscesses, and persons with abscesses caused by nonbacterial or more resistant pathogens such as fungi or *Nocardia* species. Posttraumatic abscesses are frequently multiloculated and may contain foreign bodies found at the time of injury. The advantage of excision is that it provides immediate eradication of the intracranial infection and usually involves a shortened course of postoperative medical treatment and duration of hospital stay. In cases of tuberculous brain abscesses, open excision is reserved for persons who have an expanding lesion not responsive to antituberculosis therapy.

The underlying cause of a brain abscess must be aggressively treated to prevent relapse. For example, if the brain abscess occurs from extension of infection from the mastoids or sinuses, then mastoidectomy or sinus surgery, in addition to drainage of the intracranial abscess, is warranted.

Adjunctive Therapy. Severe brain edema can develop around brain abscesses, resulting in increased intracranial pressure. This may be treated with corticosteroids, hyperventilation, and mannitol. If corticosteroids are used for a prolonged period, they may increase necrosis while delaying the encapsulation process. The ring enhancement seen on CT would then be altered, and the antibiotic penetration into the abscess would potentially be decreased.

Seizures are a frequent complication of brain abscesses. If there is no history of seizures, some experts recommend prophylactic anticonvulsants during the early stages of treatment and a minimum of 3 months after surgery. Neurology follow-up should be arranged several months after antibiotic treatment has been completed and symptoms have resolved.

There are conflicting reports about the use of corticosteroids in persons with *M. tuberculosis* brain abscesses. There is a theoretical risk of suppressing the host immune response to the mycobacterial infection. Corticosteroids may be helpful in persons who have associated cerebral edema and increased intracranial pressure. Corticosteroids are used in persons with neurocysticercosis to help control the inflammation produced as a result of cyst death. Antiepileptic drugs are frequently used in these cases to prevent seizures.

Duration of Therapy. The duration of antibiotic treatment for a brain abscess is individualized and dependent on the infecting organism, the size of the abscess, surgical drainage, and response to therapy as determined clinically and radiographically. If a susceptible etiologic organism is obtained and adequate surgical drainage can be performed, 6–8 weeks of parenteral antibiotic therapy is usually suggested. It is unclear whether additional therapy is needed after a course of intravenous antibiotics. Many will recommend 2–3 months of oral antibiotic therapy to suppress any residual infection and prevent relapses. The oral antibiotic chosen should have good absorption and central nervous system penetration (e.g., metronidazole) and should have activity against the infecting organism. Follow-up clinical examinations and CT scans every 1–2 weeks are helpful in monitoring resolution. The abscess will usually disappear on imaging, although small areas of residual enhancement may be present for a prolonged time. If this residual enhancement does not change within several weeks, antibiotic therapy may be stopped.

Nonoperative Management. In selected patients, nonoperative management with early aggressive antibiotic therapy may be effective. It is the exception rather than the rule. Candidates for such a treatment course include persons for whom the surgical risk is unacceptable, those with multiple abscesses or with abscesses in deep or otherwise difficult anatomic locations, those with small lesions considered to be in the cerebritis stage that are located in better-vascularized cortical areas, and those responding to medical therapy with decreasing abscess size visualized on CT or MRI. The risks include the need for prolonged empirical antimicrobial therapy and serious clinical deterioration including rupture of the abscess into the ventricles. Final resolution of the lesions is noted 2–14 months after therapy in the small number of persons managed in this fashion.

COMPLICATIONS

Intraventricular rupture of brain abscesses is one of the most dreaded complications of brain abscesses and carries an extremely high mortality of more than 80%. An aggressive approach is required, including open craniotomy with débridement of the abscess cavity. This can be followed by placement of a ventriculostomy catheter to permit external drainage and intrathecal administration of antibiotics if necessary.

Lateral sinus thrombosis and **cavernous sinus thrombosis** are potential complications of brain abscesses associated with chronic otitis media or mastoiditis. As the thrombus propagates and occludes the lumen, it can embolize and lead to septic infarcts throughout the body, including the lungs, bones, joints, and heart.

Neurologic sequelae from brain abscesses occur in 29–66% of cases and are common in children. These complications depend on the location of the abscess and the underlying cause and include seizures as well as hemiparesis, cranial nerve palsy, hydrocephalus, behavioral disorders, and learning disabilities. Many children will be developmentally and neurologically normal.

PROGNOSIS

The outcome of brain abscesses has improved considerably with CT and other imaging studies to aid early diagnosis. Improvements in anaerobic culture techniques, antimicrobial therapy, and surgery have also led to a better prognosis than in the past. The extent of neurologic compromise at the time of diagnosis and presentation and the rapidity of the disease progression are the most successful predictors of clinical outcome. Poor prognostic factors include age less than 1 year, concomitant meningitis, multiple foci, fungal cause, coma, and lack of available imaging studies. Rupture of the abscess into the cerebral ventricles or subarachnoid space is also a poor prognostic factor. Clinical improvement correlates well with a decrease in the size of abscesses as seen on MRI or CT scan.

In neonates, good neurologic outcome is associated with absence of initial seizures, negative CSF culture results, normal ventricles on CT scan, and early aspiration of the abscess. The capacity of the developing brain to regenerate may contribute positively to the neurologic outcome of this disease in neonates. A long period of developmental follow-up is needed to determine the final outcome.

SUBDURAL EMPYEMA AND CRANIAL EPIDURAL ABSCESS

A **subdural empyema** is a collection of pus between the cranial dura and the arachnoid membrane. A **cranial epidural abscess** is an infection between the dura mater and the inner table of the skull. It is rare in children.

ETIOLOGY

The predominant causative organisms include aerobic and anaerobic streptococci and gram-negative bacilli (Table 54–1). *S. pneumoniae* is the most common cause of subdural empyema associated with meningitis. Cranial epidural abscesses can also occur as a result of accidental or surgical trauma, and they often develop into subdural empyema, especially if untreated.

EPIDEMIOLOGY

Subdural empyemas and cranial epidural abscesses are much less common than brain abscesses and account for fewer than 20% of localized intracranial infections. These infections are most frequently seen in adolescents as a complication of frontal sinusitis and chronic middle ear disease.

PATHOGENESIS

The mechanisms that cause subdural empyema are similar to those that cause brain abscess (Table 54–2). Contiguous spread from parameningeal foci such as sinusitis, otitis media, and mastoiditis is typical, with frontal sinusitis being the leading cause. Valveless diploic veins connect intracranial and extracranial structures, allowing for retrograde extension of infection and associated thrombophlebitis into the subdural space. Cases resulting from chronic otitis media are rare and are due to contiguous spread from the middle ear to the subdural space after erosion of the bone and localized osteomyelitis. Intracranial surgery, head trauma, and occasionally bacteremia can also lead to subdural empyemas.

SYMPTOMS AND CLINICAL MANIFESTATIONS

The acute presentation of subdural empyema is in sharp contrast to the relatively nonspecific presentation of brain abscess (Table 54–3). Persons with subdural empyemas may have fever, signs of meningitis, seizures, and focal neurologic signs, especially cranial nerve palsies and hemiparesis. Increased intracranial pressure can develop quickly, with large empyemas resulting in mental status changes. Infants may have a bulging fontanelle. Thrombophlebitis can lead to focal ischemia or hemorrhagic infarction. Headaches occasionally are the only presenting sign and can be localized to the area of an accompanying sinusitis.

The presentation of cranial epidural abscess is usually a long history of nonspecific symptoms because the dura mater is closely opposed to the inner surface of the skull and the lesion enlarges slowly. Initial complaints may include fever, severe generalized headache, upper respiratory tract symptoms, or local tenderness over the frontal or mastoid sinuses. Affected persons rarely develop signs of elevated intracranial pressure, with nausea, vomiting, altered mental status, or focal neurologic signs.

DIAGNOSIS

Subdural empyema and cranial epidural abscess should be considered in any person with a predisposing condition such as chronic sinusitis or complicated meningitis. The differential diagnosis of subdural abscess, cranial epidural abscess, and brain abscess is similar and includes encephalitis, meningitis, brain abscess, subdural hematoma, epidural abscess, brain tumor, cerebral infarction, and migraine headache. The nonspecific nature of the clinical presentation requires adjunctive diagnostic imaging studies.

Laboratory Evaluation

Laboratory findings are nonspecific. The WBC count and the ESR may be elevated. As in brain abscess, lumbar puncture is usually contraindicated because of the risk of herniation and the lack of useful results from CSF analyses.

Microbiologic Evaluation

Prompt transport, including the use of anaerobic transport media, and cultures of abscess aspirate obtained at the time of surgery are crucial to the recovery of the infecting organisms. Specimens for Gram stain and for aerobic and anaerobic cultures should be obtained at the time of surgical drainage, regardless of prior antibiotic treatment. Gram stains can help guide empirical antimicrobial therapy before culture results are known. Acid-fast and fungal stains and cultures for mycobacteria and fungi should be obtained for immunocompromised persons and those with a history of exposure to tuberculosis.

Diagnostic Imaging

A subdural abscess appears as a hypodense crescent or elliptical lesion adjacent to the cranial vault or falx cerebri and can be seen on CT or MRI (Fig. 54–5). A cranial epidural abscess appears as a circumscribed hypodense area on CT or MRI (Fig. 54–6). MRI with gadolinium is superior to CT because MRI can provide better delineation between bone, CSF, and brain parenchyma. MRI is also better able to localize and characterize fluid (i.e., pus, CSF, blood) in the epidural or subdural space.

Pathologic Findings

An inflammatory exudate can be seen within the subdural space; the exudate usually remains localized but can extend throughout the entire subdural space. The location of the subdural empyema depends on the predisposing condition. Chronic otitis media usually results in accumulation of purulent material in the temporal or occipital area, whereas frontal or maxillary sinusitis usually results in frontal lobe lesions.

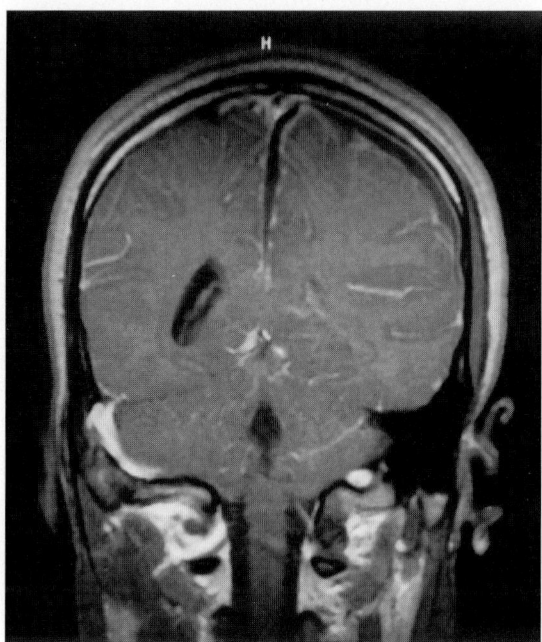

FIGURE 54–5. MRI of left subdural empyema. A crescentic lesion is seen adjacent to the cranial vault and extending to the falx cerebri.

TREATMENT

Urgent neurosurgical drainage and antibiotic use are the cornerstones of therapy. All persons should be started empirically on a regimen of intravenous antibiotic therapy. Infection associated with sinusitis should be treated with antibiotics that cover streptococci including *S. pneumoniae,* staphylococci, and anaerobes (Table 54–6). Otic and postoperative or posttraumatic infections should be treated with antibiotics that include coverage for gram-negative bacilli in addition to the organisms associated with sinusitis.

While the pus is still liquid, in the early stages, **burr hole aspiration** may provide adequate surgical drainage. Infants with an open anterior fontanelle can undergo needle aspiration if the abscess is in a frontal location. Often, subdural effusions associated with meningitis are not evacuated if the patient is neurologically stable. If the lesion is extensive or located in the posterior fossa, open craniotomy and drainage are preferred. It is unclear whether local antibiotic instillation at the time of surgery has any therapeutic value.

Vasogenic edema surrounding the subdural abscess may be much larger than the collection of pus itself, and persons with increased intracranial pressure must be treated accordingly. Many persons should undergo sinus surgery at the time of surgical drainage to treat the underlying cause of the subdural empyema.

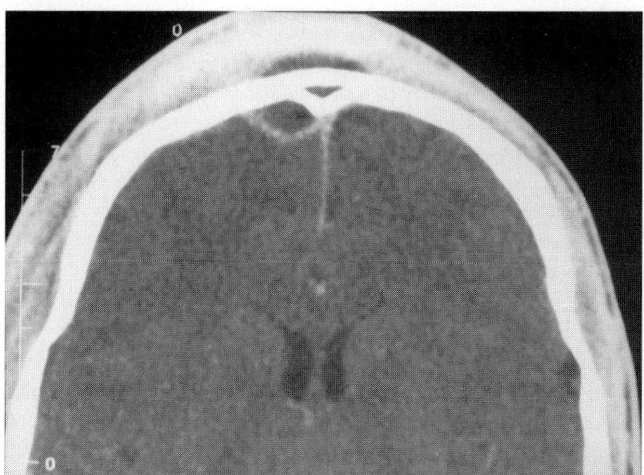

FIGURE 54–6. Right cranial epidural abscess in a 12-year-old boy as a complication of frontal sinusitis. A subperiosteal fluid collection is located superior to the cranial epidural abscess.

COMPLICATIONS

A high morbidity is associated with subdural empyema including simultaneous brain abscess, septic cortical vein thrombosis, epidural abscess, osteomyelitis, and reaccumulation of fluid along the falx cerebri. Seizures occur in approximately one third of patients. If left untreated, a cranial epidural abscess will usually develop into a subdural empyema.

PROGNOSIS

In the preantibiotic era the mortality for subdural empyemas was almost 100% even with surgical intervention. CT and MRI have facilitated earlier diagnosis and treatment. Factors that affect survival include extremes of age, level of consciousness at the time of presentation, and time to diagnosis and treatment. Persons who are obtunded or comatose at presentation are less likely to survive. Long-term complications include seizure disorder, hemiparesis, and aphasia.

SPINAL EPIDURAL ABSCESS

A **spinal epidural abscess** occurs in the spine between the bone and the dura mater, or **epidural space.** It is a true infectious disease emergency but is rare in children. This disease progresses rapidly, and complete recovery is dependent on early diagnosis and treatment.

EPIDEMIOLOGY

Spinal epidural abscesses have been reported in children of any age, with most occurring at 10–15 years. Approximately 20% of cases occur in infants.

ETIOLOGY

S. aureus is the most common etiologic agent isolated (Table 54–7). Other microorganisms include group A *Streptococcus,* other streptococci, gram-negative bacilli, and less frequently, anaerobic bacteria. Opportunistic pathogens such as *Aspergillus* and *Nocardia* have been isolated from immunocompromised persons. There are also case reports of epidural tuberculomas within the spinal cord.

PATHOGENESIS

Spinal epidural abscesses tend to occur where the epidural space is widest in the thoracic or lumbar area. The average extension is 4–7 vertebral segments. Hematogenous spread from skin and soft

TABLE 54–6. Recommended Empirical Antimicrobial Therapy for Subdural Empyema and Cranial Epidural Abscess

Source of Abscess	Microbial Flora	Empirical Antimicrobial Therapy*
Paranasal sinus and otogenic infections	Aerobic streptococci (usually *Streptococcus milleri* group)	Cefotaxime or ceftriaxone
	Streptococcus	*and*
	Anaerobic streptococci	Metronidazole
	Haemophilus	*and*
	Bacteroides (including *B. fragilis* and non-*fragilis*)	Vancomycin or penicillin G
	Enterobacteriaceae	
	Pseudomonas aeruginosa	
	Staphylococcus aureus	
Penetrating trauma *or* postoperative	*S. aureus*	Cefepime *or* ceftazidime
	Coagulase-negative staphylococci	*and*
	Clostridium species	Metronidazole
	Enterobacteriaceae	*and*
	Pseudomonas aeruginosa	Vancomycin *or* nafcillin
	Pasteurella multocida	
Meningitis		
Neonates	Group B *Streptococcus*	Cefotaxime
	Listeria monocytogenes	*and*
	Gram-negative aerobes (*Escherichia coli*)	Ampicillin
Infants, children, adolescents	*Streptococcus pneumoniae*	Cefotaxime *or* ceftriaxone
	Neisseria meningitidis	*and*
	Haemophilus influenzae type b	Vancomycin

*Suggested dosages listed in Table 54–5.

tissue infections is the leading source of spinal epidural abscesses. Direct extension from primary vertebral osteomyelitis and nonpenetrating spinal trauma are other sources of infection.

The posterior aspect of the epidural space is the most common area involved because of an extensive venous plexus and abundant adipose tissue. Granulation tissue with loculations of purulent material comprises the spinal epidural abscess.

SYMPTOMS AND CLINICAL MANIFESTATIONS

Four clinical stages have classically been described in adults. Initial complaints consist of fever and back pain. This is followed by nerve root compression with nerve root pain. Third, spinal cord compression with deficits in motor, sensory, bowel, and bladder function ensues, leading to the final stage of paralysis.

These stages are rarely present in infants and children. Local tenderness, fever, headache, and meningism are more common (Table 54–8). Irritability and fever predominate in infants. Persistent back pain may inadvertently be attributed to previous trauma. Physical examination may reveal paraspinous tenderness or a mass.

TABLE 54–7. Bacteriologic Findings in 47 Cases of Spinal Epidural Abscess*

Organism	No. (%)
Staphylococcus aureus	37 (79%)
Viridans streptococci	2 (4%)
Streptococcus pneumoniae	2 (4%)
Salmonella enteritidis	1 (2%)
Mixed culture†	4 (9%)
Sterile	1 (2%)

*Not reported in two cases.
†One culture of *S. aureus* and *Pseudomonas aeruginosa*, one of *S. aureus* and *Enterococcus faecalis*, one of *S. aureus* and *Bacillus pyocyaneus*, one of *Proteus, Escherichia coli,* and *Enterococcus*.
Adapted from Rubin GR, Michowiz SD, Ashkenasi A, et al: Spinal epidural abscess in the pediatric age group: A case report and a review of the literature. *Pediatr Infect Dis J* 1993;12:1007–11.

DIAGNOSIS

A child with fever and significant back pain should be urgently examined. The differential diagnosis includes vertebral osteomyelitis, diskitis, spinal tumors, herniated disks, transverse myelopathy, and trauma.

The WBC count and ESR may be elevated. Blood culture results are often positive for the infecting organism. A lumbar puncture should be avoided because it can lead to acute clinical decompensation and contamination of the subarachnoid space. The CSF findings are usually consistent with meningitis.

Radiographs of the spine can be normal unless vertebral osteomyelitis is present. MRI is superior to CT and has replaced myelography as the test of choice. MRI will show an epidural lesion on T2-weighted images (Fig. 54–7). Myelography shows a block of contrast material at the level of the lesion.

TREATMENT

A combination of antibiotics and surgery is the treatment of choice. Empirical antibiotic therapy should cover *S. aureus,* including MRSA if common in the community, and gram-negative organisms. Initial antibiotic choices could include vancomycin or nafcillin in combination with cefotaxime or ceftriaxone (Table 54–9). Anaerobic coverage should be added for persons with a suspected intra-abdominal, pelvic, or genitourinary tract infection. Antibiotic cov-

TABLE 54–8. Signs and Symptoms in 55 Cases of Spinal Epidural Abscess*

Signs and Symptoms	No.	%
Fever	35	64
Back pain	30	54
Paralysis	25	45
Rigor	24	44
Sphincteric disturbance	21	38
Paresis	18	33
Spinal tenderness	15	27
Sensory level	13	24
Radicular pain	11	20
Irritability	9	16
Paraspinous mass	9	16
Headache	6	11
Nausea and vomiting	5	9
Lethargy	3	5
Paresthesia	3	5
Papilledema	1	2

*Not reported in two cases.
Adapted from Rubin GR, Michowiz SD, Ashkenasi A, et al: Spinal epidural abscess in the pediatric age group: A case report and a review of the literature. *Pediatr Infect Dis J* 1993;12:1007–11.

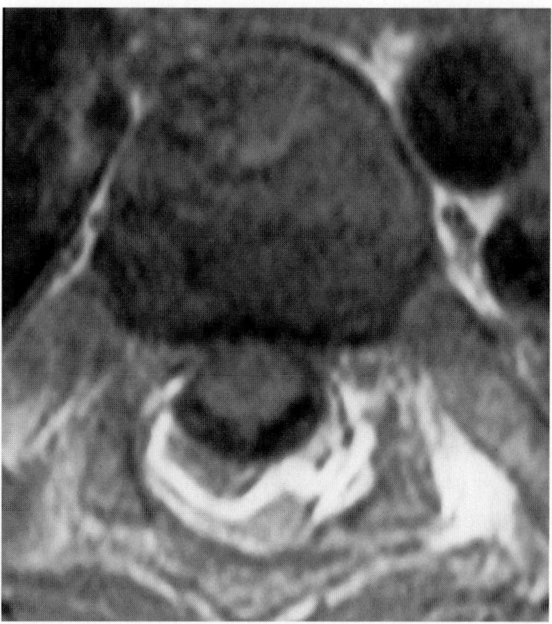

FIGURE 54–7. Spinal epidural abscess in an 11-month-old boy with MRSA bacteremia.

erage can be narrowed once a microbiologic diagnosis has been established.

Urgent neurosurgical evaluation is imperative in the management of spinal epidural abscesses. Most persons undergo surgery for removal of pus and granulation tissue. Infected bone must also be débrided. In children, laminectomy over several levels should be avoided whenever possible because of the risk of scoliosis in the future.

After surgery, patients need at least 4–6 weeks of antibiotic therapy, with a minimum of 3 weeks of parenteral antibiotic therapy. Up to 8 weeks of antibiotic therapy is needed if concomitant osteomyelitis is present.

Nonoperative management of spinal epidural abscesses has been used in some adults but has not been extensively studied in children. Medical therapy alone may be a consideration in rare circumstances when the infecting organism is known, there are no neurologic findings, and there are no underlying serious medical conditions.

COMPLICATIONS AND PROGNOSIS

The outcome is related to the neurologic condition at presentation and to the anatomic location of the abscess. Early diagnosis and prompt neurosurgical treatment are instrumental toward obtaining a good outcome, because any delay can lead to permanent paralysis and even death. Antimicrobial agent therapy should be started immediately. Approximately 90% of persons without neurologic signs or with paresis recover completely, whereas approximately 50% of persons with paralysis remain paralyzed or die, with only one third being cured of the infection. Persons with overt sepsis at presentation do poorly. Long-term neurologic sequelae include radiculopathy and motor paresis or paralysis.

TABLE 54–9. Spinal Epidural Abscess in Children: Microbiology and Recommended Empirical Antimicrobial Therapy

Source of Abscess	Microbial Flora	Empirical Antimicrobial Therapy*
Skin infection (furuncle, cellulitis)	*Staphylococcus aureus*	Vancomycin *or* nafcillin *or* oxacillin
Vertebral osteomyelitis	*S. aureus* Aerobic streptococci (viridans streptococci, *Streptococcus pneumoniae*) Anaerobic gram-negative bacteria *(Pseudomonas aeruginosa, Escherichia coli)*	Vancomycin *or* nafcillin *or* oxacillin *and* Ceftriaxone *or* cefotaxime
Spinal trauma (laminectomy, postepidural)	*S. aureus*	Vancomycin *or* nafcillin *or* oxacillin

*Suggested dosages shown in Table 54–5.

REVIEWS

Brain Abscess

Mathisen GE, Johnson JP: Brain abscess. *Clin Infect Dis* 1997;25:763–79.

Saez-Llorens XJ, Umana MA, Odio CM, et al: Brain abscess in infants and children. *Pediatr Infect Dis J* 1989;8:449–58.

Seydoux C, Francioli P: Bacterial brain abscesses: Factors influencing mortality and sequelae. *Clin Infect Dis* 1992;15:394–401.

Yogev R: Suppurative intracranial complications of upper respiratory tract infections. *Pediatr Infect Dis J* 1987;6:324–7.

Subdural Empyema and Cranial Epidural Abscess

Dill SR, Cobbs CG, McDonald CK: Subdural empyema: Analysis of 32 cases and review. *Clin Infect Dis* 1995;20:372–86.

Nathoo N, Nadvi SS, van Dellen JR, et al: Intracranial subdural empyemas in the era of computed tomography: A review of 699 cases. *Neurosurgery* 1999;44:529–35.

Sellick JA Jr: Epidural abscess and subdural empyema. *J Am Osteopath Assoc* 1989;89:806–10.

Spinal Epidural Abscess

Auletta JJ, John CC: Spinal epidural abscesses in children: A 15-year experience and review of the literature. *Clin Infect Dis* 2001;32:9–16.

Reihsaus E, Waldbaur H, Seeling W: Spinal epidural abscess: A meta-analysis of 915 patients. *Neurosurg Rev* 2000;23:175–204.

Rubin G, Michowiz SD, Ashkenasi A, et al: Spinal epidural abscess in the pediatric age group: Case report and review of literature. *Pediatr Infect Dis J* 1993;12:1007–11.

Wheeler D, Keiser P, Rigamonti D, et al: Medical management of spinal epidural abscesses: Case report and review. *Clin Infect Dis* 1992;15:22–7.

KEY ARTICLES

Brain Abscess

Anderson M: Management of cerebral infection. *J Neurol Neurosurg Psychiatry* 1993;56:1243–58.

Boom WH, Tuazon CU: Successful treatment of multiple brain abscesses with antibiotics alone. *Rev Infect Dis* 1985;7:189–99.

Brook I, Friedman EM, Rodriguez WJ, et al: Complications of sinusitis in children. *Pediatrics* 1980;66:568–72.

Brook I: Brain abscess in children: Microbiology and management. *J Child Neurol* 1995;10:283–8.

Chun CH, Johnson JD, Hofstetter M, et al: Brain abscess: A study of 45 consecutive cases. *Medicine* 1986;65:415–31.

Ciurea AV, Stoica F, Vasilescu G, et al: Neurosurgical management of brain abscesses in children. *Childs Nerv Syst* 1999;15:309–17.

Cohen LF, Dunbar SA, Sirbasku DM, et al: *Streptococcus bovis* infection of the central nervous system: Report of two cases and review. *Clin Infect Dis* 1997;25:819–23.

Garvey G: Current concepts of bacterial infections of the central nervous system. Bacterial meningitis and bacterial brain abscess. *J Neurosurg* 1983;59:735–44.

Grigoriadis E, Gold WL: Pyogenic brain abscess caused by *Streptococcus pneumoniae:* Case report and review. *Clin Infect Dis* 1997;25:1108–12.

Infection in Neurosurgery Working Party of the British Society for Antimicrobial Chemotherapy: The rational use of antibiotics in the treatment of brain abscess. *Br J Neurosurg* 2000;14:525–30.

Jadavji T, Humphreys RP, Prober CG: Brain abscesses in infants and children. *Pediatr Infect Dis* 1985;4:394–8.

Luby JP: Infections of the central nervous system. *Am J Med Sci* 1992;304:379–91.

Mampalam TJ, Rosenblum ML: Trends in the management of bacterial brain abscesses: A review of 102 cases over 17 years. *Neurosurgery* 1988;23:451–8.

Renier D, Flandin C, Hirsch E, et al: Brain abscesses in neonates. A study of 30 cases. *J Neurosurg* 1988;69:877–82.

Sable NS, Hengerer A, Powell KR: Acute frontal sinusitis with intracranial complications. *Pediatr Infect Dis* 1984;3:58–61.

Savitz MH, Dickinson T: Drug therapy for intracranial suppuration. *Am Fam Physician* 1988;37:341–4.

Snyder BD, Farmer TW: Brain abscess in children. *South Med J* 1971;64:687–90.

Stephanov S: Surgical treatment of brain abscess. *Neurosurgery* 1988;22:724–30.

Sutton DL, Ouvrier RA: Cerebral abscess in the under 6 month age group. *Arch Dis Child* 1983;58:901–5.

Tekkok IH, Erbengi A: Management of brain abscess in children: Review of 130 cases over a period of 21 years. *Childs Nerv Syst* 1992;8:411–6.

Townsend GC, Scheld WM: Infections of the central nervous system. *Adv Intern Med* 1998;43:403–47.

Yen PT, Chan ST, Huang TS: Brain abscess: With special reference to otolaryngologic sources of infection. *Otolaryngol Head Neck Surg* 1995;113:15–22.

Subdural Empyema and Cranial Epidural Abscess

Curless RG: Subdural empyema in infant meningitis: Diagnosis, therapy, and prognosis. *Childs Nerv Syst* 1985;1:211–4.

Farmer TW, Wise GR: Subdural empyema in infants, children and adults. *Neurology* 1973;23:254–61.

Miller ES, Dias PS, Uttley D: Management of subdural empyema: A series of 24 cases. *J Neurol Neurosurg Psychiatry* 1987;50:1415–8.

Smith HP, Hendrick EB: Subdural empyema and epidural abscess in children. *J Neurosurg* 1983;58:392–7.

Wackym PA, Canalis RF, Feuerman T: Subdural empyema of otorhinological origin. *J Laryngol Otol* 1990;104:118–22.

Weingarten K, Zimmerman RD, Becker RD, et al: Subdural and epidural empyemas: MR imaging. *AJR Am J Roentgenol* 1989;152:615–21.

Spinal Epidural Abscess

Angtuaco EJ, McConnell JR, Chadduck WM, et al: MR imaging of spinal epidural sepsis. *AJR Am J Roentgenol* 1987;149:1249–53.

Baker AS, Ojemann RG, Swartz MN, et al: Spinal epidural abscess. *N Engl J Med* 1975;293:463–8.

Danner RL, Hartman BJ: Update of spinal epidural abscess: 35 cases and review of the literature. *Rev Infect Dis* 1987;9:265–74.

Darouiche RO, Hamill RJ, Greenberg SB, et al: Bacterial spinal epidural abscess. Review of 43 cases and literature survey. *Medicine* 1992;71:369–85.

Del Curling O Jr, Gower DJ, McWhorter JM: Changing concepts in spinal epidural abscess: A report of 29 cases. *Neurosurgery* 1990;27:185–92.

Enberg RN, Kaplan RJ: Spinal epidural abscess in children. Early diagnosis and immediate surgical drainage is essential to forestall paralysis. *Clin Pediatr* 1974;13:247–53.

Fischer EG, Greene CS Jr, Winston KR: Spinal epidural abscess in children. *Neurosurgery* 1981;9:257–60.

Hlavin ML, Kaminski HJ, Ross JS, et al: Spinal epidural abscess: A ten-year perspective. *Neurosurgery* 1990;27:177–84.

Kaufman DM, Kaplan JG, Litman N: Infectious agents in spinal epidural abscesses. *Neurology* 1980;30:844–50.

Mackenzie AR, Laing RB, Smith CC, et al: Spinal epidural abscess: The importance of early diagnosis and treatment. *J Neurol Neurosurg Psychiatry* 1998;65:209–12.

Rockney R, Ryan R, Knuckey N: Spinal epidural abscess. An infectious emergency. Case report and review. *Clin Pediatr* 1989;28:332–4.

CHAPTER 55

Infectious Encephalitis

Philip Toltzis

Encephalitis results from inflammation of the brain parenchyma, leading to cerebral dysfunction. In general, organisms cause encephalitis by one of two mechanisms: direct infection of the brain parenchyma or an apparent immune-mediated response in the CNS that usually begins several days after the appearance of extraneural manifestations of the infection. Pathologically, immune-mediated encephalitis is characterized by perivascular demyelination and an inability to isolate the organism from either the CSF or brain tissue. Whereas some infections are clearly mediated by direct infection, as in HSV encephalitis, and others by immune-mediated responses, as in measles, the distinction is uncertain for many of the infectious encephalitides, and in others both processes may occur concomitantly.

Suggestive Symptoms and Signs. Acute infectious encephalitis is usually preceded by a prodrome of several days with nonspecific symptoms such as cough, sore throat, fever, headache, or abdominal complaints that are followed by increasing lethargy, behavioral changes, and neurologic deficits. Seizures are a common element at presentation. The diagnosis is supported by examination of the CSF, which typically demonstrates a mild lymphocytic pleocytosis, mild elevation in protein content, and normal glucose level. The EEG in infectious encephalitis commonly shows diffuse, slow-wave activity, although focal changes may be present. Neuroimaging studies may be normal or may show swelling of the parenchyma or focal abnormalities. Although most persons with infectious encephalitis in the United States recover, severe cases leading to death or substantial neurologic sequelae can occur with infection by virtually any neurotropic organism. Among survivors, symptoms usually resolve within several days to 2–3 weeks.

Differential Diagnoses. Viruses are the principal causes of acute infectious encephalitis (Table 55–1). However, encephalitis also may result from infection with bacteria, fungi, and parasites, as well as from many noninfectious diseases (Table 55–2). Currently in the United States the most common viral causes of encephalitis include the arboviruses, enteroviruses, and herpesviruses. Cases of arboviral and enteroviral encephalitis appear characteristically in clusters or epidemics that occur from midsummer to early fall. The herpesviruses and other infectious agents account for sporadic cases throughout the year.

Initial Management. With the exception of HSV and HIV, there is no specific therapy for viral encephalitis. Management is supportive and frequently requires intensive care during the initial stages until the tempo of the illness can be established. Intensive care allows aggressive therapy for seizures, timely detection of electrolyte abnormalities, and, when necessary, airway monitoring and protection and the reduction of increased intracranial pressure.

Many of the nonviral causes of encephalitis require expeditious identification and specific therapy. Therefore management must include a rigorous attempt to establish the underlying cause. Many causes are suggested by clues in the patient's history (Table 55–3). Frequently, however, the identification of the underlying cause of encephalitis requires laboratory testing that should include antibody assays for the common infectious agents, viral cultures, PCR assay for HSV and enteroviruses, an EEG, and neuroimaging studies (Table 55–4). Serologic studies should be obtained for arboviruses, Epstein-Barr virus, *Mycoplasma pneumoniae,* and Lyme disease. In addition to serologic testing, a sample of CSF and stool and a nasopharyngeal swab should be obtained for viral culture. In most cases of viral encephalitis, however, the organism is difficult to isolate from the CSF. Additionally, common nonviral causes of encephalopathy should be routinely investigated through VDRL testing, assay for antinuclear antibodies, a toxicology screen for ingestion of psychotropic medications or illicit drugs, measurement of the lead level, and a tuberculin skin test with appropriate controls. Even with extensive testing, including the employment of PCR assays, the cause of encephalitis is undetermined in one third or more of the cases.

Additional specialized tests may be pursued when clinically indicated (Table 55–4). Serologic testing for the less common

TABLE 55–1. Viral Causes of Encephalitis

Acute
- Arboviruses
- Herpesviruses
  - Herpes simplex viruses
  - Epstein-Barr virus
  - Varicella-zoster virus
  - Human herpesvirus 6
  - Human herpesvirus 7
- Enteroviruses
- Childhood-illness viruses
  - Measles virus
  - Mumps virus
  - Rubella virus
- Influenza viruses
- Lymphocytic choriomeningitis virus
- Adenoviruses
- Rabies virus

Subacute
- Human immunodeficiency virus
- JC virus
- Prion-associated encephalopathies (Creutzfeldt-Jakob disease, kuru)

TABLE 55–2. Nonviral Causes of Encephalitis

Infectious	Hypoglycemia
Bacterial	Hyponatremia
Parameningeal focus	Inborn errors of metabolism
Embolic endocarditis	Uremia
Brain abscess	Water Intoxication
Tuberculous meningitis	***Anoxic Encephalopathy***
Mycoplasma pneumoniae	***Hydrocephalus***
Cat-scratch disease	***Malignant Hypertension***
Rocky Mountain spotted fever	***Carcinomatous Meningitis***
Lyme disease	***Collagen-Vascular Disease***
Syphilis	Systemic lupus erythematosus
Shigellosis (Shiga-toxin)	Behçet's syndrome
Fungal	Sarcoidosis
Cryptococcosis	***Toxic Ingestion***
Histoplasmosis	Ethanol
Blastomycosis	Drugs
Coccidioidomycosis	***Lead Poisoning***
Amebic	***Mass Effect***
Granulomatous amebic encephalitis (*Acanthamoeba castellanii, A. culbertsoni, A. astronyxis*)	Tumor
	Hemorrhage
	Thromboembolism
Noninfectious	***Trauma***
Metabolic Disease	Contusion
Reye's syndrome	Hemorrhage
Hyperammonemia (hepatic encephalopathy)	

TABLE 55–3. Clues to the Causation of Infectious Encephalitis

Travel History	**Season**
Arboviruses	Arboviruses
Tuberculosis	Enteroviruses
Lyme borreliosis	**Associated Symptoms**
Rocky Mountain spotted fever	Rash
Rabies	Enterovirus
Community Epidemiology	Adenovirus
Arboviruses	Measles
Enteroviruses	Varicella
Measles	Rocky Mountain spotted fever
Influenza	Lyme borreliosis
Surveillance Data	Rubella
Rabies	Pneumonia
Arboviruses	*Mycoplasma pneumoniae*
Animal Exposure	Adenovirus
Rabies	Tuberculosis
Lymphocytic choriomeningitis	"Influenza-like" illness
Cat-scratch disease	Influenza
Tick Exposure	Lymphocytic choriomeningitis
Lyme borreliosis	Colorado tick fever
Rocky Mountain spotted fever	Other characteristic symptoms
Colorado tick fever	Human immunodeficiency virus
Immunization History	Epstein-Barr virus
Measles	Mumps
Mumps	Cat-scratch disease
Rubella	

Adapted from Toltzis P: Viral encephalitis. *Adv Pediatr Infect Dis* 1991; 6:130.

pathogens may be indicated if the travel, social, or medical history suggests these causes. Measurement of the serum ammonia level and other liver function tests should be performed for symptoms consistent with Reye's syndrome. Biopsy of a lymph node in a person with encephalopathy and localized lymphadenopathy may establish the diagnosis of cat-scratch disease. A skin biopsy with appropriate tissue staining for rabies, Rocky Mountain spotted fever, or varicella-zoster with an untypical-appearing rash may confirm these diagnoses. Brain biopsy may be appropriate for persons with severe encephalopathy who demonstrate no clinical improvement if the diagnosis remains obscure. HSV, rabies encephalitis, and prion-related diseases (Creutzfeldt-Jakob disease and kuru) may be routinely diagnosed by culture or pathologic examination of brain biopsy tissue. Brain biopsy may be important in identifying arbovirus and enterovirus infections, tuberculosis, and fungal infections, as well as noninfectious illnesses, particularly CNS vasculopathies. In many instances, however, culture, serologic testing, and neuroimaging studies may identify infectious causes without requiring brain biopsy.

Prognosis. Regardless of the cause, the overall mortality rate for infectious encephalitis is approximately 5%. About two thirds of patients recover fully before being discharged from the hospital. The remainder demonstrate clinically significant residua including paresis or spasticity, cognitive impairment, weakness, ataxia, and repeated seizures. Although there are few long-term follow-up studies, many persons with neurologic sequelae of infectious encephalitis at the time of hospital discharge gradually recover some or all of their function. The causative agent of encephalitis is the strongest predictive factor for the eventual outcome; HSV and *M. pneumoniae* are the common causes of encephalitides that have the worst outcomes.

HERPES SIMPLEX VIRUS ENCEPHALITIS

It is imperative in the management of a person with presumed infectious encephalitis to evaluate expeditiously the possibility of HSV encephalitis because of the availability of therapy for this potentially life-threatening infection. In comparison with herpes infection in older children and adults, neonatal herpes infections have important differences in presentation and management (Chapter 97).

ETIOLOGY

Herpes simplex virus is a large double-stranded DNA virus of the Herpesviridae family. The two subtypes, type 1 and type 2, share about 50% homology and can be distinguished genetically, biologically, and serologically. Historically, HSV-1 is regarded as the ''oral'' type and HSV-2 as the ''genital'' type, but the virus type is no longer a reliable indicator of the site of isolation. HSV infects cells of ectodermal origin. Initial infection occurs on skin in cutaneous herpes (Chapter 46) or on mucous membranes in gingivostomatitis (Chapter 60), after which the virus establishes latent infection in the sensory neural ganglia innervating the site

TABLE 55–4. Laboratory Evaluation for Acute Encephalitis

Routine Tests
Serologic tests
Arboviruses
Epstein-Barr virus
Mycoplasma pneumoniae
Lyme disease
Syphilis
Viral cultures
Stool, nasopharyngeal, cerebrospinal fluid
PCR assays
Herpes simplex virus
Enteroviruses
Tuberculin skin test
Lumbar puncture
Electroencephalogram
Neuroimaging study
Antinuclear antibodies
Toxicology screen
Lead screen
Special Cases
Serologic tests
Human immunodeficiency virus
Mumps
Lymphocytic choriomeningitis
Rubella
Adenoviruses
Rickettsia
Brucella
Bartonella henselae (cat-scratch disease)
Ammonia level and liver function tests
Lymph node biopsy
Skin biopsy
Brain biopsy

of original infection. The spread of HSV to the CNS is along neurogenic pathways. HSV-1 causes 93–96% of HSV encephalitis.

Transmission. HSV is transmitted by close contact, primarily through saliva or sexual transmission. The likelihood of transmission is increased if HSV is inoculated onto abraded or denuded skin, including burns. Under certain conditions, the virus has been identified on fomites. However, no clear evidence of indirect transmission has been found.

EPIDEMIOLOGY

HSV accounts for approximately 5–10% of all cases of encephalitis and for up to 20% of cases with a confirmed cause. HSV encephalitis may occur at any age and has no sexual predilection. During the newborn period, HSV-2 predominates (Chapter 96). However, nearly all postnatally acquired HSV encephalitis is due to HSV-1. HSV encephalitis has no seasonal pattern.

PATHOGENESIS

Approximately 30% of cases of HSV encephalitis occur during primary HSV infection, and approximately 70% occur as the result of reactivation. The mean age for encephalitis with primary infection is 15 years, compared with a mean age of approximately 50 years for reactivation. There are no distinguishing clinical characteristics between primary and reactivation HSV encephalitis. In both instances the infection has a marked predilection for the frontal and temporal lobes. In HSV encephalitis resulting from primary infection, virus cell-to-cell spread proceeds from the oral mucous membrane, through the cribriform plate, and along the olfactory nerve to the base of the brain. In HSV encephalitis associated with reactivation, disease originates from latent infection in the trigeminal ganglion. Access to the anterior and middle fossa is gained through a recurrent branch of the ophthalmic division of the trigeminal nerve, which forms perivascular plexuses at the base of the temporal and frontal lobes. Regardless of the origin, infection of the brain by HSV results in focal areas of hemorrhagic necrosis that involve the superficial cortex.

SYMPTOMS AND CLINICAL MANIFESTATIONS

HSV encephalitis is typically preceded by a prodrome of 2–4 days of increasingly severe headache. Although many cases of HSV encephalitis originate from infection of the oral mucosa, the infection in the mouth is usually subclinical, and thus the absence of overt herpes stomatitis is not a reliable indicator excluding HSV encephalitis. The hallmarks of HSV encephalitis are altered consciousness, fever, and focal abnormalities localized to the temporal or frontal lobes (Table 55–5). Within the first 2–4 days of illness, approximately 70% of patients demonstrate personality changes, and approximately one third have hemiparesis. Aphasia, cranial nerve deficits, and focal seizures also may denote focal herpetic encephalitis. Many patients with HSV encephalitis have increased intracranial pressure, which causes a global depression of sensorium. Most untreated cases progress to coma in 2–3 days.

The application of the extremely sensitive PCR assay to CSF specimens has resulted in an appreciation of a broader range of clinical presentations for herpes encephalitis. Approximately 20% of all cases of HSV CNS disease do not follow the typical pattern. Symptoms are occasionally limited to the brainstem or spinal cord. There may be no focality demonstrated by history or physical examination, or there may be mild disease. Even among atypical cases, however, most have evidence of frontal or temporal lobe disease on EEG or neuroimaging.

TABLE 55–5. Clinical and Laboratory Characteristics of Herpes Simplex Virus Encephalitis

Characteristic	Rate of Occurrence (%)
Altered consciousness	52–97
Fever	90
Focal neurologic signs	38–89
Dysphasia	46–76
Personality change	71
Seizure	67
Meningism	65
Ataxia	40
Cranial nerve palsy	32
Abnormal cerebrospinal fluid	97
Focal electroencephalogram abnormalities	81
Focal CT or MRI abnormalities	59–78

Data from Whitley RJ, Soong SJ, Linneman C Jr, et al: Herpes simplex encephalitis: Clinical assessment. *JAMA* 1982;247:317–20 and from Kennedy PG: A retrospective analysis of forty-six cases of herpes simplex encephalitis seen in Glasgow between 1962 and 1985. *Q J Med* 1988;68: 533–40.

DIAGNOSIS

Rapid diagnosis of HSV encephalitis is critical because the outcome strongly correlates with the severity of disease at the start of therapy. Unfortunately the identification of HSV encephalitis may be difficult. Any patient with severe febrile encephalopathy or evidence of focal neurologic signs should be evaluated for HSV encephalitis. Laboratory support of a diagnosis of HSV infection incorporates several techniques, and rapid performance of all of these tests is advisable. Typically an EEG reveals periodic lateralized epileptiform focal discharges over the temporal or frontal lobe against a diffuse, slow-wave background. Neuroimaging studies demonstrate local edema and contrast enhancement early in the course of the infection, followed by hemorrhagic necrosis as the disease progresses. Unfortunately the CT scan shows abnormalities in only approximately 60% of patients at the initial evaluation (see Figs. 13–4 and 13–5). However, MRI may detect early focal lesions in the temporal or frontal lobes on T2-weighted images several days before any abnormality is apparent on CT. Therefore MRI, if available, is the imaging study of choice. The characteristic findings in the CSF are a moderate monocellular pleocytosis of 100–150/mm^3 and an elevated protein level of about 80 mg/dL. The presence of red blood cells is thought to reflect the hemorrhagic nature of the viral infection, but this finding is nonspecific and inconsistent. The CSF cell count, which typically increases dramatically during the early stages of infection, can be demonstrated by repeated CSF analysis.

PCR-based assays for HSV in the CSF of persons in whom herpes encephalitis is suspected have become an important component in the initial evaluation. Most assays amplify conserved regions of the viral polymerase gene. In comparison with brain biopsy, PCR has a sensitivity and specificity exceeding 95%; however, some persons with negative biopsy results have positive PCR results, indicating that the latter assay may be the more appropriate standard. In contrast to PCR assay, viral culture and serologic tests are largely insensitive early in the course of HSV encephalitis. Virus can be isolated from the CSF in <5% of biopsy-proved cases. Routine serologic testing has limited worth; the seroprevalence of HSV is high in the general population, and although almost 70% of persons with HSV encephalitis eventually demonstrate a fourfold increase in antibody titer consistent with primary infection, seroconversion may require weeks and does not identify those with reactivation. Moreover, because stress nonspecifically stimulates reactivation of HSV, approximately 10% of persons with encephalitis from other causes also show a rise in antibody titers. Simultaneous measurement of anti-HSV antibody in the serum and CSF may yield a diagnosis without the need to wait for seroconversion, but a positive test result (serum:CSF ratio less than 20, indicating local CNS production of anti-HSV antibody) is infrequent early in the course of the disease, when therapy is most effective.

In the past, brain biopsy was routinely performed in patients with suspected HSV encephalitis. The recommendation to proceed to brain biopsy was partially based on the observation that many nonherpetic diseases that otherwise could not be distinguished from HSV encephalitis were diagnosed at biopsy, with 40% being treatable causes, including bacterial, mycobacterial, fungal, and rickettsial infections; tumors; hematomas; and lupus erythematosus. Currently the need for biopsy is less urgent, however, because (1) many of the alternative diagnoses can be established by noninvasive means, (2) PCR assays for HSV in CSF have sensitivity equivalent to that of biopsy, and (3) the excellent safety profile of acyclovir, the antiviral drug of choice, invites empirical therapy. One recommended approach is to treat the infection with a full course of acyclovir either if the CSF PCR test is positive for HSV or if the clinical presentation is characteristic, with focal findings on neurologic examination, typical CSF findings, and temporal lobe involvement by EEG or neuroimaging, in the absence of an alternative diagnosis. In the absence of these clinical characteristics, a PCR assay negative for HSV may be used to discontinue acyclovir. Biopsies are reserved for patients with uncertain diagnoses whose condition has not improved after 2–4 days of antiviral chemotherapy.

TABLE 55–6. Treatment of Herpes Simplex Virus Encephalitis (Beyond the Newborn Period*)

Recommended Regimen
Acyclovir 30 mg/mg/day divided q8hr for 14–21 days IV

Alternative Regimen
Vidarabine 15 mg/kg once daily for 14–21 days IV

*See Chapter 97 for dosing for neonatal HSV encephalitis.

TREATMENT

The drugs used most often to treat HSV encephalitis are vidarabine and acyclovir (Table 55–6). Acyclovir has been shown to be superior compared with vidarabine in controlled trials. Acyclovir is administered intravenously at a dosage of 30 mg/kg/day in three divided doses every 8 hours for a minimum of 14 days. The drug has few adverse effects; rapid administration has been associated with renal insufficiency and rarely with psychosis and other behavioral changes. The emergence of acyclovir-resistant HSV, particularly in persons with AIDS, sometimes requires alternative agents such as ganciclovir or foscarnet. Some experts have recommended repeating the lumbar puncture at the end of the planned course of therapy to determine whether virus is still present by PCR assay; consideration should be given to continuing therapy with the antiviral drug until this test is negative.

PROGNOSIS

The mortality rate for untreated HSV encephalitis is approximately 70%. Treatment with antiviral agents improves survival rates and also the clinical outcome of the survivors (Table 55–7). Factors associated with increased mortality and morbidity rates include age more than 30 years, presentation in semicoma or coma, and Glasgow coma score of <10. Early diagnosis and initiation of antiviral therapy before to progression to coma is important.

Some persons who survive the first few weeks later die or have further deterioration as a result of the damage. The mortality rate for HSV encephalitis treated with acyclovir is approximately 15–

TABLE 55–7. Prognosis at 1 Year for Persons with Herpes Simplex Virus Encephalitis

		Treatment with	
Outcome	Without Treatment	Vidarabine	Acyclovir
Mortality (%)	70	50	30
Morbidity (%)			
Severe	10	20	10
Moderate	10	15	10
Mild or none	10	15	50

20% at 1 month, 20% at 6 months, and 20–30% at 18 months. Approximately 5% of affected persons have a relapse of HSV encephalitis within several months after treatment. These persons are usually treated with another course of antiviral therapy. Some persons may have progressive deterioration of functional abilities. It is not clear whether this is the result of persistent viral replication or a postinfectious autoimmune phenomenon. There are insufficient data to recommend long-term acyclovir or other antiviral therapy for such patients.

PREVENTION

There are no specific preventive measures for HSV encephalitis, especially because 70% of cases occur with reactivation. It is unknown whether antiviral treatment of herpetic gingivostomatitis (Chapter 60) influences possible progression to HSV encephalitis.

ARBOVIRUSES

Arboviruses, or *ar*thropod*bo*rne *viruses,* are a frequent cause of epidemic encephalitis worldwide. Although they tend to be grouped together, the arboviruses actually are derived from several distinct viral families, including the two genera of togaviruses (alphaviruses and flaviviruses, both positive-stranded RNA viruses), bunyaviruses (trisegmented negative-stranded viruses), and reoviruses (segmented double-stranded viruses). The vectors for each of these viruses are species restricted, and therefore these entities are confined to distinct geographic areas and seasons (Fig. 55–1). Each of these agents must replicate in the insect before being transmitted to the next host. In temperate climates, mosquitoborne infections occur in late summer and early fall. Tickborne disease occurs from spring until the first frost.

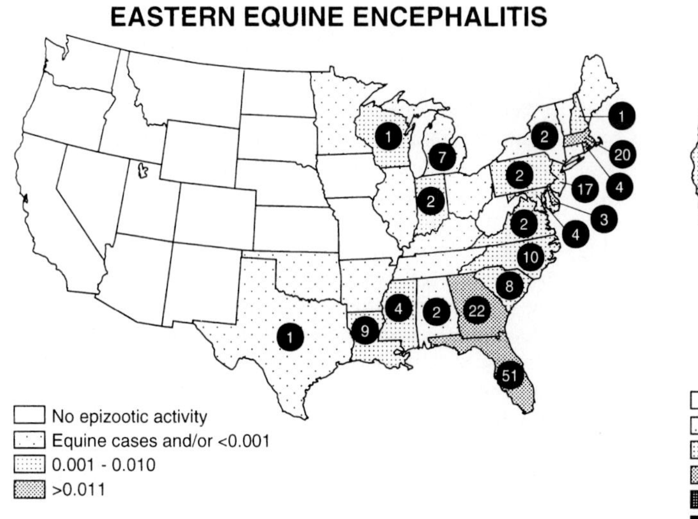

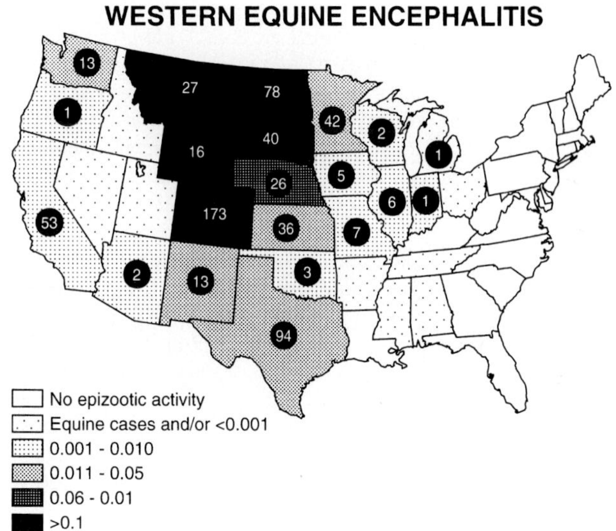

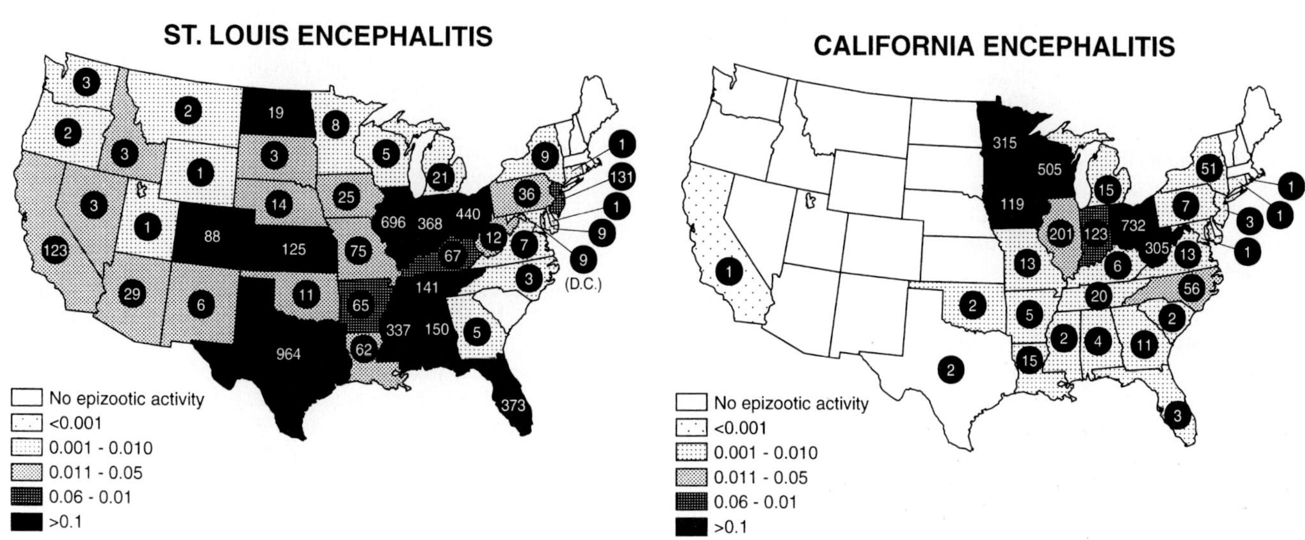

FIGURE 55–1. Reported cases (black circles) and incidence of rates per 100,000 population per year of Eastern equine encephalitis, Western equine encephalitis, St. Louis encephalitis, and California encephalitis reported to the Centers for Disease Control and Prevention by state from 1964 through 1997.

ARBOVIRUSES IN THE UNITED STATES

The most frequent arboviruses identified in the United States are those which cause St. Louis encephalitis, California encephalitis, and, less frequently, Western equine encephalitis, Colorado tick fever, and Eastern equine encephalitis virus. With the exception of the EEE virus, all produce identical, essentially nonspecific encephalitis that resolves without residua in most persons. In all instances, serologic surveys have documented a high ratio of asymptomatic to total infections.

St. Louis Encephalitis. SLE is the most frequent cause of human arbovirus encephalitis in the United States and is caused by the SLE virus, a member of the flavivirus genus of Togaviridae. SLE occurs most frequently in areas surrounding the Mississippi and Ohio Rivers, extending into the Middle Atlantic states, but infection is widespread and may occur in virtually any area in the continental United States (Fig. 55–1). In rural areas the virus is cycled and amplified principally between the *Culex tarsalis* mosquito and avian reservoirs. In urban areas the virus is found principally in *Culex pipiens* mosquitoes breeding in stagnant sewage. Usually humans serve as a dead-end host because the density of viremia in humans is insufficient to pass the infection back to uninfected mosquitoes. However, in urban epidemics a person may serve as an active intermediate host (cycling infection from person to mosquito to person), leading to rapid dissemination of infection.

The ratio of inapparent infection to disease is approximately 60:1. Usually there are no distinguishing features of SLE that allow it to be separated from other types of encephalitis. However, some persons may manifest unusual features, including opsoclonus or myoclonus, or urinary tract signs and symptoms such as incontinence, dysuria, and pyuria in the presence of normal renal function. Persons with symptomatic infections may present with aseptic meningitis without signs of CNS dysfunction, particularly in the pediatric age group; a small percentage may demonstrate only fever and headache.

The diagnosis of SLE usually is established serologically because the virus is difficult to isolate from routine clinical specimens, including CSF. Antibody levels usually begin to rise soon after the onset of clinical disease. Depending on the method used, antibodies may persist for many years; however, an IgM-specific assay has been developed that may confirm recent infection. Anti-SLE antibodies can cross-react with other flaviviruses. With the possible exception of dengue virus, however, most of these viruses are not endemic to North America.

The outcome of SLE is usually good. Occasionally the infection can be severe, and death and neurologic morbidity can occur. Descriptions of virtually all outbreaks of SLE have identified advancing age as the greatest risk factor for severe disease and death.

California Encephalitis. California encephalitis is caused by one of several members of the California serogroup of Bunyaviridae. The most common of these are La Crosse, Jamestown Canyon, and snowshoe hare viruses. Despite the name, most cases are identified in the northern midwestern and eastern states extending from Minnesota to New York. The virus is transmitted primarily by the *Aedes triseriatus* mosquito. Disease is most prevalent around communities adjacent to hardwood forests or wooden lots. The virus is transmitted from insect to insect either vertically or venereally and is amplified in small forest animals such as squirrels and chipmunks. Seroprevalence surveys of California encephalitis viruses in endemic areas indicate that inapparent infection is a common event, with ≥30% of residents in some areas having antibodies against La Crosse virus.

As with other arboviruses, most cases of encephalitis caused by the California serotypes have only nonspecific symptoms. La Crosse virus produces disease almost exclusively in children, with a peak incidence between 5 and 10 years of age. The onset may be abrupt, the temperature at presentation is typically high, and depression of the sensorium can be dramatic. Some reports have emphasized the presence in up to 20% of persons of focal neurologic signs that may be clinically indistinguishable from those of HSV encephalitis.

As with other arboviral infections, the diagnosis of California encephalitis is established by serologic techniques. Because the prevalence of antibody in the general population is high, diagnosis by conventional serologic tests requires the detection of a fourfold increase in titer from paired acute and convalescent sera. Death from La Crosse virus encephalitis is uncommon. However, some long-term disabilities, including recurrent seizures and behavioral lability, may be noted in 15–20% of affected persons.

Western Equine Encephalitis. WEE is caused by the WEE virus, a member of the alphavirus genus of Togaviridae. Cases of WEE occur over a large area extending from the Mississippi and Ohio river valleys to the Pacific Coast, peaking in the central plains states east of the Rocky Mountains. Similar to the vector for the SLE virus, the principal mosquito vector for WEE is *C. tarsalis,* although other species, including *Aedes* mosquitoes, occasionally have been infected. Breeding areas are identified most frequently around ground pools, particularly irrigation ditches. Consequently, WEE occurs most commonly near farmlands. As in the SLE virus, the WEE virus is amplified in avian and small-animal reservoirs; in addition, the WEE virus may be passed to horses and humans, both of which serve as dead-end hosts.

The clinical features of WEE are nondescript. The onset may be abrupt and the acute illness severe, but death is unusual. As with other arboviral illnesses, the diagnosis of WEE is established by serologic testing showing a fourfold increase of antibody titers. Inapparent infection with WEE is 10-fold more common in children and 1,000-fold more common in adults than disease.

Eastern Equine Encephalitis. EEE is caused by the EEE virus, a member of the alphavirus genus of Togaviridae. It is the most severe form of arthropodborne encephalitis in the United States. Fortunately the disease is uncommon, and outbreaks have been confined to limited regions of the country. Most cases have occurred in the swamps and cranberry bogs south of Boston, where the first documented outbreak was noted in 1939. Outbreaks subsequently have been recorded near the New Jersey shoreline, in Louisiana, and in the Dominican Republic.

The primary mosquito vector is *Culiseta melanura,* which breeds in freshwater swamps and feeds in adjacent open fields. Outbreaks characteristically follow climatic conditions that are necessary for the production of large larval and adult *Culiseta* populations, namely, a wet fall season followed by an unusually wet summer. With few exceptions, *C. melanura* limits its feeding to birds, which accounts for the low rates of human disease even in the presence of large numbers of infected mosquitoes. Avian reservoirs are established in species of sparrows, ducks, and pheasants, which become ill after infection and die in droves. Infection is spread to mammals, including horses and humans, only after other mosquitoes, particularly *Aedes,* carry the virus from infected birds beyond the swamplands. Outbreaks among humans can be predicted from detection of sentinel cases in pheasants and horses.

Once mammalian infection has occurred, the level of viremia is insufficient to transmit infection to uninfected mosquitoes.

Common to the other arboviral encephalitides, subclinical infections with EEE virus are more common than clinically apparent cases, but the ratios are lower, 5:1–30:1. The incidence of EEE is highest among young children, perhaps because they are frequently outdoors during the late summer months and are less likely to brush away a feeding mosquito. The characteristic clinical presentation of EEE is similar to that of other types of viral encephalitis, but it is more severe. The prodrome of EEE typically is short and the progression of encephalopathy is rapid and dramatic. Stupor or coma occurs in 90% of patients and seizures in 74%.

Unlike most other viral encephalitides, the CBC usually demonstrates a marked leukocytosis of 20,000/mm^3 or more with a shift to the left. In addition, in distinction to virtually all other forms of viral encephalitis, the CSF examination characteristically reveals a distinct polymorphonuclear pleocytosis, although the profile may shift to mononuclear leukocytes as the illness progresses. The diagnosis can be established by serologic testing. Antibodies to EEE virus usually begin to rise soon after the onset of symptoms, and therefore paired sera confirm the diagnosis. Because antibody to EEE virus is uncommon in the general population, a single positive serologic test result in a person with severe encephalitis is presumptive evidence of EEE virus infection. The virus usually cannot be isolated from CSF but can be cultured readily from brain biopsy specimens.

The mortality rate for EEE ranges from 55% to 100%, and there is a high incidence of neurologic sequelae among survivors. Although the mortality rate for this infection is lower among children than among older patients, the young are more prone to have neurologic damage. Given the severe nature of this infection, selective preventive measures have been attempted when epidemic infection has been predicted by climatic conditions and the detection of sentinel cases in animals. Public health education efforts to promote the use of insect repellent and to avoid outside activities at dusk, when many mosquitoes feed, may be effective. In addition, aerial application of malathion in Michigan in 1980 after the identification of 72 cases in horses and one in a person led to the prevention of further human disease.

West Nile Virus. West Nile virus is a neurotropic flavivirus, similar to St. Louis encephalitis virus and Japanese encephalitis virus. Infection with this organism is endemic throughout Africa and Asia. Epidemics in the Middle East, South Africa, and the Asian subcontinent were described in the mid-twentieth century. West Nile virus gained importance in Europe and North America upon outbreaks of encephalitis caused by this pathogen in Romania in 1996 and in New York City in 1999.

The principal vector for West Nile virus is the *Culex pipiens* mosquito, but the organism can be isolated in nature from a wide variety of *Culex* and *Aedes* species. A broad range of birds serves as the major reservoir for West Nile virus; in New York the virus was isolated from dead crows, hawks, and a Chilean flamingo that succumbed to the virus at the Bronx zoo. House sparrows and blue jays also can be heavily infected. Man and other mammals, particularly horses but including many feral and domestic animals, serve as dead-end hosts. The mode by which West Nile virus spread to Europe and the United States is uncertain but may have been by the natural intercontinental migration of birds, the importation of illegal birds, or the inadvertent transportation of infected mosquitoes from an area of endemicity. In both Eastern Europe and the United States, however, the animal and human populations were largely immunologically naïve for West Nile virus, which resulted in rapid spread. West Nile virus has been detected in mosquitoes and birds along the Atlantic seaboard from New England to Florida and will likely spread westward.

The majority of infections with West Nile virus are subclinical, and in endemic areas seroprevalence approaches 40% among adults. Symptoms include mild, nonspecific extraneurologic illness characterized by fever, rash, arthralgias, lymphadenopathy, gastrointestinal complaints, and conjunctivitis. Occasional cases can be complicated by hepatitis or pancreatitis. Neurologic disease can take the form of meningitis, encephalitis, or both. CNS infection is characterized by the sudden onset of fever, confusion, weakness, and stiff neck. In the American cases several patients lost their deep tendon reflexes and had EMG findings consistent with Guillain-Barré syndrome. Elderly persons are particularly susceptible to CNS disease from West Nile virus and have the highest mortality.

The diagnosis of West Nile viral infection is established serologically by IgM assay of serum or CSF. However, cross-reactivity with other flaviviruses occurs; indeed, the outbreak in New York City initially was judged to be due to St. Louis encephalitis virus. Specific serologic diagnosis is achieved by plaque-reduction neutralization. A PCR assay also has been described. Other laboratory tests, including routine tests of the CSF in patients with neurologic disease, are nonspecific, although some patients have a relative lymphocytopenia on complete blood count.

Colorado Tick Fever. CTF is caused by an orbivirus member of Reoviridae. The virus is transmitted by a wood tick, *Dermacentor andersoni,* which inhabits high elevation areas of states that extend from the Central Plains to the Pacific Coast. The tick is infected with the virus at the larval stage and remains infected for life. Squirrels and chipmunks serve as primary reservoirs. Infection of humans typically occurs in hikers and campers in indigenous areas during the spring and early summer. Most persons recall a tick bite approximately 3–5 days before the onset of illness.

Unlike most of the other arthropodborne encephalitides, CTF has a characteristic clinical appearance. Symptoms begin with the abrupt onset of an influenza-like illness, including high fever, malaise, arthralgia and myalgia, vomiting, headache, and decreased sensorium, which are sometimes accompanied by a diffuse macular rash. Despite the severity of the symptoms, the CBC usually reveals leukopenia. After 3 days of illness, the symptoms rapidly disappear. However, in many persons, a second, identical episode recurs 48 hours after the first, producing the saddle-back temperature curve that is typical of CTF. Rarely a bleeding diathesis associated with thrombocytopenia may develop in infected children. As with other arboviral encephalitides, the diagnosis may be established by serologic testing of acute and convalescent serum. The virus may be readily isolated from blood samples by using cell lines available to routine diagnostic virology laboratories.

ARBOVIRUSES OUTSIDE THE UNITED STATES

Encephalitis outside the United States may be caused by a wide variety of arboviruses, many of which remain poorly characterized (Table 55–8). Three of these entities are known to cause large-scale, severe illness in humans.

Venezuelan Equine Encephalitis. VEE occurs in South America and Central America and is caused by the VEE virus, an alphavirus of Togaviridae comprised of several serologic subtypes. Some subtypes are associated with endemic disease transmitted primarily by *Culex* mosquitoes and amplified in small swamp rodents, and

TABLE 55–8. Arboviruses That Cause Encephalitis Outside the United States

Disease	Family	Location
Venezuelan equine encephalitis	Togaviridae	Northern South America, Central America, Mexico
Rocio	Flaviviridae	Brazil
Rabies-related viral encephalitis	Rhabdoviridae	Central and South Africa
Tickborne encephalitis	Flaviviridae	Europe and Asia
Japanese encephalitis	Flaviviridae	Southeast Asia, Japan, China, Korea
Murray Valley encephalitis	Flaviviridae	Australia

other subtypes are associated with epidemic disease transmitted by a variety of mosquitoes to horses, as well as other wild and domestic mammals, and then to humans. Endemic VEE virus infection in the United States has been identified in the Florida Everglades. Epidemic subtypes have caused outbreaks affecting tens of thousands of people in Latin American countries from Peru to Mexico and occasionally extending into Texas. With either form, most persons infected with VEE virus have only influenza-like symptoms; encephalitis develops in fewer than 5% of patients. Across all age groups the mortality for CNS disease is approximately 20%, but it is highest among young children. A vaccine is available for horses, and outbreaks can be prevented by large-scale equine administration of the vaccine.

Tickborne Encephalitis. Tickborne encephalitis is caused by a complex of antigenically related members of the flavivirus genus of Togaviridae. The broad geographic distribution of these viruses is implied by their disease designations, namely, **Central European encephalitis, Russian spring-summer encephalitis,** and **Far Eastern encephalitis.** An additional member of the tickborne encephalitis complex, **Powassan virus encephalitis,** is uncommonly associated with encephalitis in Canada. Tickborne encephalitis is found in Great Britain, where it is primarily associated with **louping ill disease,** an ataxic ailment in sheep throughout most of Europe east of France and extending across Russia through Siberia. The virus is harbored in related *Ixodes* ticks that live in deciduous woodlands and is amplified in numerous forest animals. Humans are infected primarily through tick bites, but the virus also may be transmitted to humans through consumption of unpasteurized milk from an infected animal. An inactivated-virus vaccine is available in Austria.

Japanese Encephalitis. Japanese encephalitis is found throughout most of eastern Asia and is caused by Japanese encephalitis virus, a member of the flavivirus genus of Togaviridae. The virus is transmitted primarily by several species of night-feeding *Culex* mosquitoes but may be transmitted by *Aedes* as well. Amplification occurs in a wide range of mammalian hosts; in Japan, pigs bred for commercial meat production have been identified as a principal reservoir. The incidence of disease in humans is proportionate to the burden of the mosquito population.

The encephalitis follows a period of prodromal symptoms, including fever, respiratory complaints, and vomiting. CNS disease typically is very severe, manifested by fluctuating sensorium and multiple neurologic signs. The reported mortality ranges from less than 10% to 50%, with most deaths occurring among very young and elderly persons. Disease has been controlled primarily by vaccine programs for both animals and humans and by application of insecticides.

ENTEROVIRUSES

ETIOLOGY

The enteroviruses belong to the Picornaviridae, a large family of nonenveloped, single-stranded RNA viruses. Classification of viruses within the enterovirus genus was traditionally based on their growth in tissue culture and in experimental animals. Such criteria allowed the enteroviruses to be divided into four groups: **polioviruses** (types 1–3); **coxsackieviruses A** (types A1–A24, except type A23); **coxsackieviruses B** (types B1–B6); and **echoviruses** (types 1–33, except types 10 and 28). The major neurologic illness caused by polioviruses is neuropathy (Chapter 56). Because some enteroviruses do not strictly conform to the traditional criteria for classification, it is now conventional simply to designate newly discovered enterovirus strains by serotype number. Currently four such enteroviruses, named **enteroviruses 68–71,** have been characterized.

Transmission. Enteroviruses are transmitted primarily by the fecal-oral route, with replication and shedding from the intestinal tract. Enterovirus infection is most prevalent in young children, who typically transmit the infection to other household contacts.

EPIDEMIOLOGY

The enteroviruses are ubiquitous and have worldwide distribution. In tropical areas they cause endemic disease, whereas in temperate climates they are associated with yearly epidemics that occur in the summer and early fall.

Although enteroviruses account for 80–92% of cases of viral meningitis, they produce far fewer cases of encephalitis; up to 25% of cases of encephalitis of known causation are associated with enteroviruses during major epidemic years, but 10% or fewer may be caused by enteroviruses in intervening periods. Most cases of enterovirus encephalitis are caused by polioviruses, echoviruses, and several serotypes of the coxsackieviruses A and B.

PATHOGENESIS

The pathogenesis of the polioviruses serves as a model for all neurotropic enteroviral infections. Extrapolation from extensive poliovirus data indicates that 90–95% of enterovirus infections result in subclinical replication in the gastrointestinal tract. Even with asymptomatic infection, virus can be isolated from the oropharynx for several weeks and from stool samples for several months. Approximately 5–10% of infected persons have asymptomatic **primary viremia,** soon followed by **secondary viremia,** which results in fever, headache, and malaise, corresponding to the minor illness of poliovirus disease. The enteroviruses reach distant sites such as the skin, pericardium, and CNS during the secondary viremia. Neurotropic enteroviruses enter the CNS either directly through hematogenous seeding or after infection of peripheral nerves, followed by retrograde axonal transport. Once the virus enters the CNS, it spreads rapidly through neuronal pathways.

SYMPTOMS AND CLINICAL MANIFESTATIONS

The enteroviruses produce many different clinical signs and symptoms, including enteritis, respiratory tract disease, conjunctivitis, rash, myopathy, myocarditis and pericarditis, hepatitis, and neurologic disease. Each serotype tends to produce a particular clinical complex, and CNS symptoms can occur against the background of other characteristic enteroviral manifestations, particularly exanthematous illnesses such as hand, foot, and mouth disease (Chapter 46). The symptoms of enteroviral encephalitis are typically mild and short-lived but can include obtundation, seizures, and focal neurologic signs. Enteroviral infection can occasionally include cerebellar or brainstem involvement and frequently includes a meningeal component resulting in meningoencephalitis.

Hypogammaglobulinemia, either alone or in association with T-cell immune defects, predisposes the infected person to **chronic enteroviral meningoencephalitis,** which in most commonly caused by echoviruses. The infection results in a waxing and waning course, but overall there is progressive cerebral and intellectual dysfunction characterized by headaches, seizures, hearing loss, lethargy, weakness, and ataxia. Persons with hypogammaglobulinemia also may present with chronic hepatitis or a dermatomyositis-like syndrome with edema and rash; inflammatory changes are detected on biopsy of skin and muscle tissue.

DIAGNOSIS

Microbiologic Evaluation

Culture. Enteroviruses are shed in the oropharynx and stool and can be detected in blood, CSF, urine, and tissues by culture after 4–8 days. The usefulness of viral culture is limited by poor growth of some enteroviral serotypes. In addition, during epidemic years the rate of asymptomatic gastrointestinal excretion of enterovirus is so high that many cases of encephalitis associated with extraneural viral isolation probably represent coincidental dual infections. Although enteroviruses can frequently be recovered from the CSF of persons with both agammaglobulinemia and chronic meningoencephalitis, the virus usually cannot be isolated from the CSF of immunocompetent persons.

Serologic Testing. Serologic tests generally are available only for the three polioviruses, the six strains of coxsackievirus B, and a limited number of other serotypes. Enterovirus serotypes are numerous and antigenically disparate, and serologic testing is severely limited because of the large number of enteroviral serotypes, each requiring individual testing. Serologic testing is usually used only to confirm infection during an outbreak of enteroviral infection caused by a single serotype.

Polymerase Chain Reaction Testing. A commercial PCR assay for enteroviruses amplifies a conserved nucleic acid sequence that is common to almost all the known enteroviral serotypes. Early evaluation indicates that the assay's sensitivity exceeds that of viral culture, and results can be obtained in a few hours. PCR testing for enteroviruses appears superior to viral culture for the diagnosis of many enterovirus infections, particularly enteroviral meningitis. However, its utility in the diagnosis of enteroviral encephalitis is yet to be fully defined.

TREATMENT

Until recently, no specific therapy was available for enterovirus infections. **Pleconaril** is a recently developed drug that interferes with enterovirus attachment and uncoating by binding to the virus protein capsid. It has broad antiviral effects on enteroviruses, with antiviral activity against >90% of the commonly circulating serotypes. Pleconaril has been studied in enteroviral meningitis, in respiratory tract infection, and to a limited extent in enteroviral infections in immunocompromised persons. These studies suggest a benefit from pleconaril therapy and the possibility of successful therapy for enteroviral encephalitis in the future.

Antibody plays an important role in the immune response to enteroviruses, which has led to the use of IVIG as part of the therapy for serious enterovirus infections, although the benefit is uncertain.

PROGNOSIS

The prognosis of enteroviral encephalitis in immunocompetent persons is good and recovery is usually complete. Infants, however, and particularly neonates, may have clinically significant residua. Children who were infected during their first year of life tend to have slightly lower IQ scores and decreased language skills when compared carefully with age-matched control subjects. Children who acquire the infection after 12 months of age demonstrate few consequences. The prognosis for patients with hypogammaglobulinemia is poor; the progression of the neurologic illness may be slowed or reversed by the administration of immune globulin directly into the CNS through a surgically placed reservoir. Some persons ultimately die of this infection despite therapy.

PREVENTION

The enhanced-potency formalin-inactivated poliovirus vaccine and the oral poliovirus vaccine are both extremely effective in preventing infection with polioviruses. There are no vaccines for the other enteroviral serotypes. Good hygiene may contribute to decreased transmission, and standard precautions with good handwashing technique may help prevent nosocomial infections.

LYMPHOCYTIC CHORIOMENINGITIS VIRUS

LCM virus is an arenavirus, a bisegmented ambisensed RNA virus. The illness resulting from LCM virus is relatively mild. Infection may be more frequent than is recognized, accounting for 5–13% of cases from older series of encephalitis. The primary reservoir for LCM is the persistently infected house mouse, *Mus musculus,* either feral or in laboratory colonies. Pet hamsters also have been identified as sources of infection. LCM virus infection is most prevalent in rural areas during the winter months, when the mice seek shelter from the cold. Contact with rodent excreta or saliva may account for transmission to humans; human-to-human transmission of the virus does not appear to occur. In addition, infections through laboratory accidents have been well documented. In these instances the source may be chronically infected tumor cell lines or explanted tissue rather than the live animal.

The typical clinical course of LCM virus infection is biphasic. The first stage, characterized by an influenza type of illness, includes fever, myalgia, coryza, and bronchitis. This is followed by the second phase, which involves the CNS. The most common CNS manifestation is aseptic meningitis, but encephalitis with or without a meningeal component occurs in approximately one third of patients. The diagnosis can be confirmed both serologically and by viral isolation from blood or CSF. Recovery even in severe cases is the rule, and death is rare.

RABIES

Human rabies is virtually 100% fatal once symptoms develop, but the disease can be prevented with postexposure prophylaxis.

ETIOLOGY

Rabies is caused by the rabies virus, a negative-sense, single-stranded RNA virus of the Rhabdoviridae family.

Transmission. Most rabies infections occur after an overt or inapparent animal bite. In the majority of domestic cases identified in the past 20 years, the exposure was unknown. Almost all these cases were due to bat variants, suggesting that the risk of transmission from bats can be subtle. In addition to bites, rabies may be contracted through laboratory accidents or inhalation of infected aerosols, which accounts for occasional cases among people who have explored bat-infested caves. Rabies rarely has been transmitted through transplanted infected corneas, a risk reduced by the adoption of stringent guidelines for the acceptance of donor tissues.

EPIDEMIOLOGY

Worldwide, transmission of rabies from a domestic animal accounts for most human cases. In Europe and North America, however, control of stray animals and vaccination of pets have dramatically reduced the number of cases in humans. Only 36 cases of rabies diagnosed in the United States were reported to the CDC from 1981 to 1997; 12 of these cases were acquired while the patient was traveling in a developing country. Rabies infection among domestic animals in the United States is sporadic and uncommon and is identified most frequently in cats, dogs, and cattle. In contrast, rabies has been detected routinely in wild animals throughout the United States. Raccoons are the animals most commonly infected with rabies, followed by skunks, insectivorous bats, foxes, and coyotes; together, these animals account for >90% of recent cases of wild animal rabies in the United States. Animal infection has spread through epizootics, which are defined by animal group, geographic location, and viral strain (Fig. 55–2). Hawaii is the only state that currently is free of animal rabies. Raccoon rabies has been identified in many states, especially in the Southeast, the Middle Atlantic states, and New England. Skunk rabies has been found primarily throughout the central Midwestern states and parts of California. Infected foxes have been identified along the Canadian and Mexican borders. Cases among bats have been evenly distributed over the continental United States. Canada harbors significant numbers of rabid foxes, although there have been no recent cases of human rabies. In Mexico, rabies among dogs is still most prominent. The risk of rabies after an animal contact therefore varies considerably from location to location. Animal survey statistics from local and state health authorities, as well as from the CDC, can provide the most recent and accurate information regarding the presence of animal rabies in any given area.

PATHOGENESIS

A bite from an infected animal results in the direct inoculation of virus from infected saliva into the subcutaneous tissue and muscle. The virus replicates slowly, and neurologic symptoms may not appear for months. The incubation period for children is shorter than for adults and is inversely proportional to the degree of innervation of the inoculated area. Consequently bites to the face, fingers, and genitalia have the shortest incubation period. The virus infects peripheral nerves and ascends by retrograde axonal transport to the CNS, and initially it selectively infects the limbic system. Within days of reaching the CNS, the virus spreads to the entire brain and then returns to peripheral locations centrifugally through efferent nerves to infect many different tissues, including but not limited to the salivary glands, hair follicles, and heart.

SYMPTOMS AND CLINICAL MANIFESTATIONS

The clinical course of the usual case of rabies reflects the spread of virus through the peripheral nerves to the limbic system, followed by generalized brain infection and return to peripheral tissues. The first rabies-specific symptoms occur after entry of virus into the peripheral nerves and transport to the spinal cord, during which the affected person commonly has paresthesias at the site of the bite. Infection of the CNS is heralded by a prodromal phase that includes headache, malaise, difficulty in swallowing, and anorexia. Although some persons are apprehensive and anxious, objective signs referable to the CNS are few or absent at this stage and the illness may not be recognizable as rabies. With infection of the limbic system and the remainder of the brain, the patient has so-called **furious rabies,** which is characterized by intermittent periods of agitation and hyperalertness during which aggressive and bizarre behavior alternates with intervals of relatively normal mental status. Approximately half of the persons with furious rabies have painful laryngospasms when attempting to drink **(hydrophobia)** or when air or wind is blown into the face **(aerophobia);** the mere sight of water may induce subsequent spasms.

Some persons manifest an ascending paralysis with areflexia but without other neurologic manifestations, a condition labeled **dumb rabies.** Many features of dumb rabies resemble those of Guillain-Barré syndrome. In contrast to the excitability seen with furious disease, patients with dumb rabies demonstrate cranial nerve paralysis that results in a bland facial expression. In both furious and dumb rabies, alteration of consciousness and eventual coma occur preterminally, usually within 1 week of the onset of neurologic symptoms.

DIAGNOSIS

The diagnosis of rabies may be established on clinical grounds in a person with a history of animal bite who displays the characteristically severe, intermittent hyperagitated encephalopathy with hydrophobia. However, the rarity of the disease in developed countries frequently delays diagnosis. In addition, in the absence of an identified animal exposure or hydrophobia, rabies may be indistinguishable from other severe infectious encephalitides. The agitation caused by rabies may be confused with tetanus and spinal convulsions; trismus is prominent in the latter, however, and the sensorium is intact. Drug overdose or psychiatric disorders also may produce agitated states similar to those of rabies encephalitis. Dumb rabies must be distinguished from those with other paralytic peripheral neuropathies, and it may easily be mistaken for the Guillain-Barré syndrome. Unlike Guillain-Barré syndrome, however, the CSF examination in rabies usually reveals pleocytosis, with a normal protein level.

The diagnosis is confirmed by isolation of virus from saliva, CSF, or brain tissue. The diagnosis can be achieved more expeditiously by staining biopsy samples with rabies-specific fluorescent antibody. Specimens from richly innervated areas, such as cornea or skin sampled at the hairline, are the most sensitive. Results of the direct fluorescent antibody tests may be negative early in the course of the encephalitis, and repeated sampling may be necessary.

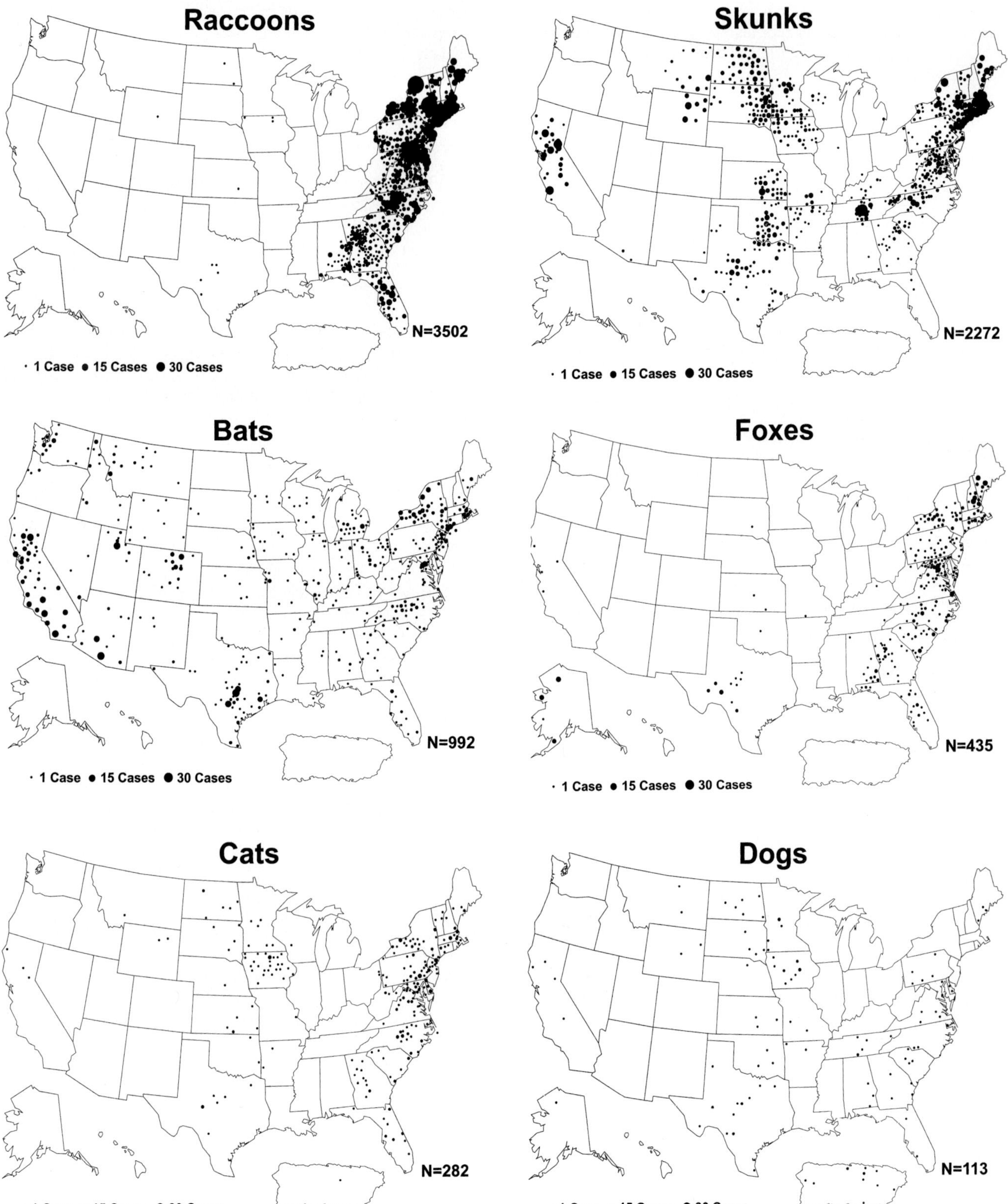

FIGURE 55–2. Reported cases of rabies by county in the United States, 1998, in raccoons, skunks, bats, foxes, cats, and dogs. (From Krebs JW, Smith JS, Rupprecht CE, et al: Rabies surveillance in the United States during 1998. *J Am Vet Med Assoc* 1999;215:1786–98.)

Serum antibodies to rabies are detectable 6–10 days after the onset of symptoms, but serologic results may be difficult to interpret in persons who received postexposure immunization with rabies vaccine. Late in the course of encephalitis, however, high antibody titers to rabies can be detected in the CSF, which is not induced by immunization.

TREATMENT

There is no specific therapy for rabies. Rabies immune globulin and human diploid cell vaccine are extremely effective for prophylaxis after exposure to rabies (Chapter 50); however, these agents are of no known benefit once symptoms have appeared. Although intensive support generally has been offered to persons with rabies, there is little convincing evidence that such support alters the grim prognosis. Virus can be cultured from saliva, tears, and urine, and therefore scrupulous body substance isolation precautions must be followed. Hospital workers do not require rabies prophylaxis unless they have been bitten by the patient or have had mucous membrane exposure to potentially infectious body fluids.

COMPLICATIONS

Both neurologic and nonneurologic complications occur in virtually all cases of rabies and frequently are the immediate cause of death. Neurologic complications include seizures, cerebral edema, dysautonomia, and sodium imbalance. In addition, persons with rabies may have cardiac dysrhythmias or sudden arrest as a result of either autonomic dysfunction or direct viral invasion of myocardial tissue. Most persons have pulmonary insufficiency because of aspiration pneumonia, pulmonary edema, or the adult respiratory distress syndrome.

PROGNOSIS

Rabies encephalitis is among the world's deadliest infections. Although rare persons survive after immune prophylaxis and aggressive intensive care, most die even when the condition is recognized and treated early in its course.

PREVENTION

Effective measures are available to prevent rabies after exposure to a rabid animal, including standard aggressive wound débridement and postexposure immune prophylaxis with rabies immune globulin and human diploid cell vaccine (see Fig. 50–2).

SYSTEMIC INFECTIONS OCCASIONALLY ASSOCIATED WITH ENCEPHALITIS

Cat-Scratch Disease. The encephalopathy associated with cat-scratch disease (Chapter 28) occurs 1–6 weeks after the appearance of the characteristic regional lymphadenopathy, which usually is still present at the onset of neurologic symptoms. Typically a rapid onset of dense encephalopathy and seizures is followed by a period of unresponsiveness for 1–4 days, after which full recovery proceeds within 1–2 days. Some persons demonstrate nuchal rigidity or movement disorders in association with the encephalopathy, but spinal cord or peripheral nerve involvement is rare. Although residual neurologic sequelae occasionally have been reported, full recovery is the rule.

Tuberculosis. Meningitis with *Mycobacterium tuberculosis* frequently is associated with an alteration of sensorium and abnormal findings on CSF examination (Chapters 35 and 52) and may be clinically indistinguishable from encephalitis. The development of a gelatinous exudate leads to a basilar meningitis complicated by intracerebral vasculitis and hydrocephalus. Symptoms begin gradually, often 1–3 weeks before medical referral. The early stage of tuberculous meningitis is characterized by personality change, anorexia, and listlessness. If the condition is untreated, nuchal rigidity, headache, and fever develop. Approximately 25% of infected children demonstrate cranial nerve palsies (most characteristically ophthalmoplegia) or hemiplegia. The most advanced stage of illness is heralded by seizures and coma. Even with antituberculosis therapy, up to 20% of patients die and as many as 30–50% of survivors have clinically significant neurologic sequelae. The outcome is directly related to the severity of symptoms at the time of initiation of treatment, and therefore it is crucial to consider the diagnosis during early stages of illness.

Confirmation of the diagnosis of tuberculous meningitis is difficult. A CSF profile of lymphocytic pleocytosis, moderately high protein level, and profound hypoglycorrhachia is characteristic but not specific, and the CSF profile in the early stages of disease may be identical to that seen in viral illnesses. Only about one third of patients have acid-fast bacilli detected on examination of the CSF, even with large or repeated samples of fluid. Similarly, only half of patients have a chest radiograph that reveals primary intrathoracic or miliary tuberculosis. However, up to 90% have positive results on a tuberculin skin test, and approximately three fourths of children have an identified infected adult contact, usually among household members.

Lyme Disease. The encephalitis of Lyme disease usually occurs during or soon after the appearance of the other early clinical manifestations (Chapter 29). Thus many patients with Lyme encephalitis have a simultaneous rash, arthralgia, chills, fatigue, myalgia, and lymphadenopathy. The encephalitis commonly is mild, consisting of headache, somnolence, emotional lability, poor concentration, or behavioral changes. Lyme encephalitis has two distinctive features: the encephalitis usually occurs concomitantly with other levels of neurologic involvement, such as meningitis, cranial neuropathies, motor or sensory radiculopathies, or cerebellar ataxia, and the neurologic symptoms follow an intermittent, waxing and waning course for weeks or months. In some persons the characteristic rash does not appear at all during the course of the encephalopathy.

Mycoplasma pneumoniae. Neurologic complications of *Mycoplasma pneumoniae* infections (Chapter 68) are noted in 7% of hospitalized persons and can be severe. The onset of neurologic symptoms occurs between 1 and 2 weeks after respiratory tract infection, although the precedent respiratory symptoms may be mild or clinically inapparent. In addition to encephalitis, several other patterns of *M. pneumoniae* neurologic involvement have been described, including meningitis, cerebellar ataxia, Guillain-Barré syndrome, transverse myelitis, and psychosis. In approximately one third of persons with neurologic manifestations, neurologic signs can be identified at more than one level. In many cases the encephalitis is profound and recovery is slow; the mortality has been estimated at 10% and the incidence of persistent sequelae at 30%. The diagnosis of *M. pneumoniae* encephalitis has been facilitated by the wide availability of serologic tests, including *Mycoplasma*-specific IgM determinations, allowing expeditious diagnosis.

Initial attempts at isolating *M. pneumoniae* from the CSF were unsuccessful, leading many to claim that the neurologic manifestations were either immune mediated or toxin mediated. However, recent reports using more sophisticated techniques increasingly have documented direct CNS invasion. Nevertheless, the benefit of antibiotics for encephalitis associated with *M. pneumoniae* remains to be established.

Rocky Mountain Spotted Fever. Infection with *Rickettsia rickettsii,* the pathogen responsible for Rocky Mountain spotted fever, may be complicated by severe meningoencephalitis (Chapter 30). CNS symptoms include severe bifrontal headaches, lethargy, confusion, and disorientation, with seizures and coma in advanced cases. Approximately one fourth of patients with Rocky Mountain spotted fever complain of neck stiffness, representing either meningeal irritation or myalgia of the neck muscles. The distinction between Rocky Mountain spotted fever and viral meningoencephalitis is relatively straightforward, with a history of tick exposure followed by the typical, centripetally spreading, petechial rash. However, 20–30% of patients with Rocky Mountain spotted fever do not have a history of a tick bite, and the exanthem may not be seen until 6 days or later into the course of the disease; up to 10% of affected persons may never have a rash at all. Moreover, the rash may appear only as erythematous papules and may not follow the characteristic distribution. Because most diagnostic tests for Rocky Mountain spotted fever require several days to 2–3 weeks of clinical illness before results are positive, presumptive treatment must be initiated.

Varicella-Zoster Virus. Both primary varicella and zoster are associated with encephalitis (Chapter 27). **Varicella encephalitis** occurs mostly among children as a complication of chickenpox. In older series, encephalitis was noted in only 0.25% of persons hospitalized with chickenpox. The onset of CNS symptoms occurs between 3 and 8 days after the onset of rash. The severity of the encephalitis is not related to the severity of the preceding exanthem. Symptoms, however, may be dramatic and include headache, vomiting, seizures, depressed mental status, and peripheral and cranial neuropathies. The diagnosis of varicella encephalitis is straightforward because CNS symptoms nearly always occur in the presence of typical exanthematous disease. The prognosis for varicella encephalitis is excellent, with virtually 100% complete recovery.

Even more common than encephalitis, varicella may be complicated by **cerebellitis** and **cerebellar ataxia,** either appearing alone or associated with changes in sensorium. The ataxia is manifested with extreme vertigo and nausea and may require hospitalization for hydration. The cerebellitis always follows a benign if somewhat uncomfortable course with gradual resolution of symptoms for several days.

Similar to varicella encephalitis, the age distribution of **zoster encephalitis** approximates that of the cutaneous disease; thus most cases are encountered in middle-aged and elderly persons, although several pediatric cases have been reported. Many cases occur in immunocompromised persons who already have cutaneous or visceral dissemination. On average, encephalitic symptoms with zoster first appear approximately 1 week after the eruption, but the rash may appear before or after the encephalitis by several weeks. An unusually severe form of CNS zoster, seen primarily in elderly persons, is associated with granulomatous arteritis of the middle cerebral artery, with ipsilateral cerebral infarcts that develop several weeks after herpes zoster ophthalmicus. Varicella-zoster viral antigens have been detected in the tunica media of the affected cerebral arteries. The diagnosis of zoster encephalitis usually is straightforward because the disease occurs concurrently with the distinctive exanthematous pattern of the cutaneous disease. Similar to varicella, the course of zoster encephalitis is usually short, with recovery in 1–3 weeks, although some persons have a prolonged recovery period. Death is unusual, but when it does occur, it is usually caused by other visceral complications of the disease.

Epstein-Barr Virus. Frank meningoencephalitis occurs in 1–7% of patients hospitalized with EBV-related infectious mononucleosis (Chapter 37). Similar to encephalitis with varicella-zoster virus, EBV encephalitis rapidly abates and the prognosis is usually good. The onset of encephalitis in persons with typical infectious mononucleosis is approximately 1–3 weeks after the appearance of other symptoms, although there is considerable variability in its timing, and CNS symptoms may precede the mononucleosis by several days. EBV infection has been associated with several other neurologic illnesses as well, including Guillain-Barré syndrome, transverse myelitis, psychosis, and cranial neuropathies. These findings may overlap in the same person. Numerous reports describe persons with serologically documented EBV encephalitis who never demonstrate any symptoms of infectious mononucleosis. The diagnosis is confirmed by an EBV antibody panel.

Human Herpesvirus 6. The T-lymphotropic HHV6 is a ubiquitous organism acquired by most persons during early childhood. It is the agent principally responsible for roseola (exanthem subitum), a benign illness of young children characterized by 2–4 days of high fever followed by spontaneous defervescence and a rash (Chapter 25). Additionally, HHV6 can be identified in approximately 15% of all children less than 2 years of age with nonspecific febrile illness. Occasionally children with roseola, as well as those with HHV6 infection but without the characteristic features of roseola, can have neurologic complications, including a febrile seizure, bulging anterior fontanel, or encephalopathy, the result of direct infection of the CNS. The seizures associated with HHV6 are usually generalized and short-lived, but status epilepticus can occur. In these cases the CSF typically is normal, although HHV6 DNA is detectable by PCR in the CSF. Overt HHV6 encephalitis characteristically is brief and benign, with prolonged residua occurring only occasionally. Like other herpesviruses, HHV6 persists in a latent stage after initial infection in peripheral blood lymphocytes and other tissues, including the brain, with CNS reactivation possibly causing recurrent febrile convulsions. Because the overwhelming majority of persons are infected with HHV6 during their first decade, cases of HHV6 encephalitis in adults are uncommon but have been reported.

HHV6 infections occur commonly in immunocompromised persons, primarily bone marrow transplant recipients and persons with AIDS. In transplant recipients, HHV6 infections usually are the result of reactivation of latent infection, but occasionally virus carried with the graft may cause infection. Most HHV6 infections occur 2–4 weeks after transplantation, resulting in fever, idiopathic marrow suppression, interstitial pneumonia, and rash. Occasionally, encephalitis also may occur. Among persons with AIDS, active HHV6 is present in many non-CNS tissues at the time of death. In at least some persons with AIDS, HHV6 acts either alone or in concert with HIV to cause demyelinating white matter disease, which is characteristic of AIDS-associated dementia. Antiviral therapy for disseminated or CNS disease in the immunocompromised person is warranted. Ganciclovir and foscarnet have superior in vitro activity against HHV6 compared with acyclovir, and cases documenting response to these two agents have been reported.

HHV6 has also been identified at autopsy in the cerebral plaques of persons with **multiple sclerosis,** but the significance of this finding is uncertain.

Measles. Measles encephalitis, a particularly severe brain infection, complicates approximately 1 in 1,000 cases of measles (Chapter 23). The age distribution of measles encephalitis reflects that seen in uncomplicated disease. Measles is a prototypical immune-mediated postinfectious encephalitis pathologically similar to experimental allergic encephalomyelitis. Virus cannot be recovered from the

CNS, and the predominant pathologic feature is a perivascular lymphocytic infiltrate with surrounding demyelination. Lymphocytic proliferative responses to myelin basic protein are found in many persons with measles encephalitis, whereas intrathecal anti-measles antibody is lacking.

The encephalitis virtually always occurs in persons with clinically apparent rubeola, with the onset of neurologic symptoms characteristically 3–6 days after the appearance of the rash. Typically the onset of the CNS illness occurs as the person is convalescing uneventfully from extraneural disease—the fever is disappearing and the exanthem is fading. Recovery is interrupted by the recrudescence of high fever with onset of delirium, depressed sensorium, and seizures. Measles encephalitis can be severe, involving a waxing and waning course marked by involuntary movement disorders, a high-pitched **cerebral cry,** hallucinations, hypotonia, or spasticity. Occasionally the encephalitis is accompanied by myelitis, cerebellar ataxia, or optic neuritis.

The diagnosis of measles encephalitis is rarely in doubt because of the presence of typical signs and symptoms of rubeola. Viral isolation from the respiratory tract or a fourfold increase of serum antibody titers in paired acute and convalescent sera confirms the diagnosis. The mortality for measles encephalitis approximates 10%, and this condition is a leading cause of measles-related deaths. Neurologic sequelae, including chronic seizures, hemiplegia, mental retardation, and behavior problems, occur in 20–50% of patients. Fever, with the temperature exceeding 40.5°C (105°F) during the course of the encephalitis, young age, a severe and long-lasting depression of sensorium, and multiple seizures have been identified as poor prognostic factors.

Mumps. The incidence of CNS infections caused by mumps (Chapter 36) has declined dramatically since the introduction of the live attenuated vaccine. Mumps virus, however, is neurotropic; in the prevaccine era 0.5–25% of cases of mumps parotitis were complicated by CNS disease. Before the introduction of the vaccine, the incidence of CNS mumps was highest among children 5–9 years of age. Similar to mumps parotitis, mumps meningitis and encephalitis occur throughout the year, but the peak incidence is during the spring and early summer. Older series consistently reported a predominance of male patients over female patients (approximately 3:1).

Although CNS infection with mumps virus traditionally had been called "meningoencephalitis," cases can usually be separated as meningitic or encephalitic on clinical grounds. In both illnesses most cases occur 1–6 days after the appearance of parotid gland swelling, although CNS disease may precede parotitis, or may follow parotitis by up to 2 weeks. Approximately half of the persons with CNS mumps have no apparent parotitis at all. Cases of predominantly mumps meningitis occur far more frequently than those of encephalitis. Mumps meningitis is a self-limiting illness with a low mortality rate and few sequelae. In contrast, mumps encephalitis typically is severe. The clinical features of mumps encephalitis include seizures, altered mental status, cranial nerve dysfunction, paresis, ataxia, and psychosis. Occasional cases of unilateral or bilateral deafness have occurred both in association with encephalitis and as isolated events. Rarely, mumps infection has resulted in myelitis or radiculitis.

The diagnosis of mumps meningoencephalitis is usually established presumptively in the presence of characteristic parotitis and neurologic symptoms. For persons without parotid swelling, the diagnosis is established by documenting a fourfold increase in mumps antibody titers. Although nearly all persons with mumps meningitis recover fully, the prognosis for those with encephalitis is more guarded. In the prevaccine era, the mortality approached 20% and sequelae occurred in 25–50% of survivors. Residua include hemiplegia, seizures, school failure, prolonged psychosis, and optic neuritis. Some cases have resulted in aqueductal stenosis. Sequelae appear to be most common in older children and adults. There is no specific therapy for CNS infection due to mumps.

Rubella. In nations offering routine immunization, rubella (Chapter 24) is an uncommon cause of encephalitis. Even in the prevaccine era, encephalitis complicated only 1:5,000 to 1:20,000 cases of rubella. As in measles and mumps, the onset of rubella encephalitis usually occurs within 1 week of the onset of systemic disease, frequently as the rash is fading. However, cases have been reported in which the CNS symptoms have preceded the exanthem.

The encephalitis associated with rubella can be severe; up to 20% of affected persons die early in the course of the illness, although survivors usually recover without neurologic sequelae. Characteristically, rubella encephalitis has a rapid onset and a short course; within 1–2 weeks the person either recovers or dies of the infection.

Adenoviruses. Adenovirus, a double-stranded DNA virus, comprises more than 40 serotypes. Approximately half of human adenovirus infections are subclinical, and most of the remainder result in respiratory disease, conjunctivitis, gastroenteritis, or, occasionally, hemorrhagic cystitis. Adenovirus also is associated with severe, disseminated infection, which usually but not always occurs in immunocompromised persons.

The most frequent serotype implicated in CNS disease is adenovirus type 7, which produces severe pulmonary disease as well. However, several other serotypes have been isolated from persons with encephalitis. Typically, adenovirus encephalitis is part of a multisystem viral sepsis that includes pneumonia, hepatitis, coagulopathy, and heart failure. In such cases, encephalitis may not be a prominent component of the clinical presentation, and death usually results from involvement of other organs. Adenovirus infection may also present with an illness similar to Reye's syndrome that conforms to the clinical criteria for Reye's syndrome but without fatty infiltration of the liver or only mild or absent mitochondrial structural abnormalities.

The diagnosis of adenoviral encephalitis is established by viral culture or by documenting a fourfold increase in antibody titer in acute and convalescent sera. Adenovirus exists in a latent form, which may occasionally be reactivated in the respiratory tract. Isolation from the nasopharynx therefore is presumptive but not definitive evidence of CNS infection. Virus has been successfully isolated from the CSF of some persons with encephalitis. Although adenoviral meningoencephalitis is uncommon, a 15–20% mortality has been estimated from available reports.

Influenza Viruses. Encephalitis is a rare complication of influenza (Chapter 68). Indeed, the association of influenza and CNS disease has been disputed. Early descriptions probably included some persons with Reye's syndrome; with the exclusion of such persons, the CNS manifestations of influenza are mild, nonspecific, and without sequelae.

SLOW INFECTIONS OF THE CENTRAL NERVOUS SYSTEM

Several agents are capable of producing slow infections of the CNS. The characteristics of slow CNS infections are a prolonged incubation period ranging from several months to many years, followed by a relatively brief, relentlessly progressive, and debilitating CNS disease that results in severe disability or death. The causes of slow viral infections of the CNS are varied. The most prominent slow viral infection in children is HIV infection. In addition, slow viral illnesses are associated with persistent measles and rubella infections and, in immunocompromised persons, with JC virus infection of the brain. Some slow CNS infections are caused by proteinaceous particles known as prions, whose biochemical structure does not conform to that commonly attributed to any previously described infectious entity.

HUMAN IMMUNODEFICIENCY VIRUS INFECTION

ETIOLOGY

HIV encephalitis and **HIV encephalopathy** are a result of HIV infection (Chapter 38). HIV-specific DNA and RNA have been identified in the brains of persons with HIV encephalopathy. In addition, virus can be isolated from the CSF, spinal cord, and peripheral nerves, and local production of anti-HIV antibody can be detected in the CSF. Moreover, persons with HIV encephalopathy usually have significantly higher CSF HIV loads than those without CNS involvement, indicating that direct invasion of the CNS by HIV is of principal importance in the pathogenesis of this complication. However, only a relatively small number of cells within the CNS are infected.

EPIDEMIOLOGY

The epidemiology of HIV encephalopathy reflects that of HIV infection in general. In both adults and children the appearance of neurologic manifestations with AIDS usually signifies advanced disease. In accordance with CDC case definitions for infected adults, HIV encephalopathy is a defining illness for AIDS. Among pediatric patients, for whom the CDC has a separate classification system, HIV encephalopathy is a class C (most severe) manifestation (see Table 38–4). Approximately 4–8% of adults and 20% of children with HIV infection develop encephalopathy at some point; this may be the first AIDS-defining complication, but it is increasingly common as the infection progresses, typically in patients with lower CD4 cell counts and higher HIV plasma viral loads than others with advanced clinical disease.

PATHOGENESIS

Virus resides in CNS monocytes and in glial and endothelial cells and is also present in monocyte-derived multinucleated giant cells noted on brain biopsies and postmortem examinations. Despite the relatively few numbers of HIV-infected cells in the CNS, the gross pathologic changes seen in HIV encephalopathy are dramatic and include severe atrophy of the cerebral mantle with secondary enlargement of the ventricles and marked pallor of the white matter. Histologically there is evidence of gliosis of the cerebral cortex and white matter, with small foci of tissue necrosis and perivascular inflammation. In children a calcific vasculopathy of small and medium-sized vessels, particularly around the basal ganglia, has been consistently noted, as has a degenerative inflammatory infiltrate of the spinal cord. Some injury may be secondary to immune-mediated destruction, because infected monocytes within the CNS produce many proinflammatory mediators, including TNF and IL-1 and such chemokines as the **macrophage inflammatory proteins** MIP-1α and MIP-1β. In addition, there is evidence that HIV-derived proteins may interfere with normal neural functioning.

SYMPTOMS AND CLINICAL MANIFESTATIONS

HIV causes relentless CNS disease in both adults and children. Occasionally an acute meningoencephalitis occurs early in the course of the illness, usually around the time of seroconversion. However, most persons with HIV-associated neurologic disease demonstrate an insidious, slowly progressive illness after a long incubation period. Although the encephalopathy may be the first manifestation of infection, characteristically persons begin to show increasingly severe nervous system dysfunction as the extraneural disease progresses. Adults have progressive cognitive impairment characterized by forgetfulness, inability to concentrate, and slowness of thought. With advancing disease the person becomes increasingly apathetic, depressed, and withdrawn. Approximately half of the adults have motor deficits, including ataxia, hypotonia, tremor, and myoclonus. Seizures may occur late in the disease. In addition to cerebral and spinal cord symptoms, adults also may have a peripheral neuropathy characterized by painful paresthesias and weakness.

Children with HIV encephalopathy also demonstrate cognitive and motor deficits, which may appear together or individually. Many children have a progressive encephalopathy marked by decline of cognitive functions. Children with HIV encephalopathy stop reaching developmental milestones and ultimately lose those already achieved. Adaptive and language function, particularly expressive language, are affected as IQ diminishes. In addition, the children may demonstrate a wide range of motor abnormalities, particularly spastic quadriparesis. Gait change, rigidity, extrapyramidal tremor, and cerebellar signs become apparent as the illness progresses. Pseudobulbar palsy and seizures may complicate late disease. As the illness progresses, head circumference measurements decrease, reflecting poor brain growth. In the final stage the child is mute, dull eyed, and quadriplegic. Progressive HIV encephalopathy typically runs a stepwise course with periods of neurologic stability. Few children, however, recover previously lost function during these periods. In addition to this progressive form of the disease, some HIV-infected children have a static encephalopathy in which skills are regularly acquired but at a slowed rate. Static encephalopathy may ultimately convert to the progressive form of the illness.

DIAGNOSIS

The principal task for diagnosis of HIV encephalopathy is to eliminate other CNS complications of HIV disease, particularly intracranial tumors and opportunistic infections such as cryptococcosis, toxoplasmosis, and neurosyphilis. These complications are uncommon in children infected with HIV and can be evaluated by neuroimaging studies and appropriate tests of the CSF. CT and MRI of persons with HIV encephalopathy reveal cerebral atrophy and secondary ventricular enlargement with abnormalities of the subcortical white matter (see Figs. 38–5 and 38–6). In addition, neuroimaging studies in children may show calcification around the basal ganglia and, less frequently, around the frontal lobe white matter. The CSF is normal in most adult and pediatric patients, although a mild lymphocytic pleocytosis with elevation of protein can be present in persons with advanced disease. High HIV viral loads in the CSF are a correlate of encephalopathy, and a decrease in the CSF viral load may be used to monitor response to antiretroviral therapy.

TREATMENT

HIV encephalopathy frequently responds to antiretroviral chemotherapy. Zidovudine has been demonstrated to slow the progression and, in some cases, improve, encephalopathic signs and symptoms in both adult and pediatric patients; children treated with zidovudine may have improvement in IQ scores concomitant with an amelioration of their CT abnormalities. However, the benefit of zidovudine monotherapy may be short-lived. Other dideoxynucleoside analogs with activity against HIV reverse transcriptase, such as didanosine, possibly may improve HIV encephalopathy, but published experience is limited. Accumulating data indicate that dramatic improvement may result after the institution of highly active antiretroviral therapy (HAART), a combination regimen usually comprising two nucleoside reverse transcriptase inhibitors and a protease inhibitor. This benefit is conferred despite the poor penetration of the protease inhibitors into the CNS. Clinical recovery may be mirrored by stabilization or improvement of findings on MRI.

PROGNOSIS

HIV encephalopathy in children is a severe manifestation of HIV infection and portends a poor prognosis. In the absence of therapy, HIV-related neurologic disease is progressive and debilitating. For children, the median survival time after diagnosis of HIV encephalopathy is <12 months in the absence of antiretroviral therapy. The prognosis for many of the severe manifestations of HIV infection has changed with HAART, however, and outcome in the face of current-day treatment has yet to be defined.

PREVENTION

There are no established measures for preventing the extension of HIV infection to the CNS. Antiretroviral chemotherapy administered to adults with HIV infection, with early or asymptomatic disease, slows the progression of illness and diminishes the occurrence of AIDS-defining illnesses. The effectiveness of early antiviral therapy in preventing neurologic disease has not been specifically studied.

SUBACUTE SCLEROSING PANENCEPHALITIS

ETIOLOGY

Subacute sclerosing panencephalitis (SSPE), a rare but uniformly fatal form of degenerative encephalitis, develops an average of 8–10 years after an apparently typical case of measles. SSPE is caused by persistent infection of the CNS by **measles virus** (Chapter 23).

EPIDEMIOLOGY

SSPE is a rare disease that occurs worldwide, with an incidence in the United States of less than 1 per million even before the introduction of the measles vaccine. Most children with SSPE have a history of having contracted measles before the age of 2 years. The average incubation period is 8–10 years after measles, and the average age at onset ranges between the late first and the early second decades.

PATHOGENESIS

The mechanism of the persistence of measles virus in the brains of patients with SSPE is poorly understood. Affected brains reveal diffuse and focal monocellular infiltrates in both white and gray matter. White matter disease is accompanied by demyelinization and astrocytosis. Intranuclear inclusions in neurons and oligodendroglia contain measles virus antigen, but budding virus, which can be readily detected in productive infection, cannot be identified (Fig. 55–3). Intracellular measles mRNAs and all viral proteins are present in SSPE brain specimens, although some investigators have detected low amounts of surface and matrix proteins in comparison with other viral components. However, the importance of these perturbations is unknown.

SYMPTOMS AND CLINICAL MANIFESTATIONS

SSPE is associated with the gradual onset of severe, generalized neurologic deterioration. Symptoms of SSPE progress for 1–3 years, sometimes relieved by periods of remission or improvement. The first signs of disease appear insidiously and are characterized by declining school performance and changes in behavior. This stage progresses to one involving frank myoclonus, dyskinesia, and hyperkinesia, with progressive intellectual deterioration often accompanied by seizures and visual disability. As the illness advances, there is progressive hyperreflexia and rigidity, leading to decorticate posturing, generalized myoclonus, and coma.

DIAGNOSIS

The CSF is normal except for increased protein, reflecting a marked elevation of measles-specific immunoglobulin within the CNS, the pathognomonic finding of SSPE. Corollary tests include an EEG, which usually reveals characteristic periodic high-amplitude slow and sharp waves. Neuroimaging studies document cortical atrophy as the disease progresses. MRI reveals lesions also in the subcortical white matter.

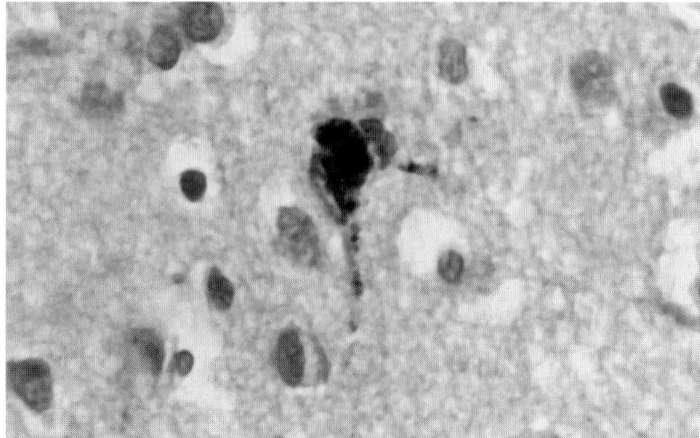

FIGURE 55–3. Section of brain from autopsy of a child with subacute sclerosing panencephalitis (SSPE) immunostained with antibody to measles virus. The neuron illustrated contains a large immunoreactive intranuclear inclusion and small immunoreactive particles in the cytoplasm of the cell body and axons (hematoxylin counterstain).

TREATMENT

Neither antiviral agents nor corticosteroids consistently result in improvement of persons with SSPE. Some studies have indicated amelioration of SSPE treated with isoprinosine, ribavirin, or α-IFN when compared with historical controls, but these results have been disputed.

PROGNOSIS

Spontaneous remission of SSPE has been reported occasionally, although survivors have been severely neurologically impaired. Death from intercurrent pulmonary infection is the eventual outcome for most children.

PROGRESSIVE RUBELLA ENCEPHALITIS

Progressive rubella encephalitis is a rare condition that has many of the characteristics of SSPE. It is believed that this illness represents persistent, slowly progressive rubella infection in the CNS. It usually occurs toward the end of the first decade of life or in the early teenage years. Some children with progressive rubella encephalitis had congenital rubella, whereas others apparently acquired rubella infection postnatally. The disease usually begins with deterioration in school performance and behavioral changes, progressing to global dementia. Ataxia and pyramidal tract signs including hyperreflexia may be prominent. The CSF examination reveals a mild monocellular pleocytosis and elevated protein levels. In addition, highly elevated titers of anti-rubella antibodies are found in the CSF.

PROGRESSIVE MULTIFOCAL LEUKOENCEPHALOPATHY

ETIOLOGY

PML is a CNS illness caused by **JC virus,** a member of the polyoma genus that is identified by the initials of the patient from whom it was first isolated. Rare cases have been associated with a virus closely related to the prototypical polyoma virus, **SV40** (Simian virus 40).

EPIDEMIOLOGY

Nearly 70% of healthy adults have serologic evidence of infection with JC virus. Nevertheless, PML is a rare disease. Nearly all patients are immunocompromised because of lymphoproliferative malignant diseases, pharmacologic suppression of the immune system, or HIV infection. Most patients are more than 40 years of age, but pediatric patients have been identified occasionally.

PATHOGENESIS

The virus may be harbored in B lymphocytes, which transport the agent to the CNS. Infection of oligodendroglia results in enlarged nuclei and altered chromatin patterns; it is presumably the dysfunction of this myelin-producing cell that results in the demyelinating lesions characteristic of this infection. Astrocytes containing JC virus DNA have bizarrely deformed nuclei. DNA homology between virus-enhancing sequences and controlling genes of susceptible cells suggests that virus-cell interactions at the molecular level are necessary for disease production.

SYMPTOMS AND CLINICAL MANIFESTATIONS

PML is a rapidly progressive illness consisting of multiple neurologic deficits, reflecting the multifocal nature of the lesions. Most commonly, patients suffer focal or generalized weakness, visual field deficits or cortical blindness, ataxia, and dysarthria or dysphagia. In addition, many patients have intellectual impairment and memory disturbances. The disease progresses relentlessly for 4–6 months, usually ending with profound generalized weakness, coma, and death. Less commonly, patients may have a more protracted course and survive for years after onset.

DIAGNOSIS

CT reveals multiple nonenhancing hypodense lesions in the white matter without mass effect. MRI may reveal earlier lesions undetected by CT. The CSF is usually normal, although occasionally the protein level is increased. Serum levels of antibodies against JC virus do not rise with the onset of PML and are not of diagnostic usefulness. The virus does not grow or produce cytopathic effects in cell lines routinely used in hospital diagnostic laboratories. Confirmation rests on characteristic pathologic findings on brain biopsy or autopsy; if the methods are available, the virus can be identified in tissue samples by in situ hybridization or immunohistochemical staining.

TREATMENT

There is no therapy for PML. Although occasional reports suggest that cytosine arabinoside or zidovudine is effective, most patients have relentless progression and death within months regardless of therapy. Preliminary evidence suggests that PML may regress in some persons with AIDS after the start of HAART if there is reconstitution of immunity.

PROGNOSIS

In most instances the illness progresses rapidly and relentlessly for 4–6 months, leading to death. Rare instances of prolonged survival or spontaneous remission of PML have been reported.

PREVENTION

There are no specific preventive measures for JC virus infection and PML.

TRANSMISSIBLE SPONGIFORM ENCEPHALOPATHIES

Three diseases of humans, **Creutzfeldt-Jakob disease (CJD), kuru,** and **new-variant Creutzfeldt-Jakob disease (nvCJD),** have been classified as sporadic prion-related encephalopathies. In addition, prions have been implicated in **Gerstmann-Sträussler syndrome** and other inherited degenerative neurologic disorders, as well as transmissible encephalopathies in animals (Table 55–9).

ETIOLOGY

Proteinaceous fibrils are noted in brain specimens from persons with CJD, kuru, and nvCJD, as well as the inherited and animal

TABLE 55–9. Transmissible Spongiform Encephalopathies

	Year First Described	Transmission	Typical Clinical and Other Features
Syndrome in Humans			
Creutzfeldt-Jakob disease (CJD)	1920	Sporadic	Dementia, myoclonus, variable ataxia; spongiform changes, variable amyloid plaques (about 15% of cases)
Familial CJD	1924	Autosomal-dominant inheritance	Dementia, myoclonus, variable ataxia; spongiform changes; longer survival, and amyloid plaques more common than in CJD
Kuru	1957	Ritual cannibalism	Ataxia, tremor, cranial nerve abnormalities; amyloid plaques common
Gerstmann-Sträussler-Scheinkes syndrome	1936	Autosomal-dominant inheritance	Ataxia, dementia; amyloid plaques universal
nvCJD	1996	Sporadic (*PRNP* codon 129 Met homozygous)	Younger age at onset; psychiatric presentation, dysesthesias, ataxia; no periodic electroencephalographic complexes; bilateral increased thalamic densities on magnetic resonance imaging; florid amyloid plaques
Fatal-familial insomnia	1986	Autosomal-dominant inheritance (mutation at *PRNP* codon 178 linked to 129 Met)	Insomnia, dysautonomia, ataxia, myoclonus, late mild dementia; minimal vacuolation, no plaques, PrP^{Sc} difficult to detect
Sporadic familial insomnia	1999	Sporadic (no mutation identified in either *PRNP* gene)	Same as fatal familial insomnia but negative family history
Syndrome in Animals			
Scrapie (sheep and goats)	ca. 1750		Ataxia, pruritus
Transmissible mink encephalopathy (mink)	1965		Ataxia, somnolence, seizures
Chronic wasting disease (deer, elk)	1980		Altered behavior, excessive salivation, wasting; florid amyloid plaques
Bovine spongiform encephalopathy (cattle, zoo ruminants)	1987		Ataxia, wasting
Feline spongiform encephalopathy (cats)	1990		Altered behavior, ataxia

nvCJD = new-variant CJD; Prp^{Sc} = scrapie-associated proteinase-resistant protein.

spongiform encephalopathies, and appear to be responsible for these diseases. These fibrils are composed of **prion,** for proteinaceous infectious agent, now known as **proteinase-resistant protein** and designated as $\mathbf{PrP^{Sc}}$ for scrapie-associated prion protein. PrP^{Sc} is an isoform of a normal cellular molecule designated as $\mathbf{PrP^{C}}$, that is encoded in humans by a gene designated as ***PRNP.*** The injection of disease-associated PrP^{Sc} into the normal brains of selected species is sufficient to induce encephalopathy; however, the disease-associated prions contain no nucleic acid and do not replicate, and therefore they constitute a novel type of transmissible agent unique in mammalian disease. In sporadic prion-associated diseases, the normal cellular PrP^{C} is conformationally altered by posttranslational events with PrP^{Sc}, which is rich in β-sheet content and relatively resistant to proteolysis compared with PrP^{C}. This conformational change is potentiated by one of a number of mutations or insertions within the prion gene, accounting for the familial prion-associated diseases, and the injection of disease-associated prions into normal brain, accounting for the transmission of some prion-associated illnesses. These agents remain infectious after treatments that inactivate most viruses and nucleic acids.

Transmission. Several forms of the spongiform encephalopathies are familial (Table 55–9). Kuru was transmitted by exposure to infected tissues during ritual cannibalization, but other human-to-human transmission has not been documented. For sporadic cases, infectivity is greatest in CNS tissues and least in peripheral tissues. CSF may be infectious, but transmission through secretions and blood, except for animals experimentally infected, has not been demonstrated.

EPIDEMIOLOGY

Classic, sporadic CJD occurs worldwide, most often between the ages of 50 and 70 years, although cases have been reported in persons in the second and third decades of life. Disease has been transmitted through corneal transplants and dura mater allographs and through the injection of growth and gonadotropic hormones purified from the pituitary glands of cadavers. Examination of these iatrogenic cases has indicated that the incubation period ranges from 15 months to more than 20 years. Familial CJD accounts for about 10% of cases, and several different point mutations and insertions in the *PRNP* gene have been identified.

Kuru is seen exclusively among the Fore highlanders of Papua, New Guinea, where it has produced disease that has devastated the indigenous population for decades. The agent of kuru is transmitted either by mucosal or subcutaneous autoinoculation or by ingestion of human brains through ritual cannibalization. The cessation of cannibalization was associated with a decreasing number of cases and now with the disappearance of kuru among the younger generations. The incubation period ranges from 5 to 30 years.

In the mid-1990s, nvCJD was described in a small number of persons, primarily from Great Britain, No cases have been diagnosed in North America. It has been hypothesized that the disease is transmitted through the ingestion of meat from cattle afflicted with **bovine spongiform encephalopathy,** or **"mad cow disease,"** which became epidemic among British herds approximately 5 years before the first cases of nvCJD were described. The bovine epidemic, in turn, may have been fostered by the addition of offal from scrapie-afflicted sheep into cattle feed as a protein supplement. The zoonotic epidemic prompted regulations concerning a ban on the feeding of nonmilk ruminant proteins to ruminants in the United Kingdom, and the number of cases among cows has subsequently declined dramatically. However, because of the prolonged incubation time for the development of nvCJD, the number of affected humans still in the incubation stage currently is unknown. Because of the cross-species transmission of bovine spongiform encephalopathy causing **feline spongiform encephalopathy,** incorporation of bovine offal into any animal feed, pet food, or fertilizer was also banned.

PATHOGENESIS

The mechanism by which the accumulation of PrP^{Sc} causes neurologic disease is unknown. Scrapie in sheep is acquired by the gastrointestinal tract, with infection in the abdominal lymph nodes followed by infection in the brain ≥12 months later. There is no associated inflammatory response.

SYMPTOMS AND CLINICAL MANIFESTATIONS

Some patients with classic CJD have a prodrome of fatigue and malaise followed by the hallmark deterioration of higher cortical functions, manifested primarily in decreased memory and reasoning ability, behavioral changes, and altered visual acuity. Nearly all persons exhibit myoclonus at some point in the course of the illness, which characteristically is induced by visual or auditory stimuli. The person's condition usually deteriorates to profound dementia within 6 months, followed by coma and death.

Persons with kuru typically have a prodrome of headache and joint pain, but in all persons the symptoms of progressive cerebellar dysfunction dominate, resulting in an inability to walk within months of onset. The ataxia is associated with a shivering tremor, giving kuru, which means "shiver" in Fore, its name. In addition, some persons have involuntary athetotic movements as the illness progresses. Dementia occurs in some but not all people with kuru.

Persons with nvCJD are distinguishable from those with classic CJD in several ways and also have been younger. These persons present with prominent behavior aberrations and have persistent paresthesias. Cerebellar signs arc uniformly present. Like the more familiar form of CJD, dementia rapidly evolves, but the mean duration of disease is relatively prolonged, slightly more than 1 year.

DIAGNOSIS

The diagnoses of CJD and kuru are most often established clinically. Classic CJD is suggested for persons 50–65 years of age with the onset of progressive dementia and myoclonus. Likewise, the diagnosis of kuru generally is established when progressive ataxia and tremors are noted in the appropriate epidemiologic setting. Prion-associated diseases do not elicit an inflammatory response, and because the putative infectious particle is similar to an endogenous human protein, the body does not mount an immune response. The CSF findings in both CJD and kuru are normal. Ultimately a definitive diagnosis requires examination of the brain tissue at biopsy or autopsy. Although differences in pathologic findings allow discrimination of the various prion-associated diseases, they all result in spongiform changes that correspond to intracytoplasmic vacuoles in neuronal and astroglial tissue.

TREATMENT

There is currently no therapy for CJD, kuru, or nvCJD.

PROGNOSIS

Both CJD and kuru are rapidly progressive encephalopathies that ultimately result in severe neurologic dysfunction and coma. Although some remissions have been reported, death within 6–12 months of onset usually results from inanition, aspiration or other forms of pneumonia, extrapulmonary infections, or respiratory insufficiency.

PREVENTION

Persons with spongiform encephalopathies require only standard precautions, especially in the handling of CSF and tissues obtained at autopsy. Although the source of infection for many persons with CJD is unknown, disease that arises from transplantation or injection of contaminated material is preventable. Careful screening of organ donors and of persons willing to donate tissue for a history of dementia or myoclonus should be effective in diminishing this risk. Kuru has virtually disappeared since the suspension of cannibalism among the Fore.

REYE'S SYNDROME

ETIOLOGY

The association between Reye's syndrome and precedent viral syndromes and the use of aspirin suggests that this illness may be triggered by a combination of infectious and toxic insults. Approximately 90% of persons with Reye's syndrome have a precedent viral prodrome. Although influenza A and B and varicella have been identified most commonly, a wide variety of viral illnesses have preceded the onset of Reye's syndrome. The association between aspirin use during the prodromal illness and the subsequent development of Reye's syndrome has been confirmed in careful prospective, case-control studies showing that aspirin use is nearly twice as prevalent among persons with Reye's syndrome than among control subjects.

EPIDEMIOLOGY

Reye's syndrome is a postinfectious illness characterized by encephalopathy and fatty degeneration of the liver. The illness was first described in 1963, and its incidence has been decreasing since the early 1980s, at least in part because of public health campaigns against the use of aspirin to treat children. The peak age group for Reye's syndrome is 5–15 years, but patients ranging from infancy to adulthood have been reported.

PATHOGENESIS

The pathogenesis of Reye's syndrome remains uncertain. Histologic changes in the brains of persons with Reye's syndrome include pale, swollen cortical neurons and astroglial cells, with a notable absence of inflammatory cells, demyelinization, and viral inclusion bodies. Biopsies of the liver reveal characteristic abundant intracytoplasmic lipid droplets within the hepatocytes; the overall fat content of the liver may be increased eightfold. Electron microscopy demonstrates pleomorphic changes in the mitochondrial structure, reflected by diminished mitochondrial enzyme activity (but not of cytoplasmic enzyme activity), as measured by histochemical staining. Fatty changes are noted in the kidney and occasionally in the heart muscle as well. It remains uncertain whether the nervous system dysfunction is secondary to the multiple metabolic abnormalities generated by hepatic dysfunction or is a result of a primary global mitochondriopathy that affects multiple organs.

SYMPTOMS AND CLINICAL MANIFESTATIONS

The clinical course of Reye's syndrome usually follows a distinctive pattern. As the affected person apparently is recovering from the prodromal viral illness, there is an abrupt onset of vomiting that lasts several hours. This period is followed by cerebral dysfunction, which generally proceeds through several stages, reflecting increasingly severe cerebral edema and heightened intracranial pressure. Many persons reach less severe stages without further progression. Illness in infants may progress directly to coma without a vomiting phase or early-stage neurologic disease.

In addition to the dramatic abnormalities in neurologic status, all patients demonstrate hepatic dysfunction. Although hepatomegaly is usually mild, hepatic aminotransferase levels are markedly elevated and serum ammonia concentrations are three times or more above the normal value during the early stages of cerebral dysfunction. Partial thromboplastin time is increased, and nearly 50% of patients have hypoglycemia. Aminoacidemia and organic fatty acid concentrations frequently are nonspecifically elevated because of increased catabolism in these severely ill persons.

DIAGNOSIS

Reye's syndrome should be suspected in any child presenting with encephalopathy and hepatic dysfunction. The diagnosis is strengthened by a history of viral illness in the recent past and episodes of vomiting immediately before a change in mental status. The case definition for Reye's syndrome established by the CDC in 1980 requires (1) a serum aspartate aminotransferase, or serum alanine aminotransferase, or serum ammonia concentration at least three times above normal, (2) typical fatty infiltration of hepatic tissue on biopsy or autopsy, (3) WBC count $<9/mm^3$ in CSF (if a measurement is obtained), and (4) exclusion of other possible diagnoses. Several conditions may have a presentation identical to that of Reye's syndrome, especially certain inborn errors of metabolism that may be silent for the first several months of life, at which point hepatic dysfunction and encephalopathy are triggered by a viral infection.

TREATMENT

The treatment of Reye's syndrome is exclusively supportive. Reye's syndrome gradually resolves spontaneously within several days. Expert intensive care is mandatory for all persons with Reye's syndrome to maintain vital functions, avoid hypoglycemia, and manage increased intracranial pressure. Invasive monitoring of intracranial pressure is required if the syndrome proceeds to stage III or beyond.

PROGNOSIS

Despite aggressive intensive management, the mortality for Reye's syndrome still approximates 30–40%. Poor prognostic factors include young age, rapid progression, severe maximal stage, and markedly elevated ammonia or creatine kinase levels at the time of admission.

PREVENTION

Avoidance of aspirin or aspirin-containing remedies during acute febrile illnesses in children appears to be effective in decreasing the risk of Reye's syndrome. It is important to ensure varicella vaccination and also annual administration of influenza vaccine for children who require long-term salicylate therapy for Kawasaki syndrome and childhood rheumatologic illnesses.

REVIEWS

Calisher CH: Medically important arboviruses of the United States and Canada. *Clin Microbiol Rev* 1994;7:89-116.

Jeffrey KJ, Read SJ, Peto TEA, et al: Diagnosis of viral infections of the central nervous system: Clinical interpretation of PCR results. *Lancet* 1997;349:313–7.

Johnson RT: Viral Infection of the Nervous System. New York, Raven Press, 1998.

Meyer HM, Johnson RT, Crawford IP, et al: Central nervous system syndromes of "viral" etiology: A study of 713 cases. *Am J Med* 1960; 29:334–47.

Nicolosi A, Hauser WA, Beghi E, et al: Epidemiology of central nervous system infections in Olmsted County, Minnesota, 1950-1981. *J Infect Dis* 1986;154:399–408.

Rautonen J, Koskiniemi M, Vaheri A: Prognostic factors in childhood acute encephalitis. *Pediatr Infect Dis J* 1991;10:441–6.

Studahl M, Bergstrom T, Hagberg L: Acute viral encephalitis in adults—a prospective study. Scand *J Infect Dis* 1998;30:215–20.

Whitley RJ: Viral encephalitis. *N Engl J Med* 1990;323:242–50.

KEY ARTICLES

Herpes Simplex Encephalitis

Cinque P, Cleator GM, Weber T, et al: The role of the laboratory investigation in the diagnosis and management of patients with suspected herpes simplex encephalitis: A consensus report. *J Neurol Neurosurg Psychiatry* 1996;61:339–45.

Domingues BR, Lakeman FD, Mayo MS, et al: Application of competitive PCR to cerebrospinal fluid samples from patients with herpes simplex encephalitis. *J Clin Microbiol* 1998;36:2229–34.

Fodor PA, Levin MJ, Weinberg A, et al: Atypical herpes simplex virus encephalitis diagnosed by PCR amplification of viral DNA from CSF. *Neurology* 1998;51:554–9.

Hanada N, Kido S, Terashima M, et al: Non-invasive method for early diagnosis of herpes simplex encephalitis. *Arch Dis Child* 1988; 63:1470–3.

Kennedy PG: A retrospective analysis of forty-six cases of herpes encephalitis seen in Glasgow between 1962 and 1985. *Q J Med* 1988:68:533–40.

Koskeniemi M, Vaheri A, Taskinen E: Cerebrospinal fluid alterations in herpes simplex encephalitis. *Rev Infect Dis* 1984;6:608–18.

Lahat E, Barr J, Barkai G, et al: Long-term neurological outcome of herpes encephalitis. *Arch Dis Child* 1999;80:69–71.

Nahmias AJ, Whitley RJ, Visintine AN, et al: Herpes simplex virus encephalitis: Laboratory evaluations and their diagnostic significance. *J Infect Dis* 1982;145:829–36.

Schroth G, Gawehn J, Thron A, et al: Early diagnosis of herpes simplex encephalitis by MRI. *Neurology* 1987;37:179.

Tebas P, Nease RF, Storch GA: Use of the polymerase chain reaction in the diagnosis of herpes simplex encephalitis: A decision analysis model. *Am J Med* 1998;105:287–95.

Whitley RJ, Soong SJ, Linneman C Jr, et al: Herpes simplex encephalitis: Clinical assessment. *JAMA* 1982:247:317–20.

St. Louis Encephalitis

Barrett FF, Yow MD, Phillips CA: St Louis encephalitis in children during the 1964 epidemic. *JAMA* 1965;193:381–5.

Brinker KR, Paulson G, Monath TP, et al: St Louis encephalitis in Ohio, September 1975: Clinical and EEG studies in 16 cases. *Arch Intern Med* 1979;139:561–6.

Lawton AH, Rich TA, McLendon S, et al: Follow-up studies of St Louis encephalitis in Florida: Reevaluation of the emotional and health status of the survivors five years after acute illness. *South Med J* 1970;63:66–71.

Southern PM Jr, Smith JW, Luby JP, et al: Clinical and laboratory features of epidemic St Louis encephalitis. *Ann Intern Med* 1969;71:681–9.

California Encephalitis

Balfour HH Jr, Siem RA, Bauer H, et al: California arbovirus (LaCrosse) infections. 1. Clinical and laboratory findings in 66 children with meningoencephalitis. *Pediatrics* 1973;52:680–91.

Cramblett HG, Stegmiller H, Spencer C: California encephalitis virus infections in children: Clinical and laboratory studies. *JAMA* 1966; 198:108–12.

Hilty MD, Haynes RE, Azimi PH, et al: California encephalitis in children. *Am J Dis Child* 1972:124:530–3.

McJunkin JE, de los Reyes EC, Irazuzta JE, et al: LaCrosse encephalitis in children. *N Engl J Med* 2001;344:801–7.

McJunkin JE, Khan R, de los Reyes EC, et al: Treatment of severe LaCrosse encephalitis with intravenous ribavirin following diagnosis by brain biopsy. *Pediatrics* 1997;99:261–7.

Western Equine Encephalitis

Earnest MP, Goolishian HA, Calverley JR, et al: Neurologic, intellectual, and psychologic sequelae following western encephalitis. A follow-up study of 35 cases. *Neurology* 1971;21:969–74.

Eklund CM: Human encephalitis of the western equine type in Minnesota in 1941: Clinical and epidemiological study of serologically positive cases. *Am J Hyg* 1946;43:171–93.

Eastern Equine Encephalitis

Faber S, Hill A, Connerly ML, et al: Encephalitis in infants and children caused by the virus of the eastern variety of equine encephalitis. *JAMA* 1940;114:1725–31.

Feemster RF: Equine encephalitis in Massachusetts. *N Engl J Med* 1957;257:701–4.

Feemster RF, Wheeler RE, Daniels JB, et al: Field and laboratory studies on equine encephalitis. *N Engl J Med* 1958;259:107–13.

Finberg RW: Case records of the Massachusetts General Hospital: Case 50-1984. *N Engl J Med* 1984;311:1559–66.

Franck PT, Johnson KM: An outbreak of Venezuelan encephalitis in man in the Panama Canal Zone. *Am J Trop Med Hyg* 1970;19:860–5.

Goldfield M, Welsh JN, Taylor BF: The 1959 outbreak of Eastern encephalitis in New Jersey. 5. The inapparent infection:disease ratio. *Am J Epidemiol* 1968;87:32–3.

West Nile Virus

Anderson JF, Andreadis TG, Vossbrinck CR, et al: Isolation of West Nile virus from mosquitoes, crows, and a Cooper's hawk in Connecticut. *Science* 1999;286:2331–3.

Asnis DS, Conetta R, Teixeira AA, et al: The West Nile virus outbreak of 1999 in New York: The Flushing Hospital experience. *Clin Infect Dis* 2000;30:413–8.

Lanciotti RS, Roehrig JT, Deubel V, et al: Origin of the West Nile virus responsible for an outbreak of encephalitis in the northeastern United States. *Science* 1999;286:2333–7.

Nash D, Mostashari F, Fine A, et al: The outbreak of West Nile virus infection in the New York City area in 1999. *N Engl J Med* 2001;344:1807–14.

Tsai TF, Popovici F, Cernescu C, et al: West Nile encephalitis epidemic in southeastern Romania. *Lancet* 1998;352:767–71.

Arboviruses Outside the United States

Aidem HP, Garagusi VF: Japanese B encephalitis: A case report from New York and a brief review of the literature. *Ann Intern Med* 1961:55:324–7.

Grascenkov NI: Tick-borne encephalitis in the USSR. *Bull World Health Organ* 1964;30:187–96.

Tigertt WD, Berge TO: Japanese B encephalitis. *Am J Public Health* 1957;47:713–8.

Enteroviruses

Hamilton MS, Jackson MA, Abel D: Clinical utility of polymerase chain reaction testing for enteroviral meningitis. *Pediatr Infect Dis J* 1999;18:533–7.

McKinney RE Jr, Katz SL, Wilfert CM: Chronic enteroviral meningoencephalitis in agammaglobulinemic patients. *Rev Infect Dis* 1987;9: 334–56.

Pevear DC, Tull TM, Seipel ME, et al: Activity of pleconaril against enteroviruses. *Antimicrob Agents Chemother* 1999;43:2109–15.

Romero JR: Reverse-transcription polymerase chain reaction detection of the enteroviruses. *Arch Pathol Lab Med* 1999;123:1161–9.

Rotbart HA: Enteroviral infections of the central nervous system. *Clin Infect Dis* 1995;20:971–81.

Rotbart HA, McCracken GH Jr, Whitley RJ, et al: Clinical significance of enteroviruses in serious summer febrile illnesses of children. *Pediatr Infect Dis J* 1999;18:869–74.

Sawyer MH, Holland D, Aintablian N, et al: Diagnosis of enteroviral central nervous system infection by polymerase chain reaction during a large community outbreak. *Pediatr Infect Dis J* 1994;13:177–82.

Sells CJ, Carpenter RL, Ray CG: Sequelae of central-nervous-system enteroviral infections. *N Engl J Med* 1975;293:1–4.

van Vliet KE, Glimaker M, Lebon P, et al: Multicenter evaluation of the Amplicor Enterovirus PCR test with cerebrospinal fluid from patients with aseptic meningitis. The European Union Concerted Action on Viral Meningitis and Encephalitis. *J Clin Microbiol* 1998;36:2652–7.

Wilfert CM, Buckley RH, Mohanakumar T, et al: Persistent and fatal central-nervous-system ECHOvirus infections in patients with agammaglobulinemia. *N Engl J Med* 1977;296:1485–9.

Lymphocytic Choriomeningitis Virus

Baum SG, Lewis AM Jr, Rowe WP, et al: Epidemic nonmeningitic lymphocytic-choriomeningitis-virus infection. An outbreak in a population of laboratory personnel. *N Engl J Med* 1966;274:934–6.

Biggar RJ, Woodall JP, Walter PD, et al: Lymphocytic choriomeningitis outbreak associated with pet hamsters: Fifty-seven cases from New York State. *JAMA* 1975;232:494–500.

Childs JE, Glass GE, Ksiazek TG, et al: Human-rodent contact and infection with lymphocytic choriomeningitis and Seoul viruses in an inner city population. *Am J Trop Med Hyg* 1991;44:117–21.

Deibel R, Woodall JP, Decher WJ, et al: Lymphocytic choriomeningitis virus in man: Serologic evidence of association with pet hamsters. *JAMA* 1975;232:501–4.

Farmer TW, Janeway CA: Infection with the virus of lymphocytic choriomeningitis. *Medicine (Baltimore)* 1942;21:1–63.

Rabies

Anderson LJ, Nicholson KG, Tauxe RV, et al: Human rabies in the United States, 1960-1979: Epidemiology, diagnosis, and prevention. *Ann Intern Med* 1984;100:728–35.

Anderson LJ, Winkler WG, Vernon AA, et al: Prophylaxis for persons in contact with patients who have rabies. *N Engl J Med* 1980;302:967–8.

Centers for Disease Control and Prevention: Human rabies prevention—United States, 1999. Recommendations of the Advisory Committee on

Immunization Practices (ACIP). *MMWR Morb Mortal Wkly Rep* 1998;48(RR-1):1–21.

DuPont JR, Earle KM: Human rabies encephalitis: A study of forty-nine fatal cases with a review of the literature. *Neurology* 1965;15:1023–34.

Krebs JW, Smith JS, Rupprecht CE, et al: Rabies surveillance in the United States during 1996. *J Am Vet Med Assoc* 1997;211:1525–39.

Krebs JW, Smith JS, Rupprecht CE, et al: Rabies surveillance in the United States during 1998. *J Am Vet Med Assoc* 1999;215:1786–98. (Published erratum appears in *J Am Vet Med Assoc* 2000;216:1223.)

Plotkin SA: Rabies. *Clin Infect Dis* 2000;30:4–12.

Smith JS, Fishbein DB, Rupprecht CE, et al: Unexplained rabies in three immigrants in the United States: A virologic investigation. *N Engl J Med* 1991;324:205–11.

Warrell DA: The clinical picture of rabies in man. *Trans R Soc Trop Med Hyg* 1976;70:188–95.

Cat-Scratch Disease

Carithers HA: Cat-scratch disease: An overview based on a study of 1,200 patients. *Am J Dis Child* 1985;139:1124–33.

Carithers HA, Margileth AM: Cat-scratch disease. Acute encephalopathy and other neurologic manifestations. *Am J Dis Child* 1991;145:98–101.

Steiner MM, Vukovitch D, Hadawi SA: Cat-scratch disease with encephalopathy. Case report and review of the literature. *J Pediatr* 1963;62: 514–20.

Tuberculosis

Idriss ZH, Sinno AA, Kronfol NM: Tuberculosis meningitis in childhood: Forty-three cases. *Am J Dis Child* 1976;130:364–7.

Sumaya CV, Simek M, Smith MH, et al: Tuberculosis meningitis in children during the isoniazid era. *J Pediatr* 1975;87:43–9.

Lyme Disease

Reik L, Steere AC, Bartenhagen NH, et al: Neurologic abnormalities of Lyme disease. *Medicine (Baltimore)* 1979;58:281–94.

Reik L Jr, Burgdorfer W, Johnson JO: Neurologic abnormalities in Lyme disease without erythema chronicum migrans. *Am J Med* 1986;81:73–8.

Mycoplasma pneumoniae infection

Clyde WA Jr: Neurological syndromes and mycoplasmal infections. *Arch Neurol* 1980;37:65–6.

Hodges GR, Fass RJ, Saslaw S: Central nervous system disease associated with *Mycoplasma pneumoniae* infection. *Arch Intern Med* 1972; 130:277–82.

Lerer RJ, Kalavsky SM: Central nervous system disease associated with *Mycoplasma pneumoniae* infection: Report of five cases and review of the literature. *Pediatrics* 1973;52:658–68.

Twomey JA, Espir ML: Neurological manifestations and *Mycoplasma pneumoniae* infection. *Br Med J* 1979;2:832–3.

Rocky Mountain Spotted Fever

Gorman RJ, Saxon S, Snead OC III: Neurologic sequelae of Rocky Mountain spotted fever. *Pediatrics* 1981;67:354–7.

Haynes RE, Sanders DY, Cramblett HG: Rocky Mountain spotted fever in children. *J Pediatr* 1970;685–93.

Helmick CG, Bernard KW, D'Angelo LJ: Rocky Mountain spotted fever: Clinical, laboratory, and epidemiological features of 262 cases. *J Infect Dis* 1984;150:480–8.

Varicella-Zoster Virus

Appelbaum E, Rachelson MH, Dolgopol VB: Varicella encephalitis. *Am J Med* 1953;15:223–30.

Appelbaum E, Kreps SI, Sunshine A: Herpes zoster encephalitis. *Am J Med* 1962;32:25–31.

Boughton C: Varicella-zoster in Sydney. II. Neurological complication of varicella. *Med J Aust* 1966;2:444–7.

Gilden DH, Kleinschmidt-DeMasters BK, LaGuardia JJ, et al: Neurologic complications of the reactivation of varicella-zoster virus. *N Engl J Med* 2000;342:635–45.

Jemsek J, Greenberg SB, Taber L, et al: Herpes zoster–associated encephalitis: Clinicopathologic report of 12 cases and review of the literature. *Medicine (Baltimore)* 1983;62:81–97.

Johnson R, Milbourn PE: Central nervous system manifestations of chickenpox. *Can Med Assoc J* 1970;102:831–4.

McCormick WF, Rodnitzky RL, Schochet SS Jr, et al: Varicella-zoster encephalomyelitis: A morphologic and virologic study. *Arch Neurol* 1969;21:559–70.

Epstein-Barr Virus

Grose C, Henle W, Henle G, et al: Primary Epstein-Barr virus infections in acute neurologic disease. *N Engl J Med* 1975;292:392–5.

Lange BJ, Berman PH, Bender J, et al: Encephalitis in infectious mononucleosis: Diagnostic considerations. *Pediatrics* 1976;58:877–80.

Schnell RG, Dyck PJ, Bowie EJ, et al: Infectious mononucleosis: Neurologic and EEG findings. *Medicine (Baltimore)* 1966;45:51–63.

Silverstein A, Steinberg G, Nathanson M: Nervous system involvement in infectious mononucleosis: The heralding and/or major manifestation. *Arch Neurol* 1972;26:353–8.

Human Herpesvirus 6

Caserta MT, Hall CB, Schnabel K, et al: Neuroinvasion and persistence of human herpesvirus 6 in children. *J Infect Dis* 1994;170:1586–9.

Pruksananonda P, Hall CB, Insel RA, et al: Primary human herpesvirus 6 infections in young children. *N Engl J Med* 1992;326:1445–50.

Singh N, Carrigan DR: Human herpesvirus-6 in transplantation: An emerging pathogen. *Ann Intern Med* 1996;124:1065–71.

Suga S, Yoshikawa T, Asano Y, et al: Clinical and virological analyses of 21 infants with exanthem subitum (roseola infantum) and central nervous system complications. *Ann Neurol* 1993;33:597–603.

Torre D, Speranza F, Martegani R, et al: Meningoencephalitis caused by human herpesvirus-6 in an immunocompetent adult patient: Case report and review of the literature. *Infection* 1998;26:402–4.

Measles

Appelbaum E, Dolgopol VB, Dolgin J: Measles encephalitis. *Am J Dis Child* 1949;77:25–48.

Boughton CR: Morbilli in Sydney. 2. Neurological sequelae of morbilli. *Med J Aust* 1964;2:908–15.

Johnson RT, Griffin DE, Hirsch RL, et al: Measles encephalomyelitis: Clinical and immunologic studies. *N Engl J Med* 1984;310:137–41.

LaBocetta AC, Tornay AS: Measles encephalitis: Report of 61 cases. *Am J Dis Child* 1964;107:247–55.

Tyler HR: Neurological complications of rubeola (measles). *Medicine (Baltimore)* 1957;36:147–67.

Mumps

Azimi PH, Cramblett HG, Haynes RE: Mumps meningoencephalitis in children. *JAMA* 1969;207:509–12.

Levitt LP, Rich TA, Kinde SW, et al: Central nervous system mumps: A review of 64 cases. *Neurology* 1970;20:829–34.

Oldfelt V: Sequelae of mumps meningoencephalitis. *Acta Med Scand* 1949;134:405–14.

Rubella

Margolis FJ, Wilson JL, Top FH: Postrubella encephalomyelitis: Report of cases in Detroit and review of the literature. *J Pediatr* 1943;23:158–65.

Sherman FE, Michaels RH, Kenny FM: Acute encephalopathy (encephalitis) complicating rubella. *JAMA* 1965;192:675–81.

Adenoviruses

Faulkner R, van Rooyen CE: Adenovirus types 3 and 5 isolated from the cerebrospinal fluid of children. *Can Med Assoc J* 1962;87:1123–5.

Gabrielson MO, Joseph C, Hsuing GD: Encephalitis associated with adenovirus type 7 occurring in a family outbreak. *J Pediatr* 1966;68:142–4.

Kelsey DS: Adenovirus meningoencephalitis. *Pediatrics* 1978;61:291–3.

Simila S, Jouppila R, Salmi A, et al: Encephalomeningitis in children associated with an adenovirus type 7 epidemic. *Acta Paediatr Scand* 1970;59:310–6.

Influenza Viruses

Delorme L, Middleton PJ: Influenza A virus associated with acute encephalopathy. *Am J Dis Child* 1979;133:822–4.

Mellman WJ: Influenza encephalitis. *J Pediatr* 1958;53:292–7.

Human Immunodeficiency Virus Infection

Ammassari A, Cingolani A, Pezzotti P, et al: AIDS-related focal brain lesions in the era of highly active antiretroviral therapy. *Neurology* 2000;55:1194–200.

Belman AL, Lantos G, Horoupian D, et al: AIDS: Calcification of the basal ganglia in infants and children. *Neurology* 1986;36:1192–9.

Belman AL, Ultmann MH, Horoupian D, et al: Neurologic complications in infants and children with acquired immunodeficiency syndrome. *Ann Intern Med* 1985;18:560–6.

Cooper ER, Hanson C, Diaz C, et al: Encephalopathy and progression of human immunodeficiency virus disease in a cohort of children with perinatally acquired human immunodeficiency virus infection. Women and Infants Transmission Study Group. *J Pediatr* 1998;132:808–12.

Epstein LG, Sharer LR, Oleske JM, et al: Neurologic manifestations of human immunodeficiency virus infection in children. *Pediatrics* 1986;78:678–87.

Filippi CG, Sze G, Farber SJ, et al: Regression of HIV encephalopathy and basal ganglia signal intensity abnormality at MR imaging in patients with AIDS after initiation of protease inhibitor therapy. *Radiology* 1998;206:491–8.

Gabuzda DH, Hirsch MS: Neurologic manifestations of infection with human immunodeficiency virus. Clinical features and pathogenesis. *Ann Intern Med* 1987;107:383–91.

Tardieu M, Le Chenadec J, Persoz A, et al: HIV-1-related encephalopathy in infants compared with children and adults. French Pediatric HIV Infection Study and the SEROCO Group. *Neurology* 2000;54:1089–95.

Thurnher MM, Schindler EG, Thurnher SA, et al: Highly active antiretroviral therapy for patients with AIDS dementia complex: Effect on MR imaging findings and clinical course. *AJNR Am J Neuroradiol* 2000;21:670–8.

Subacute Sclerosing Panencephalitis

Cutler RW, Merler E, Hammerstad JP: Production of antibody by the central nervous system in subacute sclerosing panencephalitis. *Neurology* 1968;18:129–32.

Jabbour JT, Garcia JH, Lemmi H, et al: Subacute sclerosing panencephalitis: A multidisciplinary study of eight cases. *JAMA* 1969;207:2248–54.

Markand ON, Panszi JG: The electroencephalogram in subacute sclerosing panencephalitis. *Arch Neurol* 1975;32:719–26.

Modlin JF, Halsey NA, Eddins DL, et al: Epidemiology of subacute acute sclerosing panencephalitis. *J Pediatr* 1979;94:231–6.

Progressive Rubella Encephalitis

Sever JL, South MA, Shaver KA: Delayed manifestations of congenital rubella. *Rev Infect Dis* 1985;7:S164–9.

Waxham MN, Wolinsky JS: Rubella virus and its effect on the central nervous system. *Neurol Clin* 1984;2:367–85.

Progressive Multifocal Leukoencephalopathy

Berger JR, Kaszovitz B, Post MJ, et al: Progressive multifocal leukoencephalopathy associated with human immunodeficiency virus infection. A review of the literature with a report of sixteen cases. *Ann Intern Med* 1987;107:78–87.

Berger JR, Concha M: Progressive multifocal leukoencephalopathy: The evolution of a disease once considered rare. *J Neurovirol* 1995;1:5–18.

Henson J, Rosenblum M, Armstrong D, et al: Amplification of JC virus DNA from brain and cerebrospinal fluid of patients with progressive multifocal leukoencephalopathy. *Neurology* 1991;41:1967–71.

Holman RC, Janssen RS, Buehler JW, et al: Epidemiology of progressive multifocal leukoencephalopathy in the United States: Analysis of national mortality and AIDS surveillance data. *Neurology* 1991;41:1733–6.

Houff SA, Major EO, Katz DA, et al: Involvement of JC virus–infected mononuclear cells from the bone marrow and spleen in the pathogenesis of progressive multifocal leukoencephalopathy. *N Engl J Med* 1988;318:301–5.

Transmissible Spongiform Encephalopathies

Haywood AM: Transmissible spongiform encephalopathies. *N Engl J Med* 1997;337:1821–8.

Johnson RT, Gibbs CJ Jr: Creutzfeldt-Jakob disease and related transmissible spongiform encephalopathies. *N Engl J Med* 1998;339:1994–2004.

Prusiner SB: Prion disease and the BSE crisis. *Science* 1997;278:245–51.

Scott MR, Will R, Ironside J, et al: Compelling transgenetic evidence for transmission of bovine spongiform encephalopathy prions to humans. *Proc Natl Acad Sci USA* 1999;96:15137–42.

van Duijn CM, Delasnerie-Lauprêtre N, Masullo C, et al: Case-control study of risk factors of Creutzfeldt-Jakob disease in Europe during 1993–95. European Union (EU) Collaborative Study Group of Creutzfeldt-Jakob disease (CJD). *Lancet* 1998;351:1081–5.

Whitley RJ, MacDonald N, Asher DM, et al: Transmissible spongiform encephalopathies: A review for pediatricians. Technical Report. *Pediatrics* 2000;106:1160–5.

Will RG, Matthews WB: A retrospective study of Creutzfeldt-Jakob disease in England and Wales 1970–79. *J Neurol Neurosurg Psychiatry* 1984;47:134–40.

Reye's Syndrome

Belay ED, Bresee JS, Holman RC, et al: Reye's syndrome in the United States from 1981 through 1997. *N Engl J Med* 1999;340:1377–82.

Forsyth BW, Horwitz RI, Acampora D, et al: New epidemiologic evidence confirming that bias does not explain the aspirin/Reye's syndrome association. *JAMA* 1989;261:2517–24.

Lovejoy FH Jr, Smith AL, Bresnan MJ, et al: Clinical staging in Reye's syndrome. *Am J Dis Child* 1974:128:36–41.

NIH Consensus Conference: Diagnosis and treatment of Reye's syndrome. *JAMA* 1981;246:2441–4.

CHAPTER 56

Peripheral Neuropathy and Myelopathy

Philip Toltzis

Peripheral neuropathy is an uncommon manifestation of infectious disease, but many pathogens have been associated with symptoms referable to the peripheral nervous system. The mechanism of their deleterious effects on the peripheral nerves is varied and includes induction of a destructive immune response, direct infection, and elaboration of a neurotoxin. These pathogens may be grouped into four categories depending on the clinical pattern. The first category consists of pathogens whose major manifestations are referable to the peripheral nervous system and include *Clostridium tetani, Clostridium botulinum,* and the polioviruses (Table 56–1). An additional entity, the Guillain-Barré syndrome, is not an infectious disease per se but usually follows an infectious illness. A second category consists of agents that cause peripheral neuropathy in association with multisystem, extraneural disease and includes diphtheria, leprosy, Lyme disease, and HIV infection. A third category, composed of a single entity, HTLV-I, is associated with a myelopathy.

The fourth category is composed of several infectious agents generally associated with encephalitis or aseptic meningitis but occasionally with peripheral nerve involvement. These include the nonpolio enteroviruses, several of the arthropodborne viruses, the herpesviruses other than herpes simplex virus, and *Mycoplasma pneumoniae,* which together account for a large percentage of CNS infections. In each instance the peripheral neuropathy occurs primarily in association with CNS disease and less commonly presents as an isolated clinical finding (Chapter 53).

PERIPHERAL NEUROPATHIES

TETANUS

Tetanus is an uncommon disease in the United States, occurring primarily as a complication of wound infections. Tetanus, especially neonatal tetanus, remains an important infection worldwide.

ETIOLOGY

Tetanus is caused by an exotoxin produced by *C. tetani,* an anaerobic, sporulating gram-positive bacillus. *C. tetani* is ubiquitous in nature and may be recovered routinely from samples of soil, dirt, and dust rich in organic material, particularly animal waste. In addition, *C. tetani* is a normal resident of the intestines of herbivores and less frequently of carnivores, including humans. *C. tetani* in the vegetative form is slender and motile, whereas in the sporulated form it attains a characteristic **drumstick** shape because of the presence of the **spore** at the terminal end. Spores are highly resistant to heat, light, desiccation, and antiseptics and can survive in the soil for years.

Transmission. *C. tetani* organisms are inoculated into a wound, where they proliferate and produce toxin. The infection is not spread from person to person.

EPIDEMIOLOGY

Although the incidence of tetanus has fallen dramatically in nations that offer routine immunization, the disease is endemic in many parts of the world. Tetanus most frequently follows a wound infection by *C. tetani.* Because manual labor predisposes the worker to soil-contaminated infected wounds, men are more frequently affected than women. However, tetanus also has resulted from *C. tetani* infection after a variety of other events, including abortion, intravenous or subcutaneous illicit drug use, circumcision, and ear piercing. In some cases no predisposing wound is found. Other epidemiologic risk factors worldwide include rural occupation, poor health conditions, and insufficient active immunization.

In the United States the incidence of tetanus is approximately 0.03 per 100,000 population, hundreds of times less than in countries in which tetanus remains endemic, and it occurs most frequently among elderly persons, the group with the highest case-fatality ratio. As in other parts of the world, the male:female ratio is 1.5:1. The states with the highest incidence of tetanus are in the southern Atlantic and south central areas of the country. Puncture wounds and lacerations account for more than half of the cases of tetanus in the United States, followed by infected decubiti, burns, frostbite, and dental abscesses; rare cases follow surgical procedures (frequently for a gangrenous limb), abortion, or drug use.

Neonatal Tetanus. Neonatal tetanus is endemic in many developing countries. Among vaccine-preventable diseases worldwide, tetanus is second only to measles as a cause of childhood death, with approximately 500,000 cases annually. The focus of neonatal infection is nearly always the umbilical cord. In many areas up to 10% of all live neonates may be infected, and as many as 35% of neonatal deaths may be attributed to tetanus. In regions endemic for neonatal tetanus, babies frequently are born at home, either with no medical support or with a poorly trained midwife; the infant is delivered, with the mother in a squatting position, onto a dirt floor or straw mat contaminated with *Clostridium;* and the umbilical cord is cut in a nonsterile manner.

PATHOGENESIS

C. tetani enters the wound in the sporulated form and converts to the vegetative form when exposed to the low oxygen tension found in necrotic tissue. The vegetative organisms then proliferate and elaborate toxin, which is released after autolysis of the bacteria. The tetanus toxin, or **tetanospasmin,** has a molecular mass of approximately 150 kDa and shares genetic, antigenic, and functional similarity with botulinum toxin; like the toxins associated with botulism, tetanospasmin is among the most lethal chemicals

TABLE 56–1. Comparison of the Infectious Peripheral Neuropathies and Guillain-Barré Syndrome

Feature	Tetanus	Botulism	Poliomyelitis (Paralytic)	Guillain-Barré Syndrome
Pattern of weakness	None	Symmetric Descending	Asymmetric Ascending; may be bulbar	Symmetric Ascending
Sensation	Normal	Normal	Normal	Paresthesia
Ataxia	Absent	Absent	Absent	Usually absent; may be present
Babinski sign	Present	Absent	Absent	Absent
Additional major features	Muscle rigidity and spasm	Constipation and lethargy with foodborne botulism in infants		Pain, muscle cramps, dysautonomia (constipation, hypertension)
Rate of progression	Days to 2 wk	Days to several weeks	Days to weeks	Days to weeks
Fever	Present	Absent	Present	Absent (rarely, present)
Cerebrospinal fluid				
Protein level	Normal	Normal	Elevated	Elevated
White blood cell count	Normal	Normal	Elevated	Normal
Time to recovery	Variable	Variable	Months to years, or no recovery (permanent paralysis)	Weeks to months

identified in nature. Both tetanus and the seven botulinum toxins are synthesized in the cytosol of the bacteria and activated by posttranslational modification. They share similar structural organization, containing three separate functional domains that are responsible for neurospecific binding, delivery of the toxic component to the intracellular target, and conferring toxicity through a zinc-dependent protease. Both tetanus and botulinum toxins enter the presynaptic terminus through energy-dependent endocytosis, after which they are transported to the neurotransmitter-containing vesicles. The toxin-associated peptidase activities then degrade membrane components of the neurotransmitter vesicles, inhibiting the release of the neurotransmitter into the synaptic space.

The differences in symptoms between tetanus and botulism are related primarily to the anatomic distribution of the affected nerves rather than to the biochemical activity of the toxins themselves. Tetanospasmin disseminates through the bloodstream and is taken up at the peripheral endings of motor, autonomic, and possibly sensory neurons. It is then transported in retrograde fashion within the axon to the CNS, where it is distributed primarily in the spinal cord. The physiologic effects of tetanus toxin can occur at several different levels of the nervous system, but the most prominent and characteristic effects are caused by blockage of the inhibitory neurotransmitters γ-aminobutyric acid (GABA) and glycine in interneurons. This in turn leads to an unmodulated excitatory transmission to muscle groups throughout the body, an effect similar to that produced by the poison strychnine. The clinical effects of tetanus toxin also may be seen in the autonomic nervous system and the brainstem.

SYMPTOMS AND CLINICAL MANIFESTATIONS

Most persons with tetanus are seen within 2 weeks of acquiring a tetanus-prone wound. The most characteristic clinical feature of tetanus is severe, generalized muscular rigidity and spasm of both extensor and flexor muscle groups. The position assumed by the patient is determined by the relative strengths of the opposing muscles. The rigidity increases in severity for the first 4–8 days of illness, with gradual recovery during the ensuing 2 weeks to 2 months. The pattern of rigidity tends to descend from the head downward because musculature innervated by the shortest neurons is affected first. Consequently most persons initially have rigidity of the face and neck that results in **trismus,** difficulty in swallowing, and a peculiar grinning expression, **risus sardonicus.** Excitation of the truncal musculature follows, and the predominance of the extensor muscles usually results in **opisthotonic posturing,** a form of spasm consisting of extreme hyperextension of the body with the head and the heels bent backward and the body bowed forward. The rigidity is painful. Additionally, tetanus can have dramatic effects on the autonomic nervous system, resulting in fluctuating and unpredictable changes in blood pressure, heart rate, and peripheral vascular perfusion. Serum catecholamine levels are severalfold higher than normal, which may itself lead to myocardial damage. Consciousness is not affected by tetanus toxin, and the patient is aware throughout.

Neonatal Tetanus. Neonatal tetanus has an incubation period of 3–10 days. The muscle rigidity progresses very rapidly in newborns. The first symptom usually noted is excessive crying and difficulty in feeding. Facial rigidity is reflected by closed eyes, wrinkled forehead, and a stiff upper lip. Rigidity of the trunk results in severe **opisthotonos,** the baby's head reaching close to his or her heels (Fig. 56–1). Heart rate and temperature fluctuate widely. In severe cases cyanosis is profound as a result of impairment of respiration due to truncal rigidity, uncontrolled upper airway secretions, and complicating pneumonia.

DIAGNOSIS

The diagnosis of tetanus is established exclusively on clinical grounds. Isolation of *C. tetani* from the precedent wound is helpful but not definitive, because many wounds may be contaminated with clostridia in the absence of tetanus. Moreover, clostridia may be absent on culture in more than half of persons with unequivocal clinical tetanus because of sampling error or difficulty in culturing this anaerobic organism. Furthermore, 20% of persons with tetanus have no previous wound at all.

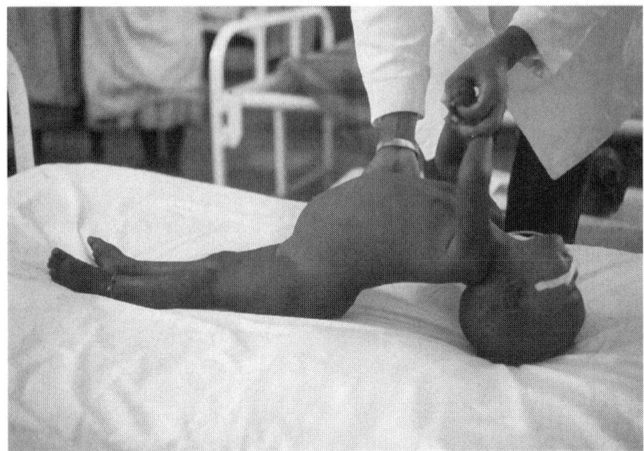

FIGURE 56–1. Typical appearance of a newborn with severe tetanus. (Photography courtesy of Kent Martin.)

Differential Diagnosis

The full-blown manifestation of tetanus is not difficult to recognize, but the clinical challenge is to arrive at the correct diagnosis during the early stages of illness. Trismus may initially be attributable to dental or oropharyngeal infections. Neck stiffness may suggest a diagnosis of meningitis. In both adults and newborns, diffuse muscle rigidity may mimic hypocalcemia. In addition, the bizarre attitudes associated with tetanus can be confused with the toxic effects of phenothiazine. Strychnine poisoning includes many of the same signs of tetanus, but the onset is more rapid and both hypotonia and rigidity may be seen. In the newborn period a brain insult from anoxia, kernicterus, or intracranial hemorrhage may cause opisthotonic posturing even though trismus is absent.

TREATMENT

The treatment of tetanus is multifactorial and complex. Persons with tetanus benefit greatly from modern intensive care, although such facilities are unavailable in areas of the world where tetanus is most common. The principles of tetanus therapy include interrupting toxin production by antibiotics, administering antitoxin, and providing supportive therapy to counteract spinal convulsions, paralysis, and autonomic dysfunction.

Definitive Treatment

Interruption of Toxin Production. The infected wound should be thoroughly débrided to lower the burden of infecting *C. tetani* and to raise the local oxygen tension, which itself decreases survival of the remaining organisms. Similarly, in neonatal disease, the cord should be cleaned and débrided. Antitoxin should be administered before débridement because toxin may be released during wound manipulation. Metronidazole (30 mg/kg/day divided every 6 hours intravenously until symptoms improve) is added adjunctively to diminish the *C. tetani* burden. Penicillin G (100,000 U/kg/day divided every 4 hours intravenously) can be used as an alternative, but its postulated central GABA antagonist activity theoretically may potentiate the activity of tetanospasmin. Because drug is distributed poorly in necrotic tissue, antibiotics should not be used as a substitute for débridement.

Antitoxin. Although administration of antitoxin is a mainstay of therapy for tetanus, its efficacy has been disputed and the ideal dose has not been determined. In general, multiple trials conducted during the past several decades indicate that antitoxin administration lowers the mortality from approximately 60–75% to 30–50%. In Haiti the administration of equine antiserum to babies with neonatal tetanus reduced the mortality by half. Antitoxin is ineffective in neutralizing tetanus toxin once the toxin has fixed to neurologic tissue. It therefore is of paramount importance to administer antitoxin at the earliest possible time. Antitoxin does not cross the blood-brain barrier; however, the effectiveness of intrathecal administration is not established and the human antitoxin available in the United States is not licensed for intrathecal use.

Both human and equine antitoxins have been developed. Recommended treatment is with a single dose of human **tetanus immune globulin (TIG),** 3,000–6,000 U intramuscularly as a single dose, with a portion of the dose administered around the wound. Although local injection makes theoretical sense, the efficacy of this approach has never been established. If human antitoxin is not available, an alternative is equine **tetanus antitoxin (TAT),** 50,000–100,000 U intramuscularly as a single dose, with a portion of the dose (20,000 U) given intravenously. As with all equine antisera, the patient must be tested for hypersensitivity and desensitized as necessary. Either a 1:10 dilution of antitoxin instilled into the conjunctival sac or a 1:10 to 1:100 dilution injected intradermally should be administered in a setting appropriate to treat any subsequent hypersensitivity reaction. Approximately 10% of patients react and require desensitization with progressively higher doses of antitoxin. If neither of the specific tetanus antitoxin preparations is available, IVIG, which contains some antitetanus toxin antibody, can be used, although the effectiveness of IVIG for tetanus is undetermined.

Supportive Therapy

Paralysis. Paralysis with nondepolarizing neuromuscular blockades effectively interrupts spinal convulsions. When available, pharmacologic paralysis and mechanical ventilation have effectively reduced mortality for tetanus. In addition to relief of muscular rigidity, this strategy enables controlled ventilation, facilitates respiratory toilet, and allows movement of the patient for nursing care without inducing convulsions. Some authors have recommended a routine tracheostomy rather than oral or nasotracheal intubation, the latter of which may induce laryngospasm.

Anticonvulsants. Several drugs have been recommended to suppress spinal convulsions. The benzodiazepines are GABA agonists and have been successfully used to block the effects of tetanospasmin. Baclofen, also a GABA agonist, has also been used similarly. Oral baclofen is not distributed well across the blood-brain barrier, but the drug has been given intrathecally to persons with tetanus with some success, although respiratory depression may result. Intravenous administration of dantrolene, which results in muscle relaxation through the interference of calcium release from the sarcoplasmic reticulum, may be introduced toward the end of therapy as the person is being weaned from neuromuscular blockade, because prolonged exposure may result in hepatotoxicity. Very large doses of these agents may be required to achieve the desired relaxation and sedation. Because these medications may affect respiration and blood pressure, caution and careful monitoring are critical to their administration, particularly in persons with autonomic lability.

Autonomic Dysfunction. Autonomic dysfunction may itself prove life threatening. Several agents have been recommended to control sympathetic and parasympathetic excitation: labetalol, which provides both α and β sympathetic blockade; phentolamine, an α blocker; clonidine, a central α_2 agonist; and magnesium sulfate and epidural bupivacaine, both of which diminish the secretion of endogenous catecholamines. Morphine, which is contraindicated for nonparalyzed patients with tetanus because of its propensity to exacerbate spasms, has been effective in controlling malignant hypertension in paralyzed persons and has the additional benefit of being readily reversible if the desired effects are not achieved. The autonomic dysfunction in tetanus is complex and multifactorial, however, and all pharmacologic measures may themselves prove life threatening and should be administered with extreme caution in intensive care settings.

General Measures. Several general measures are critical to the recovery of the person with tetanus. Stimulation, particularly tactile, may induce spinal convulsions, and nonparalyzed persons should be placed in a quiet, softly lit room and disturbed as infrequently as possible. The generalized severe muscular contractions cause enormous caloric expenditures, and replacement of calories through careful nasogastric or nasoduodenal feeding or through intravenous hyperalimentation should be vigorously pursued. Careful attention to serum electrolyte levels, scrupulous skin care, and control of constipation are important needs until the person recovers.

Vaccination. Persons with tetanus do not produce detectable antibodies against toxin, and repeated infections may occur. Therefore all persons with tetanus should receive active immunization after recovery.

COMPLICATIONS

Most of the complications of tetanus affect respiratory function and result primarily from aspiration or nosocomial pneumonia, obstruction of the upper airway, rigidity of the thoracic musculature, or pulmonary embolism. Some persons die unexpectedly and suddenly; brainstem lesions, presumably related to toxin injury, have been discovered at autopsy. Occasional persons may have adrenal insufficiency, and adrenal hemorrhages have been documented in some persons. Coinfection of the precedent wound with *Staphylococcus* or *Streptococcus* may occur, particularly in newborn omphalitis, and must be treated with appropriate antibiotics (Chapter 48).

PROGNOSIS

The overall mortality rate for tetanus is approximately 25%. Several factors that influence prognosis have been identified. A short incubation period from the time of acquisition of the wound to the first symptoms and then a rapid progression of symptoms from the time of onset of trismus to the peak period of spinal convulsions are poor prognosticators, presumably reflecting the presence of a high titer of toxin. Tetanus that originates from abortion or drug abuse is associated with poor outcome. The morbidity rate is highest among newborns and elderly persons; with neonatal tetanus, disease among premature infants is particularly deadly. Survivors of tetanus, however, appear to have a good prognosis. Even infants, who are particularly susceptible to hypoxic events, recover from tetanus with few sequelae.

PREVENTION

Prophylaxis. Prophylaxis against tetanus can be achieved effectively in persons who need care of a newly acquired wound. Injuries that contain foreign bodies or devitalized tissue should receive appropriate débridement to prevent tetanus effectively. Tetanus prophylaxis includes vaccination of persons with incomplete immunization and also TIG for wounds contaminated by dirt, fecal material, or saliva; puncture wounds; avulsions; and wounds resulting from missiles, crushing, burns, and frostbite (Table 48–5).

Vaccination. Active immunization with tetanus toxoid is a safe and extremely effective means of preventing tetanus. Although rare cases occur among adequately immunized persons, they tend to be mild. Toxoid is available in an aluminum-absorbed or fluid preparation; both induce seroconversion to protective levels of antibody, but the response is more sustained with the absorbed preparation, lasting at least 10 years (Chapter 17).

Neonatal Tetanus. Routine vaccination of women of childbearing age with two doses and tetanus vaccination of pregnant women during the last trimester of pregnancy, when material antibodies can cross the placenta, have been effective in reducing neonatal infection in developing countries. In Haiti a program of prenatal vaccination reduced the incidence of neonatal tetanus from 14% to 1.8% if the mother received two doses and to 0.2% if the mother received all three. In addition, a program of umbilical cord care, in which home-born babies who came to the clinics within the first hours or days after birth were given local cord care, antitoxin, and penicillin G, was also highly effective in preventing neonatal tetanus.

BOTULISM

Botulism is a disease characterized by a descending flaccid paralysis caused by a neurotoxin elaborated by *Clostridium botulinum.* There are three recognized clinical forms of botulism: **foodborne botulism,** resulting from consumption of food contaminated with preformed toxin; **wound botulism,** occurring after a wound becomes colonized or infected with *C. botulinum;* and **infant botulism,** occurring after gastrointestinal colonization with the organism itself.

ETIOLOGY

C. botulinum is a gram-positive anaerobic bacillus that is a common isolate in soil and marine sediment and survives most environmental stresses through spore formation. **Botulism toxin** is produced during germination and released after autolysis of the organism. Occasionally, toxin production and clinical disease have been associated with clostridial species other than *C. botulinum,* such as *C. barati* and *C. butyricum.*

Traditionally, *C. botulinum* strains have been grouped according to the toxin produced. Types C and D botulism are confined to animals, particularly fowl and cattle, and the others are associated with disease in humans. All the botulinum toxins are composed of a heavy and a light chain, have similar molecular masses of approximately 130–170 kDa, and exist in a complex with other protein molecules that protect the toxin while in the gastrointestinal tract. Most toxin is absorbed in the small intestine. The specific toxicity for the botulinum toxins is 10^7–10^8 mouse LD_{50} per milligram of protein, rendering them among the most toxic compounds in nature. Their structural organization and activity are very similar to those of tetanus toxin. Botulinum toxin acts by inhibiting the release of acetylcholine at peripheral cholinergic synapses. Toxin rapidly and tightly binds to presynaptic membranes and is internalized into the neuron, after which it prevents exocytosis of the neurotransmitter after nerve stimulation.

EPIDEMIOLOGY

C. botulinum spores can be isolated from soil worldwide, but most cases have been reported in the Northern Hemisphere. In the United States the highest incidence of botulism is detected in the Pacific

Coast states, Alaska, and the Mid-Atlantic states. The seven antigenically distinct botulinum toxins are labeled A through G, but the most common forms of botulism in the United States are caused by types A, B, and E. Type A disease is found primarily west of the Mississippi River, type B to the east of the river, and type E in the Pacific Northwest and Alaska, reflecting the distribution of *C. botulinum* spores in the environment.

Foodborne Botulism. Foodborne botulism is rare, with approximately 750 cases reported in the United States during the past 2 decades. Approximately three fourths of adult cases of foodborne botulism can be traced to ingestion of home-processed foods that have been improperly preserved and stored under anaerobic conditions. However, some cases have occurred after ingestion of commercially processed or restaurant food, and nearly 20% of cases have no identified source. In the United States, vegetables and fruits that have been contaminated with *C. tetani* from the soil account for approximately half of foodborne cases and usually are associated with type A and type B disease. However, a wide variety of foods have been linked to recent cases of botulism, including salsa, baked potatoes sealed in aluminum foil, cheese sauce, sautéed onions under a layer of butter, and garlic in oil. Most type E botulism cases result from ingestion of putrefied fish, a delicacy among some Native Americans in the Northwest.

Wound Botulism. Rarely, botulism may occur after contamination of traumatic wounds with *C. botulinum* and growth of the organism in devitalized tissues.

Infant Botulism. Infant botulism currently is the most common form of the disease in the United States, with approximately 70 cases reported annually. From 10% to 25% of cases of infant botulism can be traced to ingestion of honey; approximately 10% of randomly selected commercial containers of honey harbor botulinum spores but no toxin. Cases of infant botulism that are not associated with honey ingestion tend to occur in rural settings or in families where a parent has occupational exposure to soil. Most of these cases presumably result from infection by organisms found in the environment.

PATHOGENESIS

With few exceptions, foodborne adult botulism results from ingestion of food contaminated with preformed toxin. Wound botulism occurs from growth of *C. botulinum* in tissues and elaboration of toxin. Infant botulism follows ingestion of *C. botulinum* spores, with colonization of *C. botulinum,* luminal production of toxin, and intestinal absorption. Experiments using mice suggest that the microenvironment of the intestinal tract beyond infancy, particularly the presence of other anaerobic organisms, prevents colonization of *C. botulinum.* Therefore adult humans who ingest spores without toxin only rarely acquire botulism. In contrast, the gastrointestinal flora of infants may predispose them to *C. botulinum* colonization. The period after the introduction of solid foods to a breast-fed baby is marked by dramatic fluxes in intestinal flora and may be the most susceptible period for infant botulism.

SYMPTOMS AND CLINICAL MANIFESTATIONS

Foodborne Botulism. The incubation period for foodborne botulism is inversely proportional to the amount of toxin ingested, but the first signs of illness usually occur within hours of consumption of the contaminated food. Most persons have a prodrome of nausea and vomiting, which is followed by dizziness, light-headedness, and blurred vision. By the second to fourth day of illness, the persons begins to have dry mouth and sore throat, dysphonia, and dysphagia, and 1–2 days later has diplopia, constipation and abdominal distension, and generalized weakness. By the fifth day, persons with severe illness begin to have respiratory insufficiency.

For unknown reasons, clinical disease occurs unevenly among people who have ingested the same contaminated food. Whether the toxin is distributed unequally through a given container of contaminated food, or some persons absorb toxin poorly, or some persons are intrinsically resistant to the effects of toxin is uncertain.

Wound Botulism. The incubation period of wound botulism is 4–14 days. Historically, wound botulism has been associated with crush injuries and compound fractures, but recently it has occurred with increasing frequency in needle-using drug addicts. The wound itself may be minor and may not appear infected, but *C. botulinum* spores can be isolated on débridement. These persons do not have the gastrointestinal prodrome seen in foodborne disease, but the clinical presentation is otherwise identical.

Infant Botulism. Infant botulism usually occurs between 2–6 months of life. Some infants present with only mild hypotonia and feeding difficulties and the disease course is short and uneventful. The most severe cases of disease, however, may progress extremely rapidly, with respiratory arrest soon after the onset of illness. As in foodborne disease, the typical case of infant botulism is heralded by gastrointestinal symptoms, followed by bulbar paralysis, generalized weakness, and respiratory paralysis (Table 56–2). The disease usually begins with constipation; careful questioning of the child's caregiver may indicate that the constipation was present days to weeks before presentation. Subsequent symptoms accompanying constipation include inadequate sucking, decreased feeding, weak cry, poor head control, and floppiness. Frequently at presentation the baby has failed to thrive or is dehydrated.

Physical Examination Findings

Foodborne and Wound Botulism. The findings on physical examination reflect a progressive, descending pattern of generalized hypotonia. Unless there are complicating infections, persons typically are afebrile. Examination of the eyes demonstrates ptosis, diminished lacrimation, extraocular muscle paralysis, and, in time, poorly responsive, dilated pupils. Although hypotonia is characteristically generalized, up to 20% of persons may have asymmetric paresis. In most persons the deep tendon reflexes are normal at presentation but may disminish in time. The sensory nerves are intact.

Infant Botulism. The examination over the first several days of illness reveals drooping eyelids, a diminished gag reflex, poor suck,

TABLE 56–2. Clinical Characteristics of Infant Botulism

Characteristic	Rate of Occurrence (%)
Hypotonia	95
Poor sucking or feeding	94
Weakness	93
Facial paresis	84
Constipation	78
Decreased spontaneous movement	69
Decreased or absent deep tendon reflexes	64

Data from Long SS, Gajewski JL, Brown LW, et al: Clinical, laboratory, and environmental features of infant botulism in Southeastern Pennsylvania. *Pediatrics* 1985;75;935–41; and Schreiner MS, Field E, Ruddy R: Infant botulism: A review of 12 years' experience at the Children's Hospital of Philadelphia. *Pediatrics* 1991;87:159–65.

dysphagia, urinary retention, and poor respiratory effort. From 40% to 60% of all hospitalized infants require intubation because of either respiratory failure or loss of protective airway reflexes. Deep tendon reflexes, although present early in the course of disease, frequently diminish or disappear as the illness progresses.

DIAGNOSIS

The diagnosis of botulism is usually suspected from the clinical manifestations, especially if combined with a history of possible exposure and confirmed by identification of toxin in blood, for foodborne and wound botulism, or in stool, for infant botulism.

Differential Diagnosis

The differential diagnosis of botulism in older children and adults includes other causes of diffuse neuromuscular weakness, particularly Guillain-Barré syndrome, myasthenia gravis, intoxications, and porphyria. These diagnoses can be distinguished from botulism on the basis of sensory findings on physical examination; electromyographic tracings and nerve conduction studies; appropriate assays for heavy metals, organophosphates, and other poisons; and assays for urine porphyrin precursors. Some adults with botulism primarily have a dry, sore throat at presentation, leading to an initial diagnosis of pharyngitis before weakness becomes apparent.

The differential diagnosis of infant botulism is very broad. In some infants the weakness initially is believed to be due to failure to thrive or dehydration. The diagnoses include congenital neurologic degenerative diseases, congenital muscular dystrophy, inborn errors of metabolism, and acquired viral or bacterial infections of the CNS. Hypothyroidism, which is associated with constipation and hypotonia, may be mistaken for botulism in the early stages.

Laboratory Evaluation

Routine laboratory tests are not helpful in the diagnosis of botulism. The cerebrospinal fluid is normal.

Electromyography. Diagnostic criteria are similar for foodborne and infant botulism. Electromyography reveals low-amplitude **muscle action potentials (MAP).** Characteristically, MAP amplitudes are augmented by rapid, repetitive (≥20/sec) stimulations. This typical pattern is present in only 60% of persons at hospitalization and may require repeated testing to be detected. However, the potentiation of MAP amplitude by rapid stimulations is shared only with the Eaton-Lambert syndrome and distinguishes these diseases from myasthenia gravis and other causes of generalized weakness.

Microbiologic Evaluation

The principal diagnostic test for foodborne and wound botulism is identification of the circulating toxin. Approximately half of the persons with foodborne disease have detectable toxin in the bloodstream at the time of hospitalization and frequently for days to weeks thereafter, even after recovery. The assay entails the injection of the test serum intraperitoneally into a mouse, resulting in paralytic death of the animal. Confirmation and identification of the type of botulism require protection by monospecific antiserum in the same assay. If wound botulism is suspected, anaerobic cultures of the wound should be obtained in an to attempt to isolate *C. botulinum.*

In contrast to the diagnosis of foodborne disease, the diagnosis of infant botulism rests on the identification of *C. botulinum* or its toxin from the stool. Healthy infants and those with other neurologic diseases rarely excrete *C. botulinum.* Unlike foodborne disease, circulating toxin is identified in infant botulism only 10–20% of the time. However, toxin usually is readily identifiable in stool specimens.

TREATMENT

The mainstay treatment of foodborne and wound botulism is supportive therapy. Wound botulism also requires surgical débridement of infected and devitalized tissues. Infant botulism can be treated with human-derived botulinum antitoxin. Both adults and infants with the disease require close observation, usually in an intensive care unit. Intubation should be performed and mechanical ventilation initiated anticipatorily under controlled conditions. Enteral nutrition has proved possible, even in persons with constipation and decreased intestinal motility, by means of constant infusion through a nasojejunal or nasogastric tube. Sedatives and CNS depressants are contraindicated.

Antitoxin. Trivalent (ABE) equine antitoxin is available through many state health departments and the CDC. Before antitoxin is administered, the person must be tested for hypersensitivity to horse serum. Despite routine use in the treatment of foodborne botulism, the effectiveness of antitoxin has not been well demonstrated. Because toxin rapidly binds to neural tissue, early administration is probably critical. A survey published in 1984 indicated that the fatality rate among persons receiving antitoxin for type A botulism was 10% if the antitoxin was administered within 24 hours of onset, 15% if the antitoxin was given beyond 24 hours, and 46% if not given at all. The early-administration group also required fewer days of mechanical ventilation and had fewer days until sustained clinical improvement in comparison with the other groups. However, there is no evidence that equine antitoxin significantly alters the outcome of infant botulism. Because some newborns have had severe hypersensitivity responses, equine antitoxin is not recommended for the infant form of the disease.

Specific treatment for infant botulism is now available. In a randomized, double-blind, placebo-controlled trial, treatment of infant botulism with human-derived botulinum antitoxin, known as **botulism immune globulin (BIG),** reduced mean hospital stay from 5.5 weeks to 2.5 weeks. Treatment with BIG should be initiated as soon as possible. In the United States, BIG may be obtained from the California Department of Health Services (telephone: 510-540-2646) under an FDA-approved investigational new drug protocol.

Antibiotic Treatment. Antibiotics have no role in the treatment of foodborne and infant botulism. Because foodborne disease is only rarely associated with colonization or infection with *C. botulinum* itself, antibiotics are irrelevant. In infant botulism, penicillin therapy is ineffective in eradicating the organism from the gastrointestinal tract and does not influence the course of the illness. Although the efficacy of cathartics to purge the gastrointestinal tract of toxin or organisms has never been determined, most patients, both infant and adult, are constipated, and cathartics usually are indicated for patient comfort regardless of their influence on the toxin. However, magnesium-containing agents should be avoided because the cation may enhance the action of the botulinum toxin.

Despite unproven efficacy, wound botulism is usually treated with antibiotics in addition to antitoxin. Penicillin G 100,000 U/kg/day intravenously in divided doses every 4 hours for 10–14 days is the drug of choice. Metronidazole 30 mg/kg/day intravenously in divided doses every 8 hours is an alternative. Aminoglycoside antibiotics should be avoided because they may potentiate neuromuscular blockade by botulinum toxin.

COMPLICATIONS

Most complications of botulism result from invasive critical care such as pneumonia, urinary tract infection, and bacteremia.

Ventilator-related injuries, such as subglottic stenosis and mechanical malfunction, are occasional causes of morbidity among persons with botulism. The syndrome of inappropriate antidiuretic hormone has been reported in approximately 15% of hospitalized children with infant botulism. Some persons may have mild autonomic instability, manifested as bradycardia or tachycardia, flushing, and alterations in blood pressure. Cardiac conduction abnormalities, including bundle-branch block, have been noted occasionally in adults.

PROGNOSIS

The case fatality rate for botulism currently is less than 10%. The fatality rate for type A botulism is approximately twice that for type B or E, and death from botulism is particularly high among elderly persons. However, with the availability of appropriate intensive care, recovery from botulism can be expected within a 2-week to 2-month period. Short incubation periods and rapidity of onset directly correlate with severity of disease and duration of manifestations. Recovery is gradual and is characterized by a series of small improvements and deteriorations. Occasionally a person may be discharged and may require readmission because of recurrent weakness. Results of neurologic examination of survivors several months after illness are normal, without signs of residua.

PREVENTION

The risk of foodborne botulism can be significantly diminished by the proper preparation of preserved foods. Although the spores of *C. botulinum* are heat resistant, they can be killed by the use of a pressure cooker. In addition, a low pH is effective in inhibiting germination and toxin production, and boiling for short periods destroys the toxin. Therefore careful pressure cooking with the addition of citric acid for low-acid foods is sufficient to avoid the risk of botulism. The diagnosis of foodborne botulism may presage a common source outbreak, and expeditious notification of local health authorities is essential.

Most cases of infant botulism are unavoidable. The association of some cases with honey ingestion has led to the recommendation that infants not be fed honey until after their first birthday.

POLIOMYELITIS

Poliomyelitis is characterized by asymmetric flaccid paralysis caused by three serotypes of poliovirus. The latter half of the twentieth century witnessed dramatic events in the epidemiology of poliovirus infection, with the use of the **oral poliovirus vaccine (OPV)** and the enhanced **inactivated poliomyelitis vaccine (IPV).** Poliomyelitis has been eradicated from the Western Hemisphere and is the target of a global elimination program.

ETIOLOGY

Poliomyelitis results from infection of the CNS by polioviruses, which are members of the subgroup of enteroviruses of the group of picornaviruses. There are three antigenically distinct serotypes of poliovirus, types 1, 2, and 3. Polioviruses are nonenveloped, single-stranded, positive-sense RNA viruses. Once the virus enters the host cell, the RNA is translated into a single large protein, which is subsequently cleaved into the structural and nonstructural components of the virus. The poliovirus receptor is an integral membrane protein that is a member of the immunoglobulin superfamily.

EPIDEMIOLOGY

Poliomyelitis has probably existed since ancient times, but it was not until the late 1800s that epidemics of infantile paralysis first occurred in Western Europe and North America. These epidemics were potentiated by improvement in general hygiene and a delay of infection from infancy to late childhood, an age in which paralytic disease is more frequent. Historically, epidemics were propagated by fecal-oral spread by persons with asymptomatic infection. As with other enteroviruses, the incidence of poliovirus in temperate climates is highest in the late summer and early fall.

The cycle of epidemics in the United States was halted by the discovery of poliovirus culture methods in 1949, which allowed the rapid development of an injected IPV by 1955 and of a trivalent, attenuated live OPV that was used almost exclusively for pediatric immunization beginning in 1963. The impact of these events cannot be overstated. The incidence of reported paralytic and nonparalytic poliomyelitis in the United States in 1952 was more than 20,000 cases per year (37.5 cases per 100,000 population), accounting for more than 3,000 deaths. Through the 1980s fewer than 10 cases per year (0.002 case per 100,000 population) were recognized in the United States, and by the late 1980s no deaths from polio were recorded (Fig. 56–2). The last case of autochthonous poliomyelitis caused by wild-type virus in the United States occurred in 1979. Six additional imported cases have been reported since 1979, the last of which occurred in 1993.

In 1985 the Pan-American Health Organization established a goal to eliminate indigenous wild-type poliomyelitis from the Americas. The program consisted of concerted efforts to provide universal vaccination, bolstered by biannual "immunization days," when all children younger than 5 years of age received a dose of OPV regardless of previous immunizations. In addition, a network of 20,000 local health facilities was used to report and confirm cases expeditiously and to provide intensive house-to-house immunization in the surrounding communities. A rapid decrease ensued from the approximately 1,000 annual cases of poliomyelitis in 1986. The last case of endemic poliomyelitis in the Americas occurred in Peru in 1991. Using similar strategies, the World Health Organization has embarked on a program to eradicate poliomyelitis entirely. As a result of these efforts, worldwide immunization coverage increased from approximately 45% in 1981 to 80% by the mid-1990s. During this same period there was an 85% reduction of reported cases across 145 reporting nations. It currently is estimated that poliomyelitis will be eradicated worldwide within the first decade of the new millennium.

Vaccine-Associated Paralytic Poliomyelitis. During the 1980s, although a small number of cases were contracted outside the United States, nearly all of the remaining cases in the United States were caused by infection from the vaccine strains of virus, known as **vaccine-associated paralytic poliomyelitis (VAPP).** Most cases of VAPP are caused by spontaneous mutation of the vaccine strain, resulting in a virulent phenotype. Approximately half of the cases of VAPP occur in recipients of OPV, and of these, more than 90% occur after the first dose. The remaining cases of VAPP occur among inadequately vaccinated contacts of infants receiving the vaccine. The relative risk of VAPP in immunocompromised persons is approximately 2,000-fold higher than among infants with normal immunity. However, only a small portion of cases of VAPP have occurred in immunocompromised persons, and virtually none of these people were known to be immunocompromised before vaccination. Fortunately, the frequency of VAPP is very small, and overall there is 1 case of paralysis for every 2.5 million doses of OPV: 1 case in 700,000 after the first dose, and 1 case in 6.9 million after subsequent doses. To avoid VAPP, the United States and several Western countries have adopted vaccination policies

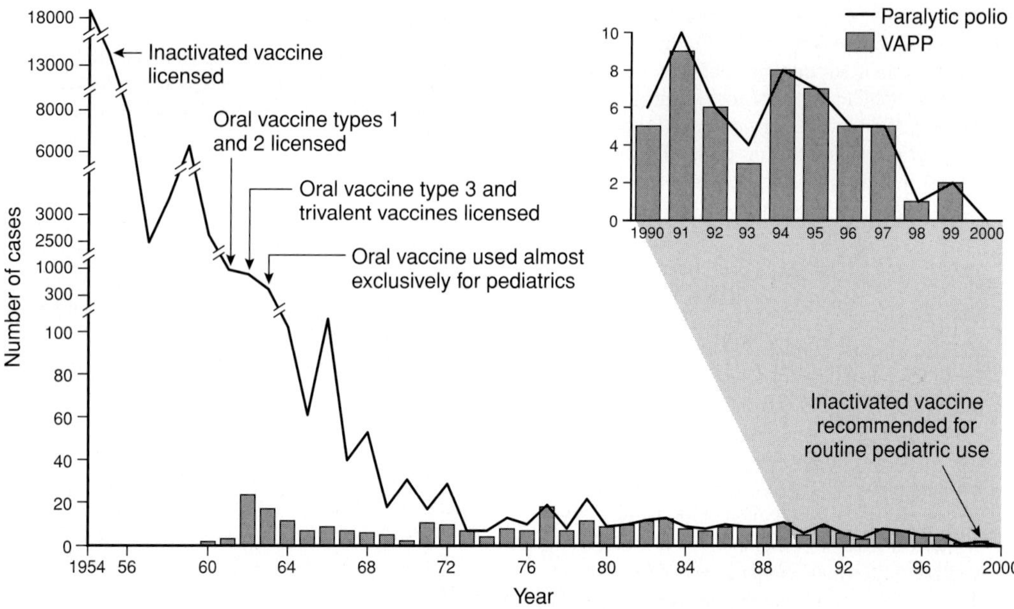

FIGURE 56–2. Reported total cases by year of paralytic poliomyelitis from 1954–2000 and of vaccine-associated paralytic poliomyelitis (VAPP) from 1960–2000 in the United States. (Data from the Centers for Disease Control and Prevention.)

using only the enhanced IPV. If global eradication is achieved, it is projected that all polio vaccination can be eliminated, as it was with smallpox, rendering the risks of VAPP moot.

PATHOGENESIS

Poliovirus initially infects the oropharynx, where it is shed and swallowed and where it replicates in the intestinal tract. Virus in both the pharynx and the intestinal tract invades local lymphatics and spreads into the bloodstream during the **primary viremic phase,** which leads to replication throughout the body, primarily in the systemic lymphatics and brown fat. From these sites a **secondary viremic phase** occurs that correlates with the onset of nonspecific systemic symptoms, known as the **minor illness.** Penetration into the CNS, leading to the **major illness,** results either directly by hematogenous spread or possibly through infection of peripheral nerves and axoplasmic transport to the spinal cord and brain. Once in the CNS, the viral infection extends along neural pathways.

Within the CNS, viral infection is confined to selected regions of the brain and spinal cord. The most intense disease is detected around the motor neurons of the **anterior horns of the spinal cord;** the cervical and lumbar segments are more severely affected than the thoracic segment. In the brain, lesions are found in the hypothalamus, thalamus, precentral motor cortex, and parts of the cerebellum and brainstem.

SYMPTOMS AND CLINICAL MANIFESTATIONS

The paradigmatic case of wild-type poliomyelitis exhibits a biphasic pattern, termed **minor illness** and **major illness.** Although biphasic disease is common in young children, monophasic disease, in which the two phases blend or the first phase is clinically inapparent, is the rule in adults. The first phase of illness, or minor illness, coincides with the period of viremia before inoculation of the CNS. The incubation period for minor illness is 2–6 days. Minor illness consists of nonspecific symptoms typical of many viral infections, including mild fever, sore throat, vomiting and gastrointestinal discomfort, malaise, and headache. Recovery occurs after 1–4 days. The illness ends at this point in most individuals and is known as **abortive poliomyelitis.**

In the 1–2% of persons in whom the disease progresses, a brief period of well-being is followed by the onset of the second phase, the major illness. This phase begins with **preparalytic poliomyelitis,** consisting of high fever, severe global headache, and vomiting. Within a day of onset the person begins to have intense stiffness and pain, especially in the lumbar region and neck but including any muscle group, which often requires movement or walking to achieve relief. Again, the illness may stop at the preparalytic stage without further progression and is then known as **nonparalytic poliomyelitis.**

Persons whose disease becomes paralytic begin to have weakness as the systemic symptoms of preparalytic poliomyelitis abate. **Paralytic poliomyelitis** has been divided into two distinct forms, **spinal poliomyelitis** and **bulbar poliomyelitis,** both of which may be present in the same person. Spinal poliomyelitis, which is the more common, is characterized by asymmetric flaccid paralysis along the trunk and extremities. The ultimate degree of paralysis is impossible to predict and may vary from mild weakness to complete quadriplegia and respiratory paralysis. As a rule, paralysis extends for 3–5 days, and progression stops when the temperature returns to normal. Deep tendon reflexes are diminished or absent in the affected limbs, and muscular atrophy usually follows.

Approximately 10–15% of persons with paralytic disease have bulbar poliomyelitis, the consequences of which are severe and life threatening. Bulbar poliomyelitis, indicating brainstem involvement, is characterized by cranial nerve palsies and respiratory and cardiovascular instability. The most common cranial nerves to be affected are the ninth and tenth, resulting in paralysis of phonation and swallowing. Involvement of the breathing and cardiovascular centers of the medulla portends a very poor prognosis. Independently of chest wall and diaphragm strength the affected person demonstrates irregular respiration and apnea, progressing to **Cheyne-Stokes** breathing and total cessation of respiratory effort. In addition, persons may have cardiac arrhythmias and blood pressure and heart rate fluctuations.

The clinical manifestations of VAPP are similar to those for wild-type virus. The incubation period for VAPP among vaccine recipients is 4–24 days; among susceptible contacts of vaccine recipients it is 11–58 days (median, 35 days) after contact. Among immunocompromised persons, the incubation period is unusually prolonged, from 12 days to 8 months; the illness may be protracted, from 2 to 3 months; and the fatality rate, exceeding 40% in one series, is much higher than that recorded for immunocompetent persons.

DIAGNOSIS

The diagnosis of a typical case of paralytic poliomyelitis may be established with confidence on clinical grounds. The combination of fever, headache, neck and back pain, asymmetric flaccid paralysis without sensory loss, and pleocytosis is not regularly seen in any other illness. In the many areas where paralytic polio is rare, the disease initially may be diagnosed as severe encephalitis because of other causes that are occasionally associated with paresis. Preparalytic disease, with fever, severe headaches, and neck pain, may resemble Rocky Mountain spotted fever or other forms of severe meningoencephalitis. The differential diagnosis also includes Guillain-Barré syndrome, transverse myelitis, and epidural abscess.

Nonpolio enteroviruses also may occasionally be associated with paralytic illness. A wide range of serotypes of coxsackieviruses and echoviruses have been implicated, but coxsackievirus A7 has been the species most commonly identified. Typically paralytic disease from nonpolio enteroviruses is mild, and recovery without residua is the rule. Bulbar disease from nonpolio enteroviruses is unusual, but occasional deaths from this manifestation have occurred.

Laboratory Evaluation

Although the CSF often is normal during the minor illness, most patients with CNS poliovirus infection demonstrate a pleocytosis of 20–300/mm^3; a polymorphonuclear response early in the disease shifts to mononuclear soon thereafter. By the second week of the major illness, the CSF pleocytosis resolves to near-normal values. In contrast, the CSF protein level is normal or only slightly elevated at the outset of CNS disease but usually rises to 50–100 mg/dL by the second week of illness.

Microbiologic Evaluation

Viral cultures of specimens from stool, pharynx, and CSF may be positive for poliovirus; culture of the CSF, however, has a low yield. Antibody titers to poliovirus in paired acute and convalescent sera regularly demonstrate a fourfold increase or greater. However, both culture and serologic tests may be confounded by the recent administration of oral polio vaccine; the vaccine strains may be shed for 3–6 weeks after vaccination. PCR sequencing of isolates is used to distinguish wild-type from vaccine strains.

TREATMENT

The treatment of poliomyelitis is entirely supportive. Preparalytic disease is treated primarily with bed rest. This recommendation stems from the observation that exertion at the onset of major illness predisposes a person to paralysis. Paralytic disease is treated according to standard rehabilitative medicine practices. Persons with early disease are placed on a firm bed with a footboard to support the back and reduce pain. Therapy with analgesia and hot packs is continued. Passive range-of-motion exercise is applied to paralyzed limbs. Once the person's condition has become stable, a vigorous program of physical therapy should be pursued in consultation with rehabilitation and orthopedic experts.

COMPLICATIONS

Respiratory impairment is the most critical complication of poliomyelitis. Respiratory failure may result from upper airway obstruction, weakness of the diaphragm and intercostal muscles, or disruption of the respiratory centers in the brainstem. When impairment results from airway obstruction or weakness of the respiratory musculature, the progression is regular and predictable. By contrast, respiratory failure from bulbar disease is less predictable. Patients may have sudden respiratory failure despite normal blood gas determinations and vital capacity measurements just before the event. In most cases, respiratory failure abates, allowing eventual weaning from mechanical ventilatory support.

Patients with paralytic poliomyelitis may have urinary retention and constipation, both of which resolve within several days. Intermittent catheterization is usually sufficient for bladder paralysis, and judicious laxative therapy provides relief from intestinal dysmotility. Older reports documented hypercalcemia resulting from immobilization and bone resorption in persons with prolonged paralysis, which is sufficient to cause renal stones in some. Hydration and acidification of the urine are recommended to prevent renal calculi.

Postpolio Syndrome. Postpolio syndrome, also called progressive **postpoliomyelitis muscular atrophy (PPMA),** is characterized by progressive muscle weakness that occurs many years after the acute illness in survivors of paralytic poliomyelitis. Most persons with PPMA have an insidious, gradual diminution of functional capacity with an increase of flaccid paralysis and a progression of muscle atrophy. The majority of persons with PPMA had paralytic poliomyelitis at a young age decades previously and were left with clinically significant residua.

The renewed paralysis is most prominent in the limbs that were left most severely affected. Sensory findings are absent. The rate of progression may be so slow that it can be detected only after several years. The mechanisms underlying this complication are not defined, and the histopathologic condition of the spinal cord and electrophysiologic findings are not significantly different from those of survivors of paralytic polio without PPMA. It is hypothesized that neuromuscular junctions, stressed by years of compensation for residual weakness, may be damaged gradually with time. Usually psychological support and additional assistance with physical therapy devices result in many additional years of self-sufficiency for patients with PPMA.

PROGNOSIS

Among persons with spinal paralytic disease, some gradual improvement in motor function is the rule. After 3 months, approximately 60% of patients with paralytic poliomyelitis demonstrate some recovery, and after 6 months, 80% show improvement. After 6 months, little additional recovery can be expected. Bulbar disease had a fatality rate of more than 80% in the epidemics in the 1940s. Ironically, bulbar paralysis rarely persists among survivors; persons with brainstem dysfunction, including cranial nerve paresis, usually recover without residua.

The strongest predictive factor for severe poliomyelitis is age. Among young children the ratio of inapparent to paralytic disease is 1,000:1, whereas among adults the same ratio is 75:1. Moreover, when paralysis occurs, it is milder in younger children. Bulbar disease and quadriplegia are uncommon in children younger than 5 years, among whom paralysis of a single extremity is the most frequent pattern.

Immunodeficiency predisposes a person to paralytic disease. Hypogammaglobulinemia and agammaglobulinemia are associated with severe, protracted paralytic poliomyelitis. Paralytic disease also occurs more commonly in children with severe combined immunodeficiency. To date, paralytic polio, particularly among recipients of the oral vaccine, has been reported only rarely in children with HIV infection.

PREVENTION

Poliovirus infection should be considered in any child with flaccid paralysis. Any possible case of poliomyelitis should be reported to the state health department and specimens collected for viral culture. Clinical isolates of poliovirus can be identified as the wild type or the vaccine type on the basis of sequence analysis. Cases of VAPP require no control measures because outbreaks of VAPP have not been recorded. Cases in which wild-type virus is documented or strongly considered possible should be contained by prompt booster vaccination of close contacts with OPV under the guidance of local or state health authorities. Nonimmunized adults have a slightly greater risk of developing VAPP than do children, and therefore, for adult contacts with no prior polio vaccination, IPV is preferable to OPV.

Vaccination. Prevention of poliomyelitis has been achieved through active vaccination. Two vaccines are currently licensed in the United States: an enhanced-potency inactivated vaccine given by injection, which is recommended for all children, and a live, attenuated oral vaccine. Both are extremely effective in preventing poliomyelitis (Chapter 17).

GUILLAIN-BARRÉ SYNDROME

The Guillain-Barré syndrome, also known as **idiopathic polyneuritis,** is characterized by an acute, nearly symmetric generalized motor and sensory polyneuropathy. There is now compelling evidence that the neuropathy results from an immune-mediated demyelinization triggered by an initial, apparently infectious, event.

ETIOLOGY

Although Guillain-Barré syndrome is not an infectious disease, many cases are preceded by an infectious illness, most frequently caused by *Campylobacter jejuni,* cytomegalovirus, Epstein-Barr virus, herpes simplex virus, *Mycoplasma pneumoniae,* HIV, or an unidentified agent that causes anicteric hepatitis. Guillain-Barré syndrome also has been associated with vaccination with an older rabies vaccine prepared from animal brain tissue contaminated with myelin and possibly with the swine influenza vaccine used in the 1970s; associations with other vaccines have not been convincingly demonstrated. Other precedent events have been less commonly identified, including surgery, epidural anesthesia, and illicit drug use. On occasion, Guillain-Barré syndrome may occur in association with other systemic diseases, most notably lupus erythematosus, lymphoma, and sarcoidosis, although the peripheral neuropathy in these conditions tends to be chronic rather than acute.

EPIDEMIOLOGY

Guillain-Barré syndrome currently is the most common cause of acute generalized paralysis in the United States, with an annual incidence of 0.75–2 cases per 100,000 population. Guillain-Barré syndrome may occur in virtually any age group, but its peak incidence is during middle age. Among children the disease occurs most commonly at 5–9 years of age.

PATHOGENESIS

Guillain-Barré syndrome represents a spectrum of pathogenetic mechanisms that vary according to the inciting event and the individual person. The pathologic findings consist of nearly symmetric inflammatory peripheral demyelination progressing symmetrically from the distal ventral and dorsal root ganglia. Nerves are infiltrated by lymphocytes with deposition of antibody and complement on the outer Schwann cell surface, leading to disruption from the outside inward. In the most severe cases, axonal degeneration occurs, presumably as an "innocent bystander," although in rare cases a primary immune attack on the axon has been detected. CNS involvement is rare, although occasional cases have been reported.

There is growing evidence that most cases of Guillain-Barré syndrome result from an autoimmune response triggered by exposure to an infectious agent that serves as a molecular mimic of one or more of the gangliosides, a class of structurally distinct glycolipids distributed throughout the nervous system. In particular, the outer core region of the LPS of selected serotypes of *C. jejuni* contains structures that are molecularly similar to the ganglioside GM_1. The connection between *C. jejuni* enteritis–associated Guillain-Barré syndrome and GM_1 antibodies has been repeatedly demonstrated. Other serotypes of *Campylobacter* lead to the development of the **Miller Fisher variant** of Guillain-Barré syndrome, characterized by ophthalmoplegia, ataxia, and areflexia. These serotypes contain an LPS that mimics the ganglioside GQ_{1b}, an antigen enriched in the oculomotor neuron, dorsal root ganglia, and cerebellum. CMV-associated Guillain-Barré syndrome has been associated with antibodies to the ganglioside GM_2.

SYMPTOMS AND CLINICAL MANIFESTATIONS

Between 25% and 40% of cases of Guillain-Barré syndrome are preceded by *Campylobacter* enteritis 1–2 weeks before the onset of neuropathy. This association is serotype specific, but the implicated *Campylobacter* serotypes vary from one geographic region to another. An additional 10–20% of cases are preceded by CMV infection. These cases tend to occur in young girls and to have prominent sensory and cranial nerve involvement.

The clinical manifestations of Guillain-Barré syndrome are extremely variable. The typical case begins with fine paraesthesias in the toes or fingers. Within 1–2 days, leg weakness develops, resulting in difficulty in climbing stairs. There is rapid ascending progression, with variable motor involvement of the upper extremities, the facial muscles, the oropharynx, and, in the most severe cases, the muscles of respiration. Pain and muscle cramps are reported by more than half of the persons with Guillain-Barré syndrome. Progression of motor disability is complete within 2 weeks of onset in 70% of persons and by 1 month in more than 90%. This is followed by a **plateau period** of variable duration and characterized by minor improvements and relapses without a noticeable net change. The plateau is followed by a slow recovery period.

Several variants of Guillain-Barré syndrome have been described. The most common and distinctive variant, **Miller Fisher syndrome,** consists of ophthalmoplegia, ataxia, and areflexia but minimal weakness. Other variants include weakness without sensory nerve involvement, pharyngeal-cervical-brachial weakness, facial paresis with paresthesias, severe ataxia or dysautonomia with sensory loss, and an axonal polyneuropathy with electrically inexcitable nerves.

Physical Examination Findings

The physical examination at presentation reveals symmetric weakness of the limbs with absent or diminished deep tendon reflexes.

Approximately half of the persons have bilateral facial weakness, the most common of the cranial neuropathies in Guillain-Barré syndrome. Despite the paresthesias, sensory loss is minimal. Severe cases of Guillain-Barré syndrome progress to paralysis of multiple cranial nerves, respiratory paralysis, and severe autonomic dysfunction. From 10% to 25% of cases require mechanical ventilation, often for only 1–2 weeks, but persons with the most severe disease may need assisted ventilation for as long as a year.

DIAGNOSIS

The diagnosis of Guillain-Barré syndrome is established clinically with support from electrophysiologic studies and lumbar puncture. The diagnostic criteria for Guillain-Barré syndrome have been formulated and revised (Table 56–3).

Laboratory Evaluation

About 90% of patients with Guillain-Barré syndrome demonstrate abnormalities in motor nerve conduction in the first week of illness, and 96% by the third week of illness. Sensory nerve conduction abnormalities are detected in 25% of patients after 1 week and in 73% after 3 weeks. The CSF demonstrates typical changes by the second week of illness. The most characteristic finding is an elevated protein concentration without pleocytosis. However, normal CSF protein values do not exclude the diagnosis, and some persons, particularly those with HIV-related Guillain-Barré syndrome, may demonstrate a mild lymphocytic pleocytosis.

TABLE 56–3. Diagnostic Criteria for Guillain-Barré Syndrome

Required
- Progressive motor weakness in more than one limb
- Areflexia or distal areflexia with proximal hyporeflexia

Supportive
- Motor weakness that progresses to maximal severity within 4 wk
- Relative symmetry of weakness
- Mild sensory abnormalities
- Cranial neuropathy
- Recovery, usually within 2–4 wk of plateau
- Autonomic dysfunction
- Afebrility
- Increased CSF protein level by second week
- CSF white blood cell count $<10/mm^3$
- Electrophysiologic features, particularly nerve conduction slowing or block

Nonsupportive
- Marked or persistent asymmetric weakness
- Persistent or early bladder or bowel dysfunction
- CSF white blood cell count $>50/mm^3$ or presence of polymorphonuclear cells
- Sharp sensory level

Diagnosis Excluded
- Hexacarbon abuse, lead neuropathy, or other toxic neuropathies
- Abnormal porphyrin metabolism
- History of diphtheria, poliomyelitis, botulism, or hysteria
- Pure sensory loss

Adapted from Asbury AK, Cornblath DR: Assessment of current diagnostic criteria for Guillain-Barré syndrome. *Ann Neurol* 1990;27:S21–24.

TREATMENT

Persons with Guillain-Barré syndrome should be hospitalized and observed closely for 1–2 weeks to establish the tempo of the illness and to confirm the diagnosis. Persons with mild disease who can still walk without support after this time require no further therapy and may be safely discharged. As with all severe neuropathies, supportive care is critical for those who have more profound disease. Passive range-of-motion exercises and frequent repositioning reduce tendon shortening and pressure sores, and pulmonary toilet lessens the incidence of complicating pneumonia. A program of active strengthening exercises initiated soon after the person demonstrates signs of recovery improves muscle tone during convalescence.

Although corticosteroids have been routinely offered to persons with Guillain-Barré syndrome in the past, there is firm evidence that they are not effective. A British study (Hughes, 1978) concluded that adult recipients of prednisolone (60 mg/day) recovered more slowly than untreated control subjects. A subsequent report from the same investigators indicated no difference in recovery when the dose was increased to 500 mg/day.

During the 1980s **plasmapheresis** was established as an effective therapy for severe Guillain-Barré syndrome. Several large multicenter international studies demonstrated that plasmapheresis significantly shortens the duration of assisted ventilation and the time required to reach a high degree of function. In the early 1990s, IVIG (400 mg/kg daily for 5 days) also was found to be effective in decreasing the severity of disease and hastening recovery. A study (Plasma Exchange/Sandglobulin Guillain-Barré Syndrome Trial Group, 1997) comparing plasmapheresis with IVIG in a large, multinational, randomized trial found no differences between the treatment groups in the degree of neurologic improvement 4 weeks after therapy. Additionally, the two treatment groups were equivalent with regard to the time required to ambulate without assistance, the duration of mechanical ventilation, the time to hospital discharge, the time to return to work, and the percentage of patients who had relapses. A third treatment arm, in which plasmapheresis was followed by IVIG, had only minimal superiority over the other two treatments. On the basis of these observations, IVIG (400 mg/kg/day daily for 5 days), which is easier to administer and better tolerated than plasmapheresis, has been established as standard therapy for Guillain-Barré syndrome.

COMPLICATIONS

The most common cause of death in Guillain-Barré syndrome is dysautonomia that results in cardiac arrhythmias. These events are usually preceded by periods of autonomic instability with fluctuations in blood pressure and heart rate. Malignant hypertension may occur in some persons on the same basis. Most other complications, including pulmonary emboli, pneumonia, sepsis, and pressure sores, are common in paralyzed persons who require long-term ventilation.

PROGNOSIS

Nearly all persons with Guillain-Barré syndrome demonstrate some motor improvement, although recovery may require weeks or months. From 60% to 85% of patients with Guillain-Barré syndrome ultimately enjoy a full or functional recovery. From 3% to 5% of patients die of complications of the disease, and 3–10% have relapses.

Several factors have been identified as predictors of poor or slow recovery from Guillain-Barré syndrome. The strongest predictor is a mean distal motor amplitude of ≤20% of normal. Elderly persons recover considerably more slowly than do younger persons, and rapid progression of disease correlates with severe disability at plateau and a prolonged convalescence. Persons with severe disease, particularly those who require mechanical ventilation, are more likely to have a prolonged or incomplete recovery; likewise, those who have a prolonged plateau period, of 2–3 weeks or longer, tend to improve slowly.

PREVENTION

There are no specific preventive measures for Guillain-Barré syndrome. Prevention of the precipitating causes, such as *C. jejuni* infection, may decrease the incidence of Guillain-Barré syndrome.

NEUROPATHIES ASSOCIATED WITH MULTISYSTEM INFECTIONS

DIPHTHERIA

Diphtheria is a multisystem disease mediated by an exotoxin produced by *Corynebacterium diphtheriae* (Chapter 58). The most characteristic sign of the disease, severe pharyngeal inflammation, and the two major complications of diphtheria outside the respiratory tract or skin, peripheral neuropathy and myocarditis, are toxin mediated. The toxin itself is an acidic globular protein with an approximate molecular weight of 63,000 kDa. It is composed of two fragments; fragment B is necessary for attachment to the cell surface, whereas fragment A possesses the toxic activity. Diphtheria toxin severely depresses cellular protein synthesis by inhibition of elongation factor 2, the intracellular molecule that facilitates the translocation of amino acids from transfer RNA to the growing peptide chain. In the small quantities that are most common in human disease, the toxin acts preferentially on myelin and striated muscle, including cardiac muscle.

The incidence of diphtheritic neuropathy is proportional to the severity of the oropharyngeal disease. Whereas 10–20% of all persons with diphtheria have some neurologic dysfunction, >50% of persons with severe respiratory tract diphtheria have neurologic disease. The peripheral neurologic manifestations of diphtheria occur locally and early, soon after the onset of respiratory tract disease, or systemically and late, several weeks after the onset of the pharyngitis. Local peripheral neuropathy is manifest primarily by weakness or paralysis of the palate, which is characterized by nasal speech and regurgitation of liquids through the nose. Ocular manifestations may develop 4–5 weeks after the onset of disease, characterized by bilateral paralysis of accommodation and resulting in complaints of blurred vision and difficulty in reading. Usually there is no alteration of extraocular movements or pupillary reflexes.

The systemic neuropathy occurs 1–2 months after the onset of disease. Bulbar manifestations are most common, with up to one third of persons having phrenic nerve paralysis, which may necessitate mechanical ventilation. Systemic polyneuropathy outside the cranial nerves occurs in only 1–2% of all cases of diphtheria. The neuropathy is bilateral, but it may be asymmetric. Sensory function is frequently more involved than motor function, resulting in paresthesias of the distal extremities and loss of vibratory sensation and stereognosis. Usually the motor effects are mild and are manifested as pelvic girdle instability, resulting in an altered gait. In unusually severe cases, paraplegia or quadriplegia may occur.

Persons with cutaneous diphtheria may have anesthesia around the lesion or, less commonly, local paresis.

LEPROSY

Leprosy is a systemic illness caused by *Mycobacterium leprae* (Chapter 46). Leprosy is rare in the United States, with fewer than 500 cases occurring annually and mostly among immigrants. However, leprosy is the most common treatable neuropathy worldwide. The neurologic manifestations of leprosy occur in nearly all cases and are manifested in areas close to the cutaneous lesions. The neuropathy of leprosy results primarily from destruction of intracutaneous nerves, but large nerve trunks containing both sensory and motor fibers as they course beneath the infected skin can be involved. Regardless of the form of illness, the cardinal sign of leprous neuropathy is sensory loss, first to temperature and pain and then to touch. The senses of position and vibration are preserved. When pain occurs, it is due to swelling of a nerve trunk because of stretching or entrapment within a bony canal or to formation of a granulomatous abscess.

The skin lesions of **tuberculoid leprosy** are hypopigmented, sharply demarcated macules, single or few in number, and asymmetrically distributed. The central area is scaly and dry with loss of hair. The neurologic manifestations of tuberculoid leprosy are characterized by sensory loss and anhydrosis well demarcated within the cutaneous lesions. Anhydrosis is due to destruction of the underlying autonomic neural tissue. Underlying nerve trunks may be sufficiently swollen to be palpable; the inflammation may result in sensory and motor loss along the distribution of affected nerves.

In contrast, the manifestations of **lepromatous leprosy** are generalized, with skin lesions that are numerous, symmetrically distributed, and polymorphic, including macules, papules, nodules, and plaques. In the most severe cases the facial skin becomes thickened, with deepened cutaneous folds and loss of eyebrows, resulting in the typical **leonine appearance.** In addition to cutaneous infection, organisms in lepromatous disease can affect the upper airway, producing chronic nasal stuffiness and epistaxis, which leads to perforation and collapse of the nasal septum. Lepromatous disease also commonly includes the anterior third of the eye, resulting in ocular pain, glaucoma, and iridocyclitis.

The neuropathy of lepromatous disease is diffuse and is less anatomically associated with overlying cutaneous disease. There is diminished sensation over the ears, hands, forearms, and eyes, which ultimately spreads to involve almost the entire surface of the distal extremities and the face. Intracutaneous nerves and nerve trunks that course through the coolest parts of the body are affected the most severely, whereas those in warmer areas are preserved. Thus, although the forehead may have greatly diminished sensation, feeling in the adjacent scalp, where the temperature is maintained by the presence of hair, is preserved. Similarly, portions of large nerves such as the ulnar, median, lateral popliteal, and posterior tibial nerves, which course near the skin surface, are commonly affected in lepromatous leprosy and are subject to paralysis and anesthesia distally. In all forms of the disease, the deep tendon reflexes are preserved.

The course of leprosy can be marked by a variety of complications, each of which may exacerbate the neurologic disease. **Reversal reactions** are characterized by the conversion of borderline to tuberculoid disease. Reversal reactions are associated with increased cell-mediated immunity against the organism and may occur either spontaneously or after the initiation of therapy. The immune response in reversal reactions typically is intense, and the granulomas are necrotizing and destructive. Conversely, **downgrading reactions** are characterized by the conversion of borderline cases in lepromatous disease, which may occur spontaneously or after the development of an unrelated immunosuppression. **Ery-**

thema nodosum leprosum occurs in approximately 50% of persons with lepromatous leprosy and is associated with high fever, malaise, and the rapid onset of painful subcutaneous nodules and focal neuritis. It is caused by the development of immune complex–associated vasculitis. Some persons with long-standing lepromatous disease have amyloidosis indistinguishable from the infiltrative amyloid disease associated with other conditions. Amyloidosis itself may be associated with peripheral neuropathy.

Leprosy can be effectively treated with one of several multidrug regimens recommended by the World Health Organization (Table 46–5). The response of the neuropathy to these regimens depends on the degree of nerve destruction suffered before the initiation of therapy. Permanent, disabling sequelae can result even when the infection is cured. Indeed, antibiotic-induced or spontaneously occurring reactions may be associated with worsening neuritis. The neurologic outcomes of these exacerbations can be modified with corticosteroids.

LYME DISEASE

Lyme disease is a systemic illness caused by infection by *Borrelia burgdorferi,* which disseminates to many tissues and may persist for years if untreated (Chapter 29). The third stage of Lyme disease develops years after the initial onset of symptoms and consists of chronic dermatologic changes, particularly acrodermatitis chronica atrophicans, chronic neuropathies and meningoencephalitis, and permanent arthritis. The course in many untreated persons is marked by periods of remissions and recurrence.

Peripheral neurologic disease is prominent in Lyme disease and occurs as a result of perivascular inflammation and axonal damage. The neurologic manifestations may assume several different patterns, including meningoencephalitis. Multiple, anatomically distinct central and peripheral nerves may be affected simultaneously. Cranial neuropathies are most typical, and involvement of each of the cranial nerves has been reported. Trigeminal and facial neuropathies are common, resulting in paresthesia and pain in the face and in **Bell's palsy.** Retinopathy, uveitis, keratoconjunctivitis, and other eye complaints occur less commonly. Lyme disease also affects the spinal nerves, most commonly as a **radiculopathy** that may affect either a single nerve or multiple nerves. The radiculopathy is painful and results in motor dysfunction and loss of reflexes along the course of the affected nerves. There may be brachial plexus palsy and, uncommonly, a presentation of a symmetric polyneuropathy clinically similar to Guillain-Barré syndrome. Acute neuropathies usually resolve with antibiotics and anti-inflammatory agents. Persons with chronic untreated infection may have a more indolent, generalized distal sensory neuropathy. In most instances this neuropathy is mild, resulting in intermittent subtle paresthesias in the distal extremities without motor deficit. Persons with chronic neurologic manifestations of Lyme disease may have slowly progressive encephalomyelitis or spastic quadriparesis.

HUMAN IMMUNODEFICIENCY VIRUS INFECTION

HIV, the cause of AIDS (Chapter 38), is associated with a variety of peripheral neurologic manifestations; 10–20% of adults with AIDS have peripheral nerve complaints. Similar complaints are infrequent in children, but the patterns of disease are similar to those observed in adults. Although most neuropathies are caused directly by HIV infection itself, others may be related to complicating opportunistic or generalized infections, CMV infection, syphilis, and zoster, or to antiretroviral therapies.

The peripheral neurologic manifestations of HIV include an acute inflammatory demyelinating polyneuropathy clinically indistinguishable from Guillain-Barré syndrome. Unlike Guillain-Barré syndrome, however, a CSF pleocytosis usually accompanies HIV infection. HIV peripheral neuropathy frequently occurs early in the course of HIV infection and usually resolves spontaneously or with plasmapheresis. Many adults have a more chronic inflammatory demyelinating polyneuropathy with sensorimotor deficits that progress for months, eventually with axonal degeneration of the peripheral nerves. This occurs most commonly during the early stages of HIV infection, and in some persons the symptoms may resolve spontaneously.

During later stages of HIV infection, many persons commonly have a distal symmetric sensorimotor neuropathy consisting of painful dysesthesias in the feet and soles, frequently making it difficult to walk. Weakness may occur but is less notable than the sensory abnormalities. With advanced disease the distal reflexes may be lost. Electrodiagnostic studies and nerve biopsies demonstrate segmental demyelination with axonal degeneration. In addition, persons with advanced HIV infection may have a **mononeuritis multiplex** that involves both the cranial and the spinal nerves. This late, chronic neuropathy is associated with high viral load and low CD4 lymphocyte count, and preliminary evidence suggests that highly active antiretroviral therapy may ameliorate the neuropathy in some persons. However, treatments including corticosteroids, amitriptyline, mexiletine, and acupuncture, that may be effective in ameliorating other forms of painful neuropathy have not been beneficial in this setting.

Antiretroviral nucleoside analogs used for the treatment of HIV infection also are associated with painful peripheral neuropathy, which is common with dideoxyinosine and dideoxycytidine, particularly when given at a high dosage. The neuropathy slowly resolves after cessation of the drug therapy.

Persons with HIV infection may have a myopathy that is manifested primarily as slowly progressive proximal weakness. Myopathy can be distinguished from neuropathy by electrodiagnostic studies and creatine kinase levels, which is severalfold higher than normal. The diagnosis can be confirmed by muscle biopsy, which shows inflammatory and necrotic changes in HIV-related myopathic disease. Zidovudine, and other antiretroviral nucleosides commonly used to treat HIV infection, may itself cause a myopathy that shares many of the clinical features of HIV-associated muscle disease. Drug-related muscle weakness abates after cessation of zidovudine therapy.

MYELOPATHY

HUMAN T-CELL LEUKEMIA/LYMPHOMA VIRUS TYPE I INFECTION

Infection with human T-cell leukemia/lymphoma virus type I (HTLV-I), a human retrovirus, may remain asymptomatic for a prolonged period, even for life, but it can lead to either of two distinct clinical situations, most commonly adult T-cell leukemia (ATL) (Chapter 4) or myelopathy. The myelopathy has been called **tropical spastic paraparesis (TSP),** a term that reflects its occurrence in tropical areas of the world and that was given before its association with HTLV-I infection was determined. An alternative name, **HTLV-I-associated myelopathy (HAM),** has been suggested.

ETIOLOGY

HTLV-I is a retrovirus endemic in many parts of the developing world, particularly southwestern Japan, the Caribbean islands, parts of South America and Central America, and areas of sub-Saharan Africa.

Transmission. Transmission of HTLV-I occurs by sexual contact, by sharing of contaminated needles or other injection paraphernalia among injection drug users, by using contaminated blood products, and perinatally by transmission from infected mother to child, either transplacentally or by breast-feeding. In endemic areas, transmission by breast-feeding is the major mode of spread, with approximately 25% of breast-fed infants born to HTLV-I-seropositive mothers acquiring infection. Intrauterine transmission occurs much less frequently, and only 5% of children born to HTLV-I-infected mothers acquire infection if they are not breast-fed. The risk of transmission from males to females by sexual contact is approximately 60% during a 10-year period, in comparison with <1% from females to males. In the United States, approximately 25–30% of sex partners of individuals who are seropositive for HTLV-I or HTLV-II are also seropositive.

EPIDEMIOLOGY

On the basis of data on volunteer blood donors, the combined seroprevalence of HTLV-I and HTLV-II in the United States is 0.016%. Most seropositive individuals in the United States are born in endemic areas or report sexual contact with individuals from such areas. Intravenous drug abusers in the United States have a seroprevalence ranging from 7% to 49%.

HAM/TSP develops in fewer than 1% of people with HTLV-I infection, is more common in women than in men, and has a much shorter median clinical latency period than HTLV-I-associated ATL, 3.3 years compared with 40–60 years. HAM/TSP and ATL (Chapter 4) almost never occur in the same person.

PATHOGENESIS

The pathogenesis of HAM/TSP has not been determined with certainty, but damage to the spinal cord by lymphocytes that have been induced by HTLV-I to produce cytokines is probably central.

SYMPTOMS AND CLINICAL MANIFESTATIONS

HAM/TSP usually occurs during middle age. The disease is characterized by the progressive, permanent evolution of lower extremity spasticity or weakness, lower back pain, and hyperreflexia of the lower extremities with an extensor plantar response. The bladder and intestines may be dysfunctional, and men may be impotent. Some persons have dysesthesias of their distal lower extremities with diminished sensation to vibration and pain. The function of the upper extremities is usually preserved, although the reflexes in the arms may be increased. Some persons have sensorineural hearing loss or optic atrophy. The symptoms and signs, unlike those of multiple sclerosis, are progressive and do not wax and wane, cranial nerves are not involved, and cognitive function is not affected.

In addition to ATL (Chapter 4), other clinical entities associated with HTLV-I infection are infective dermatitis, a diffuse eczematous condition frequently complicated by superimposed staphylococcal or streptococcal infection, and uveitis, which may predate development of HAM/TSP.

DIAGNOSIS

Typically, the CSF in persons with HAM/TSP reveals a slightly elevated protein level and, less commonly, a mild mononuclear pleocytosis. Antibodies to HTLV-I are usually detectable in the CSF, as well as the proinflammatory cytokines TNF-α, IL-1, and IL-6. There may be periventricular lesions in the white matter on neuroimaging studies, but many persons with HAM/TSP have normal imaging scans. Neuropathologic findings at autopsy have revealed axonal degeneration and myelin loss in the pyramidal tracts, most prominently at the thoracic or lumbar level.

Differential Diagnosis

Although more than half of persons with TSP have positive serologic tests for HTLV-I antibody, particularly in areas that are endemic to HTLV-I, not all persons with TSP have evidence of HTLV-I infection. In these persons, with illness that is clinically indistinguishable from HTLV-I, other causes can be identified, including chronic intoxication of cyanogenic glycosides from the consumption of cassava, amino-acid dietary deficiencies, and syphilis.

TREATMENT

Several treatments have been attempted for HAM/TSP, including anti-inflammatory agents such as corticosteroids, plasmapheresis, and the TNF antagonist pentoxifylline, as well as the antiretroviral drugs zidovudine and lamivudine. However, no therapy has proved effective.

PREVENTION

Public health policy in endemic areas of Japan advises against breast-feeding by HTLV-I-seropositive mothers to curtail transmission. Routine serologic screening of all blood for HTLV-I and HTLV-II was implemented in the United States in November 1988.

KEY ARTICLES

Tetanus

Athavale VB, Pai PN: Role of tetanus antitoxin in the treatment of tetanus in children. *J Pediatr* 1966;68:289–93.

Domenighetti M, Savary G, Stricker H: Hyperadrenergic syndrome in severe tetanus: Extreme rise in catecholamines responsive to labetalol. *BMJ* 1984;288:1483–4.

Ernst ME. Klepser ME, Fouts M, et al: Tetanus: Pathophysiology and management. *Ann Pharmacother* 1997;31:1507–13.

Marshall FN: Tetanus of the newborn: With special reference to experiences in Haiti, WI. *Adv Pediatr* 1968;15:65–110.

Pellizari R, Rosetto O, Shiavo G, et al: Tetanus and botulinum neurotoxins: Mechanism of action and therapeutic uses. *Philos Trans R Soc Lond B Biol Sci* 1999;354:259–68.

Salimpour R: Causes of death in tetanus neonatorum: Study of 233 cases with 54 necropsies. *Arch Dis Child* 1977; 52:587–94.

Weinstein L: Tetanus. *N Engl J Med* 1973;289:1293–6.

Wright DK, Lalloo UF, Nayiager S, et al: Autonomic nervous system dysfunction in severe tetanus: Current perspectives. *Crit Care Med* 1989;17:371–5.

Botulism

Arnon SS, Midura TF, Clay SA, et al: Infant botulism: Epidemiological, clinical, and laboratory aspects. *JAMA* 1977;237:1946–51.

Horwitz MA, Hughes JM, Merson MH, et al: Food-borne botulism in the United States, 1970–1975. *J Infect Dis* 1977;136:153–9.

Hughes JM, Blumenthal JR, Merson MH, et al: Clinical features of types A and B food-borne botulism. *Ann Intern Med* 1981;95:442–5.

Koenig MG, Drutz DJ, Mushlin AI, et al: Type B botulism in man. *Am J Med* 1967;42:208–19.

Long SS: Epidemiologic study of infant botulism in Pennsylvania: Report of the Infant Botulism Study Group. *Pediatrics* 1985;75:928–34.

Long SS, Gajewski JL, Brown LW, et al: Clinical, laboratory, and environmental features of infant botulism in Southeastern Pennsylvania. *Pediatrics* 1985;75:935–41.

MacDonald KL, Cohen ML, Blake PA: The changing epidemiology of adult botulism in the United States. *Am J Epidemiol* 1986;124:794–9.

Merson MH, Dowell VR Jr: Epidemiologic, clinical and laboratory aspects of wound botulism. *N Engl J Med* 1973;289:1005–10.

Schreiner MS, Field E, Ruddy R: Infant botulism: A review of 12 years' experience at the Children's Hospital of Philadelphia. *Pediatrics* 1991; 87:159–65.

Shapiro RL, Hatheway C, Swerdlow DL: Botulism in the United States: A clinical and epidemiologic review. *Ann Intern Med* 1998;129:221–8.

Spika JS, Shaffr N, Hargrett-Bean N, et al: Risk factors for infant botulism in the United States. *Am J Dis Child* 1989;143:828–32.

Tacket CO, Shandera WX, Mann JM, et al: Equine antitoxin use and other factors that predict outcome in type A foodborne botulism. *Am J Med* 1984;76:794–8.

Woodruff BA, Griffin PM, McCroskey LM, et al: Clinical and laboratory comparison of botulism from toxin types A, B, and E in the United States 1975–1988. *J Infect Dis* 1992;166:1281–6.

Poliomyelitis

Abramson H, Greenberg M: Acute poliomyelitis in infants under one year of age: Epidemiological and clinical features. *Pediatrics* 1955;16:478–88.

Chitsike I, van Furth R: Paralytic poliomyelitis associated with live oral poliomyelitis vaccine in a child with HIV infection in Zimbabwe: Case report. *BMJ* 1999;318:841–3.

Dalakas MC, Elder G, Hallett M, et al: A long-term follow-up study of patients with post-poliomyelitis neuromuscular symptoms. *N Engl J Med* 1986;314:959–63.

Horstmann DM: Epidemiology of poliomyelitis and allied diseases—1963. *Yale J Biol Med* 1963;36:5–26.

Horstmann DM: Clinical aspects of acute poliomyelitis. *Am J Med* 1949; 6:592–605.

Ogra PL: Poliomyelitis as a paradigm for investment in and success of vaccination programs. *Pediatr Infect Dis J* 1999;18:10–5.

Strebel PM, Sutter RW, Cochi SL, et al: Epidemiology of poliomyelitis in the United States one decade after the last reported case of indigenous wild virus–associated disease. *Clin Infect Dis* 1992;14:568–79.

Weinstein L, Shelokov A, Seltser R, et al: A comparison of the clinical features of poliomyelitis in adults and in children. *N Engl J Med* 1952;246:296–302.

Wright PF, Kim-Farley RJ, de Quadros CA, et al: Strategies for the global eradication of poliomyelitis by the year 2000. *N Engl J Med* 1991; 325:1774–9.

Guillain-Barré Syndrome

Asbury AK, Cornblath DR: Assessment of current diagnostic criteria for Guillain-Barré syndrome. *Ann Neurol* 1990;27:S21–4.

Eberle E, Brink J, Azen S, et al: Early predictors of incomplete recovery in children with Guillain-Barré polyneuritis. *J Pediatr* 1975;86:356–9.

Fletcher DD, Lawn ND, Wolter TD, et al: Long-term outcome in patients with Guillain-Barré syndrome requiring mechanical ventilation. *Neurology* 2000;27:2311–5.

The Guillain-Barré Syndrome Study Group: Plasmapheresis and acute Guillain-Barré syndrome. *Neurology* 1985;35:1096–104.

Hahn AF: Guillain-Barré syndrome. *Lancet* 1998;352:635–41.

Honavar M, Tharakan JK, Hughes RA, et al: A clinicopathological study of the Guillain-Barré syndrome. Nine cases and literature review. *Brain* 1991;114:1245–69.

Hughes RA, Newsom-Davis JM, Perkin GD, et al: Controlled trial of prednisolone in acute polyneuropathy. *Lancet* 1978;2:750–3.

Lasky T, Terracciano GL, Magder L, et al: The Guillain-Barré syndrome and the 1992-1993 and 1993-1994 influenza vaccines. *N Engl J Med* 1998;339:1797–802.

McKhann GM, Griffin JW, Cornblath DR, et al: Plasmapheresis and Guillain-Barré syndrome: Analysis of prognostic factors and the effect of plasmapheresis. *Ann Neurol* 1988;23:347–53.

Plasma Exchange/Sandglobulin Guillain-Barré Syndrome Trial Group: Randomized trial of plasma exchange, intravenous immunoglobulin, and combined treatments in Guillain-Barré syndrome. *Lancet* 1997;349: 225–30.

Ropper AH: The Guillain-Barré syndrome. *N Engl J Med* 1992;326:1130–6.

van der Meche FGA, Schmitz PIM, Dutch Guillain-Barré Study Group: A randomized trial comparing intravenous immune globulin and plasma exchange in Guillain-Barré syndrome. *N Engl J Med* 1992;326:1123–9.

Visser LH, van der Meche FG, Meulstee J, et al: Cytomegalovirus infection and the Guillain-Barré syndrome: The clinical, electrophysiologic, and prognostic features. *Neurology* 1996;47:668–73.

Willison HJ, O'Hanlon G, Paterson G, et al: Mechanisms of action of anti-GM_1 and anti-GQ_{1b} ganglioside antibodies in Guillain-Barré syndrome. *J Infect Dis* 1997;176:S144–9.

Winer JB, Hughes RA, Anderson MJ, et al: A prospective study of acute idiopathic neuropathy. II. Antecedent events. *J Neurol Neurosurg Psychiatry* 1988;51:613–8.

Winer JB, Hughes RA, Greenwood RJ, et al: Prognosis in Guillain-Barré syndrome. *Lancet* 1985;1:1202–3.

Neuropathies Associated with Multisystem Infections

Angerer M, Pfadenhauer K, Stohr M: Prognosis of facial palsy in *Borrelia burgdorferi* meningopolyradiculitis. *J Neurol* 1993;240:319–21.

Barohn RJ, Gronseth GS, LeForce BR, et al: Peripheral nervous system involvement in a large cohort of human immunodeficiency virus–infected individuals. *Arch Neurol* 1993;50:167–71.

Bingham PM, Galetta SL, Athreya B, et al: Neurologic manifestations in children with Lyme disease. *Pediatrics* 1995;96:1053–6.

Collier RJ: Diphtheria toxin: Mode of action and structure. *Bacteriol Rev* 1975;39:54–85.

Floeter MK, Civitello LA, Everett CR, et al: Peripheral neuropathy in children with HIV infection. *Neurology* 1997;49:207–12.

Gaskill HS: Neurologic complications of diphtheric neuritis. *Arch Neurol Psychiatry* 1947;58:639–42.

Halperin JJ: Nervous system Lyme disease. *J Neurol Sci* 1998;153:182–91.

Jacobson RR, Krahenbuhl JL: Leprosy. *Lancet* 1999;353:655–60.

Markus R, Brew BJ: HIV-1 peripheral neuropathy and combination antiretroviral therapy. *Lancet* 1998;352;1906–7.

Naiditch MJ, Bower AG: Diphtheria: A study of 1,433 cases observed during a ten-year period at the Los Angeles County Hospital. *Am J Med* 1954;17:229–45.

Reik L, Steere AC, Bartenhagen NH, et al: Neurologic abnormalities of Lyme disease. *Medicine* (*Baltimore*) 1979;58:281–94.

van Beers SM, de Wit MYL, Katser PR: The epidemiology of *Mycobacterium leprae:* Recent insight. *FEMS Microbiol Lett* 1996;136:221–30.

Simpson DM, Wolfe DE: Neuromuscular complications of HIV infection and its treatment. *AIDS* 1991;5:917–26.

Myelopathy

Bangham CR: Human T-cell leukaemia virus type I and neurological disease. *Curr Opin Neurobiol* 1993;3:773–8.

Bhagavati S, Ehrlich G, Kula RW, et al: Detection of human T-cell lymphoma/leukemia virus type I DNA and antigen in spinal fluid and blood of patients with chronic progressive myelopathy. *N Engl J Med* 1988;318:1141–7.

Bhigjee AI, Wiley CA, Wachsman W, et al: HTLV-I-associated myelopathy: Clinicopathologic correlation with localization of provirus to spinal cord. *Neurology* 1991;41:1990–2.

Bucher B, Poupard JA, Vernant JC, et al: Tropical neuromyelopathies and retroviruses: A review. *Rev Infect Dis* 1990;12:890–9.

Janssen RS, Kaplan JE, Khabbaz RF, et al: HTLV-I-associated myelopathy/ tropical spastic paraparesis in the United States. *Neurology* 1991; 41:1355–7.

Manns A, Hisada M, La Grenade L: Human T-lymphotropic virus type I infection. *Lancet* 1999;353:1951–8.

Taylor GP: Pathogenesis and treatment of HTLV-I associated myelopathy. *Sex Transm Infect* 1998;74:316–22.

CHAPTER 57

The Common Cold

Ronald B. Turner ▪ Gregory F. Hayden

The term **common cold** is used in both the lay and professional literature to refer to a variety of upper respiratory tract syndromes. The term characterizes illness in which the symptoms of rhinorrhea and nasal obstruction are prominent and systemic symptoms and signs, such as myalgia and fever, are absent or mild.

ETIOLOGY

The common cold is caused only by viral pathogens (Table 57–1). The most common pathogens are the **rhinoviruses,** members of the Picornaviridae family of small, single-stranded RNA viruses. There are 101 serologically distinct rhinoviruses, numbered 1–100 and subtype 1A. Other important causes of the common cold include coronaviruses and respiratory syncytial virus (RSV). Influenza, parainfluenza, and adenoviruses may also cause cold symptoms, although these viruses usually cause lower respiratory tract or systemic symptoms in addition to the nasal symptoms characteristic of the common cold (Chapter 68).

Transmission. Common cold viruses are spread by three general mechanisms: **small-particle aerosols, large-particle aerosols,** and **direct contact.** Some routes of transmission may be more efficient than others for particular viruses. Studies of rhinovirus colds suggest that direct contact is the most efficient mechanism of transmission, although transmission by large-particle aerosols has also been documented. Limited data indicate that direct contact is also important for the transmission of RSV, although large-particle aerosols may also play a role. In contrast to rhinoviruses and RSV, influenza viruses appear to be spread by small-particle aerosols.

EPIDEMIOLOGY

Colds account for approximately 50% of illnesses in the entire population and approximately 75% of illnesses in young infants. Colds occur year-round; however, the incidence increases from early fall until late spring. This pattern reflects the seasonal prevalence of the viral pathogens most commonly associated with cold symptoms. The highest incidence of rhinovirus infections occurs in the early fall (August–October) and in the late spring (April–May). The incidence of RSV infections usually rises from October to December and subsides from March to May. The RSV season occurs earlier in southern states than in northern states.

The average incidence of the common cold in preschool children is 6–7 illnesses per year but 10–15% of children will have at least 12 illnesses per year (Table 6–2). The incidence decreases with age, with 2–3 illnesses per year by adulthood. The number of colds experienced by young children is affected by conditions that increase exposure to the pathogens, such as contact with older children in the home or extensive contact with children outside the home, such as out-of-home child care. Children who are cared for in a child care setting during the first year of life have 50% more illnesses than children cared for at home. The difference in the incidence of illness between these groups of children decreases as the length of time spent in daycare increases; however, the incidence of illness remains higher in the daycare group through at least the first 3 years of life.

PATHOGENESIS

The first event in the pathogenesis of the common cold is viral infection of the nasal epithelium. Rhinoviruses interact with **ICAM-1,** an intercellular adhesion molecule that is present on the epithelium covering the adenoids and other epithelial cells of the nose. The infection may result in no apparent histologic damage, as with rhinovirus or coronavirus 229E infections, or there may be destruction of the nasal epithelium, as with influenza and adenovirus infections. Regardless of the histopathologic findings, infection of the nasal epithelium is associated with an infiltration of the mucosa by inflammatory cells. The subsequent steps in pathogenesis are not as clearly defined, but the release of immunologic or inflammatory mediators from the infiltrating cells or from cells present in the epithelium appears to play a role. IL-8, IL-1, TNF, and the kinins, bradykinin and lysyl-bradykinin, have all been detected in the nasal secretions of persons with common cold symptoms. Histamine does not appear to play a role in the production of cold symptoms. The release of inflammatory mediators in the nasal mucosa appears to stimulate, either directly or indirectly through neurologic mechanisms, increased glandular secretion, vasodilation, and an increase in vascular permeability. The increased glandular secretion and vascular permeability result in rhinorrhea, and the vasodilation and vascular permeability result in mucosal swelling and nasal obstruction.

The respiratory viruses use different mechanisms to avoid host defenses. Infection with the rhinoviruses and adenoviruses results in the development of serotype-specific protective immunity, but repeated infections can occur because of the large number of distinct serotypes of each virus. Similarly, influenza has the ability to change the antigens presented on the surface of the virus and thus behave as though there were multiple serotypes. In contrast, reinfections with parainfluenza viruses and RSV, each of which has a small number of distinct serotypes, occur because protective immunity to these viruses does not develop after an infection. The interaction of host immunity with coronaviruses is not well defined, but it appears that there are multiple distinct strains of coronavirus that are capable of inducing at least short-term protective immunity.

SYMPTOMS AND CLINICAL MANIFESTATIONS

Approximately 75% of rhinovirus infections are associated with symptoms, usually rhinorrhea or pharyngitis. The onset of common cold symptoms typically occurs 1–3 days after viral infection. The

TABLE 57–1. Pathogens Associated with the Common Cold

Association	Pathogen	Relative Frequency*
Agents primarily associated with common colds	Rhinovirus	Frequent
	Coronavirus	Occasional
Agents primarily associated with other clinical syndromes that also cause symptoms of common colds	Respiratory syncytial virus	Occasional
	Influenza virus	Uncommon
	Parainfluenza virus	Uncommon
	Adenovirus	Uncommon

*Relative frequency of colds caused by the agent.

first symptom noted is frequently a sore or scratchy throat, followed closely by nasal obstruction and rhinorrhea. The sore throat usually resolves quickly, and by the second or third day of illness the nasal symptoms are predominant. Cough is associated with approximately 30% of colds and usually begins after the nasal symptoms. Cough typically does not become the most bothersome symptom until the fourth or fifth day of illness, when the nasal symptoms decrease in severity. The usual cold lasts about a week, although 25% of these illnesses last at least 2 weeks.

The different common cold pathogens tend to produce slightly different clinical syndromes. Fever and other constitutional symptoms are more characteristic of influenza, RSV, and adenovirus infections than of rhinovirus or coronavirus infections. These variations in clinical presentation are not consistent enough, however, to permit accurate prediction of the pathogen on the basis of the clinical symptoms in an individual patient.

Physical Examination Findings

The physical findings of the common cold are limited to the upper respiratory tract. The increased nasal secretion is usually obvious. A change in the color or consistency of the secretions is common during the course of the illness and is not a specific indication of sinusitis or bacterial superinfection.

DIAGNOSIS

The symptoms of the common cold are so familiar that the diagnosis is usually evident to the patient or the family as well as the physician. Diagnosis of the specific viral cause is usually not possible because of the indistinguishable clinical manifestations.

Differential Diagnosis

The most important aspect of caring for a patient with a cold is to exclude other conditions that are potentially more serious or treatable. The differential diagnosis of the common cold includes noninfectious disorders as well as other upper respiratory tract infections (Table 57–2).

Allergic Rhinitis. Allergic rhinitis can usually be differentiated from the common cold by the presence of itching of the eyes and nose. Sneezing, which may be present in both illnesses, is usually more prominent in allergic rhinitis than in colds. The presence of eosinophilia (>20% of all cells) in a smear of nasal secretions is a relatively insensitive but specific finding of allergic rhinitis.

Foreign Body. Obstruction by a nasal foreign body can usually be readily differentiated from a common cold because of the unilateral nature of the symptoms. However, in some patients the unilaterality may not be obvious. Obstruction is associated with a foul odor of the nasal discharge and the presence of blood in the secretions.

Sinusitis. Bacterial sinusitis may present with common cold symptoms in some children (Chapter 65). In older children with sinusitis, the symptoms may be more severe than would be expected with a common cold and may also include fever, facial pain, and periorbital swelling. A syndrome of persistent rhinorrhea or cough has been associated with sinusitis in children. Sinusitis may also occur as a complication of the common cold.

Streptococcal Nasopharyngitis. Group A *Streptococcus* infection in children younger than 3 years of age has been associated with nasal symptoms that may be indistinguishable from the common cold. The illness, sometimes referred to as **streptococcosis,** is characterized by a mucopurulent or purulent discharge that may cause excoriation of the nares. Fever is an inconstant finding.

Pertussis. The catarrhal phase of pertussis may be indistinguishable from a common cold. The diagnosis usually becomes evident with the onset of paroxysmal coughing. A history of chronic or severe cough in an adolescent or young adult contact or the identification of other pertussis infections in the community may suggest this diagnosis before the onset of cough (Chapter 67).

Congenital Syphilis. The **snuffles** of congenital syphilis present as clear rhinorrhea beginning in the first 3 months of life, usually during the first month. A persistent or excoriating rhinorrhea in neonates or young infants should prompt an evaluation of the child and the mother for the possibility of syphilis (Chapter 95).

Laboratory Evaluation

Routine laboratory studies are generally not helpful for the diagnosis and management of the common cold. A nasal smear for eosinophils may be useful for evaluation of allergic rhinitis. A predominance of polymorphonuclear leukocytes in the nasal secretions is characteristic of uncomplicated colds and does not aid in the diagnosis of bacterial superinfection or sinusitis.

Microbiologic Evaluation

The viral pathogens associated with the common cold may be detected by culture, antigen detection, or serologic methods. In routine pediatric practice these studies are not indicated in patients with colds because a specific etiologic diagnosis is of no value in

TABLE 57–2. Conditions That May Mimic the Common Cold

Condition	Differentiating Features
Allergic rhinitis	Prominent itching and sneezing Nasal eosinophils
Foreign body	Unilateral, foul-smelling secretions Bloody nasal secretions
Sinusitis	Presence of fever, headache, or facial pain or periorbital edema or persistence of rhinorrhea or cough for longer than 14 days
Streptococcosis	Nasal discharge that excoriates the nares
Pertussis	Onset of persistent or severe cough
Congenital syphilis	Persistent rhinorrhea with onset in the first 3 months of life

their management. Bacterial cultures or antigen detection are useful only when group A *Streptococcus* (Chapter 58) or *Bordetella pertussis* (Chapter 67) infection or nasopharyngeal diphtheria (Chapter 58) are suspected. The isolation of other bacterial pathogens is not an indication of bacterial nasal infection and is not a specific predictor of the etiologic agent in sinusitis.

TREATMENT

Definitive Treatment

Specific antiviral therapy is available for both RSV infections and influenza (Chapter 14). These antiviral agents have not been studied in patients with illness limited to cold symptoms, and their use is not indicated in patients with such mild illness. In keeping with the viral cause of the common cold, antimicrobial therapy is of no benefit.

Symptomatic Treatment

The management of colds is limited to symptomatic therapy (Table 57–3). The use of symptomatic therapies in children has been the subject of some controversy. Although some of these medications have been found to be effective in adults, studies in children have been limited because they rely on subjective and objective measurements that require the cooperation of the research subject. The effects of symptomatic treatments may be similar in adults and children, but the use of these medications in children must be balanced against the potential side effects of each drug. The prominent or most bothersome symptoms of colds vary during the course of the illness and, if symptomatic treatments are used, it is reasonable to target therapy to specific symptoms.

Fever. Fever is infrequently associated with an uncomplicated common cold, and antipyretic treatment is generally not indicated.

Nasal Obstruction. Either topical or oral adrenergic agents or antihistamines may be used as nasal decongestants. Effective topical adrenergic agents with the imidazolines (e.g., 0.05% oxymetazoline and 0.1% xylometazoline) or 1% phenylephrine are available as either intranasal drops or as nasal sprays. Reduced-strength formulations of these medications are available for use in younger children, although they are not approved for use in children less than 2 years of age. Systemic absorption of the imidazolines has very rarely been associated with bradycardia, hypotension, and coma. Prolonged use of the topical adrenergic agents should be avoided to prevent the development of **rhinitis medicamentosa,** an apparent rebound effect that causes the sensation of nasal obstruction when the drug is discontinued. The oral adrenergic agents are less effective than the topical preparations at doses that can be tolerated without systemic effects. The systemic side effects of these agents are CNS stimulation, hypertension, and palpitations.

TABLE 57–3. Effective Treatments for Common Cold Symptoms

Symptom	Treatment
Fever	Acetaminophen Nonsteroidal anti-inflammatory drugs (e.g., ibuprofen)
Nasal obstruction	Topical adrenergic agents Oral adrenergic agents
Rhinorrhea	First-generation antihistamines Ipratropium bromide
Sore throat	Acetaminophen Nonsteroidal anti-inflammatory drugs (e.g., ibuprofen)
Cough	First-generation antihistamines Bronchodilators (if reactive airways disease is present)

Rhinorrhea. The first-generation antihistamines reduce rhinorrhea by 25–30%, but the second-generation or ''nonsedating'' antihistamines have no effect on common cold symptoms. The effect of the antihistamines on rhinorrhea appears to be related to the anticholinergic rather than the antihistaminic properties of these drugs. The major adverse effect associated with the use of the antihistamines is sedation. Rhinorrhea may also be treated with ipratropium bromide, a topical anticholinergic agent. This drug produces an effect comparable to that of the antihistamines but is not associated with sedation. The most common adverse effects of ipratropium are nasal irritation and bleeding.

Sore Throat. The sore throat associated with colds is generally not severe, but treatment with mild analgesics (Table 18–4) is occasionally indicated, particularly if there is associated myalgia or headache.

Cough. Cough suppression is generally not necessary in patients with colds. Cough in some patients appears to be due to upper respiratory tract irritation associated with postnasal drip. Cough in these patients is most prominent during the time of greatest nasal symptoms, and treatment with a first-generation antihistamine may be helpful. In other patients, cough may be a result of virus-induced reactive airways disease. These patients may have cough that persists for days to weeks after the acute illness, and they may benefit from bronchodilator therapy. Studies of codeine or dextromethorphan hydrobromide have failed to show an effect of these agents on cough in colds. Expectorants such as guaifenesin are not effective antitussive agents.

Ineffective Treatments. A number of common cold remedies popularized in both the lay and the medical press have no significant effect on cold symptoms in carefully controlled studies. Vitamin C, guaifenesin, and inhalation of warm, humidified air have all been found to be no more effective than placebo for the symptomatic treatment of colds. The efficacy of zinc, given in the form of oral lozenges, for the treatment of common cold symptoms has been evaluated in a number of studies. Zinc had no effect on virus replication in these studies, and the effect of zinc on symptoms has been inconsistent, with some studies reporting dramatic effects on the duration of cold symptoms and other studies finding no effect. The interpretation of these studies is difficult because of the high frequency (50–90%) of side effects in subjects who take zinc and the difficulty of producing a placebo that is as distasteful as the active preparation.

COMPLICATIONS

The most common complication of a cold is acute otitis media, which develops in 5–30% of all children who have a cold, with a higher incidence in children in a group child care setting. Sinusitis also appears to be a relatively frequent complication of the common cold and may present simply as prolonged rhinorrhea. It is reasonable to treat patients for sinusitis (Chapter 65) if rhinorrhea persists without improvement for more than 10–14 days and after other illnesses in the differential diagnosis have been excluded. Exacerbation of asthma is a relatively uncommon but potentially serious complication of colds. Approximately 85% of asthma exacerbations in children are associated with the common cold. There is no evidence that treatment of common cold symptoms prevents the development of these complications.

PROGNOSIS

The median duration of rhinovirus cold symptoms is 1 week, but in approximately one fourth of cases symptoms persist for up to 2 weeks.

PREVENTION

Chemoprophylaxis or immunoprophylaxis is generally not available for the common cold. Immunization or chemoprophylaxis against influenza may be useful for prevention of colds due to this virus, although the influenza virus is responsible for only a small proportion of all colds. Both vitamin C and echinacea have been reported to prevent the common cold, but in carefully controlled studies no significant effect has been detected.

Interruption of spread can be achieved by breaking the chain of events involved in the spread of virus by direct contact. Avoiding contact between the hands and face will prevent direct-contact spread of virus, and in the hospital setting, prevention of transmission of respiratory viruses has been achieved when personnel wore protective face shields to prevent hand-to-eye or hand-to-nose contact. Prevention of the spread of viruses by direct contact can be most readily accomplished by good hand washing on the part of the infected individual or the susceptible contact.

REVIEWS

Hendley JO, Gwaltney JM Jr: Mechanisms of transmission of rhinovirus infection. *Epidemiol Rev* 1988;10:243–58.

Turner RB: Epidemiology, pathogenesis, and treatment of the common cold. *Ann Allergy Asthma Immunol* 1997;78:531–9.

Turner RB: The role of neutrophils in the pathogenesis of rhinovirus infections. *Pediatr Infect Dis J* 1990;9:832–5.

Turner RB: The treatment of rhinovirus infections: Progress and potential. *Antiviral Res* 2001;49:1–14.

Wald ER: Purulent nasal discharge. *Pediatr Infect Dis J* 1991;10:329–33.

KEY ARTICLES

Gwaltney JM Jr, Druce HM: Efficacy of brompheniramine maleate for the treatment of rhinovirus colds. *Clin Infect Dis* 1997;25:1188–94.

Gwaltney JM Jr, Hendley JO, Simon G, et al: Rhinovirus infections in an industrial population, I. The occurrence of illness. *N Engl J Med* 1966;275:1261–8.

Gwaltney JM Jr, Moskalski PB, Hendley JO: Hand-to-hand transmission of rhinovirus colds. *Ann Intern Med* 1978;88:463–7.

Gwaltney JM Jr, Hendley JO, Simon G, et al: Rhinovirus infections in an industrial population. II. Characteristics of illness and antibody response. *JAMA* 1967;202:494–500.

Gwaltney JM Jr, Park J, Paul RA, et al: Randomized controlled trial of clemastine fumarate for treatment of experimental rhinovirus colds. *Clin Infect Dis* 1996;22:656–62.

Monto AS, Ullman BM: Acute respiratory illness in an American community: The Tecumseh Study. *JAMA* 1974;227:164–9.

Naclerio RM, Proud D, Lichtenstein LM, et al: Kinins are generated during experimental rhinovirus colds. *J Infect Dis* 1988;157:133–42.

Turner RB, Sperber SJ, Sorrentino JV, et al: Effectiveness of clemastine fumarate for treatment of rhinorrhea and sneezing associated with the common cold. *Clin Infect Dis* 1997;25:824–30.

Turner RB, Weingand KW, Yeh CH, et al: Association between interleukin-8 concentration in nasal secretions and severity of symptoms in experimental rhinovirus colds. *Clin Infect Dis* 1998;26:840–6.

Wald ER, Guerra N, Byers C: Upper respiratory tract infections in young children: Duration of and frequency of complications. *Pediatrics* 1991;87:129–33.

CHAPTER 58

Pharyngitis

Gregory F. Hayden ▪ Ronald B. Turner

Infections of the upper respiratory tract account for a substantial proportion of illnesses in children. These infections often involve more than one site, with simultaneous involvement of the mucosa of the nose, pharynx, middle ear, and paranasal sinuses. Sore throat is the primary symptom in approximately one third of such illnesses.

ETIOLOGY

A large number of infectious agents can cause pharyngitis (Table 58–1). Group A *Streptococcus* (or *Streptococcus pyogenes*) organisms are gram-positive, nonmotile cocci that are facultative anaerobes. On sheep blood agar the colonies are small (1–2 mm in diameter) and have a surrounding zone of β (or clear) hemolysis (Plate 1E). *Neisseria gonorrhoeae* organisms are gram-negative diplococci that infect noncornified epithelium. *Corynebacterium diphtheriae* organisms are club-shaped, gram-positive rods that may produce exotoxin. Other bacterial organisms associated with pharyngitis include group C β-hemolytic *Streptococcus; Arcanobacterium* (formerly *Corynebacterium*) *haemolyticum,* which is a hemolytic, gram-positive rod; and *Francisella tularensis,* the gram-negative coccobacillus that is the cause of tularemia. *Chlamydia pneumoniae,* strain TWAR, has primarily been associated with lower respiratory disease but has also been reported to cause sore throat. Other bacteria such as *Staphylococcus aureus, Haemophilus influenzae* type b, and *Streptococcus pneumoniae* are frequently cultured from the throats of children with pharyngitis, but their role in causing disease in the pharynx has not been established. *Mycoplasma pneumoniae* is most commonly associated with atypical pneumonia, but it can also cause mild pharyngitis without distinguishing clinical characteristics, especially in older children and adolescents.

EPIDEMIOLOGY

Group A Streptococcal Pharyngitis. Streptococcal pharyngitis is relatively uncommon before 2–3 years of age. Its incidence increases among young, school-age children and then declines in late adolescence and adulthood. Streptococcal pharyngitis in temperate climates occurs throughout the year but is most commonly seen during the winter and spring. The illness often spreads to siblings and classmates.

Viral Pharyngitis. Viral infections generally spread by close contact with an infected person and occur most commonly in winter and spring. A large variety of viruses can cause acute pharyngitis (Table 58–1). Some viruses, such as adenoviruses, are more likely than others to cause pharyngitis as a prominent symptom, whereas other viruses, such as rhinoviruses, are more likely to cause pharyngitis as a minor part of an illness that primarily features other symptoms, such as rhinorrhea or cough.

Gonococcal Pharyngitis. Pharyngeal infections with gonorrhea are uncommon in young children but become more frequent among sexually active adolescents and young adults. Although these infections are often asymptomatic and pose little risk of dissemination, a thorough evaluation is necessary because sites other than the pharynx are commonly involved and other sexually transmitted diseases may also be present. The incidence of gonococcal pharyngitis is highest among young, sexually active adults with a history of orogenital sexual contact. The usual source of infection is secretions from mucous surfaces of an infected sexual partner. Sexual abuse must be strongly considered if *N. gonorrhoeae* is isolated from the pharynx of a prepubertal child.

Diphtheria. Asymptomatic nasopharyngeal carriage of *C. diphtheriae* occurs in the United States in highly focal areas among unimmunized or incompletely immunized persons living in crowded conditions. Humans are the only known reservoir for *C. diphtheriae.* The mode of dissemination is contact with discharges from the nose, throat, eye, or skin lesions from an infected person. The disease is most common in the fall and winter. Widespread immunization with diphtheria toxoid has made diphtheria a rare disease in the United States, with fewer than 5 cases reported annually in the United States in recent years. In contrast, the past decade has seen a remarkable re-emergence of pandemic diphtheria in the countries of the former Soviet Union.

C. diphtheriae is also associated with chronic, nonhealing cutaneous ulcers, sometimes with a gray membrane, that are rarely associated with systemic toxicity but do induce a high antitoxin response. These lesions usually harbor *S. aureus* or group A *Streptococcus* in addition to *C. diphtheriae.* Because these cutaneous lesions do not respond to diphtheria antitoxin therapy and are associated with recognized skin pathogens, the significance of isolating *C. diphtheriae* from these lesions is unclear. Cutaneous infection may serve as a means of inducing natural immunity or as a reservoir for nasopharyngeal disease.

Other Infectious Causes of Pharyngitis. Cases of pharyngitis attributed to group C *Streptococcus* have been reported most frequently among adolescents and young adults. These cases have occurred both in localized outbreaks, often with foodborne spread, and in nonepidemic settings. Cases attributed to *A. haemolyticum* have occurred predominantly among adolescents and young adults. Tularemia is most common in the West South Central states and results primarily from contact with an infected animal (Chapter 34). In its oropharyngeal form the infection is spread by ingestion of inadequately cooked meat.

A syndrome of **periodic fever, aphthous stomatitis, pharyngitis, and cervical adenitis (PFAPA)** is an occasional cause of recurrent fever in children. The cause is, as yet, undetermined. The syndrome resolves in some children, whereas symptoms persist in

TABLE 58–1. Microbial Causes of Acute Pharyngitis

Agent	Syndrome or Disease	Estimated Occurrence (%)
Bacterial		
Group A β-hemolytic *Streptococcus* (*S. pyogenes*)	Pharyngitis/tonsillitis	15–30
Group C β-hemolytic *Streptococcus*	Pharyngitis/tonsillitis	1–5
Neisseria gonorrhoeae	Pharyngitis	<1
Arcanobacterium haemolyticum	Pharyngitis, rash	<1
Corynebacterium diphtheriae	Diphtheria	<1
Mixed anaerobic infection	Pharyngitis, gingivitis (Vincent's angina)	<1
Francisella tularensis	Oropharyngeal tularemia	<1
Viral		
Rhinovirus (100 types)	Common cold	20
Coronavirus (4 or more types)	Common cold	≥5
Adenovirus (types 3, 4, 7, 14, 21)	Pharyngoconjunctival fever, acute respiratory disease	5
Herpes simplex viruses (types 1 and 2)	Gingivitis, stomatitis, pharyngitis	4
Parainfluenza viruses (types 1–4)	Common cold, croup	2
Influenza viruses (types A and B)	Influenza	2
Coxsackieviruses (types 2, 4–6, 8, 10)	Herpangina	<1
Epstein-Barr virus	Infectious mononucleosis	<1
Cytomegalovirus	Infectious mononucleosis	<1
Other		
Mycoplasma pneumoniae	Pneumonia, bronchitis, pharyngitis	<1
Chlamydia pneumoniae	Pneumonia, pharyngitis	<1
Unknown		40

Adapted from Hayden GF, Hendley JO, Gwaltney JM Jr: Management of the ambulatory patient with a sore throat. *Curr Clin Top Infect Dis* 1988;9:63.

other children. Long-term sequelae do not develop. The syndrome is easily diagnosed when regularly recurring episodes of fever are associated with these symptoms.

PATHOGENESIS

The development of streptococcal pharyngitis requires that the organisms first adhere to epithelial cells and colonize the pharyngeal mucosa. Lipoteichoic acid on the fimbriae of the organism binds specifically to fibronectin on the surface of the epithelial cells. The ability of streptococci to adhere to pharyngeal epithelium appears related to the age of the host. The relative inability of streptococci to adhere to the pharynx of the young child may partially explain the low incidence of streptococcal pharyngitis in children younger than 2–3 years.

Colonization of the pharynx by group A *Streptococcus* may result in either active infection or asymptomatic carriage. The virulence factors of the organism are important in the development of invasive disease, but the properties of the host and the organism that result in the carrier state are poorly understood. The **M protein,** the major virulence factor of group A *Streptococcus,* provides the organisms with the ability to resist phagocytosis by polymorphonuclear neutrophils. Type-specific antibody to M protein develops during infection and is the source of protective immunity to subsequent infection with that particular M serotype. The hyaluronic acid capsule of the streptococcus also has an antiphagocytic effect.

Scarlet fever (scarlatina) is the result of pharyngeal infection with a strain of group A *Streptococcus* that produces an erythrogenic toxin. There are three **streptococcal pyrogenic exotoxins** (SPE)—A, B and C—that can induce a fine papular rash. SPE-A appears to be more virulent than SPE-B or SPE-C, and it is more strongly associated with severe scarlet fever. Exposure to each toxin confers specific immunity, limiting the number of episodes of scarlet fever in a single individual to three.

C. diphtheriae is relatively noninvasive and generally remains localized to the mucosal surfaces of the upper respiratory tract with accompanying local tissue necrosis and inflammation. *C. diphtheriae* may produce toxins locally that spread throughout the body through the bloodstream and lymphatics. Both toxigenic and nontoxigenic strains of *C. diphtheriae* can cause pharyngeal disease, but only toxigenic strains cause myocarditis and neuritis.

SYMPTOMS AND CLINICAL MANIFESTATIONS

Group A Streptococcal Pharyngitis. The onset of streptococcal pharyngitis is often rapid and associated with prominent sore throat and a moderate to high fever. A headache and gastrointestinal symptoms, including nausea, vomiting, and abdominal pain, are frequent. In a typical, florid case the pharynx is distinctly red and the tonsils are enlarged and covered with a yellow, blood-tinged exudate. There may be petechiae or "doughnut-shaped" lesions on the soft palate and posterior pharynx, and the uvula may be red, stippled, and swollen. The anterior cervical lymph nodes are enlarged and tender to touch. The clinical spectrum of disease is broad, however, and many children present with only mild pharyngeal erythema without tonsillar exudate or cervical lymphadenitis.

In addition to sore throat and fever, some patients demonstrate the stigmata of scarlet fever: circumoral pallor, strawberry tongue, and a fine papular rash (Plate 3D). The tongue initially has a white coating, but red and edematous lingual papillae later project through this coating, producing a **white strawberry tongue.** When the white coating peels off, the resulting **red strawberry tongue** is a beefy red tongue with prominent papillae. The rash commonly begins on the neck, axillae, and groin but then spreads quickly and may involve the entire body. The rash may be more prominent in natural skin folds, such as in the antecubital fossa **(Pastia's lines).** The rash is red, has a **sandpapery texture,** and resembles sunburn with goose pimples. The acute illness may be followed 1–2 weeks later by desquamation, which often progresses, like the rash, from the head downward. The severity of the desquamation generally parallels the severity of the preceding rash.

Viral Pharyngitis. Compared with classic streptococcal pharyngitis, the onset of viral pharyngitis is typically more gradual, and symptoms more often include rhinorrhea, cough, and diarrhea. Many illnesses fall in the general category of upper respiratory tract infection (URTI, URI, or common cold) in which the symptoms of rhinorrhea and nasal obstruction are prominent and systemic symptoms and signs such as myalgia and fever are absent or mild (Chapter 57).

The spectrum of illness is broad, with considerable overlap between many of the causative viruses, but certain characteristic clinical presentations may suggest a specific viral cause (Table 58–2). In adenovirus pharyngitis, there may be concurrent conjunctivitis and fever **(pharyngoconjunctival fever).** In coxsackievirus pharyngitis, there may be one or more small (1–2 mm), grayish vesicles with a surrounding erythematous rim in the posterior pharynx **(herpangina).** In contrast to the clinical situation with herpesvirus stomatitis infections in the mouth, the anterior part of the mouth is usually spared. These vesicles enlarge, rupture, and produce small, punched-out ulcers that persist for several days. The pharyngitis is frequently accompanied by fever, headache, and gastrointestinal complaints, including anorexia, vomiting, and abdominal pain. Coxsackieviruses can also produce vesicular or ulcerated lesions in the mouth as part of **hand-foot-and-mouth disease.** Infection with coxsackievirus A or B may result in an acute lymphonodular pharyngitis characterized by fever, headache, and the appearance of small (3–6 mm), yellow or whitish nodules in the posterior pharynx. These distinctive papular lesions are not vesicular and do not ulcerate. Epstein-Barr virus can cause pharyngitis characterized by prominent tonsillar enlargement with exudate or a membrane, cervical lymphadenitis, hepatosplenomegaly, rash, and generalized fatigue as part of the infectious mononucleosis syndrome (Chapter 37). Primary herpesvirus infections in infants and young children often present with high fever and gingivostomatitis (Chapter 60).

Gonococcal Pharyngitis. The incubation period for gonococcal pharyngitis is usually 2–7 days. Although most gonococcal pharyngeal infections are asymptomatic, gonococcal infections can occasionally cause acute pharyngitis or tonsillitis and be associated with fever and cervical lymphadenitis. Patients with pharyngeal gonococcal infection are at high risk of concurrent genital involvement; the pharynx is uncommonly the only infected site. These patients are likely to have other sexually transmitted diseases and should therefore be evaluated for the presence of these other infections. The risk of disseminated gonococcal infection from gonococcal pharyngitis is slight.

TABLE 58–2. Patterns of Illness Including Sore Throat Suggesting a Specific Microbial Etiology

Clinical Pattern	Etiologic Agent
Scarlet fever	Group A *Streptococcus* *Arcanobacterium haemolyticum* (rare)
Pharyngoconjunctival fever	Adenoviruses
Herpangina	Enteroviruses, especially coxsackieviruses
Hand, foot, and mouth syndrome	Coxsackieviruses
Lymphonodular pharyngitis	Coxsackieviruses
Mononucleosis syndrome	Epstein-Barr virus or cytomegalovirus
Gingivostomatitis	Herpes simplex viruses
Pharyngeal membrane and bull neck	*Corynebacterium diphtheriae*

Diphtheria. The incubation period for diphtheria is usually 2–5 days, but rarely it may be 1–8 days. The usual presentation is low-grade fever and gradual onset of mild pharyngeal symptoms over 1–2 days. Less common clinical manifestations can include malignant (or **"bull-neck"**) pharyngeal diphtheria with a more abrupt and aggressive course; nasal diphtheria with a mucoid or serosanguineous discharge but generally few constitutional symptoms; **laryngeal diphtheria** with hoarseness and loss of voice; and cutaneous diphtheria with a sharply demarcated ulcer covered with a dirty gray slough or membrane (Plate 7C). Vulvovaginal, conjunctival, and aural involvement may also be noted.

At first, the throat is only red. Over the next 24–48 hours, whitish gray spots appear and then coalesce to form a light to dark gray **pseudomembrane** that usually begins on the tonsils but then spreads to the soft palate and uvula. The membrane gradually becomes thicker, darker, and more sharply defined and may have a leatherlike appearance. It is tightly adherent to the underlying tissues, and attempts to remove it may result in bleeding. The membrane may be localized to the nasopharynx or extend deeper into the tracheobronchial tree. The bull-neck appearance results from intense tissue edema and cervical lymphadenopathy.

Although pharyngitis due to more common bacterial and viral causes may have an exudative component, the mature membrane of pharyngeal diphtheria is distinctive for a dark gray color, presence beyond the tonsils to the uvula and soft palate, and especially for hemorrhage associated with removal of the membrane. Epiglottitis caused by *H. influenzae* type b may cause difficulty in breathing similar to that of diphtheria, but on physical examination the epiglottis and supraglottic folds are intensely inflamed without a pharyngeal membrane.

Other Infectious Causes of Pharyngitis. The illnesses attributed to group C *Streptococcus* are generally indistinguishable from those caused by group A *Streptococcus.* The spectrum of illness is broad, and the physical findings are variable but again are similar to those seen with group A streptococcal pharyngitis.

The illnesses attributable to *A. haemolyticum* are likewise similar to those caused by group A *Streptococcus.* Sore throat is almost universally present, and fever is very common. The physical findings are again similar to those typical of group A streptococcal pharyngitis. The pharynx is reddened, and tonsillar exudate is frequent. These exudates are usually discrete and patchy in distribution, but confluent exudates mimicking a diphtheritic membrane have been reported. Cervical lymphadenitis is common. A scarlet fever–like presentation has also been described, with a blanching, erythematous, maculopapular rash. In contrast to classic scarlet fever, however, the rash is often pruritic, begins on the distal extremities, and rarely desquamates. In addition, strawberry tongue has not been described. Other skin findings, including urticarial rashes and erythema multiforme, have been reported.

With oropharyngeal tularemia, the sore throat may be severe out of proportion to the visible pathologic findings. Gastrointestinal symptoms may be prominent. Patients present most commonly with tonsillitis and cervical lymphadenitis. Oral ulcers may be present, and the tonsils may be covered with exudate or even with a membrane similar to that seen in diphtheria.

PFAPA is characterized by recurring nonspecific pharyngitis accompanied by fever and aphthae, which are painful solitary vesicular lesions in the mouth. The fevers begin at a young age, usually <5 years. Episodes last approximately 5 days, or less when treated with oral prednisone, with a mean of 28 days between episodes. Episodes are unresponsive to nonsteroidal anti-inflammatory agents or antibiotics.

DIAGNOSIS

The principal challenge is to distinguish episodes of pharyngitis caused by group A β-hemolytic *Streptococcus* from those caused by nonstreptococcal (and usually viral) organisms. This distinction can sometimes be made on purely clinical grounds with a great degree of confidence. For example, the cause of illness in a child with sore throat, fever, tonsillar exudate, strawberry tongue, and a scarlatiniform rash is likely to be group A *Streptococcus.* There is substantial overlap among the various syndromes, however, so that a rapid streptococcal antigen test or a throat culture or both are often performed to improve diagnostic precision and to help identify children who are most likely to benefit from antibiotic therapy.

In addition to the usual challenge of deciding whether an episode of pharyngitis is streptococcal or viral in nature, it may be necessary, in certain clinical situations, to identify less common bacterial causes such as *Neisseria gonorrhoeae* or diphtheria. Diphtheria is a rare cause of pharyngitis in the United States but demands special consideration because it can be particularly severe, requires specific diagnostic testing, and is potentially treatable with antitoxin and antimicrobial therapy.

Laboratory Evaluation

Certain routine, nonspecific laboratory studies, such as the WBC count and CRP, have some predictive value in distinguishing streptococcal from nonstreptococcal pharyngitis. The diagnostic accuracy of these tests is not sufficiently high to make them clinically useful, however, so they are not routinely recommended and more accurate microbiologic testing is advised.

A CBC in patients with infectious mononucleosis may show a predominance of atypical lymphocytes (Chapter 10). Routine laboratory studies are of little diagnostic value for the diagnosis of diphtheria or for PFAPA.

Microbiologic Evaluation

Throat Culture for Group A Streptococcus. Throat culture remains the diagnostic "gold standard" for establishing the occurrence of streptococcal pharyngitis. Unfortunately, this gold standard is flawed and imperfect. False-positive cultures can occur if other organisms are incorrectly identified as group A *Streptococcus.* Colonies of β-hemolytic staphylococci can usually be distinguished from streptococci by their larger colony size and yellowish color; in questionable cases a positive catalase test (staphylococci cause hydrogen peroxide to "bubble") quickly distinguishes the two. Certain non–group A streptococci pose another potential problem because of their similar morphologic appearance. The culture plate growth of virtually all group A organisms is inhibited around a 0.04-unit bacitracin disk, whereas most non–group A streptococci are resistant to bacitracin and will grow in the area of the disk. This technique is inexpensive and easy to use, but some non–group A streptococci are also sensitive to bacitracin and are misidentified as group A. This technique requires a moderate growth of streptococci on the culture plate to determine whether the disk is inhibiting growth. A specific latex agglutination method enables precise identification of Lancefield serogroup A, but it is more expensive and time consuming than the bacitracin method. Even when the culture technique and "positive" reading are correct in the microbiologic sense, this answer may be clinically misleading. Some such "positive" cultures occur in children who are carriers of streptococci but have acute pharyngitis caused by a different organism.

False-negative cultures constitute a more substantial problem and can be attributed to a variety of causes (Table 58–3). Studies evaluating the accuracy of throat culture testing performed in office laboratories have generally documented poor reliability. Federal regulations for office laboratories may have served to improve the standardization of test procedures and the accuracy of test results.

Rapid Tests for Group A Streptococcus. A number of rapid diagnostic techniques for streptococcal pharyngitis have been developed in recent years to provide a quicker answer and to make possible speedy institution of appropriate antimicrobial therapy. These tests begin with a chemical or enzymatic extraction of the group A antigen from the streptococcal cell wall. This frees the group-specific antigen to participate in immunologic and other reactions. With latex agglutination tests, latex particles coated with antibodies directed at the group A antigen are mixed with the treated throat swab specimen. In the presence of free group A antigen, these reagents form a latticework with visible agglutination. Rapid diagnostic kits using an enzyme immunoassay are now in widespread use and may be less vulnerable to reader bias in interpretation of the results. An optical immunoassay technique is also widely used, and in some studies, but not all, this method appears to have enhanced sensitivity.

The specificity of rapid tests is generally excellent, often 95–99%. Rapid antigen testing for group A *Streptococcus* is usually negative for patients with group C isolates. The predictive accuracy of a positive rapid test depends on the specificity but also on the prevalence of streptococcal pharyngitis in the tested population. This prevalence may vary widely according to the season of year, outbreaks of streptococcal illness in the community, and the clinical indications (such as age and physical findings) used to determine which patients are tested. If one assumes an overall test sensitivity of 85%, the positive predictive value of the test can be calculated for a variety of clinical situations. If the prevalence is as low as 10% in a particular setting, for example, and if the test specificity is 95%, then the predictive accuracy of a positive test is only 65%. In the more usual setting with a prevalence of 20–30% and a test specificity of 98–99%, the predictive accuracy of a positive rapid test is greater than 90%. Under these conditions, if the rapid test is positive, throat culture is unnecessary and appropriate antimicrobial treatment can be prescribed.

TABLE 58–3. Causes of False-Negative Throat Cultures for Group A β-Hemolytic *Streptococcus*

- Inadequate throat swab specimen (e.g., failure to sample the posterior pharynx of an unrestrained, uncooperative child)
- Inadequate culture plate (e.g., improper or outdated media)
- Poor technique of inoculating and streaking the plate
- Incorrect incubation conditions
- Incorrect "negative" reading (e.g., failure to subculture a suspicious colony on the primary plate)
- Correct culture technique and interpretation but incorrect clinical answer (e.g., patient surreptitiously taking an antibiotic left over from a previous illness)

The sensitivity of these rapid tests is more variable than the specificity and depends greatly on the number of group A streptococci present in the specimen. For specimens yielding a heavy growth on culture, the sensitivity of the rapid tests is generally very high, often exceeding 90–95%. The sensitivity of the rapid tests is much lower, however (often only 50–70%), for specimens yielding a light growth of group A streptococcal organisms on culture. Patients with low colony counts are somewhat more likely than those with high counts to be carriers of streptococci but this distinction is not sharp. A substantial proportion of patients with negative rapid tests but positive cultures have invasive infection as defined by a serologic response to streptococcal extracellular antigens. It is not safe to assume that patients with negative rapid test results but positive cultures are carriers of streptococci.

The predictive accuracy of a negative rapid test depends not only on the sensitivity of the test but also on the prevalence of streptococcal pharyngitis in the tested population. If one assumes an overall test specificity of 98%, the accuracy of a negative rapid test can likewise be calculated for a variety of clinical situations. In the usual setting with a prevalence of 20–30% and a test sensitivity of 85%, the predictive accuracy of a negative rapid test is 94–96%. If the prevalence is as high as 50% in a particular setting, however, such as a community outbreak of streptococcal disease, and if the test sensitivity is only 70%, then the predictive accuracy of a negative rapid test drops below 80%. In either setting, some patients with streptococcal pharyngitis will be missed if only a rapid test is used for diagnosis. A negative rapid test should ideally be confirmed with a negative culture, especially when the clinical suspicion of streptococcal illness is great. An algorithm for using both a rapid antigen detection method and throat culture in the approach to a child with pharyngitis is outlined in Fig. 58–1. Improvements in the rapid diagnostic methods can be anticipated, so that periodic reassessment of the predictive value and clinical usefulness of these methods is required.

Viral Culture. Viral cultures can be used to confirm a specific etiologic agent, but such cultures are generally expensive, may not be available locally, and may take too long for the results to be clinically useful. Various rapid diagnostic tests for viruses are under study and may prove more practical.

Gonococcal Pharyngitis. Gram-stained smears are not useful for the diagnosis of gonococcal pharyngitis because of the high carriage rate of nonpathogenic *Neisseria* species, which have similar morphology, in the pharynx of the young child. The organism is extremely sensitive to drying and temperature changes, so a throat swab should be inoculated immediately onto a selective culture medium, such as Thayer-Martin medium, before transport to the laboratory.

Diphtheria. A direct Gram-stained smear is unreliable, but culture of a portion of the membrane or of material obtained from beneath the membrane establishes the correct diagnosis. The nose and any lesions of the skin, eye, or ear should be cultured. The microbiology laboratory should be told that the diagnosis of diphtheria is being considered to ensure that appropriate media (Loeffler or tellurite selective medium as well as a blood agar plate) are used. All positive cultures should be evaluated for toxigenicity by a virulence test on two guinea pigs, one of which is pretreated with diphtheria antitoxin. When a broth suspension of a toxigenic organism is

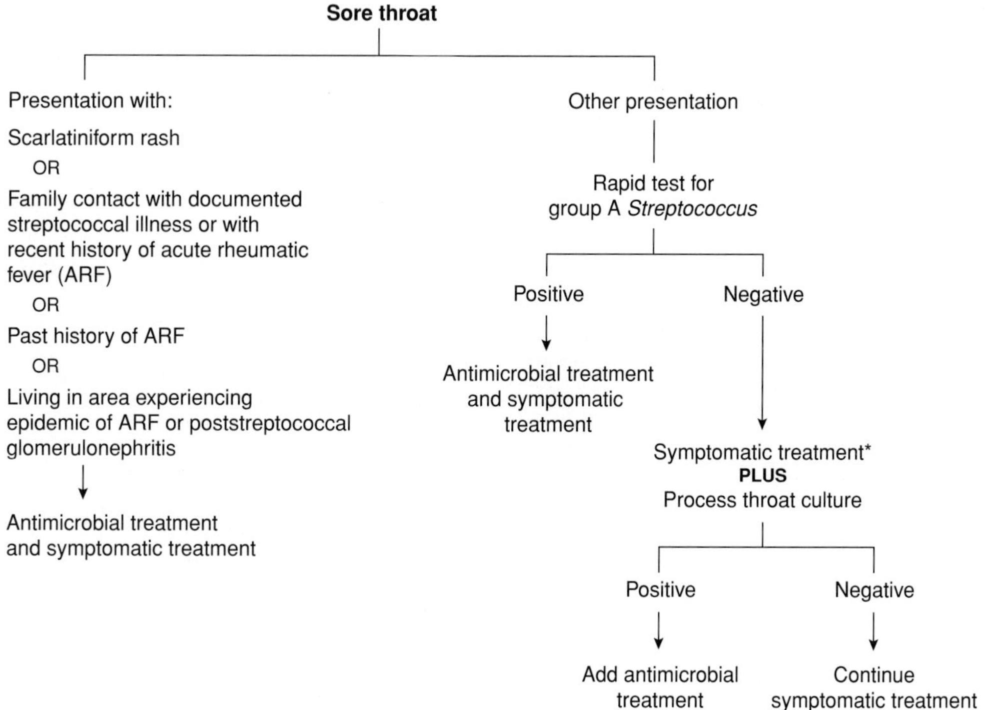

FIGURE 58–1. Management of a child older than 2 years of age whose major complaint is a sore throat. (Adapted from Hayden GF, Hendley JO, Gwaltney JM Jr: Management of the ambulatory patient with a sore throat. *Curr Clin Top Infect Dis* 1988;9:72.)

inoculated intracutaneously, the treated animal shows no skin reaction, whereas the unprotected animal has an inflammatory reaction that becomes necrotic over 24–72 hours. Because β-hemolytic *Streptococcus* may be present concurrently or secondarily in throat cultures from 20–30% of patients with diphtheria, the isolation of streptococci should not be interpreted as excluding the diagnosis of diphtheria.

Other Infectious Causes of Pharyngitis. For pharyngitis caused by group C *Streptococcus,* the culture plate is ideally incubated in a CO_2-enriched or anaerobic atmosphere. The β-hemolytic streptococcal colonies can be identified as serogroup C by means of a rapid latex agglutination technique. Some group C isolates are sensitive to bacitracin and may be mistakenly identified as group A by this presumptive grouping method. Some group C organisms (e.g., those from the species *Streptococcus equisimilis*) have large colony sizes and are roughly similar in appearance to group A isolates, whereas other group C isolates (e.g., those from the species *Streptococcus anginosus,* also known as *Streptococcus milleri*) are much smaller and more difficult to identify. Serologic studies are of limited diagnostic value because the extracellular antigens of group C *Streptococcus* are only incompletely identified. Some group C organisms produce streptolysin O, so that antistreptolysin O testing may sometimes be useful. A specific anti–group C carbohydrate antibody assay has been developed and may also have some clinical applications.

For pharyngitis associated with *A. haemolyticum,* a routine throat culture is not helpful because the hemolysis caused by colonies of *A. haemolyticum* is slow to appear and is often minimal on sheep blood agar, the medium that is generally preferred for throat cultures. If *A. haemolyticum* is suspected, the swab should be inoculated onto human or rabbit blood agar, and the culture should be held for a minimum of 72 hours to identify the small β-hemolytic colonies.

For oropharyngeal tularemia, Gram-stained smears of tonsillar exudate are not helpful, and cultures for tularemia are generally not indicated because of the risk to laboratory personnel. The diagnosis is established by a history of possible exposure, suitable clinical findings, and a rising titer of serial agglutination tests.

There are no microbiologic tests for PFAPA, although it is necessary to exclude other common causes of pharyngitis by means of appropriate diagnostic tests.

Serologic Diagnosis. Serologic tests for group A streptococcal pharyngitis are not performed routinely. They may be used to document recent inapparent group A streptococcal infection to fulfill the diagnostic criteria of rheumatic fever or poststreptococcal glomerulonephritis (Chapter 40). A variety of serologic tests are potentially useful in establishing a specific diagnosis of a viral pharyngitis, but problems of expense, availability, timing, and lack of therapeutic options diminish their clinical usefulness. An exception is the slide agglutination or spot test for mononucleosis, which is relatively inexpensive and can be performed on a single acute blood specimen. It is most useful for an older child who has been ill for a few days. If there is evidence of oropharyngeal tularemia, serial antibody tests are preferred for diagnosis.

TREATMENT

Definitive Treatment

Group A Streptococcal Pharyngitis. Even if untreated, most episodes of streptococcal pharyngitis resolve uneventfully over a few days. If instituted early in the course of illness, however, antimicrobial therapy accelerates clinical recovery by 12–24 hours. This beneficial effect has been demonstrated in several studies in which symptomatic measures were withheld. When symptomatic treatments were allowed, the additional symptomatic benefit of early antibiotic therapy was more difficult to demonstrate. Because antibiotic treatment has been shown to blunt the streptococcal serologic response, concerns have been raised that early antibiotic treatment might not allow the patient to mount a functional immune response and might therefore predispose the patient to recurrent episodes of illness. One study suggested such an effect, but a second, carefully designed study (Gerber et al., 1990) demonstrated no difference in recurrence rate for streptococcal pharyngitis, whether therapy was initiated immediately or delayed as long as 48 hours.

A second benefit of antimicrobial therapy is the prevention of acute rheumatic fever. Because the latent (or ''incubation'') period of acute rheumatic fever is relatively long (1–3 weeks), treatment instituted within 9 days of illness is almost 100% successful in preventing rheumatic fever. Treatment begun more than 9 days after the onset of illness is less than 100% successful but may still have some preventive value. It is uncertain whether antimicrobial treatment of streptococcal pharyngitis can prevent the development of acute poststreptococcal glomerulonephritis, but it is generally believed that it cannot.

For certain patients, it seems reasonable to begin antibiotic therapy immediately. These patients include children with a positive rapid test for group A *Streptococcus;* children with scarlet fever; children with symptomatic pharyngitis whose siblings are ill with documented streptococcal pharyngitis; children with symptomatic pharyngitis and a past history of rheumatic fever or a recent history of rheumatic fever in a family member; and children with symptomatic pharyngitis who are living in an area that in experiencing an epidemic of acute rheumatic fever or poststreptococcal glomerulonephritis (Fig. 58–1).

Even when treatment is begun empirically, a rapid test or throat culture to document group A *Streptococcus* as the cause may sometimes be useful. A positive test result may help to reinforce the need for compliance with the prescribed course of antimicrobial therapy and may also be helpful in directing the treatment of contacts who subsequently become ill. A negative test result may help to explain an unanticipated poor clinical response to treatment.

A variety of antimicrobial agents can be used to treat streptococcal pharyngitis (Table 58–4). The time-honored choice is

TABLE 58–4. Antimicrobial Treatment of Group A Streptococcal Pharyngitis

Penicillin
Intramuscular benzathine penicillin G (single dose)
For children <27 kg (60 lb): 600,000 U
For larger children and adults: 1,200,000 U
or
Oral penicillin V (tid or qid for 10 days)
For children <27 kg (60 lb): 125 mg per dose
For larger children and adults: 250–500 mg per dose
Erythromycin: for Persons Allergic to β-Lactams
For Larger Children and Adults
1 g/day in 2–4 divided doses for 10 days
For Smaller Children
Erythromycin ethyl succinate
40–50 mg/kg/day in 3–4 divided doses for 10 days
Erythromycin estolate
20–40 mg/kg/day in 2–4 divided doses for 10 days

Adapted from Hayden GF, Hendley JO, Gwaltney JM Jr: Management of the ambulatory patient with a sore throat. *Curr Clin Top Infect Dis* 1988;9:72.

TABLE 58–5. Treatment Regimens to Eradicate the Streptococcal Carrier State

1. Oral clindamycin, 20 mg/kg/day (max 1.2 g) in 3–4 divided doses for 10 days
2. Oral penicillin V 125 mg per dose for children <27 kg (60 lb); 250–500 mg per dose for larger children and adults, tid or qid for 10 days *or*
   Benzathine penicillin G as a single IM dose, 600,000 U for children <27 kg (60 lb); 1,200,000 U for larger children and adults
   plus
   Oral rifampin 20 mg/kg/day (max 1.2 g) in 1–2 divided doses for 4 days
3. Oral amoxicillin-clavulanate 40–45 mg amoxicillin/kg/day (max 1.5 g) in 2–3 divided doses for 10 days

penicillin, which has a narrow spectrum, is inexpensive, and has relatively few side effects. It is usually given orally three or four times daily for a full 10 days. Oral amoxicillin has been preferred over oral penicillin by some children and their parents because of its taste and its availability in the form of chewable tablets that do not require refrigeration. Previous studies had shown that oral penicillin was not as effective if given as a single daily dose or if given for less than a 10-day course. Recent studies, however, show that 750 mg of amoxicillin given as a single daily dose is as effective as 250 mg penicillin V given three times a day. Another study suggests that a shorter 6-day course of twice-a-day amoxicillin may be as effective as a 10-day course of penicillin V given three times daily. If these potential advantages are confirmed in other studies, oral amoxicillin will become an even more popular choice for treatment. A single intramuscular dose of benzathine penicillin (or a benzathine-procaine combination) is somewhat painful, but it assures compliance and will provide adequate blood levels for more than 10 days. For patients who are allergic to penicillins, erythromycin is the traditional drug of choice.

In recent years, other antibiotics have been suggested for the treatment of streptococcal pharyngitis. Because rheumatic fever is relatively uncommon, the comparative efficacy of these other agents has not been measured with respect to preventing rheumatic fever but, rather, by the proportion of treated patients in whom group A *Streptococcus* is detected in the pharynx at the completion of therapy. By this standard, some drugs (such as oral first-generation cephalosporins) appear to be as good as, or better than, penicillin. One proposed explanation is that staphylococci or anaerobes in the pharynx produce β-lactamase, which inactivates penicillin and reduces its efficacy. Another possible explanation for this apparent benefit is that these other drugs are more effective than penicillin in eradicating streptococcal carriage. Some of the newer drugs may also offer convenience, such as once-daily administration or shorter length of therapy, which may in turn translate into improved compliance. These drugs will generally be more expensive than penicillin, however, and usually have more side effects.

Follow-up cultures of treated patients generally are not necessary unless symptoms recur. Some treated patients continue to harbor group A *Streptococcus* in their pharynges and become carriers. Carriage generally poses little or no risk to patients and their contacts, but if treatment is elected, three regimens have been shown effective: clindamycin, penicillin with rifampin, and amoxicillin-clavulanate (Table 58–5).

Recurrent Group A Streptococcal Pharyngitis. Children with recurrent episodes of pharyngitis with throat cultures positive for group A *Streptococcus* pose a particular problem. The episodes may represent relapses with an identical strain, which might occur with poor compliance with the prescribed antibiotic; a strain that is resistant to or tolerant of the prescribed antibiotic; or ''protection'' of the organism by β-lactamase produced by other pharyngeal flora, especially staphylococci or anaerobes. One study (Brook and Gober, 1998) suggests that toothbrushes and removable orthodontic appliances sometimes harbor group A *Streptococcus* after penicillin treatment for streptococcal pharyngitis, but whether such occurrences contribute to relapse is uncertain. Alternatively, the recurrent episodes may be due to a different strain related to new exposures in the family setting or elsewhere. Finally, the episodes may represent pharyngitis due to another cause but accompanied by streptococcal carriage. This last possibility is likely if the illnesses are mild and otherwise atypical for streptococcal pharyngitis.

In the face of recurrent pharyngitis with positive throat cultures, several steps should be taken. First, the streptococci should be verified to be Lancefield group A by bacitracin sensitivity or latex agglutination testing. Next, an assessment should be made of poor adherence with the previously prescribed therapy as the cause for the recurrence. For nonadherence, therapy with intramuscular benzathine penicillin is recommended. Finally, any family members with symptomatic pharyngitis should be cultured and treated simultaneously as appropriate. The index patient need not have another culture unless there is a clinical relapse.

If these measures fail, an alternative antibiotic may be chosen to treat pharyngeal flora producing β-lactamase. Either amoxicillin-clavulanate or clindamycin serves the dual purpose of being an effective regimen for eliminating streptococcal carriage. Group A *Streptococcus* remains universally susceptible to penicillin, but the possibility of bacteriologic resistance to another drug, such as erythromycin, should be considered. A more likely explanation for this clinical problem is that the index patient carries group A *Streptococcus* and has experienced multiple episodes of nonstreptococcal pharyngitis. The streptococcal carrier state is not in itself harmful but may confuse the determination of etiologic agent and optimal therapy in this setting. To detect the carrier state, the clinician can perform a repeat culture a few days after treatment. If streptococcal carriage is detected, therapy to eliminate it can be recommended (Table 56–6). Performing cultures on pets and family members who do not have symptoms is rarely helpful and is not recommended.

Tonsillectomy. Referral for consideration of tonsillectomy is justified for children with well-documented histories of recurrent, culture-positive, group A streptococcal pharyngitis that has been clinically severe and very frequent, which is defined as seven or more episodes in the previous year or five or more in each of the preceding 2 years. Among such severely affected children, tonsillectomy lowers the incidence of pharyngitis during the subsequent 1–2 years. Many children who do not have the operation will spontaneously have fewer episodes over time, however, so the anticipated benefit of tonsillectomy must be balanced against the risks of anesthesia and a surgical procedure. Undocumented histories of recurrent pharyngitis do not predict subsequent experience and are not an adequate basis for recommending tonsillectomy. Referral to an otolaryngologist is advised for those few patients with acute pharyngitis who develop a suppurative complication, such as parapharyngeal abscess (Chapter 59).

Viral Pharyngitis. Specific antiviral therapy is unavailable for most cases of viral pharyngitis. Pharyngitis caused by influenza virus may potentially be improved by early antiviral treatment, but such treatment is generally reserved for patients with severe disease or with underlying conditions that put them at high risk of severe or complicated influenza (Chapter 68). Patients with primary herpetic gingivostomatitis do benefit from early treatment with oral acyclovir (Chapter 60). Acyclovir has good in vitro activity against Epstein-Barr virus, but clinical trials have not demonstrated any clinical benefit, and thus this treatment is not recommended.

Gonococcal Pharyngitis. The spontaneous cure rate within 3 months for uncomplicated pharyngeal gonococcal infection is very high. Appropriate antimicrobial therapy is nevertheless recommended to eradicate infection more quickly and prevent spread of the organism. Patients with uncomplicated gonococcal pharyngitis should receive ceftriaxone, 125 mg in a single intramuscular dose. Ciprofloxacin, 500 mg in a single oral dose, or ofloxacin, 400 mg in a single oral dose, may be used in persons ≥18 years of age. For persons who cannot take a cephalosporin or a quinolone, TMP-SMZ (720 mg trimethoprim, 3,600 mg sulfamethoxazole) given orally once a day for 5 days may be effective, although a follow-up culture should be performed to document eradication. Spectinomycin is not effective for treatment of pharyngeal gonorrhea.

Gonococcal infections of the pharynx are more difficult to eradicate than infections at urogenital and anorectal sites. Persons with uncomplicated pharyngeal gonorrhea treated with a recommended regimen do not need a follow-up culture. Persons with persistent symptoms should have a repeat culture, and any gonococci isolated should be tested for antimicrobial susceptibility. Infections after treatment with a recommended regimen usually result from reinfection rather than from treatment failure, which emphasizes the need for patient education and referral of sex partners.

Diphtheria. The most important aspect of treatment for pharyngeal diphtheria is antitoxin to neutralize the effects of diphtheria toxin. If the clinical findings are highly suggestive of pharyngeal diphtheria, a single dose of equine antitoxin should be administered immediately because of the possibility of rapid clinical deterioration if no treatment is given (Table 58–6). The antitoxin should be administered intravenously, but the patient must first be tested for possible sensitivity to horse serum (see Chapter 15).

In addition to antitoxin, antimicrobial therapy is recommended to eradicate the organism, prevent further formation of toxin, and prevent spread of the organism to other persons. Either parenteral penicillin or oral erythromycin for 14 days is acceptable therapy (Table 58–6). The patient's throat and nasopharynx should be cultured after treatment to document that the organism has been eliminated, as shown by two or three consecutive negative cultures. Active immunization against diphtheria should be carried out during convalescence because disease does not necessarily confer immunity.

Patients with severe diphtheria are often unable to swallow and require supportive treatment with intravenous fluids. Bed rest is advised for at least 2 weeks until the risk of symptomatic cardiac damage has passed.

Other Infectious Causes of Pharyngitis. The choice of specific antimicrobial therapy for pharyngitis associated with both group C *Streptococcus* and *A. haemolyticum* is unclear because no prospective, randomized clinical trials have been performed to assess the efficacy of antimicrobial therapy for pharyngitis associated with either agent. On the basis of in vitro susceptibility data and other observations, however, treatment recommendations include oral penicillin for group C *Streptococcus* and oral erythromycin for *A. haemolyticum.* The drug of choice for the treatment of tularemia is gentamicin or streptomycin (Chapter 34).

There is usually a dramatic resolution of PFAPA with one or two doses of oral prednisone, 1 mg/kg per dose, but this does not prevent recurrences. Tonsillectomy and cimetidine treatment are associated with remission in a small number of patients.

TABLE 58–6. Treatment of Nasopharyngeal Diphtheria

Antitoxin (after Testing for Hypersensitivity)*	
Pharyngeal or laryngeal disease and duration <48 hr	20,000–40,000 U
Nasopharyngeal disease	40,000–60,000 U
Extensive disease	80,000–120,000 U
Large membrane	
Soft, diffuse cervical lymphadenitis	
Toxic clinical disease	
Duration of illness longer than 48–72 hr	
Antimicrobial Therapy†	
Aqueous crystalline penicillin G 100,000–150,000 U/kg/day divided q6hr IV for 14 days	
or	
Aqueous procaine penicillin G 25,000–50,000 U/kg/day (max 1.2 MU) divided q12hr IM for 14 days	
or	
Erythromycin 40–50 mg/kg/day (max 2 g) divided q6hr PO or IV for 14 days	

*Antitoxin can be obtained from the Centers for Disease Control and Prevention. It is diluted 1:20 in normal saline solution and infused intravenously at a rate not to exceed 1 mL/min. Before intravenous administration, testing for sensitivity to horse serum should be performed by trained personnel familiar with the treatment of acute anaphylaxis. One drop of a 1:100 dilution of serum in saline solution is used for scratch, prick, or puncture testing. If this test is negative, an intradermal test is performed with 0.02 mL of a 1:1000 dilution of serum in saline solution. If negative, this test is repeated with a 1:100 dilution. If the patient is sensitive to equine antitoxin, desensitization is necessary.

†Elimination of the organism after treatment should be documented by two consecutive negative cultures.

Supportive Therapy

Symptomatic therapy can be an important part of the overall treatment plan for streptococcal pharyngitis as well as for nonstreptococcal pharyngitis. An oral antipyretic-analgesic agent (e.g., acetaminophen or ibuprofen) may help relieve fever and sore throat pain. Gargling with warm salt water is often comforting, and anesthetic sprays and lozenges (often containing benzocaine, phenol, or menthol) may provide local relief.

COMPLICATIONS AND PROGNOSIS

The complications of group A streptococcal pharyngitis include local suppurative complications, such as parapharyngeal abscess and other infections of the deep fascial spaces of the neck (Chapter 59), and later nonsuppurative problems, such as acute rheumatic fever and acute postinfectious glomerulonephritis (Chapter 40).

Viral respiratory tract infections, including those caused by influenza A virus, adenoviruses, parainfluenza type 3 virus, and rhinoviruses, may predispose to bacterial middle ear infections (Chapter 64). PFAPA eventually resolves, although episodes may recur for years, and there are no long-term sequelae.

Diphtheria. In diphtheria, respiratory obstruction by pseudomembranes may require mechanical intervention (bronchoscopy, intubation, or tracheostomy) to maintain a patent airway. Toxic complications primarily affect the heart and nervous system. The frequency and severity of complications are usually in proportion to the severity of the pharyngeal disease and most typically, but not invariably, occur in the setting of severe diphtheria with a delay in the administration of antitoxin. Administration of corticosteroids does not appear to decrease the incidence of complications.

Myocarditis may occur as early as the first week of illness, but it usually becomes evident as the pharyngeal disease is improving. Up to two thirds of patients have some evidence of myocardial toxicity, but only approximately 10% have clinical symptoms. Electrocardiographic changes may become evident as arrhythmias. Myocardial injury may result in congestive heart failure with progressive dyspnea, diminished heart sounds, and circulatory failure. Patients should have repeat ECGs and serum cardiac enzyme determinations, and a cardiologist should be consulted.

Neuritis occurs in up to three fourths of patients with diphtheria, but generally it occurs somewhat later in the course of illness, from several days to several weeks after onset. It may be manifest as paralysis of the soft palate, ocular muscles, diaphragm, or limbs. The resolution is slow but usually complete (Chapter 56).

The ultimate prognosis depends on the virulence of the particular organism, the patient's immune status, and the duration of illness before specific treatment is begun. Myocarditis is the major cause of morbidity and mortality.

PREVENTION

Attempts to develop a streptococcal vaccine have thus far been unsuccessful, but multivalent vaccines based on M protein peptides are still under development. Antimicrobial prophylaxis with daily oral penicillin prevents recurrent infections but has been recommended only to prevent recurrences of rheumatic fever (Chapter 40).

Avoidance of sexually transmitted diseases can reduce the incidence of all forms of gonococcal infection among adolescents.

Limited data suggest the value of cimetidine in preventing recurrent episodes of PFAPA, but it is unclear whether this is actually effective because studies did not exclude the possibility of spontaneous resolution, which frequently occurs.

Exposure to Pharyngeal Diphtheria. Contact tracing should begin immediately to identify household members and other persons with a history of habitual, close contact with a patient with suspected or proved pharyngeal diphtheria. The care of such exposed persons depends on their immunization status and their perceived reliability in taking prophylactic medication and returning for follow-up visits (Table 58–7). Close contacts, irrespective of their immunization status, should have their nasopharynges cultured for *C. diphtheriae* and should be given antimicrobial prophylaxis with oral erythromycin or intramuscular penicillin G (Table 56-7). The efficacy of chemoprophylaxis is presumed but not proved, so that contacts should be monitored for 7 days for evidence of disease, regardless of administration of prophylactic antibiotics. Close contacts without symptoms who are not fully immunized (fewer than 3 doses of diphtheria toxoid), who have been immunized previously but have not received a booster dose of diphtheria toxoid within 5 years, or whose immunization status is not known should receive active immunization with diphtheria toxoid (DTaP, DTP, DT, or Td, depending on age). Children who have not yet received their fourth vaccination should be vaccinated.

TABLE 58–7. Prophylaxis After Exposure to a Patient with Pharyngeal Diphtheria

Chemoprophylaxis

Erythromycin 40–50 mg/kg/day (max 2 g) divided q6hr PO for 7 days

or

Benzathine penicillin G 600,000 U for children <30 kg; 1,200,000 U for children ≥30 kg and adults as a single IM dose*

Vaccination with Diphtheria Toxoid

DTaP, DTP, DT, or Td, depending on age for:

- Close contacts not fully immunized (<3 doses of diphtheria toxoid)
- Previously immunized close contacts who have not received a booster dose of diphtheria toxoid within 5 yr
- Close contacts whose immunization status is not known
- Children who have not yet received their fourth vaccination

*Recommended for persons who cannot be kept under surveillance.

Close contacts who cannot be kept under surveillance should receive benzathine penicillin G, and not erythromycin, as chemoprophylaxis for reasons of assured compliance. The use of equine diphtheria antitoxin as prophylaxis for unimmunized close contacts who cannot be closely observed is not generally recommended because of the risk of allergic reactions to horse serum and because the efficacy of passive immunization has not been established. If antitoxin is used, the recommended dose is 5,000–10,000 U IM injected at a site separate from the site of the toxoid injection after appropriate testing for sensitivity.

Repeat pharyngeal cultures should be obtained from contacts with positive initial cultures a minimum of 2 weeks after completion of therapy. Patients with persistently positive cultures (carriers) should complete immunization or receive an additional diphtheria immunization if a booster has not been administered within 1 year. An additional 10-day course of erythromycin therapy should be given.

The **Schick test** has sometimes been used in the past to determine immunity to diphtheria. With this method, a tiny amount of diphtheria toxin is injected into the skin of one forearm. If the person being tested has toxin-neutralizing antibodies, no reaction will occur. In the absence of such antibodies, the area becomes red, swollen, and tender. This reaction cannot be interpreted for 4–5 days, however, and careful control testing is required because some immune patients are hypersensitive to the toxin or react to substances other than diphtheria toxin in the Schick reagent. For these reasons the Schick test is not clinically useful in managing persons who have been exposed to diphtheria.

Vaccination for Diphtheria. Active immunization with diphtheria toxoid is an effective preventive measure and is an important element of routine well-child care (Chapter 17). The DTaP, DTP, and DT formulations are used in the primary immunization series. The Td formulation is used for boosters at 10-year intervals, with the first booster at 12–15 years of age.

REVIEWS

Bisgard KM, Hardy IR, Popovic T, et al: Respiratory diphtheria in the United States, 1980 through 1995. *Am J Public Health* 1998;88:787–91.

Bisno AL: Acute pharyngitis. *N Engl J Med* 2001;344:205–11.

Bisno AL: Group A streptococcal infections and acute rheumatic fever. *N Engl J Med* 1991;325:783–93.

Bisno AL, Gerber MA, Gwaltney JM Jr, et al: Diagnosis and management of group A streptococcal pharyngitis: A practice guideline. *Clin Infect Dis* 1997;25:574–83.

Linder R: *Rhodococcus equi* and *Arcanobacterium haemolyticum:* Two ''coryneform'' bacteria increasingly recognized as agents of human infection. *Emerg Infect Dis* 1997;3:145–53.

Schwartz B, Marcy SM, Phillips WR, et al: Pharyngitis—Principles of judicious use of antimicrobial agents. *Pediatrics* 1998;101:171–4.

Stollerman GH: Rheumatic fever. *Lancet* 1997;349:935–42.

KEY ARTICLES

Brook I, Gober AE: Persistence of group A beta-hemolytic streptococci in toothbrushes and removable orthodontic appliances following treatment of pharyngotonsillitis. *Arch Otolaryngol Head Neck Surg* 1998;124:993–5.

Cohen R, Levy C, Doit C, et al: Six-day amoxicillin vs. ten-day penicillin V therapy for group A streptococcal tonsillopharyngitis. *Pediatr Infect Dis J* 1996;15:678–82.

Dale JB: Group A streptococcal vaccines. *Pediatr Ann* 1998;27:301–8.

Ebell MH, Smith MA, Barry HC, et al: Does this patient have strep throat? *JAMA* 2000;284:2912–8.

Farizo KM, Strebel PM, Chen RT, et al: Fatal respiratory disease due to *Corynebacterium diphtheriae:* Case report and review of guidelines for management, investigation, and control. *Clin Infect Dis* 1993;16:59–68.

Feder HM Jr, Gerber MA, Randolph MF, et al: Once-daily therapy for streptococcal pharyngitis with amoxicillin. *Pediatrics* 1999;103:47–51.

Gaston DA, Zurowski SM: *Arcanobacterium haemolyticum* pharyngitis and exanthem: Three case reports and literature review. *Arch Dermatol* 1996;132:61–4.

Gerber MA, Randolph MF, DeMeo KK, et al: Lack of impact of early antibiotic therapy for streptococcal pharyngitis on recurrence rates. *J Pediatr* 1990;117:853–8.

Gerber MA, Tanz RR, Kabat W, et al: Optical immunoassay test for group A beta-hemolytic streptococcal pharyngitis: An office-based, multicenter investigation. *JAMA* 1997;277:899–903.

Karpathios T, Drakonaki S, Zervoudaki A, et al: *Arcanobacterium haemolyticum* in children with presumed streptococcal pharyngotonsillitis or scarlet fever. *J Pediatr* 1992;121:735–7.

Kellogg JA: Suitability of throat culture procedures for detection of group A streptococci and as reference standards for evaluation of streptococcal antigen detection kits. *J Clin Microbiol* 1990;28:165–9.

Macris MH, Hartman N, Murray B, et al: Studies of the continuing susceptibility of group A streptococcal strains to penicillin during eight decades. *Pediatr Infect Dis J* 1998;17:377–81.

Markowitz M, Gerber MA, Kaplan EL: Treatment of streptococcal pharyngotonsillitis: Reports of penicillin's demise are premature. *J Pediatr* 1993;123:679–85.

Lan AJ, Colford JM, Colford JM Jr: The impact of dosing frequency on the efficacy of 10-day penicillin or amoxicillin therapy for streptococcal tonsillopharyngitis: A meta-analysis. *Pediatrics* 2000;105:E19.

Padeh S, Brezniak N, Zemer D, et al: Periodic fever, aphthous stomatitis, pharyngitis, and adenopathy syndrome: Clinical characteristics and outcome. *J Pediatr* 1999;135:98–101.

Pichichero ME, Margolis PA: A comparison of cephalosporins and penicillins in the treatment of group A beta-hemolytic streptococcal pharyngitis: A meta-analysis supporting the concept of microbial copathogenicity. *Pediatr Infect Dis J* 1991;10:275–81.

Pichichero ME, Green JL, Francis AB, et al: Recurrent group A streptococcal tonsillopharyngitis. *Pediatr Infect Dis J* 1998;17:809–15.

Schlager TA, Hayden GF, Woods WA, et al: Optical immunoassay for rapid detection of group A beta-hemolytic streptococci: Should culture be replaced? *Arch Pediatr Adolesc Med* 1996;150:245–8.

Shvartzman P, Tabenkin H, Rosentzwaig A, et al: Treatment of streptococcal pharyngitis with amoxicillin once a day. *BMJ* 1993;306:1170–2.

Tanz RR, Poncher JR, Corydon KE, et al: Clindamycin treatment of chronic pharyngeal carriage of group A streptococci. *J Pediatr* 1991;119:123–8.

Thomas KT, Feder HM Jr, Lawton AR, et al: Periodic fever syndrome in children. *J Pediatr* 1999;135:15–21

Turner JC, Hayden FG, Lobo MC, et al: Epidemiologic evidence for Lancefield group C beta-hemolytic streptococci as a cause of exudative pharyngitis in college students. *J Clin Microbiol* 1997;35:1–4.

Vitek CR, Wharton M: Diphtheria in the former Soviet Union: Reemergence of a pandemic disease. *Emerg Infect Dis* 1998;4:539–50.

Waagner DC: *Arcanobacterium haemolyticum:* Biology of the organism and diseases in man. *Pediatr Infect Dis J* 1991;10:933–9.

CHAPTER 59

Infections of the Deep Fascial Spaces of the Neck

Charles W. Gross ▪ Scott E. Harrison

Infections of the superficial and deep neck spaces in children are relatively common and include **peritonsillar abscesses,** historically known as **quinsy; parapharyngeal abscesses;** and **retropharyngeal (retroesophageal) abscesses.** Children typically present with a neck mass, fever, neck stiffness, trismus, discomfort, and occasionally airway obstruction. The incidence of deep neck abscess has decreased since antibiotic therapy has become more effective. Deep neck abscesses usually develop as a complication following an upper respiratory tract infection, such as sinusitis, pharyngitis, or tonsillitis, but may present at some time distant from the original infection. As the frequency of deep neck abscesses decreases, clinicians' familiarity with and expertise, concerning these entities dwindles. A further clinical problem is that partially treated infections may have atypical clinical presentations, often leading to difficulties in recognition.

Diagnostic imaging with CT and MRI has added greatly to the diagnostic techniques offered to physicians; however, they have not replaced the need for good clinical judgment. Thorough assessment of the initial clinical presentation and careful monitoring of the response of medical therapy are important in guiding decisions about whether to intervene surgically. Early diagnosis and treatment are the keys to successful, cost-effective treatment, which results in lower complication rates and shorter hospital stays.

ETIOLOGY

Many neck abscesses are polymicrobial, and aerobic as well as anaerobic organisms from the oropharynx and nasopharynx are present (Table 59–1). Microbial causes of abscesses at different sites in the neck have considerable overlap as far as the type of bacteria cultured is concerned. Large studies performed to isolate the most common species generally agree on the most commonly found bacteriologic causes. Aerobic pathogens are more commonly isolated, but anaerobic organisms are also frequently obtained. The gram-positive organisms *Staphylococcus aureus* and β-hemolytic *Streptococcus,* particularly group A *Streptococcus,* are the most common aerobic pathogens recovered. *Streptococcus pneumoniae* may be cultured from peritonsillar abscess. Common anaerobic bacteria include *Bacteroides,* particularly *Prevotella melaninogenica* (previously known as *Bacteroides melaninogenicus,* as well as *Peptostreptococcus, Veillonella,* and *Fusobacterium.* Notable gram-negative isolates include *Haemophilus influenzae* and *Haemophilus parainfluenzae.* Deep neck space infections frequently involve lactamase-producing organisms, which must be considered when one is determining appropriate antibiotic coverage.

EPIDEMIOLOGY

Deep neck space abscesses are usually preceded by bacterial infections of the upper respiratory tract. The initial site of infection may be the nasal cavity, paranasal sinuses, pharynx, tonsils, salivary glands, temporal bone (including the middle ear and mastoid process), or teeth. The primary infection may precede the deep neck infection by as long as 2–3 weeks, by which time the initial infection may no longer be present. Therefore it is difficult to determine with certainty the origin of many deep neck infections, although a careful history usually reveals a presumptive source of initial involvement. Patients particularly prone to these complications of upper respiratory tract infections include the very young, immunocompromised persons, and those in medically underserved areas.

Peritonsillar cellulitis and abscesses are the most frequent infections of the fascial spaces of the neck in children and most commonly arise as a complication of acute tonsillitis. Although pharyngotonsillitis is common in young children, the occurrence of a peritonsillar abscess is relatively rare. The incidence of peritonsillar abscesses is much higher among adolescents and young adults. Worsening tonsillitis in spite of adequate treatment suggests the potential for peritonsillar sepsis, especially among immunocompromised persons or persons with diabetes mellitus or other systemic disease. Peritonsillar abscesses have also reportedly been an unusual initial presentation of Kawasaki syndrome.

If left untreated, peritonsillar abscesses can enlarge to obstruct the oral airway or may rupture through the superior constrictor muscle into the parapharyngeal space. Traversing the superior constrictor muscle provides access into the retropharyngeal space, the carotid sheath, and even the mediastinum. The parapharyngeal space infections are usually not included with peritonsillar infections, but the close proximity of these two areas means that an element of the parapharyngeal space may be simultaneously involved in patients with a peritonsillar abscess. Parapharyngeal space abscesses are rare in children, but involvement implies risk to cranial nerves IX, X, XI, XII and the sympathetic chain, as well as the carotid artery and the internal jugular vein. The carotid sheath also provides a route into the mediastinum.

The retropharyngeal area contains two lymph node chains that drain the nasopharynx, adenoids, and posterior paranasal sinuses. Suppuration of these nodes can lead to abscess formation, but fortunately, progression to abscess is uncommon. Retropharyngeal abscesses are more common in infants and preschool-age children because the lymph nodes in the retropharyngeal space become obliterated with advancing age. This obliteration is believed to occur as a result of lymph node fibrosis within the retropharyngeal space due to recurrent upper respiratory infections. Children under the age of 5 years have the greatest number of active lymph nodes within retropharyngeal tissues. Another source of retropharyngeal infection in children is trauma to the posterior pharynx. Most commonly the trauma is associated with normal childhood activity, such as falling with an object such as a wooden stick, toothbrush, pen or pencil, toy, straw, or ruler in the mouth. Retropharyngeal

TABLE 59–1. Bacteriologic Findings in Abscesses of the Head and Neck

Organism	Number of Patients With Organism Isolated on Culture*			
	Peritonsillar Area (n = 42)	Superficial Neck (n = 19)	Submandibular, Submental Area (n = 20)	Retropharyngeal Area (n = 9)
Staphylococcus aureus	0	12	8	3
Streptococcus	17	3	6	7
Haemophilus influenzae, Haemophilus parainfluenzae	6	0	0	2
Moraxella catarrhalis	2	0	0	0
Anaerobic bacteria	1	3	0	0
Corynebacterium	0	0	1	0
Eikenella	0	0	1	0
Entric gram-negative bacilli	0	0	0	2
Atypical mycobacteria	0	2	0	0
Normal flora	7	0	0	0
Mixed organisms	12	3	4	5
No growth	8	0	3	0

*One or more bacteria cultured per patient.
Data from Dodds B, Maniglia AJ: Peritonsillar and neck abscesses in the pediatric age group. *Laryngoscope* 1988;98:956–9.

abscesses in these cases more commonly involve older children but have occurred in newborns after traumatic intubation.

Submandibular and submental abscesses in older children and adults originate most frequently from infectious dental conditions. In younger children, dental caries are less frequently the causative lesion. Young children more commonly have upper respiratory tract infections, impetiginous lesions, otitis media, sialadenitis, parotitis, or other regional infections that lead to abscess formation.

PATHOGENESIS

An understanding of the complex arrangement and structural relationships of neck anatomy is a prerequisite for the proper diagnosis and management of deep neck space infections (Fig. 59–1). Anatomically, the neck may be divided into a large osseomuscular portion, which includes the cervical spine and its muscular attachments, and a smaller anteriorly located visceral compartment. The visceral compartment is of greater concern, as almost all deep neck space infections are located in this area. The visceral compartment is composed of anatomically separate units divided by fascial layers. Familiarity with the specific anatomy of the fascial layers of the anterior neck enables a physician to localize infections precisely, anticipate the probable origin and direction of spread, develop an effective treatment plan, and expect and treat potential or actual complications.

Fascial Layers. The visceral compartment of the neck is divided by fascial layers that invest anatomic structures, which form boundaries and create potential spaces. Infections generally spread along fascial planes and not through them. Therefore, the route of spread may be predictable, and the fascia layers may limit the spread of infection. Infections in certain areas may be life threatening by either causing airway compromise or spreading into critical areas, such as the carotid sheath or mediastinum.

The fascia of the neck is divided into a **superficial cervical fascia** and a **deep cervical fascia,** both of which completely surround the neck and envelop anatomic structures. The superficial layer lies under the skin and extends from the base of the skull to the clavicles. Included in this fascia are the platysma muscle, muscles of facial expression, the spinal accessory nerve (cranial nerve IX), superficial lymph nodes, and the external jugular venous system. Infections and abscess formation within this fascial layer usually arise from superficial head and neck infections, such as impetigo or an infected sebaceous cyst. The sturdy deep layers of cervical fascia usually limit the inward spread of infection. If the integrity of the deep fascia has been compromised (e.g., from trauma, surgery, erosion), superficial infections may progress inward and involve structures located more deeply within the neck.

The **deep cervical fascia** is a more complicated entity comprising three distinct parts that extend from the skull base to the

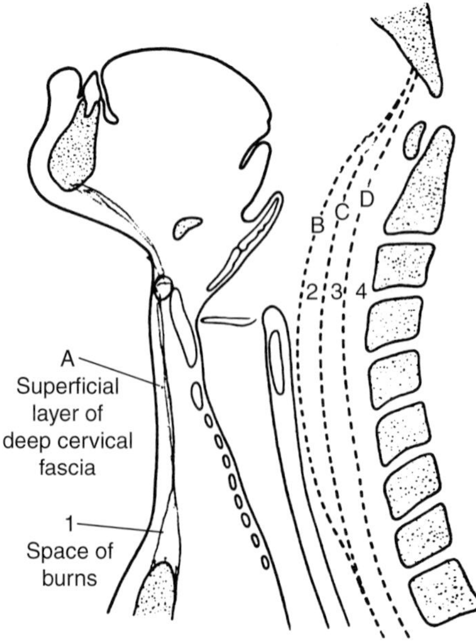

FIGURE 59–1. Midline section through the neck illustrating fascial layers *(letters)* and fascial spaces *(numbers).* The inferior limit of the retropharyngeal space is at the level of the first or second thoracic vertebra. The prevertebral space and danger space extend into the thorax. *A* = superficial layer of deep cervical fascia; *B* = visceral fascia; *C* = alar fascia; *D* = prevertebral fascia; *1* = space of Burns; *2* = retropharyngeal (retroesophageal) space; *3* = prevertebral space; *4* = danger space.

mediastinum. These parts are the superficial, middle, and deep layers of the deep cervical fascia. The **superficial layer of the deep cervical fascia** completely envelops the neck, reaching from the skull base to the chest, and attaches to the hyoid bone anteriorly. The suprahyoid portion splits to cover the submaxillary and parotid salivary glands. Special consideration must be given to the salivary glands, as the deep portion of the parotid gland in its superior aspect is devoid of fascia where it abuts the pharyngomaxillary fossa. Also, the submaxillary salivary gland extends medially and superiorly beneath the mandible where it has a close relationship with the mylohyoid muscle. This anatomic relationship forms a potential communication between the mouth and the neck, with the mylohyoid muscle forming a boundary between these two regions. This relationship is an avenue for the extension of oral or dental infections to extend from their origin into the deep neck spaces. The infrahyoid portion of the superficial layer of the deep cervical fascia splits inferiorly and attaches to the anterior and deep surfaces of the manubrium, forming the suprasternal **space of Burns.** This space contains the anterior jugular veins and several lymph nodes. Also included are the sternocleidomastoid muscles, cervical ''strap'' muscles, and muscles of mastication.

The **middle layer of the deep cervical fascia** also splits to invest the viscera of the neck including the pharynx, esophagus, larynx, trachea, thyroid, and parathyroid glands. This layer is sometimes referred to as the **visceral fascia.** The lateral aspect, sometimes called the buccopharyngeal fascia, contributes to the formation of the carotid sheath and the posterior superior portion envelops the pharyngeal constrictor muscles while forming the anterior portion of the retropharyngeal space.

The **deep layer of the deep cervical fascia** also completely surrounds the neck. Beginning in the posterior midline just anterior to the cervical bodies of the vertebrae, the fascia extends from the skull base to the coccyx. This layer envelops the deep neck muscles and covers the brachial plexus and subclavian artery. After attaching to the transverse processes of the cervical vertebrae, this deepest layer splits into two layers in front of the vertebral column, the **alar fascia** and the **prevertebral fascia,** forming the so-called **danger space.**

The carotid sheath is a condensation of all three layers of the deep cervical fascia. It encloses the carotid artery, internal jugular vein, and vagus nerve (cranial nerve X), extends from the base of the skull into the pharyngomaxillary space, and then travels into the chest. The carotid sheath, sometimes termed **Lincoln's highway,** provides direct access inferiorly into the chest and this anatomic arrangement of the deep cervical fascia makes all deep neck space infections potentially life threatening.

Potential Spaces. Certain areas within the neck are considered potential spaces located between the layers of the deep cervical fascia. The integrity of the fascia is incomplete, as perforating vessels and nerves run between the planes and provide access for infections to enter and spread. Certain neck spaces contain definite anatomic structures, whereas others, such as the retropharyngeal space, are only potential spaces that require an event such as an infection with abscess formation or bleeding between two fascial layers to ''create'' the space. The hyoid bone is the anterior point of attachment for the deep fascial layers; therefore descriptions of the neck spaces are divided into suprahyoid and infrahyoid groups.

The **parapharyngeal space** (also called the pharyngomaxillary, pterygomaxillary, carotid, or lateral pharyngeal space) has definite boundaries, but it becomes a space only when distended by purulence or blood. The space is shaped like an inverted pyramid with the base formed by the skull base and the apex formed by the fascial attachments to the hyoid bone. It is a suprahyoid potential space bounded posteriorly by the **prevertebral fascia** that contains the carotid sheath with its medial aspect in close approximation to the tonsillar fossa. The lateral aspect of the parapharyngeal space is closely approximated to the medial pterygoid muscle. The parapharyngeal space is divided into **anterior and posterior compartments** relative to the location of the styloid process **(prestyloid and poststyloid compartments).** Infection and accumulation of fluid in the anterior compartment cause inward displacement of the tonsil and may cause trismus. Inflammation of the medial pterygoid muscle from any source may cause trismus. This finding may be noted in patients with parapharyngeal space infections and peritonsillar abscesses because of their close proximity to the pterygoid musculature. When an infection develops in the poststyloid compartment, there may be little or no trismus, but there is medial bulging in the lateral pharyngeal wall and posterior tonsillar pillar. The poststyloid compartment also contains the great vessels, and therefore an infection within this area has the potential for vessel erosion with significant or life-threatening oropharyngeal hemorrhage.

The **retropharyngeal area** is subdivided anatomically into three separate spaces: the **retropharyngeal space,** the **prevertebral space,** and the **danger space.** In children younger than 5 years of age the **retropharyngeal space** contains a significant number of lymph nodes that regress and undergo fibrosis as the child ages. These nodes, sometimes referred to as the **nodes of Rouvière,** are a potential source of infection that can lead to abscess formation. The retropharyngeal space lies between the middle layer of the deep cervical fascia anteriorly and the alar fascia of the deep cervical fascia posteriorly, extending from the skull base to the mediastinum. Infections from the adenoids, nasal cavities, nasopharynx, and sinuses may spread into the retropharyngeal space through lymphatic routes, resulting in inflammation and swelling of the involved lymph nodes. Necrosis of the nodes may cause an abscess to form in the retropharyngeal space. Infections of the retropharyngeal space in infants generally remain localized. The **prevertebral space** lies deep to the retropharyngeal space and may become involved with infections originating in the cervical vertebrae, such as tuberculosis. Both the prevertebral space and the retropharyngeal space lie superficially to what is often referred to as the **danger space,** which is a potential space within the loose areolar tissue between the alar and prevertebral layers of the deep cervical fascia. It is limited laterally by the fusion of these two layers with the tips of the transverse processes of the cervical vertebrae. The danger space extends from the base of the skull into the posterior mediastinum. Infections of this space are usually the result of infectious spread from other nearby spaces, such as the retropharyngeal, prevertebral, or parapharyngeal spaces. When an infection enters this space, there is little anatomic barrier to inhibit direct extension into the chest.

Portal of Entrance. Regardless of the exact site of involvement, almost all deep neck infections are preceded by infection of the upper respiratory tract. Knowledge of these pre-existing infections and their portal of entrance enable a clinician to anticipate and recognize potential complications and to select sensible and appropriate antibiotic coverage before specific bacteriologic information is available. Infections of the nose, nasopharynx, or paranasal sinuses may drain into lymph nodes within the retropharyngeal tissues and develop into an abscess. Tonsillitis may lead to a peritonsillar abscess and can extend into the lateral pharyngeal space. Infections of the temporal bone or petrous apex can also eventually involve the lateral pharyngeal space. Oral infections or salivary gland diseases may develop abscesses that can extend into the tissue spaces around the oral cavity.

SYMPTOMS AND CLINICAL MANIFESTATIONS

The approach to diagnosis of a deep neck space abscess differs according to the location of the infection. A careful history may elicit a causative relationship between an abscess and a preceding upper respiratory tract infection, tonsillitis, sinusitis, or other infectious source. Many children with a deep neck space abscess have no localizing signs or symptoms before the development of a suppurative deep neck space collection. A fever without a focus is often the first indication of a developing abscess.

Peritonsillar cellulitis or a peritonsillar abscess is suggested clinically by a history of a sore throat with fever, unilateral neck pain, dysphagia, trismus, drooling, and voice changes such as a muffled ''hot-potato'' voice. A **hot-potato voice** is the result of a closely located infection with inflammation and edema causing dysfunction of the muscles of the soft palate with resultant velopharyngeal insufficiency. Peritonsillar abscesses are uncommon in preschool children but become increasingly more frequent in children of elementary and secondary school age.

Parapharyngeal space abscesses frequently follow a severe upper respiratory tract infection, particularly if severe tonsillitis or peritonsillar cellulitis has occurred. Parapharyngeal abscesses are characterized by greater toxicity with spiking fever, chills, and sweats. Swelling of the parotid region laterally or medial bulging into the oral cavity as the tonsil and lateral pharyngeal wall is displaced into the oropharynx is sometimes the first indicator of an abscess within the parapharyngeal space. There may also be a fullness of the retromolar trigone area. Severe neck stiffness, dysphagia, trismus, and odynophagia may indicate involvement of the deeper parapharyngeal structures.

Retropharyngeal abscesses may occur in the very young, and have been reported in neonates after traumatic intubation. Signs and symptoms of a retropharyngeal abscess may be obscure; the first symptom often is the refusal of an infant or small child to eat. Most commonly, retropharyngeal abscess follows an upper respiratory tract infection in younger children or follows oropharyngeal trauma or foreign body insertion in older children. There usually is a sore throat, with a moderate fever and often restlessness. As the swelling progresses in the posterior pharyngeal wall, the voice becomes muffled and the airway may become increasingly obstructed. Dysphagia and drooling may occur. Neck swelling is common, and neck rigidity, or torticollis, may be misinterpreted as cervical trauma or meningitis.

Physical Examination Findings

The physical examination of a child with a neck abscess may be somewhat difficult. Often the child is uncomfortable, irritable, and febrile, and the affected region may be tender to palpation. Intraoral abscess formation is often difficult to evaluate because a child may have trismus coupled with the associated discomfort and irritability. Peritonsillar cellulitis and abscess frequently cause inflammation of the muscles of mastication, particularly the pterygoid muscles, which results in trismus. There may be cervical lymphadenopathy and tenderness along the mandibular angle of the involved side. If an intraoral examination is possible, the examination reveals a pharyngotonsillar bulge that pushes the swollen and erythematous tonsil, soft palate, and uvula toward the unaffected side. In general, the degree of pharyngeal bulge and the likelihood of a muffled voice are greater among patients with an abscess than among those with cellulitis. With the exception of ''pointing'' of a clinically significant abscess, no single clinical finding can reliably differentiate between an abscess and cellulitis at the time of presentation. Most peritonsillar abscesses occur around the superior pole of the palatine tonsil, but abscess formation around the inferior pole is not uncommon. A suppurative fluid collection develops in the fascial space between the tonsillar tissue and the fibers of the superior constrictor muscle. As the abscess enlarges, the surrounding tissues become inflamed and the structures are displaced medially.

The physical findings of a parapharyngeal space abscess include systemic toxicity and bulging of the lateral pharyngeal wall. The intraoral findings are more posterior than a peritonsillar abscess and involve the lateral pharyngeal wall and the posterior pharyngeal wall, sparing the palatine tonsil and the soft palate.

The physical findings of a retropharyngeal abscess are similar to those of a parapharyngeal space abscess in that they appear as a posterior pharyngeal swelling. A retropharyngeal abscess may be difficult to detect clinically in a small child because of the small oral cavity, small airway, and tendency to pool oral secretions. Intraoral palpation and manipulation should be avoided to minimize the possibility of rupture of the abscess into the pharynx. Rupture of an intraoral abscess may lead to the aspiration of the abscess contents, leading to pulmonary complications. Cervical lymphadenopathy with tenderness and swelling may also be present with infections of these spaces.

DIAGNOSIS

The diagnosis of deep space neck infections is generally first considered on the basis of the clinical presentation. Either CT or MRI can be used to establish an accurate anatomic diagnosis. Needle aspiration may provide important bacteriologic information and confirm the diagnosis. In some situations, such as a suspected peritonsillar abscess, a fine-needle aspiration with the removal of pus from the peritonsillar space will confirm the diagnosis, obviating the need for radiographic studies. However, most deep neck abscesses are not as easily approached, and a rapid diagnosis with needle aspiration is neither safe nor specific in determining the precise anatomic limits of an abscess.

Differential Diagnosis

Many pathologic processes may present as a neck mass or neck asymmetry. Noninfectious causes of neck masses (e.g., cystic hygroma, branchial cleft cyst) are not associated with the acute clinical symptoms of fever and systemic toxicity characteristic of deep neck space abscesses.

Superficial neck abscesses that do not involve the deeper fascial spaces frequently occur in infants and children but are not as prone to complications as deeper abscesses. The more superficial infections are often preceded by upper respiratory tract infections but may also be associated with more specific causes, such as cat-scratch disease, infected lateral neck cyst, or infected thyroglossal duct cysts. Superficial infections can usually be managed by treating the primary condition by aspiration of the abscess and antibiotic therapy. Infections of congenital cysts (e.g., thyroglossal duct or branchial cleft cyst) generally respond well to antibiotic therapy, with or without aspiration, followed later by surgical excision.

Laboratory Evaluation

Laboratory studies for children with suspected deep neck space infections might include a CBC, electrolyte studies, and bleeding studies such as a prothrombin time and partial thromboplastin time if surgery is being considered. Throat culture, blood, or wound cultures may also be obtained. The WBC count is usually elevated with a predominance of polymorphonuclear leukocytes. However, laboratory studies are usually not specific for a deep space abscess and cannot differentiate the anatomic site.

Diagnostic Imaging

Plain radiography of the neck may demonstrate soft tissue swelling and airway displacement, but it cannot reliably distinguish cellulitis from abscess formation. A true lateral radiograph is required with the neck in full extension, on full inspiration if possible. The tissues of the retropharyngeal wall are very pliable, and neck flexion, swallowing, crying, or weak inspiratory effort can cause the appearance of thickened retropharyngeal tissues and may be misleading. If plain radiographs are obtained, a lateral neck radiograph is most helpful in the evaluation of a suspected retropharyngeal abscess; it reveals a convex, widened, and bulging retropharyngeal space (Fig. 59–2, *A*). Also, there is commonly a loss of the normal curvature of the cervical spine, and it appears straightened. Gas is occasionally visualized within soft tissues. A chest radiograph may also be obtained in these circumstances to evaluate for pneumonia or mediastinitis.

Improved diagnostic imaging has improved diagnostic precision in deep neck space infections and has thereby improved the manner in which management decisions are reached. Either CT or MRI may provide sharp anatomic localization of an infection and allow differentiation of cellulitis from an abscess. A CT study with intravenous contrast is the diagnostic modality of choice and will reveal a rim-enhancing lesion where the abscess periphery appears denser than the low-density center (Fig. 59–2, *B*). Contrast also improves visualization of vascular and lymphatic structures around an abscess. The CT studies are ideally performed during full inspiration with the image obtained perpendicular to the axis of the airway. These advanced studies are more frequently used in the evaluation of suspected abscesses around the carotid sheath, retropharynx, or parapharyngeal space. CT may also distinguish between peritonsillar abscess and cellulitis, which is clinically useful because fully developed abscesses are most properly treated with surgical drainage, sometimes urgently in the event of an enlarging abscess with airway compromise. In contrast, cellulitis generally responds to medical therapy, obviating unnecessary drainage procedures. However, it may be difficult or impossible to differentiate between cellulitis and tissue edema on the basis of an enhanced CT, leaving this differentiation to be made on the basis of clinical presentation and physical findings. Because CT scans are not perfectly sensitive, patients may have studies that do not reveal an abscess although the patients are clinically worse. In these situations, surgical drainage is required, even in the face of a negative or questionable CT scan.

TREATMENT

Management of deep neck abscesses includes antimicrobial therapy and otolaryngologic evaluation for incision and drainage procedures. Hospitalization is invariably required for peritonsillar abscesses in very young children and for all parapharyngeal and retropharyngeal abscesses. Because of the similarities in causative organisms, many physicians use a similar antimicrobial regimen for patients with neck abscesses involving different sites, which should provide coverage for streptococci, penicillin-resistant *S. aureus,* and anaerobic organisms, including *Bacteroides, Peptococcus,* and *Veillonella.* Most abscesses are polymicrobial, with β-lactamase production by up to 50% of organisms. A penicillinase-resistant penicillin (e.g., nafcillin or oxacillin), a penicillin-penicillinase inhibitor (e.g., ampicillin-sulbactam intravenously, or amoxicillin-clavulanate orally), or a third-generation cephalosporin are considered drugs of choice. Clindamycin is used with increasing frequency with the advent of new information that suggests a more important role of anaerobes and is an appropriate therapy for many difficult-to-treat pediatric head and neck infections, including peritonsillar, parapharyngeal, and retropharyngeal infections.

The range of possible causative organisms is broad, and therefore bacterial isolation can be extremely helpful in determining optimal therapy. At the time of surgical drainage a specimen should be obtained for aerobic and anaerobic culture. Strict anaerobic technique must be maintained for sensitive anaerobic culture. A Gram stain may provide interim information.

All deep neck space infections have the potential to cause airway obstruction, and may occur very rapidly. Continued consideration

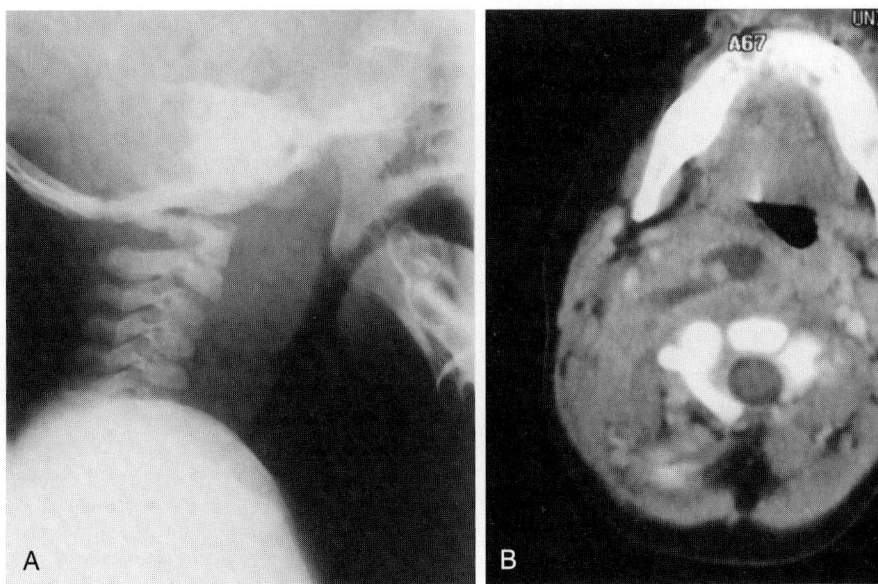

FIGURE 59–2. A, Lateral neck radiograph of a child showing marked widening of the retropharyngeal soft tissues causing narrowing and anterior displacement of the hypopharynx. The cervical spine lacks the normal lordotic curvature. The lucency inferiorly suggests an abscess. **B,** A computed tomography study with contrast in the axial view through the hypopharynx shows the same abscess illustrated in *A.* A rim-enhancing lesion with central lucency displaces the retropharyngeal structures. The hypopharyngeal airway is compromised.

to the protection of a child's airway is paramount and may require intubation or tracheotomy. If an abscess has involved the muscles of mastication, trismus may be an issue, and airway management may dictate the need for a tracheotomy. The decision to secure an artificial airway must be made before a child's condition deteriorates to the point of airway loss. Concern for the airway should also be expressed when one elects to perform radiographic studies, especially for small children who may require sedation for a CT or MRI study. If the airway is questionable because of a suspected abscess formation, sedating the child will likely increase the risk of airway compromise and may force an emergent airway procedure that might otherwise have been avoided.

Peritonsillar Cellulitis and Abscess. Peritonsillar cellulitis generally responds well to medical therapy without surgical intervention, provided the antimicrobial therapy is appropriate and the child's immune defense mechanisms are intact. Once an abscess develops, however, surgical evacuation is the standard treatment. Often it is difficult to distinguish between a peritonsillar cellulitis and a mature abscess. Historically, the inability to make a clinical distinction between the two has sometimes led to unnecessary operations and inappropriate management. Currently, the initial clinical response to parenteral antibiotic therapy, with additional information provided by CT or MRI, usually distinguishes cellulitis from an abscess and provides guidelines for management. If an abscess is not clinically obvious and if the airway is not compromised, children presenting with severe peritonsillar infections can receive a trial of intravenous hydration and parenteral antibiotic therapy. If the signs and symptoms improve, antibiotic therapy can be continued with a switch to oral medication when the patient's condition allows. If there is no improvement after 24–48 hours or if there is clinical deterioration, a CT or MRI may be performed to differentiate cellulitis from an abscess. For older children, a clinically obvious abscess can be aspirated surgically in an outpatient setting. Aspiration is followed by oral antibiotic therapy and close observation on an outpatient basis until resolution or until an unfavorable course directs a more aggressive therapy.

Surgical aspiration of peritonsillar abscesses has become increasingly popular in recent years for older children in whom this procedure can be performed without general anesthesia. General anesthesia is required in younger, uncooperative children, but the decision to use local or general anesthesia may be tailored to the maturity level of the patient. Furthermore, the risk of bleeding or of aspiration of purulent secretions is greater for younger patients, who have smaller airways and more difficulty in handling their secretions. For young children who require general anesthesia, it is generally agreed that a brief period of intravenous hydration and parenteral antibiotic therapy followed by a simultaneous tonsillectomy and drainage of the abscess (a **"quinsy tonsillectomy"**) is the appropriate treatment protocol. Most experts do not consider a single episode of peritonsillar abscess that was successfully treated by nonsurgical means to be an absolute indication for a subsequent tonsillectomy, although there is evidence to suggest that the incidence of recurrence is much greater if a tonsillectomy is not performed in the interval period. Therefore, some experts recommend interval tonsillectomy, even after a single episode of peritonsillar abscess. Tonsillectomy is clearly indicated for patients with recurring peritonsillar abscesses. When tonsillectomy is indicated for the treatment of peritonsillar abscess, bilateral tonsillectomy is usually performed because of the possibility of a peritonsillar abscess occurring on the opposite side.

Parapharyngeal Abscess. The presence of a severe parapharyngeal space abscess almost always requires surgical intervention in addition to appropriate medical therapy. Any hemorrhage associated with infections in these spaces requires emergency surgical exploration. It is desirable to avoid intraoral drainage of these abscesses, even though there may be a prominence of the glottal area, the pharyngeal wall, or the tonsillar area that may be inviting to the treating physician. The pharyngeal abscess is usually approached externally through the neck so that external drainage may be acquired and vessel ligation can be performed if required. Erosion of the carotid artery carries a significant mortality rate; therefore, the examining physician must be aware of this possibility and be aware of warning signs of possible arterial rupture. Signs of a possible hemorrhage include swelling with hematoma, neurologic alterations of cranial nerve IX, X, XI, or XII, Horner's syndrome, or systemic shock.

Retropharyngeal Abscess. Retropharyngeal abscesses must be treated aggressively because progression may lead to airway compromise, spontaneous rupture with aspiration pneumonitis, or extension inferiorly into the posterior part of the chest. Children without airway compromise or other impending complications may be treated by an initial trial of intravenous antibiotic therapy. If marked improvement is not apparent within 24 to 48 hours, however, incision and drainage is advised. Historically, the surgical approach has been an external approach with drainage to the outside, not an intraoral approach. Incision and drainage usually results in rapid resolution of the abscess. There are those who advocate surgical drainage of selected retropharyngeal and parapharyngeal abscesses by a transoral route. The proponents of this technique have shown that in selected cases transoral drainage is safe and effective, and external drainage of deep neck abscesses is reserved for abscesses that are more distant from the oral and pharyngeal walls. Transoral drainage limits the exposure of vessels and increases the risk of aspiration. The abscess itself may provide some protection to the great vessels, as the abscess tends to displace the vessels laterally, providing a margin of safety during an intraoral procedure. Some experts recommend placing a patient under general anesthesia and then performing a needle aspiration of the retropharyngeal abscess. If gross purulence is encountered, then continuation of an intraoral drainage is initiated. If blood is encountered, then a retreat is made from a transoral approach and a lateral neck approach is taken.

COMPLICATIONS

Complications are associated with a delay in diagnosis and the cervical structures involved in the infection. Edema in the surrounding airway may spread rapidly to involve the larynx; and although a tracheotomy can usually be avoided, aggressive medical or surgical treatment may be necessary to relieve airway obstruction.

Potential complications of peritonsillar cellulitis and abscess include dehydration from poor fluid intake, spontaneous rupture into the oropharynx with possible aspiration pneumonitis, and extension into other deep neck spaces or beyond. As an abscess develops, it can rupture through the tonsillar capsule (pharyngobasilar fascia) and the superior constrictor muscle, which provides access to the parapharyngeal space. From the parapharyngeal space the infection may expand into the retropharynx, carotid sheath, and eventually the mediastinum. Although commonly seen, the potential hazards of untreated or inadequately treated peritonsillar abscesses are not often considered and can be life threatening.

Parapharyngeal abscesses may extend inferiorly into the chest, resulting in mediastinitis. These infections have access to the carotid sheath area with the potential of causing thrombosis of the internal jugular vein. Worse scenarios include erosion of the internal carotid artery, which may lead to fatal hemorrhage; the external carotid artery can be ligated, when eroded, usually without complications. Parapharyngeal abscesses may extend superiorly and can even rupture into the external auditory canal. Bleeding from the external auditory canal may indicate infectious spread and vessel erosion; physical examination reveals a normal tympanic membrane in such cases.

Retropharyngeal abscesses may extend into the parapharyngeal space and spread to adjoining deep neck spaces. There may be further spread of infection inferiorly into the mediastinum as an infection moves along and ruptures through the prevertebral fascia. Atlantoaxial dislocation is a rare but recognized complication.

PROGNOSIS

Early diagnosis and treatment with appropriate antimicrobial agents, coupled with surgical incision and drainage of abscesses, result in a good prognosis. Recurrence of peritonsillar abscesses after successful treatment is unusual but may be more common after needle aspiration than after traditional surgical drainage. Some experts recommend interval tonsillectomy, even after successful medical treatment of a single episode of peritonsillar abscess.

PREVENTION

Because most infections of the deep fascial spaces of the neck follow upper respiratory tract infections, early recognition and treatment of pharyngitis and tonsillitis preclude these complications.

REVIEWS

Goldenberg D, Golz A, Joachims HZ: Retropharyngeal abscess: A clinical review. *J Laryngol Otol* 1997;111:546–50.

Hawkins DB, Austin JR: Abscesses of the neck in infants and young children: A review of 112 cases. *Ann Otol Rhinol Laryngol* 1991; 100:361–5.

Nagy M, Pizzuto M, Backstrom J, et al: Deep neck infections in children: A new approach to diagnosis and treatment. *Laryngoscope* 1997; 107:1627–34.

KEY ARTICLES

Asmar BI: Bacteriology of retropharyngeal abscess in children. *Pediatr Infect Dis J* 1990;9:595–7.

Brook I, Frazier EH, Thompson DH: Aerobic and anaerobic microbiology of peritonsillar abscess. *Laryngoscope* 1991;101:289–92.

Brechtelsbauer PB, Garetz SL, Gebarski SS, et al: Retropharyngeal abscess: Pitfalls of plain films and computed tomography. *Am J Otolaryngol* 1997;18:258–62.

Brodsky L, Sobie SR, Korwin D, et al: A clinical prospective study of peritonsillar abscess in children. *Laryngoscope* 1988;98:780–3.

Brook I: Microbiology of abscesses of the head and neck in children. *Ann Otol Rhinol Laryngol* 1987;96:429–33.

Coulthard M, Isaacs D: Neonatal retropharyngeal abscess. *Pediatr Infect Dis J* 1991;10:547–9.

Dodds B, Maniglia AJ: Peritonsillar and neck abscesses in the pediatric age group. *Laryngoscope* 1988;98:956–9.

Gaglani MJ, Moise AA, Demmler GJ: Neonatal radiology casebook: Retropharyngeal abscess in the neonate. *J Perinatol* 1996;16:231–3.

Jokipii AM, Jokipii L, Sipila P, et al: Semiquantitative culture results and pathogenic significance of obligate anaerobes in peritonsillar abscesses. *J Clin Microbiol* 1988;26:957–61.

Kronenberg J, Wolf M, Leventon G: Peritonsillar abscess: Recurrence rate and the indication for tonsillectomy. *Am J Otolaryngol* 1987;8:82–4.

Ophr D, Bawnik J, Poria Y, et al: Peritonsillar abscess: A prospective evaluation of outpatient management by needle aspiration. *Arch Otolaryngol Head Neck Surg* 1988;114:661–3.

Patel KS, Ahmad S, O'Leary G, et al: The role of computerized tomography in the management of peritonsillar abscess. *Otolaryngol Head Neck Surg* 1992;107:727–32.

Ravi KV, Brooks JR: Peritonsillar abscess—An unusual presentation of Kawaski disease. *J Laryngol Otol* 1997;111:73–4.

Sichel JY, Gomori JM, Saah D, et al: Parapharyngeal abscess in children: The role of CT for diagnosis and treatment. *Int J Ped Otolaryngol* 1996;35:213–22.

Szuhay G, Tewfik TL: Peritonsillar abscess or cellulitis? A clinical comparative pediatric study. *J Otolaryngol* 1998;27:206–12.

CHAPTER 60

Stomatitis

Celia D.C. Christie

The syndrome of stomatitis is characterized by superficial oral erosions, papules, ulcerations, or vesicles involving the vermilion border, buccal and labial mucosae, palate, tongue, floor of the mouth, and gingivae.

ETIOLOGY

Stomatitis includes several overlapping syndromes caused by *Candida albicans* and many different viruses (Table 60–1). Oral candidiasis, or **thrush,** is caused by *C. albicans*. Gingivostomatitis is often a synonym for primary herpetic stomatitis and labialis. Herpes simplex virus (HSV) type 1 is the usual etiologic agent of herpetic stomatitis and gingivostomatitis, although HSV-2 causes a small proportion of clinically indistinguishable illnesses. The mouth is the most frequent site of HSV-1 infection. Members of the family Picornaviridae cause herpangina and hand-foot-and-mouth disease. Herpangina is a characteristic pharyngeal ulceration caused by many coxsackieviruses and echoviruses. Hand-foot-and-mouth disease is a distinct illness that is usually caused by coxsackievirus A16 but that may be caused by other coxsackieviruses. Vesicular stomatitis is caused by vesicular stomatitis virus (VSV) and related vesiculoviruses, which are members of the family Rhabdoviridae. Most human infections are caused by VSV serotype New Jersey, found in the southeastern United States, Central America, and northern South America, and VSV serotype Indiana, found in Central America and northern South America.

Recurrent aphthous ulcers, also known as aphthae and canker sores, are a frequent cause of oral ulcerative conditions, affecting 10–50% of the population. Although infectious agents such as the L forms of *Streptococcus sanguis* have been implicated in the causation of recurrent aphthous ulcers, a definitive cause has not been identified. Aphthous stomatitis is especially problematic in persons with AIDS.

EPIDEMIOLOGY

Oral Candidiasis. *C. albicans* is ubiquitous in the gastrointestinal and genital tracts and is transmitted by person-to-person contact. Newborns can acquire *Candida* either perinatally, while passing through the birth canal, or postnatally. Most neonates and infants with oral candidiasis have only mild disease. Severe oral candidiasis may develop in children with congenital or acquired immunodeficiency.

Herpetic Gingivostomatitis. Primary infection with HSV-1 usually occurs in children 1–5 years of age, with the highest incidence from 9 to 36 months. Perinatally acquired HSV infection presenting in neonates is a serious, life-threatening disease (Chapter 97). Antibodies to HSV-1 develop in 90% of the population by the age of 15 years, although about 30% of children from middle- and upper-income families reach adulthood without serologic evidence of infection. Similar to other herpesviruses, HSV establishes lifelong infection in the host. It is primarily transmitted by direct contact with draining mucosal lesions or by asymptomatic shedding.

Other Forms of Stomatitis. The enteroviruses, which include coxsackieviruses and echoviruses, are common causes of febrile illnesses in children with nonspecific or overlapping symptoms, including stomatitis (Table 60–1). Humans are the only known hosts of enteroviruses. Enteroviral infections occur worldwide, with uniform prevalence year-round in tropical climates and with peaks in summer and fall in temperate climates, often in epidemics. Infection usually occurs in children 1–5 years of age, with decreasing frequency with advancing age. Enteroviral infections are uncommon in infants because of protective levels of maternal antibody.

Vesicular stomatitis is primarily a disease of livestock (e.g., horses, cattle, and pigs), and the viruses are infrequent causes of zoonotic human illness. They are harbored in the oral secretions and vesicles of infected wild and domestic animals in southern United States and Central and South America and are a common cause of epidemics of febrile infections in animals. Disease in animals is seen in the United States during the summer and fall months in the Gulf States, in the Mississippi River Valley, and in the Rocky Mountains. Because this infection is common in animals, almost all livestock handlers and veterinarians in endemic areas have antibodies to these viruses. From 25–95% of all persons in endemic areas have serologic evidence of infection, but a history of clinical illness with characteristic symptoms is uncommon.

PATHOGENESIS

Oral Candidiasis. Oral candidiasis—thrush or **acute pseudomembranous candidiasis**—in newborns possibly develops as a result of oral inoculation with *Candida* before the normal bacterial flora becomes established. Mucosal colonization is characterized by epithelial adherence of the *Candida* blastophores. Transformation to the mycelial form precedes mucosal invasion. This results in an adherent pseudomembrane composed of the components of the blastospore and pseudohyphae of *Candida*. Mucosal lesions progress to sharply demarcated ulcers, with a granulation tissue base admixed with neutrophils, *Candida,* and fibrin. In immunocompromised patients, tissue invasion occurs with hematogenous dissemination to distant sites.

Herpetic Gingivostomatitis. The pathologic changes in the epithelium for primary and recurrent HSV infection are similar but are quantitatively more severe with primary infection. HSV infects the parabasal and intermediate layers of the epithelium. Cell lysis results in accumulation of cellular debris between the epidermis and the dermis. Viremia is rare with herpetic gingivostomatitis in

TABLE 60–1. Viral Causes of Stomatitis

Oral Herpetic Gingivostomatitis and Labialis
Herpes simplex virus type 1 (herpes simplex virus type 2 less often)
Herpangina
Coxsackieviruses A16, A5, A9, A7 (A1, A2, A3, A4, A6, A8, A10, A22 less often)
Coxsackieviruses B1, B2, B3, B4, B5
Echoviruses 9, 11, 17, 20 (5, 16, 22, 25 less often)
Vesicular Stomatitis
Vesicular stomatitis virus serotypes New Jersey and Indiana (other vesiculoviruses less often)

immunocompetent persons but may occur as part of disseminated infection in immunocompromised persons.

With resolution of epidermal infection, HSV establishes latent infection in neural ganglia, such as the trigeminal, sacral, and vagal ganglia. Predisposing factors to reactivation of latent HSV include febrile infectious illnesses, psychological or physiologic stress, menstruation, mechanical trauma, exposure to sunlight and ultraviolet light, acupuncture, and others. The exact mechanism of HSV reactivation is unknown. Reactivation is associated with variable severity of oral involvement and accompanying pain, but without the fever, lymphadenopathy, and constitutional symptoms of primary infection.

Other Forms of Stomatitis. The enteroviruses are transmitted from person to person by respiratory droplet and aerosols as well as by the fecal-oral route. They gain entry to the body through the mouth, directly seed the oral mucosa and the alimentary tract, and then extend to the regional lymph nodes. Viremia then develops with extension of the infection to distant sites in approximately 7 days. Viruses continue to be shed from the intestinal tract after the infection has cleared and symptoms disappear. The pathogenicity depends on the viral inoculum and the virulence of the infecting serotypes as well as on host factors, the most common enteroviruses causing herpangina include coxsackieviruses A16, A5, and A9; coxsackieviruses B1, B2, B3, B4, and B5; and echoviruses 9, 11, 17, and 20. Coxsackievirus A16 is the principal agent of hand-foot-and-mouth disease; coxsackieviruses A9, A5, and A10 are less frequently implicated. Immunity to the enteroviruses is species- and type-specific.

Vesicular stomatitis virus and related vesiculoviruses cause an acute febrile illness in animals similar to hand-foot-and-mouth disease. Infections are transmitted among animals by insect vectors (sandflies and black flies) but are transmitted to humans by aerosols or through direct contact between conjunctivae or abrasions on the skin and the oral secretions or vesicles of infected livestock. There is a high rate of transmission on exposure. In humans these viruses rarely cause an acute febrile illness, usually with oral vesicular lesions but otherwise without distinguishing features.

The cause of aphthous ulcers is unknown. Trauma, usually inapparent, is probably a common predisposing factor in the development of aphthous ulcers. Other contributing factors that have been considered include psychosomatic causes and autoimmune phenomena. There is evidence of an immunopathogenetic basis due to altered cell-mediated immune reactions. Allergic disease, possibly food allergy, is suggested by elevated serum IgD and IgE concentrations compared with the concentrations in patients with other ulcerative mouth disorders and healthy controls. Other recognized predisposing factors are an association with transient IgA immunodeficiency of childhood and humoral immunodeficiencies.

SYMPTOMS AND CLINICAL MANIFESTATIONS

Oral Candidiasis. Oral candidiasis is the most common presentation of candidiasis in infants and children. The incubation period for oral thrush is unknown. Mucosal infection is manifest by mucocutaneous red erosions and white, ulcerative, and raised plaquelike lesions that resemble milk curds. Later the lesions coalesce to form an adherent pseudomembrane, which leaves a raw, erythematous, bleeding, denuded base if forcibly removed, **Perlèche,** or **angular cheilitis,** which results from the repetitive lip smacking, may be an associated development. **Chronic mucocutaneous candidiasis** is characterized by recurrent, severe candidiasis involving the mucosae, nails, and skin. It usually occurs in persons with severe cell-mediated immunodeficiency.

Herpetic Gingivostomatitis. The incubation period of oral HSV illness is about 7 days, with a range of 2–25 days. Primary HSV infection is more severe than recurrent illness and is usually well tolerated. Clinical features of primary HSV gingivostomatitis include high fever, anorexia for liquid and solid food, dehydration, malaise, stinging mouth pain, drooling, fetor oris (fetid breath), oropharyngeal vesicular lesions, and lymphadenopathy. Grouped lesions on an erythematous base can be seen around the stomal opening as well as on the tongue, gingivae, lips, and oral mucosa and on the soft and hard palate. The lesions usually become crusted and heal within 5–10 days, but occasionally they may last as long as 3 weeks.

Primary HSV stomatitis often involves the gingivae and the vermilion border, with extensive involvement and rapid progression of macules to vesicles over 24 hours. Extraoral lesions are present in approximately 75% of children. Individual vesicles caused by HSV are round to oval, sharply demarcated, approximately 2–4 mm in diameter, and tend to form grouped vesicles on an erythematous base. Vesicles usually last about 24 hours before they open and evolve into shallow gray ulcers with a friable gray base or pseudomembrane. The lesions are tender and bleed on contact. As they resolve, they develop a dark or black crust. There is fetor oris. Primary infection is usually accompanied by fever and tender lymphadenopathy, which are often absent with recurrent disease. The lesions persist for 12 days, with a range of 9–15 days, and heal without scarring.

Limited involvement to only a portion of the vermilion border is more characteristic of recurrent illness than primary HSV infection; this presentation is often known as **herpes labialis** (Fig. 60–1). Recurrences usually are at the same location for each individual. Recurrences are usually preceded by pain, stinging, or burning; thereafter blisters erupt on an erythematous base.

Herpangina. Symptoms of herpangina develop after an incubation period of approximately 4 days, with a range of 2–10 days. The major symptoms are sudden onset of high fever, vomiting, headache, malaise, myalgia, backache, conjunctivitis, anorexia for liquids, drooling, sore throat, and dysphagia. This presentation may be similar to the initial presentation of other serious enteroviral illnesses, including aseptic meningitis, encephalitis, and myocarditis.

The oral lesions of herpangina may be nonspecific, but classically there are one or more small, tender, papular, or pinpoint

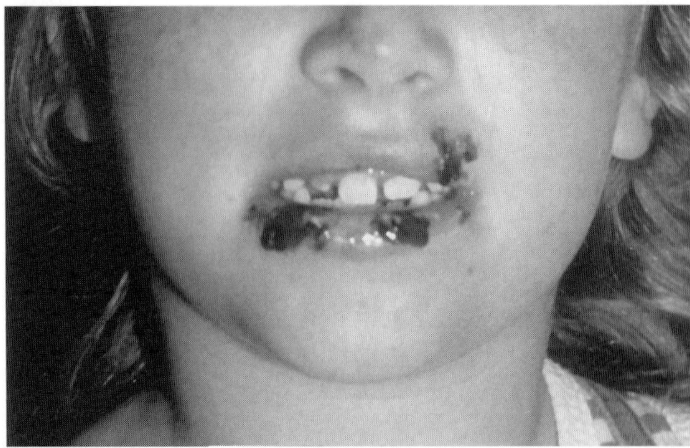

FIGURE 60–1. Herpes gingivostomatitis, or primary herpes simplex virus infection, with extensive ulceration. (Courtesy of Neil S. Prose.)

vesicular lesions on an erythematous base scattered over the soft palate, uvula, fauces, and tongue (Plate 7D). These vesicles enlarge from 1–2 to 3–4 mm over 3–4 days, rupture, and produce small, punched-out ulcers that persist for several days.

Hand-Foot-and-Mouth-Disease. The symptoms of hand-foot-and-mouth disease develop after an incubation period of 2–6 days. A cutaneous eruption with bilateral symmetrical distribution on the extremities precedes the oral exanthem. About 30 and occasionally up to 100 lesions are seen on the borders and surfaces of the palms and soles. Lesions begin as tiny, pinpoint erythematous but painful papules that evolve over about 2 days (Plate 4F). They develop into grayish vesicles that resolve spontaneously in about 10 days. Oral lesions begin as painful aphthous sores. The vesicular phase is short and may be missed. Mouth lesions are few and generally number about 10. Frequently they involve the buccal mucosa and the lips. There is minimal cervical lymphadenopathy. Constitutional symptoms of malaise, low-grade fever, and anorexia are mild.

Vesicular Stomatitis. The usual incubation period for vesicular stomatitis after contact with an infected animal is 2–8 days. Infection in humans is usually asymptomatic, but up to 50% of infected persons may experience a mild febrile illness with fever, chills, malaise, weakness, and myalgia. Up to 25% of individuals may have oral erythematous vesicular lesions that progress to discrete ulcers. Tonsillar and cervical lymphadenopathy is usually present. The disorder spontaneously resolves after about 4–7 days. No complications in humans have been reported.

Aphthous Ulcers. The clinical features of recurrent aphthous ulcers include a prodromal phase with a burning sensation at the site of mucosal ulceration. This is followed by local erythema and mucosal necrosis. Focal ulcerations with several small ulcers develop, sometimes coalescing into lesions larger than 1 cm in diameter. The lesions have a gray, exudative, shaggy, necrotic base surrounded by a raised erythematous margin. There is involvement of the lingual or buccal oral mucosa, the floor of the mouth, or the tongue; the soft palate is rarely involved. The ulcers are extremely painful and usually interfere with eating and speaking. Lesions persist for 10–14 days and then heal without scarring. Complications include recurrence of the syndrome, occasionally up to six times annually.

A syndrome of **periodic fever, aphthous stomatitis, pharyngitis, and cervical adenitis (PFAPA)** is an occasional cause of recurring nonspecific pharyngitis accompanied by fever and aphthae (Chapter 58). The fevers begin at an early age, usually <5 years. Episodes last approximately 5 days, or less if treated with oral prednisone, with a mean of 28 days between episodes. Episodes are unresponsive to nonsteroidal anti-inflammatory agents or antibiotics.

DIAGNOSIS

Candida and viral stomatitis are diagnosed on the basis of the characteristic mucocutaneous lesions. The specific cause may be suggested by the characteristic appearance of the lesions or additional symptoms as in hand-foot-and-mouth disease. In the immunocompetent person there is little benefit from fungal or viral cultures to confirm the diagnosis because oral candidiasis is easily treated and viral illnesses are self-limited and are treated symptomatically.

Vesicles on the oral mucosa in a neonate are an important indicator of perinatally acquired HSV disease, which requires further investigation (Chapter 97).

Differential Diagnosis

HSV gingivostomatitis characteristically presents with lesions in the anterior fauces, in contrast to herpangina, which involves the posterior fauces predominantly. Primary HSV stomatitis is more severe than herpangina, has a longer clinical course, and has no seasonal predilection. Oral lesions associated with enteroviral infections may be associated with a macular erythematous exanthem, unlike HSV stomatitis. HSV stomatitis may be differentiated from primary varicella (chickenpox) by the lack of systemic vesicular lesions, especially if there is a history of chickenpox or lack of exposure to chickenpox. Adolescents can sometimes incur primary HSV stomatitis that may present with exudative pharyngitis and tonsillitis resembling infectious mononucleosis (Chapter 37). The presence of painful vesicular orolabial or intraoral lesions is not characteristic of Epstein-Barr virus infection.

Illness from vesicular stomatitis virus is usually mild and clinically indistinct from enteroviral or HSV infections. The diagnosis is difficult to distinguish clinically but is suggested by the epidemiologic link of contact with infected animals or livestock.

The absence of signs of deep tissue infection differentiates these superficial infections from bacterial infections in the oral cavity (Chapter 61). **Noma,** also known as **cancrum oris** or **gangrenous stomatitis,** is a polymicrobial infection caused by mouth flora, especially anaerobes and the fusospirochetal organisms *Borrelia vincentii* and *Fusobacterium nucleatum.* The infection typically begins at the gingiva but rapidly spreads to involve the lips and cheeks with destruction of the deep tissues. The pathogenesis and management are more closely related to deeper infections in the oral cavity, such as Ludwig's angina, rather than the more superficial mucosal ulcerative or vesicular lesions of stomatitis.

Stomatitis and intraoral erosions must be differentiated from the mucosal lesions of Behçet's disease and from mucosal ulceration and mucositis commonly associated with primary immunodeficiency, cancer chemotherapy, and radiation therapy. Certain cancer chemotherapeutic drugs often cause an erythematous mucositis that develops 3–5 days after initiation of chemotherapy. Ulcerative lesions may develop after 7 days.

Microbiologic Evaluation

In immunosuppressed patients with oral thrush, yeasts and pseudohyphae are identified in infected mucosae by Gram's stain and by microscopic examination of scrapings suspended in 10% KOH. Confirmation of the specific viral cause is usually unnecessary. Viral cultures of lesions can document the specific etiologic agent for HSV stomatitis, herpangina, hand-foot-and-mouth disease, and vesicular stomatitis. A Tzanck smear for evidence of HSV infections may be performed but is only 70% as sensitive as culture for HSV. Culture is recommended for microbiologic confirmation of suspected HSV infection. Viral cultures of stool are useful in isolating the enteroviral agent of herpangina and of hand-foot-and-mouth disease.

Serologic Diagnosis. Fourfold changes in serologic antibody titer in acute and convalescent serologic samples drawn 2–4 weeks apart can be used to document primary HSV infection. Serologic testing is not useful for diagnosis of recurrences. Serologic testing to document herpangina or hand-foot-and-mouth disease is not usually recommended because these are self-limited diseases with a good prognosis and because separate serologic tests would have to be performed for each enterovirus serotype known to cause disease. Serologic testing can be used to document infection with vesicular stomatitis virus.

TABLE 60–3. Treatment of Herpes Simplex Virus Gingivostomatitis

Primary Herpetic Gingivostomatitis
Acyclovir 75 mg/kg/day divided 5 times a day (max 200 mg/dose) PO for 7 days
plus
Symptomatic therapy
Recurrent Herpetic Gingivostomatitis (Begin with First Symptoms of Recurrence)
Acyclovir 75 mg/kg/day divided 5 times a day (max 200 mg/dose) PO for 5 days
or
Penciclovir cream 1% topical application q2hr while awake for 4 consecutive days
plus
Symptomatic therapy

TREATMENT

Definitive treatment is available for oral candidiasis and herpetic gingivostomatitis. Management of viral and aphthous stomatitis is primarily supportive, directed at relief of discomfort and, especially in immunocompromised patients, decreasing the risk of secondary bacterial infection. Symptomatic treatment is usually sufficient because most illnesses are self-limited and do not have associated complications.

Definitive Treatment

Oral thrush may be treated successfully with nystatin suspension or clotrimazole troches (Table 60–2). Gentian violet is also effective but stains skin and clothing and is messy. In immunosuppressed persons or those with chronic infections, fluconazole or ketoconazole may be necessary. However, the safety and efficacy have not been established for clotrimazole in children <3 years of age, fluconazole in children <6 months of age, and ketoconazole in children <2 years of age. Amphotericin B is recommended for use in immunocompromised patients to prevent local progression to esophagitis (Chapter 74) and also hematogenous dissemination.

TABLE 60–2. Treatment of Oral Candidiasis (Thrush)

Immunocompetent Persons
Recommended Regimen
Nystatin oral suspension, 200,000–400,000 U (2–4 mL) q4–6hr for 1 week or longer
or
Clotrimazole, 10 mg tablet, dissolved in the mouth, 5–6 times daily for 1 wk or longer
Alternative Regimen
Nystatin vaginal suppository, 100,000 U dissolved in the mouth q4hr
or
Gentian violet, 0.5% or 1% solution, swabbing of the buccal mucosa, twice daily
Immunocompromised Persons
Mild Infection Limited to Oral Candidiasis
Fluconazole 6 mg/kg initial dose PO followed by 3 mg/kg/day (max 100 mg) PO for 13 more days
Severe Oral Candidiasis
Amphotericin B 0.5 mg/kg/day IV for 3–7 days
Severe Oral Candidiasis with Fever and Suspected Dissemination
Treat as for disseminated candidiasis (Chapter 99)

Treatment of primary herpetic gingivostomatitis with oral acyclovir started within 72 hours of symptoms shortens the course of viral shedding and may hasten healing (Table 60–3). Topical therapy for primary herpetic gingivostomatitis has marginal benefits and is not recommended. Oral acyclovir therapy may also be beneficial in selected cases of HSV stomatitis presenting beyond 72 hours with severe symptoms of pain and fever, especially with gingival involvement, or in infants with significant impairment of oral intake of fluids. Treatment of primary infection does not, however, prevent the development of latent herpesvirus infection and therefore does not prevent recurrent outbreaks.

Recurrences may be ameliorated if treatment with oral acyclovir or topical penciclovir cream is begun when prodromal symptoms are first experienced, with improved lesion healing, pain resolution, and cessation of viral shedding (Table 60–3). Chronic suppressive therapy with low-dose oral acyclovir is helpful in the prevention of frequent recurrences of genital infection, but similar therapy for recurrent oral HSV infection is of unproved efficacy and is rarely warranted on the basis of severity of symptoms.

Other than occasional complaints of nausea, no clinically significant short-term side effects are common with oral acyclovir. The dose of acyclovir should be altered in the presence of renal insufficiency.

In immunocompromised persons, especially solid organ or bone marrow transplant recipients who have severe oral mucositis, oral acyclovir for mild disease may be of benefit in limiting local infection. Intravenous acyclovir for at least 7 days is recommended if systemic signs of infection are present or if the infection appears to be disseminating with extraoral cutaneous lesions or respiratory symptoms suggestive of pulmonary extension. Oral or intravenous therapy should also be considered for patients with a chronic skin disorder that may predispose to development of **eczema herpeticum** (Chapter 46).

Supportive Therapy

Supportive measures include application of topical anesthetics, soothing mouthwashes and rinses, and coating agents in a variety of formulations (Table 60–4), as well as oral nonaspirin analgesics and antipyretic agents. Small children may better tolerate oral hydration with small frequent amounts of oral fluids, bland liquids, and ice slushes; nasogastric tube feedings are rarely necessary. Mouthwashes or dentifrices that contain alcohol, phenol, or aro-

TABLE 60–4. Topical Medications in the Management of Oral Mucositis

Topical Anesthetics

Viscous lidocaine, 2%: Several flavored preparations are available. Apply to the affected areas with cotton-tipped applicator. Caution: May cause burning, suppression of gag reflex, and dysphagia; may increase the risk of aspiration.

Benzocaine, 15%: Apply to the affected area with cotton-tipped applicator. Caution: May cause burning, suppression of gag reflex, and dysphagia; may increase the risk of aspiration.

Soothing Rinses

Sodium bicarbonate, 1 tsp of baking soda in 32 oz (960 mL) water or normal saline solution): Should be used initially 3 times daily to swish and spit.

Coating Agents

Diphenhydramine elixir, 12.5 mg/5 mL mixed with kaolin and pectin (e.g., Kaopectate) 50% mixture by volume: Rinse with 1 tsp for 2 min q2hr, then expectorate. An aluminum hydroxide–magnesium hydroxide antacid (e.g., Maalox) can be used as a substitute for kaolin and pectin. Dyclonine HCl 0.5% can be added for greater anesthetic efficacy.

Diphenhydramine elixir, 12.5 mg/5 mL: Rinse with 1 tsp for 2 min q2hr and before each meal.

Dyclonine HCl, 0.5% or 1%: Rinse with 1 tsp for 2 min before each meal and expectorate.

3-2-1 solution for mouthwash (3 parts kaolin and pectin, 2 parts diphenhydramine elixir, 1 part normal saline solution). Rinse with 1 tsp q2hr, then expectorate. Caution: Although kaolin and pectin may be soothing to the ulcerated mucosa, because of its white chalky consistency, it can adhere to tissue and make the diagnosis of candidal infection difficult.

Powell's mouthwash: Nystatin 1.2 MU, tetracycline suspension 500 mg, hydrocortisone 100 mg, and diphenhydramine 12.5 mg/5 mL as needed to make 250 mL.

Sucralfate, 100 mg/mL suspension: Swish liquid in the mouth, swallow, repeat q6hr for a total daily dose of 0.75 mg/kg. Administer at least 2 hr after meals and 30 min before meals.

Adapted from Herbert AA, Beng JH: Oral mucous membrane diseases of childhood: I. Mucositis and xerostomia. 2. Recurrent aphthous stomatitis. 3. Herpetic stomatitis. *Semin Dermatol* 1992;11:80–7.

matic hydrocarbons; spicy or acidic foods or foods with hard consistency; and occlusive topical ointments should all be avoided.

For recurrence of extensive aphthous stomatitis, antimicrobial mouth rinses and topical corticosteroids may be necessary. Aphthous stomatitis and pharyngitis have been effectively treated with thalidomide in patients with HIV infection, with significant healing, diminished oral pain, and improvement in the ability to eat. Minor adverse reactions included somnolence and rash; a few patients discontinued the medication because of drug toxicity.

COMPLICATIONS

Oral candidiasis remains confined to the mucosal surfaces in healthy children. Invasive *C. albicans* infection may develop with serious systemic involvement in the immunocompromised person who has HIV infection, diabetes mellitus, or neutropenia or who is receiving corticosteroids or chemotherapy.

Viral stomatitis usually resolves without complications. The primary complication is dehydration due to impaired oral intake, which may require hospitalization. Bacteremia has been reported rarely. Primary herpetic gingivostomatitis can progress to HSV encephalitis, but not with recurrent disease. Systemic enteroviral infection may be associated with involvement of other organ systems resulting in aseptic meningitis, encephalitis, hepatitis, pneumonia, pericarditis, or myocarditis. Vesicular stomatitis is occasionally accompanied by pneumonia and conjunctivitis. There are no recognized complications of aphthous ulcers.

Immunocompromised persons are at increased risk of disseminated HSV infection, which can include extensive vesiculobullous lesions involving the esophagus, perioral area, external genitalia, and fingertips. The lesions progress to necrotic plaques, erosions, and deep ulcers and may be associated with painful cervical lymphadenopathy. Dehydration may result from the accompanying high fever and anorexia for liquids. Rarely, HSV epiglottitis may be seen.

PROGNOSIS

The prognosis for the acute illness with all of these infections is generally excellent, and resolution usually occurs without sequelae. Recurrent oral candidiasis in an infant suggests the possibility of an underlying immunodeficiency, especially HIV infection.

For untreated primary herpetic gingivostomatitis, the mean duration of symptoms is 12 ± 3 days for oral lesions, 12 ± 4 days for extraoral lesions, 4 ± 2 days for fever, 9 ± 3 days for eating difficulties, and 7 ± 3 days for drinking difficulty. Viral shedding persists for 7 days (with a range of 2–12 days). Herpetic stomatitis may result in frequent recurrences of HSV labialis, but scarring is uncommon.

Both herpangina and hand-foot-and-mouth disease result in immunity to the serotype of the infecting coxsackievirus, but infection with other serotypes is still possible. Many patients with HSV stomatitis or aphthous stomatitis experience recurrent disease.

Recurrent Herpetic Stomatitis. From 20–40% of the population of the United States experiences recurrent oral episodes of HSV labialis; cold sores or fever blisters occur intermittently throughout life. Recurrent HSV cold sores represent reactivation of latent HSV residing in the trigeminal ganglion, where it has become latently established after spread of the virus from the oral mucosa during primary herpetic gingivostomatitis. Recurrences typically flare during febrile illnesses of other infectious causes, psychological or physiologic stress, menstruation, mechanical trauma, exposure to sunlight or ultraviolet light, and acupuncture and other unidentified factors. Many patients with recurrent HSV stomatitis have neutralizing antibodies at the time of their recurrence, which are not believed to be protective. Patients with virus-positive episodes of HSV stomatitis have larger lesions that heal more slowly than in virus-negative patients.

Recurrences are characteristically preceded by prodromal symptoms of burning, tingling, and itching for 1–3 days, after which grouped vesicles develop on an erythematous base. The lesions then progress through the stages of papules, vesicles, ulcers, and crusts. The clinical course is shorter than that of the primary infection; pain and tenderness are present for 2 days and are followed by crusting and complete healing, usually within 7 days. The lesions usually occur in the same site, characteristically at the border of the skin with the vermilion, the lips, and other mucocutaneous junctions. Occasionally, lesions extend to the cheeks or neck. The lesions are infectious during recurrences; patients usually carry HSV in their saliva and may transmit virus by their hands.

Episodes are usually mild and self-limited but occasionally may be severe. Treatment with oral acyclovir or topical penciclovir hastens healing and lessens clinical symptoms, but only by about 1–2 days and only if begun early in the recurrence, optimally during the prodromal phase.

PREVENTION

To prevent oral colonization and infection with *C. albicans,* prolonged antimicrobial therapy in normal and immunocompromised patients should be avoided, if at all possible.

Direct transmission of the viruses causing stomatitis is prevented by strict attention to good hygienic measures. Careful hand-washing prevents contact with infected oral secretions from patients with primary or recurrent HSV stomatitis and fecal-oral transmission of the coxsackieviruses associated with herpangina and hand-foot-and-mouth disease. Persons with recurrent HSV disease should be counseled about the possibility of transmitting infection because most are unaware of its contagious nature. Prevention of thumb-sucking is important in children with oral herpetic gingivostomatitis to prevent herpetic whitlow (Chapter 46).

Health care workers should wear gloves and wash carefully before and after providing mouth care to patients affected with stomatitis, as well as before and after contact with associated cutaneous lesions. Vesicular stomatitis can be prevented by protecting human and animal handlers from the infected vesicles of animals by practicing drainage-secretion precautions and contact isolation.

REVIEW

Herbert AA, Berg JH: Oral mucous membrane diseases of childhood. I. Mucositis and xerostomia. II. Recurrent aphthous stomatitis. III. Herpetic stomatitis. *Semin Dermatol* 1992;11:80–7.

KEY ARTICLES

Amir J, Harel L, Smetana Z, et al: Treatment of herpes simplex gingivostomatitis with aciclovir in children: A randomised double blind placebo controlled study. *BMJ* 1997;314:1800–3.

Amir J, Harel L, Smetana Z, et al: The natural history of primary herpes simplex type 1 gingivostomatitis in children. *Pediatr Dermatol* 1999;16:259–63.

Cherry JD, Jahn CL: Herpangina: The etiologic spectrum. *Pediatrics* 1965;36:632–4.

Fields BN, Hawkins K: Human infection with the virus of vesicular stomatitis during an epizoonotic. *N Engl J Med* 1967;277:989–94.

Forman ML, Cherry JD: Enanthems associated with uncommon viral syndromes. *Pediatrics* 1968;41:873–82.

Halperin SA, Shehab Z, Thacker D, et al: Absence of viremia in primary herpetic gingivostomatitis. *Pediatr Infect Dis J* 1983:2;452–3.

Jacobson JM, Greenspan JS, Spritzler J, et al: Thalidomide for the treatment of oral aphthous ulcers in patients with human immunodeficiency virus infection. *N Engl J Med* 1997;33:1487–93.

Moore M: Enteroviral disease in the United States, 1970–1979. *J Infect Dis* 1982;146:103–8.

Padeh S, Brezniak N, Zemer D, et al: Periodic fever, aphthous stomatitis, pharyngitis, and adenopathy syndrome: Clinical characteristics and outcome. *J Pediatr* 1999;135:98–101.

Parrott RH, Ross S, Burke FG, et al: Herpangina: Clinical studies of a specific infectious disease. *N Engl J Med* 1951;245:275–80.

Spruance SL, Stewart JC, Rowe NH, et al: Treatment of recurrent herpes simplex labialis with oral acyclovir. *J Infect Dis* 1990;161:185–90.

Spruance SL, Rea TL, Thoming C, et al: Penciclovir cream for the treatment of herpes simplex labialis: A randomized, multi-center, double-blind, placebo-controlled trial. *JAMA* 1997;277:1374–9.

Woo SB, Sonis ST: Recurrent aphthous ulcers: A review of diagnosis and treatment. *J Am Dent Assoc* 1996;127:1202–13.

CHAPTER 61

Dental Infections

Theodore J. Cieslak

Dental infections, or **odontogenic infections,** range in spectrum from simple caries to the common entities of pericoronitis, periodontal disease (gingivitis and periodontitis), and periapical abscess. **Vincent's infection** is a fulminant form of **acute necrotizing ulcerative gingivitis,** and the term **Vincent's angina** refers to an anaerobic pharyngitis of, perhaps, similar pathogenesis. **Noma** refers to a gangrenous stomatitis, likewise related pathogenically to **Vincent's infection,** also known as **trench mouth. Ludwig's angina** is a cellulitis of the submandibular and sublingual regions. These uncommon entities are typically odontogenic in origin.

ETIOLOGY

The normal oral flora of humans is complex and includes a dense, diverse microbiota that includes more than 250 species of aerobic and anaerobic bacteria as well as spirochetes and yeasts (Table 2–1). Anaerobic organisms outnumber aerobes tenfold and are of paramount importance in the development of odontogenic infections. The oral flora are of low virulence, but the persistence of high levels of bacteria in the oral cavity, especially in the presence of dental decay, promotes sustained, low-grade inflammation and provides continued opportunities for development of deeper infections.

In the healthy periodontium, the microflora is sparse and consists mainly of gram-positive cocci including *Streptococcus oralis* and *Streptococcus sanguis* and the gram-positive bacillus *Actinomyces. Streptococcus mutans* is etiologically linked with dental caries. A characteristic flora is associated with periodontal infections. Among patients with periodontal disease, there is a 10- to 20-fold increase in the absolute quantity of oral bacteria compared with the healthy mouth, with an increased proportion of gram-negative anaerobes. In advancing disease, *Prevotella, Porphyromonas, Fusobacterium, Capnocytophaga,* and *Treponema* predominate, while *Eikenella, Eubacterium, Lactobacillus, Leptotrichia,* and *Selenomonas* are also present in abundance. Plaques above the gingival margin contain primarily gram-positive facultative and microaerophilic cocci and bacilli, whereas plaques below the gingival margin contain primarily gram-negative bacilli and spirochetes.

Common oral spirochetes include *Treponema macrodentium, Treponema denticola,* and *Treponema orale. Candida albicans* is the most common oral yeast, which can be recovered in up to 80% of healthy persons; it causes oral candidiasis (Chapter 60) but is not associated with odontogenic infections in healthy persons. Cytomegalovirus may persist in periodontal sites and salivary glands but is asymptomatic.

The microbial pathogenesis of odontogenic infections is not straightforward and is incompletely understood. Specific bacterial species have been implicated in the pathogenesis of the various periodontitis syndromes. *Actinomyces actinomycetemcomitans* has been linked to localized juvenile periodontitis, whereas *Porphyromonas gingivalis* has been associated with generalized juvenile periodontitis. *Prevotella melaninogenicus* has been associated with periodontal disease during pregnancy. In some cases, complex interactions among multiple organisms are involved, as with **Vincent's infection,** or **trench mouth,** where synergistic infection with certain spirochetal organisms, notably *Treponema vincentii,* with anaerobic *Selenomonas* and *Fusobacterium* leads to an **acute necrotizing ulcerative gingivitis.**

Most deep odontogenic infections are mixed infections that often include microaerophilic *Streptococcus,* usually β-hemolytic in 30%; anaerobic cocci, including *Peptostreptococcus* and *Veillonella* in 20–50%; gram-negative anaerobic or facultative bacilli, including *Prevotella, Porphyromonas,* and *Fusobacterium* in 20–50%; staphylococci in 15%; *Eikenella corrodens* in 15%; and *Bacteroides fragilis* in 5–10%.

EPIDEMIOLOGY

Dental caries is principally a disorder of the pediatric age group and, until the widespread use of fluoride supplementation, was ubiquitous among American children. Until recently, its prevalence in the United States exceeded 95% by adulthood. In certain populations with limited exposure to western diets and refined sugars, however, the incidence of caries may be negligible. More recently, with the use of fluorides, the prevalence of caries has declined significantly, with 75% of 8-year-old American children now free of caries of the permanent dentition.

Gingivitis also represents one of the most common dental afflictions of humans. Roughly 50% of children exhibit some gingival inflammation, with the incidence rising with increasing age and peaking during adolescence. By 45 years of age, nearly all persons have experienced gingivitis. Neglected, long-standing gingivitis may ultimately progress to **periodontitis,** a chronic inflammation of the periodontium, which includes the gingiva and the connective tissue elements (periodontal ligament, cementum, periosteum) that secure the tooth to alveolar bone. Although caries is the most common cause of tooth loss in children, periodontitis accounts for the majority of teeth lost in adulthood. Periodontitis, however, is not rare in childhood; in some surveys, 5–9% of preadolescent children had periodontal disease extending beyond the gingiva. **Vincent's infection,** a particularly aggressive form of gingivitis, is rare in children in the developed world. It does, however, occur frequently in India and parts of Africa, especially in the setting of protein malnutrition. **Noma,** or **gangrenous stomatitis,** although also rare, tends to occur more frequently in children than in adults and may lead to significant morbidity and mortality.

Pericoronitis, principally a disease of the third mandibular molar, is not typically seen in childhood but peaks in incidence in late adolescence and early adulthood. Exceptions occur, however, and pericoronitis is occasionally seen in conjunction with eruption of other permanent teeth. **Periapical infections,** including Ludwig's angina, are also uncommon in children in developed nations but may result in significant morbidity.

PATHOGENESIS

An understanding of the pathogenesis of odontogenic infections requires a thorough knowledge of the anatomy and microbiology of the head and neck. Dental infections may be limited to the tooth itself, called **simple caries,** or may extend to involve surrounding tissues. Soft tissue involvement may be divided into three anatomic categories: pericoronal, periodontal, and periapical. Carious teeth are a common concern of all pediatricians, but most other odontogenic infections, being somewhat directly related to advancing age, are relatively uncommon in childhood. Exceptions include patients with neutrophil defects, such as cyclic neutropenia and Chédiak-Higashi disease, juvenile-onset diabetes mellitus, long-term phenytoin therapy, and hormonal perturbations such as might be seen in adolescents and pregnant females. In these groups the incidence of periodontal disease increases dramatically, and often follows a malignant course.

As in other infectious diseases, spread of infection tends to occur along the anatomic pathways of least resistance (Fig. 61–1). For this reason, pericoronal and periodontal infections, which typically gain ready access to the oral cavity by draining along the tooth surface and into the gingival sulcus, rarely lead to serious or life-threatening complications. Periapical infections, however, may spread into the adjoining mandible or maxilla, giving rise to osteomyelitis. From there, purulent material may escape the mandibular cortex and enter the various anatomic spaces of the perioral tissues and oral floor. These include the submandibular and sublingual spaces (giving rise to Ludwig's angina), the submental space (submental abscess), the buccal space (buccal cellulitis), and the canine, parotid, and masticator spaces. Infection that involves these spaces can then further progress to the lateral pharyngeal, retropharyngeal, and danger spaces and subsequently gain access to the carotid sheath and mediastinum. In the case of maxillary teeth, purulent material may escape the confines of the maxilla and again enter the buccal, canine, or parotid spaces. Furthermore, infection may gain access to the orbit through the infratemporal space or may directly enter the maxillary sinuses.

Dental Caries. The pathogenesis of caries is multifactorial, involving complex interactions among host factors (genetic predeterminants, salivary characteristics and composition, fluoride exposure), diet (principally related to sucrose content, especially when present in "sticky," retentive foodstuffs), and microbes.

Streptococcus mutans is etiologically linked with dental caries. A plausible theory of cariogenesis involves the formation of an adherent plaque that attaches to the tooth. This plaque is usually composed of viable *S. mutans* organisms encased in a protein and carbohydrate matrix formed by the action of bacterial enzymes on salivary glycoproteins. Once able to maintain close contact with the dental surface, these organisms begin the process of demineralization by producing lactic acid from dietary sucrose. Although sucrose appears to be the preferred substrate, other simple sugars may serve this function. Similarly, the cariogenic process may involve organisms other than *S. mutans,* including *Actinomyces* and *Lactobacillus.* Dental caries represents a true infectious disorder in terms of person-to-person spread; studies have demonstrated a higher incidence of caries in the offspring of carious patients directly related to transmission of large numbers of *S. mutans* organisms.

Pericoronitis. Pericoronitis is an inflammatory condition that results when food and bacteria are entrapped under the gingiva overlying a partially erupted tooth. Such entrapment is most likely to involve the mandibular third molar, especially in cases where the molar encroaches on the angle formed by the body and ramus of the mandible. The microbial cause of pericoronitis is almost exclusively anaerobic, with *Peptostreptococcus, Fusobacterium,* and *Prevotella melaninogenica* most frequently recovered.

Periodontal Disease. Although the gingiva, in general, is firmly attached to bone, a cuff of unattached gingiva surrounds each tooth. Infections and inflammatory conditions of the periodontium may be classified as either **simple gingivitis,** a localized inflammatory condition of this unattached gingiva, or as **frank periodontitis,** an infection that extends to involve other elements of the periodontium, with consequent weakening of dental supporting structures.

Gingivitis is related to poor oral hygiene. Without frequent brushing and flossing, food particles become trapped in the gingival sulcus between the free gingiva and the tooth, providing a substrate for bacterial growth and plaque formation. Bacteria within plaque may initiate a toxin-mediated inflammatory response, resulting in the characteristic swollen, erythematous, friable gingiva associated with this condition, although the gingiva itself is not infected.

Untreated gingivitis leads to an extension of plaque deeper into the gingival sulcus and ultimately to **periodontitis,** several subtypes of which are recognized. In the most common form, **chronic adult periodontitis,** there is progressive infiltration of plaque subgingivally, with destruction of the periodontal ligament and alveolar bone. The tooth then loosens, and deep pockets form in its surrounding sulcus. Ultimately, abundant calculi develop and obstruct the sulcus, permitting formation of periodontal abscesses. As these abscesses often drain freely along the tooth surface and into the sulcus, pain may be minimal or nonexistent, contributing further to a delay in seeking treatment.

In **early-onset periodontitis,** also known as **juvenile periodontitis** or **periodontosis,** the destruction of the periodontium is markedly accelerated, and rapid alveolar bone loss is seen. This condition may be generalized **(generalized juvenile periodontitis),** or it may involve principally the first molars and central incisors **(localized juvenile periodontitis).** Some patients with juvenile periodontitis appear to have subtle defects in neutrophil chemotaxis or phagocytosis, as do patients with prepubertal periodontitis, which involves the primary dentition. Whether this neutrophil dysfunction is primary or is the result of inhibition by certain oral bacteria, notably *Actinomyces actinomycetemcomitans* and *Capnocytophaga ochraceus* that are known to produce leukotoxins, has not been fully elucidated. A particularly malignant form of prepubertal periodontitis is seen in children with the Papillon-Lefevre syndrome, as well as in patients with hypophosphatasia, Chédiak-Higashi disease, cyclic neutropenia, diabetes mellitus, and certain other immunodeficiencies.

Vincent's Infection. An infrequent but particularly fulminant form of gingivitis is **acute necrotizing ulcerative gingivitis,** also known as **Vincent's infection** or **trench mouth.** In this condition, the interdental papillae are pale and eroded, and a gray pseudomembrane develops. Rarely, sites remote from the interdental papillae may be involved with a similar pathogenic process. **Vincent's angina** is the term given to a virulent form of anaerobic pharyngitis in which gray pseudomembranes are found on the tonsils, accounting for the synonym **false diphtheria.** Vincent's infection appears to occur primarily among patients under considerable stress in whom underlying gingivitis and malnutrition are present. Although

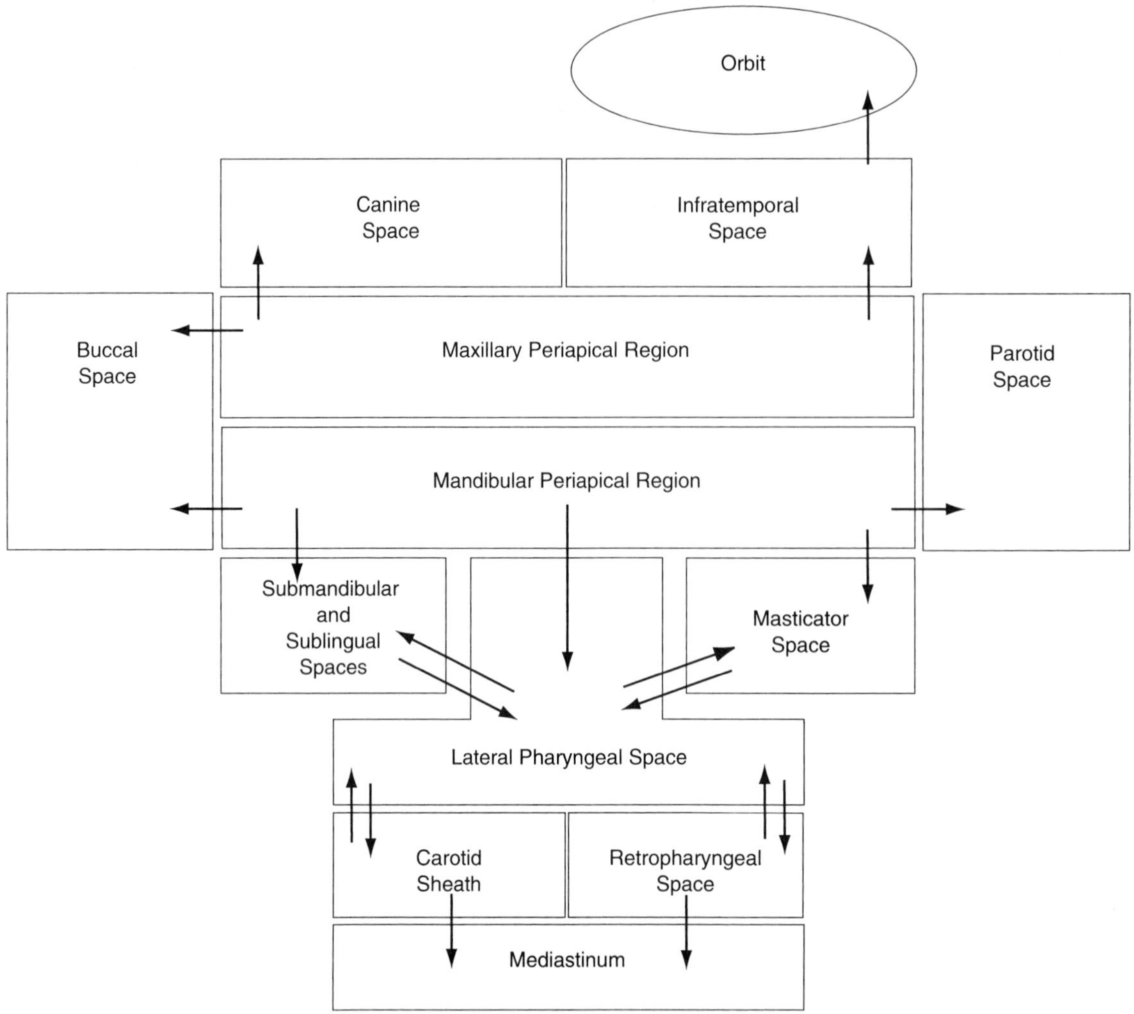

FIGURE 61–1. Potential pathways of extension in deep fascial space infections. (Adapted from: Chow AW. Infections of the oral cavity, neck, and head. In Mandell GL, Bennett JE, Dolin R (editors): *Principles and Practice of Infectious Diseases,* 5th ed. New York, Churchill-Livingstone, 2000, pp 689–702.)

the complex microbial interactions involved in its pathogenesis are incompletely understood, Vincent's infection probably involves a synergistic infection among oral spirochetes, especially *T. vincentii,* and *Fusobacterium.* Vincent's angina, or anaerobic pharyngitis, likewise involves apparent infection with fusiform anaerobes. **Lemierre's postanginal septicemia** is the term given to a septic jugular vein thrombophlebitis and secondary metastatic infection that may follow Vincent's angina and that typically is associated with infection due to *Fusobacterium necrophorum.*

Noma. Noma, also known as **cancrum oris** or **gangrenous stomatitis,** may be related pathophysiologically to Vincent's infection, but typically it begins as a focal gingival lesion and rapidly progresses to gangrene and consequent destruction of bone, teeth, and soft tissues. Mortality rates are as high as 70–90% in the absence of prompt surgical intervention. Noma has been associated with infection by *T. vincentii* and *Fusobacterium nucleatum.* Similar to Vincent's infection, noma appears related, in many cases, to severe malnutrition or to immunodeficiency states, such as advanced HIV infection or severe combined immunodeficiency disease.

Periapical Abscess. A periapical abscess develops with an extension of periodontal disease into the region of the tooth apex or, alternatively, with the implantation of bacteria into the pulp cavity and subsequent spread of the resultant pulpitis into the apex. Such implantation may occur in advanced carious disease or after dental trauma. Contrary to the usual progression seen in pericoronal and periodontal infections, periapical infections may fail to drain into the gingival sulcus, instead invading the bone of the maxilla or mandible (osteomyelitis) or perforating the bony cortex and draining into the adjacent potential spaces and fascial planes.

Periapical infections are largely anaerobic, composed of normal oral flora, and inevitably polymicrobial, with 4–6 different organisms typically isolated from individual cases. Pathogens most often implicated include *Prevotella, Fusobacterium, Veillonella, Peptococcus, Peptostreptococcus, Actinomyces,* and *Lactobacillus.*

Ludwig's Angina. The term "Ludwig's angina," although often applied to any infection of the sublingual or submandibular region, was originally reserved for a rapidly spreading bilateral cellulitis of the sublingual and submandibular spaces. It is often odontogenic in origin, typically spreading from a periapical abscess of the second or third mandibular molar. It has also been associated with tongue-piercing, and a recent dramatic increase in piercing could lead to a resurgence of this condition. A propensity for rapid spread, glottic and lingual swelling, and consequent airway obstruction make prompt intervention imperative. Ludwig's angina may also present as a cellulitis of the neck (Chapter 47).

SYMPTOMS AND CLINICAL FEATURES

Dental caries in its early stages is typically asymptomatic. As tooth enamel is first decalcified, a carious lesion appears white, progressing to cavity formation when the enamel is lost. Once this occurs, the carious process enters the dentin, which readily picks up staining material, giving the cavity a darkened appearance. Although such lesions may be readily detectable on the labial surfaces of anterior teeth, caries of the interdental or subgingival surfaces or of the posterior teeth may escape detection, even when quite advanced. Pain does not typically accompany caries until lesions have progressed into the pulp cavity and a consequent pulpitis ensues; once this occurs, the tooth is often lost. Such pain may be readily elicited by thermal changes, especially by cold liquids.

Patients with pericoronitis typically present with pain on swallowing and mastication or with a limitation of jaw opening. Physical examination reveals swollen erythematous gingiva overlying an erupting tooth; purulent exudate may often be expressed with digital pressure on the infected gingival flap.

Gingivitis is typically painless, accounting for a failure of patients to seek medical attention. The condition is manifest primarily by bleeding during brushing. Acute necrotizing ulcerative gingivitis does present with pain. Fever, malaise, cervical adenopathy, halitosis, and altered taste sensation may be present as well. The characteristic gray pseudomembranes often cover the ulcerated and necrotic-appearing gingiva. Gangrenous stomatitis typically begins as a gingival papule that rapidly progresses to a necrotic ulcer. A painful cellulitis accompanies the ulceration, and tissue destruction is rapid and extensive.

The ability of most periodontal abscesses to drain readily into the oral cavity accounts for the paucity of symptoms associated with this condition. Patients may present with a complaint of gingival bleeding or of a fetid odor to the breath. On examination, the gingiva is friable and erythematous or bluish in color. Pus may often be expressed from subgingival pockets, and the teeth may be loose in their sockets. Pain and tenderness are minimal or nonexistent.

The clinical presentation of periapical abscesses and consequent deep space infections is quite varied; many of these infections may be life threatening, however, and rapid diagnosis and treatment are thus imperative. Patients often present with fever and severe dental pain, which is exacerbated by drinking hot or cold liquids. The involved teeth are exquisitely tender to palpation, and extreme pain may also be elicited on jaw opening if the masticatory muscles are inflamed. Signs and symptoms of buccal cellulitis, orbital infection, and maxillary sinusitis should be sought, as should evidence of cervical or intraoral swelling.

DIAGNOSIS

The diagnosis of overt dental caries may be made readily by finding stained cavities, most commonly on the occlusal surfaces of molars. Unfortunately, the diagnosis of lesions that have not yet invaded the dentin is often difficult and may require careful probing by a dentist. Moreover, the discovery of interdental and subgingival caries often requires dental radiographs. For these reasons, routine dental examinations, beginning at an early age, are imperative for optimal oral health. The American Academy of Pediatric Dentistry recommends an initial well-child dental examination at no later than 18 months of age.

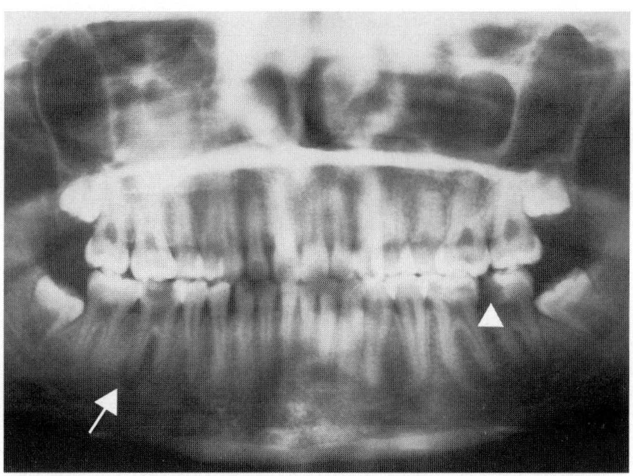

FIGURE 61–2. Panoramic radiograph (orthopantograph) of the oral cavity demonstrating a periapical abscess that appears as periapical lucency *(arrow).* Dental caries can also be identified radiographically *(arrowhead).*

A diagnosis of gingivitis is established clinically and is suggested by the finding of a friable swollen gingiva that is erythematous or bluish in color and that bleeds readily and painlessly on brushing. In Vincent's infection the ulcerative gingival lesions must be differentiated from such conditions as herpetic gingivostomatitis. This can usually be distinguished on clinical grounds, as herpetic lesions often involve the labial and other intraoral surfaces, whereas Vincent's infection is typically limited to the gingiva. A Tzanck smear, a direct fluorescent antibody test, or a viral culture may be helpful in some cases. Gangrenous stomatitis must be considered in the case of malnourished or chronically ill patients presenting with a rapidly progressive, gangrenous-appearing ulcer of the oral mucous membranes. Biopsy of the lesion may demonstrate a mat of unusual thread-like gram-negative bacteria. Cultures are rarely helpful in individual cases of gingivitis, Vincent's infection, or noma.

Periodontitis and periapical abscesses are likewise suspected on the basis of clinical findings. In the case of a periapical abscess, percussion of the tooth or exposure to cold liquids typically elicits intense pain. A panoramic radiograph, or orthopantomogram (Fig. 61–2), may be helpful in evaluating periapical abscess but should not delay treatment, especially with acute periapical infection. Cultures are rarely useful in individual cases of periodontitis or uncomplicated periapical abscess. When deep space infection is present, cultures are imperative for guiding antimicrobial therapy.

TREATMENT

Dental Caries. The treatment of caries is principally the realm of the dentist. Because many children may not visit a dentist in the first years of life, however, the pediatrician plays a primary role in appropriate referral. Fluoride, an important element in caries prevention, also has a bacteriostatic effect and may thus promote cariostasis and even reversal of early carious lesions.

Pericoronitis. Irrigation alone may provide sufficient treatment of uncomplicated pericoronitis, although tooth extraction is often necessary in severe cases. Antibiotics directed against oral anaerobes, such as penicillin, metronidazole, or clindamycin, may be indicated in selected cases, especially when concomitant cellulitis is present.

Periodontal Disease. Treatment of uncomplicated gingivitis consists of plaque removal and meticulous attention to oral hygiene; dental referral is thus imperative. Vincent's infection may be managed by dental débridement. Frequent rinsing with hydrogen peroxide appears to hasten recovery, as does the systemic administration of penicillin or metronidazole (Table 61–1). Analgesics may be necessary in the early stages of treatment. The management of gangrenous stomatitis requires prompt initiation of high-dose parenteral penicillin G therapy. In addition, débridement, removal of loose teeth and devitalized bone, and extensive cosmetic surgery are often required.

Treatment of periodontitis centers on the restoration of good dental hygiene. The removal of plaque and calculi is imperative, and dental consultation should thus be sought. Antibiotics are often useful and should be directed against oral anaerobic bacilli. Penicillin G, metronidazole, clindamycin, and the cephamycins (cefoxitin and cefotetan) represent reasonable choices in the immunocompetent host. The addition of intravenous broad-spectrum gram-negative coverage is sometimes warranted in the immunocompromised patient. Antibiotic therapy is especially important in those patients in whom a delay in obtaining dental consultation is anticipated.

Periapical Abscess. Therapy of uncomplicated pulpitis and periapical abscess involves tooth extraction and root canal procedures and is thus in the realm of the oral surgeon. Emergent surgical intervention is indicated in cases of submandibular and sublingual space infections, as well as in many other deep space infections of the head and neck. In many of these infections, airway integrity is threatened and intubation may be necessary. Antibiotic therapy should be guided by culture results, but empiric coverage should be directed largely against anaerobes. Intravenous penicillin G, clindamycin, metronidazole, or a cephamycin are reasonable choices, although an increasing number of *Prevotella* isolates are resistant to penicillin. Although *Staphylococcus aureus* is not a common isolate in odontogenic infections, the presence of gram-positive cocci in clusters on a gram-stained smear should prompt the addition of antistaphylococcal coverage.

COMPLICATIONS

Dental Caries. Premature tooth loss is the most common complication of dental caries. Loss of permanent dentition has obvious lifelong consequences, but premature loss of deciduous teeth is problematic as well. With such loss, there is a failure to reserve jaw space for permanent teeth, which may lead to a multitude of orthodontic complications. Moreover, the retention in the mouth of carious deciduous teeth probably serves to increase the intraoral burden of *S. mutans,* thereby placing erupting permanent teeth at higher risk of caries development. This may be especially true of **nursing-bottle caries,** a particularly onerous form of deciduous dental disease and a major source of morbidity in many populations. This condition, which results when toddlers are permitted to fall asleep with a bottle, leads to prolonged contact of the dentition with simple sugars. The carious lesions that result usually begin with the maxillary incisors, progress posteriorly, and may result in the loss of numerous teeth. The tendency for children with this condition to develop significant disease involving the permanent dentition is quite high. Furthermore, even properly managed carious lesions remain at high risk; recurrent caries has been reported in 18% of filled lesions. Neglected caries that is permitted to progress through the dentin may eventually enter the pulp space, giving rise to pulpitis and subsequently to periapical infection with its attendant complications.

Periodontal Disease. Complications arising from periodontal disease are frequent. Patients with neurologic impairment and periodontal disease, such as might be seen in children receiving phenytoin, are at increased risk of aspiration pneumonia. Moreover, patients with periodontitis appear to have a higher incidence of transient bacteremia after minor oral manipulations than do healthy

TABLE 61–1. Recommended Antibiotic Therapy of Odontogenic Infections

Infection	Microbiologic Etiology	Primary Therapy
Vincent's infection (trench mouth, acute necrotizing ulcerative gingivitis)	Oral spirochetes *(Treponema vincentii)* Fusobacterium	Penicillin G *or* metronidazole *plus* Débridement and peroxide rinses
Vincent's angina (false diphtheria)	Fusiform anaerobes	Penicillin G
Noma (cancrum oris, gangrenous stomatitis)	*Borrelia vincentii, Fusobacterium necrophorum, Prevotella*	Penicillin G *plus* Débridement
Ludwig's angina (sublingual and submandibular cellulitis)	Oral anaerobes	Penicillin G *and* metronidazole *or* Penicillin G *and* clindamycin *or* Ampicillin-sulbactam *and* clindamycin
Lemierre's septicemia (septic jugular vein thrombophlebitis, lateral pharyngeal space infection)	*F. necrophorum*	Penicillin G

Suggested Dosages for Patients with Normal Renal Function

ANTIBIOTIC	INTRAVENOUS DOSAGE	MAXIMUM DAILY DOSE
Ampicillin-sulbactam	200 mg/kg/day ampicillin divided q6hr	8 g
Clindamycin	40 mg/kg/day divided q8hr	2.7 g
Metronidazole	30 mg/kg/day divided q6hr	30 mg/kg/day
Penicillin G	250,000–500,000 U/kg/day divided q6hr	20–24 MU

patients. Such a finding has special implications for those with abnormal or prosthetic heart valves. Periodontitis may occasionally progress to periapical abscess formation, and from there gain access to the spaces and fascial planes of the head and neck.

Periapical Abscess. A principal determinant in the development of complications of periapical abscess involves the specific location of the individual tooth apex in relation to the adjoining bone and muscular attachments. When the apex is adjacent to the buccal cortical surface of the mandible or maxilla, infection may spread buccally, resulting in **buccal space infection** or **buccal cellulitis.** Conversely, infection of the root apices adjoining the palatal surface tends to spread in that direction. In children, maxillary root apices typically rest above the buccinator attachments (Fig. 61–3). Palatal periapical infections involving these teeth tend to spread superiorly and may extend into the canine space and into the orbit or maxillary sinus. In the case of mandibular teeth, the position of the apex in relation to the mylohyoid muscle must be considered (Fig. 61–4). Mandibular incisors, canines, premolars, and first molars have apices that rest superior to the mylohyoid attachments. Infections of these teeth thus tend to drain into the sublingual (supramylohyoid) space. The second and third molars have apices that rest inferior to the mylohyoid muscle; infections involving these teeth tend to drain into the submandibular (inframylohyoid) space. Collectively, the indurated cellulitis of the sublingual and submandibular spaces that may result from such extension is referred to as **Ludwig's angina,** a bilateral, rapidly progressive, life-threatening condition. The induration seen in Ludwig's angina is more readily apparent intraorally than externally and may lead to an upward displacement of the tongue and subsequent airway obstruction.

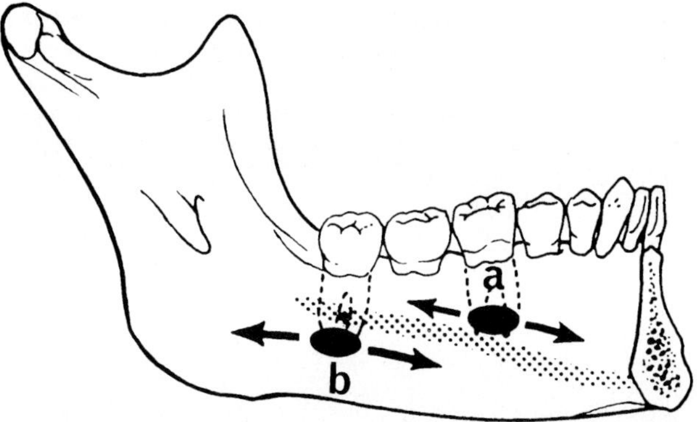

FIGURE 61–4. Lingual aspect of the mandible. *a* = apices of involved tooth above mylohyoid muscle, with spread of infection to sublingual space; *b* = apices of involved tooth below mylohyoid muscle, with spread of infection to submandibular space. (From Chow AW, Roser SM, Brady FA: Orofacial odontogenic infections. *Ann Intern Med* 1978;88:392–402.)

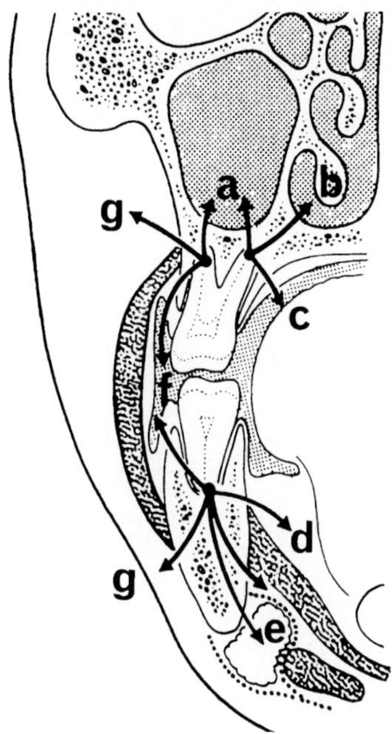

FIGURE 61–3. Coronal section in the region of the first molar teeth. *a* = maxillary antrum; *b* = nasal cavity; *c* = palatal plate; *d* = sublingual space; *e* = submandibular space; *f* = intraoral presentation with infection spreading through the buccal plates inside the attachment of the buccinator muscle; *g* = extraoral presentation to buccal space with infection spreading through the buccal plates outside the attachment of the buccinator muscle. (From Chow AW, Roser SM, Brady FA: Orofacial odontogenic infections, *Ann Intern Med* 1978;88:392–402.)

Dry socket syndrome refers to a condition that develops after dental extraction. The blood clot in the tooth socket becomes infected and disintegrates, giving rise to an alveolar osteitis. The condition is characterized by intense pain, a fetid odor in the mouth, and abnormal taste sensation. Purulent material may be visualized within the socket. Treatment consists of irrigation; packing with eugenol-soaked gauze has been recommended, and antibiotics may be of benefit.

PREVENTION

Although the treatment of caries principally involves the dentist, the pediatrician or the family physician is often instrumental in its prevention. This is especially important in the case of deciduous teeth because many children will not visit a dentist in the first few years of life. Preventive counseling might focus on the benefits of a reduction in dietary intake of simple sugars, as well as the need for the mechanical removal of plaque through brushing and flossing. Routine well-child counseling should stress the prevention of caries, particularly nursing-bottle caries. The physician can affect dental health through the prescription of fluoride supplements for those patients for whom there is inadequate municipal **water fluoridation.** Fluoride has been shown to increase the resistance of dental enamel to the effects of lactic acid. The provision of this mineral has been instrumental in the reduction of caries. Sources of dietary fluoride include fluoridated water, dentifrices, and fluoride supplements. In the United States, water is not universally or uniformly fluoridated. The physician must be familiar with the amount of fluoride present in local water supplies so that he or she can provide proper fluoride supplementation (Table 61–2). Young children may ingest variable amounts of fluoride by consuming fluoride-containing toothpaste while brushing; lower amounts of supplemental fluoride are thus recommended for children under 6 years of age to minimize the risk of fluorosis. **Dental fluorosis** may develop during tooth formation when excessive fluoride ingestion results in retention of protein within the dental enamel, with consequent disruption of crystal formation. This leads to hypomineralization of the dental enamel and dentin. Fluorosis may appear as barely perceptible striations or specks or may result in confluent

TABLE 61–2. Recommended Daily Fluoride Supplement (mg/day) Based on Concentration of Fluoride in Municipal Water Supply*

	Concentration of F (ppm) in Water Supply		
Age	**<0.3**	**0.3–0.6**	**>0.6**
Birth–6 mo	0	0	0
6 mo–3 yr	0.25	0	0
3–6 yr	0.50	0.25	0
6–16 yr	1.00	0.50	0

*Jointly endorsed by the American Academy of Pediatrics, the American Academy of Pediatric Dentistry, and the American Dental Association. Adapted from American Academy of Pediatrics, Committee on Nutrition: Fluoride supplementation for children: Interim policy recommendations. *Pediatrics* 1995;95:777.

areas of pitting and brownish gray staining. The consequences of fluorosis are chiefly cosmetic, as affected teeth apparently remain resistant to dental caries.

Of interest in the ultimate control of dental caries are prospects for a vaccine against cariogenic strains of *S. mutans.* Although preliminary results with a vaccine against *S. mutans* in animals are encouraging, widespread human application likely will require better characterization of the specific bacterial determinants of cariogenicity.

As is the case with virtually all odontogenic infections, prevention of gingivitis and periodontitis is straightforward and involves meticulous attention to oral hygiene. Regular brushing and flossing, along with routine dental examinations, will prevent most periodontal disease. Finally, because most periapical infections result either from neglected caries entering the pulp space or from advanced periodontal disease, efforts aimed at prevention of these entities will markedly diminish the risk of periapical disease and its attendant complications.

Although dental caries, periodontal disease, and other odontogenic infections are major sources of morbidity in pediatric patients, their prevention is rather straightforward. The primary care physician is in a unique position to implement such preventive measures and in so doing may have considerable impact on the overall health of children.

REVIEWS

Bimstein E: Periodontal health and disease in children and adolescents. *Pediatr Clin North Am* 1991;38:1183–207.

Creighton PR: Common pediatric dental problems. *Pediatr Clin North Am* 1998;45:1579–60.

Haug RH, Hoffman MJ, Indresano AT: An epidemiologic and anatomic survey of odontogenic infections. *J Oral Maxillofac Surg* 1991; 49:976–80.

Moenning JE, Nelson CL, Kohler RB: The microbiology and chemotherapy of odontogenic infections. *J Oral Maxillofac Surg* 1989;47:976–85.

Piecuch JF: Odontogenic infections. *Dent Clin North Am* 1982;26:129–45.

KEY ARTICLES

Enwonwu CO, Falkler WA Jr, Idigbe EO, et al: Pathogenesis of cancrum oris (noma): Confounding interactions of malnutrition with infection. *Am J Trop Med Hyg* 1999;60:223–32.

Hartmann RW Jr: Ludwig's angina in children. *Am Fam Physician* 1999;60:109–12.

Kumar JV, Green EL: Recommendations for fluoride use in children. *N Y State Dent J* 1998;64:40–7.

Kureishi A, Chow AW: The tender tooth: Dentoalveolar, pericoronal, and periodontal infections. *Infect Dis Clin North Am* 1988;2:163–82.

Perkins CS, Meisner J, Harrison JM: A complication of tongue piercing. *Br Dent J* 1997;182:147–8.

Preston AJ: A review of dentrifices. *Dent Update* 1998;25:247–53.

Tendler C, Bottone EJ: Fusospirochetal ulcerative gingivitis in children. *J Pediatr* 1987;111:400–3.

Valadas G, Leal MJ: Cancrum oris (noma) in children. *Eur J Pediatr Surg* 1998;8:47–51.

Winston AE, Bhaskar SN: Caries prevention in the 21st century. *J Am Dent Assoc* 1998;129:1579–87.

CHAPTER 62

Parotitis and Sialadenitis

Celia D.C. Christie

Inflammation accounts for more than one third of all suppurative and nonsuppurative salivary gland disorders in infancy and childhood. Distinct clinical syndromes that constitute the syndrome of **suppurative sialadenitis** include bacterial parotitis (suppurative parotitis), acute submandibular sialadenitis, chronic parotitis or sialadenitis, and recurrent parotitis or sialadenitis. **Nonsuppurative sialadenitis** is usually related to viral diseases, most commonly mumps.

ETIOLOGY

The principal etiologic agent of bacterial parotitis and submandibular sialadenitis is *Staphylococcus aureus,* which is the cause in more than two thirds of all neonatal and childhood cases (Table 62–1). In newborns, *Escherichia coli* and *Pseudomonas aeruginosa* are frequently implicated. Rarely, streptococcal species, *Moraxella catarrhalis,* and *Candida albicans* are isolated. In older children, streptococci, especially of the viridans group, and *Haemophilus influenzae* are frequently isolated. In one study (Brook et al., 1991), anaerobic bacteria were the etiologic agents in 56% of the patients evaluated, with *Prevotella melaninogenica* as the predominant anaerobic species. Nosocomial parotitis in children with underlying illnesses has been associated with gram-negative bacilli, especially *E. coli, P. aeruginosa, H. influenzae,* and *Eikenella corrodens.* Cultures of salivary secretions from infantile chronic recurrent parotitis often demonstrate *Streptococcus pneumoniae* and *H. influenzae.*

Mumps was the most common etiologic agent of parotitis before introduction of mumps vaccine, with secondary bacterial infection occasionally occurring as a complication. Parainfluenza virus and acute Epstein-Barr virus (EBV) infection usually cause bilateral parotid gland involvement.

EPIDEMIOLOGY

Historically, acute bacterial parotitis was a nosocomial postoperative staphylococcal infection in adults. It required early surgical drainage and was associated with a high rate of morbidity and mortality. The incidence declined in the antibiotic era, with a recent gradual resurgence and change in the epidemiology. Parotitis and submandibular sialadenitis are now primarily community-acquired rather than nosocomially acquired diseases. The major predisposing factors are dehydration, diuretics, and medications that reduce salivary flow.

Acute bacterial parotitis is rare in children but is the most common form of pediatric sialadenitis. The incidence is highest among newborns and adolescents, probably because of physiologic hormonal changes, and is low in other pediatric age groups. More than 100 cases of neonatal parotitis have been reported, with an incidence of 1/100,000 live births. Preterm newborns are at highest risk of sialadenitis, comprising 40% of infant cases. The disease also occurs in the presence of local or systemic illness (Table 62–2). Fever and dehydration secondary to upper respiratory tract infection, systemic viral illness, immunodeficiency, mumps, and trauma are predisposing factors. Postoperative bacterial parotitis usually occurs within 3 weeks of surgery and is rare in children.

Recurrent or chronic parotitis or sialadenitis is characterized by recurrent exacerbations of acute symptoms. Synonyms for this condition include chronic recurrent parotitis, juvenile recurrent parotitis, chronic suppuration of the parotid gland, recurrent bacterial sialadenitis, chronic sialadenitis, chronic obstructive sialadenitis, and chronic sialodochitis. Recurrent sialadenitis occurs frequently in children, usually beginning in the first decade of life with the highest incidence in children 3–6 years of age. There is a strong tendency for the disease to resolve by 15 years of age; only 8% of persons have recurrences after 20 years of age. Boys (72%) are more commonly affected than girls (28%). The disorder is bilateral in about 28–35% of patients.

PATHOGENESIS

Sialadenitis usually develops from retrograde transmission of bacteria from the oral cavity. Hematogenous spread to the salivary glands occurs rarely in neonates and with *S. aureus* in older children.

The submandibular gland is prone to sialolithiasis and ductal obstruction with calculi, whereas the parotid gland is susceptible to bacterial infection. Calculi occur in 97% of submandibular gland infections, compared with only 4% of parotid infections. Risk factors for stone formation in the submandibular ducts include the high alkalinity, high concentrations of calcium phosphate, and the viscous nature and high protein content of the submandibular fluid. The long ascending pathway of the Wharton's duct against the flow of gravity and the lack of muscular coat and external mechanical pressures to eject saliva and prevent stagnation are other contributory factors. Conversely, the buccinator muscles massage Stensen's duct repeatedly during mastication. Stenosis and strictures also cause obstruction, which predisposes to both parotitis and sialadenitis.

Mucins play a protective role and are abundant in the salivary secretions of the submandibular gland but not in the serous fluid of the parotid gland. Mucins have a bacteriostatic effect because of lysozymes, IgA antibodies, and sialic acid. These components agglutinate bacteria, competitively inhibiting their adherence to host tissues. The submandibular gland has mixed mucous and serous components, and therefore this gland is less frequently involved in bacterial infections than is the parotid gland.

Anatomic considerations related to infection include the location of the orifice of Stensen's duct directly opposite the second molar, where stagnation and heavy colonization of microbes occur, whereas the orifice of Wharton's duct is protected by the activity of the tongue. Acute bacterial parotitis develops as a result of decreased salivary flow through Stensen's duct because of dehydra-

TABLE 62–1. Infectious Causes of Parotitis and Sialadenitis

Gram-positive Organisms	*Prevotella disiens*
*Staphylococcus aureus**	*Prevotella intermedia*
Coagulase-negative staphylococci	*Prevotella magnus*
Viridans streptococci	*Actinomyces israellii*
Streptococcus pneumoniae	*Actinomyces naeslundii*
Group A *Streptococcus*	*Propionibacterium acnes*
Gram-negative Organisms	*Eubacterium lentum*
Escherichia coli	**Other Organisms**
Pseudomonas aeruginosa	*Arachnia*
Pseudomonas pseudomallei	*Mycobacterium tuberculosis*
Haemophilus influenzae	*Treponema pallidum*
Moraxella catarrhalis	*Candida albicans*
Salmonella typhi	*Histoplasma capsulatum*
Neisseria gonorrhoeae	*Blastomyces hominis*
Eikenella corrodens	**Viruses**
Salmonella enteritidis	Mumps virus
Anaerobic Organisms	Coxsackieviruses A and B
Fusobacterium nucleatum	Epstein-Barr virus
Bacteroides fragilis	Parainfluenza viruses 1 and 3
Prevotella melaninogenica	Cytomegalovirus
	Human immunodeficiency virus (AIDS)
	Lymphocytic choriomeningitis virus

**Staphylococcus aureus* is the principal cause.

tion, xerostomia, ductal obstruction, inflammation, or trauma. This reduces the mechanical flushing and cleansing effect of serous saliva. Bacteria then colonize the oral cavity, multiply, invade Stensen's duct, and cause acute parotitis. Poor oral hygiene facilitates heavy bacterial growth and xerostomia with poor salivary flow.

In recurrent parotitis and sialadenitis, the intermittent exacerbations of acute symptoms overlay the chronic low-grade infection with ongoing destruction of the salivary gland. Illnesses predisposing to recurrent sialadenitis include Sjögren's syndrome, Raynaud's disease, and other autoimmune disorders. Allergy, duct obstruction by stones, mucous plugs associated with cystic fibrosis, and congenital malformations of portions of the salivary gland are also implicated. Dehydration may exacerbate stasis and appears to promote development of ascending infection in the presence of these predisposing conditions.

Sialectasis is a uniform feature of recurrent parotitis in children. Sialectasis without obstruction has been attributed to congenital malformation, past mumps infection, viral parotitis, severe primary acute pyogenic infection, or an underlying allergic condition. Chronic submandibular sialadenitis uniformly results from calculous obstruction of the submandibular ducts.

SYMPTOMS AND CLINICAL MANIFESTATIONS

Suppurative sialadenitis presents with edema, pain, reduced function, and purulent saliva. Systemic manifestations may include a fever, rigors, and chills. In newborns, the temperature may be normal or only slightly elevated.

The clinical findings of acute parotitis include swelling of the parotid gland with induration in the preauricular area or angle of the mandible associated with pain, tenderness, warmth, and erythema of the overlying skin. Detection of fluctuance is impaired by the dense parotid capsule fibrous lobular septa. Involvement is usually unilateral but may rarely be bilateral. In approximately three fourths of cases of acute bacterial parotitis, Stensen's papilla is erythematous and Stensen's duct exudes purulent saliva that is thick and cloudy. In newborns, widespread primary or metastatic infection may be evident.

Bacterial infection of the submandibular gland causes tenderness over the area, persistent pain, and usually a purulent discharge from Wharton's duct. Systemic manifestations of fever and chills may accompany infection.

The clinical course of recurrent parotitis or sialadenitis is characterized by multiple episodes of low-grade swelling and fever, up to 12–15 occurrences per year with intervening periods of clinical remission. There may be persistent mucopurulent drainage from Stensen's duct, reflecting ongoing inflammation.

DIAGNOSIS

The diagnosis of parotitis is established by characteristic symptoms and physical findings. Stains and cultures of saliva identify the etiologic factors.

Differential Diagnosis

There are many infectious causes of parotitis and sialadenitis (Table 62–1), as well as many noninfectious causes (Table 62–3).

Mumps presents as an acute onset of parotid swelling and trismus and is bilateral in 75% of patients. It occurs after a 1- to 2-day prodrome of fever, headache, myalgia, arthralgia, sore throat, and earache on chewing. Salivary secretions are usually clear. Mumps parotitis does not usually display the exquisite tenderness to palpation and purulent discharge associated with bacterial parotitis (Chapter 36). Parainfluenza virus parotitis is a prolonged illness that typically occurs in children with a severe underlying immunodeficiency. Acute EBV infection causes bilateral parotid gland involvement.

Other infections to consider include odontogenic infections, such as Ludwig's angina (Chapter 61), facial cellulitis (Chapter 47), and anterior cervical or submandibular cervical lymphadenitis (Chapter 51). These entities can be excluded by a normal serum amylase level.

TABLE 62–2. Predisposing Factors for Sialadenitis and Parotitis

Xerostomia	Blocked Stensen's or Wharton's duct
Drugs	Mucus plugs
Anticholinergics	Sialolithiasis and calculi
Antihistamines	Strictures
β-blockers	Stenosis
Diuretics	Foreign bodies
Antiparkinson drugs	Pneumoparotitis
Phenothiazines	Trauma to salivary glands
Thiouracil	Salivary gland surgery (within 3 weeks)
Iodides	Local irradiation of salivary glands
Gentamicin aerosols	Prematurity
Systemic diseases	Malnutrition
Sjögren's syndrome	Poor oral hygiene
Diabetes mellitus	Total parenteral nutrition
Dehydration	Gastrostomy or jejunostomy tube feedings
	Allergies
	IgA deficiency
	Immune complex disease

TABLE 62–3. Noninfectious Causes of Salivary Gland Swellings

- Dehydration
- Sialolithiasis
- Collagen vascular disorders
  - Sjögren's syndrome
  - Systemic lupus erythematosus
  - Scleroderma
  - Polyarteritis nodosa
  - Polymyositis
  - Rheumatoid arthritis
- Neoplasia
  - Leukemia
  - Lymphoma
  - Hodgkin's disease
  - Parotid tumors
  - Hemangiomas
  - Lymphangiomas
  - Lipomas
  - Adenomas
- Congenital cysts
- Sarcoidosis
- Amyloidosis
- Pneumoparotitis
- Familial dysautonomia
- Ectodermal dysplasia
- Heavy metal poisons
  - Lead
  - Mercury

Chronic, painless, persistent parotitis is usually persistent benign sialadenopathy, but it may be caused by sarcoidosis, tuberculosis, actinomycosis, blastomycosis, and HIV infection (Chapter 38). The salivary glands are rarely infected in childhood tuberculosis (Chapter 35). The parotid gland is affected more commonly (70%) than the submandibular gland (25%) or the lingual glands (5%). The two forms are infiltrative disseminated tuberculosis, accounting for two thirds of cases, and circumscribed nodular tuberculosis. The infiltrative form usually presents as a painless salivary gland tumor resulting from hematogenous seeding and has a mild course. The circumscribed nodular form presents with purulence from the ducts, with pronounced or absent secretory abilities and is associated with minimal or no pain, fever, and swelling. Caseation necrosis is evident in both forms. Both presentations have minimal systemic signs and symptoms of tuberculosis. The chest radiograph usually is normal, showing no hilar adenopathy. The tonsils may occasionally be the primary focus of infection.

Laboratory Evaluation

The serum amylase level is characteristically high. There may also be an elevated ESR and leukocytosis with neutrophil predominance. However, a normal WBC count, especially in newborns, does not exclude bacterial infection.

The saliva is typically thick and cloudy, and a stained smear of saliva usually reveals many neutrophils. The saliva normally has a low sodium content and a high potassium level that is reversed in bacterial infections, which may be useful to differentiate inflammatory from noninflammatory swelling.

Microbiologic Evaluation

Appropriate stains and cultures for aerobic, acid-fast, fungal, and anaerobic organisms confirm infectious parotitis. The parotid duct may be cannulated and lavaged to obtain appropriate samples. Appropriate transport media and culture techniques should be ensured for anaerobic cultures. Blood cultures should also be obtained for newborn, immunosuppressed, and systemically ill patients.

Diagnostic Imaging

Most of the usual salivary duct obstructions are radiolucent; this is especially true of parotid calculi, which can be missed by sialography or plain roentgenography. Ultrasonography is useful to locate obstructing calculi and to identify abscess development. Sialography is usually contraindicated during acute infection because instillation of dye can rupture the terminal ducts, causing extravasation of contrast medium into acini and interstitial tissue with resultant spread of the infection. Sialography during remission of recurrent parotitis may reveal cystic cavities in the lining of the epithelium, indicating congenital abnormalities, and generalized sialectasis without anatomic obstruction. Other congenital anomalies allow stagnation of secretions, which predisposes to recurrent retrograde infection. Some patients with recurrent sialadenitis have normal sialograms.

TREATMENT

The principles of successful medical therapy involve prompt reversal of underlying risk factors and the early initiation of appropriate antibiotic therapy. Removal of calculi by ductal dilation or sialithectomy is especially important when ductal obstruction occurs secondary to stones. For acute infection or exacerbation of recurrent infection, rehydration should be instituted. Oral **sialagogues** (e.g., lemon juice, chewing gum, tamarind) should be used to stimulate salivary flow. Supportive measures include a nonaspirin analgesic and antipyretic agent, warm external compresses, and massage of the gland to encourage salivary flow.

Definitive Treatment

Systemic antibiotics are indicated for persons with fever and purulent discharge from a swollen gland. Empiric antimicrobial therapy in uncomplicated cases consists of an antistaphylococcal semisynthetic penicillin (e.g., nafcillin or oxacillin) or first-generation cephalosporin. Either clindamycin or vancomycin combined with a third-generation cephalosporin (e.g., cefotaxime or ceftriaxone), piperacillin-tazobactam, or a carbapenem (e.g., imipenem or meropenem), with or without an aminoglycoside, provide adequate empiric coverage for mixed infections with gram-positive, gram-negative, and anaerobic bacteria for nosocomial infections and for immunocompromised or severely ill persons. Definitive antimicrobial therapy is based on identification of the etiologic agent from microbiologic stains and cultures of fluid from the parotid duct. Antibiotic therapy should be continued for at least 7 days. There is usually a good clinical response within 72 hours, with a significant reduction in parotid swelling, fever, trismus, and pain.

Surgery. Surgical intervention is necessary in the presence of obstruction due to stones or other causes, if medical therapy fails, or if there is continued clinical deterioration. Additional rare indications for surgical treatment include partial airway obstruction, extreme unremitting pain, extension of infection, parotid abscess, and metastatic spread. Surgical intervention provides external surgical drainage and relieves ductal obstruction. Revision of the duct and partial parotid excision may be necessary. Ultrasonography may help determine the presence of abscess formation and the need for surgical drainage. Purulent material is often aspirated for up to 5 days in acute bacterial parotitis. A surgical complication is injury to the facial nerve, which traverses the parotid gland.

Recurrent parotitis may require parotidectomy for cure. However, a conservative approach is recommended because of potential facial nerve injury and frequent spontaneous resolution during adolescence.

Radiation Therapy. Radiation therapy was once the cornerstone of management, but the reduction in mortality was actually due to the confounding factor of concomitant rehydration. Radiation therapy is not indicated.

COMPLICATIONS

Infection may spread locally or by hematogenous spread with septicemia, especially in immunocompromised persons. Complications include parotid abscess formation, local extension of the glandular infection, massive neck swelling with airway obstruction, thrombophlebitis of the jugular vein, facial osteomyelitis, temporomandibular arthritis, aspiration pneumonia, rupture of an abscess through the auditory canal or parapharyngeal space, erysipelas, and septicemia. Noninfectious complications include extreme pain, facial nerve palsy, and sialectasis.

PROGNOSIS

The prognosis was poor in the preantibiotic era but has substantially improved with appropriate care and antibiotics. The mortality may be high among newborns and immunocompromised persons. The recurrence rate for suppurative infection of the submandibular gland is high because of associated calculi or obstruction.

Recurrent sialadenitis and parotitis usually resolves spontaneously before adulthood. Success is achieved with medical treatment of acute episodes after a complete evaluation to exclude surgically correctable obstructive lesions.

PREVENTION

The incidence of community acquired acute bacterial parotitis in children can be reduced by good oral hygiene. Nosocomial cases can be prevented by careful oral suctioning, maintenance of adequate hydration, and prevention of trauma to the parotid ducts and glands during surgical procedures.

REVIEWS

Chitre VV, Premchandra DJ: Recurrent parotitis. *Arch Dis Child* 1997; 77:359–63.

Cohen HA, Gross S, Nusinovitch M, et al: Recurrent parotitis. *Arch Dis Child* 1992;67:1036–7.

Pou AM, Johnson JT, Weissman J: Management decisions in parotitis. *Comp Ther* 1995;21:85–92.

Raad II, Sabbaugh MF, Caranosos GJ: Acute bacterial sialadenitis: A study of 29 cases and review. *Rev Infect Dis* 1990;12:591–601.

KEY ARTICLES

Brook I, Frazier EH, Thompson DH: Aerobic and anaerobic microbiology of acute suppurative parotitis. *Laryngoscope* 1991;101:170–2.

David RB, O'Connel EJ: Suppurative parotitis in children. *Am J Dis Child* 1970;119:332–5.

Ericson S, Zetterlund B, Ohman J: Recurrent parotitis and sialectasis in childhood. Clinical, radiologic, immunologic, bacteriologic, and histologic study. *Ann Otol Rhinol Laryngol* 1991;100:527–35.

Geterud A, Lindvall A, Nylen O: Follow-up study of recurrent parotitis in children. *Ann Otol Rhinol Laryngol* 1988;97:341–6.

Giglio MS, Landaeta M, Pinto ME: Microbiology of recurrent parotitis. *Pediatr Infect Dis J* 1997;16:386–90.

Goguen LA, April MM, Karmody CS, et al: Self-induced pneumoparotitis. *Arch Otolaryngol Head Neck Surg* 1995;121:1426–9.

Kaban LB, Mulliken JB, Murray JE: Sialadenitis in childhood. *Am J Surg* 1978;135:570–6.

Leake D, Leake R: Neonatal suppurative parotitis. *Pediatrics* 1970; 46:202–7.

CHAPTER 63

Otitis Externa

Paul A. Shurin

Otitis externa, also known as **swimmer's ear,** is defined by inflammation and exudation in the external auditory canal in the absence of other disorders, such as otitis media or mastoiditis, that may extend into the auditory canal and cause similar local findings. Although the pathogenesis of ordinary otitis externa is not completely clear, it appears to result from the interaction of host, environmental, and microbial factors.

ETIOLOGY

The most common bacterial pathogen is *Pseudomonas aeruginosa,* especially in cases associated with bacterial contamination from swimming in pools or lakes. *P. aeruginosa* is also associated with the more severe cases. Other common pathogens that may be present with **chronic suppurative otitis media,** which is persistent or recurrent tympanic membrane perforation with inflammation or persistent drainage, or **tympanostomy tube otorrhea,** which develops in approximately 20% of children with tympanostomy tubes, include *Staphylococcus aureus, Streptococcus pneumoniae, Moraxella catarrhalis, Proteus, Klebsiella,* and occasionally anaerobes. Coagulase-negative staphylococci and *Corynebacterium* are frequently isolated from cultures of the external canal but represent normal flora. Outbreaks of otitis externa have been associated with hot tubs contaminated with *P. aeruginosa.* Malignant otitis externa is caused by *P. aeruginosa* in immunocompromised persons.

EPIDEMIOLOGY

Otitis externa is a frequent complaint in pediatric practice. The frequency is greatest in summer, in contrast to otitis media, which occurs primarily in colder seasons in association with viral upper respiratory tract infections. Disruption of the integrity of the cutaneous lining of the ear canal and local defenses, as occurs with cleaning of the auditory canal, swimming, and, in particular, diving, predisposes to otitis externa.

PATHOGENESIS

The presence of a normal amount of cerumen and an acid pH are the major defenses against otitis externa. Removal of cerumen and changes in the normal acid environment facilitate epithelial invasion by colonizing bacteria or the introduction of more virulent bacteria that produce otitis externa. The risk from swimming correlates with the degree of bacterial contamination of pools and lakes. Infection in healthy hosts is usually limited to the superficial layers of the skin but, especially in immunocompromised persons, can progress to deeper soft tissue infection.

Malignant Otitis Externa. Malignant otitis externa, also known as **progressive necrotizing otitis externa,** is a severe, life-threatening, invasive infection of the auditory canal and temporal bone caused in most cases by *Pseudomonas aeruginosa.* There is severe pain, and granulation tissue rather than simple exudation is present in the canal. Malignant otitis externa historically was seen only in elderly patients with diabetes mellitus but is now also seen in infants and children with chronic diseases, particularly those accompanied by neutropenia or immunodeficiency. Irrigation of the auditory canal with tap water has been reported as a predisposing factor in some cases.

SYMPTOMS AND CLINICAL MANIFESTATIONS

Pain, tenderness, and aural discharge are the characteristic clinical findings of otitis externa. Fever is notably absent, and hearing is unaffected. Tenderness with movement of the pinnae, especially the tragus, and on chewing is particularly typical. This is not present in otitis media and thus is a valuable diagnostic criterion. The most common symptoms of malignant otitis externa are ear pain, tenderness on movement of the pinna, drainage from the canal, and facial nerve palsy.

Physical Examination Findings

In addition to marked tenderness on movement of the pinna and tragus, inspection usually reveals that the lining of the auditory canal is inflamed with mild to severe erythema and edema. Physical examination of the auditory canal, including attempts to examine the mobility of the tympanic membrane by insufflation, usually accentuates the pain and is often resisted by the patient. There may be a scant to copious discharge from the auditory canal, often obscuring the tympanic membrane.

In malignant otitis externa, the most common physical findings are swelling and granulation tissue in the canal, usually with a discharge from the external auditory canal. Swelling of the parotid gland and lymphadenopathy are occasionally present.

DIAGNOSIS

The diagnosis of uncomplicated otitis externa is usually established solely on the basis of the clinical symptoms and physical examination findings without the need for additional laboratory or microbiologic evaluation.

Differential Diagnosis

There are only a few entities in the differential diagnosis of otitis externa (Table 63–1). Otitis media with tympanic perforation and discharge into the auditory canal may readily be confused with otitis externa, particularly in infants in whom it may be difficult to clear the discharge and perform an adequate examination. Pain on movement of the pinnae and the tragus, which is typical of otitis externa, is not present in otitis media with tympanic perforation and discharge. Clinical symptoms suggestive of otitis media include

TABLE 63–1. Differential Diagnosis of Otitis Externa

Otitis media
Mastoiditis with extension into the auditory canal
Foreign body
Trauma
Malignancy
Tuberculous or fungal otitis media
Malignant otitis externa

fever and irritability. Local and systemic signs of mastoiditis will ordinarily indicate a process more extensive than otitis externa; these signs may be obscure, however, particularly when partially effective antimicrobial treatment has masked the overt findings. Malignant lesions presenting in the auditory canal are rare in children but may present with discharge, unusual pain, or hearing loss. Tuberculous otitis media is marked by a chronic, painless aural discharge; it is further suggested by skin testing and chest radiograph and is confirmed by acid-fast stain and culture of the discharge for mycobacteria. Large numbers of tubercle bacilli are generally present. Treatment is the same as for extrapulmonary tuberculosis involving other organs (Chapter 35).

Malignant Otitis Externa. Malignant otitis externa presents with a chronic, copious aural discharge, severe local pain, and often systemic illness. Because of invasion of the bones of the base of the skull, cranial nerve palsies may also occur, with facial nerve palsy a common presenting feature in children. An elevated ESR is a constant finding. The diagnosis requires documentation of the extent of involvement with diagnostic imaging studies such as ^{99m}Tc radionuclide bone scan, CT, or MRI. Cultures are required to identify the etiologic agent, usually *P. aeruginosa,* and the antimicrobial susceptibility.

TREATMENT

The most widely used topical otic preparations contain a quinolone antibiotic or a combination of an aminoglycoside, such as neomycin, and polymyxin B with a topical corticosteroid (Table 63–2). Neomycin is active against *S. aureus* and most gram-negative bacteria but has limited activity against *P. aeruginosa.* Polymyxin B is active against these organisms as well as *P. aeruginosa.* The quinolones ciprofloxacin and ofloxacin are active against *S. aureus* and *P. aeruginosa.* None of these have any antifungal activity. The acetic acid preparations have antibacterial and antifungal effects by acidification.

Local therapy with acetic acid preparations designed to restore the acid pH of the auditory canal with acetic acid preparations is usually effective (Table 63–2). Acetic acid (2%) solutions instilled in the auditory canal, 4 drops to fill the canal three or four times a day, should be used for several days to restore a low pH. This may be used one or two times a day for 1–2 weeks after the infection has cleared to preserve a proper pH. A 1:1 solution of water and white vinegar is an inexpensive and appropriate solution. Combinations of acetic acid in Burow's solution or with corticosteroids are frequently used to reduce local inflammation and the accompanying pain. For administration of otic solutions and suspensions, the patient should lie with the affected ear upward while the drops are instilled. This position should be maintained for 5 minutes to facilitate penetration of the drops into the auditory canal. It may be necessary to remove the aural exudate with a swab or with suction to permit instillation of the solution. The predisposing activity, such as swimming or diving, that produced the condition should be avoided until the inflammation has resolved.

There is little evidence that topical antibiotics alone are more effective than antiseptic preparations in the treatment of otitis externa. Controlled studies have indicated that local irrigation with antiseptic agents, with or without corticosteroids, and acetic acid solutions designed to restore the acid environment of the auditory canal are generally effective. In addition, these preparations lessen the risk of sensitization sometimes associated with topical antibiotic therapy, which can worsen the local inflammatory reaction and symptoms. Otic solutions containing corticosteroids are frequently used for this condition and will reduce local inflammation when there is no infection. Solutions that combine antibiotics and corticosteroids are a reasonable choice in severe cases and when therapy with acetic acid preparations has not been effective. Treatment with topical otic analgesics and cerumenolytics is usually unnecessary.

Systemic antibiotics are rarely needed in otitis externa. It is important in severe cases to obtain cultures with sensitivity testing of the bacterial isolates and to perform diagnostic studies for other conditions that might be included in the differential diagnosis.

Fungi, such as *Aspergillus, Candida,* and dermatophytes, are occasionally isolated from the external ear. It may be difficult to determine whether they represent normal skin flora or are the cause of inflammation. In most cases, local therapy and restoration of normal pH as recommended for bacterial otitis externa is sufficient.

Chronic suppurative otitis media may require both topical treatment, usually with a quinolone otic drug, and oral therapy for otitis media (Chapter 64). **Tympanostomy tube otorrhea** is best treated with a quinolone otic drug because these agents are considered less likely to be ototoxic. There are theoretical risks of ototoxicity with neomycin and polymyxin B, which should be avoided in the presence of tympanic perforation.

Malignant Otitis Externa. Malignant otitis externa is treated with parenteral antimicrobials with activity against *P. aeruginosa,* such as piperacillin-tazobactam, ceftazidime, cefepime, or meropenem with or without an aminoglycoside, in doses appropriate for sepsis.

TABLE 63–2. Topical Therapy of Otitis Externa

Composition	Trade Names
Definitive Treatment	
Acetic Acid	
Acetic acid 2% in modified Burow's solution	Otic Domeboro
Acetic Acid with Corticosteroids	
Acetic acid 2% with hydrocortisone 1%	VoSoL HC
Acetic acid 2% with desonide 0.05%	Otic Tridesilon
Antibiotics with Corticosteroids	
Ciprofloxacin with hydrocortisone 1%	Cipro HC Otic
Ofloxacin	Floxin Otic
Neomycin and polymyxin B with hydrocortisone 1%	Cortisporin, Pediotic, LazerSporin-C
Colistin, neomycin, and thonzonium with hydrocortisone 1%	Cortisporin-TC
Adjunctive Otic Drugs	
Otic Analgesics	
Benzocaine	Americaine Otic
Antipyrine, benzocaine	Auralgan
Cerumenolytics	
Triethanolamine polypeptide oleate	Cerumenex

Treatment is continued until a clinical cure is apparent, which frequently requires a total of 4–6 weeks. The duration of treatment should be at least 6 weeks if there is concomitant osteomyelitis. Invasion of the cartilage, causing chondritis or perichondritis, by *S. aureus* requires prolonged treatment with a parenteral antistaphylococcal agent (e.g., oxacillin, nafcillin, cefazolin, or cephalothin for methicillin-susceptible strains and vancomycin for methicillin-resistant strains). Surgical drainage and débridement may be necessary if there is invasion of the mastoids or auricular cartilage. Spread of infection to osseous tissue may require more extensive surgery. Recent studies report that malignant otitis externa can also be treated with prolonged oral regimens of quinolones, given alone or in combination with rifampin.

COMPLICATIONS AND PROGNOSIS

Acute otitis externa usually resolves promptly without complications within 1–2 days of initiation of treatment. Persistent pain, especially if severe or if accompanied by other symptoms such as fever, should prompt re-evaluation for other conditions.

Malignant otitis externa is frequently accompanied by complications. Invasion of the bones of the base of the skull may cause cranial nerve palsies, such as facial nerve palsy. Historically, this disease is progressive and invariably lethal, but it may now be cured with systemic antibiotic therapy. The mortality is 15–20% in adults with malignant otitis media, and relapses within the first year after treatment are common.

PREVENTION

Overly vigorous cleaning of the asymptomatic auditory canal should be avoided. Drying the auditory canals with acetic acid (2%), Burow's solution, or diluted isopropyl alcohol (rubbing alcohol) after swimming may be performed prophylactically to help prevent the maceration that may facilitate bacterial invasion. Often underwater gear, such as earplugs or diving equipment, must be avoided to prevent recurrent disease. There is no role for prophylactic otic antibiotics. Persons with diabetes mellitus or those who are otherwise immunocompromised should avoid swimming in highly contaminated waters. Hot tubs must be monitored and disinfected to prevent contamination with *P. aeruginosa.*

REVIEWS

Hannley MT, Denneny JC 3rd, Holzer SS: Use of ototopical antibiotics in treating 3 common ear diseases. *Otolaryngol Head Neck Surg* 2000;122:934–40.

Pelton SI, Klein JO: The draining ear: Otitis media and externa. *Infect Dis Clin North Am* 1988;2:117–29.

KEY ARTICLES

Angius AM, Pickles JM, Burch KL: A prospective study of otitis externa. *Clin Otolaryngol* 1992;17:150–4.

Clayton MI, Osborne JE, Rutherford D, et al: A double-blind, randomized, prospective trial of a topical antiseptic versus a topical antibiotic in the treatment of otorrhoea. *Clin Otolaryngol* 1990 Feb;15:7–10.

Dibb WL: Microbial aetiology of otitis externa. *J Infect* 1991;22:233–9.

Jones RN, Milazzo J, Seidlin M: Ofloxacin otic solution for treatment of otitis externa in children and adults. *Arch Otolaryngol Head Neck Surg* 1997;123:1193–200.

Nir D, Nir T, Danino J, et al: Malignant external otitis in an infant. *J Laryngol Otol* 1990;104:488–90.

Rubin J, Curtin HD, Yu VL, et al: Malignant external otitis: Utility of CT in diagnosis and follow-up. *Radiology* 1990;174:391–4.

Rubin J, Yu VL, Kamerer DB, et al: Aural irrigation with water: A potential pathogenic mechanism for inducing malignant external otitis? *Ann Otol Rhinol Laryngol* 1990;99:117–9.

Rubin J, Yu VL, Stool SE: Malignant external otitis in children. *J Pediatr* 1988;113:965–70.

van Asperen IA, de Rover CM, Schijven JF, et al: Risk of otitis externa after swimming in recreational fresh water lakes containing *Pseudomonas aeruginosa*. *Br Med J* 1995;311:1407–10.

CHAPTER 64

Otitis Media

Candice E. Johnson ▪ Paul A. Shurin

Otitis media is among the most frequent conditions seen by pediatricians. Diseases of the middle ear are diagnosed at approximately one third of visits to pediatrician's offices. This frequency is virtually as high for infants and young children being seen for well-child care as for those who are ill, which illustrates that clinical presentation may be asymptomatic or so severe as to require differentiation from such infections as bacteremia and meningitis. Although otitis media occurs at all ages, the disease is most frequent in early infancy. In addition to causing acute febrile illnesses, otitis media is likely to produce a conductive hearing loss that, if persistent, may result in delays in speech and cognitive development.

ETIOLOGY

Culture results are rarely available to confirm a specific bacterial or viral pathogen before the institution of therapy for acute otitis media, guide response to presumptive clinical failure, or manage persistent otologic disorders. Instead, clinical practice is based on the accumulated results of studies that include cultures from the middle ear.

Three bacterial species, *Streptococcus pneumoniae, Haemophilus influenzae,* and *Moraxella catarrhalis* (previously known as *Branhamella catarrhalis* or *Neisseria catarrhalis*), account for approximately 90% of acute otitis media episodes from which a bacterial agent can be isolated. Changing resistance patterns have become a major problem for each of these species. The choice of antibiotic therapy for initial cases of acute otitis media and for failures or recurrences is affected by the various resistance mechanisms that may be involved.

Tympanocentesis and culture of the middle ear exudate are required for identification of bacterial pathogens present in the middle ear. Although the infecting organisms are also often present in cultures of nasopharyngeal secretions, these cultures generally yield a mixed flora that is not of specific diagnostic value. Tympanic aspiration is not widely practiced in the United States but could be more widely used in children for whom identification of the specific organism would be of therapeutic value.

Respiratory viruses are involved in the pathogenesis of both bacterial and nonbacterial acute otitis media, as shown both in epidemiologic studies during outbreaks of respiratory disease and in studies of viruses and viral antigens in middle ear exudates. Specific therapy is not yet available for most such viral infections.

Bacteria are not cultured in approximately 15–30% of clinically typical acute otitis media cases. However, molecular methods, such as RT-PCR, can identify the presence of bacterial mRNA in as many as one fourth of sterile middle ear effusions. The results of cultures of both ears are frequently disparate; a frequent finding is that one middle ear effusion is bacteriologically sterile when a pathogen is present in the contralateral ear.

Streptococcus pneumoniae. *Streptococcus pneumoniae* accounts for 40% of bacterial acute otitis media. It is considered the most important agent by virtue of its association with more severe symptoms and its potential for involvement in systemic infections, such as pneumonia, bacteremia, and meningitis. Treatment of pneumococcal disease among young children is complicated by emergence of pneumococcal strains resistant to penicillin and other antibiotics. *S. pneumoniae* does not produce β-lactamase or penicillinase but is resistant because of mutational modifications of the penicillin-binding proteins of the cell wall. There is partial cross-resistance to the oral cephalosporins. High-level resistance to penicillin, indicated by a minimum inhibitory concentration (MIC) ≥ 2 μg/mL, has increased substantially during the past decade, from 1.3% in 1992 to 13.6% in 1997. In certain areas of the United States, approximately 30% of invasive isolates are **penicillin-nonsusceptible *S. pneumoniae,*** including intermediate susceptibility (MIC = 0.1–1 μg/mL) or resistant (MIC ≥ 2 μg/mL). Intermediate, or relative resistance, may be overcome with higher doses of β-lactam antibiotics although susceptibility to other classes of drugs, such as macrolides, is not dose-dependent. High-level resistance (MIC ≥ 2 μg/mL) is less common but is an even greater public health threat. Resistance to antimicrobials of other classes, such as trimethoprim-sulfamethoxazole, tetracyclines, macrolides, clindamycin, and chloramphenicol, may be present as single resistance or may accompany penicillin resistance and thus result in **multiple drug-resistant *S. pneumoniae.***

Antibiotic-resistant *S. pneumoniae* are more frequently carried by children than by adults. Risk factors associated with infection with penicillin-resistant pneumococci include younger age, attendance at a daycare center, higher socioeconomic status, recent (i.e., ≤ 3 months) antibiotic use, and recurrent episodes of acute otitis media. Recent daycare attendance and recent antibiotic treatment are associated independently with invasive disease caused by penicillin-resistant *S. pneumoniae.* Isolates from middle ear exudates are more likely than those from other infections, such as blood cultures, to be drug resistant.

Haemophilus influenzae. *Haemophilus influenzae* accounts for 30% of bacterial acute otitis media. In the past, 90% of *H. influenzae* strains from the middle ear were nontypable or did not express any of the capsular polysaccharides (types a–f) and 10% were type b. Nontypable strains cause only localized respiratory infections, such as otitis media, sinusitis, nonbacteremic pneumonia, and bronchitis. Only *H. influenzae* type b strains have significant potential to cause invasive disease and systemic infections, such as bacteremia, meningitis, and arthritis. With routine *H. influenzae* type b immunization of infants, nasopharyngeal carriage and spread of type b organisms has dramatically decreased. Thus, it may be anticipated that nontypable strains will be the only *H. influenzae* causing acute otitis media in children who live in highly immunized communities.

Production of β-lactamase is the most important mechanism of penicillin and ampicillin resistance in all types of *H. influenzae.* An estimated 45% of *H. influenzae* strains now carry β-lactamases in the United States, which varies in different geographic regions. Although drugs susceptible to hydrolysis by β-lactamase, particularly amoxicillin, are still widely used in treating acute otitis media, clinical results are not optimal when the infecting organism is resistant.

Moraxella catarrhalis. *Moraxella catarrhalis* accounts for 15% of bacterial acute otitis media, an increase from <5% in 1980. The species had previously been uniformly susceptible to penicillins, with MIC of approximately 0.001 μg/mL. The increase in frequency was accompanied by the production of β-lactamase, and an increase in MIC to 0.4–50 μg/mL. Acute otitis media caused by *M. catarrhalis* is disproportionately more frequent in the fall and winter than in the spring and summer. The clinical course of this infection does not differ greatly from that of acute otitis media caused by *S. pneumoniae* and *H. influenzae.*

Other Bacteria. Both group A *Streptococcus* and *Staphylococcus aureus* cause a small proportion of acute otitis media cases in healthy children. The role of coagulase-negative staphylococci (e.g., *Staphylococcus epidermidis* and other species) remains controversial, in part because these are frequent inhabitants of the external ear canal and may contaminate cultures of middle ear effusion. Gram-negative bacilli are frequent agents when acute otitis media occurs in infants less than 6 weeks of age (Table 64–1) but are unusual in uncomplicated acute otitis media in older children.

Respiratory Viruses and Otitis Media. The viruses associated with otitis media are the same respiratory agents that cause upper and lower respiratory tract infections (Chapter 57). Recent studies have greatly strengthened evidence of involvement of respiratory virus infection in pathogenesis of acute otitis media, in addition to the established epidemiologic link. The age distribution of acute otitis media closely parallels the distribution of respiratory tract infections. Outbreaks of the two conditions are linked temporally, both in seasonal occurrence and in observations made in individual respiratory virus outbreaks. Studies in chinchillas (Giebink, 1981) showed that influenza A virus infection markedly enhances the development of acute otitis media caused by *S. pneumoniae.* In a recent clinical study (Heikkinen et al., 1999), viruses were identified in 41% of 456 middle ear exudates of children with acute otitis media, including respiratory syncytial virus (RSV) in 74% of 65 children with RSV infection, parainfluenza viruses in 52% of 29 children with parainfluenza virus infection, influenza viruses in 42% of 24 children with influenza, 11% of 27 children with enterovirus infections, and 4% of 23 children with adenovirus infection.

There is no fixed relationship between these viral infections and bacterial otitis media. Bacterial pathogens are found as frequently in the middle ear exudates of children with or without concomitant viral respiratory tract infections, and the same bacterial species are found in both situations. It appears unlikely that a clinical form of purely viral otitis media can be identified.

Neonates. Diverse bacterial species are associated with acute otitis media in the first 6 weeks of life. Although many young infants will have infection with the *S. pneumoniae* or *Haemophilus influenzae,* it is also common to isolate *Staphylococcus,* groups A and B *Streptococcus,* and gram-negative bacilli in this age group (Table 64–1).

Immunocompromised Persons. Children with immune disorders, particularly immune globulin deficiencies or AIDS, are particularly prone to recurrent and chronic otitis media. Local factors that frequently produce a susceptibility to middle ear disorders include eustachian tube obstruction from adenoid masses and inherited disorders of ciliary function. The most frequent causes of otitis media in these children are the same bacteria as in healthy children, although it is often helpful to obtain cultures of middle ear effusion in these highly susceptible patients.

TABLE 64–1. Bacterial Pathogens Isolated from 169 Infants with Otitis Media During the First 46 Weeks of Life

Microorganism	Infants with Pathogen (%)
Respiratory bacteria	
Streptococcus pneumoniae	18.3
Haemophilus influenzae	12.4
S. pneumoniae and *H. influenzae*	3.0
Staphylococcus aureus	7.7
Streptococcus, groups A and B	3.0
Moraxella catarrhalis	5.3
Enteric bacteria	
Escherichia coli	5.9
Klebsiella and *Enterobacter*	5.3
Pseudomonas aeruginosa	1.8
Miscellaneous	5.3
None or no pathogens	32.0

Data from Berman SA, Balkany TJ, Simmons MA: Otitis media in the neonatal intensive care unit. *Pediatrics* 1978;62:198. Bland RD: Otitis media in the first six weeks of life: Diagnosis, bacteriology and management. *Pediatrics* 1972;49:187. Shurin PA, et al: Bacterial etiology of otitis media during the first six weeks of life. *J Pediatr* 1978;92:893. Tetzlaff TR, Ashworth C, Nelson JD: Otitis media in children less than 12 weeks of age. *Pediatrics* 1977; 59:827.

EPIDEMIOLOGY

In most of the United States, otitis media is a seasonal disease with a distinct peak in January and February, corresponding to the RSV and influenza season, and is uncommon from July to September.

The major risk factors for acute otitis media are young age, bottle-feeding as opposed to breast-feeding, taking a bottle to bed, parental history of ear infection, the presence of a sibling in the home, especially a sibling with a history of ear infection, sharing a room with a sibling, passive exposure to tobacco smoke from parental smoking, and increased exposure to infectious agents, such as children in daycare centers (Table 64–2). The peak incidence of acute otitis media is in the second 6 months of life. By the first birthday, 62% of children experience at least 1 episode. Few first episodes occur after 18 months of age.

Recurrent Otitis Media. Although virtually every child will experience at least one episode of acute otitis media in the first few years of life, certain children have such recurrences up to 8 years of age. There is no established definition of otitis-proneness. However, using the condition of the presence of ≥6 acute otitis media episodes in the first 6 years of life, at least 12% of children in the general population would be considered "otitis-prone." Craniofacial anomalies and immunodeficiencies are often associated with recurrent otitis media, but most children with recurrent acute otitis

TABLE 64–2. Risk Factors for the Development of Otitis Media in Children*

Anatomic (e.g., cleft palate)
Eustachian tube dysfunction (e.g., allergy)
Immune deficiency (e.g., primary antibody deficiencies, AIDS)
Male sex
Race
Native American or Inuit ancestry have increased incidence
African Americans have decreased incidence
Early age at first episode
Sibling with a history of recurrent otitis media
Lack of breast-feeding
Taking a bottle to bed
Group daycare
Parental smoking (passive tobacco smoke)
Socioeconomic status (lower socioeconomic status has increased incidence)
Pacifier use
Parental history of ear infection
Presence of a sibling in the home
Sharing a room with a sibling
Respiratory disease season (winter, fall)

*Presence of any of these factors suggests a greater than average risk of frequent otitis media.

media are otherwise healthy. In a prospective study (Marchant et al., 1984) of infants who were enrolled at birth and followed up for the first year of life, bilateral otitis media with middle ear effusions for at least 3 months developed in 8 of 15 infants (53%) who had bilateral middle ear effusions at 2 months of age, compared with 2 of 55 (4%) who did not. The onset of middle ear effusions was asymptomatic in 46% of the cases. Thus, susceptibility to persistent middle ear effusion can be detected by careful otologic examination at 2 months of life, which emphasizes the need for careful otologic examination of infants.

PATHOGENESIS

Eustachian Tube Anatomy and Function. The eustachian tube has three functions in regard to protecting the middle ear: (1) ventilation, the maintenance of air at atmospheric pressure in the middle ear cavity; (2) drainage, the function that provides for removal of exudates, inflammatory products, microorganisms, and other pathologic materials from the diseased middle ear; and (3) protection of the middle ear cavity from reflux of nasopharyngeal secretions and from acoustic damage. The occurrence of reflux has been documented radiographically during feeding in infants. Reflux of infected secretions is clearly the route of infection responsible for most acute otitis media because the infecting organisms are almost always those present in the nasopharynx. Although functional defects of eustachian tube function are involved in the pathogenesis of acute otitis media and persistent middle ear effusion, in most cases it is not feasible to test for these functions. Exceptions are the presence of eustachian tube obstruction by adenoidal or other masses, which can be evaluated clinically or radiographically, and cases of inadequate ventilation in which the persistently reduced middle ear pressure can be documented with tympanometry.

Eustachian tube dysfunction appears to be responsible for the association of otitis media with unrepaired cleft palate, trisomy 21 (Down syndrome), and craniofacial anomalies, and is thought to be involved in the predilection for severe otitis media that is found in certain populations, including Inuits, Native Americans, and Australian aborigines. Socioeconomic factors may also contribute to the apparent racial differences in disease incidence.

Host Defenses in the Upper Respiratory Tract. Maturation of host defenses provides an explanation for the decreasing frequency of otitis media during childhood. Eustachian tube dysfunction is more frequent in infants than in older children and adults. Acquired immunity and antibody production, both locally in the upper respiratory tract and systemically, develops after exposure to bacterial and viral respiratory pathogens that cause acute otitis media. The protective role of antibody against otitis media has been established in studies of pneumococcal immunization and passive protection with immunoglobulins, which prevented recurrent episodes of acute otitis media in high-risk children.

The occurrence of acute or recurrent middle ear disease may be apparent at all ages among immunodeficient children. In children older than 5 years of age who continue to have recurrences, an allergy and even an abbreviated immunologic evaluation may be useful. Atopic children have more episodes of otitis media, as do those with IgA or IgG subclass deficiencies.

SYMPTOMS AND CLINICAL MANIFESTATIONS

In infants, the most frequent symptoms of acute otitis media are nonspecific and include fever, irritability, poor feeding, and vomiting. Among older children and adolescents, acute otitis media is usually associated with fever and **otalgia,** or acute ear pain. Acute otitis media may also present with ear drainage after spontaneous rupture of the tympanic membrane. Signs of a common cold (Chapter 57), which is often present and predisposes to acute otitis media, may be present. Examination of the ears is essential for diagnosis and should be part of the physical examination of any child with fever.

Physical Examination Findings

The hallmark of otitis media is the presence of effusion in the middle ear cavity. The presence or absence of middle ear effusion should be determined at every pediatric examination. The presence of an effusion does not define its nature or potentially infectious etiology, but it does define the need for appropriate diagnosis and therapy. Otitis media without effusion, or **silent otitis media,** is rare among middle ear disorders of children and is considered primarily in the context of chronic middle ear disease.

The normal tympanic membrane has a ground-glass translucent appearance and a **pearly gray color** and maintains a **neutral position** with brisk mobility with slight negative and positive pressure (Plate 10A). Acute otitis media is characterized by **hyperemia,** or red color (but it can be pink, white, or yellow), opacification, a full to bulging position, and poor mobility in response to both negative and positive pressure (Plate 10B). The **light reflex** is lost, and the middle ear structures are obscured and difficult to distinguish. Tympanic hyperemia alone is not diagnostic of otitis media because it may occur with fever or even with crying. Otitis media with effusion is characterized by white, amber, or blue color, sometimes with visible bubbles, usually by a retracted position, and poor mobility (Plates 10C, 10D, and 10E). A hole in the tympanic membrane or purulent drainage indicates perforation (Plate 10F). Occasionally bullae are present on the lateral aspect of the tympanic membrane and are characteristically associated with severe ear pain but are not indications of *Mycoplasma pneumonia* as once believed.

Otoscopic Examination. In contrast to the diagnostic approach used for most other infectious diseases, the methods used in clinical practice for detection of acute otitis media and other middle ear disorders provide only interferential information about the condition of the middle ear. The **pneumatic otoscope,** which is a pneumatic attachment to a hermetically sealed otoscope, allows judgments about the state of ventilation of the middle ear (Fig. 64–1*A*). The air-filled middle ear will have a much more compliant tympanic membrane than a fluid-filled one, and the movement of the eardrum can be visualized directly as the external ear canal pressure is alternately increased and decreased. Pneumatic otoscopy has been adopted as a standard for clinical diagnosis by most researchers in this field and should be used in general pediatric practice.

There are several practical requirements for accurate otoscopic visualization of the tympanic membrane, including patient cooperation or restraint, and removal of excess cerumen or other foreign material from the ear canal. It is often not possible to examine the ears of an infant without some sort of restraint, such as swaddling with sheets or a restraining board. Curettage and irrigation are the most useful methods for removal of cerumen or other foreign material from the ear canal. **Curettage,** preferably through an **operating head otoscope** that has a shorter working distance than the sealed head of a diagnostic otoscope (Fig. 64–1*B*), is easily and rapidly performed but is often frightening to the patient. A small, rounded curette, size 00, is invaluable for cleaning the ear canals of infants. **Irrigation** of the ear canal with water at body temperature and a syringe or, more conveniently, a dental irrigator, is often less traumatic. Irrigation should not be performed in the presence of a tympanic perforation.

Pneumatic otoscopy or **insufflation** of the external canal extends the information available by observation of the tympanic membrane by allowing the examiner to judge whether air or fluid is present in the middle ear cavity and whether middle ear pressure is normal, reduced, or increased. The speculum of the otoscope must produce an airtight seal at its insertion into the ear canal. A rubber bulb is used to alternately increase and diminish pressure in the external ear canal. The otoscope and bulb can be tested by partially compressing the bulb and then placing a fingertip over the end of the speculum; air should not enter the system when the bulb is released. Many commercially available otoscope heads do not meet this requirement and thus are not adequate for subtle assessment of mobility of the tympanic membrane. The air leaks can in some cases be sealed with epoxy glue. In most small infants, it is also helpful to have a short sleeve of rubber tubing that can be slid onto the speculum. This serves the double purpose of giving a better airtight seal and of preventing the speculum from penetrating too far into the ear canal and impacting painfully on the tympanic membrane itself, which both obscures the upper portion of the membrane and causes direct local injury.

DIAGNOSIS

The diagnosis of acute otitis media is established by the presence of characteristic signs and symptoms of fever, irritability, pulling at the ears, or earache in the presence of middle ear effusion. The onset of acute otitis media may be virtually symptomatic, particularly in infants. Furthermore, middle ear effusion cannot be distinguished as acute or chronic from the otoscopic appearance of the tympanic membrane. A useful operational definition of acute otitis media is the presence of either a newly identified middle ear effusion with signs of inflammation, regardless of symptoms, or the onset of symptoms of acute otitis media in the presence of pre-existing middle ear effusion. This definition has been used effectively to identify illness that proved to have a very high rate of bacterial infection of the middle ear.

Laboratory Evaluation

Routine laboratory studies, including CBC and ESR, are not useful in the evaluation of otitis media. The results of these studies may also be elevated if there is a pre-existing viral infection, which often predisposes to otitis media.

Tympanometry. Tympanometry is not as useful as otoscopy in the diagnosis of acute otitis media but is used for assessing resolution to normal, ventilated, middle ear status after clinical recovery from acute otitis media. Normal tympanograms at 4–6 weeks after onset generally obviate the need for further specific follow-up.

Tympanometry provides objective acoustic measurements of the tympanic membrane–middle ear system by reflection or absorption of sound energy from the external ear canal as pressure in the canal is varied (just as in pneumatic otoscopy). Measurements of the resulting **tympanogram** correlate well with the presence or absence of middle ear effusion. Although the procedure is simple

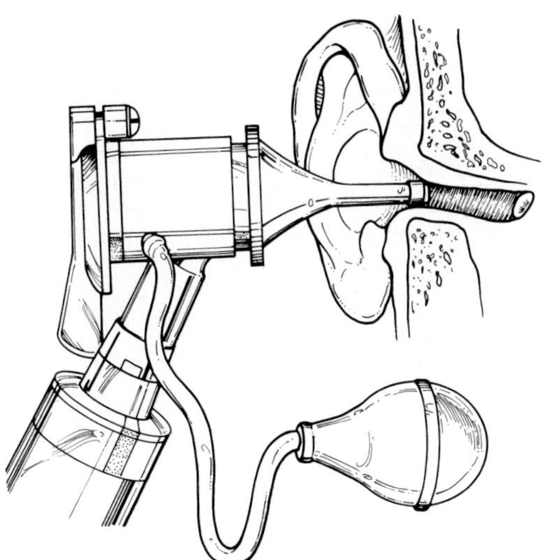

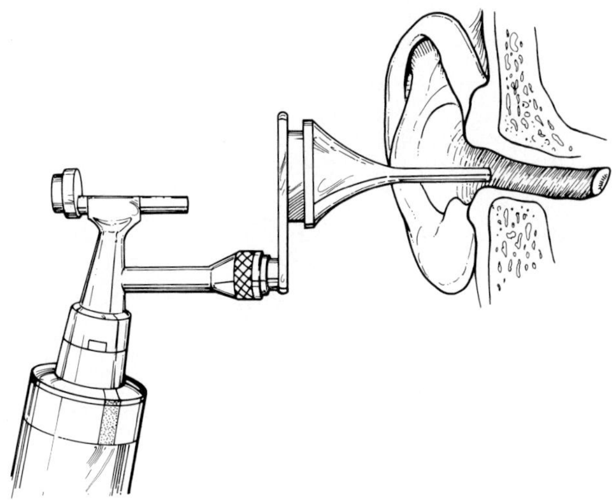

FIGURE 64–1. A diagnostic pneumatic otoscope *(left)* is required to produce an airtight seal in the external auditory canal to allow the examiner to observe the mobility of the tympanic membrane. An operating head otoscope *(right)* is ideal for the removal of cerumen with a curette and for performing tympanocentesis.

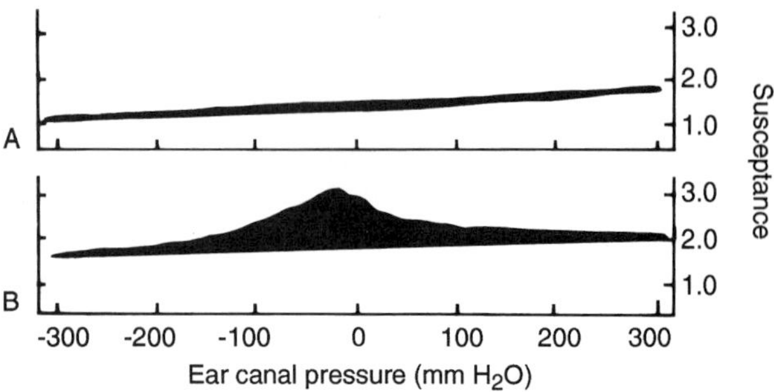

FIGURE 64–2. Tympanograms of a child with acute otitis media (shown by tympanocentesis and culture to be caused by *H. influenzae*). **A,** Flat tracing at the acute stage of the disease, indicating the lack of acoustic change with change of pressure in the fluid-filled ear. **B,** Return to normal 2 months later. The peak in susceptance at atmospheric pressure may be thought of as representing the peak in conductive function of the ear when air pressure is equal in the ear canal and in the middle ear cavity.

to perform in children of all ages, technical details of the instrumentation are critical. Tympanograms accurately reflect the presence of middle ear effusion in children as young as 2 weeks of age. Tympanometry is best performed on a quiet or sleeping child. The results are generally easy to interpret by the presence of a peak in the tracing (Fig. 64–2). The merits of tympanometry are that the procedure is painless and nontraumatic because the probe used for sound generation and signal measurement does not need to enter the external ear canal as deeply as is required for otoscopy; the test is without hazard; good results can be obtained by relatively unskilled personnel; and an objective record of the presence and course of middle ear effusion is obtained.

Acoustic Reflectometry. Instruments that use acoustic reflectometry are available for both office and home use. The instruments are easy to operate and provide rapid results in infants and children. However, acoustic reflectometry may not differentiate disorders with middle ear effusion from those with negative middle ear pressure. Use of reflectometry as a screening test for acute otitis media must be followed by examination with pneumatic otoscopy when abnormal reflectometry is identified.

Microbiologic Evaluation

Culture of pharyngeal secretions provides only indirect evidence of the bacterial cause, and is inaccurate.

Tympanocentesis and Myringotomy. Tympanocentesis and aspiration is the diagnostic method of choice when knowledge of bacterial etiology and antibiotic susceptibilities would be therapeutically useful. Such situations include therapeutic failure, otitis media in neonates and immunocompromised persons, and some cases of hypersensitivity to drugs. The procedure does not alter the course of the infection but may be useful in rapidly alleviating severe earache. Tympanocentesis is technically simple under direct vision with an operating otoscope and may be employed in office practice (Fig. 64–3). The external ear canal may be cultured with a swab before tympanocentesis is performed, which may help differentiate ear canal contaminants from pathogens in the middle ear culture. The ear canal can be sterilized by filling it with 70% ethanol for 1 minute, but this is not mandatory. The alcohol must then be completely removed by suction or drainage for several minutes. Physicians who are not trained in the technique should refer the patient to an otolaryngologist.

TREATMENT

Decisions in the management of acute otitis media include the likely causative organism and its drug susceptibilities, whether identification of the etiologic agent would be of benefit, the choice of initial oral or parenteral therapy, the plan for clinical and otologic follow-up, the use of antimicrobial drug prophylaxis after initial therapy, and subsequent referral for surgical management (Fig. 64–4). The criteria for selection of agents for treatment of acute otitis media and for prevention of recurrences are efficacy and safety documented in randomized clinical trials; good in vitro antibacterial activity against the major bacterial pathogens of acute otitis media;

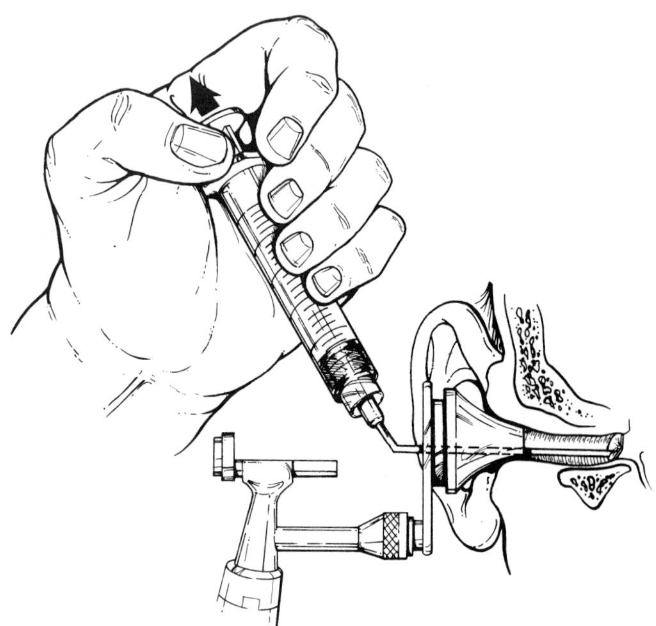

FIGURE 64–3. In an office setting, tympanocentesis is best accomplished with a spinal needle (18- or 20-gauge) bent at an angle and attached to a 1 or 3 mL syringe. The procedure should be performed through an operating otoscope. To perform the procedure, the operator's thumb is held under the plunger of the needle to allow application of suction without changing the hand position. The tympanic membrane is punctured in the inferior portion. A suction trap may be used instead of the needle and syringe but is usually not necessary. The material for Gram stain and culture may be viscous and remain in the needle; in this case, it can be recovered by flushing the needle with 1 mL of sterile culture broth.

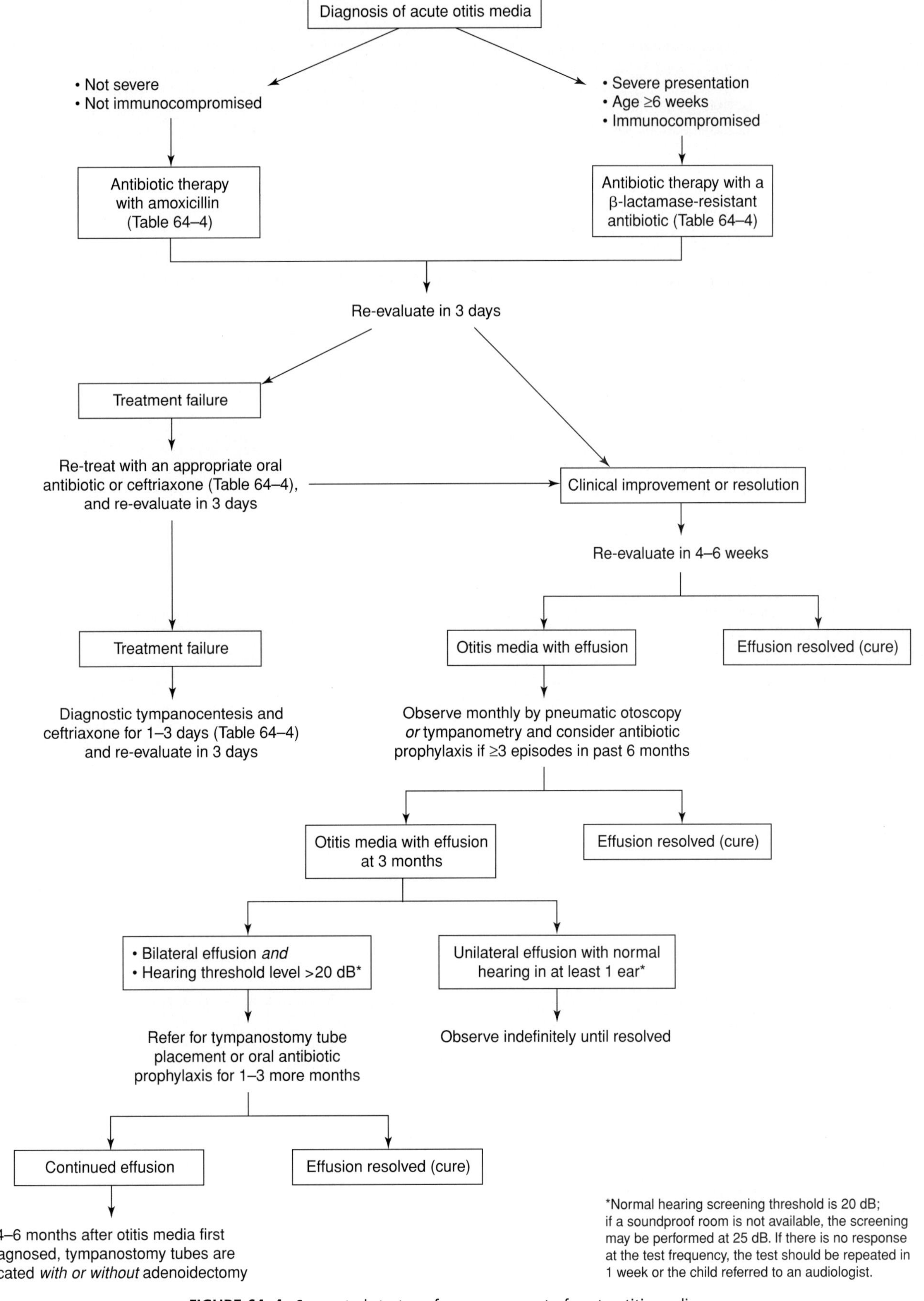

FIGURE 64–4. Suggested strategy for management of acute otitis media.

rare serious adverse effects; reliable absorption after oral administration; palatable dosage form easily administered to infants; and reasonable cost. No single agent or combination of agents currently meets all of these requirements (Table 64–3).

Several factors have led to controversy about whether all children with acute otitis media require antimicrobial therapy. Current evidence shows that antimicrobial therapy shortens the duration of symptoms in acute otitis media by an average of at least 1 day. Comparison of the frequencies of sequelae, such as mastoiditis, which were frequently observed in the preantibiotic era and are now infrequent in children with acute otitis media, leads to the conclusion that the incidence of serious complications is greatly reduced with prompt therapy. However, placebo therapy has given satisfactory clinical and microbiologic resolution in approximately 70% of treated children (Rosenfeld et al., 1994; Del Mar et al., 1997), compared with success rates with effective antibiotics of up to 90%. Clinical and bacteriologic failure in acute otitis media occurs almost entirely in children <2 years of age, and some studies using placebo or early nonantibiotic management have included only older children in whom the risk of failure is very small. A study (Damoiseaux et al, 2000) designed specifically to evaluate the outcome of antibiotic compared to nonantibiotic therapy in

TABLE 64–3. Oral Antimicrobials and Dosage Schedules for the Treatment of Acute Otitis Media in Children

		Streptococcus pneumoniae			*Haemophilus influenzae*			
Drug	**Dosage**	**Penicillin-Sensitive**	**Intermediate Resistance to Penicillin**	**Penicillin-Resistant**	**β-Lactamase-Negative**	**β-Lactamase-Positive**	***Moraxella catarrhalis***	**Adverse Effects**
Amoxicillin	60–90 mg/kg/day in 2 divided doses	+++	++	−	++	−	−	Diarrhea, rash
Amoxicillin-clavulanate*	90 mg amoxicillin/kg/day in 2 divided doses	+++	++	−	+++	+++	+++	Diarrhea, rash
Cefdinir	14 mg/kg/day in 2 divided doses or in a single daily dose	+++	+	−	+++	+++	+++	Diarrhea, rash
Cefaclor	40 mg/kg/day in 3 divided doses	++	−	−	++	+	++	Diarrhea, rash, serum-sickness-like reactions
Cefuroxime axetil	30 mg/kg/day in 2 divided doses	+++	+	−	++	++	+++	Diarrhea, rash, distaste
Cefprozil	30 mg/kg/day in 2 divided doses	+++	+	−	++	++	+++	Diarrhea, rash
Cefixime	8 mg/kg/day in a single daily dose	+	−	−	+++	+++	+++	Diarrhea, rash
Cefpodoxime	10 mg/kg/day in 2 divided doses	+++	+	−	+++	+++	+++	Diarrhea, rash, distaste
Ceftibuten	9 mg/kg/day in a single daily dose	−	−	−	+++	+++	++	Diarrhea, vomiting, abdominal pain
Loracarbef	30 mg/kg/day in 2 divided doses	++	−	−	+++	++	+++	Diarrhea, rash
Clindamycin	20 mg/kg/day in 3 divided doses	+++	++	++	−	−	−	Potentially *Clostridium difficile*-associated diarrhea
Erythromycin-sulfisoxazole	50 mg/kg erythromycin–150 mg/kg sulfisoxazole daily in 4 divided doses	++	−	−	+	+	++	Potentially severe reactions to sulfonamide (Stevens-Johnson syndrome, hematologic suppression)
Trimethoprim-sulfamethoxazole	8 mg/kg trimethoprim–40 mg/kg sulfamethoxazole daily in 2 divided doses	++	−	−	++	+	++	Potentially severe reactions to sulfonamide (Stevens-Johnson syndrome, hematologic suppression)
Azithromycin	10 mg/kg/day on day 1; 5 mg/kg/day on days 2–5, in a single daily dose	+++	±	−	+	+	++	Diarrhea, abdominal pain, rash
Clarithromycin	15 mg/kg/day in 2 divided doses	+++	±	−	+	+	++	Diarrhea, vomiting, abdominal pain, rash
Topical Therapy for Tympanostomy Tube Otorrhea								
Ofloxacin otic drops	5 drops in affected ear twice daily for 7–10 days	++	++	++	+++	+++	+++	Local discomfort
Ciprofloxacin otic drops	3 drops in affected ear twice daily for 7–10 days	++	++	++	+++	+++	+++	Local discomfort

*Using the newer formulation containing a reduced amount of clavulanate, or a combination of the older formulation of amoxicillin-clavulanate with amoxicillin alone, to provide clavulanate ~10 mg/kg/day. Higher doses of clavulanate increase the incidence of diarrhea.

toddlers <2 years of age showed 28% of placebo recipients were free of symptoms by day 4 compared with 41% of those treated with amoxicillin 40 mg/kg/day.

Antibiotic resistance is now a problem in all geographic areas. Several drugs resist hydrolysis by β-lactamase-producing strains of *H. influenzae* and *M. catarrhalis* and have good in vitro activity (Table 64–3). Drug-resistant *S. pneumoniae* frequently show cross-resistance with drugs other than penicillins and cephalosporins. Of 16 agents currently approved by the FDA for treatment of otitis media, many were licensed before 1990 and lack good evidence of efficacy in the era of drug-resistant *S. pneumoniae* (Howie, 1993). Many cephalosporins (e.g., cefaclor, cefixime, cefpodoxime, cefprozil, ceftibuten, loracarbef) and macrolides (azithromycin, clarithromycin, and the combination of erythromycin and sulfisoxazole) may not have useful activity against drug-resistant *S. pneumoniae.* In addition, azithromycin has shown poor activity clinically against *H. influenzae* otitis media.

A 10-day course of therapy is customarily used, although the duration of therapy for acute otitis media has become controversial as the cost of antibiotics and concerns about compliance have increased. A recent meta-analysis (Del Mar et al., 1997) showed no difference in outcome with 5 versus 10 days of therapy but did not differentiate results in children <2 years of age in whom bacteriologic failure is much more likely. A study (Hoberman et al., 1997) of children <2 years of age found that the success rate was twice as high after 10 days of amoxicillin-clavulanate as after 5 days. A second study (Cohen et al., 1998) of children with a mean age of 13.5 months found that 76.7% were cured after 5 days compared with 88% after 10 days ($p = .006$). Short-term therapy for 5 days appears adequate for children older than 3 years of age who have mild symptoms and do not have a history of frequent recurrent otitis media.

Initial Therapy. Amoxicillin has greater activity against drug-resistant *S. pneumoniae* than other oral antibiotics that are approved for treatment of acute otitis media. Therefore amoxicillin, alone or combined with clavulanate, remains the drug of choice for initial treatment (Table 64–4). For children at risk of infection with drug-resistant *S. pneumoniae* because of recent antibiotic use or exposure at daycare, a higher dosage of amoxicillin (80–90 mg/kg/day) increases the likelihood of eradication of the infection and is well tolerated (Dowell et al., 1999). The MIC_{90} defining susceptibility for amoxicillin against *S. pneumoniae* was recently raised from 1 μg/mL to 2 μg/mL. Dosing of amoxicillin at 90 mg/kg/day gives middle ear concentrations of 3–8 μg/mL for at least 3 hours.

Drugs stable to β-lactamases should be used for initial treatment of acute otitis media if accompanied by purulent conjunctivitis, the **otitis media-purulent conjunctivitis syndrome** that is almost always caused by *H. influenzae,* and for patients who are unusually ill at presentation, young infants, and immunocompromised persons. These drugs are also used for patients in whom initial therapy fails at 3 days with amoxicillin, which suggests that the infecting organism is likely to be β-lactamase-producing *H. influenzae* or *M. catarrhalis.* Recommended choices include high-dose amoxicillin-clavulanate (90 mg amoxicillin/kg/day), cefuroxime axetil, cefdinir, or ceftriaxone (50 mg/kg IM in 1–3 daily doses). Ceftriaxone is especially appropriate for children <3 years of age who may be bacteremic and for those whose vomiting is severe enough to preclude oral drugs. In children in whom a second course of antibiotics fails, tympanocentesis is recommended. If drug-resistant *S. pneumoniae* is found, oral clindamycin may be a good choice.

Macrolides such as clarithromycin and azithromycin, the combination of erythromycin and sulfisoxazole, and the combination of trimethoprim and sulfamethoxazole are likely to be inactive against many *S. pneumoniae, H. influenzae,* and *M. catarrhalis* organisms. These agents should therefore be considered as second-choice alternatives, primarily for use in children with hypersensitivity to β-lactams. Breakthrough pneumococcal bacteremia has been reported (Kelley et al, 2000) in patients taking a macrolide on days 3–5 of treatment.

Decongestants and Antihistamines. Clinical trials have not shown any improvement in the course of otitis media when decongestants or antihistamines have been compared with placebo. They may be used for a short period to control respiratory or allergic symptoms associated with otitis media, but they should not be used for ex-

TABLE 64–4. Treatment Recommendations for Acute Otitis Media in Children

Antibiotics in Prior Month	Day 0	Clinically Defined Treatment Failure on Day 3	Clinically Defined Treatment Failure on Days 10 to 28
No	High-dose amoxicillin (80–90 mg/kg/day) or Traditional dose amoxicillin (40–45 mg/kg/day)	High-dose amoxicillin-clavulanate (80–90 mg/kg/day of amoxicillin, ~10 mg/kg/day of clavulanate)* Cefuroxime axetil (30 mg/kg/day) or Ceftriaxone (50 mg/kg as a single injection IM)	Same as day 3
Yes	High-dose amoxicillin (80–90 mg/kg/day) High-dose amoxicillin-clavulanate (80–90 mg/kg/day of amoxicillin, ~10 mg/kg/day of clavulanate)* or Cefuroxime axetil (30 mg/kg/day)	Ceftriaxone (50 mg/kg as a single injection IM, daily for 3 days)† Clindamycin (40 mg/kg/day)‡ or Tympanocentesis	High-dose amoxicillin-clavulanate (80–90 mg/kg/day of amoxicillin, ~10 mg/kg/day of clavulanate)* Cefuroxime axetil Ceftriaxone (50 mg/kg IM) or Tympanocentesis

*Using the newer formulation containing a reduced amount of clavulanate, or a combination of the older formulation of amoxicillin-clavulanate with amoxicillin alone, to provide ~10 mg/kg/day of clavulanate. Higher doses of clavulanate increase the incidence of diarrhea.
†Ceftriaxone has documented efficacy in treatment failures if three daily doses are given.
‡Clindamycin is not effective against *Haemophilus influenzae* or *Moraxella catarrhalis.*
Adapted from Dowell SF, Butler JC, Giebink GS, et al: Acute otitis media: Management and surveillance in an era of pneumococcal resistance—A report from the Drug-Resistant *Streptococcus pneumoniae* Therapeutic Working Group. *Pediatr Infect Dis J* 1999;18:1–9.

tended periods in an attempt to promote resolution of the ear disorder.

Corticosteroids. There is a transient therapeutic effect, of 20–30%, for treatment of otitis media with short courses of corticosteroids compared with placebo, but no long-term benefit. Repeated short corticosteroid bursts have been used in some children prone to otitis media with effusion. A 3-day course of prednisolone (2 mg/kg/day orally in three divided doses) has also been shown to be effective adjuvant therapy when combined with an oral antibiotic for treatment of acute otitis media with discharge through tympanostomy tubes.

Surgical Treatment

Several surgical procedures have been shown to have efficacy in persistent or recurrent otitis media with effusion.

Myringotomy and Drainage. Myringotomy, or **tympanocentesis,** immediately relieves the severe otalgia that may occur in acute otitis media and, at the same time, allows cultures to be obtained. Studies performed to determine the outcome of acute otitis media when treated with antibiotics alone or with antibiotics and myringotomy have reached contradictory conclusions, some showing an increase in the resolution in children undergoing myringotomy and others showing no difference. Until this issue is resolved, reasonable indications for myringotomy are the presence of severe otalgia or the presence of suppurative complications of acute otitis media, including mastoiditis, meningitis, labyrinthitis, and facial paralysis. Because the external ear canal cannot be completely sterilized before surgery, it is best to perform needle aspiration for cultures before the myringotomy is performed. Myringotomy with a laser beam has recently been introduced in an attempt to produce a more persistent myringotomy without tube insertion. However, anesthesia is difficult, particularly in children, and further evaluation is needed.

Myringotomy and Insertion of Tympanostomy Tubes. In the United States, insertion of **tympanostomy tubes, pressure equalizing tubes,** or **middle ear ventilating tubes,** is the most widely used therapy for children with frequently recurrent or chronic otitis media who have failed to respond to medical strategies. Because otitis media becomes less frequent with advancing age and may respond to continued medical management, the considerations for each patient include whether the benefits from the surgical procedure are likely to outweigh both the costs and the morbidity of continued drug therapy. The beneficial effects of myringotomy and tube placement are improved hearing and reduction in frequency of acute otitis media. Restoration of normal conductive hearing is particularly important in children with language delay or school problems potentially attributable to the fluctuating hearing loss caused by otitis media. Pure-tone audiometry is of limited utility in defining the hearing loss in children with otitis media because the losses are fluctuant and frequently mild, and many affected children are too young to cooperate with these tests. Persisting otoscopic or tympanometric abnormalities may be the best clue to the likelihood of conductive loss. A study (Paradise et al, 2001) that randomized children to pressure equalization tubes early or 9 months after diagnosis found no difference in developmental outcome at 3 years of age. They concluded that tubes may be delayed indefinitely provided there are no retraction pockets or recurrence of otitis media.

Adenoidectomy. A randomized trial (Paradise et al., 1999) of adenoidectomy and adenotonsillectomy in children with severe recurrent otitis media showed only limited and short-term efficacy. Neither procedure effectively reduced subsequent manifestations of otitis media, and ordinarily they should not be considered as a first surgical intervention in children whose only indication is recurrent acute otitis media. The decision as to whether the surgical and anesthetic risks and other costs justify surgery should be determined on an individual basis. Factors that favor consideration of adenoidectomy include failure of prior ventilating tube insertion, documented conductive hearing deficit, and age >3 years. Adenoid size as assessed radiographically has not correlated with the surgical outcome. However, a nonrandomized retrospective study (Coyte et al, 2001) found a substantially lower rate of reoperation for otitis media in children over 2 years of age who had adenotonsillectomy or adenoidectomy with the first tympanostomy tube insertion.

COMPLICATIONS

The sequelae of acute otitis media are frequent, even in children given optimal antimicrobial therapy. The most frequently observed sequela is persistent middle ear effusion, but other complications do occur.

Hearing Loss and Cognitive Development. A mild to moderate **conductive hearing loss** accompanies all episodes of otitis media with effusion. In young children, the deficit may not be detectable with standard hearing tests. Sensorineural deafness is infrequent after acute otitis media, although reversible and permanent forms have been described.

The first year of life is critical for language development and is also the period of highest incidence of otitis media. Language development and language abilities are impaired by persistence of middle ear effusion in infancy.

Perforation. Acute perforations of the tympanic membrane frequently occur early with acute otitis media and are likely to be associated with virulent organisms, such as *S. pneumoniae* and group A *Streptococcus.* Treatment does not differ from that required in the absence of perforation. The external ear should be gently wiped clean of the draining exudate to avoid a local dermatitis.

Chronic Suppurative Otitis Media. **Chronic suppurative otitis media,** which is persistent or recurrent otorrhea of at least 6 weeks' duration with tympanic membrane perforation, is prevalent in certain populations, including Native Americans and Inuits, and is related in part to inadequate therapy for acute infections. Children with untreated immunologic disorders such as agammaglobulinemia are also prone to development of chronic otitis media, although the disorder may occur in otherwise healthy children. Characteristic findings are chronic aural drainage and low-grade mastoiditis. The organisms present are generally those selected by previous antimicrobial therapy, especially *S. aureus* and *P. aeruginosa.* Eardrops containing antibiotics and hydrocortisone are generally used for initial therapy. It is prudent to avoid prolonged use of eardrops containing ototoxic drugs, such as neomycin and polymyxin B. Eardrops containing the quinolone antibiotics ciprofloxacin or ofloxacin are effective and safe for this condition. Systemic antibiotics may also be used and are sometimes effective if cultures identify predominance of a susceptible organism. For better penetration of eardrops, daily suctioning of aural secretions (aural toilet) or the use of an otowick for 3-day periods between visits is recommended. Surgical consultation and therapy are needed in refractory cases.

Cholesteatoma. Cholesteatoma is an overgrowth of squamous epithelium within the middle ear cavity that is most frequently caused by chronic otitis media. Surgical resection is needed to remove the mass and restore hearing.

Intracranial Complications. Intracranial complications of otitis media include meningitis, extradural abscess, lateral sinus thrombosis, and temporal-lobe brain abscess. Intracranial complications are very uncommon because of the early antimicrobial management of acute otitis media.

Mastoiditis

The mastoid air cells and middle ear cavity are contiguous with each other. Mastoiditis is an uncommon but serious infection that usually occurs as a complication of acute or chronic otitis media and occasionally after penetrating trauma or surgery. In the preantibiotic era, this infection was extremely common and accounted for a considerable proportion of admissions to children's hospitals. The incidence of mastoiditis may be increasing, reflecting the prevalence of antibiotic-resistant organisms in acute otitis media, particularly *S. pneumoniae.*

Etiology. Because most cases of otitis media and incipient mastoiditis are treated with antibiotics before the specific diagnosis of mastoiditis is considered and cultures are obtained, there is relatively little current information about the bacterial cause of mastoiditis. In acute cases, *S. pneumoniae* is the most frequently isolated agent, group A *Streptococcus* and *S. aureus* are isolated somewhat less commonly, and other bacterial species are isolated from <5% of cases. Thus, in contrast to uncomplicated otitis media that is frequently caused by bacteria that have little invasive potential and remain localized to the mucosal cavity, highly virulent pyogenic agents generally cause mastoiditis. In **chronic mastoiditis** there is frequently a mixed population of aerobic bacteria, usually *S. aureus* or *P. aeruginosa,* and anaerobic bacteria. Tuberculosis of the mastoid is infrequent.

Symptoms and Clinical Manifestations. Mastoiditis usually presents during or after an episode of otitis media. However, a recent review (Ghaffar et al, 2001) of 17 years' experience found 39% to have had no previous occurrence of otitis media. Otoscopic signs of otitis media continue to be present as the process involves the entire middle ear–mastoid system and may include otorrhea. Postauricular swelling occurs with development of subperiosteal inflammation or abscess and may displace the external ear.

Diagnosis. In the preantibiotic era the diagnosis was made easily from the typical findings of pain and tenderness over the mastoid process, bulging into the posterior-superior portion of the external auditory canal, otorrhea, and signs of systemic toxicity. Intracranial complications of mastoiditis were frequent, and the mortality was high. Mastoiditis is currently more likely to be accompanied by low-grade fever, with few of the classic findings, because of suppression by intermittent antibiotic therapy of indolent infection.

Because of the severity of mastoiditis and its complications, cultures to identify the causative bacteria and their antibiotic susceptibilities are necessary. As in otitis media, tympanocentesis is the most suitable approach. This approach should give reliable information because the mastoid air cells and middle ear cavity are contiguous. If the tympanic membrane has been perforated, cultures of the drainage should be taken, although contaminants from the external auditory canal are likely to be present.

Plain radiographs may be helpful but are frequently normal. The diagnosis is best established by CT, which will show whether there is progression to osteitis or a subperiosteal abscess that may require mastoidectomy (Fig. 64–5).

Therapy. Mastoiditis in virtually all cases necessitates hospitalization and parenteral antibiotics to empirically treat the most frequent causative organisms. In advanced cases or in a setting of possible gram-negative bacterial infection, as with nosocomial infection, a third-generation cephalosporin or meropenem may be used empirically, with final therapy based on culture results. The duration of treatment is usually 2–4 weeks. If oral therapy is used for the latter part of treatment, it should be chosen to provide good coverage against the cultured bacteria and only if compliance can be assured.

Complications. Complications of mastoiditis include development of intracranial and extracranial abscesses, intracranial venous sinus thrombosis, facial nerve palsy, benign intracranial hypertension (otitic hydrocephalus), and osteomyelitis of the temporal bone.

PROGNOSIS

An excellent application for tympanometry is documentation of normal, ventilated, middle ear status after clinical recovery from acute otitis media. Normal tympanograms at ≥1 month after onset generally obviate the need for further follow-up.

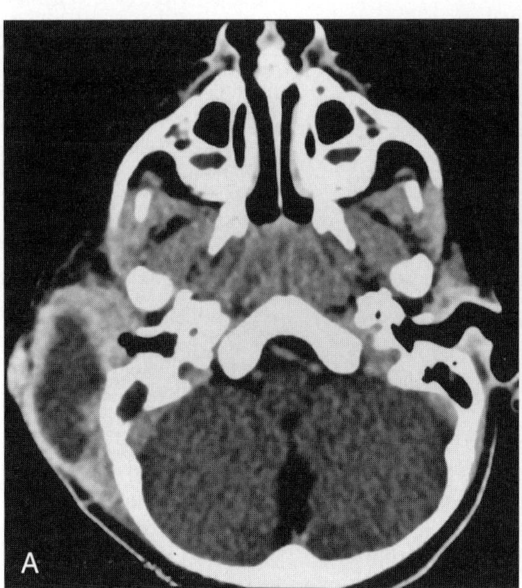

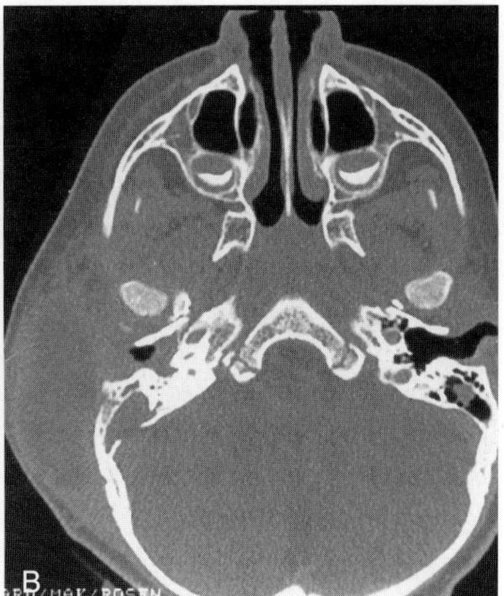

FIGURE 64–5. CT of acute mastoiditis with soft tissue abscess in a 22-month-old girl presenting with fever and swelling of the right side of the head. **A,** Postcontrast image shows an abscess on the right side superficial to the skull adjacent to the mastoid. **B,** High-resolution, thin-section bone window shows destruction of bony trabeculae within the right mastoid as well as cortical disruption laterally.

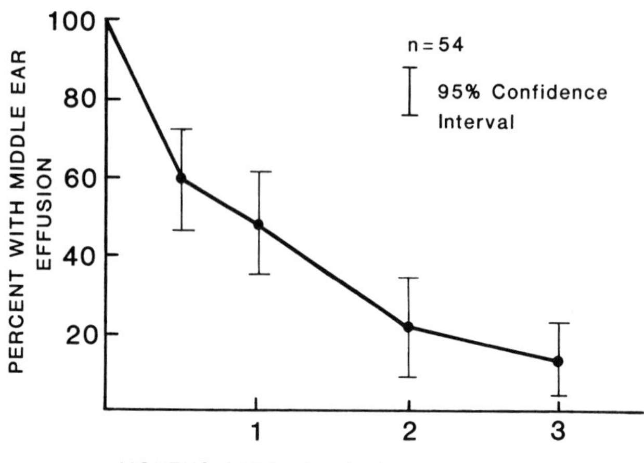

FIGURE 64–6. The time course of resolution of middle ear effusion after the presentation of acute otitis media has been similar in many studies. Approximately 50% of children have effusions after 1 month, 25% after 2 months, and at least 10% after 3 months. (From Marchant CD et al: Course and outcome of otitis media in early infancy: A prospective study. *J Pediatr* 1984;104:828.)

Persistent middle ear effusion, serous otitis media, and **otitis media with effusion** are synonymous and refer to the presence of middle ear effusion after the resolution of any symptoms related to acute otitis media. Otitis media with effusion is the most frequent sequel of acute otitis media and occurs most frequently in the first 2 years of life. Persistent middle ear effusion may last for many weeks or months in some children (Fig. 64–6). Studies have demonstrated the presence of middle ear effusion in 50% of ears at 1 month and in at least 10% at 3 months after diagnosis of acute otitis media. Clinicians should look for the condition at all well-child examinations of young children.

Conductive hearing loss should be assumed to be present in ears with persistent middle ear effusion; the loss is generally mild to moderate and often is transient or fluctuating. **Glue ear** is used to describe the presence of a very viscous, gluelike, effusion. This condition is produced when the chronically inflamed middle ear mucosa produces an excess of mucus that, because of absence of the normal clearance of the middle ear cavity, is retained for prolonged periods.

It is unclear how long middle ear effusions may persist before there is cause for clinical concern. In children who are at developmental risk and in those who are having frequent episodes of recurrent acute otitis media, 3 months of observed persistence is a reasonable indicator of need for additional therapeutic intervention (Fig. 64–4).

PREVENTION

Environmental Changes. Parents should be encouraged to continue exclusive breast-feeding as long as possible and should be cautioned about the risks of ''bottle-propping'' and of children taking a bottle to bed. The home should be a smoke-free environment. If possible, a move from a daycare to a home setting where there are fewer children may prove helpful. General hygiene practices, including good hand-washing, only one child per bed, and not sharing cups or pacifiers may help prevent spread of respiratory viruses.

Antimicrobial Prophylaxis. Children identified as being at high-risk of recurrent acute otitis media are candidates for prolonged courses of antimicrobial prophylaxis, which can significantly reduce recurrences. Many of the regimens used have employed once- or twice-daily regimens, at one half the usual daily dose used for treatment, for 3–6 months or longer. Amoxicillin (20–30 mg/kg/day) and sulfisoxazole (50 mg/kg/day), given once daily, have been the agents most widely used for prophylaxis; there have been no comparative studies indicating superiority of newer and more expensive agents. The sulfonamides, alone or in combination with trimethoprim, should be used rarely for middle ear disease because the likely causative organisms are now generally resistant to these drugs and the risk of serious drug reactions to sulfonamides is higher than with the β-lactam and macrolide drugs. Results are best among compliant patients and in children younger than 2 years of age. A reasonable strategy is to treat during the winter and spring seasons when the risk is greatest. Potential risks of antimicrobial prophylaxis include hypersensitivity reaction and the well-established role of widespread antimicrobial use in promoting the acquisition and distribution of resistant bacteria, including drug-resistant *S. pneumoniae.* Otitis media is the foremost single indication for antibiotic therapy in children, and excessive use of antibiotics must be avoided.

Vaccines. Both pneumococcal vaccine and influenza vaccine may reduce the incidence of otitis media. The conjugate pneumococcal vaccine appears to reduce pneumococcal otitis media caused by vaccine serotypes by one half, of pneumococcal otitis media by one third, and of all otitis media by 6%. The reduction in recurrences in the second year of life is more substantial, as is the reduction in pressure equalization tube placement (about 20%). The benefits of the polysaccharide pneumococcal vaccine are less because it is effective only in children ≥2 years of age. Annual immunization against influenza virus may be helpful in high-risk children. Because RSV is the most frequently identified viral agent in the respiratory tract or middle ear in children with acute otitis media and because of the severity of RSV outbreaks in children who are at the age of greatest risk for acute otitis media, it is probable that in the future control of RSV through vaccination would reduce the burden of acute otitis media in infants.

REVIEWS

Bluestone CD, Klein JO: *Otitis Media in Infants and Children,* 3rd ed. Philadelphia, WB Saunders Co, 2001.

Dowell SF, Butler JC, Giebink GS, et al: Acute otitis media: Management and surveillance in an era of pneumococcal resistance—A report from the Drug-Resistant *Streptococcus pneumoniae* Therapeutic Working Group. *Pediatr Infect Dis J* 1999;18:1–9.

Faden H, Duffy L, Boeve M: Otitis media: Back to basics. *Pediatr Infect Dis J* 1998;17:1105–12.

Rosenfeld RM, Vertrees JE, Carr J, et al: Clinical efficacy of antimicrobial drugs for acute otitis media: Metaanalysis of 5400 children from thirty-three randomized trials. *J Pediatr* 1994;124:355–67.

Teele DW, Klein JO, Rosner B, et al: Epidemiology of otitis media during the first seven years of life in children in greater Boston: A prospective, cohort study. *J Infect Dis* 1989;160:83–94.

The Otitis Media Guideline Panel: Managing otitis media with effusion in young children. *Pediatrics* 1994;94:766–73.

KEY ARTICLES

Barnett ED, Klein JO, Hawkins KA, et al: Comparison of spectral gradient acoustic reflectometry and other diagnostic techniques for detection of middle ear effusion in children with middle ear disease. *Pediatr Infect Dis J* 1998;17:556–9.

Bluestone CD: Clinical course, complications and sequelae of acute otitis media. *Pediatr Infect Dis J* 2000;19:S37–46.

Bodor FF, Marchant CD, Shurin PA, et al: Bacterial etiology of conjunctivitis-otitis media syndrome. *Pediatrics* 1985;76:26–8.

Burke P, Bain J, Robinson D, et al: Acute red ear in children: Controlled trial of non-antibiotic treatment in general practice. *BMJ* 1991;303:558–62.

Carlin SA, Marchant CD, Shurin PA, et al: Early recurrence of otitis media: Reinfection or relapse? *J Pediatr* 1987;110:20–5.

Carlin SA, Marchant CD, Shurin PA, et al: Host factors and early therapeutic response in acute otitis media. *J Pediatr* 1991;118:178–83.

Cohen D, Siegel G, Krespi J, et al: Middle ear laser office ventilation (LOV) with a CO_2 laser flashscanner. *J Clin Laser Med Surg* 1998;16:107–9.

Cohen R, Levy C, Boucherat M, et al: A multicenter, randomized, double-blind trial of 5 versus 10 days of antibiotic therapy for acute otitis media in young children. *J Pediatr* 1998;133:634–9.

Coyte PC, Croxford R, McIsaac W, et al: The role of adjuvant adenoidectomy and tonsillectomy in the outcome of the insertion of tympanostomy tubes. *N Engl J Med* 2001;344:1188–95.

Dagan R, Johnson CE, McLinn S, et al: Bacteriologic and clinical efficacy of amoxicillin/clavulanate vs. azithromycin in acute otitis media. *Pediatr Infect Dis J* 2000;19:95–104.

Damoiseaux RAMJ, van Balen FAM, Hoes AW, et al: Primary care based randomised, double blind trial of amoxicillin versus placebo for acute otitis media in children aged under 2 years. *BMJ* 2000;320:350–4.

Del Mar C, Glasziou P, Hayem M: Are antibiotics indicated as initial treatment for children with otitis media? A meta-analysis. *BMJ* 1997; 314:1526–9.

Eskola J, Kilpi T, Palmu A, et al: Efficacy of a pneumococcal conjugate vaccine against acute otitis media. *N Engl J Med* 2001;344:403–9.

Fliss DM, Leiberman A, Dagan R: Medical sequelae and complications of acute otitis media. *Pediatr Infect Dis J* 1994;13:S34–40.

Giebink GS: The pathogenesis of pneumococcal otitis media in chinchillas and the efficacy of vaccination in prophylaxis. *Rev Infect Dis* 1981;3: 342–53.

Ghaffer FA, Wordemann M, McCracken GH Jr: Acute mastoiditis in children: A seventeen-year experience in Dallas, Texas. *Pediatr Infect Dis J* 2001;20:376–80.

Heikkinen T, Ruuskanen O, Waris M, et al: Influenza vaccination in the prevention of acute otitis media in children. *Am J Dis Child* 1991; 145:445–8.

Heikkinen T, Thint M, Chonmaitree T: Prevalence of various respiratory viruses in the middle ear during acute otitis media. *N Engl J Med* 1999;340:260–4.

Howie VM: Otitis media. *Pediatr Rev* 1993;14:320–3.

Johnson CE, Carlin SA, Super DM, et al: Cefixime compared with amoxicillin for treatment of acute otitis media. *J Pediatr* 1991;119:117–22.

Kaleida PH, Casselbrant ML, Rockette HE, et al: Amoxicillin or myringotomy or both for acute otitis media: Results of a randomized clinical trial. *Pediatrics* 1991;87:466–74.

Kelley MA, Weber DJ, Gilligan P, et al: Breakthrough pneumococcal bacteremia in patients being treated with azithromycin and clarithromycin. *Clin Infect Dis* 2000;31:1008–11.

Liston TE, Foshee WS, Pierson WD: Sulfisoxazole chemoprophylaxis for frequent otitis media. *Pediatrics* 1983;71:524–30.

Marchant CD, McMillan PM, Shurin PA, et al: Objective diagnosis of otitis media in early infancy by tympanometry and ipsilateral acoustic reflex thresholds. *J Pediatr* 1986;109:590–5.

Marchant CD, Shurin PA, Turczyk VA, et al: Course and outcome of otitis media in early infancy: A prospective study. *J Pediatr* 1984;104:826–31.

Paradise JL, Bluestone CD, Colborn DK, et al: Adenoidectomy and adenotonsillectomy for recurrent acute otitis media: Parallel randomized clinical trials in children not previously treated with tympanostomy tubes. *JAMA* 1999;282:945–53.

Paradise JL, Dollaghan CA, Campbell TF, et al: Language, speech sound production, and cognition in three-year-old children in relation to otitis media in their first three years of life. *Pediatrics* 2000;105:1119–30.

Paradise JL, Feldman HM, Campbell TF, et al: Effect of early or delayed insertion of tympanostomy tubes for persistent otitis media on developmental outcomes at the age of three years. *N Engl J Med* 2001;344: 1179–86.

Rayner MG, Zhang Y, Gorry MC, et al: Evidence of bacterial metabolic activity in culture-negative otitis media with effusion. *JAMA* 1998; 28;279:296–9.

Wald ER, Guerra N, Byers C: Upper respiratory tract infections in young children: Duration of and frequency of complications. *Pediatrics* 1991; 87:129–33.

Wald ER, Mason EO Jr, Bradley JS, et al: Acute otitis media caused by *Streptococcus pneumoniae* in children's hospitals between 1994 and 1997. *Pediatr Infect Dis J* 2001;20:34–9.

CHAPTER 65

Sinusitis

Ellen R. Wald

When one is considering a diagnosis of sinusitis in a child or an adult, the major problem is to distinguish nonbacterial causes, such as simple upper respiratory tract infection or allergic inflammation, from secondary bacterial infection of the paranasal sinuses. Viral upper respiratory tract infections and allergy require prompt symptomatic treatment, whereas bacterial sinusitis requires specific antimicrobial therapy.

ETIOLOGY

Studies of children with acute maxillary sinusitis have shown the bacteria in sinus secretions to be similar to those found in the secretions of adults with maxillary sinusitis. The predominant causative organisms include *Streptococcus pneumoniae, Moraxella catarrhalis* (formerly known as *Branhamella catarrhalis*), nontypable *Haemophilus influenzae,* and occasionally viridans streptococci. Both *H. influenzae* and *M. catarrhalis* may produce β-lactamase and, consequently, may be ampicillin resistant. *Staphylococcus aureus* and anaerobic organisms are recovered most frequently from children with severe sinus symptoms requiring surgical intervention or with protracted sinusitis lasting more than 1 year. The commonly recovered anaerobes are gram-positive cocci, including *Peptococcus* and *Peptostreptococcus,* and the gram-negative bacillus *Bacteroides.* Several viruses, including adenoviruses and parainfluenzae viruses, also have been recovered.

EPIDEMIOLOGY

Both viral upper respiratory tract infections and allergic inflammation are recognized risk factors for acute sinusitis, viral infection being most common. The incidence of uncomplicated acute sinusitis generally parallels the seasonal incidence of viral upper respiratory tract infections. Host factors affect the normal function of the sinus ostia and mucociliary drainage of sinus secretions and predispose a patient to chronic symptoms. These host factors include allergic inflammation, cystic fibrosis, immunodeficiency disorders (insufficient or dysfunctional immunoglobulins), ciliary dyskinesia (immotile cilia syndrome), and anatomic abnormalities.

PATHOGENESIS

Anatomy and Development. The paranasal sinuses border the **nasal cavity,** which is divided in the midline by the nasal septum (Fig. 65–1). From the lateral wall of the nose are projected three shelflike structures designated according to their anatomic position as the **inferior and middle turbinates,** which are seen best on the sagittal view, and the **superior turbinates.** Beneath the middle and superior turbinates is a meatus that drains two or more of the paranasal sinuses. The maxillary, anterior ethmoidal, and frontal sinuses drain to the **middle meatus,** and the posterior ethmoid and sphenoidal sinuses drain to the **superior meatus.** Only the lacrimal duct drains to the **inferior meatus.**

The maxillary and ethmoidal sinuses form during the third to fourth gestational month; accordingly, although very small, they are present at birth. The awkward positioning of the outflow tract of the maxillary sinus, which sits high on the medial wall of the sinus cavity, impedes gravitational drainage, which probably predisposes to frequent bacterial infections of the maxillary sinus as a complication of viral upper respiratory tract infections.

The ethmoidal sinus comprises multiple air cells, 3–15 on each side, separated by thin bony partitions. Each air cell drains by an independent ostium, measuring 1–2 mm in diameter, into the middle meatus. The narrow caliber of these draining ostia predispose to obstruction if there is even modest inflammation of the mucosal lining as is the case in viral respiratory infection or allergies.

The frontal sinus develops from an anterior ethmoidal cell and moves to a position above the orbital ridge by the fifth or sixth birthday. Development of the frontal sinuses is not complete until late adolescence. The frontal sinus is not a frequent site of infection but may be a focus for spread of infection to the orbit or the CNS. The sphenoidal sinuses are immediately anterior to the pituitary fossa and just behind the posterior ethmoidal sinuses. Isolated involvement of the sphenoidal sinuses is unusual; they are usually infected as part of a pansinusitis.

Three key elements are important to the normal function of the paranasal sinuses: the patency of the ostia, the function of the ciliary apparatus, and, integral to the latter, the quality of secretions. Retention of secretions in the paranasal sinuses is caused by obstruction of the ostia, reduction in the number of or impaired function of the cilia, or overproduction of or a change in the viscosity of secretions.

Sinus Ostia. The ostia of the maxillary sinuses are small, tubular structures with a diameter of 2.5 mm, and therefore a cross-sectional area of approximately 5 mm^2, and a length of 6 mm. The diameter of the ostium of each of the individual ethmoidal air cells that drain independently into the middle meatus is even smaller, 1–2 mm; the ostia of the anterior cells are smaller than those of the posterior cells. The narrow caliber of the ostia sets the stage for obstruction to occur easily and often.

The factors predisposing to ostial obstruction can be classified as those that cause mucosal swelling and those that cause mechanical obstruction (Table 65–1). Although many conditions may lead to ostial closure, viral upper respiratory tract infections and allergic inflammation are by far the most frequent and the most important. If sinus ostial obstruction occurs, pressure within the sinus cavity becomes negative and the oxygen component of the inspired air is rapidly absorbed by a metabolically active mucosa. If the ostium opens again, the negative pressure favors aspiration of mucus and debris from a heavily colonized nasal chamber and nasopharynx into a presumably sterile sinus cavity. These normal flora become

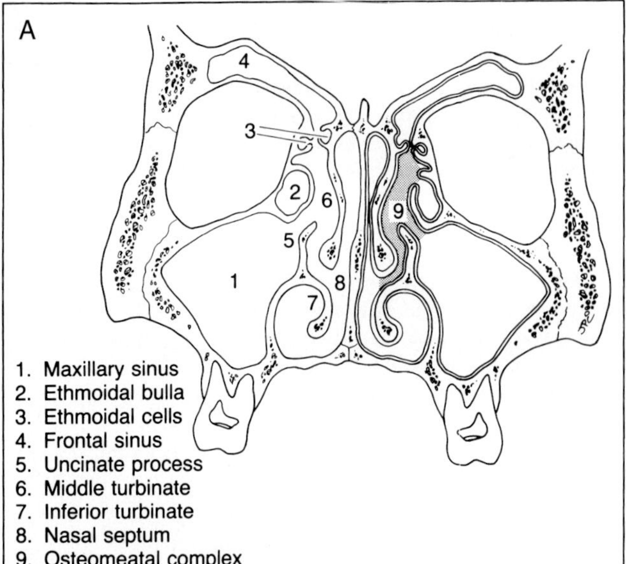

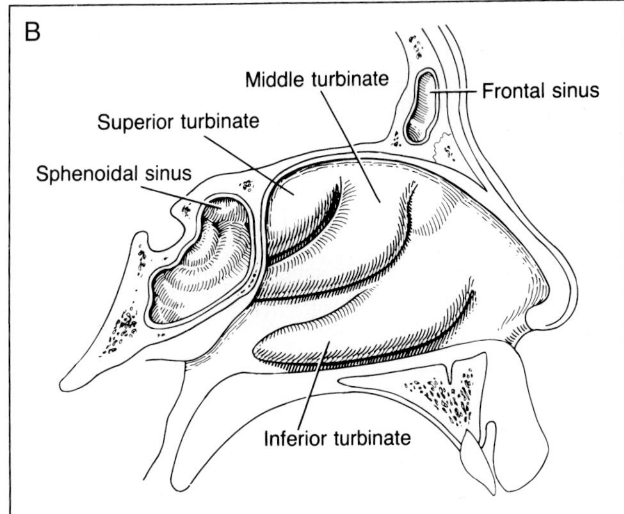

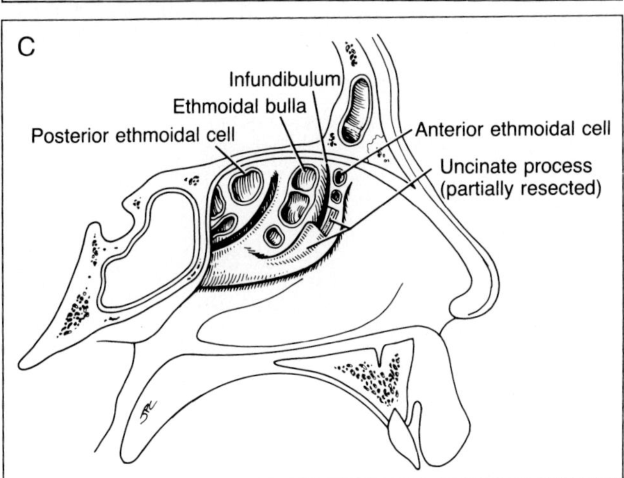

FIGURE 65–1. Coronal **(A)** and sagittal **(B)** sections of the nasal cavity and paranasal sinuses. The stippled area in **A** represents the osteomeatal complex. **C,** Parasagittal view through the middle and superior turbinates, displaying the ethmoid air cells. (From Wald ER: Sinusitis in children. *N Engl J Med* 1992;326:319–23.)

TABLE 65–1. Predisposing Factors for Obstruction of the Ostia of the Sinuses

Mucosal Swelling
Systemic Disorder
Viral upper respiratory tract infection
Allergic inflammation
Cystic fibrosis
Immune disorders
Immotile cilia syndrome
Local Insult
Facial trauma
Swimming or diving
Rhinitis medicamentosa
Mechanical Obstruction
Choanal atresia
Deviated septum
Nasal polyps
Foreign body
Tumor

pathogens when obstruction again supervenes and bacteria multiply to high density.

Interest has focused on the **osteomeatal complex,** which is the area between the middle and inferior turbinates that represents the confluence of the drainage areas of the frontal, ethmoidal, and maxillary sinuses (Fig. 65–1). In the osteomeatal complex there are several areas in which two mucosal layers come into contact and thereby are predisposed to local impairment of mucociliary clearance. This may result in the retention of secretions at the site and the potential for infection, even without actual ostial closure.

Mucociliary Apparatus. Disorders of the mucociliary apparatus in conjunction with reduced patency of the sinus ostia are major pathophysiologic events in acute sinusitis. In the posterior two thirds of the nasal cavity and within the sinuses, the epithelium is pseudostratified columnar, and most of the cells are ciliated.

Factors that may impair normal mucociliary transport include cold or dry air, alterations in mucus, chemicals and drugs, viral infection, and inborn errors such as immotile cilia syndrome. Although the cilia are hardy in withstanding ordinary variations in body temperature, humidity, and mucosal deprivation of oxygen, viral infection may cause devastating histologic alterations and, presumably, in the function of the mucosa.

Temporary acquired ciliary defects have been observed in biopsy specimens from nasal mucosa of children with acute viral upper respiratory tract infections. Presumably, these changes would also have been seen in the sinus mucosa had the area been sampled. In children with upper respiratory tract infections, nasal biopsy specimens showed mild to severe changes that tended to be patchy rather than general. In specimens obtained 2–10 weeks after onset, ciliary abnormalities were observed only occasionally, and the epithelium gradually returned to normal.

The normal motility of the cilia and the adhesive properties of the mucus layer usually protect respiratory epithelium from bacterial invasion. Viruses may have a direct cytotoxic effect on the cilia. Alteration of the number, structure, and function of the cilia may facilitate secondary bacterial invasion of the nose and the paranasal sinuses.

Sinus Secretions. Cilia can beat only in a fluid medium. There appears to be a double layer of mucus in the airways: the **gel layer (superficial viscid fluid)** and the **sol layer (underlying serous fluid).** The gel layer acts to trap particulate matter, such as bacteria and other debris. The tips of the cilia touch the gel layer during forward movement and thereby move the particulate matter along. The bodies of the cilia, however, move through the sol layer, a fluid thin enough to allow the cilia to beat. Alterations in the mucus, as in cystic fibrosis or asthma, may impair ciliary activity.

SYMPTOMS AND CLINICAL MANIFESTATIONS

Acute Sinusitis. The commonly recognized symptoms of sinusitis in adults and adolescents are unilateral or bilateral facial pain, headache, and fever. Children with acute sinusitis frequently have complaints that are less specific. During the course of apparent viral upper respiratory tract infections, the possibility of sinusitis is indicated by either persistent respiratory symptoms or severe respiratory symptoms (Table 65–2). Persistent signs and symptoms of a cold include nasal discharge and a daytime cough that last longer than 10 days and are not improving. Most uncomplicated upper respiratory tract infections last 5–7 days; although patients may not be free of symptoms by the tenth day, their condition has usually improved. The persistence of respiratory symptoms longer than 10 days without appreciable improvement suggests that a complication has developed. The nasal discharge may be of any quality (thin or thick; clear, mucoid, or purulent) and the cough, which may be dry or wet, is usually present during the daytime, although it is often noted to be worse at night. A cough that occurs only at night is a common residual symptom of an upper respiratory tract infection. When it is the only residual symptom, such a cough is usually nonspecific and does not suggest a sinus infection. Conversely, the persistence of a daytime cough is frequently the symptom that necessitates medical attention. The child may not appear ill, and if a fever is present it usually is low-grade. Parents of preschoolers often report fetid breath. Facial pain is absent, although intermittent, painless, morning periorbital swelling may have been noted by the parent. In this case, it is not the severity of the clinical symptoms but the persistence that calls for attention.

The second, less common presentation is a cold that seems more severe than usual. High fever (>39°C [102.2°F]) and purulent (thick, colored, and opaque) nasal discharge for 3–4 days constitute the critical dyad of symptoms. There may be associated unilateral or bilateral facial pain and periorbital swelling, which may involve the upper or lower periorbital areas and is gradual in onset, evolving over hours to days, and most obvious in the early morning after the patient awakes. The swelling may decrease and actually disappear during the day, only to reappear the next day. A less common complaint is a headache with a feeling of fullness or a dull ache either behind or above the eyes, which is most often reported by children older than 5 years. Occasionally, there may be dental pain, from an infection that either originates in the teeth or is referred from the sinus infection.

TABLE 65–2. Common Clinical Symptoms of Acute Sinusitis

Persistent Respiratory Symptoms
Nasal discharge of any quality, *or*
daytime cough, *or both*
for 10–30 days, *or* without clinical improvement
May be accompanied by:
Low-grade or no fever
Eye swelling
Fetid breath (children <6 yr)

Severe Respiratory Symptoms
High fever (temperature >39°C [102.2°F] *and* purulent nasal discharge for 3–4 consecutive days
May be accompanied by:
Eye swelling
Headache

Subacute Sinusitis. Subacute sinusitis is characterized by persistent respiratory symptoms for 30–90 days. These patients have nasal discharge or a daytime cough or both. Headaches are variable, and fever is intermittent and low grade.

Chronic Sinusitis. Chronic bacterial sinusitis is characterized by respiratory symptoms that persist more than 90 days. The prominent symptoms are nasal congestion, nasal discharge, or daytime cough. The patient often complains of morning sore throat and malodorous breath. Fever, headaches, and facial pain are variable complaints. Chronic sinusitis is uncommon in children. Its occurrence should prompt a search for underlying causes, such as cystic fibrosis, immunodeficiency, or an allergic diathesis.

Physical Examination Findings

On physical examination a patient with acute sinusitis may have mucopurulent discharge in the nose or posterior pharynx. The nasal mucosa is erythematous, and the throat may show moderate injection. The cervical lymph nodes are usually not greatly enlarged or tender. None of these characteristics differentiates rhinitis from sinusitis. Occasionally there is tenderness as the examiner palpates over or percusses the paranasal sinuses, appreciable periorbital edema consisting of soft, nontender swelling of the upper and lower eyelids with discoloration of the overlying skin, or both. Malodorous breath (in the absence of pharyngitis, poor dental hygiene, or a nasal foreign body) may suggest bacterial sinusitis.

Nasal endoscopy with a fiberoptic light source has been used in adults for thorough examination of the nasal chamber. This procedure allows adequate visualization of the middle turbinate and nasal septum and of structural abnormalities such as polyps. It is nearly impossible to perform this procedure on children, even if they are cooperative. Accordingly, in children, examination of the nose with a nasal speculum is all that can be accomplished from a practical point of view. Detailed examination by a pediatric otolaryngologist is appropriate for patients with protracted or frequently recurrent symptoms.

Transillumination may be helpful in diagnosing inflammation of the maxillary or frontal sinuses, but it is of limited value. The patient and the examiner must be in a darkened room. To transilluminate the maxillary sinus, the light source, shielded from the observer, is placed over the midpoint of the inferior orbital rim. The transmission of light through the hard palate is then assessed with the patient's mouth open. Light passing through the alveolar ridges should be excluded in judging light transmission. Transillumination of the frontal sinus is accomplished by placing a high-intensity light source beneath the medial border of the supraorbital ridge and evaluating the symmetry of the blush bilaterally. Transillumination is useful in adolescents and adults if light transmission is either normal or absent. "Reduced" transmission or "dull" transillumination is an assessment that correlates poorly with clinical disease. The increased thickness of both the soft tissue and the bony vault in children younger than 10 years limits the clinical usefulness of transillumination in younger children.

For most children younger than 10 years of age, the physical examination is not helpful in establishing a diagnosis of acute sinusitis. However, if the mucopurulent material can be removed from the nose and the nasal mucosa is then treated with topical vasoconstrictors, pus may be seen coming from the middle meatus. The observation of unilateral or bilateral facial tenderness or periorbital swelling, when present, is probably the most specific finding in acute sinusitis.

DIAGNOSIS

The most significant symptoms indicating sinusitis are symptoms of a common cold that are present for longer than 7–10 days without improvement, severe symptoms, fever, mucopurulent discharge for more than 7 days, and pain in the upper teeth. The most significant clinical findings are unilateral or bilateral tenderness in the midface region, intranasal pus, and purulent postnasal mucus in the pharynx. Radiographs such as a Waters' view are of variable significance, and CT imaging is not helpful. Sinus aspiration, when indicated, is the most clinically significant diagnostic test.

Differential Diagnosis

The major symptoms that prompt consideration of the diagnosis of acute sinusitis are persistent or purulent nasal discharge and persistent cough (Table 65–3). Alternative diagnostic considerations for purulent nasal discharge are simple viral upper respiratory tract infection, group A *Streptococcus* infection, adenoiditis, and nasal foreign body. In simple viral infections, the purulent nasal discharge is usually accompanied by low-grade fever and other elements of upper respiratory inflammation, such as pharyngitis and conjunctivitis. The symptoms usually begin to improve after a few days. Streptococcal infection in children younger than 3 years, so-called **streptococcosis,** may present with persistent upper respiratory tract symptoms such as nasal discharge, low-grade fever, lassitude, and poor appetite. The diagnosis can be excluded by culturing the nasopharynx or throat for group A *Streptococcus.* Adenoiditis is suggested when purulent nasal discharge persists longer than 10 days without improvement in a patient whose sinus radiographs are normal. A nasal foreign body is usually characterized by unilateral nasal discharge, which is purulent and often bloody. Most strikingly, the nasal discharge is so foul smelling that the odor is usually noticeable from the doorway of the examining room.

TABLE 65–3. Differential Diagnosis of Respiratory Symptoms of Sinusitis

Persistent or Purulent Nasal Discharge
Viral upper respiratory tract infection
Group A *Streptococcus* nasopharyngitis
Adenoiditis
Nasal foreign body
Sinusitis

Persistent Cough
Reactive airways disease
Mycoplasma pneumoniae bronchitis
Cystic fibrosis
Gastroesophageal reflux
Sinusitis

Patients who present with a persistent cough as the most troublesome symptom prompt the consideration of several diagnoses, including reactive airways disease, *Mycoplasma pneumoniae* bronchitis, cystic fibrosis, and gastroesophageal reflux. Reactive airways disease triggered by an upper respiratory tract infection may cause a dramatic cough without accompanying wheezing. This coughing may occasionally occur in conjunction with acute sinusitis but more often is a residual symptom after a viral infection that substantially prolongs the clinical course of the illness. *M. pneumoniae* bronchitis, which occurs most commonly among children 5–15 years of age, begins with a prominent sore throat and fever. As the upper respiratory symptoms subside, a cough begins and becomes prominent and persistent. Cystic fibrosis needs to be considered in children with a persistent cough, although it is unlikely to explain the symptom in a previously thriving child who presents with an intercurrent illness. Gastroesophageal reflux may be responsible for pulmonary and neurologic symptoms as well as for failure to thrive. It should be considered most seriously in children with a nighttime cough only or who have had poorly controlled asthma or previous episodes of pneumonia.

Diagnostic Imaging

Radiography has traditionally been used to determine the presence or absence of sinus disease. Standard radiographic projections include an anteroposterior, a lateral, and an occipitomental view. The anteroposterior view is optimal for evaluation of the ethmoidal sinuses, and the lateral view is best for the frontal and sphenoidal sinuses. The occipitomental view, taken after the chin is tilted upward 45 degrees to the horizontal, allows evaluation of the maxillary sinuses.

Although much has been written about the frequency of abnormal sinus radiographs in "normal" children, these studies have been flawed either by inattention to the presence of symptoms or signs of respiratory inflammation or by failure to classify abnormal radiographic findings as major (complete opacification, air-fluid level, and mucous membrane thickening of ≥4 mm) or minor (mucous membrane thickening <3 mm, diffuse haziness). A study (Kovatch et al., 1984) to determine the frequency of abnormal sinus radiographs in children without respiratory signs or symptoms reported abnormalities in only 7% of children older than 1 year.

The radiographic findings most diagnostic of bacterial sinusitis are the presence of an **air-fluid level** or **complete opacification** of the sinus cavities (Figs. 65–2 and 65–3). An air-fluid level, however, is an uncommon radiographic finding in children less than 5 years of age with acute sinusitis. In the absence of an air-fluid level or complete opacification of the sinuses, measuring the degree of mucosal swelling may be useful. If the width of the sinus mucous membrane is ≥5 mm in adults, or ≥4 mm in children, it is likely that the sinus contains pus or will yield a positive bacterial culture. When clinical signs and symptoms suggesting acute sinusitis are accompanied by abnormal radiographic findings for the maxillary sinus, bacteria are present in a sinus aspirate 70% of the time. A normal radiograph strongly suggests, but does not prove, that a sinus is free of disease.

Several studies have examined the frequency of incidental paranasal sinus abnormalities on CT and MRI of pediatric patients. There has been a failure to obtain information regarding recent

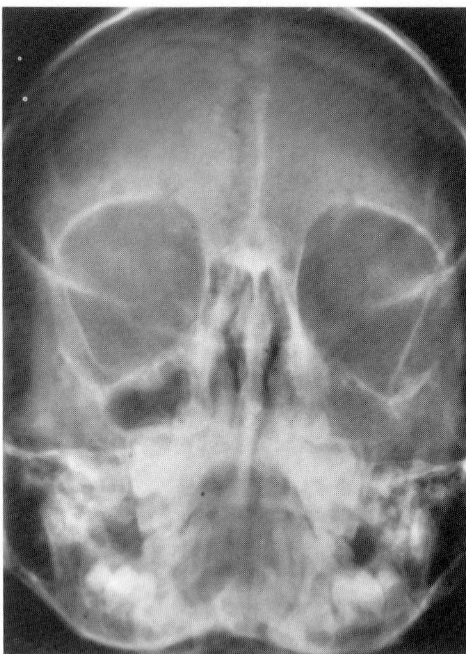

FIGURE 65–2. Complete opacification of the left maxillary sinus. Mucosal thickening along the roof of the right maxillary sinus. (From Wald ER: Acute and chronic sinusitis: Diagnosis and management. *Pediatr Rev* 1985;7:153.)

signs or symptoms of respiratory infection or to classify the degree and clinical significance of radiographic abnormalities. Some have observed that CT is superior to plain radiography in the delineation of sinus abnormalities, particularly in patients with chronic or recurrent disease. This is not surprising because plain radiographs are a summation of overlapping structures, whereas CT provides many individual images. CT and MRI are not necessary for the diagnosis of uncomplicated acute sinusitis; they should be reserved for the evaluation of complicated or chronic sinus infections (Fig. 65–4).

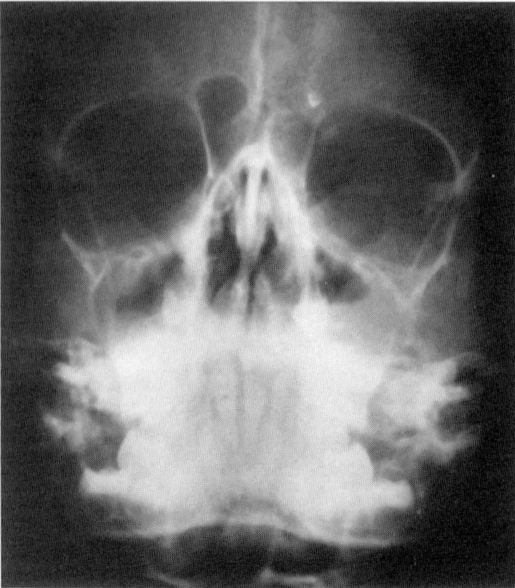

FIGURE 65–3. Marked mucosal thickening of the right maxillary sinus. An air-fluid level is present in the left maxillary sinus, and there is opacification of the left frontal sinus.

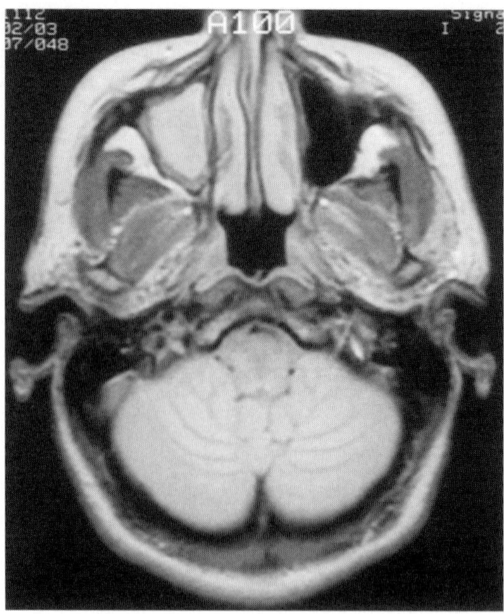

FIGURE 65–4. Left maxillary sinusitis on a magnetic resonance image.

Microbiologic Evaluation

The diagnosis of acute bacterial sinusitis is probably best proved by a biopsy of the sinus mucosa that demonstrates acute inflammation and invasion by bacteria. In practice, confirmation of the diagnosis is more often accomplished by culture of an aspirate of sinus secretions. Nonetheless, when mucosal biopsy specimens and sinus aspirates are submitted simultaneously for bacterial cultures, the biopsy specimens more frequently yield positive results.

Indications for sinus aspirations in patients believed to have sinusitis include clinical unresponsiveness to conventional therapy, sinus disease in an immunocompromised patient, severe symptoms such as headache or facial pain, and life-threatening complications such as intraorbital or intracranial suppuration at the time of clinical presentation. Although by no means a routine procedure, aspiration of the maxillary sinus, which is the most accessible of the sinuses, can be accomplished either in an outpatient setting or in the operating room. Puncture is best performed by the transnasal route with the needle directed beneath the inferior turbinate through the lateral nasal wall. This route for aspiration is preferred to avoid injury to the natural ostium and permanent dentition. Careful sterilization of the puncture site is essential to prevent contamination by nasal flora. Secretions obtained by aspiration should be submitted for Gram stain and quantitative aerobic and anaerobic cultures. All bacterial isolates should be tested for their sensitivity to various appropriate antibiotics. Bacterial counts of $>10^4$ colony-forming units per milliliter provide a high degree of assurance of actual sinus infection rather than contamination. Alternatively, examination of a Gram stain of sinus secretions may be helpful, because bacteria present in low colony counts (i.e., likely to be contaminants) are usually not observed on a smear.

TREATMENT

Therapy for acute maxillary sinusitis in the preantibiotic era consisted of sinus aspiration and irrigation. Numerous antimicrobial agents active against the bacteria commonly recovered from sinus secretions are now available. The objectives of antimicrobial therapy for acute sinus infections are achievement of a rapid clinical cure, sterilization of the sinus secretions, prevention of suppurative orbital and intracranial complications, and prevention of chronic sinus disease.

Definitive Treatment

Antimicrobials. Medical therapy with an oral antimicrobial agent is recommended for children with acute maxillary sinusitis (Table 65–4). The antimicrobial regimens recommended to treat acute sinusitis are similar in type and duration to those used to treat acute otitis media. Amoxicillin (at 40–60 mg/kg/day in 2 divided doses orally) is acceptable and recommended for the initial treatment of most cases of bacterial sinusitis in children. This is especially true if the episode of acute bacterial sinusitis is uncomplicated and mild to moderate in severity and if the patient has not been treated with antimicrobial agents within 1 month. Amoxicillin is usually effective, inexpensive, and safe. The latter characteristic is particularly important for treatment of a condition that has a high spontaneous cure rate, such as sinusitis.

Although amoxicillin is preferred in most cases, there are several clinical situations in which a broader-spectrum regimen or a higher dose of amoxicillin (90 mg/kg/day in 2 divided doses orally) is appropriate (Table 65–4). These circumstances include (1) failure to improve with treatment with lower-dose amoxicillin; (2) recent treatment with amoxicillin, within 1 month; (3) residence in a geographic area with a high prevalence of β-lactamase-producing *H. influenzae;* (4) frontal or sphenoidal sinusitis; (5) complicated ethmoidal sinusitis; and (6) presentation with very protracted symptoms, for longer than 30 days. Oral antimicrobials with the most comprehensive coverage for patients with sinusitis are amoxicillin-clavulanate, cefuroxime axetil, and cefpodoxime. For patients with chronic sinusitis, amoxicillin/potassium clavulanate is especially attractive because the mechanism for resistance of most pathogens

TABLE 65–4. Oral Antimicrobials and Dosage Schedules for the Treatment of Sinusitis in Children

		Streptococcus pneumoniae			*Haemophilus influenzae*			
Drug	**Dosage**	**Penicillin-sensitive**	**Intermediate Resistance to Penicillin**	**Penicillin-resistant**	**β-Lactamase-negative**	**β-Lactamase-positive**	***Moraxella catarrhalis***	**Adverse Effects**
Amoxicillin	60–90 mg/kg/day in 2 divided doses	+++	++	−	++	−	−	Diarrhea, rash
Amoxicillin-clavulanate*	90 mg/kg amoxicillin–6.4 mg/kg clavulanate daily in 2 divided doses	+++	++	−	+++	+++	+++	Diarrhea, rash
Cefdinir	14 mg/kg as a single daily dose	+++	+	−	+++	+++	+++	Diarrhea, rash
Cefaclor	40 mg/kg/day in 3 divided doses	++	−	−	++	+	+	Diarrhea, rash, serum-sickness–like reactions
Cefuroxime axetil	30 mg/kg/day in 2 divided doses	+++	+	−	++	++	+++	Diarrhea, distaste, rash
Cefprozil	30 mg/kg/day in 2 divided doses	+++	+	−	++	++	+++	Diarrhea, rash
Cefixime	8 mg/kg/day in a single daily dose	+	−	−	+++	+++	+++	Diarrhea, rash
Cefpodoxime	10 mg/kg/day in 2 divided doses	+++	+	−	+++	+++	+++	Diarrhea, rash
Ceftibuten	9 mg/kg/day in a single daily dose	−	−	−	+++	+++	++	Diarrhea, vomiting, abdominal pain
Loracarbef	30 mg/kg/day in 2 divided doses	++	−	−	+++	++	+++	Diarrhea
Clindamycin	20 mg/kg/day in 3 divided doses	+++	++	++	−	−	−	Potentially *C. difficile*–associated diarrhea
Erythromycin-sulfisoxazole	50 mg/kg erythromycin-150 mg/kg sulfisoxazole daily in 4 divided doses	++	−	−	+	+	++	Potentially severe reactions to sulfonamide (Stevens-Johnson syndrome, hematologic suppression)
Trimethoprim-sulfamethoxazole	8 mg/kg trimethoprim-40 mg/kg sulfamethoxazole daily in 2 divided doses	++	−	−	++	+	++	Potentially severe reactions to sulfonamide (Stevens-Johnson syndrome, hematologic suppression)
Azithromycin	10 mg/kg/day on day 1; 5 mg/kg/day on days 2–5, in a single daily dose	+++	±	−	+	+	++	Diarrhea, abdominal pain
Clarithromycin	15 mg/kg/day in 2 divided doses	+++	±	−	+	+	++	Diarrhea, vomiting, abdominal pain, rash

*The recommended formulation is the newer formulation containing a lower concentration of clavulanate.

in patients with chronic sinusitis is β-lactamase production. Eight new antimicrobial agents are available for the management of respiratory tract infections but have not been sufficiently evaluated in studies of acute bacterial sinusitis in children; these agents include cefdinir, cefixime, ceftibuten, cefprozil, cefpodoxime, loracarbef, clarithromycin, and azithromycin. Each of these antibiotics has been investigated in adults with acute sinusitis and found to be satisfactory.

The emerging problem in the management of acute or recurrent sinusitis is infection caused by penicillin- and cephalosporin-resistant *S. pneumoniae.* The prevalence of penicillin-resistant *S. pneumoniae* varies geographically. Many isolates of *S. pneumoniae* are resistant to other commonly used antimicrobials, such as trimethoprim-sulfamethoxazole. Therapeutic options include high-dose amoxicillin (80–90 mg/kg/day), azithromycin, clindamycin, or regimens that add rifampin. The optimal therapy for these infections is not known, and antibiotic selection should be guided by susceptibility results, when available.

The usual duration of oral antimicrobial therapy is 10–14 days. This recommendation is based on experience in adults, which demonstrates that 20% of sinus aspirates obtained after 7 days of antimicrobial treatment are still culture-positive. If there is only partial clinical improvement after 10–14 days of treatment, it is reasonable to continue treatment for another week. A good rule for duration of treatment is to treat until the patient is free of symptoms for 7 days.

Patients with acute sinusitis may require hospitalization because of systemic toxicity or inability to take oral antimicrobials. These patients may be treated with cefotaxime or ampicillin-sulbactam.

Surgery. There has been renewed interest regarding the role of surgical therapy for children and adults with chronic sinusitis. Early surgical efforts focused on construction of a nasoantral window within the maxillary sinus, which was thought to facilitate gravitational drainage. These procedures, however, proved to be relatively ineffective, in part because the cilia that line the maxillary sinus still transport secretions toward the natural meatus. A retrospective review (Muntz and Lusk, 1990) of the efficacy of nasal antral windows in children showed that only 27% of patients' conditions had improved at 6 months.

At present, the focus of surgical therapy is on the osteomeatal unit (Fig. 65–1). Using an endoscope, the surgeon attempts to enlarge the natural meatus of the maxillary outflow tract by excising the uncinate process and the ethmoid bullae and then performs an anterior ethmoidectomy. A pilot study (Lusk and Muntz, 1990) assessing the safety and efficacy of endoscopic sinus surgery in children with chronic sinusitis reported that 71% of patients were considered healthy by their parents 1 year postoperatively. The indications for and long-term success of functional endoscopic surgery in children requires additional study.

Supportive Therapy

Supportive therapies, including antihistamines, decongestants, and anti-inflammatory agents, for sinusitis have had little evaluation. Limited studies of systemic decongestants show that they increase the patency of the ostium of the maxillary sinus and decrease nasal airway resistance. The overall effect of these agents on the clinical course of acute sinusitis is not known. Antihistamines should be reserved for patients with recognized allergies. Topical decongestants, such as phenylephrine or oxymetazoline, shrink the nasal mucous membrane, improve ostial drainage, and provide symptomatic improvement; however, they may cause ciliostasis. Ciliary motion is an important local defense mechanism. The entire mucus covering of the maxillary antrum is normally cleared every 10 minutes. By inhibiting ciliary motion, topical decongestants may delay clearance of infected material. In addition, by decreasing blood flow to the mucosa, topical decongestants may further lower oxygen tension and impair diffusion of antimicrobial agents into the sinuses. The net effect of the various topical preparations on clinical recovery from sinusitis or the incidence of complications is unknown. Topical intranasal corticosteroids have provided only modest benefit in the second week of treatment.

COMPLICATIONS

The complications of sinus disease may cause both substantial morbidity and occasional mortality. Major complications result from either contiguous spread or hematogenous dissemination of infection (Table 65–5).

Orbital complications are the most frequent serious complication of acute sinusitis and, despite antimicrobial therapy, may lead to loss of vision and severe morbidity. Intracranial extension of infection is the second most common complication of acute sinusitis. Although the incidence of suppurative intracranial disease in patients with sinusitis is unknown, paranasal sinusitis is the source of 35–65% of subdural empyemas.

Orbital Complications and Orbital Cellulitis

Symptoms and Clinical Manifestations. The usual presenting feature of sinus-related orbital complications is a ''swollen eye.'' It is essential to establish the severity of the cellulitis clinically so that appropriate decisions can be made regarding specific therapy and the need for surgical drainage (Table 65–6). With early involvement (stage I), the inflammatory edema is confined to the medial aspect of the upper or lower eyelid. There is a gradual onset of lid swelling, minimal skin discoloration, and low-grade or no fever. There is no proptosis, visual impairment, or limitation of extraocular movement. Stage I cellulitis is not an actual infection of the orbit but is swelling caused by impedance of the local venous drainage. As such, it must be distinguished from a bacteremic form of periorbital or preseptal cellulitis caused by *H. influenzae* type b or *S. pneumoniae* (Chapter 47).

The **orbital septum** is a connective tissue reflection of periosteum that inserts into the eyelid and provides an anatomic barrier that protects the orbit. Both ''inflammatory edema'' and bacteremic preseptal infection involve tissues anterior to the orbital contents. Bacteremic periorbital cellulitis, however, is characterized by an abrupt onset, rapid progression, and severe systemic toxicity. The

TABLE 65–5. Major Complications of Sinusitis

Orbital
Inflammatory edema (preseptal or periorbital cellulitis)
Subperiosteal abscess
Orbital abscess
Orbital cellulitis
Optic neuritis
Osteomyelitis
Frontal (Pott's puffy tumor)
Maxillary
Intracranial
Epidural abscess
Subdural empyema or abscess
Cavernous or sagittal sinus thrombosis
Meningitis
Brain abscess

TABLE 65–6. Clinical Staging of Orbital Cellulitis

Stage	Description
I. Inflammatory edema	Inflammatory edema beginning in medial or lateral eyelid; usually nontender with only minimal skin changes; no induration, loss of vision, or limitation of extraocular movements
II. Subperiosteal abscess	Abscess beneath the periosteum of the ethmoid or frontal bone; proptosis down and out with varying degrees of chemosis and limitation of extraocular movement
III. Orbital posterior abscess	Abscess within the fat or muscle cone in the orbit; severe chemosis and proptosis; complete ophthalmoplegia and moderate to severe loss of vision (globe displaced forward or down and out)
IV. Orbital cellulitis	Edema of orbital contents with varying degrees of proptosis, chemosis, limitation of extraocular movement, or loss of vision
V. Cavernous sinus thrombophlebitis	Proptosis, globe fixation, severe loss of visual acuity, prostration, signs of meningitis; progress to proptosis, chemosis, and loss of vision in contralateral eye

Modified from Chandler JR, Langenbrunner DJ, Stevens ER: The pathogenesis of orbital complications in acute sinusitis. *Laryngoscope* 1970;80:1414.

markedly swollen and tender periorbital tissue has a violaceous, almost hemorrhagic discoloration, the texture of the skin is altered, and the subcutaneous tissue is indurated. *H. influenzae* type b or *S. pneumoniae* is frequently recovered from blood cultures and tissue aspirates. Because most *H. influenzae* organisms isolated from sinus aspirates are nontypable, the relationship of these acute bacteremic *H. influenzae* type b infections to sinusitis is unclear.

The presence of proptosis and ophthalmoplegia indicates that stages II to V of orbital complications must be considered. When an infection tracks backward into the cavernous sinus, the patient has signs of meningitis, focal or generalized seizures, deterioration of consciousness, and usually involvement of the opposite eye by way of the circuminfundibular communicating conduits between the two cavernous sinuses.

Diagnosis. When the infection has already infiltrated the orbital contents, the characteristic limitation of extraocular muscles, pain on eye movement, chemosis, proptosis, and vision disturbance, especially double vision, should establish the diagnosis of orbital cellulitis. If a history of sinus disease or signs and symptoms of acute sinusitis can be elicited, the origin of the cellulitis is also apparent. In stage I disease, however, when a child presents with nothing more than a swollen eye, other entities must be considered, including an infected periorbital or blepharal laceration, an insect bite, a contact allergy, conjunctivitis, dacryocystitis, and eczematoid dermatitis. If the diagnosis is in doubt, plain radiographs of the sinuses disclose partial or complete opacification, thickening of the mucous membranes, or an air-fluid level. Usually the ethmoidal and maxillary sinuses are involved together. The orbit, the paranasal sinuses, and the intracranial dural venous sinuses all can be studied simultaneously with contrast-enhanced CT. Thin CT cuts of the orbit with a multiplanar imaging technique are helpful in detecting and defining the extent of subperiosteal and orbital abscesses (Fig. 65–5).

Treatment and Prognosis. Children with stage I disease can occasionally be carefully treated as outpatients, provided the parents are cooperative and can easily return the child for re-evaluation. The antimicrobial agent selected must provide an antibacterial spectrum including β-lactamase-producing *H. influenzae* and *M. catarrhalis* and potentially penicillin-resistant *S. pneumoniae.* Amoxicillin-clavulanate (90 mg/kg amoxicillin–6.4 mg/kg clavulanate in 2 divided doses daily PO), cefuroxime axetil, or cefpodoxime is appropriate. Careful follow-up care is essential to detect progression of infection and the need for hospitalization.

If the infection does not respond promptly to oral antimicrobial therapy, hospitalization for parenteral antimicrobial therapy is appropriate. Suitable parenteral antimicrobial therapy includes cefotaxime or ampicillin-sulbactam (Table 65–7). If the infection has progressed beyond stage I, hospitalization and intravenous antimicrobial therapy are mandatory. The choice of antimicrobial agents is guided by knowledge of the bacterial agents usually found in patients with subperiosteal abscess and include the common sinus pathogens (*S. pneumoniae* and *H. influenzae*) as well as *S. aureus,* group A *Streptococcus,* and anaerobes of the upper respiratory tract (e.g., anaerobic gram-positive cocci, *Prevotella,* and *Fusobacterium*). Recommended therapies include nafcillin plus a third-generation cephalosporin (Table 65–7). Meropenem is an acceptable alternative regimen.

Blood and sinus aspirates should be obtained and cultured aerobically and anaerobically; appropriate antimicrobial drugs should be added if unsuspected organisms are observed on Gram stain or cultured from the sinus cavity or orbit. Surgical drainage is required if there is a subperiosteal or orbital abscess, but orbital cellulitis may respond to antimicrobial agents without surgical intervention. The prognosis for stage I and II disease is usually excellent if diagnosis and appropriate therapy are carried out promptly, but residual loss of vision due to infection of the optic nerve may complicate orbital abscesses. Severe neurologic sequelae or death may follow cavernous sinus thrombophlebitis.

Intracranial Complications

Four groups of symptoms and signs of intracranial involvement may be recognized, including those related to pansinusitis, increased intracranial pressure, meningeal irritation, and focal neurologic deficits.

Approximately 50–60% of patients with subdural empyema secondary to sinusitis present with symptoms of acute frontal sinusitis or an acute exacerbation of chronic pansinusitis. There are low-grade fever, malaise, frontal headache, and marked forehead and maxillary tenderness to digital pressure. On occasion, subperiosteal pus overlying the anterior wall of the frontal sinus causes dramatic epicranial edema and a painful fluctuance called **Pott's puffy tumor.**

With increased intracranial pressure, the initial headache of sinusitis worsens despite repeated doses of analgesics and oral antibiotics. Vomiting becomes intractable, and the level of consciousness deteriorates gradually. High intracranial pressure results from local cerebral edema in the area adjacent to the subdural pus and may progress rapidly to cause stupor and coma. With an isolated extradural empyema, cortical involvement is less extensive, and the patient generally remains alert.

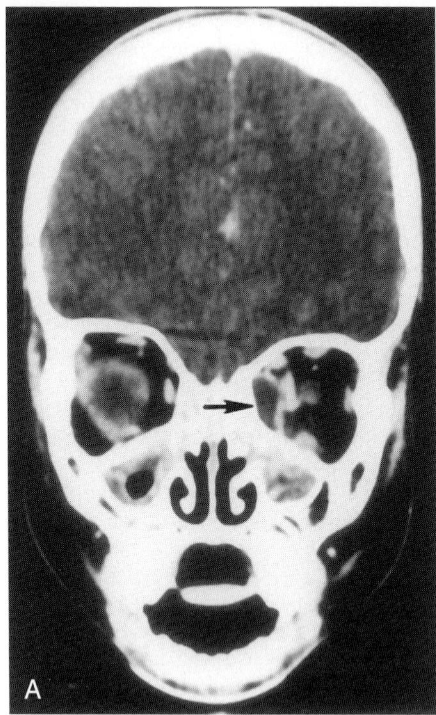

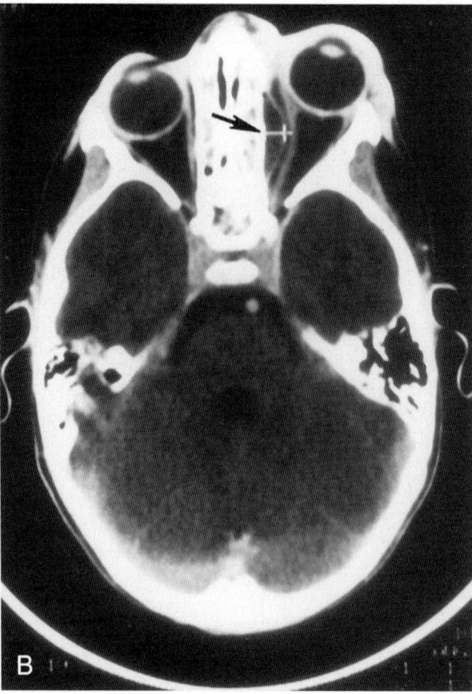

FIGURE 65–5. Coronal **(A)** and axial **(B)** CT scans of a subperiosteal abscess with thickening in the left maxillary sinus and complete opacification of the right maxillary sinus and the ethmoidal and sphenoidal sinuses bilaterally. A subperiosteal abscess is medial to the ethmoidal sinuses on the right (*arrows*). The axial view demonstrates proptosis of the right globe. (From Wald ER: Rhinitis and acute and chronic sinusitis. In Bluestone CD, Stool SE (editors): *Pediatric Otolaryngology.* Philadelphia: WB Saunders, 1990, p. 736.)

Meningeal irritation is suggested by depressed sensorium, nuchal rigidity, and photophobia. These signs represent an intense inflammatory response in the leptomeninges in contact with a subdural abscess rather than septic leptomeningitis. Because leptomeningeal inflammation is uncommon in pure extradural suppuration, subdural empyema, a much more serious lesion, should be suspected if protracted symptoms of fever and headache are accompanied by prominent signs of meningeal irritation.

Focal neurologic deficits are caused by a combination of local brain compression created by the empyema, edema, and infarction. A subdural empyema of the frontoparietal convexity causes contralateral brachiofacial weakness, contralateral conjugate gaze palsy, and expressive dysphasia. Lower limb involvement is usually late. Focal seizures that involve the arm and face occur in more than 60% of patients with dorsolateral lesions. With a parafalcine empyema, jacksonian seizures often begin in the foot and spread upward to include the trunk, arms, and face. Weakness primarily affects the leg, with sparing of speech and facial musculature. Bilateral parafalcine collections may present with paraplegia that stimulates thoracic spinal cord compression. In the terminal stage the patient is in a coma and has hemiplegia, evidence of generalized and meningeal sepsis, and finally, signs of uncal or tonsillar herniation.

Diagnosis. Intracranial infections should be considered if signs of systemic toxicity and headache do not improve with appropriate treatment for the sinusitis. Urgent diagnostic tests must be arranged if there is excruciating headache, systemic toxicity, intractable vomiting, or visual blurring. Treatment should ideally be instituted before the onset of seizures and focal neurologic findings, because these conditions signal cortical involvement by cerebritis and thrombophlebitis and may cause permanent deficits. The development of meningeal signs in a patient with sinusitis suggests meningitis or other intracranial infection. Meningitis rarely complicates sinusitis. Because the intracranial suppurative complications are primarily mass lesions that may precipitate brain herniation with lumbar puncture, this procedure should be deferred until after CT or MRI to exclude the presence of empyema and abscess.

CT and MRI are the definitive tests for the diagnosis of intracranial suppuration secondary to sinusitis and have virtually eliminated the need for cerebral angiography, radionuclide scan, and EEG. These noninvasive procedures define and exactly localize even small purulent collections, delineate associated cerebral edema, assess the amount of brain shift, and can detect concomitant brain abscess or bilateral empyema, which was often missed by angiography before CT became available. The presence of intracranial abscess as well as the extent of sinus disease can be evaluated concurrently with low axial cuts that include the ethmoidal, sphenoidal, and maxillary sinuses. A parenchymal abscess characteristically appears as a low-density center with an intensely enhancing capsule and surrounding edema (see Fig. 54–3). An extracerebral empyema always has an enhancing inner membrane, and the underlying cerebral edema often causes an impressive midline brain shift that cannot be accounted for by the amount of pus present (see Fig. 54–5). This combination of a small extracerebral collection and a disproportionate degree of brain shift distinguishes a subdural empyema from a chronic subdural hematoma, in which the severity of brain shift is determined primarily by the size of the clot.

Treatment and Prognosis. The treatment of sinusitis-related intracranial suppuration requires antimicrobials, drainage, and excellent supportive care. Because either acute sinusitis or an acute exacerbation of chronic sinusitis may precede intracranial complications, the antibiotics selected must be appropriate to include *S. pneumoniae, H. influenzae, M. catarrhalis,* respiratory anaerobes, streptococci, and *S. aureus.* A combination of vancomycin and meropenem can be used for initial therapy, with modifications as indicated by culture results.

Extradural and subdural empyemas should be drained through a generous craniotomy. An underlying brain abscess is best treated by intracapsular evacuation and catheter drainage to avoid unnecessary brain damage associated with radical excision of deep-seated lesions within eloquent areas of the brain. Results of cultures obtained at surgery should guide antimicrobial selection for continued therapy. Postoperatively, intravenous antibiotics should be main-

TABLE 65–7. Recommended Empiric Antibiotic Therapy for Severe Uncomplicated Sinusitis and Complications of Sinusitis*

Condition	Recommended Therapy
Severe uncomplicated sinusitis or stage 1 orbital cellulitis	Cefotaxime *or* Ampicillin-sulbactam
Stage II–V orbital cellulitis	Nafcillin (*or* oxacillin) *plus* cefotaxime *or* ceftriaxone *or* Vancomycin *plus* meropenem
Intracranial (including central nervous system) complications	Vancomycin *plus* meropenem *or* Nafcillin *or* oxacillin *plus* cefotaxime *or* ceftriaxone *plus* metronidazole

*Results of cultures obtained at the time of surgery may guide antimicrobial selection for continued therapy.

Suggested Dosages for Patients with Normal Renal Function

ANTIBIOTIC	DOSAGE (IV)	MAXIMUM DAILY DOSE
Ampicillin-sulbactam	200 mg/kg/day divided q6hr	12 g
Cefotaxime	200 mg/kg/day divided q6hr	12 g
Ceftriaxone	100 mg/kg/day divided every 12 hours	2–4 g
	or 80 mg/kg/day once q24hr	2–4 g
Clindamycin	40 mg/kg/day divided q6hr	2.7 g
Meropenem	100 mg/kg/day divided q6hr	2 g
Metronidazole	30 mg/kg/day divided q6hr	30 mg/kg
Nafcillin	150 mg/kg/day divided q4–6 hr	9 g
Oxacillin	150–200 mg/kg/day divided q4–6hr	12 g
Penicillin G	300,000 U/kg/day divided q4hr	20–24 MU
Vancomycin	60 mg/kg/day divided q6hr	2 g

tained for a minimum of 3–4 weeks. The shrinking of the abscess or empyema can be monitored accurately by serial CT.

Despite modern diagnostic and surgical capabilities, the mortality associated with suppurative intracranial complications of sinusitis is 7% with morbidity of 13%. The causes of death and permanent morbidity are related to delayed diagnosis, recurrent suppuration, missed concomitant lesions, extensive cortical and dural sinus thrombophlebitis, and fulminant bacterial meningitis. Early diagnosis remains the most effective way to improve survival.

PROGNOSIS AND PREVENTION

Clinical improvement is prompt in nearly all children treated with an appropriate antimicrobial agent. Fever resolves, and there is a remarkable reduction in nasal discharge and cough within 48–72 hours. If there is no improvement, or worsening, within 48 hours, clinical re-evaluation is appropriate. If the diagnosis is unchanged, sinus aspiration may be considered for precise bacteriologic information.

TABLE 65–8. Predisposing Factors for Recurrent or Chronic Sinusitis

- Recurrent viral upper respiratory tract infections
  - Day care
  - School-age siblings
- Allergic diathesis
- Immunodeficiency
  - Insufficient IgG, IgA, or IgG subclasses
  - Dysfunctional immunoglobulins
  - Acquired immunodeficiency
- Cystic fibrosis
- Ciliary dyskinesia
- Anatomic abnormalities
  - Deviated nasal septum
  - Osteomeatal complex disease
  - Nasal polyps

Some children experience recurrent or chronic episodes of sinusitis. The most common cause of recurrent sinusitis is recurrent viral upper respiratory infection, often a consequence of attending a daycare center or the presence of an older, school-age sibling in the household (Table 65–8). Other predisposing conditions include allergic inflammation, cystic fibrosis, an immunodeficiency disorder (insufficient or dysfunctional immunoglobulins), ciliary dyskinesia (immotile cilia syndrome), or an anatomic problem.

In the evaluation of children with recurrent sinusitis, considerations should include consultation with an allergist, a sweat test for cystic fibrosis, quantitative immunoglobulins and immunoglobulin subclasses, and a mucosal biopsy to assess ciliary function and structure. If specific allergens are identified or an allergic diathesis is documented, therapy might include desensitization, antihistamines, or topical intranasal steroids. If a treatable immunodeficiency is identified, specific immunoglobulin therapy should be initiated. Otherwise, a trial of antimicrobial prophylaxis until the end of the respiratory disease season may be appropriate. Although antimicrobial prophylaxis has not been studied in patients with recurrent acute sinusitis, it has proved to be a useful strategy in reducing symptomatic episodes of acute otitis media in patients with recurrent ear disease. If patients do not respond to maximal medical therapy, surgical intervention may be appropriate.

REVIEWS

Brook I, Gooch WM III, Jenkins SG, et al: Medical management of acute bacterial sinusitis. Recommendations of a Clinical Advisory Committee on Pediatric and Adult Sinusitis. *Ann Otol Rhinol Laryngol* 2000; 109(Suppl 182):1–20.

O'Brien KL, Dowell SF, Schwartz B, et al: Acute sinusitis—Principles of judicious use of antimicrobial agents. *Pediatrics* 1998;101(Suppl): 174–7.

Incaudo GA, Wooding LG: Diagnosis and treatment of acute and subacute sinusitis in children and adults. *Clin Rev Allergy Immunol* 1998; 16:157–204.

Sinus and Allergy Health Partnership: Antimicrobial treatment guidelines for acute bacterial rhinosinusitis. *Otolaryngol Head Neck Surg* 2000; 123(Suppl 1, pt 2):S1–32.

Wald ER: Sinusitis. *Pediatr Ann* 1998;27:811–8.

KEY ARTICLES

Brook I: Bacteriologic features of chronic sinusitis in children. *JAMA* 1981;246:967–9.

Carson JL, Collier AM, Hu SS: Acquired ciliary defects in nasal epithelium of children with acute viral upper respiratory infections. *N Engl J Med* 1985;312:463–8.

Evans FO Jr, Snyder JB, Moore WE, et al: Sinusitis of the maxillary antrum. *N Engl J Med* 1975;293:735–9.

Gwaltney JM Jr, Scheld WM, Sande MA, et al: The microbial etiology and antimicrobial therapy of adults with acute community-acquired sinusitis: A fifteen year experience at the University of Virginia and review of other selected studies. *J Allergy Clin Immunol* 1992;90:457–61.

Kennedy DW, Zinreich SJ, Rosenbaum AE, et al: Functional endoscopic sinus surgery: Theory and diagnostic evaluation. *Arch Otolaryngol* 1985;111:576–82.

Kovatch AL, Wald ER, Ledesma-Medina J, et al: Maxillary sinus radiographs in children with nonrespiratory complaints. *Pediatrics* 1984; 73:306–8.

Lerner DN, Choi SS, Zalzal GH, et al: Intracranial complications of sinusitis in childhood. *Ann Otol Rhinol Laryngol* 1995;104:288–93.

Lusk RP: The surgical management of chronic sinusitis in children. *Pediatr Ann* 1998;27:820–7.

Lusk RP, Muntz HR: Endoscopic sinus surgery in children with chronic sinusitis: A pilot study. *Laryngoscope* 1990;100:654–8.

McAlister WH, Lusk R, Muntz HR: Comparison of plain radiographs and coronal CT scans in infants and children with recurrent sinusitis. *AJR* 1989;153:1259–64.

Muntz HR, Lusk RP: Nasal antral windows in children: A retrospective study. *Laryngoscope* 1990;100:643–6.

Wald ER: Chronic sinusitis in children. *J Pediatr* 1995;127:339–47.

Wald ER, Byers C, Guerra N, et al: Subacute sinusitis in children. *J Pediatr* 1989;115:28–32.

Wald ER, Chiponis D, Ledesma-Medina J: Comparative effectiveness of amoxicillin and amoxicillin-clavulanate potassium in acute paranasal sinus infections in children: A double-blind, placebo-controlled trial. *Pediatrics* 1986;77:795–800.

Wald ER, Milmoe GJ, Bowen A, et al. Acute maxillary sinusitis in children. *N Engl J Med* 1981;304:749–54.

Wald ER, Reilly JS, Casselbrant M, et al: Treatment of acute maxillary sinusitis in childhood: A comparative study of amoxicillin and cefaclor. *J Pediatr* 1984;104:297–302.

CHAPTER 66

Middle Respiratory Tract Infections

Louis M. Bell

The middle respiratory tract encompasses the supraglottic structures, the glottis, and the trachea. Infections in this area include **acute laryngotracheobronchitis (LTB)**—commonly called **croup—epiglottitis,** and **bacterial tracheitis** (membranous LTB, pseudomembranous croup, bacterial croup). Although believed by some experts to be a separate clinical illness, **spasmodic or recurrent croup** is discussed with acute LTB.

Although they differ in incidence, epidemiology, pathophysiology, and approach to therapy, these infections are related through the common physical finding of inspiratory stridor. There are many different causes of stridor in children, including both infectious and noninfectious conditions (Table 66–1). Fortunately, for most children, the correct diagnosis is possible with a brief history and physical examination. Routine laboratory studies and radiographic imaging for the most part only confirm the diagnosis. The treatment and prognosis are different for each of the three middle respiratory tract infections, and therefore prompt diagnosis is vital. Acute LTB, a viral infection, is usually benign and is most frequently managed on an outpatient basis. Epiglottitis and bacterial tracheitis may lead to asphyxiating obstruction and require emergency airway management to prevent complications and death. Fortunately, immunization with *Haemophilus influenzae* type b conjugate vaccines has led to a marked reduction in epiglottitis and other invasive *Haemophilus influenzae* type b infections.

When the history and physical examination are not sufficient, laboratory studies become important. For these patients, neck radiographs are often useful. A CBC and measurement of acute phase reactants are often not helpful in establishing the diagnosis. The definitive diagnosis can be established by direct visualization of the supraglottic and subglottic structures of the larynx. Typical pathologic findings characterize each of the three infections.

Although establishment of the initial diagnosis is vital, an understanding of the expected course of illness and responses to therapy is also important (Table 66–2). Understanding that premature tracheal extubation in a child with bacterial tracheitis may be fatal or that there may be a rebound effect when nebulized racemic epinephrine is used in children with acute LTB will influence management decisions and ultimately reduce morbidity and mortality.

ACUTE LARYNGOTRACHEOBRONCHITIS

ETIOLOGY

Epidemics of acute LTB correspond to community outbreaks of respiratory viruses, namely, parainfluenza virus types 1, 2, or 3, and respiratory syncytial virus (RSV). In one study, these viruses accounted for 84% of the etiologic agents recovered from children with acute LTB. Spread among children occurs during play or close person-to-person contact or with aerosolized large-droplet spread. Other viruses and *Mycoplasma pneumoniae* may cause LTB as a component of systemic or lower respiratory tract infection. Herpes simplex virus has been reported to cause LTB in neonates (Table 66–3).

EPIDEMIOLOGY

Acute LTB is one of the most common middle and lower respiratory tract infections and accounts for as many as 20,000 hospital admissions per year in the United States. One study (Denny et al., 1983) found the incidence of croup to be highest in the second year of life, at 4.7 cases per 100 children per year, with the rate decreasing gradually until it was only 0.46 case per 100 children per year after the age of 6 years. Croup is most common between the ages of 6 months and 3 years and is unusual in infants younger than 1 month and in children older than 6 years. Boys are approximately 1.4 times more likely to have croup than girls are. Acute LTB is seasonal, occurring in fall and early winter peaks in many parts of the country.

Because severe LTB is unusual during the first 3 months of life, it has been postulated that in utero transfer of maternal virus-specific immunoglobulins may protect young infants against infection or at least ameliorate the course of the illness. Infants with high neutralizing antibody titers are less likely to have RSV infection in the first 6 months of life than infants with low titers are.

PATHOGENESIS

The respiratory viruses that cause acute LTB initially invade the epithelial cells of the pharynx and nose. As the viral pathogens replicate, the infection spreads to involve the larynx, the trachea, and in some instances the bronchi and bronchioli. Infection results in mucosal swelling, production of mucus, and the appearance of a fibrinous exudate that further obstructs the airway, leading to the

TABLE 66–1. Differential Diagnosis of Stridor

Infections	Noninfectious Conditions
Acute laryngotracheobronchitis	Foreign body aspiration
Epiglottitis	Angioneurotic edema
Pharyngitis	Spasmodic croup
Parapharyngeal abscess	Ingestion of caustic or hot fluid
Bacterial tracheitis	Trauma, smoke inhalation
Laryngopharyngeal diphtheria	Laryngomalacia
Laryngeal papillomatosis	Congenital subglottic stenosis
Extrinsic inflammatory mass compressing the trachea (e.g., tuberculosis)	Extrinsic mass compressing the trachea (e.g., cystic hygroma, hemangioma, vascular malformation)

TABLE 66–2. Clinical Features of Middle Respiratory Tract Infections

Feature	Bacterial Tracheitis	Epiglottitis	Viral Laryngotracheobronchitis	Spasmodic Croup
Viral prodromal illness	+	−	++	−
Mean age	4–5 yr	3–4 yr (25% <2 yr)	6–36 mo (60% <24 mo)	6–36 mo (60% <24 mo)
Onset of illness	Acute (1–2 days)	Acute (6–24 hr)	Gradual (2–3 days)	Sudden (at night)
Fever	+	+	±	−
Toxicity	++	±	−	−
Inspiratory stridor	Harsh	Mild	Harsh	Harsh
Drooling, neck hyperextension	−	++	−	−
Cough	++	−	++	++
Sore throat	±	++	±	−
Positive blood culture	±	+	−	−
Leukocytosis	+	+	−	−
Recurrent disease	−	−	+	++
Hospitalization and tracheal intubation	Frequent	Frequent	Rare	Rare

+ = Frequently present; − = absent; ± = may or may not be present; ++ = present and usually pronounced.

typical symptoms of stridor, cough, and hoarseness. The endoscopic appearance of acute LTB includes a reddened laryngeal mucosa and red subglottic tissue with patches of secretion or exudate that, when wiped away, leaves no ulcer or hemorrhage (Plate 8E).

On the basis of endoscopic appearance and clinical presentation, a distinction is often made between **spasmodic croup** (also called **recurrent croup**) and acute LTB. The endoscopic appearance of spasmodic croup is thought to be different from that of acute LTB in that the subglottic tissues, rather than being red in appearance, are pale and edematous. There are also clinical differences between spasmodic croup and acute LTB (Table 66–2). Classically, spasmodic croup occurs without an upper respiratory tract prodrome; it occurs usually at night with a sudden onset, but the illness has a milder course than acute LTB. Resolution of symptoms often occurs spontaneously or with the use of humidified air. The distinctions between these two illnesses are not clear, however, and it seems most likely that spasmodic croup and acute LTB are different presentations of a single disease and may be related simply to the immunologic response, involving IgE and histamine release, or to infections with RSV, parainfluenza viruses, or other viral pathogens.

SYMPTOMS AND CLINICAL MANIFESTATIONS

The onset of illness usually begins with upper respiratory symptoms, including nasal congestion, irritation, and coryza. A sore throat and a mucous cough follow soon thereafter. Fever usually appears within 24 hours of the initial symptoms; the temperature is generally mildly elevated to 38.5°C (101.5°F), but it may be higher. Because the infection involves the larynx, the cough becomes harsh and is often described as **barking** or **brassy** in nature. The classic symptoms of acute LTB are hoarseness, a barking cough, and inspiratory stridor. These symptoms are usually most severe during the evening hours and usually peak in intensity during the initial 3–4 days of illness.

Although the peak incidence of acute LTB occurs during the second year of life, school-age children with this disease have been reported. Some experts have suggested that the diagnosis of croup in a child older than 3 years should prompt consideration of the full differential diagnosis of stridor, including an underlying anatomic abnormality (Table 66–1). Similarly, crouplike symptoms in an infant less than 1 month of age should raise concern about an anatomic abnormality.

TABLE 66–3. Etiologic Agents of Acute Laryngotracheobronchitis in Children

Common	Less Common	Rare
Parainfluenza viruses 1, 2, or 3	Influenza viruses A and B	Rhinoviruses
Respiratory syncytial virus	Adenoviruses	Enteroviruses
	Mycoplasma pneumoniae	Herpes simplex virus
		Measles virus

Physical Examination Findings

A careful physical examination is important to identify findings that support the presumptive diagnosis suggested by the history and to assess the degree of respiratory distress, the need for hospitalization, and the need for an artificial airway. The physical examination should assess the degree of inspiratory stridor; the degree of suprasternal, subcostal, and intercostal retractions; air entry or exchange, as determined by auscultation; color; and level of consciousness. Children with LTB typically have inspiratory stridor only with agitation and crying, mild retractions, normal air exchange, and a pink color, and they appear alert and interactive. Stridor at rest accompanied by decreased air entry or changes in mental status necessitates hospitalization.

Marked upper airway obstruction with impending respiratory failure is a rare complication in acute LTB. Endotracheal intubation is required for only 0.2–1.3% of patients. Respiratory failure is heralded by hypotonia, marked retractions, decreased or absent breath sounds, and cyanosis. The definition of respiratory failure includes a partial pressure of arterial carbon dioxide ($Paco_2$) >60 mm Hg or a partial pressure of arterial oxygen (Pao_2) <50 mm Hg in 100% oxygen.

DIAGNOSIS

The diagnosis of acute LTB is usually suggested by history and substantiated by physical examination findings. Pulse oximetry is a reliable and noninvasive method of quickly measuring oxygen-saturated hemoglobin to assess respiratory status. Transcutaneous carbon dioxide pressure monitoring also has been recommended as a potentially reliable and objective measurement of upper airway obstruction in children with severe croup.

Laboratory Evaluation

The WBC count is usually normal, although lymphocytosis may occur as with other viral infections. In most cases, routine laboratory studies are not useful in establishing the diagnosis.

Microbiologic Evaluation

Although not indicated for most children who are treated as outpatients, rapid viral diagnosis and viral cultures for hospitalized children with acute LTB may be helpful, especially for infection control purposes. Many different indirect fluorescent antibody tests or enzyme immunosorbent assays (EIAs) have demonstrated varying degrees of sensitivity and specificity, depending on the study and the virus being tested. These rapid tests are available for all of the most common pathogens in acute LTB, including influenza viruses A and B; parainfluenza viruses 1, 2, and 3; RSV; and adenoviruses. The sensitivity of RSV indirect immunofluorescence tests using monoclonal antibodies is 75–97%; the specificity is 76–98%; and the negative predictive value is 90–97%. The sensitivity and positive predictive values for influenza virus A, parainfluenza virus, and adenovirus appear to be less than those for RSV.

Diagnostic Imaging

Radiographs may be normal (Fig. 66–1) or suggest air trapping with a widening of the hypopharynx. Lateral and posteroanterior radiographs of the neck demonstrate subglottic narrowing, the **steeple sign,** in as few as 40% of patients (Fig. 66–2). Although the lateral neck radiograph usually does not confirm the diagnosis of acute LTB, the finding of a normal epiglottis and supraglottic structures decreases concerns about possible epiglottitis. A child with a typical and mild presentation of acute LTB does not require radiographic studies.

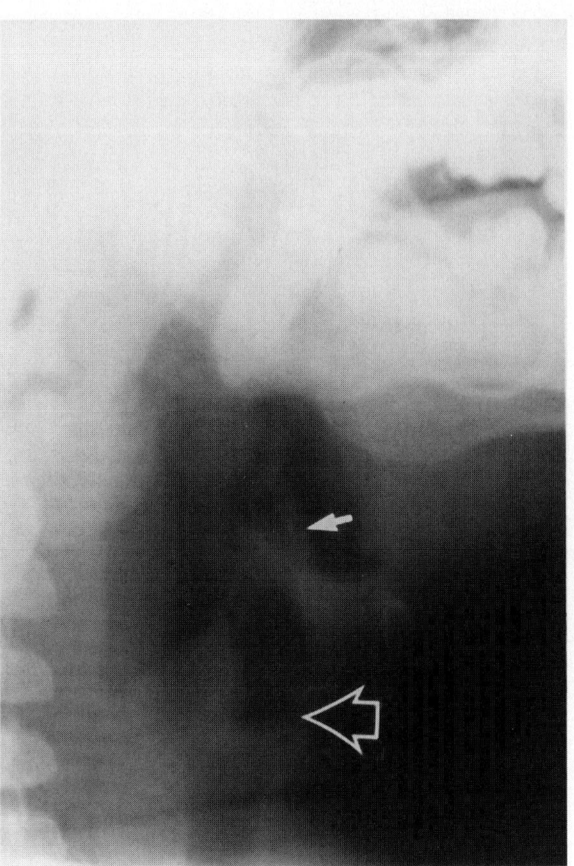

FIGURE 66–1. A lateral radiograph of a normal upper airway. A well-distended, air-filled hypopharynx outlines the normal epiglottis (*solid arrow*), aryepiglottic folds, and glottic structures (*open arrow*).

TREATMENT

Treatment of acute LTB depends on the severity of the illness (Table 66–4). If the patient is not in respiratory failure, therapy may include any or all of the following modalities: humidified air, supplemental oxygen, nebulized racemic epinephrine, and corticosteroids. Most children with acute LTB are treated as outpatients, with careful instructions regarding humidified air, oral hydration, fever control, and arrangement for follow-up visits.

The treatment of children with moderate to severe acute LTB who require hospitalization traditionally includes humidified air and oxygen. Although there is anecdotal evidence that humidified air benefits children with croup, controlled data have not supported its use. Supplemental oxygen is indicated for patients who have pulse oximetry saturation readings less than 95% and is often delivered in a mist tent apparatus.

Nebulized Adrenaline (Epinephrine). Most experts agree that **racemic epinephrine** (composed of equal amounts of D and L isomers) administered by nebulization (not by intermittent positive pressure breathing) decreases airway obstruction considerably by α-adrenergic-mediated vasoconstriction and an associated decrease in subglottic edema. The peak effect of racemic epinephrine occurs 10–30 minutes after administration. The effects of the drug dissipate within 2 hours of administration, and repeat treatments may be necessary, depending on the severity of symptoms. Racemic epinephrine in the outpatient setting should be used with caution because of concerns about a **rebound effect** in some patients, with worsening of the degree of obstruction within 2 hours of treatment. Therefore, if racemic epinephrine is used in the outpatient or emergency department, admission is indicated unless a prolonged observation period of at least 2–3 hours is planned. Although racemic epinephrine is widely used in the United States, it is not available as a pharmacologic preparation in many other countries, including the United Kingdom and Israel. A study (Waisman et al., 1992) indicates that the more readily available **L-epinephrine** (adrenaline) can be used with the same efficacy as racemic epinephrine with no risk of additional adverse effects. The dose of L-epinephrine is half that of racemic epinephrine.

Corticosteroids. The efficacy of corticosteroids in the treatment of croup has been questioned until recently. Two articles, one a meta-analysis of previous randomized trials (Kairys et al., 1989) and the other a prospective, randomized, double-blind study (Super et al., 1989), support the use of **dexamethasone** in hospitalized patients with moderate to severe acute LTB. A single parenteral dose (0.6 mg/kg) appears effective in reducing the overall severity of the disease in the first 24 hours of hospitalization and may reduce the need for racemic epinephrine and tracheal intubation. In addition, **nebulized budesonide,** a synthetic glucocorticoid with strong topical anti-inflammatory effects and little systemic activity, has been compared with intramuscular dexamethasone, oral dexamethasone, nebulized epinephrine, and placebo. A dose of nebulized budesonide (2 mg in 4 mL of normal saline solution) appears to be as effective as dexamethasone or nebulized adrenaline at reducing the need for hospitalization and shortening hospital stays. Budesonide is not approved for use in the United States. Many experts now

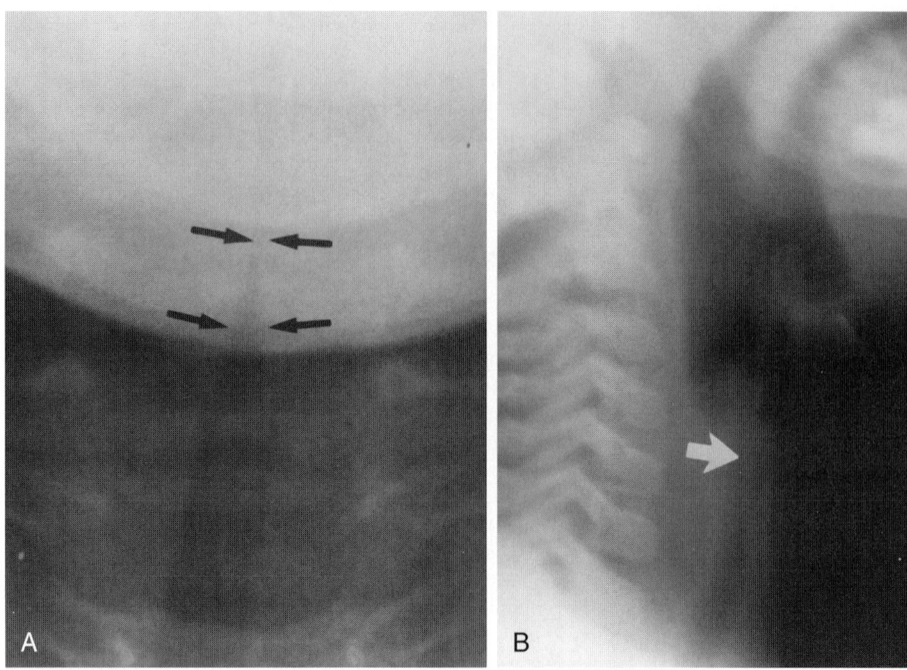

FIGURE 66–2. Croup (laryngotracheobronchitis [LTB]). **A**, Posteroanterior view of the upper airway shows the so-called steeple sign,the tapered narrowing of the immediate subglottic airway (*arrows*). **B**, Lateral view of the upper airway shows good delineation of the supraglottic anatomy. The subglottic trachea is hazy and poorly defined (*arrow*) because of the inflammatory edema that has obliterated the sharp undersurface of the vocal cords and extends down the trachea in a diminishing manner.

TABLE 66–4. Considerations for Therapy for Acute Laryngotracheobronchitis

Outpatient
Recommended Treatment
Humidified air
Oral hydration
Fever control
Plan for physician follow-up after telephone communication
Dexamethasone*
Alternative Regimens
Budesonide†
Racemic epinephrine or L-epinephrine‡ (2- to 3-hour observation time should be observed before discharge from outpatient setting)
Inpatient
Recommended
Humidified air and oxygen§
Racemic epinephrine or L-epinephrine†
Dexamethasone
Fever control
Hydration
Alternative Regimens
Budesonide†
Heliox

*May be given orally or intramuscularly (0.6 mg/kg) a single dose.
†Nebulized treatment: 2 mg in 4 ml of normal saline solution.
‡Nebulized treatment: 0.2 mL (for 5–10 kg), 0.5 mL (11–15 kg), 0.7 mL (16–20 kg), and 1 mL (≥21 kg) of a 2.25% solution in 3 mL of normal saline solution. The dose of L-epinephrine is one half the dose of racemic epinephrine.
§Based on pulse oximetry readings of <95% saturation in room air.

recommend the use of dexamethasone orally or intramuscularly in the outpatient setting for children with mild or moderate croup.

Antiviral Therapy. Although antiviral agents such as amantadine hydrochloride, rimantadine hydrochloride, and ribavirin have demonstrated in vitro or in vivo activity against most of the common viruses that cause acute LTB, no specific studies have been performed to establish efficacy.

COMPLICATIONS

The most common complication of acute LTB is spread of viral infection with concomitant upper and lower respiratory tract infection. Upper respiratory tract involvement predisposes to secondary bacterial otitis media. Involvement of the lower respiratory tract as manifested by wheezing or pneumonia occurred in 3% and 1.4%, respectively, of patients in an 11-year study (Denny et al., 1983) of acute LTB in a pediatric practice. Secondary bacterial pneumonia and airway obstruction requiring endotracheal intubation are rare. As is the case with any severe upper airway obstruction, severe croup may rarely lead to pulmonary edema.

PROGNOSIS

The outcome of acute LTB is excellent. There is possibly slightly increased bronchial reactivity in children with LTB who require hospitalization as compared with other children, but the differences are small and the clinical significance is unclear.

EPIGLOTTITIS

ETIOLOGY

Epiglottitis, especially in children, historically has almost always been caused by *Haemophilus influenzae* type b. *Streptococcus pneumoniae* is also a recognized cause, especially in immunocompromised adults. *H. parainfluenzae,* group A *Streptococcus,* and *Staphylococcus aureus* have also been reported in rare cases. These organisms are spread from person to person by secretions or large droplets.

EPIDEMIOLOGY

Historically, epiglottitis was estimated to account for approximately 1 in every 1,000 pediatric hospital admissions. Universal immunization with conjugate *H. influenzae* type b vaccine has substantially reduced the incidence of life-threatening infections caused by this organism to rates of 0.3 case per 100,000 or lower.

Approximately 75% of children with epiglottitis are 1–5 years of age; the mean age is 3.5–4 years. This infection also has been described in adults and infants as young as 6 months of age. There is a male predominance of 1.5 times the rate among female patients. Although more common in the winter months, epiglottitis has been shown to occur throughout the year.

PATHOGENESIS

Epiglottitis is a cellulitis of the supraglottic structures, which include the epiglottis, the aryepiglottic folds, and the arytenoid cartilages. It arises from either direct invasion or hematogenous seeding of these tissues by pathogens, primarily *H. influenzae* type b. After invasion, the supraglottic structures swell and tend to obstruct the glottic opening, with the resulting signs and symptoms of respiratory distress (Plate 8E). In addition, pooling saliva accumulates because of impaired swallowing, which may lead to aspiration of pharyngeal secretions and precipitate an acute respiratory arrest.

SYMPTOMS AND CLINICAL MANIFESTATIONS

The swollen epiglottis (Fig. 66–3) obstructs the glottic opening, and the swollen supraglottic tissues reduce the caliber of the airway, resulting in inspiratory stridor, the hallmark of this infection. The typical presentation is fever with sore throat and muffled voice. Stridor and respiratory distress, such as intercostal retractions and nasal flaring, soon follow. As the swelling of the supraglottic structure continues, drooling or pooling secretions in the mouth are noted in up to 70% of patients. At least 60% of children older than 2 years of age complain of a sore throat. Other frequent signs include a change in voice that is muffled but not hoarse; refusal to eat or drink; and preference for sitting, often with the head held forward, the mouth open, and the jaw thrust forward (sniffing position). The child refuses to sleep. In almost 90% of patients these symptoms develop rapidly, in less than 24 hours, and may progress in as little as 6 hours. Aphonia, cough, or hoarseness is unusual.

Approximately 25% of children with epiglottitis are younger than 2 years of age. In a study (Losek et al., 1990) comparing the signs and symptoms of epiglottitis in 58 children younger than 2 years of age with those in 178 older children, there were virtually no differences between these groups, and the signs and symptoms were the same regardless of age.

Unusual Presentations

Atypical or unusual presentations of epiglottitis frequently involve children who present early with mild symptoms or with a history or physical examination findings that are confusing and lead to the incorrect diagnosis of acute LTB or pharyngitis. In most cases, the correct diagnosis usually becomes evident over a short observation period of 3–5 hours, as the classic signs and symptoms become recognizable.

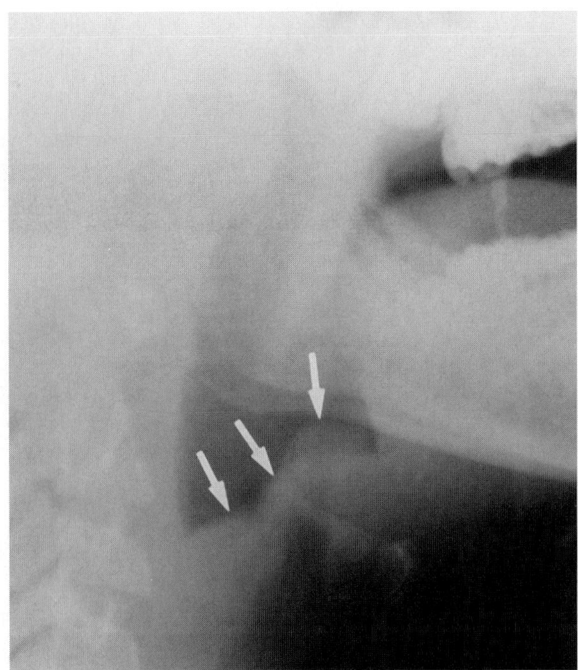

FIGURE 66–3. Epiglottitis. The lateral projection of the upper airway shows a thickened and bulging epiglottis with marked swelling of the aryepiglottic folds (*arrows*). The entrance to the glottis is severely narrowed, causing airway obstruction.

Physical Examination Findings

The diagnosis of epiglottitis can usually be established on the basis of the history and simple observation. When a child with fever is observed to be sitting anxiously in a sniffing position with mouth open, the diagnosis should be confirmed by direct laryngoscopy (Plate 8E) and tracheal intubation. The airway should be secured in the operating room by tracheal intubation performed by a skilled anesthesiologist. A qualified surgeon should be present in case an emergency tracheostomy is necessary. The most common physical findings to support the diagnosis are inspiratory stridor, intercostal and supracostal retractions, and fever. Tachycardia is usually present. The use of a tongue blade should be avoided when the posterior oropharynx is examined because of the risk of causing acute laryngeal obstruction. The pharynx should be examined if the child cooperates in opening the mouth. The pharynx is erythematous, and pooled secretions are often noted. Occasionally the swollen, erythematous epiglottis can be seen protruding above the base of the tongue.

DIAGNOSIS

The diagnosis of epiglottitis should be considered for any child of the appropriate age with a compatible history and clinical presentation, especially if the child has not received a *H. influenzae* type b vaccination. The diagnosis is usually confirmed by a physical examination in the operating room at the time of direct laryngoscopy and intubation. The microbiologic cause is confirmed by cultures of the blood and epiglottis taken *after* the airway is secured.

Differential Diagnosis

The differential diagnosis is that of stridor (Table 66–1). Although the finding of an erythematous, swollen epiglottis suggests a bacterial infection, ingestion of a caustic substance (e.g., lye) or hot fluids should also be considered in the differential diagnosis.

Laboratory Evaluation

Routine laboratory studies should not be performed on a child with suspected epiglottitis until after the airway is secured. The anxiety and pain associated with venipuncture may precipitate acute laryngeal obstruction. The WBC count is elevated above 10,000/mm^3 in 85% of patients.

Microbiologic Evaluation

Blood cultures are positive in 75–90% of cases. Cultures of the surface of the epiglottis reveal a potential pathogen in approximately half of all cases. A urine latex agglutination assay can be used to detect *H. influenzae* type b capsular antigen in patients receiving antibiotics at the time of culture or in those whose initial cultures are negative.

Diagnostic Imaging

A lateral radiograph of the neck is usually deferred for a child who has a classic presentation or whose respiratory distress is severe. In ambiguous cases, however, the lateral neck radiograph can be obtained while preparations for possible tracheal intubation are being arranged. A physician should accompany the patient to the radiology suite. There are three pathognomonic features of epiglottitis: a swollen epiglottis, thickened aryepiglottic folds, and obliteration of the vallecula (Fig. 66–3). In addition, ballooning or widening of the oropharyngeal airway is often noted.

TREATMENT

Once the diagnosis of epiglottitis is confirmed, the two goals of management are prevention of airway obstruction and eradication of the infection. The child should be left in a position of comfort, which in most instances is on the caretaker's lap. Humidified oxygen can be provided by aiming the respiratory tubing toward the child's face. The anesthesiologist and the otorhinolaryngologist should be alerted to begin preparations for endotracheal intubation or, if that fails, tracheostomy. If an acute airway obstruction occurs, resuscitation with 100% oxygen and bag-valve-mask ventilation is usually successful until emergency tracheal intubation or tracheostomy can be performed. Nasotracheal intubation is preferred.

After the airway is secure, transfer to a pediatric intensive care unit is necessary. The duration of nasotracheal intubation in a retrospective review (Gonzalez et al., 1986) of 100 children with epiglottitis revealed that most patients required intubation less than 2 days. Daily direct laryngoscopy and visualization of the supraglottic area along with resolution of fever are the most effective ways to determine when to perform tracheal extubation.

A peripheral intravenous catheter can be placed and blood cultures obtained immediately after the airway is secured. Antibiotics for empiric therapy include cefotaxime or ceftriaxone (Table 66–5). The treatment course for uncomplicated infection is usually 7 days, with antibiotics administered intravenously while the patient is intubated and until the fever and upper respiratory tract symptoms have resolved. Most patients respond rapidly to therapy and complete the final portion of treatment orally. There is no recognized role for corticosteroids in the treatment of epiglottitis.

TABLE 66–5. Recommended Antibiotic Therapy for Epiglottitis and Bacterial Tracheitis

Condition	Recommended Therapy	Alternative Therapy
Epiglottitis	Cefotaxime *or* ceftriaxone	Cefuroxime* *or* Ampicillin *plus* chloramphenicol
Bacterial tracheitis	Oxacillin *or* nafcillin *plus* cefotaxime *or* ceftriaxone	Vancomycin *plus* cefotaxime *or* ceftriaxone *or* Oxacillin *or* nafcillin *or* vancomycin *plus* chloramphenicol

*Cefuroxime should not be used if there is evidence of central nervous system infection.

Suggested Dosages for Patients with Normal Renal Function

ANTIBIOTIC	DOSAGE (IV)	MAXIMUM DAILY DOSE
Ampicillin	150–300 mg/kg/day divided q6hr	12 g
Cefotaxime	100–200 mg/kg/day divided q6hr	12 g
Ceftriaxone	50–100 mg/kg/day divided q12hr	2–4 g
	or 80 mg/kg/day once q24hr	2–4 g
Cefuroxime	100 mg/kg/day divided q8hr	12 g
Chloramphenicol	75–100 mg/kg/day divided q6hr	2–4 g
	or 75 mg/kg/day divided q6hr PO	2–4 g
Nafcillin	150 mg/kg/day divided q4–6hr	9 g
Oxacillin	150–200 mg/kg/day divided q4–6hr	12 g
Vancomycin	45–60 mg/kg/day divided q6hr	2 g

COMPLICATIONS AND PROGNOSIS

The most serious complication of epiglottitis is acute respiratory obstruction leading to death. Before recommendations for aggressive measures directed at securing an adequate airway, the mortality was 6–20%. With early recognition and therapy, this can usually be prevented, and the mortality now is approximately 1%. Pneumonia is the most commonly reported extrasupraglottic infection, which occurs in about 25% of patients. Rarely, other sites of infection with *H. influenzae* are present, although the simultaneous occurrence of epiglottitis and meningitis or pericarditis is uncommon. In a review (Bonadio and Losek, 1991) of 234 cases of epiglottitis, 2.1% of children had pulmonary edema, although all of these children had severe respiratory distress and respiratory arrest, with the pulmonary edema developing after endotracheal intubation.

PREVENTION

The routine use of conjugate *H. influenzae* type b vaccines has dramatically reduced the incidence of systemic *H. influenzae* type b infections, including epiglottitis (Chapter 17). Because of the high efficacy of conjugate vaccines, fully immunized healthy children are at minimal risk of *H. influenzae* disease even if directly exposed to an index case of invasive disease. Household contacts do not require rifampin prophylaxis when all contacts are older than 4 years or when contacts younger than 4 years are fully immunized. Rifampin postexposure prophylaxis is indicated for all household contacts if there is a contact younger than 1 year of age, regardless of the vaccination status of that infant, or if there is an immunocompromised child younger than 4 years, even if that child is fully immunized (Chapter 16).

BACTERIAL TRACHEITIS

ETIOLOGY

Bacterial tracheitis frequently represents superinfection of the trachea but not the epiglottis. *Staphylococcus aureus* is the most common cause (Table 66–6). There are cases of children with *S. aureus* bacterial tracheitis and toxic shock syndrome. Other commonly isolated bacteria include *H. influenzae* type b, group A *Streptococcus, Moraxella catarrhalis,* and *Streptococcus pneumoniae.*

EPIDEMIOLOGY

Bacterial tracheitis is a relatively rare but serious infection. In one study (Gallagher and Myer, 1991), bacterial tracheitis accounted for 0.4 episode per 1,000 pediatric admissions over a 3-year period, half as common as epiglottitis at the same children's hospital. Since 1979, approximately 160 pediatric cases of bacterial tracheitis have been reported. There is a 2:1 male-to-female predominance, similar to that for acute LTB and epiglottitis. The age range of patients with bacterial tracheitis is wide, from 3 weeks into adulthood, with a mean age of 4–5 years.

Children with anatomic abnormalities of the airway (e.g., subglottic hemangioma, tracheobronchomalacia, repaired tracheoesophageal fistula) may be at increased risk of bacterial tracheitis. Critically ill children who require endotracheal intubation or those with tracheostomies are also at risk of bacterial tracheitis.

Children with Down's syndrome appear to be at increased risk of bacterial tracheitis. Anatomic abnormalities of the upper airway, macroglossia, and poorly defined immune dysfunction related to the trisomy 21 syndrome may be the reason for this association.

PATHOGENESIS

Bacterial tracheitis usually follows a recent viral upper respiratory tract infection and therefore, in some patients, represents a bacterial superinfection in the trachea and bronchi. A mucopurulent pseudomembrane may develop. Viral upper respiratory tract infection predisposes to colonization with *S. aureus* and other potential bacterial pathogens, and infection with influenza virus A enhances adherence of *S. aureus* to epithelial cells. Viral infections caused by RSV, influenza viruses, parainfluenza viruses, measles virus, and enteroviruses have been reported as antecedents of bacterial tracheitis. Bacterial tracheitis has been described with preceding bacterial upper respiratory infections, including group A *Streptococcus* pharyngitis and *H. influenzae* type b epiglottitis.

TABLE 66–6. Bacterial Isolates From Children With Bacterial Tracheitis

Organism	Percentage (N = 169)
Staphylococcus aureus	46
Haemophilus influenzae type b	16
Viridans streptococci	11
Group A *Streptococcus*	7
Moraxella catarrhalis	5
Streptococcus pneumoniae	4
Neisseria	4
Escherichia coli	2
Klebsiella pneumoniae	2
Non-group-A streptococci	1
Pseudomonas	1
Haemophilus parainfluenzae	<1
Proteus	<1

Data from Gallagher PG, Myer CM III: An approach to the diagnosis and treatment of membranous laryngotracheobronchitis in infants and children. *Pediatr Emerg Care* 1991;7:337.

SYMPTOMS AND CLINICAL MANIFESTATIONS

The typical presentation is acute onset of respiratory distress characterized by complaints of cough and stridor. Fever is not always noted on presentation; only 9 of 18 patients in one study (Gallagher and Myer, 1991) had fever, but in other series it has been much more frequent. Other symptoms, such as congestion, sore throat, hoarseness, and wheezing, are variably reported. Patients may rarely present in cardiopulmonary arrest or in shock.

Physical Examination Findings

Physical examination findings on presentation range from mild stridor to respiratory arrest. In most cases, however, moderate to severe inspiratory stridor is present with fever. Intercostal and supraclavicular retractions, nasal flaring, and expiratory stridor are also common on examination. Pharyngitis or tonsillitis is uncommonly noted. Often the patient appears to be in a toxic condition and may show signs of shock with agitation, lethargy, cool extremities, poor capillary refill, and tachycardia.

DIAGNOSIS

The findings of fever, cough, and inspiratory stridor often lead to the initial diagnosis of viral LTB, especially if the patient does not appear to be in a toxic condition. Over a matter of hours, however, increasing respiratory distress, fever, and increasing toxicity lead to the correct diagnosis. Occasionally, patients may present in the emergency department complaining of coughing up portions of a pseudomembrane.

A definitive diagnosis is established by direct visualization of the upper airways. During direct laryngoscopy and tracheal intubation, the presence of thick mucopurulent subglottic debris or pseudomembranes is diagnostic of bacterial tracheitis. After tracheal intubation, direct laryngoscopy is both diagnostic and therapeutic if portions of the mucopurulent membrane can be removed. Endoscopy shows the subglottic area to be swollen and narrowed. The trachea contains copious amounts of mucopurulent secretions, which if left untreated, may block the airway. The tracheal mucosa is often ulcerated and hemorrhagic.

Differential Diagnosis

The differential diagnosis is that of stridor (Table 66–1), especially foreign body aspiration and epiglottitis. A diagnosis of epiglottitis is *less* likely if there is a history of a prodromal illness or if there is a cough. Drooling and neck hyperextension (sniffing position) are more commonly seen with epiglottitis and occasionally with foreign body aspiration, but they are uncommon with tracheitis.

Laboratory Evaluation

The WBC count usually shows a leukocytosis with a shift to the left, but this is inconsistent and not diagnostic.

Microbiologic Evaluation

A routine blood culture should always be obtained if bacterial tracheitis is suspected, but bacteremia is documented in less than 2% of cases. Conversely, cultures of tracheal secretions are helpful in establishing the pathogen and directing antimicrobial therapy.

Diagnostic Imaging

Roentgenographic imaging of the upper airway (lateral neck and posteroanterior views) is often helpful in diagnosis. Although the epiglottis and aryepiglottic folds usually appear normal in children with bacterial tracheitis, subglottic narrowing, irregular intratracheal densities, and clouding of the tracheal air column are indicative of the diagnosis.

TREATMENT

All patients with bacterial tracheitis should be observed in an intensive care unit, and most will require elective tracheal intubation for pulmonary toilet. Meticulous care is needed to maintain a patent airway to prevent respiratory arrest. Repeated endoscopy while the patient is intubated is often required to remove adherent mucopurulent secretions and to monitor the course of the disease. Premature removal of the endotracheal tube when mucopurulent secretions are still present may lead to an acute respiratory arrest if secretions block the trachea after tracheal extubation.

The mean duration of endotracheal intubation in one study (Kasian et al., 1989) was approximately 1 week, the mean total length of hospitalization being 10–14 days. The decision to remove the endotracheal tube should be made only after the patient no longer has a fever and when bronchoscopy reveals healing and a marked decrease in tracheal secretions.

Empiric antibiotic therapy should include coverage of the major pathogens. Cefotaxime or ceftriaxone is recommended (Table 66–5). There are no controlled studies to support the use of nebulized racemic epinephrine in the treatment of bacterial tracheitis, but anecdotal reports suggest that racemic epinephrine is of no benefit or may provide only temporary relief. There is no evidence to support the use of corticosteroids in bacterial tracheitis.

COMPLICATIONS

The most serious complications are respiratory arrest, anoxic encephalopathy, and death. These complications of bacterial tracheitis can be prevented with early recognition, elective tracheal intubation to assist in pulmonary toilet, and care in a pediatric intensive care unit. Occasionally, toxic shock syndrome or septic shock may accompany bacterial tracheitis, and multiorgan system failure and death may occur without intensive care. Other reported complications of bacterial tracheitis include pneumothorax, subglottic stenosis, retropharyngeal cellulitis, postobstructive pulmonary edema, and tracheal granuloma formation. Approximately 50% of patients with bacterial tracheitis also have evidence of an infiltrate on a chest radiograph.

PROGNOSIS

In the preantibiotic era there was an estimated 70% mortality among children with bacterial tracheitis. More recently, the mortality has been 3–4%. Respiratory arrest occurs in approximately 10% of patients who do not receive tracheal intubation.

REVIEWS

Blackstock D, Adderley RJ, Steward DJ: Epiglottitis in young infants. *Anesthesiology* 1987;67:97.

Finch RG: Epidemiological features and chemotherapy of community-acquired respiratory tract infections. *J Antimicrob Chemother* 1990; 26:53.

Gallagher PG, Myer CM III: An approach to the diagnosis and treatment of membranous laryngotracheobronchitis in infants and children. *Pediatr Emerg Care* 1991;7:337.

Rosekrans JA: Viral Group: Current diagnosis and treatment. *Mayo Clin Proc* 1998;73:1102–7.

KEY ARTICLES

Acute Laryngotracheobronchitis

Ausejo M, Saenz A, Pham B, et al: The effectiveness of glucocorticoids in treating croup: Meta-analysis. *BMJ* 1999;319:595–600.

Denny FW, Murphy TF, Clyde WA Jr, et al: Croup: An 11-year study in a pediatric practice. *Pediatrics* 1983;71:871–6.

Fitzgerald D, Mellis C, Johnson M, et al: Nebulized budesonide is as effective as nebulized adrenaline in moderately severe croup. *Pediatrics* 1996;97:772–5.

Godden CW, Campbell MJ, Hussey M, et al: Double blind placebo controlled trial of nebulised budesonide for croup. *Arch Dis Child* 1997;76:155–8.

Johnson DW, Jacobson S, Edney PC, et al: A comparison of nebulized budesonide, intramuscular dexamethasone, and placebo for moderately severe croup. *N Engl J Med* 1998;339:498–503.

Kairys SW, Olmstead EM, O'Connor GT: Steroid treatment of laryngotracheitis: A meta-analysis of the evidence from randomized trials. *Pediatrics* 1989;83:683–93.

Klassen TP, Craig WR, Moher D, et al: Nebulized budesonide and oral dexamethasone for treatment of croup: A randomized controlled trial. *JAMA* 1998;279:1629–32.

Super DM, Cartelli NA, Brooks LJ, et al: A prospective randomized double-blind study to evaluate the effect of dexamethasone in acute laryngotracheitis. *J Pediatr* 1989; 115:323–9.

Waisman Y, Klein BL, Boenning DA, et al: Prospective randomized double-blind study comparing L-epinephrine and racemic epinephrine aerosols in the treatment of laryngotracheitis (croup). *Pediatrics* 1992;89:302–6.

Welliver R, Wong DT, Choi TS, et al: Natural history of parainfluenza virus infection in childhood. *J Pediatr* 1982;101:180–7.

Epiglottitis

Bisgard KM, Kao A, Leake J, et al: *Haemophilus influenzae* invasive disease in the United States, 1994-1995: Near disappearance of a vaccine-preventable childhood disease. *Emerg Infect Dis* 1998;4:229–37.

Bonadio WA, Losek JD: The characteristics of children with epiglottitis who develop the complication of pulmonary edema. *Arch Otolaryngol Head Neck Surg* 1991;117:205–7.

Bradley JS, Ching DK, Hart CL: Invasive bacterial disease in childhood: Efficacy of oral antibiotic therapy following short course parenteral therapy in non-central nervous system infections. *Pediatr Infect Dis J* 1987;6:821–5.

Brilli RJ, Benzing G 3d, Cotcamp DH: Epiglottitis in infants less than two years of age. *Pediatr Emerg Care* 1989;5:16–21.

Fleisher G: Infectious diseases emergencies. In Fleisher G, Ludwig S (editors): *Textbook of Pediatric Emergency Medicine,* 3rd ed. Baltimore, Williams & Wilkins, 1993.

Gonzalez C, Reilly JS, Kenna MA, et al: Duration of intubation in children with acute epiglottitis. *Otolaryngol Head Neck Surg* 1986;95:477–81.

Losek JD, Dewitz-Zink BA, Melzer-Lange M, et al: Epiglottitis: Comparison of signs and symptoms in children less than two years old and older. *Ann Emerg Med* 1990;19:55–8.

Gonzalez Valdepeña H, Wald ER, Rose E, et al: Epiglottitis and *Haemophilus influenzae* immunization. The Pittsburgh experience—A five year review. *Pediatrics* 1995;96:424–7.

Bacterial Tracheitis

Britto J, Habibi P, Walters S, et al: Systemic complications associated with bacterial tracheitis. *Arch Dis Child* 1996;74:249–50.

Edwards KK, Dundon C, Altemeier WA: Bacterial tracheitis as a complication of viral croup. *Pediatr Infect Dis* 1983;2:390–1.

Jones R, Santos JI, Overall JC Jr: Bacterial tracheitis. *JAMA* 1979; 242:721–6.

Kasian GF, Bingham WT, Steinberg J, et al: Bacterial tracheitis in children. *CMAJ* 1989;140:46–50.

Liston SL, Gehrz RC, Siegel LG, et al: Bacterial tracheitis. *Am J Dis Child* 1983;137:764–7.

CHAPTER 67

Bronchitis, Bronchiolitis, and Pertussis Syndrome

Robert S. Baltimore

Bronchitis, bronchiolitis, and pertussis syndrome are infectious illnesses of children characterized primarily by a cough. Because there is considerable overlap in the clinical presentation of these three illnesses, complete separation of them is artifical and is contrary to observations in clinical practice. Considering these entities together stresses the similarities of bronchitic illnesses and emphasizes the distinctions that facilitate a specific diagnosis.

Bronchitis. The term bronchitis is clear anatomically as it refers to inflammation of the bronchi. As a clinical entity, however, bronchitis is a vague term, referring to a respiratory illness characterized by a cough, usually accompanied by the physical findings of crackles, wheezes, or rhonchi on auscultation of the chest. Acute infectious bronchitis usually is associated with some degree of fever.

Acute bronchitis as an isolated entity is rare in children. In most cases bronchitis occurs with infection and inflammation at adjacent levels of the respiratory tract, either as bronchitis-bronchiolitis, generally due to a viral infection, or as part of a middle airway infection such as the crouplike illnesses tracheobronchitis or laryngotracheobronchitis (Chapter 66). The principal symptom of bronchial involvement is cough. Some important acute diseases may present primarily as bronchitis rather than as more extensive respiratory tract inflammation, including infection with *Bordetella pertussis,* which has distinctive epidemiologic and clinical features, as well as infections with certain respiratory viruses, *Mycoplasma pneumoniae, Chlamydia pneumoniae,* and *Chlamydia trachomatis* in infants.

Chronic bronchitis is a term used by different lung disease experts to refer to different symptom complexes. In adults, it is defined as a disorder manifested by a chronic or recurrent productive cough that is present on most days for 3 months a year for 2 years. No such definition has been promoted for use with children; nor has such a definition been validated as being useful for categorizing respiratory diseases in children. A useful definition for children is chronic or recurrent cough for more than 1 month that may or may not be associated with wheezes or crackles on auscultation (Morgan and Taussig, 1984). The chest radiograph may be normal or may show changes associated with inflammation, such as peribronchial cuffing.

Chronic bronchitis is not a disorder of otherwise healthy children but is an important manifestation of several chronic respiratory conditions of children, including cystic fibrosis, bronchopulmonary dysplasia, certain immunodeficiencies and anatomic malformations, and a number of rare progressive lung diseases such as interstitial fibrosis and the ciliary dyskinesia syndromes. These conditions are marked by progressive development of bronchiectasis and pulmonary fibrosis that impair the primary host defenses against infections. Because these diseases have the same common final pathway in terms of the development of progressive pulmonary deterioration, management of the infectious aspects of these chronic diseases is similar to that of cystic fibrosis and bronchopulmonary dysplasia. Other aspects of respiratory management, such as bronchodilator therapy, anti-inflammatory agents, and respiratory exercises are important but are not specifically directed against the infectious component. In general, management is scaled to the degree of symptoms. It consists, as necessary, of vigorous bronchodilator drug therapy, pulmonary physiotherapy, early intervention with antibiotics when there is evidence of secondary bacterial infection or exacerbation of chronic bacterial infection, pneumococcal vaccination, annual influenza vaccination, and, for selected patients, long-term antibiotic therapy. Bronchitis related to cystic fibrosis is discussed separately because long-term antibiotic therapy for this disease is different from that for other childhood lung diseases.

Bronchiolitis. Acute bronchiolitis is a complex infectious respiratory disease that often presents with upper and lower respiratory tract inflammation. Its most distinctive manifestation is airway obstruction due to swelling of small bronchioles. Because this obstruction can be progressive and lead to inadequate airflow, bronchiolitis is potentially life-threatening. Most severe cases of bronchiolitis occur in infants, probably as a consequence of narrow airways and an immature immune system.

Differentiating between acute bronchitis and bronchiolitis may be difficult on clinical grounds alone. The symptoms are similar, and the infectious agents that cause primarily one disease or the other often actually cause an element of both. An element of upper respiratory tract infection also frequently occurs with each. It is reasonable to distinguish bronchitis as an acute infectious disease whose predominant respiratory manifestation is cough without respiratory obstruction and bronchiolitis as an acute infectious disease whose predominant respiratory manifestation is wheezing and lower respiratory tract obstruction. There is, of course, an anatomic differentiation between the larger and the smaller airways as the site of inflammation and swelling, but this is not appreciable in clinical practice. This differentiation is important because diseases caused by *B. pertussis, M. pneumoniae,* and *Chlamydia* often present with similar features of bronchitis and can be treated with antimicrobial agents, whereas viral bronchiolitis-bronchitis should not be treated with antibacterial agents. Agents that relieve bronchospasm may be used occasionally in treating bronchitis, whereas their use in bronchiolitis is controversial.

Pertussis Syndrome. The pertussis syndrome includes classic pertussis, the **whooping cough** syndrome, which is usually caused by *B. pertussis* and is the most important disease caused by *B. pertussis.* Other organisms cause some cases of pertussis syndrome, and some disease caused by *B. pertussis* occurs without the distinctive whooping cough syndrome. However, most of the medical literature dealing with pertussis concerns pertussis caused by *B. pertussis*.

BRONCHITIS

ETIOLOGY

The causes of acute bronchitis (Table 67–1) are primarily infectious and mostly viral. The most commonly associated infectious agents of acute bronchitis in early childhood are respiratory syncytial virus (RSV), influenza virus, and parainfluenza virus types 1 and 3. Adenoviruses may cause disease, especially in young children. After 5 years of age *M. pneumoniae* is common, becoming the most commonly isolated infectious agent causing bronchitis among persons 6–20 years of age.

Chronic bronchitis (Table 67–2), when it is not a complication of acute bronchitis, is most frequently a complication of abnormal anatomic pulmonary defenses, usually associated with an inherited immunodeficiency or as a consequence of chronic airway obstruction. Except when chronic bronchitis is associated with cystic fibrosis or immune dysfunction, the respiratory pathogens are almost exclusively viruses or *M. pneumoniae*.

EPIDEMIOLOGY

Bronchitis in children occurs most frequently in children with underlying chronic lung disease, especially bronchopulmonary dysplasia. Bronchopulmonary dysplasia is a chronic inflammatory pulmonary condition of premature infants who have had **respiratory distress syndrome** and **hyaline membrane disease** requiring prolonged assisted ventilation. Cystic fibrosis is an autosomal recessive inherited disease that affects exocrine gland secretions. It is characterized by recurrent bronchitis, intestinal malabsorption in most patients, and an elevated sweat chloride (positive sweat test), and it is frequently accompanied by a family history of cystic fibrosis.

The epidemiology of acute bronchitis is the same as that of the respiratory viral diseases. In temperate climates these infections have a peak incidence in the winter, are relatively uncommon in the summer, and have an intermediate incidence in the spring and fall. Chronic bronchitis is perennial, but exacerbations of chronic bronchitis are frequently incited by viral and *M. pneumoniae* respiratory tract infections, with possible increased incidence in the winter. Rapid climatic changes, air pollution, and air stagnation also may cause exacerbations of chronic disease.

TABLE 67–1. Causes and Differential Diagnosis of Acute Bronchitis

Infections
- *Bordetella pertussis* (pertussis syndrome)
- Adenovirus (pertussis syndrome)
- Respiratory viruses
- *Chlamydia trachomatis*
- *Chlamydia pneumoniae*
- *Mycoplasma pneumoniae*
- Measles

Other Causes
- "Silent" or "cough-equivalent" asthma
- Foreign body in the airway
- Early phase of chronic bronchitis (Table 67–2)

TABLE 67–2. Differential Diagnosis of Chronic Bronchitis

- Reactive airway disease (asthma)
- Bronchopulmonary dysplasia
- Posttraumatic or postinfectious lung injury with bronchiectasis
- Cystic fibrosis
- Chronic or recurrent aspiration
  - Associated with anatomic malformation (e.g., tracheoesophageal fistula)
  - Gastroesophageal reflux
  - Neurologic dysfunction resulting in swallowing disorder
- Airway compression
  - Enlarged lymph nodes
  - Weakened bronchial wall (tracheomalacia or bronchomalacia)
  - Vascular ring, enlarged left atrium
- Congenital heart disease with pulmonary congestion or airway edema
- Foreign body
  - Lung, airway, or esophagus
- Humoral immunodeficiency
  - IgA deficiency
  - Various combinations of isotype deficiencies or agammaglobulinemia treated primarily with IgG-containing products
- Primary ciliary dyskinesia
  - Kartagener's syndrome
  - Young's syndrome
- Alpha-1-antitrypsin deficiency
- Environmental irritation
  - Cigarette smoke (from smoking or passive exposure)
  - Air pollution
  - Use of indoor wood-burning stoves for heat
  - Indoor exposure to chemical irritants
- Infection
  - Recurrent infections with respiratory viruses
  - *Chlamydia* infection in a young infant
  - Prolonged *Mycoplasma pneumoniae* infection
  - Granulomatous infection as with tuberculosis or deep fungal infection
- Allergic bronchopulmonary aspergillosis

Varying diagnostic criteria between studies complicate the epidemiologic and clinical literature on childhood bronchitis, especially as to whether cases with wheezing are included in the definition. In a large private practice group study in North Carolina (Chapman et al., 1981), the attack rate of acute tracheobronchitis, which was defined as a deep cough and rhonchi in the large airways but without wheezing, was highest during the first and second years of life (6.47 and 6.71 cases per 100 patients, respectively) and decreased in frequency until the teenage years. The shape of the age-related epidemic curve was similar to that for all lower respiratory tract infections (see Fig. 68–1), but the decrease in rate with increasing age was not as steep because as children grow older the proportion of all lower respiratory tract infections that are tracheobronchitis increases. Cultures for respiratory viruses and *M. pneumoniae* yielded a definite diagnosis in one fourth of the 2,200 cases of bronchitis.

PATHOGENESIS

Acute Bronchitis. Acute bronchitis does not generally occur as an isolated entity in children but, rather, as one component of a complex infection of multiple sites in the airways. The pathologic lesion in viral and *M. pneumoniae* bronchitis is damage to the ciliated epithelium of the central airway and larger airway branches. Ensuing irritation from sloughed epithelium, damage to the cleansing function of the airway by impairment of ciliary function, and bronchial spasm due to airway inflammation are responsible for the clinical findings of a cough, wheezing, and rhonchi. Prolonged bronchial inflammation may lead to bacterial superinfection and hyperplasia of goblet cells, resulting in hypersecretion of respiratory mucus. This cascade of pathologic changes is the antecedent of chronic bronchitis.

Chronic Bronchitis. The epidemiologic and pathologic features of chronic bronchitis in children are not well characterized because the syndrome itself is not rigorously defined. The reported incidence, prevalence, and pathologic findings reflect heavily on how the study population is defined and differ among reports. Because the underlying cause of most cases fitting a definition of chronic bronchitis is actually **asthma (reactive airways disease),** the reported epidemiologic and pathologic data on chronic bronchitis closely approximate those of similar studies of asthma. A pathologic examination of the lungs shows findings of squamous metaplasia of the bronchial epithelium, thickened bronchial walls, and hypertrophy of mucus-producing glands. These findings are nonspecific, but they have great importance with respect to the association with infection. These findings indicate disordered clearance of mucus and increased production of sputum, which are very clearly risk factors for the development of lower respiratory tract infection with a variety of respiratory pathogens. The ensuing frequency of respiratory tract infections in children with underlying chronic bronchitis syndrome explains why many have assumed that the cause of chronic bronchitis is infection. Rather, infection may be the result of chronic bronchitis, which is mostly caused by a hyperreaction of the airways associated with asthma, environmental injury, or environmental pollution. Current approaches to asthma have emphasized the importance of consideration of the later manifestations of an attack: inflammation, edema, and production of mucus that lasts long after the acute manifestations of bronchospasm. If bronchospasm is mild and there is insufficient bronchoconstriction to cause obvious wheezing, the manifestations are cough and increased mucus production alone. This ''cough-equivalent asthma'' may be confused with some chronic infectious processes.

Bronchopulmonary Dysplasia. Bronchopulmonary dysplasia is a result of prolonged assisted ventilation, occurring as a combined consequence of the barotrauma from high ventilatory pressures and the direct toxicity of a high concentration of oxygen on immature lungs. Children with bronchopulmonary dysplasia develop chronic obstructive lung disease with loss of lung compliance and chronic hypoxia and respiratory symptoms beyond 28 days of life. Chronic care involves the use of diuretics to rid the lungs of excess fluid, bronchodilators, and supplemental oxygen. Although no conclusive studies have demonstrated an association between bronchopulmonary dysplasia and infection, recent studies link maternal colonization with *Ureaplasma urealyticum* with prematurity, respiratory distress syndrome, and bronchopulmonary dysplasia. No studies so far have demonstrated that treating mothers with antimicrobial agents for *U. urealyticum* lowers the incidence of bronchopulmonary dysplasia.

Cystic Fibrosis. Cystic fibrosis is an autosomal recessive genetic disease that results from one of a group of allelic mutants in the long arm of chromosome 7. The most common mutation, found in approximately 70% of cases, is a 3 bp deletion at the phenylalanine locus that corresponds with amino acid position 508 of the protein specified by the gene (Δ508). Other mutations, of which there are hundreds, produce a similar clinical syndrome, but typically the Δ508 form is the most severe. The cystic fibrosis locus codes for the protein **cystic fibrosis transmembrane conductance regulator (CFTR),** which is responsible for transport of chloride across cell membranes. In cystic fibrosis, the deranged ion transport associated with the abnormal protein leads to the production in exocrine glands of mucus with increased viscosity. The lung function of patients with cystic fibrosis deteriorates because the small airways become plugged with abnormally thick secretions from bronchial exocrine glands.

It is generally believed that lung disease in cystic fibrosis is ultimately attributable to the abnormally viscous lung secretions that make it difficult to cough up sputum. The stagnant sputum becomes colonized with respiratory flora, which multiply and release products that either are toxic for the lung epithelium or induce an inflammatory response that is deleterious. The bronchial epithelium in cystic fibrosis appears to specifically bind adherence factors of a limited number of bacterial species. This inflammatory response exacerbates periodically when new or more intense infection occurs, resulting in increased respiratory symptoms. This cycle leads to a chronic bronchitis-bronchiolitis, resulting in bronchiolitis obliterans and eventually fibrosis and lung scarring. The role of infection in cystic fibrosis lung disease, although secondary to the exocrine gland lesion, is an essential contributor to progressive deterioration. In addition to bacterial infection, there is evidence that exacerbations may be caused by infection with viruses or *M. pneumoniae,* and the resulting airways inflammation causes exacerbation of the chronic bronchitis and hyperirritability of the goblet cells in bronchi and bronchioles. As a result, bacteria that colonize the middle and lower airways in patients with cystic fibrosis are probably cleared even more poorly, and the chronic bronchitis worsens. This hypothetic cascade of events provides the logic for treating all exacerbations with antibiotics in an attempt to reduce the long-term consequences of inflammation: bronchiolitis obliterans, bronchiectasis, and fibrosis.

Early studies demonstrated that *Staphylococcus aureus* and *Haemophilus influenzae* were the most important pathogens colonizing the respiratory tracts of patients with cystic fibrosis. However, in the late 1950s and 1960s, along with longer survival of patients, the increasing importance of *Pseudomonas aeruginosa* was recognized. The prevalence of *P. aeruginosa* colonization is higher in older patients, in those with more advanced pulmonary disease, and in those with previous exposure to antibiotics. *P. aeruginosa* colonization in cystic fibrosis is primarily due to **mucoid** colony variants. The distinctive colonies of these variants are due to production of **alginate, an exopolysaccharide.** Mucoid *P. aeruginosa* is rarely encountered in respiratory or other specimens from patients without cystic fibrosis. Although it is not completely clear why mucoid variants of *P. aeruginosa* are specific for cystic fibrosis, it appears that the organism has increased adherence to the abnormal cell membranes. Infection may progress for decades, and infected patients cough up and swallow huge quantities of *P. aeruginosa.* Infection is virtually always limited to the lungs, localized predominantly to the lumina of small bronchioles. Bacteremia with this species is almost unknown.

A large number of other bacterial species, including *Enterobacteriaceae* and non–lactose-fermenting gram-negative bacilli, have occasionally been isolated from the sputum of patients with cystic fibrosis. The absence of a specific pattern of associated symptoms, however, has led investigators to assume that most of these are noninvasive commensal organisms. An exception is *Burkholderia* (formerly *Pseudomonas*) cepacia. Although it is encountered only occasionally at some cystic fibrosis treatment centers, this species appears to be endemic and sometimes epidemic at other centers. It appears that *B. cepacia* may spread from patient to patient. Although some patients' conditions do not appear clearly different from the baseline clinical status when *B. cepacia is* first isolated from the sputum, in other patients it may be associated with an aggressive diffuse pneumonitis quite unlike the usual course of infections by only *P. aeruginosa.* Persons with cystic fibrosis who carry *B. cepacia* should be treated aggressively with antibiotics to which it is susceptible. In clinics where *B. cepacia* is endemic or epidemic, appropriate measures should be taken to prevent spread to uninfected patients.

SYMPTOMS AND CLINICAL MANIFESTATIONS

The hallmark symptom of bronchitis is a cough. The history provides the information regarding duration of the cough that defines whether bronchitis is acute or chronic, which is differentiated by duration longer than 1 month. If coughing accompanies only upper respiratory tract symptoms that suggest rhinitis, nasopharyngitis, or sinusitis, and the lung examination findings are normal, then bronchitis probably does not exist to a clinically significant extent. If there are physical signs or radiographic evidence of pneumonia, the diagnosis is usually pneumonia and not bronchitis. In many illnesses, especially those caused by viruses and *M. pneumoniae,* bronchitis may be a stage of the disease that follows upper respiratory tract infection and possibly precedes the development of pneumonia.

Bronchopulmonary Dysplasia. Infants who are more severely affected with bronchopulmonary dysplasia may have recurrent bouts of lung decompensation during the first year or more of life. Although the role of infection in these episodes is often unproved, intercurrent infections appear to cause decompensation because the effects of minor respiratory illness are amplified by the lack of adequate pulmonary reserve. It is assumed that the agents of bronchitis or bronchopneumonia in infants with bronchopulmonary dysplasia are similar to those in healthy infants of the same age and that, if any infectious agent is responsible, respiratory viruses predominate. Because of the complexity of the disease and the difficulty of discerning subtle radiologic changes in infants with chronic lung disease, infants with bronchopulmonary dysplasia who are hospitalized with fever and an exacerbation are usually treated with antibiotics appropriate for either community- or hospital-acquired pneumonia, depending on where they previously resided.

Physical Examination Findings

A fever may or may not accompany bronchitis, depending on the etiologic agent. A physical examination of the chest usually reveals crackles and possibly scattered wheezes but not consolidation unless pneumonia is also present.

DIAGNOSIS

Bronchitis is generally a clinical diagnosis based on the history and findings of the physical exmination. Laboratory tests are of little or no value. A radiograph of the chest is often useful to exclude pneumonia, but it is frequently normal or shows minimal perihilar infiltrates or hyperinflation. Occasionally, depending on the cause of bronchitis, there may be focal atelectasis due to plugs from inspissated bronchial secretions. In chronic bronchitis there may be signs of chronic lung disease, including peribronchial thickening, bronchiectasis, focal cystic disease, hilar lymphadenopathy, and pleural thickening. These findings are especially common in cystic fibrosis and chronic lung disease associated with immunodeficiency.

TREATMENT

For acute bronchitis associated with respiratory viruses, no treatment is necessary other than rest, antipyretics, and medication for symptomatic cough (Chapter 57). Antibiotic treatment is not necessary for the treatment of acute bronchitis in healthy children. If pneumonia or sinusitis develops, antibiotic treatment appropriate for these diseases is indicated. Adults who have underlying chronic lung disease often are treated with antibiotics when they have acute bronchitis, but this is not necessary for previously healthy children. The treatment of bronchitis complicating bronchopulmonary dysplasia and cystic fibrosis may require antibiotic therapy. Chronic bronchitis associated with chronic lung conditions other than bronchopulmonary dysplasia and cystic fibrosis may be treated in a similar manner.

Cystic Fibrosis. When possible, persons with cystic fibrosis should receive their routine care at specialized regional centers, which improves their survival. Many aspects of treatment of infection in cystic fibrosis remain controversial. There are two major reasons for the controversy and the difficulty of interpreting clinical studies: (1) It is difficult to determine when infection is responsible for current symptoms because the sputum is chronically colonized with potential pathogens, and (2) it is difficult to measure end points of treatment of infection because potential pathogens remain in the sputum after the patient's condition has improved clinically. Published studies are often based on symptoms or clinical scores that may be, at best, indirect measurements of infection and are quite subjective. Therefore there is no standard treatment regimen, and antibiotic treatment regimens at cystic fibrosis centers vary considerably.

Because respiratory tract colonization with *P. aeruginosa* usually begins in midchildhood or later, infants and young children with cystic fibrosis either are not colonized with known pathogens or are colonized with *H. influenzae* or *S. aureus.* Depending on individual physicians' assessments of the value of early aggressive antibiotic treatment to prevent progressive lung disease, in the first 2 years of life children with cystic fibrosis are treated according to one of the following protocols: (1) treated continuously with antibiotics; (2) treated with antibiotics with the appropriate antibacterial spectrum when the major potential pathogens are isolated from the respiratory tract; or (3) treated with antibiotics appropriate for the organisms with which they are colonized only when a distinct deterioration (termed an exacerbation) has occurred.

An exacerbation is diagnosed when a child has most or all of the following symptoms: unexplained weight loss or failure to gain weight properly after having previously had acceptable weight gain; onset of coughing or an increase in the severity of coughing; wheezing; and decreased exercise tolerance with less motor activity. In older patients more objective measures can be used to diagnose a pulmonary exacerbation. In addition to the symptoms already described, a significant decrease in pulmonary function ($>$20%) compared with previous function is considered to be indicative of an exacerbation. Fever, leukocytosis, an elevated ESR, or a new infiltrate demonstrated by chest radiograph are not typical of an exacerbation. In younger children, an exacerbation may be associated with increased coughing alone without pneumonia or crackles. Except in preterminal patients a fever, if present, more likely represents an intercurrent infection with a virus or *M. pneumoniae* and is probably unrelated to cystic fibrosis. A patient with a mild exacerbation may be treated in the ambulatory setting. Cotrimoxazole (trimethoprim-sulfamethoxazole [TMP-SMZ]), amoxicillin-clavulanate, or an oral second-generation cephalosporin, such as cefuroxime axetil, provides appropriate coverage for the usual pathogens and is a popular option for empiric treatment. In the absence of known colonization with *H. influenzae,* an antistaphylococcal penicillin, erythromycin, or a first-generation cephalosporin, such as cephalexin, is a popular and acceptable option.

In the past, persons colonized with *P. aeruginosa* were more likely to be hospitalized and treated with parenteral antibiotics when an exacerbation was diagnosed. Exacerbations can now often be treated at home. The oral quinolone antibiotics, such as ciprofloxacin, have good activity against *P. aeruginosa,* and symptomatic improvement compares favorably with that provided by parenteral antibiotic regimens. In addition, most cystic fibrosis treatment centers recommend the use of inhaled, aerosolized tobramycin. Specific antibiotic choices are often dictated by the antibiotic susceptibility of the patient's *Pseudomonas* isolates and the need to treat other pathogens. The most frequently employed antibiotic combination is a β-lactam antibiotic, such as a third-generation cephalosporin or expanded-spectrum penicillin, plus an aminoglycoside. A recent study (Smith et al., 1999) showed that clinical responses to such a combination were more long-lasting than to a β-lactam alone. The length of therapy is usually 10–14 days but is not standardized. Longer therapy may be used for patients with far-advanced disease or when symptomatic improvement is slow. The decision regarding inpatient therapy or home antibiotic therapy is based on individual family needs, local availability of appropriately skilled home nursing, and the frequency of additional therapy such as bronchodilators, pulmonary physiotherapy, and intravenous parenteral alimentation.

Another use of antibiotics in cystic fibrosis is for pulsed intensive therapy, often termed "clean out." There is no standardized regimen, but in some centers patients with cystic fibrosis who also have demonstrable chronic bronchitis and pulmonary function abnormalities are admitted to the hospital periodically for frequent pulmonary physiotherapy, bronchodilator therapy, and perhaps hypercaloric parenteral or enteral alimentation. Selected patients may undergo clean-out regimens at home, with home intravenous therapy supported by specially trained nurses. Antibiotic therapy is usually included. The regimens are similar to those used for a pulmonary exacerbation.

The recommended regimens and doses of oral and intravenous antibiotics for treating exacerbations of bronchitis in cystic fibrosis patients vary considerably because there is a lack of studies correlating dose and clinical response (Table 67–3). The doses used are higher than the generally accepted dose range for many of the drugs for the following reasons: (1) the recognized phenomenon that patients with cystic fibrosis have an apparently larger than predicted volume of distribution and require larger doses than healthy persons of the same body weight to achieve similar blood antibiotic concentrations and (2) the need to use the highest safe levels to achieve optimal concentrations of antibiotic in lung secretions because the concentration of antibiotics in sputum is generally considerably lower than the antibiotic concentration in blood.

Patients with cystic fibrosis should have an influenza vaccination annually. Pneumococcal vaccination has not previously been recommended for children with cystic fibrosis, but they should be immunized with the new pneumococcal conjugate vaccine. Patients with cystic fibrosis may be colonized with potentially communicable organisms. Certain precaution recommendations are appropriate

TABLE 67–3. Selected Antibiotics for Treatment of Pulmonary Infection in Cystic Fibrosis

Antibiotic	Dose	Dose (Hours) Interval
Intravenous Antibiotics for Acute Exacerbations and Interval Intensive Therapy		
Aminoglycosides		
Gentamicin	7.5–10 mg/kg/day	8
Tobramycin	7.5–10 mg/kg/day	8
Amikacin	15–20 mg/kg/day	12
β-Lactam Agents		
Azlocillin	300–450 mg/kg/day	4–6
Mezlocillin	300–450 mg/kg/day	4–6
Piperacillin or piperacillin/tazobactam	300–450 mg/kg/day	4–6
Ticarcillin or ticarcillin/clavulanate	200–400 mg/kg/day	4–6
Carbenicillin	400–600 mg/kg/day	4–6
Nafcillin, oxacillin	200 mg/kg/day	4–6
Ceftazidime	150–200 mg/kg/day	6–8
Aztreonam*	90–120 mg/kg/day	6–8
Oral Antibiotics for Treatment of Exacerbations of Cystic Fibrosis		
Ciprofloxacin*	1,000–1,500 mg/day	12
Dicloxacillin	100 mg/kg/day	6
Erythromycin	30–50 mg/kg/day	6–8
Cephalexin	50–100 mg/kg/day	6–8
TMP-SMZ	8–12 mg/kg/day trimethoprim	12

*Adult dose. Ciprofloxacin is not approved at this time for growing children because of observations of joint cartilage damage in experimental animals.

(Table 67–4), although there are no official recommendations at this time.

PROGNOSIS

Acute bronchitis in otherwise healthy children is not associated with sequelae. The ultimate prognosis for bronchitis associated with chronic lung disease depends on the primary cause.

PREVENTION

Some children with chronic or recurrent bronchitis, including those with cystic fibrosis and bronchopulmonary dysplasia, appear to be sensitive to environmental irritants and allergens. Removal of specific allergens from the environment may be beneficial, as it is in asthma. Nonspecific irritants, such as cigarette smoke, chemicals, and industrial pollutants, can be reduced, or the air in the child's environment can be purified with a filtration device. Irritating smoke from wood-burning stoves and cigarette smoke should be avoided, regardless of the cause of the bronchitis. Children with chronic bronchitis from any underlying cause should be given pneumococcal vaccine beginning at 2 months of age and annual influenza vaccination beginning at 6 months of age (Chapter 17).

Except for persons with cystic fibrosis, who often continue to receive antibiotics for treatment of pulmonary infection, there is no recognized role for prophylactic antibiotics or immunoglobulin in the management of chronic bronchitis associated with other pulmonary conditions, such as bronchopulmonary dysplasia. RSV

TABLE 67–4. Recommendations for Isolation Precautions for Patients With Cystic Fibrosis Colonized With Commonly Associated Organisms

Respiratory Tract Isolate	Isolation Precaution*
Pseudomonas aeruginosa	Standard. Patients with cystic fibrosis should not come closer to each other than arm's length
P. aeruginosa (resistant†)	Contact precautions
Other resistant gram-negative rod species†	Contact precautions
Stenotrophomonas maltophilia	Standard precautions unless resistant‡
Burkholderia cepacia	Standard precautions unless resistant.† No contact with other patients with cystic fibrosis in rooms or common areas
Nontuberculous *Mycobacteria*	Standard precautions
Aspergillus	Standard precautions
Mycoplasma pneumoniae	Droplet precautions
Influenza virus	Droplet precautions
Respiratory syncytial virus	Contact precautions
Parainfluenza virus	Contact precautions
Adenovirus	Droplet and contact precautions
Methicillin-resistant *Staphylococcus aureus* (MRSA)	Contact precautions

*In general, the duration of the precaution is the duration of hospitalization.

†Resistance is defined as being susceptible to only two or fewer antibiotics tested on the standard panel. For *Enterobacter*, resistance to either TMP-SMZ or ciprofloxacin necessitates contact precautions regardless of the results of other antibiotic susceptibilities. Organisms reported as being intermediately susceptible are to be considered resistant.

‡*Stenotrophomonas maltophilia* is intrinsically resistant to multiple antibiotics. An isolate resistant to TMP-SMZ, ticarcillin-clavulanate, or piperacillin-tazobactam would be considered to be resistant and would require contact precautions.

is more severe in children with chronic lung disease, and palivizumab or RSV-IGIV should be administered prophylactically (see Bronchiolitis).

BRONCHIOLITIS

ETIOLOGY

Bronchiolitis is usually a viral infectious disorder. Although any of the respiratory viruses generally associated with acute lower respiratory tract infection in children may be implicated, one half or more of all cases of bronchiolitis necessitating hospitalization are due to RSV. When RSV is epidemic, which is frequent in the winter in temperate climates, virtually all bronchiolitis is due to this agent. Other viruses occasionally responsible for bronchiolitis include adenovirus; parainfluenza viruses 1, 2, and 3; and influenza viruses A and B. Other agents, such as rhinovirus and *M. pneumoniae,* are rare causes of bronchiolitis in infancy but are more commonly implicated in older children (Table 67–5). Bacteria other than *M. pneumoniae* do not cause bronchiolitis, and bacterial superinfection of viral bronchiolitis is distinctly uncommon.

EPIDEMIOLOGY

Like viral pneumonia, bronchiolitis is most frequently seen in the winter months. Although occasional cases are seen in late fall and early spring, studies of the incidence of bronchiolitis from several United States cities have shown a midwinter peak year after year.

Approximately 80% of cases occur in the first year of life, with a peak age of 2–6 months. The incidence falls rapidly between the ages of 1–5 years, after which bronchiolitis is uncommon. It is estimated that only 10% of healthy children with bronchiolitis and wheezing require hospitalization. Bronchopulmonary dysplasia due to prematurity and congenital heart disease is an especially important condition predisposing patients to severe wheezing and respiratory failure associated with bronchiolitis. Boys are more commonly affected than are girls in the ratio of 1.5:1.

RSV is extremely contagious and is spread by contact with infected respiratory secretions. Although coughing does produce aerosols, hand carriage of contaminated secretions is the most frequent mode of transmission.

PATHOGENESIS

Typical cases of bronchiolitis resolve within 5 days, so pathologic studies of bronchiolitis are of unusually severe cases in which specimens have been collected by biopsy or necropsy. The typical pathologic features are necrosis of ciliated epithelium with edema and mononuclear infiltration of the submucosa. Small airways become plugged with mucus, fibrin, and cellular debris. Clinical resolution of the disease is associated with complete histologic recovery.

It is not entirely clear why most cases of severe bronchiolitis occur in infants, but it is believed that immunologic as well as mechanical factors may be involved. Infants have a high proportion of small-diameter airways, and their resistance would be most severely increased by a proportional decrease in diameter from swelling associated with inflammation. Because there is little evidence that natural immunity prevents reinfection by RSV in infants and young children, there has been interest in the concept that immune responses to RSV may actually be harmful and are part of the pathogenesis of the disease. This concept was stimulated by a trial of an experimental killed-virus RSV vaccine in the late 1960s. Recipients of the vaccine had more severe disease after exposure to RSV than did controls who did not receive a vaccine. Because patients who had been vaccinated had a strong cell-mediated immune response, it has been hypothesized that these immune responses might actually trigger some of the pathologic events responsible for the symptoms of bronchiolitis. Infants also seem to have an especially strong cell-mediated immune response to either the experimental vaccine or natural infection. This may help explain why infants constitute the population most at risk of severe bronchiolitis.

Infants who have had severe bronchiolitis appear prone to recurrent bouts of bronchiolitis and asthma during later infancy and childhood. It is not clear whether residual lung inflammation from the initial infection causes a child to be more prone to recurrent bronchiolitis or whether a child who has more severe bronchiolitis is constitutionally more susceptible on the basis of hyperreactive airways or an allergy.

SYMPTOMS AND CLINICAL MANIFESTATIONS

Bronchiolitis caused by RSV has an incubation period of 4–6 days. It classically presents as a progressive respiratory illness similar

TABLE 67–5. Percentage of Wheezing Associated Respiratory Infections (Bronchiolitis) Due to Different Agents

Age (Years)	No. of Cases	% With Isolate	Percent Due to Each Agent					
			RSV	Parainfluenza 1	Parainfluenza 3	Adenoviruses	Rhinoviruses	*M. pneumonia*
0–2	909	22.3	44.3	12.8	13.8	13.3	4.4	3.0
2–5	542	21.6	30.8	12.0	17.9	10.3	4.3	11.1
5–9	275	20.7	12.3	10.5	12.3	5.3	14.0	29.8
9–15	125	15.2	10.5	15.8	5.3	0	10.5	52.6
All ages	1,851	21.4	34.1	12.4	14.4	10.6	6.1	11.6

From Henderson FW, Clyde WA Jr, Collier AM, et al: The etiologic and epidemiologic spectrum of bronchiolitis in pediatric practice. *J Pediatr* 1979;95:183–90.

to the common cold in its early phase, with a cough, coryza, and rhinorrhea, and then progresses in 3–7 days to noisy, raspy breathing and audible wheezing. There is usually a fever of 38.5–39°C (101.3–102.2°F) or higher, accompanied by irritability, which may increase with symptoms of increased respiratory effort. Most hospitalized patients show marked improvement in 2–5 days with supportive treatment alone. The course of the wheezing phase is variable, however, with some patients showing progressive improvement, some having improvement and then exacerbation, and some even having recrudescence after discharge from the hospital.

Bronchiolitis in a small number of infants progresses and may go on to respiratory failure requiring assisted ventilation. Progression from moderate to severe disease is usually accompanied by an increased respiratory rate to 60–80 breaths per minute and hypoxia. A chest radiograph frequently shows the signs of hyperexpansion of the lungs, including increased lung lucency and a depressed diaphragm. The lungs may appear normal, or there may be areas of increased density, which may represent either viral pneumonia or localized atelectasis (Fig. 67–1). One study (Shaw et al., 1991) showed that early prognostic findings, including "toxic appearance," oxygen saturation of <95% by pulse oximetry on room air, gestational age <34 weeks, respiratory rate >70 breaths per minute, atelectasis on chest radiograph, and age younger than 3 months, indicate a high probability of severe disease and the need for hospitalization. A second study (Moler and Ohmit, 1999) found that similar factors plus early use of mechanical ventilation and of ribavirin predicted extended hospitalizations, while a third study (Brooks et al., 1999) showed that extreme hypoxia and tachypnea were predictive, but with low specificity, of deterioration after hospitalization.

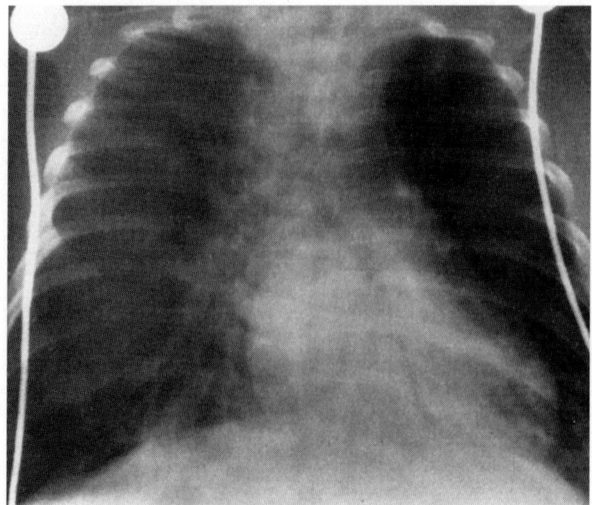

FIGURE 67–1. Chest radiograph of an infant with pneumonia caused by respiratory syncytial virus in a 5-month-old infant with fever, wheezing, and respiratory distress. A frontal chest radiograph shows diffuse pulmonary hyperinflation and peribronchial infiltrates extending into the right and left lower lobes. An air bronchogram pattern on the left behind the heart indicates more extensive consolidation of the left lower lobe. Shifting areas of atelectasis are also common in this disease because of mucous plugging of the bronchi.

An exception to the classic progression of disease over several days is seen in neonates infected with RSV, in whom a prodrome may not be noted and who may have apneic episodes as the first sign of RSV infection.

Physical Examination Findings

The diagnostic hallmarks of bronchiolitis are the physical findings evident at initial clinical presentation. The signs of bronchiolar obstruction include prolongation of the expiratory phase of breathing, intercostal retractions with indrawing of the lower ribs, and hyperexpansion of the lungs. With more severe obstruction, there may be suprasternal retractions. Tachypnea is present; monitoring the respiratory rate is one method of following the progress of the illness. During the wheezing phase of the illness, percussion of the chest usually reveals only hyperresonance, but auscultation usually reveals wheezes and crackles throughout the breathing cycle. With more severe disease, grunting and cyanosis may be present. The physical findings may vary from time to time, sometimes revealing only wheezes and at other times crackles and wheezes. Examination of the abdomen may reveal some distention, and the liver and spleen may be palpable because of their being pushed down by hyperexpanded lungs. Agitation exacerbates the dyspnea and the findings on lung examination. Some infants improve temporarily after being given oxygen or bronchodilators, with a decrease in the work of breathing and a concomitant decrease in the signs of respiratory obstruction.

DIAGNOSIS

The diagnosis of bronchiolitis with mild disease in an ambulatory setting is usually established on clinical findings. Determination of the etiologic agent is not routinely required, although some ambulatory facilities work with viral diagnostic laboratories to provide surveillance of respiratory pathogens in the community. For hospitalized patients, there are three reasons to confirm an etiologic diagnosis: (1) As with other infectious diseases, a microbiologic diagnosis more definitively excludes other infectious and noninfectious causes; (2) children with bronchiolitis due to the same specific agent may be cohorted, especially during an outbreak when hospital rooms and staff may be limited; and (3) candidates for antiviral therapy may be identified. Antigen testing for RSV, parainfluenza viruses, adenoviruses, and influenza viruses, as well as viral respiratory cultures, is useful to confirm the causative agent. In addition, if there are clinical indications for ribavirin treatment of RSV bronchiolitis, rapid confirmation of RSV infection is necessary.

Differential Diagnosis

The major difficulty in the diagnosis of bronchiolitis is to differentiate various other wheezing-associated diseases. On the basis of the physical examination findings, it may be impossible to differentiate **asthma** from bronchiolitis, but age and the presence of fever are the major differential factors. Bronchiolitis occurs mostly in the first year of life and is accompanied by a fever, whereas asthma usually begins in older children and wheezing episodes are usually not accompanied by fever unless a respiratory tract infection is the trigger for the asthma attack. Clearly there are frequent cases in which the first wheezing episode of a patient with asthma is thought to be due to viral bronchiolitis.

Wheezing may also be due to other causes, such as a foreign body in the airway, a congenital airway obstructive lesion, cystic fibrosis, exacerbation of bronchopulmonary dysplasia, viral pneumonia, and other lower respiratory tract diseases. The chest radiograph may be of help in differentiating bronchiolitis from pneumonia and other disorders. A history of recurrent wheezing episodes may suggest cystic fibrosis, bronchopulmonary dysplasia, or an anatomic obstruction. If an infant has persistent unexplained wheezing, a sweat test should be performed to exclude cystic fibrosis. **Cardiogenic asthma,** which can be confused with bronchiolitis in infants, is wheezing associated with pulmonary congestion due to left-sided heart failure.

The sudden onset of unilateral or localized wheezing without a fever or prodrome suggests a foreign body. A chest radiograph and fluoroscopy may reveal a radiodense object or a focal area of lung that does not expand or contract. Lateral decubitus chest radiographs can aid in demonstrating that the airway is blocked by a foreign body and cannot be compressed. When there is evidence of a foreign body but it is not detected by radiography, diagnostic bronchoscopy may be necessary to confirm or exclude the presence of a radiolucent object in the airway.

Laboratory Evaluation

Laboratory data are not required to confirm the diagnosis of bronchiolitis. Blood gas determinations and WBC counts are often performed in more severe cases. The WBC count is of little help because it is quite variable; a mild leukocytosis of 12,000–16,000/mm^3 is frequently encountered.

In more severe cases of bronchiolitis, it is important to assess gas exchange. One must decide whether determination of arterial blood gas tensions, an invasive test requiring arterial puncture or an indwelling arterial catheter, is needed or whether pulse oximetry, a noninvasive test, is sufficient. Visual assessment to estimate oxygenation is fraught with error and correlates poorly with actual blood gas values. However, arterial puncture performed when a child is agitated may not be representative of the values obtained when the child is in a less anxious state. More representative values of oxygen and carbon dioxide concentration in the blood come from samples taken after an arterial catheter has been inserted and the child has become calm or from transcutaneous pulse oximetry, which measures only oxygen saturation in the blood. Published data suggest that pulse oximetry is an excellent means of following arterial oxygenation in infants in whom respiratory failure may develop. Respiratory failure may develop rapidly in tired infants, even though blood gas values taken before rapid decompensation are not alarming. Frequent, regular visual assessments of infants who are unclothed above the waist to look for signs of increased work of breathing, such as flaring, retractions, and tachypnea, are important in identifying those infants in whom respiratory failure may develop.

Microbiologic Evaluation

Identification of the cause of bronchiolitis requires a suitable sample of respiratory tract secretions. A method found to be useful for obtaining high-quality secretions with plenty of infected cells is aspiration of the nasopharyngeal secretions by introduction of a small suction catheter into the nose and collection of the secretions in a syringe or a sputum trap attached to suction. If no fluid is obtained, a small amount of normal saline solution can be injected through the tube and then aspirated. Alternatively, nasal washings can be obtained by suctioning secretions by means of a tapered rubber bulb introduced into the external nares or by squirting approximately 5 mL of normal saline solution into the nose through such a device and quickly aspirating the contents. These specimens can be used both for inoculating tissue culture for virus isolation and for rapid RSV diagnostic tests.

Rapid Tests for RSV. Various rapid tests to detect RSV antigen are available. Early tests detected immunofluorescence of infected cells after incubation with the patient's secretions and commercial anti-immunoglobulin antisera (see Fig. 11–6*A*). This method is excellent and sensitive, but it requires a specimen with many cells and considerable time from an experienced technician. Newer tests use EIA and are available as kits with appropriate controls. Similar tests for influenza and parainfluenza viruses have been developed, and many laboratories offer these tests as a panel.

Viral Culture. Virus culture is necessary to confirm the specific viral diagnosis in isolated cases of bronchiolitis and in the early stages of an RSV outbreak. Routine culture of all positive rapid RSV tests may be suspended in the midst of a culture-documented outbreak.

Serologic Diagnosis. Serologic diagnosis is of limited value in bronchiolitis. In early infancy, maternal antibody may still be present, confounding serologic diagnosis. Testing of a single serum sample during acute disease is without value because no currently available test differentiates between current and past infection. Antibody to RSV may not develop in some RSV-infected infants.

TREATMENT

Management of this potentially severe, even life-threatening disease is a challenge to the practitioner. Because of the potentially rapidly changing severity of the disease and the intermittent improvement and recrudescence, an evaluation and management plan at any point in time must be viewed as temporary. Arrangements for frequent and adequate observation of the patient and for frequent reports by the caregiver to the physician are essential.

Most cases of mild bronchiolitis do not require specific treatment and can be managed at home with frequent communication with and appropriate encouragement from the physician. Caregivers must be aware of the signs of increasing severity of disease and instructed to be aware of fluid intake, which should be adequate but not forced. Hospitalization should be considered on the basis of the indicators of severe disease.

There is no evidence that bacterial agents play any role in causing bronchiolitis or to support treatment of bronchiolitis to prevent secondary bacterial infections. The likelihood that a hospital-acquired bacterial infection will develop appears to be increased among patients who receive antibiotics. The only reasons to treat with antibiotics are (1) a focus of presumed or proved bacterial infection outside the lungs, (2) development of nosocomial pneumonia, or (3) an initial diagnosis of bronchiolitis that appears to be in error, with a bacterial illness as the actual cause.

Corticosteroids have been studied for use in bronchiolitis; they do not have a demonstrated benefit and should not be used for treatment.

Definitive Treatment

The use of ribavirin has received considerable attention. Although studies in the 1980s using end points of viral concentration, oxygenation, and illness scores showed temporary improvement in high-risk patients treated with ribavirin, more recent studies (Wheeler et al., 1993; Meert et al., 1994; Moler et al., 1996; Law et al., 1997) and a meta-analysis (Randolph and Wang, 1996) failed to show benefit in the reduction of mechanical ventilation, use of supplemental oxygen, and duration of hospitalization. Earlier studies may have shown benefit because of the use of aerosolized water in the control group, which can cause bronchospasm, and also because of the choice of different end points. Because infants with mild or moderate disease are usually discharged from the hospital within 5 days, studies of ribavirin treatment have focused on infants with underlying cardiopulmonary diseases who are susceptible to severe, even life-threatening bronchiolitis, and those whose assessment in the hospital suggests impending or apparent respiratory failure. The limited size of most studies cannot exclude the possibility of moderate benefits in selected patients.

Ribavirin must be given by inhalation with the use of a special **small-particle aerosol generator (SPAG II).** Administration of ribavirin to infants who require mechanical ventilation must be done in a pediatric ICU by personnel who are experienced in the use of the drug and are aware of the need for frequent monitoring and routine changing of ventilator filters and tubing, which is necessitated by possible precipitation of the drug that may impede assisted ventilation. Ribavirin may be a teratogen in vitro, but it has not been shown to have toxicity for infants when administered by aerosolized inhalation, probably because there is little systemic absorption. There has been concern for pregnant caregivers, but high levels of drug in caregivers have not been detected.

At present, ribavirin treatment is used infrequently, if at all, in most children's hospitals. It is recommended only for infants and young children who are at high risk of severe or life-threatening RSV disease associated with underlying cardiac disease, respiratory disease, or immunodeficiency and for those with unusually severe respiratory compromise. Typical cases of bronchiolitis improve sufficiently quickly with other treatment that the expense (approximately $250 per vial) and additional medical care required to deliver the drug do not appear to be justified. The recommendations of the American Academy of Pediatrics for use of ribavirin are summarized in Table 67–6, which states that the use of ribavirin "may be considered" by individual practitioners.

Regardless of the patient's body weight, the dose of ribavirin is one 6 g vial by aerosol nebulization over 12–20 hours per day, usually for 3–5 days but sometimes for as long as 7 days. Ribavirin has been demonstrated to be effective only for RSV-associated bronchiolitis, and therefore it is recommended that a rapid diagnostic test for RSV be performed and that ribavirin be used only if the test is positive.

A report from Europe (Rimensberger and Schaad, 1994) shows improvement in RSV-infected infants with bronchiolitis treated with aerosolized immunoglobulin. Because this was only a pilot study, such therapy cannot be endorsed, but it may prove useful. Palivizumab and RSV-IVIG, used to prevent RSV infections, have failed to show benefit when used as therapy for RSV bronchiolitis.

TABLE 67–6. Suggested Indications for Ribavirin Therapy for Respiratory Syncytial Virus Infections*

Ribavirin Aerosol Therapy May Be Considered for the Following Infants and Young Children at Risk of Serious RSV Disease

- Complicated congenital heart disease, bronchopulmonary dysplasia, cystic fibrosis, and other chronic lung diseases
- Previously healthy premature infants (<37 weeks gestational age) and those less than 6 weeks of age
- Underlying immunosuppressive diseases or therapies (e.g., AIDS, severe combined immunodeficiency, or organ transplantation) associated with high mortality or prolonged RSV disease
- Severely ill with RSV infection with or without mechanical ventilation
- Hospitalized patients who may be at increased risk of progressing from mild to more severe disease because they are younger than 6 weeks of age or have an underlying condition such as multiple congenital anomalies or certain neuromuscular or metabolic diseases

*Adapted from Committee on Infectious Diseases, American Academy of Pediatrics: Reassessment of the indications for ribavirin therapy in respiratory syncytial virus infections. *Pediatrics* 1996;97:137–39.

Supportive Therapy

Bronchodilator Therapy. In the past it was believed that bronchodilator medications, such as inhaled sympathomimetic agents or atropine derivatives, that are used for patients with asthma had no appreciable effect on bronchiolitis. Some prospective studies demonstrated that wheezing and respiratory distress in an infant or young child being treated as an outpatient can be improved temporarily with the use of bronchodilators. One study (Lowell et al, 1987) demonstrated clinical improvement of respiratory distress, compared to placebo, measured by a scale in which wheezing and retractions were graded after 2 or 3 injections of epinephrine given 15 minutes apart. Another study (Alario et al, 1992) in infants given 10 mg of metaproterenol sulfate solution (0.2 mL of a 5% solution diluted in 2 mL of normal saline solution) inhaled by nebulization showed clinical benefit. Another study (Schuh et al., 1990) of 40 children 6–24 months of age randomly assigned to receive two treatments of nebulized albuterol (0.15 mg/kg per dose) 1 hour apart, or placebo, found improvement in the group given albuterol, but not placebo, in a proportion similar to that reported with the studies of epinephrine and metaproterenol. Although there is some enthusiasm and rationale for the use of bronchodilators in infants and young children with bronchiolitis, the particular agent, appropriate patient selection, and the measures to achieve the best outcome are not clear. Two recent meta-analyses (Flores and Horwitz, 1997; Kellner et al., 1996) found that diversity of study design and end points made conclusions from previous studies difficult but suggest that the overall effects are inconsequential and short term and do not appear to prevent hospitalization. Both analyses called for larger, better-designed studies. Bronchodilator therapy should be considered a temporizing measure at best while the disease runs its course. Any infant for whom improvement requires such intervention will probably require additional interventions until the disease abates.

Supplemental Oxygen. Oxygen therapy is universally agreed to be the most important initial therapy in moderately severe or severe RSV bronchiolitis. For a patient who is in distress, oxygen may be administered and adjusted by the clinical response. When blood gases or pulse oximetry are being monitored, the flow should achieve an arterial saturation percentage in the mid-90s. In general, 40% humidified oxygen is sufficient, although there does not appear to be value in using a mist tent. Mist, which is of dubious value in improving breathing, may be responsible for provoking wheezing, and it also interferes with essential observations of the infant if the mist is so thick that the child cannot be easily observed.

PROGNOSIS

For most pediatric patients with bronchiolitis, the prognosis is excellent. Although lung function tests show slight obstructive changes that may persist for months to years, the lungs appear normal histologically and tolerance of physical activity is not affected unless asthma develops. There is approximately a 1% mortality rate, generally among those with pre-existing cardiopulmonary or immunologic impairment. Recurrence is common and should be assessed and treated much like the first episode. There is a higher than normal risk that asthma will develop later in life among patients with bronchiolitis severe enough to require hospitalization. This may indicate that patients with hyperreactive airways are more likely to require hospitalization when infected with a respiratory virus.

PREVENTION

The viruses that cause bronchiolitis, especially RSV and parainfluenza virus, spread in the hospital and cause nosocomial infections. This can be extremely disruptive in units for infants, where there are likely to be many susceptible infants, including many who are ill with other diseases. These children are those most likely to have severe, even life-threatening bronchiolitis. Airborne transmission is less important than either hand carriage or transmission of contaminated secretions on soiled gowns. Identification of infected infants, use of contact isolation precautions, cohorting of those with RSV infection when there are outbreaks, and strict handwashing are of utmost importance in diminishing nosocomial transmission. If staff members become infected, their disease may not be severe but they may excrete virus that can be transmitted to susceptible young patients. The use of gowns, gloves, masks, and goggles by caretakers reduces transmission in the hospital, but the impracticality of such a routine has limited the implementation of such measures on regular hospital units.

Candidates for RSV vaccine are being investigated, but no vaccines are available at this time.

Immunoprophylaxis. Two prophylactic immunoglobulin preparations have proven to be effective in ameliorating RSV infection in infants susceptible to severe disease. **Palivizumab,** a humanized monoclonal antibody directed against the F glycoprotein of RSV, was approved in 1998. It is administered intramuscularly. Palivizumab is effective in reducing the incidence of infections that require hospitalization, days of hospitalization, ICU days, and the severity of respiratory disease (The IMpact-RSV Study Group, 1998).

RSV-IGIV (Respigam), produced from IVIG from lots having high titers of RSV neutralizing antibodies, was approved in 1996. It is administered intravenously. In multicenter studies (Groothuis et al., 1993; The PREVENT Study Group, 1997) high-risk infants who received high doses of RSV-IGIV had fewer RSV-associated hospitalizations, fewer hospital days, and fewer days in the ICU than patients in the control group. This preparation was licensed in January 1996.

TABLE 67–7. Use of Palivizumab (Preferred) and RSV-IVIG for Prophylaxis of Respiratory Syncytial Virus Infections

Indications

- Infants and children younger than 2 years of age with chronic lung disease who have required medical therapy for their chronic lung disease within 6 months before the anticipated RSV season
  - Patients with severe chronic lung disease may benefit from prophylaxis for two RSV seasons, especially those who require medical therapy
- Infants born at ≤32 weeks' gestation without chronic lung disease (decisions regarding prophylaxis should be individualized)
  - Gestational age ≤28 weeks: prophylaxis up to 12 months of age
  - Gestational age 29–32 weeks: prophylaxis up to 6 months of age
- Prophylaxis of infants 32–35 weeks' gestation should be reserved for infants with additional risk factors until more data are available
- Infants with severe immunodeficiencies, including AIDS and severe combined immunodeficiency, may benefit from prophylaxis. RSV-IGIV may be substituted for IVIG during the RSV season in children who receive IVIG.

Contraindications

- Palivizumab and RSV-IVIG are not recommended for infants with congenital heart disease, and are contraindicated for infants with cyanotic congenital heart disease. Infants with chronic lung disease and acyanotic congenital heart disease may benefit from prophylaxis.

Administration

- RSV prophylaxis should be instituted at the onset of the RSV season and terminated at the end of the RSV season (in the United States, beginning October–December and ending March–May)

RSV-IVIG = Respiratory syncytial virus intravenous immunoglobulin.
Adapted from Committee on Infectious Diseases and Committee on Fetus and Newborn, American Academy of Pediatrics: Prevention of respiratory syncytial virus infections: Indications for the use of palivizumab and update on the use of RSV-IGIV. *Pediatrics* 1998;102:1211–16.

Both preparations appear to be safe, although expensive, and are recommended (Table 67–7). Palivizumab is preferred for most high-risk children because of its ease of administration, safety, and effectiveness. The cost-effectiveness of these preparations has been debated, and recent reviews suggest that because of a lack of data showing reduced mortality, the cost benefit is small. RSV is prevented through strict observance of infection control practices; the efficacy of RSV prophylaxis for nosocomial infections has not been evaluated.

PERTUSSIS SYNDROME (WHOOPING COUGH)

Pertussis continues to be encountered despite routine vaccination against *B. pertussis.* Knowledge of the epidemiologic behavior of this syndrome is of great importance to health care providers because they must be prepared to explain to parents facets of the disease and the logic and necessity of its prevention by vaccination. Currently, much disease occurs in populations that were not formerly emphasized, such as young infants, adults, and those who choose not to be vaccinated.

ETIOLOGY

Most pertussis syndrome is caused by *B. pertussis,* with the proportion related to the degree of pertussis immunization in the population. *B. parapertussis* is closely related to *B. pertussis* and causes a similar but milder illness, but it is not affected by vaccination against *B. pertussis.* Both *B. pertussis* and *B. parapertussis* appear to have only a human reservoir and are transmitted person to person by coughing. Asymptomatic carriage is rare.

A study (Wirsing von Konig et al., 1998) of 1,179 children with pertussis-like cough, among 12.6% with no laboratory evidence of *B. pertussis* infection, showed that infections with adenovirus, parainfluenza viruses, *Mycoplasma pneumoniae,* and RSV were most common. There is confusion as to the role of adenovirus causing pertussis syndrome because dual infection with *B. pertussis* and adenovirus occurs more frequently than expected by chance. It may be that adenovirus is sometimes a cofactor in causing clinical pertussis and perhaps sometimes is reactivated by *B. pertussis.* Evidence is poor that adenovirus commonly causes the disease by itself.

EPIDEMIOLOGY

The annual rate of pertussis in the United States was approximately 100–200 cases per 100,000 population in the prevaccination era, and at present it may be higher in developing countries. This rate started falling in about 1945 when vaccine potency standards were first established and fell impressively from 15–20 per 100,000 population in the late 1950s to 1–2 per 100,000 population in the late 1960s (Fig. 67–2), probably as a consequence of intensive infant immunization programs. The rate changed little from the late 1960s until the late 1980s, when it doubled, and it has remained about the same since the late 1980s. The reported rates represent passive notifications by practitioners and are all underestimates.

Data from the United States and the United Kingdom demonstrate that in the prevaccination era the rate of pertussis was similar in both countries, but the logarithmic decline began about 10 years later in the United Kingdom than in the United States (Cherry, 1984). Routine pertussis vaccination began in the late 1940s in the United States but not until the late 1960s in the United Kingdom. In the United Kingdom there was a steady decline in the incidence of pertussis until the late 1970s, when the incidence rose again very dramatically. Immediately before this increase in incidence, there was considerable publicity in the media about the possible serious adverse effects of the vaccine, and the rate of vaccination declined. After this rise in incidence, the vaccination rate in the United Kingdom again increased and the number of cases fell. These events, a similar experience in Japan at about the same time, and the decline in the incidence of cases when vaccines were first tested are major events indicating the efficacy of pertussis vaccination.

There continues to be an interest in pertussis epidemiology for several reasons. In an unimmunized population, *B. pertussis* affects young children, who may spread it among themselves. Despite the demonstrated efficacy of the currently used killed whole-cell vaccine and acellular vaccines, some parents refuse the vaccine for their infants because of concern about adverse effects. In addition, the initial series of three immunizations is not completed until the age of 6 months, Given this pool of susceptible infants, as well as a number of adults who are susceptible on the basis of waning immunity, there is continued opportunity for pertussis transmission to persist. Active surveillance by the CDC in the United States from 1979–1981 found 1,277 cases of pertussis, with the peak incidence below the age of 4 month. Thus, although vaccination has an influence on reducing the incidence of pertussis, the age-related peak incidence has shifted to infants too young to be completely immunized. Most cases of pertussis in the United States currently occur among these unprotected children less than 1 year of age, the same group most likely to have the complications of pneumonia and overwhelming infection, which are associated with a high mortality.

Today, unlike adults in the past who had natural pertussis infection as children, adults who were vaccinated as children may not have lifelong immunity. The typical *B. pertussis*–associated illness in adults is acute bronchitis with a persistent, nonproductive, hacking cough that lasts several weeks. These adults serve as a reservoir and may transmit the disease to young infants, who are susceptible because they have not yet been fully immunized (Güris et al., 1999). Because health care providers do not commonly culture adults for *B. pertussis,* the basis for our information on pertussis in adults is confined mainly to investigations of outbreaks. Although national surveillance data do not indicate a large number of cases among adults, vaccination of adults may be a method of preventing transmission of infection to young infants before they have been fully immunized. At present, the obstacle to pertussis vaccination of adults is the perception that they have a high rate of reactions to the whole-cell vaccine. This may be overcome with the approval of acellular vaccines for use in adults.

PATHOGENESIS

Most of our knowledge about the pathogenesis of pertussis syndrome is from studies of *B. pertusis*–associated pertussis. Although there are some areas of dispute, it is generally agreed that this is a toxin-associated disease (Table 67–8). These toxins are responsible for the histologic damage to the respiratory epithelium, systemic toxicity, and hematologic changes characteristic of pertussis. These toxins act early in the disease to cause damage, which explains the lack of benefit of antibiotics once the characteristic syndrome of whooping cough has developed. Although immunity to natural infection or vaccine-induced immunity can be measured by a variety of assays, it is unclear which one of a number of immune responses is associated with resistance to infection. Antibody to **pertactin** is perhaps the most important, with some contribution by antibody to **pertussis toxin (PT),** also called lymphocytosis-promoting factor, and **fimbriae,** but no or only minimal contribution from antibody to **filamentous hemagglutinin (FHA).** This gap in our knowledge is one of the reasons for the difficulties in evaluating new candidate pertussis vaccines without full-scale field studies.

SYMPTOMS AND CLINICAL MANIFESTATIONS

One of the keys to early recognition of pertussis is knowledge of the classic signs and symptoms in different age groups. Classic pertussis is the syndrome seen in most infants beyond the neonatal period up through school age. The progression of the disease is divided into catarrhal, paroxysmal, and convalescent stages. Although the disease typically lasts 6–8 weeks, residual cough may persist for months.

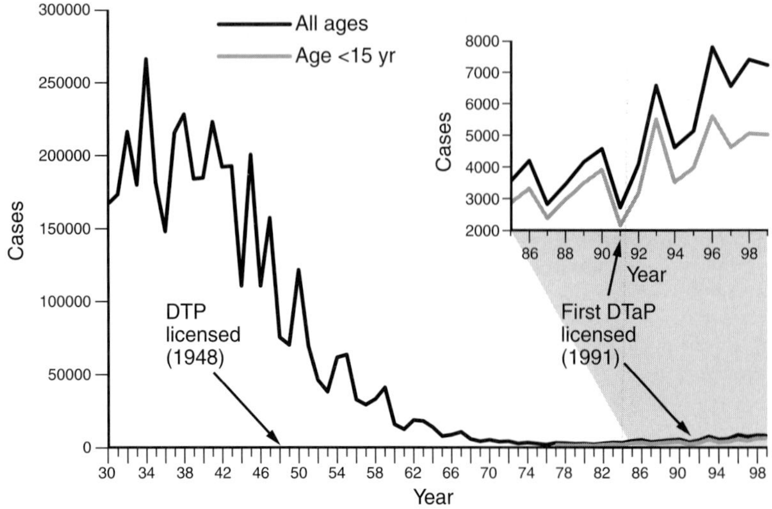

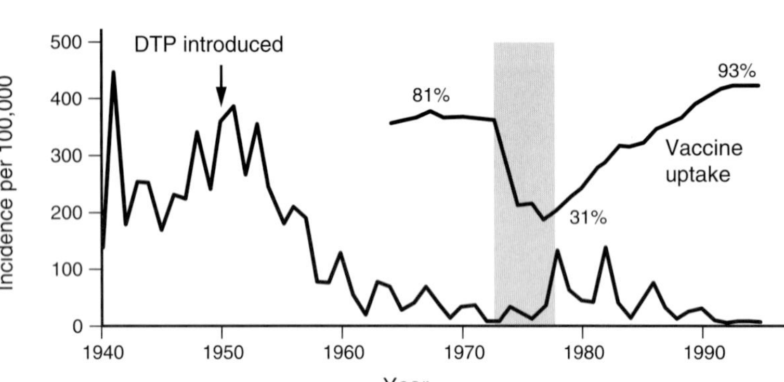

FIGURE 67–2. *Top,* Reported cases of pertussis in the United States by year from 1930 to 1999. *Bottom,* The incidence of pertussis in England and Wales and the effect of antivaccine movements during the 1970s *(shading)* on vaccine uptake. (*Top* from Centers for Disease Control and Prevention. *Bottom* from Gangarosa EJ, Galazka AM, Wolfe CR, et al: Impact of anti-vaccine movements on pertussis control: The untold story. *Lancet* 1998;351:356–61.)

TABLE 67–8. Components of *B. pertussis* and Probable Role in Disease Pathogenesis and Development of Clinical Immunity

Component	Disease Role	Immunity
Pertussis toxin (PT; also called lymphocytosis-promoting factor [LPF])	Attachment Cell damage Lymphocytosis	Yes
Filamentous hemagglutinin (FHA)	Attachment	Minimal
Agglutinogens (fimbriae, pertactin)	Attachment	Yes
Other outer membrane proteins	None known	Yes
Adenylate cyclase	Inhibits phagocytosis Cell damage	Unknown
Endotoxin	Fever and local reaction	Unknown
Tracheal cytotoxin (TC)	Ciliary stasis Cell damage	Unknown
Heat-labile toxin (HLT)	Cell damage	Unknown

Usual Presentation

Catarrhal Stage. The catarrhal period lasts 1–2 weeks and is marked by nonspecific signs and symptoms of upper respiratory tract illness. The signs include injection and excessive secretion of the membranes of the nose, throat, and conjunctivae with a mild cough and a low-grade fever.

Paroxysmal Stage. The paroxysmal stage lasts approximately 2–4 weeks and is the most distinctive stage of pertussis. Coughing occurs in paroxysms during expiration, causing young children to lose their breath. This pattern of coughing is due to the need to dislodge plugs of necrotic epithelial tissues and thick mucus. The forceful inhalation against a narrowed glottis that follows this paroxysm of cough produces the characteristic **whoop.** When these paroxysms are prolonged, there may be cyanosis, bulging of the eyes, vomiting, and petechiae. The daily pattern of these paroxysms varies among patients. Some patients have only a few or even just one paroxysm per day, and these episodes may be moderate or severe. Some have many paroxysms of varying severity. Although the whoop is characteristic, it is not present in some patients. When very young patients have many severe paroxysms, they may not be able to recover between episodes, leading to hypoxia, loss of appetite, and inanition. It is not unusual for physical and radiographic signs of segmental lung atelectasis to develop during pertussis, especially during this stage.

Convalescent Stage. The convalescent stage follows the paroxysmal stage and lasts 1–2 weeks. This term refers not to a new set of signs and symptoms but to a slow decrease in the findings that mark the paroxysmal stage. Coughing becomes less severe, and the paroxysms and whoops slowly disappear. Some degree of coughing may persist for additional months, especially with physical stress or respiratory irritants.

Unusual Presentations

Neonates and Infants. Infants in the first months of life may not display the classic pertussis syndrome. The first sign may be episodes of apnea, as is seen with RSV infection in the same age group. Neonates also may present with a progression of disease that is so compressed and severe that the classic stages may not appear to be distinct. There may be some preceding respiratory symptoms, but these symptoms may appear to be minor compared with the systemic signs of overwhelming infection. Young infants are unlikely to have the classic whoop, are more likely to have central nervous system damage as a result of hypoxia, to have a life-threatening diffuse pneumonia due to *B. pertussis,* and to have secondary bacterial pneumonia.

Adults. Because the parents of young children with pertussis may be infected with *B. pertussis* and are often the source of their children's infection, it is important to recognize the signs in them as well. Adolescents and adults with pertussis usually present with a prolonged bronchitic illness that often began as a nonspecific upper respiratory tract infection. This illness is not very different from pertussis in children, but generally adults and adolescents do not have a whoop with the cough, although they may have severe paroxysms. The cough may persist for many weeks to months. Often the patients have been to their own physician and have received prescriptions for one or more antimicrobial drugs. Because these antimicrobial agents are prescribed after toxins have already damaged the bronchial epithelium, there is usually no symptomatic response, whether or not the antimicrobial agent has activity against *B. pertussis.*

DIAGNOSIS

In general, early recognition and treatment improve the likelihood of avoiding complications and may shorten the duration of shedding of the infecting agent, thus preventing spread to other susceptible persons. Recognition of pertussis in the index patient facilitates treatment of contacts to prevent manifest disease from developing. One of the major aims of diagnosis is to avoid unnecessary treatment of other respiratory tract infections that might produce a similar disease.

Differential Diagnosis

For a young child with classic pertussis syndrome, the diagnosis based on recognition of the pattern of illness is quite accurate. The paroxysmal stage is the most distinctive part of the syndrome. Culture or serologic diagnosis is often required to confirm that *B. pertussis* rather than *B. parapertussis* or adenovirus is the infecting agent. A remarkable lymphocytosis is more characteristic of *B. pertussis.* The differential diagnosis is similar to that noted for the general syndrome of bronchitis. For an infant, respiratory viruses such as RSV, parainfluenza virus, and *Chlamydia pneumoniae* can produce bronchitic illnesses. In older children and young adults, *M. pneumoniae* may produce a prolonged bronchitic illness that is not easily distinguished from pertussis in this age group.

Laboratory Evaluation

One of the laboratory values characteristic of pertussis in patients beyond the neonatal age is an abnormally high absolute number and relative percentage of lymphocytes in the peripheral blood. Lymphocytosis may be seen not only in pertussis but also in infectious mononucleosis caused by Epstein-Barr virus or an enterovirus (Chapter 10).

In classic *B. pertussis*–associated pertussis, lymphocytosis is a characteristic finding in approximately 75–85% of patients, although in young infants the rate is much less. The total WBC count may increase from 20,000/mm^3 to more than 50,000/mm^3. Most of these cells are mature lymphocytes. A WBC count greater than 50,000/mm^3 is considered to be a **leukemoid reaction,** which may be associated with overwhelming infection by the pertussis agent or with superinfection with another bacterial pathogen.

Microbiologic Evaluation

A combination of the direct fluorescent antibody (DFA) test and culture is the most sensitive and specific strategy for the diagnosis of *B. pertussis* infection.

Direct Fluorescent Antibody (DFA). *B. pertussis* can be identified in direct smears of pharyngeal secretions with the use of a DFA technique on a nasopharyngeal smear. This test is available in many reference laboratories and in some hospitals. Appropriate specificity requires that technicians be experienced in interpreting the test, that the specimen obtained by the caregiver have a sufficient number of organisms to be visible to the technician, and that the reagents be highly specific. When performed by experienced personnel, the test has a sensitivity of approximately 60% and a specificity of approximately 90%.

Culture. *B. pertussis* and *B. parapertussis* are small gram-negative bacilli that cannot easily be isolated in the laboratory on routine culture media. With supplemented media, however, the organisms can be isolated from nasopharyngeal swab cultures in a high proportion of cases of pertussis. Calcium alginate or Dacron polyester swabs should be used, because the fatty acids in cotton swabs may inhibit the growth of *B. pertussis.* In some reports, *B. pertussis* can be isolated from nasopharyngeal swab cultures of 80–90% of patients with pertussis if samples are taken early enough in the disease. A nasopharyngeal specimen is recommended in preference to a cough plate.

The highest rate of recovery is in the first 2 weeks of the disease, during which time the syndrome is not distinctive. If one waits for classic whooping cough to develop, the rate of recovery is less. By 4 weeks it is uncommon to be able to recover the organism. It has been shown that in persons infected with the human immunodeficiency virus who contract pertussis, throat cultures may be persistently positive for *B. pertussis.*

The medium most used for isolation in the past has been **Bordet-Gengou agar (potato-glycerin-blood agar).** This medium has a short shelf life that makes optimal availability of a proper medium difficult. **Regan-Lowe medium** with kanamycin is an excellent supplemented medium that suppresses normal flora and has a longer shelf life. *B. pertussis* grows in distinctive silvery colonies that can be confirmed serologically or biochemically. *B. parapertussis* grows in much smaller colonies.

Serologic Diagnosis. Serologic diagnosis can be made with an EIA that measures antibody to certain of the extracellular toxins—pertussis toxin, filamentous hemagglutinin, and agglutinins. Serologic testing may be helpful for unimmunized patients and for those who show a rise of titer in paired sera specimens. A single specimen from immunized patients may demonstrate vaccine-induced antibodies and is nondiagnostic. Tests for IgA antipertussis antibodies may increase the specificity when single or paired specimens are tested, but these tests are not widely available.

Diagnostic Imaging

Radiographic evaluation is important in pertussis, especially for infants. Although the findings on the chest radiograph may be similar in pertussis, bronchiolitis, and viral pneumonia showing perihilar infiltrates or a bronchopneumonia pattern with hyperinflation, complications may be evident. Focal consolidations should alert one to the possibility of a secondary bacterial pneumonia. Focal atelectasis or lobar collapse may be a consequence of plugs of inspissated bronchial secretions. Diffuse multilobar pneumonia may be a sign of overwhelming disease.

TREATMENT

For pertussis syndrome caused by *B. pertussis,* there is evidence of a beneficial effect of antibiotic treatment. In sporadic pertussis the disease is rarely diagnosed before the paroxysmal phase of the disease, by which time antibiotic treatment has no symptomatic benefit. It has been shown, however, that if oral erythromycin treatment (40–50 mg/kg/day orally in four divided doses up to 2 g/day for 14 days) is used in the catarrhal stage, the duration of the whole disease process is shortened. This is important in an outbreak in which infants and children with nonspecific catarrhal illnesses are believed to have early pertussis, and it is logical to start erythromycin treatment expectantly, even before culture confirmation. Occasional patients are intolerant of erythromycin. Limited data suggest that oral TMP-SMZ (8 mg/kg/day as trimethoprim orally in two divided doses for 14 days) or clarithromycin (15 mg/kg/day in two divided doses up to 1 g/day), as well as azithromycin, is an effective substitute.

For infants with intractable paroxysms, albuterol, a β-adrenergic bronchodilator agent, has been used and has shown some efficacy. On the basis of limited data, a trial of albuterol should be considered for infants with intractable paroxysms.

In the past, pertussis immune globulin was available for therapy, but data suggesting that this product has no efficacy caused it to be withdrawn from the market. Newer, more potent immune globulin preparations are currently being tested for efficacy in infected patients.

COMPLICATIONS

In general, pertussis is a protracted infection that runs a course of about 6–8 weeks but with complete resolution. In some cases coughing may persist for several additional months. Complications are most common in young infants, especially those younger than 6 months. The most severe complications are overwhelming pneumonia, seizures, and encephalopathy. Less severe complications are due to the forceful coughing. Impaired venous return and raised intrathoracic and intra-abdominal pressure caused by forceful paroxysms of coughing can cause a petechial eruption on the mucous membranes, subconjunctival hemorrhages, pneumothorax, rectal prolapse, and hernias.

Pneumonia may be due to *B. pertussis* itself, causing diffuse bronchopneumonia or overwhelming hemorrhagic pneumonia. Despite respiratory support in an ICU the mortality rate from *B. pertussis* pneumonia in infants is high. Pneumonia also may be due to superinfection with other bacteria. Secondary staphylococcal pneumonia was common in the past, but it is rare today, and other bacterial respiratory pathogens are usually implicated. It is unclear whether convulsions and encephalopathy occasionally associated with pertussis are caused by toxins from *B. pertussis* or are the result of anoxic encephalopathy.

PROGNOSIS

Although considerable damage to the respiratory epithelium occurs during the course of pertussis, this damage eventually heals completely. Death and permanent morbidity are due to complications of pertussis and are almost completely limited to patients with pertussis in the first year of life. Since 1981, pertussis has been reported as the underlying cause of fewer than 12 deaths annually in the United States. Permanent morbidity is generally attributable to *B. pertussis*–associated encephalopathy. Proper selection of infants for management in an ICU appears to be important in preventing disability by assuring cerebral oxygenation during severe paroxysms.

PREVENTION

Vaccine. Pertussis vaccine is recommended for all children (Chapter 17). There is excellent evidence that the rate of pertussis has fallen because of the routine use of vaccination. Despite the recommendation for routine vaccination, pertussis continues to occur among older children who remain inadequately vaccinated, among infants too young to be vaccinated, and among adults with waning immunity. It is likely that there will be recommendations for reimmunization of persons older than 7 years of age with acellular pertussis vaccine.

Contacts. Hospitalized patients with pertussis syndrome should be placed on droplet precautions to prevent spread to staff and other patients. Precautions should continue for 5 days after initiation of effective antibiotic therapy or until 3 weeks after the onset of paroxysms if no antibiotic therapy is given.

Household and other close contacts of patients should be treated with erythromycin in the doses and duration used for treatment of patients. Other macrolides are recommended as an alternative, although there are scant data demonstrating their efficacy. TMP-SMZ is also an alternative. Close contacts should be treated irrespective of age and immunization status because the vaccine is not 100% effective and household exposure is virtually 100% communicable to susceptible persons. For partially or fully immunized persons with less intimate contact, close observation is appropriate with a plan for erythromycin treatment if symptoms of a respiratory illness develop.

Children younger than 7 years of age who are not fully immunized or who have not had a booster within 3 years should have a DTaP or DTP booster if they have had intimate contact with a patient. Children exposed to a patient in daycare should be managed as indicated earlier if they are well. If they are ill, they require evaluation by a physician and should be excluded from daycare either until the cause of their illness is determined or until after they have received 5 days of erythromycin treatment. Patients or contacts of patients are assumed not to have communicable disease after they have received 5 days of appropriate antimicrobial therapy.

REVIEWS

Chernick V, Boat TF (editors): *Kendig's Disorders of the Respiratory Tract in Children,* 6th ed. Philadelphia, Saunders, 1998.

Morgan WJ, Taussig LM: The chronic bronchitis complex in children. *Pediatr Clin North Am* 1984;31:851–64.

Moss RB: Cystic fibrosis: Pathogenesis, pulmonary infection, and treatment. *Clin Infect Dis* 1995;21:839–51.

Bronchitis

Bums JL, Ramsey BW, Smith AL: Clinical manifestations and treatment of pulmonary infections in cystic fibrosis. *Adv Pediatr Infect Dis* 1993;8:53–66.

Chapman RS, Henderson FW, Clyde WA Jr, et al: The epidemiology of tracheobronchitis in pediatric practice. *Am J Epidemiol* 1981;114: 786–97.

Chartrand SA, Marks MI: Pulmonary infections in cystic fibrosis: Pathogenesis and therapy. In Pennington JE (editor): *Respiratory Infections: Diagnosis and Management.* New York, Raven Press, 1989.

Ramsey BW, Pepe MS, Quan JM, et al: Intermittent administration of inhaled tobramycin in patients with cystic fibrosis: Cystic Fibrosis Inhaled Tobramycin Study Group. *N Engl J Med* 1999;340:23–30.

Smith AL, Doershuk C, Goldmann D, et al: Comparison of a beta-lactam alone versus beta-lactam and an aminoglycoside for pulmonary exacerbation in cystic fibrosis. *J. Pediatr* 1999;134:413–21.

Bronchiolitis

Alario AJ, Lewander WJ, Dennehy P, et al: The efficacy of nebulized metaproterenol in wheezing infants and young children. *Am J Dis Child* 1992;146:412–8.

Brooks AM, McBride JT, McConnochi KM, et al: Predicting deterioration in previously healthy infants hospitalized with respiratory syncytial virus infection. *Pediatrics* 1999;104:463–7.

Committee on Infectious Diseases, American Academy of Pediatrics: Reassessment of the indications for ribavirin therapy in respiratory syncytial virus infections. *Pediatrics* 1996;97:137–40.

Committee on Infectious Diseases and Committee of Fetus and Newborn, American Academy of Pediatrics: Prevention of respiratory syncytial virus infections: Indications for the use of palivizumab and update on the use of RSV-IGIV. *Pediatrics* 1998;102:1211–6.

Flores G, Horwitz RI: Efficacy of beta2-agonists in bronchiolitis: A reappraisal and meta-analysis. *Pediatrics* 1997;100:233–9.

Groothuis JR, Simoes EA, Levin MJ, et al: Prophylactic administration of respiratory syncytial virus immune globulin to high-risk infants and young children: The Respiratory Syncytial Virus Immune Globulin Study Group. *N Engl J Med* 1993;329:1524–30.

Hall CB, Douglas RG Jr: Modes of transmission of respiratory syncytial virus. *J Pediatr* 1981;99:100–3.

Henderson FW, Clyde WA Jr, Collier AM, et al: The etiologic and epidemiologic spectrum of bronchiolitis in pediatric practice. *J Pediatr* 1979; 95:183–90.

Kellner JD, Ohlsson A, Gadomski AM, et al: Efficacy of bronchodilator therapy in bronchilitis: A meta-analysis. *Arch Pediatr Adolesc Med* 1996;150:1166–72.

Law BJ, Wang EE, MacDonald N, et al: Does ribavirin impact on the hospital course of children with respiratory syncytial virus (RSV) infection? An analysis using the pediatric investigators collaborative network on infections in Canada (PICNIC) RSV database. *Pediatrics* 1997;99:E7.

Lowell DI, Lister G, Von Koss H, et al: Wheezing in infants: The response to epinephrine. *Pediatrics* 1987;79:939–45.

Meert KL, Sarnaik AP, Gelmini MJ, et al: Aerosolized ribavirin in mechanically ventilated children with respiratory syncytial virus lower respiratory tract disease: A prospective, double-blind, randomized trial. *Crit Care Med* 1994;22:566–72.

Moler FW, Ohmit SE: Severity of illness models for respiratory syncytial virus-associated hospitalization. *Am J Respir Crit Care Med* 1999; 159:1234–40.

Moler FW, Steinhart CM, Ohmit SE, et al: Effectiveness of ribavirin in otherwise well infants with respiratory syncytial virus-associated respiratory failure: Pediatric Critical Care Study Group. *J Pediatr* 1996; 128:422–8.

Randolph AG, Wang EE: Ribavirin for respiratory syncytial virus lower respiratory tract infection: A systematic overview. *Arch Pediatr Adolesc Med* 1996;150:942–7.

Rimensberger PC, Schaad UB: Clinical experience with aerosolized immunoglobulin treatment of respiratory syncytial virus infection in infants. *Pediatr Infect Dis J* 1994;13:328.

Rodriguez WJ, Gruber WC, Groothuis JR, et al: Respiratory syncytial virus immune globulin treatment of RSV lower respiratory tract infection in previously healthy children. *Pediatrics* 1997;100:937–42.

Schuh S, Canny G, Reisman JJ, et al: Nebulized albuterol in acute bronchiolitis. *J Pediatr* 1990;117:633–7.

Shaw KN, Bell LM, Sherman NH: Outpatient assessment of infants with bronchiolitis. *Am J Dis Child* 1991;145:151–5.

Smith DW, Frankel LR, Mathers LH, et al: A controlled trial of aerosolized ribavirin in infants receiving mechanical ventilation for severe respiratory syncytial virus infection. *N Engl J Med* 1991;325:24–9.

The IMpact-RSV Study Group: Palivizumab, a humanized respiratory syncytial virus monoclonal antibody, reduces hospitalization from respiratory syncytial virus infection in high-risk infants. *Pediatrics* 1998; 102:531–7.

The PREVENT Study Group: Reduction of respiratory syncytial virus hospitalization among premature infants and infants with bronchopulmonary dysplasia using respiratory syncytial virus immune globulin prophylaxis. *Pediatrics* 1997;99:93–9.

Welliver RC, Wong DT, Sun M, et al: The development of respiratory syncytial virus-specific IgE and the release of histamine in nasopharyngeal secretions after infection. *N Engl J Med* 1981;305:841–6.

Wheeler JG, Wofford J, Turner RB: Historical cohort evaluation of ribavirin efficacy in respiratory syncytial virus infection. *Pediatr Infect Dis J* 1993;12:209–13.

Pertussis Syndrome (Whooping Cough)

Baraff LJ, Wilkins J, Wehrle PF: The role of antibiotics, immunizations and adenoviruses in pertussis. *Pediatrics* 1978;61:224–30.

Bass JW: Pertussis: Current status of prevention and treatment. *Pediatr Infect Dis* 1985;4:614–9.

Cherry JD: The epidemiology of pertussis and pertussis immunization in the United Kingdom and the United States: A comparative study. *Curr Probl Pediatr* 1984;14:1–78.

Cherry JD, Olin P: The science and fiction of pertussis vaccines. *Pediatrics* 1999;104:1381–3.

Christie CD, Baltimore RS: Pertussis in neonates. *Am J Dis Child* 1989;143:1199–202.

Christie CD, Marx ML, Marchant CD, et al: The 1993 epidemic of pertussis in Cincinnati. Resurgence of disease in a highly immunized population of children. *N Engl J Med* 1994;331:16–21.

Gangarosa EJ, Galazka AM, Wolfe CR, et al: Impact of anti-vaccine movements on pertussis control: The untold story. *Lancet* 1998;351:156–61.

Güris D, Strebel PM, Bardenheier B, et al: Changing epidemiology of pertussis in the United States: Increasing reported incidence among adolescents and adults, 1990–1996. *Clin Infect Dis* 1999;28:1230–7.

Keller MA, Aftandelians R, Connor JD: Etiology of the pertussis syndrome. *Pediatrics* 1980;66:50–5.

Nelson JD: The changing epidemiology of pertussis in young infants: The role of adults as reservoirs of infection. *Am J Dis Child* 1978;132:371–3.

Pittman M: Pertussis toxin: The cause of the harmful effects and prolonged immunity of whooping cough: A hypothesis. *Rev Infect Dis* 1979; 1:401–12.

Strebel PM, Cochi SL, Farizo KM, et al: Pertussis in Missouri: Evaluation of nasopharyngeal culture, direct fluorescent antibody testing, and clinical case definitions in the diagnosis of pertussis. *Clin Infect Dis* 1993;16:276–85.

Wirsing von Konig CH, Rott H, Bogaerts H, et al: A serologic study of organisms possibly associated with pertussis-like coughing. *Pediatr Infect Dis J* 1998;17:645–9.

CHAPTER 68

Pneumonia

Robert S. Baltimore

Pneumonia is an infection of the lower respiratory tract that involves the airways and lung tissue. The term **lower respiratory tract infection** is often used in place of pneumonia to include bronchitis, bronchiolitis, pneumonia, or any combination of the three that may be difficult to distinguish clinically. Nevertheless, bronchitis, bronchiolitis, and pertussis syndrome (Chapter 67) and pneumonia have different pathologic features, etiologic agents, and progressions of disease.

INITIAL APPROACH TO PNEUMONIA

The diagnosis and treatment of lower respiratory infections in children are hampered by difficulty in obtaining material for culture that truly represents the infected tissue. In otherwise healthy children without life-threatening disease, invasive procedures to obtain lower respiratory tissue or secretions are not usually indicated, and serologic tests are useful for only a limited number of respiratory infections. Cultures of upper respiratory tract secretions, and serologic tests with paired sera are relatively accurate for the diagnosis of viral and mycoplasmal lower respiratory disease. They are not useful for the diagnosis of bacterial disease because the bacterial flora of the upper respiratory tract does not accurately reflect the species that cause acute lower respiratory tract infection. Serologic tests for the most common bacterial pathogens are not available. In addition, although examination of expectorated sputum may often be helpful for diagnosis in adults and some older children, few children are able to expectorate quality sputum on their own because they swallow their sputum. Therefore, in usual pediatric practice a diagnostic assessment is made of the child as to age, exposure history, season, predisposing factors (if any), and clinical presentation of signs and symptoms. Initial treatment decisions are made empirically on the basis of these impressions and the limited information available on comparable populations of children who have undergone intensive study or diagnostic tests. This is true of treatment in an ambulatory setting and for many patients with non-life-threatening pneumonia admitted to pediatric hospital services.

Ordinarily, empirical antibiotic treatment is sufficient for management of pneumonia in children unless there is an exceptional need to identify the specific pathogen to guide management. Such exceptional situations include lack of response to empirical therapy, unusually severe presentations, nosocomial pneumonia, and immunocompromised persons susceptible to infections with opportunistic pathogens. This includes patients with primary immunodeficiencies (Chapter 98) as well as those with acquired immunodeficiencies (Chapters 99–101), including AIDS (Chapter 38).

COMPARATIVE ETIOLOGY

The agents that commonly cause pneumonia vary according to age and whether the pneumonia is community acquired or hospital acquired (Table 68–1). The causes of hospital-acquired pneumonia include the agents of community-acquired pneumonia and also many opportunistic microorganisms. A great many other agents rarely or occasionally cause pneumonia but are limited to endemic areas or occur primarily in immunocompromised persons.

Transmission. Organisms causing pneumonia are usually spread by inhalation of **aerosols** ($\leq 5\ \mu m$ particles suspended in air) or **droplets** ($>5\ \mu m$ particles that fall to the ground or surfaces quickly) from an infected person who coughs, sneezes, or drools. Microorganisms may soil clothing or hands and be spread directly to the mucous membranes of the mouth, nose, or eyes. Inanimate objects, such as air conditioners, water fountains, and farming equipment, may also spread microorganisms through the environment and directly to individuals.

Young Infants. In young infants pneumonia may be caused by organisms that are transmitted from mother to infant, either during gestation or at birth. In most cases, infection of lung tissue before birth causes overwhelming fetal infection and results in intrauterine death. However, infants may be born with congenital pneumonia caused by rubella virus, *Treponema pallidum* (syphilis), and herpes simplex virus (HSV). Organisms that frequently cause neonatal bacterial sepsis and meningitis, such as group B *Streptococcus, Listeria, Escherichia coli,* and *Klebsiella,* may be transmitted shortly before birth, especially if there is prolonged rupture of the chorioamniotic membranes before birth or during the birth process. These pneumonias become evident within a few hours to a few days after birth (Chapter 96).

CMV, *Chlamydia trachomatis, Mycoplasma hominis,* and *Ureaplasma urealyticum* can cause a similar respiratory syndrome in the first few weeks of life, with a subacute onset of an **afebrile pneumonia** with a cough as the predominant sign. These infections are difficult to diagnose and to distinguish from each other. In adults, these organisms are spread by sexual transmission and are carried primarily as part of the genital mucosal flora. Women who harbor these agents may transmit them perinatally to newborns, and thus the epidemiology of much infant pneumonia is linked to sexually transmitted agents in adults. Of these agents *C. trachomatis* appears to be the most common.

Pneumonia that has a sudden onset and is accompanied by fever is likely to be caused by respiratory viruses or bacteria. The predominant bacterial causes of pneumonia in the first month of life are also the usual agents of neonatal sepsis and meningitis and include group B *Streptococcus, Staphylococcus aureus, E. coli, Klebsiella,* and others. Bacterial pneumonia in the first few days of life may be a focal complication of sepsis associated with bacteremia. In the 1950s and early 1960s, staphylococcal infections occurred frequently and in clusters, but currently most infants with primary staphylococcal pneumonia have an underlying defect in host resistance. Rates of staphylococcal disease among neonates

TABLE 68–1. Etiologic Agents and Empirical Antimicrobial Therapy for Pediatric Pneumonia in Otherwise Healthy Children*

Age Group	Frequent Pathogens† (in Order of Frequency)	Patients in Hospital‡	Patients in Intensive Care Unit†‡	Outpatients§
1–3 months	*Chlamydia trachomatis* Respiratory syncytial virus Other respiratory viruses	Afebrile pneumonitis: erythromycin *or* clarithromycin‖ Febrile pneumonia: cefuroxime	Afebrile pneumonitis: erythromycin *or* clarithromycin‖ Febrile pneumonia: cefuroxime *or* cefotaxime *plus* oxacillin *or* nafcillin	Initial outpatient management not recommended
3–12 months	Respiratory syncytial virus Other respiratory viruses *Streptococcus pneumoniae* *Haemophilus influenzae* (type b,¶ nontypeable) *C. trachomatis* *Mycoplasma pneumoniae*	Ampicillin *or* cefuroxime	Cefuroxime *plus* erythromycin *or* clarithromycin‖	Amoxicillin *or* erythromycin *or* clarithromycin‖
2–5 years	Respiratory viruses *S. pneumoniae* *H. influenzae* type b¶ *M. pneumoniae* *Chlamydia pneumoniae*	Same as for 3–12 months	Same as for 3–12 months	Same as for 3–12 months
5–18 years	*M. pneumoniae* *S. pneumoniae* *C. pneumoniae* *H. influenzae* type b¶ Influenza viruses A and B Adenoviruses Other respiratory viruses	Erythromycin *or* clarithromycin‖ *With or without* cefuroxime *or* ampicillin	Cefuroxime *plus* erythromycin *or* clarithromycin‖	Erythromycin *or* clarithromycin‖

*Duration of antibiotic treatment: Outpatients, 7–10 days; hospitalized, 10–14 days; ICU, 10–14 days.
†Severe pneumonia requiring admission to ICU: *S. pneumoniae, Staphylococcus aureus,* group A *Streptococcus, H. influenzae, M. pneumoniae,* adenovirus.
‡Intravenous administration, except for clarithromycin, which is given orally.
§Oral administration.
‖Azithromycin can be substituted for clarithromycin with equal safety and efficacy for treating *M. pneumoniae.*
¶*H. influenzae* type b is uncommon where there is universal *Haemophilus influenzae* type b immunization.
Adapted from Jadavji T, Lau B, Lebel MH, et al: A practical guide for the diagnosis and treatment of pediatric pneumonia. *CMAJ* 1997;156(Suppl):S703–11.

Suggested Dosages for Patients with Normal Renal Function

ANTIBIOTIC	DOSAGE	MAXIMUM DAILY DOSE
Azithromycin	10 mg/kg PO on day 1, then 5 mg/kg q24hr PO	500 mg day 1; 250 mg thereafter
Erythromycin	40 mg/kg/day divided q6hr PO or IV	4 g
Clarithromycin	15 mg/kg/day divided q12hr PO	12 g
Ampicillin	150 mg/kg/day divided q6hr IV, IM	12 g
Cefuroxime	150 mg/kg/day divided q8hr IV, IM	4.5 g

ANTIBIOTIC	DOSAGE	MAXIMUM DAILY DOSE
Cefotaxime	150–200 mg/kg/day divided q6hr IV, IM	12 g
Nafcillin	150 mg/kg/day divided q4–6hr IV, IM	9 g
Oxacillin	100–200 mg/kg/day divided q4–6hr IV, IM	12 g
Amoxicillin	40–80 mg/kg/day divided q8hr PO	1.5 g

vary considerably geographically and temporally. *Streptococcus pneumoniae* and *Haemophilus influenzae* type b may cause pneumonia at any age and are occasional causes of lower respiratory tract infections in neonates. By the age of 3 months, maternally acquired antibody to these agents has decreased to nonprotective levels, leading to an increased proportion of lower respiratory tract infections caused by these agents.

There are only limited data on the viral causes of lower respiratory tract infections in neonates. Neonates are subject to acquired pneumonia spread by droplets or hand contact from infected persons in the community, caused by the common respiratory viruses—parainfluenza virus types 1 and 3, influenza virus, adenovirus, and respiratory syncytial virus (RSV). Adenovirus has a particular predisposition to infect young infants and may produce life-threatening, explosive lower respiratory tract infections. CMV and HSV are maternally transmitted herpesviruses that may infect the lungs as well as many other organ systems in neonates.

Hospital-Acquired Pneumonia in Young Infants. Nosocomial pneumonia can be acquired shortly after birth or during subsequent hospitalizations for illness. In the first few weeks of life it may be difficult to determine whether the etiologic agent of neonatal pneumonia is transmitted from the mother, by nosocomial transmission, or by community acquisition. It is also difficult to determine the cause of pneumonia without invasive tests to culture lung tissue directly. This problem is even greater for hospitalized premature infants. Sick newborn infants frequently have changes in lung gas exchange or densities on chest radiographs, but many of these disorders have a noninfectious cause. Nevertheless, in the absence of suitable culture material, such infants are often initially treated with antibiotics. Organisms recovered from lung secretions of intubated infants represent upper airway contaminants; it is frequently unclear whether the presence of these organisms indicates infection and pneumonia, although antibiotic therapy may be directed at eradication of these species.

The range of agents associated with nosocomial pneumonia in neonates is considerable. Frequently encountered agents include those seen with maternally acquired infection, including group B *Streptococcus, E. coli,* and bacteria more frequently associated with nosocomial infection such as *S. aureus* and other gram-negative bacilli such as *Klebsiella, Pseudomonas aeruginosa,* and *Enterobacter.* Viruses, such as parainfluenza virus and RSV, may cause clusters of infection in the hospital nursery.

Community-Acquired Pneumonia in Older Infants and Children. The most common bacterial agents of pneumonia in older infants and in children are *S. pneumoniae* and *H. influenzae* type b (Table 68–1). Limited data (Mulholland et al., 1997) suggest that the incidence of *H. influenzae* type b pneumonia is reduced when conjugate vaccine is used, although pneumonia caused by *H. influenzae* non-type b and nontypable strains is not prevented by the vaccine. Group A *Streptococcus* is also an occasional agent of acute febrile pneumonia in children, with a clinical presentation similar to *S. pneumonia* and *H. influenzae* pneumonia, but it appears that such complications as empyema are more common with group A *Streptococcus* infections. In hospitalized children, *S. aureus* is also an agent of pneumonia, presumably because pneumonias caused by *S. aureus* are more severe and more likely to result in hospitalization.

Viruses, especially RSV and parainfluenza virus types 1 and 3, are the most common agents of community-acquired pneumonia in children from later infancy up to the age of 5 years. The incidence of influenza virus pneumonia varies from year to year, depending on transmission within the country and the community, as does the serotype (influenza A or B). In most cases of influenza, pneumonia is not considered although chest radiographs would be abnormal in some of these children. On occasion, otherwise healthy children have severe pneumonias caused by influenza virus, but most children with severe influenza pneumonia are either young infants or have underlying abnormalities of the immune or respiratory systems.

Hospital-Acquired Pneumonia in Older Infants and Children. Viruses predominate as causes of nosocomial respiratory tract infections in children. Transmission of RSV, especially, and also of parainfluenza viruses types 1 and 3 is frequent, resulting in considerable morbidity in hospitalized children. Carriage of viruses by hospital personnel is especially important in nosocomial transmission, which can be greatly reduced by hand-washing; the use of gloves and masks may have some additional benefit. Contact isolation generally provides an effective barrier. Because medical personnel may spread respiratory viruses to patients if they themselves are infected avoidance of infection by personnel and removal of personnel with symptoms from medical care areas reduces the incidence of nosocomial infections caused by these agents.

Bacteria are also important causes of nosocomial pneumonia, either by colonization of the upper airway followed by aspiration or by seeding of the lungs as a secondary focus after bacteremia. Bacteria may also enter the lower respiratory tract directly in patients with endotracheal tubes. Bacteria that characteristically cause nosocomial pneumonia in children include the usual agents of pneumonia, *S. pneumoniae* and *H. influenzae,* as well as organisms that spread in the hospital, such as gram-negative bacilli, including *Klebsiella, Enterobacter,* and *P. aeruginosa,* as well as gram-positive cocci, including *S. aureus,* coagulase-negative staphylococci, and viridans streptococci. Patients receiving intensive care and requiring endotracheal intubation are at risk of aspiration of the resident flora of their own upper airway, which may lead to pneumonia.

COMPARATIVE EPIDEMIOLOGY

Developing Countries. Much of the data on the causes of lower respiratory tract infections in children is limited by poor technology. In developed countries the standards of diagnosis of lower respiratory tract infections are based on reproducible methods. However, the diagnosis of pneumonia in developing countries often cannot be confirmed radiographically, and data on lower respiratory tract infections are often combined with data on all acute respiratory tract infections and thus may include upper and middle airway infections.

Each year more than 4 million deaths in developing countries are attributed to acute respiratory tract infections, which represent the major cause of preventable deaths in these countries. There is considerable variation from country to country of the most important pathogens and in the relative contribution of lower respiratory tract infections to morbidity and mortality associated with all acute respiratory tract infections. Immunization practices have a great influence on these rates. In some developing countries, tuberculosis, pertussis, diphtheria, and measles are leading causes of the morbidity and death associated with acute respiratory tract infections, whereas in other countries some or all of these diseases are controlled by the use of vaccines. In countries where vaccination programs are successful, viral acute respiratory tract infections predominate because most of these are not preventable with vaccine. Nevertheless, an annual incidence of 6–8 acute respiratory tract infections per young child is almost universal. In developing countries the interaction of diarrheal disease with acute respiratory tract infections is also recognized. As a result of repeated episodes of diarrheal disease, many young children have varying degrees of malnutrition; even moderate malnutrition causes a child to be more susceptible to many acute respiratory tract infections and their life-threatening complications. The annual incidence of acute respiratory tract infections in children can be as high as 478 (Uruguay) to 1430 (Thailand) per 100 children. The rate of lower respiratory tract infections ranges from 21 (Kenya) to 296 (Uruguay) per 100 children (Bale, 1990). These rates are much higher than in developed countries.

United States and Other Developed Countries. Pneumonia is not a notifiable disease in the United States, so there are no recent accurate national incidence reports of lower respiratory tract infections. As in developing countries, local vaccine practices regarding pertussis, diphtheria, measles, *Haemophilus influenzae* type b, and bacille Calmette Guérin (BCG) vaccines influence rates of lower respiratory tract infections. The new seven-valent conjugate pneumococcal vaccine may provide additional opportunity for significant prevention of childhood pneumonia. In the United States the CDC has estimated the rates of pneumonia and pneumococcal pneumonia (Table 68–2), but these rates are not age specific. There is a distinct age-related incidence of lower respiratory tract infections (primarily viral and mycoplasmal infections) in children (Fig. 68–1), including invasive infection with *Streptococcus pneumoniae,* the most important pathogen of bacterial pneumonia (Fig. 68–2).

TABLE 68–2. Annual Incidence of Pneumonia

Year of Report	Incidence (Cases/100,000)	Disease and Location
1935–36	558	Pneumonia, United States (population survey)
1975	130	Pneumococcal pneumonia, Seattle
1981	200–500	Pneumococcal pneumonia, U.S., estimate
1981	68–260	Pneumococcal pneumonia, U.S., CDC estimate

Estimates from Austrian R: Some observations on the pneumococcus and on the current status of pneumococcal disease and its prevention. *Rev Infect Dis* 3(Suppl 3):S1-S17, 1981; and from Centers For Disease Control: Recommendations of the Immunization Practices Advisory Committee (ACIP): Pneumococcal polysaccharide vaccine. *MMWR Morb Mortal Wkly Rep* 1981;30:410–9.

The rates of lower respiratory tract infections are higher in residential care facilities for handicapped children, just as they are in nursing homes for the elderly where crowding and neurologic compromise are risk factors. Hospitalized children may develop nosocomial lower respiratory tract infections in which the degree of risk reflects the severity and type of underlying illness. Hospitalization in intensive care units, mechanical ventilation, indwelling catheters, and administration of broad-spectrum antibiotics interfere with host resistance to infection and are risk factors for nosocomial infections, including pneumonia (Chapter 105).

COMPARATIVE PATHOGENESIS

Microorganisms may colonize only the upper airway mucosa, or they may spread to the lower respiratory tract. Viral infection of the upper and middle airway may lead to temporary derangement of the cleansing activity of the ciliated epithelium, leading in turn to bronchitis, stasis of contaminated lung secretions, and secondary bacterial pneumonia. Another mechanism of lung infection is aspiration of contaminated material, such as upper airway secretions, gastric secretions, or a contaminated foreign body. Aspiration is more likely to occur in a person with nervous system impairment, which leads to poor airway protection because the epiglottal reflex is impaired or swallowing is dysfunctional. Predisposing conditions include congenital neuromuscular disorders, cerebral palsy, impairment by alcohol or other central nervous system depressants, epilepsy, and head trauma. Pneumonia can also be due to hematogenous seeding of the lung from bacteremia of the systemic or pulmonary circulation; right-sided endocarditis results in microemboli that contain a large number of bacteria going into the pulmonary circulation, exemplifying focal pneumonia secondary to emboli from another focus.

Pathologic patterns of pneumonia have been named according to the histologic appearance of the lung and the associated radiographic findings. **Focal, lobar pneumonia, or typical pneumonia** reflects focal infiltration with organisms, inflammatory cells, and edema fluid that is limited by anatomic boundaries to one lobe of the lung or a lobar segment. This is the characteristic pattern of pneumococcal pneumonia and is also associated with pneumonia caused by *H. influenzae* type b and other bacterial pathogens. Patterns other than lobar pneumonia are termed **atypical pneumonia.** The spread of pneumonia can be along the path of the main bronchi, which is termed **bronchopneumonia,** and is caused by both bacterial and nonbacterial agents. Some agents more characteristically invade the lung tissue itself, sparing the airways and causing an **interstitial pneumonia.** Finally, organisms may be present primarily in the alveoli and not in the airways, causing an **alveolar pneumonia.**

S. pneumoniae infection is classically localized, causing lobar pneumonia, but it may also be diffuse, causing bronchopneumonia. It is characterized by alveolar fluid, infiltration with fibrin and polymorphonuclear leukocytes, and increased blood flow, which combine to bring about **consolidation,** leading to **loss of compliance** and resulting in **increased work of breathing.** Pneumonia caused by *H. influenzae* type b is similar pathologically to pneumococcal pneumonia, but the degree of edema in the tissues is especially remarkable. Pneumonia caused by group A *Streptococcus* is more necrotizing than that caused by *S. pneumoniae* and often associated with bronchial erosions and empyema. Pneumonia caused by *Staphylococcus aureus* is associated with pus-filled bronchi and abscesses in the lung parenchyma. The necrotizing quality of this pneumonia is frequently reflected by pneumatocele formation and empyema. Pneumonia caused by gram-negative bacilli has pathologic features similar to there of staphylococcal pneumonia.

Viral pneumonia is usually not an isolated entity but is associated with pathologic evidence of bronchitis, bronchiolitis, tracheitis, or any combination of these diseases. Involvement of the terminal airways and alveoli may be part of a continuum of airway inflammation. Death may be due to patchy bronchopneumonia and necrotizing bronchiolitis with extensive sloughing of bronchiolar epithelium. Adenovirus pneumonia has been characteristically associated with patchy consolidation and mucopurulent exudate within tracheobronchial lumina and severe necrotizing bronchiolitis and alveolitis. Adenovirus intranuclear inclusions are present in epithelial cells and histiocytes.

Mycoplasma pneumoniae infection rarely causes death, and therefore information on its histopathologic characteristics is not

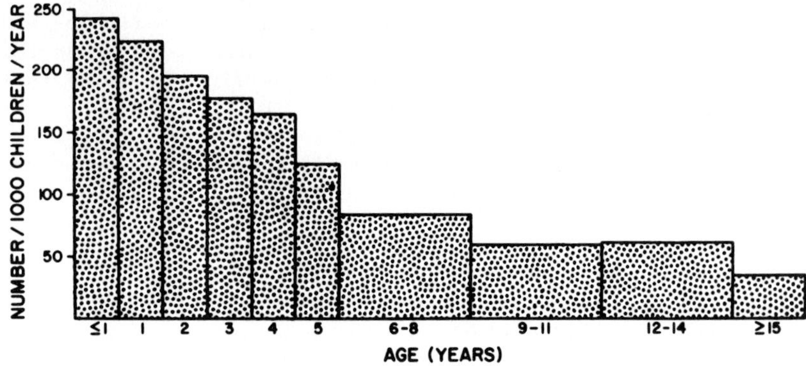

FIGURE 68–1. Incidence of lower respiratory tract infection (pneumonia, bronchiolitis, and tracheobronchitis) by age group, Chapel Hill, North Carolina. (Adapted from Glezen WP, Denny FW: Medical Progress. Epidemiology of acute lower respiratory disease in children. *N Engl J Med* 1973;288:498–505.)

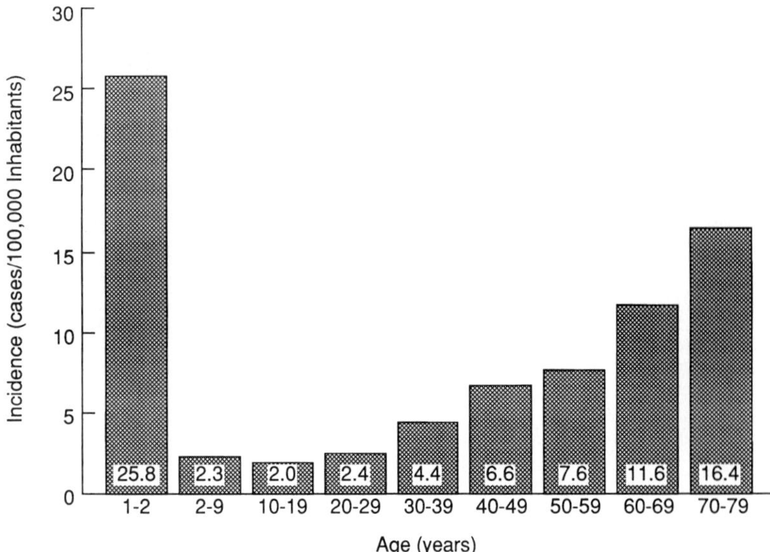

FIGURE 68–2. Incidence (cases/100,000) of invasive *Streptococcus pneumoniae* infections (pneumonia, bacteremia, and meningitis) by age group, Goteborg Sweden, 1970–80. (Data from Burman A, Norby R, Trollfors B: Invasive pneumococcal infections: Incidence, predisposing factors and prognosis. *Rev Infect Dis* 1985;7:133–42. Figure from Baltimore RS, Shapiro ED: Pneumococcal infections. In Evans AS, Brachman PS (editors): *Bacterial Infections of Humans: Epidemiology and Control,* 3rd ed. New York, Plenum Publishing Corp, 1998.)

extensive. In unusually severe infections, there are peribronchial and perivascular lymphoid infiltrates and acute bronchitis and bronchiolitis with variable consolidation of the alveoli.

Pneumonia caused by *Pneumocystis carinii,* once known as **plasma cell pneumonia,** is distinctive, with widespread alveolar infiltrates that contain plasma cells and lymphocytes. Cysts measuring 4–6 μm in diameter, observed with silver stain but not with hematoxylin and eosin, appear as negatively stained objects in fluid-filled alveolar spaces, producing a ''foamy proteinaceous'' appearance.

Host Defenses in the Lung

The airway is in contact with an atmosphere contaminated with microorganisms. Healthy persons may periodically aspirate contaminated upper respiratory tract secretions. Nevertheless, normal lower tract airways below the vocal cords and effluent are sterile, and most persons rarely have lower respiratory tract infections because of a multicomponent cleansing system.

The Ciliary Elevator System. The larger branches of the tracheobronchial airway system are lined with **ciliary columnar epithelium,** and distal branches are lined with **ciliated cuboidal epithelium.** The cilia beat synchronously in such a manner that the movement of any particles is upward and toward the central airway. This elevator system cleanses the airway by catching contaminants in the mucus secreted by the **goblet cells** and lifting the mucus up and out of the airway into the throat, where it is normally swallowed. Congenital ciliary dysmorphisms result in nonsynchronous beating of the cilia, which is ineffective, resulting in chronic infection of the airways leading to bronchiectasis and loss of elasticity and alveolar mass (Chapter 67). Of greater importance is the fact that temporary damage to the ciliary elevator system accompanies viral respiratory infections, chemical or thermal injury to the lungs, cigarette smoking, and exacerbations of chronic lung diseases, which are probably the major mechanisms responsible for bacterial lower respiratory tract infections in the general population.

Phagocytes. The two types of phagocytic cells in the lung—polymorphonuclear neutrophils from the blood and **tissue macrophages**—are able to ingest and kill microorganisms. Together they protect the lungs from less pathogenic organisms that can be phagocytosed without opsonization and the highly virulent pathogens that require antibody and complement for opsonization before ingestion. Generation of toxic radicals within the phagocyte kills the ingested microorganisms. Depletion of these cells as a result of disease or congenital granulocytic abnormalities or as an adverse effect of medication is a major risk factor for lower respiratory tract infections.

Humoral Immune System. IgA secreted into the upper airway fluid is important in the protection of mucosal surfaces against invasive infections, especially for viral neutralization. In peripheral airways, IgM and IgG are important in bacteriolysis, as opsonins, and in neutralizing toxins. Hypogammaglobulinemia, isolated IgA deficiency, and dysgammaglobulinemias are associated with an increased risk of lower respiratory tract infections. Persons with agammaglobulinemia treated with IVIG remain deficient in IgA; although they are protected against systemic infections due to virulent pathogens such as *S. pneumoniae,* they may have chronic bronchitis and progressive lung disease because of inadequate mucosal immunity.

T Lymphocytes. The lung is supplied with T cells that are produced in lymph nodes in the thoracic cavity. T-cell deficiency results in infections due to opportunistic pathogens that are usually controlled by cell-mediated immunity, including *Aspergillus, P. carinii,* CMV, and nontuberculous mycobacteria.

Host Defense Abnormalities. Certain functions of the host defense systems, if they are uncontrolled, appear to be the *cause* of lower respiratory tract infections. Many of the protective mechanisms in the lung result in the elaboration of **chemical radicals** that are toxic to invading microorganisms, activation of complement, and release of **cytokines** such as leukocyte elastase and tumor necrosis factor. Chronic lung disease can result from the toxic effect of these substances on the mucosal lining of the airway and lung parenchyma. Chronic inflammation can lead to excess production of mucus that can interfere with the ciliary cleansing function.

SUGGESTIVE SYMPTOMS AND SIGNS

The determination of the specific cause of pneumonia in children can be very difficult because diagnostic material from which to isolate an agent can be difficult to obtain. A considerable effort

TABLE 68–3. Clues to the Etiology of Pneumonia Obtained Through History Taking

Type of Contact or Prodrome	Disease or Organism
Contact with an individual with a lung infection	Tuberculosis *Mycoplasma pneumoniae* Respiratory viruses *Streptococcus pneumoniae*
Infant or young child in daycare	*Haemophilus influenzae* type b *Neisseria meningitidis* Respiratory viruses
Animal contact (see Table 3–5)	Psittacosis Tularemia Plague Q fever Hantavirus cardiopulmonary syndrome
Geographic regions	Histoplasmosis Coccidioidomycosis Rickettsial infections Hantavirus cardiopulmonary syndrome
Building construction	*Aspergillus*
Air-conditioning cooling towers	*Legionella pneumophila* Other legionelloses
Outbreak or epidemic	Group A *Streptococcus* Influenza viruses Respiratory syncytial virus
Smoker, smoking in household, wood-burning stove	Increase in all lower respiratory infections
Shorter prodrome	Bacterial agents such as *S. pneumoniae, H. influenzae,* group A *Streptococcus*
Longer prodrome	*Mycoplasma pneumoniae* *Chlamydia pneumoniae* or *Chlamydia trachomatis* Respiratory viruses
Preceding rash	Measles *N. meningitidis* *M. pneumoniae* *Staphylococcus aureus*
Preceding focal abscess (pulmonary or extrapulmonary)	*S. aureus*

Only well-established or strong associations are included.

has been made to delineate specific pneumonia syndromes characteristic of different agents or classes of agents. The problem of interpreting studies of this nature is that often the final diagnosis is suspect because of the imprecise methods used. Some studies attempt to distinguish bacterial from viral pneumonia on the basis of response to antibiotics, but the value of such studies in the absence of isolation of a specific agent is difficult to discern.

Some elements of clinical history are essential for the diagnosis of pneumonia (Table 68–3). The possibility of exposure to environmental pathogens should be sought by direct questions. Does the patient smoke, live with a smoker, or live in a house that is heated by an indoor wood-burning stove? Has the patient been in contact with metal fumes, high concentrations of other industrial pollutants, or areas of a city with an endemic smog problem? Has the patient traveled to an area where certain lower respiratory tract infections, such as histoplasmosis, coccidioidomycosis, or rickettsial infections, are endemic? Has the patient been inside a building known to be contaminated with *Legionella pneumophila?* Has the patient recently been cared for in a hospital, which raises concern about nosocomially transmitted agents?

The possibility of pathogens associated with human and animal contacts should be sought with direct questions. Has the patient been in contact with a person with a lower respiratory tract infection? Aerosols from infected persons can transmit tuberculosis, pneumococcus, respiratory viruses, and *M. pneumoniae.* In daycare situations, transmission of *H. influenzae* and *Neisseria meningitidis* may be nearly epidemic, and some of the evident infections in contacts may be lower respiratory tract infections. Animals may be the source of psittacosis (birds), hantaviruses (rodents), and the pneumonic forms of tularemia (rabbits), plague (rodents), and Q fever (sheep).

General aspects of the symptom history may help in the classification and management of lower respiratory tract infections. How long ago did symptoms begin? What were the first symptoms? How rapidly did the symptoms progress? Pneumococcal pneumonia usually has a short prodrome, and respiratory and systemic symptoms begin abruptly. *M. pneumoniae* and viral lower respiratory tract infections usually begin insidiously, and upper respiratory tract symptoms often precede the cough and breathing abnormalities. The presence of a cough, the type of cough, its productivity, the nature of the sputum if any, accompanying fever, malaise, rash, and any other focal symptoms suggesting an infection that might have spread to the lungs by a bacteremia should be elicited. Abdominal pain may be referred from lower lobe pneumonia contiguous with the diaphragm. Other areas to which pain originating in the chest cavity may be referred are the shoulders, back, and neck.

Physical Examination Findings

The physical examination is useful in suggesting possible causes of pneumonia and is essential for the assessment of severity of infection and respiratory status. Age is a determinant in the physical findings because neonates may have only the subtlest or even no physical findings of pneumonia. Many nonspecific signs and symptoms, such as fever, chills, peripheral cyanosis, and apprehension, might suggest pneumonia. Lower respiratory tract infection in infants can be diagnosed in most cases by physical examination alone using the parameters of high or very low body temperature (>39°C or <35.5°C) and by objective signs of respiratory distress (chest indrawing or retractions) or rapid breathing. Age less than 2 months, cyanosis, and stridor are additional elements that indicate greater likelihood of severe disease.

Breathing should be observed for both **respiratory pattern and rate** (Table 68–4). Faster respiratory rates could be caused by airways inflammation resulting in obstruction or by pneumonia

TABLE 68–4. Respiratory Rates (Breaths per Minute) of Healthy Children

	Normal Rate—Sleeping		Normal Rate—Awake	
Age	Mean	Range	Mean	Range
6–12 mo	27	22–31	64	58–75
1–2 yr	19	17–23	35	30–40
2–4 yr	19	16–25	31	23–42
4–6 yr	18	14–23	26	19–36
6–8 yr	17	13–23	23	15–30

Adapted from *Executive summary: Guidelines for the diagnosis and management of asthma.* US Department of Health and Human Services Publication 91-3042a, 1991, p. 25.

resulting in inadequate gas exchange and hypoxia. Nonpulmonary causes of tachypnea include metabolic disturbances and acidosis, cardiac disease, and high fever. Other signs of respiratory distress include **flaring of the alae of the nose, intercostal and subcostal retractions,** and **grunting.** In young infants, **apnea** may be the prominent or even the first sign of pneumonia. Loss of compliance results in increased **work of breathing.** Signs of obstruction, bronchospasm, or splinting due to pain are important in assessment and classification of the degree of illness.

The chest examination is critical. In addition to observation of chest movement during breathing (asymmetry or shallow breathing may be due to splinting from pain), **chest percussion** can identify areas of **dullness to percussion,** which may be due to lobar or segmental infiltrates or pleural fluid. The **level of the diaphragm** and **diaphragmatic excursion** are percussed. Low diaphragms indicate **air trapping,** which is common in asthma but also frequently accompanies viral lower respiratory infections. **Poor diaphragmatic excursion** may indicate hyperexpanded lungs or an inability to expand the lungs because a large consolidation is causing poor lung compliance. Auscultation may be normal in early or very focal pneumonia, but the presence of **crackles (rales), rhonchi,** and **wheezes** may help detect and localize pneumonia. **Distant breath sounds** may indicate pleural fluid or a large consolidated area that is not being ventilated. Additional signs that may reflect consolidation include **bronchial breath sounds** and **vocal fremitus,** which reflect air movement through smaller airways transmitted through nonaerated tissue. A pleural **friction rub** indicates pleuritis. Although these physical findings may be extremely helpful in diagnosing pneumonia, any or all of them may be absent in very young children. In general, the younger a patient, the less the chances are that pneumonia can the diagnosed on the basis of percussion and auscultation of the chest.

Examination of the heart is also important. Heart failure may accompany severe pneumonia. A flow murmur increases in intensity as the heart must increase its work because of the increased demands of fever, inflammation, and the difficulty of breathing. Pericardial effusion may be a complication of pneumonia contiguous with the pericardium and may lead to cardiac tamponade. An abdominal examination may show abnormalities related to the pneumonia. If the lungs are in a hyperinflated state, the diaphragm and viscera may be pushed down, although the liver span remains normal.

A complete examination is necessary to identify other foci of infection or associated findings that may help identify the etiologic agent. The skin should be examined to determine whether there is a focal infection, such as with *S. aureus,* which might cause bacteremic seeding of the lungs, or a rash, such as that seen in measles or *Mycoplasma* infections. Skin color is important, especially to identify **cyanosis** and determine whether it is generalized or only peripheral. Cyanosis accompanying pneumonia indicates severe and perhaps life-threatening infection, which requires intensive monitoring and treatment. Mucosal congestion and inflammation of the upper airway may suggest a viral infection.

DIAGNOSIS

The hallmark findings of pneumonia are fever, tachypnea, and malaise. Some agents, such as *C. trachomatis,* do not cause fever, but most viral, *Mycoplasma,* and bacterial pneumonias are accompanied by fever. A major point of clinical differentiation of pneumonia is that the pyogenic bacterial species have a tendency to cause focal infection that results in dense infiltrates of lung lobes or lobar segments, causing **lobar pneumonia.** Viruses and mycoplasmas are more likely to spread diffusely along the branches of the bronchial tree, causing **bronchopneumonia.** In terms of severity, bacterial pneumonia is more abrupt in onset and is associated with acute inflammation and, therefore, is more likely to be associated with blood in the sputum, high fever, air hunger, and malaise than are the other types. However, this differentiation is not absolute, as either class of agent may cause either type of pneumonia syndrome. Thus these findings cannot be considered completely specific for identifying the cause of pneumonia in an individual patient.

Wheezing is most frequently associated with viral and mycoplasmal pneumonia. In infants and young children it may be difficult to differentiate wheezing-associated lower respiratory tract infections from asthma, and it may be necessary to follow the evolution of illness for months after the initial wheezing illness to determine the prognosis. Infants who appear to have wheezing associated with infections often develop asthma later in childhood. It is still a matter of considerable debate whether an infant who intrinsically has hyperactive airways is more likely to wheeze with a viral illness or whether damage is done to the lungs by early lower respiratory tract infections, causing asthma later in life.

Laboratory Evaluation

Routine laboratory studies are of limited usefulness in the diagnosis of pneumonia. The limited literature in pediatrics suggests that pneumonia caused by bacteria, as opposed to viruses and mycoplasmas, is likely if the WBC count is $>15{,}000/mm^3$, the CRP is positive, and the ESR is elevated. These tests are not specific, however, and there is considerable overlap between bacterial, viral, and mycoplasmal pneumonias. In addition, because the diagnosis of bacterial pneumonia is difficult to confirm in studies that do not use invasive tests for culture, the standards of diagnosis in the reported studies is poor, often being based on a clinical response to antibiotics.

Microbiologic Evaluation

Attempts at etiologic diagnosis by culture are of benefit in understanding the patient's illness and in guiding therapy. Cultures from terminal airways and lung tissue afford the best chance of establishing an accurate diagnosis, but they require invasive procedures that are performed only when there is an unusually great need to know the causative organism. The need to establish a specific etiologic diagnosis of pneumonia is greater for patients who are ill enough to require hospitalization or have congenital or acquired immunodeficiencies such as AIDS, recurrent pneumonia, or pneumonia that is unresponsive to empirical therapy.

Cultures. A positive *Mycoplasma* or viral culture from the upper respiratory tract in the setting of a clinical diagnosis of pneumonia is considered to be diagnostic, whereas positive bacterial cultures of sputum require careful interpretation. Sputum, which is often of value for making an etiologic diagnosis of pneumonia in adults, is difficult to obtain from healthy children before the teenage years. **Coughed sputum** that is not heavily contaminated with upper airway secretions may be obtained from older children who are used to coughing up sputum, including those with chronic lung diseases, such as cystic fibrosis, AIDS with lymphocytic interstitial pneumonitis, or bronchiectasis. In hospitalized children, sputum may be aspirated either with a suction catheter in the trachea or through an endotracheal tube if they are intubated. **Transtracheal aspiration,** which bypasses the upper airway and is of use in diagnosing pneumonia in adults, is rarely used in children because children are unlikely to be cooperative enough for the procedure to be performed safely without anesthesia. Ideally, before a sputum is cultured, a Gram stain should be prepared and examined to ensure that there are leukocytes, fibrin, and lung cells, which confirm that the sample originated from the lungs and that squamous epithelial cells typical of upper airway secretions are absent or few in number. A particular morphology of bacteria that clearly predominates and subsequent growth in culture of a predominant species with the same morphology as the bacteria seen on the Gram stain are good evidence that the species isolated by culture is the cause of the pneumonia.

Blood cultures should be performed in an attempt to diagnose the cause of pneumonia; these are positive in 10–20% of cases. Blood cultures are considered to be diagnostic of the cause of pneumonia when positive for a recognized bacterial respiratory pathogen.

Performing a thoracentesis to obtain pleural fluid can be both diagnostic and therapeutic. Culture and Gram stain may result in a diagnosis and differentiate between empyema (Chapter 69) and a sterile parapneumonic effusion caused by irritation of the pleura contiguous with the pneumonia. If the cause of the pneumonia is unknown, the fluid should be cultured for bacteria, mycobacteria, fungi, and viruses. If the fluid is grossly infected, its removal reduces the patient's toxic condition and respiratory distress. If the accumulation is large and impairs the ability of the lung to expand, removal of the fluid improves pulmonary mechanics and gas exchange.

When there is a sufficiently great need to know the causative agent of pneumonia, as in immunocompromised persons, or when other methods have not been successful, invasive procedures can be performed to diagnose the pneumonia. **Bronchoscopy** may yield a pathogen from the lung airways or, when there is a **transbronchial needle biopsy,** from the tissues. Medical centers vary as to the expertise available for these procedures and the smallest child acceptable for the procedure. The use of bronchoscopy with **bronchoalveolar lavage** to obtain a pathogen in the lungs is increasingly being used in pediatrics. Problems with this procedure include the inability to control bleeding in the airway, the difficulty of ventilating the patient during the procedure, and contamination of the cultures with upper airway flora. The use of a shielded bronchoscopy brush increases the specificity of cultures, but such equipment is not generally available for very small children. The procedure generally requires an experienced specialist and either an appropriate procedure room or ICU for conscious sedation or general anesthesia. **Percutaneous needle aspiration** of the affected lung tissue guided by CT or ultrasonography may yield the pathogen, but the frequency of complications of hemothorax, pneumothorax, or both limits its acceptance. **Open lung biopsy** is still a favored means of culture for many specialists and is diagnostically useful in most immunocompromised persons with diffuse pulmonary infiltrates, but the need for tissue for diagnosis must justify a major surgical procedure of an ill patient. The thoracoscopic approach to open lung biopsy is somewhat less invasive than standard thoracotomy. The advantages of open lung biopsy are the ability to provide histologic and culture correlation and to isolate multiple infecting organisms, the lack of contaminating flora, and the surgeon's ability to control bleeding. One of the difficulties of the procedure is controlling air leakage after the operation in patients with poorly compliant and distended lungs who require mechanical ventilation. A recent review (Stefannuti et al, 2000) of open lung biopsy in immunocompromised pediatric patients reported a histopathologic diagnosis after all 36 biopsies, with a specific diagnosis in 61% and a nonspecific diagnosis in 39%. Review of the pediatric literature shows that open biopsy yields diagnostic information in 65–100% of cases, with a procedure-associated mortality of 0.6%.

Antigen Detection. The encapsulated bacteria, *S. pneumoniae, N. meningitidis, H. influenzae* type b, and group B *Streptococcus* all produce soluble capsular carbohydrates that diffuse in tissues and are excreted by the kidneys. They can be used for diagnosis by particle agglutination (Chapter 11). These methods have occasionally been effective in the diagnosis of pneumonia, but their value is not great enough to recommend their routine use for diagnosing pneumonia until technologic improvements result in more sensitive assays.

Serologic Studies. Serologic studies may be helpful when there is evidence that agents such as *Chlamydia, M. pneumoniae,* and some zoonotic species have caused the pneumonia (Chapter 11). Serologic studies are particularly useful in diagnosing viral pneumonia when cultures have not identified a pathogen.

Diagnostic Imaging

Radiologic assessment of pneumonia is a routine procedure in pediatric practice (Chapter 13). Both **anteroposterior and lateral views** are required to localize the diseased segments and to adequately visualize infiltrates behind structures such as the heart or the diaphragmatic leaflets. The chest radiograph may be normal in early pneumonia or in pneumonia accompanied by dehydration or severe leukopenia. In these situations an infiltrate may appear during the treatment phase of the disease, when more edema fluid is present. Although repeating the chest radiograph is not required for uncomplicated pneumonia that follows the expected clinical course in a previously well child, certain signs may require follow-up assessment. Hilar lymphadenopathy, although not unusual with many common pneumonias, suggests tuberculosis, histoplasmosis, or an underlying malignant neoplasm and may necessitate special management and follow-up care, as do multiple bouts of pneumonia in one patient. Lung abscesses, pneumatoceles, and empyema all require special management (Chapter 69). **Decubitus views** should be used to assess pleural effusions as to size and whether they consist of freely mobile fluid. CT is not used routinely but is helpful in delineating effusions, abscesses, and focal pulmonary lesions, especially in immunocompromised persons.

INITIAL MANAGEMENT AND THERAPY

Therapy for pneumonia includes specific treatment and supportive therapy. The appropriate treatment plan depends on the degree of illness, complications, and identification of the infectious agent that is causing, or probably causing, the pneumonia. In an ambulatory setting with healthy children, most cases of pneumonia can be managed on an outpatient basis. Age, severity of the illness, degree of respiratory distress, complications noted on the chest radiograph, and the ability of the family to care for the child and to assess the progression of the symptoms must all be taken into consideration in the choice of ambulatory treatment over hospitalization (Table 68–5). Infection assessed

TABLE 68–5. Factors Suggesting Need for Hospitalization of Children With Pneumonia

- Age less than 6 mo
- Toxic appearance
- Severe respiratory distress
- Requirement for supplemental oxygen
- Dehydration
- Vomiting
- No response to appropriate oral antibiotic therapy
- Immunocompromised person
- Noncompliant parents

as being caused by a virus does not require specific treatment because none is available, except for RSV pneumonia in young children with underlying cardiac or pulmonary disease or immunodeficiency (Chapter 67).

Most circumstances necessitate empirical or expectant antimicrobial treatment for a patient in whom the cause of the pneumonia has not been determined and before the results of culture or serologic testing are available. Even though most pneumonia in young children is caused by viruses, in most situations experts recommend empirical treatment for the most probable treatable bacterial causes. In the past few years many guidelines for the treatment of community-acquired pneumonia in adults and children have been developed that take into consideration the likely causes of pneumonia at different ages. Guidelines for adults (Niederman et al, 1993; Bartlett et al, 1998) are comprehensive but do not address the particular diagnostic and etiologic problems of pediatric patients. A comprehensive guide (Jadavji et al, 1997) has been developed for treatment of community-acquired pneumonias in children beyond the neonatal period in which infection due to bacteria, *Chlamydia,* or *Mycoplasma* is suspected (Table 68–1). These recommendations are based on the expected antimicrobial activity of agents against the pathogens that cause pneumonia at different ages and call for the selection of antibiotics that stress safety, moderate cost, and effectiveness against several likely pathogens. Once the specific cause of pneumonia is identified, definitive therapy can be provided (Table 68–6).

TABLE 68–6. Antimicrobial Therapy for Pneumonia in Children*

Pathogen	Recommended Treatment	Alternative Treatment
Streptococcus pneumoniae	Penicillin G *or* penicillin V	Cefuroxime *or* Cefuroxime axetil *or* Erythromycin *or* Vancomycin
Group A *Streptococcus*	Penicillin G *or* penicillin V	Cefuroxime *or* Cefuroxime axetil *or* Erythromycin
Haemophilus influenzae type b	Amoxicillin *or* ampicillin	Cefuroxime *or* Cefuroxime axetil
Mycoplasma pneumoniae	Erythromycin	Clarithromycin *or* Azithromycin *or* Doxycycline†
Group B *Streptococcus*	Penicillin G	
Gram-negative aerobic bacilli (except *Pseudomonas*)	Cefotaxime (*or* ceftriaxone) *with or without* an aminoglycoside	Ampicillin *or* piperacillin-tazobactam *plus* an aminoglycoside‡
Pseudomonas aeruginosa	Ceftazidime *with or without* an aminoglycoside‡	Piperacillin-tazobactam *plus* an aminoglycoside‡
Staphylococcus aureus	Nafcillin *or* oxacillin	Vancomycin
Legionella	Erythromycin	Azithromycin *or* clarithromycin
Chlamydia trachomatis	Erythromycin	Sulfisoxazole (*or* TMP-SMZ)
Respiratory syncytial virus	Ribavirin (see Chapter 67)	

*Oral outpatient therapy should be used for mild illness. Intravenous inpatient therapy should be used for moderate to severe illness.
†Not recommended for children younger than 9 years of age.
‡Dosing should be guided by laboratory determination of serum antibiotic concentrations once a steady state has been reached.

Suggested Dosages for Patients with Normal Renal Function

ANTIBIOTIC	DOSAGE	MAXIMUM DAILY DOSE
Amikacin	15 mg/kg/day divided q8–12hr IV	15 mg/kg
Amoxicillin	40–80 mg/kg/day divided q8hr PO	1.5 g
Ampicillin	100–200 mg/kg/day divided q6hr IV	12 g
Azithromycin	5–12 mg/kg/day once daily PO	500 mg once, then 250 mg once daily
Cefotaxime	100 mg/kg/day divided q6hr IV or IM	12 g
Cefuroxime	150 mg/kg/day divided q8hr IV	4.5 g
Cefuroxime axetil	30–40 mg/kg/day divided q12hr PO	1 g
Ceftazidime	100–150 mg/kg/day divided q8hr IV	6 g
Ceftriaxone	100 mg/kg/day divided q12hr IV	2–4 g
	or 80 mg/kg/day q24hr IV	2–4 g

ANTIBIOTIC	DOSAGE	MAXIMUM DAILY DOSE
Clarithromycin	15 mg/kg/day divided q12hr PO	1 g
Doxycycline	2–4 mg/kg/day divided q12hr PO	0.2 g
Erythromycin	25–50 mg/kg/day divided q6hr PO	2 g
Gentamicin	7.5 mg/kg/day divided q8hr IV	Adults: 5 mg/kg
Nafcillin	150 mg/kg/day q4–6hr IV	9 g
Oxacillin	150–200 mg/kg/day q4–6hr IV	12 g
Penicillin G	100,000 U/kg divided q4hr IV	12 MU
Penicillin V	50–100 mg/kg/day divided q6hr PO	2 g
Piperacillin-tazobactam	200–300 mg/kg/day divided q6hr IV	12 g
Tobramycin	7.5 mg/kg/day divided q8hr IV	Adults: 5 mg/kg
Vancomycin	45–60 mg/kg/day divided q6–8hr IV	2 g

Neonates. The most common agents of pneumonia in neonates are those that also cause neonatal sepsis and meningitis, so the usual antimicrobial therapy for neonatal sepsis is also acceptable for empirical treatment of pneumonia in the first weeks of life (Chapter 96). Ampicillin plus an aminoglycoside, such as gentamicin, is an acceptable empirical combination unless strains of bacteria resistant to these agents are known to be common in the community. An antistaphylococcal agent is added if nosocomial infection is likely or there are particular features or cultures suggesting staphylococcal pneumonia. Staphylococcal infections in infants are uncommon earlier than the second week of life. The use of a third-generation cephalosporin, such as cefotaxime, is an acceptable alternative in place of the aminoglycoside for empirical therapy for neonatal pneumonia, but routine empirical use may promote spread of resistant strains of bacteria in the neonatal ICU. Neonates in whom pneumonia develops after they leave the nursery and who are readmitted to the hospital at the age of 2–4 weeks may be infected with the same bacterial pathogens as those who have pneumonia soon after birth. The use of a third-generation cephalosporin, such as cefotaxime, as empirical therapy for bacterial pneumonia under these circumstances is acceptable because it is not likely that a neonate readmitted to the hospital with apparent pneumonia has a noninfectious lung disorder.

Older Infants to Preschool-Age Children. Infants 4–18 weeks of age without fever but with cough, excess secretions, and radiologic evidence of air trapping are likely to have *C. trachomatis* pneumonia. Erythromycin (Tables 68–1 and 68–6) is the empirical antibiotic of choice unless other findings suggest another etiologic factor.

Antibiotic therapy for likely bacterial agents of pneumonia in young children with fever should be active against the encapsulated bacteria *S. pneumoniae* and *H. influenzae.* Amoxicillin is acceptable for outpatient therapy, but ampicillin-resistant *H. influenzae* is not susceptible to this agent. There is minimal likelihood of *H. influenzae* type b pneumonia in children immunized with conjugate *H. influenzae* type b vaccine, but pneumonia due to non–type b and nontypeable strains continues to occur. Cefuroxime, oral third-generation cephalosporins such as cefpodoxime, amoxicillin-clavulanic acid, the newer macrolides, and cotrimoxazole (trimethoprim-sulfamethoxazole [TMP-SMZ]) provide activity against amoxicillin- and ampicillin-resistant strains but have not been shown to be superior to amoxicillin in the outpatient empirical treatment of childhood pneumonia. For severely ill children who require hospitalization, broader-spectrum agents are appropriate. Cefuroxime is active against *H. influenzae,* community-acquired *Staphylococcus,* group A *Streptococcus,* and *S. pneumoniae* and is of moderate cost. Chloramphenicol, either alone or with an antistaphylococcal penicillin, provides coverage similar to cefuroxime but is rarely justified for empirical therapy for childhood pneumonia in developed countries because of concerns about dose-related bone-marrow toxicity and rare bone-marrow aplasia.

Children and Adolescents. *M. pneumoniae* is a common cause of pneumonia in children, beginning at about the age of 5 years. It has become difficult to choose a single first-choice antimicrobial agent that treats *Mycoplasma* as well as the bacterial species that cause pneumonia at this age because of the rising rate of antibiotic resistance of bacterial respiratory pathogens. Azithromycin and clarithromycin have activity similar to erythromycin but with fewer gastrointestinal adverse events and easier dosing schedules. Problems with these agents include lack of evidence of efficacy against *H. influenzae* and a rising rate of resistance of *S. pneumoniae,* in some areas approximating 15%. Amoxicillin is also a time-honored choice to cover most bacterial agents in ambulatory patients, but it is not active against *Mycoplasma,* ampicillin-resistant *H. influenzae,* and penicillin/ampicillin-resistant *S. pneumoniae,* although clinical response remains good in adults with penicillin intermediate-resistant pneumococcal pneumonia (Pallares et al., 1995). On the basis of pharmacokinetic considerations, an increased dose of amoxicillin (80 mg/kg/day) may be more active against intermediate-resistant pneumococci. Clinical findings and a chest radiograph are often used to determine whether the pneumonia is likely to be bacterial or nonbacterial (viral or *Mycoplasma*), guiding the choice of a β-lactam agent for the former or a macrolide for the latter.

BACTERIAL PNEUMONIA

STREPTOCOCCUS PNEUMONIAE PNEUMONIA

ETIOLOGY

S. pneumoniae, the agent of pneumococcal pneumonia, is a gram-positive coccus in which the cocci appear on Gram stain to be **lancet shaped;** they often appear in pairs, and there are some short chains (Plate 1B). There are at least 90 serotypes based on the antigenicity and chemistry of the capsular carbohydrates. In children in developed countries, serotypes 4, 6, 14, 18, 19, and 23, known as the **pediatric serotypes,** are the most common isolates, but predominant types vary geographically and may shift over time.

S. pneumoniae isolated from the throats of healthy persons is considered to represent the asymptomatic carrier state. The carrier state is so common (present in up to one fourth of children at a given time) that isolation of *S. pneumoniae* by throat culture is not considered diagnostic of infection in children with pharyngitis, otitis media, sinusitis, pneumonia, or other infections.

Transmission. Pneumococcal pneumonia is a sporadic endemic infection, with spread of *S. pneumoniae* from person to person by droplets of respiratory secretions from close contacts. In poorly ventilated, crowded conditions, the rates of transmission are high. Thus, institutions for the elderly, poorly ventilated mines, crowded hospitals, and winter conditions are associated with high rates of transmission and infection.

EPIDEMIOLOGY

Young children are susceptible to many types of pneumococcal infections, including occult bacteremia, otitis media, sinusitis, pneumonia, and meningitis. *S. pneumoniae* is the most common cause of bacterial pneumonia beyond the neonatal period. The peak incidence of invasive infection, and pneumonia, caused by *S. pneumoniae* is in the first 2 years of life (Fig. 68–2). The incidence drops during childhood and rises continuously during adulthood and old age. Despite the high incidence during the first 2 years of life, *S. pneumoniae* is a relatively uncommon cause of infection in neonates.

Antibody-mediated immunity plays an important role in the age-specific rate phenomenon and in the pathogenesis of pneumococcal pneumonia. The specific **capsular carbohydrates,** sometimes referred to as **soluble specific substances,** are antiphagocytic. Protective antibodies are directed toward the capsular carbohydrates and are type-specific and opsonic. It was observed in the 1930s that infants are usually born with transplacentally transported IgG antibodies from the mother directed toward the specific carbohydrates; this affords considerable protection in the first few months of life. The level of maternal IgG diminishes in the first few months of life, leaving the infant relatively antibody deficient and susceptible to infection due to *S. pneumoniae* as well as other encapsulated bacteria. Throughout childhood the mean levels of antibody to *S. pneumoniae* increase until adult levels are reached in the preadolescent years. Type-specific protective antibodies develop in persons with the infection, so they can still be infected with pneumococcal strains of other serotypes. The concept of protective antibodies to the specific capsular carbohydrates led to the development of the original pneumococcal vaccine and the recently introduced conjugate pneumococcal vaccine.

It is likely that carriers of *S. pneumoniae* aspirate pneumococci, but normal hosts either expectorate them or they are ingested and killed by phagocytic macrophages in the lung. In the presence of viral respiratory tract infection, lung trauma, or immunodeficiency, however, the underlying condition predisposes the host to pneumococcal infection. Immune defects associated with repeated pneumococcal infections include severe combined immunodeficiency; agammaglobulinemia; isolated low IgG, IgA, or isotype combinations; dysgammaglobulinemias, in which large amounts of nonfunctional IgG are produced (e.g., multiple myeloma and HIV infection); and complement deficiencies. Pneumococcal infections, including pneumonia, may be the first clue of HIV infection. The spleen is important in host defense against *S. pneumoniae,* and persons with congenital absence of the spleen, who have undergone splenectomy, or who have systemic illnesses that affect the spleen, especially sickle cell disease and Hodgkin's disease, are very susceptible to pneumococcal infections. Invasive pneumococcal infections are a major problem for children younger than 5 years with sickle cell disease. Prophylactic antibiotics are used to prevent pneumococcal infections in such children. Empirical antibiotic treatment of fever, pneumonia, or overwhelming infection in such children should always include an antibiotic with excellent activity against *S. pneumoniae.*

PATHOGENESIS

S. pneumoniae infection results in inflammation of the lungs characterized by alveolar fluid, infiltration with fibrin and polymorphonuclear leukocytes, and increased blood flow, which combine to bring about consolidation. The affected areas are poorly oxygenated and stiff, resulting in some degree of respiratory compromise. Plugging of small airways and alveolar spaces with thick exudate reduces the surface for gas exchange. Severe loss of surface for gas exchange causes a reduction in oxygenation of the blood. This process is exacerbated by hyperemia of the affected lung, so there is an increase of blood flow in areas where gas exchange is poor, resulting in further hypoxia. Additional insult may occur when lymphatic spread of infection causes pleural effusion or empyema, which may further reduce tidal volume due to lung compression, and splinting because of pleuritic chest pain. The infection also may spread to the bloodstream. Breakup of the consolidated tissues is the result of intracellular digestion of phagocytosed material by macrophages, digestion by exuded cellular enzymes, and expectoration of sputum. After spontaneous resolution or treatment with antibiotics, the inflammatory processes are reversed, and normal oxygenation and compliance return to the involved tissue.

SYMPTOMS AND CLINICAL MANIFESTATIONS

The incubation period of pneumococcal pneumonia is short, only 1–3 days, often with a mild prodrome of upper respiratory symptoms. The symptoms attributable to pneumonia occur abruptly; chills, high fever, a hacking cough, and chest pain are the most common. Older children may also cough up rust-colored sputum. A physical examination may reveal evidence of consolidation in the lung, but in the small child this may not be appreciated. A chest radiograph at this time may demonstrate an area of consolidation in the lung. If not treated, the infection may spread to involve an entire lobe or several lobes. After a stormy course the infection ends in death or cessation of symptoms, sometimes termed **crisis** to describe this stage in the progression of pneumococcal pneumonia, and resolution, sometimes termed **lysis.** Antibiotic treatment dramatically shortens the clinical course. Bronchopneumonia has a less dramatic onset and is more like that of viral pneumonia. Pneumonia in the periphery of the lung may cause pleural inflammation and effusion. The effusions are often sterile and, if small, do not influence the course of the disease significantly. Effusions may be large and require drainage, and there may be a grossly purulent empyema (Chapter 69).

DIAGNOSIS

Physical findings or radiographic evidence of pneumonia accompanied by a culture of the blood, spinal fluid, percutaneous aspirate from the lung, or pleural fluid that grows *S. pneumoniae* are diagnostic. The blood culture is positive in approximately 50% of cases of pneumococcal pneumonia. A latex agglutination test that is positive for pneumococcal antigen in the blood, pleural fluid, or urine is also considered evidence of pneumococcal infection. A good-quality sputum culture that shows a predominance of gram-positive, lancet-shaped diplococci on Gram stain from which *S. pneumoniae* is the predominant organism recovered is reasonably diagnostic (Plate 1B). Latex agglutination can be used in specialized laboratories to serotype pneumococcal isolates.

Leukocytosis, high ESR, and positive CRP, either alone or in combination, have been suggested to indicate a greater likelihood of bacterial rather than viral infection, although these laboratory findings are not highly specific.

Diagnostic Imaging

The classic radiographic appearance of bacterial pneumonia in general and pneumococcal pneumonia in particular is lobar consolidation (see Figs. 13–10 and 13–11), but pneumococcal pneumonia may also present as a bronchopneumonia. Occasionally the lobar consolidation appears to result in a rounded radiographic density known as a **round pneumonia** (see Fig. 13–12).

TREATMENT

Most isolates of *S. pneumoniae* are very susceptible to all β-lactam antibiotics (e.g., penicillins, cephalosporins). Penicillin is generally considered to be the drug of choice (Table 68–6) because it is the least expensive and most active antibiotic against this species (MIC $<0.05\ \mu g/mL$) and has proven efficacy. Oral penicillin V is appropriate for mild to moderately ill children who can take an oral medication. Penicillin G, preferably given intravenously, is appropriate for children who require hospitalization. Other penicillins, such as ampicillin, amoxicillin, the antistaphylococcal penicillins, and the broad-spectrum penicillins, are also active and effective, but they offer no advantage and need not be used if the diagnosis is certain. The cephalosporins are also effective and can be used for persons with hypersensitivity to penicillins, although rare serious cross-reactions have been reported. Alternative agents with good efficacy include erythromycin, azithromycin, clarithromycin, vancomycin, and clindamycin. While not approved for use in children, the newer quinolone antibiotics are very active against pneumococci.

Antibiotic Resistance. The patterns and prevalence of drug-resistant *S. pneumoniae* vary geographically and temporally. **Intermediate-resistant strains** (MIC of 0.1—1 μg/mL of penicillin), also known as **relatively resistant strains,** have been reported with low but increasing prevalence worldwide since 1967 and were only sporadically reported until the 1980s. **High-level-resistant strains** (MIC >1 μg/mL of penicillin) have been reported since 1977, with frequent resistance to multiple antibiotics. Intermediate and high-level resistance of pneumococci has not been associated with the production of β-lactamases but with the alteration in **penicillin-binding proteins,** the cell membrane-associated enzymes that are responsible for cell wall assembly and that bind penicillin. In the past few years the incidence of infections caused by resistant strains and prevalence of resistance in colonization has increased considerably and alarmingly. Rates of resistance from 12% to >50% have been reported, with the higher rates among young children and isolates from middle ear fluid. It appears that resistant clones have spread throughout the world, although the rates of resistance vary considerably in different countries.

The cause of the increase of antibiotic resistance is unclear but is probably multifactorial. There is some evidence that prior exposure to antibiotics is a risk factor for infection caused by resistant strains and may play an important role in rising rates of resistance. The exceptional risk of children and the high prevalence of pediatric serotypes among resistant strains provide evidence that indiscriminate use of antibiotics for children with viral upper respiratory tract infections may be a major factor driving this epidemic.

In studies of patients with pneumococcal pneumonia from whom resistant strains were isolated, only strains with an MIC of penicillin of >2 μg/mL were resistant to treatment with high-dose penicillin in vivo.

All clinically significant *S. pneumoniae* isolates should be routinely checked for susceptibility. In one study of adults (Pallares et al, 1995) patients with pneumonia caused by intermediate resistant strains responded well to high-dose penicillin, and only pneumonia caused by strains with MIC >2 μg/mL did not respond clinically. Only in meningitis, where there is a borderline concentration of antibiotic killing activity in the cerebrospinal fluid, is there evidence that these less susceptible strains necessitate a change in therapy (Chapter 52). There are several alternatives to penicillin for treatment of high-level resistant *S. pneumoniae.* These strains are frequently susceptible to cephalosporins, including cefuroxime and third-generation cephalosporins such as ceftriaxone or cefotaxime. Even multiply-resistant strains have all remained susceptible to vancomycin.

COMPLICATIONS

The complications of pneumococcal pneumonia include effusion and empyema (Chapter 69), septicemia, meningitis, and rarely endocarditis. It is generally assumed that early recognition and treatment reduce the chances of complications. In very acute, virulent infections, however, the complications may be present when the patient first presents. Children whose conditions appear to deteriorate despite appropriate supportive and antibiotic therapy should be suspected of having either resistant strains of *S. pneumoniae* or one of these complications.

PROGNOSIS

Children without any underlying chronic disease usually respond well to treatment of pneumococcal pneumonia. Deaths or permanent sequelae are rare. Studies of adults with bacteremic pneumococcal infections show that the mortality in the first 4 days of treatment is not lower in the antibiotic era than it was in the preantibiotic era. It is assumed that when there is overwhelming disease, neither antibiotics nor contemporary critical care can save certain patients. There have been no similar studies of children, but septicemia, especially when accompanied by immunodeficiency or asplenia, still has a high mortality.

PREVENTION

Pneumococcal pneumonia can be prevented or minimized in certain high-risk populations with the use of vaccine and prophylactic penicillin. Pneumococcal vaccine (Chapter 17) containing the polysaccharides of 23 serotypes is effective in the elderly and in children older than 2 years of age who are predisposed to pneumococcal infection because of immunodeficiency, asplenia, or other chronic diseases. Children younger than 2 years of age do not respond to vaccination with pneumococcal polysaccharide vaccine. Recently a seven-serotype conjugate vaccine, which is highly protective against invasive disease, has been approved for universal immunization of infants. Limited data show reduction in pneumococcal pneumonia among recipients. Penicillin (125 mg penicillin V twice a day orally) has been shown to reduce the incidence of pneumococcal infections in children 3 months to 5 years of age with sickle cell disease (Chapter 101). Presumably, it is effective in other immunodeficient states.

LEGIONELLOSIS

Legionella pneumophila was determined to be the previously undiscovered agent responsible for an outbreak of pneumonia in attendees at an American Legion convention in Philadelphia in 1976; hence pneumonia caused by this species has been termed **legionnaires' disease.** Other *Legionella* may occasionally cause human disease. For reasons not yet discovered, pulmonary infection with this agent is rare in children, and there is little information about the disease in pediatrics.

ETIOLOGY

Legionella pneumophila is a small, faintly staining, aerobic gram-negative bacillus. It is found in the environment, mostly in lakes, bath water, and tap water. High concentrations of *L. pneumophila* can be found in aerosols from water tanks and from air conditioner cooling towers.

There are more than 40 species within the genus *Legionella.* Approximately 85% of legionellosis is caused by *L. pneumophila.* Many other species, such as *L. micdadei,* also known as the **Pittsburgh pneumonia agent,** have been associated with outbreaks of respiratory infection in adults. *L. bozemanii* has been isolated from human lung tissue, and outbreaks of disease due to *L. dumoffii* and *L. feeleii* have been described. No information is available about the importance of these other *Legionella* species in pediatrics.

Transmission. Because the reservoir of *L. pneumophila* is the environment and human-to-human spread is not known to occur, susceptibility factors are primarily contact with contaminated air or water.

EPIDEMIOLOGY

Epidemics of legionnaires' disease have been attributed to aerosols from cooling towers and from contaminated tap water in hotels, cruise ships, office buildings, and hospitals. As with many organisms that cause atypical (nonlobar) pneumonia, studies of the prevalence of serum antibodies show that only a small fraction of persons with antibody have recognized pneumonia or illness caused by this agent. The manifestations of disease for persons who have seroconverted without having had frank legionnaires' disease is unknown, but some have had the variant of fever and influenza-like symptoms without pneumonia, known as **Pontiac fever.** This applies especially to children, because the evidence of infection in children is mostly the presence of antibodies found in seroprevalence surveys. When paired sera of children with atypical pneumonia have been tested, fewer than 4% have shown rises in titers for *L. pneumophila.* However, simultaneous cultures for the organism have not been performed, so evidence that even this small number of infections in children is truly *Legionella* pneumonia is poor. The prevalence of antibodies in the sera of children increases with age, possibly indicating that subclinical or nonspecific mild infections due to this agent are not uncommon. Because clinical information is scarce, the possibility remains that the antibody being measured in some cases is cross-reacting antibody to the antigen of another species of microorganism.

There are few well-documented cases in children. One report (Carlson et al, 1990) documented three culture-documented cases among young children with underlying pulmonary disease and severe, complicated pneumonia and reviewed 16 culture- or antigen-positive cases in the literature, mostly among immunocompromised children. Another review (Holmberg et al., 1993) of nosocomial cases in neonates found that most had been born prematurely or were immunocompromised. Nursery outbreaks have been associated with contaminated air or water. In adults, immunosuppression is also a major risk factor for the development of *Legionella* pneumonia. Clusters of disease in hospitals show that immunocompromised patients have a much higher rate of legionellosis than other patients.

PATHOGENESIS

Legionellosis results from inhalation of aerosolized bacteria from environmental sources. The organism multiplies within monocytes in the lung and resists microbicidal oxidation within the cell. The organism produces several potential toxins, but their role in the manifestations of disease is not known.

The lung in legionnaires' disease shows a predominance of inflammation and fluid accumulation in terminal airways and alveoli. The disease may evolve to a focal or lobar pattern with consolidation similar to that seen in other bacterial pneumonias. Pulmonary cavities have been reported in severe cases. Extrapulmonary foci of infection occur almost exclusively in immunocompromised persons.

SYMPTOMS AND CLINICAL MANIFESTATIONS

The characterization of legionnaires' disease is based on experience with adult patients. The typical syndrome in children has yet to be defined because reported cases are at the severe end of the clinical spectrum.

The incubation period of *L. pneumophila* has been reported to be 2–14 days, followed by multisystem disease with considerable malaise and a characteristic respiratory disease. Atypical (nonlobar) pneumonia with a very high fever, up to 40.5°C (105°F), and tachypnea are the predominant findings. Other symptoms frequently include a cough, which may be productive or nonproductive, chills, pleuritic chest pain, and gastrointestinal symptoms such as abdominal pain and diarrhea that are reported in 20–40% of cases. Less frequent findings that may suggest the diagnosis of legionnaires' disease include such symptoms as confusion, headache, and lethargy and lack of response to treatment with β-lactam antibiotics.

Pontiac Fever. Another form of disease caused by *L. pneumophila* is fever and malaise but without pneumonia. This form is called Pontiac fever because of an epidemic of this disease in Pontiac, Michigan, where infection was diagnosed retrospectively with the use of paired sera from affected patients.

Physical Examination Findings

The physical findings are quite variable. A **pulse-temperature deficit** (the pulse rate increase does not mirror the degree of fever) is common. There may be no respiratory findings, or there may be signs of consolidation with dullness to percussion and rales, or a pleural rub. Pulmonary cavitation has been described in immunocompromised persons.

DIAGNOSIS

Routine laboratory studies are of little help in establishing the diagnosis of legionnaire's disease. There are no characteristic laboratory values. The WBC count may be high, low, or normal. Blood gas determinations may show hypoxia, which is related to the severity of the disease.

Microbiologic Evaluation

Legionnaires' disease is best diagnosed in patients with atypical pneumonia by growing the organism from culture of sputum or by visualizing the organism in a specimen using a **direct fluorescent antibody (DFA).** Culture is 100% specific but insensitive, with only approximately 40–60% sensitivity. DFA is highly specific and should be considered diagnostic if performed by experienced laboratory personnel. When inexperienced technologists perform the test, false-positive staining of other organisms may occur, so confirmation by culture is always advised. A Gram stain of the sputum should be performed if there is an adequate sample, but the organisms are sparse and stain lightly, so they may not be visualized.

Cultures are performed with the use of buffered (pH 6.9–7.0) charcoal yeast extract agar. Antibiotics may be added to the medium to suppress contaminating normal flora. The organism takes 2–7 days to grow. The organism is fastidious in its growth, and not all laboratories are able to provide culture. In such a case the specimen of sputum should be sent to a referral laboratory. DFA and culture can also be used to identify the organism in lung tissue specimens collected by biopsy or postmortem examination.

Detection of *Legionella* antigen in the urine by RIA or EIA is perhaps the most sensitive diagnostic method (approximately 60–80% sensitivity); it is specific and generally available. PCR-based tests have been developed and are available in some centers.

Serologic Testing. Serologic tests are performed mainly by means of an immunofluorescence assay, which has been used extensively in serologic surveys. Serologic testing should include both IgM and IgG responses. Serologic diagnosis can be established on paired acute and convalescent samples, taken 4–8 weeks apart, if there is a fourfold or greater rise in titer. A single convalescent titer of 1:256 is suggestive of legionellosis.

Diagnostic Imaging

There is no distinctive appearance on chest radiography. The typical radiographic finding of legionnaires' pneumonia is a patchy bronchopneumonia, which may progress to consolidation and may involve one or many lobes of the lung. Pleural effusions occur in as many as one third of patients. Uncommon manifestations include the development of nodules, abscess, cavitation, and hilar lymphadenopathy.

TREATMENT

Recommendations for antibiotic treatment are derived mainly from retrospective analyses of patients treated during outbreaks, and therefore some degree of selection bias cannot be excluded. Appropriate antibiotic treatment, however, appears to reduce the mortality from 15–20% to 5–10%. The mainstay of treatment has been erythromycin at an adult dose of 1 g every 6 hours intravenously, or 500 mg every 6 hours orally (Table 68–6). Alternative choices include azithromycin, clarithromycin, tetracycline, TMP-SMZ, and rifampin in appropriate doses for pneumonia. Quinolones, such as ciprofloxacin or levofloxacin, are recommended for adults, especially for transplant recipients, but data in children are lacking. Treatment is generally for 10–14 days, but longer treatment for 21 days is sometimes recommended in severe or complicated cases. There is no evidence that Pontiac fever, which is a self-limited disease, improves with antibiotic treatment.

PROGNOSIS

For healthy persons who are given appropriate antibiotics, the response is rapid and the prognosis is good, with the overall mortality about 5%. Legionnaires' disease is more frequently a life-threatening illness for debilitated persons who are immunosuppressed than it is for other persons. There are too few reports of pediatric cases for an evaluation of prognosis.

PREVENTION

Because *L. pneumophila* is frequently spread from a water source to humans by aerosols and causes outbreaks of infection, a considerable proportion of the disease can be prevented by disinfecting water sources, especially cooling towers, that harbor organisms found by surveillance cultures. Hospitals should institute surveillance if there is evidence of nosocomial infection. Approved methods of disinfection include treatment with calcium hypochlorite, hyperchlorination, and quaternary ammonium compounds and raising the temperature of water reservoirs to >70°C.

Antibiotic prophylaxis for exposed persons has not been rigorously tested and ordinarily would not be warranted, although erythromycin prophylaxis during outbreaks has been attempted. During outbreaks, the appropriate public health authorities should be asked to investigate the source of bacteria.

MYCOPLASMA PNEUMONIAE PNEUMONIA

ETIOLOGY

Mycoplasma species are free-living organisms that lack a cell wall and require special media for cultivation. In 1940, *M. pneumoniae* was recovered by Monroe Eaton, and the organism was referred to as **Eaton agent.** There are many species of *Mycoplasma* other than *M. pneumoniae,* but other human species do not cause respiratory disease, and humans are not subject to infection by animal *Mycoplasma* species. *M. pneumoniae* causes pneumonia as well as upper airway infections, including pharyngitis and tracheobronchitis, and central nervous system infections and is associated with rashes and a variety of syndromes in which pneumonia may or may not be present.

Transmission. *M. pneumoniae* is transmitted from person to person by inhalation of infected droplet aerosols. Because the incubation period lasts 2–3 weeks, it has been difficult to appreciate the contagious nature of this infection in sporadic community-acquired infections.

EPIDEMIOLOGY

Studies from the 1960s showed *Mycoplasma* to be the most common cause of atypical or nonlobar pneumonia. Subsequent studies showed that children older than 5 years of age and young adults were most commonly affected, with a peak at 6–21 years of age, although infection is frequently found in younger children as well. These characteristics contrast with *S. pneumoniae,* for which the peak incidence of pneumonia is in the first 2 years of life and in old age.

Although *M. pneumoniae* causes approximately 20% of all pneumonias, only about 3% of all infections due to *M. pneumoniae* result in clinically apparent pneumonia. The annual incidence of mycoplasmal pneumonia is 3 per 1,000 population. Antibody is partially protective. Infections in persons with pre-existing antibody are less severe than in those without antibody, and the attack rate among persons with pre-existing antibody with the same exposure is one third that among those without antibody. Studies of seroconversion in children demonstrate that infections are common in the preschool years but that they are not usually associated with pneumonia.

PATHOGENESIS

After inhalation, the organism attaches to and colonizes the respiratory mucosa and multiplies in the upper respiratory tract. Little is known about how the organism spreads within the respiratory tract or how spread beyond the respiratory tract results in manifestations of disease in the central nervous system, skin, and other organs. In the respiratory tract the organism injures epithelial cells and disturbs organized ciliary motility. The immune response to the organism recruits phagocytes and complement. It may be that this inflammatory response is responsible for some of the clinical signs and symptoms of *Mycoplasma* pneumonia.

SYMPTOMS AND CLINICAL MANIFESTATIONS

The most distinctive characteristic of *M. pneumoniae* is the long prodrome and incubation period. After an incubation period of 2–3 weeks there is a gradual onset of headache, sore throat, fever, and malaise for about 1 week. The disease may resolve at that point, or it may go on to involve the lower respiratory tract with a nonproductive cough, rales, and an abnormal chest radiograph. Coughing is an indicator of damage to the bronchial epithelium and dyskinesis of the cilia; it may persist for many weeks, even after the physical and radiographic findings of pneumonia have resolved. It is presumed that the cough continues because the organism develops a specific attachment to the respiratory mucosa.

In general, pneumonia caused by *M. pneumoniae,* compared with pneumonia due to *S. pneumoniae,* is more insidious in onset, less severe, and more likely to have a bronchopneumonia pattern on a chest radiograph without physical signs of consolidation. Signs and symptoms are indistinguishable from other atypical pneumonias, including those caused by *Chlamydia pneumoniae.* Some infections exhibit the common characteristics of *S. pneumoniae* pneumonia, including consolidation and pleural effusion. These cases often come to attention because they are thought to be pneumococcal pneumonia but do not respond to β-lactam antibiotics.

DIAGNOSIS

Laboratory Evaluation

The WBC count is usually normal but may be elevated. The ESR may be normal or elevated, and CRP may be present. Because T cell immunity is suppressed, skin tests for mycobacterial or fungal infection are unreliable and may yield false-negative reactions.

Microbiologic Evaluation

Examination of the sputum may show large numbers of polymorphonuclear leukocytes, but bacteria are either absent or sparse and are of mixed morphologies.

Because a long-term carrier state is not characteristic of *M. pneumoniae* infection, isolation of the agent from the throat is considered to be diagnostic of infection. Growth of the organism requires special hypertonic media, and recognition of the tiny colonies that take weeks to grow requires expertise generally found only in reference laboratories. Demonstration of the organism by PCR is reported to be both sensitive and specific and has promise, although results have been variable with a commercial test. In most practices, serologic diagnosis is more practical and rapid than a culture, although not as sensitive or specific.

Serologic Testing. Two types of serologic test are available, nonspecific and specific. The nonspecific test is **cold hemagglutination,** for detection of **cold agglutinins.** Infection with *M. pneumoniae* induces an IgM autoantibody to the I component of the red blood cell surface membrane. In the presence of these cold agglutinins, erythrocytes agglutinate at 4°C (39.2°F) but not at room temperature. A high titer of cold agglutinins is probably responsible for the hemolytic anemia that sometimes accompanies *M. pneumoniae* infections. A single cold agglutinin titer of ≥1:32 is suggestive of *M. pneumoniae* infection, although a single higher titer or a fourfold rise or fall in titer during convalescence is more specific. EBV and CMV infectious mononucleosis and other viral infections can induce cold agglutinins. A simple **bedside test for cold agglutinins** can be performed by placing four drops of whole blood in a tube with an equal volume of sodium citrate (light-blue-stopper Vacutainer tube). Before cooling, the blood forms a smooth coating of the tube. After incubation on crushed ice for 3–4 minutes, macroscopic hemagglutination is demonstrated when the tube is held up to the light and rotated by cell clumping in the thin film of blood that clings to the tube. The clumping must disappear when the tube is warmed to 37°C, as when held in the hands, and return on reincubation in ice. Although nonquantitative, this test generally correlates with a cold agglutination titer of ≥1:64.

A more specific and presumptive diagnosis is established by complement fixation, IFA, or ELISA detection of a specific antimycoplasmal antibody response, which appears later and remains elevated longer than cold agglutinin antibodies. One of these specific tests should be performed even if the cold agglutinin antibody titer is elevated. A single positive specific antibody titer and a cold hemagglutination titer of ≥1:64 or paired sera showing a fourfold or greater rise of antimycoplasmal antibody are considered diagnostic. Tests that measure specific IgM antibody, such as the IgM ELISA, correlate with recent infection but are insensitive and may be negative for the first 7–10 days of infection.

Diagnostic Imaging

The radiographic findings vary from patient to patient, but a lower lobe interstitial infiltrate or bronchopneumonia is common (Fig. 68–3). The radiographic appearance is similar to that of pneumonia caused by other agents, such as *Chlamydia pneumoniae* and respiratory viruses. Findings similar to a pneumococcal pneumonia with lobar consolidation and pleural effusion are uncommon but may occur.

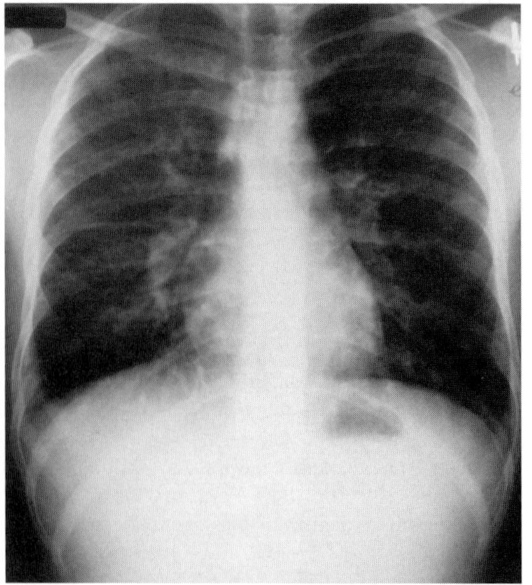

FIGURE 68–3. *Mycoplasma pneumoniae* infection (atypical pneumonia) in a 14-year-old boy with malaise, dry cough, and mild shortness of breath for 1 week. Frontal chest radiograph showing a diffuse pattern of increased interstitial markings including Kerley's lines. The heart is normal, and there are no focal infiltrates. Cold agglutinins were markedly elevated, and the patient responded to erythromycin. This radiographic pattern of reticulonodular interstitial disease is observed in 25–30% of patients with pneumonia caused by *M. pneumoniae.*

TREATMENT

M. pneumoniae is not susceptible to β-lactam antibiotics because the mode of action of these drugs is inhibition of cell wall synthesis, and mycoplasmas lack a cell wall. Erythromycin, other macrolides such as azithromycin and clarithromycin, and tetracycline and its derivatives are active in vitro. Studies in adults show a reduction in the duration of cough, fever, and hospitalization when these agents are administered early in the course of respiratory disease. Erythromycin is considered to be the drug of choice for children. There are few studies of the efficacy of treatment in children or in nonrespiratory disease caused by *M. pneumoniae.* A study of an outbreak in a summer camp (Broome et al, 1980) showed that children who were treated with erythromycin within the first 4 days of symptoms had a shorter duration of cough than those treated after more than 4 days of symptoms.

Treatment with antibiotics is usually for 2 weeks (Table 68–6). The role of corticosteroids in *Mycoplasma* pneumonia is controversial. Anecdotal literature suggests that it lessens the progression to intubation in the rare person who has respiratory failure associated with adult respiratory distress syndrome.

COMPLICATIONS

Complications of *M. pneumoniae* infection include respiratory and extrapulmonary sequelae. It is unclear whether the extrapulmonary foci of disease that accompany *M. pneumoniae* infection represent secondary spread, additional primary foci, or immunologic complications of infections. Pulmonary complications are only occasionally severe and include effusion, pneumothorax, lung abscess, and diffuse pneumonia with respiratory failure and even adult respiratory distress syndrome. Both the severity and the incidence of complications appear to be greater in immunocompromised patients, including those with sickle cell disease or who have chronic cardiopulmonary conditions, although actual incidence figures are not available.

PROGNOSIS

Complete recovery is virtually the rule in *M. pneumoniae* pneumonia, although coughing may persist for months after acute infection. There have been case reports of focal bronchiectasis, scarring, and fibrosis, but these sequelae appear to be rare.

PREVENTION

There is no licensed vaccine for the prevention of *M. pneumoniae* infection. The use of prophylactic antibiotics for exposed persons who are immunocompromised or have underlying pulmonary disease may be reasonable. Recent studies of outbreaks demonstrate the feasibility of administering macrolide antibiotics prophylactically to prevent infections. However, routine antibiotic prophylaxis is not recommended.

CHLAMYDIAL PNEUMONIA

Chlamydiae are small, obligate, intracellular, gram-negative organisms that cannot be cultured in artificial media. They were formerly considered more closely related to viruses, but they contain both DNA and RNA and have a structure similar to that of bacteria but require an intact organism, organ, or tissue culture for growth. They grow in the cytoplasm of cells and produce characteristic inclusions. These **inclusion bodies** contain small infective elementary bodies and somewhat larger, noninfectious **initial (reticulate) bodies.**

The three major chlamydial pathogens for humans all share a genus-specific lipopolysaccharide antigen, and each is capable of causing pneumonia in humans (Table 68–7). *C. trachomatis* is an agent responsible for a number of syndromes; the type of disease depends on the specific type (serovar) of *C. trachomatis.* It has been known for a long time as an agent of trachoma, lymphogranuloma venereum, and nongonococcal urethritis and cervicitis in adults and inclusion conjunctivitis and afebrile pneumonia in infants. *C. psittaci* is the agent of psittacosis, a type of acute pneumonia spread by birds. *C. pneumoniae* is an agent of acute respiratory disease, principally bronchitis and atypical pneumonia.

TABLE 68–7. Diseases Caused by *Chlamydia*

Species	Serovars	Disease
C. trachomatis	L_1–L_3	Lymphogranuloma venereum
	A, B, Ba, C	Trachoma (hyperendemic blinding)
	D–K	Inclusion conjunctivitis (newborn), neonatal pneumonia, urethritis, cervicitis, pelvic inflammatory disease
C. psittaci	Many	Acute pneumonia (psittacosis, ornithosis)
C. pneumoniae	TWAR	Acute respiratory disease

CHLAMYDIA TRACHOMATIS PNEUMONIA

ETIOLOGY

For many years there was recognition of a relationship between nongonococcal cervicitis in a mother and the development of conjunctivitis in early infancy. It was not until 1977 (Beem and Saxon, 1977) that a subacute afebrile pneumonia in young infants was recognized as another possible result of maternal transmission of serovars D–K of *C. trachomatis.* The organism is perinatally transmitted to newborns from mothers with sexually transmitted chlamydial genital infection, which is usually asymptomatic. The transmission rate from mother to infant is 50–75%.

EPIDEMIOLOGY

The demographic characteristics of infections in infants reflect those of pregnant women infected with *C. trachomatis.* In general, the prevalence of *C. trachomatis* infection among pregnant women is highest in adolescents and young women, racial minorities, women living in poverty, women with many previous sexual partners, and women with a history of sexually transmitted diseases. Among sexually active young women, carriage rates usually exceed 5%, and rates higher than 20% are reported among selected inner city populations.

The most common manifestation of disease in infants is **inclusion conjunctivitis,** which occurs in 40–50% of offspring of infected mothers (Chapter 89). The conjunctivitis may appear immediately after birth and through the first 2 weeks of life, usually from 5–14 days of age. About one half of the offspring of infected mothers have nasopharyngeal infection, but only about 30% of those exhibit the characteristic afebrile pneumonia. Thus the overall rate of symptomatic chlamydial pneumonia in offspring of infected mothers is 10–20%.

SYMPTOMS AND CLINICAL MANIFESTATIONS

The pneumonia has a gradual onset beginning at 4–18 weeks of age (median, 9 weeks). *C. trachomatis* is the most common cause of **afebrile pneumonia** in early infancy and causes 20–30% of all pneumonia among hospitalized infants younger than 6 months of age.

Chlamydial pneumonia characteristically is manifested principally by cough, congestion, and sometimes vomiting; it is slowly progressive and is not accompanied by fever. Most infants have had a prodrome lasting more than 1 week before presentation. This infection causes inflammation of all mucous membranes, with nasopharyngitis, laryngitis, tracheobronchitis, and pneumonia that may coexist or appear in any combination. There may or may not be a history of inclusion conjunctivitis.

Physical Examination Findings

Prominent signs include tachypnea and a staccato cough, often causing breathlessness, but a whoop such as that occurring with pertussis is not characteristic. Other signs frequently include crackles and findings of hyperexpanded lungs. Wheezing is rare, and fever is absent.

DIAGNOSIS

The diagnosis is usually a clinical diagnosis of a respiratory illness in infants 4–18 weeks of age, with tachypnea in the absence of fever. The diagnosis can be confirmed by culture of *C. trachomatis* from respiratory secretions, although this culture is not usually

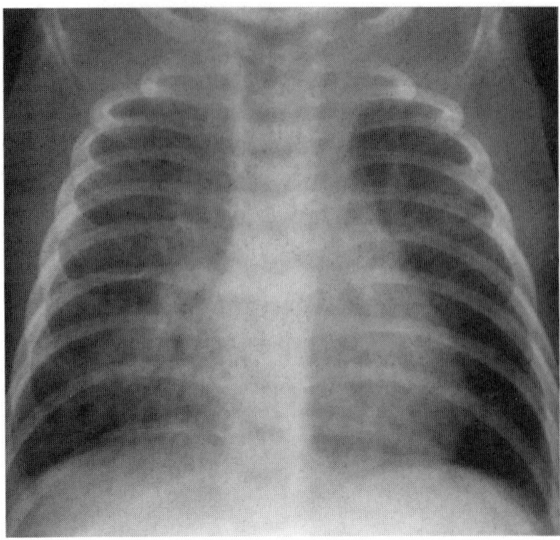

FIGURE 68–4. Frontal supine chest radiograph of a 1-month-old girl with *Chlamydia trachomatis* pneumonia. The child presented with tachypnea and cyanosis with conjunctivitis. The radiograph shows diffuse hyperinflation, bilateral interstitial infiltrates, and patchy pneumonitis of the right middle lobe.

performed. Laboratory findings may be helpful because peripheral eosinophilia, usually >300/mm^3, and hypergammaglobulinemia of all isotypes are common. No other routine laboratory tests are useful.

Microbiologic Evaluation

Culture methods require growth in an appropriately treated tissue culture. A technologist must be able to recognize the characteristic inclusions in the cytoplasm of the cells. Culture requires special transport media and special handling, is very labor intensive, requires 3–5 days of cultivation, and is not available in most clinical laboratories. Rapid (nonculture) tests for the identification of *Chlamydia* antigen have become popular. The Chlamydiazyme, an EIA test, and MicroTrak, a direct IFA, appear to be reasonably sensitive and specific for the diagnosis of chlamydial conjunctivitis when scraped conjunctival cells are tested and for chlamydial pneumonia when nasopharyngeal secretions are tested. Very high antibody titers are measurable by a highly specific IFA, but this test is rarely available at clinical facilities. PCR tests, which may be available at some clinical facilities for the diagnosis of genital infection, have not been approved for use in infant pneumonia and conjunctivitis and are not recommended.

Diagnostic Imaging

Chest radiographs show hyperexpansion of the lungs with flattened diaphragms and symmetric, patchy, ill-defined infiltrates (Fig. 68–4). Frequently the degree of infiltration in the lung appears greater than would be expected from the physical examination.

TREATMENT AND PROGNOSIS

Untreated *C. trachomatis* pneumonia of infancy rarely causes death or permanent damage to the lungs, but the disease can be quite protracted. The clinical course is shortened by treatment with erythromycin base (50 mg/kg/day divided into 4 doses orally for 10–14 days). The effectiveness of treatment with erythromycin is approximately 80%; a second course may be required. An alternative is sulfisoxazole (150 mg/kg/day divided into 4 doses orally for 10–14 days).

PREVENTION

Treatment of pregnant women who harbor *C. trachomatis* before delivery prevents transmission to their infants. The recommended treatment of infected mothers is at 36 weeks gestation with erythromycin base (500 mg 4 times a day orally for 7 days) or amoxicillin (500 mg 3 times a day orally for 7 days) (Table 85–4). Erythromycin estolate is contraindicated during pregnancy because of potential hepatotoxicity. Repeat testing of the mother is recommended, preferably by culture, because these regimens are not highly efficacious, and the frequent adverse effects of erythromycin might discourage patient adherence.

Although infants born to mothers with untreated chlamydial infections are at high risk of infection, no antibiotic regimen for infants has proven efficacy in preventing *C. trachomatis* neonatal conjunctivitis or extraocular disease, and postnatal prophylactic antibiotic treatment is not indicated. These infants should be monitored to provide appropriate treatment if symptoms develop.

The mothers (and their sex partners) of infants with chlamydial infection should be evaluated and treated for genital chlamydial infection.

CHLAMYDIA PSITTACI PNEUMONIA

ETIOLOGY

C. psittaci causes an acute pneumonia called **psittacosis, ornithosis,** or **parrot fever.** Birds are the major reservoir of *C. psittaci.* Signs of **avian chlamydiosis** include lethargy, anorexia, ruffled feathers, and serous or mucopurulent ocular or nasal discharge. Death usually results from anorexia. *C. psittaci* is excreted in the feces and nasal discharges of infected birds; it is resistant to drying and can remain infectious for several months. If infected, birds can appear healthy and shed the organism intermittently. Shedding can be activated by stress factors, including shipping, crowding, chilling, and breeding. The time between exposure to *C. psittaci* and onset of illness in birds ranges from 3 days to several weeks. However, active disease can appear years after exposure. Whether the bird exhibits acute or chronic signs of illness or dies depends on the species of bird, virulence of the strain, infectious dose, stress factors, age, and extent of treatment or prophylaxis.

Most human *C. psittaci* infections result from exposure to pet **psittacine birds** including parakeets, parrots, and macaws, especially those smuggled into the country that come from suboptimal colonies and evade examination and prophylaxis. Transmission may occur from free-ranging birds, including doves, pigeons, turkeys, birds of prey, and shore birds. Several mammalian species, including cattle, goats, sheep, and cats, as well as avian species, may become infected and develop chronic infection of the reproductive tract, leading to placental insufficiency and abortion in these animals. These strains of *C. psittaci* are transmitted to persons when they are exposed to the birth fluids and placentas of infected animals. Another strain of *C. psittaci,* **feline keratoconjunctivitis agent,** typically causes rhinitis and conjunctivitis in cats. Transmission of this strain from cats to humans rarely occurs.

Illness may also be caused by *Chlamydia pecorum,* a newly designated species formerly not distinguished from *C. psittaci.*

Transmission. Humans usually acquire *C. psittaci* by the airborne route from organisms in fecal dust of secretions of colonized birds. Person-to-person transmission from acutely ill patients, presumably via the respiratory route, has been suggested but is unproven.

EPIDEMIOLOGY

Psittacosis is worldwide in distribution and tends to occur sporadically in all seasons. Cases in the United States reported by the CDC numbered 100–200 annually in the 1980s but have decreased to fewer than 100 each year during the past decade. Some cases occur in pet store employees and among workers in poultry plants. Spread of the agent in laboratories has been reported, so isolation of this agent should not be attempted without special precautions. Infections in children are exceedingly rare because of the lack of occupational exposure.

SYMPTOMS AND CLINICAL MANIFESTATIONS

C. psittaci pneumonia usually presents after an incubation period of 1–3 weeks with a prominent, nonproductive cough, headache, malaise, chills, and fever. The severity of psittacosis ranges from inapparent illness to systemic illness with extensive interstitial pneumonia. The cough may become productive. Myalgia and arthralgia are frequent symptoms. A **pulse-temperature deficit** (the pulse rise does not mirror the degree of fever) is common. In severe cases, CNS depression, delirium, gastrointestinal symptoms, and multiorgan failure may occur. On physical examination there may be localized crackles, and occasionally there may be signs of consolidation.

DIAGNOSIS

Appropriate diagnostic tests are usually undertaken because of a history of contact with a pet bird or other bird contact. Routine laboratory tests are not helpful in establishing the diagnosis of psittacosis because there are no characteristic abnormalities. Abnormal liver function tests have been reported. A sputum examination usually shows scant cells and no bacteria.

The diagnosis of psittacosis is usually established by a serologic complement fixation test. This test is relatively specific, but rises in titer also have been reported in patients with *C. pneumoniae* infection and legionellosis. Few commercial laboratories have the capability to differentiate *Chlamydia* antibody responses. A fourfold rise in titer is considered diagnostic, or a single titer of ≥1:32 is highly suggestive of the diagnosis. Because antibiotic treatment can delay or diminish the antibody response, a third serum sample might help confirm the diagnosis. Culture of *C. psittaci* is performed by few laboratories because of technical difficulty and safety concerns of potential transmission to laboratory personnel.

Diagnostic Imaging

Chest radiographs do not differ from those of other atypical pneumonias. Patchy infiltrates are common and characteristically are more severe than would be expected from physical examination findings, but lobar involvement, though uncommon, has been reported.

TREATMENT

Tetracyclines are the drugs of choice for psittacosis. Adults are treated with doxycycline (100 mg 2 times a day orally) or tetracycline (for adults, 500 mg 4 times a day orally). For initial treatment of severely ill patients, doxycycline hyclate can be administered intravenously (4.4 mg/kg/day divided every 12 hours; maximum dose, 100 mg). Remission of symptoms usually is evident within 48–72 hours. Erythromycin is recommended for children younger than 8 years of age and for pregnant women, but there are few data on its efficacy or the optimal dosage regimen for psittacosis in children. The dosage recommended for *M. pneumoniae* pneumonia appears to be appropriate (Table 68–6). The other macrolide drugs, azithromycin and clarithromycin, as well as chloramphenicol, also are effective. Relapse can occur, and therapy should be administered for at least 10–14 days after defervescence.

COMPLICATIONS

Pericarditis, myocarditis, endocarditis, superficial thrombophlebitis, hepatitis, and encephalopathy are rare complications of psittacosis.

PROGNOSIS

With treatment the mortality for psittacosis has fallen from as high as 20% to less than 1%. Infection may not result in protective immunity.

PREVENTION

Prevention consists of elimination of the infection in birds. All birds suspected to be the source of human infection should be evaluated by a veterinarian. Birds with *C. psittaci* infection should be isolated and treated with chlortetracycline for at least 45 days. At present, imported exotic birds must undergo quarantine and treatment with chlortetracycline.

Standard infection-control precautions are sufficient for patients with psittacosis, and additional isolation procedures (e.g., private room, negative pressure air flow, and masks) are not indicated.

CHLAMYDIA PNEUMONIAE PNEUMONIA

ETIOLOGY

C. pneumoniae was first referred to as the **TWAR strain** of *C. psittaci;* TWAR was an acronym for the initials of the first two strains: TW-183 and AR-39. *C. pneumoniae* has since been determined to be distinct from other species of *Chlamydia.* Ultrastructural studies show that this species is unique in that the elementary bodies in infected cells are pear shaped, whereas other *Chlamydia* species have round elementary bodies.

Transmission. Person-to-person transmission by inhalation of infected aerosols appears to be the mode of spread. There is no known nonhuman reservoir.

EPIDEMIOLOGY

Although it has only recently been discovered, *C. pneumoniae* has emerged as a ubiquitous and important cause of respiratory disease in children and adults. It occurs throughout the year.

Serologic surveys have shown that antibody is rare in children younger than 5 years of age, but seroprevalence rises from about 10% to 30–45% during early childhood, reaching a prevalence as high as 60% among adults. The infection appears to have a wide range of clinical expressions and is especially important as a cause of pneumonia, but it may also be subclinical with asymptomatic carriage in the throat. *C. pneumoniae* is responsible for about 10–20% of cases of sporadic atypical pneumonia in children, especially in older children. It also causes exacerbations of chronic bronchitic conditions, such as childhood asthma and adult chronic obstructive pulmonary disease. Although many children have the antibody, symptomatic pneumonia appears to be a relatively uncommon expression of infection. Most infections in children younger than 5 years of age are mild or asymptomatic. Although most infections are sporadic, several outbreaks of disease have occurred among closed populations of adolescents and young adults.

A recent multicenter report (Vischinsky et al., 2000) shows that *C. pneumoniae* is the most common cause of **acute chest syndrome** in sickle cell disease, especially among older children.

SYMPTOMS AND CLINICAL MANIFESTATIONS

The incubation period has not been clearly established but is probably several weeks or longer. In otherwise healthy persons, the clinical pneumonia syndrome caused by *C. pneumoniae* resembles that of *M. pneumoniae* pneumonia. It has a prolonged prodrome of about 2 weeks that includes pharyngitis. The severity of pneumonia shows considerable variability from asymptomatic to mild to severe, but mild cases predominate in children, with severity increasing with increasing age. In some cases *M. pneumoniae* and *S. pneumoniae* have been isolated as copathogens, thus making assignment of a specific syndrome to *C. pneumoniae* even more difficult. A considerable proportion of adults with this infection have had acute bronchitis, and many have had exacerbations of chronic lung diseases, including asthma, and the acute chest syndrome of sickle cell disease. It has been reported to cause exacerbations of lung disease in persons with cystic fibrosis. Patients with pneumonia have a history of mild or no fever. Crackles may or may not be present on physical examination.

DIAGNOSIS

It is not possible to differentiate *C. pneumoniae* from other causes of atypical pneumonia on the basis of clinical findings.

Diagnostic Imaging

The radiographic abnormalities vary from small, vague infiltrates to extensive multilobar infiltrates that are similar to other causes of atypical pneumonias. A recent study (Kauppinen et al, 1996) showed lobar or sublobar pneumonia in 29% of patients with *C. pneumoniae* compared with 54% of patients with pneumonia caused by *S. pneumoniae.*

Microbiologic Evaluation

The organism can be recovered best from the nasopharynx and also from the throat, sputum, and even pleural fluid by cell culture methods with specific monoclonal antibody staining, although these tests have limited availability. Transportation must be in *Chlamydia* transport medium at room temperature, and cultures should be inoculated within 24 hours. Culture can be misleading because individuals may have prolonged asymptomatic excretion, and the current disease may be due to another agent. PCR-based assays have been developed but are not yet available commercially.

C. pneumoniae may be recovered from the oropharynges of healthy children and could be confused with *C. trachomatis,* which in the throat could indicate oral sexual transmission. This feature is of potential importance in interpreting surveillance cultures from children believed to be victims of sexual abuse and requires a laboratory that is expert at this differentiation.

Serologic Testing. The serologic test used in epidemiologic research has been a specific **microimmunofluorescence test.** The presence of specific IgM antibody that appears after 2–4 weeks indicates primary infection rather than reinfection, but antibody does not prevent subsequent attacks. A fourfold rise in IgM antibody, a fourfold rise in IgG antibody, which appears at 6–8 weeks, a single IgM titer of ≥1:16, or a single IgG titer of ≥1:512 have been suggested as diagnostic. Serologic testing is not universally available, but availability is increasing. Some studies show that younger children frequently do not develop demonstrable antibody. Complement fixation for antibody to common *Chlamydia* genus antigens may be somewhat helpful if the titer is high and there is no reason to believe *C. psittaci* is the responsible agent, but these tests are neither sensitive nor specific.

TREATMENT AND PROGNOSIS

The treatment of choice for adolescents and adults is tetracycline (1–2 g/day orally divided into 4 daily doses for 14–21 days) or doxycycline (100 mg every 12 hours orally for 14–21 days). Erythromycin (50 mg/kg/day orally divided into 4 doses for 14–21 days; maximum dose, 250 mg) is effective for children <8 years of age or as an alternative to tetracycline for older persons. Erythromycin is especially attractive as empirical therapy for atypical (nonlobar) pneumonia because it is active against the major nonviral causes including *C. pneumoniae, M. pneumoniae,* and *Legionella.* Clarithromycin (15 mg/kg/day orally divided into 2 daily doses; maximum dose, 250–500 mg) and azithromycin (5–12 mg/kg once daily orally for children, and 500 mg once on day 1 orally followed by 250 mg once on subsequent days orally for adults) are also effective. *C. pneumoniae* is resistant to penicillin, ampicillin, and sulfisoxazole. Responses to antibiotic therapy may vary, and coughing persists several weeks after therapy is begun.

FUNGAL PNEUMONIAS

Fungal pneumonias are caused by endemic pathogenic species to which healthy persons are susceptible or by opportunistic fungi that are not generally pathogenic for healthy persons (Table 68–8). Many fungi such as *Aspergillus, Histoplasma,* and *Coccidioides* cause disease in both immunocompromised persons and immunocompetent persons, but the patterns of disease are quite different. Many other fungal species have been reported to cause disease almost exclusively in severely immunocompromised patients (Chapters 98–101). Some pneumonias, such as mucormycosis, sporotrichosis, blastomycosis, and those caused by many saprophytic species, are extremely uncommon in children. Consultation and management with a specialist in infectious diseases is recommended for most children with fungal pneumonias.

TABLE 68–8. Species Causing Fungal Pneumonias

Opportunistic	Pathogenic
Aspergillosis	Histoplasmosis
Cryptococcosis	Coccidioidomycosis
Candidiasis	Blastomycosis
Zygomycosis*	Paracoccidiodomycosis*
Sporotrichosis*	

*Rare in children.
Adapted from Jacobs RF, Bradsher RW: The mycoses other than histoplasmosis. In Chernick V, Boat TF (editors): *Kendig's Disorders of the Respiratory Tract in Children,* 6th ed. Philadelphia, WB Saunders, 1998:954.

HISTOPLASMOSIS

ETIOLOGY

Histoplasmosis is caused by *Histoplasma capsulatum,* a dimorphic fungus found in soil. In humans the organism occurs in the form of budding yeast, but it occurs in the hyphal form in the soil.

Transmission. Humans become infected by inhaling spores from dirt or animal feces, especially bird and bat feces.

EPIDEMIOLOGY

Infection is endemic in the Ohio and Mississippi River valleys. The central states have the highest infection rates, including Arkansas, Missouri, Kentucky, and Tennessee. Lower rates occur in Louisiana, Texas, Illinois, Indiana, Ohio, Maryland, and Virginia. Excavation of densely contaminated soil may be responsible for epidemic outbreaks of histoplasmosis.

PATHOGENESIS

The initial infection follows inhalation and is usually in the lungs, where spores are transformed to yeast forms. Most infections in otherwise healthy persons are asymptomatic. There is evidence that there is an early self-limited dissemination, similar to that seen in tuberculosis. Primary disease is often in the form of a **Ghon complex,** with parenchymal disease and hilar lymphadenopathy similar to those of tuberculosis (see Fig. 35–8). Calcifications at the site of old disease are frequent. Reactivation of these foci after initial healing may occur if the person becomes immunosuppressed later in life. Re-exposure after primary disease produces a modified response similar to acute histoplasmosis but milder. Meningitis is rare in immunocompetent persons but may occur in immunocompromised persons, especially persons with AIDS. In endemic areas, serologic studies and routine chest radiographs demonstrate that large numbers of persons who have no specific history of histoplasmosis have humoral antibody and lung calcifications.

SYMPTOMS AND CLINICAL MANIFESTATIONS

When healthy persons are observed closely because of an environmental exposure, it appears that some have an acute, self-limited influenza-like illness that begins about 1–3 weeks after exposure. Symptoms such as a dry cough, headache, chest pain, malaise, and fever are characteristic. Rarely, erythema nodosum may accompany these symptoms.

The severity of the symptoms and the outcome depend on the inoculum and the immunocompetence of the patient (Table 68–9). In severe disease there is wheezing and tachypnea. In immunocompromised persons, including those with AIDS, dissemination probably occurs by invasion of the bloodstream after the initial pulmonary focus is established.

A syndrome of disseminated disease that follows early pulmonary infection and affects the viscera with organisms concentrated in the reticuloendothelial system and the bone marrow has been reported in children younger than 2 years of age. This syndrome may present as a chronic wasting disease manifested by fever, hepatosplenomegaly, anemia, and leukopenia. Additional sites of disseminated infection in adults and children include the eyes, the pericardium, the pleura, the adrenal glands, the skin, and the meninges. Infections at these sites are seen primarily in children with AIDS.

TABLE 68–9. Classification of Histoplasmosis

Usual benign infection of immunocompetent persons
Primary infection
Light exposure (asymptomatic)
Heavy exposure (acute primary histoplasmosis)
Reinfection
Light exposure (asymptomatic)
Heavy exposure (acute histoplasmosis, reinfection type)
Potentially progressive disease of immunocompromised persons
Childhood infection (intrinsically compromised relative to adults)
Disseminated histoplasmosis of the adult
Clinically disseminated (nonreactive)
Clinically localized (partially reactive)
Pulmonary histoplasmosis
Complications of healed primary histoplasmosis
Histoplasmomas
Mediastinal fibrosis
Broncholithiasis

Adapted from Goodwin RA, Des Prez RM: Pathogenesis and clinical spectrum of histoplasmosis. *South Med J* 1973;66:13–25.

DIAGNOSIS

Microbiologic Evaluation

In general, isolation of *H. capsulatum* from tissue or body fluids is the best way to diagnose histoplasmosis. Tissue recovered by biopsy can be stained with Gomori's methenamine silver stain. In pulmonary disease, isolation of the agent is best accomplished by recovery from the sputum or bronchoalveolar lavage during acute disease (Fig. 68–5). The fungus can be grown in most hospital laboratories, but culture may take 2–6 weeks. Laboratory personnel must be protected against inhaling spores from the agar plates. In complicated or progressive disease, invasive procedures for culture from lung tissue, lymph nodes, liver, or the CNS, especially CSF or brain abscess material, may be necessary. In disseminated disease, the fungus can be isolated from the blood and bone marrow.

Skin Testing. The **histoplasmin skin test** measures cell-mediated immunity, which develops 2–4 weeks after acute infection. Skin testing is useful in epidemiologic investigations to determine the endemicity of the disease, but it is of little use in the diagnosis of acute pneumonia because in endemic areas many persons without symptoms react to the test material. The usefulness of the skin test

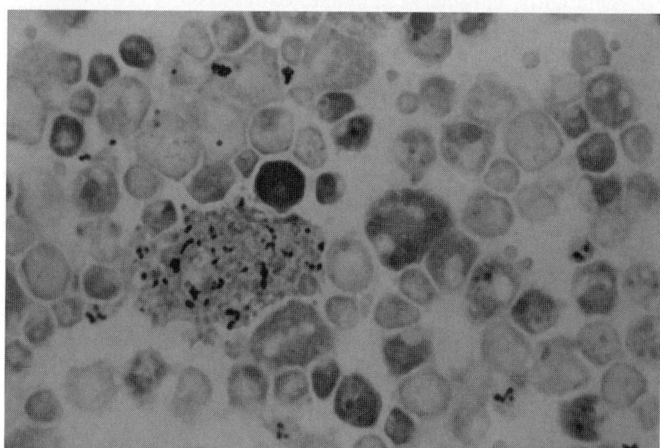

FIGURE 68–5. *Histoplasma* in the cytoplasm of a macrophage detected by Grocott staining of bronchoalveolar lavage.

is also limited by false-negative test results, which are encountered among immunocompromised persons and those with chronic infections.

Serologic Testing. The skin test antigen can produce an antibody response, so serologic tests should be performed before skin tests. A fourfold or greater rise in titer with the yeast phase complement fixation test is evidence of acute infection. Titers drop months after acute infection. Immunodiffusion tests are less sensitive and more specific and detect antibody titers longer than complement fixation.

Antigen Detection. A very specific radioimmunoassay (RIA) test for *Histoplasma* antigen, with approximately 90% sensitivity and up to 98% sensitivity in urine, is useful as a diagnostic adjunct to culture and also for monitoring response to therapy in complicated cases. This test is available only from the research laboratory of Dr. Joseph Wheat (University of Indiana, Indianapolis; telephone 317-630-6262).

Diagnostic Imaging

Pulmonary histoplasmosis has a characteristic chest radiograph. Frequently when the presentation is nonspecific and no radiograph is taken, it is a surprise many years later when a calcified lesion is detected on a routine screening radiograph of the chest. The acute primary disease has a miliary alveolar pattern primarily in the lower lobes, often with hilar lymphadenopathy (see Figs. 13–20 and 13–21). Less commonly, a lobar process may be detected.

TREATMENT

Even symptomatic disease usually requires no specific treatment, and symptoms usually abate spontaneously in 3–10 days. If an immunocompetent host does not improve within 4–6 weeks of onset of the disease, antifungal agents must be considered for the treatment of progressive disease.

For severe systemic disease, progressive pulmonary disease, or infection in immunocompromised persons, the infection is often fatal if untreated, so prompt treatment is recommended. Infants with symptomatic disease also may be treated. Amphotericin B has been standard therapy. The optimal dose of amphotericin B for children with disseminated disease is not known, but a total dose of 25–35 mg/kg has been suggested, with a daily dose of up to 1 mg/kg for 4–6 weeks (Chapter 14). Longer treatment may be necessary in immunocompromised persons, and persons with chronic cavitary disease. A shorter course of 2 weeks has been advocated for infants who show a prompt response to treatment. For meningitis, intrathecal amphotericin B may be necessary. Patients with this complication should be referred to specialists at tertiary care centers.

For immunocompetent persons there is increasing evidence of the effectiveness of the imidazoles: ketoconazole (6–8 mg/kg once daily orally; maximum dose, 200–400 mg), fluconazole (6–12 mg/kg once daily orally; maximum dose, 400 mg), and itraconazole (5–10 mg/kg orally divided in 2 daily doses; maximum dose, 200 mg).

Patients with AIDS and histoplasmosis tend to have relapses after treatment is discontinued, so maintenance therapy may have to be continued indefinitely. Histoplasmosis with severe immunodeficiency is often treated initially with amphotericin B and later with itraconazole for long term therapy.

PROGNOSIS

This disease usually clears spontaneously, but if chronic disease continues, cavitation and scarring similar to those of tuberculosis may occur. This occurs only in about 5% of infected patients and is rare in children.

ASPERGILLOSIS

ETIOLOGY

Aspergillus infections are caused primarily by *Aspergillus fumigatus,* but similar infections in humans are caused by *A. flavus, A. oryzae, A. niger,* and other less common species.

EPIDEMIOLOGY

Infection usually occurs by inhalation of spores in the air from reservoirs of spores in soil, rock, and insulation material. Disorders of immunity or neutropenia are important risk factors. Clusters of cases of nosocomial infection often occur during construction near patient rooms, causing exposure of patients to aerosols with large amounts of spores.

PATHOGENESIS

Aspergillus has a low pathogenicity for humans, and pulmonary aspergillosis is not generally considered in the differential diagnosis of lobar or bronchopneumonia in otherwise healthy persons. Invasive disease occurs primarily in immunocompromised persons. Prolonged neutropenia and neutrophil defects such as chronic granulomatous disease are important underlying conditions, with other risk factors including treatment with corticosteroids, late stages of AIDS, and organ transplantation. Adults with diabetes mellitus who are otherwise healthy and have invasive pulmonary aspergillosis have occasionally been reported.

The three well-defined types of pulmonary *Aspergillus* infections are: (1) **hypersensitivity pneumonitis,** also known as **bronchopulmonary aspergillosis;** (2) colonization of devitalized lung tissue, primarily lung cavities, also known as **aspergilloma;** and (3) invasive and disseminated infections in immunocompromised patients. Pulmonary infection in immunocompromised persons results in *Aspergillus* organisms invading blood vessels; this allows the organisms to enter and spread via the bloodstream and also may cause erosion of pulmonary blood vessels, resulting in massive hemoptysis.

SYMPTOMS AND CLINICAL MANIFESTATIONS

Aspergillus Hypersensitivity Pneumonitis. Allergic bronchopulmonary aspergillosis is an IgE-mediated hypersensitivity reaction to *Aspergillus* antigens. Symptoms are fever and bronchospasm, which may be severe. Patients may expectorate thick plugs and broncholiths. Because coughing and wheezing are the most prominent features, this condition must be considered in patients with a new onset of asthma that does not respond to conventional asthma treatment. Radiographs of the chest show a migratory pattern of lung infiltrates, and the WBC count shows eosinophilia. Elevated total serum levels of IgE, *Aspergillus*-specific IgE and IgG, and serum precipitins to *Aspergillus* antigens are usually present. Because this is not an invasive infection, the use of antifungal agents is not generally necessary, but treatment with corticosteroids is beneficial.

Aspergilloma. Aspergilloma is a saprophytic superinfection of *Aspergillus* in lung cavities or scars and does not occur in healthy lungs. A localized focus of *Aspergillus* causes a cavity to develop, and the organism continues to live in a **mycetoma (fungus ball)** inside an air-filled cavity. For immunocompetent persons, this saprophytic infection usually persists for life but without invasive infection and usually without symptoms. If immunosuppression develops, invasive pulmonary infection and even hematogenous dissemination may result. A slowly expanding cavity may erode into a blood vessel and cause hemoptysis.

Aspergillosis in Immunocompromised Persons. Aspergillosis is increasing in frequency because of the prevalence of AIDS, increases in the number of transplantations, and more aggressive chemotherapy protocols for cancer, especially leukemias. The severity and duration of neutropenia are especially important risk factors for invasive aspergillosis. Invasive aspergillosis is difficult to diagnose because of the nonspecific nature of early disease and its frequent coexistence with other pathogens. With milder forms of immunosuppression, pulmonary aspergillosis may be semi-invasive and present as a subacute or chronic infection in the lungs or sinuses. In the acute form the disease may be limited to the lung, or there may be hematogenous dissemination to almost any organ, including the skin, heart, and viscera. In the lung there is a tendency to invade blood vessels, causing hemoptysis. Rupture of a larger pulmonary arterial vessel may be fatal.

A radiograph of the chest may show only an ill-defined infiltrate or a progressive infiltrative process (see Fig. 13–15), none of which is specific unless a mycetoma within a cavity is seen. Chest CT may be more sensitive for demonstrating localized pulmonary lesions. Lack of response to antibacterial treatment, associated sinusitis, skin lesions, epistaxis, and the development of pulmonary nodules or cavities are additional clues to the diagnosis of pulmonary aspergillosis in immunocompromised persons. Skin lesions may appear anywhere, but lesions at points of pressure are characteristic. The lesions progress from macules to vesicles and then to necrotic ulcers over a variable period of time. Microscopic examination of a tissue biopsy is diagnostic.

DIAGNOSIS

Microbiologic Evaluation

The key to diagnosis of aspergillosis is recovery of the organism on culture. In pulmonary disease the sputum may yield a positive culture in only one third or fewer of cases. Nasal cultures add to both the sensitivity and the specificity of respiratory cultures to indicate invasive aspergillosis. Bronchoalveolar lavage, or biopsy, either open or through a bronchoscope, may be needed if sputum and nasal cultures do not identify the organism. When a biopsy is performed, visualization of the characteristic **septate hyphae** may precede growth of the organism in the laboratory by many days and allows rapid therapeutic decision making. It may be difficult, however, to classify the disease. In patients with aspergilloma and pneumonia of an unknown cause, *Aspergillus* may be recovered from the sputum, but it may be incidental and not the cause of the pneumonia. *Aspergillus* in isolated sputum cultures also may be a laboratory contaminant, but repeatedly positive cultures in a susceptible patient indicate a relatively high risk of invasive aspergillosis. If a lung biopsy cannot be performed in an immunocompromised patient, empirical treatment may be required if the organism is recovered repeatedly or in large numbers (2+ to 4+ in sputum). RIA and EIA have been reported to be useful in the diagnosis of disseminated aspergillosis by assaying serum for circulating antigen, but results have been inconclusive. Tests for antibody using immunoprecipitation may be helpful if serial specimens indicate a rising titer of antibody.

TREATMENT

Aspergillus Hypersensitivity Pneumonitis. Allergic bronchopulmonary aspergillosis is treated with corticosteroids. Prednisone at a dose of 0.5 mg/kg/day is given once a day for 2 weeks, which should clear the pulmonary infiltrates. Prednisone is continued every other day for 3 months and then tapered over another 3 months. Serologic tests, IgE levels, and chest radiographs must be monitored, and consultation with a specialist in allergy, pulmonology, or infectious diseases is recommended. Therapy is reinstituted if there is evidence of exacerbation of disease. A recent study (Stevens et al, 2000) demonstrated the benefit of itraconazole as an adjunct to cortisteroids for this condition.

Aspergilloma. An aspergilloma either is not treated at all or requires complete surgical excision. An aspergilloma that is a source of continued hemoptysis generally requires surgical excision. Antifungal treatment is not recommended because the likelihood of sterilizing a cavity is poor.

Aspergillosis in Immunocompromised Persons. Invasive or disseminated disease in immunocompromised persons is frequently fatal, but it is assumed that early treatment with antifungal agents increases the chance of survival. Because diagnosis may be difficult, antifungal agents are now frequently prescribed empirically for immunocompromised patients and those with severe neutropenia and fever who do not respond clinically to broad-spectrum antibiotics directed against bacteria. Amphotericin B, either the deoxycholate salt or one of the lipid formulations, is considered the drug of choice, although new imidazoles, such as itraconazole and voriconazole are useful. Success in the treatment of immunocompromised patients usually depends on reducing the degree of immunosuppression and remission of the underlying neoplastic process. The dose and duration of amphotericin B have not been established, but the guideline is long-term treatment in doses similar to those used to treat other tissue-invasive fungi (0.7–1 mg/kg/day, to an equivalent of 2 or more g total for adults) until all signs of the disease have disappeared. This may require months of therapy, with the initial therapy consisting of amphotericin B followed by oral itraconazole or voriconazole. Early institution and aggressive antifungal therapy may reduce the mortality from 80% to 50%. Some experts have suggested the addition of rifampin or flucytosine to amphotericin B, but conclusive data are lacking. For patients with chronic granulomatous disease, IFN-γ is used adjunctively with antifungal therapy.

CRYPTOCOCCAL PNEUMONIA

The fungus *Cryptococcus neoformans* is a ubiquitous saprophytic fungus resident in soil and bird feces. Humans are infected by inhalation of contaminated aerosols. Most infections in normal hosts occur as subclinical or minor localized pulmonary disease. Dissemination from a pulmonary focus is rare in normal hosts. Meningitis is one of the secondary foci that may develop from such a spreading infection. Although pneumonia has been reported in persons with normal immunity, immunosuppression caused by cancer, corticosteroid treatment, chemotherapy, or AIDS is an important predisposing risk factor. The clinical presentation is similar to that of other fungal pneumonias and to that of tuberculosis. Fever, malaise, chest pain, and later dyspnea and weight loss are the most frequent symptoms. Cough is a variable finding. The radiologic findings vary, with nodules, mass lesions, and alveolar infiltrates predominating. Widespread pulmonary involvement is more characteristic of pneumonia in immunocompromised patients than in normal hosts.

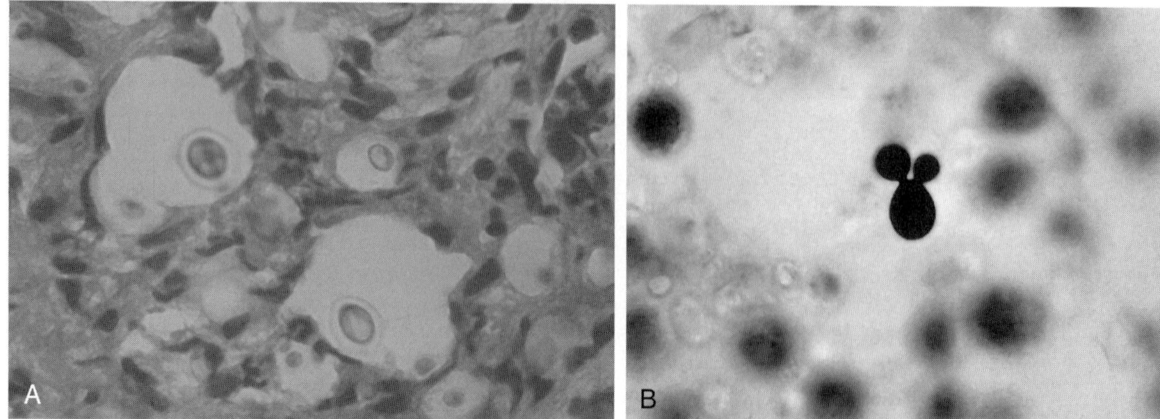

FIGURE 68–6. *Cryptococcus* pneumonia. **A,** *Cryptococcus* in lung tissue (Hematoxylin-eosin stain). **B,** *Cryptococcus* detected by Grocott staining of bronchoalveolar lavage.

The presence of *C. neoformans* in the sputum of a person with pneumonia suggests active infection. In an immunocompromised patient with pneumonia, it is nearly diagnostic. Free capsular antigen can be detected in the blood and, if present, increases the likelihood that the disease is invasive cryptococcosis, although a negative test result does not exclude this infection. The most specific diagnosis is established by visualization of the organism in tissue, but recovery of organisms with bronchoalveolar lavage is also highly suggestive (Fig. 68–6). In pneumonia the best biopsy tissue usually would be from the lung, but if dissemination has taken place, visualization of organisms or a positive culture in viscera, brain, or cerebrospinal fluid also is specific.

Immunocompetent hosts with focal pneumonia or nodular disease usually recover without treatment. Localized lesions may appear as neoplasms and often are removed surgically for diagnosis. Immunocompromised persons with cryptococcal pneumonia are treated with amphotericin B as described for *Aspergillus* pneumonia. The addition of flucytosine is also recommended. If an otherwise healthy person with cryptococcal pneumonia does not improve after several months of observation, treatment with amphotericin B should be considered. Fluconazole is also effective, especially for prevention of relapse in patients with AIDS. Ketoconazole can be used to treat focal pulmonary infections if meningitis is excluded.

COCCIDIOIDOMYCOSIS

Pneumonia due to *Coccidioides immitis* is contracted through exposure to aerosols contaminated with spores. In the United States the major focus is in the southwestern states. Pulmonary disease often occurs in clusters when excavating parties are exposed in caves, construction, or hiking. In certain highly endemic foci in California and Arizona, most permanent inhabitants are infected at some time. Symptoms, if any, develop 1–4 weeks after exposure. The duration of illness varies from days to several weeks. Children younger than 5 years and racial minorities appear to be especially susceptible.

Coccidioidomycosis is an influenza-like syndrome with a fever, cough, chest pain, and transient rash. The rash may be a nonspecific maculopapular eruption or erythema nodosum. Arthralgia may also occur. Radiographic signs vary and include patchy infiltrates, hilar lymphadenopathy, and signs of pleuritis. In rare cases in immunocompetent persons, but more commonly in immunocompromised persons, the disease may disseminate to the viscera, skeleton, or CNS. Dissemination also may occur if the onset of infection is during pregnancy. In debilitated patients the pulmonary disease may become chronic (reactivation) after the acute stage appears to be healed.

The diagnosis of coccidioidomycosis can be established by means of the **skin test** with the antigens **coccidioidin** and **spherulin.** In highly endemic areas, however, past infection is so common that the skin test may not be adequate to differentiate current disease from past exposure. Indeed, in endemic areas many patients have a positive skin test reaction in the absence of any known disease, which suggests that a large proportion of infections are asymptomatic. Antibody also can be detected in the serum by several methods. The organism can be cultured from sputum, lung biopsy specimens, and bronchoscopic samples, but serologic testing is the principal method of diagnosis in otherwise healthy persons with pulmonary disease.

Mild focal pulmonary disease usually does not require treatment, but it does respond to amphotericin B. In general, amphotericin B is reserved for severe pulmonary disease or disseminated disease. The treatment course is similar to that for *Aspergillus* pneumonia, lasting 6–8 weeks. Oral imidazoles have also been used. Ketoconazole can be used to treat focal pulmonary infections if meningitis is excluded. The newer imidazoles fluconazole and itraconazole have been shown to be useful, and fluconazole is used for meningitis.

BLASTOMYCOSIS

Pneumonia due to *Blastomyces dermatitidis,* the agent of blastomycosis, is quite uncommon in children. Similar to many of the deep fungal infections, it has a restricted geographic range and the syndrome it causes is not distinctive.

B. dermatitidis is a dimorphic fungus. The endemic areas for blastomycosis within the United States include the Mississippi, Missouri, and Ohio River valleys and the southeastern states. Outdoor recreational exposure appears to be a major risk factor, and outbreaks are often associated with soil contamination. Because of the lack of available testing for diagnosis of mild cases and the requirement for tissue to isolate the infecting organism, the number of reported cases is probably a gross underestimate of the actual number of infections. Most cases occur in men, possibly because of outdoor recreational or occupational exposure. The peak age of patients is 30–60 years. Fewer than 80 cases have been reported among pediatric patients.

Infection by *B. dermatitidis* appears to occur by inhalation of the spores, which come from environmental sources. There is little information about the natural habitat of the fungus because the organism rarely has been isolated from nonhuman reservoirs. Studies of outbreaks suggest an incubation period of 3–12 weeks for pulmonary disease.

Clinical disease associated with *B. dermatitidis* is mostly manifested as pneumonia, but other foci, including the skin, bone, joints, the genitourinary system, and the CNS (e.g., brain abscess, meningitis), have been reported. Chronic granulomatous skin lesions with verrucous hyperplasia and microabscess formation are common. Focal extrapulmonary infection probably occurs as the result of hematogenous spread from a pulmonary focus, but that focus may not be clinically evident when the patient presents with extrapulmonary disease. Although infection may occur in immunocompromised patients, most cases occur in healthy persons who have had an outdoor exposure to spores.

Pulmonary disease presents as a focal or nodular pattern or as large areas of consolidation that may appear similar to that of focal bacterial pneumonias. Nodules may suggest a tumor, so biopsies are frequently performed on the lesions. Although it appears that focal lung infections may heal without evidence of residual disease, chronic pneumonia may occur. When the pneumonia is progressive, it may be accompanied by pleuritis, pulmonary parenchymal cavitation, or spreading interstitial disease. It may appear similar to chronic tuberculosis on radiographs.

Organisms are found in both tissues and sputum. Diagnosis generally requires culturing of the organism from infected tissues. In tissues the organism appears as large refractile yeasts with a broad-based bud. The organism is easily recovered from infected tissues and body fluids with the use of appropriate fungal media such as Sabouraud's agar, although it may take up to 4 weeks to isolate the organism. It is not possible to diagnose asymptomatic or mild cases because of the lack of available specific serologic or skin tests. Skin tests (blastoplasmin) and serologic tests that have been available lack sufficient sensitivity and specificity to be recommended, but better tests are being developed and are available in research laboratories. Sometimes the organism is seen in stained tissue sections, and the diagnosis is established histologically even when appropriate cultures are not performed. It is probable that many cases of pneumonia heal spontaneously and never are correctly diagnosed because of the lack of adequate specimens.

Many mild cases heal spontaneously and require no therapy. Treatment of progressive or invasive infection is similar to that of other invasive fungal pneumonias. Amphotericin B is the most frequently used antifungal agent. Regimens such as that described for *Aspergillus* infection are recommended for progressive pulmonary blastomycosis; a total dose of at least 2 g should be administered to adolescents and adults. Among the imidazole oral antifungal agents, ketoconazole and itraconazole have been used with some success, but they should not be used for CNS infections. When ketoconazole is used, a high dose is often required. A dose of 800 mg/day for adults is effective for patients who do not respond to 400 mg/day, but toxicity is greater with the higher dose. The equivalent dose range in young children is 3.3–6.6 mg/kg/day given once a day. To prevent reactivation, some patients have been treated with long courses of imidazole oral agents (up to 6 months) following initial amphotericin B treatment.

Treatment appears to have a major impact on blastomycosis. Untreated progressive pulmonary disease has 80–90% mortality, but the cure rate is 80–100% with appropriate antifungal therapy.

CANDIDA PNEUMONIA

Candida pneumonia is seen only in ill neonates and severely immunocompromised patients. It is difficult to estimate the rate of candidal pneumonia because it is so hard to meet appropriate standards for diagnosis. Although *Candida* organisms are common inhabitants of the upper airways, true pneumonia caused by the various *Candida* species is rare. No specific signs and symptoms are known to be helpful in leading to the diagnosis. The difficulty in diagnosis is that almost any specimen—sputum, bronchoscopic lavage fluid, or transbronchial biopsy material—may be contaminated with *Candida* from the upper or middle airways and may not represent invasive disease. A lung biopsy or protected brush specimen with appropriate cultures is necessary to establish the diagnosis. No routinely available serologic tests are helpful, although this is currently an area of great research effort.

In disseminated candidal disease, the lungs may be involved as a secondary focus. Patients with advanced AIDS or neonates may have lung involvement either as an extension of upper respiratory infection or associated with fungemia. Treatment is similar to treatment of other forms of disseminated candidiasis. Amphotericin B is the drug of choice for most species, with the notable exception of *C. krusei*. This species of *Candida* has been increasingly isolated from immunocompromised patients and often has primary resistance to amphotericin B. The dosage of amphotericin B for pneumonia and systemic infection with *Candida* is similar to that for *Aspergillus* infections. In life-threatening or persistent infections, flucytosine may be added. There is little experience with the use of fluconazole, but this agent is effective in other severe candidal infections.

VIRAL PNEUMONIAS

Most pneumonias in primary care pediatric practice are caused by viruses. Epidemiologic studies of viral pneumonia in many geographic areas have documented that more than 80% of childhood pneumonias are either viral or the result of secondary bacterial infection of viral respiratory disease. In routine practice, however, it is usually not practical or feasible to identify the exact cause of pneumonia in individual cases. Many viruses cause pneumonia (Table 68–10), although the incidence of measles and influenza viruses is lower in regions where there are active immunization programs. It is important to recognize the clinical syndromes caused by these agents and to direct the appropriate type and level of care

TABLE 68–10. Relative Frequency of Respiratory Viruses in Different Pediatric Age Groups

	Age Group		
Virus Species	Infant	Preschool	School Age
Respiratory syncytial virus	+++	++	±
Parainfluenza virus type 3	++	+	+
Parainfluenza virus type 1	++	++	+
Influenza A virus	+	++	++
Influenza B virus	±	+	++
Parainfluenza type 2 virus	+	+	±
Adenoviruses	+	±	±
Measles virus	+	+	±
Cytomegalovirus	+	±	±
Picornaviruses	±	±	±

Adapted from Glezen WP: Viral pneumonia. In Chernick V, Boat TF (editors): *Kendig's Disorders of the Respiratory Tract in Children,* 6th ed. Philadelphia, WB Saunders, 1998.

toward them rather than assuming that all pneumonias should be treated with antibiotics.

Viral Pneumonias in the First 3 Months of Life. The causes of viral pneumonias in the first 3 months of life (Tables 68–1, 68–10) can be divided into those transmitted perinatally from the mother (primarily HSV and CMV) and those transmitted by inhalation of droplets from infected persons (primarily RSV, adenovirus, influenza virus, and parainfluenza viruses). Maternal HSV is a sexually transmitted infection. There is no seasonal variation in rate. CMV can be transmitted to infants by in utero infection, transfusion of blood and blood products, and possibly breast milk. Rubella was also a cause of transplacental pneumonia before universal immunization.

Transmission of the viruses that cause pneumonia in all age groups is from person to person by direct contact, by aerosols, or by droplet nuclei. Thus the predisposing factors for these respiratory viruses in young infants are related to prevalence of the viruses in members of the community, especially in the immediate household. These viruses are more prevalent in the community during the cold weather months. A study (Davies et al, 1996) of 71 infants ≤6 months of age with pneumonia found that 37% of 62 tested had a viral isolate (RSV or parainfluenza virus) and 21% of 56 tested had *Ureaplasma urealyticum* or *C. trachomatis*. Overall, in 49% of the entire group a cause was determined; only one had proven bacterial pneumonia. Influenza A virus is important mainly in epidemic years.

Infection with more than one agent at a time is not unusual. One study (Brasfield et al., 1987) reported that RSV, CMV, enterovirus, and parainfluenza virus were most frequently found. Of 145 patients in whom an identifiable agent was found as the cause of pneumonia, 32% had more than one agent, either two viruses or various combinations of viruses with other agents, including *C. trachomatis, U. urealyticum,* or *P. carinii.* Other studies that have specifically examined transmission of respiratory viruses to infants in nurseries and in the community demonstrate that RSV is the most common etiologic agent of lower respiratory tract disease, followed by the parainfluenza viruses.

Viral Pneumonias After the First 3 Months of Life. Most pneumonias that affect children 3 months to 5 years of age are caused by viruses. After 5 years of age, *M. pneumoniae* and possibly *C. pneumoniae* are more common than any single viral agent (Table 68–1). RSV and parainfluenza virus types 1 and 3 are the most common agents of viral pneumonia in young children in all regions of the United States. The incidence of influenza A and B viruses varies from year to year and from state to state, thus it is impossible to generalize about their incidence. During an influenza epidemic, however, influenza virus may be the most common agent of pneumonia, causing severe cases that may be fatal in the very young and the very old. The agents of viral pneumonia peak in incidence in the cold months of the year and are more common in children in crowded environments and in children who spend time in poorly ventilated daycare centers.

It is difficult to make distinctions between the nonbacterial pneumonias of early infancy on clinical or radiographic grounds (see Fig. 13–9*A*). Infants with viral pneumonias usually have no or low-grade fever, similar to those with *C. trachomatis* pneumonia. In neonates, however, overwhelming disease may develop rapidly. In young infants it is not unusual for apneic spells to occur as the first sign of respiratory infection, followed by respiratory failure. This is most characteristic of RSV, but it can occur with adenovirus, influenza, and parainfluenza viruses as well as with pertussis.

General Management. Viral cultures of nasopharyngeal secretions are diagnostic but are not usually indicated or required in uncomplicated cases of illness in immunocompetent, ambulatory patients. Antiviral therapy is currently available for viral respiratory infections caused by RSV (Chapter 67), influenza viruses, and for CMV and HSV pneumonia, which usually occur in immunocompromised persons (Chapter 99) and transplant recipients (Chapter 100). Antiviral therapy is not recommended for adenovirus, parainfluenza virus, or enterovirus pneumonias in otherwise healthy persons. For pneumonia caused by these agents, rest and supportive treatment, such as pain and fever control and respiratory care, are all that is currently available. Antibiotics against bacteria are of no value in viral pneumonia unless there is evidence of a secondary bacterial infection. Acetaminophen is appropriate for antipyresis and for relief of discomfort. Aspirin should not be given to children with presumed viral pneumonia because it may increase the risk of Reye's syndrome after viral illnesses, especially influenza and varicella.

The prognosis depends on the specific agent causing the pneumonia. Adenovirus pneumonia and other pneumonias in infants are associated with chronic obstructive disease and anatomic lung lesions later in childhood. Influenza virus pneumonia is a potentially fatal complication of influenza. Respiratory failure may occur rapidly and requires intubation and management in an intensive care unit.

RESPIRATORY SYNCYTIAL VIRUS

RSV is one of the agents chiefly responsible for lower respiratory tract infections worldwide. The major clinical illness caused by this agent is bronchiolitis (Chapter 67) rather than isolated pneumonia. Pneumonia may occur concomitantly with RSV bronchiolitis, with manifestations similar to those of pneumonia caused by other respiratory viruses.

PARAINFLUENZA VIRUS

Parainfluenza viruses are enveloped RNA viruses of the paramyxovirus subgroup and can be divided by surface antigens into types 1–4. Along with RSV, parainfluenza virus types 1 and 3 are the most common cause of viral pneumonia among children younger than 5 years of age and may cause pneumonia at any age. Similar to RSV, parainfluenza virus can be associated with upper respiratory tract infections, middle airway infections (especially croup), and complications of respiratory disease, including sinusitis and otitis media. Parainfluenza viruses are spread by aerosols or direct contact. The virus is shed for as long as 8–9 days, and occasionally longer.

There is nothing distinctive about pneumonia due to parainfluenza virus that allows its separation on a clinical basis from the other causes of viral pneumonia. The incubation period is 2–6 days. As with RSV pneumonia, radiographs of the lungs vary, and patchy infiltrates, hyperinflation, focal atelectasis, and even dense infiltrates may exist in any combination. The radiographic findings may change from day to day. Parainfluenza viruses may cause unusually severe and prolonged pneumonia in immunocompromised persons, often as a coinfection with opportunistic pathogens such as *P. carinii* and CMV.

A specific diagnosis is established either by recovery of the agent from viral culture or by fourfold or greater increase in antibody titers when paired sera are tested. There are also rapid identification methods using immunofluorescence or EIA on respiratory secretions. Culture is the most reliable and specific method of diagnosis.

No specific treatment is available. There have been case reports of treatment of severe infections with ribavirin, but conclusive studies of efficacy have not been reported.

ADENOVIRUS

Adenovirus is a nonenveloped DNA virus. There are 41 adenovirus types, with some specificity between the virus type and the illness it causes. Adenoviruses may cause infection of targeted organs, or they may cause severe disseminated disease. The mode of spread of respiratory disease is primarily by aerosols and droplets. Gastroenteritis (types 40, 41, and others) may be spread by the fecal-oral route, by contaminated instruments, or by water. Keratoconjunctivitis (primarily type 8 and others), pharyngoconjunctival fever (many types), and upper respiratory tract infections with fever (many types) are the most common infections caused by adenoviruses. In military recruits, adenovirus is an especially common cause of upper respiratory infections, bronchitis, and pneumonia (primarily types 4 and 7). The other target group is children younger than 5 years of age, who also may have a variety of manifestations of respiratory illness (primarily types 1, 2, 3, and 5 and also types 6 and 7). Although adenoviruses are not as common a cause of viral pneumonia in children as RSV and parainfluenza viruses, they may cause very severe pneumonia (especially with types 3, 7, and 21). In newborns they can cause a severe life-threatening disseminated infection in which pneumonia is prominent. Because of necrosis of the bronchial epithelium, these infants have considerable bleeding from the respiratory tract, and disseminated intravascular coagulation may develop.

Adenovirus pneumonia is characterized by high fever, cough, and dyspnea. In infants, coughing and wheezing similar to those of bronchiolitis are the most prominent symptoms. On auscultation, infants often have scattered crackles and wheezes. There may be concomitant involvement of the upper respiratory tract, the CNS (meningitis and encephalitis), the viscera (liver, spleen, kidney), and the heart. In older children and adults the syndrome is similar to that in atypical pneumonia of other common causes although cases of overwhelming pneumonia leading to death have been described. The chest radiographic findings can be quite variable. The infiltrates can be interstitial or have a mild to severe bronchopneumonia pattern with bilateral diffuse infiltrates.

A specific diagnosis is established by isolation of the agent from respiratory secretions placed in tissue culture. For rapid diagnosis, EIA, immunofluorescence, or PCR testing can be performed in specialized laboratories. Many serologic assays are available, with serologic diagnosis established by a fourfold or greater rise in titer in paired serum samples.

No antiviral treatment is available for adenovirus respiratory infections. Recovery from severe adenovirus pneumonia is slow, and chronic sequelae, including bronchiolitis obliterans, bronchiectasis, and unilateral hyperlucent lung, may also occur. **Bronchiolitis obliterans** is a process of subacute or chronic inflammation in which the small airways are replaced by scar tissue, resulting in a reduction in lung volume and lung compliance. The syndrome of **unilateral hyperlucent lung,** or **Swyer-James syndrome,** appears to be a focal sequela of severe necrotizing pneumonia in which all or part of a lung has increased translucency on chest radiograph, and it has been linked especially with adenovirus type 21.

Live virus oral vaccines for adenovirus types 4 and 7 are used by United States and Canadian military forces to prevent adenovirus-associated disease among recruits during basic military training. These vaccines are not available for civilian use and are not given to infants or children.

INFLUENZA VIRUS

ETIOLOGY

Influenza viruses are RNA viruses of the orthomyxovirus family. The major antigenic types are A, B, and C, although C is relatively unimportant as a cause of epidemics. Specific antibodies are directed against the **hemagglutinin (H)** and **neuraminidase (N)** antigens and are important determinants of immunity. Three immunologically distinct hemagglutinin subtypes (H1, H2, and H3) and two neuraminidase subtypes (N1 and N2) are recognized as causes of global human epidemics. H5N1 and H9N2 avian-related strains have caused regional disease in Asia. Minor changes within a subtype are termed **antigenic drift,** which occurs almost annually in influenza A and B viruses. Major changes, which result in change to another subtype such as from H1 to H2, are termed **antigenic shift** and usually occur at irregular intervals of 10 or more years. Although influenza A and B viruses continually undergo antigenic change, influenza B viruses appear only to drift and change more slowly and are not divided into subtypes. Influenza A viruses are named for the date and place of first isolation and by the H and N type (e.g., A/Shanghai/11/87 [H3N2]). In epidemic years there is usually a strain that is substantially different in antigenic composition from strains prevalent in previous years. The incidence of influenza infection is then usually higher than any other respiratory infection. Because influenza A viruses change their subtype antigens (both H and N antigens), new strains are formed by mutations and genetic reassortment, to which susceptible populations may not have antibody. Thus, although there are only three major serotypes of influenza A virus, because of reassortment, the virus behaves epidemiologically as though there were many more serotypes.

Transmission. Transmission occurs by inhalation of infected droplets and aerosols coughed by persons with the infection or by contact with contaminated objects. Spread is rapid because the incubation period is short and shedding of the virus by persons who have the infection is prolonged. Viral shedding begins 1 day before the onset of clinical illness and lasts 1–2 weeks, depending on the strain of virus.

EPIDEMIOLOGY

The incidence of infection caused by specific antigenic types varies from year to year, but overall influenza viruses are a major cause of respiratory infections in children. The worldwide epidemiology of influenza viruses demonstrates annual spread from Asia across the Pacific Ocean to North America. Sentinel viral isolations from Asia are important in predicting disease for the following season in North America.

Epidemics of influenza occur in the United States during the winter months nearly every year. Influenza viruses also can cause global epidemics of disease, known as **pandemics,** during which rates of illness and death from influenza-related complications increase dramatically. Influenza viruses cause disease in all age groups. Rates of infection are highest among children, but rates of serious illness and death are highest among persons ≥65 years of age and persons of any age who have cardiopulmonary and other medical conditions that place them at high risk of complications from influenza. The estimated overall number of influenza-associated hospitalizations in the United States ranges from approximately 20,000 to more than 300,000 annually. More than 20,000, and frequently up to 40,000, influenza-associated deaths are estimated to occur annually in the United States, either directly from influenza and pneumonia or from exacerbations of underlying cardiopulmonary conditions and other chronic diseases. In the United States, pneumonia and influenza deaths might be increasing in part because of the increasing number of elderly persons.

PATHOGENESIS

Influenza virus infects respiratory epithelium. Infected cells demonstrate pyknotic nuclei, loss of cilia, and desquamation. Severe infection may lead to sloughing of the respiratory epithelium, hemorrhage, and hyaline membrane formation. There is minimal polymorphonuclear infiltration unless secondary bacterial pneumonia develops. Secondary bacterial pneumonia occurs most frequently in the elderly and in persons with underlying cardiac, pulmonary, renal, or other chronic disease.

SYMPTOMS AND CLINICAL MANIFESTATIONS

The incubation period is usually 2–3 days, but at extremes it may be 1–7 days. Pneumonia is a relatively uncommon manifestation of this multisystem disease that otherwise has a strong respiratory component. Ciliated respiratory tract epithelium is involved with necrosis followed by healing. It is usually not possible to determine, on the basis of symptoms, the levels of the respiratory tract involved.

Classic influenza without pneumonia is usually a disease with a sudden onset of fever, headache, and general malaise. Respiratory symptoms are usually limited to a sore throat, cough, coryza, and nasal discharge. In young children the range of respiratory symptoms is similar to that of infections with other respiratory viruses. Some young infants with influenza first present with apneic episodes or with a syndrome similar to neonatal sepsis. In years with influenza epidemics, a major proportion of upper and middle respiratory tract infections are due to influenza virus. Older children and adults are likely to have fever of 39°C (102.2°F), chills, myalgias, and a prolonged illness with coughing, whereas younger children tend to have abrupt onset of fever to 39–41° with resolution in 2–5 days. Gastrointestinal complaints, including abdominal pain, diarrhea, and vomiting are quite frequent in the younger age group and accompany respiratory symptoms that frequently include cough, pharyngitis, and croup. Fever and irritability without apparent focus of infection are also characteristic of influenza in very young children.

If pneumonia follows typical influenza, it may be a **primary influenza pneumonia,** or **secondary bacterial pneumonia** due to impairment of local and systemic host defenses caused by the influenza virus. *S. aureus, H. influenzae,* and *S. pneumoniae* are common causes of secondary bacterial pneumonia. Overwhelming influenza pneumonia is a diffuse hemorrhagic pneumonia. Early in the infection hypoxia and prostration are evident, but a physical examination of the chest and a chest radiograph may be unimpressive. The disease is more severe in patients with underlying cardiac or pulmonary disease, who comprise a major portion of those admitted to the hospital or who die of influenza.

DIAGNOSIS

Routine laboratory tests are of little help in diagnosing influenza, but knowledge of current influenza infection in the community is of great help in leading one to suspect this infection. The diagnosis of influenza pneumonia can be aided by a chest radiograph, which may show little, especially early in the disease, or may show infiltrates in multiple lobes with areas of atelectasis. A WBC count and a sputum Gram stain may be helpful in the differentiation of influenza pneumonia from secondary bacterial pneumonia. If the blood cell count shows leukocytosis or a shift to the left and if the sputum shows many polymorphonuclear leukocytes and bacteria, a secondary bacterial pneumonia is likely. The WBC count in the blood with influenza pneumonia is often <5,000/mm^3.

Influenza pneumonia in children can be diagnosed by viral culture or by rapid antigen testing with immunofluorescence or ELISA. Pharyngeal swabs or nasopharyngeal aspirates or gargles provide suitable specimens for culture. Serologic testing of specimens drawn in the acute and the convalescent phases, approximately 2 weeks apart, is an alternative method of diagnosis. Serologic tests include complement fixation tests or, for both influenza and parainfluenza viruses, hemagglutination inhibition. EIA tests for antibody are being developed. In general it is best if specimens are also processed for viral culture in addition to rapid diagnostic tests, as culture may be more sensitive or may grow a different virus.

TREATMENT

Most influenza requires only symptomatic treatment. Antiviral drugs for influenza are an adjunct to, and not a substitute for, influenza vaccination for the control and prevention of influenza and are effective only if started within 48 hours of the onset of symptoms (Table 68–11). Amantadine and rimantadine are chemically related antiviral drugs with activity against influenza A viruses but not against influenza B viruses. Amantadine is approved for treatment and prophylaxis of influenza A in adults and children ≥1 year of age. Rimantadine is approved for treatment and prophylaxis of infection in adults, although many experts consider it appropriate also for treatment of children. Zanamivir and oseltamivir are neuraminidase inhibitors with activity against both influenza A and B viruses. Zanamivir is approved only for treatment of persons ≥7 years of age, and oseltamivir is approved for prophylaxis in persons ≥13 years of age, and for treatment of persons ≥1 year of age. The four drugs differ in terms of their pharmacokinetics, adverse effects, and costs.

When administered within 2 days of the onset of illness to otherwise healthy adults, amantadine and rimantadine can reduce the duration of uncomplicated influenza A illness, and zanamivir and oseltamivir can reduce the duration of uncomplicated influenza A and B illness by approximately 1 day. None of the four antiviral agents has been demonstrated to be effective in preventing serious influenza-related complications, such as bacterial or viral pneumonia or exacerbation of chronic diseases. Data are limited and inconclusive concerning the effectiveness of amantadine, rimantadine, and zanamivir for treatment of influenza in persons at high risk of serious complications of influenza. Studies of the efficacy of any of the four drugs for treatment in children are limited, and safety for infants younger than 1 year of age has not been established. To reduce the emergence of antiviral drug-resistant viruses, amantadine or rimantadine therapy for persons with influenza-like illness

TABLE 68–11. Recommended Daily Dosage of Influenza Antiviral Medications for Treatment and Prophylaxis

Antiviral Agent	Age Group			
	1–9 yr	10–13 yr	14–64 yr	≥65 yr
Amantadine[1]				
Treatment (approved for ≥1 yr of age)	5 mg/kg/day up to 150 mg[2] in two divided doses, continued for 24–48 hr after disappearance of signs and symptoms	100 mg twice daily, continued for 24–48 hr after disappearance of signs and symptoms[3]	100 mg twice daily, continued for 24–48 hr after disappearance of signs and symptoms	≤100 mg/day, continued for 24–48 hr after disappearance of signs and symptoms
Prophylaxis (approved for ≥1 yr of age)	5 mg/kg/day up to 150 mg[2] in two divided doses for at least 10 days	100 mg twice daily for at least 10 days[3]	100 mg twice daily for at least 10 days	≤100 mg/day for at least 10 days
Rimantadine[4]				
Treatment (approved for ≥18 yr of age)	Not approved	Not approved	100 mg twice daily for 7 days	100 or 200 mg/day for 7 days[5]
Prophylaxis (approved for ≥1 yr of age)	5 mg/kg/day up to 150 mg[2] in two divided doses for at least 10 days	100 mg twice daily[2] for at least 10 days	100 mg twice daily for at least 10 days	100 or 200 mg/day for at least 10 days[5]
Oseltamivir				
Treatment (approved for ≥1 yr of age)	≤15 kg: 30 mg twice daily for 5 days 16–23 kg: 45 mg twice daily for 5 days 24–40 kg: 60 mg twice daily for 5 days >40 kg: 75 mg twice daily for 5 days		75 mg[7] twice daily for 5 days	75 mg twice daily for 5 days
Prophylaxis (approved for ≥13 yr of age)	Not approved	75 mg[8] once daily for at least 7 days	75 mg[8] once daily for at least 7 days	75 mg[8] once daily for at least 7 days
Zanamivir				
Treatment[6] (approved for ≥7 yr of age)	10 mg[6] twice daily for 5 days	10 mg twice daily for 5 days	10 mg twice daily for 5 days	10 mg twice daily for 5 days
Prophylaxis (not approved for prophylaxis)	Not approved	Not approved	Not approved	Not approved

[1]Consult the drug package insert for dosage recommendations for administering amantadine to persons with creatinine clearance ≤50 mL/min/1.73 m^2.
[2]5 mg/kg of amantadine or rimantadine syrup = 1 tsp/10 kg (22 lb).
[3]Children ≥10 years of age who weigh <40 kg should be administered amantadine or rimantadine at a dosage of 5 mg/kg/day.
[4]A reduction in dosage to 100 mg/day of rimantadine is recommended for persons who have severe hepatic dysfunction or those with creatinine clearance ≤10 mL/min. Other persons with less severe hepatic or renal dysfunction taking 100 mg/day of rimantadine should be observed closely, and the dosage should be reduced or the drug discontinued, if necessary.
[5]Elderly nursing home residents should be administered only 100 mg/day of rimantadine. A reduction in dosage to 100 mg/day should be considered for all persons ≥65 years of age if they experience possible side effects when taking 200 mg/day.
[6]Zanamivir is approved for treatment for persons ≥7 years of age and is administered as two 5 mg inhalations of medicated powder twice a day (i.e., 10 mg twice a day). The medication is administered via inhalation using a plastic device included in the package with the medication. Patients will benefit from instruction and demonstration of proper use of the device. Zanamivir is not approved for prophylaxis.
[7]Oseltamivir is approved for treatment for persons ≥1 year of age. A reduction in the dose of oseltamivir is recommended for persons with creatinine clearance <30 mL/min.
[8]Oseltamivir is approved for prophylaxis for persons ≥13 years of age.
Centers for Disease Control and Prevention: Prevention and control of influenza: Recommendations of the Advisory Committee on Immunizations Practices (ACIP). *MMWR Morb Mortal Wkly Rep* 2001;50(RR-4):1–44.

should be discontinued as soon as clinically warranted, generally after 3–5 days of treatment or within 24–48 hours after the disappearance of signs and symptoms. The recommended duration of treatment with either zanamivir or oseltamivir is 5 days.

The dose of amantadine must be reduced for patients with renal insufficiency. Amantadine is associated with CNS adverse effects, such as insomnia, nervousness, and ataxia. The use of rimantadine is reported to be associated with fewer of these adverse effects and because of lower cost is often the preferred agent for treatment and prophylaxis of influenza in adults. Amantadine is an alternative for treatment of younger patients without renal dysfunction. If community surveillance indicates influenza B activity, oseltamivir or zanamivir should be used for prophylaxis. Zanamivir is administered by inhalation with a Diskhaler device, which may exacerbate underlying pulmonary disease, including asthma, and cause bronchospasm.

PREVENTION

Vaccination. Influenza vaccine is strongly recommended for any person ≥6 months of age who is at increased risk of complications of influenza (Table 17–10). In addition, health care workers and other persons (including household members) in close contact with persons in high-risk groups should be vaccinated to decrease the risk of transmitting influenza to persons at high risk. Influenza vaccine also can be administered to any person aged ≥6 months of age who wishes to reduce the chance of becoming infected with influenza.

Prophylaxis. Chemoprophylactic drugs (Table 68–11) are not a substitute for vaccination. Amantadine and rimantadine are indicated for persons ≥1 year of age for prophylaxis of influenza A virus but are not effective against influenza B virus. Both drugs are approximately 70–90% effective in preventing illness from influenza A infection. Oseltamivir is approved for prophylaxis of persons ≥13 years of age and is effective against both influenza A and B viruses. When used as prophylaxis, these antiviral agents can prevent illness while permitting subclinical infection and the development of protective antibody against circulating influenza viruses. Therefore some persons who take these drugs will develop protective immune responses to circulating influenza viruses. Chemoprophylaxis does not interfere with the antibody response to the vaccine.

To be maximally effective as prophylaxis, the drug must be continued throughout the expected influenza season; alternatively, it may be used to cover the 2 weeks immediately after vaccination during the development of protective immunity. However, to be most cost-effective, prophylaxis should be taken only during the period of peak influenza activity in a community.

PROGNOSIS

Death rates from influenza can be very high in epidemic years. The mortality is greatest among infants, the elderly, and persons of any age with a chronic debilitating underlying disease. Influenza is the only infectious disease in which the mortality in epidemic years significantly affects the raw mortality for the whole country.

ENTEROVIRUS

Enteroviruses are single-stranded RNA viruses that include coxsackieviruses, echoviruses, and polioviruses. Enteroviruses are spread primarily by the fecal-oral route and multiply in the gastrointestinal tissues. Despite their name, however, gastrointestinal symptoms are only incidental to systemic disease. Although the nonpolio enteroviruses are occasional causes of pneumonia, respiratory symptoms are among the least common symptoms of enteroviral syndromes.

Coxsackieviruses and echoviruses cause self-limited diseases notable for fever and a rash, sometimes with CNS (Chapter 55) or cardiac involvement (Chapter 72). They also may cause overwhelming perinatal infection (Chapter 97). Enterovirus 71 is a recently discovered enterovirus that is highly pathogenic. In a large outbreak in Taiwan, no cases of pneumonia were noted, although pulmonary edema and pulmonary hemorrhage were reported as complications.

In otherwise healthy children a lower respiratory tract infection, including pneumonia, that may accompany an enteroviral infection is not distinctive. Rare clusters of enteroviral pneumonia have been reported. Unlike the classic respiratory viruses (e.g., RSV, influenza virus, and parainfluenza viruses), enteroviruses are mostly dormant in the winter, with most enteroviral infection occurring during the warm weather months. Diagnosis is made by isolation of the virus from respiratory secretions or lung tissue. Isolation of enterovirus from the stool should not be considered diagnostic of pneumonia, because there are many asymptomatic stool shedders in the summer. An exception would be when paired sera demonstrate a rise in neutralizing activity against the virus isolated. Most cases of enteroviral infection are mild and self-limited. In severe overwhelming infections, intravenous immunoglobulin infusions have been used, with anecdotal reports of success mostly in neonatal infections and infections in immunocompromised hosts. At this time a new experimental antiviral agent, pleconaril, is being studied for use in overwhelming neonatal infection. The drug is available on an investigational basis.

Good hygiene is important in the prevention of enteroviral infections. Reducing contact with infected persons and meticulous hand-washing before contact with other persons are important in preventing transmission.

HANTAVIRUS CARDIOPULMONARY SYNDROME

In the southwestern United States in May 1993 an outbreak of acute febrile illness associated with respiratory failure, shock, and high mortality was identified by investigators from the CDC as being caused by a previously unrecognized hantavirus. Cases occurring since 1980 have been identified retrospectively by serologic testing.

ETIOLOGY

Several Old World hantaviruses cause hemorrhagic fever with renal syndrome, and several New World hantaviruses cause hantavirus cardiopulmonary syndrome (HCPS), most notably Sin Nombre virus in the United States (Table 68–12). Hantaviruses are single-stranded RNA viruses of the Bunyaviridae family. The prototype of the hantaviruses is **Hantaan virus,** which causes hemorrhagic fever with renal syndrome, with a 5–15% mortality. A different rodent reservoir for each hantavirus maintains the virus in nature. Severe pulmonary disease had not been recognized with hantaviruses before the outbreak in the United States in 1993.

In the United States, 95% of cases have been identified west of the Mississippi River, where *Peromyscus maniculatus* (the deer mouse) is the primary vector of Sin Nombre hantavirus (Fig. 68–7). *P. maniculatus* is found throughout Canada and the United States (except for the southeast and the Atlantic seaboard), central Mexico, and northern South America. Another hantavirus, Black Creek Canal virus, is transmitted by the rodent *Sigmondon hispidus* (the cotton rat).

Transmission. Hantavirus infection in rodents is asymptomatic and lifelong. The virus is transmitted horizontally among rodents who shed the virus in saliva, urine, and feces. Transmission to humans occurs predominantly by aerosolization and inhalation of infected rodent excreta or contaminated airborne particles. Human activities associated with hantavirus infection include cleaning of barns and other outbuildings, trapping rodents, animal herding, and farming with hand tools.

TABLE 68–12. Hantaviruses

Hantavirus	Disease	Geographic Distribution	Rodent Reservoir
Old World Hantaviruses			
Subfamily* Murinae-*Associated Viruses			
Hantaan	Hemorrhagic fever with renal syndrome (Korean hemorrhagic fever); 5–15% mortality	Rural Asia, Far East, Russia	*Apodemus agrarius* (striped field mouse)
Dobrava	Hemorrhagic fever with renal syndrome; 5–35% mortality	Balkans	*Apodemus flavicollis* (yellow-necked field mouse)
		Europe	*Apodemus agrarius* (striped field mouse)
Seoul	Hemorrhagic fever with renal syndrome (Korean hemorrhagic fever); mild to moderate in severity (1% mortality)	Worldwide	*Rattus norvegicus* *Rattus rattus* (rats)
Subfamily* Arvicolinae-*Associated Viruses			
Puumala	Hemorrhagic fever with renal syndrome (epidemic hemorrhagic fever; nephropathia epidemica); mild in severity (rare mortality)	Scandinavia, northern and eastern Europe, Balkans	*Clethrionomys glareolus* (bank vole)
New World Hantaviruses			
Subfamily* Sigmodontinae-*Associated Viruses			
Sin Nombre	Hantavirus cardiopulmonary syndrome (50% mortality)	West and Central United States and Canada	*Peromyscus maniculatus* (deer mouse)
Monongahela	Hantavirus cardiopulmonary syndrome	Eastern United States and Canada	*Peromyscus maniculatus*
New York	Hantavirus cardiopulmonary syndrome	Eastern United States	*Peromyscus leucopus*
Bayou	Hantavirus cardiopulmonary syndrome	Southeastern United States	*Oryzomys palustris*
Black Creek Canal	Hantavirus cardiopulmonary syndrome	Florida	*Sigmodon hispidus* (cotton rat)
Andes	Hantavirus cardiopulmonary syndrome	Argentina and Chile	*Oligoryzomys longicaudatus*
Oran	Hantavirus cardiopulmonary syndrome	Northwestern Argentina	*Oligorozomys longicaudatus*
Lechiguanas	Hantavirus cardiopulmonary syndrome	Central Argentina	*Oligoryzomys flavescens*
Hu39694	Hantavirus cardiopulmonary syndrome	Central Argentina	Unknown
Laguna Negra	Hantavirus cardiopulmonary syndrome	Paraguay and Bolivia	*Calomys laucha*
Juquitiba	Hantavirus cardiopulmonary syndrome	Brazil	Unknown

EPIDEMIOLOGY

Through December 2000, 277 cases in 31 states have been reported in the United States (Fig. 68–7). The states with the highest number of cases are New Mexico, Arizona, California, and Colorado. Most cases have occurred in persons 20–40 years of age (median, 31 years) who previously were healthy. There have been occasional cases in adolescents but no reports in children younger than 12 years of age or in the elderly. The virus affects both sexes equally. There is no person-to-person or nosocomial transmission of hantaviruses.

PATHOGENESIS

Hantavirus infection results from inhalation of infectious aerosols from rodent saliva or excreta. HCPS results from increased pulmo-

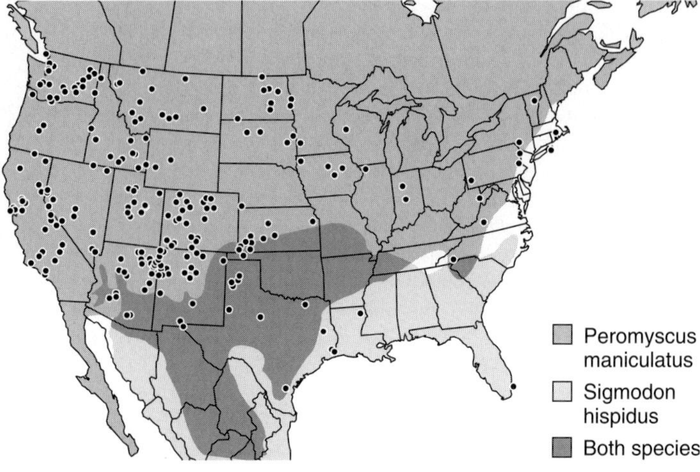

FIGURE 68–7. Distributions of known rodent hosts for hantaviruses in North America, and location of the 277 cases in 31 states of hantavirus cardiopulmonary syndrome reported in the United States through 2000. (Data from the CDC. Rodent distributions from Burt WH, Grossenheider RP: *A Field Guide to the Mammals,* 3rd ed. New York, Houghton Mifflin, 1980.)

nary vascular permeability and capillary leak syndrome, resulting in noncardiac pulmonary edema and pleural effusions and culminating in acute respiratory distress syndrome (ARDS). The liver, kidneys, heart, and brain are grossly normal. The retroperitoneal effusions that are characteristic of hemorrhagic fever with renal syndrome are absent.

SYMPTOMS AND CLINICAL MANIFESTATIONS

The incubation period following exposure is 4–42 days, with an average of 12–16 days. Asymptomatic or mild infection occurs rarely, if at all. Most affected persons have been previously healthy young adult agriculture workers or campers. The early symptoms of the prodromal phase, which lasts 3–6 days, are nonspecific. Fever and myalgia are universal, and cough, headache, and nausea or vomiting are seen in approximately 70% of patients. Chills, malaise, and diarrhea are seen in more than 50% of patients, and dizziness or light-headedness, arthralgia, back pain, abdominal pain, or chest pain are seen in 20–40%. Significant respiratory symptoms are notably absent in the early phase, and the pulmonary examination and chest radiograph are normal. During this phase most persons do not appear to be severely ill; tachypnea is the only physical finding, and patients do not appear to require hospitalization or medication. This prodrome distinguishes HCPS from ARDS, which begins as a respiratory disease with cough and dyspnea.

The cardiopulmonary phase is characterized by progressive shortness of breath with cough, tachypnea, tachycardia, and fever that are due to capillary leakage. Laboratory abnormalities develop during this phase and include leukocytosis with a shift to the left, hemoconcentration, thrombocytopenia, and prolonged partial thromboplastin time. There may be moderate proteinuria, but renal failure is not common. Progressive hypoxemia and hypotension require intubation and assisted ventilation in most patients, usually within 24 hours of hospitalization.

The convalescent phase is characterized by rapid improvement over a few days in oxygenation and hemodynamic function. Diuresis is common.

DIAGNOSIS

Distinguishing HCPS from other acute febrile illnesses, especially influenza, during the prodromal phase is difficult. The radiologic picture of HCPS is evolution of minimal bilateral pulmonary edema to severe bilateral alveolar edema, with pleural effusions commonly seen. The diagnosis of HCPS should be considered in any previously healthy person with a febrile illness (temperature of 38.3°C [101°F] or greater) characterized by unexplained ARDS or bilateral interstitial pulmonary infiltrates requiring supplemental oxygen developing within 1 week of hospitalization. It should also be considered when an unexplained respiratory illness results in death and an autopsy demonstrates noncardiogenic pulmonary edema without an identifiable specific cause of death. The differential diagnosis in the cardiopulmonary phase includes pneumococcal pneumonia, severe mycoplasmal pneumonia, influenza, respiratory syncytial virus infection in young children, legionellosis, pulmonary tularemia, pneumonic plague, leptospirosis, rickettsial infections, and disseminated fungal infections, including psittacosis and histoplasmosis.

Laboratory Diagnosis

Routine laboratory studies demonstrate nonspecific abnormalities. The WBC count is often elevated with a shift to the left (immature cells of the neutrophilic series) in approximately 90% of patients and atypical lymphocytes in approximately 25% of patients. Other frequent findings include hypoxemia, hemoconcentration due to capillary leak syndrome, a moderate degree of thrombocytopenia, clotting abnormalities, metabolic acidosis, and renal function abnormalities.

Microbiologic Diagnosis

The diagnosis of hantavirus pulmonary syndrome is usually confirmed by highly specific serologic tests for Sin Nombre virus IgM antibodies or a fourfold or greater rise in serum Sin Nombre virus IgG antibodies. The ELISA is available at the CDC, many state laboratories, and some hospitals. A Western blot test using recombinant antigens is also available. Hantavirus may also be diagnosed by detection of hantavirus antigen in tissue by immunohistochemistry, and amplification of hantavirus ribonucleic acid sequences by reverse-transcriptase PCR. Isolation of the virus from human tissue has not been reported and should not be attempted in routine laboratories because of safety issues.

TREATMENT

In patients with hantavirus pulmonary syndrome, treatment is supportive and requires intensive care and, in many cases, assisted ventilation and support for hypotension, ARDS, renal failure, and hemorrhage. Early correction of hypoxia, avoidance of excessive intravenous fluid administration, and use of inotropic and vasopressive drugs are important. Extracorporeal membrane oxygenation (ECMO) has been successful in supporting a few patients with HCPS. There is no effective specific antiviral therapy. Intravenous ribavirin has been used in some patients but with no clearly positive influence on outcome. Controlled trials have been performed without apparent dramatic improvement, and an NIH-sponsored trial is continuing.

COMPLICATIONS AND PROGNOSIS

The complications that arise are secondary to hypoxemia and hypotension. Death from intractable hypotension may occur 2–16 days after the onset of symptoms. The mortality rate is 43%. The long-term sequelae of hantavirus pulmonary syndrome are unknown, but recovery has been complete among patients who survive the cardiopulmonary phase. Laboratory predictors of mortality include severe hemoconcentration, high levels of lactate dehydrogenase, elevated WBC count, and prolonged partial thromboplastin time.

PREVENTION

There is no prophylactic agent or vaccine for hantavirus. Prevention involves avoidance of the organism by avoiding the habitat of the rodent reservoir and by control of the rodent population near homes and where people must go as part of their occupations (see Table 3–7). Campers should avoid rodent-infested areas and any food or liquid that could be contaminated with rodent excreta.

PNEUMOCYSTIS CARINII PNEUMONIA

Pneumocystis carinii pneumonia (PCP) is primarily an infection of immunocompromised persons, especially patients with AIDS. There is, however, a wide spectrum of diseases caused by this organism; these include nonpulmonary diseases and diseases in immunocompetent hosts. Nevertheless, when the diagnosis of PCP is made in a patient with no known underlying risk factor, it is necessary to evaluate immune function with appropriate tests. Extrapulmonary infections represent a small fraction of *P. carinii* infections.

ETIOLOGY

The taxonomy of *P. carinii* has not been clearly established. It behaves as a protozoan, where it is usually classified, but it has strong genetic and metabolic similarity to fungi.

EPIDEMIOLOGY

P. carinii first became known as a cause of **plasma cell interstitial pneumonia** in severely malnourished infants in Europe after World War II. It was not until the 1960s that *P. carinii* was appreciated in the United States as a cause of pneumonia in immunocompromised persons. The spectrum of immunosuppression that predisposes to PCP includes neoplasms, cancer chemotherapy, and transplant immunosuppression, but its association with AIDS since 1981 overshadows all other predisposing illnesses. Occasionally infants in the United States who were adopted from orphanages in the Far East are found to have PCP.

The importance of PCP in hosts who are not immunocompromised is the subject of some debate. Studies of infants younger than 3 months with pneumonia (Stagno et al., 1981; Brasfield et al., 1987) reported PCP as a cause of 17–18% of cases of afebrile pneumonia. The standard of diagnosis in many of these cases was measurement of an antigen in the serum by counterimmunoelectrophoresis. This test is controversial and probably not as accurate as a histologic examination, which is the standard. In these studies many patients also had evidence of coinfection with other infectious agents. A small series of healthy adults with PCP has been reported in New York City. Because empirical anti-PCP therapy is often used without diagnostic tests, the reported incidence of confirmed PCP may underestimate the actual rate.

PATHOGENESIS

Current knowledge of the pathogenesis of PCP is limited by the inability to cultivate the organism. Most information comes from histologic examinations of lungs and from the experimental model of spontaneous infection, rats treated with steroids. Evidence of person-to-person spread is lacking. One hypothesis of pathogenesis is that *P. carinii* is a ubiquitous organism that colonizes the lung but generally is not evident unless the host is immunosuppressed and its multiplication is uncontrolled. Little is known of the reservoir or transmission in nature. In the lungs *P. carinii* causes a plasma cell and lymphocytic infiltrate in the infantile form. In the immunodeficient child there are organisms and infiltrate in the alveolar spaces. With more extensive disease there is alveolar cell desquamation, alveolar wall thickening, clusters of organisms, extensive cellular infiltration, and edema in the alveolar spaces.

SYMPTOMS AND CLINICAL MANIFESTATIONS

The characteristic disease caused by *P. carinii* is pneumonia. Extrapulmonary foci have been reported in almost every tissue, including brain, bone, bone marrow, thyroid, and viscera. A high rate of extrapulmonary foci has been found in patients with AIDS who receive inhaled pentamidine prophylaxis, which protects against pulmonary PCP.

Infant PCP. PCP in premature and debilitated infants is a slowly progressive pneumonia. The symptoms are marked by a progressively increasing cough with tachypnea and the development of moderate to severe respiratory distress. Most infants are afebrile but have crackles on auscultation. Untreated, this disease has a high mortality, up to 25–50% in early reports.

PCP in Immunocompromised Patients. Although the onset of PCP can be abrupt or insidious, abrupt onset is most characteristic. In a series (Hughes et al., 1973) of 100 children with PCP and underlying cancer, nearly all children presented with a fever (<38°C [100.4°F]), tachypnea, and infiltrates on a chest radiograph, and 80% had a cough. In AIDS-associated PCP the presentation of PCP is quite variable, with a range from barely symptomatic disease with only minor tachypnea, to symptoms similar to those of bacterial pneumonia, to acute, life-threatening respiratory compromise. Fever and coughing are present in more than 80% of patients, shortness of breath in about 70%, and chills, increased sputum production, and chest pain each reported in about 25% of patients.

DIAGNOSIS

Nonspecific laboratory tests, including CBC, ESR, and CRP, are not of help in differentiating PCP from pneumonia due to other causes, especially in immunocompromised patients. Because of shunting within the lungs, clinically significant hypoxia is common with PCP, especially in comparison with focal bacterial pneumonias, and may occur very early in the clinical course. In patients with AIDS, the combination of tachypnea and decreased oxygen saturation in the blood is an early clue to the diagnosis of PCP.

Diagnostic Imaging

Typically, a chest radiograph shows bilateral diffuse markings that progress to alveolar infiltrates that spread from hilar regions to the periphery (see Fig. 38–7). Lobar patterns as well as foci that look like a nodule or an abscess are occasionally encountered. PCP has been reported in patients with chest radiographs that are normal when the diagnosis is made.

Microbiologic Evaluation

Demonstration of the organisms in smears of secretions or in tissue are essential for diagnosis because neither a culture nor tests for antigen are currently available. PCP can be diagnosed if the organism is demonstrated in coughed sputum, tracheal aspirates, bronchial washings or brushings, a transbronchial biopsy specimen, a transthoracic aspirate or biopsy specimen, or a specimen from an open-chest lung biopsy. Although less invasive studies, such as induction of sputum or bronchoscopy to obtain bronchial washings, are diagnostic when organisms are seen, negative results do not exclude PCP. An open-chest lung biopsy is the most valuable single procedure because it is definitive, is safe when performed by pediatric surgeons, and allows diagnosis of infection by other pathogens that frequently coinfect severely immunocompromised patients. Nevertheless, bronchoalveolar lavage is being used increasingly as an excellent compromise between sensitivity and safety.

The diagnosis of PCP requires that smears or tissue be examined by pathologists familiar with special stains and the morphologic features of the organism. **Gomori's methenamine-silver nitrate stain** and **toluidine blue 0** are used to stain cysts (see Fig. 8–5). Other stains, such as methylene blue, Wright's, and Giemsa, stain sporozoites and trophozoites but not cysts. Often the correct diagnosis is missed because these structures are not specific enough to be identified correctly. It is now recognized that **acellular foamy-**

appearing eosinophilic debris within alveolar spaces is consistent with PCP.

TREATMENT

There are several treatment regimens for PCP (Table 68–13). Pentamidine was the first agent found effective for PCP. Toxicities, including bone-marrow, hepatic, and renal toxicity, and hypoglycemia are common. TMP-SMZ is the treatment of choice for patients who are not intolerant to it. Adverse effects include rashes, both minor and major, bone marrow suppression, and gastrointestinal symptoms. Many patients with PCP respond slowly to either drug. Drug resistance is difficult to demonstrate, and it is not clear that resistance is a cause of clinical failure of the drug. It is recommended that switching from one drug to another be done only when drug intolerance has clearly developed or the patient continues to have pneumonia with respiratory distress after a full course of treatment. Other antimicrobial agents have been poorly studied in children and should not be considered first-choice options.

Experience with patients with AIDS shows that prednisone may be beneficial in moderate or severe PCP. The greatest benefit is achieved with early administration in addition to anti–*P. carinii* therapy (Chapter 38).

PREVENTION

A major development in the control of PCP has been the use of antimicrobial prophylaxis in patients at high risk. TMP-SMZ was first used for this purpose, and in the AIDS era additional regimens for PCP prophylaxis have been developed (Table 68–14) because intolerance to TMP-SMZ has been common in patients with AIDS. TMP-SMZ is considered to be the most effective prophylactic agent. Indications for beginning PCP prophylaxis are discussed in Chapter 38. *P. carinii* prophylaxis is indicated for all children being treated for leukemia or lymphoma, for immunosuppressed patients with transplants, and for selected patients undergoing intensive chemotherapeutic regimens for solid tumors. Prophylaxis is generally begun around the time of initiation of anticancer therapy and continued until 6 months after chemotherapy has been completed and the disease is in remission (Chapter 99).

Aerosolized pentamidine is frequently used for children, but unlike TMP-SMZ it does not prevent extrapulmonary *P. carinii* infection. The use of aerosolized pentamidine requires special nebulizers and infection containment units and is limited to specialized centers. Other regimens shown in Table 68–14 are not well studied in children, and their safety has not yet been established.

ASPIRATION PNEUMONIA AND "FOREIGN BODY" PNEUMONIA

Aspiration pneumonia is the lower respiratory tract inflammation that follows aspiration of material from the oral cavity or the stomach into the lungs. Although much of the inflammation that occurs is due to chemical irritation from the aspirated material, especially if acidic gastric contents are involved, infection is always a potential complication because of the nonsterile nature of aspirated body fluids and foreign material. **Foreign body pneumonia** is the inflammation caused by the aspiration of indigestible solid material into the tracheobronchial tree. In this case, the inflammation may be due to irritation from the foreign body or infection from contaminants carried in with the foreign body. In addition, with either type of aspiration, indigestible material wedged in the tracheobronchial tree impairs the normal host defenses afforded by the phagocytic macrophage system and the elevator effect of

TABLE 68–13. Antimicrobial Therapy for *Pneumocystis carinii* Pneumonia*

Treatment	Drug	Dosage	Route	Dose Interval*
Standard treatment	TMP-SMZ	IV: TMP 15 mg/kg/day SMZ 75 mg/kg/day	IV or PO	Divided q6hr
	or	PO: TMP 20 mg/kg/day SMZ 100 mg/kg/day		
	Pentamidine	4 mg/kg/day	IV	Once daily
	with or without			
	Prednisone	Days 1–5: 1 mg/kg/day (maximum 80 mg/day)	PO	Divided q12hr
		Days 6–10: 0.5 mg/kg/day (maximum 40 mg/day)	PO	Divided q12hr
	or	Days 11–21: 0.25 mg/kg/day (max 20 mg/day)	PO	Once daily
	Methylprednisolone	2–4 mg/kg/day	IV	q6–12hr for 5–14 days; taper for 1 additional week
Alternative treatments				
Mild to moderate disease	Dapsone	2 mg/kg/day (max 100 mg/day)	PO	Divided q6hr
	plus			
	TMP	15 mg/kg/day	PO	Divided q6hr
	Atovaquone	750 mg	PO	Divided q12hr Once daily
	Primaquine base	0.3 mg/kg/day (max 15 mg/day)	PO	
	plus			
	Clindamycin	25–40 mg/kg/day (max 2.4 g/day)	IV	Divided q6hr
Severe disease	Trimetrexate	45 $mg/m^2/day$	IV	Once per day
	plus			
	Folinic acid	80 $mg/m^2/day$	IV or PO	Divided q6hr

***Duration of antimicrobials:** 14–21 days. HIV-infected patients should be treated for 21 days.

TABLE 68–14. Primary and Secondary Prophylaxis for Preventing *Pneumocystis carinii* Pneumonia

Regimen	Drug	Dosage	Route	Dose Interval and Duration
Standard regimen Children 1 mo or older	TMP-SMZ	TMP 150 mg/m²/day; SMZ 750 mg/m²/day (max daily dose 160 mg TMP; 800 mg SMZ)	PO	Divided twice per day on 3 consecutive days each week
Alternative regimens	TMP-SMZ	Same dose as above	PO	Single dose twice daily on 3 consecutive days each week *or* Divided twice per day, daily *or* Divided twice per day, every other day, three times per week
Alternative regimens if TMP-SMZ is not tolerated				
Children 5 yr or older	Pentamidine	300 mg	Inhaled	Monthly via *Respirgard* II nebulizer
Children 1 mo or older	Dapsone *with or without*	2 mg/kg/day (max 100 mg/day) *or* 4 mg/kg/day (maximum 200 mg/day)	PO	Once daily Weekly
	Pyrimethamine	50 mg	PO	Once daily
	plus folinic acid	25 mg	PO	Weekly
Alternative regimen for children intolerant of all other regimens	Atovaquone	30–45 mg/kg/day	PO	Once daily

the ciliated epithelium. Some minor aspiration events probably occur periodically in healthy persons, but normal host defenses prevent pneumonia from developing. Unrecognized aspiration events in which potentially virulent organisms from the upper airway are transported to the small airways may be the precipitating events in the pathogenesis of pyogenic bacterial pneumonia.

ETIOLOGY

The flora associated with aspiration pneumonia reflects the normal flora of the upper airway. Anaerobic flora predominates, including anaerobic streptococci, *Fusobacterium, Bacteroides,* and *Prevotella melaninogenica,* with a smaller percentage (<20%) of *Bacteroides fragilis.* Aerobic flora also can be recovered. In addition to normal pharyngeal flora, many patients who were previously ill and hospitalized have mixed gram-negative bacilli species. In studies in which transtracheal aspiration was used to obtain cultures (Brook, 1980), an average of five different species were isolated from the lower respiratory flora of children with aspiration pneumonia. In more than 90% of the children some anaerobic species was isolated, and in more than 90% of them mixed anaerobic and aerobic species were isolated. These microbiologic isolates are similar to the isolates reported for aspiration pneumonia in adults.

EPIDEMIOLOGY AND PATHOGENESIS

The underlying predisposing factors for aspiration pneumonia are usually acute and chronic neurologic disorders that result in abnormal sucking and swallowing. In general, the types of disorders include congenital developmental disorders of the brain and genetic neuromuscular disorders that affect the state of alertness, muscle tone, coordination of swallowing, or the gag reflex. Epilepsy is associated with aspiration, as is any cardiac or traumatic disorder that involves loss of consciousness. Acquired neurologic disorders, such as brain trauma, anesthesia, binges of alcohol intake, or use of mind-altering drugs, are all associated with aspiration. Hospitalized patients who have oropharyngeal procedures, including tracheal intubation or treatment with drugs that affect the state of alertness, are predisposed to aspiration events. Gastroesophageal reflux is also associated with aspiration pneumonia. Thus, although occasional cases of aspiration pneumonia involve previously healthy persons from the community, in most patients the pneumonia develops either in the hospital or as a consequence of the acute injury or toxic ingestion that brings the patient to the hospital.

Foreign body pneumonia is much more likely to occur in previously healthy children from the community, predominantly in boys. There is some overlap with aspiration pneumonia because persons likely to have aspiration may be more likely not to be able to cough up a foreign body. Most patients are younger than 3 years and aspirate toys, coins, other small objects, or solid foods such as nuts. How the patients come to medical attention depends on the size of the object, its composition, and the location in the airway. Larger objects are more likely to lodge centrally and obstruct breathing or swallowing. These objects must be removed with a bronchoscope or a laryngoscope. Usually this is accomplished before an infectious pneumonia has had time to become established. Objects that break into many pieces do not produce dramatic acute symptoms, and pneumonia may develop later. Small objects, such as peanuts, pencil points and erasers, and foods such as seeds, may lodge peripherally and may not be noticed until pneumonia develops. One important reason to make this diagnosis quickly is that if chronic infection occurs, there may be permanent damage to the bronchus, including strictures or bronchiectasis.

SYMPTOMS AND CLINICAL MANIFESTATIONS

The actual aspiration event may or may not be witnessed. Because so many patients have either temporary or chronic mental impairment, a clear history of aspiration is often unobtainable. If, however, the event is witnessed and the aspirated material is removed promptly and adequately, subsequent pulmonary symptoms may be minimal. Other manifestations include excessive mucus production and bronchospasm as well as cough and tachypnea accompanied by fine and coarse crackles. The rapid development of fever, leukocytosis, and sputum production within hours of aspiration usually indicates noninfectious inflammation caused by chemical irritation from the material aspirated.

Bacterial pneumonia caused by aspiration usually develops relatively slowly over a period of several days. Patients usually have a low-grade fever, malaise, and increased sputum production. In patients with severe pre-existing neurologic functional abnormalities, these changes may be difficult to recognize. In later stages, complications may develop, including progressive necrotizing pneumonia, one or many lung abscesses, and empyema.

DIAGNOSIS

There are no specific diagnostic tests for aspiration pneumonia. Careful history-taking and clinical judgment are most important. Leukocytosis is frequent. If sputum is available for analysis, it shows many polymorphonuclear leukocytes and mixed morphology of bacteria. A culture of coughed sputum is of little value because the mixed aerobic flora is similar to normal throat flora. Coughed sputum is an inappropriate specimen for anaerobic culture because of the inevitable presence of upper airway anaerobes. Some sort of invasive procedure is necessary should better cultures be deemed necessary. For adults, transtracheal aspiration, which avoids contamination with upper airway flora, is useful, but this technique has not gained popularity in pediatrics. Bronchoscopy with a suction culture can be used in this circumstance, but only with a shielded instrument can contamination by upper airway flora be avoided. For these reasons, treatment of children with presumed aspiration pneumonia is usually empirical and based on a few clinical studies of efficacy. Blood cultures, cultures of pleural fluid, and specimens obtained by invasive procedures may yield information important in choosing definitive therapy.

Diagnostic Imaging

Chest radiographic findings are nonspecific. Frequently no clear change from previous baseline radiographs can be appreciated at first. The pattern of consolidation may be helpful in that consolidation usually occurs in the dependent lobes (Fig. 68–8) and may occur within 2 hours of aspiration. These are the basilar segments of the lower lobes if the patient aspirated while sitting or the posterior segments of the upper lobes if the patient aspirated while lying down.

Radiologic imaging of a foreign body may not be possible if the object is radiolucent. Use of **inspiratory and expiratory radiographs** or **fluoroscopy** to demonstrate a lobe or segment that remains either collapsed or hyperaerated throughout the breathing cycle can be a hint that a foreign body blocks a bronchus. Recurrent pneumonia in one segment or focal segmental collapse also may be a clue to the presence of a foreign body.

TREATMENT

Regardless of the type of aspiration, the most important aspect of treatment is recognition of the problem and prompt removal of the aspirated material. The management team must include radiologists and surgeons. If aspiration occurs while the patient is under medical supervision and the material is removed rapidly by suction followed by chest physiotherapy, infection is unlikely to occur, and antibiotic treatment is not indicated. Should pneumonia develop later with accompanying fever and purulent sputum with many bacteria, antibiotic treatment should be initiated. The choice of antibiotic depends on the situation leading to the aspiration. If the aspiration occurred outside the hospital or after an elective operation, penicillin or ampicillin in doses appropriate for pneumonia (Table 68–6) is generally satisfactory. Selected studies of anaerobic lung abscesses in adults suggest that adding another antibiotic for resistant gram-negative anaerobes such as clindamycin is of benefit. It is reasonable to consider this course when dealing with virulent aspiration pneumonia. Other antibiotic choices that give a similar spectrum of coverage include penicillin plus chloramphenicol, penicillin plus metronidazole, or the combination drug ampicillin-sulbactam. Numerous studies of the treatment of aspiration pneumonia in children and adults show that penicillin G is as effective as combination antibiotic therapy. The results of treatment do not always correlate with culture reports, as exemplified by the usual good response to penicillin G treatment of patients with aspiration or lung abscesses, even with isolation of penicillin-resistant *Bacteroides fragilis* from a culture that grows several bacterial species.

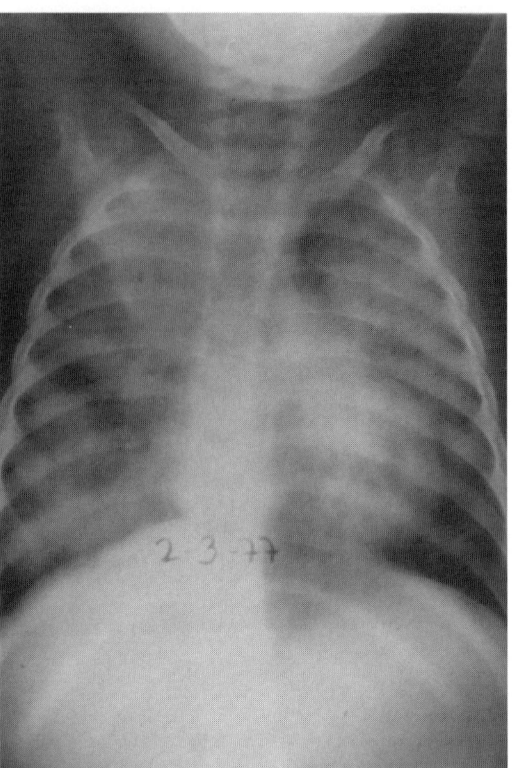

FIGURE 68–8. Aspiration pneumonia in a 4-year-old debilitated child with severe neuromuscular impairment, tachypnea, and high fever after an episode of vomiting and aspiration of stomach contents. Frontal supine chest radiograph showing widespread air-space consolidation in the dependent portions of both lungs.

The approach to a previously hospitalized patient with aspiration pneumonia requires individualization that takes into consideration underlying disease, previous respiratory cultures, the epidemiologic features of the hospital, and the toxicities of various antibiotics. Empirical therapy for hospitalized patients who are either at risk of aspirating aerobic gram-negative bacilli or in whom a sample of good-quality sputum shows predominant gram-negative bacilli, should include a third-generation cephalosporin, such as ceftazidime or cefotaxime, or the addition of an aminoglycoside, such as gentamicin. Empirical regimens may have to be individually designed to cover unusually resistant strains known to be resident in a particular hospital. Knowledge that a patient has such strains in the upper airway before the aspiration is especially important in this regard. Aspiration pneumonia can be treated for 1 week if there is a good response to therapy and if no complications such as lung abscess or necrotizing pneumonia develop. These complications necessitate longer treatment. Because so many patients with aspiration pneumonia are in a milieu such as a hospital or institution where they may become colonized with antibiotic-resistant bacterial strains, it is important to use as short a course of antibiotic therapy as possible to avoid superinfection.

Management of foreign body aspiration requires removal of the object, and experienced pediatric bronchoscopists should be consulted. The object should be removed without being shattered. If this is successful, antibiotic treatment is not necessary. If an object shatters, many procedures may be required before all of the object and fibrinous adherent tissue are removed. Prompt recognition and removal are important in reducing the chances of scarring with resultant stricture of the bronchus. The use of antibiotics for an aspirated foreign body depends on whether concomitant pneumonia develops. If it does, antibiotics directed against normal pharyngeal flora, usually with appropriate doses of a β-lactam agent such as penicillin G, ampicillin, or cefuroxime, are appropriate (Table 68–6).

NOSOCOMIAL PNEUMONIA, INCLUDING VENTILATOR-ASSOCIATED PNEUMONIA (VAP)

Diagnosis and effective treatment of ventilator-associated pneumonia (VAP) is one of the most challenging entities in infectious diseases practice. VAP is a subset of nosocomial pneumonias with risk factors similar to those of other nosocomial respiratory tract infections (Chapter 105).

ETIOLOGY

During early hospitalization nosocomial pneumonia, including VAP, is generally due to community-acquired organisms such as *S. pneumoniae, H. influenzae,* or anaerobes. After approximately 4 days of hospitalization, bacterial pneumonia is more likely to be due to gram-negative species such as *Klebsiella, Acinetobacter,* and *Pseudomonas aeruginosa,* and also *Staphylococcus aureus.* With prolonged hospitalization, especially in patients treated with antibiotics, methicillin-resistant *S. aureus* and multiply antibiotic-resistant gram-negative bacilli species are additional concerns. In addition, viral pneumonias such as those caused by RSV or parainfluenza viruses can be nosocomially transmitted and can spread in the ICU during seasonal outbreaks. However, these viruses are not particularly associated with VAP.

EPIDEMIOLOGY AND PATHOGENESIS

The major risk factor for nosocomial pneumonia is the use of mechanical ventilation. Intubation of patients bypasses the most important host defenses that prevent pneumonia: the cough reflex to expectorate respiratory secretions, the upper airway cleansing system, derangement of the ciliary elevator system, and pooled secretions that permit local multiplication of organisms from the environment, from the upper airway, and probably from the gastrointestinal tract. Organisms may enter the lower airways by direct flow of contaminated air or aerosolization of contaminated fluids from nebulizers or humidifiers. Organisms from the upper airway and stomach may leak around the cuffed end of the tube and be aspirated into the lungs. Prior antibiotic treatment appears to be an additional risk factor because environmental organisms, especially gram-negative bacilli species, may have a colonization advantage when normal flora are suppressed. The use of H_2 blockers to reduce gastric acid secretion appears to increase host susceptibility because environmental organisms may more easily colonize the stomach and later be aspirated into the lungs. Additional risk factors include durations of hospitalization, intensive care, and mechanical ventilation. In children the rate of VAP is low compared with the rate in adults, partly because of the lack of some of the risk factors but also because it is difficult to fulfill criteria used for diagnosis of VAP in adults.

DIAGNOSIS

The CDC criteria for nosocomial pneumonia require signs of rales or dullness to percussion (or, for infants, any two signs of apnea, tachypnea, bradycardia, wheezing, rhonchi, or cough) plus any one of the following: new onset of purulent sputum or change in the character of sputum; isolation of a respiratory pathogen from blood culture; or isolation of a respiratory pathogen from a lower respiratory tract specimen obtained by transtracheal aspiration, bronchoscopy, or biopsy. Also acceptable for diagnosis would be new radiographic changes consistent with an infectious process along with either sputum changes, a positive blood culture, isolation of a respiratory pathogen from a lower respiratory tract specimen, isolation of a virus from respiratory secretions, serologic evidence of infection in paired sera, or histopathologic evidence of pneumonia. The diagnosis of VAP is more difficult and frequently involves obtaining lower lung fluid by bronchoscopy with a protected specimen brush or bronchoalveolar lavage, which are not routinely performed in children. Even with these recommendations, it is generally believed that VAP is overdiagnosed.

TREATMENT

Patients require routine support, such as adequate oxygen, vigorous pulmonary toilet, and appropriate hydration. Antibiotic treatment is generally empirical but should be directed toward specific pathogens when there is either direct or indirect evidence, such as clinical history, knowledge of organisms endemic in the unit, blood culture isolates, or isolation of new pathogens from airway secretions preferably obtained by bronchoalveolar lavage or bronchoscopy. Organisms obtained by tracheal suction may or may not be evidence of a lung pathogen, as they may represent a colonization state of the middle airway.

The American Thoracic Society has recommended certain antibiotic combinations for VAP in adults, which are generally appropriate for children as well. For early-onset disease in which community-acquired organisms are the most likely cause and the patient is not in an ICU, ceftriaxone or ampicillin-sulbactam is recommended. If trauma or aspiration is present, clindamycin should be added. If there are added risk factors, such as corticosteroid use, hospitalization in an ICU, underlying pulmonary disease, or prior antibiotic use, resistant gram-negative bacilli species are a concern and a regimen of ceftazidime or imipenem plus an aminoglycoside or a quinolone (for persons $\geq$18 years of age) is recommended. Vancomycin is added if methicillin-resistant *S. aureus* is a concern. Erythromycin is added if *Legionella* is a concern.

PREVENTION

Reducing mechanical ventilation will obviate development of VAP, but this is a common life-supporting measure required in modern critical care. Several measures that can be implemented should reduce the incidence of VAP in intubated patients. Antibiotic treatment should be used only when necessary, and prophylactic antibiotics, such as perioperative antibiotics, should be minimized and used for only the minimal recommended duration. The head of the bed should be raised to 30–45 degrees to prevent aspiration. All suctioning equipment, water, and saline solution should be sterile, and all equipment should be disinfected. Hand-washing by staff before and after every patient contact and use of gloves for invasive procedures and for suctioning are important to minimize transmission of organisms to patients from staff and environment. Hospital staff who have respiratory illnesses or who are carriers of certain organisms, such as methicillin-resistant *Staphylococcus aureus,* should be masked or excluded from patient care until they are no longer contagious.

REVIEWS

Alario AJ, McCarthy PJ, Markowitz R, et al: Usefulness of chest radiographs in children with acute lower respiratory tract disease. *J Pediatr* 1987;111:187–93.

Bale JR: Creation of a research program to determine the etiology and epidemiology of acute respiratory tract infection in children in developing countries. *Rev Infect Dis* 1990;12(Suppl 8):S861–6.

Bartlett JG, Breiman RF, Mandell LA, et al: Community-acquired pneumonia in adults: Guidelines for management. The Infectious Diseases Society of America. *Clin Infect Dis* 1998;26:811–38.

Brasfield DM, Stagno S, Whitley RJ, et al: Infant pneumonitis associated with cytomegalovirus, *Chlamydia, Pneumocystis,* and *Ureaplasma:* Follow-up. *Pediatrics* 1987;79:76–83.

Chernick V, Boat TF, eds: *Kendig's Disorders of the Respiratory Tract in Children,* 6th ed. Philadelphia, WB Saunders, 1998.

Glezen PAT, Denny FW: Medical progress: Epidemiology of acute lower respiratory disease in children. *N Engl J Med* 1973;288:498–505.

Hammerschlag MR: Atypical pneumonias in children. *Adv Pediatr Infect Dis* 1995:10;1–39.

Jadavji T, Law B, Lebel MH, et al: A practical guide for the diagnosis and treatment of pediatric pneumonia. CMAJ 1997;156(Suppl):S703–11.

Klein JO: Diagnostic lung puncture in the pneumonias of infants and children. *Pediatrics* 1969;44:486–492.

Niederman MS, Bass JB Jr, Campbell GD, et al: Guidelines for the initial management of adults with community-acquired pneumonia: Diagnosis, assessment of severity and initial antimicrobial therapy. American Thoracic Society, Medical Section of the American Lung Association. *Am Rev Respir Dis* 1993;148:1418–26.

Stefanutti D, Morais L, Fournet JC, et al: Value of open lung biopsy in immunocompromised children. *J Pediatr* 2000;137:165–71.

Stagno S, Brasfield DM, Brown MB, et al: Infant pneumonitis associated with cytomegalovirus, *Chlamydia, Pneumocystis,* and *Ureaplasma:* A prospective study. *Pediatrics* 1981;68:322–9.

Streptococcus pneumoniae Pneumonia

Austrian R, Gold J: Pneumococcal bacteremia with especial reference to bacteremic pneumococcal pneumonia. *Ann Intern Med* 1964;60:759–76.

Burman LA, Norrby R, Trollfors B: Invasive pneumococcal infections: Incidence, predisposing factors and prognosis. *Rev Infect Dis* 1985;7:133–42.

Dagan R, Engelhard D, Piccard E, et al: Epidemiology of invasive childhood pneumococcal infection in Israel. The Israeli Pediatric Bacteremia and Meningitis Group. *JAMA* 1992;268:3328–32.

Eskola J, Takala AK, Kela E, et al: Epidemiology of invasive pneumococcal infections in children in Finland. *JAMA* 1992;268:3323–7.

Jacobs MR, Koornhof HJ, Robins-Browne RM, et al: Emergence of multiply resistant pneumococci. *N Engl J Med* 1978;299:735–40.

Molteni RA: Group A β-hemolytic streptococcal pneumonia: Clinical course and complications of management. *Am J Dis Child* 1977; 131:1366–1371.

Mulholland K, Hilton S, Adegbola R, et al: Randomised trial of *Haemophilus influenzae* type-b tetanus protein conjugate vaccine [corrected] for prevention of pneumonia and meningitis in Gambian infants. *Lancet* 1997;349:1191–7.

Shapiro ED, Berg AT, Austrian R, et al: The protective efficacy of polyvalent pneumococcal polysaccharide vaccine. *N Engl J Med* 1991; 325:1453–60.

Tan TQ, Mason EO Jr, Kaplan SL: Systemic infections due to *Streptococcus pneumoniae* relatively resistant to penicillin in a children's hospital: Clinical management and outcome. *Pediatrics* 1992;90:928–33.

Legionellosis

Anderson RD, Lauer BA, Fraser DW, et al: Infections with *Legionella pneumophila* in children. *J Infect Dis* 1981;143:386–90.

Carlson NC, Kuskie MR, Dobyns EL, et al: Legionellosis in children: An expanding spectrum. *Pediatr Infect Dis J* 1990;9:133–7.

Edelstein PH: Antimicrobial therapy for Legionnaire's Disease: A review. *Clin Infect Dis* 1995;21(Suppl 3):S265–76.

Hoge CW, Breiman RF: Advances in the epidemiology and control of *Legionella* infections. *Epidemiol Rev* 1991;13:329–40.

Holmberg RE Jr, Pavia AT, Montgomery D, et al: Nosocomial *Legionella* pneumonia in the neonate. *Pediatrics*. 1993;92:450–3.

Kovatch AL, Jardine DS, Dowling JN, et al: Legionellosis in children with leukemia in relapse. *Pediatrics* 1984;73:811–5.

Muldoon RL, Jaecker DL, Kiefer HK: Legionnaires' disease in children. *Pediatrics* 1981;67:329–32.

Orenstein WA, Overturf GD, Leedom JM, et al: The frequency of *Legionella* infection prospectively determined in children hospitalized with pneumonia. *J Pediatr* 1981;99:403–6.

Pallares R, Linares J, Vadillo M, et al: Resistance to penicillin and cephalosporin and mortality from severe pneumococcal pneumonia in Barcelona, Spain. *N Engl J Med* 1995;333:474–80.

Stout JT, Yu VL: Legionellosis. *N Engl J Med* 1997;337:682–7.

Tsai TF, Finn DR, Plikaytis BD, et al: Legionnaires' disease: Clinical features of the epidemic in Philadelphia. *Ann Intern Med* 1979;90:509–17.

Mycoplasma pneumoniae Pneumonia

Broome CV, LaVenture M, Kaye HS, et al: An explosive outbreak of *Mycoplasma pneumoniae* infection in a summer camp. *Pediatrics* 1980;66:884–8.

Broughton RA: Infections due to *Mycoplasma pneumoniae* in childhood. *Pediatr Infect Dis J* 1986;5:71–85.

Cassell GH, Craft JC Jr: Mycoplasmas as agents of human disease. *N Engl J Med* 1981;304:80–9.

Cherry JD, Hurwitz ES, Welliver RC: *Mycoplasma pneumoniae* infections and exanthems. *J Pediatr* 1975;87:369–73.

Denny FW, Clyde WA Jr, Glezen WP: *Mycoplasma pneumoniae* disease: Clinical spectrum, pathophysiology, epidemiology, and control. *J Infect Dis* 1971;123:74–92.

McCracken GH Jr: Current status of antibiotic treatment of *Mycoplasma pneumoniae* infections. *Pediatr Infect Dis J* 1986;5:167–71.

Principi N, Esposito S, Blasi F, et al: Role of *Mycoplasma pneumoniae* and *Chlamydia pneumoniae* in children with community-acquired lower respiratory tract infections. *Clin Infect Dis* 2001;32:1281–9.

Shulman ST, Bartlett J, Clyde WA Jr, et al: The unusual severity of mycoplasmal pneumonia in children with sickle-cell disease. *N Engl J Med* 1972;287:164–7.

Chlamydial Pneumonia

Beem MO, Saxon EM: Respiratory-tract colonization and a distinctive pneumonia syndrome in infants infected with *Chlamydia trachomatis. N Engl J Med* 1977;296:306–10.

Block S, Hedrick J, Hammerschlag MR, et al: *Mycoplasma pneumoniae* and *Chlamydia pneumoniae* in pediatric and community-acquired pneumonia: Comparitive efficacy and safety of clarithromycin vs. erythromycin ethylsuccinate. *Pediatr Infect Dis J* 1995:14:471–7.

Centers for Disease Control and Prevention: Compendium of Measures to Control *Chlamydia psittaci* Infection Among Humans (Psittacosis) and Pet Birds (Avian Chlamydiosis), 2000. *MMWR Morb Mortal Wkly Rep* 2000;49(RR-8):1–17.

Grayston JT, Kuo CC, Wang SP, et al: A new *Chlamydia psittaci* strain, TWAR, isolated in acute respiratory tract infections. *N Engl J Med* 1986;315:161–8.

Hahn DL, Dodge RW, Golubjatnikov R: Association of *Chlamydia pneumoniae* (strain TWAR) infection with wheezing, asthmatic bronchitis, and adult-onset asthma. *JAMA* 1991;266:225–30.

Harrison HR, English MG, Lee CK, et al: *Chlamydia trachomatis* infant pneumonitis: Comparison with matched controls and other infant pneumonitis. *N Engl J Med* 1978;298:702–8.

Kauppinen MT, Lähde S, Syrjälä H: Roentgenographic findings in pneumonia caused by *Chlamydia pneumoniae:* A comparison with *Streptococcus pneumoniae. Arch Intern Med* 1996;156:1851–6.

Schachter J, Grossman M, Sweet RL, et al: Prospective study of perinatal transmission of *Chlamydia trachomatis*. *JAMA* 1986;255:3374–7.

Tipple MA, Beem MO, Saxon EM: Clinical characteristics of the afebrile pneumonia associated with *Chlamydia trachomatis* infection in infants less than 6 months of age. *Pediatrics* 1979;63:192–7.

Vichinsky EP, Neumayr LD, Earles AN, et al: Causes and outcomes of the acute chest syndrome in sickle cell disease: National Acute Chest Syndrome Study Group. *N Engl J Med* 2000;342:1855–65

Fungal Pneumonias

Cameron ML, Bartlett JA, Gallis HA, et al. Manifestations of pulmonary cryptococcosis in patients with acquired immunodeficiency syndrome. *Rev Infect Dis* 1991;13:64–7.

Chesney JC, Gourley GR, Peters ME, et al: Pulmonary blastomycosis in children: Amphotericin B therapy and a review. *Am J Dis Child* 1979;133:1334–9.

Denning DW, Follansbee SE, Scolaro M, et al: Pulmonary aspergillosis in the acquired immunodeficiency syndrome. *N Engl J Med* 1991; 324:654–62.

Denning DW, Tucker RM, Hanson LH, et al: Treatment of invasive aspergillosis with itraconizole. *Am J Med* 1989;86:791–800.

Fink JN: Allergic bronchopulmonary aspergillosis. *Hosp Pract* 1988; 23:105–121.

Goodwin RA Jr, Des Prez RM: Pathogenesis and clinical spectrum of histoplasmosis. *South Med J* 1973;66:13–25.

Hammarsten JE, Hammarsten JF: Histoplasmosis: Recognition and treatment. *Hosp Pract* 1990;25:95–126.

Klein BS, Vergeront JM, Weeks RJ, et al: Isolation of *Blastomyces dermatitidis* in soil associated with a large outbreak of blastomycosis in Wisconsin. *N Engl J Med* 1986;314:529–34.

Levitz SM: The ecology of *Cryptococcus neoformans* and the epidemiology of cryptococcosis. *Rev Infect Dis* 1991;13:1163–9.

Lortholary O, Meyohas MC, Dupont B, et al: Invasive aspergillosis in patients with acquired immunodeficiency syndrome: Report of 33 cases: The French Cooperative Study Group on Aspergillosis in AIDS. *Am J Med* 1993;95:177–87.

Murphy PA: Blastomycosis. *JAMA* 1989;261:3159–62.

Stevens DA, Schwartz HJ, Lee JY, et al: A randomized trial of itraconazole in allergic bronchopulmonary aspergillosis. *N Engl J Med* 2000;342:756–62.

Werner SB, Pappagianis D, Heindl I, et al: An epidemic of coccidioidomycosis among archeology students in northern California. *N Engl J Med* 1972;286:507–12.

Young LS: Aspergillus infection in the neutropenic host. *Hosp Pract* 1989;24:37–43.

Viral Pneumonias

Avila MM, Carballal G, Rovaletti H, et al: Viral etiology in acute lower respiratory infections in children from a closed community. *Am Rev Respir Dis* 1989;140:634–7.

Belshe RB, Mendelman PM, Treanor J, et al: The efficacy of live attenuated, cold-adapted, trivalent, intranasal influenzavirus vaccine in children. *N Engl J Med* 1998:338:1405–12.

Butler JC, Peters CJ: Hantaviruses and hantavirus pulmonary syndrome. *Clin Infect Dis* 1994;19:387–95.

Centers for Disease Control and Prevention: Update: Hantavirus pulmonary syndrome—United States, 1993. *MMWR Morb Mortal Wkly Rep* 1994;43:45–8.

Centers for Disease Control and Prevention: Update: Hantavirus pulmonary syndrome—United States, 1999. *MMWR Morb Mortal Wkly Rep* 1999:48:521–5.

Centers for Disease Control and Prevention: Emerging infectious diseases: Outbreak of acute illness—Southwestern United States, 1993. *MMWR Morb Mortal Wkly Rep* 1993;42:421–24.

Centers for Disease Control and Prevention: Prevention and control of influenza: Recommendations of the Advisory Committee on Immunizations Practices (ACIP). *MMWR Morb Mortal Wkly Rep* 2001;50(RR-4):1–44.

Centers for Disease Control and Prevention: Recommendations and reports: Hantavirus infection—Southwestern United States: Interim recommendations for risk reduction. *MMWR Morb Mortal Wkly Rep* 1993;42(No. RR-11):1–13.

Couch RB: Drug therapy: Prevention and treatment of influenza. *N Engl J Med* 2000;343:1778–87.

Davies HD, Matlow A, Petric M, et al: Prospective comparative study of viral and atypical organisms identified in pneumonia and bronchiolitis in hospitalized Canadian infants. *Pediatr Infect Dis J* 1996;15:371–5.

Duchin JS, Koster FT, Peters CJ, et al: Hantavirus pulmonary syndrome: A clinical description of 17 patients with a newly recognized disease. *N Engl J Med* 1994;330:949–55.

Hall CB, Dolin R, Gala CL, et al: Children with influenza A infection: Treatment with rimantadine. *Pediatrics* 1987;80:275–82.

Kahn AS, Khabbaz RF, Armstrong LR, et al: Hantavirus pulmonary syndrome: The first 100 US cases. *J Infect Dis* 1996;173:1297–303.

Monto AS, Robinson DP, Herlocher ML, et al: Zanamivir in the prevention if influenza among healthy adults: A randomized controlled trial. *JAMA* 1999;282:31–5.

Murphy TF, Henderson FW, Clyde WA Jr, et al: Pneumonia: An eleven-year study in pediatric practice. *Am J Epidemiol* 1981;113:12–21.

Neuzil KM, Mellen BG, Wright PF, et al: The effect of influenza on hospitalizations, outpatient visits, and courses of antibiotics in children. *N Engl J Med* 2000;342:225–31.

Neuzil KM, Wright PF, Mitchel EF Jr, et al: The burden of influenza illness in children with asthma and other chronic medical conditions. *J Pediatr* 2000;137:856–64.

Wildin SR, Chonmaitree T, Swischuk LE: Roentgenographic features of common pediatric viral respiratory tract infections. *Am J Dis Child* 1988;142:43–6.

Wright PF, Ross KB, Thompson J, et al: Influenza A infections in young children: Primary natural infection and protective efficacy of live-vaccine-induced or naturally acquired immunity. *N Engl J Med* 1977; 296:829–34.

Pneumocystis carinii Pneumonia

Centers for Disease Control and Prevention: 1999 USPHS/IDSA guidelines for the prevention of opportunistic infections in persons infected with human immunodeficiency virus. *MMWR Morb Mortal Wkly Rep* 1999;48(RR-10)1–66.

Connor E, Bagarazzi M, McSherry G, et al: Clinical and laboratory correlates of *Pneumocystis carinii* pneumonia in children infected with HIV. *JAMA* 1991;265:1693–7.

Hughes WT: Trimethoprim-sulfamethoxazole therapy for *Pneumocystis carinii* pneumonitis in children. *Rev Infect Dis* 1982;4:602–7.

Hughes WT, Price RA, Kim HK, et al: *Pneumocystis carinii* pneumonitis in children with malignancies. *J Pediatr* 1973;82:404–15.

Karam GH, Griffin FM Jr: Invasive pulmonary aspergillosis in nonimmunocompromised, nonneutropenic hosts. *Rev Infect Dis* 1986;8:357–63.

Pifer LL, Hughes WT, Stagno S, et al: *Pneumocystis carinii* infection: Evidence for high prevalence in normal and immunosuppressed children. *Pediatrics* 1978;61:35–41.

Stagno S, Pifer LL, Hughes WT, et al: *Pneumocystis carinii* pneumonitis in young immunosuppressed infants. *Pediatrics* 1980;66:56–62.

Telzak EE, Cote RJ, Gold JW, et al: Extrapulmonary *Pneumocystis carinii* infections. *Rev Infect Dis* 1990;12:380–6.

Walzer PD, Schultz MG, Western KA, et al: *Pneumocystis carinii* pneumonia and primary immune deficiency diseases of infancy and childhood. *J Pediatr* 1973;82:416–22.

Aspiration Pneumonia and ''Foreign Body'' Pneumonia

Brook I: Aspiration pneumonia in institutionalized children: A retrospective comparison of treatment with penicillin G, clindamycin and carbenicillin. *Clin Pediatr* 1981;20:117–22.

Brook I, Finegold SM: Bacteriology of aspiration pneumonia in children. *Pediatrics* 1980;65:1115–20.

Nosocomial Pneumonia, Including Ventilator-Associated Pneumonia (VAP)

Craven DAE, Steger KA, LaForce FM: Pneumonia. In Bennett JV, Brachman PS (editors): *Hospital Infections,* 4th ed. Philadelphia, Lippincott-Raven, 1998.

Garner JS, Jarvis WR, Emori TG, et al: CDC definitions for nosocomial infections, 1988. *J Infect Control* 1988;16:128–40.

CHAPTER 69

Pleural Effusion, Empyema, and Lung Abscess

Robert S. Baltimore

Pleural effusion, empyema, and lung abscess generally develop as complications of underlying pneumonia. Pleural effusions and empyema are accumulations of trapped fluid between the visceral and the parietal pleura in the pleural space. A lung abscess is trapped purulent fluid or organized infection within the parenchyma of the lung. Although concurrent pneumonia is often evident, any of these conditions may occur without evidence of preceding pneumonia, either because the pneumonia was not recognized or because the infection occurred as the result of a bacteremic process. Defining the preceding infection is important in these conditions because the causative pathogens are related to the preceding condition, and management includes treatment of the underlying condition.

PLEURAL EFFUSION AND EMPYEMA

Pleural fluid frequently accompanies inflammatory or malignant conditions in the chest. In children, an infection is usually the underlying condition. With infections, pleural fluid is generally due to exudation from inflamed pleural tissue **(pleuritis)** contiguous with the pneumonia. The clinical implications of this fluid are quite variable. In many cases of pneumonia, specific signs and symptoms do not accompany a small amount of extrapulmonary fluid that may be present on a chest radiograph, and the fluid resolves with resolution of the pneumonia. In other cases the fluid may be so great in volume that it affects breathing or so purulent that it increases the severity of the lung infection. Fluid may be free flowing in the pleural space, or it may be trapped, or **loculated,** by adhesions between the pleural surfaces.

Depending on the cellular composition of the fluid, it is characterized as an **effusion,** with few leukocytes and organisms, or an **empyema,** which is frankly purulent with many leukocytes and usually organisms (Table 69–1). The protein content further partitions effusions as **transudates** (<3 g/dL of protein) or **exudates** (<3 g/dL of protein). Transudation of fluid into the pleural space occurs when hydrostatic pressure causes excess fluid accumulation in the pleural space, or when reabsorption is blocked. These processes are generally not associated with infection. Exudates are more characteristic of infectious and inflammatory processes than are transudates. During the course of an infection the composition of the fluid may change dramatically from an exudate to an empyema, which represents different stages of progressive severity but not different diseases.

Pleural Effusion. A pleural effusion is the accumulation of fluid in the potential space between the **parietal and visceral pleurae** of the thorax. Effusions can be caused by infections, malignant lesions, collagen vascular diseases, or anatomic abnormalities in which lymphatic fluid drains into the pleural space more quickly than it can be absorbed. In adults, effusions are not appreciable until they are 200–300 mL in volume; moderate-sized effusions are considered approximately 1,000 mL in volume. In children, especially very young children and infants, an effusion of a much smaller volume may be clinically significant.

A **parapneumonic effusion** is an effusion associated with pneumonia in the periphery of the lung; it may be sterile or contaminated with a low number of organisms. Parapneumonic effusions are frequently small and detected only as incidental findings on a chest radiograph, but occasionally they are large and cause significant morbidity.

Empyema. Empyema **(pyothorax)** is the accumulation of pleural fluid contaminated with a large number of organisms causing an outpouring of a large number of leukocytes and fibrin. The distinction between empyema and effusion is not rigorously defined, but in general an effusion with a WBC count of more than 50,000/mm^3 and a low pH (<7.00–7.10) is considered an empyema. Other definitions of empyema rely on the presence of grossly purulent fluid. With respect to infection, thin effusions may become purulent; therefore the artificial division may be related more to the timing of fluid sampling than to any basic difference in the disease processes.

Pleural empyema is generally associated with pulmonary infection, with the specific causes similar to those of pleural effusion. In addition, empyema may result from leakage of an abscess or of a localized collection of pus from an adjacent structure into the pleural space. Such underlying conditions include lung abscesses, mediastinitis and mediastinal abscesses, abdominal abscesses that spread upward through the diaphragm, and abscesses or fluid collections due to penetrating trauma through the chest wall or esophagus or that occur as the result of operations on the chest. Each of these conditions constitutes only a small percentage of all cases of empyema in children, but it is important to recognize the mode of spread because it suggests the most likely pathogens.

ETIOLOGY

Retrospective studies of bacterial isolates from empyema fluid (Brook, 1990; Hardie et al., 1996) and parapneumonic effusions and empyema fluid (Freij et al., 1984) in children show predominance of *Streptococcus pneumoniae* in recent years, with greatly diminished incidence of *Staphylococcus aureus* and *Haemophilus influenzae* type b (Table 69–2). The study by Brook, one of the few giving special attention to recovering anaerobic bacterial species, reported a substantial number of specimens with anaerobes, primarily from cultures containing mixed species. In this study there may have been an unusually large number of anaerobes because a number

TABLE 69–1. Characteristics of Different Types of Pleural Effusions

Clinical Condition	Type of Effusion	Predominant Cells in Effusion	Glucose	pH
Empyema	Exudate	WBC count >50,000/mm^3 (mostly neutrophils)	<30 mg/dL	<7.00
Parapneumonic effusion	Exudate	WBC count <50,000/mm^3 (mostly neutrophils)	>30 mg/dL	<7.20
Tuberculosis	Exudate	Lymphocytes	30–60 mg/dL	7.00–7.30
Congestive heart failure	Transudate	Lymphocytes	>60 mg/dL	>7.40
Hypoalbuminemia	Transudate	Lymphocytes (few)	>60 mg/dL	>7.40
Cancer, systemic lupus erythematosus	Exudate	Lymphocytes, malignant cells	Variable	Variable

of patients had aspiration pneumonia, lung abscess, or necrotizing pneumonia as the underlying infection. Anaerobes were more frequently isolated from patients older than 6 years of age, and *Staphylococcus* was found primarily in children younger than 2 years. *Haemophilus influenzae* type b was seen only in children younger than 6 years of age, with most of these infections in children younger than 2 years of age. Other studies have all shown that *S. pneumoniae, S. aureus,* group A *Streptococcus,* and *H. influenzae* type b are the most common species isolated from pleural effusions, although the percentages vary considerably from study to study. However, *H. influenzae* type b is unlikely to be encountered where the conjugate vaccine is used routinely.

TABLE 69–2. Bacterial Isolates From Effusions and Empyema Fluid in Children and Adolescents

	Percentage of Isolates		
Organism	Brook (1990) 72 Cases	Freij (1984) 227 Cases	Hardie (1996) 50 Cases
Streptococcus pneumoniae	14	22	40
Group A *Streptococcus*	3	1	2
Viridans streptococci	5	<1	6
Nonhemolytic streptococci	4		
Enterococcus faecalis	2		
Other streptococci		1	
Staphylococcus aureus	11	29	
Coagulase-negative *Staphylococcus*			4
Haemophilus influenzae	16	18	
Escherichia coli	2		
Klebsiella pneumoniae	3	1	
Pseudomonas aeruginosa	2	1	
Proteus mirabilis	1		
Actinomyces			2
Gram-positive anaerobic isolates	12		
Gram-negative rod anaerobic isolates	24		
Mixed infections		4	2
Sterile		24	44

Data from Brook I: Microbiology of empyema in children and adolescents. *Pediatrics* 1990;85:722–6; Freij BJ, Kusmiesz H, Nelson JD, et al: Parapneumonic effusions and empyema in hospitalized children: A retrospective review of 227 cases. *Pediatr Infect Dis J* 1984;3:578–91; and Hardie W, Bokulic R, Garcia VF, et al: Pneumococcal pleural empyemas in children. *Clin Infect Dis* 1996;22:1057–63.

Pneumonias due to group A *Streptococcus* and *S. aureus* have the highest rates of associated effusion (75–90%), but only when these relatively uncommon causes of pneumonia are epidemic do they represent the majority of pleural effusions. Even though only approximately 50% of pneumococcal and *H. influenzae* type b pneumonias are accompanied by effusion, these species are the most common cause of bacterial pneumonia in infants and children and therefore cause the majority of pleural effusions. Pleural effusions are associated with only approximately 20% of cases of pneumonia due to *Mycoplasma pneumoniae,* adenovirus, and other respiratory viruses.

Tuberculous empyema must be considered whenever there is a pleural effusion or empyema of undetermined cause, especially if there is a history of exposure to tuberculosis (Chapter 35). Pleural effusion associated with tuberculosis may or may not be accompanied by radiographic evidence of pulmonary tuberculosis, but pleural tuberculosis usually represents spread from a pulmonary focus or caseating mediastinal lymph nodes from a primary complex, even if a focus is not detectable on a chest radiograph.

EPIDEMIOLOGY

There are approximately 1 million cases of pleural effusion and empyema each year in the United States, with significantly more of these cases clustered in the winter months. In one study (Freij et al., 1984), 43% of the cases occurred in the first year of life, and 28% in the second year. A decreasing rate with increasing age throughout childhood is reported in most studies.

In general, epidemiologic factors are not related to effusion itself but to the underlying disease. For example, in countries where tuberculosis is common, a large proportion of effusions are caused by tuberculosis. In countries or communities where pneumonia due to pyogenic bacteria is common, these bacteria are the predominant cause of pleural effusions. In centers where children with profound neurologic diseases are treated, effusions or empyema associated with anaerobic aspiration pneumonia are common. If there is an outbreak of pneumonia due to an unusual agent, it may become the predominant cause of effusion or empyema.

PATHOGENESIS

Pleural Effusion. Effusion occurs when the pleura produces more fluid than the pleural surface can reabsorb. This can be caused by infectious as well as noninfectious conditions (Table 69–1). Under normal circumstances, fluid leaks from capillaries into the pleural space, but because the fluid is continuously removed by the pleural lymphatics, the amount of fluid in the pleural space amounts to only a few milliliters. Elevated pressure in blood and lymphatic vessels due to anatomic blockage or malformations may cause fluid to accumulate in the pleural space. Accumulation of pleural fluid associated with infection is generally due to increased production or leakage of fluid, although decreased absorption is seen in some chronic conditions.

Empyema. In its early or **exudative stage,** empyema is actually a pleural effusion. There is little change in the pleural surface, and the fluid is thin with few cells. The effusion does not interfere with lung expansion. The **fibrinopurulent stage** is the characteristic stage of empyema. In this stage, there is an outpouring of fibrin and polymorphonuclear leukocytes that thicken the fluid and restrict lung expansion. This causes fibrinous adhesions of the pleural layers and loculation of fluid. In the **organizing stage** fibroblasts adhere to the pleura in a thickened pleural membrane called a **peel.** The peel and very thick empyema fluid restrict lung expansion. This evolution is due in major part to the reaction of the pleural tissue to bacterial and cellular enzymes as well as to endogenous mediators of inflammation. Thus, although prompt treatment of empyema is desirable, it may not prevent this pathologic evolution. When empyema is due to drainage of pus from an adjacent focus (e.g., a lung abscess) or penetrating trauma, the earlier stages of evolution may not occur.

SYMPTOMS AND CLINICAL MANIFESTATIONS

Because pleural effusions associated with infection are usually caused by sympathetic exudation or transudation of fluid next to a focus of infection, a careful history is essential in identifying the proximate cause of the pleural effusion. Spontaneous empyema without spread from a contiguous focus is unusual. Thus signs and symptoms probably are referable to an underlying condition. Often the effusion is associated with pneumonia, and the predisposing factors and symptoms of pneumonia (Chapter 68) are likely to be present. Less often, the effusion is due to a subdiaphragmatic focus of infection or inflammation. Thus, when one is evaluating a pleural effusion, it is important to have a detailed history relating to current abdominal symptoms and any previous gastrointestinal disease, malignant lesion, or noninfectious inflammatory condition.

Chest pain may be due to an inflammatory effusion, although the size of the effusion may be unrelated to the degree of pain. Certain symptoms may indicate whether the pleural effusion is clinically significant and contributing to respiratory distress. Shortness of breath and tachypnea of a magnitude greater than that expected with the underlying disease may indicate that the effusion is an important contributing factor. Pneumonia that worsens after the start of empirical antibiotic treatment is another clue. The symptoms improve dramatically when the fluid is drained, but the relief is only temporary if the fluid reaccumulates.

Symptoms directly attributable to empyema are sharp chest pain and sometimes referred shoulder pain. Shortness of breath may be due to systemic toxicity and fever, underlying pneumonia, or displacement of one or both lungs by empyema fluid. Shallow breathing may be due to pain associated with expansion of the lung. Coughing and deep breathing exacerbate the pain, resulting in inhibition of deep breathing and suppression of the cough, which further diminishes host defenses in clearing infection from the respiratory tract.

Physical Examination Findings

Large pleural effusions may be diagnosed by physical examination. The physical signs of empyema are similar to those of effusion. There is dullness to percussion, often with a sharp cutoff of resonance above the level of the effusion. On auscultation, vocal sounds are transmitted as through a solid medium over the fluid, with distant breath sounds in the same area. A pleural rub is frequently heard, especially when the fluid is the result of considerable inflammation. Splinting of the chest because of pleural pain, an attempt to limit thoracic cage movement with respiration, results in shallow breathing, decreased movement on the affected side, and sometimes a lateral spinal curvature away from the involved side. In infants, only large effusions can be diagnosed by physical examination.

DIAGNOSIS

Empyema and effusion cannot be differentiated on the basis of clinical presentation alone and require analysis of the pleural fluid (Table 69–1). Diagnostic imaging studies of the chest not only aid in localizing and estimating the size of the effusion but also yield a wealth of information concerning the presence of underlying pulmonary and extrapulmonary thoracic disease. Often optimal radiography cannot be performed until the fluid is removed from the pleural space. If infection is the cause of the effusion, culture of the fluid and possibly a biopsy with culture of the pleural tissue is the best means of identifying the causative organism.

Ultrasonography and CT can be used to guide needle placement for thoracentesis. These techniques should be used when conventional thoracentesis fails to yield fluid for diagnosis or fails to evacuate sufficient fluid for relief of symptoms.

Differential Diagnosis

Because fluid in the pleural space can be associated with cardiac, vascular, pulmonary, or neoplastic disease as well as with infection and noninfectious inflammatory conditions, it is necessary to obtain a complete history and to perform a complete physical examination to acquire clues as to the cause of the effusion. The most important laboratory test to differentiate infectious (exudative) from noninfectious (transudative) effusions and to identify the organism causing the infection is complete analysis of pleural fluid obtained by thoracentesis (Table 69–3). When pleural fluid is produced by noninfectious hypersecretion or blockage of reabsorption, analysis

TABLE 69–3. Differential Diagnosis of the Etiology of Pleural Effusions

Infectious Diseases
Bacterial Infections
Streptococcus pneumoniae
Staphylococcus aureus
Haemophilus influenzae
Group A *Streptococcus*
Others (less common)
Viral Infections
Adenoviruses
Influenza viruses
Other Infections
Mycobacterium tuberculosis
Mycoplasma pneumoniae
Chlamydia pneumoniae
Fungi (*Aspergillus, Histoplasma,* others)
Parasites (*Entamoeba histolytica, Echinococcus,* others)
Noninfectious Diseases
Congestive heart failure
Malignant neoplasms
Collagen vascular disease
Hypoalbuminemia
Esophageal rupture
Other trauma including chest surgery
Anatomic abnormalities
Lymphangiomatosis

TABLE 69–4. Diagnostic Tests for Analysis of Pleural Fluid

Physical Properties
Note volume removed
Color
Clarity
Microbiologic Analysis
Gram stain, Wright stain, and stain for *Mycobacteria*
Bacterial culture (aerobic and anaerobic)
Fungal culture
Mycobacterial culture
Viral culture (optional)
Bacterial antigen tests
Chemical Analysis
Protein
Glucose
pH
Lactate dehydrogenase
Cellular Analysis
WBC count
Differential WBC count
Cytologic examination
Special Tests*
Amylase
Cholesterol
Rheumatoid factor
Antinuclear antibodies
Lupus erythematosus preparation (LE prep)

*Tests not performed routinely but that should be obtained when indicated or considered if an initial fluid analysis fails to yield a diagnosis.

of the fluid often provides the information required for specific diagnosis.

Laboratory Evaluation

Several laboratory tests should be performed on a pleural fluid sample removed by thoracentesis of an effusion of unknown cause (Table 69–4). Because pleural fluid may contain a high concentration of fibrin and clotting factors, a heparinized sample should always be collected so that the essential laboratory tests can be performed. When the cause of the effusion is already known and a therapeutic thoracentesis is performed, or when a repeat thoracentesis is performed to follow the progressive changes of specific tests, only the needed tests should be requested. Although most tests can be performed on fluid removed by the usual aseptic technique handled in a routine manner, determination of an accurate pH requires that the sample be maintained anaerobically, packed in ice in the original syringe, and transported directly to the laboratory for immediate testing.

The concentration of protein in the fluid is an important aid in the diagnosis of the cause of the effusion. The normal protein concentration of pleural fluid is 1.5 g/dL (normal range, 1–3 g/dL). Protein values in this range suggest hypersecretion of a serum filtrate (transudation). Transudates are also seen when hydrostatic pressure causes excess fluid accumulation in the pleural space or when reabsorption is blocked. These processes are generally not associated with infection. Protein concentrations exceeding 3 g/dL or a specific gravity of 1.016 or greater are characteristic of an inflammatory exudate, although these numbers are not absolute and there is some overlap with transudates. Other nonspecific indicators of an inflammatory exudate are values of lactate dehydrogenase (LDH) greater than 200 IU/L, and glucose concentrations depressed to <40 mg/dL. An elevated amylase level is seen in pleural effusions associated with gastrointestinal disorders, such as pancreatitis, esophagitis, and certain tumors. The pH determination is especially important in identifying effusions that require insertion of a chest tube. Low pH values (<7.20) are associated with an inflammatory process, and placement of a chest tube should be strongly considered to minimize the chances of a pleural reaction that interferes with expansion of the lung.

Analysis of the cellular elements in the fluid also helps in diagnosis. Exudates generally have a WBC count of more than $1,000/mm^3$, but effusions associated with pneumonia usually have a higher number of WBCs, usually greater than $50,000/mm^3$. A predominance of neutrophils is associated with bacterial pneumonia, early tuberculosis, and contiguous abdominal infections. A lymphocytic response is associated with granulomatous infections such as established tuberculosis, certain neoplasms, and sarcoidosis. The presence of erythrocytes in the fluid is nonspecific and can be associated with necrotizing infection, tumor, infarction, tuberculosis, and trauma. A small number of erythrocytes probably has no diagnostic significance.

Pleural fluid from an empyema is characterized on gross examination as thick and purulent. Fluid from an empyema has a high concentration of cells, low pH, and a low glucose concentration.

Diagnostic Imaging

Radiographic examination demonstrates effusions very well. Normal upright radiographs of the chest demonstrate small volumes of fluid by blunting of the costophrenic angles (Figs. 69–1 and 69–2*A*). Larger effusions appear as a fluid density covering the dependent portions of the lungs, generally above the diaphragm, unless the effusion is trapped in a fibrinous pocket creating a loculated collection. If the effusion is very large, an entire hemithorax may be opacified (Figs. 69–2*A* and 69–3). The volume of the effusion can be estimated by lateral decubitus radiographic

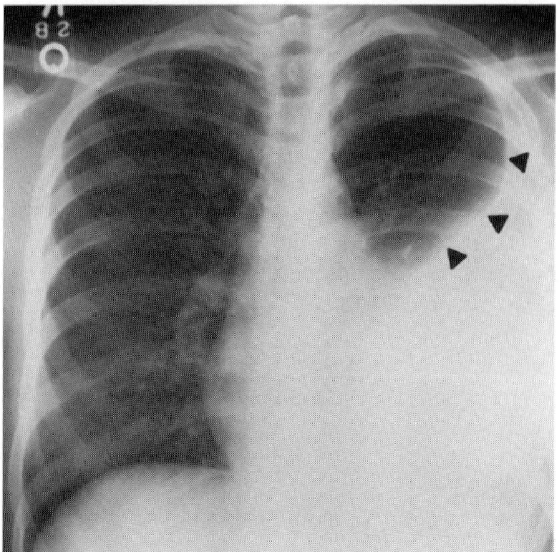

FIGURE 69–1. Primary tuberculosis with pleural effusion in a 13-year-old boy presenting with left chest pain. Frontal chest radiograph shows opacification of the lower left hemithorax with a positive meniscus sign (*arrows*) indicating a large left pleural effusion. There is no evidence of mediastinal shift, implying that the left lower lobe collapsed as the effusion developed. Left hilar lymphadenopathy cannot be excluded because of the fluid. (From Agrons GA, Markowitz RI, Kramer SS: Pulmonary tuberculosis in children. *Semin Roentgenol* 28:2,1993.)

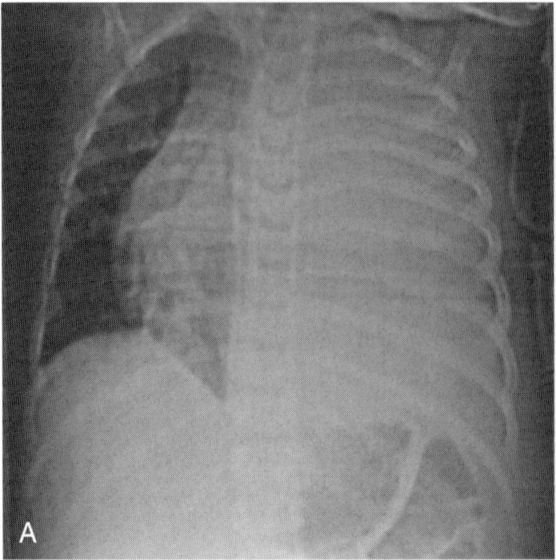

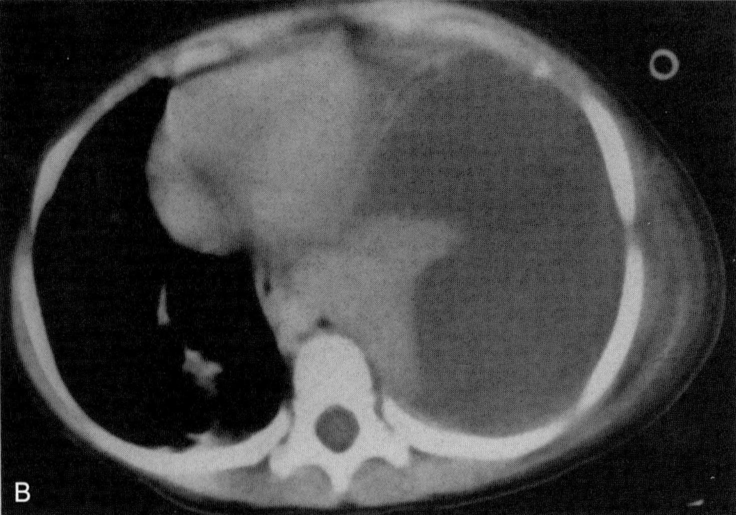

FIGURE 69–2. Bacterial pneumonia with empyema. **A,** Chest radiograph reveals opacification of the left hemithorax with mediastinal shift away from the affected side. **B,** Computed tomogram after intravenous administration of contrast medium shows the collapsed and consolidated lung medially surrounded by a large pleural effusion of lower attenuation. Chest tube drainage yielded a large amount of cloudy serosanguineous fluid. After drainage, the patient's condition improved considerably.

examinations, which also demonstrate whether the effusion is freely movable within the pleural space or is loculated. A subpulmonic effusion is fluid trapped beneath the lung above the diaphragm; it may be radiographically undetectable if it does not flow into the costophrenic spaces.

Ultrasonography may be especially useful in imaging pleural effusions and empyema and in determining whether pleural fluid is free flowing or loculated. The distinction between pleural thickening and pleural fluid may not be clear on a chest radiograph but can be distinguished by ultrasonography. Ultrasonography can be used to determine the optimum site for thoracentesis and to maximize the chance of draining a loculated effusion or a subpulmonic effusion.

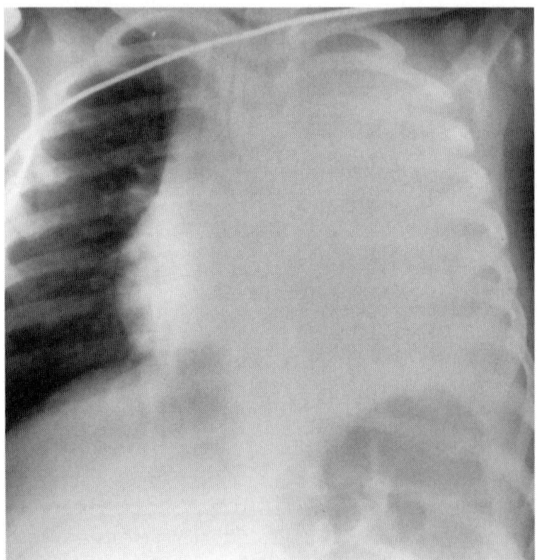

FIGURE 69–3. Consolidative pneumococcal pneumonia with empyema in a 2-year-old boy with high fever, tachypnea, and no breath sounds on the left. A frontal chest radiograph shows complete opacification of the left hemithorax with mediastinal shift toward the right. A pleural tap revealed thick pus, which grew *Streptococcus pneumoniae.*

Although it is not routinely indicated, CT is an excellent method for imaging effusion or empyema. CT is the best imaging technique to distinguish complex inflammatory disease in which there is involvement of the lung parenchyma, adjacent pleura, and pleural space (Fig. 69–2*B*). CT can also detect mediastinal lymphadenopathy, tumors, and other solid lung lesions.

Microbiologic Evaluation

Pleural fluid cultures are essential for characterization of pleural effusions (Table 69–4). Because it is often difficult to diagnose the cause of pneumonia in children, evaluation of a pleural effusion may provide a positive culture, establishing a microbiologic cause of the underlying pneumonia. This is especially true of bacterial pneumonia caused by *S. pneumoniae* and *H. influenzae* type b because they are most frequently associated with pleural effusions but cannot be diagnosed by serologic tests. Whether to perform special stains and cultures of pleural fluid for mycobacteria and fungi depends on the patient's background and risk factors and on whether another cause of the effusion has been identified.

In addition to microbiologic cultures of pleural fluid, other cultures should be performed on patients with pleural effusions. If there is evidence of underlying pneumonia, culture of an adequate specimen of sputum may be useful. Blood culture is very important and may be positive in 30–40% of patients with parapneumonic pleural effusions and empyema. Strong consideration should be given to culture of respiratory secretions for *M. pneumoniae* and respiratory viruses and to serologic tests for infection caused by these agents and by *Chlamydia trachomatis, C. pneumoniae,* and *C. psittaci.*

Latex agglutination tests for bacterial antigens may be positive. They should be performed on patients with clinically significant effusions and may be especially useful should the blood and pleural fluid cultures prove to be negative. Urine is usually the best fluid in which to detect these antigens. The common agents associated with pleural effusion for which antigen tests are widely available are *S. pneumoniae, Neisseria meningitidis, H. influenzae* type b, and group B *Streptococcus.*

Concern about infection in the pleural space due to *Mycobacterium tuberculosis* is a special aspect of the diagnosis of pleural effusion (Chapter 35). A pleural effusion may be the first sign of tuberculosis. For patients with any known or likely medical or epidemiologic predisposition to tuberculosis, stains and cultures of the pleural fluid for *M. tuberculosis* are indicated. However, these steps alone are insufficient to exclude tuberculosis as the cause, because the mycobacteria associated with pleural granulomas may not be shed into the pleural fluid. In approximately 75% of cases, cultures of tuberculous pleural effusion fluid are sterile. Thus, when the microbiologic cause of a possible pleural space infection is not found, especially if there is exposure to or risk of infection with *M. tuberculosis,* additional diagnostic tests are warranted. A biopsy of the pleura may demonstrate characteristic granulomas indicative of tuberculosis and has a high yield of *Mycobacteria* from cultures.

Pathologic Findings

A cytologic examination of a cell block from an exudate provides considerably more information about the cellular elements than a Wright stain of a smear of cells. A morphologic examination for the characteristics of malignant cells and stains for surface immunologic markers can be helpful in diagnosing malignant neoplasms. A histologic examination of pleural tissue obtained by a pleural biopsy is often used as an adjunct to a cytologic examination of the pleural fluid to diagnose malignant tumors, tuberculosis, and sarcoidosis. A histologic examination should be considered for any patient whose pleural effusion is of unknown cause or if a cytologic examination of the pleural fluid is inconclusive.

TREATMENT

Treatment of a pleural effusion consists of antimicrobial therapy for the underlying condition and drainage of fluid by thoracentesis or chest tube placement if necessary. Drainage of the effusion is necessary for relief of symptoms. It is advisable to have a surgeon participate in the care of the patient, even if chest tube placement is not initially required.

Antimicrobial Therapy. Treatment of pleural effusion requires both treatment of the underlying disease and relief of symptoms due to the effusion. For infections, antimicrobial treatment appropriate for the underlying disease is most important. The guidelines for empirical and definitive treatment of pneumonia are used (Chapter 68; Tables 68–1 and 68–7). If a Gram stain of the pleural fluid reveals a specific morphology of organism, or if a rapid test for bacterial antigen is positive, the antimicrobial regimen should include optimal activity against the putative pathogen and against the usual agents pending culture results. Empirical therapy may be necessary for patients with pneumonia and effusion if fluid is unobtainable or if the stains for bacteria are negative. For infants beyond the neonatal period and for young children who are hospitalized and moderately or severely ill, intravenous β-lactam agents with activity against *Staphylococcus, S. pneumoniae,* and *H. influenzae* type b are appropriate. Cefuroxime, a second-generation cephalosporin, is recommended. Third-generation cephalosporins also provide similar coverage but are expensive and are not as appropriate for community-acquired pneumonia. For *S. pneumoniae* that is highly resistant to penicillin and cephalosporins, the addition of vancomycin is appropriate.

Thoracentesis. Thoracentesis is recommended routinely for adequate diagnosis and relief of symptoms of pleural effusion. **Video-assisted thorascopic surgery (VATS)** performed initially decreases the number of procedures and leads to improved outcomes, and it may become the standard procedure in the future. Withdrawal of reaccumulated fluid is recommended only if the diagnosis is still in doubt or if a large amount of fluid affects breathing. In general, parapneumonic effusions do not require insertion of a chest tube for continuous drainage unless accumulation is too brisk to drain adequately by thoracentesis once or twice a day. A chest tube also is required if accumulation continues for more than a few days or if the fluid is highly inflammatory, as indicated by a very low pH (<7.00) and a high level of LDH (>1,000 IU/L). Patients with a pleural effusion pH of 7.00–7.20 should be managed individually. Chest tube drainage also is indicated for obvious empyema, as indicated by grossly purulent fluid. Reasons to avoid chest tube placement include patient discomfort and decreased mobility, the requirement for additional nursing care, and the possibility of introducing nosocomial organisms into the chest cavity.

COMPLICATIONS

There are both short-term and long-term complications of pleural effusion and empyema. The short-term complications are mostly due to the mechanical effects of the effusion on breathing. Whereas small effusions may have minor effects on the condition of a patient with pneumonia, a large effusion may increase the work of breathing by limiting diaphragmatic movement and compressing the lung. In a patient who already has compromised respiratory status from pneumonia or another underlying pulmonary condition, a large pleural effusion causes restrictive ventilatory dysfunction that may precipitate respiratory failure. Thus the presence of a large effusion may allow a moderate pneumonic illness to progress to a life-threatening condition. The presence of inflammatory proteins in the fluid may produce hyperpyrexia, further increasing the patient's metabolic demands. Fortunately, drainage of the fluid by thoracentesis usually results in a dramatic improvement in the patient's clinical condition.

The long-term consequences of untreated effusion and empyema include reduced exercise tolerance, changes in the contour of the chest, scoliosis, and chronic restrictive disease. Early effective antimicrobial treatment of the underlying condition and drainage of the effusion by thoracentesis prevent the development of these long-term complications.

Empyema fluid frequently becomes loculated because of inflammation and fibrin deposition, making drainage difficult. This process can cause thickening of the pleura, or **peel,** which entraps the lung and prevents expansion. It may be associated with local discomfort and systemic symptoms. The thickened pleura should be removed surgically. Other complications of not draining empyema fluid include burrowing of the fluid back into the lung and spontaneous drainage **(empyema necessitatis)** into a bronchus through a bronchopleural fistula that has developed or through a cutaneous fistula in the chest wall.

PROGNOSIS

The prognosis for complete recovery from pleural effusion associated with infection is excellent once the fluid is drained and appropriate antimicrobial treatment is begun. Untreated empyema is usually fatal, and infants have a considerable mortality even with appropriate treatment. The prognosis for recovery from empyema depends on how quickly appropriate treatment is begun and on whether additional complications develop.

LUNG ABSCESS

A lung abscess is a collection of purulent material in a walled-off mass within the lung parenchyma. Lung abscesses are generally diagnosed by their characteristic appearance on a chest radiograph.

They appear as radiodensities, often with air pockets within the material surrounded by a very dense wall. Lung abscesses and pneumatoceles are sometimes confused. **Pneumatoceles** are air pockets, or fluid-filled pockets, that are not surrounded by a thick wall. They represent air dissections within the lung parenchyma that may occur after a wide variety of lung injuries, including infection, hydrocarbon ingestion, and trauma.

ETIOLOGY

In a study (Brook and Finegold, 1979) of lung abscesses among children living in a state institution who were presumed to have had aspiration pneumonia as the proximate cause of the abscess, many aerobic and anaerobic bacteria causing infections were found (Table 69–5). Microbial cultures were performed by transtracheal aspiration, with special attention to anaerobic cultures. In all 10 children in the study, anaerobic organisms were recovered from the cultures, and in 9 of the 10 children the anaerobes were mixed with aerobes. These findings are similar to the microbiologic composition of lung abscesses in adults, although some reports in the pediatric literature show dissimilar data. One report (Asher et al., 1982) lists *S. aureus* as the only isolate in 14 lung abscesses; this was a review of cases, however, and did not use current technology for the recovery of anaerobic organisms. A review (Siegel and McCracken, 1979) of lung abscess in neonates reported the recovery of organisms usually associated with neonatal sepsis (e.g., *Escherichia coli,* group B *Streptococcus,* and *Klebsiella pneumoniae*) and not mixed flora or anaerobes. This finding may be due to real differences in pathogenesis and to differences between the normal respiratory flora of neonates and older children.

TABLE 69–5. Bacterial Isolates From Lung Abscess in Children and Adults

	Percentage of Isolates	
Organism	Brook (1979) Children, 10 Cases	Bartlett (1987) Adults, 93 Cases
Aerobic and Facultative Isolates	(25 Total)	(42 Total)
Gram-positive Cocci		
Streptococcus pneumoniae	3	4
Group A *Streptococcus*	6	
Group D *Streptococcus*	2	
Alpha hemolytic streptococci	8	
Staphylococcus aureus	2	8
Gram-negative Bacilli		
Escherichia coli	6	6
Klebsiella pneumoniae	6	4
Pseudomonas aeruginosa	3	4
Serratia marcescens	2	
Eikenella corrodens	2	
Anaerobic Isolates	(37 Total)	(120 Total)
Gram-positive Cocci		
Peptococcus	8	
Peptostreptococcus	13	25
Veillonella	5	
Microaerophilic streptococci	2	
Gram-positive Bacilli		
Bifidobacterium	3	
Actinomyces	2	
Gram-negative Bacilli		
Fusobacterium nucleatum	3	21
Prevotella melaninogenica	10	20
Bacteroides	15	9

Data from Brook I, Finegold SM: Bacteriology and therapy of lung abscess in children. *J Pediatr* 1979;94:10–2; and Bartlett JG: Anaerobic bacterial infections of the lung. *Chest* 1987;91:901–9.

EPIDEMIOLOGY

Lung abscess is a relatively uncommon, sporadic disease. Epidemiologcally, it is similar to the underlying diseases. Although the population-based incidence is not recorded, single reviews from large children's hospitals over several decades have yielded only 30–80 abscesses. The incidence of lung abscesses in children appears to have been declining in recent decades.

Lung abscesses in children are not as common as they were in the past because of the prompt antibiotic treatment of acute bacterial pneumonia and a decrease in the incidence of staphylococcal pneumonia. The most common antecedent illnesses for lung abscesses are aspiration pneumonia and anaerobic or aerobic necrotizing pneumonia. The conditions associated with aspiration pneumonia (Chapter 68) are therefore also associated with lung abscesses. Less commonly, organisms that produce necrotizing pneumonia, such as gram-negative aerobic bacilli, *S. aureus,* and *Aspergillus* in an immunocompromised host, also cause lung abscesses. Lung abscesses also occur as a complication of chronic pulmonary conditions such as cystic fibrosis and bronchiectasis and occasionally as a complication of operations on the chest. Less commonly in children than in adults, lung abscesses (usually multiple) can be the result of hematogenous spread, especially as a complication of infective endocarditis of the right side of the heart and venous septic thrombophlebitis.

PATHOGENESIS

Lung abscesses are almost invariably bacterial infections in immunocompetent persons; rarely are they fungal infections. Fungal lung abscesses are primarily found in severely immunocompromised patients. Most lung abscesses in adults are a complication of aspiration pneumonia, which is also a major predisposing condition in children. Compared with those that occur in adults, lung abscesses in children are more frequently a complication of necrotizing pneumonia, especially due to *S. aureus* and infections from mixed aerobic and anaerobic species.

Because aspiration is so frequently the antecedent cause of a lung abscess, the lobes of the lung that are dependent in the recumbent position (right upper lobe, left upper lobe, and apical segments of both lower lobes) are most frequently the site of lung abscesses. The basilar segments of the upper lobes are dependent when a person is upright, and these segments are often involved following aspiration while sitting or standing.

SYMPTOMS AND CLINICAL MANIFESTATIONS

Anaerobic abscesses may present insidiously. In previously healthy patients the aspiration event may have been forgotten by the time the abscess is diagnosed. A child may have had a seizure, temporarily aspirated a foreign body that was removed, or been in a coma due to alcohol or drug ingestion and appeared to fully recover. Insidious development of a cough and intermittent fever and later a putrid smell to the breath, which is caused when anaerobic organisms drain into a bronchus and are expectorated, are frequent findings in the history. Chest discomfort or chest pain may develop.

Patients with psychomotor retardation and difficulty swallowing and handling oral secretions may have frequent aspiration events, and the specific event preceding the development of a lung abscess may or may not have been noted as being unusual. In contrast, acute pneumonia may develop with a cough, fever, and prostration. What is initially diagnosed as focal pneumonia may develop into a recognizable abscess only after several days of illness when cavitation within the lesion is first seen. This can be the case in staphylococcal pneumonia as well as in aspiration pneumonia. In either, a lung abscess may develop in the periphery of the lung and, instead of draining into a bronchus, may rupture into the pleural space, resulting in empyema. In rare instances this progression can occur with a necrotizing pneumonia due to any bacterial species, but it is most clearly associated with *S. aureus* and opportunistic pneumonia due to gram-negative bacilli, which is rare in children except as a complication of nosocomial pneumonia, usually in an intensive care unit.

Physical Examination Findings

Physical findings specific to a lung abscess are uncommon in children. Occasionally a focal area of decreased breath sounds or crackles may be appreciated. Foul breath due to necrosis of tissue is associated with infection with anaerobic organisms. With a long-standing abscess, clubbing of the fingers and signs of a catabolic state, such as weight loss, may be noted. When a lung abscess is a complication of pneumonia, persistence of symptoms and signs of fever, cough, sputum production, and tachypnea may be the only findings. If the abscess ruptures into the pleural space, empyema and physical findings associated with accumulation of pleural fluid develop.

DIAGNOSIS

The diagnosis of lung abscess is usually made by chest radiography, specifically CT of the chest. The history may provide clues leading one to suspect lung abscess. The abscess cannot be confirmed by a physical examination alone.

Differential Diagnosis

In the absence of serial chest radiographs, other lung lesions may be difficult to differentiate from lung abscesses. **Pneumatoceles,** air-filled pseudocavities within the lung caused by dissection of air into the parenchyma from necrotic alveoli and small airways, can develop with pneumonia due to any organism but are particularly common with *S. aureus* pneumonia. They also may occur after hydrocarbon ingestion or trauma. They require no treatment, and they disappear spontaneously. An infected congenital cyst of the lung may be difficult to differentiate from an abscess without a biopsy of the cyst wall that demonstrates epithelium. Persistence of the cyst after signs of infection have disappeared may be a clue, but sometimes lung abscesses may persist as cystic lesions for months. Serial CT is often helpful in establishing the correct diagnosis.

Microbiologic Evaluation

What constitutes an appropriate culture representative of a lung abscess is a matter of some controversy. Coughed sputum is not useful because the organisms that are considered normal throat flora and the organisms that cause lung abscesses are frequently the same. When the contents of the abscess drain into a bronchus, transtracheal aspiration performed by an experienced practitioner yields an acceptable representation of the flora of a lung abscess, but the procedure is rarely performed on children; its safety for infants and toddlers is questionable. When bronchoscopy is performed, cultures obtained with a **shielded bronchoscope** are acceptable and reliable, but standard bronchoscopes may introduce organisms from the upper airway that cannot be distinguished from abscess flora. Percutaneous aspiration of an abscess with ultrasonographic or CT guidance is an excellent source of culture but is an invasive procedure that is potentially associated with complications, such as pneumothorax, hemothorax, or empyema. Therefore, its routine use is not recommended unless the patient is immunocompromised or fails to respond to empirical antimicrobial therapy.

Diagnostic Imaging

The typical radiographic finding of a lung abscess due to aspiration pneumonia is a single or a small number of walled masses, often with air inside and an air-fluid level. An early abscess may have a wall too thin to visualize and may appear as a solid mass. In such cases CT is beneficial in differentiating a tumor from an abscess. CT is also quite sensitive and may demonstrate additional smaller abscesses not previously visualized (Fig. 69–4). CT can be of great help in defining the location of masses near the chest wall, which may be intrapulmonary or extrapulmonary. Radionuclide scanning with indium has been reported to be helpful in visualizing abscesses but adds little to CT and is not routinely used.

TREATMENT

Antimicrobial Therapy. Initial antibiotic therapy is usually empirical, with specific recommendations depending on the underlying antecedent illness. If the abscess is likely the result of aspiration or occurs after aspiration pneumonia, the recommendations for antibiotics and dosage are similar to those for aspiration pneumonia (Chapter 68). Empirical antibiotic treatment when aspiration appears to be the underlying disorder usually consists of intravenous penicillin G until there is clinical improvement, followed by a longer course of oral penicillin for a total treatment course of 1–2 months. In a study (Weiss and Cherniack, 1974) of adults with acute anaerobic lung abscesses treated with either intravenous penicillin followed by oral penicillin, intramuscular penicillin, or only oral penicillin, the outcome was comparable in each group.

With severe disease, the entire course of treatment of approximately 1 month may be administered by the intravenous route. In complicated cases it may be better to determine duration by following chest radiographs until the lung field is clear or there is a small stable residual lesion. The routine use of additional antibiotics for anaerobic gram-negative bacilli is elective. Because clindamycin has been associated with a rapid clinical response in adults, it may be considered as a substitute for or in addition to penicillin G. Other antibiotics with similar excellent activity against penicillin-resistant anaerobes include chloramphenicol and metronidazole. The combination antibiotic drug ampicillin-sulbactam could also be considered in this situation, although there are fewer data to demonstrate efficacy.

When a lung abscess appears to be due to necrotizing pneumonia not associated with aspiration, the best approach to antibiotic management is a regimen guided by the results of appropriate cultures. If good-quality culture material is not available, empirical antibiotic therapy should be directed against both *S. aureus* and enteric gram-

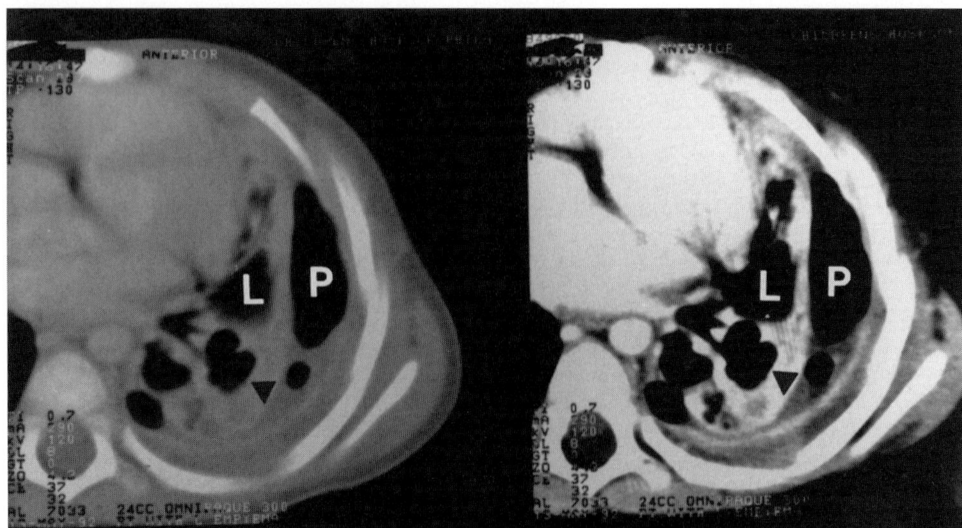

FIGURE 69–4. Lung abscess in an 8-year-old boy with fever, pulmonary consolidation, and empyema. A left pleural drainage tube had been placed before scanning. Computed tomograms (lung and mediastinal windows) of the chest after intravenous administration of contrast medium show residual air and fluid within the pleural space (*P*). Within the consolidated lung, there are areas of re-aerated lung (*L*) and necrotic air-filled holes (*arrows*), which represent abscess cavities. Communication with an adjacent bronchus is demonstrated.

negative bacilli. Appropriate empirical antibiotic choices are penicillinase-resistant penicillin, such as oxacillin, plus an aminoglycoside, such as gentamicin, or a third-generation cephalosporin, such as cefotaxime, as a single agent. An alternative is a first- or second-generation cephalosporin, such as cefazolin or cefuroxime, plus an aminoglycoside.

Recommendations regarding specific treatment of anaerobic species that may be resistant to penicillin G, such as *Bacteroides,* in mixed aerobic and anaerobic lung abscesses are based on retrospective reviews of the treatment of lung abscesses in children and in adults. This infection is unusual in that the results of the antibiotic susceptibilities of recovered isolates do not correlate well with the clinical effectiveness of antimicrobial treatment. Numerous cases of aspiration lung abscesses in which penicillin-resistant *Bacteroides* have been isolated in mixed cultures have been treated successfully with penicillin. The same is true in many cases in which a mixed flora, including *S. aureus* has been isolated. The reasons for this phenomenon are debatable, but it appears that in an immunocompetent host when drainage into a bronchus is established and the purulent material is expectorated, host defenses are adequate to eliminate the few remaining resistant organisms, especially the anaerobic organisms. In addition, the virulence of mixed-flora abscesses often depends on interaction between aerobic and anaerobic species. Elimination of some of the species with antimicrobial therapy may often be sufficient to inhibit the growth of resistant organisms and allow normal host defenses to eliminate the remainder.

Bronchoscopy, Drainage, and Surgical Treatment. Recommendations concerning the use of bronchoscopy and surgical procedures in the treatment of lung abscess vary among specialists. Bronchoscopy may facilitate the obtaining of valuable cultures and help to ensure internal drainage into a bronchus by removing any visible obstruction. Drainage of a lung abscess, however, rarely needs to be performed, although it may be necessary if the patient does not respond to medical therapy, especially if internal drainage into a bronchus does not occur spontaneously. Drainage may be established bronchoscopically or by CT-guided percutaneous drainage, which may be easier than bronchoscopy in small children. Open surgical drainage with removal of the abscess is reserved for patients who remain in a toxic condition or bacteremic after several days of appropriate empirical antibiotic therapy, usually after other attempts at drainage have proved unsuccessful.

COMPLICATIONS

Lung abscesses are usually a complication of underlying pneumonia. The major complications of lung abscesses are bacteremia and sepsis syndrome, or rarely rupture into a bronchus or into the pleural space, causing empyema.

PROGNOSIS

Lung abscesses generally have a good prognosis. In mixed aerobic and anaerobic abscesses due to aspiration, cure can be expected with antibiotics alone. When a lung abscess is associated with necrotizing pneumonia or empyema, chronic inflammation may result in restrictive lung disease. In such cases, surgical removal of the inflamed pleura and granulation tissue may be necessary to re-expand the lung, as occurs in some cases of empyema. Devitalization of a lung by necrotizing pneumonia and an abscess may result in air-filled pockets of scar tissue, which may be the sites of recurrent pneumonitis. In such cases resection of the affected area of the lung is recommended. Recurrent lung abscesses are associated with pre-existing profound neurologic disease or immunodeficiencies. Patients with underlying immunodeficiencies, especially chronic granulomatous disease, have a poor prognosis if a lung abscess occurs. They should be treated aggressively with prolonged intravenous administration of antibiotics and surgical drainage if the abscess does not respond to the antibiotics.

PREVENTION

Prevention of lung abscesses involves prevention of the underlying conditions, especially appropriate treatment of bacterial pneumonia and measures to prevent aspiration in debilitated patients.

REVIEWS

Bartlett JG: Anaerobic bacterial infections of the lung. *Chest* 1987; 91:901–9.

Bryant RE, Salmon CJ: Pleural empyema. *Clin Infect Dis* 1996;22:747–62.

Chernick V, Boat TF (editors): *Kendig's Disorders of the Respiratory Tract in Children,* 6th ed. Philadelphia, WB Saunders, 1998.

Light RW (editor): *Pleural Diseases,* 2nd ed. Philadelphia, Lea & Febiger, 1990.

Tan TQ, Seilheimer DK, Kaplan SL: Pediatric lung abscess: Clinical management and outcome. *Pediatr Infect Dis J* 1995;14:51–5.

Pleural Effusion and Empyemia

Bartlett JG, Gorbach SL, Finegold SM: The bacteriology of aspiration pneumonia. *Am J Med* 1974;56:202–7.

Brook I: Microbiology of empyema in children and adolescents. *Pediatrics* 1990;85:722–6.

Brook I: Aspiration pneumonia in institutionalized children: A retrospective comparison of treatment with penicillin G, clindamycin and carbenicillin. *Clin Pediatr* 1981;20:117–22.

Doski JJ, Lou D, Hicks BA, et al: Management of parapneumonic collections in infants and children. *J Pedatr Surg* 2000;35:265–70.

Freij BJ, Kusmiesz H, Nelson JD, et al: Parapneumonic effusions and empyema in hospitalized children: A retrospective review of 227 cases. *Pediatr Infect Dis* 1984;3:578–91.

Hardie W, Bokulic R, Garcia VF, et al: Pneumococcal pleural empyemas in children. *Clin Infect Dis* 1996;22:1057–63.

Hardie WD, Roberts NE, Reising SF, et al: Complicated parapneumonic effusions in children caused by penicillin-nonsusceptible *Streptococcus pneumoniae. Pediatrics* 1998;101:388–92.

Hoff SJ, Neblett WW, Edwards KM, et al: Parapneumonic empyema in children: Decortication hastens recovery in patients with severe pleural infections. *Pediatr Infect Dis J* 1991;10:194–9.

Ramnath RR, Heller RM, Ben-Ami T, et al: Implications of early sonographic evaluation of parapneumonic effusions in children with pneumonia. *Pediatrics* 1998;101:68–71.

Redding GJ, Walund C, Walund D, et al: Lung function in children following empyema. *Am J Dis Child* 1990;114:1337–42.

Silen ML, Weber TR: Thoracoscopic debridement of loculated empyema thoracis in children. *Ann Thorac Surg* 1995;59:1166–8.

Stovroff M, Teague G, Heiss KF, et al: Thoracoscopy in the management of pediatric empyema. *J Pediatr Surg* 1995;30:1211–5.

Valdés L, Álvarez D, San José E, et al: Tuberculous pleurisy: A study of 254 patients. *Arch Intern Med* 1998;158:2017–21.

Wolfe WG, Spock A, Bradford WD: Pleural fluid in infants and children. *Am Rev Respir Dis* 1968;98:1027–32.

Lung Abscess

Asher MI, Spier S, Beland M, et al: Primary lung abscess in childhood: The long-term outcome of conservative management. *Am J Dis Child* 1982;136:491–4.

Ball WS Jr, Bisset GS III, Towbin RB: Percutaneous drainage of chest abscesses in children. *Radiology* 1989;171:431–4.

Brook I, Finegold SM: Bacteriology and therapy of lung abscess in children. *J Pediatr* 1979;94:10–2.

Emanuel B, Shulman ST: Lung abscess in infants and children. *Clin Pediatr* 1995;34:2–6.

Levison ME, Mangura CT, Lorber B, et al: Clindamycin compared with penicillin for the treatment of anaerobic lung abscess. *Ann Intern Med* 1983;98:466–71.

Nonoyama A, Tanaka K, Osaka T, et al: Surgical treatment of pulmonary abscess in children under ten years of age. *Chest* 1984;85:358–62.

Siegel JD, McCracken GH Jr: Neonatal lung abscess: A report of six cases. *Am J Dis Child* 1979;133:947–9.

van Sonnenberg E, D'Agostino HB, Casola G, et al: Lung abscess: CT-guided drainage. *Radiology* 1991;178:347–51.

Weiss W, Cherniack NS: Acute nonspecific lung abscess: A controlled study comparing oral and parenterally administered penicillin G. *Chest* 1974;66:348–51.

Zuhdi MK, Spear RM, Worthen HM, et al: Percutaneous catheter drainage of tension pneumatocele, secondarily infected pneumatocele, and lung abscess in children. *Crit Care Med* 1996;24:330–3.

CHAPTER 70

Mediastinitis

Tod S. Russell ▪ David P. Ascher

The **mediastinum** is the extrapleural space of the thoracic cavity between the two pleural sacs. An arbitrary line from the lower manubrium to the fourth thoracic vertebra separates the mediastinum into superior and inferior portions. The **inferior mediastinum** is divided into the **anterior mediastinum,** which contains fat and lymphoid tissue; the **middle mediastinum,** which contains the heart, pericardium, aorta, bifurcation of the trachea, the main bronchi, and lymph nodes; and the **posterior mediastinum,** which contains the esophagus, descending aorta, and vagus nerve. The **superior mediastinum** contains the thymus gland, trachea, esophagus, and aortic arch. Although infections of the mediastinum are relatively uncommon, they are often difficult to diagnose and cause a serious threat to the adjacent vital structures.

Infections may be divided into two categories, acute mediastinitis and chronic mediastinitis. These infections differ in their microbiology, pathogenesis, clinical presentation, and treatment.

ETIOLOGY

The bacterial pathogens associated with mediastinitis resulting from esophageal perforation are the flora of adjacent mucosal surfaces, primarily the oral flora, which contains aerobic bacteria, including group A *Streptococcus,* and anaerobic bacteria, principally *Prevotella melaninogenica, Fusobacterium,* and *Peptostreptococcus.*

The most frequent pathogens associated with mediastinitis after thoracic surgery are *Staphylococcus aureus,* coagulase-negative staphylococci, enteric gram-negative bacilli, *Pseudomonas aeruginosa,* and *Candida albicans.*

Chronic mediastinitis is usually a complication of *Mycobacterium tuberculosis* or *Histoplasma capsulatum* infection.

EPIDEMIOLOGY

Acute mediastinitis is an aggressive infection that may complicate esophageal perforation, oropharyngeal infection, infection of contiguous structures, or thoracic surgery. **Descending cervical mediastinitis,** also called **descending necrotizing mediastinitis,** is an extension of retropharyngeal and odontogenic infections originating in the head and neck and is rarely seen in the antibiotic era. Currently most cases of mediastinitis occur as a complication of traumatic esophageal perforations or thoracic surgery. The reported incidence of mediastinitis following cardiac surgery ranges from 0.15–5%, with a mortality of approximately 8%.

Chronic mediastinitis, sometimes called **sclerosing or fibrosing mediastinitis,** is a more indolent form of mediastinitis. It can occur in any age group, but it frequently follows granulomatous infections such as tuberculosis or histoplasmosis.

PATHOGENESIS

The mediastinum is relatively protected against infection. Acute infections of the mediastinum are usually the result of direct introduction of organisms into the mediastinum by trauma or surgery or a result of pulmonary or other contiguous infection (Table 70–1).

Esophageal Perforation. Any disruption of the integrity of the esophagus, even inapparent tears, may contaminate the mediastinum with bacteria and food contents. Precipitous symptoms of mediastinitis may occur with a laceration of the esophagus that allows immediate contamination of the mediastinum with bacteria and food particles. Esophageal instrumentation, such as esophagoscopy and bougie dilation, and sharp foreign bodies, such as pins and ingested bone fragments, are the most frequent causes of transmural lacerations. Symptoms may be delayed several days when blunt objects, such as coins or large food particles become impacted in the esophagus, eventually eroding into the esophageal wall and causing suppurative necrosis. Most perforations due to instrumentation and to foreign bodies involve the **introitus,** which is the narrowest segment of the esophagus.

Extension of Infection From Contiguous Structures. Peritonsillar abscesses, Ludwig's angina, and other infections of the head and neck are infrequent causes of mediastinitis. These infections may spread through spaces formed by fascial planes that extend from the head to the thorax (Chapter 59). Mastoiditis, tracheostomy, mediastinotomy, and surgery or trauma of the oral airways may lead to acute mediastinitis. Extension of infection from vertebrae, sternum, and ribs is uncommon.

Mediastinitis following thoracic surgery is usually associated with sternal wound infections. Risk factors associated with higher rates of infection include prolonged surgery, postoperative closed-chest massage, infected tracheostomy stomas, sternal dehiscence, and emergency reoperations. The benefit of prophylactic antibiotics in the prevention of sternal wound infections is not clearly established.

Chronic Mediastinitis. Granulomatous infections, such as tuberculosis or histoplasmosis, are frequent causes of chronic, fibrosing mediastinitis, which appears to result from rupture of caseous mediastinal nodes, which provokes an intense inflammatory reaction. There may be mediastinal calcifications. Chronic mediastinitis is frequently asymptomatic. Symptoms, when present, are usually due to compression of adjacent structures, such as the superior vena cava or the tracheobronchial tree. Granulomatous and fibrous mediastinitis may account for up to 10% of all primary mediastinal masses and 20% of cases of superior vena cava syndrome. The inciting infection may precede chronic mediastinitis by months or years.

SYMPTOMS AND CLINICAL MANIFESTATIONS

Patients with acute mediastinitis are often severely ill, with substernal pain, chills, fever, and tachycardia. The infection may progress

TABLE 70–1. Pathogenesis of Acute Mediastinitis

Esophageal Perforation
Foreign body
Instrumentation
Intraoperative
Blunt or penetrating chest trauma
Direct Extension of Infections from Contiguous Structures
Postoperative thoracic wound infection, including median sternotomy
Head and neck infections (descending mediastinitis)
Subphrenic infections
Vertebral osteomyelitis
Infections of pleura, lungs, hilar lymph nodes

rapidly, and approximately 30% of patients are hypotensive or comatose on presentation. Following esophageal perforation, the predominant symptoms are neck and chest pain, respiratory distress, and dysphagia. The anatomic location of the esophageal lesion can affect the symptoms, with cervical lesions producing neck and upper anterior chest pain whereas lower esophageal lesions cause epigastric or precordial pain. Infants with acute mediastinitis may develop spasmodic and irregular breathing. Cyanosis and severe dyspnea may indicate massive pleural effusion, pneumothorax, or decreased cardiac output.

Local tenderness, erythema, purulent drainage, wound dehiscence, and persistent fevers are the main clinical features of a median sternotomy wound infection. Fever and systemic toxicity frequently precede clinical evidence of sternal wound infection.

Many patients with chronic mediastinitis have no symptoms, with infection initially detected on routine chest radiographs as a widened superior mediastinum. Symptoms may include low-grade fever, anemia, and weight loss. Compression of adjacent structures such as the superior vena cava, esophagus, or tracheobronchial tree may be present.

DIAGNOSIS

Acute mediastinitis is usually a clinical diagnosis for a patient at risk. The diagnosis is supported by abnormalities of the chest radiograph, chest CT, mediastinal tomography, or fluoroscopy. Typical findings on a chest radiograph are a widened mediastinum, subcutaneous and mediastinal emphysema, and pleural effusions. **Mediastinal emphysema** is highly suggestive of esophageal perforation in the context of compatible clinical presentation. Pneumothorax or hydropneumothorax can also occur. Radiopaque foreign bodies may be detected on plain radiographs, but CT is usually more sensitive.

The diagnostic studies of patients with possible chronic mediastinitis should include chest radiograph, CT or MRI, tuberculin skin test, and testing for *Histoplasma* antigen in serum and urine (Chapter 11). Surgical exploration of the mediastinum may be indicated for tissue biopsy for diagnosis, as well as for removal of infected tissues as part of therapy.

TREATMENT

The treatment of acute mediastinitis involves surgical débridement, antimicrobial therapy, and supportive measures. When a descending infection from the head or neck involves the mediastinum, both cervical and mediastinal drainage and irrigation are recommended. Tracheostomy is usually performed to secure the airway. If the mediastinitis progresses caudad to the fourth thoracic vertebra, transthoracic drainage is usually recommended because of an increased rate of pleural empyema. Thoracoscopic drainage and débridement of mediastinitis have recently been offered as a less invasive alternative to thoracotomy. Surgery to correct a perforation of the esophagus is necessary to prevent further contamination of the mediastinum.

Mediastinitis arising as a complication of a postsurgical sternotomy wound infection requires extensive débridement of the wound. Osteomyelitis of the sternum commonly occurs (Chapter 86).

Empiric antibiotic therapy for all cases of acute mediastinitis should be initiated immediately, with coverage for both aerobic and anaerobic bacteria, and modified as indicated by bacteriologic studies of isolates obtained from surgical specimens (Table 70–2). Mediastinitis associated with median sternotomy wound infection usually requires systemic antibiotics for a minimum of 4–6 weeks.

In chronic mediastinitis, excision of the lesion is indicated if there is evidence of compression of vital structures, especially early in the course of the disease. During the later stages, surgical resection is technically difficult and usually is only palliative. Resected tissue should be cultured, and histologic sections should be studied for evidence of *M. tuberculosis* and *H. capsulatum.* Suspected or proven *M. tuberculosis* infection requires antimycobacterial therapy (Chapter 35). The role of amphotericin B when excised tissue reveals *H. capsulatum* is controversial, but most investigators believe that antifungal treatment is unnecessary if cultures are negative.

TABLE 70–2. Recommended Empiric Antibiotic Treatment for Acute Mediastinitis

Mechanisms of Mediastinitis	Recommended Treatment
Esophageal perforation, or direct extension of infections from contiguous structures (excluding thoracic wound infection)	Clindamycin *or* Penicillin G *plus* metronidazole *or* Cefoxitin
Median sternotomy wound infection, or nosocomial mediastinitis	Vancomycin *plus* ceftazidime *or* cefepime *with or without* an aminoglycoside

Suggested Dosages for Patients with Normal Renal Function

ANTIBIOTIC	IV DOSAGE	MAXIMUM DAILY DOSE
Amikacin	15 mg/kg/day divided q8–12hr	15 mg/kg
Cefepime	100–150 mg/kg/day divided q8–12hr	4–6 g
Cefoxitin	80–160 mg/kg/day divided q6hr	12 g
Ceftazidime	100–150 mg/kg/day divided q8hr	6 g
Clindamycin	25–40 mg/kg/day divided q8hr	2.7 g
Gentamicin	7.5 mg/kg/day divided q8hr	Adults: 5 mg/kg
Metronidazole	30 mg/kg/day divided q6hr	30 mg/kg
Penicillin G	250,000–400,000 U/kg/day divided q4hr	20–24 MU
Tobramycin	7.5 mg/kg/day divided q8hr	Adults: 5 mg/kg
Vancomycin	45–60 mg/kg/day divided q6hr	2 g

COMPLICATIONS AND PROGNOSIS

The mortality that accompanies acute mediastinitis can be as high as 25%, especially if the diagnosis and appropriate treatment are delayed. Acute mediastinitis may progress to fulminating sepsis, may involve the pleura and the lungs, and may result in aortic perforation. Infrequently, acute mediastinitis can cause obstruction of the superior vena cava. Chronic mediastinitis may entrap the vessels and airways and is a frequent cause of the superior vena cava syndrome.

PREVENTION

Cognizance of the risks associated with esophageal perforation, head and neck infections, and sternal wound infections with early recognition of possible acute mediastinitis will determine the severity of this complication. The incidence of postoperative sternal wound infections can be minimized but not eliminated by strict adherence to perioperative aseptic technique, attention to hemostasis, and precise sternal closure.

REVIEWS

Bor DH, Rose RM, Modlin JF, et al: Mediastinitis after cardiovascular surgery. *Rev Infect Dis* 1983;5:885–97.

Goodwin RA, Nickell JA, Des Prez RM: Mediastinal fibrosis complicating healed primary histoplasmosis and tuberculosis. *Medicine* 1972; 51:227–46.

Kiernan PD, Hernandez A, Byrne WD, et al: Descending cervical mediastinitis. *Ann Thorac Surg* 1998;65:1483–8.

Murray PM, Finegold SM: Anaerobic mediastinitis. *Rev Infect Dis* 1984; 6(Suppl 1):S123–7.

KEY ARTICLES

Baskett RJ, MacDougall CE, Ross DB: Is mediastinitis a preventable complication? *Ann Thorac Surg* 1999;67:462–5.

Cogan IC: Necrotizing mediastinitis secondary to descending cervical cellulitis. *Oral Surg Oral Med Oral Pathol* 1973;36:307–20.

Dukes RJ, Strimlan CV, Dines DE, et al: Esophageal involvement with mediastinal granuloma. *JAMA* 1976;236:2313–5.

Levine TM, Wurster CF, Krespi YP: Mediastinitis occurring as a complication of odontogenic infections. *Laryngoscope* 1986;96:747–50.

Newman LS, Szczukowski LC, Bain RP, et al: Suppurative mediastinitis after open heart surgery: A case control study of risk factors. *Chest* 1988;94:546–53.

North J, Emanuel B: Mediastinitis in a child caused by perforation of pharynx. *Am J Dis Child* 1975;129:962–3.

Roberts JR, Smythe WR, Weber RW, et al: Thoracoscopic management of descending necrotizing mediastinitis. *Chest* 1997;112:851.

Sarr MG, Gott VL, Townsend TR: Mediastinal infection after cardiac surgery. *Ann Thorac Surg* 1984;38:415–23.

CHAPTER 71

Infective Endocarditis

Robert S. Baltimore

Infective endocarditis is an infection on the endothelial surface of the heart. The infectious endothelial lesions, called **vegetations,** usually occur on the valve leaflets. They also may occur on the mural or septal endocardium and may be associated with infectious lesions of the great vessels. The lesions are composed of microorganisms trapped in a fibrin mesh that extends into the bloodstream.

Infective endocarditis has been classified as acute or subacute on the basis of the history and epidemiologic findings. In individual cases, however, features of both types of presentations may be present and the illness may not be easily categorized. Thus the term *infective endocarditis* has generally replaced the terms *acute and subacute bacterial endocarditis.* The duration of symptoms before diagnosis is still important, however, because the prognosis for the disease is poorer in persons with a prodrome of longer than 3 months.

Historically, infectious endocarditis was most frequently a complication of congenital or rheumatic heart disease. With the decline in the incidence of acute rheumatic fever, few children now present with infective endocarditis associated with late rheumatic heart disease. Most children with infective endocarditis in tertiary care hospitals who do not have congenital heart disease tend to be acutely ill infants or children with central intravenous catheters. These catheters act as an instigating focus for the development of a clot, which becomes an infected vegetation. The factors commonly associated with infective endocarditis in adults, such as intravenous drug abuse, atherosclerosis, and degenerative heart disease, are not important predisposing factors to infective endocarditis in children. With the increasing availability of corrective or palliative surgical treatment of congenital heart disease, there is an increasing association of infective endocarditis with a previous cardiac operation or the presence of foreign material, such as vascular grafts, patches, or artificial or bioprosthetic replacement valves in the heart.

In the preantibiotic era, infective endocarditis was uniformly fatal, but today, with appropriate antibiotic and surgical management, the mortality rate is low. To some degree, infective endocarditis can be prevented by the use of appropriate prophylactic antibiotics in high-risk patients undergoing a procedure in which bacteremia is likely to occur.

ETIOLOGY

In all reports from more than 50 years of study, **viridans streptococci** have always been the leading microbial agent of infective endocarditis in children (Table 71–1). Viridans streptococci and enterococci are associated with endocarditis in children with native valves and with endocarditis occurring more than 60 days after a cardiac operation. The organisms are especially common in persons with a subacute presentation of infective endocarditis. *Staphylococcus aureus* and coagulase-negative staphylococci commonly cause endocarditis that occurs within 60 days after a cardiac operation or that is associated with intravenous drug abuse or indwelling intravenous catheters. Gram-negative bacilli and fungi are uncommon causes of infective endocarditis and most likely are associated with nosocomial catheter-related endocarditis and sepsis-related endocarditis.

Until the late 1970s, endocarditis in neonates and young infants was rare, probably because the hemodynamic abnormalities associated with congenital heart disease require a considerable period to lead to the sterile fibrin deposition that precedes the formation of infected vegetations in native, or natural, valve infective endocarditis. However, with increased survival of very low birth weight infants, the number of reports of infective endocarditis in neonates has been increasing. One study (Millard and Shulman, 1988) showed that the infecting organisms in 25 published cases of neonatal endocarditis were primarily *S. aureus,* coagulase-negative staphylococci, and group B *Streptococcus.* An increase in the use of catheters in the right side of the heart and in the number of cardiac operations performed on neonates were considered to be the causes of this increased incidence. *Candida* organisms have also been associated with neonatal infective endocarditis, with the use of indwelling intravenous lines and peripheral hyperalimentation being major risk factors. **Fungal endocarditis** is generally associated with very large vegetations. Embolus to relatively large blood vessels is a frequent serious complication that can be avoided if an operation to remove the vegetation is performed early in the disease. Although surgical removal of vegetations infected with *Candida* is generally recommended, one group (Sanchez et al, 1991) described three neonates with *Candida* endocarditis and vegetations documented by echocardiography and reported successful treatment with antifungal therapy alone.

EPIDEMIOLOGY

Currently, infective endocarditis is primarily a complication of congenital heart disease in children. It is a sporadic disease with no geographic predisposition and little gender or socioeconomic predisposition in children. This is in contradistinction to the epidemiology among adults, where there is a male preponderance linked with social and behavioral factors such as intravenous drug abuse and atherosclerotic heart disease. In the past endocarditis was often a complication of a prolonged septic process in another organ. In the antibiotic era, however, this is much less common except in the presence of an indwelling central venous catheter, which acts as a nidus for clot and vegetation formation in the right side of the heart. The average age of adults with infective endocarditis is rising, with an increase most notably among older men.

The incidence of infective endocarditis is estimated at 1.7–4 cases per 100,000 population per year in the United States and other developed countries. The rate of hospital admissions for infective endocarditis in adults has been falling during the antibiotic era, but the rate of endocarditis in children has been rising. One review (Kaye, 1992) reported an incidence of 0.55–0.78 case of

TABLE 71–1. Bacterial and Fungal Agents of Infective Endocarditis in Children and Adults

	Native Valve Endocarditis			Prosthetic Valve Endocarditis (Adults)§		
Organism	Neonates (%) 1950–1988 (n = 25)*	Children (%) 1933–1987 (n = 2,345)†	Adults (%) 1933–1987 (n = 2,345)‡	Early (%) (<3 Mo After Surgery) 1975–1994 (n = 137)	Intermediate (%) (3–12 Mo After Surgery) 1975–1994 (n = 31)	Late (%) (>12 Mo After Surgery) 1975–1994 (n = 194)
Streptococcus				1.5	10	31
Viridans streptococci		40	47‖			
Streptococcus pneumoniae		3	3			
Group B or G	16	3				
Other	4					
Enterococcus		4	6	9	13	11
Staphylococcus						
Staphylococcus aureus	48	24	19	23	13	18
Coagulase-negative staphylococci	12	5	6	31	35	11
Diphtheroids (*Corynebacterium*)				7		3
Gram-negative aerobic bacilli	8	4	6	14	3	6
Fungi	8	1	1	9	6	1
Others or mixed organisms	4	2	3	3	6	11
Culture-negative		13	9	3	13	8

*Data from Millard DD, Shulman ST: The changing spectrum of neonatal endocarditis. *Clin Perinatol* 1988;15:587–608.
†Data from Starke JR: Infective endocarditis. In Feigin RD, Cherry JD, editors: *Textbook of Pediatric Infectious Diseases,* 4th ed. Philadelphia, WB Saunders, 1998, p 324.
‡Data from Tunkel AR, Mandell GL: Infecting microorganisms. In Kaye D, editor: *Infective Endocarditis,* 2nd ed. New York, Raven Press, 1992.
§Data from Karchmer AW: Infections of prosthetic valves and intravascular devices. In Mandell GL, Bennett JE, Dolin R, editors: *Principles and Practice of Infectious Diseases,* 5th ed. Philadelphia, Churchill Livingstone, 2000, pp 903–17.
‖Includes all streptococci except *S. pneumoniae.*

infective endocarditis per 1,000 pediatric hospital admissions. The increased incidence of endocarditis in children is probably due to the improved survival of children with congenital heart disease and to advances in the surgical management of cyanotic congenital heart disease. Such surgical therapy often involves the use of indwelling prosthetic material, which is an additional risk factor for the development of endocarditis.

In the past it was rare for children younger than 2 years of age to develop infective endocarditis. Neonatal endocarditis has become more common, appearing to be a complication of severe underlying disease and the use of indwelling central venous catheters in this age group, rather than as a complication of congenital heart disease. Fewer than 30% of children younger than 2 years of age with infective endocarditis have congenital heart disease, whereas 70–90% of children older than 2 years of age with infective endocarditis have congenital heart disease.

PATHOGENESIS

The pathogenesis of most cases of infective endocarditis in children appears to be related to turbulent blood flow or the effect of a foreign body in contact with the endocardium. Turbulent blood flow is usually the result of congenital heart disease and is especially important when there is a jet of flow from high to low pressure. The jet may be across an atrial or ventricular septal defect or from regurgitation through an incompetent valve. Turbulence leads to erosion of the endothelium and deposition of platelet-fibrin thrombi on abnormal valvular or mural surfaces, allowing bacteria to implant on and become entrapped within these thrombi. The congenital cardiac lesions most frequently associated with infective endocarditis in children include tetralogy of Fallot, ventricular septal defects, aortic stenosis, aortic regurgitation, patent ductus arteriosus, and transposition of the great vessels (Table 71–2). Infective endocarditis associated with mitral valve prolapse is rare in children. In rheumatic, atheromatous, or calcific heart disease, organisms may become trapped in diseased valves or mural plaques during episodes of bacteremia or fungemia.

Although normal endocardial surfaces resist implantation of microorganisms, there has been an increase in the number of young

TABLE 71–2. Underlying Heart Disease in 266 Children with Infective Endocarditis

Type of Underlying Cardiac Disease	Patients with Infective Endocarditis (%) (n = 266)
Congenital heart disease	78
Tetralogy of Fallot	24
Ventricular septal defect	16
Congenital aortic stenosis	8
Patent ductus arteriosus	7
Transposition of the great vessels	4
Undiagnosed shunts	13
Other (pulmonic stenosis, coarctation, atrioventricular canal, atrial septal defect)	6
Rheumatic heart disease	14
No pre-existing heart disease	8

Adapted from several studies (1930–1970) reviewed in the following: Kaplan EL: Infective endocarditis in the pediatric age group. An overview. In Kaplan EL, Taranta AV, editors: *Infective Endocarditis: An American Heart Association Symposium.* American Heart Association, Dallas, 1977, pp 51–4.

children with no previous structural heart disease in whom infective endocarditis developed as the result of the presence of a central intravenous catheter that extends to the right side of the heart. An experimental animal model of endocarditis in rabbits mimics this mechanism of nosocomial endocarditis. In this model, endocarditis cannot be induced by simply injecting organisms intravenously but readily develops if bacteremia is preceded by placement of an intravenous polyethylene catheter into the right ventricle through the tricuspid valve. The catheter acts as a foreign body and also presumably causes microscopic damage by abrading endocardial and valve surfaces, causing sterile vegetations to form, which facilitates adherence of bacteria during bacteremia. This mechanism of causation appears to be clinically applicable to central venous lines, Swan-Ganz catheters, or any catheter in contact with endocardial surfaces.

Almost all bacterial genera have been known to cause infective endocarditis, but certain species are more likely to attach to endothelial surfaces than others on the basis of their physical properties. Certain species of streptococci produce **dextran,** which promotes bacterial adhesion to endothelial surfaces. Coagulase-negative staphylococci produce **extracellular polysaccharide ("slime")** that is responsible for adherence of organisms to intravascular catheters. Most gram-negative organisms adhere poorly and seldom cause endocarditis.

Once the vegetative lesion of infective endocarditis is established, most of the subsequent physical phenomena are the result of embolization of infected vegetations, either to the lungs from right-sided endocarditis or through the systemic circulation from left-sided endocarditis. Because of the large number of bacteria present and the long duration of bacterial infection in subacute infective endocarditis, some of the associated symptoms and malaise are related to immunologic phenomena associated with circulating complexes of bacterial antigens, antibodies, and complement.

A review (Kaplan, 1977) of several reported series of infective endocarditis in 266 children showed that 78% had underlying congenital heart disease with septal cardiac lesions predominating, 14% had rheumatic heart disease, and 8% had no evidence of previous heart disease (Table 71–2). In a retrospective review (Stanton et al, 1984) from Yale for 1970–1979, 23 (88%) of 26 children with infective endocarditis had had pre-existing heart disease; only one of the children had rheumatic heart disease, and three children had indwelling catheters as the risk factor. In a retrospective review (Saiman et al, 1993) from Columbia-Presbyterian Medical Center for 1977–1992, of 62 children with infective endocarditis, 40 (65%) had congenital heart disease, including 4 (6%) who had mitral valve prolapse. Only 3 children (5%) had rheumatic heart disease, and 19 (31%) had normal cardiac anatomy before the infective endocarditis. In a recent review (Stockheim et al, 1998 [for 1978–1996]), only 3 of 111 children with infective endocarditis had previous rheumatic heart disease.

Native (Natural) Valve Endocarditis. The steps in the development of native valve endocarditis are, first, the deposition of fibrin on a denuded endothelial surface, then deposition of bacteria onto this relatively rough surface, and then the growth of the vegetation with great multiplication of bacteria, implying that in each case of clinically evident infective endocarditis there is an event of preceding bacteremia. Often the exact time of the bacteremia cannot be established because the symptoms may not have been clinically significant, but bacteremia-prone events often precede the development of infective endocarditis. Whenever there is abrasion or incision of mucosal surfaces that normally harbor large numbers of bacteria or fungi, bacteremia or fungemia can occur. The most frequent site of entry is the oral cavity, with bacteremia following a dental procedure such as drainage of an abscess, operation on the gingiva, or tooth extraction. Surgical procedures that involve the upper airway, such as bronchoscopy and intubation, are also prone to cause bacteremia. Manipulation of the genitourinary tract, such as by endoscopy, urethral catheterization, or cystoscopy, is likely to cause bacteremia. The endogenous flora of these mucosal surfaces is the most common cause of native valve endocarditis. This sequence of events and the identification of bacteremia-prone events have resulted in the recommendation to treat patients susceptible to infective endocarditis with antibiotics before bacteremia-prone procedures.

Prosthetic Valve Endocarditis. Endovascular infection associated with valve homografts and artificial heart valves is referred to as prosthetic valve endocarditis. The pathogenesis and infecting organisms causing prosthetic valve endocarditis differ between endocarditis occurring within 2 months of surgery, known as **early prosthetic endocarditis,** and endocarditis occurring later than 2 months, known as **late prosthetic endocarditis** (Table 71–1).

In the immediate postoperative period there are areas of denuded epithelium near the sites of prosthetic material and exposed sutures. During this time endocarditis may develop after bacteremia induced by contamination of intravenous solutions, contamination from the cardiac bypass pump, surgical wound infection, catheter-associated infection, or direct implantation of bacteria intraoperatively. Host defenses against bacteria work poorly at the site of a foreign body, and there may also be host factors predisposing the person to infection, such as immunosuppression and poor nutrition. In early prosthetic endocarditis the most common bacterial causes of endocarditis are coagulase-negative staphylococci, followed by *S. aureus,* diphtheroids, and gram-negative bacilli (Table 71–1). Less commonly, streptococci, enterococci, and, rarely, fungi may be isolated.

Late prosthetic valve endocarditis occurs after re-endothelialization of cardiac and vascular incisions, which usually occurs 2–4 months after placement of an artificial valve, graft, or conduit. A smooth endothelial surface develops, and then both the natural history of infective endocarditis and the causative organisms resemble those of native valve endocarditis. In adults, in whom there is much greater experience with prosthetic valve endocarditis, late prosthetic valve endocarditis is due primarily to streptococci and coagulase-negative staphylococci (Table 71–1).

SYMPTOMS AND CLINICAL MANIFESTATIONS

The most frequent symptoms and signs of infective endocarditis emphasize the presentation of the classic subacute presentation (Table 71–3). Symptomatic disease, however, may present from as short a time as a few days after the causative bacteremia to several months after the start of infection. Because the most common early symptoms of infective endocarditis (e.g., fever, malaise, and weight loss) are nonspecific and can be confused with ordinary viral or other influenza-like illnesses, subacute endocarditis may continue for weeks or even months with symptoms and even physician evaluation but without diagnosis. If such persons are treated empirically for a bacterial infection with a short course of oral antibiotics, they may have temporary improvement, only to have a relapse because more intensive treatment is required to cure infective endocarditis. If a person initially complains of chest pain or has symptoms indicative of heart failure, such as shortness of breath or exercise intolerance, it is likely that endocarditis will be considered more strongly as the underlying cause and a correct diagnosis be made early. Endocarditis in children with congenital heart disease

TABLE 71–3. Symptoms, Signs, and Laboratory Findings Associated with Infective Endocarditis in Children

	Frequency*
Symptoms	
Fever	++++
Malaise	+++
Anorexia, weight loss	++
Heart failure	++
Myalgia/arthralgia	++
Chest pain	+
Neurologic symptoms (e.g., focal neurologic deficit, aseptic meningitis)	+
Gastrointestinal symptoms	+
Signs	
Fever	++++
Splenomegaly	+++
Petechiae	++
Embolic phenomenon	++
New or changed murmur	++
Clubbing	+
Osler's nodes	+
Roth's spots	+
Janeway lesions	+
Splinter hemorrhages	+
Conjunctival hemorrhages	+
Laboratory Findings	
Positive blood culture result	++++
Elevated ESR	++++
Anemia	++
Positive rheumatoid factor	++
Hematuria	++

*Legend: ++++, 75–100% of patients; +++, 50–75% of patients; ++, 25–50% of patients; +, 0–25% of patients.

may first appear with subtle and nonspecific findings, underscoring the need to obtain blood cultures at this stage so that the diagnosis can be established early.

Some persons with infective endocarditis have a more acute onset of the disease, similar to that of bacterial sepsis. These persons generally have a high fever and may or may not have recognizably new cardiac symptoms. Persons who do not have underlying structural heart defects usually have an intravenous catheter or other indwelling device, or they have recently had an episode of documented bacteremia. For these persons it is important to consider the diagnosis of infective endocarditis in an investigation of the cause of sepsis or of a lack of response to the usual treatment of sepsis.

Physical Examination Findings

Findings of the physical examination may play an important role in confirming the diagnosis of infective endocarditis. Fever is the most common symptom (Table 71–3). Prolonged fever or unexplained malaise or weight loss in a person with structural heart disease suggests endocarditis. Although some persons may lack any of the specific physical features of endocarditis, most persons with a long illness have specific findings associated with endocarditis. The relatively common signs of splenomegaly, arthralgia, and petechiae are infrequently associated with common viral infections in children and suggest the possibility of endocarditis. A change in murmur, especially if suggestive of valvular insufficiency, indicates possible endocarditis. Dramatic embolic findings that are specific for endocarditis include sudden loss of pulses in a limb; central nervous system signs such as cranial nerve deficits, seizure, or strokelike symptoms; petechiae or hemorrhage on mucosal surfaces such as the conjunctiva or oral mucosa; and embolic pneumonia from right-sided endocarditis.

Although becoming uncommon in recent years, some classic findings are specific for endocarditis. **Osler's nodes** are small (2–15 mm), purplish, painful lesions in the pulp of the fingers or toes that may persist for hours or days. **Janeway lesions** (Plate 8C) are painless hemorrhagic macular plaques on the palms or soles. They are due to emboli and may persist for days. **Roth's spots** are small, hemorrhagic lesions with a pale center found on the retina, usually near the optic disk. **Splinter hemorrhages** are dark, linear streaks in the nail beds that are due to microemboli and increased capillary fragility. Because splinter hemorrhages can also be caused by local trauma, they are less specific than Osler's nodes, Janeway lesions, or Roth's spots.

In acute infective endocarditis the physical examination may or may not be helpful in establishing the diagnosis. It may not be possible to discern a change in murmur from previous examinations by auscultation for persons with pre-existing cardiac murmurs or recent cardiac surgery. Signs of emboli in the lungs or in the peripheral circulation suggest endocarditis, but the other infectious and noninfectious conditions that predispose a person to acute endocarditis (e.g., recovery from an operation, intravenous drug abuse, postpartum state) may also be the cause of pulmonary or systemic emboli.

DIAGNOSIS

The diagnosis is most obvious for persons with pre-existing heart lesions who clearly have new valvular vegetations and also blood cultures that are positive for an organism that commonly causes endocarditis. In complex clinical situations the presentation may not be clear. Diagnostic criteria are important when the diagnosis is considered in the absence of an image of a vegetation or positive blood culture results (Tables 71–4 and 71–5). Von Reyn and associates (1981) proposed a strict case definition for definite, probable, or possible cases of infective endocarditis for the purpose of retrospective analysis of cases (Beth Israel criteria). These case definitions, suitably modified, may be used for analyzing the strength of the diagnosis in specific cases. Subsequently, Durack and associates (1994) developed a modified set of criteria that incorporate newer developments in echocardiograhy as well as additional clinical criteria (Duke criteria). Subsequent clinical studies in adults and children (Stockheim et al, 1998) have consistently demonstrated the superiority of the Duke criteria. It is sometimes extremely difficult to diagnose infective endocarditis, and a decision frequently is made to treat as if endocarditis were present even though the diagnosis is uncertain—the ''possible'' category by the Beth Israel and the Duke criteria.

Laboratory Evaluation. An elevated ESR is usually present unless there is either congestive heart failure or polycythemia with pre-existing cyanotic heart disease. A leukocytosis is present in only approximately 50% of persons. Anemia, hypergammaglobulinemia, microscopic hematuria, and a positive rheumatoid factor and immune complexes frequently are found.

Microbiologic Evaluation

The most useful laboratory test for the diagnosis of infective endocarditis is a blood culture. Failure to obtain blood culture specimens from persons with infective endocarditis who have a subacute presentation is the prime reason for failure to make a timely diagnosis. Blood culture specimens should be obtained from a child with

TABLE 71–4. Duke Clinical Criteria for Diagnosis of Infective Endocarditis

Definite Infective Endocarditis

Pathologic Criteria

Microorganisms demonstrated by culture or histologic findings in a vegetation *or* in a vegetation that has embolized, *or* in an intracardiac abscess *or*

Pathologic lesion: vegetation or intracardiac abscess present, confirmed by histologic findings showing active endocarditis

Clinical Criteria, Using Specific Definitions (Listed in Table 71–5)

2 Major criteria *or*

1 Major and 3 minor criteria *or*

5 Minor criteria

Possible Infective Endocarditis

Findings consistent with infective endocarditis that fall short of "definite" but not "rejected"

Rejected

Firm alternate diagnosis for manifestations of endocarditis *or*

Resolution of manifestations of endocarditis, with antibiotic therapy for 4 days or less *or*

No pathologic evidence of endocarditis at surgery or autopsy, after antibiotic therapy of 4 days or less

From Durack DT, Lukes AS, Bright DK, et al: New criteria for diagnosis of infective endocarditis: Utilization of specific echocardiographic findings. Duke Endocarditis Services. *Am J Med* 1994;96:200–9.

risk factors for infective endocarditis as part of the medical evaluation of a fever, especially for fever associated with symptoms or signs suggestive of endocarditis (Table 71–3). Because the bacteremia of infective endocarditis is continuous, usually all or nearly all blood culture results are positive. Although the optimal number of blood cultures recommended varies, three separate venipunctures for blood culture represents near-maximal sensitivity (about 95%) among persons who have not recently been treated with antibiotics. Persons who have been treated with antibiotics recently or who are currently receiving antibiotics should have additional culture specimens taken initially. All persons believed to have infective endocarditis should have additional blood cultures obtained if the first cultures fail to grow an organism and symptoms persist.

When blood culture specimens are obtained, it is important always to obtain more than one blood culture specimen from persons with risk factors for infective endocarditis to account for possible contamination of the culture. A clinical dilemma arises when the sole blood culture specimen obtained from a child who has risk factors for infective endocarditis yields an organism that might be considered part of the normal skin flora, such as coagulase-negative staphylococci. If all other cultures are sterile, it is plausible that the single isolate is a contaminant. The diagnosis of probable or possible infective endocarditis (Table 71–4) may require demonstration of persistent bacteremia. Depending on the degree of certainty of the clinical diagnosis of infective endocarditis and the cardiovascular status of the person, several blood cultures for a 1- to 2-day period may be advised before the initiation of empirical antimicrobial therapy. Many persons with infective endocarditis have had blood culture specimens obtained as part of an outpatient evaluation for fever, and the infecting organism may already be known at the time of admission to the hospital. Nevertheless, it is prudent to have additional blood cultures before initiating antimicrobial therapy to demonstrate the persistent bacteremia characteristic of infective endocarditis. Generally there is no urgent need to start antibiotic therapy, and repeated culture specimens can be obtained during the first hospital day. An exception would be the uncommon occurrence of a "septic appearing" person with rapidly evolving disease.

Diagnostic Imaging

Echocardiography for noninvasive imaging of endocardial vegetations has become a major diagnostic technique for diagnosing endocarditis. As technology has improved and methods have advanced from M-mode to two-dimensional echocardiography to Doppler echocardiography, sensitivity and diagnostic accuracy have improved, although some very small lesions still cannot be imaged. Given ideal contrast to surrounding structures, lesions as small as 2 mm in diameter can usually be visualized.

TABLE 71–5. Definition of Terms Used in the Duke Criteria for the Diagnosis of Infective Endocarditis

Major Criteria

Blood Culture Positive for Infective Endocarditis

Typical microorganisms for infective endocarditis from two separate blood cultures

Viridans streptococci,* *Streptococcus bovis,* HACEK group, *or*

Community-acquired *Staphylococcus aureus,* or *Enterococcus* in the absence of a primary focus *or*

Persistently positive blood culture result, defined as recovery of a microorganism consistent with endocarditis from:

- Blood culture specimens drawn more than 12 hours apart *or*
- All of three or a majority of four or more separate blood culture specimens, with first and last drawn at least 1 hour apart

Evidence of Endocardial Involvement

Echocardiogram positive for infective endocarditis

- Oscillating intracardiac mass, on valve or supporting structures *or* in path of regurgitant jets, *or* on implanted material, in the absence of an alternative anatomic explanation, *or*
- Abscess *or*
- New partial dehiscence of prosthetic valve *or*
- New valvular regurgitation (increase or change in pre-existing murmur not sufficient)

Minor Criteria

Predisposition: predisposing heart condition *or* intravenous drug use

Fever ≥38°C (100.4°F)

Vascular phenomena: major arterial emboli, septic pulmonary infarcts, mycotic aneurysm, intracranial hemorrhage, conjunctival hemorrhages, Janeway lesions

Immunologic phenomena: glomerulonephritis, Osler's nodes, Roth's spots, rheumatoid factor

Microbiologic evidence: positive blood culture result but not meeting major criteria as noted previously† *or* serologic evidence of active infection with organism consistent with infective endocarditis

Echocardiogram: consistent with infective endocarditis but not meeting major criterion as noted previously

*Including nutritionally variant strains.

†Excluding single cultures positive for coagulase-negative staphylococci and organisms that do not cause endocarditis.

From Durack DT, Lukas AS, Bright DK, et al: New criteria for diagnosis of infective endocarditis: Utilization of specific echocardiographic findings. Duke Endocarditis Services. *Am J Med* 1994;96:200–9.

The earliest echocardiographic finding in infective endocarditis is **valve leaflet thickening** followed by irregularly shaped lesions on the valve leaflets, chordae, and base of the valves. Doppler flow imaging, which uses pulse waves to identify and quantitate flow through intracardiac and extracardiac vascular structures, can demonstrate the hemodynamic consequences of valvular lesions. Blood flow is displayed as a color map with flow toward the transducer probe, represented in red, and flow away from the transducer in blue (Plate 8D). Serial Doppler flow studies detect new regurgitation and turbulence. Similarly, once the diagnosis of infective endocarditis is made, regression of a vegetation may be followed by echocardiography, although reduction in physical size may lag long after bacteriologic cure with antibiotics. The sudden disappearance of a lesion previously imaged usually indicates embolization. It thus demonstrates the cause of new embolic findings, such as petechiae and new neurologic signs, which may develop during the course of treatment of infective endocarditis as caused by embolizaton of vegetations.

In the early 1980s the reported diagnostic sensitivity of echocardiography varied from 13% to 83%; patient preselection and sonographer bias made these studies difficult to interpret. The information from an abnormal test result was helpful, with a specificity of 96% among 138 persons in one study of adults (Come, 1982). In this study, lesions detectable by ultrasonography had a poor prognosis because persons whose lesions could be imaged had more complications and deaths than those with undetectable lesions. Further studies of the prognostic implications of echocardiographic findings have yielded conflicting results for adults. Later studies did not show a worse prognosis if lesions could be identified by echocardiography. It is speculated that although having large vegetations probably is a poor prognostic finding, diagnostic sensitivity has increased and many small vegetations are now being imaged. In the past these persons might have been classified as not having an imageable lesion.

There is not as much experience with echocardiography for the diagnosis of infective endocarditis in children as there is in adults. A study (Kavey et al, 1983) using two-dimensional echocardiography found vegetations in 9 (82%) of 11 children with a diagnosis of endocarditis. Complications of infective endocarditis occurred in 7 of 9 of the patients with vegetations but in neither of the 2 patients without vegetations. A study (Bricker et al, 1985) of children reported that M-mode echocardiography revealed vegetations in 7 (20%) of 35 children, and two-dimensional echocardiography revealed vegetations in 16 (75%) of 28 children. In this relatively small series, complications requiring surgical treatment were unrelated to the demonstration of a vegetation by echocardiography.

A recent advance in cardiac imaging is **transesophageal echocardiography,** which uses an endoscopic esophageal lead and has increased sensitivity over **transthoracic echocardiography** in imaging cardiac vegetations. In a study (Mugge et al, 1989) notable for confirmation of all cases by direct inspection either during operation or at autopsy, transesophageal echocardiography demonstrated a lesion in 90% of persons with infective endocarditis, in comparison with 58% with a lesion demonstrated by M-mode or two-dimensional echocardiography. Transesophageal echocardiography was especially useful for evaluation of prosthetic valves. No similar comparative studies involving a pediatric population have been reported. This technique is more difficult in young children and usually requires general anesthesia for placement of the esophageal lead. Although the specificity of echocardiographic techniques is excellent, a negative examination result does not have sufficient sensitivity in high-risk persons to exclude endocarditis. In a recent study (Aly et al, 1999) transthoracic echocardiography had poor sensitivity (46%), which emphasizes the lack of usefulness in poorly selected persons with fever but without other specific risk factors for endocarditis. Transesophageal echocardiography should be considered in persons without a lesion demonstrated by transthoracic echocardiography who have persistent bacteremia (5–7 days or more), unexplained fever with a prosthetic valve, new murmur of aortic insufficiency or mitral insufficiency, or evidence of a left-sided cardiac lesion.

TREATMENT

Treatment of infective endocarditis requires attention to multiple facets of the illness and in many cases the cooperative efforts of a number of specialists. The initial evaluation of the patient should include assessment of cardiac status including evidence of clinical sepsis and identification of complications caused by septic emboli. Septic emboli may have manifestations as diverse as absence of peripheral pulses, focal neurologic symptoms and signs, and other vascular phenomena, such as mycotic aneurysms or coronary artery thrombosis. Persons with evidence of infective endocarditis should be hospitalized for initial antimicrobial treatment, and unless the illness is subacute and the person's condition is obviously stable, consideration should be given to admission to an intensive care unit until it is clear that the treatment is effective. Specialists in cardiology, neurology, and infectious diseases are frequently required to assess the status and to plan appropriate therapy. If heart failure is florid or not easily controlled with medication, or if there is obvious impending failure as a result of valvular damage, it is imperative to involve a cardiac surgeon early to assess the need and optimal timing for surgery. Neurologic findings may require consultation with a neurosurgeon regarding imaging studies and possible surgery for an abscess or aneurysm. Although antibiotic therapy is important for a microbiologic cure, the survival of critically ill persons with infective endocarditis may depend in the initial stages on support of vital functions and treatment of the cardiovascular phenomena.

Definitive Treatment

Antimicrobial Treatment. In many cases of infective endocarditis it is not necessary to begin antibiotic treatment before a microbiologic diagnosis is made. If the disease has a subacute presentation and the person is neither critically ill nor in obvious sepsis, it is reasonable to obtain blood culture specimens and determine the most appropriate antibiotic therapy after an organism has been isolated from the blood. For an acutely ill person, empirical antimicrobial therapy is advised immediately after initial blood culture specimens are obtained from at least three separate venipunctures.

Empirical therapy for infective endocarditis in children begun before isolation of the causative agent is based on the likely causative microorganisms (Table 71–6). Each of the antibiotics recommended is bactericidal. Bacteriostatic agents are considered to be less effective than bactericidal drugs in the treatment of infective endocarditis. The efficacy of therapy should be documented by repeated blood cultures to document blood sterilization.

Alternative antimicrobial regimens for persons allergic to the recommended antibiotics may require a judgment whether a person allergic to penicillins should be treated with cephalosporin because cross allergy to these β-lactam agents may exist (Table 71–6). Vancomycin does not cross-react but is more expensive than the first-generation cephalosporins and causes more adverse effects. The alternative agents recommended are those for which there are clinical data indicating excellent efficacy. Newer agents may be

TABLE 71–6. Antibiotic Treatment of the Most Common Bacterial Causes of Infective Endocarditis in Children and Young Adults

Infective Agent or Condition	Recommended Antibiotic Regimen	Alternative Antibiotic Regimen
Unknown Agent (Presumptive Therapy or Culture-Negative Endocarditis)		
Native valve (community acquired) or "late" prosthetic valve (>60 days after surgery) infection	Penicillinase-resistant penicillin (oxacillin *or* nafcillin; with or without penicillin *or* ampicillin) *plus* Gentamicin	Vancomycin *plus* Gentamicin
Nosocomial endocarditis associated with vascular cannulas or "early" prosthetic valve endocarditis (≤60 days after surgery)	Vancomycin *plus* Gentamicin (with or without rifampin if prosthetic material present)	
Streptococci		
Highly susceptible to penicillin G (MBC ≤0.1 μg/mL; includes most viridans, groups A, B, C, G and nonenterococcal group D streptococci [*S. bovis, S. equinus*])	Penicillin G (4-wk regimen) *or* Penicillin G *plus* Streptomycin (*or* gentamicin) (2-wk regimen)*	Vancomycin *or* First-generation cephalosporin *or* Ceftriaxone
Relatively resistant to penicillin (MBC ≥0.2 μg/mL; includes enterococci and less susceptible viridans streptococci)	Penicillin G (*or* ampicillin) *plus* Gentamicin (for first 2 wks, *or* entire course for *Enterococcus*)	Vancomycin (*plus* gentamicin for *Enterococcus*)
Staphylococci (*S. aureus* or Coagulase-Negative Staphylococci)		
Susceptible to ≤1 μg/mL penicillin G	Penicillin G	Oxacillin *or* First-generation cephalosporin *or* Vancomycin
Resistant to 0.1 μg/mL penicillin G	Penicillinase-resistant penicillin (oxacillin or nafcillin) *with or without* gentamicin for first 3–5 days	Vancomycin *or* First-generation cephalosporin
Resistant to 4 μg/mL oxacillin (MRSA)	Vancomycin	Vancomycin
For all *Staphylococcus aureus* strains: Gentamicin (*or* tobramycin *or* amikacin) should be added for first 2 wk if prosthetic material is present. Rifampin is an option that can be added to any regimen.		
HACEK Group[†]	Ceftriaxone *or* cefotaxime	Ampicillin (for susceptible organisms) *plus* Gentamicin (*or* tobramycin *or* amikacin)
Gram-Negative Enteric Bacilli	Ceftazidime *or* cefotaxime *or* Ceftriaxone *plus* gentamicin (*or* tobramycin *or* amikacin, depending on susceptibility)	Broad-spectrum penicillin *plus* Gentamicin (*or* tobramycin *or* amikacin)
Fungi		
Candida *Aspergillus*	Surgical resection *plus* amphotericin B *with or without* flucytosine	Amphotericin B followed by imidazole (e.g., itraconazole) suppression if surgery cannot be performed

*Published experience only with adults.

[†]HACEK organisms include *Haemophilus parainfluenzae, Haemophilus aphrophilus, Actinobacillus actinomycetemcomitans, Cardiobacterium hominis, Eikenella corrodens,* and *Kingella kingii.*

Table continued on following page

TABLE 71–6. Antibiotic Treatment of the Most Common Bacterial Causes of Infective Endocarditis in Children and Young Adults *(Continued)*

Suggested Dosages for Persons with Normal Renal Function

ANTIBIOTIC	DOSAGE	MAXIMUM DAILY DOSE
Amikacin*	15 mg/kg/day divided q8–12hr IV	15 mg/kg
Ampicillin	200–300 mg/kg/day divided q4–6hr IV	12 g
Cephalothin	100 mg/kg/day divided q4–6hr IV	12 g
Cefazolin	100 mg/kg/day divided q8hr IV	6 g
Cefotaxime	200 mg/kg/day divided q6hr IV	12 g
Ceftazidime	100–150 mg/kg/day divided q8hr IV	6 g
Ceftriaxone	100 mg/kg/day divided q12hr IV *or* 80 mg/kg/day q24hr IV	4 g
Gentamicin*	5–6 mg/kg/day divided q8hr IV	Adults: 3–5 mg/kg
Nafcillin	150 mg/kg/day divided q4–6hr IV	9–12 g
Oxacillin	150–200 mg/kg/day divided q4–6hr IV	12 g
Penicillin G	200,000–300,000 units/kg/day, continuously or divided q4hr IV (use high end of range for *Enterococcus*)	18–24 MU
Rifampin	10–20 mg/kg once daily PO	600 mg
S. aureus prosthetic valve endocarditis	10–20 mg/kg divided q8hr IV	900 mg
Streptomycin	20–40 mg/kg/day divided q12hr IV	1 g
Tobramycin*	5–6 mg/kg/day divided q8hr IV	Adults: 3–5 mg/kg
Vancomycin*	30–40 mg/kg/day divided q6–12hr IV	2 g
ANTIFUNGAL AGENTS		
Amphotericin B	1 mg/kg/day administered for 3–4hr IV	
Flucytosine*	150 mg/kg/day divided q6hr PO	

*Dosage adjustment is necessary with renal insufficiency.

effective, but data regarding their use are insufficient to allow a recommendation. Infective endocarditis is such a serious infection that persons allergic to penicillin should be desensitized (Chapter 14) to one of the penicillins if response to an alternative agent appears to be suboptimal.

Treatment of infective endocarditis requires a conservative approach. Infective endocarditis is a difficult infection to eradicate because the microorganisms are enmeshed in avascular fibrinous material. Antibiotics must diffuse through a barrier, so a high concentration of antibiotic in blood must be maintained for at least several weeks to ensure sterilization of vegetations. In the early days of antibiotic treatment, lack of appreciation of these concerns resulted in many recurrences after what appeared to be a good initial clinical response.

The intravenous route is recommended for antibiotic treatment, although intramuscular administration of aminoglycoside antibiotics (gentamicin, tobramycin, and amikacin) and of ceftriaxone is effective. Streptomycin is generally administered intramuscularly. Experience has shown that certain organisms are more difficult to treat, so treatment-specific schedules are based on the infecting species and whether prosthetic cardiac material is present. A longer duration of disease before treatment is begun suggests greater deposition of fibrin in vegetations and the necessity for a longer course of antibiotics.

Infective endocarditis due to viridans streptococci on a native valve is the simplest situation and has an excellent prognosis. A 2-week regimen of penicillin G plus an aminoglycoside has been shown to be effective in adults. Traditional monotherapy with penicillin G alone for 4 weeks is also effective and is preferred by most pediatric infectious disease specialists because of the lack of experience with the 2-week regimen in children. A longer treatment course of 4–6 weeks is recommended in high-risk situations, including infection with relatively resistant streptococci, *Enterococcus, Staphylococcus,* or gram-negative bacilli, and a course of at least 6 weeks in any case of infective endocarditis in a person with implanted prosthetic cardiac material.

Although rarely encountered in children, endocarditis with the fastidious, small gram-negative organisms of the **HACEK group** (*Haemophilus aphrophilus, Actinobacillus actinomycetemcomitans, Cardiobacterium hominis, Eikenella corrodens,* and *Kingella kingii*) has been treated with penicillin or ampicillin alone or in combination with an aminoglycoside, but recently either ceftriaxone or cefotaxime has been recommended as a first choice because of increased antibiotic resistance of these species. Infective endocarditis caused by enteric gram-negative bacilli is uncommon in children. It should be treated with two bactericidal agents chosen on the basis of the antibiotic susceptibility of the infecting organism, usually a combination of an expanded-spectrum β-lactam agent and an aminoglycoside. The newer third-generation cephalosporins have not been well studied in the treatment of infective endocarditis in children, but ceftriaxone has been used in adults with excellent results.

Vancomycin and aminoglycosides are nephrotoxic and ototoxic, and drug levels of these agents must be monitored and adjusted to avoid potentially toxic concentrations. Doses of antibiotics must be individualized, especially for low birth weight neonates, and adjusted on the basis of blood level monitoring.

The use of the **serum bactericidal titer (SBT; Schlichter assay)** to monitor antibiotic efficacy has been popular for many years, but a review of this practice (Coleman, 1982) demonstrated that the association between these assay results and success in the eradication of infective endocarditis is doubtful. It had been proposed that antibiotic dosing should be adjusted to provide a concentration of antibiotic in the blood that was bactericidal at a serum dilution of ≥1:8. In recent studies, high ratios were associated with excellent cure rates, but low ratios are usually associated with nonstreptococcal organisms and it is unclear whether intrinsic properties of the organism, the lack of susceptibility to β-lactam antibiotics, or a low blood level was most important. Few hospital clinical laboratories, however, can provide a reproducible serum bactericidal assay. The ratio of the measured serum concentration of antibiotic to the minimum bactericidal concentration of antibiotic required to kill the organism in vitro is often substituted.

Surgical Treatment. The outcome in persons with infective endocarditis has improved with a better understanding of the optimal time to intervene with surgical removal of infected tissue and possible replacement of destroyed heart valves with grafts or prostheses. In the absence of complications, and with a good clinical response to antibiotic therapy, no surgical intervention is needed. If the person's condition is stable, valve replacement can await completion of antibiotic therapy to sterilize the vegetation. Early surgical intervention is indicated for (1) inability to sterilize the blood despite a conventional medical regimen for a person with a vegetation localized to a heart valve, a valve annulus, or the mural surface of the heart; (2) a large abscess of the valve annulus or the myocardium or extension of the abscess during treatment; (3) recurrent serious extracardiac embolic events during treatment; (4) rupture of a valve leaflet or chordae or acute valvular insufficiency with intractable cardiac failure; (5) progressive cardiac failure incompletely controlled by medical management (usually because of mitral or aortic valve insufficiency); and (6) fungal endocarditis, which only rarely can be sterilized by antifungal agents alone. It is often difficult to determine whether surgical excision of infected foreign bodies is needed for a person with infective endocarditis associated with prosthetic material, such as an artificial heart valve, patch, or conduit. The rate of success of treatment without removal of foreign material is low among adults. However, one study (Stanton et al, 1984) reported a successful outcome among most children receiving medical treatment alone. In general, surgical intervention can be withheld if the person responds to a medical regimen. Surgery is necessary if the clinical response is poor, if cardiac status deteriorates, or if a microbiologic cure is not achieved.

COMPLICATIONS

The major complications of infective endocarditis are direct damage to the heart and heart valves and distant complications due to sterile and septic emboli from vegetations.

Damage to the heart and heart valves can be monitored by physical examination and echocardiography. Complications include regurgitation due to vegetations on the edges of the leaflets or actual defects in the leaflets due to embolization of the leaflet tissue. Flail leaflets can be the result of rupture of the chordae. A more difficult diagnosis is abscess of the valve ring or myocardial abscess. Such an abscess may be evident from echocardiography, but the diagnosis may be made at the time of surgery, which is usually required because of continued bacteremia that does not resolve with antimicrobial therapy.

In general, right-sided endocarditis is likely to be associated with embolization to the lungs and with septic foci to the lung parenchyma, and left-sided endocarditis is likely to be associated with systemic emboli to the brain, viscera, limbs, and perhaps the coronary arteries. Emboli to the central nervous system can also cause a stroke. In the viscera, septic emboli may cause hemorrhage, infarction, or an abscess. Delayed splenic rupture due to emboli is a potentially fatal complication of endocarditis. A **mycotic aneurysm** caused by infection of the wall of a vessel can cause vascular compromise or life-threatening bleeding and requires emergency attention from a vascular surgeon.

Anticoagulation is contraindicated because of the possible development of cerebral hemorrhage at the site of infarction in the brain. Unfortunately, anticoagulation may be necessary for surgical management, so the physician is required to balance the risks and benefits.

PROGNOSIS

In the preantibiotic era, infective endocarditis was a uniformly fatal disease. Today, with appropriate treatment, the outcome of infective endocarditis due to the most common organisms is good. In uncomplicated endocarditis due to viridans streptococci on a native valve, the cure rate is greater than 90%. The cure rates for enterococcal endocarditis treated by a synergistic combination of antibiotics are almost as good, 75–90%. The presentation and course of *S. aureus* endocarditis may be acute and severe, with a cure rate of 60–75%. The prognosis for endocarditis due to gram-negative bacilli and other infrequent organisms is poor. Fungal endocarditis has the poorest prognosis, with a cure rate of about 50% even with routine valve replacement. A poorer prognosis is associated with endocarditis in persons with prosthetic cardiac material, especially artificial heart valves; in persons of advanced age; and possibly in those with larger vegetations. The prognosis improves when expert cardiac surgery is available and intervention is performed in a timely manner.

PREVENTION

Experience has shown that a large number of persons with infective endocarditis frequently have undergone a procedure known to have a high risk of causing bacteremia. Persons who do not have predisposing factors for infective endocarditis, such as structural heart abnormalities or intravascular prosthetic appliances, clear these bacteremias by natural host defenses. In persons with pre-existing endothelial or endocardial lesions, these bacteria may adhere to heart valves or other endothelial surfaces and not be eradicated by normal host defenses. Such bacteremia-associated procedures (Table 71–7) include invasive dental procedures, colonoscopy, and urinary tract instrumentation in persons who have bacteriuria. In response to this information, there has been a general recommendation to use prophylactic antibiotics aimed at the bacterial species known to cause infective endocarditis. The drugs are administered close to the time of the bacteremia-associated procedures for persons predisposed to infective endocarditis (Tables 71–8 and 71–9). It has not proved efficacious to give prolonged or continuous antibiotic prophylaxis to such persons. As with surgical prophylaxis (Chapter 16), antibiotic administration just before the procedure is most effective.

The American Heart Association provides specific guidelines that identify procedures (Table 71–7) and cardiac conditions (Table 71–10) for which prophylaxis is indicated. Persons with cardiac conditions that place them at risk of acquiring infective endocarditis should receive prophylactic antibiotic therapy according to these guidelines for dental, oral, respiratory tract, or esophageal procedures (Table 71–8) and for genitourinary and gastrointestinal (excluding esophageal) procedures (Table 71–9).

TABLE 71–7. Dental or Other Procedures*

Endocarditis Prophylaxis Recommended	Endocarditis Prophylaxis Not Recommended
Dental Procedures	***Dental Procedures***
Dental extractions	Restorative dentistry[‡] (operative and prosthodontic) with or without retraction cord[§]
Periodontal procedures including surgery, scaling and root planing, probing, and recall maintenance	Local anesthetic injections (nonintraligamentary)
Dental implant placement and reimplantation of avulsed teeth	Intracanal endodontic treatment; post placement and buildup
Endodontic (root canal) instrumentation or surgery only beyond the apex	Placement of rubber dams
Subgingival placement of antibiotic fibers or strips	Postoperative suture removal
Initial placement of orthodontic bands but not brackets	Placement of removable prosthodontic or orthodontic appliances
Intraligamentary local anesthetic injections	Taking of oral impressions
Prophylactic cleaning of teeth or implants where bleeding is anticipated	Fluoride treatments
	Taking of oral radiographs
	Orthodontic appliance adjustments
	Shedding of primary teeth
Other Procedures	***Other Procedures***
Respiratory	*Respiratory Tract*
Tonsillectomy or adenoidectomy or both	Tympanostomy tube insertion
Surgical operations that involve respiratory mucosa	Endotracheal intubation
Bronchoscopy with a rigid bronchoscope	Bronchoscopy with a flexible bronchoscope, with or without biopsy[‖]
Gastrointestinal Tract[†]	*Gastrointestinal Tract*
Sclerotherapy for esophageal varices	Endoscopy with or without gastrointestinal biopsy[‖]
Esophageal stricture dilation	Transesophageal echocardiography[‖]
Endoscopic retrograde cholangiography with biliary obstruction	*Genitourinary Tract*
Biliary tract surgery	Vaginal hysterectomy[‖]
Surgical operations that involve intestinal mucosa	Vaginal delivery
Genitourinary Tract	Cesarean section
Prostatic surgery	In uninfected tissue:
Cystoscopy	Urethral catheterization
Urethral dilation	Uterine dilation and curettage
	Therapeutic abortion
	Sterilization procedures
	Insertion or removal of intrauterine devices
	Other
	Cardiac catheterization including balloon angioplasty
	Implanted cardiac pacemakers, implanted defibrillators and coronary stents
	Incision or biopsy of surgically scrubbed skin
	Circumcision

*Prophylaxis is recommended for persons with high- and moderate-risk cardiac conditions.
[†]Prophylaxis is recommended for high-risk patients and is optional for medium-risk patients.
[‡]This includes restoration of decayed teeth (filling cavities) and replacement of missing teeth.
[§]Clinical judgment may indicate antibiotic use in selected circumstances that may create significant bleeding.
[‖]Prophylaxis is optional for high-risk patients.
Adapted from Dajani AS, Taubert KA, Wilson W, et al: Prevention of bacterial endocarditis. Recommendations by the American Heart Association. *JAMA* 1997;277:1794–801.

TABLE 71–8. Prophylactic Regimens for Dental, Oral, Respiratory Tract, or Esophageal Procedures*

Situation	Agent	Regimen*
Standard general prophylaxis	Amoxicillin	Adults: 2 g; children: 50 mg/kg 1 hr before procedure PO
Unable to take oral medications	Ampicillin	Adults: 2 g; children: 50 mg/kg within 30 min before procedure IM or IV
Allergic to penicillin	Clindamycin *or*	Adults: 600 mg; children: 20 mg/kg 1 hr before procedure PO
	Cephalexin† *or* cefadroxil† *or*	Adults: 2 g; children: 50 mg/kg 1 hr before procedure PO
	Azithromycin *or* clarithromycin	Adults: 500 mg; children: 15 mg/kg 1 hr before procedure PO
Allergic to penicillin and unable to take oral medication	Clindamycin *or*	Adults: 600 mg; children: 20 mg/kg within 30 min before procedure IV
	Cefazolin†	Adults: 1 g; children: 25 mg/kg within 30 min before procedure IM or IV

*Total children's dose should not exceed adult dose.

†Cephalosporins should not be used in persons with immediate-type hypersensitivity reaction (urticaria, angioedema, or anaphylaxis) to penicillins.

Adapted from Dajani AS, Taubert KA, Wilson W, et al: Prevention of bacterial endocarditis. Recommendations by the American Heart Association. *JAMA* 1997;277:1794–801.

TABLE 71–9. Prophylactic Regimens for Genitourinary and Gastrointestinal (Excluding Esophageal) Procedures

Situation	Agents*	Regimen†
High-risk patients	Ampicillin *plus* Gentamicin	Adults: ampicillin 2 g IV or IM *plus* gentamicin 1.5 mg/kg (not to exceed 120 mg) within 30 min of start of procedure; 6 hr later, ampicillin 1 g IV or IM *or* amoxicillin 1 g PO Children: ampicillin 50 mg/kg IV or IM (not to exceed 2 g) *plus* gentamicin 1.5 mg/kg within 30 min of start of procedure; 6 hr later, ampicillin 25 mg/kg IV or IM *or* amoxicillin 25 mg/kg PO
High-risk patients allergic to ampicillin/amoxicillin	Vancomycin *plus* Gentamicin	Adults: vancomycin 1 g over 1–2 hr IV *plus* gentamicin 1.5 mg/kg IV or IM (not to exceed 120 mg); complete injection/infusion within 30 min of start of procedure Children: vancomycin 20 mg/kg over 1–2 hr IV *plus* gentamicin 1.5 mg/kg; complete injection/infusion within 30 min of start of procedure
Moderate-risk patients	Amoxicillin *or* Ampicillin	Adults: amoxicillin 2 g 1 hr before procedure PO, *or* ampicillin 2 g within 30 min of start of procedure IV or IM Children: amoxicillin 50 mg/kg 1 hr before procedure PO *or* ampicillin 50 mg/kg within 30 min of start of procedure IV or IM
Moderate-risk patients allergic to ampicillin/amoxicillin	Vancomycin	Adults: vancomycin 1 g over 1–2 hr IV; complete infusion within 30 min of start of procedure Children: vancomycin 20 mg/kg over 1–2 hr IV; complete infusion within 30 min of start of procedure

*Total children's dose should not exceed adult dose.

†No second dose of vancomycin or gentamicin is recommended.

Adapted from Dajani AS, Taubert KA, Wilson W, et al: Prevention of bacterial endocarditis. Recommendations by the American Heart Association. *JAMA* 1997;277:1794–801.

TABLE 71–10. Cardiac Conditions Associated with Endocarditis*

Endocarditis Prophylaxis Recommended

High-Risk Category

Prosthetic cardiac valves, including bioprosthetic and homograft valves

Previous bacterial endocarditis

Complex cyanotic congenital heart disease (e.g., single ventricle states, transposition of the great arteries, tetralogy of Fallot)

Surgically constructed systemic pulmonary shunts or conduits

Moderate-Risk Category

Most other congenital cardiac malformations (other than those listed elsewhere)

Acquired valvular dysfunction (e.g., rheumatic heart disease)

Hypertrophic cardiomyopathy

Mitral valve prolapse with valvular regurgitation or thickened leaflets or both

Endocarditis Prophylaxis Not Recommended

Negligible-Risk Category (No Greater Risk than for General Population)

Isolated secundum atrial septal defect

Surgical repair without residua beyond 6 mo of atrial septal defect, ventricular septal defect, or patent ductus arteriosus

Previous coronary artery bypass graft surgery

Mitral valve prolapse without valvular regurgitation

Physiologic, functional, or innocent heart murmur

Previous Kawasaki disease without valvular dysfunction

Previous rheumatic fever without valvular dysfunction

Cardiac pacemakers (intravascular and epicardial) and implanted defibrillators

*This table lists selected conditions but is not meant to be all inclusive. Adapted from Dajani AS, Taubert KA, Wilson W, et al: Prevention of bacterial endocarditis. Recommendations by the American Heart Association. *JAMA* 1997;277:1794–801.

REVIEWS

Baltimore RS: Infective endocarditis in children. *Pediatr Infect Dis J* 1992;11:907–12.

Bayer AS, Bolger AF, Taubert KA, et al: Diagnosis and management of infective endocarditis and its complications. *Circulation* 1998;98: 2936–48.

Dajani AS, Taubert KA, Wilson W, et al: Prevention of bacterial endocarditis. Recommendations by the American Heart Association. *JAMA* 1997;277:1794–801.

Kaye D (editor): *Infective Endocarditis,* 2nd ed. New York, Raven Press, 1992.

Millard DD, Shulman ST: The changing spectrum of neonatal endocarditis. *Clin Perinatol* 1988;15:587–608.

Wilson WR, Karchmer AW, Dajani AS, et al: Antibiotic treatment of adults with infective endocarditis due to streptococci, enterococci, staphylococci, and HACEK microorganisms. American Heart Association. *JAMA* 1995;274:1706–13.

KEY ARTICLES

Aly AM, Simpson PM, Humes RA: The role of transthoracic echocardiography in the diagnosis of infective endocarditis in children. *Arch Pediatr Adolesc Med* 1999;153:950–4.

Bricker JT, Latson CA, Huhta JC, et al: Echocardiographic evaluation of infective endocarditis in children. *Clin Pediatr* 1985;24:312–7.

Coleman DL, Horwitz RI, Andriole VT: Association between serum inhibitory and bactericidal concentrations and therapeutic outcome in bacterial endocarditis. *Am J Med* 1982;73:260–7.

Come PC, Isaacs RE, Riley MR: Diagnostic accuracy of M-mode echocardiography in active infective endocarditis and prognostic implications of ultrasound-detectable vegetations. *Am Heart J* 1982;103:839–47.

Durack DT, Lukes AS, Bright DK, et al: New criteria for diagnosis of infective endocarditis: Utilization of specific echocardiographic findings. Duke Endocarditis Services. *Am J Med* 1994;96:200–9.

Johnson DH, Rosenthal A, Nadas AS: A forty-year review of bacterial endocarditis in infancy and childhood. *Circulation* 1975;51:581–8.

Kaplan EL: Infective endocarditis in the pediatric age group: An overview. In Kaplan EL, Taranta AV (editors): *Infective Endocarditis: An American Heart Association Symposium.* American Heart Association, Dallas, 1977.

Kavey RE, Frank DM, Byrum CJ, et al: Two-dimensional echocardiographic assessment of infective endocarditis in children. *Am J Dis Child* 1983;137:851–6.

Mayayo E, Moralejo J, Camps J, et al: Fungal endocarditis in premature infants: Case report and review. *Clin Infect Dis* 1996;22:366–8.

Mugge A, Daniel WG, Frank G, et al: Echocardiography in infective endocarditis: Reassessment of prognostic implications of vegetation size determined by the transthoracic and the transesophageal approach. *J Am Coll Cardiol* 1989;14:631–8.

Saiman L, Prince A, Gersony WM: Pediatric infective endocarditis in the modern era. *J Pediatr* 1993;122:847–53.

Sanchez PJ, Siegel JD, Fishbein J: *Candida* endocarditis: Successful medical management in three preterm infants and review of the literature. *Pediatr Infect Dis J* 1991;10:239–43.

Stanton BF, Baltimore RS, Clemens JD: Changing spectrum of infective endocarditis in children. Analysis of 26 cases, 1970–1979. *Am J Dis Child* 1984;138:720–5.

Stockheim JA, Chadwick EG, Kessler S, et al: Are the Duke criteria superior to the Beth Israel criteria for the diagnosis of infective endocarditis in children? *Clin Infect Dis* 1998;27:1451–6.

Von Reyn CF, Levy BS, Arbeit RD, et al: Infective endocarditis: An analysis based on strict case definitions. *Ann Intern Med* 1981; 94:505–18.

CHAPTER 72

Acute Myocarditis

Michael Cappello

Acute myocarditis refers to an inflammatory condition that primarily and directly involves the cardiac muscle, although it is not unusual for inflammatory processes to also involve the pericardium and endocardium. The spectrum of illness associated with acute myocarditis is broad, ranging from asymptomatic disease to fulminant heart failure complicated by life-threatening arrhythmia. Although myocarditis may occur at any age, children, and particularly newborns, appear to be at higher risk than adults.

ETIOLOGY

The list of potential infectious causes of acute myocarditis is extensive and includes viruses, which are the most common etiology, as well as bacteria, fungi, and parasites (Table 72–1). However, in most cases a definitive microbiologic diagnosis is not established, and thus there remains considerable controversy as to the appropriate diagnostic and therapeutic interventions for this relatively common clinical entity. Moreover, the natural history of the disease suggests that most children do not develop long-term sequelae following myocarditis, and therefore the role of antimicrobial or immunosuppressive therapy in most circumstances remains undefined.

EPIDEMIOLOGY

Most cases of acute myocarditis occur in the warmer months, overlapping considerably with the peak incidence of enterovirus, specifically coxsackievirus, infections. Because of this overlap, it is thought that many cases of idiopathic myocarditis might also be attributable to enteroviral infection. Therefore conditions that favor the fecal-oral spread of enteroviruses may also increase risk for the development of myocarditis. Protection from enteroviral myocarditis is thought to be associated with circulating protective antibodies, and therefore neonates and young children are at higher risk of developing this complication following enteroviral infection. Clusters of neonatal myocarditis, which have been documented by viral culture or serology, have been identified in children born to women who lacked protective antibody, and have generally been associated with high mortality rates in infected babies. For reasons that are not completely understood, pregnancy itself also appears to predispose women to enteroviral myocarditis. Infection late in gestation may be associated with clinical signs in the fetus that may develop in utero or soon after delivery.

Most persons who acquire coxsackievirus infections do not develop clinically significant myocarditis, although subclinical involvement of the myocardium may be present. The estimated risk of myocarditis following coxsackievirus infection is 34.6/1,000 cases. The strains of coxsackievirus that are more likely to cause myocarditis include coxsackie B3 and B4 viruses, presumably because of an increased ability to directly infect myocardial tissue. Other viruses that cause myocarditis include influenza A and B viruses, echoviruses, adenoviruses, cytomegalovirus, and HIV.

Myocarditis in immunocompromised hosts may not exhibit the same seasonal variation, and the list of potential pathogens is considerably broad. In persons infected with HIV, up to 8% may develop dilated cardiomyopathy that is frequently associated with evidence of HIV or other cardiotropic viruses present in endomyocardial tissue. Carditis is a relatively common complication of Lyme disease (Chapter 29), occurring in as many as 10% of all patients. Myocarditis is a major manifestation of rheumatic fever (Chapter 40). In parts of the world where diphtheria is endemic, the toxin produced by *Corynebacterium diphtheriae* is a major cause of myocarditis. In South America, up to 20 million people may be infected with the protozoan parasite *Trypanosoma cruzi.* Many of those infected with *T. cruzi,* particularly children, develop clinical signs of **Chagas' disease,** or **American trypanosomiasis.** Cardiac manifestations include an acute myocarditis that is characteristic of early infection, and a chronic dilated cardiomyopathy that develops decades later. Because most persons are identified years after infection, Chagas' disease is increasingly being diagnosed in adults with cardiomyopathy who have previously emigrated from endemic areas. Although uncommon, *T. cruzi* is present in the southwestern United States, and in rare instances, acute infection with *T. cruzi* has been acquired in the United States by blood transfusion.

PATHOGENESIS

The mechanisms underlying the pathogenesis of viral myocarditis has not been fully elucidated. Much of our understanding is derived from a murine model of coxsackievirus infection, which exhibits many of the histologic features of myocarditis in humans. The myocardium is damaged by at least two distinct mechanisms in the course of viral infection: direct viral infection of myocytes, and the characteristic diffuse inflammation that results from the concerted effects of components of both the humoral and cellular immune system, often in response to circulating cytokines and other inflammatory mediators. It appears that myocardial damage is primarily the result of the inflammatory response that occurs in response to infection and that continues well beyond the time that viral replication has ceased.

During the first 3 days after infection, the virus directly invades the myocardium, resulting in cell death. The early histologic features of disease include focal myonecrosis in the absence of significant inflammatory cell infiltrates. Despite the relative lack of histologic evidence of inflammation at this time, upregulation of cytokine transcription by myocytes has already begun. At approximately 4 days after infection, mononuclear cells begin to infiltrate the damaged myocardium, starting with NK cells that presumably act in concert with rising levels of neutralizing antibodies to inhibit further viral replication. During the ensuing days or weeks, chronic inflammation persists, mediated primarily by cytotoxic T lymphocytes that recognize infected myocytes via interaction with MHC

TABLE 72–1. Infectious Causes of Myocarditis

Viruses	Mycobacteria
Coxsackie A viruses	*Mycobacterium tuberculosis*
Coxsackie B viruses	*Mycobacterium avium* complex
Echoviruses	**Fungi**
Respiratory syncytial virus	Actinomycosis
Rubella virus	Blastomycosis
Measles virus	Cryptococcosis
Adenoviruses	Coccidioidomycosis
Polioviruses	Histoplasmosis
Mumps virus	Candidiasis
Herpes simplex virus	Aspergillosis
Epstein-Barr virus	Mucormycosis
Cytomegalovirus	**Protozoa**
Hepatitis A virus	Chagas' disease *(Trypanosoma cruzi)*
Hepatitis B virus	Toxoplasmosis *(Toxoplasma gondii)*
Arboviruses	Malaria *(Plasmodium)*
Influenza viruses	Visceral leishmaniasis (kala-azar)
Varicella-zoster virus	**Other Parasites**
Human immunodeficiency virus	Amebiasis
Bacteria	Echinococcosis
Corynebacterium diphtheriae (toxin mediated)	Visceral larva migrans *(Toxocara canis)*
Neisseria meningitidis	Trichinellosis
Staphylococcus	Ascariasis
Haemophilus influenzae type b	Paragonimiasis
Group A *Streptococcus*	Strongyloidiasis (disseminated)
Salmonella typhi	
Brucella (brucellosis)	
Mycoplasma pneumoniae	
Spirochetes	
Lyme disease *(Borrelia burgdorferi)*	
Relapsing fever *(Borrelia recurrentis)*	
Syphilis *(Treponema pallidum)*	
Leptospirosis *(Leptospira)*	

class I antigens. Peak T-cell infiltration generally occurs at approximately 7–14 days after infection.

In animal models, virus can no longer be cultured from the myocardium by approximately 14 days after infection. This perhaps explains why viral cultures from patients with acute myocarditis are rarely positive. However, methods that rely on detection of viral RNA, including PCR and in situ hybridization, have effectively been used to demonstrate that pieces of the viral genome are present for weeks to months postinfection. The significance of this finding is unclear, but suggests that ongoing, low-level viral replication may play a role in the persistent immune mediated inflammation characteristic of chronic myocarditis.

The pathogenesis of carditis caused by the Lyme spirochete *Borrelia burgdorferi* is also mediated by initial invasion of myocytes, followed by a sustained inflammatory response that causes further tissue damage. For reasons that are not well understood, the conduction system seems to be particularly vulnerable to damage after infection with *B. burgdorferi.* In persons with acute Chagas' disease, replication of *T. cruzi* amastigotes occurs at high levels in the cardiac muscle, leading to significant damage of both myocardium as well as the various components of the conduction system. Persistent inflammation beyond the period of active parasite replication may, like other types of myocarditis, be mediated by autoimmune phenomena directed at antigens shared by *T. cruzi* and myocytes. Diphtheritic myocarditis is caused primarily by diphtheria toxin released by *C. diphtheriae,* which exerts a direct effect on the cardiac muscle. Myocarditis caused by suppurative bacteria is generally a result of bacteremic spread of organisms, which can lead to multiple metastatic foci of replication within the myocardium.

SYMPTOMS AND CLINICAL MANIFESTATIONS

Symptoms of myocarditis may be subtle and of gradual onset, which frequently delays diagnosis (Table 72–2). Often exercise tolerance is decreased, with shortness of breath associated with even mild exertion. Chest pain may be present if there is associated pericarditis. Congestive heart failure can result in mild to severe pulmonary edema, which should be suspected in patients with a non-productive cough. Palpitations suggest conduction disturbances and intermittent cardiac arrhythmia. Symptoms of concurrent systemic enteroviral infection, including aseptic meningitis or meningoencephalitis, may also be present.

In newborns, the diagnosis of myocarditis may be particularly difficult. The clinical features of myocarditis in the newborn resemble those of other acute, life threatening conditions, including sepsis and congenital cyanotic heart disease. These babies will generally exhibit signs of compromised systemic perfusion, as well as tachypnea and poor feeding. End-organ damage may lead to prerenal azotemia, hepatic insufficiency manifested by elevated transaminases or coagulopathy, and neurologic abnormalities. Older infants will often present with tachypnea leading to poor oral intake. If hypoxia is severe, there will be signs of significant respiratory distress, including nasal flaring and retractions.

Patients with Lyme disease carditis frequently present with heart block, which is usually manifested by reduced exercise tolerance secondary to bradyarrhythmias. Other signs or symptoms of early-disseminated Lyme disease may also be present, including multiple lesions of erythema migrans, cranial nerve palsy, or aseptic meningitis. In acute Chagas' disease, persons may also complain of fevers, sweats, myalgias, and abdominal pain due to liver and spleen enlargement. Unilateral periorbital edema **(Romaña's sign)** or a painless cutaneous ulcer **(chagoma)** indicate the site at which the parasites invaded the mucosal surface or skin. The trypanosomes may also damage the conduction system in the acute phase

TABLE 72–2. Clinical Manifestations and ECG Findings of Acute Infectious Myocarditis

Clinical Manifestations
Malaise
Easy fatigability
Fever
Dyspnea
Tachypnea
Tachycardia
Abdominal pain
Pallor
Cardiomegaly
Muffled heart sounds
Congestive heart failure
ECG Findings
Prolonged PR interval
Low-voltage QRS complexes
Premature atrial and ventricular complexes
ST and T wave abnormalities

of disease, leading to bradyarrhythmias, although tachycardia on presentation is much more common.

Myocarditis caused by bacteria is generally a consequence of bacteremia and direct myocardial invasion. Therefore these persons generally show signs and symptoms of disseminated or suppurative bacterial infections, including fever, tachycardia, and possibly evidence of systemic vasodilatation in response to overwhelming infection.

Physical Examination Findings

Examination of the heart may reveal findings consistent with congestive heart failure including a **ventricular S_3 (third heart sound) gallop,** diffuse pulmonary crackles that suggest pulmonary edema, and a murmur of mitral regurgitation that suggests significant left ventricular dilation. There may also be evidence of volume overload, including hepatic enlargement due to passive congestion, pedal edema, and elevated jugular venous pulses in adolescents and adults.

DIAGNOSIS

The diagnosis of myocarditis is difficult because of the subtle clinical manifestations. While the diagnosis of acute myocarditis can be suspected based on clinical grounds of circulatory compromise or acute heart failure (Table 72–2), definitive diagnosis requires histologic evidence of inflammation or PCR identification of viral DNA on **endomyocardial biopsy.** However, because most patients with acute viral myocarditis will improve without specific therapy, it remains controversial as to which patients should have this invasive and potentially dangerous procedure.

Differential Diagnosis

There are many noninfectious causes of myocarditis (Table 72–3). The presence of a friction rub, acute chest pain, and the absence of a gallop help differentiate pericarditis (Chapter 73) from myocarditis, although these may occur simultaneously.

Laboratory Evaluation

The WBC count and ESR are usually normal or slightly elevated. **Creatine phosphokinase (MB fraction)** and **cardiac troponin T** levels may also be elevated, which are nonspecific markers of cardiac muscle damage.

Electrocardiography and Echocardiography

The ECG may show a variety of abnormalities (Table 72–2). The most characteristic ECG changes with myocarditis are low-voltage QRS complexes (<5 mm total amplitude) with low amplitude or even absent Q waves in leads V_5 and V_6. Prolonged PR interval and ST- and T-wave abnormalities are frequently seen but are less specific of myocardial involvement. Atrial and ventricular premature complexes may be seen with intraventricular conduction defects. Electrocardiographic evidence of acute coronary ischemia has also been reported in a child with acute myocarditis. **Heart block** (first, second, or third degree) at the level of the atrioventricular node is the most common electrocardiographic finding in persons with Lyme disease carditis. Nearly all of these persons will exhibit some degree of heart block, and up to half may have transient complete block, occasionally requiring temporary pacemaker placement. **Wenckebach periodicity** and fluctuating right or left **bundle-branch block** may also be seen in Lyme disease carditis, while atrial or ventricular tachyarrhythmias are less commonly encountered.

Echocardiography is an extremely useful modality for assessing global myocardial function, as well as evaluating alternative diagnoses such as congenital heart malformations, pericarditis, or endocarditis. Persons with acute myocarditis may have reduced left ventricular function with decreased **ejection fraction,** as well as evidence of cardiac dilatation. Occasionally the wall motion abnormalities may be focal or regional. Mitral regurgitation may result from progressive dilatation of the left ventricle. Small pericardial effusions may be present as well.

TABLE 72–3. Noninfectious Causes of Myocarditis

Collagen-Vascular Disease
Systemic lupus erythematosus
Juvenile rheumatoid arthritis (Still's disease)
Scleroderma
Sarcoidosis
Thyrotoxicosis
Radiation induced
Pheochromocytoma
Drugs (Direct Toxic Effect)
Alcohol
Cocaine
Arsenic
Catecholamines
Cyclophosphamide
Doxorubicin
Amphetamines
Drug Induced (Hypersensitivity)
Methyldopa
Sulfonamides
Tetracycline
Chloramphenicol
Streptomycin
Other Causes
Scorpion stings, spider bites, bee and wasp stings
Acute rheumatic fever
Kawasaki disease
Idiopathic causes

Microbiologic Evaluation

Persons with suspected myocarditis should be evaluated for concurrent or recent viral infections using both culture and serologic methods. Viral cultures of the nasopharynx, throat, urine, and rectum should be obtained. If signs of aseptic meningitis or meningoencephalitis are present, a lumbar puncture should be performed and cerebrospinal fluid sent for bacterial and viral cultures, as well as routine studies. Blood cultures should be obtained for patients with fever and hemodynamic instability. In the setting of meningitis, cerebrospinal fluid can also be tested by PCR to detect enterovirus and *B. burgdorferi.*

Endomyocardial biopsy specimens should routinely be sent for viral and bacterial culture, although the diagnostic yield of viral culture is generally poor. Although not used routinely, PCR is the most sensitive technique for detecting a viral etiology for myocarditis. One study (Martin et al, 1994) of 34 children with suspected acute viral myocarditis found that 26 of 38 (68%) endomyocardial biopsy specimens were positive by PCR for viral DNA (15 adenovirus, 8 enterovirus, 2 herpes simplex virus, 1 cytomegalovirus), compared to only 4 (12%) children with positive viral cultures. More recently, the same research group has reported that PCR of tracheal aspirates from intubated children with myocarditis can also be used to identify a viral cause. In this study, the viral DNA amplified from tracheal aspirates matched that found by PCR using endomyocardial biopsy specimens, suggesting that in patients with concomitant respiratory disease, biopsy may not be necessary.

Serologic Testing. Antibody titers can be measured for *B. burgdorferi* to diagnose Lyme disease carditis. Serologic diagnosis of enteroviral infection requires acute and convalescent sera (4 weeks later). Demonstration of a fourfold rise in virus-specific neutralizing titer can be used to confirm infection, but is generally useful only when a specific enterovirus is suspected or has been previously identified during a community outbreak. Because of the large number of enteroviruses, serologic screening is not generally performed.

Pathologic Findings

Definitive diagnosis of myocarditis requires evidence of endomyocardial inflammation found on biopsy, which also permits PCR testing of myocardial tissue. However, the histologic findings of myocarditis may be patchy or focal, requiring multiple biopsy specimens to establish the diagnosis accurately (Fig. 72–1). The advantage of endomyocardial biopsy is that the nature of the inflammatory infiltration can be more clearly defined, which may aid in the diagnosis. Lymphocytic infiltrates suggest a viral cause, whereas a predominance of neutrophils is consistent with an acute bacterial infection. Lyme disease carditis is characterized by transmural infiltrate of lymphocytes and plasma cells, and may show evidence of small and large vessel vasculitis. In cases of Lyme disease carditis, *B. burgdorferi* has been detected in endomyocardial biopsy specimens using a modified silver staining technique.

The most widely recognized system for interpreting myocardial biopsy specimens is the **Dallas Classification System,** which was first proposed in 1986 by a panel of cardiac pathologists. According to the Dallas criteria, an initial biopsy must show myocyte necrosis or degeneration in association with an inflammatory infiltrate. Subsequent biopsy specimens are held to slightly different standards that allow for the identification of persistent, healing, or healed myocarditis. Unfortunately, the Dallas criteria are subject to prohibitive interobserver variability in routine clinical practice.

Diagnostic Imaging

A chest radiograph will frequently show enlargement of the cardiac silhouette (Fig. 72–2), although in the acute stage of disease the heart size may be normal. Evidence of pulmonary edema with or without effusions may also be present.

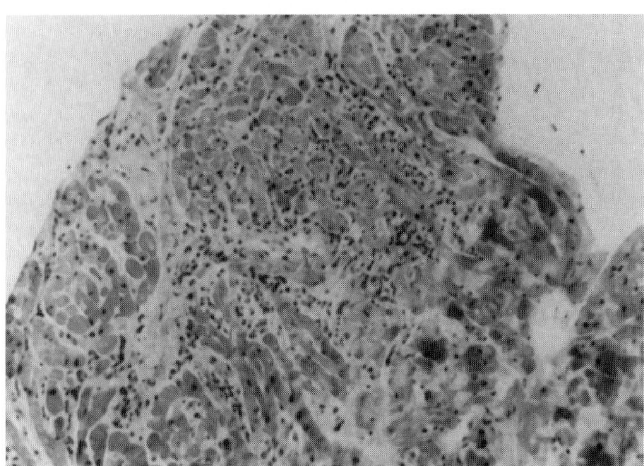

FIGURE 72–1. Acute myocarditis in 7-year-old child. Endomyocardial biopsy shows interstitial infiltrate, intercellular edema, and focal myocyte necrosis. (×100.) (From Hoyer MH, Fischer DR: Acute myocarditis simulating myocardial infarction in a child. *Pediatrics* 1991;87:250–3.)

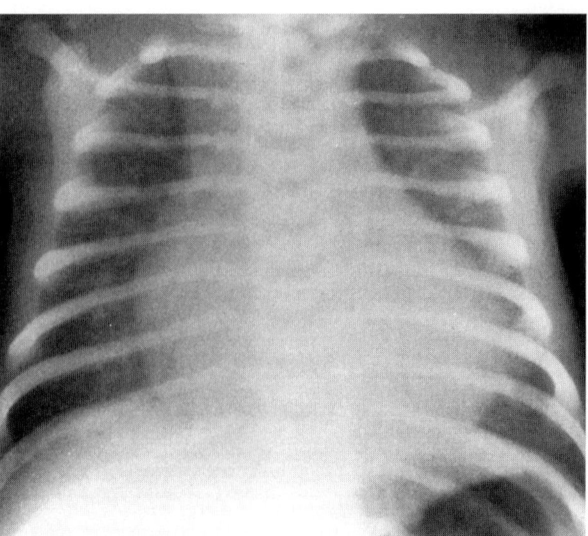

FIGURE 72–2. Acute viral myocarditis in 4-week-old infant with new onset of tachypnea and difficulty in feeding. Frontal supine chest radiograph shows moderate cardiomegaly, diffuse pulmonary hyperinflation, and a pattern of mild vascular congestion due to congestive heart failure.

Nuclear medicine studies have also been evaluated as a means of diagnosing acute myocarditis. In one study (O'Connell et al, 1984), 5 of 6 persons with biopsy-documented myocarditis showed increased uptake of gallium-67 in the heart, and 5 of 14 persons with a positive nuclear scan had a positive biopsy. Only 1 (2%) of 57 persons with a negative gallium scan result had myocarditis, demonstrating a high negative predictive value. Indium 111–labeled antimyosin monoclonal antibody scans, which can detect areas of myocardial necrosis, have also been used as a diagnostic tool for myocarditis. Unfortunately, nuclear scans lack specificity for myocarditis, as extramyocardial diseases (e.g., endocarditis, pericarditis, and hilar lymphadenopathy) may be associated with positive scans.

More recently, contrast enhanced MRI has been shown to effectively visualize changes in the myocardium during the course of biopsy proven viral myocarditis. Although it also lacks specificity, this non-isotopic, noninvasive modality holds promise as a potential tool for the diagnosis and follow-up of patients with acute myocarditis.

TREATMENT

Supportive care and limited physical activity remain the cornerstones of therapy for acute myocarditis. Patients should be monitored initially for cardiac rhythm disturbances, and if necessary, receive anti-arrhythmic agents. In the setting of compromised cardiac function, inotropic support, afterload reduction, and diuretics may also be needed to manage congestive heart failure and volume overload.

Although the majority of cases of acute myocarditis are most likely caused by viruses, there does not appear to be any role for empirical antiviral therapy. This is most likely due to the fact that at the time of clinical presentation, much of the ongoing inflammation is due to chronic immune mediated processes in the absence of significant viral replication. A possible exception is myocarditis caused by herpesviruses in a severely immunocompromised host, in which case antiviral therapy is most likely warranted.

Because of a paucity of randomized, controlled trials of immunosuppressive therapy for the treatment of acute myocarditis, there is no clear consensus as to how these patients should be managed. The results of small, uncontrolled studies (Chan et al, 1991; Juhl et al, 1994; Kleinert et al, 1997) suggest that therapy with immunosuppressive agents may preserve cardiac function in some persons. The fundamental difficulty in extrapolating these data to individual patient management is that these studies lacked appropriate control groups for comparison. Two prospective, randomized trials have been conducted to evaluate the role of immunosuppressive therapy in persons with myocarditis. One study (Parillo et al, 1989) of 60 patients with dilated cardiomyopathy who had evidence of ongoing inflammation by endomyocardial biopsy randomized to receive prednisone or no immunosuppressive therapy the prednisone treated group showed greater improvement at 3 months in left ventricular ejection fraction, the primary end point, as well as exercise tolerance. Another study (Mason et al, 1995) of 111 patients with biopsy-proved myocarditis randomized to receive either prednisone with cyclosporine or azathioprine, or no immunosuppressive therapy showed no differences in survival or improvement in left ventricular ejection fraction at 28 weeks between the two groups. There appears to be no clear benefit of immunosuppressive therapy for acute viral myocarditis. Immunosuppressive therapy is recommended for viral myocarditis only in the context of clinical studies.

A retrospective study (Drucker, 1994) of 21 children with acute myocarditis suggested that IVIG (2 g/kg over 24 hours) improved recovery of left ventricular function compared with recent historical controls. Another study (McNamara et al, 1997) reported that 9 of 10 adults with new-onset cardiomyopathy treated with high doses of IVIG showed marked improvement in left ventricular function at 1 year. These two studies suggest that the potential efficacy of IVIG in myocarditis should be more closely evaluated using randomized, controlled trials. Other agents currently being evaluated for the treatment of myocarditis include IL-2, IFN-α, and monoclonal antibodies TNF-α.

Although Lyme disease carditis generally resolves spontaneously, persons with Lyme disease and evidence of heart block should receive appropriate antibiotic therapy, and should be hospitalized and undergo cardiac monitoring for at least 24 hours to identify those with progression to complete heart block (Chapter 29). There are no data to support the use of corticosteroids or other anti-inflammatory agents in the management of Lyme disease carditis.

COMPLICATIONS

The most serious complications resulting from acute myocarditis include sudden death from arrhythmia and congestive heart failure. Fortunately, these conditions are relatively rare, and most patients with myocarditis respond to conservative medical management and supportive care. A few persons with acute myocarditis will experience chronic inflammation, ultimately progressing to dilated cardiomyopathy that may require cardiac transplantation.

PROGNOSIS

Complete and uneventful recovery is usual for most patients with acute myocarditis, regardless of cause, except for enteroviral myocarditis in the newborn, which carries a very high mortality despite aggressive care. The risk factors for progression to dilated cardiomyopathy have not been identified, making it difficult to predict outcome in all cases. Although *B. burgdorferi* has been identified as a potential cause of chronic dilated cardiomyopathy, persons treated for Lyme disease do not appear to be at increased risk of future cardiac disease.

PREVENTION

Because of the sporadic nature and multiple causes of acute myocarditis, it is unlikely that any uniform control measures will have a significant effect on its epidemiology. Standard measures to prevent the spread of enteroviruses, particularly in newborn nurseries, may help prevent outbreaks of viral myocarditis in this selected population. Treatment of early *B. burgdorferi* infection with antibiotics, or immunization to prevent infection entirely, should both reduce the risk of developing Lyme disease carditis. Screening of blood donors who have lived in areas endemic for Chagas' disease by questioning and for antibodies to *T. cruzi* should prevent the rare transmission by transfusion. Controlling the triatomine insect vector of *T. cruzi* most likely represents the best means of preventing Chagas' disease in rural South America and Central America.

REVIEWS

Anandasabapathy S, Frishman WH: Innovative drug treatments for viral and autoimmune myocarditis. *J Clin Pharmacol* 1998;38:295–308.

Brodison A, Swann JW: Myocarditis: A review. *J Infect* 1998;37:99–103.

Drucker NA, Newburger JW: Viral myocarditis: Diagnosis and management. *Adv Pediatr* 1997;44:141–71.

Kawai C: From myocarditis to cardiomyopathy: Mechanisms of inflammation and cell death: Learning from the past for the future. *Circulation* 1999;99:1091–100.

Kirchhoff LV: Chagas disease. American trypanosomiasis. *Infect Dis Clin North Am* 1993;7:487–502.

Parillo JE: Myocarditis: How should we treat in 1998? *J Heart Lung Transplant* 1998;17:941–4.

KEY ARTICLES

Akhtar N, Ni J, Stromberg D, et al: Tracheal aspirate as a substrate for polymerase chain reaction detection of viral genome in childhood pneumonia and myocarditis. *Circulation* 1999;99:2011–8.

Basso NG, Fonseca ME, Garza AG, et al: Enterovirus isolation from foetal and placental tissues. *Acta Virol* 1990;34:49–57.

Chan KY, Iwahara M, Benson LN, et al: Immunosuppressive therapy in the management of acute myocarditis in children: A clinical trial. *J Am Coll Cardiol* 1991;17:458–60.

Drucker NA, Colan SD, Lewis AB, et al: Gamma-globulin treatment of acute myocarditis in the pediatric population. *Circulation* 1994:89: 252–7.

Fenoglio JJ Jr, Ursell PC, Kellogg CF, et al: Diagnosis and classification of myocarditis by endomyocardial biopsy. *N Engl J Med* 1983; 308:12–8.

Friedrich MG, Strohm O, Schulz-Menger J, et al: Contrast media–enhanced magnetic resonance imaging visualizes myocardial changes in the course of viral myocarditis. *Circulation* 1998;97:1802–9.

Garg A, Shiau J, Guyatt G: The ineffectiveness of immunosuppressive therapy in lymphocytic myocarditis: An overview. *Ann Intern Med* 1998;129:317–22.

Grant IH, Gold JW, Wittner M, et al: Transfusion-associated acute Chagas disease acquired in the United States. *Ann Intern Med* 1989; 111:849–51.

Haddad J, Gut JP, Wendling MJ, et al: Enterovirus infections in neonates. A retrospective study of 21 cases. *Eur J Med* 1993;2:209–14.

Hoyer MH, Fischer DR: Acute myocarditis simulating myocardial infarction in a child. *Pediatrics* 1991;87:250–3.

Juhl U, Strauer BE, Schultheiss HP: Methylprednisolone in chronic myocarditis. *Postgrad Med J* 1994;70:S35–42.

Kibrick S, Benirschke K: Acute aseptic myocarditis and meningoencephalitis in the newborn child infected with Coxsackie virus group B, type 3. *N Engl J Med* 1956; 255:883–9.

Kleinert S, Weintraub RG, Wilkinson JL, et al: Myocarditis in children with dilated cardiomyopathy: Incidence and outcome after dual therapy immunosuppression. *J Heart Lung Transplant* 1997;16:1248–54.

Martin AB, Webber S, Fricker FJ, et al: Acute myocarditis. Rapid diagnosis by PCR in children. *Circulation* 1994;90:330–9.

Mason JW, O'Connell JB, Herskowitz A, et al: A clinical trial of immunosuppressive therapy for myocarditis. *N Engl J Med* 1995;333:269–75.

McNamara DM, Rosenblum WD, Janosko KM, et al: Intravenous immune globulin in the therapy of myocarditis and acute cardiomyopathy. *Circulation* 1997;95:2476–8.

Midttun M, Labech AM, Hansen K, et al: Lyme carditis: A clinical presentation and long time follow-up. *Scand J Infect Dis* 1997;29:153–7.

O'Connell JB, Henkin RE, Robinson JA, et al: Gallium-67 imaging in patients with dilated cardiomyopathy and biopsy-proven myocarditis. *Circulation* 1984;70:58–62.

Parillo JE, Cunnion RE, Epstein SE, et al: A prospective, randomized, controlled trial of prednisone for dilated cardiomyopathy. *N Engl J Med* 1989;321:1061–8.

Sangha O, Phillips B, Fleischmann KE, et al: Lack of cardiac manifestations among patients with previously treated Lyme disease. *Ann Intern Med* 1998;128:346–53.

Stanek G, Klein J, Bittner R, et al: Isolation of *Borrelia burgdorferi* from the myocardium of a patient with longstanding cardiomyopathy. *N Engl J Med* 1990;322:249–52.

CHAPTER 73

Acute Pericarditis

Michael Cappello

The pericardium encloses the heart and the proximal portion of the great vessels. Either infectious or noninfectious processes may cause pericarditis, which can be the sole manifestation of a disease or an element of a systemic inflammatory or infectious disease. Viral pericarditis is seen more frequently in adults than children and is usually a benign self-limited disease. **Bacterial (purulent) pericarditis** refers to a bacterial infection of the pericardium and is most frequently seen in infants and children.

ETIOLOGY

Numerous infectious agents can cause acute pericarditis (Table 73–1). Enteroviruses, especially the coxsackie B viruses, are the most common cause in developed nations. Bacterial pericarditis is most commonly caused by *Staphylococcus aureus,* infrequently by *Haemophilus influenzae* type b and *Neisseria meningitidis,* and by *Mycobacterium tuberculosis* in groups at high risk of tuberculosis (Chapter 35). The range of potential pathogens that can cause pericarditis in immunocompromised persons is especially broad and includes viruses, bacteria, fungi and yeast, and parasites. Cardiac involvement with HIV infection occurs frequently and may be the result of direct cardiac infection with HIV, as well as a manifestation of secondary opportunistic infections.

EPIDEMIOLOGY

Acute pericarditis affects all age groups and occurs more commonly in children, particularly those less than 2 years of age. Retrospective reviews, in the absence of population-based studies, suggest that pericarditis occurs at a rate of approximately 2–3/1,000 admissions to children's hospitals. Because viruses cause the majority of cases of infectious pericarditis, most cases present in the spring and summer months, overlapping with the peak enterovirus season. Cases occurring in the winter months are more likely to be caused by influenza virus. Bacterial pericarditis caused by bacterial pathogens occurs throughout the year. Pericarditis due to unusual pathogens such as fungi and parasites is less likely to exhibit seasonal variation.

Individuals at high risk of tuberculosis are also more likely to develop **tuberculous pericarditis.** High-risk groups include recent immigrants and adoptees from developing nations and children from economically depressed urban centers in the United States. In areas of the world where tuberculosis is endemic, this represents a major cause of bacterial pericarditis in all age groups. A recent retrospective study (Chen et al, 1999) found that 40 (33%) of 122 consecutive adults with pericardial effusion at an inner city hospital were HIV infected. In this population, as shown in other studies, mycobacteria were the most commonly isolated pathogens responsible for pericardial disease.

Pericarditis may follow cardiothoracic surgery as a postoperative infectious complication caused by pyogenic bacteria. Symptoms of pericarditis also occur with the **postpericardiotomy syndrome,** a noninfectious inflammatory condition that generally occurs 2–6 months after cardiac surgery.

PATHOGENESIS

Enteroviruses most likely seed the pericardium as a result of viremia, and therefore pericarditis may occur concomitantly with other manifestations of enteroviral infections, including aseptic meningitis. Occasionally myocarditis and pericarditis will coexist, a condition referred to as **myopericarditis.** However, it is possible that many cases of so-called "idiopathic" pericarditis are caused by isolated enteroviral infection. Certain enteroviruses, particularly the **coxsackie B viruses,** are cardiotropic in animal models and may be a frequent cause of isolated pericarditis or myocarditis (Chapter 72) in humans. In contrast to enteroviral pericarditis, influenza pericarditis most likely develops as a sequela of influenza pneumonia by contiguous spread of the virus from the lungs to the adjacent pericardium.

Bacterial pericarditis is usually the result of hematogenous spread or direct extension from infected tissues; it occurs as an isolated infection in only 10% of cases. Pericarditis caused by *S. aureus* or *H. influenzae* type b is most often associated with pneumonia, osteomyelitis, and cellulitis as primary sites of infection. Pericarditis caused by *N. meningitidis* is more likely to be associated with concomitant meningitis. Because these infections are all frequently associated with bacteremia, it is likely that hematogenous seeding of the pericardial space is the most likely pathogenic mechanism of bacterial pericarditis.

The pathogenesis of postoperative bacterial pericarditis mimics that of mediastinitis after cardiothoracic surgery and may occur as a result of early or late infection with bacteria introduced at the time of surgery. Alternatively, poststernotomy pericarditis may be a manifestation of deep wound infection acquired postoperatively. Tuberculous pericarditis usually occurs in the absence of identifiable pulmonary disease, which suggests that the pathogenesis of this condition involves the spread of mycobacteria from adjacent mediastinal lymph nodes into the pericardium. Pericardial involvement associated with HIV infection most likely occurs by direct invasion of the pericardium by the virus itself, usually associated with HIV infection of the myocardium as well.

The **pericardial space** normally contains approximately 10–20 mL of serous fluid that separates the **visceral pericardium** from the **parietal pericardium.** The visceral pericardium essentially forms the outermost layer of the myocardium itself, whereas the parietal pericardium surrounds the various structures contained within the mediastinum. The pericardial fluid acts primarily as a lubricant but also protects the heart from physiologic changes in intracardiac pressure related to respiration and postural change. When microorganisms invade the pericardial space, an inflammatory response quickly ensues and then leads to extravasation of

TABLE 73–1. Infectious Causes of Acute Pericarditis

Viruses	Mycobacteria
Coxsackie A viruses	*Mycobacterium tuberculosis*
Coxsackie B viruses*	*Mycobacterium avium* complex
Echoviruses	
Adenovirus	***Mycoplasma pneumoniae***
Influenza viruses	**Fungi**
Cytomegalovirus	*Histoplasma capsulatum*
Herpes simplex virus	*Coccidioides immitis*
Hepatitis B virus	*Blastomyces dermatitidis*
Measles virus	*Candida*
Mumps virus	*Aspergillus*
Bacteria	*Cryptococcus neoformans*
*Staphylococcus aureus**	**Parasites**
Streptococcus pneumoniae	*Toxoplasma gondii*
Group A *Streptococcus*	*Entamoeba histolytica*
Other streptococci	*Toxocara canis*
*Neisseria meningitidis**	*Schistosoma*
Haemophilus influenzae type b	
Klebsiella	
Pseudomonas aeruginosa	
Escherichia coli	
Salmonella	
Anaerobes	
Listeria monocytogenes	
Neisseria gonorrhoeae	
Coxiella burnetii	
Actinomyces	
Nocardia	

*Indicates the most common causes of pericarditis in North America.

additional pericardial fluid and an influx of polymorphonuclear WBCs and monocytes. These inflammatory cells mediate fibrin generation, which leads to loculation of fluid, scarring, and ultimately fibrosis. The pericardial space may eventually lose its compliance, compromising ventricular filling and resulting in **constrictive pericarditis.**

A small volume of fluid developing within the pericardial space as a result of pericarditis can generally be tolerated without significant symptoms; it is eventually resorbed. Similarly, if fluid accumulates for a period of weeks or months, then even relatively large volumes can be tolerated without cardiac compromise. However, if pericardial fluid accumulates rapidly, then even moderate volumes will result in symptomatic filling defects and reduced cardiac output. **Cardiac tamponade** occurs when increased fluid within the pericardial space prevents adequate right atrial filling, which leads to reduced stroke volume, low output cardiac failure, and shock.

SYMPTOMS AND CLINICAL MANIFESTATIONS

Chest pain is commonly reported in adults with pericarditis, although this symptom is often difficult to elicit from children. In infants and small children, fever and irritability during or shortly after a respiratory illness may be the most prominent feature of the disease. As a result, the diagnosis may be delayed in children, particularly those with an underlying viral infection. In the summer months, cardiorespiratory symptoms after a viral syndrome, perhaps in association with a characteristic rash, suggest possible enterovirus infection. One study (Carmichael, 1951) found that more than half of the persons reviewed with ''nonspecific'' pericarditis of presumed viral origin had a preceding respiratory illness. In this setting, pericarditis generally develops 2–3 weeks after the respiratory symptoms.

More pronounced symptoms of persistent nonproductive cough, tachypnea, dyspnea, and chest pain in the presence of fever after an untreated respiratory tract infection may indicate bacterial pericarditis. Bacterial pericarditis may also complicate pneumonia, osteomyelitis, and meningitis, which predispose a person to bacterial pericardial disease.

A study (Fowler, 1973) of 19 persons with tuberculous pericarditis found that the most common symptoms included cough (94%), dyspnea (88%), chest pain (76%), and night sweats (58%). Hemoptysis suggestive of active cavitary lung disease was an infrequent finding, which was present in only 2 of 14 subjects. Persons with constrictive pericarditis will most likely develop symptoms consistent with chronic right-sided congestive heart failure including dyspnea on exertion, orthopnea, dependent edema, and eventually weight gain due to fluid retention.

Physical Examination Findings

Nearly all persons with pericarditis, regardless of cause, have tachycardia. Bacterial pericarditis is more likely to be associated with fever and tachypnea and with possible evidence of at least one additional site of infection (e.g., pneumonia, meningitis, and osteomyelitis). The most characteristic physical finding in acute pericarditis is the presence of a **friction rub** heard on cardiac auscultation. The rub may be confused with a high-pitched murmur, particularly when it is present only in systole. In general, however, the pericardial friction rub is diphasic or even triphasic in quality and can be heard throughout the precordium. It may be best appreciated with the patient leaning forward or even in the knee-chest position. It is important to remember that even persons with large pericardial effusions may have a prominent rub.

The presence of a **pulsus paradoxus,** or **paradoxical pulse,** suggests the possibility of **cardiac tamponade,** which may require emergent intervention. Pulsus paradoxus is defined as a drop in systolic blood pressure greater than 10 mm Hg on inspiration, indicative of reduced right atrial filling. This condition is most frequently found in the presence of a large or rapidly accumulating pericardial effusion or in constrictive disease from long-standing pericarditis with fibrosis. Pulsus paradoxus can also be found in persons with long-standing lung disease, such as chronic obstructive pulmonary disease (e.g., emphysema), asthma, or pulmonary hypertension.

DIAGNOSIS

Findings of a combination of cough, tachypnea, dyspnea, chest pain, fever, or tachycardia or the solitary finding of a friction rub, pulsus paradoxus, or characteristic electrocardiographic changes suggests the possibility of pericarditis. The diagnosis usually requires diagnostic imaging, especially two-dimensional echocardiography to confirm the presence of pericardial fluid and diagnostic pericardiocentesis to identify the cause.

Electrocardiography. The classic electrocardiographic changes associated with pericarditis include nonspecific ST-T wave abnormalities, either elevation or depression (Fig. 73–1). Low-voltage QRS complexes may also be present in association with a large pericardial effusion and may occur in the absence of acute myocardial ischemia or prior myocardial infarction. The initial electrocardiographic abnormality in acute pericarditis may be PR-segment deviation, particularly depression, which is seen primarily in the first 2 days after the onset of symptoms. Late electrocardiographic changes in pericarditis include flat or inverted T waves.

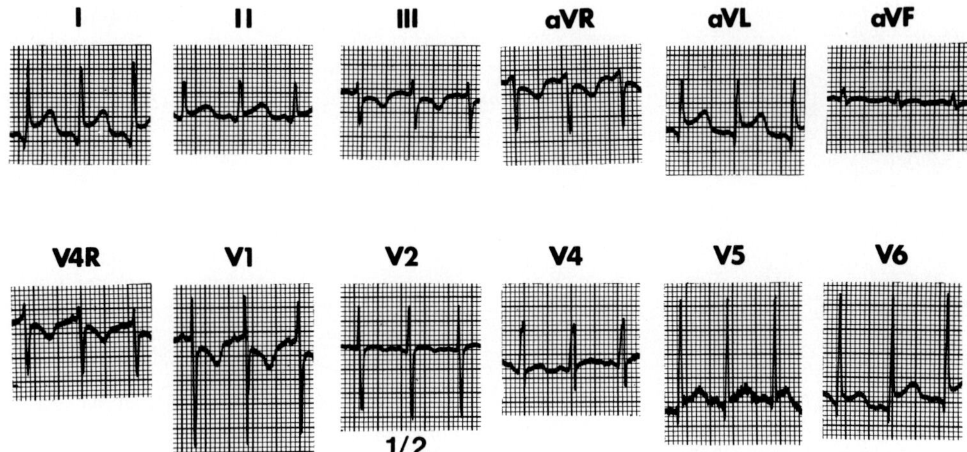

FIGURE 73–1. Electrocardiogram of 10-year-old child with acute pericarditis. Elevated or depressed ST segments in most leads are greatest in the limb leads. The QRS voltages are not low and the T waves are normal, suggesting that the process is in the early stages. (Courtesy of Myung K. Park.)

Differential Diagnosis

A substantial proportion of pericarditis is noninfectious (Table 73–2). Culture of pericardial fluid obtained by **pericardiocentesis** is the most reliable means to differentiate infectious pericarditis from other causes. An experienced physician should perform pericardiocentesis, usually under echocardiographic guidance. Recurrent, unexplained pericardial effusion may indicate the rare cardiac or pericardial tumor.

Diagnostic Imaging

An acutely enlarged cardiac silhouette on chest radiography, particularly in the absence of increased pulmonary vascularity, suggests the presence of pericardial effusion. However, there may be no radiographic abnormalities detected in persons with small but rapidly accumulating effusions or in those with constrictive disease.

Echocardiography. Echocardiography is the diagnostic study of choice for detecting the presence of pericardial fluid and should be performed in all persons with suspected pericarditis. Both **M-mode** and **two-dimensional echocardiography** (Fig. 73–2) are useful for detecting effusions, and serial studies are helpful in follow-up of persons in whom the diagnosis has been established. In persons with poststernotomy pericarditis, CT and MRI are both extremely useful for identifying additional mediastinal fluid collections and abscesses.

TABLE 73–2. Major Noninfectious Causes of Acute Pericarditis

Collagen Vascular Diseases
Systemic lupus erythematosus
Rheumatoid arthritis
Scleroderma
Rheumatic fever
Drugs
Procainamide
Hydralazine
Injury
Acute myocardial infarction
Chest trauma (penetrating or blunt)
Postpericardiotomy syndrome
Chylopericardium
Metabolic-Endocrine
Hypothyroidism
Uremia
Neoplasia
Primary
Metastatic
Other Causes
Bleeding diathesis
Familial Mediterranean fever
Sarcoidosis
Radiotherapy

Microbiologic Evaluation

Pericardial fluid obtained by pericardiocentesis should be transported quickly to the microbiology laboratory for Gram stain, acid-fast stain, and silver stain; cultures to identify bacteria (aerobic and anaerobic), mycobacteria, fungi, and viruses; and total and differential cell counts, glucose and total protein determinations, and cytologic analyses. Analysis of pericardial fluid from a person with bacterial pericarditis reveals a markedly elevated WBC count with a neutrophilic predominance, usually with organisms observed on Gram stain.

For suspected viral pericarditis, swabs from the nasopharynx, throat, and rectum should also be cultured for viruses because these sites are more likely to yield a culture positive for enteroviruses. In the presence of pneumonia, sputum or tracheal aspirates should be cultured for influenza A and B viruses. An acute serum sample should be saved to provide for performing acute and convalescent antibody titers later.

Blood culture results are frequently positive when children have bacterial pericarditis. Other foci of infection should also be examined, especially for pneumonia, osteomyelitis, and meningitis. A positive result on bacterial culture of a specimen from one of these sites in the presence of pericarditis is strongly suggestive of the cause of the pericardial infection.

The diagnosis of tuberculous pericarditis can be particularly challenging (Chapter 35). Culture of pericardial fluid shows positive results in 75% of suspected cases of tuberculous pericarditis, although the results may not be available for weeks. **Pericardial biopsy** may provide a more rapid diagnosis for *M. tuberculosis*

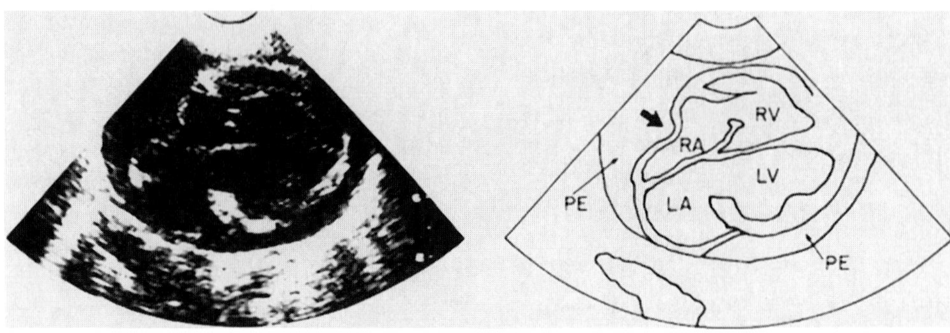

FIGURE 73–2. Subcostal four-chamber view of two-dimensional echocardiogram demonstrating pericardial effusion and collapse of the right atrial wall *(arrow)*, a sign of cardiac tamponade. PE = pericardial effusion; RA = right atrium; LA = left atrium; RV = right ventricle; LV = left ventricle. (From Park MK: *Pediatric Cardiology for Practitioners,* 3rd ed. St Louis, Mosby, 1996, p 293.)

infection, particularly if the characteristic granulomatous changes are present. One study (Cigielski et al, 1997) showed that PCR analysis was nearly as sensitive as culture (81% vs 93%) for detecting *M. tuberculosis* in pericardial biopsy specimens.

TREATMENT

Persons with presumed viral pericarditis should be considered for a drainage procedure (therapeutic pericardiocentesis) if the amount of effusion is large, rapidly accumulating, or causing cardiac tamponade. No specific antiviral therapy is recommended for enteroviral pericarditis, which is generally self-limited. Bed rest and monitoring for the development of hemodynamic compromise are important. Symptomatic therapy for pain is with nonsteroidal anti-inflammatory drugs. Corticosteroids for acute viral pericarditis should be avoided because they may exacerbate viral myocarditis (Chapter 72), which usually accompanies viral pericarditis.

Drainage of pericardial fluid should be considered an urgent necessity in any person with a diagnosis of bacterial pericarditis. Outcome is generally poor without surgical drainage, even with appropriate antibiotic therapy. A review (Feldman, 1979) of 162 cases showed that only 6 (18%) of 34 children with bacterial pericarditis survived without surgical intervention, despite antibiotic therapy. In contrast, 90 (78%) of 115 persons treated with surgical drainage and antibiotics survived. Therefore, if diagnostic pericardiocentesis reveals a markedly elevated WBC count with a predominance of neutrophils, the person should be evaluated promptly for more definitive surgical exploration of the pericardial space, possibly to include placement of a **pericardial drain or window.** Administration of intrapericardial streptokinase may facilitate drainage of fluid (Juneja et al, 1999).

If analysis and Gram stain of pericardial fluid do not suggest the etiologic agent in the setting of bacterial pericarditis, empirical antibiotic coverage should be initiated while the results of cultures are awaited (Table 73–3). Initial therapy for community-acquired bacterial pericarditis should include an agent with activity against *S. aureus* because this is the most common pathogen. Semisynthetic penicillins (e.g., oxacillin or nafcillin) are the drugs of choice for community-acquired staphylococcal infections. A third-generation cephalosporin should be added for activity against *Streptococcus pneumoniae, N. meningitidis,* and the rare cases caused by *H. influenzae* type b. Empirical antibiotic therapy is continued until the identification and susceptibilities of the infecting organism are known (Table 73–3).

Tuberculous pericarditis should be treated with at least three drugs, including isoniazid, rifampin, and pyrazinamide (Table 73–3). If the patient is at risk of an infection with an organism resistant to several drugs, then a fourth agent, ethambutol, may be added pending the results of culture and susceptibility testing. The recommended duration of therapy for pericarditis caused by *M. tuberculosis* is 6 months. The addition of corticosteroids to the initial antituberculosis regimen leads to more rapid resolution of effusion and may reduce the risk of developing late constrictive disease.

COMPLICATIONS

Cardiac tamponade with compromised cardiac output is an acute complication of bacterial pericarditis. Sepsis and septic shock may also occur.

Constrictive Pericarditis. Persons with pericarditis from any cause are at risk of developing **constrictive pericarditis,** even if treated appropriately. Persons with tuberculous pericarditis are at particularly high risk of progressing to constrictive pericarditis. The time interval between the initial episode and the development of constriction is variable, ranging from a few weeks to years. In many cases of constrictive pericarditis, no specific antecedent episode can be discerned.

The diagnosis of constrictive pericarditis may be suspected on the basis of a chest x-ray film and an echocardiogram, but definitive diagnosis requires analysis of the hemodynamic tracings obtained at cardiac catheterization. The classic finding in persons with constrictive pericarditis is an equalization of pressure (i.e., a difference of less than 5 mm) between atrial and ventricular pressures during diastole.

The definitive treatment of constrictive pericarditis is surgical **pericardiectomy,** in which the pericardium itself is removed, or "stripped." This is generally associated with dramatic improvement in hemodynamic status and with resolution of symptoms of impaired cardiac filling. However, some persons, particularly late in the course of the disease, may not have substantial improvement despite adequate surgical removal of fibrotic pericardium. Abnormalities in left ventricular diastolic filling are common after pericardiectomy and may persist for months postoperatively.

PROGNOSIS

Viral or idiopathic pericarditis has a relatively benign prognosis, with complete resolution of symptoms generally occurring within a few weeks. There have been a number of reports of "recurrent" disease, suggesting postviral autoimmunity as a potential pathogenic mechanism.

The prognosis for children with bacterial pericarditis is dependent on prompt diagnosis and a combination of surgical and medical treatment. The overall mortality ranges from 25% to 75% for bacterial pericarditis, with the youngest patients (less than 1 year of age) faring most poorly. In the absence of surgical drainage,

TABLE 73–3. Recommended Antibiotic Therapy for Pericarditis According to Etiologic Agent

Etiologic Agent	Recommended Therapy	Alternative Therapy
Viral	No specific therapy	
Bacterial		
Initial empirical for community acquired	Oxacillin *or* nafcillin *and* Cefotaxime *or* ceftriaxone	
Initial empirical for nosocomially acquired	Vancomycin *and* Ceftazidime *with or without* an aminoglycoside	
Staphylococcus aureus	Oxacillin *or* nafcillin	Vancomycin (for patients allergic to β-lactams)
Coagulase-negative staphylococci		
Methicillin sensitive	Oxacillin *or* nafcillin	Vancomycin
Methicillin resistant	Vancomycin	
Streptococcus pneumoniae		
Penicillin susceptible (MIC ≤0.06 μg/mL)	Penicillin G	Cefotaxime *or* ceftriaxone
Penicillin resistant (intermediate [MIC 0.1–1 μg/mL] or absolute [MIC ≥2 μg/mL]) and cefotaxime susceptible (MIC ≤0.5 μg/mL)	Cefotaxime *or* ceftriaxone	Vancomycin *or* chloramphenicol
Penicillin resistant (intermediate [MIC 0.1–1 μg/mL] or absolute [MIC ≥2 μg/mL]) and cefotaxime resistant (intermediate [MIC 1 μg/mL] or absolute [MIC ≥2 μg/mL])	Vancomycin *with or without* cefotaxime *or* ceftriaxone	Vancomycin *and* Rifampin *with or without* ceftriaxone *or* cefotaxime
Group A *Streptococcus*	Penicillin G	Ampicillin *or* cefotaxime *or* ceftriaxone
Neisseria meningitidis	Penicillin G	Ampicillin *or* cefotaxime *or* ceftriaxone *or* chloramphenicol (for penicillin-resistant strains)
Haemophilus influenzae type b	Ampicillin (if susceptible) *or* cefotaxime *or* ceftriaxone	Chloramphenicol
Mycobacterium tuberculosis	Isoniazid *and* rifampin *and* pyrazinamide *and* prednisone (see Chapter 35)	

Suggested Dosages for Persons with Normal Renal and Hepatic Function*

ANTIBIOTIC	DOSAGE	MAXIMUM DAILY DOSE	ANTIBIOTIC	DOSAGE	MAXIMUM DAILY DOSE
Amikacin	15 mg/kg/day divided q8–12hr IV	15 mg/kg	Gentamicin	7.5 mg/kg/day divided q8hr IV	Adults: 5 mg/kg
Ampicillin	300–400 mg/kg/day divided q6hr IV	12 g	Nafcillin	150 mg/kg/day divided q4–6hr IV	9 g
Cefotaxime	200 mg/kg/day divided q6hr IV or IM	12 g	Oxacillin	150–200 mg/kg/day divided q4–6hr IV	12 g
Ceftriaxone	100 mg/kg/day divided q12hr IV	2–4 g	Penicillin G	250,000–400,000 U/kg/day divided q4hr IV	20–24 MU
	or 80 mg/kg/day q24hr IV	2–4 g	Tobramycin	7.5 mg/kg/day divided q8hr IV	Adults: 5 mg/kg
Chloramphenicol	75–100 mg/kg/day divided q6hr IV	2–4 g	Vancomycin	45–60 mg/kg/day divided q6hr IV	2 g
	or 75 mg/kg/day divided q6hr PO	2–4 g			

*See Table 96–4 and Chapter 14 for doses for neonates and for persons with impaired renal or hepatic function.

bacterial pericarditis is fatal in up to 80% of cases. The outcome for tuberculous pericarditis is dependent on adequate drainage and appropriate antituberculosis therapy.

REVIEWS

Fowler NO, Manitsas GT: Infectious pericarditis. *Prog Cardiovasc Dis* 1973;16:323–36.

Osterberg L, Vagelos R, Atwood JE: Case presentation and review: Constrictive pericarditis. *West J Med* 1998;169:232–9.

Park S, Bayer AS: Purulent pericarditis. *Curr Clin Top Infect Dis* 1992;12:56–82.

Skiest DJ, Steiner D, Werner M, et al: Anaerobic pericarditis: Case report and review. *Clin Infect Dis* 1994;19:435–40.

Strang JI: Tuberculous pericarditis. *J Infect* 1997;35:215–9.

KEY ARTICLES

Baljepally R, Spodick DH: PR-segment deviation as the initial electrocardiographic response in acute pericarditis. *Am J Cardiol* 1998;81:1505–6.

Benzing G III, Kaplan S: Purulent pericarditis. *Am J Dis Child* 1963; 106:289–94.

Carmichael DB, et al: Acute non-specific pericarditis. *Circulation* 1951; 3:321–31.

Cayler GG, Taybi H, Riley HD Jr, et al: Pericarditis with effusion in infants and children. *J Pediatr* 1963;63:264–72.

Chen Y, Brennessel D, Walters J, et al: Human immunodeficiency virus–associated pericardial effusion: Report of 40 cases and review of the literature. *Am Heart J* 1999;137:516–21.

Cigielski JP, Devlin BH, Morris AJ, et al: Comparison of PCR, culture, and histopathology for diagnosis of tuberculous pericarditis. *J Clin Microbiol* 1997;35:3254–7.

Corey GR, Campbell PT, Van Trigt P, et al: Etiology of large pericardial effusions. *Am J Med* 1993;95:209–13.

Desai HN: Tuberculous pericarditis. A review of 100 cases. *S Afr Med J* 1979;55:877–80.

Feldman WE: Bacterial etiology and mortality of purulent pericarditis in pediatric patients. Review of 162 cases. *Am J Dis Child* 1979;133:641–4.

Gersony WM, McCracken GH Jr: Purulent pericarditis in infancy. *Pediatrics* 1967;40:224–32.

Juneja R, Kothari SS, Saxena A, et al: Intrapericardial streptokinase in purulent pericarditis. *Arch Dis Child* 1999;80:275–7.

Senni M, Redfield MM, Ling LH, et al: Left ventricular systolic and diastolic function after pericardiectomy in patients with constrictive pericarditis: Doppler echocardiographic findings and correlation with clinical status. *J Am Coll Cardiol* 1999;33:1182–8.

Spodick DM: Electrocardiogram in acute pericarditis: Distributions of morphologic and axial changes by stages. *Am J Cardiol* 1974;33:470–4.

Strang G, Latouf S, Commerford P, et al: Bedside culture to confirm tuberculous pericarditis. *Lancet* 1991;338:1600–1.

Strang JI: Rapid resolution of tuberculous pericardial effusions with high dose prednisone and anti-tuberculous drugs. *J Infect* 1994;28:251–4.

Strauss AW, Santa-Maria M, Goldring D: Constrictive pericarditis in children. *Am J Dis Child* 1975;129:822–6.

Weir EK, Joffe HS: Purulent pericarditis in children: An analysis of 28 cases. *Thorax* 1977;32:438–43.

CHAPTER 74

Esophagitis

Tod S. Russell ▪ David P. Ascher

Many infectious agents have been found to cause acute and chronic esophagitis, most commonly *Candida albicans* and herpes simplex virus (HSV). Most cases of esophagitis occur in persons with a combination of altered systemic immune defenses and also another predisposing factor that affects local defenses, such as trauma.

ETIOLOGY

C. albicans and HSV are the most common pathogens associated with esophagitis, but many organisms can cause esophagitis, including other *Candida* species and cytomegalovirus (CMV). Rarely causing esophagitis are varicella-zoster virus, *Aspergillus, Mycobacterium tuberculosis,* gram-negative bacilli, and gram-positive cocci. Esophagitis due to *Helicobacter pylori* may occur as an extension of *H. pylori* gastritis and peptic ulcer disease (Chapter 75).

EPIDEMIOLOGY

Esophagitis resulting from gastroesophageal reflux is commonly encountered in pediatrics, but infectious esophagitis is uncommon in immunocompetent persons. HSV, which is the most common cause of infectious esophagitis in immunocompetent persons, can cause esophagitis as an extension of primary oral herpes stomatitis (Chapter 60). *Candida* esophagitis can occur in immunocompetent persons, especially with broad-spectrum antimicrobial treatment for an unrelated bacterial infection, and in newborns.

The reported prevalence of infectious esophagitis in persons with cancer is 2.8–13%; the most common cause is *C. albicans.* Other fungal species reported as causes of esophagitis include *Candida tropicalis, Candida parapsilosis,* and *Candida glabrata.* The prevalence of esophagitis is 4–46% for bone marrow transplant recipients, 2–24% for kidney transplant recipients, and 11% for liver transplant recipients. Viral causes predominate in bone marrow and liver transplant recipients, and candidiasis predominates in persons with renal transplants. From 33% to 75% of persons with AIDS have symptoms attributable to esophageal infection sometime during the course of their disease.

HSV esophagitis usually begins as a cluster of discrete vesicles in the lower third of the esophagus and in immunocompromised persons has a predilection for traumatized areas. CMV esophagitis, which does not occur in immunocompetent persons, occurs in persons with AIDS, and in approximately 10% of renal and hepatic transplant recipients. Esophagitis caused by varicella-zoster virus has been reported in association with thoracic dermatomal zoster but is rare. The necrotic esophageal ulcers of viral esophagitis are prone to superinfection and colonization with *Candida.*

Bacterial esophagitis is a recently described entity that is defined as bacterial invasion of the mucosa without evidence of *Candida* or other fungal or viral infections. Bacterial esophagitis most often occurs in persons with profound neutropenia, probably as a result of esophageal injury (e.g., nasogastric tube, radiation, reflux esophagitis). In one study (Walsh et al, 1986), 11% of endoscopic biopsy specimens and 16% of autopsy specimens fulfilled the criteria of bacterial esophagitis. Most of these persons had symptoms, although fever and occult bacteremia may be the only manifestations of esophageal infection. The organisms are for the most part representative of oral flora, particularly gram-positive bacteria including viridans streptococci, *Staphylococcus,* and *Bacillus.*

Tuberculous esophagitis is rare and usually indicates infection of an adjacent organ, usually mediastinal lymphadenitis, with spread into and secondary involvement of the esophagus. Esophagitis caused by *Histoplasma capsulatum* or *Blastomyces dermatitidis* represents secondary esophageal involvement originating from paraesophageal nodes. Aspergillosis is uncommon but should be considered in cases of apparent *Candida* esophagitis that are resistant to appropriate antifungal therapy. Other unusual causes of infectious esophagitis include *Actinomyces israelii, Trypanosoma cruzi,* diphtheria, and scarlet fever. Esophagitis with syphilis, caused by *Treponema pallidum,* has not been reported since 1961. Esophageal pathogens in persons with AIDS may also include *Mycobacterium avium* complex, *Cryptosporidium parvum,* Epstein-Barr virus, and *Pneumocystis carinii.*

PATHOGENESIS

The risk factors most often associated with infectious esophagitis are the combination of immunosuppression and trauma to the mucosa. Many persons with esophagitis also have impaired humoral or cellular immunity from cancer and from cancer chemotherapy, posttransplantation immunosuppression, prolonged corticosteroid use, or AIDS. Gastroesophageal reflux, decreased peristalsis, mechanical obstruction, radiation therapy, prolonged antibiotic therapy allowing for overgrowth or colonization of a pathogen, ulcerations caused by pills that stick to the esophagus, and nasogastric tubes have all been implicated as conditions that may facilitate initiation of an opportunistic infection by damaging local mucosal defenses.

SYMPTOMS AND CLINICAL MANIFESTATIONS

Acute infectious esophagitis often presents with odynophagia, or severe pain in swallowing, dysphagia, and retrosternal chest pain. Fever, nausea, vomiting, melena, and hematemesis may occur but are uncommon. HSV esophagitis typically presents with the sudden onset of severe odynophagia.

Oral candidiasis is commonly a marker for *Candida* esophagitis, especially in immunocompromised persons, but it may be absent in as many as half of the cases. Fungal esophagitis often presents with painful swallowing and retrosternal pain. Fungal esophagitis may be asymptomatic, as demonstrated by its incidental discovery during routine endoscopy and its high prevalence at autopsy in immunocompromised persons.

DIAGNOSIS

An **esophagogram** with a contrast medium is often the initial step in evaluating esophagitis. It can show obstruction, abnormal motility and peristalsis, and ulcerations and plaques suggestive of esophagitis. Nevertheless, many persons with esophagitis have normal or nondiagnostic esophagograms because the mucosal abnormalities, especially early in the course of the disease, are subtle. A **double-contrast study,** performed by having the patient swallow gas-producing effervescent crystals to inflate or dilate the esophagus, is necessary to see fine mucosal detail.

Endoscopy, or esophagoscopy, is the best means to make a definitive diagnosis. Through the endoscope, the lesions can be directly visualized, brushings can be obtained for cytologic examination and culture, and biopsy specimens can be obtained for histologic examination and culture. A sleeve can be used over the brush to prevent contamination by commensal oral flora. Brushings may have a higher diagnostic yield than biopsies because more of the mucosa is sampled.

Candidal Esophagitis. In persons with AIDS the combination of thrush and esophageal symptoms has a >95% predictive value for the diagnosis of *Candida* esophagitis. Nevertheless, only 50% of persons with AIDS and *Candida* esophagitis have thrush.

Single-contrast studies for *Candida* esophagitis have a sensitivity of 55%, whereas double-contrast studies have a sensitivity of 88%. Mild to moderate cases are associated with a shaggy, or moth-eaten, irregular mucosal pattern (see Fig. 13–24). Ulcers, longitudinally oriented plaques, pseudomembranes, abnormal motility, and a cobblestone pattern are also seen. The changes shown on contrast studies are not always specific for fungal infection. Radiographic studies are most helpful in establishing the diagnosis when endoscopy is contraindicated because of thrombocytopenia or neutropenia. Endoscopic brushings and biopsies are the most accurate diagnostic method. The endoscopic appearance of the mucosa varies from moderate erythema and friability, to ulcers covered with a thick white exudate, to a black membrane. The classic finding is multiple white, raised lesions, usually <1 cm in diameter. The exudate may contain yeast and hyphae. Culture specimens may be contaminated by the presence of oropharyngeal candidiasis and must be interpreted appropriately. The diagnosis is unequivocal if invading hyphal forms are seen on a biopsy specimen.

Viral Esophagitis. A double-contrast, barium-swallow study for viral esophagitis can be helpful by showing ulcerations (punctate, linear, or stellate), plaques, a cobblestone pattern, or a diffusely shaggy mucosa. These findings may be clinically indistinguishable from those of *Candida* esophagitis, so endoscopy is often necessary to obtain brushings for cytology and to obtain culture and biopsy specimens for culture and histologic examination. HSV and varicella-zoster virus characteristically cause epithelial necrosis, and CMV affects the submucosal tissues. A viral cytopathic effect can be identified on mucosal biopsy specimens of HSV or CMV esophageal ulcerations.

On endoscopy, HSV esophagitis may have vesicular lesions but more commonly appears as a bumpy, eroded esophagus with punched-out ulcerations approximately 5 mm in diameter. A **volcano ulcer** with a yellow rim has been regarded as typical of HSV infection. Biopsy specimens of HSV esophagitis should be obtained from the edge of the ulcer. The presence of HSV may be demonstrated by immunohistochemical staining or by the characteristic intranuclear inclusion bodies in squamous cells. In one study (Bonacini et al, 1991) of persons with AIDS, the yield was 10% for histologic examination, 30% for cytologic examination, 100% for viral culture of endoscopic brushings, and 90% for viral culture of biopsy specimens.

The diagnosis of CMV esophagitis requires a biopsy of the center of the ulcer. The most prominent feature of CMV esophagitis is giant mucosal ulcerations that may exceed 2–3 cm in length. Esophageal infection occurs within submucosal fibroblasts and endothelial cells, not in the epithelium, and is usually part of a widespread visceral infection. These findings are most commonly found at the base of the ulcers in the granulation tissue. CMV causes basophilic intranuclear inclusions and positive-staining periodic acid–Schiff cytoplasmic inclusions in endothelial cells. Immunoperoxidase staining for CMV antigen has helped maximize diagnostic yield. In one study (Bonacini et al, 1991) of persons with AIDS, the yield was 42% for histologic examination, 3% for cytologic examination, 58% for viral culture of endoscopic brushing specimens, and 52% for viral culture of biopsy specimens. The diagnosis of CMV esophagitis ideally would be based on typical histologic changes, together with a positive tissue culture result. Culture of CMV from secretions is probably not sufficiently specific to be used as a basis for therapy.

TREATMENT

Candidal Esophagitis. Candidal esophagitis responds to topical therapy (nystatin or clotrimazole), oral therapy (ketoconazole or fluconazole), or intravenous therapy (amphotericin B). In immunocompetent persons and in persons with AIDS, there is usually no urgency in initiating the administration of amphotericin B because esophagitis is rarely associated with bleeding, perforation, fungemia, or disseminated fungal disease. The mode of treatment depends on the severity of the disease and the degree of immunocompromise. Mild oropharyngeal and esophageal candidiasis in immunocompetent persons usually responds to oral nystatin (500,000 U [5 mL] four times a day) or clotrimazole troches (10 mg five times a day) for 10–14 days, although these drugs are rarely effective in immunocompromised persons. As an alternative systemic treatment for immunocompetent persons or, initially, for immunocompromised persons, fluconazole (3–6 mg/kg/day once daily orally; maximum: 100–200 mg), ketoconazole (3.3–6.6 mg/kg/day once daily orally; maximum: 200–400 mg), or itraconazole (5 mg/kg/day once daily orally; maximum: 200–400 mg) can be used. Fluconazole appears to be less toxic and better tolerated, does not require an acid environment for absorption, and has potentially greater efficacy than ketoconazole. *Candida krusei* is usually resistant, and *C. glabrata* is often resistant, to fluconazole. Itraconazole is the most potent of the available oral azole agents. The oral solution of itraconazole is more effective than the itraconazole capsules for oropharyngeal candidiasis. Severe disease and disease that does not respond in 1 week should be treated with amphotericin B. Low-dose amphotericin B therapy (0.3–0.5 mg/kg/day intravenously in children; 10 mg/day intravenously in adults) is definitive for most cases of *Candida* esophagitis, including azole-resistant *Candida,* but the adverse effects of amphotericin B warrant cautious use.

Persons with AIDS and oral candidiasis with mild esophageal symptoms are often given empirical antifungal therapy without further evaluation. Endoscopy is reserved for persons who do not respond to antifungal therapy within 7–10 days. One study (Laine et al, 1992) demonstrated that fluconazole, 100 mg daily, resulted in significantly greater endoscopic and clinical cure rates than ketoconazole, 200 mg daily, in persons with AIDS and *Candida* esophagitis. Therapy was continued for 2 weeks after resolution of symptoms, with a total treatment duration of 3–8 weeks. For persons with AIDS after treatment of *Candida* esophagitis, maintenance or intermittent therapy with daily fluconazole or ketoconazole is usually necessary to prevent relapse.

Viral Esophagitis. The treatment of viral esophagitis is probably less effective than treatment of *Candida* esophagitis. Immunocompromised persons with HSV esophagitis may be treated with acyclovir, famciclovir, valacyclovir, or foscarnet. The treatment of HSV esophagitis with acyclovir has been successful with the use of 750 mg/m^2/day in three divided doses daily intravenously, for 7–10 days. Immunocompetent persons with HSV esophagitis may require no specific antiviral therapy, only symptomatic treatment with analgesics and antacids.

Ganciclovir appears to be an effective drug against CMV infections, at a dosage of 5 mg/kg every 12 hours intravenously for 12–14 days. CMV esophagitis in persons with AIDS may respond to ganciclovir therapy, but adverse effects may limit treatment. Ganciclovir may suppress or eradicate CMV from some immunocompromised persons, but many of these persons will have relapses. Long-term, low-dose suppressive therapy with ganciclovir or foscarnet may be required.

COMPLICATIONS

Fungal esophagitis in immunocompetent persons is rarely associated with complications. *Candida* esophagitis in immunocompromised persons may lead to several complications including abnormal esophageal motility, intramural diverticula, bands, esophageal obstruction, perforation, fistulas, life-threatening hemorrhage, systemic candidiasis, and secondary bacterial infection with sepsis. Often concomitant infection with HSV or a bacterium occurs.

Complications of viral esophagitis include hemorrhage, disseminated viral infection, fistula formation, and bacterial superinfection. Late complications such as strictures are rare. *Candida* is often found in association with HSV esophageal ulcerations and probably is a colonizer of the herpetic ulcerations.

PROGNOSIS

An immunocompetent person with *Candida* or HSV esophagitis has an excellent prognosis. An immunocompromised, neutropenic person or transplant recipient with *Candida* or HSV esophagitis usually responds to appropriate therapy and usually does not have esophageal relapses, especially if therapy with immunosuppressive drugs is discontinued. Persons with AIDS and *Candida* or HSV esophagitis typically take longer to respond to appropriate therapy and often have oropharyngeal or esophageal relapses.

PREVENTION

Routine prophylaxis for *Candida* esophagitis is not currently recommended. Because of the risk of developing drug-resistant organisms, the low morbidity associated with mucosal candidiasis, and the relative efficacy of treatment, prophylaxis is not justified in most instances. If the severity or frequency of relapses warrants long-term prophylaxis, either fluconazole or clotrimazole can be used.

Acyclovir prophylaxis for reactivation of HSV infection is of clinical value in severely immunocompromised persons, especially those undergoing induction chemotherapy or transplantation. A sequential regimen of intravenous acyclovir therapy, followed by oral acyclovir therapy for 3–6 months, markedly reduces the incidence of symptomatic HSV infection in transplant recipients. There is currently no role for the use of prophylactic topical antiviral agents to prevent oral HSV infections in immunocompromised persons, although topical penciclovir is effective in treating recurrent herpetic gingivostomatitis (Chapter 60). Acyclovir is not effective in the treatment of CMV infections, but its prophylactic administration decreases the frequency of symptomatic CMV disease in bone marrow and renal transplant recipients (Chapter 100).

REVIEWS

Génédreau T, Rozenberg F, Bouchaud O, et al: Herpes esophagitis. A comprehensive review. *Clin Microbiol Infect* 1997;3:397–407.

Minamoto GY, Rosenberg AS: Fungal infections in patients with acquired immunodeficiency syndrome. *Med Clin North Am* 1997;81:381–409.

Noyer CM, Simon D: HIV infection and the gastrointestinal tract. *Gastroenterol Clin North Am* 1997;26:241–57.

KEY ARTICLES

Alexander JA, Brouillette DE, Chien MC, et al: Infectious esophagitis following liver and renal transplant. *Dig Dis Sci* 1988;33:1121–6.

Bonacini M, Young T, Laine L: The causes of esophageal symptoms in human immunodeficiency virus infection. A prospective study of 110 patients. *Arch Intern Med* 1991;151:1567–72.

Galbraith JC, Shafran SD: Herpes simplex esophagitis in the immunocompetent patient: Report of four cases and review. *Clin Infect Dis* 1992; 14:894–901.

Laine L, Dretler RH, Conteas CN, et al: Fluconazole compared with ketoconazole for the treatment of *Candida* esophagitis in AIDS. A randomized trial. *Ann Intern Med* 1992;117:655–60.

Levine MS, Macones AJ Jr, Laufer I: *Candida* esophagitis: Accuracy of radiographic diagnosis. *Radiology* 1985;154:581–7.

Porro GB, Parente F, Cernuschi M: The diagnosis of esophageal candidiasis in patients with acquired immune deficiency syndrome: Is endoscopy always necessary? *Am J Gastroenterol* 1989;84:143–6.

Walsh TJ, Belitsos NJ, Hamilton SR: Bacterial esophagitis in immunocompromised patients. *Arch Intern Med* 1986;146:1345–8.

Wilcox CM: Esophageal disease in the acquired immunodeficiency syndrome: Etiology, diagnosis, and management. *Am J Med* 1992;92: 412–21.

Wilcox CM, Straub RF, Schwartz DA: Cytomegalovirus esophagitis in AIDS: A prospective evaluation of clinical response to ganciclovir therapy, relapse rate, and long-term outcome. *Am J Med* 1995;98:169–76.

CHAPTER 75

Gastritis

M. Susan Moyer ▪ Hal B. Jenson

Gastritis and **peptic ulcer disease** can be viewed as a continuum of compromise of the gastroduodenal mucosa from superficial diffuse inflammation to discrete ulcerations. **Ulcers** are defined as deep lesions that extend through the muscularis mucosa. Understanding of the cause and pathogenesis of these disorders has been greatly enhanced by recognition of the role of *Helicobacter pylori* in the development of gastritis and mucosal ulcers. Three distinct causes of peptic ulcer disease are now recognized: *H. pylori* infection, use of nonsteroidal anti-inflammatory drugs, and pathologic hypersecretory states such as the Zollinger-Ellison syndrome. The latter two are extremely uncommon causes of gastritis in children. Infection with *H. pylori* is strongly associated with histologic gastritis and duodenal ulcer disease and is the most common recognized cause of gastroduodenal disease. Although the pathogenic mechanisms of ulcer formation are not well-defined, it is clear that peptic ulcer disease associated with *H. pylori* is an infectious disorder that can often be cured with appropriate antimicrobial therapy.

It is now well established that *H. pylori* causes peptic ulcer disease. *H. pylori* has also been implicated in the pathogenesis of gastroduodenal carcinomas and in certain types of gastric and intestinal lymphomas. However, its role in **nonulcer dyspepsia,** which is defined as persistent or recurrent upper abdominal discomfort of at least 3 months' duration without evidence of organic disease, remains controversial.

ETIOLOGY

H. pylori, formerly called *Campylobacter pylori,* is a catalase-negative, oxidase-negative, **urease-positive,** microaerophilic, gram-negative spiral- or comma-shaped microbe first isolated in 1983. It is possible that the first report of visualization dates from 1938, when spiral-shaped microbes overlying the gastric epithelium of humans were reported. *H. pylori* has multiple powerful flagella that enable movement through viscous material. The organism is found only on **gastric-type epithelial cells** and resides in the mucus layer overlying gastric epithelium (Fig. 75–1), which may explain the survival of this acid-susceptible microbe. Two other species of *Helicobacter, H. felis* and *H. heilmanii (Gastrospirillum hominis),* have also been identified in human stomachs, but their association with disease is uncertain.

Several putative *H. pylori* virulence factors have been identified, including ***cagA*** (cytokine-associated gene A), ***vacA*** (vacuolating cytotoxin), and ***iceA.*** Although *cagA*$^+$ strains do seem to be associated with more intense gastric inflammation and increased mucosal concentrations of inflammatory cytokines, including IL-8, their presence does not necessarily predict the development of more severe disease. There is currently reasonable evidence to conclude that none of the putative virulence factors have disease specificity and that virulence may be a host-dependent factor.

Transmission. The natural reservoir of *H. pylori* is probably humans. There is no other known environmental reservoir. The organism is transmitted from person to person, principally by fecal-oral and perhaps oral-oral spread and occasionally through contaminated endoscopic equipment. *H. pylori* has been cultured from stool, and *H. pylori* DNA has been identified in oral secretions. Intrafamilial clustering is common, usually with identical strains of the organism. Parents, especially infected mothers, may have a key role in transmission of *H. pylori* within families.

EPIDEMIOLOGY

H. pylori can be isolated worldwide from humans with gastritis and peptic ulcer disease and is associated with 85% of cases of gastritis, 65% of cases of gastric ulcer, and almost all cases of duodenal ulceration. Prevalence rates of 13–25% have been observed in young persons with histologic evidence of gastritis. Prevalence as high as 80% is found among children in developing countries. The prevalence of *H. pylori* in developed countries increases with age from <10% in children to as high as 60% in adults older than 60 years. There is increased prevalence among institutionalized persons and among children of lower socioeconomic status living in crowded conditions. In the United States the major risk factor for acquiring *H. pylori* is low socioeconomic status. The higher prevalence in minority groups, including African American and Hispanic groups, that was reported in early studies may be related largely to their socioeconomic status and not to race or ethnicity.

The incidence of gastritis in the pediatric population correlates highly with the presence of *H. pylori* infection. Once infection occurs, microbes may persist for months to years and perhaps even decades, causing continuous inflammation. Recovery of *H. pylori* from the stomach has been reported with increasing frequency in antral chronic gastritis, peptic ulcer disease, episodic hypochlorhydria, and nonulcer dyspepsia.

PATHOGENESIS

H. pylori does not appear to invade the gastric epithelium but is found more commonly at tight epithelial junctions in intimate contact with the surface mucus cell (Fig. 75–1). Several factors contribute to the ability of *H. pylori* to colonize gastric mucosa. The urease, **urea amidohydrolase,** produced by *H. pylori* neutralizes the acidic microenvironment by breaking down urea in the gastric fluid to ammonia and carbon dioxide, thus creating a more hospitable environment for bacteria and providing a source of nitrogen. The spiral shape, the presence of the polar flagella, and the production of proteases that are mucinolytic and that decrease local viscosity facilitate movement of the organism through the mucus layer. Finally, although the majority of organisms exist freely in the mucus layer, some can adhere to gastric mucosal cells by producing **adhesins** specific for gastric-type mucosa. *H. pylori* is also associated with ectopic islands of gastric mucosa in the duodenum, known as gastric metaplasia.

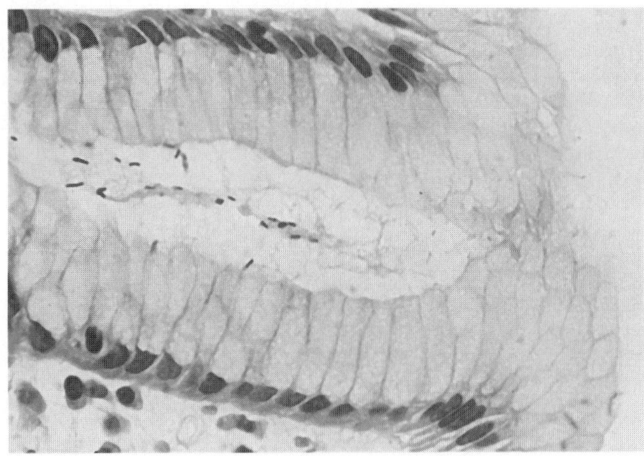

FIGURE 75–1. *Helicobacter pylori* in the gastric mucosa. The organisms lie on the luminal surface of the epithelial cells and in the mucous coat. (Genta modification of the Warthin-Starry stain: magnification: ×300.)

The precise pathogenesis of *H. pylori*–induced gastrointestinal injury is still not clearly defined. Several substances released by *H. pylori* can potentially mediate local tissue injury, including urease, cytotoxin, mucinase, phospholipase, and platelet-activating factor. The organism induces a mucosal immune response that may result in epithelial damage. Chemotactic factors produced by *H. pylori* recruit inflammatory cells, specifically neutrophils and monocytes, which then release other inflammatory mediators. In addition, *H. pylori* appears to directly induce IL-8 production by gastric epithelial cells. There is also a host B cell response that results in production of specific IgM, IgG, and secretory IgA antibodies. IgG antibodies promote complement-dependent phagocytosis by neutrophils. Histologically the acute inflammatory infiltrate of polymorphonuclear leukocytes is followed during the second week of infection by infiltration with chronic inflammatory mononuclear cells. Destruction of epithelial cells is associated with marked depletion of mucus. In children, the inflammatory infiltrate is composed mainly of lymphocytes and plasma cells and is usually localized to the gastric antrum.

Regardless of the mechanism of tissue injury, compromise of mucosa in the presence of acid and pepsin results in ongoing mucosal inflammation, leading to clinical symptoms of gastritis or development of ulcers. Acid production may actually be higher in the setting of *H. pylori* infection, particularly in persons with duodenal ulcers. A decrease in **antral D cells,** which produce somatostatin, an inhibitor of gastrin production, has been demonstrated with *H. pylori* infection. This disinhibition of gastrin production is reflected in increased basal and stimulated gastrin levels and, potentially, in an increase in acid production. The increased acid, as well as other, as-yet-undefined factors, may contribute to gastric metaplasia in the duodenum. Further colonization of metaplastic gastric epithelium can then lead to local inflammation, mucosal injury, and ulcer formation.

Glandular atrophy may develop as a result of the chronic inflammatory process. Achlorhydria develops by the beginning of the third week of infection. The determinants of host susceptibility that lead to the development of a chronic process are not known. Infectious *H. pylori* gastritis persists despite local and systemic immune responses.

On endoscopy the appearance of the gastric mucosa does not consistently correlate with the histopathologic findings. Gastric mucosa that appears to be healthy by endoscopy is often found to be inflamed on histopathologic examination. Gastric inflammation may or may not be reflected in clinical symptoms.

Gastritis resolves spontaneously in fewer than 5% of individuals infected with *H. pylori* (Fig. 75–2). In the majority, there is persistence of a diffuse, predominantly antral gastritis that may or may not be associated with clinical symptoms. Of chronically infected individuals, 10–15% develop peptic ulcer disease; 1–2% develop a diffuse atrophic gastritis, intestinal metaplasia, or both, which are risk factors for **gastric adenocarcinoma;** and fewer than 1% develop **mucosa-associated lymphoid tissue (MALT) lymphoma,** which has been definitively linked to chronic *H. pylori* infection.

The IgG response to *H. pylori* remains elevated for months or years after the onset of infection. If untreated, infectious gastritis persists in the presence of a specific humoral immune response. However, once a person is treated for *H. pylori,* the rate of reinfection is low, <1% per year. This appears to be true for both children and adults. Relapse may occur and is related to failure of eradication.

SYMPTOMS AND CLINICAL MANIFESTATIONS

H. pylori infection may or may not be symptomatic. There is no single pathognomonic symptom, and attempts to identify a symptom complex that supports the underlying diagnosis of *H. pylori*–related disease have been unsuccessful (Table 75–1). Dyspeptic symptoms of acute infection develop 7 days after ingestion of the microorganism and may include pain in the epigastrium, nausea, and vomiting. These symptoms may be accompanied by borborygmi, halitosis, and bloating, but fever is absent. Symptoms may persist a few days or as long as a few weeks and then spontaneously disappear. Achlorhydria or hypochlorhydria has been demonstrated after the acute infection.

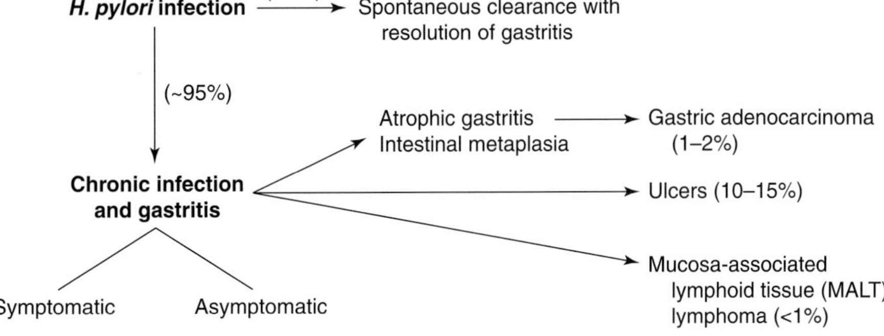

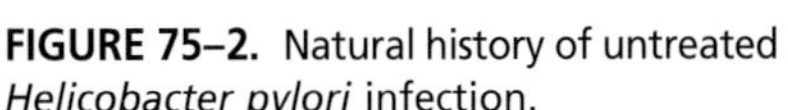

FIGURE 75–2. Natural history of untreated *Helicobacter pylori* infection.

TABLE 75–1. Clinical Presentations of *Helicobacter pylori* Infection

Acute Infection

Children and Adults
Epigastric pain
Nausea
Vomiting
Borborygmi
Halitosis
Achlorhydria

Infants
Poor feeding
Hematemesis

Symptomatic Chronic Infection

Gastritis and Peptic Ulcer Disease
Epigastric pain
Nausea
Vomiting
Nocturnal pain (awakens at night)
Hematemesis
Weight loss

Complicated Peptic Ulcer Disease
Gastric outlet obstruction
Perforation
Significant gastrointestinal bleeding (hematemesis; melena)

Gastric Adenocarcinoma (Adults)
Anemia
Fatigue
Hematemesis

MALT Lymphoma
Symptoms vary according to disease location

H. pylori infections should be considered likely in persons with acute symptoms lasting longer than 1 month, indicating progression into a chronic stage. Symptoms are similar to those manifested during the acute period but are of varying severity. In infants and young children the chronic loss of appetite and chronic vomiting may lead to failure to thrive. Young infants may also develop severe iron deficiency anemia, which is particularly prevalent in developing countries, where acquisition of *H. pylori* infection commonly occurs in infancy and early childhood. Recurrent severe abdominal pain and occasionally hematemesis have been reported.

Gastritis caused by *H. pylori* is not self-limiting in the majority of cases. Evaluation for underlying *H. pylori* infection should be considered for persons with chronic abdominal symptoms suggestive of chronic gastritis or peptic ulcer disease.

DIAGNOSIS

The diagnosis of *H. pylori* infection is supported or confirmed by both invasive and noninvasive tests (Table 75–2). The diagnosis may be suggested by noninvasive tests, which include serologic testing, detection of exhaled radiolabeled carbon after a urea liquid meal labeled with carbon 13 or carbon 14 **(urea breath test),** or a stool test for the presence of a specific *H. pylori* antigen. Definitive diagnosis is established by identification of the organism in biopsy specimens obtained at endoscopy, which is invasive. The organism may be identified in gastric biopsy specimens by culture, histologic examination, or a **rapid urease test.** There is still controversy regarding indications (Table 75–3) for testing for *H. pylori* infection in both adults and children (Gold et al, 2000).

TABLE 75–2. Currently Available Tests for *Helicobacter pylori*

Noninvasive
Serologic studies (serum and whole blood antibodies)
Stool antigen
Urea breath testing

Invasive (Endoscopic)
Biopsy with histologic analysis
Rapid urease test
Bacterial culture
PCR assay for *H. pylori*

Endoscopy, followed by identification of *H. pylori* by culture, histologic analysis, and rapid urease testing, remains the gold standard for diagnosis of *H. pylori* infection and disease but is invasive and expensive. Endoscopy may reveal duodenitis, antral gastritis, and ulceration of either the duodenum or the stomach (Plate 8A). In children the gastric mucosa may have a nodular, **cobblestone appearance,** which is suggestive of *H. pylori*–associated gastritis. Although serologic assays are reasonably sensitive and specific in adults, they have significant limitations in children, particularly those less than 10 years of age, and are currently considered unreliable for screening in infants and children. Both the urea breath test and the stool antigen assay appear to be sensitive and specific tests for *H. pylori* in both adults and children. The urea breath test is more expensive, and there are technical difficulties associated with performing this test in younger children. More information, as well as standardization of testing, in children will be necessary before these tests can replace endoscopic diagnosis.

Microbiologic Evaluation

H. pylori can be cultured by inoculation of gastric mucosal tissue within 2 hours after endoscopy. A semiselective medium (Skirrow medium) and a nonselective blood-and-chocolate agar incubated at 37°C (98.6°F) under humid microaerobic conditions for 3–5 days yield the organism in about 90% of cases when the histologic examination demonstrates organisms with morphologic features consistent with *H. pylori.* Diagnosis of *H. pylori* by culture is not widely used clinically and is reserved for research purposes or to identify resistant strains, particularly in the setting of recurrent infection.

At endoscopy at least two biopsy specimens of gastric mucosa should be obtained, one from the antrum and one from the body

TABLE 75–3. Guidelines for Testing Children for *Helicobacter pylori*

Manifestation	Test
Duodenal and gastric ulcers	Yes
Recurrent abdominal pain (without ulcers)	No
No symptoms	No
Routine screening	
No symptoms	No
Family history of recurrent peptic ulcers or gastric cancer	No
MALT lymphoma	Yes
After therapy for *H. pylori* with:	
Complicated peptic ulcer disease (bleeding, perforation, gastric outlet obstruction)	Yes
Persistent symptoms	Yes*
Uncomplicated ulcer	No

*Endoscopy with biopsy.

of the stomach. The presence of neutrophils in the gastric mucosa strongly suggests *H. pylori* infection. Detection of microorganisms after special staining of the specimen (e.g., Warthin-Starry stain) is characteristic (Fig. 75–1) and almost 100% sensitive and specific for the diagnosis. *H. pylori* is usually found in the areas of normal-appearing gastric mucosa and is present in smaller numbers in eroded and denuded mucosa. The gastric mucosa is usually colonized with fewer organisms in infected children than in infected adults.

A rapid and inexpensive test for detection of *H. pylori* urease enzyme is performed at endoscopy by placing a small piece of the gastric biopsy sample into a semisolid test well containing urea and a color indicator. If urease enzyme is present in the inserted tissue sample, the resulting degradation of urea causes the pH to rise and the color of the gel to turn from yellow to a bright magenta (Plate 8A). Many commercially available tests are available. This test has a 91% positive predictive value and a 73% negative predictive value for chronic gastritis related to *H. pylori.* Tests for gastric urease are specific for *H. pylori* because mammalian cells do not produce urease and, except for *H. pylori,* the stomach is usually sterile. False-positive test results may be obtained for persons with pernicious anemia, hypochlorhydria, or achlorhydria or for persons taking antacids or other acid suppression therapy, including **histamine 2 (H_2)–receptor antagonists** and **proton pump (H^+-K^+-ATPase) inhibitors.** Diminished production of stomach acid permits colonization of the stomach with other urease-producing commensal organisms, such as *Proteus.* False-negative test results may be obtained if the person has taken antibiotics or bismuth in the 3 weeks before biopsy, because the growth of *H. pylori* may be patchy after partial therapy. In addition, the color change may take up to 24 hours in children, who tend to be colonized with fewer organisms. Additional gastric biopsies may be of benefit under such circumstances.

Serologic Testing. Serum antibodies in an untreated person persist at high stable titers. They may be more sensitive for diagnosis than biopsy, which may miss patchy disease; however, they are not specific. Serologic testing may be less sensitive in children than in adults. Mean antibody levels are lower, and in infected children, specific antibody levels do not appear to reach their maximum level until 7–9 years of age. The result may be more false-negative findings in younger children. No cutoff values for children have been established for the commercially available assays, which may also add to the lack of sensitivity in testing of the pediatric patient. In general, a rapid decrease in serum IgG antibodies to *H. pylori* has been noted after treatment and eradication of *H. pylori* in biopsy-proved gastritis in adults. Little information is available on the rate of decline of antibodies in treated children, and monitoring the response to therapy with serologic testing in children is currently not recommended.

Many tests using ELISA are commercially available and are reported to have high sensitivity and specificity for the serologic diagnosis of *H. pylori* chronic gastritis in adults. Determinations of levels of serum IgG, IgA, and IgM antibodies against *H. pylori* using these tests are relatively inexpensive and easy to implement. However, these tests have been shown to have lower sensitivity and specificity when used outside the populations in which they were initially developed. This is also true in children. In one study (Khanna et al, 1998) a research immunoassay developed to detect specific IgG antibody to *H. pylori* was 91% sensitive, in comparison with a sensitivity of less than 70% for three commercially available assays. Improvement is necessary if these methods are to replace culture and histologic examination of gastric material for diagnosis.

Urea Breath Testing. Urea breath tests (UBTs) both are noninvasive and have high sensitivity and specificity, of >95%. The test is performed by ingestion of urea labeled with either carbon 14 or the stable isotope carbon 13. In the presence of *H. pylori,* urease splits the labeled urea into ammonia and labeled bicarbonate. The bicarbonate is absorbed, and labeled carbon dioxide content is measured in an expired breath. This method is more reliable than serologic testing for determining response to therapy and recurrence of disease.

In children, urea breath tests using carbon 13–labeled urea have a reported sensitivity of 98–100% and a specificity of 92–96%. Use of the stable isotope is recommended in children. The test is technically more difficult to perform in infants and younger children, and there is limited experience in children less than 5 years of age. Test parameters including dose, cutoff values, period of fasting, use of a test meal, and sample timing have not been standardized in children, which also limits the usefulness of these tests in the clinical setting at the present time.

Stool Antigen. Recently an ELISA that detects a specific *H. pylori* antigen in the stool has been developed and is commercially available. The precise antigen identified is unknown. Initial reports suggest that this assay holds promise as an accurate noninvasive test for the initial diagnosis of *H. pylori* infection and for monitoring the response to therapy and reinfection. There have been few studies in the pediatric population; however, two recently published reports support the reliability and accuracy of this test compared with the urea breath test (Braden, 2000) and with endoscopic diagnosis (Oderda et al, 2000). As with the urea breath test, additional studies are needed before this assay can replace the more invasive diagnostic tests in the pediatric population.

TREATMENT

Initial therapeutic trials to eradicate *H. pylori* used bismuth salts in combination with antibiotics with in vitro efficacy against *H. pylori.* These antibiotics included metronidazole, amoxicillin, erythromycin, rifampin, tetracycline, penicillin, cefoxitin, quinolones, clindamycin, third-generation cephalosporins, chloramphenicol, and aminoglycosides. In vitro susceptibility results for *H. pylori* did not always correlate with in vivo efficacy in various studies. Poor antibiotic penetration at the site of infection and low gastric pH decrease the in vivo effectiveness of many antimicrobial agents. Dual- or multiple-agent therapy was usually recommended because of the rapid development of antibiotic resistance by *H. pylori,* especially to metronidazole. Triple-agent therapy with bismuth subsalicylate, metronidazole, and tetracycline or amoxicillin for 2 weeks was well tolerated and resulted in good clearance and eradication rates of more than 80%.

Newer regimens have incorporated the use of **proton pump inhibitors,** such as omeprazole or lansoprazole. Antisecretory therapy enhances the efficacy of the antibiotics by neutralizing gastric pH and ameliorates the clinical symptoms associated with gastritis or ulcer disease. In addition, the proton pump inhibitors have intrinsic in vitro inhibitory activity against *H. pylori.* Most current regimens for initial therapy combine a proton pump inhibitor with at least two antibiotics active against *H. pylori.* These therapeutic regimens result in eradication rates of 80% or higher, which is considered to be effective treatment. The medications are given twice daily to improve compliance and for 10–14 days. Regimens for 7 days have been proposed, but the highest eradication rates are obtained with treatment for at least 10 days. The most commonly used combinations in adults are a proton pump inhibitor with two antibiotics—amoxicillin and clarithromycin, amoxicillin and metronidazole, or clarithromycin and metronidazole (Table 75–4).

The data on the efficacy of these therapies is much more limited in children, and the majority of published trials are open-labeled,

TABLE 75–4. Guidelines for Treatment of *Helicobacter pylori* in Children

Recommended Therapy*
Proton pump inhibitor:
Omeprazole 1 mg/kg/day divided twice daily PO (max dose 20 mg) (or equivalent dose of another proton pump inhibitor)
plus two of the following antibiotics:
Amoxicillin 50 mg/kg/day divided twice daily PO (max dose 1 g)
Metronidazole 20 mg/kg/day divided twice daily PO (max dose 500 mg)
Clarithromycin 15 mg/kg/day divided twice daily PO (max dose 500 mg)
Alternative Therapy
Bismuth subsalicylate 1 tablet (262 mg) *or* 15 mL (17.6 mg/mL) 4 times daily PO
Metronidazole 20 mg/kg/day divided twice daily PO (max dose 500 mg)
Proton pump inhibitor:
Omeprazole 1 mg/kg/day divided twice daily PO (max dose 20 mg) (or equivalent dose of another proton pump inhibitor)
plus one of the following antibiotics:
Amoxicillin 50 mg/kg/day divided twice daily PO (max dose 1 g)
Tetracycline† 50 mg/kg/day divided twice daily PO (max dose 1 g)
Clarithromycin 15 mg/kg/day divided twice daily PO (max dose 500 mg)
or
Ranitidine bismuth-citrate (RBC) 1 tablet 4 times daily PO
Clarithromycin 15 mg/kg/day divided twice daily PO (max dose 500 mg)
Metronidazole 20 mg/kg/day divided twice daily PO (max dose 500 mg)

*Therapy is given for 7–14 days. In adult studies, eradication rates are higher for the duration of treatment ≥10 days. Twice-daily dosing regimens enhance compliance.

†Tetracycline is not recommended for treatment of *H. pylori* gastritis in children <8 years of age because of the potential for permanent dental discoloration.

uncontrolled case series. Large, well-constructed clinical trials in children are needed to verify the effectiveness of these treatment regimens. Until then, physicians dealing with *H. pylori* in children must translate treatment strategies from adult studies.

The efficacy of therapy may be measured by clinical, microbiologic, and histologic criteria. A clinical cure is defined as the relief of symptoms of dyspepsia and the healing of any associated ulcer. Microbiologic eradication is defined as no growth of *H. pylori* in subsequent cultures of tissue specimens, a significant decrease in antibody titer 10–14 weeks after completion of antimicrobial therapy, or a normal urea breath test result. Histologic improvement is measured by the degree of inflammation recorded with a standardized scoring system of biopsy specimens. In general, clearance of *H. pylori* correlates with resolution of gastritis and healing of ulceration. Recurrence of symptoms after treatment is associated with demonstrable gastric mucosal inflammation and usually represents relapse rather than reinfection. If the first attempt at microbiologic eradication fails, triple-drug therapy using a different combination of antibiotics may be used (Table 75–4). There are also alternative regimens for treatment failures. One commonly used regimen is bismuth subsalicylate, metronidazole, and a proton pump inhibitor plus an additional antibiotic: amoxicillin, tetracycline, or clarithromycin. Generally it is recommended that persons who do not respond either to an initial or to a secondary course of anti–*H. pylori* therapy be referred to a gastroenterologist. In children, the lack of reliability of serologic testing may necessitate referral to the gastroenterologist to aid in the initial diagnosis.

Nonulcer Dyspepsia. The association between *H. pylori* infection and nonulcer dyspepsia in adults remains controversial. Recommendations for screening of adults include screening persons with dyspeptic symptoms who are less than 50 years of age. In published series, 30–60% of persons with nonulcer dyspepsia may have *H. pylori*–induced gastritis, and yet eradication of *H. pylori* has not consistently resulted in relief of symptoms in as many as 70% of persons treated. This finding suggests that *H. pylori* infection may not play a significant role in this disorder. A recent meta-analysis (Moayyedi et al, 2000) that used symptom relief at 12 months as the primary outcome showed a small but significant benefit of *H. pylori* eradication in these persons. However, to relieve one person of symptoms, 15 patients needed to be treated, which raises the issue of cost-effectiveness. There is even less information in children, but available data do not currently support treatment of *H. pylori* infection in children in the setting of nonulcer dyspepsia or **functional recurrent abdominal pain.**

COMPLICATIONS

Infection with *H. pylori* is associated not only with acute gastritis but also with **chronic gastritis,** which may lead to peptic ulcer disease, atrophic gastritis, and intestinal metaplasia. Both atrophic gastritis and intestinal metaplasia are risk factors for gastric adenocarcinoma (Chapter 4). Prevalence rates of *H. pylori* infection among persons with gastric cancer have been as high as 80%, and the relative risk of gastric cancer is estimated to be 2.1–8.7 times greater in adults infected with *H. pylori* than in uninfected control subjects. The International Agency for Research on Cancer and the World Health Organization have classified *H. pylori* as a group I carcinogen (sufficient evidence exists to determine that the agent is carcinogenic in humans). Non-Hodgkin's lymphoma has also been associated with previous infection with *H. pylori.* These lymphomas include both low-grade MALT lymphomas and, more significantly, high-grade gastric lymphomas. It is unknown whether eradication of *H. pylori* in persons without symptoms, or even in persons with symptoms, reduces the risk of gastric cancer, although remissions in persons with biopsy-proved, low-grade MALT gastric lymphomas have been reported after antimicrobial treatment and subsequent eradication of *H. pylori.* Although decision analyses have suggested that screening for *H. pylori* to prevent gastric cancer may be cost-effective, no clinical trials or prospective studies have been performed that document a decreased risk of developing gastric cancer after eradication of *H. pylori.* There may be other, as-yet-unidentified cofactors that contribute to the development of gastric cancer in these individuals and are independent of, or in association with, chronic *H. pylori* infection. Therefore routine population-based screening for *H. pylori* in either adults or children is not recommended at this time.

PROGNOSIS

The most important factors related to the cure rate for these regimens are compliance and the presence of resistant strains of the organism. Attempts have been made to enhance compliance with twice-daily dosage regimens and prepackaged treatment regimens. Adherence to the treatment regimen may be a particular problem in children who refuse, or are intolerant of, the medications. In addition, those agents that do not come in a liquid form may need to be compounded. Poor compliance with therapy not only affects cure rates but also may lead to antimicrobial resistance. In the United States, primary resistance of *H. pylori* to metronidazole is 28–39%, and the rate of clarithromycin resistance is reported to be as high as 11%.

Although more experience is needed to determine the optimal and long-term efficacy of treatment regimens for peptic ulcer disease associated with *H. pylori* infection, treatment studies have reported increased healing, improvement in symptoms, and a decreased recurrence rate. Optimum therapy results in eradication of *H. pylori* in ≥80% of cases, with a very low rate of reinfection. Eradication of *H. pylori* favorably alters the natural course of peptic ulcer disease; the recurrence rate significantly diminished to <5%. Elimination of infection will potentially decrease the incidence of gastric cancer.

PREVENTION

No recognized methods or vaccines are currently available to prevent gastroduodenal disease caused by *H. pylori.* Treatment of household or casual contacts is not recommended. Standard precautions are sufficient for hospitalized persons. Endoscopic equipment should be thoroughly disinfected between uses (Chapter 105).

REVIEWS

Blecker U, Gold BD: Treatment of *Helicobacter pylori* infection: A review. *Pediatr Infect Dis J* 1997;16:391–9.

Dooley CP, Cohen H, Fitzgibbons PL, et al: Prevalence of *Helicobacter pylori* infection and histologic gastritis in asymptomatic persons. *N Engl J Med* 1989;321:1562–6.

Gold BD, Colletti RB, Abbott M, et al: *Helicobacter pylori* infection in children: Recommendations for diagnosis and treatment. *J Pediatr Gastroenterol Nutr* 2000;31:490–7.

Peterson WL, Fendrick AM, Cave DR, et al. *Helicobacter pylori*–related disease: Guidelines for testing and treatment. *Arch Intern Med* 2000; 160:1285–91.

Salcedo JA, Al-Kawas F: Treatment of *Helicobacter pylori* infection. *Arch Intern Med* 1998;158:842–51.

KEY ARTICLES

Alm RA, Trust TJ: Analysis of the genetic diversity of *Helicobacter pylori:* The tale of two genomes. *J Mol Med* 1999;77:834–46.

Bode G, Rothenbacher D, Brenner H, et al: *Helicobacter pylori* and abdominal symptoms: A population-based study among preschool children in southern Germany. *Pediatrics* 1998;101:634–7.

Braden B, Posselt HG, Ahrens P, et al: New immunoassay in stool provides an accurate noninvasive diagnostic method for *Helicobacter pylori* screening in children. *Pediatrics* 2000;106:115–7.

Breslin NP, O'Morain CA: Noninvasive diagnosis of *Helicobacter pylori:* A review. *Helicobacter* 1997;2:111–7.

Corvaglia L, Bontems P, Devaster JM, et al: Accuracy of serology and ^{13}C-urea breath test for detection of *Helicobacter pylori* in children. *Pediatr Infect Dis J* 1999;18:976–9.

Drumm B, Peraz-Peraz GI, Blaser MJ, et al: Intrafamilial clustering of *Helicobacter pylori* infection. *N Engl J Med* 1990;322:359–63.

Graham DY, Yamaoka Y: Disease-specific *Helicobacter pylori* virulence factors: The unfulfilled promise. *Helicobacter* 2000;5(Suppl 1):S3–9; discussion S27–31.

Feldman M, Cryer B, Lee E, et al: Role of seroconversion in confirming cure of *Helicobacter pylori* infection. *JAMA* 1998;280:363–5.

Fendrick AM, Chernew ME, Hirth RA, et al: Clinical and economic effects of population-based *H. pylori* screening to prevent gastric cancer. *Arch Intern Med* 1999;159:142–8.

Forbes GM, Glaser ME, Cullen DJ, et al: Duodenal ulcer treated with *Helicobacter pylori* eradication: Seven-year follow-up. *Lancet* 1994; 343:258–60.

Friedman LS: *Helicobacter pylori* and nonulcer dyspepsia. *N Engl J Med* 1998;339:1928–30.

Ganga-Zandzou PS, Michaud L, Vincent P, et al: Natural outcome of *Helicobacter* infection in asymptomatic children: A two-year follow-up study. *Pediatrics* 1999;104:216–21.

Imrie C, Rowland M, Bourke B, et al: Is *Helicobacter pylori* infection in childhood a risk factor for gastric cancer? *Pediatrics* 2001;107:373–80.

Khanna B, Cutler A, Israel NR: Use caution with serologic testing for *Helicobacter pylori* infection in children. *J Infect Dis* 1998;178:460–5.

Macarthur C: *Helicobacter pylori* infection and childhood recurrent abdominal pain: Lack of evidence for a cause and effect relationship. *Can J Gastroenterol* 1999;13:607–10.

McColl K, Murray L, El-Omar E, et al: Symptomatic benefit from eradicating *Helicobacter pylori* infection in patients with nonulcer dyspepsia. *N Engl J Med* 1998;339:1869–74.

Moayyedi P, Soo S, Deeks J, et al: Systematic review and economic evaluation of *Helicobacter pylori* eradication treatment for non-ulcer dyspepsia. *BMJ* 2000;321:659–64.

Oderda G, Rapa A, Ronchi B, et al: Detection of *Helicobacter pylori* in stool specimens by non-invasive antigen enzyme immunoassay in children: Multicentre Italian study. *BMJ* 2000;320:347–8.

Ofman JJ, Etchason J, Fullerton S, et al: Management strategies for *Helicobacter pylori*–seropositive patients with dyspepsia: Clinical and economic consequences. *Ann Intern Med* 1997;126:280–91.

Parsonnet J, Friedman GD, Vandersteen DP, et al: *Helicobacter pylori* infection and the risk of gastric carcinoma. *N Engl J Med* 1991; 325:1127–31.

Parsonnet J, Hansen S, Rodriguez L, et al: *Helicobacter pylori* infection and gastric lymphoma. *N Engl J Med* 1994;330:1267–71.

Parsonnet J, Shmuely H, Haggerty T: Fecal and oral shedding of *Helicobacter pylori* from healthy infected adults. *JAMA* 1999;282:2240–5.

Raymond J, Sauvestre C, Kalach N, et al: Immunoblotting and serology for diagnosis of *Helicobacter pylori* infection in children. *Pediatr Infect Dis J* 2000;19:118–21.

Rothenbacher D, Bode G, Berg G, et al: *Helicobacter pylori* among preschool children and their parents: Evidence of parent-child transmission. *J Infect Dis* 1999;179:398–402.

Rowland M, Lambert I, Gormally S, et al: Carbon 13–labeled urea breath test for the diagnosis of *Helicobacter pylori* infection in children. *J Pediatr* 1997;131:815–20.

van der Hulst RW, Rauws EA, Koycu B, et al: *Helicobacter pylori* reinfection is virtually absent after successful eradication. *J Infect Dis* 1997; 176:196–200.

Villako K, Maards H, Tammur R, et al: *Helicobacter* (*Campylobacter*) *pylori* infestation and the development and progression of chronic gastritis: Results of long-term follow-up examination of a random sample. *Endoscopy* 1990;22:114–7.

Yamagata H, Kiyohara Y, Aoyagi K, et al: Impact of *Helicobacter pylori* infection on gastric cancer incidence in a general Japanese population: The Hisayama study. *Arch Intern Med* 2000;160:1962–8.

CHAPTER 76

Acute Enteritis

Nalini Singh ▪ William J. Rodriguez*

Acute enteritis is the leading cause of morbidity and the second most common disease among children in the United States, accounting for 16% of the illnesses in children. It is useful to consider enteritis in terms of pathophysiology, grouping the infectious agents of enteritis by those that cause symptoms primarily by invasive mechanisms, those that interfere with either absorption or digestion, and those that produce enterotoxins and have minimal or no invasive capabilities. Some infectious agents cause disease by a combination of these mechanisms, and the overall clinical picture may reflect the result of the overall aggregate effect.

COMPARATIVE ETIOLOGY

There are numerous bacterial, viral, and parasitic causes of infectious enteritis (Table 76–1). The manifestations of acute enteritis can be classified according to pathogenic mechanisms of disease and principal clinical manifestations (Table 76–2).

Invasive disease is characteristic of **dysentery-like disease,** with *Shigella* as the prototype, in which, in addition to gastrointestinal symptoms, fever and other systemic symptoms such as headache and myalgia may appear. Another form of invasive disease is **typhoid fever,** caused by *Salmonella typhi* and *Salmonella paratyphi.* Systemic invasion, fever, and constipation usually precede the final enteric phase. **Enterotoxigenic disease** is caused by agents that produce enterotoxins, with *Vibrio cholerae* being the prototype.

Viral gastroenteritis is responsible for approximately one third of all cases of gastroenteritis, exceeding bacterial and parasitic causes. Six major categories of viruses are responsible for viral gastroenteritis: rotavirus, enteric adenoviruses, caliciviruses (Norwalk virus), astroviruses, and coronaviruses. Rotavirus is the leading cause of viral gastroenteritis, accounting for 3.5 million cases annually in the United States.

Common-source diarrhea is usually associated with ingestion of contaminated food. This includes ingestion of **preformed enterotoxins** produced by bacteria such as *Staphylococcus aureus* and *Bacillus cereus* that multiply in contaminated foods or toxins, such as from fish, shellfish, and mushrooms. The incubation period after ingestion is usually very short. Vomiting and cramps are the prominent symptoms, and diarrhea may or may not be present.

Heavy metals that leach into canned food or drinks, leading to gastric irritation and emetic syndromes, and preformed toxins found in shellfish and mushrooms are other agents that may mimic symptoms of acute infectious enteritis.

COMPARATIVE PATHOGENESIS

The invasive organisms of dysentery-like disease characteristically cause lesions in the intestinal mucosa and typically involve the

*The views expressed represent those of the author. No official support or endorsement by the U.S. Food and Drug Administration is provided or should be inferred.

TABLE 76–1. Acute Enteritis in the United States

Disease or Agent	Estimated Total Cases Annually	% Foodborne Transmission
Bacteria		
*Aeromonas**		
Bacillus cereus	27,360	100
Campylobacter	2,453,926	80
*Entamoeba histolytica**		
Escherichia coli O157:H7	73,480	85
Escherichia coli, enterotoxigenic	79,420	70
Escherichia coli, non-O157:H7 EHEC	36,740	85
Escherichia coli, other diarrheogenic	79,420	30
Listeria monocytogenes	2,518	99
Salmonella typhi†	824	80
Salmonella, nontyphoidal	1,412,498	95
Shigella	448,240	20
Staphylococcus aureus	185,060	100
Streptococcus	50,920	100
Vibrio cholerae	54	90
Vibrio vulnificus	94	50
Vibrio, other	7,880	65
Yersinia enterocolitica	96,368	90
Viruses		
Astroviruses	3,900,000	1
Caliciviruses*		
Coronaviruses*		
Enteric adenoviruses*		
Norwalk virus	23,000,000	40
Rotavirus	3,900,000	1
Parasites		
Cryptosporidium parvum	300,000	10
Cyclospora cayetanensis	16,264	90
*Dientamoeba fragilis**		
*Entamoeba histolytica**		
Giardia lamblia	2,000,000	10
*Isospora belli**		
Microsporidia*		
Antibiotic-associated		
*Clostridium difficile**		
*Staphylococcus aureus**		

*Insufficient surveillance data to provide estimates.
†More than 70% of cases are acquired abroad.
From Mead PS, Slutsker L, Dietz V, et al: Food-related illness and death in the United States. *Emerg Infect Dis* 1999;5:607–25.

TABLE 76–2. Distinguishing Characteristics of Enteritis Syndromes

Primarily Dysenteric
Fever
Systemic symptoms or malaise
Stool with mucus or blood, possibly foul smelling

Primarily Toxigenic
Usually no or low-grade fever
Dehydration varying with length and severity of symptoms
Watery stools with no mucus or blood, usually not foul smelling

Viral
Fever
May have vomiting, malaise; dehydration may be prominent
Watery stools, no mucus or blood, not foul-smelling

Parasitic
Usually no fever
Watery or mucoid stool, possibly foul-smelling or bloody
Entamoeba histolytica may behave as a dysenteric agent, with bloating and protracted mild diarrhea

Antibiotic-associated Diarrhea
History of current or recent exposure to antimicrobial drugs
Watery to bloody diarrhea with abdominal pain and cramps

Traveler's Diarrhea
Variable symptoms depending on etiology
History of recent travel
Onset of symptoms commonly <72 hours of ingestion
Fever is uncommon
Profuse diarrhea; vomiting is not common
Self-limited, with recovery within 5 days except with dysentery-like syndrome

Common Source
Variable symptoms depending on etiology
Ingestion of food or water in common with others with similar symptoms
Onset of symptoms <72 hours, sometimes minutes, after ingestion
Fever uncommon except with dysentery-like microorganisms
Vomiting is common

terminal ileum or colon, resulting in bloody, foul-smelling diarrhea with leukocytes and erythrocytes in the stools. Enterotoxin-producing organisms typically alter the digestive and absorptive capability at the villous tips, primarily affecting the upper part of the small intestine. They disrupt the electrophysiologic systems responsible for homeostasis, resulting in a net loss of fluid and electrolytes. They produce essentially no mucosal lesions and cause vomiting and diarrhea without inflammatory elements, such as leukocytes in the stools. Some organisms, such as enteropathogenic *Escherichia coli,* alter the digestive and absorptive capability at the villous tips. Viruses cause enteritis by noncytotoxic mechanisms, with stools that are watery, nonmucoid, and nonbloody.

Deaths due to diarrhea reflect the principal problem of disruption of fluid and electrolyte homeostasis, which leads to dehydration, electrolyte imbalance, vascular instability, and shock. In the United States approximately 75–150 deaths occur annually from diarrheal disease, primarily among children <1 year of age born to young mothers who have had little or no prenatal care or education. These deaths occur in a seasonal pattern between October and February, concurrent with the rotavirus season. Early recognition of enteric illness and appropriate supportive care with rehydration are key steps to reducing these deaths.

DYSENTERIC SYNDROMES

NONTYPHOIDAL SALMONELLA

ETIOLOGY

Salmonella species are gram-negative enteric bacteria, named after D. E. Salmon, who first isolated *Salmonella choleraesuis.* There are more than 2400 antigenically distinct **serotypes,** or **serovars,** of *Salmonella* in nature. Typing systems use the flagellar or **H antigen,** and the somatic or polysaccharide **O antigen.** Historically, the serotype name has been written as the species, such as *S. typhimurium,* but the nomenclature is changing. Currently, all *Salmonella* serotypes belong to two species: *S. bongori* and *S. enterica,* also known as *S. choleraesuis. S. bongori* contains fewer than 10 rare serovars. *S. enterica* is subdivided into 6 subspecies: *S. arizonae, S. choleraesuis, S. gallinarum, S. paratyphi, S. pullorum,* and *S. typhi.* In a study (Olsen et al., 2001) of salmonellosis in the United States from 1987–97, the most common *Salmonella* serotypes were Typhimurium (24%), Enteritidis (22%), Heidelberg (8%), Newport (5%), and Hadar (4%). *Salmonella* Typhimurium is associated with most chronic carriers in the United States. *S. typhi* and *S. paratyphi* are highly adapted to human hosts, whereas other *Salmonella* species are adapted to nonhuman hosts or are not adapted to any specific host. *Salmonella* survives within macrophages, and can harbor many a variety of plasmids that encode virulence factors or confer antimicrobial resistance.

Transmission. The primary source of *Salmonella* infections, 95% of cases, is foodborne transmission, especially from dairy and poultry products contaminated by food handlers or by the animals themselves. Methods of mass production, storage, and distribution of foods make it easier to disseminate *Salmonella* if contamination occurs. Contaminated eggshells of raw eggs have been specifically implicated as a source. In addition, infected persons without symptoms, or **chronic carriers,** serve as reservoirs and sources of continuous spread. Intrafamilial spread to infants can occur through contaminated food, although person-to-person spread is unusual outside of nurseries or hospitals because of the large number of organisms required for infection of healthy persons.

Salmonella infections associated with reptile exposure are becoming more common, with approximately 7% of all cases of salmonellosis in humans associated with pet reptile or amphibian contact. Many reptiles are colonized with *Salmonella* and intermittently shed organisms in their feces. Persons become infected by ingesting *Salmonella* after handling a reptile or objects contaminated by a reptile and then failing to wash their hands properly. Pet turtles were an important source of salmonellosis in the United States until commercial distribution of pet turtles <4 inches long was banned in 1975. The popularity of other reptiles as pets is growing, and an estimated 3% of households in the United States now have a reptile. Rare *Salmonella* serotypes, such as Java, Marina, Stanley, Poona, and Chameleon, which are associated with reptiles, are increasingly isolated from humans.

EPIDEMIOLOGY

Salmonella causes approximately 1.4 million illnesses and 600 deaths annually in the United States. Recent declines in food-

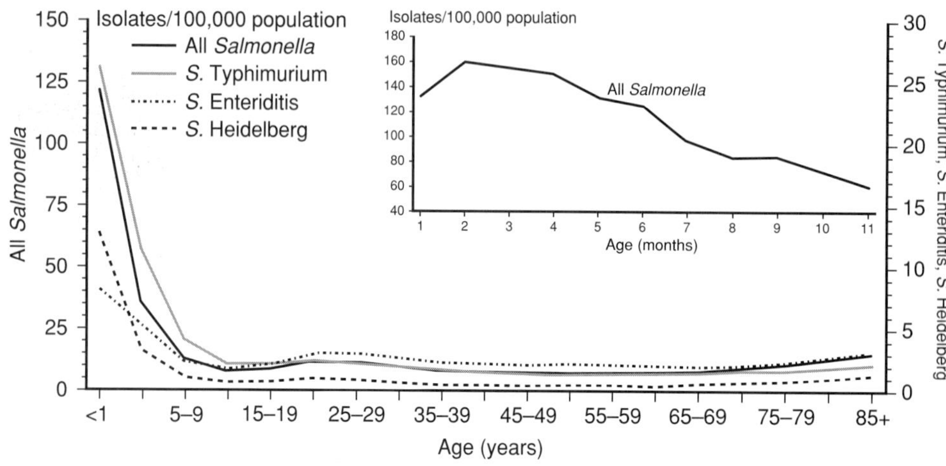

FIGURE 76–1. Isolation rates by age and sex for all *Salmonella* and *Salmonella* serogroups Typhimurium, Enteritidis, and Heidelberg in the United States, 1987–1997. Inset shows isolation rate for all *Salmonella* among infants. (From Olsen SJ, Bishop R, Brenner FW, et al: The changing epidemiology of *Salmonella:* Trends in serotypes isolated from humans in the United States, 1987–1997. *J Infect Dis* 2001;183: 753–61.)

associated outbreaks may reflect changes in the meat, poultry, and egg industries. Most cases do not occur in recognized outbreaks but, rather, as sporadic infections. The annual isolation rate from stool cultures is 3 per 100,000 persons, but the peak is 159.5 per 100,000 persons in the second month of life (Fig. 76–1). Rates decline abruptly after infancy and remain stable throughout life, with a slight increase after the age of 70 years. There is a marked seasonality, with the number of cases approximately doubling in warm summer months.

Most cases of reptile-associated salmonellosis occur in infants and young children. In 1994, 413 (81%) of 513 *Salmonella* Marina cases occurred in children <1 year of age, whereas only 4301 (14%) of 30,723 reported cases of salmonellosis occurred in children <1 year of age. During 1989–1998, 516 (24%) of 2150 *Salmonella* isolates with reptile-associated serotypes were from children <4 years of age, whereas 50,755 (19%) of 267,131 other serotypes were from this age group. Because infants and immunocompromised persons have increased susceptibility, many reptile-associated *Salmonella* infections involve serious complications, including septicemia and meningitis.

PATHOGENESIS

Most *Salmonella* infections are asymptomatic or mild. Oral ingestion of at least 100,000 viable organisms is required to cause enteritis. Natural defenses, such as a gastric pH of ≤2.0, and other nonspecific mechanisms, such as the normal intestinal flora and intestinal flow, may protect against infection. Conditions that cause achlorhydria (e.g., antacids, H_2 blockers), alter normal intestinal flora (e.g., broad-spectrum antibiotics), or decrease intestinal transit (e.g., surgery, opiates) may predispose to *Salmonella* infection.

Once the organisms survive transit through the stomach, facilitated in some instances by the rapidity of gastric emptying, they multiply and may penetrate the epithelium and invade **Peyer's patches.** The specialized ileal **M cells** overlying Peyer's patches internalize particles from the lumen and transfer them to underlying macrophages and may facilitate *Salmonella* penetration of epithelium. The predominant clinical manifestations depend on either the production of a **cytotoxin** that results in cell destruction and dysentery-like diarrhea or production of an **enterotoxin** that leads to increased prostaglandin synthesis and elevated levels of cyclic adenosine monophosphate, resulting in enterotoxigenic diarrhea that is clear, without blood or mucus. If bacteria invade the intestinal endothelium, a polymorphonuclear leukocyte response in the lamina propria protects against further invasion. Additional manifestations depend on whether bacteremia occurs.

SYMPTOMS AND CLINICAL MANIFESTATIONS

Ingestion of a large inoculum is associated with a short incubation period of <1 week, usually 24–48 hours. A prodromal phase in young children may include behavioral changes, such as listlessness and decreased feeding. The highest incidence of symptomatic enteritis occurs among infants, whereas older children and adults may have asymptomatic infection. Symptoms are variable but are usually self-limited and include colicky abdominal pain, nausea, vomiting, loose stools, and a low-grade fever. Illness among infants usually begins suddenly with diarrhea and vomiting (Table 76–3). A low-grade fever is observed in many infants, although this is not useful in differentiating uncomplicated gastroenteritis from invasive *Salmonella* infection, particularly in infants <6 months of age. Diarrhea is often described as green (reflecting the rapidity of the intestinal transit time) and foul smelling. Blood may or may not be present.

Usually the disease is self-limited, with resolution in 1–3 weeks. Healthy older children generally are free of symptoms in 2–5 days. Bacteremia occurs in >5% of infants with salmonellosis and also

TABLE 76–3. Epidemiology and Clinical Manifestations of Non-typhoidal *Salmonella* Infections

Season	Year-round
Vectors	Food, other humans, reptiles
Primary age	<1 yr, >60 yr
Incubation	<1 wk usually 24–48 hr
Symptoms	Fever (++++)
	Malaise (++++)
	Abdominal pain (++++)
	Diarrhea (++++)
	Nausea (+++)
	Vomiting (++)
	Headache (+)
	Constipation (+)
	Encephalopathy (+)
Duration of symptoms	2–7 days
Differential diagnosis	Enterotoxigenic agents
	Dysenteric agents
	Food-associated agents or toxins
	Viruses

++++ = Very common; +++ = common; ++ = sometimes occurs; + = uncommon.

among immunocompromised persons, such as those who have cancer, are taking corticosteroids, or have hemoglobinopathies.

Physical Examination Findings

Many patients, especially older persons, have no symptoms and no physical manifestations. Illness among infants is more likely to cause a fever and listlessness. Abdominal findings include tenderness with increased bowel sounds and abdominal cramps. The state of hydration, tearing, mucous membrane moisture, and skin turgor usually reflects the severity and the duration of the enteritis. A fever, with or without enteric symptoms, may be the only manifestation of illness. An enteric fever–like syndrome not unlike that seen with *S. typhi,* with a fever to 41°C (105.8 °F), can occur with nontyphoidal *Salmonella* infections. Extra-abdominal findings may reflect bacteremia and foci, such as arthritis with bony tenderness or inability to move an extremity, and meningitis with extreme irritability, lethargy, or bulging fontanelles.

DIAGNOSIS

Differential Diagnosis

The differential diagnosis includes *Shigella,* enterotoxigenic *E. coli, Yersinia enterocolitica,* and *Campylobacter* infections. The patient usually has a more acutely toxic condition with shigellosis. Confirmation of *Salmonella* infection in other persons exposed to the same food suggests foodborne disease. Toxigenic diarrhea, such as that caused by enterotoxigenic *S. aureus, B. cereus,* and *Clostridium perfringens,* is associated with food contamination and seldom has significant fever.

Laboratory Evaluation

The peripheral WBC count may be normal, depressed, or, more commonly, increased. Occult blood is reported in 83% and fecal leukocytes in 54% of children with *Salmonella* enteritis, with relatively fewer leukocytes than in children with shigellosis. The presence of mononuclear cells in the stool suggests typhoid fever.

Microbiologic Evaluation

Stool cultures are positive in more than 90% of cases with three stool cultures obtained at 24-hour intervals. Serologic testing, as with **febrile agglutinins** or the **Widal test,** is not recommended for diagnosis. The serologic response to *S. typhi* O and H antigens characteristically is minimal and may not reach titers indicative of infection. There is a high frequency of cross-reactions with other bacteria and serotypes of *Salmonella.* Properly performed cultures of blood and stool are far superior to serologic testing for the diagnosis of *Salmonella* infection.

Because of the increased risk of bacteremia, blood cultures are recommended for children <3 months of age who are believed to have a *Salmonella* infection regardless of the presence or absence of a fever, for children 3–12 months of age with fever ≥39°C (102.2°F), or for children who appear lethargic or moderately ill.

TREATMENT

Salmonellosis is generally self-limited in patients ≥3 months of age, and only supportive therapy is indicated for infection localized to the intestinal tract. Specific antimicrobial therapy is indicated for patients with bacteremia or extraintestinal dissemination and for high-risk patients with noninvasive gastroenteritis, including infants <3 months of age, immunocompromised persons, and persons with hemoglobinopathies or chronic gastrointestinal disease. Ampicillin, TMP-SMZ, and third-generation cephalosporins have been effective. The quinolones, which are not recommended for use in persons <18 years of age or in pregnant women, and chloramphenicol may also be effective alternatives. However, even antibiotics with good bile levels may fail to eradicate *Salmonella* from the intestinal tracts of infants. About one third of *Salmonella* Typhimurium were reported to be resistant to ampicillin, chloramphenicol, streptomycin, sulfonamides, and tetracycline.

Infections with *S. typhi* (typhoid fever) and *S. choleraesuis* subspecies *choleraesuis* are exceptional because of the increased risk of systemic infection. These infections should be treated with antimicrobial agents, even if symptoms are localized to the intestine. If the blood culture is positive for *Salmonella,* antimicrobial treatment should be considered, even if no identifiable extraintestinal focus is found (Table 76–4). In many cases the patient returns to medical care because of a positive blood culture 24–48 hours after the initial presentation, but with spontaneous resolution of clinical symptoms. These patients do not require treatment, but a blood culture should be repeated to document resolution of bacteremia. Patients with continuing symptoms or persistent bacteremia should be treated. Oral antimicrobial therapy for uncomplicated enteric illness is ineffective. There also has been a controversy about such treatment prolonging the shedding and ultimately promoting chronic carriage as well as the development of antimicrobial resistance.

COMPLICATIONS

Salmonellosis, particularly in the very young, immunocompromised, or elderly patient, can be associated with invasive disease such as bacteremia. Estimates of such complications have been as high as 15%, particularly in high-risk groups.

Salmonellosis is usually a self-limited disease in persons >3 months of age with no risk factors. When bacteremia occurs, it may be intermittent or continuous. The ability to cause extraintestinal intravascular and extravascular complications seems to be determined not only by the host but also by the type of *Salmonella. S. choleraesuis* subspecies *choleraesuis* frequently invades the blood but also invades extravascular sites such as the bones and joints. Stool cultures may be negative, and several blood cultures may be necessary to document infection. Reactive arthritis may also occur.

Among the nontyphoidal *Salmonella, Salmonella* Heidelberg has been associated with a high rate of sepsis among infants, with mortality as high as 20%. Meningitis, liver abscesses or nodules, and pulmonary involvement have been reported. Approximately 40% of infants with meningitis have died, and survivors have a high rate of neurologic impairment.

PROGNOSIS

Approximately 45% of patients continue to excrete *Salmonella* in the stool 12 weeks after an acute infection, and 5% excrete *Salmonella* 5 months after the infection. Thus there is usually no need for routine follow-up cultures. Approximately 1% of patients asymptomatically excrete *Salmonella* in the stool for >12 months after infection and are considered **chronic carriers.**

PREVENTION

No vaccine is available for the prevention of *Salmonella* infections. Good handwashing with soap and water and hygienic measures are the best means of controlling the large inoculum of *Salmonella* needed for person-to-person spread. Similarly, poultry products such as eggs should be considered potentially contaminated and should be handled and cooked appropriately.

TABLE 76–4. Therapy for Nontyphoidal *Salmonella* Infection

Condition	Suggested Regimen	Alternative Regimen
Acute *Salmonella* enteritis in a patient >3 months of age	Usually no treatment is needed	
Acute *Salmonella* enteritis in a patient <3 months of age	Ampicillin 200 mg/kg/day divided q6hr IV for 5–7 days *or* Cefotaxime 150 mg/kg/day divided q6hr IV for 5–7 days	
Acute *Salmonella* enteritis in a patient with a hemoglobinopathy or immunosuppression	Ampicillin *or* cefotaxime for 5–7 days	Chloramphenicol 75 mg/kg/day divided q6hr IV for 5–7 days
Bacteremia	Ampicillin *or* cefotaxime for 10 days	HIV-infected patients should be treated for 4–6 wk
Extraintestinal complications	Ampicillin or cefotaxime, duration and doses dictated by system involved	—
Chronic carrier state (>1 year)	Usually no treatment is required. If eradication is necessary, i.e., for public health measures, amoxicillin 50–100 mg/kg/day (max 6 g) divided q6hr PO for 6 wk; if cholelithiasis, begin treatment 10 days before cholecystectomy and continue for 4 weeks after cholecystectomy	Adult carriers can be given ciprofloxacin 500 mg bid PO *or* norfloxacin 400 mg bid PO for 4 wk

Changes in the food industry, such as provision of chlorinated drinking water to turkeys, have contributed to the decline in salmonellosis. In 1998 the USDA began routine testing for *Salmonella* in large, federally inspected raw meat and poultry plants.

Families should be aware of the risk of acquiring salmonellosis from reptiles. Transmission of *Salmonella* from reptiles can be prevented by thorough handwashing with soap and water after handling of reptiles or reptile cages. Children <5 years of age and immunocompromised persons should avoid contact with reptiles. Pet reptiles should not be allowed to roam freely in the home or living areas and should be kept out of kitchens and food preparation areas to prevent contamination. Sinks or bathtubs used to bathe reptiles or to wash their dishes should be thoroughly disinfected. Reptiles should not be kept in childcare centers.

SALMONELLA TYPHI (TYPHOID FEVER)

Typhoid fever, or **enteric fever,** is distinguished from other diseases caused by *Salmonella* because of the potential for extraintestinal manifestations, complications, and the likelihood of a prolonged fever.

ETIOLOGY

S. typhi and *S. paratyphi* are separate subspecies of *S. enterica.* The Vi antigen of *S. typhi* and *S. paratyphi* can inhibit O antigen agglutination because it is so abundant. The Vi antigen is a homopolymer of *N*-acetylgalactosaminouronic acid, and is identical to that of *Citrobacter freundii.*

Transmission. *S. typhi* and *S. paratyphi* colonize only humans, and therefore transmission requires close contact with a person who has typhoid fever or is a chronic carrier. Foodborne transmission accounts for about 80% of all cases.

EPIDEMIOLOGY

The incidence of typhoid fever has decreased in the United States from more than 1 case per 100,000 population in 1955 to 0.16 case per 100,000 in 1992. Approximately 350–400 cases occur annually in the United States. The disease, though well documented, is rare in children <12 months of age. Most cases in recent years are reported among Latin Americans, Asians, and Pacific Islanders, suggesting the predilection for contact with sources outside the United States. The disease is endemic in Asia, Africa, and Central and South America, where in some countries rates 100-fold greater than those reported in the United States are common. The incidence of typhoid is 3–30 cases per 100,000 travelers to developing countries per month. Humans are the only reservoir and source of *S. typhi.* Those infected shed the bacteria, even while being treated, increasing the risk of spread. Many persons who shed *S. typhi* have had no identifiable episode of illness.

PATHOGENESIS

When a large number of virulent, typhoid bacilli (about 10^7 from studies of volunteers) are ingested, they multiply in the intestinal tract, penetrate the mucosa of the intestine, and use the lymphatics in the mesentery to reach the reticuloendothelial system. These strains inhibit the postphagocytic oxidative metabolism by polymorphonuclear leukocytes. Monocytes not only are inefficient in destroying the bacilli but also help disseminate the microbe into the mesenteric lymph nodes and other organs of the reticuloendothelial system. Low-grade bacteremia and bacteriuria precede the ultimate appearance of the typhoid bacilli in the stools as the infection reaches the biliary tract.

In contrast to nontyphoidal *Salmonella,* acute infection with *S. typhi* usually follows ingestion of a small inoculum. Approximately 4% of patients continue to shed *S. typhi* asymptomatically in the stool for >1 year and are considered chronic carriers. Patients with previous conditions that affect the urinary tract, such as tuberculosis or *Schistosoma haematobium* infection, may continue to shed *S. typhi* in their urine. Patients with *Schistosoma mansoni* infection may have prolonged bacteremia with *S. typhi* as well as with *S. choleraesuis.*

SYMPTOMS AND CLINICAL MANIFESTATIONS

The incubation period of typhoid fever is 3–60 days, usually 7–14 days. During the first week the patient has a fever, headache, and abdominal pain that worsen over 48–72 hours (Table 76–5). Nausea, a decrease in appetite, and constipation are observed during this phase.

The untreated disease runs its course over a period of 2–3 weeks, marked by weight loss. If abdominal rigidity ensues, perforation is likely; this complication is rare in children and common in adults. Occasionally, hematochezia or melena may be present. Among 94 children in one series (Colon et al., 1975), the symptoms included temperature >37.8°C (100.0 °F) in 79 (84%), lethargy in 49 (52%), diarrhea in 47 (50%), vomiting in 43 (46%), lower abdominal pain in 36 (38.8%), anorexia in 21 (22%), nausea in 17 (18.3%), cough in 11 (12.2%), and headache in 6 (7%). Encephalopathy manifested by psychosis or mania also may occur.

Physical Examination Findings

A fever as high as 41°C (105.8°F) is not uncommon. The skin feels hot and dry, and the conjunctivae are injected. Worsening abdominal tenderness occurs during the second week, and there is a paucity of bowel sounds. The patient may manifest pain on abdominal palpation. The spleen is often enlarged, and hepatomegaly, seen in approximately 23% of children, is present along with generalized lymphadenopathy. The patient may appear confused.

TABLE 76–5. Epidemiologic and Clinical Manifestations of *Salmonella typhi* Infections

Season	Year-round
Primary age	All
Incubation period	1–4 weeks
Symptoms	Fever (++++)
	Malaise (++++)
	Abdominal pain (+++)
	Diarrhea (+++)
	Vomiting (+++)
	Nausea (++)
	Constipation (++)
	Encephalopathy (++)
	Headache (+)
Duration of symptoms	3–4 weeks
Vector	Other humans, food
Differential diagnosis	Epstein-Barr virus
	Cytomegalovirus
	Rickettsia
	Francisella
	Leptospira
	Brucella

++++ = Very common; +++ = common; ++ = sometimes occurs; + = uncommon.

A disassociation between pulse and fever has been described, that is, relative bradycardia in the presence of a fever. **Rose spots,** discrete salmon-colored macular papules 2–4 mm in diameter on the trunk, are seen in approximately 20% of patients.

DIAGNOSIS

The diagnosis of typhoid fever should be considered for patients with fevers lasting longer than 1 week who have a recent history of travel to an endemic area or known exposure to *S. typhi.*

Differential Diagnosis

Other potential causes of symptoms similar to typhoid fever include sepsis with agents such as *Brucella, Francisella, Leptospira,* rickettsial infection, infection with Epstein-Barr virus (EBV), or cytomegalovirus (CMV), tuberculosis, or a lymphoproliferative disorder.

Laboratory Evaluation

Anemia exacerbated by intestinal blood loss is common, and thrombocytopenia may occur. The peripheral WBC count may be decreased, commonly with granulocytosis, especially in children, from 65% to more than 95%. Hepatic transaminase enzyme levels may be mildly elevated.

Microbiologic Diagnosis

In the course of typhoid fever, bacteremias occur at two distinct stages. A primary transient bacteremia occurs within hours of ingestion of the pathogen and is quickly cleared by the reticuloendothelial system. A secondary bacteremia occurs after an incubation period of 2 weeks as bacteria re-enter the bloodstream from reticuloendothelial areas in the liver, spleen, and bone marrow. This second, sustained bacteremia accompanies the onset of clinical typhoid fever. The rate of positive blood culture drops from 90% during the first week of illness to about 50% during the third week. A urine culture may be helpful; 15% of patients may shed *S. typhi* in the urine during the second week of illness. A bone marrow culture may be very useful for diagnosis as the disease evolves. Early in the illness, culture of the rose spots may also yield the bacterium.

The bacterium is detected by growth in special agars, such as MacConkey, eosin–methylene blue, and *Salmonella-Shigella* agar. Isolates believed to be *S. typhi* are identified by biochemical tests and confirmed by serologic tests, which detect somatic (O) and flagellar (H) antigens. Tests that employ DNA probes and monoclonal antibodies against protein antigens of *S. typhi* are being evaluated.

Serologic Diagnosis. Fourfold or greater rises in *Salmonella* agglutinins by serologic tests as the **Widal test** may be useful epidemiologically, although they are not useful for clinical diagnosis or management. EIA tests with *S. typhi* protein or lipopolysaccharide antigen have been reported to have superior sensitivity to the Widal test for the diagnosis of typhoid fever. Food handlers have been found to be carriers of *S. typhi* by indirect hemagglutination tests using highly purified Vi antigen. The procedure is 79% sensitive compared with culture. Similar experience has been noted with Vi indirect fluorescent antibody tests.

TREATMENT

Initial care involves appropriate fluid and blood replacement. Definitive antimicrobial therapy depends on susceptibility of the or-

TABLE 76–6. Therapy for *Salmonella typhi* Infection

Recommended Regimen	Alternative Regimen
Ampicillin 200 mg/kg/day divided q6hr IV	Chloramphenicol 75–100 mg/kg/day divided q6hr IV
or	*or*
Cefotaxime 150 mg/kg/day divided q6hr IV	Chloramphenicol 75 mg/kg/day divided q6hr PO
or	
Ceftriaxone 100 mg/kg/day divided q12hr IV or IM	

For treatment of carrier state, see Table 76–4.

ganisms (Table 76–6). For susceptible *S. typhi,* ampicillin, chloramphenicol, or TMP-SMZ for at least 2 weeks is adequate. For multiply antimicrobial-resistant *S. typhi* acquired in Asia (India, Pakistan), and Africa (Egypt), ceftriaxone or ofloxacin or ciprofloxacin should be considered. Furazolidone has also been used.

Chloramphenicol reduces the mortality from 12% to 4%, and most patients become afebrile within 5 days after the onset of therapy. Some strains of *S. typhi* have been found resistant to chloramphenicol; the most notorious of such strains was described in a 1972 epidemic of typhoid fever in Mexico. Other resistant strains have been reported from Africa and Southeast Asia. Many of these epidemics have been self-limited, however. Response of susceptible strains to parenteral ampicillin is predictable. The third-generation cephalosporins have an overall relapse rate of about 7%. In vitro strain susceptibility should be interpreted with caution because clinical failure has been reported with aminoglycosides, furazolidone, and first- and second-generation cephalosporins.

Patients with intestinal perforation need immediate surgery and should be treated with a third-generation cephalosporin, ampicillin, or chloramphenicol as part of a regimen active against facultative aerobic and anaerobic enteric flora, such as that provided by the addition of an aminoglycoside along with either clindamycin or metronidazole (Chapter 77). For patients with severe enteric fever, toxemia or shock, at presentation and no evidence of perforation, dexamethasone 3 mg/kg followed by 1 mg/kg/day for at least 2 days can be lifesaving.

Chronic Carriers. Chronic carriers who have cholelithiasis and *Salmonella* infection susceptible to ampicillin may be treated with high-dose ampicillin or high-dose amoxicillin combined with probenecid for at least 7–10 days or cholecystectomy (Table 76–4). Carriers without demonstrable gallbladder or biliary tract disease can be treated for 6 weeks with parenteral ampicillin. Ciprofloxacin is the drug of choice for adult carriers with persistent *Salmonella* excretion.

COMPLICATIONS

At least 10% of patients who have typhoid fever shed *S. typhi* for about 3 months, and 4% become chronic carriers. The biliary tract constitutes a harbor for *Salmonella,* particularly if there is previous scarring or concomitant gallstones.

Other complications include intestinal perforation, seen in 3% of all patients but more commonly in those 11 years of age or older. Bacterial multiplication leads directly to necrosis of the intestinal wall. The perforation usually involves the distal ileum and rarely the proximal colon. It is most likely to occur during the second week of untreated illness. These patients require a team approach that often includes surgical intervention, especially to limit blood loss through intestinal hemorrhage. Antimicrobial treatment of this complication should provide at least 10 days of broad-spectrum antimicrobial therapy for enteric flora in addition to antimicrobial coverage for *S. typhi.*

Coagulation abnormalities documented by laboratory tests are common but are usually self-limited. Approximately 10% of patients experience a hemorrhage. The thrombocytopenia and partial coagulopathy may dictate the need for appropriate replacement of blood, platelets, and clotting factors.

Pneumonia secondary to either the *S. typhi* infection or superinfection with exogenous (usually nosocomial) flora occurs mostly among children up to 5 years of age, affecting approximately 15% of children with these infections. Pneumonia is more common during the second to the third week of illness. Treatment consists of broadening the antimicrobial spectrum, depending on the known or likely resident nosocomial flora.

Anemia is common among patients <10 years of age, probably because of infection and intestinal blood loss. The hemoglobin level may drop to as low as 5.2 g/dL and may require blood replacement. Enzymatic deficiencies such as G6PD deficiency are prevalent in some ethnic groups, such as patients of Chinese or Mediterranean origin. Chloramphenicol or sulfonamides may aggravate hemolysis.

Encephalopathy, manifest as mania or psychosis or as cerebellar signs, has been found in untreated patients; the onset is during the second to the third week of illness. Encephalopathy is an ominous sign that is associated with high death rates, especially if the level of consciousness is affected. Once treated, the neurologic symptoms improve over the subsequent week. Seizures have been reported frequently in children up to 10 years of age; they are managed with conventional anticonvulsant therapy.

Myocarditis, although commonly detected by an ECG, is usually asymptomatic, but it may progress to frank cardiac failure necessitating appropriate cardiovascular support.

Glomerulonephritis and pyelonephritis are usually self-limited and require no treatment. Fifteen percent of patients may have urine cultures positive for *S. typhi* during the second week of illness. If renal failure occurs, appropriate support should be instituted.

Hepatitis, when present, is usually subclinical and requires no specific treatment. Elevation of hepatic enzyme levels to up to $2\frac{1}{2}$ times normal have been reported at the time of presentation.

Suppurative complications need to be managed with consultative support and appropriate antimicrobial drugs. Osteomyelitis of the spine or long bones, septic arthritis, soft-tissue abscesses, nodular hepatic lesions with frank abscesses, and mycotic aneurysms of the distal aorta and femoral arteries have been described. There are relatively few cases in the literature of suppurative typhoidal meningitis. Although both meningitis and encephalitis are recognized as complications and sequelae of typhoid fever, *S. typhi* meningitis without enteric symptoms is also known. Reactive arthritis and Reiter's syndrome have been reported occasionally with typhoid fever, although urethritis usually does not occur in these patients.

PROGNOSIS

More than 99% of patients respond rapidly to treatment. Although the overall mortality is $<1\%$, children <1 year of age and adults >30 years of age have a mortality as high as 10%. Death is more commonly associated with complications of pneumonia and intestinal perforation. Approximately 4% of patients continue to shed *S. typhi* asymptomatically in the stool for >1 year; they are chronic carriers.

PREVENTION

Good hygienic and sanitary measures are important, especially for those living in endemic areas, household contacts with *S. typhi* carriers, laboratory workers who have frequent contact with *S. typhi,* and travelers to endemic areas (Chapter 104). Three different types of typhoid vaccine have been licensed in the United States: (1) an oral live-attenuated vaccine, Ty 21a; (2) a parenteral heat-phenol-inactivated, killed whole-cell vaccine; and (3) a parenteral capsular polysaccharide vaccine, Vi CPS. The efficacy of the three vaccines ranges from 17% to 66%. In the United States, targeted immunization is recommended for travelers to developing countries in South Asia, North and West Africa, and the impoverished areas of Latin America; long-term (2–4 weeks) travelers and backpackers; and travelers staying with families in developing countries. However, immunization is not a substitute for consumption of purified water and food that has been prepared properly because vaccines are not 100% effective. Vaccination should also be given to immunocompromised persons or persons with cholelithiasis; such persons are likely to have complications from enteric fever. The vaccine's protection can be overwhelmed by a large inoculum of *S. typhi.* Immunization is also indicated for persons with intimate exposure (e.g., household contact) to a documented *S. typhi* carrier and for laboratory technicians with repeated exposure to *S. typhi.* Routine immunization of schoolchildren with typhoid vaccine also is practiced in some countries with substantial typhoid risk. Typhoid vaccine is not indicated for prevention of secondary cases in common-source outbreaks or after natural disasters, including floods. Routine vaccination of sewage sanitation workers is not indicated in the United States, but may be implemented in typhoid-endemic areas.

SHIGELLA

ETIOLOGY

Shigella is a gram-negative enteric rod with a worldwide distribution. It is a major cause of enteric illness in the United States. Four serologic groups of this non-lactose-fermenting bacillus (some are slow, lactose-fermenting) and more than 40 serotypes have been identified. These groups and representative serotypes are group A (*Shigella dysenteriae*), group B (*Shigella flexneri*), group C (*Shigella boydii*), and group D (*Shigella sonnei*). *S. dysenteriae* type I causes the most severe disease; *S. flexneri* strains are less virulent. *S. boydii* and *S. sonnei* generally cause self-limited disease. In the United States, *S. sonnei* causes 60–80% of cases, followed by *S. flexneri. S. sonnei* has been the predominant serotype recovered in developed countries; *S. flexneri* is most commonly reported in developing countries. *S. dysenteriae* type I (the Shiga bacillus) is rare in the United States but is widespread in rural Africa and the Indian subcontinent. *S. boydii* is also uncommon in the United States.

Transmission. Shigellosis is highly communicable. Foodborne transmission accounts for about 20% of cases. An attack rate of approximately 50% has been reported in food outbreaks. The bacteria are easily transmitted by the fecal-oral route from person to person, particularly by inadequate handwashing by food handlers, or in contaminated food or water in which the bacteria can survive for months. Rodents, cockroaches, and flies may carry the organism on their legs and in their feces and mechanically transfer the bacteria and serve as reservoirs of disease.

EPIDEMIOLOGY

Humans are the only known natural host of *Shigella,* although experimental infection has been established in rhesus monkeys. The highest infection rate occurs among children 1–4 years of age. Approximately 450,000 cases of shigellosis occur annually in the United States. Factors contributing to spread of infection are poor sanitary conditions, crowded environments, and use of contaminated water for human consumption or washing of vegetables. High rates of shigellosis are found in daycare centers, long-term care facilities, and on Native American reservations.

PATHOGENESIS

As few as 200 cfu of some strains of *Shigella* can establish an infection. After a period of 12–48 hours, and sometimes up to 1 week, the organisms that attach to and multiply in the small intestine cause local damage by invasion or production of enterotoxins. Once ingested, *Shigella* organisms are almost always confined to the intestine. A virulence plasmid is critical for ability of *Shigella* to invade epithelial cells. Other chromosomal regions may also influence invasiveness. Most *Shigella* species other than *S. dysenteriae* produce a chromosomally mediated cytotoxin, usually in small amounts, which plays a role in the clinical manifestations. Although the **Shiga toxin** produced by *S. dysenteriae* has been called a neurotoxin because of its adverse neurologic effect on experimental animals, its effect appears to be mediated primarily through endothelial cell damage. Even microscopic myocardial hemorrhages have been observed in experimental animals exposed to this toxin. When the cytotoxin is used in the rabbit ileal loop model, the intraluminal intestinal fluid is characteristically bloody. Impairment of absorptive, rather than secretive, mechanisms is considered to be the causative mechanism of fluid loss after damage to the villous epithelium.

SYMPTOMS AND CLINICAL MANIFESTATIONS

Patients present with an abrupt, high fever, changes in affect, or even seizures (Table 76–7). Occasionally vomiting is described.

TABLE 76–7. Epidemiologic and Clinical Manifestations of *Shigella* Infection

Season	Summer
Primary age	<4 years
Incubation period	12–48 hr, maybe 1 wk
Symptoms	High fever (++++)
	Abdominal tenderness (++++)
	Dysentery (+++)
	Fever (+++)
	Headache (++)
	Diarrhea (++)
	Cramps (++)
	Seizures (+)
	Nausea (+)
	Vomiting (+)
	Respiratory symptoms (+)
	Confusion (+)
	Loss of rectal tone (+)
Duration of symptoms	1 wk
Vector	Person to person

++++ = Very common; +++ = common; ++ = sometimes occurs; + = uncommon.

Voluminous diarrhea stools follow. This presentation may be self-limited and resolve within 3 days or progress to the classic dysenteric syndrome. The latter occurs as the bacilli multiply in the large intestine and cause damage to the colonic epithelium. On colonoscopy, a diffuse colitis is observed, and the mucosa is covered with neutrophils and blood. A fever, which can range from low to moderately high, accompanies the presentation. Rose spots, though rare, have been seen with *S. flexneri* and *S. dysenteriae* and have been reported in a patient with *S. sonnei.*

In other children dysentery is the presenting complaint, with fever, abdominal pain with cramps, frequent stools, a small volume of mucoid bloody stool, tenesmus, and even a loss of anal sphincter tone. Abdominal pain may be periumbilical initially and may subsequently localize in the right lower quadrant, which can lead to a spurious diagnosis of appendicitis. The natural length of illness with this presentation of shigellosis is 1 week or longer with subsequent malaise. Shigellosis in patients who have mild diarrhea may be diagnosed only within the context of evaluation of an outbreak. Patients with moderate to severe diarrhea may present with dehydration. Respiratory symptoms, such as a cough or runny nose, are observed in approximately 10% of the patients. Protein-losing enteropathy can have a serious impact on patients who are malnourished. In the Japanese literature, **ekiri** is described in association with *Shigella* infection. This is a fulminating presentation of diarrhea, vomiting, fever, seizure, delirium, and shock with a fatal outcome, even for patients who have been treated with aggressive fluid replacement.

Physical Examination Findings

Clinical findings depend on the stage of development of the dysenteric symptoms and are particularly related to the state of hydration. Changes in mentation and affect have been noted in some patients. Increased bowel sounds and abdominal tenderness may be more pronounced over both lower quadrants. Loss of rectal tone after profuse diarrhea and even prolapse of the rectum have been noted. Seizures, which occur particularly among the very young with high fevers, have been noted early in the disease preceding or accompanying the diarrhea and are usually self-limited. The cerebrospinal fluid analysis in such instances is within normal limits.

DIAGNOSIS

Shigellosis should be considered in cases of acute diarrheal illness associated with systemic symptoms or if blood or mucus is present in stools. Stool cultures should be considered for children who have diarrhea with fever or blood or mucus in the stools, who are <4 years of age, who attend daycare centers, or who have a history of recent travel or institutionalization. A stool examination for neutrophils supports a diagnosis of shigellosis or other enteroinvasive infections (Plate 2E). Blood cultures should be obtained for severely ill, immunocompromised, or malnourished children, although bacteremia is rare. The WBC count may be elevated to as high as 50,000/mm^3 with increased immature forms.

Differential Diagnosis

The differential diagnosis of shigellosis is extensive. It includes not only other conditions associated with enteroinvasive agents, such as *Yersinia, Salmonella, E. coli* (enteroinvasive as well as enterohemorrhagic), *Campylobacter,* and *Entamoeba histolytica,* but also surgical conditions, such as intussusception (particularly if changes in mental status are present), volvulus, acute appendicitis, and central nervous system infections in patients with seizures and changes in mental status.

TABLE 76–8. Therapy for Shigellosis

Recommended Regimens

If susceptible to ampicillin, ampicillin 50 mg/kg/day divided q6hr PO for 5–7 days

or

TMP-SMZ 6–10 mg/kg/TMP divided bid PO for 5–7 days

Alternative Regimens for Strains Resistant to TMP-SMZ

Ceftriaxone 50 mg/kg/day as a single daily dose IM or IV for 5 days

or

Quinolones (No pediatric indication, although effective in adults with *Shigella* infections with strains resistant to traditional therapy.)

For adolescents ≥18 yr

Ciprofloxacin 500 mg q12hr PO for 3 doses

or

Ofloxacin 300 mg q12hr PO for 3 doses

TREATMENT

Antimicrobial therapy shortens the clinical illness and reduces the excretion of *Shigella.* Persons with the potential to spread the organism, such as institutionalized patients or those attending daycare, should especially be treated. No treatment is recommended in self-limited cases when symptoms have resolved by the time the microbiologic diagnosis is established.

For susceptible strains of *Shigella,* ampicillin and TMP-SMZ are effective, with a duration of treatment of at least 5 days (Table 76–8). Amoxicillin is less effective. For treatment of cases before susceptibilities are known or when strains resistant to ampicillin and TMP-SMZ are prevalent, ceftriaxone, an oral third-generation cephalosporin, or a quinolone such as ciprofloxacin or ofloxacin may be given. Quinolones are not approved for use in persons <18 years of age or in pregnant or lactating women.

Drugs that inhibit gastrointestinal motility, such as opiates, may worsen the disease and prolong the diarrhea and thus are contraindicated. As for all enteric diseases, rehydration is mandatory. Oral rehydration is very effective because fluid loss is not as dramatic as in the secretory diarrheas.

COMPLICATIONS

Convulsions, usually self-limited, and changes in mental status have been described not only with *S. dysenteriae,* which putatively produces Shiga toxin, but also with other species, such as *S. sonnei,* in which no Shiga toxin has been demonstrated. Seizures with shigellosis do not appear to place patients at higher risk of subsequent seizures. Rarely, bacteremia occurs in severely malnourished patients, either primary bacteremia with *Shigella* or bacteremia secondary to intestinal invasion by normal enteric organisms. Fulminating, rapidly fatal *Shigella* infections due to *S. sonnei, S. flexneri,* and *Shigella paradysenteriae* have been described in the United States. Rarely, systemic disease with extravascular abscesses has been seen with *S. flexneri. Shigella* vaginitis associated with a bloody vaginal discharge has been observed either as an isolated finding or, less commonly, in patients with a history of previous diarrhea. Rarely, hemolytic-uremic syndrome has been reported with renal failure at the end of the first week of illness. Prior treatment with antimicrobial agents and markedly elevated WBC counts, including a leukemoid reaction, have been reported as risk factors for the development of the hemolytic uremic syndrome

(HUS). As with many other bacterial enteric agents, reactive arthritis may occur in association with shigellosis.

PROGNOSIS

In contrast to *Salmonella,* the carrier state for *Shigella* is unusual. *Shigella* is shed in stools for 1–4 weeks and rarely longer. If antimicrobial drugs are used, this period is reduced to 1–4 days, with an average of 2 days.

Most cases of shigellosis are self-limited. Death occurs in fewer than 1% of cases; it occurs among young children secondary to dehydration. Malnourished children and neonates have a higher incidence of bacteremia and a higher mortality than other patients.

PREVENTION

Good hygiene, especially good handwashing, prevents spread. Children should complete at least 5 days of antimicrobial therapy and should have at least two consecutive stool cultures taken 24 hours apart that are negative for *Shigella* after antibiotics are discontinued before they return to school or daycare. It has been recommended that children who are convalescing be isolated while receiving antimicrobial therapy to control shigellosis in daycare centers.

No vaccine is currently available. Recent efforts include development of a live, attenuated vaccine by transfection of the plasmid of *S. sonnei* encoding somatic (O) antigen into *S. typhi* 21a, which is currently used in the live oral typhoid vaccine, so that it expresses both *S. typhi* and *S. sonnei* lipopolysaccharides.

YERSINIA ENTEROCOLITICA

ETIOLOGY

Yersinia is an enteric, non-lactose-fermenting gram-negative coccobacillus of the family Enterobacteriaceae. The organism is able to reproduce at 4°C (39.2°F). **Yersiniosis** is an enteric disease caused by *Yersinia enterocolitica* and *Yersinia pseudotuberculosis. Y. enterocolitica* has 34 distinguishable O serotypes, and *Y. pseudotuberculosis* has 5 serotypes. *Y. enterocolitica* serotypes O:3 and O:9 are the most common causes of diarrhea.

Transmission. Sources of *Y. enterocolitica* human infections are food, especially refrigerated milk, and water contaminated by feces or urine. The reservoirs of *Yersinia* are animals and birds. Dogs and cats, especially those from animal shelters, pig chitterlings (*Y. enterocolitica*), cows, goats, horses, rabbits, squirrels, fish, domestic fowl, and birds (*Y. pseudotuberculosis*) have all been implicated as carriers. Contact with wild animals or infected household pets and poor hygiene are other risk factors. Foodborne transmission accounts for 90% of cases.

EPIDEMIOLOGY

Yersinia causes approximately 100,000 cases of diarrhea annually in the United States, accounting for 5% of diarrheal disease. *Y. enterocolitica* infections occur more frequently in cooler climates and more frequently in winter than in summer. Patients with excessive iron storage syndromes such as β-thalassemia, patients who are undergoing iron chelation therapy with deferoxamine for iron overload, and immunocompromised patients are at particularly high risk of serious infections.

PATHOGENESIS

After *Yersinia* is ingested, the microbe attaches to intestinal epithelial cells. A cytotoxic heat-stable enterotoxin may be responsible for the enteric symptoms. Plasmids encode for factors that confer virulence and invasiveness. As *Yersinia* multiply, they may invade the intestinal lymphoid tissue, and infiltration by polymorphonuclear leukocytes leading to mesenteric lymphadenitis and terminal ileitis may ensue. In some instances, attachment occurs without penetration or epithelial damage and heat-stable enterotoxin is produced, which is ultimately responsible for secretory diarrhea. *Yersinia* is also capable of producing a cytotoxin that damages the intestinal epithelium of the large intestine and the terminal ileum, leading to a classic dysenteric stool.

Yersinia may invade the bloodstream subacutely with minimal or no gastrointestinal findings or may cause septicemia with fever, neutrophilia, jaundice, and abdominal pain. Extraintestinal spread, bacteremia, and shock are special problems of yersiniosis in persons who have chronic illnesses, especially iron overload (hemochromatosis and thalassemia major) and cirrhosis.

SYMPTOMS AND CLINICAL MANIFESTATIONS

The incubation period is usually 5 days, but it can be as long as 3 weeks. Diarrhea is the most common symptom of *Y. enterocolitica* infection, often with fever of up to 40°C (104°F). Persons >4 years of age are more likely to have accompanying abdominal pain and vomiting (Table 76–9). Bloody diarrhea occurs in approximately 30% of persons ≤18 years of age and is uncommon in persons between 19–29 years of age; it is not found in patients ≥30 years of age. Stools may be watery but are most often mucoid. Invasive infections are more likely in persons with predisposing conditions such as excessive iron storage. *Y. pseudotuberculosis* may present with a triad of fever, scarlatiniform rash, and abdominal symptoms suggestive of mesenteric adenitis, terminal ileitis, and appendicitis. Approximately 5% of older children with yersiniosis have diarrhea with a **pseudoappendicitis syndrome** in which pain progresses from the periumbilical or epigastric area to the right upper quadrant. Older patients may have postinfectious manifestations of reactive arthritis and erythema nodosum. Erythema nodosum occurs in up to 30% of adult patients with yersiniosis, primarily women, and resolves in a few weeks.

TABLE 76–9. Epidemiologic and Clinical Manifestations of *Yersinia* Infection

Season	No definite pattern, sometimes fall (also sometimes spring)
Primary age	>2 yr (5–15 yr most common)
Incubation period	2–11 days (usually 5 days)
Symptoms	Age-dependent fever (++++)
	Severe diarrhea (+++)
	Abdominal tenderness (+++)
	Vomiting (+++)
	Bloody diarrhea (++)
	Pseudoappendicitis (+)
	Arthritis (+)
	Pharyngitis (+)
Duration of symptoms	A few days to 4 wk
Vector	Animals, food

++++ = Very common; +++ = common; ++ = sometimes occurs; + = uncommon.

Physical Examination Findings

Fever and abdominal tenderness are common. Fever, abdominal pain, tenderness in the right lower abdominal quadrant, and leukocytosis may be confused with appendicitis. Fullness and tenderness on rectal examination of the right rectal shelf have been noted.

DIAGNOSIS

The diarrheal syndrome may be indistinguishable from that caused by other enteric agents. Bloody diarrhea, abdominal pain, and fever in a child whose condition appears otherwise stable should suggest *Yersinia* infection.

Mesenteric lymphadenitis caused by *Y. pseudotuberculosis* is a major differential diagnosis of appendicitis. *Y. pseudotuberculosis* should be suspected if, at the time of appendectomy, the appendix appears normal or only slightly inflamed and inflammation and suppuration are noted in the mesenteric nodes.

Laboratory Evaluation

The WBC count is frequently elevated, with a neutrophil predominance. Fecal leukocytes are typically present (Plate 2E).

Microbiologic Evaluation

Stool cultures with the use of enteric media (as described for *Salmonella* and *Shigella* infections) incubated at room temperature are usually sufficient for detection. Although "cold enrichment" with incubation at 4–6°C (39.2–42.8 °F) for a few weeks enhances recovery, it is too time-consuming to be considered practical for routine use. In cases of mesenteric lymphadenitis, the stool culture may not yield the microbe, particularly in patients infected with *Y. pseudotuberculosis.* In disseminated infection, *Yersinia* can be readily recovered from blood, cerebrospinal fluid, mesenteric lymph nodes, and peritoneal fluid with standard media such as blood agar.

Serologic Tests. Both EIA and RIA have been used to measure antibodies against *Y. enterocolitica,* but these tests are available only from reference laboratories. A fourfold rise in antibody titer between acute and convalescent titers to the specific offending serotype is diagnostic.

TREATMENT

Antibiotic therapy has not been proved to be definitely effective against *Y. enterocolitica* enterocolitis, but therapy is recommended for patients with pseudoappendicitis syndrome, mesenteric adenitis, or invasive disease and for immunocompromised patients with severe or protracted gastrointestinal symptoms (Table 76–10). In one study (Pai et al., 1984), shedding of microorganisms after antimicrobial treatment was less frequent than in untreated cases, although bacteriologic relapse may occur. *Y. enterocolitica* and *Y. pseudotuberculosis* are usually susceptible to aminoglycosides, cefotaxime, chloramphenicol, TMP-SMZ, and tetracycline, which is not recommended for children <9 years of age. No treatment is recommended in self-limited cases when symptoms have resolved by the time the microbiologic diagnosis is established, except in patients with hemoglobinopathies, iron overload, or cirrhosis. Extraintestinal infection may require at least 3 weeks of therapy.

TABLE 76–10. Therapy for *Yersinia* Infection

Usually none in uncomplicated cases
6 mg/kg TMP–30 mg/kg SMZ divided bid PO for 5–7 days
or
Gentamicin 7.5 mg/kg/day divided q8hr IV for extraintestinal disease
or
Cefotaxime 150 mg/kg/day divided q6hr IV for extraintestinal disease for as long as 3 wk

COMPLICATIONS

Intestinal perforation has been reported. Extraintestinal suppurative infections occur almost exclusively in patients with underlying disease, especially in those with disorders of iron excess but also in those with cirrhosis, cancer, or immunosuppressive therapy. Bacteremia, pneumonia, meningitis, osteomyelitis, arthritis, and pyomyositis have been seen. The most common extraintestinal manifestation of *Y. enterocolitica* infection is reactive arthritis. Approximately 10–30% of adults and 5% of children of Northern European or Scandinavian descent develop postinfectious polyarticular arthritis, which characteristically involves the knees, ankles, and wrists. The arthritis typically develops a few days to 1 month after onset of diarrhea and usually resolves in 4–6 months but may become chronic. Patients with HLA B27 antigen are particularly predisposed to development of ankylosing spondylitis after *Yersinia* infection.

PROGNOSIS

The natural course is for the illness to last for a few days to 1 month, but usually less than 10 days. Most disease is self-limited. The microorganism may persist in stool for 4–79 days (mean, 27 days) after the symptoms resolve, regardless of treatment, although patients are less likely to shed *Yersinia* after antimicrobial treatment. Although uncommon, death due to intestinal perforation has occurred in infants.

PREVENTION

No vaccine is available. Because patients may shed the organism for prolonged periods after resolution, even with antimicrobial therapy, appropriate hygienic measures are indicated to prevent transmission.

CAMPYLOBACTER

ETIOLOGY

Campylobacter is a microaerophilic, curved, gram-negative rod. *Campylobacter jejuni* causes diarrhea, whereas *Campylobacter fetus* rarely causes invasive disease but may be responsible for sepsis and meningitis in neonates.

Transmission. Domestic and wild animals and birds are the reservoir of infection. *C. jejuni* has been isolated from feces of 30–90% of chickens and turkeys. Many farm animals, including sheep, goats, and cattle, as well as shelter dogs and cats and household pets, have been infected. Ingestion of undercooked foods and unpasteurized milk, a contaminated water supply, and poor hygiene contribute to transmission of *C. jejuni.* Foodborne transmission accounts for 80% of cases.

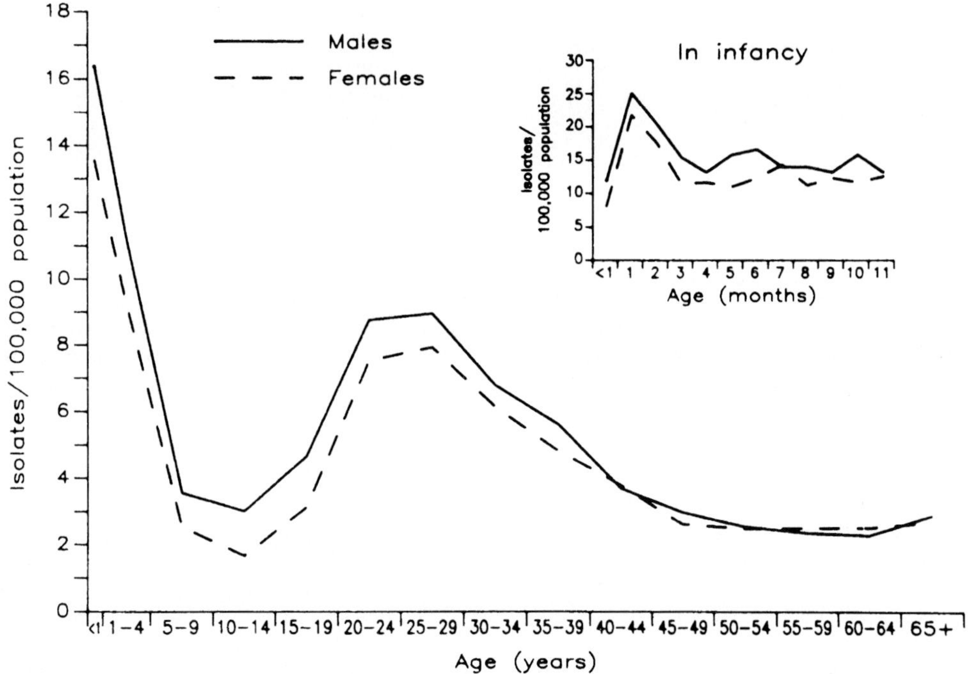

FIGURE 76–2. Isolation rates by age and sex for all *Campylobacter* in the United States, 1982–1986. Insert shows isolation rate among infants. (From Centers for Disease Control: *Campylobacter* Isolates in the United States, 1982–1986. *MMWR* 1988;37(SS-2):1–13.)

EPIDEMIOLOGY

Campylobacter is the most common cause of bacterial diarrhea in the United States, causing approximately 2,500,000 cases annually. Most instances of infection are symptomatic. *Campylobacter jejuni* is more prevalent during the summer months and in the early fall. The highest rate occurs in the first year of life (Fig. 76–2).

PATHOGENESIS

Campylobacter produces a cytotoxin and a heat-labile enterotoxin, which has homology to *E. coli* enterotoxin. The sites of infection are the ileum and the jejunum, and mesenteric lymph node enlargement is sometimes present. Disease is facilitated by the ability of the pathogen to penetrate the mucosa, the heat-labile enterotoxin that mediates the fluid accumulation, and the cytotoxin that produces the inflammatory aspects of the diarrhea as well as the capability of *Campylobacter* to invade either locally or systemically. If the microbe invades the lamina propria and mesenteric nodes, it may multiply there and then disseminate. This dissemination gives rise to the extraintestinal manifestation of *Campylobacter* infection, and it may occur with minimal local intestinal inflammatory reaction. Neonates and immunocompromised patients are at risk of extraintestinal complications.

SYMPTOMS AND CLINICAL MANIFESTATIONS

The incubation period of *Campylobacter* can be as long as 7 days, usually 2–4 days. The usual symptoms involve colicky abdominal pain (88%), diarrhea (83%), fever (52%), headache (54%), backache, aching limbs, and nausea that is seldom associated with vomiting (Table 76–11). The diarrhea may be watery at the start but can frequently appear bloody or mucosanguineous. The onset may be gradual, or it may be explosive and associated with fecal incontinence, without tenesmus. Intermittent central or upper abdominal pain is usually noted and is often described as severe. Mild illness lasts 1–2 days, although 20% of the patients have a prolonged or severe illness.

Physical Examination Findings

Fever is present in approximately one half of cases. Abdominal tenderness on deep palpation is common and at times is sufficiently severe in the lower quadrant to mimic appendicitis. The degree of dehydration parallels the profusion of diarrhea. Severe persistent illness may be confused with acute inflammatory disease.

TABLE 76–11. Epidemiologic and Clinical Manifestations of *Campylobacter* Infection

Season	Epidemic (increases in summer and early fall)
Primary age	2–24 mo
Incubation period	2–11 days (usually 3–4 days)
Symptoms	Diarrhea (++++)
	Abdominal cramps lasting several days (++++)
	Mucosanguineous stools (++++)
	Abdominal tenderness (+++)
	Fever (++)
	Headache (++)
	Muscle aches (++)
	Splenomegaly (+)
Duration of symptoms	3 days to 3 wk
Vector	Animals, food

++++ = Very common; +++ = common; ++ = sometimes occurs; + = uncommon.

DIAGNOSIS

When *Campylobacter* infection presents as a dysenteric syndrome, it may be clinically indistinguishable from other causes of this syndrome. The disease has been confused with ulcerative colitis, appendicitis, pseudoappendicitis caused by *Yersinia,* and severe ileitis simulating Crohn's disease.

Laboratory Evaluation

Stool examination usually demonstrates many leukocytes and erythrocytes (Plate 2E). Light microscopic examination of a fecal smear stained with 1% aqueous carbolfuchsin demonstrates the characteristic **seagull morphology** of the organism and can detect approximately two thirds of acute infections. This is useful for patients with diarrhea that exceeds 4–5 days in duration, especially if the stools are bloody or mucopurulent.

Microbiologic Evaluation

Stool culture should be performed in a microaerophilic environment (5% O_2, 10% CO_2) in a selective medium, such as *Campylobacter* blood agar, and incubated at 42°C (107.6°F).

TREATMENT

Disease caused by *Campylobacter* is usually self-limited. Because the impact of antibiotic therapy depends on the rapidity of initiation, prompt recognition by fecal smear examination is important. Treatment is recommended if it can be started within 5 days of the onset of illness. Treatment is also recommended for patients who continue to have a high fever or severe diarrhea, particularly if it remains bloody longer than 5 days. *Campylobacter* is resistant to TMP-SMZ, penicillins, cephalosporins, and vancomycin; it is susceptible to aminoglycosides, furazolidone, chloramphenicol, quinolones, tetracyclines, erythromycin, and azithromycin. Erythromycin and azithromycin have been demonstrated to be effective in eradicating *Campylobacter* from the stools and are the recommended treatment agents (Table 76–12). Of patients treated early, 86% have fewer stools and marked reduction of fever and abdominal pain within 24–36 hours, and the diarrhea subsides within 48 hours of the initiation of therapy. The total duration of therapy is 5–7 days. For children ≥8 years of age, tetracycline is effective. For patients ≥18 years of age, quinolones, such as ciprofloxacin, are effective. Bacteremia should be treated with aminoglycosides and either imipenem or meropenem pending determination of antimicrobial susceptibilities.

COMPLICATIONS

In one series (Lerner et al., 1984), 29% of children 3–36 months of age had febrile seizures but with no sequelae, Extraintestinal complications are more likely to occur in neonates, among whom bacteremia secondary to *C. fetus* is a well-known complication, and in patients with chronic underlying conditions that affect the immune response. Reactive arthritis, erythema nodosum, and idiopathic polyneuritis (Guillain-Barré syndrome) have been reported after *Campylobacter* infections.

TABLE 76–12. Therapy for *Campylobacter* Infection

Erythromycin 40 mg/kg/day divided q6hr PO for 7 days
or
Azithromycin 5–10 mg/kg once daily
Children >8 yr of Age
Tetracycline 10–25 mg/kg/day divided bid or qid
Children >18 yr of Age
Ciprofloxacin 30 mg/kg/day divided bid

PROGNOSIS

Campylobacter infection is usually a self-limited disease. The symptoms resolve in 1–2 weeks if untreated or 2 days after treatment has begun. Untreated patients may shed *Campylobacter* for 3 days to several months. Treatment with erythromycin for 10 days usually reduces stool excretion, with cessation of shedding occurring in 48 hours. However, antibiotic-resistant strains of *Campylobacter* have been recovered during therapy. Symptoms in most pediatric patients tend to disappear by the end of the first week of disease. As a group, adults have a more prolonged convalescence than children, some as long as 3 weeks.

PREVENTION

Breast-feeding may be protective against infection and helpful in decreasing the length of illness. Control of spread of infection depends on proper hygienic technique and avoidance of contamination of cooked foods with uncooked food. Pasteurization of milk and chlorination of water supplies are important preventive measures. Infected personnel should not handle food preparation in childcare centers and in health care environments. There is no vaccine.

AEROMONAS

ETIOLOGY

Aeromonas are gram-negative bacteria of the family Vibrionaceae. *Aeromonas caviae* and *Aeromonas hydrophila,* as well as the related species *Plesiomonas shigelloides,* have been implicated as causes of enteritis. *Aeromonas* is oxidase positive when grown in nonselective medium and is a late-lactose or nonlactose fermenter.

EPIDEMIOLOGY

Aeromonas are found worldwide in water and soil. Estuarial areas, rivers, and lakes constitute fertile ground for their growth. These bacteria are occasionally isolated from the stool cultures of persons without symptoms. *Aeromonas* are pathogens for fish, amphibians, and reptiles as well as for humans. Human enteric illness caused by these agents is most commonly seen during spring and summer, with a peak in the midsummer. Enteric illness appears to be more common in children 2 years of age or younger. Rectal or oral administration of *P. shigelloides* to volunteers has not resulted in gastrointestinal symptoms.

PATHOGENESIS

The clinical manifestations of *Aeromonas* illness suggest production of enterotoxin, with stools that are usually watery and nonbloody. Cholera-like disease has been reported in India and Africa, associated with heat-labile and acid-labile enterotoxins. However, not all *Aeromonas* strains recovered from infected patients produce enterotoxin.

TABLE 76–13. Epidemiologic and Clinical Manifestations of *Aeromonas* Infection

Season	Spring and summer
Primary age	All ages (primarily <10 and >60 yr)
Incubation period	1 wk or less
Symptoms	Fever (++)
	Vomiting (++)
	Watery stool (++)
	Dysentery (++)
	Abdominal tenderness (++)
	Dehydration (+)
Duration of symptoms	About 15 days, rarely months
Vector	Estuarial water, seafood

++ = Sometimes occurs; + = uncommon.

SYMPTOMS AND CLINICAL MANIFESTATIONS

Three patterns of presentation have been reported (Table 76–13). Approximately 60% of patients have mild fever and vomiting accompanied by watery diarrhea. Older children usually have no vomiting. Symptoms last ≤1 week, and no specific therapy is necessary. Approximately 20% of patients have mucoid, bloody diarrhea that usually lasts ≤1 week. Proctitis may be seen on sigmoidoscopy. Approximately 20% of patients have diarrhea that lasts >2 weeks, and approximately one half of these have diarrhea that persists >1 month. It is in this latter group that ulcerative colitis is particularly entertained as a possible diagnosis. The mean overall duration of diarrhea in all patients is usually 15 days. In all hosts, *Aeromonas* is capable of causing cellulitis, as well as cutaneous abscess formation, and of systemic dissemination into bones, joints, meninges, and other sites. A history of traumatic inoculation with contaminated soil or water is usually found.

Physical Examination Findings

Patients with predominantly gastrointestinal symptoms have increased bowel sounds and diffuse abdominal pain. A fever is not usual, although it is consistently present when there is dissemination from the gastrointestinal area. Findings of dehydration are also unusual.

DIAGNOSIS

In their early presentation, *Aeromonas* intestinal infections produce mild symptoms and watery diarrhea. In approximately 20% of cases, features of dysentery may predominate and may be indistinguishable from those caused by other microorganisms in the dysenteric group. If disease persists for longer than 1 week, *Aeromonas* infection is likely.

Laboratory Evaluation

Usually no invasive diagnostic procedures are indicated. If the dysenteric presentation predominates, stool should be examined for leukocytes (Plate 2E). Depending on the presence of systemic symptoms, a blood culture may be indicated.

Microbiologic Evaluation

Stools can be inoculated for isolation in blood agar containing 10 μg/mL ampicillin. The colonies are easily recognized as gray colonies surrounded by β-hemolysis, which has good correlation with enterotoxin production.

TABLE 76–14. Therapy for *Aeromonas* Infection

TMP-SMZ as for *Shigella* infection (Table 76–8); 6–10 mg/kg TMP divided bid PO for 5–7 days
or
Cefotaxime 150 mg/kg/day divided q6hr IV for systemic disease or extravascular localized processes
or
Gentamicin 5–7.5 mg/kg/day divided q8hr IV for systemic diseases or extravascular localized processes
or
Quinolones (No pediatric indications, but effective in vitro.)

TREATMENT

Diarrhea due to *Aeromonas* is usually mild and requires no specific treatment. Patients with persistent diarrhea or dysentery may benefit from trimethoprim or TMP-SMZ (Table 76–14). Most strains are also susceptible to chloramphenicol, tetracycline (not recommended for children <8 years of age), nitrofurantoin, and third-generation cephalosporins, aminoglycosides, and quinolones. The penicillins are ineffective, and the first- and second-generation cephalosporins and erythromycin have variable activity. If systemic dissemination or extraintestinal focal infection occurs, parenteral therapy should be initiated with a third-generation cephalosporin and an aminoglycoside. The duration of therapy should be appropriate for the site involved.

COMPLICATIONS

Peritonitis caused by *Aeromonas* has occurred after rupture of the appendix. Extraintestinal complications are more common among immunocompromised persons.

PROGNOSIS

Aeromonas infection is generally a self-limited disease, and in immunocompetent persons it usually remains localized to the gastrointestinal tract. Focal infection responds well to appropriate antimicrobial treatment and surgical drainage if indicated.

PREVENTION

Persons, especially immunocompromised persons, in contact with estuarial water and streams and with reptiles, amphibians, and fish should be aware of the possible risk. No vaccine is available.

AMEBIASIS

ETIOLOGY

Amebiasis is caused by the mobile protozoan *Entamoeba histolytica.* Amebic trophozoites (60 μm) are found worldwide. These cysts exist in the alkaline small intestine and produce trophozoites that infect colonic mucosa. Trophozoites produce cysts (10–20 μm) that are shed in the stool. *E. histolytica* cysts survive outside the host for weeks to months in a moist environment and are resistant to digestion by gastric acid and enzymes.

Transmission. Organisms are transmitted by the fecal-oral route, including ingestion of contaminated food or water. Infected persons can excrete cysts intermittently, and persons without symptoms are important reservoirs of infection.

EPIDEMIOLOGY

E. histolytica is present in approximately 10% of the world population with manifestations from asymptomatic shedding of cysts, to mild diarrhea, to fulminant enterocolitis. Infection with *E. histolytica* is more prevalent in persons of lower socioeconomic status living under poor sanitary conditions in developing countries. Travelers to these countries where the infection is endemic are at increased risk of acquiring this infection. Among other intestinal parasites, *E. histolytica* was isolated in 0.29% of stools in a daycare center in Toronto. In the United States, the prevalence is 1–10% of cases of diarrhea, depending on the population studied. An increasing incidence of amebiasis is being seen among young men who have sex with men.

PATHOGENESIS

The ascending colon, sigmoid, and rectum can be involved with the progression of the disease. After a variable period of time, which can range from a few days to years, trophozoites appear and invade the intestinal mucosa to form ulcers. These ulcers extend laterally into the submucosa and occasionally perforate the serosa, allowing the development of bacterial peritonitis by enteric organisms. Abundant amoebae are present in the intestinal ulcer, although the intestinal mucosa between ulcers remains normal.

Several substances such as proteolytic enzymes, including trypsin and hyaluronidase, have been proposed as virulence factors for *E. histolytica*. Another proposed virulence mechanism is resistance to lysis through complement. Characterization of amebic enzymes reveals a distinct difference in pattern among pathogenic and nonpathogenic strains. An immune response to both intestinal and extraintestinal infection due to *E. histolytica* occurs. IgG is the major antibody in the immune response to invasive amebiasis that persists in a high titer despite successful treatment. *E. histolytica* does not stimulate an appreciable IgM antibody response.

SYMPTOMS AND CLINICAL MANIFESTATIONS

The incubation period ranges from a few days to months; usually it is 1–4 weeks. The clinical manifestations of intestinal amebiasis vary from asymptomatic shedding of cysts, to noninvasive intestinal infection with mild diarrhea, to fulminant enterocolitis and liver abscess. An amebic dysenteric syndrome can manifest not only with severe diarrhea but also with bloody or bloody and mucoid stools. Dehydration is uncommon. Asymptomatic or mildly symptomatic intraluminal amebiasis is perhaps the most common type, presenting as vague abdominal pain, nausea, fatigue, and epigastric fullness (Table 76–15). Amebic dysentery causes severe diarrhea and blood and mucus in the stool. Severe abdominal pain is very common in children. Fever occurs in about one third of children.

TABLE 76–15. Epidemiologic and Clinical Manifestations of *Entamoeba histolytica* Infection

Season	Year-round
Primary age	Malnourished pediatric patients Immunosuppressed patients of any age
Incubation period	3 wk or less
Symptoms	Abdominal pain (++++) Diarrhea (++++) Dysentery (++++) Hepatomegaly (+++)* Fever (++) Nausea (++) Fatigue (++)
Duration of symptoms	Variable, usually 10 days or longer
Vector	Fecal-oral contact, contaminated equipment, contaminated food

*In invasive disease.
++++ = Very common; +++ = common; ++ = sometimes occurs.

DIAGNOSIS

Amebiasis should be considered in children who present with dysentery who were born in developing countries or who attend daycare centers. Other causes of dysenteric syndrome due to bacterial enteritis or inflammatory bowel disease must be excluded. Proctoscopy or sigmoidoscopy with visual and histologic evaluation is helpful in excluding the latter. In some cases of amebic dysentery associated with abdominal pain, the diagnosis of appendicitis may be considered

Microbiologic Evaluation

Examination of multiple (at least three) consecutive daily stool specimens increases the diagnostic yield to 60–70%. *Entamoeba* should be differentiated from nonpathogenic human amoebae, including *Entamoeba coli, Entamoeba hartmanni,* and *Endolimax nana.* Fresh stool specimens should be examined within 30 minutes of collection to avoid disintegration of the trophozoites. Media that contain polyvinyl alcohol (PVA) or formalin enable identification of amebic trophozoites in the laboratory when fresh specimens cannot be examined. These trophozoites may contain ingested erythrocytes, which help confirm the diagnosis. A normal stool specimen does not exclude the diagnosis of amebiasis. In such cases, proctoscopic, or sigmoidoscopic, or colonoscopic examination should be performed. Examination of the intestinal mucosa reveals ulcers and mucus-containing trophozoites. Biopsy specimens should be stained by appropriate histologic techniques to highlight tissue trophozoites.

Diagnostic Imaging

Radiography is seldom needed to diagnose intestinal amebiasis. A laboratory examination to exclude *E. histolytica* should be performed before a contrast agent such as barium is administered, because contrast media may interfere with stool examination. Ultrasonography, technetium-99m liver scanning, and CT are helpful in the evaluation of hepatic abscesses (Chapter 79). Because of the lack of leukocytes in amebic abscesses, a gallium scan is not useful.

TREATMENT

The treatment of amebiasis is determined in part by the degree of tissue invasion (Table 76–16). For patients in nonendemic areas who have no symptoms but are passing cysts, iodoquinol (diiodohydroxyquin), 30–40 mg/kg/day in three divided doses for 20 days, is recommended. Only a small fraction of this drug is absorbed. The adverse effects include abdominal pain, nausea, vomiting, and diarrhea. The drug is contraindicated for patients with hepatic disease or those who are allergic to iodine. Paromomycin, a broad-spectrum antibiotic, in doses of 25–30 mg/kg/day in three divided

TABLE 76–16. Therapy for *Entamoeba histolytica* Infection

Disease	Recommended Regimen	Alternative Regimens
Asymptomatic cyst passers	Iodoquinol	Paromomycin *or* Diloxanide furoate
Mild to moderate intestinal symptoms with no dysentery*	Metronidazole	
Dysentery or extraintestinal disease (including hepatic abscess)*	Metronidazole	Dehydroemetine followed by chloroquine phosphate

*Treatment should be followed by a course of iodoquinol or one of the other intraluminal drugs used to treat asymptomatic amebiasis.

Suggested Dosages for Patients with Normal Renal Function

ANTIBIOTIC	DOSAGE	MAXIMUM DAILY DOSE
Chloroquine phosphate	20 mg/kg base (33 mg salt) daily for 2 days, then 10 mg/kg base (17 mg salt) daily for 2–3 weeks	600 mg base (1 g salt); 300 base (500 mg salt)
Dehydroemetine	1–1.5 mg/kg/day IM for 5 days	90 mg
(available from the CDC Drug Service, telephone (404) 639-3670 [evenings, weekends, and holidays: (404) 639-2888])		
Diloxanide furoate	20 mg/kg/day divided q8hr PO for 10 days	1500 mg
Iodoquinol	30–40 mg/kg/day divided q8hr PO for 20 days	2 g
Metronidazole	35–50 mg/kg/day divided q8hr PO for 10 days	2250 mg
Paromomycin	25–30 mg/kg/day divided q8hr PO for 7 days	30 mg/kg

doses for 7 days, has been used for patients who excrete cysts asymptomatically. Loose stools are seen frequently with this agent. Diloxanide furoate is an alternative intraluminal agent. The reported efficacy rates are 33–100%; the actual rate is probably more than 90%. Patients who have symptomatic intestinal amebiasis with dysentery should receive therapy with metronidazole followed by a luminal agent such as iodoquinol (Table 76–16).

COMPLICATIONS

The complications of intestinal amebiasis include cutaneous extension into the perianal area and amebic liver abscesses, which are the second most common type of invasive amebiasis (Chapter 79). A liver abscess is a more common complication in adults than in children; among adults, men are most frequently infected. Affected children present with a high fever, irritability, tachypnea, abdominal distention, and frequently hepatomegaly. However, <50% of patients with subacute disease have an actual or low-grade fever. More important, they may not have abdominal pain. Pediatric patients may have diarrhea or a cough or both in the absence of pulmonary findings. Extra-abdominal amebiasis occurs as a result of seeding from a liver abscess. Symptoms depend on organ involvement (e.g., pleuropulmonary abscess, pericardial amebiasis, cerebral abscess). The use of corticosteroids may result in severe complications of intestinal amebiasis. Hence, if these agents are to be used, one should exclude *E. histolytica* as a cause of inflammatory bowel disease.

PROGNOSIS

Most infections progress to a cure or an asymptomatic carrier state. Death is unusual and occurs in only about 5% of patients who have extraintestinal involvement. It is usually secondary to perforation of the intestine at the site of amebic ulceration. Involvement of the liver, pleural area, pericardium, or central nervous system results in an increase in mortality even with therapy.

PREVENTION

The risk of infection can be reduced in endemic areas by good hygienic practices, such as meticulous handwashing, avoidance of raw fruits and vegetables, and decontamination (filtering or boiling) of potable water. Treatment of carriers to eradicate spread of the organism is also important.

ENTEROTOXIGENIC SYNDROMES

The enterotoxigenic enteritides are syndromes caused by agents whose pathogenic potentials are derived predominantly from the production of enteric toxins that ultimately disrupt absorptive mechanisms. The classic representatives are *V. cholerae* and enterotoxigenic *E. coli.* The *E. coli* strains may also cause diarrhea by other mechanisms; however, for simplicity and because of the clinical similarities, the discussion of *E. coli* infections is included in this section.

VIBRIO CHOLERAE (CHOLERA)

ETIOLOGY

Cholera is a diarrheal disease caused by hemolytic strains of enterotoxin-producing *Vibrio cholerae,* which is present worldwide. *V. cholerae* can be separated by somatic group antigens into O group 1 strains **(O1)** and **non-O1** strains. *V. cholerae* O1 can further be classified by serotyping into subtypes **Ogawa** and **Inaba** and can be independently grouped by physiologic properties into one of two biotypes, **El Tor** or **classic.** Only toxigenic *V. cholerae* with the O group 1 antigen (O1) is associated with the epidemic severe diarrheal illness that is cholera, although nontoxigenic *V. cholerae* O1 and *V. cholerae* non-O1 can cause nonepidemic cholera-like diarrheal illness. The classic biotype appears restricted to Bangladesh. The El Tor biotype has caused the most recent major outbreaks in the western hemisphere. Epidemic cholera-like illness in India and Bangladesh has been linked to non-O1 *V. cholerae* strains. These strains, unlike O1 strains, were encapsulated. They were all toxigenic.

Transmission. The organism is transmitted by the fecal-oral route. Risk factors noted in the recent South American epidemics continue to reflect traditional problems, such as contamination of water sources or food. Lack of a sanitary water supply, private toilet facilities, refrigeration, and trash collection are frequently present. Isolates of the South American strains have been detected in shellfish off the Gulf States, although no known indigenous human cases caused by these strains have been described in the United States.

EPIDEMIOLOGY

From 4 to 103 cases of cholera have been reported annually in the United States since 1992. Most cases are acquired during international travel and involve either a United States resident returning from a visit or a visitor to the United States. It is a rare infection among the travelers to the developing countries (0.2 reported cases per 100,000 travelers per month). *V. cholerae* O1 biotype El Tor has spread from Asia to Africa, southern Europe, and the Pacific Islands. The organism has spread unabated to more than 20 countries of South and Central America, and there have been several hundred thousand reported cases of cholera. Once the disease is introduced in a community, adults are affected first and then children. By virtue of their occupational or behavioral activity, men and boys are at higher risk than women and girls.

In the United States an endemic source of *V. cholerae* has been described on the Gulf Coast. The disease is usually associated with consumption of seafood harvested from the Gulf of Mexico coastal waters, especially raw oysters and shrimp. The most frequent *Vibrio* infections from this area are unique strains of *V. cholerae* O1 and *Vibrio parahaemolyticus,* which primarily causes diarrheal illness, and *Vibrio vulnificus,* which causes wound infections and can cause septicemia in immunocompromised patients.

PATHOGENESIS

Natural protective mechanisms, especially normal gastric acidity, play an important role in protection from *Vibrio* infection. Hypochlorhydria and chronic gastritis place patients at increased risk. Patients of blood group O Rh+ also appear to be at greater risk. Ingestion of between 10^8 and 10^{10} *V. cholerae* microorganisms is necessary to cause infection in volunteers. Most *V. cholerae* organisms do not survive transit across the acid milieu of the stomach. Once attachment to the epithelial cells of the intestine occurs through a pilus, known as TapA, *V. cholerae* produces an 84 kDa enterotoxin composed of an A and a B subunit. This toxin mediates disease by noninflammatory mechanisms with no invasion or destruction of the mucosa. The **A subunit** activates adenyl cyclase with production of cyclic adenosine monophosphate (cAMP), and the **B subunit** is important in attachment. This subunit becomes attached to a membrane receptor monosialosyl ganglioside-GM_1 in the intestinal epithelium. Thus the heat-labile enterotoxin in most cases affects cells of the villi as well as the crypts and causes an isotonic loss of water, sodium, and other electrolytes. The toxin is closely related to the heat-labile enterotoxin of enterotoxigenic *E. coli.* This consideration is important in the management of rehydration.

SYMPTOMS AND CLINICAL MANIFESTATIONS

The incubation period is 1–3 days, although symptoms have started as early as a few hours after exposure to as late as 5 days after exposure (Table 76–17). Classically there is no fever, and the symptoms can be ascribed totally to fluid depletion and dehydration. Diarrhea may start explosively, ranging to as high as 20 stools a day in some pediatric patients with severe diarrhea, resulting in a loss of fluid of more than 400 mL/hr. Vomiting may or may not be present. Infection with *V. cholerae* El Tor generally leads to unreported infection in approximately 75% of cases; mild disease in 20%, with <5% dehydration; moderate disease in 4%; and severe disease in 2%.

The stools are watery in 70% of patients and mucosanguineous in 3%, with the remainder having yellow, rice-water stools. Abdominal cramps occur in approximately three fourths of symptomatic cases. Painful cramping of the legs may occur because of electrolyte imbalances. In children, hypoglycemia, seizures, and coma occur if rapid fluid replacement is not provided.

TABLE 76–17. Epidemiologic and Clinical Manifestations of Cholera

Season	Variable
Primary age	In outbreaks, adults first, then children
Incubation period	5–10 days
Symptoms	Watery stools (++++)
	Mucus in stool (++)
	Fever (+)
	Headache (+)
	Blood in stool (+)
Duration of symptoms	About 1 wk
Vector	Seafood contaminated with bacilli

++++ = Very common; ++ = sometimes occurs; + = uncommon.

Physical Examination Findings

The findings generally reflect the degree of dehydration, usually without fever even in severe disease.

DIAGNOSIS

When symptomatic, the profound severity of the watery diarrhea and the rapidity of progression to dehydration suggest cholera as a likely diagnosis. The presence of similar illness in others in the community also suggests cholera. Enterotoxigenic *E. coli,* especially in travelers, and rotavirus are other possible causes.

Microbiologic Evaluation

Most laboratories do not routinely culture *V. cholerae.* In suspected cases, a confirmatory laboratory diagnosis is established by recovery of *V. cholerae* from stools in a thiosulfate citrate bile salt source (TCBS) agar, in which most strains are sucrose-fermenting. Other laboratory methods to confirm the culture include agglutination by specific *Vibrio* antisera. Darkfield examination of the fluid stools demonstrates vibrios whose motility is affected negatively by the addition of specific *Vibrio* antisera. If *V. cholerae* is isolated, it should be sent for serotyping to the CDC through the local health department. However, a clinical diagnosis is most critical and depends on elucidation of possible exposure by history and awareness of the physician of current epidemiologic reports.

TREATMENT

Adequate supportive treatment with oral or intravenous hydration is essential in the management of cholera. Rice-based oral rehydration solution in adults with cholera decreases stool output by 41% during the first 24 hours. Oral rehydration solutions containing amylase-resistant starch need to be evaluated for their efficacy. Antibiotic treatment reduces the duration of diarrhea and accompanying fluid loss and abbreviates the shedding of *V. cholerae* (Table 76–18). Antibiotic therapy reduces stool output by 65% during the second 24 hours, and diarrhea resolves within 48 hours. Tetracycline and doxycycline are drugs of choice for *V. cholerae* O1 and 139 Bengal. Tetracyclines are generally contraindicated in children ≤8 years of age because of adverse effects of dental staining, but in cases of severe cholera the benefits outweigh the risks. If the *V. cholerae*

TABLE 76–18. Therapy for Cholera in Children

Severe Cases and Children >8 yr of Age
Tetracycline 50 mg/kg/day divided q6hr for 3 days
Doxycycline 6 mg/kg in one dose
Ciprofloxacin 30 mg/kg/day divided bid
For Resistant to Tetracycline
TMP-SMZ: TMP 8 mg/kg/day divided bid for 3 days
Furazolidone, 5 to 8 mg/kg/day divided q6hr for 3 days
Erythromycin 40 mg/kg/day divided tid for 3 days

is resistant to tetracycline, TMP-SMZ, erythromycin, furazolidone, or ciprofloxacin or ofloxacin can be used.

COMPLICATIONS

Severe dehydration, sometimes accompanied by hypoglycemia and hypokalemia, is the major complication of cholera. It is readily managed with appropriate carbohydrate- and electrolyte-containing solutions.

PROGNOSIS

The key to good outcome is early diagnosis and appropriate fluid replacement. Rehydration, either parenteral or oral, has been the main contributor to an improved outcome. The prognosis for survival without sequelae is excellent. Fewer than 1% of severely dehydrated patients die if appropriately treated with intravenous fluid and electrolytes.

PREVENTION

To reduce the risk of cholera during travel to developing countries with inadequate sanitation, avoidance of uncooked or undercooked seafood, vegetables, fruit, and contaminated water in any form, including ice, is the best prevention.

Coprimary and secondary cases of cholera may be prevented by administration of TMP-SMZ, tetracycline, or doxycycline to household contacts within 24 hours of identification of the index case. Prophylaxis usually is not necessary in the United States unless poor sanitary and hygiene conditions indicate the likelihood of secondary transmission.

Vaccine. A killed vaccine (heat or phenol inactivation) provides poor protection, with at best 50% protection for about 6 months. An oral inactivated vaccine of the B subunit may provide 50% protection for 5 years after three doses. These vaccines are inefficient for controlling cholera and may provide a false sense of security. Travelers rarely need vaccination against cholera.

Live attenuated oral vaccines that express the B subunit genes have yielded results compatible with vibriocidal antibody, which could result in protection for more than 90% of those immunized. Good antibody activity, immunogenicity, and tolerance have been reported in some patients given a recombinant preparation. This vaccine has demonstrated a 100% seroconversion rate with doses of 10^6 microorganisms, as compared with the 56–89% seroconversion rate observed among patients immunized with dead preparations or a combination of dead preparations and the B subunit.

ESCHERICHIA COLI SYNDROMES

E. coli can cause prolonged symptoms in young children. These strains may play a role in diarrhea of the traveler.

ETIOLOGY

Much has been learned about *E. coli* and gastrointestinal illness since Bray and coworkers first described *E. coli neapolitanum* in the early 1940s. Gastrointestinal disease due to *E. coli* is now divided according to mechanisms of disease as well as to signs and symptoms. There are five types of diarrhea-producing *E. coli:* enterotoxigenic (ETEC) strains, enteroinvasive (EIEC) strains, enterohemorrhagic (EHEC) strains (Shiga toxin–producing *E. coli*), enteropathogenic (EPEC) strains, and some enteroaggregative (EAEC) strains with enteroadherent capability have been identified as an important cause of diarrhea in young children in South America.

Transmission. Fecal-oral spread through consumption of contaminated water and foods represents the major route of spread for *E. coli* gastroenteritides. Food borne transmission accounts for 85% of cases.

EPIDEMIOLOGY

Enterotoxigenic E. coli (ETEC). The classic strains of ETEC are those that produce enterotoxins and adherence factors and are associated with episodes of travelers' diarrhea and infantile diarrhea in the developing countries. These strains are a rare cause of diarrhea in developed countries, although there have been reports from Native American reservations in the United States.

Enteroinvasive E. coli (EIEC). Enteroinvasive strains are closely related to Shigella and have been associated with infection from consumption of contaminated foods such as cheeses. They are rare in the United States and have been reported more frequently in Europe and Africa.

Enterohemorrhagic E. coli (EHEC). Enterohemorrhagic strains are Shiga toxin– or verotoxin-producing *E. coli* strains that have been described in food-related outbreaks in the United States, such as those involving hamburgers and unpasteurized apple cider. In the United States *E. coli* **O157:H7** is the major representative, but in other locales strains O157:H−, O26:H11, and many others are found. These strains are recovered primarily in late summer and early fall.

Enteropathogenic E. coli (EPEC). Enteropathogenic strains belong to well-characterized serotypes. During the 1940s and the 1950s, these strains contributed to outbreaks of diarrhea among infants throughout the world. Failure to demonstrate invasive or enterotoxic characteristics led to disregard of their pathogenic potential. EPEC strains produce adherence factors and cytotoxin, and this may well correlate with pathogenicity. This disease occurs in the developing parts of the world.

Enteroaggregative E. coli (EAEC). Enteroaggregative strains have been described as common causes of acute watery diarrhea. EAEC, when fed to volunteers in experimental challenge, have resulted in diarrheal illness without fecal blood or neutrophils. They are an important cause of diarrhea among young children in South America. These strains were isolated more often from patients with acute gastroenteritis who lived in India and whose diarrhea lasted longer than 14 days.

PATHOGENESIS

Enterotoxigenic E. coli (ETEC). After ingestion, the enterotoxigenic strains adhere by colonization factors. They colonize the small intestine and damage mucosa but do not invade. They produce enterotoxins, including **heat-labile (cholera-like) enterotoxins, heat-stable enterotoxins,** or both. Approximately 48 hours after exposure, most human illness is caused by heat-stable enterotoxins that act by causing a derangement of the absorption mechanisms for electrolytes in the small intestine. These mechanisms are mediated through adenyl cyclase (for the heat-labile enterotoxin) and guanyl cyclase (for the heat-stable enterotoxin).

Enteroinvasive E. coli (EIEC). These strains, which belong to restricted serotypes, share a plasmid with *Shigella flexneri.* They colonize the colon and distal part of the small intestine and are capable of invading and proliferating within the epithelium of the large intestine.

Enterohemorrhagic E. coli (EHEC). These strains adhere by novel colonization fimbriae and form effacing lesions. The process is responsible for secretory diarrhea in the patients. This is followed by production of specific cytotoxins, **Shiga-like toxins I and II (SLT-I and SLT-II),** which have been demonstrated in *E. coli* O157:H7, as well as other strains. SLT-I is almost identical to **Shiga toxin** produced by *Shigella dysenteriae,* and SLT-II has 60% homology. These cytotoxins efface the microvilli of intestinal epithelium, leading to hemorrhagic colitis. Systemic spread of toxin may lead to HUS. Strains of *E. coli* that produce toxin, which include many *E. coli* O157:H7 strains, are referred to as **Shiga toxin–producing E. coli (STEC).**

Enteropathogenic E. coli (EPEC). After ingestion, these EPEC (nonenteroinvasive, nonenterotoxigenic) strains adhere to the small intestine, multiply, destroy microvilli, lower disaccharidase levels, and cause localized inflammatory changes and malabsorption but do not produce Shiga toxin. There are 12 O serogroups of EPEC. They possess adherence factors, such as **EAF.** Expression of these genes has been demonstrated by localized adherence to Hep2 cells.

Enteroaggregative E. coli (EAEC). EAEC strains belong to new O groups, and are associated with characteristic histopathologic intestinal lesions distinct from the enteropathogenic strains. One strain produces a stable toxin that fails to produce a reaction in suckling mouse models or hybridize with the ST probes. EAEC strains produce enterotoxins and damage the mucosa.

SYMPTOMS AND CLINICAL MANIFESTATIONS

The symptoms and clinical manifestations of *E. coli* syndromes vary according to the mechanism of the infecting strain (Table 76–19).

Enterotoxigenic E. coli (ETEC). The symptoms consist almost exclusively of cramps and voluminous watery stools, sometimes with mucus. The symptoms usually start about 48 hours after ingestion. These episodes of diarrhea are self-limited and are of moderate severity with watery stools and cramps. Symptoms usually last about 5 days and rarely as long as 10 days. Fever, headaches, or myalgia, and upper gastrointestinal symptoms, such as nausea and vomiting, are uncommon.

Enteroinvasive E. coli (EIEC). EIEC diarrhea is usually watery without blood or mucus, although dysenteric stools are seen in 7% of cases. Children usually have fever, and stools may show leukocytes (Plate 2E). Within 24 hours of ingestion or sometimes as long as 72 hours after ingestion, a *Shigella*-like syndrome may commence. Other symptoms include fever, headache, malaise, myalgia, nausea, vomiting, and abdominal pain. The diarrhea is less in volume than that seen in infection with enterotoxigenic strains. Rarely, there have been toxemia and hypotension with blood invasion. The duration of the illness is usually 7–10 days.

Enterohemorrhagic E. coli (EHEC). The incubation period of enterohemorrhagic *E. coli* is 2–9 days. Patients experience abdominal cramps, no fever or a low-grade fever, nausea, vomiting, and grossly bloody diarrhea. EHEC infection begins with nonbloody diarrhea but usually progresses to hemorrhagic colitis occasionally leading to development of HUS. Fever occasionally occurs, and there are severe abdominal pains. The bloody intestinal discharge resembles lower gastrointestinal bleeding. Symptoms are usually self-limited and last 7–10 days. Shigellosis, amebiasis, campylobacteriosis, and enteroinvasive *E. coli* infection are excluded by lack of fever and by the nature of the bloody stool, which resembles lower gastrointestinal bleeding.

Enteropathogenic E. coli (EPEC). Diarrhea develops approximately 48 hours after ingestion. The diarrhea of older children and adults is usually self-limited, whereas infants may have protracted

TABLE 76–19. Epidemiologic and Clinical Manifestations of *Escherichia coli* Infections

Factor	ETEC	EIEC	EHEC	EPEC	EAggEC
Season	Year-round	Summer (usually)	Late summer, early fall	Epidemic	Year-round, some from outbreaks
Primary age	Beyond infancy	Beyond infancy	1–10 yr	0–1 yr	0–6 mo, also travelers' diarrhea
Incubation period	2 days	24–72 hr	2–9 days	2 days	Variable
Symptoms	Diarrhea (+++) Fever (++)	Dysentery (+++) Diarrhea (+) Fever (+)	Vomiting (++) Diarrhea (+) Hematochezia (+)	Diarrhea (+++) Fever (++) Mucus in stool (++) Blood in stool (+)	Diarrhea (+++) Fever (++)
Duration of symptoms	5 days	7–10 days	7–10 days	1 wk, may last 3 wk	≥2 wk
Vector	Food, water	Food	Food	People	Food

ETEC = Enterotoxigenic *E. coli;* EIEC = enteroinvasive *E. coli;* EHEC = enterohemorrhagic *E. coli;* EPEC = enteropathogenic *E. coli;* EAggEC = enteroaggregative *E. coli.*
+++ = Common; ++ = sometimes occurs; + = uncommon.

diarrhea that lasts 2 weeks or longer. EPEC causes severe diarrhea with dehydration. Chronic infection has led to growth retardation in neonates and children <2 years of age.

Enteroaggregative E. coli (EAEC). In experimental studies, adult volunteers have had purely diarrheal illness. These strains may account for acute watery diarrhea, although sometimes protracted diarrhea of >14 days in infants and travelers can occur. Occasionally, bloody stools have been reported.

DIAGNOSIS

Diarrhea-associated *E. coli* is difficult to differentiate in most clinical microbiology laboratories from *E. coli* normally present in the stool. Clinical and epidemiologic correlation helps to elucidate the association with the diarrhea. Enterotoxigenic strains should be considered likely in disease associated with travel. The self-limited nature of this disease makes the need for diagnosis primarily of epidemiologic interest. Therapy is readily available for infection due to enteroinvasive strains, although these strains are not highly prevalent in the United States. Enterohemorrhagic strains have been associated with foodborne infection. Infection due to an enterohemorrhagic strain should be documented by culture in the first week of illness; stool cultures tend to become negative soon after the first week, even as the symptoms persist. The association of enteropathogenic strains with protracted diarrhea in infants and the ability to detect these organisms in small-intestine biopsy specimens, coupled with the availability of effective treatment, make it of paramount importance to be aware that these organisms may be responsible for prolonged diarrhea of infancy.

Enterotoxigenic E. coli (ETEC). No fecal leukocytes are demonstrated in the stools, and the peripheral WBC count shows no immature forms. Laboratory assays include tissue culture in a (Y-1) adrenal cell carcinoma or the rabbit ileal loop assay for heat-labile toxin as well as suckling mouse assays for heat-stabile toxin.

Enteroinvasive E. coli (EIEC). Laboratory tests have included the Serinje test (corneal ulceration of a guinea pig eye after inoculation with viable organisms).

Enterohemorrhagic E. coli (EHEC). Stool samples should be obtained early in the course of disease. EHEC O157:H7 can be detected by MacConkey agar base with sorbitol. Any sorbitol-negative *E. coli* recovered under these circumstances should be sent to a reliable reference laboratory. Demonstration of SLT-I or SLT-II (Shigalike toxin) by nucleic acid probes also confirms the diagnosis.

Enteropathogenic E. coli (EPEC). Patients have no fecal leukocytes in the stools. Examination of the contents of the small intestine by biopsy, microscopic evaluation, and culture confirms the diagnosis. Strains capable of causing disease also have the capability of localized adhesion in tissue culture (HeLa) cells.

Enteroaggregative E. coli (EAEC). These strains can be identified because they adhere to Hep2 cells. Their unusual pattern of adherence is different from the localized or diffuse adherence shown by other strains of *E. coli* and produces a stacked-brick appearance. The organisms also attach in clusters to the glass.

TREATMENT

The treatment of *E. coli* syndromes varies according to the mechanism of the infecting strain (Table 76–20). Antimotility agents should not be used in children with bloody diarrhea and fever, but these patients should be followed up carefully for development of HUS. If there is no evidence of hemolysis, thrombocytopenia, or nephropathy 3 days after the resolution of diarrhea, then the risk of development of HUS is low.

TABLE 76–20. Therapy for Enteric *Escherichia coli* Infections

Type of *E. coli*	Antimicrobial Treatment
Enterotoxigenic	None recommended, although TMP-SMZ PO has shown efficacy in adults
Enteroinvasive	TMP-SMZ as for shigellosis: 6–10 mg/kg/day TMP divided bid PO for 5 days should be effective with susceptible strains. Ampicillin should also be effective with susceptible strains
Enterohemorrhagic	None usually
Enteropathogenic	TMP-SMZ 6–10 mg/kg/day divided bid PO for 5–7 days *or* Neomycin 50–100 mg/kg/day *or* Gentamicin divided q6–8hr PO
Enteroaggregative	TMP-SMZ or aminoglycoside

Enterotoxigenic E. coli (ETEC). The preferred management is supportive only by oral rehydration. Antimicrobial agents such as TMP-SMZ have shown effectiveness in shortening the course of the disease in adults.

Enteroinvasive E. coli (EIEC). The treatment of enteroinvasive *E. coli* is similar to that recommended for *Shigella* infections. TMP-SMZ, given orally or intravenously for 5 days, is recommended. Ampicillin could be used for susceptible strains.

Enterohemorrhagic E. coli (EHEC). The illness runs its course in 2–9 days, requiring only symptomatic treatment. There is a significantly increased risk of HUS in patients with *E. coli* O157:H7 treated with antibiotics. Although death has been reported in fewer than 10% of patients with HUS, sequelae in the form of hypertension or abnormalities in renal function may occur in as many as 50% of patients.

Enteropathogenic E. coli (EPEC). Treatment of infection due to EPEC in infants should include nonabsorbable antibiotics, such as neomycin or gentamicin. TMP-SMZ should be considered if diarrhea is intractable and if the organisms are susceptible.

Enteroaggregative E. coli (EAEC). Treatment of these strains should be reserved for protracted cases, although the effect of antimicrobial therapy for this syndrome has not been studied. Either TMP-SMZ or an aminoglycoside could be used. Supportive management with lactose-free diets may have to be used, as well as elemental diets in protracted cases.

COMPLICATIONS AND PROGNOSIS

The disease in most instances is self-limited. Dehydration and electrolyte imbalance represent the major complications of enterotoxigenic enteritis. Thus, with appropriate supportive fluids the typical patient should recover fully. Infants who have protracted diarrhea due to enteroaggregative strains of *E. coli* may demonstrate failure to thrive. Children in whom HUS develops after an enterohemorrhagic *E. coli* infection usually recover if the renal failure and neurologic manifestations are managed properly.

PREVENTION

Good hygienic practices in all instances, especially in the care of newborns, and avoidance of raw, unpeeled vegetables and tap water, including ice, while traveling are important in preventing enterotoxigenic *E. coli* disease. Hot food should be eaten while it is still hot. Antimicrobial prophylaxis is not recommended for prevention of traveler's diarrhea. Antibiotics, including TMP-SMZ, doxycycline, and ciprofloxacin, although effective for prophylaxis to reduce the incidence of traveler's diarrhea, should not be used routinely because the potential risks outweigh the benefits. The adverse effects include an allergic reaction, antibiotic-associated colitis, and the potential of inducing antibiotic-resistant pathogens. Human milk has been reported to contain a *Shigella*-like toxin receptor glycolipid Gb3, which could exert a protective effect in those diarrheal illnesses of infancy mediated by the *Shigella*-like toxins (SLT-I and SLT-II).

VIRAL ENTERITIS

Viral gastroenteritis is responsible for up to 40% of all cases of infectious gastroenteritis in the United States, outnumbering the 20% of enteritis caused by bacterial and parasitic agents. The remaining 40% of cases are presumed to be infectious, but no etiologic agent has been isolated from them.

Five major categories of viruses are responsible for viral gastroenteritis: rotavirus, enteric adenoviruses, caliciviruses (Norwalk virus), astroviruses, and coronaviruses (Table 76–21). **Rotavirus** is the leading cause of viral gastroenteritis worldwide. In the developing world it is the major cause of death, resulting in 600,000 deaths among children because of dehydration and lack of medical care. In the United States, most deaths due to diarrhea in children younger than 1 year are attributable to dehydration, electrolyte imbalance, and shock. These 75–100 deaths occur in an annual seasonal pattern between October and February, simultaneous with the rotavirus season, primarily among children living in the southern United States who are born to young mothers who have had little or no prenatal care or education.

There is no specific treatment for any of the viral enteritides, although new modalities of treatment may be on the horizon because the pathogenesis of infection has been recently elucidated. At present, appropriate management of fluid and electrolyte balance is fundamental in minimizing morbidity and mortality. This is especially critical for young infants, for patients with associated vomiting, and for those with pre-existing conditions who have limited capability to withstand additional acute illness.

Methods to prevent the spread of viral gastroenteritis are limited to meticulous handwashing and appropriate handling of the stool of a person with the infection. Rotavirus vaccines are under development, but none is available currently.

ROTAVIRUS

ETIOLOGY

Rotavirus measures 70 μm in diameter and resembles a wheel. It belongs to the Reoviridae family, which contains segmented, double-stranded RNA with 11 gene segments. This genome is capable of genetic reassortment with the potential for antigenic changes. Unlike the influenza virus, there is no evidence to indicate that new pathogenic strains of rotavirus are introduced into the community by genetic mechanisms. There are at least seven distinct serotypes (A to G) of human rotavirus. Group A is the major cause of diarrhea, and groups B and C have also been identified as being of clinical significance in humans.

The serotype specificity of the rotavirus is determined by the VP7 glycoprotein. VP7 and VP4 are two outer capsid proteins responsible for induction of neutralizing antibodies against the virus, providing protective humoral immunity. VP4 is also important in the establishment of viral infection. It is cleaved into VP5 and VP4 by proteolytic activity of pancreatic trypsin, which initiates viral replication in the small intestine. There are also two major

TABLE 76–21. Epidemiologic and Clinical Manifestations and Diagnosis of Viral Gastroenteritis

Virus	Epidemiologic Features	Clinical Manifestations	Laboratory Diagnosis
Rotavirus	Major cause of endemic severe diarrhea in infants and young children worldwide (in winter in temperate zone)	Dehydration, vomiting, and diarrhea for 5–7 days; fever	Immunoassay, electron microscopy, polymerase chain reaction
Enteric adenoviruses	Second most important cause of endemic diarrhea among infants and young children	Prolonged diarrhea lasting 5–12 days; occasional vomiting and fever	Immunoassay, electron microscopy
Caliciviruses (Norwalk virus)	Epidemics of vomiting and diarrhea in older children and adults; occurs in school and is often associated with shellfish, other food, or water or ice	Acute vomiting, diarrhea, fever, myalgia for 1–2 days; self-limited	Immunoassay
Astroviruses	Diarrhea in children and the elderly	Watery diarrhea often lasting 2–3 days	Immunoassay, electron microscopy
Coronavirus	Few cases of neonatal enterocolitis	Necrotizing enterocolitis	Electron microscopy

inner-capsid polypeptides, VP6 and VP2. VP6 contains the domain for the common group–subgroup antigen shared by most human and animal rotaviruses. It is also the most immunogenic rotavirus protein.

Transmission. Rotavirus is transmitted by fecal-oral spread. Infected persons serve as a reservoir for infection. Rotavirus has been detected in the stool before the development of symptoms and is shed in the stool in high titers for 10–12 days after the diarrhea. Respiratory spread may also play a role in transmission of the virus. Common-source outbreaks due to rotavirus have been reported. Transmission of rotavirus in childcare centers and among families is common. Nosocomial spread of rotavirus has been reported, leading to prolongation of hospital stays.

EPIDEMIOLOGY

Rotavirus is the leading cause of viral gastroenteritis, accounting for 3.5 million cases a year in the United States, of which 1.1 million cases require hospitalization. Rotavirus accounts for 50% of total diarrheal episodes during the winter among infants and toddlers in childcare centers. The annual epidemic starts in the southwest area of the United States and reaches Canada by spring (Fig. 76–3).

Symptomatic rotavirus infection occurs in infants <3 years, with a peak at 4–24 months of age. Mild reinfection is common. About 30–40% of exposed adults have mild infection. Neonates may have asymptomatic infection or mild disease because of maternal antibody and breast-feeding that provide protection in infants younger than 3 months.

PATHOGENESIS

Rotavirus infection is established in the small intestine after the virus is activated by pancreatic trypsin. Viral replication occurs in enterocytes on the tips of the villi, resulting in villous shortening and blunting. There is patchy and selective destruction of the tip of the small-intestine villi, leaving the crypt of the intestinal epithelium and its secretory functions intact. In mice, the virus activates the enteric nervous system, which controls intestinal motility, fluid absorption, and secretion resulting in diarrhea. Rotavirus infection in the intestines releases chemicals in the gut that stimulate nerve endings in the intestines, and this affects secretory reflexes of intestinal cells with efflux of chloride ions into the intestine. This, in turn draws water into the intestine. This pathogenesis is similar to that of *V. cholerae* and enterotoxigenic *E. coli.*

Immunity to rotavirus has been associated in part with the presence of serum-neutralizing antibody to the specific serotype. In children younger than 6 months of age who have not had prior exposure to rotavirus, infection is associated with serotype-specific responses (homotypic antibody response) and not a heterotypic response to other serotypes. In older children with previous asymptomatic primary infection, subsequent exposure to rotavirus may result in a broad heterotypic antibody response and heterotypic immunity. Some human rotavirus strains also share common neutralizing epitopes on VP4, which also can account for a heterotypic response.

During both primary and secondary infections, IgM, IgG, and IgA immune responses to VP4 and VP7 have been seen. There is an apparent correlation between clinical immunity and the high antibody titer. The role of cellular immunity, that is, cytotoxic T cells, in the prevention of rotavirus infections has been demonstrated in animals. These immune cytotoxic T cells can prevent or clear rotavirus infection in mice. Local intestinal immunity also plays a major role in resistance to rotavirus in animals.

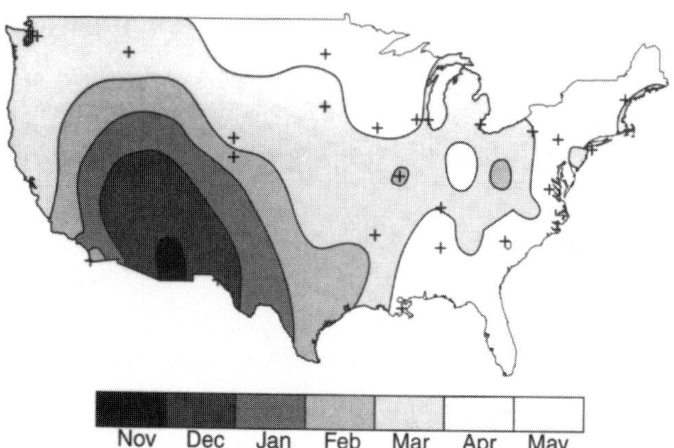

FIGURE 76–3. Peak rotavirus activity by month in the United States from July 1996 to June 1997. This pattern is typical of the annual rotavirus activity each year. (From Centers for Disease Control and Prevention: Laboratory-based surveillance for rotavirus—United States, July 1996–June 1997. *MMWR Morb Mortal Wkly Rep* 1997; 46:1092–4.)

SYMPTOMS AND CLINICAL MANIFESTATIONS

The incubation period of rotavirus diarrhea is 1–3 days. The illness usually lasts 5–7 days. Vomiting is a prominent clinical feature associated with the diarrhea leading to early dehydration. Fever is also observed in some patients.

Otitis media and upper respiratory tract symptoms are also seen occasionally. Neonates with rotavirus infection have mild or no symptoms, although rotavirus is shed in the stool and is capable of infecting other children and adults.

DIAGNOSIS

Laboratory diagnosis of rotavirus infection is indicated for patients with gastroenteritis for whom a definitive diagnosis needs to be established, such as patients who are hospitalized or patients in whom possible bacterial enteritis is suspected. Laboratory diagnosis is also necessary as part of an epidemiologic investigation, as in daycare center outbreaks in which bacterial and parasitic causes must be excluded.

Several specific and sensitive assays to detect rotavirus antigen in stool are commercially available and are the diagnostic methods of choice for routine clinical use. The EIA is rapid and sensitive, although false-positive reactions can occur in neonates. The virus is readily visualized in stool by electron microscopy and by specific nucleic acid amplification methods. Viral RNA can be extracted directly from fecal specimens and identified on gel electrophoresis. The rotavirus can be further serotyped and subgrouped by specific monoclonal antibodies or PCR.

TREATMENT

There is no specific treatment of rotavirus infections. Rotavirus diarrhea associated with loss of water and electrolytes can be treated by oral rehydration, especially because the glucose-coupled sodium transport system in unaffected cells in the small intestine remains intact. A non-lactose-containing formula can also be used initially until the tips of the villi have had an opportunity to regenerate for about 2 weeks.

COMPLICATIONS AND PROGNOSIS

Acute loss of fluid and electrolytes in rotavirus gastroenteritis can lead to severe dehydration and death. For marginally nourished children, diarrhea coupled with poor intake can aggravate the poor nutritional status. The infection is self-limited in most persons.

PREVENTION

Young children with diarrhea who are not toilet trained are a potential source of rotavirus infection in a childcare center and should not attend until the diarrhea resolves. Diapering areas of childcare centers should be disinfected between diaper changes.

Vaccine. Various rotavirus vaccines initially showed promise. A tetravalent rhesus-human reassortant rotavirus vaccine capable of eliciting broad heterotypic responses to rotaviruses was approved for use in the United States in 1998, but postmarketing surveillance showed that it was associated with a 21.7-fold increased incidence of intussusception. This vaccine was voluntarily withdrawn from the market in October 1999. Other rotavirus vaccine candidates, such as bovine rotavirus, are being evaluated.

ENTERIC ADENOVIRUSES

ETIOLOGY

Enteric adenovirus types 40 and 41, which belong to subgroup F, are 70–80 μm viruses that contain double-stranded DNA. They have fastidious growth characteristics distinguishable from those of respiratory adenoviruses that cause keratoconjunctivitis and nasopharyngitis. These two enteric adenoviruses have 62–69% DNA homology.

EPIDEMIOLOGY

Enteric adenoviruses are responsible for 4–10% of cases of pediatric diarrheal enteritis and are important pathogens of diarrhea that persists for >2 weeks. Enteric adenovirus gastroenteritis is endemic and occurs throughout the year, although outbreaks occur. Antibodies to enteric adenovirus, indicative of infection, are acquired early in infancy. By early adolescence, 41% of the population has serologic evidence of past exposure.

SYMPTOMS AND CLINICAL MANIFESTATIONS

The incubation period of adenoviral gastroenteritis is 8–10 days, and the illness lasts for about 2 weeks. Children present primarily with prolonged watery diarrhea. A few have vomiting and a low-grade fever (Table 76–21). Virus is shed in the stool, although none of the family contacts shed adenovirus in the stool, unlike the situation with rotavirus infection.

DIAGNOSIS

Laboratory confirmation of enteric adenovirus should be considered for persons with prolonged diarrhea and as a part of the evaluation during an outbreak of gastroenteritis among young children who are negative for rotavirus. Numerous diagnostic methods are available in research laboratories that use DNA-based hybridization techniques. An EIA using Ad40- and Ad41-specific monoclonal antibodies can detect enteric strains of adenovirus with high specificity and sensitivity.

COMPLICATIONS AND PROGNOSIS

Adenovirus infections are self-limited in most patients, but diarrhea can last up to 1 month, possibly exacerbating pre-existing malnutrition or malabsorptive states.

NORWALK VIRUS

ETIOLOGY

Norwalk virus is a small, round, 27 μm virus classified as an RNA virus belonging to the family of Caliciviridae. The Norwalk virus is the prototype strain of a group of 26–35 mm nonenveloped viruses that cause gastroenteritis. These viruses have been named after the location of the outbreak. There are five distinct groups: Norwalk, Montgomery County, Hawaii, Snow Mountain, and Tauton. These viruses have a single-stranded RNA genome, lack distinctive morphologic characteristics on electron microscopy, and are unable to grow in cell culture. These viruses have a classic six-pointed surface star with a hollow center and a cup-like depression on the outer surface that is distinguishable from the cultivatable astroviruses that have a five- or six-pointed surface star with a stained center. The Norwalk virus has been characterized from the cloned cDNA and has been sequenced.

Transmission. Norwalk virus is excreted in the stool, and fecal-oral transmission is the most common route of spread. In some outbreaks, airborne transmission by means of droplets in vomitus causing secondary cases from person-to-person transmission has been suggested. Vehicles of transmission in common-source food-borne outbreaks are contaminated food items, such as frosting, salad, potato salad, coleslaw, celery, melon, consommé, sandwiches, cold cooked ham, water, and commercial ice.

EPIDEMIOLOGY

The prevalence of antibodies to Norwalk virus increases with age, with a rapid increase during adolescence to the 60% prevalence seen in adults. Young children from developing countries with inadequate sanitation are exposed to the virus and develop antibodies beginning in infancy. In one study (Ryder et al, 1985) 35% of children <5 years of age from Panamanian Islands were seropositive.

Outbreaks occur throughout the year in various settings, such as families, communities, schools, colleges, camps, military populations in different parts of the world, and cruise ships.

PATHOGENESIS

Pre-existing serum antibody to Norwalk virus does not correlate with protective immunity and long-term resistance to infection. Short-term protective immunity after repeated exposure is observed, although long-term immunity to Norwalk virus appears to be related to nonimmune factors or host response. A Norwalk-specific IgM response is seen in the acute phase, and an IgG response is seen in the convalescent phase. A specific serum IgA response to Norwalk virus is also seen in the acute phase of illness. Much information has been obtained from adult volunteers who ingested Norwalk virus. Nausea and vomiting accompanying Norwalk viral gastroenteritis result from abnormal gastric motor function with marked delay in gastric emptying. Other gastric secretory function remains normal, although there is transient malabsorption of D-xylose, lactose, and fat. Jejunal biopsies at the height of illness reveal partial villous flattening, broadening of the villi, and disorganization of the epithelial lining cells. There is a mononuclear cellular infiltration of the lamina propria, although no definite viral particles are seen. Repeat biopsies 2 weeks after the height of illness show normal mucosa.

SYMPTOMS AND CLINICAL MANIFESTATIONS

After an incubation period of 10–48 hours following the ingestion of contaminated food or water, acute nausea (79%) and vomiting (69%) are followed by abdominal cramps (30%) and diarrhea (60%). Fever (37%), chills (32%), myalgia (26%), and headache (22%) are usually present (Table 76–21). The disease is generally mild and self-limited. The duration of symptoms is between 12 and 60 hours.

DIAGNOSIS

Illness caused by Norwalk virus is indistinguishable from other foodborne diarrheal syndromes. Presumptive diagnosis of Norwalk virus infection can be established as a part of an investigation of an outbreak by the following criteria: (1) stool cultures fail to detect a bacterial pathogen or parasite; (2) vomiting occurs in 50% of cases; and (3) the median duration of illness is between 12–60 hours. A virologic diagnosis can be established in research laboratories by detection of antigen in the stool and by acute and convalescent serum antibody tests.

ASTROVIRUSES

Astroviruses are small, round viruses, 27–32 μm in diameter. They have three structural proteins and a single-stranded RNA. The astroviruses are infrequently associated with gastroenteritis outbreaks and do not cause illness serious enough to require hospitalization. They cause a rotavirus-like illness in infants, young children, and the elderly. The illness has an incubation period of 1–2 days with clinical symptoms predominantly of watery diarrhea (Table 76–21). The virus is shed in the stool. Outbreaks of astrovirus gastroenteritis have been reported, especially among children. Most children have antibodies to astrovirus by the age of 4 years. In the United States, pooled immunoglobulin contains antibody to all five astrovirus serotypes. The diagnosis is established only by electron microscopic examination of stool specimens.

CORONAVIRUSES

Coronaviruses are positive-stranded RNA viruses, approximately 80–150 μm in diameter. These viruses are often detected in persons from developing countries who live with poor sanitary conditions. Human coronavirus has been isolated from the stools of neonates with necrotizing enterocolitis (Table 76–21). These infants also developed coronavirus-specific antibodies. Enteric coronavirus was detected in epithelial cells of the ileum in a fatal case of severe enteritis in an infant. The definitive role of coronavirus infantile gastroenteritis remains to be elucidated.

CHRONIC INFECTIOUS DIARRHEA

GIARDIASIS

ETIOLOGY

Giardia is a flagellated protozoan. There are at least three species: *Giardia muris* in rodents, birds, and reptiles; *Giardia agilis* in amphibians; and *Giardia lamblia* in humans. Even among *G. lamblia* isolates there are different strains as determined by isoenzyme analysis, restriction fragment length polymorphisms, and surface antigens.

Transmission. *Giardia* is transmitted from person to person and from animals to humans in the cyst stage by the fecal-oral route. The infectious dose of *Giardia* is low: 10 cysts can infect a human. Persons at highest risk are children in daycare centers who are not toilet trained, their close contacts, men who have sex with men, and campers drinking unfiltered water. Diarrhea commonly occurs in the families of children who attend daycare during a *Giardia* outbreak, with a secondary attack rate of 17–30%.

EPIDEMIOLOGY

Giardia is found worldwide and is the most common intestinal parasite. The prevalence varies from 1% to 7%, and is higher in developing countries. The seasonal peak occurs in the summer along with increased use of communal swimming pools and water parks.

Large community-wide outbreaks of infection have been seen after contamination of water or food either by infected persons or by domestic and wild animals. Because of the proximity between domestic animals and humans, *Giardia* cysts can be introduced into the environment by the infected host and can spread by waterborne (unfiltered, unchlorinated water) or direct contact. There is also a high prevalence of *Giardia* in sheep and cattle, which may be important reservoirs of human infection in an enzootic cycle. Beavers are also believed to be vectors for water contamination in the Rocky Mountain region.

PATHOGENESIS

Variation in strains is probably responsible for the differences in ability to colonize and establish infection. No specific markers responsible for virulence have been identified.

The development of protective immunity to *Giardia* may be achieved in part by host immune defense mechanisms that are responsible for controlling acute infection. There is epidemiologic evidence of acquisition of protective immunity with advancing age; the prevalence of giardiasis decreases, beginning at adolescence. This immunity is probably acquired by multiple exposures. Anti-*Giardia* IgG, IgM, and IgA responses are seen in patients with giardiasis. An IgG response is seen in 80% of patients with symptomatic infections. It appears to be persistent and does not allow a distinction between past or present infection. An IgM response develops within 2–3 weeks after the onset of infection and may help in differentiating current from previous infection. There appears to be a correlation between persistent cases of giardiasis and low levels of antibodies to *Giardia* plasma membrane. Anti-*Giardia* IgA is also detected in acute infection in approximately one third of patients. Local secretory IgA antibody within the intestinal lumen is probably responsible for clearance of *Giardia* from the intestines. Patients with a secretory IgA deficiency are especially susceptible to intestinal giardiasis. They have a predominantly nodular lymphoid hyperplasia with an increased number of IgM-containing plasma cells.

Evidence also suggests that neonates born to immune mothers acquire a passive immunity during breast-feeding. Infants born to mothers with high levels of secretory IgA (sIgA) in their milk have lower rates of *Giardia* infection (16%) than infants born to mothers with low sIgA levels (63%).

Colonization of the duodenum and proximal jejunum occurs in three steps: (1) encystation, (2) attachment to the intestinal epithelium, and (3) multiplication by binary fission. The mechanism by which *Giardia* produces diarrhea and malabsorption is not clearly established. The condition of the mucosa varies from normal mucosa to villous atrophy. Crypt-cell hyperplasia occurs with the reduction of villous height. The degree of mucosal damage correlates with the extent of functional impairment of the intestine. *Giardia* rarely directly invades the mucosa, although lymphocytes do infiltrate the lamina propria. There is a good correlation between the intensity of mucosal infiltration and the severity of intestinal malabsorption.

SYMPTOMS AND CLINICAL MANIFESTATIONS

The incubation period of giardiasis is 3–42 days, with an average of 8 days. The clinical manifestations vary and may be related to the virulence of the parasite as well as to the host factors (Table 76–22). It causes a spectrum of illness from asymptomatic excretion of *G. lamblia* cysts to acute and chronic diarrhea associated with intestinal malabsorption. The most common symptoms are a brief diarrheal illness with or without a low-grade fever, anorexia, nausea, abdominal cramps, pain, bloating, and flatulence. Protracted diarrhea with or without malabsorption may lead to weight loss. Occasionally patients with giardiasis present with oral aphthous ulcers, urticaria, and salt-and-pepper degeneration of the optic discs. Severe giardiasis has been seen in immunosuppressed patients, such as those who have had a bone marrow transplant. Giardiasis should be considered in patients who have had contact with a young child who attends a daycare center and those who have traveled to an endemic area if they have unexplained gastrointestinal symptoms, failure to thrive, and weight loss. From 1997 to 1998, an estimated 4600 hospitalizations occurred annually in the United States because of severe giardiasis and its complications of dehydration and failure to thrive.

DIAGNOSIS

Both trophozoites and cysts can be identified in fresh stool by direct smear. *Giardia* cysts can be excreted in the stool intermittently for weeks or months. Trophozoites are present more frequently in unformed stool as a result of a rapid intestinal transit time. *Giardia* is often difficult to identify because of its intermittent excretion. The sensitivity of a single direct stool smear is 50–75%, which increases to 95% with three specimens. If repeat stool specimens are negative for *Giardia* but the diagnosis is still considered likely, aspiration or biopsy of the duodenum or upper jejunum should be performed. An alternative to obtaining duodenal fluid by endoscopy is the commercially available Entero-Test (HDC-Corporation, San Jose, California). In this test a nylon string is affixed to a gelatin capsule, which is swallowed. After several hours, the string is withdrawn and duodenal contents are examined for *G. lamblia* trophozoites. An EIA has been developed for the rapid detection of *G. lamblia* and *Cryptosporidium parvum* in the stool with a sensitivity of 75%.

TREATMENT

Children with acute diarrhea or chronic diarrhea with malabsorption and failure to thrive should be treated (Table 76–22). The drug of choice is metronidazole, which has a cure rate of 80–90%. Adverse effects of metronidazole include a metallic taste. Several other drugs are available for treatment of giardiasis. Tinidazole has a 90–100% cure rate, but the safety and efficacy in children are not established. Furazolidone has a cure rate of 72–100%. Adverse effects include nausea, vomiting, mild hemolysis in patients with glucose-6-phosphate dehydrogenase (G-6-PD) deficiency, and a disulfiram-like reaction with alcohol. Albendazole has been shown to be effective in children >2 years of age. Paromomycin is also effective in 50–70% of cases, and is the treatment of choice for pregnant women. Quinacrine can also be used. Adverse effects of quinacrine include bitter taste, yellow discoloration of skin and sclera, nausea, vomiting, toxic psychosis, exfoliative dermatitis, exacerbation of psoriasis, and a disulfiram-like reaction with alcohol. Immunocompromised patients may require prolonged treatment and combination therapy.

Treatment of symptom-free carriers who are incidentally found to excrete *G. lamblia* is generally not recommended. Possible exceptions, principally to prevent transmission, are excreters without symptoms who are household contacts of persons with hypogammaglobulinemia or cystic fibrosis. Toddlers with asymptomatic cyst excretion in a household with a pregnant woman should be treated to prevent transmission in the household.

DIENTAMOEBA FRAGILIS

ETIOLOGY

Dientamoeba fragilis is an intestinal protozoan frequently isolated from children.

EPIDEMIOLOGY

Acquisition of this parasite has been associated with contact with cats. After *Giardia, Dientamoeba* is the most frequent parasite isolated in daycare centers and has been found in up to 8.6% of children and 4% of staff. Trophozoites of *D. fragilis* have been detected within the ova of the pinworm *Enterobius vermicularis* and appear to be transmitted with the pinworm eggs, resulting in simultaneous infection with both parasites. Under poor hygienic and sanitary conditions, fecal-oral transmission probably occurs among close contacts.

SYMPTOMS AND CLINICAL MANIFESTATIONS

The clinical manifestations of *D. fragilis* infection include nausea, vomiting, diarrhea, flatulence, and abdominal pain. Headache, fever, weight loss, and fatigue may occur infrequently as well.

TABLE 76–22. Clinical Manifestations and Treatment for Chronic Infectious Diarrhea

Pathogen	Symptoms and Clinical Features	Treatment
Giardia lamblia	Transmission is fecal-oral, water-borne zoonosis, and childcare center contacts. In acute cases diarrhea is associated with abdominal cramps, bloating, and flatulence. In chronic cases protracted diarrhea occurs with malabsorption and weight loss	***Recommended Regimen*** Metronidazole 20 mg/kg/day (max 250 mg) divided tid PO for 7 days ***Alternative Regimens*** Furazolidone 6–8 mg/kg/day (max 100 mg) divided tid or qid PO for 10 days *or* Albendazole 400 mg/day PO for 5 days *or* Tinidazole 50 mg/kg/day (max 2 g) PO* *or* Quinacrine 6 mg/kg/day (max 100 mg) divided tid PO for 5 days* ***Pregnant Women*** Paromomycin 30 mg/kg/day (max 500 mg) divided tid or qid PO for 7 days ***Refractory Cases*** Metronidazole 20 mg/kg/day (max 250 mg) divided tid PO *and* quinacrine 6 mg/kg/day (max 100 mg) divided tid PO for 14 days*
Dientamoeba fragilis	Probably fecal-oral transmission, and childcare center contacts; patients present with nausea, vomiting, diarrhea, flatulence, abdominal pain	***Recommended Regimen*** Iodoquinol 30–40 mg/kg/day (max 2 g) divided tid PO for 20 days ***Alternative Regimens*** Paromomycin 25–35 mg/kg/day divided tid PO for 7 days *or* Tetracycline 40 mg/kg/day (max 2 g) divided qid PO for 10 days
Cryptosporidium parvum	Transmission is through infected mammals, birds and reptiles. Waterborne outbreaks and childcare contacts. Acute cases present with watery, foul-smelling diarrhea, vomiting, and abdominal cramps. Chronic cases present with a persistence of symptoms associated with weight loss, malaise, and biliary tract involvement	Paromomycin 25–35 mg/kg/day divided bid, tid, qid PO (Infection is self-limited in immunocompetent persons. Treatment is not curative in immunocompromised persons; combination therapy with azithromycin [600 mg/day in adults] may be beneficial.)
Isospora belli	Same as *Cryptosporidium parvum*	***Recommended Regimen*** TMP 5 mg–SMZ 25 mg (max TMP 160 mg–SMZ 800 mg) qid PO for 10 days, then bid for 3 wk ***Alternative Regimens*** Sulfadoxine-pyrimethamine *or* Pyrimethamine and folic acid
Cyclospora cayetanensis	Endemic in countries such as Haiti, Nepal, and Peru. Diarrhea, weight loss, fatigue, abdominal pain, and nausea are reported by more than 75% of those with symptoms	TMP 5 mg–SMZ 25 mg (max TMP 160 mg–SMZ 800 mg) bid PO for 7 days (HIV-infected persons may require higher dosage and longer maintenance.)
Microsporida	Watery diarrhea without fever aggravated by food intake with wasting, abdominal pain are the more common findings in AIDS patients	***Recommended Regimen*** Albendazole 400 mg bid PO ***Alternative Regimens*** Metronidazole *or* atovaquone (HAART may lead to clinical and microbiologic response in HIV-infected persons.)

*Not commercially available in the United States.

TREATMENT

Treatment regimens are investigational. Iodoquinol (diiodohydroxyquin) or paromomycin, an oral aminoglycoside, are the drugs of choice (Table 76–22). Persons >8 years of age can also be treated with tetracycline.

INTESTINAL SPORE-FORMING COCCIDIAN PROTOZOA

ETIOLOGY AND EPIDEMIOLOGY

Cryptosporidium and Isospora. The coccidial protozoans *Cryptosporidium parvum* and *Isospora belli* are closely related and are increasingly being identified as important causes of waterborne outbreaks of enteritis and of enteritis associated with outdoor swimming. *C. parvum* oocysts are spherical and measure 2–5 μm in diameter. *Isospora* oocysts are ellipsoid and large, measuring 20–30 μm by 10–20 μm. *C. parvum* is found in mammals, birds, and reptiles. *C. parvum* is associated with outbreaks of diarrhea among infants and toddlers in daycare centers, particularly children who wear diapers and are not toilet trained. *I. belli* occasionally is associated with travelers' diarrhea and can also cause severe chronic diarrhea in immunocompromised persons. For pediatric patients with AIDS, the prevalence of *C. parvum* is 5.1%. These rates have probably been underestimated, however, because not all patients with AIDS are routinely examined for these particular parasites. Because chronic diarrhea can be especially devastating for patients with AIDS, causing continuous and severe fluid and electrolyte disturbances, malnutrition, and severe weight loss, identification of these parasitic infections may have a marked effect on patient management, especially with respect to isosporiasis, for which an effective treatment is available. In immunocompetent hosts with cryptosporidiosis and isosporiasis, the nutritional consequences of the diarrhea are much less severe because the diseases are self-limited.

Both of these organisms are transmitted from infected animals, through contaminated water supplies, and by person-to-person contact (e.g., diaper changing and placing of shared objects among infants and toddlers in the mouth). Transmission in childcare centers may reach rates of 30–60%. These parasites are resistant to chlorine, and sand filters used for swimming pools are ineffective for removing oocysts from contaminated water. Cryptosporidiosis may be spread through aerosolization, fomites, food, and sexual activity (Table 76–22).

Cyclospora. *Cyclospora cayetanensis,* previously called cyanobacterium-like body, is a coccidian parasite that is increasingly recognized as a causative agent of diarrheal diseases. *Cyclospora* oocysts measure 8–10 μm in diameter. The parasite has worldwide distribution, and disease is endemic in countries such as Haiti, Nepal, and Peru. The prevalence varies from as high as 11% in Katmandu to as low as 0.2% in the United States. Infection is rare in children <18 months of age. Cases in the United States are associated with travel or immunocompromise, with outbreaks associated with contaminated food or water. A large outbreak of *Cyclospora* in the United States in 1997 was associated with contaminated frozen raspberries. Other fresh produce has also been associated with transmission.

Microsporida. More than 700 species in at least six genera belong to the order Microsporida. The organisms best associated with enteritis are *Enterocytozoon bieneusi* and *Septata intestinalis.* These intracellular, obligate protozoa are ubiquitous and have gained attention by their ability to cause illness in immunocompromised persons. Transmission occurs through ingestion of contaminated food or water (Table 76–22). In dogs, pigs, rabbits, and parakeets, transmission occurs by ingestion of microsporida spores in food or present in the environment through stool and urine.

PATHOGENESIS

Cryptosporidium and Isospora. Cryptosporidiosis and isosporiasis are acquired by ingestion of infective sporulated oocysts. Both parasites undergo asexual schizogony and sexual gametogeny almost exclusively in the parasitophorous vacuoles in epithelial cells of the intestinal villi. These vacuoles are located in the microvillar region of the cytoplasm for *C. parvum,* and deep within the cytoplasm for *I. belli. C. parvum* completes its life cycle in the mucosal epithelium of a variety of organs, including the respiratory tract and the biliary tract and gallbladder (Fig. 76–4). The major difference

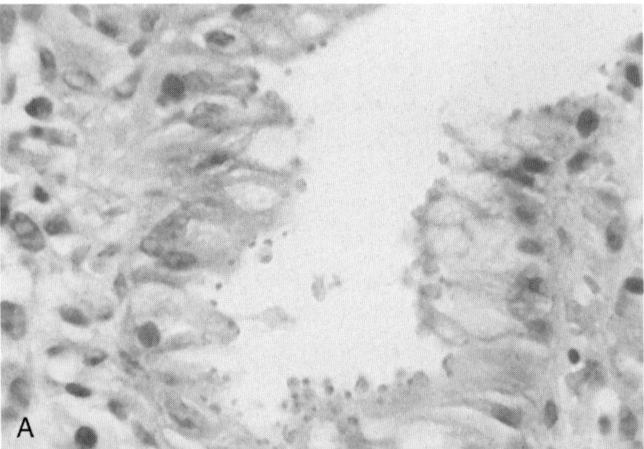

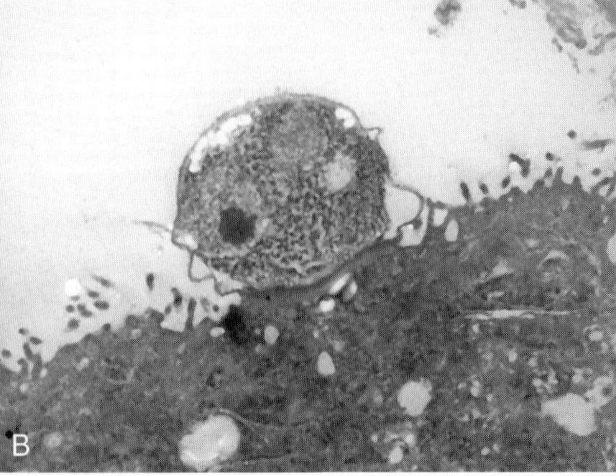

FIGURE 76–4. Cryptosporidiosis in a patient with the acquired immunodeficiency syndrome (AIDS). **A,** Round, hematoxophilic organisms 2–4 μm in diameter are seen attached to the apical surface of the epithelial cells of the gallbladder. The epithelium on the left is ragged in comparison with the less heavily infected area on the right (hematoxylin and eosin stain). **B,** Electron micrograph of a 4 μm diameter *Cryptosporidium* oocyst located on the apical surface of a colonocyte. At first sight, the organism appears to be extracellular, but it is enclosed in a space bounded by the host cell membrane and is therefore intracellular.

between the cycles of the parasites is in their periods of infectivity. Thin-walled oocysts produced during the asexual schizogony in cryptosporidiosis may be released into the intestinal lumen, where they are free to invade other host cells and thereby reinitiate the developmental cycle. This is why low infecting doses of *C. parvum* oocysts can cause quite persistent infections, even in the absence of repeated oral exposure to the thick-walled infectious oocysts. This phenomenon does not occur with *I. belli.* In addition, the oocysts of *C. parvum* sporulate within the host cells and are immediately infectious on passage of the stool, whereas the oocysts of *I. belli* sporulate only outside the host when exposed to increased oxygen concentrations and temperatures below 37°C (98.6°F). Limited data suggest that both humoral and cellular immunity play a role in limiting the infection of cryptosporidiosis. Prolonged shedding is eliminated once the immune function has been restored.

The mechanisms whereby both parasites cause diarrhea are poorly defined. The cholera-like symptoms of cryptosporidiosis suggest a mechanism of hypersecretion into the intestine or toxin production, but malabsorption is also plausible. *Isospora* intestinal lesions are characterized by villous atrophy or fused villi, focal necrosis of epithelial cells, crypt hyperplasia, and infiltration of the lamina propria by eosinophils, mononuclear cells, and inflammatory cells. These conditions could be a result of parasite entry or exit, a parasite toxin, or hypersensitivity to parasite antigens.

Cyclospora. *Cyclospora* affects the upper part of the small bowel. Intracellular parasites lead to villous atrophy and hyperplasia of crypts in the jejunum. The actual mechanisms of clinical illness remain to be determined.

Microsporida. Disease caused by this opportunistic protozoan is directly linked to immunodeficiency. Organisms have been found in intestinal epithelial cells of HIV-infected patients without diarrhea. Other members of the group, such as *Encephalitozoon cuniculi,* have been reported to disseminate to various body sites, including pulmonary and conjunctival sites. The actual mechanisms of clinical illness remain to be determined.

SYMPTOMS AND CLINICAL MANIFESTATIONS

Cryptosporidium and Isospora. The incubation period is 2–14 days. In immunocompetent hosts, the signs and symptoms of self-limiting cryptosporidiosis include watery, foul-smelling diarrhea, anorexia, vomiting, abdominal cramps, and a fever and cough lasting 7–10 days (Table 76–22). The symptoms of self-limiting isosporiasis include an acute onset with diarrhea, steatorrhea, colicky abdominal pain, headache, and asthenia that last 6 weeks to a few months.

In immunocompromised hosts the clinical manifestations of chronic cryptosporidiosis and isosporiasis are virtually indistinguishable, and their severity increases as immune function deteriorates. Symptoms in adults include voluminous, watery, noninflammatory diarrhea, abdominal pain usually made worse by food ingestion, flatulence, dehydration, nausea, vomiting, anorexia, malaise, and weight loss. Fever is uncommon. If *C. parvum* infection spreads to the respiratory tract, chronic cough, dyspnea, bronchiolitis, and pneumonitis may occur.

Cyclospora. The incubation period is approximately 1 week, with a range of 2–10 days. Illness may last days to weeks. The duration of illness in one study (Shlim et al, 1991) of immunocompetent patients was 43 ± 24 days. Diarrhea, weight loss, fatigue, abdominal pain, and nausea are reported by >75%, and bloating, myalgias, and chills occur in two thirds of persons with symptoms. Stools are typically frequent and watery, with mucus or blood infrequently. Symptoms may remit and relapse. This etiology should be considered in patients with prolonged diarrheal illness. As the symptoms resolve, shedding decreases and ultimately ceases, although there are reports of asymptomatic shedding. Patients with AIDS experience symptoms that may be indistinguishable from cryptosporidiosis and isosporiasis. Infection of the biliary tree has been reported in some of these patients.

Microsporida. Watery diarrhea without fever that is aggravated by food intake and associated with wasting and abdominal pain is the common finding in patients with AIDS infected by one of these parasites. Coinfection with *C. parvum* is not uncommon and should be considered. The parasite may infect the biliary tree and cause cholangitis and cholecystitis. Extension beyond the intestinal tract to kidneys, muscle, respiratory tract, and rarely the central nervous system has been reported in severely immunocompromised patients.

DIAGNOSIS

Because these infections are infrequent and self-limited in immunocompetent hosts, their diagnosis usually is not sought except in immunocompromised patients with severe or prolonged symptoms. The diagnosis is most often based on the identification of oocysts in a stained fecal smear.

Laboratory Evaluation

Lactose intolerance and fat malabsorption occur with both *C. parvum* and *I. belli.* In cases of chronic cryptosporidiosis involving the biliary tract, serum levels of alkaline phosphatase and glutamyl transpeptidase are elevated, whereas serum transaminases and bilirubin levels are usually normal.

Microbiologic Evaluation

C. parvum and *I. belli* oocysts are acid-fast and are therefore easily distinguished from morphologically similar yeasts that are not acid-fast. *C. parvum* can be identified in the stool by concentrating the stool oocysts before staining it with modified Kinyoun acid-fast stain (Plate 2F). The oocysts of *I. belli* can be distinguished from those of *C. parvum* by their five times larger size and their oval shape with the use of modified Kinyoun acid-fast stain and auramine-rhodamine stains. In addition, a method for detecting *C. parvum* oocysts using fluorescein-labeled IgG monoclonal antibodies is available commercially. This method may be more sensitive and specific than the acid-fast staining technique, but it does not allow for a simultaneous diagnosis of isosporiasis.

Cyclospora is identified by examining stool specimens and staining with phenosafranin or modified acid-fast stains and by autofluorescence. The parasite is not visualized by other staining methods, such as Gram, hematoxylin-eosin, or Giemsa stains.

Microsporida can be detected in formalin-fixed stool specimens or duodenal aspirates by modified trichrome stain viewed with light microscopy. Identification for classification purposes requires electron microscopy to differentiate among the various genera. Microsporida can also be identified in biopsy specimens of the small intestine.

Serologic Tests. Although IgG, IgM, and IgA antibodies to *C. parvum* have been detected by immunofluorescent assays and EIA, serologic tests are not useful in the diagnosis of acute cryptosporidiosis because elevated antibody titers are not detectable until

6–8 weeks after the onset of illness. There is no serologic test for isosporiasis.

Diagnostic Imaging

The radiographic abnormalities of the intestine are nonspecific and include prominent mucosal folds, thickened intestinal walls, and disordered mobility. In cases of chronic cryptosporidiosis involving the biliary tract, radiographic analysis reveals a thickened gallbladder, dilated bile ducts, distal bile duct structures, and luminal irregularities suggestive of cholangitis. These radiographic findings are also associated with cytomegalovirus infection.

TREATMENT

Cryptosporidium and Isospora. Cryptosporidiosis is usually self-limited with serious consequences for immunocompetent persons, but the effects of chronic cryptosporidial diarrhea can be life threatening for immunocompromised persons. Paromomycin, clarithromycin, or nitazoxanide may offer some hope for therapy. Supportive care with oral or intravenous hydration and avoidance of gastrointestinal stimulants such as caffeine are recommended. In addition, parenteral alimentation is advised on an individual basis to optimize and offset limitations on oral uptake (Table 76–22).

In contrast to cryptosporidiosis, there is readily available therapy for isosporiasis. A 10-day course of TMP-SMZ, 10 mg TMP–50 mg SMZ/kg/day, and pyrimethamine-sulfadoxine is effective (Table 76–22). Immunocompromised persons usually require secondary prophylaxis with TMP-SMZ and sulfadoxine-pyrimethamine, or pyrimethamine and folic acid for patients who are allergic to sulfonamides.

Cyclospora. Cyclosporiasis shows striking improvement after treatment with TMP-SMZ, although immunocompromised persons may require secondary prophylaxis (Table 76–22).

Microsporida. There is no standard treatment for organisms of the class Microsporida. Albendazole, metronidazole, and atovaquone have led to improvement of the diarrhea but without eradication of the organisms. Symptoms may recur with cessation of treatment, and thus long-term suppressive therapy may be necessary.

PREVENTION

Immunocompromised persons should avoid untreated water and raw vegetables. Standard enteric precautions should be used in patient care. Daycare staff should practice good handwashing before and after changing diapers and when handling food and bottles. During outbreaks, daycare centers should be closed to new admissions and children with symptoms should be kept together.

TRAVELERS' DIARRHEA

Most of the information about travelers' diarrhea is derived from observations of adults. Although illness usually occurs within weeks of arrival in the foreign country, travelers' diarrhea can start several days after a person has been infected. Thus the physician should ask the family about foreign travel whenever treating a child with diarrhea. This entity must also be considered in patients arriving in the United States from travel overseas.

ETIOLOGY

Infectious agents that may be the cause of endemic diarrhea usually cause travelers' diarrhea (Table 76–23). In 20–40% of cases the cause is unknown.

TABLE 76–23. Etiologic Agents of Travelers' Diarrhea

Agent	Average Frequency (%)
Bacterial Agents	
Enterotoxigenic *Escherichia coli*	40–60
Salmonella	<5
Shigella	10
Campylobacter	<5
Vibrio parahaemolyticus	<2
Other *E. coli*	15
Viral Agents	
Rotavirus	<5
Norwalk virus	<5
Parasitic Agents	
Giardia lamblia	<5
Entamoeba histolytica	<3
Cryptosporidium, Isospora belli, Strongyloides	<1
Unknown	20–40

Bacteria. Enterotoxigenic *E. coli* (ETEC) are implicated in approximately 50% of cases in which a cause is detected. *Campylobacter* accounts for approximately 10% of cases. *Salmonella* and *V. cholerae,* although rare in the United States, are common in some geographic areas such as Asia. *Shigella* are recovered from approximately 15% of patients with travelers' diarrhea, mostly from Mexico. *V. parahaemolyticus* has been associated with ingestion of raw or poorly cooked seafood and has caused illness in passengers on Caribbean cruise ships. Other less common bacterial pathogens include *Y. enterocolitica, V. cholerae* O1, O139, and other non-O1 *V. cholerae, V. fluvialis, A. hydrophila,* and *P. shigelloides.*

Viral Agents. Rotaviruses and Norwalk-like viruses cause approximately 10–36% of cases. Viruses probably constitute a high percentage of the causative agents of travelers' diarrhea in children. Seasonal differences between the northern and southern hemispheres should be taken into consideration when rotavirus and other viral causes of enteritis are considered.

Parasitic Agents. Few studies of travelers' diarrhea have included examination for parasites. *E. histolytica* and *G. lamblia* each cause 6% of cases of travelers' diarrhea. *C. parvum, I. belli, Cyclospora, D. fragilis, Balantidium coli,* and *Strongyloides stercoralis* cause occasional cases and should be considered with persistent diarrhea.

EPIDEMIOLOGY

Estimates are that each year at least 100 million of 250 million persons who travel from one country to another develop travelers' diarrhea. Although the cause is uncertain in 20–50% of cases, even patients with travelers' diarrhea of unknown cause are likely to respond to antimicrobial therapy. Travelers who become ill have usually ingested an inoculum of virulent pathogens sufficiently large to overcome individual defense mechanisms, resulting in symptoms.

SYMPTOMS AND CLINICAL MANIFESTATIONS

Travelers' diarrhea is an intestinal syndrome, usually acute and self-limited, caused by one or more of multiple enteric infectious agents. There is a more than twofold increase in frequency over baseline of unformed bowel movements that assume the form of the container. About 15% of persons with diarrhea have vomiting, and 2–10% have fever or bloody stool or both. The typical clinical situation of diarrhea without fever reflects the predominant contribution of the toxigenic bacteria. Other causative agents usually manifest in a manner characteristic of illness caused by the specific agent.

DIAGNOSIS

The epidemiologic background of travel, along with a history of consumption of improperly processed food (especially raw or unpeeled) or ice or tap water, is helpful in suggesting the syndrome. Predisposing conditions, such as achlorhydria and T-cell dysfunction associated with immunosuppression, are not a prerequisite for acquisition of disease but may allow for more severe symptoms and a more dramatic presentation.

Culture of the stool is recommended for patients with fever, with or without dysentery, or with profuse diarrhea and dehydration. A rapid diagnostic test for rotavirus should be performed if the patient returns during the winter season. Stool evaluation for parasitic agents should be considered for acute dysenteric illness or in protracted cases of diarrhea in which no bacterial agent can be identified.

TREATMENT

The management of travelers' diarrhea includes hydration, use of nonspecific absorptive agents such as kaolin and pectin and bismuth subsalicylate, other nonspecific methods with the potential for a higher toxicity such as administration of loperamide, and antimicrobial agents (Table 76–24). Children without fever can be treated conservatively with oral fluids to ensure hydration and other measures of supportive therapy. Children with dysentery symptoms with fever ≥38.5°C (101.5°F), or blood or mucus in the stool, can be treated empirically for *Shigella* with a 5-day course of TMP-SMZ (Table 76–24). Furazolidone can be used for patients who do not respond to or who are allergic to TMP-SMZ. In addition, furazolidone has activity against other agents, such as *G. lamblia.* The quinolones, which are not recommended for use in persons <18 years of age or in pregnant women, are effective against the predominant bacterial pathogens associated with travelers' diarrhea, including multiply-resistant strains.

COMPLICATIONS

Complications are those related to the particular etiologic agent. Approximately 10% of travelers sustain chronic diarrhea. In these patients, a concerted clinical evaluation is needed to explore the possibility of parasitic infection or other conditions, such as tropical

TABLE 76–24. Therapy for Travelers' Diarrhea

Presumptive Self-Treatment*	Symptomatic Treatment	Prophylaxis
Children 6–10 mg/kg/day TMP, 30–50 mg/kg/day SMZ (max TMP 160 mg, SMZ 800 mg) divided bid PO for 3 days Alternative: Furazolidone 5 mg/kg/day divided qid PO **Adults** Ciprofloxacin 500 mg bid PO for 3 days *or* Norfloxacin 400 mg bid PO for 3 days *or* Ofloxacin 300 mg bid PO for 3 days *or* TMP 160 mg–SMZ 800 mg divided bid PO for 3 days	Replacement of fluids and salts lost in diarrheal stools WHO Oral Rehydration Solution (ORS) packets are available at stores or pharmacies in almost all developing countries Prompt medical evaluation is indicated for disease persisting >3 days, bloody stools, fever >38.8°C (>102°F) or chills, persistent vomiting, or moderate to severe dehydration, especially in young children or pregnant women Loperamide (Imodium) reduces diarrhea by 80%; bismuth subsalicylate (Pepto-Bismol) reduces diarrhea by 50%. These are not recommended for young children, or high fever, or blood in the stools Loperamide ≥12 yr 4 mg, then 2 mg after each unformed stool, not to exceed 8 mg/day 9–11 yr 2 mg, then 1 mg after each unformed stool, not to exceed 6 mg/day 6–8 yr 1 mg then 1 mg after each unformed stool, not to exceed 4 mg/day < 6 yr Not recommended Bismuth subsalicylate† ≥12 yr 30 mL or 2 tablets as often as q30min for 8 doses, with no more than 8 doses in 24 hr 9–11 yr 15 mL or 1 tablet, as above 6–8 yr 10 mL or $\frac{2}{3}$ tablet, as above 3–5 yr 5 mL or $\frac{1}{3}$ tablet, as above < 3 yr Not recommended	Not routinely recommended Bismuth subsalicylate (Pepto-Bismol) 2 oz or 2 tablets orally qid may be effective for prevention but is not recommended for periods of >3 wk or in children, adolescents, or pregnant women†

*Initiated at first symptoms of diarrhea, nausea, bloating, or urgency.

†There is concern about taking such large amounts of bismuth and salicylate. This should not be used by persons with intolerance to salicylates, renal insufficiency, or gout; persons taking anticoagulants, probenecid, or methotrexate; or persons who take salicylates for other reasons.

sprue, bacterial overgrowth of the small intestine, and inflammatory bowel disease, in relation to the acute episode.

PROGNOSIS

Travelers' diarrhea is generally self-limiting, typically resulting in 4–5 loose stools per day. The median duration of diarrhea is 3–4 days. Diarrhea lasts for >1 week in 10%, >1 month in 2%, and >3 months in <1%.

PREVENTION

Travelers should receive careful instructions regarding precautions for food and beverage consumption (Table 104–5). Immunization for typhoid fever should be provided when indicated (Chapter 104). There are no clear guidelines for the use of nonantimicrobial medications, such as bismuth subsalicylate (Pepto-Bismol), and prophylactic antimicrobial drugs such as SMP-TMZ, doxycycline, or quinolones in children. Most experts advise against prophylaxis, reserving antibiotics for presumptive self-treatment along with oral rehydration.

FOODBORNE AND WATERBORNE INFECTIONS

Foodborne and waterborne illnesses are an important public health concern. Foodborne and waterborne illnesses should be reported to local and state health agencies, which are responsible for investigating and reporting the illness to the CDC. Reporting is voluntary, and only a fraction of such outbreaks are thoroughly investigated and reported. The **FoodNet** program, initiated in 1996, is an active surveillance network at seven sites nationally. According to information from FoodNet there are an estimated 360 million cases of diarrheal illness per year. Most foodborne illnesses are neither laboratory confirmed nor reported to state health departments. The extent of underreporting is unknown.

ETIOLOGY

FoodNet tracks infections caused by seven bacterial pathogens (*Campylobacter, E. coli* O157:H7, *Listeria, Salmonella, Shigella, Vibrio,* and *Yersinia*) and two parasitic (*C. parvum* and *Cyclospora*) pathogens. *Campylobacter* was the most frequently identified cause of diarrhea.

EPIDEMIOLOGY

Foodborne Infections. The CDC surveillance system defines an outbreak of foodborne disease as an incident in which (1) ≥2 persons experience a similar illness after ingestion of a common food and (2) epidemiologic analysis implicates the food as the source of the illness. A few exceptions exist; for example, one case of botulism or chemical poisoning is considered to constitute an outbreak. It is estimated that 28 million medical visits annually are associated with foodborne disease and that the cost for all foodborne illness in the United States ranges from $8 billion to $12.3 billion annually.

Several factors contribute to the current epidemiologic nature of foodborne illness. These include changes in the type of foods consumed, improper storage or holding temperature, poor personal hygiene on the part of food handlers, inadequate cooking, and contaminated cooking equipment. Many fruits and vegetables are harvested outside the United States and are delivered to supermarkets in the United States within days. Although cautions are given about consumption of raw fruits and vegetables during travel in developing countries to prevent travelers' diarrhea, the risk of consumption of food shipped from such countries is not widely appreciated.

In 1999, among bacterial cases of foodborne infection were 4553 cases due to *Salmonella,* 3794 due to *Campylobacter,* 1031 due to *Shigella,* 530 due to *E. coli* O157:H7, 163 due to *Yersinia,* 113 due to *Listeria,* and 45 due to *Vibrio.* Among parasitic infections there were 474 cases of *C. parvum* and 14 cases of *Cyclospora* infection. Among all cases, 15% of infected persons were hospitalized; the rate was highest with *Listeria* infections (88%) followed by *E. coli* O157:H7 (29%), *Salmonella* (21%), *Yersinia* (15%), *Shigella* (13%), *Campylobacter* (10%), and *Vibrio* (10%) infections. There were 33 deaths; the highest case-fatality rate was in case of *Listeria* infection. *Escherichia coli* O157:H7 is the most common cause of foodborne outbreaks in northern United States, and undercooked ground beef was the major source of *E. coli* O157:H7 infections. Most foodborne *Vibrio* infections are caused by *V. parahaemolyticus, V. cholerae* non-O1, or *V. vulnificus.* Most of these infections occur as a result of eating contaminated crabs or raw oysters. *V. vulnificus* is associated with deaths of patients with underlying liver disease or with some degree of immunocompromise. *V. cholerae* O1 is the cause of epidemic cholera, which is the most important foodborne and waterborne *Vibrio* infection.

In summer months (June-August), 66% of the *Vibrio,* 52% of the *E. coli* O157:H7, 35% of the *Campylobacter,* and 32% of th Salmonella infections were isolated in 1999. For children <1 year of age, the *Salmonella* infection rate was 112 cases/100,000 population, and the *Campylobacter* infection rate was 57 cases/100,000 population, which is higher than for other age groups. The incidence rate was higher in males than in females; males accounted for 100% of *Vibrio* infections.

Epidemics of *Listeria monocytogenes* foodborne illness have been associated with ingestion of contaminated food such as coleslaw, milk, and Mexican-style soft cheese. This organism is frequently cultured from raw poultry and from meat that has been processed and is ready to eat. The source of these organisms in sporadic cases has been uncertain. Approximately 90% of patients with invasive listeriosis have underlying immunosuppression. This organism also causes perinatal infections in neonates.

Among viral pathogens, hepatitis A virus causes 71% of virus-associated outbreaks. The number of outbreaks due to Norwalk and other viruses is low, probably because of limitations of laboratory methods to identify these pathogens. The actual number of cases is underreported.

Waterborne Infections. Outbreaks of waterborne illness are defined by two criteria: (1) ≥2 persons with similar illness after ingestion of drinking water or exposure to water used for recreational purposes and (2) epidemiologic evidence implicating water as the source of the illness. Exceptions are a single case of laboratory-confirmed primary amebic meningoencephalitis and a single case of chemical poisoning in which water-quality data indicated chemical contamination. Although not considered to be a type of waterborne gastrointestinal illness, whirlpool-associated outbreaks of folliculitis caused by *Pseudomonas* are included in the surveillance system, but wound infections caused by water-related organisms, such as *Aeromonas,* are not. Outbreaks of Pontiac fever caused by *Legionella* in whirlpool baths are listed, but outbreaks of Legionnaires' disease are not included.

TABLE 76–25. Outbreaks of Waterborne Disease Associated with Water Intended for Drinking—United States, 1995–1996 (N = 22)

Etiologic Agent	No. of Cases	Type of Illness	Type of System
Acute gastrointestinal illness of unknown etiology	684	Acute gastroenteritis	Community (spring, well, lake) and individual
Giardia lamblia	1,459	Gastroenteritis	Community and noncommunity (reservoir, river, or lake supplies water to lodge and resort)
Shigella sonnei	93	NS*	Noncommunity
Copper	37	NS	Community
Nitrite	9	NS	Community
Small round structured virus	148	NS	Community
Plesiomonas shigelloides	60	NS	Noncommunity
Escherichia coli O157:H7	33	Bloody gastroenteritis, hemolytic uremic syndrome	Noncommunity
Sodium hydroxide	30	NS	Community
Concentrated liquid soap	13	NS	Community
Chlorine	1	NS	Community
Total	2,567	NS	

*NS, not specified.
From Centers for Disease Control and Prevention: Surveillance for waterborne-disease outbreaks—United States, 1995–1996. *MMWR Morb Mortal Wkly Rep* 1998;47(SS-5):1–34.

For the period 1995–1996, 22 outbreaks associated with drinking water were reported. Fifteen (68.2%) of the 22 outbreaks were of infectious origin, and seven (31.8%) were attributed to chemical poisoning (Table 76–25). Four outbreaks were caused by bacteria (two by *S. sonnei,* one by *E. coli* O157:H7, and one by *P. shigelloides*); two were caused by *Giardia;* one was caused by a virus; and eight were of unknown origin. Many of the unknown outbreak illnesses were consistent with viral syndromes. Seven outbreaks due to chemical poisoning were caused by chlorine, nitrite, and sodium hydroxide. Ten (45.5%) of the 22 outbreaks were associated with community water systems, 10 (45.5%) with noncommunity systems, and 2 (9.1%) with individual systems. Approximately 10% of the United States population use noncommunity or semipublic water systems, as opposed to community or municipal systems, which are used by approximately 90% of the population.

For the period 1995–1996, 37 outbreaks associated with recreational water were reported (Table 76–26). With exception of one outbreak, all of the outbreaks occurred during summer and early fall. These outbreaks caused illnesses in 9129 persons. There were six cases of amoebic meningoencephalitis, all of which were fatal. Thirty-three (89.2%) outbreaks were of infectious origin. Of these, 10 (45.5%) were caused by bacteria (six *E. coli* O157:H7, three *S. sonnei,* one *Salmonella* serotype Java), seven (31.8%) by parasites (six *Cryptosporidum* and one *Giardia*), one (4.5%) by Norwalk virus, and four (18.2%) were of unknown origin. There were nine outbreaks of dermatitis that were associated with hot tubs or lakes. *Pseudomonas aeruginosa* was isolated from four outbreaks, and in one outbreak it was suspected on the basis of the clinical illness. Two outbreaks were suspected to be caused by *Schistosoma* species.

SYMPTOMS AND CLINICAL MANIFESTATIONS

Outbreaks of unknown causation are those for which epidemiologic evidence implicates a food source, but adequate laboratory confirmation is not obtained and these can be divided into four subgroups by incubation period of the illness (Table 76–27). In general, the pathogenesis and clinical features of these illnesses depend on the causative agent (Table 76–28).

CLINICAL MANIFESTATIONS

Symptoms of foodborne and waterborne enteric illnesses may range from those that are rather inapparent to severe disease. Among the most common manifestations are abdominal pain, nausea, loss of appetite, vomiting, diarrhea, fever, fatigue, chills, and rash. The diarrhea may have mucus, leukocytes, or blood.

TABLE 76–26. Outbreaks of Waterborne Disease Associated with Recreational Water Use (N = 37)

Etiologic Agent	No. of Cases	Type of Illness	Type of System
Cryptosporidium parvum	3025	NS*	Pool, lake
Shigella sonnei	120	NS	Lake
Giardia lamblia	77	Gastroenteritis	Pool
Escherichia coli O157:H7	24	Bloody gastroenteritis Hemolytic uremic syndrome	Pool, lake
Norwalk-like virus	55	Acute gastroenteritis	Hot spring
Acute gastrointestinal illness	36	Acute gastroenteritis	Lake
Total	3337		

*NS, not specified.
From Centers for Disease Control and Prevention: Surveillance for Waterborne-Disease Outbreaks—United States, 1995–1996. *MMWR Morb Mortal Wkly Rep* 1998;47(SS-5):1–34.

TABLE 76–27. Food Poisoning Syndromes

Symptoms	Incubation Period (hr)	Possible Agents
Acute gastrointestinal symptoms	6	Chemical
Acute upper gastrointestinal symptoms	1	Preformed heat-stable toxins of *Staphylococcus aureus, Bacillus cereus;* also *Diphyllobothrium latum,* anisakiasis, heavy metals
Upper small-intestinal symptoms; watery noninflammatory diarrhea	8–72	*Clostridium perfringens* type A, *B. cereus,* enterotoxigenic *Escherichia coli, Vibrio cholerae, Giardia lamblia,* Norwalk-like virus
Inflammatory ileocolitis	14–72	*Salmonella, Shigella, Campylobacter jejuni, Vibrio parahaemolyticus,* enteroinvasive *E. coli, Yersinia, Aeromonas*
Sensory or motor neurologic symptoms with or without gastrointestinal symptoms, suggesting toxins associated with *Clostridium,* seafood, or food additives	Variable	Neurotoxin, histamine-like scombroid toxin (mackerel), dinoflagellate neurotoxins (snapper and grouper), shellfish, monosodium glutamate, mushroom

TABLE 76–28. Confirmed Outbreaks of Foodborne Disease

Etiologic Agent	No. of Cases	Deaths	Vehicle
Bacterial	50,304 (92%)*	132 (96%)	
Brucella	38†	1†	Cheese
Bacillus cereus	261†	0	Beef, fried rice
Campylobacter	727 (1%)	1†	Raw milk consumed on school outings
Clostridium botulinum	140†	10 (7%)	Meats and stews, fish, turkey
Clostridium perfringens	2,743 (5%)	2†	Beef, chick, turkey
Escherichia coli	640 (1%)	4	Uncooked hamburger
Salmonella	31,245 (57%)	39	Contaminated cheese; poultry, hamburger, raw fruits and vegetables; ice cream
Shigella	9,971 (18%)	2	Food handler–contaminated foods
Staphylococcus aureus	3,181 (6%)	0	Custards and cream filling; sliced and chopped meats
Group A *Streptococcus*	1,001 (25%)	0	Potato salad, egg salad, poultry, or fish
Streptococcus (other)	85†	3	Cheese
Vibrio cholerae (non 01)	2†	0	Fish
Vibrio parahaemolyticus	11†	0	Contaminated crab or raw oysters
Other bacterial	259†	70 (51%)	
Chemical	1,244 (2%)	3 (2%)	
Ciguatoxin	332†	0	Fish
Heavy metal	176†	0	
Monosodium glutamate	7†	0	
Mushrooms	49†	2	
Scombrotoxin	306†	0	
Shellfish	3†	0	
Other chemical	371†	3 (2%)	
Parasitic	203†	1†	
Giardia lamblia	41†	0	Food handler–contaminated cold foods, e.g., pork, sausages
Trichinella spiralis	162†	1†	Same as *Giardia lamblia*
Viral	2,789 (5%)	1†	
Hepatitis A	1,067	0 (2%)	Food handler–contaminated cold foods; ham, raw fruits and vegetables, shellfish
Norwalk-like viruses	1,164 (2%)	0	Same as hepatitis A
Other viruses	558 (1%)	0	
	54,540 (100%)		
Total		137 (100%)	

*Figure in parentheses is percent of total of foodborne outbreaks.
†Less than 1%.
Adapted from Centers for Disease Control: Foodborne disease outbreaks, 5-year summary, 1983–1987. *MMWR Morb Mortal Wkly Rep* 1990;39(SS-1):25–29.

TABLE 76–29. Prevention Methods for Foodborne Disease

- Avoid raw and cracked eggs
- Use pasteurized milk
- Cook foods thoroughly, especially foods of animal origin
- Don't place cooked meat in the pan with the meat's raw juices
- Wash hands, cutting board, and utensils with soap and water immediately after chopping raw meat, or heat wooden cutting board in the microwave oven
- Refrigerate foods within an hour of preparation
- Do not store raw meat and poultry above ready-to-eat foods (i.e., salads) in the refrigerator
- Clean the inside of the refrigerator frequently
- Wash hands before handling food and after using the toilet
- Wash hands after handling diapers, sheets, and clothing soiled by stool
- Dispose stool-soiled items in a place safe from human contact
- Keep fingernails clean

COMPLICATIONS

The most common complication is dehydration, particularly in the very young or very old, as well as in those who are immunocompromised.

PREVENTION

There are several measures that can help prevent foodborne diseases (Table 76–29).

TOXIN-ASSOCIATED ILLNESS

Sensory or motor neurologic symptoms are evidence of disease due to a preformed toxin of *Clostridium botulinum,* ciguatera, scombroids, mushrooms, or pesticides. These neurologic symptoms can occur with or without gastrointestinal symptoms. Ciguatera fish poisoning is caused by ciguatoxin, a poorly characterized lipid-soluble toxin accumulated by fish through the food chain, and is associated with approximately 75% of outbreaks of illness due to chemical agents.

In patients other than neonates, the classic *C. botulinum* gastrointestinal syndrome has an incubation period of 12–36 hours, although incubation periods up to 1 week have been reported. Eight antigenically distinct neurotoxins affect the presynaptic release of acetylcholine. The classic gastrointestinal syndrome is caused by a preformed toxin found in improperly canned foods, usually due to types A, B, or E. Patients initially have xerostomia, diplopia, and loss of the pupillary light reflex. About one half of patients then have nausea, vomiting, and abdominal cramps; some have diarrhea. As the disease progresses, constipation occurs. Less commonly, the gastrointestinal symptoms may precede the onset of neurologic symptoms. The recuperative period is prolonged and ranges from weeks to months. *C. botulinum* infection in infants can cause a syndrome in which toxin is made in the intestine. The neurotoxins belong primarily to antigenic types A, B, and rarely F. The clinical spectrum of botulism in infants ranges from asymptomatic carriage of organisms, to mild hypotonia and failure to thrive, to constipation, bulbar weakness, and profound hypotonia.

Another member of the clostridial species, *C. perfringens,* has been associated with diarrhea. After a person ingests meat contaminated with *C. perfringens,* the bacteria promptly produce a heat-sensitive enterotoxin that works through the adenyl cyclase system. Ingestion of contaminated foods is followed by the abrupt onset of colicky abdominal pain with foul-smelling diarrhea, generally without mucus or blood. Vomiting is not a part of this syndrome. This is a self-limited illness that resolves in about 1 day.

Seafood. Toxins associated with seafood are primarily reported from the tropical or subtropical coastal areas in the Caribbean and rarely from Hawaii. Outbreaks usually occur from February to September. Fish such as snapper and grouper, among others, have been implicated. The fish become toxic through ingestion of **dinoflagellates** (*Gambierdiscus toxicus*), which contain either the toxin or its precursor. Classically, the perioral region and distant extremities are affected by paresthesias and dysesthesias (cold-hot). Diarrhea occurs in two thirds of those intoxicated, 2–30 hours after ingestion. The other one third initially experience emetic symptoms. Lower-extremity myalgia or pruritus may be presenting symptoms. One third to one half of patients experience headache, confusion, weakness, dyspepsia, and diaphoresis. An unusually painful sensitivity of the teeth has been reported. The neurologic muscular symptoms are usually severe, although cranial nerve paralysis, respiratory failure, or cardiovascular symptoms are unusual. The acute illness usually lasts a few days, although the convalescent period may be as long as 6 months for those with severe symptoms.

A second fish-associated syndrome is that caused by **scombroid toxin,** produced by bacteria in fish of the mackerel family (such as tuna), although dolphins and bluefish have also been implicated. The fish characteristically has a peppery taste. Symptoms are caused by histamine, thereby producing clinical symptoms outside the gastrointestinal tract that begin soon after consumption. Initially patients may complain of a burning sensation in the mouth. Headache, flushing, urticaria, vomiting, diarrhea, intestinal cramping, and dizziness are frequently seen. Scombroid poisoning is self-limited and runs its course in a few hours to a few days.

Consumption of shellfish that have concentrated **neurotoxins,** such as saxitoxin, from dinoflagellates (*Gonyaulax tamarensis* or *Gonyaulax catenella*) can cause either a paralytic syndrome that occurs less than 4 hours after consumption and lasts at most a few days or a neurotoxic shellfish poisoning syndrome with a similar incubation period and symptoms of diarrhea. The patients experience paresthesias of the extremities and ocular facial muscle weakness. Although paralysis may occur, it is associated only with paralytic shellfish poisoning.

Consumption of mussels contaminated with *Nitzschia pungens* can lead **to domoic acid poisoning.** Domoic acid is a heat-stable substance that acts as an excitatory neurotransmitter. The most common symptoms are vomiting (76%), abdominal cramps (50%), diarrhea (42%), headache (often described as incapacitating) (43%), and loss of short-term memory (25%). The onset of gastrointestinal symptoms has ranged from 15 minutes to 38 hours after ingestion, with a median of 5.5 hours. Neurologic symptoms occur within 48 hours. Cognitive and short-term memory losses may persist for prolonged periods of time. Patients who are elderly or who have an underlying condition such as chronic renal failure or diabetes mellitus are predisposed to more severe symptoms.

Mushroom Poisoning. At least seven groups of mushroom toxins have been described. The intoxications are grouped according to the target organ system affected and the rapidity of onset of symptoms after ingestion. Those that produce self-limited neurologic or gastrointestinal illness usually cause symptoms within 15 minutes of ingestion and have a favorable outcome. The toxins capable of causing death induce symptoms 6–18 hours after ingestion.

Food Additives. Symptoms resulting from ingestion of food additives, including monosodium glutamate, which classically has been associated with consumption of Chinese food, are usually self-limited. Symptoms include a burning sensation of the trunk and neck, headache, nausea, abdominal cramps, and a feeling of tightness over the face, chest, and throat. Symptoms usually begin within 1 hour of ingestion of the food and may last a few hours.

Heavy Metal Poisoning. Acute intoxication with lead and other heavy metals in water causes an abrupt onset of symptoms that suggest gastric irritation. The symptoms usually occur within 15 minutes of ingestion. Copper and cadmium, among other metals, have been implicated. There is frequently a history of ingestion of a carbonated or acidic drink such as lemonade, which may have corroded its metal container. Symptoms are usually self-limited but may last as long as 3 hours.

CLOSTRIDIUM DIFFICILE–ASSOCIATED DIARRHEA

ETIOLOGY

The principal cause is toxigenic *C. difficile.* The association with antibiotic administration and the presence of whitish yellow plaques, or pseudomembranes, have led to alternate names for *Clostridium difficile*–associated diarrhea, including **antibiotic associated diarrhea** and **pseudomembranous colitis.**

Evaluation of healthy adults has shown that 1–3% of persons carry this microbe, without toxin production, in the stool. *C. difficile* colonization and toxin production can occur in both healthy infants and those with symptoms. Healthy neonates without symptoms may carry *C. difficile* that produce toxin but not disease. Up to 80% of healthy neonates carry the organism asymptomatically, and up to 40% of these strains produce toxin A or toxin B. Normal adult carrier levels are reached by around 6 months of age.

EPIDEMIOLOGY

Alteration of normal bowel flora, usually by administration of antibiotics, facilitates the emergence of resistant organisms such as *C. difficile* that produce toxins that affect mucosal function. The severity of *C. difficile*–associated diarrhea may range from self-limited illness to diarrhea with dehydration, pseudomembranous colitis, toxic megacolon, or even death. Reports of pseudomembranous colitis have been extant in the literature since the end of the 19th century, but the disease has become better recognized and characterized since the introduction of antimicrobial agents. The source of infection is generally endogenous, although the almost epidemic nature described by some centers suggests nosocomial spread because *C. difficile* can be cultured from fomites in the rooms of affected patients.

PATHOGENESIS

C. difficile produces two toxins: **toxin A,** an enterotoxin associated with diarrhea, and **toxin B,** a cytotoxin associated with colitis. Toxin A is also cytotoxic but considerably less so than toxin B. In some series, *C. difficile* was present in virtually all patients with pseudomembranous colitis confirmed by the presence of toxin B. Toxin B is a heat-labile toxin that is rapidly lethal to hamsters, causes increased vascular permeability to rabbit skin, is cytotoxic to cells in tissue culture, and is neutralized by antitoxin directed against *Clostridium sordelli.*

Pseudomembranous colitis is more commonly reported among patients receiving clindamycin, penicillin, and cephalosporins. It usually occurs after oral therapy but can occur after parenteral therapy. Virtually all known antibiotics have been implicated, with the exception of vancomycin.

In the appropriate clinical setting, the presence of either toxin A or toxin B constitutes supportive evidence for *C. difficile*–induced disease. Although the illness usually starts after 4–9 days of antibiotic therapy, cases have occurred weeks to months after a course of antimicrobial drugs.

SYMPTOMS AND CLINICAL MANIFESTATIONS

C. difficile–associated diarrhea is characterized by abrupt onset of diarrhea in patients who are taking antibiotics. Diarrhea occurs frequently in patients taking antibiotics, and the cause is often unknown. *C. difficile*–associated diarrhea has a wide spectrum of clinical presentations (Table 76–30). Most patients usually have a mild, self-limiting diarrhea without pseudomembranes, explosive watery diarrhea with occult blood and extraintestinal symptoms, or the classic situation of pseudomembranous colitis with blood and mucus, profuse stools, fever, cramps, abdominal pain, nausea, and vomiting.

DIAGNOSIS

The clinical setting of diarrhea after exposure to antibiotics, as well as exclusion of other enteric agents, suggests the diagnosis. Although most patients with *C. difficile*–associated diarrhea do not develop pseudomembranous colitis, the syndrome should be considered for patients with diarrhea, fever, leukocytosis, and blood in the stools. Other abdominal findings, including distention and tenderness on palpation, often occur while the patient is taking antibiotics. Although a clinical diagnosis may be confirmed by endoscopic demonstration of discrete and elevated fibrinous yellow or white plaques on the colonic mucosa, endoscopy is unnecessary in uncomplicated cases. A favorable response to oral vancomycin or metronidazole supports the diagnosis.

TABLE 76–30. Epidemiologic and Clinical Manifestations of *Clostridium difficile* Infection

Season	Year-round
Primary age	3 months to 18 years
Incubation period	Days to months
Symptoms	Watery diarrhea (++) Fever (++) Colitis (++) Nausea (++) Vomiting (+) Blood in stool (+)
Duration of symptoms	1–2 days after stopping of antibiotics or within days of starting therapy
Vector	Person-to-person transmission

++ = Sometimes occurs; + = uncommon.

Microbiologic Evaluation

Stool must be submitted for culture of *C. difficile* and for demonstration of its preformed toxins. Samples should not be submitted for culture or latex agglutination for *C. difficile* alone because these tests do not differentiate toxin-producing strains from others. A selective differential medium for recovery of *C. difficile* in anaerobic culture contains cycloserine, cefoxitin, and fructose and is sensitive and selective. Colonies of *C. difficile* growing on this medium have distinctive morphologic features and are fluorescent, properties that speed identification by a trained microbiologist. An EIA or counterimmunoelectrophoresis (CIE) is used to detect the toxins. Toxin B may be demonstrated by tissue culture, and both toxin A and toxin B may be demonstrated by EIA. It is recommended that tissue culture and EIA be used in conjunction. Although cumbersome, colitis can be induced in hamsters for a confirmatory pathologic examination.

TREATMENT

The first and essential step in treatment is the discontinuation of the offending antibiotic(s). In most instances, this course combined with appropriate fluid and electrolyte replacement is sufficient. Patients with pseudomembranous colitis should be treated with antibiotics such as metronidazole.

Various approaches have been advocated for children whose symptoms continue but who must continue to take the offending antibiotics. For mild cases, some authors have advocated the use of resins such as cholestyramine, which acts by binding the toxin and preventing its effect. Another approach is to eradicate the causative agent by administering oral metronidazole for 10 days. Alternatives include oral vancomycin or oral bacitracin. If the child cannot tolerate oral administration, intravenous metronidazole should be used. Metronidazole is preferred to vancomycin, especially for hospitalized patients, to minimize selection of vancomycin-resistant *Enterococcus.*

Relapses of diarrhea have occurred in 10–20% of patients after discontinuation of treatment with antibiotics or cholestyramine therapy. If a relapse occurs after a second course of oral antimicrobial therapy, the patient should take cholestyramine for 2 weeks. A repeat stool sample for toxins should be taken at the end of the first week to help gauge the risk of relapse. Relapses also can be managed with second and even third courses of the same antimicrobial drug. These patients could benefit from a subsequent course of cholestyramine, the major side effect of which is constipation. Because cholestyramine also binds vancomycin, these two drugs should not be administered concurrently.

COMPLICATIONS AND PROGNOSIS

Mortality as high as 28% was once reported for pseudomembranous colitis; however, with early recognition and institution of vancomycin therapy the mortality has become negligible. Rare patients may have toxic megacolon and need to be treated surgically. One of every six patients has a relapse regardless of the antimicrobial regimen responsible for inducing disease.

PREVENTION

Lactobacillus acidophilus has been recommended as a **probiotic** to prevent antibiotic-associated diarrhea. Recently two studies have demonstrated the value of *Lactobacillus* in reducing the incidence of antibiotic-associated diarrhea in children treated with oral antibiotics for other infectious diseases. The beneficial effect might be mediated by several mechanisms of probiotics: production of an antimicrobial substance, local competition of adhesion receptors and nutrients, and stimulation of intestinal antigen-specific and nonspecific immune responses.

HEMOLYTIC UREMIC SYNDROME

The clinical spectrum of HUS varies from subclinical illness to fulminating life-threatening disease. HUS is characterized by acute onset of the classic triad of microangiopathic hemolytic anemia, thrombocytopenia, and acute renal insufficiency.

ETIOLOGY

There are several major predisposing causes of HUS, including bacterial and viral infections, systemic lupus erythematosus, cancer, transplant rejection, glomerulonephritis, pregnancy, and exposure to toxins. A familial form accounts for 5% of cases of HUS and is associated with recurrent HUS. Both autosomal dominant and autosomal recessive inheritance patterns have been described.

In children the primary cause in 90% of cases of HUS is preceding infectious enteritis. Enterohemorrhagic strains of *E. coli* are responsible for 72% of HUS in the United States, and *E. coli* O157:H7 was the responsible strain in >80% of those cases. *Shigella dysenteriae* type 1 is also clearly associated with HUS, especially in developing countries, and several other intestinal pathogens are suspected of being linked to HUS (Table 76–31). In one study (Wong et al., 2000) the risk of developing HUS increased to 14% after TMP-SMZ treatment of *E. coli* serotype O157:H7 enteritis.

EPIDEMIOLOGY

HUS occurs throughout the world and causes sporadic and epidemic gastrointestinal infections. In the United States the incidence is 0.3–10 cases per 100,000 children. The incidence in South America may be as high as 30 cases per 100,000 children. Most epidemic cases of HUS in the United States occur during the summer and early fall, peaking in July, paralleling the incidence of enterohemorrhagic *E. coli* O157:H7 enteritis (Fig. 76–5). HUS typically occurs in outbreaks following epidemics of diarrheal illness and common-source food exposure to undercooked ground beef, which accounts for 40% of outbreaks, and unpasteurized milk and cheese. Epidemic cases may occur from the neonatal period to adulthood but occur predominantly in children 6–48 months of age, with an equal

TABLE 76–31. Infectious Agents Associated with Hemolytic Uremic Syndrome

Cases Associated with Diarrhea
Recognized association
Escherichia coli O157:H7
Shigella dysenteriae (producing Shiga toxin)
Possible association
Salmonella
Campylobacter jejuni
Yersinia
Aeromonas hydrophila
Coxsackieviruses
Cases Not Associated with Diarrhea
Streptococcus pneumoniae

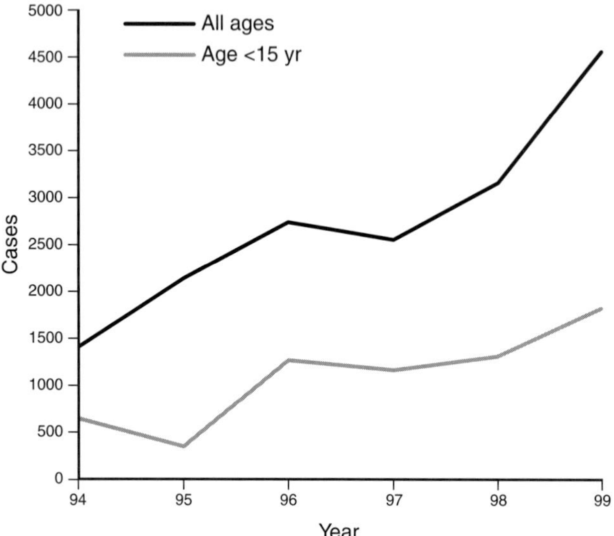

FIGURE 76–5. The incidence of hemolytic uremic syndrome (HUS) in the United States from 1994 to 1999. The incidence of HUS parallels the incidence of enterohemorrhagic *E. coli* enteritis. (Data from the Centers for Disease Control and Prevention.)

occurrence in the two sexes. All races are affected, but the incidence may be lower among blacks. Epidemics have been reported in daycare centers. There is no seasonal variation or age predisposition for sporadic cases.

Sporadic cases have been reported with infection caused by neuraminidase-producing *S. pneumoniae,* a variety of drugs, and cancer, organ transplantation, and pregnancy. Cases associated with pregnancy are frequently familial forms.

Transmission. *E. coli* O157:H7 is transmitted by ingestion of beef and other foods contaminated with cattle feces. *E. coli* is killed by thorough cooking, and most outbreaks are associated with undercooked beef. This organism can be recovered from the intestines of approximately 1% of cattle. *E. coli* O157:H7, and *S. dysenteriae* may also be transmitted person to person by the fecal-oral route.

PATHOGENESIS

The pathogenesis of HUS associated with *E. coli* serotype O157:H7 is related to elaboration of **Shiga toxin,** although many factors influence this development of the syndrome. The bacteria colonize the intestine after ingestion. There are several virulence factors. **Intimin** is a protein necessary for attachment. **Hemolysin** is a protein that affects the growth of other bacteria and may hemolyze cells and cause the release of **Shiga-like toxin,** which can initiate apoptosis in endothelial and epithelial cells. Shiga toxins have a similar structure of a central subunit **(A subunit)** surrounded by five peripheral subunits **(B subunits)**. After absorption from the gastrointestinal tract, the peripheral subunit binds endothelial cell surface glycoproteins **(Gb3)** and facilitates internalization by endocytosis. The central subunit is then released and cleaved into a fragment **(A_2)** that binds to ribosomes and inhibits RNA transcription. Cell injury or cell death leads to a loss of the antithrombotic properties of the endothelium, resulting in platelet aggregation and white blood cell activation and culminating in localized coagulation, fibrin deposition, and formation of thrombi. This **thrombotic microangiopathy** occurs in the endothelium of many organs but is most pronounced in the kidney, probably because of the abundant expression of Gb3 on glomerular endothelium. Children appear to have increased Gb3 expression, which may partially explain the age-related epidemiology of HUS.

Erythrocytes become damaged as they transit the damaged renal glomeruli, and thrombocytopenia results from platelet consumption. The pathologic changes in the glomeruli account for the reduction in the glomerular filtration rate and renal insufficiency. This pathology results in the characteristic clinical findings of microangiopathic hemolytic anemia, thrombocytopenia, and renal insufficiency. In vitro, TMP-SMZ increases the release of Shiga toxin in cultures of *E. coli,* and in one study (Wong et al., 2000) children who received TMP-SMZ or β-lactam antibiotics during the diarrheal prodrome had a significantly higher risk (relative risk of 17.3, confidence interval 2.2 to 137) of HUS than those who did not receive antibiotics. Other factors, such as factor H–von Willebrand factor, in addition to antibiotic must be involved. Mutation or deficiency of factor H appears to increase the risk of HUS.

The pathogenesis of noninfectious causes of many sporadic cases has not been defined. Sporadic cases of HUS associated with *S. pneumoniae* infection have a distinct initial mechanism of pathogenesis in comparison with epidemic cases but a similar final pathway and clinical manifestations. Streptococcal **neuraminidase** cleaves N-acetylneuraminic acid (a sialic acid) from cell surface glycoproteins, exposing a cellular antigen **(Thomsen-Friedenreich antigen)** of endothelial cells, erythrocytes, and platelets that is normally hidden. Once exposed, this antigen binds IgM antibodies normally present in serum and initiates an inflammatory response leading to platelet and erythrocyte agglutination and endothelial cell damage. Platelet deposition and activation follow, resulting in similar glomerular damage that leads to the same clinical findings seen in HUS associated with diarrheal illness.

SYMPTOMS AND CLINICAL MANIFESTATIONS

In typical cases the episode of enteritis precedes the onset of HUS by 3–12 days. Enteritis caused by *E. coli* O157:H7 is characteristically associated with abdominal cramps, no fever or low-grade fever, nausea, vomiting, and grossly bloody watery diarrhea. After or near the resolution of the diarrheal illness, nonspecific symptoms of irritability, restlessness, confusion, or lethargy are followed by decreased urine output or even anuria. Hypertension is variable but suggests more severe disease. The degree of pallor may be variable, depending on the rate of hemolysis, and icterus may be apparent. The hemolytic anemia may occur without significant clinical renal involvement. Sporadic cases of HUS are not associated with any prodrome.

Physical Examination Findings

Physical examination usually reveals a patient who appears ill with evidence of peripheral edema and some degree of pallor. Abdominal tenderness and hepatosplenomegaly may be present. Hypertension and signs of pulmonary edema may result if intravenous fluids are given in an attempt to increase urinary output.

DIAGNOSIS

The diagnosis should be considered in any patient with a compatible preceding diarrheal illness or in an ill patient with symptoms or signs of thrombocytopenia, anemia, and renal compromise. The diagnosis is usually established by clinical findings supported by routine blood test results.

Differential Diagnosis

Thrombotic thrombocytopenic purpura (TTP) closely simulates the fever and microangiopathic hemolytic anemia but typically has less severe renal involvement and more severe neurologic involvement. TTP occurs mainly in adults and without preceding enteric infection. TTP is associated with deficient activity of a circulating metalloprotease that cleaves von Willebrand factor in a shear stress–dependent manner. Low levels of von Willebrand factor–cleaving protease activity, which are normal in HUS, can distinguish TTP from HUS. A decrease in large von Willebrand factor multimers occurs in HUS, presumably caused by abnormal shear stress in the microcirculation.

Sepsis and disseminated intravascular coagulopathy (DIC) is not usually accompanied by severe anemia but is typically differentiated from HUS by prolonged prothrombin time and partial thromboplastin time coagulation tests. The patient with Henoch-Schönlein purpura usually has a normal platelet count. Several causes of acute renal failure may mimic HUS: poststreptococcal glomerulonephritis (Chapter 40), noninfectious glomerulonephritis, systemic lupus erythematosus, and other collagen-vascular diseases associated with systemic vasculitis.

Laboratory Evaluation

Routine laboratory tests are essential and are usually sufficient in confirming the diagnosis. A red blood cell smear and CBC invariably demonstrate evidence of a microangiopathic hemolytic anemia with fragmented red blood cells (e.g., schistocytes, burr cells, helmet cells, and spherocytes). The anemia is usually moderate to severe and accompanied by an increased reticulocyte count, decreased serum haptoglobin, and increased serum bilirubin. The direct and indirect Coombs' tests are usually negative. The platelet count is decreased to as low as 20,000/mm^3, and an increased platelet size indicates accelerated platelet formation and release of young platelets from the bone marrow. The PT and PTT are normal. The fibrinogen and fibrin degradation products are often increased, and the C3 and C4 components of complement are often decreased. The WBC count is frequently elevated with an increase in immature forms (e.g., bands, metamyelocytes); the degree of leukocytosis correlates with severity. The BUN and creatinine levels are elevated and reflect the degree of renal compromise. The bicarbonate and serum sodium levels are usually decreased. The serum potassium level is characteristically low but may be elevated. Urinalysis usually reveals proteinuria with microscopic hematuria and pyuria with hyaline, granular, and epithelial casts. Liver enzyme (e.g., alanine aminotransferase [ALT], aspartate aminotransferase [AST]) levels and the serum bilirubin level are frequently mildly increased. There is an elevated lactate dehydrogenase (LDH) level from cellular destruction.

Microbiologic Evaluation

Stool should be cultured for *E. coli* O157:H7 as early as possible in the illness, and if this pathogen does not grow, other EHEC should be sought. A negative stool culture for EHEC does not preclude the diagnosis of EHEC-associated HUS. The frequency of isolation decreases with the interval from the diarrheal illness. The combination of stool culture, stool toxin, and serologic testing demonstrates *E. coli* in up to 75% of cases of HUS.

Pathologic Findings

Renal biopsy is not necessary to confirm the diagnosis. If performed, the biopsy demonstrates variable changes of microangiopathic injury to the glomerular endothelium. Capillary lumina are occluded with microthrombi of platelets and fibrin. The glomerular membrane is thickened with deposition of periodic acid-Schiff (PAS)–positive material in the subendothelial spaces.

TREATMENT

The treatment of HUS is supportive. Management for renal insufficiency, anemia, thrombocytopenia, hypertension, and nutritional support are essential components. The management of acute renal insufficiency requires fluid restriction, diuretics, and peritoneal dialysis for severe fluid overload, hyperkalemia, acidosis, hyponatremia, severe hypertension, or anuria for >48 hours. Packed red blood cell transfusions and platelet transfusions may be necessary for anemia and thrombocytopenia. Early dialysis may be beneficial in lowering levels of plasminogen-activating factor (PAF) inhibitor type 1, which correlates with improvement in renal function. Management of HUS should be under the direction of an experienced pediatric nephrologist.

There is no evidence that heparin therapy, fibrinolytic agents (e.g., streptokinase, urokinase), aspirin, dipyridamole, corticosteroids, vitamin E, furosemide, plasmapheresis, or IVIG have any therapeutic efficacy for HUS. Plasma infusion is contraindicated in cases of HUS associated with *S. pneumoniae* because the antibodies to Thomsen-Friedenreich antigen may exacerbate the illness.

COMPLICATIONS

Central nervous system involvement may become pronounced, with ataxia, seizures, decreased level of consciousness, or coma. These symptoms may be due in part to the microangiopathic process and in part to fluid and electrolyte imbalances, especially hyponatremia, as well as uremia and hypertension. Major neurologic complications are present in approximately one half of cases and are more pronounced in cases of HUS that are not associated with diarrhea. CT of the brain may demonstrate cerebral edema or evidence of thrombosis or hemorrhage.

PROGNOSIS

The oliguria or anuria typically continues for 4–12 days but may last as long as 30 days. The platelet count usually returns to normal before the oliguria resolves. Poor prognostic factors for diarrhea-associated cases of HUS include age <1 year or >5 years, severe prodromal illness, initial anuria for >8 days, severe hypertension, central nervous system involvement, and a WBC count of >20,000/mm^3 at presentation. The overall mortality is <5%. Approximately 50% of the deaths occurring during the acute phase are secondary to central nervous system involvement either as a principal component of HUS or secondary to renal failure. The prognosis for HUS associated with *S. dysenteriae* is more guarded.

The long-term prognosis for persons with HUS associated with *E. coli* O157:H7 is generally good for full recovery of renal function and no subsequent relapses. The outcome correlates with the severity of the initial episode. Persons with HUS should have lifelong follow-up for blood pressure and renal function. Hypertension and decreased glomerular filtration rate occur in 30% of patients with severe disease, compared with 10% with mild initial disease. Approximately 5% of all patients surviving the acute illness will eventually have end-stage renal failure. Renal transplantation for renal failure following HUS can be performed, but HUS has been documented to occur in the transplanted kidney. End-stage renal disease and death are much more likely in the 10% of cases that are not associated with diarrhea, especially if there is a familial history of HUS; in these circumstances the mortality rate during the acute phase may be as high as 70–90%. The microangiopathic process continues to progress with relapses, development of severe hypertension, and eventually end-stage renal disease.

PREVENTION

Antimicrobial therapy should be avoided in children with enterohemorrhagic *E. coli* infection because of the increased risk of HUS. *E. coli* O157:H7 and *S. dysenteriae* may also be transmitted person to person by the fecal-oral route, and standard precautions with meticulous handwashing and appropriate disposal of soiled diapers and garments is necessary. Ill children should not be allowed to attend childcare centers. *E. coli* O157:H7 enteritis is a notifiable disease and should be reported to the public health department.

Beef products should be thoroughly cooked (to an internal temperature of at least 68°C [155°F]) before ingestion. This is especially true of hamburger because meat from many animals may contribute to a single hamburger. Cross-contamination may be minimized by washing hands and surfaces after contact with raw ground beef, storing raw beef to ensure that drippings do not contaminate other foods, and using different utensils to handle raw and cooked meat. This is especially important in commercial food preparation because the potential for outbreaks is much greater.

US Department of Agriculture regulations require only gross inspection of animal carcasses. More comprehensive regulations, including guidelines for microbiologic testing of meat, have been proposed and have been implemented by some meat producers. Feeding hay to cattle for 5 days before slaughter reduces the burden of acid-resistant *E. coli,* including *E. coli* O157:H7. Complete implementation of microbiologic testing should decrease *E. coli* O157:H7 contamination of the meat supply.

Fresh juice processors may be required to implement practices to reduce the number of microbes in the finished products. Warning labels on packaged juice products that have not been pasteurized or otherwise treated to eliminate microbes may be required. Unpasteurized milk and diary products and juices should not be consumed.

WHIPPLE'S DISEASE

Whipple's disease is a systemic bacterial illness caused by *Tropheryma whippleii,* and predominantly affects white, middle-aged men. In 1961 visualization of the organism by electron microscopy confirmed the bacterial origin of the disease. In 1991 the amplification and sequencing of a portion of 16S ribosomal RNA classified the bacterium as a gram-positive actinomycete. PCR has been a useful tool for detecting this organism.

The illness is characterized by gradual onset of diarrhea, abdominal pain, arthralgias, and weight loss accompanied by fever, mesenteric and peripheral lymphadenopathy, and hyperpigmentation of the skin. Arthralgias, usually of the large joints, may precede gastrointestinal symptoms by years to decades. Whipple's disease of the central nervous system has been reported in the absence of gastrointestinal symptoms.

The diagnosis traditionally has been confirmed by duodenal biopsy with macrophages that are positive on PAS staining. Similar macrophages may be detected in other involved tissues.

The illness responds clinically to many antibiotics, although prolonged treatment is necessary. TMP-SMZ or, alternatively, penicillin V, given orally in usual doses for 1 year is recommended, although relapses may occur. Many patients are severely malnourished and require vitamin and mineral supplementation.

SUPPORTIVE TREATMENT OF ACUTE ENTERITIS

FLUID AND ELECTROLYTES

Most cases of diarrhea are self-limited and require only simple replacement of fluids and salt lost in the stools. The best way to achieve this is by use of an oral rehydration solution such as World Health Organization (WHO) Oral Rehydration Salt (ORS) solution (Table 76–32). The WHO preparation is available for initial rehy-

TABLE 76–32. Composition of Some Oral Electrolyte Solutions and Clear Liquids

Solution	Sodium	Potassium	Base (mmol/L)	Carbohydrate (mmol/L)	Osmolality (mOsm/L)
Rehydration					
WHO oral rehydration salts*	90	20	30	111 (glucose)	310
Maintenance†					
Lytren	50	25	10	111 (glucose)	290
Naturalyte	45	20	48	140 (glucose)	265
Pediatric electrolyte	45	20	30	140 (glucose)	250
Infalyte (formerly Rice-Lyte)	50	25	30	70 (glucose)	200
Rehydrate	75	20	30	140 (glucose)	310
Pedialyte	45	20	10	140 (glucose)	250
Clear Liquids Not Appropriate for Oral Rehydration					
Apple juice	3	32	0	690 (fructose, glucose, sucrose)	730
Chicken broth	250	8	0	0	500
Cola	2	0.1	13	700 (fructose, glucose)	750
Ginger ale	3	1	4	500 (fructose and/or glucose)	540
Sports beverage	20	3	3	255 (sucrose, glucose)	330
Tea	0	0	0	0	5

*Available from Jaianas Bros Packaging Company, 2533 SW Blvd, Kansas City, MO 64108.
†These products are best suited for use as maintenance solutions but can be used for rehydration of healthy children with mild to moderate dehydration.

dration worldwide. It contains 3.5 g/L of sodium (90 mEq), 1.5 g/L of potassium chloride (20 mEq), and 20 g/L of glucose (111 mEq). The 3.5 g/L of sodium is sufficient for acute dehydration caused not only by choleralike agents but also by other enteric pathogens. This preparation can be used for treating as well as preventing dehydration. ORS packets are available at stores or pharmacies in almost all developing countries. ORS is prepared by adding one packet to boiled or treated water. ORS solution should be consumed or discarded within 12 hours if held at room temperature or 24 hours if kept refrigerated.

Once a patient's dehydration status has been assessed, the caregiver should estimate the deficit and ongoing losses and calculate the daily requirement to replenish the intravascular fluid and replace other deficits. Management of mild to moderate dehydration caused by viral or other diarrhea with a normal serum sodium concentration and mild acidosis consists of symptomatic treatment with oral rehydration solution. Dehydration can be managed with the WHO preparation in the first 4 hours, followed by a solution containing less sodium (45–50 mEq/L), such as Pedialyte or Lytren. Because lactose intolerance in patients with acute diarrhea can be present and may last for weeks, lactose feeding should not be reintroduced immediately after initial oral hydration. Most patients tolerate reintroduction of formula at the end of the first day of therapy. Breast-feeding should be restarted as soon as is feasible.

The prototype of fluid management of enteritis is that of cholera, with fluid replacement using the intestinal route with *one-to-one* fluid replacement of stool volume losses. This is particularly effective during the early course of illness. In Peru, patients with less than 5% dehydration were treated by oral hydration at outpatient health centers. Those with moderate dehydration (up to 10%) were treated in emergency departments. For patients with 10–15% dehydration, an initial intravenous rehydration was administered and followed by oral rehydration if the patients were not vomiting and if their mental status allowed. Patients with severe dehydration (15% or greater) were hospitalized for intravenous rehydration.

For patients in shock, either Ringer's lactate or an appropriate electrolyte solution (90–120 mEq/L sodium, 20 mEq/L potassium, 25–30 mEq/L bicarbonate, and 2–5% glucose) at 20 mL/kg can be used for resuscitation. The rate of fluid administration for severe dehydration usually is at least 25 mL/kg/hr for 4 hours followed by oral rehydration as tolerated. Careful monitoring of input and output and for hyperkalemia and hypoglycemia is critical. Hyperkalemia is common, and hypoglycemia may be seen in up to 10% of children, which emphasizes the need for 2% glucose in the oral rehydration fluid.

It has been reported that hydrating solutions containing starch or cereal improve the rate of absorption of sodium and water. When digested, these long-chain glucose polymers provide an excess of glucose molecules directly to the intestinal wall for absorption, resulting in an overall low osmolar concentration. In a recent study of children with cholera (Ramakrishna et al., 2000) substitution of amylase-resistant starch for rice in oral rehydrating solution reduced the volume and duration of diarrheal stools.

The American Academy of Pediatrics Committee on Nutrition recommends initial oral rehydration therapy for gastroenteritis. It is important to remember that an oral rehydration solution containing glucose does not decrease the amount of stool. However, a rice-based oral rehydration solution does decrease stool output. Feeding during diarrhea is an essential component. Breast-feeding has been shown to shorten the duration of illness and should be encouraged. Children who received oral rehydration solution and early feeding with a full-strength diet have better absorption of nitrogen, carbohydrate, and fat than children with delayed feeding after oral rehydration or intravenous therapy. Therefore early feeding enables these children to grow normally.

Homemade salt preparations are not to be given to children because these solutions may contain too much sodium, which could lead to hypernatremia. Commercially available beverages or sodas contain rather small amounts of sodium and potassium and also have too much carbohydrate, which could result in even more diarrhea. With children, careful attention should be paid to the presence of such signs as tearing, urination, and moistness of mucous membranes, which are good indicators of the state of hydration. Parents should be cautioned to contact a physician if they have any concerns.

NONSPECIFIC TREATMENT

A variety of **absorbents** have been used to stem the flow of fluid from the gastrointestinal tract. Activated charcoal has been found to be ineffective in the treatment of diarrhea. Agents such as kaolin and pectin (e.g., Kaopectate) increase the consistency of the stool but have not been shown to decrease cramps and frequency of stool or shorten the course of infectious diarrhea. *Lactobacillus* preparations and yogurt have also been advocated, and there is evidence that supports the use of these treatments in traveler's diarrhea.

Bismuth subsalicylate (e.g., Pepto-Bismol) 1 ounce or two 262 mg tablets every 30 minutes for eight doses is known to decrease stool frequency for adult travelers in several placebo-controlled studies but is not recommended for children (Table 76–33). It should be used with caution, and only in children older than 2 years, because the salicylate load could conceivably lead to intoxication. Patients should not consume this preparation if they have an allergy to aspirin or a bleeding diathesis. Prophylaxis with a bismuth

TABLE 76–33. Treatment of Diarrhea with Nonspecific Antidiarrheals in Children

Mode of Action	Agent	Pediatric Application
Absorbent, firmer stool	Kaolin and pectin (Kaopectate)	Safe; efficacy uncertain
Inhibitor of secretory function (decreases cramps and diarrhea)	Bismuth subsalicylate (Pepto-Bismol)	Effective in travelers' diarrhea Beware of salicylate intoxication potential (use only in children ≥2 yr of age)*
Inhibitor of intestinal motility†	Paregoric (tincture of opium)	Not used in children
	Diphenoxylate (Lomotil)	Efficacy uncertain; use only in children ≥3 yr of age
	Loperamide hydrochloride (Imodium)	Use only in children ≥3 yr of age
Alteration of intestinal microflora	*Lactobacillus*	Uncertain

*In a 3-year-old child a 40 mL total daily dose (5 mL single dose) is equivalent to 344 mg of salicylate and 404 mg of bismuth. If tablets are used, the total daily dose is 2⅔ tablets (⅓ tablet single dose), resulting in a total dose of 272 mg salicylate and 404 mg bismuth.

†Infection with dysenteric agents such as *Shigella* could be worsened.

subsalicylate tablet preparation is effective and may ultimately provide a more convenient way to medicate both adults and children. The protection rate against diarrhea in adults who take the tablet has been reported to be 65% for a large dosage regimen consisting of two tablets (524 mg of bismuth subsalicylate) four times a day. This regimen is well tolerated when used for 3 weeks. The most common adverse effects are black stools, a black tongue, and a small incidence of tinnitus. This preparation is not approved for children. The salicylate content must be considered and appropriately calculated if the drug is prescribed for use in children.

Antimotility agents, such as the natural opiates (paregoric), should *not* be used in children. Their use in patients with infection due to dysenteric agents such as *Shigella* can result in aggravation of clinical symptoms and increased toxicity. Diphenoxylate (Lomotil) or loperamide (Imodium) should not be used in children younger than 3 years of age. Diphenoxylate has been associated with respiratory depression and coma in very young children. In a study (Karrar et al., 1987) conducted in Egypt, loperamide, 0.24 mg/kg/day divided in three doses, was given to children younger than 2 years of age with diarrhea. The beneficial result did not differ significantly from that in children who received a placebo.

A recent study (Salazar-Lindo et al., 2000) of boys with diarrhea and dehydration in Peru showed that oral rehydration with the addition of racecadotril, which inhibits intestinal enkephalinase and decreases intestinal hypersecretion without affecting intestinal motility, significantly reduced the volume of stool and the duration of diarrhea compared with oral rehydration plus placebo given to controls.

REVIEWS

Centers for Disease Control and Prevention: Preliminary FoodNet data on the incidence of foodborne illnesses—Selected sites, United States, 1999. *MMWR Morb Mortal Wkly Rep* 2000;49:201–5.

Cohen MB: Etiology and mechanisms of acute infectious diarrhea in infants in the United States. *J Pediatr* 1991;118:S34–9.

Guerrant RL, Bobak DA: Bacterial and protozoal gastroenteritis. *N Engl J Med* 1991;325:327–40.

Guerrant RL, Van Gilder T, Steiner TS, et al: Practice guidelines for the management of infectious diarrhea. *Clin Infect Dis* 2001;32:331–51.

Guerrant RL, Lohr JA, Williams EK: Acute infectious diarrhea. 1. Epidemiology, etiology and pathogenesis. *Pediatr Infect Dis J* 1986;5:353–9.

Ho MS, Glass PI, Pinsky PI, et al: Diarrhea deaths in American children: Are they preventable? *JAMA* 1988;260:3281–5.

Mead PS, Slutsker L, Dietz V, et al: Food-related illness and death in the United States. *Emerg Infect Dis* 2000;5:607–25.

KEY ARTICLES

Nontyphoidal *Salmonella*

Carroll WL, Balistreri WF, Brilli R, et al: Spectrum of *Salmonella* associated arthritis. *Pediatrics* 1981;68:717–20.

Goldberg MB, Rubin RH: The spectrum of *Salmonella* infection. *Infect Dis Clin North Am* 1988;2:571–98.

Meadow WL, Schneider H, Beem MO: *Salmonella enteritidis* bacteremia in childhood. *J Infect Dis* 1985;152;185–9.

Olsen SJ, Bishop R, Brenner FW, et al: The changing epidemiology of *Salmonella:* Trends in serotypes isolated from humans in the United States, 1987–1997. *J Infect Dis* 2001;183:753–61.

Nelson S, Granoff D: *Salmonella* gastroenteritis in the first three months of life: A review of management and complications. *Clin Pediatr* 1982:21:709–12.

St. Louis ME, Morse DL, Potter ME, et al: The emergence of grade A eggs as a major source of *Salmonella enteritidis* infections: New implications for the control of salmonellosis. *JAMA* 1988;259:2103–7.

Torrey S, Fleisher G, Jaffe D: Incidence of *Salmonella* bacteremia in infants with *Salmonella* gastroenteritis. *J Pediatr* 1986;108:718–21.

Mermin J, Hoar B, Angulo FJ: Iguanas and *Salmonella marina* infection in children: A reflection of the increasing incidence of reptile-associated salmonellosis in the United States. *Pediatrics* 1997;99:399–402.

Woodward DL, Khakhria R, Johnson WM: Human salmonellosis associated with exotic pets. *J Clin Microbiol* 1997;11:2786–90.

Salmonella typhi (Typhoid Fever)

Centers for Disease Control and Prevention: Typhoid immunization: Recommendations of the Advisory Committee on Immunization Practices (ACIP). *MMWR* 1994;43(RR-14):1–7.

Colon AR, Gross DR, Tamer MA: Typhoid fever in children. *Pediatrics* 1975:56:606–9.

Farid Z, Bassily S, Kent DC, et al: Chronic urinary *Salmonella* carriers with intermittent bacteremia. *J Trop Med Hyg* 1970;73:153–6.

Ferreccio C, Levine MM, Manterola A, et al: Benign bacteremia caused by *Salmonella typhi* and *paratyphi* in children younger than two years. *J Pediatr* 1984;104:899–901.

Goldberg MP, Rubin RH: The spectrum of *Salmonella* infection. *Infect Dis Clin North Am* 1988;2:571–98.

Hoffmann SL, Punjabi NH, Kumala S, et al: Reduction of mortality in chloramphenicol-treated severe typhoid fever by high-dose dexamethasone. *N Engl J Med* 1984;310:82–8.

Nourmand A, Ziai M: Typhoid and paratyphoid fever in children: Review of symptoms and therapy in 165 cases. *Clin Pediatr (Phila)* 1969;8:235–8.

Ryan CA, Hargrett-Bean NT, Blake PA: *Salmonella typhi* infections in the United States, 1975–1984: Increasing role of foreign travel. *Rev Infect Dis* 1989;11:1–8.

Sinha A, Sazawal S, Kumar R, et al: Typhoid fever in children aged less than 5 years. *Lancet* 1999;354:734–7.

Shigella

Bennish ML, Harris JR, Wojtyniak, et al: Death in shigellosis: Incidence and risk factors in hospitalized patients. *J Infect Dis* 1990:161:500–6.

DuPont HL: *Shigella. Infect Dis Clin North Am* 1988;2:599–605.

Keusch GT, Bennish ML: Shigellosis: Recent progress, persisting problems and research issues. *Pediatr Infect Dis J* 1989;8:713–9.

Varsano I, Eidlitz-Marcus T, Nussinovitch M, et al: Comparative efficacy of ceftriaxone and ampicillin for treatment of severe shigellosis in children. *J Pediatr* 1991;I18:627–32.

Zvulunov A, Lerman M, Ashkenazi S, et al: The prognosis of convulsions during childhood shigellosis. *Eur J Pediatr* 1990;149:293–4.

Yersinia enterocolitica

Black RE, Slome S: *Yersinia enterocolitica. Infect Dis Clin North Am* 1988;2:625–41.

Kelly D, Price E, Jani B, et al: *Yersinia* enterocolitis in iron overload. *J Pediatr Gastroenterol Nutr* 1987;6:643–5.

Kohl S, Jacobson JA, Nahmias A: *Yersinia enterocolitica* infections in children. *J Pediatr* 1976;89:77–9.

Osuoff SM, et al: Clinical features of sporadic *Yersinia enterocolitica* infections in Norway. *J Infect Dis* 1992;166:812.

Pai CH, Gillis F, Tuomanen E, et al: Placebo-controlled double-blind evaluation of trimethoprim-sulfamethoxazole treatment of *Yersinia enterocolitica* gastroenteritis. *J Pediatr* 1984;104:308–11.

Rodriguez WJ, Controni G, Cohen GJ: *Yersinia enterocolitica* enteritis in children. *JAMA* 1979:242:1978–80.

Campylobacter

Cornick NA, Gorbach SL: *Campylobacter. Infect Dis Clin North Am* 1988;2:643–54.

Ebright JR, Ryan LM: Acute erosive reactive arthritis associated with *Campylobacter jejuni*–induced colitis. *Am J Med* 1984;76:321–3.

Griffiths PL, Park RW: Campylobacters associated with human diarrhoeal disease. *J Appl Bacteriol* 1990;69:281–301.

Lerner A, Ianco TC, Landoy Z, et al: Seizures associated with *Campylobacter jejuni* enteritis. *Pediatr Infect Dis* 1984;3:281.

Ruiz-Palacios GM, Calva JJ, Pickering LK: Protection of breast fed infants against *Campylobacter* diarrhea by antibodies in human milk. *J Pediatr* 1990:116:707–13.

Ruiz-Palacios GM, Torres J, Torres NI, et al: Cholera-like enterotoxin produced by *Campylobacter jejuni. Lancet* 1983;112:250–3.

Salazar-Lindo E, Sack RB, Chea-Woo E, et al: Early treatment with erythromycin of *Campylobacter jejuni*–associated dysentery in children. *J Pediatr* 1986;109:355–60.

Aeromonas

Agger WA, McCormick JD, Gurwith MJ: Clinical and microbiologic features of *Aeromonas hydrophila*–associated diarrhea. *J Clin Microbiol* 1985:2 I:909–13.

Brenden RA, Miller MA, Janda JM: Clinical disease spectrum and pathogenic factors associated with *Plesiomonas shigelloides* infections in humans. *Rev Infect Dis* 1988;10:303–16.

Holmberg SD: *Vibrios* and *Aeromonas. Infect Dis Clin North Am* 1988;2:655–76.

Holmberg S, Farmer JJ: *Aeromonas hydrophila* and *Plesiomonas shigelloides* as causes of intestinal infection. *Rev Infect Dis* 1984;6:633–9.

Kipperman H, Ephrds M, Lambden M, et al: *Aeromonas hydrophila:* A treatable cause of diarrhea. *Pediatrics* 1984;73:253–4.

Wadstrom T, Ljungh A: *Aeromonas* and *Plesiomonas* as food- and waterborne pathogens. *Int J Food Microbiol* 1991;12:303–11.

Amebiasis

Dykes AC, Ruebush TK, Gorelkin L, et al: Extraintestinal amebiasis in infancy: Report of three patients and epidemiologic investigations of their families. *Pediatrics* 1980; 65:799–803.

Krogstad DJ, Spencer HC, Healy GR: Current concepts in parasitology: Amebiasis. *N Engl J Med* 1978;298:262–5.

McAuley JB, Herwaldt BL, Stokes SL, et al: Diloxanide furoate for treating asymptomatic *Entamoeba histolytica* cyst passers: 14 years' experience in the United States. *Clin Infect Dis* 1992;15:464–8.

Panosian CB: Parasitic diarrhea. *Infect Dis Clin North Am* 1988;2:685–703.

Reed SL: Amebiasis: An update. *Clin Infect Dis* 1992:14:385–93.

Rimsza ME, Berg RA: Cutaneous amebiasis. *Pediatrics* 1983;71:595–8.

Vibrio cholerae (Cholera)

Holmberg S: *Vibrios* and *Aeromonas. Infect Dis Clin North Am* 1988; 2:655–76.

Hunt MD, Woodward WE, Keswick BN, et al: Seroepidemiology of cholera in Gulf Coastal Texas. *Appl Environ Microbiol* 1988;54:1673–7.

Ries AA, Vugia DJ, Beingolea L, et al: Cholera in Piura, Peru: A modern urban epidemic. *J Infect Dis* 1992;166:1429–33.

Ramakrishna BS, Venkataraman S, Srinivasan P, et al: Amylase-resistant starch plus oral rehydration solution for cholera. *N Engl J Med* 2000;342:308–313.

Sack DA: Cholera in pediatric travelers. *Semin Pediatr Infect Dis* 1992;3:54.

Swerdlow DL, Ries AA: Cholera in the Americas: Guidelines for the clinician. *JAMA* 1992;267:1495–9.

Tauxe RV, Blake PA: Epidemic cholera in Latin America. *JAMA* 1992; 267:1388–90.

Escherichia coli Syndromes

Griffin PM, Ostroff SM, Tauxe RV, et al: Illnesses associated with *Escherichia coli* O157:H7 infections: A broad clinical spectrum. *Ann Intern Med* 1988;109:705–12.

Levine MM: *Escherichia coli* that cause diarrhea: Enterotoxigenic. enteropathogenic, enteroinvasive, enterohemmorhagic, and enteroadherent. *J Infect Dis* 1987;155:377–89.

Robins-Browne RM: Traditional enteropathogenic *Escherichia coli* of infantile diarrhea. *Rev Infect Dis* 1987;9:28–53.

Schlager TA, Guerrant RL: Seven possible mechanisms for *Escherichia coli* diarrhea. *Infect Dis Clin North Am* 1988;2:607–24.

Willshaw GA, Scotland SM, Smith HR, et al: Properties of vero cytotoxin producing *Escherichia coli* of human origin of O serogroups other than O157. *J Infect Dis* 1992;166:797–802.

Slutsker L, Ries AA, Greene KD: *Escherichia coli* O157:H7 diarrhea in the United States: Clinical and epidemiologic features. *Ann Intern Med* 1997;126:505–13.

Viral Gastroenteritis

Bartlett AV, Reves RR, Pickering LK: Rotavirus in infant-toddler day care centers: Epidemiology relevant to disease control strategies. *J Pediatr* 1988;113:435–41.

Becker KM, Moe CL, Southwick KL, et al: Transmission of Norwalk virus during a football game. *N Engl J Med* 2000;343:1223–7.

Centers for Disease Control and Prevention: ''Norwalk-like viruses.'' Public health consequences and outbreak management. *MMWR Morb Mortal Wkly Rep* 2001;50(RR-9):1–17.

Dinulos MB, Matson DO: Recent developments with human caliciviruses. *Pediatr Infect Dis J* 1994;13:998–1003.

Fankhauser RL, Noel JS, Monroe SS, et al: Molecular epidemiology of ''Norwalk-like viruses'' in outbreaks of gastroenteritis in the United States. *J Infect Dis* 1998;178:1571–8.

Ho M, Glass RI, Pinsky PF, et al: Rotavirus as a cause of diarrheal morbidity and morality in the United States. *J Infect Dis* 1988:158:1112–6.

Kapikian AZ, Flores J, Hoshino Y, et al: Prospects for development of a rotavirus vaccine against rotavirus diarrhea in infants and young children. *Rev Infect Dis* 1989;11:S539–46.

Koopmans MP, Goosen ES, Lema AA, et al: Association of torovirus with acute and persistent diarrhea in children. *Pediatr Infect Dis J* 1997; 16:504–7.

Lew JF, Valdesuso J, Vesikari T, et al: Detection of Norwalk virus or Norwalk-like infections in Finnish infants and young children. *J Infect Dis* 1994;169:1364–7.

Ryder RW, Singh N, Reeves WC, et al: Evidence of immunity induced by naturally acquired rotavirus and Norwalk virus infection on two remote Panamanian islands. *J Infect Dis* 1985;151:99–105.

Uhnoo I, Wadell G, Svensson L, et al: Importance of enteric adenoviruses 40 and 41 in acute gastroenteritis in infants and young children. *J Clin Microbiol* 1984;20:365–72.

Wickelgren I: How rotavirus causes diarrhea. *Science* 2000;287:409–11.

Chronic Infectious Diarrhea

Alpert G, Bell LM, Kirkpatrick CE, et al: Outbreak of cryptosporidiosis in a daycare center. *Pediatrics* 1986;77:152–7.

Centers for Disease Control and Prevention: Giardiasis surveillance United States, 1992–1997. *MMWR Morb Mortal Wkly Rep* 2000; 49(SS-7):1–13.

Farthing M: Host-parasitic interactions in human giardiasis. *Q J Med* 1989;70:191–204.

Keystone JS, Yang J, Grisdale D, et al: Intestinal parasites in metropolitan Toronto day-care centres. *Can Med Assoc J* 1984;131:733–5.

Ortega YR, Adam RD: *Giardia:* Overview and update. *Clin Infect Dis* 1997;25:545–50.

Shlim DR, Cohen MT, Eaton M, et al: An alga-like organism associated with an outbreak of prolonged diarrhea among foreigners in Nepal. *Am J Trop Med Hyg* 1991;45:383–9.

Soave R, Johnson WD: *Cryptosporidium* and *Isospora belli* infections. *J Infect Dis* 1988;157:225–9.

Wolfe MS: Giardiasis. *Clin Microbiol Rev* 1992;5:93–100.

Travelers' Diarrhea

Banwell JG: Treatment of travelers' diarrhea: Fluid and dietary management. *Rev Infect Dis* 1986;8:S182–7.

Baqui A, Sack RB, Black RE, et al: Enteropathogens associated with acute and persistent diarrhea in Bangladeshi children <5 years of age. *J Infect Dis* 1992;166:792–6.

Black RE: Epidemiology of travelers' diarrhea and relative importance of various pathogens. *Rev Infect Dis* 1990;12:S73–9.

Gianella RA: Chronic diarrhea in travelers: Diagnostic and therapeutic consideration. *Rev Infect Dis* 1986:8:S223–6.

Sack RB: Travelers' diarrhea: Microbiologic bases for prevention and treatment. *Rev Infect Dis* 1990;12:S59–63.

Steffen R: Worldwide efficacy of bismuth subsalicylate in the treatment of travelers' diarrhea. *Rev Infect Dis* 1990;12:S80–6.

Wiström J, Jertborn M, Ekevall E: Empiric treatment of acute diarrheal disease with norfloxacin: A randomized, placebo controlled study: A Swedish Study Group. *Ann Intern Med* 1992;117:202–8.

Common Source Diarrhea

Centers for Disease Control and Prevention: Diagnosis and management of foodborne illnesses: A primer for physicians. *MMWR Morb Mortal Wkly Rep* 2001;50(RR-2):1–67.

Centers for Disease Control and Prevention: Surveillance for foodborne-disease outbreaks—United States, 1996. *MMWR Morb Mortal Wkly Rep* 1996;45(SS-5):1–55.

Centers for Disease Control and Prevention: Surveillance for water-borne disease outbreaks—United States. *MMWR Morb Mortal Wkly Rep* 1998;47(SS-5):1–34.

Hayes EB, Matte TD, O'Brien TR, et al: Large community outbreak of Cryptosporidiosis due to contamination of a filtered public water supply. *N Engl J Med* 1989;320:1372–6.

Mead PS, Slutsker L, Griffin PM, et al: Food-related illness and death in the United States. *Emerg Infect Dis* 1999;5:841–2.

Antibiotic-Associated Diarrhea

Adler SP, Chandrika T, Berman WF: *Clostridium difficile* associated with *pseudomonas* colitis: Occurrence in a 12-week-old infant without prior antibiotic therapy. *Am J Dis Child* 1981;135:820–2.

Arvola T, Laiho K, Torkkeli S, et al: Prophylactic *Lactobacillus* GG reduces antibiotic-associated diarrhea in children with respiratory infections: A randomized study. *Pediatrics* 1999;104:e64.

Johnson S, Samore MH, Farrow KA,: Epidemics of diarrhea caused by a clindamycin-resistant strain of *Clostridium difficile* in four hospitals. *N Engl J Med* 1999;341:1645–51.

McFarland LV, Surawicz CM, Stamm WE: Risk factors for *Clostridium difficile* carriage and *C. difficile* associated diarrhea in a cohort of hospitalized patients. *J Infect Dis* 1990;162:678–84.

Viscidi RP, Bartlett JG: Antibiotic-associated pseudomembranous colitis in children. *Pediatrics* 1981;67:381–6.

Vanderhoof JA, Whitney DB, Antonson DL, et al: *Lactobacillus* GG in the prevention of antibiotic-associated diarrhea in children. *J Pediatr* 1999;135:564–8.

Hemolytic Uremic Syndrome

Banatvala N, Griffin PM, Greene KD, et al: The United States National Perspective Hemolytic Uremic Syndrome Study: Microbiologic, serologic, clinical, and epidemiologic findings. *J Infect Dis* 2001;183: 1063–70.

Butler T, Islam MR, Azad MA, et al: Risk factors for development of hemolytic uremic syndrome during shigellosis. *J Pediatr* 1987;110: 894–7.

Cimolai N, Carter JE, Morrison BJ, et al: Risk factors for the progression of *Escherichia coli* O157:H7 enteritis to hemolytic uremic syndrome. *J Pediatr* 1990;116:589–92.

Griffin PM, Tauxe RV: The epidemiology of infections caused by *Escherichia coli* O157:H7, other enterohemorrhagic *E. coli,* and the associated hemolytic uremic syndrome. *Epidemiol Rev* 1991;13:60–98.

Pickering LK, Obrig TG, Stapleton FB: Hemolytic-uremic syndrome and enterohemorrhagic *Escherichia coli. Pediatr Infect Dis J* 1994;13: 459–76.

Proulx F, Turgean JP, Delage G, et al: Randomized controlled trial of antibiotic therapy for *Escherichia coli* O157:H7 enteritis. *J Pediatr* 1992;121:299–303.

Robson WL, Leung AKC, Kaplan BS: Hemolytic-uremic syndrome. *Curr Probl Pediatr* 1993;23:16–33.

Siegler RL: Management of hemolytic-uremic syndrome. *J Pediatr* 1988;112:1014–20.

Tarr PI, Neill MA, Clausen CR, et al: *Escherichia coli* O157:H7 and the hemolytic uremic syndrome: Importance of early cultures in establishing the etiology. *J Infect Dis* 1990;162:553–6.

Wong CS, Jelacic S, Habeeb RL, et al: The risk of the hemolytic-uremic syndrome after antibiotic treatment of *Escherichia coli* O157:H7 infections. *N Engl J Med* 2000;342:1930–6.

Zimmerhackl LB: *E. coli,* antibiotics and the hemolytic-uremic syndrome. *N Engl J Med* 2000;342;1990–1.

Whipple's Disease

Donaldson RM: Whipple's disease—Rare malady with uncommon potential. *N Engl J Med* 1992;327:346–8.

Fleming JL, Wiesner RH, Shorter RG: Whipple's disease: Clinical, biochemical, and histopathologic features and assessment of treatment in 29 patients. *Mayo Clin Proc* 1988;63;539–51.

Lowsky R, Archer GL, Fyles G, et al: Diagnosis of Whipple's disease by molecular analysis of peripheral blood. *N Engl J Med* 1994;331:1343–6.

Raoult D, Birg ML, LaScola B, et al: Cultivation of the bacillus of Whipple's disease. *N Engl J Med* 2000.342:620–5.

Supportive Therapy of Acute Enteritis

American Academy of Pediatrics, Provisional Committee on Quality Improvement, Subcommittee on Acute Gastroenteritis: Practice parameter: The management of acute gastroenteritis in young children. *Pediatrics* 1996;97:424–35.

Di John D, Levine MM: Treatment of diarrhea. *Infect Dis Clin North Am* 1988;2:719–45.

Isolauri E, Vesikari T, Saha P, et al: Milk versus no milk in rapid refeeding after acute gastroenteritis. *J Pediatr Gastroenterol Nutr* 1986;5:254–61.

Karrar ZA, Abdulla MA, Moody JB: Loperamide in acute diarrhea in childhood: Results of a double blind placebo controlled clinical trial. *Ann Trop Med* 1987;7:122–7.

Mohan M, Sethi JS, Daral TS: Controlled trial of rice powder and glucose rehydration solutions as oral therapy for acute dehydrating diarrhea in infants. *J Pediatr Gastroenterol Nutr* 1986;5:423–7.

Molla AM, Molla A, Rohde J: Turning off the diarrhea: The role of food and ORS. *J Pediatr Gastroenterol Nutr* 1989;8:81–4.

Pizarro D, Posado G, Sandi L, et al: Rice based oral electrolyte solutions for the management of infantile diarrhea. *N Engl J Med* 1991;324:517–21.

Ramakrishna BS, Venkataraman S, Srinivasan P, et al: Amylase-resistant starch plus oral rehydration solution for cholera. *N Engl J Med* 2000;342:308–13.

Salazar-Lindo E, Santisteban-Ponce J, Chea-Woo E, et al: Racecadotril in the treatment of acute watery diarrhea in children. *N Engl J Med* 2000;343:463–7.

CHAPTER 77

Intra-abdominal and Retroperitoneal Infections

Edward J. O'Rourke

Intra-abdominal infections are an important cause of morbidity in the pediatric population. During the past century, advances in diagnostic imaging, surgical management, intensive care, and antibiotic therapy have markedly reduced the mortality rate; yet these infections remain serious threats. New antibiotics and minimally invasive surgical techniques may allow additional management options, but neither is likely to improve current treatment outcomes substantially. Further advances in management are likely to result from earlier diagnosis, an elusive goal that depends on the skill of the primary clinician. The early symptoms of intra-abdominal infections, typically nonfocal abdominal pain, with or without fever, are frustratingly similar to the presenting symptoms of many common minor illnesses. Thus early recognition requires great clinical acumen. The clinician must obtain a thorough history, make a careful physical examination, and observe the disease progression closely to determine whether additional diagnostic evaluation is indicated. Although new imaging tools are useful in confirming or localizing infection, diagnosis depends on the suspicion of the alert primary clinician.

Most intra-abdominal infections are the result of indigenous gastrointestinal organisms that escaped their normal anatomic confines when the integrity of the intestinal wall was compromised. Perforation and spillage of gastrointestinal contents into the peritoneal cavity result in peritonitis. Microorganisms may seed adjacent areas through the blood supply or as a consequence of local spread within the abdominal cavity. Infection of the intra-abdominal cavity can also occur when microorganisms gain entry into the abdominal cavity through the bloodstream during episodes of bacteremia, by extension of infection from the uterine cavity and fallopian tubes, or by extension through the abdominal wall.

Although many infections remain localized, infection becomes generalized when microorganisms are carried to various intraperitoneal locations by the flow of peritoneal fluid within the intra-abdominal cavity. The history and physical findings often enable the physician to determine the location and extent of infection in older children. Identification of infection in neonates and toddlers is more difficult because young patients are frequently unable to localize pain and communicate their symptoms. Diagnostic imaging can be invaluable in these settings. Arguably, diagnostic and interventional radiology has had a greater influence on the changes in diagnosis and management of intra-abdominal infection during the past two decades than any other therapeutic or diagnostic measure. Currently, it is unusual in modern pediatric facilities to proceed to exploratory surgery without prior imaging studies, and often the findings allow surgery to be avoided altogether. The delineation of the type, location, and extent of the intra-abdominal process by imaging studies may also permit increasing use of laparoscopic techniques. When imaging data reveal a possible infection, percutaneous drainage or limited surgery, with the collection of microbiologic specimens, may be possible.

Anatomy of the Abdominal Cavity. The abdominal cavity and the pelvic cavity are bounded anteriorly and posteriorly by the walls of the abdomen, superiorly by the diaphragm, and inferiorly by the lower limits of the pelvis. Within the abdominal cavity are the digestive organs, the spleen, liver, kidneys, adrenal glands, and the reproductive organs.

Most of the abdominal organs are encased or covered by the **peritoneum,** a serous membrane that forms a sac within the abdominal cavity. The reflection of peritoneum that lines the walls of the abdominal cavity is the **parietal peritoneum;** the visceral reflection of the peritoneal sac encases the abdominal organs. A small amount of sterile fluid is normally present within the peritoneal cavity.

Early in embryologic development, the peritoneum forms a simple cavity. As the abdominal viscera undergo complex rotation during fetal development, the simple peritoneal cavity becomes compartmentalized by the mesenteric attachments and peritoneal reflections of these organs (Fig. 77–1). The rotation of the abdominal viscera thus forms recesses within the peritoneal cavity, which may collect and sequester infected fluid, and pathways, which allow movement of fluid from one area of the abdomen to another, thereby allowing the spread of infection.

The organs encased by the peritoneum, the **intraperitoneal viscera,** are suspended within the peritoneal sac by folds of peritoneum called **mesenteries,** if they are suspended from the body wall itself, or **ligaments,** if they are suspended from another organ (Fig. 77–1*B*). The mesenteries of the intestine suspend the small intestine and portions of the colon from the posterior abdominal wall and deliver its blood supply. An **omentum** is a ligament that joins the stomach to another structure. The **lesser omentum (hepatogastric ligament)** joins the liver to the stomach. The **greater omentum** connects the greater curvature of the stomach to the transverse colon and then descends toward the pelvis, forming an apron over the small intestine. Several abdominal structures, including the liver, spleen, ascending and descending colon, and rectum, are only partially encased by peritoneum (Fig. 77–1*A*). The bare area of the liver comes in direct contact with the diaphragm. The pancreas and duodenum are covered by peritoneum but are located within the retroperitoneal area. In men and boys, the peritoneum is a closed sac. In women and girls, however, the peritoneum has continuity with the mucous membranes of the fallopian tubes, thereby allowing communication between the abdominal cavity and the external environment through the female genital tract.

The subphrenic space is divided anatomically into right and left spaces by the falciform ligament of the liver. This ligament is a peritoneal fold that attaches the liver to the anterior abdominal wall and to the underside of the diaphragm. The falciform ligament (Fig. 77–1*A*) can act as a barrier to small amounts of fluid, accounting for the low incidence of bilateral subphrenic abscesses.

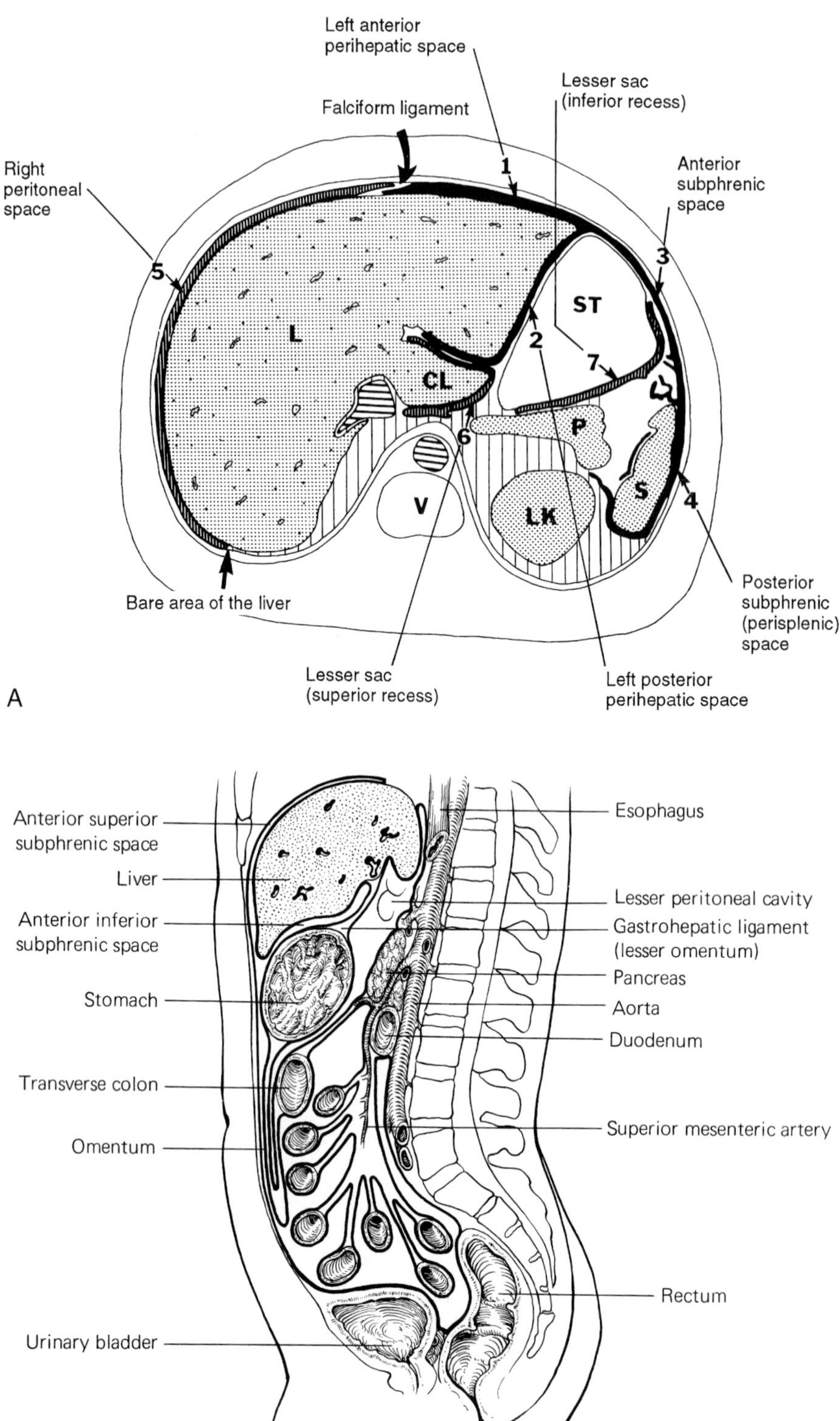

FIGURE 77–1. **A,** Peritoneal spaces of the upper abdomen. Heavy black lines indicate left peritoneal spaces. Right peritoneal spaces are indicated by vertical hatching. The left peritoneal space has four divisions. Anterior to the liver, limited medially by the falciform ligament *(curved arrow)*, is the left anterior perihepatic space *(1)*. Curving posteriorly to cover the visceral hepatic surface is the left posterior perihepatic space *(2)*. The anterior subphrenic space *(3)* separates the gastric fundus *(ST)* from the diaphragm, and the posterior subphrenic (perisplenic) space *(4)* surrounds the spleen *(S)*. The right peritoneal space consists of the perihepatic space and the lesser sac. The diaphragmatic surface of the lesser sac *(5)* is limited on the left by the falciform ligament and posteromedially by the hepatic bare area (*arrow* marks the peritoneal reflection). The lesser sac has two components. The superior recess of the lesser sac *(6)* surrounds the caudate lobe of the liver *(CL)* and is separated from the inferior recess *(7)* by the lesser omentum. *L,* Liver; *V,* vertebral body; *P,* pancreas; *LK,* left kidney. **B,** The peritoneal reflections and location of the lesser peritoneal cavity. (*A* modified from Lee JK, Sagel SS, Stanley RJ: *Computed Body Tomography with MRI Correlation,* 2nd ed. New York, Raven Press, Ltd., 1989, p 425; *B* from Dunphy JE, Way LW [editors]: *Current Surgical Diagnosis and Treatment,* 5th ed. San Diego, Calif., Lange Medical Publications, 1981, p 395.)

The **hepatorenal recess (Morison's pouch)** is located between the liver and the right kidney. It is the most dependent portion of the subhepatic space when the body is in the supine position and plays an important role in the containment and spread of infected intraperitoneal fluid. Collections of fluid in this area can come from the right lobe of the liver, the gallbladder, the descending portion of the duodenum, and the colon or from the pelvis through the right paracolic gutter.

The **lesser peritoneal cavity (sac)** is the largest recess of the peritoneal cavity and is an area where inflammatory fluid collects in the abdominal cavity. It consists of the posterior subphrenic space and the entire space posterior and inferior to the liver. The lesser cavity is separated from the **greater peritoneal cavity** by the **gastrohepatic ligament (lesser omentum)** (Fig. 77–1*B*). The lesser peritoneal cavity communicates with the greater peritoneal cavity only by a small opening between the inferior vena cava and the medial free margin of the lesser omentum called the **epiploic foramen (of Winslow).** Because the lesser peritoneal cavity is separated from the remainder of the peritoneal cavity, a fluid collection within this space may not involve the rest of the peritoneal cavity. Abscesses within the lesser peritoneal cavity can spread through the epiploic foramen to the right subhepatic area or may become sequestered if the epiploic foramen closes because of inflammation. Although fluid collections in the lesser peritoneal cavity are uncommon, knowledge of them is important clinically because they are difficult to detect.

The pelvic recess consists of the lateral paravesical spaces and the midline space, called the **pouch of Douglas** (also known as the **rectouterine pouch** in women and girls and the **rectovesicular pouch** in men and boys). The midline space, because of its dependent position, often collects inflammatory fluid.

INTRA-ABDOMINAL AND PELVIC ABSCESSES

ETIOLOGY

Most intra-abdominal abscesses resulting from intestinal spillage are polymicrobial and contain both anaerobic and aerobic bacteria. The anaerobic bacteria usually found in these abscesses are *Bacteroides fragilis, Prevotella melaninogenica, Peptococcus, Peptostreptococcus, Fusobacterium,* and *Clostridium* species. The aerobic organisms and facultative anaerobes cultured most commonly are *Escherichia coli, Enterococcus* species, *Klebsiella pneumoniae,* and *Pseudomonas aeruginosa.* Most *B. fragilis* strains and many isolates of *E. coli* produce β-lactamases. In hospitalized patients, antibiotic-resistant pathogens and yeast are seen more commonly.

In newborn infants the bacteria found in intra-abdominal abscesses after perforation of the intestine as a result of necrotizing enterocolitis are the usual intestinal colonizers of neonates as well as resistant pathogens acquired in the neonatal nursery or intensive care unit. In these infants there is predominance of aerobic bacteria, including *K. pneumoniae, Enterobacter, Streptococcus,* and, in some patients, coagulase-negative *Staphylococcus*. Anaerobes, including *Clostridium difficile,* also are found.

In patients with a **ventriculoperitoneal shunt,** an intra-abdominal abscess may form at the abdominal tip of the shunt from infected cerebrospinal fluid. Coagulase-negative *Staphylococcus* is the usual offending organism, although more virulent pathogens are also seen in this setting.

EPIDEMIOLOGY

Appendicitis is the most common cause of intra-abdominal and pelvic abscesses in pediatrics. Perforation of the appendix occurs in one third of pediatric patients with appendicitis before diagnosis. In approximately 5% of these patients, intraperitoneal abscesses will develop, most commonly in the pelvis. Intra-abdominal abscesses following uncontaminated abdominal surgery, although uncommon, may occur. Operations on the colon are responsible for about one half of the subphrenic abscesses on the left side.

PATHOGENESIS

Intra-abdominal infection occurs when the integrity of the intestinal wall is compromised by a pathologic condition, allowing spillage of pathogenic microorganisms into the peritoneum. The conditions include ischemia or necrosis of the intestinal wall due to necrotizing enterocolitis, intussusception, volvulus, or an incarcerated hernia; perforation of the intestine due to rupture of an inflamed appendix, perforation of Meckel's diverticulum, Crohn's disease, or ulcerative colitis; trauma to the intestine; or an operation on the gastrointestinal tract.

An abscess, which is a localized collection of bacteria, pus, and necrotic material, may occur after incomplete resolution of diffuse peritonitis, or it may originate from a perforation with intestinal spillage that was successfully localized but not sterilized and resorbed by the peritoneal defenses. It contains viable pathogens that can cause continued enlargement of the abscess. If not walled off completely, an abscess can serve as a continuous source of infection, seeding other areas of the body.

Three forms of host defense attempt to combat bacterial contamination in the peritoneum: lymphatic clearance, phagocytosis, and sequestration by fibrin. Lymphatic clearance of bacteria is very efficient, and abscess formation occurs only when large numbers of bacteria are spilled or when substances such as hemoglobin, barium, or necrotic tissue are present. These substances inhibit bacterial clearance by blocking lymphatic vessels, providing bacterial nutrients, or impairing bacterial killing. Peritoneal macrophages are the predominant phagocytic cells early in host defense. As bacteria proliferate, polymorphonuclear leukocytes invade and become more numerous. The peritoneal inflammation increases splanchnic blood flow with resultant protein and fluid exudation into the peritoneal cavity. Fibrin deposition entraps bacteria and localizes infection, allowing abscesses to form within several days after perforation of a viscus or several weeks after diffuse peritonitis.

Abscesses form within the abdomen when bacteria enter the normally sterile peritoneal space and cannot be eliminated by the defense mechanisms of the peritoneum, as discussed. Several conditions must exist within the abdomen to permit abscess formation. Contaminated debris or foreign materials encourage the growth of anaerobes by establishing a microenvironment with a low oxygen concentration that interferes with phagocytosis and chemotaxis. The environment within the growing abscess cavity diminishes host defenses. Neutrophils, which depend on oxidative metabolism, cannot kill bacteria in an anaerobic environment. Synergy between aerobic and anaerobic bacteria may interfere with host defenses. For example, *B. fragilis* and *P. melaninogenica* inhibit the phagocytosis of *E. coli. B. fragilis* also interferes with the alternative complement pathway. These bacteria produce several chemicals that destroy tissue and promote abscess formation. In addition, many antibiotics are rendered inactive or less active in anaerobic environments. Because aminoglycoside antibiotics require oxygen-dependent transport to penetrate the bacterial cell envelope, they are ineffectual within the abscess. Antibiotics, such as β-lactams that work by preventing cell wall formation in actively growing bacteria, are less efficient in killing bacteria in an abscess because much of the bacterial population has achieved a stationary phase of growth. In addition, the lack of blood supply to the center of an abscess prevents antibiotics from being delivered efficiently to the core of the abscess.

Primary peritonitis, also known as **spontaneous bacterial peritonitis,** is often caused by pneumococcus in children. It rarely results in abscess formation. More commonly, intra-abdominal abscesses form as a complication of **secondary peritonitis,** defined as loss of integrity of the gastrointestinal tract. Each part of the gastrointestinal tract contains its own resident bacteria that are normally not pathogenic if contained within the gastrointestinal tract. The stomach normally contains no resident microflora but is intermittently seeded with bacteria contained in food and in nasopharyngeal drainage and saliva. Abscesses arising from the stomach, liver, and biliary tract have a predominance of coliform bacteria, sometimes accompanied by anaerobic bacteria. The lower gastrointestinal tract has an anaerobic environment; the ratio of obligate anaerobes to facultative anaerobes ranges from 100:1 to 10,000:1. Therefore, abscesses arising from the ileum and colon have a predominance of anaerobes with some aerobic organisms present. Although 400–500 species of microorganisms are found in the colon, only a few of these species are pathogenic and able to survive within an abscess cavity. Some organisms, such as enterococci, rarely cause abscesses alone but may be found in polymicrobial abscesses.

A pelvic abscess caused by rupture of a tubo-ovarian abscess secondary to pelvic inflammatory disease contains mixed aerobic and anaerobic organisms representative of the pelvic flora and may include pathogenic genital flora such as *Neisseria gonorrhea.* Abscesses caused by direct spread of a pyogenic process within the liver and spleen can be found in the subphrenic areas. The organisms are those that caused the infection in the viscus.

Occasionally, patients with percutaneous gastric feeding tubes develop abscesses when reinsertion accidentally perforates the stomach or creates a new track outside the stomach. Infecting organisms reflect those colonizing the catheter exit site or in infused fluids.

Once an abscess has formed within the peritoneal cavity, the infected material can be disseminated to distal intraperitoneal sites by the normal flow of fluid within the cavity. This flow is determined by the presence of an unobstructed pathway, by gravity, and by changes in intra-abdominal pressure due to movement of the diaphragm during respiration. Normally, the right paracolic gutter provides a freely communicating pathway between right subhepatic and subphrenic spaces and the pelvis. Fluid in the right upper peritoneal cavity moves into Morison's pouch, to the right subphrenic space, and then caudally into the pelvis through the right paracolic gutter. Fluid in the left upper peritoneal space collects in the left subphrenic space but does not travel caudally because the phrenicocolic ligament, which attaches the left flexure of the colon to the diaphragm, limits flow. Fluid within the lower peritoneal cavity often collects in the pelvic recess. Although the pelvic recess is the most dependent space of the peritoneal cavity in both the erect and supine positions, fluid can travel cephalad independently of position through the right paracolic gutter to the right subhepatic space. It often collects in Morison's pouch and then travels around the lateral border of the liver to the right subphrenic space. In addition, abscesses can develop in the paracolic gutters or between the loops and mesentery of the small intestine.

In general, the location of abscess formation often depends on the source of the contaminating bacteria and the flow of peritoneal fluid. Contaminated material that originates in the lower abdomen, such as after rupture of the appendix or of a tubo-ovarian abscess, usually remains within the pelvic area. Such infected material, however, may become distributed from the pelvic area to the subphrenic and subhepatic spaces through the right paracolic gutter.

SYMPTOMS AND CLINICAL MANIFESTATIONS

The clinical presentation of an intra-abdominal abscess depends to some extent on its location. Subphrenic abscesses often develop insidiously. A patient may have mild, nonlocalizing abdominal pain. Because the abscess is directly under the diaphragm, signs attributable to chest disease are often prominent. These include dyspnea, chest pain, and rapid, shallow breathing due to pain on motion of the diaphragm. If the abscess is between the liver and the diaphragm, referred ipsilateral shoulder pain may be present. The patient usually has anorexia, nausea, and vomiting. If the abscess is posterior to the liver within the lesser peritoneal cavity, the patient may have vomiting and upper and mid abdominal pain that radiates to the back. The initial symptoms of a pelvic abscess are fever, nonspecific lower abdominal pain, rectal pain, diarrhea due to irritation of the rectum, and urinary urgency due to pressure on the bladder.

Patients who develop postoperative abscesses typically present with a new fever 1–2 weeks after an operation. When an abscess is present, the onset of chills implies bacteremia, seeding to a secondary focus, or impending perforation or extension of the abscess into adjacent organs.

Physical Examination Findings

Many of the physical signs of intra-abdominal abscesses also depend on the location. The abdominal peritoneum is segmentally innervated by the lower sixth thoracic to first lumbar spinal nerves, which also innervate the overlying muscles and skin. Irritation of the parietal abdominal peritoneum produces pain and abdominal rigidity. Although it is often difficult to determine the location of an abscess by the physical findings alone, certain signs are helpful. Subphrenic abscesses cause decreased breath sounds and dullness to percussion at the base of the lung because of pleural effusion, atelectasis, pneumonitis, or empyema. An anterior subphrenic abscess produces upper abdominal tenderness and peritoneal signs. A subphrenic abscess in the lesser peritoneal cavity, which is posterior to the liver, is not palpable through the anterior abdominal wall. Physical examination of a patient with such an abscess may reveal upper abdominal tenderness without peritoneal irritation until the abscess is very large. Patients with intermesenteric abscesses may have a fever but often do not have localizing signs. Most patients with intra-abdominal abscesses have signs of a paralytic ileus with decreased bowel sounds and abdominal distention.

A pelvic abscess may become large before it can be localized. This is because the parietal peritoneum in the pelvis is supplied by the obturator nerve, which does not innervate the overlying pelvic abdominal musculature. Thus a pelvic inflammatory process does not produce lower abdominal rigidity, and examination of the lower abdomen reveals few signs. There may be tenderness only to deep palpation. The most important part of the physical examination of a child believed to have a pelvic infection is the rectal or vaginal examination. A bimanual examination palpates a mass in the pelvis through the anterior abdominal wall and the rectum. A tender, bulging mass may be felt through the anterior rectal wall. Repeated daily rectal or vaginal examinations may have to be done to distinguish a nonfluctuant pelvic inflammatory mass, such as an appendiceal phlegmon, from a pelvic abscess that requires drainage.

DIAGNOSIS

An intra-abdominal abscess is highly likely if a patient has abdominal pain, tenderness to palpation, distention, diaphragmatic symptoms, and a fever and has recently undergone any abdominal procedure or has an underlying abdominal disease, such as regional enteritis or ulcerative colitis. An elevated leukocyte count is a common but nonspecific finding. Suspicion of an intra-abdominal abscess warrants further diagnostic imaging. Special attention needs to be paid to children with a fever and nonlocalized abdominal findings who are taking corticosteroids. Otherwise, these abscesses may be overlooked until sepsis has occurred.

Differential Diagnosis

A number of pathologic conditions in the lower abdominal cavity that cause fever and vague abdominal pain may be confused with a pelvic abscess. These conditions include pelvic appendicitis, pelvic tumors or hematomas, salpingitis, and tubo-ovarian abscesses. It is important to differentiate between pelvic inflammatory cellulitis (phlegmon) and an abscess because the latter requires drainage, whereas a phlegmon cannot be drained and responds to appropriate antibiotic therapy.

Laboratory Evaluation

A CBC usually reveals leukocytosis. A severely ill patient believed to have sepsis due to a focal intra-abdominal infection should have a complete fluid, electrolyte, and hematologic evaluation. Renal and liver function should be assessed.

Microbiologic Evaluation

Aerobic and anaerobic blood cultures should be performed for any child believed to have an intra-abdominal infection. Aerobic and anaerobic specimens obtained at the time of abscess drainage should be placed in a syringe that is tightly capped after the air is removed. Because anaerobic bacteria are killed when exposed to atmospheric concentrations of oxygen for more than 1–2 hours, these specimens should be transported immediately to a microbiology laboratory for anaerobic and aerobic culturing. A common error is to use a cotton swab to absorb pus and transport it in an air-filled tube.

In addition, patients who have been taking broad-spectrum antibiotics and immunocompromised patients should have fungal cultures. Antibiotic sensitivity tests should be performed on all isolates to determine the presence of antibiotic resistance and to guide antibiotic treatment.

Diagnostic Imaging

Plain **radiographs** of the chest and abdomen can be helpful in determining the presence of a subphrenic abscess. Images of the chest should include anteroposterior and lateral views, to look for a basal pneumonic process or pleural effusion and determine whether the abscess is anterior or posterior. Fixed elevation of the diaphragm may be seen. In advanced abscesses, an air-fluid level below the diaphragm not attributable to the gastric air bubble can be seen. Unfortunately, if the history is incomplete, plain chest radiographs may lead to the misdiagnosis of a primary pneumonic process and the appropriate abdominal source of infection may not be sought. Abdominal radiographs may be helpful in showing displacement of the intestine if an intermesenteric abscess is large. Plain abdominal radiographs are not helpful in determining the presence of a pelvic abscess.

Ultrasonography is highly accurate and sensitive in the detection of abscesses, especially in upper quadrants and in the pelvis (Fig. 77–2). It may be difficult to detect abscesses in the mid abdomen and the pelvis because of intestinal gas, which does not transmit ultrasonic waves, especially if the abdomen is distended. Ultrasonography can be done at the bedside of a patient who is too ill to be transported for CT or MRI or who cannot wait 24–72 hours for the results of a radionuclide scan. In addition, ultrasonography uses no ionizing radiation and is less expensive than gallium or indium scanning. However, it may be difficult to perform an ultrasonic study on a patient who has recently undergone an abdominal operation because the probe must make contact with the skin, and the patient may have incisional pain or there may be bandages or staples in place.

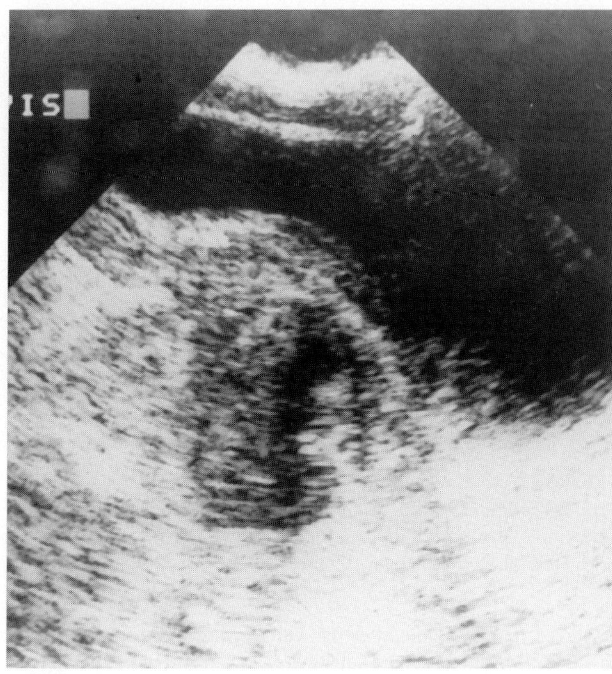

FIGURE 77–2. Pelvic abscess. A sagittal midline sonogram through the distended bladder reveals an irregular mass of mixed echogenicity behind the bladder. Surgical exploration revealed a pelvic abscess caused by a ruptured appendix.

Although radionuclide scanning can be useful in determining the presence and location of intra-abdominal abscesses, it has largely been replaced by ultrasonography, CT, and MRI. Both ^{67}Ga- and ^{111}In-labeled leukocytes are taken up in areas of inflammation. However, a chronic abscess may not be revealed because it is surrounded by a well-defined wall and has minimal inflammatory activity. These tests are not useful in the first 2 weeks of a peritoneal infection or within 2 weeks of an operation because the isotopes localize to the inflamed peritoneum and all areas of incision. After this period, however, these studies may be helpful. ^{67}Ga imaging has the additional disadvantage of being taken up by certain tumors and excreted by the colon, possibly masking the presence of a focal intra-abdominal infection. In addition, a patient in unstable condition may not be able to wait the day or more required for interpretation of the images. ^{111}In imaging takes less time than ^{67}Ga imaging, and the radionuclide is not excreted by the colon. However, the leukocytes that have been removed and labeled have a decreased ability to accumulate at sites of inflammation.

CT and MRI are the diagnostic methods of choice for patients believed to have intra-abdominal or pelvic abscesses, including tubo-ovarian abscesses (Fig. 77–3). These imaging techniques give superb anatomic detail with a diagnostic accuracy approaching 95% in determining the presence of an abscess. It is important,

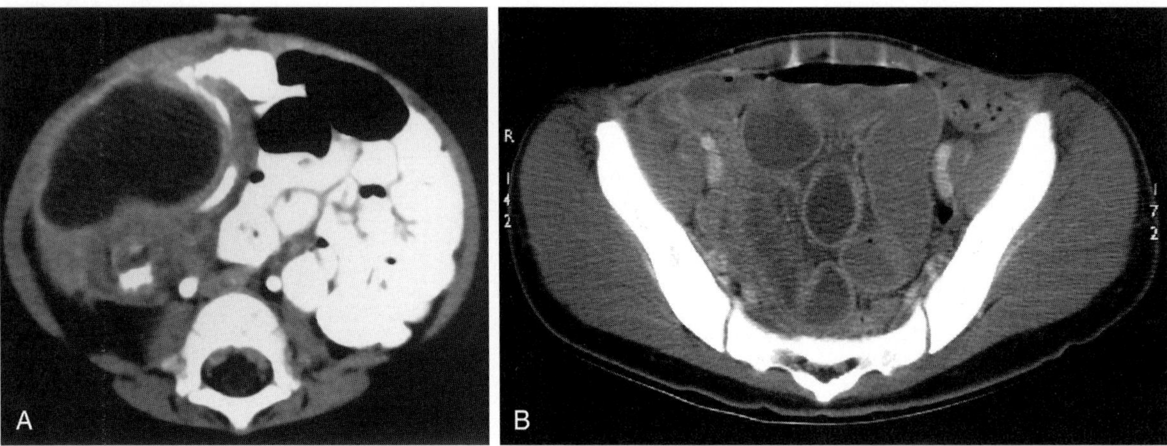

FIGURE 77–3. **A,** Abdominal abscess in a 12-year-old boy with Crohn's disease and recent onset of fever and abdominal pain. After intravenous and oral administration of contrast medium, CT of abdomen reveals a large abscess in the right lower abdomen adjacent to the anterior abdominal wall and displacing loops of intestine medially. Because of the size and location of the abscess, percutaneous drainage by catheter is feasible. **B,** Tubo-ovarian abscess.

however, to opacify the intestine with an oral contrast agent so that air-fluid levels in the gastrointestinal tract can be distinguished from those within an abscess cavity. A water-soluble contrast agent is preferred if there is clinical suspicion of a perforation. In the postsurgical period it is often important to differentiate an abscess from a hematoma. Inability to administer bowel contrast can limit the diagnostic ability of CT. If the patient is unable to drink contrast medium, it can be administered through a nasogastric tube or another enteric tube. Rectal contrast may also be administered if initial images are equivocal. Administration of intravenous contrast is useful to demonstrate the enhancing wall of an abscess and to clearly define adjacent vascular anatomy. Intravenous contrast is also needed for complete evaluation of hepatic, splenic, or renal abscess.

The diagnosis of abdominal abscess by CT scan depends on the identification of a fluid density that cannot be attributed to bowel or another known structure. The presence of an enhancing wall and adjacent inflammatory changes favors the diagnosis of infected fluid collections over noninfected ones. Any low-density fluid collection visualized by CT should be differentiated from unopacified bowel. Delayed images are often necessary to allow the bowel to opacify fully with contrast. Intra-abdominal inflammatory cellulitis (phlegmon) does not exhibit fluid density but, instead, looks like solid tissue with inhomogeneous enhancement.

Sometimes the CT appearance can suggest the cause of the abscess. Periappendiceal abscesses typically occur in the right lower quadrant adjacent to the cecum, often with an appendicolith visible (Fig. 77–4). Abscesses associated with Crohn's disease may demonstrate adjacent thickened small bowel.

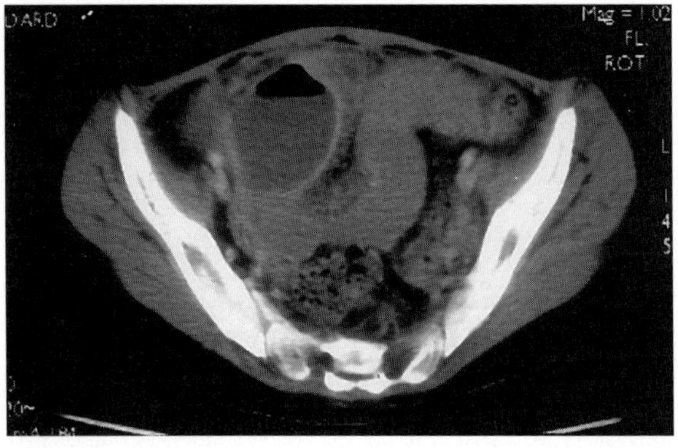

FIGURE 77–4. Periappendiceal abscess. (Courtesy of George A. Taylor, M.D.)

Although the CT appearance may strongly suggest an abscess, definitive diagnosis is made by testing a sample of the fluid by either diagnostic aspiration or a surgical procedure. CT scanning can guide diagnostic aspiration or percutaneous abscess drainage and provides the best visualization of intervening structures. Frequently CT-guided percutaneous drainage eliminates the need for surgery.

Figure 77–5 presents an algorithm for the radiologic diagnosis of an abdominal abscess. The type and order of the studies to be performed vary according to the stability of the patient's condition. In some cases, surgical exploration may be required before an objective diagnosis is made on the basis of clinical presentation and progression of signs and symptoms.

TREATMENT

Empirically chosen antimicrobial drugs should be administered before a drainage procedure to help prevent dissemination of the bacteria from the abscess. Because they most often occur after colonic perforation, intra-abdominal abscesses are typically polymicrobial in nature. Therefore the antimicrobial agents should be active against the organisms most likely to be involved in the formation of an intra-abdominal abscess. Gram-negative enteric bacilli include *E. coli, Klebsiella, Enterobacter, Proteus,* and *P. aeruginosa.* Gram-positive aerobic bacteria found in intra-abdominal abscesses include *Enterococcus* and α- and β-hemolytic streptococci. The predominant anaerobic bacteria include *Bacteroides, Peptococcus, Peptostreptococcus, Fusobacterium,* and *Clostridium.* Many of the *Bacteroides* and gram-negative enteric bacteria produce β-lactamases, which render β-lactam antibiotics (such as the penicillins and some of the cephalosporins) inactive unless combined with β-lactamase inhibitor.

In general, antibiotics are effective only in conjunction with **drainage of an abscess.** Antibiotic therapy without abscess drainage can fail for a number of reasons, including poor penetration of antibiotics into abscess cavities and the acidic environment and low oxygen tension in the necrotic tissue of the abscess. After drainage, the initial antibiotic regimen should be based on the Gram stain of the abscess fluid and clinical setting. Once the organisms are identified and sensitivities are reported, antibiotic selections

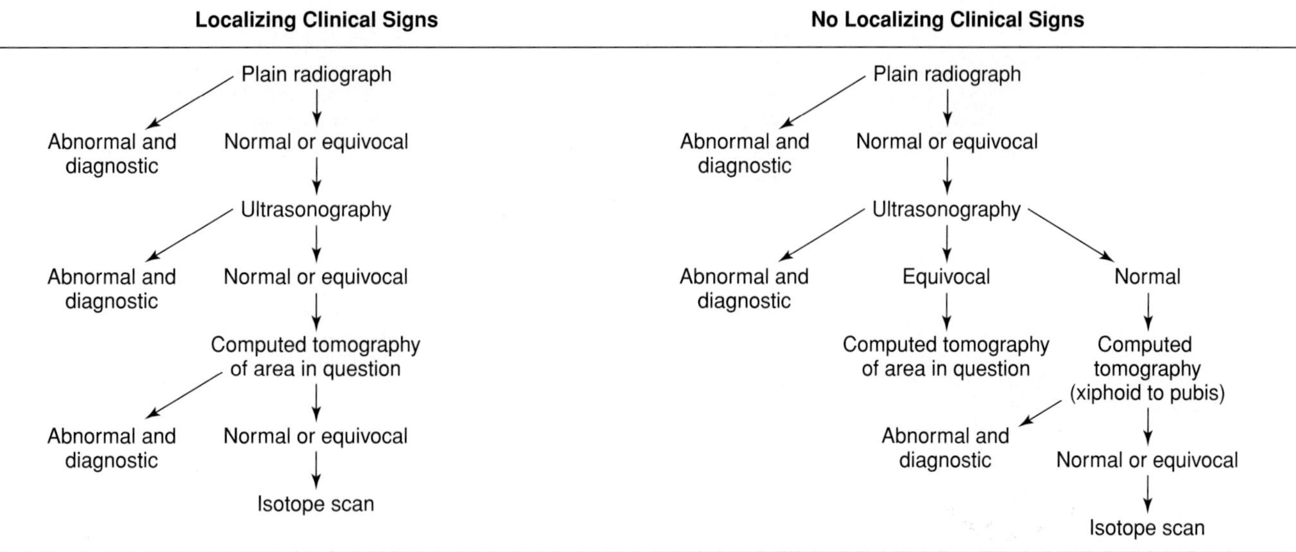

FIGURE 77–5. Diagnostic algorithm for abdominal abscess.

can be modified to optimize coverage. Antimicrobial treatment of intra-abdominal abscess should be continued until the patient has a normal leukocyte count and is afebrile.

Antibiotic selection is directed to the common organisms isolated from each type of abscess, primarily coliforms such as *E. coli* and anaerobes such as *B. fragilis* in the case of abdominal abscess. Multiple active regimens are available and have roughly equivalent efficacy, although comparable studies in children are limited. Possible antibiotic resistance should be considered for patients who develop abscesses or peritonitis after lengthy stays in the intensive care unit or hospital. There are several acceptable empirical antibiotic regimens in the management of intra-abdominal infection.

An aminoglycoside can be combined with a second antibiotic that provides good coverage for intestinal anaerobes. Gentamicin or another aminoglycoside combined with either clindamycin or metronidazole is such a commonly used regimen. The aminoglycoside provides good empiric coverage against gram-negative bacilli. Clindamycin provides excellent coverage for most anaerobes. Metronidazole is also very active against intestinal anaerobic bacteria and is active against isolates of *B. fragilis* resistant to clindamycin. Neither regimen is active against *Enterococcus. Enterococcus* is usually not considered a significant pathogen alone or even in a polymicrobial infection if other pathogens are eradicated. By contrast, immunocompromised patients and those who have resided in an intensive care unit for any length of time may require ampicillin for optimal enterococcal coverage. The triple combination of ampicillin, gentamicin, and clindamycin is often considered standard therapy and remains the best-studied regimen in children. However, this regimen requires frequent dosing, with up to 10 separate infusions daily.

A broad-spectrum β-lactam antibiotic combined with a β-lactam inhibitor can be used as single agent for empiric therapy. These include a combination of ampicillin and sulbactam (Unasyn), ticarcillin and clavulanate (Timentin), or piperacillin and tazobactam (Zosyn). All three provide good aerobic and excellent anaerobic coverage and are active against *B. fragilis.* Piperacillin- and ticarcillin-containing regimens provide greater gram-negative coverage, especially for *P. aeruginosa,* than ampicillin. The β-lactam-inhibitor combinations have been successfully used, though not well studied, in children.

Cefoxitin or cefotetan can be used alone or in combination with an aminoglycoside and ampicillin. Both cefoxitin and cefotetan are resistant to β-lactamases produced by resistant gram-negative rods and therefore have good activity against many of these organisms. However, *Enterobacter* organisms are resistant to these antibiotics. Although cefoxitin and cefotetan are active against many anaerobes, approximately 10% of *B. fragilis* and approximately 33% of *Clostridium* organisms are resistant to them. These two antibiotics have not been approved for use in children.

Carbapenem monotherapy with either imipenem or meropenem provides excellent gram-negative, gram-positive, and anaerobic activity and is effective as a single agent in management of peritonitis or abdominal abscess. Limited data are available on its use in children.

Most abscesses do not resolve with antibiotic treatment alone and must be adequately drained. In certain instances, abscesses within the mesentery of the small intestine may resolve without drainage because of the rich blood supply to this region. The preferred drainage procedure depends on the location and number of abscesses.

Percutaneous drainage of intra-abdominal abscesses under ultrasonic or CT guidance is possible for many patients. In many institutions the standard initial treatment is percutaneous drainage in combination with antibiotics. Percutaneous abscess drainage has been increasingly accepted for initial management of sepsis associated with a periappendiceal abscess, allowing the surgeon to perform appendectomy subsequently on an elective basis. Percutaneous drainage requires that the abscess is accessible, its location precisely defined, that no hollow viscus or vascular structure impedes access, and that the patient's clinical condition is stable. The initial diagnostic imaging study and the percutaneous drainage procedure can often be performed in a single session. In the past, patients with multiple separate abscesses have been considered poor candidates for percutaneous drainage; however, multiple drainage catheters may be used for management of multiple separate abdominal abscesses. Some small fluid collections may not accommodate a catheter. Such collections can be managed by percutaneous aspiration for diagnosis followed by antibiotic therapy. Surgical exploration may be required if the abscesses are inaccessible to percutaneous catheter drainage or if perforated bowel is suspected.

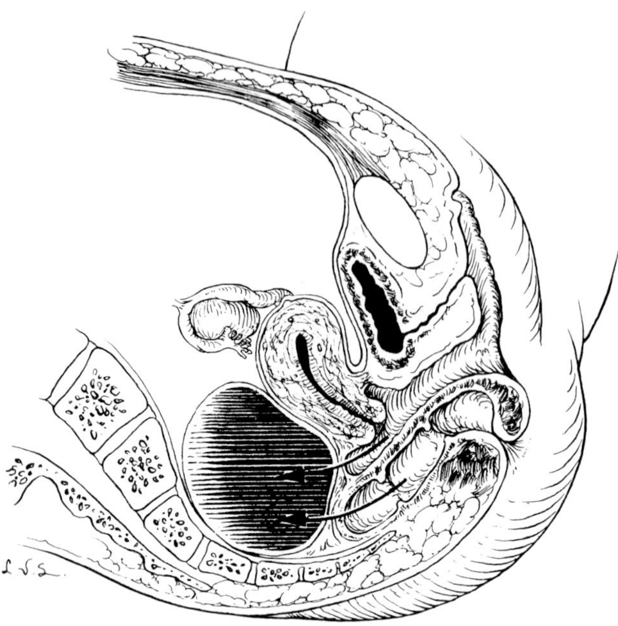

FIGURE 77–6. A pelvic abscess may be drained through the rectum or the vagina. (From Way LW [editor]: *Current Surgical Diagnosis and Treatment,* 10th ed. San Diego, Calif., Lange Medical Publications, 1994, p 405.)

For patients with signs of intra-abdominal sepsis, exploration of the abdomen may be needed to determine whether multiple abscesses, a perforated viscus, or leakage from an intestinal anastomosis is present.

An established pelvic abscess can be drained adequately by aspiration of the pus with a syringe through the anterior rectal wall or the posterior vaginal vault (Fig. 77–6). All septa within the abscess cavity must be disrupted so that drainage is complete. A drain should remain in the abscess cavity. Antibiotics should be continued for several days after complete drainage of the abscess.

The choice of antibiotics after abscess drainage should be determined by the organisms isolated at the time of drainage and their antibiotic sensitivities. Empiric therapy pending culture results should be given as discussed earlier. Recent hospitalization and antibiotic treatment increase the risk of infection by multiply resistant bacteria and fungal agents, usually *Candida.* Table 77–1 lists the antibiotics and pediatric doses that can be administered to provide adequate coverage for organisms associated with abdominal infections.

COMPLICATIONS

Untreated intra-abdominal abscesses may extend into adjacent structures. A subphrenic abscess can rupture through the diaphragm into the pleura, or an abscess can perforate into a hollow viscus. In addition, the abscess can serve as a source of ongoing intra-abdominal sepsis and peritonitis, causing septic shock, multiple-system organ failure, and death. A long-term subacute abscess can be associated with weight loss and chronic malnutrition leading to cachexia and even death.

Pelvic abscesses can spread along various fascial planes to cause retroperitoneal and ischiorectal abscesses as well as infections in the buttocks, hips, and thighs. Necrotizing fasciitis in the thigh can occur because of the spread of the infecting material from the pelvis. Pelvic abscesses involving the uterine tubes or ovaries may result in the formation of adhesions, which may cause infertility.

PROGNOSIS

The prognosis for intra-abdominal and pelvic abscesses depends on the underlying illness, the location and number of abscesses, the occurrence of complications, and the rapidity with which the diagnosis is made and appropriate treatment instituted. Uncomplicated abscesses that are diagnosed and treated early have a favorable outcome. Subphrenic abscesses and abscesses of the lesser peritoneal sac are difficult to diagnose because of their location, resulting in a delay in treatment. In the past, these abscesses had a mortality approaching 30%, even after institution of treatment. More recent data on outcome are lacking. Pelvic abscesses also may have an increased morbidity if there is a delay in diagnosis. Abscesses that extend to adjacent structures or are associated with peritonitis are associated with a higher mortality.

PREVENTION

The only way to prevent abscess formation is to diagnose and treat an intra-abdominal or pelvic pathologic process before the intraperitoneal cavity becomes contaminated. Once contamination occurs, as with a perforated appendix, prompt surgery with intraperitoneal lavage and antibiotic treatment often prevents abscesses from developing. With early recognition and treatment of these abscesses, the risk of complications is lessened.

PERITONITIS

The **peritoneum** is a specialized organ with a surface area in an adult of about 2 m^2. It lubricates the abdominal viscera and clears the cavity of invading bacteria. Mesothelial cells line the visceral and parietal surfaces. These mesothelial cells lie on a layer of loose connective tissue that is capable of accumulating a large amount of fluid during peritoneal inflammation. The mesothelial cells that line the diaphragmatic surface have a special configuration that aids in the clearing of contaminating particles and fluid from the cavity. This cell layer has many **stomata,** which communicate with the lymphatic channels within the diaphragm. These channels eventually drain into the substernal lymph nodes and, ultimately, the thoracic duct. Thus diaphragmatic movement aids in the removal of intra-abdominal fluid.

ETIOLOGY

The microorganisms found to cause peritonitis depend on the source of infection. Infections of the peritoneal cavity secondary to rupture of an abdominal viscus most often involve bacteria found in the gastrointestinal tract, including the aerobic and anaerobic organisms that cause intra-abdominal abscesses.

In young girls, primary peritoneal infection is monomicrobial, most often associated with *Streptococcus pneumoniae* and group A *Streptococcus*. Children with nephrotic syndrome have peritonitis due to such organisms as *Staphylococcus, Streptococcus*, and gram-negative bacteria. Patients with cirrhosis who have preexisting ascites may have peritoneal infections with such gastrointestinal bacteria as *E. coli, Bacteroides*, and *Clostridium.* Children who have undergone a splenectomy are at risk of peritonitis because of encapsulated bacteria such as *S. pneumoniae* and *Haemophilus influenzae* type b. Immunocompromised persons with lymphoma or leukemia and children who are receiving high doses of corticosteroids may have peritonitis due to gram-negative enteric bacteria, such as *Klebsiella, Enterobacter, Serratia, P. aeruginosa,* and by *Streptococcus, Enterococcus, Candida*, and other fungi.

TABLE 77–1. Recommended Empirical Antibiotic Therapy for Intra-abdominal Infections

Condition	Recommended Regimen	Alternative Regimens
Intra-abdominal infections ▪ including anorectal abscess ▪ with or without peritonitis	Appropriate surgical drainage *plus* An aminoglycoside *plus* Clindamycin *or* metronidazole *with or without* Ampicillin	Appropriate surgical drainage *plus* Cefoxitin *or* cefotetan *or* ampicillin-sulbactam *or* piperacillin-tazobactam *with or without* An aminoglycoside *or* Imipenem *or* meropenem
Peritonitis associated with peritoneal dialysis catheter, or spontaneous bacterial peritonitis with nephrotic syndrome	Ceftazidime *or* an aminoglycoside *plus* Vancomycin	Piperacillin-tazobactam *plus* Vancomycin *with or without* An aminoglycoside
Appendicitis ▪ perioperative (discontinue after surgery if there is no perforation or abscess)	Cefoxitin *or* cefotetan	Cefotaxime *or* ceftriaxone *or* an aminoglycoside *plus* Clindamycin
▪ associated with perforation or abscess (continue for 5–10 days if abscess is found and drained; continue for 4–6 weeks for established appendiceal abscess and delayed or no appendectomy)	An aminoglycoside *plus* Clindamycin *or* metronidazole *with or without* Ampicillin	Cefoxitin *or* cefotetan *or* ampicillin-sulbactam *or* piperacillin-tazobactam *with or without* An aminoglycoside *or* Imipenem *or* meropenem
Retroperitoneal abscess	Oxacillin *or* nafcillin *plus* An aminoglycoside *plus* Clindamycin *or* metronidazole	Vancomycin *plus* An aminoglycoside *plus* Metronidazole

Suggested Dosages for Patients with Normal Renal Function

ANTIBIOTIC	INTRAVENOUS DOSAGE	MAXIMUM DAILY DOSE
Amikacin	15 mg/kg/day divided q8–12hr	15 mg/kg
Ampicillin	150–300 mg/kg/day divided q6hr	12 g
Ampicillin-sulbactam	150–300 mg ampicillin/kg/day divided q6hr	12 g
Cefotaxime	100–180 mg/kg/day divided q6hr	12 g
Cefotetan	40–80 mg/kg/day divided q12hr	4 g
Cefoxitin	80–160 mg/kg/day divided q6hr	4 g
Ceftriaxone	50–100 mg/kg/day divided q12hr	2–4 g
	or 80 mg/kg/day once q24hr	2–4 g
Clindamycin	40 mg/kg/day divided q6hr	2.4 g
Gentamicin	5–7.5 mg/kg/day divided q8hr	Adults: 5 mg/kg/day
Imipenem	60–100 mg/kg/day divided q6hr	4 g
Meropenem	60–120 mg/kg/day divided q8hr	6 g
Metronidazole	30 mg/kg/day divided q6hr	30 mg/kg
Nafcillin	150 mg/kg/day divided q4–6hr	9 g
Oxacillin	150–200 mg/kg/day divided q4–6hr	12 g
Piperacillin-tazobactam	200–300 mg piperacillin/kg/day divided q6hr	18 g
Tobramycin	5–7.5 mg/kg/day divided q8hr	Adults: 5 mg/kg/day
Vancomycin	45 mg/kg/day divided q6hr	2 g

Gonococcal peritonitis can occur in adolescent girls if gonococcal pelvic inflammatory disease extends to the peritoneum. Tuberculous peritonitis is an uncommon cause of peritonitis in children but should be considered in the appropriate clinical setting, especially if a child has been exposed to a person with tuberculosis.

Peritonitis that occurs in the setting of peritoneal dialysis is often due to infection by skin flora, enteric bacteria, or environmental organisms. Most often *Staphylococcus aureus*, coagulase-negative staphylococci, and streptococci are isolated from the dialysate fluid. Gram-negative bacteria, such as *E. coli* and *Candida*, and, less commonly, atypical mycobacteria may be found.

EPIDEMIOLOGY

Peritonitis is caused by any intra-abdominal process that induces an inflammatory response of the peritoneal lining. It is a common complication after perforation of any abdominal organ, such as the appendix, or after leakage of gastrointestinal contents after an abdominal operation. Peritonitis can also occur when an infection extends from an organ within the peritoneal cavity or after perforating abdominal trauma. In neonates, peritonitis is most often due to perforation of an intra-abdominal viscus, often associated with necrotizing enterocolitis. In older children, peritonitis is most commonly seen with perforating appendicitis.

Peritonitis is the most common infectious complication of peritoneal dialysis and can occur as often as several times a year in prolonged peritoneal dialysis.

Spontaneous primary peritonitis may occur in infant girls, usually those younger than 2 months, and in both boys and girls between the ages of 5 and 9 years. Such cases account for approximately 10% of cases of generalized peritonitis in children.

Immunocompromised patients are at greater risk than the general population for the development of primary peritonitis. These patients include those with nephrotic syndrome and those with cirrhosis who have pre-existing ascites.

PATHOGENESIS

Processes that introduce bacteria, foreign material, and fluid into the peritoneal cavity and that prevent clearing of this material predispose to the development of peritonitis. Thus perforation of the intestine contaminates the peritoneal cavity. In addition, the diaphragmatic paralysis caused by general anesthesia given during an operation markedly reduces clearing of the contaminating material.

The early responses of the peritoneum to infection include nonspecific inflammation, which results in vasodilation, increased capillary permeability, edema, and fluid transudation into the peritoneal cavity, followed by an influx of neutrophils. The diaphragmatic lymphatic system, the peritoneal macrophages, and the incoming neutrophils all work to eliminate the invading microorganisms from the peritoneal cavity. Bacteria and their toxins are often absorbed by the lymphatic vessels and capillaries, causing bacteremia and toxemia.

Such products as complement, immunoglobulins, clotting factors, and fibrin accumulate in the peritoneal cavity. The fibrin forms adhesions in an attempt to localize the infection. As the infection continues, massive amounts of fluid are lost because of the third space effect. Extensive transudation of fluid from the plasma space into the layer of connective tissue beneath the mesothelial cell layer, the peritoneal cavity, and the lumen of the paralytic intestine occur. The extent of the translocation of this fluid depends, in part, on the surface area of the peritoneum. In adults with untreated peritonitis, as much as 4 liters of fluid can be translocated in 24 hours. Thus hemodynamic and electrolyte abnormalities may occur rapidly. If not corrected, these abnormalities can cause severe hemodynamic instability and death.

In neonates most cases of peritonitis are caused by conditions that cause intestinal ischemia or perforation, including necrotizing enterocolitis, intestinal obstruction due to atresia or stenosis, meconium ileus, and Hirschsprung's disease. Bacterial seeding of the peritoneum secondary to bacteremia, as in group B *Streptococcus* disease, and extension of omphalitis is less common.

Primary (spontaneous) peritonitis may occur in both immunocompetent and immunocompromised children. Peritonitis probably results most often from hematogenous spread of bacteria to the peritoneal cavity.

SYMPTOMS AND CLINICAL MANIFESTATIONS

Peritonitis in a neonate often presents within the first few days of life because the predisposing conditions, such as intestinal obstruction and subsequent perforation, are present at birth. The usual symptoms are vomiting and abdominal distention, with or without a fever. Shock may be present, as well as other signs and symptoms of the underlying condition.

Older children and adults with peritonitis present with abdominal pain, nausea and vomiting, distention, high fever, and toxemia. Tachycardia, tachypnea, and a decreased pulse pressure are present. As the disease progresses, shock ensues. Other clinical features are determined by the underlying condition. A girl with gonococcal peritonitis may have right upper quadrant pain due to **gonococcal perihepatitis (Fitz-Hugh-Curtis syndrome).**

Patients who are receiving high doses of corticosteroids or who have severe neutropenia may have mild symptoms that often are not attributable to the severe underlying abdominal disorder. This phenomenon occurs because of the lack of inflammatory cells within the peritoneal cavity. However, abdominal pain and tenderness are still present. Children receiving high doses of corticosteroids may not exhibit high fevers.

A child with tuberculous peritonitis usually has an insidious onset of fever, night sweats, fatigue, abdominal pain, and diarrhea. There is usually a history of exposure to a family member with tuberculosis.

Physical Examination Findings

The diagnosis of peritonitis may be difficult in a neonate because of the paucity of localizing signs. The infant appears ill with prominent abdominal distention, often with hypothermia, and may have signs of shock. If the peritoneal cavity has been grossly contaminated, the abdominal wall may be inflamed.

Early in the disease process, an older child has diffuse abdominal guarding, rigidity and rebound tenderness, a tympanitic abdomen, and decreased bowel sounds. Localized peritonitis, which may occur in uncomplicated appendicitis, presents with local abdominal tenderness. However, there is diffuse abdominal tenderness and rebound tenderness if contaminated material has been dispersed throughout the peritoneal cavity. In these cases, rectal or vaginal examination reveals signs of pelvic tenderness. Right upper quadrant tenderness should also make the clinician think of gonococcal peritonitis in girls. Peritonitis due to contamination of a dialysis catheter presents with tachycardia, hyperventilation, fever, and oliguria and is accompanied by cloudy peritoneal dialysate fluid. As the disease progresses, multiple-system organ failure and septic shock occur.

A child receiving corticosteroids may have little or no abdominal tenderness. Lack of bowel activity is noted by auscultation. The physical signs of sepsis may be present.

DIAGNOSIS

Differential Diagnosis

In the neonate, meconium peritonitis, which causes peritoneal inflammation that is not infectious in origin, is not easily distinguished clinically from bacterial peritonitis. In addition, other abdominal processes, such as necrotizing enterocolitis not accompanied by peritonitis, may present with the same symptoms and signs.

Processes that cause peritoneal irritation and therefore abdominal pain can mimic peritonitis. These include familial Mediterranean fever, porphyria, lead toxicity, and chylous ascites.

Laboratory Evaluation

In a patient with normal immune function, generalized peritonitis is associated with a WBC count that often exceeds 20,000/mm^3, with a predominance of neutrophils. In the later stages of disease, the presence of septic shock is associated with a low WBC count, anemia, and signs of disseminated intravascular coagulation. Fluid and electrolyte studies reveal dehydration, and urine output is decreased.

Cardiovascular abnormalities depend on the stage of disease. Early in the course of illness there is increased cardiac output, normal central venous pressure, and decreased peripheral vascular resistance. If left untreated, there will be a depression of cardiac function and vasoconstriction with decreased perfusion of peripheral tissues, resulting in metabolic acidosis.

Respiratory alkalosis is usually present because of hyperventilation. However, as the disease progresses, a capillary leak syndrome occurs, leading to fluid in the lungs. This results in pulmonary edema and decreased ventilatory ability. Shock lung may occur if disease progresses.

The peritoneal fluid of patients with peritonitis may provide clues about the cause of the peritonitis. Examination of fluid obtained during paracentesis or during an operation, in the case of secondary or primary peritonitis, or of dialysate fluid, if the patient is undergoing continuous ambulatory peritoneal dialysis, reveals cloudy fluid that contains many neutrophils, if immune function is normal, and bacteria. Tuberculous peritonitis is accompanied by a protein level greater than 2.5 g/dL, a predominance of lymphocytes, and a glucose concentration less than 30 mg/dL.

Microbiologic Evaluation

Both anaerobic and aerobic blood cultures should be performed. If ascites is present or if peritoneal lavage is performed, the fluid obtained should be transported and processed within 2 hours of collection for culture of aerobic and anaerobic bacteria and fungi. The sample obtained for anaerobic culture must be transported in the same manner as indicated for intra-abdominal abscesses. A Gram stain and fungal stain should be done in all cases, and a mycobacterial stain and cultures should be considered if the patient is undergoing peritoneal dialysis or has been exposed to a person with tuberculosis. If tuberculous peritonitis is suspected, a peritoneal biopsy to search for granulomas and tuberculous organisms may be necessary if special stains and cultures of peritoneal fluid are negative. All organisms isolated should be tested for antimicrobial sensitivities to guide antibiotic treatment.

Diagnostic Imaging

Plain radiographs of the abdomen, including upright, supine, and left lateral decubitus positions, may be helpful in demonstrating free air in the peritoneal cavity. The air is seen under the diaphragm on an upright radiograph and between the right lobe of the liver and the right diaphragm on a left lateral decubitus radiograph. Paralytic ileus and fluid between loops of intestine may also be seen. The radiographic studies discussed for intra-abdominal abscesses should be performed if an intra-abdominal source of contamination is likely, and chest radiographs should be obtained to assess lung involvement.

TREATMENT

The source of the peritoneal contamination must be sought and controlled by surgical intervention if a viscus has perforated or if leakage from a recent abdominal anastomosis has occurred. Contaminated intraperitoneal material and foreign bodies must be removed, with débridement of necrotic tissue. Intraoperative peritoneal irrigation with saline solution has been shown to decrease the bacterial burden.

The empirical choice of antimicrobial agents should be based on the likely source of contamination, that is, secondary bacterial peritonitis, primary peritonitis, or peritonitis secondary to contamination of an intraperitoneal foreign body. The results of a Gram stain of the peritoneal fluid, if peritoneal lavage is performed, and the age and underlying medical condition of the patient (e.g., immunosuppression, on peritoneal dialysis) should be used in determining the proper antibiotic(s) to administer. Peritonitis due to intestinal contamination should be treated with the same antimicrobial agents as discussed for intra-abdominal abscesses. An immunocompromised child who has undergone multiple hospitalizations and who has peritonitis because of a ruptured abdominal organ may have such microorganisms as *Pseudomonas*. Therefore, the antimicrobial regimen should be adjusted as soon as the organisms are identified and their antibiotic sensitivities known. A regimen of vancomycin, gentamicin, and clindamycin should be considered for neonates with necrotizing enterocolitis and peritonitis.

A child with primary peritonitis should be treated with antimicrobial agents active against the most likely organisms. For an immunocompetent child, these include *Staphylococcus, S. pneumoniae*, and gram-negative enteric organisms. Acceptable regimens are oxacillin with gentamicin or, alternatively, a third-generation cephalosporin alone. An immunocompromised child with primary peritonitis should have additional coverage for anaerobic bacteria and enterococci. Ampicillin, gentamicin and clindamycin, and a third-generation cephalosporin plus clindamycin are acceptable choices. Vancomycin should be included in the antimicrobial regimen for a child with peritonitis secondary to peritoneal dialysis to cover methicillin-resistant staphylococci. Final modifications of the antimicrobial regimen should be based on the susceptibility profile of organisms isolated from the blood and peritoneal fluid.

Fungi and yeast isolated from peritoneal fluid and indicative of infection should be treated with amphotericin B. The treatment of atypical mycobacterial infection should be guided by the specific organism and its sensitivity. Amikacin and cefoxitin are reasonable choices initially for the species of mycobacteria that are usually involved in dialysis-associated peritonitis. Treatment of tuberculous peritonitis is the same as that of other tuberculosis of extrapulmonary causes (Chapter 35).

Appropriate hemodynamic and respiratory management must be instituted promptly. Aggressive fluid resuscitation must be performed because of the substantial loss of fluid into the peritoneal cavity.

COMPLICATIONS

Peritonitis is fraught with numerous life-threatening complications, including septic shock, multiple-system organ failure, intra-abdominal abscesses necessitating a reoperation and repeated drainage procedures, and postsurgical abdominal wound infections. Adhesions and a prolonged hospital stay are important but less severe complications.

PROGNOSIS

Before antibiotics became available, the mortality of secondary bacterial peritonitis following intestinal perforation was 70%. With proper surgical intervention and administration of antibiotics, the mortality has decreased to about 30%. By contrast, primary peritonitis has a mortality of less than 10% among children and 50% among neonates when treated with antibiotics. Peritonitis in an immunocompromised patient carries a high mortality because of delays in making the diagnosis and instituting appropriate treatment.

ACUTE APPENDICITIS

EPIDEMIOLOGY

Acute appendicitis is the most common acute surgical disease of the abdomen. In the United States, about 75,000 cases occur each year in the pediatric population. Most cases of appendicitis occur between the ages of 12 and 20 years. Incidence in boys peaks during the preteen and early teenage years, and in girls the highest rates occur between the ages of 15 and 19 years. Appendicitis is found in children of all ages but is rare during the first year of life and unusual during the second and third years of life.

ETIOLOGY

Polymicrobial flora, predominantly anaerobes, are usually found in an inflamed appendix. In appendiceal rupture the most common anaerobic organisms isolated are *B. fragilis, Peptococcus, Peptostreptococcus, Fusobacterium, P. melaninogenica,* and *Clostridium.* The aerobic bacteria usually isolated are *E. coli*, α- and β-hemolytic *Streptococcus, Enterococcus*, and *P. aeruginosa*.

PATHOGENESIS

The appendix is an outpouching of the cecum and has the same bacterial content as the colon. In adults it is 5–10 cm long and has a very narrow lumen. Although the cause of appendicitis is unknown, obstruction of the narrow appendiceal lumen predisposes to this condition. Appendicitis may be unusual in the first few years of life because the lumen of the appendix is large and is less likely to become obstructed. After the first 10 years of life, the muscular layer becomes more developed, narrowing the lumen. The most common cause of obstruction is the development of a **fecalith** (a concretion of fecal material) within the lumen. In addition, lymphoid tissue within the appendix can become hypertrophied because of a concurrent viral infection. Adenovirus and measles virus have been found in the lymphoid follicles of the appendix and the mesenteric lymph nodes in acute and chronic appendicitis. Other obstructing agents include ingested foreign material, such as seeds of vegetables and fruits, and possibly intestinal parasites such as *Ascaris*, pinworm (*Enterobius vermicularis*), and whipworm (*Trichuris trichiura*). Once obstruction occurs, mucosal secretions accumulate, causing a rapid increase in intraluminal pressure. This results in venous congestion with compression of the end arteries that supply the distal appendix. Luminal bacteria multiply, leading to invasion of the already ischemic wall of the appendix. Left untreated, the wall may eventually rupture and the intraluminal contents spill into the peritoneal cavity. About 20% of patients with acute appendicitis have a perforation within the first 24 hours and 80% in the first 48 hours after the onset of symptoms.

If the process evolves slowly, the inflammatory process may be controlled by formation of adhesions between the cecum and the ileum and by migration of part of the greater omentum to the inflamed appendix, where it wraps itself around the appendix, localizing the infection. In children younger than 2 years, the greater omentum is poorly developed and thus is less protective.

SYMPTOMS AND CLINICAL MANIFESTATIONS

Usual Presentation

Infants and toddlers with appendicitis usually present with an acute abdomen. The diagnosis is very difficult to make in this age group and may be missed because of its infrequency and its nonspecific presentation. Parents give a history of irritability and decreased food intake by the child, with subsequent development of fever and bilious vomiting, diarrhea, or both. Some children may draw up their legs. As the disease progresses, diaphragmatic movement becomes painful because of diffuse peritoneal inflammation. This manifests itself as rapid, shallow respirations. An important clue to the diagnosis of appendicitis is that diarrhea, when present, begins with the onset of abdominal pain and vomiting.

In older children the diagnosis of appendicitis is less difficult to make. Colicky or diffuse abdominal pain is the most constant feature of acute appendicitis. The pain usually begins in the region of the abdomen innervated by the tenth thoracic nerve in the periumbilical or epigastric region. The pain is caused by distention of the appendix, which stimulates the stretch receptors within the appendix. Within several hours, the pain usually shifts to the right lower quadrant, becoming more constant and severe. This area, known as **McBurney's point,** is just below the middle of a line from the umbilicus to the right anterior superior iliac spine. The pain may occasionally begin in the right lower quadrant. Pain in the right lower quadrant is caused by local peritoneal irritation (the parietal peritoneum is somatically innervated) secondary to inflammation that has spread from the appendiceal mucosa through the wall of the appendix. Loss of appetite, nausea, and vomiting are common symptoms. Vomiting in appendicitis generally begins after abdominal pain, a finding that may be helpful in distinguishing it from gastroenteritis, where vomiting is often the presenting symptom. A fever may not be present at the onset of appendicular distention, but it usually appears within 24 hours. Diarrhea or constipation is occasionally present. Diarrhea, when present, usually indicates a pelvic appendix and is caused by irritation of the overlying rectal mucosa. It is important to remember this symptom because the appendicitis can be misdiagnosed as gastroenteritis. Diarrhea in appendicitis is typically of low volume and frequency. A rectal or vaginal examination is essential to reveal right pelvic tenderness, which is specific for a pelvic inflammatory lesion.

Late in the course of appendicitis, an ominous sign is a sudden decrease in abdominal pain, lasting for about an hour. This indicates rupture of the appendix.

Unusual Presentations

The appendix is usually located in the right iliac fossa behind the cecum. It arises from the left dorsal surface of the cecum about 2.5 cm distal to the ileocecal junction. Its tip is usually directed upward. In this position, its relation to the anterior abdominal wall is such that its base is situated 4–5 cm from the right anterior superior iliac spine along a line extending to the umbilicus. However, the appendix varies in position from person to person. The tip of the appendix has a considerable range of movement and can be intraperitoneal or extraperitoneal (Fig. 77–7). Two variations in position can make the diagnosis of appendicitis especially difficult: if the appendix lies in the right iliac fossa behind the ileum or if the appendix is directed downward to the pelvis. Both of these positions cause an atypical presentation of appendiceal inflammation, which may lead to a delay in diagnosis and to rupture of the appendix. Although the early symptoms of appendiceal distention are the same, the pain is not usually localized. An appendix located behind the ileum gives fewer localizing symptoms because it is masked by the ileum and does not contact the anterior parietal peritoneum. Pyuria may be present because the right ureter lies close to an inflamed appendix in this position. Psoas irritation also is present. Inflammation of an appendix that is directed toward the pelvis does not localize pain to the right iliac fossa because the appendix is not in contact with the parietal peritoneum. The symptoms of appendiceal distention persist, and no localization of pain occurs until the appendix ruptures. Diagnosis of appendicitis when the appendix is located in the pelvis requires a great deal of awareness. Diarrhea may be present because of rectal irritation, and pyuria may be present as a result of bladder irritation.

Physical Examination Findings

An infant with appendicitis appears ill, with a fever and elevated pulse and respiratory rate (Table 77–2). Examination of the abdomen usually reveals distention, tenderness, and, occasionally,

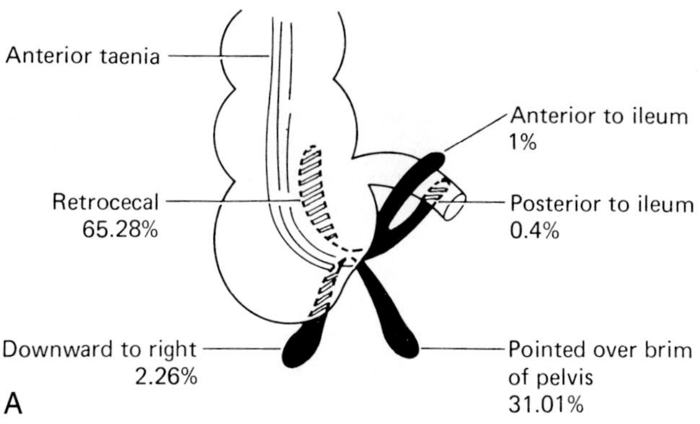

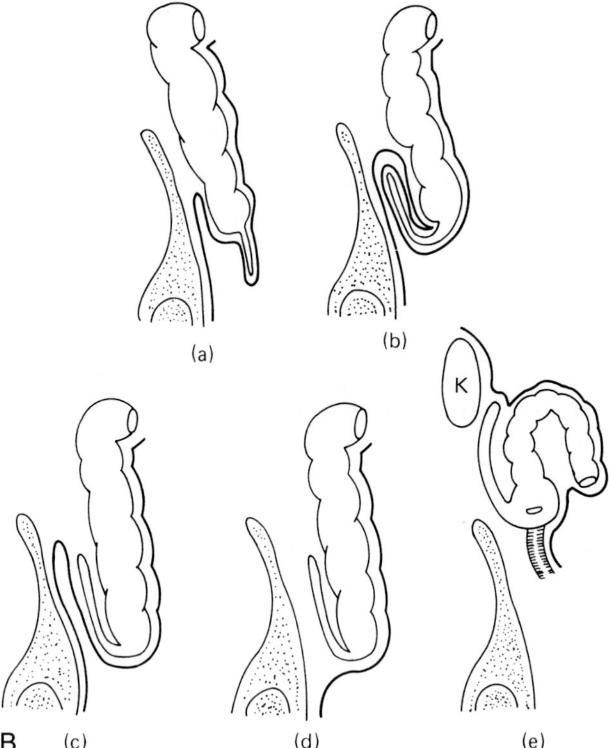

FIGURE 77–7. **A,** Incidence of variations in position of the appendix. **B,** Normal variations in the position and peritoneal fixation of the appendix. *a,* Intraperitoneal, pointing over the brim of the pelvis. *b,* Intraperitoneal, ascending retrocecal. *c,* Extraperitoneal, ascending retrocecal. A paracecal fossa is present. *d,* Extraperitoneal, ascending retrocecal. e, Extraperitoneal, ascending retrocecal, lying anterior to the right kidney (*K*) deep to the liver, associated with an undescended subhepatic cecum. The terminal ileum, also extraperitoneal, enters the cecum from behind. (*A* modified from Wakeley CPG: The position of the vermiform appendix as ascertained by analysis of 10,000 cases. *J Anat* 1933;67:277–83. *B* modified from Meyers MA, Oliphant M: Ascending retrocecal appendicitis. *Radiology* 1974; 110:295–9.)

guarding. Erythema, edema, or cellulitis over the right lower quadrant may be present, as may a palpable mass in that region.

A child or adolescent may have a fever, especially as the disease progresses. The pulse rate is not elevated unless peritonitis is present. Pain on movement and coughing often occur, causing the patient to move with extreme caution. Shallow, rapid breathing may be due to pain on diaphragmatic movement. A careful lung examination should be performed to determine whether a pneumonic process is present. Tenderness and guarding localized to the right iliac fossa are often present if the appendix is in its most common location, the retrocecal position. The iliopsoas muscle becomes secondarily irritated, causing the patient to experience pain on extension of the right thigh when lying on the left side (the psoas test). A tender, palpable mass in the right lower quardrant may be present if a localized abscess is forming around the appendix. Rebound tenderness, if present, heightens concern for appendicitis. If peritonitis becomes diffuse, generalized tenderness with guarding is found.

If a patient has acute abdominal symptoms and few of the typical signs of appendicitis, pelvic or retroileal appendicitis requires careful consideration, and a rectal or vaginal examination must be performed. If the appendix is in the pelvis, there is tenderness and often a mass against the pelvic wall on the right. Because the overlying inflamed appendix affects the obturator internus muscle, a positive obturator test can be elicited (internal rotation of the flexed thigh with referred pain to the hypogastrium). However, because retroileal appendicitis is difficult to diagnose on the basis of localizing signs, additional diagnostic imaging is necessary to confirm the diagnosis and to avoid perforation of the appendix.

TABLE 77–2. Physical Findings of Appendicitis

Frequent
General
Pain on movement or coughing
Shallow, rapid breathing
Abdominal Examination
Tenderness and guarding in right lower quadrant
Rebound tenderness
Other
Positive psoas test
Atypical (Pelvic Appendicitis)
Abdominal Examination
Usual signs not present
Pelvic and Rectal Examination
Tenderness and occasional palpable mass against right pelvic wall
Other
Positive obdurator test
Infant
General
Ill-appearing
Fever
Tachycardia
Abdominal Examination
Distention
Tenderness
Occasionally guarding present
Erythema, edema, cellulitis over right lower quadrant
Occasional palpable mass in right lower quadrant

DIAGNOSIS

Making the diagnosis of appendicitis before perforation occurs is difficult. Although many parents are aware that the child is experiencing abdominal pain, they may delay contacting a physician because they do not know the seriousness of the illness. If a child is younger than 3 years, referral to a surgeon is often delayed because the symptoms are nonspecific and because it is difficult to perform a thorough examination. Eighty percent of these children have a perforated appendix and either generalized peritonitis or an appendiceal abscess at the time the disease is recognized. Therefore, it is advisable to closely observe any child with abdominal pain that has lasted longer than 6 hours for the continuation of or worsening of these symptoms. The preliminary laboratory studies should be done in the physician's office, and the physician should keep in close contact with the patient. If the symptoms persist, the child should have abdominal imaging studies and a prompt surgical evaluation.

Differential Diagnosis

Many illnesses mimic appendicitis (Table 77–3). Enteritis due to infection with *Campylobacter jejuni* may cause periumbilical and right-sided abdominal pain. Respiratory infections that cause right lower lobe pneumonia may cause right-sided abdominal pain and rigidity.

Mesenteric Lymphadenitis. Bacterial and, less commonly, viral infections of the ileocecal lymph nodes (acute mesenteric adenitis) are most often seen in children and young adults. Although acute mesenteric adenitis is usually a self-limited disease, some patients undergo operations because of the difficulty of distinguishing this entity from appendicitis. A number of etiologic agents have been associated with this syndrome, most frequently *Yersinia enterocolitica* and less frequently *Yersinia pseudotuberculosis, Streptococcus,* and *Staphylococcus aureus.* Outbreaks of acute mesenteric adenitis due to *Yersinia* have been reported. Clinically, mesenteric lymphadenitis is indistinguishable from acute appendicitis. Abdominal pain, fever, diarrhea, nausea, anorexia, and vomiting are the most common clinical signs. Right-sided abdominal tenderness and rebound tenderness are found on physical examination. Often leukocytosis is present, and neutrophils may be seen in the stool if the disease is due to *Yersinia.* Stool cultures may be positive for these organisms. If ileitis is present, a radiographic contrast study of the intestine may reveal mucosal abnormalities in the terminal ileum. These findings may allow the differentiation of acute mesenteric adenitis from appendicitis.

Renal Infections. Infections of the right kidney and perirenal area, such as perinephric abscesses, pyelonephritis, and pyonephrosis, can usually be distinguished from appendicitis by a history of dysuria and urinary frequency and the presence of pyuria and bacteriuria. Occasionally, an inflamed appendix may lie over the region of the renal pelvis, causing renal inflammation and symptoms attributable to renal disease. In this case, there are leukocytes but no bacteria in the urine. Infrequently, perinephric abscess can mimic, and be caused by, retrocecal appendicitis.

Gynecologic Infections. In adolescent girls, acute salpingitis and tubo-ovarian abscesses can be confused with pelvic appendicitis. Salpingitis usually presents with a cervical discharge for several days before the patient appears with a high fever and pain in both lower quadrants. In some cases, the pain is limited to the right lower quadrant. It is worth noting that cervical motion tenderness may not distinguish salpingitis from pelvic appendicitis once the appendix has ruptured. Complicating the diagnosis is the fact that salpingitis can cause periappendicitis of a pelvic appendix.

Typhlitis (Cecitis). In children with profound neutropenia and immunosuppression from underlying diseases and associated treatment, such as acute myelogenous leukemia, acute lymphocytic

TABLE 77–3. Differential Diagnosis of Appendicitis

Syndrome	Causative Agent	Clinical Manifestations
Gastroenteritis	*Campylobacter jejuni*	Periumbilical and right-sided abdominal pain
Acute mesenteric lymphadenitis	*Yersinia pseudotuberculosis, Yersinia enterocolitica*, adenoviruses, *Mycobacterium tuberculosis* (if these lymph nodes are involved)	Mimics retroileal appendicitis
Respiratory infections	Bacterial pneumonias involving right lower lobe	Often associated with right-sided abdominal pain and rigidity
	Influenza viruses	Usually diffuse abdominal pain occasionally in right iliac fossa
	Enteroviruses	Pleurodynia
Kidney disease (pyelonephritis or perinephric abscess, especially right-sided)	Gram-negative enteric bacteria, *Staphylococcus aureus*	Mimics appendicitis; usually history of dysuria, urinary frequency, pyuria
Psoas abscess	*S. aureus*	Mimics retroileal appendicitis
Hepatitis A and B	Hepatitis A and B viruses	Occasionally right-sided abdominal pain in early preicteric stage
Crohn's disease of terminal ileum		Mimics retroileal appendicitis
Surgical complications (inflammation or perforation of Meckel diverticulum, incarcerated inguinal hernia, torsion of testis, torsion of greater omentum, intussusception)		Mimics appendicitis; most can be distinguished with use of proper physical examination and diagnostic tests (i.e., Meckel scan, bariuim enema)
Conditions affecting female adolescents (acute salpingitis, tubo-ovarian abscess, rupture of graafian follicle, torsion of ovarian cyst, ectopic pregnancy, incomplete abortion)		Mimics appendicitis; most can be distinguished with use of proper physical examination and diagnostic tests (i.e., ultrasonography)

leukemia, lymphoma, aplastic anemia, cyclic neutropenia, renal transplantation, and AIDS, typhlitis may be difficult to distinguish from appendicitis. Typhlitis (also known as neutropenic colitis, necrotizing enteropathy, cecal necrosis, and cecitis) is an uncommon infection. It is characterized by invasion of a damaged cecal, ileal, or colonic wall by bacteria, fungi, or virus, resulting in edema and induration of the wall with a minimal inflammatory response. These children are at risk of infection because the intestinal mucosa is damaged by chemotherapeutic agents and corticosteroids and there is often overgrowth of resistant bacteria and fungi from prior use of broad-spectrum antibiotics. Accordingly, *Pseudomonas* and *Candida* have been associated with typhlitis. In children with AIDS, cytomegalovirus has been associated with mucosal lesions in the cecum as well as in the rest of the colon. A CT scan may be helpful in distinguishing appendicitis from typhlitis. Diffuse thickening of the cecal wall is suggestive but not specific for the diagnosis because it can also be seen with leukemic infiltrates of the cecal wall, periappendiceal abscesses, and intramural hemorrhage.

Typhlitis not complicated by perforation should be treated medically with antibiotics active against *Pseudomonas* and other aerobic and anaerobic intestinal flora. Antifungal therapy should be instituted if *Candida* organisms have been isolated from the blood or if the patient has not responded to antibacterial therapy. Antiviral therapy with ganciclovir should be considered if cytomegalovirus infection is proved by biopsy.

Laboratory Evaluation

A complete WBC count with a predominance of neutrophils may be helpful in determining whether an infection is present, although the neutrophil count may not be elevated in one third of the cases. A considerable rise in the number of leukocytes shown by serial WBC counts may indicate perforation.

Examination of the urine for the presence of pyuria and especially bacteriuria may be helpful in distinguishing a urinary tract infection from appendicitis. Because appendicitis causes decreased oral intake, vomiting, and occasionally diarrhea, and because rupture with secondary peritonitis can cause severe derangements of fluid and electrolyte balance, it is crucial to evaluate the fluid and electrolyte status of the patient. If there is evidence of acidosis, arterial blood gas studies should be done to determine blood pH.

Microbiologic Evaluation

Although traditional recommendations include sending aerobic and anaerobic cultures from peritoneal fluid or swabs during surgery, more recent studies suggest that these cultures rarely influence therapeutic decisions.

Diagnostic Imaging

Developments in radiologic imaging, particularly the radial CT scan, have improved sensitivity and specificity of diagnosis in the patient with an acute abdomen. Imaging studies are especially useful in diagnosing appendicitis if the clinical presentation is atypical. Plain abdominal radiographs are of limited value but may be helpful in showing a calcified appendicolith or a mass displacing the intestine (see Fig. 13–26). However, if CT is readily available, it is preferable to perform this study without delay. A barium enema often shows nonfilling of the appendix and an extrinsic mass effect on the cecum, terminal ileum, and ascending colon if appendicitis is present. The availability of ultrasonography and especially helical CT with rectal contrast has diminished the role of barium enema in evaluation of appendicitis. Helical CT has higher sensitivity and accuracy than graded compression sonography for the diagnosis of appendicitis in a pediatric and young adult population. Ultrasonography can be useful in settings where it can be performed more rapidly or when CT is not available (Fig. 77–8*A*).

CT is now the most sensitive and specific method of visualizing the inflamed appendix (Fig. 77–8*B*). Helical appendiceal CT with rectal contrast has very high positive and negative predictive values for appendicitis. In experienced hands, the CT scan is more than 95% sensitive and, when negative, reliably rules out appendicitis. Imaging can facilitate prompt surgery or, when imaging reveals a normal appendix, allows nonsurgical management. Thickening and dilatation of the appendix and surrounding inflammation can be seen directly. CT is also used to determine whether an appendiceal abscess is present, to differentiate the abscess from a phlegmon, and to determine whether the abscess is amenable to percutaneous drainage under CT guidance. High-resolution ultrasonography with graded compression also has a very good sensitivity and specificity, but its value is operator dependent, and there is a limited field of view (see Fig. 13–27).

If respiratory symptoms are present, it is advisable to obtain a chest radiograph to determine whether a focal pneumonia is present.

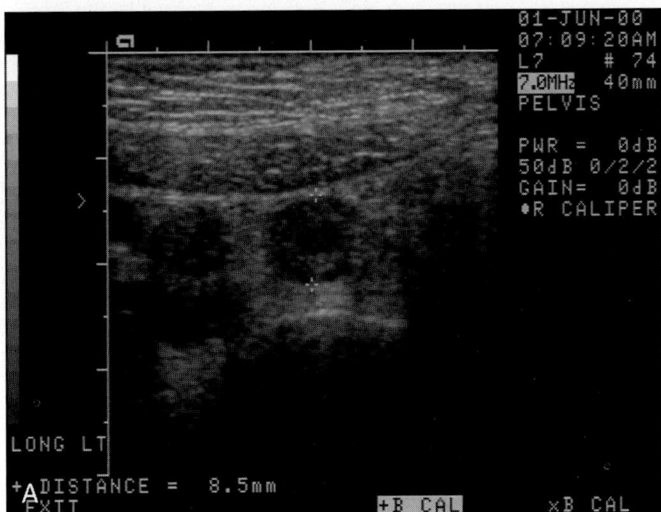

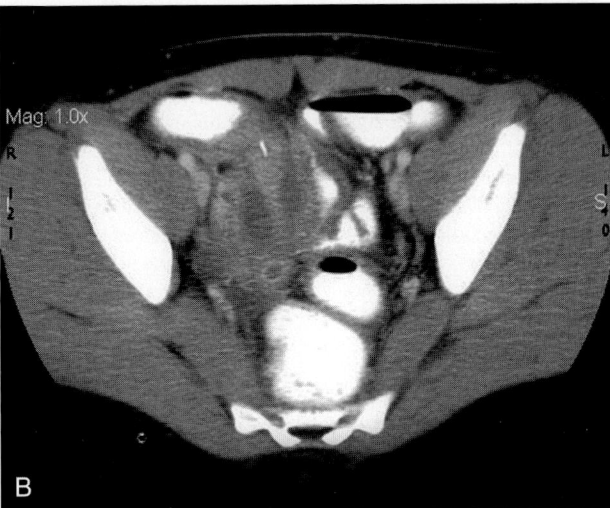

FIGURE 77–8. **A,** Ultrasound image of an inflamed appendix. **B,** CT scan showing an inflamed appendix.

TREATMENT

An appendectomy should be performed if the findings are strongly suggestive of acute appendicitis, and yet the decision to perform an appendectomy may be difficult to make because of nonspecific findings. Because the consequences of perforation of the appendix are so serious, additional evaluation is indicated in equivocal cases. Protocols or pathways that use imaging studies are often helpful if ultrasonography and CT are available. Children with equivocal clinical presentations of acute appendicitis may be promptly evaluated with ultrasonography. Patients with findings that are positive for acute appendicitis on ultrasonography proceed to laparotomy, whereas patients with negative or equivocal ultrasonographic findings should undergo a limited CT scan with rectal contrast. Limited helical CT with rectal contrast is 95% sensitive for detection of an abnormal appendix. The use of CT in equivocal cases may reduce the number of unnecessary appendectomies or hospital admissions.

A brief course of perioperative prophylactic antibiotics has been shown to decrease the rate of postoperative wound infections. An appropriate regimen is clindamycin in combination with an aminoglycoside or cephalosporin. Cefoxitin alone is also acceptable. The timing of administration of these prophylactic antibiotics is crucial because the antibiotics must have high tissue concentrations at the time of inoculation of bacteria in the incision site. Therefore, these antibiotics should be given approximately 30 minutes before the operation and discontinued postoperatively if there is no appendiceal rupture or phlegmon.

Antibiotics should be given preoperatively to patients believed to have a perforation or abscess. The combination of clindamycin, gentamicin, and ampicillin is an effective antibiotic regimen. Alternative regimens as discussed previously for management of intra-abdominal abscess may also be used. Duration of therapy is typically 5–10 days if perforation has occurred. Duration of therapy if abscess or phlegmon are present may be longer.

There is much controversy regarding the treatment of an appendiceal mass in a child with a history of appendicitis for more than 5 days. An appendiceal mass may be a phlegmon, an inflammatory lesion caused by appendicitis but well localized by adherent omentum and intestine, or it may be an abscess, a collection of pus, bacteria, and necrotic debris (Fig. 77–4). An appendiceal phlegmon may progress to abscess formation, which may resolve over time with or without antibiotic treatment as the inflammatory lesion continues to coalesce. The patient must be observed carefully in a hospital for possible abscess formation and spread of infection and may be discharged home only when all signs of disease have resolved. An appendectomy is then performed in 2 to 3 months.

Patients with an appendiceal mass due to abscess formation around the appendix are at risk of rupture of the abscess into the peritoneal cavity and generalized sepsis. Although many surgeons believe that surgical removal of the abscess is the treatment of choice, the complication rate is approximately 30% if the operation is performed. These complications include wound infection, fecal fistula, obstruction of the small intestine, prolonged ileus, and recurrent abscess. Conservative management is practiced in some cases of appendiceal abscess. The patients are treated by intravenous fluid and antibiotic thereapy followed by an appendectomy within 4–6 weeks. About one half of the patients treated this way improve. An alternative to surgical removal and conservative management is percutaneous catheter drainage of the appendiceal abscess under ultrasonic or CT guidance. This technique has been shown to be safe and effective for treating select appendiceal abscesses.

Correction of fluid and electrolyte disturbances by intravenous therapy must be done as needed to correct hypovolemia and acidosis. Fever control and nasogastric suctioning also may be needed. In advanced disease, sepsis and shock may be present, requiring aggressive life-support measures.

COMPLICATIONS

Complications are rare when an unruptured appendix is removed. However, unrecognized appendicitis can lead to appendiceal perforation, resulting in diffuse peritonitis or abscess formation. Perforation occurs in 15–37% of children. Higher rates occur among young children and among patients with pelvic or retroileal appendicitis in whom the diagnosis was delayed. When the appendix perforates, leakage of the fecal contents of the cecum into the peritoneal cavity is often prevented by newly forming adhesions and the presence of omentum. However, in children younger than 2 years, diffuse peritonitis usually occurs because the omentum is poorly developed. On release of fecal contents, with or without diffuse peritonitis, infected material may travel to the intraperitoneal recesses, forming abscesses in the pelvis and subhepatic and subphrenic spaces.

Wound infections complicate the surgical treatment of appendicitis. They occur in approximately 5% of cases of uncomplicated appendicitis and in 30% of cases if rupture has occurred. A life-threatening infection due to synergistic gangrene may occur in a closed, infected surgical wound.

Other complications include bacteremia and fistula formation between the appendix and the bladder. Portal vein thrombophlebitis and subsequent development of pyogenic liver abscesses and cholangitis may occur if appendicitis remains untreated. In fact, before complicated cases of appendicitis were treated with early removal of the inflamed appendix and effective antibiotics, appendicitis was the most common cause of portal vein thrombophlebitis. Fortunately this complication is now rare.

PROGNOSIS

With early removal of the appendix, before it has perforated, the morbidity is limited and the patient is usually discharged within a few days. Convalescence is normally rapid and complete. With complications such as rupture and either formation of an abscess or peritonitis, repeated operations and a long convalescence may follow. When the diagnosis of acute appendicitis is made promptly and the unruptured appendix is removed, the mortality is approximately 0.1%. Even in complicated cases of appendicitis, death is rare with current antibiotic, surgical, and ICU resources. Death is due to generalized peritonitis and the resulting multiple-system organ failure.

SPLENIC ABSCESS

ETIOLOGY

The most common bacteria isolated from splenic abscesses are *Streptococcus* and *Staphylococcus*. *Salmonella* may be found in the splenic abscesses of patients with diseases such as sickle cell anemia. These diseases predispose a patient to splenic infarction due to decreased phagocytosis and opsonization. If it is an extension of a subphrenic abscess, the abscess reflects the aerobic and anaerobic organisms found in the subphrenic abscess. In immunosuppressed patients, cultures of splenic abscesses may yield *Candida* and *Aspergillus*. Rarely, *Brucella* can cause splenic abscesses. In these cases, the organism can be isolated from splenic tissue, and a rise in serum antibody titers can be demonstrated. Splenic abscesses can also be caused by *Mycobactrium tuberculosis*.

EPIDEMIOLOGY

Abscesses in the spleen are uncommon in the general population; the estimated incidence is 0.2–0.7%, according to several autopsy studies. Children with underlying diseases that cause an immunocompromised state, especially those with leukemia who are undergoing treatment with chemotherapeutic and antimicrobial agents, are at risk of developing splenic abscesses due to fungi. Multiple small splenic abscesses can be seen as a finding in cat-scratch disease (bartonellosis).

PATHOGENESIS

Splenic abscesses are uncommon in healthy persons. However, persons with an abnormal spleen that has necrotic areas because of embolism or that contains a hematoma due to trauma and those with an immunodeficiency that prevents the spleen from performing its normal role of clearing organisms are predisposed to splenic abscesses. Such diseases as sickle cell anemia can cause bland infarcts within the spleen, and endocarditis or sepsis originating at a distant site, such as the tonsils, urinary tract, abdomen, or skin, can send infected emboli to the spleen. In addition, splenic abscesses can occur postoperatively, most likely because of seeding of the spleen with pathogenic organisms during the operation. The most common route of splenic infection is the splenic artery, through which organisms, primarily bacteria, seed the spleen and proliferate within the areas of infarction or hematoma. The infection also can spread from a contiguous focus, such as a subpulmonic abscess. *M. tuberculosis* seeds the spleen during the initial lymphohematogenous spread but rarely causes large splenic granulomas. Impaired immunity predisposes to the development of a splenic abscess from a distant site. Disseminated fungal infections such as those due to *Candida* and *Aspergillus* may cause microabscesses in the spleen, as well as in many other organs, in children with hematologic malignancies. Similarly, *Bartonella* infection is thought to cause multiple small abscesses after hematogenous spread from the primary infection site.

SYMPTOMS AND CLINICAL MANIFESTATIONS

A patient with a subphrenic abscess often has a history of a fever. Abscesses that are small and deep within the spleen have few clinical manifestations directly attributable to infection of the spleen. Many abscesses enlarge, however, producing splenomegaly, and as the lesions extend to the splenic capsule, localizing signs appear. These include left-sided pleuritic pain, usually in the lower chest, upper abdomen, or costovertebral angle. The pain may radiate to the left shoulder. Many of the symptoms of a splenic abscess overlap those of the disease that caused the seeding of the spleen (i.e., endocarditis). Many patients with splenic abscess will have no localizing signs other than abdominal pain.

Physical Examination Findings

The patient usually has a fever. Depending on the extent of splenic involvement, there is splenomegaly and left upper quadrant tenderness. In advanced disease, the patient may have cachexia, tachycardia, and constant pain.

DIAGNOSIS

Patients with a history of fever and of pain in the left chest, upper abdomen, flank, or shoulder, especially those who have had possible splenic trauma, abnormal heart valves, or sickle cell anemia, should have a complete evaluation for the presence of splenic abscesses.

In approximately 75% of patients with infection of the spleen, multiple abscesses are found in other organs, including the liver, brain, and kidneys. Therefore, a search for the original source of sepsis is essential.

Laboratory Evaluation

A CBC often shows leukocytosis, unless an underlying disease suppresses bone marrow production.

Microbiologic Evaluation

Aerobic and anaerobic blood cultures should be performed. These may be positive if the splenic abscess is serving as a source of continued bacteremia. Blood cultures are less helpful in immunocompromised children with candidal splenic abscesses, only 25% of whom have positive blood cultures. Specimens of splenic abscesses should be transported to the microbiology laboratory as soon as they are obtained. They should be cultured for aerobic and anaerobic bacteria and for acid-fast bacilli. Cultures for fungi should also be performed. Serologic studies are useful for *Bartonella*.

Diagnostic Imaging

Plain radiographs may reveal elevation of the left diaphragm, a left pleural effusion, a soft-tissue mass with or without air in the left upper quadrant of the abdomen, and displacement of the stomach, colon, and kidney. CT with contrast is effective in demonstrating splenic abscesses of a wide range of sizes and shows abscesses as focal lesions with a lower density than the surrounding tissue. Fungal microabscesses have a characteristic appearance on CT. Scattered punctate calcifications can be seen in patients with tuberculosis. Abscesses associated with brucellosis appear as large, thin-rimmed, concentrically laminated calcifications. MRI is also a sensitive test for the presence of splenic abscesses. Ultrasonography will detect larger abscesses but may miss smaller microabscesses. With bartonellosis, multiple small abscesses may be visualized on CT or MRI and can involve both the liver and the spleen.

TREATMENT

An effort must be made to determine the source of the pathogens causing the abscess and to find any extrasplenic foci of infection that are extensions from the infected spleen. Treatment of the underlying disease and the source of the organisms is essential.

Splenectomy has been the treatment of choice for an isolated splenic abscess. However, CT-guided catheter drainage may be an effective method of diagnosis and treatment of splenic abscesses. Empiric administration of systemic antibiotics should be started promptly. Coverage should be provided for the most likely organisms on the basis of the patient's clinical history and presentation. For example, for a splenic abscess secondary to trauma, the antibiotics should cover *S. aureus* and *Streptococcus*; those secondary to abdominal operations should provide coverage for gram-negative enteric organisms and anaerobic bacteria; those occurring in a patient with hemoglobinopathy should provide additional coverage for *Salmonella*. Antifungal therapy with amphotericin B should be considered for abscesses in patients with a hematologic malignancy. Antibiotics should then be directed at the organism isolated from the blood and splenic lesions. In bartonellosis, debate continues regarding the need for antibiotic therapy, and although symptoms may persist for weeks, the condition is self-limited in a normal host.

COMPLICATIONS

Most splenic abscesses remain localized in the spleen. However, bacteremia due to release of the organisms from the infected focus can occur intermittently. Hemorrhage into an abscess cavity can occur. In addition, abscesses can rupture, and the infectious fluid can spread through the diaphragm into the pleural space, causing thoracic empyema. Abscesses that rupture into the abdomen can cause a subphrenic abscess or generalized peritonitis.

PROGNOSIS

Untreated splenic abscesses carry a high mortality because of the many serious complications that can result. With appropriate surgical and antimicrobial treatment, patients generally do well. A solitary splenic abscess carries the best prognosis because about two thirds of patients with such an abscess do not have lesions outside the spleen. The prognosis for splenic abscess due to *Bartonella* infection is excellent.

PREVENTION

Recognition of underlying disorders that predispose to splenic abscesses and prompt treatment of bacteremia are important in preventing splenic abscesses. A high degree of awareness in treating patients with predisposing conditions is important for early recognition and treatment to prevent complications.

RETROPERITONEAL AND PSOAS INFECTIONS

ETIOLOGY

The organisms involved in retroperitoneal abscesses reflect the source of infection. *S. aureus* is the most frequent cause of perinephric abscesses when seeding is hematogenous from a remote site. Most perinephric abscesses, however, are due to direct extension from an intrarenal abscess caused by gram-negative organisms such as *E. coli* and *Proteus*. Abscesses due to perforation of the appendix contain intestinal flora, including anaerobes. Before the incidence of tuberculous infection of the spine (Pott's disease) decreased, psoas abscesses were often due to *Mycobacterium tuberculosis*.

EPIDEMIOLOGY

Retroperitoneal abscesses are uncommon in all age groups. They are most often caused by perforation of a retroperitoneal appendix or by renal disease. The diagnosis is difficult to make, resulting in a substantial delay in treatment with attendant morbidity and mortality. **Psoas abscesses** are uncommon in children. When they do occur, primary infections of the psoas muscle most often affect children younger than 15 years, are more frequent in boys than in girls, and present more often on the left side than on the right.

PATHOGENESIS

The retroperitoneum is a complex anatomic region that consists of the potential spaces between the posterior parietal peritoneum and the posterior portion of the transversalis fascia (Fig. 77–9). Posterior to the transversalis fascia are the vertebral column and the psoas, iliacus, and quadratus lumborum muscles. The posterior limit of the retroperitoneum, the transversalis fascia, separates the retroperitoneum from the retrofascial space. The superior limit of the retroperitoneum is the undersurface of the diaphragm, and the inferior limit is the pelvic rim within the retroperitoneum; this space is in continuity with the posterior mediastinum. Because the space containing these vessels and lymph nodes is not enclosed in a fascial sheath, inflammatory processes can extend from this space to other retroperitoneal spaces.

The retroperitoneum is anatomically divided into three potential spaces—the space anterior to the kidneys (the anterior retroperito-

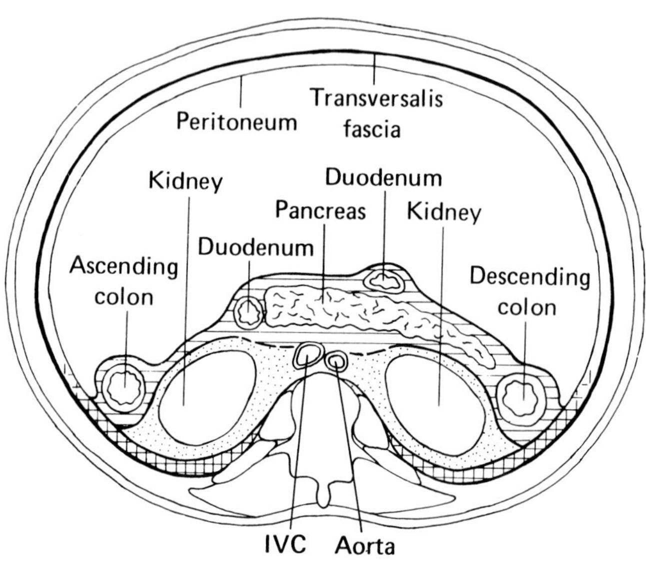

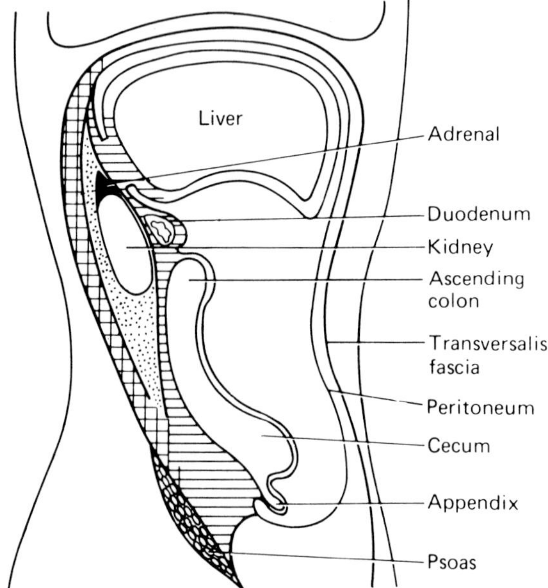

FIGURE 77–9. The three retroperitoneal compartments. *Striped areas* are the anterior pararenal space; *stippled areas* are the perirenal space; and *cross-hatched areas* are the posterior pararenal space. *IVC*, Inferior vena cava. (Modified from Meyers MA: Acute extraperitoneal infection. *Semin Roentgenol* 1973;8:445–64.)

neal or pararenal space), the perirenal space, and the space posterior to the kidneys (the posterior retroperitoneal or pararenal space). Abscesses in the perirenal space usually are due to extension of an intrarenal infection secondary to pyelonephritis or are due to hematogenous spread from a distant site that has extended beyond the renal capsule. They may also be due to hematogenous spread of bacteria directly to the perirenal space or to direct extension from an adjacent inflammatory process, such as a perforated retrocecal appendix.

The psoas muscle is invested in fascia through most of its course. The fascia forms a compartment in the space posterior to the retroperitoneal structures that is in direct communication with the posterior retroperitoneal (posterior pararenal) space. This relationship allows infections within the retroperitoneum to spread to the psoas muscle. This is the most common route of spread of infection to the psoas muscle, other than by hematogenous seeding. In children, often no source of the psoas abscess can be found. Some children may have a history of skin infection or upper respiratory illness. A primary psoas abscess or a psoas abscess that originates from a vertebral, sacroiliac, or perirenal infection is often due to *S. aureus.* Abscesses secondary to perirenal disease with obstructive pyelonephritis may be caused by gram-negative bacteria such as *E. coli* and *Proteus,* whereas abscesses due to perforations of retroperitoneal abdominal structures often contain intestinal flora, which includes anaerobic organisms. Suppurating bacterial infection of the inguinal nodes also has been reported to extend to the underlying psoas muscle.

SYMPTOMS AND CLINICAL MANIFESTATIONS

There are few localizing symptoms of retroperitoneal infections and psoas abscesses. The patients usually appear ill out of proportion to the complaints and physical findings. Abdominal pain, which is not localized, is often accompanied by flank pain, abdominal distention, weakness and pain in the ipsilateral hip, thigh, or knee, and psoas spasm. The patient may also have a fever, chills, anorexia, weight loss, and malaise. If the psoas muscle is involved, the patient often has a limp and keeps the hip flexed and externally rotated because this position releases tension on the psoas muscle. Pain may be present in the abdomen, flank, back, or iliac fossa or over the groin and the thigh. Symptoms may be present for weeks before a diagnosis is made.

Physical Examination Findings

Both retroperitoneal and psoas abscesses are often difficult to diagnose because of the lack of localizing signs. A tender mass in the flank representing a retrofascial abscess, if sufficiently large, may be felt. In the case of a psoas muscle abscess, the mass may be present in the iliac fossa or the abdomen. Scoliosis is often present because the patient leans toward the side of the infected psoas muscle in an attempt to relieve the pain. The patient usually has a fever and has a hip flexion deformity and pain on extension of the ipsilateral thigh (psoas sign).

DIAGNOSIS

Differential Diagnosis

The differential diagnosis of retroperitoneal and psoas abscesses includes septic arthritis of the hip, osteomyelitis of the femoral head or ilium, sacroiliitis, vertebral osteomyelitis (pyogenic or tuberculous), diskitis, paraspinal abscess, and noninfectious diseases, including aseptic necrosis of the hip (Perthes' disease) and hip dislocation.

Laboratory Evaluation

The WBC count and erythrocyte sedimentation rate are often elevated. Anemia is usually present if the disease is of long standing. A urinalysis should be performed, especially if the patient has flank pain or has a history of urinary tract infections. Because the ureter lies over the psoas muscle, an inflammatory process involving the psoas muscle may cause ureteral irritation and sterile pyuria. If there is a perinephric abscess, leukocytes, bacteria, and often protein are usually present in the urine. If the patient has been exposed to tuberculosis, a skin test with purified protein derivative (PPD) with appropriate control antigens and a chest radiograph should be performed.

Microbiologic Evaluation

Blood cultures may be positive in children with a retroperitoneal or psoas abscess. Material obtained by aspiration or drainage of the abscess should be transported to the microbiology laboratory in two different receptacles for culture and Gram stain. Material for aerobic culture should be sent in a syringe or sterile transport swab. Samples for anaerobic culture should be sent in a capped syringe with all air removed and should be processed for culture within 2 hours. If a tuberculous psoas abscess is likely, stains and culture for acid-fast bacilli should be obtained.

Diagnostic Imaging

Plain radiographs of the abdomen may show a bulging or obliterated psoas shadow, if the psoas muscle is involved, as well as scoliosis secondary to sympathetic posturing. Gas within the abscess, if present, can also be seen. If the infection has originated from the vertebral column, bony changes may be seen. An intravenous pyelogram may be helpful in determining whether the kidneys are involved. If a psoas abscess is present, an intravenous pyelogram is often normal but may show medial deviation of the lower third of the ureter on the affected side. Gallium- and indium-labeled WBC scanning is helpful in localizing the lesion, but there is a delay in obtaining results, especially with gallium scanning. Ultrasonography is useful in establishing the presence of an abscess or of renal involvement, especially for a child who is too ill for CT. CT or MRI is the procedure of choice in evaluation of psoas abscess; either of these gives clear anatomic details of the psoas muscle and the structures in the retroperitoneal space and may even help to identify the source of the infection. Giving intravenous contrast medium before CT may enhance visualization of the rim of the abscess wall. CT can be used to guide drainage of these abscesses.

TREATMENT

If a patient has a fever and appears ill, antibiotics active against the most common organisms associated with these abscesses in children should be given. The antibiotics should provide initial coverage for *S. aureus* and gram-negative and anaerobic intestinal flora until further microbiologic data and information on the possible source of infection are available. An appropriate initial antibiotic regimen is oxacillin, gentamicin, and clindamycin. Fluid, electrolyte, and hematologic abnormalities should be corrected.

The retroperitoneal abscess or psoas muscle abscess should be drained, either surgically or by CT-guided percutaneous aspiration. Parenterally administered antibiotics directed against the organisms isolated from the blood and the abscess should be continued for 2–3 weeks. An underlying source of the abscess, such as renal or gastrointestinal disease or osteomyelitis, should be sought and corrected.

COMPLICATIONS

Untreated abscesses can rupture into the peritoneal space. Retroperitoneal abscesses can also extend long distances along the fascial plane superior to the subdiaphragmatic space, mediastinum, and thoracic cavity; laterally to the anterior abdominal wall and subcutaneous tissue of the flank; and inferiorly to the thigh, hip, and psoas muscle. Infection can spread within the fascial plane of the psoas muscle to cause osteomyelitis of the vertebrae or the hip. These complications are rarely seen because of improved diagnostic techniques and early intervention.

PROGNOSIS

The prognosis is favorable in uncomplicated retroperitoneal and psoas infections when detected and treated early. Diagnostic delays, however, often result in complications, including sepsis.

PREVENTION

No true preventive strategies are practical for these rare infections. Clinicians should focus on early diagnosis and prompt therapy.

ANORECTAL ABSCESS

ETIOLOGY

Most anorectal abscesses contain multiple intestinal and skin organisms, with anaerobic bacteria predominating, particularly *Bacteroides* (especially *B. fragilis*), *P. melaninogenica*, *Peptostreptococcus,* and *Fusobacterium.* The predominant aerobic bacteria are *E. coli*, *K. pneumoniae*, and *Staphylococcus aureus.*

EPIDEMIOLOGY

Anorectal abscesses are not common in pediatrics. They occur more frequently in children younger than 2 years; the greatest incidence is in neonates and infants. Boys are more predisposed to anorectal abscesses than are girls. The risk of anorectal abscess is greatest in immunosuppressed and neutropenic children. Children with ulcerative colitis and Crohn's disease, diabetes mellitus, chronic granulomatous disease, those who have had a recent rectal operation, and those receiving high doses of corticosteroids are also at increased risk.

PATHOGENESIS

The anorectal region consists of the anal canal and the inferior portion of the rectum. Superficial abscesses occur in the anal epithelium, and deep abscesses occur in the ischiorectal fossa. Although several pathologic conditions predispose to the formation of anorectal abscesses, often no inciting factor can be found. The abscesses may occur by extension of bacteria through small tears, abrasions, or fissures in the anal epithelium during bouts of diarrhea or constipation, which cause abrasions. In addition, the anal crypts may become occluded, leading to infection and to the formation of abscesses anywhere along the path of the anal ducts from the anal epithelium to the space between the internal and external sphincters. Once infection begins in the anal crypts, extension can occur laterally through the external sphincter into the fat contained within the ischiorectal fossa or inferiorly to form a perianal abscess, which exits through a fistula in ano at the anal skin. Infection can also spread superiorly to the space between the internal sphincter and the levator ani muscles, a deep space lying immediately inferior to the pelvic peritoneum.

SYMPTOMS AND CLINICAL MANIFESTATIONS

The clinical features of anorectal abscesses depend on the location of the abscess and the age of the child. Children younger than 2 years often have a recent history of diarrhea. On occasion constipation may be present. An older child with a superficial abscess (perianal abscess) usually has a history of pain on sitting and walking, manifested as a refusal to walk or an abnormal gait, and a history of redness and swelling in the perianal area. An enlarging perianal abscess may produce pain with defecation, coughing, and sneezing. Abscesses in the deeper anorectal tissue, such as those in the ischiorectal fossa or in the pelvirectal region, often cause poorly localized, deep, throbbing pain. They are usually associated with rigors, fever, malaise, a decreased appetite, and lower abdominal pain.

Physical Examination Findings

Perianal abscesses produce an erythematous, tender, indurated region that is fluctuant near the anus. There is no pain in the anal canal on digital anorectal examination beyond the superficial lesion. A perianal abscess can be confused with an anorectal fistula, which results from drainage of an anorectal abscess with formation of a fistulous tract. In neutropenic patients, evidence of abscess may be less striking because of the paucity of polymorphonuclear leukocytes available to contribute to local inflammation.

Deep abscesses are often difficult to diagnose, leading to a delay in treatment. These patients appear ill and have a fever. Evidence of an anorectal abscess is often not seen on external examination of the anus, although there may be brawny edema of the perianal area on the affected side. Rectal examination demonstrates a tender mass deep to the rectal wall. Rectal examination should not be performed in neutropenic patients.

DIAGNOSIS

Differential Diagnosis

Cellulitis of the perianal skin due to group A *Streptococcus* can be confused with early perianal abscess formation. An anorectal fistula, a complication of an anorectal abscess that drains pus or mucus through the perianal region, can be confused with a perianal abscess. Hidradenitis suppurativa should be considered. This condition occurs in adolescents and adults and is characterized by acute inflammation of the apocrine sweat glands located in the perianal region, the axilla, the perineum, and the buttocks.

Laboratory Evaluation

A CBC often shows leukocytosis, unless an underlying disease suppresses bone marrow production.

Microbiologic Evaluation

Aerobic and anaerobic blood cultures should be obtained if the patient has signs of systemic toxicity. Material obtained from drainage or aspiration of the abscesses should be evaluated by performing a Gram stain and aerobic and anaerobic culture.

Diagnostic Imaging

Once it is considered, the diagnosis of an anorectal abscess can be made by the clinical history and a thorough anorectal examination.

Therefore, imaging studies are usually not indicated unless the patient is neutropenic, in which case imaging studies with CT or ultrasonography can substitute for a digital rectal examination.

TREATMENT

In an immunocompetent child, prompt and adequate surgical drainage and exploration of the abscess followed by antibiotics is appropriate treatment. The surgeon may opt to aspirate the abscess if adequate drainage can be achieved. Adjunctive therapy includes antimicrobial agents active against β-lactamase-resistant anaerobic bacteria, gram-negative enteric organisms, and *S. aureus*. A combination of clindamycin (which is active against *S. aureus* and β-lactamase–producing anaerobes) and an aminoglycoside (to provide coverage for gram-negative enteric bacteria) is appropriate. Other effective antimicrobial regimens are (1) cefoxitin as a single agent, (2) a β-lactam plus β-lactamase inhibitor combination, and (3) a combination of metronidazole with either an aminoglycoside or a third-generation cephalosporin. Once the infecting bacteria have been identified, therapy can be focused. Although the length of treatment has not been defined, an antibiotic course of 7–10 days is generally adequate except in neutopenic patients.

Treatment of anorectal abscesses in immunocompromised hosts remains difficult. These patients often have little suppurative material to drain and are at risk of postoperative complications because of their underlying disease. These complications include poor wound healing, increased bleeding, and the spread of infection. For an immunocompromised patient without a fluctuant mass, extensive infection, or sepsis, a trial of parenterally administered antibiotics can be given initially. The antibiotic regimen should cover anaerobes as well as organisms of concern in neutropenia. Progression of the disease on appropriate antibiotics will necessitate reconsideration of surgery both for microbiologic diagnosis and for management.

COMPLICATIONS

Complications of anorectal abscesses relate to underlying conditions. The most common complications are anorectal fistulas, recurrence of the abscess, and bacteremia. Infants are at risk of fistula formation after drainage of an abscess. Fistulas may develop even when appropriate surgical and antibiotic treatment is given. The rate of these complications is much higher among immunocompromised children than among those with normal immunity. Life-threatening septicemia and necrotizing fasciitis can occur in all patients but are especially of concern in neutropenic patients.

PROGNOSIS

Early surgical drainage in combination with antibiotic therapy has decreased the incidence of sepsis due to these abscesses. However, there is still a high complication rate, especially in immunocompromised children.

REVIEW

McClean KL, Sheehan GJ, Harding GK: Intraabdominal infection: A review. *Clin Infect Dis* 1994;19:100–16.

KEY ARTICLES

Intra-abdominal and Pelvic Abscesses

Brook I: Microbiology of intra-abdominal abscesses in children. *Am J Dis Child* 1987;141:1148–9.

Churchill RJ: CT of intra-abdominal fluid collections. *Radiol Clin North Am* 1989;27:653–66.

John SD: Trends in pediatric emergency imaging. *Radiol Clin North Am* 1999;37:995–1034.

Joseph AE, MacVicar D: Ultrasound in the diagnosis of abdominal abscesses. *Clin Radiol* 1990;42:154–6.

Saini S, Kellum JM, O'Leary MP, et al: Improved localization and survival in patients with intra-abdominal abscesses. *Am J Surg* 1983;145:136–42.

Stanley P, Atkinson JB, Reed BS, et al: Percutaneous drainage of abdominal fluid collections in children. *AJR Am J Roentgenol* 1984;142:813–6.

von Sonnenberg E, D'Agostino HB, Casola G, et al: Percutaneous abscess drainage: Current concepts. *Radiology* 1991;181:627.

Wiesenfeld HC, Sweet RL: Progress in the management of tuboovarian abscesses. *Clin Obstet Gynecol* 1993;36:433–44.

Peritonitis

Bell MJ: Peritonitis in the newborn—Current concepts. *Pediatr Clin North Am* 1985;32:1181–201.

Chadwick EG, Shulman ST, Yagev R: Peritonitis as a late manifestation of Group B streptococcal disease in newborns. *Pediatr Infect Dis J* 1983;2:142–3.

Clark JH, Fitzgerald JF, Kleinman MB: Spontaneous bacterial peritonitis. *J Pediatr* 1984;104:495–500.

Johnson CC, Baldessarre J, Levinson ME: Peritonitis: Update on pathophysiology, clinical manifestations, and management. *Clin Infect Dis* 1997;24:1035–47.

Maddaus MA, Ahrenholz D, Simmons RL: The biology of peritonitis and implications for treatment. *Surg Clin North Am* 1988;68:431–43.

McDougal WS, Izant RJ, Zollinger RM: Primary peritonitis in infancy and childhood. *Ann Surg* 1975;181:310–3.

Mocan H, Murphy AV, Beattie TJ, et al: Peritonitis in children on continuous ambulatory peritoneal dialysis. *J Infect* 1988;16:243–51.

Gorensek MJ, Lebel MH, Nelson JD: Peritonitis in children with nephrotic syndrome. *Pediatrics* 1988;81:849–56.

Warady BA, Bashir M, Donaldson LA: Fungal peritonitis in children receiving peritoneal dialysis: A report of the NAPRTCS. *Kidney Int* 2000;58:384–9.

Woolf A, Christie D, Wilson CB: Tuberculous peritonitis in an infant. *Pediatr Infect Dis J* 1985;4:684–6.

Acute Appendicitis

Bauer T, Vennits B, Holm B, et al: Antibiotic prophylaxis in acute nonperforated appendicitis. The Danish Multicenter Study Group III. *Ann Surg* 1989;209:307–11.

Bilik R, Burnweit C, Shandling B: Is abdominal cavity culture of any value in appendicitis? *Am J Surg* 1998;175:267–70.

Blakely ML, Spurbeck W, Lakshman S, et al: Current status of laparoscopic appendectomy in children. *Curr Opin Pediatr* 1998;10:315–7.

Blewett CJ, Krummel TM: Perforated appendicitis: Past and future controversies. *Semin Pediatr Surg* 1995;4:234–8.

Elmore JR, Dibbins AW, Curci MR: The treatment of complicated appendicitis in children: What is the gold standard? *Arch Surg* 1987; 122:424–7.

Fishman SJ, Pelosi L, Klavon SL, et al: Perforated appendicitis: Prospective outcome analysis for 150 children. *J Pediatr Surg* 2000;35:923–6.

Haecker FM, Bergr D, Schumacher U, et al: Peritonitis in childhood: Aspects of pathogenesis and therapy. *Pediatr Surg Int* 2000;16: 182–8.

Hoelzer DJ, Zabel DD, Zern JT: Determining duration of antibiotic use in children with complicated appendicitis. *Pediatr Infect Dis J* 1999;18: 979–82.

Jelloul LB, et al: Mesenteric adenitis caused by *Yersinia pseudotuberculosis* presenting as an abdominal mass. *Eur J Pediatr Surg* 1997;7:180.

Kaplan S: Antibiotic usage in appendicitis in children. *Pediatr Infect Dis J* 1998;17:1047–8.

Kokoska ER, Silen ML, Tracy TF Jr, et al: The impact of intraoperative culture on treatment and outcome in children with perforated appendicitis. *J Pediatr Surg* 1999;34:749–53.

Knight PJ, Vassy LE: Specific diseases mimicking appendicitis in childhood. *Arch Surg* 1981;116:744–6.

Lund DP, Murphy EU: Management of perforated appendicitis in children: A decade of aggressive treatment. *J Pediatr Surg* 1994;29:1130–3.

Nance ML, Adamson WT, Hedrick HL: Appendicitis in the young child: A continuing diagnostic challenge. *Pediatr Emerg Care* 2000; 16:160–2.

Pena BM, Taylor GA: Radiologists' confidence in interpretation of sonography and CT in suspected pediatric appendicitis. *AJR Am J Roentgenol* 2001;175:71–4.

Pena BM, Taylor GA, Fishman SJ, et al: Costs and effectiveness of ultrasonography and limited computed tomography for diagnosing appendicitis in children. *Pediatrics* 2000;106:672–6.

Pena BM, Taylor GA, Lund DP, et al: Effect of computed tomography on patient management and costs in children with suspected appendicitis. *Pediatrics* 1999;104:440–6.

Rao PM, Rhea JT, et al: Helical CT technique for the diagnosis of appendicitis: Prospective evaluation of a focused appendix CT examination. *Radiology* 1997;202:139–44.

Rautio M, Saxén H, Siitonen A, et al: Bacteriology of histopathologically defined appendicitis in children. *Pediatr Infect Dis J* 2000;19: 1078–83.

Rhea JT, Rao PM, Novelline RA, et al: A focused appendiceal CT technique to reduce the cost of caring for patients with clinically suspected appendicitis. *AJR Am J Roentgenol* 1997;169:113–8.

Soderquist-Elinder CK, Hirsch K, Bergdahl S, et al: Prophylactic antibiotics in uncomplicated appendicitis during childhood—A prospective randomised study. *Eur J Pediatr Surg* 1995;5:282–5.

Snyder WH, Chaffin L: Appendicitis during the first two years of life: Report on twenty-one cases and review of four hundred forty-seven cases from the literature. *Arch Surg* 1952;64:549–60.

Splenic Abscess

Allal R, Kastler B, Gangi A, et al: Splenic abscesses in typhoid fever: US and CT studies. *J Comput Assist Tomogr* 1993;17:90–3.

Brook I, Frazier EH: Microbiology of liver and spleen abscesses. *J Med Microbiol* 1998;47:1075–80.

Dunn MW, Berkowitz FE, Miller JJ, et al: Hepatosplenic cat-scratch disease and abdominal pain. *Pediatr Infect Dis J* 1997;16:269–72.

Berkman WA, Harris SA, Bernardino ME: Nonsurgical drainage of splenic abscesses. *AJR Am J Roentgenol* 1983;141:395–6.

Fernandes ET, Tavares PB, Garcette CB, et al: Conservative management of splenic abscesses in children. *J Pediatr Surg* 1992;27:1578–9.

Hatley RM, Donaldson JS, Raffensperger JG: Splenic microabscesses in the immune-compromised patient. *J Pediatr Surg* 1989;24:697–9.

Phillips GS, Radosevich MD, Lipsett PA, et al: Splenic abscess: Another look at an old disease. *Arch Surg* 1997;132:1331–6.

Smith MD, Nio M, Camel JE, et al: Management of splenic abscess in immunocompromised children. *J Pediatr Surg* 1993;28:823–6.

Vallejo JG, Stevens AM, Dutton RV, et al: Hepatosplenic abscesses due to *Brucella melitensis:* Report of a case involving a child and review of the literature. *Clin Infect Dis* 1996;22:485–9.

Retroperitoneal and Psoas Infections

Altemeier WA, Alexander JW: Retroperitoneal abscess. *Arch Surg* 1961; 83:512–24.

Andreou A, Karasavvidou A, Papadopoulou F, et al: Ilio-psoas abscess in a neonate. *Am J Perinatol* 1997;14:519–21.

Bresee JS, Edwards MS: Psoas abscess in children. *Pediatr Infect Dis J* 1990;9:201–6.

Brook I: Microbiology of retroperitoneal abscesses in children. *J Med Microbiol* 1999;48:697–700.

Cybulsky IJ, Tam P: Intra-abdominal abscesses in Crohn's disease. *Am Surg* 1990;56:678–82.

Kang M, Gupta S, Gulati M, et al: Ilio-psoas abcess in the paediatric population: Treatment by US-guided percutaneous drainage. *Pediatr Radiol* 1998;28:478–81.

Parbhoo A, Govender S: Acute pyogenic psoas abscess in children. *J Pediatr Orthop* 1992;12:663–6.

Tong CW, Griffith JF, Lam TP, et al: The conservative management of acute pyogenic iliopsoas abscess in children. *J Bone Joint Surg Br* 1998;80:83–5.

Simons GW, Sty JR, Starshak RJ: Retroperitoneal and retrofascial abscesses: A review. *J Bone Joint Surg Am* 1983;65:1041–58.

Stephenson CA, Seibert JJ, Golladay ES, et al: Abscess of the iliopsoas muscle diagnosed by magnetic resonance imaging and ultrasonography. *South Med J* 1991; 84:509–11.

Anorectal Abscess

Arditi M, Yogev R: Perirectal abscess in infants and children: Report of 52 cases and review of literature. *Pediatr Infect Dis J* 1990;9:411–5.

Brook I, Martin WJ: Aerobic and anaerobic bacteriology of perirectal abscess in children. *Pediatrics* 1980;66:282–4.

Enberg RN, Cox RH, Burry VF: Perirectal abscess in children. *Am J Dis Child* 1974;128:360–1.

Glenn J, Cotton D, Wesley R, et al: Anorectal infections in patients with malignant diseases. *Rev Infect Dis* 1988;10:42–52.

Krieger RW, Chusid MJ: Perirectal abscess in childhood: A review of 29 cases. *Am J Dis Child* 1979;133:411–2.

CHAPTER 78

Viral Hepatitis

M. Susan Moyer ▪ Hal B. Jenson

Infectious hepatitis was first described more than 2,000 years ago and remains an important cause of acute and chronic infection. Five distinct hepatotropic viruses—hepatitis viruses A through E (HAV, HBV, HCV, HDV, and HEV)—from five different virus families, and two new potential agents—hepatitis G virus (HGV) and TT virus (TTV)—have recently been identified (Table 78–1). These agents cause overlapping clinical illnesses that cannot be distinguished on clinical or epidemiologic features but can be diagnosed by serologic testing. Specific serologic markers permit precise diagnosis, determination of resolution or progression of disease, response to therapy, and epidemiologic studies to identify populations at risk. All five viruses are associated with acute hepatitis, but only HBV, HCV, and HDV are associated with chronic hepatitis or a chronic carrier state. The chronic hepatic inflammation of hepatitis B and hepatitis C also has been shown to be an important risk factor in the development of cirrhosis and hepatocellular carcinoma (Chapter 4). Hepatitis B and C are of particular importance in pediatrics because of the potential for vertical transmission.

ETIOLOGY

The five primary hepatotropic viruses differ in their biophysical characteristics and classification (Table 78–2). Two viruses from patients with **non-A-E hepatitis** have recently been isolated and characterized: HGV, which is similar to HCV, and TT virus (TTV), which is thought to represent a new family of viruses, the Circinoviridae. Their role in causing acute and chronic liver disease has yet to be defined. Epidemiologic evidence suggests that there are additional hepatotropic viruses that have yet to be identified. None of the known viruses are present in 10–15% of cases of sporadic, community-acquired acute hepatitis and in 15–20% of cases of posttransfusion hepatitis. In addition, 30–50% of persons with fulminant hepatic failure, hepatitis-associated aplastic anemia, and cryptogenic cirrhosis have no identified cause for their illness.

Other viruses that are not primarily hepatotropic may occasionally cause inflammation of the liver as part of a systemic illness (Table 78–3).

Hepatitis A Virus. HAV is a spherical, nonenveloped virus approximately 27 nm in diameter that contains a single-stranded molecule of RNA. It is in the Hepatovirus genus of the Picornaviridae and is also known as **enterovirus 72.**

Transmission is by the fecal-oral route and by oral ingestion. Most cases occur from person-to-person transmission during community-wide outbreaks. Parenteral transmission is extremely rare but has been reported. The most frequently reported sources are household or sexual contact with a person with acute hepatitis A (in 12–26% of cases), international travel, water or food contaminated by sewage, cyclic outbreaks among users of injecting and noninjecting drugs, and contact among men who have sex with men. The source is not identified in approximately 50% of cases of hepatitis A.

Hepatitis A is highly contagious. A considerable burden of virus is shed in the stool toward the end of the incubation period of 2–7 weeks, during the preicteric phase. Infectivity decreases considerably by the end of the first week of jaundice, with the period of greatest contagiousness just before the onset of clinical symptoms. The secondary attack rate among household members of a person with hepatitis A is 10–20%. The difficulty in recognizing HAV infection in infants and children is a risk factor, especially among children in nursery or primary school or daycare centers and among children in long-term care facilities who do not adhere to optimal hygienic practices.

Hepatitis B Virus. HBV, formerly designated the **Australia antigen,** is a complex virion that represents a new family of viruses, the Hepadnaviridae, which require reverse transcriptase activity to replicate through RNA intermediates. The intact virus, or **Dane particle,** is spherical, approximately 42 nm in diameter, and contains a double shell. The outer surface and inner core are immunologically distinct, and the antigenic components are designated **hepatitis B surface antigen (HBsAg)** and **hepatitis B core antigen (HBcAg).** The core contains the genomic partially double-stranded DNA, with one incomplete strand forming a gap region. Other components of the core include DNA-dependent **DNA polymerase** and **hepatitis B e antigen (HBeAg).** The core of the virus is assembled in the nucleus of the infected hepatocyte, whereas the surface antigen–associated particles are produced in the cytoplasm. During viral replication, HBsAg is synthesized in excess and can be detected in the blood as spherical or tubular particles approximately 22 nm in diameter. HBeAg, but not HBcAg, also can be identified in the circulation and correlates with virus synthesis and

TABLE 78–1. Terminology of Hepatitis Viruses

Disease	Viral Agent	Synonyms
Hepatitis A	Hepatitis A virus	Infectious hepatitis Short-incubation hepatitis Epidemic jaundice
Hepatitis B	Hepatitis B virus	Serum hepatitis Transfusion hepatitis Long-incubation hepatitis Homologous serum jaundice
Hepatitis C	Hepatitis C virus	Parenterally transmitted non-A, non-B hepatitis
Hepatitis D	Hepatitis D virus	Delta hepatitis
Hepatitis E	Hepatitis E virus	Enterically transmitted non-A, non-B hepatitis
Hepatitis G	Hepatitis G virus; GB virus type C	No synonym

TABLE 78–2. Comparison of the Causes of Viral Hepatitis

Attribute	Hepatitis A	Hepatitis B	Hepatitis C	Hepatitis D	Hepatitis E	Hepatitis G	TT Virus
Virus Characteristics							
Name	Hepatitis A virus (HAV)	Hepatitis B virus (HBV)	Hepatitis C virus (HCV)	Hepatitis D virus (HDV)	Hepatitis E virus (HEV)	Hepatitis G virus GB virus type C (HGV, GBV-C)	TT virus (TTV)
Family	Picornavirus	Hepadnavirus	Flavivirus	Satellite	Calicivirus	Flavivirus	? Circinoviridae
Size (nm)	27	42	45	36	32	50–100	30–50
Nucleic acid	ssRNA	dsDNA	ssRNA	ssRNA	ssRNA	ssRNA	ssDNA
Genome size (kb)	7.8	3.2	10.5	1.7	8.2	9.3	3.8
Epidemiology							
Incubation period (average)	4 wk	4 mo	7–9 wk	Coinfection: same as HBV Superinfection: 4–8 wk	6 wk	Unknown	Unknown
Incubation period (range)	2–7 wk	2–6 mo	2–20 wk		2–8 wk		
Predominant mode of spread of infection	Fecal-oral	Parenteral, sexual, perinatal	Parenteral, sexual, perinatal	Parenteral, sexual (coinfection with hepatitis B)	Fecal-oral	Parenteral, sexual, perinatal	Parenteral, perinatal, ? sexual
Occurs in epidemics	Yes	No	No	No	Yes	No	No
Clinical Manifestations							
Onset	Usually acute	Usually insidious	Insidious	Insidious	Acute	See text	See text
Duration of elevated transaminases	2–6 wk	2–6 mo or longer	2–6 mo or longer	2–6 mo or longer	Several weeks		
Acute mortality rate (%)	0.2	0.2–1	0.2	2–20	0.2 (20% in the third trimester of pregnancy)		
Rate of chronic infection (%)	None	5–10 (60–90% in infection acquired perinatally or during infancy)	50–70	2–70	None		
Duration of immunity	Lifelong	Lifelong	Unknown	Unknown	Unknown		
Diagnostic Tests							
Antigens*	HAV Ag	HBsAg HBeAg	HCV Ag	HDV Ag	HEV Ag		
Antibodies*	Anti-HAV IgM anti-HAV	Anti-HBs Anti-HBc IgM anti-HBc Anti-HBe	Anti-HCV	Anti-HDV	Anti-HEV	Anti-HGV	
Viral markers	HAV RNA	HBV DNA DNA polymerase	HCV RNA	HDV RNA	HEV RNA	HGV RNA	TTV DNA

ssRNA = single-stranded RNA; dsDNA = double-stranded DNA.
*See Table 78–8 for serologic terminology.

infectivity. In addition, the DNA polymerase can be detected in serum, as can circulating HBV DNA, which is measured directly by a molecular hybridization test.

HBV is transmitted by contact with infected blood, by intimate (usually sexual) contact with acutely infected persons or with chronic carriers, or perinatally from a mother to her newborn. Rarely, HBV may be transmitted in blood products or transplanted organs. Saliva and urine may contain small amounts of virus, but these fluids are not efficient means of transmission. Transmission among children in the same household may occur by exposure to mucous membranes, abraded skin, or unrecognized wounds. Transmission in the daycare environment is extremely rare and has been recognized only with aggressive behavior such as biting. HBV is not transmitted by the fecal-oral route or by water.

Vertical transmission to infants occurs from mothers who are chronic carriers or who have acute infection in the third trimester. The risk of infection correlates with maternal markers of infectivity, including high HBsAg titer; presence of HBeAg, HBV DNA, or

TABLE 78–3. Other Viruses that May Cause Hepatitis as Part of Systemic Infection

Epstein-Barr virus
Cytomegalovirus
Varicella-zoster virus (chickenpox)
Herpes simplex virus
Human herpesvirus 6 (roseola infantum)
Adenoviruses
Enteroviruses
Rubella virus
Arboviruses

polymerase; HBsAg in the cord blood; and siblings with HBsAg positivity. From 60% to 90% of offspring born to HBsAg-positive mothers acquire infection at birth and become chronic carriers. These infants usually have no symptoms but by 1–3 months of age have biochemical evidence of acute infection. Infection only rarely is acquired prenatally across the placenta or postnatally in breast milk.

Hepatitis C Virus. HCV is the major etiologic agent of posttransfusion hepatitis. It is 30–60 nm in diameter, contains single-stranded RNA, and is classified with HGV in the Hepacivirus genus of the Flaviviridae family. There are six major genotypes having <60% sequence identity, with 75% of isolates in the U.S. genotype 1/subtype 1a or 1b. Frequent mutation results in multiple HCV variants, or **quasispecies,** with a single individual. The **E2** outer envelope protein of genotype 1, which more closely resembles RNA-activated protein kinase than that of other genotypes, confers interferon resistance and is associated with a poorer prognosis.

HCV is transmitted primarily by injection drug use and high-risk sexual behaviors, especially having multiple sex partners. The risk that hepatitis C will develop after needle-stick exposure or intimate contact is considerably lower than for HBV. In the United States before 1986, transfusion-associated hepatitis occurred in 5–13% of recipients. From 1986 to 1990, exclusion of persons with risk factors from the donor pool and surrogate testing decreased the rate to 1.5%. With anti-HCV screening introduced in 1990, the risk of posttransfusion hepatitis has decreased to ≤0.1% per recipient and to 0.01–0.001% per unit transfused. Vertical transmission from mother to infant does occur, but the risk is relatively small, estimated to be 5–7%. The risk of transmission correlates with maternal viral load and is 14% with maternal HIV coinfection. HCV has been identified in breast milk, although transmission by breast-feeding has not been documented. Breast-feeding is not contraindicated for offspring of HCV-infected mothers. The first outbreak of HCV transmission by IVIG occurred in 1994, but all immune globulin products must now undergo an inactivation step, such as solvent-detergent inactivation, or be HCV RNA-negative (Chapter 15).

Hepatitis D Virus. HDV, also known as the **delta agent,** is classified in the Deltavirus genus of the **satellite** group of **subviral agents.** HDV is a **defective virus** that cannot cause infection by itself but requires the presence of HBV. HDV is transmitted simultaneously with HBV, causing **coinfection,** or it infects chronic HBsAg carriers, causing **superinfection.** HDV is a double-shelled particle that measures 35–37 nm in diameter and resembles HBV on electron microscopy. The external coat is composed of the HBsAg, which is derived from the HBV genome, and the delta antigen, provided by the HDV genome, constitutes the inner shell. The HDV genome itself is a small, circular molecule of single-stranded RNA that shares no homologic features with HBV DNA. The structure of this virus and its unique replicative cycle are distinct from those of other families of animal viruses.

HDV is usually transmitted through familial or intimate contact, especially in developing countries, where the prevalence is highest. In contrast, transmission by the percutaneous route is more important in areas of low prevalence, such as the United States.

Hepatitis E Virus. HEV is a single-stranded RNA virus classified in the Caliciviridae family. The virus particles were first isolated, and subsequently characterized, from the stool of a volunteer who ingested the fecal supernatant from a patient with non-A, non-B, non-C acute hepatitis. HEV is a labile, nonenveloped virus approximately 32 nm in diameter.

HEV is transmitted by the fecal-oral route. Hepatitis E has a low secondary attack rate of 0.7–2.2% among household contacts. During outbreaks of hepatitis E, the attack rate and the mortality are particularly high among pregnant women, approaching 25%. Vertical transmission from mother to infant has been documented. No chronic carrier state has been identified.

Hepatitis G Virus. Two laboratories independently isolated the virus that is now generally termed HGV. Initially, two novel RNA viruses, GB virus A and GB virus B (named after the person from whom the original serum was obtained), were isolated and characterized. These viruses did not appear to be responsible for acute or chronic hepatitis in humans, but, with the use of reverse-transcriptase PCR (RT-PCR) in sera that contained antibodies to these viruses, a third novel RNA virus, GB virus C, was subsequently characterized. GB virus C was found to be nearly identical by nucleotide (85%) and amino acid sequence (100%) to the hepatitis G virus (HGV), which had been isolated by another laboratory. HGV and GB virus C are considered to be separate isolates of the same virus and are classified with HCV in the Hepacivirus genus of the Flaviviridae family. HGV and GB genes encoding nonstructural proteins are similar to HCV, but there are numerous differences in the genes encoding structural proteins. The mutation rate of HGV appears to be low.

HGV is transmitted parenterally, mainly through blood and blood products. Sexual transmission is probable, and mother-to-infant transmission has been documented. There is evidence of a high frequency of infection in populations repeatedly exposed to blood products, injecting drug use, and HCV infection.

TT Virus. TTV, a novel single-stranded DNA virus originally isolated from a Japanese patient (TT), has variably been termed **transfusion-associated virus** and **transfusion-transmitted virus.** The viral genome is circular and negative stranded, with an estimated viral size of 30–50 nm. The virus is similar to the Circoviridae, members of which are known to infect plants and vertebrates such as birds and swine, but the distinct biophysical and molecular characteristics suggest that it is a member of a new family of viruses, the Circinoviridae.

The route of TTV transmission appears to be parenteral, although the high prevalence of TTV in individuals without a history of exposure supports the probability of a nonparenteral route as well. Domesticated farm animals may represent a reservoir of infection, with evidence of TTV DNA in 19–30%.

EPIDEMIOLOGY

The prevalence of the various types of hepatitis varies by age and by geographic location. In children in the United States, approximately 70–80% of all cases of viral hepatitis are related to HAV, 5–30%

to HBV, and 5–15% to HCV. In adults, approximately 30% of all cases of viral hepatitis are related to HAV, 40–50% to HBV, 25% to HCV, and 1% to HDV. Hepatitis caused by HEV occurs only in persons who have traveled to endemic areas (outside the United States). All five viruses cause acute hepatitis of variable clinical severity. HBV, HCV, and HDV infections can result in **chronic hepatitis,** or a **chronic carrier** state, which contributes significantly to morbidity and mortality rates and to the perpetuation and dissemination of the virus within a susceptible population. Definitive correlation of HGV and TTV infection with significant acute or chronic liver disease remains speculative.

Hepatitis A. HAV causes acute hepatitis that occurs in outbreaks as well as sporadically without seasonal variation. Chronic hepatitis with persistent viremia does not occur. The incidence of hepatitis A infection is highest among children 5–14 years of age, but most children have asymptomatic or unrecognized infections. Children shed HAV for longer periods than do adults and are important reservoirs of infection among adults, who are more likely to develop symptomatic disease with infection. HAV prevalence is directly related to age and inversely related to income and household size. The prevalence of HAV antibody in the United States is 9% among children 6–11 years of age, 19% among persons 20–29 years of age, 33% among persons 40–49 years of age, and 75% among those >70 years of age. Prevalence is 70% among Mexican Americans, 39% among non-Hispanic black persons, and 23% among non-Hispanic white persons. The national incidence is 10 cases per 100,000 population, with approximately 50% of cases occurring in 11 Western states that represent approximately 22% of the U.S. population (Fig. 78–1).

Hepatitis A is endemic worldwide except in the United States, Canada, Western Europe, Scandinavia, Australia, New Zealand, and Japan; its endemicity is of particular importance to travelers (Chapter 104). In developing countries, infection is most common in the first decade of life.

Hepatitis B. HBV causes both acute and chronic hepatitis and has the highest morbidity and mortality of the hepatotropic viruses. The disease is infectious if HBsAg is present in serum, either because of acute infection or as chronic carriage, which is defined as having HBsAg in the serum for ≥6 months. Worldwide, 5% of the population has chronic HBV infection. The prevalence rates are up to 15% in endemic areas of eastern Asia and sub-Saharan Africa and among Alaskan Eskimos and Pacific Islanders.

Populations at particular risk of postnatal acquisition of HBV infection include household contacts and sex partners of chronic carriers of HBsAg; health care professionals and other persons exposed to blood and body fluids; persons with hemophilia or requiring hemodialysis; clients and staff of institutions for developmentally disabled persons; residents of, travelers to, or refugees and adoptees from endemic areas; and persons with high-risk social behaviors such as having sexual relations with multiple partners or injecting illicit drugs. The relative risk among these groups is reflected in an increased prevalence of serologic markers for HBV infection (Table 78–4). In the general population, the prevalence of hepatitis B infection begins to increase steadily beginning at 12–18 years of age. In approximately one third of acute cases, no risk factor is identified.

Chronic hepatitis B infection occurs in approximately 5–10% of adults with acute HBV infections, compared with 60–90% of infants born to HBsAg-positive mothers. These chronic carriers constitute the major reservoir of HBV. **Carriers** with no symptoms have positive results on tests for HBsAg but no other biochemical evidence or serologic markers of active viral replication. Unless there is reactivation of the HBV or superinfection with HDV, the clinical course is usually uncomplicated. Cirrhosis develops in 25%

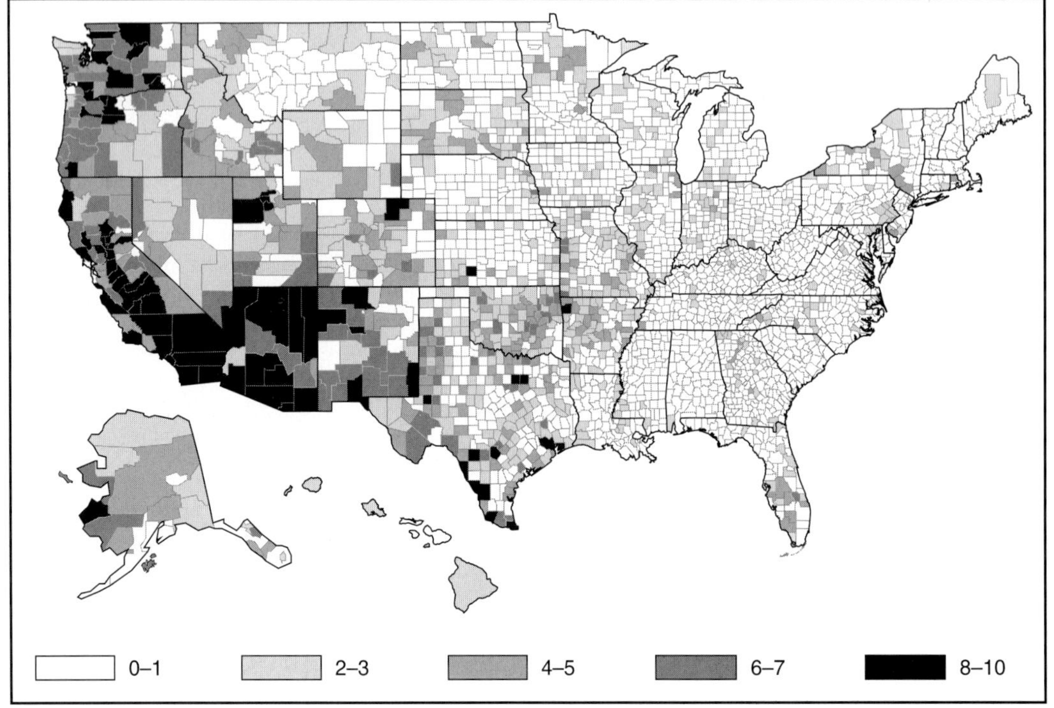

FIGURE 78–1. Incidence of hepatitis A in the United States, shown by the number of years from 1987 to 1997 that the incidence by county exceeded the national average of 10 cases per 100,000 population. (From National Notifiable Diseases Surveillance System.)

TABLE 78–4. Prevalence of Hepatitis B Serologic Markers in Various Population Groups

Population Group	Prevalence of Serologic Markers of HBV Infection	
	HBsAg (%)	Any Marker (%)
Immigrants and refugees from areas of high HBV endemicity	13	70–85
Alaskan Natives, Pacific Islanders	5–15	40–70
Clients in institutions for developmentally disabled persons	10–20	35–80
Users of illicit parenterally taken drugs	7	60–80
Sexually active men who have sex with men	6	35–80
Household contacts of HBV carriers	3–6	30–60
Patients in hemodialysis units	3–10	20–80
Health care workers with frequent contact with blood	1–2	15–30
Prisoners (male)	1–8	10–80
Staff of institutions for developmentally disabled persons	1	10–25
Heterosexuals with multiple partners	0.5	5–20
Health care workers with no or infrequent contact with blood	0.3	3–10
General population of black persons	0.9	14
General population of white persons	0.2	3

Adapted from Centers for Disease Control and Prevention: Protection against viral hepatitis: Recommendations of the Immunization Practices Advisory Committee (ACIP). *MMWR Morb Mortal Wkly Rep* 1990;39 (RR-2):5.

of HBsAg-positive persons who have evidence of chronic hepatitis; these persons are also at risk of developing hepatocellular carcinoma. This risk is of particular concern in perinatally acquired infections because of the lifelong risk of developing cancer. Childhood hepatitis B vaccination in Taiwan has already been shown (Chang, 1997) to decrease the incidence of hepatocellular carcinoma in vaccinees.

Hepatitis C. HCV is contracted largely through parenteral exposure and is historically responsible for most cases of posttransfusion hepatitis. In the United States, HCV has been implicated in 20–40% of cases of acute infectious hepatitis and as many as 85% of cases classified as non-A, non-B hepatitis. This estimate may be low because variants of HCV are not detected by existing immunoassays. From 0.5% to 2% of the adult population, or about 4 million persons, in the United States are seropositive for antibodies to HCV, with two thirds among persons 30–50 years of age. Infection is infrequent among children, with a seroprevalence of 0.2% in children <12 years of age and of 0.4% in adolescents 12–19 years of age. Risk factors include use of injecting drugs, needle-stick exposure, transfusion, chronic hemodialysis, and occupational or sexual exposure. Approximately 10% of persons with HCV infections have no identified risk factor.

Approximately 85% of infected persons become chronically infected, with an estimated 100 million carriers worldwide. The incidence of ongoing hepatitis among persons who are chronically infected with HCV may be as high as 50%, but there may be a period of 10–20 years of clinical quiescence before the development of symptomatic cirrhosis, which occurs in approximately 20% of persons with chronic HCV infection. There are approximately 20,000–30,000 new cases diagnosed each year in the United States. HCV infection and cirrhosis are significant risk factors for hepatocellular carcinoma (Chapter 4).

Hepatitis D. HDV infection cannot occur without the coexistence of HBV. Simultaneous acute coinfection is more common in developing countries. Superinfection with HDV in association with chronic HBV infection can exacerbate previously stable HBV liver disease or induce a more fulminant course. The incidence of HDV infection is higher in persons with fulminant hepatitis B than in those with a less aggressive course. In contrast to coinfection, superinfection with HDV frequently leads to chronic HDV hepatitis, which can progress to cirrhosis. Persons at risk include those with injecting drug use and those with hemophilia. HDV is associated with approximately 6% of all cases of chronic viral hepatitis in the United States. Perinatal HDV infection, although rare, has been described. Epidemics of HDV-associated fulminant hepatitis have been reported in Brazil, Venezuela, and Colombia. A particularly severe form of childhood hepatitis in the Amazon basin and in northern Colombia has been associated with HDV superinfection.

Hepatitis E. HEV infection is generally limited to certain developing geographic areas. Areas of high prevalence include Africa, Central America, the subcontinent of India, and central and southeastern Asia, where epidemics may result from contamination of drinking water. Hepatitis E is much more common in adults than in children. In endemic areas the seroprevalence is about 5% in children and 10–40% in adults, although these rates may vary among different geographic locations.

Endemic hepatitis E has not been recognized in the United States or Western Europe, but cases have been reported in the United States in travelers returning from endemic areas. In the nonendemic regions, HEV accounts for fewer than 1% of cases of acute viral hepatitis.

Hepatitis G. Epidemiologic studies are ongoing to define the role of HGV in clinical liver disease, but HGV is probably not an important etiologic agent in acute non-A-E hepatitis. Although this virus has been identified in about 20% of cases of posttransfusion non-A-E hepatitis, the disease is usually mild, with elevated aminotransferase values in only a few cases and with clearance of virus in the majority of immunocompetent persons. HGV has also been detected in persons with fulminant hepatitis, but confirmation as the causative agent is lacking. The role of HGV in other diseases such as hepatitis-associated aplastic anemia, hepatocellular carcinoma, and non-Hodgkin's lymphoma is also under investigation.

Currently it appears that HGV is not a classic hepatitis virus and is responsible for significant liver disease in only a small percentage of infected individuals. Also poorly defined is the role of HGV in the progression of liver disease in persons with chronic HBV or HCV infection.

TT Virus. Evidence of TTV infection is frequent in the general population. Direct evidence of an association of TTV infection with acute or chronic liver disease is currently lacking.

PATHOGENESIS

Viral hepatitis is associated with prolific virus production, with $>10^9$ virions produced per day for HBV and $>10^{12}$ virions produced per day with HCV. The hepatocellular damage caused by infection with the hepatitis viruses is related more to the immune response than to a direct cytopathic effect of the virus. In acute hepatitis with recovery from infection with hepatitis A, B, C, or D virus, an efficient immune response eradicates the virus, most likely through cytotoxic T-cell lysis. In chronic hepatitis a defective or inefficient immune response may allow the virus to persist with ongoing hepatocellular necrosis, which reflects various degrees of T-lymphocyte cytolysis of those hepatocytes with viral replication. With chronic hepatitis B, the viral DNA may become incorporated into the host genome. A superimposed insult, such as HDV infection, can cause reactivation of HBV, which has a high mutation rate from errors in reverse transcription of RNA from the viral DNA during viral replication. As an RNA virus with RNA-dependent DNA polymerase, HCV is also prone to mutations. Mutant variants may evade the immune response and may persist, contributing to the development of chronic infection even if wild-type virus is effectively cleared.

The precise pathogenic mechanism for the extremely high incidence, 60–90%, of chronicity of perinatally acquired hepatitis B remains unclear but may be the result of the immaturity of the neonatal immune system, the immunosuppressive effects of α-fetoprotein, a state of immune tolerance to the HBcAg and HBeAg induced by prenatal transplacental exposure to the HBeAg, or a combination of these phenomena. The propensity for chronic hepatitis B to develop also appears to be higher among immunocompromised persons, such as renal transplant recipients, than among other groups.

SYMPTOMS AND CLINICAL MANIFESTATIONS

There is considerable overlap in the clinical hepatitis caused by the five viruses. Manifestations can range from asymptomatic infection with seroconversion, to subacute anicteric illness, to acute icteric illness, and to fulminant illness, which may be fatal. Icteric disease accounts for only 20–50% of all infections. In general, infection is mild or asymptomatic in infants and younger children. Jaundice may or may not be apparent and when present may wax and wane or may persist for weeks. The clinical course is divided into preicteric and icteric phases. Symptoms during the **preicteric phase** are often nonspecific and include fever, headache, fatigue, anorexia, vomiting, and abdominal discomfort. Hepatomegaly with or without splenomegaly may be present. Dark urine may be noted before clinical jaundice. The **icteric phase** is usually accompanied by an abatement of symptoms, particularly in children. Adults may have a brief exacerbation of preicteric symptoms. Other signs and symptoms variably seen during the icteric phase include persistent lassitude, pruritus, acholic stools, and weight loss. This phase is often shorter in children, lasting 1–2 weeks, compared with 3–4 weeks in adults.

Fulminant hepatitis is uncommon either at presentation or as a sequela of infection with the hepatotropic viruses, but when it occurs, it is associated with a very high mortality rate. A fulminant clinical course with severely compromised hepatic function may be manifested clinically as hepatic encephalopathy, gastrointestinal bleeding from esophageal varices and coagulopathy, and profound jaundice.

Chronic hepatitis, which occurs with HBV and HCV infection, may result in vague symptoms of fatigue and anorexia or may be asymptomatic. Jaundice is variable, but the incidence increases with progressive disease. With the development of fibrosis and eventually cirrhosis, other signs of chronic liver disease, such as telangiectasia and palmar erythema, become apparent. Eventually, evidence of portal hypertension, including ascites and splenomegaly, may develop.

Hepatitis A. The clinical course of hepatitis A may last a few weeks or months (Fig. 78–2). The incubation period is relatively short, 2–7 weeks, with an average of 4 weeks. Infection in infants and children is asymptomatic in 70% of cases. Symptomatic disease includes abrupt onset of nonspecific symptoms of fever, malaise, anorexia, nausea, abdominal discomfort, and a mild anicteric course. Jaundice develops in <10% of children <6 years of age, 40–50% of children 6–14 years of age, and 70–80% of children >14 years of age. The duration of jaundice is brief in children but in adults is more prolonged and is associated with more severe and prolonged constitutional symptoms. The acute illness usually resolves within 2 months without chronic sequelae. Approximately 10–15% of adults will have prolonged cholestatic hepatitis, or relapsing hepatitis, lasting up to 6 months. Although HAV rarely causes fulminant hepatitis in individuals without underlying chronic

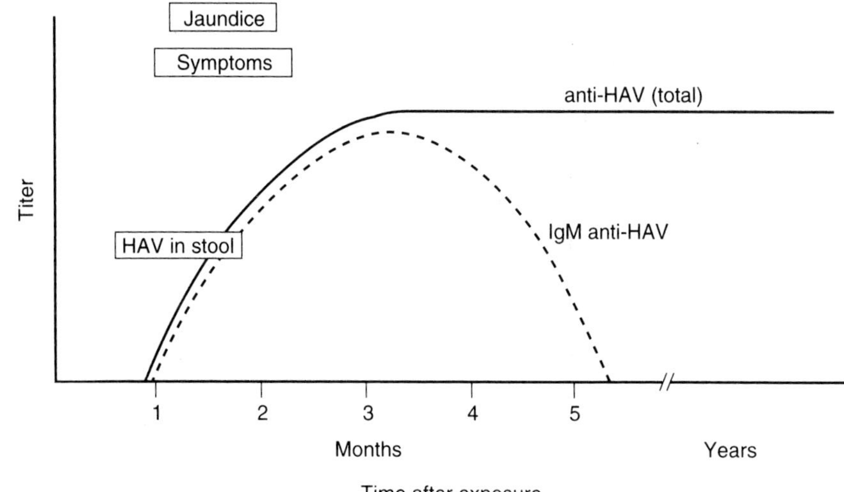

FIGURE 78–2. Acute hepatitis A infection. (See Table 78-5 for serologic terminology.)

liver disease, those with chronic HCV infection appear to have a substantial risk of fulminant hepatitis and death associated with HAV superinfection.

Hepatitis B. The incubation period in hepatitis B is 2–6 months, with an average of 4 months. Prodromal symptoms suggestive of hepatitis B include urticaria, arthritis, and arthralgia. The presence and duration of clinical jaundice vary and may persist for weeks or months. In contrast to HAV infection, in which symptoms develop acutely, hepatitis B is characterized by an insidious onset. The clinical outcome can be resolution (Fig. 78–3*A*), chronic HBV infection (Fig. 78–3*B*), or, in a small percentage of cases, fulminant hepatitis. Chronic hepatitis B may be clinically inapparent, or nonspecific symptoms may persist.

Hepatitis C. The incubation period of hepatitis C is 2–20 weeks, with an average of 7–9 weeks. The onset of clinical features is insidious and variable, and the disease is usually anicteric with only mild and nonspecific symptoms. Frequently there is only biochemical evidence of infection with elevated aminotransferase levels. Symptomatic hepatitis occurs occasionally, and fulminant hepatitis and hepatic failure related to acute HCV infection have been reported. The development of chronic infection, which may occur in as many as 85% of persons with acute hepatitis C, is often asymptomatic or accompanied by mild complaints, as in hepatitis B.

Hepatitis D. Hepatitis D occurs as coinfection with acute hepatitis B (Fig. 78–4*A*) or as superinfection in a person with HBsAg positivity (Fig. 78–4*B*). In the presence of HDV infection, the HBV-associated liver disease typically progresses more rapidly than when HBV infection occurs alone, and chronic hepatitis and fulminant hepatitis are more likely to develop. Coinfection has an incubation period similar to that of hepatitis B, with more severe clinical symptoms than with HBV alone, although it usually is self-limited and resolves. The rate of chronic HBV infection is increased to 70%, compared with 5–10% with HBV infection alone, and the mortality rate is increased to 2–20%, compared with 0.2–1% with HBV infection alone. **Superinfection** with HDV has an incubation period of 4–8 weeks and may result in exacerbation of the underlying HBV infection with recurrence of clinical hepatitis.

Hepatitis E. The incubation period of hepatitis E is 2–8 weeks, with an average of 6 weeks. The clinical presentation of HEV infection is similar to that of hepatitis A, with fever, malaise,

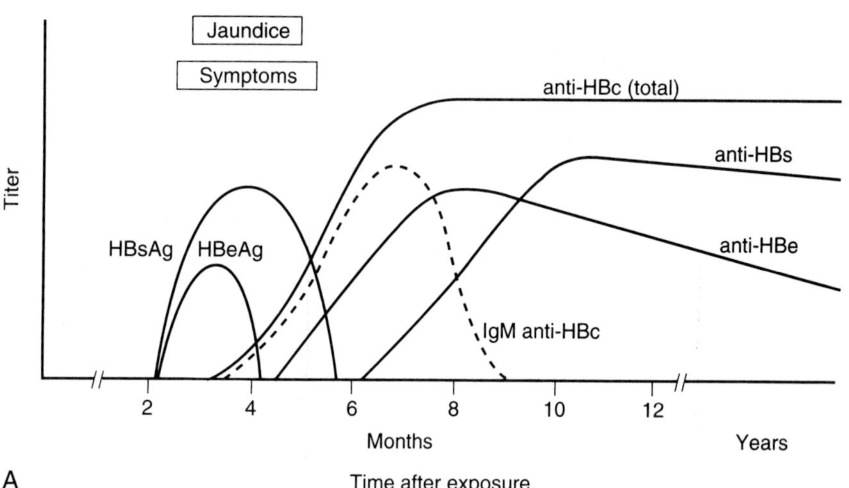

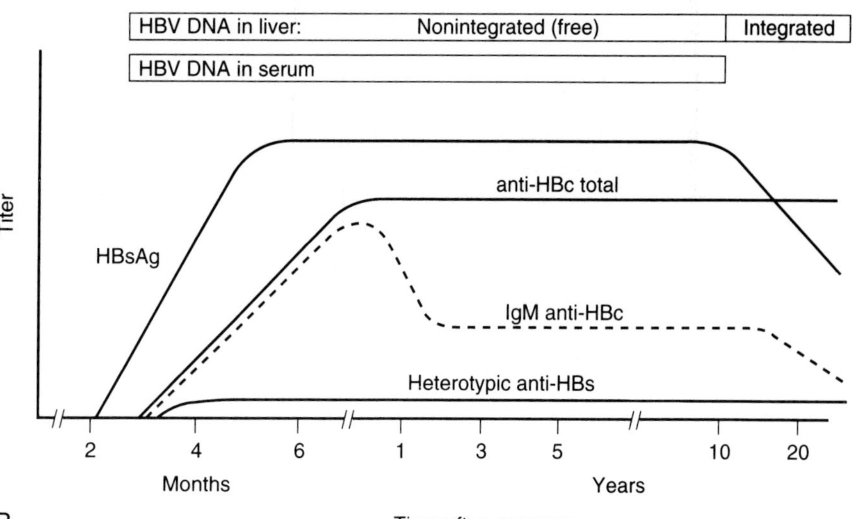

FIGURE 78–3. A, Acute hepatitis B infection. **B,** Acute hepatitis B infection leading to a chronic carrier state. (See Table 78–5 for serologic terminology.)

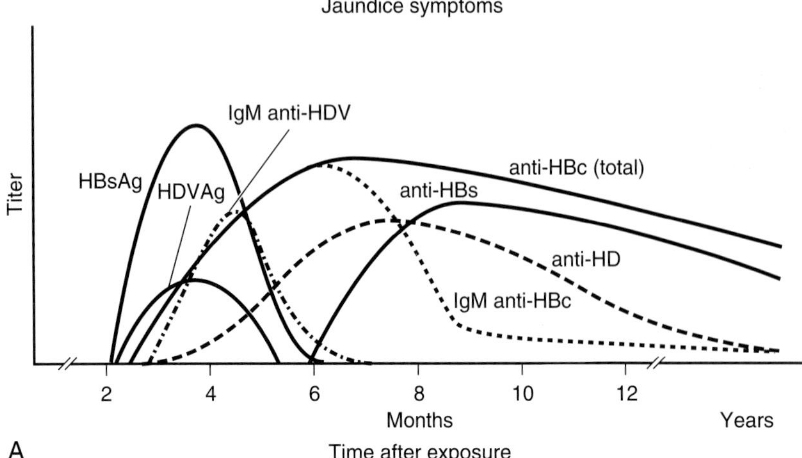

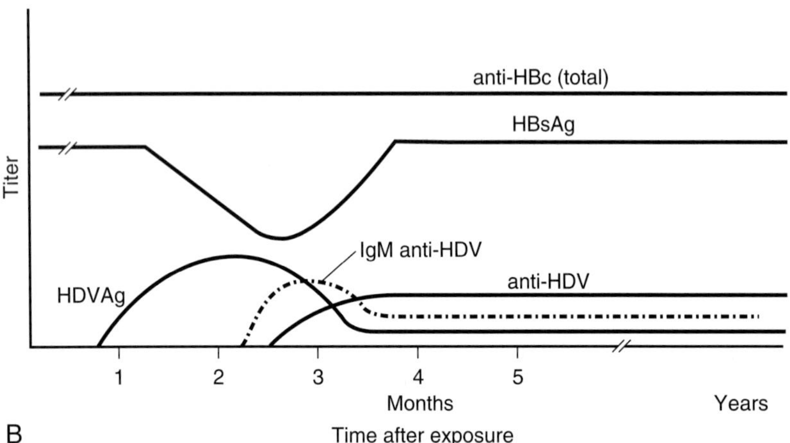

FIGURE 78–4. A, Simultaneous hepatitis D virus and hepatitis B virus infection. **B,** Superinfection of hepatitis B virus carrier leading to persistent hepatitis D virus coinfection. (See Table 78–5 for serologic terminology.)

anorexia, abdominal pain, and jaundice (Fig. 78–5). It is usually seen in adolescents and adults and is self-limited. Although no carrier state has been identified, fulminant hepatitis has been described, particularly in pregnant women, with a mortality rate during the third trimester that can reach 25%, compared with a mortality of much less than 1% among nonpregnant women and among men.

DIAGNOSIS

These five viruses cause hepatitis with overlapping manifestations that cannot be distinguished on clinical or epidemiologic grounds but can be diagnosed by serologic testing. Most cases of hepatitis remain undiagnosed, especially in children, because the symptoms are relatively mild and often nonspecific and therefore diagnostic testing is not performed. Asymptomatic cases may be evident only by elevated aminotransferase levels and by seroconversion.

In children especially, the asymptomatic or insidious onset of both acute and chronic hepatitis requires a high degree of awareness for diagnosis. Recognition of which children are at risk may be the most important aspect of diagnosis. Fatigue is the most common symptom. Varying degrees of anorexia, nausea, abdominal discomfort, or any degree of hepatomegaly or jaundice should prompt laboratory evaluation of aminotransferase levels, which are usually abnormal during acute infection (Fig. 78–6).

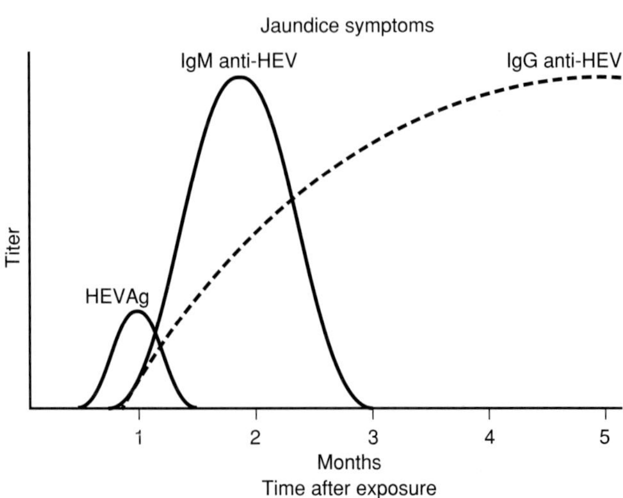

FIGURE 78–5. Acute hepatitis E infection. (See Table 78–5 for serologic terminology.)

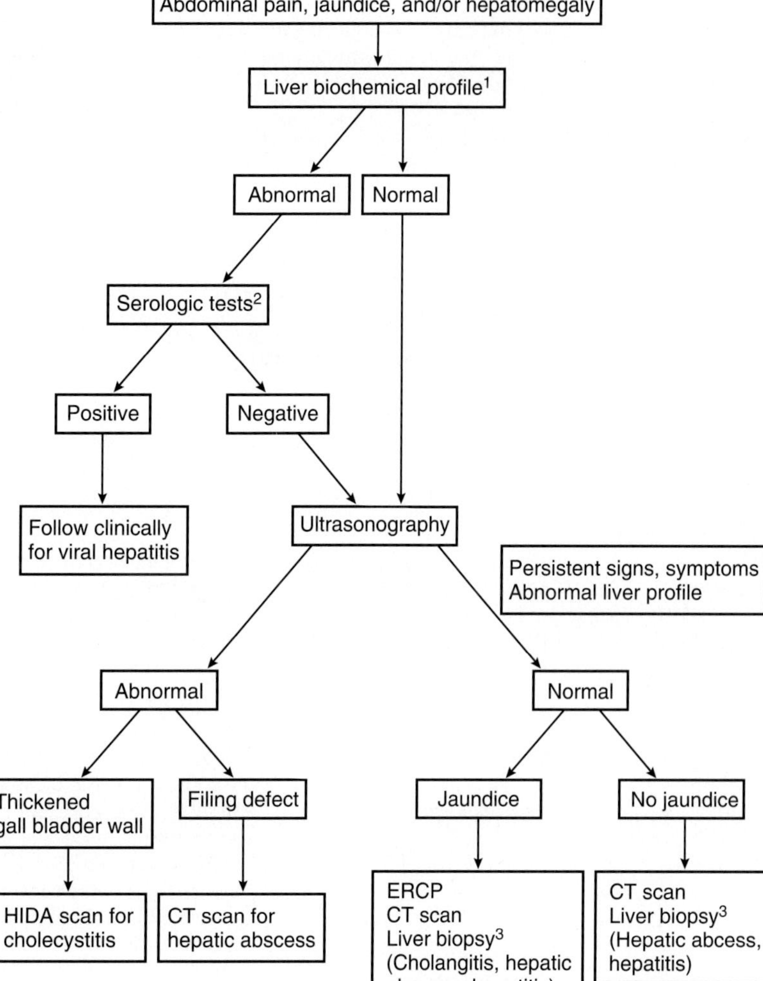

FIGURE 78–6. Evaluation for hepatobiliary disease related to infection. HIDA = hepato-iminodiacetic acid (scan); ERCP = endoscopic retrograde cholangiopancreatography.

Differential Diagnosis

The differential diagnosis of acute viral hepatitis includes other hepatobiliary infections and conditions, specifically cholecystitis, cholangitis, and choledocholithiasis, which usually have an acute presentation. They are diagnosed by specific imaging studies, such as ultrasonography and radioisotopic scanning (Chapter 80). Many viruses may cause mild and usually self-limited hepatic inflammation as part of systemic infection (Table 78–3). If the clinical presentation is insidious in onset or the person presents with chronic indolent hepatitis, one must consider other causes of chronic or subclinical hepatic inflammation, including drug- or toxin-induced hepatitis, autoimmune hepatitis, or metabolic liver diseases such as α_1-antitrypsin deficiency or Wilson's disease. The presence of hepatic inflammation (hepatitis) with or without cholestasis is established by routine biochemical tests, whereas serologic markers identify the specific viral etiologic agent. Viral cultures are not used in the diagnosis of viral hepatitis. Histopathologic assessment of liver biopsy material is usually reserved for management decisions and to determine prognosis in chronic hepatitis.

Laboratory Evaluation

The initial laboratory evaluation should include biochemical tests for hepatic inflammation and tests of liver function, CBC with WBC count differential, and urinalysis. **Alanine aminotransferase (ALT [SGPT])** and **aspartate aminotransferase (AST [SGOT])** levels are elevated and roughly reflect the degree of parenchymal inflammation. Elevated **alkaline phosphatase, 5′-nucleotidase,** and **total and direct (conjugated) bilirubin** levels are indicators of the degree of cholestasis, which may be a result of hepatocellular and bile duct damage or of biliary tract disease. Screening hepatic function tests include determinations of serum ammonia albumin levels and of prothrombin time (PT). If the PT is prolonged, clotting factor levels, specifically factors V and VII, provide a sensitive indicator of hepatic synthetic function and have prognostic significance in severe hepatitis. If the degree of cellular injury is severe, as suggested by extreme elevation of aminotransferase levels, an increased serum ammonia level, prolonged PT, or a depressed serum albumin level, then clinical and laboratory parameters should be monitored closely for possible progression to fulminant hepatic failure.

Microbiologic Evaluation

Serologic markers are useful not only in establishing the cause but also in monitoring the clinical course and assessing the response to treatment of chronic hepatitis (Tables 78–5 and 78–6).

Hepatitis A. **Anti-HAV** is detected early in the course of the disease (Fig. 78–2). During acute infection most anti-HAV is IgM. The IgM anti-HAV may persist for up to 20 weeks and then wanes, whereas IgG anti-HAV persists for life as a serologic marker for past infection and provides protective immunity to HAV.

Hepatitis B. Several antigen and antibody markers for HBV aid in diagnosis and in defining the stage of illness and the degree of chronicity and infectivity (Fig. 78–7). HBsAg indicates HBV infection and is present in approximately 90% of persons at the time of initial presentation. It may be detectable 1–4 weeks after parenteral exposure and approximately 8 weeks after oral exposure, during the incubation period and several weeks before an increase in aminotransferase levels or clinical jaundice is noted. In acute, resolving hepatitis B infection, a test for HBsAg shows negative results soon after the onset of jaundice.

Anti-HBc is the first detectable antibody (Fig. 78–3*A*). The IgM antibody appears 1 week or longer after the onset of hepatitis, and the level remains elevated for several months before declining. IgG anti-HBc persists for years. The presence of IgM anti-HBc can differentiate recent from remote HBV infection and may be the only detectable marker during the **window phase** of acute infection, when tests for HBsAg show negative results and **anti-**

TABLE 78–5. Terminology of Serologic Markers for the Diagnosis of Viral Hepatitis

Abbreviation	Name	Clinical Significance
Hepatitis A Virus		
HAV	Hepatitis A virus	The etiologic agent of hepatitis A
Anti-HAV	Total antibody to HAV	Detectable at onset of symptoms (IgM) Lifetime persistence (IgG)
IgM anti-HAV	IgM antibody to HAV	Detectable at onset of symptoms Indicates recent HAV infection Detectable up to 4–6 mo after infection
Hepatitis B Virus		
HBV	Hepatitis B virus	Etiologic agent of hepatitis B Also known as the Dane particle
HBsAg	Hepatitis B surface antigen	Major envelope protein of HBV (formerly known as Australia antigen) Detectable in large quantities in serum of acutely infected people or chronic HBsAg carriers Several subtypes identified
HBeAg	Hepatitis B e antigen	Soluble HBV antigen Associated with HBV replication, high titer of HBsAg, high infectivity of serum, and chronic HBsAg carriage with chronic active hepatitis
HBcAg	Hepatitis B core antigen	Major structural protein of the HBV capsid No commercial test available
Anti-HBs	Antibody to HBsAg	Indicates past infection with immunity to HBV, passive antibody from HBIG, or immune response from hepatitis B vaccine
Anti-HBe	Antibody to HBeAg	Presence in serum of chronic HBsAg carrier indicates a lower titer of HBsAg and lower risk of infectivity
Anti-HBc	Antibody to HBcAg	Indicates prior infection with HBV at some undefined time
IgM anti-HBc	IgM antibodies to HBcAg	Indicates recent infection with HBV Detectable up to 4–6 mo after infection
Hepatitis C Virus		
HCV	Hepatitis C virus	Etiologic agent of parenterally transmitted non-A, non-B hepatitis
Anti-HCV	Antibody to HCV	Indicates past infection with HCV
Hepatitis D Virus		
HDV	Hepatitis D virus	Etiologic agent of hepatitis D Indicates acute coinfection or superinfection
Anti-HDV	Antibody to HDV	Indicates superinfection or chronic infection with HDV
IgM anti-HDV	IgM antibodies to HDV	Indicates acute or chronic HDV infection
Hepatitis E Virus		
HEV	Hepatitis E virus	Etiologic agent of hepatitis E
Anti-HEV	Antibody to HEV	Indicates past HEV infection
IgM anti-HEV	IgM antibodies to HEV	Indicates recent HEV infection
Hepatitis G Virus		
HGV	Hepatitis G virus	Etiologic agent of hepatitis G
GBV-C	GB virus type C	
Anti-HGV	Antibody to HGV	Indicates recent or past HGV infection
Anti-HGV-E2	Antibody to E2	Antibody to recombinant envelope protein and associated with viral clearance

There are no commercially available tests for hepatitis E virus.

TABLE 78–6. Interpretation of Serologic Markers for Viral Hepatitis

Viral Infection and Clinical Setting	Serologic Marker						
			anti-HBc		anti-HAV		
	HBsAg	anti-HBs	Total	IgM	Total	IgM	anti-HCV
Hepatitis A							
Recent acute infection					+	+	
Past infection					+	–	
Hepatitis B							
Early acute infection	+	–	–	–			
Acute infection	+	–	+	+			
Acute infection ("core window")	–	–	+	+			
Past infection (immune)	–	+	+	–			
Chronic hepatitis B carrier	+	–	+	–			
Immunization without infection	–	+	–	–			
Hepatitis C							
Acute, past, or chronic infection*							+
Other NANBNC hepatitis	–	–	–	–			–

+ = present; – = not present; NANBNC = non-A, non-B, non-C.
*Interpretation depends on the clinical setting and liver biochemical profile.

HBs has not yet appeared. A low titer of IgG anti-HBc in the presence of anti-HBs suggests remote infection. The persistence of IgM anti-HBc or high titers of IgG anti-HBc, usually with persistent HBsAg and in the absence of anti-HBs, implies an ongoing viral infection. Healthy carriers of HBsAg generally have negative results on tests for anti-HBc. Anti-HBs appears later in the course of the illness, often 2–8 weeks after HBsAg is no longer detectable, and suggests both recovery from infection and immunity. Anti-HBs is present in approximately 80% of persons with acute hepatitis B who eventually become HBsAg-negative. In the other 20%, the anti-HBs titer may be too low for detection. From 5% to 10% of chronic carriers of HBsAg may have positive anti-HBs test results as well.

HBeAg and **anti-HBe** reflect infectivity and are not used routinely for diagnosis. The presence of HBeAg correlates with viral replication, is a marker for infectivity, and, if detectable for >10 weeks, suggests chronicity. The presence of anti-HBe and the disappearance of HBeAg imply low infectivity. Other serum markers that reflect the degree of viral replication include HBV DNA and DNA polymerase.

The persistence of HBsAg for >3 months, usually in the absence of anti-HBs, suggests the development of chronic hepatitis (Fig. 78–3*B*). Chronic carriers without symptoms typically have a normal liver biochemical profile and absent or low levels of serum markers of viral replication, such as HBeAg, HBV DNA, and DNA polymerase. Patients with ongoing hepatitis demonstrate variable elevations in aminotransferase and bilirubin levels and the presence of serologic markers of viral synthesis and infectivity.

Amplification of the HBV DNA genome by using PCR provides a sensitive assay for HBV in both serum and liver tissue, even in the presence of anti-HBc and anti-HBs. This assay has been particularly useful in studying the epidemiology of hepatocellular carcinoma in persons with persistent HBV infection.

Hepatitis C. **Anti-HCV** is an antibody to a nonstructural peptide of the virus. There is a long lag time from infection to seroconversion, so results of tests for anti-HCV are usually negative during the acute illness. Anti-HCV first appears as late as 3–6 months after infection and 5–20 weeks after the onset of clinical symptoms. In posttransfusion hepatitis C, the mean interval from exposure to the detection of antibody is 15 weeks, with a range of 4–32 weeks. Therefore this serologic marker is more useful for diagnosis of chronic rather than acute HCV infection. The presence of anti-HCV signals past infection and possible infectivity but does not necessarily indicate continuing viral replication. Anti-HCV is not protective and does not confer immunity. Anti-HCV may wane after acute infection resolves.

Since the first EIA for anti-HCV came into use, several more sensitive assays have been developed. False-positive test results have been obtained for persons with autoimmune hepatitis and high levels of immunoglobulin. A **recombinant immunoblot assay (RIBA),** a variant of the immunoblot (Chapter 11), is currently in use as a confirmatory test. If the EIA result is positive and the RIBA result is negative, the person is considered to have a false-positive EIA result.

RT-PCR assay allows detection of even very small quantities of the HCV RNA genome, which would otherwise be undetectable, similar to the situation for HBV. Measurements of HCV RNA are now available commercially and are used for diagnosis and to monitor response to therapy.

Hepatitis D. The diagnosis of HDV infection can be established by serologic tests including those for anti-HDV IgM and IgG, HDV antigen, and HDV RNA. With HDV and HBV coinfection (Fig. 78–4*A*), both HBsAg and HDV antigen appear simultaneously, before an increase in aminotransferase levels and the onset of clinical disease. The elevations in aminotransferase levels may be biphasic. IgM anti-HDV is detectable soon after the appearance of clinical disease, followed by a rise in IgG anti-HDV levels. Although the hepatitis may be severe, HDV coinfection is usually self-limited, as verified by the development of IgM anti-HBc and subsequently anti-HBs, as well as by the disappearance of HDV antigen.

Superinfection with HDV in association with chronic HBV infection is usually heralded by an exacerbation of clinical symptoms or a sudden deterioration in results of biochemical or functional liver tests (Fig. 78–4*B*). During the acute phase, both HDV antigen and HBsAg are detectable, but IgM anti-HBc is absent. In

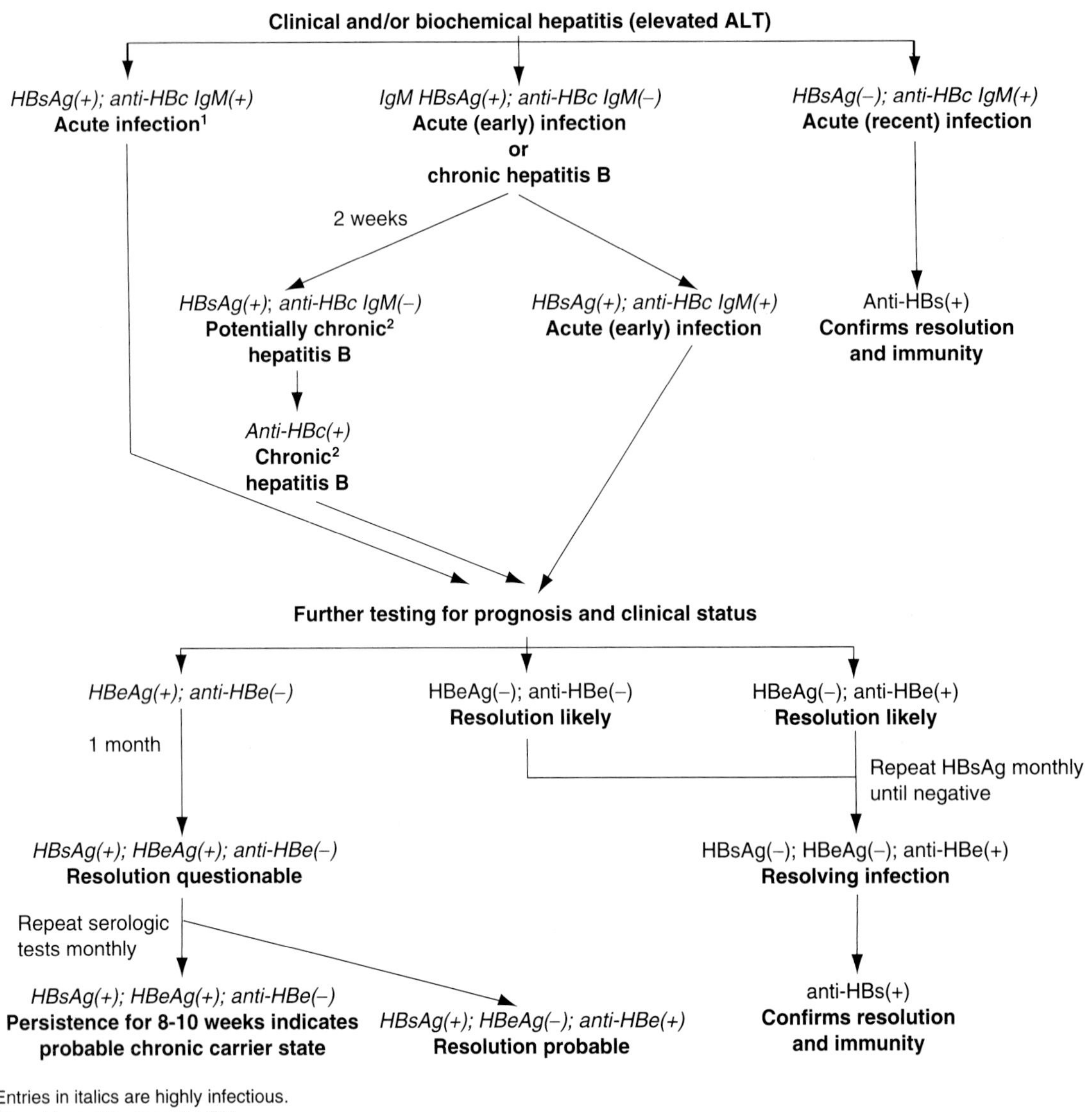

FIGURE 78–7. Serologic testing to distinguish acute and chronic hepatitis B infection. ALT = alanine aminotransferase; + = positive; – = negative. (See Table 78–5 for serologic terminology.)

contrast to coinfection, superinfection with HDV commonly leads to chronic HDV hepatitis characterized by persistence of HDV antigen and by high titers of anti-HDV (both IgM and IgG). Superinfection can usually be distinguished from coinfection by the absence of IgM anti-HBc, which suggests HDV superinfection in association with an earlier or chronic HBV infection.

Hepatitis E. Diagnostic tests for HEV infection include serologic assays for anti-HEV IgM and IgG antibodies and detection of HEV-RNA in serum using RT-PCR (Fig. 78–5). There are also methods for molecular and immune electron microscopy detection of the virus in stool, but these are tedious and rarely used for clinical diagnosis. HEV antigen can be detected in the liver, but the test is not used in the clinical diagnosis of HEV infection.

The most commonly used serologic test is an EIA for antibodies targeted against structural proteins of the virus. IgM anti-HEV appears early in the illness and precedes anti-HEV IgG by a few days. The IgM antibody usually disappears by 4–5 months, whereas the IgG antibody can persist for years.

Hepatitis G. HGV genomic RNA can be detected by commercially available RT-PCR assays. Anti-HGV antibodies against nonstructural and structural proteins of the virus have been identified. Most currently available immunodiagnostic assays use antigens derived from structural genes such as a recombinant membrane protein E2, a surface protein that may also be a target for host humoral immune response. The appearance of these antibodies is often associated with clearance of detectable HGV.

TT Virus. Currently the presence of TT virus is determined by identifying the viral DNA in serum using PCR.

Diagnostic Imaging

Diagnostic imaging studies are not frequently used in the evaluation of viral hepatitis, with the exception of ultrasonography, which is useful in excluding biliary tract disease (Chapter 80) from the differential diagnosis.

Pathologic Findings

A liver biopsy is usually not indicated in acute viral hepatitis because the histopathologic findings are nonspecific and of little diagnostic or prognostic value. In general, there is a necrotizing inflammatory process characterized by various degrees of diffuse lobular and portal tract inflammation and degenerating hepatocytes. The mononuclear cell infiltrate in the sinusoids and portal tracts is predominantly lymphocytic, and the limiting plate is usually well defined. The exception is hepatitis A, which is characterized histologically by a plasma cell infiltrate and **piecemeal necrosis,** an inflammatory necrosis that violates the limiting plate of the portal area. **Confluent necrosis** is associated with increased morbidity and mortality, and **bridging necrosis,** from portal tract to portal tract, may suggest progression to chronic hepatitis.

A liver biopsy is indicated in the evaluation of chronic hepatitis if the etiologic agent is in question or if therapeutic intervention is anticipated for chronic hepatitis B or hepatitis C. Histologically, chronic hepatitis may be generally classified as **chronic persistent,** having portal inflammation without piecemeal necrosis; **chronic lobular,** having lobular inflammation with liver cell necrosis but with minimal portal inflammation; or **chronic active,** having both portal and periportal inflammation with piecemeal necrosis. Specific histologic findings associated with hepatitis C include the presence of lymphoid follicles and aggregates in the portal tracts and microvesicular fat. In hepatitis B, hepatocytes may have a ground-glass appearance in which intracellular inclusions represent HBsAg. HBsAg appears brownish black with orcein staining. Immunoperoxidase staining can be used to demonstrate HBcAg in the hepatocyte nucleus and to demonstrate HBsAg in the cytoplasm (Plate 2H).

TREATMENT

There is no curative therapy for acute infectious hepatitis. General management includes early detection, supportive therapy, monitoring during the acute illness, determining resolution or persistence of the viral infection, and identifying others at risk to control spread of the virus. Hospitalization may be required for person with a clinically significant coagulopathy or pronounced clinical symptoms such as protracted vomiting and is indicated for those who have, or whose disease is progressing to, fulminant hepatic failure. After resolution of the clinical symptoms, periodic biochemical and serologic studies should be performed to document both biochemical resolution of the hepatitis and the convalescent serologic profile, particularly for HBV and HDV infections.

The results of initial trials using corticosteroids to suppress the inflammatory response have shown variable efficacy and a tendency toward enhanced viral replication with long-term use.

Interferon therapy has proved beneficial for HBV, HCV, and HDV chronic hepatitis, although the initial response rates and potential for relapse differ. Since the earlier trials, treatment regimens have been refined and other agents have been added to the therapeutic armamentarium. The overall goal of therapy is normalization of the biochemical profile (e.g., ALT value), a decrease in the necroinflammatory activity on biopsy, and clearance of the viremia. Response to therapy is categorized as follows: **sustained,** with no evidence of virus 6 months after the end of therapy; **relapse,** with recurrence of viremia, usually with a concurrent increase in the ALT value; and **no response.** Contraindications to interferon therapy include decompensated cirrhosis, cardiopulmonary disease, clinically significant psychiatric illness, and uncorrected thyroid disease. The adverse effects, including fever, headache, and myalgia, are usually self-limited. Unfortunately, although the sustained response is excellent in selected subpopulations of persons with chronic hepatitis, the overall response is still discouraging and supports the need for more effective treatments.

Hepatitis B. In chronic HBV infection, response is defined as loss of HBeAg, seroconversion to anti-HBe, and clearance of HBV DNA. Persons with a sustained response may also acquire anti-HBs as well. Interferon alfa-2b treatment (5 MU daily, or 10 MU three times a week for 16 weeks) of chronic hepatitis B infection in adults resulted in the loss of HBeAg and HBV DNA from the serum in 30–40% of persons. This result was associated with a transient increase in aminotransferase levels, eventually followed by a return to normal levels, improvement in liver histologic findings, and frequently clearance of HBsAg from the serum. Recurrence of infection in persons with a good initial response was unusual. In general, the best predictors of response were serum aminotransferase levels greater than twice normal and serologic markers of viral replication, including low to moderate levels of HBV DNA and the presence of HBeAg (Table 78–7). Longer treatment did not appear to increase the response rate. The current FDA-approved regimen for treatment of chronic hepatitis B is interferon alfa-2b 5 MU three times a week for 16 weeks.

Initial controlled trials (Lai et al, 1987) of recombinant interferon alfa-2b therapy for chronic hepatitis B in children in China demonstrated only a poor response as measured by seroconversion and decreased aminotransferase levels. In these series, however, most of the children were symptom-free HBV carriers who had acquired HBV infection early in life and had normal or low serum aminotransferase levels or high HBV DNA levels, both predictors of a poor response in adults. Results were more promising in a subsequent study (Ruiz-Moreno et al, 1991) of children in Spain with histologically verified chronic hepatitis, abnormal aminotransferase levels, and detectable HBeAg and HBV DNA. In the groups treated with interferon alfa-2b 5 or 10 MU/m^2 three times a week for 6 months, 50% showed HBV DNA negativity and had seroconversion to anti-HBe, in comparison with 17% of the control group. The responders also had an appreciable improvement in histologic activity. The children in this series most likely acquired the infection later in infancy or childhood, as reflected by a more active hepatitis and higher aminotransferase levels. This later acquisition of HBV infection, along with a higher dosage and longer duration of treatment, may explain the more favorable results. In a more recent multicenter study (Sokal et al, 1998) involving 144 children treated with interferon alfa-2b 6 MU/m^2 three times a week for 6 months, 26% of treated children lost HBeAg at 1 year, in comparison with 11% of untreated children. At 18 months, 33% of treated children lost HBeAg. This response rate is similar to that of adults.

TABLE 78–7. Predictors of Favorable Response to Interferon alfa Therapy for Chronic Hepatitis B (HBV) Infection

Infection acquired in adulthood
Female sex
Aminotransferase levels >2 times normal
Low-to-moderate levels of HBV DNA
HBeAg in serum
Active hepatitis on liver biopsy
Absence of HDV infection
Absence of HIV infection

An alternative therapy for chronic HBV infection is now available for persons who do not respond or who have a contraindication to interferon therapy. Lamivudine, a nucleoside analog that inhibits replication of the virus by interfering with DNA polymerase, given to adults as 100 mg daily orally results in seroconversion in 16–32% of persons, with significantly fewer side effects than interferon alfa-2b. Viral clearance is not as abrupt and is not usually accompanied by an increase in the ALT value. If anti-HBe does not develop during therapy, relapse may occur once lamivudine therapy is discontinued. In 15–35% of persons taking lamivudine, genotypic mutants in the **YMDD** (tyrosine, methionine, aspartate, aspartate) region of HBV DNA may develop, resulting in reduced sensitivity and reappearance of viremia. Neither the usefulness of continuing therapy in the presence of these escape mutants nor the optimal duration of therapy in general is known. The recommended dosage for children is 3 mg/kg daily, although published clinical trials are lacking. Studies of the efficacy and safety of long-term lamivudine therapy in children are ongoing.

Hepatitis C. The clinical efficacy of interferon alfa has also been demonstrated for chronic HCV infection, and HCV appears to be more sensitive than HBV to interferon. There are currently three forms of interferon available for the treatment of chronic HCV infection: interferon alfa-2a and alfa-2b (3 MU subcutaneously or intramuscularly three times a week) and consensus interferon (9 μg subcutaneously three times a week). Trials in adults using interferon alfa-2b 3 MU three times a week for 6 months have shown considerable improvement in aminotransferase levels and histologic activity in the liver in approximately 50% of subjects. Unfortunately, only 15–20% of persons have a sustained biochemical response, and the sustained viral response is only 10–20%. The biochemical sustained response increases to 20–30% with 12 months of therapy. Response to therapy can be predicted as early as 3 months into therapy. If the ALT value has not normalized and HCV RNA is still detectable, the person can be considered a nonresponder. Factors that predict a poor response include a high HCV RNA level, infection with HCV genotype 1, and the presence of cirrhosis. Genotype 1 is the most common genotype in the United States.

Recent trials have evaluated the efficacy of combination therapy using interferon alfa-2b and oral ribavirin. Therapy with ribavirin alone has no effect on HCV infection but in combination with interferon results in a sustained response rate of 49% when used for relapse during interferon therapy and a rate of 38% when used as the initial therapy. For genotypes 2 and 3, the sustained response rate for initial therapy is as high as 68%. Combination therapy with interferon and ribavirin (1,000–1,200 mg orally daily) is now the treatment of choice for chronic HCV infection (Fig. 78–8). This regimen may be further optimized by the use of pegylated interferon (attached to polyethylene glycol), which is currently under study. Attachment of interferon to polyethylene glycol allows for more sustained release, delivery of a greater amount of drug, and higher response rates.

Very few studies of the efficacy of interferon in children, and none evaluating combination therapy, have been published, and those reported in the literature were small and uncontrolled. The results of these studies have not been encouraging, with sustained response rates of 12–19%. In general, because chronic HCV infection seems to be a milder disease in children and the impact of therapy requiring multiple injections can be significant, the decision to treat at all is a difficult one. There is currently no evidence that treatment in childhood significantly alters disease progression in adulthood. Children with evidence of aggressive disease and documented histologic deterioration, as well as those with significant constitutional symptoms, should be offered treatment. Until controlled trials involving a sufficient number of subjects are performed, many issues will remain unanswered.

Hepatitis D. High doses of interferon alfa-2a (9 MU three times a week) have been used to treat HDV infection in adults. Approximately 50% of patients have a complete clinical response with return of aminotransferase levels to normal and clearance of HDV RNA from the serum, but only about 20% are free of disease 6 months after therapy has been discontinued. Studies with interferon alfa-2b also showed its effectiveness in lowering aminotransferases values, but, again, relapse was common after discontinuation of therapy.

COMPLICATIONS

The most serious complication of acute hepatitis caused by any of the five viruses is the development of fulminant hepatic failure. Although the incidence of fulminant hepatic failure is <1%, the mortality remains high. The incidence of hepatic failure is higher with HDV infections and with HEV in pregnant women than it is with the other types of hepatitis. **Hepatic failure** is defined by evidence of hepatic encephalopathy, which may range from subtle changes in mentation or personality to coma. Other signs of hepatic failure include rapidly progressive symptoms, decreasing liver size, increasing jaundice, leukocytosis, increasing serum ammonia levels, and a coagulopathy with a prolonged PT unresponsive to vitamin K therapy, with low factor V and factor VII levels. Hepatic failure may be acute, occurring within a few days to 1 month after the onset of hepatitis, or subacute, following a more prolonged deterioration of 1–3 months.

Some conditions are specifically associated with acute hepatitis B and are probably related to a systemic immune-complex type of vasculitis. These conditions include a serum sickness–like prodrome that occurs late in the incubation period and is composed of polyarthralgia, arthritis, urticaria, and a maculopapular, erythematous rash; polyarteritis nodosa with manifestations of acute vasculitis, which may evolve for months and is associated with persistent HBV antigenemia; and renal disease, including membranous nephropathy, mesangiocapillary glomerulonephritis, and mesangial proliferative glomerulonephritis.

An infrequent complication of acute infectious hepatitis, particularly HCV infection, is aplastic anemia, which usually occurs within 1 year of the hepatitis with an average interval of 8–10 weeks from the onset of hepatitis. HCV infection also may be associated with mixed cryoglobulinemia, which contributes to glomerular deposition of immune complexes and the development of membranoproliferative glomerulonephritis.

PROGNOSIS

The immediate prognosis for full recovery in acute viral hepatitis is usually very good. Death is related primarily to the development of fulminant hepatitis during the acute infection. The overall acute mortality for viral hepatitis is generally <1%, but the mortality is 2–20% for acute HDV and HBV coinfection and may reach 25% for HEV infection in the third trimester of pregnancy.

HAV and HEV cause only acute infection. Although chronic infection with persistent viremia does not occur, sequelae of acute infection with HAV include a protracted or relapsing course in 10–15% of cases, lasting for up to 6 months, induction of autoimmune chronic active hepatitis, and, rarely, fulminating hepatitis with liver failure.

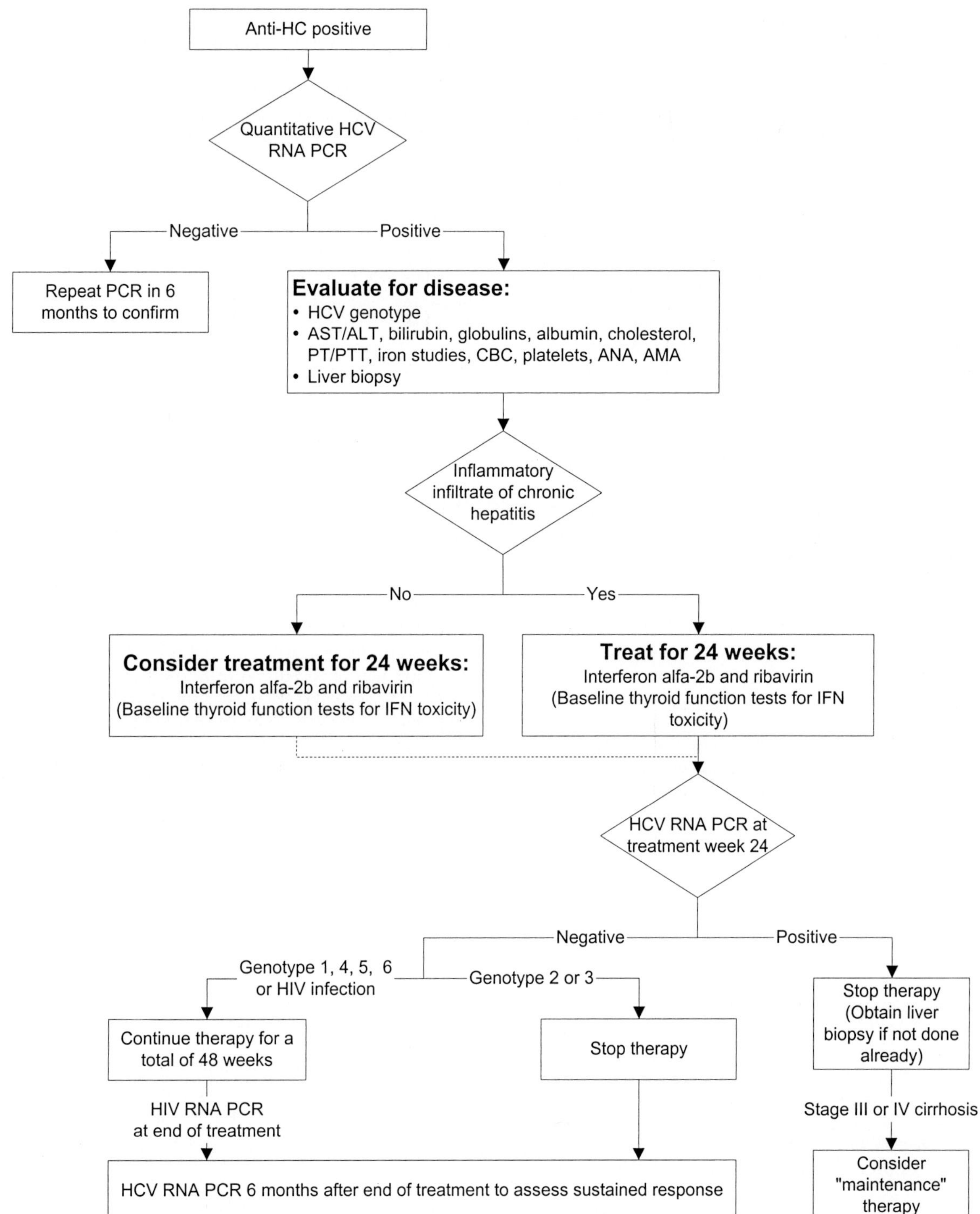

FIGURE 78–8. Evaluation and management of chronic HCV infection. PTT = partial thromboplastin time; AMA = antimitochondrial antibody; ANA = antinuclear antibody; IFN = interferon.

Chronic infection is associated with HBV, HCV, and HDV. The long-term morbidity and mortality for these viral infections depend on the degree of chronic hepatic inflammation, the development of cirrhosis, and the associated risk of hepatocellular carcinoma.

The incidence of chronic HBV infection varies largely according to age at acquisition. From 5% to 10% of adults with hepatitis B become chronic carriers of HBsAg, defined by persistence of HBsAg in the blood for >6 months, in comparison with 20% of children who become chronic carriers. The incidence of persistent infection may reach 70% in the presence of superinfection with HDV and 60–90% in infection acquired perinatally or during infancy. Persistent infection may result in an asymptomatic **chronic carrier state** in which there is no clinical, biochemical, or serologic evidence of active viral replication or hepatitis. Histologically the liver is normal or exhibits only mild nonspecific changes on biopsy. Chronic carriers of HBV are usually HBeAg-negative, often have no history of clinical hepatitis, and rarely demonstrate clinical deterioration. From 10% to 15% eventually clear HBsAg. Unless there is reactivation of the HBV or superinfection with HDV, the clinical course is usually uncomplicated. Chronic hepatitis B may be associated with varying degrees of ongoing hepatic inflammation, which may eventually progress to cirrhosis and end-stage liver disease. Persons with chronic HBV infection are at risk of superinfection with HDV and the development of hepatocellular carcinoma (Chapter 4), regardless of the presence or absence of ongoing hepatic inflammation.

Approximately 85% of persons infected with HCV retain the virus, and those with chronic hepatitis may have progressive liver disease (Fig. 78–9). In chronic infection, there is poor correlation between the symptoms and the extent of ongoing liver damage. Persons with no symptoms may have advanced liver disease. Approximately 20% of persons with chronic infection may develop cirrhosis with a concomitant risk of hepatocellular carcinoma (Chapter 4), similar to that seen in chronic HBV infection.

Chronic HDV infection frequently progresses to cirrhosis. This may occur rapidly in the space of a few years or have a more insidious course in which hepatic cirrhosis develops for 10–15 years. In some cases, chronic HDV infection is nonprogressive, reverting to an inactive carrier state. Chronic hepatitis D infection is responsible for approximately 6% of all cases of chronic viral hepatitis in the United States.

PREVENTION

Implementation of good hygienic measures is important in preventing fecal-oral spread of HAV and other enteric pathogens. All donated blood is screened by using specific tests for evidence of HBV infection (HBsAg and anti-HBc) and, since 1990, HCV infection (anti-HCV), as well as for evidence of elevated ALT as a surrogate marker of viral hepatic inflammation from other causes of viral hepatitis, known and unknown. The practice of universal precautions (Chapter 105) for exposure to blood and body fluids is important for health care workers to minimize transmission of viral agents of hepatitis, especially bloodborne pathogens such as HBV and HCV.

Passive immunization for prophylaxis is available for both HAV and HBV infection. A vaccine against HBV is recommended for universal immunization of newborns (Chapter 17). No effective immunoprophylaxis exists for HCV, HDV, or HEV infection, and therefore prevention is directed at recognizing and reducing the risk of exposure. Prevention of HBV infection will effectively prevent infection with HDV. Immunoglobulin prophylaxis has not been demonstrated to be effective after accidental exposure to blood containing HCV or after enteric exposure to HEV. Chronic carriers of HBsAg should refrain from activities that might expose them to HDV.

Hepatitis A. Two inactivated HAV vaccines are available. Immunization consists of two doses administered intramuscularly 6–12 months apart, and immunity is induced within 14 days after the first dose. Vaccination is recommended for all children who live in states where the average annual hepatitis A rate is 20 cases per 100,000 population (i.e., approximately twice the national average of 10 cases per 100,000 population), including Arizona, Alaska, Oregon, New Mexico, Utah, Washington, Oklahoma, South Dakota, Idaho, Nevada, and California. Vaccination should be considered for all children in states where the average annual rate of hepatitis A is 10–20 cases per 100,000 population, including Missouri, Texas, Colorado, Arkansas, Montana, and Wyoming. Hepatitis A vaccination is also recommended for children in communities with high rates of hepatitis A (e.g., American Indian reservations, Alaskan Native villages) and for susceptible persons who travel to countries with intermediate or high endemicity of hepatitis A (all countries except Canada, the Western Europe countries, the Scandinavian countries, Japan, Australia, and New Zealand), men who have sex with men, injection drug users, laboratory workers who work with HAV, persons who use clotting factor concentrates, and persons with chronic liver disease.

Unvaccinated household and sexual contacts of persons who have serologically confirmed hepatitis A should be given IG (0.02 mL/kg) intramuscularly as soon as possible but not >2 weeks

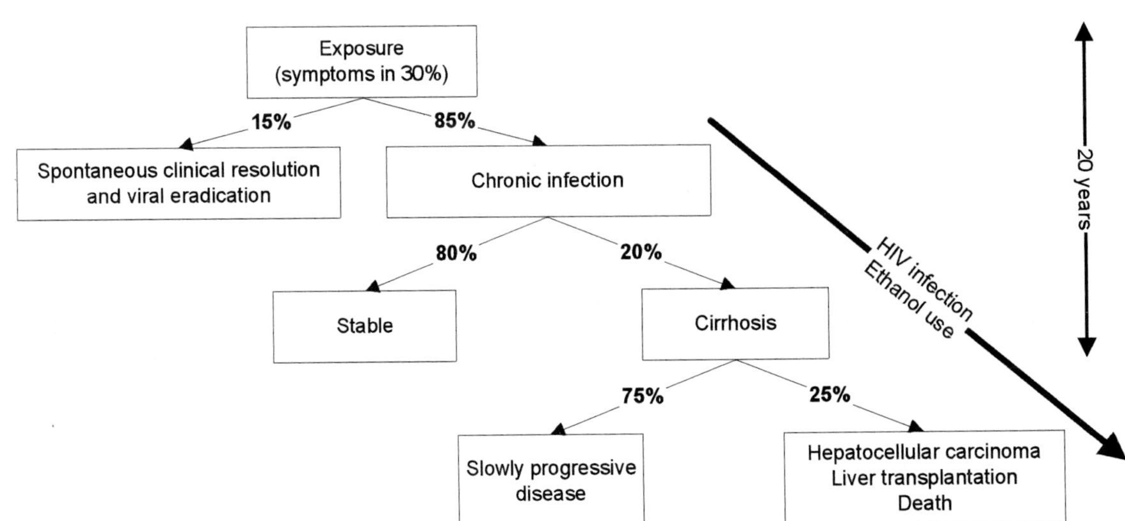

FIGURE 78–9. Natural history of hepatitis C. HIV infection and ethanol use predispose the person with hepatitis C to progression to cirrhosis and hepatocellular carcinoma.

after the last exposure (Table 78–8). IG should be administered to all previously unvaccinated staff and attendees of daycare centers or homes if one or more cases of hepatitis A occur in children or employees or if cases are recognized in two or more households of center attendees. In centers that do not provide care to children who wear diapers, IG is needed only for classroom contacts of the person with the index case. When an outbreak occurs (i.e., hepatitis cases in three or more families), IG also should be considered for members of households that have center attendees in diapers. In those communities where routine vaccination is recommended, hepatitis A vaccine can be administered at the same time as IG in children receiving postexposure prophylaxis in daycare centers. IG is not routinely indicated when a single case occurs in an elementary or secondary school or in an office or other work setting if the source of infection is outside the school or work setting, a newborn of an infected mother, or hepatitis A occurring in an institution or hospital if proper hygienic measures are followed.

If hepatitis A is diagnosed in a food handler, IG should be administered to other food handlers at the same establishment. Because common-source transmission to patrons is unlikely, IG administration to patrons is usually not recommended but can be considered if the food handler both directly handled uncooked foods or cooked foods and had diarrhea or poor hygienic practices and if patrons can be identified and treated within 2 weeks after exposure. In settings where repeated exposure to HAV might have occurred (e.g., institutional cafeterias), stronger consideration of IG use might be warranted. In the event of a common-source outbreak, IG should not be administered to exposed persons after cases have begun to occur because the 2-week period during which IG is effective will have expired.

Persons who have received one dose of hepatitis A vaccine at least 1 month before exposure to HAV do not need IG. Serologic confirmation of HAV infection in the index patient by IgM anti-HAV testing is recommended before postexposure treatment of contacts. Screening of contacts for HAV infection is not recommended because screening is likely to be more costly than IG and would delay its administration. Hepatitis A vaccine can be administered simultaneously with IG, at a separate anatomic injection site. The use of hepatitis A vaccine alone is not recommended for postexposure prophylaxis.

Children should be excluded from school or daycare for 1 week after the onset of symptoms and until jaundice, if present, disappears or until IG has been administered to appropriate individuals.

Travelers to developing countries should receive hepatitis A vaccine if travel does not begin within 14 days, with the booster dose given 6–12 months later. Alternatively, travelers can be tested for anti-HAV to determine the need for hepatitis A prophylaxis. If the antibody status is negative or unknown and if protection within 14 days is needed, the traveler should receive IG prophylaxis (see Chapter 104).

Hepatitis B. HBV vaccine is recommended for routine immunization of all infants, beginning at 0–2 months of age, and of all children and adolescents through 18 years of age, at any visit, who have not been previously immunized. It is also recommended as a pre-exposure vaccination for older children and adults at substantial risk of having hepatitis B (Table 78–9).

Postexposure prophylaxis is recommended for infants born to mothers with HBsAg positivity, for intimate and sexual contacts of people with acute hepatitis B or chronic carriers of HBsAg, and for those who have had percutaneous or permucosal exposure to the virus (Table 78–10). Both passive immunoprophylaxis and vaccination are available for postexposure prophylaxis.

Routine prenatal screening for HBsAg is recommended for all pregnant women in the United States. In certain circumstances of continuing high-risk behavior (e.g., injection drug users) or acute hepatitis during pregnancy, a repeated HBsAg test should be performed late in pregnancy. Infants, including preterm infants, born to HBsAg-positive mothers should receive, at separate sites, vaccine and HBIG 0.5 mL within 12 hours of birth. The second dose

TABLE 78–8. Indications for Immune Globulin Prophylaxis (0.02 mL/kg Intramuscularly) for Hepatitis A Virus Infection

Situation	Recipients of Prophylaxis
Pre-exposure (consider testing for anti-HAV or HAV vaccination if travel is not within 15 days)	Traveler to endemic area (if staying >3 mo, give 0.06 mL/kg and repeat every 5 mo)
Postexposure Setting	
Individual Patient	Household and sexual contacts who have not been vaccinated ≥1 mo before exposure Not indicated for casual or school-room contacts
Daycare Facilities	
All children older than 2 yr or toilet trained *with* 1 case in staff or enrolled child	Staff in contact with index patient and enrolled children in same room as index patient
All children not yet toilet trained *with* 1 case in staff or enrolled child *or* 2 cases in household contacts of two enrolled children	All staff and all enrolled children
3 or more cases *or* Cases over a period of ≥3 wk	All staff, all enrolled children, and household contacts of all enrolled children in diapers
Foodborne or Waterborne Outbreak	All exposed individuals (if within 2 wk of last exposure)

TABLE 78–9. Individuals Who Should Receive Pre-exposure Hepatitis B Immunization

Routine Vaccination
All infants (beginning at 0–2 mo of age)*
All unvaccinated children by or before 11 or 12 yr of age

Persons at Increased Risk of Severe Disease
Persons with chronic liver disease

Adolescents and Adults at Substantial Risk of HBV Infection

Household and Other Close Contacts of HBsAg-Positive Individuals
Household contacts and sex partners of persons with acute HBV infection, or HBsAg-carriers
Household contacts of HBsAg-positive adoptees
International travelers who will live for >6 mo in areas of high HBV endemicity and who will have close contact with the local population
Unvaccinated children <11 yr of age who are Pacific Islanders or who reside in households of first-generation immigrants from countries where HBV is of high or intermediate endemicity

Populations at Increased Risk of Exposure
Persons undergoing hemodialysis
Persons with hemophilia and other recipients of certain blood products (clotting factor concentrates)
Residents (and staff) of institutions for developmentally disabled persons
Attendees of nonresidential daycare and school programs for developmentally disabled persons if attended by a known HBsAg-positive carrier who behaves aggressively

Persons at Increased Risk of Exposure Because of Sexual or Social Habits
Sexually active persons diagnosed with a sexually transmitted disease, who are prostitutes, or who have a history of sexual activity with >1 sex partner in previous 6 mo
Sexually active men who have sex with men
Injection drug users
Inmates of juvenile detention and other correctional facilities

Health Care Providers
Health care workers and others with exposure to blood or body fluids
Staff (and residents) of institutions for developmentally disabled persons
Staff of nonresidential daycare and school programs for developmentally disabled persons if attended by a known HBsAg-positive carrier (and attendees of such institutions if a child behaves aggressively)

*For premature infants with birth weights <2,000 g born to HBsAg-negative women, it is advisable to delay initiation of hepatitis B vaccination until just before hospital discharge, providing the infant weighs ≥2,000 g, or until about 2 mo of age, when other immunizations are given.

is recommended at 1–2 months of age and the third dose at 6 months of age. Infants born to mothers whose HBsAg status is unknown should receive vaccine within 12 hours of birth. Maternal blood should be drawn at delivery to determine the mother's HBsAg status; if the HBsAg test result is positive, the infant should receive HBIG as soon as possible but no later than 1 week of age. These infants should be tested for HBsAg and anti-HBsAg 1–3 months after completion of the vaccination series to demonstrate the efficacy of the immunoprophylaxis. Children with HBsAg positivity should have follow-up testing 6 months after the first test. If the follow-up test result is positive, the child has become chronically infected with hepatitis B and will be a chronic carrier of HBsAg. Further vaccination is of no benefit. Children who are negative for HBsAg and anti-HBs should receive one to three additional doses of vaccine, with testing for anti-HBs after each dose, or a second three-dose series of vaccine at intervals of 1–2 months. The efficacy of the combination of HBIG and vaccination in preventing vertical transmission is 98–99%. Vaccination alone without HBIG may prevent up to 75% of cases of perinatal HBV transmission and approximately 95% of cases of symptomatic childhood HBV infection.

Children who carry HBsAg but have no behavioral risk factors, such as biting and scratching, and no medical risk factors, such as cutaneous wounds or bleeding disorders, pose a negligible risk of disease transmission and may attend daycare and school without restriction. The management of children with special risk factors should be individualized to minimize exposure. Routine HBsAg screening is not warranted.

Postexposure prophylaxis of household contacts of persons with acute hepatitis B, using both HBIG and vaccine, is recommended for sex partners who have had relations within the previous 14 days and for household members with intimate contact with the index patient. Intimate contact most commonly denotes sexual contact, but it also includes the sharing of toothbrushes and razors and exposure to the blood of the index patient through wounds. Prophylaxis should also be given to children younger than 12 months if the parent or primary care provider has acute hepatitis. Prophylaxis is not indicated for other household members unless the index patient becomes a chronic HBsAg carrier.

Postexposure prophylaxis of household contacts of chronic carriers of HBsAg, using HBIG and vaccine, is recommended for sex partners who have had relations within the previous 14 days. Vaccination is recommended for all household contacts.

The need for and the type of postexposure prophylaxis after percutaneous or permucosal contact depend on the hepatitis B vaccination history of the exposed person, on whether the response is known, and on the likelihood of exposure to HBsAg (Table 78–10).

Refugees and adoptees from areas in which hepatitis B is endemic should be screened for past infection and chronic carriage of HBsAg (Chapter 103). Household contacts of adoptees who are from countries where HBV is endemic and who are HBsAg carriers should receive hepatitis B vaccination.

TABLE 78–10. Postexposure Prophylaxis for Hepatitis B Virus Infection

Exposure	Prophylaxis*		
Perinatal Exposure			
Newborn of HBsAg-positive mother	HBIG 0.5 mL IM as soon as possible (within 12 hr of birth) and begin immunization with first dose, preferably within 12 hr of birth (no later than 7 days), and at 1 mo and 6 mo		
Contacts of a Person with Acute Hepatitis B			
Unimmunized household contact	Begin immunization; if sharing toothbrushes or razors, prophylaxis is indicated for permucosal contact		
Unimmunized children <12 mo of age with index case in parent or primary care provider	HBIG 0.5 mL IM as soon as possible and initiate hepatitis B vaccine series		
Unimmunized sexual contact (within 14 days)	HBIG 0.06 mL/kg IM as soon as possible and initiate hepatitis B vaccine series		
Casual contact	No prophylaxis unless routine immunization is otherwise recommended (Table 78–9)		
Contacts of a Person Who Is a Chronic HBsAg Carrier			
Household contact	Initiate hepatitis B vaccine series		
Sexual contact	Initiate hepatitis B vaccine series		
Casual contact	No prophylaxis unless routine immunization otherwise recommended (Table 78–9)		
Percutaneous or Permucosal Contact			
	HBsAg-positive Source	**HBsAg-negative Source**	**Source Unknown or Not Tested**
Unvaccinated person	HBIG 0.06 mL/kg IM and initiate hepatitis B vaccine series	Initiate hepatitis B vaccine series	Initiate hepatitis B vaccine series
Previously vaccinated *and*			
Known responder	No prophylaxis	No prophylaxis	No prophylaxis
Known nonresponder	HBIG 0.06 mL/kg IM as soon as possible and at 1 mo† *or* HBIG 0.06 mL/kg IM as soon as possible and 1 dose of hepatitis B vaccine	No prophylaxis	If known high-risk source, may treat as if source were HBsAg-positive
Response unknown	Test exposed person for anti-HBs‡: ■ If inadequate response, HBIG 0.06 mL IM and 1 dose of hepatitis B vaccine ■ If adequate response, no prophylaxis	No prophylaxis	Test exposed person for anti-HBs‡: ■ If inadequate response, 1 dose of hepatitis B vaccine ■ If adequate response, no prophylaxis

*HBIG and hepatitis B vaccine can be given at the same time but at different anatomic sites.
†Recommended for persons who have not responded to a three-dose vaccine series and to reimmunization with three additional doses.
‡An adequate response to hepatitis B immunization is anti-HBs ≥10 mIU/mL.

REVIEWS

Aggarwal R, Krawczynski K: Hepatitis E: An overview and recent advances in clinical and laboratory research. *J Gastroenterol Hepatol* 2000;15: 9–20.

American Academy of Pediatrics, Committee on Infectious Diseases: Prevention of hepatitis A infections: Guidelines for the use of hepatitis vaccine and immune globulin. *Pediatrics* 1996;98:1207–15.

American Academy of Pediatrics, Committee on Infectious Diseases: Hepatitis C virus infection. *Pediatrics* 1998;101:481–5.

Centers for Disease Control and Prevention: Hepatitis B virus: A comprehensive strategy for eliminating transmission in the United States through universal childhood vaccination. Recommendations of the Immunization Practices Advisory Committee (ACIP). *MMWR Morb Mortal Wkly Rep* 1991;40(RR-13):1–25.

Centers for Disease Control and Prevention: Recommendations for prevention and control of hepatitis C virus (HCV) infection and HCV-related chronic disease. *MMWR Morb Mortal Wkly Rep* 1998;47(RR-19):1–39.

Centers for Disease Control and Prevention: Prevention of hepatitis A through active or passive immunization: Recommendations of the Advisory Committee on Immunization Practices (ACIP). *MMWR Morb Mortal Wkly Rep* 1999;48(RR-12):1–37.

Lee WM: Hepatitis B virus infection. *N Engl J Med* 1997;337;1733–45.

Liang TJ, Rehermann B, Seeff LB, et al: Pathogenesis, natural history, treatment and prevention of hepatitis C. *Ann Intern Med* 2000;132: 296–305.

Robaczewska M, Cova L, Podhajska AJ, et al: Hepatitis G virus: Molecular organization, methods of detection, prevalence, and disease association. *Int J Infect Dis* 1999;3:220–33.

Sokal EM, Bortolotti F: Update on prevention and treatment of viral hepatitis in children. *Curr Opin Pediatr* 1999;11:384–9.

KEY ARTICLES

Alter MJ, Ahtone J, Weisfuse I, et al: The effect of underreporting on the apparent incidence and epidemiology of acute viral hepatitis. *Am J Epidemiol* 1987;125:133–9.

Alter MJ, Margolis HS, Krawezynski K, et al: The natural history of community-acquired hepatitis C in the United States. *N Engl J Med* 1992;327:1899–905.

Bell BP, Shapiro CN, Alter MJ, et al: The diverse patterns of hepatitis A epidemiology in the United States—Implications for vaccination strategies. *J Infect Dis* 1998;178:1579–84.

Bjøro K, Froland SS, Yun Z, et al: Hepatitis C infection in patients with primary hypogammaglobulinemia after treatment with contaminated immune globulin. *N Engl J Med* 1994;331:1607–11.

Bortolotti F, Cadrobbi P, Crivellaro C, et al: Long-term outcome of chronic type B hepatitis in patients who acquire hepatitis B virus infection in childhood. *Gastroenterology* 1990;99:805–10.

Bortolotti F, Resti M, Giacchino R, et al: Changing epidemiologic pattern of chronic hepatitis C virus infection in Italian children. *J Pediatr* 1998;133:378–81.

Brook MG, Karayiannis P, Thomas HC: Which patients with chronic hepatitis B virus infection will respond to α-interferon therapy? A statistical analysis of predictive factors. *Hepatology* 1989;l0:761–3.

Chang MH, Chen CJ, Lai MS, et al: Universal hepatitis B vaccination in Taiwan and the incidence of hepatocellular carcinoma in children. Taiwan Childhood Hepatoma Study Group. *N Engl J Med* 1997;336:1855–9.

Chayama K, Suzuki Y, Kobayashi M, et al: Emergence and takeover of YMDD motif mutant hepatitis B virus during long-term lamivudine therapy and re-takeover by wild type after cessation of therapy. *Hepatology* 1998;27:1711–6.

Davis GL, Esteban-Mur R, Rustgi V, et al: Interferon alpha-2b alone or in combination with ribavirin for the treatment of relapse of chronic hepatitis C. *N Engl J Med* 1998;339:1493–9.

Debray D, Cullifi P, Devictor D, et al: Liver failure in children with hepatitis A. *Hepatology* 1997;26:1018–22.

Farci P, Barbera C, Navone C, et al: Infection with the delta agent in children. *Gut* 1985;26:4–7.

Farci P, Mandas A, Coiana A, et al: Treatment of chronic hepatitis D with interferon alfa-2a. *N Engl J Med* 1994;330:88–94.

Hagler L, Pastore RA, Bergen JJ, et al: Aplastic anemia following viral hepatitis: Report of two fatal cases and literature review. *Medicine* 1975;54:139–64.

Lai CL, Lok AS, Lin JH, et al: Placebo-controlled trial of recombinant α_2-interferon in Chinese HbsAg-carrier children. *Lancet* 1987;2:877–80.

Lai CL, Chien RN, Lueng NW, et al: A one year trial of lamivudine for chronic hepatitis B. Asia Hepatitis Lamivudine Study Group. *N Engl J Med* 1998;339:61–8.

Linnen J, Wages J, Zhang-Keck ZY, et al: Molecular cloning and disease association of hepatitis G virus: A transfusion-transmissable agent. *Science* 1996;271:505–8.

Malay S, Tizer K, Lutwick LI: Current update of pediatric hepatitis vaccine use. *Pediatr Clin North Am* 2000;47:395–406.

McHutchison JG, Gordon SC, Schiff ER, et al: Interferon alfa-2b alone or in combination with ribavirin as initial treatment for chronic hepatitis C. *N Engl J Med* 1998;339:1485–92.

McMahon BJ, Alward WL, Hall DB, et al: Acute hepatitis B virus infection: Relation of age to the clinical expression of disease and subsequent development of the carrier state. *J Infect Dis* 1985;151:599–603.

Mushahwar IK, Erker JC, Muerhoff AS, et al: Molecular and biophysical characterization of TT virus: Evidence for a new virus family infecting humans. *Proc Natl Acad Sci USA* 1999;96:3177–82.

Nishizawa T, Okamoto H, Konishi K, et al: A novel DNA virus (TTV) associated with elevated transaminase levels in posttransfusion hepatitis of unknown etiology. *Biochem Biophys Res Commun* 1997;241:92–7.

Prescott LE, Simmonds P: Global distribution of transfusion-transmitted virus. *N Engl J Med* 1998;339:776–7.

Ruiz-Moreno M, Rua MJ, Carreno V, et al: Prospective, randomized controlled trial of interferon-α in children with chronic hepatitis B. *Hepatology* 1991;13:1035–9.

Sokal EM, Conjeevaram HS, Roberts EA, et al: Interferon alpha therapy for chronic hepatitis B in children: A multinational randomized controlled trial. *Gastroenterology* 1998;114:988–95.

Tang JR, Hsu HY, Lin HH, et al: Hepatitis B surface antigenemia at birth: A long-term follow-up study. *J Pediatr* 1998;133:374–7.

Taylor JM: Hepatitis delta virus. *Intervirology* 1999;42:173–8.

Vento S, Garofano T, Renzini C, et al: Fulminant hepatitis associated with hepatitis A virus superinfection in patients with chronic hepatitis C. *N Engl J Med* 1998;338:286–90.

Vogt M, Lang T, Frosnr G, et al: Prevalence and clinical outcome of hepatitis C infection in children who underwent cardiac surgery before the implementation of blood-donor screening. *N Engl J Med* 1999; 341:866–70.

Werzberger A, Mensch B, Kuter B, et al: A controlled trial of a formalin-inactivated hepatitis A vaccine in healthy children. *N Engl J Med* 1992;327:453–7.

Zanetti AR, Furoni P, Magliano EM, et al: Perinatal transmission of the hepatitis B virus and of the HBV-associated delta agent from mothers to offspring in northern Italy. *J Med Virol* 1982;9:139–48.

CHAPTER 79

Hepatic Abscess

M. Susan Moyer ▪ Hal B. Jenson

Hepatic abscesses are rare in the United States, especially in children, but they are important because early recognition and treatment prevents the severe complications historically associated with them. Because hepatic abscesses rarely have specific clinical manifestations, a high degree of awareness is required, especially for children with predisposing risk factors.

ETIOLOGY

Pyogenic, or bacterial, hepatic abscesses are usually polymicrobial in origin, including gram-negative and anaerobic bacteria of colonic origin and occasionally *Staphylococcus aureus* (Table 79–1). Fungal hepatic abscesses, caused primarily by *Candida albicans,* may occur in immunocompromised persons, especially those treated with broad-spectrum antimicrobial agents for extended periods. **Amebic liver abscesses,** caused by the protozoan *Entamoeba histolytica,* are much more common worldwide than pyogenic abscesses but are less frequently seen in the United States than in other countries. **Hydatid cysts,** caused by infection of the larval stage of *Echinococcus,* are a relatively uncommon infectious cause of hepatic cavitation, although 60% of all hydatid cysts occur in the liver (Chapter 44). Hydatid cysts may also become secondarily infected with bacteria.

In developed countries, where amebiasis is not endemic, 85% of hepatic abscesses are bacterial, 10% are fungal, and 5% are amebic. Up to 50% of amebic abscesses are also infected with bacteria or fungi. In regions where amebiasis is endemic, approximately 80% of hepatic abscesses are amebic, 18% are bacterial, and fewer than 2% are fungal.

EPIDEMIOLOGY

Many forms of biliary tract disease associated with stasis predispose affected persons to hepatic abscess, notably common bile duct stones, malignant neoplasms, cirrhosis, and alcoholism. Crohn's disease is associated with an increased incidence of pyogenic hepatic abscess, probably because of mucosal ulceration and loss of the normal protective barrier. Persons with diabetes mellitus are predisposed to hepatic abscess, although the mechanism is unclear. Biliary tract complications typically occur in the advanced stages of these diseases and are uncommon in childhood. Pyogenic hepatic abscesses are rare in healthy children and occur primarily in immunocompromised children, especially with chronic granulomatous disease, or in children who have previously undergone a biliary operation, such as repair of extrahepatic biliary atresia or after liver transplantation. Any operation that modifies the normal unobstructed flow of bile or circumvents the protective function of the sphincter of Oddi may result in a predisposition to ascending biliary infection and hepatic abscess.

After amebic dysentery, amebic liver abscess is the second most common form of invasive amebiasis caused by *E. histolytica.* It occurs in 1–5% of children and 10–50% of adults with invasive intestinal amebiasis. Hepatic abscesses and their complications account for up to 40% of deaths associated with amebiasis. Untreated intestinal carriers of *E. histolytica* have a 25% lifetime risk of developing an amebic hepatic abscess, with the highest incidence in endemic areas during the third and fourth decades of life. In the United States, persons with pyogenic abscesses tend to be older, typically in the fifth and sixth decades of life. Persons with amebic abscesses often have emigrated from or traveled to Mexico or to Central or South America.

PATHOGENESIS

A **hepatic abscess** is a localized collection of pus that occurs with destruction of the local parenchyma and stroma. Pyogenic abscesses can be 1–20 cm or more in diameter. Fungal abscesses tend to be multiple and small, 1–2 cm in diameter. Amebic abscesses tend to be solitary and can be small or large. Multiple hepatic abscesses, occurring in approximately one third of cases,

TABLE 79–1. Microbiologic Causes of Hepatic Abscesses

Bacterial (Pyogenic)
Polymicrobial with Enteric Organisms
Gram-negative aerobes
Escherichia coli
Klebsiella
Proteus
Enterobacter
Serratia
Pseudomonas
Gram-positive aerobes
Enterococcus faecalis
Anaerobes
Fusobacterium
Bacteroides fragilis
Streptococcus milleri
Peptostreptococcus
Other Organisms
Staphylococcus aureus
Group A *Streptococcus*
Salmonella
Yersinia enterocolitica
Listeria monocytogenes
Fungal
Candida albicans
Parasitic
Entamoeba histolytica (amebic abscess)
Echinococcus (hydatid cyst)
Ascaris

are more common with bacterial or fungal abscesses rather than amebic abscesses. Frequently, persons with solitary hepatic abscesses are found to have additional microscopic foci at the time of autopsy. Hydatid cysts may be solitary or multiple, and they may be small or large.

Organisms can spread to the liver by ascending from the gastrointestinal tract through the biliary tree, by direct extension of a contiguous infection, by spread of gastrointestinal infection through the portal vein, by hematogenous spread through the hepatic artery, or by penetrating trauma. Hepatic abscess may complicate umbilical vein catheterization in newborns. Although localized "bacterial hepatitis" must precede development of an abscess cavity, this has only rarely been identified as a clinical entity. The right lobe of the liver, especially the periphery, is more commonly affected, probably because it is larger than the left lobe.

The rich blood supply and the reticuloendothelial functions of the liver militate against the development of hepatic abscesses. However, because children have fewer predisposing conditions than do adults, systemic bacteremia with hematogenous seeding of the liver is historically responsible for a relatively high percentage of hepatic abscesses in children. The classic organism associated with this mode is *S. aureus,* although such abscesses are uncommon because most primary *S. aureus* infections are recognized and treated early, with less chance of systemic spread than in historical controls. Abscesses caused by *C. albicans* usually occur in immunocompromised persons and probably also result from hematogenous spread.

Amebic abscesses develop as a complication of amebic dysentery and spread to the liver through the portal venous system, with a predominance of peripheral lesions. Less frequently, amebic abscesses develop from direct extension of infection from the hepatic flexure of the colon. Amebic abscesses develop over several months or years and have a subacute onset of symptoms.

SYMPTOMS AND CLINICAL MANIFESTATIONS

The clinical features of hepatic abscesses are usually nonspecific, with onset that is insidious for several days or several weeks (Table 79–2). A low-grade fever, malaise, anorexia, and abdominal pain and discomfort are the most typical symptoms. Approximately 10–30% of patients do not have fever. Amebic abscesses cause less severe illness than pyogenic abscesses. Although right upper quadrant abdominal pain or, less commonly, epigastric pain is typically associated with hepatic disease, this characterization of pain is more common in adults than in children, who complain mostly of diffuse abdominal pain. Pain may be referred to the right shoulder or right side of the chest. Nausea and vomiting, weight loss, diarrhea, chills and sweats, and hiccups are occasionally present. Extension of infection to the pleural space or lungs may result in tachypnea or dyspnea.

Because there are few specific clinical symptoms, hepatic abscesses should be considered in the evaluation of children with a prolonged fever of unknown origin, obscure abdominal pain, or unexplained weight loss.

Physical Examination Findings

Hepatomegaly and hepatic or diffuse abdominal tenderness are present in up to 70% of patients (Table 79–2). Abdominal distention and pain on deep inspiration or movement may also be present. Jaundice is not an expected finding but may be present if the hepatic abscess is accompanied by biliary tract obstruction.

TABLE 79–2. Symptoms and Signs of a Hepatic Abscess

Finding	Incidence (%)
Symptoms	
Common	
Fever	70–90
Malaise	5–90
Anorexia	5–90
Chills	50
Abdominal pain	50
Weight loss	50
Infrequent	
Nausea	Up to 50
Vomiting	Up to 50
Diarrhea	Occasional
Sweating	Occasional
Signs	
Common	
Hepatomegaly	50–70
Right-upper quadrant tenderness	50–70
Infrequent	
Respiratory symptoms	20
Abdominal distention	10–20
Jaundice	10–20
Laboratory Findings	
Common	
Elevated ESR	90
Leukocytosis	70
Elevated alkaline phosphatase level	70
Anemia	50
Hypoalbuminemia	50
Elevated hepatic aminotransferase values (ALT, AST)	50
Elevated γ-GT value	50
Infrequent	
Hyperbilirubinemia	<25

ALT = alanine aminotransferase; AST = aspartate aminotransferase; γ-GT = γ-glutamyltransferase.

DIAGNOSIS

The subtle presenting symptoms of hepatic abscesses often contribute to a delay in diagnosis. The symptoms and signs, although sometimes impressive, are nonspecific. There is a trend toward an increased prominence of symptoms associated with multiple hepatic abscesses, although there is sufficient overlap that this finding cannot be reliably determined without appropriate diagnostic imaging. There are no distinctive clinical features of pyogenic as opposed to amebic hepatic abscesses, and therefore specific serologic and imaging tests are necessary for diagnosis (Fig. 79–1).

Differential Diagnosis

Because the symptoms and signs of a hepatic abscess are nonspecific, almost any condition that causes abdominal pain may be included in the differential diagnosis. Appropriate diagnostic imaging quickly indicates or excludes the possibility of a hepatic abscess, although the specific etiologic agent often cannot be determined without appropriate culture of the abscess material. Tumors and cysts are the primary noninfectious considerations (Table 79–3).

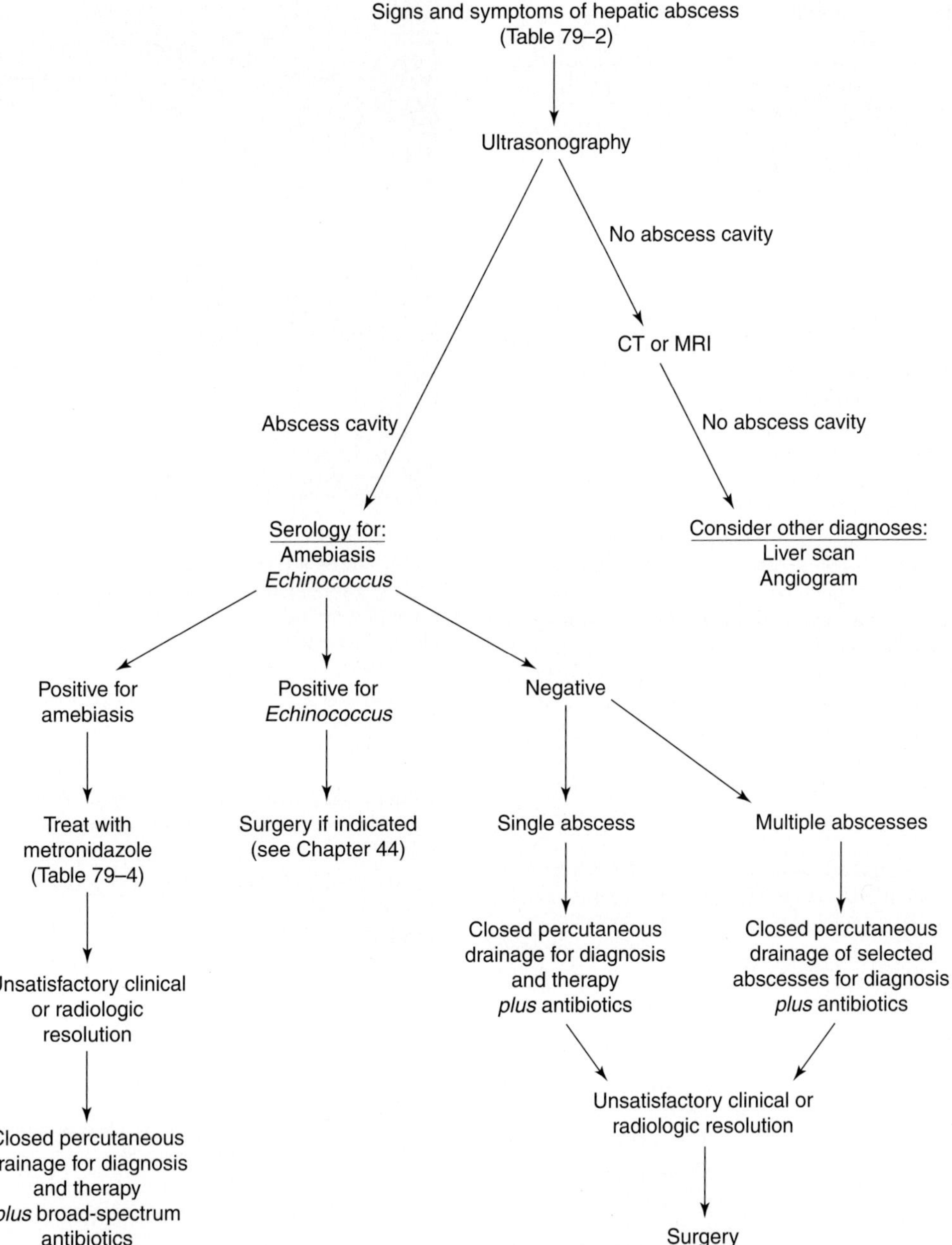

FIGURE 79–1. Algorithm for the diagnosis and management of hepatic abscess.

Laboratory Evaluation

Routine laboratory tests are usually not helpful in the evaluation of a hepatic abscess. Anemia, leukocytosis, and an elevated serum alkaline phosphatase level are present in most cases (Table 79–2). Serum levels of alanine aminotransferase (ALT) and aspartate aminotransferase (AST) are normal to mildly elevated. Hypoalbuminemia is sometimes present. Hyperbilirubinemia, either direct or indirect, is uncommon unless biliary tract obstruction is also present. Eosinophilia is not usually present with amebic abscesses and is variably present with echinococcal cysts.

Microbiologic Evaluation

Pyogenic and Fungal Abscesses. Bacterial and fungal organisms can usually be recovered from abscess cavities at the time of drainage, even if there has been anti-infective therapy. Blood cultures should routinely be obtained before antibiotic therapy is begun, although culture results are positive in only approximately half of the cases. Approximately two thirds of pyogenic hepatic abscesses are polymicrobial in origin, caused by enteric gram-negative and anaerobic organisms, but this is not usually reflected in the blood culture. *C. albicans* in immunocompromised persons are frequently associated with fungemia and disseminated infection.

Amebic Abscess. Although serologic studies for *E. histolytica* are not helpful in the diagnosis of amebiasis limited to the colon, antibodies to this organism are usually present in persons with extraintestinal amebiasis, including liver disease with or without a hepatic abscess. The sensitivity of available serologic tests for amebiasis is 90–100%, although antibodies detected by indirect immunofluorescence and indirect hemagglutination persist for

TABLE 79–3. Differential Diagnosis of Space-Occupying Hepatic Lesions

Hepatic abscess
Bacterial (pyogenic)
Fungal
Amebic *(Entamoeba histolytica)*
Hydatid cyst *(Echinococcus)*
Hepatocellular adenoma
Hepatocellular carcinoma
Metastatic tumor
Hematoma
Hemangioma
Biloma
Bile duct cyst(s)
Caroli's disease
Adult polycystic kidney disease
Extrapancreatic pseudocysts

years after an infection and are therefore of limited usefulness in endemic areas.

Culture of the abscess may be negative for *E. histolytica* because viable organisms are in the periphery of the lesion and difficult to retrieve, especially by percutaneous drainage. Stool examination for ova and parasites demonstrates *E. histolytica* trophozoites in only approximately 10% of persons with an amebic hepatic abscess. As many as 50% of amebic abscesses that occur in the United States are also infected with bacteria or, much less commonly, with fungi.

Hydatid Cysts. Sensitive and specific serologic tests for *Echinococcus* are available and should be performed if a hydatid cyst is suspected on the basis of internal septa on diagnostic imaging or on the basis of epidemiologic exposure, such as among Native Americans in New Mexico, persons of Basque descent living in California, and the families of sheep ranchers in Utah (Chapter 44). Diagnostic aspiration of intact hydatid cysts should not be performed because of the danger of protoscolex dissemination within the abdominal cavity and because of possible anaphylaxis.

Diagnostic Imaging

Diagnostic imaging is very sensitive in the detection of space-occupying hepatic lesions but is often nondiagnostic because many lesions, including primary hepatocellular carcinoma and metastatic malignant tumors, appear similar to hepatic abscesses. Although pyogenic abscesses are more likely to have a honeycomb appearance and ill-defined margins than are amebic abscesses, it is impossible to reliably distinguish these entities with ultrasonography, CT, or MRI. The diagnostic modality of choice for hepatic abscess is CT or MRI, which can detect lesions as small as 1 cm in diameter. These studies most accurately identify the number, exact location, and size of abscesses as well as involvement of perihepatic tissues. The CT appearance of a hepatic abscess classically is a nonloculated, although sometimes loculated, low-density area within the liver parenchyma that may be smooth or poorly defined, usually without rim enhancement with contrast (Fig. 79–2). Use of contrast material does not appear to aid in the identification of large lesions but may be helpful in identifying smaller, adjacent abscesses and is therefore recommended. Approximately 20% of hepatic abscesses demonstrate gas. Ultrasonography is useful in screening for hepatic abscess because it is readily available, is very sensitive, and does not involve ionizing radiation, but abnormalities on sonograms require further imaging by CT or MRI. Demonstration of **internal septa** or **daughter cysts** by CT, MRI, or ultrasonography is pathognomonic for hydatid cysts. These findings are present in approximately 50% of unilocular liver cysts (Chapter 44).

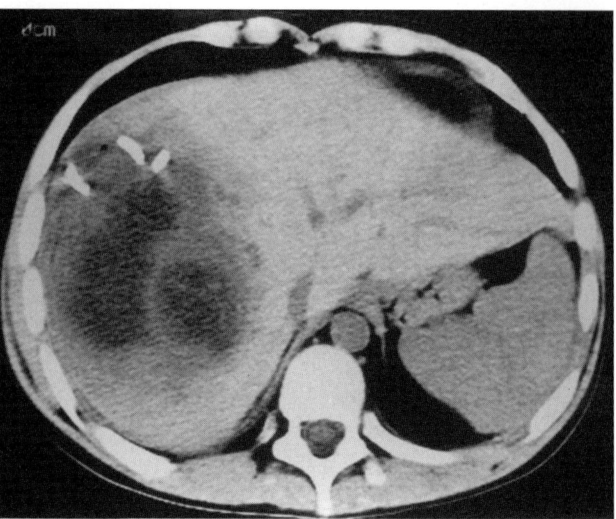

FIGURE 79–2. CT of hepatic abscess. A 14-year-old person with Crohn's disease treated with prednisone later had persistent fever and right shoulder pain without gastrointestinal symptoms. Ultrasonography showed a hepatic abscess. CT demonstrated a multiloculated abscess with surrounding edema. A percutaneous catheter is in place. This polymicrobial bacterial abscess was treated by percutaneous drainage and antimicrobial agents intravenously administered for 3 weeks.

Radionuclide liver-spleen scintigraphy using ^{67}Ga or ^{99m}Tc shows abscesses as hepatic lucencies, but it cannot detect abscesses smaller than 2 cm in diameter and is limited in distinguishing primary from metastatic tumors. Endoscopic retrograde cholangiopancreatography (ERCP), transhepatic cholangiography, and hepatic angiography are seldom necessary and do not add to the diagnostic usefulness of CT or MRI. Hepatic angiography is most often used to plan partial hepatic resection of lesions refractory to drainage and antimicrobial therapy.

Abdominal plain radiographs may show intrahepatic air if gas-forming organisms are involved or if a fistula has formed. Because of their low sensitivity, however, plain radiographs are not routinely recommended in place of CT or MRI. A chest radiograph more often shows abnormalities than do plain radiographs of the abdomen. Approximately 40% of patients demonstrate changes in the right lung, including elevation of the right hemidiaphragm, pleural effusion, subsegmental or linear atelectasis in the right pulmonary base, and lower lung infiltrate. These radiographic findings suggest possible hepatic disease if not already considered in the differential diagnosis. Fungal abscesses tend to be small and are rarely associated with pulmonary findings.

Pathologic Findings

The contents of amebic abscesses have been reported classically to have an anchovy paste consistency, although this finding is inconsistent. Trophozoites are demonstrated in only approximately 20% of amebic abscesses. The wall of an echinococcal cyst contains calcium.

TREATMENT

The most important components in the treatment of pyogenic hepatic abscesses are adequate drainage and appropriate anti-infective therapy, which is usually begun empirically before culture results are known (Table 79–4). No controlled trial has compared antibiotic therapy alone with the combination of a drainage procedure plus antibiotic therapy. Pyogenic abscesses require an initial drainage procedure, which besides being important for diagnosis and identification of the infecting organisms may also be therapeutic. The drainage procedure is followed by appropriate antimicrobial therapy. Solitary hepatic abscesses are best managed by both drainage and antibiotics; the approach to multiple hepatic abscesses is more problematic because adequate drainage of all cavities may not be feasible, necessitating an individualized approach, often using selective drainage and prolonged antimicrobial therapy.

TABLE 79–4. Recommended Antibiotic Therapy for Hepatic Abscess

Infection	Recommended Regimen	Alternative Regimen
Empirical Treatment	Piperacillin-tazobactam *or* cefepime *or* cefotaxime *or* mezlocillin *plus* metronidazole *or* clindamycin *with or without* gentamicin (*or* another aminoglycoside)	
Definitive Treatment		
Polymicrobial pyogenic abscess (mixed gram-negative and anaerobic organisms)	Piperacillin-tazobactam *or* cefepime *or* cefotaxime *or* mezlocillin *plus* metronidazole *or* clindamycin *with or without* gentamicin (*or* another aminoglycoside)	
Staphylococcus aureus	Nafcillin *with or without* gentamicin (*or* another aminoglycoside)	Oxacillin *or* vancomycin *with or without* gentamicin (*or* another aminoglycoside)
Candida albicans	Amphotericin B	
Entamoeba histolytica (amebic abscess)	Metronidazole (for 10 days) *followed by* iodoquinol (for 20 days)	Dehydroemetine (for 5 days) *followed by* chloroquine phosphate (for 2–3 wk) *plus* iodoquinol (for 20 days)
Echinococcus (hydatid cyst)	See Table 44–5	

Suggested Dosages for Persons with Normal Renal Function

ANTIBIOTIC	DOSAGE	MAXIMUM DAILY DOSE
Amikacin	15 mg/kg/day divided q8–12hr IV	15 mg/kg
Cefepime	100–150 mg/kg/day divided q8–12hr IV	4–6 g
Cefoperazone	100–150 mg/kg/day divided q8–12hr IV	6 g
Cefotaxime	200 mg/kg/day divided q6hr IV	12 g
Ceftazidime	150 mg/kg/day divided q8hr IV	6 g
Chloroquine phosphate	20 mg/kg base (33 mg salt) daily for 2 days, then 10 mg/kg base (17 mg salt) daily for 2–3 wk	600 mg base (1 g salt); 300 mg base (500 mg salt)
Clindamycin	40 mg/kg/day divided q6hr IV	2.7 g
Dehydroemetine*	1–1.5 mg/kg/day for 5 days IM	90 mg
Gentamicin	7.5 mg/kg/day divided q8hr IV	Adults: 5 mg/kg
Iodoquinol	30–40 mg/kg/day divided q8hr PO	2 g
Metronidazole	35–50 mg/kg/day divided q6hr IV	30 mg/kg (adults)
Mezlocillin	200–300 mg/kg/day divided q4–6hr IV	18–24 g
Piperacillin-tazobactam	200–300 mg piperacillin/kg/day divided q4–6hr IV	18 g
Nafcillin	150 mg/kg/day divided q16hr IV	9 g
Oxacillin	150–200 mg/kg/day divided q4–6hr IV	12 g
Tobramycin	7.5 mg/kg/day divided q8hr IV	Adults: 5 mg/kg
Vancomycin	40 mg/kg/day divided q6hr IV	2 g
ANTIFUNGAL AGENT		
Amphotericin B	1 mg/kg/day for 3–4 hr IV (to 40 mg/kg total dose)	

*Available from the CDC Drug Service, telephone (404) 639-3670 (evenings, weekends, and holidays: [404] 639-2888).

Uncomplicated amebic abscesses usually respond well to medical therapy alone. Echinococcal cysts usually cause no local or systemic inflammatory response and respond well to surgical resection and albendazole. After drainage and during antimicrobial therapy, repeated ultrasonography, CT, or MRI is important to confirm appropriate resolution and to detect complications.

Definitive Treatment

Pyogenic and Fungal Abscesses. Evidence by CT or MRI of a pyogenic hepatic abscess necessitates appropriate surgical consultation. The surgical approach to hepatic abscesses must be individualized. The number, size, and location of abscesses are evaluated to determine the appropriate procedure, which may include drainage and catheter placement by closed percutaneous aspiration guided by ultrasonography or CT, laparoscopy, or open laparotomy with either extraserous or transperitoneal surgical drainage. Although laparotomy has been used historically, the results of percutaneous drainage appear to be comparable to those of an open operation. Open drainage is preferable if the contents of the cyst are too viscous to allow evacuation by drainage, the anatomic location precludes a safe percutaneous approach, or an additional abdominal surgical procedure is necessary. The drainage catheter should be withdrawn gradually if the cavity shows radiographic evidence of becoming obliterated. Either closed percutaneous drainage or open drainage with placement of a catheter is effective, although repeated drainage procedures, which usually necessitate an open laparotomy, may be necessary.

It may not be possible to drain multiple hepatic abscesses, although these cavities often communicate and can be drained by a single catheter. Alternatively, multiple catheters may be used or selective drainage of larger abscesses may be performed. The latter procedure is especially helpful in obtaining cultures to guide antibiotic therapy. Hepatic resection may sometimes be required for infections resistant to drainage and antimicrobial therapy, although resection is much less frequently required than it was previously.

Empirical antimicrobial therapy can be initiated before drainage on the basis of the likely route of infection and the organisms most commonly responsible for infection (Table 79–4). Definitive antimicrobial therapy should be directed by Gram stain, culture, and susceptibilities of the organisms recovered by the drainage procedure. Certain antibiotics exhibit better hepatic penetration and biliary excretion and are preferred for hepatic and biliary tract disease. These antibiotics include the extended-spectrum penicillins (e.g., piperacillin) and cefoperazone for gram-negative enteric organisms, metronidazole and clindamycin for anaerobic organisms, and nafcillin for *S. aureus.* Empirical therapy with an extended-spectrum penicillin or cefoperazone, plus metronidazole or clindamycin, is recommended, although results of comparative trials of these newer agents for hepatic abscesses are unavailable.

Antimicrobial therapy should be administered intravenously until defervescence and until radiographic evidence is obtained that drainage is complete, usually at least 1–3 weeks. The total duration of therapy is usually at least 4–6 weeks, until there is a good clinical response and radiographic evidence that the abscess has collapsed, although the antimicrobials may be given orally for the final 2–3 weeks. A longer duration of treatment is indicated for multiple abscesses that cannot be drained or if the clinical response is slow.

Although several cases have been reported that demonstrate the possibility of treating pyogenic abscesses by antimicrobial therapy alone, usually because of a malignant neoplasm or other complicating factor, the overall mortality is very high and therefore this treatment is not routinely recommended.

Fungal liver abscesses should be treated by drainage, repeated aspiration if necessary, and amphotericin B, possibly with the addition of flucytosine. The duration of antifungal therapy is usually as long as 6 months, as indicated by clinical and radiographic resolution.

Amebic Abscess. More than 90% of amebic abscesses respond to medical therapy with metronidazole (Table 79–4), which should be initiated without waiting for the results of serologic studies. A favorable clinical response is usually evident within a few days. Ultrasonography usually shows a decrease in the size of the abscess within 7–10 days, although the abscess may be detectable for months. Aspiration is necessary only if a concomitant bacterial infection cannot be excluded for persons who do not respond to metronidazole. Mixed bacterial and pyogenic abscesses should be treated by drainage and an antimicrobial regimen that includes metronidazole. Treatment of amebic hepatic abscess should be followed by a course of iodoquinol.

Hydatid Cysts. The preferred therapy for hydatid cysts has been surgical removal and albendazole (Table 44–5). Closed percutaneous aspiration of hydatid cysts was considered contraindicated because of the possibility of rupture, which would lead to protoscolex dissemination within the abdominal cavity or possible anaphylaxis. However, several reports indicate that percutaneous drainage combined with albendazole therapy may be an effective and safe treatment of uncomplicated hydatid liver cysts (Chapter 44).

Supportive Therapy. Appropriate intravenous fluid management, with parenteral nutrition, is necessary in the early stages of management. Occasionally, biliary obstruction may necessitate relief by endoscopic papillotomy or laparotomy for surgical drainage.

COMPLICATIONS

Untreated pyogenic hepatic abscesses can result in bacterial infection, sepsis, and death. Early diagnosis and appropriate therapy have greatly diminished these complications. Complications that can occur even during treatment include rupture, extrahepatic extension of infection, and septic emboli with secondary foci of infection. Extension of infection into the peritoneal, pleural, or pericardial cavity can cause subphrenic or subhepatic abscesses, pleural effusion or empyema, bronchohepatic fistula, and right lung infiltrate. Pericardial extension is classically associated with hepatic abscesses in the left lobe of the liver. Most foci of amebiasis outside the abdominal cavity are the result of dissemination from hepatic abscesses rather than direct dissemination from the intestinal tract.

PROGNOSIS

Pyogenic Abscesses. Much of the experience with hepatic abscesses was before the widespread availability of CT and MRI. The presence of a pyogenic hepatic abscess is a serious, life-threatening condition with almost 100% mortality rate if left untreated. Death is caused by rupture of the abscess into the peritoneal space, extension of infection into the pleural space or pericardium, associated sepsis, or, less commonly, extensive hepatic damage and hepatic failure. Since the 1940s the overall mortality has decreased dramatically, from more than 80% to less than 5%. Persons with multiple abscesses have historically had the highest mortality, although more recent experience suggests that there is not a significant difference in mortality rates between persons with one abscess and those with more than one.

Amebic Abscesses. Amebic abscesses respond well to medical management with metronidazole, with resolution of symptoms within 2–3 weeks. Larger abscesses, however, especially those larger than 10 cm in diameter, may remain detectable by ultrasonography for well over a year.

PREVENTION

Most pyogenic liver abscesses in children result from ascending biliary infections associated with underlying biliary stasis or occur after hepatobiliary operation or liver transplantation. Prompt recognition and aggressive treatment of cholangitis in these patients at risk should reduce the possibility of hepatic abscess. Use of ultrasonography, CT, or MRI for early diagnosis of hepatic abscess should lead to earlier recognition and treatment, with decreased morbidity and mortality rates.

REVIEWS

Adams EB, MacLeod IN: Invasive amebiasis. II. Amebic liver abscess and its complications. *Medicine* 1977;56:325–34.

Fujihara T, Nagai Y, Kubo T, et al: Amebic liver abscess. *J Gastroenterol* 1996;31:659–63.

Kays DW: Pediatric liver cysts and abscesses. *Semin Pediatr Surg* 1992; 1:107–14.

McDonald MI, Corey GR, Gallis HA, et al: Single and multiple pyogenic liver abscesses. Natural history, diagnosis and treatment, with emphasis on percutaneous drainage. *Medicine* 1984;63:291–302.

Seeto RK, Rockey DC: Pyogenic liver abscess. Changes in etiology, management, and outcome. *Medicine* 1996;75:99–113.

KEY ARTICLES

Bartley DL, Hughes WT, Parvey LS, et al: Computed tomography of hepatic and splenic fungal abscesses in leukemic children. *Pediatr Infect Dis* 1982;1:317–21.

Bertel CK, van Heerden JA, Sheedy PF II: Treatment of pyogenic hepatic abscesses. Surgical vs. percutaneous drainage. *Arch Surg* 1986;121: 554–8.

Brans YW, Ceballos R, Cassady G: Umbilical catheters and hepatic abscesses. *Pediatrics* 1974;53:264–6.

Brook I, Frazier EH: Microbiology of liver and spleen abscesses. *J Med Microbiol* 1998;47:1075–80.

Dehner LP, Kissane JM: Pyogenic hepatic abscesses in infancy and childhood. *J Pediatr* 1969;74:763–73.

Farges O, Leese T, Bismuth H: Pyogenic liver abscess: An improvement in prognosis. *Br J Surg* 1988;75:862–5.

Frider B, Larrieu E, Odriozola M: Long-term outcome of asymptomatic liver hydatidosis. *J Hepatol* 1999;30:228–31.

Halvorsen RA, Korobkin M, Foster WL, et al: The variable CT appearance of hepatic abscesses. *AJR Am J Roentgenol* 1984;142:941–6.

Johnston RB Jr, Baehner RL: Chronic granulomatous disease: Correlation between pathogenesis and clinical findings. *Pediatrics* 1971;48:730–9.

Kabaalioglu A, Karaali K, Apaydin A, et al: Ultrasound-guided percutaneous sclerotherapy of hydatid liver cysts in children. *Pediatr Surg Int* 2000;16:346–50.

Khuroo MS, Wani NA, Javid G, et al: Percutaneous drainage compared with surgery for hepatic hydatid cysts. *N Engl J Med* 1997;337:881–7.

Kubo S, Kinoshita H, Hirohashi K, et al: Risk factors for and clinical findings of liver abscess after biliary-intestinal anastomosis. *Hepatogastroenterology* 1999;46:116–20.

Miedema BW, Dineen P: The diagnosis and treatment of pyogenic liver abscesses. *Ann Surg* 1984;200:328–35.

Narayanan S, Madda JP, Johny M, et al: Crohn's disease presenting as pyogenic liver abscess with review of previous case reports. *Am J Gastroenterol* 1998;93:2607–9.

Oleszczuk-Raszke K, Cremin BJ, Fisher RM, et al: Ultrasonic features of pyogenic and amoebic hepatic abscesses. *Pediatr Radiol* 1989;19:230–3.

Reynolds TB: Medical treatment of pyogenic liver abscess. *Ann Intern Med* 1982;96:373–4.

Shulman ST, Beem MO: A unique presentation of sickle cell disease: Pyogenic hepatic abscess. *Pediatrics* 1971;47:1019–22.

Tashjian LS, Abramson JS, Peacock JE Jr: Focal hepatic candidiasis: A distinct clinical variant of candidiasis in immunocompromised patients. *Rev Infect Dis* 1984;6:689–703.

Tazawa J, Sakai Y, Maekawa S, et al: Solitary and multiple pyogenic liver abscesses: Characteristics of the patients and efficacy of percutaneous drainage. *Am J Gastroenterol* 1997;92:271–4.

Thaler M, Pastakia B, Shawker TH, et al: Hepatic candidiasis in cancer patients: The evolving picture of the syndrome. *Ann Intern Med* 1988; 108;88–100.

Weinberg JJ, Cohen P, Malhotra R: Primary tuberculous liver abscess associated with the human immunodeficiency virus. *Tubercle* 1988; 69:145–7.

CHAPTER 80

Infections of the Biliary Tract

M. Susan Moyer ▪ Hal B. Jenson

Inflammation of the gallbladder and biliary tract—cholecystitis and cholangitis—is uncommon in children. In adults the most common cause of cholecystitis is gallstones (calculous cholecystitis), and the inflammation is initially chemically induced rather than the result of infection. Cholelithiasis and its associated complications in the gallbladder or biliary tract are often the cause of the ductal obstruction that results in cholangitis. Because gallstones are uncommon in the pediatric age group, cholecystitis and cholangitis are encountered much less frequently than in adults and in somewhat different clinical settings. When inflammation is complicated by infection, the microbiologic agents of cholecystitis and cholangitis are usually intestinal flora or enteric pathogens, although both cholecystitis and cholangitis have been described as sequelae of systemic streptococcal infections.

CHOLECYSTITIS

Cholecystitis, or inflammation of the gallbladder, can be acute or can be associated with a more chronic course of repeated episodes of abdominal pain occurring for several months or years. It is infrequently infectious in origin, but infection is a significant complication of many cases of cholecystitis.

ETIOLOGY

Although bacteria can be cultured from bile in approximately 10% of cases of chronic cholecystitis, infection per se is not believed to be the cause of either the symptoms or the disease in this condition. The frequency of bacteria in bile increases with longer duration and severity of symptoms, age >60 years, jaundice, acute cholecystitis compared with chronic cholecystitis, and obstruction of the common bile duct. Bacteria ascend from the duodenum, which normally has sparse bacteria. The usual bacteria that may be found in bile include the enteric gram-negative organisms *Escherichia coli, Klebsiella, Enterobacter,* and *Proteus,* as well as *Enterococcus* and anaerobes.

Primary infections of the gallbladder that present as acute cholecystitis have been described in the setting of enteric bacterial infections *(Salmonella, Shigella, E. coli, Vibrio cholerae)* and as a complication of group A *Streptococcus* infections associated with bacteremia. Cholecystitis complicating bacterial enteric infections and bacteremia may be more common in immunocompromised persons, particularly those with AIDS.

EPIDEMIOLOGY

Acute cholecystitis is almost always associated with a predisposing condition. In adults, cholelithiasis is the underlying cause of most acute episodes, referred to as **calculous cholecystitis.** Only 10% of cases of cholecystitis occur in the absence of stones, referred to as **acalculous cholecystitis,** and of these, very few are related to primary infection of the bile or gallbladder. In children, more than half of the cases of acute cholecystitis are acalculous. The inflammation, as in adults, is not usually secondary to an infectious agent but may be related to trauma, ischemia, or stasis associated with an underlying congenital anomaly of the biliary ductal or vascular systems.

Acalculous cholecystitis usually occurs when normal gallbladder filling is disrupted, as in hospitalized patients who are relatively immobile, not enterally fed, and receiving parenteral long-term nutritional support. This condition is most commonly found in elderly persons and, although often associated with secondary sepsis, is not primarily an infectious disorder. Premature infants and neonates with chronic medical or surgical conditions that limit enteral intake and necessitate parenteral nutrition are also at increased risk for cholecystitis. The lack of enteral stimulation of gallbladder contraction, along with other factors such as the use of diuretics, contributes to the development of biliary sludge or stones in these persons. Severely ill, hospitalized children receiving parenteral nutrition are also at increased risk.

PATHOGENESIS

The pathogenic mechanisms implicated in acute inflammation of the gallbladder include stasis, ischemia, and infection. In calculous cholecystitis and most cases of acalculous cholecystitis, inflammation results from inflammatory mediators acting chemically rather than from infection. This occurs with stasis or obstruction of normal gallbladder filling and emptying, whether mechanical (e.g., by biliary stones) or functional (e.g., in illness or immobilization without enteral modulation of gallbladder function). Calculi in adults usually consist of cholesterol or mixed stones, whereas in children they are usually pigment stones associated with chronic hemolysis associated with hereditary spherocytosis or sickle cell disease.

Bile is normally sterile, but it provides an excellent growth medium for bacteria. Although acute cholecystitis is usually not infectious, results of gallbladder bile cultures are positive early in the course of disease in most persons, and in approximately 20% of persons the conditions in the bile support continued bacterial proliferation. This proliferation may ultimately lead to infectious complications such as **suppurative cholecystitis (empyema)** or perforation with abscess formation. Early in the course of cholecystitis the gallbladder wall becomes hyperemic and edematous. Subsequently an inflammatory exudate develops and cellular infiltrates are apparent histologically. With resolution of the episode, the mucosal surface usually heals, but residual scarring compromises the absorptive capacity of the gallbladder, eventually resulting in loss of function.

In persons with enteric infection, contamination of the gallbladder by the infectious agent is common; however, actual inflammation resulting in clinical symptoms, although reported, is rare. Intestinal bacteria usually reach the gallbladder by ascending infection but occasionally are spread hematogenously, as is common in *Salmonella typhi* infection and group A *Streptococcus* cholecystitis.

Hydrops of the gallbladder, defined as acute distention and characterized by marked gallbladder wall edema, usually results from a stone in the cystic duct. It has been reported in Kawasaki syndrome and in streptococcal infections in the absence of gallstones.

SYMPTOMS AND CLINICAL MANIFESTATIONS

The clinical presentation of cholecystitis is usually acute right-upper-quadrant abdominal pain and fever with or without jaundice. Other symptoms may include nausea, vomiting, and anorexia. Although abdominal pain is common, fever may be the only presenting symptom but does not imply infection. The pain may be localized to the right upper quadrant or referred to the shoulder or back. It may be continuous or intermittent (''colicky'') but is frequently generalized or obscured if the child is seriously ill. Because the symptoms may be nonspecific, it is important to recognize the clinical setting in which acute cholecystitis can occur, especially hospitalization with a requirement for total parenteral nutrition, the presence of a bacterial enteric or streptococcal infection, or immunocompromise, including that caused by AIDS.

Physical Examination Findings

Abdominal tenderness and guarding, either diffuse or localized to the right upper quadrant, may be present. A tender mass is palpable if the gallbladder is greatly enlarged, a finding in approximately 10% of affected children. **Murphy's sign** is the arrest of inspiration as the patient takes a deep breath when the inflamed gallbladder comes in contact with the examiner's fingers placed at the right costal margin below the liver edge. Abdominal distention and diminished or absent bowel sounds are also common clinical findings. The patient may have a fever. Jaundice is present in approximately 20% of cases.

DIAGNOSIS

Differential Diagnosis

The differential diagnosis of acute cholecystitis includes other inflammatory and infectious disorders of the abdomen, especially acute appendicitis, and conditions involving the right pleural space (Table 80–1). In children with sickle cell anemia the symptoms may closely mimic acute abdominal pain crisis. Because these children also are predisposed to the development of gallstones, differentiating between a pain crisis and acute cholecystitis is of particular importance.

TABLE 80–1. Differential Diagnosis of Acute Cholecystitis

Cholangitis
Acute appendicitis
Acute pancreatitis
Acute viral hepatitis
Peptic ulcer disease
Intestinal obstruction
Hepatic abscess
Hepatic tumor
Gonococcal perihepatitis (Fitz-Hugh–Curtis syndrome)
Renal disease
Pleurisy, pneumonitis
Sickle cell disease pain crisis

Laboratory Evaluation

Leukocytosis is common but not universal. Results of liver biochemical tests (e.g., determinations of aminotransferase, γ-glutamyl transferase, bilirubin, and alkaline phosphatase values) may be normal; if values are abnormal, they are usually only mildly elevated and are not specific for acute cholecystitis. Hyperbilirubinemia, when present, includes both direct and indirect fractions. An elevated serum amylase or lipase level may indicate concomitant pancreatitis, which is more commonly seen with cholangitis than with cholecystitis.

Microbiologic Evaluation

Blood culture results are rarely positive but may be positive with systemic streptococcal infection. Bile is not routinely sampled for culture unless it is obtained at the time of either percutaneous drainage for decompression or therapeutic cholecystectomy. A positive bile culture result does not necessarily indicate that the cultured organisms are responsible for the inflammation. Stool cultures to establish the specific etiologic agent in enteric infections can indicate the causative agent of associated acute cholecystitis.

Diagnostic Imaging

The diagnosis of acute cholecystitis is usually established by ultrasonography in conjunction with cholescintigraphy using ^{99m}Tc-labeled derivatives of **iminodiacetic acid** (e.g., **hepato-iminodiacetic acid [HIDA] scan**) that are taken up by the liver and excreted in the gallbladder and biliary tract. On ultrasonography the gallbladder is distended and the wall thickened. In acalculous cholecystitis, no stones are present, but there may be sludge in the lumen and subserosal edema. Ultrasonography is useful in identifying pericholecystic collections of fluid or abscesses. **Cholescintigraphy** outlines a normal gallbladder and bile ducts 15–30 minutes after intravenous injection of the radionuclide, with subsequent excretion into the proximal duodenum. Persons with cholecystitis demonstrate good hepatic uptake and emptying into the duodenum, but the gallbladder is not visualized. In acute cholecystitis this finding reflects compromise of gallbladder mucosal function from inflammation. In chronic cholecystitis, mucosal scarring leads to nonfunction and therefore to nonvisualization on scintigraphic scanning. Unfortunately, these scans are more sensitive in calculous cholecystitis, and scans may show no abnormalities in 20% of cases of acalculous cholecystitis. In addition, false-positive scanning results can be obtained in persons with acute pancreatitis, those with neoplasms of the liver or gallbladder (uncommon in children), and in those receiving parenteral nutrition. Equivocal scans may result from poor hepatic uptake of the radionuclide, which can occur in the presence of underlying liver disease.

When ultrasonography is not diagnostic, cholescintigraphy findings are equivocal or negative, and the possibility of cholecystitis is still considered, scanning may be repeated once the initial radioisotope has cleared. If results of repeated scintigraphy are negative, transhepatic aspiration of the gallbladder under ultrasonographic guidance for analysis of the bile, including Gram stain and culture, can be performed. This procedure may be preferable to exploratory laparotomy, particularly for persons who are seriously ill.

There is no longer a role for intravenous cholangiography or oral cholecystography. Although pigment stones are radiopaque, an ultrasonographic examination is preferred because it is very sensitive and also detects radiolucent (cholesterol) stones.

TREATMENT

Calculous cholecystitis is usually managed by supportive therapy, including administration of intravenous fluids, correction of electrolyte imbalances, administration of antipyretics, and cholecystectomy. Cholecystectomy may be performed early in the course of the disease, particularly if clinical deterioration is noted, or after the initial attack has resolved. Alternatively, persons who are deemed too ill for cholecystectomy may undergo percutaneous or surgical cholecystostomy and drainage; cholecystectomy can then be performed at a later time. Although the primary cause of inflammation is chemical and not infectious, antibiotics are generally recommended because of the early and prevalent contamination of the bile with bacteria in a setting where perforation and septic complications are possible. However, empirical antibiotic treatment has not been demonstrated to decrease the incidence of suppurative cholecystitis. The main benefits may be to prevent bacteremia and to provide prophylaxis in the perioperative period.

The management of acalculous cholecystitis is similar to that of calculous disease, with initial efforts directed at fluid resuscitation and stabilization. Because this disorder tends to be rapidly progressive, particularly in elderly persons, prompt diagnosis and therapeutic intervention with early surgical cholecystectomy, cholecystostomy, or percutaneous transhepatic cholecystostomy are important. Empirical administration of antibiotics is recommended. A single agent such as cefoxitin may be used. For seriously ill persons or those whose condition is septic or deteriorating, a combination of piperacillin-tazobactam, an aminoglycoside, and an antibiotic effective against *Bacteroides fragilis* and other anaerobic bacteria, such as metronidazole or clindamycin, should be used (Table 80–2). If the cholecystitis has developed in association with an identified enteric bacterial infection, antibiotic therapy directed at that organism should be included as part of the broad coverage against other intestinal bacteria that may colonize an inflamed gallbladder. Aerobic and anaerobic cultures of bile should be taken during the surgical procedure to guide subsequent antimicrobial therapy.

TABLE 80–2. Recommended Empirical Antibiotic Therapy for Infections of the Biliary Tract

Piperacillin-tazobactam or cefoperazone *plus*
gentamicin (or another aminoglycoside)
with or without
metronidazole or clindamycin

Suggested Dosages for Persons with Normal Renal Function

ANTIBIOTIC	INTRAVENOUS DOSAGE	MAXIMUM DAILY DOSE
Amikacin	15 mg/kg/day divided q8–12hr	15 mg/kg
Cefoperazone (safety and efficacy have not been established in children)	150 mg/kg/day divided q8hr	12 g
Clindamycin	40 mg/kg/day divided q6hr	2.7 g
Gentamicin	7.5 mg/kg/day divided q8hr	Adults: 5 mg/kg
Metronidazole	30 mg/kg/day divided q6hr	30 mg/kg
Piperacillin-tazobactam	200–300 mg/kg/day divided q4–6hr	18 g
Tobramycin	7.5 mg/kg/day divided q8hr	Adults: 5 mg/kg

COMPLICATIONS

Complications associated with acute cholecystitis include empyema (suppurative cholecystitis with an intraluminal abscess) and necrosis or gangrene of the wall of the gallbladder, followed by perforation. These complications are usually accompanied by bacteremia with heightened systemic signs and symptoms. Local perforation may lead to a hepatic abscess. In addition, the perforation may be into the intestine, forming a cholecystenteric fistula into the abdominal cavity and causing generalized peritonitis, with an associated mortality rate of approximately 30%. These complications are particularly common in acalculous cholecystitis. In adults, they may be present in 75% at the time of the operation, which emphasizes the need for early diagnosis and surgical intervention. Pancreatitis as a complication of cholecystitis usually occurs concomitantly with the gallbladder disease and is due to the presence of stones.

PROGNOSIS

The prognosis for an acute episode of uncomplicated calculous cholecystitis is very good. Acalculous cholecystitis tends to be more severe and is associated with a 10% mortality rate in persons who are elderly or seriously ill or in those who have complications. Subsequent episodes are precluded by cholecystectomy.

PREVENTION

There are no specific measures to prevent acute cholecystitis. Recognition of the population at risk, expeditious diagnosis, and early institution of appropriate therapy will decrease the incidence of complications and thereby the overall morbidity and mortality. In infants and children with cholelithiasis, cholecystectomy is recommended, regardless of age, when disease is symptomatic. In addition, cholecystectomy is also considered for children younger than 3 years with asymptomatic disease if the stones have been present for at least 12 months or are radiopaque. Older children who have no symptoms with an incidental finding of gallstones but no evidence of biliary tract obstruction or hepatic dysfunction, and who do not have an underlying hemolytic disorder, may be followed up clinically with periodic ultrasonographic examinations and laboratory tests.

Oral therapy for dissolution of gallstones, such as the administration of ursodeoxycholate, is not effective for pigment stones and therefore is rarely of use in children.

CHOLANGITIS

Cholangitis, or inflammation of the biliary tract, implies bacterial infection and is usually encountered in the presence of mechanical or functional biliary tract obstruction that predisposes the patient to contamination of bile with enteric organisms.

ETIOLOGY

Enteric bacteria that ascend from the duodenum are the most common organisms implicated in cholangitis. The usual bacteria found in bile and liver biopsies of cases of cholangitis include the gram-negative organisms *E. coli, Klebsiella, Enterobacter,* and *Proteus,* as well as *Pseudomonas aeruginosa* and anaerobes. Anaerobes, especially *B. fragilis* and *Clostridium perfringens,* are involved in 15–39% of cases. Less frequently cultured organisms include *Enterococcus,* streptococci, and staphylococci. In immunocompromised persons, abnormal immune function is a predisposing factor for infection with fungi such as *Candida* and *Cryptococcus,* viruses such as cytomegalovirus, and other opportunistic organisms such as *Cryptosporidium,* but bile stasis or compromise of the physiologic barrier to ascent of organisms into the ductal system is still important in the pathogenesis of cholangitis.

Rarely, other infections or infestations may result in clinical cholangitis. *Echinococcus* hepatic cysts may rupture into the biliary tract. Cholangitis may also develop with ascariasis if the worms migrate from the duodenum, through the sphincter of Oddi, into the bile ducts.

EPIDEMIOLOGY

Cholangitis is more common in adults than in children and is usually seen in association with choledocholithiasis. Cholangitis is also associated with bile duct strictures caused by neoplasms, biliary tract operations, or abdominal trauma (Table 80–3). In children, biliary tract stones, neoplasms of the bile ducts, and operations on the biliary tract are uncommon.

The most common clinical setting of cholangitis among children is that following **hepatoportoenterostomy** (the **Kasai procedure**) for surgical repair of extrahepatic biliary atresia. This procedure involves resecting the extrahepatic biliary tract to the level in the porta hepatis where bile flow is evident and then anastomosing the liver directly to a segment of intestine that has been made into a Roux-en-Y loop. Infection of the biliary tract, a frequent complication of this surgical procedure, develops in 50–100% of persons postoperatively. Most episodes occur within the first 2 years after the operation, although cholangitis may occur more than 5 years postoperatively. Cholangitis is usually seen in persons with effectively functioning portoenterostomies and well-established bile flow. The abnormal anatomy, with loss of the protective function of the sphincter of Oddi and direct contact of the biliary system with the intestinal contents, predisposes the person to bacterial overgrowth and the development of clinically apparent ascending cholangitis.

TABLE 80–3. Conditions that Predispose a Child to Cholangitis

Hepatoportoenterostomy (Kasai procedure)
Congenital anomalies of the biliary tract
Choledochal cysts
Caroli's disease
Biliary tract strictures
Surgical
Traumatic
Neoplastic
Liver transplantation
Choledocholithiasis
Pancreatitis
Acquired immunodeficiency syndrome (AIDS)
Other infections or infestations
Echinococcosis (rare)
Ascariasis (rare)

Cholangitis is also a complication of congenital anomalies of the biliary tract, specifically choledochal cysts and Caroli's disease. **Choledochal cysts** may involve intrahepatic ducts, extrahepatic ducts, or both. Although the clinical presentation varies, nearly half of the cases occur at a later age, beginning in adolescence, with cholangitis. **Caroli's disease** involves multiple cystic dilatations of the intrahepatic bile ducts and may be seen in association with congenital hepatic fibrosis and medullary sponge kidney. Persons with cystic disease of the intrahepatic ducts alone most commonly have cholangitis.

Cholangitis is also a frequent complication of liver transplantation, occurring in 26–88% of adult liver transplant recipients. The biliary tract reconstruction and indwelling stents can predispose the person to bacterial colonization, obstruction of normal bile flow, and ascending infection. Presurgical debilitation and postsurgical immunocompromise are also risk factors, particularly for infection by less commonly associated pathogens such as *Cryptosporidium, Candida, Cryptococcus,* and cytomegalovirus. These infectious agents also cause cholangitis in other immunocompromised persons, particularly those with AIDS.

PATHOGENESIS

Conditions that result in either functional or mechanical obstruction to normal biliary flow or that bypass the mechanical barrier to ascending infection result in a predisposition to bacterial infection of bile. Compromise of the normal physiologic barrier to retrograde colonization of the biliary tract by intestinal bacteria is another predisposing factor in the development of cholangitis. After the Kasai procedure, the abnormal anatomy and the proximity of the porta hepatis to the intestine without an interposed physical barrier to bacterial contamination account for the frequent occurrence of postsurgical cholangitis. Similarly, bile stasis related to the abnormal biliary tract anatomy seen in congenital choledochal cysts and Caroli's disease allows the development of clinically significant bacterial infections of these cysts and bile ducts. Mechanical obstruction from a stricture or stone similarly results in a pathophysiologic predisposition to infection.

Recurrent pyogenic cholangitis (Oriental cholangiohepatitis), although not a disorder that occurs in childhood, has a presumed infectious cause. This disease is characterized by chronic infection and stone formation in the bile ducts. Prevalent in Southeast Asia, this disorder usually occurs in adulthood, between the ages of 25 and 80 years; in virtually all cases, *E. coli* is cultured from the bile. This organism produces β-glucuronidase, which unconjugates bilirubin, predisposing the patient to stone formation. Although the precise pathophysiology of this infection is unclear, the initial event is thought to be portal phlebitis resulting in portal bacteremia. Approximately half of these persons are also infested with the parasitic fluke *Clonorchis sinensis,* found in raw freshwater fish; the fluke can migrate from the duodenum into the biliary tract. Definitive treatment of this disorder usually involves biliary drainage, which may be accomplished surgically or by endoscopic sphincterotomy.

SYMPTOMS AND CLINICAL MANIFESTATIONS

The most common presenting symptoms of cholangitis are abdominal pain, fever and chills resulting from bacteremia, and jaundice. This constellation of clinical symptoms is known as **Charcot's triad.** Pain and fever are present in approximately 90% of patients, although jaundice is less common, occurring in approximately 20%. Jaundice may be related to mechanical obstruction or intrahepatic cholestasis caused by sepsis. In the absence of jaundice the clinical presentation may be nonspecific, particularly in infants and younger children, who may merely manifest fever and irritability. Other associated symptoms may include abdominal distention, nausea and vomiting, dark urine, and **acholic** (pale) stools.

In some persons, symptoms may be transient and self-limited. In more severe cases the presentation may be one of septic shock, which can obscure the symptoms of biliary tract disease.

Physical Examination Findings

On physical examination the person usually is febrile and may appear to be in a toxic or septic state. Jaundice may be present, as may abdominal tenderness, distention, and diminished or absent bowel sounds because of an adynamic ileus. Abdominal pain may be diffuse or localized to the right upper quadrant, and peritoneal signs such as rebound tenderness may be elicited. Hepatomegaly is commonly present in persons with extrahepatic biliary atresia and in some children with congenital cystic biliary tract disease; therefore it is not a helpful differentiating diagnostic sign. In other persons an enlarged liver may suggest the presence of a hepatic abscess, a late complication of cholangitis.

DIAGNOSIS

The diagnosis of cholangitis is usually established by compatible clinical symptoms in a person at risk of having cholangitis, supported by evidence of biliary obstruction, and confirmed by identification of the causative organisms by culture of blood, bile, or liver tissue. Culture results are frequently negative, however, often necessitating empirical treatment.

Differential Diagnosis

The differential diagnosis of cholangitis varies, depending on the clinical setting, but includes many other infections and inflammatory disorders of the hepatobiliary system and abdomen (Table 80–4).

Laboratory Evaluation

Routine laboratory tests may be helpful but, as with cholecystitis, are usually nonspecific. Common abnormalities include elevated levels of bilirubin (total and direct), serum aminotransferases, and alkaline phosphatase, accompanied by leukocytosis with a left shift and an elevated ESR. Infants who have had a Kasai procedure may continue to have abnormal findings on liver biochemistry tests for a variable period postoperatively, and therefore it is important to compare values obtained during acute illness with previous values.

TABLE 80–4. Differential Diagnosis of Cholangitis*

Cholecystitis
Acute viral hepatitis
Appendicitis
Pancreatitis
Peritonitis
Intra-abdominal infections
Hepatic abscess
Urinary tract infections
Renal disease
Sickle cell disease pain crisis
Allograft rejection after liver transplantation

*Varies depending on clinical setting.

Elevated amylase or lipase levels may indicate acute pancreatitis as a complication of cholangitis.

Microbiologic Evaluation

The specific organisms responsible for infection may be identified by culture of blood, bile, and liver tissue. Because bacteremia is common in cholangitis, blood culture results may be positive, particularly if obtained during fever spikes. The bacteremia is most likely related to the forced entry of bacteria into the hepatic system by increased biliary pressure, which, in turn, is related to the degree of obstruction. Culture of hepatic tissue obtained by **percutaneous liver biopsy** is perhaps more sensitive and specific but is usually reserved for specific clinical situations, such as recurrent cholangitis after a portoenterostomy or fever or worsening serum aminotransferase values in a liver transplant recipient or an immunocompromised child. In a report (Piccoli, 1986) comparing blood culture results with liver biopsy culture results in an evaluation of 32 episodes of cholangitis in persons who had undergone a Kasai procedure, 68% of the tissue cultures showed positive results, whereas only 31% of the blood cultures yielded an organism. In infants and children in whom cholangitis develops after a portoenterostomy or liver transplantation, isolation of an organism from blood or liver tissue is particularly helpful because many of these persons receive multiple courses of antibiotics and resistant gastrointestinal flora may develop. In addition to tissue culture, a liver biopsy allows histologic support for the diagnosis of cholangitis, which is important in differentiating a biliary tract infection from allograft rejection in a liver transplant recipient and from other causes of hepatobiliary dysfunction in an immunocompromised person. Specific immunohistochemical stains for organisms such as cytomegalovirus may also be of diagnostic assistance.

Obtaining bile for culture from persons who have undergone a Kasai procedure is difficult. The bile ducts are usually not dilated, making percutaneous transhepatic cannulation problematic, and the anatomy of the Roux-en-Y intestinal loop generally precludes endoscopic assessment. In persons who do have a dilated biliary tract, bile for culture can be obtained either by percutaneous transhepatic catheterization or by endoscopic cannulation of the common bile duct. Culture specimens are usually obtained when a procedure is performed specifically to decompress the biliary tract. In adults, bile culture results are positive for two organisms in approximately half of the cases, whereas blood cultures usually contain only one organism. Whether this implies that more than one agent is involved in the pathogenesis of cholangitis, implies the propensity of some organisms to spread by bacteremia, or merely reflects the profile of contaminating intestinal flora is unclear.

Blood, bile, and liver tissue should be cultured for routine bacteria and also for anaerobes. In immunocompromised persons, cultures for fungal pathogens (e.g., *Candida, Cryptococcus*), viruses (e.g., cytomegalovirus), and opportunistic organisms (e.g., *Cryptosporidium*) should be obtained.

Diagnostic Imaging

Imaging studies are helpful in determining the presence of obstruction. Ultrasonography can demonstrate dilated ducts proximal to the level of obstruction and can document the presence of stones or sludge in the biliary tract. Ultrasonography also can show the presence of intrahepatic or extrahepatic cysts. Cholangiography, either transhepatic or endoscopic, helps localize the site of obstruction and may help identify the cause as well.

Pathologic Findings

Histologic findings consistent with cholangitis on liver biopsy include neutrophilic infiltration of the wall and lumen of portal bile ducts, focal necrosis of bile duct epithelial cells, and microabscesses adjacent to bile duct walls. With extrahepatic obstruction, bile duct proliferation may be present. In cholangitis related to cytomegalovirus infection, viral inclusions may be evident in bile duct epithelium.

TREATMENT

Management involves appropriate antibiotic coverage, decompression of acute obstruction, and definitive treatment of the underlying cause of obstruction or bile stasis. Empirical antibiotic treatment should include antimicrobial agents effective against the common gram-negative, gram-positive, and anaerobic organisms known to cause cholangitis and should preferably have good biliary penetration (Table 80–2). None of the cephalosporins provide coverage against *Enterococcus,* and only cefoperazone and ceftazidime provide good coverage against *Pseudomonas* but do not reliably cover *B. fragilis.* Many penicillins and cefoperazone have good hepatic excretion, but the bile-to-serum ratio for aminoglycosides is very low. Ceftriaxone is usually avoided because of its propensity to cause biliary sludge and stones, which can complicate the clinical situation.

The extended-spectrum penicillins, such as piperacillin-tazobactam, have good coverage of gram-negative bacilli including *Pseudomonas, Enterococcus,* and anaerobes. In addition, the biliary concentration is on the order of 30-fold higher than the serum concentration. These antibiotics are susceptible to β-lactamases and are usually combined with an aminoglycoside to minimize development of resistance. Cefoperazone is an alternative for persons who are allergic to penicillin.

In general, empirical coverage with piperacillin-tazobactam or cefoperazone and an aminoglycoside may be sufficient when the presentation is mild and uncomplicated. For moderately to severely ill persons, an antibiotic effective against anaerobes, such as metronidazole or clindamycin, may be added. Because of the high incidence of resistant isolates in persons who have undergone a Kasai procedure, at least two agents should be used (e.g., piperacillin-tazobactam and gentamicin) until definitive sensitivities can be established. Clinical improvement is usually evident within 6–12 hours of the initiation of antibiotic therapy.

Identification of the organism by culture allows determination of the antibiotic susceptibilities and permits narrowing of antibiotic therapy, which reduces the risk that resistant organisms will develop because of broad-coverage antimicrobial therapy. Avoiding this risk is particularly important in infants with a portoenterostomy, who often require multiple or prolonged courses of therapy for persistent or recurrent cholangitis.

Biliary Decompression. A person with an identified site of obstruction who has a "toxic" presentation or fails to improve after receiving antibiotics should undergo biliary tract decompression. It is virtually impossible to attain therapeutic levels of antibiotics in the biliary tract in the presence of obstruction. Increased biliary pressure also contributes to the bacteremia commonly seen with cholangitis. Decompression can be accomplished endoscopically or by percutaneous transhepatic catheterization, depending on the level of obstruction and the condition of the patient. In extreme circumstances the obstruction must be relieved surgically. The common bile duct can be cannulated endoscopically to allow visualization of the biliary tract, bile sampling, and decompression by sphincterotomy, removal of stones, dilation of strictures, or placement of stents or catheters, depending on the site and cause of obstruction. With the transhepatic approach, a sample of bile can be obtained for culture, the biliary tract can be imaged by injection of contrast material, and the catheter can be left in place for decompression. Either endoscopy or catheterization provides temporary decompression until the condition of a person who requires definitive surgical therapy, for removal of large bile duct stones or resection of neoplasms or strictures, is clinically stable.

Infants or children with portoenterostomies or those with congenital bile duct anomalies do not usually have a specific site of acute obstruction. If a child has persistent or recurrent cholangitis after a Kasai procedure, evaluation for other predisposing conditions, such as an infected bile lake, hepatic abscess, or stasis in a Roux-en-Y intestinal loop, should be undertaken. Ultrasonography or CT can identify fluid collections or abscesses, and guided percutaneous aspiration can then determine the presence of infection. Stasis in a Roux-en-Y loop, which may predispose a person to bacterial overgrowth and ascending infection, is suggested on a HIDA scan when the radioisotope is concentrated in the area of the loop and does not quickly pass into the contiguous intestine. In selected cases, surgical drainage or revision of the portoenterostomy may be necessary. Choledochal cysts have considerable malignant potential and should be resected after treatment of the cholangitis. In Caroli's disease the diffuse intrahepatic involvement of the biliary tract precludes surgical excision of cysts.

COMPLICATIONS

The most significant complications of cholangitis are bacteremia and the development of a pyogenic hepatic abscess (Chapter 79). In children with hepatoportoenterostomy for extrahepatic biliary atresia, episodes of cholangitis tend to accelerate the progression of the underlying hepatobiliary disease and can hasten the development of biliary cirrhosis.

PROGNOSIS

Ultimately the prognosis depends on the underlying disorder, or the cause of the biliary obstruction. In individual episodes of biliary tract infection, the immediate prognosis is good with prompt initiation of appropriate antibiotic therapy and with decompression when indicated. Cholangitis can cause temporary or permanent damage to the liver in persons with portoenterostomies, which emphasizes the importance of prompt diagnosis and aggressive therapy.

PREVENTION

The use of prophylactic antibiotics is an issue that arises in the treatment of infants who have undergone hepatoportoenterostomy, because of the prevalence of postsurgical cholangitis, and in the treatment of patients with Caroli's disease. Antibiotics such as trimethoprim-sulfamethoxazole have been used prophylactically but have not been shown to decrease substantially the incidence of cholangitis. Theoretically, prophylactic antibiotics could also contribute to the development of resistant organisms. For these reasons the use of antibiotics for prophylaxis is not routinely recommended.

REVIEWS

Lillemoe KD: Surgical treatment of biliary tract infections. *Am Surg* 2000; 66:138–44.

Nash JA, Cohen SA: Gallbladder and biliary tract disease in AIDS. *Gastroenterol Clin North Am* 1997;26:323–35.

Rescorla FJ: Cholelithiasis, cholecystitis, and common bile duct stones. *Curr Opin Pediatr* 1997;9:276–82.

Westphal JF, Brogard JM: Biliary tract infections: A guide to drug treatment. *Drugs* 1999;57:81–91.

KEY ARTICLES

Blumberg RS, Kelsey P, Perrone T, et al: Cytomegalovirus- and *Cryptosporidium*-associated acalculous gangrenous cholecystitis. *Am J Med* 1984; 76:1118–23.

Dickinson SJ, Corley G, Santulli TV: Acute cholecystitis as a sequel of scarlet fever. *Am J Dis Child* 1971;121:331–3.

Howlett SA, Schulman ST, Ayoub EM, et al: Cholangitis complicating congenital hepatic fibrosis. *Am J Dig Dis* 1975;20:790–5.

Jacobson MA, Cello JP, Sande MA: Cholestasis and disseminated cytomegalovirus disease in patients with the acquired immunodeficiency syndrome. *Am J Med* 1988;84:218–24.

Kuhls TL, Jackson MA: Diagnosis and treatment of the febrile child following hepatic portoenterostomy. *Pediatr Infect Dis* 1985;4:487–90.

Kuzu MA, Kale IT, Col C, et al: Obstructive jaundice promotes bacterial translocation in humans. *Hepatogastroenterology* 1999;46:2159–64.

Lopez-Santamaria M, Martinez L, Hierro C, et al: Late biliary complications in pediatric liver transplantation. *J Pediatr Surg* 1999;34:316–20.

Lunzmann K, Schweizer P: The influence of cholangitis on the prognosis of extrahepatic biliary atresia. *Eur J Pediatr Surg* 1999;9:19–23.

Misra SP, Dwivedi M: Clinical features and management of biliary ascariasis in a nonendemic area. *Postgrad Med J* 2000;76:29–32.

Nakaysma F, Soloway RD, Nakama T, et al: Hepatolithiasis in East Asia. Retrospective study. *Dig Dis Sci* 1986;31:21–6.

Piccoli DA, Mohan P, McConnie RM: Cholangitis post-Kasai: Diagnostic value of blood cultures and liver biopsy [abstract]. *Pediatr Res* 1986; 20:247A.

Rha SY, Stovroff MC, Glick PL, et al: Choledochal cysts: A ten-year experience. *Am Surg* 1996;62:30–4.

Skummerfield JA, Nagafuchi Y, Sherlock S, et al: Hepatobiliary fibropolycystic diseases. A clinical and histologic review of 51 patients. *J Hepatol* 1986;2:141–56.

Zaidi E, Bachur R, Harper M: Non-typhi *Salmonella* bacteremia in children. *Pediatr Infect Dis J* 1999:18;1073–7.

CHAPTER 81

Acute Pancreatitis

M. Susan Moyer ▪ Hal B. Jenson

Pancreatitis, although not a common disease in infants and children, is recognized with increasing frequency but is not usually associated with infection. Pancreatitis is classified clinically as either acute or chronic. **Acute pancreatitis** implies the likelihood of resolution of pancreatic inflammation with restoration of function and includes clinically relapsing or **recurrent acute pancreatitis.** Acute pancreatitis may also be classified as **interstitial pancreatitis** or as **necrotizing pancreatitis.** Necrotizing pancreatitis may be complicated by bacterial infection, requiring antimicrobial therapy and surgical débridement. **Chronic pancreatitis** indicates ongoing inflammation and damage, often associated with eventual compromise of endocrine and exocrine pancreatic function, and is usually not complicated by infection. In adults, cholelithiasis and alcohol abuse are the most common causes of pancreatitis, accounting for 70–80% of cases. The causes of acute pancreatitis in the pediatric population are varied and rarely include alcohol or biliary tract stones.

ETIOLOGY

Pancreatitis implies inflammation but is not usually associated with infection. Noninfectious causes of acute pancreatitis include mechanical or structural abnormalities, trauma, metabolic and inherited disorders, drugs and toxins, and multisystem diseases (Table 81–1). Numerous infectious agents have been associated with acute pancreatitis (Table 81–2), but whether each has a direct effect on the pancreas or incites pancreatic inflammation as a result of generalized systemic effects (e.g., hypotension, shock) is not always clear. In most pediatric series, primary infection accounts for only 3–5% of cases of pancreatitis. Secondary bacterial infection is an important complication of necrotizing pancreatitis. Approximately 25% of cases of acute pancreatitis in children are classified as **idiopathic pancreatitis,** and no predisposing condition is identified.

Secondary bacterial infection complicating necrotizing pancreatitis occurs from spread of enteric bacteria from the colon and is associated with high morbidity and mortality. Other bacterial infections associated with pancreatitis are rare but may complicate acute bacterial enteritis caused by *Salmonella, Yersinia,* and *Campylobacter.* Pancreatitis may complicate hemolytic uremic syndrome, a systemic disorder caused by *E. coli* serotype O157:H7 producing verotoxin. Both influenza B virus and varicella-zoster virus have been causally associated with Reye's syndrome, another systemic disorder associated with acute hemorrhagic pancreatitis in as many as 50% of those persons with moderate to severe neurologic symptoms. Mumps has been implicated historically as one of the more common causes of acute pancreatitis in children, but the incidence may be overestimated. Abdominal pain is a frequent complaint in children with mumps, and the serum amylase level is commonly elevated because of parotid gland inflammation. Unless the hyperamylasemia is attributed to the pancreatic isoenzyme or there is additional evidence of pancreatic inflammation, the presence of pancreatitis with mumps should not be assumed.

EPIDEMIOLOGY

The epidemiology of acute pancreatitis reflects the diverse underlying causes, which are primarily noninfectious (Table 81–1). Because the pathogenic mechanisms for initiation of pancreatic inflammation remain unclear, an etiologic relationship between a clinical condition and the development of pancreatitis is often defined by epidemiologic observations. Mechanical or structural factors include congenital anomalies of the biliary tract (e.g., choledochal cysts) or pancreatic ducts (e.g., pancreas divisum) and acquired disorders. **Pancreas divisum** is the failure of the dorsal and ventral pancreatic ducts to fuse during development, resulting in drainage of the pancreas through the dorsal duct, which obstructs outflow. Although this anomaly may be a normal variant, it is a cause of recurrent acute pancreatitis. Migration of parasites such as *Ascaris lumbricoides* and *Clonorchis sinensis* into the biliary or pancreatic ducts may also in-

TABLE 81–1. Conditions Associated with Acute Pancreatitis

Mechanical or Structural	Drug- or Toxin-Induced
Trauma	*Drugs*
Blunt, nonpenetrating	Sulfonamides
Postsurgical	Tetracyclines
Post–endoscopic retrograde cholangiopancreatography (ERCP)	Estrogens
Pancreatic Outflow Obstruction (Congenital or Acquired)	Furosemide
Ductal anomalies (pancreas divisum)	Thiazides
Strictures	6-Mercaptopurine
Cholelithiasis	Azathioprine
Ascaris lumbricoides	L-Asparaginase
Clonorchis sinensis	Valproic acid
Bile Reflux (Congenital or Acquired)	Pentamidine
Ductal anomalies (choledochal cyst)	*Toxins*
Strictures	Ethanol
Choledocholithiasis	Borates
Duodenopancreatic Reflux (Congenital or Acquired)	Organophosphates
Duodenal obstruction	Carbamates
Metabolic	Yellow scorpion venom
Hypercalcemia	**Multisystem Disorders**
Hyperlipidemia (types I, IV, and V)	Infections (Table 81–2)
Hypothermia	Sepsis
Uremia	Shock
Malnutrition with refeeding	Vasculitis and inflammatory disorders
α_1-Antitrypsin deficiency	Reye's syndrome
Cystic fibrosis	
Diabetes mellitus	
Hereditary (familial) pancreatitis	

TABLE 81–2. Infectious Causes of Acute Pancreatitis

Viruses	Bacteria
Mumps virus	*Salmonella typhi*
Enteroviruses	*Escherichia coli* serotype O157:H7 (verotoxin-producing serotype)
Coxsackievirus B	*Mycoplasma pneumoniae*
Echovirus	*Treponema pallidum* (including congenital syphilis)
Influenza A virus	*Leptospira*
Influenza B virus	**Parasites**
Varicella-zoster virus	*Plasmodium* (malaria)
Epstein-Barr virus	*Ascaris lumbricoides*
Hepatitis A virus	*Clonorchis sinensis*
Hepatitis B virus	
Hepatitis E virus	
Measles virus (rubeola)	
Rubella virus (including congenital rubella syndrome)	
Congenital syphilis	
Rotavirus	

duce pancreatitis by obstruction but without infection of pancreatic parenchyma. Metabolic and inherited disorders associated with pancreatitis include cystic fibrosis if there is residual function of the gland. Recently a genotype of cystic fibrosis has been identified that presents clinically as recurrent acute pancreatitis. The predominant genetic mutation for **hereditary (familial) pancreatitis,** another condition of recurrent bouts of acute pancreatitis, has also been identified. Numerous drugs and toxins have a well-established correlation with the development of acute pancreatitis, although definitive evidence of a cause-and-effect relationship is lacking for many. A varied and diverse group of multisystem disorders with severe or widespread systemic involvement compose the largest etiologic subdivision of acute pancreatitis, although the development of clinical pancreatitis in each disorder may be rare. Many of the infectious agents associated with pancreatitis (Table 81–2) are characterized by systemic involvement and may induce pancreatitis by systemic effects of hypotension and shock.

PATHOGENESIS

Pancreatic inflammation results from premature activation of pancreatic enzymes either within the acinar cells or in the pancreatic ducts. Many diverse processes may merge into this final common event, although the exact mechanism initiating this activation is not known. Several protective mechanisms in the pancreas itself and in the systemic circulation prevent or modify the effects of prematurely activated digestive enzymes. Within the acinar cell, digestive enzymes are synthesized in an inactive form and packaged in **zymogen granules,** which are physically separated from **lysosomal hydrolases** (e.g., cathepsin B) that could activate **trypsinogen** to **trypsin.** In addition, a trypsin inhibitor accompanies the digestive enzymes to inactivate any trypsin that may be released. Pancreatic enzymes do not normally become active until they reach the intestinal lumen. To prevent systemic effects, circulating active proteases form a complex with α_1-antiprotease and are transferred to α_2-macroglobulin, which are rapidly cleared by monocytes. In pancreatitis, premature activation of trypsinogen to trypsin results in activation of other digestive enzymes, which initiates a cascade of local pancreatic autodigestion and systemic injury. This injury may be compounded by the local generation of oxygen free radicals. In moderate or severe pancreatitis the systemic pathway of protease inactivation is overwhelmed, exacerbating the systemic effects of circulating active enzymes. The genetic mutation identified in hereditary pancreatitis renders trypsin resistant to hydrolysis by pancreatic enzymes designed to degrade excess trypsin and protect the pancreas from autodigestion.

Interstitial pancreatitis is mild pancreatic inflammation characterized by edema and infiltration of inflammatory cells but with preservation of pancreatic architecture. **Necrotizing pancreatitis** is more severe inflammation that results in destruction of pancreatic acini and one or more diffuse or focal areas of nonviable pancreatic parenchyma. CT with contrast enhancement is used to make this distinction because tissue for histologic examination is rarely available. The risk of secondary bacterial infection is significantly greater in necrotizing pancreatitis (30–50%) than in interstitial pancreatitis (<1%).

SYMPTOMS AND CLINICAL MANIFESTATIONS

The presenting symptoms of pancreatitis in children are variable, but they usually include abdominal pain and vomiting (Table 81–3). The pain is often sudden in onset, sharp in nature, severe, constant, and frequently located in the epigastrium. Eating is often an aggravating factor. Radiation of the pain to the back, chest, or other parts of the abdomen may be noted. Vomiting accompanies the pain in as many as 70% of cases and may be bilious. Other symptoms include nausea, loss of appetite, and, rarely, altered mental status. Occasionally, pain may be mild or even absent.

Physical Examination Findings

The most common finding is epigastric tenderness, which may be accompanied by guarding and rebound tenderness (Table 81–3). The abdomen may be distended, and bowel sounds are frequently decreased or absent, reflecting an underlying ileus. Fever, when present, is usually low grade. If vomiting has been protracted and oral intake poor, there may be signs of dehydration with tachycardia, hypotension, and decreased urine output. In cases of more severe pancreatic inflammation, the presentation may include respiratory distress or cardiovascular shock or both. Hemorrhagic pancreatitis may result in dissection of blood along the fascial plains of the abdominal wall, with ecchymoses noted along the flanks **(Turner's sign)** or in the periumbilical area **(Cullen's sign).**

DIAGNOSIS

The diagnosis depends on a careful history to determine the presence of predisposing factors, compatible signs and symptoms, and supportive laboratory and imaging studies. Distinguishing **severe acute pancreatitis** is important for management and is established by the following clinical criteria: a score of ≥3 on **Ranson's criteria** (Table

TABLE 81–3. Signs and Symptoms of Acute Pancreatitis

Symptoms	Signs
Abdominal pain	Abdominal tenderness (epigastric)
Vomiting	Peritoneal signs
Nausea	Guarding
Anorexia	Rebound tenderness
	Abdominal distention
	Decreased or absent bowel sounds
	Fever (usually low grade)
	Hypotension, shock
	Pleural effusion
	Ascites
	Respiratory distress
	Oliguria or anuria
	Cullen's sign
	Turner's sign

TABLE 81–4. Ranson's Criteria for Severe Acute Pancreatitis (Ranson Score ≥3)

At Presentation
Age ≥55 yr
Leukocyte count >16,000/mm^3
Blood glucose level >200 mg/dL
Serum lactate dehydrogenase (LDH) level >350 IU/L
Serum aspartate aminotransferase (AST) level >250 IU/L
During Initial 48 Hr
Hematocrit decrease >10%
Blood urea nitrogen increase >5 mg/dL
Serum calcium <8 mg/dL
Arterial Pao_2 <60 mm Hg
Base deficit >4 mEq/L
Fluid sequestration >6 L (for adults)

Adapted from Ranson JHC, Rifkind KM, Roses DF, et al: Prognostic signs and the role of operative management in acute pancreatitis. *Surg Gynecol Obstet* 1974;139:69–81.

81–4), which include five risk factors on presentation and six risk factors assessed during the first 2 days of observation; **APACHE II** score ≥8; organ failure; or pancreatic necrosis, pseudocysts, or abscess (Fig. 81–1). Pancreatic necrosis indicates areas of nonviable pancreatic parenchyma, which are infected in 30–50% of cases. Because secondary bacterial infection increases the morbidity and mortality for acute pancreatitis, identifying the process as necrotizing and ascertaining the presence of infection by CT-guided percutaneous aspiration of fluid collections, phlegmon, or necrotic tissue are important for guiding antimicrobial treatment and determining the need for débridement of infected necrosis.

TABLE 81–5. Differential Diagnosis of Acute Pancreatitis

Hepatobiliary Disease	Intestinal Disease
Hepatitis	Obstruction
Hepatic abscess	Perforation
Cholecystitis	Appendicitis
Cholangitis	**Renal Disease**
Biliary colic (choledocholithiasis)	Nephrolithiasis
Peptic Acid Disease	Pyelonephritis
Gastritis	
Duodenitis	
Ulcers	

Differential Diagnosis

The differential diagnosis of pancreatitis includes a wide variety of disorders that cause abdominal pain and tenderness. Depending on the severity of the presentation, the differential diagnosis ranges from mild gastritis to small intestinal obstruction or perforation (Table 81–5). Persons with recurrent bouts of pancreatitis should be evaluated for cystic fibrosis and hereditary pancreatitis.

Laboratory Evaluation

Evaluation includes both specific laboratory tests to support the diagnosis of pancreatitis and nonspecific tests to assess the clinical condition of the patient and predict the severity of the illness. Although there is no definitive diagnostic test for acute pancreatitis, serum amylase and lipase determinations are the most frequently used.

Amylase is produced largely in the pancreas and salivary glands. Approximately 33–45% of amylase isoforms in normal serum are of pancreatic origin. The amylase level is often elevated in pancreatic inflammation, but it may be normal, particularly in the acute

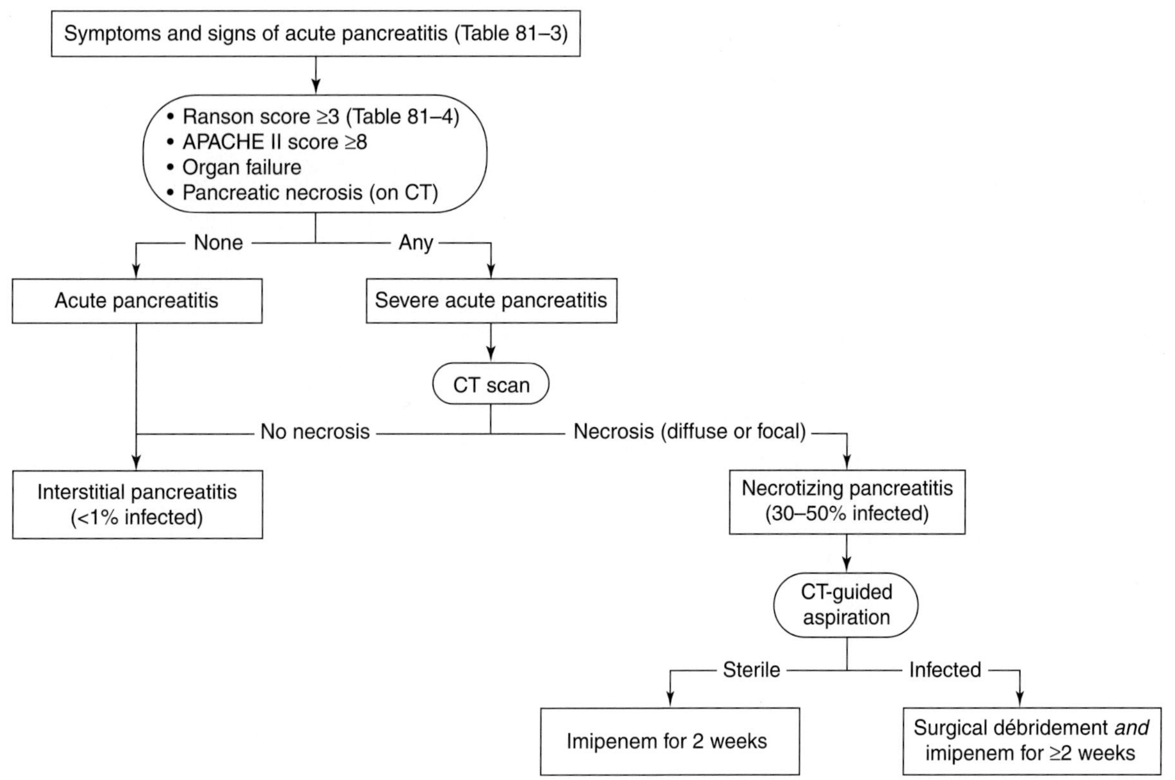

FIGURE 81–1. Diagnosis of acute pancreatitis.

phase of the illness. The degree of hyperamylasemia does not correlate well with the severity of the disease. In addition, many conditions other than pancreatitis are associated with hyperamylasemia (Table 81–6). Techniques are available to measure amylase isoforms, and these levels are more sensitive and specific than total serum amylase levels for pancreatitis, especially if the amylase level is elevated and the source is in question. The amylase:creatinine clearance ratio was thought to be a more specific diagnostic test, but this ratio is increased in any condition associated with elevated serum amylase levels and has not been shown to have diagnostic superiority over a serum amylase determination.

Lipase exists in two isoforms that are immunologically identical. Nonpancreatic lipase is found in the salivary glands, the stomach, and breast milk. Although elevation of the serum lipase level has been considered more specific and sensitive for pancreatic inflammation than hyperamylasemia, comparative studies remain inconclusive. Serum lipase activity may remain elevated somewhat longer during the clinical course of the illness (5–6 days) than amylase levels (4 days) and therefore may be more useful in persons who have had symptoms for several days.

Recent interest has focused on immunoassays for a variety of pancreatic proteases, including trypsin-trypsinogen, elastase, chymotrypsin, and carboxypeptidases. Of these, the immunoassay for cationic trypsin-trypsinogen has been more extensively evaluated in both adults and children and appears to be both specific and sensitive for acute pancreatic inflammation. These assays are relatively expensive, however, and are still not widely used in clinical practice.

Nonspecific tests for pancreatitis include a CBC and determinations of blood urea nitrogen, creatinine, glucose, electrolytes, calcium, and magnesium. As clinically indicated, other helpful tests may include a liver biochemical profile, a serum lipid level, and arterial or venous blood gas measurements. These laboratory parameters are useful in the initial assessment and management of pancreatitis, particularly to identify severe acute pancreatitis (Table 81–4). They also have some value in predicting the severity of the clinical course.

Microbiologic Evaluation

Secondary bacterial infection of necrotic pancreatic tissue or of peripancreatic fluid collections is a serious complication of pancreatitis and requires prompt diagnosis and intervention (Fig. 81–1). Evaluation of severe acute pancreatitis with contrast-enhanced CT is used to identify the presence of necrosis. Approximately 30–50% of cases of acute necrotizing pancreatitis are complicated by infection, but distinguishing sterile from infected necrotizing pancreatitis is difficult. Pancreatic infection is relatively uncommon in the first week of illness and has a peak incidence at approximately 3 weeks. The presence of infection is determined by **CT-guided fine-needle aspiration** of fluid collections, phlegmon, or necrotic tissue for Gram stain and culture. This approach has a sensitivity of 96% and a specificity of 99%. Ultrasound-guided aspiration may have lower sensitivity and specificity but can be performed at the bedside.

In cases of systemic infection associated with pancreatitis, culture of other sites or serologic studies may add supportive evidence to a specific infectious cause.

TABLE 81–6. Causes of Hyperamylasemia

Pancreatic	Salivary Gland*
Pancreatitis	Parotitis (mumps)
Pancreatic tumors	Trauma
Pseudocysts	Salivary duct obstruction
Cystic fibrosis	Tubo-ovarian disease
Biliary obstruction	**Mixed**
Intestinal obstruction	Renal insufficiency
Intestinal perforation	Diabetic ketoacidosis
Trauma	Radiation
Appendicitis	Macroamylasemia
Mesenteric ischemia	
Endoscopic retrograde cholangiopancreatography (ERCP)	

*Hyperamylasemia with a normal serum lipase level.

Diagnostic Imaging

Plain radiographs of the abdomen are of limited diagnostic value but may reveal findings consistent with acute pancreatic inflammation such as radiographic evidence of an ileus and diffuse haziness that may indicate the presence of ascites. Two radiographic signs that are suggestive of, but not specific for, acute pancreatitis are the **sentinel loop** (a distended loop of small intestine near the pancreas) and the **colon cutoff sign** (dilatation of the transverse colon, abrupt termination of the gas pattern at about the level of the splenic flexure, and lack of colonic gas distally). The presence of pancreatic calcifications on an abdominal radiograph suggests the presence of chronic pancreatitis.

Ultrasonography is the most frequently used imaging modality for the initial assessment of suspected pancreatitis. This technique is useful not only in establishing the initial diagnosis of acute pancreatitis but also in the diagnosis, management, and monitoring of complications such as pancreatic abscesses and pseudocysts. Ultrasonographic visualization of the biliary and pancreatic ducts can establish the presence of ductal obstruction or stones, which may contribute to the development of pancreatitis. In acute pancreatitis, inflammation and edema result in an increase in the size, an alteration in the contour, and a decrease in the echodensity of the pancreas. The inflammation may be diffuse or localized. In healthy children, there is wide variation in the size and contour of the pancreas as determined by ultrasonography, resulting in overlap with parameters suggestive of pancreatitis. Therefore other sonographic findings such as dilatation of the main pancreatic duct may be helpful. The tail of the pancreas may be difficult to image by ultrasonography; therefore, and because inflammation may be localized, the diagnosis of acute pancreatitis should not be excluded unless the entire gland can be visualized.

CT with contrast enhancement is used to determine the severity of pancreatic inflammation and establish prognostic indicators. CT is especially helpful if the findings of ultrasonography are normal or nondiagnostic, if better anatomic definition is necessary, such as for assessing inflammation in the tail of the pancreas, and if it is necessary to identify and quantitate the presence of necrosis. CT can differentiate between interstitial inflammation, usually representing relatively mild pancreatitis, and the more severe necrotizing pancreatitis. CT is also used to monitor pancreatic abscesses and pseudocysts and to guide drainage procedures related to these complications.

Endoscopic retrograde cholangiopancreatography (ERCP) is not routinely used to establish the diagnosis of acute pancreatitis. Pancreatitis is a well-recognized complication of ERCP, and ongoing acute pancreatic inflammation is a relative contraindication unless endoscopy is being used therapeutically to relieve an obstruction in the biliary or pancreatic ducts. ERCP may be most helpful in establishing the cause of recurrent pancreatitis and is usually performed when the inflammation is quiescent.

Pathologic Findings

Pancreatic tissue is not routinely obtained to aid in establishing the diagnosis or determining the severity of the pancreatitis unless a surgical procedure is performed for débridement or drainage.

Histologic findings of interstitial pancreatitis include periacinar and interstitial edema accompanied by an inflammatory cell infiltrate, which may involve the ductules as well. Acinar cells are well preserved. In necrotizing pancreatitis, there is loss of pancreatic architecture, destruction of acini, and parenchymal necrosis with diffuse or focal areas of nonviable pancreatic parenchyma.

TREATMENT

Treatment of acute pancreatitis involves supportive care, reduction of inflammation, and assessment for and treatment of complications. Interstitial pancreatitis is not usually treated with antimicrobial therapy because secondary bacterial infection occurs only in <1% of cases. Necrotizing pancreatitis includes phlegmon, fluid collections, and areas of pancreatic necrosis that may be sterile or infected. Infected necrotizing pancreatitis requires both antimicrobial treatment and surgical débridement. It is uniformly fatal without intervention and is the most common cause of death from pancreatitis among adults. In the presence of clinically severe acute pancreatitis (Fig. 81–1), CT-guided aspiration of fluid should be performed to obtain specimens for Gram stain and culture to identify the presence of infection. ERCP should be considered for pancreatitis associated with gallstones in the presence of jaundice or cholangitis.

The treatment of infected necrotizing pancreatitis requires initiation of appropriate antimicrobial therapy for polymicrobial infection with enteric organisms and, in addition, urgent surgical débridement. The recommended antimicrobial treatment is imipenem or meropenem (Table 81–7).

If the aspirate is sterile, continued clinical observation and supportive therapy are important. The use of antibiotics as prophylaxis for infection and the use of surgical débridement for sterile necrotizing pancreatitis are controversial but are frequently instituted. A study (Pederzoli, 1993) of empirical treatment of 74 adults with necrotizing pancreatitis with imipenem for 2 weeks showed a significant decrease in sepsis but no difference in the development of organ failure. Repeated aspiration rarely shows infection if the initial aspiration was sterile, but it may be indicated if there is clinical deterioration. The impact of selective gut decontamination on the incidence of infection has also been studied, and although the results are encouraging, the practical issue related to the oral and rectal administration of medications during acute pancreatitis remains an obstacle. The timing and type of surgical intervention for sterile necrotizing pancreatitis are controversial. Some experts advocate débridement for persons who remain systemically ill after 4–6 weeks, with inability to eat or intractable abdominal pain. The longer interval may facilitate surgical demarcation between viable and nonviable tissue. Other experts do not advocate débridement if the process remains sterile.

Supportive Therapy

Supportive measures include close clinical monitoring, minimizing pancreatic exocrine function by eliminating oral intake of food and liquid, gastrointestinal decompression with a nasogastric tube in the presence of protracted vomiting or an ileus, intravenous fluid hydration and correction of electrolyte imbalances, nutritional support, and pain management. There may be abundant third-space fluid losses and associated electrolyte derangements because of pancreatic inflammation, necessitating aggressive fluid management and frequent laboratory monitoring. Although limiting oral intake has been the traditional approach, there is emerging enthusiasm for supplementing nutrition enterally by nasojejunal tube feedings in persons with severe or prolonged pancreatitis once they are clinically stabilized and there is no significant ileus. Enteral feeding by nasoenteric tube beyond the ligament of Treitz may be used if there is no significant ileus. Parenteral nutrition should be instituted if oral or enteral feedings cannot be tolerated for more than a few days. There is no exacerbation of pancreatitis by any component of parenterally administered nutrition, including lipid emulsions. Narcotics may be necessary for adequate control of pain. Meperidine causes less contraction of the sphincter of Oddi than do other narcotics and is recommended in the treatment of acute pancreatitis. Measures directed toward ''resting'' the pancreas by decreasing secretion, including administration of such agents as histamine antagonists, glucagon, anticholinergics, and somatostatin, have not been shown to have clinically significant benefit. In the presence of an ileus or more severe clinical disease, gastric decompression, along with prophylactic therapy for gastric stress ulceration, is indicated.

Eliminating factors that may cause or perpetuate inflammation, such as drugs or impacted gallstones, reduces inflammation. Specific measures directed at reduction or inhibition of pancreatic and systemic inflammation have generally been unsuccessful. Therapeutic agents that stabilize cell walls, remove or inhibit circulating proteases, or remove oxygen-derived free radicals have not shown efficacy in clinical trials.

TABLE 81–7. Antimicrobial Treatment for Pancreatitis

Diagnosis	Recommended Treatment	Alternative Regimen
Interstitial pancreatitis	None recommended	
Necrotizing pancreatitis		
Sterile	Imipenem *or* meropenem for 2 wk	Piperacillin-tazobactam *plus* an aminoglycoside for 2 wk
Infected	Surgical débridement *and* Imipenem *or* meropenem for ≥2 wk	Surgical débridement *and* Piperacillin-tazobactam *plus* an aminoglycoside for ≥2 wk

Recommended Dosages for Persons with Normal Renal Function

ANTIBIOTIC	INTRAVENOUS DOSAGE	MAXIMUM DAILY DOSE
Amikacin	15–20 mg/kg/day divided q8–12hr	(same)
Gentamicin	7.5 mg/kg/day divided q8hr	5 mg/kg (adult dose)
Imipenem	40–60 mg/kg/day divided q6hr	2 g
Meropenem	60–120 mg/kg/day divided q8hr	3 g
Piperacillin-tazobactam	200–300 mg/kg/day divided q6hr	18 g
Tobramycin	7.5 mg/kg/day divided q8hr	5 mg/kg (adult dose)

COMPLICATIONS

Although both pancreatic exocrine and endocrine insufficiency may be present during acute pancreatitis, the values normalize with resolution of the inflammation.

Hypocalcemia. Hypocalcemia is an early complication that usually results from extravasation of nonionized, albumin-bound calcium with third-space fluids. If the serum ionized calcium value is normal and there are no symptoms, specific therapy is not necessary. Ionized calcium also may be decreased by saponification within areas of fat necrosis by forming a complex with fatty acids in serum or ascitic fluid. Low levels of ionized calcium are manifested clinically as neuromuscular irritability **(Chvostek's and Trousseau's signs)** and require correction with intravenous calcium therapy.

Pseudocysts. Pseudocysts are collections of fluid and debris that are encapsulated but do not contain an epithelial lining. They are best identified by ultrasonography or CT. Pseudocysts are associated with varying degrees of pancreatic inflammation, occur in 10–20% of persons with pancreatitis, and are particularly common in traumatic pancreatitis. Many of these cysts resolve spontaneously, although resolution is unlikely and the incidence of complications increases if they persist for more than 1–2 months. Complications of pseudocysts include severe pain, obstruction of the common bile duct or duodenum, bleeding into the cysts or peritoneum, infection, and leakage or frank rupture. An infected pseudocyst may not present with systemic signs of infection, and there are no reliable findings suggestive of pseudocyst infection on imaging studies. Definitive diagnosis is made with aspiration and analysis of fluid from the pseudocyst. An infected pseudocyst should be drained, either percutaneously or surgically. Other indications for interventional management of pseudocysts are size greater than 5 cm, persistence longer than 16 weeks, intractable pain, rapid expansion, or the presence of a complication.

PROGNOSIS

In general, mild interstitial pancreatitis has an excellent prognosis with low associated morbidity and mortality. Interstitial pancreatitis, based on CT criteria, is associated with a mortality of less than 1%. The mortality for sterile necrotizing pancreatitis is approximately 10%, but it increases to 30% in the presence of infection. Early deaths are caused by the release of inflammatory mediators and cytokines. Late deaths result from local or systemic infection. Various prognostic criteria have been used to predict the severity of acute pancreatitis, including Ranson's criteria (Table 81–4) and APACHE II. Persons whose disease fulfills only 1–2 of Ranson's criteria have a mortality of less than 1%, whereas the presence of 9–11 criteria predicts an 80% mortality. The APACHE II appears to have greater sensitivity and specificity and, combined with CT classification and grading, may provide the most accurate prognostic information. These criteria have not been systematically applied to pediatric patients with pancreatitis.

PREVENTION

There are no specific measures to prevent pancreatitis. Surgical or endoscopic correction of mechanical or obstructive causes of pancreatitis precludes additional attacks. In other clinical settings, early diagnosis and aggressive supportive management optimize outcome.

REVIEWS

Baron TH, Norgan DE: Acute necrotizing pancreatitis. *N Engl J Med* 1999; 340:1412–7.

Dassopoulus T, Ehrenpreis ED: Acute pancreatis in human immunodeficiency virus–infected patients: A review. *Am J Med* 1999;107:78–84.

Goldberg DM: Proteases in the valuation of pancreatic function and pancreatic disease. *Clin Chim Acta* 2000;291:201–21.

McKay CJ, Imrie CW: Staging of acute pancreatitis. Is it important? *Surg Clin North Am* 1999;79:733–43.

Sakorafas GH, Tsiotou AG: Etiology and pathogenesis of acute pancreatitis. *J Clin Gastroenterol* 2000;30:343–56.

KEY ARTICLES

Balthazar EJ, Robinson DL, Megibow AJ, et al: Acute pancreatitis: Value of CT in establishing prognosis. *Radiology* 1990;174:331–6.

Banks PA, Gerzof SG, Chong FK, et al: Bacteriologic status of necrotic tissue in necrotizing pancreatitis. *Pancreas* 1990;5:330–3.

Cohn JA, Friedman KJ, Noone PG, et al: Relation between mutations of the cystic fibrosis gene and idiopathic pancreatitis. *N Engl J Med* 1998; 339:653–8.

De La Rubia L, Herrara MI, Cebrero M, et al: Acute pancreatitis associated with rotavirus infection. *Pancreas* 1996;12:98–9.

Durie PR, Gaskin KJ, Ogilvie JE, et al: Serial alterations in the forms of immunoreactive pancreatic cationic trypsin in plasma from patients with acute pancreatitis. *J Pediatr Gastroenterol Nutr* 1985;4:199–207.

Ellis GH, Mirkin CD, Mills MC: Pancreatitis and Reye's syndrome. *Am J Dis Child* 1979;133:1014–6.

Gorry MC, Gabbaizedeh D, Furey W, et al: Mutations in the cationic trypsinogen gene are associated with recurrent acute and chronic pancreatitis. *Gastroenterology* 1997;113:1063–8.

Gumaste V: Prophylactic antibiotic therapy in the management of acute pancreatitis. *J Clin Gastroenterol* 2000;31:6–10.

Hill MC, Huntington DK: Computed tomography and acute pancreatitis. *Gastroenterol Clin North Am* 1990;19:811–42.

Ho HS, Frey CF: The role of antibiotic prophylaxis in severe acute pancreatitis. *Arch Surg* 1997;132:487–92.

Kale-Pradhan PB, Elnabtity MH, Park NJ, et al: Enteral nutrition in patients with pancreatitis. *Pharmacotherapy* 1999;19:1036–41.

Luiten EJ, Hop WC, Lange JF, et al: Differential prognosis of gram-negative versus gram-positive infected and sterile pancreatic necrosis: Results of a randomized trial in patients with severe acute pancreatitis treated with adjuvant selective decontamination. *Clin Infect Dis* 1997;25:811–6.

Mardh PA, Ursing B: The occurrence of acute pancreatitis in *Mycoplasma pneumoniae* infection. *Scand J Infect Dis* 1974;6:167–71.

Mishra A, Saigal S, Gupta R, et al: Acute pancreatitis associated with viral hepatitis: A report of six cases with review of literature. *Am J Gastroenterol* 1999;94:2292–5.

Naficy K, Nategh R, Ghadimi H: Mumps pancreatitis without parotitis. *BMJ* 1973;1:529.

Pederzoli P, Bassi C, Vesentini S, et al: A randomized multicenter clinical trial of antibiotic prophylaxis of septic complications in acute necrotizing pancreatitis with imipenem. *Surg Gynecol Obstet* 1993;176:480–3.

Ranson JC, Rifkind KM, Roses DF, et al: Prognostic signs and the role of operative management in acute pancreatitis. *Surg Gynecol Obstet* 1974;139:69–81.

Ratschko M, Fenner T, Lankisch PG: The role of antibiotic prophylaxis in the treatment of acute pancreatitis. *Gastroenterol Clin North Am* 1999;28:641–59.

Sharer N, Schwarz M, Malone G, et al: Mutations of the cystic fibrosis gene in patients with chronic pancreatitis. *N Engl J Med* 1998;339;645–52.

Siegel MJ, Martin KW, Worthington JL: Normal and abnormal pancreas in children: US studies. *Radiology* 1987;165:15–8.

Steinberg WM: Predictors of severity of acute pancreatitis. *Gastroenterol Clin North Am* 1990;19:849–61.

Steiner E, Mueller PR, Hahn RF, et al: Complicated pancreatic abscesses: Problems in interventional management. *Radiology* 1988;167:443–6.

Whitcomb DC, Gorry MC, Preston RA, et al: Hereditary pancreatitis is caused by a mutation in the cationic trypsinogen gene. *Nat Genet* 1996;14:141–5.

Wilson C, Heath DI, Imrie CW: Prediction of outcome in acute pancreatitis: A comparative study of APACHE II, clinical assessment and multiple factor scoring systems. *Br J Surg* 1990;77:1260–4.

CHAPTER 82

Urinary Tract Infections

Gary D. Overturf

Urinary tract infection (UTI) includes cystitis, with infection localized to the bladder; pyelonephritis, with infection of the renal parenchyma, calyces, and renal pelvis; and renal abscess, which may be intrarenal or perinephric. **Chronic cystitis or pyelonephritis** is rarely due to persistent infection but implies repeated episodes of acute infection. **Lobar nephronia** refers to pyelonephritis localized to a region of the kidney. UTI is protean in clinical presentation (depending on age and other host factors), is inconsistent in response to treatment, and may be recurrent. The clinical approach to the child with UTI is predicated on the knowledge that infection may be the first manifestation of significant genitourinary congenital anomalies and that, in those children with normal anatomy, recurrence is frequent and often associated with vesicourethral reflux of infected urine, resulting in renal scarring. Management of the pediatric UTI is directed at eliminating or minimizing the potential for continuing renal damage.

ETIOLOGY

The most common agent causing first episodes of UTI in children is *Escherichia coli,* which accounts for approximately 80% of all isolates (Table 82–1). Many other Enterobacteriaceae account for most other UTIs. With recurrent episodes of UTI, the bacterial strains are more likely to be antibiotic resistant, probably as a result of repeated selective antibiotic pressure on colonizing bowel flora. Thus, in subsequent infections, *Enterobacter, Pseudomonas,* and antibiotic-resistant strains of *E. coli, Klebsiella,* and *Proteus* become more common causes of UTI. *Enterococcus* may also cause UTI, particularly in children with a long-term indwelling urinary catheter or in children with recurrent episodes. *Staphylococcus* is an unusual cause of UTI, with the exception of coagulase-negative staphylococci, which have been associated with at least 50% of infections in sexually active female adolescents. Coagulase-negative staphylococci, along with *Chlamydia trachomatis* and *E. coli,* are the chief causes of the **acute urethral syndrome,** or **postcoital urethritis,** which typically occurs 12–72 hours after sexual intercourse.

Nosocomial infections are more likely to be caused by antibiotic-resistant pathogens such as *Pseudomonas, Citrobacter, Enterobacter, Proteus, Providencia,* or *Enterococcus.* From 67% to 85% of nosocomial UTIs are associated with urinary tract instrumentation or catheterization. UTI is the second most frequent cause of nosocomial infection in children, occurring chiefly in intensive care units. Infection rates in children with long-term catheterization approach 100% after 4 days with open drainage systems; the rate can be reduced to approximately 20% with carefully maintained closed drainage systems.

Candida has also become a major UTI pathogen in intensive care units, primarily in catheterized children. *Candida albicans* is the most frequent yeast pathogen, but infection with antifungal-resistant yeast such as *Candida tropicalis* has become increasingly more frequent. *Candida* can cause UTI by ascending from colonized urinary catheters or by hematogenous dissemination from other infected sites.

EPIDEMIOLOGY

The incidence of UTI is not known precisely. Approximately 5% of girls will have at least one UTI by grade 12. The lifetime incidence of UTI in females is about 30%, whereas it is only about 1% in males, although more male than female infants have UTI during the first year of life. Approximately 75% of children with bacteriuria at less than 3 months of age are male, whereas only 10% between the ages of 3 and 8 months are male. After 12 months of age, UTI is almost entirely confined to girls.

Infection of the urinary tract is the cause of fever without apparent source in 4.6% of infants less than 2 months of age and causes 5.9% of fevers in children greater than 2 months of age in whom UTI is suspected. Although the prevalence of UTI does not vary with age, the incidence is higher in girls than boys and higher in white than in African American children. The degree of fever is generally not predictive of UTI, but children with the highest temperatures (>39°C) are more likely to have UTI. White girls with temperatures of >39°C without another focus have a 17% prevalence of UTI.

Asymptomatic bacteriuria is identified by isolation of significant numbers of bacteria of a single species from properly collected urine, in the absence of any symptoms. Use of the term *asymptomatic bacteriuria* to describe a condition in children with significant bacteriuria and no complaints may be inaccurate because 35% of subjects with so-called asymptomatic bacteriuria in some surveys had urinary tract symptoms such as dysuria, frequency, or urgency at the time of the survey or had had at least one prior symptomatic UTI. Prospective studies report asymptomatic bacteriuria in ap-

TABLE 82–1. Microbiologic Etiology of Urinary Tract Infections

Species	Total (%) (n = 4176)	First Infection (%) (n = 1428)	Recurrence (%) (n = 2748)
Escherichia coli	79.5	88.6	74.7
Klebsiella	3.5	2.0	4.3
Proteus	3.3	3.4	3.2
Pseudomonas	0.5	0.1	0.6
Enterococcus	2.6	2.9	2.5
Staphylococcus	2.6	0.6	3.6
Others or unknown	8.0	2.4	11.1

From Edén C, de Man P: Bacterial virulence in urinary tract infection. *Infect Dis Clin North Am* 1987;1:732.

proximately 2.2–2.7% of neonates, 1.5% of school-age girls, and 0.7% of 13- and 14-year-old girls.

PATHOGENESIS

The urinary tract is normally protected by several anatomic, physiologic, and antibacterial mechanisms. The longer length of the male urethra is credited with a protective role. However, the preputial skin appears to account for a high number of UTIs in male neonates: as many as 95% of male neonates with a UTI are uncircumcised. Uncircumcised boys have a 5- to 12-fold increased incidence of UTI in comparison with circumcised boys.

Urine (except at the extremes of osmolality) supports bacterial growth, although urea, organic acids, and the extremes of pH inhibit bacterial multiplication. Mucopolysaccharides lining the bladder inhibit bacterial adherence in animal models. Immunoglobulins in urine from persons with pyelonephritis prevent bacterial attachment to uroepithelial cells in vitro. There are conflicting reports of the role of secretory IgA in protecting the host from bacterial colonization. Although phagocytic cells may prevent the spread of infection, persons with neutropenia do not have more UTIs than healthy persons except with instrumentration or obstruction of the urinary tract. Persons with functional phagocytic defects, such as chronic granulomatous disease, may have renal staphylococcal abscesses as a result of bacteremia.

An important defense against bacterial colonization of the bladder is the flushing action of voiding, providing complete emptying of the bladder. Obstruction to the flow of urine by anatomic stricture or functional abnormality, as in neurologic disease, is a major risk factor for UTI. **Vesicoureteral reflux (VUR),** whether primary (about 70% of cases) or secondary to obstruction of the urinary tract, predisposes persons to pyelonephritis. Obstruction may be due to congenital anomalies (e.g., ureteropelvic junction obstruction, megaureter) or acquired conditions (e.g., calculi, extrinsic compression, pregnancy). In animal models, even transient ureteral obstruction leads to infection. Severe grades of VUR with marked dilatation of the ureters and large volumes of residual urine are associated with renal scarring. Animal studies suggest that ongoing antigen-antibody reactions in the kidney lead to chronic interstitial pyelonephritis and end-stage renal disease.

Of the two possible routes of infection, hematogenous or ascending, the latter is far more common. The commonest bacterial species isolated from persons with UTI is *E. coli,* which sequentially colonizes the bowel, perineum, and periurethral area and thereafter ascends the urethra to the bladder. Relatively few *E. coli* serotypes make up the isolates from pyelonephritis and are thus deemed **pyelonephritic.** As many as 90% of these isolates possess surface **P-fimbriae,** which enables them to adhere to uroepithelial cells with surface receptors recognized by the bacteria. Adherence is the prerequisite in establishing colonization leading to subsequent infection. After colonization the release of bacterial products, such as endotoxin, initiates an inflammatory response that may account for fever and many of the constitutional symptoms of UTI.

Cell surface receptors of the host are genetically determined. The best studied receptor is the disaccharide **α-Gal(14)β-Gal** (gal-gal) receptor on host cells, which binds to the adhesion molecule PapG of *E. coli.* Host receptors such as those related to the P blood group are genetically determined. The specific adhesion molecules are present in greater than 90% of *E. coli* strains associated with acute pyelonephritis, 20% of cystitis strains, 15% of asymptomatic bacteriuria strains, and 7% of fecal strains. Additional evidence of the importance of the role of the P-fimbria-receptor interaction in UTI is the observation that P-fimbriated bacteria do not adhere to uroepithelial cells of P-negative individuals who lack the receptor group.

Renal and Perinephric Abscess. Renal and perinephric abscesses are caused by direct invasion of the renal parenchyma or the perinephric or retroperitoneal space. **Intrarenal abscesses** are confined to the renal capsule and the contiguous urinary tract. Bacteria may invade the renal parenchyma and subsequently spread to the perinephric space by first ascending the urinary tract, by hematogenous dissemination from a distantly infected site, or by contiguous spread of infection in continuity with the retroperitoneal space (e.g., the peritoneum or lumbar spine). Renal and perinephric abscesses are rare complications of UTI, usually occurring in children with chronic UTI or pyelonephritis and often in the presence of structural urinary tract disease resulting in obstruction. Abscesses characteristically develop in four settings: (1) a minor abscess incidental to a recent symptomatic or asymptomatic bacteremia, commonly in the collecting system; (2) a renal and perinephric abscess in a child with an obstructed urinary tract; (3) an abscess in a child with a renal abnormality other than obstruction; and (4) an abscess in a child with an underlying immunodeficiency. Gram-positive organisms such as *Staphylococcus* frequently cause the first abscess, and gram-negative bacteria typically cause the second; the causes of subsequent abscesses are often unpredictable.

SYMPTOMS AND CLINICAL MANIFESTATIONS

The clinical features of UTI vary depending on age, clinical setting, and sex of the child (Table 82–2). In neonates, failure to thrive and feeding disorders are the only consistent symptoms. Parents may report symptoms of poor feeding, vomiting, lethargy, or abdominal symptoms, such as diarrhea, loose stools, abdominal distention, jaundice, or a change in the color or odor of urine on the diaper. Although fever is an infrequent manifestation of UTI among children less than 2 years of age, infection of the urinary tract is the most commonly identified bacterial infection among children less than 2 years of age who have fever. Thus UTI should be considered in all children less than 2 years of age with unexplained fever at presentation. UTI in infancy is more frequently associated with bacteremia, and thus infants may initially have signs and symptoms of sepsis.

TABLE 82–2. Symptoms and Signs of Urinary Tract Infection in Children

	Frequency of Occurrence (%) by Age			
Symptom or Sign	0–1 Mo	1–24 Mo	2–5 Yr	5–12 Yr
Failure to thrive	53	36	7	0
Jaundice	44	0	0	0
Vomiting	24	29	16	3
Diarrhea	18	16	0	3
Fever	11	38	57	50
Convulsions	2	7	9	5
Irritability	0	13	7	0
Changes in urine	0	9	13	0
Hematuria	0	7	16	8
Frequency, dysuria	0	4	34	41
Enuresis	0	0	27	29
Abdominal pain	0	0	23	0
Flank pain	0	0	0	0

Adapted from Smellie JM, Hodson CJ, Edwards D, et al: Clinical and radiological features of urinary tract infection in childhood. *Br Med J* 1964; 2:1222–6.

In young children, parents may report vague symptoms of abdominal pain, vomiting, decreased appetite, and changes in the color or odor of the urine. Children are more likely to complain of nonspecific back or abdominal pain, rather than pain localized to the kidneys. As children become older, the presenting signs and symptoms of infection typically become more localized to the urinary tract. In preschool children, complaints of urgency and frequency may be manifested as a loss of previously gained continence. Most cases of enuresis, however, are not the result of UTI unless there is a change from previous nighttime continence to new episodes of nocturnal enuresis. Symptoms of dysuria, frequency, and urgency are progressively more common, particularly among children who are toilet trained. Flank pain is often noted in adolescents and adults but is uncommon in children. Fever as a symptom of UTI is more likely as children become a little older and may be the only clue to UTI in toddlers.

For adolescents the occurrence of UTI often coincides with the onset of sexual activity. The onset of both classic UTI and a more limited syndrome of **acute urethral syndrome,** or **postcoital urethritis,** may occur within 12–72 hours after sexual intercourse, with symptoms of dysuria, frequency, and urgency with or without fever. The acute urethral syndrome is frequently caused by *C. trachomatis, E. coli,* and coagulase-negative staphylococci and is associated with pyuria, although there may be fewer organisms in urine ($<10^5$/mL).

Physical Examination Findings

The physical examination should focus on the urogenital anatomy. Children with renal abscess or pyelonephritis may have generalized abdominal pain or tenderness on direct renal palpation or percussion. Bladder tenderness may be present on direct palpation. However, classic **costovertebral tenderness** elicited by gentle to vigorous percussion is frequently present in adolescents and adults but is unusual in infants and young children. Attempts should be made to palpate the kidneys bilaterally to assess size, cystic changes, or tenderness. Fever should be recorded and the blood pressure should be accurately measured. Older children and adolescents should have a complete genital examination, including visualization of the vaginal mucosa and cervix in the female patient. The perineal structures of both sexes should be examined carefully to exclude periurethral inflammation or trauma.

The physical examination should also document anomalies associated with renal dysgenesis syndromes: (1) facial dysplasia; (2) limb anomalies, particularly of the distal small extremities, such as polydactyly, clinodactyly, and syndactyly; (3) abnormalities of the external genitalia, such as hypogonadism, hypospadias, cryptorchidism, and vaginal or uterine atresia or dysplasia; (4) anal atresia or imperforate anus; (5) anomalies of the external ears, such as low-set, posteriorly rotated, small, large, or dysplastic ears, or preauricular pits with or without deafness; (6) abnormalities of the ribs, particularly short dysplastic ribs resulting in a narrowed thorax; and (7) anomalies of the vertebrae.

DIAGNOSIS

The diagnosis of UTI is suggested by symptoms and signs and must be confirmed by urine culture. Infants and young children with unexplained fever who are assessed as being sufficiently ill to warrant immediate antibiotic therapy should have a urine specimen obtained by catheterization or suprapubic percutaneous aspiration.

A history of urinary tract anomalies or previous UTIs is important because infection occurs with increased frequency both in children with known urinary tract anatomic abnormalities and in those with a history of UTI even with normal anatomy. Recurrences of UTI occur at a rate of about 30% per year for each of the 3 years after a first UTI. A history of maternal oligohydramnios is significant in young infants with UTI because it may indicate an intrinsic or obstructive renal abnormality.

In children with chronic bladder catheterization, changes in the urinary WBC count, in association with systemic signs of infection, are sufficient to suspect UTI. Colonization of an indwelling catheter resulting in urine cultures with a relatively low number of bacteria frequently occurs after 3–5 days of continuous catheterization, with a progressively increased incidence after this time. Careful catheter care and closed system techniques may extend the period of urine sterility to 7–14 days.

Differentiation of Upper from Lower UTI. Systemic signs and symptoms do not reliably distinguish upper tract from lower tract infection, nor do they reliably predict the presence of concurrent sepsis. Although fever, chills, nausea, and vomiting may be more frequent in children with upper tract disease, such symptoms may also be present in children with cystitis alone. With the use of sensitive techniques such as renal scans, as many as 25% of children without signs and symptoms commonly associated with pyelonephritis have been shown to have infections of the renal parenchyma.

Renal and Perinephric Abscess. Abscesses are suggested by persistent signs or symptoms of UTI, continued abnormalities in urinalysis, or continued positive urine culture findings despite treatment, especially if accompanied by systemic or other local signs of infection such as flank pain or back pain. Infection of the perinephric tissues may spread to adjacent structures within the retroperitoneal space; thus signs and symptoms may be referable to infections of the psoas muscle and other soft tissues.

Differential Diagnosis

The signs and symptoms of UTI overlap with those of generalized sepsis, particularly in infants, and with focal or diffuse abdominal disease or other systemic infections in the older children. Acute appendicitis and infectious gastroenteritis can usually be excluded on the basis of history, specific physical findings, and laboratory examination of the urine and stool. Abdominal pain with fever may also be associated with appendicitis, bacteremia, and lobar pneumonias or pleuritis. Dysuria, urgency, or frequency may be related to UTI but may also be caused by urethral irritation resulting from trauma, perineal irritation, masturbation, pinworm infection, direct chemical injury or hypersensitivity (e.g., to soaps, detergents), or sexual abuse with or without concomitant sexually transmitted infections.

In young girls the clinical presentation of vaginitis may be indistinguishable from UTI and often is caused by contamination with fecal flora or chemical agents. In older girls, dysuria may be associated with vaginitis or with specific sexually transmitted infections. Similarly, infection of the urethra with sexually transmitted diseases or urethral trauma may cause comparable symptoms in the male. A history of spontaneous urethral discharge or the eliciting of discharge by urethral stripping will usually confirm a specific sexually transmitted disease as the cause of urethral symptoms. In the female adolescent, ectopic pregnancy, tubal ovarian abscess, and cystic ovarian disease should be considered when lower abdominal pain is present with or without fever and with or without normal urinary examination findings.

Pyuria or hematuria, alone or in combination, without bacteriuria has been described in a variety of other conditions, including dehydration, vaginitis, urethritis, renal stones, renal tubular acidosis, interstitial nephritis, cystic renal disease, glomerulonephritis, and appendicitis.

Failure to thrive may be the result of chronic infection or the associated renal insufficiency caused by congenital or acquired renal parenchymal disease. Abdominal masses may be felt and may be the result of urinary tract obstruction (e.g., posterior urethral valves in boys), leading to an enlarged bladder or to cystic or diffusely swollen kidneys. Alternatively, such a mass may be caused by the presence of an obstructive mass that is extrinsic (e.g., Wilms' tumor or other intra-abdominal tumor) or intrinsic (e.g., ureterocele, duplication of the urethra) to the urinary tract.

Laboratory Examination

The WBC count, polymorphonuclear leukocyte count, ESR, and CRP concentration do not reliably distinguish upper from lower tract disease, although all these values tend to be elevated more frequently in pyelonephritis. Serum electrolyte, creatinine, and blood urea nitrogen concentrations may be measured to assess renal function or associated symptoms of UTI such as vomiting or diarrhea.

Urine Collection. Examination of the urinary sediment and urine culture are central to the diagnosis of acute UTI. Adequate collection and prompt transport of urine samples to the laboratory are essential in obtaining adequate results. All collected samples, regardless of the method of collection, should be cultured within 20 minutes or promptly refrigerated (at 4°C) until cultured. Most children with UTI will have $>10^5$ colony forming units of a single bacterial species per milliliter of an adequately collected specimen. Cultures of urine obtained by catheterization may be considered significant if >10,000 cfu/mL are present, whereas cultures of specimens obtained by suprapubic percutaneous aspiration may be considered significant if >1,000 cfu/mL are present.

In continent children, adolescents, and adults, the midstream clean-catch urine sample is preferred for culture. For toilet-trained children beyond 3–5 years of age, clean-voided specimens are adequate provided competent medical personnel directly supervise the collection. Teenagers and older children can usually provide adequate clean-voided samples with minimal instruction or parental assistance. Exceptions are those children with neurologic or other spontaneous voiding problems, who will require catheterization.

The standard for urine culture in children too young to provide an adequate clean-catch specimen must be either urine collection by simple catheterization after careful perineal disinfection or percutaneous suprapubic aspiration of urine. **Catheterization** of infants and children should use the smallest possible straight feeding tube (e.g., No. 5 to No. 10 French). After thorough antiseptic cleansing of the perineum, the catheter can be gently passed into the bladder. For infants younger than 24 months with fever alone at presentation, for whom other causes of fever have been excluded by history and physical examination, the routine standard of urine collection should be catheterization.

Suprapubic percutaneous aspiration of urine is generally safe and reliable but is best suited for the very young infant who has not voided for 1–3 hours and whose bladder is palpable. After antiseptic preparation of the skin, a 21- to 25-gauge needle attached to a 10 mL syringe is inserted percutaneously at about one fingerbreadth above the symphysis pubis, at an angle 70–80 degrees to the abdominal wall, and directed toward the symphysis. The needle should be advanced with continuous gentle suction applied to the syringe until slight resistance is encountered with passage through the bladder wall. Aspirated urine should be sent immediately to the laboratory for urinalysis and culture. Bladder urine can be obtained in more than 90% of children, and complications are rare, with only a 3% incidence of transient hematuria.

Although a **perineal bag** is a convenient method of collection in noncontinent infants, unfortunately it is often inadequate to confirm the diagnosis of UTI because of frequent contamination of the urine sample with perineal or fecal flora and because of the intrinsic delay in culturing urine when the time of voiding is not known. Preparative perineal antisepsis deteriorates with time; therefore, if a bag remains on an infant for longer than 30 minutes before the infant voids, the perineum requires repeated antiseptic preparation. As many as 75% of bag cultures with $>10^5$ cfu/mL cannot be confirmed by subsequent cultures of urine obtained by catheter or suprapubic aspiration. However, a negative culture result does exclude UTI. Because the subsequent evaluation and follow-up of a UTI are expensive and invasive, the diagnosis should be confirmed by an accurate method rather than by culture of urine obtained with a perineal bag.

Urinalysis. The presence of WBCs, proteinuria, and bacteria on urinalysis supports the diagnosis of UTI. **Pyuria,** defined as ≥5 leukocytes per high powered field (uncentrifuged) of urinary sediment, is not uniformly reliable in the diagnosis of UTI because as many as two thirds of children with UTI may not have pyuria, particularly infants younger than 12 months. Older children with UTI typically have greater than 5–10 WBCs hpf in uncentrifuged urinary sediment. The lack of standardization for the definition of pyuria may explain some differences in the reported incidence of pyuria, from less than 30% to more than 90% in children with UTI. The use of enhanced urinalysis, performed on uncentrifuged urine with a hemocytometer chamber, and the finding of ≥10 WBCs/mL appear to provide greater diagnostic accuracy. In children, enhanced urinalysis has a sensitivity and a positive predictive value for UTI of 84.5% and 93.1%, respectively, compared with 65.6% and 80.8% for standard urinalysis. The absence of pyuria does not exclude the diagnosis of UTI.

Children with UTI may have microscopic hematuria as well as pyuria, and some may have gross hematuria at presentation. WBC casts, also present in some children, are indicative of upper tract disease but are relatively rare in children with UTI; WBC casts also may be seen in some other noninfectious inflammatory disorders of the renal parenchyma. Proteinuria of variable degrees is frequently present in acute UTI, but neither its presence nor its absence is reliable diagnostically.

A Gram stain of uncentrifuged urine showing one organism per oil-immersion field has a high correlation with the presence of bacteria at $>10^5$ cfu/mL.

Rapid Diagnostic Tests. The use of quick tests such as measurement of urinary **leukocyte esterase** or **urinary nitrite** has been better evaluated for adults than for children. A positive leukocyte esterase value correlates with >10 WBCs/hpf, with a sensitivity of only 48% but a specificity of >99% in children. The leukocyte esterase test is inadequate as a diagnostic test in children because of the infrequency of pyuria in some children and the occasional presence of leukocytes from other causes such as vaginitis or urethritis. Therefore a positive leukocyte esterase test result must be correlated with the clinical picture, and neither a positive nor a negative test result proves the presence or absence of UTI.

Nitrite test results are generally positive with bacterial counts of $>10^5$ cfu/mL, but the ability to perform the test depends on the detection of nitrite produced by bacterial enzymatic reduction (nitrate reductase) of urinary nitrates. Sensitivity is approximately 30% in children, with a specificity of 99%. Poor sensitivity may be caused by insufficient bacterial enzyme, insufficient time for reduction of nitrates in urine, or the presence of urinary tract pathogens that lack nitrate reductase (e.g., *Pseudomonas*). The first morning voided urine (e.g., an overnight urine specimen) provides the most accurate sample for nitrite testing, a requirement that may contribute to decreased sensitivity in young children with nighttime incontinence.

Urine Culture. In most children the diagnosis of UTI is confirmed by the presence of pure culture of $\geq 10^5$ cfu/mL of urine collected by the clean-catch method, $\geq 10^4$ cfu/mL of urine collected by catheterization, and $\geq 10^3$ cfu/mL of urine collected by suprapubic aspiration. If there are convincing signs and symptoms of UTI, then lower numbers of bacteria may be considered diagnostic. Mixed bacterial cultures, even when two or more species are present, each at $>10^5$ cfu/mL, should be reassessed by repeated culture because infections with two bacterial agents are rare. Most mixed cultures reflect contamination of the urine sample.

A variety of urine culture kits designed for physician office use, such as the dip-slide, filter paper, pad, and inverted-cup (roll-tube) culture systems, have been marketed. The dip-slide test is the most accurate and easiest to use and has few false-negative or false-positive results. Although these tests are inexpensive and expedient, they necessitate quality control in the office laboratory practice and generally will not be useful or accurate unless a large number of patients are regularly tested. In addition, when organisms are isolated, the isolates will need to be submitted to a referral laboratory for speciation and susceptibility testing.

Diagnostic Imaging

Ultrasonography, voiding cystourethrography (VCUG), radionuclide cystography (RNC), renal nucleotide scans, intravenous pyelography, and CT or MRI can be used for anatomic and functional assessment of the child with UTI. Anatomic or structural abnormalities of the genitourinary tract occur in approximately 15% of the otherwise normal population, but approximately 30% of children with a single episode of UTI will be found to have an anatomic or functional abnormality and as many as 50% of children less than 3 months of age with UTI will have reflux demonstrated at the time of radiographic study.

Ultrasonography provides a noninvasive evaluation of renal size and some aspects of parenchymal structure, and it can provide limited information about obstructive lesions. Gross dilatation of the renal pelvic structures and collecting system or cystic changes of the kidney can be detected by ultrasonography. Thus most clinicians agree that ultrasonography should be performed as a first screening examination in all first episodes of UTI in children.

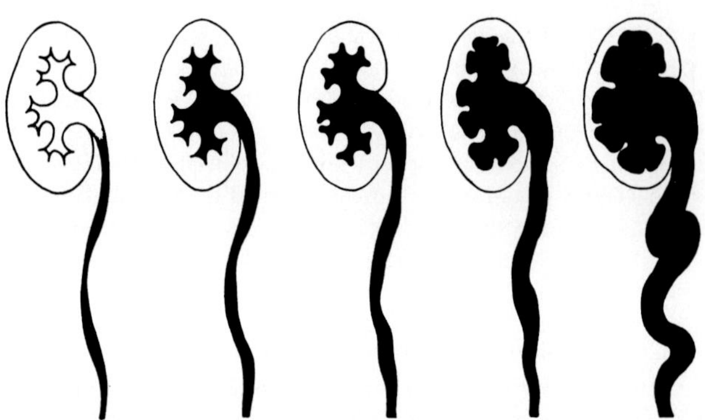

FIGURE 82–2. International classification of vesicoureteral reflux, which is usually determined by voiding cystourethrography or radionuclide cystography. *Left to right:* grades I, II, III, IV, and V. (From Fowler JE Jr: Urinary Tract Infection and Inflammation. Chicago, Year Book Medical Publishers, 1989.)

VCUG and RNC are usually the best imaging studies for demonstrating obstructive lesions of the urinary tract, defining upper tract anatomy, and determining the presence or absence of reflux (Fig. 82–1). The degree of reflux and alteration in anatomy is graded from I–V on the basis of the international system of classification (Fig. 82–2). Grade I reflux involves the ureter only. Grade II reflux involves the ureter and the intrarenal collecting system. Grades III through V include collecting system dilatation, beginning with mild ureteral and pelvic dilatation (grade III) and progressing to obliteration of the caliceal fornices (grade IV) and thereafter to complete gross dilatation of the ureter and obliteration of caliceal and pelvic anatomy on the image (grade V). Any degree of abnormality on VCUG should prompt consultation with a pediatric urologist or nephrologist to assist in further management and follow-up care.

Either ^{99m}Tc **dimercaptosuccinic acid (DMSA)** or ^{99m}Tc **glucoheptonate (GHA) renal cortical scintigraphy** can reliably predict the presence of pyelonephritis (Fig. 82–3). DMSA binds to proximal renal tubular cells and accumulates in functioning renal cortex but does not filter through the glomerulus, whereas GHA does

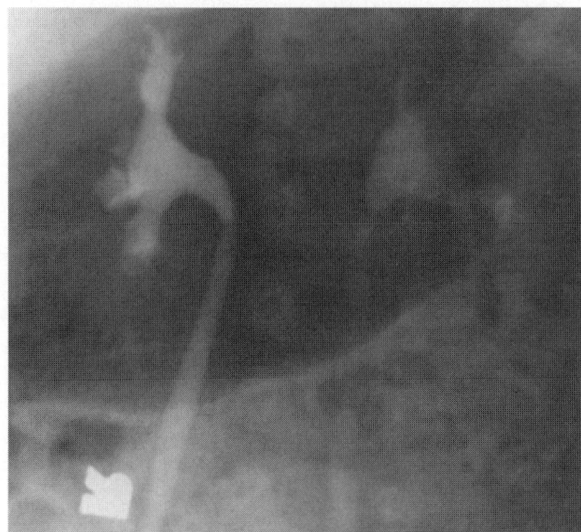

FIGURE 82–1. Grade III vesicoureteral reflux demonstrated by voiding cystourethrography in a 3-year-old child with recurrent urinary tract infections.

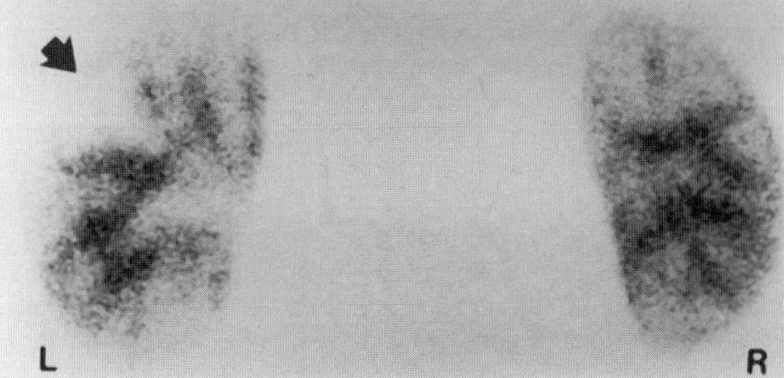

FIGURE 82–3. ^{99m}Tc dimercaptosuccinic acid (DMSA) renal scan *(posterior view)* in a 4-year-old girl presenting with fever for 3 weeks, demonstrating a focal, wedge-shaped photopenic defect *(arrow)* involving the upper and midpolar regions of the left kidney and extending to the cortex, consistent with pyelonephritis. (Courtesy of Sydney Heyman.)

both. In animal studies, renal scans have 91% sensitivity and 99% specificity in the diagnosis of acute pyelonephritis. In children with UTI followed prospectively, 42% have been shown by DMSA scan to have developed renal scars. Thus renal cortical scans may be the optimal tool to define upper tract disease in children. However, the decisions regarding early treatment and management of UTI are not affected by these findings because it is not clear that therapy should differ in children with upper tract versus lower tract disease. Therefore the DMSA scan should be reserved for children with suggestive signs of pyelonephritis or as a follow-up examination to define the presence or absence of renal scars.

Intravenous pyelography is primarily a functional test that provides few anatomic data for most pediatric patients with UTI. The DMSA or GHA scans are useful in assessing function, documenting the involvement of the renal parenchyma by infection, and assisting in the diagnosis of neoplastic lesions or other mass lesions such as renal abscess. Renal abscesses are best visualized on abdominal CT or MRI or, alternatively, by radionuclide scanning using ^{67}Ga-labeled citrate or ^{111}In-labeled WBCs. CT remains the single best imaging study for abscesses largely because of availability. However, MRI may provide better soft tissue resolution and sensitivity of diagnosis. Renal or perinephric abscesses are problematic in newborn infants because the small size and frequently fragile clinical status of the newborns make the performance of imaging studies more difficult.

Recommendations regarding the timing and frequency of radiographic studies to assess urinary tract anatomy vary from center to center. The American Academy of Pediatrics recommends that all children with UTI undergo ultrasonography promptly and either VCUG or RNC at the earliest convenient time, although some experts delay any further radiographic evaluation beyond ultrasonography until the second occurrence of UTI. VCUG and RNC for evaluating the extent of renal parenchymal involvement in the first episodes of UTI are particularly important in the following: neonates; males of any age; girls less than 5 years of age; children with UTI and positive blood culture results, high fever, localizing symptoms of pyelonephritis, or severe toxicity; and children with abnormal ultrasonographic findings, a second episode of UTI after 2 years of age, evidence of prior missed infections, or renal dysfunction such as an elevated serum creatinine concentration. VCUG should be completed after culture confirmation that the urine is sterile and is often performed after successful completion of a therapeutic course of antibiotics when follow-up urine cultures have been shown to be sterile. Usually VCUG or RNC can be scheduled for 2–6 weeks after the first day of treatment. A prophylactic antibiotic regimen should be continued after completion of therapy and until 48–72 hours after the procedure. Children with VUR demonstrated on VCUG or RNC are candidates for continued prophylaxis.

TREATMENT

The overall principles and evidence of treatment of UTI with antibiotics have recently been summarized in a practice guideline published by the American Academy of Pediatrics (Table 82–3). Children and adolescents with a urine culture confirming a UTI should have either oral or parenteral antibiotic therapy. Children or adolescents with a suspected UTI who are assessed as toxic, dehydrated, or unable to retain oral intake should have parenteral therapy initially, and hospitalization should be considered.

Definitive Treatment

Most antibiotics used for UTI are well absorbed and well tolerated when given orally and are excreted unchanged in the urine. Laboratory reporting of susceptibility to some antibiotics (e.g., nalidixic acid, nitrofurantoin, trimethoprim, carbenicillin, sulfisoxazole, and quinolones) recognizes the inherently higher urine concentration of antibiotics. Antibiotics to which organisms have only intermediate or moderate susceptibility are nevertheless often adequate for the treatment of UTIs because the isolates are often susceptible to concentrations of antibiotics achievable in urine. Many antibiotics, including ampicillin, amoxicillin, many oral cephalosporins, trimethoprim-sulfamethoxazole (TMP-SMZ), and nitrofurantoin, will be efficacious for treatment of UTI with susceptible organisms when given in moderate or low doses (see Table 82–4). In recent years the incidence of resistance to ampicillin or amoxicillin among urinary isolates of enteric bacteria has significantly increased, and therefore neither can be considered a drug of choice in the treatment of UTI. In the United States, most isolates remain susceptible to TMP-SMZ, and although resistance is also increasing to this agent,

TABLE 82–3. Summary of American Academy of Pediatrics Practice Guidelines for Diagnosis, Treatment, and Evaluation of Initial Urinary Tract Infection in Febrile Infants and Children 2 Months to 2 Years of Age

- The presence of UTI should be suspected in infants and young children with unexplained fever.
- The degree of toxicity, dehydration, and ability to retain oral intake should be carefully assessed.
- In infants and young children with unexplained fever who are assessed as being sufficiently ill to warrant immediate antibiotic therapy, a urine specimen should be obtained by catheterization or suprapubic percutaneous aspiration.
- If a child with unexplained fever who is assessed as not being too ill to require antibiotics, the options are (1) obtain and culture a urine specimen by catheterization or suprapubic aspiration or (2) obtain a urine by the most convenient method and repeat the urine collection by catheterization or suprapubic aspiration if the urinalysis suggests a UTI.
- Diagnosis of UTI requires a culture of the urine.
- If the child with suspected UTI is assessed as having a toxic appearance, being dehydrated, or being unable to retain oral intake, initial antibiotics should be administered parenterally and hospitalization should be considered.
- In a child who may not appear ill but who has a urine culture confirming the presence of UTI, antibiotic therapy should be initiated parenterally or orally.
- Infants and children who do not demonstrate the expected clinical response within 2 days of antimicrobial therapy should be re-evaluated, and another urine specimen should be cultured.
- Infants and children who do not demonstrate the expected clinical response within 2 days of antimicrobial therapy should undergo ultrasonography promptly, and either VCUG or RNC should be performed at the earliest convenient time.
- Infants and young children should complete a 7- to 14-day antimicrobial course (parenteral plus oral).
- After a 7- to 14-day course of antimicrobial therapy and sterilization of the urine, infants and young children should receive prophylactic antimicrobial dosages until the imaging studies are completed.

it is presently the preferred oral drug for primary and recurrent UTI. Many oral cephalosporins (e.g., cefixime and cefpodoxime) are also excellent candidate agents for the treatment of UTI because of their enhanced gram-negative activity, but these agents are more expensive alternatives to TMP-SMZ. Therefore they are usually used in situations where there is intolerance, hypersensitivity, or antimicrobial resistance to TMP-SMZ. A prospective randomized clinical trial (Hoberman et al, 1999) demonstrated that a regimen of oral cefixime (16 mg/kg/day on day 1, followed by 8 mg/kg/day for 13 days) was equivalent to a regimen of 3 days of cefotaxime intravenously followed by oral cefixime for 11 days.

Parenterally administered third-generation cephalosporins and aminoglycosides remain effective agents for UTI but are generally used in situations where there is no effective oral treatment, such as infection with *Pseudomonas* or antibiotic-resistant pathogen or hospitalization deemed necessary because of suspected upper tract disease (i.e., pyelonephritis) or because of symptoms suggestive of possible bacterial sepsis. The third-generation cephalosporins, aminoglycosides, parenteral preparations of TMP-SMZ, and newer β-lactam–β-lactamase inhibitor combinations are especially useful agents for hospitalized children, who may have infection caused by bacteria resistant to conventional antibiotics. A study (Carapetis et al, 2001) of gentamicin using age-appropriate dosing (2.5 mg/kg for children <5 years; 6 mg/kg for children 5–10 years; 4.5 mg/kg for children ≥11 years) and measurement of serum trough concentrations before the second dose demonstrated that once daily gentamicin was as safe and effective as dosing gentamicin three times daily.

Hospitalization and treatment with intravenously administered antibiotics is appropriate for selected children. All neonates and most infants less than 6 months of age with first episodes of UTI should be hospitalized and treated with parenteral antibiotics until the presence of significant urinary tract abnormalities or septicemia has been excluded and a parenteral antibiotic has been given for a minimum of 5 days. Children with known complex urinary tract abnormalities predisposing them to UTI and those with a prior history of recurrent UTI also may be appropriate candidates for initial hospitalization until the response to therapy is ensured and the presence of antibiotic-resistant organisms is excluded.

Children with suspected pyelonephritis should be hospitalized. However, because there is considerable clinical overlap between presumptive lower and upper tract disease, clinicians have to judge the likelihood of pyelonephritis on the basis of the degree of severity of clinical toxicity, fever, chills, and other systemic symptoms; the presence or absence of flank pain; prior history of UTI; and ancillary laboratory data, including ESR, CRP concentration, leukocytosis, or the presence of WBC casts. DMSA or GHA scanning may be useful in defining the presence of pyelonephritis and subsequent scarring, but these tests have not been evaluated completely as tools in the acute phase of infection to determine the need for hospitalization and parenteral antibiotics.

Asymptomatic Bacteriuria. The significance of asymptomatic bacteriuria is unknown. It may represent a sequela of prior partially treated but unrecognized UTI, or it has been postulated that it may be a marker for a predisposition to UTI with subsequent renal scarring. Screening of symptom-free children for bacteriuria has been suggested, but the yield is small and it is uncertain what treatment or follow-up is necessary for children.

Antibiotic treatment of asymptomatic bacteriuria in children undergoing long-term catheterization or in those with neurologic dysfunction is not generally recommended. Treatment of asymptomatic bacteriuria in this clinical setting leads to the selection of antibiotic-resistant flora that will make treatment of symptomatic episodes difficult or impossible. Antibiotic prophylaxis is also less effective in these children because of the extended periods that the antibiotics are used. Emphasis should be placed on appropriate techniques to provide adequate bladder evacuation (e.g., programs of self-catheterization) in consultation with a urologist or pediatric nephrologist.

Acute Urethral Syndrome. Treatment of the acute urethral syndrome in sexually active adolescents must provide coverage for the major pathogens, which include *C. trachomatis, E. coli,* and coagulase-negative staphylococci. The best-evaluated regimen is doxycycline 100 mg twice daily for 7–10 days.

Duration of Therapy. Early studies documented lower reinfection or relapse rates with treatment durations of 7–10 days, but no advantage has been proved for a duration of therapy longer than 10 days, and therefore a period of 7–10 days has become the conventional duration of treatment in most children with acute UTI. A longer duration of treatment may be indicated for certain children with known structural abnormalities of the urinary tract, antibiotic-resistant isolates, or a history of frequent relapse or reinfection.

The recommendation for 7- to 10-day regimens in children is in contradistinction to the more frequent recommendations for shorter regimens in adults. One reason is that many children are treated at a time when knowledge regarding reflux or another possible anatomic abnormality is unknown, whereas in adult women with UTI the majority have been evaluated and are known to have an anatomically normal urinary tract (e.g., an "uncomplicated UTI"). Thus shorter courses of antibiotics, ranging from a single large dose to 3–5 days of oral therapy, have been better evaluated in women with UTI. In women it can be concluded that all regimens shorter than 5 days and those using β-lactam antibiotics instead of TMP-SMZ are inferior, resulting in higher rates of persistence and relapse of infection (Norrby, 1990). In a review (Shapiro, 1982) of eight studies of abbreviated antibiotic therapy in children, conflicting results were observed with cure rates for single-dose regimens ranging from 63% to 95%. For certain older children and adolescents with UTI, shorter courses of antibiotics may be effective. Short courses of therapy should be considered for older children with normal urinary tracts who are noncompliant with longer courses of antibiotic therapy. The most successful single-dose regimen is TMP-SMZ given as a single dose of 320 mg TMP plus 1,600 mg SMZ; other regimens that have been less well evaluated include kanamycin (500 mg intramuscularly) and amoxicillin (3 g orally). Some long-acting oral cephalosporins have been used in single-dose regimens (e.g., cefadroxil 30 mg/kg orally) or 3-day regimens (e.g., cefadroxil 30 mg/kg divided twice daily orally) with success rates comparable to that of TMP-SMZ.

Renal and Perinephric Abscesses. Management of renal and perinephric abscesses necessitates a cooperative effort between the primary care or infectious disease physician and a nephrologist or urologic surgeon. Antibiotic treatment of abscesses will depend on the antibiotic susceptibility of pathogens recovered from urine, blood, or direct aspiration of the abscess or other contiguous site. Abscesses occurring in the renal collecting system, particularly those that are incidental to sepsis, often drain spontaneously. For abscesses involving the renal cortex, perinephric spaces, or contiguous tissues, decisions regarding the need for surgical drainage and the mode of drainage will need to be individualized on the basis of the initial response to antimicrobial therapy. Both direct surgical drainage and percutaneous radiographically assisted aspiration or drainage may be feasible, depending on the anatomic location. In most cases, it will be desirable to drain perinephric and renal cortical abscesses to facilitate earlier recovery and prevent spread to contiguous tissues or further damage of renal parenchyma. Limited surgery may also be necessary to relieve associated obstructive lesions. The duration of antibiotic therapy must be individualized and should be extended several days after drainage has ceased, wound and radiographic healing is evident, and cultures of specimens from draining sites are sterile.

Supportive Therapy

The degree of toxicity and dehydration and the ability to retain oral intake should be carefully assessed. Provision of adequate hydration, by either the intravenous or oral route, to maintain an adequate urine output is important but not curative. Serum electrolyte abnormalities caused by vomiting or poor oral intake should be corrected. Acidification of the urine, such as with cranberry juice ingested orally, does not accelerate the response to antibiotics or reduce the likelihood of relapse or reinfection.

COMPLICATIONS

Pyelonephritis is estimated to be present in 3–40% of children at the time of first UTI. UTI is complicated by positive blood culture results in 2–5% of episodes. Sepsis is far more likely in infants than in older chilren: 31% of neonates <1 month of age have bacteremia, compared with 18% of those 1–3 months of age and 6% of those 3–8 months of age.

The incidence of focal infections, including renal and perinephric abscesses, is unknown. Focal renal abscesses may complicate 1–5% of episodes of staphylococcal bacteremia but seem to be far less common with bacteremia caused by enteric organisms. An abscess is more likely with ascending infection in an obstructed urinary tract.

PROGNOSIS

Response to Therapy and Follow-up. The recurrence rate of UTI in children with or without demonstrated urinary tract abnormalities is high, 25–40% within 12 months of the first episode. The majority of relapses occur within 2–3 weeks after the end of treatment of the acute episode, whereas reinfection may occur much later.

Most children will have resolution of clinical symptoms and signs, and negative urine culture results within 48–72 hours of the start of active antibiotic therapy. Infants and children who do not demonstrate the expected clinical response within 48 hours of the start of antimicrobial therapy should be re-evaluated with repeated urinalysis and culture and with prompt ultrasonography. Failure to obtain sterile urine cultures may indicate an antibiotic-resistant pathogen, a renal or perinephric abscess, or an obstructed urinary tract. Late follow-up urine cultures should be obtained at 1–2 weeks after the cessation of therapy to document sterility of the urine in anticipation of the scheduled VCUG. In children in whom VCUG will be performed, prophylactic antibiotics should be administered until the study has been completed and it is known whether reflux is present. Further urine cultures should be obtained even for children without a demonstrated urinary tract abnormality. Some experts recommend that urine cultures be obtained monthly for 3 months and then at 3-month intervals for the next 6 months and yearly for 2–3 years. Variations in this regimen of cultures may be justifiable, but clinical follow-up lasting at least 2–3 years is prudent.

Persistence, Relapse, and Reinfection. Persistence of infection is rare with first episodes of UTI because the risk is directly related to the number of prior infections and to the emergence of infection with resistant organisms selected by exposure to antibiotics in prior episodes. Antibiotic efficacy is >95% for first episodes of UTI. Approximately two thirds of reinfections occur during the first year, with the highest incidence within the first 3 months. The tendency for UTI to recur persists until 5–6 years of age. Approximately 40% of girls and 32% of boys with UTI beyond the first year of life have recurrences.

Renal Scarring. The management recommended for UTI in children is based on the prevention of progressive renal disease. VUR is present in 30–50% of children with UTI, with the frequency inversely proportional to age. The natural history of reflux favors self-resolution as the child becomes older. Approximately 30–60% of children with reflux will develop renal scarring, which is thought to be the direct result of reflux of infected urine into the upper urinary tract. Children younger than 5 years are particularly susceptible to the development of VUR with acute infection and reflux and to subsequent scarring of the renal parenchyma.

PREVENTION

Chronic constipation and encopresis are also risk factors for UTI. Daytime and nighttime urinary incontinence is frequent, and UTI may occur in more than 10% of these children, especially girls, with rates 10-fold that of boys (33% vs 3%). Treatment is directed toward relief of the underlying constipation, with disimpaction and bowel maintenance programs, and includes the use of antibiotics for UTI.

Prophylaxis. Prophylaxis is based on the principal of maintaining sterile urine, providing prolonged symptom-free intervals, and aborting the progression to renal scarring and chronic pyelonephritis. A recent meta-analysis (Williams et al, 2001) of five randomized controlled trials from more than 900 published reports of low-dose antibiotic administration for prevention of recurrent UTI showed approximately two-thirds reduction in risk of recurrence (relative risk 0.31, 95% confidence interval 0.10–1.00), although significant study heterogeneity limited these findings. There appears to be no sustained benefit once antibiotics are discontinued. TMP-SMZ, nitrofurantoin, and methenamine mandelate have all proved successful as prophylactic agents and are associated with low rates of progressive antibiotic resistance. A single daily bedtime dose of these drugs is usually successful in children with urinary continence (Table 82–4). Nitrofurantoin may occasionally be associated with symptoms of peripheral neuropathy or with nausea and vomiting in young children. Both hypersensitivity to SMZ and (occasionally) leukopenia may complicate TMP-SMZ prophylaxis. Oral β-lactam antibiotics, such as cephalosporins and amoxicillin, facilitate the selection of resistant bowel flora and should be avoided as prophylactic agents.

Urinary tract prophylaxis should be considered for all children with demonstrated VUR and those with known abnormal obstructive urinary tract anatomy who have had a UTI. Children with normal anatomy and without demonstrated VUR, but with at least two recurrences of UTI, should also be considered for prophylaxis. The optimal duration of prophylaxis is unknown, but the regimen should continue until at least 6 years of age in children with VUR or until reflux has resolved spontaneously or has been surgically corrected and the child has been free of symptoms and bacteriuria for at least 1 year. In children with a normal urinary tract, recommendations have been made for the duration of prophylaxis ranging from 3 months to 1 year after a second episode, with careful surveillance after antibiotic therapy is discontinued. Unfortunately, only older children with urinary continence have been evaluated for the efficacy of bedtime prophylactic regimens. The efficacy of

TABLE 82-4. Antibiotics for Treatment and Prophylaxis in Children with Urinary Tract Infection

Drug	Treatment Regimen	Prophylaxis Regimen
Parenteral Therapy		
Ampicillin	100 mg/kg/day divided q6hr	
Cefotaxime	100–150 mg/kg/day divided q8hr	
Ceftazidime	100–150 mg/kg/day divided q8hr	
Cefepime	100–150 mg/kg/day divided q8–12hr	
Gentamicin	5–7.5 mg/kg/day divided q8hr	
Amikacin	15–22.5 mg/kg/day divided q8hr	
Ampicillin-sulbactam	100–200 mg/kg/day ampicillin divided q6hr	
TMP-SMZ	8–12 mg/kg/day TMP with 40–60 mg/kg/day SMZ divided q12hr	
Oral Therapy		
Amoxicillin	30–40 mg/kg/day divided q12hr	10–15 mg/kg once daily hs
Amoxicillin-clavulanate	30 mg/kg/day divided q12hr	25 mg/kg once daily hs
Cephalexin	40–50 mg/kg/day divided q6–8hr	12–15 mg/kg once daily hs
Cefixime	8–16 mg/kg/day once daily or divided q12hr	
Cefpodoxime	10 mg/kg/day divided q12hr	
Methenamine mandelate	40–50 mg/kg/day divided q8–12hr	
Nitrofurantoin	5–7 mg/kg/day divided q6hr	1–2 mg/kg once daily hs
Sulfisoxazole	150 mg/kg/day divided q6hr	50 mg/kg once daily hs
TMP-SMZ	6–12 mg/kg/day TMP with 30–60 mg/kg/day SMZ divided q8–12hr	2 mg/kg TMP with 10 mg/kg SMZ once daily hs

prophylactic antibiotics for infants with smaller bladder capacities and more frequent voiding has never been studied, so the benefits of prophylaxis, if any, in this setting are unknown.

There are inconsistent results among studies of the efficacy of drinking cranberry juice for prevention of UTI. A randomized study (Kontiokari et al, 2001) of adult women with a prior UTI reported a 16% incidence of UTI over 6 months among women who drank 50 mL of cranberry-lingonberry juice concentrate daily, compared to a 36% incidence in the control group. Cranberry juice is not recommended as the sole means for prevention of UTI among susceptible children.

REVIEWS

American Academy of Pediatrics, Committee on Quality Improvement, Subcommittee on Urinary Tract Infections: Practice parameter: The diagnosis, treatment, and evaluation of the initial urinary tract infection in febrile infants and young children. *Pediatrics* 1999;103:843–52. [Published errata appear in *Pediatrics* 1999;103:1052; *Pediatrics* 1999;104:118; and *Pediatrics* 2000;105:141.]

Hansson S, Martinell J, Stokland E, et al: The natural history of bacteriuria in childhood. *Infect Dis Clin North Am* 1997;11:499–512.

Hoberman A, Wald ER: Urinary tract infections in young febrile children. *Pediatr Infect Dis J* 1997;16:11–7.

Svanborg Edén C, de Man P: Bacterial virulence in urinary tract infection. *Infect Dis Clin North Am* 1987;1:731–50.

KEY ARTICLES

Andrich MP, Majd M: Diagnostic imaging in the evaluation of the first urinary tract infection in infants and young children. *Pediatrics* 1992;90:436–41.

Carapetis JR, Jaquiery AL, Buttery JP, et al: Randomized, controlled trial comparing once daily and three times daily gentamicin in children with urinary tract infections. *Pediatr Infect Dis J* 2001;20:240–6.

Ginsburg CM, McCracken GH Jr: Urinary tract infections in young infants. *Pediatrics* 1982;69:409–12.

Hoberman A, Wald ER, Hickey RW, et al: Oral versus initial intravenous therapy for urinary tract infections in young febrile children. *Pediatrics* 1999;104:79–86.

Honkinen O, Lehtonen OP, Ruuskanen O, et al: Cohort study of bacterial species causing urinary tract infection and urinary tract abnormalities in children. *BMJ* 1999;318:770–1.

Hooton TM: Pathogenesis of urinary tract infections: An update. *J Antimicrob Chemother* 2000;46(Suppl A):1–7.

Jakobsson B, Esbjorner E, Hansson S: Minimum incidence and diagnostic rate of first urinary tract infection. *Pediatrics* 1999;104:222–6.

Kontiokari T, Sundqvist K, Nuutinen M, et al: Randomised trial of cranberry-lingonberry juice and *Lactobacillus* GG drink for the prevention of urinary tract infections in women. *Br Med J* 2001;322:1571–3.

Kunin CM, Deutscher R, Paquin A Jr: Urinary tract infection in schoolchildren: An epidemiologic, clinical, and laboratory study. *Medicine* 1964;43:91–130.

Kunin CM: The natural history of recurrent bacteriuria in schoolgirls. *N Engl J Med* 1970;282:1443–8.

Lin DS, Huang SH, Lin CC, et al: Urinary tract infection in febrile infants younger than eight weeks of age. *Pediatrics* 2000;105:E20.

Majd M, Rushton HG, Jantausch B, et al: Relationship among vesicoureteral reflux, P-fimbriated *Escherichia coli*, and acute pyelonephritis in children with febrile urinary tract infection. *J Pediatr* 1991;119:578–85.

Nelson JD, Peters PC: Suprapubic aspiration of urine in premature and term infants. *Pediatrics* 1965;36:132–44.

Norrby SR: Short-term treatment of uncomplicated lower urinary tract infection in women. *Rev Infect Dis* 1990;12:458.

Schlager TA, Anderson S, Trudell J, et al: Effect of cranberry juice on bacteriuria in children with neurogenic bladder receiving intermittent catheterization. *J Pediatr* 1999;135:698–702.

Shapiro ED: Short course antimicrobial treatment of urinary tract infections in children: A critical analysis. *Pediatr Infect Dis* 1982;1:294–7.

Smellie JM, Prescod NP, Shaw PJ, et al: Childhood reflux and urinary infection: A follow-up of 10–41 years in 226 adults. *Pediatr Nephrol* 1198;12:727–36.

Wennerström M, Hansson S, Jodal U, et al: Disappearance of vesicoureteral reflux in children. *Arch Pediatr Adolesc Med* 1998;152:879–83.

Wennerström M, Hansson S, Jodal U, et al: Primary and acquired renal scarring in boys and girls with urinary tract infection. *J Pediatr* 2000;136:30–4.

Williams G, Lee A, Craig J: Antibiotics for the prevention of urinary tract infection in children: A systematic review of randomized controlled trials. *J Pediatr* 2001;138:868–74.

Winberg J, Anderson HJ, Bergstrom T, et al: Epidemiology of symptomatic urinary tract infection in childhood. *Acta Paediatr Scand* 1974;252:1–20.

Wiswell TE, Smith FR, Bass JW: Decreased incidence of urinary tract infections in circumcised male infants. *Pediatrics* 1985;75:901–3.

CHAPTER 83

Infections of the Lower Genitourinary Tract

Gary D. Overturf

Infections of the lower genitourinary tract are usually considered in the presence of local symptoms or as part of the differential diagnosis of urinary tract infections (Chapter 82) and sexually transmitted diseases (Chapter 85). Because of the intra-abdominal location, the syndromes of salpingitis and oophoritis are difficult to diagnose and do not characteristically have localized findings at presentation. These syndromes are distinctly uncommon as isolated entities and most commonly occur with cervicitis as a manifestation of sexually transmitted infections. Prostatitis, epididymitis, and orchitis occur in men and boys. Urethritis occurs in both sexes. Genital infections are not necessarily transmitted by sexual contact, and many sexually transmitted infections involve anatomic areas other than the genitalia.

PROSTATITIS

Prostatitis is inflammation or infection of the prostate gland. It may be acute or chronic. It usually occurs in sexually active men and is rare in prepubertal boys but may occur even in infants. **Prostatism** and **prostatodynia** are used to describe chronic symptoms of perianal pain and voiding dysfunction suggestive of prostatitis but with negative bacterial culture results and no objective evidence of prostatic inflammation.

ETIOLOGY, EPIDEMIOLOGY, AND PATHOGENESIS

Prostatitis is rare in children. Conditions recognized to predispose a person to acute prostatitis include a foreign body in the genitourinary tract, urethral instrumentation, surgical procedures, immunosuppression, and diabetes mellitus, primarily in adults.

The organisms commonly responsible for urinary tract infections, the gram-negative enteric bacilli, are the usual causes of acute bacterial prostatitis. Gram-positive organisms such as *Staphylococcus aureus* (especially in newborn infants), coagulase-negative staphylococci, α- and β-hemolytic *Streptococcus,* and *Enterococcus* also may cause bacterial prostatitis in children. The role of anaerobic bacteria in acute bacterial prostatitis has not been established. *Neisseria gonorrhoeae* and other sexually transmitted organisms such as *Chlamydia trachomatis, Ureaplasma urealyticum, Treponema pallidum,* and *Trichomonas vaginalis* can cause acute prostatitis. In addition, systemic brucellosis may involve the prostate.

The bacteria associated with acute prostatitis may also cause chronic prostatitis. Uncommon causes include *Mycobacterium tuberculosis,* which is usually associated with tuberculosis at another site such as the kidney. Atypical mycobacteria, especially *Mycobacterium fortuitum* and *Mycobacterium kansasii,* have been associated with prostatitis in adults. *Actinomycosis* rarely has been associated with prostatitis.

Rare causes of prostatitis include fungi such as *Candida albicans* and endemic fungal species such as *Cryptococcus neoformans, Histoplasma capsulatum, Blastomyces dermatitidis,* and *Coccidioides immitis,* especially in immunocompromised persons and usually as part of disseminated infections. Echoviruses and varicella-zoster virus, during an attack of sacral zoster, have also been implicated circumstantially as causes of prostatitis.

SYMPTOMS AND CLINICAL MANIFESTATIONS

The symptoms of acute prostatitis in children are variable and may be vague. They usually include perineal, suprapubic, perirectal, or low back pain; urinary symptoms such as dysuria, urgency, frequency, and acute urinary retention; and urethral discharge. In addition, systemic symptoms such as fever, irritability, chills, and myalgia may be present. Men with chronic bacterial prostatitis are generally free of symptoms between episodes of recurrent bacterial infections of the urinary tract caused by the same organism.

Physical Examination Findings

In acute prostatitis the prostate gland is very tender, tense, boggy, and swollen on examination. If a prostatic abscess is present, a bulging mass may be palpable in the prostate gland. A rectal examination of the prostate of prepubertal boys and infants may be very difficult to perform and interpret. Fever, hypotension, and systemic toxicity may be present if prostatitis is complicated by bacteremia or sepsis. In chronic prostatitis the prostate gland is usually normal on rectal examination.

DIAGNOSIS

The diagnosis of acute bacterial prostatitis is supported by the presence of pyuria and bacteriuria. Examination for leukocytes and culture of segmented urine (e.g., the first 10 mL of urine) and expressed prostatic fluid obtained after prostatic massage (e.g., expressed prostatic fluid or the first 10 mL of urine after massage) are important in establishing the diagnosis as well as the etiologic agent. Care should be taken in performing prostatic massage if acute bacterial prostatitis is suspected, because the procedure may precipitate bacteremia. A Gram-stained smear of the urine and fluid should be performed and the samples cultured for bacteria. If the prostatitis is chronic or if the patient is immunocompromised, cultures for mycobacteria and fungi are also needed. Viral cultures also can be obtained if a virus is suspected. Biopsy of the prostate can be performed in unusual circumstances or if cancer is suspected.

Imaging of the prostate by ultrasonography or CT should be performed if there is clinical evidence or suspicion of a prostatic abscess.

TREATMENT

Persons with acute prostatitis should be treated with antibiotics active against the likely etiologic agents. Ampicillin or a third-generation cephalosporin plus an aminoglycoside, such as gentamicin, are appropriate in most cases where enteric organisms are likely. A semisynthetic penicillin, such as nafcillin or oxacillin, is appropriate for treating prostatitis caused by *S. aureus,* which may occur in young infants. Most antibiotics diffuse poorly into prostatic secretions because of the acidic pH of prostatic fluid, which is usually 6.8–7.2. In general, nonpolar, lipid-soluble drugs are preferred. TMP-SMZ provides good prostatic tissue concentrations and may be particularly useful in the oral treatment of prostatitis. Quinolone antibiotics, such as ciprofloxacin, norfloxacin, and levofloxacin, may be used in postpubertal adolescents, and tetracycline antibiotics may be used in children 9 years or older. The treatment of prostatitis associated with sexually transmitted infections is discussed in Chapter 85.

In addition to specific antibiotic therapy, supportive and symptomatic treatment with bed rest, hydration, stool softeners, and analgesics may be helpful. If urinary retention is present or there is evidence of a prostatic abscess, urologic consultation should be obtained. Suprapubic drainage may be required if urinary retention is severe, and surgical aspiration or drainage of an abscess may be necessary.

COMPLICATIONS AND PROGNOSIS

The complications of acute prostatitis include abscess formation and urinary retention. Chronic prostatitis also may develop, although this is unusual. Persons with chronic bacterial prostatitis may require suppressive antimicrobial therapy to prevent recurrent symptomatic episodes; the bacteria usually remain sensitive to most antibiotics. Low doses of penicillins, nitrofurantoin, or TMP-SMZ (Table 82–4) may prevent symptomatic bladder infection despite the persistence of bacteria in the prostate gland.

EPIDIDYMITIS

Epididymitis is inflammation or infection of the epididymis. It may be acute or chronic, unilateral or bilateral, and even recurrent in nature. It can occur in both prepubertal and pubertal boys. Epididymitis commonly accompanies orchitis **(epididymo-orchitis)** or prostatitis.

ETIOLOGY, EPIDEMIOLOGY, AND PATHOGENESIS

In children less than 2 years of age, epididymitis is often associated with congenital anomalies of the urinary tract, including vesicoureteral reflux, urethral valve disorders, urethral diverticulum or stricture, and ectopic ureteral openings. In older children, conditions associated with epididymitis include trauma and prior instrumentation or operations on the genitourinary tract. In postpubertal boys, epididymitis is associated with sexually transmitted pathogens.

The organisms commonly responsible for urinary tract infections, the gram-negative enteric bacilli, usually cause acute epididymitis, especially in older men or after urologic instrumentation. Occasionally, gram-positive organisms, such as *S. aureus,* coagulase-negative staphylococci, *Streptococcus pneumoniae,* and *Enterococcus,* may cause epididymitis. *Haemophilus influenzae* type b, *Brucella, Salmonella, Shigella,* and *Neisseria meningitidis* are rare causes of epididymitis. In adolescents, sexually transmitted organisms such as *N. gonorrhea, C. trachomatis,* and *U. urealyticum* are the most common causes of epididymitis. Epididymitis is a rare manifestation of congenital syphilis in infants.

Tuberculosis of the epididymis occasionally occurs and usually produces a chronic, painless scrotal swelling or a mass lesion, although acute symptoms also may develop. Tuberculous epididymitis most often occurs in older men as a manifestation of generalized tuberculosis or in association with renal tuberculosis. Atypical mycobacteria, including *M. kansasii, M. avium-intracellulare, M. xenopi,* and *M. fortuitum,* may also cause epididymitis. *Mycobacterium leprae* may involve the epididymis in persons with leprosy. *Actinomyces israelii* has been rarely cited as a cause of epididymitis.

Viral causes of epididymitis usually may occur in association with orchitis from infection with mumps virus, Epstein-Barr virus, enteroviruses (especially group B coxsackieviruses), herpes simplex virus, cytomegalovirus, adenovirus, lymphocytic choriomeningitis virus, and arboviruses. Congenital rubella infection has been associated with abnormalities of the epididymis.

Fungal agents causing epididymitis include the disseminated endemic mycoses of *B. dermatitidis, C. immitis,* and *H. capsulatum.* Parasites, including *T. vaginalis, Schistosoma mansoni,* amebae, and filariae, all have reportedly caused epididymitis. Sarcoidosis is an unusual cause of epididymitis.

SYMPTOMS AND CLINICAL MANIFESTATIONS

Acute epididymitis is characterized by acute scrotal pain accompanied by dysuria and dripping of urine for days to weeks. Epididymitis is usually unilateral. Fever is uncommon, occurring in only 10–15% of patients. Other systemic symptoms include nausea, vomiting, lower abdominal pain, and irritability. Young infants may cry with diaper changes, and toddlers may refuse to walk because of pain associated with epididymitis. Chronic epididymitis may be difficult to diagnose and may have minimal symptoms.

Physical Examination Findings

Erythema and swelling of the scrotum are present with swelling and tenderness of the epididymis. The ipsilateral testicle may be tender. Occasionally a bluish discoloration may occur (the **blue dot sign**). Induration of the posterior-lying epididymis may be appreciated, although local or general anesthesia may be required to perform this detailed examination on an acutely ill person. The **cremasteric reflex,** seen as elevation of the scrotal sac elicited by gentle stroking of the medial proximal aspect of the thigh, is usually preserved in epididymitis but may be absent in many healthy adolescents. Chronic epididymitis may be manifested as a painless scrotal mass, an enlarged epididymis, irregular nodularity of the epididymis, or a hydrocele. Classic **beading of the vas deferens** can be palpated if tuberculous epididymitis is present.

DIAGNOSIS

It is crucial to differentiate acute epididymitis from the most common cause of acute scrotal pain, testicular torsion, because the latter is a surgical emergency and delay in diagnosis and treatment may result in loss of the testicle. Relief of pain usually occurs when the testis is elevated (e.g., supported) in epididymitis **(Prehn's sign),** whereas elevation increases pain if torsion of the testis is present. The cremasteric reflex is usually present in epididymitis but classically is absent in torsion. Other causes of acute painful scrotal masses include torsion of the spermatic cord, torsion of the testicular appendage, orchitis, and, rarely, tumors. The small-vessel vasculitis associated with Henoch-Schönlein purpura also may involve the epididymis, and in rare instances, epididymitis may be the only presenting symptom. Epididymitis has been reported with other vasculitis syndromes such as Kawasaki syndrome. Behçet's syndrome also may involve the epididymis. Occasionally the cause of the epididymitis is not found and the term *idiopathic* or *nonspecific epididymitis* is used.

The differential diagnosis of chronic epididymitis in the presence of a painless scrotal mass includes neoplasm, varicocele, hydrocele, and spermatocele. Varicoceles cannot be transilluminated, unlike hydroceles and spermatoceles. Hydroceles are usually localized in the tunica vaginalis anterior and inferior to the testes, and spermatoceles are localized to the efferent ductal system superior to the testes.

The diagnosis of acute epididymitis is supported by the presence of peripheral leukocytosis, an elevated CRP concentration or ESR, pyuria and bacteriuria, or bacteremia. Culture of the urine reveals the etiologic organism in concentrations greater than 10^5/mL in approximately one third of cases. Children less than 2 years of age are likely to have an underlying anomaly of the urinary tract. If a urethral discharge is present, especially in adolescents, it should be cultured for *N. gonorrhoeae,* and specimens should be cultured for *Chlamydia* or nucleic acid testing should be performed. Blood should be obtained for culture if systemic toxicity or an epididymal abscess is found.

The diagnosis of chronic epididymitis may be difficult. Urine and urethral discharge should be sent for routine culture and for culture of *Brucella,* mycobacteria, fungi, and viruses, and appropriate PCR testing (e.g., for *C. trachomatis*) should be performed. An epididymal aspiration or biopsy may be necessary to establish the cause of chronic epididymitis and to differentiate an infectious cause from a noninfectious cause (e.g., tumor). Tuberculous epididymitis is suggested by a history of household exposure to an adult with active tuberculosis. Sterile pyuria, positive acid-fast stain of the urine sediment, or a urine culture positive for *M. tuberculosis* may be obtained. A chest radiograph and a tuberculin skin test may help establish the diagnosis.

Noninvasive imaging procedures, such as nuclear imaging using ^{99m}Tc pertechnetate, continuous-wave Doppler ultrasonography, and real-time ultrasonography of the scrotum, establish the diagnosis in more than 80% of children. In epididymitis, the epididymis is enlarged and hypoechoic areas are seen on the ultrasonographic examination; increased blood flow is present on Doppler ultrasonography; and a scrotal nuclear scan demonstrates increased uptake of the tracer. If the epididymitis is chronic, scrotal ultrasonography may show an enlarged epididymis surrounded by reactive fluid. In young children with epididymitis, excretory urography, voiding cystourethrography, and abdominal and scrotal ultrasonography should be performed when acute symptoms have resolved, because of the common association of epididymitis with other urogenital anomalies.

TREATMENT

Acute epididymitis is treated with antibiotics directed against the proved or suspected etiologic organisms. If the patient has a systemic illness or is an infant younger than 24 months, parenteral administration of a third-generation cephalosporin plus an aminoglycoside is usually indicated. If the person is older and not acutely ill, oral TMP-SMZ may be efficacious and should be continued until symptoms resolve, which may be several weeks. Tuberculous epididymitis is treated as for other forms of extrapulmonary tuberculosis (Table 35–5). Scrotal exploration should be considered if the diagnosis remains in doubt after noninvasive examination or after failure of response to antibiotic treatment.

Scrotal support, bed rest, and analgesics may provide symptomatic relief of pain. If an abscess is present, surgical drainage or aspiration may be indicated. Urologic or surgical consultation is recommended for all children with epididymitis because most have underlying anatomic anomalies and because an abscess or testicular torsion may be present.

COMPLICATIONS AND PROGNOSIS

The most common complication of acute epididymitis is abscess formation. In long-standing epididymitis a scrotal fistula or discharge may be present. Moreover, especially with immunocompromise, epididymitis may progress to Fournier's gangrene, a rapidly synergistic, necrotizing fasciitis of the scrotal wall that often is fatal (Chapter 48).

ORCHITIS

Orchitis is an inflammation or infection of the testes. It most commonly is associated with systemic viral illness. Bacterial orchitis usually results from extension of infection of the epididymis **(epididymo-orchitis),** although it also may result from hematogenous or lymphatic spread of bacteria.

ETIOLOGY, EPIDEMIOLOGY, AND PATHOGENESIS

Unlike prostatitis and epididymitis, orchitis more likely is due to a viral illness than to infection with gram-negative enteric organisms. Mumps virus is the most common cause of isolated orchitis, which develops in approximately 20% of postpubertal boys with mumps virus infection; oophoritis occurs in 5–10% of postpubertal girls with mumps. Mumps orchitis is rare in prepubertal boys. Mumps orchitis is usually unilateral but is bilateral in 15–30% of cases and typically develops 5–7 days after the onset of parotitis, although rarely it develops before or without clinical parotitis. Other viruses occasionally associated with orchitis include enteroviruses, especially coxsackieviruses and echoviruses, varicella-zoster virus, influenza virus, lymphocytic choriomeningitis virus, dengue virus, and Epstein-Barr virus.

When gram-negative enteric organisms do cause orchitis, it usually is associated with epididymitis. Gram-positive bacteria causing orchitis include *S. aureus* and group A *Streptococcus,* as an element of scarlet fever. Unusual causes of orchitis include *Brucella,* rickettsiae, and diphtheria. Orchitis may also accompany acute appendicitis or cholecystitis. Unusual causes of orchitis include tuberculosis, fungi, parasites (amebae, schistosomiasis, malaria, and filariae), and syphilis.

SYMPTOMS AND CLINICAL MANIFESTATIONS

Orchitis presents with pain and swelling of the scrotum, and it may be unilateral or bilateral. Systemic signs and symptoms such as fever, chills, nausea, vomiting, and irritability also may be present. Young infants may cry with diaper changes, and toddlers may refuse to walk because of the pain associated with orchitis.

Physical Examination Findings

The testicle and scrotum demonstrate swelling and erythema. Petechiae or bluish discoloration of the scrotum may also be present.

DIAGNOSIS

The diagnosis of orchitis is established by clinical manifestations. Other causes of acute scrotal pain and swelling include testicular torsion, trauma, tumor, and epididymitis.

Scrotal ultrasonography usually reveals a testis that is enlarged with a heterogeneous decrease in echogenicity. The surrounding soft tissue may be thickened, and reactive fluid collection may be present. A focal anechoic, hypoechoic, or mixed echoic area may indicate abscess formation. If gas-producing organisms are present in the testis or scrotum, bright echogenic shadowing areas and fluid levels may be seen. Color-flow Doppler ultrasonography may show a decrease in perfusion of the involved testis. Testicular nuclear scans using ^{99m}Tc pertechnetate may help differentiate orchitis from other conditions, especially testicular torsion.

TREATMENT

Viral orchitis is treated with supportive treatment only. Broad-spectrum antibiotics are indicated for bacterial orchitis and should be continued until the signs and symptoms resolve, which may take several days to weeks. Serial scrotal sonograms are helpful in evaluating resolution and in excluding chronic inflammation, testicular atrophy, or testicular neoplasm, especially if symptoms do not resolve. Supportive treatment is indicated for both bacterial and viral orchitis and includes bed rest, scrotal support, hot or cold compresses, and analgesics.

COMPLICATIONS AND PROGNOSIS

Mumps orchitis, as well as other forms of viral orchitis, usually resolves in 7–10 days with symptomatic treatment. Secondary atrophy of the testicle, with fibrosis and possible sterility, is more common after pyogenic orchitis but may accompany any form of orchitis. However, sterility is rare because the orchitis is usually unilateral. Testicular atrophy occurs in 10–20% of affected testes, and therefore bilateral atrophy occurs in fewer than 5% of cases. Complications of bacterial orchitis include testicular infarction, abscess formation, and pyocele of the scrotum. Fournier's gangrene, a synergistic infection that causes a rapidly progressive, necrotizing fasciitis of the scrotum and perineum, may complicate orchitis, especially if anaerobes are involved or the person is immunocompromised (Chapter 48).

PREVENTION

Mumps vaccine is highly effective in preventing mumps infection and mumps orchitis.

URETHRITIS

Urethritis is inflammation of the anterior urethra and may occur in boys, girls, men, and women. It is caused by a variety of infectious and noninfectious agents. Infectious urethritis is usually classified as gonococcal or nongonococcal **(nonspecific urethritis).** This condition is uncommon in prepubertal children.

ETIOLOGY, EPIDEMIOLOGY, AND PATHOGENESIS

The common etiologic agents associated with urethritis vary according to age. Urethritis is much more common in adolescents, who are likely to be sexually active, and is usually caused by sexually transmitted organisms such as *N. gonorrhoeae, C. trachomatis, U. urealyticum,* or *T. vaginalis.* In infants and young children, urethritis is commonly caused by fecal contamination, poor hygiene, irritation from physical or chemical substances (e.g., bubble baths, soap), or the introduction of a foreign body.

Uncommon bacterial causes of urethritis include *Staphylococcus saprophyticus,* especially in females, and gram-negative enteric organisms, especially in males with phimosis. Urethral trauma or urologic instrumentation also may induce bacterial urethritis. Rarely, *H. influenzae* type b, *N. meningitidis, Moraxella catarrhalis,* anaerobic organisms, *Mycoplasma pneumoniae,* or *Mycoplasma hominis* may be associated with urethritis.

Viruses, most commonly herpes simplex virus, may cause vesicular lesions and ulcers on the genitalia and produce urethritis. Although the most common form of transmission is sexual contact, newborns may be inoculated with herpes simplex virus during passage through the birth canal, or children with primary herpetic gingivostomatitis may autoinoculate their genitalia. Coxsackieviruses and varicella-zoster virus may cause papulovesicular lesions in the genital area that may involve the urethra. Adenovirus, a common cause of conjunctivitis and pharyngitis, also may cause hemorrhagic cystitis and urethritis.

C. albicans may produce urethritis, but other fungal etiologic agents are exceedingly rare. Parasites, especially pinworms (*Enterobius vermicularis*), are a common cause of urethritis in young boys and girls. Pinworm infestation in boys or girls is frequently associated with concomitant perianal pruritus or, rarely, vaginitis in girls.

SYMPTOMS AND CLINICAL MANIFESTATIONS

The symptoms of urethritis include dysuria, pruritus, and urethral discharge. Although urethritis may occur as an isolated syndrome, it may also occur as a part of an infectious or noninfectious syndrome or symptom complex, such as Kawasaki syndrome, Wegener's granulomatosis, or Stevens-Johnson syndrome.

The urethral meatus may be erythematous and inflamed. A urethral discharge is usually present and may be thick and purulent, or it may be clear, thin, and watery. The discharge may be more apparent in males than in females. Ulcers or vesicles around the urethra or in the perineum may be present, especially if a virus is the etiologic agent.

DIAGNOSIS

The diagnosis of urethritis is established by clinical manifestations and supported by findings of pyuria and hematuria and by urethral discharge. The etiologic agent can be confirmed by tests of urethral discharge, which can be expressed and collected on a swab. A Gram-stained smear may show polymorphonuclear leukocytes and bacteria or yeast. If no organisms are seen, *Chlamydia* or *Ureaplasma* should be considered, and appropriate cultures should be grown or antigen testing performed. If a viral cause is considered, specimens should be obtained from lesions for viral culture.

TREATMENT

Urethritis from gonococci, herpes simplex virus, and other sexually transmitted pathogens is treated as a sexually transmitted infection (Chapter 85). Neonates should have complete evaluation for systemic infection with herpes simplex virus (Chapter 97). A diagnosis of urethritis caused by other organisms is based on the identification and susceptibility of the suspected or confirmed etiologic agent. For gram-negative enteric organisms such as *E. coli* associated with phimosis, amoxicillin, an oral third-generation cephalosporin, or TMP-SMZ is usually adequate. Treatment of urethritis due to *C. albicans* includes topical treatment with nystatin. Urethritis associated with pinworm infection should be treated with mebendazole (Chapter 42).

All persons with urethritis should have local including genital cleansing, appropriate diaper or underwear changes, and zinc oxide or bacitracin ointment applied to the meatus if it appears inflamed.

MEATITIS

Meatitis is inflammation of the urethral meatus. It occurs most commonly in infant boys who have just been circumcised.

ETIOLOGY, EPIDEMIOLOGY, AND PATHOGENESIS

Meatitis is primarily caused by mechanical irritation from a diaper or chemical irritation from the child's urine. Occasionally, however, secondary bacterial infection with skin or fecal flora occurs. In older children or adolescents, meatitis is usually accompanied by urethritis, and the etiologic agents associated with urethritis should be considered.

SYMPTOMS, CLINICAL MANIFESTATIONS, AND DIAGNOSIS

The diagnosis of meatitis is established by clinical findings. The urethral meatus appears red and edematous. A clear, serosanguineous or slightly purulent discharge or exudate may be present or may appear on the circumcision dressing or the diaper. If the discharge appears purulent, a Gram stain and bacterial culture should be performed.

TREATMENT

Local care is usually all that is necessary to alleviate meatitis. Appropriate care includes gentle genital cleansing to remove the exudate and topical application of bacitracin ointment or zinc oxide. A petrolatum gauze dressing also may help prevent local irritation from the diaper. If symptoms are severe or persistent, urologic consultation should be considered because meatal stenosis can cause urinary obstruction that may require meatotomy.

BALANITIS

Balanitis is inflammation or infection of the glans penis. **Balanoposthitis** refers to inflammation of both the glans penis and the penile foreskin.

ETIOLOGY, EPIDEMIOLOGY, AND PATHOGENESIS

Balanitis is usually associated with poor hygiene and is caused by accumulation of desquamated epithelial cells, glandular secretions, and urine under the foreskin. This environment allows overgrowth of bacteria normally present on the genitalia and perineum, especially gram-negative enteric organisms or the atypical mycobacteria, primarily *Mycobacterium smegmatis.* Rarely, gram-positive organisms such as *S. aureus* or group A or B *Streptococcus* cause balanitis.

If the patient has a sexual partner with vaginitis, then *C. albicans* and other vaginal flora should be considered as etiologic agents of the male partner's balanitis. *C. albicans* and herpes simplex virus may cause severe, recurrent balanitis in immunocompromised persons, including persons with AIDS. Children with a **condom catheter** may have balanitis caused by gram-negative enteric organisms. Rarely, in immunocompromised persons, anaerobic bacteria may cause gangrenous balanitis or balanoposthitis, a potentially serious infection that can cause necrosis of the penis.

Occasionally, especially in infants or small children, a circumferential foreign body, such as a hair or thread, may constrict the penis and cause erythema and swelling similar to balanitis. Careful inspection for a foreign body is therefore indicated for all young persons with balanitis.

SYMPTOMS, CLINICAL MANIFESTATIONS, AND DIAGNOSIS

The symptoms of balanitis include pain and pruritus of the penis. On examination the penis and foreskin are edematous, indurated, and erythematous. Occasionally, vesicles, ulcerations, papules, and other lesions may be present on the penis. Rarely a urethral discharge may be noted.

In uncomplicated balanitis the diagnosis is established by clinical findings. However, if the condition is severe, persistent, or recurrent, or if the patient is immunocompromised, a specific diagnosis should be sought by Gram stain and routine anaerobic and viral culture of specimens from the lesions and penile discharge, if present.

TREATMENT

A constricting foreign body such as a hair or thread, if present, should be removed. Good penile hygiene with warm, soapy water, sitz baths, and gentle retraction of the foreskin usually alleviates balanitis. If local care is not effective and if a specific etiologic organism is identified, then treatment directed against that organism is indicated. If the condition is severe or recurrent, or if phimosis is present, urologic consultation should be considered because circumcision may be indicated.

Balanitis due to *C. albicans* usually resolves with topical administration of nystatin or oral fluconazole. Immunocompromised persons with *Candida,* herpes simplex virus, or anaerobic infections require infectious diseases and urologic consultation. A temporizing dorsal slit of the foreskin may be necessary for anaerobic gangrenous balanoposthitis to release pressure and expose the anaerobic organisms to air. Later, circumcision is usually performed.

REVIEWS

Dominique GJ Sr, Hellstrom WJ: Prostatitis. *Clin Microbiol Rev* 1998; 11:604–13.

Edelsberg JS, Surh YS: The acute scrotum. *Emerg Med Clin North Am* 1988;6:521–46.

Edwards S: Balanitis and balanoposthitis: A review. *Genitourin Med* 1996; 72:155–9.

Likitunukul S, McCracken GH Jr, Nelson JD, et al: Epididymitis in children and adolescents. A 20-year retrospective study. *Am J Dis Child* 1987; 141:41–4.

Meares EM Jr: Prostatitis syndromes: New perspectives about old woes. *J Urol* 1980;123:141–7.

Rushton HG, Greenfield SP: Pediatric urology. *Pediatr Clin North Am* 1997;44:1065–348.

KEY ARTICLES

Gorse GJ, Belshe RB: Male genital tuberculosis: A review of the literature with instructive case reports. *Rev Infect Dis* 1985;7:511–24.

Greenberg RN, Rein MF, Sanders CV, et al: Urethral syndrome in women. *JAMA* 1981;245:923.

Harrison SC, Whitaker RH: Idiopathic urethritis in male children. *Br J Urol* 1987;59:258–60.

Hermansen MC, Chusid MJ, Sty JR: Bacterial epididymo-orchitis in children and adolescents. *Clin Pediatr* 1980;19:812–5.

Horstman WG, Middleton WD, Melson GL: Scrotal inflammatory disease: Color Doppler US findings. *Radiology* 1991;179:55–9.

Kadish HA, Bolte RG: A retrospective review of pediatric patients with epididymitis, testicular torsion, and torsion of testicular appendages. *Pediatrics* 1998;102:73–6.

McAlister WH, Sisler CL: Scrotal sonography in infants and children. *Curr Probl Diagn Radiol* 1990;19:201–42.

Melekos MD, Asbach HW, Markou SA: Etiology of acute scrotum in 100 boys with regard to age distribution. *J Urol* 1988;139:1023–5.

Orland SM, Hanno PM, Wein AJ: Prostatitis, prostatosis, prostatodynia. *Urology* 1985;25:439–59.

Schwartz RH, Rushton HG: Acute balanoposthitis in young boys. *Pediatr Infect Dis J* 1996;15:176–7.

Siegel A, Snyder H, Duckett JW: Epididymitis in infants and boys: Underlying urogenital anomalies and efficacy of imaging modalities. *J Urol* 1987;138:1100–3.

Stamm WE, Wagner KF, Amsel R, et al: Causes of the acute urethral syndrome in women. *N Engl J Med* 1980;303:409–15.

CHAPTER 84

Vulvovaginitis

Sarah A. Rawstron

Vulvovaginitis is the most common gynecologic problem in children, with vaginal discharge the most common symptom. **Vulvovaginitis** includes inflammation of the vulva or the vagina or sometimes both. There are a multitude of causes of vulvovaginitis in addition to sexually transmitted diseases such as infections with *Neisseria gonorrhoeae* and *Trichomonas* (Chapter 85), which are actually uncommon causes. Vulvovaginitis in young girls usually occurs in the absence of sexual intercourse and includes many infectious and noninfectious causes.

ETIOLOGY

Etiologic studies of vulvovaginitis have led to some changes in terminology. What was once called nonspecific vaginitis is now, through a greater understanding of this infection, renamed **bacterial vaginosis.** The entity was first described by Gardner and Dukes (1955), who associated the presence of *Gardnerella vaginalis* with vaginitis. However, McCormack et al (1981) found no association between *G. vaginalis* and an abnormal discharge and concluded that isolation of *G. vaginalis* in an individual person was of no clinical significance. Subsequent studies have shown that bacterial vaginosis is a polymicrobial infection in which bacterial anaerobes interact synergistically with *G. vaginalis* (formerly named *Haemophilus vaginalis*), resulting in changes in the vaginal flora.

In contrast, what is now called **nonspecific vaginitis** is so called because the vaginal flora is essentially the same as in healthy girls and includes lactobacilli, diphtheroids, coagulase-negative staphylococci, and α-hemolytic streptococci. Sometimes there is a preponderance of gram-negative organisms such as *Escherichia coli,* which also can be considered to be part of the normal flora. Nonspecific vaginitis is associated with poor hygiene and is the most common cause of vulvovaginitis in most studies.

In addition to *G. vaginalis,* which is associated with bacterial vaginosis, other common specific causes of vulvovaginitis include *Candida* and pinworms (*Enterobius vermicularis*), especially in prepubertal girls. Less common causes include many bacteria that can be roughly divided into respiratory pathogens and enteric pathogens. The respiratory pathogens most commonly responsible for causing vulvovaginitis are group A *Streptococcus, Haemophilus influenzae* (typeable and nontypeable), and *Neisseria meningitidis* (meningococcus). The mode of spread of bacterial respiratory pathogens (group A *Streptococcus, H. influenzae,* and *N. meningitidis*) is believed to be from the nose and throat by the fingers to the perineal area. In addition, in some cases of streptococcal infection, skin lesions of impetigo are the primary source of transmission, with spread to the vulval area by the fingers. The enteric pathogens causing vulvovaginitis are *Shigella* and *Yersinia enterocolitica,* which are probably spread by contaminated fecal material onto the vagina, with subsequent vaginal infection.

Vulvovaginitis can occur as part of HSV infection or genital herpes (Chapter 85). There have been few well-documented cases of vulvovaginitis associated with viruses other than HSV. A study (Heller et al, 1969) described two young children with vulvovaginitis, one with adenovirus type 12 on vaginal and rectal cultures and one with echovirus on vaginal and rectal cultures. For another five girls with vulvovaginitis, cultures grew echovirus and group B coxsackieviruses from rectal but not vaginal specimens. None of the control group had any cultures positive for virus. Many studies of girls with vulvovaginitis have not included viral cultures. Vulvovaginitis has been described as part of the general skin manifestations associated with varicella-zoster virus and measles infections.

Vulvovaginitis in children has also been reported in association with other bacteria, such as *Streptococcus pneumoniae, Staphylococcus aureus,* and *Corynebacterium diphtheriae.* Vulvovaginitis has also been described in association with some respiratory and enteric viruses, such as adenoviruses and echoviruses. Information on vulvovaginitis in association with these organisms is scanty.

Vulvovaginitis has been described in girls in whom *S. aureus* was the only probable pathogen isolated, although *S. aureus* can be part of the normal vaginal flora in some girls. Toxic shock syndrome is a multisystem disease that occurs in menstruating women and is associated with tampon use and toxin-producing *S. aureus* (Chapter 22). However, persons with this syndrome do not usually present with a vaginal discharge or isolated vulvovaginal findings, and fewer than half have any abnormal genital signs on examination.

EPIDEMIOLOGY

Nonspecific Vulvovaginitis. Probably the most common cause of vulvovaginitis in young girls is nonspecific vulvovaginitis (not to be confused with bacterial vaginosis, which formerly was called nonspecific vaginitis). Nonspecific vulvovaginitis is a mixed bacterial infection with overgrowth of normal aerobic vaginal flora. One study (Emans, 1986) found that 20 of 38 cases of vulvovaginitis in prepubertal children were nonspecific vaginitis, with either normal flora, *E. coli,* or other gram-negative organisms found on culture.

Bacterial Vaginosis. Bacterial vaginosis, which previously was called nonspecific vaginitis, now refers to a polymicrobial infection in which vaginal anaerobes act synergistically with *G. vaginalis.* There are few data on the prevalence of bacterial vaginosis in preadolescent children. The isolation of *G. vaginalis* from vaginal specimens does not correlate with the presence of bacterial vaginosis. Unfortunately, most studies in children have simply evaluated the prevalence of *G. vaginalis* in vaginal cultures rather than using accepted diagnostic criteria for bacterial vaginosis. The prevalence of *G. vaginalis* in vaginal cultures of specimens from girls without symptoms in one study (Hammerschlag et al, 1978a) was 13.5%. Another study (Bartley et al, 1987) found the prevalence of *G. vaginalis* to be 14.6% in sexually abused girls and 4.2% in nonabused girls. A third study (Bump et al, 1986) found the prevalence of *G. vaginalis* in sexually active adolescents to be 34%, compared with 17% in girls who were not sexually active. Thus *G. vaginalis* can be seen as part of the normal vaginal flora in preadolescent girls but appears increased in girls who have been abused or are sexually active. Isolation of *G. vaginalis* in most of these girls was not associated with a vaginal discharge or any other symptoms. Cultures of *G. vaginalis* should not be performed to diagnose bacterial vaginosis.

Bacterial vaginosis has been described in girls with and without a history of sexual abuse. A study (Samuels et al, 1985) found bacterial vaginosis in 8 (33%) of 25 girls with vaginitis and was the most common identifiable cause of vaginitis. Only two of these eight girls had a history of sexual abuse. That bacterial vaginosis can follow an episode of sexual abuse has been documented. A study (Hammerschlag et al, 1985) found that 4 (13%) of 31 girls had definite bacterial vaginosis more than 7 days after an episode of abuse or rape. The ages of the girls with bacterial vaginosis in these studies ranged from 5 to 12 years.

Candida. *Candida* vulvovaginitis is much less common in preadolescent girls than in adult women, in whom it is frequently seen. *Candida albicans* and other *Candida* species can be cultured as part of the normal flora in young girls. The most common species isolated are *C. albicans* and *Candida tropicalis,* but other *Candida* species are occasionally isolated. A study (Hammerschlag et al, 1978a) of healthy children found that 28% had yeast isolated from vaginal cultures, with colonization being more prevalent among infants and teenagers. Colonization by yeasts appeared to be related to a higher prevalence of abnormal discharge in the colonized children, 30% of those colonized having had abnormal discharges. In another study (Emans and Goldstein, 1980) of girls with vulvovaginitis, 3 of 38 episodes were due to *Candida.*

Pinworms. Pinworm (*E. vermicularis*) infestations occur worldwide and are seen among adults and children of all socioeconomic classes. Pinworms are a fairly common cause of vulvovaginitis in prepubertal children, with reported prevalences of 2% (Heller et al, 1969), 6% (Paradise et al, 1982), and 23% (Pierce and Hart, 1992) in girls with vulvovaginitis.

Other Specific Infectious Agents. Group A *Streptococcus* is responsible for approximately 14% of vulvovaginitis in prepubertal girls, but the incidence varies from 0 to 20%, probably because of seasonal variation. Most cases occur in the fall and winter months, from November to April. The mean age of persons with group A *Streptococcus* vulvovaginitis is 5 years, with a range of 2–12 years. This infection is seen in all racial and socioeconomic groups.

The clinical significance of culturing *H. influenzae* from the vagina of a young girl is not clear. *H. influenzae,* both typeable and nontypeable, is a normal commensal in the vagina and can be cultured from the vagina of 5–12% of healthy girls, but it is also capable of causing disease. A study (Macfarlane and Sharma, 1987) found the average age of girls with *H. influenzae* vulvovaginitis to be 4.7 years, with a range of 2–10 years. Four *H. influenzae* isolates were type b, two were type a, two were type c, and two isolates were nontypeable. The geographic distribution is unknown but is presumed to be worldwide.

Meningococcal vulvovaginitis is rare among prepubertal girls. *Shigella* vulvovaginitis is responsible for 2–4% of cases of vulvovaginitis, with no seasonal pattern in the incidence. Approximately 90% of cases of *Shigella* vulvovaginitis are caused by *Shigella flexneri,* with the remainder being caused by *Shigella sonnei* and rarely *Shigella boydii.* There is only one documented case of vulvovaginitis caused by *Y. enterocolitica.*

PATHOGENESIS

Normal Physiologic Changes from Birth Through Puberty. At birth the vagina physiologically resembles that of an adult because it has been exposed to estrogen in utero. The vaginal mucous membrane is thick, about 40 cells, and there is abundant vaginal glycogen as a result of stimulation from maternal estrogen. The fetal vagina is sterile until delivery, when it is seeded with microorganisms from the maternal birth canal. Within a few days of birth there is *Lactobacillus* colonization and the pH drops to 4.0–5.0.

After birth the lack of maternal estrogen causes the vaginal mucosa to become thin, red, atrophic, and dry in a few weeks. The lactobacilli largely disappear because of the lack of glycogen, and the pH rises to 6.5–7.5. This physiologic condition remains fairly constant until puberty, when again under the influence of estrogen the vagina develops a thick mucosal epithelium, cellular glycogen increases, pH decreases, and lactobacilli again predominate in the vaginal flora.

Physiologic Vaginal Discharge. Twice in a girl's development she may have a physiologically normal vaginal discharge. First, soon after birth there may be a physiologic vaginal discharge lasting for about 1 week and consisting of desquamated vaginal cells and endocervical mucus. It is a white, mucoid discharge with few pus cells and may become blood tinged, although rarely is there gross blood. The discharge is a result of uterine withdrawal bleeding caused by maternal estrogen stimulation in utero.

Second, a physiologic discharge may occur about 6 months to 1 year before the first menstrual period. It consists of desquamated vaginal cells, vaginal transudate, and endocervical mucus and may contain a few white blood cells but no pathogens (Fig. 84–1). The discharge is gray-white, has no odor, and is nonirritating. No therapy is necessary except reassurance and local cleansing.

Normal Vaginal Flora. The vaginal flora changes from birth through puberty, reflecting the physiologic changes. At delivery, neonates become colonized with maternal vaginal flora, and as soon as 12 hours after delivery, bacteria may be visible on a vaginal smear. Cultures of specimens taken within 24 hours of birth are no longer sterile in most infants. Soon after delivery there is a preponderance of lactobacilli in vaginal cultures because the vagina is estrogenized at this time. However, once the effect of maternal estrogen diminishes, the vaginal flora changes and lactobacilli no longer predominate. A study (Hammerschlag et al, 1978b) of the vaginal flora of healthy girls 2 months to 14 years of age found a

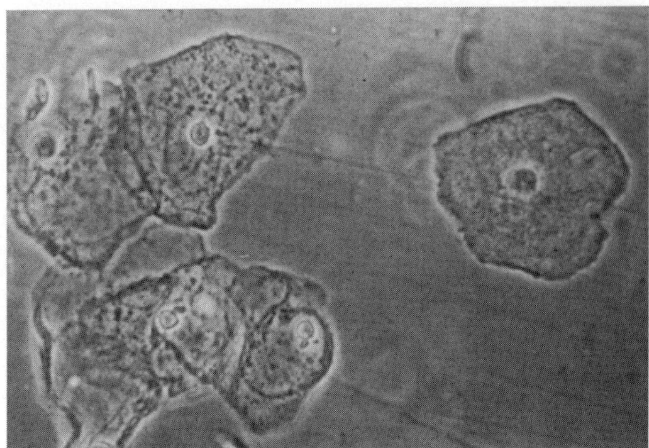

FIGURE 84–1. Photomicrograph of a wet mount demonstrating normal desquamated vaginal epithelial cells. (Courtesy of Michael Rein.)

great variety of organisms (Table 84–1). There was a mean of 8.7 species per specimen, with a mean of 3.7 aerobic and facultatively anaerobic specimens per specimen and a mean of 5.3 obligate anaerobic species per specimen.

Few studies of the vaginal flora of postpubertal girls have been performed. Approximately three fourths of postpubertal girls harbor lactobacilli, and *G. vaginalis* is present in 34–60% of those who are sexually active and in 17–33% of those who are not. The vaginal flora begins to resemble that of adults as the physiologic changes of puberty change the vaginal environment. Sexual activity may also influence the vaginal flora. A study (Shafer et al, 1985) found a mean of 6.1 isolates among sexually active adolescents, compared with 3.1 in those not sexually active.

After menarche the flora of the vagina is dominated by lactobacilli, which constitutes 95% of the total microbial burden, but it also contains diphtheroids, *G. vaginalis,* coagulase-negative staphylococci, and α-hemolytic and nonhemolytic streptococci. Gram-negative organisms are less common after menarche. Anaerobic organisms also constitute the usual vaginal flora after menarche.

It is believed that the normal predominance of *Lactobacillus* in the vaginal flora of women acts as a primary defense against infection by genital pathogens. Lactobacilli produce **hydrogen peroxide,** which appears to decrease the likelihood that adult women will acquire bacterial vaginosis and *Trichomonas vaginalis* and may also decrease the likelihood of acquisition of gonorrheal and chlamydial infections. No studies have evaluated the role of hydrogen peroxide–producing lactobacilli in the vagina of children.

TABLE 84–1. Vaginal Flora of Girls

Organism	Patients (%)
Aerobic and Facultatively Anaerobic Bacteria	
Diphtheroids	78
Coagulase-negative staphylococci	73
α-Hemolytic streptococci	39
Lactobacillus	39
Nonhemolytic streptococci	34
Escherichia coli	34
Klebsiella	15
Gardnerella vaginalis	13.5
Group B *Streptococcus*	11
Group D *Streptococcus*	8.5
Staphylococcus aureus	7
Haemophilus influenzae (typeable and nontypeable)	5
Pseudomonas aeruginosa	5
Proteus	5
Acinetobacter	3
Genital Mycoplasmas	
Ureaplasma urealyticum	27
Mycoplasma hominis	6
Yeast	
Candida	28
Anaerobic Bacteria	
Peptococcus	76
Peptostreptococcus	56
Eubacterium	32
Clostridium	48
Bacteroides fragilis	24
Prevotella melaninogenica	56

Data from Hammerschlag MR, Alpert S, Rosner I, et al: Microbiology of the vagina in children: Normal and potentially pathogenic organisms. *Pediatrics* 1978;62:57–62; Hammerschlag MR, Alpert S, Onderdonk AB, et al: Anaerobic microflora of the vagina in children. *Am J Obstet Gynecol* 1978;131:853–6; and Hammerschlag MR, Baker CJ, Alpert S, et al: Colonization with group B streptococci in girls under 16 years of age. *Pediatrics* 1977;60:473–6.

Nonspecific Vulvovaginitis. Young girls are susceptible to vulvovaginitis for several reasons. Children tend to have poor personal hygiene, and after urinating or defecating often wipe the perineum from back to front, spreading fecal flora onto the vulva and vagina. In young girls the vulva is unprotected because it lacks the labial fat pads and pubic hair of adults. The vulva in young girls has only small labia minora, which tend to open as the child squats. The vulvar skin is also thin and delicate and easily traumatized and inflamed. The vagina in young girls is an excellent culture medium for bacteria because it is warm, moist, and has a neutral pH, unlike the adult vagina, which is acidic. Vaginal cultures of specimens from patients with nonspecific vulvovaginitis usually grow mixed normal flora, sometimes with a predominance of enteric organisms such as *E. coli.*

Bacterial Vaginosis. Bacterial vaginosis is associated with a change in the vaginal flora in adults. In adults with bacterial vaginosis, *G. vaginalis* and a mixed, predominantly anaerobic flora replace lactobacilli, which normally predominate in the vaginal flora. The anaerobic bacteria associated with bacterial vaginosis include *Bacteroides, Eubacterium, Fusobacterium, Mobiluncus, Peptostreptococcus,* and *Veillonella parvula.* The predominant anaerobic gram-negative rods are *Prevotella bivia, Prevotella disiens,* and *Porphyromonas. Mycoplasma hominis* and *Ureaplasma urealyticum* have also been associated with bacterial vaginosis.

Candida. Because *Candida* can be part of the normal flora in the absence of symptoms, it is probable that a change in host resistance or altered bacterial flora plays a part in the development of *Candida* vulvovaginitis. *Candida* grows well in an estrogenized environment, with the associated increase in glycogen, and therefore *Candida* vulvovaginitis is more commonly seen in neonates and adolescents. Factors that create a predisposition to *Candida* vulvovaginitis are those that increase vaginal glycogen, such as diabetes mellitus, pregnancy, use of oral contraceptives, and estrogen therapy. Use of antibiotics and immunodeficiency may result in a predisposition to *Candida* vulvovaginitis by altering the bacterial vaginal flora. *Candida* diaper dermatitis is frequently seen among children, but usually affects the vulva only. Although *Candida* diaper dermatitis may be seen in healthy children, it can also be seen in association with pre-existing eczema or seborrhea.

Pinworms. The female pinworm migrates from the anus to lay her eggs at night. Fecal bacteria are carried with her onto the perineum. Occasionally the pinworm actually migrates into the vagina, where a foreign body reaction may ensue. The deposited ova cause pruritus of the vulval area, and vulvitis and vulvovaginitis may occur.

SYMPTOMS AND CLINICAL MANIFESTATIONS

The most common presenting complaint with all causes of vulvovaginitis is a vaginal discharge (Table 84–2).

Nonspecific Vulvovaginitis. The symptoms of nonspecific vulvovaginitis are usually a vaginal discharge with or without discomfort. In one case (Touloukian, 1974) a girl had acute salpingitis with gram-negative enteric bacilli in association with severe vulvovaginitis.

Bacterial Vaginosis. In adults, bacterial vaginosis is manifested by a vaginal discharge that is usually thin, gray, and homogeneous.

TABLE 84–2. Symptoms and Signs of Vulvovaginitis

Cause	History	Physical Findings
Nonspecific vaginitis	Vaginal discharge, dysuria, itching	Fecal soiling of underwear; evidence of poor hygiene
Bacterial vaginosis	Often no symptoms; possible thin vaginal discharge with a "fishy" odor	Thin, homogeneous vaginal discharge with "fishy" odor
Candida	Itching, dysuria, vaginal discharge	White "cottage cheese" vaginal discharge; possible white plaques adhering to vaginal walls
Pinworms	Itching, especially at night; parents (rarely) may have seen threadworms	Excoriation from scratching
Group A *Streptococcus*	Vaginal discharge often serosanguineous, sometimes frankly bloody; possible history of sore throat or skin rash	Vaginal discharge, possibly bloody; occasionally with rash of scarlet fever
Haemophilus influenzae	Vaginal discharge; sometimes upper respiratory tract infection, otitis media, conjunctivitis	No distinguishing findings
Neisseria meningitidis	No characteristic history	No distinguishing findings
Shigella	Vaginal discharge bloody in approximately 50% of cases; possible history of diarrhea	Bloody vaginal discharge
Yersinia enterocolitica	Possible history of gastrointestinal complaints	No distinguishing findings
Foreign body	Foul-smelling vaginal discharge	Vaginal discharge with offensive odor; sometimes blood-tinged discharge

An abnormal vaginal odor or vulvar irritation may also be present. However, more than half of women with bacterial vaginosis have no symptoms. There are few data on children, but the presentation appears to be similar. The incubation period is not clearly defined, but girls who acquired bacterial vaginosis from an episode of sexual abuse had the disease 7 or more days after the episode of abuse.

Candida. In young girls and adolescents with *Candida* vulvovaginitis, the vaginal discharge is thick and white, similar in appearance to cottage cheese. This discharge is often associated with pruritus and dysuria because of the vulvar irritation. Sexually active girls may complain of dyspareunia. Young children with diaper dermatitis usually are brought for treatment because the mother notices the obvious visible dermatitis, which is painful and irritating.

Pinworms. Children with pinworms usually present with nocturnal perianal or vulvar itching, which may progress to symptoms of a vaginal discharge. Rarely a child will present with abdominal pain that mimics appendicitis.

Other Specific Infectious Agents. Group A *Streptococcus* may have a slightly uncommon presentation in that the vaginal discharge is usually described as serosanguineous, but it may be blood tinged or frankly bloody. Dysuria is the second most common complaint with group A *Streptococcus* infection. The symptoms are usually abrupt in onset, and the patients usually seek medical care within a week of the onset of illness. Most children have no fever. In one series (Straumanis, 1990) few patients gave a history of preceding respiratory symptoms, although 75% had throat or nasopharyngeal cultures positive for group A *Streptococcus*. Group A *Streptococcus* vulvovaginitis can also be seen in association with scarlet fever; 14% of girls with scarlet fever in one series had concomitant vulvovaginitis. Untreated, the infection can last for several months. Complications of group A *Streptococcus* vulvovaginitis are rare but include proctitis, peritonitis, and pelvic abscess.

Girls with *H. influenzae* vulvovaginitis present with a vaginal discharge that is mucoid or mucopurulent and odorless. Some have concomitant otitis media or conjunctivitis. Meningococcal vulvovaginitis has presented as a vaginal discharge associated with itching and excoriation.

Shigella vulvovaginitis usually presents as a vaginal discharge that generally is not accompanied by pain, pruritus, or dysuria. The vaginal discharge is bloody in approximately 50% of girls with *Shigella* vulvovaginitis and can persist for 1 week to several months. In one series (Murphy, 1979) diarrhea was present in approximately only one fourth of persons with *Shigella* vulvovaginitis. The diarrhea usually preceded vulvovaginitis by 6–12 days but in some cases was concurrent with or followed vulvovaginitis.

Physical Examination Findings

Examination of the external genitalia should be part of the routine examination of every girl who visits a pediatrician for normal health care. The examination of a girl with vulvovaginitis is no different from the examination of the genitalia of any girl except that it may be necessary to obtain culture specimens from the former.

Examination of the genitalia should be reserved until the other elements of the physical examination have been performed. This approach may be useful in terms of diagnosis because clues to the cause of the vulvovaginitis may be found, but it is also important in placing the child at ease. Three main methods are used to examine the genitalia of young prepubertal girls (Fig. 84–2). The classic position for examining the female genitalia is the **frog-leg position.** In this position the child lies on her back on the examining table with her feet together and her knees apart. This is the best position for collecting specimens because the child can observe what the examiner is doing and avoid becoming overly anxious. The second method is the **knee-chest position.** With the child in this position the examiner can usually obtain a good view of the vagina and cervix, in many cases without the need for instrumentation. The girl is asked to lie on her abdomen on the examining table with her knees on the table and her bottom in the air. After the child takes a few deep breaths, the vaginal orifice falls open and the vagina and cervix are easily seen. This is not a good position for obtaining specimens, however, because the child cannot see what is happening and may become frightened. A third method is to place the child on her mother's lap. After a general physical examination, the child is placed in a semirecumbent position on the mother's lap, facing the examiner, with the examiner supporting the feet, which should be placed with the soles together, in a variation on the frog-leg position. The labia majora are then drawn outward to expose the vaginal introitus.

In many cases adequate visualization of the vagina and cervix can be achieved without the use of a speculum. However, one sometimes needs to visualize the entire vagina and cervix, particu-

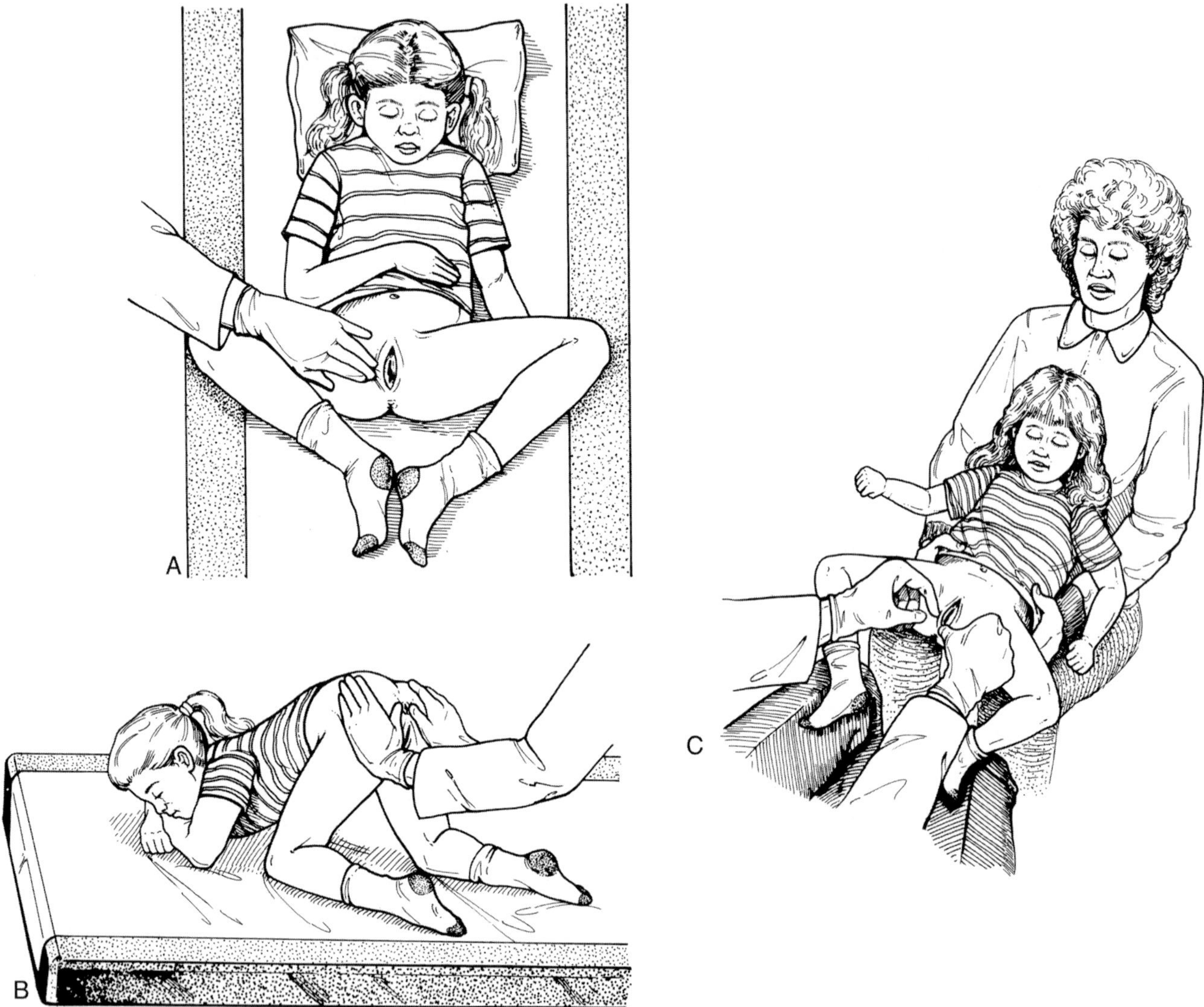

FIGURE 84–2. The three principal methods of examining the genitalia of young prepubertal girls. **A,** Frog-leg position. **B,** Knee-chest position. **C,** On the mother's lap.

larly with a possible foreign body or tumor. In many cases an ordinary otoscope (without a speculum) may be adequate to provide light and magnification. A pediatric otoscope with the addition of a veterinary otoscopic speculum to improve visualization may also be used. Physicians who frequently see girls with genital complaints often use a special pediatric vaginoscope or a special vaginal speculum for instrumentation, but this is not necessary in a typical pediatric practice. A **bimanual rectal examination** may be performed on prepubertal girls, particularly if there is suspicion of a foreign body. A **bimanual vaginal examination** can be done only on older girls who are already menstruating.

Nonspecific Vaginitis. A physical examination does not usually reveal clinically significant erythema of the vulva or vagina. The only abnormal finding is the vaginal discharge. On examination there may be fecal material on the underpants, on the perineum, or in the vagina.

Bacterial Vaginosis. A physical examination does not usually reveal clinically significant erythema of the vulva or vagina. The only abnormal finding is the vaginal discharge and concomitant odor, which is often described as **fishy.**

Candida. The physical examination of an older child with *Candida* infection may show a diffusely red and swollen vulva. The vagina is also erythematous and often has visible white patches on the vaginal wall. Young children with diaper dermatitis present with red, macerated lesions on the vulva that are often weeping; satellite lesions are also frequently present. *Candida* infection in young children is usually confined to the perineum.

Pinworms. A physical examination for pinworms during the day usually reveals only signs of vulvitis with erythema and excoriations from the scratching.

Other Specific Infectious Agents. The physical findings of group A *Streptococcus* infections are usually limited to the vaginal area, unless the vulvovaginitis is associated with scarlet fever, in which case the systemic cutaneous signs of scarlet fever are present (Chapter 58). Most girls with vulvovaginitis have an obvious vaginal discharge and vulval erythema. Sometimes local excoriation is present. The physical findings of vulvovaginitis caused by pinworms, *H. influenzae,* meningococcus, and *Shigella* are usually confined to vulval erythema and inflammation.

DIAGNOSIS

No clinical features of any of the causes of vulvovaginitis can accurately distinguish one cause from another. Wet mount microscopic examination, made by mixing vaginal secretions with normal saline solution, and culture are the only means to confirm the definitive diagnosis.

The history is usually obtained from the child if she is old enough. If she is not, the parents provide the history. Often there is a history of a vaginal discharge, with or without odor, that stains the underwear. Sometimes this discharge is bloody. The child may complain of itching or simply pain or burning in the genital area. She may also complain of dysuria without any urinary frequency. Children who are too young to describe complaints may present with irritability, a new onset of walking awkwardly, or a history of rubbing or scratching the vulva. The history should include recent respiratory, ear, or skin infections; diarrhea; trauma; bathing with bubble bath; or playing in sandboxes.

Nonspecific Vulvovaginitis. The diagnosis of nonspecific vulvovaginitis is usually established on the basis of history, physical examination, and culture results. There is usually a history consistent with poor perineal hygiene, and on examination there may be fecal material on the underpants, on the perineum, or in the vagina. Cultures do not reveal any pathogenic organisms but merely reveal mixed vaginal flora consisting mostly of enteric gram-negative bacteria.

Bacterial Vaginosis. In adults the diagnosis of bacterial vaginosis is established by the presence of at least three of the following four criteria: (1) thin, homogeneous vaginal discharge; (2) vaginal pH ≥4.5; (3) the release of a **fishy odor** of volatile amines on the addition of a drop of 10% potassium hydroxide to a drop of vaginal discharge (the **whiff test**); and (4) the presence of clue cells on a **saline wet mount** of vaginal discharge. **Clue cells** are vaginal epithelial cells that are covered with bacteria and have a granular appearance (see Fig. 84–4). For children, because of a lack of information on normal ranges of pH, the diagnosis of bacterial vaginosis is usually established by a positive whiff test result and the presence of clue cells. For adults, diagnosis also can be established from a Gram stain of the vaginal discharge, although there are no data on the efficacy of this procedure for children. The Gram stain for adults with bacterial vaginosis reveals a mixed flora of *Gardnerella* morphotype (small, gram-variable bacilli), other gram-negative and gram-positive bacteria, and few *Lactobacillus* morphotype organisms (large, gram-positive bacilli).

Candida. The diagnosis of *Candida* vulvovaginitis is based on the typical history and physical findings and the demonstration of *Candida* on a **saline wet mount** (Fig. 84–3) or by culture.

Pinworms. Occasionally the diagnosis of pinworms can be made in a child when the parents report finding the white, pin-sized worms on the perianal area at night. Rarely a worm may be discovered on examination of the vagina. The diagnosis should be confirmed with an early-morning cellophane tape test performed at home by a parent (see Fig. 8–1).

Other Specific Infectious Agents. Other specific agents of vulvovaginitis may be considered on the basis of systemic, respiratory, or gastrointestinal symptoms and confirmed by culture of the vaginal discharge.

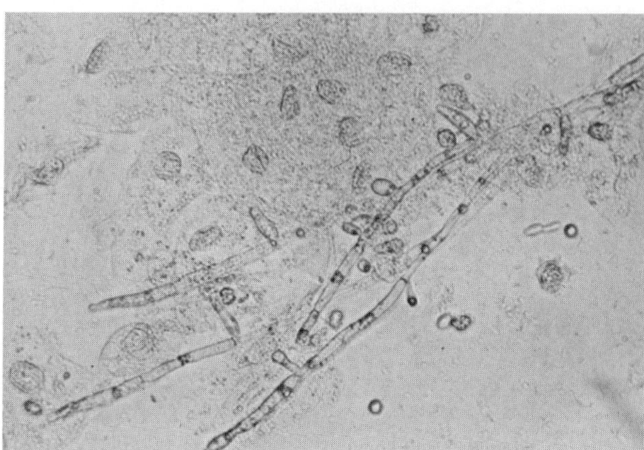

FIGURE 84–3. Photomicrograph of a wet mount preparation demonstrating vulvovaginal candidiasis. (Courtesy of William McCormack.)

Differential Diagnosis

The differential diagnosis of vulvovaginitis includes many infectious as well as noninfectious causes (Table 84–3).

Foreign Bodies. Foreign bodies in the vagina are a well-recognized cause of vaginal discharge in girls. Emans (1986) found that 5 of 38 episodes of vulvovaginitis were caused by foreign bodies. Foreign bodies can be found in girls of any age, including adolescents. Many objects have been found, the most common being pieces of toilet paper or cloth. However, coins, pencils, safety pins, beads, stones, and many other objects have been found. In postmenarchal girls a forgotten tampon is probably the most common foreign body.

Physical examination usually reveals a **foul-smelling vaginal discharge,** which is highly suggestive of the presence of a foreign

TABLE 84–3. Causes of Vulvovaginitis

Infectious Causes	Noninfectious Causes
Respiratory and Skin Pathogens	**Physical Agents**
Group A *Streptococcus*	Sand
Streptococcus pneumoniae	**Chemical Agents**
Neisseria meningitidis	Bubble bath
Staphylococcus aureus	Medications
Haemophilus influenzae (typeable and nontypeable)	Antiperspirants
Respiratory viruses	**Allergenic Agents**
Enteric Pathogens	Soaps, laundry detergents
Shigella	Medications
Yersinia enterocolitica	Synthetic fabrics
Sexually Transmitted Pathogens	**Gynecologic Conditions**
Neisseria gonorrhoeae	Rhabdomyosarcoma
Trichomonas vaginalis	**Urologic Conditions**
Herpes simplex virus	Urethral prolapse
Alterations in Vaginal Flora	Ectopic ureter
Nonspecific vaginitis	**Vulvar Skin Disease**
Bacterial vaginosis	Seborrhea
Candida	Atopic dermatitis
Pinworms	Psoriasis
Foreign bodies	

body. When the diagnosis of foreign body is being considered, it is imperative to obtain adequate visualization of all of the vagina and cervix. The foreign body can then be removed with forceps or sometimes by irrigation. Culture of vaginal discharge or the foreign body usually reveals only vaginal flora with a predominance of enteric organisms, as is typical of nonspecific vulvovaginitis.

Chemical, Physical, and Allergenic Irritants. Many of the common causes of vulvovaginitis in girls can be discovered by obtaining an adequate history. Noninfectious causes to be considered include chemical or contact irritants such as bubble bath, perfume, antiperspirants, deodorants, synthetic or dyed fabrics, residual laundry detergent in clothing, and medications. Vulvovaginitis associated with these causes abates when the offending irritant is removed. Physical agents, particularly sand, also can be responsible for vulvovaginitis. Girls who play in sandboxes may have sand introduced into the vagina, resulting in physical irritation. Children should wear tight-fitting underwear or a bathing suit when playing in sand to minimize this cause of vulvovaginitis.

Sexually Transmitted Infections. Sexually transmitted pathogens cause few cases of vulvovaginitis among prepubertal girls, although this diagnosis is often entertained. The sexually transmitted organisms that can cause vulvovaginitis are *N. gonorrhoeae, T. vaginalis,* and HSV (Chapter 85), which cause vulvovaginitis in both prepubertal and postpubertal girls. Once the diagnosis of a sexually transmitted infection is established, a thorough investigation should be undertaken regarding sexual abuse; such an investigation is not necessary for the older adolescent or adult who is sexually active.

The prevalence of gonococcal vulvovaginitis is low, ranging from 0 to 8%. *T. vaginalis* is an infrequent cause of vulvovaginitis among prepubertal children, in part because nonestrogenized epithelium is much less favorable for the growth of *T. vaginalis* than is estrogenized vaginal epithelium. *T. vaginalis* is therefore more commonly seen in neonates and infants, who have estrogenized mucosa as a result of maternal estrogen stimulation, and in postmenarchal girls, in whom an estrogenized mucosa has developed. Neonates can become colonized by maternal trichomonads during delivery. Symptoms do not always develop, although the infant may present with a vaginal discharge. A wet mount of the vaginal discharge may demonstrate the organism. Genital HSV infection usually presents with vulval pain, dysuria, and obvious vesicles on examination of the vulva. Although genital HSV can be transmitted sexually, it can also be transmitted nonsexually. The usual scenario for nonsexual transmission is that a child with herpes gingivostomatitis or a herpetic cold sore transmits the virus to the genitalia on her hands. Toddlers are more likely than older children to transmit HSV nonsexually; however, toddlers can also have genital HSV infections as a result of sexual abuse.

Although girls with condylomata acuminata (venereal warts) do not usually have a vaginal discharge at presentation, they do present with complaints referable to the vulvovaginal area. Occasionally they may present with a discharge if the warts become secondarily infected. *Chlamydia trachomatis* does not cause symptoms of vulvovaginitis. A child with vulvovaginitis should be evaluated for *Chlamydia* only if sexual abuse is also suspected.

Gynecologic Conditions. Rhabdomyosarcoma of the vagina is rare, but a child may present because of a polypoid mass protruding through the vagina, sometimes accompanied by a bloody vaginal discharge.

Urologic Conditions. Urethral prolapse presents as a tender, friable, and often bleeding vulvar mass. The diagnosis can usually be established by physical examination. Ectopic ureter can present as a persistent, watery vaginal discharge. The diagnosis is established by intravenous pyelography.

Vulvar Skin Disease. Some skin diseases may be manifested primarily in the vulvar area, although similar lesions are present elsewhere. Vulvar skin disease tends to affect the outer labia minora, the labia majora, and the genitocrural folds. Seborrheic vulvitis is common, and the vulva may become secondarily infected with *Candida.* Psoriasis and atopic dermatitis (eczema) also can be seen in the vulvar area. Labial adhesions may present as vulvovaginitis, predominantly with symptoms of soreness and dysuria. Lichen sclerosus is a rare condition in children. It presents with atrophy and fissuring; girls with this condition have an increased susceptibility to trauma.

Laboratory Evaluation

Routine laboratory tests such as a CBC and urinalysis are not useful in the evaluation of vulvovaginitis. A urine dipstick test should be performed on any girl with *Candida* vulvovaginitis to screen for the possibility of diabetes mellitus.

Microbiologic Evaluation

Specimens for microscopic examination and culture (Table 84–4) are best taken with the patient in the supine frog-leg position (see Fig. 84–2*A*). The most common method is to obtain cultures by using cotton-tipped or calcium-alginate swabs. Simply inserting the dry cotton-tipped swab into the vagina can be very uncomfortable for young girls with a dry and atrophic vagina. It is preferable to moisten the swab with sterile nonbacteriostatic saline solution before inserting it into the vagina. Calcium-alginate swabs are smaller than cotton-tipped swabs and thus are less traumatic.

A second method is to obtain cultures with a sterile plastic or glass dropper, which can be used to aspirate vaginal secretions. If there is scanty discharge, sterile nonbacteriostatic saline solution may be instilled into the vagina with the dropper and then aspirated and sent for culture.

Nonspecific Vulvovaginitis. Cultures of the vaginal discharge do not reveal any pathogenic organisms but merely show mixed vaginal flora consisting mostly of enteric gram-negative bacteria.

Bacterial Vaginosis. The presence of clue cells on a saline wet mount, made by mixing vaginal secretions with normal saline

TABLE 84–4. Suggested Tests for Evaluating Vaginal Discharges

Wet Mount Preparations
Saline solution for *Trichomonas, Candida,* clue cells
10% KOH (whiff test) for bacterial vaginosis, *Candida*

Gram Stain
Neisseria gonorrhoeae, bacterial vaginosis

Cultures
Sheep blood agar for most organisms, especially group A *Streptococcus, Shigella*
Chocolate agar for *Haemophilus influenzae*
Thayer-Martin or other selective media for *N. gonorrhoeae*
MacConkey agar or other selective media for gram-negative enteric organisms

Cellophane Tape Test
Pinworms

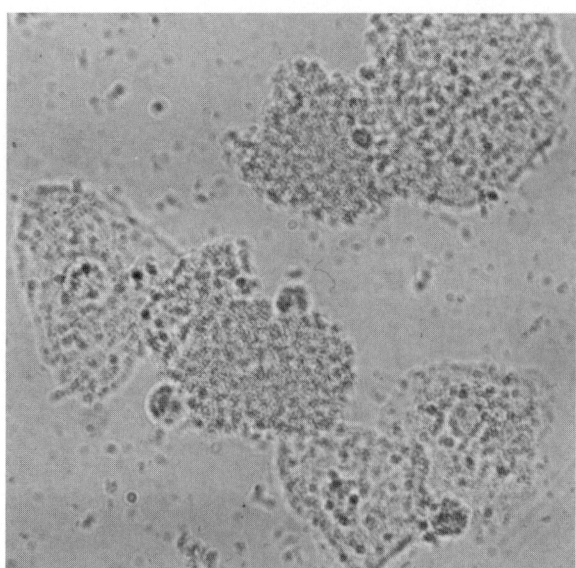

FIGURE 84–4. Photomicrograph of a wet mount demonstrating clue cells, which are epithelial cells covered with bacteria. Clue cells are diagnostic of bacterial vaginosis. (Courtesy of William McCormack.)

solution, of the vaginal discharge is diagnostic of bacterial vaginosis (Fig. 84–4). Vaginal cultures for *G. vaginalis* are not useful for establishing or confirming the diagnosis.

Candida. The diagnosis of *Candida* vulvovaginitis is based on the history and physical examination and confirmed by the demonstration of *Candida* either microscopically or by culture. A wet mount usually demonstrates mycelia (see Fig. 84–3). Alternatively, mixing the vaginal secretions with 10% potassium hydroxide may be useful for dissolving extraneous cellular material and may reveal the fungi more easily. Gram stains also show the organism, which is gram-positive. Cultures are usually grown on Sabouraud dextrose agar.

Pinworms. A cellophane tape test performed in the early morning by a parent can confirm the diagnosis (see Fig. 8–1). This test is accomplished by attaching sticky cellophane tape to a tongue depressor, sticky side out, and swabbing the perianal area first thing in the morning, before the child gets out of bed. The tape and tongue depressor are then pressed to a glass slide, and together they are sent to the laboratory to determine whether pinworm ova are present.

Other Specific Infectious Agents. Specialized growth media may be necessary for culturing suspected group A *Streptococcus* (5% sheep blood agar), *H. influenzae* (chocolate agar supplemented with bacitracin), meningococcus (modified Thayer-Martin medium incubated in a humid environment of 3–10% carbon dioxide), and *Shigella* (blood agar or MacConkey agar). The yield improves if the medium is inoculated and streaked immediately after the sample is taken, although placing the swab in transport medium is acceptable.

Diagnostic Imaging

Radiographs have been used historically to identify vaginal foreign bodies, but they are not recommended because most foreign bodies are not visualized as radiopaque.

TREATMENT

The treatment of vulvovaginitis depends greatly on the presumed or documented microbiologic cause (Table 84–5). The use of douches or vaginal irrigation is not recommended as therapy for any form of vulvovaginitis. Normal vaginal flora, which play a large part in protection against pathogenic organisms, are removed by douching, and the protective function is thus decreased. In addition, douching may be traumatic for small children.

Nonspecific Vulvovaginitis. Treatment should consist of general advice about routine perineal hygiene. Parent and child should be instructed that after defecation the perineum should always be wiped from front to back. In addition, while the child has the acute symptoms of vulvovaginitis, daily warm **sitz baths** relieve the symptoms. The sitz baths can be with plain water or with water and cornstarch, colloidal oatmeal, or baking soda. The perineum should be patted dry after the bath. The sitz baths can be given two or three times a day or as frequently as every 4 hours for severe symptoms. Gentle washing of the perineum after defecation with soap and water also hastens recovery. After the acute symptoms have subsided, the child and parent should be instructed on preventive measures that can be taken to prevent recurrences, such as regular bathing with supervision. The vulva should be washed at least once or twice a day with bland, nonperfumed, nonmedicated soap, after which the vulva should be patted dry. Loose-fitting cotton underpants should be worn, and tights, tight jeans, and leotards should be avoided if possible. Many girls show improvement with this conservative regimen, but some girls continue to have symptoms regardless of the improvement in hygiene.

There have been no controlled trials regarding therapy for nonspecific vulvovaginitis, but there is anecdotal experience with other treatments. Altchek (1984) recommends that if a careful investigation shows no abnormal findings and there is persistent or recurrent nonspecific vulvovaginitis, the following treatments be tried. Topical estrogen cream applied sparingly on the introitus at night for 1–3 weeks thickens the vaginal mucosa and possibly cures nonspecific vulvovaginitis. Prolonged use of topical estrogen creams, however, may cause systemic effects, so the duration of therapy should be as short as possible. Another possible treatment is the use of broad-spectrum antibiotics active against *E. coli,* such as amoxicillin or oral cephalosporins. These regimens have not been fully evaluated, however, and are not routinely recommended.

Bacterial Vaginosis. Data on the treatment of bacterial vaginosis in children are limited, and recommendations are based on data from adult women. However, recommended adult therapies in appropriate pediatric doses are reasonable choices. The recommended regimen for the treatment of bacterial vaginosis is oral metronidazole for 7 days (see Table 84–5). Alternative recommended therapies with proven clinical efficacy in adults but limited experience in children include intravaginal clindamycin cream or metronidazole gel. The intravaginal cream is sometimes preferred because of a lack of systemic adverse effects. Other alternative regimens include a single dose of metronidazole or oral clindamycin for 7 days. Pregnant women with bacterial vaginosis are treated with oral medications, but in lower doses, such as metronidazole 250 mg three times a day instead of 500 mg three times a day. Clindamycin vaginal cream is no longer recommended for the treatment of pregnant women with bacterial vaginosis because two randomized trials indicated an increase in preterm deliveries in women treated with this regimen.

Candida. Imidazole creams and vaginal tablets and suppositories are all effective for the treatment of acute vulvovaginal candidiasis

TABLE 84–5. Antibiotic Regimens Recommended for Vulvovaginitis

Cause	Treatment
Nonspecific Vaginitis	Advice about perineal hygiene Warm sitz baths with water, cornstarch, or colloidal oatmeal 2–3 times daily or q4hr for severe symptoms If symptoms do not respond to conservative treatment, treat with amoxicillin orally for 7–10 days If no response to above measures, consider topical low-dose estrogen cream for 1–3 wk
Bacterial Vaginosis	
Adolescents and adults	Metronidazole 500 mg bid PO for 7 days *or* Clindamycin cream 2%, one full applicator (5 g) hs intravaginally for 7 days *or* Metronidazole gel 0.75%, one full applicator (5 g) bid intravaginally for 5 days *or* Metronidazole 2 g in a single dose PO *or* Clindamycin 300 mg bid PO for 7 days
Younger children	Metronidazole 15–20 mg/kg/day divided q8hr PO for 7 days *or* Clindamycin 20–30 mg/kg/day divided q6hr PO
Candida	
Adolescents	Butoconazole 2% cream 5 g intravaginally for 3 days* *or* Clotrimazole 1% cream 5 g intravaginally for 7–14 days* *or* Clotrimazole 100 mg vaginal tablet, 1 tablet for 7 days *or* Clotrimazole 100 mg vaginal tablet, 2 tablets for 3 days *or* Clotrimazole 500 mg vaginal tablet, single application *or* Miconazole 2% cream 5 g intravaginally for 7 days* *or* Miconazole 200 mg vaginal suppository, 1 suppository for 3 days* *or* Miconazole 100 mg vaginal suppository, 1 suppository for 7 days* *or* Nystatin 100,000 U vaginal tablet, 1 tablet for 14 days *or* Tioconazole 6.5% ointment 5 g intravaginally in a single application* *or* Terconazole 0.4% cream 5 g intravaginally for 7 days *or* Terconazole 0.8% cream 5 g intravaginally for 3 days
Candida Adolescents *(Continued)*	*or* Terconazole 80 mg vaginal suppository, 1 suppository for 3 days *or* Fluconazole 150 mg oral tablet, 1 tablet in a single dose
Younger children	Miconazole 2% cream 5 g applied intravaginally for 7 days *or* Any of the above suppositories divided into halves or quarters lengthwise and given according to adolescent dose
***Candida* Diaper Dermatitis**	Topical miconazole 2% cream applied twice a day for 7–14 days *or* Nystatin cream (100,000 U/g) applied bid–qid for 7–14 days
Group A *Streptococcus*	Penicillin V 25–50 mg/kg/day divided q6hr PO *or* Amoxicillin 40 mg/kg/day divided q8hr PO *or* Cefaclor 40 mg/kg/day divided q8hr PO *or* Cephalexin 25–50 mg/kg/day divided q6hr PO *or* Erythromycin 40 mg/kg/day divided q6hr PO
Pinworms *(Enterobius vermicularis)*	See Table 42–15
***Haemophilus influenzae* (Typeable and Nontypeable)**	
Non-β-lactamase producing	Amoxicillin 40 mg/kg/day divided q8hr PO
β-Lactamase producing	Amoxicillin-clavulanate 40 mg/kg/day divided q8hr PO *or* TMP-SMZ: TMP 8–10 mg/kg/day divided q12hr PO *or* Cefaclor 40 mg/kg/day divided q8hr PO
Neisseria meningitidis	Penicillin V 25–50 mg/kg/day divided q6hr PO *or* Amoxicillin 40 mg/kg/day divided q8hr PO
Shigella	TMP-SMZ: TMP 8–10 mg/kg/day divided q12hr PO *or* Ampicillin 50–100 mg/kg/day divided q6hr PO (*not amoxicillin*)
Yersinia enterocolitica	TMP-SMZ: TMP 8–10 mg/kg/day divided q12hr PO
Foreign Body	Remove foreign body with direct visualization, using forceps or with irrigation. If necessary, perform examination with patient under general anesthesia for diagnosis and foreign body removal.

*Over-the-counter medication.

in adolescents and adults (see Table 84–5). No advantage in efficacy has been demonstrated for any particular regimen, and recurrences are frequent after all regimens. There have been no well-conducted clinical trials of the use of these agents in young girls to determine the optimal treatment. Intravaginal instillation of one of the creams recommended for adults, such as miconazole 2% cream, can be applied by the parent at bedtime with a small syringe and attached tubing. Vaginal suppositories may not be practical because of their size, but they could be cut in halves or quarters lengthwise and used as alternative therapy. A single dose of fluconazole orally is often preferred. Adolescents and adults with recurrent vulvovaginal candidiasis who are immunocompromised, such as those with diabetes mellitus, may require longer therapy, for 10–14 days, with either topical or oral azoles. Therapy for *Candida* diaper dermatitis is with a topical agent such as miconazole or clotrimazole (see Table 84–5).

Pinworms. Once the diagnosis of pinworm infestation has been made, it is important to treat not only the patient but also the entire family. Therapy is with albendazole, mebendazole, or pyrantel pamoate, with two doses given 2 weeks apart (see Table 42–15). Children with enterobiasis with vulvovaginitis may benefit from warm sitz baths and washing with soap and water after defecation for a few days to clear the vulvovaginitis.

Other Specific Infectious Agents. Treatment of group A *Streptococcus* vulvovaginitis should be with oral antibiotics for 10 days (see Table 84–5). Penicillin is the preferred choice, but amoxicillin, oral cephalosporins, and erythromycin are all acceptable alternatives. Treatment of *H. influenzae* vulvovaginitis with oral antibiotics is necessary only when the child has symptoms of vulvovaginitis with a culture growing *H. influenzae.* Asymptomatic colonization does not necessarily need to be treated. Amoxicillin for 7–10 days is appropriate for sensitive strains. Alternatives for β-lactamase-producing strains are amoxicillin-clavulanic acid, cefuroxime, or cefpodoxime. At least two girls with meningococcal vulvovaginitis had resolution of their illness, including negative repeat cultures, without any therapy (Fallon, 1974). Nevertheless, treatment of meningococcal vulvovaginitis with either penicillin or amoxicillin for 7–10 days is usually recommended (see Table 84–5).

Treatment of *Shigella* vulvovaginitis is with 5–7 days of oral antibiotics to which the *Shigella* strain is susceptible. Antimicrobial resistance of *Shigella* is an increasing problem, with 60–70% resistance to amoxicillin and 30–40% resistance to TMP-SMZ. For empirical treatment, or for *Shigella* strains resistant to both ampicillin and TMP-SMZ, or for empirical treatment in areas of high levels of resistance to both, a third-generation cephalosporin is recommended. Ciprofloxacin or another quinolone antibiotic may be used for adolescents 18 years of age or older.

COMPLICATIONS

There are few serious complications of vulvovaginitis. Group A *Streptococcus* infections have rarely been complicated by proctitis, peritonitis, and pelvic abscesses. Pyosalpinx has been described in a young girl with *S. pneumoniae* vaginal infection, and acute salpingitis with gram-negative enteric bacilli has been described in a girl with severe nonspecific vulvovaginitis. All these complications are extremely unusual.

PROGNOSIS

The prognosis is excellent for most girls with vulvovaginitis. Many episodes of vulvovaginitis are self-limiting without any specific therapy. The prognosis is better if a specific cause of the vulvovaginitis is found, such as pinworms or group A *Streptococcus.* In these cases, treatment usually results in rapid resolution of symptoms. However, in documented cases of *H. influenzae* vulvovaginitis with positive culture results, therapy with appropriate antibiotics did not result in improvement. The reason may be that *H. influenzae* was not the cause of the symptoms and the vaginal flora was normal.

The prognosis for vulvovaginitis associated with nonspecific vaginitis is variable. Some persons respond well to improving their perineal hygiene, but others continue to have symptoms and require further therapy.

Vulvovaginitis due to *Candida* may become recurrent in adolescents and women, especially in women with specific risk factors (Table 84–6). Oral fluconazole, 150 mg given orally once weekly or once monthly, or ketoconazole, 100 mg given orally once daily, for up to 6 months has been effective in some women with persistent or frequently recurring candidiasis.

TABLE 84–6. Risk Factors for Recurrent Vulvovaginal Candidiasis

Hormonal Factors
Pregnancy
Oral contraceptives
Physical Factors
Tight-fitting clothing
Synthetic clothing
Contact irritation (e.g., douch)
Alteration of Normal Flora
Corticosteroids
Antibiotics
Compromised Immunity
Diabetes mellitus
HIV infection

PREVENTION

There is no means to prevent many of these infections. Increased awareness among girls and their caregivers about the importance of perineal hygiene could prevent some cases of vulvovaginitis. However, it is not conceivable that most cases of vulvovaginitis associated with specific causes can be prevented. Douching is not effective for the prevention of any vaginal infection. It reduces the normal flora, which plays a significant role in protection against pathogenic organisms. Douching may be a risk factor for upper genital tract infection and may be traumatic for small children.

REVIEWS

Altchek A: Pediatric vulvovaginitis. *J Reprod Med* 1984;29:359–75.

Altchek A: Pediatric and adolescent gynecology. *Compr Ther* 1995; 21:235–41.

Emans PF: Vulvovaginitis in the child and adolescent. *Pediatr Rev* 1986; 8:12–9.

Farrington PM: Pediatric vulvo-vaginitis. *Clin Obstet Gynecol* 1997; 40:135–40.

Sobel JD: Vaginitis. *N Engl J Med* 1997;337:1896–903.

Vandeven AM, Emans SJ: Vulvovaginitis in the child and adolescent. *Pediatr Rev* 1993;14:141–7.

Williams TS, Callen JP, Owen LG: Vulvar disorders in the prepubertal female. *Pediatr Ann* 1986;15:588–9.

KEY ARTICLES

Bartley DL, Morgan L, Rimsza ME: *Gardnerella vaginalis* in prepubertal girls. *Am J Dis Child* 1987;141:1014–7.

Bump RC, Sachs LA, Buesching WJ III: Sexually transmissible infectious agents in sexually active and virginal asymptomatic adolescent girls. *Pediatrics* 1986;77:488–94.

Cox RA: *Haemophilus influenzae:* An underrated cause of vulvovaginitis in young girls. *J Clin Pathol* 1997;50:765–8.

Emans SJ, Goldstein DP: The gynecologic examination of the prepubertal child with vulvovaginitis: Use of the knee-chest position. *Pediatrics* 1980;65:758–60.

Fallon RJ, Robinson ET: Meningococcal vulvovaginitis. *Scand J Infect Dis* 1974;6:295–6.

Ferris DG, Litaker MS, Woodward L, et al: Treatment of bacterial vaginosis: A comparison of oral metronidazole, metronidazole vaginal gel, and clindamycin vaginal cream. *J Fam Pract* 1995;41:443–9.

Gardner HL, Dukes CD: *Haemophilus vaginalis* vaginitis: A newly defined specific infection previously classified ''nonspecific'' vaginitis. *Am J Obstet Gynecol* 1955;69:962–76.

Hammerschlag MR, Alpert S, Onderdonk AB, et al: Anaerobic microflora of the vagina in children. *Am J Obstet Gynecol* 1978b;131:853–6.

Hammerschlag MR, Alpert S, Rosner I, et al: Microbiology of the vagina in children: Normal and potentially pathogenic organisms. *Pediatrics* 1978a;62:57–62.

Hammerschlag MR, Cummings M, Doraiswamy B, et al: Nonspecific vaginitis following sexual abuse in children. *Pediatrics* 1985;75: 1028–31.

Hawes SE, Hillier SL, Benedetti J, et al. Hydrogen peroxide–producing lactobacilli and acquisition of vaginal infections. *J Infect Dis* 1996; 174:1058–63.

Heller RH, Joseph JM, Davis HJ: Vulvovaginitis in the premenarcheal child. *J Pediatr* 1969;74:370–7.

Macfarlane DE, Sharma DP: *Haemophilus influenzae* and genital tract infections in children. *Acta Paediatr Scand* 1987;76:363–4.

McCormack WM, Evrard JR, Laughlin CF, et al: Sexually transmitted conditions among women college students. *Am J Obstet Gynecol* 1981;139:130–3.

Meis JF, Festen C, Hoogkamp-Korstanje JA: Pyosalpinx caused by *Streptococcus pneumoniae* in a young girl. *Pediatr Infect Dis J* 1993;12:539–40.

Murphy TV, Nelson JD: *Shigella* vaginitis: Report of 38 patients and review of the literature. *Pediatrics* 1979;63:511–6.

Paradise JE, Campos JM, Friedman HM, et al: Vulvovaginitis in premenarchal girls: Clinical features and diagnostic evaluation. *Pediatrics* 1982; 70:193–8.

Pierce AM, Hart CA: Vulvovaginitis: Causes and management. *Arch Dis Child* 1992;67:509–12.

Redondo-Lopez V, Cook RL, Sobel JD: Emerging role of lactobacilli in the control and maintenance of the vaginal bacterial microflora. *Rev Infect Dis* 1990;12:856–72.

Samuels P, Hammerschlag MR, Cummings M, et al: Nonspecific vaginitis (NSV) is an important cause of vaginitis in children. Interscience Conference on Antimicrobial Agents and Chemotherapy, 1985, Minneapolis, MN.

Shafer MA, Sweet RL, Ohm-Smith MJ, et al: Microbiology of the lower genital tract in postmenarchal adolescent girls: Differences by sexual activity, contraception, and presence of nonspecific vaginitis. *J Pediatr* 1985;107:974–81.

Spiegel CA: Bacterial vaginosis. *Clin Microbiol Rev* 1991;4:485–502.

Straumanis JP, Bocchini JA Jr: Group A beta-hemolytic streptococcal vulvovaginitis in prepubertal girls: A case report and review of the past twenty years. *Pediatr Infect Dis J* 1990;9:845–8.

Touloukian RJ: Acute coliform salpingitis in a premenstrual child with severe vulvovaginitis. *J Pediatr* 1974;85:281.

Watkins S, Quan L: Vulvovaginitis caused by *Yersinia enterocolitica*. *Pediatr Infect Dis* 1984;3:444–5.

CHAPTER 85

Sexually Transmitted Infections

Margaret R. Hammerschlag ▪ Sarah A. Rawstron

Sexually transmitted diseases (STDs) encompass a variety of infections that are transmitted primarily by sexual activity. These infections may be asymptomatic or may present with a spectrum of genital and extragenital manifestations. Several infections not generally traditionally considered STDs can be transmitted through sexual contact. Many of these infections occur simultaneously and may contribute to concurrent transmission, as indicated by the increased rate of transmission of HIV infection among persons with concomitant genital sores or ulcers. The classic STDs, gonorrhea and syphilis, are now being overshadowed by other STDs, which not only are more common but also are more difficult to diagnose and treat. The newer STDs include bacterial vaginosis and infections due to *Chlamydia trachomatis,* human papillomavirus (HPV), and HIV.

In addition to the classic STDs, several agents capable of systemic infection may be transmitted by sexual contact. Hepatitis B virus (HBV) can be sexually transmitted, and infection may occur as a complication of sexual abuse. It has been recommended that male victims of homosexual rape be screened for HBV infection.

INITIAL APPROACH TO SEXUALLY TRANSMITTED DISEASES

COMPARATIVE EPIDEMIOLOGY

STDs include some of the most common of all infections. In 1996, genital *C. trachomatis* infection was the most frequent infectious disease in the United States. Infections with STDs are most prevalent among adolescents and young adults. Three million teenagers, roughly one in eight aged 13–18 years and one in four of those who have had sexual intercourse, acquire an STD each year, accounting for a substantial portion of the 20 million cases of STDs reported annually in the United States. The age group of 15–19 years has the highest rate of STDs, two to three times higher than persons older than 20 years. The STD prevalence rates among sexually active teenagers in the general population are 5–15% for asymptomatic *C. trachomatis* infection among female adolescents and 10% among male adolescents, 1–5% for asymptomatic gonorrhea among female adolescents, 20% for genital herpes, and 15% for HPV infection. More than 4 million cases of *C. trachomatis* infection, approximately 3 million cases of trichomoniasis, 1.1 million cases of gonorrhea, 120,000 cases of syphilis, and 3,500 cases of chancroid are reported annually in the United States. Approximately 500,000–1 million cases of HPV infection, 200,000–500,000 cases of genital herpes, 100,000–200,000 cases of hepatitis B, and 40,000 cases of HIV infection occur annually.

STDs can be transmitted during child sexual abuse and assault, although the exact risks are unknown. Although men who have sex with men are at increased risk of HBV infection, there is also a similar increased risk among heterosexuals with multiple sex partners. Screening for hepatitis B probably should be included in the medical evaluation of child victims of sexual assault.

SUGGESTIVE SYMPTOMS AND SIGNS

The major STDs may be grouped by their primary clinical presentation (Table 85–1). Primary infection with the most common STDs, *C. trachomatis* infection and gonorrhea, presents with **urethritis** and **cervicitis,** or more correctly, **endocervicitis.** However, more than 70% of genital chlamydial infections in women are asymptomatic. **Genital ulcers** are characteristic of chancroid *(Haemophilus ducreyi),* syphilis *(Treponema pallidum),* lymphogranuloma venereum (serotypes L_1, L_2, and L_3 of *C. trachomatis*), and genital herpes simplex virus (HSV) infections. **Vaginal discharge** is a symptom of trichomoniasis (*Trichomonas vaginalis*) and is part of the spectrum of vulvovaginitis (Chapter 84), which is not always associated with sexual intercourse. HPVs cause **condylomata acuminata,** the genital counterparts of the common warts, flat warts, and plantar warts also caused by papillomavirus infection. **Proctitis** is most common in men who have sex with men by receptive anal intercourse, but it also may occur in women and is due to infection with classic STD organisms (e.g., *Neisseria gonorrhoeae, C. trachomatis, T. pallidum,* and HSV) and with enteric organisms (e.g., *Shigella, Campylobacter, Entamoeba histolytica,* and *Giardia lamblia*).

The clinical manifestations of some STDs may not become apparent until acute life-threatening complications or late consequences develop. Most STDs have sequelae. The most serious complications occur in women and include infertility and ectopic pregnancy. Certain STDs during pregnancy may affect the fetus and newborn, causing stillbirth, infant death, growth retardation, or a myriad of other sequelae (Chapters 94 and 95). HPV is a recognized cofactor in the development of cervical cancer (Chapter 4).

DIAGNOSIS

The type of signs and symptoms may suggest the differential diagnosis in many persons. However, there is significant overlap in presentations among the various pathogens responsible, many patients will be infected with more than one organism, and many will also have asymptomatic infection.

INITIAL MANAGEMENT

The suspicion of an STD is frequently based on epidemiologic factors such as young age, new sexual partner, and various high-risk behaviors. It is important to make a specific microbiologic diagnosis. Only the nonviral STDs (e.g., gonorrhea, *C. trachomatis* infection, syphilis, chancroid, and trichomoniasis) are cur-

TABLE 85–1. **Infections that May Be Sexually Transmitted**

Organism	Genital Disease
Genital Manifestations	
Urethritis and cervicitis	
Neisseria gonorrhoeae	Gonorrhea
Chlamydia trachomatis	Nongonococcal urethritis
Genital ulcers	
Treponema pallidum	Syphilis
Herpes simplex virus type 2 (HSV type 1 less often)	Genital herpes
Haemophilus ducreyi	Chancroid
Calymmatobacterium granulomatis	Donovanosis
C. trachomatis serovars L_1, L_2, and L_3	Lymphogranuloma venereum
Vaginal discharge	
Trichomonas vaginalis	Trichomoniasis
Gardnerella vaginalis	Bacterial vaginosis
Candida albicans	Vulvovaginal candidiasis
Genital warts	
Human papillomaviruses	Condylomata acuminata
Ectoparasitic infestation	
Phthirus pubis	Pubic lice
Extragenital Manifestations	
Proctitis and proctocolitis	
N. gonorrhoeae	
C. trachomatis serovars L_1, L_2, and L_3	
T. pallidum	
HSVs	
Enterocolitis	
Giardia lamblia	
Systemic infections	
Human immunodeficiency virus	
Human T-cell leukemia/lymphoma virus types I and II	
Cytomegalovirus	
Epstein-Barr virus	
Human herpesvirus type 6	
Human herpesvirus type 8	
Hepatitis B virus	
Hepatitis C virus	
Superficial cutaneous infection	
Molluscum contagiosum virus	
Ectoparasitic infestation	
Sarcoptes scabei	

able. The viral STDs (e.g., HPV infection, genital herpes, hepatitis B, and HIV disease) are incurable. HSV infection can be suppressed but not eliminated. Because STDs may produce only mild symptoms, or even none at all, a specific microbiologic diagnosis is necessary for appropriate treatment. All STDs are preventable. It is important for health care providers to recognize the patient groups at risk, to screen persons in those risk groups who do not have symptoms, to treat documented infections in patients and their sexual partners, and to counsel them regarding preventive strategies. Persons being treated for an STD should be instructed to delay sexual activity until treatment has been completed and all of their sexual partners have been evaluated and, if necessary, treated.

URETHRITIS AND CERVICITIS

GONORRHEA

ETIOLOGY

Gonorrhea, an inflammatory disease of the mucous membranes of the genitourinary tract, occurs only in humans. It is caused by the **gonococcus** *N. gonorrhoeae,* which was first described by Neisser in 1879. *N. gonorrhoeae* is a nonmotile, gram-negative coccus that characteristically grows in pairs with flattened adjacent sides, in the configuration of coffee beans. All *Neisseria* organisms are oxidase positive and have a cell envelope similar to that of other gram-negative bacteria. Specific surface components of the envelope have been related to adherence, tissue and cellular penetration, cytotoxicity, and evasion of host defenses both systemically and at the mucosal level. One component of the gonococcal surface is **pili,** which are filamentous projections that traverse the outer membrane of the organism and are composed of repeating protein subunits. Pili are a virulence factor; organisms without pili are avirulent.

Many strains of *N. gonorrhoeae* possess a plasmid that encodes high-level resistance to tetracycline, defined as an MIC of >16 μg/mL, which can be readily transferred to other gonococci. This resistance factor, called the **tetM determinant,** encodes a protein that protects ribosomes from the effects of tetracycline. Antibiotic resistance in *N. gonorrhoeae* can also be mediated by chromosomal mutations. Chromosomally mediated resistance to β-lactam antibiotics and the tetracyclines appears to result from a series of minor mutations that reduce the permeability of the outer membrane or alter penicillin-binding protein-2, reducing its affinity for penicillin. These strains have an MIC to penicillin of >1 μg/mL, and 75% have an MIC of >2 μg/mL. Resistance to quinolones has been associated with mutations in the *gyr*A subunit of DNA gyrase and in the *par*C subunit of DNA topoisomerase.

Transmission. The most common portal of entry is the genital tract. Newborns may acquire the organism during delivery through direct contact with contaminated vaginal secretions, which leads to conjunctivitis.

EPIDEMIOLOGY

The CDC reported 690,169 new infections with *N. gonorrhoeae* in the United States in 1990, with a decrease to 360,076 in 1999 (Fig. 85–1). Approximately 24–30% of the reported cases of gonorrhea occur in adolescents. Rates among African Americans have tended to be higher but have also decreased dramatically during the past decade. In 1997 the rate of infection with *N. gonorrhoeae* among males decreased slightly, from 128.5 to 125.4 in 100,000. However, in women the rate went up slightly, to 119.3 from 118.3. Higher rates in adolescents have been associated with younger age at sexual debut, multiple partners, and failure to use condoms. In girls, older age of the sexual partner has also been associated with an increased risk of acquiring gonorrhea and other STDs.

N. gonorrhoeae has been found in approximately 2–3% of children believed to have been sexually abused. *N. gonorrhoeae* may rarely be spread by sexual play among children, but the index patient is likely to be a victim of abuse.

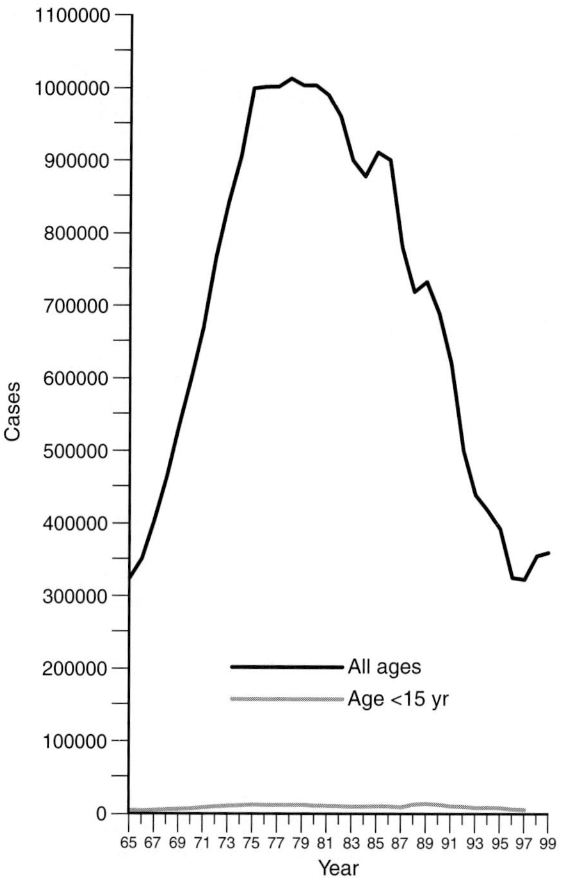

FIGURE 85–1. Reported cases of gonorrhea by year in the United States from 1965 to 1999. The number of cases among persons <15 years of age is no longer reported by the CDC. (Data from the Centers for Disease Control and Prevention.)

PATHOGENESIS

Stratified squamous epithelium can resist invasion by the gonococcus, whereas columnar epithelium is susceptible. The susceptibility of columnar epithelium facilitates infection of the urethra, prostate, seminal vesicles, and epididymis in males; the urethra, Skene's and Bartholin's glands, cervix, and fallopian tubes in females; and the rectum, pharynx, and conjunctivae in both sexes. The alkaline pH of secreted mucus and the lack of estrogenization allow vaginal infections with overt vulvovaginitis to occur in prepubertal girls.

Gonococci penetrate the surface cell layers through the intracellular spaces and reach the subepithelial connective tissue by the third or fourth day of infection. An inflammatory exudate quickly forms beneath the epithelium. In the acute phase of infection, numerous leukocytes, many with phagocytosed gonococci, are present in the lumen of the urethra, causing a characteristic profuse yellow-white discharge in males. In the absence of specific treatment, the inflammatory exudate in the subepithelial connective tissue is replaced by fibroblasts and eventually by fibrous tissue around the urethra, with ensuing stricture of the urethra. Direct extension occurs through the lymphatic vessels and less often through the blood vessels. In males, infection spreads to the posterior urethra, Cowper's glands, seminal vesicles, prostate, and epididymis, which leads to perineal, perianal, ischiorectal, or periprostatic abscesses. In females, primary infection most frequently affects the columnar epithelium of the postpubertal cervix, and the histopathologic appearance resembles that of the male urethra. Bacteremia may occur and most often causes cutaneous lesions, arthritis, and, rarely, endocarditis or meningitis.

Vaginal infections in female adolescents or younger girls may progress to involve the fallopian tubes, causing **salpingitis,** which may be subacute without specific signs and symptoms or acute. The condition is sometimes extremely difficult to recognize. Salpingitis or endometritis or both are encompassed by the term **pelvic inflammatory disease (PID).** Approximately 15% of cases of gonorrhea in teenagers progresses to PID, which comprises a spectrum of inflammatory disorders of the upper genital tract in women and may include endometritis, salpingitis, tubo-ovarian abscess, and pelvic peritonitis. *N. gonorrhoeae* and *C. trachomatis* are implicated in most cases; however, endogenous organisms such as gram-negative enteric bacilli, streptococci, anaerobic bacteria, and *Mycoplasma hominis* may be involved as etiologic agents. Cultures of endocervical specimens from women with acute PID show *N. gonorrhoeae* in 35–80% of cases, and the organism is found in a smaller proportion of cultures of fallopian tube aspirates. Risk factors for PID and acute salpingitis include young age at acquisition of gonococcal disease, a history of PID, multiple sex partners, and the use of an intrauterine device for contraception.

SYMPTOMS AND CLINICAL MANIFESTATIONS

Gonorrhea may occur in males or females without signs or symptoms. The principal signs of early disease in postpubertal women are dysuria, vaginal discharge, and abdominal pain. Spread of gonococcal infection from the cervix into the fallopian tubes is characterized by lower abdominal pain and may progress to acute salpingitis or PID. In females, direct intraperitoneal spread of the organism to the capsule of the liver may result in gonococcal perihepatitis, known as Fitz-Hugh–Curtis syndrome. The onset of these manifestations may be abrupt, without prior symptoms of lower genital tract infection.

Ascending pelvic infection may occur in prepubertal girls and may occur in the absence of clinically significant vaginal discharge. In males the most important manifestation of gonococcal infection is sudden burning on urination that occurs 2 days to 2 weeks after sexual exposure. This is followed by a mucopurulent discharge from the urethra. Involvement of the prostate is manifested by retention of urine, pain, and fever. Epididymitis is characterized by severe pain, tenderness, and swelling of the testes (Chapter 83).

Gonococcal perihepatitis, or **Fitz-Hugh–Curtis syndrome,** results from direct extension of infection from salpingitis to the capsule and outer surface of the liver. It should be considered in females with right upper quadrant abdominal pain, a palpable liver, abnormal liver function, and adnexal and uterine cervical tenderness. An endocervical culture positive for *N. gonorrhoeae* supports the diagnosis.

Gonococcal pharyngitis is common among men who have sex with men. Infection follows orogenital contact and may be asymptomatic or may simulate streptococcal pharyngitis, with swollen tonsils, exudate, and enlarged cervical lymph nodes. Temporomandibular arthritis is an uncommon complication of gonococcal pharyngitis.

Conjunctivitis after the newborn period follows direct spread, usually by fingers contaminated with genital secretions. It rarely results from gonococcemia.

Young Children. *N. gonorrhoeae* infection may cause purulent vulvovaginitis in girls or urethritis in boys, and it may cause gonococcal proctitis and pharyngitis in both sexes. However, as many as 20–25% of children with genital cultures containing *N. gonorrhoeae* have no symptoms. An even greater percentage of rectal and pharyngeal infections are asymptomatic. Gonococcal ophthalmia may be due to autoinoculation from a genital site.

N. gonorrhoeae has been found in approximately 2–3% of children believed to have been sexually abused. A culture positive for *N. gonorrhoeae* from any site in a child without prior peer sexual activity is strongly suggestive of sexual abuse. *N. gonorrhoeae* may rarely be spread by sexual play among children, but the index patient is usually a victim of abuse.

Disseminated Gonococcal Infection. In addition to direct spread of the organisms in females locally to the peritoneal cavity and the hepatic capsule, extragenital manifestations of *N. gonorrhoeae* infection may result from bacteremia. They include dermatitis with petechial or pustular acral skin lesions, tenosynovitis, septic arthritis, occasionally hepatitis, and rarely endocarditis and meningitis. Disseminated gonococcal infection (DGI) results from gonococcal bacteremia and occurs in 0.5–3% of persons with gonorrhea. Most of the clinical manifestations of DGI are secondary to the bacteremia, although immune complexes and other immunologic mechanisms may contribute to arthralgia and tenosynovitis in some persons. Patients usually have a fever and some systemic toxicity, which is frequently mild but may be absent.

The particular strains of *N. gonorrhoeae* associated with DGI tend to cause minimal genital inflammation, are very susceptible to penicillin, are resistant to the bactericidal action of nonimmune serum, and belong to the nutritionally deficient small-colony AHU auxotype, to the 1A serogroup based on characterization of the outer membrane protein 1, and to specific serotypes. These strains have become much less common in the United States since the early 1980s. Persons with deficiency of the terminal components of complement (C5, C6, C7, or C8) are more susceptible to DGI and meningococcal bacteremia; approximately 5% of persons with DGI have such a deficiency.

The most common clinical manifestation of DGI is the **arthritis-dermatitis syndrome.** The first complaint is arthralgia, which may be migratory. The knees, elbows, and distal joints are usually involved. Physical examination demonstrates arthritis or tenosynovitis, or periarticular inflammation, in two or more joints. A characteristic rash, present on 75% of patients, consists of discrete papules and pustules, often with a hemorrhagic or necrotic component. Usually 5–40 lesions are present, primarily on the extremities. The polyarthropathy and dermatitis frequently resolve spontaneously if not treated. However, arthritis may persist and progress, usually in one or two joints, most commonly the knee, ankle, elbow, or wrist. At this stage the clinical features resemble those of septic arthritis. Studies of septic arthritis in children have found *N. gonorrhoeae* to be the third most frequent organism in children >3 years of age and the most frequent cause in children >11 years of age. Some persons can have gonococcal septic arthritis without prior polyarthritis or dermatitis.

Infection During Pregnancy and in Newborns. Gonorrhea during pregnancy has been associated with a greater risk of premature rupture of the membranes, prolonged rupture of the membranes, and premature delivery. In addition to the effect on the fetus, postpartum complications in the mother are common. Recurrent infection after an initial episode during pregnancy is common. Mothers infected in early pregnancy should have a repeated culture in later pregnancy, as in any other high-risk situation.

Gonococcal ophthalmia is the most common form of gonorrhea in infants. It results from perinatal transmission from an infected mother during parturition (Chapter 89). After an initially nonspecific conjunctivitis, serosanguineous discharge is rapidly replaced by a thick, purulent exudate. Corneal ulceration and iridocyclitis are unilateral or bilateral. Unless therapy is initiated promptly, perforation of the cornea may occur and lead to blindness.

DIAGNOSIS

The clinical diagnosis of gonorrhea is relatively easy in men because most have the typical manifestations of mucopurulent urethritis. In women the clinical features are variable. The early studies suggesting that gonorrhea is always symptomatic in men and usually asymptomatic in women were completed in populations from STD clinics, where the women were usually symptom-free contacts of men with symptomatic infections. However, most women with gonorrhea have nonspecific complaints, including lower abdominal pain and dysuria, and are more likely to obtain medical care from a gynecologist or internist than at an STD clinic. Acute gonococcal salpingitis or PID must be differentiated from acute appendicitis, cystitis, pyelonephritis, cholecystitis, and ectopic pregnancy. Prepubertal children often have purulent vaginitis or urethritis at presentation. Pharyngeal and rectal infections, usually seen in sexually abused children, are frequently asymptomatic.

In young children, because of medicolegal implications, an accurate microbiologic diagnosis is essential. A culture positive for *N. gonorrhoeae* from any site in a child without prior peer sexual activity is strongly suggestive of sexual abuse.

The differential diagnosis of DGI includes meningococcemia, other infectious arthritides, and an entire range of inflammatory arthritides. Infrequent but serious complications of DGI include infective endocarditis, meningitis, osteomyelitis, and pneumonia.

Pelvic Inflammatory Disease. The diagnosis of PID may be difficult. Some women have few or no symptoms. The three minimum criteria for diagnosis of PID are lower abdominal tenderness, adnexal tenderness, and cervical motion tenderness. In the absence of another cause, these findings are sufficient to warrant empirical therapy. Other findings may include oral temperature >38.3°C (>101°F), abnormal cervical or vaginal discharge, elevated ESR, elevated CRP concentration, and laboratory documentation of cervical infection with *N. gonorrhoeae* or *C. trachomatis.* The definitive criteria for diagnosing PID, which may be warranted in selected cases, include histopathologic evidence of endometritis on endometrial biopsy, transvaginal ultrasonography or other imaging techniques showing thickened fluid-filled tubes with or without free pelvic fluid or tubo-ovarian complex, and laparoscopic abnormalities consistent with PID.

The differential diagnosis includes numerous other conditions of the lower abdomen and pelvis, including acute appendicitis, ectopic pregnancy, cholecystitis, mesenteric lymphadenitis, cystitis, pyelonephritis, and septic abortion. Misdiagnosis of PID is common, and it is one of the more common causes of medically nonindicated laparotomy.

Microbiologic Evaluation

A Gram stain of a urethral discharge from a male adult or adolescent has a positive predictive value of >99% in the diagnosis of gonorrhea, but Gram stain of a vaginal discharge from a child is not accurate and has a poor predictive value. Diagnostic culture specimens from the pharynx, rectum, vagina, and urethra should be taken and immediately plated onto selective media appropriate for isolation of *N. gonorrhoeae.* The media that may be used include

chocolate blood agar and **Thayer-Martin agar.** The plates should then be placed in an atmosphere enriched with carbon dioxide, the easiest method being the use of an extinction candle jar. *N. gonorrhoeae* organisms are gram-negative, oxidase-positive diplococci, and their presence should be confirmed with additional tests, including rapid carbohydrate tests, enzyme-substrate tests, and rapid serologic tests. Failure to perform appropriate confirmatory tests may lead to misidentification of other organisms, such as other *Neisseria, Moraxella catarrhalis,* and *Kingella,* as *N. gonorrhoeae.* At least two procedures that use different principles (e.g., biochemical, enzyme substrate, serologic, or DNA probe) should be used to confirm identification of *N. gonorrhoeae.*

Gonococci frequently can be cultured from blood during the arthritis-dermatitis phase of DGI. The organism also may be detected by immunochemical tests on biopsy specimens of the skin lesions, but results of Gram stains and cultures of specimens from pustular skin lesions are usually negative. Overall, only about 50% of persons with DGI have positive results on blood or synovial fluid cultures, but *N. gonorrhoeae* can be recovered from a mucosal site (e.g., pharynx, rectum) in at least 80% of patients.

Nonculture Tests. Several nonculture antigen detection tests using EIA for detection of *N. gonorrhoeae* were introduced in the 1980s but had unsatisfactory sensitivity or specificity. In the late 1980s a nonamplified DNA probe assay was introduced (PACE, Gen-Probe), with an overall sensitivity, in comparison with culture of endocervical specimens, of approximately 95%. Data are similar for male urethral specimens, with sensitivities of 98.8–100% and specificities >99% compared with culture. However, neither the DNA probe nor EIA is sufficiently sensitive for use with urine specimens from males or females.

Several nucleic acid amplification tests for detection of *N. gonorrhoeae* have been approved by the FDA. These include assays based on PCR, ligase chain reaction (LCR), transcription-mediated amplification (TMA), RNA amplification, and strand displacement amplification (SDA). All have FDA approval for detection of *N. gonorrhoeae* in endocervical and urethral specimens as well as urine for men and women. TMA is an RNA amplification method that uses reverse transcriptase and T7 RNA polymerase and that can produce 1 million to 1 billion copies of an RNA target. One test is a coamplification PCR assay that detects both *N. gonorrhoeae* and *C. trachomatis* from a single specimen. This assay does not distinguish between the two organisms but indicates whether one or both are present in a specimen. It is often used to screen for infections among populations with a low prevalence of STDs. These nonculture tests perform best in high-prevalence populations. The positive predictive values for these tests in low-prevalence groups, such as children, have not been determined. Culture of *N. gonorrhoeae* remains the only appropriate test for children being evaluated for suspected sexual abuse.

TREATMENT

The development of antibiotic resistance has greatly affected the treatment of gonorrhea (Table 85–2). Antibiotic-sensitive and antibiotic-resistant strains cause the same spectrum of illness. In the United States, >40% of *N. gonorrhoeae* isolates are penicillin resistant. Resistance is both chromosomally and plasmid mediated. There has also been a similar increase in tetracycline-resistant *N. gonorrhoeae* strains. Resistance to the quinolones has become established in Japan, Thailand, the Philippines, Africa, and Australia, where it is now as high as 70%. Quinolone-resistant *N. gonorrhoeae* has been identified only rarely in the United States, with <0.05% of isolates collected by the CDC during 1996 having an MIC ≥1.0 μg/mL to ciprofloxacin. The CDC recommends that as long as quinolone-resistant strains comprise <1% of all *N. gonorrhoeae* strains, quinolone treatment regimens can be used. The resistance of *N. gonorrhoeae* to ceftriaxone has not as yet been reported, but strains with reduced susceptibility have been found in some areas.

Some agents (e.g., oral cephalosporins, spectinomycin) are relatively ineffective against pharyngeal gonorrhea. Only ceftriaxone, ciprofloxacin, and ofloxacin are recommended for the treatment of pharyngeal gonococcal infection.

Definitive Treatment

Children. It is especially important, in cases of gonococcal infection in children, to identify the source of infection. Children with genital gonorrhea should be hospitalized and treated with ceftriaxone 125 mg as a single intramuscular injection (see Table 85–2). Children who cannot tolerate ceftriaxone may be treated with spectinomycin as a single injection. Spectinomycin is not as effective in the treatment of rectal or pharyngeal gonorrhea. Quinolones are not approved for use in children. The newer expanded-spectrum oral cephalosporins such as cefixime have been shown to be effective as a single oral dose in adults, but they have not yet been evaluated in children.

Children with gonococcal bacteremia or arthritis should be treated with ceftriaxone for 7 days. All children with rectogenital gonorrhea should be evaluated for coinfection with *C. trachomatis.*

Adolescents and Adults. The efficacy of single-dose therapy is an important consideration in the treatment of gonococcal infections, especially in adolescents. For adolescents >12 years of age, treatment should follow the recommended regimens for adults (see Table 85–2). The first-line regimen recommended by the CDC is either ceftriaxone 125 mg as a single intramuscular dose or an oral quinolone as a single dose, plus either azithromycin 1 g in a single oral dose or doxycycline 100 mg orally twice a day for 7 days. Azithromycin or doxycycline is administered because *C. trachomatis* coinfection with *N. gonorrhoeae* is common, occurring in up to 45% of adolescents with gonorrhea in some populations. Among adolescents, treatment of gonorrhea with drug regimens effective against gonococci but not *C. trachomatis* has led to a high incidence of residual salpingitis in females and urethritis in males, both associated with continued disease due to *C. trachomatis.* Several alternative regimens that incorporate intramuscular or oral cephalosporins or oral quinolones are available but do not offer clear advantages (see Table 85–2). Ciprofloxacin or ofloxacin in a single dose may be used if the patient is 18 years of age or older. All these regimens should be followed by single-dose azithromycin therapy or by a 7-day course of doxycycline or another tetracycline for possible coinfection with *C. trachomatis.* Spectinomycin can be used to treat pregnant women allergic to β-lactam antibiotics, but it is relatively ineffective against pharyngeal gonococcal infection and is ineffective against incubating syphilis. If pharyngeal infection is a concern, the person should be treated with either ceftriaxone or ciprofloxacin. There is less experience with many of these alternative regimens than with the recommended regimens.

Neonates. An infant born to a mother with untreated gonorrhea should have orogastric and rectal culture specimens taken routinely, and blood culture specimens should be taken if the infection is symptomatic. A term infant should receive a single intravenous or intramuscular injection of ceftriaxone (see Table 85–2). A neonate with gonococcal ophthalmia should be hospitalized. The CDC recommends that uncomplicated gonococcal ophthalmia be treated

TABLE 85–2. Recommended Regimens for the Treatment of Gonococcal Infection

Uncomplicated Gonococcal Infections of the Cervix, Urethra, and Rectum in Adults and Adolescents

Recommended Regimens

Cefixime 400 mg in a single dose PO
or
Ceftriaxone 125 mg in a single dose IM
or
Ciprofloxacin* 500 mg in a single dose PO
or
Ofloxacin* 400 mg in a single dose PO
plus
Azithromycin 1 g in a single dose PO
or
Doxycycline 100 mg bid PO for 7 days

Alternative Regimens

Spectinomycin 2 g in a single dose IM
or
Ceftizoxime 500 mg IM in a single dose†
or
Cefotaxime 500 mg IM in a single dose†
or
Cefotetan 1 g IM in a single dose†
or
Cefoxitin 2 g IM with probenecid 1 g PO in a single dose†
or
Enoxacin 400 mg PO in a single dose‡
or
Lomefloxacin 400 mg PO in a single dose‡
or
Norfloxacin 800 mg PO in a single dose‡

Uncomplicated Gonococcal Infection of the Pharynx

Ceftriaxone 125 mg in a single dose IM
or
Ciprofloxacin 500 mg in a single dose PO
or
Ofloxacin 400 mg in a single dose PO
plus
Azithromycin 1 g in a single dose PO
or
Doxycycline 100 mg bid PO for 7 days

Uncomplicated Gonococcal Vulvovaginitis, Cervicitis, Urethritis, Pharyngitis, or Proctitis Infection in Children Who Weigh $<$45 kg

Recommended Regimen

Ceftriaxone 125 mg in a single dose IM

Alternative Regimen

Spectinomycin 40 mg/kg (max 2 g) in a single dose IM (unreliable for pharyngeal infection)

Uncomplicated Genital Infection in Children Who Weigh $\geq$45 kg

These children should be treated with one of the regimens recommended for adults

Bacteremia or Arthritis for Children Who Weigh $<$45 kg

Ceftriaxone 50 mg/kg (max 1 g) in a single daily dose IM or IV for 7 days

Bacteremia or Arthritis for Children Who Weigh $\geq$45 kg

Ceftriaxone 50 mg/kg (max 2 g) in a single daily dose IM or IV for 10–14 days

Gonococcal Conjunctivitis

Ceftriaxone 1 g in a single dose IM; lavage of infected eye with buffered saline solution once daily until discharge clears

Ophthalmia Neonatorum Caused by *Neisseria gonorrhoeae*

Ceftriaxone 25–50 mg/kg (max 125 mg) in a single dose IM or IV

Disseminated Gonococcal Infection (DGI) and Gonococcal Scalp Abscess in Newborns

Ceftriaxone 25 mg/kg in a single daily dose IM or IV for 7 days (duration of 10–14 days if infant has meningitis)
or
Cefotaxime 25–50 mg/kg q12hr IM or IV for 7 days (duration of 10–14 days if infant has meningitis)

Prophylactic Treatment for Infants Whose Mothers Have Untreated Gonococcal Infection

(in Absence of Signs of Gonococcal Infection)

Ceftriaxone 25–50 mg/kg (max 125 mg) in a single dose IM or IV

Disseminated Gonococcal Infection (DGI)

Recommended Initial Regimen

Ceftriaxone 1 g q24hr IM or IV

Alternative Initial Regimens

Cefotaxime *or* ceftizoxime 1 g every q8hr IV

Regimen for Persons with Hypersensitivity to β-lactam Antibiotics

Ciprofloxacin 500 mg q12hr IV
or
Ofloxacin 400 mg q12hr IV
or
Spectinomycin 2 g q12hr IM

NOTE: All regimens should be continued for 24–48 hr after improvement begins, at which time therapy may be switched to one of the following to complete a full week of antimicrobial therapy:

Cefixime 400 mg bid PO
or
Ciprofloxacin 500 mg bid PO
or
Ofloxacin 400 mg bid PO

Gonococcal Meningitis and Endocarditis

Ceftriaxone 1–2 g q12hr IV; duration of therapy for meningitis should be 10–14 days and for endocarditis at least 4 wk

*Ciprofloxacin, ofloxacin, and other quinolone antibiotics are contraindicated for pregnant and lactating women, for children, and for adolescents younger than 18 years.
†This regimen offers no advantage over ceftriaxone.
‡This regimen offers no advantage over ciprofloxacin or ofloxacin.

with a single intravenous or intramuscular injection of ceftriaxone (Chapter 89). Infants with gonococcal ophthalmia should receive eye irrigation with buffered saline solution one time until the discharge clears. Additional topical antimicrobial therapy is not indicated. Simultaneous infection with *C. trachomatis* has been reported and should be considered in infants who do not respond satisfactorily. Both the mother and infant should be tested for chlamydial infection.

Complicated neonatal infections such as septicemia, arthritis, or other focal infections should be treated by hospitalization and administration of ceftriaxone for 7 days. Meningitis should be treated with ceftriaxone for 10–14 days.

Disseminated Gonococcal Infection. Persons with DGI should be hospitalized for initial therapy for 24–48 hours. Reliable persons with uncomplicated disease and complete resolution of symptoms may complete therapy on an outpatient basis, using an oral antibiotic to complete a total of 1 week of therapy.

Pelvic Inflammatory Disease. The regimens for PID recommended by the CDC—cefotetan plus doxycycline *or* clindamycin plus gentamicin—are active against the polymicrobial etiologic agents of PID, including *N. gonorrhoeae,* enteric gram-negative bacteria, anaerobic bacteria, and *C. trachomatis* infection (Table 85–3). Current opinion suggests that it is not mandatory to admit every person, or even every adolescent, with PID for treatment. Indications for inpatient therapy for PID include surgical emergencies, such as appendicitis, in which PID cannot be excluded; no response to oral antimicrobial therapy; pregnancy; noncompliance with an oral outpatient regimen; severe illness with nausea, vomiting, or high fever; tubo-ovarian abscess; and immunodeficiency (i.e., HIV infection with low CD4 counts; immunosuppressive therapy).

Supportive Therapy

Persons with genital gonorrhea or with extragenital gonorrhea originating with a genital infection should be treated presumptively for concurrent *C. trachomatis* infection (Table 85–4). They should also be screened for syphilis by serologic testing. Many gonorrhea treatment regimens (e.g., ceftriaxone or doxycycline or erythromycin for 7 days) may cure incubating syphilis. Spectinomycin is ineffective against incubating syphilis, and the effectiveness of azithromycin has not been established. However, persons should receive specific antisyphilis therapy if serologic test results are positive.

Sexual Partners. Persons with gonorrhea should be instructed to refer sexual partners for evaluation and treatment. Sexual partners of patients with symptomatic infection should be evaluated and treated if the last sexual contact was within 30 days of the onset of the patients' symptoms. Sexual partners of patients without symptoms should be evaluated and treated if the last sexual contact was within 60 days. If the last sexual contact occurred more than 60 days before the onset of the patients' symptoms, the partners should be treated presumptively. Patients should avoid sexual intercourse until they and all sexual partners have been treated and are either free of symptoms or have negative culture results.

COMPLICATIONS

Persons with uncomplicated gonorrhea treated with a recommended regimen who have resolution of symptoms do not require repeated cultures to document cure. Repeated cultures are indicated for persons with persistent symptoms. Repeated positive culture results usually indicate reinfection and failure of referral and treatment of the sexual partner, but any gonococcal isolates after treatment should be submitted to a reference laboratory for susceptibility testing. The infected person should be re-treated with another regimen pending results of susceptibility testing.

PROGNOSIS

The recommended regimens cure more than 95% of cases of anal and genital gonorrhea. Persistent urethritis, cervicitis, or proctitis may represent infection with another organism, such as *C. tracho-*

TABLE 85–3. Regimens for the Treatment of Pelvic Inflammatory Disease

Parenteral Treatment
Parenteral Regimen A
Cefotetan 2 g q12hr IV
or
Cefoxitin 2 g q6hr IV
plus
Doxycycline 100 mg q12hr IV or PO
NOTE: Parenteral therapy may be discontinued 24 hr after the patient's condition improves clinically; oral doxycycline should continue for a total of 14 days. When a tubo-ovarian abscess is present, many health care providers use clindamycin or metronidazole with doxycycline for continued therapy, rather than doxycycline alone, as the combination provides better anaerobic coverage.
Parenteral Regimen B
Clindamycin 900 mg q8hr IV
plus
Gentamicin (loading dose 2 mg/kg, followed by 1.5 mg/kg q8hr IV or IM; alternatively, single daily dosing may be substituted.)
NOTE: Parenteral therapy may be discontinued 24 hr after the patient's condition improves clinically; continuing oral therapy should consist of doxycycline 100 mg q12hr PO or clindamycin 450 mg qid PO, to complete a total of 14 days.
*Alternative Parenteral Regimens**
Ofloxacin† 400 mg q12hr IV
plus
Metronidazole 500 mg q8hr IV
or
Ampicillin-sulbactam 3 g q6hr IV
plus
Doxycycline 100 mg q12hr IV or PO
or
Ciprofloxacin 200 mg q12hr IV
plus
Doxycycline 100 mg q12hr IV or PO
plus
Metronidazole 500 mg q8hr IV

Oral Treatment
Oral Regimen A
Ofloxacin† 400 mg bid PO for 14 days
plus
Metronidazole 500 mg bid PO for 14 days
Oral Regimen B
Ceftriaxone 125 mg once IM
or
Cefoxitin 2 g IM plus probenecid 1 g in a single dose PO concurrently
or
Other parenteral third-generation cephalosporin (e.g., ceftizoxime or cefotaxime)
plus
Doxycycline 100 mg bid PO for 14 days

*Ampicillin-sulbactam plus doxycycline has good coverage against *C. trachomatis, N. gonorrhoeae,* and anaerobes. Because ciprofloxacin has poor coverage for *C. trachomatis* and anaerobes, doxycycline and metronidazole should be added routinely.
†Ofloxacin and other quinolone antibiotics are contraindicated for pregnant and lactating women, for children, and for adolescents younger than 18 years.

TABLE 85–4. Regimens for the Treatment of *Chlamydia trachomatis* Infection

Uncomplicated Genital Infection in Children ≥8 Years of Age, Adolescents, Adult Men, and Adult Nonpregnant Women *Recommended Regimens* Azithromycin 1 g in a single dose PO *or* Doxycycline 100 mg bid PO for 7 days *Alternative Regimens* Erythromycin base 50 mg/kg/day (max 500 mg) qid PO for 7 days *or* Erythromycin ethylsuccinate 800 mg qid PO for 7 days *or* Ofloxacin 300 mg qid PO for 7 days*	**Uncomplicated Genital Infection in Pregnant Women** *Recommended Regimen* Erythromycin base 500 mg qid PO for 7 days *or* Amoxicillin 500 mg tid PO for 7–10 days *Alternative Regimens* Erythromycin base 250 mg qid PO for 14 days *or* Erythromycin ethylsuccinate 800 mg qid PO for 7 days *or* Erythromycin ethylsuccinate 400 mg qid PO for 14 days *or* Azithromycin 1 g in a single dose PO
Uncomplicated Genital Infection in Children Who Weigh <45 kg Erythromycin base 50 mg/kg/day (max 500 mg) in 4 divided doses PO for 10–14 days†	**Infants with Conjunctivitis** Erythromycin ethylsuccinate 50 mg/kg/day (max 500 mg) in 4 divided doses PO for 10–14 days
Uncomplicated Genital Infection in Children Who Weigh ≥45 kg but Are <8 yr of Age Azithromycin 1 g in a single dose PO	**Infants with Pneumonia** Erythromycin ethylsuccinate 50 mg/kg/day (max 500 mg) in 4 divided doses PO for 2–3 wk

*Ofloxacin and other quinolone antibiotics are contraindicated for pregnant and lactating women, for children, and for adolescents younger than 18 years.
†The effectiveness of treatment with erythromycin is approximately 80%; a second course of therapy may be required.

matis. Pharyngeal infection can be cured in >90% of cases with ceftriaxone or ciprofloxacin. PID has been linked to ectopic pregnancy and infertility, which occurs in approximately one fourth of infected women as a consequence of scarring of the fallopian tubes. It is probable that the risk of infertility after PID is lessened with prompt appropriate therapy.

PREVENTION

Treatment of gonorrhea in pregnant women is the best means to prevent neonatal gonococcal disease. Many mothers conceive their first children while they are teenagers, a time of life in which gonococcal disease has a high prevalence and when the women may turn to their pediatricians for medical care. All pregnant women should have endocervical cultures for *N. gonorrhoeae* as an integral part of prenatal care at the first prenatal visit. A second culture late in pregnancy should be obtained from women who are at high risk of having gonococcal infection.

Newborns should receive prophylactic treatment with topical therapy to prevent gonococcal neonatal ophthalmia; such treatment is required in most states. Topical therapy is effective in preventing ocular infections and is especially important for pregnant women who do not receive adequate prenatal care. Gonococcal neonatal ophthalmia may be prevented by a single application of silver nitrate 1% aqueous solution, erythromycin 0.5% ophthalmic ointment, or tetracycline 1% ophthalmic ointment (Chapter 89). The infant may be more likely to acquire the infection despite prophylaxis if there has been premature rupture of the membranes. Prophylactic treatment of *N. gonorrhoeae* may not affect neonatal conjunctivitis from *C. trachomatis* and does not prevent nasopharyngeal colonization with this organism.

CHLAMYDIA TRACHOMATIS INFECTION

ETIOLOGY

The genus *Chlamydia* is a group of obligate intracellular parasites with a unique developmental cycle with morphologically distinct infectious and reproductive forms. All members of the genus have a gram-negative envelope without peptidoglycan, share a genus-specific lipopolysaccharide antigen, and use host adenosine triphosphate for the synthesis of chlamydial protein. The genus contains four species: *C. trachomatis, C. psittaci, C. pneumoniae,* and *C. pecorum.* There are 15 known serotypes of *C. trachomatis* (Table 68–7). The other two species cause lower respiratory tract infections (Chapter 68).

Transmission. The most common portal of entry is the genital tract. Newborns may acquire the organism during delivery through direct contact with contaminated vaginal secretions, which leads to conjunctivitis. Pregnant women who have cervical infection with *C. trachomatis* can transmit the infection to their infants. Approximately 50–75% of infants born to infected women have infections at one or more anatomic sites, including the conjunctiva, nasopharynx, rectum, and vagina, and may subsequently develop neonatal conjunctivitis (Chapter 89) and pneumonia (Chapter 68). Transmission after cesarean delivery is rare and usually occurs after early rupture of the amniotic membrane.

EPIDEMIOLOGY

C. trachomatis is probably the most prevalent sexually transmitted infection in the United States today. *C. trachomatis* infection has been a reportable disease since 1995. In contrast to gonococcal infections, infections with *C. trachomatis* appear to be increasing, with 477,638 cases reported in 1995 and 604,420 reported in 1998. However, the number of cases is underreported; the CDC estimated that in 1996 the point prevalence of *C. trachomatis* infections among persons 15–44 years of age was 1.6 million, with an annual incidence of 2.4 million cases per year. Among males, *C. trachomatis* is the single most frequently identifiable cause of nongonococcal urethritis. It accounts for 30–40% of all episodes of urethritis, or 1.5 million episodes annually. The prevalence of chlamydial infection is more weakly associated with socioeconomic status, urban or rural residence, and race and ethnicity than is the prevalence of gonorrhea and syphilis. The prevalence of *C. trachomatis* infection is consistently greater than 5% among sexually active, adolescent, and young adult women who attend outpatient clinics, regardless of the region of the country, location of the clinic (urban or rural), or race or ethnicity of the population. In many locales the prevalence commonly exceeds 10%. Adolescent women have the highest reported rates of chlamydial infection, often exceeding 15%. The prevalence of infection among pregnant women has been reported to range from 2% to 30%, depending on the population studied.

In rare cases, children may acquire chlamydial infection as a result of sexual abuse. Vaginal infection with *C. trachomatis* was reported uncommonly in prepubertal children before 1980. The possibility of sexual contact frequently was not discussed. Recent studies identified rectogenital chlamydial infection in 2–3% of sexually abused children after routine culture of the organism. Most chlamydial infections are asymptomatic.

PATHOGENESIS

The chlamydial developmental cycle involves an infectious, metabolically inactive extracellular form **(elementary body)** and a noninfectious, metabolically active intracellular form **(reticulate body).** The elementary body, which is 200–400 nm in diameter, attaches to the host cell by electrostatic binding or to attachment proteins and is taken into the cell by endocytosis, which does not depend on the microtubule system. Within the host cell, the elementary body remains within a membrane-lined phagosome, and phagosomal-lysosomal fusion is inhibited. The elementary bodies then differentiate into reticulate bodies, which undergo binary fission. After approximately 36 hours, the reticulate bodies differentiate into elementary bodies. At about 48 hours, release may occur by cytolysis or by a process of exocytosis or extrusion of the whole inclusion, leaving the host cell intact (Fig. 85–2).

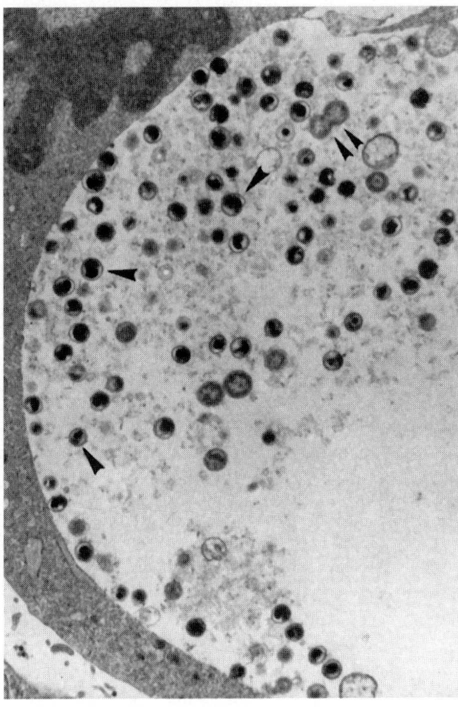

FIGURE 85–2. Electron micrograph of *Chlamydia trachomatis* inclusion in McCoy cell at 72 hours after infection, demonstrating elementary bodies *(single arrowheads)* and reticulate body undergoing binary fission *(double arrowhead)*.

SYMPTOMS AND CLINICAL MANIFESTATIONS

C. trachomatis causes **nongonococcal urethritis,** epididymitis, mucopurulent cervicitis, and PID. Infection is typically of long duration, with few or no symptoms in both women and men. The incubation period is usually 5–10 days. Nongonococcal urethritis usually causes much less dysuria and less profuse, less purulent urethral exudate than gonorrhea. However, in a person with symptoms, it may be difficult to differentiate between chlamydial and gonococcal infections. Most men have acute symptoms after *C. trachomatis* infection, but some may have a prolonged, clinically inapparent infection. The presence of ≥5 polymorphonuclear leukocytes per high-power field on Gram stain of a urethral secretion, a positive leukocyte esterase test result on first-voided urine, or the presence of ≥10 polymorphonuclear leukocytes per high-power field in the sediment of a first-voided urine specimen is evidence of urethritis even in the absence of frank discharge.

C. trachomatis is also the most frequent cause of epididymitis in young men (Chapter 83). It has been estimated that one diagnosed case of epididymitis caused by *C. trachomatis* occurs for every 18 diagnosed episodes of uncomplicated chlamydial urethritis in men 15–34 years of age. Overall, *C. trachomatis* causes 50% of cases of epididymitis among men 15–34 years of age. *C. trachomatis* may also cause proctitis among men who have sex with men. If the infection is due to a lymphogranuloma venereum (LGV) strain, a proctocolitis may develop that may be difficult to differentiate from Crohn's disease both clinically and histopathologically.

In women, cervical infections with *C. trachomatis* are frequently asymptomatic and often of long duration. It has been estimated that >70% of cervical infections in women are asymptomatic. *C. trachomatis* can cause mucopurulent cervicitis (MPC), which is also frequently asymptomatic. Some women may have an abnormal vaginal discharge and vaginal bleeding (i.e., after sexual intercourse). Although some experts consider an increased number of polymorphonuclear leukocytes on endocervical Gram stain to be useful in the diagnosis of MPC, this criterion has not been standardized and has a low positive predictive value. MPC can also be caused by *N. gonorrhoeae.*

DIAGNOSIS

The definitive diagnosis of genital chlamydial infections in adolescents and adults is isolation of the organism in tissue cultures or detection of *C. trachomatis* nucleic acids in specimens from the urethra in men and from the endocervix in women. Because of medicolegal implications, culture is the only approved method of diagnosiing rectal and genital chlamydial infections in prepubertal children. Culture means isolation of the organism in tissue culture with confirmation by visual identification of the characteristic inclusions, preferably with fluorescent staining. However, culture methods are not standardized and performance may vary greatly from laboratory to laboratory. Nonculture methods cannot be used in this setting. Few data are available on the use of these tests in rectal and genital specimens from prepubertal children, and what is available suggests that the tests are neither sensitive nor specific.

Microbiologic Evaluation

Care should be taken in obtaining culture specimens to obtain cells and not discharge. Dacron polyester–tipped swabs with either wire or plastic shafts are preferred. The most commonly used tissue culture system uses cycloheximide-treated McCoy cells and has high sensitivity (70–90%) and specificity (100%). However, culture of *C. trachomatis* is not standardized and performance may vary significantly from laboratory to laboratory. After 48–72 hours of incubation, the culture results are confirmed by microscopic identification of the characteristic intracytoplasmic inclusions by staining of the inclusions, preferably with a fluorescein-conjugated species-specific monoclonal antibody. EIA should not be used for culture confirmation because of the possibility of false-positive results.

Nonculture Tests. Several nonculture methods for direct testing of specimens for chlamydial antigen or nucleic acids have been developed. The first such assay to be developed was a direct fluorescent antibody test in which chlamydial elementary bodies are identified directly on a specimen smear stained with a fluorescein-conjugated antichlamydial monoclonal antibody. This test is now used infrequently; it was labor intensive, had a significant subjective component, and was not suitable for screening large numbers of specimens. A series of EIAs were introduced in the 1980s that offered a semiautomated format but had sensitivities of only 70–80% compared with culture. A DNA probe–based test was also introduced at this time, but its performance was similar to that of the EIAs.

The development of nucleic acid amplification tests has resulted in a significant increase in sensitivity. The most widely used nucleic amplification technologies are PCR, LCR, TMA, and SDA. EIA can detect a minimum of 10^{4-5} organisms, culture can detect 10–100 organisms, and DNA amplification tests can detect 1–10 organisms. The nucleic acid amplification tests are more sensitive than culture for the detection of *C. trachomatis* in genital specimens, detecting an additional 25–30% more than culture. Multiple studies have demonstrated that each has a sensitivity of 80–100%, compared with 65–88% for culture, while maintaining high specificities of 95–100%. Amplification tests are more sensitive than currently available EIA and nonamplification DNA-probe assays. However, these tests are not all equivalent. False-negative results obtained because of inhibitors of DNA polymerase is a greater problem than false-positive results because of amplicon carryover. Inhibitors appear to be more frequent in cervical specimens. The LCR test appears to be less susceptible to inhibitors than the PCR test. Of note, there are no inhibition controls included with any of the currently available kits. Moreover, there are rare strains of *C. trachomatis* that lack the cryptic plasmid and thus would not be detected by PCR or LCR.

Because of false-positive results, antigen and nucleic acid amplification tests for chlamydial infection should not be used to diagnose chlamydial infections for legal purposes; only cultures should be used in such circumstances. These tests are not approved for any site in prepubertal children. However, the PCR assay has been demonstrated to be sensitive and specific for the detection of *C. trachomatis* in infants with neonatal conjunctivitis.

Serologic Testing. Serologic testing is not helpful in the diagnosis of chlamydial infections in adults because most infections in adolescents and adults are asymptomatic. Serologic surveys of sexually active adult populations have found the prevalence of antichlamydial antibody to be >20% in these persons. The most widely available serologic test is the complement fixation test, which is a genus-specific test and is most useful in the diagnosis of LGV. Unfortunately it is not sufficiently sensitive for use in the diagnosis of oculogenital infections caused by the trachoma biovar in adults or children. The microimmunofluorescence test is species specific and species sensitive but is available only at a limited number of research laboratories.

TREATMENT

Treatment of chlamydial infections is hampered by the long growth cycle of the organism. However, the long half-life in tissue of azithromycin makes single-dose treatment feasible. The current recommended regimen for the treatment of uncomplicated urethral, endocervical, or rectal infections in adolescent and adult men and in nonpregnant women is single-dose azithromycin or doxycycline therapy for 7 days (see Table 85–4). Chlamydial infections in children should be treated with erythromycin orally for 7–14 days. Children older than 8 years may be treated with tetracycline orally for 7 days. Infections in infants should be treated with erythromycin ethylsuccinate for 14 days. However, this regimen has a 20% failure rate, often requiring re-treatment. Azithromycin suspension, 20 mg/kg as a single oral dose per day for 3 days, appeared to be at least as effective as erythromycin for the treatment of chlamydial conjunctivitis in one small study.

Treatment During Pregnancy. The CDC currently recommends several different regimens, including the use of erythromycin, during pregnancy, but none of them has been extensively evaluated. Poor gastrointestinal tolerance may reduce compliance to 50% or less in some populations. The current recommended regimen is either erythromycin base 500 mg four times a day orally for 7 days or amoxicillin 500 mg three times a day orally for 7 days. The latter regimen is as effective as erythromycin in the eradication of the organism and is associated with fewer side effects. Preliminary data indicate that azithromycin 1 g in a single oral dose may also be safe and effective, but available data are insufficient to recommend the routine use of azithromycin during pregnancy.

Supportive Therapy

Patients with *C. trachomatis* infections should be treated presumptively for concurrent gonorrhea (see Table 85–2). They should also be screened for syphilis by serologic testing.

Sexual Partners. Persons with *C. trachomatis* infections should be instructed to refer sexual partners for evaluation and treatment. Sexual partners of patients with symptomatic infections should be evaluated and treated if the last sexual contact was within 30 days of the onset of the patients' symptoms. Sexual partners of patients without symptoms should be evaluated and treated if the last sexual contact was within 60 days. If the last sexual contact occurred more than 60 days before the onset of the patients' symptoms, the partners should be treated presumptively. Patients should avoid sexual intercourse until they and all sexual partners are treated and are either free of symptoms or have negative culture results.

COMPLICATIONS

Among many possible complications of chlamydial infection, the most important in females is acute salpingitis. Several studies from Scandinavia, as well as histopathologic reports, indicate a strong causal association between *C. trachomatis* infection and salpingitis. Later clinical and animal studies from the United States, using aggressive culture methods including cultures of specimens from the fallopian tubes, have confirmed the European experience. The organism is probably responsible for at least 20% of cases of salpingitis in the United States. Studies from Sweden and the United States indicate that approximately one in four persons admitted to the hospital with acute salpingitis has an upper genital tract infection with *C. trachomatis* confirmed by isolation of the organism from the fallopian tubes. The presence of *C. trachomatis* in the cervix of a woman with PID does not necessarily imply that the organism is present in the tubes, but it is suggestive. The reason that ascending infection develops in some women with cervical infections is not known. Salpingitis may be 10 times more likely in a sexually active 15-year-old girl than in a sexually active 25-year-old woman.

Chlamydial salpingitis can cause permanent tubal dysfunction leading to infertility. Infertility rates of 13% after one episode of salpingitis, 36% after two episodes, and 75% after three or more episodes have been reported. In addition to a higher prevalence than gonococcal infections, chlamydial salpingitis appears to have a more severe clinical outcome. Compared with persons who have gonococcal salpingitis or nonchlamydial, nongonococcal salpingitis, persons with chlamydial salpingitis have a less acute presentation, have fevers less often, have a longer history of symptoms, have a higher erythrocyte sedimentation rate, and have more tubal inflammation. In addition, chlamydial salpingitis appears to be more likely to lead to infertility. Case-control studies have documented a consistent association between high titers of antibody to *C. trachomatis* and tubal obstruction.

Another serious complication of chlamydial salpingitis is an increased risk of ectopic pregnancy, which is related directly to the damage to the oviducts. Many women who have had an ectopic pregnancy give no history of PID, but more than 20% have histopathologic and serologic evidence of chlamydial infection.

Chlamydial infection during pregnancy has been inconsistently linked to premature birth. The overall relationship, when found, has been weak and the mechanism is not understood. Late endometritis, occurring 72 hours or more after the procedure, occurs consistently in 10–30% of women with chlamydial infections who undergo induced abortion. *C. trachomatis* appears to be an important cause of postabortion complications.

Perinatal maternal-infant transmission of *C. trachomatis* can lead to neonatal inclusion conjunctivitis (Chapter 89) and pneumonia in infants (Chapter 68). The transmission rate from mother to newborn is 50–75%. Conjunctivitis occurs in 40–50% of newborns of infected mothers. The conjunctivitis may appear immediately after birth or at any time until the infant is 2 weeks of age, usually between 5 and 14 days of age. Approximately 50% of newborns of infected mothers have nasopharyngeal infections, but only about 30% of those newborns have the characteristic pneumonia (overall about 10–20% of the newborns of all infected mothers). The pneumonia has a gradual onset beginning at 4–18 weeks of age (median: 9 weeks). Pharyngeal infection for up to 3 years has been documented. Subclinical rectal and vaginal infections have been detected in 14% of infants born to *C. trachomatis*–infected women.

PROGNOSIS

Untreated *C. trachomatis* can persist for months in the female genital tract. Antimicrobial therapy is highly effective, and patients do not need to be routinely retested after completing treatment unless symptoms persist or reinfection is suspected. Results of nonculture tests may remain positive for up to 3 weeks after completion of therapy because of continued excretion of dead organisms. Some studies have reported high rates of infection among women tested several months after treatment, presumably because of reinfection. Screening high-risk populations, such as adolescents, several months after treatment may be appropriate.

PREVENTION

Ocular prophylaxis with silver nitrate solution or erythromycin or tetracycline ointments is not effective in the prevention of neonatal chlamydial conjunctivitis or pneumonia. Prenatal screening and treatment of pregnant women can prevent chlamydial infection among neonates. Pregnant women who are <25 years of age or who have new or multiple sex partners should be targeted for screening.

The mothers, and their sex partners, of infants who have chlamydial infection should be evaluated and treated for genital *C. trachomatis* infection.

GENITAL ULCERS

SYPHILIS

ETIOLOGY

Treponema pallidum, the causative agent of syphilis, is a thin, delicate organism. It varies in length from 5 to 15 μm, with a width of 0.15 μm, and is not visible by light microscopy. *T. pallidum* has tight spirals every 1.1 g along its length, giving the appearance of a helix. When seen through darkfield microscopy, the organism exhibits a spiral movement with flexion about its mid portion (Fig. 7–1). The organism divides slowly, only every 30 hours, and cannot be cultured on artificial media. Tissue culture does not sustain the growth of *T. pallidum* for long periods, and inoculation into rabbits is the only reliable means of cultivating this organism. Humans are the only natural host, although several mammals (including rabbits and monkeys) can be infected.

EPIDEMIOLOGY

Although most recognized syphilitic disease of children is congenital (Chapter 95), syphilis can be acquired by sexual contact at any age. Acquired syphilis in preadolescent children almost always is the result of sexual abuse or assault, although sexually active adolescents may acquire the disease through consensual sexual activity.

The 6,657 cases of primary and secondary syphilis reported in the United States in 1999 is the lowest number ever reported for 1 year and represents an 87% decrease from the peak of 50,223 cases reported in 1990 (Fig. 85–3). The disease has become increasingly concentrated, with rising rates in several states and cities. In 1999, half of all cases occurred in <1% of counties, with 79% of counties reporting no cases of syphilis. Rates are highest in the South. Syphilis continues to disproportionately affect minority populations, although this difference is narrowing. In 1999 the rate among blacks (15.2 cases/100,000 population) was approximately 30 times higher than for non-Hispanic whites (0.5 cases/100,000 population), in part because of poverty and lack of access to health care services, especially in the rural South. The rate among Hispanics was 1.8 cases/100,000 population. Rates historically have been higher for men, with a male-to-female ratio that peaked at 3.5:1 in 1980. This decreased to 1:1 in 1994, but rates of syphilis recently have been increasing among males, which may be attributable to outbreaks among men who have sex with men. The number of babies with congenital syphilis is known to closely parallel the rates of primary and secondary syphilis among women of childbearing age. It has risen steadily from a low of 115 cases in 1978 to a peak of 4,410 cases in 1991, followed by a decline to 529 cases in 2000 (see Fig. 95–2).

Syphilis has not been commonly reported among sexually abused children. In one study (White et al, 1983) of 409 children believed to be sexually abused, 108 had serologic tests for syphilis and 6 children had evidence of syphilis. Five children had no symptoms and had an additional STD; only one child had chancres. A subsequent study (Ingram et al, 1992a) found that only 1 of 1,263 abused children had a serologic test positive for syphilis. Children can have the same signs and symptoms as adults with syphilis, including the rashes and condylomata lata of secondary syphilis. A serologic test for syphilis should be performed for every child believed to have been sexually abused and should be repeated 12 weeks later.

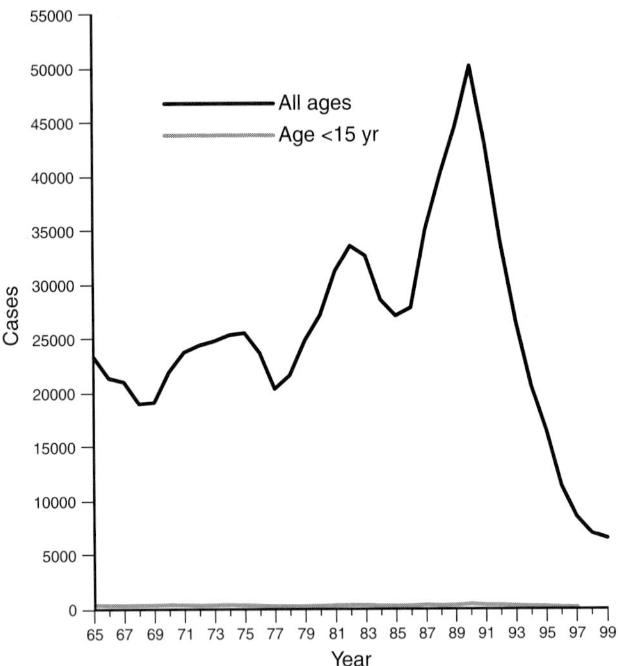

FIGURE 85–3. Reported cases of primary and secondary syphilis in the United States from 1965 to 1999. The number of cases among persons <15 years of age is no longer reported by the CDC. (Data from the Centers for Disease Control and Prevention.)

PATHOGENESIS

The central problem in understanding the pathogenesis of syphilis is that despite a vigorous host response to infection, treated disease has a minimal effect on resistance to reinfection and the infection may persist for life. Treponemes initially invade the body through microscopic abrasions produced by sexual intercourse. About one third of persons who have sex with infected partners become infected. The treponemes attach to the epithelial cells by one end, and once inside the epithelial layer, the organisms replicate locally. The host response is an influx of polymorphonuclear cells. The treponeme undergoes rapid phagocytosis, probably because host IgG is present on the surface of the organism. Lymphocytes soon replace the neutrophils. By the time the patient comes to clinical attention, a variety of antibodies are usually detected. However, the occurrence of secondary syphilis at the same time that the antibody titers are at their highest indicates that the host response to infection is not effective, because the localized disease comes under control at the same time that the manifestations of generalized infection appear. However, at this time the host is immune to intradermal challenge with *T. pallidum.* The host eventually suppresses the infection, and there are no clinically apparent lesions, although the organism is not necessarily eradicated from the body because *T. pallidum* can be isolated from patients years after acquisition.

SYMPTOMS AND CLINICAL MANIFESTATIONS

Syphilis acquired in childhood follows a course similar to that in adults. **Primary syphilis** is characterized by a painless skin lesion, known as a **chancre,** which appears at the site of contact 10–90 days (average: 21 days) after exposure (Plate 7A). Chancres are rounded, firm ulcers with a rubbery base and well-defined margins. The lesion is usually single and is most commonly found on the glans penis of the male and on the cervix or external genitalia of the female. It can also be found on the scrotum, on the anus or rectum, and on the lips, tongue, tonsils, nipples, and fingers. Primary lesions in women often go unnoticed because they may not be visible. Chancres persist for 3–6 weeks and then heal spontaneously. They are usually accompanied by early spirochetemia and regional lymphadenopathy. The lymph nodes are painless, nonfluctuant, nontender, and rubbery in consistency and often are bilaterally enlarged with genital lesions.

Manifestations of **secondary syphilis** usually appear about 3–6 weeks after the appearance of the chancre and about 6 weeks to several months after the initial contact. The primary lesion may still be evident or may have healed when the secondary lesions appear. Signs and symptoms commonly include a local or generalized rash, generalized lymphadenopathy, malaise, fever, headache, and pharyngitis. Less common manifestations are **condylomata lata** (Fig. 85–4), mucous patches of the mouth, and alopecia. This is a systemic infection with spirochetemia. It is not unusual to find pleocytosis or increased protein levels in the CSF of persons with secondary syphilis.

The skin rash is usually macular or maculopapular and rarely is pustular. The rose-pink rash spreads to involve the whole body, including the palms and soles, darkens to a dull red, and is usually not pruritic (Plate 7B). The secondary manifestations of syphilis usually resolve in 3–12 weeks.

After the secondary lesions resolve, the stage of **latent syphilis** begins. This stage is arbitrarily divided into **early latency** (syphilis <1 year's duration) and **late latency** (syphilis >1 year's duration) on the basis of the interval from diagnosis, the first symptoms of primary or secondary syphilis, or sexual contact with a partner with syphilis. During early latency about 25% of persons with untreated syphilis have relapses of secondary syphilis. By definition, latent syphilis is clinically inapparent, and the diagnosis is established only by a positive serologic test result in the absence of any primary or secondary symptoms. All untreated cases of syphilis are latent at some time during the course of the disease, and indeed the disease may be latent for the duration of the infection or the life of the patient.

Late syphilis, or **tertiary syphilis,** is an uncommon entity among adults in the antibiotic era and is extremely uncommon in children. Late syphilis is asymptomatic in most cases, but it may

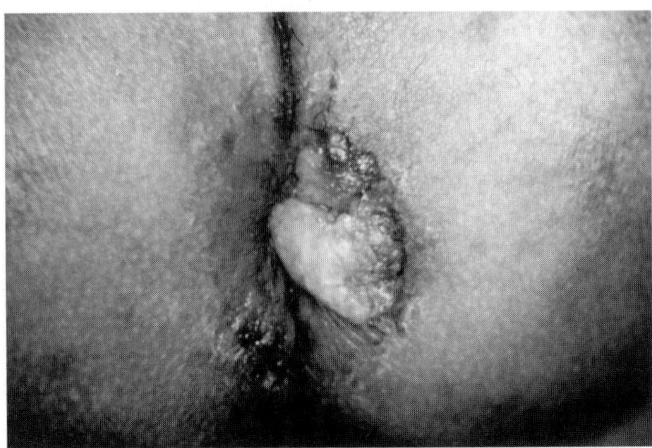

FIGURE 85–4. Perianal condylomata lata in a 3-year-old girl with syphilis. These lesions initially were thought to be condylomata acuminata. (Courtesy of Martin Finkel, MD.)

be manifested as neurosyphilis, cardiovascular syphilis, or gummas. Patients can have more than one late manifestation of syphilis. The essential pathologic process of all types of neurosyphilis is **obliterative endarteritis,** usually of terminal vessels, with associated parenchymal degeneration.

Optic atrophy, a serious complication of neurosyphilis, is detected by examination of the peripheral visual fields. Pupillary changes may be seen in late neurosyphilis. The classic change is the **Argyll Robertson pupil,** which is small and irregular and responds normally to accommodation but fails to react to light.

Acute syphilitic meningitis usually presents within a year of infection as acute hydrocephalus, cranial nerve palsies, or focal cerebral involvement. The CSF shows pleocytosis, increased protein level, and a positive VDRL test result.

In meningovascular neurosyphilis, definite signs and symptoms of central nervous system damage are present, indicating cerebrovascular occlusion, infarction, and encephalomalacia with focal neurologic signs, depending on the size and location of the lesion. The CSF is always abnormal, with pleocytosis, increased protein level, and a positive VDRL test result.

Parenchymal neurosyphilis appears as paresis or **tabes dorsalis.** The manifestations of paresis may be myriad and are always indicative of widespread damage to the parenchyma. Personality changes range from minor ones to obvious psychosis. Focal neurologic signs are uncommon. The CSF is always abnormal, with pleocytosis, increased protein level, and a positive VDRL test result.

The damage in cardiovascular syphilis is caused by medial necrosis of the aorta, with aortic dilatation often extending into the valve commissures. The essential signs are those of aortic insufficiency or saccular aneurysm of the thoracic aorta.

Gummas are nonspecific granuloma-like lesions that may represent a hypersensitivity syndrome. They are found most commonly in skin or bone and less commonly in mucosa, viscera, and muscle. The lesions are usually benign, although they may cause serious problems if located in vital areas.

DIAGNOSIS

The diagnosis of primary syphilis can be definitively established by positive results on a darkfield examination or on a direct fluorescent antibody test for *T. pallidum.* Serologic tests for syphilis are the principle means of diagnosis. However, nontreponemal serologic test results are positive for only about 80% of persons who present with primary syphilis. The treponemal test results become positive earlier than those of nontreponemal tests; about 90% of persons who present with primary syphilis have positive treponemal test results. Therefore, if primary syphilis is being considered as a diagnosis, the laboratory should be instructed to perform the treponemal test even if the nontreponemal test is nonreactive.

During secondary syphilis, *T. pallidum* can be demonstrated in any mucous or cutaneous lesion, but it is found most easily in moist lesions. The diagnosis is usually established by serologic testing during this stage, and serologic test results are virtually always positive with high titers (>1:16). In one study (Lukehart, 1988) *T. pallidum* was isolated from the CSF in 30% of persons with secondary syphilis; one third of the persons with treponemes in the CSF had normal CSF values. Nevertheless, it is not routine or recommended that lumbar punctures be performed on persons with secondary syphilis because central nervous system involvement is so common as to be considered a part of the disease.

Laboratory Evaluation

After the newborn period, all children with syphilis should have a lumbar puncture performed to evaluate central nervous system involvement. The CSF in neurosyphilis shows an increase in the number of cells, an increased protein level, and a positive VDRL test result.

Microbiologic Evaluation

Syphilis may be confirmed by the direct detection of treponemes during a darkfield or immunofluorescence examination of material obtained from lesions. It may also be confirmed with serologic nontreponemal and treponemal antibody tests to detect antibodies formed in response to a treponemal infection.

Darkfield Examination. The diagnosis of syphilis can be confirmed when treponemes are found on darkfield examination of appropriate specimens (see Fig. 7–1). This test requires a compound microscope equipped with a darkfield condenser, which illuminates the specimen by reflected light against a dark background. An experienced technician can establish a positive diagnosis on the basis of characteristic morphologic and motility features. Darkfield examination is most useful during primary, secondary, and early congenital syphilis when lesions are present. Gloves should be worn when one is examining lesions believed to be syphilitic and when one is performing darkfield examinations. Lesions should be cleaned thoroughly with physiologic saline solution with no additives. The lesion should then be squeezed and scraped firmly to collect serum rather than blood. Aspirated material from involved regional lymph nodes can also be examined for *T. pallidum,* but the specimen must be viewed within 5–10 minutes after collection to detect motile treponemes. If the initial darkfield examination has a negative result, it should be repeated on at least 2 successive days to confirm the negative result.

Immunofluorescent Antigen Detection. Alternative methods to detect *T. pallidum* in lesions are direct and indirect fluorescent antibody tests for *T. pallidum.* In these tests, either monoclonal or polyclonal antibodies directed against *T. pallidum* are directly fluorescein tagged, or a second fluorescence-tagged antibody is used to detect the antigen-antibody complex. The advantage of this method is that slides are permanent and can be mailed to reference laboratories for review by experts if the patient population is too small to warrant purchase of a darkfield microscope.

Serologic Testing. The serologic diagnosis of syphilis uses two general types of tests: **reaginic, or nontreponemal, tests** and **treponemal tests** (Table 85–5). When reaginic tests are used, serologic findings are positive for approximately 80% of persons with primary syphilis, 100% of persons with secondary syphilis, and 95% of those with early latent syphilis, but the findings are positive for only 70% of persons with late latent or late (tertiary) syphilis. Thus false-negative results on serologic reaginic tests are a problem in very early and late stages of untreated syphilis. Serologic tests for syphilis are accurate and reliable in most persons infected with HIV.

The reaginic tests use **cardiolipid lecithin** as the antigen. The antibody measured has been called **reagin,** which has no relation to the reaginic IgE in allergic persons. Antibody appears in the blood 1–3 weeks after the chancre appears, or approximately 4–6 weeks after infection. The reaginic tests commonly used are the **rapid plasma reagin (RPR) test,** the **Veneral Disease Research Laboratories (VDRL) test,** and the **automated reagin test (ART).** The RPR test and ART use a modified VDRL antigen. These two tests are useful when large numbers of sera are screened and speed is essential. The tests are inexpensive, can be well controlled, and can be quantitated. Sequential serologic tests should use the same method by the same laboratory. The VDRL and RPR tests are equally valid, but quantitative results cannot be compared directly because RPR titers are often slightly higher than VDRL titers. The

TABLE 85–5. Sensitivity of Serologic Tests for Syphilis

Test	Primary Syphilis; Secondary Syphilis; Early Latent Syphilis	Late Latent Syphilis; Tertiary Syphilis
Reaginic (Nontreponemal) Tests Rapid plasma reagin (RPR) test Veneral Disease Research Laboratories (VDRL) test Automated reagin test (ART)	80–100%	70–98%
Treponemal Tests Fluorescent treponemal antibody-absorbed (FTA-ABS) test Microhemagglutination assay for antibodies to *T. pallidum* (MHA-TP)	50–90%	98–100%

height of the titer tends to correlate with disease activity, rising with new infection and falling after treatment. A change of one doubling dilution is within laboratory error and therefore is not significant. Changes of two dilutions (fourfold changes) are considered to be significant when disease activity is assessed. These tests are not specific for syphilis and may also be reactive in persons with collagen vascular disease, liver disease, and other conditions. With adequate treatment the reaginic tests should become nonreactive 6–12 months after primary syphilis and 12–24 months after secondary syphilis. The titers of persons with later stages of syphilis who are treated take a long time to fall, and their nontreponemal tests may never revert to nonreactive. These so-called **serofast** individuals may have low titers for life.

Specific treponemal tests include the **fluorescent treponemal antibody absorption (FTA-ABS) test** and the **microhemagglutination assay for antibodies to *T. pallidum* (MHA-TP).** The MHA-TP test has essentially replaced the FTA-ABS test in most laboratories, although clinicians often use the now-obsolete term. The FTA-ABS test is an indirect antibody test that uses *T. pallidum* as the antigen; it is sensitive and specific. The MHA-TP test is technically more difficult than the nontreponemal tests and is used for confirmation of positive nontreponemal test results. The results of the MHA-TP test are reported as positive or negative, and they are not quantitated. The treponemal tests become reactive earlier in primary syphilis than do nontreponemal tests, and once results are positive, they normally remain so for life, even after appropriate therapy.

The MHA-TP test is a qualitative hemagglutination test that uses sheep erythrocytes as carriers of the *T. pallidum* antigen. False-positive results are uncommon with both the FTA-ABS and MHA-TP tests. However, persons with systemic lupus erythematosus may have false-positive results on FTA-ABS and MHA-TP tests as well as false-positive nontreponemal test results.

Another treponemal test, the ***T. pallidum* immobilization test,** has been used in the past but at present is available for research purposes only. The test uses live *T. pallidum* organisms and complement. When serum containing *T. pallidum*–specific antibody is present, the *T. pallidum* is immobilized.

For antibody testing of CSF, only a nonquantitative VDRL test should be performed. The CSF VDRL test is highly specific but is relatively insensitive (22–69%) for neurosyphilis. Use of either the RPR or FTA-ABS test for CSF is not recommended because of the high incidence of false-positive results.

TREATMENT

Parenteral penicillin G remains the drug of choice for treating all stages of syphilis (Table 85–6). There has been no evidence that *T. pallidum* is resistant to penicillin, and the drug has minimal toxicity and established efficacy. *T. pallidum* is exquisitely sensitive

TABLE 85–6. Regimens for the Treatment of Syphilis

Primary and Secondary Syphilis and Early Latent Syphilis (<1 yr in Duration)

Benzathine penicillin G 50,000 U/kg (max 2.4 MU) in a single dose IM

*Nonpregnant Adolescents and Adults with Hypersensitivity to β-lactam Antibiotics**

Doxycycline 100 mg bid PO for 2 wk

or

Tetracycline 500 mg qid PO for 2 wk

Late Latent Syphilis (≥1 yr in Duration), Latent Syphilis of Unknown Duration, Late Syphilis

Benzathine penicillin G 50,000 U/kg (max 2.4 MU) once a week IM for 3 successive doses

*Nonpregnant Adolescents and Adults with Hypersensitivity to β-lactam Antibiotics**

Doxycycline 100 mg bid PO 4 wk

or

Tetracycline 500 mg qid PO for 4 wk

Neurosyphilis

Recommended Regimen

Aqueous crystalline penicillin G 50,000 U/kg (usual adult dose: 2–4 MU; max 4 MU) q4hr IV for 10–14 days

Alternative Regimen

Procaine penicillin G 2.4 MU once daily IM plus probenecid 500 mg bid PO, both for 10–14 days

NOTE: Some experts recommend that either regimen for neurosyphilis be followed by benzathine penicillin G 50,000 U/kg (max 2.4 MU) in a single dose IM.

Pregnant Patients Allergic to β-lactam Antibiotics

NOTE: Hospitalization for desensitization and treatment with a penicillin regimen appropriate for the woman's stage of syphilis. Some experts recommend a second dose of benzathine penicillin G 2.4 MU/wk IM after the initial dose for women in the third trimester of pregnancy and for women who have secondary syphilis during pregnancy.

*There is less clinical experience with doxycycline than with tetracycline, but compliance may be better with doxycycline. Patients infected with HIV should be desensitized and treated with penicillin.

to penicillin, with an MIC of 0.0050–0.01 μg/mL. Effective therapy for syphilis has been aimed at maintaining a minimum concentration of 0.03 U/mL (0.018 μg/mL) in serum for 7–10 days because of the slow dividing time of *T. pallidum* (every 30 hours). Thus therapy is designed to achieve and maintain several times the necessary inhibitory levels. Penicillin is the only recommended treatment for syphilis in children and in pregnant women. Therefore, if there is a history of hypersensitivity to penicillin, children and pregnant women should undergo skin testing and desensitization if necessary.

Primary, secondary, and early latent syphilis of <1 year's duration in persons with normal findings on neurologic examination should be treated with benzathine penicillin G 50,000 U/kg (maximum dose: 2.4 MU) in one intramuscular dose. An alternative regimen for persons with hypersensitivity to penicillin is either doxycycline 100 mg twice a day orally for 2 weeks or tetracycline 500 mg four times a day orally for 2 weeks.

Persons with latent syphilis of more than 1 year's duration or of unknown duration who have normal findings on neurologic examination should be treated with three doses of benzathine penicillin G 50,000 U/kg (maximum dose: 2.4 MU) at weekly intervals intramuscularly for 3 consecutive weeks. Alternative therapy for persons allergic to penicillin is with doxycycline or tetracycline in the same doses used for early syphilis but given for 4 weeks instead of 2 weeks.

Any person who is thought to have neurologic involvement, including children with congenital syphilis (Chapter 95), should be treated with aqueous crystalline penicillin G 50,000 U/kg (maximum dose: 4 MU) every 4–6 hours intramuscularly for 10–14 days. Alternative therapy is procaine penicillin G 2.4 MU daily intramuscularly with probenecid 500 mg 4 times a day orally for 10–14 days. This regimen can be given on an outpatient basis if compliance can be ensured. Many experts also recommend a regimen of benzathine penicillin G 2.4 MU once intramuscularly after either of the preceding treatment regimens is completed.

Patients should be re-examined for clinical symptoms and should have repeated serologic testing at 3 and 6 months after the completion of treatment. All persons with syphilis should be strongly encouraged to have tests for infection with HIV. Persons infected with HIV who also have early syphilis have a small but appreciable increased risk of disease progression to neurosyphilis and of treatment failure; treatment of syphilis with penicillin regimens is recommended. Close clinical and serologic follow-up evaluations are essential and should be performed at 1, 2, 3, 6, 9, and 12 months after the completion of treatment.

COMPLICATIONS

There are so few data on acquired syphilis in children and adolescents that any information has to be extrapolated from experience with adults. Complications of untreated syphilis in adults consist of all the manifestations of primary, secondary, and tertiary syphilis, although this progression appears to be extremely uncommon in children. In addition, for women of childbearing age there is the possibility that their children may contract congenital syphilis and have all of its sequelae (Chapter 95).

Complications of the treatment of syphilis include drug reactions, mostly to penicillin, and the **Jarisch-Herxheimer reaction,** which is an acute febrile reaction that may occur after any effective therapy for syphilis but occurs most commonly after penicillin therapy because it is used most often. The reaction is caused by the release of pyrogen from spirochetes and starts 1–2 hours after treatment is begun. Fever, usually accompanied by headache and myalgia, usually lasts less than 24 hours. Pregnant women may develop contractions and should be warned of this possibility. No specific treatment is recommended, except the use of antipyretics if necessary.

PROGNOSIS

The prognosis for treated syphilis is excellent. Penicillin treatment of early syphilis prevents late complications of the disease. There have been a few reports of adults who have had progression to central nervous system disease after conventional therapy with benzathine penicillin for early and latent syphilis. However, only a few cases have been well documented.

The prognosis for treated syphilis among persons with HIV infection is also excellent. However, there have also been some well-documented treatment failures among HIV-infected persons treated for early and latent syphilis. The CDC has no recommendations to modify therapy for HIV-infected persons, but it is recommended that penicillin regimens be used in these persons if possible. Some experts also advise lumbar punctures or treatment with regimens appropriate for neurosyphilis in all persons with HIV infection. Persons who have both HIV and syphilis should undergo careful follow-up for early detection of treatment failure or reinfection.

Approximately one third of infected and untreated persons have late manifestations of syphilis, with characteristic central nervous system, cardiovascular, or gummatous lesions. About two thirds of untreated, infected people do not have problems later, although more than half remain seropositive. However, these persons have a shorter-than-normal life expectancy. Persons who have latent syphilis for more than 4 years rarely pass the infection to their sexual partners, but pregnant women can transmit the disease to a fetus even after having latent syphilis for many years. A pregnant woman with untreated syphilis may transmit the infection to the fetus at any clinical stage of the disease, but transmission is more likely when infection occurs early in pregnancy.

HERPES SIMPLEX VIRUS INFECTION

Infection due to HSV, although not the most prevalent sexually transmitted infection in the United States, is perhaps the most notorious. HSV infection is ubiquitous, and most people in most populations have serologic evidence of infection by adulthood. Genital herpes may be chronic and recurrent. The epidemiologic character of HSV infection is symptomatic or asymptomatic infection that is transmitted, resulting in a huge pool of latently infected individuals.

ETIOLOGY

HSV, a member of the Herpesviridae family of viruses, has a double-stranded DNA genome of 150 kilobase pairs. The two types, HSV-1 and HSV-2, differ in their antigenic and biologic properties. They share many features with the other herpesviruses, including the ability to cause latent infection with recurrence.

Transmission. The principal mode of spread is direct contact, with transmission through infected secretions. HSV-1 is transmitted primarily by contact with oral secretions, whereas HSV-2 is transmitted primarily by contact with genital secretions. However, as many as 5–30% of genital herpes infections can be caused by HSV-1, and conversely HSV-2 can cause 10–20% of cases of herpes labialis. HSV can be transmitted congenitally (Chapter 95) and perinatally to infants from mothers with genital infection (Chapter 96).

EPIDEMIOLOGY

HSV has a worldwide distribution. Humans appear to be the only natural reservoir. All ages are susceptible to infection. Currently the prevalence of HSV-2 infection is >20% among adults in the United States. Seroprevalence rates are higher in African Americans. HSV-2 seroprevalence is as high as 50% among women attending STD clinics. Most infections with HSV-2 appear to be acquired in the third decade of life, correlating with the onset of sexual activity, but recent seroprevalence studies point to a shift toward earlier acquisition. HSV-2 seroprevalence among teenagers is now >5% (4.5% among white teenagers and 9% among African Americans). HSV-2 seroprevalence has quintupled in white teenagers and has doubled among young adults in their twenties during the past 2 decades.

Fewer than 20 cases of genital herpes infections have been reported in prepubertal children. As with many of the other STDs, the possibility of sexual abuse was not mentioned in any of the cases reported before 1968. In the cases reported later, sexual abuse of most of the children was documented. HSV-1 infections in children may be acquired by nonsexual transmission, typically autoinoculation to the genital area from an oral infection, such as gingivostomatitis. Because culture specimens are usually taken only from children with a clinical presentation suggestive of genital herpes, it is not known whether a genital reservoir of HSV exists in healthy children. The risk of acquisition of HSV after sexual abuse has not been accurately determined.

PATHOGENESIS

After HSV enters the skin, it replicates locally in parabasal and intermediate epithelial cells, resulting in lysis of the infected cells and production of a local inflammatory response. The characteristic lesion of superficial HSV infection is a thin-walled vesicle on an inflammatory base. Multinucleated giant cells are formed with ballooning degeneration, marked edema, and **Cowdry type I inclusion bodies,** which are characteristic. Lymphatics and regional lymph nodes may become involved. Viremia and visceral dissemination may occur, depending on the immunocompetence of the infected person.

After primary infection, HSV may become latent within sensory nerve ganglia. Latency has been demonstrated in the trigeminal, sacral, and vagal ganglia; reactivated virus appears to spread peripherally by the sensory nerves. Recurrences of both HSV-1 and HSV-2 infections are frequent; they appear to be mostly reactivations rather than reinfections. Recurrent infections of the lips or perioral areas occur in 20–40% of the population. HSV-2 orolabial lesions recur less frequently than do HSV-1 orolabial lesions. The frequency of recurrences of genital herpes depends on the sex of the individual, the type of HSV, and both the presence and the titer of neutralizing antibody. Recurrences are more likely to develop in men than in women; are more frequent with HSV-2 than HSV-1; and develop in persons with high titers of neutralizing antibody. HSV may be transmitted during primary infections or recurrences whether or not symptoms or signs are present.

SYMPTOMS AND CLINICAL MANIFESTATIONS

Primary genital herpes infection is caused by HSV-2 in 70–95% of cases. Adolescents and young adults have the highest incidence of primary infection. The incubation period of genital herpes is 2–14 days after exposure. In males the characteristic vesicles on an erythematous base usually occur on the glans penis or penile shaft. In women the lesions may occur on the vulva, perineum, buttocks, cervix, or vagina. Persons with vaginal lesions may have a vaginal discharge. Primary genital infection is frequently associated with systemic symptoms, including fever, malaise, anorexia, and tender inguinal lymphadenopathy. Vesicles may persist in men but ulcerate rapidly in women. These lesions may be exquisitely tender. Urethral involvement can result in urinary retention. The lesions may persist for several weeks before they heal. Primary perianal and anal HSV-2 infection also can occur, particularly in men who have sex with men. Symptoms include pain, itching, tenesmus, and discharge.

The current clinical strategy for diagnosing genital HSV infection in women, which relies on clinical findings plus the selective use of viral culture, misses many cases. Asymptomatic viral shedding is common. Characteristic ulcerations of the external genitalia may be present in only two thirds of women with positive HSV culture results.

Recurrent genital herpes is generally associated with less severe systemic symptoms, less extensive local involvement, and a shorter duration of symptoms than is true of the primary infection. There may be a prodrome of tenderness, itching, burning, or tingling for several hours before the recurrence. Of the cases of genital HSV infection in abused children that were reported in the literature, more than half recurred.

DIAGNOSIS

Genital herpes, especially in young children, must be differentiated from other vesicular rashes, especially those caused by varicella-zoster virus. In older, sexually active adolescents, genital ulcers due to HSV are often difficult to differentiate from syphilis and chancroid. Coinfection is not uncommon. Detection of virus should be used in persons with lesions. The most sensitive means of diagnosis is isolation of the virus in tissue culture. Antigen tests are nearly as sensitive as culture; however, the sensitivity of these tests declines as lesions heal and is lower in persons with recurrent lesions than in those with first episodes. PCR assays are currently being evaluated but are not available commercially. Serologic testing is useful as a backup, providing one is looking for seroconversion with a type-specific test. Rises in antibody titer are not usually demonstrable during recurrences. Commercially available tests for HSV antibody do not differentiate between antibody to HSV-1 and antibody to HSV-2 in children. These tests are based on whole-virus antigen preparations, and because HSV-2 and HSV-1 are closely related antigenically and both cause lifelong infections with intermittent reactivation, differentiation by serologic testing is difficult. These tests can identify antibody to HSV only and thus are not useful as diagnostic tools. If a serologic test is performed to exclude genital herpes in a person with mild symptoms, a positive result with these tests could be due to a past oral infection with HSV-1. Several research laboratories offer tests that reliably differentiate HSV-I from HSV-2 antibodies, if necessary; these include immunoblot and assays based on the type-specific glycoprotein G (gG-2) from HSV-2 and either glycoprotein C (gC-1) or glycoprotein G (gG-1) from HSV-1. Immunoblot is expensive to perform and requires 2–5 days for screening and confirmation. Several commercial gG-based assays have been developed but are not as yet approved by the FDA. Only cultures for HSV should be used as forensic evidence of HSV infection in children who are believed to be victims of sexual abuse.

TREATMENT

Genital herpes infection is a chronic, recurrent viral disease for which no known cure exists. There are no data on the efficacy of antiviral therapy for genital herpes in children.

First Clinical Episode of Genital Herpes. Antiviral therapy for primary genital herpes with oral acyclovir in adults (Table 85–7) shortens the duration of symptoms, promotes healing, and decreases viral shedding but does not eliminate the virus from the body. For the first clinical episode in adults, the preferred regimen is oral acyclovir 400 mg three times a day for 7–10 days, initiated within 6 days of the onset of lesions; this regimen shortens the median duration of eruptions by 3–5 days and may reduce systemic symptoms. Therapy with oral acyclovir does not affect the subsequent risk, rate, or severity of recurrences. Alternative regimens include the use of famciclovir and valacyclovir. Treatment may be extended if healing is incomplete after 10 days of therapy.

Recurrent Episodes of HSV Disease. Treatment started during the prodrome or within 1 day after onset of lesions is often helpful. Daily suppressive therapy reduces the frequency of recurrences by ≥75% in persons who are subject to frequent recurrences. Safety and efficacy of daily treatment with acyclovir have been documented for as long as 6 years. Experience with famciclovir and valacyclovir is less, but these drugs also appear to be safe and well tolerated. Daily suppressive therapy has not been associated with the emergence of clinically significant acyclovir resistance among immunocompetent persons, although resistance has occurred in individuals with AIDS. Suppressive treatment with acyclovir can reduce the frequency of subclinical shedding of HSV from the genital tract by as much as 94%. Suppression of clinical and subclinical viral shedding may reduce HSV transmission, but because viral excretion may still occur at low frequency and titer during suppressive treatment, the extent to which transmission has been reduced or interrupted is not known. Patients should still use protection.

TABLE 85–7. Recommended Regimens for the Treatment of Genital Herpes Simplex Virus Infections

First Clinical Episode of Genital Herpes
Acyclovir 400 mg tid PO for 7–10 days
or
Acyclovir 200 mg 5 times daily PO for 7–10 days
or
Famciclovir 250 mg tid PO for 7–10 days
or
Valacyclovir 1 g bid PO for 7–10 days

Episodic Recurrent Infections
Acyclovir 400 mg tid PO for 5 days
or
Acyclovir 200 mg 5 times daily PO for 5 days
or
Acyclovir 800 mg bid PO for 5 days
or
Famciclovir 125 mg bid PO for 5 days
or
Valacyclovir 500 mg bid PO for 5 days

Daily Suppressive Therapy
Acyclovir 400 mg bid PO
or
Famciclovir 250 mg bid PO
or
Valacyclovir 500 mg once daily PO
or
Valacyclovir 1 g once daily PO

Severe Disease
Acyclovir 5–10 mg/kg q8hr IV for 5–7 days or until clinical resolution

Intravenous therapy should be used for persons who have severe disease or complications necessitating hospitalization, such as disseminated infection, pneumonitis, hepatitis, meningitis, or encephalitis.

COMPLICATIONS

HSV is capable of spreading to extragenital cutaneous sites, causing lesions on the groin, hands, and face (Chapter 46), and of hematogenous spread, causing systemic illnesses, including encephalitis (Chapter 55). Systemic illness is seen almost exclusively in immunocompromised persons. Women with active genital herpes at the time of delivery may transmit the agent to newborns (Chapter 97). It is estimated that the risk of transmittal of HSV to newborns is as high as 50% for women during a first episode of genital herpes; it is >3% for women with recurrent genital infections. In a large study (Brown et al, 1997) of pregnant women, 2.3% of seronegative women showed conversion to HSV-1 and 1.4% showed conversion to HSV-2 during pregnancy. Seronegative women whose sexual partners were seropositive for HSV-2 were at the highest risk: 33% showed seroconversion. Acquisition of infection with seroconversion completed before labor did not appear to affect the outcome of pregnancy, but among the infants born to nine women who acquired genital HSV infection shortly before labor, neonatal HSV infection developed in four infants, of whom one died.

PROGNOSIS

Genital herpes is a chronic remitting illness. The recurrence rate for genital herpes varies greatly, but in time clinically significant reductions in episodes occur in a majority of patients. Approximately 90% of persons with HSV-2 and 60% of persons with HSV-1 infections have recurrences within 12 months of primary infection, and approximately one third will have frequent recurrences (≥6 per year). The median number of recurrences after HSV-2 infection is approximately five episodes per year. Recurrences may be presaged by a range of symptoms, from a mild tingling sensation that occurs only hours before lesions erupt to severe pain that lasts 1–3 days before the episode. The area of involvement with recurrence is usually unilateral and is limited to a small area compared with the area of primary infection. The symptoms are usually mild, but they seem to be more severe in women than in men.

CHANCROID

ETIOLOGY

Chancroid is caused by *Haemophilus ducreyi,* a small nonmotile, gram-negative, non-spore-forming rod.

EPIDEMIOLOGY

Chancroid is prevalent in some countries but occurs with relatively low frequency in the adult population in several areas of the United

States. It also occurs in outbreaks, several of which occurred in the 1980s, especially in urban areas including Los Angeles, New York, and Miami. A total of 4,000 cases of chancroid were reported in 1990, and only 243 cases were reported in 1997. No cases of chancroid in children have been reported. Up to 10% of persons with chancroid have concomitant syphilis or HSV infection. Chancroid, like other STDs that cause genital ulcers, is also a cofactor for transmission of HIV. High rates of coinfection with HIV have been reported among individuals who have chancroid in the United States and other countries.

SYMPTOMS AND CLINICAL MANIFESTATIONS

The incubation period is usually 7 days, with a range of 3–10 days. The lesion is manifested clinically by a small inflammatory papule on the preputial orifice or frenulum in men and on the labia, fourchette, or perineal region in women. The lesion becomes pustular, eroded, and ulcerated within 2–3 days. There is also an associated painful, tender inguinal lymphadenopathy in more than 50% of cases. Unlike lymphogranuloma venereum, the ulcer of chancroid is concurrent with lymphadenopathy. Untreated infection resolves slowly for several weeks or months, or it may cause a protracted illness for several years with incomplete resolution.

DIAGNOSIS

Diagnosis of chancroid is usually made clinically by the presence of one or more painful genital ulcers that are not typical of genital herpes, together with culture of a lesion specimen that is negative for HSV and either normal darkfield examination findings of the exudate for *T. pallidum* or a serologic test negative for *T. pallidum* at least 7 days after the onset of the ulcers. Clinically the combination of a painful ulcer and suppurative inguinal lymphadenopathy is practically pathognomonic. The definitive diagnosis requires culture of *H. ducreyi* on special culture media that are not widely available commercially. Even using these media, the sensitivity is 80% or less.

TREATMENT

Treatment with several different antimicrobial agents is curative of chancroid, although scarring may result. The treatment of choice is azithromycin in a single oral dose (Table 85–8). Alternatives are ceftriaxone, ciprofloxacin, and erythromycin. Intermediate resistance to ciprofloxacin and erythromycin has been reported. All four regimens are effective for the treatment of chancroid in HIV-infected persons, although they are at increased risk of treatment failure with single-dose regimens and may require multiple doses.

TABLE 85–8. Recommended Regimens for the Treatment of Chancroid (*Haemophilus ducreyi* Infection)

Azithromycin 1 g in a single dose PO
or
Ceftriaxone 250 mg in a single dose IM
or
Ciprofloxacin* 500 mg bid PO for 3 days
or
Erythromycin base 500 mg qid PO for 7 days

*Ciprofloxacin and other quinolone antibiotics are contraindicated for pregnant and lactating women, for children, and for adolescents younger than 18 years.

Some experts recommend a 7-day course of erythromycin for chancroid in HIV-infected persons.

PROGNOSIS

Patients should be re-examined 3–7 days after the start of therapy. Ulcers will usually improve symptomatically and objectively within 3–7 days after the initiation of treatment. The time required for complete healing is dependent on the size of the ulcer; large ulcers may take up to 2 weeks to heal. Resolution of fluctuant lymphadenopathy is slower than that of ulcers, and surgical drainage may be required.

Because of the high rate of coinfection, persons with chancroid should be tested for HIV at the time of diagnosis and 3 months later if the initial HIV test result is negative.

DONOVANOSIS

ETIOLOGY

Donovanosis, also known as **granuloma inguinale** or **granuloma venereum,** is caused by an intracellular gram-negative bacterium, *Calymmatobacterium granulomatis,* formerly known as *Donovania granulomatis.* The organism cannot be cultured on standard media.

EPIDEMIOLOGY

Donovanosis is rare in the United States and developed countries. The disease is endemic in certain tropical and developing areas, including India, Papua New Guinea, central Australia, and southern Africa.

SYMPTOMS AND CLINICAL MANIFESTATIONS

The infection is only mildly contagious and causes indolent infection. The disease involves the external genitalia in approximately 90% of cases, indicating that sexual transmission is an important means of spread, although the infection may occur after close nonsexual contact and may be spread from the genitalia to the mouth.

The incubation period is 1–12 weeks. The illness begins with one or more painless ulcerative lesions without regional lymphadenopathy. The lesions are highly vascular, often with a beefy, red appearance, which bleed easily on contact. Secondary bacterial infections of the lesions can occur.

DIAGNOSIS

The diagnosis is established from the characteristic appearance of lesions in endemic areas. A Wright stain, Gram stain, or Papanicolaou smear of granulation tissue from a lesion demonstrates **Donovan bodies,** the blue- or black-staining organisms with a safety-pin appearance in the cytoplasm of mononuclear cells.

TREATMENT

Two recommended regimens are TMP-SMZ, 160 mg TMP with 800 mg SMZ twice a day orally, and doxycycline, 100 mg twice a day orally, both for a minimum of 3 weeks or until the lesions are healed. Alternative regimens include ciprofloxacin, 750 mg

TABLE 85–9. Regimens for the Treatment of Lymphogranuloma Venereum

Recommended Regimen
Doxycycline 100 mg bid PO for 21 days
Alternative Regimen
Erythromycin base 500 mg qid PO for 21 days

twice a day orally, and erythromycin base, 500 mg four times a day orally, also for a minimum of 3 weeks. An aminoglycoside, such as gentamicin 1 mg/kg every 8 hours intravenously, should be added to one of these regimens if lesions do not respond within the first few days of treatment. Treatment halts the progressive destruction of tissue, although prolonged therapy is often required for granulation and re-epithelialization of the ulcerated area. Relapses can occur 6–18 months later, despite what appears to be a good response to initial therapy, and may require re-treatment.

Sexual partners of patients with donovanosis should be evaluated, and treatment should be given if the partners have clinical signs and symptoms of infection or if the last sexual contact was within 60 days of the onset of the patients' symptoms.

LYMPHOGRANULOMA VENEREUM

Lymphogranuloma venereum (LGV) is a systemic STD caused by the **LGV biovars** of *C. trachomatis* (L_1, L_2, L_3). Approximately 20 cases of LGV have been reported in children. Fewer than 500 cases are reported in adults in the United States each year. Unlike the trachoma biovar, LGV strains have a predilection for lymph node involvement. The clinical course of LGV can be divided into three stages. The first stage is manifested by a primary lesion at the site of inoculation, a painless papule on the genitals that usually is transient. Most patients present during the second stage of lymphadenitis or lymphadenopathy with enlarging, painful buboes, usually in the groin. The nodes may break down and drain, especially in males. In females, the lymphatic drainage of the vulva is to the retroperitoneal nodes. Fever, myalgia, and headache are also common. The tertiary stage is a **genitoanorectal syndrome** with rectovaginal fistulas, rectal strictures, and urethral destruction.

The diagnosis of LGV can be established by culture of *C. trachomatis* from a bubo aspirate or by serologic testing. Most persons with LGV have complement fixation titers of >1:16. An important distinction of the clinical presentation is that in LGV the ulcer is not concurrent with the lymphadenopathy. If an ulcer is present, other conditions such as chancroid or HSV infection are more likely. The recommended therapy is doxycycline orally for 3 weeks, with erythromycin as an alternative, which is recommended for pregnant women (Table 85–9). Azithromycin may also be effective, but clinical data are lacking.

Sexual partners of patients with LGV should be evaluated, and treatment should be given if the partners have clinical signs and symptoms of infection or if the last sexual contact was within 30 days of the onset of the patients' symptoms.

VAGINAL DISCHARGE

Most cases of vulvovaginitis and vaginal discharge in children are not the result of a sexually transmitted infection. The most common causes are bacterial vaginosis or vulvovaginal candidiasis (Chapter 84). The sexually transmitted organisms that can cause vulvovaginitis are *N. gonorrhoeae, T. vaginalis,* and HSV. These are important causes of vulvovaginitis in both prepubertal and postpubertal girls. Of these STDs, trichomoniasis is typically associated with vaginal discharge.

TRICHOMONIASIS

ETIOLOGY

T. vaginalis is a flagellated, highly motile protozoan. The trophozoites of *T. vaginalis,* the only stage in the life cycle, are found in the urine of both sexes, in vaginal secretions, and in prostatic secretions. The organism is widespread in nature and was previously thought to be a harmless commensal of humans.

Transmission. Sexual transmission is most important. The organism survives for several hours in moist environments, and there is potential for nonvenereal transmission. Although nonsexual transmission of *T. vaginalis* has been reported between infected mothers and their infants at delivery, the exact risk of an infant's acquiring the infection is unknown. The presence of this organism in vaginal specimens from prepubertal girls strongly suggests sexual abuse. As with other STDs, however, perinatally acquired infection can be an important confounding variable. The duration of perinatally acquired trichomoniasis has been assumed to be very short, 2–3 months after birth, although in the authors' own experience there have been two infants with well-documented neonatal trichomonal infection that persisted for 6 and 9 months before treatment. In most reports of infection with *T. vaginalis* in prepubertal children published before 1978, the possibility of sexual activity or abuse is not discussed.

EPIDEMIOLOGY

Approximately 3 million women develop trichomoniasis in the United States annually. The incidence appears to be declining, possibly because of the frequent use of metronidazole for bacterial vaginosis. *T. vaginalis* may be associated with some cases of nongonococcal urethritis in men.

PATHOGENESIS

The organism attaches to the mucosal membranes of the urogenital tract exclusively. Trichomonal infection in women usually results in an inflammatory response with large numbers of polymorphonuclear leukocytes in the vaginal secretions. Symptoms develop within 6 months in only about one third of women with asymptomatic infections. Infections in men are usually asymptomatic.

SYMPTOMS AND CLINICAL MANIFESTATIONS

Trichomoniasis in women ranges from an asymptomatic carrier state to florid vaginal inflammation. After an incubation period of 5–38 days, most women with symptoms have a yellow-green vaginal discharge accompanied by vulvovaginal irritation and pruritus. The discharge may be malodorous and frothy, similar to that seen in bacterial vaginosis. Mild dysuria, dyspareunia, and lower abdominal pain may be present in some women with symptomatic infection. Most men infected with *T. vaginalis* are free of symptoms and present for treatment only because they are sexual partners of women with symptomatic disease. A minority of men with *T. vaginalis* infection will have nonspecific urethritis.

Infected women usually have visibly frothy, malodorous vaginal discharge with diffuse vulvar erythema and vaginal wall inflammation. On colposcopy, approximately half of infected women will have punctate hemorrhages over the cervix **(strawberry cervix)** that strongly suggest trichomoniasis.

DIAGNOSIS

Clinical diagnosis of trichomoniasis is difficult because the "classic" symptoms are similar to those of other STDs. Traditionally diagnosis of *T. vaginalis* infection has depended on the microscopic observation of motile protozoa in vaginal secretions. However, the sensitivity of this technique can vary from 38% to 82% (Fig. 85–5). Low sensitivity may be a result of the loss of motility after the organism has been removed from body temperature, which would be expected to occur during transport of the specimen to the laboratory.

Trichomonads can sometimes be seen in fresh urine sediment in urine samples collected for other purposes. Specimens can be cross-contaminated by fecal matter with a commensal species such as *Trichomonas hominis,* particularly if the specimen was obtained with a urine collection bag, as is done frequently for young girls. The only means to differentiate the two species is by the presence of an undulating membrane that extends most of the length of the organism in *T. hominis* but only half of the length of the organism in *T. vaginalis.* In addition, old urine specimens may also be contaminated with free-living flagellates, especially if the urine-collection vessel is open to the air and not sterile. The presence of trichomonads in a vaginal specimen has greater significance than trichomonads in urine.

In most reported studies, wet-mount preparations are infrequently used in the evaluation of children without symptoms who have been sexually abused and often are not used if an abused girl does not have a vaginal discharge.

Microbiologic Evaluation

Cultivation of the organism in broth media is the current gold standard. It is simple and requires as few as 300–500 trichomonads/mL of inoculum to initiate growth, but it requires 2–7 days and is not widely available to clinicians. Tissue culture has also been used and appears to be superior to both wet-mount and broth culture and detects as few as 3 organisms/mL.

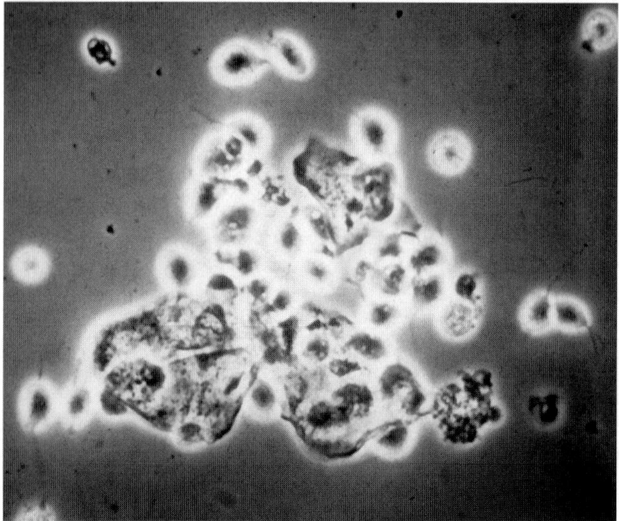

FIGURE 85–5. Photomicrograph of wet mount of vaginal secretions, demonstrating *Trichomonas vaginalis* trophozoites.

TABLE 85–10. Regimens for the Treatment of Trichomoniasis

Adult Women
Recommended Regimen
Metronidazole 2 g in a single dose PO
Alternative Regimen
Metronidazole 500 mg bid PO for 7 days
Prepubertal Girls
Metronidazole 15–35 mg/kg/day divided bid PO for 7 days

Nonculture antibody-based assays have also been developed and hold promise as rapid diagnostic tests. These include a conjugated monoclonal antibody stain, EIA, and PCR assay. None of these assays has been approved by the FDA or is available commercially.

TREATMENT

Although there are no published studies of trichomoniasis in children, trichomoniasis in adult women can be successfully treated with a single dose of metronidazole (Table 85–10). The few cases of trichomoniasis in prepubertal girls reported in the literature were treated with oral metronidazole 15–35 mg/kg/day divided twice a day for 7 days. Treatment results in microbiologic eradication, reduction of transmission, and relief of symptoms. Treatment is approximately 95% effective. There are no effective alternatives to therapy with metronidazole. Strains of *T. vaginalis* with decreased susceptibility to metronidazole have been reported. If treatment fails, the patient should be re-treated; second failures in adults may respond to a 2 g dose once a day for 3–5 days. Metronidazole should be avoided during the first trimester of pregnancy, but a single dose of 2 g in adult women may be used for those with severe symptoms after the first trimester. Lactating mothers should be given a single 2 g dose and instructed to continue to pump and discard their milk for 24 hours and then resume nursing. Metronidazole gel has been approved for the treatment of bacterial vaginosis but has not been evaluated for the treatment of vaginal trichomoniasis. Douching has no role in therapy for trichomoniasis or any other form of vulvovaginitis. Sex partners should be treated. Patients should avoid sex until they and their sex partners have completed therapy and symptoms have resolved.

COMPLICATIONS

No complications of trichomoniasis have been documented.

PROGNOSIS

The relapse rate when the 7-day course of therapy is used is very low. Occasional relapses have been observed with strains of *T. vaginalis* that have a decreased susceptibility to metronidazole. Repeated relapses may require determination of the susceptibility of *T. vaginalis* to metronidazole and should be evaluated in consultation with an infectious diseases specialist.

PREVENTION

The treatment of sex partners without symptoms, in addition to those with symptoms, is important. Douching is not effective in the prevention of any vaginal infection and may be a risk factor for upper genital tract infection. The normal vaginal flora, which plays a large part in protection against pathogenic organisms, is removed by douching and its protective efficacy is thus decreased. In addition, douching may be traumatic for small children.

HUMAN PAPILLOMAVIRUS INFECTION

ETIOLOGY

HPV, a double-stranded DNA virus, is responsible for a variety of benign proliferations, including common warts (Chapter 46) and **venereal warts,** or **condylomata acuminata.** Most of these infections are caused by HPV types 6 and 11, and smaller numbers are caused by HPV types 16 and 18. Common warts, plantar warts, and flat warts are associated with HPV types different from those that cause genital warts (see Table 46–11).

Transmission. HPV infections that cause genital papillomas in adults are transmitted by sexual intercourse and may affect the vulva, perineum, vaginal introitus, and periurethral area.

EPIDEMIOLOGY

HPV infection is the most common viral STD and is becoming recognized as one of the most frequent of all STDs; 18–33% of sexually active female adolescents have tested positive for HPV DNA in several studies. More than 80% of male partners of females with HPV are also infected with HPV; most of these infections are subclinical. Girls seem to be affected twice as frequently as boys, although this may reflect a difference in patterns of reporting rather than a true epidemiologic observation. From 24 million to 40 million people in the United States may be infected with HPV.

The causation of genital papillomas in children is less well studied, but sexual abuse by an infected adult or, less likely, contact with warts at other body sites has been suggested. The risk of genital warts in sexually abused children has not been adequately assessed because no studies include long-term follow-up data. The most important confounding variable in linking genital warts in children to sexual abuse is the possibility of perinatal acquisition. Maternal HPV infection may be more common than previously thought, and it is likely that most infections in women are asymptomatic, without macroscopically visible warts. The prolonged period of latency before the appearance of visibly detectable genital warts further complicates this issue. It is impossible to define the longest latency period between viral infection at delivery and the presence of clinical disease. When visible warts develop, the average latency period appears to be approximately 3 months, but it may be as long as 1 year or longer. Children also may have visually undetectable genital or perianal condylomata for months before close inspection such as colposcopy is performed.

There have been several published studies of anogenital warts in children and the potential relation of the warts to sexual abuse. The general conclusion reached in these studies is that anogenital warts in children may contain either skin or genital wart HPV types. Although the type of HPV may give some indication of the likely mode of transmission, the data can be interpreted only in conjunction with all available clinical and social information. The type of virus does not confirm or exclude transmission by sexual contact. The data also suggest that nonsexual transmission, including perinatal acquisition, is common, especially among children younger than 3 years. HPV can be transmitted from maternal lesions to infants at birth, causing laryngeal papillomas. However, the rate of transmission is not known.

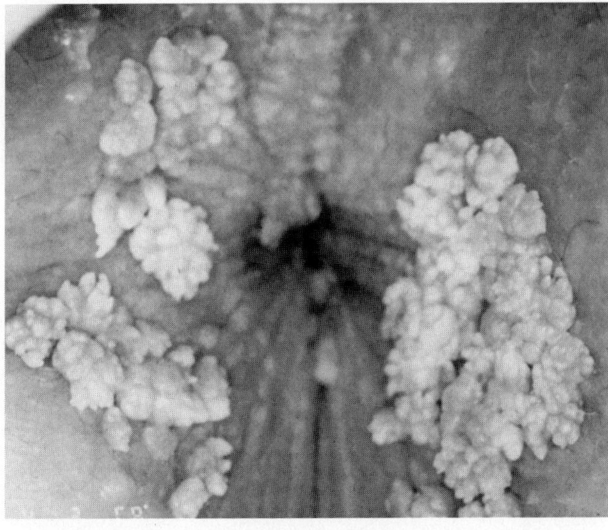

FIGURE 85–6. Perianal condylomata acuminata with multiple papillomatous lesions in an 8-year-old girl. (Courtesy of Martin Finkel, MD.)

SYMPTOMS AND CLINICAL MANIFESTATIONS

The lesions of condylomata acuminata are usually flesh-colored to purple papillomatous growths. These warts are often multiple and commonly coalesce into large masses (Fig. 85–6). In females, condylomata acuminata usually occur at the posterior part of the introitus, the adjacent labia minora, and the rest of the vestibule. Less commonly, they can be found on the clitoris, perineum, vagina, cervix, anus, and rectum. In males, venereal warts are usually localized to the penis, including the shaft, prepuce, frenulum, corona, and glans. The meatus, anus, and scrotum also may be involved. Anal warts are more commonly seen in persons who engage in anal intercourse. In contrast, many women with anal warts report no history of anal sex, suggesting autoinoculation as a mode of transmission.

The anatomic distribution may be different in prepubertal children, especially boys. Boys are less likely to have involvement of the penile shaft, prepuce, or glans, 3% as opposed to 18–52%, and are more likely to have perianal disease, 77% as opposed to 8%. Disease patterns among female patients show fewer age-related differences.

Subclinical HPV infection of the genital skin appears to be common. These lesions, known as **condylomata plana,** cannot be seen with the naked eye and require colposcopy, development of white lesions after application of acetic acid **(acetowhitening),** or cytologic studies for diagnosis. They may occur anywhere in the anogenital tract. In women they occur predominantly on the cervix, and in men they may occur anywhere on the penis, as well as on the perianal area, scrotum, and urethra.

DIAGNOSIS

Until the recent recognition that HPV infection may present subclinically, the diagnosis of condylomata acuminata was usually based on the history and appearance of the lesions. Anogenital warts must be differentiated from other papillomatous lesions, including benign and malignant neoplasms, anatomic variants, and other infectious conditions, of which the most important lesions to differentiate are condylomata lata of secondary syphilis. Because both types of lesions may coexist, serologic tests for syphilis and darkfield microscopy of likely or ulcerating lesions are necessary. Genital lesions of molluscum contagiosum can be confused with genital warts.

In adolescents and women the Papanicolaou smear is commonly used to diagnose HPV infection. The koilocyte (''balloon cell'') may be seen on a Papanicolaou smear and is pathognomonic for HPV. However, there is a subjective component to reading smears and the problem of sampling error. A normal Papanicolaou smear does not exclude HPV infection. A biopsy should be considered for any puzzling lesion.

Electron microscopy can be used to identify HPV particles in biopsy specimens. It may be especially useful in identifying lesions in children. Antigen detection and molecular hybridization techniques have shown promise in detecting HPV in scrapings and biopsy specimens from lesions. However, the same problems encountered with Papanicolaou smears are seen with these newer methods. Their diagnostic utility may be compromised by sampling error, insufficient material, or interference with large numbers of red or white blood cells that obscure visualization of the cervical epithelial cells. None of these methods has been evaluated for use with prepubertal children.

TREATMENT

None of the currently available therapies for genital warts in adults has been shown to eradicate the virus, and no single form of treatment is uniformly effective in eliminating warts and preventing recurrence. Little information is available regarding infection in children. The most commonly used treatments are topical application of podophyllin (10–25% in compound tincture of benzoin) and cryotherapy with liquid nitrogen or a cryoprobe. Podophyllin therapy is inexpensive and safe but usually requires a large number of treatments. Cryotherapy is also inexpensive but requires special equipment and training. Only about two thirds of patients respond, and about one fourth of those who respond have a recurrence. Other treatment modalities that have been used include topical 80–90% trichloroacetic acid, electrodesiccation, electrocautery, fluorouracil, and surgical removal. IFN-α has been tried but has no demonstrated advantages over other treatment modalities for condylomata acuminata. Intralesional IFN-α may be helpful for some persons. Treatment of genital warts in children can be complicated and should be carried out in consultation with a dermatologist.

Asymptomatic genital HPV infection without exophytic warts is very common. Infection may be suggested by Papanicolaou smear, but this finding does not correlate very well with the presence of HPV DNA in cervical cells. The importance of HPV DNA in cervical cells is uncertain, but screening and initiation of therapy based on such findings are not recommended.

COMPLICATIONS AND PROGNOSIS

HPV types 16 and 18 have been associated with genital carcinomas, particularly cervical carcinoma (Chapter 4). HPV structural antigens and DNA have been found in the lesions of cervical intraepithelial neoplasia, which precedes the development of frank cervical carcinoma. HPV antigens and DNA have been found in specimens of invasive carcinoma and in specimens of anal, vulvar, vaginal, and penile carcinomas. Numerous HPV types have been cultured from skin carcinomas, usually occurring at sun-exposed sites, in persons with epidermodysplasia verruciformis.

SEXUALLY TRANSMITTED INFECTIONS AND SEXUAL ASSAULT

Sexual assault is a violent crime that affects men, women, and children of all ages. Every state has laws requiring the reporting of child abuse if there is reasonable suspicion, but the exact requirements vary from state to state. Any STD may be transmitted during sexual assault, but the risk varies considerably (Table 85–11). In children, the isolation of a sexually transmitted organism may be the first indication that abuse has occurred. Most sexually abused children do not present with genital complaints initially, and typically they have normal findings on physical examination.

The identification of a sexually transmissible agent from a child older than a newborn suggests sexual abuse, but exceptions do exist. The most notable exception is rectal and genital infection with *C. trachomatis,* which may be due to a persistent perinatally acquired infection that may continue for as long as 3 years. Bacterial vaginosis has been identified in both abused and nonabused children. *Gardnerella vaginalis* may be isolated from vaginal specimens in as many as 37% of postmenarchal girls who are not sexually active (median age: 15.9 years; range: 13–21 years). The finding of genital warts, although suggestive of abuse, is nonspecific without supportive findings.

The incidence and prevalence of sexual abuse of children are difficult to estimate because much sexual abuse of children escapes detection. Several relatively extensive studies of sexual abuse of children in the United States have examined sex, race, and age-dependent variables. Patterns of sexual abuse of children appear to depend on the sex and age of the victim. About 80–90% of abused children are girls, with a mean age of 7–8 years, and 75–85% were abused by a male assailant, adult or minor, known to the child. This assailant is most likely to be a family member, especially the father or father substitute (e.g., stepfather, mother's boyfriend), uncle, or other male relative. Victims of strangers or unknown assailants tend to be older than the children abused by a known person, and usually only a single episode of abuse occurs. In contrast, abuse by family members or acquaintances usually involves multiple episodes for periods ranging from 1 week to years.

Most victims describe a single type of sexual activity, but more than 20% have experienced multiple types of forced sexual acts. Vaginal penetration has been reported to occur in approximately 50% and anal penetration in 33% of female victims. More than

TABLE 85–11. Approximate Risk (%) of Becoming Infected During One Act of Unprotected Intercourse with an Infected Person

Organism	Male-to-Female Transmission	Female-to-Male Transmission
Neisseria gonorrhoeae	50	25
Chlamydia trachomatis	40	20
Treponema pallidum (syphilis)	30	20
Herpes simplex virus	30	30
Haemophilus ducreyi (chancroid)	30	15
Human papillomaviruses (genital warts)	10	10
Hepatitis B virus	10	5
Human immunodeficiency virus (AIDS)	1	<1

50% of male victims have experienced anal penetration. Other types of sexual activity include orogenital contact in 20–50% of victims, and fondling. Children who are abused by a known assailant usually have less physical trauma than victims of assault by a stranger.

An accurate determination of the risk of sexually transmitted conditions in victims of sexual abuse has been hindered by a variety of factors. The prevalence of sexually transmitted infections may vary regionally. It is frequently difficult to differentiate between infections existing before the abuse and those resulting from the abuse. The presence of pre-existing infection in adults is usually related to prior sexual activity. In children, pre-existing infection may be related to prolonged colonization after perinatal acquisition, inadvertent nonsexual spread, prior peer sexual activity, or prior sexual abuse. The incubation periods for STDs range from a few days for *N. gonorrhoeae* to several months for HPV. The incubation periods and the timing of an examination after an episode of abuse are critical in detecting infections.

Multiple episodes of sexual abuse have been found to increase the risk of infection, probably by increasing the number of contacts with an infected person. In most cases the site of infection is consistent with the child's history of assault. Rates of infection also vary with respect to the type of assault initially described. Vaginal or rectal penetration is more likely to lead to detectable infection than is fondling. However, most children who are abused have no physical complaints related either to trauma or to infection. The reported incidence of specific STDs among sexually abused children is 5–20% for gonorrhea, approximately 2–3% for *C. trachomatis* infection, and <1% for syphilis.

A team of professionals experienced in dealing with the special needs of sexually abused children best treats them. Because a child's report of abuse may not be complete, cultures for *N. gonorrhoeae* should be obtained from the pharynx and rectum as well as from the vagina (girls) or urethra (boys) (Table 85–12). Cultures for *C. trachomatis* should also be obtained from the rectum but not from the pharynx because the latter site correlates poorly with sexual activity. Testing should be done by culture using standard methods; identification of inclusions by microscopic examination should be used only as an ancillary test. An internal pelvic examination is usually not necessary unless a foreign body or trauma is suspected. Testing for hepatitis B and HIV should be based on the prevalence of infection in the population and on the probable risk for the individual patient. Testing for these infections must be immediate to document seronegative status at the time of the sexual assault. The tests should be repeated 6 months after the initial tests to document or exclude infection. Seropositivity at the time of initial presentation represents past infection, sexually transmitted or otherwise. Seroconversion in the few months after the episode of sexual assault may suggest infection by sexual transmission, but it does not exclude acquisition by a nonsexual route.

Consideration should also be given to screening for HIV infection in victims of sexual assault, including children. Although no studies have documented the risks of transmission in this situation, there have been individual reports in which acquisition through sexual assault seemed likely. Because HIV, like hepatitis B, can be transmitted through homosexual or heterosexual activity, screening for infection may be indicated in any form of sexual assault, which should be considered an epidemiologic risk factor for HIV infection.

TABLE 85–12. Recommended Laboratory Testing of Sexually Abused Children

Cultures for *Neisseria gonorrhoeae*
Vagina (girls)
Urethra (boys)
Throat
Rectum
Cultures for *Chlamydia trachomatis*
Vagina (girls)
Urethra (boys)
Rectum
Culture of cutaneous lesions (if any) for herpes simplex virus
Examination of wet mount of vaginal wash
Trichomonads (trichomoniasis)
Clue cells (bacterial vaginosis)
Serum syphilis serologic tests (RPR or VDRL)
Serum HBsAg and anti-HBs
Serum HIV antibody
Serum sample saved (frozen) for later serologic testing, if needed

REVIEWS

Centers for Disease Control and Prevention: 1998 Guidelines for the treatment of sexually transmitted diseases. *MMWR Morb Mortal Wkly Rep* 1998;47(RR-1):1–116.

Chernesky MA: Nucleic acid tests for the diagnosis of sexually transmitted diseases. *FEMS Immunol Med Microbiol* 1999;24:437–46.

Holmes KK, Sparling PF, Mårdh P-A, et al (editors): *Sexually Transmitted Diseases,* 3rd ed. New York, McGraw-Hill, 1999.

KEY ARTICLES

Gonorrhea

American Academy of Pediatrics, Committee on Child Abuse and Neglect: Gonorrhea in prepubertal children. *Pediatrics* 1998;101:134–5.

Ingram DL, Everett VD, Flick LA, et al: Vaginal gonococcal cultures in sexual abuse evaluations: Evaluation of selective criteria for preteenaged girls. *Pediatrics* 1997;99:E8.

Ison CA, Dillon JA, Tapsall JW: The epidemiology of global antibiotic resistance among *Neisseria gonorrhoeae* and *Haemophilus ducreyi. Lancet* 1998;351:8–11.

McClure EM, Stack MR, Tanner T, et al: Pharyngeal culturing and reporting of pediatric gonorrhea in Connecticut. *Pediatrics* 1986;78:509–10.

Rawstron SA, Hammerschlag MR, Gullans C, et al: Ceftriaxone treatment of penicillinase-producing *Neisseria gonorrhoeae* infections in children. *Pediatr Infect Dis J* 1989;8:445–8.

Shafer MA, Irwin CE, Sweet RL: Acute salpingitis in the adolescent female. *J Pediatr* 1982;100:339–50.

Walker CK, Workowski KA, Washington AE, et al: Anaerobes in pelvic inflammatory disease: Implications for the Centers for Disease Control and Prevention's guidelines for the treatment of sexually transmitted diseases. *Clin Infect Dis* 1999;28:S29–36.

Whittington WL, Rice RJ, Biddle JW, et al: Incorrect identification of *Neisseria gonorrhoeae* from infants and children. *Pediatr Infect Dis J* 1988;7:3–10.

Chlamydia trachomatis Infection

Beck-Sague CM, Farshy CE, Jackson TK, et al: Detection of *Chlamydia trachomatis* cervical infection by urine tests among adolescents clinics. *J Adolesc Health* 1998;22:197–204.

Black CM: Current methods of laboratory diagnosis of *Chlamydia trachomatis* infections. *Clin Microbiol Rev* 1997;10:160–84.

Burstein GR, Gaydos CA, Diener-West M, et al: Incident *Chlamydia trachomatis* infections among inner-city adolescent females. *JAMA* 1998; 280:521–6.

Burstein GR, Zenilman JM: Nongonococcal urethritis—a new paradigm. *Clin Infect Dis* 1999;28:S66–73.

Centers for Disease Control and Prevention: Recommendations for the prevention and management of *Chlamydia trachomatis* infections, 1993. *MMWR Morb Mortal Wkly Rep* 1993;42(RR-12):1–39.

Cohen DA, Nsuami M, Etame RB, et al: A school-based *Chlamydia* control program using DNA amplification technology. *Pediatrics* 1998;101:E1.

Gaydos CA, Crotchfelt KA, Howell MR, et al: Molecular amplification assays to detect chlamydial infections in urine specimens from high school female students and to monitor the persistence of chlamydial DNA after therapy. *J Infect Dis* 1998;177:417–24.

Hammerschlag MR, Ajl S, Laraque D: Inappropriate use of nonculture tests for the detection of *Chlamydia trachomatis* in suspected victims of child sexual abuse: A continuing problem. *Pediatrics* 1999;104:1137–9.

Porder K, Sanchez N, Roblin PM, et al: Lack of specificity of Chlamydiazyme for detection of vaginal chlamydial infection in prepubertal girls. *Pediatr Infect Dis J* 1989;8:358–60.

Rietmeijer CA, Yamaguchi KJ, Ortiz CG, et al: Feasibility and yield of screening urine for *Chlamydia trachomatis* by polymerase chain reaction among high-risk male youth in field-based and other nonclinic settings. A new strategy for sexually transmitted disease control. *Sex Transm Dis* 1997;24:429–35.

Syphilis

Berry CD, Hooten TM, Collier AC, et al: Neurologic relapse after benzathine penicillin therapy for secondary syphilis in a patient with HIV infection. *N Engl J Med* 1987;316:1587–9.

Centers for Disease Control and Prevention: Primary and secondary syphilis—United States, 1999. *MMWR Morb Mortal Wkly Rep* 2001;50:113–7.

Davis LE, Schmitt JW: Clinical significance of cerebrospinal fluid tests for neurosyphilis. *Ann Neurol* 1989;25:50–5.

Hart G: Syphilis tests in diagnostic and therapeutic decision making. *Ann Intern Med* 1986;104:368–76.

Hook EW III, Marra CM: Acquired syphilis in adults. *N Engl J Med* 1992;326:1060–9.

Jaffe HW, Kabins SA: Examination of cerebrospinal fluid in patients with syphilis. *Rev Infect Dis* 1982;4:S842–7.

Johns DR, Tierney M, Felsenstein D: Alteration in the natural history of neurosyphilis by concurrent infection with the human immunodeficiency virus. *N Engl J Med* 1987;316:1569–72.

Klein VR, Cox SM, Mitchell MD, et al: The Jarisch-Herxheimer reaction complicating syphilotherapy in pregnancy. *Obstet Gynecol* 1990; 75:375–80.

Lukehart SA, Hook EW, Baker-Zander SA, et al: Invasion of the central nervous system by *Treponema pallidum:* Implications for diagnosis and treatment. *Ann Intern Med* 1988;109:855–62.

Mohr JA, Griffiths W, Jackson R, et al: Neurosyphilis and penicillin levels in cerebrospinal fluid. *JAMA* 1976;236:2208–9.

Schroeter AL, Turner RH, Lucas JB, et al: Therapy for incubating syphilis. Effectiveness of gonorrhea treatment. *JAMA* 1971;218:711–3.

Tramont EC: Syphilis in the AIDS era. *N Engl J Med* 1987;316:1600–1.

Herpes Simplex Virus Infection

Ashley RL, Wald A: Genital herpes: Review of the epidemic and potential use of type-specific serology. *Clin Microbiol Rev* 1999;12:1–8.

Benedetti J, Corey L, Ashley R: Recurrence rates in genital herpes after symptomatic first-episode infection. *Ann Intern Med* 1994;121:847–54.

Brock BV, Selke S, Benedetti J, et al: Frequency of asymptomatic shedding of herpes simplex virus in women with genital herpes. *JAMA* 1990;263:418–20.

Brown ZA, Selke S, Zeh J, et al: The acquisition of herpes simplex virus during pregnancy. *N Engl J Med* 1997;337:509–15.

Bryson Y, Dillon M, Bernstein DI, et al: Risk of acquisition of genital herpes simplex virus type 2 in sex partners of persons with genital herpes: A prospective couple study. *J Infect Dis* 1993;167:942–6.

Fleming DT, McQuillan GM, Johnson RE, et al: Herpes simplex virus type 2 in the United States, 1976 to 1994. *N Engl J Med* 1997;337:1105–11.

Kaplan KM, Fleisher GR, Paradise JE, et al: Social relevance of genital herpes simplex in children. *Am J Dis Child* 1984;138:872–4.

Koelle DM, Benedetti J, Langenberg A, et al: Asymptomatic reactivation of herpes simplex virus in women after the first episode of genital herpes. *Ann Intern Med* 1992;116:433–7.

Koutsky LA, Stevens CE, Holmes KK, et al: Underdiagnosis of genital herpes by current clinical and viral-isolation procedures. *N Engl J Med* 1992;326:1533–9.

Wald A: New therapies and prevention strategies for genital herpes. *Clin Infect Dis* 1999;28:S4–13.

Chancroid

Haydock AK, Martin DH, Morse SA, et al: Molecular characterization of *Haemophilus ducreyi* strains from Jackson, Mississippi, and New Orleans, Louisiana. *J Infect Dis* 1999;179:1423–32.

Kunimoto DY, Plummer FA, Namaara W, et al: Urethral infection with *Haemophilus ducreyi* in men. *Sex Transm Dis* 1988;15:37–9.

Schmid GP: Treatment of chancroid, 1997. *Clin Infect Dis* 1999;28:S14–20.

Schmid GP, Sanders LL Jr, Blount JH, et al: Chancroid in the United States. Reestablishment of an old disease. *JAMA* 1987;258:3265–8.

Trees DL, Morse SA: Chancroid and *Haemophilus ducreyi:* An update. *Clin Microbiol Rev* 1995;8:357–75.

Donovanosis

Lal S, Nicholas C: Epidemiological and clinical features in 165 cases of granuloma inguinale. *Br J Venereal Dis* 1970;46:461–3.

Rosen T, Tschen JA, Ramsdell W, et al: Granuloma inguinale. *J Am Acad Dermatol* 1984;11:433–7.

Lymphogranuloma Venereum

Abrams AJ: Lymphogranuloma venereum. *JAMA* 1968;205:199–202.

Schachter J, Osoba AO: Lymphogranuloma venereum. *Br Med Bull* 1983;39:151–4.

Trichomoniasis

Jones JG, Yamauchi T, Lambert B: Trichomonas vaginalis infestation in sexually abused girls. *Am J Dis Child* 1985;139:846–7.

Krieger JN, Tam MR, Stevens CE, et al: Diagnosis of trichomoniasis. Comparison of conventional wet-mount examination with cytologic studies, cultures, and monoclonal antibody staining of direct specimens. *JAMA* 1988;259:1223–7.

Petrin D, Delgaty K, Bhatt R, et al: Clinical and microbiological aspects of *Trichomonas vaginalis. Clin Microbiol Rev* 1998;11:300–17.

Wolner-Hanssen P, Krieger JN, Stevens CE, et al: Clinical manifestations of vaginal trichomoniasis. *JAMA* 1989;261:571–6.

Human Papillomavirus Infection

Beutner KR, Wiley DJ, Douglas JM, et al: Genital warts and their treatment. *Clin Infect Dis* 1999;28:S37–56.

Boyd AS: Condylomata acuminata in the pediatric population. *Am J Dis Child* 1990;144:817–24.

Cohen BA, Honig P, Androphy E: Anogenital warts in children. Clinical and virologic evaluation for sexual abuse. *Arch Dermatol* 1990;126:1575–80.

Cripe TP: Human papillomaviruses: Pediatric perspectives on a family of multifaceted tumorigenic pathogens. *Pediatr Infect Dis J* 1990;9:836–44.

Gutman LT, St Claire K, Herman-Giddens ME, et al: Evaluation of sexually abused and nonabused young girls for intravaginal papillomavirus infection. *Am J Dis Child* 1992;146:694–9.

Ho GY, Bierman R, Beardsley L, et al: Natural history of cervicovaginal papillomavirus infection in young women. *N Engl J Med* 1998;338: 423–8.

Moscicki AB, Palefsky J, Gonzales J, et al: Human papillomavirus infection in sexually active adolescent females: Prevalence and risk factors. *Pediatr Res* 1990;28:507–13.

Moscicki AB, Shiboski S, Broering J, et al: The natural history of human papillomavirus infection as measured by repeated DNA testing in adolescent and young women. *J Pediatr* 1998;132:277–84.

Obalek S, Jablonska S, Favre M, et al: Condylomata acuminata in children: Frequent association with human papillomaviruses responsible for cutaneous warts. *J Am Acad Dermatol* 1990;23:205–13.

Sedlacek TV: Advances in the diagnosis and treatment of human papillomavirus infections. *Clin Obstet Gynecol* 1999;42:206–20.

Siegfried E, Rasnik-Conley J, Cook S, et al: Human papillomavirus screening in pediatric victims of sexual abuse. *Pediatrics* 1998;101:43–7.

Watts DH, Koutsky KL, Holmes KK, et al: Low risk of perinatal transmission of human papillomavirus: Results from a prospective cohort study. *Am J Obstet Gynecol* 1998;178:365–73.

Sexually Transmitted Infections and Sexual Assault

Beck-Sague CM, Solomon F: Sexually transmitted diseases in abused children and adolescent and adult victims of rape: Review of selected literature. *Clin Infect Dis* 1999;28:S74–83.

Gardner JJ: Comparison of the vaginal flora in sexually abused and non-abused girls. *J Pediatr* 1992;120:872–7.

Gellert GA, Durfee MJ, Berkowitz CD: Developing guidelines for HIV antibody testing among victims of pediatric sexual abuse. *Child Abuse Negl* 1990;14:9–17.

Glaser JB, Hammerschlag MR, McCormack WM: Epidemiology of sexually transmitted diseases in rape victims. *Rev Infect Dis* 1989;11:246–54.

Hammerschlag MR: Sexually transmitted diseases in sexually abused children: Medical and legal implications. *Sex Transm Infect* 1998;74:167–74.

Hampton HL: Care of the woman who has been raped. *N Engl J Med* 1995:332:234–7.

Ingram DL, Everett VD, Lyna PR, et al: Epidemiology of adult sexually transmitted disease agents in children being evaluated for sexual abuse. *Pediatr Infect Dis J* 1992a;11:945–50.

Ingram DL, White ST, Lyna PR, et al: *Gardnerella vaginalis* infection and sexual contact in female children. *Child Abuse Negl* 1992b;16:847–53.

Jenny C, Hooten TM, Bowers A, et al: Sexually transmitted diseases in victims of rape. *N Engl J Med* 1990;322:713–6.

Neinstein LS, Goldenring J, Carpenter S: Non-sexual transmission of sexually transmitted diseases: An infrequent occurrence. *Pediatrics* 1984;74:67–76.

Seigel RM, Schubert CJ, Myers PA, et al: The prevalence of sexually transmitted diseases in children and adolescents evaluated for sexual abuse in Cincinnati: Rationale for limited STD testing in prepubertal girls. *Pediatrics* 1995;96:1090–4.

White ST, Loda FA, Ingram DL, et al: Sexually transmitted diseases in sexually abused children. *Pediatrics* 1983;72:16–21.

CHAPTER 86

Osteomyelitis

Kathryn S. Moffett ▪ Stephen C. Aronoff

Osseous infections in childhood frequently present a distinct diagnostic challenge to the clinician. The bacterial causes, clinical manifestations, and initial management vary with the patient's age, the pathogenesis of the infection, the duration of infection, and the presence of specific predisposing factors. There are five discernible syndromes of pediatric osteomyelitis: (1) acute systemic disease, or **hematogenous osteomyelitis,** characterized by systemic symptoms and often accompanied by bacteremia; (2) subacute focal disease that usually follows local inoculation and is devoid of systemic symptoms; (3) chronic osteomyelitis that is the result of an untreated or inadequately treated bone infection; (4) sternal infection after a cardiac operation; and (5) neonatal osteomyelitis.

ETIOLOGY

In infancy and childhood, acute systemic disease is the most common form of osteomyelitis (Table 86–1). Although *Staphylococcus aureus* is the most common cause of this form of the disease in otherwise healthy children, group A *Streptococcus* and *Streptococcus pneumoniae* are frequently encountered in young children, particularly those with concomitant suppurative arthritis. The incidence of osteomyelitis due to *Haemophilus influenzae* has been virtually eliminated since the introduction of the conjugate vaccine. Persons with hemoglobinopathies, typically sickle cell disease, have an increased risk of infections, including osteomyelitis, caused by *Salmonella.*

Subacute focal infections usually occur in ambulatory persons who sustain **puncture wounds** of the feet. *Pseudomonas aeruginosa* and *S. aureus* are the most common pathogens in this clinical setting. Anaerobic species are also encountered but in a different clinical setting. Chronic disease may result from infection with any pathogen. In most cases *S. aureus* is recovered, although *P. aeruginosa* has also been implicated. **Multifocal recurrent osteomyelitis** is a poorly understood syndrome characterized by recurrent episodes of fever, bone pain, and radiographic findings of osteomyelitis; no pathogen has been identified as the cause of this syndrome.

Osseous infections after cardiac operations may be caused by a variety of pathogens. In most series, *S. aureus* and *P. aeruginosa* predominate, although coagulase-negative staphylococci have been encountered after a common-source outbreak. These same pathogens occur in sporadic cases of sternal osteomyelitis.

Neonatal osteomyelitis is caused by the same pathogens responsible for neonatal sepsis (Chapter 96). In most series, group B *Streptococcus* is the predominant pathogen, although *S. aureus, Escherichia coli,* and *Candida* account for many infections. Premature infants and infants requiring indwelling catheters or undergoing repeated instrumentation, particularly blood sampling from the heel, are at increased risk of having bacteremia and hematogenous skeletal infections. Neonatal bone infections in neonates are usually acquired nosocomially rather than vertically, and they usually become clinically apparent after the first 2 weeks of life.

EPIDEMIOLOGY

Osteomyelitis is an uncommon disease of childhood. Accurate prevalence data, particularly nationwide, are unavailable. The majority of children with acute systemic disease are younger than 5 years. Osteomyelitis accounts for approximately 0.015% of hospitalized children.

PATHOGENESIS

Acute systemic disease is the result of osseous seeding from a hematogenous source. Most healthy children younger than 10 years in whom osteomyelitis develops have an antecedent or concurrent episode of bacteremia. Although a history of penetrating trauma

TABLE 86–1. Infectious Causes of Osteomyelitis in Children

Disease Type	Frequency
Acute Systemic	
Staphylococcus aureus	25–60
Haemophilus influenzae type b*	4–12
Streptococcus pneumoniae	2–5
Group A *Streptococcus*	2–4
Mycobacterium tuberculosis	<1
Neisseria meningitidis	<1
Salmonella†	<1
None identified	10–15
Subacute Focal	
Pseudomonas aeruginosa	ND
S. aureus	ND
Sternal Osteomyelitis‡	
P. aeruginosa	37
Staphylococci	30
Enterobacteriaceae	18
Enterococcus	1
Neonatal Osteomyelitis§	
S. aureus	53
Group B *Streptococcus*	23
Enterobacteriaceae	13
None identified	11

ND = insufficient data.
*Incidence greatly reduced since introduction of the conjugate vaccine.
†Particularly in persons with hemoglobinopathies.
‡Adapted from Siegman-Igra Y, Shafir R, Weiss J, et al: Serious infectious complications of midsternotomy: A review of bacteriology and antimicrobial therapy. *Scand J Infect Dis* 1990;22:633–43.
§Adapted from Nelson JD: Skeletal infections in children. *Adv Pediatr Infect Dis* 1991;6:59–78.

is rare in acute systemic disease, blunt trauma frequently precedes clinical manifestations of bone infection, but the causal relationship is uncertain. Because *S. aureus* expresses a unique receptor for fibronectin, it has been suggested that blunt trauma exposes collagenous fibronectin, enhancing bacterial adherence. In children beyond the newborn period and without hemoglobinopathies, bone infections are found almost exclusively in the metaphysis. Sluggish blood flow through tortuous vascular loops unique to this site in long bones is one explanation for this phenomenon. Osseous infections in children with sickle cell disease occur in the diaphyseal portion of the long bones, probably as a consequence of antecedent focal infarction.

Group A *Streptococcus* is the most frequent cause of osteomyelitis in children with varicella. Osteomyelitis caused by *H. influenzae* type b and *S. pneumoniae* in young children with concomitant adjacent suppurative arthritis most likely represents initial hematogenous seeding of the joint space, with subsequent spread to underlying bone. In older children osteomyelitis is typically unifocal, without accompanying joint-space infection. A unique syndrome of **flat bone osteomyelitis** (skull, vertebrae, and ribs) has been identified in persons with indwelling venous catheters and among abusers of intravenous drugs. In these persons, bone infection is believed to follow repeated episodes of low inoculum bacteremia.

Subacute focal disease follows direct inoculation of bone or spread of infection from an adjacent, nonosseous focus. The most commonly encountered example of this form of infection occurs in older children and adolescents and follows penetrating trauma of the foot through an athletic shoe with a foam innersole. Under these circumstances, *P. aeruginosa* is directly inoculated into bone or cartilage from the foam padding of the shoe. The resulting infection develops as **osteochondritis** involving both bone and cartilage with accompanying erythema and swelling. Osteomyelitis of the hand after human bites or closed-fist injuries or after animal bites usually results from either direct inoculation of bone or spread of infection from adjacent soft tissue. Osteomyelitis of the skull is usually the result of localized spread from adjacent infected sinuses or dental abscesses.

Sternal Osteomyelitis. Sternal osteomyelitis after cardiac operation represents extension of a severe wound infection into bone. The soft tissue infections may follow intraoperative contamination, usually resulting in coagulase-negative staphylococcal infections, or may follow perioperative contamination with endogenous flora, as occurs in persons requiring prolonged hospitalization. Persons with diabetes mellitus or those receiving corticosteroid therapy in the immediate postoperative period are at increased risk of having sternal osteomyelitis.

Neonatal Osteomyelitis. Neonatal osteomyelitis appears to be a late sequela of recognized or occult bacteremia. Unlike containment of acute hematogenous osteomyelitis in older children, communication in neonates of metaphyseal and epiphyseal vessels across the cartilage precursor of the ossification nucleus permits epiphyseal involvement and destruction of the epiphysis, leading to involvement of adjacent bone spaces and concomitant suppurative arthritis. Approximately 40% of cases of neonatal osteomyelitis have multiple osseous foci of infection with involvement of the adjacent joint spaces.

Chronic Osteomyelitis. Chronic osteomyelitis is the end result of long-standing untreated or inadequately treated osseous infection. With time the products of infection gradually destroy bone, producing focal necrosis. **Sequestra,** or portions of avascular bone that have separated from adjacent bone, are frequently covered with a thickened sheath, or an **involucrum.**

SYMPTOMS AND CLINICAL MANIFESTATIONS

Focal pain and decreased use of an affected extremity are the most common presenting complaints among neonates, infants, children, and adolescents with osteomyelitis (Table 86–2). The femur, tibia, or humerus is affected in approximately 67% of patients. In this same population infections of the bones of the hands or feet account for an additional 15% of cases. Flat bone infections, including the bones of the pelvis, account for approximately 10% of pediatric osseous infections.

Symptoms in children with acute systemic osteomyelitis reflect the accompanying bacteremia and bone involvement. The abrupt onset of fever and, less commonly, anorexia, irritability, lethargy, and vomiting accompanies focal tenderness of the involved bone, pain on passive motion of an extremity, or a limp. Soft-tissue swelling, local erythema, and drainage are not seen in the early stages of this form of the disease but may be present in subacute focal, sternal, or chronic osteomyelitis. After the newborn period, most otherwise healthy children older than 3 years with the acute systemic form of osteomyelitis have unifocal disease without accompanying joint space infection. In children younger than 3 years, osteomyelitis due to *H. influenzae* or *S. pneumoniae* is often accompanied by an adjacent joint space infection. With *H. influenzae,* multiple osseous sites of infection occur in approximately 25% of cases. Young children with *H. influenzae* type b osteomyelitis should be examined closely for evidence of other focal infections, such as meningitis, pericarditis, or epiglottitis. Young children with *S. pneumoniae* osteomyelitis often have a history of chest wall abscesses. Bone infection should be suspected in any child with varicella who has joint pain, refuses to bear weight, or has fever or re-emergence of fever beyond the first 3 days of varicella illness.

In contradistinction, the subacute focal form of osteomyelitis is characterized by the insidious onset of local symptoms without systemic manifestations of infection. Adolescents who have had puncture wounds of the foot may have persistent or intermittent pain for months before seeking medical advice. Fever may be present, but other systemic signs are typically absent in these persons, whereas localized soft-tissue swelling, erythema, and occasionally drainage may be found. Among persons in whom osteomyelitis develops after an animal or human bite, as a complication of a sinus or dental infection, or after a gunshot wound, the signs and symptoms of local soft-tissue infection often mask the signs of underlying bone involvement. An unusually long duration of focal symptoms is often the first clue to bone infection in these cases.

Although definitions vary depending on the series, chronic osteomyelitis represents recurrent or persistent symptoms of localized bone infection extending for a period of months or years. Two clinical patterns of staphylococcal disease have been described. The least common form of the disease is manifested by persistent localized pain and swelling, often limiting use of the affected limb. The more common form of chronic staphylococcal osteomyelitis is characterized by intermittent exacerbations of localized pain. In both conditions the same site is recurrently or persistently involved in time. Persons with recurrent multifocal osteomyelitis have intermittent symptoms that may include acute episodes of fever but that differ from chronic staphylococcal osteomyelitis in that (1) multiple sites of involvement are identified clinically or radiographically, (2) the lesions are sterile, and (3) draining sinuses are rarely seen.

TABLE 86–2. Comparison of Osteomyelitis in Children

	Neonates and Young Infants* (<3 mo)	Acute Systemic Osteomyelitis in Children†	*Pseudomonas* Osteochondritis‡
Signs and Symptoms at Presentation			
Pain, swelling, tenderness	64%	94%	100% met at least 3 of 4 criteria being present
Fever	45%	85%	
Cellulitis or deep soft tissue infection	NR	NR	
Laboratory or radiographic evidence of skeletal infection			
Erythrocyte sedimentation rate ≥20 mm/hr	70%	89%	91%
Bone destruction by radiography	NR	6%	14%
Increased uptake on bone scan	32–84%	99%	95%
White blood cell count >11,000/mm³	NR	31%	NR
Local changes, erythema	30%	69%	NR
Irritability, lethargy	36%	4–12%	0%
Anorexia	Common	10%	NR
Vomiting	NR	3%	NR
Puncture wound to foot	Rare association with heel sticks	NR	100%
Bone Sites	Femur>humerus>tibia	Femur>tibia>humerus	Metatarsal>calcaneus>small bones of feet
Multifocal	22–47%	3.7%	None
Positive Culture Results			
Blood	71%	30%	NR
Bone	90%	51%	100%
Contiguous Joint Involved	28–76%	18%	22%
Risk Factors	Abnormal delivery Prematurity Invasive catherization	Blunt trauma Sickle cell disease	Puncture wound through shoe (especially rubber-soled shoes)
Male:Female Ratio	1:1.2	1.5:1	1.9:1

NR = not reported.
*Data from Asmar BI: Osteomyelitis in the neonate. *Infect Dis Clin North Am* 1992;6:117–32.
†Data from Faden H, Grossi M: Acute osteomyelitis in children. Reassessment of etiologic agents and their clinical characteristics. *Am J Dis Child* 1991;145:65–9.
‡Data from Jacobs RF, McCarthy RE, Elser JM: *Pseudomonas* osteochondritis complicating puncture wounds of the foot in children: A 10-year evaluation. *J Infect Dis* 1989;160:657–61.

Sternal Osteomyelitis. Sternal osteomyelitis after an open-chest operation is a relatively early complication of sternal wound infection. Clinically, bone involvement is indistinguishable from the wound infection except by radiographic evaluation. Fever is common, as are purulent wound drainage and localized pain.

Neonatal Osteomyelitis. Neonatal osteomyelitis typically occurs in infants 2–8 weeks of age and is often unaccompanied by systemic signs of infection such as fever or irritability. In these cases, bone infection is considered likely by the presence of pseudoparesis or pseudoparalysis of an extremity, which is partial or complete loss of spontaneous movement of the affected extremity. Joint space involvement with effusion, limitation of motion, warmth, and pain on passive movement accompanies bone infection in most cases. Radiographic or clinical evaluation often demonstrates multiple bone sites.

Pelvic Osteomyelitis. Pelvic osteomyelitis is rare in children. The principal manifestations are fever and gait disturbance. Physical examination may reveal focal tenderness and pain with hip abduction. Radiographs of the pelvis demonstrate bone destruction within several weeks of the onset of illness.

Vertebral Osteomyelitis. Vertebral osteomyelitis is rare in children and is typically a complication of diskitis (Chapter 88). Pott's disease is a form of cervical vertebral osteomyelitis caused by *Mycobacterium tuberculosis.*

DIAGNOSIS

The diagnosis of osteomyelitis should be considered for any child with acute or chronic pain of bone origin. In most cases of acute systemic disease, the onset of symptoms is abrupt and includes systemic manifestations of the disease. Besides fever, a single focus of point tenderness at the site of infection is typically elicited. The differential diagnosis (Table 86–3) of hematogenous osteomyelitis includes bacterial sepsis, occult bacteremia in children younger than 2 years, leukemia, cancer of bone origin, and collagen vascular

TABLE 86–3. Differential Diagnosis of Osteomyelitis in Children

Other Infectious Syndromes
Bacteremia or sepsis
Cellulitis
Wound infection
Fasciitis
Pyomyositis
Septic arthritis
Diskitis
Parameningeal abscess
Mediastinitis
Iliopsoas abscess
Malignant Neoplasms
Primary or metastatic bone tumors
Acute leukemia
Rheumatic Diseases
Juvenile rheumatoid arthritis
Other collagen vascular diseases
Other Conditions
Trauma (subacute focal)
Congenital bone cysts
Neuropathies (neonates)

diseases, particularly juvenile rheumatoid arthritis. Because persons with subacute focal and chronic osteomyelitis present with focal pain and tenderness in the absence of systemic symptoms, these forms of osteomyelitis must be differentiated from soft-tissue infections, bone cysts, malignant neoplasms, trauma, and recurrent, multifocal osteomyelitis. Postoperative sternal osteomyelitis often heralds bacterial mediastinitis. Neonatal osteomyelitis often presents as lack of movement of an extremity without systemic manifestations and must be distinguished from birth trauma.

Laboratory Evaluation

Laboratory testing frequently occurs during an initial evaluation of suspected osteomyelitis, and normal values may be found. An elevated WBC count is helpful; however, 60% of children with proven acute hematogenous osteomyelitis have a total WBC count less than 10,000/mm^3 at presentation. Therefore a normal WBC count does not exclude the diagnosis of osteomyelitis.

Elevated acute-phase reactants, including ESR and CRP, are sensitive but nonspecific findings of osteomyelitis. The ESR and CRP values are elevated in 92% and 98%, respectively, of persons with acute systemic osteomyelitis at presentation, reaching a peak on days 3–5 and day 2, respectively. An increase in ESR of ≥20 mm/hr is usually seen 24 hours or more after the onset of signs and symptoms of acute disease. The CRP value has proved to be an especially useful marker in invasive bacterial infections of childhood, especially osteomyelitis. Sequential determination of ESR and CRP are of clinical value in monitoring the course of the illness. The CRP levels tend to rise faster and also diminish faster with effective therapy, compared with the ESR, which may remain elevated for several days after clinical improvement resulting from effective therapy.

Microbiologic Evaluation

Direct subperiosteal or metaphyseal aspiration with a needle is the definitive procedure for establishing the diagnosis of osteomyelitis. Needle aspirates of possible sites not only confirm the diagnosis but provide bacteriologic culture and drainage of pus. Identification of bacteria in aspirated material by Gram stain may establish the diagnosis within hours of clinical presentation.

Cultures from closed aspirates of bone at the site of infection show positive results in 70–85% of cases, and blood culture results are positive in approximately 50–66% of cases. Adequate surgical drainage should follow bone aspiration if significant pus accumulation is found at the site of closed aspiration. Surgical drainage and débridement is recommended in the following situations: (1) presence of grossly purulent material at the time of diagnostic bone tap, (2) persistence of bacteremia after 48 hours of adequate parenteral therapy, (3) extension of pain along the shaft of the bone in the presence of adequate therapy, (4) extension of the infection to the adjacent joint, and (5) failure of acute systemic symptoms and laboratory markers to resolve in a reasonable amount of time despite adequate therapy. In young children with osteomyelitis caused by *H. influenzae* type b or *S. pneumoniae,* cultures of other potentially infectious foci (cerebrospinal fluid, joint fluid, and chest wall abscesses) may also yield the pathogen. In the other forms of childhood osteomyelitis, acute-phase reactants are often normal, and only cultures of bone yield the offending pathogen.

Diagnostic Imaging

Plain radiographs are a useful initial study for confirming the site of osseous infection in preparation for needle aspiration or open débridement (Figs. 86–1 and 86–2; Fig. 13–32). Although the earliest radiographic finding of acute systemic osteomyelitis is **loss of the periosteal fat line,** focal osseous destruction is the most common finding in persons with this form of osteomyelitis and with symptoms that last more than 2–3 weeks. **Periosteal elevation** and **periosteal destruction** are late findings in bone infections. **Brodie's abscess** is a subacute intraosseous abscess that does not drain into the subperiosteal space, clasically located in the distal tibia. **Involucra** and **sequestra** are hallmarks of chronic disease (Fig. 13–34).

Early in the course of osteomyelitis, plain radiographs may be normal. ^{99m}Tc bone scans are useful for confirming the site of osteomyelitis in persons who have had symptoms for less than 2 weeks, and the scans are particularly helpful in establishing the diagnosis of multifocal disease. These scans may be falsely negative in neonates and in persons with long-standing infection and devitalized bone. In questionable cases, subsequent total body or focused scans with ^{67}Ga or ^{111}In may be used to confirm the diagnosis (Fig. 13–32). In most cases, follow-up plain radiographs obtained well into therapy demonstrate bone changes consistent with infection and confirm the diagnosis. MRI detects change in the bone marrow, reflecting the inflammation of osteomyelitis, and is very sensitive, especially in the early stages of infection. MRI is especially useful for identifying adjacent soft-tissue infections, differentiating diskitis and disk-space infections (Chapter 88) and paraspinal infections from vertebral osteomyelitis, and diagnosing osteomyelitis of the pelvis (Fig. 13–31). CT can demonstrate bone changes in most cases of osteomyelitis but is not as sensitive as MRI.

Because malignant disease is often a concern in children with focal bone pain and radiographic evidence of destruction, a bone biopsy is often required to establish the final diagnosis. In children with acute systemic disease, evidence of acute inflammation is usually seen. In long-standing disease, neutrophil and monocyte infiltration and localized necrosis may be demonstrated; periosteal involvement and devitalized, separated bone (sequestrum) is often seen in chronic infections. Necrotizing granulomas are characteristic of chronic disease caused by *M. tuberculosis.*

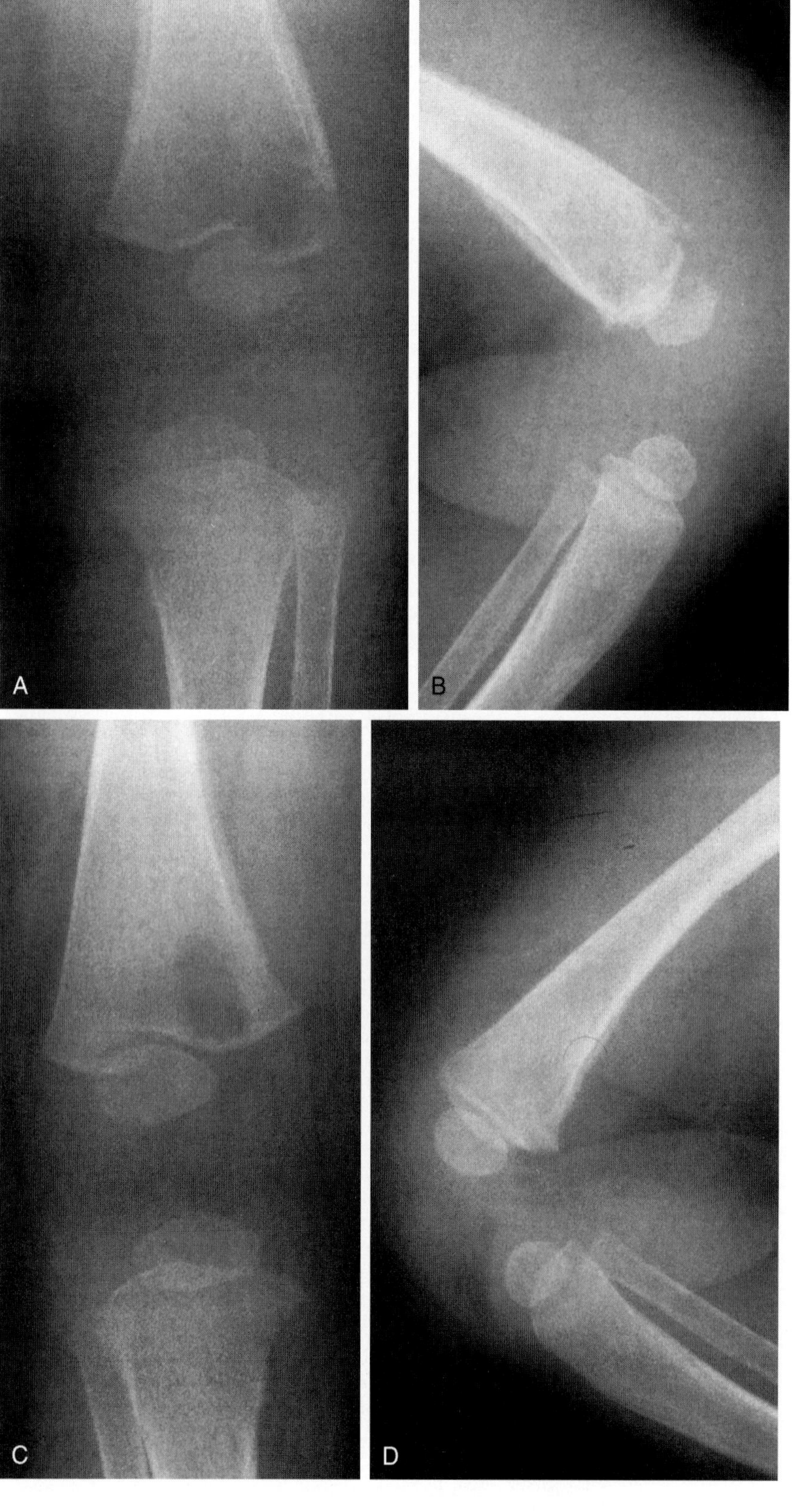

FIGURE 86–1. Multifocal acute osteomyelitis in a 3-week-old infant with multiple joint swelling and generalized malaise. Frontal **(A)** and lateral **(B)** radiographs of the left knee show focal destruction of the distal femoral metaphysis with periosteal reaction and generalized soft tissue swelling. Frontal **(C)** and lateral **(D)** views of the right knee show an area of focal bone destruction at the distal femoral metaphysis with periosteal reaction and medial soft-tissue swelling. Needle aspiration of multiple sites revealed *Staphylococcus aureus.*

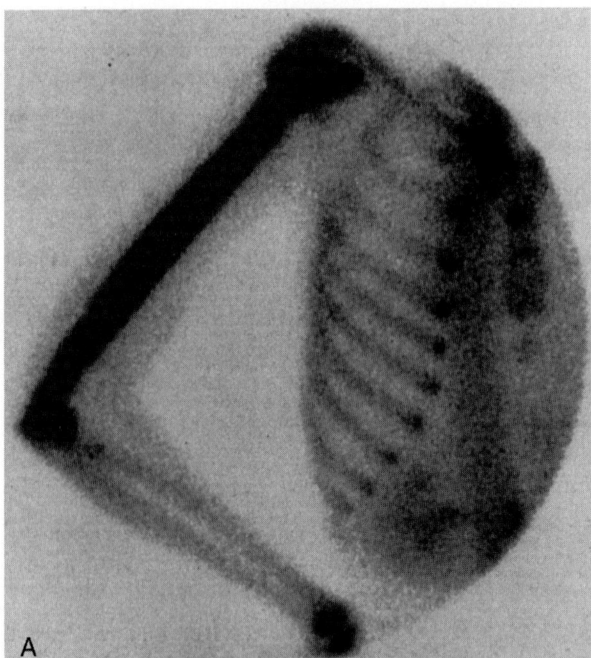

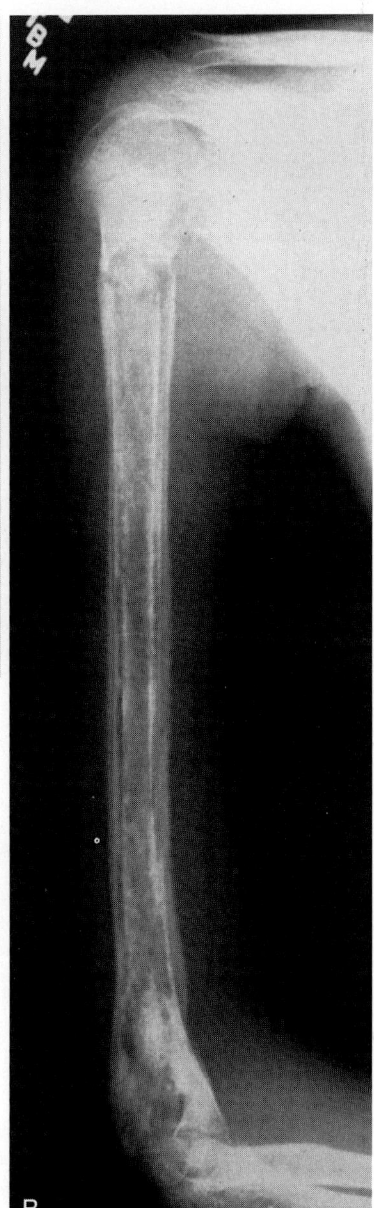

FIGURE 86–2. Chronic osteomyelitis due to *Salmonella* in a patient with sickle cell anemia. Teenaged girl with several months of pain and swelling of the right arm. **A,** ^{99m}Tc radionuclide bone scan shows strong uptake of radionuclide by the entire right humerus. **B,** Corresponding radiograph of the right humerus shows extensive periosteal reaction and destruction of bone throughout the diaphysis. It is interesting that the ends of the bone are relatively spared, considering the considerable involvement of the shaft.

TREATMENT

Management of pediatric bone infections requires close cooperation and communication between the pediatrician or infectious disease specialist and the orthopedist. In persons with all forms of childhood osteomyelitis, blood cultures and often bone cultures should be obtained before the initiation of antimicrobial therapy. Closed aspiration of bone is frequently necessary for establishing the diagnosis, identifying the bacterial pathogen, and determining the need for further surgical intervention. Definitive antimicrobial therapy for all forms of childhood osteomyelitis consists of antimicrobial therapy directed against the identified pathogen (Table 86–4).

Definitive Treatment

Initial antibiotic treatment is based on the likelihood of specific pathogens, given the patient's clinical presentation and the results of Gram stain of aspirated material. Older children with acute systemic disease should receive empirical parenteral therapy directed against *S. aureus,* such as a semisynthetic antistaphylococcal penicillin (oxacillin or nafcillin) or first-generation cephalosporin (cefazolin). For persons with β-lactam hypersensitivity, clindamycin is recommended because vancomycin achieves poor intraosseous drug concentrations. For osteomyelitis in children younger than 3 years and in persons with hemoglobinopathy, empirical treatment needs to be broadened to include *S. pneumoniae,* such as with cefotaxime or ceftriaxone. In a child who has been fully immunized for *H. influenzae* type b, empirical coverage for *H. influenzae* type b is not necessary.

Limited data exist as to the optimal treatment of osteomyelitis due to strains of *Streptococcus pneumoniae* not susceptible to penicillin, in comparison with penicillin-susceptible strains. A recent prospective study (Bradley et al, 1998) of 21 children with acute hematogenous osteomyelitis due to *S. pneumoniae,* included nine children with strains not susceptible to penicillin. Parenteral antibiotic treatment for nonsusceptible strains did not differ from treat-

TABLE 86–4. Recommended Antibiotic Therapy for Osteomyelitis in Children

	(Initial) Parenteral Therapy		Oral Therapy*	
Etiologic Agent	Recommended	Alternative	Recommended	Alternative
Acute Hematogenous Osteomyelitis				
Staphylococcus aureus	Nafcillin (*or* oxacillin) *or* cefazolin	Clindamycin	Cephalexin *or* dicloxacillin	Clindamycin
Streptococcus pneumoniae	Penicillin *or* ceftriaxone (*or* cefotaxime)	Clindamycin (*or* vancomycin)	Amoxicillin	Clindamycin
Group A *Streptococcus*	Penicillin G	Clindamycin	Amoxicillin	Clindamycin
Haemophilus influenzae type b†	Ceftriaxone (*or* cefotaxime)	Chloramphenicol	Chloramphenicol	—
Subacute Focal Osteomyelitis				
Pseudomonas aeruginosa (puncture wound osteomyelitis)	Ceftazidime *or* piperacillin-tazobactam *and* aminoglycoside	Aztreonam	—	—
S. aureus	Nafcillin (*or* oxacillin) *or* cefazolin	Clindamycin	Cephalexin *or* dicloxacillin	Clindamycin
Sternal Osteomyelitis				
P. aeruginosa	Ceftazidime *or* piperacillin-tazobactam and aminoglycoside	Aztreonam	—	—
S. aureus	Nafcillin (*or* oxacillin) *or* cefazolin	Clindamycin	—	—
Neonatal Osteomyelitis‡	Nafcillin (*or* oxacillin) *and* cefotaxime (*or* ceftriaxone)§	Cefotaxime	—	—

*Change to oral therapy only after clinical and laboratory response to parenteral therapy.
†Incidence greatly reduced since introduction of conjugate vaccine.
‡Use lower dose and longer dosing interval for neonates, especially for those younger than 7 days; see Chapter 14 and Table 96–5).
§Should not be administered in presence of hyperbilirubinemia, especially to premature neonates.

Suggested Dosages for Persons with Normal Renal Function

ANTIBIOTIC	DOSAGE	MAXIMUM DAILY DOSE
Parenteral Therapy		
Amikacin	22.5 mg/kg/day divided q8–12hr IV	750–900 mg
Aztreonam	90–120 mg/kg/day divided q6–8hr IV	6 g
Cefotaxime	200 mg/kg/day divided q6hr IV	12 g
Ceftriaxone	100 mg/kg/day divided q12hr IV or IM	3–4 g
	or 80 mg/kg/day divided q24hr IV or IM	3–4 g
Chloramphenicol	75–100 mg/kg/day divided q6hr IV	2–4 g
Gentamicin	7.5 mg/kg/day divided q8hr IV	250–300 mg
Nafcillin	150–200 mg/kg/day divided q6hr IV	9 g
Oxacillin	150–200 mg/kg/day divided q6hr IV	12 g
Penicillin G	250,000–500,000 units/kg/day divided q6hr IV	20–24 MU
Tobramycin	7.5 mg/kg/day divided q8hr IV	250–300 mg
Vancomycin	45–60 mg/kg/day divided q6hr IV	2 g
Oral Therapy		
Amoxicillin	90 mg/kg/day divided three times a day PO	1.5 g
Cephalexin	100–150 mg/kg/day divided q6hr PO	2 g
Chloramphenicol	75 mg/kg/day divided q6hr PO	2–4 g
Clindamycin	30 mg/kg/day divided q6hr PO	1.2 g
Dicloxacillin	100 mg/kg/day divided q6hr PO	2 g

ment for penicillin-susceptible strains. There were no microbiologic failures, and there were similar clinical responses to therapy, with no differences in complications or long-term sequelae. In contrast, a retrospective study (Abbasi et al, 1996) of pneumococcal bone and joint infections reported that two thirds of children with pneumococcal infections due to non-penicillin-susceptible strains had slow clinical response to antimicrobial therapy. Because penicillin, clindamycin, and β-lactam antibiotics achieve excellent penetration into bone and joints, they remain the treatment of choice for pneumococcal infections.

Initial therapy is administered parenterally and is continued until clinical symptoms resolve. Since the mid-1980s it has become conventional to complete therapy for hematogenous osteomyelitis by the oral route on an outpatient basis. Because of the serious complications of inadequately treated osteomyelitis and because the outcome of parenteral therapy is generally excellent, oral therapy should be considered only if the following criteria can be fulfilled: (1) a pathogen has been isolated or the person is in a group in which *S. aureus is* the most likely pathogen; (2) most of the presenting symptoms have responded to parenteral therapy; (3) an effective oral agent is available and is tolerated by the person; (4) compliance is ensured; and (5) the CRP level has returned to normal.

Once oral therapy is begun, peak and trough **serum bactericidal titers,** or **Schlichter titers,** may be determined by using a fixed inoculum of the person's own isolate or reference strain of *S. aureus* and serial dilutions of the persons's serum. A reliable laboratory should perform this test. Studies in children have demonstrated that a peak titer ≥1:8 constitutes effective dosing. Conversely, in adults trough titers ≤1:2 have been associated with an increased risk of treatment failure. Thus peak titers ≥1:8 with demonstrated trough activity should provide adequate dosing for children with osteomyelitis.

The authors of one study (Peltola et al, 1997) have recommended that treatment of childhood osteomyelitis be simplified by keeping surgery to a minimum, shortening hospitalization and the course of antimicrobials, switching to the oral route early, and not monitoring serum bactericidal activity. No failure rate or long-term sequelae were described, although caution must be used in universally adopting such recommendations. Unless all five criteria are met, completion of therapy should be by the parenteral route. In most of these cases, parenteral therapy may be completed outside the hospital under adequate supervision, such as by a home intravenous therapy technician or the experienced personnel of a specialty clinic.

Quinolones have been used in adults for treatment of osteomyelitis but are not currently recommended for persons <18 years of age. The once-daily administration of ceftriaxone suggests its use for treatment of acute hematogenous osteomyelitis. However, treatment of *S. aureus* infection with ceftriaxone has not been adequately studied for efficacy or long-term sequelae, and many superior antistaphylococcal agents with proven efficacy are available.

The optimal duration of antimicrobial therapy for acute systemic disease is controversial. An early retrospective study (Dich et al, 1975) demonstrated an increased risk of recurrence in children who received therapy for less than 3 weeks. In another retrospective study (Syrogiannopoulos and Nelson, 1988) of osteomyelitis caused by *S. aureus,* the median treatment duration ranged from 24 days for staphylococcal and streptococcal infections to 17 days for bone infections caused by *H. influenzae* type b. In a recent prospective study (Peltola et al, 1997) by the Finnish Study Group, the mean duration of antimicrobial treatment was 23 days. The mean or median duration of intravenous therapy was not stated, but the change from intravenous to oral therapy was 4 days or less in 85% of patients.

In general, a period of 24–28 days of therapy is reasonable in a person whose symptoms have resolved rapidly during therapy and who has had a normal ESR, CRP level, and peripheral WBC count for at least 1 week before to discontinuation of therapy. In the Finnish Study Group trial (Peltola et al, 1997) the CRP value normalized in 9 days and the ESR normalized in 21–29 days. The measurement of ESR and CRP values may be useful every 2–3 days during initial diagnosis and management and weekly until normalization. These acute-phase reactants are not meant to replace the clinical examination but are meant as an aid to guide treatment duration.

Early normalization of CRP values is encouraging information and may be a good prediction of appropriate treatment and response to therapy. Prolonged elevation of CRP values has been shown to distinguish a complicated course of acute systemic osteomyelitis. In the child hospitalized for suppurative arthritis, a delay in normalization of CRP values should prompt suspicion of a contiguous osteomyelitis. Young infants with hip or shoulder infection and those with a slow clinical response to therapy should be considered at high risk of having osteomyelitis. Treatment in these children may need longer therapy (4–6 weeks) to ensure adequate treatment. Waiting for normalization of the ESR is a conservative end point. However, because potential lifelong disability can occur with relapse of infection, treatment should be continued until normalization of the ESR for at least 1 week before therapy is discontinued.

Plain radiographs may not reveal bone changes in acute systemic disease until at least 7–14 days after symptoms develop. In the Finnish Study Group trial (Peltola et al, 1997), lytic x-ray changes were found in 19% of cases on admission; 68% had positive radiologic findings by day 29. Radiographic findings were still positive in 52% at 3 months and in 23% at 1 year after hospitalization, with no correlation to patient outcome.

Puncture Wound Osteomyelitis. Bone infections complicating puncture wounds of the foot require empirical coverage for *P. aeruginosa* and *S. aureus.* Although a variety of options are available for empirical coverage of these organisms, the combination of clindamycin, piperacillin-tazobactam, or ceftazidime and an aminoglycoside is recommended. For pseudomonal puncture-wound osteomyelitis or osteochondritis of the foot, meticulous surgical débridement, followed by 7–10 days of parenteral therapy with piperacillin or ceftazidime and an aminoglycoside, is therapeutically definitive. Conversely, a period of parenteral therapy as long as 8 weeks has been recommended for children with puncture-wound osteomyelitis who do not undergo surgical débridement. Oral therapy with ciprofloxacin has been evaluated only in a small number of cases. Because of the potential for cartilaginous injury in children <18 years of age receiving quinolones and because *Pseudomonas* appears to develop resistance to these agents rapidly, quinolones are not recommended for *Pseudomonas* osteochondritis.

Osteomyelitis of the hand after human bites or osteomyelitis complicating sinusitis or odontogenic infections requires antistaphylococcal and antianaerobic therapy. Empirical treatment with cefoxitin or clindamycin is recommended. Anaerobic osteomyelitis complicating human or animal bites should be treated parenterally for 4–6 weeks. The lack of applicable data coupled with the technical difficulty of performing serum bactericidal titers against anaerobic organisms precludes the use of oral therapy in this patient population.

Osteomyelitis complicating cat or dog bites is often caused by *Pasteurella multocida,* an organism sensitive to penicillin G.

Sternal Osteomyelitis. Osteomyelitis of the sternum is a difficult disease to treat; it requires aggressive surgical and medical management. Initially the sternal wound is opened and all sutures and wires are removed. The need for definitive surgical intervention is based on the extent of disease. Limited infections require local débridement, and moderate infections require resection of usually less than half of the sternum. In severe cases, extensive resection of the sternum and portions of the attached ribs is required to remove all devitalized tissue. After the appropriate surgical procedure, the chest wall is reconstructed with autologous muscle flaps.

Sternal osteomyelitis may be caused by a variety of pathogens; however, *S. aureus,* coagulase-negative staphylococci, and *P. aeruginosa* predominate. Vancomycin provides adequate initial coverage against both *Staphylococcus* species, with nafcillin or oxacillin recommended susceptible strains. In the case of possible *Pseudomonas* infections, administration of piperacillin-tazobactam or ceftazidime combined with an aminoglycoside is appropriate. Aztreonam may be substituted for the β-lactam component of therapy for persons with β-lactam hypersensitivity. In the rare cases in which *Enterococcus faecalis* or *Enterococcus faecium* is believed to be causative, ampicillin with an aminoglycoside is recommended.

Identification of the causative organism directs the selection of antimicrobial agents, although the route and duration of therapy are largely empirical. Persons with uncomplicated mild or moderate sternal osteomyelitis may be treated successfully with 3–6 weeks of parenteral antimicrobial therapy. Persons with extensive bone infection or accompanying mediastinitis require an extensive course of therapy. For infections caused by *S. aureus,* 2 weeks of parenteral oxacillin or nafcillin, followed by 3 months of oral therapy with cephalexin or clindamycin, may be necessary. For *Pseudomonas* infections, parenteral therapy may need to be continued for a total of 3–4 months. Completion of therapy with oral quinolones is not recommended because few data are available and because these agents are not currently approved for use in persons <18 years of age.

Neonatal Osteomyelitis. Neonatal osteomyelitis may be treated empirically with oxacillin or nafcillin plus cefotaxime, or with cefotaxime alone, although few comparative data are available regarding the treatment of neonatal skeletal infections. Definitive antimicrobial therapy is based on the culture results. Because no data are available that address oral therapy for this entity, the 4- to 6-week course of treatment is usually administered intravenously. Because of the absence of comparative data, surgical débridement remains an integral component of the management of these infections.

Chronic Osteomyelitis. The definitive treatment of chronic staphylococcal osteomyelitis requires extensive débridement with resection of involucrum, sequestrum, and all devitalized bone. Effective treatment of this infection requires a prolonged course of antimicrobial therapy. Several authorities recommend at least 1 month of parenteral drug administration followed by an additional 6–10 months of effective oral therapy (defined by the criteria outlined previously). Although chronic, recurrent, multifocal osteomyelitis is believed to be of noninfectious origin, at least one reported instance was caused by *Mycoplasma hominis* and responded to antimicrobial therapy. Most cases are also treated symptomatically with nonsteroidal anti-inflammatory agents.

COMPLICATIONS

Recurrent infection and loss of function of the affected extremity are the most common complications of childhood osteomyelitis. Recurrent infection with development of chronic osteomyelitis, manifested by a pattern of constant or intermittent symptoms, occurs in approximately 4% of acute systemic infections despite adequate therapy. Of these cases, approximately 25% fail to respond to extensive surgical débridement and prolonged antimicrobial therapy, resulting in ultimate bone loss or sinus tract formation. Extensive resection and bone grafting may eliminate the infection at the expense of extremity function. In rare instances, amputation may be required.

Sequelae of skeletal infections may not be apparent for months or years because children are in a dynamic state of growth. Therefore long-term follow-up is important. Because the metaphyseal growth plate is involved in most patients with the common childhood form of osteomyelitis and in neonates, loss of longitudinal bone growth with ultimate limb shortening is an unpreventable, well-identified complication.

Comparison of rates of complications of osteomyelitis in the literature is difficult because the definition of the term *complication* varies widely from study to study, there is no obvious method of separating complications of osteomyelitis from complications of inadequate treatment, and inadequate long-term follow-up results in a lack of information on sequelae. Most studies report a complication rate in children of 4–10%. In neonates, severe sequelae related to retarded growth of an affected bone may reach 40–50%. There is essentially no mortality rate for persons who receive treatment.

Children with recurrent multifocal osteomyelitis often have recurrences of focal symptoms. Although this entity was originally believed to be benign and self-limited, in one series (Jurik, 1988), five of eight patients continued to have recurrences 3–7 years after onset. Permanent complications of this disorder included persistent or progressive bone lesions, leading to thoracic outlet obstruction, premature epiphyseal closure, pathologic fractures, and valgus deformities.

PROGNOSIS

Prompt diagnosis, surgical drainage if necessary, and antimicrobial therapy are each important in the treatment of osteomyelitis. It is often difficult to predict at diagnosis and treatment which children will develop sequelae. The age of the patient and the site of infection influence the long-term outcome. In children with acute systemic osteomyelitis, the poorest results are in neonates and in infants with involvement of the hip or shoulder joints. An older study (Dunkle and Brock, 1982) of long-term follow-up of osteomyelitis suggested that duration of symptoms longer than 7 days before diagnosis and treatment was associated with a poorer prognosis. This poor outcome was not related to a shorter duration of parenteral or oral therapy but was significantly associated with infection due to *S. aureus*.

Follow-up of children in one study (Jackson et al, 1992) with concomitant osteomyelitis and joint infections indicated long-term sequelae in 57% of children. Compared with a group of children who had suppurative arthritis without osteomyelitis, these patients were younger (median age, 10 vs 22 months) and had had symptoms longer (≥1 week) before hospital admission. Most of the patients had a delay in diagnosis of the bone infection because of misleading results of diagnostic studies, with management focusing on further joint compression rather than exploration for a contiguous osteomyelitis. Most patients displayed a slow clinical response to therapy, promoting subsequent evaluation of bone sites.

In a recent study (Roine, 1995) the CRP value normalized earlier in children with acute systemic osteomyelitis and asymptomatic versus symptomatic outcome after acute systemic osteomyelitis. The outcome in this series was evaluated at 1–2 months after discharge, with a symptomatic outcome defined as having pain, edema, or limited mobility of the adjoining joint. Longer-term outcomes were not reported.

Treatment failures occur in a high percentage of cases of sternal osteomyelitis, particularly among persons with extensive infection. Mediastinitis may be lethal in some cases. In one series (Siegman-Igra, 1990) of adults, 6% of the persons died of noninfectious complications after definitive operations, and 2% had chronic sinus tract infections.

PREVENTION

Acute systemic osteomyelitis in children is of hematogenous origin, making prevention difficult. Since the advent of universal immunization of infants with the *H. influenzae* type b vaccine, serious bacterial infections due to *H. influenzae* type b, including bone and joint infections, have been practically eliminated. Because the serotypes of *S. pneumoniae* causing joint infections are represented in the new conjugate pneumococcal vaccine, the incidence of pneumococcal bone infections should decrease after widespread immunization.

Puncture Wounds. Children with puncture wounds to the foot should receive prompt irrigation, cleansing, débridement, and removal of any visible foreign body or debris. Tetanus prophylaxis is also important (Chapter 48). The decision to administer oral antibiotic therapy is based on the age of the wound and the degree of contamination at initial evaluation. Antibiotics that could be considered for use in this setting include semisynthetic antistaphylococcal penicillin, first- or second-generation cephalosporins, and amoxicillin-clavulanate. An oral fluoroquinolone may be an alternative choice for persons older than 18 years. *Pseudomonas* osteochondritis has occurred in persons who received initial ciprofloxacin as antimicrobial prophylaxis. The development of redness, tenderness, pain, or fever requires immediate medical attention despite the prophylactic use of antibiotics.

Surgery. Prophylactic antimicrobial agents have been shown to lower the rate of wound infection after surgery, although recommendations for optimal timing, duration, and agents used may vary (Table 16–6). In a prospective study (Dellinger et al, 1988) the necessary duration of antibiotic administration after open fracture showed that a brief course (24 hours) of cefonicid was equivalent to a prolonged course of antibiotics for prevention of postoperative fracture site infections. A more recent prospective study (Boxma et al, 1996) of closed fractures in adults showed that a single preoperative dose of ceftriaxone was superior to placebo in preventing the incidence of wound infections and early nosocomial infections after surgery.

REVIEWS

Lew DP, Waldvogel FA: Osteomyelitis. *N Engl J Med* 1997;336:999–1007.

Nelson JD: Acute osteomyelitis in children. *Infect Dis Clin North Am* 1990; 4:513–22.

Nelson JD: Skeletal infections in children. *Adv Pediatr Infect Dis* 1991; 6:59–78.

KEY ARTICLES

Abbasi S, Orlicek SL, Almohsen I, et al: Septic arthritis and osteomyelitis caused by penicillin and cephalosporin-resistant *Streptococcus pneumoniae* in a children's hospital. *Pediatr Infect Dis J* 1996;15:78–83.

Adeyokunnu AA, Hendrickse RG: Salmonella osteomyelitis in childhood. A report of 63 cases seen in Nigerian children of whom 57 had sickle cell anaemia. *Arch Dis Child* 1980;55:175–84.

Asmar BI: Osteomyelitis in the neonate. *Infect Dis Clin North Am* 1992; 6:117–32.

Bergdahl S, Ekengren K, Eriksson M: Neonatal hematogenous osteomyelitis: Risk factors for long-term sequelae. *J Pediatr Orthop* 1985;5:564–8.

Bolivar R, Kohl S, Pickering LK: Vertebral osteomyelitis in children: Report of four cases. *Pediatrics* 1978;62:549–53.

Boxma H, Broekhuizen T, Patka P, et al: Randomised controlled trial of single-dose antibiotic prophylaxis in surgical treatment of closed fractures: The Dutch Trauma Trial. *Lancet* 1996;347:1133–7.

Bradley JS, Kaplan SL, Tan TQ, et al: Pediatric pneumococcal bone and joint infections. The Pediatric Multicenter Pneumococcal Surveillance Study Group (PMPSG). *Pediatrics* 1998;102:1376–82.

Burnett MW, Bass JW, Cook BA: Etiology of osteomyelitis complicating sickle cell disease. *Pediatrics* 1998;101:296–7.

Chandrasekar PH, Narula AP: Bone and joint infections in intravenous drug abusers. *Rev Infect Dis* 1986;8:904–11.

Correa AG, Edwards MS, Baker CJ: Vertebral osteomyelitis in children. *Pediatr Infect Dis J* 1993;12:228–33.

Dellinger EP, Caplan ES, Weaver LD, et al: Duration of preventive antibiotic administration for open extremity fractures. *Arch Surg* 1988;123: 333–9.

Demopulos GA, Bleck EE, McDougall IR: Role of radionuclide imaging in the diagnosis of acute osteomyelitis. *J Pediatr Orthop* 1988;8:558–65.

Dich VQ, Nelson JD, Haltalin KC: Osteomyelitis in infants and children. A review of 163 cases. *Am J Dis Child* 1975;129:1273–8.

Dunkle LM, Brock N: Long-term follow-up of ambulatory management of osteomyelitis. *Clin Pediatr* 1982;21:650–5.

Edwards MS, Baker CJ, Granberry WM, et al: Pelvic osteomyelitis in children. *Pediatrics* 1978;61:62–7.

Elliott SJ, Aronoff SC: Clinical presentation and management of *Pseudomonas* osteomyelitis. *Clin Pediatr* 1985;24:566–70.

Erdman WA, Tamburro F, Jayson HT, et al: Osteomyelitis: Characteristics and pitfalls of diagnosis with MR imaging. *Radiology* 1991;180:533–9.

Faden H, Grossi M: Acute osteomyelitis in children. Reassessment of etiologic agents and their clinical characteristics. *Am J Dis Child* 1991; 145:65–9.

Fernandez M, Carrol CL, Baker CJ: Discitis and vertebral osteomyelitis in children: An 18-year review. *Pediatrics* 2000;105:1299–304.

Givner LB, Luddy RE, Schwartz AD: Etiology of osteomyelitis in patients with major sickle hemoglobinopathies. *J Pediatr* 1981;99:411–3.

Gold RH, Hawkins RA, Katz RD: Bacterial osteomyelitis: Findings on plain radiography, CT, MR, and scintigraphy. *AJR Am J Roentgenol* 1991;157:365–70.

Hummel DS, Anderson SJ, Wright PF, et al: Chronic recurrent multifocal osteomyelitis: Are mycoplasmas involved? *N Engl J Med* 1987; 317:510–1.

Jackson MA, Burry VF, Olson LC: Pyogenic arthritis associated with adjacent osteomyelitis: Identification of the sequelae-prone child. *Pediatr Infec Dis J* 1992;11:9–13.

Jacobs NM: Pneumococcal osteomyelitis and arthritis in children. A hospital series and literature review. *Am J Dis Child* 1991;145:70–4.

Jacobs RF, McCarthy RE, Elser JM: *Pseudomonas* osteochondritis complicating puncture wounds of the foot in children: A 10-year evaluation. *J Infect Dis* 1989;160:657–61.

Jurik AG, Helmig O, Ternowitz T, et al: Chronic recurrent multifocal osteomyelitis: A follow-up study. *J Pediatr Orthop* 1988;8:49–58.

Karwowska A, Davies HD, Jadavji T: Epidemiology and outcome of osteomyelitis in the era of sequential intravenous-oral therapy. *Pediatr Infect Dis J* 1998;17:1021–6.

Kim HC, Alavi A, Russell MV, et al: Differentiation of bone and bone marrow infarcts from osteomyelitis in sickle cell disorders. *Clin Nucl Med* 1989;14:249–54.

Nelson JD: Bone and joint infections. *Pediatr Infect Dis* 1983;2:S45–50.

Nelson JD: Toward simple but safe management of osteomyelitis. *Pediatrics* 1997;99:883–4.

Norden CW: Antibiotic prophylaxis in orthopedic surgery. *Rev Infect Dis* 1991;13:S842–6.

Pelkonen P, Ryoppy S, Jaaskelainen J, et al: Chronic osteomyelitislike disease with negative bacterial cultures. *Am J Dis Child* 1988;142: 1167–73.

Peltola H, Unkila-Kallio L, Kallio MJ: Simplified treatment of acute staphylococcal osteomyelitis of childhood. The Finnish Study Group. *Pediatrics* 1997;99:846–50.

Roine I, Fainqezicht I, Arguedas A, et al: Serial serum C-reactive protein to monitor recovery from acute hematogenous osteomyelitis in children. *Pediatr Infect Dis J* 1995;14:40–4.

Schreck P, Schreck P, Bradley J, et al: Musculoskeletal complications of varicella. *J Bone Joint Surg Am* 1996;78:1713–9.

Siegman-Igra Y, Shafir R, Weiss J, et al: Serious infectious complications of midsternotomy: A review of bacteriology and antimicrobial therapy. *Scand J Infect Dis* 1990;22:633–43.

Syrogiannopoulos GA, Nelson JD: Duration of antimicrobial therapy for acute suppurative osteoarticular infections. *Lancet* 1988;1:37–40.

Unkila-Kallio L, Kallio MJ, Eskola J, et al: Serum C-reactive protein, erythrocyte sedimentation rate, and white blood cell count in acute hematogenous osteomyelitis of children. *Pediatrics* 1994;93:59–62.

CHAPTER 87

Infectious Arthritis

Kathryn S. Moffett ▪ Stephen C. Aronoff

Four infectious clinical syndromes are associated with arthritis in children and adolescents: **suppurative arthritis,** an acute bacterial infection of the joint space that is also known as **septic arthritis** or **pyogenic arthritis;** disseminated gonococcal infections; reactive arthritis; and fungal arthritis. Lyme disease is an infection associated with arthritis as part of a systemic illness (Chapter 29).

ETIOLOGY

Suppurative arthritis is the most common serious form of infectious arthritis encountered in children. In the first 2 months of life, group B *Streptococcus* and *Staphylococcus aureus* are the most common causes of joint infections (Table 87–1). *Candida* is an important cause of nosocomial neonatal joint infections. Beyond this extended neonatal period, *Streptococcus pneumoniae, S. aureus,* and *Haemophilus influenzae* type b are the most common causes of suppurative arthritis in young children up to 2 years of age. *H. influenzae* type b was once the leading cause of suppurative arthritis in children, but the incidence of invasive *H. influenzae* type b infections has diminished greatly since implementation of the conjugate vaccine. After 2 years of age, *S. aureus* is the most common joint pathogen. Musculoskeletal infections are caused by group A *Streptococcus* in children with varicella and streptococcal bacteremia. Anaerobic streptococci, *Fusobacterium,* and *Eikenella corrodens* are pathogens in joint infections of the hands, after closed-fist injuries. *Mycobacterium tuberculosis,* an unusual cause of joint infections in children, has resurfaced as a clinically significant pathogen, primarily in children with HIV infection.

Disseminated gonococcal infections are most often caused by nutritionally deficient strains of *Neisseria gonorrhoeae.* Disseminated infection with joint involvement due to penicillin-resistant strains has occurred rarely.

Reactive arthritis in children typically complicates gastrointestinal infections caused by *Yersinia enterocolitica, Campylobacter, Shigella flexneri,* or *Salmonella.* Nondiarrheal diseases associated with reactive arthritis include *Chlamydia* urethritis, localized or systemic infections due to group A *Streptococcus,* and late complications of *Neisseria meningitidis* infections. Naturally acquired rubella, rubella vaccination, and enteroviral infections are associated rarely with reactive arthritis. Some cases of joint symptoms associated with *H. influenzae* type b may represent reactive arthritis rather than invasive suppurative infections. *Chlamydia* urethritis has been implicated as the cause of Reiter's syndrome, which consists of nongonococcal urethritis, conjunctivitis, and nonsuppurative arthritis.

Joint infections caused by fungi are uncommon among immunocompetent children. *Candida albicans* arthritis occurs in premature neonates and in immunocompromised children. Disseminated histoplasmosis, which occurs in young infants and immunocompromised persons, may include joint infection; reactive arthritis has been described in some immunocompetent persons with systemic histoplasmosis. Infections with *Sporothrix schenckii* typically produce a cutaneous or lymphocutaneous infection in immunocompetent persons, although fungal arthritis may complicate cutaneous infections. Otherwise healthy girls and women with an exaggerated immune response to a primary infection with *Coccidioides immitis* may develop a rheumatoid disease that includes joint swelling (valley fever). Other systemic mycoses, such as blastomycosis and cryptococcosis, may have joint involvement as part of the clinical expression of systemic disease.

EPIDEMIOLOGY

Although the exact incidence of infectious arthritis in children is unknown, several retrospective reviews demonstrate the uncommon nature of this pediatric infection. Suppurative arthritis accounts for approximately 0.25% of hospitalized children. In the largest series reported (Nelson, 1991), approximately 80% of the cases of suppurative arthritis occurred in children younger than 5 years, and half of these cases occurred in children younger than 2 years.

The prevalence of disseminated gonococcal infection in sexually active females is higher than in males, and this infection often complicates pregnancy or menses.

TABLE 87–1. Infectious Causes of Arthritis in Children

Young Infants (age <2 mo)	Adults
Common	***Common***
Group B *Streptococcus*	*S. aureus*
Staphylococcus aureus	*S. pneumoniae*
Escherichia coli	Group A *Streptococcus*
Klebsiella pneumoniae	Enterobacteriaceae
Uncommon	**Reactive Arthritis**
Neisseria gonorrhoeae	*Yersinia enterocolitica*
Candida	*Campylobacter jejuni*
Older Infants and Children (age 2 mo to Adulthood)	*Shigella flexneri*
	Salmonella
Common	Group A *Streptococcus*
Streptococcus pneumoniae	*Neisseria meningitidis*
S. aureus	*Coccidioides immitis*
Haemophilus influenzae type b*	Rubella virus
Kingella kingae	
N. gonorrhoeae	
Uncommon	
Anaerobic bacteria	
Pseudomonas aeruginosa	
Group A *Streptococcus*	
Enterobacteriaceae	
Mycobacterium tuberculosis	

*The incidence of invasive infections caused by *H. influenzae* type b has greatly diminished since introduction of conjugate vaccine.

Reactive arthritis complicates *Yersinia* and *Campylobacter* gastroenteritis in approximately 1% of cases.

PATHOGENESIS

Bacteremia with hematogenous seeding of the synovium is the most common cause of suppurative arthritis in children. Other foci such as meningitis may be manifested well in advance of suppurative arthritis. Less commonly, joint infections arise from contiguous sites of infection or from penetrating injury. It is estimated that 13–16% of children and 70% of neonates with joint infection have concomitant osteomyelitis. *S. aureus* or anaerobic bacteria may infect a joint after a penetrating injury with direct inoculation into the joint space. Penetration of the joint space with sharp plant thorns **(blackthorn arthritis)** gives rise to a syndrome of arthritis and synovial fluid that suggests bacterial infection, but this foreign body arthritis typically fails to yield a pathogen.

Disseminated gonococcal infections are unique because the early and late arthritides associated with this illness represent reactive and suppurative forms of arthritis, respectively. After an untreated (and presumably asymptomatic) primary infection with auxotrophic variant strains of *N. gonorrhoeae,* a febrile illness develops in association with rash and polyarticular, symmetric arthritis, typically described as periarthritis involving the joints of the hands and the feet. Bacterial cultures of the synovium are sterile at this stage despite a relatively high prevalence of bacteremia. If left untreated, this acute illness subsides, and days to weeks later a monoarticular arthritis of large, weight-bearing joints appears. In this stage of the illness, cultures of affected synovial fluid often yield the pathogen.

Reactive arthritis follows an antecedent local or systemic infection. The mechanism of synovial inflammation is immune mediated. In most cases it is assumed that antibodies against specific bacterial epitopes, most likely pili, cross-react with an expressed antigen on synovial cells. The antibodies bind and activate complement and also initiate various cytokine cascades, resulting in influx of polymorphonuclear leukocytes; degranulation of these cells produces inflammation. Involvement of the hip joint in children 3–6 years of age is a notable presentation and has been known as **toxic synovitis** or **transient synovitis** of the hip. Patients with Reiter's syndrome complicating gastrointestinal or urethral infection often have a genetic predisposition; more than 90% have an HLA-B27 haplotype.

SYMPTOMS AND CLINICAL MANIFESTATIONS

Typically, fever and joint effusion accompanied by **pseudoparesis** or **pseudoparalysis** (i.e., partial or complete loss of spontaneous movement of the affected extremity) and by painful movement of the affected joint are the hallmarks of infectious arthritis in children (Table 87–2). The joints of the lower extremity are most often involved, the knees in 40% of the cases, the hips in 20%, and the ankles in 14%. Small joints, such as those of the hand, are more often involved after penetrating trauma and closed-fist injuries. Antecedent infections such as gastroenteritis, meningitis, urethritis, or sepsis precede the reactive types of arthritis. In neonates, suppurative arthritis commonly follows spread of osteomyelitis from adjacent bone through metaphyseal and epiphyseal vessels across the cartilage precursor of the ossification nucleus (Chapter 86).

Minor genitourinary symptoms that have been ignored by a patient may precede development of the early **arthritis-dermatitis syndrome** associated with disseminated gonococcal infection. A history of febrile illness antedating the development of monoarticular arthritis is characteristic of late gonococcal arthritis.

Reactive arthritis may occur soon after the systemic bacterial infections, typically within 3 weeks of the onset of gastroenteritis. The arthritis is typically symmetric and polyarticular and involves the large joints. Occasionally symptoms of conjunctivitis and urethritis suggest Reiter's syndrome, but other mucosal and skin manifestations are rare in children.

Fungal arthritis is rare in the pediatric age group and typically accompanies systemic mycoses. In very ill neonates, prolonged ventilation, long-standing indwelling catheters, and hyperalimentation may antedate the insidious onset of localized erythema, joint swelling, irritability, and pseudoparesis or pseudoparalysis. Beyond the newborn period, fungal joint infections occur primarily among immunocompromised persons treated with broad-spectrum antibiotics for prolonged periods and are often manifestations of disseminated mycoses. Joint infections in sporotrichosis usually occur in immunocompromised persons but may complicate cutaneous infections or lymphocutaneous infections in otherwise healthy persons. In most cases of sporotrichosis, helpful diagnostic clues are exposure to plant products or sphagnum moss and the development of a cutaneous papule that becomes necrotic and forms an eschar (Chapter 46).

Physical Examination Findings

The physical findings in infectious arthritis are similar regardless of the cause. Overlying erythema, joint effusion, limitation of joint movement, and pain on joint movement are characteristic findings. When large, weight-bearing joints are involved, a limp or an inability to walk may be apparent. The physical findings in neonates are often subtle.

Suppurative arthritis of the hip is difficult to diagnose by physical examination. Pain on internal hip rotation and on extension, when present, is a helpful sign. Young children often hold the hip in the position of maximum comfort, which is externally rotated and flexed.

DIAGNOSIS

The diagnosis of suppurative arthritis is usually considered because of the clinical symptoms and physical findings. Diagnostic imaging, such as ultrasonography, is most helpful in identifying the presence of a joint effusion, especially in joints such as the hip, because of the difficulty in determining the presence of an effusion by physical examination. Definitive diagnosis of a joint-space infection requires analysis and culture of joint fluid, obtained by simple aspiration, by ultrasound-guided aspiration, or by an open operation. Blood cultures are also useful in identifying the causative organism.

Differential Diagnosis

The differential diagnosis of arthritis in infants, children, and adolescents includes other infectious diseases (e.g., Lyme disease), rheumatologic disorders, rheumatic fever (Chapter 40), and trauma. Suppurative arthritis must be distinguished from osteomyelitis, suppurative bursitis, fasciitis, myositis, cellulitis, and soft tissue abscesses, which may mimic the signs and symptoms of infectious arthritis. Abscesses of the psoas muscle, which often present with fever and with pain on hip flexion and rotation, must be distinguished from infections of the hip. Juvenile rheumatoid arthritis, Kawasaki syndrome, Henoch-Schönlein purpura, Crohn's disease, and other rheumatologic disorders must be differentiated from infectious arthritis. In most cases the presence of symmetric joint involvement or of effusions of multiple joints excludes infectious

TABLE 87–2. Comparison of Infectious Arthritis in Children and Adults

	Neonates	Children	Adults: Nongonococcal Arthritis	Adults: Disseminated Gonococcal Infections
Symptoms at Presentation				
Fever ≥38.3°C	48%	65%	78%	67%
Septic/toxic	8%	Rare	Rare	NA
White blood cell count >10,000/mm^3	NA	30–60%	50%	NA
Shift-to-the-left	NA	65%	NA	NA
Erythrocyte sedimentation rate ≥20 mm/hr	NA	>90%	Common	NA
C-reactive protein ≥20 mg/L	NA	95%	NA	NA
Associated symptoms	Pseudoparesis or pseudoparalysis	Limp Painful movement of joint	NA	Dermatitis Tenosynovitis
Contiguous Osteomyelitis	70%	12–16%	NA	NA
Male:Female Ratio	1:1.2	2:1	NA	Female more common
Joint Involvement	Hip	Knee>hip>ankle	Knee	Hands, feet
Number involved	40% Multifocal	94% Monoarticular	>85% Monoarticular	>50% Migratory polyarthritis
Risk Factors	Prematurity Invasive procedures Delivery trauma	Blunt trauma Hemophilia	Elderly Immunocompromised Chronic arthritis Recent or past joint damage Joint surgery Intravenous drug use	Young, healthy, and sexually active Complement deficiency Pregnancy After menses
Positive Culture Results				
Joint fluid	NA	60–80%	85–95%	25%*
Blood	NA	29–63%	10–60%	<10%
Both	NA	43%	NA	NA

NA = not available.
*May also have genital, rectal, pharyngeal, or skin scraping culture positive for *Neisseria gonorrhoeae.*

causes. Gastrointestinal or renal involvement is more likely to be manifested in rheumatologic disorders. A history of injury, penetrating trauma, or bleeding dyscrasia is usually elicited in hemarthrosis.

Suppurative Bursitis. Infections of the bursae are infrequent in children. Suppurative bursitis occurs most often in older boys and adult men and is usually a consequence of trauma. Less commonly, suppurative bursitis occurs as a complication of bacteremia. Although data on children are lacking, the incidence of acute suppurative bursitis has been estimated at 0.6–1.2 cases per 1,000 hospital admissions. Most persons with suppurative bursitis have either a history of superficial or penetrating trauma to the area overlying the bursa or an occupation that predisposes them to repeated bursal trauma, such as gardener, carpet layer, or athletic instructor.

S. aureus appears to be the most common etiologic agent, although group A *Streptococcus,* group G *Streptococcus,* and *S. pneumoniae* occasionally have been recovered from infected bursal fluid.

Approximately half of the cases of suppurative bursitis present abruptly, with rapid onset of localized, focal pain, swelling, redness, and tenderness. The remaining persons have an insidious onset of symptoms after a recent cutaneous injury near the affected bursa. Almost all cases of suppurative bursitis involve either the olecranon or the prepatellar bursa. Suppurative bursitis must be distinguished from noninfectious bursitis and from osteomyelitis and suppurative arthritis. The diagnosis of suppurative bursitis can be confirmed by evaluation and culture of bursal fluid. Suppurative bursitis requires local care, antimicrobial therapy, and effective drainage, similar to the management of suppurative arthritis. Most cases resolved without sequelae.

A syndrome called **postinfectious bursitis** consists of recurrent, sterile, bursal effusions, often reappearing after minimal trauma. Orally administered nonsteroidal anti-inflammatory agents are the drugs of choice for this complication.

Laboratory Evaluation

Elevated WBC count, ESR, and CRP levels are common in children with joint-space infections, but these findings are nonspecific. Arthrocentesis and synovial fluid analysis and culture are the most useful studies for establishing the diagnosis of suppurative arthritis and should be performed before initial treatment. The recovery of grossly purulent fluid with a WBC count of >50,000/mm^3, with a predominance of polymorphonuclear leukocytes, high protein content, and low glucose concentration, usually approximately 33% of serum glucose, is characteristic of suppurative arthritis. The recovery of fluid with fewer inflammatory cells is consistent with rheumatologic disorders, whereas the recovery of grossly bloody

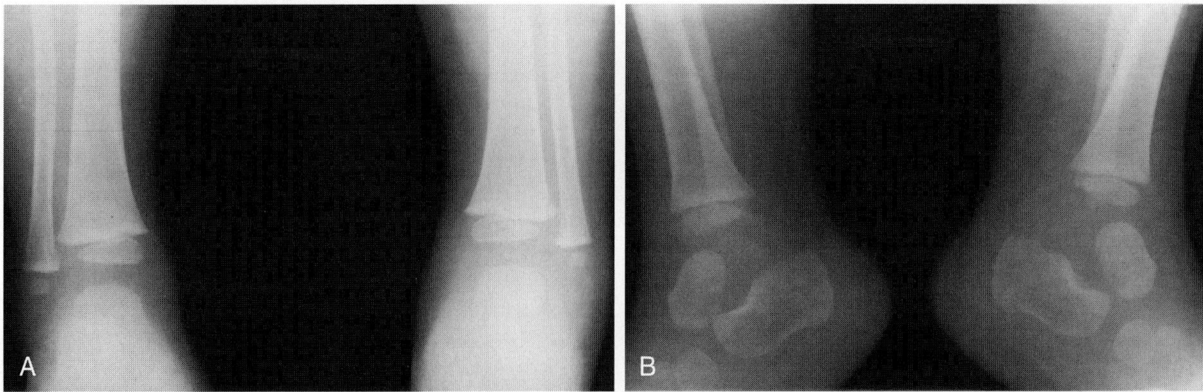

FIGURE 87–1. Septic arthritis of left ankle in a 4-year-old boy with swollen and painful left ankle. **A,** Frontal view of both ankles shows diffuse swelling of the soft tissues in and around the left ankle joint. **B,** Lateral view of both ankles shows the swelling of the deep tissues around the joints with displacement or obliteration of the adjacent fat planes.

fluid is highly suggestive of hemarthrosis. Joint effusions associated with rheumatologic disorders typically have a WBC count of 10,000–20,000/mm^3, with an almost equal distribution between polymorphonuclear and lymphocytic leukocytes and with a glucose concentration 66–75% that of serum.

Microbiologic Evaluation

Definitive diagnosis of suppurative arthritis is confirmed by either the recovery of a bacterial pathogen from purulent synovial fluid or the recovery of a bacterial pathogen from the blood of a person with purulent synovial fluid. In most studies the bacterial recovery rate from infected synovial fluid is less than 50%, which is due to the bactericidal activity of joint fluid. The yield from joint fluid can be improved by culture of samples in broth and on agar so that bactericidal factors present in the infected fluid are diluted out. Among all children with suppurative arthritis, approximately one third have a positive blood culture result.

Diagnostic Imaging

Plain radiographs typically are not a helpful addition to the physical findings in the diagnosis of early suppurative arthritis. Typical radiographic findings can include swelling of the joint capsule, a widened joint space, and displacement of adjacent normal fat lines (Fig. 87–1). Later radiographic findings include evidence of synovial thickening. Radionuclide scans are of limited use for establishing the diagnosis of suppurative arthritis, although ^{67}Ga scans, ^{111}In-tagged WBC scans, and ^{99m}Tc scans may be required to exclude concurrent bone infection distant from the infected joint. Ultrasonography is useful not only for establishing the presence of fluid in hip infections but also as a guide for closed arthrocentesis of the joint (see Fig. 13–33). MRI is useful in distinguishing joint infections from cellulitis or deep abscesses, detecting Legg-Calvé-Perthes disease, and identifying concomitant osteomyelitis.

TREATMENT

The effective treatment of infectious arthritis in children requires a multidisciplinary approach. The establishment of the diagnosis requires, at the very least, closed arthrocentesis. Repeated closed arthrocenteses are recommended for the control of effusions in cases of suppurative arthritis complicated by early fluid reaccumulation. Arthroscopy or open arthrotomy for diagnosis and drainage is recommended for suppurative arthritis of the hip, suppurative arthritis complicated by adjacent osteomyelitis, fungal arthritis, recurrent joint effusions unresponsive to repeated arthrocenteses, persistence of systemic symptoms, or persistent bacteremia. In blackthorn arthritis, débridement with or without synovectomy is curative.

Suppurative Arthritis of the Hip. Because the metaphysis of the head of the femur is encompassed by the extension of the joint capsule, the increased pressure in the hip-joint space accompanying suppurative arthritis of the hip may impede vascular flow across nutrient vessels to the head of the femur, rendering the area particularly susceptible to ischemic injury and possibly avascular necrosis. As a result, prompt open surgical drainage of a hip joint that may be infected is generally considered imperative. Because the shoulder joint is also a ball-and-socket joint similar in structure to the hip, many experts recommend open surgical drainage for suppurative arthritis of the shoulder.

Neonatal Suppurative Arthritis. The treatment of neonatal arthritis is largely empirical because results of large, comparative trials are not available. Because most cases are multifocal and involve both joint and adjacent bone, surgical débridement continues to be a mainstay of therapy. Closed or open drainage in addition to antimicrobial therapy is recommended for all cases of isolated neonatal infectious arthritis.

Definitive Treatment

A variety of antimicrobial agents are potentially useful for the treatment of infectious arthritis in children because of the high concentrations these agents achieve in infected synovial fluid when administered parenterally (Table 87–3). Intra-articular drug instillation is not required and may, in fact, provoke synovial damage. Initial empirical antimicrobial therapy for neonates should include nafcillin or oxacillin plus cefotaxime, with or without an aminoglycoside. In uncomplicated infectious arthritis beyond the newborn period, initial therapy must provide coverage against both gram-positive cocci and *Kingella kingae.* The use of a penicillinase-resistant penicillin (nafcillin or oxacillin) provides adequate empirical coverage. Clindamycin may be used for persons with β-lactam hypersensitivity. In a child who has been fully immunized for *H. influenzae* type b, empirical coverage for *H. influenzae* type b is not necessary unless gram-negative rods are visualized in synovial fluid analysis.

Limited data are available on the optimal treatment of infectious arthritis due to penicillin-nonsusceptible strains of *S. pneumoniae*

TABLE 87–3. Recommended Antibiotic Therapy for Infectious Arthritis

Age	Common Pathogens	Parenteral Therapy		Oral Therapy	
		Recommended	Alternative	Recommended	Alternative
Infants (<2 mo of age)*	Group B *Streptococcus*	Ampicillin *plus* Aminoglycoside†	Cefotaxime (*or* ceftriaxone‡)	—	—
	Escherichia coli *Klebsiella pneumoniae*	Cefotaxime (*or* ceftriaxone‡) *plus* Aminoglycoside		—	—
	Staphylococcus aureus	Nafcillin (*or* oxacillin)	Clindamycin	—	—
Older infants and children (2 mo of age to adulthood)	*S. aureus*	Nafcillin (*or* oxacillin)	Clindamycin	Cephaloxin *or* dicloxacillin	Clindamycin
	Streptococcus pneumoniae	Penicillin G *or* cefotaxime (*or* ceftriaxone)	Clindamycin	Amoxicillin	Clindamycin
	Kingella kingae	Penicillin G *or* nafcillin (*or* oxacillin)	Cefazolin	Penicillin G *or* amoxicillin	Cephalexin *or* dicloxacillin
	Group A *Streptococcus*	Penicillin G	Clindamycin	Amoxicillin	Clindamycin
	Haemophilus influenzae type b§	Cefuroxime (*or* cefotaxime *or* ceftriaxone)	Chloramphenicol†	—	—
Disseminated gonococcal infections	*Neisseria gonorrhoeae*	Ceftriaxone‡	Cefotaxime *or* ceftriaxone	See Table 85–2	

*Use lower dose and longer dosing interval for neonates, especially for those younger than 7 days (see Chapter 14 and Table 96–5).
†Dosing should be guided by laboratory determination of serum antibiotic concentrations once a steady state has been reached.
‡Should not be administered to neonates with hyperbilirubinemia, especially those born prematurely.
§The incidence of invasive infections caused by *H. influenzae* type b has greatly diminished since introduction of conjugate vaccine.

Suggested Dosages for Persons with Normal Renal Function

ANTIBIOTIC	DOSAGE	MAXIMUM DAILY DOSE
Parenteral Therapy		
Amikacin	22.5 mg/kg/day divided q8–12hr IV	750–900 mg
Cefotaxime	200 mg/kg/day divided q6hr IV	12 g
Ceftriaxone	100 mg/kg/day divided q12hr IV or IM	3–4 g
	or	
	80 mg/kg/day divided q24hr IV or IM	3–4 g
Chloramphenicol	75–100 mg/kg/day divided q6hr IV	2–4 g
Gentamicin	7.5 mg/kg/day divided q8hr IV	250–300 mg
Nafcillin	150–200 mg/kg/day divided q6hr IV	9 g
Oxacillin	150–200 mg/kg/day divided q6hr IV	12 g
***Parenteral Therapy** (Continued)*		
Penicillin G	250,000–500,000 units/kg/day divided q6hr IV	20–24 MU
Tobramycin	7.5 mg/kg/day divided q8hr IV	250–300 mg
Vancomycin	45–60 mg/kg/day divided q6hr IV	2 g
Oral Therapy		
Amoxicillin	90 mg/kg/day divided three times a day PO	1.5 g
Cephalexin	100–150 mg/kg/day divided q6hr PO	2 g
Chloramphenicol	75 mg/kg/day divided q6hr PO	2–4 g
Clindamycin	30 mg/kg/day divided q6hr PO	1.2 g
Dicloxacillin	100 mg/kg/day divided q6hr PO	2 g

compared with treatment of infectious arthritis due to penicillin-susceptible strains. A recent prospective study (Bradley et al, 1998) of 21 children with infectious arthritis due to *S. pneumoniae* revealed that 5 of 21 children were infected with nonsusceptible strains. Parenteral antibiotic treatment of infection with penicillin-nonsusceptible strains did not differ from treatment of infection with penicillin-susceptible strains. There were no treatment failures by microbiologic criteria, and there were similar clinical responses to therapy, with no differences in complications or long-term sequelae. Because β-lactam antibiotics achieve excellent penetration into bone and joints, they remain the treatment of choice.

The appropriate duration of antimicrobial therapy for suppurative arthritis is unsettled and not defined by comparative clinical trials. Joint infections caused by *S. pneumoniae* or *H. influenzae* type b should be treated for 14 days, and infections caused by *S. aureus* or gram-negative bacilli should be treated for 3–4 weeks. These are recommendations for minimum duration provided that the patient's signs and symptoms of infection have resolved, the CRP level has returned to normal, and the ESR is normal for at least 1 week before therapy is discontinued. In cases in which the signs and symptoms of infection persist beyond 1 week, concomitant osteomyelitis should be considered. Therapy should be continued for a minimum of 4 weeks or for at least 1 week after the resolution of all clinical symptoms.

Infectious arthritis due to *M. tuberculosis* is unusual in an immunocompetent person and suggests the possibility of HIV infection. Treatment is as recommended for extrapulmonary tuberculosis (Chapter 35). Fungal arthritis usually occurs in immunocompromised persons with disseminated infection and usually requires surgical drainage as well as antifungal therapy (Chapter 99).

Disseminated Gonococcal Infections. Gonococcal arthritis with or without bacteremia is treated by ceftriaxone (50 mg/kg/day [maximum daily dose: 1 g] intravenously or intramuscularly for 7 days). Treatment of persons with disseminated gonococcal infection initially should include ceftriaxone given intravenously or intramuscularly as inpatient therapy for 24–48 hours. The symptoms in persons with disseminated gonococcal infections resolve dramatically after the initiation of therapy. Reliable persons with uncomplicated disease and complete resolution of symptoms may complete therapy on an outpatient basis for a total of 1 week of oral therapy (see Table 85–2). Doxycycline or azithromycin should also be administered for the treatment of presumed concurrent *Chlamydia trachomatis* genital infection (Chapter 85).

Reactive Arthritis. Reactive arthritis is often a self-limited illness in children, particularly when the precipitating infection is treated appropriately. Additional treatment with aspirin or nonsteroidal anti-inflammatory agents often provides symptomatic relief of joint symptoms.

COMPLICATIONS

The major complications of neonatal, childhood, and gonococcal arthritis are loss of joint function due to damage to the articular surface and foreshortening of the extremity caused by destruction of the growth plate. The highest incidence of these complications occurs with hip infections, presumably as a result of ischemic injury to the head of the femur. As a result, most experts recommend prompt open drainage of infected hip joints. Similar arguments have been extended to infected shoulder joints. The high incidence of concurrent suppurative arthritis and adjacent osteomyelitis in neonates places the epiphyseal growth plate at great risk, and thus the incidence of limb abnormalities is greater among neonates than among older children. Most authorities therefore recommend open surgical drainage of infected joints in neonates. The major complications of fungal arthritis include risks to limb function and complications of disseminated infection.

PROGNOSIS

In general the prognosis for the common forms of infectious arthritis encountered in infants and children is excellent, but it is often difficult to predict at diagnosis which children will develop sequelae. The age of the patient and the site of the infection influence the long-term outcome. Neonates with concomitant osteomyelitis have a high likelihood, approximately 40–50%, of growth disturbances with loss of longitudinal bone growth and ultimate limb shortening. The poorest outcome in infants and children is for those with suppurative arthritis of the hip or shoulder. Severe overall functional deterioration is usually associated with infection in elderly adults, pre-existing joint disease, or joints containing synthetic material.

Follow-up of children in one study (Jackson et al, 1992) with concomitant bone and joint infections indicates long-term sequelae in 57% of children. In comparison with a group of children who had suppurative arthritis without osteomyelitis, these children were younger (median age 10 vs 22 months) and had had symptoms for more than 1 week before hospital admission. Most of the study subjects had a significant delay in diagnosis of the bone infection and a slow clinical response to therapy, promoting subsequent evaluation for bone site involvement.

PREVENTION

Since the advent of universal immunization of infants with the *H. influenzae* type b vaccine, serious bacterial infections due to *H. influenzae* type b, including bone and joint infections, have been practically eliminated. Because the serotypes of *S. pneumoniae* causing joint infections are represented in the new conjugate pneumococcal vaccine, the incidence of pneumococcal joint infections should decrease after widespread immunization.

REVIEWS

Barton LL, Dunkle LM, Habib FH: Septic arthritis in childhood. A 13-year review. *Am J Dis Child* 1987;141:898–900.

Green NE, Edward K: Bone and joint infections in children. *Orthop Clin North Am* 1987;18:555–76.

Nelson JD: Skeletal infections in children. *Adv Pediatr Infect Dis* 1991; 6:59–78.

Trujillo M, Nelson JD: Suppurative and reactive arthritis in children. *Semin Pediatr Infect Dis* 1997;8:242–9.

Welkon CJ, Long SS, Fisher MC, et al: Pyogenic arthritis in infants and children: A review of 95 cases. *Pediatr Infect Dis* 1986;5:669–76.

KEY ARTICLES

Bradley JS, Kaplan SL, Tan TQ, et al: Pediatric pneumococcal bone and joint infections. The Pediatric Multicenter Pneumococcal Surveillance Study Group (PMPSSG). *Pediatrics* 1998;102:1376–82.

Dan M: Septic arthritis in young infants: Clinical and microbiologic correlations and therapeutic implications. *Rev Infect Dis* 1984;6:147–55.

De Cunto CL, Giannini EH, Fink CW, et al: Prognosis of children with poststreptococcal reactive arthritis. *Pediatr Infect Dis J* 1988;7:683–6.

Feigin RD, Pickering LK, Anderson D: Clindamycin treatment of osteomyelitis and septic arthritis in children. *Pediatrics* 1975;55:213–23.

Fink CW: Reactive arthritis. *Pediatr Infect Dis J* 1988;7:58–65.

Goldenberg DL, Brandt KD, Cohen AS, et al: Treatment of septic arthritis: Comparison of needle aspiration and surgery as initial modes of joint drainage. *Arthritis Rheum* 1975;18:83–90.

Greenwood BM, Mohammed I, Whittle HC: Immune complexes and the pathogenesis of meningococcal arthritis. *Clin Exp Immunol* 1985:59: 513–9.

Ho G Jr, Tice AD: Comparison of nonseptic and septic bursitis: Further observations on the treatment of septic bursitis. *Arch Intern Med* 1979; 139:1269–73.

Jackson MA, Burry VF, Olson LC: Pyogenic arthritis associated with adjacent osteomyelitis: Identification of the sequela-prone child. *Pediatr Infect Dis J* 1992;11:9–13.

Jacobs NM: Pneumococcal osteomyelitis and arthritis in children. A hospital series and literature review. *Am J Dis Child* 1991;145:70–4.

Kaandorp CJ, Krijnen P, Moens HJ, et al: The outcome of bacterial arthritis: A prospective community-based study. *Arthritis Rheum* 1997;40: 884–92.

Kallio MJ, Unkila-Kallio L, Aalto K, et al: Serum C-reactive protein, erythrocyte sedimentation rate and white blood cell count in septic arthritis of children. *Pediatr Infect Dis J* 1997;16:411–3.

Nelson JD: Antibiotic concentrations in septic joint effusions. *N Engl J Med* 1971;284:349–53.

Nelson JD, Howard JB, Shelton S: Oral antibiotic therapy for skeletal infections of children. I. Antibiotic concentrations in suppurative synovial fluid. *J Pediatr* 1978;92:131–4.

Peters W, Irving J, Letts M: Long-term effects of neonatal bone and joint infection on adjacent growth plates. *J Pediatr Orthop* 1992; 12:806–10.

Petty RE, Tingle AJ: Arthritis and viral infection. *J Pediatr* 1988;113: 948–9.

Rush PJ, Shore A, Inman R, et al: Arthritis associated with *Haemophilus influenzae* meningitis: Septic or reactive? *J Pediatr* 1986;109:412–5.

Schreck P, Schreck P, Bradley J, et al: Musculoskeletal complications of varicella. *J Bone Joint Surg Am* 1996;78:1713–9.

Syrogiannopoulos GA, Nelson JD: Duration of antimicrobial therapy for acute suppurative osteoarticular infections. *Lancet* 1988;1:37–40.

Tetzlaff IR, McCracken GH Jr, Nelson JD: Oral antibiotic therapy for skeletal infections of children. II. Therapy of osteomyelitis and suppurative arthritis. *J Pediatr* 1978;92:485–90.

Yagupsky P, Bur-Ziv Y, Howard CB, et al: Epidemiology, etiology, and clinical features of septic arthritis in children younger than 24 months. *Arch Pediatr Adolesc Med* 1995;149:537–40.

CHAPTER 88

Diskitis

Kathryn S. Moffett ▪ Stephen C. Aronoff

Diskitis is an inflammation or infection of the vertebral end plates. When diskitis is caused by bacterial infection, it is sometimes referred to as **pyogenic infectious spondylitis.** Clinically, diskitis ranges from a benign inflammatory process to a frank pyogenic disk-space infection accompanied by vertebral osteomyelitis. Most cases occur in children.

ETIOLOGY

The cause of diskitis is unclear, and both infectious and traumatic causes have been proposed. Although diskitis is considered an infectious disease, most of the cultures are sterile, and many persons recover without antimicrobial therapy. The organism most commonly recovered from infectious diskitis is *Staphylococcus aureus. Pseudomonas aeruginosa* has been associated with disk-space infections in heroin users. Other organisms, such as streptococci, diphtheroids, and *Klebsiella,* have been infrequently reported.

EPIDEMIOLOGY

Diskitis is uncommon in both adults and children and was estimated (Cushing, 1993) to occur in one or two children per year in a hospital that evaluated 32,500 children per year. This disorder occurs primarily in children 1–7 years of age, with an average of approximately 3 years of age. Boys are affected almost twice as often as girls. A history of trauma or recent upper respiratory or urinary tract infection is often present. The most common area of involvement is the lumbar region of the spine, especially the L3–4 and L4–5 disk spaces, followed by the thoracic and cervical regions.

PATHOGENESIS

The pathophysiology is poorly understood, but differences in the blood supply to the intervertebral disk by age appear to be important. Vascular channels present during the first 3 decades of life may provide a vascular conduit for seeding of the disk space during bacteremia. A recent cadaveric study (Rudert and Tillman, 1993) of lymph and blood supply to the intervertebral disk revealed vessels penetrating into the cartilage end plate and emerging from the marrow space of the adjacent vertebral bodies in children up to 7 years of age. The vessels accumulated toward the margins of the cartilage, with lymphatics detected in the area where small vessels supplied blood to the disk and adjacent tissues. Thus the persisting presence of vessels in the outer annulus fibrosis and in the cartilage end plates in infants and children as a site of entry for septic microemboli may explain the higher incidence of diskitis in children. In children, diskitis may represent either secondary reactive inflammatory changes of the disk space, in association with vertebral bacterial osteomyelitis, or pyogenic infection of the disk space itself.

SYMPTOMS AND CLINICAL MANIFESTATIONS

Although diskitis usually is manifested predominantly as back pain, it may present with a variety of complaints, such as limp, limited weight bearing, hip irritability, and abdominal pain. Children may refuse to stand, walk, or sit. A history of febrile illness, mild upper respiratory tract infection, or trauma may precede the skeletal symptoms by several weeks. Children usually do not appear acutely ill, and only approximately 28% are febrile. Constitutional symptoms including anorexia, irritability, and malaise may be present for several weeks.

Children 3 years of age and younger commonly present with refusal to walk or with hip irritability. These children may also have localized tenderness in the lumbar spine region or abdominal pain. In contrast, children 3–7 years of age often present with refusal to walk and have limp, back pain, spinal tenderness, and abdominal pain. Older children and adolescents usually present with back pain alone and are less likely to complain of associated problems such as abdominal pain or to refuse to walk.

Physical Examination Findings

The physical findings in diskitis are variable, ranging from decreased lumbar lordosis and positive results on a **straight leg raise test** (pain on flexion of the hip with knee fully extended) to positive findings on a **log roll test** (pain on internal and external hip rotation of the straight leg in the supine position) and paravertebral muscle spasm. Hamstring tightness, decreased motion of the spine, localized tenderness, and a mildly elevated temperature also may occur. Palpation of the spine variably reproduces symptoms. Postexercise soreness and herniated disks are seen infrequently in children compared with adults.

DIAGNOSIS

The diagnosis of diskitis is usually suspected on the basis of symptoms and physical findings and is confirmed by diagnostic imaging, usually plain radiographs and MRI. A blood culture should be obtained, but culture of blood and the disk, if obtained, are frequently sterile.

Differential Diagnosis

The differential diagnosis for diskitis varies with the presenting complaint. Back pain may also indicate vertebral osteomyelitis, tumor, Scheuermann's kyphosis, spondylolysis, or spondylolisthesis. Poor posture and idiopathic scoliosis rarely cause back pain in children. Scheuermann's kyphosis is a condition that develops during puberty and is associated with adjacent vertebral wedging. The pars interarticularis of L5 may undergo stress fracture and may be nondisplaced (spondylolysis), or the L5 vertebra may move forward (spondylolisthesis). This can result in low back pain, pain in the gluteal area, and pain in the sciatic distribution. Spondylolysis and spondylolisthesis may be seen in children from 10 years of age through adolescence, with symptoms that are aggravated by activity and diminished with rest. Vertebral osteomyelitis, including *Mycobacterium tuberculosis* infection, occurs most often in older children, adolescents, and adults and is accompanied by local tenderness, spasm, and kyphotic deformity. Ankylosing spondylitis may be seen in adolescents. Tumors such as osteoid osteoma, osteoblastoma, hemangioma, giant cell tumor, eosinophilic granuloma, and aneurysmal bone cysts may present with back pain. Prominent abdominal pain suggests appendicitis or urinary tract infection.

Laboratory Evaluation

In most cases the WBC count is normal to slightly elevated and the ESR is elevated.

Microbiologic Evaluation

It is often difficult to distinguish bacterial diskitis from noninfectious disk necrosis clinically, and therefore isolation of a bacterial organism is usually necessary to confirm a bacterial cause. Blood cultures are usually sterile, but results may be positive in cases with short duration of symptoms. Biopsy of the affected disks usually shows nonspecific inflammatory tissue. Disk culture results are positive in 25–66% of cases and are more likely to be positive with chronic disease. Biopsy and culture are important to identifying the bacterial cause if MRI suggests vertebral osteomyelitis.

Diagnostic Imaging

Plain radiographs, technetium 99m and gallium 67 radionuclide scans, CT, and MRI all have been used for the diagnosis of diskitis. Plain radiographs of the spine show abnormalities in approximately 75% of children with diskitis, with decreased height of the disk space and erosion of adjacent vertebral end plates (Fig. 88–1). Findings of radionuclide bone scans are positive in 72–90% of cases. These scans are most useful in very young children in whom a skeletal or abdominal infection is suspected but cannot be localized on physical examination. Normal plain radiographs and ^{99m}Tc bone scans do not exclude a diagnosis of diskitis early in the course of the disease. MRI is the imaging technique of choice, especially if the plain films are normal (Fig. 88–2). MRI is also useful in excluding the diagnosis of vertebral osteomyelitis.

Radiographic evaluation identifies recognizable phases of diskitis. Radiographs appear normal during the onset of symptoms, but 2–4 weeks after the onset of symptoms, radiographically demonstrated narrowing of an isolated intervertebral disk space becomes evident, accompanied by decreased vertebral height, demineralization, and localized erosion of the vertebral margins. Approximately 2–3 months after the appearance of initial radiographic changes, remineralization with sclerosis is seen at the margins of the adjacent vertebral bodies. The involved disk space remains narrowed, and occasionally the adjacent vertebrae enlarge. The posterior vertebral elements are never involved, and abscess formation is rarely seen. Because patients are often first seen after symptoms have been present for several weeks, the radiographic findings at presentation typically consist of a narrowed disk space, end plate irregularities of at least one contiguous vertebra, and loss of lumbar lordosis. Results of the ^{99m}Tc and ^{67}Ga scans may be positive early in the disease, before radiographic evidence of disk narrowing appears. Results of a ^{67}Ga scan may be abnormal even with normal findings on a ^{99m}Tc scan if there is no concomitant bone involvement. MRI is sensitive for the evaluation of diskitis and confirms disk-space

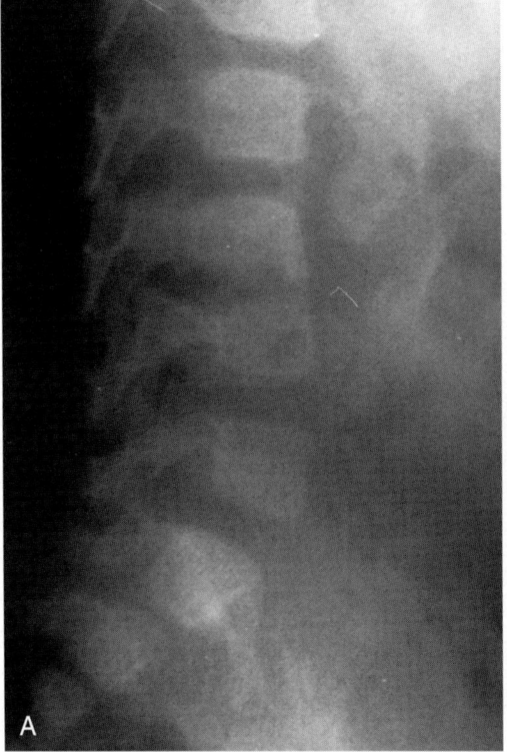

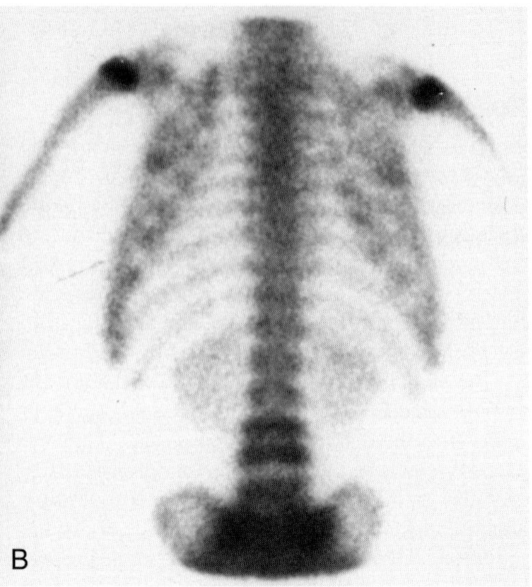

FIGURE 88–1. Diskitis in a 9-month-old girl with a history of refusing to sit up or bear weight and mild fever of several weeks' duration. **A,** Lateral radiograph of lumbar spine shows narrowing of the L3–4 disk space and irregularity of the involved vertebral-body end plates. **B,** Radionuclide scan (^{99m}Tc) shows increased uptake by the L3 and L4 vertebral bodies.

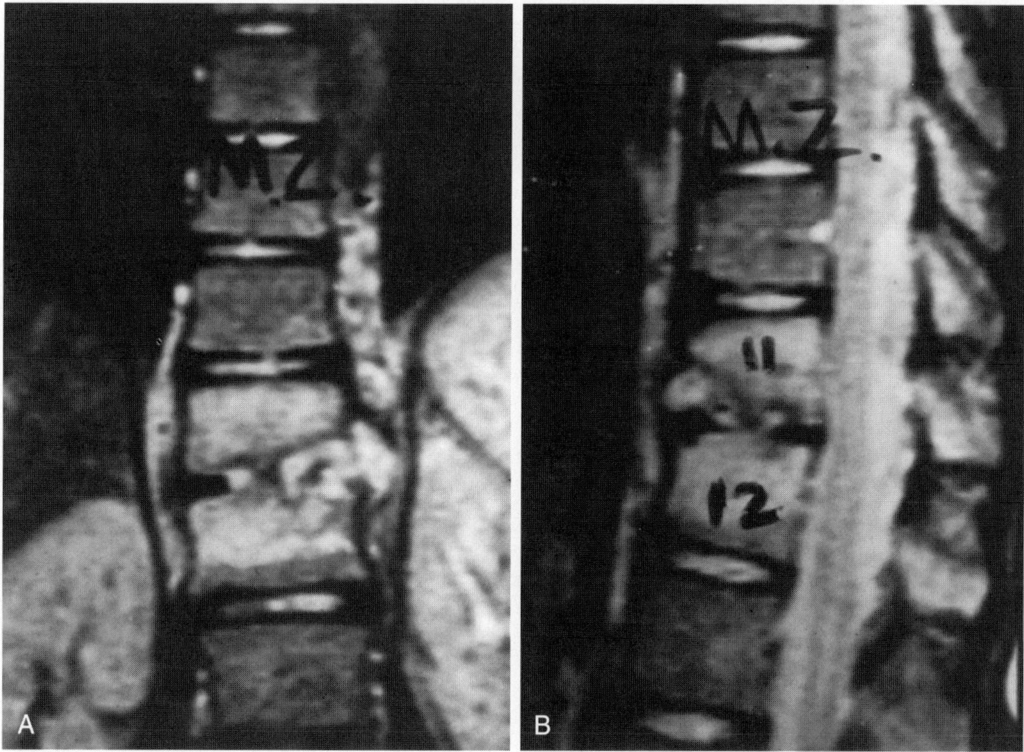

FIGURE 88–2. MRI of diskitis in a 7-year-old boy with a history of fever, irritability, and back pain. **A,** Coronal T2-weighted image of the lower thoracic spine shows increased signal intensity within the T11 and T12 vertebral bodies. The intervening disk contents are enlarged and have extruded into the paraspinal space on the left side. **B,** Lateral midline image likewise reveals extrusion of disk material anteriorly with destruction of the normal disk material (compared with the disk spaces above and below). Vertebral tuberculosis cannot be excluded from the differential diagnosis on the basis of this study.

narrowing and irregularities in the vertebral end plate early in the course of the disease. MRI readily demonstrates the extent of the inflammatory process and infection, as well as the condition of the surrounding soft tissue. MRI often shows relative loss of disk height, irregular contour, and increased signal from adjacent vertebral bodies (Fig. 88–2).

TREATMENT

Bed rest with or without traction is used when pain is present, the ESR is elevated, and radiographs show abnormalities. If the diskitis is refractory to these measures, immobilization with a plaster jacket or pantaloon cast may be necessary.

Antimicrobial therapy directed against the infecting organism is indicated for cases of diskitis associated with bacteremia or a positive disk culture result. Biopsy or disk aspiration should be reserved for cases of recurrence when the clinical situation dictates the need, when the person still has continued back pain or pain on walking after immobilization, or when vertebral osteomyelitis is evident by diagnostic imaging. Antibiotic regimens should be directed by cultures of blood and biopsy material, if results are positive. In the absence of a positive blood or disk culture result, antimicrobial agents have not been shown to be of value in treating diskitis. Recommendations for the empirical use of antibiotics are controversial because there are no controlled studies of therapy, including the route of administration and duration of treatment. Antibiotic use does not appear to alter the disease process in cases of undocumented infection. Nevertheless, there appears to be a basis for the empirical treatment of this condition with antistaphylococcal antibiotics in doses used for osteomyelitis if biopsy results are nondiagnostic but suggest an infection. Oral therapy for 4–6 months has been advocated, although the optimal route and duration of empirical treatment remain undetermined.

COMPLICATIONS

Most persons have resolution of their symptoms without complications, especially those with negative bacterial culture results. Recurrences are infrequent. Radiographic changes tend to develop regardless of treatment.

PROGNOSIS

The prognosis for persons with this disease is excellent, with most having complete clinical recovery. Long-term follow-up of children has documented disk space narrowing but without significant impairment or pain. One study (Jansen, 1993) reported follow-up of 35 children, on average 17 years after treatment of diskitis. Frequent or daily backache was present in 10%. Flexion of the low back was normal in 90%, whereas extension was markedly restricted in 85%. Narrowing of the vertebral canal was present in 80%. The mode of treatment of the diskitis did not appear to affect the eventual outcome. A longer period of follow-up will be needed to determine back pain and disability in later adulthood. Comparison with similar populations who did not have diskitis in childhood is also needed.

PREVENTION

There are no recognized specific measures to prevent diskitis.

REVIEWS

Crawford AH, Kucharzyk DW, Ruda R, et al: Diskitis in children. *Clin Orthop* 1991;266:70–9.

Cushing AH: Diskitis in children. *Clin Infect Dis* 1993;17:1–6.

Fernandez M, Carrol CL, Baker CJ: Discitis and vertebral osteomyelitis in children: An 18-year review. *Pediatrics* 2000;105:1299–304.

Ring D, Wenger DR: Pyogenic infectious spondylitis in children. The evolution to current thought. *Am J Orthop* 1996;25:342–8.

Scoles PV, Quinn TP: Intervertebral discitis in children and adolescents. *Clin Orthop* 1982;162:31–6.

KEY ARTICLES

Bunnell WP: Back pain in children. *Orthop Clin North Am* 1982; 13:587–604.

Fischer GW, Popich GA, Sullivan DE, et al: Diskitis: A prospective diagnostic analysis. *Pediatrics* 1978;62:543–8.

Heller RM, Szalay EA, Green NE, et al: Disc space infection in children: Magnetic resonance imaging. *Radiol Clin North Am* 1988;26:207–9.

Jansen BHR, Hart W, Schreuder O: Diskitis in childhood: 12–35 year follow-up of 35 patients. *Acta Orthop Scand* 1993;64(1):33–6.

King HA: Back pain in children. *Pediatr Clin North Am* 1984;31:1083–95.

Littleton HR, Rhoades ER: Septic diskitis: Report of case and review of the literature. *J Am Osteopath Assoc* 1980;79:544–6.

Magera BE, Klein SG, Derrick CW Jr: Radiological cases of the month. Diskitis. *Am J Dis Child* 1989;143:1479–80.

Norris S, Ehrlich MG, Keim DE, et al: Early diagnosis of disc-space infection using gallium-67. *J Nucl Med* 1978;19:384–6.

Rudert M, Tillman B: Lymph and blood supply of the human intervetebral disc: Cadaver study of correlation to diskitis. *Acta Orthop Scand* 1993;64(1):37–40.

Sartoris DJ, Moskowitz PS, Kaufman RA, et al: Childhood diskitis: Computed tomographic findings. *Radiology* 1983;149:701–7.

Wenger DR, Bobechko WP, Gilday DL: The spectrum of intervertebral disc space infection in children. *J Bone Joint Surg Am* 1978;60:100–8.

CHAPTER 89

Bacterial and Viral Conjunctivitis

Albert W. Biglan ▪ Hal B. Jenson

The **conjunctiva** is a thin mucous membrane that lines the eyelids **(palpebral conjunctiva)** and covers the anterior surface of the globe **(bulbar conjunctiva)**. It consists of an epithelial layer and a deeper substantia propria. Conjunctivitis refers to a diverse group of diseases or conditions, both infectious and noninfectious, that primarily affect the conjunctivae. Conjunctivitis may be associated with systemic conditions, or it can be limited, involving only the conjunctival tissue. Infections of the conjunctiva are frequently self-limiting, but associated complications can occur and damage adjacent ocular structures such as the cornea, eyelids, and deeper orbital structures.

Neonatal conjunctivitis includes several distinct infections that may be acquired perinatally. Conjunctivitis in older children, adolescents, and adults is caused by both bacterial and viral agents with overlapping clinical findings.

NEONATAL CONJUNCTIVITIS

Neonatal conjunctivitis, or **ophthalmia neonatorum,** refers to purulent conjunctivitis during the first 10 days of life, usually acquired during birth. Historically this term referred only to gonococcal infection. Ophthalmia neonatorum is most common in countries or regions of the world where prophylaxis for gonococcal ophthalmia neonatorum is not routinely practiced.

ETIOLOGY

The common causes of neonatal conjunctivitis, in order of decreasing prevalence, include chemical in nurseries where silver nitrate 1% is used for gonococcal prophylaxis; *Chlamydia trachomatis;* common bacterial causes of conjunctivitis, including viridans streptococci, *Staphylococcus aureus, Haemophilus influenzae,* group D *Streptococcus, Moraxella catarrhalis, Escherichia coli,* and other gram-negative enteric bacilli; and *Neisseria gonorrhoeae,* which can also be associated with disseminated neonatal infections. Neonatal conjunctivitis can also occur as a component of perinatal herpes simplex virus infection (Chapter 96).

Transmission. Expectant mothers, especially those who receive inadequate prenatal care and screening for gonococcal and chlamydial genital infections, may harbor organisms in the cervix and birth canal that may be transmitted to the eyes during birth. Prolonged rupture of the amniotic membranes may permit organisms in the lower birth canal to ascend into the amniotic fluid and infect the external structures of the eye. In both nurseries and home environments, bacteria and viruses may be transmitted postnatally to the eyes by unwashed hands.

EPIDEMIOLOGY

Neonatal conjunctivitis occurs in 1–12% of neonates. A mild to moderate chemical conjunctivitis commonly occurs within 24–48 hours of age in newborns who receive silver nitrate 1% applied to the eyes for gonococcal prophylaxis. The prevalence of *N. gonorrhoeae* and *C. trachomatis* neonatal infections is related directly to the prevalence of maternal genital infections and screening of pregnant women for gonorrhea and chlamydial infections (Chapter 85). Nasopharyngeal and conjunctival acquisition of *C. trachomatis* occurs perinatally in approximately 50% of infants born vaginally to infected mothers and in some infants delivered by cesarean section with intact membranes. Among those infants who acquire *C. trachomatis,* the risk of conjunctivitis is 25–50% and that of pneumonia is 5–20% (Chapter 68).

PATHOGENESIS

The conjunctiva provides a favorable environment for local proliferation of pathogenic bacteria, producing the associated signs of inflammation and purulent discharge.

SYMPTOMS AND CLINICAL MANIFESTATIONS

The timing of development of clinical manifestations and the presence and type of discharge can be helpful in identifying the organism or agent causing the conjunctivitis (Table 89–1). Premature rupture of the amniotic membranes may cause the onset a day or more earlier. Chemical conjunctivitis develops within the first 24–48 hours after application; it then rapidly subsides and produces a watery discharge. *N. gonorrhoeae* conjunctivitis typically emerges 3 days after birth, with a range of 2–7 days, and has a copious purulent discharge that, when wiped away, returns quickly, sometimes within 10–15 minutes (Fig. 89–1). *C. trachomatis* conjunctivitis typically emerges 7 days after birth, with a range of 5–14 days, and has a scanty mucopurulent discharge with mild swelling of the eyelids and conjunctivae. Affected children may also develop chlamydial pneumonia between 3 weeks and 3 months of age. Herpes simplex virus predominantly involves the conjunctiva and periocular skin of the eyelid, with significant periocular swelling. The onset usual occurs between 3 and 21 days—and typically between 6 and 14 days. Common bacterial causes of conjunctivitis show the mild to moderate purulent discharge that is also seen in older children.

DIAGNOSIS

Although the clinical criteria listed are helpful in differential diagnosis and in guiding initial therapy, laboratory diagnosis is essential.

TABLE 89–1. Clinical Manifestations and Treatment of Neonatal Conjunctivitis

Organism	Percentage of Cases	Discharge and External Examination	Age at Onset	Diagnosis*	Associated Manifestations	Treatment
Neisseria gonorrhoeae (Fig. 89–1)	<1%	Copious, purulent discharge Severe swelling of lids and conjunctivae Cornea involvement common Risk for perforation and corneal scar	1–7 days	Gram stain (gram-negative intracellular diplococci [Plate 1C]) Culture on chocolate agar	May be associated with disseminated gonococcal infection	Ceftriaxone 50 mg/kg (max 125 mg) IV or IM *or* Penicillin G 50,000 U IV or IM *plus* Saline lavage of conjunctivae
Chlamydia trachomatis	2–40%	Scant discharge Mild swelling Hyperemia Follicular response (Fig. 89–5) Late corneal staining	4–19 days	Giemsa stain of scraping (purple intracytoplasmic inclusions near nucleus [Fig. 89–2]) Direct determination with direct immunofluorescent antibody test Direct determination with PCR	May presage *C. trachomatis* pneumonia at 3 wk to 3 mo of age (Chapter 68)	Erythromycin ethylsuccinate 50 mg/kg/day in 4 divided doses PO for 2 wk
Herpes simplex virus	<1%	Clear or serosanguineous discharge Lid swelling Keratitis with cloudy cornea Dendrite formation	3 days to 3 wk	Giemsa stain of scraping (multinucleate giant cells with intranuclear inclusions) Viral culture	May be associated with disseminated perinatal herpes simplex virus infection (Chapter 97)	Systemic acyclovir for systemic involvement (Chapter 97) *plus* trifluridine 1% ophthalmic solution 5–6 times a day
Bacterial *Staphylococcus* *Streptococcus* *Pseudomonas*	30–50%	Purulent moderate discharge Mild lid and conjunctival swelling Corneal involvement with risk for perforation	2–7 days	Gram stain Culture on blood agar		Topical therapy (Table 89–4)
Chemical Silver nitrate 1%	Variable, depending on use of silver nitrate	Watery discharge	1–3 days	No organisms on smear or culture		None

*All cases of suspected infectious neonatal conjunctivitis should be Gram stained and cultured for bacteria.

Laboratory evaluation should include smears of the secretions stained with Gram and Giemsa stains. *N. gonorrhoeae* appears as gram-negative intracellular diplococci on Gram stain. Because this infection can rapidly damage the eye, all neonates with purulent conjunctivitis should have Gram stain and bacterial culture. Newborns with suspected gonococcal ophthalmia should be hospitalized and evaluated for signs of disseminated infection. Giemsa stain of conjunctival scrapings with *C. trachomatis* conjunctivitis reveals intracytoplasmic inclusions near the nucleus (Fig. 89–2). Newborns with *C. trachomatis* conjunctivitis should be evaluated for chlamydial pneumonia (Chapter 68). The presence of multinucleated giant cells with intranuclear inclusions suggests infection with herpes simplex virus, which can be confirmed by PCR assay or virus culture. Children with conjunctivitis from sexually transmitted organisms should be tested for other sexually transmitted diseases such as syphilis.

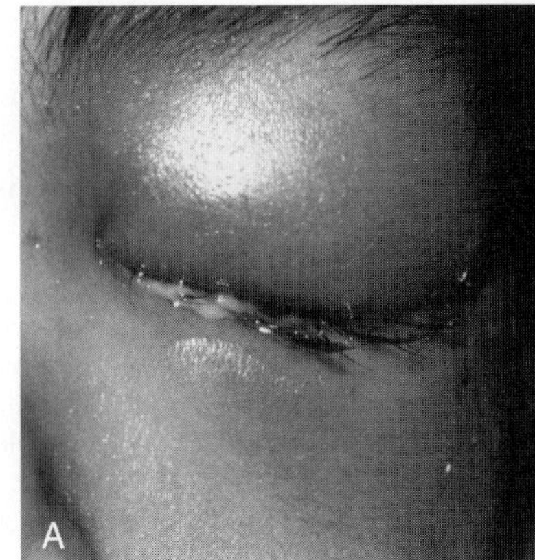

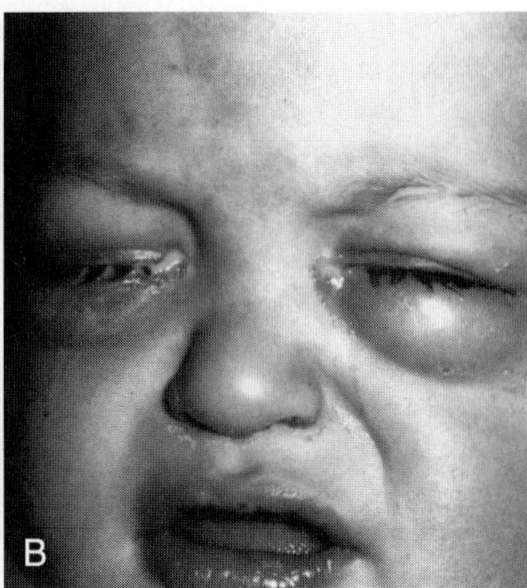

FIGURE 89–1. *Neisseria gonorrhoeae* conjunctivitis with severe lid edema, and a copious yellowish green purulent discharge. **A,** Four-year-old child. **B,** Two-month-old child.

TREATMENT

Conjunctivitis caused by *N. gonorrhoeae* or *C. trachomatis* should be treated systemically (Table 89–1). Treatment of gonococcal conjunctivitis includes ceftriaxone (25–50 mg/kg; maximum dose: 125 mg) given once intravenously or intramuscularly or cefotaxime (100 mg/kg) given once intravenously or intramuscularly, combined with frequent saline ophthalmic lavages, as often as hourly initially and continued until the discharge is eliminated, with care to avoid disrupting the corneal epithelium. Erythromycin 0.5% or tetracycline 1% ophthalmic ointment applied three times daily may be used to supplement systemic treatment and will speed resolution of the discharge. *C. trachomatis* conjunctivitis should be treated with erythromycin 50 mg/kg/day given orally and divided in four daily doses for 14 days. *C. trachomatis* conjunctivitis can be treated with erythromycin 0.5% ophthalmic ointment applied four times a day, but topical therapy will not adequately treat the >50% of infants with chlamydial conjunctivitis who also have nasopharyngeal colonization. Systemic therapy is recommended to minimize progression to chlamydial pneumonia; topical therapy is not necessary with oral therapy. The mother and her sexual partners should also receive empirical treatment for chlamydial genital infection (Table 85–4).

Other causes of bacterial conjunctivitis are treated with topical application of a broad-spectrum antibiotic such as tobramycin or erythromycin ophthalmic ointment applied to the eyes three or four times daily until resolution. Chemical conjunctivitis requires only supportive measures such as compresses. Newborns with perinatal herpes simplex virus conjunctivitis should be treated systemically with acyclovir (Chapter 97) and also with topical trifluridine 1% solution every 2 hours (9 times daily) for 7 days. Ophthalmologic consultation is recommended for conjunctivitis with ocular involvement, which may be indicated by eye pain, severe photophobia, or decreased visual acuity.

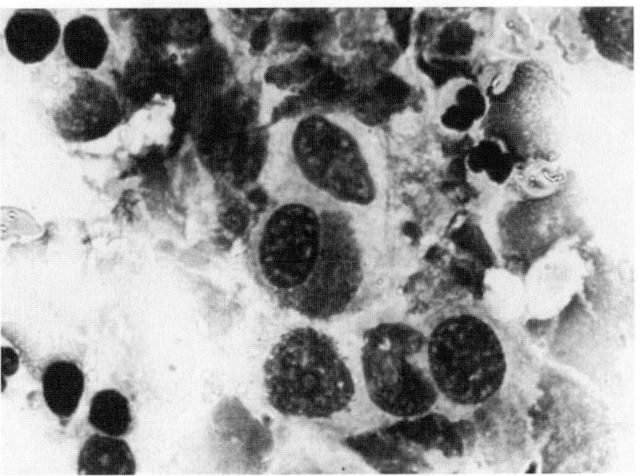

FIGURE 89–2. Conjunctival scraping and Giemsa staining of cells shows the characteristic intracellular inclusions near the nucleus in *Chlamydia trachomatis* conjunctivitis.

COMPLICATIONS AND PROGNOSIS

Ocular complications of neonatal conjunctivitis are uncommon, except with *N. gonorrhoeae* and herpes simplex virus infections. Corneal and conjunctival scarring, corneal perforation, especially with *N. gonorrhoeae,* and orbital cellulitis can occur. Herpes simplex keratitis can be recurrent, with each attack increasing the likelihood of visual impairment resulting from scarring of the cornea.

Oral erythromycin therapy has been associated with **infantile hypertrophic pyloric stenosis** in children <6 weeks of age. The risk with other macrolides is unknown. Erythromycin continues to be recommended for *C. trachomatis* neonatal infections.

PREVENTION

Infected infants should be isolated from other newborns. Strict hygiene, isolation measures, and good hand-washing techniques should be enforced in all nurseries. Parents should receive instruction on using similar measures at home. Prenatal care can establish a diagnosis of chlamydial or gonococcal cervicitis and other sexually transmitted diseases. Appropriate treatment of the mother should be instituted before delivery. Infants born to mothers with untreated gonococcal infection should be treated with a single dose of ceftriaxone (25–50 mg) or cefotaxime (100 mg/kg) in addition to ocular prophylaxis. Infants born to mothers with untreated chlamydial infections are at high risk of having a neonatal infection, but prophylactic treatment is not routinely recommended because the efficacy is unknown. These infants should have close follow-up for *C. trachomatis* conjunctivitis and pneumonia.

Neonatal Gonococcal Prophylaxis. All infants should receive prophylaxis for gonococcal ophthalmia neonatorum. The traditional **Credé prophylaxis,** instilling silver nitrate 1%, is common. Alternative methods may be equally effective and less irritating; either erythromycin 0.5% ointment or tetracycline 1% ointment can be used. There is no standard regimen for prophylaxis. Povidone-iodine 2.5% solution is also effective, but there is no commercial ophthalmic preparation available in the United States. If applied correctly, these methods are approximately equally effective for gonococcal prophylaxis, but none appear effective in preventing chlamydial conjunctivitis or nasopharyngeal colonization. Silver nitrate 1% is associated with chemical conjunctivitis more commonly than the other agents.

Each eyelid should be wiped gently with sterile cotton before administration. Two drops of 1% silver nitrate solution or a 1 cm ($\frac{1}{2}$ inch) ribbon of antibiotic ointment (erythromycin 0.5% or tetracycline 1% ointment) is placed in each lower conjunctival sac; the eyelids are then massaged gently to spread the medication. After 1 minute, excess solution or ointment may be wiped away with sterile cotton. The eyes should not be rinsed or flushed with normal saline solution after administration because doing so may reduce the effectiveness and does not reduce the incidence of chemical conjunctivitis. All infants should receive prophylaxis, including those born by cesarean delivery. Prophylaxis should be given shortly after birth. Some experts suggest that prophylaxis may be administered more effectively in the nursery than in the delivery room, although delaying prophylaxis for as long as 1 hour after birth to facilitate parent-infant bonding is unlikely to influence efficacy.

BACTERIAL AND VIRAL CONJUNCTIVITIS

ETIOLOGY

The rapidity of onset, the duration, and the recurrence of conjunctivitis are used to classify conjunctivitis. **Acute conjunctivitis** is characterized by a rapid onset of symptoms and signs for 1–2 days and usually has a bacterial or viral cause. The most common causes of bacterial conjunctivitis in children include *H. influenzae* (usually nontypeable), *Streptococcus pneumoniae,* and *M. catarrhalis* (Table 89–2). *N. gonorrhoeae* and *Neisseria meningitidis* are less common causes. Other bacteria occasionally isolated include *Staphylococcus,* group A *Streptococcus, E. coli, Klebsiella pneumoniae,* and *Pseudomonas aeruginosa.* Normal ocular bacterial flora includes *S. aureus,* coagulase-negative staphylococci, viridans streptococci, and *Corynebacterium.* Viral conjunctivitis is most commonly caused by adenoviruses and less frequently by coxsackieviruses and other enteroviruses. Acute conjunctivitis usually resolves within 7–14 days. **Chronic conjunctivitis** indicates persistence for >14 days. Chronic infectious conjunctivitis is com-

TABLE 89–2. Acute Conjunctivitis in Children

	Common Organisms	
	Bacterial	Viral
	Haemophilus influenzae (usually nontypeable) *Streptococcus pneumoniae* *Moraxella catarrhalis*	Adenoviruses type 8, 19 Enteroviruses Herpes simplex virus
Incubation	24–72 hr	1–14 days
Symptoms		
Photophobia	Mild	Moderate to severe
Blurred vision	Common with discharge	If keratitis is present
Foreign body sensation	Unusual	Yes
Signs	See Plate 9A	See Plate 9B
Discharge	Purulent discharge	Watery discharge
Palpebral reaction	Papillary response	Follicular response (Fig. 89–5)
Preauricular node	Unusual for acute (<10%)	More common (20%)
Chemosis	Moderate	Mild
Hemorrhagic conjunctiva	Occasionally with *Streptococcus*	Frequent with enteroviruses
Cornea stain	Unusual	Frequent
Subepithelial opacity	Unusual	Frequent
Phlyctenule (Fig. 89–3)	Common with *Staphylococcus*	No
Associated defects	Contaminated eye solutions Allergic conjunctivitis Blepharitis Nasolacrimal duct obstruction Eyelid or blink abnormalities Eczema Contact lens use Otitis media	Upper respiratory tract infection, especially pharyngitis Rash Gastroenteritis
Treatment	See Table 89–4	Adenovirus: self-limited
Topical	Sulfacetamide 10% *or* Polymyxin B–trimethoprim *or* Erythromycin	Herpes simplex virus: trifluridine 1% solution or vidarabine 3% ointment, with ophthalmologic consultation
End of contagious period	24 hr after start of effective treatment	7 days after onset of symptoms

monly caused by *Moraxella lacunata,* viral or chlamydial infections, or an unrecognized foreign body with an accompanying secondary infection. **Recurrent conjunctivitis** usually has a noninfectious cause, such as conjunctival exposure as a result of **lagophthalmos,** a condition in which the eye cannot be closed; exposure to a chemical or an allergen; or eye rubbing. It also may be due to recurrence associated with dry eye or lacrimal duct obstruction or to infection with herpes simplex virus or varicella-zoster virus. Herpes simplex virus predominantly affects the cornea, and conjunctivitis is usually a secondary manifestation (Chapter 90).

EPIDEMIOLOGY

Bacterial conjunctivitis is common in young children with congenital nasolacrimal duct obstruction, sinus disease, ear infection, or allergic conjunctivitis and in children with upper respiratory tract infection who rub nasal secretions into their eyes. Bacterial conjunctivitis frequently occurs in children who are in contact with other infected children.

There are no reliable figures of the prevalence of viral conjunctivitis. However, in some communities, infection with **epidemic keratoconjunctivitis** associated with adenovirus types 8 and 19 has reached epidemic portions.

Transmission. The most common method of spreading bacterial and viral conjunctivitis is person-to-person transmission of infected secretions to the eye, facilitated by failure to wash hands and other lapses in personal hygiene. Viral conjunctivitis is usually contracted by exposure to an infected individual, with spread by aerosol or direct transmission.

PATHOGENESIS

The conjunctiva provides a favorable environment for local proliferation of pathogenic bacteria that produce a **purulent conjunctivitis** with moderate signs of inflammation of red or pink conjunctivae and purulent discharge. Viral conjunctivitis is characterized as **nonpurulent conjunctivitis** with less inflammation, with a pink conjunctiva, and with a clear, watery eye discharge. Bilateral disease occurs in 75–90% of bacterial and viral conjunctivitis.

The conjunctiva responds acutely to infection by development of papillae and follicles. Bacterial conjunctivitis usually results in a papillary or nonspecific conjunctival reaction, whereas viral conjunctivitis usually results in a follicular reaction. **Follicles** have a network of blood vessels covering their surface, whereas **papillae** have a vessel at the core. Histologically, follicles are really germinal centers composed of masses of lymphoid cells, whereas papillae represent a growth of small vessels in the conjunctiva that have been infiltrated by lymphocytes and other inflammatory cells, without organization into a germinal center. Conjunctival follicles are uncommon in children <2 years of age and do not develop in the neonate, presumably because of the immaturity of the lymphoid system. Papillae are usually smaller than follicles and more commonly occur on the upper tarsal conjunctiva. A granulomatous conjunctivitis may be seen with many chronic infecting agents, such as *Mycobacterium tuberculosis,* or with fungi such as *Aspergillus, Candida,* or *Fusarium.*

SYMPTOMS AND CLINICAL MANIFESTATIONS

Bacterial Conjunctivitis. Bacterial conjunctivitis typically has an incubation period of 24–72 hours. Symptoms include mild photophobia, redness, and discharge (Plate 9A). The eyelids are frequently matted after sleep because of drying of the thick, purulent discharge. The cornea is usually not involved. Physical findings include chemosis, red injection of the conjunctiva, and mild to moderate edema of the eyelids. Hemorrhages in the conjunctiva may occur with *Streptococcus* species and are also seen in children who vigorously rub their eyes. Children with bacterial conjunctivitis are more likely to have concomitant otitis media, the **conjunctivitis-otitis syndrome.**

Patients with *Staphylococcus* infection of the lid margins, or blepharitis (Chapter 91), frequently develop conjunctivitis and occasionally have infiltrates at the corneal limbus. Typically there is an interval of clear cornea between the infiltrates and the corneal limbus. The infiltrates can lead to scarring and vascularization of the marginal cornea; the resulting vesicles and nodules are known as **phlyctenules** (Fig. 89–3). Phlyctenules can also occur on the conjunctiva adjacent to the cornea, where they appear as a white, raised patch, which stains with fluorescein. Phlyctenules may also be caused by tuberculosis. Chronic infection of the conjunctiva with *Staphylococcus* can cause punctate staining of the cornea and marginal ulcers (Fig. 89–4).

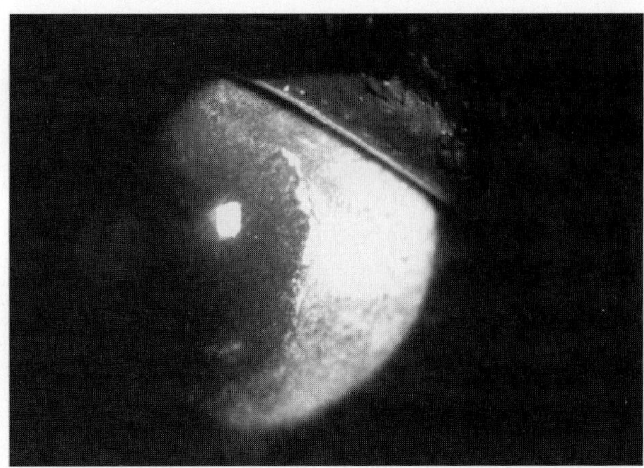

FIGURE 89–3. Fluorescein stain of the conjunctiva, demonstrating a phlyctenule of the conjunctiva. (Courtesy of Department of Ophthalmic Photography, Eye and Ear Institute, Pittsburgh, Penn.)

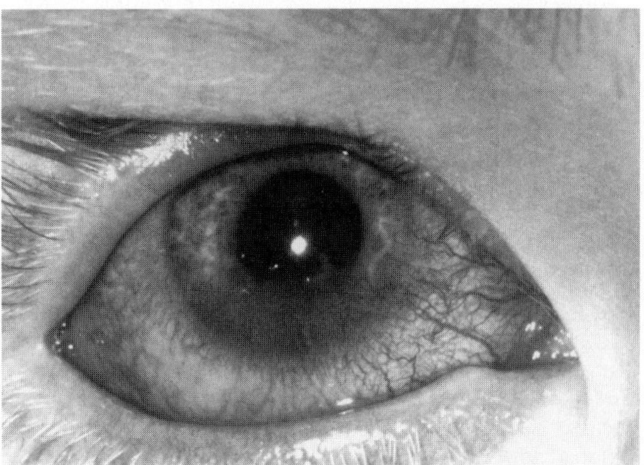

FIGURE 89–4. Chronic staphylococcal blepharoconjunctivitis may result in punctate stains and marginal ulcers of the cornea. Prolonged infection can cause blood vessel invasion of the cornea and pannus formation. (Courtesy of Department of Ophthalmic Photography, Eye and Ear Institute, Pittsburgh, Penn.)

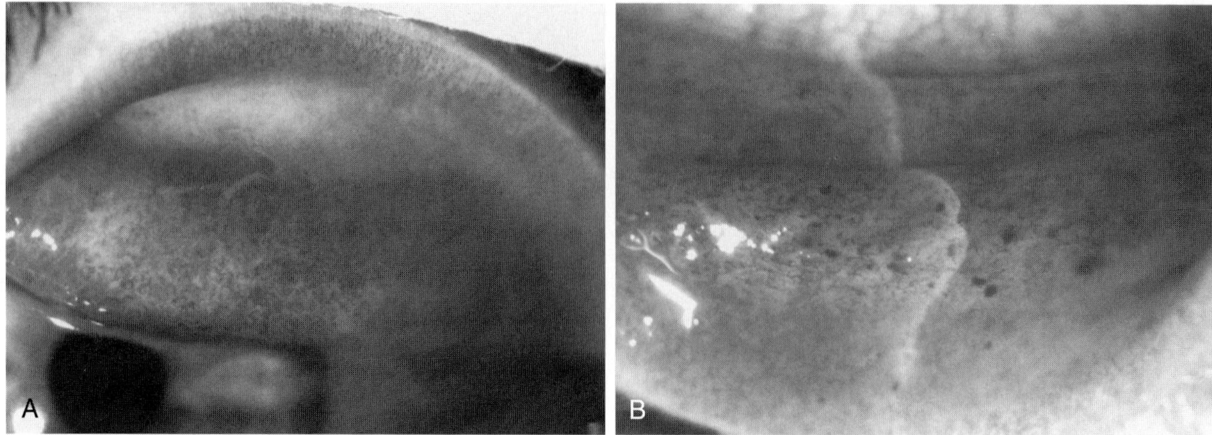

FIGURE 89–5. Viral conjunctivitis, demonstrating the follicular response under the everted upper eyelid (**A**) and the appearance of the conjunctiva behind the everted lower eyelid (**B**). (Courtesy of Department of Ophthalmic Photography, Eye and Ear Institute, Pittsburgh, Penn.)

An inflammatory membrane can develop over the palpebral conjunctiva and cul-de-sac with severe infections, particularly those associated with *Corynebacterium diphtheriae.* These membranes adhere to the palpebral conjunctiva, which may bleed when the membrane is removed.

Viral Conjunctivitis. Adenoviral keratoconjunctivitis typically has an incubation period of 7–10 days. Viral conjunctivitis begins with a watery discharge and is accompanied by a scratchy sensation and mild chemosis with a pink injection of the conjunctiva (Plate 9B). Involvement of the cornea is associated with extreme light sensitivity. There may be a palpable preauricular lymph node that may be tender but is usually nontender with adenovirus infection. The inferior fornix and conjunctiva usually demonstrate a follicular response (Fig. 89–5). Conjunctival hemorrhages may be present, especially with enterovirus infections. The cornea may develop punctate keratitis, followed in 1–2 weeks by subepithelial infiltrates. Punctate keratitis can be demonstrated by placing a drop of fluorescein stain in the conjunctival sac and illuminating the cornea with a cobalt blue light. A slit lamp facilitates examination. Viral conjunctivitis is more frequently associated with upper respiratory tract infection and pharyngitis than is bacterial conjunctivitis.

DIAGNOSIS

Distinguishing bacterial from viral conjunctivitis on the basis of clinical examination alone is difficult. Examination reveals red, edematous conjunctiva and purulent discharge with bacterial conjunctivitis or pink conjunctiva and serous discharge with viral conjunctivitis (Table 89–2). In one study (Weiss, 1993), slit-lamp examination showed a papillary or mixed conjunctival response in 72% of bacterial infections and a follicular response in 88% of viral infections, but this examination is difficult to perform successfully in most young children. Bacterial conjunctivitis is more often associated with otitis media, and viral conjunctivitis with pharyngitis.

TABLE 89–3. Differential Diagnosis of Bacterial and Viral Conjunctivitis

Allergic conjunctivitis	Anterior uveitis (iritis)
Vernal keratoconjunctivitis	Scleritis or episcleritis
Chemical conjunctivitis	Dry eye
Conjunctival or corneal foreign body	Contact dermatitis
Nasolacrimal duct obstruction	Ultraviolet keratitis
Stevens-Johnson syndrome	Arteriovenous malformations or fistulas
Giant papillary conjunctivitis	Kawasaki syndrome
Eye rubbing	Corneal abrasion/erosion
Medicamentosa	Blepharitis

Differential Diagnosis

There are many noninfectious causes that can mimic bacterial and viral conjunctivitis (Table 89–3), especially eye rubbing, corneal abrasion, conjunctival foreign body, vernal keratoconjunctivitis, anterior uveitis, and ultraviolet keratitis. Both allergic conjunctivitis and vernal conjunctivitis produce a chronic red eye.

Microbiologic Evaluation

Because bacterial conjunctivitis is usually self-limited or responds readily to topical treatment, cultures are not routinely grown. Cultures are reserved for cases of severe purulent discharge, delayed spontaneous resolution, lack of response to antibiotic treatment, or recurrence. Smears of the discharge placed on slides and stained with Gram and Giemsa stains may assist in identification of organisms.

Virus culture and PCR assay to detect adenovirus are not routinely obtained but may be useful in epidemics to confirm the presence of a particular agent for epidemiologic studies.

TREATMENT

The lids should be treated frequently with warm compresses to remove the accumulated discharge. The lashes are cleansed with cotton-tipped swabs moistened with tap water. The child and caregiver should be instructed to perform careful hand washing before and after treatment.

Bacterial Conjunctivitis. Acute bacterial conjunctivitis is frequently a self-limiting condition, but the use of antibiotics is associated with significantly improved rates of early clinical remission and of early and late microbiologic remission. Antibiotics that suppress bacterial proliferation are instilled between the eyelids four times a day until the discharge subsides and the chemosis resolves. Frequently used antibiotics include sulfacetamide 10% solution, trimethoprim–polymyxin B solution, and erythromycin ointment (Table 89–4). Ointments prolong the contact of the drug

TABLE 89–4. Commonly Used Ophthalmic Antibiotics for Bacterial Conjunctivitis in Children*

Drug and Formulation	Trade Names	Solution	Ointment
Recommended Regimens			
Polymyxin B–trimethoprim	Polytrim, generic	10,000 U/mL–1 mg/mL	Not available
Sulfacetamide†	AK-Sulf, Bleph-10, Cetamide, Sulamyd, Sulf-10, generic	10%	10%
Erythromycin	Ilotycin, generic	Not available	0.5%
Alternative Regimens			
Gentamicin	Garamycin, Genoptic, Gentacidin, Gentak, generic	0.3%	0.3%
Tobramycin	Tobrex, generic	0.3%	0.3%
Ciprofloxacin	Ciloxan	0.3%	0.3%
Norfloxacin	Chibroxin	0.3%	Not available
Ofloxacin	Ocuflox	0.3%	Not available
Other Formulations			
Bacitracin	AK-Tracin	Not available	500 U/g
Chloramphenicol	AK-Chlor, Chloromycetin, Chloroptic, generic	0.5% (also available as 0.16% [Chloromycetin])	1% (Chloromycetin, Chloroptic)
Polymyxin B–bacitracin	AK-Poly-Bac, Polysporin, generic	Not available	10,000 U/g–500 U/g
Polymyxin B–neomycin–bacitracin	AK-Spore, Neosporin, generic	Not available	10,000 U/g–3.5 mg/g–400 U/g
Polymyxin B–neomycin–gramicidin	AK-Spore, Neosporin, generic	10,000 U/mL–1.75 mg/mL–0.025 mg/mL	Not available
Polymyxin B–oxytetracycline	Terramycin, Terak	Not available	10,000 U/g–5 mg/g

*In general, solutions (eyedrops) are instilled in the conjunctival sac(s) as 1–2 drops every 2 hours while awake for 2 days, then every 4 hours while awake for 5 days. Ointments are applied as a ½-inch ribbon into the conjunctival sac(s) three times a day for 2 days, then two times a day for 5 days.
†Sulfacetamide is also available as 15% solution (Isopto Cetamide) and 30% solution (Sulamyd, generic) but these are not routinely recommended.

with the conjunctiva, but tend to blur vision, so solutions as eyedrops are preferred. Aminoglycoside and newer quinolone antibiotics should be reserved for more serious ocular infections. Reports of resistant strains of bacteria are emerging, and these agents should be reserved for treatment of keratitis and endophthalmitis. Children with conjunctivitis-otitis syndrome require oral therapy as for otitis media (Chapter 64).

Viral Conjunctivitis. Symptoms usually persist for 7–14 days. Cool compresses and oral analgesics are the mainstay of treatment. During this period some ophthalmologists recommend a topical antibiotic solution, such as sulfacetamide 10% or polymyxin B–trimethoprim three or four times daily, to suppress bacterial growth. Persons with persistent symptoms with punctate keratitis and associated subepithelial infiltrates will have blurred vision, which may decrease visual acuity to 20/40 if the keratitis involves the visual axis. Acute hemorrhagic conjunctivitis also occurs with many systemic viral infections such as measles, chickenpox, and mumps. Recommended treatment is with weak topical solutions of corticosteroids such as medrysone 1% (HMS Liquifilm) or rimexolone 1% (Vexol) applied three or four times daily. Treatment with corticosteroids will alleviate symptoms of photophobia and improve vision but may prolong the time to resolution. Children should be referred for ophthalmologic consultation if there is decreased visual acuity, marked pain, marked light sensitivity, or development of purulent discharge. Viral conjunctivitis caused by herpes simplex virus can be treated with trifluridine 1% solution five or six times daily or vidarabine 3% ointment four times daily, in combination with systemic acyclovir. Corticosteroids should be avoided if herpetic infection is suspected, and immediate ophthalmologic consultation is recommended.

COMPLICATIONS

If the corneal epithelium is abraded, bacterial conjunctivitis can lead to corneal ulceration. Ulceration can occur in the absence of abrasion with *N. gonorrhoeae* infection. Organisms can invade the eyelid tissues and cause a preseptal cellulitis.

Children with nasolacrimal duct obstruction have repeated episodes of bacterial conjunctivitis and chronic dacryocystitis that will not resolve until the obstruction is relieved with a probe-and-irrigation procedure. This procedure is usually performed after 6 months of age. Recurrent bouts of conjunctivitis complicating nasolacrimal duct obstruction may contribute to the slight decline in effectiveness of the probe-and-irrigation procedure when it is performed after 1 year of age.

PROGNOSIS

The prognosis for bacterial and viral conjunctivitis is excellent. Recurrences are to be expected if the child is re-exposed to infected individuals or if an underlying condition such as nasolacrimal duct obstruction is not treated. Viral conjunctivitis is a self-limited condition. Viral shedding may continue for 7–14 days after onset, during which the condition is contagious.

PREVENTION

Careful hand washing and good hygiene measures, including proper disposal of nasal secretions to prevent their coming in contact with other persons, should be taught to all children to reduce the transmission of bacterial conjunctivitis. Sharing of washcloths, linens, pillows, and sheets should be discouraged. Children with conditions that tempt them to rub their eyes, such as allergic conjunctivitis and blepharitis, should receive treatment to reduce the behavior.

The contagious period for bacterial conjunctivitis is considered to be 24 hours after effective treatment measures have been started. Children may return to school, but treatment measures must be continued until there is complete clinical resolution. Nonpurulent conjunctivitis does not require exclusion.

REVIEWS

Alessandrini EA: The case of the red eye. *Pediatr Ann* 2000;29:112–6.

Wald ER: Conjunctivitis in infants and children. *Pediatr Infect Dis J* 1997;16:S17–20.

Weiss A, Brinser JH, Nazar-Stewart V: Acute conjunctivitis in childhood. *J Pediatr* 1993;122:10–4.

KEY ARTICLES

Bialasiewicz AA, Jahn GJ: Evaluation of diagnostic tools for adult chlamydial keratoconjunctivitis. *Ophthalmology* 1987;94:532–7.

Credé CSF: Reports from the obstetrical clinic in Leipzig: Prevention of eye inflammation in the newborn. *Am J Dis Child* 1971;121:3–4. (Translated from *Arch Gynecol* 1881;71:50–3.)

Dawson CR, Hanna L, Wood TR, et al: Adenovirus type 8 keratoconjunctivitis in the United States. 3. Epidemiologic, clinical, and microbiologic features. *Am J Ophthalmol* 1970;60:473–80.

Gigliotti F, Hendley JO, Morgan J, et al: Efficacy of topical antibiotic therapy in acute conjunctivitis in children. *J Pediatr* 1984;104: 623–6.

Gross R, Hoffman RO, Lindsay RN: A comparison of ciprofloxacin and tobramycin in bacterial conjunctivitis in children. *Clin Pediatr (Phila)* 1997;36:435–44.

Holland GN: Infectious diseases of the eye. In Isenberg SJ (editor): *Infancy,* 2nd ed. St. Louis, Mosby, 1994, pp 493–521.

Isenberg SJ, Apt L, Wood M: A controlled trial of povidone-iodine as prophylaxis against ophthalmia neonatorum. *N Engl J Med* 1995; 332:562–6.

Isenberg SJ, Apt L, Wood M: The influence of perinatal infective factors on ophthalmia neonatorum. *J Pediatr Ophthalmol Strabismus* 1996; 33:185–8.

Isenberg SJ, Apt L, Yoshimori R, et al: Povidone-iodine for ophthalmia neonatorum prophylaxis. *Am J Ophthalmol* 1994;118:701–6.

Lomholt JA, Moller JK, Ehlers N: Prolonged persistence on the ocular surface of fortified gentamicin ointment as compared to fortified gentamicin eye drops. *Acta Ophthalmol Scand* 2000;78:34–6.

Rapoza PA, Quinn TC, Kiessling LA, et al: Assessment of neonatal conjunctivitis with a direct immunofluorescent monoclonal antibody stain for chlamydia. *JAMA* 1986a;255:3369–73.

Rapoza PA, Quinn TC, Kiessling LA, et al: Epidemiology of neonatal conjunctivitis. *Ophthalmology* 1986b;93:456–61.

Retin JB, Robin SB: Gonococcal ocular disease. In Frauenfelder FT, Roy FH, Grove J (editors): *Current Ocular Therapy,* 4th ed. Philadelphia, WB Saunders, 1995, p 23.

Stenson S, Newman R, Fedukowicz H: Conjunctivitis in the newborn: Observations on incidence, cause and prophylaxis. *Ann Ophthalmol* 1981;13:329–34.

Talley AR, Garcia-Ferrer F, Laycoch KA, et al: Comparative diagnosis of neonatal chlamydial conjunctivitis by polymerase chain reaction and McCoy cell culture. *Am J Ophthalmol* 1994;117:50–7.

Tullo AB: Clinical and epidemiological features of adenovirus keratoconjunctivitis. *Trans Ophthalmol Soc U K* 1980;100:263–7.

Watson PG, Gairdner D: TRIC agent as a cause of neonatal eye sepsis. *BMJ* 1968;3:527–8.

CHAPTER 90

Keratitis

Albert W. Biglan ▪ Hal B. Jenson

Keratitis is inflammation of the cornea. The cornea, because of its unique structure and function, demonstrates characteristic symptoms and signs of disease. Infections that affect the cornea are vision threatening and should prompt immediate consultation with an ophthalmologist, preferably one who specializes in cornea and external eye diseases.

ETIOLOGY

Keratitis or corneal ulcers can be caused by bacterial, viral, fungal, and parasitic microorganisms. Agents causing conjunctivitis (Chapter 89) may also cause keratitis. The most common pathogen causing keratitis and corneal ulceration in neonates is *Neisseria gonorrhoeae.* In older children, *Staphylococcus aureus, Streptococcus pneumoniae, Pseudomonas aeruginosa,* and *Klebsiella pneumoniae* are commonly cultured. *P. aeruginosa* causes more than 50% of corneal ulcers among wearers of extended-wear soft contact lenses. Less common pathogens include *Bacillus cereus, Mycobacterium fortuitum, Mycobacterium chelonae,* and *Mycobacterium lacunata.*

Viral causes of keratitis include herpes simplex virus types 1 and 2, varicella-zoster virus, and adenoviruses, especially serotypes 8, 11, and 19. Approximately 7% of newborns with perinatal herpes simplex virus infection have keratitis. Infection with varicella-zoster virus, or chickenpox, usually involves only the lids but may also cause conjunctivitis and keratitis. Adenovirus serotype 8 is the cause of **epidemic keratoconjunctivitis,** which is highly contagious. Serotypes 19 and 37 have also caused epidemics, but other serotypes cause only sporadic cases of keratoconjunctivitis.

Fungal keratitis is rare in children but causes 5–10% of corneal ulcers in adults. Immunocompromised persons, as a result of AIDS or transplant medications, are at greatest risk. Fungal keratitis occurs more frequently in the warmer regions of North America. Risk factors include mild injury or abrasion of the cornea, especially by a twig or vegetable matter, compromised immunity, topical corticosteroid therapy, and wearing improperly maintained contact lenses. *Candida* is the most common cause of fungal keratitis in northern North America. In Southern states, filamentous fungal species, including *Fusarium, Aspergillus, Curvularia,* and *Penicillium,* are more common.

Acanthamoeba organisms are free-living amebas that exist as a uninucleated, motile trophozoite and, under adverse conditions, both in the environment and in the cornea, revert to an inactive, double-walled cyst that is extremely hardy. *A. polyphaga* and *A. castellanii* are the most common isolates. *Onchocerca volvulus,* the cause of river blindness, causes sclerosing keratitis in Africa and Central and South America. *Leishmania* also causes keratitis in tropical regions.

Transmission. Bacterial and fungal pathogens are primarily transmitted by direct inoculation to the eye, either by person-to-person spread or with minor trauma and contaminated foreign bodies.

TABLE 90–1. Clinical Manifestations of Infectious Keratitis

	Bacterial	Viral	Fungal	Amoebic
Pathogens	*Neisseria gonorrhoeae* *Staphylococcus aureus* *Streptococcus aureus* *Pseudomonas aeruginosa*	Herpes simplex virus Varicella-zoster virus Adenoviruses	*Candida* *Fusarium* *Aspergillus* *Curvularia* *Penicillium*	*Acanthamoeba*
Symptoms				
Pain	Severe	Mild to moderate	Severe	Severe
Injection	Severe	Severe	Severe	Severe
Signs				
Opacity	Mild to severe	Mild (disciform)	Mild	Severe
Dendritic ulcer	No	Yes	No	Rare
Corneal vessels	Rare	Mild (chronic-recurrent)	Mild	Severe
Conjunctivitis	Yes, with lid involvement	Mild bulbar	No	No
Discharge	Purulent	Watery	Watery	Watery
Sensation	Present	Absent	Present	Present
Diagnosis	Gram stain, and bacterial culture (of corneal scrapings)	Giemsa stain, and viral culture (of corneal scrapings) PCR (for HSV)	Methenamine silver stain, and fungal culture (of corneal scrapings)	Calcofluor white stain, and culture on nonnutrient agar (of corneal scrapings)

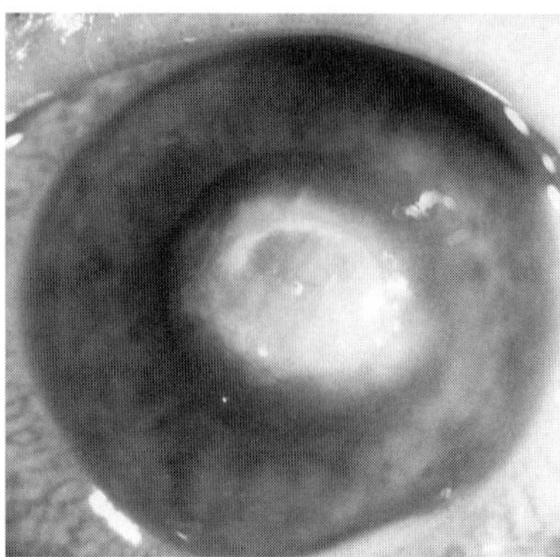

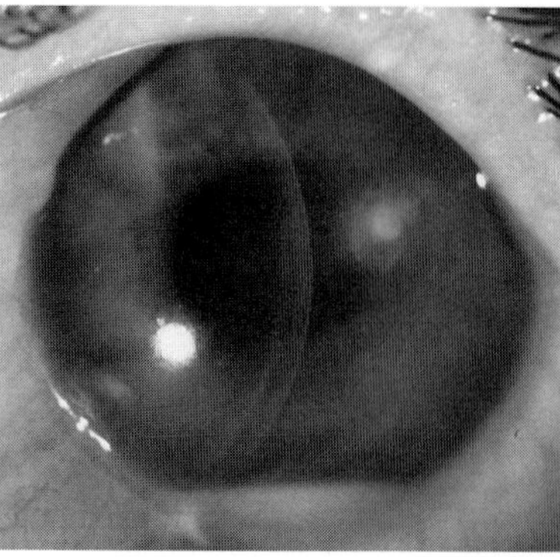

FIGURE 90–1. *Left:* Large bacterial corneal ulcer with an associated hypopyon. The ulcer has a distinct border with a white center. There is moderate chemosis and mild injection. *Right:* Small corneal bacterial ulcer with an associated hypopyon. (Courtesy of Department of Ophthalmic Photography, Eye and Ear Institute, Pittsburgh, Penn.)

Herpes simplex viruses can be transmitted perinatally during birth. Adenoviruses are highly communicable and may be spread by droplets or by direct contact with secretions. *Acanthamoeba* organisms are free-living amebas that are found in freshwater, well water, brackish water, and soil; in humans they are frequently found in oral secretions.

EPIDEMIOLOGY

Herpes simplex virus is the most common cause of keratitis in developed countries, and bacterial and fungal causes are more common in developing countries, where keratitis often occurs as a result of trauma or trachoma. Keratitis caused by herpes simplex virus can occur as a complication of herpetic conjunctivitis (Chapter 89) and also with perinatal infection (Chapter 97). Keratitis caused by varicella-zoster virus occurs principally with disseminated disease in immunocompromised persons (Chapter 27). Adenovirus types 3, 7, and 8 can cause epidemics of keratitis associated with an upper respiratory tract infection. Health care providers, particularly eye care providers, can spread adenoviruses in epidemic proportions.

The corneal changes in trachoma conjunctivitis, caused by *Chlamydia trachomatis,* affect approximately 500 million persons worldwide and are a major health problem in developing countries. **Trachoma** begins as a follicular conjunctivitis but with chronic infection progresses to conjunctival cicatrization with inward-turned eyelashes, or **trichiasis,** infolding of the eyelid margins, or **entropion,** and destruction of conjunctival goblet cells. The result is dry eye, which, with the abrasive effect of the inward-turned eyelid margin, causes corneal scarring and vascularization, or **pannus,** eventually leading to blindness. Secondary bacterial keratitis further increases the risk of blindness.

Conditions that decrease tear production (e.g., congenital alacrima, dysautonomia), increase evaporation (e.g., exophthalmos), alter the immune response (e.g., effects of topical corticosteroids, radiation), or cause decreased corneal sensation (e.g., neurotrophic keratitis and compromised blink reflex) lead to drying and exposure of the cornea and a predisposition to bacterial infection. Minor trauma, especially with vegetable matter, may introduce organisms into the stroma. Contact lenses are unsterile, foreign objects that rest on the tear film of the cornea and increase the risk of corneal infection, especially with *P. aeruginosa.*

Acanthamoeba causes keratitis worldwide but is a rare cause among children. The highest prevalence is among young, healthy adolescents who wear improperly maintained contact lenses. Exposure to the parasite is associated with swimming, hot tubs, and contaminated contact lens solution.

PATHOGENESIS

The **cornea** is a smooth, transparent, domelike structure approximately 0.6 mm thick, which forms the anterior surface of the eye. The interface of the air and cornea forms an important optical structure that is responsible for refracting light entering the eye. The cornea is rich in sensory nerves, and any disease process that causes swelling will produce extreme pain and will also produce symptoms of rainbows or halos around illuminated objects. When the corneal surface becomes irregular, it will cause light sensitivity, or **photophobia,** and **reflex blepharospasm.** Processes that involve the corneal stroma can cause opacification resulting from stromal swelling or scarring. Scarring of the visual axis of the cornea can cause a permanent decrease in vision.

SYMPTOMS AND CLINICAL MANIFESTATIONS

The manifestations of infectious keratitis vary according to the cause (Table 90–1). Unlike conjunctivitis, keratitis is characterized by a variable decrease in vision.

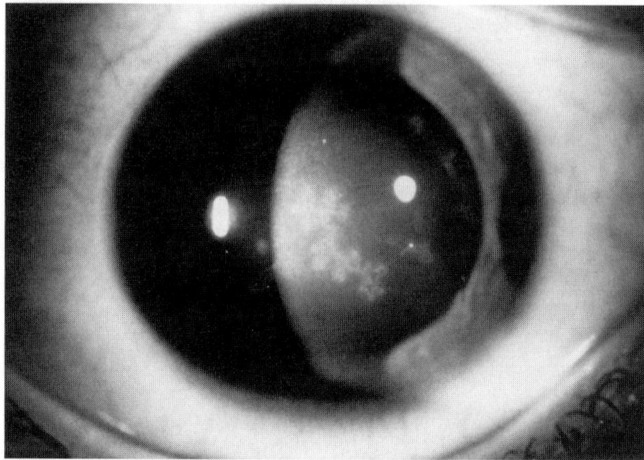

FIGURE 90–2. Dendritic ulcer of herpes simplex virus keratitis demonstrated by fluorescein stain and a cobalt blue light source.

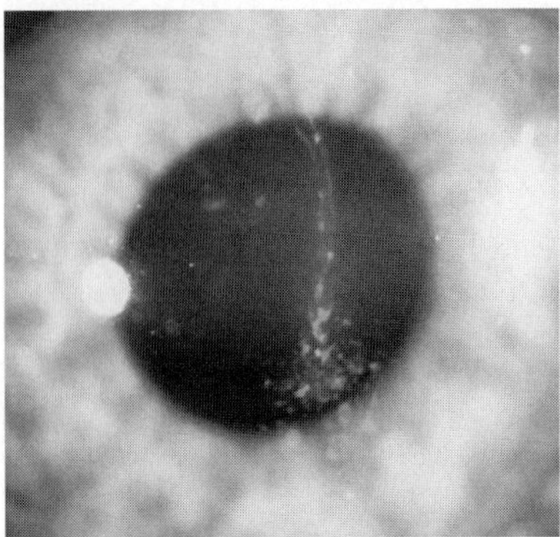
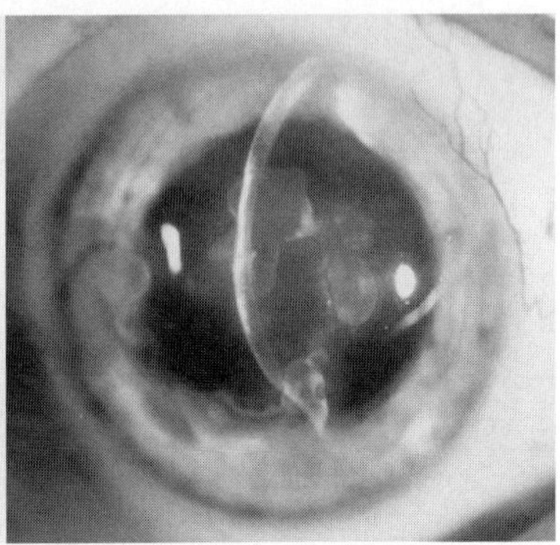

FIGURE 90–3. *Left:* Dendritic ulcer of varicella-zoster virus keratitis, demonstrated by fluorescein stain and a cobalt blue light source. *Right:* Nummular keratitis occurs less commonly with varicella-zoster virus keratitis.

Bacterial keratitis is suggested by signs of chemosis and injection of the bulbar conjunctiva, ciliary injection, photophobia, severe pain, increased lacrimation, blepharospasm, and a focal area of haziness or opacification of the cornea, with or without a foreign body. Bacterial keratitis is often associated with unilateral or bilateral purulent conjunctivitis. In children a bacterial corneal ulcer (Fig. 90–1) will cause limbal blood vessels to invade the clear corneal stroma rapidly, sometimes within 24–48 hours. In severe cases an ulcer will cause a hypopyon, which may be sterile or may contain organisms.

Keratitis from herpes simplex virus causes decreased corneal sensation. Defects in the corneal epithelium, which can be demonstrated with fluorescein staining and a cobalt blue light source, demonstrate a characteristic **dendritic ulcer** with a fine, delicate branching pattern (Fig. 90–2; Plate 9C). The dendritic ulcer caused by varicella-zoster virus has a more coarse appearance and may have a nodular swelling at the site of branching. Varicella-zoster virus may also cause **nummular keratitis** (Fig. 90–3). Unrecognized herpes simplex keratitis that is treated with topical corticosteroids results in proliferation of the virus and invasion of the corneal stroma, causing a disciform or hazy opacification of the cornea (Fig. 90–4). This may be associated with a slowly healing geographic, or shieldlike, defect in the epithelium. Severe keratitis can cause an anterior chamber reaction or anterior uveitis.

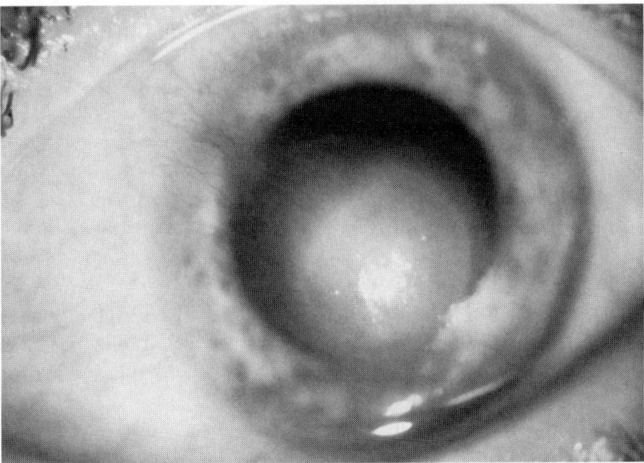

FIGURE 90–4. Disciform lesion of the cornea caused by herpes simplex virus, which was treated inappropriately with topical corticosteroids. The corneal stroma is edematous and hazy. The epithelium may not be intact over the area of stromal swelling. (Courtesy of Department of Ophthalmic Photography, Eye and Ear Institute, Pittsburgh, Penn.)

Adenovirus has an incubation period of 5–14 days, after which one eye will typically develop a pink hyperemia of the conjunctiva in association with a clear, watery discharge (Fig. 90–5). This may be followed by photophobia and a diffuse punctate keratitis, which can be demonstrated with fluorescein staining. Spread to the other eye is common. The acute phase of keratitis lasts about 10–15 days and is followed by emergence of subepithelial infiltrates, which may persist for weeks or months.

Fungal keratitis may present as a slowly enlarging corneal ulcer with a fine, feathery margin. There may be a history of poor response to antibacterial treatment. The cornea may have central or paracentral opacity with or without conjunctival hyperemia. With chronic infection, vessels may invade the corneal stroma. *Candida* is typically associated with a yellowish white microabscess in the corneal stroma.

Acanthamoeba keratitis is characterized by a slowly enlarging, exquisitely painful central or paracentral **ring ulcer,** with a dense ring of opacification surrounding a central area of relative clearness (Fig. 90–6). Corneal vessels encroach from the limbus, and the cornea develops a haze.

DIAGNOSIS

The presence of extreme pain and hyperemia, often with copious purulent discharge, suggests a bacterial corneal ulcer, which is a medical emergency and necessitates prompt evaluation of the cornea with a slit lamp, cultures, and empirical treatment. Photophobia and reflex blepharospasm make examination very difficult, especially of children, and may require general anesthesia. If foreign material is present, it should be removed and cultured.

The diagnosis of viral keratitis is established by clinical features and slit-lamp examination of the cornea and confirmed by viral culture. The presence of an enlarged, not necessarily tender, preauricular lymph node suggests adenovirus.

Differential Diagnosis

The differential diagnosis includes noninfected corneal foreign body, healing corneal abrasion, and the presence of organic or inorganic matter beneath the upper lid, including insect structures such as caterpillar hairs. Foreign material can cause symptoms and signs similar to those of infectious keratitis. Examination of the

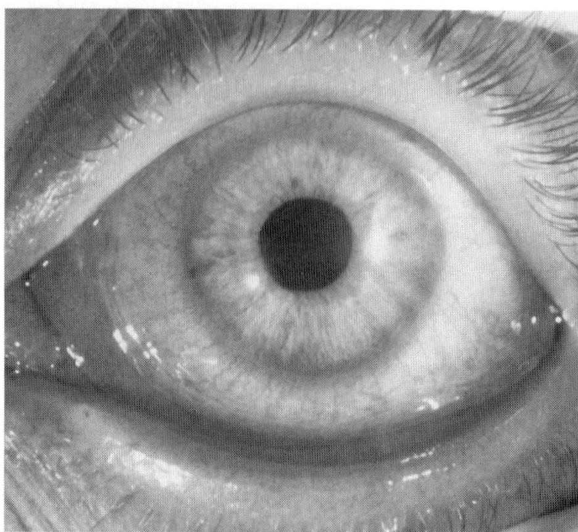
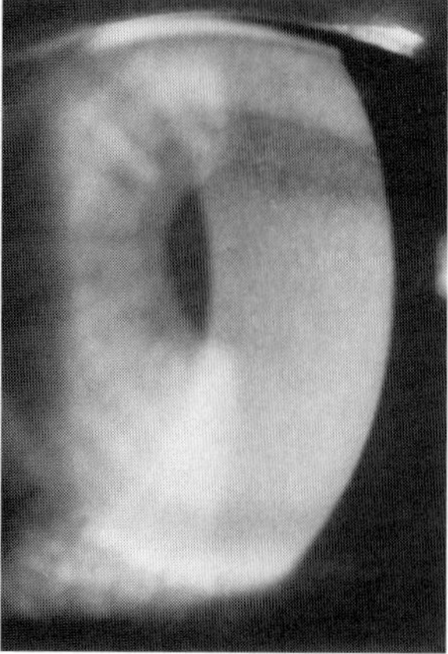

FIGURE 90–5. *Left:* Adenovirus (epidemic keratoconjunctivitis) produces a watery discharge and a pink hyperemia of the conjunctiva. *Right:* Cornea has a punctate keratitis demonstrated with fluorescein stain and a cobalt blue light source. Photophobia is extreme during this phase.

palpebral conjunctiva by everting the upper and lower eyelids may be necessary to localize the offending material. This can be accomplished by using cotton-tipped swabs or eyelid retractors, combined with examination by means of a Wood's lamp with fluorescein or with loupe magnification. A slit-lamp examination may be necessary if the foreign body is small. Eye rubbing may cause a keratitis that may have a staining pattern similar to that of adenovirus.

Noninfectious conditions such as glaucoma and inherited corneal dystrophies should also be considered in an evaluation of a hazy cornea. These conditions, especially glaucoma, cause photophobia and tearing but do not exhibit other signs of infection.

Microbiologic Evaluation

Corneal scrapings, and in some instances a biopsy specimen, must be obtained to identify the cause of the infection. A recommended culture technique for a corneal ulcer is to anesthetize the cornea with topical applications of proparacaine. If the child is young or uncooperative, general anesthesia may be required.

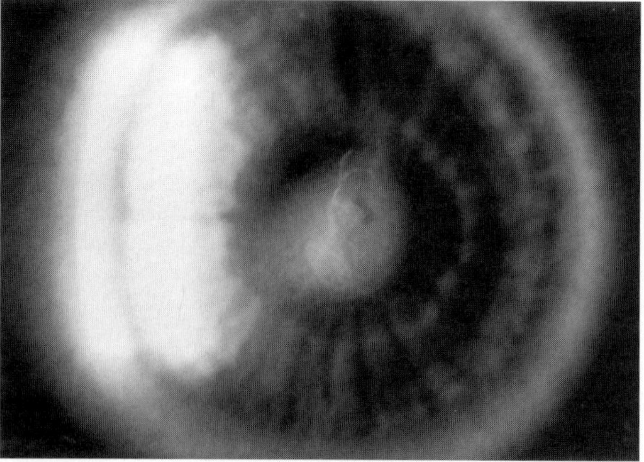

FIGURE 90–6. *Acanthamoeba* keratitis with a central corneal ulcer. The edge of the ulcer is indistinct. An advanced phase of this infection will develop a relatively clear center with a dense, large ring of opacification and invasion of blood vessels into the cornea. (Courtesy of Department of Ophthalmic Photography, Eye and Ear Institute, Pittsburgh, Penn.)

The conjunctival surfaces are first swabbed with a cotton-tipped swab moistened with transfer broth, and the swab is then streaked onto blood agar, Sabouraud without cycloheximide (which inhibits growth of filamentous species), thioglycolate, and chocolate agar. The chocolate agar is incubated in a 10% CO_2 environment.

After conjunctival and lid cultures are obtained, the corneal epithelium is scraped with the blunt edge of a sterile Kimura spatula, and cells and necrotic corneal material are placed on slides. Slides are stained with Gram and Giemsa stains. Potassium hydroxide and methenamine silver stains are also prepared if fungi are suspected. A calcofluor white stain may be useful for both fungi and *Acanthamoeba.* Scrapings of the central and marginal portions of the ulcer are plated directly onto the media for culture. Viral cultures of discharge and corneal scrapings should be obtained if viral keratitis is suspected. PCR assay may be used to confirm keratitis caused by herpes simplex virus.

If the patient wears contact lenses, the contact lens and cleaning solution should also be cultured for bacteria and fungi and examined for *Acanthamoeba.*

TREATMENT

Corneal ulcers should be referred immediately to an ophthalmologist who specializes in corneal and external eye diseases. Administration of antibiotic drops or ointments should be avoided until smears and culture specimens have been obtained, after which treatment should be initiated promptly, with initial selection of antibiotics guided by the organisms found on slides. Broad-spectrum treatment should be administered if the organism cannot be identified presumptively and modified according to the results of culture and susceptibility testing.

Definitive Treatment

Bacterial Keratitis. The choice of antibiotic and route of administration will depend on the severity of the ulcer. Except for the quinolone eyedrops, commercially available preparations are not as effective as the **fortified,** or high-concentration, solutions that hospital pharmacies can prepare from parenteral antibiotic formulations.

Small ulcers (<1–2 mm) in which *P. aeruginosa* is not suspected and that are not vision-threatening may be treated with topical ofloxacin 0.3% or ciprofloxacin 0.3%, with careful monitoring for progression or regression of the ulcer. An alternative is topical cefazolin 50 mg/mL. If the ulcer is large or there is a suggestion of intraocular involvement, subconjunctival injection of ceftazidime 100 mg in 0.5 mL can be used.

If *P. aeruginosa* or another gram-negative organism is suspected (e.g., because of contact lens use), topical tobramycin 9–14 mg/mL, or alternatively gentamicin 10 mg/mL, is administered in combination with cefazolin. Subconjunctival injection of tobramycin 20 mg in 0.5 mL, or alternatively gentamicin 20 mg in 0.5 mL, is administered if the ulcer is large and threatens penetration of the cornea.

Topical cycloplegics, such as homatropine 5% three times daily, are often used to reduce ciliary spasm and photophobia. The use of a soft contact lens or corneal shields has been used in adults to protect the corneal surface from mechanical trauma during re-epithelialization, but no comparative studies of safety and efficacy have been performed. Treatment of a visually immature child, <8 years of age, with prolonged use of occlusive dressings or ointments that interfere with vision or with unilateral use of strong cycloplegic agents such as atropine can lead to iatrogenic **deprivation amblyopia** and is discouraged.

Herpes Simplex Keratitis. Treatment of the dendritic form of herpes simplex keratitis is with topical vidarabine ointment 3% five times a day. Alternatively, topical trifluridine 1% drops are applied to the affected eye every 2 hours while the patient is awake. Both of these drugs can produce a toxic reaction of the cornea and conjunctiva. Courses longer than 7–10 days may cause conjunctival chemosis and a punctate or a filamentary keratitis. The addition of acyclovir 400 mg orally three times daily can reduce the recurrence rate of herpes simplex keratitis by 45%.

Topical cycloplegics, such as homatropine 5% three times daily, are often used to reduce ciliary spasm and photophobia. If the patient has decreased vision related to a disciform lesion of the cornea, topical corticosteroids, such as fluorometholone (FML) or prednisolone acetate 0.1%, can be used cautiously in conjunction with antiviral drops or ointment. Prolonged use of a pressure patch may be needed to facilitate healing of the epithelium but is avoided in visually immature children.

Varicella-Zoster Keratitis. Varicella-zoster keratitis has a self-limited course, and management is directed toward prevention of secondary bacterial infection. Broad-spectrum antibiotic drops, such as sulfacetamide 10% or polymyxin B–trimethoprim, are used topically three or four times daily. Treatment with systemic drugs such as acyclovir, valacyclovir, or famciclovir can be considered, especially with severe keratitis or disseminated disease in immunocompromised persons (Chapter 27). If stromal keratitis or disciform keratitis with iritis caused by varicella-zoster virus is present, topical corticosteroids, such as FML or prednisolone acetate 0.1%, can be used.

Adenovirus Keratitis. Adenovirus keratitis has a self-limited course, and management is focused on relief of symptoms. Artificial tears and oral analgesics are somewhat helpful until the keratitis resolves, which may take 1–2 weeks. If subepithelial infiltrates develop and involve the visual axis, a mild topical corticosteroid preparation may be used, but use of corticosteroids will delay resolution of the infiltrates and prolong recovery.

Fungal Keratitis. Agents used to treat fungal ulcers include natamycin 5%, which is active against 70–90% of the fungi that infect the cornea. Natamycin 5% is administered topically as 1 drop every 15 minutes for 3 hours, then hourly for 1 week. Alternative treatments for fungal ulcers include topical amphotericin B 0.15–1%, topical fluconazole using a 1% intravenous solution, or miconazole 10 mg/mL using the intravenous solution applied topically. Higher concentrations of amphotericin B (1–5%) are irritating and may damage the cornea.

Acanthamoeba Keratitis. Treatment of *Acanthamoeba* keratitis is with topical dibromopropamidine 0.15% ointment or propamidine 0.1% solution administered hourly for 5–7 days, with gradually decreasing frequency for several weeks as the keratitis resolves. Ketoconazole and itraconazole have also been used to treat this condition. *Acanthamoeba* ulcers are very slow to respond to treatment. Medical therapy in combination with keratoplasty to remove cysts from the corneal tissue may be necessary. Corneal transplant, if necessary, is performed after the ulcer has been treated and shows no recurrence for 6–12 months.

COMPLICATIONS

Infections caused by *P. aeruginosa* and *N. gonorrhoeae* can penetrate the cornea within 24–48 hours and infect the internal ocular structures, causing endophthalmitis (Chapter 92). Delay in treatment or suboptimal antibiotic treatment can lead to corneal perforation.

PROGNOSIS

Prompt and effective treatment of a bacterial corneal ulcer can result in a clear cornea with no visual impairment. Irregularity of the refracting surface of the cornea may cause a commensurate decrease in visual acuity. Invasion of the corneal stroma will leave a temporary haze or permanent opacity. If the haze or opacity lies in the central visual axis, it can reduce visual acuity. Poor resolution may lead to corneal changes that permanently reduce the clarity of vision. If a child is <2 years of age and resolution takes longer than 2–3 weeks, **deprivation amblyopia** may occur.

If there is no underlying predisposing condition, recurrence of bacterial keratitis is unusual. Both herpes simplex keratitis and varicella-zoster keratitis tend to recur. Recurrence of herpes simplex keratitis occurs in approximately one fourth to one third of patients within 2 years. Persons with stromal herpes simplex keratitis with recurrent episodes are candidates for long-term acyclovir prophylaxis. Corneal anesthesia, pannus formation, vascularization of the corneal stroma, and anterior uveitis may occur as complications of herpes simplex and varicella-zoster keratitis. Disciform lesions of the cornea are considered to represent an immune response.

Subepithelial infiltrates associated with adenovirus may take weeks to months to resolve (Fig. 90–7).

Fungal ulcers of the cornea are difficult to treat and respond slowly to medications. Some degree of corneal scarring or irregularity of the cornea usually persists. The optical distortion may cause astigmatism, decreased vision, and amblyopia. Surgical removal of the diseased cornea, followed by corneal transplant, may be required. Corticosteroids used to suppress graft rejection and the poor response of children to keratoplasty contribute to a poor prognosis for advanced forms of fungal keratitis.

PREVENTION

Children with foreign material under the eyelids and those with a corneal foreign body should have the foreign material removed promptly. Children and young adults who wear contact lenses must be instructed on careful hand-washing techniques and proper care of their lenses. Overwearing of contact lenses, or wearing contact lenses beyond their recommended lifespan, is discouraged.

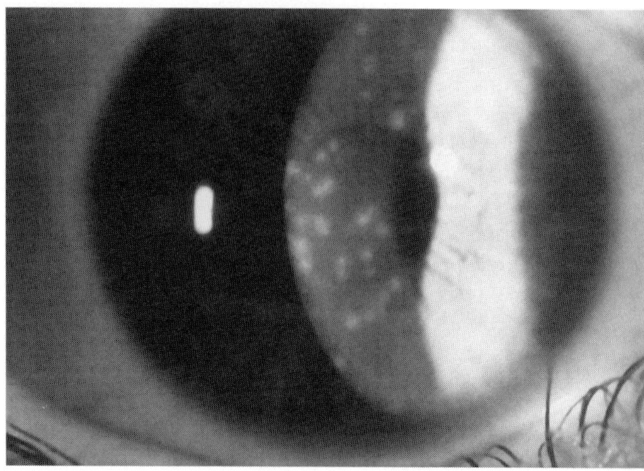

FIGURE 90–7. Subepithelial infiltrates of adenovirus (epidemic keratoconjunctivitis) after 4 weeks. (Courtesy of Department of Ophthalmic Photography, Eye and Ear Institute, Pittsburgh, Penn.)

Children in intensive care units and those with a decreased blink reflex should receive preventive care. Daily cleansing of the lids and surrounding skin structures with a 5% povidone-iodine solution and use of lubricating ointments will help prevent keratitis. Children with conjunctivitis should receive topical antibiotic drops, such as sulfacetamide 10% or polymyxin B–trimethoprim eyedrops administered three or four times each day, to suppress bacterial flora.

The risk of herpes simplex keratitis can be reduced by avoiding contact with primary herpetic lesions and by practicing good hand-washing technique and good hygiene. Persons with primary herpetic lid lesions are treated with trifluridine eyedrops every 2 hours for 5 days to prevent infection of the corneal epithelium. Recurrences are reduced by avoidance of sunlight, stress, and minor trauma. Persons with recurrent herpes keratitis should be provided with a prescription for trifluridine drops for initiation of treatment with the onset of symptoms; the drops are administered every 2 hours until the recurrence can be evaluated by an ophthalmologist.

The risk of adenovirus infections can be reduced by avoiding infected children, exercising good hand-washing technique, and using proper sanitizing measures for equipment and medical instruments.

Tap water and oral secretions can harbor *Acanthamoeba.* Providing meticulous care of contact lenses, with sterile saline solutions and avoiding tap water for contact lens preparations can reduce the possibility of *Acanthamoeba* keratitis. All persons who wear contact lenses, especially those who wear rigid gas-permeable lenses, should use meticulous hygiene for their contact lenses and the storage cases. Users of soft contact lenses should use heat sterilization whenever possible because chemical sterilization is less effective against *Acanthamoeba.*

REVIEWS

Clinch TE, Palmon FE, Robinson MJ, et al: Microbial keratitis in children. *Am J Ophthalmol* 1994;117:65–71.

Limberg MB: A review of bacterial keratitis and bacterial conjunctivitis. *Am J Ophthalmol* 1991;112:2S–9S.

Wang AG, Wu CC, Liu JH: Bacterial corneal ulcer: A multivariate study. *Ophthalmologica* 1998;212:126–32.

KEY ARTICLES

Chern KC, Conrad D, Holland GN, et al: Chronic varicella-zoster virus epithelial keratitis in patients with acquired immunodeficiency syndrome. *Arch Ophthalmol* 1998;116:1011–7.

Cooper RJ, Yeo AC, Bailey AS, et al: Adenovirus polymerase chain reaction assay for rapid diagnosis of conjunctivitis. *Invest Ophthalmol Vis Sci* 1999;40:90–5.

Gardner LM, Mathers WD, Folberg R: New technique for cytologic identification of presumed *Acanthamoeba* from cornea epithelial scrapings. *Am J Ophthalmol* 1999;127:207–9.

Herpetic Eye Disease Study Group: Acyclovir for the prevention of recurrent herpes simplex virus eye disease. *N Engl J Med* 1998;339:300–6.

Hyndiuk RA, Eiferman RA, Caldwell DR, et al: Comparison of ciprofloxacin ophthalmic solution 0.3% to fortified tobramycin-cefazolin in treating bacterial corneal ulcers. Ciprofloxacin Bacterial Keratitis Study Group. *Ophthalmology* 1996;103:1854–62.

Jabs DA: Acyclovir for recurrent herpes simplex virus ocular disease. *N Engl J Med* 1998;339:340–1.

Kinchington PR, Turse SE, Kowalski RP, et al: Use of polymerase chain amplification reaction for detection of adenovirus in ocular swab specimens. *Invest Ophthalmol Vis Sci* 1994;35:4126–34.

Kowalski RP, Gordon YJ, Romanowski EG, et al: A comparison of enzyme immunoassay and polymerase chain reaction with the clinical examination for diagnosing ocular herpetic disease. *Ophthalmology* 1993;100: 530–3.

Kunimoto DY, Sharma S, Garg P, et al: In vitro susceptibility of bacterial keratitis pathogens to ciprofloxacin. *Ophthalmology* 1999;106:80–5.

Langston DP: Oral acyclovir suppresses recurrent epithelial and stromal herpes simplex. *Arch Ophthalmol* 1999:177:391–2.

O'Brien TP, Maguire MG, Fink NE, et al: Efficacy of ofloxacin vs cefazolin and tobramycin in the therapy for bacterial keratitis. Report from the Bacterial Keratitis Study Research Group. *Arch Ophthalmol* 1995; 113:1257–65.

Radford CF, Lehmann OJ, Dart JK: *Acanthamoeba* keratitis: Multicentre survey in England 1992–6. National Acanthamoeba Keratitis Study Group. *Br J Ophthalmol* 1998;82:1387–92.

Schein OD, Glynn RJ, Poggio EC, et al: The incidence of ulcerative keratitis among users of daily-wear and extended-wear soft contact lenses. A case-control study. Microbial Keratitis Study Group. *N Engl J Med* 1989;321:773–8.

Schwartz GS, Holland EJ: Oral acyclovir for the management of herpes simplex virus keratitis in children. *Ophthalmology* 2000;107:278–82.

CHAPTER 91

Infections of the Eyelids and Ocular Adnexa

Albert W. Biglan ▪ Hal B. Jenson

Common infections of the eyelids and their surrounding tissues can be classified as infections of the eyelid margin **(blepharitis),** glandular structures **(hordeola),** and the lacrimal collecting apparatus **(dacryocystitis).** In addition, children's eyelids have a propensity for infection with molluscum contagiosum virus (Chapter 46), and the base of the cilia may harbor pediculosis (Chapter 46). Impetigo or secondary bacterial infection of the vesicular eruption of primary herpes simplex or varicella-zoster infection may be present on the skin of the eyelids (Chapter 46). The eyelids may also develop a deeper infection, or cellulitis. It occurs most commonly anterior to the orbital septum and is then called preseptal cellulitis (Chapter 47); less frequently it occurs behind the orbital septum and is called orbital cellulitis (Chapter 65). Orbital cellulitis results in edema, hyperemia, and restriction of motility of the globe.

Eyelids are unique to vertebrates. The eyelids remove debris from the ocular surface, protect the globe, and serve as the area of transition between the keratinized facial skin and the nonkeratinized squamous epithelium of the conjunctiva. These two epithelial tissues meet at the **eyelid margin.** At this junction, extending along the upper and lower eyelid margins, are the orifices of the meibomian glands. These oil-secreting glands, oriented perpendicular to the eyelid margin, are located within the **tarsal plate,** which provides rigidity for the upper and lower eyelids. The two other glands of the eyelids are apocrine glands. **Moll's glands** are modified sweat glands, and the **glands of Zeis** are sebum-secreting glands located at the base of the eyelashes, or cilia.

Beyond the mucocutaneous junction, on the internal portion on the eyelid, conjunctiva is reflected posteriorly to line the underside of the tarsal plates. The **palpebral and bulbar conjunctivae** join in the **superior and inferior conjunctival cul-de-sacs.** In the superior cul-de-sac, **Krause's glands** and the **glands of Wolfring** produce an aqueous secretion that forms the **basal tear secretions,** which combine with the **reflex secretions** produced by the **lacrimal gland** to form the aqueous portion of the **tear film.**

Tears act as a lubricant between the globe and the eyelids and serve as a cleansing medium for the external ocular structures. The mucous layer of the tear film promotes equal distribution of the tears over the cornea, and the lipid layer helps to retard tear evaporation. Tears provide the cornea with a clear and optically smooth surface. Tears contain lysozymes, which have a bactericidal property.

After formation and circulation over the cornea and conjunctiva, tears are collected by the **upper and lower lacrimal puncta,** located in the **inner (medial) canthus.** Tears then flow into the lacrimal **canaliculus** and empty into the **lacrimal sac.** The sac collects tears, which then flow through the **nasolacrimal duct** and exit beneath the inferior turbinate in the nasal cavity.

BLEPHARITIS

ETIOLOGY

Marginal blepharitis is associated with *Staphylococcus* infections, seborrhea, and meibomian gland dysfunction. Both *Staphylococcus aureus* and coagulase-negative staphylococci are commonly cultured from persons with excessive crusting or ulceration of the eyelid margin.

Transmission. Because hordeola are caused by normal flora, they are not considered contagious.

EPIDEMIOLOGY

Marginal blepharitis is a commonly occurring infection of the eyelid margin that affects both children and adults. Approximately 5% of children have some degree of this condition. Children with trisomy 21 and immune or nutritional compromise have a predilection for this condition. Blepharitis in children is more prevalent during the winter months. There is no unique geographic distribution.

PATHOGENESIS

Blepharitis is associated with eczema and seborrheic changes of the scalp and the lid margin. With seborrhea, there is greasy scaling of the skin of the anterior lid margin. The meibomian glands are plugged, and their orifices may appear dilated.

SYMPTOMS AND CLINICAL MANIFESTATIONS

Blepharitis has an insidious onset. Children of all ages complain of light sensitivity, burning, and irritation, and some may complain of a foreign body sensation. These symptoms cause the child to rub his or her eyes. Clinical findings include dry, crusty flakes or greasy scaling at the base of the lashes and the eyelid margin (Fig. 91–1). Without treatment, the eyelid margin becomes red and somewhat thickened. In severe or chronic cases, there is an increase in the number and diameter of blood vessels on the eyelid margin. *Staphylococcus* liberates an exotoxin that can cause a **punctate keratitis,** which is best visualized by placing fluorescein stain into the conjunctival cul-de-sac and examining the cornea with the cobalt blue light source of a slit lamp or a Wood's lamp with magnification. The corneal stain pattern has a horizontal and inferior distribution and is located on the interpalpebral space of the cornea.

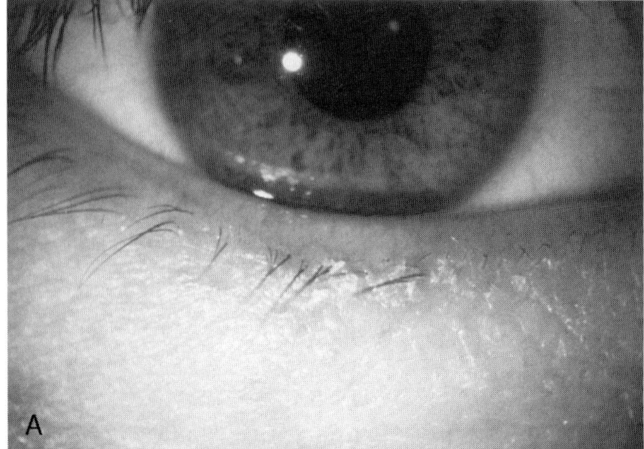

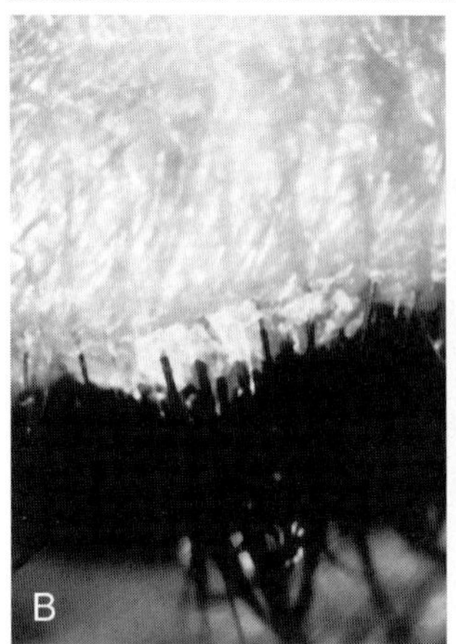

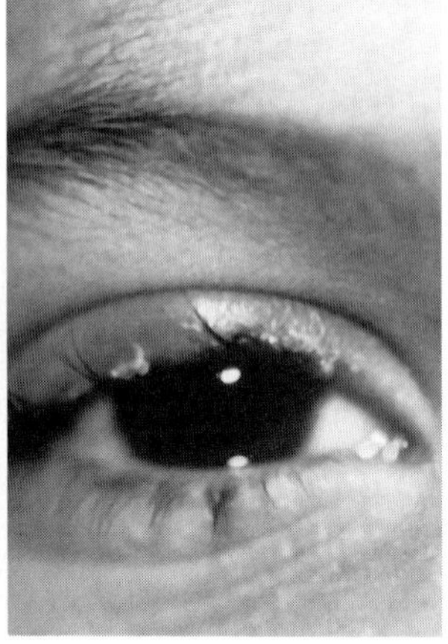

FIGURE 91–1. **A,** Common appearance of blepharitis with minimal crusting. There is slight thickening and hyperemia of the lid margin. **B,** Crusting and serous accumulation with matting of the cilia of the eyelids in a child with untreated staphylococcal blepharitis.

DIAGNOSIS

The diagnosis is established by symptoms and clinical findings. Ancillary laboratory studies are seldom requested. Cultures, if grown, commonly reveal *S. aureus,* coagulase-negative staphylococci, and other normal skin flora. The differential diagnosis includes impetigo, eczema, herpes simplex virus infection, and *Phthirus pubis* infestation.

TREATMENT

Eyelid hygiene with an **eyelid scrub** routine is the initial step in treatment. Moist, warm compresses are applied four times a day for 3–5 minutes, which softens the adherent crusts on the lid and warms the meibomian glands. The inspissated meibomian gland secretions become soft and will exude from the gland aperture. The eyelid margin is then cleansed with a cotton swab moistened with tap water. If the lids have a greasy film, the addition of a dilute solution of a nonirritating soap solution, such as baby shampoo, to the eyelid scrub should be considered. There are also commercially available eyelid cleansers that perform equally well. This eyelid cleansing routine should be performed twice daily for moderate symptoms and more frequently for severe symptoms. Once the lid scaling and crusting have resolved, the number of lid scrubs can be reduced to daily or less frequent scrubs, according to symptoms.

Occasionally a low-grade infection of the lids will be resistant to eyelid hygiene measures. In these cases, erythromycin ophthalmic ointment can be applied twice daily to the eyelid margins with a cotton swab, similar to the eyelid scrub routine. In severe cases, in which the cornea has punctate staining and the patient is light sensitive or complains of ocular irritation or burning, a brief course of an antibiotic-corticosteroid eyedrop preparation can be used for 3 or 4 days. This solution can be instilled into the lower conjunctival cul-de-sac, or the drop can be applied directly to the eyelid with a cotton swab saturated with the antibiotic-corticosteroid eyedrop. Medications such as the combination of 10% sodium sulfacetamide and prednisolone acetate 0.1% (Blephamide) and the combination of tobramycin and dexamethasone (TobraDex) are some commonly used treatment options.

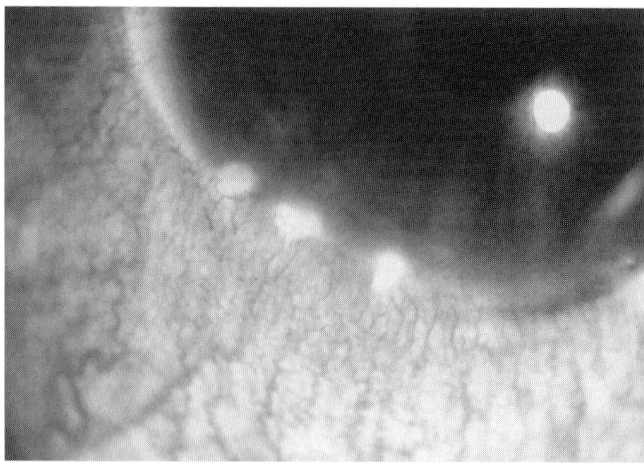

FIGURE 91–2. Severe blepharitis, causing a staphylococcal hypersensitivity reaction with an associated phlyctenular or immune response at the limbus.

COMPLICATIONS

Chronic eyelid inflammation can cause the glands of Zeis and Moll and the meibomian glands to malfunction and become infected. Infection or inflammation of these glands may produce a hordeolum or form a chalazion. A **chalazion** is a chronic lipogranulomatous reaction of the meibomian gland and is not a true infection, although the gland can become infected secondarily. If blepharitis is untreated for many years, it will lead to thickening of the eyelid margin, stunting, misdirection, and poliosis of the lashes. Chronic punctate keratitis can lead to corneal vascularization. A phlyctenular keratoconjunctivitis may develop as a result of hypersensitivity or an immune response to ***Staphylococcus*** (Fig. 91–2).

PROGNOSIS

Blepharitis is a chronic condition that can be controlled but is seldom cured. Recurrence is common when lid hygiene is suspended. Young children frequently suspend or discontinue lid hygiene measures.

PREVENTION

There is no known prevention for blepharitis.

HORDEOLUM

ETIOLOGY

Hordeola are acute suppurative nodular inflammatory lesions of the eyelids associated with pain and redness (Fig. 91–3). Hordeola

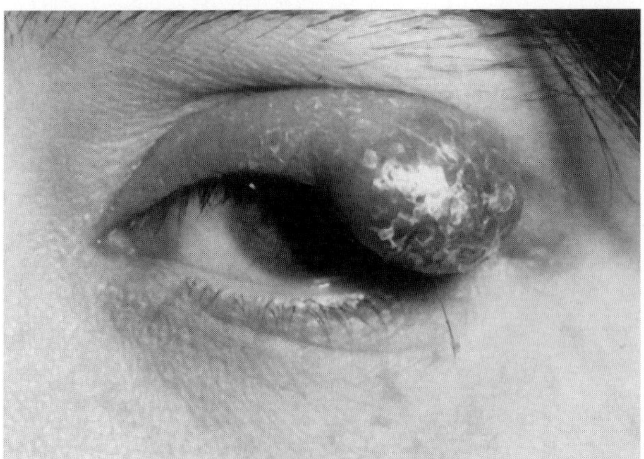

FIGURE 91–3. Large external hordeolum. (Courtesy of Department of Ophthalmic Photography, Eye and Ear Institute, Pittsburgh, Penn.)

that occur on the anterior eyelid, in the glands of Zeis or in the lash follicles, are termed **external hordeola** or **styes** and are usually caused by *Staphylococcus*. Hordeola that occur in the meibomian glands are termed **internal hordeola,** and these may be infected with *Staphylococcus* or may be sterile. If the meibomian gland becomes obstructed, the gland secretions will accumulate and a **chalazion** will develop. Hordeola will frequently localize and form a purulent abscess at the lid margin.

Transmission. Because blepharitis is caused by normal flora, it is not considered contagious.

EPIDEMIOLOGY

Hordeola occur infrequently in children. They are associated with blepharitis and with any conditions that compromise the immune system.

SYMPTOMS AND CLINICAL MANIFESTATIONS

A hordeolum usually presents as a single isolated pustular lesion on the lid margin that appears during a 2–3 day period. Hordeola are frequently associated with blepharitis. Spontaneous resolution is common. An internal hordeolum will form a suppurative nodular swelling within the meibomian gland (Fig. 91–4). It will have an undulating course of swelling, followed by resolution within 1 or more weeks. The hordeolum may drain spontaneously to the conjunctival surface of the eyelid. Internal hordeola may elevate the internal layer of the palpebral conjunctiva. During the early stages, it is often termed an **acute chalazion.**

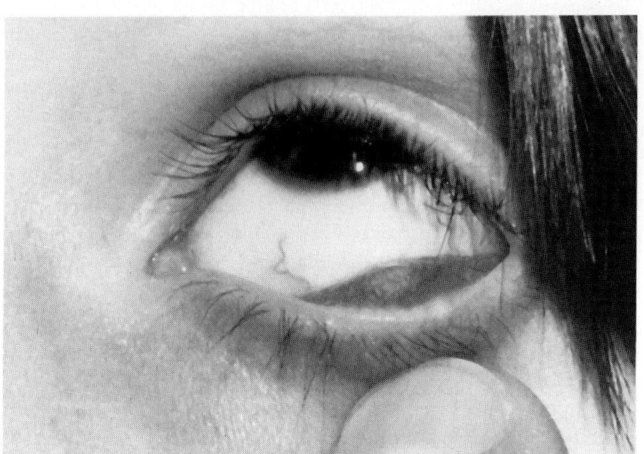

FIGURE 91–4. Internal hordeolum in the acute stage, also known as an acute chalazion.

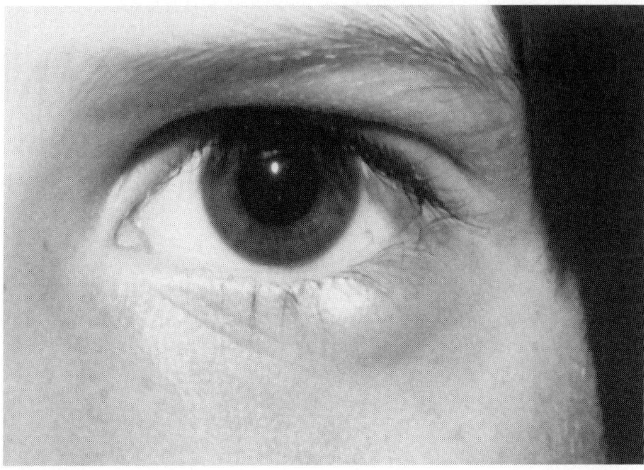

FIGURE 91–5. Chalazion, which can mimic an external hordeolum. A chalazion has less erythema and more induration than a hordeolum.

DIAGNOSIS

The diagnosis is established by symptoms and clinical findings. Ancillary laboratory studies are seldom requested. Cultures, if grown, commonly reveal *S. aureus,* coagulase-negative staphylococci, and other normal skin flora. Several small internal hordeola with surrounding eyelid swelling and edema can be confused with early preseptal cellulitis. During early states, a chalazion may simulate the swelling produced by a hordeolum (Fig. 91–5).

TREATMENT

Hordeola are self-limited and respond to moist, warm compresses applied four times a day for 3–5 minutes. In young children, this treatment may be difficult to achieve. Application of heat to the eyelid by using a hot-water bottle or sealable plastic bag (Ziploc) filled with warm water and placed over a clean, warm, moist washcloth is an effective measure. Topical antibiotics may be used to treat associated blepharitis. Systemic antibiotics may be used if extension suggests progression to preseptal cellulitis.

COMPLICATIONS

Extension of a hordeolum to preseptal cellulitis or orbital cellulitis can occur rarely.

PROGNOSIS

Hordeola usually respond spontaneously to local treatment measures but may recur.

PREVENTION

If blepharitis is present, lid hygiene measures are recommended. Repeated bouts of hordeola in children >8 years of age may be treated with oral tetracycline, but this treatment is not recommended for younger children because of the possibility of staining of the permanent teeth. Tetracycline decreases *Staphylococcus* lipase production and seems to alter the composition of the secretions of the meibomian glands.

DACRYOCYSTITIS

ETIOLOGY

Dacryocystitis is an infection or inflammation of the lacrimal sac and may be acute or chronic. Bacterial infection in children is most commonly caused by *S. aureus,* by coagulase-negative staphylococci, or, less commonly, by *Streptococcus pneumoniae, Klebsiella,* or *Pseudomonas.*

Transmission. Because dacryocystitis is caused by normal flora, it is not considered contagious.

EPIDEMIOLOGY

With few exceptions, dacryocystitis develops because of an obstruction of the nasolacrimal duct. It may be acute or chronic. Congenital obstruction of the nasolacrimal duct may lead to recurrent or chronic dacryocystitis in infancy. Dacryocystitis in the teens to the thirties is more commonly due to dacryoliths or to midline facial fractures involving the nasolacrimal duct.

PATHOGENESIS

Dacryocystitis results from obstruction of the normal tear passages within the nasolacrimal sac and duct, causing stasis and stagnation of tears and mucus and predisposing the patient to infection with flora normally present in the conjunctival sac. The mucosal barrier and the bacteriostatic action of the tears offer some protection but are soon overwhelmed with persistent stasis.

A **nasolacrimal sac mucocele,** evident as a **blue dome cyst,** predisposes neonates to dacryocystitis (Fig. 91–6). The mucoid secretions within the distended nasolacrimal sac become infected, causing acute dacryocystitis.

Children with a persistent, or imperforate, membrane at the lower end of the nasolacrimal duct may develop a discharge, usually during the first month of life (Fig. 91–7), with chronic, low-grade dacryocystitis. Older children usually will have a history of several months of a chronic mucopurulent discharge on the affected side. Reflux of mucopurulent material can be elicited by placing gentle pressure over the nasolacrimal sac. Repeated bouts of infection are common until the membrane obstruction of the nasolacrimal duct becomes patent spontaneously or until it is opened with a probe.

Orbital or facial trauma with or without fracture of facial bones, craniofacial syndromes in children, and immune compromise all result in a predisposition to acute dacryocystitis.

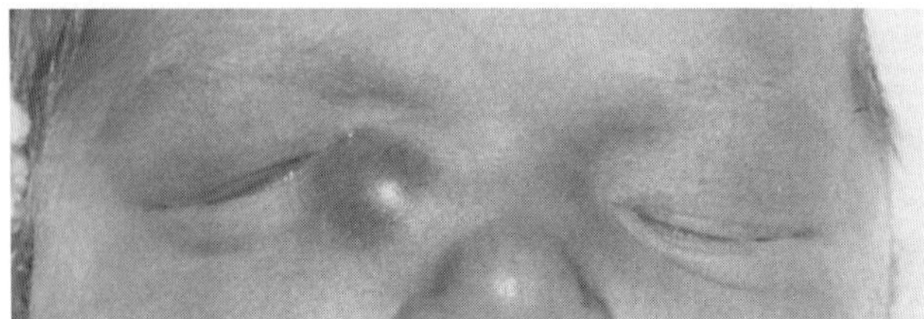

FIGURE 91–6. Nasolacrimal sac mucocele, or blue dome cyst, in a newborn. The cyst is caused by congenital obstruction of the upper and lower portions of the nasolacrimal collecting system.

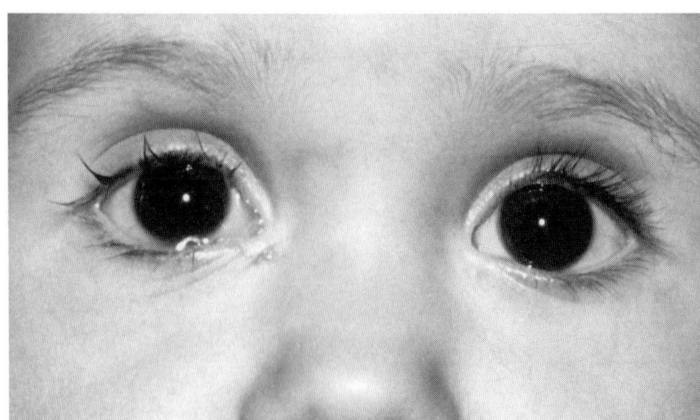

FIGURE 91–7. Congenital nasolacrimal duct obstruction with chronic, low-grade dacryocystitis, characterized by persistent tearing and the presence of a chronic mucopurulent discharge.

SYMPTOMS AND CLINICAL MANIFESTATIONS

Infants with a nasolacrimal sac mucocele will have a **blue dome cyst,** which is usually recognized at birth and increases in size. Gentle pressure applied to the dome of the cyst results in reflux expression of a mucoid material. If the mucoid material becomes contaminated, the surrounding area will become warm, erythematous, and swollen.

Frequent bouts of dacryocystitis with large amounts of mucopurulent discharge in children 1–12 months of age suggest the presence of a membrane obstructing the nasolacrimal duct.

The swelling and induration of dacryocystitis may extend onto the upper and lower eyelids. If the condition is untreated, the cystic lacrimal sac can form an abscess and drain externally. In older children with dacryocystitis, the nasolacrimal sac is usually not distended. The infection can produce cellulitis of the surrounding tissues.

DIAGNOSIS

The diagnosis is established by symptoms and clinical findings. Neonates and children with acute dacryocystitis, with associated redness, swelling, and induration of the surrounding tissues, should have culture specimens taken. Blood cultures are indicated if there is fever. The differential diagnosis includes preseptal cellulitis, lymphangioma, hemangioma, and frontal para-midline encephalocele. Diagnostic imaging with a **dacryocystogram** and imaging of the nasolacrimal duct and surrounding structures are useful in adults, although these studies are usually not performed in children because of lack of cooperation.

TREATMENT

Treatment of a congenital nasolacrimal sac mucocele with acute dacryocystitis consists of probing the nasolacrimal system to establish communication of the sac externally via the lacrimal puncta and internally to the nasal cavity. To obtain accurate control of passage of the probe and to ensure passage of the probe through the nasolacrimal duct into the nose, one must often use general anesthesia. Some ophthalmologists prefer to perform this procedure in an office setting. If the infection is extensive, oral antibiotics should be administered in combination with frequent application of gentle pressure to the dome of the cystic nasolacrimal sac in an attempt to evacuate the mucopurulent material into the canaliculi. Severe infections may produce swelling, induration, and erythema and may require intravenous antibiotics. The addition of topical antibiotic drops such as tobramycin or gentamicin, applied to the conjunctival cul-de-sac four times a day, will help to decrease the bacterial composition of the discharge. Some nasolacrimal sac mucoceles have a cystic structure extending into the nasal cavity and communicating with the distended, infected nasolacrimal sac. This cystic structure, if bilateral, may be of sufficient size to reduce the passage of air through the nose and interrupt normal respiration. Once communication with the nasal cavity has been established, copious irrigation of the mucopurulent discharge with simultaneous suctioning of the nasal cavity should be performed and should then be repeated until clear irrigation fluid is recovered. The saline solution used for irrigation may have 3 or 4 drops of tobramycin or gentamicin ophthalmic solution added to a volume of 30 mL of normal saline solution. Higher concentrations of antibiotics may be toxic if systemically absorbed. If maintenance of a free communication between the lacrimal canaliculi and the opening of the nasolacrimal duct in the nose is in doubt, placement of a Silastic tube stent in the nasolacrimal collecting system for 1–3 months should be considered. After placement of the Silastic stent, the patient should be treated with topical antibiotic-corticosteroid solutions four times daily for the first 7–10 days. Afterward, intermittent treatment with topical antibiotic drops such as 10% sodium sulfacetamide can be used to suppress bacterial proliferation and reduce the amount of discharge. Once the Silastic stent has been removed, free communication is usually maintained between the lacrimal puncta and the nasal cavity.

Frequent bouts of dacryocystitis in children 1–12 months of age is treated by massage of the nasolacrimal sac three or four times a day to express the mucopurulent material from the sac and by cleansing of the surrounding area, followed by application of antibiotics such as 10% sodium sulfacetamide or trimethoprim. The goal of massage of the nasolacrimal sac is to reduce the amount of discharge. Attempts to massage the contents downward to force the membrane open are usually unsuccessful. The diameter of the nasolacrimal duct is small, and the amount of pressure required to rupture the membrane would be great. **Laplace's law** states that the pressure required to distend the surface of the membrane is inversely proportional to the radius of curvature. It is best to attempt to express the secretions upward, rather than to attempt to rupture the membrane in the duct. When the membrane does not spontaneously open by 6–12 months of age, a probing of the nasolacrimal duct will cure the condition in 95–97% of affected children.

Persons with a history of facial trauma, nasal fractures, or craniofacial abnormalities may have bone defects in the region of the lacrimal sac or the nasolacrimal duct. Dacryocystitis associated with these defects may be treated by canalizing the lacrimal collecting system with Silastic stents or, in severe cases, by performing a dacryocystorhinostomy.

COMPLICATIONS

Dacryocystitis can extend into the surrounding lid tissues and progress to preseptal cellulitis. Severe infections can extend posteriorly into the orbit and cause orbital cellulitis. Failure to treat chronic dacryocystitis related to congenital nasolacrimal duct obstruction by 1 year of age may result in a decrease in the ultimate success rate.

PROGNOSIS

Recurrence of congenital nasolacrimal sac mucoceles is uncommon. If they do recur, intubation with a Silastic tube stent, with the tube left in the collecting system for 3–6 months, is recommended. Recurrent dacryocystitis indicates a malformation or dysfunction of the lacrimal collecting system. From 95% to 97% of children who have a probe-and-irrigation procedure performed between 6 and 12 months of age will be cured.

PREVENTION

Recurrence should prompt evaluation with CT or MRI to identify abnormalities in the structures of the nasolacrimal collecting system.

REVIEWS

Brown DD, McCulley JP: Staphylococcal and mixed staphylococcal seborrheic blepharoconjunctivitis. In Fraunfelder FT, Roy FH, Grove J (editors): *Current Ocular Therapy,* 4th ed. Philadelphia, WB Saunders, 1995, pp 596–7.

Dailey RA: Dacryocystitis. In Fraunfelder FT, Roy FH, Grove J (editors): *Current Ocular Therapy,* 4th ed. Philadelphia, WB Saunders, 1995, pp 687–8.

Hussein N, Schwab I, Ostler HB: Blepharitis. In Tasman W, Jaeger EA (editors): *Duane's Clinical Ophthalmology,* Vol 4. Philadelphia, Lippincott, Williams & Wilkins, 1994, pp 1–9.

Matoba AY (Chair): *Blepharitis.* Preferred Practice Pattern, American Academy of Ophthalmology. San Francisco, American Academy of Ophthalmology, 1998.

CHAPTER 92

Endophthalmitis

Albert W. Biglan ▪ Hal B. Jenson

Endophthalmitis is an inflammatory reaction that involves the intraocular fluids and ocular structures and is one of the most serious, sight-threatening, and emergent conditions that can affect the eye. **Panophthalmitis** indicates that the inflammatory process extends beyond the sclera and involves the extraocular orbital contents. Endophthalmitis can be classified as infectious, which is the most common, or noninfectious (Table 92–1). The difference between noninfectious endophthalmitis and uveitis is in the lesser degree of the inflammatory response in uveitis.

Exogenous endophthalmitis results from inoculation during trauma or surgery and occurs after penetrating trauma or ocular surgery. **Endogenous endophthalmitis** results from bacteremia and most often occurs in persons receiving hyperalimentation or in persons with immunocompromise. Infectious endophthalmitis is most common in children and most frequently follows penetrating trauma related to accidental injury. Endophthalmitis should be suspected when inflammatory signs after trauma or surgery exceed the expected response or when they persist longer than expected in a particular clinical setting.

Endophthalmitis is an emergency and requires prompt recognition and involvement of an ophthalmologist, preferably a vitreoretinal specialist who can obtain culture specimens and initiate treatment. Delays in treatment can adversely affect outcome.

ETIOLOGY

Many bacterial species, even those ordinarily considered to be of low virulence or pathogenicity, can cause endophthalmitis (Table 92–2). **Acute postoperative endophthalmitis** usually develops within 24–72 hours after a surgical procedure but may develop as late as 6 weeks afterward. **Late postoperative endophthalmitis,** or **delayed postoperative endophthalmitis,** occurs >6 weeks after the procedure. The specific organisms vary according to the source or cause of the infection. Gram-positive organisms are cultured more frequently than gram-negative organisms. *Candida,* by far, is the most common fungal organism causing endophthalmitis. Polymicrobial infection occurs in approximately 20% of cases of posttraumatic endophthalmitis and is reported in 0–10% of cases of postoperative endophthalmitis.

EPIDEMIOLOGY

Trauma is the most common cause of endophthalmitis in children. In a report (Weinstein, 1979) of 22 consecutive cases of endophthalmitis in children, 86% followed accidental trauma. In another series (Brinton, 1984) conducted for 8 years, 7.4% of 257 children with penetrating trauma of the globe developed endophthalmitis. Children, especially boys between 4 and 8 years of age, are the most susceptible to trauma and penetrating injuries of the eye. Risk factors for posttraumatic endophthalmitis include penetrating injury, disruption of the lens, presence of an intraocular foreign body, soil-related injury, injury occurring in a rural environment, delayed primary repair, and penetration of the globe by an obviously contaminated device.

Endophthalmitis occurs infrequently after surgical procedures. A study (Good, 1990) of 671 children after cataract surgery reported an incidence of postoperative endophthalmitis of 0.45%. In adults the incidence is 0.07–1.2%, with a slightly higher incidence after secondary intraocular lens implantation. The incidence of endophthalmitis after glaucoma filtering procedures in adults is 0.06–1.8%. The incidence in children is probably higher. The relatively low occurrence of postoperative endophthalmitis in children reflects the infrequent requirement for intraocular surgery in this population compared with that in adults, rather than a protective effect of age. Risk factors for developing postoperative endophthalmitis in children include blepharitis, conjunctivitis, canaliculitis, dacryocystitis, nasolacrimal duct obstruction, contact lens use, immunosuppression, upper respiratory tract infection, placement of foreign material such as a seton for glaucoma control or an intraocular lens, and any procedure that leaves a nonabsorbable suture retained in the sclera or cornea.

The incidence of endogenous endophthalmitis in children is unknown. Endogenous endophthalmitis is associated with cardiac anomalies, renal failure, prematurity, leukemia, immunosuppression, hyperalimentation, indwelling catheters, and surgical procedures performed on other parts of the body.

PATHOGENESIS

The offending organism enters the eye by an exogenous or an endogenous route. Penetrating trauma, either accidental or surgical, may lead to the introduction of bacteria through an ocular wound or with a retained contaminated foreign body.

Endogenous endophthalmitis occurs as a result of metastatic septic embolism from a distant focus or foci of infection. The infectious emboli lodge in the choriocapillaris underlying the retina or enter through the retinal circulation. Organisms proliferate and

TABLE 92–1. Classification of Endophthalmitis

Infectious Endophthalmitis
Posttraumatic
Postoperative
Acute postoperative endophthalmitis (onset <6 wk)
Delayed-onset endophthalmitis (onset >6 wk)
Endogenous
Noninfectious Endophthalmitis
Posttraumatic
Sterile uveitis
Sympathetic ophthalmia

TABLE 92–2. Microbiologic Etiology of Endophthalmitis

Postoperative			
Acute Onset	**Delayed Onset**	**Traumatic**	**Endogenous**
Coagulase-negative staphylococci	Coagulase-negative staphylococci	Coagulase-negative staphylococci	*Streptococcus pneumoniae*
Staphylococcus aureus	*Propionibacterium acnes*	*Streptococcus*	Other *Streptococcus*
Streptococcus	*Candida*	*S. aureus*	*Staphylococcus*
Pseudomonas	*Aspergillus*	*B. cereus*	*Candida*
Bacillus cereus		*Pseudomonas*	*Neisseria meningitidis*
Candida		Other gram-negative bacilli	*B. cereus*
Aspergillus		Fungi (various)	Enteric gram-negative bacilli

extend into the retina and vitreous cavity. The inflammatory process can range from a localized suppurative uveitis to endophthalmitis involving all structures of the eye. An impaired immune response may delay recognition or alter the response of the eye to an infectious agent.

SYMPTOMS AND CLINICAL MANIFESTATIONS

The clinical features of endophthalmitis are determined by the route of entry, quantity of bacteria in the inoculum, virulence of the infecting organism, and defense mechanisms of the host. The symptoms of endophthalmitis include decreased visual acuity, light sensitivity, eye pain, lid edema, and bulbar conjunctival edema. In children the presence of endophthalmitis may be associated with irritability, combativeness, pain, extreme light sensitivity, and severe blepharospasm. Obtaining an adequate examination of the eye may be challenging. If penetrating trauma is suspected, forcible opening of the eyes may extend the severity of the injury. If this is a concern, an examination with the patient under anesthesia should be considered.

The clinical setting and the history may heighten the suspicion for endophthalmitis. Children with ocular trauma should be questioned carefully regarding the cause and type of trauma. Children will fear parental repercussions when they suffer trauma in an unsupervised environment or while engaged in unapproved activities. Children who have a prolonged or aberrant recovery period after a surgical procedure should also be closely observed for postoperative endophthalmitis (Fig. 92–1). Children with bacteremia or fungemia, who are debilitated or immunocompromised, who have an indwelling catheter, who are undergoing hyperalimentation, or who were born prematurely are at risk of having endogenous endophthalmitis.

Posttraumatic Endophthalmitis. The onset of traumatic endophthalmitis may be difficult to detect if trauma causes disruption of the lens capsule or in the presence of severe traumatic iritis or hyphema. Eyes of children produce an exuberant fibrinoid response to trauma, and this sterile response may be difficult to differentiate from an infectious inflammatory process. The admixture of lens remnants, the fibrinoid response, and blood can create a confusing clinical presentation, especially for a child who is resistant to examination. The onset of endophthalmitis after trauma usually occurs within 48–72 hours, although delayed onset may occur within 6 weeks with organisms of low virulence or with fungi.

Postoperative Endophthalmitis. Postoperative endophthalmitis usually develops within 1–3 days after the surgical procedure but may occur any time in the postoperative period. The degree of reaction of the eye depends on the duration and type of procedure performed. The ocular inflammatory response after most surgical trauma is usually during a phase of resolution, at 2–3 days after surgery. Delayed endophthalmitis may occur 6 or more weeks after the operation. Eyes that are treated for glaucoma with filtering procedures can present with endophthalmitis months or even years after the procedure. A persistent intraocular inflammatory response after any surgical procedure should raise suspicion for infectious endophthalmitis. Pain, light sensitivity, lid edema, and increasing chemosis are signs that raise concern. Examination of the eyes with a table-mounted or hand-held slit lamp is ideal, but it may be difficult to accomplish in a young child who is in pain. Visualization of the anterior chamber can be achieved by using the magnification provided by an illuminated magnification source such as a Wood's light or by using an indirect ophthalmoscope, holding the condensing lens close to the globe and using it as a magnifying lens.

Endogenous Endophthalmitis. Endogenous endophthalmitis may occur coincident with a systemic infection or sepsis, or its occurrence may be unrelated to any infectious event. Clinical features include reduced visual acuity, diminished red reflex, and chorioretinitis observed on fundus examination. Hypopyon, haze of the cor-

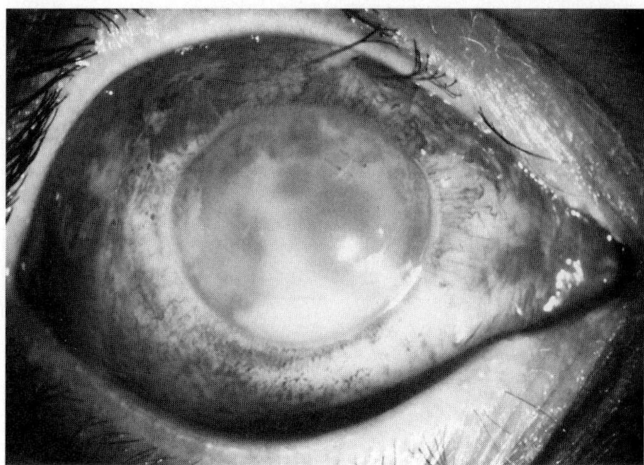

FIGURE 92–1. Acute endophthalmitis with pain, hemorrhagic conjunctivae, and lid edema 48 hours after an intraocular surgical procedure. There is a 2 mm hypopyon, obscuration of the anterior chamber structures, and purulent material within the eye.

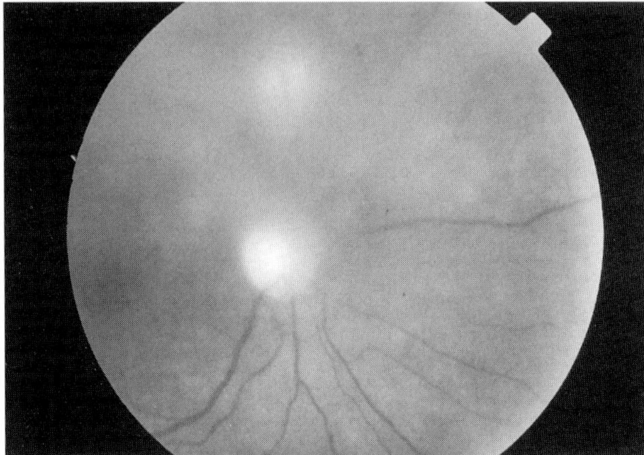

FIGURE 92–2. Vitreitis associated with *Candida* sepsis. The optic nerve and the emanating retinal blood vessels are visualized clearly inferiorly, but the superior fundus shows obscuration of the vessels, with a wispy, cotton-like nidus strongly suggesting *Candida* endophthalmitis. (Courtesy of Department of Ophthalmic Photography, Eye and Ear Institute, Pittsburgh, Penn.)

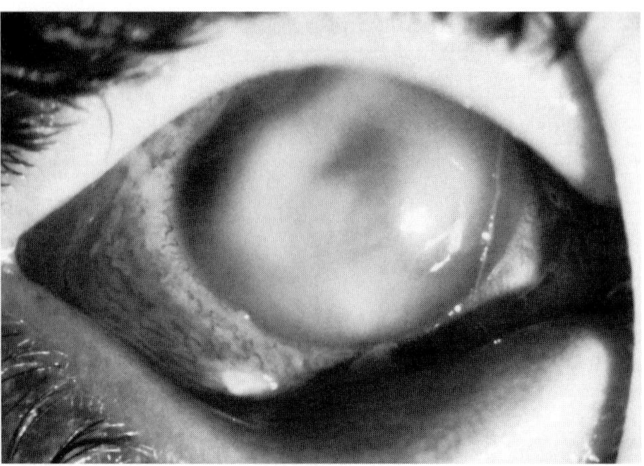

FIGURE 92–4. Endophthalmitis caused by *Staphylococcus aureus.* There is complete obscuration of the iris after a penetrating wound of the eye at the right (*white area*).

nea, and lid edema may be late findings. Severe vitreous inflammation with an underlying vasculitis suggests an infectious cause for the problem. Flame-shaped retinal hemorrhages, with or without white centers, and a vitreous cellular reaction resembling a cotton ball or snowball are characteristic features of *Candida* (Fig. 92–2).

Physical Examination Findings

The physical findings of endophthalmitis include decreased visual acuity; photophobia; decreased red reflex; afferent pupillary defect; upper eyelid edema; hypopyon (Fig. 92–1), which is a leukocytic exudate in the anterior chamber of the eye; corneal edema or infiltrates; fibrinoid anterior chamber response (Fig. 92–3); obscuration of the anterior chamber structures (Fig. 92–4); vitreous inflammatory response; **chemosis,** which is edema of the ocular conjunctiva; and ciliary injection after surgery or accidental trauma.

DIAGNOSIS

Because of the seriousness of delaying the diagnosis of endophthalmitis, a person with risk factors and suggestive clinical findings should be presumed to have infectious endophthalmitis until it can be proved otherwise. Frequent evaluations may be needed until the diagnosis is either proved or excluded.

Differential Diagnosis

Other conditions that can mimic or masquerade as endophthalmitis include posttraumatic severe inflammatory response; rupture of the lens capsule with dispersion of white, fluffy lens material throughout the anterior chamber; retained lens fragments after surgery; sterile uveitis associated with sympathetic ophthalmia; hypopyon uveitis associated with rifabutin, metipranolol, and cidofovir; and a khaki-colored hyphema. A corneal ulcer with extreme pain, blepharospasm, and hypopyon can also mimic endophthalmitis (Fig. 92–5). Tumors such as an exfoliating retinoblastoma, large cell lymphoma, and leukemia can also simulate endogenous endophthalmitis.

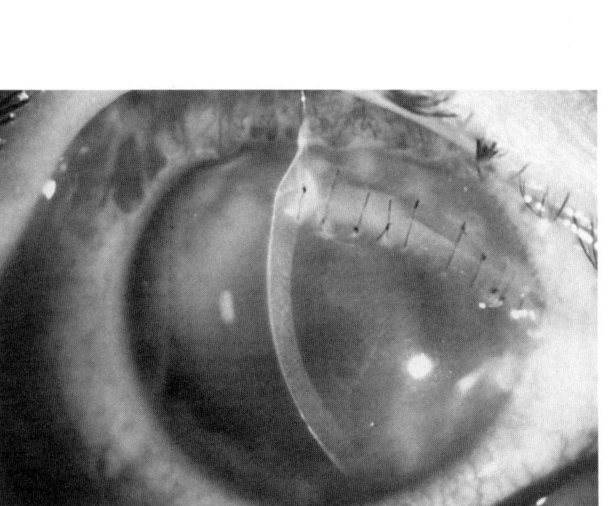

FIGURE 92–3. Penetrating trauma: 5 days after laceration of the cornea with a piece of glass. The degree of fibrinoid reaction obscures the iris, and the reaction is excessive. *Streptococcus* was cultured from the aqueous and vitreous humors.

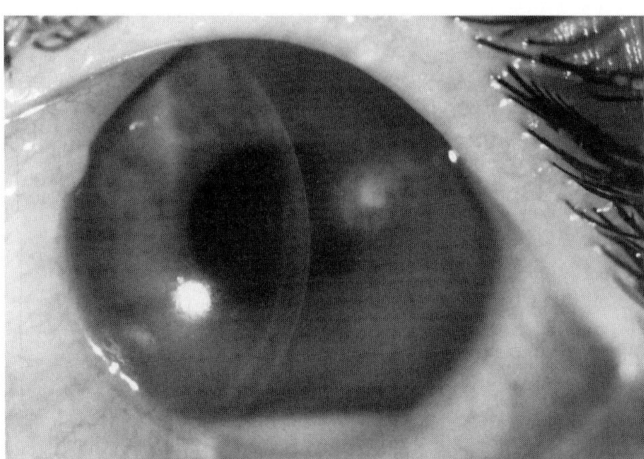

FIGURE 92–5. A corneal ulcer can cause a sterile (or noninfectious) hypopyon that may suggest endophthalmitis. (Courtesy of Department of Ophthalmic Photography, Eye and Ear Institute, Pittsburgh, Penn.)

Microbiologic Evaluation

Cultures of the aqueous, vitreous, lids, and conjunctiva must be obtained to diagnose endophthalmitis. Obtaining only an aqueous aspirate or lid cultures is not sufficient because more than half the cultures of aqueous are sterile in cases of infectious postoperative endophthalmitis, and lid cultures may not yield the pathogen. Cultures should be obtained with the patient under general anesthesia. Indications for ocular cultures include the presence of a hypopyon after intraocular surgery, an infected filtering bleb after glaucoma surgery, the presence of a white plaque on an intraocular lens, the presence of intraocular foreign material, chronic intraocular inflammation unresponsive to corticosteroids, and the presence of beaded opacities and haze in the vitreous.

If intraocular foreign material is present, it should be removed and cultured for bacteria and fungi. An aliquot of ocular fluids should be placed directly on slides and stained with Gram and Giemsa stains. A potassium hydroxide preparation may be included if fungi are a consideration.

Persons with endogenous endophthalmitis should also undergo a systemic evaluation to identify a source of infection. The extent and focus of the search should be based on the history and the results of the physical examination. Additional cultures of blood, urine, cerebrospinal fluid, and wound specimens may be indicated.

Diagnostic Imaging

If an intraocular foreign body is suspected or present, diagnostic imaging to detect and localize the foreign body is conducted by using either CT or B-scan ultrasonography. A routine skull series is also necessary because CT and B-scan ultrasonography can miss a small foreign body. An MRI should be requested only if the foreign body is known to be nonmagnetic.

TREATMENT

Prompt diagnosis and early therapeutic intervention are critical if the eye and vision are to be preserved. Persons with suspected endophthalmitis should be transferred to the combined care of an ophthalmologist and a pediatric infectious disease specialist. The ophthalmologist should be involved early to provide aqueous and vitreous specimens for culture and to perform the vitreous biopsy.

The organism present on smears should be used to guide initial therapy, but because of the serious nature of endophthalmitis, broad-spectrum treatment should be used to cover both gram-positive and gram-negative organisms. Antifungal treatment should be added if a fungus is considered. After the aqueous tap and the diagnostic vitrectomy, intravitreal, periocular, and topical antibiotics are administered. The selection of antibiotics, routes, and frequency of administration is based on the presumed pathogens and their antibiotic susceptibilities. The mainstay of treatment is intravitreal and subconjunctival antibiotics supplemented by topical therapy (Table 92–3). Penetration of systemically administered antibiotics into the aqueous and vitreous humor is unreliable and generally poor. A therapeutic or extensive vitrectomy is performed in eyes with signs of profound visual loss, evidenced by light perception only; rapid onset of inflammation after surgery; purulent material in the vitreous humor; posttraumatic endophthalmitis; and endophthalmitis suspected to be caused by virulent bacteria such as *Staphylococcus aureus, Streptococcus, Bacillus cereus,* and gram-negative bacilli; or suspected fungal endophthalmitis. Eyes with hand motions or better vision do equally well with immediate vitrectomy or immediate tap and biopsy for culture.

The Endophthalmitis Vitrectomy Study Group (1995) has established guidelines for the treatment of acute postoperative endophthalmitis after cataract surgery in adults. This national collaborative study recommended intravitreal administration of amikacin and vancomycin (Table 92–4). Aminoglycosides such as amikacin can be toxic to the retina and retinal pigment epithelium at therapeutic doses. For this reason, some ophthalmologists favor ceftazidime for gram-negative coverage because of its broad antimicrobial activity,

TABLE 92–3. Empirical Therapy for Endophthalmitis

Surgical Therapy
Aqueous humor aspiration for culture and smear
Vitreous humor biopsy for culture and smear
Culture of specimens from lids and conjunctivae
Culture of any foreign material
Therapeutic vitrectomy

Antibiotic Therapy
Intravitreal antibiotic
Subconjunctival antibiotic
Topical antibiotic
Systemic antibiotic

Adjunctive Therapy
Topical
Cycloplegic agents: homatropine 5% 3 times a day or atropine 1% twice daily
Corticosteroids: prednisolone acetate, 1 drop every 1–2 hr, reduced to q4hr as inflammation subsides
Systemic
Corticosteroids: prednisone 1–2 mg/kg/day, 24 hr after appropriate antimicrobial therapy has been started
Follow-up
Adjust antibiotic therapy according to culture and susceptibility results, response to treatment, and virulence of organism
Repeat vitrectomy for failure to respond after 48–72 hr

TABLE 92–4. Recommended Antibiotic Treatment of Bacterial Endophthalmitis

Route of Administration	Drug	Dose
Intravitreal	Amikacin	400 μg in 0.1 mL
	or	
	Ceftazidime	2.25 mg in 0.1 mL
	Vancomycin	1 mg in 0.1 mL
	Dexamethasone	400 mg in 0.1 mL
plus		
Subconjunctival	Vancomycin	25 mg in 0.5 mL
	Ceftazidime	100 mg in 0.5 mL
	Dexamethasone	6 mg in 0.25 mL
plus		
Topical	Vancomycin	50 mg/mL drops every hour
	Ceftazidime	100 mg/mL drops every hour
with or without		
Systemic	Ceftazidime	
	Children	150 mg/kg/day divided q8hr IV
	Adults	2 g q8hr IV
	Vancomycin	1 g q12hr IV
	Prednisone	1 mg/kg for 5–10 days PO

wide safety margin, lower risk of retinal toxic effects. However, ceftazidime is incompatible with vancomycin, which will coprecipitate. When these two agents are used, they are injected with separate syringes at separate locations. Subconjunctival antibiotics penetrate into the vitreous and aqueous humor better than topical medications, but the use of subconjunctival antibiotics alone is inadequate because the MIC is not achieved within the vitreous cavity.

The inflammatory reaction caused by infection within the vitreous cavity may generate fibrovascular proliferation that may lead to a traction retinal detachment. In addition, the inflammatory process may lead to retinal necrosis and possibly secondary retinal detachment. The addition of dexamethasone, administered both into the vitreous cavity and orally, may reduce the inflammatory response, hasten resolution, and thereby reduce the risk of late retinal detachment. There is insufficient evidence for or against the use of intravitreal corticosteroids for infective endophthalmitis. The use of corticosteroids is best assessed on a case-by-case basis.

The use of systemic antibiotics for postoperative endophthalmitis is controversial. The Endophthalmitis Vitrectomy Study Group (1995) showed that intravenously administered antibiotics in most cases are not useful adjuncts in the treatment of postoperative endophthalmitis. The use of systemic antibiotics must be based on the clinical circumstances on a case-by-case basis.

Fungal endophthalmitis is usually caused by *Candida,* and a vitrectomy for culture should be performed. If the cultures confirm the presence of fungi, injection of intravitreal and periocular amphotericin B is recommended. Antifungal agents such as fluconazole and itraconazole have less toxicity when used systemically, but intravitreal use has not been well studied. Fungal endophthalmitis tends to be less acute and usually responds to antifungal therapy. Ophthalmologic examination may be indicated in persons with fungemia for evaluation of the presence of fungal ophthalmic infection.

Endogenous endophthalmitis with intraocular inflammation severe enough to obscure visualization of the optic nerve or macula should be managed as for acute postoperative infectious endophthalmitis, with systemic antibiotics.

All persons with endophthalmitis should be hospitalized for their biopsy or culture and to ensure proper administration of antimicrobial therapy and close observation. During treatment, severe pain may require systemic narcotics to provide comfort. If the eye is not responding after 3 days of therapy, a repeated vitreous biopsy or vitrectomy, or both, may be considered, in combination with additional intravitreal and periocular antibiotics.

The treatment of presumed sterile uveitis includes high doses of systemic and topical corticosteroids, with the administration of a topical cycloplegic agent such as homatropine 5% or atropine 1% solutions applied two or three times daily. Prolonged treatment with either systemic or periocular corticosteroids may cause undesirable side effects in children. If extended treatment is necessary, more potent immunosuppressive drugs such as cyclosporine may be substituted or used in combination with systemic corticosteroids.

COMPLICATIONS

Numerous complications of endophthalmitis can occur, especially corneal edema and glaucoma. Additionally, the iris may become atrophic, the pupil may adhere to the anterior lens capsule, cataracts may form as a result of trauma or as a result of treatment, and the vitreous may organize and develop a cyclitic membrane that can pull the retinal structures centrally, causing a traction retinal detachment. The retina may become necrotic because of toxins liberated by the bacteria or because of adverse events related to antibiotic use. With excessive scarring and subsequent loss of function, the eye may become blind and develop **phthisis bulbi,** or shrinking and wasting of the globe.

Infection may rarely spread from the confines of the globe to the orbit, causing panophthalmitis and an orbital abscess. The cavernous sinus, because of its proximity, may develop a thrombus, resulting in a life-threatening infection.

PROGNOSIS

The prognosis after endophthalmitis correlates with the speed of recognition, virulence of the organism, size of the inoculum, effectiveness of the antibiotic treatment, and any concomitant disease or process that alters the immune response. In a study (Weinstein, 1979) of 22 consecutive cases of endophthalmitis in children, only five eyes had visual acuity better than 20/200, and seven eyes required enucleation or evisceration.

The Endophthalmitis Vitrectomy Study Group (1995) found no difference in visual outcome, whether or not an immediate vitrectomy was performed for persons whose initial visual acuity was hand motions or better. However, in the subgroup of persons with initial light perception–only vision, vitrectomy was significantly associated with improved prognosis, with 33% achieving visual acuity of 20/40 or better, 56% achieving 20/100 or better, and 20% having severe visual loss, in comparison with persons who did not have vitrectomy.

PREVENTION

The prevention of endophthalmitis after penetrating ocular trauma requires prompt repair of adnexal lacerations and prompt re-establishment of the integrity of the globe. Cultures of foreign material should be obtained, and the wound and cul-de-sac should be bathed with a 5% povidone-iodine solution. Topical, subconjunctival, and systemic antibiotics may be used to prevent infection after penetrating injuries to the globe. Persons with penetrating trauma should have ophthalmologic consultation.

For persons undergoing elective surgery, meticulous preparation of the surrounding ocular structures with a 5% povidone-iodine solution, followed by isolation of the cilia from the surgical field with an adhesive drape, is recommended. These measures minimize the number of bacteria in the conjunctival sac. The use of preoperative antibiotics for 1–2 days preceding surgery has not been proved to lower the frequency of endophthalmitis effectively. Most surgeons at the completion of a surgical procedure inject cefazolin (50–100 mg) subconjunctivally and administer dexamethasone (1–2 mg) subconjunctivally, with topical antibiotics such as tobramycin, gentamicin, or a quinolone for 2–24 hours after surgery (Table 16–6). Patients with severe blepharitis, nasolacrimal duct obstruction, or an upper respiratory tract infection should have elective ophthalmologic surgery postponed.

Prevention of endogenous endophthalmitis is difficult unless there is an obvious source of infection such as an infected heart valve or abscess. Posttraumatic, non-infectious endophthalmitis most commonly is due to **sympathetic ophthalmia.** The incidence of sympathetic ophthalmia can be prevented or reduced by using meticulous surgical technique to repair penetrating ocular trauma, followed by administration of topical and periocular corticosteroids. Topical prednisolone acetate is also used until the ocular inflammatory reaction related to trauma has subsided.

REVIEWS

Brod RD, Flynn HW Jr: Infectious endophthalmitis. *Curr Opin Infect Dis* 1997;10:153–62.

Doft BH: Endophthalmitis Vitrectomy Study. *Arch Ophthalmol* 1991; 109:487–9.

Kresloff MS, Castellarin AA, Zarbin MA: Endophthalmitis. *Surv Ophthalmol* 1998;43:193–224.

Okada AA, Johnson RP, Liles WC: Endogenous bacterial endophthalmitis. Report of a ten-year retrospective study. *Ophthalmology* 1994;101: 832–8.

Wilson FM II: Causes and prevention of endophthalmitis. *Int Ophthalmol Clin* 1987;27:67–73.

KEY ARTICLES

Aaberg TM, Flynn HW, Schiffman J, et al: Nosocomial acute-onset postoperative endophthalmitis. A 10-year review of incidence and outcomes. *Surv Ophthalmol* 1998;105:1004–10.

Alfaro DV, Roth DB, Laughlin RM, et al: Pediatric post-traumatic endophthalmitis. *Br J Ophthalmol* 1995;79:888–91.

Allen HF, Mangiaracine AB: Bacterial endophthalmitis after cataract extraction. *Arch Ophthalmol* 1964;72:454–62.

Baley JE, Annable WL, Kliegman RM: *Candida* endophthalmitis in the premature infant. *J Pediatr* 1981;98:458–61.

Bohigian GM, Olk RJ: Factors associated with a poor visual result in endophthalmitis. *Am J Ophthalmol* 1986;101:332–41.

Brinton GS, Topping TM, Hyndiuk RA, et al: Posttraumatic endophthalmitis. *Arch Ophthalmol* 1984;102:547–50.

Brod RD, Flynn HW, Clarkson JG, et al: Endogenous *Candida* endophthalmitis: Management without intravenous amphotericin B. *Ophthalmology* 1990;97:666–72.

D'Amico DJ, Caspers-Velu L, Libert J, et al: Comparative toxicity of intravitreal aminoglycoside antibiotics. *Am J Ophthalmol* 1985;100: 264–75.

Davis JL: Intravenous antibiotics for endophthalmitis. *Am J Ophthalmol* 1996;122:724–6.

de Courten C, Sancho P, BenEzra D: Metastatic *Serratia marcescens* endophthalmitis. *J Pediatr Ophthalmol Strabismus* 1988;25:45–7.

Donahue SP, Kowalski RP, Jewart BH, et al: Vitreous cultures in suspected endophthalmitis. Biopsy or vitrectomy. *Ophthalmology* 1993;100: 452–5.

Endophthalmitis Vitrectomy Study Group: Microbiologic factors and visual outcomes in the Endophthalmitis Vitrectomy Study. *Arch Ophthalmol* 1996;122:830–46.

Endophthalmitis Vitrectomy Study Group: Results of the Endophthalmitis Vitrectomy Study: A randomized trial of immediate vitrectomy and of intravenous antibiotics for the treatment of postoperative bacterial endophthalmitis. *Arch Ophthalmol* 1995;113:1479–96.

Forster RK: Etiology and diagnosis of bacterial postoperative endophthalmitis. *Ophthalmology* 1978;85:320–6.

Forster RK, Abbott RL, Gelender H: Management of infectious endophthalmitis. *Ophthalmology* 1980;87:313–9.

Good WV, Hing S, Irvine AR, et al: Postoperative endophthalmitis in children following cataract surgery. *J Pediatr Ophthalmol Strabismus* 1990;27:283–5.

Jewelewicz DA, Schiff WM, Brown S, et al: Rifabutin-associated uveitis in an immunosuppressed pediatric patient without acquired immunodeficiency. *Am J Ophthalmol* 1998;125:872–3.

Johnson MW, Doft BH, Kelsey SF, et al: The Endophthalmitis Vitrectomy Study Group. Relationship between clinical presentation and microbiologic spectrum. *Ophthalmology* 1997;104:261–72.

Mandelbaum S, Forster RK, Gelender H, et al: Late onset endophthalmitis associated with filtering blebs. *Ophthalmology* 1985;92:964–72.

Nelsen PT, Marcus DA, Bovino JA: Retinal detachment following endophthalmitis. *Ophthalmology* 1985;92:1112–7.

Puliafito CA, Baker AS, Haaf J, et al: Infectious endophthalmitis. Review of 36 cases. *Ophthalmology* 1982;89:921–9.

Rifai A, Peyman GA, Daun M, et al: Rifabutin-associated uveitis during prophylaxis for *Mycobacterium avium* complex infection. *Arch Ophthalmol* 1995;113:707.

Rowsey JJ, Newsom DL, Sexton DJ, et al: Endophthalmitis: Current approaches. *Ophthalmology* 1982;89:1055–66.

Scherer WJ, Lee K: Implications of early systemic therapy on the incidence of endogenous fungal endophthalmitis. *Ophthalmology* 1997;104: 1593–8.

Tervo T, Ljungberg P, Kautiaien T, et al: Prospective evaluation of external ocular microbial growth and aqueous humor contamination during cataract surgery. *J Cataract Refract Surg* 1999;25:65–71.

Weinstein GS, Mondino BJ, Weinberg RJ, et al: Endophthalmitis in a pediatric population. *Ann Ophthalmol* 1979;11:935–43.

Wheeler DT, Stager DR, Weakley DR : Endophthalmitis following pediatric intraocular surgery for congenital cataracts and congenital glaucoma. *J Pediatr Ophthalmol Strabismus* 1992;29:139–41.

CHAPTER

93

Uveitis and Retinitis

Albert W. Biglan ▪ Hal B. Jenson

Uveitis, retinitis, and optic neuritis are inflammatory conditions that affect the internal structures of the eye. Uveitis is not usually the result of an infectious process. However, when the inflammation is granulomatous, an infectious cause should be investigated. Retinitis is often associated with viral and parasitic infections but may also be caused by a nonspecific inflammatory process. Optic neuritis, or inflammation of the optic nerve, almost never has an infectious cause.

UVEITIS

Uvea refers to the pigmented ocular tissue that extends posteriorly from the pupillary border of the iris, the ciliary body, and the choroid. The uvea helps the eye to absorb light energy, supplies the retina with some of its nutrition, and helps to fulfill its oxygen requirement.

Uveitis is a nonspecific term that refers to inflammation of the uvea and surrounding structures. **Anterior uveitis** refers to **iritis** or **keratouveitis. Intermediate uveitis,** or **cyclitis,** involves the ciliary body and pars plana. **Posterior uveitis** involves the choroid or the overlying retinal tissue. **Panuveitis** refers to involvement of all of the ocular uveal tissue. Uveitis may be acute, lasting days or weeks, or chronic, lasting for years.

Uveitis may be nongranulomatous or granulomatous. Nongranulomatous uveitis, which usually has a noninfectious cause, is characterized by inflammation consisting of cells and flare, or protein, which have leaked into the anterior chamber of the eye. The inflammation leads to delicate keratic precipitates on the corneal endothelium. Granulomatous uveitis is characterized by larger cells and clumps of macrophages and epithelioid cells and may have an infectious cause.

ETIOLOGY

Most forms of uveitis do not have an infectious cause. The most common cause in children is trauma, as in traumatic iritis. Other causes include juvenile rheumatoid arthritis, Behçet's syndrome, ankylosing spondylitis, and sarcoidosis. Infectious causes that have been associated with uveitis in children include tuberculosis caused by *Mycobacterium tuberculosis,* Lyme disease caused by *Borrelia burgdorferi,* infection with herpes simplex virus, zoster caused by reactivation of varicella-zoster virus, toxoplasmosis caused by *Toxoplasma gondii,* rubella, cat-scratch disease caused by *Bartonella henselae,* and syphilis. Toxoplasmosis may cause uveitis but more commonly causes **chorioretinitis** which is considered as part of retinitis. Histoplasmosis affects adults who reside in the Mississippi and upper Ohio river valleys, although symptomatic histoplasmosis in children is uncommon. Uveitis has been reported to be caused by Whipple's bacillus *(Tropheryma whippelii).*

EPIDEMIOLOGY

Uveitis affects children of all ages and has an equal sex distribution. Noninfectious causes such as sarcoid have a predilection for the African American population. Persons receiving immunosuppressive drugs or those with immunodeficiency, including AIDS, are at greater risk of having uveitis and chorioretinitis.

PATHOGENESIS

The hallmark of anterior uveitis is the development of **keratic precipitates,** which consist of epithelioid and mononuclear cells attached to the internal surface of the cornea (Fig. 93–1). Inflammatory nodules at the iris margin **(Koeppe nodules)** and the iris surface **(Busacca nodules)** may coexist. The inflammatory cells in the anterior chamber flow in a vertical convection current, which causes cells to adhere to the corneal endothelium, producing a **vertical pigmented zone (Krukenberg's spindle).** Vascular wall integrity is disrupted, and blood vessels will leak protein, causing a **flare reaction.**

SYMPTOMS AND CLINICAL MANIFESTATIONS

Children present with an insidious onset of irritation of one or both eyes, manifested by dilatation of the fine mesh of vessels located at the corneal-conjunctival junction, or limbus, and known as a **limbal flush.** Ocular discomfort due to spasm of the ciliary body, light sensitivity, and blurred visual acuity are signs of uveitis.

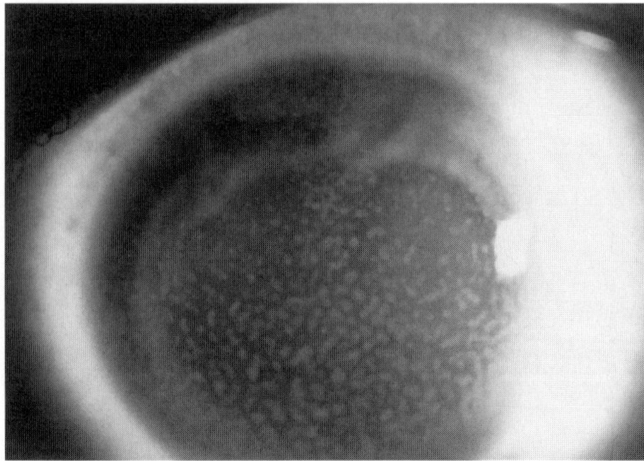

FIGURE 93–1. Keratitic precipitates, which consist of epithelioid and mononuclear cells attached to the internal surface of the cornea, are the hallmark of anterior uveitis.

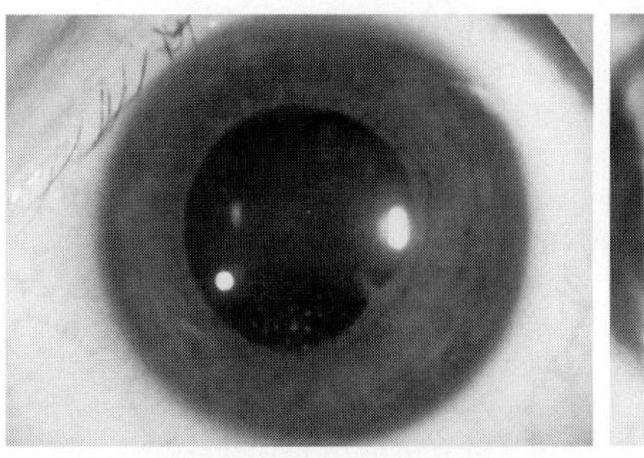
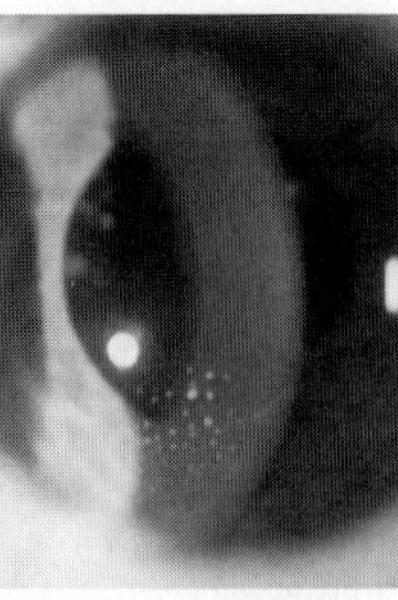

FIGURE 93–2. An 8-year-old child with an irregular pupil due to a posterior synechia *(left).* Slit-lamp examination showed granulomatous "mutton fat" keratic precipitates and a Krukenberg's spindle, which is a vertical pigmented zone *(right).*

Chronic forms cause a fibrovascular pannus on the surface of the cornea, which may acquire calcium, resulting in **band keratopathy.**

Physical Examination Findings

Examination should include measurement of the best-corrected visual acuity and an assessment of the lymph nodes, lacrimal gland, eyelids, and conjunctiva. A slit-lamp examination of the cornea, anterior chamber, iris, lens, retrolental space, and vitreous should be performed. An indirect ophthalmoscope is used to view the retina and choroid and to assess the optic nerve for inflammation and swelling. When possible, intraocular pressure should be measured with applanation tonometry (Tono-Pen tonometer). Physical examination should include the lungs, heart, skin, liver, and lymph nodes.

Keratic precipitates are microscopic collections of lymphocytes on the internal surface of the cornea and are the hallmark of noninfectious anterior uveitis (Fig. 93–1). In granulomatous uveitis, the precipitates will appear larger and will have a greasy or **mutton fat appearance** (Fig. 93–2). This form of uveitis is more likely to have an infectious cause. The iris may adhere to the anterior lens capsule, causing the pupil to be irregular. Cataracts and vitreous haze may occur.

DIAGNOSIS

The history should assess the patient's immune status, use of immunosuppressive drugs, exposure to tuberculosis, cat scratches, tick bites (suggestive of Lyme disease), and ingestion of raw meat (suggestive of toxoplasmosis).

The differential diagnosis includes Kawasaki syndrome, Vogt-Koyanagi-Harada syndrome, juvenile rheumatoid arthritis, ankylosing spondylitis, Behçet's syndrome, sarcoidosis, sympathetic ophthalmia, retinoblastoma, juvenile xanthogranuloma, and low-grade bacterial endophthalmitis (Chapter 92). **Vogt-Koyanagi-Harada syndrome,** a systemic, noninfectious form of anterior uveitis occurring at higher frequency among Asians, is associated with poliosis and dysacusis.

Laboratory evaluation for infectious uveitis should include CBC and WBC differential counts, chest x-ray examination, and serologic testing for herpes simplex viruses, rubella, syphilis, and Lyme disease. A PPD skin test is placed to evaluate for tuberculosis. Additional tests include antinuclear antibody for juvenile rheumatoid arthritis, angiotensin-converting enzyme titer for sarcoidosis, and HLA-B27 for ankylosing spondylitis.

TREATMENT

The management of uveitis should include evaluation and treatment by a qualified ophthalmologist. The goal of treatment should be to identify, if possible, the causative agent and specifically to treat the underlying infection, to suppress the inflammation, and to minimize ocular and systemic adverse effects. It is essential to monitor the response to treatment by repeated ophthalmologic examination. Specific treatment of the infectious agent causing uveitis may not cure the uveitis.

Uveitis that is a manifestation of systemic infection, such as in tuberculosis (Chapter 35) and Lyme disease (Chapter 29), is treated as one of the elements of the systemic disease. Herpes simplex virus and varicella-zoster virus may cause infection limited to keratouveitis, or occasionally in association with central nervous system involvement, and should be treated with systemic acyclovir in doses appropriate for central nervous system infection (Chapter 55). The treatment of uveitis caused by rubella virus is supportive. Toxoplasmosis is treated primarily as a retinitis.

Treatment of nonspecific uveitis is supportive. Malnourished persons should establish a healthy diet with vitamin supplementation. Topical applications to the eye of short-acting cycloplegic agents such as homatropine 5% or cyclopentolate 1% or 2% are used two or three times daily to dilate the pupil, which will help prevent posterior synechiae. Cycloplegic agents reduce the cellular inflammatory response, symptoms of light sensitivity, and ocular discomfort. Caution should be exercised when these agents are used in children <8 years of age because of the risk of amblyopia. Oral corticosteroids, such as prednisone 1 mg/kg/day, are administered daily until inflammation is suppressed, and then alternate-day dosage should be used to minimize the adverse effects.

Topical corticosteroids are used to treat mild and severe forms of anterior uveitis. Prednisolone acetate 1% is applied to the eye every 2 hours, with later applications limited to four times a day or less until the cellular reaction in the anterior chamber is reduced to "rare or trace" cells. Residual flare reaction is not specifically treated.

Intermediate uveitis is treated with periocular injections of triamcinolone 0.5 mL or methylprednisolone 0.5 mL in 40 mg/mL suspension. Persons with refractory cases and persons with chronic uveitis can be treated with oral doses of cyclosporine 250–350 mg daily in conjunction with oral prednisone. Methotrexate 12.5 mg/wk is also used. Periocular sustained-release corticosteroids should not be used in infectious uveitis without identification and specific treatment of the infectious agent.

COMPLICATIONS

The complications of uveitis include deposition of cellular components on the iris, formation of synechiae between the iris and the anterior lens capsule, posterior subcapsular and/or cortical cataract, and band keratopathy. The filtration angle may become obstructed with cellular debris and may block the egress of the aqueous, which can cause elevation of the intraocular pressure. It may be difficult to distinguish elevated intraocular pressure caused by topical or systemic corticosteroids from angle closure or obstruction. Chronic uveitis may cause cystoid macular edema, which can cause a permanent decrease in central visual acuity. Chronic uveitis may cause the ciliary processes, which produce the aqueous humor, to become fibrotic, causing a reduced production of aqueous humor, hypotonis oculi, and, in advanced stages, phthisis bulbi.

Prolonged use of oral corticosteroids in children may result in sequelae of aseptic necrosis of the femoral head, reduction in growth, hypertension, Cushing's syndrome, acne, mood changes, and increased intraocular pressure.

PROGNOSIS

The prognosis is extremely variable. Some forms of uveitis may affect one eye exclusively, whereas other forms will affect both eyes. Some children may have a single episode of uveitis. Others will have recurrent episodes. Protracted courses of months to years are not uncommon. Fortunately, uveitis in children is rare. Some eyes will become blind as a result of uveitis.

PREVENTION

Prevention of infectious uveitis includes avoidance of exposure to tuberculosis and, in areas endemic for Lyme disease, to wildlife environments and ticks. The avoidance of cats will prevent cat-scratch disease, and avoiding the eating of uncooked meats will prevent ingestion of *T. gondii.* Rubella uveitis can be prevented by rubella vaccination.

RETINITIS

Retinitis is an inflammatory or infectious condition that involves the retina or underlying choroid or a combination of both of these tissues, causing **chorioretinitis.** Retinitis may extend into the vitreous, causing **vitreitis.** Disease may be limited to one or both eyes, or it may be a manifestation of a systemic disease. Retinitis that involves the macula can cause blindness. If retinitis is limited to the peripheral retina, good vision may be preserved but peripheral vision may be reduced.

ETIOLOGY

The most common infectious causes of retinitis are herpes simplex virus, varicella-zoster virus, cytomegalovirus (CMV), rubella virus, cat-scratch disease caused by *Bartonella henselae,* toxoplasmosis caused by *T. gondii,* and toxocariasis caused by the ascarid *Toxocara canis,* also known as the **dog roundworm.** Tertiary syphilis, caused by *Treponema pallidum,* can also cause uveitis.

Transmission. The viruses causing retinitis may be acquired perinatally by maternal transmission or acquired later in life. In immunocompetent persons, *T. gondii* retinitis usually occurs as a reactivation of congenital infection (Chapter 95), which is acquired by maternal ingestion or inhalation of oocysts in cat feces or by ingestion of undercooked meat. Acquired toxoplasmosis rarely involves the eye. *T. canis* is usually acquired by pica or by direct exposure to puppies and their excrement.

EPIDEMIOLOGY

Herpes simplex virus, varicella-zoster virus, and CMV are endemic and may be acquired at any age, as well as by perinatal transmission. Congenital toxoplasmosis has an incidence of 1 in 1,000 to 1 in 8,000 live births, with ocular symptoms developing in 10% of infected individuals. Ocular disease caused by *T. canis* usually has an onset around 4 years of age, in association with contact with puppies.

PATHOGENESIS

The herpes simplex viruses types 1 and 2, varicella-zoster virus, and CMV infect epithelial cells and also exhibit neurotropism, which includes the retina.

Retinitis caused by *T. gondii* usually represents reactivation of congenital infection and can occur at any age.

The eggs of *T. canis* of the worm are ingested orally, and the larvae penetrate the gastrointestinal tract and migrate to the liver and lungs, causing **visceral larva migrans,** which typically occurs in children 2–4 years of age. Occasionally the larvae migrate to other sites, including the central nervous system and the eyes, causing **ocular larva migrans,** which typically occurs in older children and young adults. The larvae do not develop beyond this stage in human hosts. Inflammation occurs as a result of the intraocular death of the larvae, which elicits an intense eosinophilic and mononuclear inflammatory response in the liver and lungs but a much less intense response in the eyes, primarily consisting of mononuclear cells and a few eosinophils (Fig. 93–3).

SYMPTOMS AND CLINICAL MANIFESTATIONS

Ocular symptoms and signs of retinitis include decreased visual acuity, light sensitivity, diminished red reflex, **ocular floaters,** and **photopsia,** or the appearance of flashes. Ophthalmoscopic examination shows patchy areas of white or hemorrhagic retina

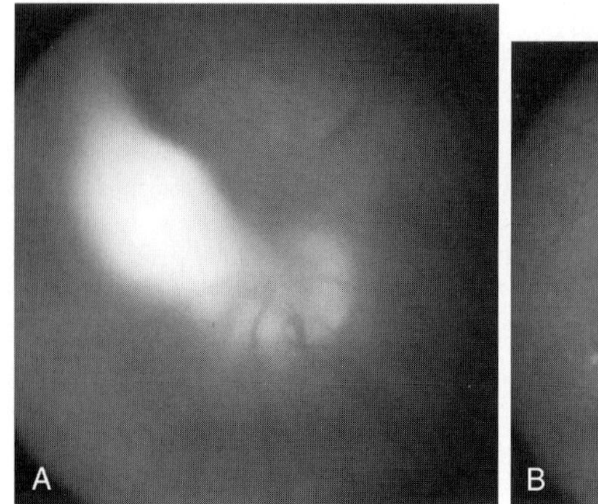

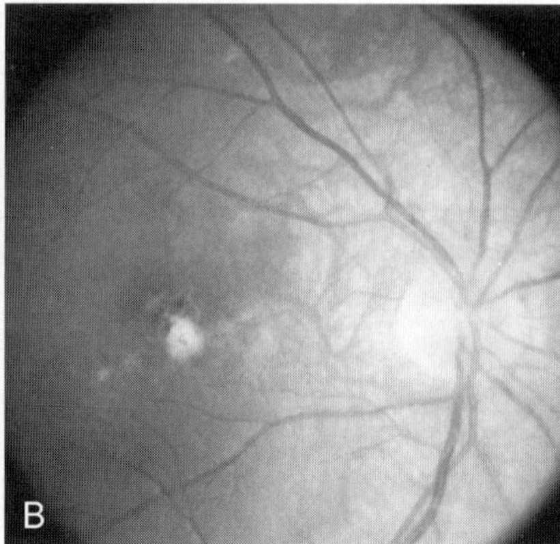

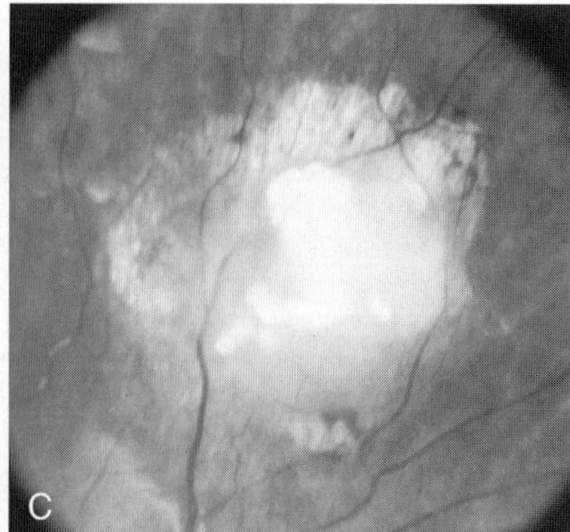

FIGURE 93–3. A, *T. canis* infection with an inflammatory vitreitis. The wispy edges of the granuloma overlie the optic nerve. **B,** Inactive *T. canis* infection that is resolving. **C,** A small, perimacular scar is presumed to have been caused by *T. canis.*

with overlying vitreous haze. These conditions may be indolent and focal or may be fulminant and involve the retinal tissue of both eyes. Extraocular and systemic symptoms of conditions causing retinitis may also be present. Interstitial keratitis and retinitis suggest syphilis.

DIAGNOSIS

The diagnosis of retinitis is usually established by using indirect ophthalmoscopy with visualization of the retina through a dilated pupil. Serologic testing is useful for confirming the cause.

Acute phases of herpes simplex virus and CMV present as a hemorrhagic retinitis with patches of yellow and as a blanched retina with patches of hemorrhage (Plate 9D). Retinitis, with a **macular star** or **stellate retinopathy** pattern (Plate 9D) is reported with cat-scratch disease, which is caused by *B. henselae* (Chapter 28). Toxoplasmosis presents as a retinochoroiditis with focal necrotizing retinitis, with varying degrees of vitreitis and anterior chamber inflammation. After a period of activity, the chorioretinal pigment will clump and deposit around the peripheral zone of inflammation (Plate 9D). Congenital toxoplasmosis may also cause calcification of the central nervous system, along with other manifestations (Chapter 95). *T. canis* presents as a unifocal, elevated granulomatous mass on the retinal surface; this mass is approximately the same size as the optic nerve and is frequently associated with intense vitreitis (Fig. 93–2).

The differential diagnosis of retinitis includes retinal hemorrhages that occur at birth and that usually clear within 2–3 weeks. Child abuse can cause a hemorrhagic retinitis, **Coats' disease,** which may involve either the peripheral or central retina and is characterized by retinal vascular abnormalities and a yellow exudate in the macula. The absence of retinal tissue or coloboma can be seen as a small or large white patch involving one or both eyes. Systemic lupus erythematosus or AIDS retinopathy can present as a hemorrhagic vasculitis. Toxoplasmosis must be differentiated from **North Carolina macular dystrophy,** which is an autosomal recessive areolar pigmentary dystrophy. **Aicardi's syndrome** is suggested by the presence of punched-out retinal lesions in multiple locations that are associated with infantile spasms and retardation. Infection with *T. canis* can appear similar to a raised elevation of the retina or similar to retinoblastoma, although the presentation of retinoblastoma is usually before 2 years of age, whereas the presentation of ocular larva migrans is usually in children older than 4 years. Both toxoplasmosis and toxocariasis should be included in the differential diagnosis of **leukokoria,** which is the observation of a white pupil.

Retinitis caused by infection with herpes simplex virus, CMV (Plate 9D), or *T. gondii* (Plate 9D) is suggested by the ophthalmologic appearance and can be confirmed by serologic testing of serum and also samples from the aqueous or vitreous humors. Syphilis can cause retinitis and interstitial keratitis (Fig. 93–4) and is confirmed by serologic testing (Chapter 85). There are also PCR tests for herpes simplex virus and for *T. gondii* infection. Toxoplasmosis may also be identified by the encysted form of the parasite found in the retina when a specimen is stained with hematoxylin and eosin. *T. canis* infection is confirmed by serum antibody titers of ≥1:64. Rubella is detected by a rise in the IgG titers and by the presence of IgM antibodies. Children with *T. canis* may have eosinophilia.

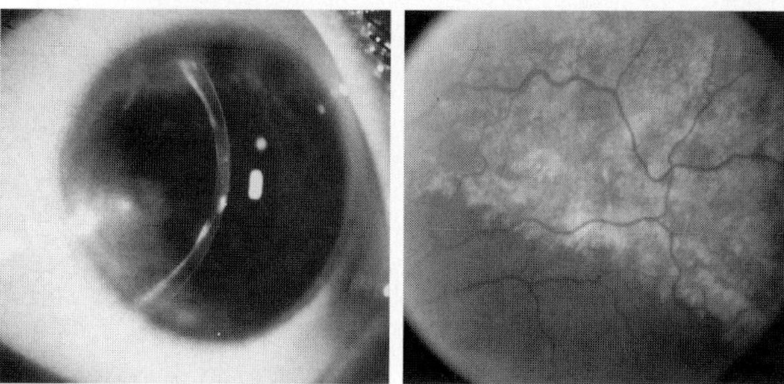

FIGURE 93–4. Syphilis can cause interstitial keratitis *(left)* and retinitis *(right).*

TREATMENT

Retinitis caused by herpes simplex virus or varicella-zoster virus is treated with intravenous acyclovir, which reduces the risk of involvement of the second eye by 50%. The usual adult dose is 1,500 mg/m^2/day divided every 8 hours intravenously for 5–10 days, followed by oral acyclovir 400 mg five times a day and continued for up to 4–6 weeks.

Infection with CMV is treated with ganciclovir, foscarnet, or cidofovir. These drugs are virostatic. Induction-dose systemic therapy consists of 2 weeks of ganciclovir 10 mg/kg divided twice daily intravenously, foscarnet 90 mg/kg twice daily intravenously, or cidofovir 5 mg/kg once weekly intravenously, followed by maintenance therapy. Ganciclovir can be implanted as a sustained-release intraocular delivery system designed to last 6–8 months. The implant contains 4.5 mg of ganciclovir with a release rate of approximately 1 μg/hr. Oral ganciclovir has limited bioavailability and is not recommended as sole maintenance therapy.

There is no specific treatment of rubella retinitis; only supportive treatment can be offered. Antimicrobial therapy for cat-scratch disease with neuroretinitis should be considered (Chapter 28). Retinitis with syphilis is treated as tertiary syphilis (Table 85–6).

Newborn infants with congenital toxoplasmosis should be treated with pyrimethamine and sulfadiazine, with leucovorin, for 1 year (Table 95–9). Some experts recommend the addition of prednisone for congenital toxoplasmosis with chorioretinitis. Treatment of toxoplasmosis in older children and adults remains controversial. The combination of pyrimethamine and sulfadiazine, which act synergistically, is recommended, especially if the lesion is near the macula or optic nerve, if significant hemorrhage or inflammation is present, or if the person is immunocompromised. Lesions in the periphery can usually be followed up without treatment.

Systemic treatment of ocular larva migrans is usually not administered because it does not alter the ocular prognosis. The visual acuity is affected by the granulomatous inflammatory reaction in response to the death of the larvae. Direct photocoagulation of the larvae has been beneficial. Systemic visceral larva migrans is treated with diethylcarbamazine 0.5 mg/kg or thiabendazole 50 mg/kg/day.

COMPLICATIONS

The complications involving vision are determined by the location and extent of the infection and its associated inflammatory reaction and may include chronic iridocyclitis, cataract, glaucoma, and retinal detachment. Decreased vision may be caused by focal involvement of the retinal tissue or by systemic involvement of the visual cortex if encephalitis complicates the presentation. In immunocompromised persons, fulminant forms of retinitis may occur, with acute vasculitis that leads to ischemia and **acute retinal necrosis** and eventually to retinal detachment. Acute retinal necrosis is frequently associated with varicella-zoster virus and less often with herpes simplex virus. Treatment with acyclovir reduces involvement of the contralateral eye in approximately half the cases.

PROGNOSIS

Retinitis caused by rubella is self-limited and will usually not affect visual acuity. Toxoplasmosis is generally self-limited, often involutes without treatment, but may recur years later. Ocular larva migrans, from *T. canis,* does not recur.

For immunocompromised persons, reduction of immunosuppression or treatment of the underlying immunodeficiency may help to reduce the likelihood of recurrence.

PREVENTION

Avoidance of exposure to the infectious causes of retinitis will minimize the risk of retinitis. Herpes simplex viruses type 1 and type 2 and CMV, because of their high prevalence, are difficult to avoid. Rubella vaccination will prevent rubella infections in vaccinees, as well as congenital rubella syndrome in newborns of immunized women. Intrauterine toxoplasmosis can be greatly minimized by mothers' eliminating exposure to cats and avoiding ingestion of raw meat. Exposure to *T. canis* can be minimized if young children wash their hands after playing, avoid playing in areas exposed to feces from dogs, and avoid geophagia. Syphilis is avoided by exercising safe sexual practices.

REVIEWS

Bernadino VB, Naidoff MA: Retinal inflammatory diseases. In Tasman W, Jaeger EA, editors: *Duane's Clinical Ophthalmology.* Philadelphia, Lippincott Williams & Wilkins, 2000: vol 3, pp 1–12.

Fujikawa LS: Advances in immunology and uveitis. *Ophthalmology* 1989;96:1115–20.

Knox DL: Uveitis. *Pediatr Clin North Am* 1987;34:1467–85.

Tugal-Tutkun I, Havrlikova K, Power WJ, et al: Changing patterns in uveitis of childhood. *Ophthalmology* 1996;103:375–83.

Weinberg RS: Uveitis, update on therapy. *Ophthalmol Clin North Am* 1999;12:71–81.

KEY ARTICLES

Baarsma GS, LaHey E, Glassius E, et al: The predictive value of serum angiotensin converting enzyme and lysozyme levels in the diagnosis of ocular sarcoidosis. *Am J Ophthalmol* 1987;104:211–7.

Baumal CR, Levin AV, Read SE: Cytomegalovirus retinitis in immunosuppressed children. *Am J Ophthalmol* 1999;127:550–8.

Biglan AW, Glickman LT, Lobes LA Jr: Serum and vitreous *Toxocara* antibody in nematode endophthalmitis. *Am J Ophthalmol* 1979; 88:898–901.

Colin J, Prisant O, Cochener B, et al: Comparison of the efficacy and safety of valacyclovir and acyclovir for the treatment of herpes zoster ophthalmicus. *Ophthalmology* 2000;107:1507–11.

George RK, Walton RC, Whitcup SM, et al: Primary retinal vasculitis. Systemic associations and diagnostic evaluation. *Ophthalmology* 1996; 103:384–9.

Giles CL: Pediatric intermediate uveitis. *J Pediatr Ophthalmol Strabismus* 1989;26:136–9.

Helm C, Holland GN: The effects of posterior subtenon injection of triamcinolone acetonide in patients with intermediate uveitis. *Am J Ophthalmol* 1995;120:55–64.

Herpetic Eye Disease Group: Oral acyclovir for herpes simplex virus eye disease. Effect on prevention of epithelial and stromal heredities. *Arch Ophthalmol* 2000;118:1030–6.

Jabs DA, Enger C, Dunn JP, et al: Cytomegalovirus retinitis and viral resistance. 3. Culture results. CMV Retinitis and Viral Resistence Study Group. *Am J Ophthalmol* 1998;126:543–9.

Kanski JJ, Shun-Shin GA: Systemic uveitis syndromes in childhood: An analysis of 340 cases. *Ophthalmology* 1984;91:1247–52.

Martin DF, Dunn JP, Davis JL, et al: Use of the ganciclovir implant for treatment of cytomegalovirus retinitis in the era of potent antiretroviral therapy: Recommendations of the International AIDS Society—USA Panel. *Am J Ophthalmol* 1999a;127:329–39.

Martin DF, Kuppermann BD, Wolitz RA, et al: Oral ganciclovir for patients with cytomegalovirus retinitis treated with a ganciclovir implant. *N Engl J Med* 1999b;340:1063–70.

Nussenblatt RB, Palestine AG, Chan CC, et al: Randomized double-masked study of cyclosporine compared to prednisolone in the treatment of endogenous uveitis. *Am J Ophthalmol* 1991;112:138–46.

Rickman LS, Freeman WR, Green WR, et al: Brief report: Uveitis caused by *Tropheryma whippelii* (Whipple's bacillus). *N Engl J Med* 1995; 332:363–6.

Ronday MJ, Ongkosuwito JU, Rothova A, et al: Intraocular anti–*Toxoplasma gondii* IgA antibody production in patients with ocular toxoplasmosis. *Am J Ophthalmol* 1999;127:294–300.

Rothova A, van Veenedaal MS, Linssen A, et al: Clinical features of acute anterior uveitis. *Am J Ophthalmol* 1987;103:137–45.

Shah SS, Lowder CY, Schmitt MA, et al: Low-dose methotrexate therapy for ocular inflammatory disease. *Ophthalmology* 1992;99:1419–23.

Small KW, Hermsen V, Gurney N, et al: North Carolina macular dystrophy and central areolar pigment epithelial dystrophy. One family, one disease. *Arch Ophthalmol* 1992;110:515–8.

CHAPTER 94

Pediatric Implications of Maternal Infection

Kenneth M. Boyer

A fetus in utero is sterile, as is its placental and amniotic fluid environment. The maternal immune system, fetal immune system, placenta and membrane barriers, and, to a degree that varies with gestational age, transplacentally acquired maternal IgG antibodies preserve fetal sterility. At birth, a newborn infant abruptly confronts a contaminated environment, and surface colonization by maternal and environmental organisms rapidly ensues. During the birth process and the newborn period, transplacental antibodies, breast milk antibodies and lymphocytes, the baby's integument and immune system, and the ecologic balance established among the various organisms in the baby's emerging normal flora protect the baby against invasion by pathogenic organisms.

To the extent that protective mechanisms are inadequate, maternal infections in pregnancy may be transmitted from the mother to the fetus or newborn infant, a process known as **transplacental or vertical transmission.** Transplacental transmission during gestation results in **congenital infection** of the fetus. Vertical transmission at the time of birth or shortly thereafter results in **perinatal infection** of the newborn (Table 94–1).Either type of infection may cause self-limited conditions in an infant that resolve without sequelae; silent infections with symptoms or consequences that may not appear until later in life; clinically apparent infections that develop into handicapping chronic conditions; life-threatening acute disease necessitating immediate therapy; or spontaneous abortion, stillbirth, or perinatal death (Table 94–2). Even if a fetus is not infected, maternal infection during pregnancy may have indirect consequences, including enhanced severity of the mother's illness; triggering of spontaneous abortion, premature delivery, or stillbirth; and adverse effects of maternal antimicrobial therapy on the mother as well as the fetus. In addition, preterm delivery, in many instances the consequence of maternal infection, places a newborn at greater risk of diseases of prematurity as well as nosocomial infection in the neonatal intensive care unit environment.

Some perinatal conditions, such as puerperal sepsis, neonatal tetanus, and neonatal gonococcal ophthalmia, have been drastically reduced in incidence by aseptic and antiseptic approaches to obstetric and newborn care initiated more than a century ago. Recent decades have seen the dramatic decline of other conditions, such as congenital rubella, through the use of universal immunization. Still other diseases, such as congenital syphilis, have been reduced in incidence by the use of antibiotics, but they remain disturbingly common. Pediatric AIDS from vertical transmission has emerged as one of the major public health threats of our era.

Pediatricians and pediatric subspecialists in infectious diseases, neonatology, and genetics bring unique expertise to the care of pregnant women with possible or proved infections. A spirit of collaboration with obstetric providers optimizes management. The focus of the pediatrician should be on the baby, for whom the pediatrician should be an advocate. Correct diagnosis of infection in a mother, a fetus, or a newborn infant may not be simple or routine, and specialized tests or unusual specimens often are necessary. Differentiation between physiologically normal and diagnostically meaningful test results may be difficult. Empirical treatment may be required before test results are available. Pregnancy termination and related ethical issues may be involved and have strong emotional overtones. All these factors contribute to making the management of maternal, fetal, and neonatal infections challenging.

Maternal Chorioamnionitis. In addition to leading to direct infection of the fetus and newborn, maternal infection can have indirect adverse effects on the newborn. A meta-analysis (Wu and Colford, 2000) showed that clinical chorioamnionitis was significantly associated with both cerebral palsy (RR, 1.9; 95% CI, 1.4–2.5) and cystic periventricular leukomalacia (RR, 3.0; 95% CI, 2.2–4.0) in premature infants. Among full-term infants a positive association was found between clinical chorioamnionitis and cerebral palsy (RR, 4.7; 95% CI, 1.3–16.2). There is growing evidence in animal models that fetal inflammation caused by maternal infection results in elevated blood and brain cytokine levels leading to central nervous system damage in the fetus and subsequent cerebral palsy.

TABLE 94–1. Vertical Transmission of Infection: Relative Frequency of Congenital and Perinatal Infection According to Pathogen

Pathogen	Congenital	Perinatal
Parvovirus B19	++++	–
Rubella virus	+++	+
Toxoplasma gondii	+++	+
Treponema pallidum	+++	+
Varicella-zoster virus	++	++
Listeria monocytogenes	++	++
Mycobacterium tuberculosis	+	+++
Herpes simplex virus	+	+++
Cytomegalovirus	+	+++
Enteroviruses (coxsackieviruses and echoviruses)	+	+++
Hepatitis B virus	+	+++
Hepatitis C virus	Unknown	Unknown
Human immunodeficiency virus type 1	+	+++
Human papillomaviruses	–	++++
Chlamydia trachomatis	–	++++
Group B *Streptococcus*	–	++++
Neisseria gonorrhoeae	–	++++

++++ = Most frequent; + = least frequent; – = organism not transmitted this way.

TABLE 94–2. Pediatric Consequences of Maternal Infection: Pathogenic Mechanisms, Important Causative Organisms, and Typical Clinical Manifestations

Maternal Infection	Pediatric Consequence	Pathogenic Mechanism	Important Causative Organisms	Typical Clinical Manifestations
Systemic Infection during pregnancy	Congenital infection (chronic)	Transplacental infection	Cytomegalovirus	Microcephaly, thrombocytopenia, deafness
			Toxoplasma gondii	Hydrocephalus, chorioretinitis, encephalitis
			Treponema pallidum	Snuffles, skin rash, osteitis
			Rubella virus	Cataracts, deafness, heart defects
			Varicella-zoster virus	Limb reduction defects
Systemic infection during pregnancy	Congenital infection (fulminant or fatal)	Transplacental infection	Parvovirus B19	Nonimmune fetal hydrops
			Listeria monocytogenes	Miliary granulomatosis, pneumonia
			Mycobacterium tuberculosis	Hepatitis, miliary tuberculosis
			Varicella-zoster virus	Disseminated varicella
Systemic infection during pregnancy	Stillbirth, spontaneous abortion, or premature delivery (without fetal infection)	Enhanced severity of maternal disease during pregnancy; placental insufficiency; premature labor	*Plasmodium falciparum*	Severe malaria (maternal)
			Measles virus	Measles pneumonia (maternal)
			Varicella-zoster virus	Varicella pneumonia (maternal)
Genital infection at delivery	Perinatal infection	Ascending infection of amniotic fluid	Group B *Streptococcus*	Pneumonia, septic shock
			Escherichia coli K1	Sepsis, meningitis
Genital infection at delivery	Perinatal infection	Inoculation during passage through birth canal	Herpes simplex virus	Skin vesicles, hepatitis, disseminated intravascular coagulopathy, pneumonia
			Group B *Streptococcus*	Sepsis, meningitis, osteomyelitis
			Neisseria gonorrhoeae	Conjunctivitis
			Chlamydia trachomatis	Conjunctivitis, pneumonia
			Human papillomavirus	Laryngeal papilloma
Enteric infection at delivery	Perinatal infection	Ingestion during passage through birth canal	Enteroviruses	Hepatitis, myocarditis
			Salmonella	Colitis, sepsis, meningitis
Systemic infection at delivery	Perinatal infection	Maternal-fetal transfusion	Hepatitis B virus	Chronic infection with hepatitis B virus
			Human immunodeficiency virus	Chronic infection with HIV-1, AIDS
			Hepatitis C virus	Chronic infection with hepatitis C virus
Latent systemic infection after delivery	Perinatal infection	Breast-feeding	Cytomegalovirus	Asymptomatic; latent infection
			Human T cell leukemia virus	Asymptomatic; latent infection
			Human immunodeficiency virus	Chronic infection with HIV-1, AIDS
Respiratory infection after delivery	Perinatal infection	Inhalation during close contact	*Mycobacterium tuberculosis*	Miliary tuberculosis
			Respiratory viruses (influenza viruses, respiratory syncytial virus)	Pneumonia, apnea

Children with cerebral palsy have elevated neonatal blood and amniotic fluid cytokine levels, indicating that cerebral palsy is preceded by perinatal inflammation.

PREVENTION OF MATERNAL INFECTION

Prevention of infection in a fetus and newborn begins with prevention of maternal infection **(primary prevention)** and is one of the first responsibilities of parenthood. All obstetricians and midwives should provide prepregnancy and prenatal counseling about infection. Much relevant information for prospective parents can be found in manuals published by the American College of Obstetrics and Gynecology (ACOG) and the American Academy of Pediatrics (AAP). Many health care providers recommend these materials.

Because many pathogens that may infect an infant are sexually transmitted, sexual promiscuity on the part of either the mother or the father should be avoided. Barrier prophylactic techniques can work but are a much less appropriate option than avoiding relations with multiple partners. Injection drug use is an important mechanism of transmission of hepatitis B virus and HIV and may also be secondarily associated with most sexually transmitted pathogens. Counseling and referral to drug treatment programs should be offered to pregnant women with drug dependency.

Congenital toxoplasmosis, although relatively rare in the United States, can be prevented by limiting contact with cats, particularly disposing of cat box filler. Because many uncooked meats, particularly pork and lamb but also beef, may contain encysted bradyzoites of *Toxoplasma gondii,* sampling uncooked meat during preparation and eating dishes containing raw or undercooked meat should also be avoided. Educational programs that emphasize these two basic mechanisms of transmission have reduced the incidence of congenital toxoplasmosis by 50% over the past decade in France and Austria, countries with a high incidence of congenital toxoplasmosis.

Currently available immunizations are capable of preventing several of the most important causes of congenital and perinatal infection. The incidence of congenital rubella in the United States, for example, has been reduced more than 100-fold by universal infant and selective adult immunization. Chronic hepatitis B in mothers and its consequent vertical transmission is the major mode of persistence of hepatitis B in the populations of many developing countries. Universal childhood immunization for hepatitis B, recommended for children in the United States since 1991, is the long-term solution to this public health problem, but full realization of its benefits remains at least a generation away.

Immunization of pregnant women with tetanus toxoid during pregnancy is a standard component of prenatal care in many developing countries. By passively immunizing the fetus, this program has the proved benefit of reducing the incidence of neonatal tetanus. Similar in concept are current investigations into the use of group B *Streptococcus* conjugate vaccines for pregnant women or women of childbearing age in the United States.

RECOGNITION OF MATERNAL INFECTION DURING PREGNANCY

Asymptomatic Infection

Many of the maternal infections that can profoundly affect a fetus are trivial or asymptomatic for the mother, and the only possible approaches for detection, therefore, are screening laboratory tests. Recommendations regarding maternal screening for infection during pregnancy are determined by the nature of the maternal infection, as either acute or chronic infection; its prevalence and incidence; whether infection can be accurately diagnosed and characterized; the severity or long-term effects of fetal involvement; whether there are effective preventive or therapeutic interventions; and the financial cost. **Universal screening** of pregnant women in the United States is currently recommended for *Treponema pallidum, Neisseria gonorrhoeae,* hepatitis B, rubella virus, group B *Streptococcus,* and HIV (Table 94–3).

Group B Streptococcus. Universal screening for carriage of group B *Streptococcus* can be justified because maternal carriage is asymptomatic, chronic, and reliably detected at 35–37 weeks' gestation. Approximately 20% of pregnant women are colonized with group B *Streptococcus.* Life-threatening neonatal infection develops in 1% of exposed infants at delivery, and 4% of those infants with infection have the perinatal risk factors of prematurity, prolonged rupture of membranes, or intrapartum fever. Invasive neonatal infection causes death in approximately 5% of the infected neonates and permanent disability in 15–30% of the survivors. Selective antimicrobial prophylaxis during labor has almost 100% preventive efficacy against early-onset disease in high-risk deliveries. Economic analysis reveals that the strategy of maternal screening and selective intrapartum chemoprophylaxis is cost-effective. Intrapartum antibiotic prophylaxis does not appear to delay the onset of early-onset disease and has had no effect on late-onset disease, and the rates of maternal bacteremic infections have declined only moderately.

HIV. Universal screening for HIV is now recommended because maternal infection is generally asymptomatic and can be reliably detected. Pretest counseling and informed consent are necessary because a positive result indicates the presence of an ultimately fatal maternal disease, a diagnosis with profound exposure implications not only for the fetus but also for the mother's sexual partners and older children. Positive results with the EIA test, which must be confirmed by immunoblot or RT-PCR, can be misleading to the patient, to health care providers who have had limited experience with HIV, and to insurers. The mother's confidentiality must be protected, but because of measures to promote confidentiality, a positive result can occasionally be overlooked. Thus meticulous record keeping is essential. The preventive benefit of antiretroviral therapy for the fetus and newborn is now well established and justifies the complex process involved in HIV screening.

Targeted Screening. Prenatal maternal screening of selected populations is recommended in the United States for infections by *Mycobacterium tuberculosis,* herpes simplex virus (HSV), and *T. gondii.* Perinatal infections such as these are less frequent than those for which universal screening is recommended. Cost-effectiveness generally determines the screening recommendations. In France, for example, screening for seroconversion to *T. gondii* during pregnancy is mandated. Such a program is appropriate because only approximately 20% of women of childbearing age in France are seronegative and are therefore susceptible, which markedly reduces the pool of mothers for whom paired serologic determinations are necessary. This, in effect, makes the program somewhat selective. Seroconversion occurs in about 1% of pregnancies among susceptible women in France. Intervention has proved to be possible and effective in these pregnancies. In the United States, where 70–97% of pregnant women are susceptible to toxoplasmosis and seroconversion occurs in only approximately 0.1% of pregnancies, a comparable program would have substantially higher cost and lower yield. Thus screening laboratory tests are presently recommended only for asymptomatic women who report possible exposure to *T. gondii.*

The complex biology of HSV infections makes even selective screening difficult in many cases. Most cases of neonatal HSV infection occur in the newborn infants of women who do not have

TABLE 94–3. Recommended Screening of Pregnant Women for Asymptomatic Infectious Diseases with Pediatric Consequences

Organism	Current Screening Recommendation	Criteria for Selection	Best Current Screening Test	Confirmatory Test
Treponema palliidum	All	None	Reagin serology (RPR or VDRL)	Treponemal serology (MHA-TP or FTA)
Neisseria gonorrhoeae	All	None	DNA probe on vaginal swab	Culture on Thayer-Martin with organism susceptibilities
Hepatitis B virus	All	None	HBsAg serology	Liver functions (enzymes); HBeAg serology
Group B *Streptococcus*	All*	None	Vaginal and rectal culture with selective broth enrichment at 36 weeks' gestation	Vaginal and rectal culture at presentation in labor
Rubella virus	All	None	IgG; IgG and IgM following possible exposure	None necessary
Human immunodeficiency virus	All†	Drug abuse; high-risk sex partners; multiple sex partners; syphilis	EIA	Western blot
Mycobacterium tuberculosis	Selective	Population groups with high endemicity; exposure to active case of tuberculosis	Intradermal tuberculin (Mantoux) test	Chest radiograph, gastric cultures, tuberculin tests of extended family, organism susceptibilities
Herpes simplex virus	Selective	History of genital herpes; exposure to genital herpes	Vaginal culture in susceptible cell lines during late gestation	Vaginal culture at delivery
Toxoplasma gondii	Selective	Exposure to cats; ingestion of raw meat; positive HIV serology	Paired IgG specific serology; double-sandwich IgM EIA serology	Reference laboratory serologic tests (AC/HS differential agglutination test, IgM ISAGA, IgA [EIA], IgE [EIA])
Chlamydia trachomatis	Selective	Multiple sex partners	Vaginal culture, EIA, or DNA probe	None necessary
Cytomegalovirus	Not recommended	See Table 94–4	Urine culture (virus)	Paired IgG serology; IgM serology
Listeria monocytogenes	Not recommended	See Table 94–4	Blood culture	None necessary
Varicella-zoster virus	Not recommended	See Table 94–4	Clinical diagnosis, especially with known contact	Immunofluorescence; culture; paired IgG serology
Parvovirus B19	Not recommended	See Table 94–4	Clinical diagnosis, especially with known contact	Paired IgG serology, IgM serology, polymerase chain reaction
Enteroviruses	Not recommended	See Table 94–4	Clinical diagnosis in summer months	Stool or throat culture
Ureaplasma urealyticum	Not recommended	See Table 94–4	Culture of vaginal swab	None necessary
Human papillomaviruses	Not recommended	See Table 94–4	Clinical diagnosis	DNA probe or immunoperoxidase stain of biopsy specimens

RPR = Rapid plasma reagin; VDRL = Venereal Disease Research Laboratories; MHA-TP = microhemagglutination assay–*Treponema pallidum;* FTA = fluorescent treponema antibody; HBsAg = hepatitis B surface antigen; HBeAg = hepatitis B e antigen; EIA = enzyme immunoassay; HSV = herpes simplex virus; ISAGA = immunosorbent agglutination assay.

*Using the culture and risk factor–based prevention strategy (Fig. 94–2).

†With pretest counseling and informed consent.

TABLE 94–4. Clinically Significant Transplacental or Perinatal Pathogens in Pregnant Women or Parturients with Symptoms According to Presenting Maternal Symptoms

Symptom in Mother	Causative Pathogens That May Be Transmitted
Fever of undetermined origin	Cytomegalovirus, *Toxoplasma gondii,* hepatitis B virus, *Mycobacterium tuberculosis, Plasmodium, Salmonella, Listeria monocytogenes*
Exanthem	Rubella virus, varicella-zoster virus, measles virus, *Treponema pallidum, Neisseria gonorrhoeae,* parvovirus B19, enteroviruses
Lymphadenopathy	*T. gondii,* human immunodeficiency virus, *T. pallidum,* rubella virus
Upper respiratory tract infection	Influenza viruses, respiratory syncytial virus
Lower respiratory tract infection	*M. tuberculosis,* influenza viruses, respiratory syncytial virus, measles virus, varicella-zoster virus
Diarrhea	*Salmonella,* enteroviruses
Vaginal discharge	*N. gonorrhoeae, Chlamydia trachomatis, Ureaplasma urealyticum, T. pallidum*
Vaginal or perineal lesion	*T. pallidum,* herpes simplex virus, human papillomaviruses
Urinary tract infection	Gram-negative enteric organisms, group B *Streptococcus*
Arthritis	Rubella virus, *N. gonorrhoeae,* parvovirus B19
Amnionitis; postpartum endometritis	Group B *Streptococcus,* gram-negative enteric organisms, group A *Streptococcus,* other streptococci, anaerobes

a long-term history of recurrent genital lesions. Thus selective screening of mothers with a history of genital lesions is aimed at a population that has a relatively low risk of neonatal involvement. Other approaches, such as combined culture and serologic screening at delivery, may be determined to be more appropriate in the future, even though they may not allow cesarean delivery, currently the only established preventive intervention.

On the basis of similar analyses, maternal screening for cytomegalovirus (CMV), parvovirus B19, and many other pathogens is not routinely recommended (Table 94–3).

Symptomatic Infection

Symptomatic maternal infection during pregnancy can affect the fetus directly by transplacental transmission or indirectly by adverse effects on the mother. Both physically and immunologically, a pregnant woman may not respond to some acute infections as well as when she is not pregnant. The differential diagnosis of many common symptoms of illness during pregnancy includes infections that may affect the fetus or newborn infant (Table 94–4). Symptomatic maternal illness is more likely to represent primary than recurrent infection, and it is primary maternal infection, with hematogenous spread, that poses the greatest risk to a fetus. Depending on the pathogen, an etiologic diagnosis may allow specific prophylactic or therapeutic measures to be instituted.

Equally, if not more, important is the etiologic diagnosis of maternal infection occurring at or soon after delivery. Because most neonatal infections are transmitted vertically, knowledge of the cause of a maternal infection can be valuable in the care of a sick newborn infant and must be communicated to the pediatrician. The converse situation is also important, and infection in a newborn should be communicated to the obstetrician.

RECOGNITION OF INFECTION IN UTERO

Fetal Exposure

Only a fraction of mothers with proved infections during pregnancy transmit the pathogen transplacentally to the developing fetus (Table 94–5). The rates differ, depending on the pathogenicity of the infecting organism, the stage of gestation, and whether the maternal infection is primary or recurrent. The clinical severity of infection in the fetus tends to vary inversely with postconceptional age, which reflects the immature fetus's incomplete organ development and limited immune response (Table 94–5). An exception occurs with maternal infection in the immediately perinatal period, such

TABLE 94–5. Probability of Transplacental Infection and Severity of Fetal Involvement in Maternal Infection During Pregnancy in Relation to Time of Primary Infection

	Early Gestation		Late Gestation	
Pathogen*	Probability of Transmission (%)	Degree of Severity	Probability of Transmission (%)	Degree of Severity
Rubella virus	High (80–100)	High	Medium (50)	Low
Treponema pallidum	High (50–100)	High†	High (50–100)	Medium†
Cytomegalovirus	Medium (20–50)	High	Medium (20–50)	Medium
Toxoplasma gondii	Medium (15)	High†	High (50–60)	Medium†
Parvovirus B19	Low (10)	High	Low (10)	Medium
Varicella-zoster virus	Low (1–2)	High	High (50–100)	Low‡

*Data are lacking on the comparative risks associated with maternal human immunodeficiency virus infection (overall vertical transmission rate is approximately 25% if the mother is not treated).

†Reduced with maternal treatment.

‡High in maternal infection manifested 5 days before and up to 2 days after delivery (risk of neonatal infection decreased by administration of specific immune globulin [VZIG] after birth).

as with primary varicella-zoster virus infection (chickenpox). In this circumstance, maternal infection at or shortly before delivery transmits a large virus inoculum to the near-term fetus hematogenously. If the baby is separated from the mother before transplacental passage of specific maternal antibody can occur, life-threatening disseminated varicella-zoster virus infection may develop (Chapter 97).

Two key issues for the clinician regarding maternal infection are determination of when the infection occurred during gestation and whether it is a primary infection or a reactivation. The timing of infection and its primary nature may be apparent from clinical features alone, as in the case of maternal chickenpox in the perinatal period, but less obvious infections require a high degree of awareness by the obstetrician. The only clues may be screening laboratory tests (Table 94–3) or subtle clinical presentations (Table 94–4). In these circumstances, recognition of a specific immune response by a single IgM serologic test or paired IgG serologic tests is the most useful way to establish the time of infection. If the timing of infection is consistent with disease activity during gestation, the magnitude of the antibody response, combined with selected additional testing, can usually establish whether the infection is primary, recrudescent, or remote. An example of such an additional test is the AC/HS differential agglutination test for infection with *T. gondii* (Chapter 11).

All infants born to mothers with untreated syphilis are at risk for congenital infection, although untreated latent syphilis constitutes a lower risk to the baby than untreated primary or secondary syphilis. Staging of maternal syphilis and determination of treatment status are best established by the mother's titer of serum reagin antibodies and by history. Maternal infection with HIV also carries a risk of congenital infection; approximately one third of HIV-infected infants acquire infection in utero, and two thirds acquire infection perinatally.

Fetal Infection

Proof of maternal infection is not proof of fetal infection. Fetal infection can sometimes be inferred from noninvasive approaches such as elevated maternal levels of α-fetoprotein or ultrasonography, which may reveal intracranial calcifications, hydrocephalus, organomegaly, intrauterine growth retardation, or fetal hydrops. However, fetal involvement can be established early and with certainty only by invasive techniques, all of which have attendant risks. The techniques that have been used to sample fetal tissue, blood, or biologic fluids include amniocentesis, placentocentesis, fetoscopy, chorionic villus sampling, and cordocentesis. Amniocentesis and cordocentesis have been the most widely used methods to diagnose fetal infections antenatally. The optimal point for sampling during gestation is determined by the time frame necessary to establish maternal infection with certainty (e.g., paired serum samples), the safety of the procedure (in general, the later in gestation, the safer the procedure), the method and accuracy of fetal diagnosis (e.g., the fetus reliably synthesizes IgM antibodies only after 20 weeks' gestation), and the options for intervention (e.g., pregnancy termination, intrauterine transfusion, or maternal therapy).

Molecular biologic techniques, such as in situ hybridization and PCR (Chapter 12), are gradually replacing conventional serologic tests (e.g., IgM serology) for the diagnosis of intrauterine infection and permit accurate fetal diagnosis with less risky sampling techniques. A good example of this is the development of intrauterine diagnosis of congenital toxoplasmosis. Before the mid-1970s, fetal involvement could not be directly tested but was simply inferred from the results of maternal serologic testing. Because of the uncertainty of the diagnosis, maternal treatment was limited to relatively nontoxic drugs such as spiramycin. With the development of cordocentesis, fetal blood sampling in mothers with confirmed infections became possible. Fetal infection could be identified by mouse inoculation of fetal blood and amniotic fluid, in conjunction with cord blood IgM serology. This diagnostic advance made possible selective and more aggressive maternal antiparasitic treatment and improved outcome for the infected fetus. More recently, PCR amplification of *T. gondii* sequences in exfoliated fetal cells obtained by amniocentesis has proved to be more sensitive than fetal blood sampling, with a comparable specificity. This advance now allows substitution of amniocentesis for cordocentesis, with greater safety and flexibility in gestational ages for sampling. After diagnosis, monitoring the fetus by serial ultrasonographic examinations allows additional assessment of severity of fetal involvement and response to treatment.

Diagnostic Evaluation After Birth

Knowledge of a mother's infection during gestation with a pathogen capable of producing a congenital infection, regardless of whether fetal diagnosis was attempted, allows a directed approach to the diagnostic evaluation of the baby in the nursery. The classic physical features of congenital infection include intrauterine growth retardation; ocular findings, such as cataracts or microphthalmia; abnormalities in head circumference reflecting microcephaly or hydrocephalus; hepatosplenomegaly; and thrombocytopenic purpura. Other findings may be missed on a routine neonatal examination; these include sensorineural deafness with congenital rubella or CMV infection, macular chorioretinitis in congenital toxoplasmosis, and neurologic involvement in congenital toxoplasmosis, rubella, syphilis, and CMV infection. Formal evaluations, such as indirect ophthalmoscopic examination, auditory evoked potentials, echocardiography, skeletal radiographs, lumbar puncture, ultrasonography of the head, or CT, may be justified.

For many pathogens, the opportunity to definitively diagnose a congenital infection after birth exists for only a brief window of time. Placental histopathologic examinations and cultures (e.g., culture or mouse inoculation of placental tissue for proof of *T. gondii* infection) are generally practical only if the need is anticipated before delivery. Viral cultures, although likely to remain positive for prolonged periods with congenital infection, can differentiate congenital rubella, CMV, or HIV infection from infection acquired postnatally only if they are performed in the immediate neonatal period. Elevated levels of specific IgM antibodies can be specific indicators of congenital infection, but available tests lack sensitivity and specificity for many pathogens. The use of IgG antibody levels is limited by the impossibility of distinguishing maternal antibodies acquired transplacentally from endogenous antibodies. Detection of antibody-dissociated antigens and PCR detection of DNA or RNA genomes are new approaches that can detect circulating viral pathogens at the time of delivery. At this time, however, these studies remain investigational diagnostic approaches for most organisms other than hepatitis C and HIV.

RECOGNITION OF PERINATAL INFECTION

As with congenitally transmitted pathogens, knowledge that a neonate has been exposed to a maternal infection at the time of delivery should suggest the possibility of the infant's having or developing a perinatal infection. Many factors affect the likelihood of perinatal transmission and the severity of infection, including the route of transmission, inoculum size, virulence of the organism, and the baby's passively acquired humoral immunity (Table 94–6). Severity varies from completely asymptomatic infection to fulminant and fatal disease. HSV and group B *Streptococcus* infections are

TABLE 94–6. Probability of Perinatal Infection and Severity in the Newborn of a Mother with Infection at Delivery

Pathogen	Probability (%)	Degree of Severity
Cytomegalovirus	High (90–100) (breast-feeding)	Asymptomatic
Hepatitis B virus	High (60–90)*	Low†
Human immunodeficiency virus	Medium (13–39)	High
Chlamydia trachomatis	Medium (5–30)	Low
Neisseria gonorrhoeae	Medium (25)‡	Moderate
Mycobacterium tuberculosis	Medium (20)	High
Herpes simplex virus	Low (3–50)§	High
Hepatitis C virus	Low (5)	Low†
Group B *Streptococcus*	Low (0.5–4)‖	High

*The probability is higher if the mother is HBeAg-positive.
†Usually asymptomatic in infancy, although infected infants may develop chronic hepatitis with susceptibility to cirrhosis and hepatocellular carcinoma as adults.
‡Without mandated topical ophthalmic prophylaxis.
§The higher figure (50%) with maternal primary infection at vaginal delivery.
‖The higher figure (4%) in mothers with intrapartum fever, premature labor, or prolonged rupture of membranes.

the two most common perinatally acquired infections that lead to fulminant neonatal disease.

Group B Streptococcus. Early-onset group B *Streptococcus* infections are invariably perinatal in their acquisition. Babies whose mothers are colonized with group B *Streptococcus* may acquire the organism during passage through the birth canal and develop early-onset infection (Chapter 96). Awareness of maternal colonization with group B *Streptococcus* allows selective chemoprophylaxis or prompt postnatal intervention against early-onset disease. It may also identify an older baby who deserves a careful evaluation for relatively minor symptoms. Perinatal or postnatal nosocomial or community-acquired transmission may lead to late-onset infections, which less frequently involve a history of obstetric complications and are more likely to be insidious in their onset, a reflection of their less frequent pulmonary involvement (Chapter 96).

Herpes Simplex Virus. Perinatally acquired HSV infections most often present at 1–2 weeks of age. Skin vesicles suggest HSV infection, but many infected newborns do not have cutaneous involvement, and the infections may present similar to bacterial sepsis (Chapter 97).

Varicella-Zoster Virus and Enteroviruses. Acute maternal viral infections in the immediate perinatal period may result in hematogenous transmission of virus to the fetus. Although maternal virus-specific IgG antibody may be transferred to the fetus, providing some protection when maternal viral infection occurs close to term, there may not be sufficient time before birth for synthesis and passage of antibody to the infant. In these special circumstances, varicella-zoster virus and the enteroviruses that usually cause limited illness in older children may produce life-threatening infection in the newborn (Chapter 97).

Hepatitis B. Maternal-fetal hepatitis B transmission is determined primarily by the state of maternal immunity. Transmission rates range from 12% when the mother is HBsAg-positive, HBeAg-negative, and anti-HBeAg-positive; to 90% when the mother is HBsAg-positive, HBeAg-positive, and anti-HBeAg-negative. Nearly all babies with perinatal hepatitis B have no symptoms in infancy, but the 60–90% who go on to be chronic carriers of HBsAg are at high risk in adulthood of liver disease in the form of chronic active hepatitis and cirrhosis (Chapter 78) and hepatocellular carcinoma (Chapter 4). Diagnostic studies of the neonate are not of value. Preventive intervention, which includes hepatitis B vaccine and HBIG, are determined solely on the basis of the mother being positive for HBsAg.

HIV. HIV-infected infants generally have clinically inapparent infection that is detectable only by laboratory means. Maternal HIV antibodies may persist until 12–18 months of age. Optimal early diagnosis is based on detection of HIV DNA or RNA by PCR (Chapter 38). The diagnosis can be established by PCR in 90–95% of infected babies by 1 month of age and in nearly all infants by 4 months of age. Although many babies remain without symptoms, persistent oral candidiasis, hepatosplenomegaly, and failure to thrive suggest HIV infection. In the absence of prophylaxis, *Pneumocystis carinii* pneumonia is the most common AIDS-defining condition in infancy.

PREVENTION OF TRANSPLACENTAL TRANSMISSION AND INTRAUTERINE TREATMENT OF INFECTION IN A FETUS

A definitive diagnosis of infection in a pregnant woman immediately raises the question of whether fetal involvement can be prevented **(secondary prevention)** or altered. In some instances, the precise timing of maternal infection is not known with certainty, but the risk for the fetus continues for a prolonged period, as with syphilis and toxoplasmosis (Table 94–7). For both of these conditions, there are effective therapies with sufficient transplacental passage to benefit the fetus.

Adequate treatment of maternal syphilis is adequate treatment of fetal syphilis. Current treatment guidelines emphasize staging of infection and documentation of response by monthly posttreatment reagin serologic testing. A fourfold or greater decline in titer indicates therapeutic adequacy. There is the possibility of a Jarisch-Herxheimer reaction following treatment; such a reaction could trigger premature labor or fetal distress, although this is not an indication for delay of treatment. Because tetracycline is contraindicated during pregnancy, the preferred therapy for a woman with penicillin hypersensitivity is desensitization to penicillin by the oral route. For maternal syphilis treated during the third trimester, there may not be sufficient time to document a decline in reagin serologic results before delivery. In such circumstances, inadequate therapy should be assumed and the newborn should be evaluated and treated after birth as if no maternal treatment had been given (Chapter 95).

Congenital toxoplasmosis can be prevented with the the use of spiramycin in acutely infected pregnant women. Spiramycin is available in the United States only on request from the Food and Drug Administration (telephone: 301-827-2349), and is reserved for pregnant women with well-documented acute infection but without fetal infection as demonstrated by analysis of fetal blood or amniotic fluid. Acute maternal infection with proved fetal involvement should be treated with a combination of pyrimethamine and sulfadiazine with supplemental folinic acid (leucovorin) to minimize suppression of hematopoiesis. This regimen is recom-

TABLE 94–7. Measures for Prevention of Infection by Transplacental Pathogens During Pregnancy and Treatment of Mother and Fetus with Infection

Pathogen	Prevention of Maternal Infection	Prevention of Transplacental Transmission	In Utero Therapy
Rubella virus	Immunization	No method established	No method established
Treponema pallidum	Prepregnancy serologic screening and penicillin treatment; avoidance of sexually transmitted diseases	Maternal penicillin treatment	Maternal penicillin treatment
Cytomegalovirus	Secretion precautions	No method established	No method established
Toxoplasma gondii	Avoidance of cat feces and raw meat	Maternal spiramycin treatment	Maternal pyrimethamine-sulfadiazine treatment, alternating with spiramycin
Parvovirus B19	No method established	IVIG by umbilical vein*	Fetal transfusion*
Varicella-zoster virus	Postexposure VZIG; immunization	No method established	VZIG immediately after delivery†

IVIG = Intravenous immune globulin; VZIG = varicella-zoster immune globulin.
*Anecdotal experience only.
†If mother ill 5 days before and up to 2 days after delivery.

mended in an alternating 3-week schedule with spiramycin. Although this approach has not been subjected to a rigorous controlled trial of efficacy, the results in one large study from France (Hohlfeld et al., 1989) have been highly encouraging. In this series, only 1 of 53 infants whose mothers were treated with the alternating regimen had signs of severe congenital infection. The others were either subclinically infected (41 infants) or had asymptomatic signs, such as a retinal scar with normal vision or cerebral calcifications with normal neurologic status (12 infants). Because the optimal treatment regimen has not been defined, consultation with a specialist in infectious diseases is recommended.

The possibilities of intervening to prevent other congenital infections, particularly those with an acute course that occur early in gestation, are limited. Administration of immune globulin to the mother, for example, is ineffective in preventing fetal varicella-zoster virus, rubella virus, or parvovirus B19 infection once maternal infection is established. In part, this is because transplacental passage of immunoglobulin is extremely limited before the middle of the second trimester. Administration of immune globulin directly into the umbilical vein has been reported to be successful in preventing parvovirus B19 infection in a few instances. In this circumstance, however, there is no risk of congenital malformation, so

TABLE 94–8. Measures for Prevention of Infection by Perinatal Pathogens at Delivery

Pathogen	Prevention of Maternal Infection	Prevention of Perinatal Infection
Cytomegalovirus	Secretion precautions	Not necessary under ordinary circumstances; use of CMV-negative blood products if transfusions required
Hepatitis B virus	Immunization	Passive-active neonatal immunization with HBIG and HBV vaccine
Human immunodeficiency virus	Avoidance of sexually transmitted diseases	Combined regimen of prenatal, intrapartum, and neonatal antiretroviral therapy
Chlamydia trachomatis	Avoidance of sexually transmitted diseases	Maternal erythromycin treatment
Neisseria gonorrhoeae	Avoidance of sexually transmitted diseases	Maternal ceftriaxone treatment before delivery; neonatal topical ophthalmic prophylaxis; penicillin or ceftriaxone for infant whose mother has a positive culture or DNA probe test result at delivery
Mycobacterium tuberculosis	Prepregnancy screening with antimycobacterial prophylaxis or treatment	Maternal antituberculous chemotherapy; neonatal prophylaxis with isoniazid or BCG
Herpes simplex virus	Avoidance of sexually transmitted diseases	Cesarean section; ophthalmic prophylaxis; systemic prophylaxis with acyclovir is controversial
Group B *Streptococcus*	No method established	Selective intrapartum chemoprophylaxis with penicillin or ampicillin (for ascending infection of amniotic fluid); postnatal penicillin chemoprophylaxis (for birth canal inoculation)

HBIG = Hepatitis B immune globulin; HBV = hepatitis B virus; BCG = bacille Calmette-Guérin.

the risk of in utero manipulation must be weighed against the risk of fetal death from nonimmune hydrops.

PREVENTION OF PERINATAL TRANSMISSION OF INFECTION

Diseases that are transmitted perinatally have the greatest potential for prevention by immunoprophylaxis and chemoprophylaxis (Table 94–8).

Neisseria gonorrhoeae. Topical gonococcal ophthalmic prophylaxis, instituted by Crede in 1881, is currently mandated by law in most states regardless of maternal carriage of *N. gonorrhoeae* (Chapter 89). However, knowledge of maternal carriage or infection is a component of preventive strategies for most other organisms.

Group B Streptococcus. Group B *Streptococcus* disease has, until recently, been the most frequent life-threatening neonatal infection in the United States. Strategies for selective **intrapartum antimicrobial prophylaxis** recommended by the CDC, ACOG, and AAP have resulted in dramatic reductions in incidence of early-onset disease. Two strategies have been recommended, one based only on risk factors (Fig. 94–1) and the second based on the combination of prenatal culture screening at 35–37 weeks' gestation and risk factors (Fig. 94–2). The **risk factor–based prevention strategy** has the advantage of simplicity but has the potential to prevent only about 60% of infections. Full implementation of the **culture and risk factor–based prevention strategy,** including prophylaxis of colonized parturients without risk factors, has the potential to prevent at least 90% of infections.

The recommended maternal regimen of intrapartum prophylaxis is penicillin G 5 MU (alternative: ampicillin 2 g) at the onset of labor intravenously, followed by penicillin G 2.5 MU (alternative: ampicillin 1 g) every 4 hours intravenously until delivery. Clindamycin (900 mg every 8 hours) or erythromycin (500 mg every 6 hours) intravenously until delivery is recommended as an alternative for women with hypersensitivity to penicillin. Maternal fever during labor, suggesting chorioamnionitis, in addition to being a risk factor for neonatal disease, requires broad-spectrum antibiotic therapy of the mother. If the mother is receiving treatment for chorioamnionitis with antibiotics that are effective against group B *Streptococcus,* additional prophylactic antibiotics are not needed.

Infants born to mothers who are receiving intrapartum antimicrobial treatment or prophylaxis require special consideration based on the presence or absence of signs compatible with systemic infection at birth; the ability to assess signs, according to gestational age; the number of doses of maternal chemoprophylaxis before delivery; and the likelihood that features of early-onset group B *Streptococcus* disease will occur within 48 hours of delivery (Fig. 94–3). Routine administration of antibiotics to all newborns born to mothers who receive intrapartum antibiotics is not recommended. Neonates with signs of sepsis should have a complete diagnostic evaluation and initiation of empirical antimicrobial therapy (Chapter 96). Neutropenia (ANC $<1{,}500/mm^3$) and an elevated **immature-to-total (I:T) neutrophil ratio** of >0.20 are the most useful indicators of sepsis, whereas the WBC count and differential are usually not helpful as single indicators (Chapter 10). A normal I:T ratio has a 98% negative predictive value. The duration of empiric antibiotic therapy, when initiated, depends on laboratory and culture results, and the clinical course of the infant. If the laboratory evaluation and clinical course suggest that invasive infection is unlikely, therapy should be discontinued after 48–72 hours. All symptom-free infants <35 weeks of gestation and symptom-free newborns ≥35 weeks of gestation whose mothers received <2 doses of antibiotics before delivery should be evaluated, which could be limited to a CBC and WBC differential count and blood culture, and observed in the hospital for at least 48 hours without empirical antimicrobial therapy. If the initial laboratory tests or clinical course suggest systemic infection, a complete diagnostic evaluation and empirical antibiotic treatment are indicated. Symptom free infants ≥35 weeks of gestation whose mothers received ≥2 doses of antibiotics before delivery should be managed as healthy newborns, with hospital observation for at least 48 hours.

Mycobacterium tuberculosis. Prevention of congenital and neonatal tuberculosis requires antenatal detection and treatment of the mother. Although transplacental transmission can occur, the principal means of transmission of *M. tuberculosis* is droplet spread after delivery. Isoniazid given in the first 3 months of life protects an exposed infant, assuming the mother complies with her treatment

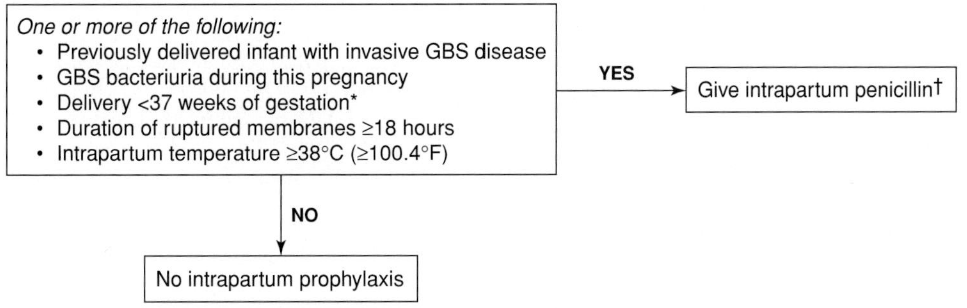

One or more of the following:
• Previously delivered infant with invasive GBS disease
• GBS bacteriuria during this pregnancy
• Delivery <37 weeks of gestation*
• Duration of ruptured membranes ≥18 hours
• Intrapartum temperature ≥38°C (≥100.4°F)
YES
Give intrapartum penicillin†
NO
No intrapartum prophylaxis

*If membranes ruptured at <37 weeks of gestation and the mother has not begun labor, collect group B *Streptococcus* culture and either (1) administer antibiotics until cultures are complete and the results are negative or (2) begin antibiotics only with positive culture results.

†Broad-spectrum antibiotics may be considered at the discretion of the physician on the basis of the clinical indications.

FIGURE 94–1. Risk factor–based prevention strategy for early-onset GBS disease. (Adapted from Centers for Disease Control and Prevention: Prevention of perinatal group B streptococcal disease: A public health perspective. *MMWR Morb Mortal Wkly Rept* 1996;45(RR-7):1–24; and American Academy of Pediatrics, Committee on Infectious Diseases and Committee on Fetus and Newborn: Revised guidelines for prevention of group B streptococcal (GBS) infection by chemoprophylaxis. *Pediatrics* 1997;99:489–96.)

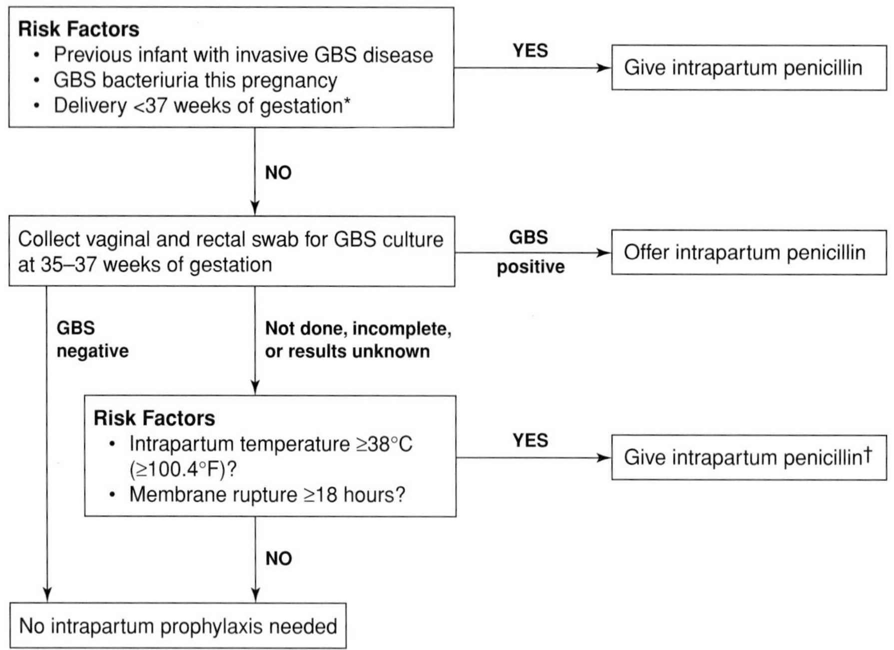

*If membranes ruptured at <37 weeks of gestation and the mother has not begun labor, collect group B *Streptococcus* culture and either (1) administer antibiotics until cultures are complete and the results are negative or (2) begin antibiotics only with positive culture results. No prophylaxis is needed if culture result at 35–37 weeks is known to be negative.

†Broad-spectrum antibiotics may be considered at the discretion of the physician on the basis of the clinical indications.

FIGURE 94–2. Culture and risk factor–based prevention strategy for early-onset GBS disease. (Adapted from Centers for Disease Control and Prevention: Prevention of perinatal group B streptococcal disease: A public health perspective. *MMWR Morb Mortal Wkly Rept* 1996;45(RR-7):1–24; and American Academy of Pediatrics, Committee on Infectious Diseases and Committee on Fetus and Newborn: Revised guidelines for prevention of group B streptococcal (GBS) infection by chemoprophylaxis. *Pediatrics* 1997;99:489–96.)

and household exposure is eliminated. Bacille Calmette-Guerin (BCG) immunization, widely used in developing countries, is generally reserved in the United States for the infants of mothers with drug-resistant infections or a high likelihood of noncompliance (Chapter 35).

Herpes Simplex Virus. Cesarean section is the established means of prevention of neonatal HSV infection if the mother has active genital lesions at the time of delivery. However, the strategy of prenatal culturing of women with a history of genital herpes infections and cesarean delivery for those with positive results has proved to be problematic for several reasons. Infants born to mothers with recurrent genital herpes infections who have viral shedding at the time of a vaginal delivery have only a 3% chance of having a neonatal HSV infection. In contrast, the attack rate is 50% among infants of mothers with primary infection at delivery. This dramatic difference in risk reflects a lower inoculum and shorter duration of shedding in women with recurrent disease as well as transplacental passage of their serum neutralizing antibodies. Thus, it is not surprising that many mothers of infants with neonatal HSV infections lack a history of prior genital HSV infection. Uncovering these important epidemiologic facts in recent years has led to a gradual decline in aggressive third-trimester culture programs for mothers with a history of recurrent genital herpes and greater use of maternal chemoprophylaxis with acyclovir. Care of a neonate whose mother has a culture-positive lesion at delivery but who has delivered the baby vaginally is somewhat controversial. Most authorities now recommend obtaining **surface cultures** from the oropharynx, nasopharynx, urine, and stool or rectum of the neonate at 24–48 hours of age and reserving acyclovir treatment for those with positive culture results or overt clinical symptoms (Chapter 97).

Hepatitis B. With universal maternal screening for carriage of HBsAg and with neonatal hepatitis B vaccination, it is now possible to eliminate most perinatal acquisition of hepatitis B, which is the greatest risk factor for becoming a chronic carrier of HBsAg. Combined passive immunization with HBIG combined with vaccination is more than 95% effective in preventing perinatal acquisition of infection. All infants who are born to HBsAg-positive mothers should be tested for HBsAg and anti-HBsAg 1–3 months after completion of the vaccination series to document successful immunization (Chapter 78).

HIV. Several risk factors influence the rate of vertical HIV transmission. Rupture of membranes for >4 hours is the major risk factor, which doubles the transmission rate. Other risk factors include gestation <34 weeks, low birth weight, low maternal antenatal CD4 count, and injection drug use during pregnancy. Rates of vertical HIV transmission from infected mothers can be reduced by a sequential regimen of prenatal, intrapartum, and postpartum therapy with zidovudine (see Table 38–10). In the epochal PACTG 076 trial (Connor et al., 1994), HIV was acquired by only 15 (8.3%) of 180 infants in the treatment group, compared with 47 (25.5%) of 184 recipients of the placebo regimen, a 67% reduction. Adverse effects of treatment were inconsequential and have remained so with long-term follow-up. More aggressive maternal combination

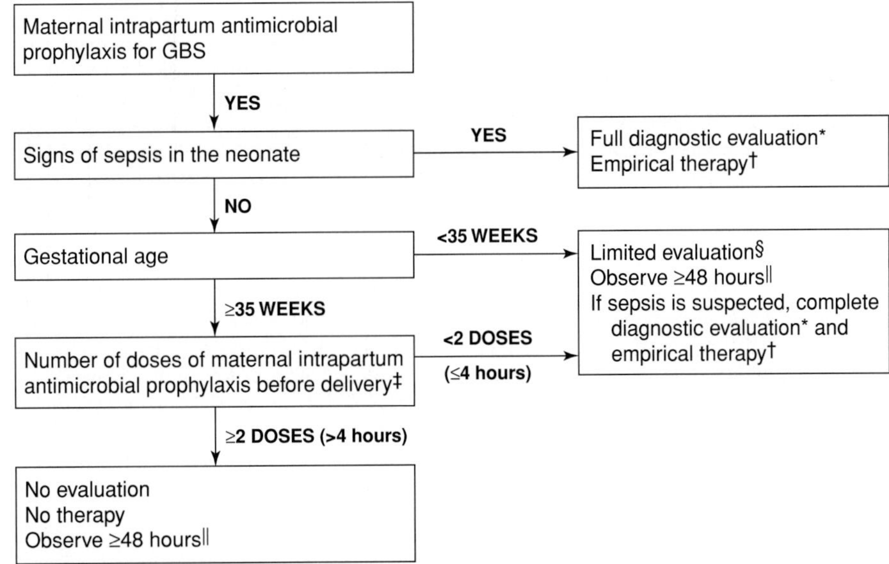

*Includes CBC and WBC differential counts, blood culture, and chest radiograph if the neonate has respiratory symptoms. A lumbar puncture is performed at the discretion of the physician.

†Duration of therapy will vary depending on results of blood culture and CSF results (if obtained), as well as on the clinical course of the infant. If laboratory results and clinical course are unremarkable, duration may be as short as 48–72 hours.

‡Applies to penicillin or ampicillin chemoprophylaxis.

§CBC and WBC differential counts, blood culture.

||Does *not* allow early discharge.

FIGURE 94–3. Suggested algorithm for empiric management of neonate born to a mother who received intrapartum antimicrobial prophylaxis for prevention of early-onset GBS disease. (Adapted from Centers for Disease Control and Prevention: Prevention of perinatal group B streptococcal disease: A public health perspective: *MMWR Morb Mortal Wkly Rept* 1996;45(RR-7):1–24; and American Academy of Pediatrics, Committee on Infectious Diseases and Committee on Fetus and Newborn: Revised guidelines for prevention of group B streptococcal (GBS) infection by chemoprophylaxis. *Pediatrics* 1997;99:489–96.)

treatment, aimed at reducing plasma viral loads to undetectable levels, has been associated with even greater reductions in vertical transmission rates. Short-term administration of nevirapine also appears to be capable of reducing transmission and provides a useful intrapartum intervention for mothers who have not received prenatal treatment. Widespread application of these regimens has had a profound effect on decreasing the incidence of pediatric HIV infection in the United States.

Multiple prospective studies have demonstrated that elective cesarean section reduces vertical HIV transmission by as much as 50%, either without zidovudine prophylaxis or in addition to the reduction offered by zidovudine. The role of cesarean section in HIV-infected mothers is evolving but offers an additional intervention in preventing vertical transmission of HIV, especially among women who do not receive prophylaxis and if they also refrain from breast-feeding.

TRANSMISSION OF INFECTION BY BREAST-FEEDING

Breast milk has excellent nutritional value and is generally free of contamination by environmental pathogens. Breast milk contains IgG and IgA antibodies and lymphocytes that also provide the infant with local and intraluminal immunity against infection. The preventive value of breast milk against infection is well established for gastrointestinal tract infections, especially in underdeveloped countries with poor sanitation and frequent environmental contamination. Breast milk may also provide some protection against respiratory tract infections, including otitis media. Human infants acquire the majority of their passive humoral immunity before birth by passive as well as active transport of IgG across the placenta. Immunoglobulin present in human breast milk is not absorbed in quantity and contributes little or nothing to serum immunoglobulin levels, a circumstance that is reversed in some other vertebrate animals.

Certain maternal infections may be transmitted by breast milk (Table 94–9). Decisions regarding feeding of breast milk during

TABLE 94–9. Infectious Agents with the Potential To Be Transmitted by Breast-Feeding

Bacteria (Mastitis, Breast Abscess)
Staphylococcus aureus
Streptococcus
Mycobacterium tuberculosis
Viruses
Viruses causing acute systemic viral infections or viremia
Lifelong viral infections
Cytomegalovirus
Herpes simplex virus
Hepatitis B virus
Human immunodeficiency virus
Human T cell leukemia/lymphoma virus types I and II

maternal infection, especially of premature infants, should balance the benefits of human milk with the risk of disease transmission. Viruses causing systemic viral infections or viremia may be shed into breast milk during acute maternal infection. Primary infection during lactation poses the greatest risk to the infant because maternal virus levels are high, the infant has not received any protective antibody transplacentally, and specific maternal antibody is not present in the breast milk during the initial phases of infection. However, most viral infections are more likely to be transmitted to the infant by direct contact or by contaminated respiratory secretions. Breast-feeding appears to pose little added risk. In addition to acute viral infections, those viruses that cause lifelong viral infections (e.g., herpes viruses, retroviruses, viral hepatitis) may be shed intermittently in bodily secretions, including breast milk. For these viruses, primary maternal infection during lactation is more likely to result in transmission by breast-feeding. Preterm infants may be at greater risk of acquisition of these viruses by breast-feeding because premature newborn infants have acquired less transplacental maternal antibody prior to delivery.

Maternal Mastitis. Maternal mastitis and breast abscess, most commonly caused by *Staphylococcus aureus* and less commonly by streptococci, may contaminate breast milk with bacteria. Mothers with mastitis being treated with an appropriate antibiotic may continue to breast-feed their infants. Breast abscesses have the potential to rupture with the release of large numbers of organisms into breast milk. A mother with a breast abscess may resume feeding from the affected breast once the abscess is appropriately drained and the mother is being treated with antibiotics.

Mycobacterium tuberculosis. Mothers with active respiratory tuberculosis suspected to be contagious at the time of delivery should be discouraged from breast-feeding to minimize the potential for transmission by respiratory droplets during close contact until the mothers have been treated for ≥2 weeks or are confirmed to be noncontagious. Chronic tuberculous mastitis is rare but could result in contamination of milk with *M. tuberculosis.*

Herpes Simplex Virus. Cutaneous HSV infections of the breast areola are uncommon, but they potentially shed large amounts of virus into breast milk. Mothers with active HSV breast lesions should not breast-feed until the lesions are healed. Recurrent cutaneous lesions not involving the breast should be covered during breast-feeding. HSV has been recovered in breast milk during primary maternal HSV infection, even in the absence of breast lesions. Because viremia and extragenital spread is more likely during primary infection, mothers with primary HSV infection should refrain from breast-feeding until all lesions have healed.

Cytomegalovirus. CMV is commonly found in breast milk. Breast-fed infants whose mothers have latent CMV infection have a high probability of acquiring CMV infection, which is virtually always asymptomatic and remains so, a reflection, at least in part, of passive humoral immunity acquired transplacentally. Diagnostic efforts to document such transmission, therefore, are unnecessary. Premature infants may be at higher risk of symptomatic disease because of acquisition of less maternal CMV antibody prior to birth. **Holder pasteurization** (62.5°C [144.5°F] for 30 minutes) of breast milk inactivates CMV; freezing at −20°C (−68°F) for 7 days diminishes the titer of CMV.

Hepatitis B. Hepatitis B virus from HBsAg-positive mothers is usually transmitted to their infants during birth but may be transmitted postnatally by breast-feeding. Breast-feeding does not appear to increase the risk of transmission, however. Infants born to HBsAg-positive women should receive both HBIG and hepatitis B vaccine, which essentially eliminates the potential risk of transmission by breast-feeding (see Table 78–10).

HIV. HIV is found in the breast milk of some HIV-infected mothers. In a controlled trial in Kenya (Nduati et al., 2000; John et al., 2001), HIV-infected mothers who breast-fed had a 1.7-fold higher risk of transmitting HIV vertically than mothers whose infants were formula-fed. Breast-feeding, especially during early infancy, accounted for 16% of vertical HIV transmission. In contrast to HIV, the major mode of transmission of HTLV-I/II is from mother to infant by breast-feeding. In the United States, breast-feeding is not recommended for women who are seropositive for HIV or HTLV-I/II. In areas of the world where gastrointestinal infections and malnutrition cause substantial morbidity and mortality during infancy, the World Health Organization (WHO) currently recommends that infants be breast-fed regardless of the mother's HIV status.

Antibiotics During Breast-Feeding. Infections requiring the administration of antimicrobial agents to a lactating mother do not usually preclude breast-feeding. Although several exceptions exist, a general guideline is that drugs approved for use and safe for administration to infants are safe for administration to lactating mothers (Table 94–10). The amount of drug the infant ingests in breast milk is usually less than a recommended dose for the infant; therefore maternal treatment should not be considered to achieve therapeutic doses in the breast-fed infant, although there is the potential for adverse drug interactions. The infant will not absorb drugs administered parenterally to the mother that are not orally bioavailable. Administration of tetracycline to the mother is usually compatible with breast-feeding despite the potential for dental staining because most of the drug complexes with the calcium of milk and is not bioavailable to the infant.

Immunization During Breast-Feeding. Lactating mothers of term or preterm infants may be immunized as indicated for other adults without any interruption of the feeding schedule. Breast-feeding does not adversely affect immunization and is not a contraindication to any vaccine, including vaccination with inactivated poliovirus vaccine and live virus vaccines. Most vaccine viruses of live viral vaccines have not been detected in breast milk. Rubella vaccine virus may be transmitted in breast milk following maternal immunization but has not been associated with infection or harm to the infant. Breast-fed infants of mothers receiving vaccination should be immunized according to the schedule recommended for other infants. Although high concentrations of antipoliovirus antibody may be found in breast milk following maternal polio immunization, there is no evidence of interference of the immunogenicity of the oral polio vaccine in the infant after maternal immunization.

Donor Breast Milk. Human breast milk from the infant's mother or a donor may be collected and used for feeding premature infants. Freezing at −20°C (−68°F) before use limits growth of bacteria and reduces viability of CMV. Some centers use donor human breast milk from an unrelated donor or pooled from several donors using the guidelines for collection, processing, storage, and evaluation for contamination established by the Human Milk Bank Association of North America. However, **Holder pasteurization** (62.5°C [144.5°F] for 30 minutes) of donor milk to inactivate CMV, HIV, and other viruses also destroys much of the immunologic advantage of human milk over commercial infant formulas. If used, donors of human breast milk should be screened as if they were blood

TABLE 94–10. Antimicrobial Agents and Breast-Feeding

Antimicrobial Agent	Comments
Generally Compatible with Breast-Feeding	
Antibacterial drugs	
Penicillins (including β-lactamase inhibitor combinations)	
Cephalosporins	
Aztreonam	
Aminoglycosides	
Macrolides and azalides	
Clindamycin	
Tetracycline	
Trimethoprim-sulfamethoxazole (TMP-SMZ)	
Antimycobacterial drugs	
Isoniazid	May be hepatotoxic
Rifampin	
Dapsone	
Antiviral drugs	
Acyclovir, valacyclovir, famciclovir	
Antiparasitic drugs	
Chloroquine	
Quinine sulfate	
Usually Compatible with Breast-Feeding (Use with Caution)	
Antibacterial drugs	
Nalidixic acid	Hemolysis in infants with G6PD deficiency
Nitrofurantoin	Hemolysis in infants with G6PD deficiency
Sulfisoxazole	Hemolysis in infants with G6PD deficiency and in ill, stressed, or premature infants
Usually Not Compatible with Breast-Feeding	
Antibacterial drugs	
Quinolones	May affect cartilage development
Chloramphenicol	May cause reversible bone marrow suppression, and irreversible (idiosyncratic) bone marrow aplasia
Metronidazole*	Mutagenic in vitro

G6PD = glucose-6-phosphate dehydrogenase.
*Lactating mothers treated with a single 2 g dose for vaginal trichomoniasis should continue to pump and discard their milk for 24 hours after the administration of metronidazle, then resume nursing.

donors, with exclusion of milk from women seropositive for syphilis, CMV, hepatitis B virus, hepatitis C virus, HIV, or HTLV-I/II.

COUNSELING

Counseling a family about the possible and probable consequences of a maternal infection is both complex and time-consuming. Each situation is different. The diseases differ, and the levels of sophistication, motivation, and mores of the families differ. Counseling also has complex legal, economic, and insurance implications. All of these issues should be taken seriously. Counseling is often more appropriate in person than by telephone and should be conducted by persons with experience and expertise, preferably with both parents present.

The fundamental issues in counseling involve weighing the risks of the disease, the diagnostic tests, and the adverse effects of treatment against the benefits of accurate diagnosis, treatment, or prophylaxis. These issues should be covered in sufficient clinical and mathematical detail to allow informed decisions, but it is generally considered best for the physician to be nonjudgmental. In this regard, the counselor should convey concern and compassion but make no guarantees of outcome.

Decisions regarding termination of a pregnancy, in particular, should be left to the family. Several critical issues should always be addressed in discussions: whether this infection and particular situation could happen again; the likelihood that the mother may achieve another pregnancy; how late in gestation a termination can be carried out without legal restrictions or increased risk to the mother; and, if the family elects to carry an at-risk pregnancy to term, whether the insurance carrier will consider the baby to have a pre-existing condition and deny coverage for medical care after birth.

These issues clearly are of profound importance to a family. Regardless of outcome, provision of information in an honest and compassionate way is considered by most patients to be extremely helpful and gives them a sense of having some control over the situation. It also assures the physician that the family's expectations are both informed and realistic.

REVIEWS

American Academy of Pediatrics, Committee on Infectious Diseases and Committee on Fetus and Newborn: Revised guidelines for prevention of group B streptococcal (GBS) infection by chemoprophylaxis. *Pediatrics* 1997;99:489–96.

American College of Obstetricians and Gynecologists: Management of herpes in pregnancy. *Int J Gynaecol Obstet* 2000;68:165–73.

Centers for Disease Control and Prevention: 1998 guidelines for treatment of sexually transmitted diseases *MMWR Morb Mortal Wkly Rep* 1998;47(RR-1):1–111.

Centers for Disease Control and Prevention: Prevention of perinatal group B streptococcal disease: A public health perspective. *MMWR Morb Mortal Wkly Rep* 1996;45(RR-7):1–24.

Perinatal HIV Guidelines Working Group: Public Health Service Task Force Recommendations for Use of Antiretroviral Drugs in Pregnant HIV-1 Infected Women for Maternal Health and Interventions to Reduce Perinatal HIV-1 Transmission in the United States. HIV/AIDS Treatment Information Service: http://www.hivatis.org

Remington JS, Klein JO (editors): *Infectious Diseases of the Fetus and Newborn Infant,* 5th ed. Philadelphia, WB Saunders, 2001.

KEY ARTICLES

American Academy of Pediatrics, Committee on Drugs: The transfer of drugs and other chemicals into human milk. *Pediatrics* 1994;93:137–50.

Boyer KM, Gotoff SP: Prevention of early-onset neonatal group B streptococcal disease with selective intrapartum chemoprophylaxis. *N Engl J Med* 1986;314:1665–9.

Brown ZA, Selke S, Zeh J, et al: The acquisition of herpes simplex virus during pregnancy. *N Engl J Med* 1997;337:509–15.

Centers for Disease Control and Prevention: Hepatitis B virus: A comprehensive strategy for eliminating transmission in the United States through universal childhood vaccination. *MMWR* 1991;40(RR-13):1.

Centers for Disease Control and Prevention: Rubella and congenital rubella syndrome—United States, January 1, 1991—May 7, 1994. *MMWR* 1994;43:391.

Centers for Disease Control and Prevention: Zidovudine for the prevention of HIV transmission from mother to infant. *MMWR* 1994;43:285.

Connor EM, Sperling RS, Gelber R, et al: Reduction of maternal-infant transmission of HIV-1 with zidovudine treatment. Pediatric AIDS Clinical Trials Group Protocol 076 Study Group. *N Engl J Med* 1994; 331:1173–80.

Goldenberg RL, Hauth JC, Andrews WW: Intrauterine infection and preterm delivery. *N Engl J Med* 2000;342:1500–7.

Hamadeh MA, Glassroth J: Tuberculosis and pregnancy. *Chest* 1992; 101:1114–20.

Hohlfeld P, Daffos F, Costa JM, et al: Fetal toxoplasmosis: Outcome of pregnancy and infant follow-up after in utero treatment. *J Pediatr* 1989;115:765–9.

Hohlfeld P, Daffos F, Costa JM, et al: Prenatal diagnosis of congenital toxoplasmosis with a polymerase chain reaction test of amniotic fluid. *N Engl J Med* 1994;331:695–9.

International Perinatal HIV Group: The mode of delivery and the risk of vertical transmission of human immunodeficiency virus type 1—A meta-analysis of 15 prospective cohort studies. *N Engl J Med* 1999; 340:977–87.

John GC, Nduati RW, Mbori-Ngacha DA, et al: Correlates of mother-to-child human immunodeficiency virus type 1 (HIV-1) transmission: Association with maternal plasma HIV-1 RNA load, genital HIV-1 DNA shedding, and breast infections. *J Infect Dis* 2001;183:206–12.

Meyers JD: Congenital varicella in term infants: Risk reconsidered. *J Infect Dis* 1974;129:215–7.

Nduanti R, John G, Mbori-Ngach D, et al: Effect of breastfeeding and formula feeding on transmission of HIV-1: A randomized clinical trial. *JAMA* 2000;283:1167–74.

Prober CG, Sullender WM, Yasukawa LL, et al: Low risk of herpes virus infection in neonates exposed to the virus at the time of vaginal delivery to mothers with recurrent genital herpes simplex virus infections. *N Engl J Med* 1987;316:240–4.

Schrag SJ, Zywicki S, Farley MM, et al: Group B streptococcal disease in the era of intrapartum antibiotic prophylaxis. *N Engl J Med* 2000;342:15–20.

Stagno S, Reynolds DW, Pass RF, et al: Breast milk and the risk of cytomegalovirus infection. *N Engl J Med* 1980;302:1073–6.

Wong SY, Remington JS: Toxoplasmosis in pregnancy. *Clin Infect Dis* 1994;18:853–62.

Wu YW, Colford JM Jr: Chorioamnionitis as a risk factor for cerebral palsy: A meta-analysis. *JAMA* 2000;284:1417–24.

CHAPTER 95

Intrauterine Infections

Stuart P. Adler

The microorganisms that characteristically cause intrauterine infections of the fetus include the spirochete *Treponema pallidum;* the viruses cytomegalovirus (CMV), herpes simplex virus (HSV), varicella-zoster virus (VZV), rubella, human parvovirus B19 (B19), and lymphocytic choriomeningitis virus; and the coccidian, *Toxoplasma gondii.*

With the exception of HSV that ascends the genital tract and may cause fetal infection with recurrent maternal infection, these organisms can produce severe fetal disease after primary infection during pregnancy when, in the absence of maternal immunity, they are transported through the bloodstream across the placenta to the fetus. Primary maternal infection by these or other microorganisms during pregnancy does not always result in intrauterine infection of the fetus; when intrauterine infection does occur, symptomatic fetal disease does not always follow. Most commonly, infants infected in utero appear normal at birth. Chronic persistent infection by most of these organisms, however, causes progressive disease with significant developmental abnormalities that may become apparent over the first several years of life. Examples of such abnormalities are postnatal blindness associated with persistent infection by *T. gondii* or progressive hearing deficit or mental retardation that may occur with *T. pallidum* or CMV infection.

In general, infection of the mother by these microbes and development of immunity before conception protects the fetus from either infection or the severe consequences of intrauterine infection, both in utero and in the immediate postnatal period. For example, women with immunity to CMV before pregnancy frequently deliver infants with intrauterine infection, but with rare exceptions congenital CMV disease occurs only as the result of a primary infection during pregnancy.

Along with maternal immunity, another important factor that affects both the frequency of transplacental transmission and the severity of disease is the gestational age at the time the woman becomes infected. For example, intrauterine rubella infections are most devastating when maternal infection occurs in the first trimester of pregnancy. *T. gondii* infections can be transmitted from mother to fetus at any time during gestation, but the most severe intrauterine disease occurs early in pregnancy, and the mildest occurs late in pregnancy. In contrast, congenital infection with syphilis most commonly occurs with maternal infection in the last half of pregnancy.

Another influence on the severity and the manifestations of an intrauterine infection is the tissue tropism, or the affinity of a particular microbe for specific cell types or tissues. Most of the organisms that cause intrauterine infections such as CMV and *T. pallidum* replicate in all organs and tissues, hence causing disease in many or all organs or tissues. Other organisms are more tissue tropic; for example, VZV is tropic for neural tissue, and many of the manifestations of severe intrauterine infection with VZV arise from effects on the developing nervous system. Regardless of tissue tropism, fetal infection with any of the microbes may cause stillbirth or spontaneous abortion, or **intrauterine growth retardation,** defined as small size for gestational age. **Prematurity,** defined as birth ≤37 weeks of gestation, is not often caused by intrauterine infection alone.

Until recently, possible intrauterine infection was commonly referred to as **TORCH syndrome,** an acronym for some of the microorganisms causing intrauterine infection. This term obscures the reality that these congenital infections differ significantly in pathogenesis, clinical manifestations, diagnosis, and therapy. Considering congenital infection as a single syndrome often triggers a senseless diagnostic search with the use of inappropriate or unnecessary tests. Many neonatologists and infectious disease specialists consider the use of the term *TORCH syndrome* inappropriate for categorizing infants with intrauterine infections. The diagnostic evaluation of a congenital infection does not begin with a rote battery of diagnostic tests.

Suggestive Findings. For infants with symptoms of intrauterine infection at birth, each of these causative microbes causes different characteristic manifestations that are typical and have diagnostic significance (Table 95–1). A rational evaluation begins with a careful history, including history obtained from the mother and the mother's chart, and complete physical examination, including ophthalmologic examination, searching for clues to congenital infection and the particular characteristics of each of the possible intrauterine infections (Fig. 95–1).

Many diagnostic tests are useful in the evaluation of congenital infection (Table 95–2). As a nonspecific screening test, an elevated **total IgM** concentration in cord or infant serum suggests intrauterine infection, although many infected infants have normal total IgM concentrations of IgM at birth. Maternal IgM does not cross the placenta, but the fetus synthesizes IgM antibodies in response to foreign antigens. The normal IgM concentration increases from a mean of about 6 mg/dL in premature infants of <28 weeks' gestation to about 11 mg/dL at term. Infants infected in utero may have an IgM concentration in cord serum at term of >20 mg/dL. Unlike IgM, the active transport from the mother to the fetus of all four subclasses of IgG increases with gestational age. IgG is present in fetal blood in very small amounts beginning as early as 8 weeks of gestation, but levels remain low until about 17–20 weeks of gestation when IgG transport across the placenta accelerates. At birth the IgG levels are usually 5–10% higher in the newborn than in the mother. Unlike IgM, the presence of organism-specific IgG in cord or infant serum does not discriminate between congenital infection and pre-existing maternal seropositivity.

TABLE 95–1. Possible Consequences of Intrauterine Infections Present at Birth

	Microorganism						
Clinical Sign	**Rubella Virus**	**Cytomegalovirus**	***Toxoplasma gondii***	**Intrauterine Herpes Simplex Virus**	***Treponema pallidum***	**Varicella**	**Lymphocytic Choriomeningitis Virus**
Prematurity	−	−	+	+	+	−	−
Intrauterine growth retardation	+	++++	+	+	+	−	−
Hepatosplenomegaly	+	++	+	−	+	−	−
Jaundice	+	++	+	−	+	−	−
Lymphadenopathy	+	−	+	−	+	−	−
Pneumonitis	+	+	+	+	+	−	−
Lesions of skin or mucous membranes							
Petechiae or purpura	+	+	+	−	+	−	−
Vesicles	−	+	−	+	+	−	−
Maculopapular exanthems	−	−	+	+	++	+	−
Scarring	−	−	−	++	−	++	−
Lesions of nervous system							
Meningoencephalitis	+	+	+	+	+	+	+
Microcephaly	−	++	+	++	−	++	+
Hydrocephaly	+	+	++	+	−	++	++
Intracranial calcifications	−	++	++	+	−	+	++
Paralysis	−	−	−	−	−	++	−
Hearing deficits	+	++	−	−	+	−	+
Hydrancephaly	−	−	−	++	−	−	−
Lesions of heart							
Myocarditis	+	−	+	+	−	−	−
Congenital defects	++	−	−	−	−	−	−
Bone lesions	++	−	+	−	++	−	−
Eye lesions							
Glaucoma	−	−	−	−	+	−	−
Chorioretinitis or retinopathy	++	+	++	++	+	++	++
Cataracts	++	−	+		−	+	−
Optic atrophy	−	+	+	−	−	++	−
Microphthalmia	+	−	+	−	−	+	−
Uveitis	−	−	+	−	+	−	−
Conjunctivitis or keratoconjunctivitis	−	−	−	++	−	+	

− = Rare or absent; + = uncommon (<20% of cases); ++ = common (>20% of cases).

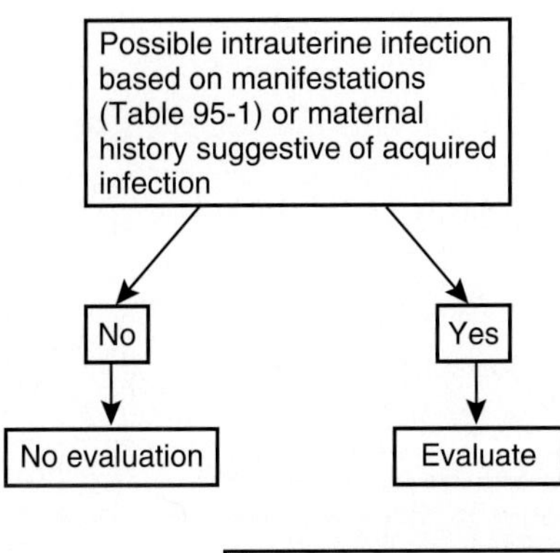

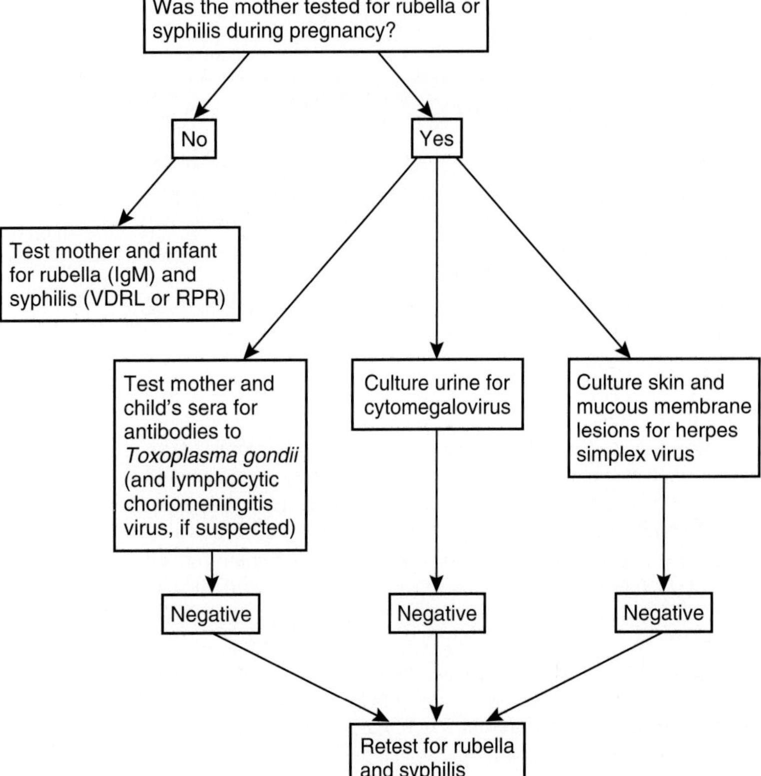

FIGURE 95–1. Simplified algorithm for screening for congenital infection.

TABLE 95–2. Laboratory Approach to the Diagnosis of Intrauterine Infection

Test	Specimens	For
Viral culture	Urine	CMV, HSV, rubella, LCM
	Skin vesicles	HSV, VZV
	Throat swabs	CMV, HSV, rubella
Placental histology	Placenta	Syphilis, *Toxoplasma,* CMV (inclusion cells)
Dark-field examination	Placenta Snuffles Skin lesions Nasal discharge	Syphilis
IgG-specific antibody (negative tests generally exclude diagnosis)	Maternal and infant sera	Syphilis, CMV, HSV (types 1 and 2), LCM, *Toxoplasma*
IgM-specific antibody		Reliable for rubella, LCM, and *Toxoplasma* only

CMV = Cytomegalovirus; HSV = herpes simplex virus; VZV = varicella-zoster virus; LCM = lymphocytic choriomeningitis virus.

TREPONEMA PALLIDUM

The most common dilemma currently posed by syphilis is the management of symptom-free infants born to mothers with positive serologic tests for syphilis. The effectiveness of the maternal syphilis treatment regimen must be assessed for adequacy of treatment of infection in the fetus, and the need to treat an infection that may not be clinically apparent in the newborn infant must be determined.

ETIOLOGY

Syphilis was first described in detail in 1498 and is caused by *T. pallidum,* a pathogenic spirochete that is transmitted primarily by sexual contact. Humans are the main hosts for *T. pallidum,* and maternal infection during pregnancy results in fetal infection. *Treponema* is one of five genera of the order Spirochaetales, which are difficult to cultivate in vitro, although *T. pallidum* can be maintained for days to weeks in artificial media or cultivated in experimental animals. Typical lesions may develop in guinea pigs infected with *T. pallidum.* Rabbits are readily infected with *T. pallidum,* developing lesions that resemble those that occur in humans with progressive secondary infection. Currently the best assay for detection of *T. pallidum* in biologic material is infection of rabbit testicles followed by the development of orchitis.

Transmission. An infant can acquire syphilis by vertical transmission either in utero, across the placenta and often associated with placentitis, or by contact with active maternal lesions, or **chancres,** if present in the maternal cervical-vaginal tract at birth. It was previously thought that infection of the placenta, and hence transmission to fetus, did not occur before the fourth month of pregnancy because the Langhans cell layer, which atrophies in the fourth month of pregnancy, was impermeable to spirochetes. A few cases of fetal infections with *T. pallidum* do occur in early pregnancy. The fetus can be infected at any stage during pregnancy, but the risk of infection increases with gestational age. Handling of infected placentas may transmit the spirochetes to health care providers; therefore standard precautions are recommended in the handling of infected placentas.

Fetal transmission rates were studied in the early 1950s. For women with primary and secondary syphilis during late pregnancy, there was a 90% rate of transmission of the spirochete to the fetus. For women with early syphilis there was a 40% transmission rate, and for women with late latent disease there was a 10% rate of transmission. Current data are not available; in general, however, most infants with symptomatic congenital syphilis are infected after the fifth month of pregnancy.

EPIDEMIOLOGY

The incidence of congenital syphilis parallels the incidence of primary and secondary syphilis in women. Determination of the actual number of cases of congenital syphilis is complicated by syphilis-associated stillbirths that are unrecognized and unreported, the difficulties of identifying infection in the newborn that is often not accompanied by disease, and the need for follow-up serologic testing to confirm the presence of congenital infection, especially in patient groups characterized by inconstant use of health care. The true incidence of congenital syphilis is probably underestimated. The greatest risk factors for congenital syphilis are lack of prenatal care and cocaine drug abuse, which is associated with prostitution, unprotected sex, and trading of sex for drugs in addition to inadequate prenatal care of pregnant addicts.

After a recent epidemic of primary and secondary syphilis that peaked in 1990 (see Fig. 85–3), with a peak of 4,410 cases of congenital syphilis in 1991, the incidence of primary and secondary syphilis and of congenital syphilis fell dramatically, with 529 congenital cases in 2000 (Fig. 95–2). Several factors contributed to the decrease in syphilis in the United States during the 1990s including increased allocation of federal and state resources for clinical services and community-based screening and outreach programs instituted spe-

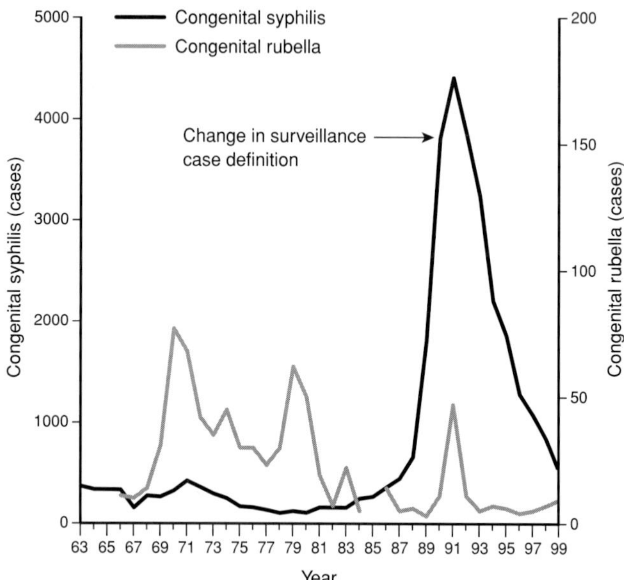

FIGURE 95–2. Incidence of congenital syphilis (reported cases in infants younger than 1 year of age) and primary and secondary syphilis by year in the United States, 1965–2000. The surveillance case definition for congenital syphilis changed in 1989. (Data from the Centers for Disease Control and Prevention.)

cifically for control of syphilis, HIV, and other sexually transmitted diseases. Use of crack cocaine and trading of sex for drugs were major contributors to the syphilis epidemic and have declined. Development of acquired immunity to syphilis after infection in the populations at risk may have also contributed to the decline. Despite these declines, syphilis remains endemic in parts of the South where it is many times more common (6.6 per 100,000 population) than in the Midwest (2.0), Northeast (1.1), and West (1.0).

Before 1989, **confirmed cases** were defined only by identification of spirochetes by microscopic or dark-field examination of infected tissue. **Presumed cases** were defined as those with signs and symptoms of congenital infections and supporting serologic data. **Asymptomatic** cases in infants of mothers with untreated syphilis were not considered to be infections. The revised guidelines in 1989, however, now require that all three categories of infants be reported as cases of congenital infection. Regardless of the change in case definition, the resurgence of maternal infections paralleled the increased rate of congenital infections (Fig. 95–2), suggesting a true increase in the rate of congenital syphilis.

PATHOGENESIS

Similar to CMV, rubella, and *T. gondii, T. pallidum* infects all organs and tissues, producing a chronic inflammatory reaction. *T. pallidum* infection of the fetus, because it occurs late in gestation, is not teratogenic. Placental infection with *T. pallidum* typically produces a large placenta that is pale and thick and histologically has inflamed villi. Spirochetes can be detected in the placenta by silver stain or dark-field examination, and can be recovered by a biologic assay.

SYMPTOMS AND CLINICAL MANIFESTATIONS

Intrauterine infection with syphilis is also associated with a 25–50% rate of miscarriage or stillbirth, particularly if acquired early in pregnancy. Approximately two thirds of infected newborns have no symptoms at birth, and their infections are identified only by mandatory screening. Congenital syphilis is separated into two stages, early and late (Table 95–3). **Early manifestations** are those that appear in the first 2 years of life, and **late manifestations** are those that appear after the age of 24 months. Most infants congenitally infected with *T. pallidum* have no symptoms. The late manifestations may reflect either a chronic progressive infection or intrauterine damage. Congenital syphilis should be considered in any infant with unexplained prematurity, especially if the prematurity is associated with hydrops or an enlarged placenta.

Early Manifestations. In early infancy, clues to congenital syphilis may be failure to thrive, persistent rhinitis known as **snuffles,** unusual rashes (particularly in the diaper area), unexplained jaundice or hepatosplenomegaly, and anemia. Hepatosplenomegaly is present in most infants with congenital syphilis and is one of the hallmarks of congenital syphilis. Only about one third of the patients with hepatosplenomegaly have prolonged neonatal jaundice with elevated direct or indirect bilirubin levels. Frequently, the only manifestation of congenital syphilis is hepatosplenomegaly, with or without jaundice. Congenital syphilis and human parvovirus B19 are the two frequent infectious causes of hydrops fetalis; anemia without hemolysis in hydropic infants suggests these two infections.

About one half of infected infants may have some degree of neonatal lymphadenopathy, which is usually generalized. Any unusual lymphadenopathy in early infancy should raise the concern about possible congenital syphilis. Epitrochlear nodes are often involved.

TABLE 95–3. Common Early and Late Manifestations of Congenital Syphilis

Early	Late
Intrauterine growth retardation	Dentition
Hepatomegaly, splenomegaly	Hutchinson's teeth
Jaundice	Mulberry molars
Generalized lymphadenopathy	Eye
Osteochondritis, periostitis, osteomyelitis	Interstitial keratitis
	Healed chorioretinitis
Snuffles	Uveitis
Condylomata lata	Glaucoma
Bullous lesions	Corneal scarring
Palmar or plantar rash	Ear
Elevated CSF cell count or protein	Eighth nerve deafness
Hemolytic anemia	Nose and face
Intravascular coagulopathy	Saddle nose
Pseudoparalysis	Frontal bossing
Pneumonitis	Protuberant mandible
Nonimmune hydrops	Skin
Nephrotic syndrome	Rhagades
Enlarged placenta	Central nervous system
Failure to thrive	Mental retardation
	Arrested hydrocephalus
	Seizures

A variety of hematologic abnormalities are common in congenital syphilis, including anemia, leukopenia or leukocytosis, and thrombocytopenia. Neonatal Coombs'-negative hemolytic anemia should be considered secondary to congenital syphilis until proven otherwise. The basis for the abnormal hemolytic manifestations, including lymphocytosis or monocytosis, is unknown.

Many infants with symptomatic congenital syphilis will have skin manifestations. A maculopapular rash classically appears at 2 weeks of age and lasts 1–3 months if untreated. The lesions are oval, pink, and red and may subsequently become a copper-brown color. The rash may occur on all body surfaces, but the buttocks, back, thighs and soles appear to be the most common sites. Another characteristic rash is **disseminated vesicular bullae** that typically involve the palms and soles. These bullous lesions may contain hemorrhagic fluid with many hundreds of thousands of spirochetes. When they rupture they release these organisms, leaving a denuded area that will become macerated and crusted. These lesions and the typical snuffles that develop in infants with congenital syphilis are highly infectious, which should be emphasized to health care providers. **Condylomata lata** are later manifestations of syphilis, usually occurring at 2–3 months of life. These occur in the perioral area around the nose and angles of the mouth and may also occur in the perianal area. They are large, flat, wartlike areas that are moist and may have single or multiple fissures.

Characteristic bone lesions are the most frequently encountered abnormalities of early congenital syphilis (Fig. 95–3). Radiographs show signs of **osteochondritis, periostitis,** or even osteomyelitis. The tibia, humerus, and femur are most commonly involved. Lesions are seen most often at the metaphysis, often along the lateral surfaces. **Wimberger's sign,** although not specific for congenital syphilis, is a bilateral lesion of the metaphysis along the medial surfaces of the tibiae. Clinically, a characteristic **pseudoparalysis,** also known as **pseudoparalysis of Parrot** or **postnatal Erb palsy,** may develop in infants that is characterized by irritability and refusal to move the limb because of an osteochondritis or periostitis

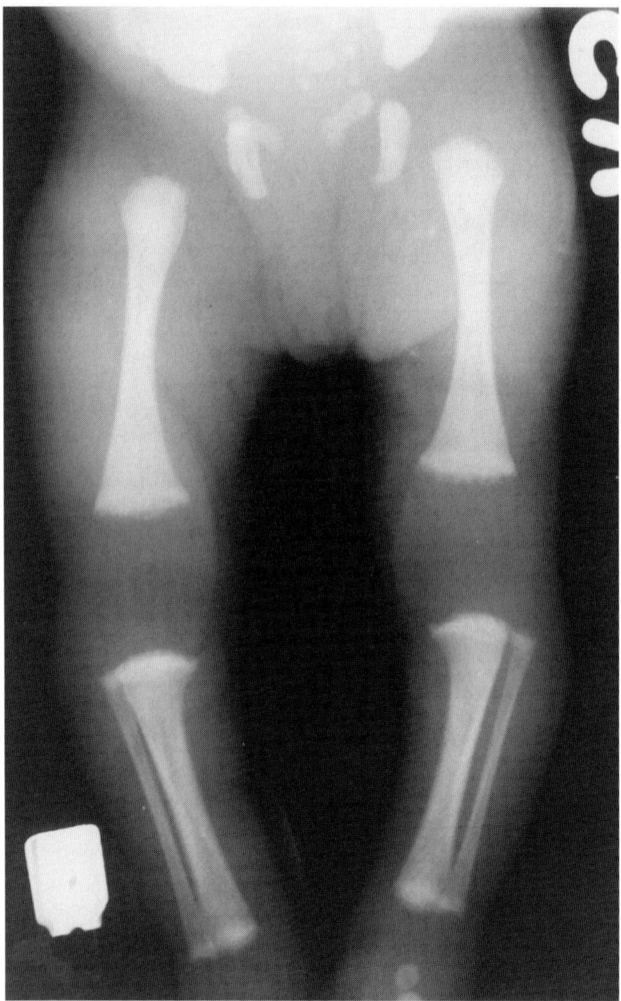

FIGURE 95–3. Radiographic abnormalities of the long bones in an infant with congenital syphilis. Radiograph of the distal femur and proximal tibia shows typical irregular metaphyses associated with periosteal new bone formation. (Photograph courtesy of Das Narla.)

of the long bones. The upper limbs may be affected more frequently than the lower limbs. There is a poor correlation between radiographic findings and symptoms.

Renal manifestations, particularly nephrotic syndrome, may develop at 2–3 months of age.

The most significant and devastating effects of congenital syphilis occur in the CNS. At birth there is usually aseptic meningitis, with >60% of children with symptomatic congenital syphilis having pleocytosis and an elevated protein concentration in the cerebrospinal fluid. If frank meningitis is not present at birth, subacute or chronic **syphilitic meningitis** may appear later, often between 3–6 months of age. The initial signs and symptoms of syphilitic meningitis are similar to those of bacterial meningitis, including a positive Kernig's sign, bulging fontanelles, and separation of the sutures. Evaluation of the cerebrospinal fluid is mandatory in cases of suspected congenital syphilis and should include cell count, protein, glucose, and VDRL determinations. A positive CSF VDRL is evidence of CNS infection of the newborn.

The eye is infrequently involved in congenital syphilis and may include chancres of the eyelids, chorioretinitis, uveitis, and glaucoma secondary to uveitis.

Late Manifestations. The late manifestations are usually observed in untreated infants whose mothers were also untreated during pregnancy. The late manifestations can probably be prevented if congenital syphilis is treated promptly at birth.

Dental changes presumably occur as a result of a vasculitis at birth that damages the tooth buds, primarily of the permanent teeth. **Hutchinson's teeth** are peg-shaped or notched permanent upper central incisors that become widely spaced and shorter than the lateral incisors, sometimes with discoloration of the enamel. **Moon's molar,** or **Fournier teeth** or **mulberry molar,** usually affects the lower first molar, resulting in a narrow grinding surface and small cuspids with poor enamel. Dental abnormalities can be prevented if infants are treated in the first 3 months of life.

Ocular changes include interstitial keratitis, healed chorioretinitis, and secondary glaucoma with or without corneal scarring. These manifestations are preventable if treatment is given early.

Eighth nerve deafness occurs in about 3% of the patients with late congenital syphilis. There may be an associated vertigo, and deafness may be bilateral or unilateral.

Characteristic rhinitis may be present at birth and last for many weeks or months. In addition, as the child grows, changes in the shape of the nose and face include a concave shape to the middle section of the face with a protruding mandible and a high, arched palate. There may be inflammation of cartilage and bone, leading to the destruction of underlying bone in the nasal septum and the **saddle nose deformity.**

There may be linear scars, or **rhagades,** that result from fissures and ulcerations around body orifices, including the mouth and nose.

Neurologic manifestations of late congenital syphilis include mental retardation, hydrocephalus, convulsive disorders, blindness, and deafness. Early treatment may prevent these late sequelae.

Chronic inflammation of the bones and joints may occur in late congenital syphilis. Periosteal inflammation may involve any of the bones, including the skull. Involvement of the skull may cause **frontal bossing.** Involvement of the tibia may result in so-called **saber shins,** and thickening of sternoclavicular portion of the clavicle is seen radiographically as **Higouménakis' sign. Clutton's joints** are a rare manifestation, most frequently involving the knee and characterized by synovitis with hydrarthrosis and local pain and tenderness. On radiographic examination the joints may appear normal, but examination of joint fluid reveals an inflammatory response with mononuclear cells.

DIAGNOSIS

The diagnosis of congenital syphilis is suspected on the basis of maternal history of syphilis, whether treated or not, or clinical findings in the infant, and is confirmed by serologic testing (Fig. 95–4).

Serologic tests of cord serum of infants born to women who acquired syphilis during pregnancy may be positive not as a result of intrauterine infection but because of transfer of maternal IgG antibodies. Determining whether an infant was infected in utero or only acquired passive antibody can sometimes be difficult. Infants should be treated if (1) the baby's RPR titer is fourfold or higher than the mother's; (2) the baby has signs of congenital infection and a positive RPR or VDRL; or (3) the baby has rising RPR or VDRL titers on serum obtained several weeks or months apart. In all infants believed to have congenital syphilis, cerebrospinal fluid should be tested for antibodies using the VDRL test, which, if positive, is a presumptive diagnosis of neurosyphilis.

Assessment of Maternal Treatment. Mothers in whom serologic tests are positive for syphilis should be considered infected unless

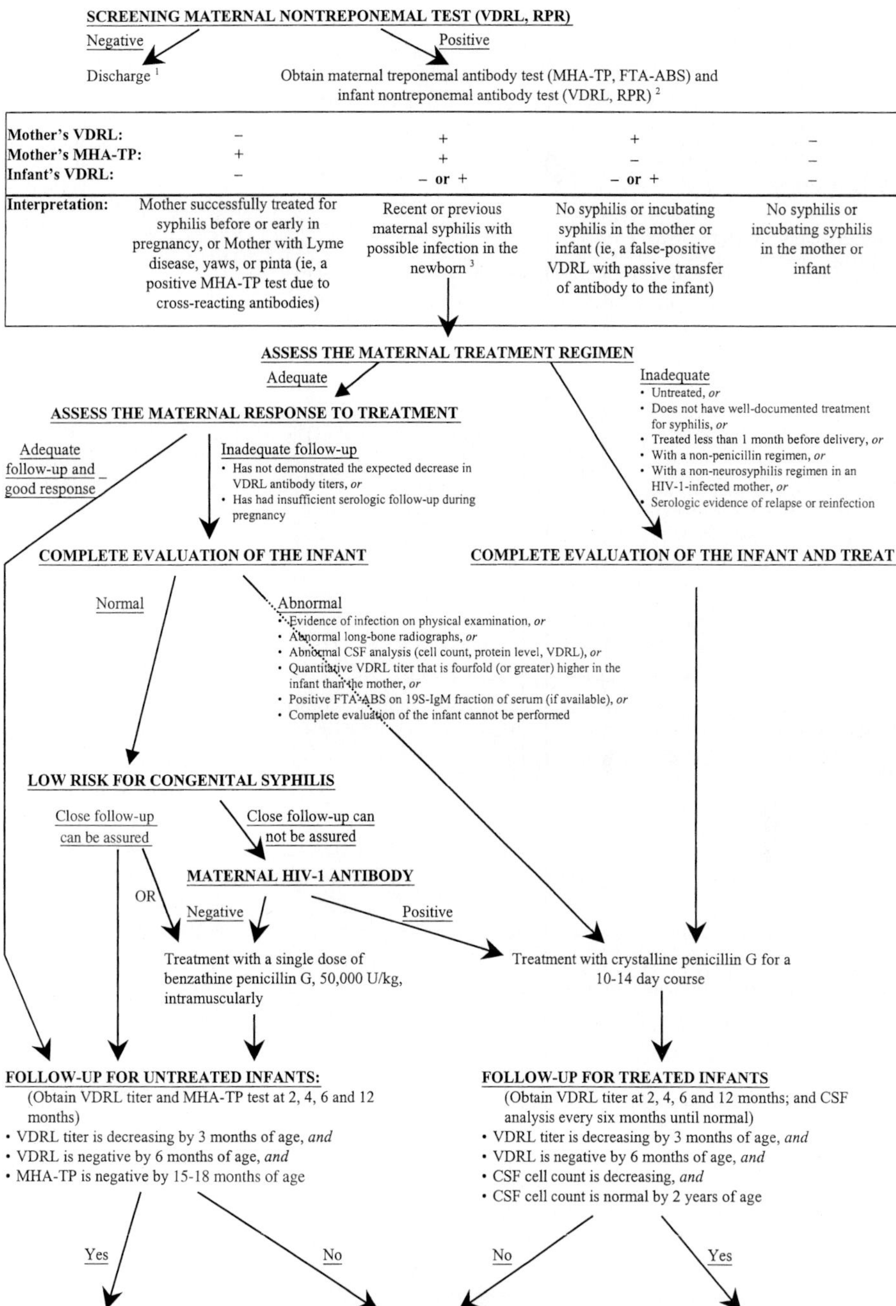

FIGURE 95–4. Algorithm for the management and follow-up of infants born to mothers with positive nontreponemal serologic tests for syphilis (VDRL, RPR).

[1]If the mother is noted to have a chancre or has a history of recent sexual contact with another person with syphilis, the infant should be completely evaluated and treated for congenital syphilis.

[2]A treponemal antibody test (MHA-TP, FTA-ABS) of the infant is not necessary.

[3]A mother with latent syphilis may have nonreactive nontreponemal test results.

an adequate treatment is clearly documented in the medical records and sequential nontreponemal antibody (VDRL, RPR) titers have declined. Treatment of syphilis during pregnancy that did not include penicillin G in the regimen recommended for the stage of maternal syphilis (Table 85–6) should be presumptively considered inadequate for the fetus. Treatment failures are higher in women with secondary syphilis, possibly because of the greater number of organisms, and in women treated during the last trimester of pregnancy, possibly because of diminishing placental transfer of antimicrobial agents. Benzathine penicillin G regimens appear adequate to treat syphilis during pregnancy before 20 weeks of gestation but may be less effective after 20 weeks of gestation. Maternal syphilis treated less than 4 weeks before delivery, even with an appropriate penicillin regimen, is a significant risk factor for congenital syphilis.

Microbiologic Evaluation

Serologic Testing. There are two types of serologic test for syphilis (Chapter 11). The **nontreponemal tests** for syphilis, **RPR (rapid plasma reagin)** and **VDRL (Venereal Disease Research Laboratory),** do not use antigens from *T. pallidum* but rather use **cardiolipid,** which is extracted from beef hearts. These serologic tests are quantitative and are highly sensitive; either test is positive in 95% of cases of primary syphilis and in 100% of cases of secondary syphilis. After adequate therapy, these tests become negative. The **treponemal tests** for syphilis, **microhemagglutination–*Treponema pallidum* (MHA-TP)** and **fluorescent treponemal antibody (FTA),** which is seldom performed, use membrane proteins from *T. pallidum.* These tests detect antibodies to *T. pallidum,* are not quantitative, and remain positive for life even after appropriate treatment.

Histologic Evaluation

A specific diagnosis of *T. pallidum* infection may be confirmed by identification of spirochetes by dark-field examination (see Fig. 7–1) of the placenta, discharge from rhinitis or snuffles, and skin lesions.

TREATMENT

Treatment is recommended for all infants with a positive VDRL or RPR test at birth whose mothers did not receive adequate therapy during pregnancy (Table 95–4). Newborns of mothers who were adequately treated during pregnancy may have positive test responses because of maternally acquired IgG. If such infants have symptoms at birth (Table 94–3), a VDRL or RPR titer that is fourfold or higher than the mother's, or a positive CSF VDRL, they also require therapy. Symptom-free infants with a VDRL or RPR titer equal to or lower than the maternal titer require serial postnatal titers over the first 6 months of life to exclude congenital infection. Rising or persistent titers indicate congenital infection.

Follow-up. All infants, untreated or treated, with positive serologic tests for syphilis or infants born to mothers with positive serologic tests for syphilis require careful follow-up examinations and serial VDRL or RPR tests at a minimum of 2, 4, 6, and 12 months of age to confirm decreasing titers, which should be undetectable by 6–12 months of age (Fig. 95–4). Positive VDRL or RPR tests in the newborn from transplacental maternal IgG antibody, in the absence of fetal infection, should be declining by 3 months of age and should be undetectable by 6 months of age. Approximately 16% of uninfected infants will have a positive VDRL or RPR test at 6 months of age but a negative test on repeat testing at 12 months of age.

Untreated infants who develop clinical signs or symptoms of congenital syphilis (Table 95–3), have a fourfold increase in VDRL or RPR titers, stable titers at 6–12 months of age, or a positive MHA-TP test after 12 months of age should be reevaluated (including CSF examination) and treated for possible neurosyphilis with a 10-day course of aqueous crystalline penicillin G (Table 95–4).

PROGNOSIS

Treated infants should not have MHA-TP or FTA-ABS tests to evaluate response to therapy because these tests can remain positive despite effective therapy. Organ systems with evidence of involvement in the neonatal period need to be monitored through childhood, particularly if there are neurologic, auditory, and ophthalmologic abnormalities. Infants whose CSF evaluation at birth was abnormal should have repeat CSF evaluation every 6 months until the CSF findings are normal. A positive CSF VDRL finding at 6 months or other abnormal CSF indices that cannot be attributed to another process that are still abnormal at 2 years of age require re-evaluation and re-treatment for possible neurosyphilis with a 10-day course of aqueous crystalline penicillin G (Table 95–4). Treated infants who show persistent or recurrent clinical signs or symptoms of congenital syphilis, a fourfold increase in nontreponemal antibody titers, an absence of decline in the nontreponemal antibody titers by 12 months of age, a positive CSF VDRL at 6 months of age, or other abnormal CSF indices (cell count, protein level) at 2 years of age that cannot be attributed to another process should be re-treated. The serologic test findings may remain positive longer for children treated for syphilis after the neonatal period. It is possible that in the future the follow-up of these infants will include PCR tests of serum and CSF to confirm absence or eradication of congenital infection.

Re-treatment of Early and Treatment of Late Congenital Syphilis. The lack of definitive diagnostic criteria and the difficulty of excluding neurosyphilis necessitate that a regimen for neurosyphilis be used for all patients treated beyond the neonatal period for congenital syphilis. These children should be treated with aqueous crystalline penicillin G 200,000–300,000 U/kg/day, divided into four doses given every 6 hours, intravenously for 10–14 days. The three-dose regimen of benzathine penicillin G, 50,000 U/kg (not to exceed 2.4 million U), given every week intramuscularly for 3 successive weeks, may be considered for infants with normal CSF analysis, including negative CSF VDRL.

PREVENTION

Prenatal screening remains the most important factor in the identification of infants at risk of development of congenital syphilis and ideally results in diagnosis and treatment during pregnancy. Routine maternal serologic testing for syphilis is legally required at the beginning of prenatal care in all states. In pregnant women without optimal prenatal care, serologic screening for syphilis should be performed at the time pregnancy is diagnosed. Any

TABLE 95–4. Therapy for Neonates (≤4 wk of Age) Born of Mothers with Syphilis

Maternal Therapy	Clinical Findings in the Infant	Recommended Regimen*†
None, inadequate, or undocumented	Present or absent	Aqueous crystalline penicillin G 100,000–150,000 U/kg/day divided q12hr IV for the first week of life, and q8hr thereafter for a total of 10 days *or* Procaine penicillin G 50,000 U/kg/day once daily IV for 10 days
Adequate, but <1 mo before birth, or insufficient serologic follow-up during pregnancy	Absent	Benzathine penicillin G 50,000 U/kg once IV

*With clinical and serologic follow-up (Fig. 95–4).
†If more than 1 day of therapy is missed, the entire course should be restarted.

woman who delivers a stillborn infant after 20 weeks of pregnancy should be tested for syphilis. In communities and populations with a high prevalence of syphilis, or for patients at high risk, testing should be performed at least two additional times, at the beginning of the third trimester (28 weeks) and at delivery. Some states mandate repeat testing of all women at delivery. Testing is indicated at any time for women with suspicious lesions or a history of recent sexual exposure to a person with syphilis. Women at high risk of syphilis should possibly be screened more frequently, either monthly or, pragmatically because of inconsistent prenatal care, at every medical encounter because they may have repeat infections during pregnancy or infection late in pregnancy.

Testing of the mother's serum is preferred to testing of cord blood or of the infant's serum because the titers are frequently lower in the infant and may be nonreactive if the mother was infected late in pregnancy. No newborn infant should be discharged from the hospital without the serologic status of the mother having been determined at least once during pregnancy.

CYTOMEGALOVIRUS

ETIOLOGY

Human CMV, a member of the Herpesviridae family, has a double-stranded DNA genome of 230 kbp containing more than 200 genes. It shares many features with the other herpesviruses, including the ability to cause persistent and latent infection.

EPIDEMIOLOGY

CMV infects 50–80% of the population and infrequently causes disease, but it causes serious disease in immunocompromised persons, including persons with AIDS and with intrauterine infection. In undeveloped areas or among lower socioeconomic groups of developed countries 0.5–2% of all newborns are congenitally infected with CMV. By 5 years of age, most children have acquired CMV infection. Acquired CMV infection usually occurs in the first year of life, and is transmitted perinatally by contact with maternal cervical-vaginal secretions or postnatally from seropositive mothers via breast milk. From 6–12% of infants of seropositive mothers acquire CMV through maternal cervical-vaginal secretions, and approximately 50% acquire CMV through breast milk. After primary infection, infants and young children shed CMV in saliva and urine for many months or years, whereas adults shed the virus for the first several weeks or months and intermittently thereafter. Thus young children who do not acquire CMV from their mothers presumably acquire the infection from frequent contact with other children, or possibly adults, who are shedding CMV. In developing areas where infection is acquired postnatally early in life, CMV rarely causes clinically apparent disease.

In developed countries, among persons in middle or upper socioeconomic groups, infection may occur later in life, although most persons eventually acquire CMV infection. In the United States, infection rates average between 1–2% per year. Between 40–70% of women 15–45 years of age are seropositive, although specific seropositivity rates vary with location and race. Seroprevalence rates are significantly higher among African Americans than among white persons.

PATHOGENESIS

Worldwide, approximately 1% of newborns are infected with CMV in utero and excrete virus at birth, but fewer than 10% of these infants have congenital CMV disease at birth or develop postnatal sequelae such as mental retardation and deafness. Of the 90% of congenitally infected infants who have no symptoms at birth, approximately 85% develop normally. The reason only 10% of infants congenitally infected with CMV have symptoms at birth and only approximately 15% of infants without symptoms at birth develop postnatal sequelae is that, with rare exceptions, it is the offspring of women who acquire primary CMV infection during pregnancy who are at risk of congenital disease. Approximately 40% of women who acquire primary CMV infection at any time during pregnancy transmit CMV to the fetus, compared with only 0.5–2% of women infected before pregnancy. Of congenitally infected newborns whose mothers acquired a primary CMV infection during pregnancy, approximately one third will have disease at birth or will develop significant sequelae (Fig. 95–5). The risk of symptomatic infection appears to be greatest when primary maternal infection occurs in the first half of pregnancy, but congenital disease also occurs among infants born to mothers who have a primary infection in the second half of pregnancy.

Because primary maternal infection is responsible for the majority of congenital CMV disease, symptomatic infection is most frequent in areas with a high proportion of seronegative women who are frequently exposed to the virus. In the United States, primary maternal CMV infections during pregnancy are seldom recognized, and many infants in whom neurologic sequelae develop after primary maternal infection in early pregnancy have no symptoms at birth. Thus the precise number of affected infants born annually in this country is unknown. Estimates are that each year 1–4% of 4 million pregnant women in the United States acquire

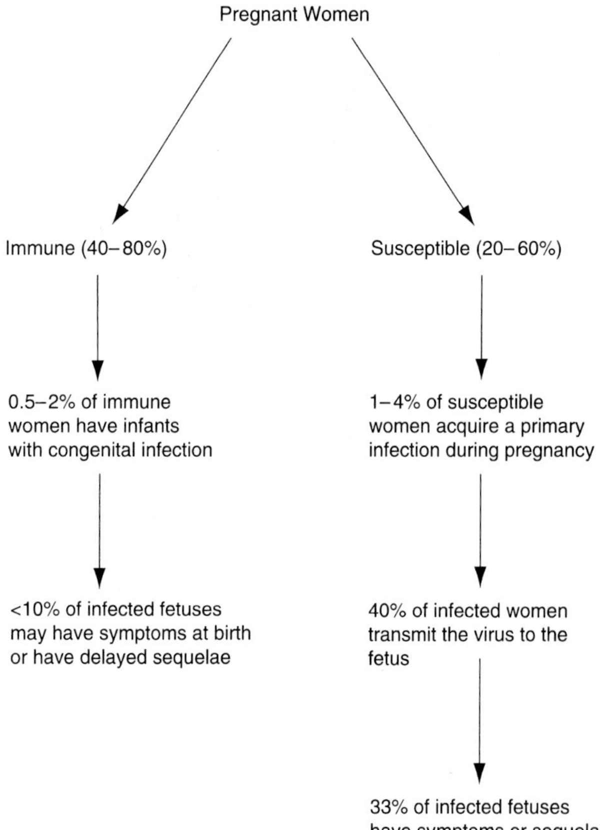

FIGURE 95–5. Relationship of maternal immunity to disease caused by congenital infection with cytomegalovirus.

primary CMV infection and that up to 8,000 newborns annually may develop significant handicaps caused by congenital CMV infection.

SYMPTOMS AND CLINICAL MANIFESTATIONS

Cytomegalovirus replicates in all organs and tissues, and therefore the manifestations of congenital CMV infections are protean (Table 95–5). Congenital CMV infection should be considered in any newborn with one or more of the characteristic manifestations. The reticuloendothelial system and the CNS are most frequently involved. Reticuloendothelial manifestations commonly include hepatosplenomegaly, hepatitis, direct hyperbilirubinemia, hemolytic anemia, and thrombocytopenia. CNS involvement is often manifested by microcephaly and intracranial calcifications, which are typically periventricular (Fig. 95–6). Chorioretinitis at birth or intracranial calcifications or other abnormalities on CT scan of the head are frequently associated with a poor neurologic prognosis, but none of the other manifestations of congenital infection accurately predict the severity of mental retardation or hearing deficit.

Approximately 15% of infants who have no symptoms at birth develop significant mental retardation or hearing deficit within the first 5 years of life. Children with symptomatic infections often have viremia at birth, which may persist for the first few months of life. Children with and children without symptoms excrete CMV in urine or saliva for up to 5 years postnatally. Children with symptomatic infections shed higher titers of virus, up to 10^6 pfu/mL of urine, than infants without symptoms. Hearing deficit, either mild or absent at birth, may develop or progressively worsen over the first several years of life, perhaps as a result of the chronic CMV infection. Profound hearing deficits are not generally reversible. The severity of mental retardation and developmental delay, which are the most serious neurologic sequelae of this infection, is difficult to predict at birth. Most children with symptoms at birth have some degree of mental retardation or developmental delay, although IQ scores may approach 100 in these children, and the level of functional impairment may be relatively mild or inapparent. Therefore, parents of congenitally infected children, including those without symptoms, should not be given a firm prognosis at birth.

TABLE 95–5. Common Manifestations of Symptomatic Congenital CMV Infection

Unexplained hepatomegaly with abnormal liver function tests
Unexplained splenomegaly
Unexplained hyperbilirubinemia (usually direct > indirect)
Ocular findings
Chorioretinitis
Strabismus
Optic atrophy
Microphthalmia
Cataracts
Retinal necrosis
Microcephaly
Cerebral calcifications
Hemolytic anemia

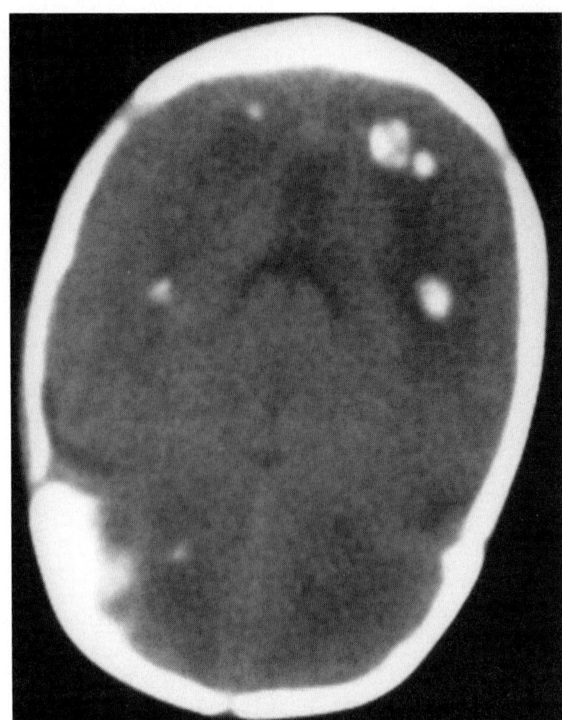

FIGURE 95–6. CT image of the brain of a newborn showing periventricular calcification typical of symptomatic congenital cytomegalovirus infection.

DIAGNOSIS

The diagnosis of congenital CMV infection is based chiefly on a positive urine culture within the first 3 weeks of life. A common practice is to test up to three urine samples to assure detection, although a single positive culture is diagnostic. With **shell vial culture assay** (Chapter 9), a diagnosis of congenital CMV infection can usually be established within 3 days. Because congenital infection with CMV occurs in up to 2% of all newborns and because 90% of these infants will develop normally, a positive urine culture alone is inadequate to establish a diagnosis of symptomatic congenital CMV infection. Antibody testing in the mother is helpful only if the mother is seronegative for antibodies to CMV, which excludes the diagnosis.

Similar manifestations in the newborn may be caused by congenital toxoplasmosis and congenital syphilis (Table 95–1).

TREATMENT

No specific therapy exists for congenital infection with CMV. A study (Whitley et al., 1997) of infants with symptoms of congenital CMV infection who were given ganciclovir daily for 6 weeks showed that viruria quantitatively decreased during treatment but later returned to near pretreatment levels. Hearing improvement or stabilization occurred in 16% of 30 babies at ≥6 months of age. Ganciclovir treatment of congenital CMV infection appears to offer only minimal to moderate benefits in a small proportion of infants.

PREVENTION

Women of childbearing age who work with young children, especially in a hospital or daycare setting, should be informed of the potential risks of CMV infection and should practice good hand-washing and hygiene. However, most older children and adults are already immune to CMV. Routine serologic screening is not recommended.

Hospitalized Patients. Patients with congenital CMV infection shed virus in high titers, especially in the urine. However, nosocomial transmission, other than potential transmission by blood transfusion, is not a significant problem in hospital nurseries. There are no documented instances of CMV transmission from infants to personnel, and therefore no special isolation precautions are necessary. Occasionally, infant-to-infant transmission of CMV occurs among children who are hospitalized side by side for prolonged periods. Standard precautions with good hand-washing are the only necessary control measures (Chapter 105); no special isolation measures are necessary.

HERPES SIMPLEX VIRUS

ETIOLOGY

Herpes simplex (HSV), a member of the Herpesviridae family of viruses, has a double-stranded DNA genome of 150 kbp. There are 2 types—HSV-1 and HSV-2—which differ in their antigenic and biologic properties. They share many features with the other herpesviruses, including the ability to cause latent infection with recurrence.

EPIDEMIOLOGY

Approximately 5% of all neonatal infections with HSV are acquired in utero, 85% are acquired peripartum through contact with infected maternal lesions or asymptomatic cervical shedding of HSV (Chapter 97), and 10% are acquired postpartum from environmental sources, such as persons with oral HSV infections (Chapter 46). Intrauterine infections with HSV occur with a frequency of 1 in 200,000–300,000 live births, compared with 1 in 3000 live births for peripartum HSV infections. Intrauterine infections may occur with primary maternal HSV infection or reactivation of a latent maternal HSV infection at any time during gestation. In utero infection during the first 20 weeks of pregnancy is associated with the highest infant morbidity and mortality, including stillbirths and spontaneous abortions.

PATHOGENESIS

Although the exact route by which infants acquire intrauterine HSV infections is not known, several observations suggest that most infants become infected by virus ascending through the chorioamnionic membrane rather than from a maternal viremia and transplacental passage of HSV to the fetus. The first observation is that maternal viremia does not occur with either primary or recurrent HSV infections. The second observation is that HSV is commonly present in the cervicovaginal tract, and this is the usual site of primary or recurrent HSV infections in women who deliver infants with intrauterine HSV infection. Although women with primary HSV infection deliver infants with the most severe form of intrauterine HSV infection, these primary infections are still in the cervicovaginal tract, and viremia does not occur. The third observation is that even when a woman with viremia has disseminated HSV disease during pregnancy, most fetuses born of these women die because of maternal complications, not directly as a consequence of intrauterine HSV infection. Surviving fetuses of women with widely disseminated maternal disease usually have no evidence of HSV disease at delivery. The fourth observation is that most infants born with intrauterine HSV infection have evidence of cutaneous disease, often manifested by scarring. The chronicity of the skin infection suggests that with intrauterine HSV infections, as with peripartum and postpartum acquired infections, the skin or the mucous membranes are the first sites of HSV infection, followed by fetal viremia and subsequent CNS infection. The fifth observation suggesting an ascending route of infections is that when HSV is found within the placenta, there is usually extensive concomitant fetal involvement, suggesting that passage of the virus was from fetus to placenta. Infants who survive placental infection usually have evidence of disseminated organ dysfunction.

SYMPTOMS AND CLINICAL MANIFESTATIONS

Diagnosis of intrauterine HSV infection requires clinical evidence of HSV infection at birth and virologic confirmation by recovery of the virus from the newborn within the first 48 hours of life. The classic triad of symptoms is cutaneous scarring, hydranencephaly, and chorioretinitis. Depending on the time of intrauterine HSV infection, skin lesions may include erythematous macules that progress to vesicles, areas of aplastic or denuded skin, and finally scars. Skin lesions may occur at sites of trauma (e.g., sites of fetal scalp electrode) and often recur, but they do not usually progress to other sites. Dissemination with multiorgan system involvement, if present, is usually manifest by hepatic, renal, and hematologic disorders. Intrauterine growth retardation and subsequent postnatal growth retardation are also relatively common.

When hydranencephaly is absent, microcephaly, intracranial calcifications, hydrocephalus, porencephaly and subdural or epidural cysts may occur, with subsequent development of blindness, deafness, and mental retardation. Involvement of the eye, particularly chorioretinitis with a concomitant strabismus, is common. This occurs more frequently with intrauterine HSV infection than with HSV infection acquired peripartum or postpartum.

DIAGNOSIS

Intrauterine HSV infections are diagnosed by recovery of virus from the infant within the first 48 hours of life. Cultures obtained for HSV isolation within 48 hours of birth from infants who have none of the manifestations of intrauterine HSV infection may merely reflect perinatal HSV colonization. HSV should be recoverable from bullous lesions or vesicles, if present at birth. A Tzanck test or Wright's stain of epithelial cells scraped from cutaneous lesions may reveal multinucleated giant cells, which are associated either with HSV or VZV lesions.

TREATMENT

Antiviral therapy with acyclovir should be initiated promptly for newborns with suspected intrauterine HSV infection, according to treatment guidelines for perinatally acquired HSV infections (Chapter 97). There is a high incidence of recurrence of HSV after therapy, particularly of skin lesions, and consultation with a pediatric infectious diseases specialist is recommended.

PROGNOSIS

Intrauterine HSV infection often leads to disseminated disease, resulting in spontaneous abortion or stillbirth. Infants born alive with intrauterine HSV infection are more likely to have localized cutaneous infection. The morbidity and mortality associated with intrauterine HSV infections parallel disease acquired peripartum or postpartum. If the infection is untreated, the mortality is about 70%, and treatment with acyclovir reduces it to about 30%. The effect of antiviral therapy on morbidity is unknown, and many treated infants, particularly those with CNS involvement, will be blind, deaf, or profoundly retarded.

VARICELLA-ZOSTER VIRUS

ETIOLOGY

Varicella-zoster virus (VZV), a member of the Herpesviridae family and the cause of chickenpox (Chapter 27), has a double-stranded DNA genome of 125 kbp. It shares many features with the other herpesviruses, including the ability to cause latent infection with recurrence.

EPIDEMIOLOGY

Women who have had chickenpox or the vaccine before pregnancy are immune, and their fetuses are not at risk of intrauterine infection. However, approximately 5% of women in the United States have not had chickenpox or the vaccine before conception. The overall risk of intrauterine disease after maternal chickenpox in susceptible mothers is about 4%, with risk of infection of the infant and development of a varicella syndrome up to the twenty sixth week of pregnancy. This is much lower than with primary varicella in a pregnant women that occurs within a few days of delivery, with an associated risk of approximately 20% (Chapter 97). Maternal zoster, or shingles, during pregnancy poses virtually no risk to the fetus for intrauterine infection.

PATHOGENESIS

VZV causes both primary chickenpox and also recurrences months to years later, known as shingles or zoster. The natural history of VZV infection is characterized by two episodes of viremia: **primary viremia,** which follows the replication of the virus at a local site such as a regional lymph node in the head or neck that results in the seeding and replication of VZV at multiple body sites, and **secondary viremia,** which after viral replication infects epithelial cells throughout the body and produces the characteristic skin lesions of chickenpox. Transmission to the fetus may occur with either primary or secondary viremia. Infection after a primary maternal viremia usually causes fetal disease within 1–2 days after the appearance of skin lesions in the mother. If, however, fetal infection occurs after the secondary maternal viremia, fetal skin lesions do not appear until 10–14 days after the appearance of lesions in the mother.

Maternal acquisition of chickenpox late in gestation may be associated with a higher fetal mortality rate but is not associated with dysgenesis. Intrauterine infection with VZV that develops within the first 20 weeks of pregnancy may lead to severe teratogenesis because the fetal organs are developing morphologically. Intrauterine VZV infections are commonly associated with stillbirth. In liveborn infants, common manifestations include chorioretinitis, optic atrophy, limb atrophy, skin scarring, and mental retardation.

SYMPTOMS AND CLINICAL MANIFESTATIONS

VZV has a tropism for peripheral and central neural tissue. Major manifestations of intrauterine varicella infections are those related to the nervous system and include zigzag skin lesions and hypopigmented areas; damage to sensory nerves; microphthalmia, cataracts, chorioretinitis, and optic atrophy; damage to the cervical lumbar spinal cord with hypoplasia of the upper and lower extremities with motor and sensory deficits; absence of dependent reflexes; anal dysfunction; and Horner's syndrome. Cortical damage includes encephalitis with microcephaly, hydrocephaly, intracranial calcifications, and cerebral aplasia. All of the manifestations are the direct consequence of viral infection and inflammation of central and peripheral neural tissue and skin.

In addition to disease, infants may develop immunologic evidence of intrauterine infection without symptoms. A study (Paryani and Arvin, 1986) of 33 infants whose mothers had varicella during pregnancy found only one infant with clinical manifestations of intrauterine varicella infection. However, 8 of the 33 infants had immunologic evidence of intrauterine exposure to VZV, as indicated by the detection of IgM antibodies or by the persistence of IgG antibodies to VZV. This suggests that intrauterine infection is more common than fetal disease due to VZV. The developmental effects of asymptomatic intrauterine infection with VZV are unknown.

TREATMENT

Antiviral therapy for intrauterine varicella is not recommended. Infants whose mothers develop chickenpox at or within a few days of delivery should receive prophylactic treatment with VZIG (Chapter 97). Newborns who develop disease should be treated with acyclovir (Chapter 97).

PREVENTION

Maternal VZV infections can be either prevented or ameliorated if VZIG is used for postexposure prophylaxis. Pregnant women without a history of chickenpox who have household exposure to chickenpox should receive VZIG promptly or be tested immediately for immunity, with VZIG administered if they are seronegative. Most adults who do not recall having had chickenpox are immune, but delaying the administration of VZIG while awaiting a test result is usually inappropriate for pregnant women. Although VZIG is very effective in preventing or reducing the severity of maternal disease, its effectiveness in preventing intrauterine infection is unknown.

Varicella vaccine is recommended for immunocompetent children ≥12 months of age and for adults who have not had chickenpox. Pregnant women should not be immunized because of the potential risk for fetal infection. Women inadvertently immunized 3 months prior to pregnancy or during pregnancy should be reassured about the low risk. The vaccine manufacturer (Merck) maintains a pregnancy registry to monitor fetal outcome of pregnant women immunized with varicella vaccine, and health care providers are encouraged to report any exposures (telephone: 800-986-8999). Administration of VZIG is an option for women who are inadvertently immunized with varicella vaccine in the first half of pregnancy.

RUBELLA VIRUS

In 1941 a landmark publication by Gregg reported an association between maternal rubella infection during pregnancy with cataracts and heart disease discovered in infants born to these mothers. The classic triad of findings of **congenital rubella syndrome** consists of congenital heart disease, cataracts, and deafness. Mental retardation and other defects involving every organ system have also been described.

ETIOLOGY

Rubella virus is a togavirus, from the Latin word *toga* meaning cloak, a single-stranded RNA virus in the Togaviridae family. There is only one type of rubella virus, and humans are the only hosts.

The virus was first isolated in 1962, and by 1969 a live attenuated strain of rubella vaccine was developed and licensed. The rubella vaccine has been extraordinarily effective in reducing the incidence of maternal infection in the United States (see Fig. 24–1).

EPIDEMIOLOGY

Rubella infections occur worldwide. The virus circulates throughout a nonimmune population year-round, but endemic infections are more common in late winter and spring. Besides the constant and low-level endemic transmission of the virus, there are major worldwide epidemics every 6–9 years, although in various parts of the world the intervals between major epidemics may be up to 30 years.

Similar to most viral infections, there is a high rate of inapparent infection. Disease, when it does occur in pregnant women, is often mild and characterized by a mild rash, arthralgia, or simply malaise. Given the paucity of clinical findings associated with rubella, it is difficult to determine the exact incidence in a particular population. In the United States, because of the nearly complete immunization of the population, clinical disease due to rubella is uncommon (see Fig. 24–1). During the 1962–64 period there were 11,000 estimated fetal deaths and approximately 20,000 infants born with defects from rubella. Currently in the United States, fewer than 20 infants are born each year with a congenital rubella syndrome associated with a primary maternal infection (Fig. 95–2).

PATHOGENESIS

Maternal viremia, which occurs regardless of the presence of maternal symptoms, leads to placental infection and subsequent fetal infection. Congenital infection occurs only during primary maternal infection; recurrent infection with rubella is rare. Therefore, maternal immunity, whether acquired after natural infection or by vaccination, is protective against fetal infection. Infants infected in utero develop both IgG and IgM antibodies to rubella postnatally.

During maternal rubella infection, placental infection occurs in 50–70% and fetal infection in 20–30% of cases. Placental or fetal infection may lead to stillbirth or spontaneous abortion. The frequency of placental and fetal infection is related to the gestational age at the time of maternal infection. The rate of fetal infection is up to 80% with maternal infection during the first trimester and declines throughout the middle period of pregnancy to as low as 7%. The lowest rates of fetal infection following primary maternal rubella occur between 12–28 weeks of pregnancy. After the 36th week of pregnancy, infection rates for the fetus may actually increase to as high as 60–100%.

The risk of congenital defects and disease is greatest when the pregnant woman acquires infection during the first trimester. Overall, congenital defects occur in about 90% of infants whose mothers have infection before the 11th week of pregnancy, about 33% during weeks 11–12, about 10% during weeks 13–14, and about 24% during weeks 15–16. Therefore, during the first trimester the overall risk that an infant will be live-born with severe congenital defects is about 70%. If a mother acquires a primary infection after the 16th week of pregnancy, infection of the fetus may occur, although the risk of congenital defects is low.

Unlike primary rubella in adults or older children intrauterine infection results in a chronic infection with prolonged viremia and viral shedding in pharyngeal secretions, urine, tears, and feces. Infection may occur in many organs or in only a few. The virus has been recovered from CSF, bone marrow, and circulating leukocytes. Pharyngeal shedding of the virus is most common and persists for many months but usually ends by 2 years of age. The chronic persistent postnatal infection may cause the evolution of sequelae, such as hearing deficit and mental retardation, in many infants who are apparently unaffected at birth.

Similar to many of the other organisms that cause severe intrauterine infections, the rubella virus infects all organs and tissues. Autopsies of infected infants show inflammation in virtually every organ system, with hypoplasia a common finding. The placenta is also extensively involved with many inflammatory foci that may be edematous and necrotic.

SYMPTOMS AND CLINICAL MANIFESTATIONS

Congenital rubella syndrome classically consists of multiple defects usually involving some combination of congenital heart disease, eye and hearing abnormalities with or without retardation, and microcephaly in addition to intrauterine growth retardation (Table 95–6). As many as 71% of infants with no symptoms at birth may develop manifestations of disease within the first 5 years of life, including hearing deficits; developmental problems, including poor motor, intellectual, and language development; visual problems, including glaucoma and corneal and lens defects; mental retardation; and progressive encephalitis. Cardiac manifestations of con-

TABLE 95–6. Common Early and Late Manifestations of Congenital Rubella Syndrome

Early	Late
Lymphadenopathy	Neurologic
Bone radiolucencies	Peripheral and central hearing deficit
Encephalitis	Mental retardation with developmental delays in:
Pulmonary arterial hyperplasia	Motor
Patent ductus arteriosus	Speech
Severe hearing defects	Intellect
Cataracts	Behavior
Intrauterine growth retardation	Endocrine
Hepatitis	Diabetes mellitus
Hepatosplenomegaly	Thyroid disease
Hyperbilirubinemia	Growth hormone deficiency
Thrombocytopenia	Precocious puberty
	Eye
	Glaucoma
	Retinal lens
	Corneal abnormalities
	Keratic abnormalities

genital rubella infection are usually apparent at birth; the most common of these are patent ductus arterious and pulmonary arterial hyperplasia.

Deafness is the most common manifestation of congenital rubella syndrome, occurring in >80% of cases, and may be the sole manifestation of infection. CNS dysgenesis may occur when maternal infection occurs before week 8 of pregnancy, but the organ of Corti is vulnerable up to weeks 16–20 of pregnancy, and therefore either peripheral or central sensorineural hearing loss may occur. Bilateral hearing deficit is common.

Some of the most important consequences and late complications of congenital rubella are endocrinopathies, including **insulin-dependent diabetes,** which is the most common. It occurs in approximately 20% of these children at some time before adulthood, an incidence 100–200 times greater than in the general population. The mechanism by which congenital rubella syndrome causes diabetes is unknown, but it may be an autoimmune disease stimulated by chronic, persistent infection with the rubella virus. Hypothyroidism or hyperthyroidism occurs in about 5% of children. Other endocrinopathies occasionally associated with congenital rubella infection are growth hormone deficiency and precocious puberty.

The hearing deficit that occurs with rubella worsens with age and may become symptomatic after years of apparently normal hearing. Other late manifestations of congenital infection that may not be manifest at birth include glaucoma and retinopathies, as well as a subretinal neovascularization.

DIAGNOSIS

The diagnosis is usually established by virus isolation or the detection of rubella-specific IgM antibody in the presence of clinical signs and symptoms (Table 95–7). A history and review of the mother's chart revealing that rubella exposure was unlikely during pregnancy and that the mother had IgG antibodies to rubella at the beginning of pregnancy is usually all that is necessary to exclude intrauterine rubella infection. Occasionally, if there is a compatible syndrome and other causes of congenital infection are inapparent, it may be appropriate to obtain urine and throat swabs for the isolation of rubella virus or to obtain maternal and infant sera for IgG and IgM assays for antibodies to rubella.

TABLE 95–7. Diagnostic Criteria for Congenital Rubella Syndrome (CRS)

Confirmed case of CRS: At least one defect in category A or B below plus laboratory confirmation of rubella infection
Compatible case of CRS: Two defects from category A or one from A and one from B without laboratory confirmation

Category A
Cataract, congenital glaucoma (either one or both count as one)
Congenital heart disease
Loss of hearing
Pigmentary retinopathy

Category B
Purpura
Splenomegaly
Jaundice
Microcephaly
Mental retardation
Meningoencephalitis
Radiolucent bone disease

Laboratory Confirmation
Viral isolation
Cord IgM to rubella virus
Persistent or increasing levels of IgG antibodies to rubella virus over the first 6 mo of life

From Centers for Disease Control and Prevention: Rubella prevention. Recommendations of the Immunization Practices Advisory Committee (ACIP). *MMWR Morb Mortal Wkly Rep* 1990;39(RR–15):1–18.

Diagnostic Imaging

Radiographs of long bones are often recommended in the evaluation of suspected congenital rubella as well as congenital syphilis. Osseous lesions associated with congenital rubella infection consist of longitudinal radiolucent streaks that have been characterized as **celery stalking** (Fig. 95–7), and are sometimes associated with pathologic fractures. These lesions are not pathognomonic for congenital rubella and can also be seen with congenital CMV infection.

The bone lesions of both congenital rubella and congenital CMV infection take the radiologic appearance of ovoid and linear radiolucent streaks in the metaphyses of the long bones, particularly in the distal femur and the proximal tibia. Histologically, in congenital rubella infection there is focal metaphyseal osteoporosis, corre-

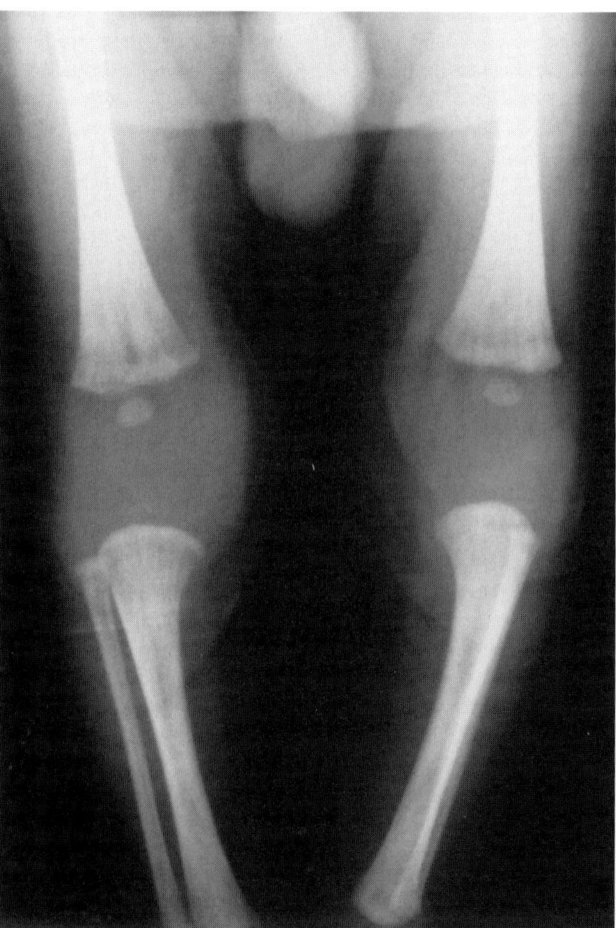

FIGURE 95–7. Congenital rubella in a neonate with a history of maternal rubella infection during pregnancy. A frontal radiograph of both lower extremities shows demineralization at the metaphyses of the long bones along with a pattern of vertical linear striations, known as celery-stalking, which is characteristic of in utero infection but is not specific for rubella.

sponding to areas of radiolucency, which is likely due to an insult in complex bone formation during the period of viremia. Bone lesions are associated with congenital rubella in more than one half of the cases.

TREATMENT

No specific therapy exists for congenital infection with rubella.

PREVENTION

Rubella immunization during childhood is the best preventive measure against congenital rubella syndrome. Passive immunization with standard immune globulin is ineffective in postexposure prophylaxis but, if given before exposure, should be effective in preventing maternal infection. For pregnant women exposed to rubella, postexposure immune globulin may be administered to attempt to prevent or ameliorate infection, but fetal protection cannot be assured (Chapter 24).

Although pregnant women should not receive rubella vaccine, inadvertent immunization of pregnant women with the rubella vaccine does not constitute a significant risk to the fetus and ordinarily should not be considered a reason to interrupt the pregnancy.

HUMAN PARVOVIRUS B19

ETIOLOGY

Human parvovirus B19 is a single-stranded DNA virus with 5,500 basepairs in the Parvoviridae family. The designation ''B19'' refers to the laboratory number used to identify the first clinical isolate. It is endemic among humans and is the causative agent of **erythema infectiosum,** acute self-limited arthralgias in adults, and an acute aplastic crisis in patients with a shortened erythrocyte survival, such as persons with sickle cell disease (Chapter 26). A primary viremia leads to replication in and lysis of erythroblastic progenitor cells, causing a transient anemia.

Transmission. Human parvovirus B19 is probably transmitted person to person in respiratory droplets and can also be transmitted transplacentally to the fetus. Human parvovirus B19 is not acquired from or transmitted to animals.

EPIDEMIOLOGY

Most persons acquire B19 between 5–17 years of age. Infection before conception produces immunity, which protects against intrauterine infection. Approximately 70% of women are immune. From 2–8% of susceptible women may become infected with human parvovirus B19 during pregnancy. Several factors increase the risk of maternal infection during pregnancy, including exposure to children, with school personnel and parents of school-age children at highest risk, and prevalence increases during late winter and early spring. There is also often an infectious cycle in communities, with major outbreaks of human parvovirus B19 occurring every 4–5 years.

PATHOGENESIS

During pregnancy, viremia during primary infection leads to transplacental passage of human parvovirus B19 and fetal infection. The fetal bone marrow and liver are sites of fetal erythroid progenitor cells, which are lysed by human parvovirus B19 infection. In affected fetuses, anemia occurs and leads to fetal heart failure and **hydrops fetalis,** which may develop at any time during pregnancy, and ultimately to fetal death, either spontaneous abortion or stillbirth with or without hydrops.

DIAGNOSIS

Congenital human parvovirus B19 infection is diagnosed by detecting IgM to the virus in the mother and demonstrating human parvovirus B19 DNA in either fetal tissues or neonatal serum or urine by PCR.

TREATMENT

Neither specific antiviral therapy nor prophylactic therapy is available for women exposed to human parvovirus B19 during pregnancy. Prophylactic administration of IVIG to prevent human parvovirus B19 infection is not recommended.

PROGNOSIS

The outlook for fetal survival is good, even if a susceptible woman acquires human parvovirus B19 infection during pregnancy. Regardless of the gestational age when maternal infection occurs, fetal death occurs in $\leq$2% of such pregnancies.

On the basis of detection of viremia or the presence of IgM antibodies to human parvovirus B19 at birth, approximately one half of live-born infants born to women with human parvovirus B19 infection during pregnancy may have had intrauterine human parvovirus B19 infection. These infants are apparently healthy at birth. It is not known whether apparently asymptomatic intrauterine infection with human parvovirus B19 causes any long-term sequelae.

PREVENTION

The greatest risk to pregnant women is from children in the household. There is occupational risk to daycare workers and teachers, especially those in contact with children 5–7 years of age. Effective measures for control of B19 infection in homes, daycare centers, and schools are limited. Because children are generally not infectious by the time the rash is present, exclusion of affected children from school is not reasonable. Good hand-washing and prompt disposal of facial tissues are practical measures that should help reduce transmission.

LYMPHOCYTIC CHORIOMENINGITIS VIRUS

LCM is a rare cause of congenital infection, with only 26 cases described in the medical literature since 1955. LCM is an arenavirus that infects primarily rodents. Infected mice and hamsters have no symptoms but shed LCM for prolonged periods of time (up to several months), primarily in urine, and transmit the virus to humans. Human-to-human transmission does not occur, which accounts for the low incidence of human infection.

Although most primary LCM infections of humans are probably asymptomatic, acute primary LCM infection may be accompanied by influenza-like symptoms consisting of fever, headache, nausea, and myalgias lasting up to 2 weeks. The diagnosis of infection with LCM can be established by isolation of the virus or by serologic testing. Serologic assays include an indirect immunofluorescence antibody test that may be positive as early as the first day of symptoms and a complement fixation test that may not be positive until 10 days or longer after the onset of illness. Neutralizing antibodies appear late, usually after the fourth week of infection, but persist for many years.

LCM infections in pregnant women have been associated with abortion and stillbirth, intrauterine infection, and perinatal infection. Intrauterine infection of the fetus may cause congenital hydrocephalus, chorioretinitis, and microcephaly with intracranial calcifications. Severe neurologic sequelae and neonatal death are common. Intrauterine disease due to LCM is usually suspected on the basis of a history of maternal contact with rodents during pregnancy, a compatible maternal illness, and an infant with symptoms. The diagnosis of intrauterine LCM infection is confirmed by viral isolation from CSF, blood, or urine or by the presence of IgM antibodies to LCM in the newborn. Persistence of IgG antibodies in an infant with symptoms beyond 6 months of age is also suggestive of intrauterine LCM infection. There is no treatment.

Because mice and hamsters may consistently shed LCM, pregnant women should avoid direct contact with rodents as well as with aerosolized excreta. Unless laboratory rodents are known to be free of LCM, pregnant laboratory workers should take special precautions to avoid infection during pregnancy.

TOXOPLASMA GONDII

ETIOLOGY

Toxoplasma gondii is a coccidian parasite of cats, with humans and other warm-blooded animals as intermediate hosts. The organism that has three forms: (1) an oocyst that produces sporozoites, (2) a proliferative form called a trophozoite, endozoite, or tachyzoite, and (3) a tissue cyst with an intracytoplasmic form called a cytozoite or bradyzoite. This organism is ubiquitous in nature and causes a variety of illnesses in humans. The reproductive cycle of the organism occurs in the intestines of all types of cats. It is only in the small intestine of cats that **oocysts** are formed, usually over a 5- to 24-day period after ingestion of *T. gondii* cysts. Oocysts are passed in cat feces, with peak oocyst production occurring 5–8 days after infection and up to 10 million oocysts shed daily. Once shed, the oocysts sporulate after 1–5 days in the soil and may remain infectious in warm, moist soils for as long as 12–18 months. **Sporulated oocysts** contain 2 **sporocysts,** each of which contains 4 **sporozoites.** The oocysts deposited in the soil are disseminated widely and eventually are ingested by humans and other mammals. Oocysts may be inactivated by simple measures, such as freezing or heating to a temperature of 45–55°C (113–131°F).

Ingestion of infectious spores by humans or other mammals results in the formation of **trophozoites,** the proliferative form of the organism during the acute stage of mammalian infection that invade many types of cells. Trophozoites can be cultivated in either tissue culture or mice. Both IgG and IgM antibodies develop during this stage. In the cells the trophozoites multiply within **vacuoles** approximately every 4–6 hours. The cytoplasm of infected cells becomes filled with trophozoites, and eventually the cells rupture, releasing trophozoites to invade contiguous cells by either phagocytosis or direct invasion. Infected tissue trophozoites may undergo **encystation** and the formation of **tissue cysts,** which may vary in size from very small cysts with only a few organisms to very large cysts of >100 μm containing more than 3,000 organisms. These cysts can be stained and readily identified in tissues. The cyst wall is usually identified with a periodic acid–Schiff stain in an infected host as early as 8 days after infection. Cysts can be typically found in the brain, eye, and heart and skeletal muscles. The tissue cysts are a latent form of the coccidian and may persist for life in an infected mammal and therefore are not an indication of recent infection.

Transmission. Humans are only incidental hosts in this zoonotic infection. Humans acquire infections with *T. gondii* by two principal routes, either by contact with soil or other objects contaminated with cat feces that contain sporulated oocysts or by eating poorly cooked meat that contains latent cysts.

EPIDEMIOLOGY

Infection rates with *T. gondii* vary worldwide depending on the risk of exposure. High rates of infection are found among persons living in France, where up to 80% of pregnant women have antibodies to *T. gondii* compared with 16–40% among pregnant women in the United States and London. Infection in France occurs primarily by ingestion of inadequately heated meats.

The highest risk for fetal infection with *T. gondii* occurs with primary infection during pregnancy, although several infected infants have been reported born to mothers who were seropositive before becoming pregnant. Reactivation of *T. gondii* after a primary infection occurs only in persons who become immunosuppressed. It is not known whether maternal HIV infection causes reactivation of *T. gondii* during pregnancy.

More than 99% of infants with congenital *T. gondii* infection have probably been infected after a primary maternal infection during pregnancy. Approximately 1 in 9,000 women in the United States acquires primary infection with *T. gondii* during pregnancy. This rate appears to have decreased about tenfold over the last 20 years. Primary infection rates in other areas of the world are generally between 0.25–2 infections per 1,000 live births.

PATHOGENESIS

Most primary infections with *T. gondii* in children and adults are asymptomatic. Symptoms, when present, usually include diffuse lymphadenopathy, most often without fever and occasionally accompanied by fatigue, malaise, headache, and sore throat. Toxoplasmosis is a benign and self-limited illness that may cause an infectious mononucleosis-like illness (Chapter 37).

During primary infection in a pregnant woman, the rate of transmission of *T. gondii* through the placenta to the fetus is related to gestational age. The highest rates of transplacental transmission occur during primary maternal infection late in pregnancy, with up to 80% of infants infected in utero, compared with <15% of infants in whose mothers primary maternal infection occurred during the first trimester of pregnancy. As expected, however, the severity of fetal disease is greatest among infants infected in early gestation. Infection during late gestation generally causes the lowest rate of disease, with fewer than 17% showing signs or symptoms of infection at birth, although as many as one half of the fetuses infected in the third trimester may have a subclinical infection that is progressive after birth. Of women infected during the second trimester, approximately 20% will transmit the infection to the fetus and about one half of the infected infants will have symptoms at birth. Infection during the first trimester produces the lowest rate of transmission to the fetus (<15%) but the highest rate of severe disease, with about 80% of infected infants exhibiting symptoms at birth.

SYMPTOMS AND CLINICAL MANIFESTATIONS

Most infected newborns have no symptoms or recognizable signs of infection at birth. The spectrum of manifestations that may be present at birth is very broad, ranging from nearly normal to severe hydrops fetalis, which complicates diagnosis based on specific signs and symptoms. The triad of hydrocephalus, chorioretinitis, and intracranial calcifications is typical in severely affected infants (Table 95–8). *T. gondii,* similar to CMV, *T. pallidum,* and rubella replicate in all organs and tissues, resulting in potential dysfunction of any organ. *T. gondii,* however, also has a tropism for neuronal tissue, and neurologic signs of disease are frequently more extensive than initially suspected. Particularly important neurologic signs that are diagnostic clues include convulsions, bulging fontanelles, nystagmus, an abnormal increase in the head circumference, or an elevated CSF protein level.

As in congenital CMV and rubella infections, late sequelae are important complications of congenital disease. In most cases, they are neurologic in nature and include severe mental retardation and blindness. Mild cases may not be recognized at birth, but the disease progresses and symptoms are recognized later. Chorioretinitis, often not apparent at birth, is a major problem postnatally because chorioretinal scars may lead to decreased visual acuity and blindness. Neurologic damage or eye lesions may appear in the first 3 months of life, particularly in infants without signs of generalized infection at birth, such as hepatosplenomegaly, hyperbilirubinemia, and lymphadenopathy.

DIAGNOSIS

The diagnosis of congenital toxoplasmosis is difficult. The diagnosis is usually established by serologic testing but can also be established by PCR or demonstration of trophozoites in tissues, such as a brain biopsy specimen, bone marrow aspirate, body fluids, or placental tissue. It is frequently difficult, however, to identify trophozoites in tissues by the usual histopathologic methods, and immunofluorescence antibody techniques may be necessary. *T. gondii* can also be cultured from infected tissues or blood with the use of either mouse inoculation or infection of appropriate cells in tissue culture. PCR performed on amniotic fluid has been shown to be useful for diagnosis of intrauterine infection.

TABLE 95–8. Common Early and Late Manifestations of Congenital Toxoplasmosis

Early	Late
Chorioretinitis	Mental retardation
Elevated CSF protein	Convulsions
Anemia	Spasticity and palsies
Convulsions	Severely impaired vision
Intracranial calcifications	Hydrocephalus or microcephaly
Jaundice	Deafness
Hydrocephalus	
Splenomegaly	
Lymphadenopathy	
Hepatomegaly	
Microcephaly	

Serologic Diagnosis. The serologic diagnosis of congenital toxoplasmosis is complicated by the high seroprevalence in most populations and the persistence of both IgM and IgG antibody at high levels for years after infection. Serologic diagnosis generally relies on one of several different tests to detect antibodies to *T. gondii,* including **Sabin-Feldman dye test** for IgG antibodies; IgM-, IgA-, and IgG-ELISA; IgM- and IgG-IFA; **agglutination test** for IgG; **IgM-immunosorbent agglutination assay (IgM-ISAGA);** and the **differential agglutination test (AC/HS test).** The Sabin-Feldman dye test is the reference standard, but it requires live organisms and is not widely available. The IgG-ELISA is the most widely used test. The agglutination test uses formalin-preserved whole tachyzoites and is inexpensive. The AC/HS test can be used to distinguish acute from chronic stages of infection.

A serologic diagnosis of congenital toxoplasmosis is established by positive tests for IgM or IgA antibodies in the newborn or by an IgG titer in the newborn that is equal to or greater than the mother's titer at birth and that either rises or fails to fall during infancy. High titers of IgG antibodies to *T. gondii* may inhibit the IgM reaction, and the presence of rheumatoid factor may produce false-positive results. The IgM-IFA detects only approximately 25% of infected newborns, and the IgM-ELISA detects only approximately 80%. The IgM-ISAGA test is recommended. These tests should be performed or confirmed in a laboratory that employs experienced personnel because false-negative and false-positive results can occur. Testing for specific *T. gondii* IgA antibody is more sensitive than IgM testing for detecting congenital toxoplasmosis in the neonatal period but is available only in research laboratories. Interpretation of serologic tests for infants born of women treated for toxoplasmosis during pregnancy is difficult because infection before the 20th week of pregnancy, or treatment of maternal infection may diminish both IgG and IgM antibody responses.

Diagnostic Imaging

In utero infection with toxoplasmosis or CMV may produce dystrophic calcification within the brain that can be detected on plain radiographs (Fig. 13–8). A CT scan shows the calcification in greater detail with finer anatomic localization (Fig. 95–8).

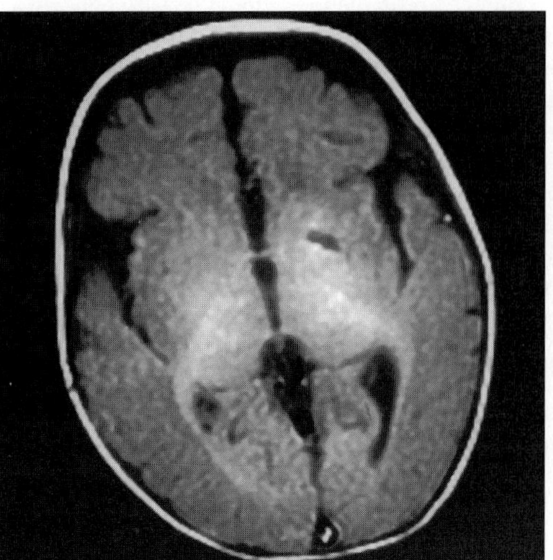

FIGURE 95–8. CT image of the brain of a 2-month-old infant showing parenchymal and subependymal punctate calcifications throughout the cerebral hemispheres typical of symptomatic congenital *T. gondii* infection. The ventricles and cortical sulci are slightly prominent, suggesting a mild degree of diffuse cerebral atrophy.

TABLE 95–9. Therapy for Congenital Toxoplasmosis

First 6 Months
Pyrimethamine 15 mg/m²/day or 1 mg/kg/day (max 25 mg) once daily PO following an initial loading dose of 2 mg/kg/day for 2 days
and
Sulfadiazine 100 mg/kg/day divided bid PO
and
Leucovorin 5–10 mg 3 times a week PO*
NOTE: Consider adding corticosteroids (prednisone 1 mg/kg/day divided bid) for infants and chorioretinitis, high concentrations of CSF protein (≥1000 mg/dL), or systemic or generalized infection until resolution of elevated CSF protein or improvement of chorioretinitis

Next 6 Months
Pyrimethamine 15 mg/m²/day or 1 mg/kg/day (max 25 mg) three times per week PO
and
Sulfadiazine 100 mg/kg/day divided bid PO
and
Leucovorin 10 mg 3 times a week PO*

*The dosage may be adjusted for megaloblastic anemia, granulocytopenia, or thrombocytopenia. Complete blood counts should be monitored.

TREATMENT

Specific therapies are available for congenital toxoplasmosis (Table 95–9). In infants with congenital toxoplasmosis a prospective trial (Roizen et al., 1995) of treatment using pyrimethamine and sulfadiazine for 1 year showed that neurologic and developmental outcomes were significantly improved for children treated for 1 year compared with children treated for only 1 month or with untreated children. Therapy is indicated for congenital *T. gondii* infection and should be undertaken after contacting the primary investigator for a major study now in progress in the United States, Dr. Rima McLeod at the University of Chicago Medical Center (telephone 773-834-4152).

Prednisone, 1 mg/kg/day in two divided doses orally, may be beneficial for children with active chorioretinitis or CSF protein levels ≥1 g/dL. Corticosteroids should be used only with specific treatment and should be tapered and discontinued once active inflammation subsides, as demonstrated by improvement of chorioretinitis by serial ophthalmologic examinations or a fall in CSF protein level to <1 g/dL.

Leucovorin (folic acid) is administered during and for 1 week after pyrimethamine therapy. The CBC and platelet counts should be monitored during therapy, and the dosage of leucovorin should be adjusted for megaloblastic anemia, granulocytopenia, or thrombocytopenia.

PROGNOSIS

There is considerable variability in outcome even with treatment. Children without hydrocephalus or with obstructive hydrocephalus responsive to CSF shunting who are treated for 1 year have had normal or near-normal neurologic and developmental outcomes. Treated children have impaired cognitive function compared with uninfected siblings but do not demonstrate progressive neurologic or developmental deterioration. Poor prognostic factors include hydrocephalus ex vacuo present at birth, high CSF protein level (>300 mg/dL), and lack of response to shunting.

Visual loss is the most frequent sequela of congenital toxoplasmosis. Chorioretinitis in one or both eyes is present in approximately two thirds of infected infants, with lesions affecting the macula in approximately one half of these infants. Treatment does not appear to improve retinal damage present at the initiation of therapy but does appear to prevent progression of visual loss. There is little correlation of visual loss with neurologic and developmental outcome.

Seizures in the perinatal period require anticonvulsant therapy that can often be discontinued within the first few months of life. In some children there may be an onset of convulsive disorders later in childhood. Tone and motor abnormalities resolve in approximately 60% of neonates with such abnormalities at birth.

PREVENTION

Simple hygienic measures should prevent maternal infection during pregnancy. All seronegative pregnant women and all pregnant women in the United States should be advised to (1) eat only well-cooked meats, (2) wash hands frequently after handling uncooked meats, (3) prevent access to food by flies and roaches, which may transmit the parasite, (4) avoid contact with materials contaminated with cat feces, (5) always wear gloves when working in the garden or soil or when handling materials that have been contaminated with feces, and (6) change cat litter daily to avoid an accumulation of infectious oocysts, because the oocysts require 1–5 days to sporulate and become infectious following shedding by the cat.

Pregnant women can be tested for antibodies to *T. gondii* at the beginning of pregnancy. This would not be cost-effective in the United States because approximately 80% of women are seronegative, but it has been advocated. Prenatal antibiotic therapy after toxoplasmosis during pregnancy has no apparent impact on the fetomaternal transmission rate but reduces the rate of sequelae among the infected infants. The benefit is greater with earlier initiation of therapy.

REVIEW

Remington JS, Klein JO (editors): *Infectious Diseases of the Fetus and Newborn Infant,* 5th ed. Philadelphia, WB Saunders, 2001.

Treponema pallidum

Beck-Sague C, Alexander ER: Failure of benzathine penicillin G therapy in early congenital syphilis. *Pediatr Infect Dis J* 1987;6:1061–4.

Beeram MR, Chopde N, Dawood Y, et al: Lumbar puncture in the evaluation of possible asymptomatic congenital syphilis in neonates. *J Pediatr* 1996; 128:125–9.

Centers for Disease Control and Prevention: Congenital syphilis—United States, 2000. *MMWR Morb Mortal Wkly Rep* 2001;50:273–7.

Chhabra RS, Brion LP, Castro M, et al: Comparison of maternal sera, cord blood neonatal sera for detecting presumptive congenital syphilis: Relationship with maternal treatment. *Pediatrics* 1993;91:88–91.

Dorfman DH, Glaser JH: Congenital syphilis presenting in infants after the newborn period. *N Engl J Med* 1990;323:1299–302.

Dunn RA, Zenker PN: Why radiographs are useful in evaluation of neonates suspected of having congenital syphilis. *Radiology* 1992;182:639–40.

Hira SK, Bhat GJ, Patel JB, et al: Early congenital syphilis: Clinico-radiologic features in 202 patients. *Sex Transm Dis* 1985;12:177–83.

Larsen SA, Steiner BM, Rudolph AH: Laboratory diagnosis and interpretation of tests for syphilis. *Clin Microbiol Rev* 1995;8:1–21.

Litwin CM, Hill HR: Serologic and DNA-based testing for congenital and perinatal infections. *Pediatr Infect Dis J* 1997;16:1166–75.

Mobley JA, McKeown RE, Jackson KL, et al: Risk factors for congenital syphilis in infants of women with syphilis in South Carolina. *Am J Public Health* 1998;88:597–602.

Moyer VA, Schneider V, Yetman R, et al: Contribution of long-bone radiographs to the management of congenital syphilis in the newborn infant. *Arch Pediatr Adolesc Med* 1998;152:353–7.

Paryani SG, Vaughn AJ, Crosby M, et al: Treatment of asymptomatic congenital syphilis: Benzathine versus procaine penicillin G therapy. *J Pediatr* 1994;125:471–5.

Rawstron SA, Vetrano J, Tannis G, et al: Congenital syphilis: Detection of *Treponema pallidum* in stillborns. *Clin Infect Dis* 1997;24:24–7.

Risser WL, Hwang LY: Problems in the current case definitions of congenital syphilis. *J Pediatr* 1996;129:499–505.

Sanchez PJ: Laboratory tests for congenital syphilis. *Pediatr Infect Dis J* 1998;17:70–1.

Sison CG, Ostrea EMJ, Reyes MP, et al: The resurgence of congenital syphilis: A cocaine-related problem. *J Pediatr* 1997;130:289–92.

Stamos JK, Rowley AH: Timely diagnosis of congenital infections. *Pediatr Clin North Am* 1994;41:1017–33.

Stoll BJ: Congenital syphilis: Evaluation and management of neonates born to mothers with reactive serologic tests for syphilis. *Pediatr Infect Dis J* 1994;13:845–52.

Cytomegalovirus

Barbi M, Binda S, Primache V, et al: Cytomegalovirus in peripheral blood leukocytes of infants with congenital or postnatal infection. *Pediatr Infect Dis J* 1996;898–903.

Boppana SB, Fowler KB, Vaid Y, et al: Neuroradiographic findings in the newborn period and long-term outcome in children with symptomatic congenital cytomegalovirus infection. *Pediatrics* 1997;99:409–14.

Demmler GJ: Congenital cytomegalovirus infection. *Semin Pediatr Neurol* 1994;1:36–42.

Demmler GJ: Congenital cytomegalovirus infection and disease. *Adv Pediatr Infect Dis* 1996;11:135–62.

Fowler KB, McCollister FP, Dahle AJ, et al: Progressive and fluctuating sensorineural hearing loss in children with asymptomatic congenital cytomegalovirus infection. *J Pediatr* 1997;130:624–30.

Fowler KB, Stagno S, Pass RF, et al: The outcome of congenital cytomegalovirus infection in relation to maternal antibody status. *N Engl J Med* 1992;326:663–7.

Istas AS, Demmler GJ, Dobbins JG, et al: Surveillance for congenital cytomegalovirus disease: A report from the National Congenital Cytomegalovirus Disease Registry. *Clin Infect Dis* 1995;20:665–70.

Ivarsson SA, Lernmark B, Svanberg L: Ten-year clinical, developmental, and intellectual follow-up of children with congenital cytomegalovirus infection without neurologic symptoms at one year of age. *Pediatrics* 1997;99:800–3.

Kashden J, Frison S, Fowler K, et al: Intellectual assessment of children with asymptomatic congenital cytomegalovirus infection. *J Dev Behav Pediatr* 1998;19:254–9.

Murph JR, Souza IE, Dawson JD, et al: Epidemiology of congenital cytomegalovirus infection: Maternal risk factors and molecular analysis of cytomegalovirus strains. *Am J Epidemiol* 1998;147:940–7.

Mussi-Pinhata MM, Yamamoto AY, Figueiredo LT, et al: Congenital and perinatal cytomegalovirus infection in infants born to mothers infected with human immunodeficiency virus. *J Pediatr* 1998;132:285–90.

Stagno S, Pass RF, Cloud G, et al: Primary cytomegalovirus infection in pregnancy: Incidence, transmission to fetus, and clinical outcome. *JAMA* 1986;256:1904–8.

Whitley RJ, Cloud G, Gruber W, et al: Ganciclovir treatment of symptomatic congenital cytomegalovirus infection: Results of a phase II study. National Institute of Allergy and Infectious Diseases Collaborative Antiviral Study Group. *J Infect Dis* 1997;175:1080–6.

Herpes Simplex Virus

Baldwin S, Whitley RJ: Intrauterine herpes simplex virus infection. *Teratology* 1989;39:1–10.

Brown ZA, Selke S, Zeh J, et al: The acquisition of herpes simplex virus during pregnancy. *N Engl J Med* 1997;337:509–15.

Hutto C, Arvin A, Jacobs R, et al: Intrauterine herpes simplex virus infections. *J Pediatr* 1987;110:97–101.

Parish WR: Intrauterine herpes simplex virus infection hydranencephaly and a nonvesicular rash in an infant. *Int J Dermatol* 1989;28:397–401.

Prober CG, Hensleigh PA, Boucher FD, et al: Use of routine viral cultures at delivery to identify neonates exposed to herpes simplex virus infection. *N Engl J Med* 1988;318:887–91.

Robb JA, Benirschke K, Barmeyer R: Intrauterine latent herpes simplex virus infection: I. Spontaneous abortion. *Hum Pathol* 1986;17:1196–1209.

Whitley R, Arvin A, Prober C, et al: A controlled trial comparing vidarabine with acyclovir in neonatal herpes simplex virus infection. The National Institute of Allergy and Infectious Diseases Collaborative Antiviral Study Group. *N Engl J Med* 1991;324:444–9.

Whitley R, Arvin A, Prober C: Predictors of morbidity and mortality in neonates with herpes simplex virus infections. The National Institute of Allergy and Infectious Diseases Collaborative Antiviral Study Group. *N Engl J Med* 1991;324:450–4.

Varicella-Zoster Virus

Chapman SJ: Varicella in pregnancy. *Semin Perinatol* 1998;22:339–46.

Enders G: Management of varicella-zoster contact and infection in pregnancy using a standardized varicella-zoster ELISA test. *Postgrad Med J* 1985;61:23–30.

Figueroa-Damian R, Arredondo-Garcia JL: Perinatal outcome of pregnancies complicated with varicella infection during the first 20 weeks of gestation. *Am J Perinatol* 1997;14:411–4.

Miller E, Cradock-Watson JE, Ridehalgh MK: Outcome in newborn babies given anti-varicella-zoster immunoglobulin after perinatal maternal infection with varicella-zoster virus. *Lancet* 1989;2:371–3.

Mouly F, Mirlesse V, Meritet JF, et al: Prenatal diagnosis of fetal varicella-zoster virus infection with polymerase chain reaction of amniotic fluid in 107 cases. *Am J Obstet Gynecol* 1997;177:894–8.

Paryani SG, Arvin AM: Intrauterine infection with varicella-zoster virus after maternal varicella. *N Engl J Med* 1986;314:1542–6.

Scharf A, Scherr O, Enders G, et al: Virus detection in the fetal tissue of a premature delivery with a congenital varicella syndrome: A case report. *J Perinat Med* 1990;18:317–22.

Rubella Virus

Centers for Disease Control and Prevention: Control and prevention of rubella: Evaluation and management of suspected outbreaks, rubella in pregnant women, and surveillance for congenital rubella syndrome. *MMWR Morb Mortal Wkly Rep* 2001;50(RR-12):1–23.

Cullen A, Brown S, Cafferkey M, et al: Current use of the TORCH screen in the diagnosis of congenital infection. *J Infect* 1998;36:185–8.

Frey TK: Neurological aspects of rubella virus infection. *Intervirology* 1997;40:167–75.

Gregg N: Congenital cataract following German measles in the mother. *Trans Ophthalmol Soc Aust* 1941;3:35–46.

Grillner L, Forsgren M, Barr B, et al: Outcome of rubella during pregnancy with special reference to the 17th and 24th weeks of gestation. *Scand J Infect Dis* 1983;15:321–5.

Gyorkos TW, Tannenbaum TN, Abrahamowicz M, et al: Evaluation of rubella screening in pregnant women. *CMAJ* 1998;159:1091–7.

Kaplan KM, Cochi SL, Edmonds LD, et al: A profile of mothers giving birth to infants with congenital rubella syndrome: An assessment of risk factors. *Am J Dis Child* 1990;144:118–23.

Katow S: Rubella virus genome diagnosis during pregnancy and mechanism of congenital rubella. *Intervirology* 1998;41:163–9.

Lindegren ML, Fehrs LJ, Hadler SC, et al: Update: Rubella and congenital rubella syndrome, 1980–1990. *Epidemiol Rev* 1991;13:341–8.

Murph JR: Rubella and syphilis: Continuing causes of congenital infection in the 1990s. *Semin Pediatr Neurol* 1994;1:26–35.

O'Neill JF: The ocular manifestations of congenital infection: A study of the early effect and long-term outcome of maternally transmitted rubella and toxoplasmosis. *Trans Am Ophthalmol Soc* 1998;96:813–79.

Pustowoit B, Liebert UG: Predictive value of serological tests in rubella virus infection during pregnancy. *Intervirology* 1998;41:170–7.

Revello MG, Baldanti F, Sarasini A, et al: Prenatal diagnosis of rubella virus infection by direct detection and semiquantitation of viral RNA in clinical samples by reverse transcription-PCR. *J Clin Microbiol* 1997;35:708–13.

Rubella and congenital rubella syndrome—United States, 1994–1997. *MMWR Morb Mortal Wkly Rep* 1997;46:350–4.

Schluter WW, Reef SE, Redd SC, et al: Changing epidemiology of congenital rubella syndrome in the United States. *J Infect Dis* 1998;178:636–41.

Watson JC, Hadler SC, Dykewicz CA, et al: Measles, mumps, and rubella—vaccine use and strategies for elimination of measles, rubella, and congenital rubella syndrome and control of mumps: Recommendations of the Advisory Committee on Immunization Practices (ACIP). *MMWR Morb Mortal Wkly Rep* 1998;47:1–57.

Human Parvovirus B19

Brown KE, Young NS: Human parvovirus B19 infections in infants and children. *Adv Pediatr Infect Dis* 1997;13:101–26.

Brown KE, Young NS: Parvovirus B19 in human disease. *Ann Rev Med* 1997;48:59–67.

Forestier F, Tissot JD, Vial Y, et al: Haematological parameters of parvovirus B19 infection in 13 fetuses with hydrops foetalis. *Br J Haematol* 1999;104:925–7.

Harger JH, Adler SP, Koch WC, et al: Prospective evaluation of 618 pregnant women exposed to parvovirus B19: Risks and symptoms. *Obstet Gynecol* 1998;91:413–20.

Koch WC, Adler SP: Human parvovirus B19 infections in women of childbearing age and within families. *Pediatr Infect Dis J* 1989;8:83–7.

Koch WC, Harger JH, Barnstein B, et al: Serologic and virologic evidence for frequent intrauterine transmission of human parvovirus B19 with a primary maternal infection during pregnancy. *Pediatr Infect Dis J* 1998; 17:489–94.

Levy R, Weissman A, Blomberg G, et al: Infection by parvovirus B19 during pregnancy: A review. *Obstet Gynecol Surv* 1997;52:254–9.

Miller E, Fairley CK, Cohen BJ, et al: Immediate and long term outcome of human parvovirus B19 infection in pregnancy. *Br J Obstet Gynaecol* 1998;105:174–8.

Plachouras N, Stefanidis K, Andronikou S, et al: Severe nonimmune hydrops fetalis and congenital corneal opacification secondary to human parvovirus B19 infection. A case report. *J Reprod Med* 1999;44:377–80.

Rodis JF, Rodner C, Hansen AA, et al: Long-term outcome of children following maternal human parvovirus B19 infection. *Obstet Gynecol* 1998;91:125–8.

Skjoldebrand-Sparre L, Fridell E, Nyman M, et al: A prospective study of antibodies against parvovirus B19 in pregnancy. *Acta Obstet Gynecol Scand* 1996;75:336–9.

Lymphocytic Choriomeningitis Virus

Barton LL, Budd SC, Morfitt WS: Congenital lymphocytic choriomeningitis virus infection in twins. *Pediatr Infect Dis J* 1993;12:942–6.

Larsen PD, Chartrand SA, Tomashek KM, et al: Hydrocephalus complicating lymphocytic choriomeningitis virus infection. *Pediatr Infect Dis J* 1993;12:528–31.

Wright R, Johnson D, Neumann M, et al: Congenital lymphocytic choriomeningitis virus syndrome: A disease that mimics congenital toxoplasmosis or cytomegalovirus infection. *Pediatrics* 1997;100(1):E9.

Toxoplasma gondii

Boyer KM: Diagnosis and treatment of congenital toxoplasmosis. *Adv Pediatr Infect Dis* 1996;11:449–67.

Centers for Disease Control and Prevention: Preventing congenital toxoplasmosis. *MMWR Morb Mortal Wkly Rep* 2000;49(RR-2):57–75.

Daffos F, Forestier F, Capella-Pavlovsky M, et al: Prenatal management of 746 pregnancies at risk for congenital toxoplasmosis. *N Engl J Med* 1988;318:271–5.

Foulon W, Pinon JM, Stray-Pedersen B, et al: Prenatal diagnosis of congenital toxoplasmosis: A multicenter evaluation of different diagnostic parameters. *Am J Obstet Gynecol* 1999;181:843–7.

Foulon W, Villena I, Stray-Pedersen B, et al: Treatment of toxoplasmosis during pregnancy: A multicenter study of impact on fetal transmission and children's sequelae at age 1 year. *Am J Obstet Gynecol* 1999; 180:410–5.

Friedman S, Ford-Jones LE, Toi A, et al: Congenital toxoplasmosis: Prenatal diagnosis, treatment and postnatal outcome. *Prenat Diagn* 1999;19: 330–3.

McCabe R, Remington JS: Toxoplasmosis: The time has come. *N Engl J Med* 1988;318:313–5.

McLeod R, Johnson J, Estes R, et al: Immunogenetics in pathogenesis of and protection against toxoplasmosis. *Curr Top Microbiol Immunol* 1996;219:95–112.

Naessens A, Jenum PA, Pollak A, et al: Diagnosis of congenital toxoplasmosis in the neonatal period: A multicenter evaluation. *J Pediatr* 1999; 135:714–9.

O'Neill JF: The ocular manifestations of congenital infection: A study of the early effect and long-term outcome of maternally transmitted rubella and toxoplasmosis. *Trans Am Ophthalmol Soc* 1998;96:813–79.

Roizen N, Swisher CN, Stein MA, et al: Neurologic and developmental outcome in treated congenital toxoplasmosis. *Pediatrics* 1995;95:11–20.

Sever JL, Ellenberg JH, Ley AC, et al: Toxoplasmosis: Maternal and pediatric findings in 23,000 pregnancies. *Pediatrics* 1988;82:181–92.

Stray-Pedersen B: Infants potentially at risk for congenital toxoplasmosis: A prospective study. *Am J Dis Child* 1980;134:638–42.

Villena I, Aubert D, Leroux B, et al: Pyrimethamine-sulfadoxine treatment of congenital toxoplasmosis: Follow-up of 78 cases between 1980 and 1997. Reims Toxoplasmosis Group. *Scand J Infect Dis* 1998;30: 295–300.

Vogel N, Kirisits M, Michael E, et al: Congenital toxoplasmosis transmitted from an immunologically competent mother infected before conception. *Clin Infect Dis* 1996;23:1055–60.

Wallon M, Caudie C, Rubio S, et al: Value of cerebrospinal fluid cytochemical examination for the diagnosis of congenital toxoplasmosis at birth in France. *Pediatr Infect Dis J* 1998;17:705–10.

CHAPTER 96

Perinatal Bacterial and Fungal Infections

Robert S. Baltimore

Infections or suspected infections in neonates represent a large proportion of the practice of pediatric infectious diseases. Perinatal bacterial and fungal infections in newborns often present with sepsis and usually without focal signs of infection. The term **neonatal sepsis** generally refers to systemic symptomatic bacterial, fungal, and viral infections that, on earliest presentation, may be associated with any gradation of symptoms from only subtle feeding disturbances to frank septic shock.

Many focal infections such as meningitis, pneumonia, and urinary tract infections that can occur in other age groups may occur in neonates as well, but infections in neonates have unique elements that differ from those in older age groups. However, in neonates, focal signs and symptoms due to localized infections may be clinically imperceptible and thus difficult to differentiate on initial presentation from generalized or bloodstream infections. Some distinctive focal bacterial infections in neonates, such as scalp abscesses, mastitis, and omphalitis, have special epidemiologic and clinical features. These focal infections may or may not be associated with bacteremia or sepsis. Necrotizing enterocolitis, although perhaps not primarily an infectious disease, is often complicated by bacterial invasion of the intestinal wall and secondary bacteremia and is a special problem of the stressed neonate.

Neonatal infections may be caused by bacterial species resident in the maternal vagina, bacterial species transmitted from persons or the environment, or bacterial or fungal species resident on the infant's skin. Some perinatally transmitted viral infections can also present as neonatal sepsis (Chapter 97). In addition, some microbial species cause intrauterine infections that present as congenital infections in the newborn (Chapter 95).

SEPSIS

ETIOLOGY

Several bacterial and fungal species are particularly associated with neonatal sepsis. The organisms that cause neonatal sepsis are the same species that cause neonatal meningitis (Chapter 52). Since the early 1970s, when group B *Streptococcus* emerged as a major cause of neonatal sepsis and meningitis, group B *Streptococcus* and *Escherichia coli* have accounted for approximately 60–80% of cases of early-onset neonatal sepsis and meningitis (Table 96–1). Since perinatal prophylaxis has been encouraged, the rate of group B *Streptococcus* infections has fallen; the CDC has predicted that an 80% drop is possible. All of the major types of group B *Streptococcus* **(types Ia, Ib, Ia/c, II, III, IV, and V)** may colonize women and may cause early-onset sepsis in the neonate, with clinical presentations distributed among sepsis, meningitis, and pneumonia. Type III strains appear to have special virulence properties for the development of meningitis and cause >85% of cases of early-onset meningitis and most late-onset group B streptococcal infections, which most often present as meningitis and sepsis.

There are >100 capsular serotypes of *E. coli,* but **K1 serotype** strains cause >75% of cases of *E. coli* neonatal meningitis and are the most common cause of neonatal *E. coli* sepsis. *E. coli* neonatal infections due to serotype K1 strains are also more severe than *E. coli* infections due to non-KI strains. Thus the K1 carbohydrate is a virulence factor, and it is probable that lack of anti-K1 antibody in the newborn is a susceptibility factor for severe infection due to these strains. Extrapolation from in vitro and animal studies suggests that the transplacentally passed IgG antibodies for group B *Streptococcus* and *E. coli* act as opsonins. It is unclear why the susceptibility for either of these organisms is so much greater in the neonatal period than later in infancy. It is less clear what the pathogenic mechanisms and susceptibility factors are for other organisms that cause early-onset sepsis, but immunologic immaturity is certainly important.

The microbiologic epidemiology of late-onset neonatal sepsis has changed over time. It is important to recognize these trends because they provide the basis for rational empirical antibiotic therapy. There is a tendency for certain species to emerge and cause an increased proportion of infections for a limited period of time, such as the increase in *Staphylococcus aureus* in the late 1950s and early 1960s and the emergence of group B *Streptococcus* in the early 1970s, which continues still. An increase in coagulase-negative staphylococci and *Candida* over the past two decades appears to be due to the increased survival among extremely premature infants, the use of parenteral nutrition, and the frequent use of broad-spectrum antibiotics. In many institutions coagulase-negative staphylococci are now the most common cause of all cases of neonatal bacteremia. Continuous surveillance of the microbiologic epidemiology and the antimicrobial susceptibilities should be routine for all neonatal intensive care units.

EPIDEMIOLOGY

The rate of sepsis in infants born at any hospital varies according to the perinatal risk factors in the community of women who deliver there. Economic standards, availability of prenatal care, geographic variations, and outbreaks of cases caused by particular species of pathogens may each play a role in determining the overall rate. Although there is some year-to-year variation, the rate of neonatal sepsis has been 2–4 per 1,000 live births since 1980 in the United States, with a worldwide range of 1–8 per 1,000 live births; higher rates are reported in developing countries. The incidence of sepsis among infant boys is greater, sometimes double, that among infant girls. Low birth weight is associated with a much higher rate of sepsis (Table 96–2).

Neonatal infections are usually classified according to time and mode of onset (Table 96–3). They are grouped into three categories: (1) **congenital infection,** acquired in utero by **vertical transmis-**

TABLE 96–1. Bacteria and Fungi Causing Neonatal Sepsis at Yale–New Haven Hospital, 1928–1988

Organism	Percent in Each Study Period*					
	1928–1932	1933–1943	1944–1957	1958–1965	1966–1978	1979–1988
Gram-positive bacterial species						
Group B *Streptococcus*	—	5	6	1	32	37
Group D *Streptococcus*	—	—	2	10	4	8
Nongrouped and other streptococci	38	36	10	—	—	—
Viridans streptococci	—	2	—	3	1	3
Streptococcus pneumoniae	5	11	5	3	1	1
Staphylococcus aureus	28	9	13	3	5	3
Coagulase-negative staphylococci	—	—	—	1	1	8
Listeria monocytogenes	—	2	2	—	1	1
Gram-negative aerobic bacteria						
Escherichia coli	26	25	37	45	32	20
Klebsiella and *Enterobacter*	—	—	—	11	12	3
Pseudomonas aeruginosa	3	—	21	15	2	3
Haemophilus	—	—	—	1	4	5
Salmonella	—	—	2	—	1	1
Gram-negative anaerobic bacteria	—	—	—	—	1	3
Fungi	—	—	—	—	2	1
Others	—	9	3	5	5	1
Total number of cases	39	44	62	73	239	147
Mortality rate	87%	90%	67%	45%	26%	16%

— = none.
*Percentages do not always equal 100% because of rounding. Only infants born at Yale–New Haven Hospital with sepsis occurring within the first 30 days of life are included.
Adapted from Gladstone IM, Ehrenkranz RA, Edberg SC, et al: A ten-year review of neonatal sepsis and comparison with the previous fifty-year experience. *Pediatr Infect Dis J* 1990;9:819–25.

sion with onset before birth; (2) **early-onset neonatal infections,** acquired by **vertical transmission** in the perinatal period, either shortly before or during the process of birth; and (3) **late-onset neonatal infections,** acquired by **horizontal transmission** in the nursery. Opinion differs as to the appropriate age for dividing early-onset from late-onset infections; the range is 2–7 days of age. Because most early-onset bacterial infections manifest within the first 2 days of life, a substantial amount of the literature divides early from late onset at 2 days of age.

A **neonate** is defined as an infant in the first month of life, so traditionally infections that have an onset within the first month of life are considered to be neonatal infections. A change in practice since approximately 1980 is that neonatal intensive care units now frequently provide continuing care for severely premature and chronically ill infants up to several months of age, frequently up to 1 year of age. The term **late, late-onset infections** may be used to indicate nosocomial infections acquired in a neonatal intensive care unit with onset at age greater than 1 month.

TABLE 96–2. Birth Weight–Specific Sepsis Rate Within the First 30 Days of Life for Infants Born at Yale–New Haven Hospital, 1978–1988

Birth Weight (g)	No. of Infants	No. of Cases of Sepsis per 1,000 Live Births
600–999	406	86
1,000–1,499	618	45
1,500–2,499	2,269	14
>2,500	50,280	1
All infants >600	53,573	2.7

Adapted from Gladstone IM, Ehrenkranz RA, Edberg SC, et al: A ten-year review of neonatal sepsis and comparison with the previous fifty-year experience. *Pediatr Infect Dis J* 1990;9:819–25.

Prenatal-Onset and Early-Onset Infections. Bacterial infections caused by rapidly dividing highly pathogenic organisms that have an onset long before birth usually result in intrauterine death. It is not usually possible to distinguish between infections acquired shortly before birth and those acquired as a result of contact with maternal flora during the process of delivery. It is generally assumed, however, that early-onset infections that are manifest within the first few hours of life, especially if pneumonia is already present, probably result from contamination of the fetus through defects or rupture of the fetal membranes before delivery.

Several risk factors for early-onset postnatal infections have a very strong influence on infection rates (Table 96–3). Healthy full-term infants born without incident or complications actually have the lowest incidence of infection, including nosocomial infections, of any population of hospitalized patients (Table 96–2). Infants at increased risk of early-onset postnatal infections are those with risk factors, including prematurity, birth to a mother with an infection, birth to a mother who has had stress because of a complication of the pregnancy or the delivery, and rupture of membranes for >6 hours. Prolonged premature rupture of the membranes often results in amnionitis, with the risk of early-onset infection increasing with longer duration of rupture. Otherwise healthy full-term infants born to mothers with amnionitis have a rate of infection of only approximately 1%, compared with 20–25% for premature infants born to mothers with amnionitis, probably because premature infants have relatively poor immune protective mechanisms with disability roughly proportional to the degree of prematurity

TABLE 96–3. Relationship of Time of Onset of Neonatal Infection and Mode of Transmission of Infection

Time of Onset	Age at Onset of Infection	Mode of Transmission of Infection	Major Risk Factors	Most Common Organisms
Prenatal	Prior to birth	Transplacental or ascending	Maternal infection, usually primary infection Prolonged premature rupture of membranes	Cytomegalovirus Syphilis Toxoplasmosis Maternal vaginal flora Human immunodeficiency virus
Early onset	Birth to 2–5 days	Maternal flora transmitted peripartum	Prolonged premature rupture of membranes Prematurity Septic or traumatic delivery Fetal anoxia Male sex Maternal infection (especially urogenital) Maternal poverty, pre-eclampsia, cardiac disease, diabetes mellitus	*Escherichia coli* Group B *Streptococcus* *Klebsiella pneumoniae* *Enterococcus* *Listeria monocytogenes* Other enteric gram-negative bacilli species
Late onset	>2–5 to 30 days	Nosocomial	Intravascular catheters Endotracheal intubation Assisted ventilation Surgery (including necrotizing enterocolitis) Contact with hands of colonized personnel Contact with contaminated equipment	Those causing early onset sepsis *Staphylococcus aureus* Coagulase-negative staphylococci *Pseudomonas aeruginosa* *Candida*
Late, late onset	≥30 days	Nosocomial	Indwelling intravascular devices Extreme prematurity Bronchopulmonary dysplasia Short-gut syndrome Complex congenital malformations Previous broad-spectrum antibiotic therapy	*Staphylococcus aureus* Coagulase-negative staphylococci *Pseudomonas aeruginosa* *Candida* Antibiotic-resistant gram-negative bacilli species

(Chapter 5). Similarly, compared with full-term infants, premature infants are at a greater risk of an invasive infection if born to a mother with a peripartum infection. Maternal factors that relate to poverty and poor prenatal care and chronic diseases, such as cardiac disease and diabetes mellitus, appear to have some independent effect on neonatal infection rates, but they are also risks for premature birth.

Late-Onset Infections. Nosocomial infection in the nursery is an important and growing problem. As the technology for treating very premature and very sick infants advances, there is a commensurate increase in the population of surviving immunocompromised infants who require invasive life support measures such as mechanical ventilation, intravascular catheters, total parenteral nutrition, and surgical drains, each of which carries a substantial risk of infection (Table 96–3). The liberal use of broad-spectrum antibiotics increases the risk of acquisition of pathogens by interfering with the development of normal flora. Recently there has been a reduction of early-onset infections as a result of perinatal prophylaxis of mothers with suspected amnionitis or colonization with group B *Streptococcus,* but in highly specialized referral neonatal intensive care units there is an increase in late-onset nosocomial infections (Philip, 1994).

In contrast to the risk factors for sepsis due to bacterial infections, the risk of acquiring nosocomial viral infections appears to depend mostly on the chances of contact with another person infected with the virus. Therefore, community activity of respiratory and gastrointestinal viruses and the absence of barriers to prevent spread within the unit appear to be the most important risk factors; maternal health problems and perinatal history are much less important. Infection rates in referral neonatal intensive care units are similar to those for other intensive care units (approximately 20 per 100 discharges). This number includes sepsis, focal infections, and various viral infections.

Any condition that causes a newborn to have a long stay in the nursery increases the opportunity for late-onset nosocomial infections. Therefore, the risk factors for late-onset infections cannot be separated from those for early-onset infections because the most common reason for prolonged neonatal hospitalization is prematurity. These infants require more intravenous lines and life support apparatus, and thus the risk factors for early-onset infections also indirectly predispose an infant to late-onset infections.

PATHOGENESIS

The pathogenesis of sepsis in a newborn, like the epidemiologic characteristics, is grossly divided into two categories: infections transmitted from mother to infant and nosocomial infections transmitted to an infant after birth by contact with contaminated personnel or hospital equipment.

Prenatal-Onset and Early-Onset Infections. The fetus and the environment within the amniotic membranes are normally sterile. Transmission of infection from mother to infant before birth can be bloodborne, but the effectiveness of the placental barrier makes this mode of transmission unusual. Infection of the fetus as an extension of maternal sepsis long before birth usually results in fetal death but may also result in premature labor. In practice it is uncommon to be able to prove that this was the route of bacterial or fungal infection other than in cases of congenital syphilis. More commonly, there is ascending infection by contamination of the amniotic fluid with organisms from the mother's bacterial vaginal flora. This is the opposite of virus and protozoan infections, in which transplacental infection is more likely (Chapters 95 and 97). Vertical transmission of bacteria may occur at any time from several hours to days before delivery. It may occur as a consequence of frank rupture of the membranes or inapparent tears that later seal. If the fetus ingests these organisms by swallowing amniotic fluid, the organisms may contaminate the upper and lower respiratory tract and gastrointestinal tract before birth. Signs of infection following ascending infection may be present at delivery, within hours of birth, or, less commonly, within several days.

Perinatal transmission of pathogens may take place in the absence of prolonged rupture of the membranes. The skin and upper respiratory tract of a neonate may become contaminated with organisms from the mother's cervical, vaginal, or fecal flora by contact or aspiration during the process of delivery. The mechanisms by which colonization, which is common, becomes invasive infection, which is less common, are not well understood. Occasionally the route of infection is apparent, as when the umbilical cord stump is contaminated and omphalitis accompanies sepsis or when instruments are used in the respiratory tract, as in endotracheal intubation.

It is presumed that the major susceptibility factor for invasive infection is the weaker immune function of neonates, especially premature neonates, compared with older children or adults. Humoral immunity, cellular immunity, and inflammation are all weaker (Chapter 5). Maternally derived IgG antibody is an important component of protection. Late in the third trimester, IgG antibody is actively transported from the mother across the placenta, resulting in a concentration of IgG in the blood of the newborn slightly higher than that of the mother. The specificities of the antibodies and the protection afforded are similar to the mother's. If the infant is born prematurely, the transmission of IgG antibodies is decreased and the neonate is susceptible to those pathogens. Serologic studies of mother-infant pairs have shown that a major susceptibility factor to infection with group B *Streptococcus* type III, the cause of most group B streptococcal neonatal sepsis and almost all group B streptococcal meningitis, is lack of antibody to major virulence antigen, the type III capsular carbohydrate. From 15–30% of delivering mothers have rectal or vaginal colonization with strains of group B *Streptococcus,* and 50% or more of the infants born to these mothers have colonization of the skin, mucous membranes, or gastrointestinal tract (Chapter 94). It appears that newborns who are heavily colonized with group B *Streptococcus* at multiple sites are more likely to develop invasive infection than newborns with limited colonization. However, only approximately 0.1% will have invasive group B streptococcal infection, and these infants clearly have a lower concentration of antibody to the capsular carbohydrates than the 99.9% who do not have invasive infections.

Additional risk factors may affect certain maternal-fetal pairs. Unusual pathogens that colonize or infect the vagina or other parts of the mother's genital tract may be the cause of neonatal sepsis. This appears to be the case in neonatal infections caused by *Haemophilus influenzae, Streptococcus pneumoniae, Listeria monocytogenes, Salmonella* species, *Mycoplasma hominis, Candida,* and others. Introduction of pathogens into the lower genital tract from the outside can occur shortly before or during birth. Faulty examining technique may introduce organisms during an obstetric examination or when monitoring equipment is used. Scalp electrodes as well as vaginal organisms have been determined to be the mode of introduction of new pathogens to the tissues of the emerging newborn, even when there has been no apparent deviation from accepted techniques.

Late-Onset Infections. Late-onset neonatal infections appear to be similar in mode of acquisition and in foci of infection to nosocomial infections involving patients of all ages. A major conceptual difference, however, is that whereas many nosocomial infections in older children and adults involve the individual's own skin, respiratory, and gastrointestinal flora, a neonate is born sterile and acquires surface flora in the nursery. Normal flora confers resistance to colonization with new organisms and is an important constituent of host resistance to infection. A long hospitalization, especially with prolonged or repeated exposure to antibiotics, may have an influence on the nature of this flora. Some experts believe that in a neonatal intensive care unit a newborn acquires atypical flora that make him or her more susceptible to invasive infection. Colonization of the skin and gastrointestinal and respiratory tracts with flora acquired from the mother at birth or later on from nursery personnel or inanimate objects precedes late-onset infections. In addition, some cases of late-onset sepsis may be caused by organisms that cause early-onset sepsis, such as group B *Streptococcus, Listeria monocytogenes, E. coli,* and *Klebsiella pneumoniae.* It is often impossible to determine whether the organisms were acquired from the mother or from the nursery environment. It is unclear why infants colonized with these organisms at birth may suddenly develop severe infections caused by these organisms many days or weeks later.

Late-onset infections caused by organisms commonly found on the skin, such as *S. aureus,* coagulase-negative staphylococci, viridans streptococci, and *Candida* may follow colonization either at birth or after birth. The major risk factors for infections caused by these species are the use of intravascular catheters, the presence of surgical wounds and drains, congenital malformations, and use of invasive life-support equipment. Although these medical and surgical support measures are responsible for the improvement in survival of low-birth-weight and otherwise ill neonates, they predispose to infection by interfering with normal barriers.

Another risk factor for late-onset infections is the use of intravenous hyperalimentation fluids, especially with lipid emulsions. Use of this therapy is common in neonatal intensive care units for delivering needed nutrition to growing very-low-birth-weight infants and to infants who have had gastrointestinal operations. Indwelling catheters allow for a pathway between the skin and the cannulated blood vessel. The infusion fluid is a medium that facilitates the growth of certain organisms, which may normally be of low pathogenicity. There is evidence that the use of these fluids is a risk factor for infections due to coagulase-negative staphylococci as well as certain fungi. *Malassezia furfur,* a lipophilic yeast that frequently colonizes infants in newborn intensive care units, occasionally has been encountered in neonates receiving lipid emulsion intravenously. Other lipophilic fungi have rarely been isolated from the blood of infants receiving intravenous lipid emulsion.

SYMPTOMS AND CLINICAL MANIFESTATIONS

The clinical history is quite important in raising the suspicion of sepsis and in the evaluation of a newborn believed to have sepsis. A complete history of the pregnancy and the perinatal events, the postnatal obstetric course of the mother, and the need for any surgical procedures on mother or child are most important. Endometritis, sepsis, pneumonia, and serologic evidence of an infection such as syphilis have great implications in the assessment of the newborn. Although such findings should influence the assessment of a neonate at any time, the older the postnatal age of neonate, the less likely that the perinatal events will be helpful in assessing whether nonspecific new clinical features represent the development of sepsis. A relevant history should include such risk factors as use of intravenous catheters, hyperalimentation, life-support equipment, previous antimicrobial treatment, presence of surgical wounds or drains, and unusual clustering of infections in the unit.

One of the most important aspects of the clinical presentation of neonatal sepsis is that newborns frequently do not manifest specific signs of sepsis or even of focal infections. In fact, the greatest challenge in providing care for newborns is recognition of the variety of illnesses that may present with similar signs. Thus alterations of breathing rate, heart rate, blood circulation to the extremities and skin, and laboratory findings may indicate such diverse disorders as congenital or acquired metabolic disturbances, anoxic brain damage, transient tachypnea of the newborn, hemolytic disease of the newborn, respiratory distress syndrome, or sepsis. In practice, a large number of infants with similar homeostatic derangements are treated with antibiotics until appropriate tests and cultures have revealed the true cause of the signs or at least have excluded infection as the likely cause. Occasionally, blood cultures obtained as part of "routine" tests in neonates who have no homeostatic alterations grow a pathogen. Although some of these findings represent transient bacteremia, it appears that some infants early in the course of sepsis have no early signs at all.

The nonspecific signs of sepsis in newborns that correlate best with sepsis include impaired temperature regulation reflected as temperature instability with hyperthermia or hypothermia alone or sometimes alternating, respiratory distress, jaundice, lethargy, irritability, anorexia, and vomiting. The appearance of any of these signs without evidence of another cause should raise the question of sepsis or another invasive infection. The greater the number of these signs that are present, the higher should be the suspicion. The early signs of meningitis are often not different from those of sepsis without meningitis, and only examination of cerebrospinal fluid obtained by lumbar puncture identifies the presence of meningitis. Occasionally convulsions, a bulging fontanelle, or nuchal rigidity will suggest a clinical diagnosis of meningitis, but these are inconsistently present, especially early in the neonatal period.

Physical Examination Findings

Notable physical findings of neonatal sepsis include abnormalities in general appearance, respiratory status, feeding status, vital signs, and temperature. A fever in the few first days of life may be the sole sign of an acquired viral or bacterial infection. The signs of systemic neonatal infection may be obvious and resemble shock with tachycardia, poor perfusion, respiratory distress, and diminished gastrointestinal motility with poor feeding. Such signs can be seen at birth or at any time during the neonatal period. More often, however, subtle symptoms such as low-grade fever or hypothermia, poor feeding, and irritability precede manifest sepsis, although the presence and extent of these symptoms are quite variable and nonspecific. Change in respiratory status, especially respiratory distress, is often an early nonspecific sign of sepsis. Abdominal tenderness and increased abdominal girth may suggest necrotizing enterocolitis. Anatomic anomalies, especially along the craniospinal axis, may be important because they provide a direct entrance for microorganisms to the cerebrospinal fluid.

DIAGNOSIS

The diagnosis of neonatal sepsis is considered likely on the basis of one or more abnormal findings on physical examination or of a combination of risk factors plus abnormal laboratory data that indicate that sepsis is highly likely. The diagnosis of sepsis is confirmed by isolation of the infecting organism from cultures of the appropriate bodily fluids and sites. Empirical antimicrobial therapy directed against the common organisms and against other likely organisms on the basis of individual findings is begun immediately after cultures are obtained. Antibiotic therapy is discontinued or adjusted after culture results are known in 2–3 days. In contemporary diagnostic microbiology laboratories, the key cultures of blood, cerebrospinal fluid, and urine are generally positive within 48 hours of incubation if infection is due to any of the usual neonatal bacterial or fungal pathogens.

Laboratory Evaluation

Leukocyte Counts. The WBC total count and differential count are important in assessing a neonate for the possibility of sepsis and for evaluating a neonate being treated for proved sepsis. The marrow reserves of leukocytes in a newborn are relatively smaller than those of older children and adults, and leukopenia occurs more frequently as a sign of overwhelming infection. Although the diagnosis of sepsis should not be based solely on the results of the WBC total count and differential count, this information is important and can be added to other clinical and epidemiologic information to determine which infants should be empirically treated because of the strong likelihood of sepsis. There is a wide range in the peripheral WBC count of normal newborns, from 5,000–20,000/mm^3, but even values outside this range still have a poor specificity for predicting sepsis. Although it is controversial, there is some evidence that the **absolute neutrophil count,** determined by the WBC total count multiplied by the fraction of neutrophils, is more predictive of sepsis than is the total WBC count. Although not specific for sepsis, neutrophil concentrations outside the normal range support an impression of sepsis or a high risk of sepsis. It is important in the interpretation of WBC count and the absolute neutrophil count to use the normal range for age, especially in the neonatal period when normal values change greatly (see Fig. 10–1).

In an attempt to increase the specificity of the WBC count as an indicator of sepsis, parameters have been evaluated, such as the concentration of immature cells of the neutrophil series (bands, metamyelocytes, and myelocytes) and the ratio of immature to total cells of the neutrophil series, known the **I:T ratio.** An increased concentration of immature neutrophil series cells and an I:T ratio of >0.2 have been reported to have moderately increased specificity for sepsis. The I:T ratio takes into consideration the normative values over the first days of life (Chapter 10). It is frequently used and has only moderate sensitivity but good negative predictive value if normal.

Other Screening Laboratory Tests. In practice, so many low-birth-weight infants who do not have infection receive antibiotics that there is concern about the deleterious effects of so much unnecessary antibiotic use. It is expensive, there are adverse drug effects, and it fosters development of antibiotic-resistant organisms in newborn nurseries. These concerns have led to attempts to develop screening systems to target those newborns who are much more likely to benefit from antibiotic treatment. Newborns who have symptoms consistent with sepsis should be treated empirically after appropriate cultures, chest radiograph, and laboratory tests have been performed. For newborns with symptoms, laboratory tests need not be used in making the decision for treatment, which should not be withheld while waiting for the results of tests that have been ordered.

Acute-phase reactants (Chapter 10) such as CRP, ESR, and concentrations of certain cytokines, have each been reported to have moderate positive and negative predictive values. The use of the quantitative CRP test has been studied extensively, primarily outside the United States. It is moderately sensitive for bacteremia if there are serial determinations in the first days of life. Several studies also have suggested that decrease in the CRP level during treatment for sepsis is a good determinant of effectiveness of treatment and can be used to shorten the length of therapy. Recent studies have shown that IL-6, IL-8, and CD11b, which is a member of the β-integrin family of adhesion proteins, are moderately sensitive assays for neonatal bacteremia but have great potential for use as screening tests to exclude bacteremia. Although all of these tests of acute-phase reactants may be useful, it is not clear which test is the most useful in the first hours after birth when decisions to begin empirical antibiotic treatment are usually necessary, but their use may allow shortened antibiotic courses.

Sepsis Screening Panels. An interesting addition to the use of single tests for determining which newborns would benefit from empirical treatment for sepsis has been the use of a panel of tests, which are useful only for newborns without any symptoms. For newborns who have no symptoms, some experts advocate the use of standard blood, urine, and CSF cultures plus a radiograph of the chest, a WBC count, I:T ratio, and CRP, ESR, and serum haptoglobin levels as a sepsis screen. One study (Philip and Hewitt, 1980) showed that of 30 proven cases of sepsis among 376 newborns, 28 occurred among the 71 newborns with positive screens, and only 2 newborns with proven sepsis had negative screens, giving a screen sensitivity of 93%, a specificity of 88%, and a positive predictive accuracy of 39%. Newborns with a negative screen were at low risk and did not need to be empirically treated with antibiotics (Philip, 1981). Some neonatologists use laboratory screens, and others have been unwilling to withhold antibiotic treatment from newborns with risk factors such as low birth weight, perinatal asphyxia, or prolonged rupture of the membranes. There is no clear standard of practice at this time.

Microbiologic Evaluation

Cultures of a newborn being evaluated for sepsis should routinely include one or more blood cultures, a urine culture, and a CSF culture. Other cultures, such as joint fluid, bone, and peritoneal fluid, are not performed routinely but should be performed if there is evidence of focal infection. None of the ''routine'' cultures for the evaluation of sepsis is without some controversy. Although a single blood culture is fairly sensitive for diagnosing sepsis, the chances of a contaminant growing in a blood culture are high enough that concordance or discordance between two cultures is helpful to determine whether the organism was a true cause of sepsis. Concordant positive results indicate a higher probability of sepsis, and discordant results indicate a higher probablility that the isolate is a contaminant. Therefore, two blood cultures obtained by venipuncture from separate sites are recommended if this will not delay treatment.

The use of superficial cultures, such as cultures of skin, umbilicus, and gastric contents **(surface cultures),** may be helpful if obtained immediately after birth in determining whether organisms have been transferred from mother to newborn. These cultures may indicate that the infant is colonized and is at risk of sepsis because of these organisms. However, positive superficial cultures demonstrate only colonization and should not be interpreted as indicating invasive infection. Furthermore, cultures may be negative because of a poor-quality specimen, inappropriate handling or transport, or inappropriate culture technique, and therefore negative surface cultures do not indicate absence of risk. The value of such cultures, especially if taken after a few days of life, is dubious, and they are not recommended in ordinary circumstances.

Urine. Although some perinatologists have questioned the value of urine cultures or CSF cultures in the routine evaluation of newborns for sepsis, these tests are useful, especially when a blood culture grows a pathogen and the specific focus of infection needs to be clarified. Cultures of urine or CSF taken during the course of antibiotic treatment are not useful for determining whether a focus existed at the time antibiotic treatment was begun. There is little question that cultures of blood, urine, and CSF are the minimal cultures for the evaluation of a neonate older than 2 days or who develops new signs of infection.

Urine cultures should be obtained by urethral catheterization or suprapubic bladder aspiration. Bagged urine from a neonate is frequently contaminated by skin flora, making the culture result uninterpretable. Compared with urethral catheterization, suprapubic aspiration has the advantage of causing less trauma and introducing fewer organisms into the bladder when performed by an experienced physician.

Cerebrospinal Fluid. Recent studies have demonstrated the low incidence of meningitis in infants undergoing ''routine'' evaluation for sepsis in the first 72 hours of life who have no specific signs of infection, and some perinatologists have suggested that a lumbar puncture is unnecessary in this situation. A small number of cases of meningitis will be missed. Evaluation and interpretation of CSF should be a routine part of the evaluation of a neonate for possible sepsis. Approximately one fourth to one third of neonates with proved bacterial sepsis also have meningitis, but most often they do not appear different from infants with symptoms of sepsis but without meningitis. It is important to document meningitis because antibiotic treatment may have to be altered, evaluation during the course of treatment is altered, and the prognosis is different. Interpretation of the CSF from a newborn requires knowledge of normal values for this age group because the range of normal values for cells and protein differs from those for an older child (Table 52–11).

Tests for Bacterial Antigens. It is possible with particle agglutination to detect the free soluble antigens produced by bacteria multiplying in bodily fluids such as blood, urine, and CSF (Chapter 7). Attempts to detect *E. coli* and group B *Streptococcus* in neonatal infections have looked promising in some studies, but recent data suggest that the tests have sufficiently poor sensitivity and specificity to render treatment decisions on the basis of their results alone unwise. At this time they have been de-emphasized in management strategies until improved tests that are currently under study become available.

Viral Cultures. The use of viral cultures in the evaluation of an ill newborn varies considerably from institution to institution. Either congenital viral infection (Chapter 95) or perinatally acquired viral infection with HSV, VZV, and enteroviruses (Chapter 97) may present as neonatal sepsis. Postnatal community-acquired viral infections may occur in newborns in the first few days of life and in neonates with chronic underlying illnesses, who may be resident in the hospital for many weeks. Respiratory viruses such as adenoviruses, RSV, influenza viruses, and parainfluenza viruses may be transmitted by respiratory spread to newborns from the mother or health care workers. Viral cultures are indicated whenever there is an outbreak of a nonbacterial respiratory infection in a nursery. They are also useful in the routine evaluation of infants with suspected respiratory tract infection. Viral diarrheal agents may also affect neonates, but the availability of tests for these agents and their applicability for infants is limited (Chapter 76).

Diagnostic Imaging

Radiologic examination of neonates is important in the evaluation of the lower respiratory tract for evidence of pneumonia and of the gastrointestinal tract for evidence of necrotizing enterocolitis. A chest radiograph is important in the evaluation for congenital heart disease, which may cause congestive heart failure and symptoms suggestive of sepsis. Infants believed to have clinically significant congenital cardiac disease should also have a cardiac ultrasonographic examination interpreted by a pediatric cardiologist.

Radiologic examination of the abdomen with plain radiography as well as cross-table lateral images may reveal the nonspecific finding of **fixed, dilated loops** of intestine. **Pneumatosis intestinalis** with or without the finding of **intrahepatic portal air,** which is seen most easily on cross-table lateral images, confirms the diagnosis of necrotizing enterocolitis, but it is not always present and is not necessary for the diagnosis.

TREATMENT

Treatment of neonatal sepsis encompasses three major forms of therapy: antimicrobial therapy, adjunctive therapy, and supportive therapy. The antibiotics chosen, either empirically before the isolation of an infecting agent or definitively on the basis of culture results, should be the most efficacious and specific drug that is safe for neonates. Adjunctive pharmaceutical agents to enhance host defenses against infection may also be used. Sustaining organ function by treating shock and acidosis and by life-support measures such as assisted ventilation, fluid resuscitation, and inotropic agents as a part of aggressive neonatal care is critical. Advances in this area are probably responsible for the dramatic decrease in mortality from neonatal sepsis seen since the mid-1970s. At this time the standard of care requires treatment in a specialized neonatal intensive care unit.

Definitive Treatment

The approach to rational antibiotic therapy for presumed or proved sepsis in a newborn relies on principles similar to those for the use of antibiotics in any population of susceptible patients, but with certain modifications. Some of the special aspects of treating neonates are the limited information available concerning neonatal dosing and safety of many antimicrobial agents and the epidemiologic concerns of housing a large number of ill infants receiving antibiotics in an enclosed unit. The ratio of infants believed to have sepsis and being empirically treated to the number who are actually proved to have sepsis is very high (10–20:1 and sometimes higher). Because there is little evidence that routine culture methods frequently fail to confirm sepsis in infants who actually have sepsis, it appears that a large number of infants are treated with antibiotics who receive no benefit from them. Antibiotic use should be designed to minimize undesirable adverse effects in uninfected infants and to maximize efficacy in those who have infections. For this reason the number of antibiotics frequently used for the treatment of neonatal sepsis is relatively small, and an attempt is made to use agents that appear to be least associated with inducing antibiotic resistance in the bacterial flora of the patient population.

Antimicrobial Therapy for Early-Onset Sepsis. It is reasonable to treat newborns who have risk factors because the predicted incidence of sepsis is up to 20–30% in newborns with certain risk factors (Table 96–3). Accordingly, administration of antibiotics for early-onset infections is frequently begun before the infecting organism is identified (Tables 96–4 and 96–5). Neonates, especially those who are premature, typically do not manifest classic signs and symptoms of infection early in the infection. Symptoms develop so late in the course of the infection that waiting results in unacceptably high morbidity and mortality. Thus many schemas have been developed for empirical antibiotic treatment of infants with multiple epidemiologic risk factors alone or with nonspecific signs and laboratory test abnormalities plus epidemiologic risk factors. The common features of these schema are recognition of known risk factors (Table 96–3); the possibility that severe infection may present as temperature instability or other subtle changes in vital signs, unexplained hyperbilirubinemia, vomiting, or changes in feeding; and the fact that even a short delay in treatment may result in overwhelming sepsis and death. Empirical treatment is designed to provide adequate antimicrobial activity against the likely organisms (Table 96–1). Often the primary focus of infection is not identified, but for an infant without focal signs therapy is directed at bacteremia and meningitis because experience demonstrates that these are the most likely types of infection to present without focal findings. If pneumonia or a urinary tract infection is present, the usual physical examination or screening tests, including chest radiographs and urinalysis, demonstrate these foci.

Empirical treatment of sepsis is generally accomplished by a combination of a broad-spectrum penicillin and an aminoglycoside or a broad-spectrum penicillin and an extended-spectrum (third-generation) cephalosporin (Table 96–4). Most experts continue to recommend the combination of a penicillin, usually ampicillin, and an aminoglycoside, usually gentamicin. The advantages of this combination are low cost, considerable experience, low rate of

TABLE 96–4. Guidelines for Empirical Antibiotic Treatment for Presumed Neonatal Sepsis (With or Without Meningitis) in the First Month of Life

Clinical Setting	Recommended Antibiotic Regimen	Alternative Regimens
Early-onset sepsis	Ampicillin *plus* gentamicin*	Ampicillin *plus* cefotaxime
Late-onset sepsis (up to 1 month)		
Readmission to the hospital from the community	Ampicillin *plus* cefotaxime (or ceftriaxone†)	Ampicillin *plus* gentamicin* *with or without* cefotaxime (or ceftriaxone†)
Occurring in the hospital, with no intravenous catheter(s)	Ampicillin *plus* gentamicin*	Ampicillin *plus* cefotaxime (or ceftriaxone†)
Occurring in the hospital with intravascular catheter(s) in place	Oxacillin *or* vancomycin* *plus* gentamicin*	Vancomycin* *plus* cefotaxime (*or* ceftriaxone†)

*Adjust dose according to concentration of the antibiotic in the blood once a steady state has been achieved.
†Ceftriaxone can displace bilirubin from albumin, thus intensifying hyperbilirubinemia and may also cause deposition of sludge in the gallbladder, so it should be used with caution in newborns.

TABLE 96–5. Dosages and Dosing Intervals of Antibiotics by Patient Weight and Age for the Treatment of Neonatal Infections

Antibiotic	Dosage (mg/kg/dose)[1] Birth Weight <1,200 g Age 0–4 wk	Birth Weight 1,200–2,000 g Age 0–7 Days	Birth Weight 1,200–2,000 g Age >7 Days	Birth Weight >2,000 g Age 0–7 Days	Birth Weight >2,000 g Age >7 Days
Penicillins					
Penicillin G					
Meningitis	50,000 U q12hr	50,000 U q12hr	75,000 U q8hr	50,000 U q8hr	50,000 U q6hr
Other infections	25,000 U q12hr	25,000 U q12hr	25,000 U q8hr	25,000 U q8hr	25,000 U q6hr
Ampicillin[2]					
Meningitis	50 q12hr	50 q12hr	50 q8hr	50 q8hr	50 q6hr
Other infections	25 q12hr	25 q12hr	25 q8hr	25 q8hr	25 q6hr
Ticarcillin	75 q12hr	75 q12hr	75 q8hr	75 q8hr	75 q6hr
Mezlocillin, piperacillin[3]	75 q12hr	75 q12hr	75 q8hr	75 q12hr	75 q8hr
Penicillinase-resistant penicillins (nafcillin, oxacillin)					
Meningitis	50 q12hr	50 q12hr	50 q8hr	50 q8hr	50 q6hr
Other infections	25 q12hr	25 q12hr	25 q8hr	25 q8hr	25 q6hr
Cephalosporins					
Cephalothin	20 q12hr	20 q12hr	20 q8hr	20 q8hr	20 q6hr
Cefazolin	20 q12hr	20 q12hr	20 q12hr	20 q12hr	20 q8hr
Cefotaxime	50 q12hr	50 q12hr	50 q8hr	50 q12hr	50 q8hr
Ceftazidime	50 q12hr	50 q12hr	50 q8hr	50 q12hr	50 q8hr
Ceftriaxone[4]	50 q24hr	50 q24hr	50 q24hr	50 q24hr	75 q24hr
Other β-lactams					
Aztreonam[5]	30 q12hr	30 q12hr	30 q8hr	30 q8hr	30 q6hr
Imipenem[3]	20 q18–24hr	20 q12hr	20 q12hr	20 q12hr	20 q8hr
Meropenem	—	20 q12hr	20 q12hr	20 q12hr	20 q8hr
Aminoglycosides					
Gentamicin[6]	2.5 q18–24hr	2.5 q12–18hr	2.5 q8–12hr	2.5 q12hr	2.5 q8hr
Tobramycin[6]	2.5 q18–24hr	2.5 q12–18hr	2.5 q8–12hr	2.5 q12hr	2.5 q8hr
Amikacin[6]	7.5 q18–24hr	7.5 q18–24hr	7.5 q8–12hr	10 q12hr	10 q8hr
Others					
Clindamycin	5 q12hr	5 q12hr	5 q8hr	5 q8hr	5 q6hr
Metronidazole[3]	7.5 q48hr	7.5 q24hr	7.5 q12hr	7.5 q12hr	15 q12hr
Vancomycin[6]	15 q24hr	15 q12–18hr	15 q8–12hr	15 q12hr	15 q8hr
Chloramphenicol[4,6]	25 q24hr	25 q24hr	25 q24hr	25 q24hr	25 q12hr
Antifungal Agents					
Amphotericin B		1 mg/kg once daily (see Tables 14–71 and 14–72)			
Flucytosine[7]		150 mg/kg/day divided q6hr			
Fluconazole[8]		3–6 mg/kg once daily			

[1]These dosages are for parenteral (intravenous or intramuscular) administration.
[2]Dosing of ampicillin-sulbactam and ticarcillin-tazobactam is determined by the ampicillin and ticarcillin component, respectively.
[3]Safety and efficacy in infants and children younger than 12 years of age have not been established.
[4]Should not be administered to neonates with hyperbilirubinemia, especially those born prematurely.
[5]Safety and efficacy in infants younger than 9 months of age have not been established.
[6]Dosing should be guided by laboratory determination of serum antibiotic concentrations once a steady state has been reached.
[7]Safety and efficacy in infants and children younger than 12 years of age have not been established. There are limited data on dosing for neonates. The dose for older infants is indicated.
[8]Efficacy in infants and children younger than 12 years of age has not been established. There are limited data on dosing for neonates. The dose for older infants is indicated.
Dosages for neonates less than 1200 g adapted from Prober CG, Stevenson DK, Benitz WE: The use of antibiotics in neonates weighing less than 1200 grams. *Pediatr Infect Dis J* 1990;9:111–21.

development of antibiotic resistance, and low toxicity when there is proper monitoring of blood aminoglycoside levels. Of the common bacterial agents that cause neonatal sepsis, group B *Streptococcus* and *Listeria* are susceptible to ampicillin, as are many strains of *E. coli* and *Proteus.* In nurseries where gram-negative bacilli with acquired plasmid or chromosomal resistance to the aminoglycosides are not prevalent, gentamicin is active against *E. coli, Klebsiella, Proteus,* most *Enterobacter,* and *Pseudomonas aeruginosa.* Species commonly resistant to gentamicin include *Acinetobacter,* many strains of *Enterobacter cloacae,* some strains of *Serratia,* and *Flavobacterium.* These resistant species are rarely associated with early-onset sepsis, but if a cluster of cases of sepsis caused by these organisms is known to be occurring, alternative empirical therapy regimens should be considered.

The advantages of the extended-spectrum cephalosporins are greater activity against many of the pathogens and good activity against strains of gram-negative bacilli resistant to gentamicin. The third-generation cephalosporins most used in neonates, cefotaxime and ceftriaxone, have excellent CNS penetration in the presence of inflammation. Several properties of the extended-spectrum cephalosporins that may militate against the routine use of these drugs for empirical therapy for neonatal sepsis must be considered. Extended-spectrum cephalosporins are less active than the first- or second-generation cephalosporins against gram-positive cocci, and their activity against group B *Streptococcus* is not as good as that of penicillin or ampicillin. The extended-spectrum cephalosporins are inactive against *Enterococcus* and *Listeria,* which are not infrequent causes of neonatal sepsis in many large centers. For these reasons, ampicillin is added to the cephalosporin when it is used empirically for neonatal sepsis or meningitis. Ceftriaxone, which has a similar spectrum of activity to cefotaxime but a longer half-life, has the potential to displace bilirubin from albumin-binding sites and should not be used in infants with hyperbilirubinemia. Experience has shown that when there is a high rate of use of these broad-spectrum cephalosporin agents, the prevalent flora in the neonatal intensive care unit may include strains of bacteria resistant to cephalosporins, so there is an advantage in using them only when they are of proved or theoretical superiority. If a diagnosis of gram-negative bacillary meningitis is based on Gram stain or culture of the CSF, it is reasonable to use the combination of ampicillin and an extended-spectrum cephalosporin empirically as a first choice, although it has not been shown that this combination results in a better outcome for neonatal meningitis than ampicillin and gentamicin do.

Sometimes the aminoglycoside of choice should be an agent other than gentamicin. Tobramycin has greater activity against *P. aeruginosa,* but this is an uncommon cause of neonatal infections. The third-generation cephalosporin ceftazidime can be used safely for neonates and generally has excellent activity against *P. aeruginosa.* If it is known that there have been infections in the community or in the nursery caused by gentamicin-resistant gram-negative bacilli, amikacin should be the aminoglycoside added to ampicillin for empirical treatment of neonatal sepsis. Amikacin is considerably more expensive than gentamicin and has no better activity against gentamicin-susceptible organisms. It is resistant to most of the aminoglycoside-inactivating enzymes produced by gram-negative bacilli. Although in most large centers gram-negative bacilli are sufficiently resistant to kanamycin that it is rarely used, in some communities resistance to kanamycin is so rare that kanamycin continues to be safe and effective, as well as low in cost.

Antimicrobial Therapy for Late-Onset Sepsis. Infants likely to have late-onset infections are most likely to be residents of the intensive care nursery with risk factors (Table 96–3). Empirical antibiotic therapy for late-onset neonatal sepsis should take into consideration the resident flora of the nursery, especially isolates from previously infected neonates and the particular risk factors of the individual patient (Tables 96–4 and 96–5). If intravascular catheters have not been used, the infant has not been treated for a previous infection, and there have not been isolates of gentamicin-resistant gram-negative aerobic bacilli, it is appropriate to use the same empirical treatment as for early-onset sepsis, such as ampicillin plus an aminoglycoside. In fact, many infants believed to have late-onset sepsis usually have specific risk factors, and another regimen is often more appropriate. Infants who are ill frequently have intravascular catheters in place, which may be the focus of infection. The most common bacterial species causing catheter-associated infections are *S. aureus* and coagulase-negative staphylococci (Chapter 105). Although penicillinase-resistant semisynthetic penicillins (e.g., oxacillin and nafcillin) are usually the agents of choice against staphylococci, resistance to this class, commonly referred to as **methicillin-resistant *S. aureus* or MRSA,** is occurring more commonly in many institutions. In addition, coagulase-negative staphylococci more commonly cause symptomatic infection of very-low-birth-weight infants, and this species is more likely to have methicillin resistance. Therefore, in institutions with large numbers of methicillin-resistant staphylococci, it is reasonable to use vancomycin for empirical treatment of late-onset infections that are likely to be associated with catheter use. Generally an aminoglycoside, usually gentamicin, is added for empirical coverage of gram-negative bacilli. If new symptoms of infection develop while the infant is receiving gentamicin, either amikacin or an expanded spectrum (third-generation) cephalosporin is substituted for gentamicin. Blanket use of vancomycin for all cases of late-onset sepsis is generally not warranted because this agent is expensive; is toxic compared with the penicillins, including the penicillinase-resistant penicillins; and has activity only against aerobic gram-positive bacteria. Similarly, antibiotics active against gentamicin-resistant bacteria should be used only when there is a high risk of resistant pathogens. Frequent use of such agents in an enclosed nursery population promotes the emergence and persistence of even more resistant strains of bacteria. Thus the recommendations for empirical therapy (Table 96–5) should be followed only when there are no unusual factors or clues to the cause of infection, but many patients require individualization.

Neonates who have been discharged from the hospital and are readmitted for treatment of presumed sepsis or sepsis with meningitis should be treated empirically with a third-generation cephalosporin (usually cefotaxime or ceftriaxone) plus ampicillin. This combination is active against the usual causes of non-hospital-acquired sepsis, group B *Streptococcus,* enterococci, *Listeria, S. aureus,* and gram-negative bacilli. If these infants are hospitalized in a regular infant unit as opposed to a neonatal intensive care unit, there is a lower prevalence of antibiotic use, and there should be less antibiotic pressure for the development of resistant strains of bacteria on the unit.

Duration of Antibiotic Treatment. The optimal duration of therapy for neonatal sepsis has not been determined, but a number of useful guidelines exist. Cultures of blood, urine, and CSF are usually positive by 2 days after incubation, only occasionally becoming positive during the third day. Empirical antibiotic therapy for sepsis should be stopped if cultures are sterile 2–3 days after initiation if the infant or the mother was not treated with antibiotics that might interfere with recovery of an organism from a culture and there is no evidence of a focal infection. For infants with bacteremia without meningitis or another focus of infection but with a prompt bacteriologic and clinical response to therapy, 7–10 days of antibiotic treatment are sufficient. If there is bacteremia and a focus exists, the duration of therapy is generally 7–10 days or that which is appropriate for the focus of infection, whichever is longer. When meningitis accompanies sepsis, 2–3 weeks of antibiotic therapy is recommended for meningitis caused by group B *Streptococcus* or *Listeria.* For meningitis caused by gram-negative bacilli, a minimum of 3 weeks of antibiotic therapy is recommended.

Occasionally an infant in whom antibiotic treatment is started empirically will continue to have symptoms after 2–3 days, with convincing evidence of sepsis despite all cultures being sterile. Such cases should be analyzed individually, and in some cases it will be appropriate to continue antibiotic treatment for 7–10 days for presumed sepsis. Although blood cultures are usually positive in neonatal bacterial sepsis, false-negative results can result (if antibiotics were given prenatally to the mother) from a small volume of blood drawn for culture with a low concentration of bacteria in the blood or with poor handling of the specimen.

Supportive Therapy. The use of agents to support or enhance the immune system during treatment of neonatal sepsis is controversial. Some clinical studies show a number of agents to be beneficial, and in others there is either no benefit or no statistical difference. Small studies have suggested that exchange transfusion, WBC transfusion when there is severe neutropenia and bone marrow failure, IVIG, and specific immune serum globulin preparations reduce mortality in neonatal sepsis, but clear-cut efficacy of most of these agents is lacking. Although WBC transfusions appear to reduce the mortality in some studies, the logistics of providing them in a safe and timely manner has been difficult at most centers. The use of hematopoietic growth factors such as G-CSF (Miura et al., 2001) and GM-CSF (Bilgin et al., 2001) in newborns with sepsis and neutropenia appears potentially promising, but data are limited and results are inconclusive. A meta-analysis (Jenson and Pollock, 1997) suggests that IVIG (750 mg/kg as a single dose) is beneficial in decreasing the morbidity of neonatal sepsis. Immune system enhancers and cell transfusion have not been widely adopted, and if any adjunct is used in the treatment of overwhelming sepsis, the one with which a facility has the most experience may be the best inasmuch as complications are known to occur with each agent.

Infants Born to Mothers Who Received Peripartum Antibiotics. Current obstetric practice emphasizes antibiotic treatment of mothers with evidence of chorioamnionitis or other urogenital tract infections at parturition, which reduces the incidence of early-onset sepsis in newborns. In addition, many mothers who are colonized with group B *Streptococcus* receive perinatal prophylaxis with penicillin or ampicillin (Chapter 94). Antibiotics administered to the mother cross the placenta and give rise to significant blood and tissue concentrations of antibiotic in the infant. This practice presents the physician treating newborns with several challenges. For infants with symptoms born to mothers receiving antibiotics, should the usual antibiotics be used for empirical treatment? Or should alternatives be used? If infants with symptoms are treated with antibiotics and show clinical improvement but all cultures are sterile, can antibiotics be discontinued? Or should they be continued for some predetermined duration because maternal antibiotics may have interfered with the isolation of pathogens in the blood, urine, or CSF of the infant? Should healthy-appearing infants of mothers being treated with antibiotics have postnatal antibiotics continued for some predetermined period because an infection may have been only partially suppressed, resulting in a lack of noticeable symptoms?

Because of the lack of controlled studies, there is a range of opinion among neonatologists and infectious diseases specialists concerning treatment in these situations. At the extremes, some experts recommend treating only infants with symptoms, whereas others recommend treating all infants for presumed sepsis with a full course of 7–10 days of broad-spectrum antibiotics. A compromise recommended by many experts is based on the presence of symptoms and risk factors. Infants with signs or symptoms of sepsis, or gestation of <35 weeks, should have a complete evaluation for sepsis, including CBC, cultures of the blood, urine, and CSF, and be treated as for sepsis for 7–10 days even if cultures are negative. Symptom-free infants who have risk factors for sepsis (e.g., fever, prematurity, prolonged premature rupture of membranes, maternal infection) should have a complete sepsis evaluation, including CBC, cultures of the blood, urine, and CSF (at the discretion of the physician), and treatment with broad-spectrum antibiotics for 48 hours. After 48 hours, a decision about length of treatment should be made on the basis of initial evaluation, culture reports, and clinical course. Symptom-free infants with no risk factors should be observed for 48 hours without antibiotic treatment and should be evaluated and treated if symptoms develop. These guidelines are consistent with the recommendations for group B *Streptococcus* prophylaxis (Chapter 94).

COMPLICATIONS

Sepsis is a major cause of death among neonates. The overall mortality from neonatal sepsis is 15–20%, whereas it had been approximately 90% in the preantibiotic era (Table 96–1). Undoubtedly the severity of the sepsis syndrome affects this rate. It will be difficult to lower the rate because many cases of sepsis are in very-low-birth-weight neonates, who are already quite fragile before the development of sepsis.

PROGNOSIS

For infants who survive sepsis a major determinant of quality of survival is whether the infection included meningitis. For those with meningitis the likelihood of neurologic disability is quite high, with 20–30% or more of the survivors having serious developmental and learning handicaps.

Relapses of neonatal sepsis and meningitis occur infrequently. Relapses of group B *Streptococcus* meningitis have been reported in patients treated with less than the recommended dosage of penicillin or for less than 14 days and in patients with in vitro **tolerance** of the organism to penicillin. Recurrence of meningitis should prompt investigation for the possibility of an anatomic defect along the craniospinal axis, such as a communicating tract at the lower end of the sacrum, which has the external appearance of a simple pilonidal dimple. This is especially true in recurrent meningitis caused by gram-negative bacilli.

PREVENTION

The most successful techniques for the prevention of early-onset sepsis involve interruption of the spread of pathogens from the mother to the newborn infant. Efforts to eradicate maternal carriage of group B *Streptococcus* during pregnancy have been ineffective. The efficacy of treatment after the birth of infants who have been colonized but who have no symptoms remains controversial, and empirical treatment is not recommended. Intrapartum treatment of mothers colonized with group B *Streptococcus* with risk factors such as prematurity, prolonged rupture of the membranes, or chorioamnionitis reduces the newborn colonization rate from 51% to 9% and is very effective in the prevention of early-onset neonatal group B streptococcal infections (Chapter 94). Treatment of mothers with signs and symptoms of chorioamnionitis, endometritis, or prolonged premature rupture of membranes independent of colonization status is also effective in reducing the rate of neonatal sepsis (Mercer et al., 1997).

Attempts have been made to prevent late-onset neonatal infections by administration of IVIG prophylactically. Because a high proportion of neonatal infections arise in infants who have long stays in neonatal intensive care units, and because a large proportion of these infants are so premature that they have acquired little IgG from their mothers, it seems logical that prophylactic IVIG, which contains mostly IgG isotype antibodies, might benefit tiny newborns. The results of prophylactic IVIG have been inconsistent, with some studies reporting some benefit and others reporting little or no benefit. Overall, the benefit appears to be minimal, especially in consideration of the cost, and this method of prevention has not been widely recommended.

In the past, bathing of newborns with a hexachlorophene-containing solution was done regularly as a method of reducing colonization with staphylococci. This practice has been largely discontinued since the demonstration of vacuolation of the brain in some exposed infants. During outbreaks of staphylococcal infection in nurseries, this may be an effective control method if used carefully.

Topical application of **triple dye** to the umbilical stump has been used for decades to prevent colonization with gram-positive organisms, especially *S. aureus.* Triple dye is composed of brilliant green (2.29 mg/mL), gentian violet (2.29 mg/mL), and proflavin hemisulfate (neutral acriflavine, 1.14 mg/mL). It is applied in a single application, painted on the umbilical stump and the surrounding 1–2 cm of skin shortly after birth. Alternative agents, such as mupirocin, have been proposed, but the proven efficacy, lack of toxicity, and low cost of triple dye makes it the preferred agent. Noninfectious umbilical stump exudate may be managed by the application of isopropyl alcohol to the stump with a cotton-tipped swab as needed until the umbilical stump spontaneously falls off. Recent analyses of umbilical cord care show not only lack of superiority of any specific care regimen but also lack of data showing that microbicides are necessary at all. Many newborn nurseries now just keep the cord clean and dry.

FOCAL BACTERIAL INFECTIONS

Cutaneous and Subcutaneous Abscesses. Neonates are susceptible to **scalp abscesses** or cellulitis of the scalp during the first week of life. The abscesses are commonly associated with the use of intrauterine fetal monitoring with scalp electrodes during labor or forceps during delivery. Scalp electrodes also may introduce organisms into a cephalohematoma. **Soft-tissue abscesses** and cellulitis may develop at the site of peripheral intravenous catheters or at any site of disruption of the integrity of the cutaneous barrier. The organisms involved can be quite diverse, but they are similar to those that cause early-onset sepsis such as *E. coli* and group B *Streptococcus,* as well as *S. aureus,* group A *Streptococcus,* herpes simplex virus, and *Candida* because they are acquired by contact with the vaginal and skin flora.

The most useful laboratory tests are Gram stain and culture of the abscess contents, in addition to a blood culture for evidence of secondary bacteremia. Methods of obtaining material to examine include gentle expression of discharge from the abscess, percutaneous needle aspiration directly from the abscess, and aspiration from the dermal tissue involved in cellulitis.

If the Gram stain demonstrates a large number of bacteria of a single morphology, antibiotic treatment against the probable pathogen can be started. A penicillinase-resistant penicillin (e.g., nafcillin or oxacillin) can be used if there are gram-positive cocci in clusters; penicillin or ampicillin if there are gram-positive cocci in chains; and ampicillin and an aminoglycoside (e.g., gentamicin) or a third-generation cephalosporin (e.g., cefotaxime) if there are gram-negative bacilli. In the absence of any evidence of a specific etiologic agent, a combination of oxacillin plus either an aminoglycoside (e.g., gentamicin) or a third-generation cephalosporin (e.g., cefotaxime) is reasonable empirical coverage. Doses appropriate for sepsis should be used (Table 96–5). Therapy may have to be modified after the results of the culture become available.

Cellulitis. Cellulitis without a discernible abscess is treated similarly to an abscess. Although cellulitis as well as some early abscesses can be treated with antibiotics alone, drainage of an abscess is often necessary. Initially there should be an attempt at aspiration to remove the pus. If there is fluctuance, a surgeon should be consulted about incision and drainage. Although there is not much information on the duration of antibiotic treatment, 10–14 days of treatment is adequate when there is no other focus of infection. If an abscess is drained and the inflammation resolves quickly, an even shorter course (5–7 days) is reasonable.

Neonatal Mastitis. Neonatal mastitis is a special entity that usually appears in full-term infants after the first week of life and within the first 5–7 weeks. Girls are more commonly affected than boys in a ratio of about 2:1. This infection appears to occur only in full-term infants, probably because of underdevelopment of the mammary glands in premature infants. The fetus in utero is under the influence of maternal estrogens that cause glandular hypertrophy of the breast, and there may even be some milk secretion in the early weeks of life. The pathogen most commonly reported to cause cellulitis and abscess of the breast is *S. aureus,* but gram-negative bacilli, especially *E. coli,* as well as group B *Streptococcus, Enterococcus,* and *Salmonella* are also causes of neonatal breast infections (Table 96–6). Breast abscess may be more common during outbreaks of staphylococcal disease in the nursery.

TABLE 96–6. Results of Culture in 36 Cases of Neonatal Mastitis

	Procedure to Obtain Culture				
Species of Pathogen	Incision and Drainage	Nipple Discharge	Needle Aspiration	Uncertain Procedure	Total Infants
S. aureus	24	3	3	2	30*
S. aureus plus another organism	1†	1‡	0	0	2
Coagulase-negative staphylococci	1	0	0	0	1
Other	1§	1‖	0	0	2
No growth	0	0	1	0	1
Total	27	5	4	2	36

*Several infants had more than one procedure.
†*S. aureus* and viridans streptococci.
‡*S. aureus* and coagulase-negative staphylococci.
§Coagulase-negative staphylococci and *Peptostreptococcus.*
‖Group B *Streptococcus.*
Table adapted from Walsh M, McIntosh K: Neonatal mastitis. *Clin Pediatr* 1986;25:395–9. No infant received antibiotics before all cultures were obtained.

The most frequent sign of neonatal breast abscess is swelling of the affected breast, with redness and warmth reported in many cases. Unilateral involvement is usual, although there have been rare reports of bilateral infection. The disease may be manifest as cellulitis without obvious abscess formation, as a discrete abscess, or as a spreading abscess that may involve tissues adjacent to the breast. Fever may or may not occur.

The most useful laboratory tests are Gram stain and culture of the abscess contents, in addition to a blood culture for evidence of secondary bacteremia. Methods of obtaining material to examine include gentle expression of discharge from the abscess or nipple, percutaneous needle aspiration directly from the abscess, and aspiration from the dermal tissue involved in cellulitis.

Empirical therapy should include drainage of any abscess and antimicrobial therapy against *S. aureus,* group B *Streptococcus,* and enteric gram-negative bacilli, adjusted according to culture results. Doses appropriate for sepsis should be used (Table 96–5). Therapy may have to be modified after the results of culture become available. Treatment of uncomplicated neonatal mastitis is usually continued for 10–14 days. With appropriate antimicrobial therapy, the prognosis for neonatal mastitis is excellent, but cosmetic defects may develop, including scars and depressions. In rare cases of neonatal mastitis, a decrease in ultimate breast size compared with the unaffected breast has been reported.

Omphalitis. Omphalitis may develop at the umbilical cord stump and progress to life-threatening necrotizing fasciitis because the devitalized tissue is an excellent medium for bacterial growth (Chapter 48). Limited inflammation at the base of the umbilical cord remnant is the earliest finding of omphalitis (see Fig. 48–1), and it is usually controlled with local antisepsis. Invasive infection, due to either unusually aggressive superficial infection or lack of recognition of early infection, may involve the periumbilical tissues and the umbilical vessel remnants, resulting in a necrotizing fasciitis that leads to a life-threatening systemic infection. Once invasive infection occurs, therapy consists of a combination of antibiotic treatment appropriate for neonatal sepsis but including coverage for *S. aureus, Clostridia,* and enteric gram-negative bacilli, with local surgical débridement and drainage and physiologic support to avoid septic shock.

NECROTIZING ENTEROCOLITIS

EPIDEMIOLOGY

Even though neonatal necrotizing enterocolitis (NEC) has been familiar since the 1960s, many aspects of this entity remain unclear. Before the routine survival of very-low-birth-weight infants, this was a much rarer disease than it is today. NEC usually occurs in the first week of life and is more common among infants with the lowest birth weight, although it may also appear later and may even occur as an unexpected event in growing neonates. In neonatal care units the incidence rate is about 5% overall. In a multicenter study (Uauy et al., 1991), the incidence of proved NEC was 10.1% among very-low-birth-weight infants (501–1,500 g), with considerable variation from 4% to 22% at different medical centers. Male infants are significantly more likely to have NEC than females.

There have been numerous reports of clusters of NEC in neonatal intensive care units. In some cases certain microbes have been isolated from the enteric contents of a high proportion of the infants involved in these clusters, but at this time there is no convincing evidence that these organisms were responsible for NEC or the high frequency of cases. No single pathogen has been implicated in multiple clusters.

PATHOGENESIS

Although many of the essential aspects of the pathogenesis of NEC are unknown, it appears that intestinal ischemia associated with stress events is an essential early step in its pathogenesis. Although NEC may occur during a period when a premature infant appears to be in clinically stable condition, it is often preceded by circulatory instability associated with polycythemia and often metabolic, surgical, cardiac, or pulmonary crises. It may also be associated with neonatal sepsis, usually as a secondary consequence of intestinal mucosal ischemia and bacterial invasion, although sepsis from another source may predispose to the development of NEC if the intestine becomes hypoperfused and ischemic. Generalized edema and areas of intestinal necrosis are present. Air in the intestinal wall leads to the hallmark radiologic finding of a linear pattern of air between the lumen and the serosa of the intestine, known as **pneumatosis intestinalis** (Fig. 96–1). Surgical findings do not always correlate with the radiologic findings because considerably more or, in varying degrees, less abnormal intestine may be identified at surgery compared with the amount of intestine showing submucosal air radiographically.

Breast-feeding has been associated with a lower incidence of NEC. The early introduction and rapid advancement of formula feeding in premature infants appear to be risk factors for NEC.

It appears that when there is intestinal ischemia, bacteria from the intraluminal contents of the intestine may cross the mucosa and invade the intestinal wall **(bacterial translocation).** When there is transmural necrosis of the intestine, perforation occurs, and microorganisms and enteric secretions leak out, causing peritonitis. Aerobic and anaerobic bacteria as well as fungi, principally *Candida,* may be involved in peritonitis associated with intestinal perforation, but anaerobes appear to play a less important role in peritonitis in newborns than in older children and adults.

SYMPTOMS AND CLINICAL MANIFESTATIONS

The initial symptoms of NEC may be subtle, with poor tolerance of oral or gavage feedings because of delayed gastric emptying and distention of the abdomen, usually in the first week of life. Evidence of frank gastrointestinal bleeding may be present. Cases with a more fulminant onset can appear to be similar to sepsis, with disorders of temperature regulation, sometimes evidence of peritonitis, clotting abnormalities, and shock. Unfortunately this latter presentation is associated with intestinal perforation, peritonitis, and a high mortality rate.

Physical Examination Findings

In addition to the physical findings suggestive of sepsis, abdominal tenderness and increased abdominal girth may suggest NEC. Retention of gastric contents and gastrointestinal bleeding are frequent early findings. This may progress to apnea and bradycardia, paleness, and mottled skin indicating poor perfusion. In advanced peritonitis there may be redness and edema of the abdominal wall, which is a grave sign.

DIAGNOSIS

Signs of NEC may not be easily differentiated from signs of generalized sepsis in a newborn, which may include only distention and ileus. A persistent dilated section of bowel that is fixed in position is suggestive of NEC. The specific diagnosis is often based on the

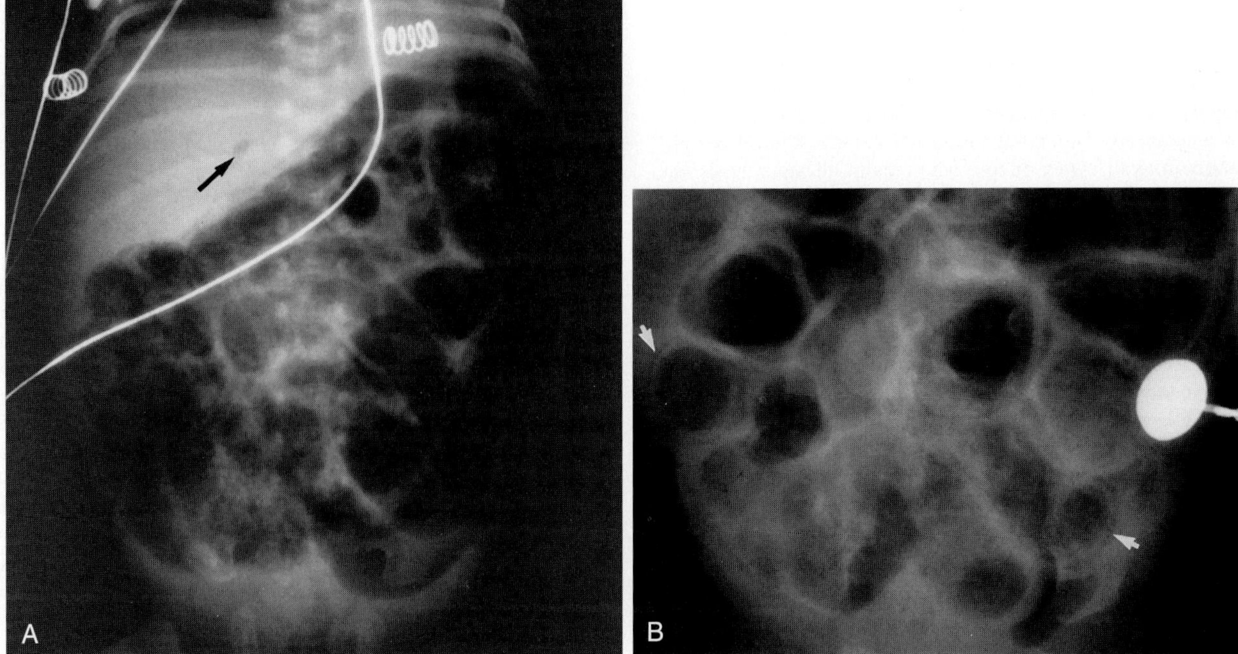

FIGURE 96–1. Necrotizing enterocolitis in two premature newborns. **A,** A frontal supine abdominal radiograph shows diffuse gaseous distention of the intestine with areas of bubblelike pneumatosis intestinalis, especially in the right lower quadrant. Note branching lucencies *(arrow)* within the liver, which represent portal venous gas. All of these signs are indicative of necrotizing enterocolitis. **B,** Detail of supine abdominal radiograph shows circular lucencies *(arrows)* surrounding several loops of air-filled intestine, signifying pneumatosis intestinalis.

clinical presentation of symptoms and signs of sepsis in association with a variable combination of feeding intolerance evidenced by poor gastric emptying with residual gastric contents, abdominal distention, emesis, bilious emesis, positive reducing substances in the stool, and occult or frank gastrointestinal bleeding. Signs of complicated disease, such as peritoneal fluid and free abdominal gas, may be present and indicate impending or frank perforation. This assessment may be aided by abdominal paracentesis and examination of the peritoneal fluid for leukocytes and bacteria, which are indicators of peritonitis and the need for immediate surgical intervention. The diagnosis may be confirmed by the demonstration of pneumatosis intestinalis or air in the biliary tree (Fig. 96–1), or by findings of ischemic intestine at laparotomy.

Infants suspected of having NEC should have a complete evaluation for sepsis. Blood cultures are positive in about one third of the cases and may help in directing antibiotic therapy. Organisms commonly recovered include enteric gram-negative bacilli and infrequently *Pseudomonas aeruginosa* and *S. aureus.*

Diagnostic Imaging

Radiologic examination of the abdomen with a plain anteroposterior radiograph as well as a cross-table lateral view may reveal the nonspecific finding of **fixed, dilated loops of intestine. Pneumatosis intestinalis** with or without the finding of **intrahepatic portal air,** seen most easily on cross-table lateral images, confirms the diagnosis of NEC (Fig. 96–1). These radiographic findings are not always present and are not necessary for the diagnosis of NEC.

TREATMENT

The treatment of NEC depends on its severity. Mild disease without perforation requires observation in a skilled neonatal intensive care unit with surgical expertise available, if needed. Intravenous fluid treatment is begun, and the intestine is rested and decompressed with a nasogastric tube. The use of antibiotics at this stage is controversial, but most experts recommend empirical administration of antibiotics similar to the treatment of early-onset neonatal sepsis (Tables 96–4 and 96–5). If there is evidence of toxicity (which indicates intestinal gangrene) or of perforation, surgical intervention is necessary, and it must be assumed that there are extraintestinal microorganisms. Perforation occurs in about one third of infants with NEC. Surgical treatment generally involves resection of the gangrenous intestine and an enterostomy. Empirical antibiotic therapy is chosen to cover enteric gram-negative and gram-positive (e.g., *Enterococcus*) aerobes. Continuing therapy should take into consideration the results of blood, peritoneal fluid, and surgical cultures and should be modified as necessary. For infants not known to harbor antibiotic-resistant organisms, a combination of ampicillin and gentamicin is effective against most intestinal pathogens (Table 96–5). Nafcillin, oxacillin, or vancomycin may be added if there is evidence of *Staphylococcus.* Some pediatric surgeons routinely treat peritonitis associated with NEC with an antibiotic active against gram-negative anaerobic bacilli. Clindamycin is often added in this situation because it is active against most intestinal anaerobes and is also active against most strains of *S. aureus,* but there is an absence of proof that an anti-anaerobic antibiotic improves outcome.

Infants with NEC should be treated at an institution with expertise in pediatric surgery and anesthesia that can provide for controlled medical treatment of shock, including volume expanders and inotropic agents. Experienced specialists who have been observing the infant patient as long as possible can best decide the need for surgery.

COMPLICATIONS AND PROGNOSIS

The prognosis for NEC depends on the severity of the disease and the underlying medical condition of the infant. Infants with very low birth weight, congenital malformations, and sepsis have a high mortality. Those who require surgical intervention usually have severe NEC with signs of perforation and have a poorer prognosis. Early complications of NEC include overwhelming sepsis with leukopenia and disseminated intravascular coagulation. Among those who survive, infants who did not require surgical therapy generally do well. Among those who require intestinal resection, the ultimate prognosis depends on the length and location of the resected intestine. Infants who require a large resection may have **short-gut syndrome,** in which the absorptive surface of the remaining intestine is insufficient for adequate absorption of nutrients fed by mouth. Other problems associated with intestinal operations, such as abscesses, peritoneal adhesions, anastomotic leakage, and intestinal stenosis may complicate the recovery period and may be life threatening in fragile neonates. Overall the mortality is 20–40%, although the rate varies depending on the standards used to confirm the diagnosis. There has been a trend toward improved survival rates, except among infants with overwhelming intestinal necrosis and sepsis, whose chances of survival remain poor.

PREVENTION

The use of oral antibiotics to prevent NEC may have some theoretical benefit in eliminating flora that participate in the development of pneumatosis and intestinal injury. Clinical studies have been inconclusive as to benefit, so prophylactic oral antibiotics cannot be recommended, especially because they may encourage carriage of antibiotic-resistant organisms. The inability to prove that any particular species of microorganism in the intestine is the cause of NEC indicates that neither the use of surveillance cultures nor the treatment of selected infants who harbor certain species is of proven benefit. Studies of the feeding of breast milk to premature neonates, the use of orally administered immune globulin preparations, and special early feeding regimens have shown inconsistent benefit.

FUNGAL INFECTIONS

Candida species are the major cause of fungal infections in the neonate. Environmental fungi are uncommon pathogens in neonates. Increasingly, normal skin flora dermatophytes are being recognized as possible causes of fungemia in very-low-birth-weight infants with central catheters placed for parenteral alimentation.

EPIDEMIOLOGY

Oral candidiasis (thrush) and ***Candida*** **diaper dermatitis** are common in neonates, especially if broad-spectrum antibiotics are administered, and are similar to oral thrush and diaper rash in older infants (Chapter 46). Neonates may have superficial cutaneous infections caused by several dermatophytic fungal species such as *Epidermophyton, Microsporum,* and *Trichophyton,* although such infections are uncommon. When the skin is involved, these species cause cutaneous tinea, or ringworm, and can be treated as in older children (Chapter 46).

Although superficial cutaneous fungal infections are relatively common among neonates, disseminated fungal infections were rarely reported in neonates until the early 1980s. The increase in invasive fungal infections is primarily among very low-birth-weight infants (<1,500 g) and is related to the increased survival rates of these infants associated with prolonged hospitalization, long-term use of indwelling intravenous catheters, intravenous hyperalimentation (especially with lipid emulsion), and often multiple courses of broad-spectrum antibiotics for possible bacterial infections. Invasive fungal infections caused by species other than *Candida* are uncommon in neonates because many fungal infections, such as aspergillosis, cryptococcosis, coccidioidomycosis, blastomycosis, and histoplasmosis, are generally contracted from the environment, and neonates are unlikely to be exposed. In utero exposure may occur in very rare instances.

PATHOGENESIS

During birth newborns are often contaminated with *Candida* from maternal vaginal colonization. Transmission to an infant after birth could occur from the skin of the mother or other caregiver. *Candida* is a frequent and normal flora of the skin and upper respiratory and gastrointestinal tracts. Proliferation of *Candida* on the mucous membranes of the mouth and intertriginous areas of normal infants is common and is responsible for oral thrush and a common form of diaper dermatitis. Inhibition of normal bacterial flora with the use of antibiotics and also with immunosuppression, especially of cell-mediated immunity, allows the organism to proliferate abnormally. Premature infants often have both risk factors as a result of their relatively poor immunologic function (Chapter 5). Both the frequent use of broad-spectrum antibiotics in premature infants and the use of steroids for respiratory distress and prevention of bronchopulmonary dysplasia magnify the risk of *Candida* infection.

Most serious neonatal fungal infections are caused by *Candida.* In addition to *C. albicans,* less common species include *C. tropicalis, C. parapsilosis,* and *C. lusitaniae.* Infections due to *C. krusei* are uncommon but are notable because many strains of this species are not susceptible to amphotericin B. *Candida* infection may rarely occur before birth from ascending infection in the genital tract, which presents as widespread **mucocutaneous candidiasis** at birth. A syndrome of disseminated papular and vesicular superficial skin lesions has been reported. It appears to be benign in many cases because the lesions heal without sequelae without the use of antifungal agents. However, recently there have been reports of superficial dermatitis leading to disseminated disease in premature infants.

SYMPTOMS AND CLINICAL MANIFESTATIONS

Candida infections must be considered in tiny premature infants who have evidence of systemic infection after they have survived the first few weeks of life, especially those who have been treated with repeated or prolonged courses of broad-spectrum antibiotics for presumed or proven bacterial infections. The clinical manifestations of candidemia or disseminated candidiasis may include evidence of local infection, such as mucocutaneous lesions or a macular rash, or the symptoms may be nonspecific, such as temperature irregularity, poor feeding, irritability, and altered respiratory pattern. Growth of *Candida* from a culture of the blood, even without evidence of focal infection in any organ, is considered diagnostic of candidemia and should not be dismissed as a contaminated blood culture. The diagnosis of **disseminated candidiasis** is confirmed if there is candidemia with local infection in viscera, including the renal system, the brain, CSF, heart valves, lungs, skeletal tissue, or the vitreous humor of the eye, or if pseudohyphae are seen in the urine or in biopsy specimens of tissue. *Candida* pneumonia is probably very rare (Chapter 68), but it is exceedingly difficult to confirm the diagnosis of lower respiratory tract infection with *Candida* because of the inability to culture the lungs without contamination with upper respiratory secretions.

The clinical manifestations of **mucocutaneous candidiasis** are the characteristic whitish gray plaques on the mucous membranes of the oral mucosa and vesicular and pustular lesions on the skin, generally in moist intertriginous areas of the body.

DIAGNOSIS

Mucocutaneous *Candida* infections are usually diagnosed by the characteristic appearance of the lesions and confirmed by Gram stain and culture of scrapings from the skin or mucous membranes. Disseminated disease is usually first detected in neonates by a positive blood culture, but other signs of dissemination include masses in visceral organs that may be detected by CT or MRI; debris in the renal collecting system that may be detected by ultrasonography; central nervous system disease detected by analysis and culture of the CSF and CT; and ocular disease detected by ophthalmologic examination. Biopsy and culture of organs must be individualized and often depend on whether the infection is in doubt and requires confirmation.

TREATMENT

Candidemia with or without evidence of invasive focal candidiasis in a newborn is treated with amphotericin B (Chapter 14). The principles are similar to those of treatment of older children with candidiasis, but less is known about the pharmacologic aspects and toxicity. In general, an initial treatment dose of 0.2–0.3 mg/kg once daily is recommended with the dose increased by 0.25 mg/kg each day over 2–3 days to a maximum of 0.5–1.0 mg/kg/day (van den Anker et al., 1995). Many infants with candidemia respond to a dose lower than 1 mg/kg/day, with doses of 0.3–0.4 mg/kg/day reported to result in successful eradication of the organism. The maximum dose should be used for infants with evidence of focal infection in organs, especially those with meningitis. If there is evidence of endocarditis, the lesion may have to be excised from the cardiac valve (Chapter 71). The optimal duration of treatment of neonatal candidemia has not been determined, and experts differ in their recommendations. Although amphotericin B is often dosed by the total amount of amphotericin B per kilogram of body weight for the treatment of deep-tissue fungal infections, candidemia often can be treated according to the duration of the dose effective in eliminating the candidemia. Treatment for 2 weeks beyond the last positive blood culture is usually curative. When infection has disseminated to organs or there has been meningitis, a longer duration will be necessary, and a total dose of 25–30 mg/kg is recommended; this will require treatment for about 1 month at a dosage of 1 mg/kg/day. If the organism is relatively resistant to amphotericin B or if eradication is unsuccessful with 1 mg/kg/day, the use of higher doses (up to 1.5 mg/kg/day) or the use of liposomal amphotericin B (5 mg/kg/day) has been reported anecdotally. For the treatment of meningitis, the addition of flucytosine (50–150 mg/kg/day divided in four doses orally) is recommended, but experience is limited in neonates. In some cases, intrathecal amphotericin B may be required to eradicate the organism. Infants with disseminated candidiasis should be treated at centers familiar with management of the sickest newborns, and consultation with an infectious diseases specialist is desirable.

It is unclear whether antifungal agents are at all effective against *Malassezia furfur,* a dermatophyte frequently recovered from blood cultures of premature infants who have central indwelling catheters. Removal of the intravascular catheter and discontinuation of intravenous lipid emulsion are essential and usually curative. If treatment is necessary, griseofulvin can be used, although griseofulvin alone is not sufficient for cure of infection by this or other lipophilic organisms.

Oral candidiasis (thrush) is generally treated with nystatin solution, 100,000–400,000 units 4–6 times a day orally for 1 week (Chapter 46). The higher dose is used if the infection is not cured with the lower dose. Candidiasis of the skin may be treated by exposure to light to dry the skin and aid healing, a drying ointment or powder such as zinc oxide, or nystatin ointment applied 3–4 times per day. Persistent mucocutaneous candidiasis that resists several attempts at treatment may be an early sign of immunodeficiency, including neonatal AIDS. Before therapy with other antifungal agents is attempted an immune function evaluation should be performed.

Treatment of superficial candidiasis that appears to have developed in utero is quite different from treatment of disseminated fungal disease. The prognosis is generally excellent, and in most cases the condition is self-limited and in a term infant does not require antifungal therapy.

In the rare case of infection due to environmental fungi, including *Aspergillus,* a long course of amphotericin B is required, and consultation with an infectious diseases specialist is advised.

PROGNOSIS

The prognosis for superficial cutaneous or mucous membrane candidiasis in newborns is excellent. Response to treatment can be expected within several days; many cases resolve without any specific treatment. In otherwise healthy infants, relapses are common and may be treated similarly to the first infection.

Although candidemia may be transient and disappear without treatment, especially infection associated with an intravascular catheter that is removed, there is a tendency for candidemia to persist in premature infants. Therefore, treatment should always be started. Untreated disseminated candidal disease is usually fatal, but if antifungal treatment is initiated early the prognosis is similar to that for infection with bacteria. If meningitis occurs, the prognosis is considerably worse, and many survivors have neurologic sequelae. Endocarditis caused by *Candida* in older children or adults usually requires surgical removal of the vegetation for cure. This may be necessary for some neonates as well, but cure using only amphotericin B and medical management has been reported. One review (Sanchez et al., 1991) reported that although the historical survival rate of neonates with *Candida* endocarditis was only 39%, many infants never received definitive treatment, and the diagnosis was made only at autopsy.

REVIEWS

Baltimore RS: Neonatal nosocomial infections. *Semin Perinatol* 1998; 22:25–32.

Kaftan H, Kinney JS: Early onset neonatal bacterial infections. *Semin Perinatol* 1998;22:15–24.

Klein JO, Marcy SM: Bacterial sepsis and meningitis. In Remington JS, Klein JO (editors): *Infectious Diseases of the Fetus and Newborn Infant,* 5th ed. Philadelphia, WB Saunders, 2000.

Sepsis

American Academy of Pediatrics, Committee on Infectious Diseases and Committee on Fetus and Newborn: Revised guidelines for prevention of early-onset group B streptococcal (GBS) infection. *Pediatrics* 1997; 99:489–96.

Baker CJ, Kasper DL: Correlation of maternal antibody deficiency with susceptibility to neonatal group B streptococcal infection. *N Engl J Med* 1976;294:753–6.

Baltimore RS: Late, late-onset infections in the nursery. *Yale J Biol Med* 1988;61:501–6.

Berger M: Use of intravenously administered immune globulin in newborn infants: Prophylaxis, treatment, both, or neither? *J Pediatr* 1991; 118:557–9.

Bilgin K, Yaramis A, Haspolat K, et al: A randomized trial of granulocyte-macrophage colony-stimulating factor in neonates with sepsis and neutropenia. *Pediatrics* 2001;107:36–41.

Bromberger P, Lawrence JM, Braun D, et al: The influence of intrapartum antibiotics on the clinical spectrum of early-onset group B streptococcal infection in term infants. *Pediatrics* 2000;106:244–50.

Cairo MS, Worcester CC, Rucker RW, et al: Randomized trial of granulocyte transfusion versus intravenous immune globulin therapy for neonatal neutropenia and sepsis. *J Pediatr* 1992;120:281–5.

Centers for Disease Control and Prevention: Prevention of perinatal group B streptococcal disease: A public health perspective. *MMWR Morb Mortal Wkly Rep* 1996;45(RR-7):1–24.

Gladstone IM, Ehrenkranz RA, Edberg SC, et al: A ten-year review of neonatal sepsis and comparison with the previous fifty-year experience. *Pediatr Infect Dis J* 1990;9:819–25.

Gregory J, Hey E: Blood neutrophil response to bacterial infection in the first month of life. *Arch Dis Child* 1972;47:747–53.

Jenson HB, Pollock BH: Meta-analyses of the effectiveness of intravenous immune globulin for the prevention and treatment of neonatal sepsis. *Pediatrics* 1997;99:E2.

Kosloske AM: Sepsis and infection in the neonate. In Fonkalsrud EW, Krummel TM (editors): *Infections and Immunologic Disorders in Pediatric Surgery.* Philadelphia, WB Saunders, 1993.

Manroe BL, Weinberg AG, Rosenfeld CR, et al: The neonatal blood count in health and disease. I. Reference values for neutrophilic cells. *J Pediatr* 1979;95:89–98.

Mercer BM, Miodovnik M, Thurnau GR, et al: Antibiotic therapy for reduction of infant morbidity after preterm premature rupture of the membranes: A randomized controlled trial. National Institute of Child Health and Human Development, Maternal-Fetal Medicine Units Network. *JAMA* 1997;278:989–95.

Miura E, Procianoy RS, Bittar C, et al: A randomized, double-masked, placebo-controlled trial of recombinant granulocyte colony-stimulating factor administration to preterm infants with the clinical diagnosis of early-onset sepsis. *Pediatrics* 2001;107:30–5.

Patrick CC, Kaplan SL, Baker CJ, et al: Persistent bacteria due to coagulase-negative staphylococci in low birth weight neonates. *Pediatrics* 1989; 84:977–85.

Philip AG: Decreased use of antibiotics using a neonatal screening technique. *J Pediatr* 1981;98:795–9.

Philip AG: The changing face of neonatal infection: Experience at a regional medical center. *Pediatr Infect Dis J* 1994;13:1098–102.

Philip AG, Hewitt JR: Early diagnosis of neonatal sepsis. *Pediatrics* 1980;65:1036–41.

Robbins JB, McCracken GH Jr, Gotschlich EC, et al: *Escherichia coli* KI capsular polysaccharide associated with neonatal meningitis. *N Engl J Med* 1974;290:1216–20.

Schrag SJ, Zywicki S, Farley MM, et al: Group B streptococcal disease in the era of intrapartum antibiotic prophylaxis. *N Engl J Med* 2000; 342:15–20.

Focal Bacterial Infections

Burry VF, Beezley M: Infant mastitis due to gram-negative organisms. *Am J Dis Child* 1972; 124:736–7.

Feder HM Jr, MacLean Jr, Moxon R: Scalp abscess secondary to fetal scalp electrode. *J Pediatr* 1976;89:808–9.

Gladstone IM, Clapper L, Thorp JW, et al: Randomized study of six umbilical cord care regimens: Comparing length of attachment, microbial control, and satisfaction. *Clin Pediatr* 1988;27:127–9.

Hsieh WS, Yang PH, Chao HC, et al: Neonatal necrotizing fasciitis: A report of three cases and review of the literature. *Pediatrics* 1999;103:e53.

Mason WH, Andrews R, Ross LA, et al: Omphalitis in newborn infant. *Pediatr Infect Dis J* 1989;8:521–5.

Nelson J: Suppurative mastitis in infants. *Am J Dis Child* 1973;123:458–9.

Walsh M, McIntosh K: Neonatal mastitis. *Clin Pediatr* 1986;25:395–9.

Necrotizing Enterocolitis

Albanese CT, Rowe MI: Necrotizing enterocolitis. In Fonkalsrud EW, Krummel TM (editors): *Infections and Immunologic Disorders in Pediatric Surgery.* Philadelphia, WB Saunders, 1993.

Books LS, Overall JC Jr, Herbst JJ, et al: Clustering of necrotizing enterocolitis: Interruption by infection-control measure. *N Engl J Med* 1977; 297:984–6.

Edelson MB, Bagwell CE, Rozycki HJ: Circulating pro- and counterinflammatory cytokine levels and severity in necrotizing enterocolitis. *Pediatrics* 1999;103:766–71.

Eibl MM, Wolf HM, Fürnkranz H, et al: Prevention of necrotizing enterocolitis in low-birth-weight infants by IgA-IgG feeding. *N Engl J Med* 1988;319:1–7.

Kliegman RM, Fanaroff AA: Necrotizing enterocolitis. *N Engl J Med* 1984;310:1093–103.

Lucas A, Cole TJ: Breast milk and neonatal necrotising enterocolitis. *Lancet* 1990;336:1519–23.

McClead RE Jr (editor): Neonatal necrotizing enterocolitis: Current concepts and controversies. *J Pediatr* 1990;117(Suppl):S1–S74.

Uauy RD, Fanaroff AA, Korones SB, et al: Necrotizing enterocolitis in very low birth weight infants: Biodemographic and clinical correlates. National Institute of Child Health and Human Development Neonatal Research Network. *J Pediatr* 1991;119:630–8

Fungal Infections

Baley JE: Neonatal candidiasis: The current challenge. *Clin Perinatol* 1991;18:263–80.

Baley JE, Kliegman M, Fanaroff AA: Disseminated fungal infections in very low-birth-weight infants: Clinical manifestations and epidemiology. *Pediatrics* 1984;73:144–52.

Baley JE, Kliegman RM, Fanaroff AA: Disseminated fungal infections in very low-birth-weight infants: Therapeutic toxicity. *Pediatrics* 1984; 73:153–7.

Botas CM, Kurlat I, Young SM, et al: Disseminated candidal infections and intravenous hydrocortisone in preterm infants. *Pediatrics* 1995; 95:883–7.

Butler KM, Rench MA, Baker CJ: Amphotericin B as a single agent in the treatment of systemic candidiasis in neonates. *Pediatr Infect Dis J* 1990;9:51–6.

Chapman RL, Faix RG: Persistently positive cultures and outcome in invasive neonatal candidiasis. *Pediatr Infect Dis J* 2000;19:822–7.

Darmstadt GL, Dinulos JG, Miller Z: Congenital cutaneous candidiasis: Clinical presentation, pathogenesis, and management guidelines. *Pediatrics* 2000;105:438–44.

Faix RG: Systemic *Candida* infections in infants in intensive care nurseries: High incidence of central nervous system involvement. *J Pediatr* 1984;105:616–22.

Huttova M, Hartmanova I, Kralinsky K, et al: *Candida* fungemia in neonates treated with fluconazole: Report of forty cases, including eight with meningitis. *Pediatr Infect Dis J* 1998;17:1012–5.

Kam LA, Giacoia GP: Congenital cutaneous candidiasis. *Am J Dis Child* 1975;129:1215–8.

Kossoff EH, Buescher S, Karlowicz MG: Candidemia in a neonatal intensive care unit: Trends during fifteen years and clinical features of 111 cases. *Pediatr Infect Dis J* 1998;17:504–8.

Makhoul IR, Kassis I, Smolkin T, et al: Review of 49 neonates with acquired fungal sepsis: Further characterization. *Pediatrics* 2001;107:61–6.

Sanchez PJ, Siegel JD, Fishbein J: *Candida* endocarditis: Successful medical management in three preterm infants and review of the literature. *Pediatr Infect Dis J* 1991;10:239–43.

Van den Anker JN, van Popele NM, Sauer PJ: Antifungal agents in neonatal systemic candidiasis. *Antimicrob Agents Chemother* 1995;39:1391–7.

CHAPTER 97

Perinatal Viral Infections

Rebecca C. Brady ▪ Lawrence R. Stanberry

Perinatal viral infections are infections of the fetus and newborn infant that are acquired in utero, during delivery, or in the postpartum period. The clinical course and outcome of perinatal viral infections are influenced by the stage of development when infection occurs and the pathogenicity of the virus (Table 97–1). An infection early in gestation, during organ development, may produce extensive tissue destruction resulting in malformation, intrauterine growth retardation, or stillbirth. The same virus causing infection late in gestation may produce no apparent injury. Similarly, viruses with greater virulence tend to cause more severe perinatal disease. For example, a lytic virus such as measles may cause fetal death, whereas infection by a less destructive virus such as rubella is generally not fatal but may produce congenital anomalies.

Perinatal viral infections may be asymptomatic or may produce clinically evident illness. Unrecognized infections are common with some viruses, such as cytomegalovirus (CMV), which may produce few or no acute symptoms but can also cause injury that results in sequelae, such as hearing loss, later in life. Symptomatic perinatal viral infections can be placed into one of the three following categories on the basis of the age of the infant at the onset of symptoms: (1) the infant may have evidence of infection at the time of delivery; (2) the newborn may appear healthy at birth but become ill during the neonatal period; (3) the infant may appear well throughout the neonatal period only to manifest sequelae of a perinatally acquired infection months to years after delivery. Although not all congenital infections result in symptoms in newborns, all infants who have symptoms at birth acquired the infection in utero. Healthy newborns who become ill days, weeks, or months after birth are typical of those whose infections were acquired at delivery or in the postpartum period. The most important factor influencing the age at onset of clinical disease is the incubation period of the virus (Table 97–2). Viruses with short incubation periods, such as herpes simplex virus (HSV), cause perinatally acquired infections that present in the neonatal period, whereas infections that present later in infancy are caused by viruses with longer incubation periods, such as hepatitis B virus (HBV).

Only a few viruses result in the scenario of a healthy newborn becoming ill in the first month of life with a severe and potentially life-threatening infection. Neonates are also susceptible to acquisition of and infection by the same viruses that produce infections in older children and adults, such as rhinoviruses. As in older patients, infections are generally self-limited, and the young infant recovers without complication. However, with some perinatal viral infections there are unique circumstances whereby a virus that causes limited illness in older children may produce life-threatening

TABLE 97–1. Viruses That Cause Perinatal Infection and Their Effect on the Fetus and Newborn

	Maternal Infection						Postnatal Infection		
Virus	In Utero Transmission	Persistent Fetal Infection	Fetal Death	Growth Retardation	Prematurity	Malformation	Acute Infection	Persistent Infection	Neonatal or Infant Death
Cytomegalovirus	+	+	+	+	+	+	+	+	Rare
Enteroviruses (nonpolio)	Rare	–	–	–	–	–	+	–	Rare
Epstein-Barr virus	+	+	±	±	+	±	Rare	+	–
Hepatitis B virus	Rare	+	–	–	+	–	+	+	+
Herpes simplex virus	Rare	+	+	+	+	+	+	+	+
Human immunodeficiency virus	+	+	–	+	±	±	+	+	+
Human papillomavirus	–	–	–	–	–	–	Rare	Rare	±
Influenza virus	–	–	–	–	–	–	+	–	+
Measles virus	+	–	Rare	+	+	±	+	–	–
Mumps virus	±	–	Rare	–	–	±	Rare	–	–
Parvovirus	+	–	+	±	–	–	?	–	–
Polio virus	+	–	+	–	+	–	+	–	Rare
Rabies virus	–	–	–	–	–	–	+	–	+
Respiratory syncytial virus	–	–	–	–	–	–	+	–	+
Rubella virus	+	–	+	+	+	+	+	–	–
Smallpox virus	+	–	+	+	+	–	+	–	+
Varicella-zoster virus	+	+	Rare	+	+	+	+	+	+

+ = Established effect; – = effect not noted; ± = effect believed to occur on basis of case reports; ? = inadequate data.

TABLE 97–2. Time From Exposure to Onset of Clinical Disease Due to Perinatally Acquired Viral Infections

Virus	Incubation Period
Cytomegalovirus	3–12 wk (typically 4–8 wk)
Enteroviruses	2–14 days (typically 3–5 days)
Hepatitis B virus	2–5 mo to onset of hepatitis
Herpes simplex virus	2–20 days (typically 2–12 days)
Human immunodeficiency virus	1 mo to 5 yr to clinical recognition of infection
Human papillomavirus	<6 mo to development of laryngeal papillomatosis
Influenza virus	1–7 days (typically 1–2 days)
Measles virus	9–19 days (typically 10–14 days)
Mumps virus	7–25 days (typically 16–20 days)
Respiratory syncytial virus	2–8 days (typically 5 days)
Rubella virus	12–23 days (typically 16–20 days)
Varicella-zoster virus	8–21 days (typically 12–16 days)

infection in a fetus or newborn. These circumstances include (1) the potential for acquiring the infection by an unusual route of transmission (e.g., transplacentally as a consequence of maternal viremia), (2) the potential for being exposed to a higher inoculum than typically occurs with older patients (e.g., exposure resulting from prolonged labor or from maternal viremia), and (3) the relative immunologic immaturity of the fetus and neonate. Although maternal virus-specific IgG antibody may be transferred to the fetus, providing some protection, maternal viral infection close to term may preclude maternal synthesis and transfer of antibody to the infant. The net effect of maternal infection around the time of delivery can be a fetus or newborn who is exposed to a very high inoculum by an unusual route without benefit of maternal antibody. These potentially deadly neonatal infections are caused by HSV, varicella-zoster virus (VZV), and the enteroviruses. They are distinctly different from the *intrauterine* infections caused by HSV (Chapter 95), other congenital intrauterine infections, and perinatally acquired infections due to viruses with long clinical incubation periods such as HBV and human immunodeficiency virus (HIV).

HERPES SIMPLEX VIRUS

ETIOLOGY

HSV, a member of the Herpesviridae family, is a large, enveloped, double-stranded DNA virus. Alpha herpesviruses, including HSV, are neurotropic human pathogens capable of entering and traversing within peripheral nerves. During initial infection these viruses are transported to sensory ganglia, where they establish latent infection with only limited transcription of the viral genome and no replication of the viral DNA. Therefore, antiviral drugs such as acyclovir, which act by inhibiting the replication of virus, have no effect on latent viral infection. The nonreplicating latent virus persists within sensory neuronal ganglia throughout the life of the host. By mechanisms that are not understood, latent virus can be reactivated to a replication-competent form by tissue damage, ultraviolet light, immunosuppression, or physical or emotional stress. This reactivated virus is responsible for causing recurrent infections such as herpes labialis (fever blisters) and herpes genitalis (genital herpes).

There are two serologically and genetically distinct subtypes of HSV, type 1 (**HSV-1**), also known as human herpesvirus 1, and type 2 (**HSV-2**), also known as human herpesvirus 2. Historically, these two viruses were distinguished from each other by the anatomic location of lesions in adult patients from whom they were isolated. HSV-1 was purported to cause disease above the waist (herpes labialis), whereas HSV-2 was purported to cause disease below the waist (genital herpes). With recent changes in sexual mores, adults have been cross-infecting mucous membranes and as a consequence HSV-1 is now a common cause of genital herpes, and HSV-2 has been documented to produce infection of the oral cavity. Both HSV-1 and HSV-2 can cause neonatal infection.

EPIDEMIOLOGY

Neonatal HSV infection occurs in an estimated 2–7 infants per 10,000 live births. It is expected that 700–2500 newborns have neonatal HSV infection annually in the United States. Intrauterine HSV infection does occur but is rare (Chapter 95). Most cases of neonatal infection are acquired during labor and delivery or in the postpartum period. From 70–85% of neonatal cases are due to HSV-2, and the remainder are caused by HSV-1. Cases of neonatal HSV infection may also result from the postpartum transmission of virus. Although HSV-1 can produce genital infection in adults, more frequently it causes infection of the lip and oral cavity, and it can be incidentally transferred to a susceptible newborn. The source of the virus may be the mother, but it can be any close contact.

Neonatal herpes due to HSV-2 is usually contracted during passage through an infected birth canal. Genital HSV replication is estimated to occur in approximately 1% of pregnant women at some time during gestation. Most cases of genital herpes in pregnant women are recurrent infections that are clinically inapparent or asymptomatic in at least 40% of women. For women with a history of recurrent genital herpes before pregnancy, the mean number of clinically recognized episodes of recurrent infections increases from 0.97 in the first trimester, to 1.26 in the second trimester, and 1.63 in the third trimester. Shedding of virus from the genital tract in the absence of recognized lesions can also occur, with recovery of HSV found in 0.65–3.03% of genital cultures collected during gestation. When shedding of the virus occurs around the time of delivery, HSV may be transmitted to the infant during birth. It is estimated that 0.1–0.39% of all pregnant women shed HSV at the time of delivery, with a frequency that increases to 1.3% during the week before delivery for women with a history of recurrent genital herpes. Although HSV is frequently present in the genital tracts of women with a history of recurrent infections, it is usually present for only a short time (1.5 days for women who are not pregnant). Thus cultures that are collected from the mother's genital tract days to weeks before delivery do not predict the infant's risk of exposure to HSV at the time of delivery.

Considering the high incidence of recurrent genital herpes in pregnant women, it is surprising that so few infants develop neonatal HSV infections. Two factors may account for this apparent contradiction. First, women who experience primary genital HSV-2 infection before pregnancy develop antibodies to the virus, some of which are passively transferred to the fetus. These transplacentally acquired neutralizing antibodies have been shown to confer at least partial protection to the newborn, thus preventing or modifying infection. Second, compared with primary genital herpes, at least 100-fold fewer infectious virions are present in the genital tract during a recurrent infection, and consequently infants born to women with recurrent genital herpes are exposed to considerably less viral burden than infants born to women with a primary infection. It is estimated that the risk of acquiring neonatal herpes is as high as 50% for women experiencing a first episode of genital herpes at the time of delivery, and less than 3% for women with

TABLE 97–3. Risk Factors Associated with Perinatally Acquired Viral Infections

Herpes Simplex Virus Infections
Active genital infection at the time of delivery
Risk is greater with primary than with recurrent genital herpes
History of genital herpes in mother or her sexual partner or partners
Delivery through an infected birth canal
Delivery by cesarean section 6 or more hours after rupture of membranes
Instrumented delivery (scalp electrode) in the HSV-2 seropositive woman
Varicella-Zoster Virus Infections
Active maternal chickenpox within 7 days before and 21 days after delivery
Maternal history negative for chickenpox
Enterovirus Infections
Maternal infection at delivery
Lower socioeconomic status
Lack of breast-feeding

recurrent genital infections. Several risk factors associated with perinatally acquired HSV infections have been identified (Table 97–3).

PATHOGENESIS

Infection begins with the transmission of virus from a contagious person to a portal of entry or site of inoculation of a susceptible neonate. The source of virus in most cases of perinatal disease is the mother. Any mucous membrane may serve as a portal of entry, especially the conjunctival sacs and the epithelial lining of the mouth and nose. Skin may also serve as a portal of entry if the integrity of the skin has been damaged by trauma, as in a forceps delivery or placement of a scalp electrode. Virus replication may be restricted to the site of inoculation, in which case the infection is limited to the skin, eye, or mouth. Unfortunately, virus may also spread beyond the portal of entry by local extension, intraneuronal transport, and hematogenous spread to produce pneumonia, central nervous system (CNS) infection, or disseminated disease. In survivors the intraneuronal spread of virus allows the establishment of latent infection in nerves innervating the portal of entry. Reactivation of latent virus may result in recurrent cutaneous or neural infections throughout infancy. Several factors may influence the extent and severity of neonatal HSV infection, including the portal of entry, the amount of virus to which the infant is exposed, the virulence of the virus strain, the gestational age of the infant, the presence of maternally derived antibodies specific to the virus causing infection, the immunocompetence of the infant, and possibly genetic determinants of susceptibility to infection.

SYMPTOMS AND CLINICAL MANIFESTATIONS

The clinical spectrum of neonatal HSV infection varies greatly (Table 97–4). The infection is rarely asymptomatic and should always be considered a potentially life-threatening illness. In some newborns there is evidence of infection at birth, but more commonly clinical signs of neonatal herpes develop when the infant is 1–3 weeks of age. On the basis of physical findings and diagnostic tests, three categories of neonatal disease have been described:

TABLE 97–4. Signs and Symptoms Associated with Neonatal Herpes Simplex Virus Infection

Disease Category	Signs and Symptoms
Localized disease	
Skin disease	Vesicles
Eye disease	Keratoconjunctivitis, chorioretinitis
Mouth disease	Vesicles, ulcers
Encephalitis	Seizures (focal or generalized)
	Tremors
	Irritability
	Lethargy
	Coma
	Posturing
	Paralysis (flaccid or spastic)
	Bulging fontanelle
	Temperature instability
	Poor feeding
Disseminated disease	
Without central nervous system involvement	Hypothermia or hyperthermia
	Feeding intolerance
	Lethargy
	Purpura
	Respiratory distress
	Jaundice
	Hepatomegaly
	Keratoconjunctivitis
	Skin vesicles
	Vesicles or ulcers in the oral cavity
With central nervous system involvement	Signs of disseminated infection *plus*
	Irritability
	Seizures
	Posturing
	Paralysis
	Coma

(1) skin, eye, and mouth (SEM) disease; (2) disseminated disease involving multiple organs; and (3) disease limited to the CNS. Infants with **SEM disease** typically present with vesicular skin or mucous membrane lesions in the first or second week of life. These vesicles are usually 1–2 mm in diameter and may be surrounded by an erythematous base. The vesicles may be limited to a defined region, such as the site of a scalp electrode or a single dermatome (zosteriform distribution), or the lesions may be generalized, involving distant anatomic regions. Occasionally the vesicles progress to form bullous lesions. These infants do not appear ill, and their infections may be misdiagnosed as superficial bacterial infections. Without prompt institution of intravenous antiviral therapy, this localized infection usually progresses to encephalitis or disseminated infection.

Infants with **disseminated disease** classically present in the first 2 weeks (mean, day 11 of life) with a sepsislike illness. These infants may exhibit hyperthermia or hypothermia, irritability or lethargy, respiratory distress, cyanosis, feeding intolerance, and seizures. Involvement of the CNS is common in these patients. When skin vesicles are present, HSV infection is considered high in the differential diagnosis. Unfortunately, 20–30% of infants with neonatal herpes do not have skin vesicles, reducing the likelihood that HSV infection will be considered in the differential diagnosis.

Infants with **CNS disease** only often present during the second and third weeks (mean, day 17 of life) with lethargy or irritability and focal or generalized seizures. Neonatal encephalitis due to HSV-2 is reported to be more severe than that caused by HSV-1. There is a higher frequency of seizures and CNS structural damage and greater pleocytosis and higher protein concentrations in the CSF than with HSV-1 infections. Interestingly, a large percentage of infants infected with HSV are born prematurely.

Physical Examination Findings

The physical findings with neonatal infection depend on whether the infant has localized infection, disseminated disease, or CNS disease only. Neonates with infection localized to the skin, eye, or mouth may have a fever and skin or mucous membrane vesicles without findings indicative of systemic disease. Neonates with disseminated infection may have a fever or hypothermia, hypotension, cutaneous herpetic vesicles, hepatomegaly, pneumonia, or disseminated intravascular coagulation. CNS infection, either alone or with disseminated infection, may result in hypotonia or hypertonia, loss of suck and gag reflexes, and seizures.

DIAGNOSIS

A history of exposure to HSV is useful when one is considering the diagnosis of neonatal HSV infection. Unfortunately, most infants with neonatal herpes have had no recognized exposure to the virus. A history of genital herpes occurring at any time in the mother's past is obtained in fewer than 20% of the cases of neonatal disease. Furthermore, a history of active genital infection during pregnancy is noted in only approximately 5% of cases. Hence, a negative medical history for genital herpes does not exclude the diagnosis of neonatal infection. In obtaining exposure history, it is also important to determine whether the mother's sexual partner or partners have a history of genital herpes and whether the infant has been exposed to any friend or family member with active orolabial herpes (fever blisters).

Differential Diagnosis

The differential diagnosis of neonatal herpes is influenced by whether the infant has localized infection, encephalitis, or disseminated disease (Table 97–5). For infants who present with infection limited to the skin and mouth, the differential diagnosis includes VZV infection, hand-foot-and-mouth disease caused by coxsackievirus A, bullous lesions resulting from streptococcal or staphylococcal infections, and a variety of dermatologic conditions, including pustular melanosis, erythema toxicum, and acrodermatitis enteropathica. Keratoconjunctivitis or chorioretinitis due to HSV may be confused with ocular disease of other causes, such as CMV or adenovirus infection or toxoplasmosis. For encephalitis the differential diagnosis includes bacterial meningitis caused by group B *Streptococcus* and *Listeria monocytogenes,* brain abscesses caused by *Citrobacter* and other bacteria, enteroviral meningoencephalitis, neurosyphilis, toxoplasmosis, and noninfectious conditions such as metabolic disorders and intraventricular hemorrhage. Disseminated infection without skin lesions may be mistaken for bacterial sepsis, enteroviral infection, and syphilis. HSV pneumonitis may mimic hyaline membrane disease or respiratory infections caused by other viruses and bacteria.

TABLE 97–5. Differential Diagnosis of Neonatal Herpes Simplex Virus Infection

Disease Category	Differential Diagnosis
Localized disease	
Skin or mouth	Varicella-zoster virus infection
	Hand-foot-and-mouth disease (coxsackievirus A)
	Bullous impetigo
	Pustular melanosis
	Erythema toxicum
	Acrodermatitis enteropathica
Eye	Cytomegalovirus chorioretinitis
	Adenovirus keratoconjunctivitis
	Toxoplasmosis chorioretinitis
Encephalitis	Bacterial meningitis
	Brain abscesses
	Enterovirus meningoencephalitis
	Neurosyphilis
	Toxoplasmosis
	Metabolic disorders
	Intraventricular hemorrhage
Disseminated disease	Bacterial sepsis
	Enterovirus infection
	Syphilis
Pneumonitis	Respiratory syncytial virus infection
	Influenza virus infection
	Parainfluenza virus infection
	Adenovirus infection
	Bacterial pneumonia
	Hyaline membrane disease

Laboratory Evaluation

Routine laboratory studies may demonstrate hypoglycemia, elevated liver enzyme levels, direct hyperbilirubinemia, neutropenia, eosinophilia, thrombocytopenia, and prolonged thrombin and partial thromboplastin times. With encephalitis, analysis of the CSF may reveal mild lymphocytic pleocytosis with mild to marked (>500 mg/dL) elevation of protein concentration.

Microbiologic Evaluation

Special laboratory studies are often needed to establish the diagnosis of neonatal HSV infection. The gold standard test remains the viral culture. HSV grows rapidly in cell culture, with virus typically isolated from clinical specimens in 24–72 hours. Multiple culture specimens are desirable and may include nasopharyngeal washes, conjunctival swabs, vesicle fluid or swab specimens taken from the base of the vesicle or herpetic ulcer, urine, CSF, buffy coat or whole blood, and biopsy material. Recovery of virus is greatest from vesicular lesions. If the lesion is crusted, the crust should be lifted and the base of the lesion gently scraped to obtain cellular debris. Although CSF cultures are often negative, they should be considered for all infants believed to have neonatal HSV infection, especially those with positive CNS findings. Specimens should be placed on ice or refrigerated if they cannot be transported immediately and processed.

Rapid and specific diagnostic tests have been developed for specimens obtained from mucocutaneous lesions. The most commonly used method is a **direct immunofluorescence** assay using fluorescein-conjugated monoclonal anti-HSV antibodies. This method is very specific and is 80–90% as sensitive as culture. The **Tzanck smear** is a cytologic examination of skin lesions prepared from cellular debris collected by scraping the base or roof of a vesicle. The material is stained with Giemsa or Papanicolaou's or Wright's stain and then examined for multinucleated giant cells and intranuclear inclusions. This method is only approximately

50% as sensitive as culture and does not distinguish between HSV and VZV.

A recent major advance has been the use of the PCR to detect HSV DNA, especially in the CSF, in which cultures are often negative. Because PCR detects viral DNA, a positive result does not prove that replicating virus is present. Indeed, in neonates with CNS HSV disease, PCR of the CSF may remain positive for 1–2 weeks after the onset of appropriate antiviral therapy. Evaluation of all infants with suspected or proven neonatal HSV infection should include collection of CSF for evaluation by PCR if this test is available.

The serologic diagnosis of HSV infection generally relies on demonstration of an increase in antibody titer over a period of several weeks, and thus it is not useful in the care of an acutely ill neonate. Serologic testing in neonates is further complicated by the presence of transplacentally acquired maternal IgG antibodies to HSV. In addition, reliable type-specific assays for HSV antibodies are not commercially available.

Diagnostic Imaging

Infants with herpes encephalitis may show electroencephalographic changes, such as bitemporal spike and slow-wave activity. CT images may appear normal early in encephalitis or may reveal multifocal areas of low attenuation consistent with edema and ischemia. Regions of delayed myelination and destructive cystic encephalomalacia may be evident later in the course of the disease. MRI demonstrates decreased signal on T1-weighted images and increased signal on T2-weighted images in the region of infection. The progression to cystic encephalomalacia is seen on MRI as developing cavities filled with fluid with a density identical to that of CSF.

Pathologic Findings

HSV is a highly lytic pathogen that produces extensive tissue destruction. Herpes encephalitis results in cortical hemorrhagic necrosis. Disseminated infection may produce necrosis, multinucleated giant cells, and intranuclear inclusions in liver, lungs, and adrenal glands.

TREATMENT

There is general agreement that antiviral therapy should be initiated for the following patients: (1) newborns with culture-proven HSV infection; (2) infants believed to have neonatal HSV infection on the basis of clinical findings and from whom appropriate cultures have been collected; (3) neonates with nonspecific illnesses born to women with active genital herpes at the time of delivery; and (4) infants who have a relapse of CNS or disseminated infection after cessation of therapy. Antiviral therapy should be considered for apparently healthy infants delivered to women with active *primary* (first episode) genital herpes **(anticipatory treatment).**

The risk of neonatal infection in apparently healthy infants born to mothers with primary HSV infection is as high as 50%. Because of the high attack rate, it is prudent and preferable not to delay the treatment of infants born to women with active primary genital herpes but, rather, to collect **surface cultures** (e.g., swabs or specimens of the oropharynx, nasopharynx, urine, and stool or rectum) from the newborn after delivery and initiate anticipatory treatment immediately. Some experts argue that, for apparently healthy infants, treatment should be delayed until a second set of cultures can be collected 36–48 hours after delivery, because recovery of virus from cultures collected at delivery may reflect exposure (i.e., contamination rather than infection), whereas positive viral cultures or specimens obtained 36–48 hours after delivery indicate infection. The rationale for the aggressive approach is based on animal studies that demonstrate that HSV spreads to the CNS of a newborn within 48 hours of virus inoculation; thus virus may be in the brain even before cutaneous lesions develop. Although some infants will be treated unnecessarily, for others early treatment may prevent or reduce spread of the virus to the CNS. Although antiviral drug therapy is not without toxicity, allowing HSV to replicate and spread for 36–48 hours is believed to pose a greater risk to these infants than does antiviral treatment.

Anticipatory treatment of infants without symptoms who are born to women with active *recurrent* genital herpes is not recommended because the risk of neonatal infection in this setting is less than 3%. Cultures may be performed on specimens obtained when these infants are 36–48 hours of age, or earlier if symptoms develop. Antiviral therapy should be started if the culture is positive.

Definitive Treatment

Two antiviral drugs, vidarabine and acyclovir, have proven efficacy in the treatment of neonatal HSV infection. Acyclovir is generally preferred because it can be delivered in smaller volumes and is better tolerated. Acyclovir at a dose of 30 mg/kg/day has been shown to be equivalent to vidarabine in the treatment of neonatal herpes. However, recent research has shown that treatment of neonates with CNS or disseminated HSV infection with acyclovir at a higher dose of 60 mg/kg/day in three divided doses for 21 days provides better outcome with regard to both mortality and morbidity than lower-dose and shorter-duration therapy does. Consequently, the current recommendation is for acyclovir at a dose of 60 mg/kg/day in three divided doses. Infants with SEM disease should be treated for 14 days, and infants with suspected or proven CNS or disseminated disease should be treated for 21 days. Neonates with ocular infections should receive topical ophthalmic treatment in addition to intravenous antiviral therapy. Treatment with topical trifluridine, iododeoxyuridine, or vidarabine should be initiated with the assistance of an ophthalmologist.

Supportive Therapy

Supportive care is important. Concurrent bacterial infections with group A *Streptococcus* or gram-negative organisms occur commonly and require appropriate antibiotic therapy. Many infants with neonatal HSV infection are born prematurely, and their care may be complicated by pulmonary and intestinal immaturity and the risk of intraventricular hemorrhage. Infants may have inappropriate secretion of antidiuretic hormone, necessitating careful fluid management. Oral feeding may not be possible, in which case parenteral nutrition becomes necessary. Bleeding diathesis, pneumonitis, and seizures may require specialized management. Psychosocial support for the family is important, particularly when there is a component of guilt associated with the acquisition of infection.

The decision regarding whether to treat or refer an infant with neonatal HSV infection to a tertiary care center depends largely on the facilities available to the physician. Infants with SEM disease can be treated in a hospital capable of caring for neonates with bacterial sepsis. Infants with disseminated disease or CNS involvement should usually be transferred to a tertiary care center.

COMPLICATIONS

Localized infection may disseminate to either the CNS or other organs. Untreated, localized infection progresses in approximately 70% of neonates. Infections of the skin or mouth that remain localized are generally uncomplicated, but CNS involvement may be recognized only later in life, even with neonatal disease limited to the skin and mucous membranes. Herpes keratoconjunctivitis may progress to involve the retina with chorioretinitis and retinal detachment and cataracts. Multiple organ failure and shock may complicate disseminated infection. Hydrocephalus and hyponatremia secondary to inappropriate secretion of antidiuretic hormone may complicate CNS infection.

PROGNOSIS

The following factors are associated with poor outcome for infants with neonatal HSV infection: prematurity, pneumonitis and disseminated intravascular coagulopathy, coma or semicoma at initiation of antiviral treatment, seizures, long duration of symptoms before initiation of therapy, and infection due to HSV-2. The extent of spread of infection also greatly influences outcome (Table 97–6). Death is rare if infants with localized infection receive effective antiviral therapy. Clinically significant morbidity, including cataract formation, retinal detachment, and neurologic sequelae, may occur but is uncommon. Very commonly survivors of localized infections later have recurrent cutaneous infections. Even with effective antiviral therapy, more than half of infants who survive infection of the CNS exhibit neurologic sequelae, including seizures, microcephaly, hydrocephalus, paralysis, spasticity, developmental delay, and mental retardation. Infants with disseminated infection are at greatest risk of dying, usually of pneumonitis or disseminated intravascular coagulation. Before antiviral drugs became available, the mortality exceeded 80%; even with treatment, more than 50% of infants with disseminated infection die. More than 50% of the survivors recover completely, with the remainder developing neurologic sequelae similar to those seen with encephalitis.

Recurrence. Infants with neonatal HSV infection are at risk of relapse after cessation of antiviral therapy. A report (Whitley et al., 1991a) indicated that 8% of infants who survived encephalitis or disseminated infection had a recurrence of CNS disease within 1 month after completing therapy. Cutaneous recurrences were noted within the first month after cessation of therapy in 27% of survivors. The risk of recurrent skin lesions was similar for all disease categories. Infants experiencing the first episode of recurrent cutaneous disease should be evaluated carefully for evidence of systemic infection. Those with evidence of CNS or systemic disease should be re-treated with acyclovir intravenously. Recurrences limited to the skin may be treated with a course of acyclovir orally.

Infants with SEM disease who have three or more episodes of recurrent cutaneous infection in the first 6 months of life are more likely to be neurologically impaired than infants who have fewer than three cutaneous recurrences. A study (Kimberlin et al., 1996b) of **suppressive therapy** on cutaneous recurrences after SEM disease among 26 neonates found that fewer than 20% of the infants who received oral acyclovir therapy (300 mg/m^2 given 2–3 times per day) for 6 months after completion of intravenous acyclovir had cutaneous recurrences. Approximately 50% of those treated with suppressive acyclovir had drug-related neutropenia. This study did not have adequate power to assess the effect of suppressive oral acyclovir therapy on neurologic outcome; therefore, additional studies are needed before the routine use of suppressive acyclovir therapy after neonatal SEM disease can be recommended.

TABLE 97–6. Short-term Outcome for Infants Treated for Herpes Simplex Virus Infection

		Neurologic Outcome of Survivors (%)	
Disease Category	Mortality (%)	Impaired	Normal
Localized infection	0	6	94
Encephalitis	14	68	32
Disseminated disease	54	41	59

PREVENTION

Most strategies designed to prevent neonatal HSV infection have targeted women with genital herpes. Pregnant women with active genital lesions during labor should undergo cesarean section to decrease the likelihood of exposing the infant to the virus. Even with intact membranes, cesarean delivery is not completely effective in preventing transmission; therefore, these infants still require careful observation. It has been suggested that acyclovir could be used to prevent recurrent genital herpes during the last few weeks of pregnancy. This strategy has not been carefully studied, and acyclovir is not currently approved for use during pregnancy. Women with a history of genital herpes or who are known to be seropositive for HSV-2 should not have an instrumented delivery (i.e., delivery should be without use of scalp electrode or forceps).

Vaccination. A more promising strategy is the development of safe and effective HSV vaccines. A variety of vaccines, including inactivated whole-virus preparations, subunit vaccines, and genetically engineered viruses, are currently being developed. Clinical evaluation of several candidate vaccines is under way. The hope is that vaccines not only will prevent genital herpes in women of childbearing age but also will induce antibodies that can be passed transplacentally to a fetus, providing protection against postnatally acquired HSV disease.

Isolation. Currently, prevention of postnatal transmission depends on **effective isolation techniques.** Infants with cutaneous lesions or proven infections should be placed in contact isolation, ideally in a private room. Isolation should be maintained for the duration of the illness. Medical personnel with active herpes labialis should not participate in the care of neonates. Mothers with fever blisters should be educated about the dangers posed by their infection and should wash their hands before and use disposable masks while handling their infants. Women with herpetic infections may breastfeed if there are no herpetic lesions on the breast.

VARICELLA-ZOSTER VIRUS

ETIOLOGY

Varicella-zoster virus (VZV), or human herpesvirus 3, is a member of the Herpesviridae family that is a neurotropic alphaherpesvirus capable of spread within neurons by intra-axonal transport. Initial infection results in varicella, commonly called chickenpox (Chapter 27). After recovery from chickenpox, the virus persists throughout the life of the host, as evidenced by the detection of viral nucleic acids within sensory ganglia. There is only limited transcription of the latent viral genome; hence, antiviral drugs such as acyclovir, which act by inhibiting the replication of virus, have no effect on the persistent latent infection. Reactivation of the latent virus can result in zoster (shingles), the clinical manifestation of recurrent VZV infection. It is not known how often latent VZV is reactivated, but recurrent infection due to reactivated virus is an uncommon event that occurs mostly in elderly or immunocompromised patients. Patients with chickenpox and, to a lesser degree, zoster may transmit VZV to susceptible neonates.

EPIDEMIOLOGY

VZV is one of the most contagious of human pathogens. In the United States in the prevaccine era, chickenpox occurred primarily during the school year with a dramatic decrease in the number of cases during the summer months. More than 90% of cases occur in children, and fewer than 1% of cases occur in women of childbearing age. The estimated incidence of chickenpox during pregnancy is 1–5 cases per 10,000 pregnancies. Because there are only a few cases in pregnant women each year, it is difficult to estimate the incidence of perinatally acquired varicella. Postnatal exposure of newborns to siblings with varicella occurs frequently but only occasionally results in neonatal chickenpox, probably because of the protective effect of maternally derived, virus-specific antibody. Several risk factors are associated with perinatal acquisition of VZV infection (Table 97–3).

PATHOGENESIS

VZV infection of the newborn may be acquired in utero or as a consequence of postnatal exposure. Neonatal infection that develops within 10 days of birth may be due to in utero transmission. VZV infection produces viremia, which in pregnant women may result in transplacental transmission of the virus. Once VZV reaches the fetus, further replication and hematogenous dissemination ensue. When maternal chickenpox occurs between 21 days before delivery and 17 days after delivery, the risk of neonatal varicella is 17–33%. If a mother develops symptoms of varicella infection 5–21 days before delivery, the infected infant typically has lesions within the first 4 days of life. Neonatal varicella in these infants is self-limiting, presumably because there was adequate time before delivery for the mother to produce and transplacentally pass virus-specific antibodies. When symptoms of maternal infection occur 4 days before to 17 days after delivery, there appears to be insufficient time for the mother to make and transfer virus-specific antibodies after transmitting the virus. In the absence of maternally-derived antibody, neonatal varicella may be severe, particularly in cases in which maternal infection occurred 4 days before to 2 days after birth. In this setting a fatal, generalized infection may be seen in as many as 31% of untreated newborns.

Neonatal varicella may be acquired postnatally from exposure of a susceptible newborn to a person with either chickenpox or zoster. The typical incubation period for postnatally acquired varicella is 11–20 days. This is usually a community-acquired infection, although nosocomial infection resulting from exposure in the newborn nursery has been reported. The pathogenesis of postnatally acquired neonatal varicella is the same as that for varicella in older children (Chapter 27). Postnatally acquired neonatal chickenpox typically results in a self-limited infection similar to that seen in older infants and children. However, the infection may be severe in newborns delivered to women who have not had chickenpox and hence do not have antibodies and in premature infants delivered before they acquire maternally derived antibodies.

SYMPTOMS AND CLINICAL MANIFESTATIONS

The clinical features of postnatally acquired VZV infection are the same as those seen in older infants and children (Table 97–7).

TABLE 97–7. Signs and Symptoms Associated with Neonatal Varicella-Zoster Virus Infection

Disease Category	Signs and Symptoms
Postnatally acquired chickenpox	Hyperthermia Maculovesicular rash
In utero acquired chickenpox	
5 or more days before delivery	Typical chickenpox
4 or fewer days before delivery	Progressive varicella, including Hyperthermia Poor feeding Maculovesicular rash Hemorrhagic rash Respiratory distress Hepatomegaly Irritability Seizures

Fever and rash occur simultaneously, the rash beginning as discrete macules that rapidly progress to vesicles, which subsequently umbilicate and crust (Fig. 97–1). From macular stage to crusting takes 5–7 days, with new lesions developing over 2–5 days. The number of lesions varies greatly. Except for a fever, there are rarely signs of systemic illness.

VZV infection acquired in utero may be mild if the transmission of virus occurred 5 or more days before delivery. However, infants infected in utero but delivered before they can acquire maternally derived, virus-specific antibodies may have severe, potentially fatal disease. The infants exhibit fever, poor feeding, and a maculovesicular rash that occasionally becomes hemorrhagic. The virus may disseminate to lungs, liver, kidney, brain, and adrenal glands, producing multiple organ failure and death.

Physical Examination Findings

The most important physical finding in neonatal varicella is the classic chickenpox rash, which consists of small **vesicles on an erythematous base** characterized as a ''dewdrop on a rose petal.'' Hepatosplenomegaly, respiratory distress, hemorrhagic rash, and clinical evidence of meningoencephalitis may be seen in infants with severe progressive (malignant) varicella.

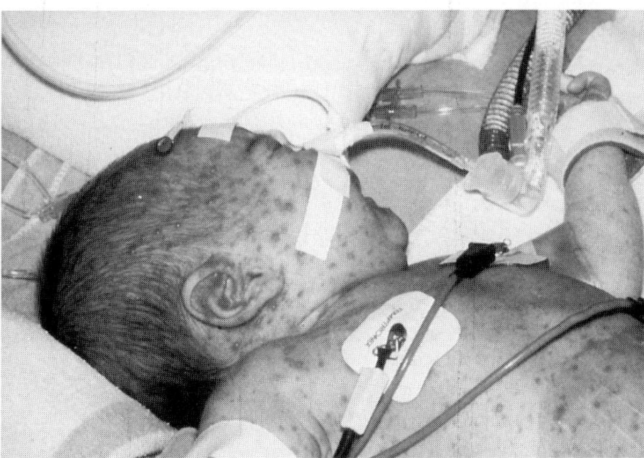

FIGURE 97–1. Varicella-zoster virus infection of a newborn. (Courtesy of Thomas F. Murphy, M.D.)

DIAGNOSIS

Maternal chickenpox near the time of delivery suggests the possibility of in utero transmission of virus from mother to infant. Unrecognized chickenpox in a mother is highly unlikely because asymptomatic varicella in adults probably does not occur. Exposure of a newborn to anyone with active chickenpox or shingles (zoster) places the infant at risk of primary VZV infection. In eliciting exposure history, it is important to remember that patients with chickenpox are contagious 24–48 hours before the first cutaneous lesions occur.

Differential Diagnosis

Of the possibilities in the differential diagnosis (Table 97–8), it is important to consider neonatal herpes if there is no history of exposure of the infant or mother to chickenpox or zoster. Vesicles with hand-foot-and-mouth disease caused by coxsackieviruses, usually coxsackievirus A16, are generally limited to the palms, soles, and oral cavity. Vesicles or pustules may be seen in cases of contact dermatitis resulting from exposure of the infant to irritants. Pustules are also present on infants with pustular melanosis. Neither of these conditions is associated with systemic signs such as fever. Bullous impetigo may produce cutaneous lesions and systemic signs of sepsis; however, the lesions are large and should not be confused with the small vesicles seen with chickenpox. Smallpox and disseminated vaccinia may mimic neonatal varicella. Smallpox has been eradicated, and the routine use of vaccinia for immunization against smallpox is no longer required in the United States.

Laboratory Evaluation

In infants with mild varicella, routine laboratory studies are generally unremarkable. Initially there may be mild leukopenia followed by absolute lymphocytosis. There also may be a transient elevation in serum transaminases. In patients with CNS disease, the cerebrospinal fluid may show a modest lymphocytic pleocytosis and mild elevation of protein level. Infants with progressive (malignant) varicella may have cerebrospinal fluid leukocytosis, thrombocytopenia, prolonged thrombin and partial thromboplastin times, and greatly elevated liver enzyme concentrations.

Microbiologic Evaluation

The clinical diagnosis is confirmed by isolation of the virus from vesicle fluid or by demonstration of viral antigen in scrapings collected from the base of a vesicle. Detection of virus-specific IgM or demonstration of a rise in virus-specific IgG over a period of 4–6 weeks also supports the diagnosis of primary VZV infection.

Pathologic Findings

Most cases of neonatal varicella are self-limiting, and therefore little is known about the pathologic findings associated with nonfatal infection. Autopsy findings from cases of severe fatal infection have shown that VZV produces punctate lesions in the skin, liver, lungs, and, less commonly, the adrenal glands, spleen, thymus, kidneys, heart, pancreas, and gastrointestinal tract. The lesions are necrotic and surrounded by epithelioid cells. Mild inflammatory changes are present, and both multinucleated giant cells and intranuclear inclusion bodies are present.

TABLE 97–8. Differential Diagnosis of Neonatal Varicella-Zoster Virus Infection

Neonatal herpes simplex virus infection
Hand-foot-and-mouth disease due to enterovirus infection
Contact dermatitis
Pustular melanosis
Impetigo, staphylococcal sepsis
Smallpox virus infection (not seen in current era)

TREATMENT

The management of infected infants includes a combination of observation, immunoprophylaxis, and antiviral therapy (Table 97–9).

Definitive Treatment

Intravenous acyclovir is safe and effective in the treatment of neonatal varicella (Table 97–9). A dose of 500 mg/m^2 every 8 hours for 5 days has been used safely, although controlled trials have not been conducted. The decision to treat an infant with neonatal chickenpox is based on the risk of severe disease. If the newborn's mother had chickenpox between 4 days before and up to 17 days after delivery, transmission of virus may have occurred in utero without sufficient time for the infant to acquire maternally derived antibodies. In this setting the infant is at increased risk of severe varicella. A neonate whose mother's chickenpox develops more than 2 days after delivery is probably at relatively low risk of severe varicella; however, there have been case reports of severe infection in such infants. Consequently, neonates who develop active varicella as a result of maternal chickenpox occurring anytime after 4 days before delivery should be considered candidates for antiviral therapy. Premature infants are immunologically imma-

TABLE 97–9. Prophylactic and Therapeutic Management of Neonatal Varicella-Zoster Virus Infection

Clinical Setting	Management Strategy
Exposed Infants	
Due to maternal varicella	
More than 5 days before delivery	Observe; no VZIG
Less than 5 days before delivery	VZIG at birth or as soon as maternal infection is observed
Due to postnatal exposure	
Term infant of mother immune to varicella	Observe; no VZIG
Term infant of mother susceptible to varicella	Observe; no VZIG
Premature infant	VZIG as early as possible
Infected Infants	
Due to maternal varicella	
More than 5 days before delivery	Observe; no acyclovir
Less than 5 days before delivery	Acyclovir
Due to postnatal exposure	
Term infant of mother immune to varicella	Observe; no acyclovir
Term infant of mother susceptible to varicella	Observe; no acyclovir
Premature infant	Acyclovir
Severe infection (pneumonitis or disseminated infection)	Acyclovir

VZIG (varicella-zoster immune globulin) dose = 125 U. Acyclovir dose = 500 mg/m^2 q8h IV for 5 days.

ture and have decreased levels of maternal antibodies. Therefore, premature infants with active varicella should also be considered candidates for antiviral therapy.

Infection in term infants born to mothers who are immune or susceptible to chickenpox rarely results in severe disease; therefore, these infants may be carefully observed and treated only if infection becomes severe. This includes varicella acquired in utero if symptoms of chickenpox developed in the mother 5 or more days before delivery.

Supportive Therapy

Supportive care includes keeping the lesions clean and dry. When secondary infection occurs, cultures of blood and lesions should be obtained and empirical antibiotic therapy initiated. In general, treatment with a first-generation cephalosporin, such as cephalothin or cefazolin, provides adequate streptococcal and staphylococcal coverage.

The decision to transport a newborn with VZV infection to a tertiary care center depends largely on the facilities available to the physician. Mild cases of varicella in term infants generally can be managed in any hospital capable of caring for neonates with bacterial sepsis. Premature infants with chickenpox or any infant with severe disseminated varicella should be referred to a tertiary care center.

COMPLICATIONS

The most common complication of varicella is **secondary bacterial infection** of skin lesions, which may progress to bacteremia or sepsis. The usual pathogens are *Staphylococcus aureus* and group A *Streptococcus*. Viral pneumonia is also a well-recognized problem. Prolonged fever and the development of lesions, which often become hemorrhagic, characterize progressive malignant varicella. Less common complications of varicella include encephalitis, transverse myelitis, aseptic meningitis, uveitis, hepatitis, glomerulonephritis, myocarditis, disseminated intravascular coagulation, and Reye's syndrome.

PROGNOSIS

Infants at risk of fatal infection include those who have acquired their infection in utero (less than 4 days before delivery) and newborns who lack maternally derived anti-VZV antibodies, such as premature infants or newborns whose mothers have never had chickenpox. Fortunately, such susceptible infants are uncommon. Children with pneumonia, encephalitis, or Reye's syndrome are at high risk of death. With the advent of effective antiviral therapy, death due to neonatal varicella has become a rare event. Most infants show complete recovery, and sequelae are rare.

PREVENTION

Varicella-Zoster Immune Globulin (VZIG). Primary VZV infection can be prevented or modified by the timely administration of VZIG (Table 97–9). Infants born to women who develop chickenpox more than 2 days after delivery are at relatively low risk of severe varicella and therefore do not require VZIG prophylaxis. Because there are documented cases of severe varicella developing in such infants, it may be prudent to administer VZIG to all infants whose mothers develop chickenpox 4 days before to 17 days after delivery. Traditionally, infants born to mothers in whom chickenpox developed 5 or more days before delivery have been thought to be at low risk of severe varicella. One study (Miller et al., 1989) showed that some infants whose mothers had chickenpox 7 days before delivery were born with little or no virus-specific antibody. Hence, it may be reasonable to extend the recommended use of VZIG to infants whose mothers had chickenpox within 7 days of birth. VZIG is most effective when administered within 3 days of exposure, although it is worthwhile to administer VZIG at any time during the incubation period. VZIG may also be useful as an adjunct to antiviral therapy for infected infants at high risk of complications.

The fetus may be protected from in utero infection by administration of VZIG to the susceptible pregnant woman. In this setting, VZIG should be administered to the woman as soon as possible, preferably within 2 days but no more than 4 days after maternal exposure. The dosage for postexposure prophylaxis is 125 U/10 kg of body weight up to a maximum of 625 U.

Vaccination. A live, attenuated VZV vaccine has been licensed in the United States since 1995. It should be given to all infants at 12 months of age, as well as to all healthy adolescents past the age of 13 who have not been immunized previously and who have no history of chickenpox. The vaccine is safe and effective in protecting healthy as well as immunocompromised children from chickenpox. Immunization of susceptible women before they become pregnant may be a useful strategy until girls immunized in childhood as part of universal immunization attain childbearing age.

Prevention of Exposure. Hospitalized infants with chickenpox should be placed in strict isolation in negative-pressure rooms, and all health care providers should be immune to varicella. Studies have shown that viral DNA can be detected in the nasopharynges of immune adults and children after exposure to an active case of chickenpox. Hence, health care providers should wear masks to reduce the remote risk that they could transmit virus to a susceptible patient. Susceptible hospitalized infants who have been exposed to persons with either chickenpox or zoster should be isolated, beginning 8 days after the exposure and continuing for the entire possible incubation period, which is usually up to 21 days. For infants receiving postexposure prophylaxis with VZIG, however, the incubation period may be as long as 28 days.

A frequent dilemma is presented by the newborn infant who has siblings at home with active chickenpox. Full-term infants born to women immune to chickenpox may be discharged home because they are not at increased risk of severe varicella. Infants born to women who are susceptible to varicella should not be exposed to an infected sibling. Similarly, the mother should avoid contact with the infected child. This is usually accomplished by sending the infected child to the home of a neighbor or a relative until the chickenpox is no longer contagious. If this is impractical, both newborn and mother can be given VZIG and discharged home. The efficacy of prophylactic administration of antiviral drugs to infants exposed to VZV has not been established, and the use of such prophylaxis has not been recommended.

ENTEROVIRUSES

ETIOLOGY

The enteroviruses belong to the Picornaviridae family, a large group of nonenveloped, single-stranded RNA viruses. Classification of viruses within the enterovirus genus was traditionally based on their growth in tissue culture and in experimental animals. Such criteria allowed the enteroviruses to be divided into four groups: polioviruses (types 1–3); coxsackieviruses A (types A1–A24, except type A23); coxsackieviruses B (types B1–B6); and echoviruses (types 1–33, except types 10 and 28). Because some viruses do not strictly conform to the criteria for classification, it is now convention to simply designate newly discovered enterovirus strains by serotype number. Currently four viruses named enterovirus 68–71 have been characterized.

EPIDEMIOLOGY

Enteroviruses are ubiquitous, and infection occurs commonly. These viruses may cause disease at any time during the year, but in temperate climates infections are more prevalent in the summer and fall months. There are only limited data on the incidence of enterovirus infections in neonates. A study of newborns (Jenista et al., 1984) in one community found that during the summer and early fall 12.8% of infants acquired a nonpolio enterovirus infection within the first month of life. No virus was isolated from the mother or infant at the time of delivery; therefore, it is likely that these cases represent postnatally acquired infection. Of the infants with positive cultures, 21% were admitted to the hospital in the first month of life. All the infected neonates in this study survived the infection, but other reports have documented a fatal outcome for neonates with postnatally acquired enterovirus infection. Infection was associated with low socioeconomic status and lack of breast-feeding (Table 97–3). For infants less than 2 months of age with symptoms, there was a male-to-female ratio of 1.4:1, with viral isolates being echoviruses in 51% of the infants, coxsackieviruses B in 45%, and coxsackieviruses A in 4%.

PATHOGENESIS

Neonatal enterovirus infection can be acquired in utero, during delivery, or in the postnatal period. Most infected infants are probably exposed during or shortly after delivery, and the mother is the most likely source of the virus. However, postnatal transmission of enteroviruses from health care personnel to susceptible newborns has been documented. The transmission of enteroviruses probably occurs through ingestion or inhalation of contaminated stool, genital tract secretions, or respiratory secretions. The virus is thought to replicate at the portal of entry and spread to local lymphoid tissue, where further replication results in the **first (or minor) viremia.** Virus is then disseminated to multiple organs (e.g., heart, CNS), where it further replicates, producing local injury (e.g., myocarditis, meningitis) and a **secondary (or major) viremia.** Because enteroviruses produce viremia, enterovirus infection in a pregnant woman can result in transplacental spread of virus to the fetus and in utero transmission of infection. Termination of viremia is temporally related to the development of serum antibody. Thus maternally derived, transplacentally passed antibodies may provide an infant with passive protection against specific enteroviruses. The importance of secretory antibody and cell-mediated immune responses in controlling enteroviral disease is poorly understood.

SYMPTOMS AND CLINICAL MANIFESTATIONS

The spectrum of illness caused by enterovirus infection of a newborn may range from asymptomatic to fulminant fatal disease (Table 97–10). Three clinical syndromes are typically seen in newborns infected with enteroviruses. The most common presentation is a nonspecific febrile illness, with fever often >38.8°C (102°F), occasionally associated with an exanthem. The illness may be mild, and the infant's condition may appear nontoxic, but because the physical examination fails to reveal a source of the fever, the infant commonly undergoes evaluation for bacterial sepsis.

TABLE 97–10. Signs and Symptoms Associated with Neonatal Enterovirus Infection

Disease Category	Signs and Symptoms
Nonspecific febrile illness	Hyperthermia Exanthem, enanthem Poor feeding Vomiting Diarrhea Irritability Lethargy
Meningitis, meningoencephalitis	Hyperthermia Poor feeding Lethargy Tremors Seizures Coma Exanthem
Severe infection with multiple organ involvement	Hyperthermia Feeding intolerance Exanthem Lethargy Hypotonia Apnea Hepatomegaly Splenomegaly Cyanosis Respiratory distress Cardiac abnormalities Meningitis Jaundice Bleeding diathesis

The second most common presentation of neonatal enterovirus infection is meningitis or meningoencephalitis. Infants with enterovirus infection of the CNS may present with fever, irritability or lethargy, tremors, seizures, and sometimes coma. Less commonly, focal neurologic signs or spasticity may be present. Occasionally an exanthem is also noted.

A less common but more dramatic clinical syndrome is the sepsis like illness produced by enteroviruses. Infection may be limited to a single organ, such as the liver or heart, but more commonly involves multiple organs. The initial presentation may be indistinguishable from that of bacterial sepsis; it may include fever, lethargy, anorexia, and hypotonia. Echoviruses and less commonly the coxsackieviruses may produce fulminant hepatitis with little or no involvement of other organs. Findings suggestive of echovirus hepatitis include hepatosplenomegaly, jaundice, and disseminated intravascular coagulation. Enteroviruses may produce infection limited to the heart (myopericarditis), resulting in cyanosis, respiratory distress, transient pericardial friction rub, and symptoms indicative of congestive heart failure. Enteroviruses may also produce disseminated infection in which the infant has signs of multiple organ failure, including myocarditis, hepatitis, meningoencephalitis, pneumonitis, and pancreatitis. The cutaneous manifestations of neonatal enterovirus infection include macular and maculopapular rashes and occasionally petechial rashes (Plate 5B). Vesicular rashes are uncommon but can be seen with hand-foot-and-mouth disease due to coxsackievirus, usually coxsackievirus A16. Less common manifestations of enterovirus infection include poliomyelitis, sudden infant death syndrome, gastroenteritis, necrotizing enterocolitis, and upper respiratory tract symptoms.

Physical Examination Findings

No pathognomonic physical findings are associated with neonatal enterovirus infection. Infants with nonspecific febrile illnesses, those with clinical syndromes suggestive of bacterial sepsis, and those with evidence of meningitis, myocarditis, hepatitis, or disseminated intravascular coagulation may have an enterovirus infection. A generalized maculopapular rash, with or without associated manifestations, suggests an enterovirus infection (Plate 5B).

DIAGNOSIS

The diagnosis of enterovirus infection should be considered in any neonate for whom the diagnosis of bacterial sepsis is being entertained, inasmuch as the clinical features of enterovirus infection and bacterial sepsis may be indistinguishable. The epidemiologic characteristics of enterovirus infection may assist in establishing the diagnosis. Enteroviruses circulate principally in warm weather; therefore, in temperate climates enterovirus infections more commonly occur during the summer and fall and are less likely during the winter. In tropical climates enterovirus infections are seen throughout the year.

The family history may also assist in establishing the diagnosis. A nonspecific febrile illness during the summer or fall, especially in the mother, should suggest the possibility of perinatal enteroviral infection. The history should include possible exposure to anyone (family member or nursery staff) with specific symptoms suggestive of enterovirus infection, including aseptic meningitis, myocarditis, herpangina, pleurodynia, or hand-foot-and-mouth disease. A history of compatible illness in the mother warrants further evaluation for evidence of enterovirus infection in the neonate.

Differential Diagnosis

The differential diagnosis of enterovirus infections depends on the clinical findings (Table 97–11). For infants with nonspecific febrile illnesses, the most important differential diagnosis is bacterial sepsis. Other congenital and perinatal infections, including rubella, CMV, HSV, and syphilis, should be considered. For infants presenting with meningitis or meningoencephalitis, the differential diagnosis includes bacterial meningitis as well as congenital syphilis, toxoplasmosis, and infection due to HSV or *Mycobacterium tuberculosis.* The differential diagnosis of disseminated enteroviral disease includes overwhelming bacterial sepsis as well as infection by other microorganisms known to produce multiorgan disease, such as HSV, CMV, and *Mycobacterium tuberculosis.* In the case of myocarditis it is important to exclude congenital heart disease. For enteroviral hepatitis the differential diagnosis includes infection due to HSV and CMV as well as biliary atresia.

TABLE 97–11. Differential Diagnosis of Neonatal Enterovirus Infection

Disease Category	Differential Diagnosis
Nonspecific febrile illness	Bacterial sepsis Herpes simplex virus infection Cytomegalovirus infection Syphilis
Meningitis, meningo-encephalitis	Bacterial meningitis Herpes simplex virus infection Toxoplasmosis Tuberculosis Syphilis
Severe single or multiple organ disease	Bacterial sepsis Cytomegalovirus infection Herpes simplex virus infection Tuberculosis Congenital heart disease

Laboratory Evaluation

Various routine laboratory studies may yield abnormal findings. There is usually a leukocytosis, as well as increased numbers of mature and immature (band form) neutrophils. This may be of limited value because similar elevations are often noted in bacterial sepsis. In most cases of CNS infection, the CSF protein concentration is modestly increased. The concentration of glucose in the CSF is generally about one half that found in serum, although occasionally severe hypoglycorrhachia (values <20 mg/dL) has been reported. Both neutrophils and lymphocytes may be present in the CSF. Most patients have a leukocyte count $<500/mm^3$, although counts of $>4000/mm^3$ occasionally have been noted. Infants with hepatic involvement exhibit mild to marked elevation of serum transaminase concentrations, and both the prothrombin and partial thromboplastin times are prolonged. Patients with cardiac involvement demonstrate electrocardiographic changes, which may include evidence of low voltage, ST segment depression, and tachyarrhythmias. Echocardiograms may show evidence of poor cardiac contractility, and elevation of cardiac enzyme levels (creatine phosphokinase and lactate dehydrogenase) reflects destruction of the myocardium.

Microbiologic Evaluation

Virus isolation in culture is the standard for establishing the diagnosis of enteroviral infection, although viral culture is limited by its relatively low sensitivity ($<75\%$ for the diagnosis of meningitis) as well as the poor growth of some coxsackieviruses A in cell culture. Isolation of an enterovirus from clinical specimens usually takes 3–7 days, whereas identification of the specific virus type may take longer, depending on the identification methods available. Because enteroviruses cause disseminated infection in a newborn, it is preferable to collect culture specimens from multiple sites, including nasal wash, throat swab, serum, buffy coat, cerebrospinal fluid, urine, stool, and biopsy or autopsy material. Specimens should be transported on ice and processed as soon as possible. If there is a lengthy delay between collection and processing, the specimens should be stored frozen at $-20°C$ ($-4°F$).

The most promising recent development in diagnostic techniques for enteroviral infections is the polymerase chain reaction (PCR). A study (Abzug et al., 1995b) demonstrated that a 5-hour colorimetric PCR assay of serum and urine samples from neonates in whom enteroviral infection was suspected was more sensitive than cell culture and 100% specific. This PCR method will likely become commercially available in the near future and may facilitate the management of acutely ill neonates.

Pathologic Findings

Most enterovirus infections are self-limiting. Little is known about the pathologic findings associated with nonfatal infections. Autopsy findings have shown that echoviruses may cause necrosis of the liver, kidney, and myocardium as well as hemorrhagic changes in a variety of organs, including the liver, kidney, adrenal glands, and cerebellum. The coxsackieviruses B produce inflammatory changes in the heart, liver, pancreas, adrenal glands, brain, and spinal cord.

Polioviruses have been shown to destroy anterior horn cells and produce myofibril necrosis and subsequent paralysis. Numerous enteroviruses have been noted to cause focal or diffuse pneumonitis.

TREATMENT

Definitive Treatment

Until very recently, no specific therapy was available for enterovirus infections. The molecular characterization of enteroviruses has led to the development of drugs, such as pleconaril, that interfere with enterovirus attachment and uncoating by binding to the virus protein capsid. Pleconaril has broad antiviral effects on enteroviruses and is being studied for treatment of neonatal enteroviral sepsis in a multicenter collaborative study.

Antibody plays an important role in the immune response to enteroviruses, which has led to the use of IVIG as part of the therapy for serious enterovirus infections. A small, randomized study (Abzug et al., 1995a) of administration of IVIG (750 mg/kg) to neonates with enteroviral infections revealed a modest increase in serum neutralization titers but did not reduce the daily incidence of viremia and viruria compared with controls. However, receipt of IVIG containing high neutralizing antibody titers to the infant's specific viral isolate was associated with more rapid cessation of viremia and viruria. Larger controlled trials are needed before the widespread use of IVIG for neonates with suspected or proven enterovirus infection can be recommended. The use of IVIG is not indicated for short-lived, non-life-threatening infections.

Supportive Therapy

Supportive therapy is the mainstay of treatment of enterovirus infections. Respiratory support, cardiovascular pharmacotherapy, and blood product administration may be required in infants with a sepsislike illness. Extracorporeal membrane oxygenation (ECMO) has been used in the care of patients with presumed enteroviral myocarditis, although the usefulness of ECMO has not been established. Oral neomycin has been used to suppress intestinal flora in patients with hepatitis.

The decision regarding whether to refer an infant with enteroviral disease to a tertiary care center depends largely on the facilities available. Infants with mild, nonspecific, febrile illnesses or uncomplicated viral meningitis can generally be treated in a hospital capable of treating neonates with bacterial sepsis. Infants with evidence of meningoencephalitis, sepsislike illness, myocarditis, hepatitis, or multiple organ involvement should be referred to a tertiary care center.

COMPLICATIONS

The complications of enteroviral disease depend on the organ systems involved. Complications associated with CNS infection include seizures, spasticity, and hyponatremia secondary to inappropriate antidiuretic hormone secretion. Complications of enteroviral myocarditis include arrhythmias and circulatory failure. Shock, adrenal failure, necrotizing enterocolitis, uncontrollable bleeding, hepatic failure, and respiratory distress may complicate disseminated enteroviral disease.

PROGNOSIS

Most infants with mild, nonspecific febrile illnesses due to nonpolio enteroviruses recover without sequelae. Infants with symptomatic poliovirus infections may later have mild to severe poliomyelitis, possibly resulting in paralysis or death. Newborns with enteroviral meningitis usually survive the infection. Some follow-up studies of infants with enteroviral meningitis have reported long-term sequelae, including speech and language delay, whereas other studies have failed to demonstrate any evidence of neurologic sequelae in these patients.

The prognosis for infants with enteroviral encephalitis, hepatitis, myocarditis, or disseminated disease is poor; the mortality is high. Little has been reported on the long-term outcome of infants who survive severe enteroviral infections, although case reports indicate that some infants recover without apparent residua.

PREVENTION

As with all enteric pathogens, patients with enterovirus infections require isolation by procedures that minimize spread of the virus to other susceptible hosts. Good hand-washing hygiene is the single most important procedure for protecting patients and staff from acquiring an enterovirus infection.

The use of polio vaccine has eliminated poliomyelitis in the Western hemisphere. There are no current plans for the development of vaccines effective against other enteroviruses. Postexposure prophylaxis has not been studied but would probably be of limited use.

REVIEWS

Modlin JF: Update on enterovirus infections in infants and children. *Adv Pediatr Infect Dis* 1996;12:155–80.

Remington JS, Klein JO (editors): *Infectious Diseases of the Fetus and Newborn Infant,* 4th ed. Philadelphia, WB Saunders, 1995.

Rotbart HA (editor): *Human Enterovirus Infections.* Washington, DC, American Society of Microbiology Press, 1995.

Scott LL, Hollier LM, Dias K: Perinatal herpesvirus infections: Herpes simplex, varicella, and cytomegalovirus. *Infect Dis Clin North Am* 1997;11:27–53.

Stoll BJ, Weisman LE (editors): *Infections in Perinatology.* Philadelphia, WB Saunders, 1997.

Herpes Simplex Virus

Ashley RL, Dalessio J, Burchett S, et al: Herpes simplex virus-2 (HSV-2) type-specific antibody correlates of protection in infants exposed to HSV-2 at birth. *J Clin Invest* 1992;90:511–4.

Brown ZA, Benedetti J, Ashley R, et al: Neonatal herpes simplex virus infection in relation to asymptomatic maternal infection at the time of labor. *N Engl J Med* 1991;324:1247–52.

Brown ZA, Benedetti J, Selke S, et al: Asymptomatic maternal shedding of herpes simplex virus at the onset of labor: Relationship to preterm labor. *Obstet Gynecol* 1996;87:483–8.

Brown ZA, Selke S, Zeh J, et al: The acquisition of herpes simplex virus during pregnancy. *N Engl J Med* 1997;337:509–15.

Catalano PM, Merritt AO, Mead PB: Incidence of genital herpes simplex virus at the time of delivery in women with known risk factors. *Am J Obstet Gynecol* 1991;164:1303–6.

Corey L, Whitley RJ, Stone EF, et al: Difference between herpes simplex virus type 1 and type 2 neonatal encephalitis in neurological outcome. *Lancet* 1988;1:1–4.

Gutierrez KM, Falkovitz Halpern MS, Maldonado Y, et al: The epidemiology of neonatal herpes simplex virus infections in California from 1985 to 1995. *J Infect Dis* 1999;180:199–202.

Kimberlin D, Powell D, Gruber W, et al: Administration of oral acyclovir suppressive therapy after neonatal herpes simplex virus disease limited to the skin, eyes and mouth: Results of a phase I/II trial. *Pediatr Infect Dis J* 1996;15:247–54.

Kimberlin DW, Lakeman FD, Arvin AM, et al: Application of the polymerase chain reaction to the diagnosis and management of neonatal herpes simplex virus disease. National Institute of Allergy and Infectious Diseases Collaborative Antiviral Study Group. *J Infect Dis* 1996; 174:1162–7.

Malm G, Forsgren M, el Azazi M, et al: A follow-up study of children with neonatal herpes simplex virus infections with particular regard to late nervous disturbances. *Acta Paediatr Scand* 1991;80:226–34.

Prober CG, Sullender WM, Yasukawa LL, et al: Low risk of herpes simplex virus infections in neonates exposed to the virus at the time of vaginal delivery to mothers with recurrent genital herpes simplex virus infections. *N Engl J Med* 1987;316:240–4.

Stanberry LR, Floyd-Reising SA, Connelly BL, et al: Herpes simplex viremia: Report of eight pediatric cases and review of the literature. *Clin Infect Dis* 1994;18:401–7.

Whitley R, Arvin A, Prober C, et al: A controlled trial comparing vidarabine with acyclovir in neonatal herpes simplex virus infection. Infectious Diseases Collaborative Antiviral Study Group. *N Engl J Med* 1991; 324:444–9.

Whitley R, Arvin A, Prober C, et al: Predictors of morbidity and mortality in neonates with herpes simplex virus infections. The National Institute of Allergy and Infectious Diseases Collaborative Antiviral Study Group. *N Engl J Med* 1991;324:450–4.

Whitley RJ, Corey L, Arvin A, et al: Changing presentation of herpes simplex virus infection in neonates. *J Infect Dis* 1988;158:109–16.

Varicella-Zoster Virus

American Academy of Pediatrics Committee on Infectious Diseases: The use of oral acyclovir in otherwise healthy children with varicella. *Pediatrics* 1993;91:674–6.

Brunell PA: Varicella in pregnancy, the fetus, and the newborn: Problems in management. *J Infect Dis* 1992;166:S42–7.

Connelly BL, Stanberry LR, Bernstein DI: Detection of varicella-zoster virus DNA in nasopharyngeal secretions of immune household contacts of varicella. *J Infect Dis* 1993;168:1253–5.

Enders G, Miller E, Cradock-Watson J, et al: Consequences of varicella and herpes zoster in pregnancy: Prospective study of 1739 cases. *Lancet* 1994;343:1548–51.

Friedman CA, Temple DM, Robbins KK, et al: Outbreak and control of varicella in a neonatal intensive care unit. *Pediatr Infect Dis J* 1994;13:152–4.

Gershon AA, LaRussa P, Hardy I, et al: Varicella vaccine: The American experience. *J Infect Dis* 1992;166:S63–8.

Gustafson TL, Shehab Z, Brunell PA: Outbreak of varicella in a newborn intensive care nursery. *Am J Dis Child* 1984;138:548–50.

Miller E, Cradock-Watson JE, Ridehalgh MK: Outcome in newborn babies given anti-varicella-zoster immunoglobulin after perinatal maternal infection with varicella-zoster virus. *Lancet* 1989;2:371–3.

Myers MG: Viremia caused by varicella-zoster virus: Association with malignant progressive varicella. *J Infect Dis* 1979;140:229–33.

Rubin L, Leggiadro R, Elie MT, et al: Disseminated varicella in a neonate: Implications for immunoprophylaxis of neonates postnatally exposed to varicella. *Pediatr Infect Dis* 1986;5:100–2.

Williams H, Latif A, Morgan J, et al: Acyclovir in the treatment of neonatal varicella. *J Infect* 1987;15:65–7.

Enteroviruses

Abzug MJ, Keyserling HL, Lee ML, et al: Neonatal enterovirus infection: Virology, serology, and effects of intravenous immune globulin. *Clin Infect Dis* 1995;20:1201–6.

Abzug MJ, Levin MJ, Rotbart HA: Profile of enterovirus disease in the first two weeks of life. *Pediatr Infect Dis J* 1993;12:820–4.

Abzug MJ, Loeffelholz M, Rotbart HA: Diagnosis of neonatal enterovirus infection by polymerase chain reaction. *J Pediatr* 1995;126:447–50.

Ahmed A, Brito F, Goto C, et al: Clinical utility of the polymerase chain reaction for diagnosis of enteroviral meningitis in infancy. *J Pediatr* 1997;131:393–7.

Arnon R, Naor N, Davidson S, et al: Fatal outcome of neonatal echovirus 19 infection. *Pediatr Infect Dis J* 1991;10:788–9.

Jenista JA, Powell KR, Menegus MA: Epidemiology of neonatal enterovirus infection. *J Pediatr* 1984;104:685–90.

Johnston JM, Overall JC Jr: Intravenous immunoglobulin in disseminated neonatal echovirus 11 infection. *Pediatr Infect Dis J* 1989;8:254–6.

Kaplan MH, Klein SW, McPhee J, et al: Group B coxsackievirus infections in infants younger than three months of age: A serious childhood illness. *Rev Infect Dis* 1983;5:1019–32.

Lake AM, Lauer BA, Clark JC, et al: Enterovirus infections in neonates. *J Pediatr* 1976;89:787–91.

Morens DM: Enteroviral disease in early infancy. *J Pediatr* 1978;92:374–7.

CHAPTER 98

Primary Immune Deficiency Disorders

Anthony J. Infante ▪ Naynesh Kamani

Children presenting with recurrent or unusual infections can usually be classified into one of three broad groups with the help of a diagnostic evaluation (Chapter 6). The first group consists of children who have no identifiable factor known to be associated with increased susceptibility to infection and whose immune system appears to function normally according to currently available immunologic tests. Although the possibility of subtle immune defects that are currently undetectable remains open, prevailing opinion asserts that these are normal children. The other two groups of children either have a nonspecific predisposition to infection or have a recognized primary immune deficiency.

NONSPECIFIC CAUSES OF INCREASED SUSCEPTIBILITY TO INFECTION

The vast majority of patients with increased susceptibility to infection do not have a primary immune deficiency disorder, that is, an intrinsic mechanism leading to dysfunction of all or part of the immune system. Excluding the physiologic causes of susceptibility to infection operative in neonates and very young infants (Chapter 5), many patients with recurrent infection will have nonspecific or nonimmunologic factors contributing to their conditions. These factors can be further split into two subcategories (Table 98–1). In the first group are conditions, usually localized in nature, that lead to increased infections but that are not associated with a decrease in immunologic function. The second group includes conditions that are often systemic or constitutional and that lead to suppression of immune function by an extrinsic mechanism. These latter conditions are often called **secondary immune deficiencies,** which include several clinically relevant nonspecific causes of increased susceptibility to infection. Where any of these conditions are known to be operative, diagnostic evaluation of the immune system should be limited until the effects of these nonspecific causes have been carefully addressed. In cases of secondary immune deficiency, unless there is damage to bone marrow stem cells, reconstitution of immune function usually follows correction of the underlying cause of immune suppression.

Anatomic Factors

Various anatomic factors result in chronic or recurrent infection, which includes some of the most common disorders seen in pediatric practice. These conditions all have in common some local alteration that delays the clearance of microorganisms, primarily bacteria, from specific anatomic sites or regions. Although many of these conditions do not lead to life-threatening infection, they are a significant source of long-term morbidity.

By far the most common problems in this group involve children who have asthma and allergic rhinitis. In addition to mimicking the signs and symptoms of infection of the upper respiratory tract, these illnesses predispose to secondary bacterial infection of the middle ear and sinuses by obstructing drainage of the eustachian tubes and sinus ostia. Resolution of the vicious cycle that perpetuates these infections may require treatment of allergic symptoms and mechanical drainage of the middle ear and maxillary sinuses, as well as appropriate antibiotic therapy. Recurrent urinary tract infections are almost always due to local anatomic factors rather than a defect in host defense, and correction of anatomic anomalies is usually curative. Less common anatomic factors leading to recurrent infection include cystic fibrosis and ciliary dysfunction. A sweat chloride analysis for cystic fibrosis and an appropriate test

TABLE 98–1. Nonspecific Causes of Increased Susceptibility to Infection

Group 1. Nonimmunologically Mediated		Group 2. Immunologically Mediated (Secondary Immune Deficiency)	
Class	**Example**	**Class**	**Example**
Anatomic	Asthma, allergic rhinitis, cystic fibrosis, foreign bodies, burns, ciliary immotility, urinary tract stenosis, cardiac defects	Anatomic	Asplenia
Metabolic	Diabetes mellitus, nephrotic syndrome	Metabolic	Malnutrition, micronutrient deficiencies, uremia
Environmental	Contaminated food or water	Environmental	Radiation
Therapeutic	Shunts, catheters, heart valves, broad-spectrum antibiotics	Therapeutic	Radiation, cancer therapy, systemic corticosteroids, splenectomy
		Infection	Human immunodeficiency virus (HIV), cytomegalovirus (CMV), measles virus
		Related diseases	Leukemia, lymphoma, myeloma, aplastic anemia

of ciliary motility or ultrastructure should be performed for children with recurrent pneumonia.

Absence of a functioning spleen increases the risk of sepsis due to pyogenic bacteria, principally *Streptococcus pneumoniae.* Asplenia may be a developmental defect occurring alone or, more commonly, associated with complex congenital heart defects. Splenectomy is sometimes indicated for the control of traumatic bleeding or as therapy for thrombocytopenia. Certain hematologic disorders such as sickle cell disease and thalassemia, progressively lead to functional asplenia by infarction or other means. The mechanism by which anatomic or functional asplenia results in increased risk of sepsis is probably related to the ability of the spleen to remove particulate material, especially opsonized (antibody and complement coated) particles, from the blood stream. A decreased ability to produce antibodies after challenge with antigen may also play a role. Antibiotic prophylaxis with penicillin or amoxicillin is highly recommended for young children with disorders such as sickle cell disease, although its benefit in patients splenectomized after trauma is controversial (Chapter 101). All asplenic children require prompt evaluation of signs and symptoms consistent with infection.

Metabolic Factors

The major metabolic factor resulting in increased susceptibility to infection on a worldwide basis is malnutrition. Malnutrition, especially deficiencies of protein and certain trace nutrients, causes significant reductions in immune reactivity, particularly of T-lymphocyte function. Thus malnutrition is a true secondary immune deficiency. Although the incidence of malnutrition in the general population of developed nations is low, it may be a factor in susceptibility to infection in special populations such as the chronically ill, the institutionalized, and the aged. Correction of malnutrition usually leads to rapid normalization of immune dysfunction. However, there is little objective evidence to support claims that immune function can be "boosted" by specific dietary manipulation.

Whether there is immune dysfunction in diabetes mellitus has long been debated. Increased infections of the lower extremities may reflect microvascular complications of long-term disease. A direct inhibitory effect of ketoacidosis on energy-dependent phagocytic cell functions has been proposed. Renal diseases, including chronic renal failure and the nephrotic syndrome, have also been implicated in increased susceptibility to infection. Although various defects in T-cell, B-cell, phagocyte, and complement function have been described, the evidence is contradictory.

Environmental Factors

Contaminated water remains a significant source of recurrent gastrointestinal infection, particularly in underdeveloped countries. This may be complicated by malabsorption, diarrhea, and malnutrition, further compromising immune function. Nosocomial infections are a special group of environmentally influenced infections.

Ionizing radiation can clearly cause immunosuppression at doses that are able to disrupt lymphocyte replication or function or damage bone marrow stem cells. Whether low-level radiation, including electromagnetic field (EMF) radiation, is capable of causing symptomatic illness by alteration of immune function is currently under intense study. Interesting effects of EMF radiation on cell-mediated immunity have been reported under research conditions.

Adverse Effects of Medical Therapy

Physicians knowingly and unknowingly increase susceptibility to infection by a variety of therapeutic maneuvers. Catheters and related devices serve as foreign bodies that predispose a person to local infection. Broad-spectrum antibiotic therapy alters normal microbiologic flora, disturbing the normal equilibrium dominated by nonpathogenic bacterial strains. Increased susceptibility to infection is an unavoidable consequence of immunosuppressive therapy for rheumatologic and autoimmune disease and an adverse effect of cancer therapy. Limited prophylactic options to attenuate these adverse effects are available, including IVIG, antimicrobials, and isolation. Two new approaches may lead to a decrease in these undesired adverse effects. Specific targeting of clones of cells involved in autoimmune and malignant disorders with monoclonal antibodies may reduce or eliminate the need for broadly immunosuppressive modalities. Augmentation of hematopoietic recovery after myelosuppressive cancer therapy using recombinant colony stimulating factors (CSFs) and other hematopoietic growth factors has decreased infectious complications.

PRIMARY IMMUNE DEFICIENCY DISEASES

More than 50 individual primary immune deficiency disorders are currently recognized by the working group of the World Health Organization (WHO). Although many of these disorders are clinically well defined and have had specific defects identified at the cellular and molecular level, quite a few are clinically heterogeneous and probably represent similar manifestations of separate defects in a particular cellular or molecular pathway. Given the current limited number of treatment options for immune deficiency, it is pragmatic to "lump" patients into a few major groups rather than to split them further on the basis of perceived differences in clinical presentation or laboratory information. In recent years significant progress has been made in defining these diseases at the molecular level, and specific gene replacement therapy has been attempted for a few of these entities. The list of primary immune deficiency diseases is likely to undergo dramatic revision as molecular defects are further identified. Early identification and proper classification of these patients is necessary for the institution of potentially life-saving therapy. For this reason, all patients suspected of having a primary immune deficiency after initial laboratory screening should be further evaluated by a clinical immune deficiency specialist.

Classification. It is useful to classify the primary immune deficiencies according to the cellular or molecular pathway that expresses the predominant, clinically important defect, that is, T cells, B cells, phagocytes, or complement (Table 98–2). This is consistent with the clinical and laboratory evaluation of suspected immunodeficiency (Chapter 6). This scheme has inherent limitations. It classifies certain patients with common variable immune deficiency (CVID) whose underlying defect appears to be in the T-cell compartment as patients with antibody deficiencies. Also, severe combined immune deficiency (SCID) is classified as a T-cell defect, even when B cells and antibodies are absent. As much as any factor, these two examples reflect the fact that patients with CVID do well with antibody replacement therapy, whereas patients with SCID require hematopoietic stem cell transplantation.

Incidence. Many of the primary immune deficiency conditions listed in Table 98–2 are rare, including some based on less than a handful of literature reports. The difficulty of definitive diagnosis, clinical heterogeneity, and early death in some of the syndromes makes estimates of incidence difficult. The overall incidence of primary immune deficiency has been estimated at about 1 in 5,000–10,000 individuals in the population (this estimate excludes patients with asymptomatic IgA deficiency). For comparison, the incidence

TABLE 98–2. World Health Organization (WHO) Classification of Primary Immune Deficiency Diseases

Predominant Defect in Antibody Production	
X-linked (Bruton's) agammaglobulinemia	
X-linked hypogammaglobulinemia with growth hormone deficiency	
Autosomal recessive agammaglobulinemia	
Non X-linked hyper-IgM syndrome	
Ig heavy-chain gene deletion	
Selective IgA deficiency	
Selective IgG subclass deficiency with or without IgA deficiency	
Kappa-chain deficiency	
Antibody deficiency with normal immunoglobulin levels	
Transient hypogammaglobulinemia of infancy	
Common variable immunodeficiency (CVID) with predominant defect in B cells	
Combined Immunodeficiencies	
T-B+ SCID syndromes	ZAP-70 deficiency
T-B− SCID syndromes	Purine nucleoside phosphorylase deficiency
X-linked hyper-IgM syndrome	Adenosine deaminase deficiency
MHC class II deficiency	CVID with predominant T-cell defect
CD3γ or CD3ε deficiency	X-linked lymphoproliferative syndrome
Other Defects or Syndromes	
Wiskott-Aldrich syndrome	DiGeorge syndrome
Hyper-IgE syndrome	Ataxia-telangiectasia
Autoimmune polyendocrinopathy with chronic mucocutaneous candidiasis	
Complement Deficiencies	
C1q deficiency	C8 β deficiency
C1r deficiency	C9 deficiency
C2 deficiency	C1 inhibitor deficiency (hereditary angioedema)
C3 deficiency	Factor I deficiency
C4 deficiency	Factor H deficiency
C5 deficiency	Factor D deficiency
C6 deficiency	Properdin deficiency
C7 deficiency	
C8 α deficiency	
Phagocytic Cell Defects (Excludes Neutropenias)	
Chronic granulomatous disease	Specific granule deficiency
Leukocyte adhesion deficiency 1	Schwachman syndrome
Leukocyte adhesion deficiency 2	Myeloperoxidase deficiency
Chédiak-Higashi syndrome	IFN-γ receptor deficiency
Neutrophil G6PD deficiency	

of cystic fibrosis is 1 in 2,500 population and that of phenylketonuria is 1 in 14,000. The incidence of some of the more common individual disorders, including x-linked agammaglobulinemia (XLA), CVID, and SCID, is 1 in 50,000–150,000. According to the national birth rate, there should be about 400 new cases of primary immune deficiency per year in the United States, and a city of 1 million should yield 1–2 new cases per year.

Another useful way to analyze the incidence of immune deficiency disease is to give the relative frequency of the major subgroups of defects. By this measurement, antibody deficiencies constitute about 50% of the immune deficiencies, T-cell defects constitute about 30–40%, phagocytic cell defects about 10–20%, and complement deficiencies only 2–5% of the total. These figures can be used to judge the adequacy of local referral patterns.

ANTIBODY DEFICIENCY

The underlying pathophysiology of antibody deficiency syndromes includes abnormalities of B-cell development, differentiation, and activation. Interestingly, deletion of Ig genes is rarely, if ever, identified as a cause of immune deficiency. Antibody deficiency syndromes are classified by analyzing peripheral blood for the presence of cells of the B-lymphocyte lineage. Mature B cells are identified by the presence of surface Ig and by B-cell lineage–specific surface antigens such as CD19 or CD20. The presence of mature B cells indicates that the antigen-independent, genetically programmed development of B cells has occurred. Failure to make antibodies under this circumstance must be due to activation defects or failure of T-cell help. The absence of mature B cells and the presence of normal-appearing pre-B cells, which are marked by B-cell molecules other than surface Ig and containing μ heavy chains in the cytoplasm, represent a developmental arrest. Two scenarios account for the majority of B cell defects.

X-linked Agammaglobulinemia

In 1952, Ogden Bruton described boys who had repeated serious bacterial infections and lacked the gamma fraction on serum protein electrophoresis analysis, known to contain the majority of antibody activity. Thus the first immune deficiency disease, X-linked agammaglobulinemia (XLA), was described and its genetics, pathophysiology, diagnosis, and treatment were suggested. Further analysis revealed that this syndrome, often called **Bruton's agammaglobulinemia,** was characterized by an arrest of B-cell development at the pre-B-cell level. The gene affected in XLA, located on the long arm of the X chromosome at locus Xq21.3, encodes a cytoplasmic tyrosine kinase designated as Bruton's tyrosine kinase or Btk. Btk plays an essential role in signal transduction from several B-cell receptors, including surface Ig, CD38, and IL-5. How defects in signal transduction secondary to loss of Btk function lead to B-cell differentiation arrest has not been elucidated.

As expected, these boys are susceptible to repeated serious infections including otitis media, sinusitis, pneumonia, septic arthritis, sepsis, and meningitis due to the "common" pathogens of these infections in childhood: *Haemophilus influenzae* type b, *Staphylococcus aureus,* and *S. pneumoniae.* In general, these illnesses strike after maternal antibody has been catabolized, after the age of 4–6 months. Diarrheal illness, commonly a *Giardia lamblia* infection, and skin infections occur less frequently. Although patients with XLA handle most viral and mycobacterial infections well, enteroviral infections, especially with echovirus, may cause chronic meningoencephalitis that is often refractory to treatment. *Pneumocystis carinii* pneumonia is rare but may occur. Occasional children may have concomitant neutropenia, either persistent or cyclical. The reason for this association is unclear, but it may significantly complicate treatment.

Absence or low levels of serum antibodies of all classes suggest the diagnosis of XLA. The lower the level of IgG, especially if less than 200 mg/dL, the less the need to confirm the diagnosis with response to immunization. Lymphopenia is not present, even when peripheral blood B cells are absent. Plasma cells are absent from biopsy specimens of lymph nodes or mucosal sites.

Management calls for immediate, aggressive treatment with intravenous preparations of IVIG. Delay in diagnosis or inadequate treatment is usually associated with chronic pulmonary disease, including bronchiectasis and *Pseudomonas* colonization. Conversely, prompt recognition and aggressive management are associated with normal growth and development, freedom from infection, and survival into adulthood. The improvement in long-term health with the use of IVIG compared with intramuscular Ig replacement has been substantial. Although there is an increased risk of lymphoid cancer in these patients compared with the general population, it is far less than that in T-cell deficiency disorders. The impact of IVIG on this long-term complication is uncertain.

X-linked Hyper IgM Syndrome

X-linked hyper IgM syndrome (XHIM) presents in males in a manner similar to that with XLA but can be distinguished by the presence of B cells in the peripheral blood and the gradual attainment of quite elevated levels of serum IgM. This suggests a problem with B cells ''switching'' from synthesis of IgM to IgG and other isotypes, a process requiring T cell–B cell communication. For a long time it was unclear whether the underlying defect was expressed in T cells or B cells. The majority of patients with the XHIM syndrome were eventually found to have mutations in the X chromosome gene encoding the T-cell surface activation molecule CD154. CD154 is the so-called CD40 ligand (CD40L), triggering isotype switching through interaction with CD40 on the surface of B cells. A few patients, males and females, have been documented to have mutations in other genes, defining so-called ''non-X-linked'' HIM. The treatment and prognosis are similar to those of XLA.

Although the disorder was initially described as a form of hypogammaglobulinemia, patients with XHIM have more recently been recognized to have variable defects in cell-mediated immunity, such as increased susceptibility to opportunistic infections and lymphoid cancers. This has resulted in increased consideration of these patients as candidates for stem cell transplantation, particularly those who do not achieve an acceptable clinical response to IVIG replacement alone.

Common Variable Immunodeficiency

CVID is a collection of disorders with the common feature of hypogammaglobulinemia with low IgG and IgA levels. Up to half of the patients also have low IgM levels; elevated IgM levels are not seen. Although CVID may present at any age with symptoms of recurrent infection, there is a bimodal distribution with peaks of onset of disease at the ages of 1–5 years and 16–20 years. Some patients have clearly been shown to lose immune function over time, but in the majority of older children and adults the ''late onset'' of hypogammaglobulinemia is presumptive. When studied, patients may have one of a number of defects. Most patients will have circulating mature B cells that fail to become activated by antigen-specific or nonspecific agents. A few patients will have increased numbers or activity of CD8 T cells that can suppress in vitro antibody production. Others will have defects in CD4 T helper cells. Patients with CVID may, therefore, also present with symptoms of mild T-cell deficiency, but the diagnosis of CVID indicates that antibody deficiency is predominant. In general, patients with CVID present with recurrent sinopulmonary infections with common pathogens. Gastrointestinal abnormalities, including infection with *G. lamblia,* and autoimmune symptoms, including sterile arthritis and cytopenias, are common. The treatment and prognosis are similar to those for XLA.

Selective IgA Deficiency

The issue of IgA deficiency is confusing for the specialist as well as for the generalist. IgA deficiency is defined as <0.05 g/L of serum IgA. Serum IgA is absent in as many as 1 in 500 persons in the general population and in up to 1 in 200 atopic persons. Most, if not all, of these persons are presumed to also lack IgA in secretions. The vast majority of IgA-deficient persons have no symptoms, which may reflect the fact that although IgA is the predominant Ig in secretions, it is not the sole antibody class present. Nonetheless, among patients referred with recurrent infections, many will have IgA deficiency as their only immunologic abnormality and are said to have selective IgA deficiency. More recently, an association of deficiencies of IgA, IgG2, and IgG4 has been described. Patients in both IgA-deficient groups, with or without an IgG subclass deficiency, have chronic sinopulmonary infections. Asthma, other forms of lung disease, including chronic obstructive pulmonary disease, and autoimmune symptoms are frequent. Treatment is problematic, since IVIG contains only trace amounts of IgA. In fact, IVIG is contraindicated in patients with selective IgA deficiency because patients with normal levels of total IgG who lack IgA have a peculiar tendency to develop anaphylaxis due to anti-IgA antibodies of the IgE class. Patients with IgA-IgG subclass deficiency may be carefully treated with IVIG. The use of IVIG formulations with ''ultra-low'' IgE levels may be helpful. This caution does not apply to patients with XLA or CVID who may lack IgA.

IgG Subclass Deficiencies

When measurement of IgG subclasses became routinely available a few years ago, there was some enthusiastic belief that deficiencies of one or more subclasses might explain a large percentage of children with recurrent sinopulmonary infection and normal or near-normal IgG levels. This has not proven to be the case, and bona fide IgG subclass deficiency appears to be as uncommon as other antibody deficiency syndromes. Most specialists would now require the following diagnostic criteria: (1) recurrent upper and lower respiratory tract infections, (2) a normal or near-normal level of total IgG, (3) at least two separate IgG subclass determinations showing low levels of one or two subclasses, and (4) failure to adequately respond to immunization with protein (for IgG1 and IgG3 deficiency) or polysaccharide (for IgG2 and IgG4 deficiency) antigens. IVIG replacement therapy is usually advocated for these patients. Because the IgG2 subclass value seems to reach normal adult levels more slowly than the others, IVIG replacement in children with IgG2 or other subclass deficiency should be suspended periodically in order to judge the necessity of continued treatment.

Transient Hypogammaglobulinemia of Infancy

Some infants present with IgG levels low for their age and a history of recurrent infections, most of which are not serious or life threatening. If there is evidence of adequate response to immunization, these infants can be observed to eventually reach normal IgG levels, usually by 3–4 years of age. IVIG treatment is not routinely recommended.

T-CELL AND COMBINED IMMUNE DEFICIENCY

Although a few patients may present with severely defective T-cell function but with nearly normal IgG levels, antibody responses to T cell–dependent antigens are severely impaired. Thus there is always some element of combined deficiency in patients with T-cell disorders, even when intrinsic B-cell function appears normal. From a pragmatic standpoint, treatment is directed at correcting the T-cell defect, usually through hematopoietic stem cell transplantation. IVIG replacement can be a valuable adjunct to pretransplant treatment but will not affect the long-term outcome for these patients.

Severe Combined Immune Deficiency

SCID is a collection of distinct syndromes affecting both T and B cells and characterized by a common presentation. Affected children usually have symptoms in early infancy, and death invariably occurs by the second or third year. Many of these infants fail to thrive. Infection with *Candida* in the form of persistent thrush is common and difficult to treat. Interstitial pneumonitis is frequent and may be due to *P. carinii* or viruses. Bacterial infections become prevalent after maternal antibody has waned but may be inapparent in those children whose B cells retain intrinsic function. Fungal infection of the scalp and nails occurs. Peculiar skin manifestations, including seborrhea-like changes or graft-versus-host-like erythroderma may occur. Although absence of tonsils, lymph nodes, and thymic shadow on radiographs is common, some patients with SCID may also present with lymphoid hyperplasia, a complex called **Omenn's syndrome.**

Adenosine deaminase (ADA) enzyme deficiency is a well-defined cause of SCID. Toxic metabolites of deoxyadenosine are specifically lethal for lymphocytes, which lack the salvage pathway present in most tissue. Lymphopenia is usually present, and ADA activity measured in erythrocytes is low or absent. This defect represents 20–30% of patients with SCID in the United States. ADA-deficiency SCID was the first disease to be approved for clinical application of specific gene replacement therapy. Although the results of therapy with gene-modified autologous T lymphocytes have been encouraging, bone marrow transplant is still the therapy of choice for these patients.

X-linked SCID, which accounts for about 40–45% of all SCID cases, is characterized by T-cell lymphopenia, decreased NK cell number and function, and normal to increased numbers of functionally impaired B cells (T^-, B^+, NK^-). The molecular basis for X-SCID is a defect in *IL2RG,* the gene encoding the γ-chain of the IL-2 receptor. The γ-chain is common to several cytokine receptors, including IL-4, IL-7, IL-9, and IL-15, hence the name *common γ-chain* (γc). Because IL-7 is a critical cytokine in T-cell precursor maturation and IL-15 is critical for NK cell development, abnormal expression of the IL-7 and IL-15 receptors is thought to be the key defect. A genetic defect of JAK3, the signaling kinase that interacts intracellularly with γc, results in a phenotype similar to X-SCID, except that both males and females are affected because the *JAK3* gene is autosomal. Several other gene defects resulting in the SCID phenotype have recently been identified (Table 98–3).

Despite the multiple phenotypes, SCID should be strongly suspected in infants who present clinically as described and with laboratory evidence of (1) lymphopenia, (2) abnormal numbers of T cells, especially low levels of CD4 cells, or (3) reduced in vitro T-cell function. Patients should be aggressively treated for ongoing infections, including initiation of *P. carinii* prophylaxis (Table 68–14), and, if needed, IVIG. Transplantation of bone marrow or cord blood from an HLA-matched sibling or matched unrelated donor or transplantation with a T-cell-depleted, haplotype-mismatched (parental) bone marrow should be accomplished as soon as possible. Early diagnosis and prompt institution of therapy significantly improve outcome after hematopoietic stem cell transplantation. The long-term survival of patients who receive transplants when free of serious infection exceeds 70%.

DiGeorge Syndrome

DiGeorge syndrome (DGS) is characterized clinically by congenital heart disease, congenital hypoparathyroidism, dysmorphic facial features, and immune dysfunction. The major immune defect is

TABLE 98–3. Severe Combined Immune Deficiency Syndromes (SCID)

Name	Genetic Defect/ Pathogenesis	Immunologic Features
X-linked SCID	IL-2 receptor common γ chain	T^-, B^+, NK^-, lymphopenia
Autosomal recessive	JAK3 mutation	T^-, B^+, NK^-, lymphopenia
SCID	RAG-1/RAG-2 defect	T^-, B^-, NK^+, lymphopenia
	Adenosine deaminase deficiency	T^-, $B^{\pm}$, NK^+, lymphopenia
	Purine phosphorylase deficiency	T^-, B^+, NK^+, lymphopenia
	ZAP-70 defect	CD8 deficiency, normal TLC
MHC class II deficiency	Defect in MHC II gene transcription	CD4 deficiency, normal TLC
Omenn's syndrome	?Partial RAG-1/RAG-2 defect	Normal to ↑ T cells, ↓ B, ↓ Igs
CD3 deficiencies	CD3γ or CD3ε gene defect	↓ CD3, variable CD4, CD8

absence or hypoplasia of the thymus. These defects can be explained by abnormal embryonic development of the third and fourth pharyngeal pouches. Most cases are sporadic, although some familial occurrence has been reported. Although no definitive toxic, infectious, or other environmental factor has been implicated in pathogenesis, it is now known that DGS is caused by deletion of chromosomal region 22q11.2. Hemizygosity for the gene *Ufd-1,* encoding a ubiquitin-dependent protease involved in neural crest development, has been proposed as the key to pathogenesis. Similar deletions of 22q11 have been detected in patients with the velocardiofacial and the conotruncal anomaly face syndromes. DGS has a wide spectrum of severity, particularly immunologically. Most patients have a mild and transient T-cell immunodeficiency. Immunologic reconstitution of severely affected children has been accomplished by fetal thymus transplantation as well as bone marrow transplantation.

Wiskott-Aldrich Syndrome

Wiskott-Aldrich syndrome (WAS) is an X-linked syndrome of combined immunodeficiency, thrombocytopenia, and eczemalike skin rash. Immune deficiency may be severe and thrombocytopenia profound. Defective T-cell function, poor in vivo antibody production to polysaccharide antigens, and a characteristic pattern of low IgM and high IgA and IgE are usually present. WAS is caused by mutations in a gene in the Xp11.22 region encoding a 54 kDa protein called the **WAS protein** (WASP). The exact function of WASP is unknown, but a resultant pleiotropic defect in cell membrane ultrastructure has been implicated. Infants typically die of bleeding or infection. Later in their course patients may experience severe autoimmune problems or develop lymphoid cancer. Survival into adulthood is exceptional. Splenectomy has been advocated to alleviate thrombocytopenia and control the bleeding tendency, but the potential benefit must be balanced against the risk of postsplenectomy sepsis, which further complicates immunologic management. Long-term survival and correction of immunologic and hematologic abnormalities can be accomplished with allogeneic bone marrow transplantation. Stem cell transplantation during early childhood with a matched sibling donor or a matched unrelated bone marrow or cord blood donor results in survival rates exceeding 70%.

PHAGOCYTIC CELL DISORDERS

Disorders of various intracellular pathways can affect the ability of monocytes/macrophages, polymorphonuclear neutrophils, or both to kill bacteria. These disorders commonly present with recurrent bacterial infections at sites that are usually protected by these phagocytic cells, such as the lungs, skin, and gums (periodontium). Because these intracellular pathways generate many of the adverse effects of acute infection (e.g., pain, erythema, warmth), a cardinal sign of phagocytic cell disorders is the **cold abscess,** defined as an abscess that is devoid of erythema and warmth. In addition, patients with these disorders often have hypergammaglobulinemia because failure to kill the pathogen results in continuous immune stimulation.

Chronic Granulomatous Disease

Chronic granulomatous disease (CGD) is the most common functional phagocytic cell defect. Children with this defect present with recurrent pneumonia, lymphadenitis, and skin abscesses. Characteristic organisms isolated from these sites include *S. aureus, Aspergillus, Pseudomonas,* and *Serratia marcescens.* Diagnosis is established by finding normal phagocyte ingestion but reduced intracellular killing of bacteria and reduced activity of oxidative enzymes that generate reactive compounds capable of killing bacteria. The latter can be measured by reduction of the dye **nitroblue tetrazolium (NBT)** or by recently developed flow cytometric assays. The most common molecular defect in CGD, accounting for all of the X-linked cases and about 65% of all CGD cases, is a mutation in the gene encoding gp91, which is a membrane component of the NADPH oxidase enzyme (phox), the enzyme that catalyzes the oxidative burst. Most of the remaining CGD patients have defects in the gene for p47, a cytosolic component of phox. Mutations in the genes for the phox components p67 and p22 are rare, accounting for fewer than 10% of cases.

Recombinant IFN-γ recently has been shown to decrease the incidence of infections in CGD, presumably by enhancing nonoxidative pathways of bactericidal activity. Therapy with IFN-γ, along with daily trimethoprim-sulfamethoxazole prophylaxis, decreases the number of infections. Although bone marrow transplantation is potentially curative, it has not gained wide acceptance in the treatment of CGD because of its associated morbidity and mortality compared with more conservative therapy.

Chédiak-Higashi Syndrome

Chédiak-Higashi syndrome is a rare disorder that is notable for the ease with which it is diagnosed. Leukocytes from these patients with recurrent, serious bacterial infections characteristically contain large cytoplasmic inclusions, known as **giant granules.** Partial albinism and increased susceptibility to lymphoma and leukemia are also present. NK cell function is impaired. There is no specific treatment available, although successful bone marrow transplantation reverses the immunologic abnormalities.

Leukocyte Adhesion Deficiency

Several kindreds have been described with **leukocyte adhesion deficiency type 1 (LAD-1)** where affected members have recurrent bacterial infections of the skin and periodontal tissues. Omphalitis, intramural infection of the bowel (cecitis/typhlitis), and intraabdominal abscesses have been reported. Hyperleukocytosis is a key finding, routinely exceeding 50,000/mm^3. Monocytes, granulocytes, and lymphocytes from these patients exhibit reduced expression of cell surface molecules, called β_2 integrins, involved in cell-cell and cell-tissue interactions and reduced adhesive properties in vitro. The molecular defect in LAD-1 is a mutation in the gene encoding the β_2 subunit (CD18) common to the three leukocyte integrins (Mac-1, LFA-1, and p150,95). In patients with the severe phenotype, expression of CD18 is low to absent. These patients invariably die during the first few years of life. Those with the moderate phenotype have 5–30% surface expression of CD18 and usually survive into adulthood. Allogeneic hematopoietic SCT is curative. A few patients with **LAD type 2,** who have a generalized defect in fucose metabolism resulting in an absence of SLeX, a ligand for selectins, have recently been described.

COMPLEMENT DEFICIENCIES

Complement deficiencies are rare and may be more frequent causes of rheumatologic disease than of recurrent infections. Most known deficiencies involve the components of the classical, antibody-dependent pathway, whereas a few are due to alternate pathway or regulatory components.

C2 Deficiency

C2 deficiency is the most common of the complete complement deficiencies, with an estimated prevalence of 1 in 10,000 persons. Almost 40% of affected patients develop systemic or discoid lupus erythematosus; about 50% suffer from recurrent infections; and a few affected persons remain free of symptoms.

C3 Deficiency

The best understood complement deficiency leading to recurrent infections is deficiency in the central component of both the classical and alternate pathways, C3. These patients present much like those with hypogammaglobulinemia, except that infections may begin earlier in life. There is some evidence that when antibody titers are high enough, opsonization of bacteria is less dependent on C3. Thus immunization of C3-deficient persons with pneumococcal, *Haemophilus influenzae* type b, and meningococcal vaccines has been recommended.

Deficiency of C6, C7, C8, or C9

Patients with deficiency of one of the terminal components of the classical pathway—C6, C7, C8, and C9—have a peculiar susceptibility to *Neisseria* infections. This suggests a particular requirement for membrane lysis in protection against *Neisseria,* which is not completely understood.

Complement Deficiency and Noninfectious Disease

Many patients present with rheumatologic symptoms and complement abnormalities. Although active systemic lupus erythematosus causes complement consumption, a few patients have permanent depression of complement activity, even when in remission. Rare patients with other autoimmune disorders, not normally associated with complement consumption, also are found to have low complement levels. Finally, complement deficiencies in such patients can be confirmed at the nucleic acid level. The most common deficiencies of this type are those of C2 and C4. The proposed mechanism of rheumatologic signs and symptoms in complement deficiency is the failure to solubilize and clear antigen-antibody complexes from the circulation.

Deficiencies of complement components are also responsible for other noninfectious diseases. Deficiency of the regulatory protein C1 inhibitor (C1INH), which reduces the spontaneous activation of the classical pathway, leads to hereditary angioedema. This disorder is marked by recurrent episodes of painless swelling without itching or urticaria. Laryngeal edema may be fatal, whereas swelling of the bowel wall may cause intense cramping pain. Paroxysmal nocturnal hemoglobinuria (PNH) is associated with acquired deficiency of decay-accelerating factor (DAF), a cell membrane protein that normally limits complement pathway activity. Uninhibited deposition of C3 and the membrane attack complex leads to episodes of erythrocyte destruction.

MISCELLANEOUS SYNDROMES

Ataxia-Telangiectasia

As the name of the syndrome suggests, these patients present with oculocutaneous telangiectasia and progressive cerebellar ataxia and also exhibit neurologic deterioration and a high incidence of cancer. Recurrent sinopulmonary infection is common, but opportunistic infections are not seen. Common laboratory findings include low IgA and IgE levels and high serum α-fetoprotein levels. Some patients have low IgG subclass 2 levels and significant T-cell lymphopenia with decreased T-cell function. The disease gene in ataxia-telangiectasia, designated *ATM* (A-T mutated), is located on chromosome 11q23. The gene product, ATM protein, is a member of the phosphatidyl inositol (PI)-3 kinaselike protein family. A role in the repair of double-stranded DNA breaks is postulated and correlates with increased in vitro susceptibility of A-T cells to damage by x-rays. The cause of immune deficiency is proposed to be defective T-cell receptor and Ig gene rearrangement.

Hyper-IgE Syndrome

A peculiar syndrome of recurrent staphylococcal abscesses and strikingly elevated levels of serum IgE (>2,000 IU/mL) has been described. Abscess formation usually involves the skin, where it may be confused with severe atopic dermatitis. Abscesses may also form in the lungs or joints. The underlying immune defect and, indeed, the relationship of the elevated IgE to the abscess formation is unclear. The causative gene for this syndrome has not been identified. Infection with *Staphylococcus aureus* is characteristic, but other gram-positive abscesses and *Candida* granulomas may occur. Lifelong therapy with penicillinase-resistant penicillins is clearly beneficial and appears indicated. Persistent abscesses may require surgical treatment.

MANAGEMENT OF PRIMARY IMMUNE DEFICIENCY DISEASES

Until very recently, treatment of the underlying immunologic abnormalities of the immune deficiencies was limited to two strategies: (1) replacement therapy with pooled antibodies from normal donors and (2) bone marrow transplantation. Advances in molecular medicine now make it possible to envision the addition of gene therapy and cytokines to the medical armamentarium available to treat these disorders.

Antibody Replacement Therapy

Patients with antibody deficiency disorders can be adequately treated with monthly intravenous infusions of a purified IgG fraction, as IVIG, derived from the pooled plasma of screened, healthy blood donors. Replacement therapy is aimed at prophylaxis of acute infections and prevention of chronic local infection. The usual dose is 400 mg/kg every 3–4 weeks, but more may be required in select patients to keep them free of symptoms. Alternatively, the frequency of administration may be increased. In patients with agammaglobulinemia, this dose will usually produce trough (preinfusion) IgG levels at the lower limit of normal. Although it is useful to measure trough IgG levels, the goal is clinical improvement and not necessarily the attainment of a specific IgG level. IVIG contains only trace quantities of IgM and IgA, and these levels will not increase. Most patients require up to 6 months of IVIG treatment to reach maximum benefit, presumably due to eradication of chronic infection and altered catabolism. Significant improvement, however, is usually noted immediately. A ''wearing-off'' of the beneficial effect in the week preceding the next infusion is a reliable indicator of suboptimal dosage.

There are two principal adverse effects of IVIG. Anaphylaxis is rare but potentially fatal, and therefore all new patients should be treated in a physician-attended setting with emergency capability. Transfusionlike reactions are common, occurring in 10–20% of patients and can consist of fever, chills, muscle aches, abdominal cramps, and headache. Presumably, these symptoms are due to Ig aggregates in the preparation or combination of IVIG with minute amounts of circulating antigens in the bloodstream, which cause the release of inflammatory mediators. Acetaminophen, antihistamines, and, if needed, corticosteroid pretreatment along with slower administration will eliminate most such side effects. The biologic safety record of IVIG and its intramuscular predecessor are impressive, and the risk of acquiring hepatitis B or HIV infection is exceedingly remote. HIV transmission with IVIG has never been reported, even in immune-deficient patients infused with IVIG known to contain anti-HIV antibodies. Transmission of hepatitis C virus occurred before the use of current solvent-detergent IVIG preparative methods. Many immunology centers have active home IVIG therapy programs, which is feasible in clinically stable patients with no history of serious adverse reactions.

Stem Cell Transplantation

Most, if not all, diseases affecting T, B, and phagocytic cells are potentially curable with stem cell transplantation. In practice, the risks of stem cell transplantation limit its routine use to patients with severe disorders of T-cell function (e.g., SCID, Wiskott-Aldrich syndrome) at the present time. Despite the defects in cellular immunity demonstrated by these patients, extensive experience has demonstrated the need for ''conditioning'' the recipient with marrow ablative therapy except in the few SCID patients with no T-, B-, and NK-cell function. It has been repeatedly shown that infection present at the time of stem cell transplantation, especially acute or chronic pulmonary infection, is the single most important factor in transplant failure. Thus prompt diagnosis is critical to success. The use of alternative sources of stem cells, such as cord blood–derived hematopoietic stem cells, will allow the implementation of this approach in greater numbers of patients.

Supportive Therapy

Antibiotics. In general, patients with primary immune deficiencies will require antibiotic therapy frequently unless curative therapy, such as bone marrow transplantation, is successfully instituted. Although it may be argued that patients who lack certain immune functions may not resolve acute infections as rapidly as other persons, there is no general rule for extending the duration of currently accepted antibiotic therapy for serious infections in these patients. This may reflect the probability that many treatment regimens could be much shorter in normal hosts. Whatever the case, routine extension of indicated antimicrobial therapy is not recommended, and treatment of chronic infection should be individualized. A tendency to be more aggressive in diagnosis and follow-up, including the appropriate use of invasive procedures, in the management of chronic infections should be encouraged.

Prophylactic antibiotics are a difficult issue in the case of children with immune deficiency. In general, prophylactic antibiotics should be avoided. Most patients with antibody deficiency who are receiving adequate doses of IVIG should not require antibiotics for prophylaxis. However, IgA deficiency, phagocyte deficiency (other than CGD), and complement component deficiency have no convenient, effective means for immunologic prophylaxis. Cautious use of prophylactic antibiotics may outweigh the risk of colonization with antibiotic-resistant bacteria in the more seriously affected persons in these categories. Several schemes of antibiotic administration (e.g., low doses, ''pulse'' therapy, rotation of drug classes) have been promulgated but have not been subjected to controlled evaluation.

Immunization. Live virus vaccines, including polio (OPV), measles/mumps/rubella (MMR), and varicella-zoster, are contraindicated because of the risk of vaccine-induced illness in children with T-cell deficiency. In practice these vaccines should also be avoided in children with significant antibody deficiency. OPV also should not be given to family members of children with immune deficiency because of viral shedding from the gastrointestinal tract and the possibility of transmission to the patient. Routine childhood immunizations likely will not produce protective antibody response, but IVIG probably confers adequate passive protection against the illnesses covered by these vaccines.

Avoidance Measures. In addition to avoiding certain vaccines as cited, patients with cellular immune deficiency should avoid transfusions with nonirradiated cellular blood products, which may cause fatal graft-versus-host disease. Allogeneic T lymphocytes capable of mediating graft-versus-host disease will be inactivated by irradiation. The increasingly routine use of efficient leukodepletion may eventually render irradiation unnecessary. Patients with immune deficiencies should avoid close contact with persons who have obvious signs of contagious illness. Once treatment with IVIG or successful bone marrow transplantation has been accomplished, however, these patients can attend school and function in society. IVIG-treated patients have been cautiously allowed to attend well-supervised daycare centers. Parents need considerable education and support in living with these children on an everyday basis. The Immune Deficiency Foundation (P.O. Box 508, Columbia, MD 21045; www.primaryimmune.org) is a valuable source of information and support for families.

Pulmonary Management. In addition to acute pneumonia, chronic lung infection is a leading cause of morbidity and premature death in immune deficiency. Asthma (reactive airways disease) also appears to be overrepresented in these patients. Scrupulous attention should be paid to pulmonary management, with annual pulmonary function testing in older children and adults. Home physiotherapy and aerosolized bronchodilator or antibiotic treatment (similar to that in cystic fibrosis) may be indicated.

Role of the Primary Care Physician. Partnership between the primary physician and the specialist provides optimal care for these complicated patients. Despite their special conditions, they have many of the same problems of growth, development, and acute illness as normal children. In addition, administration of IVIG at a local clinic may save the family considerable time and expense if they live far from the referral center. Patients who tolerate two or three doses of IVIG at the immunology clinic can usually be referred to their local physician for routine monthly infusion. In selected patients, the physician can also supervise home infusion. Annual or semiannual immunology follow-up is adequate for stable patients. At these times, laboratory studies can be updated and new knowledge of pathogenesis, genetics, or treatment options can be shared with the family.

REVIEWS

Buckley RH, Schiff RI, Schiff SE, et al: Human severe combined immunodeficiency: Genetic, phenotypic, and functional diversity in one hundred eight infants. *J Pediatr* 1997;130:378–87.

Candotti F, Blaese RM: Gene therapy for primary immunodeficiencies. *Springer Semin Immunopathol* 1998;19:493–508.

Fischer A, Cavazzana-Calvo M, De Saint Basile G, et al: Naturally occurring primary deficiencies of the immune system. *Annu Rev Immunol* 1997;15:93–124.

Kapoor N, Crooks G, Kohn DB, et al: Hematopoietic stem cell transplantation for primary lymphoid immunodeficiencies. *Semin Hematol* 1998; 35:346–53.

Malech HL, Nauseef WM: Primary inherited defects in neutrophil function: Etiology and treatment. *Semin Hematol* 1997;34:279–90.

Ochs HD, Smith CIE, Puck JM (editors): *Primary Immunodeficiency Diseases: A Molecular and Genetic Approach.* New York, Oxford University Press, 1999.

Puck JM: Primary immunodeficiency diseases. *JAMA* 1997;278:1835–41.

Stiehm ER: Human intravenous immunoglobulin in primary and secondary antibody deficiencies. *Pediatr Infect Dis J* 1997;16:696–707.

Stiehm ER (editor): *Immunologic Disorders in Infants and Children,* 4th ed. Philadelphia, WB Saunders, 1996.

WHO Scientific Group: Primary immunodeficiency diseases: Report of a WHO scientific group. *Clin Exp Immunol* 1997;109:1–28.

Winkelstein JA, Marino MC, Johnston RB Jr, et al: Chronic granulomatous disease: Report on a national registry of 368 patients. *Medicine* (*Baltimore*) 2000;79:155–69.

CHAPTER 99

Patients with Cancer

Dennis A. Conrad

Patients with cancer are at increased risk of infection, both as a consequence of certain types of primary cancer and as a complication of anticancer treatment. Knowledge of this fact and recognition of the most likely causes (Table 99–1) forearm the practitioner in managing the care of these special patients.

EPIDEMIOLOGY

The relative rate of infection in adult patients with cancer at the time of admission or during hospitalization is 10–15%, which results in an overall rate of approximately 6 infective episodes per 1,000 patient days of hospitalization. The highest individual rates of infection occur in patients with acute myelogenous leukemia, skeletal cancers, and hepatic carcinomas. The most frequent infected sites, in descending order, are the respiratory tract, the bloodstream, surgical wounds, and the urinary tract. *Staphylococcus aureus, Escherichia coli, Pseudomonas aeruginosa, Klebsiella pneumoniae,* and coagulase-negative staphylococci are the most commonly identified pathogens. The data for pediatric cancer patients are comparable to those for adult patients.

Bacterial Infections. In the United States over the past decade, trends in the most commonly identified bacterial pathogens causing infections in patients with cancer reveal a decline in the frequency of infections due to *P. aeruginosa* and the Enterobacteriaceae, with a concomitant rise in the frequency of infection due to gram-positive organisms, especially *Staphylococcus, Streptococcus,* and *Enterococcus.* However, gram-negative bacillary infections predominate in less well-developed countries. The reasons for trend differences in species recovery are unproved. Intuitively, increased use of central venous catheters and increasing *Staphylococcus* and *Enterococcus* resistance to broad-spectrum β-lactam antimicrobials potent against gram-negative organisms may account for the changes in the United States, whereas reduced access to medical care, limited availability of the newer extended-spectrum antimicrobials, and greater environmental contamination may influence the trends seen in less well-developed countries.

Fungal Infections. Approximately 40% of deaths from infection in patients with cancer are due to fungal or mixed fungal-bacterial infections, largely occurring during the remission-induction phase of chemotherapy. Factors contributing to the propensity for fungal infections include cancer- or therapy-associated cellular immunity defects, cutaneous ulcerations and oropharyngeal or gastrointestinal mucosal lesions permitting systemic invasion, and the presence of long-term indwelling intravascular catheters. Moreover, broad-spectrum antibacterial therapy promotes fungal colonization as a precursor to infection. Concomitant diabetes mellitus, intermittent periods of acidosis, use of parenteral nutrition, and surgical procedures also increase the risk of fungal infection. On the basis of autopsy findings, disseminated candidiasis and disseminated aspergillosis have proven to be the two most common infections not suspected antemortem; approximately 15% of all cases of disseminated aspergillosis will have been earlier misdiagnosed as bacterial infections.

The predominant deficiency in host defense determines the fungal pathogens most likely to cause infection. Defective phagocytic defenses, as in the case of neutropenia, predispose persons to infection due to opportunistic mycoses such as *Aspergillus, Mucor, Rhizopus, Absidia, Pseudallescheria boydii, Candida,* and *Trichosporon.* These opportunistic fungi are unlikely causes of significant tissue-invasive or disseminated infection in immunocompetent hosts. By comparison the fungal pathogens *Coccidioides immitis, Histoplasma capsulatum, Blastomyces dermatitidis,* and *Sporothrix schenckii* are more prone to infect hosts with defective cell-mediated immunity but may also cause significant infections in apparently healthy hosts. *Cryptococcus neoformans* may cause infections in hosts with defective cell-mediated immunity, but it almost never causes infection in either the healthy or the neutropenic host.

Parasitic Infections. Infections with *Pneumocystis carinii* and *Toxoplasma gondii* represent reactivation of quiescent infection facilitated by cancer- or therapy-associated cellular immunodeficiency. *P. carinii* primarily causes pneumonitis, mostly in patients with leukemia or lymphoma, but it can also cause extrapulmonary disease such as sinusitis and otitis media.

Viral Infections. Viral opportunistic infections in patients with cancer usually represent symptomatic reactivation from latency facilitated by cancer- or therapy-associated cellular immunodeficiency. Herpes simplex virus can cause severe and prolonged mucocutaneous infection, especially in patients with mucosal injury from another source, such as mucositis or irradiation injury. Varicella-zoster virus can cause serious primary infection in susceptible persons, often with accompanying encephalitis, hepatitis, or, most ominously, pneumonitis. Zoster can also reactivate during chemotherapy and may occur in dermatomes within irradiation fields of patients undergoing radiotherapy. Patients with Hodgkin's lymphoma are particularly prone to eruption of zoster, largely because of the abnormalities in T lymphocyte–mediated immunity that characterizes this cancer. Cytomegalovirus can cause focal disease in immunocompromised patients, being most likely to occur in patients receiving allogeneic bone marrow transplantation as treatment of hematologic cancer (Chapter 100). Manifestations of cytomegalovirus disease include hepatitis, pneumonitis, and ulcerations of the gastrointestinal mucosa.

PATHOGENESIS

Cancers That Predispose to Infection

Leukemia. Infection remains the leading cause of morbidity and mortality associated with leukemia. The increased risk of infection

TABLE 99–1. Selected Pathogens of Importance in Patients with Cancer

Organism	Comment
Bacteria	
Bacteroides fragilis	Most common in hematogenous, gastrointestinal, genitourinary cancers; bacteremia often associated with abscess
Campylobacter hyointestinalis	Newly recognized cause of diarrhea in hematogenous cancer
Clostridium difficile	*Clostridium difficile*-associated diarrhea (antibiotic-associated diarrhea)
Clostridium septicum, Clostridium perfringens	Septicemia in hematogenous, gastrointestinal cancer; associated with mucositis, gastrointestinal obstruction
Comamonas acidovorans	Catheter-associated bacteremia in children with non-Hodgkin's lymphoma and neuroblastoma
Enterobacter cloacae	Multiple antibiotic-resistant bacteremias in leukemia; may be due to prior β-lactam exposures
Escherichia coli	Death in children associated with neutropenia, pressor need, presence of central venous catheter
Haemophilus influenzae	Bacteremia risk 6 times greater in children with cancer; vaccine response if given ≤1 year after chemotherapy begun
Klebsiella pneumoniae	Second only to *Escherichia coli* as cause of bacteremia by Enterobacteriaceae in cancer; most infections acquired nosocomially
Listeria monocytogenes	Septicemia and meningitis in patients with lymphoma or receiving corticosteroids
Moraxella catarrhalis	Septicemia in leukemia; most strains β-lactamase producers
Mycobacterium avium complex	Septicemia, mycotic aneurysm, disseminated disease; high risk in hairy cell leukemia
Mycobacterium chelonae	Skin, soft tissue, bone infections; majority of patients receiving corticosteroids, immunosuppressants
Mycobacterium haemophilum	Fastidious organism requiring hemin for growth in cooler environment; causes skin ulcers, septic arthritis
Nocardia asteroides	Pneumonia, empyema, brain abscess; occurs in patient with solid tumors, hematologic cancer
Pediococcus acidilactici	Septicemia in leukemia; gram-positive cocci resistant to vancomycin
Propionibacterium granulosum	Skin colonizer; septicemia in hepatic carcinoma
Pseudomonas aeruginosa	Septicemia during neutropenia; environmental acquisition, with few strains causing most infections
Pseudomonas pseudomallei	Melioidosis; septicemia/disseminated disease in leukemia/lymphoma in tropics
β-hemolytic streptococci, Viridans streptococci, *Enterococcus*	Increasing cause of septicemia in hematogenous cancer; infections associated with intravenous catheters, disruption of oral/gastrointestinal mucosa
Coagulase-negative staphylococci	Becoming most prevalent organism recovered during febrile neutropenia; most catheter-associated
Staphylococcus aureus	Catheter-associated; skin/soft tissue/bone infections; pneumonia in neutropenic leukemia
Vibrio vulnificus	Soft tissue infections/septicemia in leukemia following punctures in seawater
Fungi	
Aspergillus flavus, Aspergillus fumigatus, Aspergillus niger	Pneumonia, sinusitis, disseminated disease; most common in hematogenous cancer with neutropenia; aspergillus pneumonia most common cause of fatal hemoptysis in leukemia/lymphoma; successful treatment more dependent on correction of underlying immunosuppression
Blastoschizomyces capitis	Former names: *Trichosporon capitium, Geotrichum capitatum;* pneumonia, hepatitis in leukemia
Candida albicans, Candida parapsilosis, Candida tropicalis, Candida glabrata, Candida krusei, Candida lusitaniae	Mucocutaneous, oral, esophageal, laryngotracheal, fungemia, retinitis, hepatosplenic, renal, skeletal infections; most common fungal pathogen in hematogenous cancer; increasing prevalence due to fluconazole resistance
Chrysosporium	Nose/paranasal fungal infection in leukemia
Cryptococcus neoformans	Hodgkin's lymphoma, corticosteroid therapy most common associations; less frequent in leukemia than would be predicted
Cunninghamella bertholletiae	Pneumonia in leukemia
Fusarium proliferatum, Fusarium solani	Cutaneous and disseminated infections in leukemia; more often with positive blood culture than other fungi; relatively resistant to amphotericin B
Geotrichum candidum	Disseminated disease in leukemia; may be incorrectly assumed to be saprophyte
Hansenula anomala	Catheter-associated fungemia in leukemia
Malassezia furfur	Fungemia/disseminated disease in hematogenous cancer associated with central venous catheters, lipid hyperalimentation
Scopulariopsis	Sinusitis, otitis externa, disseminated disease in hematogenous cancer
Trichosporon beigelii	Disseminated disease in agranulocytopenia; cross-reactive with cryptococcus-latex agglutination test

Table continued on following page

TABLE 99–1. Selected Pathogens of Importance in Patients with Cancer *(Continued)*

Organism	Comment
Protozoa	
Cryptosporidium parvum, Isospora belli, Giardia lamblia, Cyclospora cayetanensis, Enterocytozoon bieneusi, Septata intestinalis	Chronic diarrhea in immunocompromised patients
Leishmania donovani	Cutaneous and visceral disease in hematogenous cancer in endemic areas; more likely fatal than in healthy hosts
Viruses	
Adenoviruses	Prolonged fever, gastroenteritis, hemorrhagic cystis, conjunctivitis, interstitial pneumonitis in immunocompromised patients
Cytomegalovirus	Pneumonitis, oral/gastrointestinal ulcers, hepatitis, retinitis, fever/wasting syndrome; pneumonitis most life-threatening
Echoviruses	Disseminated disease in hematogenous cancer; immunity may be immunoglobulin-dependent
Hepatitis A virus	Hepatitis in hematogenous cancer
Herpes simplex viruses	Mucocutaneous disease during chemotherapy of leukemia/lymphoma
Influenza A virus	Hemophagocytic syndrome cluster in children with leukemia
Parvovirus B19	Anemia, neutropenia, hemophagocytic syndrome, hemolysis, aplastic crisis in hematogenous cancer
Respiratory syncytial virus	Interstitial pneumonia; progressive severe respiratory distress in immunocompromised patients
Varicella zoster virus	Severe primary infection, zoster, cutaneous, disseminated, pulmonary, hepatic, central nervous system disease; lymphoma, corticosteroid therapy at greatest risk

is due to the reduced numbers of circulating functional granulocytes and to disruption in cell-mediated immunity.

Granulocytopenia is defined as fewer than 1,000 polymorphonuclear leukocytes per cubic millimeter of blood. The risk of infection is inversely proportional to the **absolute neutrophil count (ANC),** with the greatest risk of infection associated with absolute neutrophil counts less than $100/mm^3$. Although granulocytopenia more often arises from cytotoxic chemotherapy administered as treatment for the leukemia, acute leukemias can also be associated with a profound granulocytopenia at the time of presentation.

The most common infections associated with granulocytopenia are bacterial and fungal infections that arise from gastrointestinal flora. *Enterobacteriaceae* and *P. aeruginosa* traditionally have been regarded as the most important causes of bacteremia in neutropenic patients, although *Streptococcus, Enterococcus,* and *Staphylococcus* are becoming increasingly significant. *Candida* are the most important pathologic yeasts in patients with granulocytopenia, and *Aspergillus* and *Fusarium* are the most important molds. Although many viruses and some parasites can cause infection in patients with cancer, granulocytopenia is not a significant risk factor.

Lymphoma. Certain cancers, especially the lymphomas, are associated with a primary defect in cell-mediated immunity. Bacterial infections do not occur as prominently in patients with abnormalities in cell-mediated immunity as in patients with granulocytopenia, although *Streptococcus pneumoniae, Haemophilus influenzae,* and *Neisseria meningitidis* remain important potential pathogens. *Salmonella, Mycobacterium,* and *Legionella* are potential pathogens of special concern, especially in environments of increased endemicity. The yeast *C. neoformans* is an important cause of fungal infection in patients with abnormal cell-mediated immunity. Disease most commonly occurs as meningitis, but *C. neoformans* may also manifest as pneumonia and cutaneous infection. The herpesviruses are significant causes of infection in patients with abnormalities in cell-mediated immunity. Herpes simplex virus most commonly causes orolabial and esophageal lesions but may also cause mucocutaneous or cutaneous lesions at other sites. Varicella-zoster virus can cause severe primary (chickenpox) and reactivated (zoster or shingles) infections. Zoster can be complicated by cutaneous dissemination involving more than two contiguous dermatomes and visceral dissemination, most ominously manifesting as pneumonitis, hepatitis, or meningoencephalitis. Cytomegalovirus, either as primary or reactivated infection, can cause prolonged viremia and fever, pneumonitis, hepatitis, gastroenteritis, and chorioretinitis. The spectrum of infection is broad, ranging from apparently asymptomatic viruria to rapidly progressive, fatal pneumonitis. The protozoans *P. carinii, T. gondii,* and *Cryptosporidium parvum* are important parasitic pathogens in patients with defects in cell-mediated immunity. *P. carinii* pneumonia most often presents as fever with progressive dyspnea, usually associated with radiographic evidence of interstitial pneumonitis. Primary infection with *T. gondii* usually presents as lymphadenopathy or an infectious mononucleosis–like syndrome, and reactivation most often presents as an encephalopathy with focal brain lesions. Central nervous system infection with *T. gondii* occurs more commonly in persons with AIDS than in patients with cancer. *C. parvum* can occasionally cause a chronic enteropathy in cancer patients.

Solid-Tissue Cancers. Solid-tissue carcinomas do not predispose persons to infection as greatly as do hematologic cancers. The mechanisms of infection for patients with solid-tissue tumors tend to arise either from disruption of primary barriers to infection by destructive extension of the tumor or from a mechanical obstruction—tumor mass effect—producing stasis. The pathogens most likely to cause infections when the tumor mass causes disruption of structural integrity or function are those species that colonize contiguous surfaces. Hence, in the case of pneumonia, oral and upper respiratory tract flora are potential pathogens, whereas *Enterobacteriaceae* and *Pseudomonas* are important in infections arising from the gastrointestinal tract and in urinary tract infection. Septicemia due to *Clostridium septicum* occurs in patients with gastrointestinal carcinomas, a situation arising from obstruction, microbial overgrowth, and disruption of gastrointestinal luminal surfaces. Patients with Wilms' tumor or pelvic rhabdomyosarcoma are predisposed to recurrent urinary tract infection because of urinary stasis caused by disruption of the normal emptying of the urinary collecting system by obstructing tumor. Endobronchial tumors and tumors metastatic to lung parenchyma can occlude bronchioles, promoting atelectasis and pneumonia.

Anticancer Treatments That Predispose to Infection

Chemotherapy. Treatment of cancer can increase the risk of infection (Table 99–2). Cytolytic chemotherapy, which acts on rapidly dividing cells, can produce significant granulocytopenia, the nadir occurring approximately 7–10 days after exposure to the drug, with return to baseline values an additional 1–3 weeks later. Granulocytopenia, whether due to primary cancer or induced by chemotherapy, potentiates bacterial and fungal infections.

In addition to granulocytopenia, chemotherapy can produce a desquamative mucositis involving the gastrointestinal tract from the oropharynx to the anus. Desquamation of mucosal surfaces exposes vascularized underlying tissues vulnerable to both surface infection and direct invasion by pathogens. Denuded luminal surfaces in the gastrointestinal tract are the predominant source for gram-negative bacteremia in patients undergoing treatment for cancer. *Candida* can establish mucosal surface infections in patients with mucositis, most prominently presenting as oropharyngeal and esophageal candidiasis but also less frequently as perineal mucocutaneous candidiasis. Broad-spectrum antibacterial therapy, xerostomia, and prior *Candida* colonization are contributing risk factors. Herpes simplex virus can cause symptomatic recurrence of orolabial and gingival stomatitis, especially in patients with antecedent mucositis.

Catheter-Associated Infections. Indwelling intravascular catheters are commonly used for cancer treatment, especially in childhood hematogenous cancers. The indwelling device can also become the entrance point for bacteria and fungi. The majority of isolates obtained in catheter-associated infections are those that colonize the skin surface contiguous to the exit site of these catheters, especially coagulase-negative staphylococci but also *S. aureus* and *Enterococcus.* Enterobacteriaceae collectively cause appropriately 20% of catheter-associated infections, with the remainder caused by *P. aeruginosa, Candida,* and *Bacillus.*

Virtually all catheter-associated fungal infections are caused by *Candida,* with *Candida albicans* and *Candida tropicalis* the two most commonly isolated species. Approximately 80% of all cases of disseminated, tissue-invasive candidiasis are characterized by fever, neutropenia, the long-term presence of an indwelling catheter, and persistently positive blood cultures. Catheter-associated fungemia should be treated with amphotericin B or another appropriate antifungal agent and by prompt catheter removal.

Corticosteroid Treatment. Corticosteroids, which are part of the treatment regimens for some cancers, can predispose to infection because of their immunosuppressive effects. Corticosteroids are lympholytic, affecting both T-cell and B-cell lymphocytes. The cell-mediated immune response shows impaired skin test reactivity, potentially apparent within 2 weeks of therapy initiation. Corticosteroids also decrease serum IgG concentrations by increasing ca-

TABLE 99–2. Cancer Treatments That Predispose to Opportunistic Infection

Treatment	Mode of Action	Adverse Effect Predisposing to Infection	Pathogens
Cytolytic chemotherapy	Inhibits cellular division	Granulocytopenia	Encapsulated bacteria *Candida* *Fusarium* *Aspergillus*
		Mucositis	Viridans-streptococci *Clostridium septicum* *Candida* Herpes simplex virus Enterobacteriaceae
Indwelling vascular catheter	Intravascular foreign body communicating with external environment	Breaches primary barrier to infection	Coagulase-negative staphylococci *Staphylococcus aureus* *Enterococcus* *Bacillus* Enterobacteriaceae *Candida*
Corticosteroids	Lympholytic response	Marrow sequestration of T lymphocytes	Encapsulated bacteria *Listeria monocytogenes*
	Increased catabolism	Reduction in response to antigenic stimulation Prevention of lymphokine release	*Mycobacterium* *Candida* *Cryptococcus neoformans* *Aspergillus*
	Stabilization of cellular membranes	Diminished granulocyte migration and killing	Herpes simplex virus Varicella-zoster virus Cytomegalovirus
Immunomodulating agents	Inhibition of nucleic acid and protein synthesis	Toxic reaction against large lymphocytes Suppression of proliferation of B lymphocytes Mucositis	Encapsulated bacteria *Mycobacterium* *Pneumocystis carinii* *Listeria monocytogenes* *Cryptococcus neoformans*

tabolism and inhibiting synthesis and depress polymorphonuclear leukocyte killing by preventing release of lysosomal enzymes. The blood neutrophil concentration increases transiently upon immediate exposure to corticosteroid treatment by release from the **marginating pool** and increased discharge from the marrow, which may reduce later ability to respond to antigenic stimulation. Furthermore, corticosteroids reduce the functional response of neutrophils and macrophages to inflammation, partially by stabilization of cellular membranes, which prevents the release of vasoactive mediators.

Bacteria that require intracellular killing as the primary host defense against infection have greater pathogenic potential in patients receiving corticosteroid therapy. Infections due to intracellular pathogens such as *Listeria monocytogenes, Salmonella,* and *Mycobacterium tuberculosis* occur with increased frequency in patients on long-term corticosteroid treatment regimens. Corticosteroid therapy in patients with cancer also increases the risk of fungal infections, ranging from mucocutaneous candidiasis to fungemia and tissue-invasive fungal infections due to *Candida, C. neoformans, Aspergillus,* agents of zygomycosis, and similar fungi. Corticosteroid therapy can potentiate the severity of certain viral infections, especially those caused by varicella-zoster virus, herpes simplex virus, cytomegalovirus, and measles virus.

Immunomodulating Agents. Therapeutic immunosuppression in cancer patients can promote infection because it disrupts normal lymphocytic function. Purine antagonists, such as mercaptopurine and azathioprine, inhibit synthesis of inosinic acid and have a primary lymphocytotoxic effect against rapidly replicating cells. These agents are toxic against large lymphocytes and can reduce neutrophil and monocyte concentrations in peripheral blood through cytotoxic action on hematopoietic precursors. Cyclophosphamide is an alkylating agent with significant cytotoxic action against B-cell lymphocytes. Cyclophosphamide therapy can produce lymphopenia and reduce the ability of residual lymphocytes to proliferate in vitro. Methotrexate is an immunosuppressive agent that inhibits cellular folate metabolism, resulting in suppression of both cellular and humoral immunity. In addition to increasing the risk of infection by direct cytotoxic effect, methotrexate produces mucositis, disrupting the primary barrier to tissue invasion by oropharyngeal and gastrointestinal colonizing microorganisms, thereby increasing the risk of opportunistic infection.

Blood Transfusions. Allogeneic blood transfusions can be immunosuppressive, impairing host defense against bacterial infections. The actual mechanism of this action is unclear, although the homologous IgG contained in infused plasma will inhibit host macrophage function.

CLINICAL SYMPTOMS AND DIAGNOSIS

The presence of fever during a time of neutropenia, even in the absence of other signs or symptoms, demands prompt evaluation of the patient because of the potential for life-threatening infection (Fig. 99–1). Initially, the patient should have a complete physical examination, including careful scrutiny of the oropharynx, nares, external auditory canals, skin and axilla, groin and perineum, and rectal area. The exit site and subcutaneous tunnel of any indwelling vascular catheter should be closely examined and palpated for tenderness and expression of purulent material. Quantitative blood cultures for bacterial and fungal pathogens should be obtained by peripheral venipuncture and from all lumina of any indwelling vascular catheter. Obtaining surveillance cultures from the anterior nares, oropharynx, and anus are procedures of low predictive value to establish the cause of the current presumptive infection, but knowledge of antibacterial susceptibility patterns of colonizing bacteria can help direct selection of an appropriate empirical antimicrobial regimen. Chest radiographs are important to assess for presence of pulmonary infiltrates. Specialized imaging studies, such as computed tomography or magnetic resonance, can be useful in selected cases, as when sinusitis or intra-abdominal pathology is suspected. Radioisotopic studies such as ^{67}Ga or ^{111}In may be useful in selected cases but generally are unrewarding. Selected serologic studies, such as detection of urinary bacterial antigens or serum cryptococcal antigen, may help establish a diagnosis. Any presumptive infection source that may be identified during patient evaluation will help tailor anti-infective therapy (Fig. 99–2).

Pulmonary Infections. Pulmonary infections account for the greatest number of cancer-associated infections for those in whom a source can be identified. Pulmonary infiltrates in patients with leukemia are problematic, inasmuch as the majority of cases will have a noninfectious cause (e.g., hemorrhage, congestive heart failure, leukemic infiltrate), although infection will account for 30–40% of all cases, with 90% of these infections due to opportunistic pathogens.

In patients with lymphoma, *S. pneumoniae* is the most commonly isolated pathogen, although the expanded differential includes *L. monocytogenes, Nocardia, P. carinii, Mycobacterium, T. gondii,* varicella-zoster virus, and cytomegalovirus. As the development of pulmonary infiltrates in patients with cancer could herald the onset of infection due to any one of a number of pathogens, procedures to establish a definitive diagnosis should be performed. Unfortunately, because blood culture results are often negative and the serologic diagnosis of acute infection often lacks the desired sensitivity, the best single diagnostic method is lung biopsy, which identifies the cause in 40–70% of all cases. However, the procedure is associated with potential complications, especially in patients with significant respiratory distress or a bleeding diathesis.

Bronchoalveolar lavage has been advocated as a procedure that is less risky than open lung biopsy, with a comparable diagnostic yield of approximately 30–40% in identifying the cause of pulmonary infiltrates. The small size of airways in infants will preclude this procedure, restricting its use to larger children. A bleeding diathesis is also a contraindication.

Empirical anti-infective therapy with regimens active against gram-positive and gram-negative bacteria, including trimethoprim-sulfamethoxazole for treatment of *P. carinii* infection, should be initiated before any invasive procedure when a pulmonary infection occurs in a patient with cancer. A macrolide, such as erythromycin, clarithromycin, or azithromycin, should be added for treatment of legionellosis if this has been previously identified as an endemic nosocomial pathogen. Bronchoalveolar lavage or lung biopsy should be reserved for those patients who fail to improve with empirical treatment. Empirical anti-infective regimens are changed in only 10–20% of all cases after an invasive diagnostic procedure, as either the definitive cause is already being appropriately treated by one of the administered agents or the procedure identifies a condition for which no specific treatment exists.

Otolaryngologic Infections. Approximately 60% of patients undergoing prolonged myelosuppression for treatment of cancer experience an otolaryngologic complication during the period of neutropenia. Oral microbiologic flora are an important source of infections in patients with cancer. Serial determination of oral flora in patients undergoing treatment for cancer has documented the simultaneous appearance of potentially pathogenic bacteria in supragingival and subgingival plaques with the onset of granulocytopenia. Disruption

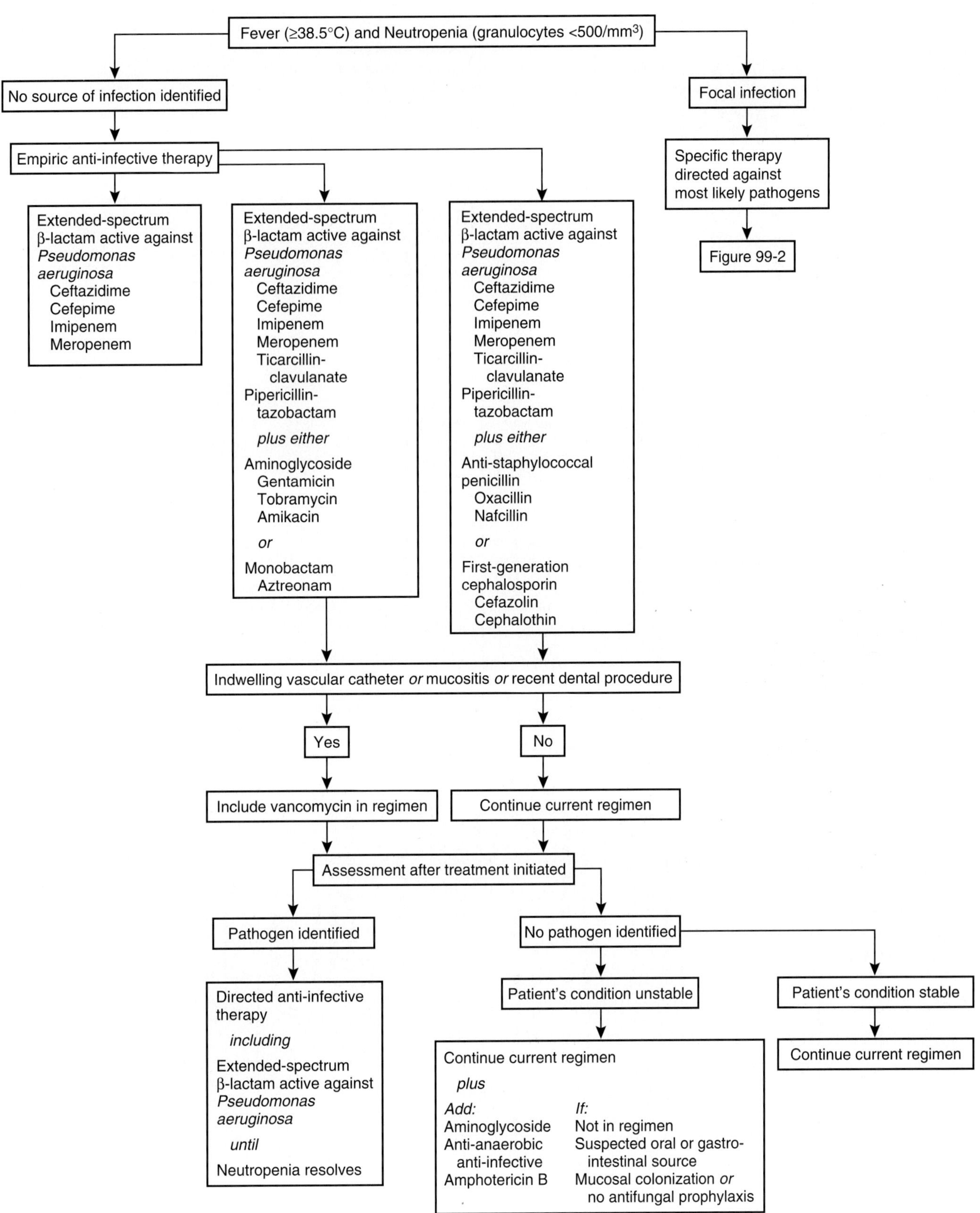

FIGURE 99–1. Initial management of fever and possible infection without an identified source in patients with cancer.

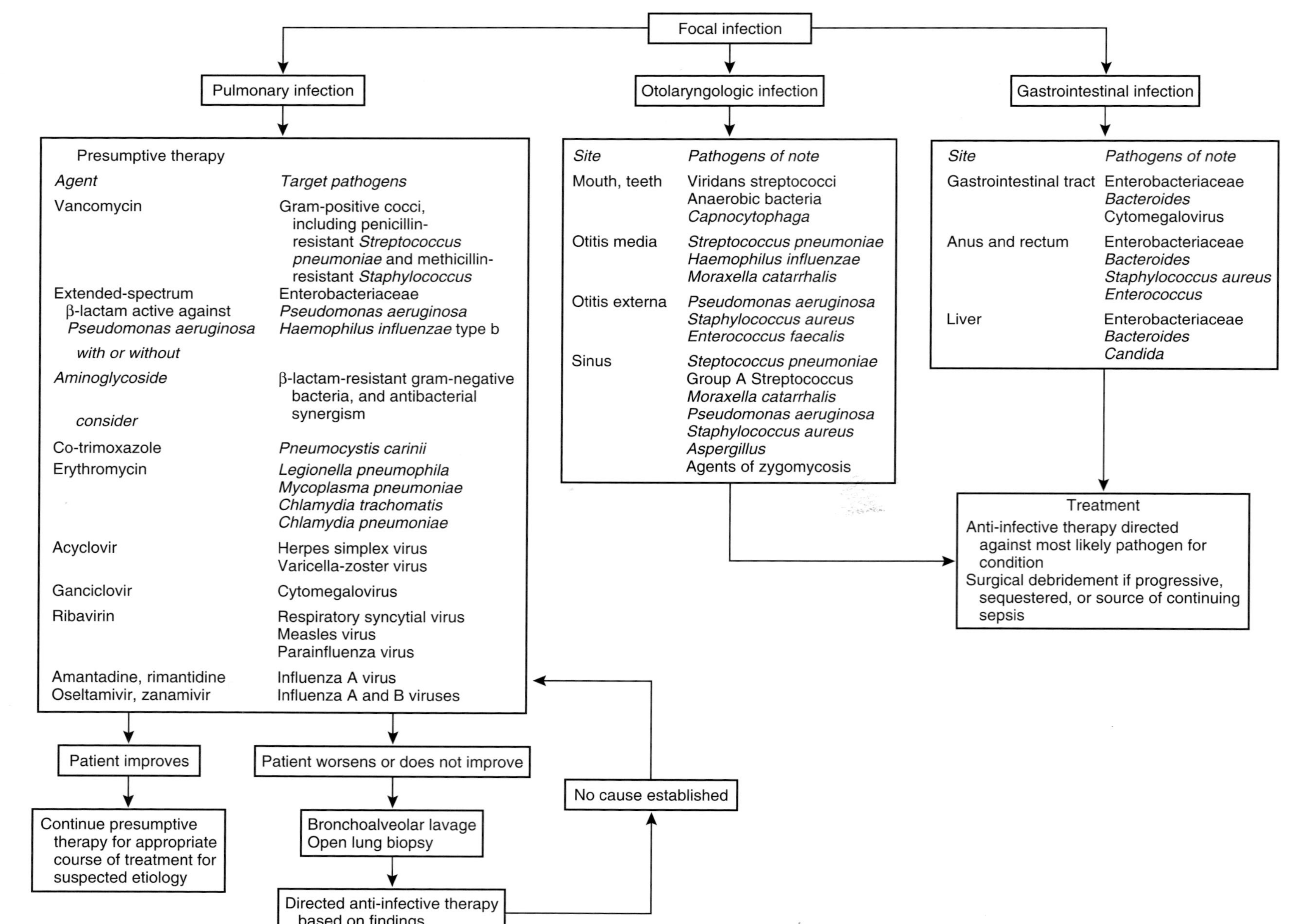

FIGURE 99–2. Management of possible infection with an identified source in patients with cancer.

of mucosal barriers by inflammatory mucositis induced by cytotoxic therapy or the presence of periodontal disease allows a portal of entry for systemic invasion by these organisms.

Sinusitis in patients with leukemia can be a particularly devastating disease. Fully 40% of patients with leukemia will have abnormal sinus radiographs, encompassing infectious and noninfectious causes. Differentiation of cause is based on clinical signs; infection will be associated with fever and facial pain plus the abnormal sinus radiographs. Although traditional bacterial causes, such as *S. pneumoniae, H. influenzae,* and *Moraxella catarrhalis* must be considered, infection by *P. aeruginosa,* group A *Streptococcus,* and *S. aureus* also occurs. Of special concern is fungal sinusitis, caused by *Aspergillus,* agents of zygomycosis, and selected dematiaceous fungi, especially in patients with acute myelocytic or lymphocytic leukemia having an absolute neutrophil count below $100/mm^3$. A high index of suspicion, prompt antifungal therapy with amphotericin B, and aggressive sinus irrigation and surgical débridement of devitalized tissue are imperative for successful treatment. Approximately 80% of patients so treated during a time of remission will survive, whereas fewer than 10% will survive if in leukemic relapse. Necrotizing otitis externa may occur in children during treatment of acute lymphocytic leukemia, caused most commonly by *P. aeruginosa, S. aureus,* and *Enterococcus faecalis.* Risk factors include pre-existing bacterial colonization and instrumentation of the ear canal during periods of neutropenia.

Gastrointestinal Infections. An acute abdomen may develop in patients with cancer during periods of neutropenia. Although the usual differential diagnoses of acute appendicitis and similar conditions remain, **neutropenic enterocolitis,** also known as **cecitis/typhlitis,** bears special mention. Neutropenic enterocolitis presents as fever and abdominal pain, often with tenderness in the right lower quadrant. This condition begins as a locally invasive infection due to disruption of gastrointestinal mucosal surfaces, with systemic host defense further reduced by neutropenia. Often pathogens can disseminate systemically from this site, with a resultant significant mortality. Typhlitis is one of the conditions most commonly present in patients who die during treatment of cancer and not diagnosed until postmortem examination. A high index of suspicion, imaging studies such as CT or MRI, broad-spectrum antibiotic therapy with agents active against Enterobacteriaceae and anaerobic bacteria, and judicious surgical intervention in selected cases are necessary to treat this condition successfully.

Anorectal infections manifesting as perirectal ulceration, cellulitis, or cutaneous abscess can be potentially serious in patients with cancer. The occurrence best correlates with a prolonged period of antecedent neutropenia, and the total length of neutropenia is directly proportional to the probability of an unsuccessful treatment outcome and patient death. The most effective antibacterial regimens include a broad-spectrum β-lactam antibiotic, an aminoglycoside, and an agent active against anaerobic bacteria; the expected cure rate is approximately 90%. Surgical intervention, in addition to antibiotics, should be considered if anorectal lesions have a palpable fluctuance, necrotic tissue is present, the infection is locally progressive despite antimicrobial treatment, or the patient experiences continuing bacteremia from the infection site.

The prolonged periods of neutropenia predispose to a special form of disseminated candidiasis called **hepatosplenocandidiasis.** The typical patient will have received a protracted course of empirical antibacterial therapy but will still be febrile. Sometimes these patients will have right upper quadrant tenderness, elevation of the serum hepatic enzyme levels, and possibly hepatic or splenic enlargement. A CT of the abdomen, when positive, most often reveals either a circular hypodense lesion surrounded by a rim of increased density in the liver or a diffuse nodular infiltrate. Aspiration of large lesions may yield fungal elements. Treatment requires prolonged administration of antifungal therapy; on occasion, concomitant splenectomy is also necessary, especially if splenic lesions are also apparent on CT or at laparotomy.

Cytomegalovirus infection can present as cholecystitis, hepatitis, pancreatitis, and gastrointestinal mucosal ulceration in patients with cancer, more commonly after prolonged immunosuppression than during periods of neutropenia.

TREATMENT

Antibacterial Treatment. Fever without an identified source and identified focal infections in neutropenic patients should be promptly evaluated and treated with a broad-spectrum antibacterial regimen. The primary regimen should at least include an extended-spectrum penicillin or cephalosporin with activity against Enterobacteriaceae and *P. aeruginosa.* Acceptable regimens include any antipseudomonal penicillin such as piperacillin-tazobactam, extended-spectrum cephalosporins with activity against *P. aeruginosa* such as ceftazidime or cefepime, plus an aminoglycoside for synergistic activity against Enterobacteriaceae and *P. aeruginosa.* Currently ceftazidime is the agent most commonly used when monotherapy is chosen. The carbapenems, imipenem and meropenem, or the quinolone ciprofloxacin can also be used as monotherapy.

Empirical antibacterial treatment for patients without indwelling central catheters is directed primarily against gram-negative bacterial pathogens. Mortality is low among neutropenic patients infected with gram-positive organisms, even if empirical therapy does not include an antibiotic highly active against the pathogen. The combination of an antipseudomonal β-lactam with an aminoglycoside is an attractive empirical regimen despite the potential for renal toxicity and ototoxicity and the need to monitor the aminoglycoside serum concentration, because of the complementary extension of the antimicrobial spectrum and the potential for synergy against Enterobacteriaceae and *P. aeruginosa.* The monobactam aztreonam could be substituted for the aminoglycoside in this regimen, resulting in reduced probability of renal toxicity and ototoxicity and no requirement for serum concentration determinations, but the potential for antibacterial synergy is reduced.

An agent active against gram-positive organisms, such as an antistaphylococcal penicillin, first-generation cephalosporin, or vancomycin can be included as part of the empirical antibacterial regimen in fever and neutropenia, especially for patients with indwelling vascular catheters. Vancomycin is the preferred agent because of the increasing prevalence of methicillin-resistant staphylococci and ampicillin-resistant enterococci. However, no significant morbidity or mortality has occurred in neutropenic patients infected with gram-positive organisms when treatment with vancomycin was deferred until after the organism was first identified in blood cultures. This approach of withholding vancomycin until a gram-positive pathogen is identified is further justified by the cost of the agent and potential adverse drug effects. Despite this rationale, initiation of an empirical antibacterial regimen that includes vancomycin may provide symptomatic improvement in patients by the time culture results are known. If a gram-positive isolate is not identified after 48–72 hours of treatment, the vancomycin should be discontinued because of cost, potential toxicity, and selection for vancomycin-resistant organisms. If continuing empirical gram-positive antibacterial therapy is deemed necessary, then an antistaphylococcal penicillin or first-generation cephalosporin could be substituted for vancomycin at that time.

Once initiated, the duration of empirical antibacterial treatment of fever and neutropenia is determined by the time until resolution of the neutropenia. Treatment directed against gram-negative bacteria should never be discontinued while neutropenia persists, even with negative cultures, because of the continued potential for rapidly progressive gram-negative bacillary infection. Should bacterial infection be confirmed during the treatment course, then the duration of therapy should be at least the period traditionally appropriate to treat that specific infection. As the patient will remain vulnerable to second infective events while neutropenic, therapy should be continued beyond the traditional treatment period for that infection for as long as the patient remains neutropenic. The risk of a second, rapidly progressive gram-negative bacillary infection exists in those neutropenic patients with a documented gram-positive bacterial infection; therefore broad-spectrum antibiotic therapy should continue until the neutropenia resolves.

Often no pathogen is identified. In those cases in which fever resolves by the seventh day of antibacterial therapy, treatment should continue until the neutropenia resolves or until the patient has had at least 14 days of antibacterial treatment. Approximately 40% of patients with persistent neutropenia in whom antibacterial therapy is discontinued after 7 days of treatment because of defervescence will subsequently have relapse of fever, often associated with clinical deterioration. By comparison, approximately 30% of patients who receive at least 14 days of antibacterial therapy because of persisting neutropenia will have relapse of fever, regardless of whether antibiotics are continued beyond 2 weeks. Thus a continued therapeutic benefit to the persistently neutropenic but afebrile patient is provided by 2 weeks of empirical therapy, beyond which no further advantage occurs. The risk of subsequent fever and infection once defervescence is achieved by empirical antibacterial treatment appears to be quite small for patients with an absolute neutrophil count of $\geq$100/mm^3, especially if the count is rising rapidly, which indicates postchemotherapy bone marrow recovery and allows treatment cessation at that time. Final decisions pertaining to duration of treatment should be individualized by the patient's clinical appearance, anticipation of when resolution of neutropenia should occur, and the ability to promptly reassess a relapse of fever after cessation of antimicrobial therapy (Fig. 99–3).

Despite the unqualified requirement to treat febrile neutropenic patients promptly with a comprehensive antibacterial regimen, problems may occur. There is a direct correlation between the total number of antimicrobial agents used to treat a patient with febrile neutropenia and the probability that renal and hepatic toxicity will occur during therapy. For this reason, persistence of fever during empirical antibiotic treatment is an insufficient reason alone to warrant changing antibacterial agents.

Antifungal Treatment. The possibility of a disseminated fungal infection must be considered in a patient with neutropenia and fever that persists despite empirical broad-spectrum antibacterial therapy. Before the practice of empirical antifungal treatment, autopsy findings for patients with hematogenous cancer who died despite broad-spectrum antibacterial therapy during febrile neutropenia revealed that 60% of all patients with fever persisting $\geq$8 days had tissue-invasive fungal disease, largely caused by *Candida*. Virtually none of these patients had documented fungemia before death.

The childhood cancer infection rate is approximately four infections per 1,000 patient days, with fungal pathogens accounting for approximately 10% of all infections. *Candida* causes 60% of all fungal infections, with *Aspergillus fumigatus, Aspergillus flavus,* agents of zygomycosis (*Rhizopus, Mucor, Rhizomucor, Absidia,* and *Cunninghamella*), *Fusarium, Trichosporon,* and dematiaceous fungi (*Bipolaris, Cladosporium,* and *Dactylaria*) constituting the remaining 40%.

Amphotericin B therapy should be instituted empirically in patients who have neutropenia and persistent fever despite broad-spectrum antibacterial therapy. Fever that continues through the seventh day of antibacterial therapy is generally regarded as the critical indication for institution of amphotericin B therapy. Empirical amphotericin B therapy should be instituted as early as the fourth day of fever in selected patients, especially in those patients shown to have mucosal fungal colonization or infiltrates on chest radiograph. Recommended dosages are amphotericin B deoxycholate 0.6–1 mg/kg/day (max 50 mg/day) once daily intravenously, and lipid amphotericin B 3–5 mg/kg/day once daily intravenously. The recommended duration of empirical antifungal therapy is variable; a minimum treatment duration of 2 weeks should be considered, with reassessment after that time to determine whether therapy should be extended. Treatment should continue at least until the patient is afebrile and has an absolute granulocyte count that exceeds 500/mm^3 for 2 successive days.

Amphotericin B therapy does have shortcomings in empirical treatment of suspected fungal infection. The agent is fairly toxic, with immediate self-limited adverse reactions associated with infusion (e.g., fever, chills, hypotension, rigors) and dose-dependent organic toxicity, most significantly renal injury manifesting as hypokalemia, diminished creatinine clearance, and tubular electrolyte wasting. Immediate infusion-related reactions can be reduced by pretreating the patient with acetaminophen, diphenhydramine, and meperidine, and corticosteroids can be mixed with the infusate during amphotericin B administration. Hypokalemia may be corrected with daily potassium supplementation, and renal tubular toxicity may be mitigated by **salt-loading:** increasing daily sodium supplementation to 5–8 mEq/kg/day. Renal toxicity often limits the dose of amphotericin B that can be given during empirical therapy. The lipid-complex, lipid colloidal dispersion, and liposomal formulations are associated with fewer infusion-related adverse effects as well as reduced cumulative renal toxicity but must be administered in higher daily doses and are substantially more expensive.

Amphotericin B is active against most fungi, especially *Candida,* the most probable opportunistic fungal pathogen in neutropenic patients. However, *Aspergillus* can be relatively resistant to amphotericin B, with disseminated aspergillosis occurring in patients receiving empirical amphotericin B therapy. *Fusarium* can also be resistant to amphotericin B at standard therapeutic doses. When *Aspergillus* or disseminated *Fusarium* is recognized, the relative resistance may be partially compensated by increasing the daily amphotericin B dose to 1.5–2 mg/kg/day, although renal toxicity at this higher dose often requires further modification of therapy. Because of the potential toxicity associated with these high daily doses of amphotericin B, the lipid formulations may be initiated at onset of treatment and administered in daily doses of 5–7.5 mg/kg/day. *P. boydii* is particularly resistant to amphotericin B; parenteral miconazole or itraconazole is often substituted to treat this infection. Fluconazole has proven efficacy for treatment of mucocutaneous and disseminated candidiasis and cryptococcosis. Itraconazole has demonstrated clinical efficacy for treatment of candidiasis, cryptococcosis, and disseminated infections due to *Aspergillus,* dimorphic fungi, and dematiaceous fungi. These agents may selectively be substituted for amphotericin B in the empirical treatment of febrile neutropenia on the basis of the reduced drug toxicity and feasibility of oral administration, although clinical trials supporting this have demonstrated selection for resistant fungal isolates, occasionally resulting in breakthrough infection.

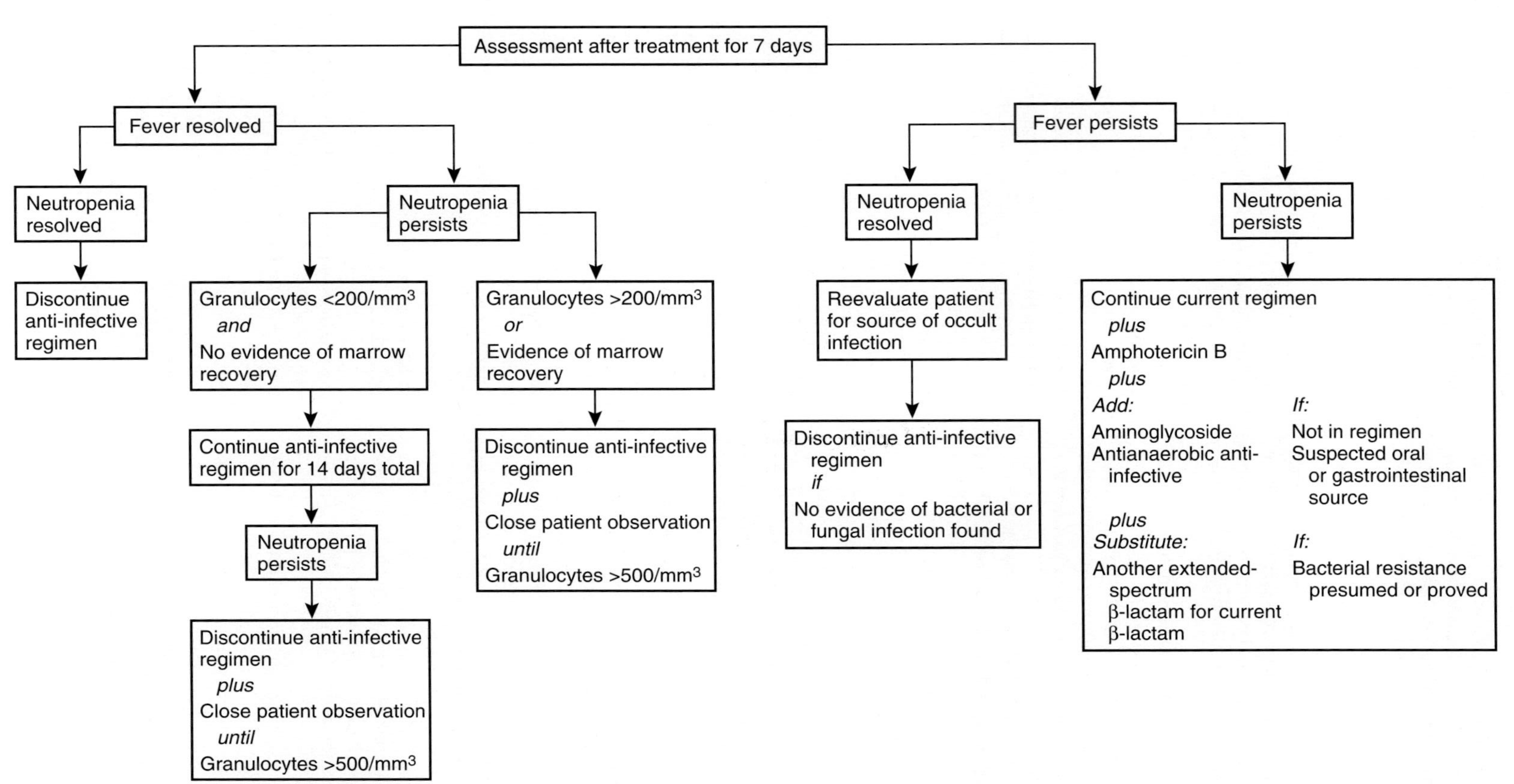

FIGURE 99–3. Continuing management of possible infection after 7 days of fever without an identified source in patients with cancer.

Newer agents, such as voriconazole, appear promising, especially because of their activity against *Aspergillus*.

Antiviral Treatment. Viral infections in patients with cancer are best treated by prevention. Acyclovir can be given prophylactically to prevent mucocutaneous herpes simplex virus infection and therapeutically to treat symptomatic infection. Varicella-zoster virus infections can be prevented by vaccination and by postexposure prophylaxis with VZIG, which should be provided for all susceptible immunocompromised persons following exposure to chickenpox. Acyclovir is also used to treat varicella-zoster virus infections. Cytomegalovirus infection can be prevented by administering only serologically negative blood products, although ganciclovir and foscarnet and CMV-IG and high-dose IVIG have been used alone or in combination for prophylaxis of seronegative persons.

Empirical Treatment for Pulmonary Infections. Simultaneous empirical treatment of many potential pulmonary pathogens is occasionally given to selected patients with febrile neutropenia, especially those presenting in respiratory distress with an interstitial infiltrate on chest radiographs. In addition to the broad-spectrum antibacterial regimen, the empirical institution of trimethoprim-sulfamethoxazole (20 mg/kg/day TMP–100 mg/kg/day SMZ [max 980 mg TMP/4,900 mg SMZ]) should be added, especially in institutions where bronchoalveolar lavage is not available or when poor patient condition precludes this procedure. Moreover, if *Legionella* is suspected, empirical treatment with a macrolide should be added. More problematic is determining the appropriate duration of empirical trimethoprim-sulfamethoxazole and macrolide therapy. Pragmatically, if the patient improves during empirical treatment and if no specific microbiologic diagnosis is established, the total duration of therapy is 2–3 weeks for treatment of *Pneumocystis carinii* pneumonia, followed by prophylaxis until the immunocompromising condition has resolved, and 2–4 weeks for legionellosis.

Persistent Fever. Neutropenic patients with fever should receive anti-infective treatment; yet not all fevers are due to infection. Approximately 60% of all fevers in patients with cancer are attributed to infection, and the remaining 40% can be ultimately attributed to a noninfectious cause. Causes of fever in neutropenic patients, in addition to infection, include blood transfusions, central nervous system metastasis, effects of radiation, adrenal crisis, and adverse drug effects, especially of the chemotherapeutic drugs bleomycin, daunorubicin, cisplatin, L-asparaginase, or interferon. Fever may even be caused directly by the cancer (the so-called neoplastic fever). Despite the fact that fever may be due to a noninfectious cause, empirical antibiotic therapy should be continued until either the fever resolves or improvement in absolute neutrophil count allows discontinuation of empirical therapy.

PREVENTION

Cancer patients are at risk of both **exogenous infection,** from contact with infected persons directly or through infected fomites, and **endogenous infection,** which usually originates from oropharyngeal and gastrointestinal mucosal surfaces. Moreover, the normal oropharyngeal and gastrointestinal microbiologic flora of patients hospitalized for any length of time may have been replaced by nosocomial organisms that are resistant to multiple antibiotics. Therefore, methods that reduce these risks may reduce the incidence and severity of infection.

Mucosal Surface Antisepsis. Attempts to reduce mucosal colonization through administration of nonabsorbable antibiotics such as colistin, neomycin, and nystatin were effective when first employed but more recently have been shown to be increasingly ineffective. However, systemically absorbable antimicrobials have a demonstrated efficacy in preventing infection, with amoxicillin-clavulanate, trimethoprim-sulfamethoxazole, and the quinolones the most extensively used. Prophylactic administration of these antimicrobials reduces the incidence of gram-negative bacillary infections, although no improvement in patient mortality rates has been demonstrated.

Patient Isolation. Isolation of the patient during hospitalization has been attempted to reduce contact with potential pathogens. Isolation techniques include simple hand washing by health care personnel before and after patient contact, gown-mask-and-glove isolation before visits to patients hospitalized in private rooms, and patient sequestration in rooms with high-efficiency particulate air (HEPA) filtration maintaining air pressure in the room greater than that externally. The latter is the setting for **total protective isolation,** which also includes daily decontamination of room surfaces, patient diets with low microbial content, administration of nonabsorbable antimicrobials, daily skin cleaning, and mouth and perineal care with topical antimicrobial cleansers. Atmospheric filtration, room surface decontamination, and low-microbial diets do reduce the risk of *Aspergillus* infections, although the procedures are not considered cost-effective in terms of infections prevented. Granting the fact that these labor-intensive, costly procedures have reduced the number of infective episodes and febrile periods in neutropenic patients as compared with simple hand washing and private room isolation, overall patient survival still has not improved despite the use of these techniques. A more pragmatic approach is private room isolation, good hand washing, exclusion of any potentially infected health care worker from patient care, and daily cleansing of the patient's mouth, skin, and perineum.

Antibacterial Prophylaxis. The prolonged neutropenia associated with chemotherapy, with incumbent increased risk of bacterial infection, has been the rationale for employment of antimicrobial prophylaxis. Various regimens, including trimethoprim-sulfamethoxazole, quinolones, amoxicillin-clavulanate, and nonabsorbed broad-spectrum topical antimicrobials (e.g., erythromycin base and neomycin) have been used in an attempt to prevent or reduce the frequency of bacteremia during chemotherapy-induced neutropenia. Despite the fact that relatively short-term treatment for 1–3 months has on occasion been effective in selected patient groups, the overall risks of emergence of antibiotic-resistant bacterial strains, oral mucosal and gastrointestinal fungal overgrowth, adverse drug effects, and additional treatment costs outweigh the potential benefits.

Postexposure Prophylaxis Against VZV. Postexposure prophylaxis with VZIG following exposure to chickenpox is warranted for immunocompromised patients undergoing anticancer chemotherapy (Table 27–6). The timing of exposure should be within 2 days before the onset of rash until up to 5 days after the onset of rash in the index case. Modified infection after VZIG may not result in protective immunity; therefore, persons who receive VZIG prophylaxis should be considered at risk with any subsequent exposures.

VZIG contains 10–18% globulin and is available in vials of 125 U in a volume of approximately 1.25 mL. Prophylaxis is administered as a single intramuscular injection in a dose of 125 U (the minimum dose) for each 10 kg increment of body weight, to a maximum dose of 625 U (5 vials). VZIG should be administered within 96 hours after exposure, preferably beginning as soon as possible.

The use of IVIG may either prevent or ameliorate symptomatic illness. Patients routinely receiving IVIG (100–400 mg/kg) are considered protected and do not require specific postexposure prophylaxis if the last infusion was administered within 3 weeks of exposure to VZV.

Prophylaxis Against Infection with Pneumocystis carinii. Administration of trimethoprim-sulfamethoxazole to prevent *P. carinii* infection has become a mainstay in patients with leukemia or lymphoma and for selected patients undergoing intensive chemotherapy for solid tumors. Prophylaxis is generally begun around the time of initiation of anticancer therapy and continued until 6 months after chemotherapy has been completed. Several different dosing regimens are used, but the recommended regimen is twice daily by mouth (150 mg/m^2/day TMP–750 mg/m^2/day SMZ [max 320 mg TMP and 1,600 mg SMZ]) on 3 consecutive days each week (Table 67–13). Other prophylactic regimens have also been used, especially aerosolized pentamidine, although the risk of extrapulmonary disease increases because of the lack of significant systemic concentration of the drug when administered by inhalation.

Granulocyte Transfusion and Cytokines. Because neutropenia is a significant risk factor for bacterial and fungal infections, granulocyte transfusions have been attempted for neutropenic patients with documented infection. Despite initial success, the practice is now generally regarded as having limited efficacy. A newer modality is administration of hematopoietic cytokines, granulocyte-colony stimulating factor (G-CSF) and granulocyte-monocyte colony stimulating factor (GM-CSF), to reduce the period of neutropenia and thus lessen the risk of infection. Selected chemotherapeutic protocols for the treatment of solid tumors that result in prolonged neutropenia now incorporate hematopoietic cytokine therapy as part of the treatment protocol.

REVIEWS

Anaissie E: Opportunistic mycoses in the immunocompromised host: Experience at a cancer center and review. *Clin Infect Dis* 1992;14(S1):S43–53.

Hildebrand FL, Rosenow EC 3rd, Habermann TM, et al: Pulmonary complications of leukemia. *Chest* 1990;98:1233–9.

Hughes WT, Armstrong D, Bodey GP, et al: 1997 Guidelines for the use of antimicrobial agents in neutropenic patients with unexplained fever. Infectious Diseases Society of America. *Clin Infect Dis* 1997;25:551–73.

Pizzo PA: Fever in immunocompromised patients. *N Engl J Med* 1999; 341:893–900.

Pizzo PA, Rubin M, Freifeld A, et al: The child with cancer and infection. I. Empiric therapy for fever and neutropenia, and preventive strategies. *J Pediatr* 1991;119:679–94.

Pizzo PA, Rubin M, Freifeld A, et al: The child with cancer and infection. II. Nonbacterial infections. *J Pediatr* 1991;119:845–57.

KEY ARTICLES

Bergmann OJ: Oral infections and septicemia in immunocompromised patients with hematologic malignancies. *J Clin Microbiol* 1988; 26:2105–9.

Glenn J, Cotton D, Wesley R, et al: Anorectal infections in patients with malignant disease. *Rev Infect Dis* 1988;10:42–52.

Hathorn JW, Rubin M, Pizzo P: Empirical antibiotic therapy in the febrile neutropenic cancer patient: Clinical efficacy and impact of monotherapy. *Antimicrob Agents Chemother* 1987;31:971–7.

Klastersky J: Empiric antimicrobial therapy for febrile granulocytopenic cancer patients: Lessons from four EORTC trials. *Acta Oncol* 1988; 5:497–502.

Lecciones JA, Lee JW, Navarro EE, et al: Vascular catheter-associated fungemia in patients with cancer: Analysis of 155 episodes. *Clin Infect Dis* 1992;14:875–83.

O'Brien S, Kantarjian HM, Anaissie E, et al: Successful medical management of neutropenic enterocolitis in adults with acute leukemia. *South Med J* 1987;80:1233–5.

Pizzo PA: Considerations for the prevention of infectious complications in patients with cancer. *Rev Infect Dis* 1989;11(Suppl 7):S1551–63.

Sugar AM: Empiric treatment of fungal infections in the neutropenic host. *Arch Intern Med* 1990;150:2258–64.

CHAPTER 100

Transplant Recipients

Dennis A. Conrad

The increasing number of stem cell (bone marrow) and organ transplantations performed annually has created an ever-enlarging pediatric population at increased risk of opportunistic infections. Before the introduction of the selective immunosuppressant cyclosporine, patients undergoing transplantation often faced a potentially lethal outcome from engraftment rejection and transplanted organ failure, graft-versus-host disease, or severe opportunistic infection. Cyclosporine and the newer agent tacrolimus, which suppress cytotoxic T-lymphocyte proliferation and function without significantly disrupting helper and suppressor T-lymphocyte number and activity, have increased the probability of successful transplant outcome and prolonged patient survival. Although lessened, the risk of opportunistic infectious complications in the posttransplantation period still exists.

In view of the potential risk of transmitted infection, donors are screened as extensively as is practical for the presence of infection. Many donors are rejected outright if they are febrile, acutely infected, or show serologic evidence of infection with hepatitis B, hepatitis C, or HIV. Those donors who are accepted are then matched, whenever possible, to recipients on the basis of serologic status for cytomegalovirus, Epstein-Barr virus, and *Toxoplasma gondii* infection. Although donor infection with any of these latter pathogens is not an absolute contraindication to transplantation, the potential for transmission of infection from donor to recipient by transplanted tissue remains a significant risk.

The immunosuppression necessary to prevent allograft rejection affects T-lymphocyte function, increasing the probability of infection by pathogens preferentially defended against by lymphocytes, including cytomegalovirus, herpes simplex virus, *Listeria monocytogenes*, *Legionella pneumophila*, *Mycobacterium tuberculosis*, atypical mycobacteria, *Nocardia asteroides*, *Pneumocystis carinii*, and *T. gondii.* The risk of infection with one of these pathogens is substantially increased with the use of pulsed high-dose corticosteroid therapy, antithymocyte immunoglobulin, or one of the monoclonal antibodies directed against CD3 T lymphocytes. In addition, azathioprine and corticosteroids adversely affect B lymphocytes, and corticosteroids also disrupt polymorphonuclear leukocyte and macrophage function.

The risk of fatal infections in transplant recipients directly attributed to immunosuppressive therapy is 0–3% for renal transplantation, 15% for heart transplantation, 25% for hepatic transplantation, and 45% for heart-lung transplantation. Because of this risk, aggressive evaluation of any potential infection in the posttransplantation period is necessary to maximize patient survival.

STEM CELL TRANSPLANTATION

Most stem cell (bone marrow) transplants performed are for treatment of cancer, serving either as allogeneic or syngeneic reconstitution of bone marrow ablated in an attempt to eradicate hematogenous cancer in the recipient or as autologous or allogeneic bone marrow rescue after aggressive treatment of solid tumors. Stem cell transplantation has also been employed to treat nonmalignant conditions, supplying a stem cell source for correction of aplastic anemia syndromes or for clonal expansion of normal cell lines to compensate for selected inborn errors of metabolism.

Mechanisms of Increased Susceptibility to Infection

Immediately after transplantation during the time before marrow engraftment, neutropenia and mucositis are the greatest risk factors for patient infection. Endogenous bacteria and fungi colonizing the intestinal tract are the important opportunistic pathogens. Indwelling intravascular devices predispose to catheter-associated bacteremia and fungemia with skin flora. The most significant viral infections occurring in the pre-engraftment transplant period are oral and esophageal infection due to herpes simplex virus reactivation, especially in patients with mucositis, and zoster, especially in patients who received irradiation during the conditioning regimen.

Allogeneic bone marrow transplant recipients may have IgG2 and IgG4 deficiency that persists for months after the transplantation as a result of disordered T-lymphocyte subset reconstitution. The IgG subclass deficiency increases the risk of septicemia and tissue-invasive infections due to encapsulated bacteria, especially *Streptococcus pneumoniae,* which may develop as late as 1 year after the transplant. Because of the IgG subclass deficiency and also a functional asplenia that may further complicate allogeneic bone marrow transplantation, which is most likely to occur in the presence of chronic graft-versus-host disease with splenic involvement, allogeneic bone marrow transplant recipients remain highly susceptible to bacterial infections beyond the initial period of neutropenia. Approximately 30% of infections that occur ≥6 months after bone marrow transplantation are bacterial, with gram-positive bacteria, especially *S. pneumoniae,* predominating. In addition to IgG subclass deficiency and functional asplenia, these patients are also more prone to have impaired granulocyte function in vitro, decreased serum opsonic activity, and, especially in the face of chronic graft-versus-host disease, an impaired T-lymphocyte-dependent B-lymphocyte immune response, which further increases the probability of serious infection due to encapsulated bacteria.

Although autologous bone marrow transplant recipients have subtle abnormalities in T-lymphocyte and B-lymphocyte function that may persist for 6–12 months after transplantation, the risk of infection in autologous bone marrow transplantation is substantially decreased once correction of the granulocytopenia and recovery from the adverse affects of the conditioning regimen have occurred. However, allogeneic bone marrow transplantation is associated with an increased risk of opportunistic infection beyond the initial period of neutropenia before engraftment, as prolonged immunosuppression is usually required to prevent graft-versus-host disease once the donor bone marrow reconstitutes.

Site-Specific Infections

Lower Respiratory Tract. Nosocomial pneumonia in the bone marrow transplant recipient is the most significant life-threatening clinical condition and shares many features of the illness that occurs in the patient with leukemia (Chapter 99). The bone marrow transplant recipients most likely to develop nosocomial pneumonia are those with a history of prior nosocomial infection, allogeneic bone marrow transplantation, or treatment with methotrexate. In almost every case, an initial disruption in mucosal and cutaneous integrity leads to an infectious process that precedes the pneumonia. Occasionally, acute and chronic graft-versus-host disease can cause small-airway disease ranging in severity from early bronchiolar wall damage to bronchiolitis obliterans. This pulmonary injury predisposes the patient to subsequent respiratory tract infection caused by *P. carinii*, *Candida*, and CMV.

Because of the extensive differential diagnosis of a pulmonary infiltrate occurring in bone marrow transplant recipients, an attempt to establish a tissue diagnosis should be made whenever possible. In the case in which open lung biopsy is performed, tissue should be sent for Gram stain (for bacteria), potassium hydroxide preparation (for fungi), modified acid-fast stain (for *Nocardia*), auramine-rhodamine stain (for *Mycobacterium*), direct fluorescent antibody stain (*L. pneumophila*), silver or calcofluor white stain (*P. carinii*), or Giemsa stain (*T. gondii*) and cultured appropriately for bacteria, fungi, mycobacteria, *Nocardia*, *L. pneumophila,* and CMV and respiratory viruses.

Aspergillus is the most frequent cause of fatal pneumonia in hospitalized bone marrow transplant recipients, accounting for approximately 40% of all fatal cases. The rates of *Aspergillus* infection vary by institution, and outbreaks tend to be episodic. Construction, especially digging in soil or disturbing ventilation systems, is a notorious cause of nosocomial epidemics. In addition, live plants and certain foods, especially black pepper, have been implicated in nosocomial infections. Overall, bone marrow transplant recipients have a tenfold greater risk of developing nosocomial aspergillosis than do other immunocompromised patients, especially when hospitalized outside of a high-efficiency particulate air (HEPA) filtration environment. The diagnosis of pulmonary aspergillosis in bone marrow transplant recipients by noninvasive means is problematic, and the chest radiographs will often appear normal because of the subtle nature of early infection. Imaging by CT or MRI of the chest increases the sensitivity of detection, especially in identifying the small pulmonary nodules that often characterize early disease. It is not necessary to confirm the diagnosis of pulmonary aspergillosis before initiating antifungal therapy in bone marrow transplant recipients. Persistent fever despite antibacterial therapy, especially in the patient who is neutropenic, is adequate justification to begin empiric antifungal treatment. Infection with *Aspergillus* is difficult to treat and unlikely to be cured. The best outcomes are achieved with amphotericin B (deoxycholate: 1–2 mg/kg/day, to a cumulative dose of 30–45 mg/kg; liposomal: 5–7.5 mg/kg/day to a cumulative dose of 150–225 mg/kg) plus surgical débridement of devitalized tissue. The antifungal agent voriconazole has demonstrated activity against *Aspergillus* in vitro and in vivo, but therapeutic superiority to amphotericin B remains to be proven in clinical practice.

The most important event leading to a successful outcome in the treatment of lower respiratory tract aspergillosis remains correction of neutropenia after bone marrow recovery.

Upper Respiratory Tract. The oropharynx can be a portal for local tissue invasion and bacteremia by mouth flora, most frequently α-streptococci. Oral microorganisms have been reported to cause septicemia in as many as 40% of patients during the period of neutropenia that follows bone marrow transplantation. *Capnocytophaga* is the organism most likely to cause bacteremia during neutropenia complicated by mucositis, especially if gingival bleeding is also present. *Capnocytophaga* is resistant to vancomycin and has varying susceptibilities to the cephalosporins, although most isolates are susceptible to penicillin, with clindamycin the antibacterial agent of choice. This organism should be considered in bone marrow transplant recipients with febrile neutropenia, especially if fever persists despite empiric therapy with vancomycin and a third-generation cephalosporin. *Streptococcus mitis* is also becoming an increasingly important cause of bacteremia in bone marrow transplant recipients. The presence of mucositis is a risk factor, even more so if the patient has concurrent herpes stomatitis. Most *S. mitis* isolates are susceptible to vancomycin.

The use of methotrexate as prophylaxis for graft-versus-host disease, with subsequent development of mucositis and oral ulceration as adverse drug effects, is the single most important risk factor promoting invasive disease by oral flora. In addition, reactivation of latent herpes simplex virus infection resulting in stomatitis, which occurs more commonly in patients receiving total-body irradiation as a conditioning regimen, further increases the risk of septicemia due to oral microorganisms. Those patients receiving acyclovir prophylaxis during the first 30 days after bone marrow transplantation, which is given to lessen the probability of herpes simplex virus reactivation and subsequent gingivolabial stomatitis, will also have a lower incidence of α-streptococcal septicemia than those patients who do not receive acyclovir prophylaxis.

Gastrointestinal Tract. The common causes of enteritis in bone marrow transplant recipients are either a gastrointestinal manifestation of graft-versus-host disease or infection, usually viral (e.g., CMV, rotaviruses, adenoviruses, enteroviruses, coronaviruses) or bacterial (e.g., *Clostridium difficile*, *Campylobacter*, *Salmonella*). Parasitic infection, specifically *Cryptosporidium parvum,* has caused nosocomial outbreaks of diarrhea in bone marrow transplant units, with rapid spread and high infectivity rates. Many patients will continue to have symptoms despite therapy until improvement in their immunodeficiency and healing of their mucositis occurs.

Common Pathogens

Bacteria. During the period of neutropenia that immediately follows bone marrow transplantation, the most significant bacterial pathogens are Enterobacteriaceae, *Pseudomonas aeruginosa*, *Streptococcus*, *Staphylococcus*, and *Enterococcus.* The management of bone marrow transplant recipients with neutropenia in whom fever develops is similar to that of cancer patients with febrile neutropenia (Chapter 99).

After marrow engraftment, the risk of invasive gram-negative enteric bacterial infection declines, and the predominant pathogens become those associated with indwelling intravascular devices, including coagulase-negative staphylococci, *Enterococcus*, and *Bacillus.* During the period beyond 100 days after transplantation, *S. pneumoniae*, *Staphylococcus aureus*, and the re-emergent *P. aeruginosa* are the pathogens of greatest significance.

Fungi. More than 40% of all bone marrow transplant recipients will have a significant fungal infection if they are granulocytopenic for more than 20 consecutive days, with 70% of all fatal fungal infections caused by *Candida* and 30% caused by *Aspergillus.* Intestinal colonization resistance is disrupted by broad-spectrum antibiotic use, leading to increased intestinal fungal growth. Primary barriers that are breached by indwelling intravascular catheters and mucositis facilitate fungemia and invasive fungal infections.

Viruses. Viral infections are a significant problem in bone marrow transplant recipients (Table 100–1). After bone marrow transplantation, children have the same risk of viral infections as adults, although the time of peak occurrence may be somewhat different. Cutaneous zoster occurs earlier in children, with more than one half of all cases occurring within the first 100 days after transplantation and 90% within the first year.

Symptomatic CMV infection occurs in 40% of bone marrow transplant recipients, with CMV pneumonitis, the most severe focal form of infection, in 20% of these patients. Severe graft-versus-host disease is the greatest risk factor for development of CMV disease and the one most likely to contribute to patient death. Ganciclovir, initiated at the time of bone marrow engraftment and administered at 10 mg/kg/day divided every 12 hours intravenously for the first 5 days, then at 5 mg/kg/day until day 100 after transplantation, effectively suppresses CMV infection and disease in CMV-seropositive patients. Unfortunately, ganciclovir prophylaxis is also associated with an increased risk of bacterial infection due to drug-induced neutropenia. Therefore, in CMV-seropositive patients with severe graft-versus-host disease, ganciclovir should be given prophylactically. However, in patients who have no or only mild graft-verus-host disease, monitoring the viral load in blood by weekly CMV antigen determinations allows the delay of ganciclovir therapy until the demonstration of significant CMV antigenemia as a predictor of subsequent disease. At the threshold of at least two CMV-positive blood polymorphonuclear cells per slide, ganciclovir therapy can then be initiated at 10 mg/kg/day divided every 12 hours intravenously for 14–21 days and continued at 5 mg/kg/day until day 100 after transplantation.

The incidence of Epstein-Barr virus–associated lymphoproliferative disorders, primarily non-Hodgkin's lymphoma and angioimmunoblastic lymphadenopathy, after bone marrow transplantation is approximately 0.6%. Use of antilymphocyte immunoglobulin for treatment of acute graft-versus-host disease, and T-lymphocyte depletion from donor marrow before transplantation are significant risk factors. Concomitant acute graft-versus-host disease, especially in the case of human leukocyte-antigen-disparate donor-recipient mismatch, is most likely to result in uncontrolled, fatal lymphoproliferation. Although many of the lymphoproliferative disorders that follow bone marrow transplantation often prove fatal, clinical improvement in most cases results from reduction of immunosuppression and from interferon-α therapy in selected cases.

Prevention of Infection

Cytokines. The cytokine granulocyte-macrophage colony stimulating factor (GM-CSF) has been used to hasten neutrophil recovery after autologous bone marrow transplantation. Patients given GM-CSF achieve an absolute neutrophil count exceeding 500/mm^3 7 days earlier than would occur without GM-CSF. Patients treated with GM-CSF tend to have fewer infective episodes, require less antibiotic therapy, and can be discharged from the hospital earlier, but there has not been any increase in survival rates at 100 days after transplantation.

Prevention of Graft-Versus-Host Disease. For transplants involving HLA mismatched donor and recipient, harvested marrow can be depleted of mature T lymphocytes by the use of monoclonal antibody or soybean protein agglutination with sheep erythrocyte rosette formation ex vivo. Recipients of T-lymphocyte-depleted bone marrow experience a lower infection-related mortality than non-T-lymphocyte-depleted marrow recipients, largely because of a reduced incidence of pneumonia, which appears to be directly associated with reduced incidence and severity of acute graft-versus-host disease and CMV pneumonitis. However, these patients have also experienced an increased frequency of central venous intravascular catheter infections due to abnormal T-lymphocyte-

TABLE 100–1. Viral Infections Occurring in Bone Marrow Transplantation

Virus	Clinical Manifestations	Peak Occurrence (Months after Transplantation)	Treatment/Prophylaxis
Herpes simplex viruses	Gingivolabial stomatitis	0–1	Acyclovir, famciclovir, valacyclovir
Human herpesvirus 6	Fever Skin rash Pneumonitis	0–1	None
Polyomaviruses	Hemorrhagic cystitis	1–2	None
Cytomegalovirus	Pneumonitis Prolonged fever Enterocolitis	1–4	Ganciclovir, foscarnet, cidofovir, immunotherapy
Respiratory viruses	Pneumonitis Irreversible respiratory failure	1–4	Amantadine and rimantidine (influenza A virus); oseltamivir and zanamivir (influenza A and B viruses); ribavirin (respiratory syncytial virus, parainfluenza viruses)
Parvovirus	Anemia Delayed engraftment	2–4	None
Adenoviruses	Pneumonitis Hepatitis Enterocolitis Meningoencephalitis	2–6	None
Enteroviruses	Pneumonitis Myocarditis Meningocephalitis	2–6	None
Varicella-zoster virus	Cutaneous zoster	2–12	Acyclovir, famciclovir, valacyclovir

dependent polymorphonuclear leukocyte function and have experienced increased cancer relapses as a result of reduction in the beneficial graft-versus-malignant-host-cell activity of mature T lymphocytes.

Enteric Decontamination. Many bone marrow transplantation centers attempt enteric decontamination with orally administered antimicrobial agents as a component of prophylaxis during periods of increased vulnerability. Most regimens used are either nonabsorbable antibacterial agents, such as neomycin, bacitracin, or erythromycin base, or absorbable antibacterial agents, such as trimethoprim-sulfamethoxazole, amoxicillin-clavulanate, norfloxacin, or ciprofloxacin, plus an antifungal agent, such as nystatin, clotrimazole, orally administered amphotericin B, fluconazole, or itraconazole. Benefits of enteric decontamination include a reduced incidence of bacteremia in the first month after transplantation and a reduction in the incidence and severity of acute graft-versus-host disease. The disadvantages of enteric decontamination include cost, patient compliance, and selection of resistant microorganisms.

Antifungal Prophylaxis. Antifungal prophylaxis can be given to bone marrow transplant recipients to reduce the incidence of fungal infections, but the efficacy is often disappointing. The use of nystatin or orally administered amphotericin B as part of an enteric decontamination regimen has not always prevented invasive candidiasis; in most cases, the agents do not eradicate oropharyngeal or gastrointestinal colonization. Prophylaxis with fluconazole can reduce the frequency of invasive candidiasis due to *Candida albicans* and *Candida tropicalis,* but this can significantly increase colonization and infection caused by the more resistant *Candida krusei.* The empirical use of parenteral amphotericin B for neutropenic patients with fever persisting after 7–10 days of broad-spectrum antibacterial therapy remains the most cost-effective way to combat fungal infections.

Antiviral Prophylaxis. Herpes simplex virus infection at one time was the most prevalent viral infection occurring in the immediate posttransplant period. It is most commonly manifested as orolabial gingivostomatitis and less frequently causes esophagitis, pneumonitis, and hepatitis. The institution of routine acyclovir prophylaxis, usually administered at 750 mg/m^2 divided every 8 hours orally or intravenously beginning 1 week before transplantation and continued until 1 month after transplantation, significantly reduces the incidence of symptomatic infection.

Immunoprophylaxis. IVIG has been serially administered to recipients of bone marrow transplants as prophylaxis against infection during the posttransplantation period. Patients who receive intravenous immunoglobulin (500 mg/kg/wk for the first 3 months, then monthly until 1 year after transplantation) demonstrate a reduction in the frequency of episodes of gram-negative septicemia, focal bacterial infections, and CMV pneumonitis. Moreover, patients receiving intravenous immunoglobulin require less platelet support, probably because of mechanisms similar to those that occur in the treatment of idiopathic thrombocytopenic purpura. Overall, immunoprophylaxis with IVIG provides measurable short-term benefit with few adverse consequences, although no long-term improvement in survival has been shown.

Reimmunization. Patients who successfully undergo allogeneic bone marrow transplantation should be reimmunized because of the potential for loss of immunologic memory, which is dependent on donor immune status, degree of host immunosuppressive therapy, period of time since transplantation, and presence of graft-versus-host disease. Reimmunization against pertussis, tetanus, and *Haemophilus influenzae* type b using the 3-dose series for each vaccine should occur 1 year after transplantation. Pneumococcal, influenza, hepatitis B, and measles-mumps-rubella vaccination should be initiated approximately 2 years after transplantation. Those patients with chronic graft-versus-host disease should not receive measles-mumps-rubella vaccine because of concern about promoting chronic latent viral infection. The decision to immunize against poliovirus should be based on perceived risk of exposure; if vaccine is given, the patient and all family members should receive only the parenteral inactivated polio vaccine.

RENAL TRANSPLANTATION

Infection is the major cause of early morbidity and death in renal allograft recipients, especially in elderly recipients and those who receive renal transplantation because of diabetic nephropathy, and during the time immediately following augmented antiallograft rejection therapy. Infections adversely affect patient and renal allograft survival rates; 1-year and 3-year survival rates of both organ and patient are approximately 5% lower when infection occurs during the posttransplantation period. About 7% of all renal transplant recipients will die because of infection, and 85% of these deaths will occur in the 6 months after transplantation.

Most infectious episodes in renal allograft recipients will occur in the 4 months after transplantation, with approximately 65% of all febrile episodes occurring between the second and third weeks. As a general rule, infections occurring fairly early after transplantation are bacterial, most often due to *Staphylococcus*, *Streptococcus*, and gram-negative bacilli, and usually arise from the urinary tract, the lower respiratory tract, the operative wound site, or an intravascular catheter. Later infections are more commonly due to *L. pneumophila*, *P. aeruginosa*, *Mycobacterium*, and *N. asteroides. Listeria monocytogenes* can also cause meningitis during this time.

Fungal pathogens include *Candida*, which usually presents early in the posttransplantation period as mucocutaneous candidiasis; disseminated candidiasis is rare. The fungal pathogens more likely to cause deep mycosis include *Cryptococcus neoformans*, *Aspergillus*, *Histoplasma capsulatum*, *Coccidioides immitis*, and the agents of zygomycosis. These infections seldom occur within the first month after transplantation.

P. carinii, presenting almost always as pneumonitis, has a peak incidence approximately 2–4 months after renal transplantation.

Patients can experience reactivation of latent viral infection with CMV, herpes simplex virus, Epstein-Barr virus, and varicella-zoster virus. Primary CMV infection in susceptible persons or reactivated infection in seropositive patients can cause renal allograft dysfunction by direct viral glomerulopathy and by triggering acute allograft rejection. CMV antigenemia of more than 10 CMV-positive cells per slide predicts which renal transplant recipients are at high risk of subsequent development of CMV-associated disease. Empirical treatment with ganciclovir at this threshold of CMV antigenemia may prevent development of overt disease.

Mechanisms of Increased Susceptibility to Infection

Overall, the risk of infection in renal allograft recipients is increased by a cadaveric source of the renal allograft, one or more prior organ rejection episodes, combined renal and pancreatic allograft transplantations, and female gender. The source of the kidney for transplantation is an important determinant of subsequent infection during the posttransplantation period. The lowest rates of infection are associated with the transplantation of allografts from living related donors, with an increased infection risk associated with the use of cadaveric allografts. The risk factors that increase the probability of urinary tract and wound infections are prolonged postoperative bladder catheterization, inadequate perioperative antimicrobial prophylaxis, and increased empirical use of antibiotics postoperatively, especially with prolonged treatment. Requirement of a prolonged period of hemodialysis before hospitalization predicts an increased likelihood for the subsequent development of posttransplant urinary tract infection, and a high serum creatinine concentration directly correlates with an increased risk of postoperative wound infection. Both urinary tract and wound infections are often due to exposure of sutured tissue to postoperative urine extravasation at surgical anastomosis sites.

Site-Specific Infections

Wound. Surgical wound infections are largely due to technical factors and complicate approximately 6% of renal transplant procedures (Table 100–2). The single greatest practice that has deceased the frequency of wound infections is perioperative antimicrobial prophylaxis; before adaption of this routine, some institutions had posttransplantation wound infection rates of 25%. With the use of intraoperatively administered antibacterials and irrigation of the operative field and bladder with topical antibiotics, the incidence of posttransplant wound infections can be reduced to as low as 1%.

Urinary Tract. Urinary tract infections are common after renal allograft transplantation; they occur with greater frequency when ureteral stents are employed, and they tend to manifest within the first 2 weeks postoperatively. The simple practice of prompt removal of the bladder catheter postoperatively can significantly reduce the incidence of urinary tract infection.

Recurrent urinary tract infections and postoperative pyelonephritis occur in approximately 4% of all renal allograft recipients, caused largely by technical factors such as postoperative urinary and ureteral stump reflux, reflux into a remaining native kidney, and incomplete emptying of the bladder during micturition. Although most infections are fairly inconsequential in terms of overall patient and allograft survival, the site of infection is important, with upper tract or recurrent infections more likely to result in serious morbidity and premature patient death.

Respiratory Tract. Pulmonary infection is uncommon but potentially life threatening in renal allograft recipients, especially in those patients receiving cyclosporine or tacrolimus immunosuppression and concomitant corticosteroids. The peak occurrence is 1–5 months after transplantation. Although invasive procedures may be necessary to establish a definitive cause, initial radiographic evaluation may provide a clue as to the most probable cause. Focal air-space disease is generally caused by bacterial or fungal pathogens, and the presence of pleural effusion strongly suggests a bacterial pathogen. An interstitial or reticulonodular pattern is consistent with early *P. carinii* or viral infection, both of which progress to diffuse air-space disease with advanced infection. Pulmonary nodules, with or without cavitation, are most consistent with fungal pneumonia or pneumonia due to *N. asteroides.*

The bacterial pathogens tend to be nosocomially acquired gram-negative bacteria or *L. pneumophila*, with a peak incidence within the first months after transplantation. Risk factors for bacterial pneumonia include malnutrition and prior pulmonary disease. During the later posttransplantation period, community-acquired pneumonia tends to be more commonly caused by gram-positive bacteria and *H. influenzae.*

Mycobacterial infection has an incidence of approximately 0.5–2.5% in renal transplant recipients, although the rate may be as high as 10% in those regions with an increased prevalence of tuberculosis in the general population. Pulmonary infections due to mycobacteria have a peak onset approximately 1 year after transplantation, with atypical mycobacteria accounting for 20–40% of all cases. Reactivation of tuberculosis after renal transplantation is relatively uncommon, occurring in only 2% of all cases.

Fungal pneumonia remains a significant problem in renal transplant recipients, with risk of infection directly related to number of augmented immunosuppressive treatments of acute allograft rejection episodes. Important pathogens include *Aspergillus*, *Candida*, *C. neoformans*, *H. capsulatum*, and *C. immitis.* Fungal pneumonia usually occurs within the first 4 months after transplantation but may become manifest as late as 1 year after transplantation. Pulmonary aspergillosis can present as nodules, as single or multiple focal cavitary lesions, or as diffuse parenchymal disease. Approximately 75% of all cases of coccidioidomycosis and histoplasmosis will present as disseminated disease.

P. carinii pneumonitis occurs in <5% of all renal transplant recipients, largely because of trimethoprim-sulfamethoxazole prophylaxis in the first year after transplantation. The addition of

TABLE 100–2. Site Infections Following Renal Transplantation

Site of Infection	Peak Occurrence (After Transplantation)	Pathogens	Comments
Postsurgical wound	1–2 wk	*Staphylococcus aureus* Enterobacteriaceae	Occurs in 6% of patients; perioperative prophylaxis effective prevention
Urinary tract	1–2 wk	Enterobacteriaceae *Enterococcus* *Mycoplasma hominis*	Associated with technical problems and prolonged bladder catheterization; recurrent in 4% of patients
Pulmonary	1–4 mo	Cytomegalovirus	Symptoms in 20% of patients
	2–3 mo	*Pneumocystis carinii*	Reduced incidence with chemoprophylaxis
	1–5 mo	*Legionella pneumophila*	Patients unusually susceptible to pathogen
	1–5 mo	*Nocardia asteroides*	Mimics fungal pneumonia
	1–5 mo	Agents of zygomycosis	High mortality
Cutaneous	4–24 mo	*Mycobacterium chelonae*	Usually of low morbidity
Ocular	1–3 mo	Herpes simplex virus	Poor response to treatment
Gastrointestinal/Pulmonary	3–4 mo	*Strongyloides stercoralis*	Travel to/residence in endemic areas

cyclosporine in immunosuppressive regimens is associated with an increased incidence of *P. carinii* pneumonitis, a more acute onset of respiratory symptoms than typically occurs, and widely varying mortality rates that can be as high as 80%.

CMV is the most common cause of pneumonia in renal allograft recipients, usually occurring 1–4 months after transplantation. Infected patients occasionally may have normal chest radiographs and normal arterial oxygenation. The presumptive diagnosis is suggested by CT or MRI or by an ^{111}In-labeled leukocyte scan, in which a diffuse pulmonary uptake suggests that the lungs are the site of occult disease. The definitive cause is established by bronchoalveolar lavage or transtracheal biopsy yielding the virus in respiratory secretions or tissue and by cytopathologic evidence of basophilic intranuclear and cytoplasmic inclusions in pneumonocytes or detection of intracellular virus-associated antigens.

Vascular Aneurysm. Aneurysm of the grafted vessel is an unusual but serious infectious complication after renal transplantation, especially in patients who have experienced suppuration at the graft site earlier in the posttransplantation period. Bacterial pathogens, especially *S. aureus* and the Enterobacteriaceae, predominate. The risk of this complication is substantially increased if foreign arterial material is used to construct the vascular graft.

Common Pathogens

Bacteria. Epidemic outbreaks of nosocomial legionnaires' disease has been reported in renal transplantation centers, with the attack rate as high as 10%. Beyond the institutional risk, renal allograft recipients and patients with chronic renal failure undergoing dialysis have an unusual susceptibility to *L. pneumophila* infection, with a relative risk as much as 50 times greater than that of other immunocompromised persons. Attempts to eradicate colonization of hospital water sources with shock chlorination and superheating of water-holding tanks may not always prove entirely successful. Prophylaxis with a macrolide antibiotic against nosocomial *Legionella* infection during hospitalization may be selectively used.

Mycobacterium chelonae is an opportunistic pathogen with a propensity to cause skin and subcutaneous tissue infections in renal transplant recipients; these infections present most commonly as indolent, mildly tender, nodular lesions occurring on the extremities, especially the lower legs. There are generally no systemic symptoms, and the CBC count is normal. Treatment includes excision, with cultures requiring incubation for 1 month before visible growth of the organism, and long-term antibiotic therapy, usually with clarithromycin and amikacin. Despite treatment, some patients will experience a chronic, relapsing course.

Mycoplasma hominis, a genitourinary tract colonizer of low pathogenicity, may establish opportunistic infection in renal allograft recipients that can threaten allograft survival. Postoperative wound infection and urinary tract infection caused by *M. hominis* have occurred in patients receiving cadaveric allografts. *M. hominis* is not isolated by routine culture methods, and suspicion of this organism as the cause of ''culture-negative'' infection is necessary to establish the diagnosis. Either a macrolide antibiotic or tetracycline is appropriate therapy.

Fungi. Renal transplant recipients are vulnerable to the development of deep mycotic infections due to the agents of zygomycosis, especially patients with diabetes mellitus receiving corticosteroid immunosuppression during the posttransplantation period. Clinical manifestations of zygomycosis in renal transplant recipients are rhinocerebral disease (70%), cutaneous disease (15%), pulmonary disease (10%), and hepatic disease (5%). The best treatment outcomes have been achieved with long-term parenteral amphotericin B therapy, plus surgical resection of all involved tissue, but the majority of deep mycotic infections in renal allograft recipients prove fatal.

The transplanted kidney can be a source of fungal infection in the allograft recipient. Infections acquired from infected kidney allografts have been caused by *Scedosporium apiospermum, Histoplasma, Cryptococcus,* and *Candida.*

Viruses. In renal transplant recipients, keratitis may develop as a focal manifestation of herpes simplex virus infection during the posttransplantation period. The infection usually appears in the form of epithelial herpetic lesions in the periphery of the cornea, without the stromal involvement that characterizes herpetic keratitis in other patients.

The polyomaviruses, BK virus and JC virus, can cause primary and reactivation infection in renal allograft recipients. The majority of infections are due to viral reactivation, with approximately 20% of renal allograft recipients showing serologic evidence of BK virus infection and 10% showing serologic evidence of JC virus infection during the posttransplantation period. Infection with polyomavirus is not associated with an adverse patient outcome in the early posttransplantation period, although BK and JC viruses have been implicated in pancreatitis and transient renal dysfunction in individual patients. However, the actual pathogenicity of these viruses remains to be proven; most probably, reactivation is merely a marker of host immunosuppression and not evidence of focal disease.

Rotavirus can cause nosocomial infection in the renal transplant unit, which can result in acute hypovolemia and malabsorption of orally administered immunosuppressive agents, subsequently promoting acute allograft rejection.

Parasites. Opportunistic infection with the nematode *Strongyloides stercoralis* can occur in renal allograft recipients, with most infections occurring within 3–4 months after transplantation. Strongyloidiasis is most likely to manifest as severe gastrointestinal symptoms or as progressive pulmonary infection. Secondary bacterial and fungal infections can arise from translocation of intestinal flora through injured gastrointestinal mucosa. Primary infection could have occurred as remotely as 30 years previously, remaining quiescent as occult intestinal infection until the patient became immunocompromised. Localized infection may progress to **disseminated infection,** with extension of filariform larvae beyond the gastrointestinal and pulmonary systems. In addition, larvae may reinvade the same host in an **autoinfective cycle,** which may lead to **hyperinfection.**

The diagnosis of strongyloidiasis should be considered for renal transplant recipients with unexplained peripheral eosinophilia, especially with travel or residence in endemic regions. It is confirmed by microscopic examination of stool, sputum, and duodenal secretions. The treatment of choice is thiabendazole (50 mg/kg/day divided every 12 hours orally; maximum daily dose, 3 g/day) given therapeutically until stool and sputum examinations are negative for parasites, then prophylactically at the same daily dose given for 2 days each month to prevent new infection.

Prevention of Infection

Prophylactic use of trimethoprim-sulfamethoxazole, given routinely to prevent *P. carinii* infection, is cost-effective for the prevention of bacterial infection in renal allograft recipients during the first year after transplantation. Continued prophylaxis may be cost-effective for a longer period of time, especially in high-risk patients such as those who have diabetes mellitus, a history of infection during the immediate posttransplantation period, or recurrent urinary tract infections, who are receiving cyclophosphamide or high-dose corticosteroids, or who are treated in institutions where there is a higher frequency of *P. carinii* infections as a late complication of renal transplantation.

The best preventive measure to reduce the incidence of significant CMV infection in renal transplant recipients is careful selection of the donor. It is most critical to match a seronegative recipient with a seronegative donor whenever feasible. Pretransplant immunization of seronegative allograft recipients with an experimental CMV vaccine (Towne strain) shows no difference in rates of either CMV infection or symptomatic disease, but seronegative vaccine recipients have had decreased severity of symptomatic CMV infection and enhanced 1-year and 5-year posttransplant survival.

The use of acyclovir or valacyclovir in kidney transplant recipients for the first 90 days after transplantation as prophylaxis against herpes simplex virus reactivation in the posttransplantation period has had additional benefit in reducing the incidence of CMV and varicella-zoster virus infections, but this unanticipated benefit appears to be limited specifically to renal transplantation.

HEPATIC TRANSPLANTATION

The two most significant determinants of patient and hepatic allograft survival are organ rejection and opportunistic infection. Before the use of cyclosporine, the 1-year posttransplantation patient survival rate was approximately 30%. With the use of cyclosporine and tacrolimus, 1-year survival rates have dramatically improved to 65–85%. However, infections remain a significant problem, arising largely from postoperative surgical complications, reactivation of latent virus infections, and as an adverse consequence of immunosuppressive regimens meant to prevent allograft rejection. Most patient deaths occur within 6 months after hepatic transplantation, with 90% of all deaths within this time period attributable to infection. Approximately 15% of all patients receiving orthotopic liver transplantation will die of infection during the first year after transplantation.

Overall, 50–75% of all orthotopic liver transplant recipients become infected after transplantation and experience an average of 1.5–3 episodes of infection. Bacterial infections account for 50–65% of all infections, viral infections for 20–40%, and fungal infections for 5–15%. Retransplantation because of initial hepatic allograft dysfunction is even more likely to be complicated by infection during the second posttransplantation period; virtually all patients will experience at least one infection during that time. During retransplantation, viral infection, especially caused by CMV, becomes increasingly important and may account for the majority of infection episodes. Fungal infections also increase in proportional significance after retransplantation, although they account for only a minority of infections.

P. carinii and *T. gondii* are the more important pathogens causing late opportunistic infections in orthotopic liver transplant recipients. The peak incidence of *P. carinii* pneumonia is 2–3 months after transplantation and is often associated with CMV coinfection. The mortality rate is 10%.

Mechanisms of Increased Susceptibility to Infection

Risk factors for infection include adult age, elevated serum aminotransferase and bilirubin concentrations, depression of normal CD4 T-lymphocyte counts with inverted helper-to-cytotoxic/suppressor T-lymphocyte ratio, prolonged intraoperative time and increased operative blood transfusion requirements, requirement of more than one abdominal operation and prior hepatobiliary surgery, dialysis in the early postoperative period, liver transplantation to correct biliary atresia, postoperative biliary tract complications, and hepatic artery occlusion. Hepatic artery thrombosis, which occurs in approximately 40% of all pediatric orthotopic liver transplants and for which 75% of the cases will require a second-liver retransplantation, can cause vascular occlusion that leads to hepatic necrosis and abscess formation and bile duct ischemia that leads to the formation of bile lakes. Intestinal microorganisms, ascending through biliary-enteric anastomoses, can infect these bile lakes, causing intrahepatic abscesses that promote allograft dysfunction.

Site-Specific Infections

Intra-abdominal, perihepatic, and wound infections occur primarily as a consequence of abdominal surgery and are usually caused by skin and bowel flora (Table 100–3). The incidence, especially in the first weeks after transplantation, is similar to that associated with other intra-abdominal operative procedures. However, most of the fatal infections in the immediate posttransplantation period

TABLE 100–3. Site Infections Following Hepatic Transplantation

Infection	Peak Time of Occurrence (After Transplantation)	Pathogens
Pneumonia	First month	*Streptococcus pneumoniae*
		Staphylococcus aureus
		Pseudomonas aeruginosa
		Enterobacteriaceae
	1–2 mo	*Nocardia asteroides*
		Aspergillus
	2–3 mo	*Pneumocystis carinii*
Intra-abdominal	First month	Enterobacteriaceae
Postsurgical wound		*P. aeruginosa*
Hepatic abscess		*S. aureus*
Urinary tract		*Enterococcus*
		Anaerobic bacteria
Septicemia	First month	*S. pneumoniae*
		Enterobacteriaceae
	1–12 mo	*P. aeruginosa*
	1–2 mo	*Candida*
Meningitis	4–24 mo	*Cryptococcus neoformans*

have a pulmonary component. Bacterial pneumonia occurs in 2–25% of all orthotopic hepatic transplants, accounting for 12–50% of pulmonary infections. Bacterial pneumonia due to gram-negative bacteria has a 40% case-fatality rate. The advent of selective bowel decontamination by the administration of nonabsorbable antibacterials and antifungal agents has decreased the incidence of bacterial pneumonia, but the frequency of pneumonia due to gram-positive bacteria has increased. Risk factors for the development of bacterial pneumonia include endotracheal intubation, pulmonary atelectasis, aspiration of oral secretions, and mechanical ventilation.

Common Pathogens

Bacteria. Bacterial infections predominate in the first 2 months after transplantation, especially within the first month, and appear as pneumonia and septicemia (*S. pneumoniae*, *S. aureus*, Enterobacteriaceae, *P. aeruginosa*), intra-abdominal infections (Enterobacteriaceae, *P. aeruginosa*, *S. aureus*, *Enterococcus*, anaerobic bacteria), urinary tract infections, and postoperative wound infections. Approximately 80% of intra-abdominal infections and 40% of septicemia episodes arise from intra-abdominal complications of the surgical procedure. Infection caused by *L. pneumophila*, *Nocardia*, *L. monocytogenes*, or *Mycobacterium* occurs less commonly during the immediate posttransplantation period. *Nocardia* can cause pneumonia, appearing radiographically as pleural consolidation, cavitating lesions, intraparenchymal nodules, or pleural effusion. Lesional biopsy with CT guidance may be required to establish the diagnosis. Recognizing nocardiosis that presents as pleural effusion can be especially tricky because of the common postoperative occurrence of a rightsided pleural effusion after orthotopic liver transplantation.

Fungal Infections

Fungal pneumonia once accounted for 40% of all lower respiratory tract infections occurring in recipients of orthotopic hepatic transplants, but more recently the incidence of fungal pneumonia has declined, partly because of improved surgical technique, decreased operative time, more selective immunosuppressive regimens, and selective bowel decontamination. The fungal pathogens most likely to cause infection in hepatic transplant recipients include *Candida*, *Aspergillus*, *C. neoformans*, *Trichosporon beigelii*, *Pseudallescheria boydii*, and the agents of zygomycosis. Approximately 25% of liver transplant recipients will have fungal infection during the posttransplantation period, with approximately 80% of the cases caused by *Candida* and 13% caused by *Aspergillus*. Fungal infections are most frequent in the first 2 months after liver transplantation and most often occur in those patients who are receiving broad-spectrum antibacterial therapy or those who are experiencing a postoperative intra-abdominal complication. Moreover, the transient disruption in the hepatic reticuloendothelial system that occurs in the newly transplanted liver, with temporary loss of an important defense against systemic invasion by fungal bowel flora, also contributes to the increased risk of early fungal infections.

C. neoformans tends to cause infection later in the posttransplantation period. Infection most commonly presents as a subacute, chronic meningitis occurring more than 4 months postoperatively, but it may also present as cutaneous lesions, either occurring early in the posttransplantation period as a manifestation of disseminated disease or occurring later as a disease limited to the skin.

Viruses. The most important viruses causing infections in hepatic allograft recipients are CMV, herpes simplex virus, varicella-zoster virus, Epstein-Barr virus, and adenoviruses (Table 100–4).

CMV causes infection in 40–80% of all patients undergoing orthotopic liver transplantation, with approximately 30% occurring as primary infection and 70% as reactivation of latent virus. CMV infections have an associated mortality rate of 20%, with virtually all deaths occurring in patients primarily infected after transplantation. Peak occurrence of disease is 3–7 weeks after transplantation. The most frequent site of CMV infection in primary hepatic allograft recipients is the liver, but extrahepatic sites are frequently involved. CMV antigenemia exceeding 100 positive cells per slide is the threshold defining high risk of subsequent disease and identifies the need for institution of ganciclovir therapy.

Herpes simplex virus infection, most likely to manifest as orolabial gingivostomatitis, occurs somewhat earlier than symptomatic CMV infection, with peak occurrence 1–4 weeks after transplantation.

Varicella-zoster virus infection, which most frequently presents as a cutaneous infection, affects 5–10% of all hepatic transplant recipients, and tends to manifest later than either herpes simplex virus or CMV infections.

Epstein-Barr virus infection reactivates in approximately 25% of adult patients and 50% of pediatric patients during the posttransplantation period. Approximately two thirds of seronegative chil-

TABLE 100–4. Viral Infections Following Hepatic Transplantation

Virus	Peak Time of Occurrence (After Transplantation)	Incidence (Percentage of Recipients)	Clinical Manifestations
Herpes simplex viruses	1–4 wk	<10*	Orolabial stomatitis Pneumonitis
Respiratory syncytial virus	First month	0–3	Bronchiolitis
Adenoviruses	4 wk	10	Hepatitis Pneumonia Gastroenteritis
Cytomegalovirus	3–7 wk	40–80	Serologic reactivation Hepatitis Pneumonitis
Epstein-Barr virus	4–12 mo	25–50 2–3	Serologic reactivation Lymphoproliferative disorder
Varicella-zoster virus	6–24 mo	5–10	Cutaneous zoster Pneumonitis Hepatitis

*Reduced incidence due to use of acyclovir prophylaxis.

dren will experience primary infection when given livers from seropositive donors, manifesting as illness ranging from asymptomatic infection with seroconversion, through prolonged allograft dysfunction and infectious mononucleosis, to the most serious with malignant lymphoproliferative disease. Most patients will have mild disease.

Epstein-Barr virus–associated **posttransplantation lymphoproliferative disease** occurs in approximately 3% of hepatic allograft patients who receive an immunosuppressive regimen of cyclosporine or tacrolimus and corticosteroid therapy during the posttransplantation period and tends to occur within the first 6 months. Lymphoproliferative disorders often involve the gastrointestinal tract and may manifest clinically in lymphadenopathic, systemic, or lymphomatous forms. Treatment consists of reduction of immunosuppression and sometimes excision of tumor. The survival rate is 50–60% with therapy.

In approximately 10% of patients receiving hepatic allografts, adenovirus infection develops during the posttransplantation period, with the peak incidence of symptomatic disease occurring at 4 weeks after transplantation. Most commonly, presentation is as a mild respiratory tract infection, although adenovirus types 1, 2, and 5 have caused fatal pneumonia, and adenovirus type 5 has caused serious, sometimes fatal hepatitis in the transplanted liver.

Human herpesvirus 6 has recently been recognized as a significant cause of fever due to viral infection during the posttransplant period. Infections most commonly occur between 2 and 12 weeks after transplantation, are often associated with leukopenia, and generally resolve without significant consequence to the patient.

Patients with irreversible hepatic injury from hepatitis B virus infection have received orthotopic liver transplants in an attempt to prevent or forestall impending death from liver failure. On some occasions, these patients have even received infected but less diseased livers from donors who also had hepatitis B virus infection. The posttransplantation survival rates of patients receiving hepatic allografts under such circumstances are 80% at 1 year and 70% at 3 years. The increased mortality rate in these patients is attributable to hepatitis B virus infection of the hepatic allograft. Use of HBIG, hepatitis B vaccine, and α-interferon therapy has had no effect in modifying development of recurring hepatitis B virus infection in the transplanted liver. Approximately 80% of patients with hepatitis B and hepatitis D virus who receive liver transplants have recurrent viral infection with hepatitis D virus. Recurrence of hepatitis due to hepatitis C virus infection has also been observed in liver transplant recipients, and in these patients it may be the most important cause of fever due to an infection occurring beyond the first year after transplantation.

Nosocomial infection with respiratory syncytial virus can cause significant morbidity and death in children undergoing orthotopic liver transplantation. Death due to progressive pulmonary disease may occur in 10% of infected children. Risk factors include the requirement of endotracheal intubation before the onset of infection, pre-existing lung disease, and young patient age.

Parasites. Pneumonitis due to *P. carinii* has declined in frequency with the widespread use of trimethoprim-sulfamethoxazole prophylaxis. As opposed to pneumonia due to fungi, the time of occurrence after liver transplantation tends to be more delayed, with the peak incidence of occurrence 3–5 months after transplantation.

Prevention of Infection

Technical prowess in surgical technique may be more important in hepatic transplantation than in any other solid-organ transplantation in preventing infection and death in the posttransplantation period. The immediate postoperative death rate has been halved by intraoperative use of venovenous bypass. Surgical times exceeding 12 hours are associated with an increased risk of bacterial and fungal infections, with liver implantation involving choledochojejunostomy for biliary drainage more likely to be associated with postoperative infections. As many as three fourths of all deaths occurring early in the posttransplantation period are directly referable to the technical problems encountered during orthotopic liver transplantation.

Prophylaxis. Risk of infection can be reduced by selective bowel decontamination with nonabsorbable antimicrobial agents and cleansing enemas preoperatively, perioperative and limited postoperative broad-spectrum antibacterial prophylaxis, prophylactic trimethoprim-sulfamethoxazole and acyclovir therapy during the posttransplantation period, and use of cyclosporine or tacrolimus alone for selective immunosuppression.

Liver transplant recipients may undergo weekly percutaneous liver biopsies during the immediate posttransplantation period for evaluation of acute allograft rejection, ischemic injury, or viral hepatitis. However, the liver biopsy procedure has the potential for introducing infection. Enteric bacteria cause virtually all intra-abdominal infections induced by liver biopsy. Therefore, appropriate antibacterial prophylaxis at the time of biopsy will significantly reduce the risk of procedure-associated infection.

The prophylactic use of weekly infusions of IVIG for the first month and acyclovir chemoprophylaxis for the first 3 months has caused a reduction in the increased incidence of herpes simplex virus and Epstein-Barr virus infections that traditionally accompany the immunotherapy given to prevent acute hepatic allograft rejection. An unanticipated benefit of this prophylactic regimen has been the reduction in the number of fungal infections and patient deaths due to sepsis because of passive protection provided by IVIG. However, this has not changed the increased incidence of CMV infection. The use of CMV-IG has had no effect in modifying CMV infection or disease that may occur when a seronegative patient receives a liver allograft from a seropositive donor.

CARDIAC AND PULMONARY TRANSPLANTATION

Cardiac Transplantation. Isolated pediatric cardiac transplantation is a procedure with a generally good outcome, with survival rates >90% at 1 year after transplantation and approximately 80% at 3 years after transplantation. Increased pulmonary vascular resistance and noncardiac organ-system failure significantly jeopardize survival in the immediate posttransplantation period. Beyond the immediate posttransplantation period, opportunistic infections and allograft rejection are the major risks to patient survival, with approximately 50% of deaths being due to infection, 20% to allograft rejection, 10% to pulmonary hemorrhage, 10% to secondary neoplasm, and 5% to myocardial infarction. Nonsurvivors are more likely to have had episodes of rejection and infection during the posttransplantation period, although death due to rejection is uncommon after approximately 8 months after transplantation. A complex interrelationship exists between infection and rejection episodes as a major determinant of patient survival after the first posttransplantation year; aggressive immunosuppressive treatment of late rejection episodes predisposes to opportunistic infection. Therefore, overall patient survival after cardiac allograft transplantation has been improved by less aggressive treatment of rejection episodes. Infection risks are reduced by the use of selective immunosuppressants, such as cyclosporine or tacrolimus, CMV-negative blood products, and acyclovir and trimethoprim-sulfamethoxazole prophylaxis.

The largest single reduction in deaths due to infection has occurred with the introduction of cyclosporine as a selective immunosuppressant, with a decline in mortality rates from more than 50% to less than 40%. Before the use of cyclosporine, bacterial infections were the most common infections affecting the cardiac allograft recipient. Since the introduction of cyclosporine, viral and bacterial infections now occur with similar frequency, followed by fungal and parasitic infections.

Cardiopulmonary Transplantation. Infections account for one half of all deaths after combined heart-lung transplantation, with the majority of these infections occurring within the first 3 months after transplantation. The most significant complication affecting long-term survival in combined heart-lung transplant recipients is **bronchiolitis obliterans** in the pulmonary allograft. Combined heart-lung transplant recipients experience more opportunistic infections than do isolated cardiac allograft recipients, largely because of vulnerability of the transplanted lung. Transplanted lungs demonstrate decreased mucociliary function, lack protective clearance because of a diminished or absent cough reflex, experience frequent acute rejection episodes with incumbent requirement for augmented immunosuppression, and have depletion of bronchus-associated lymphoid tissue.

Pulmonary Transplantation. The survival rate of patients with isolated lung transplants is approximately 70% at 1 year after transplantation, which declines to approximately 55% by the third year. Approximately 40% of lung transplant recipients are alive 5 years after transplantation, compared with 70% of patients receiving either a heart or a liver transplant. Longer patient survival and the need of prolonged immunosuppression have been associated with an increased risk of opportunistic infections occurring later in the posttransplant period.

Mechanisms of Increased Susceptibility to Infection

The condition of the patient before cardiac transplantation predicts the risk of infection in the postoperative period. The need for invasive support, such as an intra-aortic balloon pump, a left ventricular assist device, or a total artificial heart before transplantation increases the risk of perioperative infection, and the use of preoperative mechanical support (left ventricular assist device or total artificial heart) increases the risk of an infection-associated death. Perioperative infections associated with cardiac transplantation are most commonly urinary tract infections and intravascular catheter-associated bacteremia. If either a left ventricular assist device or a total artificial heart is employed, mediastinitis and thoracic cavity infections due to gram-negative bacilli predominate, with an associated mortality rate exceeding 65%. Most of the deaths that occur within the first 3 months after cardiac transplantation that employed preoperative or perioperative mechanical support will be due to infection associated with such devices.

Site-Specific Infections

Respiratory Tract. The most frequent infection that occurs in isolated lung transplantation is pneumonia, due largely to impaired mucociliary function and poor lymphatic drainage in the allograft. Rates of infection range from approximately 1.5 times greater than that in other solid-organ transplant recipients receiving the same degree of immunosuppression to 10 times greater than that in renal transplant recipients. Infections occur more frequently in cases of double-lung transplantation than in cases of single-lung transplantation. Overall, 60% of all lung transplant recipients have infections during the posttransplantation period; of these, 50% have pneumonia and 30% have purulent bronchitis. Three fourths of all cases of pneumonia will occur within 2 months after transplantation.

Approximately 30% of all cases of pneumonia are due to bacterial infections, usually gram-negative bacteria, especially *P. aeruginosa*, and tend to occur within the first 10 days after transplantation. The most common causes of purulent bronchitis are *S. aureus* and *P. aeruginosa.*

Combined heart-lung transplant recipients are prone to selected opportunistic infections arising from pre-existing allograft injury and immunosuppression. *Mycobacterium tuberculosis* and atypical mycobacteria can cause progressive pulmonary infection, which may require transbronchial biopsy to establish the diagnosis. Pulmonary infections due to *Mycobacterium* are most likely to occur when obliterative bronchiolitis is present as a pre-existing condition. Fungal pneumonia is less frequent than is bacterial pneumonia, but fungal pneumonia more often proves fatal and has a mortality rate that exceeds 40%. *Candida* and *Aspergillus* are the predominant pathogens.

Infection with *Aspergillus* occurs more frequently in isolated lung and combined heart-lung transplantation than in isolated cardiac transplantation. Infection usually arises from prior colonization of bronchiectatic airways in the pulmonary allograft, especially when chronic lung rejection is also present, and leads to bronchocentric granulomatous mycosis, cavitating pneumonia, and disseminated disease.

Herpes simplex virus and CMV are the most important causes of viral pneumonia, generally occurring within 4 months after lung transplantation. In addition to immediate respiratory insufficiency due to the effects of active infection, viral pneumonia can also promote allograft rejection leading to bronchiolitis obliterans, often resulting in the requirement for retransplantation with a second pulmonary allograft to prevent the patient's death from pulmonary insufficiency.

Chest radiographs can be used to evaluate infection and rejection in heart-lung allograft recipients during the posttransplantation period, but 3 months after transplantation, radiographs have reduced sensitivity in detecting rejection and pulmonary infection. A more sensitive screening test to identify rejection and infection is pulmonary function testing performed serially. A significant decline in the 1-second forced expiratory volume, vital capacity, and carbon monoxide diffusion coefficient has a specificity of 75% in identifying allograft rejection and infection. Pulmonary function testing may best serve as a screening test to identify candidates for transbronchial lung biopsy.

The diagnosis of opportunistic infection in heart-lung transplant recipients may require invasive pulmonary diagnostic procedures to establish the specific cause. Specific bacterial and fungal pathogens may be identified by bronchoalveolar lavage, whereas viral and *P. carinii* pneumonia may be diagnosed only from lung tissue specimens obtained by transbronchial biopsy. Bronchiolitis obliterans may be diagnosed by transbronchial biopsy and may be a consequence of chronic pulmonary allograft rejection, although infection with either CMV or Epstein-Barr virus may be a cofactor in promoting the condition.

Children tolerate transbronchial biopsy fairly well. A biopsy specimen has a sensitivity of 90% and a specificity of 70% in identifying allograft rejection and may be used to distinguish opportunistic infection from rejection. Pneumothorax is the most common complication of transbronchial biopsy in children, occurring in approximately 5%; hemorrhage is the second most frequent complication, occurring in 1–3%. These risks are justified, rejection and infection have significantly dissimilar treatment requirements.

Central Nervous System. One third of patients experience a central nervous system complication during the posttransplantation period, with 10% of the complications being central nervous system infections, primarily meningitis, encephalitis, and brain abscess. Opportunistic pathogens are prevalent causes of the central nervous system infections. Meningitis caused by *L. monocytogenes* and *C. neoformans,* encephalitis caused by *Aspergillus, T. gondii, Candida,* and JC virus, and brain abscesses caused by *N. asteroides* are the most common central nervous system infections. Fewer than one half of central nervous system infections have an identified cause before the patients' death.

Virtually every patient with meningitis will have headache. More than one half of the patients with central nervous system infection present with seizures, and 60% of these patients will progress to irreversible coma. Diagnostic imaging with CT or MRI is the procedure of choice to identify brain abscesses. Hematogenous dissemination of *N. asteroides* to the central nervous system occurs in 20–45% of infected heart-lung transplant recipients, with a mortality rate of 50–70%. From 75% to 80% of these patients have pre-existing pulmonary lesions, an association that should raise the suspicion of *N. asteroides* infection.

Common Pathogens

A few bacterial, fungal, and viral microbes constitute the majority of pathogens in cardiac and pulmonary transplant recipients (Table 100–5). Cardiac failure during the posttransplantation period is usually due to allograft dysfunction caused by acute rejection, although infection of the transplanted heart may also be the cause. *L. monocytogenes* specifically targets the donor heart and can cause an isolated myocarditis, with microscopic abscess formation and necrosis mimicking rejection. Most infections occur between 2 weeks and 7 months after transplantation. The majority of cases of listeriosis have also involved the central nervous system, usually as meningitis or meningoencephalitis, and thus may be suspected on the basis of these simultaneous manifestations. *L. monocytogenes* myocarditis requires prolonged treatment with ampicillin plus an aminoglycoside or with trimethoprim-sulfamethoxazole. The severity of cardiac involvement is such that retransplantation is often required.

CMV infection develops in about one third of all cardiac transplant recipients. The use of corticosteroids as part of the immunosuppressive regimen increases the risk of symptomatic infection. CMV antigenemia exceeding 100 positive cells per slide is predictive of high risk of subsequent disease and is the threshold for which ganciclovir therapy should be initiated. CMV-dependent depression of cellular immunity also predisposes to the development of serious secondary infections. Infections that have occurred in cardiac allograft recipients immediately after CMV infection include gram-negative bacillary pneumonia and septicemia; *N. asteroides* vertebral osteomyelitis, pneumonia, and cerebral abscess; pulmonary aspergillosis; *P. carinii* pneumonia; and *Streptococcus pneumoniae* pneumonia.

Approximately one fourth of cardiac transplant recipients demonstrate significant changes in Epstein-Barr virus serum antibodies during the posttransplantation period, but most patients remain free of symptoms. Occasionally, Epstein-Barr virus–associated **posttransplantation lymphoproliferative disorder** occurs in cardiac transplant recipients, involving the lungs, lymph nodes, spleen, kidney, and even the intima of the coronary arteries in the transplanted heart. Posttransplantation lymphoproliferative disorder occurs in 1–2% of all cardiac transplantations, increasing to 10% if antilymphocyte immunotherapy is employed.

Approximately one half of cardiac transplant recipients will experience herpes simplex virus reactivation during the posttransplantation period; this usually manifests as a recurrence of orolabial gingivostomatitis, but esophagitis can also occur. Esophagitis is best evaluated by upper gastrointestinal endoscopy. The differential diagnosis of herpes simplex esophagitis includes CMV esophagitis and gastritis. The presence of an actively bleeding duodenal ulcer does not exclude the presence of concomitant viral infection.

TABLE 100–5. Selected Infections Following Cardiac and Pulmonary Transplantation

Pathogens	Clinical Manifestations
Bacterial	
Enterobacteriaceae	Urinary tract infection, catheter-associated infection, pneumonia, septicemia
Listeria monocytogenes	Myocarditis, pneumonia, meningitis
Mycobacterium tuberculosis	Pneumonia
Nocardia asteroides	Pneumonia, brain abscess
Pseudomonas aeruginosa	Pneumonia, bronchitis, septicemia
Staphylococcus aureus	Bronchitis, postsurgical wound infection, catheter-associated infection
Fungal	
Aspergillus	Pneumonia, septicemia, encephalitis
Candida	Pneumonia, septicemia
Cryptococcus neoformans	Meningitis
Parasitic	
Pneumocystis carinii	Pneumonitis
Toxoplasma gondii	Myocarditis, pneumonitis, encephalitis
Viral	
Cytomegalovirus	Pneumonitis, myocarditis, gastroenteritis
Epstein-Barr virus	Serologic reactivation, lymphoproliferative disorder
Herpes simplex viruses	Stomatitis, esophagitis, pneumonitis
JC virus	Serologic reactivation, encephalitis

The serologic status of donor and recipient for *T. gondii* and CMV helps predict the likelihood of infection during the posttransplantation period. The risk of primary toxoplasmosis in a seronegative patient receiving a heart from a seropositive donor is approximately 15%, being the most frequent donor-to-host transplantation-transmitted parasitic infection in the United States. Infection is most likely to occur within the first month after transplantation. *P. carinii* and *T. gondii* can cause necrotizing encephalitis, progressive pneumonitis, and myocarditis in cardiac-pulmonary allograft recipients, manifesting as primary infection in susceptible persons who receive infected organs, as well as reactivation of latent infection during immunosuppressive therapy.

Primary CMV infection after transplantation in seronegative recipients may present as pneumonitis, gastrointestinal infection, or myocarditis in the transplanted heart. Reactivation of latent infection can also occur during the posttransplantation period, with focal infection usually manifesting as pneumonitis. Pulmonary CMV infection occurs in approximately one third of all heart-lung transplant recipients. The combination of seropositive donor and seronegative recipient is the best predictor of the development of CMV pneumonitis, which develops in approximately 65% of this combination of patients, with a mortality rate that exceeds 50%. Disease is most likely to manifest within the first 4 months after transplantation.

Herpes simplex virus may reactivate during the first month after transplantation, usually as mucocutaneous lesions, but systemic dissemination may occur, as well as focal, necrotizing tracheobronchitis and pneumonia in the pulmonary allograft.

Combined heart-lung transplant recipients are most likely to manifest Epstein-Barr virus–associated **posttransplant lymphoproliferative disease** in cervical lymph nodes, tonsils, lungs, and the gastrointestinal tract, with involvement of the lung allograft in approximately 60% of cases. Bronchiolitis obliterans develops in 50–60% of transplant recipients with pulmonary allograft involvement. Histologically, the tumors that occur in combined cardiac-pulmonary transplant recipients are similar to those that occur in other solid-organ transplantation, characterized as lymphoid and immunoblastic proliferations ranging from diffuse hyperplasia to malignant lymphoma of immunoblastic or large-cell type. Recipients who are Epstein-Barr virus-seronegative and receive heart and lung allografts from a seropositive donor and who also receive intensive immunosuppressive regimens during the posttransplantation period are most likely to develop Epstein-Barr virus–associated posttransplant lymphoproliferative disease.

Prevention of Infection

Early postoperative care of cardiac allograft recipients that reduces the incidence of postsurgical wound infections includes preoperative and postoperative antimicrobial prophylaxis with a second-generation cephalosporin plus perioperative vancomycin administered intravenously and as a wound irrigant during surgery.

Whenever possible, the CMV serologic status of donor and recipient should be matched. When this is not practical, seronegative recipients receiving a heart from a seropositive donor should receive CMV-IG as immunoprophylaxis and should be monitored weekly for CMV antigenemia to identify early manifestations of active infection.

Trimethoprim-sulfamethoxazole prophylaxis against *P. carinii* infection is instituted after transplantation, to be continued for at least the first year, and perhaps for the lifetime of the patient. Nystatin can be administered orally and intranasally for the first 3 months after transplantation to reduce fungal mucosal colonization. Ketoconazole (5–10 mg/kg/day; maximum 200 mg/day) initiated immediately after cardiac transplantation will provide antifungal prophylaxis and reduce the need for cyclosporine because of inhibition of cyclosporine metabolism, reducing the rates of both rejection and infection without appreciable toxicity. Ketoconazole is continued for at least 1 year, if not indefinitely.

Protective isolation, with the patient in a private room and all persons in direct contact with the patient wearing hat, mask, gloves, grown, and does not lessen the overall infection rate, the number of infection-related deaths, or the types of infection and does not influence overall patient outcome during the posttransplantation period. There is an increased risk of minor fungal infections in patients hospitalized in an unprotected environment, but these infections generally lack clinical significance. Therefore, most patients can be hospitalized under standard infection control procedures.

REVIEWS

Craig FE, Gulley ML, Banks PM: Post-transplantation lymphoproliferative disorders. *Am J Clin Pathol* 1993;99:265–76.

Fishman JA, Rubin RH: Infection in organ transplant recipients. *N Engl J Med* 1998;338:1741–51.

Gottesdiener KM: Transplanted infections: Donor-to-host transmission with the allograft. *Ann Intern Med* 1989;110:1001–16.

Kim JH, Perfect JR: Infection and cyclosporine. *Rev Infect Dis* 1989; 11:677–90.

Patel R, Paya CV: Infections in solid-organ transplant recipients. *Clin Microbiol Rev* 1997;10:86–124.

Bone Marrow Transplantation

Boeckh M, Boivin G: Quantitation of cytomegalovirus: Methologic aspects and clinical applications. *Clin Microbiol Rev* 1998;11:533–54.

Goodrich JM, Bowden RA, Fisher L, et al: Ganciclovir phophylaxis to prevent cytomegalovirus disease after allogeneic marrow transplant. *Ann Intern Med* 1993;118:173–8.

Heimdahl A, Mattsson T, Dahllöf G, et al: The oral cavity as a port of entry for early infections in patients treated with bone marrow transplantation. *Oral Surg Oral Med Oral Pathol* 1989;68:711–6.

Henning KJ, White MH, Sepkowitz KA, et al: A national survey of immunization practices following allogeneic bone marrow transplantation. *JAMA* 1997;277:1148–51.

Kalhs P, Panzer S, Kletter K, et al: Functional asplenia after bone marrow transplantation. A late complication related to extensive chronic graft-versus-host disease. *Ann Intern Med* 1988;109:461–4.

Milliken ST, Powles RL: Antifungal prophylaxis in bone marrow transplantation. *Rev Infect Dis* 1990;12:S374–9.

Sable CA, Donowitz GR: Infections in bone marrow transplant recipients. *Clin Infect Dis* 1994;18:273–84.

Sheridan JF, Tutschka PJ, Sedmak DD, et al: Immunoglobulin G subclass deficiency and pneumococcal infection after allogeneic bone marrow transplantation. *Blood* 1990;75:1583–6.

Sullivan KM, Kopecky KJ, Jocom J, et al: Immunomodulatory and antimicrobial efficacy of intravenous immunoglobulin in bone marrow transplantation. *N Engl J Med* 1990;323:705–12.

Wald A, Leisenring W, van Burik JA, et al: Epidemiology of *Aspergillus* infections in a large cohort of patients undergoing bone marrow transplantation. *J Infect Dis* 1997;175:1459–66.

Renal Transplantation

Brayman KL, Stephanian E, Matas AJ, et al: Analysis of infectious complications occurring after solid-organ transplantation. *Arch Surg* 1992; 127:38–48.

Fox BC, Sollinger HW, Belzer FO, et al: A prospective, randomized, double-blind study of trimethoprim-sulfamethoxazole for prophylaxis of infection in renal transplantation: Clinical efficacy, absorption of trimethoprim-sulfamethoxazole, effects on the microflora, and the cost-benefit of prophylaxis. *Am J Med* 1990;89:255–74.

Lapchik MS, Castelo Filho A, Pestana JO, et al: Risk factors for nosocomial urinary tract and postoperative wound infection in renal transplant patients: A matched-pair case-control study. *J Urol* 1992;147:994–8.

Lowance D, Neumayer HH, Legendre CM, et al: Valacyclovir for the prevention of cytomegalovirus disease after renal transplantation. International Valacyclovir Cytomegalovirus Prophylaxis Transplantation Study Group. *N Engl J Med* 1999;340:1462–70.

Yoshimura N, Oka T: Medical and surgical complications of renal transplantation: Diagnosis and management. *Med Clin North Am* 1990; 74:1025–37.

Hepatic Transplantation

Chang FY, Singh N, Gayowski T, et al: Fever in liver transplant recipients: Changing spectrum of etiologic agents. *Clin Infect Dis* 1998;26:59–65.

Colonna JO 2nd, Winston DJ, Brill JE, et al: Infectious complications in liver transplantation. *Arch Surg* 1988;123:360–4.

Falagas ME, Snydman DR, Werner BG: Effect of cytomegalovirus infection status on first-year mortality rates among orthotopic liver transplant recipients. The Boston Center for Liver Transplantation CMVIG Study Group. *Ann Intern Med* 1997;126:275–9.

George DL, Arnow PM, Fox A, et al: Patterns of infection after pediatric liver transplantation. *Am J Dis Child* 1992;146:924–9.

George DL, Arnow PM, Fox AS, et al: Bacterial infection as a complication of liver transplantation: Epidemiology and risk factors. *Rev Infect Dis* 1991;13:387–96.

Kusne S, Dummer JS, Singh N, et al: Infections after liver transplantation: An analysis of 101 consecutive cases. *Medicine* 1988;67:132–43.

Winston DJ, Emmanouilides C, Busuttil RW: Infections in liver transplant recipients. *Clin Infect Dis* 1995;21:1077–91.

Cardiac and Pulmonary Transplantation

Arcasoy SM, Kotloff RM: Lung transplantation. *N Engl J Med* 1999; 340:1081–91.

Bolman RM, Saffitz JE: Early postoperative care of the cardiac transplantation patient: Routine consideration and immunosuppressive therapy. *Prog Cardiovasc Dis* 1990;33:137–148.

Braunlin EA, Canter CE, Olivari MT, et al: Rejection and infection after pediatric cardiac transplantation. *Ann Thorac Surg* 1990;49:385–90.

Cisneros JM, Munoz P, Torres-Cisneros J, et al: Pneumonia after heart transplantation: A multiinstitutional study. Spanish Transplantation Infection Study Group. *Clin Infect Dis* 1998;27:324–31.

Hall WA, Martinez AJ, Dummer JS, et al: Central nervous system infections in heart and heart-lung transplant recipients. *Arch Neurol* 1989;46:173–7.

Haydock DA, Trulock EP, Kaiser LR, et al: Lung transplantation. *J Thorac Cardiovasc Surg* 1992;103:329–40.

Maurer JR, Tullis E, Grossman RF, et al: Infectious complications following isolated lung transplantation. *Chest* 1992;101:1056–9.

Petri WA Jr: Infections in heart transplant recipients. *Clin Infect Dis* 1994;18:141–8.

Sable CA, Donowitz GR: Infections in bone marrow transplant recipients. *Clin Infect Dis* 1994;18:273–84.

Scott JP, Higenbottam TW, Smyth RL, et al: Transbronchial biopsies in children after heart-lung transplantation. *Pediatrics* 1990;86:698–702.

CHAPTER 101

The Vulnerable Host

Dennis A. Conrad

Congenital and acquired abnormalities in the structure and function of the major organ systems of the body can impair physiologic function and contribute to vulnerability to infection. Certain medical conditions are strongly associated with increased risk of infection by specific pathogens. These predisposing conditions include asplenia and polysplenia syndromes, homozygous S hemoglobinopathy (sickle cell disease), diabetes mellitus, trisomy 21, protein-energy malnutrition, iron-overload syndrome, and nephrotic syndrome (Table 101–1).

ASPLENIA AND POLYSPLENIA

Asplenia is the congenital absence of any splenic tissue. **Polysplenia** is a condition of multiple, anatomically displaced, dysfunctional splenic-tissue remnants. Both conditions are usually associated with complex congenital heart disease; asplenia is associated with right isomerism, and polysplenia is associated with left isomerism. In addition to congenital abnormalities, asplenia may also result from either splenectomy secondary to trauma or gradual loss of functional splenic tissue, as is seen after multiple infarction episodes in the sickling hemoglobinopathies. As the spleen is an important immunologic organ, functioning by opsonization and reticuloendothelial clearance of encapsulated bacteria, absence diminishes host response to invasive disease.

All patients who lack a spleen are at increased risk of bacteremia caused by encapsulated bacteria, with an overall risk of septicemia that is approximately 10 times that of the general population. Those patients who have lost a spleen secondary to trauma are the least likely to suffer septicemia with encapsulated bacteria because the previous functional spleen allowed appropriate processing of bacterial antigens and production of specific antibodies. Persons with congenital splenic absence are at the greatest risk of septicemia, and persons with sickle cell disease are at intermediate risk.

Streptococcus pneumoniae is the most significant pathogen in patients who lack a functional spleen, accounting for 50–90% of all bacteremic episodes. Other important pathogens in asplenia include *Haemophilus influenzae*, *Neisseria meningitidis*, and *Salmonella.* Septicemia due to *Capnocytophaga canimorsus* in asplenic persons can follow soft tissue infection arising from animal bites. Although it does not increase the risk of infection, asplenia increases the severity of malaria and babesiosis.

Vaccination

Children with sickle cell disease and asplenia should receive routine vaccines, including the conjugate pneumococcal and *H. influenzae* vaccines, and also the pneumococcal and quadrivalent meningococcal polysaccharide vaccines at 2 years of age. Older children and adults with asplenia who were not immunized or were partially immunized should receive conjugate pneumococcal and *H. influenzae* type b vaccines and polysaccharide pneumococcal and meningococcal vaccines according to age (Chapter 17).

Patients who are anticipated to undergo elective splenectomy, such as for treatment of hereditary spherocytosis, should receive these vaccines as soon as possible and at least one dose of these vaccines more than 2 weeks before splenectomy in order to optimize host response. Patients immunized with polyvalent polysaccharide pneumococcal vaccine during childhood should be reimmunized with a second dose 3–5 years later and before the age of 10 years to boost waning humoral immunity. Adult patients should also receive a second pneumococcal vaccination 6 years after primary immunization to increase specific antipneumococcal serum antibody, in spite of a slight risk of severe local or systemic reaction to reimmunization.

Penicillin Prophylaxis. Daily administration of oral penicillin (penicillin V, 125 mg orally twice daily for children less than 5 years of age; 250 mg orally twice daily for older children and adults) or parenteral administration of long-acting penicillin (penicillin G benzathine, 600,000 U intramuscularly every 3–4 weeks for children <60 pounds; 1,200,000 U intramuscularly every 3–4 weeks for children ≥60 pounds) is recommended to diminish the risk of pneumococcal bacteremia in patients with asplenia and is effective, especially in conjunction with immunization (Table 101–2). Unfortunately the optimal duration of penicillin chemoprophylaxis is undetermined, and defining an appropriate antibacterial alternative for populations with increased prevalence of penicillin-resistant *S. pneumoniae* has not been resolved. Penicillin prophylaxis should be continued indefinitely for patients with sickle cell disease who have had a prior episode of pneumococcal sepsis. Penicillin prophylaxis may be discontinued at 5 years of age in children who have not had a prior severe pneumococcal infection or splenectomy. These children must continue to have ready access to comprehensive medical care, and all febrile episodes should receive prompt medical evaluation. In circumstances in which this is not feasible, penicillin prophylaxis should continue. Similarly, penicillin prophylaxis may be discontinued after 2 years following posttraumatic splenectomy in adults. For those persons at highest risk of severe pneumococcal infection, such as congenital asplenia, penicillin prophylaxis should continue throughout life.

Febrile Illnesses. Immunoprophylaxis and chemoprophylaxis reduce, but do not eliminate, the risk of bacteremia in these patients. Febrile episodes must be promptly evaluated. *S. pneumoniae* remains the principal pathogen, regardless of immunization status or compliant penicillin prophylaxis. All patients with fever should be promptly evaluated by history, physical examination, CBC count, blood culture, and chest radiograph. Urinalysis, urine culture, lumbar puncture, and other specific evaluations should be individualized on the basis of patient age, history, physical examination, and physician concern. Empirical therapy with an agent active against *S. pneumoniae, H. influenzae* type b, and *N. meningitidis* should be initiated after evaluation of the patient. Depending on the patient's

TABLE 101–1. Organ System Dysfunction Predisposing to Infection

Abnormal Condition	Important Pathogens	Clinical Infections
Facial		
Cleft lip and palate	*Streptococcus pneumoniae* *Haemophilus influenzae* *Moraxella catarrhalis*	Otitis media
Cardiopulmonary		
Valvular heart disease	Viridans streptococci *Staphylococcus aureus* *Enterococcus*	Endocarditis
Cyanotic heart disease with right-to-left shunt	Viridans-streptococci *S. aureus* *Nocardia asteroides* Anaerobic bacteria	Brain abscess
Pulmonary hypertension	Respiratory syncytial virus	Severe bronchiolitis
Pulmonary edema	*S. pneumoniae* *H. influenzae* *Klebsiella pneumoniae*	Pneumonia
Cystic fibrosis	*Pseudomonas aeruginosa* *S. aureus* *H. influenzae*	Chronic pneumonitis, progressive respiratory failure
Gastrointestinal		
Achlorhydria	*Salmonella typhi* Nontyphoidal *Salmonella*	Enterocolitis, enteric fever
Inflammatory bowel disease	Nontyphoidal *Salmonella* *Shigella*	Enterocolitis
Cirrhosis	*S. pneumoniae* *Vibrio vulnificus* *Listeria monocytogenes* *Yersinia enterocolitica*	Septicemia, pneumonia, enterocolitis, hepatic abscess
Neuromuscular		
Werdnig-Hoffmann disease	Viridans streptococci Anaerobic bacteria *S. pneumoniae* *H. influenzae*	Pneumonia
Meningomyelocele	*Escherichia coli* *S. aureus* Coagulase negative-staphylococci	Urinary tract infection, meningitis, ventriculitis
Encephalocele	*S. pneumoniae* Group A *Streptococcus* Viridans streptococci	Meningitis
Paralysis	*S. aureus* *Bacteroides fragilis* Enterobacteriaceae	Infected decubitus ulcers
Cutaneous		
Scaling dermatitides	*S. aureus* Group A *Streptococcus* *Candida*	Impetigo, pyoderma Mucocutaneous candidiasis
Thermal injury	*P. aeruginosa* *S. aureus* *Candida* *Aspergillus*	Septicemia Cellulitis
Hematopoietic		
Iron-overload syndrome	*Y. enterocolitica* *Yersinia pseudotuberculosis* *V. vulnificus*	Enterocolitis, hepatic abscess, septicemia
Asplenia, polysplenia, sickle cell disease	*S. pneumoniae* *H. influenzae* *Neisseria meningitidis* Non-typhoidal *Salmonella*	Septicemia Pneumonia, skeletal infections
Glucose-6-phosphate dehydrogenase deficiency	*S. aureus* *E. coli* *Serratia marcescens* *Rickettsia rickettsii*	Septicemia, pneumonia, cellulitis

TABLE 101–1. Organ System Dysfunction Predisposing to Infection *(Continued)*

Abnormal Condition	Important Pathogens	Clinical Infections
Renal		
Nephrotic syndrome	*S. pneumoniae* *E. coli* *H. influenzae*	Peritonitis, septicemia, pneumonia
Endocrine		
Diabetes mellitus	*S. aureus* *K. pneumoniae* *B. fragilis* *Candida* species Agents of zygomycosis	Septicemia, pneumonia, urinary tract infection, pyomyositis, sinusitis
Multiorgan		
Trisomy 21	*S. pneumoniae* *H. influenzae* *Mycoplasma pneumoniae*	Pneumonia, sinusitis, tracheitis
Malnutrition	*L. monocytogenes* *Mycobacterium tuberculosis* *Pneumocystis carinii* *Salmonella* *Candida* Coxsackie B virus	Septicemia, pneumonia, enteric fever, disseminated disease

appearance, clinical suspicion, and estimate of the patient's compliance, therapy may be administered on an inpatient or outpatient basis, pending culture results and clinical course. Older patients who appear to be clinically stable, have not had an episode of pneumococcal sepsis previously, and are known to be compliant may be treated with a single dose of ceftriaxone (50–100 mg/kg intramuscularly) as outpatients, returning the next day for re-evaluation and culture review. Under any other circumstance, febrile patients with asplenia should be hospitalized for empirical therapy, even if for only 24–72 hours until culture results are known. Recommended regimens include cefotaxime (100–200 mg/kg/day divided every 6–8 hours intravenously) or ceftriaxone (50–100 mg/kg/day divided every 12–24 hours intravenously), with the addition of vancomycin (60 mg/kg/day divided every 6–8 hours intravenously) if pneumococcal meningitis is suspected.

SICKLE CELL DISEASE

Children with sickle cell disease, especially if homozygous S, are at increased risk of infection, largely as the result of functional asplenia. The risk of invasive *S. pneumoniae* infection is 30–100 times that of the general population and tends to occur primarily in children younger than 5 years of age. The leading cause of death in patients 1–3 years of age with homozygous hemoglobin S disease is infection. The risk among children with hemoglobin SC disease is lower than among those with sickle cell disease, but higher than in healthy children.

The high risk of pneumococcal infections among persons with sickle cell disease is caused by the combination of low levels of circulating antibodies, splenic dysfunction, and complement deficiency, resulting in decreased clearance of encapsulated bacteria from the bloodstream. In addition, tissue microinfarcts occur during vaso-occlusive episodes that predispose to infection. Splenic dysfunction and bone infarctions account for the high incidence of bacterial osteomyelitis seen in these patients. In addition to *Staphylococcus aureus, Salmonella* and *Proteus mirabilis* are important pathogens. The risk of salmonella osteomyelitis in patients with sickle cell disease may be more than 400 times that of the general population. The risk of enteric fever is also greatly increased, and the infection is more severe in this population; septicemia and salmonellosis can result in a mortality rate as high as 25%.

Acute chest syndrome is defined as fever and newly abnormal chest radiograph findings in a patient with sickle cell disease. Pulmonary infarction is a cause of the syndrome and occurs with a greater frequency in adult patients; infection is the more probable cause in children. Significant pathogens include *S. pneumoniae, Mycoplasma pneumoniae, Chlamydia pneumoniae,* and the respiratory viruses. *M. pneumoniae* may account for 15% of all episodes of acute chest syndrome, producing disproportionately severe illness compared with infection in the general population. Although parvovirus B19 infection has been associated with acute chest syndrome, the more significant manifestation of the disease is aplastic crisis (Chapter 26).

Acute pain crisis, arising from a vaso-occlusive episode leading to tissue hypoperfusion, ischemia, and infarction, can be precipitated by occult infection, especially pneumonia and urinary tract infection.

Like patients with asplenia, children with sickle cell disease, especially homozygous hemoglobin S disease, should receive bacterial vaccinations, penicillin prophylaxis, and evaluation of febrile illnesses.

GLUCOSE-6-PHOSPHATE DEHYDROGENASE DEFICIENCY

Glucose-6-phosphate dehydrogenase (G6PD) deficiency, largely occurring in the United States in African Americans and often coincident with sickle cell disease, is associated with increased risk of infection, especially in severe deficiency (less than 10% activity), through a defect in intracellular killing by polymorphonuclear leukocytes. Patients are at increased risk of infection due to *S. aureus, Salmonella, Escherichia coli, Klebsiella pneumoniae,*

TABLE 101–2. Prophylaxis for Individuals With Anatomic and Functional Asplenia

Immunoprophylaxis	
Vaccine	**Regimen**
Conjugated pneumococcal vaccine	Initial: Infants: routine childhood immunization Children ≥12 mo and adults: 2 doses 2 mo apart Reimmunization: not established
Polyvalent polysaccharide pneumococcal vaccine	Initial: High risk children: ≥2 years of age Reimmunization: 3–5 years after primary immunization and before 10 years of age (children); 6 years after primary immunization (adults)
Quadrivalent meningococcal vaccine	Initial: High risk children: ≥2 years of age Reimmunization: 2–3 years after primary immunization
Conjugated *Haemophilus influenzae* type b vaccine	Initial: Infants: routine childhood immunization Children ≥12 mo and adults: 2 doses 2 mo apart Reimmunization: not recommended
Chemoprophylaxis	
Antibotic	**Regimen**
Penicillin V	125 mg bid PO (children <5 years of age) 250 mg bid PO (children ≥5 years of age)
Penicillin G benzathine	600,000 U every 3–4 weeks IM (<27.21 kg [60 lb]) 1,200,000 U every 3–4 weeks IM (≥27.21 kg [60 lb])

Serratia marcescens, and *Chromobacterium violaceum.* When Rocky Mountain spotted fever occurs in these patients, the illness may be of significantly greater severity.

IRON-OVERLOAD SYNDROME

Bacteria require iron as an essential factor for growth and multiplication. The host normally restricts the amount of ionic iron available in body fluids by forming complexes with the binding proteins **transferrin** and **lactoferrin,** resulting in iron concentrations that are too low to readily support bacterial growth. When this balance is upset in the iron-overload syndrome, excess iron becomes available to supplement bacterial metabolism, which in turn can increase the virulence of the organism. This condition can be further complicated when iron-overload syndrome is treated with an iron-chelator such as deferoxamine, which is a siderophore that binds ferric iron, converting the inorganic iron into a compound available for bacterial incorporation. Some bacteria, such as *Yersinia enterocolitica,* cannot synthesize a siderophore; the presence of iron bound to deferoxamine allows use by this organism, substantially increasing pathogenicity.

The virulence of certain microorganisms, such as *Y. enterocolitica, Yersinia pseudotuberculosis, Listeria monocytogenes, Vibrio vulnificus, Candida albicans,* and *Brucella* increases significantly in the presence of iron-overload syndrome, especially if associated with chelation therapy. However, confounding variables such as hepatic failure and cirrhosis, cardiac dysfunction, and diabetes mellitus are also present in these patients. The strongest independent association specifically between the iron-overload syndrome and opportunistic infection occurs for *Y. enterocolitica.*

The most common clinical manifestations of infections in iron-overload syndrome are bacteremia, enterocolitis, and hepatic abscess, the latter often presenting as multiple liver lesions. The other gastrointestinal manifestations, which occur less frequently, include ileal perforation, mesenteric lymphadenitis, and peritonitis. Organisms are usually acquired by ingestion of contaminated food, such as *Yersinia* in contaminated dairy products and meat, *L. monocytogenes* in unpasteurized cheese and unwashed vegetables, *V. vulnificus* in uncooked shellfish, and *Brucella* in dairy products and also by direct animal contact. The host ingests the organism, and the underlying iron-overload syndrome promotes invasive disease. Previously healthy children accidentally ingesting an amount of iron sufficiently large to require deferoxamine treatment have subsequently developed invasive disease due to *Y. enterocolitica* arising from prior gastrointestinal colonization.

Recognition of the conditions that predispose to the iron-overload syndrome, such as β-thalassemia, hemochromatosis, or receipt of multiple blood transfusions, is most important in reducing the risk of these infections. Persons with these conditions should avoid unpasteurized or improperly pasteurized dairy products, incompletely cooked meats (internal temperatures ≤76.6°C [170°F]), and uncooked shellfish. Fever, especially associated with gastrointestinal symptoms, should be promptly evaluated. When the cause of the infection is unclear, empirical antibiotic therapy directed against *Yersinia* and *V. vulnificus* should be instituted pending culture results and clinical course.

DIABETES MELLITUS

The increased risk of infection seen in diabetes mellitus occurs most prominently in adult patients, although adolescents also have an increased, albeit somewhat less pronounced risk. The primary defect is one of abnormal polymorphonuclear function involving adherence, chemotaxis, phagocytosis, and intracellular killing. Hyperglycemia, especially if associated with glucosuria, increases the frequency of mucocutaneous candidiasis, especially perineal candidiasis.

Infections that occur with increased frequency and severity with diabetes mellitus include urinary tract infections, septicemia due to gram-negative bacteria, soft tissue infections, tuberculosis, superficial and deep mycosis, and malignant otitis externa. Pyomyositis of the legs (with >90% of episodes caused by *S. aureus*) and feet (with *Bacteroides fragilis* the most important pathogen causing diabetic foot infections) is a focal musculoskeletal infection of particular importance.

Patients with diabetes mellitus have an increased frequency of sinusitis, with *S. aureus* and viridans streptococci the most important bacterial causes. The agents of zygomycosis, including *Mucor, Rhizopus,* and *Aspergillus* species, can cause a devastating, locally aggressive fungal sinusitis that may be fatal. These patients have a risk three times greater than that of the general population of gastrointestinal salmonellosis and enteric fever, which is promoted by decreased gastric acidity and prolonged gastrointestinal transient time due to autonomic neuropathy. *K. pneumoniae* infections occur with greater frequency because of global polymorphonuclear leukocyte dysfunction. This pathogen is especially prone to cause pneumonia, myonecrosis, urinary tract infection, and septicemia in these patients.

The most effective therapy that reduces the frequency of infection in patients with diabetes mellitus is strict serum glucose control, maintenance of euglycemia, and avoidance of ketoacidosis.

NEPHROTIC SYNDROME

Nephrotic syndrome results in diminished complement and IgG serum concentrations, with resultant increased risk of infection, especially bacterial peritonitis and bacterial pneumonia. The incidence of **primary** or **spontaneous bacterial peritonitis** in children with nephrotic syndrome is 6–17%, with 80% of episodes occurring during disease relapse or corticosteroid therapy. *S. pneumoniae* and *E. coli* are the pathogens of greatest importance in this infection.

Respiratory infection and septicemia due to *H. influenzae* occur with increased frequency in patients with nephrotic syndrome. Immunization with *H. influenzae* type b vaccine appears to provide incomplete protection against systemic infection in these patients.

Children with nephrotic syndrome should receive routine vaccines, including the conjugate pneumococcal and *H. influenzae* vaccines, and also the pneumococcal polysaccharide vaccine at 2 years of age. Protection against subsequent infection is incomplete, and reimmunization with the polysaccharide pneumococcal vaccine should be given 3–6 years after primary immunization, despite the slight risk of adverse reaction to a second dose of vaccine.

Penicillin prophylaxis has also been employed in patients with nephrotic syndrome, although the benefit is less well established than in patients with asplenia. Moreover, an increased frequency of systemic infection with penicillin-resistant *S. pneumoniae* has occurred when penicillin chemoprophylaxis had been used in communities with an increased prevalence of penicillin-resistant *S. pneumoniae* strains.

TRISOMY 21

Trisomy 21 (Down syndrome) is associated with abnormal cell-mediated and humoral immunity, abnormal inflammatory response, diminished interferon production, and reduced production of IgG subclasses IgG2 and IgG4. The net effect of the immunodeficiency associated with trisomy 21 is a significantly increased rate of bacterial respiratory infections, especially sinusitis, tracheitis, and pneumonia. Important pathogens include *S. pneumoniae* and *H. influenzae*. Unusually severe pneumonia due to *M. pneumoniae* has occurred in patients with trisomy 21.

One study (Annerén et al, 1990) showed that IgG subclass deficiency can be partially corrected with selenium supplementation (10 μg/kg orally daily for 6 months), resulting in a decreased frequency of recurrent respiratory tract infections in selected patients. Children with trisomy 21 should receive routine vaccines, including the conjugate pneumococcal and *H. influenzae* vaccines, and also the pneumococcal polysaccharide vaccine at 2 years of age and should be immunized annually against influenza.

MALNUTRITION

The most significant detriment to the health of children worldwide is total-calorie protein-deficient malnutrition. The United States is largely spared from the same prevalence of human malnutrition that is currently occurring in developing nations, but severe malnutrition still occurs in selected population groups in this country. Malnourishment affects cellular and humoral immune response, causing diminished T-lymphocyte activity that results in anergy, reduced secretory IgA production, impaired host response to polysaccharide antigens, defective complement activation, and dysfunctional phagocytosis. Malnutrition increases the mortality from respiratory tract infections, especially pneumonia, to three times that of a well-nourished population.

Pathogens of significant importance in malnourished populations include *L. monocytogenes, Salmonella,* coxsackie B virus, *Mycobacterium tuberculosis, P. carinii,* and *Candida.* Shigellosis, occurring with the same incidence as in well-nourished populations of similar hygienic standards, more often results in death in a malnourished population, especially in young children. Measles virus, influenza virus, and other respiratory viruses exact an increased lethal toll in malnourished populations.

Correction of the immunodeficiencies associated with malnutrition is achieved by adequate daily consumption of requisite calories and minimal protein requirements. Vitamin A supplementation significantly reduces the risk of death associated with measles infection. In addition to dietary correction, improvement in commu-

TABLE 101–3. Special Vaccination Requirements for the Vulnerable Host

Vaccine	Underlying Medical Condition for Which Immunization Is Recommended
Pneumococcal conjugate and polysaccharide vaccines	Routine childhood immunization (conjugate pneumococcal vaccine)
	Diabetes mellitus
	Alcoholic cirrhosis
	Asplenia or polysplenia*
	Postsplenectomy*
	Sickle cell disease (hemoglobin SS)*
	Nephrotic syndrome*
	Cerebrospinal fluid leakage syndromes
	Medical immunosuppression
	Chronic renal failure or uremia*
	Cardiovascular disease
	Pulmonary disease
	Bone marrow or solid organ transplantation*
Quadrivalent meningococcal vaccine	Asplenia or polysplenia
	Terminal complement component deficiency
Haemophilus influenzae type b vaccine	Routine childhood immunization
	Asplenia or polysplenia*
	Postsplenectomy*
	Sickle cell disease (hemoglobin SS)†
Influenza virus vaccine‡	Diabetes mellitus
	Alcoholic cirrhosis
	Chronic renal failure or uremia
	Cardiovascular disease
	Pulmonary disease
Hepatitis A virus vaccine	Chronic liver disease
Hepatitis B virus vaccine	Routine childhood immunization
	Chronic renal failure or uremia
	Hemodialysis

*Reimmunize children 3–5 years after initial vaccination by the age of 10 years at time of second immunization; reimmunize adults 6 or more years after initial vaccination.
†May require reimmunization after the age of 5 years.
‡Given annually regardless of underlying condition.

nity sanitation practices, reduction in population habitation density, and universal childhood immunization against vaccine-preventable diseases will reduce the prevalence of infection to match that of developed nations.

SPECIAL VACCINATION REQUIREMENTS FOR THE VULNERABLE HOST

Exceptions to routine immunization procedures must be made when vaccinating the vulnerable host, defined as those with primary or secondary immunodeficiency (excluding specifically persons infected with the human immunodeficiency virus), those immunosuppressed by virtue of cancer or therapy, or those who are at increased risk of infections because of an underlying condition.

Immunocompromised patients should not be immunized with live-virus vaccines, with the exceptions of measles and varicella vaccinations for children with HIV infection who have no symptoms. Oral polio vaccine should not be given to immunocompromised persons or any household contacts because of the risk of transmission. Similarly, oral typhoid vaccine should not be administered to immunocompromised persons. For patients receiving cancer chemotherapy or any immunosuppressive agent, vaccination should preferably precede these treatments by at least 2 weeks. Patients with hematogenous cancer in remission who have received no anticancer chemotherapy within the preceding 3 months should not be considered immunocompromised for immunization purposes.

Immunocompromising conditions, such as chronic renal failure, diabetes mellitus, alcoholic cirrhosis, and asplenia, warrant use of selected vaccines in addition to those given routinely to all children (Table 101–3).

REVIEWS

Advisory Committee on Immunization Practices: Use of vaccines and immune globulins in persons with altered immunocompetence. *MMWR Morb Mortal Wkly Rep* 1993;42:1–18.

Hershko C, Peto TEA, Weatherall DJ: Iron and infection. *Br Med J* 1988;296:660–4.

Styrt B: Infection associated with asplenia: Risks, mechanisms, and prevention. *Am J Med* 1990;88:33N–42N.

KEY ARTICLES

Wright J, Thomas P, Serjeant GR: Septicemia caused by *Salmonella* infection: An overlooked complication of sickle cell disease. *J* Pediatr 1997;130:394–9.

Anderson B, Goldsmith GH, Spagnuolo PJ: Neutrophil adhesive dysfunction in diabetes mellitus: The role of cellular and plasma factors. *J Lab Clin Med* 1988;111:275–85.

Anneréen G, Magnusson CG, Lilja G, et al: Abnormal serum lgG subclass pattern in children with Down's syndrome. *Arch Dis Child* 1992; 67:628–31.

Anneréen G, Magnusson CG, Nordvall SL: Increase in serum concentrations of IgG_2 and IgG_4 by selenium supplementation in children with Down's syndrome. *Arch Dis Child* 1990;65:1353–5.

Berkowitz FE: Infections in children with severe protein-energy malnutrition. *Pediatr Infect Dis J* 1992;11:750–9.

Bernard DB: Extrarenal complications of the nephrotic syndrome. *Kidney Int* 1988;33:1184–202.

Chandra RK: Protein-energy malnutrition and immunological responses. *J Nutr* 1992;122:597–600.

Cullingford GL, Watkins DN, Watts ADJ, et al: Severe late postsplenectomy infection. *Br J Surg* 1991;78:716–21.

Desenclos JA, Klontz KC, Wolfe LE, et al: The risk of *Vibrio* illness in the Florida raw oyster eating population, 1981–1988. *Am J Epidemiol* 1991;134:290–7.

Falletta JM, Woods GM, Verter JI, et al: Discontinuing penicillin prophylaxis in children with sickle cell anemia. *J Pediatr* 1995;127:685–90.

Hongeng S, Wilimas JA, Harris S, et al: Recurrent *Streptococcus pneumoniae* sepsis in children with sickle cell disease. *J Pediatr* 1997;130:814–6.

Johnston JM, Becker SF, McFarland LM: *Vibrio vulnificus:* Man and the sea. *JAMA* 1985;253:2850–3.

Mazzoleni G, deSa D, Gately J, et al: *Yersinia enterocolitica* infection with ileal perforation associated with iron overload and deferoxamine therapy. *Digest Dis Sci* 1991;36:1154–60.

Rogers ZR, Morrison RA, Vedro DA, et al: Outpatient management of febrile illness in infants and young children with sickle cell anemia. *J Pediatr* 1990;117:736–9.

Wong WY, Overturf GD, Powars DR: Infection caused by *Streptococcus pneumoniae* in children with sickle cell disease: Epidemiology, immunologic mechanisms, prophylaxis, and vaccination. *Clin Infect Dis* 1992;14:1124–36.

Wright J, Thomas P, Serjeant GR: Septicemia caused by *Salmonella* infection: An overlooked complication in sickle cell disease. *J Pediatr* 1997;130:394–9.

CHAPTER 102

Infections in Daycare Environments

Ellen R. Wald

Approximately 75% of the mothers of children younger than 5 years work outside the home; the 12 million children of these women receive some form of daycare outside of the home. Many factors contribute to the transmission of infectious agents in the daycare setting. Most important are host factors relating to the immunologic susceptibility of young children. Once an infection is established it is easily transmitted because of the natural tendency for intimacy in an age group that has not established mature toileting practices and is ignorant of basic hygienic practices. Toys become contaminated with respiratory and gastrointestinal pathogens. Caregivers may be insufficiently trained in infection control practices. A lack of policy regarding immunization and health care screening for employees may contribute to the spread of infection.

Overcrowding, understaffing, and poorly designed physical environments contribute to the transmission of illness in daycare. It is important to separate children who wear diapers from those who are older to limit transmission of enteric illnesses. It is essential to separate meal preparation areas from toilet areas. If food is brought from home, it should be properly transported and stored to avoid spoilage. Lack of attention to this issue may result in additional illness. Finally, parents sometimes do not voluntarily withdraw ill children from daycare because of the expense and inconvenience of making alternative care arrangements.

MODES OF DAYCARE TRANSMISSION OF INFECTIOUS DISEASES

Many pathogens and modes of transmission are associated with infections in daycare environments. (Table 102–1) Respiratory infections are by far the most common cause of illness among infants, toddlers, and preschoolers, whether or not they attend daycare.

Respiratory Transmission of Infection

Many microbiologic species that cause infection are spread by **airborne transmission.** For these agents, the organism is **aerosolized** and remains in the air like cigarette smoke. Direct contact with the infected person is not necessary for airborne spread of the infection. Agents that are transmitted in this way include measles, varicella, and tuberculosis.

More commonly, respiratory organisms are spread by **droplet transmission,** with the production of droplets laden with infective particles. These droplets may be transmitted directly from mucosa to mucosa (nasal, oropharyngeal, or conjunctival) when there is close physical contact. More often, droplets land on nonporous surfaces (cribs, tables, chairs) or on fomites (clothes and paper) and remain infective from minutes to hours. Hand contact with contaminated surfaces and fomites may then result in infection if the hands touch the nasal or conjunctival mucosa. Agents that can be transmitted by droplet spread (mucosa to mucosa), by finger-to-mucosa contact, or by fomites include most respiratory viruses (RSV, rhinoviruses, influenza viruses, parainfluenza viruses, adenoviruses, measles, mumps, rubella, and varicella-zoster virus), *Streptococcus pneumoniae, Haemophilus influenzae* type b, *Neisseria meningitidis,* and group A *Streptococcus.* Finger-to-mucosa spread of respiratory pathogens is the most important and common mechanism for transmission of viral and bacterial infection. Consequently, hand washing is essential to preventing the spread of infection.

Gastrointestinal Transmission of Infection

Spread of gastrointestinal organisms is by **fecal-oral transmission.** The inoculum of organisms required to produce an infection (Table 3–4) influences whether infection occurs by person-to-person spread or whether a food or fluid intermediary is required. Rotavirus, *Giardia lamblia,* and *Shigella* infections are readily transmitted by very small numbers of organisms found on the hands after person-to-person contact or after touching infected surfaces, even without obvious gross contamination. In contrast, *Salmonella,* rarely a cause of diarrheal outbreaks in the daycare setting, requires large numbers of organisms to produce infection. Accordingly, an intermediary step of food or beverage contamination is required to allow organisms to replicate up to the necessary inocula.

Numerous studies in daycare centers have demonstrated fecal organisms on environmental surfaces with which infants and toddlers have had contact. The contamination of the environment is highest when the children are younger than 3 years of age. This age predilection correlates with the number of children still wearing diapers. Important pathogens, including rotavirus, hepatitis A virus, and *G. lamblia* cysts are able to survive on environmental surfaces for periods ranging from hours to weeks.

Skin Disease and Transmission of Infection by Direct Contact

Bacterial, viral, and parasitic infections can be transmitted from person to person by **direct contact.** Bacterial pathogens such as group A *Streptococcus* and *Staphylococcus aureus* are usually not primarily invasive unless there is a break in the integument as might occur with minor trauma such as insect bites. Herpes simplex virus (HSV) may be transmitted from skin or mucosa to skin by direct contact, again only if the skin is broken. Infestations such as scabies and lice and the superficial dermatophytes responsible for tinea infections (*Trichophyton, Microsporum,* and *Epidermophyton*) are transmitted from person to person or by contact with infected fomites, such as combs, hairbrushes, and hats.

Blood, Saliva, and Urine Transmission of Infection

Hepatitis B virus, hepatitis C virus, and human immunodeficiency virus (HIV) are **bloodborne pathogens** that are usually transmitted from adult to adult by **bloodborne transmission.** This includes intravenous drug use and sharing of contaminated syringes and needles and sexual activity, which presumably causes mild trauma, thereby leading to exposure to blood. Although both HBV and HIV can be detected in urine and saliva, exchange of these body

TABLE 102–1. Pathogens and Modes of Transmission of Infections in Daycare

Mode of Transmission	Bacteria	Viruses	Others
Respiratory	*Streptococcus pneumoniae*	Adenovirus	
	Haemophilus influenzae type b	Influenzae A and B viruses	
	Neisseria meningitidis	Measles	
	Group A *Streptococcus*	Mumps	
	Bordetella pertussis	Parainfluenza viruses	
	Corynebacterium diphtheriae	Parvovirus B19	
	Mycobacterium tuberculosis	Respiratory syncytial virus	
		Rhinoviruses	
		Varicella-zoster virus	
Fecal-oral	*Salmonella*	Enteroviruses	*Cryptosporidium parvum*
	Shigella	Rotaviruses	*Giardia lamblia*
	Campylobacter jejuni	Norwalk virus	*Enterobius vermicularis*
	Yersinia enterocolitica	Enteric adenoviruses	
	Escherichia coli O157:H7	Caliciviruses	
	Clostridium difficile	Astroviruses	
		Hepatitis A viruses	
Person to person by direct contact	Group A *Streptococcus*	Herpes simplex virus	*Pediculus humanus capitis*
	Staphylococcus aureus	Varicella-zoster virus	*Pediculus humanus*
			Sarcoptes scabiei (scabies)
			Trichophyton
			Microsporum
Contact with blood		Hepatitis B virus	
		Hepatitis C virus	
		Human immunodeficiency virus	
Contact with saliva		Cytomegalovirus	
		Hepatitis B virus	
		Herpes simplex types 1 and 2	
		Human herpesvirus type 6	
		Human herpesvirus type 7	
		Human herpesvirus type 8	
Contact with urine		Cytomegalovirus	

Modified with permission from American Academy of Pediatrics: Recommendations for care of children in special circumstances: Children in out-of-home child care. In *2000 Red Book: Report of the Committee on Infectious Diseases*, 25th ed. American Academy of Pediatrics, 2000.

fluids is highly unlikely to transmit infection. In daycare, CMV is probably transmitted by contamination of toys with saliva. Mothers and daycare providers may become infected with CMV by the finger-to-mucosa route after hand contamination by urine and saliva. HHV6, HHV7, and HHV8 are also shed in the oral cavity and may be transmitted by saliva from infected persons. CMV may also be transmitted by contaminated urine.

RISK FACTORS FOR INFECTION

The risk factors for spread of infection relate to the age of the participants, the number of children, and the ratio of staff to children (Table 102–2). The staff-to-child ratio is determined in part by the age of the children and the experience of the daycare provider. In overcrowded situations with inadequate staffing, infection is easily spread because of inadequate hand washing and lack of attention to other facets of infection control. An inadequate number of hand washing facilities for both children and providers is an almost insurmountable barrier to infection control.

Factors identified as particularly important in the spread of gastrointestinal organisms are large numbers of diaper-age children in centers where staff members who diaper children are also responsible for food preparation. Likewise, the proximity of diaper-changing stations and food-preparation areas facilitates contamination and spread of disease. Daycare centers that have low staff-to-children ratios are also at high risk of outbreaks of infectious disease; this problem appears to be greatest in centers that operate

TABLE 102–2. Risk Factors for Infectious Disease in the Daycare Setting

Children
- Immunologic susceptibility to infectious agents
- Lack of toilet training
- Natural tendency to intimacy
- Frequent oral contact with environment
- Lack of awareness and practice of good hygiene

Caregivers
- Insufficient training in infection control
- Inadequate screening for chronic infectious diseases

Environmental and Economic Problems
- Inappropriate staff-to-child ratios
- Overcrowding
- Failure to separate age groups
- Poorly designed physical plant
  - Inadequate or poorly placed sinks
  - Failure to separate toilet areas from areas of food preparation
- Parental pressure to admit sick children to daycare

TABLE 102–3. Patterns of Occurrence of Infections in Daycare

Pattern of Occurrence	Example
Clinical manifestation of infection primarily in children	*Haemophilus influenzae* type b Respiratory syncytial virus
Infection affects children, daycare staff, and close family members	*Shigella* *Giardia lamblia* *Neisseria meningitidis*
Inapparent infection in children with clinically apparent disease in adult contacts	Hepatitis A
Inapparent or mild infection in children and adults but may have serious consequences for fetus in pregnant contact	Cytomegalovirus Rubella Parvovirus B19

Modified from Goodman RA, Osterholm MT, Granoff DM, et al: Infectious diseases and child day care. *Pediatrics* 1984;74:134–9.

for profit. Inadequate in-service training and supervision of daycare employees regarding infection control policies are also risk factors for infection.

PATTERNS OF INFECTION IN DAYCARE

Several different patterns of occurrence of infection are experienced by children in daycare (Table 102–3). The children themselves, rather than the staff, experience most of the infectious disease burden in daycare centers. They have an increase in respiratory and gastrointestinal infections above those experienced by children who are cared for entirely at home. Certain agents, such as *H. influenzae* type b, rotavirus, and RSV, infect children almost exclusively. However, adult personnel sometimes experience some of the same respiratory and gastrointestinal infections as the children.

Several infections barely recognizable in a child because they are mild or asymptomatic become serious when they are spread to adults (either parents or daycare providers). The most notable of these is hepatitis A, which in adults is a moderately severe illness that often leads to extended time lost from work. Some infections that are mild in adults are potentially harmful to a fetus, which raises concern if a parent of a daycare attendee or a childcare provider is pregnant. CMV and rubella are associated with severe birth defects if infection occurs in the first trimester. Infection with parvovirus B19 during pregnancy poses a risk of nonimmune hydrops and fetal death.

INFECTIOUS AGENTS IN DAYCARE

Infections Spread by the Respiratory Tract

Infectious agents from the respiratory tract may be spread by direct contact with large droplets, small particles, and fine particles that have been aerosolized. These media may transmit viruses that primarily infect the upper respiratory tract; viruses that cause systemic viral infection (CMV and varicella-zoster virus); group A *Streptococcus,* which causes streptococcal pharyngitis; and bacteria, such as *S. pneumoniae, H. influenzae* type b, and *N. meningitidis,* which can colonize the nasopharynx and may cause systemic disease in susceptible persons.

Streptococcus pneumoniae. Children in daycare have increased rates of pharyngeal pneumococcal carriage from 21–59%, especially of pneumococcal serotypes 14, 23F, and 12F. Daycare attendance increases the risk of invasive pneumococcal infections (2.6-fold risk in children 2–11 months of age, 2.3-fold risk in children 12–23 months of age, and 3.3-fold risk in children 24–59 months of age). Factors associated with carriage of antibiotic-resistant pneumococci include age younger than 2 years, frequent upper respiratory tract infections, frequent use of antibiotics, and history of acute otitis media unresponsive to antibiotic treatment. Childhood immunization with the conjugate pneumococcal vaccine should decrease incidence of invasive disease and may also affect pharyngeal carriage rates.

Haemophilus influenzae Type b. Before routine immunization with the conjugate vaccine, *H. influenzae* type b was the most important bacterial pathogen of children less than 5 years of age, with a risk of disease that was considerably higher in children attending daycare than in those who stayed at home. Appreciation of the potential for spread of this organism among age-susceptible family and daycare contacts led to recommendations for rifampin prophylaxis to prevent secondary or associated cases (Chapter 16). The availability of conjugate vaccine administered in early infancy has already resulted in a markedly decreased incidence of serious disease caused by *H. influenzae* type b and also a decreased rate of pharyngeal carriage.

Neisseria meningitidis. *N. meningitidis* frequently colonizes the nasopharynx, which may lead to sepsis or meningitis in susceptible persons. The attack rate is highest among children 6–12 months of age. Secondary spread of infection with *N. meningitidis* has been recognized as a risk, especially in crowded conditions such as in military barracks, college dormitories (especially among incoming freshmen), and large-group daycare centers. Prompt institution of rifampin prophylaxis to prevent secondary infections is the recommended strategy for management of all intimate contacts of a person with invasive *N. meningitidis* infection (Chapter 16). It is not recommended that throat cultures be performed to identify persons who require rifampin prophylaxis. The cultures may be insensitive, and waiting for results may delay appropriate management. Meningococcal vaccination is recommended for new military recruits and for matriculating college freshmen. The vaccine is recommended only for persons ≥2 years of age and is not routinely recommended for children in daycare.

Group A Streptococcus. Group A *Streptococcus* is a common cause of respiratory and skin infections. Children with group A *Streptococcus* infections of the throat or skin should be excluded from daycare for 24 hours after the initiation of appropriate antibiotic treatment.

Viral Upper Respiratory Tract Infections. Respiratory viruses (rhinoviruses, RSV, parainfluenza viruses, influenza viruses, adenoviruses, and Epstein-Barr virus [EBV]) are the most common causes of infection in preschool children. The range of clinical manifestations includes asymptomatic infection, simple upper respiratory tract infections (rhinitis) sometimes with nonpurulent conjunctivitis, pharyngitis, croup, tracheitis, bronchiolitis, and pneumonitis. Disease may be mild or severe and may involve single or multiple levels of the respiratory tree. Children may experience multiple infections with each agent because of antigenic diversity within virus subtypes (e.g., influenza A), the presence of multiple subtypes (e.g., rhinoviruses), and failure of immunity to develop after a single exposure (e.g., RSV). Viruses are shed from the site of infection (conjunctiva, nose, throat) even before clinical symptoms develop, making it difficult to control the spread of these infections in daycare. There is ample documentation that children in daycare (family or large daycare centers), experience more respiratory infections than children in home care. As the frequency of viral respiratory infections increases in children attending daycare, these children experience a notable increase in the frequency of both otitis media and sinusitis.

It is not recommended that children with mild respiratory tract infections be excluded from daycare or separated from the group of well children. This strategy has not been shown to achieve an overall reduction in the number of infections among children in daycare.

Cytomegalovirus. CMV is a common cause of infection in preschool children, which is usually completely asymptomatic. Rarely a child may experience a febrile illness with lymphadenopathy and hepatosplenomegaly. The source of CMV in the daycare setting is infants and children who have been infected by their mothers by vertical transmission in utero (1–2%), at delivery, or through breastfeeding (approximately 6%). The incidence of infection peaks among children 1–3 years of age, with viral excretion in as many as 70% of children in this age group who attend daycare.

CMV infection poses a risk to the fetus if transmitted to the fetus during early pregnancy as part of the infection of a pregnant daycare provider or mother of a child who attends daycare. The virus may cause clinically evident congenital CMV infection (microcephaly, hepatosplenomegaly, chorioretinitis, psychomotor retardation, and deafness) in approximately 5% of infected children. Another 10–15% of infants experience an occult but potentially damaging infection that causes a mild hearing loss and learning disabilities.

Infection in preschoolers leads to viral shedding documented by positive CMV cultures obtained from swabs of the throat and urine. Transmission probably occurs by respiratory spread or by fomites (e.g., toys and blankets) contaminated with saliva.

Varicella-Zoster Virus. Chickenpox, or primary varicella-zoster virus infection, is a highly contagious infection that affects more than 80% of the population by the age of 10 years. A child with chickenpox should be excluded from daycare and may return 6 days after the onset of the rash, or when all the lesions have dried and crusted.

Lesions of zoster (shingles) are potentially contagious for varicella-zoster virus but pose minimal risk to normal children and staff unless there is direct contact with fluid or drainage. Children with zoster may attend daycare if a dressing can be used to cover the lesions. If the lesions cannot be covered, the child should be excluded from daycare until all the lesions are dried and crusted.

Infections Spread by Gastrointestinal Tract

Salmonella. *Salmonella* is the most common cause of bacterial diarrhea in many parts of the United States, but it is an uncommon cause of outbreaks of gastroenteritis in daycare. Person-to-person spread is very uncommon except in infancy, when the infective dose is small. Exclusion from daycare is recommended until the diarrhea resolves.

Shigella. Infection with *Shigella* causes an illness of variable severity but easy transmissibility. Accordingly, *Shigella* is one of the most common causes of outbreaks of diarrhea in the daycare population. Infection can be caused by as few as 10–100 organisms. Treatment of shigellosis with an appropriate antimicrobial agent effectively terminates the illness.

Campylobacter jejuni. *Campylobacter jejuni* is a more common cause of diarrhea in children than *Shigella,* but it is less likely than *Shigella* to cause outbreaks of diarrheal disease in daycare centers. This phenomenon relates to the usual inoculum required to produce infection. Most often a high inoculum is required to produce infection with *Campylobacter,* necessitating a food or water vehicle. Less often, transmission can occur by person-to-person spread of smaller numbers of organisms. Erythromycin is effective in terminating excretion of the infective organism; this may be important in controlling epidemics or outbreaks. The impact of erythromycin on the clinical course of disease is variable.

Clostridium difficile. *Clostridium difficile* is the classic cause of pseudomembranous colitis in patients who have received or are receiving antimicrobial agents. It rarely causes disease not associated with the use of antimicrobials. Hospital environments and daycare facilities are a reservoir for the organism. Children and personnel should be excluded from daycare until free of symptoms.

Other Bacteria. Outbreaks of diarrheal disease caused by *Escherichia coli* O157:H7 and *Aeromonas* have also been reported to occur in children attending daycare.

Rotavirus. Rotavirus is the most common cause of gastroenteritis in infants and children and the leading cause of hospitalization due to gastroenteritis in industrialized countries, including the United States. It is an important cause of diarrhea in developing countries and contributes substantially to the worldwide mortality figures for gastroenteritis.

Spread of rotavirus infections is extremely common in hospitals; not surprisingly, transmission within a daycare center is very rapid. Treatment is supportive, and exclusion from daycare is recommended until diarrhea resolves. Other viral agents that have been associated with outbreaks of diarrhea in children attending daycare centers are astroviruses and adenoviruses.

Hepatitis A Virus. Hepatitis A virus, an enterovirus, is the most common cause of acute hepatitis in children. Similar to other enteric pathogens, hepatitis A virus is transmitted by the fecal-oral route and is shed in high density in the stool of infected persons from 2 weeks before until 1 week after the onset of clinical symptoms. Transmission is primarily from person to person, but fomites may play an important role because the organism can persist and remain infective in the dried state for months.

Hepatitis A virus can be spread easily in daycare centers with diaper-age children because of the facility of person-to-person transmission. Spread of infection is barely noticeable until an adult contact, usually a parent or daycare worker, has symptomatic hepatitis A. Clusters of cases of hepatitis A in communities have been traced to a single daycare center. Illness in contacts can be prevented with intramuscular immune serum globulin. Hepatitis A vaccine might be useful for parents of children in daycare and those who work as daycare providers.

Giardia lamblia. *G. lamblia* is one of the most common causes of diarrhea in the daycare setting. This parasite infects the duodenum and proximal jejunum, which may result in asymptomatic carriage or clinical disease. After the symptoms resolve either by treatment or by spontaneous cure, the patient may continue to shed cysts for a very long time. Treatment is not recommended for asymptomatic shedding of *G. lamblia* cysts. For patients with symptoms, treatment with metronidazole or albendazole may be given (Table 76–22). Relapses occur in approximately 15% of patients.

Cryptosporidium. *Cryptosporidium* is a cause of severe diarrhea in immunocompromised hosts, but it usually causes a self-limited illness in immunocompetent children or adults. The parasite may be spread from person to person or by food or water. Exclusion from daycare is recommended until the symptoms resolve.

Infections Spread by Skin Contact

Group A Streptococcus. Group A *Streptococcus* has become a less common cause of impetigo and pyoderma in children since 1980, but there has been a concomitant rise in cases caused by *Staphylococcus aureus.* Group A *Streptococcus* can cause infections of traumatized skin (e.g., insect bites, scratches) such as erysipelas and cellulitis that result in the abrupt onset of fever and dramatic cutaneous erythema and tenderness, often accompanied by regional lymphadenopathy. The diagnosis can be established by careful performance of cultures of specimens obtained after careful cleansing of the wound area or of tissue aspirates. The spread of typical impetigo is common within families and presumably also occurs within daycare centers. Children should be excluded from daycare until 24 hours of appropriate antimicrobial therapy (of a 10-day course) has been completed.

Lice. Head lice infestation is common in daycare and school-age children consequent to infection with *Pediculus humanus capitis.* Transmission is by direct contact or by fomite spread of live lice, which is facilitated by common storage of hats and coats.

Scabies. Scabies is an infection of the skin caused by infestation with the female mite *Sarcoptes scabiei.* Transmitted from person to person by an infested person, the mite buries itself beneath the stratum corneum and burrows along for its 30-day life span, laying two to three eggs per day. Transmission of scabies within the daycare setting has only rarely occurred. An infected child should be excluded from daycare for 24 hours after treatment is undertaken. Transmission usually occurs within the family setting.

Infections Spread by Contact with Blood, Saliva, and Urine

Hepatitis B Virus. Transmission of hepatitis B within the daycare setting has been documented on several occasions in the United States. The probable sources were biting by a child who was a carrier of hepatitis B in combination with exudative skin lesions in the child who was bitten. In Japan, where the background prevalence of HBsAg carriage is higher than in the United States, there are data to suggest that transmission of hepatitis B most probably occurs among children in nursery schools. Nonsexual horizontal spread of hepatitis B in an Asian community in Atlanta also supports concern regarding transmission of HBV in daycare settings. Furthermore, studies in the Middle East, China, and Africa also support the nonsexual horizontal transmission of hepatitis B. The current recommendation to screen all parturients for hepatitis B and to provide universal immunization against hepatitis B in infancy should curtail spread of this infection among children in daycare centers in the future.

Human Immunodeficiency Virus. To date, transmission of HIV infection in a daycare center has not been reported. In light of its rare horizontal transmission to nonsexual contacts within households with an infected member, HIV would not be expected to spread easily in daycare centers. The risk of transmission of HIV is less than 1 in 500 exposures, even when there is direct inoculation with HIV-infected blood by needlestick injury to a health care worker. The risk of exposures other than by direct inoculation is far less than 1 in 500. The risk in daycare is even lower. Potential risk factors that might necessitate exclusion from daycare include persistent biting, extensive weeping skin lesions, or bleeding diatheses. Adults who have HIV infection but do not have open and uncoverable skin lesions or other transmissible infections may provide care for children in childcare programs.

Other Viruses. Hepatitis C virus is also a significant bloodborne pathogen, but the low prevalence of hepatitis C virus in children reduces the likelihood of transmission. The risk of transmission of hepatitis C virus from percutaneous exposure is estimated to be 10 times greater than that of HIV, but lower than that of hepatitis B virus. The herpesviruses, including CMV, HHV6, HHV7, and HHV8, are potentially transmissible by contact with blood but are more likely to be transmitted by contact with saliva. CMV can also be transmitted by contact with urine.

Vaccine-Preventable Diseases

Routine childhood immunization programs have eliminated poliomyelitis from the United States and have virtually eliminated pertussis, diptheria, *H. influenzae* type b infection, measles, rubella, and mumps. Routine immunization with the varicella vaccine, hepatitis B vaccine, and the conjugate pneumococcal vaccine should similarly decrease the incidence of these infections in daycare settings. Vaccine-preventable infections may still occur, especially in persons who have not been immunized and in infants and young children who have not been fully vaccinated.

Rubella during the first or early second trimester of pregnancy may cause a severe fetal infection, known as **congential rubella syndrome,** resulting in microcephaly, deafness, congenital heart defects, eye disorders, and psychomotor retardation. Chickenpox acquired early in pregnancy may lead to **varicella embryopathy** with limb bands or amputation in a small fraction of offspring. Acquisition of these infections during pregnancy is a potential hazard for daycare personnel and mothers of children who attend daycare. There is no definitive intervention for the management of susceptible pregnant contacts after exposure to rubella. Immune globulin has been used, but its efficacy is unproved. Rubella and the congenital rubella syndrome and varicella and varicella embryopathy can be eliminated by appropriate immunization of children and personnel.

MANAGEMENT OF INFECTIONS

Exclusion Policy. The American Academy of Pediatrics and the American Public Health Association have reached consensus regarding exclusion policies for children attending daycare (Table 102–4). These recommendations reflect the understanding that children with moderate to severe illnesses should not be allowed to participate in usual activities or may require more individualized care than is available and that the spread of certain communicable diseases within the daycare centers will be reduced by the exclusion of children with infections. This means that children known to have highly infectious illnesses should not be allowed to attend daycare until treatment is initiated, as for head lice or group A *Streptococcus* infections, or until transmissibility has waned, as in pertussis, varicella, measles, and mumps. In addition, children should be excluded if the contagiousness of their illness is uncertain, for example, if a child has a high fever and a rash.

Important conditions that do not necessarily require exclusion from daycare include (1) asymptomatic excretion of an enteropathogen, (2) nonpurulent conjunctivitis, (3) a rash without a fever or behavioral change, (4) CMV infection, (5) the carrier state of HBV, and (6) HIV infection. Any exceptions to this statement are found in the individual discussions of the infectious agents.

Postexposure Prophylaxis. Postexposure prophylaxis is a strategy that may be helpful in the management of some infections that

TABLE 102–4. Recommendations for Exclusion From Daycare

Symptoms

- The illness prevents the child from participating comfortably in program activities.
- The illness results in a greater care need than the childcare staff can provide without compromising the health and safety of the other children.
- The child has any of the following conditions: fever, unusual lethargy, irritability, persistent crying, difficult breathing, or other signs of possible severe illness.
- Diarrhea (defined as an increased number of stools compared with the child's normal pattern, with increased stool water or decreased form) that is not contained by diapers or toilet use.
- Vomiting two or more times in the previous 24 hours unless the vomiting is determined to be due to a noncommunicable condition and the child is not in danger of dehydration.
- Mouth sores associated with an inability of the child to control his or her saliva, unless the child's physician or local health department authority states that the child's condition is noninfectious.
- Rash with fever or behavior change until a physician has determined the illness not to be a communicable disease.

Specific Diseases

- Purulent conjunctivitis (defined as pink or red conjunctivitis with white or yellow eye discharge, often with matted eyelids after sleep and eye pain or redness of the eyelids or skin surrounding the eye), until examination by a physician and approved by a physician for readmission, with or without treatment.
- Tuberculosis, until the child's physician or local health department authority states that the child is noninfectious.
- Impetigo, until 24 hours after treatment has been initiated.
- Ringworm, until the morning after topical or systemic therapy has been started.
- Streptococcal pharyngitis, until 24 hours after treatment has been initiated, and until the child has had no fever for 24 hours.
- Pinworms, until the morning after topical or systemic therapy has been given.
- Head lice (pediculosis), until the morning after the first treatment.
- Scabies, until after treatment has been completed.
- Chickenpox, until the sixth day after onset of rash or sooner, if all lesions have dried and crusted.
- Pertussis (confirmed by laboratory or presumed on the basis of symptoms of the illness or because of onset of a cough within 14 days or having face-to-face contact with a person in a household or classroom who has a laboratory-confirmed case of pertussis), until 5 days of appropriate antibiotic therapy (erythromycin) has been completed (total course of treatment is 14 days).
- Measles, until 5 days after the onset of rash.
- Mumps, until 9 days after the onset of parotid gland swelling.
- Hepatitis A, until 1 week after onset of illness and jaundice, if present, has disappeared or until passive immunoprophylaxis (immune globulin) has been administered to appropriate children and staff in the program, as directed by the responsible health department.

occur in daycare centers (Table 16–2). Daycare contacts of persons with invasive disease caused by *H. influenzae* type b or *N. meningitidis* should receive rifampin prophylaxis to prevent secondary cases. Contacts of children with pertussis should receive erythromycin for 14 days for prophylaxis and may require a booster immunization. Prophylaxis has a negligible clinical effect after the paroxysmal stage begins. Intramuscular immune globulin may be used to provide short-term prophylaxis of susceptible contacts after exposure to measles or hepatitis A, although vaccination is important for long-term protection. In persons found to harbor *Corynebacterium diphtheriae,* which causes diphtheria, in the nasopharynx, prophylaxis with erythromycin or penicillin can reduce transmission. When measles is diagnosed in a household or within a daycare center after many days of exposure, intramuscular immune globulin for susceptible contacts is the most effective way to prevent secondary cases. When there has been a single recent exposure to a case of measles, administration of measles-mumps-rubella (MMR) vaccine should be effective in preventing infection.

Vaccination. Vaccination can be used as a strategy to prevent infection during epidemics in a community. Immunization with MMR vaccine is usually successful in terminating epidemics of measles in elementary or high school. However, if exposure to measles occurs in a daycare center, use of immune globulin is a more certain intervention if there has been prolonged contact with the index patient. HBV vaccination protects against transmission of infection if a carrier of HBV is identified in the daycare center. Routine immunization with varicella and conjugate pneumococcal vaccines should substantially reduce the spread of these organisms in the daycare setting.

PREVENTION

Vaccination. There are several vaccine-preventable infections for preschool children: diphtheria, tetanus, pertussis, polio, measles, mumps, rubella, varicella, *H. influenzae* type b, *S. pneumoniae,* and hepatitis B. Selective or mandatory immunization with hepatitis A vaccine may control this infection in the daycare environment. The timely and appropriate use of these immunizations will successfully eliminate or reduce these problems from the daycare setting (Chapter 17). Children who attend registered daycare facilities are more likely to be up to date in their immunizations than children cared for at home.

Education. An integral part of the control of infection within a daycare center is education of staff and families. It is essential that the staff understand the general principles of infection transmission and control. Education before job placement and frequent in-service seminars reinforce the importance of some basic techniques, especially hand washing. Supervision is essential to ensure compliance with policies. Parents should be educated regarding recognition of illness, especially illnesses that are best cared for at home. The rationale and importance of compliance with daycare center rules should be emphasized. The childcare program should inform parents of the need to share information about communicable illnesses, in the child or a family member.

TABLE 102–5. Immunizations for Daycare Employees

Vaccine	Personnel	Schedule
Tetanus-diphtheria (TD)	All employees	Every 10 years
Measles-mumps-rubella (MMR)	All employees	If born after 1955, evidence of prior infection or two doses at least 1 month apart
Poliovirus	All employees	Primary immunization with inactivated poliomyelitis vaccine if needed; consider booster if previously immunized
Influenza	Recommended	Annually
Varicella-zoster virus	Recommended if nonimmune	Two doses 4–8 weeks apart for persons older than 12 years of age
Hepatitis A	Recommended	Two doses 6 months apart
Hepatitis B	Not required	

Written Policies. Each daycare facility should have written policies for managing child and employee illness. There should be written procedures for hand washing, personal hygiene policies, environmental sanitation policies and procedures, and policies for filing and updating immunization records. Employees should be screened for tuberculosis by skin testing, with a chest radiograph if the skin test is positive, and should have appropriate immunizations (Table 102–5). There is no indication to screen daycare attendees or employees for hepatitis B, hepatitis C, CMV, or HIV.

Physical Plant Characteristics. In the planning of daycare facilities, areas for infants and toddlers should be separated from those for older children. The kitchen and food-storage areas should be separated from the toilet space. Because hand contamination represents the most critical factor in transmission of infection, hand washing facilities must be available to staff and children. This is especially important in the diaper changing and food preparation areas. The hand washing facility is preferably pedal operated and in easy reach of soap and towel dispensers.

Because fecal contamination is strongly and inversely related to age, it is important to have a physical plant large enough to separate children younger than 3 years from older children. If this is not possible, an age restriction should be placed on admission.

When construction materials are selected, the choice should be based on durability and ease of cleaning. Diaper changing areas should be easily cleaned and light in color so that soilage can be detected. A pedal-operated, closed receptacle is ideal for the disposal of soiled diapers. The toddler area should be equipped with training toilets and junior-sized toilets. These areas must be frequently cleaned, and hand washing facilities should be appropriate in size and preferably pedal-operated.

REVIEWS

Crosson FJ, Black SB, Trumpp CE, et al: Infections in day-care centers. *Curr Probl Pediatr* 1986;16:121–84.

National Health and Safety Performance Standards: Guidelines for out-of-home child care programs. In *Caring for Our Children. National Health and Safety Performance Standards: Guidelines for Out-of-Home Child Care Programs.* Washington, DC, American Public Health Association, 2000.

Thompson SC: Infectious diarrhea in children: Controlling transmission in the child care setting. *J Paediatr Child Health* 1994;30:210–9.

Wald ER, Dashefsky B, Byers C, et al: Frequency and severity of infections in daycare. *J Pediatr* 1998;112:540–6.

KEY ARTICLES

Adler SP: Cytomegalovirus transmission and child daycare. *Adv Pediatr Infect Dis* 1992;7:109–22.

Boken DJ, Chartrand SA, Goerin RV, et al: Colonization with penicillin-nonsusceptible *Streptococcus pneumoniae* in urban and rural child-care centers. *Pediatr Infect Dis J* 1996;15:667–72.

Cordell RL, Thor PM, Addiss DG, et al: Impact of a massive waterborne cryptosporidiosis outbreak on child care facilities in metropolitan Milwaukee, Wisconsin. *Pediatr Infect Dis J* 1997;16:639–44.

Craig AS, Erwin PC, Schaffner W, et al: Carriage of multidrug-resistant *Streptococcus pneumoniae* and impact of chemoprophylaxis during an outbreak of meningitis at a day care center. *Clin Infect Dis* 1999;29: 1257–64.

David E, McIntosh G, Bek MK, et al: Molecular evidence of transmission of hepatitis B in a daycare center. *Lancet* 1996;347:118–9.

Giebink GS: National standards for infection control in out-of-town child care. *Semin Pediatr Infect Dis* 1990;1:184.

Gillespie SM, Cartter ML, Asch S, et al: Occupational risk of human parvovirus B19 infection for school and day-care personnel during an outbreak of erythema infectiosum. *JAMA* 1990;263:2061–5.

Goodman RA, Osterholm MT, Granoff DM, et al: Infectious disease and child day care. *Pediatrics* 1984;74:134–9.

Hadler SC, McFarland L: Hepatitis in day care centers: Epidemiology and prevention. *Rev Infect Dis* 1986;8:548–57.

Kotch JB, Weigle KA, Weber DJ, et al: Evaluation of an hygienic intervention in child day-care centers. *Pediatrics* 1994;94:991–4.

Louhiala PJ, Jaakkola N, Ruotsalainen R, et al: Day-care centers and diarrhea: A public health perspective. *J Pediatr* 1997;131:476–9.

MacDonald KL, White KA, Heiser J, et al: Evaluation of a sick child day care program: Lack of detected increased risk of subsequent infections. *Pediatr Infect Dis J* 1990;9:15–20.

Nafstad P, Hagen JA, Oie L, et al: Day care centers and respiratory health. *Pediatrics* 1999;103:753–8.

Uhari M, Mottonen M: An open randomized controlled trial of infection prevention in child day-care centers. *Pediatr Infect Dis J* 1999;18:672–7.

Wald ER, Guerra N, Byers C: Frequency and severity of infections in daycare: Three year follow-up. *J Pediatr* 1991;118:509–14.

CHAPTER 103

The Immigrant, Refugee, or Internationally Adopted Child

Jerri Ann Jenista

Every pediatrician treats children whose health care has been influenced by residence in another country. Careful history taking is the clue to recognizing such children. Pediatric immigrants come from many diverse groups. Certain long-term travelers have medical needs similar to those of immigrants. Other children are born in the United States and yet are at risk of the diseases of immigrants. The effect of foreign residence is not always obvious (Table 103–1).

The routine infectious disease evaluation of the healthy child who has lived in another country need not be complicated or time-consuming. The most common error is to ignore or leave out parts of a comprehensive evaluation soon after arrival because of perceived barriers of language or culture. However, the time spent in obtaining complete information early on will address most serious infectious diseases quickly and will make later evaluations far simpler. Careful attention to detail soon after immigration will relieve children of most infectious disease threats acquired in their former lives.

POPULATIONS AT RISK

Immigration is dramatically changing the composition of the U.S. population. In the year 2000, more than 28 million persons born in other countries were living in the United States, a 43% increase during the past decade. Immigrants currently constitute more than 10% of the entire population of the United States. Foreign-born residents are disproportionately concentrated in various parts of the country. For example, immigrants constitute 26% of the population of California and 43% of the Miami metropolitan area. Immigrants arriving in the 1990s (11.2 million) and children born to immigrants during the same period (6.4 million) accounted for almost 70% of the population growth in the United States during the last decade of the 20th century. There are many groups of immigrants at risk of infectious diseases (Table 103–2).

Immigrants. Almost 200,000 children entered the United States in 1998 as various types of permanent residents, usually as relatives of persons already living in the United States. The majority of these immigrants came from the former Soviet Union, North America, especially Mexico, and various Asian countries, primarily China, India, and the Philippines. Very few arrived from Africa or Oceania. Two thirds of immigrant families intended to live in California, New York, Florida, Texas, New Jersey, or Illinois. North Dakota, South Dakota, West Virginia, Wyoming, and Montana each typically receive fewer than 400 new foreign-born permanent residents annually.

Illegal or Undocumented Immigrants. The total population of illegal immigrants in the United States was estimated at about 6 million in 2000. Some situations are as uncomplicated as those involving students or travelers who have overstayed their visas, but most involve persons who crossed U.S. borders, usually from Mexico, the Caribbean, or Central America, without the necessary legal documents. The Immigration and Naturalization Service (INS) estimates that more than 30,000 such children enter the United States with their families each year; most live in California, Texas, or other border states. The parents often work in domestic situations, on farms, in factories, or in other poorly paid positions with little or no access to health care for themselves or their children.

Refugees and Persons Seeking Asylum. In 1998, 14,221 children less than 20 years of age entered the United States as refugees or seeking asylum. Such children usually accompany relatives, but many, especially adolescents, enter alone, most often from Central America. Although some families arrive from various types of refugee camps, most individuals immigrate without ever having been detained in a refugee center.

In the 1980s and early 1990s, the majority of refugees originated in Asia, Central America, and the Caribbean. More recently, there has been a marked increase in the number of refugees from Bosnia-Herzegovina, the republics of the former Soviet Union and the former Yugoslavia, Vietnam, and various African nations, including Somalia, Liberia, and Sudan. At entry, at least 60% of the refugees or those seeking asylum head for the major metropolitan areas of Florida, California, New York, Washington, and Illinois.

TABLE 103–1. Children Whose Healthcare May Be Affected by Residence in a Foreign Country

Immigrant families
Illegal or undocumented immigrants
Refugee families and those seeking asylum
Unaccompanied minors
Amerasians and their families
Visitors, including tourists, temporary workers, students, and long-term residents such as diplomatic families
Internationally adopted children
Medical foster children
U.S. households with:
- ties to traditional ethnic communities
- contact with international travelers
- employment of household workers from other countries

U.S. citizens:
- born or raised abroad
- traveling abroad for longer than 3 months
- long-term students returning from abroad

TABLE 103–2. Populations at Risk of Diseases of Travelers and Immigrants*

Population	Definition	Number of Children <20 Years Entering the United States in 1998	Most Frequent Country of Birth	Most Frequently Intended States of Residence
Immigrants	Children granted permanent legal residence in the United States, most often joining relatives who are already U.S. citizens	197,610 (2457 of whom were married at the time of immigration)	Mexico, China, Philippines, former Soviet Union, India, Dominican Republic	California, Texas, New York, Florida, Illinois, New Jersey
Illegal or undocumented immigrants	Children living in the United States without permanent residency visas; includes students or other visitors who overstay temporary visas	Unknown, probably 30,000 annually	Mexico, El Salvador, Guatemala, Canada, Haiti	California, Texas, New York, Florida, Illinois, New Jersey, Arizona
Refugees and seekers of asylum	Persons who have suffered or fear persecution in their country of origin; includes children traveling with relatives and unaccompanied minors	14,221	Bosnia-Herzegovina, Croatia, former Soviet Union, Vietnam, Somalia, Iran, Cuba, Liberia, Sudan	California, New York, Florida, Washington
Amerasians	Children fathered by U.S. servicemen during the Vietnamese War; includes their children and other relatives	347	Vietnam	
Adoptees	Includes children already adopted abroad or to be adopted in the United States	14,867	Former Soviet Union, China, Korea, Guatemala, Vietnam, India, Cambodia, Romania	New York, California, Pennsylvania, Illinois, Texas, New Jersey, Minnesota, Michigan
Nonimmigrants	Includes tourists, foster children with medical visas, children accompanying their working parents for long-term stays, and all others not granted a permanent residency visa	4,147,536 (does not include most Canadians and Mexicans, who do not require visas)	Japan, United Kingdom, Mexico, Germany, Canada, India	Florida, California, New York, Hawaii, Texas
Students	Admitted to complete a specific course of education or training	564,683	Japan, China, Korea, India	California, New York, Massachusetts, Florida, Texas, Pennsylvania

*From *1998 Statistical Yearbook of the Immigration and Naturalization Service,* U.S. Government Printing Office: Washington, DC, November 2000.

Virtually none claim residency in Wyoming, West Virginia, or Hawaii at the time they are granted permanent residency.

Amerasians. Amerasians are children fathered by U.S. servicemen during the Korean and Vietnamese wars. Special laws allow these children to immigrate with their parents, spouses, and children. However, by 1998, only 347 Amerasians and family members entered the United States.

Adoptees. U.S. citizens adopt more than 15,000 foreign-born children each year. Between 1960 and 1990, most internationally adopted children came from Korea, Latin America, and various Asian nations. Since 1990, markedly increased numbers of children have entered the United States under orphan visas from Eastern European countries, especially Romania and Bulgaria; from the republics of the former Soviet Union, particularly Russia, Kazakhstan, and Ukraine; and from China, Cambodia, and Vietnam.

Only 46% of the adoptees are <1 year of age at the time of arrival. Almost two thirds are girls because 98% of the 5000 children adopted annually from China are girls. The greatest numbers of internationally adopted children reside in New York, California, New Jersey, Michigan, Minnesota, Pennsylvania, Illinois, and Texas, but even North Dakota, South Dakota, Nevada, and Wyoming had at least 15 new adoptees each in 1998.

Long-Term Visitors. More than 4 million children younger than 20 years of age entered the United States in 1998 as tourists or other temporary visitors. Of these, more than 50,000 were children accompanying their families for long-term stays in the United States. Their parents were temporary workers, businessmen, researchers, diplomats, or other professionals. Most of these visitors are from Europe, North America, and Japan.

Approximately 565,000 students arrive annually to study academic or vocational courses or as household childcare **(au pair)** workers. Most of these students or workers are from Japan, China, Korea, India, and Europe.

Foster Children. A special group consists of those children holding medical visas sponsored by philanthropic organizations. Although the intent is for the children to return to their native countries, many will live with U.S. foster families for weeks or months while recovering from surgery or undergoing rehabilitation. For example, in 2000, the Spokane-based organization, Healing the Children, sponsored more than 200 new arrivals from more than 20 countries, primarily Central American nations. The children stayed an average of 3–6 months, living with families all over the United States, especially in the Northeast and Mid-Atlantic States.

United States Households. Some children who have never left this country may be at risk of diseases that usually affect immigrants. Close-knit ethnic communities may provide environments that allow transmission of infections prevalent in the original immigrants, such as hepatitis B among Hmong families in Wisconsin. Visitors from the native country may bring gifts of food contaminated with organisms epidemic in the native country, such as seafood from Ecuador contaminated with *Vibrio cholerae.* Foreign visitors may import common childhood illness into susceptible populations, such as rubella in unvaccinated Hispanic communities.

Those U.S. households that employ domestic helpers from other countries are at possible risk of exotic diseases. For example, an epidemic of neurocysticercosis among orthodox Jews in New York City was traced to household workers from Latin America who were asymptomatically infected with *Taenia solium.*

United States Expatriates. Children who are U.S. citizens but who have lived in other countries for at least 3 months are also at risk of diseases of immigrants. Examples are children who accompany their diplomatic, professional, military, or missionary parents, as well as teenage exchange students or volunteer workers. These long-term visitors are at risk of both the diseases of travelers (Chapter 104) and those of immigrants.

DIFFERENCES IN DISEASES BETWEEN IMMIGRANTS AND TRAVELERS

Children who were born in or who have lived in another country, especially a developing nation, may have very different infectious disease problems than short-term travelers returning from the same country (Table 103–3).

Past Exposure. Living in a developing or tropical country, a child is exposed more frequently and at a younger age to a broader spectrum of infectious disease agents. Exposure and infection with hepatitis A, EBV, CMV, and numerous enteric pathogens occur early in life. Repeated exposures to the agents that cause malaria, giardiasis, scabies, and other diseases may decrease the severity of or alter the typical symptoms associated with those organisms. The classic descriptions of diseases may not apply to the child with repeated exposures.

TABLE 103–3. Reasons for Differences in Infectious Disease Problems of Immigrants From Those of Travelers

Past exposure to infectious disease
Immunization history
Presence of subclinical or incubating infection
Organisms with unusual resistance patterns
Maternal transfer of infection
Genetic differences
Food choices or methods of preparation
Incomplete history due to cultural or language differences

Data from Wilson (1991).

Past Immunizations. Children who live outside the United States may receive different vaccinations, or none at all. *Haemophilus influenzae* type b vaccine is not available worldwide. Japanese children may have received Japanese encephalitis virus vaccine but not pertussis vaccine. Measles-mumps-rubella vaccine is not used in many regions of the world because of lack of refrigeration, and in some countries the vaccine is given at much older ages than in the United States. Different strains of bacille Calmette-Guérin (BCG) vaccine are used worldwide with various degrees of efficacy.

Even a child who is apparently fully vaccinated against an agent may have little or no response to the immunization, depending on the potency of the vaccine, age at immunization, and underlying immunosuppression induced by severe malnutrition or chronic infection.

Subclinical Infections. Some infections acquired outside the United States, such as tuberculosis, malaria, or echinococcosis, may remain latent or asymptomatic for many years. When an immigrant is evaluated for an exotic infection of long incubation, diseases prevalent at the time the child lived in the other country must be considered. For example, a region may be free of malaria now but not when the child emigrated. Occasionally, subclinical infections are recognized only many years after immigration when a complication arises, such as neurocysticercosis in a child presenting with seizures or chronic hepatitis B virus infection in an internationally adopted child whose parent has an unexplained hepatitis.

Microbial Resistance. Children from countries other than the United States may have easily diagnosed disease, and yet standard therapy may fail because of unusual drug resistance patterns, as with multiple-drug resistant tuberculosis in a Russian child or chloramphenicol-resistant typhoid fever imported from India.

Maternal Transmission. The legacy of foreign residence may be transmitted at birth to a child born in the United States. Examples of infections acquired elsewhere but transmitted by immigrant mothers to the their U.S.-born offspring include hepatitis B, HTLV-1, malaria, and rubella.

Genetic Differences. Symptoms related to genetic differences from the general U.S. population may masquerade as infectious disease. For example, a lactose-intolerant Chinese or Asian Indian child may react to a milk-rich Western diet by developing chronic diarrhea, abdominal pain, and weight loss leading to fruitless studies for nonexistent intestinal pathogens.

Dietary Habits. Traditional ethnic cooking methods may not be safe, even when North American ingredients are used. Religious dietary precautions may call for the use of unpasteurized milk, as in certain Indian desserts. Game, pork, or fish eaten raw or marinated without cooking may lead to infection with *Trichinella* or *Diphyllobothrium latum* (fish tapeworm). Mushrooms collected in the wild may look exactly like those that are a delicacy in Korea and yet may be severely toxic.

Inadequate History. The family of an immigrant child may be unwilling or unable to give a complete history because of language or cultural barriers. A parent whose English-speaking child acts as a translator may be too embarrassed to report past risky behaviors or family medical secrets. An immigrant may not report symptoms or past exposures because these are not perceived as unusual, such as treatment with nonsterile acupuncture needles, herbal medicines, or traditional remedies. Unaccompanied minors, internationally adopted children, and others for whom no translator can be found may present with little or no medical history available.

MEDICAL ASSESSMENT BEFORE ARRIVAL IN THE UNITED STATES

All Immigrants and Refugees. Children who enter the United States as permanent residents must undergo a medical examination by a physician approved by the U.S. consul, usually in the country of origin. The minimum requirements for all people for this **visa examination** include a medical history and physical examination emphasizing excludable conditions. Serologic testing for syphilis and HIV infection and a chest radiograph are required for applicants ≥15 years of age. Excludable conditions that may result in denial of a visa are "communicable diseases of public health importance," including syphilis, lymphogranuloma venereum, gonorrhea, chancroid, granuloma inguinale, HIV infection, active tuberculosis, or infectious leprosy; any physical, mental, or behavioral disorder that poses a threat to the safety or welfare of the alien or others; drug abuse or addiction or any condition that may result in the immigrant's becoming a public charge. The medical officer may request additional testing on the basis of the initial examination findings or local conditions. Thus children with known exposure to tuberculosis may be required to have tuberculin skin testing or a chest radiograph or both. The examination of a child adopted from a Romanian orphanage will almost certainly include HIV testing.

In addition, all applicants for a permanent residency visa except internationally adopted children <10 years of age must show proof of complete immunization against measles, mumps, rubella, polio, diphtheria, pertussis, tetanus, *Haemophilus influenzae* type b, varicella, pneumococcus, and influenza. If the person has an incomplete immunization record, he must show reasonable proof of immunity from the disease or receive a single dose of each missing vaccine at the time of the visa examination. Certain exceptions are allowed if the vaccine is not indicated for the age group of the individual, is unavailable in the country of origin, is medically contraindicated, or is given only seasonally. An applicant may also request a waiver for one or more vaccines for religious or moral reasons.

The excludable condition requirement is waived for a child whose parent is a U.S. citizen or is an immigrant who already holds a permanent residency visa. Other children with an excludable condition may appeal a medical examination determination after further evaluation or treatment. Guardians may apply for a **waiver of excludability** by showing that they understand the extent and severity of the condition, have adequate medical resources to care for the child, and have adequate financial resources to prevent the child from becoming a public liability. With such waivers, severely medically or mentally impaired children and HIV-infected children have been granted permanent residency in the United States.

In general, the visa examination must be completed before arrival in the United States. Refugees or persons seeking asylum admitted to the United States under emergency conditions may complete the examination in the United States under the supervision of the Public Health Service. Other persons, such as undocumented immigrants or visitors already residing in the United States, must undergo the examination at the time they apply for readjustment of their immigration status.

The quality and completeness of the visa medical examination are highly variable, depending on the expertise and experience of the medical officer and the available medical resources. The reports of the examination, including radiographs, are sealed in an envelope and handed to the INS officer at the port of entry. The pediatrician providing subsequent care may not have access to the results unless the child is a refugee or is holding a waiver of excludability. Thus the visa medical examination does not substitute for a thorough medical evaluation after arrival in the United States.

Special Groups of Refugees. Some children, especially from East Africa and the former Yugoslavia, may arrive from refugee or displaced persons camps managed by the United Nations, governmental authorities, or humanitarian organizations. Medical evaluation and care are variable, depending on the needs and resources of the particular population. Children immigrating to the United States must have the standard visa examination, but treatment or immunizations given in the camp may not be documented in that examination.

Haitian refugee children may arrive from the large migrant camp at the U.S. Naval Base at Guantánamo Bay, Cuba. All children receive at least the standard visa medical examination. In addition, some receive more extensive evaluations for tuberculosis, malaria, filariasis, or intestinal parasites if signs or symptoms indicate possible infection. Attempts are made to bring immunizations up to date, including immunization against *H. influenzae* type b.

The federal **Office of Refugee Resettlement (ORR)** also manages a program for unaccompanied minor refugees. These are typically adolescents, although some are members of sibling groups with younger children. Most are from Central America, although a large number of teenagers arrived from Sudan in 2000. Although some of these children are cared for in group homes while awaiting disposition of their immigration status, most are currently placed with foster families.

Occasionally, special processing centers are established to manage a large influx of refugees over a short period. For example, in 1999, Fort Dix, New Jersey, served as a temporary refugee center for more than 4000 Kosovar refugees. Standard medical screening and care were provided, and arrangements were made for long-term follow-up after resettlement in other parts of the country.

Visa medical records for *all* refugees, whether or not they ever resided in a refugee camp, are forwarded to the state and local health departments where the refugees intend to live. The local health department is responsible for contacting the refugees and assuring follow-up care for documented medical conditions, such as partially treated tuberculosis. Most refugees qualify for Medicaid, and all are eligible for care financed by the ORR at designated clinics for at least the first 8 months after the date of arrival in the United States. In regions where there are very few refugees, the refugees' sponsor, often a church or other civic organization, may arrange for follow-up medical care, usually by private physicians.

Undocumented Immigrants. Most undocumented immigrant children come from Mexico or Central American countries. If the family applies for temporary or permanent residency under amnesty programs, the children undergo the standard visa medical examination. Otherwise, medical care is variable, entirely dependent on the resources of the parents and the policies of the local public health care facilities.

Amerasians. There are no special guidelines beyond the standard visa medical examination. Medical records are not routinely forwarded to the local health department unless there is an active medical condition such as tuberculosis under treatment. After arrival, however, Amerasians are eligible for ORR-funded care.

International Adoptees. Children who apply for orphan visas must undergo the standard visa medical examination. Unlike refugee children, there is no provision for follow-up care after arrival.

Adoption agencies, foreign childcare institutions, and lawyers abroad may develop their own guidelines for evaluation before adoption, but quality and documentation are highly variable.

Temporary Visitors. Tourists, visitors, students, medical foster children, and other nonimmigrants do not routinely have to undergo a medical examination, although the U.S. consul always has the option to require an examination of any person believed to have an excludable condition. The only medical restriction to admission to the United States is HIV infection. No medical examination or proof of testing is required, although the visitor must answer questions about HIV status on the visa application. A person with a positive HIV test must apply for a waiver to enter the United States.

INFECTIOUS DISEASE ASSESSMENT AT ARRIVAL

Timing of the Consultation. The physician rarely has the opportunity to schedule or plan the medical evaluation of an immigrant child in advance of the child's arrival in the United States. Exceptions are refugee children and those granted waivers of excludability for known medical conditions. For these groups, the Public Health Service forwards the medical records to the state and local health departments, where arrangements are made for follow-up care. Other exceptions are children coming to the United States for medical care or for adoption. The majority of adoptive or foster families have a ''prearrival'' consultation with a physician, most often to review the medical information presented in the child's referral paperwork. At such a visit, the pediatrician has the chance to assess the child's basic health status. Depending on the completeness of the records, the practitioner can often anticipate common infectious disease problems, such as inadequate immunization, intestinal parasites, or lice. In addition, such a consultation allows the physician to outline to the parent the routine infectious disease evaluation for most immigrant children (Fig. 103–1).

Any child who appears acutely ill upon arrival or is known to have a chronic medical or physical condition should be seen within a few days for a symptom-oriented evaluation. New adoptive parents may need reassurance within a day or two that the child is basically healthy. The comprehensive medical evaluation for all children should be delayed until about 1 month after arrival. It is much more productive to examine a child after jet lag and the initial anxiety of moving to a new culture have subsided.

Obtaining the History. One of the major tasks of a comprehensive evaluation is to obtain a thorough medical history. Decoding medical records may present a formidable challenge. For the most part, it is not particularly helpful to have extensive records translated

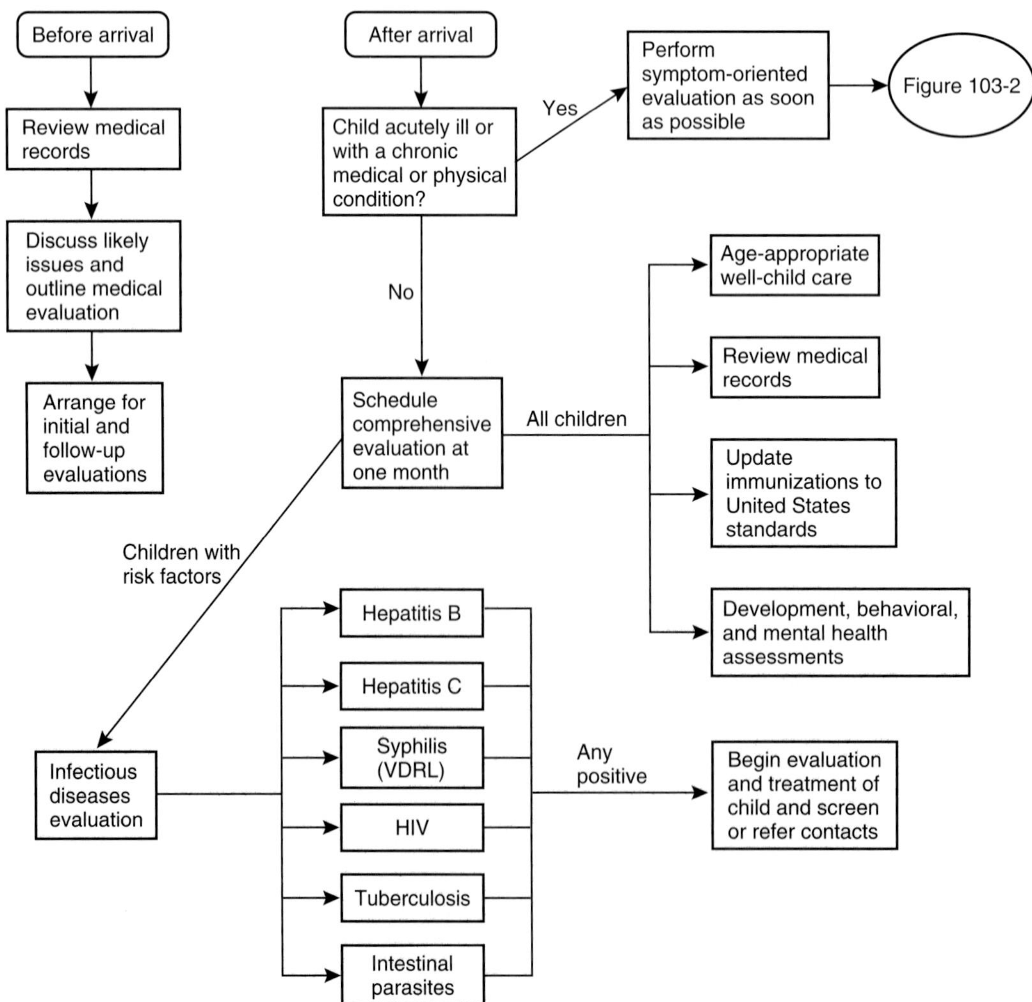

FIGURE 103–1. Routine infectious disease evaluation of the immigrant child.

unless the child has an unexplained or unstable medical condition. Translation, if not performed by a person experienced in medical terminology and abbreviations, may be more confusing than informative. Even accurate translation may be perplexing if the pediatrician is not familiar with the terminology of other medical cultures, such as the British ''calipers'' for orthopedic leg braces or the Russian ''perinatal encephalopathy'' loosely referring to maternal or infant risk factors for poor developmental outcome.

Interpretation of the medical record may be essential for children with chronic medical conditions, prolonged hospitalization periods, or unexplained illness soon after arrival. Even if a translation service is not available locally, almost any practitioner can obtain a translation quickly by facsimile message. Good resources are modern language departments of universities, embassies or consulates, ethnic cultural associations, language schools, and professional medical translators. The most useful information can usually be gleaned from records, even without translation. Growth charts are often self-explanatory, and immunization records are easily recognized by the typical array of acronyms and dates.

Most immigrant children are accompanied by an adult who can shed light on the past medical history. Even for adoptees and unaccompanied minors, certain questions are important in planning a subsequent infectious disease evaluation (Table 103–4). Although a child may appear healthy, the comprehensive evaluation soon after arrival may be the best or only chance to obtain information on past exposure to disease. As the time from immigration increases, details are often lost, forgotten, or deliberately ignored as the immigrant assimilates.

The physician should determine how well the informant knows the child and attempt to establish the reliability of the information provided. The informant should be able to verify or tell the physician how to verify written medical records and the child's personal and family medical history. Medical records that are ''too neat'' may be fraudulent, but they may merely reflect precise attention to well-child care. For instance, immunization cards from institutions may record that vaccines were given at exactly 1- or 2-month intervals.

The physician needs to know whether the informant is familiar with the medical care, customs, and beliefs of the child's culture. Traditional medical practices, such as Vietnamese *cao-gío* (coin-rubbing of the skin) or Asian burning of *moxa* (herbs) on the skin, may be interpreted as child abuse by inexperienced observers. Certain forms, colors, or even temperatures of medication or treatment may not be accepted if they clash with cultural perceptions of health or illness.

Adoptive or foster parents may have no particular knowledge of the child. Often medical records are scanty, completely missing, or too out of date to be useful. Occasionally, agencies will provide information about the general type of care received by a child before travel. If a child's condition seems far more serious than the medical records or the parent's expectations indicate, it is sometimes helpful to consult with the agency directly for information about the typical condition of children placed from a particular orphanage or country.

Ascertaining why the child came to the United States is helpful. A child accompanying his professional father from Japan for a

TABLE 103–4. Questions in the Comprehensive Infectious Disease Evaluation of an Immigrant Child

Question	Relevance
Who is providing the history? Is it a relative or guardian of the same culture, a U.S. sponsor, adoptive or foster parents, the child himself?	Relatives or others who have accompanied the child through the emigration process may be better able to verify any medical history or records. Adoptive parents or sponsors may have no specific knowledge of the child and often must depend on general information from an adoption agency or childcare institution.
In which countries or what regions has the child lived? For how long? Were there any transit stops in other countries or in refugee or displaced person camps?	Potential disease exposure varies widely, even within the same country with region, climate, season, altitude, and length of residence. Unless questioned, guardians may not report stays, even of many months' duration, in temporary settings such as refugee or cultural training camps.
Under what circumstances has the child emigrated? Is it abandonment, war, poverty, political or religious persecution, for medical care or adoption, to join relatives, for educational purposes, to accompany professional parents?	Involuntary emigration is almost always under stressful and medically inadequate circumstances. Voluntary emigrants leave variable backgrounds ranging from extreme poverty to highly privileged urban lifestyles.
What were the living circumstances in the other countries? Did the child live in a refugee camp, orphanage, foster home, privileged urban setting?	Disease exposure risk increases with increasing poverty of living circumstances, regardless of the country of origin. Communal living, as in camps or institutions, increases the risk of exposure to common childhood infectious diseases.
What were the quality and quantity of diet, housing and medical care available to the child? Were they above or below the standards or norm of the country of origin?	Children with a chronically deprived background have different health problems than those who suffered only a brief period of inadequate medical care.
What is the child's exposure history? Has the child undergone blood transfusions, operations, injections, traditional healing, occupational hazards, sexual or physical abuse, torture?	Many exposures, such as giving all medications by injection, are the standards of medical care other than in the United States and thus may not be reported. Occupational hazards, especially for children, may not be recognized as such unless details of the work are sought.
Has the child taken or is he or she still taking any medications? Who prescribed them, and for what condition? Is the drug or container available for review?	Traditional remedies may not be reported or considered as "medication." Therapy for tuberculosis, leprosy, malaria, or intestinal parasites may be in progress at the time of immigration. Drugs not available in the United States may be difficult to identify without the container or tablet.

2-year stay in the United States likely has had excellent medical care with no more risk of unusual infectious diseases than if that same child had been born and raised in California. A child adopted from a Filipino orphanage after years of street living, the Sudanese teen who spent the last 10 years in refugee centers in three different countries, and the middle-class Russian Jewish family joining relatives in the United States all have dramatically different risks of infectious diseases. In general, the more involuntary the choice to emigrate, the more inadequate the health conditions before travel and en route.

The history should determine in which regions or countries the child has lived and for how long. Interim stops in institutions, refugee or displaced persons camps, and other temporary residences should be noted. Season, climate, altitude, duration of residence, and specific region of the country all may play a role in determining exposure to infectious diseases. For example, a child who has always lived at high altitude in Nepal will have no malaria risk, whereas a child who has lived during the rainy season on the *terai* (flatlands) of Nepal adjacent to India almost certainly has been exposed to malaria.

The physician should ascertain the living circumstances in the other countries. Privileged urban living, even in a country with few medical resources, poses far fewer risks of infectious diseases than does communal living, as in institutions or camps. Informants may not report exposures to measles, varicella, lice, scabies, malaria, or others if these diseases were conditions of daily life.

The examiner should determine whether the child received adequate housing, food, water, and medical care and whether these were above or below the standards of the country of origin. The examiner needs to know whether conditions recently changed for the worse or for the better for the child. Chronic deprivation poses health problems different from those of only a brief period of inadequate medical care. Similarly, a period of rehabilitation may mask a severely inadequate past medical environment.

The child's history of exposure to disease should be determined. The examiner needs to determine whether the child has had any transfusions, injections, or dental or surgical procedures. An informant may not report practices considered the standard of medical care in the original country, such as the administration of all medications to children by injection. Reuse of needles is common in developing countries, resulting in epidemics of hepatitis B or C or even HIV infection in childcare institutions.

The examiner needs to determine whether the child has received any traditional healing methods such as acupuncture, has been physically abused or tortured, or has performed labor in the household or community. Occupational hazards may not be recognized unless details of the work are sought. For example, the child helping his or her family transplant rice may have been exposed to a variety of water-associated or insectborne diseases, whereas the child working a few miles away in a weaving household is more likely to have respiratory illness as a result of chronic exposure to cotton fibers.

A medication history should be elicited. Traditional remedies may not be considered medication. In addition, remedies purchased at ethnic pharmacies may be herbal extracts, pharmaceuticals packaged to resemble herbal mixtures, contaminated with pharmaceutical drugs or heavy metals, or simply neither drugs nor herbs at all. Therapy for malaria, tuberculosis, leprosy, or parasitic diseases may be in progress at the time of immigration. Although the tendency is to rewrite prescriptions or to replace them with drugs manufactured in the United States, some foreign-made formulations are easier to give children and may not be available in the United States. Commonly encountered examples are rifampin or chloroquine in suspension. Examination of the original packaging is often helpful. Drugs or other substances that are not easily recognized, even in translation, may be identified with help from a regional poison control center or with use of the publication *Unlisted Drugs*, published monthly with periodic indices by Pharmaco-Medical Documentation, Inc., Chatham, NJ 07928.

Immunizations. An unsupported statement that the child's immunizations are up to date is inadequate. A child may be fully immunized by the standards of another country and yet be considered incompletely immunized according to the recommendations used in the United States. Additional vaccines, such as Japanese encephalitis virus or plague vaccines, or alternate vaccines, such as oral instead of killed polio vaccine, may have been administered. A child may have received more than the usual number of doses of a vaccine under ''National Immunization Day'' campaigns to eliminate certain agents such as polio. Immunization records are usually easily interpreted, but several questions must be addressed:

1. Is the record valid? Records that consist of one or more pages in a ''health booklet'' or written in different inks and hands as part of a growth chart are usually reliable.
2. Does the record pertain to this child? Records for a sibling who died or of another child are sometimes substituted. If the immunizations are part of a health card, the growth chart can be checked. Weights discrepant with the weight of the child in the office are a good clue to switched records.
3. Were the vaccines listed actually available in that country on the dates indicated? For developing nations the best clue is the date of availability in the United States. For example, *Haemophilus influenzae* type b vaccine was not available in most countries before U.S. licensure in 1985. In contrast, some vaccines were available in other industrial nations before they were in the United States, such as acellular pertussis and varicella vaccines in Japan.
4. Were the vaccines used effective? If the vaccine requires continuous refrigeration from manufacturer to vaccinee, especially if electricity was not available in the region where the child lived, oral polio, measles-mumps-rubella, and varicella vaccines may not have been potent when administered.
5. Is it likely that the child was able to respond immunologically to the vaccine? A severely malnourished or otherwise chronically ill child may not have responded fully to vaccines administered. For instance, some severely malnourished Asian Indian children fully immunized against hepatitis B while awaiting adoption proceedings have had no detectable hepatitis B surface antibody after arrival in the adoptive home.
6. Did the child receive all his or her vaccines in an institutional setting, such as a hospital or orphanage? Some children from Russian and Chinese institutions have no detectable antibody despite complete immunization records, whereas children who have received medical care in community settings in the same countries have adequate antibody levels on testing.

If there is any doubt about the veracity or accuracy of the records or the effectiveness of the vaccines used, the best plan is usually to repeat at least a single dose of all the common childhood vaccines. For older children, an alternative is to assess serologic titers for immunity. Children who have received no vaccines or who have no verification of administration should receive a full course of childhood immunizations, following the modified scheme recommended for older children (Chapter 17).

A common error is to delay starting or catching-up immunizations until all evaluations are complete or until nutritional deficiencies are fully corrected. Except for a child with an acute illness, such as measles, possible HIV infection, or life-threatening malnutrition, there is no justification for delaying immunizations. Indeed, immigrant children, especially refugees, may be at higher risk of many vaccine-preventable diseases because later arrivals and fellow travelers import infections such as measles and pertussis.

Some immigrant children should receive additional vaccines beyond those recommended for U.S. children. For example, children living in states or migrant communities with endemic hepatitis A and children with chronic hepatitis B or C should receive hepatitis A vaccine. Children who will return to a developing country should receive a five-dose series of polio vaccine instead of the four-dose U.S. schedule.

Well-Child Care. Although the concern when one is first evaluating a child born outside the United States is usually for exotic infectious diseases, routine well-child care should not be ignored. It is especially tempting to delay age-appropriate hearing, vision, and developmental screenings because of language or cultural barriers. However, many immigrant children have common pediatric problems that should be addressed early. Often the evaluation of other problems uncovers an infectious disease, such as unsuspected giardiasis in an infant with failure to thrive or recurrent abdominal pain in an adolescent refugee with *Helicobacter pylori*–associated gastritis. Conversely, resolving some issues, such as milk intolerance due to lactase deficiency, will eliminate the need for an extensive parasitologic investigation.

The Asymptomatic Immigrant Child

Immigrant or long-term visiting children from privileged backgrounds, especially from western Europe, Australia, New Zealand, Canada, or Japan, do not need any special infectious disease evaluation unless the children have an unusual personal history, such as having lived in a refugee camp or mission setting with their volunteer-worker parents. For children who come from most other countries, for those with an unknown past history, and for those who have lived on the street, in refugee camps, or in orphanages, certain evaluations should be routine, regardless of symptoms or findings on examination. These evaluations are used to detect endemic infections (Table 103–5), especially hepatitis, syphilis, tuberculosis, intestinal parasites, and HIV if there are risk factors for infection.

Up to 15% of Indochinese and eastern African refugees are chronic HBsAg carriers, and 53% of unselected Romanian adoptees show evidence of past or current hepatitis B infection. Chronic infection rates for adoptees range from 5–20%, depending on the country of origin and previous living circumstances. Hepatitis B serologic screening should include at least HBsAg and anti-Hbc and anti-HBs determinations. Results of tests done in other countries may not be reliable. Screening for hepatitis B should be performed at arrival and again in 6 months, the maximum incubation period for hepatitis B, for any child who is not clearly immune or infected at the first screening. Children who are HBsAg carriers should also be screened for delta hepatitis, especially if they come from endemic areas such as the Mediterranean basin, the Amazon, or certain tropical regions.

Routine screening for hepatitis C virus is controversial. Reported prevalence rates for various settings vary widely, with small clusters of hepatitis C infection reported among Chinese adoptees, probably secondary to the reuse of needles for drawing blood. Children who have received medical care or undergone invasive medical procedures in institutions or in developing nations are candidates for hepatitis C screening.

Syphilis screening may have been performed as part of a visa medical evaluation, especially if the child came from a refugee camp. However, all children should be screened at least once after arrival. Infants with probable congenital syphilis must be followed serologically, even if appropriately treated, until the screening test reverts to negative. Congenital syphilis is endemic in Eastern Europe and the countries of the former Soviet Union, with rates up 1000 times higher than in the United States. Children originating from certain areas may have positive screening tests because of nonvenereal (endemic) syphilis, yaws, or pinta. If adequate treatment is not documented, these children should receive an appropriate course of therapy.

Tuberculosis is an often-overlooked condition, especially if the child has received BCG vaccine. The most common mistakes are to omit testing because of the presence of a BCG scar or to fail to read the test result correctly if at all. In a recent case, a 9-year-old boy from the Marshall Islands transmitted tuberculosis to 56 (20%) of his contacts in North Dakota; a Mantoux test had been placed at arrival but never read. In the United States, 42% of new cases of tuberculosis are diagnosed in foreign-born persons. Annual infection rates for immigrant children and adoptees are as high as 150 times the yearly incidence rate in the general U.S. population. Even children without symptoms should be screened for tuberculosis with a PPD skin test (Mantoux test), regardless of BCG history. A healthy child with a healing BCG vaccine administration site may be screened with a chest radiograph initially and followed up with a PPD skin test 1 year later.

Recommendations for interpretation of tuberculin skin tests have changed because of concurrent increases in HIV and *Mycobacterium tuberculosis* infections worldwide. Almost certainly, reactions of <5 mm in healthy persons are due to BCG vaccine or exposure to nontuberculosis mycobacteria; reactions of >20 mm are due to exposure to *M. tuberculosis.* Children with reactions of >10 mm should start a regimen of either prophylaxis or treatment, depending on the results of a chest radiograph (Chapter 35). HIV-infected children with reactions of 5–10 mm should be treated similarly. Severely malnourished children and PPD-negative children with a known history of tuberculosis exposure close to the time of immigration should undergo repeat screening within 6–12 months after arrival in the United States.

Intestinal parasites are common and are often unsuspected. A minimum of three stool specimens separated by at least 1 week between samples is preferred. Infection by multiple organisms is not uncommon, with the number of organisms increasing with the age of the child and the poverty level of the previous living conditions. Samples collected into preservative are convenient because the specimens can be saved and submitted all at once, even by mail if necessary. Reported infection rates range from none among adopted Korean infants who arrive from middle-class foster homes to 40% among Latin American immigrants, Romanian adoptees, and adolescent Somali refugees. Any treatment course should be followed by at least one stool examination to confirm eradication. It is not unusual for treatment of the predominant organism to uncover lighter infestations by other parasites. Some immigrant health clinics treat all immigrants from developing countries with an empiric course of albendazole, regardless of screening test results; this strategy has not been evaluated in children.

HIV screening is controversial and probably is not routinely indicated for children from countries of low prevalence, such as Korea, unless there are personal risk factors for infection. However, the current trend is to screen all children at least once, especially those with an unknown medical background. In children adopted from Romania, Russia, Vietnam, and Cambodia HIV infection has been diagnosed after arrival in the United States, despite reportedly negative HIV screening in the country of origin.

Many other diseases are common in immigrant children but do not require routine screening in children who have no symptoms. For example, CMV infection is ubiquitous in most developing nations, with virtually all children being infected by the age of 10 years. There is no benefit from confirming CMV infection in an otherwise healthy child. In the case of a potentially nonimmune mother who is considering pregnancy subsequent to adoption, it is more useful to determine maternal CMV status.

Similarly, serologic tests for hepatitis A or stool cultures for *Salmonella* may be positive but usually have no implications for the health of the child. Parents of immigrant or refugee children are likely to be immune or similarly infected themselves. Adoptive and foster families should be counseled to practice good hygiene and hand washing techniques with all recent arrivals.

Some conditions, such as filariasis or malaria, may not be detected except during clinical relapse, and therefore routine screening is frequently fruitless and falsely reassuring. The rates of HTLV-I, HTLV-II, and hepatitis C infections have not been extensively studied in immigrant compared with nonimmigrant children. The cost of screening otherwise healthy children at this time far outweighs any clinical benefit.

Follow-up Evaluation After Positive Screening Tests. Any positive screening test should trigger a more thorough evaluation and treatment of the presumed condition. Members of the family or household should be screened or referred for appropriate evaluation. The child is often the index patient who leads to identification of infection in adult caretakers. In some situations, such as chronic hepatitis B infection or tuberculosis, other household members may require immunization or chemoprophylaxis.

The Symptomatic Immigrant Child

Unlike their immigrant parents, children may not yet have become immune by means of naturally occurring infections or immunizations to all the common pathogens found in their environment. Thus a recently arrived immigrant child is similar to a traveler returning from that same country (Chapter 104). Within the first month after arrival, as many as one half of immigrant children will have an infectious disease, usually a simple pediatric condition such as otitis media, an upper respiratory tract infection, or gastrointestinal disease (Fig. 103–2).

As the date of immigration becomes more remote, children are far less likely to have the diseases of travelers unless they have

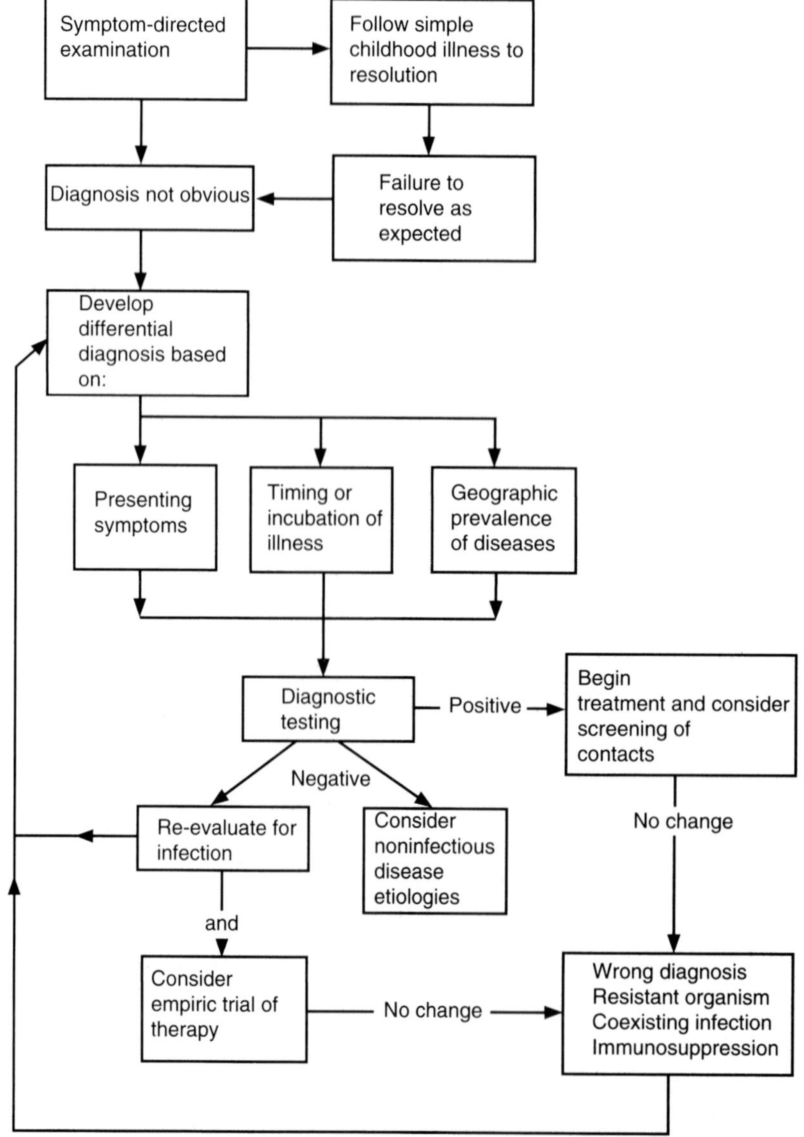

FIGURE 103–2. Infectious disease evaluation of the symptomatic immigrant child.

had continued new exposure because of return trips to or contact with household visitors from the country of origin. For most infectious disease evaluations of immigrant children, the time interval since immigration is the first and often the most important consideration in determining the cause of an illness (see Table 104–9).

Within 1 Month of Arrival. Diseases with short (<1 week) and intermediate (1–4 weeks) incubation periods include most of the vaccine-preventable and common childhood illnesses, all of which are found worldwide. The most frequent diagnoses in newly arrived immigrant children include viral gastroenteritis, measles, rubella, varicella, hepatitis A, pertussis, mumps, lice, scabies, upper respiratory tract infection, impetigo, giardiasis, bacterial enteritis, otitis media, urinary tract infection, and cutaneous candidiasis.

Evaluation should begin with a physical examination to determine the presenting signs and symptoms. The next step is to develop a differential diagnosis list that considers routine childhood illnesses and other diseases, eliminating conditions that do not exist in the geographic areas where the child has recently lived or traveled (Table 103–5 and Fig. 103–3). It should be determined whether any diagnostic testing is required immediately or should be deferred until later if the condition does not resolve. If the child does not appear ill enough to require laboratory evaluation, hospitalization, or empiric treatment, a reasonable plan might be to send the child home on a regimen of symptomatic treatment and provide follow-up by telephone or an office visit within a day or two.

Some literature suggests that drug doses should be revised downward for severely malnourished children, especially for compounds with primarily hepatic excretion. However, pharmacokinetic studies show that alterations in dosage are not necessary for most classes of antimicrobial agents, including antimalarial agents, aminoglycosides, penicillins, and antituberculosis drugs. The exception is chloramphenicol, which may reach high serum concentrations in the severely malnourished child with hepatic compromise.

All acute illnesses, even apparently simple conditions such as otitis media, should be followed to complete resolution. If the illness does not resolve as expected, re-evaluation is necessary to determine whether the original diagnosis was correct, whether the illness is attributable to another process, whether infection is caused by an antibiotic-resistant organism, and whether the family has adhered to antibiotic administration. The symptoms might be attributed to a noninfectious disease, toxin or poison, food intolerance, allergy, or psychological stress. A coexisting acute or chronic infection may complicate the child's recovery. For example, a poorly resolving pneumonia may be the first indication of active pulmonary tuberculosis. Immunosuppression from another chronic infection or malnutrition may impair the response to treatment. The widespread use of over-the-counter antimicrobial agents in other countries has led to multiple drug resistance for many common organisms. In such circumstances, re-treating with an alternate drug should be considered. The physician must also determine whether the child has actually received the prescribed treatment. Some apparent treatment failures are due to incorrect administration of the drug, such as application of oral amoxicillin suspension to the external ear canal for otitis media. Occasionally, the child has not received the medication because it is being used for another family member or the parent has cultural biases about the color, temperature, or mode of administration of the drug. It is often helpful to have a culturally sensitive translator explore the family's medical customs and beliefs, the parent's opinion about what is wrong, and how he or she believes the condition might best be treated.

Within 6 Months of Arrival. Most infectious diseases in immigrant children will present within the first 6 months in the United States (see Table 104–9). After the immediate arrival period is past, the most common conditions recognized include malaria, intestinal and other parasites, hepatitis B, tuberculosis, typhoid or other enteric fevers, and skin diseases. Less frequent in children are exotic mycoses, trachoma, rickettsial diseases, and sexually transmitted diseases.

For a child whose symptoms develop soon after travel to the United States, a differential diagnosis is developed (Fig. 103–2). Most illnesses with long incubation periods (1–6 months) are not easily transmitted to others because of the usual standards of hygiene in the United States, which permits time for thoughtful evaluation.

There is no recommended routine screening list after the initial arrival evaluation is completed. However, the initial step for many

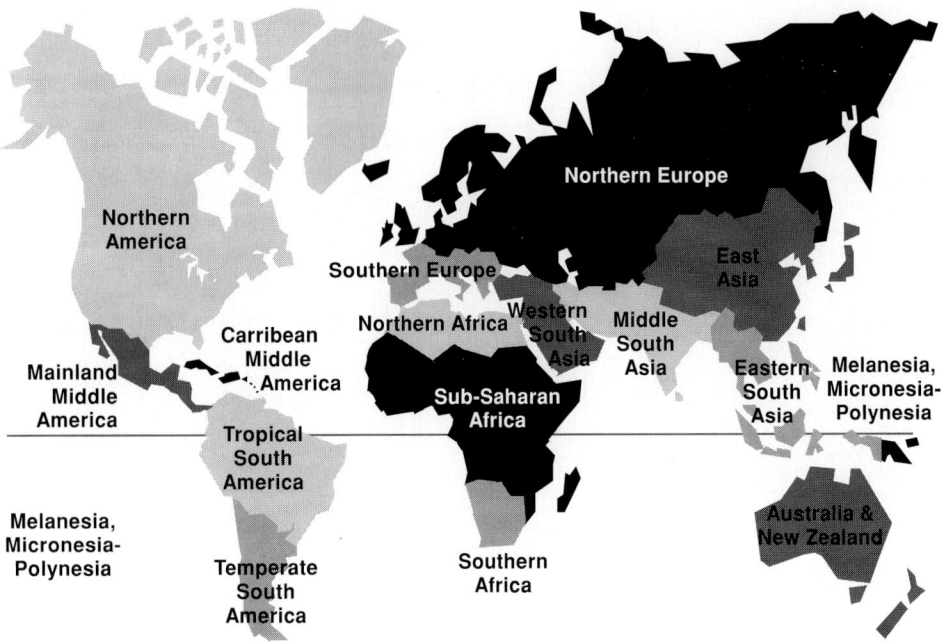

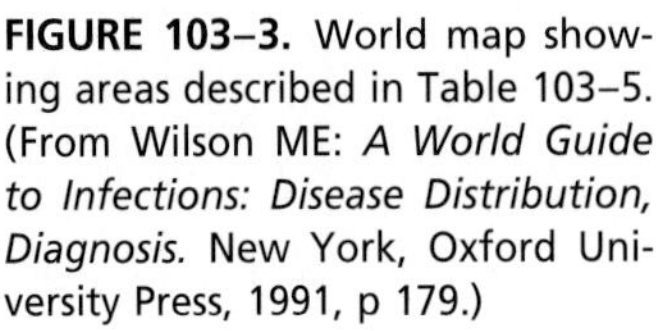
FIGURE 103–3. World map showing areas described in Table 103–5. (From Wilson ME: *A World Guide to Infections: Disease Distribution, Diagnosis.* New York, Oxford University Press, 1991, p 179.)

TABLE 103–5. Infectious Diseases by Worldwide Location (see Fig. 103–3)

Disease	Worldwide*	Africa			Americas					Asia				Europe		Oceania	
		Northern	Sub-Saharan	Southern	Northern	Mainland Middle	Caribbean	Tropical South	Temperate South	East	Eastern South	Middle South	Western South	Northern	Southern	Australia, New Zealand	Melanesia, Micronesia, Polynesia
AIDS	X	X	X	X	X	X	X	X	X	X	X	X	X	X	X	X	X
Acute hemorrhagic conjunctivitis	X	X	X	X	X	X	X	X		X	X	X	X	X	X	(X)	X
Amebiasis	X	X	X	X	X	X	X	X	X	X	X	X	X	X	X	X	X
Angiostrongyliasis		(X)	(X)		X	X	X	X	X	X	X	X				X	X
Anisakiasis					X				X	X	X			X		X	X
Anthrax		X	X	X	X	X	X	X	X	X	X	X	X	X	X	X	X
Ascariasis	X	X	X	X	X	X	X	X	X	X	X	X	X	X	X	X	X
Blastomycosis		X	X	X	X	X		(X)			X	X	X	X			
Brucellosis	X	X	X	X	X	X	X	X	X	X	X	X	X	X	X	X	X
Chagas' disease					X	X	X	X	X								
Chancroid		X	X	X	X	X	X	X	X	X	X	X	X	X	X	X	X
Chikungunya virus			X	X						X	X	X					(X)
Chlamydia	X	X	X	X	X	X	X	X	X	X	X	X	X	X	X	X	X
Cholera		X	X	X	X	(X)		X		X	X	X	X	X	X	X	X
Ciguatera poisoning					X	(X)	X	X			(X)	X				X	X
Clonorchiasis										X	X		(X)				
Coccidioidomycosis					X	X		X	X								
Creutzfeldt-Jakob disease, new variant (nvCJD)														X			
Crimean-Congo hemorrhagic fever		X	X	X						X	X	X	X	X	X		
Cryptosporidiosis	X	X	X	X	X	X	X	X		X	X	X	X	X	X	X	X
Cyclosporiasis	X																
Cysticercosis		X	X	X	X	X	X	X	X	X	X	X	X	X		(X)	(X)
Dengue		X	X	(X)	(X)	X	X	X	X	X	X	X	X			X	X
Diphtheria														X			
Ebola-Marburg virus			X	X							(X)						
Echinococcosis		X	X	X	X	X	(X)	X	X	X	X	X	X	X	X	X	
Enterobiasis	X	X	X	X	X	X	X	X	X	X	X	X	X	X	X	X	X
Escherichia coli O157:H7	X	X	X	X	X	X	X	X	X	X	X	X	X	X	X	X	X
Filariasis		X	X		X	X	X	X		X	X	X	X			(X)	X
Giardiasis	X	X	X	X	X	X	X	X	X	X	X	X	X	X	X	X	X
Gnathostomiasis			X			X				X	X	X	X	X	X	X	
Gonococcal infections	X	X	X	X	X	X	X	X	X	X	X	X	X	X	X	X	X
Hantavirus cardiopulmonary syndrome						X			X								
Hemorrhagic fever with renal syndrome		(X)	(X)	(X)	(X)	(X)		(X)	(X)	X	X	X	(X)	X	X	(X)	(X)
Hepatitis A	X	X	X	X	X	X	X	X	X	X	X	X	X	X	X	X	X
Hepatitis B	X	X	X	X	X	X	X	X	X	X	X	X	X	X	X	X	X
Hepatitis C	X	X	X	X	X	X	X	X	X	X	X	X	X	X	X	X	X
Hepatitis D		X	X	X	X	X	X	X	X	X	X	X	X	X	X	X	X
Hepatitis E		X	X	X		X				X	X	X	X	X			
Histoplasmosis		X	X	X	X	X	X	X	X	X	X	X	X	X	X		(X)
Hookworm		X	X	X	X	X	X	X	X	X	X	X		X	X	X	X
HTLV-1					X		X	X	X								
Japanese encephalitis										X	X	X		X			X
Lassa fever			X	(X)													
Legionellosis		X	X	X	X	X	X		X	X	X	X	X	X	X	X	
Leishmaniasis, cutaneous		X	X	X	X	X	X	X	X	(X)	(X)	X	X	X	X		
Leishmaniasis, visceral		X	X			X	X	X	(X)	X	X	X	X	X	X		
Leprosy		X	X	X	X	X	X	X	X	X	X	X	X	X	X	X	X
Leptospirosis	X	X	X	X	X	X	X	X	X	X	X	X	X	X	X	X	X
Loiasis			X														
Lyme disease		(X)	(X)		X	X				X				X	X		
Lymphogranuloma venereum		X	X	X	X	X	X	X	X	X	X	X	X	X	X	X	X
Malaria		X	X	X	(X)	X	X	X	X	X	X	X	X	X	X	(X)	X
Measles	X	X	X	X	X	X	X	X	X	X	X	X	X	X	X	X	X
Melioidosis			X		(X)	X	X	X		X	X	X	X			X	X
Meningococcus	X	X	X		X			X		X	X	X	X			X	X

TABLE 103–5. Infectious Diseases by Worldwide Location (see Fig. 103–3) *(Continued)*

		Africa			Americas					Asia				Europe		Oceania	
Disease	**Worldwide***	**Northern**	**Sub-Saharan**	**Southern**	**Northern**	**Mainland Middle**	**Caribbean**	**Tropical South**	**Temperate South**	**East**	**Eastern South**	**Middle South**	**Western South**	**Northern**	**Southern**	**Australia, New Zealand**	**Melanesia, Micronesia, Polynesia**
Mumps	X	X	X	X	X	X	X	X	X	X	X	X	X	X	X		X
Onchocercosis		X	X			X		X					X				
Paragonimiasis			X	X	X	X	X	X		X	X	X		X	X		X
Parvovirus	X	X	X	X	X	X	X	X	X	X	X	X	X	X	X	X	X
Pertussis	X	X	X	X	X	X	X	X	X	X	X	X	X	X	X	X	X
Pinta						X	(X)	X									
Plague		X	X	X	X	(X)		X	X	X	X	X	(X)	X			
Poliomyelitis	X	X	X	(X)	(X)	(X)	(X)	(X)	X	X	X	X	X	(X)	(X)	(X)	(X)
Rabies		X	X	X	X	X	X	X	X	X	X	X	X				
Relapsing fever		X	X	X	X	X		X	X	X	X	X	X	X	X		
Rift Valley fever			X										X				
Rocky Mountain spotted fever						X											
Rubella	X	X	X	X	X	X	X	X	X	X	X	X	X	X	X	X	X
St. Louis encephalitis						X											
Salmonellosis	X	X	X	X	X	X	X	X	X	X	X	X	X	X	X	X	X
Scabies	X	X	X	X	X	X	X	X	X	X	X	X	X	X	X	X	X
Schistosomiasis		X	X	X			X	X		X	X	X	X		(X)		
Scombroid fish poisoning	X																
Shigellosis	X	X	X	X	X	X	X	X	X	X	X	X	X	X	X	X	X
Strongyloidiasis		X	X	X	X	X	X	X	X	X	X	X	X	X	X	X	X
Syphilis, nonvenereal		(X)	(X)	(X)								X	X			(X)	
Syphilis, venereal	X	X	X	X	X	X	X	X	X	X	X	X	X	X	X	X	X
Taeniasis		X	X	X	X	X	X	X	X	X	X	X	X	X	X	X	X
Tetanus	X	X	X	X	X	X	X	X	X	X	X	X	X	X	X	X	X
Tickborne encephalitis														X	X		
Toxoplasmosis	X	X	X	X	X	X	X	X	X	X	X	X	X	X	X	X	
Trachoma		X	X	X	X	X	X	X	X	X	X	X	X	X	X	X	X
Trichinellosis		X	X	X	X	X	(X)	X	X	X	X	X	X	X	X	(X)	(X)
Trichuriasis		X	X	X	X	X	X	X	X	X	X	X	X	X	X	X	X
Trypanosomiasis, African			X	X													
Tuberculosis	X	X	X	X	X	X	X	X	X	X	X	X	X	X	X	X	X
Typhoid fever	X	X	X	X	X	X	X	X	X	X	X	X	X	X	X	X	X
Typhus, louseborne		X	X	X	X	X	X	X	X	X	X	X	X	X	X	(X)	X
Typhus, scrub										X	X	X		X		X	X
Typhus, murine	X	X	X	X	X	X	X	X	X	X	X	X	X	X	X	X	X
West Nile virus		X	X	X	X								X	X			
Yaws			X	(X)		X	X	X		(X)	X	X				(X)	X
Yellow fever			X	(X)		X	X	X	(X)								

*Under Worldwide, X = disease agent found in all countries of the world.
X = Disease present in at least part of area.
(X) = Presence of disease in past, uncertain, or poorly documented.
Modified from Wilson ME: *A World Guide to Infections: Disease, Distribution, Diagnosis.* New York, Oxford University Press, 1991, pp 180–203.

of the diseases of long incubation is to review the results of arrival screening tests and to repeat any test that was equivocal or negative. Other useful information is occasionally obtained from a WBC count with a total eosinophil count, chest radiograph, urinalysis, and a thick blood smear for malaria if the child came from an endemic area. Diseases that may no longer exist in the country of origin but were present when the child lived in that country should be included in the differential diagnosis (Table 103–5). Most diagnoses can be eliminated by lack of exposure history or lack of compatible symptoms. Diagnostic tests for many exotic or rare conditions, such as hepatitis E, strongyloidiasis, and rickettsial diseases, are available through state health departments or the CDC. It is usually advisable to discuss the possible differential diagnosis and evaluation with a travel or tropical medicine expert before embarking on an extensive serologic evaluation. If there is doubt, a few milliliters of serum can be saved for antibody titers to be determined later.

As time since immigration lengthens, infectious diseases become less important and other chronic health conditions become more apparent. The temptation is to consider an exotic disease first for an immigrant child, but other common pediatric problems should not be ignored. In a survey of adoptive families, the most common conditions that parents listed that were misdiagnosed, addressed late, or caused the family or child significant distress included abnormal growth, recurrent otitis media, skin disease, food intolerance, allergies, vision or hearing loss, developmental delay, emotional or behavioral difficulties, anemia, nutritional deficiencies, and unrecognized previous physical or sexual abuse.

The physician must also guard against the tendency to attribute all problems to foreign residence. Long-term studies of adoptees and refugees show that the issues relating to adoption, abandonment, war, or cultural transplantation may never be completely resolved, even in persons who moved as infants. Infectious diseases rarely play a role in these circumstances.

Six Months or More After Arrival. Infectious disease issues are far less common 6 months or more after immigration to the United States. Usual pediatric problems, depression, and cultural issues assume more importance as time passes. However, the pediatrician should keep in mind that some diseases have very long incubation periods (2 months to 2 years). Usually these diseases manifest as long-term complications of the underlying disease rather than with the signs and symptoms of the disease itself. The most common diagnoses in this category are neurocysticercosis presenting as seizures, chronic hepatitis B presenting as nephrotic syndrome or glomerulonephritis, echinococcosis presenting as peritonitis or pleural effusion following rupture of a hydatid cyst, and various long-term parasitic infections such as liver flukes or schistosomiasis presenting as liver or central nervous system disease. Chagas' disease may present in adulthood as heart failure. Tuberculosis or leprosy may become recrudescent after other stresses, such as immunosuppression or pregnancy. AIDS is not yet a major issue in immigrant children because of restrictive U.S. admission policies, but it will become more important as HIV infection spreads in Southeast Asian countries, where a large percentage of immigrant children originate.

REVIEWS

Centers for Disease Control and Prevention: *Health Information for International Travel, 2001–2002.* Atlanta, US Department of Health and Human Services, Public Health Service, 2001. (Available at www.cdc.gov/travel/yellowbook.pdf)

Jenista JA (editor): Medical issues in international adoptions. *Pediatr Ann* 2000;29:204–52.

Wilson ME: *A World Guide to Infections: Disease, Distribution, Diagnosis.* New York, Oxford University Press, 1991.

KEY ARTICLES

Albers LH, Johnson DE, Hostetter MK, et al: Health of children adopted from the former Soviet Union and Eastern Europe: Comparison with preadoptive medical records. *JAMA* 1997;278:922–4.

American Thoracic Society: Targeted tuberculin testing and treatment of latent tuberculosis infection. *Am J Respir Crit Care Med* 2000; 161:S221–47.

Centers for Disease Control and Prevention: Health status of and intervention for U.S.-bound Kosovar refugees–Fort Dix, New Jersey, May-July 1999. *MMWR Morb Mortal Wkly Rep* 48:729–32, 1999.

Centers for Disease Control and Prevention: Measles—United States—1999. *MMWR Morb Mortal Wkly Rep* 49:557–60, 2000.

Committee on the Health and Adjustment of Immigrant Children and Families, National Research Council and Institute of Medicine: In Hernandez DJ, Charney E, editors: *From Generation to Generation: The Health and Well-Being of Children in Immigrant Families.* Washington, DC, National Academy Press, 1998. (May be downloaded from www.nap.edu)

DeRiemer K, Chin DP, Schecter GF, et al: Tuberculosis among immigrants and refugees. *Arch Intern Med* 1998;158:753–60.

Dreskin SC: A prescription drug packaged in China and sold as an ethnic remedy. *JAMA* 2000;283:2393.

Dwelle TL: Inadequate basic preventive health measures: Survey of missionary children in sub-Saharan Africa. *Pediatrics* 1995;95:733–7.

Espinal MA, Kim SJ, Suarez PG, et al: Standard short-course chemotherapy for drug-resistant tuberculosis: Treatment outcomes in 6 countries. *JAMA* 2000;283:2537–45.

Fadiman A: *The Spirit Catches You and You Fall Down: A Hmong Child, Her American Doctors, and the Collision of Two Cultures.* New York, Farrar, Straus and Giroux, 1997.

Flores G: Culture and the patient-physician relationship: Achieving cultural competency in health care. *J Pediatr* 2000;136:14–23.

Halfon N, Wood DL, Valdez RB, et al: Medicaid enrollment and health services access by Latino children in inner-city Los Angeles. *JAMA* 1997;277:636–41.

Hoge CW, Shlim DR, Echeverria P, et al: Epidemiology of diarrhea among expatriate residents living in a highly endemic environment. *JAMA* 1996;275:533–8.

Humphrey JH, Rice AL: Vitamin A supplementation of young infants. *Lancet* 2000;356:422–4.

Hurie MB, Gennis MA, Hernandez LV, et al: Prevalence of hepatitis B markers and measles, mumps and rubella antibodies among Jewish refugees from the former Soviet Union. *JAMA* 1995;273:954–6.

Lobato MN, Hopewell PC: *Mycobacterium tuberculosis* infection after travel to or contact with visitors from countries with a high prevalence of tuberculosis. *Am J Respir Crit Care Med* 1998;158:1871–5.

Meropol SB: Health status of pediatric refugees in Buffalo, NY. *Arch Pediatr Adolesc Med* 1995;149:887–92.

Miller LC: Internationally adopted children—immunization status. *Pediatrics* 1999;103:1078.

Muennig P, Pallin D, Sell RL, et al: The cost effectiveness of strategies for the treatment of intestinal parasites in immigrants. *N Engl J Med* 1999;340:773–9.

Pastore DR, Diaz A: Cultural and medical issues of Latino adolescents. *Adolesc Med* 1998;9:315–22.

Pollack RJ, Kiszewski A, Armstrong P, et al: Differential permethrin susceptibility of head lice sampled in the United States and Borneo. *Arch Pediatr Adolesc Med* 1999;153:969–73.

Statistical Yearbook of the Immigration and Naturalization Service, 1998. Washington, DC, US Government Printing Office, 2000. (May also be downloaded from www.ins.usdoj.gov/graphics/aboutins/statistics/index.htm)

Talbot EA, Moore M, McCray E, et al: Tuberculosis among foreign-born persons in the United Sates, 1993–1998. *JAMA* 2000;284:2894–900.

World Health Organization: *International Travel and Health: Vaccination Requirements and Health Advice—Situation as on 1 January 2001.* WHO, 2001. (May also be downloaded from www.who.int/ith/index.html)

CHAPTER 104

The International Child Traveler

Jerri Ann Jenista

Almost every pediatric practitioner will be faced with questions about international travel. Children of all ages travel widely, with or without parents. Parents are often unaware of specific health precautions for children, especially if the parents travel infrequently. Medical information from travel agencies, embassies, consulates, or national airlines is inconsistent, often out of date, and rarely specific for children. Even traveler's clinics, which care primarily for adults, may not be fully aware of differing recommendations for children in many aspects of travel health: routine and special immunizations, immunoglobulin injections, pediatric doses of prophylactic medications, and anticipatory guidance for the maintenance of health and the care of childhood illnesses abroad.

Most children can travel quite safely if they have a thorough health consultation before they depart. Prophylactic measures and education about dietary precautions are the best insurance for a healthy trip. Parental flexibility, a sense of humor, planning for the worst, and a relaxed travel itinerary will make for the most enjoyable trip for all.

POPULATION AT RISK

Statistics are not kept separately for children, but more than 30 million U.S. citizens travel abroad each year, one half of them to developing nations. In a study (Pitzinger et al, 1991) of 363 Swiss children traveling to tropical regions, 6% were <3 years of age, 13% were 3–6 years of age, 13% were 7–14 years of age, and 69% were 15–20 years of age. About one third of the children, including the very young, were making repeat visits. In this study, although most children visited a single hotel or a resort, 17%, including 9% of child travelers <7 years of age, took adventure tours and lived under primitive conditions. Apart from tourism, older children, especially adolescents, may travel without parents or even alone as exchange students, on school trips, or as volunteer workers.

Immigrant parents may not consider themselves tourists when taking their children to visit extended family in their native country. Since the travel is not "exotic," there may be a tendency to reduce or ignore health precautions in one's own home. The notion that the parent had a perfectly healthy childhood in the native country may not apply to offspring born and reared in the United States.

In a special class with regard to medical needs are children who accompany their parents for military duty, long-term business, educational or diplomatic tours, or missionary or foreign aid work. Stays of longer than 3 months may place such children at risk not only of the problems of travelers but also those of immigrants. Evaluation of these groups must be designed carefully on the basis of both the living circumstances and the duration of the foreign residence.

BEFORE THE TRIP

Brief travel to Western Europe, Japan, Canada, Australia, or New Zealand poses little or no more health risk to the pediatric tourist than staying in the United States. All other traveling children need a careful and comprehensive evaluation. Military, public health, university, or private international health clinics should be used where available. Travel recommendations change so frequently that it is nearly impossible for the individual practitioner to keep current. Some corporations, student programs, and aid or volunteer organizations require an orientation at a central location before travel. Health evaluation and education are frequently major components of that preparation.

However, even the most experienced centers deal primarily with adults. The pediatrician may still have to determine drug dosages and schedules peculiar to children and to alter the routine immunization schedule for very young children. Fortunately, there are now many easily available and useful resources for the physician treating such patients (Table 104–1).

Timing a Travel Consultation. There are several components of travel health (Table 104–2). If possible, the first travel consultation visit should be at least 6–8 weeks before the proposed trip. It may take several weeks to complete a compressed immunization schedule for the very young child or certain special vaccine series for travelers of all ages. An office visit 3 weeks before travel may be sufficient for children who have completed their primary immunization series and do not need any special vaccines. A visit during the week before travel is necessary for the administration of immunoglobulin injections for some travelers. Last-minute visits, except by frequent travelers who have had good travel health care in the past, should be discouraged.

Reviewing the Itinerary. The first step of any travel consultation should be a general evaluation of risk of any particular trip (Table 104–3). Long stays with young children in primitive conditions with several intermediate stops present more chances for disease exposure than does a brief single hotel stay with an older child. Mingling with the local population is different from traveling with a tour group.

HIV Testing. More than 50 countries or territories, including the United States, contrary to World Health Organization guidelines, require HIV- or AIDS-free certificates to admit certain travelers. Young children are usually exempt from these rules, but it is wise to inquire at the time of any visa application.

Routine Childhood Immunizations

Routine childhood immunizations are an important element of travel health (Table 104–4).

Measles. Measles is endemic throughout much of the developing world and remains a risk even in some developed nations of Europe and Asia. Some industrialized countries do not require vaccine or require that it be administered at later ages than in the United

TABLE 104–1. Resources on Pediatric Travel Health

Health Information for International Travel (the "Yellow Book")

Published by the Centers for Disease Control and Prevention and updated annually, this excellent resource is essential for the management of any travel evaluation. Most helpful are the country-by-country lists of vaccines and malaria prophylaxis recommendations and detailed instructions on immunizations for children. You can download the full version for free at www.cdc.gov/travel/yellowbook.pdf or order from:

Public Health Foundation
877-252-1200
bookstore.phf.org/prod159.htm

CDC Travelers' Health Home
www.cdc.gov/travel

This is the CDC website on travel health with links to many other services, such as lists of travel clinics and immunization guidelines. All the information available in CDC printed materials and by fax is available here. Most helpful are the destination-specific recommendations and disease descriptions. Also, the site posts daily updated information on disease outbreaks, rumors, and hoaxes.

International Travel and Health: Vaccination Requirements and Health Advice

Updated annually by the World Health Organization and published a few months in advance of the CDC version, this is also an excellent resource for country-by-country lists of disease risks. The parts relevant to U.S. travelers are usually reprinted in the CDC version. The full document can be downloaded for free from www.who.int/ith/index.html or order from:

WHO Publications Center USA
49 Sheridan Ave.
Albany, NY 12210
518-436-9686

World Health Organization Website
www.who.int

This website contains updated information on travel health, including the above book. However, this is one of the best resources on disease outbreaks (www.who.int/emc/outbreak_news/) and emerging infectious diseases worldwide. There are also links to other helpful services, such as physicians and clinics.

CDC International Traveler's Information Line
877-FYI-TRIP (877-394-8747)

This is an automated telephone version of the CDC book listed above. It is updated regularly and is available 24 hours a day, 7 days a week. You must use a touch-tone telephone, and it is best to have pencil and paper handy. A typical phone call addressing all the travel precautions for a trip to India for a child takes about 15–20 minutes. A shorter version, dispensing with the disease descriptions, takes about 10 minutes. Specific questions, such as the dose of an antimalarial drug for a 2-year old, can be accessed in less than 3 minutes. There is no live consultant, but health care providers may ask CDC experts for malaria-specific questions during working hours at 770-488-7788 or 888-232-3228.

CDC Information Line
800-311-3435

Open during working hours, this line will allow you access to all CDC travel services, including consultants who speak Spanish.

CDC Fax Information Service
888-232-3299

You must first call to receive a directory. Numerous directories of CDC information are available, including Travel Health. Callers should have the telephone number of their fax machine readily available. Once callers have received the directory, sent immediately by return fax, they may call back and receive documents of interest. Up to 5 documents may be ordered during one call.

United States State Department Travel Warnings and Consular Sheets
travel.state.gov/travel_warnings.html

This excellent website provides information updated daily on health, social, and physical warnings about travel, including natural disasters, political unrest, and disease outbreaks. This site is a must for any traveler going to a nontourist destination.

International Society for Travel Medicine
www.istm.org

This professional organization offers travel health information and links to other sites. They also sponsor a biennial conference and lists of member practitioners and travel clinics worldwide. The reader may search back issues of the *Journal of Travel Medicine* with many articles and abstracts directly accessed directly from the site.

American Society for Tropical Medicine and Hygiene
www.astmh.org

This is an excellent site for up-to-date information on tropical diseases. Readers can search abstracts of the upcoming annual meeting for both research and clinical topics.

TABLE 104–1. Resources on Pediatric Travel Health *(Continued)*

International Association for Medical Assistance to Travelers
Provides complete "health packets" of information for travelers, including worldwide directories of English-speaking physicians experienced in travel medicine. The website www.sentex.net/~iamat/ provides ordering information.

IAMAT
736 Center Street
Lewiston, NY 14092
716-754-4883

United States Environmental Protection Agency Office of Pesticide Programs
www.epa.gov/pesticides/citizens/deet.htm
www.epa.gov/pesticides/citizens/insectrp.htm
These pages provide practical information on the use and safety of DEET (N,N-diethyl-3-methylbenzamide) and other insect repellants. The EPA also sponsors the National Pesticide Telecommunications Network to answer professional and consumer questions at 800-858-7378 or via the Internet at www.ace.orst.edu/info/nptn

Wilderness Medicine Institute
This private group provides education for medical professionals, travel organizers, and lay persons on preventive and emergency medical care in wilderness settings, including at high altitudes. They also sponsor a number of helpful handbooks and guides to be used in the field or in the office. Order through the website wmi.nols.edu

WMI
413 Main Street
Pitkin, CO 81241
970-641-3572

TABLE 104–2. Checklist for Travel Health Consultation

Prophylactic Infectious Disease Measures
Routine childhood immunizations
Special-risk immunizations
Immunoglobulin injections
Chemoprophylaxis for malaria

Counseling for General Health
Diet
Hygiene
Sexual contacts
Wilderness or high-altitude travel
Injury prevention

Counseling for Potential Illness
Where to seek medical care
General precautions for medical care abroad
Specific advice for:
- Diarrhea
- Fever
- Otitis media
- Respiratory or rash illness

Travel Health Documents
International Certificate of Vaccination or waiver
HIV- or AIDS-free certificate
Written prescriptions for medications, eyeglasses, medical equipment
Health insurance information
List of medical contacts
Routine and special immunization and immunoglobulin injection records
Summary of condition and treatment for any chronic or recurring health problem
Personal identification on the child

States. Because measles can be severe in very young children, it is best to assure immunity before travel. In the United States, the first dose of MMR is given at 12–15 months of age. The second dose is routinely given at 4–6 years of age but may be given at any visit, provided that at least 4 weeks have elapsed since the first dose and that both doses are given when the child is ≥12 months of age. Any child who is to travel, even if of preschool age, should receive the second dose of MMR before travel.

An unimmunized child should receive a single dose of MMR before departure and a second dose 1 month later if he or she remains in the high-risk area. If the child returns to the United States within that month, the second dose can be given at the recommended 4–6 years of age.

Infants 6–11 months of age should receive measles vaccine alone, with MMR at 12–15 months of age and a third dose at 4–6 years of age. If simple measles vaccine is not available, MMR can be used. Infants remaining in high-risk areas should be reimmunized with MMR at 12 months of age. Infants <6 months of age are protected by maternal antibody, but if they remain in an endemic area beyond 6 months of age, MMR immunization is given as for an infant 6–11 months of age.

All MMR doses should be administered at least 2 weeks before any anticipated injection of immunoglobulin. There are no data on the efficacy of immunoglobulin injection in preventing infection or disease when given before exposure. If measles or MMR vaccine is contraindicated, the child can be given postexposure prophylaxis, if needed, with intramuscular IG (0.25 mL/kg for immunocompetent children; 0.5 mL/kg for immunocompromised children) up to 6 days after an exposure. Immunoglobulin produced in developing nations may carry risks of disease transmission, as may the administration itself, especially if poorly sterilized injection equipment is used.

Mumps and Rubella. Mumps or rubella infection carries little risk to an otherwise healthy child. MMR vaccine is given according to routine schedules as early as the age of 12–15 months. Susceptible parents should be immunized to avoid contracting either infection from their children.

TABLE 104–3. Questions to Determine the General Risk of Travel

Questions	Relevance
Which countries will the child visit? Will there be any transit stops in the itinerary?	Western Europe, Canada, United States, Australia, and Japan are generally low-risk areas. Transit stops may impose further entry requirements upon arrival in the destination country.
What is the purpose of this trip? • Tourism or family visit? • Educational visit or exchange? • Long-term residence or emigration? • Adventure or volunteer work?	Resort tourism, business, or family visits present less risk for infectious disease exposure than adventure tours, volunteer work, or long-term residence.
What types of activities are anticipated? • Camping or trekking? • Extensive contact with the local population, especially children? • Involvement in medical or refugee work?	The more intimate or prolonged the contact with the environment or the local population, the greater the chance of exposure to disease. Medical or refugee work may be particularly high risk.
With whom will the child travel? • Relatives, school, or other leaders? • Will the adults be familiar with the child's medical history? • Will they be familiar with the medical system of the region visited?	Unaccompanied children, children traveling with unfamiliar adults, and adolescents traveling in groups or alone are at higher risk of disease because of the difficulty of supervising their behavior and hygiene.
Where will the child be staying? • Hotels, hostels, resorts, family homes, or camping?	Family homes and international-class urban or resort hotels present lower risk of exposure than youth hostels, campgrounds, or other traveler accommodations. Meals from a regular source are generally safer than those obtained from a different kitchen each day.
What is the expected duration of the total trip? Of each stop?	Stays of hours to <3 weeks present low risk for exposure to disease except for waterborne and foodborne pathogens.
Will any stay be longer than 3 months?	Residence of >3 months increases the disease risk closer to that of the local population.
What is the child's ability to supervise his or her own diet and hygiene? Will infants be breast-fed exclusively?	Adolescents are at high risk of foodborne and waterborne illness, as are toddlers and infants. Exclusive breast-feeding is optimal when possible.
What is the medical history of the child? Are there problems likely to recur or deteriorate during travel?	Recurrent problems such as otitis media or chronic conditions such as diabetes, asthma, or immune deficiency may necessitate special planning and provision of medications or medical equipment.

TABLE 104–4. Immunizations and Immunoglobulin for Traveling Children

Routine Childhood Immunizations	Special Immunizations	Immunoglobulins
Measles*	Rabies	Standard (IG)§
Mumps*	Hepatitis A	Rabies (RIG)
Rubella*	Typhoid	Hepatitis B (HBIG)
OPV or IPV	Yellow fever†‡	
Diphtheria	Japanese encephalitis	
Pertussis	Meningococcus	
Tetanus	BCG	
Hepatitis B	Influenza virus	
Haemophilus influenzae type b	Tickborne encephalitis	
Pneumococcus		
Varicella*		

*Give at least 2 weeks before anticipated immunoglobulin injection.
†Avoid giving cholera vaccine within 3 weeks of yellow fever vaccine.
‡The only vaccine that may be required for entry into a country under WHO guidelines.
§For pre-exposure hepatitis A prophylaxis if hepatitis A immunization is not given or if immediate protection (within 14 days) is necessary. IG is also used for postexposure hepatitis A and measles prophylaxis.

Poliomyelitis. For travel to all developing countries and to any country that has a polio epidemic, children should have a full primary series of polio vaccine. In the United States, a primary series is three doses of IPV given at the ages of 2, 4, and 6–18 months. A booster dose is given at the age of 4–6 years. Previously unimmunized children traveling to high-risk areas should receive three doses of IPV at 6- to 8-week intervals. A booster dose, if time permits, may be given 8–12 months after the primary series is completed. If the time to travel is short, the primary immunization schedule can be compressed to three doses given at 4-week intervals. If the time to travel is less than 4 weeks, a single dose of OPV should be given.

School-age children and adults who have completed a three- or four-dose primary series of IPV or OPV should receive a once-per-lifetime booster dose of IPV before traveling to a developing country.

Infants who have received only one or two doses of IPV should receive another dose before travel if it has been at least 4 weeks since the last dose. If the infant remains in the high-risk area, he or she should complete a primary series of three doses at 4-week intervals, followed by a fourth dose 6 weeks after the third dose. If the infant returns to the United States before the series is complete, the standard immunization schedule may be resumed.

Infants <6 weeks of age should receive a "newborn" dose of OPV before travel. This "newborn" dose does not count as part of a primary series. For infants remaining in high-risk areas, the three-dose primary series should be started with the first dose 4 weeks after the ''newborn'' dose, the second and third doses at 4-week intervals, and a fourth dose at least 6 weeks after the last of the primary series. The standard schedule can be resumed if the child returns to the United States at any point in the primary series.

If OPV is contraindicated or unavailable, IPV can be substituted in these schedules. IPV may be given to infants as young as 6 weeks of age; efficacy before 6 weeks of age has not been studied.

***Haemophilus influenzae* Type b.** *H. influenzae* type b is found worldwide. All children <5 years of age should receive a full series of conjugate vaccine. The number and timing of doses depend on which vaccine is used (Chapter 17). Any child <15 months of age should have at least two doses given at a minimum interval of 4 weeks. After 15 months of age, a single dose of any licensed conjugate vaccine is sufficient, even in a previously unimmunized child.

Diphtheria, Pertussis, and Tetanus. Compared with the United States, children are at higher risk of contracting diphtheria or pertussis in many areas of the world, including certain developed nations where the vaccines are not mandatory. Tetanus is found worldwide. Thus all traveling children should be protected from these infections as fully as possible.

All children should receive DTP, starting at the age of 6–8 weeks and repeated every 6–8 weeks, with a fourth dose at the age of 15–18 months and a booster at the age of 4–6 years. If necessary for travel, immunization can begin when the child is as young as 4 weeks of age and be repeated at 4-week intervals. A single dose provides little or no protection; two doses may be sufficient protection against tetanus or diphtheria but not against pertussis. The fourth dose of acellular DTaP should be given about 12 months after the third dose but can be given as soon as the age of 12 months, provided at least 6 months have elapsed since the third dose, if the child travels to or remains in a high-risk area.

Unimmunized children >7 years of age should receive a primary series of three doses of the adult formulation of tetanus and diphtheria toxoids (Td). The first two doses are given 4–8 weeks apart, and the third dose 6–12 months after the second dose. All immunized children and adults, whether traveling or not, after receiving the full primary series should receive a Td booster every 10 years.

Hepatitis B. All children should receive a three-dose series of hepatitis B vaccine, beginning at birth or by the age of 2 months. Vaccination is recommended for unimmunized persons who will be living in a high-risk country for >6 months, who expect to receive medical or dental care, who may have exposure to blood or bodily fluids, who expect to have sexual relations, or who may have prolonged intimate contact with young children in the endemic country. This includes children in families working in refugee camps or orphanages or making extended visits to relatives in countries where there is a high prevalence of hepatitis B. Regions endemic for hepatitis B include most of South and Southeast Asia, Oceania, and sub-Saharan Africa. Areas of intermediate risk include most of South and Central America and the countries surrounding the Mediterranean Sea.

Immunization against hepatitis B requires three doses, with the second dose 1–2 months and the third dose 4–12 months after the first dose. Parents may wish to bring vaccine and injection equipment to complete the series while traveling if the risk of exposure will be high. There is no contraindication to finishing a series with a vaccine from a different manufacturer as long as the correct dose for age is used. If the time to travel is short and there is expected to be a high risk of exposure to hepatitis B, alternative schedules of 0, 1, 2 and 12 months, or 0, 1, 3 weeks and 6–12 months may be used.

Hepatitis B immunoglobulin (HBIG) provides only temporary protection against disease and should never be substituted for vaccination. The primary use of HBIG is for postexposure prophylaxis of unimmunized persons.

Varicella. All children 12 months to 13 years of age should receive one dose of varicella vaccine. Vaccination should be considered for international travelers who do not have serologic evidence of immunity to VZV, especially if they expect to have close personal contact with local populations, because varicella is endemic in most countries. Nonimmune children ≥13 years of age and adults should receive two doses given ≥4 weeks apart.

Pneumococcus. All children 2–23 months of age should receive pneumococcal conjugate vaccine. Vaccination is also recommended for children 24–59 months of age who are at increased risk of pneumococcal disease, including children with sickle cell disease, HIV infection, and other immunocompromising or chronic medical conditions. There are no specific recommendations for travelers.

Influenza. Influenza vaccines should be given annually to persons ≥6 months of age who, because of age or underlying medical condition, are at increased risk of complications of influenza. Household members in close contact with persons in high-risk groups should be vaccinated to decrease the risk of transmitting influenza to persons at high risk. Influenza vaccine also can be administered to any person ≥6 months of age to reduce the chance of infection with influenza, including travelers with likely exposure. The risk of exposure to influenza during travel depends on the time of year and the destination. In the tropics, influenza can occur throughout the year. In the temperate regions of the Southern Hemisphere, most influenza activity occurs from April through September. In temperate climate zones of the Northern and Southern Hemispheres, travelers also can be exposed to influenza during the summer, especially when traveling as part of large organized tourist groups that include persons from areas of the world where influenza viruses are circulating. Persons at high risk of complications of influenza who were not vaccinated with influenza vaccine during the preceding fall or winter should consider receiving influenza vaccine before travel if they plan to go to the tropics, to travel with large organized tourist groups at any time of year, or to travel to the Southern Hemisphere from April through September.

No information is available regarding the benefits of revaccinating persons before summer travel who were already vaccinated in the preceding fall. Persons at high risk who received the previous season's vaccine before travel should be revaccinated with the current vaccine in the following fall or winter. Persons at high risk, including those >50 years of age, embarking on travel during the summer might be advised to carry antiviral medications for either prophylaxis or treatment of influenza because many of these drugs are unavailable outside the United States (Table 68–11).

Special Immunizations

For all special use vaccines, the risk of actual exposure to the disease must be weighed carefully against the cost, adverse effects, and efficacy of the vaccine (Table 104–4).

Cholera. Despite the current pandemic of cholera, the disease is unusual in travelers from the United States. Most imported cases have been traced to improperly prepared or contaminated imported foods. Careful attention to food preparation and water purity is the best protection for most children. Families should be counseled carefully about how to use **oral rehydration solution (ORS)** if symptoms of cholera occur.

Cholera vaccine is not required for entry or exit by any country. Cholera vaccine is of questionable efficacy and is not recommended for any traveler. Currently, it is not manufactured in or available for use in the United States. Cholera vaccine may interfere with the efficacy of yellow fever vaccine; if given in another country, the two vaccines should be given at least 3 weeks apart.

Rabies. Rabies vaccine should be seriously considered for travelers with occupational risk of exposure or for persons with children who will be living for longer than 1 month in regions where rabies in dogs is endemic, which includes most of South and Central America, South and Southeast Asia, and Africa. A list of rabies-free countries is available on the CDC Travel Health website (Table 104–1).

The rabies pre-exposure vaccination schedule is the same for children and adults: three doses given either intramuscularly (1 mL) or intradermally (0.1 mL) on days 0, 7, and 28. The larger intramuscular dose is strongly preferred to maximize the immune response and may be especially important for travelers who will also be taking chloroquine or related antimalarial drugs that may interfere with rabies antibody production.

Children are attracted to animals and are at far higher risk of being bitten than are adults. Families should be counseled carefully about the need to avoid strange animals, especially dogs and monkeys. All animal bites in a rabies-endemic area should be treated immediately. An immunized person requires two postexposure doses of vaccine (days 0 and 3), whereas an unimmunized person needs five postexposure doses of vaccine (days 0, 3, 7, 14, and 28) in addition to RIG.

Typhoid. Typhoid vaccines are not a substitute for careful food and water precautions. Children traveling to the Indian subcontinent or to the western regions of South America should receive a primary typhoid series if exposure to contaminated foods or water seems likely. However, typhoid vaccine is not an entry requirement for any country. There are two vaccines available. Both have been shown to protect 50–80% of recipients.

The oral live attenuated typhoid vaccine, manufactured from the **TY21a strain** of *Salmonella typhi,* is given as a capsule every other day for four doses, beginning at least 2 weeks before travel. It has few or no side effects but is licensed for use in persons ≥6 years of age. The series is repeated every 5 years if there will be continued exposure. The Ty21a vaccine should not be used for immunocompromised persons or persons who are taking antibiotics.

An injectable capsular polysaccharide typhoid vaccine **(ViCPS)** is indicated for persons ≥2 years of age. A full immune response follows a single injection within 4 weeks, but there is substantial protection even at 2 weeks. Adverse effects are reportedly far less frequent and less severe than with the heat-phenol–inactivated vaccine, which is no longer manufactured. A booster dose is recommended every 2 years if there will be continued exposure.

Meningococcus. Meningococcal disease is found worldwide. A single dose of meningococcal vaccine is recommended for travelers to sub-Saharan Africa or to any country reporting epidemic disease. Saudi Arabia requires a certificate of meningococcal immunization for pilgrims traveling to Mecca.

Meningococcal vaccine consists of capsular polysaccharide extracted from whole bacteria. The vaccine available in the United States covers serogroups A, C, Y, and W-135. There is no vaccine for serogroup B. The response to the quadrivalent vaccine or to any individual component is unpredictable in children <2 years of age, especially in infants <3 months of age. Any child who received the vaccine when younger than 4 years of age should receive a booster dose 2–3 years after the initial dose if there will be continued or new exposure. The *H. influenzae* type b vaccine conjugated to meningococcal outer membrane protein does *not* substitute for meningococcal vaccine.

Japanese Encephalitis. Japanese encephalitis virus is a mosquitoborne arbovirus found throughout Japan, eastern Asia, and the Indian subcontinent. The disease now occurs rarely on the main islands of Japan or in Hong Kong. In endemic areas most infections are subclinical, although in symptomatic cases the fatality rate approaches 50%; many survivors have neurologic sequelae. An effective inactivated virus vaccine is available and should be considered for children who will live ≥4 weeks in endemic regions either during the rainy seasons in tropical areas or during the summer or autumn in temperate countries. Travel outside these seasons or confined to urban areas poses little risk of transmission. Fewer than 10 confirmed cases have occurred among U.S. travelers in the past 10 years, primarily among military personnel. Details of risk by country, region, and season are listed on the CDC Travel Health website (Table 104–1).

The WHO recommends that the vaccine be given only to persons ≥1 of age because most infants in endemic areas are protected by maternal antibody. However, children, regardless of age, traveling from nonendemic countries should receive Japanese encephalitis vaccine if the travel itinerary indicates that exposure to mosquitoes in high-risk areas is unavoidable. For most travelers, however, mosquito nets, insect repellents, protective clothing, room insecticides, and sleeping in air-conditioned or screened rooms are sufficient protection.

Japanese encephalitis vaccine, a formalin-inactivated, purified mouse-brain-derived vaccine, is now available in the United States for travelers to high-risk regions of Asia. Those whose travel itinerary suggests a high risk of exposure to the mosquito vector of the virus should receive a primary series of three doses of vaccine given on days 0, 7, and 30, with the last dose ≥10 days before travel to the endemic area. The dose is 0.5 mL for children 1–3 years of age and 1 mL for older children and adults, given subcutaneously. An abbreviated schedule of 0, 7, and 14 days can be used if necessitated by time constraints. Two doses given 1 week apart induce antibodies in approximately 80% of vaccinees but should not be used except under unusual circumstances. A booster dose may be recommended 2–3 years after the primary series if exposure is recurring. Reactions to the vaccine are usually mild to moderate. Allergic reactions, including urticaria and angioedema, are among the more serious. Local side effects, such as redness or swelling, occur in 20% of vaccine recipients. A few patients report systemic symptoms, such as fever, malaise, nausea, or abdominal pain.

Yellow Fever. Yellow fever is endemic in a belt across mid-Africa and the Amazon basin of South America. However, the countries reporting disease change frequently. Yellow fever is the *only* disease for which countries may require an International Certificate of Vaccination under WHO guidelines. In general, a vaccine certificate is required for any person traveling to or from a country reporting transmission. The CDC Travelers' Health website provides a current country listing.

Yellow fever vaccine is an attenuated live-virus preparation. A single dose probably provides lifetime immunity, but vaccine certificates are good for only 10 years. Vaccine is available solely through official Yellow Fever Vaccination Centers, designated by each state health department, and should be administered at least 10 days before travel to endemic areas. The vaccine certificate is acceptable only if filled out correctly, validated by a Uniform Stamp, and verified by an original signature.

The most serious complication of yellow fever vaccine is viral encephalitis, which occurs exclusively in infants. Thus the vaccine is contraindicated in any infant <4 months of age. Infants 4–9 months of age should be immunized only if the risk of exposure will be high and other means of preventing mosquitoborne disease (e.g., mosquito nets, repellants) cannot be used. Children >9 months of age and adults should be immunized if they will be visiting or residing in countries with current outbreaks or in rural areas of any country lying in endemic areas, even if no cases of yellow fever have been reported from that country.

For travel to some countries, unvaccinated children <12 months of age, or for other countries, children <6 months of age, must obtain a signed and dated medical waiver written on letterhead stationery. The itinerary of any child traveling through South America or Africa should be reviewed carefully because transit stops of even a few hours may necessitate a vaccine certificate or waiver to enter the country of final destination. Travelers who arrive without the proper documents may be detained in isolation, denied entry, or vaccinated at the point of entry.

Tickborne Encephalitis. The tick vector of the virus of tickborne encephalitis is found throughout Europe and the countries of the former Soviet Union. The disease occurs most frequently in the spring and summer. It occurs among persons working in forest and farmland and is also transmitted by consumption of unpasteurized dairy products from infected goats, sheep, or cows. There is a vaccine available in Europe, but it is not recommended for routine use in travelers. Backpackers and campers should follow standard measures, such as protective clothing and insect repellant, to avoid exposure to ticks (Table 3–8).

Tuberculosis. Tuberculosis is an increasing risk worldwide. Children who will live in prolonged contact with the local population in high-prevalence localities or who will live or work in health care settings may be at risk of exposure. Even so, vaccination with bacille Calmette-Guérin vaccine is not recommended for travelers from the United States. Before travel, any child who may have had prior exposure to tuberculosis should be skin-tested with PPD, and prophylaxis should be started if indicated. Previously unexposed and PPD-negative children who live in high-risk situations abroad should be tested with PPD upon return to the United States or any time that symptoms develop.

Immunoglobulin

Hepatitis A. Hepatitis A is endemic worldwide except in the United States, Canada, western Europe, Scandinavia, Australia, New Zealand, and Japan. The best protection against infection is scrupulous attention to food preparation and water purity; however, travel-related hepatitis A is reported even with good tourist accommodations and precautions. Travelers living in rural areas, who are trekking, or living in close contact with young children are at especially high risk.

Hepatitis A vaccine is recommended for travelers ≥2 years of age if it can be given at least 2 weeks before travel. For infants <2 years of age and others who plan to travel within 2 weeks, immune globulin provides immediate protection. For a stay of less than 3 months, a single intramuscular dose of immunoglobulin of 0.02 mL/kg is sufficient. For prolonged travel, a dose of 0.06 mL/kg is given and repeated every 5 months.

Hepatitis E. The efficacy of immunoglobulin injection in the prevention of enterically acquired hepatitis E is unknown. However, the prevalence of antibody to hepatitis E is very low in the United States; therefore, it is likely that immunoglobulin produced in this country would have correspondingly low antibody titers. Travelers should consider themselves at risk, regardless of any immunoglobulin injection.

Scheduling of Testing, Immunizations, and Immunoglobulin

Almost any combination of live and inactivated vaccines (except cholera and yellow fever vaccines) can be given on the same day at different anatomic sites without a reduction in antibody titers or an increase in the severity of adverse effects. Yellow fever and cholera vaccines may interfere with each other and should be separated by 3 weeks, if possible. Injectable cholera and typhoid vaccines given together may accentuate the adverse effects of either and should be given separately, if time permits.

In general, inactivated vaccines can be given at any time in relation to any other inactivated or live vaccine. Injected live vaccines are best all given on the same day or else separated by at least 4 weeks to avoid the theoretical possibility of interference with viral replication and antibody response. Oral polio vaccine, however, can be given at any time in relation to any other vaccine.

Except for oral typhoid vaccine, it is not necessary to restart the series or to give extra doses if a vaccine series is interrupted.

PPD testing should be done on the day live virus vaccines are given or delayed for 4–6 weeks because these vaccines may depress the cell-mediated immunity necessary to produce a reaction to PPD. Immunoglobulin does not interfere with the immune response to inactivated vaccines, yellow fever vaccine, or OPV. The first dose of hepatitis A vaccine may be administered with immunoglobulin without a reduction in the efficacy of protection. Other parenterally administered live virus vaccines should be given at least 2 weeks before immunoglobulin. Administration of measles and varicella vaccines must be delayed for 3–11 months after administration of immunoglobulin, depending on the type and dose given (Table 17–4).

Breast-feeding does not interfere with any of the vaccines recommended for the very young infant. Vaccines administered to a breast-feeding mother, including yellow fever vaccine, are either not transmitted or pose little risk to the infant. Breast-feeding should be strongly encouraged because it protects against cholera, typhoid, giardiasis, and many other enterically transmitted pathogens.

HIV-infected or Immunocompromised Children. Although the response to vaccines may not be adequate, a traveling child with HIV infection or other immunocompromising conditions should receive all the inactivated vaccines recommended for healthy children. Children with asymptomatic HIV infection should receive MMR because the morbidity from measles is far higher than any morbidity recognized from vaccine. Children with CD4 counts ≥25% of normal for age should receive varicella vaccine after consideration of the expected risk of exposure. BCG should not be given because this live organism can cause disseminated or invasive infection in the immunocompromised child. The safety and efficacy of typhoid, hepatitis A, or yellow fever vaccines have not been evaluated in adults or children with HIV infection. Pneumococcal and influenza vaccinations should be given as recommended. It is advisable to carry antiviral medications for either prophylaxis or treatment of influenza (Table 68–11) because many of these drugs are unavailable outside the United States. All HIV-infected children should probably undergo routine PPD testing.

Malaria Chemoprophylaxis

Transmission of malaria occurs in many parts of the world, especially Central and South America, sub-Saharan Africa, the Indian subcontinent, Southeast Asia, and Oceania. The risk of transmission in each area depends on the season, altitude, living conditions, use of antimalarial prophylaxis, and use of measures to avoid exposure to mosquito bites. Rural areas present a high risk, probably because it is so much more difficult to avoid mosquitoes in such areas. Most cases of malaria imported to the United States originate in Africa and the Indian subcontinent

Parents of all children traveling to areas endemic for malaria, especially if they are staying for >3 weeks, should be advised about the signs and symptoms of malaria. Adults most often complain of an influenza-like illness with myalgia, headache, fever, chills, and malaise. Signs in children are usually nonspecific, but they include fever, irritability, vomiting, diarrhea, and respiratory symptoms. Delaying therapy may lead to severe and even fatal complications in children. Malaria can develop as early as 8 days after the first exposure and for many months after the last exposure, even after appropriate chemoprophylaxis. Parents should seek medical attention *immediately* for any child in whom a febrile illness occurs during travel in a region endemic for malaria.

Parents should have a thorough understanding of antimosquito measures, such as use of mosquito nets, sleeping in screened or air-conditioned rooms, and dressing in clothes with long sleeves and long pant legs to cover exposed skin from dusk until dawn. Insect repellents such as **DEET (N,N-diethyl-meta-toluamide)** should be used cautiously in children because these agents may cause severe neurologic symptoms. To minimize such toxicity, repellent should be used sparingly only on exposed skin or clothing; high-concentration products (such as 95% DEET) should not be used on the skin. Repellents should not be inhaled or ingested, and children's hands should be kept clean of repellents. Repellent should not be used on injured or irritated skin. If a repellent reaction occurs, contaminated clothing should be removed, the skin washed, and medical care sought. **Pyrethrum**-containing sprays are useful against flying insects in sleeping areas in the evening and at night. **Permethrin** sprays are available for use on clothing and bedding. Practical advice for the safe use of DEET and other repellants is available (Fradin, 1998), and on the Environmental Protection Agency website (Table 104–1).

No chemoprophylaxis regimen against malaria is totally protective (see Table 32–7). Worse yet, fewer than one half of surveyed U.S. travelers returning from Africa report full compliance with prophylaxis. Before prescribing any drug regimen, the physician must carefully review the child's itinerary to determine any area of malaria risk, check with current WHO or CDC listings on regions reporting drug-resistant malaria, and question the family about any past history of reactions to antimalarial or sulfonamide drugs or the possibility of glucose-6-phosphate-dehydrogenase (G-6-PD) deficiency. If prophylaxis is necessary, it should be started as early as 1–2 weeks before travel and continued for as long as 4 weeks after travelers leave the malarious area, depending on the drug regimen used.

In regions with low-level or no chloroquine resistance, chloroquine or hydroxychloroquine is the drug of choice, given orally once a week (see Table 32–7). In the United States, these two drugs come in tablet form only and taste very bitter. The dose should be calculated exactly on a per-weight basis, because chloroquine compounds are quite toxic in overdose. It is usually best to have the pharmacist grind the tablets to powder and measure an exact dose into gelatin capsules. If the child cannot swallow the capsule, the powder can be combined with a small amount of food to disguise the taste. Inexpensive suspensions are available outside the United Sates. If parents intend to use these suspensions, they must be careful to calculate an exact dose after checking the concentration because the available suspensions vary.

For persons visiting areas where malaria with known chloroquine resistance is endemic, there are several choices for chemoprophylaxis. One choice is mefloquine, given orally once a week, starting 1 week before travel and continuing for 4 weeks after return. A newly licensed combination of atovaquone and proguanil (Malarone) given once daily, starting 1–2 days before travel and continuing for 7 days after leaving the malarious area, is available for heavier (≥11 kg) children. An alternative for the child >8 years of age is doxycycline, given daily beginning 1–2 days before travel and continuing for 4 weeks after departing the region of malaria risk. If the child cannot take any of these choices, chloroquine can be used alone. An older chloroquine-proguanil regimen is no longer recommended for travelers from the United States.

Multi-drug-resistant malaria is present in the rural parts of Thailand, Cambodia, and Myanmar. Parents with children too young for doxycycline or Malarone should be strongly discouraged from taking their children to those areas.

All persons traveling to areas with chloroquine-resistant malaria should be provided with a single treatment dose of pyrimethamine-sulfadoxine (Fansidar) or Malarone. This should be administered if a febrile illness develops and medical care is not available within 24 hours. This is only a temporary measure, and medical care should not be delayed. Chemoprophylaxis should be continued, even after a treatment dose of Fansidar or Malarone. Fansidar should be used as presumptive treatment when Malarone was used as the prophylactic agent. Fansidar should not be given to persons with a history of intolerance to sulfa drugs or G-6-PD deficiency or to infants <2 months of age. Patients should avoid presumptive self-treatment with mefloquine or with mefloquine-Fansidar combinations sold outside the United States, because of serious adverse reactions (e.g., psychoses, convulsions) at the higher doses used for treatment.

Rapid dipstick tests for the self-diagnosis of malaria exist but are not recommended for the typical traveler because they require specialized training and practice for reliable performance and interpretation of the results. Only tiny amounts of most antimalarial drugs are excreted into breast milk. Thus breast-fed babies should be given full doses, based on weight, of any indicated chemoprophylactic or therapeutic drugs.

DURING TRAVEL

After assuring adequate routine childhood immunization, probably the best service a pediatric practitioner can provide a traveling family is counseling on appropriate health habits. Most traveling children will leave home in good health; maintaining that health is the best form of infection resistance.

Counseling for Health

Diet. The most difficult task of almost any traveler is assuring the safety and purity of food and water. Traveling children usually do not understand or choose to ignore dietary precautions (Table 104–5).

Except in areas with high standards of water purity, the traveler's adage **"Boil it, cook it, peel it, or forget it"** still holds true. Breast-feeding, boiled water, and bottled carbonated beverages without ice are usually the safest for children. Tap water too hot to run over a hand is a last resort. Packets of dry presweetened drink mix are lightweight to pack and may make beverages more palatable. Baby formula reconstituted with boiled water is preferable to unpasteurized or questionable milk products.

Travelers living in primitive conditions or those who take wilderness or high-altitude tours may require special water-purification methods. Disinfectant tablets or solutions and filters are available

TABLE 104–5. Guide to Safe Foods and Beverages

Recommended Choices	Generally Safe	To Be Avoided
Breast milk	Meals prepared in family homes	Cloudy or tap water
Boiled water stored in a clean container	Jams, jellies, or honey	Unpasteurized milk or dairy products
Bottled or canned carbonated beverages with the outside of the container wiped clean	Preserved dried, salted, or pickled foods	Ice or ice products, such as flavored ice desserts
Drink mixes, tea, coffee, or powdered formula made with boiled water	Tap water too hot to run over a hand	Raw or undercooked fruits or vegetables
Personally peeled fruits or vegetables	Water purified with disinfectant tablets or solutions or by filter systems	Reheated foods
Freshly prepared hot foods and cereals		Undercooked or raw meat, fish, or shellfish
Breads and dry baked goods		Salads
Hot noodles, rice, or pasta		Fish or shellfish in regions with known outbreaks of biotoxins, such as ciguatoxin
Well-cooked meat or fish		Food from street vendors

from many camping outfitters in the United States. Osmotic filtration systems are available in Western Europe; these are lightweight and easy to use but are expensive and time consuming. Parents should practice with any such products before travel and should carry detailed instructions for proper use under varying conditions of altitude, temperature, and water cloudiness.

Raw fruits or vegetables are to be avoided unless they can be peeled. Freshly prepared steaming hot food, breads and other dry baked goods, hot rice, noodles, or pasta, and well-cooked meat or fish are usually safe. Meals prepared in family homes are less risky than those made by street vendors. A supply of dry crackers and a plastic tub of peanut butter will pass through almost any customs inspection and are good to keep available for a hungry child when there is doubt about the food supply.

Neither the CDC nor a National Institutes of Health Consensus Panel recommends antibiotics or bismuth subsalicylate for the prevention of traveler's diarrhea in children.

Hygiene. After diet, hygiene is probably the most difficult problem to manage in small children. Sanitary diaper-changing facilities are difficult to find. Toddlers put water in their mouths while they take baths. Children wade in puddles on hot days. Teenagers turn on the bathroom tap to rinse out a toothbrush. A supply of boiled or bottled water should be kept readily available. Collapsible plastic water containers pack small and are useful when the opportunity arises to obtain a supply of safe water.

In general, children should wear sandals or shoes when outdoors. Swimming in filtered and chlorinated pools or in seawater is usually safe. Wading or swimming in freshwater bodies in developing countries should be avoided unless the water is known to be clean. However, what is safe for the repeatedly exposed local population may not be benign for an immunologically naive tourist.

Sexual Contact. Adolescents, especially those traveling without parents, should be advised specifically against sexual contacts with unknown persons. Nearly one third of American college students studied in the 1980s who traveled in the tropics reported sexual contact with a new partner while traveling. Almost one half of these contacts were without condom protection. Although HIV is the most serious infectious consequence of sexual encounters with strangers, hepatitis B, gonorrhea, and syphilis are among the most common sexually transmitted diseases reported in travelers.

Skin-Piercing Procedures. Travelers should be counseled to avoid any procedures involving invasion of the skin, including acupuncture, tattoos, piercing of various body parts, or blood or plasma donation, to minimize risk of exposure to hepatitis B, hepatitis C, and HIV.

Wilderness and High-Altitude Exposure. Wilderness or adventure travel and trips to high altitudes pose additional health risks, most related to injury, heat or cold stress, bites and stings, and acute mountain sickness with its most serious sequelae, pulmonary or cerebral edema. A prudent parent can avoid or manage most problems with some advance planning. A wilderness medical kit and a carry-along medical guide are strongly recommended for any excursion beyond 1–2 days (Table 104–1).

Other Concerns. Other conditions of concern to a long-distance child traveler are motion sickness and jet lag. An antinausea drug or patch may be given to the child who is susceptible to vomiting during travel. Many remedies exist for jet lag. The best is probably rest, allowing 1 day for each 1 hour of time change for full adjustment.

Severe sunburn can be avoided by use of sunscreen creams or ointments appropriate for the child's age and skin type. In the tropics, sunburn can occur with a shorter exposure time than in temperate zones.

Persons with diabetes who travel across >6 time zones must readjust their insulin schedules. A simple algorithm is available for east- or west-bound travel (Barry and Bia 1989). Sufficient insulin, syringes, and needles should be packed to last the entire trip. Customs agents usually do not question a small supply of medical equipment, but it is always best to have a statement on letterhead explaining that the items are for personal use for a legitimate medical condition.

Counseling for Illness

Health Documents. Health documents are at least as important as a passport or plane ticket and should be kept in as safe a place (Table 104–2). Immunizations may be recorded on an **International Certificate of Vaccination** (PHS-731). This certificate is acceptable only if complete in every detail and validated by a physician who has a Uniform Stamp obtained from a state health department. The only vaccine that *must* be recorded on an International Certificate of Vaccine is yellow fever vaccine. No other vaccines are required under WHO guidelines. In all other situations, a record of immunizations and immunoglobulin injections, the product names, manufacturers, and dates of administration listed on letterhead stationery and signed by a physician is acceptable.

TABLE 104–6. Precautions When Obtaining Medical Care Abroad

Avoid transfusions of blood or blood products unless absolutely necessary. Insist on products screened for HIV and hepatitis B and C, if at all possible.
Avoid injections, infusions, blood drawing, acupuncture, tattoos, or medical or dental procedures using unsterilized equipment. Reusable items should be boiled or autoclaved. Disposable items should come from freshly opened intact packages.
Avoid unlabeled, over-the-counter, or folk remedies. Many traditional medicines contain harmful substances, such as lead or actual pharmaceutical agents. Some pharmaceuticals may be fraudulent.
Ask for a written copy of any diagnosis or treatment regimen. Ask for the name, dose, and purpose of each drug prescribed.
Obtain a copy of the results of any laboratory tests performed.
Keep recommended follow-up appointments, both while continuing to travel and after return home.

Children should carry some form of identification, even if only a plastic name bracelet.

Seeking Medical Care. Caution should be exercised when obtaining any medical care outside the United States (Table 104–6). If emergency medical care is needed for a child during travel, the parent may be forced to accept whatever professional help is available. If the option exists, the parent should choose an English-speaking or North American–trained physician, not so much for expertise, but to avoid the language and cultural nuances of translating symptoms. For long trips, medical contacts should be identified before travel (Table 104–1). The United States embassy or consulate can provide a list of local physicians or clinics.

Many book and travel stores carry pocket-sized guides to signs and symptoms in various languages. The best of these include the word or phrase in the original script of the language and a phonetic rendering for the traveler. Also useful are diagrams of parts of the body and pictograms of symptoms. It is particularly important to report any such treatment after arrival home because some illnesses, such as malaria, may require immediate or long-term treatment.

Traveler's Diarrhea. More than half of tourists to developing countries suffer some health problem during or after travel. At least half of the reported illnesses are gastrointestinal. In one study (Pitzinger et al., 1991), 31% of Swiss children visiting developing nations had at least one attack of diarrhea during or within 2 weeks of travel despite dietary precautions. Attack rates were highest in children <3 years of age (40%) and in adolescents 15–20 years (36%). Nearly one third of the children had repeat episodes. The median duration of illness was 3 days for all children, but 18 days for the youngest group. More recent studies in various cohorts show similar results, with the risk of illness increasing by 3–4% for each day of travel.

The most common causes of traveler's diarrhea are infection with enterotoxigenic *Escherichia coli* and rotaviruses. Even a single incident of dietary indiscretion can lead to the acquisition of several pathogens of different incubation periods—for example, *Shigella*, hepatitis A virus, and *Giardia lamblia* (Table 76–22). Thus apparent recovery from a first episode of diarrhea does not guarantee continued health, even without further exposure.

When diarrheal illness occurs in a child, the treatment of choice is **oral rehydration solution (ORS).** Many inexpensive formulations of ORS are readily available worldwide in pharmacies and grocery stores. Premixed U.S. formulation solutions (e.g., Infalyte, Pedialyte, Kaolyte) are too heavy to pack for travel. Packets of ORS are available in the United States (Jianas Brothers, Kansas City, MO; telephone: 816-421-2880). One powdered formulation (CeraLyte) with osmolality intermediate between WHO-ORS and the premixed solutions is also available (Cera Products, Columbia, MD; telephone: 410-997-2334). Solutions made from household ingredients are discouraged because the final concentrations are extremely variable. The composition of a particular ORS is not nearly as significant a problem as the failure to use any ORS at all. Parents should be instructed carefully on the use of ORS (Table 104–7). The purpose of ORS is to prevent the serious complications of dehydration; its use does not decrease the number of stools or shorten the duration of the illness.

Antimotility drugs, including over-the-counter drugs such as loperamide (Imodium) or diphenoxylate (Lomotil), are not recommended for treatment of diarrhea in children, especially infants. For adults, loperamide (4 mg loading dose, then 2 mg after each loose stool, to a maximum of 16 mg/day) can relieve symptoms of mild traveler's diarrhea. The use of antibiotics to treat traveler's diarrhea in adults is controversial; there have been no studies of

TABLE 104–7. Instructions for the Use of Oral Rehydration Solution (ORS)*

- Do not wait for signs of dehydration (decreased urination or tears, dry mouth, increased thirst, weight loss, sunken eyes, or lethargy).
- Begin ORS with any episode of watery stools or with any vomiting episode that is not an isolated event.
- Mix one packet of ORS solution with 1 L of boiled water in a clean container. Discard leftover solution 12 hours after mixing if at room temperature and 24 hours after mixing if refrigerated.
- Give 120–240 mL (4–8 oz) of ORS for each diarrheal stool in the nondehydrated child. Continue breast milk, milk, or formula and solids except for foods high in simple sugars (e.g., soft drinks, fruit juice, Jell-O) or fats. Lactose-free milk or formula is not necessary with an acute diarrheal illness unless it is part of the child's normal diet.
- If the child is mildly dehydrated, give ORS replacement of at least 50–100 mL/kg (1 ounce/pound) over 4 hours. Continue stool replacement doses of ORS and the diet as above.
- If the child is vomiting, continue to offer ORS but in small frequent sips, for example, 5 mL (1 teaspoon) every 15–20 minutes.
- Avoid antidiarrheal agents. Do not use antimicrobial agents except for a diagnosed pathogen.
- Continue ORS but seek immediate medical attention for a child with bloody diarrhea, intractable vomiting, high stool output (>12 stools a day or frequent watery stools of large volume), high fever, or illness lasting longer than 3 days.

*Packets of ORS are available in the United States (Jianas Brothers, Kansas City, MO; telephone: 816-421-2880). One powdered formulation (CeraLyte) with osmolality intermediate between WHO-ORS and the premixed solutions (e.g., Infalyte, Pedialyte, Kaolyte) is also available (Cera Products, Columbia, MD; telephone: 410-997-2334).

children. It may be possible to modify mild disease in the child ≥2 months of age with trimethoprim-sulfamethoxazole (4 mg trimethoprim/kg; maximum dose 160 mg) twice a day orally for up to 3 days. Resistance of *E. coli* to trimethoprim-sulfamethoxazole is common in many areas. For persons ≥18 years of age, ciprofloxacin (500 mg), norfloxacin (400 mg), or ofloxacin (300 mg) orally twice a day for up to 3 days may be used. Severe disease with high fever, bloody stools, moderate or severe dehydration, or lasting >3 days requires prompt medical consultation, especially in the very young child.

Febrile Illness. Fever is a frequent nonspecific symptom in children but should not be treated lightly in the traveling child. In regions where malaria is endemic, especially where chloroquine resistance is prevalent, the child should be seen by a medical professional as soon as possible. Parents should avoid self-treatment with antibiotics because most illnesses are viral. Antibiotic resistance is widespread in regions where antibacterial agents are sold over the counter.

One exception to self-treatment may be recurrent otitis media in a child who has typical symptoms or pus draining from the ear. For a child with such a history, the parent may wish to bring from home a supply of chewable antibiotic tablets or a suspension such as azithromycin that does not require reconstitution or refrigeration.

Parents should pack an antipyretic medication for travel. Chewable tablets are a better choice than bottled suspensions, which are heavy and may become contaminated, especially if a dropper is used to measure the dose. Tablets can also be crushed between two spoons and mixed with food. The traveler should be wary of unknown or unlabeled "fever" medications sold over the counter. In some areas, these are actually antimalarial or antibacterial agents.

Colds and Rashes. Respiratory and rash illnesses are not unusual in traveling children. Most are inconsequential, self-limited infections, but some, such as measles, may be severe in the very young. Other infections, such as rubella or CMV or parvovirus infections, may pose a risk to the nonimmune pregnant parent. Medical care should be sought for any unusual or severe episode, especially if long-distance airplane travel is imminent. Some international airlines do not allow obviously ill children or children with a noticeable rash to board a flight.

Airline and Cruise Ship Travel and Infection. Transmission of foodborne diseases, including cholera, staphylococcal food poisoning, salmonellosis, shigellosis, Norwalk virus, enterotoxigenic *E. coli* infection, and illness caused by many other gastrointestinal pathogens, on aircraft and on cruise ships is well documented. The CDC Vessel Sanitation Program reduced the rate of outbreaks of gastrointestinal disease on cruise ships operating from the United States from an average of 12–15 episodes per year in the 1970s to 3 per year by 2000.

Numerous outbreaks of diseases transmitted via respiratory droplets, including legionellosis, rubella, measles, and influenza, have been reported on cruise ships. The CDC has recently implemented guidelines for the control of epidemics of influenza and other respiratory diseases on cruise ships. Outbreaks of airborne diseases transmitted on aircraft, including influenza, measles, and tuberculosis, are recognized. Some of these outbreaks occurred because of poor air circulation during prolonged stays on the ground, but most have been traced to sitting within one row of a passenger or working with a crew member with active infection. Investigations of flights carrying persons with meningococcal and Ebola virus infections have not noted any evidence of transmission to other passengers. However, both the WHO and the CDC have developed guidelines for tracing and testing or treating contacts of passengers with meningococcal disease or active tuberculosis.

In general, there are few precautions that an individual passenger can take to avoid transmission of infectious agents while traveling except to avoid obviously ill fellow passengers.

TABLE 104–8. Injury Prevention for Travelers

Use seat belts and car seats whenever available.
Avoid motorcycles and other small vehicles; choose a large vehicle over a small one.
Do not ride in the back of an open truck.
Use bicycle or motorcycle helmets.
Avoid small and nonscheduled airplanes.
Do not travel alone.
Choose sensible locations to swim; do not drink alcohol while swimming.
Do not travel or drive at night, if possible.

Modified from Hargarten SW, Baker TD, Guptill K: Overseas fatalities of United States citizen travelers: An analysis of deaths related to international travel. *Ann Emerg Med* 1991;20:622–6.

Death Due to Travel. Although travelers worry most about acquiring an exotic infection while away from home, the greatest risks to life are actually cardiovascular disease and unintentional injury, accounting for 49% and 22%, respectively, of deaths of U.S. citizens traveling abroad. Infectious diseases (excluding pneumonia) account for only 1% of the deaths across all age groups. Injury deaths include motor vehicle and airplane crashes, drowning, isolated episodes of animal mauling, and falls from mountains.

Men and persons traveling to developing countries have the highest death rates among travelers. Only 2% of U.S. citizen deaths abroad involve children <15 years of age. Suggestions for avoiding injury developed for Peace Corps volunteers seem reasonable for families with children (Table 104–8). A travel health evaluation may be the only opportunity most families have to hear this type of advice.

AFTER THE TRIP

Scheduling the Follow-up Visit. Any child who was ill or who received medical treatment during travel should be seen within 1 week of returning home. Children who become ill on the return trip or at any time in the first weeks at home should be seen within 1 day. Travelers who make brief visits to developed countries and who are otherwise well need not have a routinely scheduled posttravel visit. Children returning from developing nations or from prolonged stays abroad should be scheduled for a health evaluation 4–8 weeks after travel unless illness develops before that time.

Posttravel Evaluation. At any posttravel health consultation, the physician should review carefully the actual travel itinerary, activities, illnesses and treatments, accidents, and recognized exposures. Any acute or continuing symptoms should be determined. Although no data for children are reported, returning adult travelers most frequently complain of diarrhea, respiratory tract symptoms, fever, abdominal pain, malaise, skin lesions, accidents, and genital discharge. The physician should examine the child meticulously, looking especially for weight loss, skin lesions, jaundice, fever, or abdominal findings.

Travel-related illness most frequently occurs within weeks of travel. Even diseases of long incubation usually manifest themselves within 6 months. The most likely exceptions are malaria and some intestinal parasite infections. The differential diagnosis list should be based on the actual probability of exposure in light of current symptoms or findings, prevalence in the geographic area (Table 103–5), and the incubation period (Table 104–9).

Most children have nonexotic diagnoses, such as otitis media or viral upper respiratory tract infections. The most common infectious disease diagnoses in adults are traveler's diarrhea (all causes), acute upper respiratory tract infections, giardiasis, viral hepatitis, amebiasis, gonorrhea, and malaria (Table 104–10). Children who have lived in developing countries for longer than 1 year should have an evaluation similar to that for immigrants (Chapter 103).

For sick children, most posttravel laboratory evaluations should be performed in a stepwise manner, examining for the most likely disease on the basis of exposure and symptoms. In general, besides the physical examination, the tests most likely to yield a clue to a diagnosis include a CBC count, particularly to identify eosinophilia; thin and thick blood smears for malaria; stool examination for bacteria, ova, and parasites; and serologic tests for hepatitis A and hepatitis E. A second series of diagnostic tests should be performed only after consulting a microbiology laboratory, the CDC, or a travel health expert on the best means of diagnosis. If there is doubt, a few milliliters of serum can be saved for possible serologic titers that may be desired later.

Few common traveler's diseases, with the exception of malaria, are immediately life threatening for children. Others, such as cholera, may cause severe illness, but treatment is generally supportive while the diagnostic evaluation proceeds.

TABLE 104–9. Incubation Periods of Diseases of Travelers and Immigrants

Short (<1 wk)	Intermediate (1–4 wk)	Long (1–6 mo)	Very Long (2 mo to 2 yr)
Acute hemorrhagic conjunctivitis	Amebiasis	Ascariasis	AIDS
Anthrax	Brucellosis	Blastomycosis	Cysticercosis
Arboviruses	Chagas' disease	Hepatitis B	Echinococcosis
Boutonneuse fever	Chicken pox	Hepatitis C	Filariasis
Chancroid	Cryptosporidiosis	Hepatitis D	Fluke infections
Chikungunya	Enterobiasis	Filariasis	Leishmaniasis, visceral
Chlamydial infections	Enterovirus infections	Leishmaniasis, cutaneous	Leprosy
Ciguatera poisoning	Giardiasis	Loiasis	Schistosomiasis
Cholera	Hemorrhagic fever with renal syndrome	Malaria	Trypanosomiasis, African (Gambian; *T. brucei gambiense*)
Congo-Crimean hemorrhagic fever	Hepatitis A	Melioidosis	Tuberculosis
Cyclosporiasis	Hepatitis E	Pinta	Variant Creutzfeldt-Jakob disease
Dengue	Katayama fever	Rabies	
Diarrhea, acute	Lassa fever	Taeniasis	
Diphtheria	Leptospirosis	Trachoma, scarring	
Ebola-Marburg hemorrhagic fever	Lyme disease	Trichuriasis	
Encephalitis viruses	Lymphogranuloma venereum	Tropical sprue	
Food poisoning	Malaria	Tuberculosis	
Gonorrhea	Measles	Yaws	
Hantavirus pulmonary syndrome	Mumps		
Herpes simplex virus infection	Nonspecific urethritis		
Histoplasmosis	Parvovirus infection		
Legionellosis	Pertussis		
Meningococcus	Poliomyelitis		
Plague	Q fever		
Psittacosis	Rocky Mountain spotted fever		
Relapsing fever	Rubella		
Salmonellosis	Scabies		
Shigellosis	Strongyloidiasis		
Tetanus	Syphilis		
Trypanosomiasis, African (chancre)	Trypanosomiasis, African (sleeping sickness; *T. brucei rhodesiense*)		
Upper respiratory tract infection	Typhoid fever		
Viral gastroenteritis	Typhus, louseborne		
West Nile virus	Typhus, murine		
Yellow fever	Typhus, scrub		

Modified from Halstead SB, Warren KS: Diseases of travelers and immigrants. Kalamazoo, Mich, Upjohn, 1987.

TABLE 104–10. Traveler's Relative Risk of Acquiring Infectious Disease in a Developing Country

High: >1 Case in 10 Travelers	Moderate: >1 Case in 200 Travelers but <1 Case in 10 Travelers	Low: >1 Case in 1,000 Travelers but <1 Case in 200 Travelers	Very Low: <1 Case in 1,000 Travelers	
Diarrhea	Dengue	Acute hemorrhagic conjunctivitis	Actinomycosis	Leishmaniasis, cutaneous*
Upper respiratory tract infection	Enterovirus infections	Amebiasis	AIDS	Leishmaniasis, visceral*
	Food poisoning	Ascariasis	Angiostrongyliasis	Legionellosis
	Gastroenteritis	Chickenpox	Anisakiasis	Leprosy*
	Giardiasis	Enterobiasis	Anthrax	Loiasis*
	Hepatitis A	Hepatitis B	Arboviruses	Lyme disease*
	Malaria (without prophylaxis)	Hepatitis C	Blastomycosis	Lymphogranuloma venereum
	Salmonellosis	Hepatitis E	Boutonneuse fever	Malaria (with prophylaxis)
	Chlamydial infection	Leptospirosis	Brucellosis*	Melioidosis
	Gonorrhea	Measles	Chagas' disease	Meningococcus
	Herpes simplex	Mumps	Chikungunya	Paragonimiasis
	Nonspecific urethritis	Poliomyelitis	Cholera	Pertussis
	Shigellosis	Scabies	Ciguatera poisoning	Pinta
		Chancroid	Clonorchiasis	Plague
		Syphilis	Coccidioidomycosis	Poliomyelitis
		Strongyloidiasis	Congo-Crimean hemorrhagic fever	Psittacosis
		Trichuriasis	Cryptosporidiosis	Q fever
		Tropical sprue	Cysticercosis*	Rabies
		Tuberculosis	Diphtheria	Relapsing fever
		Typhoid fever	Ebola-Marburg hemorrhagic fever	Rocky Mountain spotted fever
			Echinococcosis	Schistosomiasis
			Encephalitis viruses	Taeniasis*
			Filariasis	Tetanus*
			Gnathostomiasis	Toxocariasis
			Hantavirus pulmonary syndrome	Trachoma
			Hemorrhagic fever with renal syndrome*	Trichinosis
			Histoplasmosis	Trypanosomiasis
			Hookworm	Typhus
			Japanese encephalitis virus	Yaws
			Katayama fever*	Yellow fever
			Lassa fever*	West Nile virus

*Anecdotal reports only or not well studied.
Modified from Halstead SB, Warren KS: Diseases of travelers and immigrants. Kalamazoo, Mich, Upjohn, 1987; and Steffen R, DuPont HL: *Manual of Travel Medicine and Health.* Hamilton, Ontario, BD Decker, 1999.

REVIEWS

Centers for Disease Control and Prevention: *Health Information for the International Traveler 2001–2002.* Atlanta, US Department of Health and Human Services, Public Health Service, 2001. (Available at www.cdc.gov/travel/yellowbook.pdf)

Ryan ET, Kain KC: Health advice and immunizations for travelers. *N Engl J Med* 2000;342:1716–24.

Sood SK: Immunization for children traveling abroad. *Pediatr Clin North Am* 2000;47:435–48.

Steffen R, DuPont HL: *Manual of Travel Medicine and Health.* Hamilton, Ontario, BD Decker, 1999.

Wilson ME: *A World Guide to Infections: Disease, Distribution, Diagnosis.* New York, Oxford University Press, 1991.

World Health Organization: *International Travel and Health: Vaccination Requirements and Health Advice—Situation as on 1 January 2001.* WHO, 2001. (May also be downloaded from www.who.int/ith/index.html)

KEY ARTICLES

Barry M, Bia F: Advice for the traveling diabetic. *JAMA* 1989;261:1799.

Bruni M, Steffen R: Impact of travel-related health impairments. *J Travel Med* 1997;4:61–4.

Centers for Disease Control and Prevention: *Preliminary Guidelines for the Prevention and Control of Influenza-like Illness Among Passengers and Crew Members on Cruise Ships.* CDC, August, 1999.

Cobelens FG, van Deutekom H, Draayer-Jansen IW, et al: Risk of infection with *Mycobacterium tuberculosis* in travellers to areas of high tuberculosis endemicity. *Lancet* 2000;356:461–5.

Edwards BJ, Atkinson G, Waterhouse J, et al: Use of melatonin in recovery from jet-lag following an eastward flight across 10 time-zones. *Ergonomics* 2000;43:1501–13.

Forgey WW (editor): *Wilderness Medical Society Practice Guidelines for Wilderness Emergency Care.* Pitkin, Colo., Wilderness Medical Society, 2000.

Fradin MS: Mosquitoes and mosquito repellants: A clinician's guide. *Ann Intern Med* 1998;128:931–40.

Hargarten SW, Baker TD, Guptill K: Overseas fatalities of United States citizen travelers: An analysis of deaths related to international travel. *Ann Emerg Med* 1991;20:622–6.

Hill DR: Health problems in a large cohort of Americans traveling to developing countries. *J Travel Med* 2000;7:259–66.

Jelinek T, Grobusch MP, Nothdurft HD: Use of dipstick tests for the rapid diagnosis of malaria in nonimmune travelers. *J Travel Med* 2000;7:175–9.

Kemmerer TP, Cetron M, Harper L, et al: Health problems of corporate travelers: Risk factors and management. *J Travel Med* 1998;5:184–7.

Lobato MN, Hopewell PC: *Mycobacterium tuberculosis* infection after travel to or contact with visitors from countries with a high prevalence of tuberculosis. *Am J Respir Crit Care Med* 1998;158:1871–5.

Lobel HO, Kozarsky PE: Update on prevention of malaria for travelers. *JAMA* 1997;278:1767–71.

MacPherson DW, Guérillot F, Streiner DL, et al: Death and dying abroad: The Canadian experience. *J Travel Med* 2000;7:227–33.

Minooee A, Rickman LS: Infectious diseases on cruise ships. *Clin Infect Dis* 1999;29:737–43.

Pitzinger B, Steffen R, Tschopp A: Incidence and clinical features of traveler's diarrhea in infants and children. *Pediatr Infect Dis J* 1991;10:719–23.

Steffen R, Collard F, Tornieporth N, et al: Epidemiology, etiology, and impact of travelers' diarrhea in Jamaica. *JAMA* 1999;281:811–7.

Valway S, Watson J, Bisgard C, et al: *Tuberculosis and Air Travel: Guidelines for Prevention and Control.* Geneva, World Health Organization, 2000. (May also be downloaded from www.who.int/gtb/publications/aircraft/index.html)

Viani RM, Bromberg K: Pediatric imported malaria in New York: Delayed diagnosis. *Clin Pediatr (Phila)* 1999;38:333–7.

von Sonnenburg F, Tornieporth N, Waiyaki P, et al: Risk and aetiology of diarrhoea at various tourist destinations. *Lancet* 2000;356:133–4.

Wilks J: International tourists, motor vehicles and road safety: A review of the literature leading up to the Sydney 2000 Olympics. *J Travel Med* 1999;6:115–21.

CHAPTER 105

Nosocomial Infections and Infection Control

Margaret C. Fisher

Infection control is an integral part of pediatric practice. Nosocomial infections prolong hospital stays by an average of 10–15 days per infection and contribute significantly to the morbidity, mortality, and costs of hospitalization. Infection is a major cause of death in immunocompromised persons, persons with multiple organ failure, burn victims, and persons who undergo major surgical procedures. Nosocomial infections often form the basis for litigation against physicians, nurses, and hospitals.

A **nosocomial infection** is an infection that is acquired during hospitalization and may also be acquired in physicians' offices, emergency departments, and outpatient clinics. It is neither present nor incubating at the time of admission, although community-acquired infection can serve as a source of nosocomial infection by transmission in the hospital. Most nosocomial infections are not preventable, even when recommended precautions are followed. **Infection** is defined as replication of organisms within tissues; **colonization** is growth and multiplication of microorganisms in or on a host, without evidence of disease or immune reaction. Hospital-acquired infections may become symptomatic only after a person has been discharged from the hospital, but they may not be recognized as nosocomial infections unless there is special postdischarge surveillance.

Incidence. The incidence of nosocomial infection varies by hospital and by hospital service (Table 105–1). Rates are computed in a variety of ways, such as infections per hospital admission or per hospital discharge, infections per hospital day, and infections per catheter or device day. Rates for pediatric services are generally in the range of 1–3%, lower than community hospital general services with rates of nosocomial infection between 2–5%, that is, 2–5 infections per 100 hospital discharges. Rates of infection are influenced by host factors, type and duration of medical care, and the skill of the health care providers. In a comparison of nosocomial infection rates among hospitals, it is essential to adjust the data for specific infection risks, which can be accomplished by using device-associated or device-day rate rather than crude overall rate or even site-specific rate. In general, hospitals or services that serve more critically ill patients and use more risk-associated devices have higher nosocomial infection rates.

There is less information regarding rates of infection after care in an outpatient setting. Numerous outbreaks of infection from outpatient sites have been reported. However, studies show that persons who visit physicians' offices for routine care are less likely to become ill in the subsequent weeks than persons who do not receive such care.

Pathogens. Bacteria, viruses, fungi, and parasites are potentially nosocomial pathogens (Table 105–2). In pediatric units, viruses are major causes of hospital-acquired infections. Nosocomial bacterial pathogens vary by age group. The most common nosocomial isolate recovered from adults is *Escherichia coli,* which is less common in children than adults because urinary tract infections are less common in children. Nosocomial pathogens vary by season. The source of a child's hospital-acquired infection frequently is a visitor with a community-acquired infection.

Device-related infections have increased in frequency as the use of certain devices has increased. Medical devices are foreign bodies, which greatly increase the risk of infection. Nosocomial pathogens vary depending on the type of device. In general, flora of the surrounding skin or mucosa colonizes the device, and the device provides a pathway that results in a local or systemic infection.

Notifiable Diseases. A **notifiable** or **reportable disease** is one for which regular, frequent, and timely information on individual cases is considered necessary for the prevention of the disease. It is the legal duty of a physician who cares for a person with a notifiable disease to report the infection. Regulations regarding reportable illness vary by state. In general, reporting starts with a written or telephoned report to the local health department. Reports are forwarded from the local department to the state. Reporting is

TABLE 105–1. Average Rates of Nosocomial Infection

	Rate (% of Hospital Discharges)	
Service	Nonteaching Hospital	Teaching Hospital
Adult	3–5	5–10
Pediatric	1–3	3–5
Newborn	5–10	10–20
Intensive care unit	—	10–30

TABLE 105–2. Common Nosocomial Pathogens

Adults	Children	Neonates
Escherichia coli	*Staphylococcus*	*Staphylococcus*
Pseudomonas aeruginosa	*E. coli*	*E. coli*
Enterococcus	*P. aeruginosa*	*P. aeruginosa*
Staphylococcus	*Candida*	*Klebsiella*
Klebsiella	*Klebsiella*	*Candida*

mandated only at the state level; reporting of nationally notifiable diseases to the CDC by the states is voluntary. In addition to the infectious diseases that should be reported nationally (Table 105–3), states or municipalities may include additional illnesses. Diseases are added to the list as new pathogens emerge, and they are deleted as their incidence declines. Tallies of reported infections appear weekly and annually in the *Morbidity and Mortality Weekly Report,* published by the CDC. Clusters of communicable diseases and outbreaks associated with food or water contamination also should be reported to state health departments.

Host Factors and Increased Risk. Host factors are probably the most important risk factors for the development of hospital-acquired infections (Table 105–4). Most nosocomial infections are caused by endogenous flora. Normal flora is altered by illness and medical therapy during hospitalization; for example, replacement of oral gram-positive streptococci are by gram-negative bacilli. The presence of anatomic abnormalities, particularly those that cause stasis of body fluids, increases the risk of infection. Abnormal communications also increase the risk of infection; for example, cleft palate increases the risk of otitis media. Metabolic disorders also influence host defense; for example, persons with uremia have abnormalities of both cellular and antibody-mediated immunity, and persons with diabetes mellitus have an increased risk of a variety of infections. The greater the number of affected organ systems, the higher the rate of hospital-acquired infection. Abnormalities of the immune system, congenital or acquired, greatly increase the chances of infection. A variety of injuries adversely affect the immune system; for example, extensive body burns or major trauma suppresses immune function.

Organ dysfunction acts in a variety of ways to increase the rate of infection (Table 105–5). For example, children with congestive

TABLE 105–3. Infectious Diseases Designated as Notifiable at the National Level in the United States, 2000

Acquired immunodeficiency syndrome (AIDS)	Legionellosis
Anthrax	Listeriosis
Botulism	Lyme disease
Brucellosis	Malaria
Chancroid	Measles
Chlamydia trachomatis, genital infections	Meningococcal disease
Cholera	Mumps
Coccidioidomycosis	Pertussis
Cryptosporidiosis	Plague
Cyclosporiasis	Poliomyelitis, paralytic
Diphtheria	Psittacosis
Ehrlichiosis, human granulocytic	Q fever
Ehrlichiosis, human monocytic	Rabies, animal
Encephalitis, California serogroup	Rabies, human
Encephalitis, eastern equine	Rocky Mountain spotted fever
Encephalitis, St. Louis	Rubella
Encephalitis, western equine	Rubella, congenital syndrome
Escherichia coli O157:H7	Salmonellosis
Gonorrhea	Shigellosis
Haemophilus influenzae, invasive disease	Streptococcal disease, invasive, group A
Hansen's disease (leprosy)	Streptococcal toxic-shock syndrome
Hantavirus pulmonary syndrome	*Streptococcus pneumoniae,* drug-resistant invasive disease
Hemolytic-uremic syndrome, postdiarrheal	Syphilis
Hepatitis A	Syphilis, congenital
Hepatitis B	Tetanus
Hepatitis C/non-A, non-B	Toxic-shock syndrome
Human immunodeficiency virus infection, adult (≥13 yr of age)	Trichinosis
Human immunodeficiency virus infection, pediatric (<13 yr of age)	Tuberculosis
	Tularemia
	Typhoid fever
	Varicella (deaths only)*
	Yellow fever

*Although not a nationally notifiable disease, the Council of State and Territorial Epidemiologists recommends reporting cases of varicella (chickenpox) through the National Notifiable Diseases Surveillance System.

From the Centers for Disease Control and Prevention: Changes in national notifiable diseases data presentation. *MMWR Morb Mortal Wkly Rep* 2000;49:892–3.

TABLE 105–4. Risks for Nosocomial Infection

Anatomic Abnormality	**Underlying Disease or Comorbidity**
Dermoid sinus	Cystic fibrosis
Cleft palate	Nephrosis
Obstructive uropathy	Diabetes mellitus
Alteration of Flora	**Catheterization**
Antibiotic therapy	Bladder
Newborn status	Blood vessels
Critical illness	Central nervous system
Organ Dysfunction	**Respiratory Support**
Renal failure	Intubation
Respiratory failure	Ventilation
Damage to Skin	**Season of the Year**
Incisions	Seasonal viruses
Burns	
Malnutrition	
Chronic illness	
Chemotherapy	

TABLE 105–5. Consequences of Organ Dysfunction

Organ System Failure	Adverse Outcome
Central nervous system	Aspiration
	Immobility leading to pressure sores and edema
Respiratory	Atelectasis
	Bronchiectasis
	Ciliary dysfunction
Cardiac	Pulmonary edema
	Collapse of bronchus by enlarged heart
	Hypoxemia
Gastrointestinal	Bacteremia
	Cholangitis
Genitourinary	Uremia causing immune suppression
Musculoskeletal	Immobility leading to pressure sores and edema
Bone marrow	Neutropenia
	Anemia

TABLE 105–6. Catheters as Risk Factors for Infection

Bypass anatomic host defenses
Occlude normal ostia (middle ears, sinuses)
Provide direct access to sterile sites
Provide adherence site for microbes
Increased risk with increased duration
Increased risk with increased manipulation
Increased risk with stopcocks or monitoring devices

heart failure due to congenital heart disease are at increased risk of having pneumonia because of pulmonary atelectasis due to enlarged heart chambers that impinge on bronchi, diminished ciliary clearance due to edema fluid, ciliary dysfunction due to medications, and altered flora due to frequent antibiotic therapy. Studies in intensive care units have confirmed that persons with multiple organ failure are at high risk of infection. In addition, infection is a frequent cause of or cofactor leading to death.

The use of catheters and tubes drastically increases the risk of infections (Table 105–6). Catheters bypass normal host defenses and give microbes direct access to host tissues. Not all catheters carry the same risk of infection. Higher rates of infection correlate with a longer duration of catheterization and increased manipulation of the catheter. Catheters also increase the risk of infection by occluding or damaging mucosal surfaces. For example, nasogastric tubes occlude the ostia of sinuses and interfere with normal function of the eustachian tubes, resulting in a predisposition to otitis media, sinusitis, or both. In addition, these tubes damage the esophagus, increasing the risk of esophagitis. Some data suggest that nasogastric tubes increase the incidence of gastroesophageal reflux. This in turn increases the risk of pulmonary aspiration, followed by bacterial pneumonia.

TABLE 105–7. Determinants of Relative Risk of Postoperative Infection

Type of Operation
Clean
Uninfected
No inflammation
No entry into respiratory, alimentary, or genitourinary tract
Clean contaminated
Controlled entry into respiratory, alimentary, or genitourinary tract
Contaminated
Accidental wounds
Operative wounds in which there has been gross spillage from the gastrointestinal tract or a major break in sterile technique
Dirty and infected
Old traumatic wounds
Wounds with existing clinical infection
Wounds with perforated viscera
Duration of Operation
Comorbidities
Burns
Neutropenia
Cancer
Organ failure
Use of Antibiotics

TABLE 105–8. Drugs as Risk Factors for Nosocomial Infection

Antibiotics	**Chemotherapy**
Alter normal microbial flora	Cause neutropenia
Suppress bone marrow	Cause anemia
Cause skin exfoliation	Cause lymphopenia
Cause organ dysfunction	**Immunosuppressants**
Encourage colonization by resistant flora	Cause lymphocyte dysfunction
	Blunt inflammatory response
Antacids	Cause cytokine dysfunction
Alter gastric acidity and flora	**Sedatives**
Narcotics	Impair mentation
Cause ciliary dysfunction	**Other Drugs**
Impair pulmonary macrophages	Affect neutrophil function
Impair mentation	Affect lymphocyte function
	Affect cytokine production and release

Burns increase the risk of infection by damaging the skin, normally a superb barrier to local and systemic infection. The higher the percentage of burned skin, the higher the rate of infection and the greater the risk of death due to infection.

Surgical procedures increase risk in many ways: skin is incised; tissues are exposed to airborne, handborne, and instrumentborne agents; damaged tissue has an altered pH; blood supply to the area operated on is altered; tubes and catheters are often used during and after the operation; anesthetics and analgesics alter normal host defenses and have adverse effects that include organ dysfunction; hospitalization exposes the patient to hospital flora; and perioperative antibiotics alter endogenous flora (Table 105–7).

Drugs often alter normal host defenses (Table 105–8). For example, morphine and other narcotics alter consciousness, increasing the chance of pulmonary aspiration, and interfere with normal ciliary function and with normal behaviors such as eating and personal hygiene. Antibiotics alter the normal microbial flora. This alteration in the normal flora increases the risk of colonization by hospital flora. Immunosuppressants are even more important in increasing a person's risk of infection by altering normal defenses.

NOSOCOMIAL INFECTIONS

RESPIRATORY TRACT INFECTIONS

Nosocomial infections of the upper and lower portions of the respiratory tract include rhinitis, pharyngitis, otitis media, sinusitis, tracheitis, and pneumonia (Table 105–9). The season of the year determines which viruses are circulating in the community, which can be transmitted to other patients by hospitalized contacts or by visitors. Hands are the most important carriers of viruses, with the usual route of respiratory viral infection either indirectly from the mucous membranes of a child to that child's hands and to the environment or directly to another set of hands and from there to that child's mucous membranes.

Multiple studies have demonstrated the importance of hands in the transmission of rhinoviruses, which is true for other respiratory

TABLE 105–9. Nosocomial Respiratory Infections

Types	Risk Factors	Etiologic Agents	Diagnostic Tests	Preventive Measures
Otitis media Sinusitis Tracheitis Bronchitis Bronchiolitis Pneumonia	Antibiotic therapy Aspiration Feeding tube Impaired consciousness Immunosuppression Poor nutritional status Pulmonary edema Tracheostomy Intubation Mechanical ventilation Contaminated equipment Underlying disease Prior operation Season of the year Antacid therapy	**Nasopharyngeal Flora** *Streptococcus pneumoniae* *Haemophilus influenzae* *Moraxella catarrhalis* *Staphylococcus aureus* Group A *Streptococcus* **Acquired and Enteric Flora** *Escherichia coli* *Klebsiella* *Serratia marcescens* *Pseudomonas aeruginosa* Other hospital-acquired, gram-negative bacilli **Fungi** *Candida albicans* *Aspergillus* **Viruses** Respiratory syncytial virus Influenza viruses A and B Parainfluenza viruses Adenoviruses Herpes simplex virus **Mycobacteria** *Mycobacterium tuberculosis*	Physical examination Tympanocentesis Nasopharyngeal wash for antigen detection and culture Sputum Gram stain and culture Radiography and other imaging Bronchoscopy Bronchoalveolar lavage Analysis of pleural fluid Culture of pleural fluid Culture of lung aspirate Lung biopsy	Use good hand washing technique Isolate patients with contagious disease Limit visiting; restrict ill visitors Remove nasogastric or nasotracheal tubes as soon as possible Avoid antacids Provide pulmonary toilet by patient positioning, incentive spirometry, cough, deep breathing, ambulation Use meticulous ventilator care; do not allow condensation in tubing to enter patient Suction as needed, using no-touch technique and sterile catheters Perform meticulous care and cleaning of all respiratory equipment

viruses as well. An early study (Hall and Douglas, 1981) showed transmission of respiratory syncytial virus (RSV) by hands and fomites. Three groups of volunteers were studied: sitters, touchers, and cuddlers. Sitters sat in a room with a child infected with RSV but did not touch the child or anything around the child. Touchers entered the room after the child was removed and touched crib rails and items on the bed and then inoculated their eyes and noses by rubbing them with their fingers. Cuddlers gave care directly to the child, which included feeding, handling, and playing with the child. None of the sitters contracted RSV infection, which suggests that RSV is neither airborne nor effectively transmitted by this route. However, 40% of touchers contracted infections by handling fomites and then self-inoculating the mucous membranes, and 70% of cuddlers contracted infections through the close interactions. This study demonstrated that community-acquired viruses are likely to be transmitted to staff by close contact with patients. In addition, hands are capable of transmitting virus not only to staff but also to other patients. It is obvious that hand washing is essential in decreasing transmission of respiratory viruses.

Intubation of the airway provides direct access to the lungs and bypasses normal host defenses. Organisms enter the trachea directly through the tube or by descending around the tube, which may result in ventilator-associated pneumonia (Chapter 68). The tube keeps the upper airway open, increasing the risk of aspiration of oropharyngeal flora and refluxed gastric contents and interfering with clearance of the airway by coughing, because an effective cough requires a closed glottis.

Contamination of respiratory therapy equipment or humidification systems introduces bacteria directly into lower airways. Fluid that condenses in the tubing that connects the airway to the ventilator supports the growth of a variety of bacterial species. If equipment is not properly decontaminated, condensate entering the airway carries these bacteria. Nasotracheal tubes obstruct the ostia of the paranasal sinuses and of the eustachian tubes, increasing the risk of otitis media and sinusitis.

Etiology. Agents that cause nosocomial respiratory tract infections include viruses, bacteria, and fungi (Table 105–9). Organisms in the nasopharynx enter the middle ear and sinuses. Hospital-acquired sinusitis and otitis are due to normal flora of the nasopharynx or due to hospital-acquired flora. A study of hospitalized premature infants revealed that otitis media occurred in intubated infants. Pathogens recovered from these hospitalized infants were much more likely to be gram-negative enteric organisms than were pathogens recovered from outpatients of similar age. Nosocomial sinusitis due to fungi occurs in immunocompromised hospitalized persons. Rhinitis and pharyngitis are usually due to agents circulating in the community. Hospital-acquired viruses, especially RSV and influenza viruses, are frequent causes of fevers and respiratory infections in hospitalized children and adults. In addition, viral infections result in a predisposition to bacterial superinfections. Tracheitis due to staphylococci or streptococci occasionally complicates the course of croup. In some instances the pathogens are acquired in the hospital, whereas in other cases the child has tracheal involvement at presentation.

Viral, bacterial, and fungal agents cause nosocomial pneumonia. Lower respiratory involvement by viruses is most common in immunocompromised persons. Viruses include RSV, influenza, and herpes simplex virus (HSV). Bacterial pathogens superinfect viral pneumonitis, areas of atelectasis, and areas damaged by aspiration of gastric acids or other foreign materials. Both normal flora and hospital-acquired flora may be involved. Oral anaerobes, *Staphylococcus aureus,* and gram-negative enteric bacilli are common pathogens. The flora of a patient is rapidly altered by the underlying illness and by medical treatment, especially with the use of antimicrobial agents. The normal flora is replaced by gram-negative enteric organisms such as *E. coli* and *Klebsiella,* as well as *S. aureus* and fungi. All these agents can cause pneumonia. Gram-negative bacilli enter the lungs through the upper airways, whereas fungi often enter via the bloodstream.

Unusual causes of nosocomial infection of the lungs include *Mycobacterium tuberculosis* and *Aspergillus. M. tuberculosis* is an unusual cause of nosocomial disease in children. However, outbreaks due to infections in health care providers and secondary spread from patients with infections have been reported. Most children with tuberculosis are not contagious. Adults with cavitary disease are most likely to transmit tuberculosis. The parent of children with tuberculosis should be questioned about whether the parent has a cough. The parent should not visit until or unless it is demonstrated that he or she does not have an active infection. In the 1990s the incidence of nosocomial tuberculosis increased dramatically in hospitals with patients coinfected with *M. tuberculosis* and human immunodeficiency virus (HIV). These patients should be isolated in rooms with negative air pressure until stains of sputum indicate that the infection is not contagious. Pulmonary aspergillosis occurs primarily in persons with severe immunocompromise. *Aspergillus* spores are transported by air currents. Contamination of air is most common during building construction and renovation. *Aspergillus* species grow well in air ducts. Overgrowth in these areas leads to dissemination of fungus through the air supply of a room or hospital ward to the mucous membranes of a patient.

Diagnosis. The diagnosis of a respiratory tract infection is not always easy or straightforward. Otitis is best diagnosed by a physical examination. Tympanocentesis should be performed if identification of the infecting organism is necessary for therapy, that is, in the care of an immunocompromised person or to exclude fungal infection. Sinusitis is often difficult to diagnose, particularly in obtunded patients. Plain radiographs are notoriously difficult to interpret. In addition, sinuses sometimes become filled with fluid because of the position of the patient; fluid-filled or cloudy sinuses are not necessarily infected. CT is useful but expensive, and it requires transport of the patient. Rhinitis and pharyngitis are clinical diagnoses. Bronchitis and tracheitis are best diagnosed by direct visualization, which often is not practical. Infiltrates in the lung may represent areas of atelectasis, infection, edema, inflammation, or malignant infiltration. Distinguishing among these possibilities requires consideration of the patient's underlying problem, of the treatments given for that problem, and of exposures that have occurred during hospitalization. A definitive diagnosis sometimes requires bronchoalveolar lavage or a lung biopsy. The need to establish the specific cause of a nosocomial infection depends on the degree of illness in the patient, the availability of specific therapy, and the hospital setting. It is often important to define specific agents to determine whether an outbreak has occurred. Although most outpatients with respiratory infections are given empirical treatment because the specific infective agent is unknown, it is often important to determine the cause of a nosocomial infection so that specific measures can be employed to identify other infected patients and to prevent additional transmission of the agent.

Prevention. Complete prevention of a respiratory infection is not possible, but reduction in rates of infection is a reasonable aim. Endotracheal tubes should be removed as soon as medically possible. No data show that the incidence of infection is related to the frequency of tube change. For example, it is not known whether it is beneficial to change a nasogastric tube from one nostril to the other. It seems reasonable to decrease the chance of erosion of the nares and to allow the ostia of the sinuses and middle ear to aerate more effectively. However, the optimal frequency and efficacy of tube changes have not been established. Antibiotic therapy has been shown to be useful in preventing recurrent otitis media in the outpatient setting. In a hospitalized child, antibiotic therapy alters the flora and thus increases the risk of infection by resistant flora. There is no information about the overall incidence of otitis or sinusitis in antibiotic-treated inpatients as opposed to untreated control subjects. The incidence of viral infection can be decreased by enforcement of hand-washing policies and isolation of persons whose infection is contagious.

Children who have transmissible infections at the time of admission or who acquire such infections during hospitalization should be cared for in rooms that do not house children who do not have the same infections. In general, children with infections can be placed with other children who have the same infection. The air in most hospital rooms is at positive pressure with respect to the hallways, and thus airflow goes from the room to the hall. This airflow is not appropriate for patients with infections that are transmitted through the air in small, aerosolized particles or for patients who are receiving aerosolized agents that could escape into the hall. **Negative-pressure rooms** are needed for the management of these patients. Negative-pressure rooms are necessary for children with varicella and measles and should be used for the rare child who has cavitary lung disease or draining adenitis due to *M. tuberculosis.*

The use of gloves and gowns has not uniformly decreased the transmission of respiratory viruses. In one study (Gala et al, 1986) the use of goggles and masks was effective in decreasing the transmission of RSV. It is difficult to educate hospital visitors regarding infection control, and therefore consideration should be given to implementing policies to restrict visits by adults and children with influenza or upper respiratory tract infections.

GASTROINTESTINAL TRACT AND HEPATIC INFECTIONS

Nosocomial infections of the gastrointestinal tract include esophagitis, enteritis, colitis, and hepatitis (Table 105–10). Risk factors include season of the year, intubation, medications, and ingestion of contaminated foods. During winter there is a high incidence of community-acquired rotavirus infection, whereas during summer there is frequent infection with enteroviruses. Intubation of the stomach or jejunum with tubes passed through the nose places a patient at risk of obstruction of the ostia of the sinuses and eustachian tubes. Percutaneous gastrostomy tubes provide direct access to the stomach from the skin surface and expose abdominal skin to gastric secretions. The ostomy site is rapidly colonized by fecal flora and skin flora. Gastric acid often irritates the surrounding skin, increasing the incidence of cellulitis due to skin or enteric flora. Jejunostomy tubes, whether placed through the nose, percutaneously, or through a gastrostomy, permit fluids to bypass the stomach and the antimicrobial action of gastric acid and, if contaminated, can more easily cause infection.

Contamination of hospital food has caused a variety of outbreaks of gastroenteritis caused by viruses (Norwalk and Norwalk-like viruses), bacteria (*Salmonella, Shigella,* and *S. aureus*), and parasites (*Giardia lamblia*). Normal gastric acidity destroys most bacte-

TABLE 105–10. Nosocomial Gastrointestinal and Hepatic Infections

Types	Risk Factors	Etiologic Agents	Diagnostic Tests	Preventive Measures
Stomatitis Esophagitis Gastroenteritis Colitis Hepatitis	Prior antibiotic therapy Antacid therapy Ingestion of contaminated food or water Irritation of mucosa by indwelling tubes Contact with an infected patient Epidemic season of the year	*Clostridium difficile* *Candida albicans* *Salmonella* *Shigella* Rotaviruses Enteroviruses Hepatitis A, B, and C viruses Cytomegalovirus	Culture of stool Assays for rotavirus Stool smear for fecal leukocytes Endoscopy Assays for cytotoxin of *C. difficile* Liver enzyme analysis Serologic testing for hepatitis viruses and cytomegalovirus	Use good hand washing technique Isolate patients with contagious disease Prepare food and formula properly Use antibiotics appropriately Screen blood donors for hepatitis viruses

ria but has no effect on Norwalk viruses. The most common cause of foodborne outbreaks is contamination of food during handling. *Salmonella* outbreaks most often result from contamination of foods before delivery to the kitchen, especially from contaminated poultry products. Cross-contamination of salads or sandwiches occurs when cutting boards are improperly cleaned or poultry products are prepared in the same areas as salads or other uncooked foods. Eggs are contaminated on their shells, and often inside the shells, because the ovaries of hens are sometimes infected chronically with *Salmonella.* In many areas the use of raw eggs is prohibited within hospital cafeterias. Thorough cooking of food, including poultry and eggs, destroys *Salmonella.*

Enteral feedings and formulas must be prepared in an aseptic manner. Many liquid formulas are infused for hours at room temperature, allowing for overgrowth of any contaminants introduced during preparation. Several outbreaks have been traced to contamination of infant formula. Many cities and states often have specific health codes that address preparation and testing of formulas.

Drugs such as antacids or H_2 blockers decrease gastric acidity and in turn decrease the amount of ingested bacteria needed to cause infection. The combination of antacids and antimicrobial agents increases colonization and invasion of the intestinal wall by *Candida,* which can serve as a source for dissemination of *Candida.* Enteral tubes irritate the intestinal wall, leading to inflammation and possibly to ulceration, which results in perforation and extension of local flora into adjacent tissues. Ulcerated intestinal walls are often colonized by hospital-acquired bacteria and fungi.

Etiology. Agents that cause nosocomial gastrointestinal infections include viruses, bacteria, fungi, and parasites (Table 105–10). Community-acquired viruses are often transmitted from one child to another. Thus viral nosocomial infections are a reflection of the prevalence of viral infections in the community. In one study (Champsaur et al, 1984) almost half of the children admitted to the hospital during the winter months were shedding rotaviruses, although about half of these children had no symptoms. During spring, summer, and early fall, enteroviruses are the major causes of community-acquired infections that necessitate hospitalization.

Bacteria involved in gastrointestinal infections include enterotoxin-producing *S. aureus, Salmonella, Shigella,* and toxin-producing *Clostridium difficile. C. difficile* is a spore-forming anaerobe; spores contaminate the environment around a person who is colonized and are resistant to detergents. The carriage rate of *C. difficile* in healthy adults and children is approximately 4%. Transmission of the organism from a patient to an environmental source to hands and on to the next patient occurs frequently. *C. difficile* causes disease by production of enterotoxins, which occurs when the normal flora is altered, as by stress or antibiotic therapy.

Foods are sometimes contaminated by enterotoxin-producing strains of *S. aureus.* Ingestion of preformed toxin causes nausea, vomiting, and diarrhea. *Salmonella* and *Shigella* are also transmitted directly from patient to patient or from patient to the health care provider. The inoculum of *Shigella* required to cause disease is low; thus person-to-person transmission is common. *Salmonella* organisms are not usually transmitted from person to person because a large inoculum is required to cause infection. However, the inoculum needed to cause disease is lowered in an infant or child without normal gastric acidity or in one who is receiving antibiotics. Under these circumstances, outbreaks and person-to-person and often baby-to-baby transmission have been reported.

Fungi that colonize the intestine are usually present at the time of hospitalization as part of the endogenous flora. Under certain conditions, fungi are transmitted, usually by the hands of health care providers, from patient to patent. Fungi can also be acquired from food sources. Hospital-acquired fungi colonize the intestine or skin and at times enter the bloodstream or adjacent tissues to cause hospital-acquired infection.

Transmission of parasites within a hospital is uncommon. Roundworms and flatworms are not transmitted directly from patient to patient because intermediate hosts or incubation time in soil are required to complete the life cycles. Protozoa such as *Giardia* and *Cryptosporidium* are transmitted directly by the fecal-oral route. Children, especially those in diapers, often contaminate their fingers and hands with feces and transmit parasites directly to other children or indirectly to fomites, which are then handled by other hands. Children's hands spend much time in their mouths, and young children tend to explore the environment with their mouths. A study (Hutto, 1986) conducted in a daycare center documented the frequencies with which children of various ages put objects into their mouths. Children younger than 1 year put objects into their mouths 64 times each hour; those 1–2 years of age, 34 times each hour; those 2–3 years of age, 16 times each hour; and those 3–4 years of age, 10 times each hour. Thus there is ample opportunity for effective fecal-oral spread of pathogens among young children.

Infectious hepatitis can be acquired from transfusions of blood or blood products. Approximately 80% of cases are caused by hepatitis C virus (HCV), with the remainder caused by hepatitis A virus (HAV), hepatitis B virus (HBV), cytomegalovirus (CMV), or Epstein-Barr virus (EBV). Hepatitis due to viruses is often clinically indistinguishable from toxic hepatitis or damage due to hypoperfusion or hypoxemia.

Diagnosis. The diagnosis of hospital-acquired gastroenteritis is often established on clinical grounds. Not all cases of diarrhea are related to infection. Laboratory studies are used to confirm specific etiologic agents. Enzyme immunoassays (EIAs) are available for detection of rotaviruses in stool samples. Culture of stool is used to recover agents such as enteroviruses, *Salmonella,* and *Shigella.* Toxin assays and EIA-based tests to identify the toxin of *C. difficile* are commercially available.

Hepatitis is suggested by clinical symptoms and confirmed by measurement of liver enzymes and bilirubin; the specific etiologic agent of hepatitis is determined by the clinical setting and by serologic testing. A biopsy is sometimes needed to define the extent of disease and to determine the cause of hepatic dysfunction.

Prevention. Prevention of gastrointestinal infection involves many of the methods used to prevent respiratory infection. Hand washing before and after every patient contact is critical. Hand washing before preparation of foods is essential. The temperature at which foods are held is important. Hot foods must be uniformly heated and thoroughly cooked to inactivate microbes. Cold foods must be kept cold, and care must be taken to prevent contamination of foods during and after preparation. Education of all members of the dietary service is important. Policies regarding formula preparation must be appropriate and must be enforced. Samples of hospital-prepared formulas should be cultured on a regular basis; this allows for identification and correction of breaks in technique, which could lead to an outbreak. The potentially adverse effects of antacid therapy and of antimicrobial therapy should be considered in the care of each patient. The use of tubes should be discontinued as soon as medically possible. When tubes are needed to ensure optimal nutrition, however, the benefit of adequate nutrition outweighs the risk of infection and irritation.

Blood products are currently screened for a variety of infectious agents, including many that cause hepatitis, such as HBV and HCV.

SKIN INFECTIONS

Nosocomial infections of skin include cellulitis, wound infections, and soft-tissue abscesses (Table 105–11). The major predisposing factor is injury to the skin. Incisions or wounds become colonized at the time of injury or before healing is complete. Sutures serve as foreign bodies that increase the risk of infection. Skin, a natural barrier, is bypassed by the insertion of catheters. Skin is broken down by pressure, and pressure sores are rapidly colonized by pathogenic flora. The area is usually inflamed and often superinfected, leading to local cellulitis and occasionally to lymphangitis, lymphadenitis, or bacteremia. Both gram-positive and gram-negative bacteria rapidly colonize burned skin. Infection and burn-wound sepsis is a major cause of morbidity and death among burn victims.

Etiology. The most common infectious agents of hospital-acquired wound and skin infections are *S. aureus* and group A *Streptococcus* (Table 105–11). Burns and damaged skin are frequently colonized by enteric gram-negative flora such as Enterobacteriaceae, *Enterococcus,* and group B *Streptococcus.* Anaerobic bacteria are present within the margins of pressure sores but rarely cause invasive disease. Burn-wound infection is manifested by fever, inflammation, and failure of grafts to adhere. Quantitative culture of a biopsy sample of burned skin has been used in some centers for better differentiation of colonization from infection. Pathogens that infect burned skin include *S. aureus,* group A *Streptococcus, E. coli* and other gram-negative enteric bacilli, *Pseudomonas aeruginosa,* and other waterborne gram-negative bacilli.

Diagnosis. The diagnosis of cellulitis or wound infection is made on clinical grounds by the presence of erythema, heat, pain, and discharge. It is more difficult to determine when a burn or pressure sore has become infected; quantitative cultures are sometimes helpful. The presence of systemic signs of infection or bacteremia confirms that the infection has spread beyond the wound. The ideal culture specimen of a wound infection or area of cellulitis is an aspirate. The point of maximal induration or the area of fluctuance should be prepared and aspirated with a large-gauge needle for optimal recovery of pathogens, including anaerobes.

Prevention. Prevention of a skin infection requires meticulous attention to aseptic technique when skin is incised or entered with tubes. Wounds are usually seeded at the time of an operation with the endogenous flora of the patient or contaminating flora from the surgical team. Necrotic or contaminated tissues should be débrided carefully, with attention to good hemostasis. The prophylactic use of antibiotics decreases the incidence of infection after surgical procedures (Tables 105–7 and 105–12). This has been proved for clean-contaminated operations and also appears to be true for some clean procedures. Contaminated wounds are at highest risk of infection; in these circumstances, antibiotics are considered to be part of therapy rather than prophylaxis only.

The timing of antibiotic administration for prophylaxis against wound infection is important. The first dose of antibiotic should be administered at 30 minutes before the skin incision to ensure adequate tissue levels of drug at the time of entry. If the operation

TABLE 105–11. Nosocomial Skin Infections

Types	Risk Factors	Etiologic Agents	Diagnostic Tests	Preventive Measures
Cellulitis Wound infections Surgical incision Site of catheterization Abscess Burn wound sepsis	Incisions Operation Catheterization Burns Premature birth Abnormal skin Eczema Ichthyosis Obesity	*Staphylococcus aureus* Group A *Streptococcus* *Pseudomonas aeruginosa* *Candida albicans* Hospital-acquired, gram-negative bacilli	Gram stain of drainage Culture of drainage Aspiration of infected site for Gram stain and culture Blood culture	Use good hand washing technique Provide meticulous care of catheters Use topical agents for burn care Débride burned skin Graft burns early Use prophylactic perioperative antibiotics appropriately Use optimal surgical technique Provide optimal nutrition

TABLE 105–12. Surgical Prophylaxis

Indications for Prophylaxis
High risk of postoperative infection (see Table 105–7)
Consequences of infection catastrophic

Timing
First dose administered immediately as a single dose ~30 min before procedure
Repeat doses q6hr during long operative procedures
Limit antimicrobial therapy after surgery completed

Choice
Based on the surgical procedure and likely pathogens (see Table 16–5)
Broad-spectrum antimicrobial agents should be avoided

is prolonged, repeated doses of antibiotics should be given intraoperatively to maintain therapeutic concentrations of antibiotic in blood and tissue. Antibiotic therapy is often continued after skin closure but is probably not needed. In any case, antibiotics should not be continued beyond 24 hours after the operation. The choice of prophylactic antibiotic depends on the surgical site and the patient's flora (see Table 16–5). It is not necessary to provide prophylaxis against every possible nosocomial pathogen, but it is preferable to use narrow-spectrum drugs aimed at the most likely and most virulent bacteria. The first-generation cephalosporins remain the drugs of choice for surgical prophylaxis.

Surgical technique is even more important than antibiotic prophylaxis. Necrotic tissue, hematomas, or foreign bodies left in the surgical field greatly increase the risk of infection. Aseptic technique should be used for insertion of all catheters.

In some studies the use of occlusive transparent dressing was associated with increased infection. Hand washing and the use of gloves for dressing changes are essential to decrease the risk of secondary contamination of wounds and damaged skin. Pressure sores should be treated promptly. Every effort should be made to avoid the formation of pressure sores, including frequent turning, use of special mattress, and special beds. Prevention of burn-wound infection begins with aseptic technique during dressing changes. Topical agents are very useful to decrease colony counts of colonizing bacteria. Débridement of necrotic tissue is essential; early grafting decreases the incidence of infection.

URINARY TRACT INFECTIONS

Nosocomial infections of the urinary tract include urethritis, cystitis, and pyelonephritis (Table 105–13); secondary bacteremia is an occasional complication. Important risk factors for infection of the urinary tract are the presence of catheters, instrumentation, and anatomic abnormalities. Any anomaly of the urinary tract that results in urinary stasis sets the stage for infection. Bacteria are introduced by catheterization. After simple straight catheterization, the incidence of infection is 1–2%. Indwelling catheters provide access to the bladder and should have a closed drainage system. Closed systems become infected at a rate of 5% per day. Rates are much higher if the drainage system is left open; 100% of catheters in open systems are infected within 48 hours. Organisms enter the bladder either through the catheter by instillation of contaminated irrigation fluids, by back flow of contaminated urine in the drainage bag, or by ascent around the outside of the catheter from the area around the urethra. Bacteremia occurs in approximately 1% of persons with indwelling urinary catheters. Diarrhea predisposes a person to urinary tract infection, probably because the colony counts of perineal flora increase during episodes of diarrhea. Perineal bacteria ascend into the bladder and cause infection.

Etiology. Organisms that cause urinary tract infections include fecal flora such as *Enterococcus* and gram-negative enteric bacilli (see Table 105–13); *E. coli* is the most common cause of urinary tract infections. If a patient has been treated with antibiotics, resistant organisms predominate and fungi emerge as pathogens.

Diagnosis. The diagnosis is established by urinalysis and urine culture. For patients with long-term indwelling catheters, it is expected that the catheter will become colonized, which places the patient at risk of having upper tract infection. Routine cultures of urine are not recommended, but urine and blood cultures should be obtained if a patient with an indwelling catheter has fever, pain in the back or kidneys, or evidence of decreased renal function. Infection is defined as more than 100,000 organisms per milliliter

TABLE 105–13. Nosocomial Urinary Tract Infections

Types	Risk Factors	Etiologic Agents	Diagnostic Tests	Preventive Measures
Cystitis: lower tract infection Pyelonephritis: ascending or following bacteremic spread	Anatomic abnormality Female sex Catheterization Surgical procedure Diarrhea Underlying illness	*Escherichia coli* *Klebsiella* *Proteus* *Enterobacter* *Enterococcus* *Pseudomonas* *Staphylococcus* *Candida albicans*	Urine culture Urinalysis Blood culture	Use good hand washing technique Limit use of catheters Maintain a closed sterile drainage system Limit duration of catheterization Limit manipulation of indwelling catheters Secure the catheter to minimize movement Maintain drainage tubes and bags below level of bladder Use aseptic technique for insertion of catheters Use aseptic technique when accessing the drainage system Use antibiotics appropriately

of voided urine, 1,000 or more organisms per milliliter of urine obtained by catheterization, or any number of organisms in urine obtained by bladder aspiration. Usually only a single species is involved; however, polymicrobial infections occur when catheters are in place or after an operation or instrumentation of the urinary tract.

Prevention. The most important aspect of prevention is to minimize the duration and use of catheterization and to avoid urinary stasis. Insertion of catheters must be performed with aseptic technique. Perineal care should be minimized because the less the catheter is manipulated, the lower the risk of nosocomial infection. The drainage system must remain closed at all times, with sterile technique used whenever the system is entered. The drainage bag must be lower than the bladder to ensure proper drainage and to avoid backflow of urine into the bladder. Attention to hand washing before handling the drainage bag is important in preventing the spread of multiresistant organisms from one bag to another and thus from one person to another. The use of detergents in the collection bag has not been effective in decreasing the incidence of infection, nor has bladder irrigation with antibiotics been effective. Parenteral antibiotic therapy protects the patient for a short time. However, the use of antibiotics leads to replacement of normal flora and increases the risk of infection with resistant organisms. Intermittent catheterization is preferred over indwelling catheter drainage.

CENTRAL NERVOUS SYSTEM INFECTIONS

Nosocomial infections of the central nervous system include ventriculitis and meningitis (Table 105–14). Important risks of infection are surgical intervention, placement of ventriculoperitoneal shunts, and the presence of spinal fluid leaks. Infection related to ventriculoperitoneal shunts arises from contamination of the system with skin flora at the time of placement (Chapter 53). Devices used to monitor intracranial pressure include subdural bolts and intraventricular catheters, which allow skin bacteria to gain direct access into the spinal fluid. Rates of infection increase with the duration of catheterization.

Etiology. The most common pathogens that contaminate shunts are coagulase-negative staphylococci and *S. aureus.* After head trauma or surgical trauma to the dura, there can be a connection between the ear or nose and the cerebrospinal fluid that permits ascending infection, which in almost all such cases is caused by *Streptococcus pneumoniae.* Intracranial infection sometimes follows neurosurgical procedures. Brain abscesses or infected collections of blood or spinal fluid and infection of the skull rarely occur.

Diagnosis. Signs of increased intracranial pressure and fever suggest infection of central nervous system catheters. Examination and culture of cerebrospinal fluid confirm the diagnosis. Imaging studies are useful in confirming the presence of infected fluid collections and in confirming shunt malfunction.

Prevention. Antibiotics are frequently used perioperatively during placement of shunts and after neurosurgical procedures. There is no proof that antibiotics decrease infection rates in these clean procedures. Although many surgeons flush the shunt with antibiotic solutions, there are no controlled trials proving efficacy. Meticulous surgical technique with attention to hemostasis is probably most important. The use of external drainage tubes such as ventriculostomies should be minimized, and catheters should be removed as soon as possible. Pressure monitoring devices must be inserted under conditions of asepsis, tubing handled with care, the use of stopcocks kept to a minimum, and sterile technique used when entering the system is essential. Hand washing is essential to prevent transmission of organisms from patient to patient or from one drainage bag to another.

EYE INFECTIONS

Nosocomial infections of the eye include conjunctivitis, keratitis, endophthalmitis, and uveitis (Table 105–15). Risks of infection include trauma to the eye, exposure of the cornea, and exposure of the patient to seasonal viruses. Outbreaks of viral conjunctivitis have occurred because of hand-to-eye transmission and because of contamination of ophthalmic equipment. **Exposure keratitis** is common in paralyzed or incapacitated persons. The exposed cornea is inflamed and easily colonized by bacteria. Corneal ulcers predispose a person to corneal perforation and contamination of the interior of the globe. Infection also follows surgical intervention, including intraocular procedures.

Etiology. Viral pathogens causing nosocomial eye infections include enteroviruses and adenoviruses. Bacterial agents include skin flora and gram-negative enteric bacilli as well as *Pseudomonas* species.

Diagnosis. The diagnosis of an eye infection is made by clinical inspection. A slit-lamp examination helps to determine the extent of the infection. The agent is confirmed by culture of the conjunctiva, cornea, or contents of the globe.

Prevention. Hand washing is the key to preventing viral infection. Equipment must be cleaned after every patient encounter. Attention

TABLE 105–14. Nosocomial Central Nervous System Infections

Types	Risk Factors	Etiologic Agents	Diagnostic Tests	Preventive Measures
Meningitis Ventriculitis	Trauma with spinal fluid leak Surgical procedure Intracranial monitoring device Ventriculoperitoneal shunt Intracranial reservoir	*Staphylococcus* *Corynebacterium* Gram-negative enteric bacilli *Pseudomonas aeruginosa*	Spinal fluid analysis Spinal fluid culture	Use good hand-washing technique Use aseptic technique for insertion of intracranial monitoring devices Limit use of monitoring devices and drainage systems Limit duration of monitoring and external drainage Use aseptic technique for accessing monitoring devices or drainage systems

TABLE 105–15. Nosocomial Eye Infections

Types	Risk Factors	Etiologic Agents	Diagnostic Tests	Preventive Measures
Conjunctivitis Corneal ulceration Endophthalmitis Chorioretinitis	Contamination of ophthalmic equipment Epidemic season of year Trauma to cornea Exposure keratitis Bacteremia Fungemia	Adenoviruses *Staphylococcus aureus* *Pseudomonas aeruginosa* *Candida albicans* Herpes simplex virus	Culture of conjunctival scrapings Slit-lamp examination Ophthalmoscopic examination Culture of orbital contents	Use good hand-washing technique Decontaminate equipment before and after use Use proper technique for suctioning the airway Avoid exposure keratitis Isolate patients and staff with contagious disease

to detail in the operating room and aseptic technique are important in minimizing postoperative infection. Exposure keratitis must be avoided. Eye shields and artificial tears should be used as needed for obtunded persons. Care must be taken to avoid inoculating the conjunctivae while suctioning the respiratory tract.

PERITONEAL DIALYSIS–ASSOCIATED INFECTIONS

Peritoneal dialysis requires the placement of an indwelling catheter with possible infectious complications including exit site infection, tunnel infection, and peritonitis (Table 105–16). The usual route of infection is from the skin surface along the tunnel and into the peritoneum. Other routes of infection are perforation of the intestine or translocation of bacteria across the intestinal wall.

Patients with end-stage renal disease frequently receive transfusions and are thus at risk of acquiring hepatitis and other bloodborne pathogens. The use of recombinant erythropoietin diminishes the need for blood transfusion.

Etiology. The most common pathogens are skin flora such as *Staphylococcus,* organisms that contaminate water such as *Pseudomonas* and *Acinetobacter,* enteric flora such as *E. coli* and *Klebsiella,* and fungi such as *Candida albicans.*

Diagnosis. The diagnosis is established on clinical grounds and confirmed by culture of the dialysate.

Prevention. Prevention depends on hand washing, aseptic insertion of the catheter, planning of the location of the exit site, meticulous care of the catheter site, securing of the catheter to avoid motion, and aseptic technique when bags of dialysate are attached.

INFECTIONS AFTER TRANSFUSION AND TRANSPLANTATION

Many infectious agents have been transmitted by blood transfusion (Table 105–17). Contamination of blood products during collection, storage, or transfusion is usually due to bacteria. The skin flora of the donor is a minor problem. Collection of blood from a donor with inapparent bacteremia due to *Yersinia* or *Salmonella* occasionally occurs, and both agents survive at refrigerator temperatures. Malaria also has been transmitted in blood, and therefore donors who have been to areas of the world where malaria is endemic are excluded. Donors are screened for antibody to *Treponema pallidum,* HBV, HCV, HIV (starting March 1985), and HTLV-I and HTLV-II (starting November 1988) (Table 105–18). In one study (Schreiber, 1996) the risk of infection from a person donating blood who passed all screening tests but was infectious (i.e., the donor was in the window period, when the serologic screening result was not yet positive) was 1 in 103,000 for hepatitis C (non-A, non-B hepatitis), 1 in 63,000 for hepatitis B, and 1 in 493,000 for HIV. Donors with antibody that suggests prior infection are eliminated from the donor pool and their blood is not used. In addition to serologic screening, donors are asked a variety of questions regarding recent immunizations, travel, exposure to infected persons, and behaviors or lifestyles that would put a person at risk of infection by bloodborne pathogens (Table 105–19).

Blood collected from volunteer Red Cross donors is the safest blood available. Directed donors are not necessarily safe donors.

TABLE 105–16. Peritoneal Dialysis-Related Infections

Types	Risk Factors	Etiologic Agents	Diagnostic Tests	Preventive Measures
Entry-site infection Tunnel infection Hepatitis	Peritoneal dialysis Transfusion	*Staphylococcus* *Pseudomonas* *Streptococcus* *Escherichia coli* *Pseudomonas aeruginosa* *Acinetobacter* Environmental mycobacteria *Candida albicans* Hepatitis B and C viruses Cytomegalovirus Epstein-Barr virus	Skin or soft-tissue aspiration Analysis of dialysate Culture of dialysate	Use good hand-washing technique Use aseptic technique for insertion of all catheters Meticulously prepare graft site or catheter before insertion Use aseptic technique whenever accessing bloodstream catheter or peritoneal catheter Secure catheters to avoid motion Choose an appropriate location for catheter exit sites Screen blood products Immunize against hepatitis B virus Use erythropoietin therapy

TABLE 105–17. Pathogens Transmissible by Blood or Transplanted Tissues

Viruses	Bacteria
Cytomegalovirus	*Bartonella bacilliformis*
Epstein-Barr virus	*Bartonella quintana*
Varicella-zoster virus	*Borrelia*
Human herpesvirus type 6	*Brucella*
Human herpesvirus type 7	*Salmonella*
Hepatitis A virus	*Yersinia*
Hepatitis B virus	**Mycobacteria**
Hepatitis C virus	*Mycobacterium leprae*
Human immunodeficiency virus type 1	**Spirochetes**
Human immunodeficiency virus type 2	*Leptospira interrogans*
Human T-cell lymphotropic virus type 1	*Treponema pallidum*
Human T-cell lymphotropic virus type 2	**Rickettsiae**
Colorado tick virus	*Coxiella burnetii*
Parvovirus B19	*Rickettsia rickettsii*
Rabies virus	**Parasites**
Subviruses	*Leishmania donovani*
Prions (Agents of spongiform encephalopathies)	*Plasmodium*
Satellite Viruses	*Babesia*
Hepatitis D virus	*Toxoplasma gondii*
	Trypanosoma

TABLE 105–18. Serologic Studies for Prospective Blood Donors

- Hepatitis B surface antigen
- Hepatitis B core antibody
- Antibody to human immunodeficiency virus type 1
- Antibody to human immunodeficiency virus type 2
- Antibody to hepatitis C virus
- Antibody to human T-cell lymphotropic virus type I
- Antibody to human T-cell lymphotropic virus type II
- Test for syphilis

Volunteer donors are more likely to be repeated donors; their blood has been screened and used safely in the past. Directed or designated donors may be unwilling to admit to risks of viral infection. Studies to date have revealed that the rate of HIV antibody positivity is not lower in designated donors than in volunteer donors. Autologous transfusions are even safer than transfusions of blood from volunteer donors. However, it is not always possible for children or ill persons to donate their own blood for later use. In some cases, other volume expanders can replace transfusion of blood or blood products. Risks and benefits must be considered before transfusion of any blood product.

Persons seropositive for HIV, HTLV-I, or HTLV-II should be counseled not to donate blood, semen, body organs, or other tissues; not to share drug needles or syringes; to refrain from breastfeeding; to inform their sex partners of their infection; and to use latex condoms, especially if there have been multiple sex partners, nonmutually monogamous sexual relationships, or a monogamous relationship with a seronegative individual.

Organs used in transplantation contain blood and tissue that are sometimes infected with bacteria, parasites, or viruses. Potential donors are screened before transplantation like blood donors and by history to eliminate possible acute bacterial infections. Organs are usually sampled at the time of transplantation and the samples are cultured for bacteria. The major viruses transmitted by organs are CMV and EBV. HIV has occasionally been transmitted by organ transplantation. Rabies has been transmitted by corneal transplantation. Creutzfeldt-Jakob disease has been transmitted by corneal tissue, pituitary extract, and cadaveric dura mater grafts. *Toxoplasma gondii* encysts in muscles and has been transmitted by heart transplantation. Transplant recipients are at increased risk of having disease due to these agents because of the immunosuppression required for successful transplantation and because of underly-

TABLE 105–19. Screening of Prospective Blood Donors

General Appearance
Ask questions about how donor feels
Inspect venipuncture site; it must be free of lesions

Temperature
Obtain oral temperature; must be below 37.5°C (98.6°F)

Recent Immunizations
Toxoids and killed vaccines acceptable
Live attenuated vaccine
  For measles, mumps, poliomyelitis, or yellow fever vaccination: defer donation for 2 wk
  For rubella vaccination: defer donation for 4 wk
Hepatitis B immune globulin: defer donation for 12 mo

Recent Transfusion
Exclude donors who have received blood or blood components or derivatives that are possible sources of hepatitis

Infectious Diseases
Exclude donors with history of viral hepatitis, infection with human immunodeficiency viruses, infection with human T-cell lymphotropic viruses, elevated alanine aminotransferase levels, receipt of pituitary growth hormone of human origin, babesiosis, or Chagas' disease
Treatment of syphilis or gonorrhea: Defer donation for 12 mo

Lifestyle
Exclude donors with stigmata of drug or alcohol abuse
Exclude donors who admit to behaviors putting them at risk of acquiring the human immunodeficiency viruses
Question donors regarding history
  Positive test result for the AIDS virus
  Use of illegal drugs
  Receipt of clotting factor concentrates
  Money or drugs taken for sex
  Sex with a person who has had AIDS or a positive test result for the AIDS virus
  Sex with a person who has taken illegal drugs with a needle
  Money given to anyone for sex
  Sex with anyone who has taken money or drugs for sex
  Diagnosis of syphilis or gonorrhea
  Receipt of blood or blood products
Ask male donors about having had sex with another man
Ask female donors about having had sex with a man who has had sex with another man
Ask donors about recent tattoos

Travel History
Exclude donors who have traveled to areas where malaria is endemic
Exclude donors who have lived in Great Britain for ≥6 mo

TABLE 105–20. Prevention of Blood-Borne and Transplantation-Related Infection

Screen donors for acute infection
Screen donors for prior infection with latent viruses
Use aseptic technique for collection of blood and blood products
Screen blood products for antibodies
Immunize recipients of transplanted tissues, when possible, before transplantation
Give chemoprophylaxis to transplant recipients (antibiotics, antiviral agents)
Use immunoprophylaxis for transplant recipients (immunoglobulins after transplantation, specific immunoglobulins after exposure)
Use blood products selectively
Use autologous blood for transfusion
Use erythropoietin therapy

ing organ dysfunction leading to the procedure. The diagnosis depends on the pathogen and organ system involved. Prevention of infection requires screening of donors, immunization of recipients, and the use of immunoprophylaxis and chemoprophylaxis (Table 105–20).

SYSTEMIC VIRAL INFECTIONS

Additional nosocomial agents of concern include varicella, measles, rubella, and parvovirus, which are spread by airborne transmission and direct contact. Children with community-acquired disease usually serve as reservoirs. Outbreaks have occurred when hospital personnel acquired these infections and exposed their contacts. The diagnosis is based on clinical manifestations, with confirmation by serologic testing. Prevention requires hand washing and isolation in a room with negative airflow for measles and varicella. Varicella, measles, rubella, and parvovirus infections are contagious before the onset of skin lesions. It is essential to include questions regarding exposure to contagious disease in the history of all hospitalized children. If a child has been exposed in the community or during hospitalization, that child should be placed into isolation during the period when the infection is likely to develop. For example, a child exposed to varicella should be isolated for 10–21 days after exposure, that is, from the end of the earliest to the end of the latest possible incubation period. All hospital personnel should be immune to measles, rubella, and varicella. The varicella vaccine, licensed in 1995, should be offered to hospital employees who are not immune to varicella. Nonimmune employees who are exposed to varicella should refrain from patient care on day 10 to day 21 after exposure. If exposed personnel or patients have received varicella-zoster immune globulin (VZIG), the incubation period can be prolonged to 28 days; subsequent infection is often subclinical or mild. People with mild and subclinical varicella are capable of transmitting the virus; thus they should be isolated from day 10 to day 28 after exposure. Zoster is also contagious, and children or employees with zoster should be isolated and removed from patient care activities until the disease is no longer contagious.

VASCULAR INFECTIONS

Nosocomial vascular infections include bacteremia, fungemia, and phlebitis. The bloodstream can be the primary focus of infection, as in infection of an indwelling vascular catheter (Chapter 106), or hematogenous spread can occur from any other site of infection. The most important risk factor is the presence of a catheter. Other risks include primary sites of infection, use of antibiotics, and damage to mucous membranes or skin.

PREVENTION OF NOSOCOMIAL INFECTIONS

Infection control involves all members of the health care team in the goal of preventing infection. Education of all health care providers (i.e., medical or nonmedical, paid or volunteer, full-time or part-time, student or nonstudent, with or without patient-care responsibilities) in infection control strategies (Table 105–21) must begin during orientation and continue throughout employment.

HAND WASHING

The importance of good hand-washing technique cannot be overemphasized (Table 105–22). Unfortunately, hand washing is often forgotten or ignored. In studies of intensive care units and outpatient facilities, physicians washed their hands less than 50% of the time before and after examination of a child. There are often concerns about the type of soap used, but this is a minor consideration. Some soaps are more effective in decreasing colonization of hands, but to be effective, the soap and sink must be used. Thus it seems more relevant to concentrate on methods to encourage hand washing than to study the nuances of different soaps. An important consideration is the location of sinks, which must be readily available and always in good operating condition.

Educational efforts should focus on the importance of hand washing; peer review is an underutilized tool. Hand washing is essential even when gloves are used. Gloves increase hand temperature and moisture and allow growth of resident flora. Gloves are often torn, and these breaks usually go unrecognized. Gloves must be changed between patients. There is good evidence that gloves cannot be effectively decontaminated by simple washing. Thus gloves must be available at each bedside and a new pair used for each patient.

The extent of hand washing varies depending on the clinical situation. Before an operation, surgeons and nurses perform a 10-minute surgical scrub. A soft brush and a manicure stick are used to clean the nails, and hands and forearms are scrubbed to the elbows. A shorter scrub is recommended for those providing care in the newborn nursery and in intensive care units. Between patients, a shorter wash is appropriate; a 15-second wash is sufficient to reduce transient skin bacteria.

Hands should be washed at the start of the day; before and after each patient contact; before contact with the face and mouth of a

TABLE 105–21. Prevention of Nosocomial Infection

Hand washing
In-service training
Isolation and cohorting
Employee health services
Policies for catheter care
Infection surveillance and control
Disinfection
Education
Standard precautions
Aseptic technique
Policies for visitors
Appropriate use of antibiotics
Optimal patient nutrition
Sterilization

TABLE 105–22. Hand Washing

When
Before and after every patient contact
After use of bathroom facilities
Before eating
After contact with laboratory specimens
Whenever hands are contaminated

With What
Water for at least 15 seconds
Soap provides some additional protection
Antiseptic soaps are provided in intensive care units and nurseries
Hand-rub antiseptics are appropriate in certain areas

Where
Sinks must be located conveniently to areas of patient care

patient; after handling of used dressings, soiled urinals, bedpans, or used specimen containers; whenever hands are soiled; before eating; after use of the toilet; after blowing or wiping of the nose; and at the end of the workday.

A variety of alternative hand-washing methods have been described. The most promising and effective alternative method is the **hand rub** with an alcohol-based product. In some European countries the hand rub has replaced hand washing because of claims of superior compliance and timesaving. Hand rubs are clearly appropriate in areas where sinks do not exist, such as in ambulances. In intensive care areas, hand rubs save time over the 15-second hand wash. Hand rubs are not appropriate if there is soiling of the hands because the rubs are not effective in the presence of organic debris.

ASEPTIC TECHNIQUE

Aseptic technique should be used whenever body defenses are being breached. Skin should be prepared appropriately before entry, either as an incision or as a puncture. The type of preparation depends on the procedure. If the skin is being punctured to obtain blood for study, a simple preparation with alcohol is sufficient. If a catheter is to be left in place, more thorough preparation is recommended. **Povidone-iodine** or **tincture of iodine** scrub inactivates skin flora. Tincture of iodine has the advantage that it kills on contact, whereas povidone-iodine must become dry to release active iodine. Aseptic technique is appropriate for placement of all catheters and for any surgical intervention.

Suctioning of the respiratory tract or mouth does not require aseptic technique because there is a high background of normal flora in this area. Clean technique rather than sterile technique is appropriate. Suction catheters that reach the lower airways must be sterile and are designed for single use, whereas bulbs used to suction oral secretions are designed to be used several times. The potential exists for overgrowth of flora within the bulb, and the safety of reusing bulbs has not been demonstrated. These bulbs are probably safe for home use, but they are of limited use in the hospital setting. For persons who require intermittent catheterization of the bladder, clean technique has been shown to be safe and cost-effective. These patients reuse catheters after cleaning, and they use clean rather than aseptic technique for catheterization.

ISOLATION

Children with presumed or proved contagious disease should be separated from children who do not have infections. A child with a contagious disease should be isolated until the disease is no longer contagious. Duration of isolation varies depending on the infecting organism and on the immunocompetence of the child. Children with similar infections can usually be isolated together or grouped together.

Standard precautions have been defined by the CDC (Table 105–23). These precautions should be used in the care of all patients. Standard precautions include hand washing; use of protective gear such as gloves, masks, eye protection, face shields, and gowns; safe handling of equipment and linen; avoidance of bloodborne pathogens; and use of mouthpieces, resuscitation bags, and other devices instead of mouth-to mouth resuscitation. Gloves are worn when one is touching blood, body fluids, secretions, excretions, and items contaminated with these fluids. Masks and eye and face shields are used to protect mucous membranes during procedures

TABLE 105–23. Standard Precautions: To Be Used Consistently for All Patients

Barrier Precautions to Prevent Skin and Mucous Membrane Exposure
Gloves for touching blood and body fluids, mucous membranes, nonintact skin, items or surfaces soiled with blood or body fluids
Gloves when performing venipuncture and other vascular access procedures
Masks and protective eyewear or face shields during procedures that are likely to generate droplets of blood or other body fluids
Gowns or aprons during procedures that are likely to generate splashes of blood or other body fluids

Hand Washing
Hands and other body surfaces should be washed immediately and thoroughly if contaminated with blood or other body fluids
Hands should be washed after removal of gloves

Handling of Sharp Instruments
Needles must not be recapped, bent, broken, removed by hand from syringes, or manipulated by hand
Sharp instruments including needles must be placed in puncture-resistant containers for disposal
Disposal containers should be as close as practical to the use area
Reusable sharp instruments should be placed in puncture-resistant containers for transport to processing areas

Resuscitation Equipment
Available for use in areas in which the need for resuscitation is predictable
Mouth-to-mouth resuscitation should be avoided

Health Care Workers with Exudative Lesions
Refrain from direct patient care

Pregnant Health Care Workers
Must be aware of and adhere to these precautions

TABLE 105–24. Categories of Disease Transmission–Based Precautions

Category	Private Room	Gowns	Gloves	Masks	Hand Washing
Airborne	Yes, can cohort	If soiling likely	If touching infective material	Yes	Yes
Droplet	Yes, can cohort	If soiling likely	If touching infective material	For close contact	Yes
Contact	Yes, can cohort	If soiling likely or for certain pathogens	If touching infective material	For close contact	Yes

likely to generate splashes or sprays of blood or body fluids. Gowns are used to prevent soiling of clothing. Needles, scalpels, and sharp instruments and devices should be handled with great care. Needles should not be recapped. All sharp materials should be disposed of into impermeable containers. Such containers must be available in all areas where needles and sharp instruments are in use.

Transmission-based isolation precautions are designed to prevent the transmission of pathogens from patient to patient. Categories of transmission are airborne, droplet, and contact (Table 105–24). Most pathogens are transmitted by contact. **Airborne transmission** occurs by airborne droplets from one room to another without a physical vector. Only a few pathogens, such as varicella and tuberculosis, are truly spread by airborne transmission. Thus airflow must be altered to ensure that air from the room of a child hospitalized with varicella stays in the room or exits to the outside and not to the hallway. These rooms should have negative air pressure with 6–12 air changes per hour; the air should be externally exhausted or, if recycled, passed through a high-efficiency particulate air (**HEPA**) filter. If infectious tuberculosis is suspected or proved, all health care providers should wear specially fitted masks. **Droplet transmission** occurs during close contact when pathogens are present in droplets generated by patients or procedures. Masks are used during close patient contact. **Contact transmission** is the most common route of transmission, with pathogens being transmitted by direct and indirect contact. Single-room isolation is desirable but not always possible; cohorting is acceptable. The use of curtained-off areas in intensive care units, for contact and droplet isolation, is acceptable if single rooms are not available; however, this is not adequate for airborne precautions (Table 105–25).

All employees must be educated regarding proper and improper use of protective equipment. Federal regulations regarding protection of employees against bloodborne pathogens went into effect in May 1992. The American Academy of Pediatrics has published *Materials to Assist the Pediatric Office in Implementing the Blood-*

TABLE 105–25. Type and Duration of Isolation Precautions

Infection/Condition	Precautions: Type[1]	Precautions: Duration[2]
Abscess		
Draining, major[3]	C	DI
Draining, minor or limited[4]	S	
Acquired immunodeficiency syndrome (AIDS)[5]	S	
Actinomycosis	S	
Adenovirus infection in infants and young children	D, C	DI
Amebiasis	S	
Anthrax		
Cutaneous	S	
Pulmonary	S	
Antibiotic-associated colitis (*see Clostridium difficile*)		
Arthropodborne viral encephalitides (eastern, western, Venezuelan equine encephalomyelitis; St. Louis, California encephalitis)	S[6]	
Arthropodborne viral fevers (dengue, yellow fever, Colorado tick fever)	S[6]	
Ascariasis	S	
Aspergillosis	S	
Babesiosis	S	
Blastomycosis, North American (cutaneous or pulmonary)	S	
Botulism	S	
Bronchiolitis (*see* Respiratory infectious disease in infants and young children)		
Brucellosis (undulant, Malta, Mediterranean fever)	S	
Campylobacter gastroenteritis (*see* Gastroenteritis)		
Candidiasis, all forms including mucocutaneous	S	
Cat-scratch fever (benign inoculation lymphoreticulosis)	S	
Cellulitis, uncontrolled drainage	C	DI
Chancroid (soft chancre)	S	
Chickenpox (varicella; *see* F[7] for varicella exposure)	A, C	F[7]

[1]A = airborne; C = contact; D = droplet; S = standard; when A, C, and D are specified, also use S.
[2]CN = until off antibiotics and culture result is negative; DH = duration of hospitalization; DI = duration of illness (with wound lesions, DI means until they stop draining); U = until time specified in hours after initiation of effective therapy; F = see footnote number.
[3]No dressing or dressing does not contain drainage adequately.
[4]Dressing covers and contains drainage adequately.
[5]Pulmonary tuberculosis should be suspected in an HIV-infected person or a person at high risk of HIV infection with cough, fever, and pulmonary infiltrate in any lung location.
[6]Install screens in windows and doors in endemic areas.
[7]Maintain precautions until all lesions are crusted. The average incubation for varicella is 10 to 16 days, with a range of 10 to 21 days. After exposure, use varicella-zoster immune globulin (VZIG) when appropriate, and discharge susceptible persons if possible. Place exposed susceptible persons on Airborne Precautions beginning 10 days after exposure and continuing until 21 days after last exposure (up to 28 days if VZIG has been given). Susceptible persons should not enter the room of patients on precautions if other, immune caregivers are available.

TABLE 105–25. Type and Duration of Isolation Precautions *(Continued)*

Infection/Condition	Precautions Type[1]	Precautions Duration[2]
Chlamydia trachomatis		
Conjunctivitis	S	
Genital	S	
Respiratory	S	
Cholera (*see* Gastroenteritis)		
Closed-cavity infection		
Draining, limited or minor	S	
Not draining	S	
Clostridium		
C. botulinum	S	
C. difficile	C	DI
C. perfringens		
Food poisoning	S	
Gas gangrene	S	
Coccidiodomycosis (valley fever)		
Draining lesions	S	
Pneumonia	S	
Colorado tick fever	S	
Congenital rubella	C	F[8]
Conjunctivitis		
Acute bacterial	S	
Acute viral (acute hemorrhagic)	C	DI
Chlamydia	S	
Gonococcal	S	
Coxsackievirus disease (*see* Enteroviral infections)		
Creutzfeldt-Jakob disease	S[9]	
Croup (*see* Respiratory infectious disease in infants and young children)		
Cryptococcosis	S	
Cryptosporidiosis (*see* Gastroenteritis)		
Cysticercosis	S	
Cytomegalovirus infection, neonatal or immunocompromised	S	
Decubitus ulcer, infected		
Major[3]	C	DI
Minor or limited[4]	S	
Dengue	S[6]	
Diarrhea, acute—infective cause suspected (*see* Gastroenteritis)		
Diphtheria		
Cutaneous	C	CN[10]
Pharyngeal	D	CN[10]
Ebola viral hemorrhagic fever	C[11]	DI
Echinococcosis (hydatidosis)	S	
Echovirus (*see* Enteroviral infections)		
Encephalitis or encephalomyelitis (*see* specific etiologic agents)		
Endometritis	S	
Enterobiasis (pinworm disease, oxyuriasis)	S	
Enterococcus species (*see* Multidrug-resistant organisms if epidemiologically significant or vancomycin resistant)		
Enterocolitis, *C. difficile*	C	DI
Enteroviral infections		
Adults	S	
Infants and young children	C	DI
Epiglottitis caused by *Haemophilus influenzae* type b	D	U[24 hr]
Epstein-Barr virus infection, including infectious mononucleosis	S	
Erythema infectiosum (*see also* Parvovirus B19)	S	
Escherichia coli gastroenteritis (*see* Gastroenteritis)		
Food poisoning		
Botulism	S	
C. perfringens or *C. welchii*	S	
Staphylococcal	S	
Furunculosis—staphylococcal		
Infants and young children	C	DI
Gangrene (gas gangrene)	S	
Gastroenteritis		
Campylobacter species	S[12]	
Cholera	S[12]	
C. difficile	C	DI
Cryptosporidium parrum	S[12]	
Escherichia coli		
Enterohemorrhagic O157:H7	S[12]	
Diapered or incontinent	C	DI
Other species	S[12]	
Giardia lamblia	S[12]	
Rotavirus	S[12]	
Diapered or incontinent	C	DI
Salmonella species (including *S. typhi*)	S[12]	
Shigella species	S[12]	
Diapered or incontinent	C	DI
Vibrio parahaemolyticus	S[12]	
Viral (if not covered elsewhere)	S[12]	
Yersinia enterocolitica	S[12]	
German measles (rubella)	D	F[13]
Giardiasis (*see* Gastroenteritis)		
Gonococcal ophthalmia neonatorum (gonorrheal ophthalmia, acute conjunctivitis of newborn)	S	
Gonorrhea	S	
Granuloma inguinale (donovanosis, granuloma venerum)	S	
Guillain-Barré syndrome	S	
Hand, foot, and mouth disease (*see* Enteroviral infections)		
Hantavirus cardiopulmonary syndrome	S	
Helicobacter pylori	S	
Hemorrhagic fevers (e.g., Lassa, Ebola)	C[11]	DI

[8]Place infant on precautions during any admission until 1 year of age, unless nasopharyngeal and urine cultures are negative for virus after 3 months of age.

[9]Additional special precautions are necessary for handling and decontamination of blood, body fluids and tissues, and contaminated items from persons with confirmed or suspected disease. See latest College of American Pathologists (Northfield, Illinois) guidelines (www.cap.org/html/publications/cjd.html) or other references.

[10]Until results of two cultures of specimens taken at least 24 hours apart are negative.

[11]Call state health department and CDC for specific advice about management of a suspected case. See Centers for Disease Control and Prevention: Update: management of patients with suspected viral hemorrhagic fever—United States. *MMWR Morb Mortal Wkly Rep* 1995;44:475–9.

[12]Use Contact Precautions for diapered or incontinent children <6 years of age for duration of illness.

[13]Until 7 days after onset of rash.

Table continued on following page

TABLE 105–25. Type and Duration of Isolation Precautions *(Continued)*

Infection/Condition	Precautions	
	Type[1]	Duration[2]
Hepatitis, viral		
Hepatitis A	S	
Diapered or incontinent	C	F[14]
Hepatitis B—HBsAg positive	S	
Hepatitis C and other unspecified non-A, non-B	S	
Hepatitis E	S	
Herpangina (*see* Enteroviral infections)		
Herpes simplex (*Herpesvirus hominis*)		
Encephalitis	S	
Mucocutaneous, disseminated or primary, severe	C	DI
Mucocutaneous, recurrent (skin, oral, genital)	S	
Neonatal[15] (*see* F[15] for perinatal exposure)	C	DI
Herpes zoster (varicella-zoster)		
Localized in immunocompromised patient, or disseminated	A, C	DI[16]
Localized in normal patient	S[16]	
Histoplasmosis	S	
Hookworm disease (ancylostomiasis, uncinariasis)	S	
Human immunodeficiency virus infection[5]	S	
Impetigo	C	U$^{24 \text{ hr}}$
Infectious mononucleosis	S	
Influenza	D[17]	DI
Kawasaki syndrome	S	
Lassa fever	C[11]	DI
Legionnaires' disease	S	
Leprosy	S	
Leptospirosis	S	
Lice (pediculosis)	C	U$^{24 \text{ hr}}$
Listeriosis	S	
Lyme disease	S	
Lymphocytic choriomeningitis	S	
Lymphogranuloma venereum	S	
Malaria	S[6]	
Marburg virus disease	C[11]	DI
Measles (rubeola), all presentations	A	DI
Melioidosis, all forms	S	
Meningitis		
Aseptic (nonbacterial or viral meningitis [*see* Enteroviral infections])	S	
Meningitis *(Continued)*		
Bacterial, gram-negative enteric, in neonates	S	
Other diagnosed bacterial	S	
Fungal	S	
Haemophilus influenzae, known or suspected	D	U$^{24 \text{ hr}}$
Listeria monocytogenes	S	
Neisseria meningitidis (meningococcal), known or suspected	D	U$^{24 \text{ hr}}$
Pneumococcal	S	
Tuberculosis[18]	S	
Meningococcal pneumonia	D	U$^{24 \text{ hr}}$
Meningococcemia (meningococcal sepsis)	D	U$^{24 \text{ hr}}$
Molluscum contagiosum	S	
Mucormycosis (*see* Zygomycosis)		
Multidrug-resistant organisms, infection or colonization[19]		
Gastrointestinal	C	CN
Respiratory	C	CN
Pneumococcal	S	
Skin, wound, or burn	C	CN
Mumps (infectious parotitis)	D	F[20]
Mycobacteria, nontuberculosis (atypical)		
Pulmonary	S	
Wound	S	
Mycoplasma pneumonia	D	DI
Necrotizing enterocolitis	S	
Nocardiosis, draining lesions or other presentations	S	
Norwalk agent gastroenteritis (*see* Gastroenteritis, viral)		
Orf	S	
Parainfluenza virus infection, respiratory, in infants and young children	C	DI
Parvovirus B19	D	F[21]
Pediculosis (lice)	C	U$^{24 \text{ hr}}$
Pertussis (whooping cough)	D	F[22]
Pinworm infection	S	
Plague		
Bubonic	S	
Pneumonic	D	U$^{72 \text{ hr}}$
Pleurodynia (*see* Enteroviral infections)		

[14]Maintain precautions in infants and children <3 years of age for duration of hospitalization; in children 3 to 14 years of age, until 2 weeks after onset of symptoms; and in others, until 1 week after onset of symptoms.

[15]For infants delivered vaginally or by cesarean procedure and if mother has active infection and membranes have been ruptured for more than 4 to 6 hours.

[16]Persons susceptible to varicella are also at risk of varicella when exposed to persons with herpes zoster lesions; therefore susceptible persons should not enter the room if other, immune caregivers are available.

[17]The "Guideline for Prevention of Nosocomial Pneumonia" recommends surveillance, vaccination, antiviral agents, and use of private rooms with negative air pressure as much as feasible for persons with suspected or diagnosed influenza. Many hospitals encounter logistical difficulties and physical plant limitations when admitting several persons with suspected influenza during community outbreaks. If sufficient private rooms are unavailable, consider cohorting patients; at the least, avoid room sharing with high-risk patients. *See:* Tablan OC, Anderson LG, Arden NH, et al: Guideline for prevention of nosocomial pneumonia. The Hospital Infection Control Practices Advisory Committee, Centers for Disease Control and Prevention. *Am J Infect Control* 1994;22:247–92. (Published errata appear in *Am J Infect Control* 1994;22:324 and 1994;22:351.)

[18]Patients should be examined for evidence of current (active) pulmonary tuberculosis. If evidence exists, additional precautions are necessary (*see* Tuberculosis).

[19]Resistant bacteria judged by the infection control program, on the basis of current state, regional, or national recommendations, to be of special clinical and epidemiologic significance.

[20]For 9 days after onset of swelling.

[21]Maintain precautions for duration of hospitalization when chronic disease occurs in an immunodeficient person. For persons with transient aplastic crisis or red-cell crisis, maintain precautions for 7 days.

[22]Maintain precautions until 5 days after effective therapy is begun.

TABLE 105–25. Type and Duration of Isolation Precautions *(Continued)*

Infection/Condition	Precautions Type[1]	Precautions Duration[2]
Pneumonia		
Adenovirus	D, C	DI
Bacterial not listed elsewhere (including gram-negative bacterial)	S	
Burkholderia cepacia in patients with cystic fibrosis, including respiratory tract colonization	S[23]	
Chylamydia	S	
Fungal	S	
H. influenzae		
Adults	S	
Infants and children (any age)	D	U[24 hr]
Legionella	S	
Meningococcal	D	U[24 hr]
Multidrug-resistant bacterial (*see* Multidrug-resistant organisms)	S	
Mycoplasma (primary atypical pneumonia)	D	DI
Pneumococcal	S	
Multidrug-resistant (*see* Multidrug-resistant organisms)		
Pneumocystis carinii	S[24]	
Pseudomonas cepacia (*see Burkholderia cepacia*, under Pneumonia)	S[23]	
Staphylococcus aureus	S	
Streptococcus, group A		
Adults	S	
Infants and young children	D	U[24 hr]
Viral		
Adults	S	
Infants and young children[5]	C	DI
Poliomyelitis	S	
Psittacosis (ornithosis)	S	
Q fever	S	
Rabies	S	
Rat-bite fever (*Streptobacillus moniliformis* disease, *Spirillum minus* disease)	S	
Relapsing fever	S	
Resistant bacterial infection or colonization (*see* Multidrug-resistant organisms)		
Respiratory infectious disease, acute (if not covered elsewhere)		
Adults	S	
Infants and young children[5]	C	DI
Respiratory syncytial virus infection in infants, young children, and immunocompromised adults	C	DI
Reye's syndrome	S	
Rheumatic fever	S	
Rickettsial fevers, tickborne (Rocky Mountain spotted fever, tickborne typhus fever)	S	
Rickettsialpox (vesicular rickettsiosis)	S	
Ringworm (dermatophytosis, dermatomycosis, tinea)	S	
Ritter's disease (staphylococcal scalded skin syndrome)	S	
Rocky Mountain spotted fever	S	
Roseola infantum (exanthema subitum)	S	
Rotavirus infection (*see* Gastroenteritis)		
Rubella (German measles: *see also* Congenital rubella)	D	F[13]
Salmonellosis (*see* Gastroenteritis)		
Scabies	C	U[24 hr]
Scalded skin syndrome, staphylococcal (Ritter's disease)	S	
Schistosomiasis (bilharziasis)	S	
Shigellosis (*see* Gastroenteritis)		
Spirillum minus disease (rat-bite fever)	S	
Sporotrichosis	S	
Staphylococcal disease (*S. aureus*)		
Skin, wound, or burn		
Major[3]	C	DI
Minor or limited[4]	S	
Enterocolitis	S[12]	
Multidrug-resistant (*see* Multidrug-resistant organisms)		
Pneumonia	S	
Scalded skin syndrome	S	
Toxic shock syndrome	S	
Streptobacillus moniliformis disease (rat-bite fever)	S	
Streptococcal disease (group A *Streptococcus*)		
Endometritis (puerperal sepsis)	S	
Pharyngitis in infants and young children	D	U[24 hr]
Pneumonia in infants and young children	D	U[24 hr]
Scarlet fever in infants and young children	D	U[24 hr]
Skin, wound or burn		
Major[3]	C	U[24 hr]
Minor or limited[4]	S	
Streptococcal disease (group B *Streptococcus*), neonatal	S	
Streptococcal disease (not group A or B) unless covered elsewhere	S	
Multidrug-resistant (*see* Multidrug-resistant organisms)		
Strongyloidiasis	S	
Syphilis		
Skin and mucous membrane, including congenital, primary, secondary	S	
Latent (tertiary) and seropositivity without lesions	S	
Tapeworm disease		
Hymenolepis nana	S	
Taenia solium (pork tapeworm)	S	
Other	S	
Tetanus	S	
Tinea (fungus infection, dermatophytosis, dermatomycosis, ringworm)	S	
Toxic shock syndrome (staphylococcal disease)	S	
Toxoplasmosis	S	
Trachoma, acute	S	
Trench mouth (Vincent's angina)	S	
Trichinosis	S	

[23]Avoid cohorting or placement in the same room with a person with cystic fibrosis who is not infected or colonized with *B. cepacia*. Persons with cystic fibrosis who visit or provide care and are not infected or colonized with *B. cepacia* may elect to wear a mask when within 3 feet of a colonized or infected patient.

[24]Avoid placement in the same room with an immunocompromised person.

Table continued on following page

TABLE 105–25. Type and Duration of Isolation Precautions *(Continued)*

Infection/Condition	Precautions Type[1]	Precautions Duration[2]
Trichomoniasis	S	
Trichuriasis (whipworm disease)	S	
Tuberculosis		
Extrapulmonary, draining lesion (including scorfula)	S	
Extrapulmonary, meningitis[18]	S	
Pulmonary (confirmed or suspected) or laryngeal disease	A	F[25]
Skin test positive with no evidence of current pulmonary disease	S	
Tularemia		
Draining lesion	S	
Pulmonary	S	
Typhoid (*Salmonella typhi*) fever (*see* Gastroenteritis)		
Typhus, endemic and epidemic	S	
Urinary tract infection (including pyelonephritis), with or without urinary catheter	S	
Varicella (chickenpox)	A, C	F[7]
Vibrio parahaemolyticus (*see* Gastroenteritis)		
Vincent's angina (trench mouth)	S	
Viral diseases		
Respiratory (if not covered elsewhere)		
Adults	S	
Infants and young children[5]	C	DI
Whooping cough (pertussis)	D	F[22]
Wound infections		
Major[3]	C	DI
Minor or limited[4]	S	
Yersinia enterocolitica gastroenteritis (*see* Gastroenteritis)		
Zygomycosis (phycomycosis, mucormycosis)	S	
Zoster (varcella-zoster)		
Localized in immunocompromised patient, disseminated	A, C	DI[16]
Localized in normal person	S[16]	

[25]Discontinue precautions *only* when the patient is receiving effective therapy, is improving clinically, and has three consecutive negative sputum smears collected on different days or tuberculosis ruled out. *See*: Centers for Disease Control and Prevention: Guidelines for preventing the transmission of tuberculosis in health-care facilities, 1994. *MMWR Morb Mortal Wkly Rep* 1994;43(RR-13):1–132.

Adapted from Garner JS, the Hospital Infection Control Practices Advisory Committee. Guideline for isolation precautions in hospitals. *Infect Control Hosp Epidemiol* 1996;17:73–80.

borne Pathogen, Hazard Communication, and Other OSHA Standards, relating to these and other federal standards; the publication is updated on a regular basis.

CATHETER CARE

The most important aspect of catheter care is prompt removal of the catheter when it is no longer needed for patient care. Aseptic technique is critical during placement of catheters. There is little information regarding optimal times for changing tubing used in ventriculostomies and for changing of collection bags. Collection bags should be maintained so that the system remains closed at all times. Aseptic technique is used to enter any drainage system. Drainage bags should always be dependent to avoid reflux of fluid into the patient.

ANTIBIOTICS

The use and abuse of antibiotics are important factors in infection control. Antibiotics are used to treat infection and to decrease infectivity in a patient, and antibiotic prophylaxis is effective in certain cases in preventing acquisition of new organisms and in decreasing the rate of infection by endogenous flora. Unfortunately, overuse or misuse of antibiotics facilitates the emergence of drug-resistant pathogens.

Antibiotic therapy alters endogenous flora. Antibiotic treatment may eradicate the causative agent, but the normal flora is also altered or eliminated. Normal flora is important in protecting a person from colonization by new bacteria. Thus persons who receive antibiotics are at risk of eradication of the normal flora and recolonization with more virulent or antibiotic-resistant flora. Different antibiotics have differing effects on normal flora. The expanded-spectrum cephalosporins are especially effective in eliminating flora because all are excreted into bile and act directly on aerobic and to a lesser extent on anaerobic flora. Thus, after a single dose of cefoxitin or ceftriaxone, there is a marked decrease in the usual aerobic gram-negative intestinal flora. This sets the scene for overgrowth of yeasts and gram-positive bacteria such as *Enterococcus* and *Staphylococcus.*

Prophylactic antibiotic therapy is useful in preventing perioperative infections (Chapter 16). Its value has been proved in so-called dirty operations, and it is of probable value in many so-called clean operations. The timing of administration of perioperative antibiotics is critical. The drugs should be given 30 minutes before skin incision to ensure appropriate tissue levels at the time of the surgical procedure, and doses should be repeated during the operation if the procedure is prolonged. There is little evidence that continuing antibiotic therapy after an operation is helpful, and there is some evidence that it is harmful because of the effect on flora. Similarly, perioperative therapy should not be given too early because it alters the flora before the operation. Continuation of perioperative antibiotics while chest tubes or drains are in place is not useful; this practice should be abandoned.

ENVIRONMENTAL ISSUES

In general, the role of the environment in transmission of infectious agents is overrated. Most hospital-acquired infections result from endogenous flora or from agents transmitted by the hands of health care providers or visitors. On occasion, airborne infections occur. There are standards for the number of air circulations required per hour in operating theaters, isolation rooms, and offices. Within offices and clinics, care should be taken to ensure that there are areas with separate airflow in which persons infected with measles or varicella can be safely examined.

Cover Gowns. Although a great deal of money and effort have gone into laundry, linens, and gowns, there is little evidence that laundry plays a role in the transmission of pathogens. Any pathogens present on laundry would have to be ingested or deposited onto mucous membranes to cause disease. Gowns have often been used to cover clothing, but there is no evidence that pathogens are transmitted from a visitor's or health care provider's clothes to a patient. In addition, it has been shown that the act of gowning does not increase the frequency of hand washing. Thus the use of cover gowns for admission to an intensive care unit has not been helpful in encouraging the use of sinks. Gowns should be available in all patient care areas as part of supplies sometimes needed for standard precautions and contact isolation.

Medical Equipment. Equipment that comes into contact with patients must be properly cleaned between uses. The type of decontamination needed varies depending on the use of the equipment. Stethoscopes should be disinfected with alcohol or soap and water between uses. Tape measures are usually disposable; if cloth or metal tapes are used, they should be wiped off between patients. Thermometers must be cleaned properly between uses. Electronic thermometers have single-use shields that are discarded after each use. Users of electronic thermometers should take care to avoid contaminating the box during use. If the box is contaminated with patients' secretions, it should be wiped off immediately to prevent transfer of the patient's secretions onto equipment from room to room. Similarly, precautions should be taken to prevent pulse oximetry equipment and machines used to obtain electrocardiograms, electroencephalograms, radiographs, and sonograms from becoming contaminated by a patient's secretions. Equipment should be inspected before and after use and should be wiped down whenever there is the possibility that the patient's secretions or those of the operator have contaminated the equipment. Soap and water are effective for wiping equipment. Bleach or alcohol should be used if blood is being removed. Equipment that enters a body cavity such as the mouth must be decontaminated to a high level of disinfection (Table 105–26). Equipment that enters body tissues or vessels must be sterile before use. Policies for disinfection and

TABLE 105–26. Disinfection and Sterilization

Agents

A. Ethyl or isopropyl alcohol (70–90%)
B. Ethyl alcohol (70–90%)
C. Formaldehyde (8%) and alcohol (70%) solution
D. Quaternary ammonium germicidal detergent solution (2% aqueous solution of concentrate)
E. Iodophor germicidal detergent (100 ppm available iodine)
F. Iodophor (500 ppm available iodine)
G. Phenolic germicidal detergent solution (1% aqueous solution of concentrate)
H. Phenolic solutions (3% aqueous solution of concentrate)
I. Sodium hypochlorite (100 ppm available chlorine)
J. Sodium hypochlorite (1000 ppm available chlorine); not recommended for metal instruments
K. Ethylene oxide gas (see manufacturer's recommendations for times)
L. Aqueous formaline (40% formaldehyde)
M. Glutaraldehyde (2% aqueous solution)
N. Wet pasteurization at 75°C (167°F) after detergent cleaning
O. Heat sterilization (see manufacturer's recommendations)

Disinfection: Appropriate for Articles that Come in Contact with Skin or Mucous Membranes but Do Not Enter Tissue or the Vascular System

Smooth, hard-surfaced objects that will not come in contact with skin or tissue can be disinfected with agent A, D, E, G, or I for ≥10 min

Smooth, hard-surfaced objects that will come in contact with skin or mucous membranes can be disinfected with agent A, C, F, H, J, L, M, or N for ≥30 min

Rubber tubing and catheters that will come in contact with skin or mucous membranes can be disinfected with agent F, H, M, or N for ≥30 min

Polyethylene tubing and catheters that will come in contact with skin or mucous membranes can be disinfected with agent A, F, H, M, N, or L for ≥30 min (polyethylene tubing must be completely filled for disinfection; thermostability should be investigated when indicated)

Lensed instruments that will come into contact with skin or mucous membranes can be disinfected with agent L or M for ≥30 min

Thermometers (oral and rectal) must be thoroughly wiped, preferably with soap and water before disinfection. Thermometers that will come in contact with skin or mucous membranes can be disinfected with agent B or M for ≥30 min

Sterilization: Appropriate for Articles that Will Enter Tissue or the Vascular System

Smooth, hard-surfaced objects can be sterilized with agent C for 18 hr, agent L for 12 hr, agent M for 10 hr, or agent K or P for times recommended by manufacturer

Rubber tubing and catheters can be sterilized with agent K or P for times recommended by manufacturer

Polyethylene tubing and catheters can be sterilized with agent C for 18 hr, agent L for 12 hr, agent M for 10 hr, or agent K or P for times recommended by manufacturer

Lensed instruments can be sterilized with agent K for time recommended by manufacturer or agent L or M for 12 hr

Thermometers must be thoroughly wiped, preferably with soap and water, before sterilization; thermometers can be sterilized with agent C for 18 hours, agent K for time recommended by manufacturer, agent L for 12 hr, or agent M for 10 hr

Hinged instruments can be sterilized with agent L for 12 hr, agent M for 10 hr, or agent K or P for times recommended by manufacturer

Modified from U.S. Department of Health, Education, and Welfare: *Isolation Techniques for Use in Hospitals,* 2nd ed. DHEW Publication No. (CDC) 78-8314. Atlanta, Centers for Disease Control, 1975.

TABLE 105–27. Personal Protective Equipment

Gloves: use whenever contact with blood or body fluids is anticipated
Gowns: use to protect clothing
Masks: use if splash or spray of blood or body fluids is anticipated
Eye protection: use if splash or spray of blood or body fluids is anticipated
Respirators: use during resuscitation

sterilization of equipment should be written and enforced in the hospital and in the office.

Medical Waste. Medical waste has attracted a great deal of attention. Although it is unpleasant to see waste on beaches or in public areas, there is relatively little danger of infection from these wastes. Waste must be ingested, injected, or applied to mucous membranes or nonintact skin to transmit disease. Nonetheless, it is appropriate to dispose of all waste properly, especially medical waste. Legislation has been passed to address the disposal of waste generated in health care settings and in most circumstances is based on public fear of infection rather than on risk of infection. Medical waste handling is important. Contaminated products should be discarded in such a way that people cannot be exposed to pathogenic wastes. Laboratory wastes that contain microorganisms are generally disinfected or sterilized before disposal. Sharp objects such as blades and needles are important causes of puncture wounds and lacerations. Used needles and blades must be discarded into puncture-resistant containers. The practice of recapping needles should be stopped. If it is essential to cap a used needle, this should be done by placing the needle on a flat surface and bringing the cover toward the needle. Products have been developed that incorporate needle guards in the design of the product. Needle-free systems should be used whenever possible. Gloves do not prevent needle-stick injuries. Gloves do, however, decrease the amount of blood or fluid that enters the finger and thus may decrease transmission of bloodborne pathogens.

Toys. Play is an important part of childhood and has an important role in recovery from disease. Toys and other play equipment should be available for inpatients, but toys can serve as fomites. If a toy goes from one infant's mouth to another's mouth, organisms will be transferred. Similarly, if a child has an upper respiratory tract infection, the offending virus is frequently on the child's hands. These hands transmit virus to toys, and from there the next set of hands acquires the virus. If those hands pick a nose or rub an eye, virus is effectively transmitted to a new host. Thus toys must be washed between uses by different children. Few studies document toys as transmitters of disease, and yet it is logical that they serve as vectors for infectious diseases. It may not be wise to have small toys in office waiting rooms. Fish tanks, blackboards, and movies entertain and are less likely to spread infectious agents.

EMPLOYEE HEALTH

The most common route of acquisition of infection by health care providers is by direct contact. Unwashed hands are the primary culprits in the spread of pathogens from patient to patient and from patient to health care provider. Other routes of infection include needle or blade injuries, splashes of body secretions onto mucous membranes, and ingestion of contaminated foods.

PREVENTION OF EMPLOYEE INFECTIONS

The most important means to prevent infection is the use of good hand-washing technique before and after every patient encounter (Table 105–22). Sinks must be readily available in all patient care areas. The type of soap is not nearly as important as the regular use of water. Rinsing the hands for 15 seconds is effective in washing off pathogens that have been acquired from a patient encounter. Hands should be washed even if gloves have been used. Breaks in the gloves are frequent and often go unnoticed.

Standard precautions are designed to protect the health care provider from contact with body fluids and must be used during every patient encounter (Tables 105–23 and 105–27). No special precautions are needed to talk with people, shake hands, or perform routine physical examinations. Gloves should be worn whenever it is anticipated that hands will be in contact with body fluids. Gowns, masks, and eye protection should be worn whenever the possibility of splashing or aerosolization is anticipated.

Proper use of standard precautions is essential. All health care providers must be aware of the risky and nonrisky situations involved in providing health care. Training must be given at the time of employment and must be regularly reinforced. The physician must serve as a role model, especially for the use of standard precautions and hand washing.

Employee Immunizations

Health care providers should receive the appropriate immunizations before beginning patient care (Table 105–28). All health care providers (i.e., medical or nonmedical, paid or volunteer, full-time or part-time, student or nonstudent, with or without patient-care responsibilities) who work in health care institutions (i.e., inpatient and outpatient, public and private) should be immune to measles,

TABLE 105–28. Immunizations for Employees

Vaccine	Personnel	Schedule
Diphtheria, tetanus (dT)	All employees	Every 10 yr
Measles-mumps-rubella (MMR)	All employees	Evidence of prior infection or two doses ≥1 mo apart
Poliomyelitis	Laboratory or health care providers likely to be exposed	Primary immunization if needed or complete series; consider booster
Hepatitis A virus	Laboratory or health care providers likely to be exposed	Two doses 6–12 mo apart (adults)
Hepatitis B virus	Employees exposed to blood	Series of three injections
Influenza	All employees	Annually
Varicella-zoster virus	Nonimmune employees	Two doses 4–8 wk apart

rubella, and varicella. Adults should receive diphtheria-tetanus combination vaccine every 10 years. All adults should have received two immunizing doses of measles-mumps-rubella vaccine unless they have had the diseases naturally or can show proof of antibody to these agents. Adults who have no history of varicella infection should be tested for the presence of antibody. If the person is susceptible to varicella, two immunizing doses of vaccine should be given. All employees whose tasks place them at risk of exposure to blood should be vaccinated against hepatitis B during training before potential contact with blood. Determination of an antibody response to hepatitis B vaccine in the health care provider is recommended to assist in the management of subsequent inadvertent percutaneous or permucosal contact with blood or body fluids (see Table 78–10). Yearly vaccination against influenza is recommended for all health care providers, primarily to prevent spread to susceptible patients, because the health care providers are likely to be exposed and are capable of transmitting the virus to patients.

Employee Health Care Services

Health care services should be readily available for employees. Health maintenance and health screening should be emphasized and provisions made for regular health care visits. Procedures and policies regarding on-the-job injuries, including needle-stick injuries, must be in place (Table 105–29). Employees should be aware of the policies and should be encouraged to report injuries. The type of injury dictates the appropriate response.

Bloodborne Pathogens

Injuries due to needles or sharp instruments and to splash exposures often cause immediate anxiety and unnecessary panic. The following questions must be asked: Did an injury occur, for example, was the skin punctured or did material splash onto a mucous membrane? What type of body fluid was involved? Did the patient have an infection? Is the employee immune to that infection?

In some cases the source of the needle is unknown. This is especially true of needle-stick injuries that occur outside a hospital. In these cases the decision to initiate testing and prophylaxis must be based on the likelihood that the needle contains an infectious agent. For example, if a person is stuck by a needle on the sidewalk in front of a drug house, it should be considered likely that HBV is contaminating the needle. It is much less likely that HIV would survive in a needle left out on a sidewalk. Thus prophylaxis against hepatitis B (Table 105–29) and counseling regarding HIV transmission would be appropriate. If a person is stuck with an unused needle or a needle that has been used to add an agent to intravenous fluid, no prophylaxis is needed.

Hepatitis B. The risk of acquiring hepatitis B after percutaneous exposure to blood from a person with HBsAg positivity varies

TABLE 105–29. Needle-Stick Injury

Report Injury to Personnel Health Service or Designee
Complete appropriate forms to document injury and circumstances

Determine Source Patient
If this is not possible, base actions on likelihood of exposure, considering source of needle and type of exposure
Obtain permission and determine serologic status of source of hepatitis B virus (HBV), hepatitis C virus (HCV), and human immunodeficiency virus (HIV)

Determine Serologic Status of Injured Person (Employee)
Determine Vaccination History for HBV
If response is unknown, test for anti-HBsAg
Obtain Permission and Test for Antibody to HCV and HIV

Give Postexposure Prophylaxis for HBV After Percutaneous or Permucosal Exposure
Unvaccinated Exposed Person
Source HBsAg-positive: one dose (0.06 mL/kg; max 5 mL) of HBIG intramuscularly and initiate HBV vaccine series
Source HBsAg-negative: initiate HBV vaccine series
Source not tested or unknown: initiate HBV vaccine series
Previously Vaccinated and Known Responder
Source HBsAg-positive: test exposed person for anti-HBsAg; if adequate (at least 10 mIU/mL), no treatment other than educational counseling; if inadequate, HBV vaccine booster dose
Source HBsAg-negative: no treatment other than educational counseling
Source not tested or unknown: no treatment other than educational counseling
Previously Vaccinated and Known Nonresponder
Source HBsAg-positive: HBIG immediately and repeat in 1 mo, or HBIG immediately plus a booster dose of HBV vaccine
Source HBsAg-negative: no treatment other than educational counseling
Source not tested or unknown: if high-risk source, consider treatment as for HBsAg-positive source

Give Postexposure Prophylaxis for HBV After Percutaneous or Permucosal Exposure *(Continued)*
Previously Vaccinated and Response Unknown
Source HBsAg-positive: test exposed for anti-HBsAg; if adequate (at least 10 mIU/mL), no treatment other than educational counseling; if inadequate, one dose (0.06 mL/kg; max 5 mL) of HBIG and a booster dose of HBV vaccine

Postexposure Management for Hepatitis C
Provide educational counseling regarding risks of infection, symptoms, and methods of transmission of the virus
Inform person that currently there is no effective postexposure prophylaxis
Retest patient at 6 mo; some experts recommend PCR testing for HCV at 6 wk, 3 mo, and 6 mo

Postexposure Prophylaxis for HIV After Percutaneous or Permucosal Exposure
Provide educational counseling regarding risks of infection, symptoms of early infection, and methods of transmission of the virus (see Table 105–30)
Provide clinical and serologic evaluation for evidence of HIV infection as soon as possible after exposure; if health care worker is seronegative, retesting should be done 6 wk, 3 mo, and 6 mo after exposure; some experts recommend screening 12 mo after exposure
Inform and educate health care worker regarding any possible effective chemoprophylaxis; if prophylaxis is appropriate, provide it as soon as possible after exposure; current protocols for postexposure therapy are available at the CDC website (see Table 105–31)

Counseling and Education
Information should include but not be limited to the risk of exposure, safe handling of sharp instruments, safe disposal of sharp instruments, immunizations, standard precautions, and safe work practices

from 5% to 43%. The risk is highest if the source patient is positive for e antigen. The immune status of the injured person is also important. Prior vaccination will protect the person. The need for postexposure prophylaxis is determined by the immune status of the injured person and the source of the blood (Table 105–29).

Hepatitis C. The risk of acquiring hepatitis C virus after needle-stick injury is less well established, but rates are estimated to be 3–10% after percutaneous exposure to blood of a patient with antibody to HCV. There is no role for postexposure prophylaxis with immune globulin because donors with antibody to HCV are eliminated from the donor pool. Furthermore, studies of immune globulin performed before HCV screening showed no protection. Use of antiviral agents for HCV has limited efficacy for treatment; data regarding the use of antivirals for prophylaxis are limited. The injured person should be counseled and tested for antibody at baseline and again at 6 months. Some experts recommend PCR testing for HCV at 6 weeks, 3 months, and 6 months. Employees with a positive PCR test result or seroconversion should be referred to a hepatologist for possible IFN-α therapy.

Human Immunodeficiency Virus. Several factors should be considered in the determination of whether to initiate postexposure chemoprophylaxis after a needle-stick injury from a patient infected with HIV (Table 105–30). These factors include the HIV status of the injured person; the availability of serologic testing to determine or confirm HIV status in a timely manner; the type of exposure and the type and volume of body fluids involved; the rapidity with which postexposure prophylaxis can be started; the availability of counseling about, and the need for informed consent for, unproved therapies with drugs that may have potential adverse effects; the possible risk of transmission to sexual partners; and the potential teratogenicity of antiviral agents. The overall risk of transmission of HIV after percutaneous exposure to blood or body fluids from a patient infected with HIV is approximately 0.3% per injury. The risk of transmission is higher when the injury involves exposure to a larger volume of virus (Table 105–30), as when a hollow-bore needle of large caliber is used or when blood is actually injected. The viral titer in the source patient is also a risk factor; viral titers are highest during the acute seroconversion phase and in persons with end-stage HIV disease. Children with perinatally acquired HIV often have high viral loads.

Chemoprophylaxis is recommended for health care providers with an exposure to HIV-contaminated blood, in conjunction with counseling about the risk of infection, the potential benefits and risks of prophylaxis, and the need for retesting. The choice of drugs depends on the type of exposure (Table 105–31).

TABLE 105–30. Risk Factors for HIV Transmission Associated with Needle-Stick Injury

Risk Factor	Adjusted Odds Ratio	95% Confidence Interval
Deep puncture or wound	16.1	6.1–44.6
Visible blood on device	5.2	1.8–17.7
Procedure involving needle placed directly in vein or artery	5.1	1.9–14.8
Terminal illness in source patient	6.4	2.2–18.9
Postexposure use of zidovudine	0.2	0.1–0.6

From Centers for Disease Control and Prevention: Case-control study of HIV seroconversion in health-care workers after percutaneous exposure to HIV-infected blood—France, United Kingdom, and United States, January 1988–August 1994. *MMWR Morb Mortal Wkly Rep* 1995;44:929–33.

The need for prophylaxis depends on the type and degree of exposure (Table 105–31). If the source person's HIV infection status is unknown at the time of exposure, the decision to use prophylaxis should be made on a case-by-case basis after consideration is given to the type of exposure and the clinical or epidemiologic likelihood of HIV infection in the source (Table 105–31). If there is a possibility of HIV transmission and HIV testing of the source person is pending, initiating a basic prophylaxis regimen is reasonable until laboratory results have been obtained, with discontinuation of prophylaxis if the source person is determined to be HIV-negative.

Two regimens for postexposure prophylaxis are recommended: (1) a **basic two-drug regimen** of nucleoside analogues that should be appropriate for most HIV exposures and (2) an **expanded three-drug regimen** that should be used for exposures that pose an increased risk for transmission (Table 105–32). Prophylaxis should be implemented in consultation with persons who have expertise in antiretroviral treatment and HIV transmission whenever this is possible. Health care facilities should have drugs for an initial prophylaxis regimen selected and available for use. Confidentiality following occupational exposure should be ensured.

Prophylaxis should be initiated as soon as possible. The maximum interval from exposure to initiation of prophylaxis during which optimal efficacy can be achieved is not known, but prophylaxis is probably substantially less effective when started more than 24–36 hours after exposure. Initiating therapy after a period as long as a week, however, might be considered for exposures that represent an increased risk for transmission. The optimal duration to continue prophylaxis is unknown, but it should be administered for 4 weeks if tolerated. Reevaluation of the exposed person should be considered within 72 hours after exposure, especially as additional information about the exposure or source person becomes available.

The evaluation is similar if the exposed person is pregnant, but the decision to use any antiretroviral drug during pregnancy requires discussion between the woman and her health care provider regarding the potential benefits and risks to her and her fetus. Certain drugs should be avoided in pregnant women. Efavirenz is teratogenic in primates, and the combination of stavudine and lamivudine has been associated with fatal lactic acidosis in pregnant women. Because of the risk of hyperbilirubinemia in newborns, indinavir should not be administered to pregnant women shortly before delivery.

All persons with occupational exposure to HIV should receive follow-up counseling, postexposure testing, and medical evaluation, regardless of whether prophylaxis was administered. HIV-antibody testing with EIA should be performed for at least 6 months after exposure (e.g., at 6 weeks, 12 weeks, and 6 months). Direct virus assays for routine follow-up are not recommended. Extended HIV follow-up is recommended for health care providers who become infected with HCV following exposure to a source coinfected with HIV and HCV. HIV testing should be performed on any exposed person who has an illness compatible with acute retroviral syndrome. If HIV infection is identified, the person should be referred to a specialist in HIV treatment and counseling.

Other Infectious Agents

Employees are often exposed to infectious agents while caring for patients. Hand washing is the most important infection control practice. The use of standard precautions and protective equipment is essential. Some exposures cannot be avoided. An employee who is not immune to varicella should not care for a child with active varicella. If the employee is exposed in the hospital or outside the

TABLE 105–31. Recommendations for HIV Postexposure Prophylaxis After Occupational Exposure

	Infection Status of Source				
Exposure Type	**HIV-Positive Class 1**[1]	**HIV-Positive Class 2**[1]	**Source of Unknown HIV Status**[2]	**Unknown Source**[3]	**HIV-Negative**
Percutaneous Injuries					
Less severe[4]	Recommend basic 2-drug prophylaxis	Recommend expanded 3-drug prophylaxis	Generally, no prophylaxis warranted; however, consider basic 2-drug prophylaxis[5] for source with HIV risk factors[6]	Generally, no prophylaxis warranted; however, consider basic 2-drug prophylaxis[5] in settings where exposure to HIV-infected persons is likely	No prophylaxis warranted
More severe[7]	Recommend expanded 3-drug prophylaxis	Recommend expanded 3-drug prophylaxis	Generally, no prophylaxis warranted; however, consider basic 2-drug prophylaxis[5] for source with HIV risk factors[6]	Generally, no prophylaxis warranted; however, consider basic 2-drug prophylaxis[5] in settings where exposure to HIV-infected persons is likely	No prophylaxis warranted
Mucous Membrane and Nonintant Skin Exposures[8]					
Small volume[9]	Consider basic 2-drug prophylaxis[5]	Recommend basic 2-drug prophylaxis	Generally, no prophylaxis warranted; however, consider basic 2-drug prophylaxis[5] for source with HIV risk factors[6]	Generally, no prophylaxis warranted; however, consider basic 2-drug prophylaxis[5] in settings where exposure to HIV-infected persons is likely	No prophylaxis warranted
Large volume[10]	Recommend basic 2-drug prophylaxis	Recommend expanded 3-drug prophylaxis	Generally, no prophylaxis warranted; however, consider basic 2-drug prophylaxis[5] for source with HIV risk factors[6]	Generally, no prophylaxis warranted; however, consider basic 2-drug prophylaxis[5] in settings where exposure to HIV-infected persons is likely	No prophylaxis warranted

[1]HIV-positive, class 1: asymptomatic HIV infection or known low viral load (e.g., <1,500 RNA copies/mL); HIV-positive, class 2: symptomatic HIV infection, AIDS, acute seroconversion, or known high viral load. If drug resistance is a concern, obtain expert consultation. Initiation of postexposure prophylaxis should not be delayed pending expert consultation, and because expert consultation alone cannot substitute for face-to-face counseling, resources should be available to provide immediate evaluation and follow-up care for all exposures.
[2]Source of unknown HIV status (e.g., deceased source person with no samples available for HIV testing).
[3]Unknown source (e.g., a needle from a sharps disposal container; splash from inappropriately disposed of blood).
[4]Less severe (e.g., solid needle and superficial injury).
[5]The designation "consider prophylaxis" indicates that prophylaxis is optional and should be based on an individualized decision between the exposed person and the treating clinician.
[6]If prophylaxis is offered and taken and the source is later determined to be HIV-negative, prophylaxis should be discontinued.
[7]More severe (e.g., large-bore hollow needle, deep puncture, visible blood on device, or needle used in patient's artery or vein).
[8]For skin exposures, follow-up is indicated only if there is evidence of compromised skin integrity (e.g., dermatitis, abrasion, or open wound).
[9]Small volume (i.e., a few drops).
[10]Large volume (i.e., major blood splash).
From Centers for Disease Control and Prevention: Updated U.S. Public Health Service guidelines for the management of occupational exposures to HBV, HCV, and HIV and recommendations for postexposure prophylaxis. *MMWR Morb Mortal Wkly Rep* 2001;50(RR11):1–42.

hospital, consideration should be given to removing the employee from patient care responsibilities from day 10 until day 21 after exposure. Ideally all employees should be immune to varicella, as well as rubella and measles. If an employee is not immune and is exposed to rubella or measles, the employee should be released from patient care activities for 5–21 days after exposure.

Tuberculosis in children is rarely contagious. Thus it is unusual for an employee to be exposed to *M. tuberculosis* in a pediatric hospital. Infected adult visitors are a concern if their disease is contagious (e.g., if they are coughing). Infected hospital staff are a risk to patients and visitors if their disease is contagious (e.g., if an employee has cavitary lung disease). All hospital staff should be screened for tuberculosis at the time of employment; the frequency of repeated skin testing should be based on the incidence of infectious tuberculosis in the hospital and in the geographic area. Screening is done by Mantoux testing. If the skin test is positive, the employee is evaluated for the presence of tuberculosis. A chest radiograph is done to determine whether the disease is contagious. The decision to begin preventive therapy is based on the size of the reaction and the age of the employee. Repeated

TABLE 105–32. Basic and Expanded HIV Postexposure Prophylaxis Regimens*

Basic Regimen
Zidovudine *and* lamivudine†
Alternative basic regimens
Lamivudine *and* stavudine
Didanosine *and* stavudine

Expanded Regimen
Basic regimen *plus* one of the following:
Indinavir *or* nelfinavir *or* efavirenz *or* abacavir

Antiretroviral Agents for Use as Postexposure Prophylaxis Only with Expert Consultation
Ritonavir
Saquinavir
Amprenavir
Delavirdine
Lopinavir-Ritonavir

Antiretroviral Agent Generally Not Recommended for Use as Postexposure Prophylaxis
Nevirapine

*See Table 38–13 for adverse effects, drug-drug interactions, and instructions for administration.
†Zidovudine *and* lamivudine are available in a single formulation as Combivir.
From Centers for Disease Control and Prevention: Updated U.S. Public Health Service guidelines for the management of occupational exposures to HBV, HCV, and HIV and recommendations for postexposure prophylaxis. *MMWR Morb Mortal Wkly Rep* 2001;50(RR11):1–42.

Suggested Dosages for Adults with Normal Renal Function

ANTIVIRAL	DOSAGE
Abacavir	300 mg twice daily PO
Didanosine	400 mg once daily PO (125 mg twice daily PO if body weight is <60 kg)
Efavirenz	600 mg once daily PO at bedtime
Indinavir	800 mg q8hr PO
Lamivudine	150 mg bid PO
Nelfinavir	750 mg tid PO or 1250 mg bid PO
Stavudine	40 mg bid PO (30 mg bid PO if body weight is <60 kg)
Zidovudine	600 mg/day divided bid or tid PO

testing is done to detect recent skin test conversion. Prophylaxis is recommended for all people with recent conversion because the risk of tuberculosis is greatest in the first few years after infection. The benefit of prophylaxis for a person of any age whose skin test result has recently converted exceeds the possible adverse effects of isoniazid (Chapter 35).

Infected Employees

Employees with infections pose a risk to patients. An employee with a viral respiratory infection must be careful to use and dispose of tissues properly and must be meticulous about hand washing. Employees with conjunctivitis pose a risk to children and to their fellow employees. Consideration should be given to restricting patient care activities of providers with viral conjunctivitis. Food handlers with colitis or hepatitis A should also be excluded until their disease is deemed noncontagious.

There is no evidence that HIV is spread from person to person by casual contact. A health care provider with HIV infection should use common sense and should be meticulous in avoiding injuries by needle sticks or by sharp objects. A provider with HIV infection should consult his or her own physician regarding protection from infectious agents encountered on the job. Screening of health care providers for antibody to HIV is not recommended. Each hospital should develop policies regarding activities of employees with HIV infections and the care of patients with the infection.

Education

Education regarding infection control begins during orientation and continues throughout employment. In-service training should include information regarding hand washing, exposure control plans, standard precautions, safe handling of sharp instruments, appropriate use of protective equipment, the rationale for and use of isolation, and immunizations for employees. Educational sessions should be presented at least once a year. Attendance should be mandatory. Peer review of hand washing and other infection control practices is an underused tool. The use of signs as reminders can be helpful; however, signs must not infringe on patient confidentiality.

REVIEWS

Abrutyn E (editor): *Saunders Infection Control Reference Service,* 2nd ed. Philadelphia, WB Saunders, 2001.

American Academy of Pediatrics: *Materials to Assist the Pediatric Office in Implementing the Bloodborne Pathogen, Hazard Communication, and Other OSHA Standards,* 2nd ed. Elk Grove Village, Ill., American Academy of Pediatrics, 1994.

Bennett JV, Brachman PS (editors): *Hospital Infections,* 4th ed. Boston, Little, Brown, 1998.

Ford-Jones EL, Mindorff CM, Langley JM, et al: Epidemiologic study of 4684 hospital-acquired infections in pediatric patients. *Pediatr Infect Dis J* 1989;8:668–75.

Gaynes RP, Edwards JR, Jarvis WR, et al: Nosocomial infections among neonates in high-risk nurseries in the United States. National Nosocomial Infections Surveillance System. *Pediatrics* 1996;98:357–61.

Goodman RA, Solomon SL: Transmission of infectious diseases in outpatient health care settings. *JAMA* 1991;265:2377–81.

Herwaldt LA (editor): *The Society for Healthcare Epidemiology of America: A Practical Handbook for Hospital Epidemiologists.* Thorofare, NJ, Slack Inc, 1998.

Richards MJ, Edwards JR, Culver DH, et al: Nosocomial infections in pediatric intensive care units in the United States. National Nosocomial Infections Surveillance System. *Pediatrics* 1999;103:e39.

Sepkowitz KA: Occupationally acquired infections in health care workers. Part I. *Ann Intern Med* 1996a;125:826–34.

Sepkowitz KA: Occupationally acquired infections in health care workers. Part II. *Ann Intern Med* 1996b;125:917–28.

KEY ARTICLES

American Academy of Pediatrics Committee on Infectious Diseases and Committee on Practice and Ambulatory Medicine: Infection control in physicians' offices. *Pediatrics* 2000;105:1361–9.

American Thoracic Society/CDC Statement Committee on Latent Tuberculosis Infection: Targeted tuberculin testing and treatment of latent tuberculosis infection. *MMWR Morb Mortal Wkly Rep* 2000;49(RR-6):1–51.

Archibald LK, Manning ML, Bell LM, et al: Patient density, nurse-to-patient ratio and nosocomial infection risk in a pediatric cardiac intensive care unit. *Pediatr Infect Dis J* 1997;16:1045–8.

Avila-Aguero ML, Umana MA, Jimenez AL, et al: Handwashing practices in a tertiary-care, pediatric hospital and the effect on an educational program. *Clin Perform Qual Health Care* 1998;6:70–2.

Bernard L, Kereveur A, Durand D, et al: Bacterial contamination of hospital physicians' stethoscopes. *Infect Control Hosp Epidemiol* 1999;20:626–8.

Bolyard EA, Tablan OC, Williams WW, et al: Guideline for infection control in healthcare personnel, 1998. Hospital Infection Control Practices Advisory Committee. *Infect Control Hosp Epidemiol* 1998;19: 407–63.

Centers for Disease Control and Prevention: Guidelines for preventing the transmission of tuberculosis in health-care facilities, 1994. *MMWR Morb Mortal Wkly Rep* 1994;43(RR-13):1–132.

Centers for Disease Control and Prevention: Guidelines for prevention of nosocomial pneumonia. *MMWR Morb Mortal Wkly Rep* 1997; 46(RR-1):1–79.

Centers for Disease Control and Prevention: Updated U.S. Public Health Service guidelines for the management of occupational exposures to HBV, HCV, and HIV and recommendations for postexposure prophylaxis. *MMWR Morb Mortal Wkly Rep* 2001;50(RR-11):1–42.

Champsaur H, Questiau E, Prevot J, et al: Rotavirus carriage, asymptomatic infection, and disease in the first two years of life. I. Virus shedding. *J Infect Dis* 1984;149:667–74.

Classen DC, Evans RS, Pestotnik SL, et al: The timing of prophylactic administration of antibiotics and the risk of surgical-wound infection. *N Engl J Med* 1992;326:281–6.

Davies MW, Mehrs S, Garland ST, et al: Bacterial colonization of toys in neonatal intensive care cots. *Pediatrics* 2000;106:E18.

Friedman C, Barnette M, Buck AS, et al: Requirements for infrastructure and essential activities of infection control and epidemiology in out-of-hospital settings: A consensus panel report. Association for Professionals in Infection Control and Epidemiology and Society for Healthcare Epidemiology of America. *Infect Control Hosp Epidemiol* 1999;20: 695–705.

Gala CL, Hall CB, Schnabel KC, et al: The use of eye-nose goggles to control nosocomial respiratory syncytial virus infection. *JAMA* 1986; 256:2706–8.

Garner JS: Guideline for isolation precautions in hospitals. The Hospital Infection Control Practices Advisory Committee. *Infect Control Hosp Epidemiol* 1996;17:53–80.

George DL, Falk PS, Umberto Meduri G, et al: Nosocomial sinusitis inpatients in the medical intensive care unit: A prospective epidemiological study. Clin Infect Dis 1998;27:463–70.

Hall CB, Douglas RG Jr: Modes of transmission of respiratory syncytial virus. *J Pediatr* 1981;99:100–3.

Herwaldt LA, Smith SD, Carter CD: Infection control in the outpatient setting. *Infect Control Hosp Epidemiol* 1998;19:41–74.

Hutto C, Little EA, Ricks R, et al: Isolation of cytomegalovirus from toys and hands in a day care center. *J Infect Dis* 1986;154:527–30.

Larson EL: APIC guideline for handwashing and hand antisepsis in health care settings. *Am J Infect Control* 1995;23:251–69.

Mangram AJ, Horan TC, Pearson ML, et al: Guideline for prevention of surgical site infection, 1999. Hospital Infection Control Practices Advisory Committee. *Infect Control Hosp Epidemiol* 1999;20:250–78.

Pfaller MA, Herwaldt LA: The clinical microbiology laboratory and infection control: Emerging pathogens, antimicrobial resistance, and new technology. *Clin Infect Dis* 1997;25:858–70.

Rutala WA: Disinfection and sterilization of patient-care items. *Infect Control Hosp Epidemiol* 1996;17:377–84.

Scheckler WE, Brimhall D, Bucks AS, et al: Requirements for infrastructure and essential activities of infection control and epidemiology in hospitals: A consensus panel report. Society for Healthcare Epidemiology of America. *Infect Control Hosp Epidemiol* 1998;19:114–24.

Schreiber GB, Busch MP, Kleinman SA, et al: The risk of transfusion-transmitted viral infections. The Retrovirus Epidemiology Donor Study. *N Engl J Med* 1996;334:1685–90.

Tablan OC, Anderson LG, Arden NH, et al: Guideline for prevention of nosocomial pneumonia. The Hospital Infection Control Practices Advisory Committee, Centers for Disease Control and Prevention. *Am J Infect Control* 1994;22:247–92. (Published errata appear in *Am J Infect Control* 1994;22:324 and 1994;22:351.)

Widmer AF: Replace hand washing with use of a waterless alcohol hand rub? *Clin Infect Dis* 2000;31:136–43.

CHAPTER 106

Infections Involving Intravascular Devices

Margaret C. Fisher

Intravascular devices are often required for patient care. Vascular catheters are inserted in most inpatients and are also used in many outpatients. The use of **central catheters** for long-term access to the bloodstream has been an important advance for the care of persons who require parenteral nutrition, chemotherapy, or long-term parenteral antibiotic therapy. The major complication of catheters is infection.

A **catheter-related bloodstream infection** implies isolation of the same organism from a semiquantitative or quantitative culture of a sample from a catheter segment and from blood of a patient with clinical symptoms of bacteremia and no other apparent source of infection. An **infusate-related bloodstream infection** implies isolation of the same organism from infusate and from separate percutaneous blood cultures with no other identifiable source of infection. **Exit-site infection** is inflammation or drainage of purulent fluid from the catheter's entry site through the skin. **Pocket infection** is inflammation of skin around a totally implanted device or purulent exudate in the subcutaneous pocket surrounding the device. **Tunnel infection** is inflammation in the tissues overlying the catheter's subcutaneous route.

Types of Intravascular Catheters. Short peripheral catheters are used for short-term access in physiologically stable patients. Percutaneously placed plastic (Teflon) central venous catheters inserted into a central vein, such as the jugular or subclavian vein, and threaded into the superior vena cava are by far the most commonly used central venous access devices for short-term situations. For persons requiring prolonged central venous access such as for chemotherapy or total parenteral nutrition, cuffed, tunneled silicone elastomer catheters (e.g., Broviac or Hickman catheters) have become indispensable. These catheters are inserted into a central vein and passed through a subcutaneous tunnel before exiting the skin, usually medially to the nipple. Totally implanted venous access systems (e.g., Port-a-Cath, Infuse-a-Port) consisting of a silicone elastomer catheter tunneled beneath the skin to a subcutaneous pocket, in which a reservoir is implanted, can also be used. The resultant system is totally intracorporeal, and infusions are administered by percutaneous injection of the reservoir.

ETIOLOGY

Many classes of microorganisms cause catheter-related infections (Table 106–1). The most common organisms causing bloodstream infections are *Staphylococcus aureus,* coagulase-negative staphylococci, *Candida,* and *Enterococcus* (Table 106–2). Other skin flora are sometimes involved, including diphtheroids and *Bacillus.* Oral streptococci enter the bloodstream during chewing and during brushing of the teeth, and they may become trapped in thrombosed areas around catheters or on the intravascular fibrin sheath. Gram-negative bacilli such as *Escherichia coli, Klebsiella,* and *Pseudomonas* were relatively common causes of such infections in the past but are less common currently. Fungi such as *Candida albicans* are most common in persons who are receiving broad-spectrum antibiotics or parenteral nutrition. *Malassezia furfur* is an unusual but important pathogen associated with infusion of intravenous fat emulsions as part of parenteral nutrition. Atypical mycobacteria are occasionally involved in catheter-related infections.

The density and type of. bacteria on the skin vary in different anatomic areas. In adults the beard area is heavily colonized, whereas in children this area is less heavily colonized. Although resident flora on the neck may be less, oral secretions contaminate the area, especially in drooling or obtunded patients. Organisms colonizing the femoral area include gram-negative bacilli and yeast, in addition to the usual gram-positive skin organisms. Climate and room temperature may influence infection rates. If the hospitalized patient or home care patient is sweating, there is a greater chance of contaminating the entrance site and dressings.

EPIDEMIOLOGY

Catheter-related infections increase morbidity and mortality and health care costs. The incidence of catheter-related infection varies according to patient risk factors, type and location of the catheter (Table 106–3), site of catheterization, duration of catheterization, amount of use of the catheter, skill and aseptic technique during initial insertion, and care of the catheter. The rates of bloodstream infection due to peripheral venous catheters are 0–2/1,000 catheter-days and for central catheters from <2–30/1,000 catheter-days. Infection rates are higher in persons who require intensive care and when patient care units are overcrowded or understaffed. Infec-

TABLE 106–1. Percentage of Catheter-Related Infections Caused by Various Classes of Microorganisms

Classification of Pathogen	Septic Infection: Bacteremia and Sepsis (%)*	Local Infection: Tunnel and Exit Site (%)*
Gram-positive cocci	71	52
Gram-negative bacilli	20	40
Fungi	6	2
Candida albicans, other *Candida*		
Malassezia furfur		
Miscellaneous uncommon bacterial species	3	6
Bacillus species, *Neisseria meningitidis, Micrococcus,* others		

*Percentage of total infections for type of infection (septic or local).

TABLE 106–2. Organisms Causing Catheter-Related Infection

Common Isolates
Coagulase-negative staphylococci
Staphylococcus aureus
Enterococcus
Candida albicans
Occasional Isolates
Escherichia coli
Klebsiella
Pseudomonas aeruginosa
Malassezia furfur
Candida parapsilosis
Candida glabrata
Candida tropicalis
Acinetobacter
Enterobacter
Nontuberculous *Mycobacterium*

tion rates are lower for tunneled and implanted catheters. In most series, bacteremia was more common when catheters were placed in the femoral area than in the subclavian area. The number of lumens is also important. A higher number of lumens increase opportunities for contamination of the system. In most studies, there is a higher infection rate in multilumen catheters than in single-lumen catheters.

Outbreaks of catheter-related infection have occurred because of contamination of infused fluids, medications, and in-line attachment devices. In some cases, substances to be infused, such as flush solutions or medications, were drawn into syringes in advance and became contaminated before use. In some needleless systems, a locking or connecting device is used to attach the intravenous tubing to the catheter hub. Contamination of the locking device with nonsterile water can lead to contamination of the hub or intravenous fluids.

Persons receiving home parenteral therapy are possibly at greater risk of infection. Home care providers and parents must follow the same precautions as for hospitalized patients.

Infection is more common in younger and sicker children and in immunocompromised persons. Premature infants, burn victims, and persons with underlying skin disorders have the highest risk of catheter-related infection because all lack normal skin as a barrier to invasion by microorganisms. Neutropenia is an independent risk factor for catheter-related infection. Catheters inserted in emergency settings are more likely to be infected than those placed electively.

TABLE 106–3. Bloodstream Infection Rates for Intravascular Devices

Device	Bloodstream Infection Rates (per 1,000 Catheter Days)
Peripheral catheter	0–1
Percutaneously inserted central catheter	0–1
Jugular catheter	2.4
Subclavian catheter	4.6
Femoral catheter	10.2
Tunneled catheter	0–3
Subcutaneous implanted port	0.96–1.5
Umbilical arterial catheter	5–30
Arterial catheter	0–1

TABLE 106–4. Distribution of Specific Type of Catheter-Related Infection (Broviac and Hickman Catheters)

Type of Infection	Overall Proportion of Infections (%)	Proportion of Infections with Bacteremia (%)
Exit-site infection	46	20
Tunnel infection	20	50
Septic thrombophlebitis	4	100
Septic infection (septicemia)	31	100

Catheters used for hemodialysis have a higher rate of infection. Contamination of these catheters occurs during dialysis as a result of manipulation of the catheters, inadequate disinfection of dialyzers, leaks in dialyzer membranes, and contamination of dialysate.

PATHOGENESIS

Pathogens enter catheters and the bloodstream by two major routes: (1) entry at the skin site, either during insertion of the catheter or during manipulation of the catheter during use, dressing change, and everyday activity, and (2) entry via infused fluids. Organisms gain access to infused fluids at the time the fluids are prepared and when the tubing is entered. Contamination of the hub of the catheter or the hub of the intravenous tubing is common and is considered to be a major predisposition to infection. Implanted catheters or ports decrease but do not eliminate the opportunity for microbial entry at the skin site.

The most frequent clinical problems are **bacteremic infection** and **septic infection,** which are infections related to the central venous line itself that are complicated by bacteremia or occasionally by sepsis. Other types of infections include **exit-site infection,** or local infection of the tissue at the point where the catheter exits the skin, and **tunnel infection,** or local infection of the subcutaneous tract that extends proximally from the skin exit site to the site of central vein entry (Table 106–4).

Catheter-related thrombosis and catheter-related infection can develop separately or together. **Thrombophlebitis** consists of inflammation and thrombosis, and if it is associated with infection, known as **septic thrombophlebitis,** colonies of organisms may be embedded in the clot. Invasion of the intima of the vessel wall leads to extravascular spread of the infection. Seeding of organs or distal sites from emboli can occur. Infection of the heart valves or the endomyocardium results in the typical findings of infective endocarditis (Chapter 71).

Scanning electron microscopic views of infected catheter tips reveal a complex matrix of fibrin, organisms, and products of the organism. Certain organisms such as coagulase-negative staphylococci produce a loose polysaccharide capsule, or **slime layer,** that interferes with opsonophagocytosis. The complex matrix about the organisms creates a microenvironment beneficial to the organism. The pH and biophysical characteristics of this microenvironment are thought to protect the microbes from antibiotics and host defenses.

SYMPTOMS AND CLINICAL MANIFESTATIONS

Usual Presentation

Clinical signs of catheter-associated bacteremia or fungemia range from mild fever to overwhelming sepsis. The rate of progression of illness depends on the organism and the host risk factors. Infection with organisms of low virulence often is manifested by fever alone, and removal of the catheter frequently is followed by prompt clearance of the bacteremia and rapid full recovery. Infection with highly virulent organisms or infection in immunocompromised persons is often accompanied by signs of sepsis and progressive clinical deterioration.

Infection at the catheter entrance site is manifested as a local wound infection or cellulitis. Warmth, tenderness, swelling, erythema, and discharge are common. Tunnel infections are manifested by similar findings along the course of the catheter tunnel.

Phlebitis classically is manifested as a hot, red, tender cord arising from an intravenous catheter site. Phlebitis also may be subclinical or manifested by fever without obvious signs of local inflammation. Phlebitis should be considered as a source of fever in any hospitalized patient with an indwelling catheter, particularly if the catheter has been in place for >72 hours. Phlebitis of deep veins can lead to thrombosis and partial or complete obstruction to venous drainage. Subclavian obstruction is manifested by swelling of the neck, arm, and face. Partial obstruction is common and often subclinical.

Physical Examination Findings

Fever is the most common and often the only finding of catheter-related infection. The insertion site and tunnel should be examined for signs of inflammation, redness, warmth, swelling, and purulent drainage. Tenderness and swelling are signs of phlebitis. Signs of catheter-related endocarditis are similar to those of spontaneous endocarditis. Chorioretinitis may accompany fungal infection and occasionally complicates bacterial endocarditis.

DIAGNOSIS

The diagnosis of infection related to an intravascular device should be suspected in any person with an indwelling catheter who develops fever or local signs of infection. The diagnosis is confirmed only by culture, usually of the blood. Special techniques are occasionally needed, such as special media to support the growth of *M. furfur.*

Repeated clinical examination, serial blood cultures, and imaging studies are used to determine the presence and extent of infection. In the sicker person, the immunocompromised person, or the person whose condition fails to improve after removal of the catheter, extension of infection to a second focus must be suspected. Persistently positive blood culture results signify ongoing infection with persistent colonization of the catheter, a thrombus, the blood vessel, or a heart valve. Ultrasonography is useful in detecting thrombophlebitis and endocarditis.

Differential Diagnosis

Fever may be caused by a variety of other infections or medications. Bacteremia or fungemia can be primary and catheter related, secondary to intercurrent infection elsewhere, or seeding from the respiratory or gastrointestinal tract.

Laboratory Evaluation

Routine laboratory tests are of limited use in the diagnosis of catheter-related infections. The CBC may be normal or elevated, the ESR may be normal or elevated, and CRP may be present. Many of these infections occur in premature neonates or immunocompromised persons with an impaired immunologic response.

Microbiologic Evaluation

Cultures of blood taken from the catheter or from another vein are needed to establish the diagnosis of bacteremia or fungemia. If cultures of blood taken from the catheter show positive results while peripheral blood culture results are negative, the diagnosis of catheter-related infection is likely. Removal of the catheter and culture of a sample from the catheter tip will confirm the diagnosis. Determining the extent of infection involves follow-up cultures and ultrasonography or venography to determine whether intraluminal infection persists.

Quantitative blood culture by means of the **lysis centrifugation method** (Isolator) or by direct inoculation of 0.5 mL of blood onto an agar plate to permit counting can also be useful in identifying the catheter as the source of bacteremia. If the concentration of bacteria in the blood obtained via the catheter is significantly greater, or 5–10 times higher, than that in the blood obtained peripherally, a catheter infection is likely.

Certain techniques have been proposed to diagnose catheter sepsis without removing the line. Surveillance blood or skin cultures have been shown to correlate with subsequent infection, but the predictive value of such culture is so low that they are of little practical use. Recently the **acridine-orange leukocyte cytospin test** of blood drawn through the catheter has shown promise in combination with Gram stain (Kite, 1999); it has a sensitivity of 96% and a specificity of 92%. These results need to be confirmed before this test could be routinely recommended.

Gram stain and culture of a specimen from the exit site is useful to confirm a local infection. The exit site will be colonized with normal skin flora, and therefore identifying a pathogen in the absence of inflammation does not alone establish that an infection is present.

Culture of organisms on the catheter tip is helpful in confirming that the infection is catheter related. The exit site should be prepared before removal of the catheter. The catheter tip is rolled across culture media for **semiquantitative culture,** by the **method of Maki** (Maki, 1977), and then is also placed into broth. Other methods of processing catheter tips include sonication of the tip and culture in liquid media. If the roll plate technique is used, growth of >15 colonies is considered significant and indicates catheter-associated infection. Fewer colonies likely represent contamination of the catheter as the catheter was removed. The positive predictive value of a catheter tip culture alone is low.

Standard methods for culture of blood specimens will detect almost all episodes of catheter-related infection. Certain agents such as fungi and atypical mycobacteria require special media. The laboratory should be informed if *M. furfur* is suspected, as when patients, especially neonates, have received emulsified lipid as a component of parenteral nutrition.

Diagnostic Imaging

Echocardiography is useful for identifying endocarditis as a complication of catheter-related infection (Chapter 71). Ultrasonography of peripheral blood vessels is useful for determining the presence of thrombosis and thrombophlebitis. Doppler studies can also be used to determine the presence or absence of blood flow.

TREATMENT

The treatment of catheter-related infection depends on the site of the infection and the pathogen involved. Catheters that are no longer necessary should be removed if infection is suspected. Other indications for catheter removal include sepsis, clinical deterioration with appropriate therapy, persistently positive blood culture results after 48–72 hours of appropriate antimicrobial therapy, septic thrombophlebitis, embolic lesions, fungal infection, and *Bacillus* infection.

Some superficial exit-site infections can be managed with local care and topical antibiotics. In immunocompromised persons, infection at the exit site often precedes dissemination of the pathogen, especially with local fungal infections that have a propensity to invade the skin, eventually leading to local necrosis. Removal of the catheter speeds healing.

Infection of the tunneled area of the catheter is difficult to manage without catheter removal. In general these infections are managed by removal followed by combination antimicrobial therapy. Similarly, infection of the pocket around an implanted port is unlikely to respond to antibiotics, and removal of the foreign body is usually needed.

Eradication of the organism causing sepsis can be accomplished without removal of the central line in approximately 89% of bacteremic infections, 94% of exit-site infections, and 25% of tunnel infections. Thus catheter-associated bacteremia can be treated with simple catheter removal, removal plus antibiotics, or an attempt of antibiotic therapy alone. The choice of management depends on the patient risk factors and the specific pathogen. If the patient is not critically ill and the pathogen is likely to be killed by antibiotic therapy, a trial of antibiotics is given through the infected catheter. Daily cultures should be obtained to confirm sterilization of the blood. If the culture results remain positive after 48–72 hours, even if the patient is clinically stable, the catheter should be removed and antibiotic therapy continued.

The total duration of therapy depends on the pathogens and the duration of positive culture results. No studies have compared shorter with longer therapy. Most experts recommend continuing antibiotic therapy for 7–14 days after sterilization of the bloodstream. The need for combination antibiotics is unclear, but combinations are often used for synergy. Most β-lactams are less active in the presence of foreign material, while rifampin and clindamycin are notable for activity in the presence of catheters or implanted materials. The need for bactericidal combinations is also unclear. For endocarditis therapy, it seems clear that bacteriocidal antibiotics are needed for cure. This is almost certainly true for septic thrombophlebitis, and it is probably true for catheter-related infections in which the catheter remains in place. Surgical excision of infected clots or valves may be required for management of septic thrombophlebitis or endocarditis.

In immunocompetent persons, initial empirical therapy should include antibiotics active against staphylococci (oxacillin, nafcillin, or vancomycin, depending on the prevalence of methicillin-resistant staphylococci) plus an agent active against hospital-acquired gram-negative rod species (usually a third-generation cephalosporin, such as cefotaxime, ceftriaxone, or ceftazidime, or an aminoglycoside, such as tobramycin or gentamicin). For immunocompromised persons, some experts recommend both a cephalosporin and an aminoglycoside for better activity against gram-negative bacilli. For assessment of the efficacy of treatment, peripheral and catheter blood cultures should be repeated 24–48 hours after the institution of therapy. Antimicrobial therapy should be adjusted on identification and susceptibility testing of the causative pathogen(s).

Catheter-related infections caused by fungi and associated with fungemia rarely responds to antifungal agents alone. Thus, as soon as fungemia is detected, the catheter should be removed and antifungal therapy begun. Antifungal therapy may not be necessary for all immunocompetent hosts, but unfortunately it is difficult to determine the extent of infection and fungal abscesses may not appear for days to weeks. Amphotericin B is the drug of choice in most cases; however, fluconazole and other azoles are active against most species of *Candida* and have much less toxicity. Optimal duration of therapy is unknown, but 2 weeks is considered sufficient provided there is no evidence of ongoing infection or organ involvement. The eyes should be examined for evidence of fungal retinitis.

Antibiotic-lock technique is a method of sterilizing intravascular catheters by using high concentrations of antibiotics infused into the portion of the catheter between the hub and the vessel entry. The solution is allowed to dwell within the catheter segment for several hours. High rates of sterilization have been reported with this technique; fungal infections have been suppressed but not eliminated with this technique.

Supportive Therapy

Maintaining and enhancing the immune function of the host is important as supportive therapy. Nutrition should be maintained; enteral nutrition is generally safer than and superior to parenteral nutrition. The use of growth factors should be considered to limit neutropenia. Macrophage growth factor also has shown promise as adjunctive therapy for fungal infection.

COMPLICATIONS

Complications of vascular catheters include hemorrhage, damage to the vessel, phlebitis, thrombosis, displacement of the catheter, breakage of the catheter, allergic reaction to the catheter, and infection (Table 106–5). Reactions to catheters have been described in adults managed with one brand of midline catheters. Reactions included dyspnea, urticaria, skin changes, acute onset of abdominal or back pain, hypotension, and anaphylaxis. This type of catheter was not widely used in children. Minor reactions to catheter materials often go unnoticed.

Thrombosis of catheterized vessels is common and usually asymptomatic and unrecognized. Examination during autopsy and Doppler ultrasonography during life in persons with indwelling central catheters show that more than 20% of vessels are partially or completely filled with thrombus. In many cases the thrombi are infected with bacteria or fungi.

The major complication of catheter-related infection is spread of the infection. Infection within a blood vessel results in inflammation and thrombosis of the vessel. If the catheter is within the heart, infection may involve the valves or endocardium. Hematogenous spread of the infection to organs of the body results in local infection and organ dysfunction. Eventually this results in multiorgan system failure and death. Infection is most common in the most immunocompromised persons. It is not always possible to determine whether deterioration and death are due to infection or due to the underlying illness. Infection leads to increased morbidity, death, prolonged hospitalization, and increased medical costs.

TABLE 106–5. Complications of Vascular Catheters

Noninfectious Complications
Hemorrhage
Thrombosis
Phlebitis
Perforation of the vessel
Displacement of the catheter
Allergic reaction to catheter
Infectious Complications
Exit-site infection
Tunnel infection
Pocket infection
Septic phlebitis
Catheter-tip colonization
Bacteremia
Fungemia
Endocarditis
Metastatic abscesses
Sepsis
Multiorgan system dysfunction

PROGNOSIS

The prognosis varies greatly. In the immunocompetent person who has a catheter for hydration or for the infusion of medications, a catheter-related infection with skin organisms is often a minor problem that is easily managed by simple removal of the catheter. In the immunocompromised person with disseminated cancer or in the very small premature neonate with multiorgan system failure, infection with skin flora is more significant and may result in death. Delay of recognition of the infection and thus delay of therapy may result in spread of the infection to organs or through the vessel or into a clot. These infections are more difficult to manage.

Recurrence. Bacteremia recurs in about 20% of catheters managed in situ. Recurrence is also very high in children with short gut syndrome, presumably associated with frequent bacteremia, which is probably due to local overgrowth of bacteria in stagnant loops of bowel or to translocation of bacteria through inflamed loops of bowel. The bacteria adhere to fibrin clots on the catheters and multiply locally.

PREVENTION

Prevention of bacteremia involves preventing infection at the catheter site and minimizing the use of catheters (Table 106–6). Aseptic technique is essential during catheter insertion. Skin should be prepared with 1% iodine, 70% alcohol, 10% povidone-iodine, or 2% chlorhexidine. If an iodophor is used, the area must dry to release enough active iodine to kill bacteria. Maximal barrier precautions, including large drapes, masks, gowns, and gloves, should be used for insertion of long-term catheters. Catheters that are placed during emergency situations should be replaced as soon as medically feasible. A vascular catheter should be removed as soon as its use is no longer necessary. An idle indwelling catheter is an invitation to infection. Bloodstream infection rates in persons undergoing hemodialysis can be decreased by use of vascular fistulas instead of central catheters.

Care of indwelling catheters involves meticulous attention to sterile technique whenever the system is entered. Hand washing before and after manipulation of the catheter is essential. The use of stopcocks should be minimized. All access ports must be capped, and sterile technique must be used whenever injection ports or stopcocks are entered. The use of **inline filters** has had only a small impact on rates of catheter infection because contamination of intravenous fluids is an infrequent manner of infection. The use of multidose vials increases the possibility for contamination of flush solutions. Similarly, flush solutions and medications should not be prepared in advance unless preparation is done under sterile conditions and the sterility can be maintained during the interval before infusion.

Care of the catheter entry site commonly involves a topical antibiotic or disinfectant, although data regarding efficacy of such therapy in preventing infection are lacking. Frequency of dressing changes should be limited; in general, less manipulation is better. Weekly dressing changes are adequate provided the dressing remains dry and intact. The ideal dressing is unclear. Initial studies and meta-analysis found that transparent, occlusive dressings increased the risk of infection, but subsequent studies failed to reveal differences. Gauze and tape are less expensive than occlusive dressings. The need for any dressing is unproved. Outbreaks of bacteremia caused by gram-negative bacilli have occurred in persons who swim or bathe with an indwelling catheter. Care of catheters by infusion therapy teams has been associated with lower rates of infection. In several studies the introduction of needleless intravascular systems was associated with an increase in the incidence of bloodstream infection. The inability or failure to prepare hubs before insertion of a needleless device is one problem; slits in the hub surface and designs in which the needleless device enters a recessed portal provide areas that cannot be prepared and where growth of bacteria may occur.

Cuffed catheters have somewhat lower infection rates; presumably, cuffs anchor the catheter. Silver-impregnated cuffs have been studied in adults; the silver is slowly released into the tunnel area. Initial studies found lower infection rates in short-term catheters but not in long-term catheters. Extrusion of the silver cuff from the entry site and inflammation due to the silver ion have been reported. Antiseptic- and antibiotic-impregnated catheters have been associated with lower rates of colonization and bacteremia. Although these catheters are more expensive than untreated catheters, there was a net savings if the incidence of bacteremia was at least 3 in 1,000 catheter-days.

Although infection rates increase with an increasing duration of catheterization, it is not appropriate to change catheter sites on a regular basis. Studies comparing routine catheter replacement every 72 hours, either over a guidewire or to a new site, have not demonstrated any decrease in infection rates but have demonstrated increases in mechanical complications related to catheter placement. Although studies in adults have suggested that peripheral catheters should be rotated every 72 hours, this has not been confirmed in children. It is important to remove catheters that are no longer necessary for care.

Infection rates are increased in persons with thrombosis around the catheter tip. Staphylococci and *Candida* adhere to components within the thrombus, and thrombosis also increases the incidence of catheter occlusion. Thus it has become common practice to add heparin to infusions or to use heparin flush solutions. However,

TABLE 106–6. Prevention of Catheter-Related Infection

General
- Choose sites likely to have minimal bacterial flora
- Avoid femoral vessels in all patients and avoid leg vessels in older adolescents and adults
- Remove catheter as soon as medically possible
- Limit manipulation of the catheter
- Limit use of stopcocks and monitoring devices
- Ensure that surveillance for catheter-related infection occurs in hospitalized patients and in outpatients

Insertion
- Prepare the skin with tincture of iodine, chlorhexidine, or povidone-iodine
- Use maximal barrier protection for insertion of central catheters and long-term catheters
- Use peripheral placement or subcutaneous tunnels for long-term catheters

Maintenance
- Wash hands before and after manipulation of any part of the catheter
- Prepare catheter hubs before entry
- Ensure adequate nurse-patient ratios
- Use specially trained teams to maintain catheters and educate providers, patients, and families
- Limit access and manipulation
- Change dressings when they are wet or contaminated
- Limit exposure of catheter entry site and catheter hubs to nonsterile water

although early studies showed a decrease in the incidence of infection in heparin-infused catheters, later studies have not confirmed this finding. In neonates the risk of bleeding outweighs the possible benefit of heparin added to infusions. Thus there is no consensus regarding the use of heparin for prevention of infection.

Antibiotic prophylaxis at the time of catheterization has not been shown to decrease the incidence of catheter-related infection. Likewise the ongoing use of systemic antibiotics does not prevent catheter infection; it does, however, alter flora and increases the risk of infection due to resistant bacteria or fungi.

Surveillance for catheter-related infection is essential in both hospitalized and home care patients. Identification of clusters of infection should lead to formal outbreak investigations.

REVIEWS

Darouiche RO: Anti-infective efficacy of silver-coated medical prostheses. *Clin Infect Dis* 1999;29:1371–8.

Hoffmann KK, Weber DJ, Samsa GP, et al: Transparent polyurethane film as an intravenous catheter dressing. A meta-analysis of the infection risks. *JAMA* 1992;267:2072–6.

Mermel LA: Prevention of intravascular catheter–related infections. *Ann Intern Med* 2000;132:391–402.

Pearson ML: Guideline for prevention of intravascular-device–related infections. Hospital Infection Control Practices Advisory Committee. *Infect Control and Hosp Epidemiol* 1996;17:438–73.

Raad II, Bodey GP: Infectious complications of indwelling vascular catheters. *Clin Infect Dis* 1992a;15:197–208.

Raad II, Sabbagh MF: Optimal duration of therapy for catheter-related *Staphylococcus aureus* bacteremia: A study of 55 cases and review. *Clin Infect Dis* 1992b;14:75–82.

Veenstra DL, Saint S, Saha S, et al: Efficacy of antiseptic-impregnated central venous catheters in preventing catheter-related bloodstream infection. A meta-analysis. *JAMA* 1999a;281:261–7.

Veenstra DL, Saint S, Sullivan SD: Cost-effectiveness of antiseptic-impregnated central venous catheters for the prevention of catheter-related bloodstream infection. *JAMA* 1999b;282:554–60.

KEY ARTICLES

Arnow PM, Garcia-Houchins S, Neagle MB, et al: An outbreak of bloodstream infections arising from hemodialysis equipment. *J Infect Dis* 1998;178:783–91.

Beck C, Dubois J, Grignon A, et al: Incidence and risk factors of catheter-related deep vein thrombosis in a pediatric intensive care unit: A prospective study. *J Pediatr* 1998;133:237–41.

Benoit JL, Carandang G, Sitrin M, et al: Intraluminal antibiotic treatment of central venous catheter infections in patients receiving parenteral nutrition at home. *Clin Infect Dis* 1995;21:1286–8.

Bertone SA, Fisher MC, Mortensen JE: Quantitative skin cultures at potential catheter sites in neonates. *Infect Control Hosp Epidemiol* 1994; 15:315–8.

Cobb DK, High KP, Sawyer RG, et al: A controlled trial of scheduled replacement of central venous and pulmonary-artery catheters. *N Engl J Med* 1992;327:1062–8.

Do AN, Ray BJ, Banerjee SN, et al: Bloodstream infection associated with needleless device use and the importance of infection-control practices in the home health care setting. *J Infect Dis* 1999;179:422–8.

Douard MC, Arlet G, Longuet P, et al: Diagnosis of venous access port–related infections. *Clin Infect Dis* 1999;29:1197–1202.

Edmond MB, Wallace SE, McClish DK, et al: Nosocomial bloodstream infections in United States hospitals: A three-year analysis. *Clin Infect Dis* 1999;29:239–44.

Eyer S, Brummitt C, Crossley K, et al: Catheter-related sepsis: Prospective, randomized study of three methods of long-term catheter maintenance. *Crit Care Med* 1990;18:1073–9.

Fridkin SK, Pear SM, Williamson TH, et al: The role of understaffing in central venous catheter–associated bloodstream infections. *Infect Control Hosp Epidemiol* 1996;17:150–8.

Furfaro S, Gauthier M, Lacroix J, et al: Arterial catheter–related infections in children. A 1-year cohort analysis. *Am J Dis Child* 1991;145:1037–43.

Garland JS, Dunne WM Jr, Havens P, et al: Peripheral intravenous catheter complications in critically ill children: A prospective study. *Pediatrics* 1992;89:1145–50.

Garland JS, Buck RK, Maloney P, et al: Comparison of 10% povidone-iodine and 0.5% chlorhexidine gluconate for the prevention of peripheral intravenous catheter colonization in neonates: A prospective trial. *Pediatr Infect Dis J* 1995;14:510–6.

Goetz AM, Wagener MM, Miller JM, et al: Risk of infection due to central venous catheters: Effect of site or placement and catheter type. *Infect Control Hosp Epidemiol* 1998;19:842–5.

Kellerman S, Shay DK, Howard J, et al: Bloodstream infections in home infusion patients: The influence of race and needleless intravascular access devices. *J Pediatr* 1996;129:711–7.

Kite P, Dobbins BM, Wilcox MH, et al: Rapid diagnosis of central-venous-catheter–related bloodstream infection without catheter removal. *Lancet* 1999;354:1504–7.

Lange BJ, Weiman M, Feuer EJ, et al: Impact of changes in catheter management on infectious complications among children with central venous catheters. *Infect Control Hosp Epidemiol* 1997;18:326–32.

Lederle FA, Parenti CM, Berskow LC, et al: The idle intravenous catheter. *Ann Intern Med* 1992;116:737–8.

Maki DG, Weise CE, Sarafin HW: A semiquantitative culture method for identifying intravenous-catheter–related infection. *N Engl J Med* 1977; 296:1305–9.

Maki DG, Stolz SM, Wheeler S, et al: Prevention of central venous catheter–related bloodstream infection by use of an antiseptic-impregnated catheter. A randomized, controlled trial. *Ann Intern Med* 1997;127:257–66.

Marr KA, Sexton DJ, Conlon PJ, et al: Catheter-related bacteremia and outcome of attempted catheter salvage in patients undergoing hemodialysis. *Ann Intern Med* 1997;127:275–80.

McDonald LC, Banerjee SN, Jarvis WR: Line-associated bloodstream infections in pediatric intensive-care-unit patients associated with a needleless device and intermittent intravenous therapy. *Infect Control Hosp Epidemiol* 1998;19:772–7.

Mermel LA, Parenteau S, Tow SM: The risk of midline catheterization in hospitalized patients. A prospective study. *Ann Intern Med* 1995; 123:841–4.

Raad I, Darouiche R, Dupuis J, et al: Central venous catheters coated with minocycline and rifampin for the prevention of catheter-related colonization and bloodstream infections. A randomized, double-blind trial. The Texas Medical Center Catheter Study Group. *Ann Intern Med* 1997;127:267–74.

Rudnick JR, Beck-Sague CM, Anderson RL, et al: Gram-negative bacteremia in open-heart-surgery patients traced to probable tap-water contamination of pressure-monitoring equipment. *Infect Control Hosp Epidemiol* 1996;17:281–5.

Sotir MJ, Lewis C, Bisher EW, et al: Epidemiology of device-associated infections related to a long-term implantable vascular access device. *Infect Control Hosp Epidemiol* 1999;20:187–91.

Taylor GD, McKenzie M, Buchanan-Chell M, et al: Central venous catheters as a source of hemodialysis-related bacteremia. *Infect Control Hosp Epidemiol* 1998;19:643–6.

Timsit JF, Bruneel F, Cheval C, et al: Use of tunneled femoral catheters to prevent catheter-related infection. A randomized, controlled trial. *Ann Intern Med* 1999;130:729–35.

Yeung CY, Lee HC, Huang FY, et al: Sepsis during total parenteral nutrition: Exploration of risk factors and determination of the effectiveness of peripherally inserted central venous catheters. *Pediatr Infect Dis J* 1998;17:135–42.

Index

Note: Page numbers followed by f refer to figures; page numbers followed by t refer to tables.

A

Abacavir, 152t, 203t, 205t
  in HIV infection, 456, 457t, 458t, 460t
Abdominal cavity, anatomy of, 921–923, 922f
Abortion, fetal infection and, 1099
Abscess
  anorectal, 940–941
    clinical manifestations of, 940
    complications of, 941
    diagnosis of, 940–941
    epidemiology of, 940
    etiology of, 940
    pathogenesis of, 940
    prognosis for, 941
    treatment of, 941
  appendiceal. *See* Appendicitis.
  brain, 657–664
    biopsy in, 663
    clinical manifestations of, 659, 659t
    complications of, 663
    computed tomography in, 128f, 660, 661f
    culture in, 659
    diagnosis of, 659–660, 659t, 660f, 661f
    differential diagnosis of, 659t
    epidemiology of, 657
    etiology of, 657, 658t
    fungal, 662
    magnetic resonance imaging in, 130f, 660, 661f
    needle aspiration in, 663
    pathogenesis of, 657–659, 658f, 658t
    prognosis for, 663–664
    rupture of, 659, 663
    surgery in, 663
    treatment of, 660–663, 662t
    tuberculous, 657, 662, 663
  breast, in neonate, 1129–1130, 1129t
  cerebellar, 658
  dental. *See* Abscess, neck; Dental infection.
  epidural
    cranial, 657, 664–665, 665f, 666t
    spinal, 657, 665–667, 666t, 667f, 667t
  hepatic, 963–969
    amebic, 965–966, 968–969
    chest radiography in, 966
    clinical manifestations of, 964, 964t
    complications of, 968
    computed tomography in, 966, 966f
    culture in, 964–965
    diagnosis of, 964–966, 965f, 966t
    differential diagnosis of, 964, 966t
    epidemiology of, 963
    etiology of, 963, 963t
    fungal, 965, 967t, 968

Abscess *(Continued)*
  hepatic *(Continued)*
    imaging in, 966, 966f
    pathogenesis of, 963–964
    prevention of, 969
    prognosis for, 968–969
    treatment of, 965f, 966–968, 967t
  in hyper-IgE syndrome, 1154
  in neonate, 1129–1130, 1129t
  intra-abdominal, 923–928
    clinical manifestations of, 924
    complications of, 928
    computed tomography in, 925–926, 926f
    diagnosis of, 925–926, 927f
    differential diagnosis of, 925
    drainage of, 928, 928f
    epidemiology of, 923
    etiology of, 923
    imaging in, 925–926, 925f–927f
    pathogenesis of, 923–924
    periappendiceal, 926, 926f
    physical examination in, 924
    prevention of, 928
    prognosis for, 928
    radionuclide scan in, 925
    treatment of, 926–928, 929t
    ultrasonography in, 925, 925f
    ventriculoperitoneal shunt and, 923
  lung, 837–840
    bronchoscopy in, 839, 840
    clinical manifestations of, 838–839
    complications of, 840
    computed tomography in, 839, 840f
    culture in, 839
    diagnosis of, 839
    differential diagnosis of, 839
    drainage of, 840
    epidemiology of, 838
    etiology of, 838, 838t
    pathogenesis of, 838
    prevention of, 840
    prognosis for, 840
    treatment of, 839–840
  neck, 721–727
    airway management in, 725–726
    clinical manifestations of, 724
    complications of, 726–727
    computed tomography in, 725, 725f
    diagnosis of, 724–725, 725f
    differential diagnosis of, 724
    epidemiology of, 721–722
    etiology of, 721, 722t
    hot-potato voice in, 724
    imaging in, 725, 725f

Abscess *(Continued)*
  neck *(Continued)*
    laboratory evaluation in, 724
    pathogenesis of, 722–723, 722f
    physical examination in, 724
    prognosis for, 727
    respiratory tract infection in, 723
    surgery in, 726
    treatment of, 725–726
  pelvic. *See also* Abscess, intra-abdominal.
    complications of, 928
    drainage of, 928, 928f
    pathogenesis of, 924
    physical examination in, 924
    prognosis for, 928
    ultrasonography in, 925–926, 925f
  perinephric, 983, 984, 985, 989–990. *See also* Urinary tract infection.
    vs. appendicitis, 934, 934t
  psoas, 938–940
    clinical manifestations of, 939
    diagnosis of, 939
    epidemiology of, 938
    pathogenesis of, 938–939
  renal, 983, 984, 985, 989–990. *See also* Urinary tract infection.
  retroperitoneal, 938–940
    clinical manifestations of, 939
    diagnosis of, 939
    epidemiology of, 938
    etiology of, 938
    pathogenesis of, 938–939, 938f
  specimen collection from, 62t
  splenic, 936–937
  tubo-ovarian, vs. appendicitis, 934, 934t
  vs. inguinal lymphadenopathy, 618
Absolute lymphocyte count, 93–94
Absolute neutrophil count, 92
  in cancer, 1158
  in fever evaluation, 265, 266
  in neonatal sepsis, 1123
  in occult bacteremia evaluation, 269
Acanthamoeba infection, 13, 1063, 1063t, 1065, 1066f, 1067, 1068
Accident prevention, for international travel, 1217, 1217t
Acetaminophen, in fever, 266, 267t
Acetowhitening, in human papillomavirus infection, 1029
Achlorhydria, 1182t
AC/HS test, in toxoplasmosis, 109
Acid-fast stains, 68–69, 68t, 69t
Acne fulminans, 548, 548t
Acne vulgaris, 547–549

Acne vulgaris *(Continued)*
clinical manifestations of, 548, 548t
pathogenesis of, 547–548
treatment of, 548–549, 549t
Acoustic reflectometry, in otitis media, 752
Acquired immunodeficiency syndrome (AIDS), 437–476. *See also* Human immunodeficiency virus (HIV) infection.
adenovirus infection in, 469
amebiasis in, 472
anemia in, 473–474
antibiotic prophylaxis in, 460–461, 461t, 462t
aphthous ulcers in, 470
aspergillosis in, 452t, 469, 814–815
bacillary angiomatosis in, 474
bacterial infections in, 450t, 466–467
Bartonella infection in, 474
campylobacteriosis in, 450t, 471
candidiasis in, 452t–453t, 462t, 463, 469, 470, 471, 475, 870–871
cat-scratch disease in, 474
CD4 cell count in, 444, 444t, 460–461, 461t
chickenpox in, 461, 462t
classification of, 443–444, 444t, 445t
coccidiomycosis in, 451t, 468
cryptococcosis in, 451t–452t, 462t, 469, 475
cryptosporidiosis in, 472, 473, 904, 904f
cytomegalovirus infection in, 463, 470, 472, 473
dental caries in, 470
drug reactions in, 475, 476t
encephalopathy in, 463–465, 464f, 683–684
Enterocytozoon bieneusi infection in, 472
Epstein-Barr virus infection in, 25, 427–428, 430
esophagitis in, 471
fungal infection in, 452t–453t, 468–469, 475
gastrointestinal tract disease in, 450t, 470–472
Haemophilus influenzae type b infection in, 450t, 467
heart disease in, 470
hepatic disease in, 472–473
hepatitis in, 473
hepatomegaly in, 472–473
herpes simplex virus infection in, 461, 470, 474
histoplasmosis in, 452t, 462t, 468–469
human herpes virus 6 infection in, 681
influenza in, 469
information sources for, 454t
Isospora belli infection in, 472
Kaposi's sarcoma in, 24t, 25–26, 475
leukopenia in, 474
lymphoid interstitial pneumonitis in, 466, 467f
malignancy in, 472
measles in, 461, 469
molluscum contagiosum in, 475
mononeuritis multiplex in, 704
Mycobacterium avium complex infection in, 451t, 461, 461t, 462t, 471–472
oral disease in, 470–471
oral hairy leukoplakia in, 470
otitis media in, 749
parainfluenza virus infection in, 469
parotitis in, 470–471
peripheral neuropathy in, 704–705
Pneumocystis carinii infection in, 453t, 454, 461, 461t, 462t, 465–466, 465f
prognosis for, 475–476
Acquired immunodeficiency syndrome (AIDS) *(Continued)*
Pseudomonas aeruginosa infection in, 474
psychosocial support services in, 463
respiratory syncytial virus infection in, 469
respiratory tract infections in, 461, 469–470
salmonellosis in, 471
Septata intestinalis infection in, 472
shigellosis in, 450t, 471
skin disease in, 474–475
Staphylococcus aureus infection in, 474
Streptococcus pneumoniae infection in, 450t, 467
strongyloidiasis in, 472
thrombocytopenia in, 474
tinea in, 475
toxoplasmosis in, 453t, 461, 461t, 462t, 465, 663
tuberculosis in, 450t–451t, 461, 462t, 467–468
urinary tract infection in, 473
varicella-zoster virus infection in, 334, 461, 462t, 469–470, 474–475
viral infections in, 469–470, 474–475
Acridine orange stain, 67, 68t
Acrodermatitis chronica atrophicans, in Lyme disease, 350
Actinomycetes infection, 57–59, 58t
antimicrobial susceptibility testing in, 76
bite-wound, 602–603, 603t, 607t, 608t. *See also* Bite-wound infection.
Acute cerebellar ataxia, in varicella-zoster virus infection, 338
Acute chest syndrome, 1183
Acute Illness Observation Scale, 264, 265t
in fever evaluation, 264, 265t, 286, 286t
in sepsis evaluation, 285, 286
Acute retroviral syndrome, in HIV infection, 444
Acute urethral syndrome, 983, 985, 989
Acute-phase reactants, 96–97, 97t
Acute-phase response, 35
Acyclovir, 152t, 196–197, 198t
dosing for, 198t
in burn wound infection, 599
in congenital herpes simplex virus infection, 1109
in genital herpes simplex virus infection, 1024t
in herpes simplex encephalitis, 672, 672t
in herpetic gingivostomatitis, 731, 731t
in perinatal herpes simplex virus, 1139
in varicella-zoster virus infection, 335–337, 336t, 1142t
in viral esophagitis, 871
Adenoidectomy, in otitis media, 756
Adenosine arabinoside. *See* Vidarabine.
Adenovirus infection, 819
diagnosis of, 88t, 90, 90f
electron microscopy in, 90, 90f
encephalitic, 682
enteric, 898t, 900
exanthem in, 537
in AIDS, 469
keratoconjunctival, 1059, 1063, 1065, 1066f, 1067, 1068f
meningeal, 631, 631t. *See also* Meningitis, viral.
Adherence, 1
Adhesins, 1
Adhesion, granulocyte, 33
Adopted children, 1194–1206. *See also* Foreign-born children.
Adult respiratory distress syndrome, in Rocky Mountain spotted fever, 357
Adult T-cell leukemia, 27
Aedes aegypti, in dengue fever, 392
Aedes triseriatus, in California encephalitis, 673
Aerobacter infection. *See Enterobacter* infection.
Aerobes, 57, 58t
Aeromonas infection, 588, 590, 890–891
clinical manifestations of, 891, 891t
complications of, 891
diagnosis of, 891
epidemiology of, 890
pathogenesis of, 890
prevention of, 891
prognosis for, 891
toxins of, 4t
treatment of, 891, 891t
Aerosols, in pathogen transmission, 13
Afipia felis infection, 343
African tick-bite fever, 355t
Agammaglobulinemia, X-linked, 1150–1151
Agar diffusion method, in antimicrobial susceptibility testing, 75–76
Agar dilution method, in antimicrobial susceptibility testing, 76
Age
bacteremia and, 281
fever and, 265
immune response and, 49–50
Agglutination assay, for antibody detection, 102
Aicardi's syndrome, vs. toxoplasmosis, 1083
Airborne disease, 13
Airway obstruction, in infectious mononucleosis, 434
Albendazole, 153t, 209–210, 209t, 210t
in cutaneous larva migrans, 506t
in cysticercosis, 526–527, 527t
in echinococcosis, 529–530, 529t
in enterobiasis, 515, 515t
in giardiasis, 902, 903t
in hookworm infection, 506, 506t
in microsporida infection, 903t
in trichinellosis, 516, 517t
in trichuriasis, 508, 508t
in visceral larva migrans, 512, 512t
Alcohol, metronidazole interaction with, 189
Alertness, in fever evaluation, 264, 265t
Alice-in-Wonderland syndrome, in infectious mononucleosis, 428
Allergic rhinitis, vs. common cold, 708, 708t
Allergy
cephalosporin, 165
in chronic fatigue syndrome, 499
penicillin, 156, 160t
to animal antisera, 221, 221t
vs. vulvovaginitis, 1004
Allopurinol, vidarabine interaction with, 200
Alopecia, 542–543, 557, 557f
Alveolar hydatid disease, 528, 529, 529t, 530
Amantadine, 152t, 201–202, 201t
adverse effects of, 201–202, 202t
in influenza virus infection, 820–821, 821t
Amblyomma americanum, 21t
in ehrlichiosis, 359
in tularemia, 382

Amblyomma maculatum, 21t
Amblyopia, deprivation, in keratitis, 1067
Amebiasis, 891–893. *See also Entamoeba histolytica* infection (amebiasis).
Amikacin, 151t, 167–172, 168t
  adverse effects of, 170–171
  clinical indications for, 168–169
  dosing for, 169–170, 170t
  in acute pancreatitis, 981, 981t
  in acute pericarditis, 867t
  in burn wound infection, 600t
  in cholecystitis, 972, 972t
  in endophthalmitis, 1077t
  in hepatic abscess, 967t
  in infectious arthritis, 1048t
  in infective endocarditis, 851t–852t
  in intra-abdominal abscess, 929t
  in meningitis, 646t
  in neonatal sepsis, 1126t
  in osteomyelitis, 1040t
  in sepsis, 291t, 1126t
  in shunt-related infection, 655t
  in urinary tract infection, 991t
  spectrum of activity of, 167–168, 168t
Aminoglycosides, 167–172
  adverse effects of, 170–171
  clinical indications for, 168–169
  dosing for, 169–170, 169t
  drug interactions with, 171–172, 171t
  metabolism of, 169
  neuromuscular blockade with, 171
  ototoxicity of, 170–171
  penicillin interaction with, 157, 160t
  spectrum of activity of, 167–168, 168t
Aminopenicillins, 151t
Aminosalicylic acid, 152t
Amoxicillin, 151t
  dosing for, 158t, 159t
  formulations of, 157t
  in bite-wound infection, 606, 606t, 607t
  in cellulitis, 580t, 585t
  in erysipelas, 580t
  in gastritis, 875–876, 876t
  in gonococcal vulvovaginitis, 1006t
  in group A streptococcal vulvovaginal infection, 1006t
  in *Haemophilus influenzae* vulvovaginal infection, 1006t
  in infectious arthritis, 1048t
  in occult bacteremia, 271
  in osteomyelitis, 1040t
  in otitis media, 754t, 755t
  in sinusitis, 765, 765t
  in streptococcal pharyngitis, 717, 717t
  in urinary tract infection, 991t
  pathogen susceptibility to, 155t
Amphotericin B, 152t, 190–192, 191t, 192t
  adverse effects of, 190–192
  dosing for, 190, 191t, 192t
  in aspergillosis, 815
  in blastomycosis, 817
  in burn wound infection, 599
  in candidiasis, 731, 731t, 870, 1133
  in coccidioidomycosis, 816
  in hepatic abscess, 967t
  in histoplasmosis, 814
  in meningitis, 645t–646t
Amphotericin B *(Continued)*
  in neonatal candidiasis, 1133
  in neonatal sepsis, 1126t
  in shunt-related infection, 655t
  in sporotrichosis, 563
  metabolism of, 190
  pathogen susceptibility to, 191t
Ampicillin, 151t
  dosing for, 158t
  formulations of, 157t
  in acute pericarditis, 867t
  in bite-wound infection, 606, 606t, 607t
  in burn wound infection, 600t
  in cellulitis, 585t
  in cranial epidural abscess, 666t
  in infective endocarditis, 851t–852t
  in intra-abdominal abscess, 929t
  in meningitis, 643t, 644, 645t, 646t
  in neonatal sepsis, 1125t, 1126t
  in pelvic inflammatory disease, 1015t
  in salmonellosis, 881, 882t
  in sepsis, 291t, 1125t, 1126t
  in shigellosis, 886, 886t, 1006t
  in shunt-related infection, 655t
  in subdural empyema, 666t
  in typhoid, 884, 884t
  in urinary tract infection, 991t
  pathogen susceptibility to, 155t
Ampicillin rash, in infectious mononucleosis, 428
Amprenavir, 152t, 204t, 205t
  in HIV infection, 456, 457t, 459t
Amylase, in acute pancreatitis, 979–980, 980t
Amyloidosis, in leprosy, 704
Anaerobes, 57, 58t
Analytic study, 11
Anaphylactic reaction, penicillin-induced, 156, 160t
Anatomic barriers, in host defense, 6
Ancylostoma braziliense infection (cutaneous larva migrans), 20t, 504, 505, 569–570, 570f
  treatment of, 506t
Ancylostoma ceylanicum infection, 504
Ancylostoma duodenale, life cycle of, 504, 505f
Ancylostoma duodenale infection, 504–507. *See also* Hookworm infection.
Anemia, 98
  amphotericin B–related, 192
  chloramphenicol-related, 180
  in AIDS, 473–474
  in hookworm infection, 506, 507
  in infectious mononucleosis, 428, 434
  in malaria, 364
  in *Salmonella typhi* infection, 884
  in whipworm infection, 507
Aneurysm
  in Kawasaki syndrome, 484
  mycotic, 853
Angina, Ludwig's, 582, 583, 584, 734, 736–737, 738t, 739
Angiography, 127t
Angiostrongyliasis, 517–518, 517t
Angiostrongylus cantonensis infection, 517–518, 517t
  meningeal, 631, 632t
Angiostrongylus costaricensis infection (angiostrongyliasis), 517–518, 517t
Angular cheilitis, in candidiasis, 562
Animal bite, 602–608. *See also* Bite-wound infection.
Anisakis simplex infection (anisakiasis), 20t
Anogenital warts, 567, 567t, 568f, 1029–1030, 1029f
  sexual abuse and, 568
  treatment of, 568
Anorectal abscess, 940–941. *See also* Abscess, anorectal.
Anthelmintics, 153t, 209–211, 209t, 210t
  in angiostrongyliasis, 517, 517t
  in cysticercosis, 526–527, 527t
  in enterobiasis, 515, 515t
  in hookworm, 506–507, 506t
  in strongyloidiasis, 514, 514t
  in toxocariasis, 512, 512t
  in trichinellosis, 516, 517t
  in trichuriasis, 508, 508t
Anthrax, 4t, 18t, 551–552
  cutaneous, 551
  immunization against, 245t
  pulmonary, 551
Antibiotics, 153–190. *See also specific antibiotics.*
  additive effects of, 77, 78f
  aminoglycoside, 167–172
    adverse effects of, 170–171
    clinical indications for, 168–169
    dosing for, 169–170, 169t
    drug interactions with, 171–172, 171t
    metabolism of, 169
    neuromuscular blockade with, 171
    spectrum of activity of, 167–168, 168t
  antagonistic effects of, 77, 78f
  azalide, 175–178, 176t
    adverse effects of, 177–178
    dosing for, 177, 178t
    formulation of, 177
    mechanism of action of, 176
    metabolism of, 176–177, 177t
  before meningitis diagnosis, 643
  blood levels of, 78–79
  carbapenem, 166–167, 166t, 167t
  cephalosporin, 151t–152t, 157, 159–165, 161t, 162t
    adverse effects of, 165
    clinical indications for, 160, 163t
    dosing for, 163–165, 164t
    drug interactions with, 165
    formulations of, 163
    fourth-generation, 159–160
    metabolism of, 162–163, 163t
    pharmacokinetics of, 162–163, 163t
    second-generation, 159
    spectrum of activity of, 157, 159–160, 162t
    third-generation, 159
  for febrile infant, 266, 274
  glycopeptide, 172–175, 173t, 174t, 175t
  β-lactam, 151t, 153–157, 155t
    adverse effects of, 156, 160t
    clinical indications for, 154–155
    desensitization to, 160t
    dosing for, 156, 158t–159t
    drug interactions with, 156–157, 160t
    metabolism of, 155–156, 156t
    pharmacokinetics of, 151t, 155–156, 156t
    spectrum of activity of, 154, 155t
  levels of, 78–79

Antibiotics *(Continued)*
lincosamide, 187, 187t, 188t
macrolide, 175–178, 176t
adverse effects of, 177–178
dosing for, 177, 178t
drug interactions with, 178, 179t
formulation of, 177
mechanism of action of, 176
metabolism of, 176–177, 177t
minimum bactericidal concentration of, 76
minimum inhibitory concentration of, 76
monobactam, 165–166, 165t, 166t
oxazolidinone, 172–175, 173t, 174t, 175t
perioperative, 588, 655, 1238
quinolone, 184–187, 185t, 186t
resistance to, 3, 6–7
selection of, 150, 151t–152t, 153t
serum bactericidal tests of, 77–78
streptogramin, 172–175, 173t, 174t, 175t
sulfonamide, 182–184, 183t, 184t
susceptibility testing for, 75–79, 75t, 78f
synergistic effects of, 77, 78f
tetracycline, 180–182, 181t, 182t
Antibiotic-associated colitis. *See Clostridium difficile–*associated diarrhea.
Antibiotics, perioperative, 1227, 1228t
Antibody (antibodies), 41–45, 99–111. *See also at* Immunoglobulin(s).
anti-*Babesia,* 376–377
anti-*Bartonella,* 346
anti–*Borrelia burgdorferi,* 108, 350–351
anti-*Brucella,* 381
anti–*Chlamydia pneumoniae,* 812
anti–*Chlamydia psittaci,* 811
anti–*Chlamydia trachomatis,* 810
anti-*Coltivirus,* 394
anti–*Coxiella burnetii,* 390
anti-dengue virus, 393
antideoxyribonuclease B, 491
anti–Epstein-Barr virus, 431–433, 431f, 432t
anti–*Francisella tularensis,* 383
anti–*Helicobacter pylori,* 875
anti–herpes simplex virus, 1024
anti–*Histoplasma capsulatum,* 813–814
anti-HIV, 448, 448t
antihyaluronidase, 491
anti-interleukin-1, in septic shock, 292
anti–*Legionella pneumophila,* 806
anti-*Leptospira,* 387
anti-lipopolysaccharide, in septic shock, 290, 292
anti-measles, 310
anti-mumps, 423
anti–*Mycoplasma pneumoniae,* 808
anti–*Neisseria gonorrhoeae,* 1013
anti–parvovirus B19, 328
anti–*Rickettsia rickettsii,* 108, 355–356
anti–*Rickettsia typhi,* 389
anti-roseola, 323
anti-rubella, 318
antistreptolysin, 491
anti–*Toxoplasma gondii,* 1115
anti–*Treponema pallidum,* 105, 108, 1021–1022, 1022t
anti-TSST-1, 297
anti–tumor necrosis factor, in septic shock, 292
anti–varicella-zoster virus, 110, 335

Antibody (antibodies) *(Continued)*
anti–*Yersinia pestis,* 384
C gene of, 43–44, 43f
classes of, 44–45, 44t
D genes of, 44
detection of, 99–111
agglutination assays for, 102
bacteria-specific tests for, 104–105, 106t, 108
competitive inhibition assay for, 101, 102f
complement fixation assay for, 102–103
direct sandwich assay for, 101–102
fungus-specific tests for, 106t, 108–109
hemagglutination inhibition assay for, 103
immunoblotting for, 103–104, 104f
in newborn, 100
indirect sandwich assay for, 101–101, 101f
labeled-antibody techniques for, 100–102, 101f, 102f
mycoplasma-specific tests for, 108
neutralization assay for, 103
parasite-specific tests for, 106t–107t, 109–110
particle agglutination inhibition assay for, 102
precipitation assays for, 103
radioimmunoprecipitation assay for, 104
reverse class capture assay for, 101, 102f
Rickettsia-specific tests for, 106t, 108
test panels for, 104, 106t–107t
virus-specific tests for, 107t, 110–111
diversity of, 43–44, 43f
Forssman, 431–432, 431f
in antibody-dependent cellular cytotoxicity, 35f, 44t, 45
in complement activation, 34f, 44t, 45
J genes of, 43–44, 43f
light chain classes in, 45
natural, 32
Paul-Bunnell, 431–432, 431f
primary deficiency of, 1150–1151
structure of, 42–43, 42f, 43f
subclasses of, 44–45, 44t
V genes of, 43–44, 43f
X-linked deficiency of, 1150–1151
Antibody class switching, 42
Antibody test panels, 104, 106t–107t
Antibody-dependent cellular cytotoxicity, 35f, 44t, 45
Anticipatory therapy, vs. prophylactic therapy, 225
Anticomplement immunofluorescence assay, 101, 101f
Anticonvulsants
in meningitis, 647
in tetanus, 694
Anti-deoxyribonuclease B (anti-DNase B) assay, 105
Antidiuretic hormone, syndrome of inappropriate secretion of, in meningitis, 646
Antifungals, 152t, 190–196. *See also specific drugs.*
Antigen(s). *See also* Antibody (antibodies).
detection of, 111–115
bacteria-specific assays for, 112t
fungus-specific assays for, 112t
immunoprecipitation assays for, 115
in sepsis, 288
labeled-antibody techniques for, 111, 113f–115f
parasite-specific assays for, 112t

Antigen(s) *(Continued)*
detection of *(Continued)*
particle agglutination assays for, 111, 115
toxin neutralization assay for, 115
virus-specific assays for, 112t
persistence of, 46
Antigen presentation, 38, 39f
Antigen processing, 37–41, 37f, 39f, 39t, 40t
antigen presentation and, 38, 39f
cytokines in, 40–41, 40t
T-cell activation in, 39–40
T-cell receptors in, 38, 40f
Antigen-presenting cells, 38, 39f
Antihistamines
in common cold, 709, 709t
in otitis media, 755–756
Antihyaluronidase assay, 105
Anti-infective therapy, 147–213. *See also specific drugs and classes of drugs.*
agent selection in, 150, 151t–153t
area under the drug concentration time curve in, 148–149, 149t
combination, 150, 153, 154t
elimination half-life in, 149
ideal agent in, 149–150, 149t, 150f
mechanisms of, 147, 148t
minimum bactericidal concentration in, 148
minimum inhibitory concentration in, 148
monitoring of, 153
pharmaceutics in, 149
pharmacodynamics in, 147–149, 149t, 150f
pharmacokinetics in, 149, 150f
prophylactic, 225–231, 226t, 227t, 228t, 229t–230t
selectivity in, 147, 148t
therapeutics of, 147, 148f, 148t
Antimalarials, 153t, 211–213, 212t, 213t
Antimicrobial susceptibility testing, 75–79, 75t, 78f
agar diffusion in, 75
agar dilution in, 76
broth dilution in, 76
β-lactamase testing in, 76–77
serum bactericidal tests in, 77–78
synergy testing in, 77, 78f
Antimotility agents, in acute enteritis, 917–918, 917t
Antimycobacterials, 152t, 205–208, 206t, 207t, 208t
Antiprotozoal drugs, 152t, 208–209, 209t
Antipyretic therapy, 266, 267t
in bacteremia evaluation, 268–269, 269t
Antiretroviral drugs, 152t, 202–205, 203t–204t, 205t. *See also specific drugs.*
Antistreptolysin O test, 105
Antitoxins, 220–221, 221t
in botulism, 697
in tetanus, 694
Antitussive agents, in common cold, 709, 709t
Antiviral drugs, 152t, 196–202. *See also specific drugs.*
Antiviral susceptibility testing, 90–91
Aphthous ulcer (canker sore)
clinical manifestations of, 730
etiology of, 729
in AIDS, 470
pathogenesis of, 729

Aplastic anemia, in infectious mononucleosis, 434
Aplastic crisis, transient, in erythema infectiosum, 327, 328
Apnea, in pneumonia, 800
Appendectomy, 936
Appendicitis, 923, 931–936. *See also* Abscess, intra-abdominal.
  anatomy in, 932, 933f
  clinical manifestations of, 932–933
  complications of, 936
  computed tomography in, 935–936, 935f
  diagnosis of, 933–935, 934t
  diarrhea in, 932
  differential diagnosis of, 934–935, 934t
  enterobiasis and, 515
  epidemiology of, 931–932
  etiology of, 932
  imaging in, 137, 138f, 139f, 935, 935f
  laboratory evaluation in, 935
  pain in, 932
  pathogenesis of, 932
  pelvic, 934
  perforation with, 936
  physical examination in, 932–933, 933t
  prognosis for, 936
  retroileal, 934
  treatment of, 936
  vs. urinary tract infection, 985
  vs. yersiniosis, 888
Appendix
  anatomy of, 932, 933f
  imaging of, 137, 138f, 139f
  inflammation of. *See* Appendicitis.
Ara-A. *See* Vidarabine.
Arabinosyl hypoxanthine, 199–200
Arbovirus infection, 88t, 673–676, 674f, 676t. *See also specific infections.*
  meningeal, 631, 631t. *See also* Meningitis, viral.
Arcanobacterium haemolyticum infection, pharyngeal, 712t, 713, 716, 718
Area under the drug concentration time curve, 148–149, 149t
Argyll Robertson pupil, in neurosyphilis, 1021
Arthralgia, in Kawasaki syndrome, 481
Arthritis
  blackthorn, 1045
  foreign body, 1045
  in brucellosis, 381
  in erythema infectiosum, 326
  in Kawasaki syndrome, 481
  in mumps, 422
  in rheumatic fever, 488–489, 491
  in rubella, 319
  infectious, 1044–1049
    clinical manifestations of, 1045, 1046t
    complications of, 1049
    culture in, 1047
    diagnosis of, 1045–1047, 1047f
    differential diagnosis of, 1045–1046
    epidemiology of, 1044–1045
    etiology of, 1044, 1044t
    fungal, 1044, 1045
    gonococcal, 1044, 1045, 1046t, 1049
    imaging in, 1047, 1047f
    laboratory evaluation in, 1046–1047
    of hip, 1047
    pathogenesis of, 1045
Arthritis *(Continued)*
  infectious *(Continued)*
    physical examination in, 1045
    prevention of, 1049
    prognosis for, 1049
    treatment of, 1047–1049, 1048t
  reactive. *See* Reactive arthritis.
  septic. *See* Suppurative arthritis.
Arthritis-dermatitis syndrome, 1045
  in gonococcal infection, 541, 542f, 1012
Ascaris lumbricoides, life cycle of, 508–509, 509f
Ascaris lumbricoides infection (ascariasis), 508–510
  clinical manifestations of, 509, 509t
  complications of, 510
  diagnosis of, 509–510, 510f
  epidemiology of, 509
  pathogenesis of, 509, 509f
  treatment of, 510, 510t
Aschoff body, in rheumatic fever, 491
Aseptic technique, 1233
Aspergilloma, 814, 815
Aspergillosis, 814–815
  bronchopulmonary, 814
  culture in, 815
  disseminated, 814
  epidemiology of, 814
  etiology of, 814
  imaging in, 131, 134f
  in AIDS, 452t, 469
  pathogenesis of, 814
  serologic testing in, 108
Aspiration pneumonia, 826–829. *See also* Pneumonia, aspiration.
Aspirin
  in Kawasaki syndrome, 482, 482t, 483
  in rheumatic fever, 491, 492t
  long-term, immunization and, 241t
  Reye's syndrome and, 687–688
Asplenia, 282–283, 1181, 1182t, 1183
  immunization in, 1181, 1184t
Asthma, vs. bronchiolitis, 786
Astrovirus infection, enteric, 898t, 901
Asymmetrical periflexural exanthem. *See* Unilateral laterothoracic exanthem.
Ataxia
  after meningitis, 648
  cerebellar
    acute, in varicella-zoster virus infection, 338
    encephalitis with, 681
Ataxia-telangiectasia, 1154
Atovaquone, 152t
  in babesiosis, 377, 377t
  in malaria, 370, 371t
  in malaria prophylaxis, 373t, 374
  in *Pneumocystis carinii* infection, 826, 826t
Attachment factors, 1, 3t
Attack rate, 12
Atypical mycobacteria. *See at specific mycobacterial species.*
Australia antigen. *See* Hepatitis B surface antigen.
Automated reagin test, 1021–1022, 1022t
Azalide antibiotics, 175–178, 176t
  adverse effects of, 177–178
  dosing for, 177, 178t
  formulation of, 177
  mechanism of action of, 176
  metabolism of, 176–177, 177t
Azidothymidine. *See* Zidovudine.
Azithromycin, 151t, 175–178, 176t, 177t
  dosing for, 178t
  in babesiosis, 377, 377t
  in *Campylobacter jejuni* infection, 890, 890t
  in cat-scratch disease, 346
  in *Chlamydia trachomatis* infection, 1018
  in gonorrhea, 1014t
  in *Haemophilus ducreyi* infection, 1026t
  in otitis media, 754t
  in sinusitis, 765t
Azlocillin, 151t
  dosing for, 159t
  formulations of, 157t
  pathogen susceptibility to, 155t
AZT. *See* Zidovudine.
Aztreonam, 151t, 165–166, 165t, 166t
  dosing for, 166t
  in neonatal sepsis, 1126t
  in osteomyelitis, 1040t
  pathogen susceptibility to, 165t
  probenecid interaction with, 166

B

B cells, 36–37, 36t, 37f, 41–45, 42f, 43f, 44t. *See also* Antibody (antibodies).
  evaluation of, 51, 52t, 54, 54t, 55
  in neonate, 48–49
  properties of, 36–37, 36t, 37f
  regulation of, 45–47
  surface markers of, 36, 36t
B virus infection, 602, 605, 608
Babesia spp., 375
  life cycle of, 375, 376f
Babesia spp. infection (babesiosis), 375–377
  blood smear in, 376, 377f
  clinical manifestations of, 376, 376t
  complications of, 377
  diagnosis of, 376–377, 376t, 377f
  epidemiology of, 20t, 375
  etiology of, 375, 376f
  incubation period of, 376
  pathogenesis of, 375–376
  prevention of, 377
  prognosis for, 377
  transmission of, 375
  treatment of, 377, 377t
Bacampicillin, 151t
Bacillary angiomatosis
  in AIDS, 474
  in cat-scratch disease, 343, 344t, 345, 346
Bacillary peliosis, in cat-scratch disease, 345, 346
Bacille Calmette-Guérin vaccine, 243, 243t, 245t, 246, 417–418, 418f
Bacillus anthracis infection (anthrax), 18t, 551–552
  cutaneous, 551
  immunization against, 245t
  pulmonary, 551
  toxins in, 4t
Bacillus cereus infection, 4t, 16t
Baclofen, in tetanus, 694
Bacteremia, 279–294
  anatomic defects and, 282
  asplenia and, 282
  blood specimen collection in, 60t, 62–63, 62t, 63t

Bacteremia *(Continued)*
burn-related, 282
catheter-related, 281. *See also* Catheter-related infection.
clinical manifestations of, 285
complications of, 293–294, 293t, 294t
culture in, 271, 288
definition of, 279, 280t
epidemiology of, 281, 281t
etiology of, 279, 280t
fever in, 265
imaging in, 288
in cancer patient, 283
in cat-scratch disease, 344t
in hemoglobinopathy, 283
in immunocompromised host, 281–282, 282t
in malignancy, 283
in sickle cell disease, 283, 293–294
microbiologic evaluation in, 288
nosocomial, 1232
occult, 268–274
complications of, 270–272, 270t, 271t, 272t
culture in, 271
fever peak in, 269
follow-up of, 271–272
Haemophilus influenzae type b in, 272, 272t, 293
in children over 8 weeks, 268–270, 269t, 270t, 271t, 272t
in children under 8 weeks, 272–274, 272t, 273f
treatment of, 270–272, 270t, 271t, 272t
WBC count in, 269, 271
pathogenesis of, 283
postsplenectomy, 282–283
prevention of, 294
secondary, 281, 282t
treatment, 289, 291t
WBC count in, 286–287
Bacteria. *See also specific infections.*
classification of, 57, 58t
gram-negative, 57, 58t
gram-positive, 57, 58t
oxygen requirements of, 57, 58t
specimen collection of, 59–66, 60t–62t
Bacterial endocarditis. *See* Infective endocarditis.
Bactericidal test, serum, 77–78
Bacteriocins, 6, 31
Bacteriuria, asymptomatic, 983–984, 989. *See also* Urinary tract infection.
Bacteroides fragilis infection, 923–928. *See also* Abscess, intra-abdominal.
Bacteroides gingivalis. See Porphyromonas gingivalis infection.
Bacteroides melaninogenicus. See Prevotella melaninogenica infection.
Bacteroides spp. infection, bite-wound, 602–608, 603t, 606t, 607t
Baermann technique, in strongyloidiasis, 513
Balanitis, 996
Balanoposthitis, 996
Band keratopathy, in uveitis, 1081
Bannwarth's syndrome, in Lyme disease, 350
Barium enema, in appendicitis, 137, 138f
Barium esophagraphy, in fungal esophagitis, 137, 137f
Bartonella bacilliformis infection (bartonellosis), 18t
Bartonella henselae infection (cat-scratch disease), 343–347, 602
bite-wound, 602–608, 603t, 606t, 607t
clinical manifestations of, 344–345, 345f, 604–605, Plate 9D
complications of, 346
culture in, 346
diagnosis of, 345–346, 605
differential diagnosis of, 346
encephalitis in, 680
epidemiology of, 18t, 343, 602, 603t
etiology of, 343, 344t
imaging in, 345f
in AIDS, 474
lymphadenopathy in, 615, 616
microbiologic evaluation in, 346
ophthalmic, 344–345, 345f
pathogenesis of, 343–344, 604
prevention of, 346
prognosis for, 346
serologic testing in, 346
skin test in, 346
stains for, 346
transmission of, 343
treatment of, 346, 605
Baylisascaris procyonis infection (baylisascariasis), 20t, 510–512, 511f, 511t
Beau's lines, in Kawasaki syndrome, 481
Bed rest, in rheumatic fever, 491
Beef tapeworm infection, 530t, 531
Behavior, in fever evaluation, 264, 265t
Bell's palsy, in Lyme disease, 704
Benzocaine, in stomatitis, 732t
Benzodiazepines, in tetanus, 694
Beta-lactam antibiotics, 151t, 153–157, 155t. *See also* Aztreonam; Cephalosporins; Penicillin(s).
adverse effects of, 156, 160t
clinical indications for, 154–155
desensitization to, 160t
dosing for, 156, 158t–159t
drug interactions with, 156–157, 160t
metabolism of, 155–156, 156t
pharmacokinetics of, 151t, 155–156, 156t
resistance to, 154
spectrum of activity of, 154, 155t
Beta-lactamase testing, 76–77
Bilharziasis. *See Schistosoma* spp. infection (schistosomiasis).
Biliary tract. *See also* Gallbladder; Liver.
ascariasis of, 510
inflammation of, 972–975. *See also* Cholangitis.
Biopsy. *See also* Pathology.
in acute myocarditis, 859
in aspergillosis, 815
in brain abscess, 663
in burn wound infection, 598
in cervical lymphadenopathy, 625
in cholangitis, 974
in encephalitis, 669, 672
in inguinal lymphadenopathy, 619
in lymphadenopathy, 614–615
in osteomyelitis, 1037
in pneumonia, 801
in poststreptococcal glomerulonephritis, 595
Bismuth subsalicylate
in acute enteritis, 917–918, 917t
Bismuth subsalicylate *(Continued)*
in gastritis, 875–876, 876t
in travelers' diarrhea, 907t
Bite-wound infections, 602–608
clinical manifestations of, 604–605, 604f
complications of, 607–608
culture in, 605
diagnosis of, 605
epidemiology of, 602–603
etiology of, 602, 603t
in immunocompromised host, 608
pathogenesis of, 603–604
prevention of, 608, 608t
rabies immune globulin therapy in, 607–608
risk factors for, 604, 608, 608t
severity of, 604
tetanus immunization in, 607
treatment of, 605–607, 606t, 607t
Black dot, in tinea capitis, 556, 557, 557f
Blackflies, 15
Blackheads, 548
Blackwater fever, 368, 372
Bladder carcinoma, *Schistosoma haematobium* in, 29
Blastomyces dermatitidis infection (blastomycosis), 13, 816–817
serologic testing in, 108–109
Blepharitis, 1069–1070, 1070f, 1071f
complications of, 1070, 1071f
culture in, 1070
treatment of, 1070
Blepharospasm, in keratitis, 1064
Blistering distal dactylitis, 549–550, 550f
Blood, collection of, 60t, 62–64, 62t, 63t
for parasites, 80
quantity of, 63
technique of, 63, 63t
timing of, 63
Blood flow, in septic shock, 285
Blood transfusion
donation screening for, 1231t
in cancer-associated infection, 1160
infection after, 1230–1231, 1231t 1232t
Blue dome cyst, 1072–1073, 1072f
Blue dot sign, in epididymitis, 993
Blue macules, 574
Body fluids
bactericidal activity in, 77–78
collection of, 60t, 64
in pathogen transmission, 13
Body lice, 573–574
Boil, 545–547, 546t, 547f
Bone
biopsy of, 61t, 66
infection of, 1034–1043. *See also* Osteomyelitis.
Bone marrow
chloramphenicol-induced aplasia of, 180
examination of
in erythema infectiosum, 328, 329f
in fever of unknown origin, 277
flucytosine toxicity to, 193
hypoplasia of, 98
transplantation of. *See* Transplantation, bone marrow.
Bone scan. *See* Radionuclide scan.
Bordetella pertussis
lymphocytosis-promoting factor of, 94

Bordetella pertussis (Continued)
toxins of, 4t
Bordetella pertussis infection (pertussis syndrome), 4t, 18t, 788–792
catarrhal stage of, 790
clinical manifestations of, 789–791
complications of, 792
convalescent stage of, 791
culture in, 791
diagnosis of, 131, 132f, 791–792
differential diagnosis of, 791
direct fluorescent antibody test in, 791
epidemiology of, 789, 790f
etiology of, 789
imaging in, 131, 132f
immunization against, 245t, 248–249. *See also* Diphtheria, tetanus toxoids, pertussis (DTP) vaccine.
postexposure, 242t
in adult, 791
in neonate, 791
lymphocytosis in, 791
paroxysmal stage of, 790
pathogenesis of, 789, 790t
prevention of, 792
prognosis for, 792
radiography in, 792
treatment of, 792
vs. common cold, 708, 708t
Borrelia burgdorferi infection (Lyme disease), 348–353
age distribution of, 348
carditis in, 857, 858, 860, 861
clinical manifestations of, 349–351, 350t
congenital, 350–351
diagnosis of, 351–352, 351t
differential diagnosis of, 351, 351t
early disseminated manifestations of, 350
early localized manifestations of, 350, Plate 6B
encephalitis in, 680
epidemiology of, 18t, 348–349, 349f
erythema migrans in, 349, 350
etiology of, 348
geographic distribution of, 348, 349f
immunization against, 247, 353
laboratory evaluation of, 351
late manifestations of, 350
meningitis in, 633
meningopolyneuritis in, 350
microbiologic evaluation of, 351–352
neuropathy in, 704
pathogenesis of, 349
prevention of, 353
prognosis for, 352–353
seasonal distribution of, 348
serologic testing in, 108, 351–352
seventh-nerve palsy in, 350
transmission of, 348, Plate 9E
treatment of, 352, 352t
Borrelia hermsii infection (tickborne relapsing fever), 387–388, 388t
Borrelia recurrentis infection (louseborne relapsing fever), 19t, 387–388, 388t
Borrelia vincentii infection, 730
Borreliosis, Lyme. *See Borrelia burgdorferi* infection (Lyme disease).
Botfly infestation, 571, 571f
Botulinum antitoxin, 218t
Botulism. *See Clostridium botulinum* infection (botulism).
Boutonneuse fever, 355t
Bowel, antisepsis regimen for, 231
Brain
abscess of, 657–664. *See also* Abscess, brain.
calcifications in, 130, 131f
imaging of, 126–130, 128f–130f
in rheumatic fever, 491
Brainstem herniation, with lumbar puncture, 659
Branchial cleft cyst, 624
Branhamella catarrhalis. See Moraxella catarrhalis infection.
Breast abscess, in neonate, 1129–1130, 1129t
Breast-feeding
antibiotic therapy during, 1096, 1097t
immunization during, 1096
infection transmission with, 1095–1097, 1095t
Breath sounds, in pneumonia, 800
Brill-Zinsser disease, 388–389, 389t
Bronchiolitis, 784–788
bronchodilator therapy in, 787
chest radiography in, 785, 785f
clinical manifestations of, 784–785, 785f
culture in, 786
diagnosis of, 785–786
differential diagnosis of, 786
epidemiology of, 784
etiology of, 784, 785t
gas exchange assessment in, 786
immunoprophylaxis in, 788, 788t
oxygen therapy in, 788
pathogenesis of, 784
physical findings in, 785
prevention of, 788, 788t
prognosis for, 788
ribavirin in, 787, 787f
treatment of, 786–788, 787f
vs. bronchitis, 779
Bronchiolitis obliterans
in adenovirus infection, 819
in measles pneumonia, 312
Bronchitis, 780–784
acute, 779
epidemiology of, 780
etiology of, 780, 780t
pathogenesis of, 780–781
treatment of, 782–783
chronic, 779
epidemiology of, 780
etiology of, 780, 780t
pathogenesis of, 781
cough in, 782
diagnosis of, 782
epidemiology of, 780
etiology of, 780, 780t
pathogenesis of, 780–782
prevention of, 783–784
vs. bronchiolitis, 779
Bronchoalveolar lavage
in *Pneumocystis carinii* infection, 80
in pneumonia, 801
Bronchodilator therapy, in bronchiolitis, 787
Bronchogenic carcinoma, *Mycobacterium tuberculosis* infection and, 29
Bronchopneumonia, 797. *See also* Pneumonia.
Bronchopulmonary dysplasia, 781, 782
Bronchoscopy
in lung abscess, 839, 840
in pneumonia, 801
in tuberculosis, 406
Bronchospasm
pentamidine-associated, 209
ribavirin-associated, 200
Broth dilution method, in antimicrobial susceptibility testing, 76
Brucella spp. infection (brucellosis), 16t, 379–382
clinical manifestations of, 379, 380t
complications of, 381
diagnosis of, 380–381
differential diagnosis of, 380
epidemiology of, 18t, 379
etiology of, 379
lymphadenopathy in, 617
meningeal, 633
pathogenesis of, 379
prevention of, 381–382
prognosis for, 381
serologic testing in, 381
species in, 379
transmission of, 379
treatment of, 381, 381t
Brudzinski's sign, in meningitis, 638–639
Brugia malayi infection (filariasis), 20t, 518
Bubonic plague, 383–385, 385t, 615, 616. *See also Yersinia pestis* infection (plague).
Buccal cellulitis, 581–585, 585t, Plate 7F. *See also* Cellulitis, head and neck.
Budesonide, in laryngotracheobronchitis, 773–774
Bullae, definition of, 533
Burkitt's lymphoma, Epstein-Barr virus in, 23, 24t, 25
Burns, infection of, 282, 596–601
antibiotics in, 598–599, 599t, 600t
antifungals in, 599
antivirals in, 599
clinical manifestations of, 597–598, 597t
complications of, 600–601
culture in, 65, 598
diagnosis of, 598
epidemiology of, 596
etiology of, 596, 597t
immune globulin in, 599
mortality from, 601
nosocomial, 1223
pathogenesis of, 596–597, 597f
prevention of, 601
prognosis for, 601
specimen collection from, 65
supportive therapy in, 599
surgery in, 598
treatment of, 598–600, 599t, 600t
Burr hole aspiration, in cranial epidural abscess, 665
Bursitis
postinfectious, 1046
vs. infectious arthritis, 1046
Burton's agammaglobulinemia, 1150–1151
Buruli ulcer, 555
Busacca nodules, in uveitis, 1080
Butoconazole, 152t
in vulvovaginal candidiasis, 1006t

C

C2 deficiency, 1153
C3 deficiency, 1153
C6 deficiency, 1153
C7 deficiency, 1153
C8 deficiency, 1153
C9 deficiency, 1153
Cachexin. *See* Tumor necrosis factor.
Calcifications
  brain, 130, 131f
  in tuberculosis, 408, 410f
Calcofluor white stain, 69, 70f, 70t
California encephalitis, 673, 674f
Calitroga americana infestation, 571
Calymmatobacterium granulomatis infection, lymphadenopathy in, 616, 617
Campylobacter jejuni infection (campylobacteriosis), 16t, 17t, 888–890
  clinical manifestations of, 889, 889t
  complications of, 890
  culture in, 890
  diagnosis of, 890
  epidemiology of, 18t, 889, 889f
  foodborne, 908–911, 910t, 911t
  Guillain-Barré syndrome and, 701–702
  in AIDS, 450t, 471
  in day care environment, 1190
  pathogenesis of, 889
  prevention of, 890
  prognosis for, 890
  seagull morphology in, 890
  toxins in, 4t
  transmission of, 888
  treatment of, 890, 890t
Campylobacter pylori. See Helicobacter pylori infection.
Cancer, 23–28
  absolute neutrophil count in, 1158
  bacteremia with, 283
  Chlamydia trachomatis and, 24t, 29
  cytokines in, 1167
  Epstein-Barr virus and, 23–25, 24t, 25t, 428, 435
  fever of unknown origin and, 276t, 277
  granulocyte transfusion n, 1167
  granulocytopenia in, 1158
  Helicobacter pylori and, 24t, 28–29
  hepatitis B virus and, 24t, 26
  hepatitis C virus and, 24t, 26
  human herpesvirus 8 and, 24t, 25–26
  human papillomaviruses and, 24t, 28, 1030
  infection and, 1156–1167, 1157t–1158t
    antibacterial prophylaxis against, 1166
    antibacterial treatment of, 1163–1164, 1165f
    antifungal treatment of, 1164, 1166
    antiviral treatment of, 1166
    bacterial, 1156, 1157t
    blood transfusion and, 1160
    catheter and, 1159
    chemotherapy and, 1159, 1159t
    clinical manifestations of, 1160, 1163
    corticosteroid therapy and, 1158t, 1159–1160
    epidemiology of, 1156
    etiology of, 1157t–1158t
    fever in, 1166
    fungal, 1156, 1157t
    gastrointestinal, 1162f, 1163
    immunomodulating agents and, 1159t, 1160
Cancer *(Continued)*
  infection and *(Continued)*
    leukemia and, 1156, 1158
    lymphoma and, 1158
    mucosal surface antisepsis in, 1166
    otolaryngologic, 1160, 1162f, 1163
    parasitic, 1156, 1158t
    pathogenesis of, 159t, 1156, 1158–1160
    patient isolation in, 1166
    prevention of, 1166–1167
    pulmonary, 1160, 1162f, 1166
    treatment of, 1161f, 1162f, 1163–1166, 1165f
    viral, 1156, 1158t
  lymphadenopathy in, 613, 623
  Mycobacterium tuberculosis and, 24t, 29
  parasites and, 24t, 29
  Pneumocystis carinii infection prophylaxis in, 1167
  polyomaviruses and, 24t, 28
  postexposure varicella-zoster prophylaxis in, 1166–1167
  retroviruses and, 24t, 26–27
  Salmonella paratyphi and, 24t, 29
  Salmonella typhi and, 24t, 29
Cancrum oris, 730, 736, 737
Candida spp. infection (candidiasis)
  abdominal computed tomography in, 137, 139f
  chronic, 562, 562f
  cutaneous manifestations of, 536t, 537–538
  disseminated, neonatal, 1132, 1133
  enzyme assay in, 75
  esophageal, 869–871
    clinical manifestations of, 869–870
    complications of, 871
    culture in, 65
    diagnosis of, 870
    epidemiology of, 869
    prevention of, 871
    prognosis for, 871
    treatment of, 870–871
  host defense against, 561–562
  in AIDS, 452t–453t, 462t, 463, 469, 470, 471, 475
  in septic shock, 281
  magnetic resonance imaging in, 140, 140f
  meningeal, 633
  mucocutaneous, 560–563, 562f
    chronic, 562, 562f, 729
    neonatal, 1132–1133
  neonatal, 562, 1132–1133
  of diaper area, 562
  of hands, 562, 562f
  oral, 562, 728–733
    clinical manifestations of, 729
    complications of, 732
    diagnosis of, 730
    epidemiology of, 728
    etiology of, 728
    neonatal, 1132, 1133
    pathogenesis of, 728
    prevention of, 733
    prognosis for, 732
    supportive treatment of, 731–732, 732t
    treatment of, 731, 731t
  pathogenesis of, 561–562
  penile, 996
  pulmonary, 817
  serologic testing in, 108
Candida spp. infection *(Continued)*
  stool culture in, 65
  treatment of, 562–563
  ultrasonography in, 140, 140f
  urinary tract, 983
  vulvovaginal, 1002, 1003, 1003f, 1005
    clinical manifestations of, 1001, 1001t
    culture in, 61t, 65
    diagnosis of, 1003, 1003f
    epidemiology of, 999
    pathogenesis of, 1000
    physical examination in, 1002
    prognosis for, 1007, 1007t
    treatment of, 1005–1007, 1006t
Capillary leak syndrome, in dengue fever, 393
Capnocytophaga canimorsus infection, 18t, 608
  bite-wound, 602–608, 603t, 606t, 607t
  in sepsis, 283
Capture assay
  for antibody detection, 101, 102f
  for antigen detection, 111, 114f
Carbacephem, 151t
Carbapenems, 166–167, 166t, 167t
Carbenicillin, 151t
  dosing for, 158t
  formulations of, 157t
  pathogen susceptibility to, 155t
Carbuncles, 545–547, 546t
Cardiac tamponade, 864
Cardiothoracic surgery, pericarditis after, 863
Cardiotoxicity
  erythromycin-induced, 178
  quinolone-induced, 185
Carditis, in rheumatic fever, 488, 492
Carey Coombs murmur, in rheumatic fever, 488
Caries, dental, 734
  clinical manifestations of, 737
  complications of, 738
  diagnosis of, 737
  in AIDS, 470
  nursing-bottle, 738
  pathogenesis of, 735
  prevention of, 739–740, 740t
  treatment of, 737
Caroli's disease, 973
Carrier, 1, 12
Carrión's disease, 344t
Case definition, 11
Case-control study, 11
Case-fatality rate, 12
Caspofungin, 152t, 194
Castleman's disease, human herpesvirus 8 in, 26
Cat bite, 602–608. *See also Bartonella henselae* infection (cat-scratch disease); Bite-wound infection.
Catalase, 57
Catheter-related infection, 1246–1251
  antibiotic-lock technique treatment in, 1249
  bacteremia with, 281
  clinical manifestations of, 1247–1248
  complications of, 1249, 1249t
  cuffed catheter and, 1250
  culture for, 62t, 66
  culture in, 1248
  diagnosis of, 1248
  differential diagnosis of, 1248
  epidemiology of, 1247, 1247t

Catheter-related infection *(Continued)*
  etiology of, 1246–1247, 1246t, 1247t
  fungal, 1249
  imaging in, 1248
  in burn injury patient, 601
  in cancer patient, 1159, 1159t
  inline filters and, 1250
  pathogenesis of, 1247, 1247t
  prevention of, 1250, 1250t
  prognosis for, 1250
  recurrence of, 1250
  risk for, 1223t, 1223t
  specimen collection from, 62t, 66
  supportive treatment in, 1249
  treatment of, 1248–1249
    algorithm for, 289f, 291t
Cat-scratch disease, 343–347. *See also Bartonella henselae* infection (cat-scratch disease).
Cavernous sinus thrombosis, with brain abscess, 663
CDC group DF-2. *See Capnocytophaga canimorsus.*
CD4:CD8 ratio, 95
  in AIDS, 444, 444t, 460–461, 461t
CD95/Fas pathway, 46–47
Cecitis, 1163
  vs. appendicitis, 934–935, 935t
Cefaclor, 151t
  dosing for, 164t
  formulations of, 162t
  in group A streptococcal vulvovaginal infection, 1006t
  in otitis media, 754t
  in sinusitis, 765t
  pathogen susceptibility to, 161t
  pharmacokinetics of, 163t
Cefadroxil, 151t
  dosing for, 164t
  formulations of, 162t
  pathogen susceptibility to, 161t
  pharmacokinetics of, 163t
Cefamandole, 151t
  dosing for, 164t
  formulations of, 162t
  pathogen susceptibility to, 161t
  pharmacokinetics of, 163t
Cefazolin, 151t
  dosing for, 164t
  formulations of, 162t
  in bite-wound infection, 606, 606t, 607t
  in burn wound infection, 600t
  in cellulitis, 580t, 585t
  in erysipelas, 580t
  in infective endocarditis, 851t–852t
  in neonatal sepsis, 1126t
  in wound infection, 593t
  pathogen susceptibility to, 161t
  pharmacokinetics of, 163t
Cefdinir, 151t
  in cellulitis, 585t
  in otitis media, 754t
  in sinusitis, 765t
Cefepime, 151t
  dosing for, 164t
  formulations of, 162t
  in brain abscess, 662t
  in burn wound infection, 600t
Cefepime *(Continued)*
  in cranial epidural abscess, 666t
  in ecthyma gangrenosum, 580t
  in hepatic abscess, 967t
  in mediastinitis, 843, 843t
  in subdural empyema, 666t
  in urinary tract infection, 991t
  in wound infection, 593t
  pathogen susceptibility to, 161t
  pharmacokinetics of, 163t
Cefixime, 151t
  dosing for, 164t
  formulations of, 162t
  in gonorrhea, 1014t
  in otitis media, 754t
  in sinusitis, 765t
  in urinary tract infection, 991t
  pathogen susceptibility to, 161t
  pharmacokinetics of, 163t
  probenecid interaction with, 165
Cefonicid, 151t
Cefoperazone, 151t
  dosing for, 164t
  formulations of, 162t
  in cholecystitis, 972, 972t
  in hepatic abscess, 967t
  pharmacokinetics of, 163t
Ceforanide, 151t
Cefotaxime, 151t
  dosing for, 164t
  formulations of, 162t
  in acute pericarditis, 867t
  in *Aeromonas* infection, 891, 891t
  in bite-wound infection, 606, 606t, 607t
  in brain abscess, 661, 662t
  in burn wound infection, 600t
  in cellulitis, 585t
  in cranial epidural abscess, 666t
  in epiglottitis, 776t
  in gonorrhea, 1014t
  in hepatic abscess, 967t
  in infectious arthritis, 1048t
  in infective endocarditis, 851t–852t
  in intra-abdominal abscess, 929t
  in meningitis, 643t, 644, 645t, 646t
  in neonatal sepsis, 1125t, 1126t
  in osteomyelitis, 1040t
  in salmonellosis, 881, 882t
  in sepsis, 291t
  in shunt-related infection, 655t
  in spinal epidural abscess, 667t
  in subdural empyema, 666t
  in tracheitis, 776t
  in typhoid, 884, 884t
  in urinary tract infection, 991t
  in wound infection, 593t
  in yersiniosis, 888, 888t
  pathogen susceptibility to, 161t
  pharmacokinetics of, 163t
Cefotetan, 151t
  dosing for, 164t
  formulations of, 162t
  in gonorrhea, 1014t
  in intra-abdominal abscess, 929t
  in pelvic inflammatory disease, 1015t
  pathogen susceptibility to, 161t
  pharmacokinetics of, 163t
Cefoxitin, 151t
  dosing for, 164t
  formulations of, 162t
  in bite-wound infection, 607t
  in gonorrhea, 1014t
  in intra-abdominal abscess, 929t
  in mediastinitis, 843, 843t
  in pelvic inflammatory disease, 1015t
  pathogen susceptibility to, 161t
  pharmacokinetics of, 163t
Cefpodoxime, 151t
  dosing for, 164t
  formulations of, 162t
  in cellulitis, 585t
  in otitis media, 754t
  in sinusitis, 765t
  in urinary tract infection, 991t
  pathogen susceptibility to, 161t
  pharmacokinetics of, 163t
Cefprozil, 151t
  formulations of, 162t
  in cellulitis, 585t
  in otitis media, 754t
  in sinusitis, 765t
  pathogen susceptibility to, 161t
  pharmacokinetics of, 163t
Ceftazidime, 151t
  dosing for, 164t
  formulations of, 162t
  in bite-wound infection, 607t
  in brain abscess, 662t
  in burn wound infection, 600t
  in cranial epidural abscess, 666t
  in ecthyma gangrenosum, 580t
  in endophthalmitis, 1077t
  in hepatic abscess, 967t
  in infective endocarditis, 851t–852t
  in mediastinitis, 843, 843t
  in meningitis, 643t, 644, 645t
  in neonatal sepsis, 1126t
  in sepsis, 291t
  in shunt-related infection, 655t
  in subdural empyema, 666t
  in urinary tract infection, 991t
  pathogen susceptibility to, 161t, 162t
  pharmacokinetics of, 163t
Ceftibuten, 151t
  dosing for, 164t
  formulations of, 162t
  in otitis media, 754t
  in sinusitis, 765t
  pathogen susceptibility to, 161t
  pharmacokinetics of, 163t
Ceftizoxime, 151t
  dosing for, 164t
  formulations of, 162t
  in gonorrhea, 1014t
  pathogen susceptibility to, 161t
  pharmacokinetics of, 163t
Ceftriaxone, 151t
  dosing for, 164t
  formulations of, 162t
  in acute pericarditis, 867t
  in bite-wound infection, 606, 606t, 607t
  in brain abscess, 661, 662t
  in burn wound infection, 600t
  in cellulitis, 585t

Ceftriaxone *(Continued)*
in cranial epidural abscess, 666t
in epiglottitis, 776t
in gonorrhea, 1013, 1014t
in *Haemophilus ducreyi* infection, 1026t
in infectious arthritis, 1048t
in infective endocarditis, 851t–852t
in intra-abdominal abscess, 929t
in Lyme disease, 352, 352t
in meningitis, 643t, 644, 645t, 646t
in meningococcal meningitis prophylaxis, 225, 228t
in neonatal sepsis, 1125t, 1126t
in occult bacteremia, 271
in osteomyelitis, 1040t
in otitis media, 755t
in pelvic inflammatory disease, 1015t
in sepsis, 291t
in shigellosis, 886, 886t
in shunt-related infection, 655t
in spinal epidural abscess, 667t
in subdural empyema, 666t
in tracheitis, 776t
in typhoid, 884, 884t
in wound infection, 593t
pathogen susceptibility to, 161t
pharmacokinetics of, 163t
phenytoin interaction with, 165
warfarin interaction with, 165
Cefuroxime, 151t
dosing for, 164t
formulations of, 162t
in bite-wound infection, 606, 606t, 607t
in cellulitis, 585t
in otitis media, 754t, 755t
in sepsis, 291t
in sinusitis, 765t
pathogen susceptibility to, 161t
pharmacokinetics of, 163t
Celery stalk appearance
in congenital rubella infection, 1112, 1112f
in syphilis, 141, 145f
Cellophane tape preparation, for *Enterobius vermicularis* collection, 80, 82, 82f, 515
Cellulitis, 578–585. *See also* Wound infection.
aspiration in, 579
culture in, 579, 583
extremity and trunk, 578–581
clinical manifestations of, 578–579, Plate 8A
complications of, 581
diagnosis of, 579, Plate 8B
epidemiology of, 578
etiology of, 578
pathogenesis of, 578
prevention of, 581
prognosis for, 581
treatment of, 579–581, 580t
head and neck, 581–585, 581f
clinical manifestations of, 581f, 582–583, 583f, Plate 7E, Plate 7F
complications of, 584
epidemiology of, 581
etiology of, 581
imaging in, 583, 584f
in sinusitis, 766–767, 767t, 768f, 769t
pathogenesis of, 582
prevention of, 584

Cellulitis *(Continued)*
head and neck *(Continued)*
prognosis for, 584
treatment of, 583–584, 585t
in neonate, 1129–1130, 1129t
periorbital. *See* Cellulitis, head and neck.
peritonsillar, 721. *See also* Abscess, neck.
clinical manifestations of, 724
complications of, 726
diagnosis of, 724–725
treatment of, 726
Central European encephalitis, 676
Cephalexin, 151t
dosing for, 164t
formulations of, 162t
in bite-wound infection, 606, 606t, 607t
in cellulitis, 580t, 585t
in group A streptococcal vulvovaginal infection, 1006t
in infectious arthritis, 1048t
in osteomyelitis, 1040t
in urinary tract infection, 991t
pathogen susceptibility to, 161t
pharmacokinetics of, 163t
Cephalosporins, 151t–152t, 157, 159–165, 161t, 162t. *See also specific drugs.*
adverse effects of, 165
clinical indications for, 160, 163t
dosing for, 163–165, 164t
drug interactions with, 165
first-generation, 151t, 157, 159
formulations of, 162t, 163
fourth-generation, 151t, 159–160
metabolism of, 162–163, 163t
pathogen susceptibility to, 161t
pharmacokinetics of, 162–163, 163t
second-generation, 151t, 159
spectrum of activity of, 157, 159–160, 162t
third-generation, 151t, 159
Cephalothin, 151t
in infective endocarditis, 851t–852t
in neonatal sepsis, 1126t
Cephamycins, 151t
Cephapirin, 151t
Cephradine, 151t
Cercarial dermatitis, 523
Cercopithecine herpesvirus 1 (B virus), 602, 605, 608
Cerebellar ataxia, acute, in varicella-zoster virus infection, 338
Cerebellitis, encephalitis with, 681
Cerebral palsy, maternal chorioamnionitis and, 1085, 1087
Cerebritis, 657, 658. *See also* Abscess, brain.
Cerebrospinal fluid (CSF)
chloride in, 642
collection of, 60t, 64, 66–67, 66t
bleeding after, 640
complications of, 639–640
for parasites, 80
traumatic, 640
C-reactive protein in, 642
culture of, 642
examination of
in cellulitis, 583
in fever evaluation, 265, 288
in herpes simplex encephalitis, 672

Cerebrospinal fluid (CSF) *(Continued)*
examination of *(Continued)*
in HTLV-I infection, 705
in infectious mononucleosis, 431
in meningitis, 288, 639–643, 640t, 642t. *See also* Meningitis, cerebrospinal fluid examination in.
in mumps, 423
in neonatal sepsis, 1124
in poliovirus infection, 700
in rubella, 319
in shunt-related infection, 652, 653–654, 654f
in tuberculosis, 406–407
glucose in, 640, 641t
Gram stain of, 641, 642t
immunoglobulin G in, 100
lactic acid of, 642
polymerase chain reaction testing of, 642
protein in, 640–641, 642t
shunt for, 651–655. *See also* Shunt-related infection.
stains of, 641–642, 642t
white blood cells in, 640, 641t
xanthochromic, 640
Cerumen, removal of, 751, 751f
Cervical lymphadenitis, 619–626, 620f. *See also* Lymphadenitis, cervical.
Cervicitis, 1009, 1010t. *See also* Sexually transmitted infections.
chlamydial, 1017
Cervix
carcinoma of
Chlamydia trachomatis in, 29
human papillomavirus in, 24t, 28, 1030
tuberculosis of, 404
Cestode infection, 525–531. *See also Echinococcus granulosus* infection (echinococcosis); *Taenia solium* infection (cysticercosis).
Chagas' disease, 857, 858–859
Chalazion, 1070, 1071, 1071f
Chancroid, 1025–1026, 1026t
diagnosis of, 618
lymphadenopathy in, 616, 617
Charcot's fever, 275
Charcot's triad, in cholangitis, 973–974
Checkerboard titration method, in antimicrobial synergy testing, 77
Chédiak-Higashi syndrome, 1153
Cheilitis, angular, in candidiasis, 562, 729
Chemical irritants, vs. vulvovaginitis, 1004
Chemokines, in innate immunity, 32, 33t
Chemotherapy. *See also* Cancer.
infection with, 1159, 1159t
Chest radiography, 131–136, 131f–137f
in acute viral myocarditis, 860, 860f
in aspergillosis, 815
in *Aspergillus* infection, 131, 134f
in aspiration pneumonia, 828, 828f
in bacterial pneumonia, 131, 132f
in chickenpox, 335
in *Chlamydia pneumoniae* pneumonia, 812
in *Chlamydia psittaci* pneumonia, 811
in *Chlamydia trachomatis* pneumonia, 810, 810f
in diffuse necrotizing pneumonia, 131, 133f
in echinococcosis, 529, 529f
in empyema, 835–836, 836f

Chest radiography *(Continued)*
in fever of unknown origin, 277
in fungal pneumonia, 131, 134f
in hepatic abscess, 966
in herpes simplex virus infection, 131, 134f
in histoplasmosis, 136, 136f, 137f, 814
in infectious mononucleosis, 131, 131f
in *Legionella pneumophila* infection, 806–807
in lymphocytic interstitial pneumonitis, 136, 136f, 466, 467f
in lymphoid interstitial pneumonitis, 466, 467f
in measles, 310–311, 311f
in murine typhus, 389
in *Mycobacterium tuberculosis* infection, 131, 135f, 136f
in *Mycoplasma pneumoniae* infection, 808, 808f
in necrotizing pneumonia, 131, 133f
in pertussis pneumonia, 131, 132f
in pleural effusion, 835–836, 835f
in pneumococcal pneumonia, 131, 133f
in *Pneumocystis carinii* infection, 465, 465f, 825
in pneumonia, 131, 132f–134f, 801
in *Pseudomonas aeruginosa* infection, 131, 133f
in round pneumonia, 131, 133f
in sepsis, 288
in viral pneumonia, 131, 132f, 134f
Cheyne-Stokes respiration, in poliovirus infection, 700
Chickenpox, 331–341
acute cerebellar ataxia with, 338
aseptic meningitis with, 338–339
chest radiography in, 335
clinical manifestations of, 331–334, 332f, 333f
complications of, 337–339, 338t, 339f
congenital, 1110
culture in, 335
diagnosis of, 334–335, 334t
differential diagnosis of, 334, 334t
encephalitis with, 338–339, 681
epidemiology of, 331
etiology of, 331
hepatitis with, 339
in AIDS, 461, 462t
isolation in, 340
laboratory evaluation in, 334–335
pathogenesis of, 331
perinatal, 1140–1143, 1141f, 1142t
physical examination in, 333
pneumonia with, 338, 339f
postexposure prophylaxis in, 340–341, 340t
prevention of, 339–341
prognosis for, 339
Reye's syndrome with, 339
secondary bacterial infection with, 338
serologic testing in, 335
transmission of, 331
treatment of, 335–337, 336t
vesicles of, 541, 541t
Child abuse, sexually transmitted disease and, 1030–1031, 1030t, 1031t
Chinese liver fluke infection, 522t
Chlamydia pneumoniae infection, 73, 795t, 811–812
Chlamydia psittaci infection (psittacosis), 19t, 810–811
Chlamydia trachomatis infection, 1016–1019
clinical manifestations of, 1017
Chlamydia trachomatis infection *(Continued)*
complications of, 1018–1019
conjunctival, 1055–1058, 1056t, 1057f
corneal, 1063
culture in, 73, 1017–1018
diagnosis of, 1017–120
epidemiology of, 1016–1017
etiology of, 1016
genital, 1016–1019, 1016t, 1017f
in oncogenesis, 29
maternal, 1016t, 1018, 1019, 1088t, 1092t
neonatal, 1019, 1056t, 1057f
pathogenesis of, 1017, 1017f
prevention of, 1019
prognosis for, 1019
pulmonary, 795t, 809–810. *See also* Pneumonia, *Chlamydia trachomatis.*
sexual partner evaluation in, 1018
specimen collection in, 65
systemic, 1027, 1027t
transmission of, 1016, 1019
treatment of, 1016t, 1018
Chloramphenicol, 152t, 179–180, 179t, 180t
adverse effects of, 180
dosing for, 179, 179t
drug interactions with, 180, 180t
formulations of, 180
in acute pericarditis, 867t
in brain abscess, 661
in ehrlichiosis, 361
in infectious arthritis, 1048t
in meningitis, 643t, 645t, 646t
in neonatal sepsis, 1126t
in osteomyelitis, 1040t
in plague, 385t
in rickettsialpox, 391t
in Rocky Mountain spotted fever, 356–357, 356t
in salmonellosis, 881, 882t
in shunt-related infection, 655t
in typhoid, 884, 884t
metabolism of, 179
pathogen susceptibility to, 179, 179t
serum monitoring for, 180
Chloride, in cerebrospinal fluid, 642
Chloroform, in wound myiasis, 571
Chloroquine, 153t, 211–213, 212t
dosing for, 212t
in malaria, 370, 371t
in malaria prophylaxis, 373t, 374
Chloroquine phosphate
in amebiasis, 893t
in hepatic abscess, 967t
Chlorosis, in hookworm infection, 506
Chlortetracycline, 151t
Cholangiocarcinoma, *Opisthorchis* in, 29
Cholangitis, 972–975
biliary decompression in, 975
biopsy in, 974
clinical manifestations of, 973–974
complications of, 975
culture in, 974
diagnosis of, 974–975, 974t
differential diagnosis of, 974, 974t
epidemiology of, 973, 973t
etiology of, 972–973
Kasai procedure and, 973, 973t
Cholangitis *(Continued)*
Oriental, 973
pathogenesis of, 973
physical examination in, 974
prevention of, 975
prognosis for, 975
recurrent, 973
treatment of, 975
Cholecystitis, 970–972
acalculous, 970
calculous, 970
clinical manifestations of, 971
complications of, 972
diagnosis of, 971–972, 971t
differential diagnosis of, 971, 971t
epidemiology of, 970
etiology of, 970
imaging in, 971–972
pathogenesis of, 970–971
prevention of, 972
prognosis for, 972
suppurative, 970
treatment of, 972, 972t
Choledochal cyst, 973
Cholera, 893–895. *See also Vibrio cholerae* infection (cholera).
Cholescintigraphy, 971
Cholesteatoma, in otitis media, 756–757
Chorea, in rheumatic fever, 488, 489, 492
Chorioamnionitis, 1085, 1087. *See also* Maternal infection.
Chorioretinitis, 1080, 1082. *See also* Retinitis.
nosocomial, 1229–1230, 1230t
with congenital toxoplasmosis, 1116
Chronic fatigue syndrome, 497–502
clinical manifestations of, 498–499, 498t
complications of, 502
diagnosis of, 499–501, 499f, 501t
differential diagnosis of, 500, 500t
epidemiology of, 497
etiology of, 497
immune disorders and, 498
in infectious mononucleosis, 434
infectious disease and, 497
pathogenesis of, 497–498
prognosis for, 502
psychological disorders and, 498, 501
treatment of, 501–502
Chronic granulomatous disease, 1153
interferons in, 223
Chronic progressive myelopathy. *See* Tropical spastic paraparesis.
Chvostek's sign, in acute pancreatitis, 982
Cidofovir, 152t
Ciguatoxin, 16t
Cilastatin, with imipenem, 167
Cilia
beating action of, 31
of respiratory tract, 798
Cinchonism, 213
Cinoxacin, 151t
Ciprofloxacin, 151t, 184–187, 185t, 186t
dosing for, 186t
in *Campylobacter jejuni* infection, 890, 890t
in cholera, 894–895, 895t
in gonorrhea, 1013, 1014t
in *Haemophilus ducreyi* infection, 1026t

Ciprofloxacin *(Continued)*
in meningococcal meningitis prophylaxis, 225, 228t
in pelvic inflammatory disease, 1015t
in shigellosis, 886, 886t
in travelers' diarrhea, 907t
in tularemia, 383, 383t
Cirrhosis, 1182t
Citrobacter diversus infection, meningeal, 631. *See also* Meningitis, bacterial.
Citrobacter freundii infection, meningeal, 631. *See also* Meningitis, bacterial.
Clam-digger's itch, 523
Clarithromycin, 151t, 175–178, 176t, 177t
dosing for, 178t
drug interactions with, 178, 179t
in gastritis, 875–876, 876t
in otitis media, 754t
in sinusitis, 765t
Cleft lip, 1182t
Cleft palate, 1182t
Clenched-fist injury, 603, 604. *See also* Bite-wound infection.
Clindamycin, 152t, 187, 187t, 188t
dosing for, 188t
in babesiosis, 377, 377t
in bacterial vaginosis, 1006t
in cellulitis, 580t, 585t
in cholecystitis, 972, 972t
in hepatic abscess, 967t
in impetigo, 545, 546t
in infectious arthritis, 1048t
in intra-abdominal abscess, 929t
in malaria, 370
in mediastinitis, 843, 843t
in neonatal sepsis, 1126t
in osteomyelitis, 1040t
in otitis media, 754t, 755t
in pelvic inflammatory disease, 1015t
in *Pneumocystis carinii* infection, 826, 826t
in sinusitis, 765t
in staphylococcal toxic shock syndrome, 302, 302t
in streptococcal pharyngitis, 717t
in streptococcal toxic shock syndrome, 303
in wound infection, 592, 593t
Clofazimine, 152t
in leprosy, 554, 554t
Clonorchis sinensis infection (clonorchiasis), 20t, 522t
Clostridium botulinum infection (botulism), 16t, 693t, 695–698, 911
antibiotics in, 697
antitoxin in, 697
clinical manifestations of, 696–697, 696t
complications of, 697–698
diagnosis of, 115, 697
differential diagnosis of, 697
electromyography in, 697
epidemiology of, 695–696
etiology of, 695
foodborne, 696, 697, 698
in infant, 696–697, 696t
pathogenesis of, 696
physical examination in, 694f, 696–697
prevention of, 698
prognosis for, 698
Clostridium botulinum infection (botulism) *(Continued)*
suckling mouse assay in, 71
toxin in, 4t, 695
treatment of, 697–698
wound, 696, 697
Clostridium difficile infection
cytotoxin assay in, 71
in day care environment, 1190
toxins in, 4t
Clostridium difficile–associated diarrhea, 187, 912–913, 912f
clinical manifestations of, 912, 913t
complications of, 913
culture in, 913
diagnosis of, 912–913
epidemiology of, 912
lincosamide-induced, 187
metronidazole-induced, 189
pathogenesis of, 912
prevention of, 913
toxins in, 912
treatment of, 913
Clostridium perfringens infection, 16t, 911
deep-tissue, 587–595. *See also* Gangrene, gas (clostridial myonecrosis); Myonecrosis.
toxins in, 4t, 589
Clostridium spp. infection, 923–928. *See also* Abscess, intra-abdominal.
Clostridium tetani infection (tetanus), 692–695, 693t
anticonvulsants in, 694
autonomic dysfunction in, 694–695
bite-wound, 602–608, 603t, 606t, 607t
clinical manifestations of, 693
complications of, 695
diagnosis of, 693–523
differential diagnosis of, 694
epidemiology of, 692
etiology of, 692
immunization against, 245t, 250–251, 695. *See also* Diphtheria, tetanus toxoids, pertussis (DTP) vaccine.
in pregnancy, 238, 695
postexposure, 242t
in burn injury patient, 600–601
neonatal, 588, 692, 693, 694f, 695
nutrition in, 695
opisthotonic posturing in, 693
pathogenesis of, 589, 692–693
prevention of, 695
prognosis for, 695
risus sardonicus in, 693
toxins in, 4t
treatment of, 694–695
trismus in, 693, 694
Clotrimazole, 152t
in oral candidiasis, 731, 731t
in vulvovaginal candidiasis, 1006t
Cloxacillin, 151t
dosing for, 158t
formulations of, 157t
pathogen susceptibility to, 155t
Clue cells, in vulvovaginitis, 1003, 1005f
Clustering, 12
Clutton's joints, in congenital syphilis, 1104
Coats' disease, vs. retinitis, 1083
Coccidioides immitis infection (coccidioidomycosis), 13
in AIDS, 451t, 468
lymphadenopathy in, 613
meningeal, 633
pulmonary, 816
serologic testing in, 109
Cohort study, 11
Cold. *See* Common cold.
Cold agglutinins, 97–98
Cold hemagglutination test, in *Mycoplasma pneumoniae* infection, 808
Colistimethate, 152t
Colistin (polymyxin E), 152t
Colitis
neutropenic. *See* Typhlitis.
pseudomembranous. *See Clostridium difficile*–associated diarrhea.
trichuris, 507, 508
Collagen vascular disease, in fever of unknown origin, 276, 276t
Colon cutoff sign, in acute pancreatitis, 980
Colonization, 1
vs. infection, 6
Colonization resistance, 31
Colony-stimulating factors, therapeutic, 223–224
Colorado tick fever, 19t, 393–394, 394t, 537, 675
Colorectal cancer, *Schistosoma japonicum* in, 29
Coltivirus infection, 393–394, 394t
Comedones, 547–548
Commensal organism, 1, 6. *See also* Normal flora.
Common cold, 707–710
clinical manifestations of, 707–708
complications of, 709–710
diagnosis of, 708–709
differential diagnosis of, 708, 708t
epidemiology of, 707
etiology of, 707, 708t
in international child traveler, 1217
in sinusitis, 762
pathogenesis of, 707
prevention of, 710
prognosis for, 710
transmission of, 707
treatment of, 709, 709t
Common variable immunodeficiency, 1151
Competitive inhibition assay, for antibody detection, 101, 102f
Complement, 32, 32f
alternative pathway of, 32, 32f, 34, 34f
antibody activation of, 34f, 44t, 45
classical pathway of, 32, 32f, 34, 34f
deficiencies of, 1153–1154
evaluation of, 51, 52t, 54, 56
in innate immunity, 34–35, 34f, 34t, 35f
Complement fixation assay, for antibody detection, 102–103
Computed tomography, 127t
in acute pancreatitis, 980
in AIDS encephalopathy, 464, 482f
in appendicitis, 935–936, 935f
in brain abscess, 128f, 659–660, 661f
in candidiasis, 137, 139f
in cat-scratch disease, 345, 345f
in cellulitis, 583, 584f
in central nervous system infection, 126–127, 128f–130f

Computed tomography *(Continued)*
in CMV-related hydrocephalus, 130f
in congenital cytomegalovirus infection, 1108, 1108f
in cysticercosis, 525, 526f
in echinococcosis, 529
in epidural abscess, 664, 665f
in hepatic abscess, 966, 966f
in herpes simplex virus encephalitis, 129f
in intra-abdominal abscess, 925–926, 926f
in lung abscess, 839, 840f
in lymphoid interstitial pneumonitis, 466, 467f
in mastoiditis, 757, 757f
in meningitis, 639, 643
in *Mucor* infection, 131, 134f
in neck abscess, 725, 725f
in necrotizing pneumonia, 134f
in nephritis, 140, 140f
in psoas abscess, 939
in sinusitis, 130, 767, 768, 768f
in splenic abscess, 937
in toxoplasmosis, 1115, 1115f
in tuberculosis, 408, 409f–412f
in urinary tract infection, 988
of abdominal organs, 137, 139f, 140f
Condom catheter, infection with, 996
Condylomata acuminata, 567, 567t, 568f, 1009, 1029–1030, 1029f
vs. vulvovaginitis, 1004
Condylomata lata, 1020, 1020f, 1103
Condylomata plana, 1029
Congenital cytomegalic inclusion disease. *See* Cytomegalovirus (CMV) infection, congenital.
Congenital infection. *See* Intrauterine infection; Maternal infection; Perinatal infection.
Congenital malformations, bacteremia and, 282
Conjunctiva
injection of, in Kawasaki syndrome, 480
normal flora of, 9t
Conjunctivitis
bacterial, 1056t, 1058–1062, 1058t
acute, 1058
chronic, 1058–1059
clinical manifestations of, 1059–1060, 1059f, Plate 9A
complications of, 1061
diagnosis of, 66, 1060, 1060t
discharge in, 1059
epidemiology of, 1059
etiology of, 1055, 1056t
nasolacrimal duct obstruction with, 1061
pathogenesis of, 1059
prevention of, 1061–1062
prognosis for, 1061
purulent, 1059
recurrent, 1059
transmission of, 1059
treatment of, 1060–1061, 1061t
chronic, 1058–1059
in health care providers, 1244
neonatal, 1055–1058
chemical (silver nitrate), 1055, 1056t
Chlamydia trachomatis in, 1019, 1056t, 1057, 1057f
clinical manifestations of, 1055, 1056t, 1057f
complications of, 1057
Conjunctivitis *(Continued)*
neonatal *(Continued)*
Credé prophylaxis in, 1057–1058
diagnosis of, 66, 1055–1056
discharge with, 1055, 1056t, 1057f
epidemiology of, 1055
etiology of, 1055, 1056t
herpes simplex virus in, 1056t
Neisseria gonorrhoeae in, 1011, 1012, 1013–1014, 1014t, 1016, 1056t, 1057, 1057f
pathogenesis of, 1055
prevention of, 1057–1058
transmission of, 1055
treatment of, 1056t, 1057, 1057t
nosocomial, 1229–1230, 1230t
specimen collection in, 62t, 66
viral, 1058–1062, 1058t
acute, 1058
chronic, 1058–1059
clinical manifestations of, 1059–1060, 1060f, 1060t, Plate 9B
complications of, 1061
diagnosis of, 66, 1060, 1060t
discharge in, 1059
epidemiology of, 1059
nonpurulent, 1059
pathogenesis of, 1059
prevention of, 1061–1062
prognosis for, 1061
recurrent, 1059
transmission of, 1059
treatment of, 1061
Conjunctivitis-otitis syndrome, 1059
Consolability, in fever evaluation, 264
Contagious disease, 1
Cooling, in fever, 266
Copper penny lesions, in syphilis, 537
Co-primary case, 12
Cornea
inflammation of, 1063–1068. *See also* Keratitis.
specimen collection from, 62t, 66
ulcer of, 1065, 1064f–1066f
vs. endophthalmitis, 1076, 1076f
Coronary arteries, in Kawasaki syndrome, 484
Coronary artery bypass surgery, in Kawasaki syndrome, 483
Coronavirus infection, 898t, 901
Corticosteroids, 221, 222t
acne with, 548
immunization and, 239t
immunosuppressive effects of, 1159–1160, 1159t
in brain abscess, 663
in cysticercosis, 527
in infectious mononucleosis, 433
in Kawasaki syndrome, 483
in laryngotracheobronchitis, 773–774
in meningitis, 646–647
in otitis media, 756
in rheumatic fever, 491–492, 492t
in septic shock, 290
in trichinellosis, 516–517, 516t
in tuberculosis, 415
in uveitis, 1081–1082
Corynebacterium diphtheriae infection (diphtheria)
false (Vincent's angina), 735, 736, 738t
laryngeal, 712, Plate 7C
Corynebacterium diphtheriae infection (diphtheria) *(Continued)*
neuropathy in, 703
pathogenesis of, 589–590
pharyngeal, 711, 712
clinical manifestations of, 713, Plate 7C
complications of, 718–719
diagnosis of, 715
myocarditis after, 719
neuritis after, 719
pathogenesis of, 712
postexposure prophylaxis for, 719, 719t
prevention of, 719, 719t
pseudomembrane in, 712
treatment of, 718, 718t
Schick test in, 719
toxin in, 4t, 703
Corynebacterium haemolyticum. See Arcanobacterium haemolyticum infection.
Corynebacterium infection
bite-wound, 602–608, 603t, 606t, 607t
cutaneous, 549, 549f
Corynebacterium jeikeium infection, in cancer patient, 283
Corynebacterium vaginalis. See Gardnerella vaginalis infection.
Cough. *See also Bordetella pertussis* infection (pertussis syndrome); Bronchiolitis; Bronchitis.
differential diagnosis of, 763, 763t
in bacterial tracheitis, 777
in bronchitis, 782
in laryngotracheobronchitis, 772
in pertussis syndrome, 790
Counterimmunoelectrophoresis
for antibody detection, 103
for bacterial and fungal antigens, 70
Cowdry type I inclusion bodies, in herpes simplex virus infection, 1024
Coxiella burnetii infection (Q fever), 13, 19t, 390–391, 390t
Coxsackievirus infection
encephalitic, 676–677
meningeal, 631. *See also* Meningitis, viral.
vesicles of, 541, 541f, 541t
Cranberry juice, in urinary tract infection prevention, 991
C-reactive protein, 35, 97, 97t
in cerebrospinal fluid, 642
in neonatal sepsis, 1123–1124
in osteomyelitis, 1037, 1041, 1042
Credé prophylaxis, 1057–1058
Cremasteric reflex, in epididymitis, 993
Creutzfeldt-Jakob disease, 685–687, 686t
Croup. *See* Laryngotracheobronchitis.
Cryotherapy, in human papillomavirus infection, 568, 1030
Cryptococcus neoformans infection (cryptococcosis)
epidemiology of, 19t
in AIDS, 451t–452t, 462t, 469, 475
India ink preparation in, 69, 69f, 69t
meningeal, 633
pulmonary, 815–816, 816f
Cryptosporidium parvum infection, 15, 17t, 903t, 904–906, 904f
acid-fast stains in, 82–83

Cryptosporidium parvum infection *(Continued)*
clinical manifestations of, 905
diagnosis of, 905–906
in AIDS, 472, 473, 904, 904f
in day care environment, 1190–1191
pathogenesis of, 904–905, 904f
treatment of, 903t, 906
Ctenocephalides felis, in cat-scratch disease, 343
Culex spp.
in Japanese encephalitis, 676
in St. Louis encephalitis, 673
in Venezuelan equine encephalitis, 676
in West Nile virus infection, 675
in Western equine encephalitis, 673–674
Culiseta spp., in Eastern equine encephalitis, 674–675
Culture, 72–75. *See also at specific infections.*
anaerobic glove box for, 73
colony-count streaking method for, 72, 72f
four-quadrant streaking method for, 72, 72f
in viral infection, 84, 89, 89f
incubation period for, 72
incubation temperature for, 72
laked blood media in, 73
media for, 72, 72t, 73–74, 74t
of anaerobic organisms, 72–73
of chlamydiae, 73
of fungi, 74–75, 74t, 75f
of mycobacteria, 73–75, 74t, 75f
of mycoplasmas, 73
surveillance, 10
Cutaneous larva migrans, 20t, 504, 505, 569–570, 570f
treatment of, 506t, 570
Cyanobacterium-like body. *See Cyclospora cayetanensis* infection.
Cyanosis, in pneumonia, 800
Cycloserine, 152t
Cyclospora cayetanensis infection, 903t, 904–906
clinical manifestations of, 905
diagnosis of, 905
pathogenesis of, 905
treatment of, 903t, 906
Cyst(s)
branchial cleft, 624
choledochal, 973
hydatid, 527–530, 966, 968, 969t. *See also Echinococcus granulosus* infection (echinococcosis).
thyroglossal, 624
Cystic fibrosis, 1182t
bronchitis-bronchiolitis in, 781–782
treatment of, 782–783, 783t, 784t
Cystic hygroma, 624
Cysticercosis, 525–527. *See also Taenia solium* infection (cysticercosis).
Cystitis, 983–991. *See also* Urinary tract infection.
Cytocentrifugation, for Gram stain, 66
Cytochrome-*c*-oxidase, 57
Cytokine(s)
in antigen processing, 40–41, 40t
in cancer patient, 1167
in immune response, 36
in meningitis, 636–637, 636f
in respiratory tract infection, 798
in septic shock, 284
therapeutic, 221–224, 223t
Cytokine storm, 38
Cytomegalovirus (CMV) infection
computed tomography in, 130f
congenital, 1107–1109
clinical manifestations of, 1108, 1108f, 1108t
diagnosis of, 1108
epidemiology of, 1107
in hospitalized patients, 1109
pathogenesis of, 1107–1108, 1107f
prevention of, 1108–1109
treatment of, 1108
cutaneous eruptions in, 536
diagnosis of, 88t, 89, 90f
esophageal, 870, 871
hydrocephalus in, 130f
in AIDS, 463, 470, 472, 473
in burn injury, 596, 598, 599
in day care environment, 1190
in situ hybridization assay in, 121f
lymphadenopathy in, 612
maternal, 1088t, 1089t, 1092t, 1096
owl eyes in, 90
retinal, 1082, 1083, 1084
serologic testing in, 110
shell vial assay in, 89, 90f
vs. infectious mononucleosis, 430
Cytomegalovirus immune globulin, 218t, 220
Cytopathic (cytoproliferative) reaction, 116, 118f, 118t
Cytoplasmic granularity, 116, 119t

D

D cells, in gastritis, 873
Dacryocystitis, 1072–1073, 1072f
Dactylitis
distal, blistering, 549–550, 550f
tuberculous, 403
Dalfopristin-quinupristin, 151t, 172–175, 173t, 174t, 175t
Dapsone, 152t
in leprosy, 554, 554t
in *Pneumocystis carinii* infection, 826, 826t
Dark-field examination, in syphilis, 65, 68, 68f
Day care environment
exclusion from, 1191, 1192t
infections in, 1187–1193
blood transmission of, 1188, 1188t, 1191
Campylobacter jejuni in, 1190
Clostridium difficile in, 1190
contact transmission of, 1188, 1188t, 1191
Cryptosporidium in, 1190–1191
cytomegalovirus in, 1190
education about, 1192–1193
gastrointestinal transmission of, 1187–1188, 1188t, 1190–1191
Giardia lamblia in, 1190
group A *Streptococcus* in, 1189, 1191
Haemophilus influenzae type b in, 1189
hepatitis A virus in, 1190
hepatitis B virus in, 1191
hepatitis C virus in, 1191
human immunodeficiency virus in, 1191
immunization against, 1192, 1193t
lice, 1191
management of, 1191–1192, 1192t
Neisseria meningitidis in, 1189
Day care environment *(Continued)*
infections in *(Continued)*
patterns of, 1189, 1189t
postexposure prophylaxis in, 1191–1192
prevention of, 1191, 1192–1193
respiratory transmission of, 1187, 1188t, 1189–1190
risk factors for, 1188–1189
rotavirus in, 1190
saliva transmission of, 1188, 1188t, 1191
Salmonella in, 1190
Sarcoptes scabiei in, 1191
Shigella in, 1190
Streptococcus pneumoniae in, 1189
transmission of, 1187–1188, 1187t
urine transmission of, 1188, 1188t, 1191
vaccine-preventable, 1191
varicella-zoster virus in, 1190
viral, 1189–1190
written policy on, 1193
planning for, 1193
ddC. *See* Zalcitabine.
ddI. *See* Didanosine.
Dead-end host, 15
Débridement
in bite-wound infection, 605
in burn injury, 598
in necrotizing fasciitis, 592, 592f
Decongestants
in common cold, 709, 709t
in otitis media, 755–756
Decubitus ulcers, 550–551, 551f
Deer tick
in ehrlichiosis, 359, 361f, Plate 9E
in Lyme disease, 348, Plate 9E
DEET, 17, 374
in babesiosis prevention, 377
in malaria prevention, 374
Definitive host, 15
Dehydroemetine
in amebiasis, 893t
in hepatic abscess, 967t
Delavirdine, 152t, 203t, 205t
in HIV infection, 456, 457t, 459t
Delta hepatitis. *See* Hepatitis D virus infection.
Demeclocycline, 151t, 180–182, 181t, 182t
adverse effects of, 182, 182t
dosing for, 181–182, 182t
drug interactions with, 182, 182t
pharmacokinetics of, 181, 181t
Demodex infestation, 573
Dendritic cells, 35–36
Dengue fever, 19t, 392–393, 392t
Dental infection, 734–740
cellulitis with, 582, 583, 585t
clinical manifestations of, 737
complications of, 738–739, 739f
diagnosis of, 737, 737f
epidemiology of, 734–735
etiology of, 734
in dry socket syndrome, 739
pathogenesis of, 735–737, 736f
periapical, 736, 737, 737f
complications of, 739, 739f
treatment of, 738
prevention of, 739–740, 740t
radiography in, 737, 737f

Dental infection *(Continued)*
treatment of, 737–738, 738t
vs. lymphadenopathy, 624
Depression, in chronic fatigue syndrome, 498, 499, 501
Deprivation amblyopia, in keratitis, 1067
Dermacentor andersoni, 15, 21t
in Colorado tick fever, 393, 675
in Rocky Mountain spotted fever, 354
in tularemia, 382
Dermacentor variabilis, 15, 21t
in Rocky Mountain spotted fever, 354
in tularemia, 382
Dermanyssidae infestation, 573
Dermatitides, scaling, 1182t
Dermatobia hominis infestation, 571, 571f
Dermatophyte infections
of non-hair-bearing skin, 558–560, 559f, 559t, 560f, 561t
of scalp, 556–558, 556t, 557f, 558t
potassium hydroxide preparation for, 69, 69t, 70f, 557
Dermatophyte test medium (DTM), for tinea capitis diagnosis, 557
Descriptive study, 11
Desensitization
for animal antisera, 221, 221t
for penicillin, 160t
Dexamethasone
in cysticercosis, 527
in endophthalmitis, 1077t
in laryngotracheobronchitis, 773
in meningitis, 636–637
Diabetes mellitus, 1183t
immunization in, 241t
with congenital rubella infection, 1112
Diagnosis
imaging in, 126–146. *See also specific imaging modalities.*
microbiology in, 57–79. *See also at* Specimen.
parasitology in, 80–83, 81t, 82f, 83f
pathology in, 116–124. *See also* Pathology.
serology in, 99–115. *See also* Antibody (antibodies); Antigen(s).
virology in, 84–91, 85t–86t, 87t, 88t, 89f, 90f
Dialysis, infection with, 1230, 1230t
Diapedesis, 33
Diaper dermatitis, *Candida* in, 562, 563
Diarrhea
acute. *See* Enteritis.
chronic
in *Cryptosporidium parvum* infection, 903t, 904–906, 904f
in *Cyclospora cayetanensis* infection, 903t, 904–906
in *Dientamoeba fragilis* infection, 902, 903t, 904
in *Escherichia coli* infection, 906–908, 906t, 907t
in giardiasis, 901–902, 903t
in *Isospora belli* infection, 903t, 904–906
in microsporida infection, 903t, 904–906
Clostridium difficile–associated. *See Clostridium difficile*–associated diarrhea.
in appendicitis, 932
in measles, 312
lincosamide-induced, 187
Diarrhea *(Continued)*
travelers', 906–908, 906t, 907t, 1216–1217, 1216t. *See also* Travelers' diarrhea.
Dicloxacillin, 151t
dosing for, 158t
formulations of, 157t
in bite-wound infection, 606, 606t, 607t
in cellulitis, 580t, 585t
in infectious arthritis, 1048t
in osteomyelitis, 1040t
pathogen susceptibility to, 155t
Didanosine, 152t, 203t, 205t
in HIV infection, 456, 457t, 458t, 460t
Dientamoeba fragilis infection, 515, 902, 903t, 904
Dietary precautions, for international travel, 1214–1215, 1215t
Diethylcarbamazine, 153t
in filariasis, 518
DiGeorge syndrome, 1152
Diiodohydroxyquin. *See* Iodoquinol.
Diloxanide furoate, in amebiasis, 893, 893t
Dimercaptosuccinic acid scan, 987–988, 987f
Diphenhydramine elixir, in stomatitis, 732t
Diphenoxylate, in acute enteritis, 917t, 918
Diphtheria, 589–590, 703. *See also Corynebacterium diphtheriae* infection (diphtheria).
Diphtheria, tetanus toxoids, pertussis (DTP, DTaP) vaccine, 233t, 235t–236t, 245t, 246, 248–249
for international travel, 244t, 1211
in pregnancy, 238
postexposure, 242t
Diphtheria antitoxin, 218t
Diphyllobothrium latum (diphyllobothriasis), 20t, 530, 530t
Dipylidium caninum infection (dipylidiasis), 20t, 530–531, 530t
Direct sandwich assay
for antibody detection, 101–102, 102f
for antigen detection, 111, 113f
Dirithromycin, 151t
Discitis. *See* Diskitis.
Disease, pathogenesis of, 1, 2f. *See also at specific infections.*
Disinfection, 1239–1240, 1239t
Diskitis, 1051–1053
clinical manifestations of, 1051
complications of, 1053
culture in, 1052
diagnosis of, 1051–1053, 1052f, 1053f
differential diagnosis of, 1051–1052
epidemiology of, 1051
etiology of, 1051
imaging in, 1052–1053, 1052f, 1053f
log roll test in, 1051
pathogenesis of, 1051
prognosis for, 1053
straight leg raise test in, 1051
treatment of, 1053
Disseminated intravascular coagulation (DIC), purpura in, 539t, 540
DMSA (^{99m}Tc dimercaptosuccinic acid) scan, 987–988, 987f
DNA microarray assay, 123
organism-specific, 124
Dobutamine, in septic shock, 292t
Dog bite, 602–608. *See also* Bite-wound infection.
Dog tapeworm infection, 530–531, 530t
Dog tick
in Rocky Mountain spotted fever, 354
in tularemia, 382
Döhle bodies, 93
in infectious mononucleosis, 429
Domoic acid poisoning, 911
Donovan bodies, 1026
Donovanosis, 616, 617, 1026–1027, 1027t
Dopamine, in septic shock, 292t
Doppler ultrasonography, transcranial, 130
Douglas, pouch of, 923
Doxycycline, 151t, 180–182, 181t, 182t
adverse effects of, 182, 182t
dosing for, 181–182, 182t
drug interactions with, 182, 182t
in acne vulgaris, 548–549
in brucellosis, 381, 381t
in *Chlamydia trachomatis* infection, 1018
in cholera, 894–895, 895t
in donovanosis, 1026–1027
in ehrlichiosis, 361
in gonorrhea, 1013, 1014t
in Lyme disease, 352, 352t
in malaria, 370
in malaria prophylaxis, 373t, 374
in murine typhus, 389, 389t
in pelvic inflammatory disease, 1015t
in relapsing fever, 388t
in rickettsialpox, 391t
in Rocky Mountain spotted fever, 356–357, 356t
in *Yersinia pestis* prophylaxis, 385t
pathogen susceptibility to, 181t
pharmacokinetics of, 181, 181t
Dracunculus medinensis infection (dracunculiasis), 20t
Dressing, in burn injury, 598
Droplets, in pathogen transmission, 13
Drotrecogin alfa, in septic shock, 292–293
Drug(s). *See also specific drugs.*
antibiotic, 153–190. *See also* Antibiotics *and specific drugs.*
antifungal, 152t, 190–196
antimalarial, 153t, 211–213, 212t, 213t
antiretroviral, 152t, 202–205, 203t–204t, 205t
antiviral, 152t, 196–202
eosinophilia with, 96, 96t
lymphadenopathy with, 613
nosocomial infection and, 1223, 1223t
Stevens-Johnson syndrome/toxic epidermal necrolysis and, 539
Drug eruption, vs. roseola, 323
Drug interactions
with abacavir, 205t
with acyclovir, 198
with albendazole, 210
with amantadine, 202
with aminoglycoside antibiotics, 171–172, 171t
with amprenavir, 205t
with antiretroviral drugs, 205t
with cephalosporin antibiotics, 165
with chloramphenicol, 180, 180t
with delavirdine, 205t
with didanosine, 205t
with efavirenz, 205t
with ethambutol, 208t

Drug interactions *(Continued)*
with fluconazole, 194, 194t
with flucytosine, 193, 193t
with foscarnet, 199
with griseofulvin, 195, 195t
with indinavir, 205t
with isoniazid, 208t
with ketoconazole, 196
with β-lactam antibiotics, 156–157, 160t
with lamivudine, 205t
with linezolid, 175, 175t
with macrolide antibiotics, 178, 179t
with mebendazole, 210
with metronidazole, 189, 189t
with nelfinavir, 205t
with nevirapine, 205t
with penicillin, 156–157, 160t
with praziquantel, 211
with quinine, 213
with quinupristin-dalfopristin, 175, 175t
with rifampin, 208t
with rimantadine, 202
with ritonavir, 205t
with saquinavir, 205t
with stavudine, 205t
with thiabendazole, 210
with trimethoprim-sulfamethoxazole, 184
with vancomycin, 175, 175t
with vidarabine, 200
with zalcitabine, 205t
with zidovudine, 205t
Drug rash, vs. erythema infectiosum, 328
Drug reaction, in AIDS, 475, 476t
Dry socket syndrome, 739
d4T. *See* Stavudine.
DTP. *See* Diphtheria, tetanus toxoids, pertussis (DTP) vaccine.
Dubos Tween albumin broth, 74
Duncan's syndrome, 427–428
Dust mask, 13
Dyclonine HCl, in stomatitis, 732t
Dysentery, 879–893. *See also* Diarrhea; Enteritis.
Aeromonas, 890–891, 891t
Campylobacter, 888–890, 889f, 889t, 890t
Entamoeba histolytica, 891–893, 892t, 893t
nontyphoidal, 879–882, 880f, 880t, 882t
Salmonella typhi, 882–885, 883t, 884t
Shigella, 885–887, 885t, 886t
Trichuris trichiuria, 508
Yersinia, 887–888, 887t, 888t
Dyspepsia
nonulcer, 872, 876
ulcer. *See* Gastritis.
Dysrhythmias, erythromycin-induced, 178

E

Eagle effect, 303, 592
Ear
aminoglycoside toxicity to, 170–171
cerumen removal from, 751, 751f
erythromycin toxicity to, 178
infection of. *See* Otitis media.
normal flora of, 9t
specimen collection from, 62t, 66
tuberculosis of, 404
Eastern equine encephalitis, 674–675, 674f
Eaton agent. *See Mycoplasma pneumoniae.*
Ecchymoses, definition of, 533
Echinocandins, 194
Echinococcus granulosus, life cycle of, 528, 528f
Echinococcus granulosus infection (echinococcosis), 527–530
chest radiography in, 529, 529f
clinical manifestations of, 528–529, 528t
complications of, 530
diagnosis of, 529, 529f
epidemiology of, 20t, 527–528
etiology of, 527, 528t
pathogenesis of, 528, 528f
prevention of, 530
prognosis for, 530
serologic testing in, 109
specimen collection in, 81
surgical therapy of, 530
treatment of, 529–530, 529t
Echinococcus multilocularis infection, 20t, 528, 528t, 529, 529t, 530. *See also Echinococcus granulosus* infection (echinococcosis).
Echocardiography, 136–137
in acute myocarditis, 859
in infective endocarditis, 849–850, Plate 8D
in Kawasaki syndrome, 482, 483
in pericarditis, 865, 866f
in rheumatic fever, 491
Echovirus infection
encephalitic, 676–677
exanthem in, 536t, 537
meningoencephalitic, 677
Ecthyma, 578
Ecthyma gangrenosum, 286, 540, 578–579
purpura in, 539t, 540
treatment of, 579, 580t
Ectopic pregnancy, *Chalmydia trachomatis* infection and, 1019
Eczema herpeticum, 541, 564–565, 565f, 566
vs. chickenpox, 334
Eczema vaccinatum, 334
Edema
presternal, in mumps, 421, 422f
pulmonary, 1182t
in malaria, 372
subcutaneous, in *Onchocerca volvulus* infection, 518
with Ludwig's angina, 584
Edema toxin, in anthrax, 551
Efavirenz, 152t, 203t, 205t
in HIV infection, 456, 457t, 459t, 460t
Ehrlichia spp. infection (ehrlichiosis), 355t, 359–362, 360t
culture in, 361
epidemiology of, 19t, 359
etiology of, 359, 360f, 361f
geographical distribution of, 359
granulocytic, 359, 360f
monocytic, 359, 360f
morulae in, 360f, 361
pathogenesis of, 359–360
prevention of, 362
prognosis for, 362
seasonal distribution of, 359
vs. Rocky Mountain spotted fever, 355
Eikenella corrodens infection, bite-wound, 602–608, 603t, 606t, 607t
Electrocardiography
in acute myocarditis, 859
in pericarditis, 864, 865f
Electrocautery, for warts, 568
Electroencepahlography, in rubella, 319
Electroimmunodiffusion assay, for antibody detection, 103
Electrolytes, in septic shock, 287
Electromyography, in botulism, 697
Electron microscopy, 119
in viral infection, 90, 90f
Elementary body, in *Chlamydia trachomatis* infection, 1017, 1017f
Elephantiasis, 518
Elimination half-life, 149
ELISA. *See* Enzyme immunoassay.
Empyema, 832–837
chest radiography in, 835–836, 836f
clinical manifestations of, 834
complications of, 837
diagnosis of, 834–837
epidemiology of, 833
etiology of, 832–833, 833t
pathogenesis of, 834
prognosis for, 837
subdural, 657, 664–665, 665f, 666t
in meningitis, 648
in sinusitis, 767–769
treatment of, 837
Empyema necessitatis, 837
Enanthem. *See also* Exanthem.
in measles, 306, 308, 535, 536t, Plate 3B
in rubella, 317
Encephalitis, 669–688
adenoviral, 682
amebic, granulomatous, 632
arbovirus, 673–676, 674f, 676t
bacterial, 669, 670t
California, 673, 674f
Colorado tick fever, 675
cysticercosis, 526, 526t
diagnosis of, 669, 670t, 671t
differential diagnosis of, 669, 670t
Eastern Equine, 674–675, 674f
enterovirus, 676–677
herpes simplex virus, 670–673
clinical manifestations of, 671, 671t
computed tomography in, 129f
diagnosis of, 672
epidemiology of, 671
etiology of, 670–671
pathogenesis of, 671
prevention of, 673
prognosis for, 672–673, 672t
treatment of, 672, 672t
HIV, 683–684
in cat-scratch disease, 680
in human herpesvirus 6 infection, 681
in infectious mononucleosis, 428, 431
in Lyme disease, 680
in Rocky Mountain spotted fever, 357, 681
in varicella-zoster virus infection, 338–339, 338t
influenza, 682
Japanese, 244t, 253t, 255, 676, 676t
lymphocytic choriomeningitis virus, 677
measles, 307, 311, 312–313, 681–682, 684–685, 684f

Encephalitis *(Continued)*
mumps, 421, 424, 682
prognosis for, 669–670
rabies, 678–680
clinical manifestations of, 678
complications of, 680
diagnosis of, 678, 680
epidemiology of, 678, 679f
pathogenesis of, 678
prevention of, 680
prognosis for, 680
treatment of, 680
rubella, 319, 682
progressive, 685
St. Louis, 673, 674f
symptoms and signs of, 669
tickborne, 676, 676t
treatment of, 669, 670t
tuberculous, 680
varicella, 681
Venezuelan equine, 675–676, 676t
viral, 669, 670t
West Nile virus, 675
Western equine, 673–674, 674f
zoster, 681
Encephalocele, 1182t
Encephalopathy
HIV, 463–465, 464f, 683–684
JC virus, 685
rubella, 319
spongiform, 685–687, 686t
with *Salmonella typhi* infection, 884
Endemic disease, 12
Endocardial fibroelastosis, mumps virus in, 424
Endocarditis, 282, 1182t
bacterial. *See* Infective endocarditis.
gonococcal, 1014t
in cat-scratch disease, 344t
natural valve. *See* Native valve endocarditis.
Endocervicitis, 1009, 1010t. *See also* Sexually transmitted infections.
Endometrium, tuberculosis of, 404
Endophthalmitis, 1074–1078
classification of, 1074, 1074t
clinical manifestations of, 1075–1076, 1075f, 1076f
complications of, 1078
culture in, 1077, 1078
diagnosis of, 1076–1077, 1076f
differential diagnosis of, 1076, 1076f
endogenous, 1074, 1075–1076, 1077, 1078
prevention of, 1078
epidemiology of, 1074
etiology of, 1074, 1075t
exogenous, 1074
fungal, 1078
imaging in, 1077
nosocomial, 1229–1230, 1230t
pathogenesis of, 1074–1075
physical examination in, 1076, 1076f
postoperative, 1074, 1075, 1075f
prevention of, 1078
posttraumatic, 1074, 1075
prevention of, 1078
prognosis for, 1078
retinal detachment with, 1078
treatment of, 1077–1078, 1077t
Endoscopic retrograde cholangiopancreatography, in acute pancreatitis, 980
Endostreptosin, 594
Endothelial cells, in innate immunity, 32, 33t
Endotoxins, 3, 4t, 284
in meningitis, 636
in septic shock, 284
Enoxacin, 151t
in gonorrhea, 1014t
Entamoeba histolytica infection (amebiasis), 17t, 891–893
clinical manifestations of, 892, 892t
complications of, 893
diagnosis of, 892
encephalitic, 632
epidemiology of, 892
in AIDS, 472
meningoencephalitic, 632
pathogenesis of, 892
prevention of, 893
prognosis for, 893
serologic testing in, 109
transmission of, 891–892
treatment of, 892–893, 893t
Enteritis, acute, 4t, 878–918
absorbent therapy in, 917–918, 918t
dysenteric, 879–893
Aeromonas in, 890–891, 891t
Campylobacter in, 888–890, 889f, 889t, 890t
Entamoeba histolytica in, 891–893, 892t, 893t
nontyphoidal, 879–882, 880f, 880t, 882t
Salmonella typhi in, 882–885, 883t, 884t
Shigella in, 885–887, 885t, 886t
Yersinia in, 887–888, 887t, 888t
etiology of, 878, 878t, 879t
fluid therapy in, 916–917, 916t
hemolytic uremic syndrome and, 913–916. *See also* Hemolytic uremic syndrome.
in AIDS, 450t, 471
nosocomial, 1225–1227, 1226t
diagnosis of, 1227
etiology of, 1226, 1226t
prevention of, 1227
pathogenesis of, 878–879
supportive treatment in, 916–918, 916t, 917t
toxigenic, 893–898
Escherichia coli in, 895–898, 896t, 897t
Vibrio cholerae in, 893–895, 894t, 895t
tuberculous, 403–404
viral, 898–901
adenovirus in, 898t, 900
astrovirus in, 898t, 901
coronavirus in, 898t, 901
Norwalk virus in, 898t, 900–901
rotavirus in, 898–900, 898t, 899f
vs. urinary tract infection, 985
waterborne, 909, 909t
Enterobacter infection
in sepsis, 279
in septic shock, 281
meningeal, 630, 630t. *See also* Meningitis, bacterial.
Enterobius vermicularis infection (enterobiasis, pinworms), 514–515
cellophane tape preparation in, 80, 82, 82f, 515
clinical manifestations of, 514–515, 514t
treatment of, 515, 515t
Enterobius vermicularis infection (enterobiasis, pinworms) *(Continued)*
vulvovaginal
clinical manifestations of, 1001, 1001t
diagnosis of, 1003
epidemiology of, 999
pathogenesis of, 1000
physical examination in, 1002
treatment of, 1005, 1006t, 1007
Enterococcus spp. infection
cardiac, 845, 846. *See also* Infective endocarditis.
in sepsis, 279
in septic shock, 281
intra-abdominal, 923–928. *See also* Abscess, intra-abdominal.
urinary tract, 983, 983t. *See also* Urinary tract infection.
Enterocolitis, neutropenic, 1163. *See* Typhlitis.
Enterocytozoon bieneusi infection, in AIDS, 472
Enterotest (string test), 80–81
Enterotoxins, 5
Enterovirus infection, 676–677. *See also* Coxsackievirus infection; Echovirus infection; Poliovirus infection.
clinical manifestations of, 677
diagnosis of, 88t, 677
epidemiology of, 676
maternal, 1088t, 1091
meningeal, 631, 631t. *See also* Meningitis, viral.
oral, 728
epidemiology of, 728
pathogenesis of, 729
pathogenesis of, 676, 729
perinatal, 1135t, 1136t, 1143–1146
clinical manifestations of, 1144–1145, 1144t
complications of, 1146
culture in, 1145
cutaneous manifestations of, 1144, Plate 5B
diagnosis of, 1145–1146, 1145t
differential diagnosis of, 1145, 1145t
epidemiology of, 1144
fever in, 1144
pathogenesis of, 1144
pathology of, 1145–1146
physical examination, 1145
polymerase chain reaction in, 1145
prevention of, 1146
prognosis for, 1146
sepsis-like syndrome in, 1144
treatment of, 1146
prevention of, 677
prognosis for, 677
pulmonary, 822
treatment of, 677
Entropion, in trachoma conjunctivitis, 1063
env, of HIV, 437, 439t
Environment, 12f, 13–22
food, 15, 16t, 17t
soil, 13, 14t
vector, 15, 17, 18t–20t, 21f, 21t, 22, 22t
water, 13–15, 14f, 15t
zoonotic, 15, 17, 18t–20t, 21f, 21t, 22t
Enzootic cycle, 12
Enzootic disease, 12
Enzyme immunoassay (enzyme-linked immunosorbent assay)
for antibody detection, 100

Enzyme immunoassay (enzyme-linked immunosorbent assay) *(Continued)*
for antigen detection, 111, 114f
for bacterial and fungal antigens, 71
Eosinophil count, 93t
Eosinophilia, 95–96, 95t, 96t
CSF, 652
drug-induced, 96, 96t
in systemic disease, 96, 96t
Eosinophilic granuloma, in toxocariasis, 511
Eosinophilic meningitis, 517, 517t, 631, 632t
Epidemic, 12
Epidemiology, 11–22, 12f. *See also at specific infections.*
basic concepts of, 11–12
of foodborne pathogens, 15, 16t, 17t
of soilborne pathogens, 13, 14t
of vectorborne pathogens, 15, 17, 18t–20t, 21t, 22t
of waterborne pathogens, 13–15, 14t, 15t
of zoonotic pathogens, 15, 17, 18t–20t, 21t, 22t
statistics in, 11
terminology for, 11–12
Epidermodysplasia verruciformis, 28
Epidermophyton floccosum infection, 19t, 558–560, 559t, 560f, 561t
Epididymitis, 993–994
chlamydial, 1017
culture in, 994
mumps, 420–421
tuberculous, 404
Epididymo-orchitis, 994–995
Epidural abscess
cranial, 657, 664–665, 665f, 666t
spinal, 657, 665–667, 666t, 667f, 667t
Epiglottitis, 774–776
atypical, 775
clinical manifestations of, 771t, 775, 775f
complications of, 776
diagnosis of, 775–776
epidemiology of, 775
etiology of, 774–775
pathogenesis of, 775, Plate 8E
prevention of, 776
treatment of, 776, 776t
Epinephrine
in laryngotracheobronchitis, 773
in septic shock, 292t
Epiploic foramen of Winslow, 923
Epizootic disease, 12
Epstein-Barr nuclear antigen, 110–111, 426, 432–433, 432t
Epstein-Barr virus, 426
in oncogenesis, 23–26, 24t, 428
transmission of, 426
Epstein-Barr virus infection. *See also* Infectious mononucleosis.
cancer and, 23–25, 24t, 25t, 428, 435
cutaneous eruptions in, 536, 536t, 537f
in AIDS, 25, 427–428, 430
posttransplantation, 429–430, 1176, 1179
Equine encephalitis
Eastern, 674–675, 674f
Western, 673–674, 674f
Equipment, cleaning of, 1239–1240, 1239t
Erb palsy, in congenital syphilis, 1103–1104
Erisipela del la costa, 518
Erosions, definition of, 533
Erysipelas, 578, Plate 8A
gangrenous, 587
treatment of, 579–581, 580t
Erysipelothrix rhusiopathiae infection (erysipeloid), 18t, 578, 579, 580t
Erythema, macular, 534–535, 534t, 535f, 536f
Erythema chronicum migrans. *See* Erythema migrans.
Erythema infectiosum (fifth disease), 325–330, 326t, 1113
bone marrow evaluation in, 328, 329f
clinical manifestations of, 325–328, 327t
complications of, 329
diagnosis of, 88t, 328–329, 329f
differential diagnosis of, 328
epidemiology of, 325
etiology of, 325
exanthem of, 326–327, 536, 536t, Plate 4A, Plate 4B
hospital isolation in, 329–330
imaging in, 328–329
immunization against, 328
laboratory evaluation in, 328
maternal, 1088t, 1089t, 1092t
outbreak control for, 329
pathogenesis of, 325, 326f
physical examination in, 326–327
prevention of, 329–330
prognosis for, 329
pure red cell aplasia in, 327–328
serologic diagnosis of, 328
transient aplastic crisis in, 327, 328
treatment of, 329
Erythema marginatum, in rheumatic fever, 488, 489, 489f
Erythema migrans, in Lyme disease, 349, 350
Erythema multiforme, 538, 539t
Erythema nodosum, 542, 542t
Erythema nodosum leprosum, 554, 703–704
Erythematous macular rash, 534–535, 534t, 535f, 536f
Erythrasma, 549
Erythrocyte sedimentation rate (ESR), 35, 96–97, 97t
in fever evaluation, 265
in fever of unknown origin, 276
in neonatal sepsis, 1123–1124
in osteomyelitis, 1037, 1041
Erythromycin, 151t, 152t, 175–178, 176t, 177t
dosing for, 178t
drug interactions with, 178, 179t
hypertrophic pyloric stenosis with, 1057
in bite-wound infection, 606, 606t
in blistering distal dactylitis, 549
in *Campylobacter jejuni* infection, 890, 890t
in *Chlamydia trachomatis* infection, 1018
in cholera, 894–895, 895t
in erythrasma, 549
in group A streptococcal vulvovaginal infection, 1006t
in *Haemophilus ducreyi* infection, 1026t
in perianal dermatitis, 550
in relapsing fever, 388t
in rheumatic fever prevention, 493, 493t
in streptococcal pharyngitis, 716t
ophthalmic prophylaxis with, 1057, 1058
Erythromycin-sulfisoxazole
in otitis media, 754t
in sinusitis, 765t
Escherichia coli infection
culture in, 897
enteroaggregative strains in, 895–898, 896t, 897t
enterohemorrhagic strains in, 895–898, 896t, 897t
enteroinvasive strains in, 895–898, 896t, 897t
enteropathogenic strains in, 895–898, 896t, 897t
enterotoxigenic, 895–898, 896t, 897t
gastrointestinal, 15, 16t, 17t, 91t, 895–898, 908–911, 910t
clinical manifestations of, 896–897, 896t
complications of, 897–898
diagnosis of, 897
epidemiology of, 895
etiology of, 895
pathogenesis of, 895–896, 896t
prevention of, 898
transmission of, 895
treatment of, 897, 897t
in cancer patient, 283
in hemolytic uremic syndrome, 913–916, 914t. *See also* Hemolytic uremic syndrome.
in sepsis, 279
in septic shock, 281
intra-abdominal, 923–928. *See also* Abscess, intra-abdominal.
meningeal, 630, 630t, 631t, 634. *See also* Meningitis, bacterial.
rabbit ileal loop assay in, 72
suckling mouse assay in, 72
toxins in, 4t, 72
urinary tract, 983, 984. *See also* Urinary tract infection.
Vero cell assay in, 72
waterborne, 15, 908, 909, 909t
Esophagitis, 869–871
candidal, 870–871
clinical manifestations of, 869–870
complications of, 871
cytomegalovirus, 870, 871
diagnosis of, 870
endoscopy in, 870
epidemiology of, 869
esophagography in, 870
etiology of, 869
fungal, 137, 137f
herpes simplex virus, 870, 871
in AIDS, 471
pathogenesis of, 869
prevention of, 871
prognosis for, 871
viral, 870, 871
Esophagography, in esophagitis, 870
E-Test, in antimicrobial susceptibility testing, 75
Ethambutol, 152t, 205–206, 206t, 207t, 208t
Ethionamide, 152t
Eustachian tube, in otitis media, 750
Exanthem
in echovirus infection, 537
in erythema infectiosum (fifth disease), 326–327, 536, 536t, Plate 4A, Plate 4B
in Kawasaki syndrome, 535, Plate 5E
in measles, 308, Plate 3A

Exanthem *(Continued)*
in *Mycoplasma pneumoniae* infection, 537
in roseola, 321, 322, 535–536, 536t, Plate 3E
in rubella, 316–317, 535, 536t, Plate 3C
in scarlet fever, 534, Plate 3D
in staphylococcal scalded skin syndrome, 534–535, 534f, 535f
in toxic shock syndrome, 535, Plate 6A
laterothoracic, unilateral, 537
Exanthem subitum. *See* Roseola.
Exchange transfusion
in babesiosis, 377
in septic shock, 293
Exfoliatin, 5, 534
Exotoxins, 3–5, 4t
Extraventricular device, in shunt-related infection, 652, 653, 654
Exudative reaction, 116, 118f, 120t
Eye
ethambutol toxicity to, 206
infection of. *See* Conjunctivitis; Keratitis.
nosocomial infections of, 1229–1230, 1230t
specimen collection from, 62t, 66
tuberculosis of, 404
Eyelid, infection of, 1069–1072. *See also* Blepharitis; Hordeolum.
Eyelid scrub, 1070

F

Facial cellulitis, 581–585, 583f, 585t. *See also* Cellulitis, head and neck.
FACS. *See* Flow cytometry.
Fallopian tube
inflammation of
chlamydial, 1018–1019
gonococcal, 1011
vs. appendicitis, 934, 934t
tuberculosis of, 404
Famciclovir, 152t, 196–197
in genital herpes simplex virus infection, 1024t
Far Eastern encephalitis, 676
Fasciola hepatica infection (fascioliasis), 20t, 522t
Fasciolopsis buski infection (fasciolopsiasis), 20t, 522t
Fatigue, 498. *See also* Chronic fatigue syndrome.
5-FC. *See* Flucytosine.
Febrile agglutinin tests, 104
Febrile seizures, 639
Fecalith, 932
Feline keratoconjunctivitis agent, 810
Fetus
immunity in, 47–49, 48f, 48t
infection in, 1089–1090, 1089t, 1099–1116. *See also* Intrauterine infection; Maternal infection; Perinatal infection.
prevention of, 1091–1093, 1092t
Fever, 35, 263–267
age and, 265
blood culture in, 266
bone marrow aspiration in, 277
breakbone, in dengue fever, 392
Charcot's, 275
culture in, 266
diagnosis of, 263–266, 264t, 265t
Boston screening criteria for, 272t, 273–274
Fever *(Continued)*
diagnosis of *(Continued)*
Philadelphia screening criteria for, 273–274, 273f
double-quotidian, 275
factitious, 275
follow-up for, 266
hectic, 275
hospitalization for, 266
imaging in, 277
in asplenic patient, 1181, 1183
in children over 8 weeks, 268–270, 269t, 270t, 271t, 272t
in infants under 8 weeks, 272–274, 272t, 273f
in international child traveler, 1217
in Kawasaki syndrome, 480
in malaria, 364, 366
in measles, 307
in meningitis, 647–648, 647t
intermittent, 275
laboratory evaluation of, 265, 276–277
observational assessment of, 264, 265t
of unknown origin, 275–277, 276t, 277t
patient history in, 264–265
Pel-Ebstein, 275
physical examination in, 264–265
quartan, 275
quotidian, 275
relapsing, 19t, 275, 387–388, 388t
remittent, 275
saddleback
in Colorado tick fever, 393
in dengue fever, 392
seizures with, 639
septic, 275
sustained (continuous), 275
tertian, 275
thermoregulatory center in, 263
treatment of, 266, 267t, 277
urine culture in, 266
without localizing signs, 275
Fibrin ring granuloma, 120t
Fibroelastosis, endocardial, mumps virus in, 424
Fibromyalgia, 500
Fifth disease. *See* Erythema infectiosum (fifth disease).
Filarial fever, 518
Filariasis, 20t, 518
Fimbriae, 1
Finger, herpetic whitlow of, 564, 565f
Fish tank granuloma, 555
Fish tapeworm infection, 530, 530t
Fish toxins, 911
Fitz-Hugh–Curtis syndrome, 930, 1011
Flare reaction, in uveitis, 1080
Fleaborne disease, 15
prevention of, 17, 21t
Fleaborne typhus, 388–389, 389t
Fleroxacin, 151t
Floaters, in retinitis, 1082
Flora, normal (indigenous), 6–10. *See also* Normal flora.
Flow cytometry (florescence-activated cell sorter), 54
Fluconazole, 152t, 193–194
adverse effects of, 193, 194t
dosing for, 193, 194t
Fluconazole *(Continued)*
drug interactions with, 194, 194t
in candidiasis, 562, 731, 731t, 870–871, 1006t
in histoplasmosis, 814
in neonatal sepsis, 1126t
metabolism of, 193, 193t
spectrum of activity of, 193
Flucytosine, 152t, 192–193, 193t
adverse effects of, 193, 193t
drug interactions with, 193, 193t
in meningitis, 645t
in neonatal sepsis, 1126t
Fluid therapy
in acute enteritis, 916–917, 917t
in enteritis, 916–917, 916t
in septic shock, 290, 292t
in staphylococcal toxic shock syndrome, 302, 302t
in travelers' diarrhea, 907t
Fluke infection, 521–524, 522t, 523f, 523t, 524t
Fluorescence immunoassay, for antibody detection, 100
Fluorescent antibody to membrane antigen (FAMA) test, in varicella-zoster virus infection, 101, 335
Fluorescent treponemal antibody test absorbed with nonpallidum treponemes (FTA-ABS), 105, 108, 1021–1022, 1022t
Fluoride, in caries prevention, 739–740, 740t
Fluorochrome stain, 68–69, 68t
5-Fluorocytosine. *See* Flucytosine.
Fluoroquinolone. *See* Quinolone.
Fluorosis, dental, 739–740
Fly infestation, 571, 571f
Foam cell reaction, 116, 118f, 119t, 120t
Folinic acid, in *Pneumocystis carinii* infection, 826, 826t
Folliculitis, 545–547, 546f, 546t
dissecting, 543
gram-negative, 548, 548t
Folliculitis decalvans, 543
Fomite, 12
Fontanelle, bulging, in meningitis, 639
Food additives, 912
Foodborne infection, 908–911
clinical manifestations of, 909, 910t
epidemiology of, 12, 15, 16t, 17t, 908
in traveler, 1217
prevention of, 911, 911t
FoodNet program, 908
Foot (feet)
pitted keratolysis of, 549, 549f
tinea of, 558–560, 559t, 561t
Forchheimer spots, 535
Foreign body
vs. bronchiolitis, 786
vs. common cold, 708, 708t
vs. vulvovaginitis, 1003–1004
Foreign body pneumonia, 826–829
clinical manifestations of, 827–828
diagnosis of, 828
pathogenesis of, 827
treatment of, 829
Foreign-born children, 1194–1206
adopted, 1195, 1195t
medical assessment of, 1197–1198
Amerasian, 1195, 1195t
medical assessment of, 1197

Foreign-born children *(Continued)*
dietary habits of, 1196
drug-resistant infection in, 1196
expatriate, 1196
foster, 1196
immigrant, 1194, 1195t
visa examination in, 1197
immunizations in, 1196, 1200–1201
infectious disease assessment in, 1198–1206, 1198f
after six months, 1206
immunization history in, 1200–1201
in asymptomatic child, 1201–1202
in symptomatic child, 1202–1206, 1202f, 1203f, 1204t–1205t
medication history in, 1200
patient history in, 1198–1200, 1199t
within 1 month of arrival, 1203, 1203f, 1204t–1205t
within 6 months of arrival, 1203, 1206–1207
medical assessment in, 1196–1198
refugee, 1194–1195, 1195t
medical assessment of, 1197
subclinical infections in, 1196
tourist, 1195–1196, 1195t
medical assessment of, 1198
vs. traveler, 1196–1197, 1196t
well-child care for, 1201
Formalin–ethyl acetate concentration procedure, for parasite examination, 81
Forssman antibodies, 431–432, 431f
Foscarnet, 152t, 197, 199, 199t
adverse effects of, 199, 199t
Four Corners virus infection. *See* Hantavirus cardiopulmonary syndrome.
Fournier teeth, in congenital syphilis, 1104
Fournier's gangrene, 587, 589, 591
Francisella tularensis infection (tularemia), 18t, 382–383, 382t
immunization against, 245t
oropharyngeal, 712t, 713–714, 715, 718
treatment of, 383, 383t
ulceroglandular, 615–616, 618
Friction rub
in pericarditis, 864
in pneumonia, 800
Frontal bossing, in congenital syphilis, 1104
Frostbite, 590
Fungal infections, 59, 60t. *See also specific infections.*
antimicrobial susceptibility testing in, 76
blood specimen collection in, 63–64
catheter-related, 66
corneal, 1064t, 1065, 1067
culture in, 74–75, 74t, 75f
cutaneous, 556–564. *See also specific infections.*
eosinophilia in, 95–96, 95t
imaging in, 131, 134f
in AIDS, 452t–453t, 468–469, 475
lymphadenopathy in, 613
meningeal, 634–635, 634t, 645t–646t, 646, 649
molecular tests in, 124
pulmonary, 812–817, 812t. *See also at* Pneumonia.
serologic testing in, 108–109
sputum collection in, 64
Fungemia
nosocomial, 1232
specimen collection in, 63–64
Funisitis, 589
Furazolidone, 152t
in cholera, 894–895, 895t
in giardiasis, 902, 903t
in travelers' diarrhea, 907t
Furuncles, 545–547, 546t, 547f
Furuncular myiasis, 571, 571f
Fusobacterium infection, 923–928. *See also* Abscess, intra-abdominal.
bite-wound, 603t, 607t. *See also* Bite-wound infection.
Fusobacterium nucleatum infection, 730

G

^{67}Ga scan. *See* Radionuclide scan.
gag, of HIV, 437, 439t
Gallbladder
cancer of, *Salmonella* in, 29
hydrops of, 971
inflammation of, 970–972. *See also* Cholecystitis.
Gamasidae infestation, 573
Ganciclovir, 152t, 196–197, 198t
dosing for, 198t
in burn wound infection, 599
in viral esophagitis, 871
Gangrene
dry, 587
Fournier's, 587, 589, 591
gas (clostridial myonecrosis), 587, 589
clinical manifestations of, 591
complications of, 593
diagnosis of, 591–592
prevention of, 595
prognosis for, 593–595
treatment of, 592–593, 593t
in Kawasaki syndrome, 484
streptococcal, 587, 589
Gardnerella vaginalis infection, 998–1007. *See also* Vaginosis; Vulvovaginitis.
Gastric carcinoma
gastritis and, 873, 876
Helicobacter pylori in, 28
Gastric lymphoma, *Helicobacter pylori* in, 29
Gastritis, 28, 872–877
bacterial toxin–induced, 4t
clinical manifestations of, 873–874, 874t
cobblestone mucosa in, 874
complications of, 876
culture in, 874–875
diagnosis of, 874–875, 874t, Plate 8A
endoscopy in, 874, Plate 8A
epidemiology of, 872
etiology of, 872, 873f
pathogenesis of, 872–873, 873f
prevention of, 877
prognosis for, 876–877
stool antigen test in, 875
treatment of, 875–876, 876t
urea breath test in, 875
Gastroenteritis. *See* Enteritis.
Gastrointestinal tract
anthrax of, 551
imaging of, 137, 137f, 138f
Gastrointestinal tract *(Continued)*
infection of. *See* Enteritis; Gastritis.
nosocomial, 1225–1227, 1226t
normal flora infection of, 7
normal flora of, 8t
specimen collection from, 61t, 64–65
Gatifloxacin, 151t, 184–187, 185t, 186t
Gaucher's disease, lymphadenopathy in, 614
Genitoanorectal syndrome, in lymphogranuloma venereum, 1027
Genitourinary tract
imaging of, 140–141, 140f, 141f
infection of. *See* Sexually transmitted infections; Urinary tract infection.
normal flora infection of, 7
normal flora of, 9t
specimen collection from, 61t, 65
Gentamicin, 151t, 167–172, 168t
adverse effects of, 170–171
clinical indications for, 168–169
dosing for, 169–170, 169t, 170t
in acute pancreatitis, 981, 981t
in acute pericarditis, 867t
in *Aeromonas* infection, 891, 891t
in burn wound infection, 600t
in cholecystitis, 972, 972t
in donovanosis, 1027
in hepatic abscess, 967t
in infectious arthritis, 1048t
in infective endocarditis, 851t–852t
in intra-abdominal abscess, 929t
in meningitis, 643t, 646t
in neonatal sepsis, 1125t, 1126t
in osteomyelitis, 1040t
in pelvic inflammatory disease, 1015t
in plague, 384–385, 385t
in sepsis, 291t
in shunt-related infection, 655t
in tularemia, 383, 383t
in urinary tract infection, 991t
in yersiniosis, 888, 888t
spectrum of activity of, 167–168, 168t
Gentian violet, in oral candidiasis, 731, 731t
German measles. *See* Rubella.
Gerstmann-Strässler syndrome, 685–687, 686t
Ghon's complex, 407, 813
Gianotti-Crosti syndrome, 536, 537f
Giant cell (Hecht's) pneumonia, 312
Giardia infection (giardiasis), 16t, 17t, 901–902, 903t
clinical manifestations of, 902, 903t
diagnosis of, 902
Enterotest (string test) in, 80–81
epidemiology of, 901
etiology of, 901
in day care environment, 1190
pathogenesis of, 901–902
transmission of, 901
treatment of, 902, 903t
waterborne, 15, 908, 909, 909t
Gingiva, cystic mass of, in *Streptococcus pneumoniae* bacteremia, 286
Gingivitis
clinical manifestations of, 737
diagnosis of, 737
etiology of, 734
pathogenesis of, 735

Gingivitis *(Continued)*
ulcerative, necrotizing, 734, 735–736, 738t, 7373
Gingivostomatitis, herpetic. *See* Herpes simplex virus infection, oral (gingivostomatitis).
Glandular fever. *See* Infectious mononucleosis.
Glandular tularemia, 382, 382t
Glans penis, inflammation of, 996
Glasgow Meningococcal Septicemia Prognostic Score, 293, 294t
Glomerulonephritis
impetigo and, 545
poststreptococcal, 493–495
clinical manifestations of, 494
complications of, 495
diagnosis of, 494–495, 495t
epidemiology of, 493–494
etiology of, 493
pathogenesis of, 494
pathology of, 495
prevention of, 495
prognosis for, 495
treatment of, 495
with *Salmonella typhi* infection, 884
Gloves and socks syndrome, in erythema infectiosum, 327
Glucose, in cerebrospinal fluid, 640t, 641
Glucose-6-phosphate dehydrogenase deficiency, 1182t, 1183–1184
Glue ear, 758
Glycopeptide antibiotics, 172–175, 173t, 174t, 175t
Glycoproteins, of HIV, 437, 438f
Goblet cells, 798
Gonorrhea, 1010–1016. *See also Neisseria gonorrhoeae* infection (gonorrhea).
Gonyaulax toxins, 911
gp120, 3t
Graft-versus-host disease, in bone marrow transplantation, 1170–1171
Gram stain, 67, 67t
cytocentrifugation for, 66
in meningitis, 641, 642t
in *Pneumocystis carinii* infection, 82
of cerebrospinal fluid, 641–642, 642t
Granulocyte, in innate immunity, 32–33
Granulocyte colony-stimulating factor, 223t
therapeutic, 223–224
Granulocyte transfusion
in cancer patient, 1167
in septic shock, 293
Granulocyte-macrophage colony-stimulating factor, 223t
therapeutic, 223–224
Granulocytopenia, in cancer, 1158
Granuloma, enterobiasis and, 515
Granuloma inguinale (donovanosis), 617, 1026–1027
lymphadenopathy in, 616
Granuloma venereum, 1026–1027
Granulomatous reaction, 116, 118f, 119, 120t
Gray syndrome, chloramphenicol-induced, 180
Griseofulvin, 152t, 194–195, 195t
in tinea capitis, 557–558, 558t
Ground itch, 505
Group A *Streptococcus*
Lancefield carbohydrate C of, 486
M protein of, 486
Group A *Streptococcus (Continued)*
nephritogenic strains of, 494
rheumatogenic strains of, 487
Group A *Streptococcus* infection, 486–495. *See also* Glomerulonephritis, poststreptococcal; Rheumatic fever.
bone, 1034, 1034t. *See also* Osteomyelitis.
cervical lymphadenitis in, 621–626. *See also* Lymphadenitis, cervical.
cutaneous, 544–545, 545f, 545t
in day care environment, 1189, 1191
in foodborne disease, 16t
in sepsis, 279
in toxic shock syndrome, 296–304. *See also* Streptococcal toxic shock syndrome.
meningeal, 630, 630t. *See also* Meningitis, bacterial.
of digital fat pad, 549–550
of lymphatic channels, 626–628
perianal, 550, 550f
pharyngeal, 711–717. *See also* Streptococcal pharyngitis.
serologic testing in, 104–105, 106t
vs. common cold, 708, 708t
vs. sinusitis, 763, 763t
vulvovaginal, 999, 1001, 1001t, 1002, 1005
treatment of, 1006t, 1007
with chickenpox, 338
Group B *Streptococcus* infection
in neonatal cellulitis-adenitis, 622
in sepsis, 279
maternal, 1087, 1088t, 1091, 1092t, 1093, 1093f–1095f
meningeal, 630, 630t. *See also* Meningitis, bacterial.
of bone, 1034, 1034t. *See also* Osteomyelitis.
of digital fat pad, 549–550
Growth factors, 2, 3t
Guillain-Barré syndrome, 693t, 701–703
clinical manifestations of, 701–702
complications of, 702
diagnosis of, 702, 702t
epidemiology of, 701
etiology of, 701
Miller Fisher variant of, 701
pathogenesis of, 701
physical examination in, 701–702
plasmapheresis in, 702
prevention of, 703
prognosis for, 702–703
treatment of, 702
Gumma, in syphilis, 1021

H

Haemophilus ducreyi infection, 1025–1026, 1026t
lymphadenopathy in, 616
Haemophilus influenzae infection
conjunctival, 1058, 1058t. *See also* Conjunctivitis, bacterial.
otologic, 748–749. *See also* Otitis media.
sinus, 760. *See also* Sinusitis.
vulvovaginal, 999, 1001, 1001t, 1005
treatment of, 1006t, 1007
Haemophilus influenzae type b infection
immunization against, 233t, 235t–236t, 246–247, 649
Haemophilus influenzae type b infection *(Continued)*
immunization against *(Continued)*
adverse reactions to, 237t
for international travel, 1211
in epiglottitis prevention, 776
meningococcal protein conjugate for, 247
protein conjugates for, 246–247
tetanus conjugate for, 247
in AIDS, 450t, 467
in bacteremia, 270–272, 270t, 272t, 282t, 283, 293
in day care environment, 1189
in sepsis, 279, 285
in septic shock, 280–281, 280t
meningeal, 630–649. *See also* Meningitis, bacterial.
prophylactic therapy against, 226, 228t
rapid diagnosis of, 288
Haemophilus spp. infection, bite-wound, 602–608, 603t, 606t, 607t
Haemophilus vaginalis. See Gardnerella vaginalis infection.
Hair loss, 542–543
Hairy leukoplakia, in AIDS, 427, 430
Hand hygiene. *See* Handwashing.
Hand, tinea of, 558–560, 559t, 561t
Hand-foot-and-mouth disease, 713, 713t
clinical manifestations of, 730, Plate 4f
vesicles of, 541, 541f, 541t
vs. chickenpox, 334
Handwashing, 1232–1233, 1233t
Hanger-Rose test, in cat-scratch disease, 346
Hansen's disease, 552–554, 552f, 553f, 553t, 554t. *See also* Leprosy.
Hantavirus cardiopulmonary syndrome, 822–824
clinical manifestations of, 824
diagnosis of, 824
epidemiology of, 19t, 823, 823f
etiology of, 822, 823t, 824f
pathogenesis of, 823–824
prevention of, 21t
transmission of, 822
Haverhill fever, 602
Head lice, 573–574, 573f
Health care–associated infection. *See* Nosocomial infections.
Health care providers, 1240–1244
conjunctivitis in, 1244
education of, 1244
health services for, 1241, 1241t
hepatitis B infection in, 1241–1242, 1241t
hepatitis C virus infection in, 1241t, 1242
HIV infection in, 1242, 1242t, 1243t, 1244
immunization for, 241, 1040t, 1240–1241
infection prevention for, 1240–1244, 1240t, 1241t, 1242t
needle-stick injury in, 1241–1242, 1241t
postexposure varicella-zoster virus infection prophylaxis for, 340t, 341
protective equipment for, 1240t
standard precautions for, 1233t, 1240t
tuberculosis in, 1243–1244
varicella-zoster virus infection in, 1242–1243
Hearing loss
with congenital cytomegalovirus infection, 1108
with congenital rubella infection, 1112
with congenital syphilis, 1104

Hearing loss *(Continued)*
  with Kawasaki syndrome, 484
  with meningitis, 648
  with otitis media, 756, 758
Heart
  erythromycin toxicity to, 178
  in infectious mononucleosis, 434
  quinolone toxicity to, 185
  transplantation of, 1176–1179, 1178t
Heart disease, 1182t
  in AIDS, 470
Heart failure, in pneumonia, 800
Heart sounds, in acute myocarditis, 859
Heavy metal poisoning, 16t, 912
Helicobacter pylori infection, 28, 872–877. *See also* Gastritis.
  clinical manifestations of, 873–874, 873f, 874t
  complications of, 876
  cutlure in, 874–875
  diagnosis of, 874–875, 874t, Plate 8A
  epidemiology of, 872
  in oncogenesis, 24t, 28–29, 876
  pathogenesis of, 872–873, 873f
  prognosis for, 876–877
  serologic testing in, 105, 875
  toxins of, 4t
  treatment of, 875–876, 876t
Helminth infection, 14t, 21t, 80, 81t. *See also specific helminth infections.*
  eosinophilia in, 95, 95t
  specimen collection in, 80–83, 82f
Hemagglutination inhibition assay, for antibody detection, 103
Hemagglutinin, 3t
Hemangioma, 624
Hematopoietic stem cell transplantation. *See* Transplantation, bone marrow.
Hematuria, 986. *See also* Urinary tract infection.
Hemolysins, 35
Hemolytic anemia, 98
Hemolytic uremic syndrome, 913–916
  clinical manifestations of, 914
  complications of, 915
  culture in, 915
  diagnosis of, 914–915
  epidemiology of, 913–914, 914f
  etiology of, 913
  pathogenesis of, 914
  prevention of, 916
  prognosis for, 915–916
  treatment of, 915
Hemoperfusion, in septic shock, 293
Hemophagocytic lymphohistiocytosis, in infectious mononucleosis, 434
Hemophagocytosis, in infectious mononucleosis, 434
Hemorrhage
  retinal, vs. retinitis, 1083
  splinter, in infective endocarditis, 540, 848
Hepatitis
  in AIDS, 473
  in infectious mononucleosis, 429
  in varicella-zoster virus infection, 339
  isoniazid-induced, 206
  rifampin-associated, 208
  viral, 943–961, 943t. *See also specific hepatitis virus infections.*
    biopsy in, 955
Hepatitis *(Continued)*
  viral *(Continued)*
    chronic, 955
    clinical manifestations of, 948–950, 948f–950f
    complications of, 956
    diagnosis of, 950–955, 951f
    differential diagnosis of, 951
    epidemiology of, 945–947, 946f, 947t
    etiology of, 943–945, 943t, 944t, 945t
    hepatic failure with, 956
    imaging in, 954–955
    laboratory evaluation in, 951
    microbiologic evaluation in, 952–954, 952t, 953t, 954f
    nosocomial, 1225–1227, 1226t
    pathogenesis of, 948
    pathologic findings in, 955
    prevention of, 958–961, 959t
    prognosis for, 956–958, 958f
    treatment of, 955–956, 955t
  with *Salmonella typhi* infection, 884
Hepatitis A virus infection, 16t, 943, 943t, 944t
  biopsy in, 955
  clinical manifestations of, 948–949, 948f
  complications of, 956
  diagnosis of, 88t, 950–952, 951f, 952t, 953t
  epidemiology of, 946, 946f
  immune globulin in, 216–217
  immunization against, 233t, 252–253, 253t, 254t, 958–959, 959t
    for international travel, 244t, 1213
  in day care environment, 1190
  maculopapular rash in, 536–537, 536t
  pathogenesis of, 948
  prognosis for, 956–958
Hepatitis B immune globulin, 218t, 220
Hepatitis B surface antigen, 943
Hepatitis B virus infection, 943–945, 943t, 944t
  biopsy in, 955
  clinical manifestations of, 949, 949f
  complications of, 956
  diagnosis of, 88t, 950–953, 951f, 952t, 953t, 954f
  epidemiology of, 946–947, 947t
  immunization against, 233t, 253–254, 253t, 254t
    adverse reactions to, 237t
    for international travel, 244t, 1211
    in residential institutions, 238
    postexposure, 242t, 959–960, 960t, 961t
  in AIDS, 473
  in day care environment, 1191
  in health care providers, 1241–1242, 1241t
  in oncogenesis, 24t, 26
  interferon alfa-2b in, 955, 955t
  lamivudine in, 956
  maternal, 1088t, 1091, 1092t, 1094, 1096
  pathogenesis of, 948
  prognosis for, 956–958
  treatment of, 955–956, 955t, 957f
    interferons in, 222–223
Hepatitis C virus infection, 943t, 944t, 945
  biopsy in, 955
  clinical manifestations of, 949
  complications of, 956
  diagnosis of, 88t, 950–951, 951f, 952t, 953, 953t
  epidemiology of, 947
  in AIDS, 473
  in day care environment, 1191
  in health care providers, 1241t, 1242
Hepatitis C virus infection *(Continued)*
  in oncogenesis, 24t, 26
  interferon alfa-2b in, 956, 957f
  pathogenesis of, 948
  prognosis for, 956–958, 958f
  treatment of, 956, 957f
    interferons in, 223
Hepatitis D virus infection, 943t, 944t, 945
  clinical manifestations of, 949, 950f
  complications of, 956
  diagnosis of, 88t, 950–951, 951f, 952t, 953–954
  epidemiology of, 947
  pathogenesis of, 948
  prognosis for, 956–958
  treatment of, 956
Hepatitis E virus infection, 943t, 944t, 945
  clinical manifestations of, 949–950, 950f
  complications of, 956
  diagnosis of, 950–951, 951f, 952t, 954
  epidemiology of, 947
  in international child traveler, 1213
  prognosis for, 956–958
Hepatitis G virus infection, 943t, 944t, 945
  diagnosis of, 950–951, 951f, 952t, 954
  epidemiology of, 947
Hepatocellular carcinoma, hepatitis B virus in, 24t, 26
Hepatomegaly, in AIDS, 472–473
Hepatoportoenterostomy, cholangitis and, 973, 973t
Hepatorenal recess, 923
Hepatosplenocandidiasis, 1163
Hepatotoxicity, erythromycin-induced, 178
Herpangina, 541, 541t, 713, 713t, 729–730, Plate 7D
Herpes gladiatorum, 564
Herpes labialis, 729, 730f. *See also* Herpes simplex virus infection, oral (gingivostomatitis).
Herpes simplex virus infection
  congenital, 1109–1110
  corneal, 566, 1063t, 1064, 1065, 1065f, 1067, 1068
  culture in, 565
  diagnosis of, 88t, 90, 90f
  electron microscopy in, 90, 90f
  encephalitic, 670–673
    brain biopsy in, 672
    clinical manifestations of, 671, 671t
    computed tomography in, 129f, 672
    CSF examination in, 672
    diagnosis of, 672
    epidemiology of, 671
    etiology of, 670–671
    magnetic resonance imaging of, 672
    pathogenesis of, 671
    prevention of, 673
    prognosis for, 672–673, 672t
    treatment of, 672, 672t
  esophageal, 869–871
    clinical manifestations of, 869
    complications of, 871
    diagnosis of, 870
    epidemiology of, 869
    prevention of, 871
    prognosis for, 871
    treatment of, 871
  genital, 1023–1025
    clinical manifestations of, 1024

Herpes simplex virus infection *(Continued)*
genital *(Continued)*
complications of, 1025
diagnosis of, 1024
epidemiology of, 1024
etiology of, 1023–1024
lymphadenopathy in, 616, 617
pathogenesis of, 1024
primary, 1024
prognosis for, 1025
recurrence of, 1024, 1025, 1025t
transmission of, 1023–1024
treatment of, 1025, 1025t
imaging in, 131, 134f
in AIDS, 461, 470, 474
in burn injury, 596, 598, 599
latent, 1024
maternal, 1024, 1088t, 1091, 1092t, 1094, 1096
mucocutaneous, 564–566
clinical manifestations of, 564–565, 564f–566f
complications of, 566
diagnosis of, 565–566, 566f
epidemiology of, 564
pathogenesis of, 564
prevention of, 566
prognosis for, 566
transmission of, 564
treatment of, 566
oral (gingivostomatitis), 728–733
clinical manifestations of, 729–730, 730f
complications of, 732
diagnosis of, 730–731
epidemiology of, 728
etiology of, 728
pathogenesis of, 728–729
prevention of, 733
prognosis for, 732–733
recurrent, 732–733
supportive therapy in, 731–732, 732t
treatment of, 731, 731t
perinatal, 1135t, 1136–1140
clinical manifestations of, 1137–1138, 1137t
CNS, 1137–1138
complications of, 1139–1140
culture in, 1138
diagnosis of, 1138–1139, 1138t
differential diagnosis of, 1138, 1138t
disseminated, 1137
epidemiology of, 1136–1137, 1137t
etiology of, 1136
imaging in, 1139
isolation precautions for, 1140
pathogenesis of, 1137
polymerase chain reaction test in, 1139
prevention of, 1140
prognosis for, 1140, 1140t
recurrence of, 1140
SEM, 1137
treatment of, 1139
Tzanck smear in, 1138–1139
retinal, 1082, 1083, 1084
serologic testing in, 110, 565–566
Tzanck smear in, 566, 566f
vesicles of, 541, 541t
Herpes zoster. *See* Zoster.
Herpesvirus hominis. *See* Herpes simplex virus infection.
Herpesvirus simiae (herpes B virus) infection, 19t, 602, 603t, 605, 608
Herpetic whitlow, 564, 565f
Heterophile antibody test, 110
Heterophydiasis, 522t
Heterophyes heterophyes infection, 522t
Hib. *See Haemophilus influenzae* type b.
Hidradenitis suppurativa, 547
vs. abscess, 940
High-altitude exposure, travel and, 1215
Higouménakis' sign, in congenital syphilis, 1104
Hip joint effusion, ultrasonography in, 144f
Histiocytic disorders, lymphadenopathy in, 614
Histiocytosis, sinus, lymphadenopathy in, 623
Histoplasmin skin test, 813
Histoplasmosis, 13, 812–814, 813t
culture in, 813
disseminated, 813
epidemiology of, 19t
Ghon complex in, 813
imaging in, 136, 136f, 137f
in AIDS, 452t, 462t, 468–469
lymphadenopathy in, 613
meningeal, 633
serologic testing in, 109
HIV infection. *See* Human immunodeficiency virus (HIV) infection.
HLA typing, 56
HLA-G, in fetus, 47
Hodgkin's disease
Epstein-Barr virus in, 24t, 25
immunization in, 239t
lymphadenopathy in, 613
Holder pasteurization, of breast milk, 1096
Hookworm infection, 504–507
clinical manifestations of, 505–506, 506t
complications of, 507
diagnosis of, 506
epidemiology of, 505
etiology of, 504–505, 505f, 505t
infantile, 506
pathogenesis of, 505
prevention of, 507
prognosis for, 507
treatment of, 506–507, 506t
Hordeolum, 1070–1072, 1071f
Host defenses, 6
Hot-potato voice, 724
HTLV-I. *See* Human T-cell leukemia/lymphoma virus type I (HTLV-I).
HTLV-I-associated myelopathy. *See* Tropical spastic paraparesis.
HTLV-II. *See* Human T-cell leukemia/lymphoma virus type II (HTLV-II).
HTLV-III. *See* Human immunodeficiency virus type 1 (HIV-1).
HTLV-IV. *See* Human immunodeficiency virus type 2 (HIV-2).
Human bite, 602–608. *See also* Bite-wound infection.
Human foamy virus, 26–27
Human granulocytic agent infection, 19t
Human granulocytic ehrlichiosis, 359–362. *See also Ehrlichia* spp. infection (ehrlichiosis).
Human herpesvirus type 8, in oncogenesis, 24t, 25–26
Human herpesvirus type 6 infection. *See* Roseola.
Human herpesvirus type 7 infection. *See* Roseola.
Human immunodeficiency virus (HIV) infection, 437–476. *See also* Acquired immunodeficiency syndrome (AIDS).
acute retroviral syndrome in, 444
antibiotic prophylaxis in, 460–461, 461t, 462t
breast-feeding and, 446
cellular targets in, 437–439, 440f
classification of, 443–444, 444t, 445t
clinical manifestations of, 443–447, 444t, 445t
diagnosis of, 88t, 447–449, 448t
drug use and, 441, 442
encephalopathy in, 463–465, 464f, 683–684
epidemiology of, 438–439, 441–442
herpes simplex virus infection with, 565, 565f
immunization in, 240t, 460
in adolescents, 441–442
in children <13 years, 441
in day care environment, 1191
in Europe, 439
in health care providers, 1242, 1242t, 1243t, 1244
in international child traveler, 1213
in Latin America, 439
in neonate, 449, 454–455, 454t
in Southeast Asia, 439
in sub-Saharan Africa, 438–439
in United States, 439, 441
in women, 441
indeterminate test result in, 448
information sources for, 454t
initial clinical presentation of, 446–447, 447t
intravenous immune globulin in, 294
maternal, 441, 446, 1091, 1092t, 1094–1095, 1096
screening for, 1087, 1088t
mononeuritis multiplex in, 704
mucocutaneous manifestations of, 543
nutrition in, 460
oncogenesis and, 24t, 27
p24 protein antigen test in, 449
pathogenesis of, 442–443, 443f
peripheral neuropathy in, 704
polymerase chain reaction assay in, 448–449
postexposure prophylaxis for, 476
prevention of, 441, 476
progression of, 444–446, 444t, 445t
serologic testing in, 448, 448t
sexual abuse and, 476, 1031
testing for, 447–449, 448t
in international child traveler, 1207
transfusion transmission of, 442
treatment of, 188t–191t, 449–463, 454t
combination therapy in, 455–456, 457t, 458t–459t, 460t
initiation of, 455
monitoring of, 456, 459
supportive, 460–463, 461t, 462t
tuberculosis in, 398, 405, 414–415, 460
universal precautions for, 454
vertical transmission of, 446, 1091, 1092t, 1096
prevention of, 441, 1092t, 1094–1095
viral load assay in, 456
Human immunodeficiency virus type 1 (HIV-1), 437–438, 438f, 439t
Human immunodeficiency virus type 2 (HIV-2), 437, 442
Human leukocyte antigens, 37–38

Human monocytic ehrlichiosis, 359–362. *See also Ehrlichia* spp. infection (ehrlichiosis).
Human papillomavirus infection
diagnosis of, 88t, 567, 1029–1030
genital, 1029–1030, 1029f
clinical manifestations of, 567, 568f, 1029, 1029f
complications of, 1030
diagnosis of, 1029–1030
epidemiology of, 1029
treatment of, 1030
in oncogenesis, 24t, 28, 1030
interferons in, 223
maternal, 1029, 1088t
nongenital, 566–568, 568f
clinical manifestations of, 566, 567f
diagnosis of, 567
epidemiology of, 566
etiology of, 566, 567t
laryngeal, 567, 568
treatment of, 568
Human T cell lymphotropic virus. *See* Human immunodeficiency virus (HIV) infection.
Human T-cell leukemia/lymphoma virus type I (HTLV-I) infection, 24t, 27
diagnosis of, 88t
myelopathy of, 705
serologic testing in, 111
Human T-cell leukemia/lymphoma virus type II (HTLV-II) infection, 24t, 27–28
diagnosis of, 88t
serologic testing in, 111
Hutchinson's teeth, 1104
Hydatid cyst, 527–530. *See also Echinococcus granulosus* infection (echinococcosis).
Hydatidosis. *See Echinococcus granulosus* infection (echinococcosis).
Hydrocephalus, in cytomegalovirus infection, 130f
Hydrops, of gallbladder, 971
Hydroxychloroquine, 153t
14-Hydroxyclarithromycin, 175–178, 176t, 177t
Hygroma, cystic, 624
Hymenolepis spp. infection (hymenolepiasis), 20t, 530t, 531
Hyperalimentation, intravenous, sepsis and, 1122
Hyperbaric oxygen therapy
in streptococcal toxic shock syndrome, 303
in wound infection, 594
Hyper-IgE syndrome, 1154
Hyperinfection syndrome, in strongyloidiasis, 513, 514
Hypersensitivity reaction. *See also* Allergy.
rifampin-induced, 208
T cells in, 41
Hypertension
in poststreptococcal glomerulonephritis, 595
pulmonary, 1182t
Hyperthermic therapy
in lymphangitis, 627
in sporotrichosis, 563
Hypocalcemia, in acute pancreatitis, 982
Hypogammaglobulinemia, transient, of infancy, 1151
Hypoglycemia
in malaria, 372
pentamidine-associated, 209
Hypoglycorrhachia, in meningitis, 640, 641t
Hypokalemia, penicillin-related, 156
Hypoprothrombinemia, with cephalosporins, 165
Hypotension
in hantavirus cardiopulmonary syndrome, 824
in staphylococcal toxic shock syndrome, 298
pentamidine-associated, 209

I

Ibuprofen
in fever, 266, 267t
in septic shock, 290
Idiotypic network, in immune response, 47, 47f
Idoxuridine, 152t
Ileocecal syndrome. *See* Typhlitis.
Imaging, 126–146. *See also specific imaging modalities.*
interpretation of, 146
of abdomen, 137–140, 137f–140f
of airway and chest, 131–136, 131–137f
of genitourinary tract, 140–141, 140f, 141f
of head and neck, 126–131, 128f–131f
of heart, 136–137
of musculoskeletal system, 141–145, 141f–145f
Imipenem, 151t, 166–167, 166t, 167t
in acute pancreatitis, 981, 981t
in brain abscess, 661
in intra-abdominal abscess, 929t
in neonatal sepsis, 1126t
in wound infection, 593t
Immigrant children, 1194–1206. *See also* Foreign-born children.
Immune deficiency disorders
acquired. *See* Acquired immunodeficiency syndrome (AIDS).
clinical manifestations of, 51–53, 52t
intravenous immune globulin in, 217
primary, 1148–1155. *See also specific disorders.*
antibody-deficient, 1150–1151
classification of, 1149, 1150t
complement-related, 1153–1154
immunization and, 239t
incidence of, 1149–1150
infection in, 283, 1148–1155
anatomic factors in, 1148–1149, 1148t
asplenia and, 1149
environmental factors in, 1148t, 1149
ionizing radiation and, 1149
metabolic factors in, 1148t, 1149
therapeutic factors in, 1148t, 1149
water contamination and, 1149
management of, 1154–1155
phagocytic, 1153
T-cell, 1151–1153, 1152t
Immune globulin, 216–220
botulism, 697
cytomegalovirus, 218t, 220
for hepatitis A prophylaxis, 216–217
for postexposure measles prophylaxis, 217, 314
for postexposure rubella prophylaxis, 320
hepatitis B, 218t, 220
intravenous, 216, 217–220, 218t, 219t
in acute myocarditis, 861
in AIDS, 474
in bone marrow transplantation, 1171
in burn injury, 599
in HIV infection, 294
Immune globulin *(Continued)*
intravenous *(Continued)*
in immunodeficiency, 217
in Kawasaki syndrome, 482–483, 482t, 484
in neonatal infections, 219–220
in neonatal prophylaxis, 217–219
in neonatal sepsis prevention, 1128–1129
in neonate, 217–219
in postexposure measles prophylaxis, 314
in primary immune deficiencies, 1154, 1155
in respiratory syncytial virus infection, 788, 788t
in septic shock, 293
in streptococcal toxic shock syndrome, 303
in tetanus, 694
preparations of, 216, 218t, 219f, 219t, 220
rabies, 218t, 220, 607–608
respiratory syncytial virus, 218t, 220, 788, 788t
tetanus, 218t, 220, 251, 594, 595t, 694
varicella-zoster, 218t, 220
for cancer patient, 1166–1167
for pregnant woman, 1110
in perinatal varicella-zoster virus infection, 1142t
in varicella-zoster virus infection prevention, 339–341, 340t, 1143
with immunization, 234, 236t
Immune response. *See also* Immunity; Immunization.
antigen persistence and, 46
body temperature and, 263
evaluation of, 51–56
ancillary studies in, 56
B-cell function in, 54, 54t, 55
clinical, 51–53, 52t
cold agglutins in, 97–98
complement function in, 54, 56
eosinophil count in, 95–96, 95t
HLA typing in, 56
illness patterns in, 51, 52t
infection history in, 51–52, 52t
laboratory, 53–56, 53t, 54t, 55t, 92–98, 93t, 94f
lymphocyte count in, 93–95
neutrophil count in, 92–93, 93t, 94f
phagocytic cell function in, 54, 56
physical examination in, 52–53, 52t
screening studies in, 53–54, 53t
T-cell function in, 53–55, 53t, 55t
idiotypic network in, 47, 47f
in burn injury, 597
in chronic fatigue syndrome, 498
in malaria, 365–366
in measles, 307
in neonate, 48–49, 48f
in rheumatic fever, 487
in tuberculosis, 400
of respiratory tract, 798
virulence factors and, 1, 2f
Immune serum globulin. *See* Immune globulin.
Immunity, 12, 31–50
adaptive, 36–47
B cells in, 36–37, 36t, 37f, 41–45, 42f, 43f, 44t. *See also* B cells.
innate immunity interface with, 35–36
memory in, 36–37
regulation of, 45–47, 46f, 47f

Immunity *(Continued)*
adaptive *(Continued)*
T cells in, 36–41, 36t, 37f, 39f, 39t, 40f, 40t, 41t. *See also* T cells.
aging and, 49–50
cytokine-producing cells in, 36
dendritic cells in, 35–36
in fetus, 47–49, 48f, 48t
in newborn, 48–49, 48f
innate, 31–35
adaptive immunity interface with, 35–36
cellular components of, 32–35, 32f, 33t
complement in, 34–35, 34f, 34t, 35f
endothelial cells in, 32, 32f, 33t
granulocytes in, 32–32, 32f
macrophages in, 32f, 34
mononuclear phagocytes in, 32f, 33–34
mucous membrane barriers in, 31
neutrophils in, 33, 33t
normal flora in, 31–32
skin barriers in, 31
vs. adaptive, 32t
malnutrition and, 49, 49t
natural killer cells in, 36
nonspecific. *See* Immunity, innate.
physiologic changes in, 49–50, 49t
principles of, 31
specific. *See* Immunity, adaptive.
stress and, 49
Immunization, 232–260
adenovirus, 819
adverse reactions to, 234, 237t
after bone marrow transplantation, 240t
after splenectomy, 240t–241t
after transplantation, 240t
anthrax, 245t
before splenectomy, 240t–241t
cholera, 245t, 246, 895
for international travel, 244t, 1211–1212
contraindications to, 234, 236, 238
delayed, 232, 235t–236t
diphtheria, tetanus toxoids, pertussis, 233t, 235t–236t, 245t, 246
during pregnancy, 238
for international travel, 244t
postexposure, 242t
during breast-feeding, 1096
during corticosteroid therapy, 239t
during immunosuppressive therapy, 239t
during long-term aspirin therapy, 241t
during pregnancy, 238
for day care personnel, 1192, 1193t
for health care workers, 1240–1241, 1240t
for international travel, 243, 243t–244t, 1207, 1209–1211, 1210t, 1213
Haemophilus influenzae type b, 233t, 235t–236t, 246–247, 649
adverse reactions to, 237t
for international travel, 1211
in epiglottitis prevention, 776
hepatitis A, 233t, 252–253, 253t, 254t, 958–961, 959t
for international travel, 244t, 1213
hepatitis B, 233t, 253–254, 253t, 254t, 959–960, 960t, 961t
adverse reactions to, 237t
for international travel, 244t, 1211

Immunization *(Continued)*
hepatitis B *(Continued)*
in residential institutions, 238
postexposure, 242t
herpes simplex virus, 1140
idiotype-anti-idiotype principles in, 47, 47f
immune globulin administration with, 234, 236t
in adolescents, 238, 241
in asplenia, 1181
in bone marrow transplantation patient, 1171
in chronic illness, 241t
in college students, 238, 241
in congenital immunodeficiency, 239t
in diabetes mellitus, 241t
in foreign-born children, 1200–1201
in health care workers, 241
in HIV infection, 240t, 460
in Hodgkin's disease, 239t
in immunocompromised persons, 238, 239t–241t
in Kawasaki syndrome, 483
in metabolic disease, 241t
in nephrotic syndrome, 241t
in otitis media prevention, 758
in preterm infant, 238
in primary immune deficiencies, 1155
in residential institutions, 238
in sickle cell disease, 240t–241t
in thalassemia, 240t–241t
in vulnerable host, 1185t, 1186
influenza, 253t, 254–255, 255t, 822
for international travel, 1211
informed consent for, 232, 234
Japanese encephalitis, 253t, 255
for international travel, 244t, 1212
Lyme disease, 247, 353
measles, 255–256, 313–314, 315
for international travel, 244t, 1207, 1209
postexposure, 242t
measles-mumps-rubella, 233t, 235t–236t, 253t
adverse reactions to, 233t, 235t–236t
meningococcal, for international travel, 1212
mumps, 256, 424
for international travel, 1209
postexposure, 242t
Neisseria meningitidis, 245t, 247–248, 649
for international travel, 244t
parvovirus B19, 328
pertussis, 245t, 248–249, 792
postexposure, 242t
plague, 245t
pneumococcal, 233t, 235t–236t, 245t, 249–250
for international travel, 1211
polysaccharide, 249–250
protein conjugates for, 250
polio, 233t, 235t–236t, 253t, 256–257
adverse reactions to, 237t
for international travel, 244t, 1210–1211
paralytic poliomyelitis with, 257
postexposure, 241–243, 242t–243t
rabies, 253t, 257
for international travel, 244t, 1212
postexposure, 243t
rotavirus, 258, 900
adverse reactions to, 237t
route of administration for, 234
routine, 232, 233t, 234t

Immunization *(Continued)*
rubella, 258, 319, 1113
for international travel, 1209
simultaneous, 234
streptococcal, 493
tetanus, 245t, 250–251
during pregnancy, 238
in wound infection, 594, 595t, 607
postexposure, 242t
tuberculosis, 243, 245t, 246, 417–418, 418f
postexposure, 243t
tularemia, 245t
typhoid, 245t, 251–252, 885
for international travel, 244t, 1212
heat-phenol-inactivated, 252
live-attenuated, 251–252
polysaccharide, 252
vaccinia, 258–259
varicella-zoster virus, 233t, 235t–236t, 253t, 259, 339–340, 1110, 1143
adverse reactions to, 237t
for international travel, 245t, 1211
web site for, 233t, 243
WHO schedule for, 234t
yellow fever, 253t, 260
for international travel, 244t–245t, 1212–1213
Immunoassay
for bacterial and fungal antigens, 69–71, 70t
in viral infection, 89
Immunoblotting, 103–104, 104f
Immunochromatography, for bacterial and fungal antigens, 71
Immunocompromised persons. *See also* Acquired immunodeficiency syndrome (AIDS); Cancer; Imunodeficiency disorders; Transplantation.
bacteremia in, 281–282, 282t
bite-wound infection in, 608
immunization in, 238, 239t–241t
measles in, 309
postexposure varicella-zoster virus infection prophylaxis for, 340t, 341
roseola in, 322
sepsis in, 281–282, 282t
septic shock in, 281–282
varicella-zoster virus infection in, 337
Immunodiffusion assay, for antibody detection, 103
Immunofluorescence assay
for antibody detection, 100, 101f
for bacterial and fungal antigens, 70
in pertussis syndrome, 791
in *Pneumocystis carinii* infection, 82
Immunoglobulin(s). *See also* Antibody (antibodies); Antigen(s).
normal levels of, 54, 54t
structure of, 42–43, 42f, 43f
Immunoglobulin A (IgA), 44t, 45, 100
normal levels of, 54, 54t
of respiratory tract, 798
selective deficiency of, 1151
Immunoglobulin D (gD), 44, 44t
Immunoglobulin E (IgE), 44t, 45
elevated levels of, 1154
Immunoglobulin G (IgG), 44–45, 44t, 99–100
CSF, 100
in viral infection, 90
maternal, 48, 48f, 1122

Immunoglobulin G (IgG) *(Continued)*
normal levels of, 54, 54t
subclass deficiencies of, 1151
Immunoglobulin M (IgM), 44, 44t, 99
fetal, 1099
in viral infection, 90
maternal, 1099
normal levels of, 54, 54t
X-linked elevated levels of, 1151
Immunoglobulin M (IgM) immunosorbent agglutination assay, in toxoplasmosis, 109
Immunohistochemistry, 119, 121t
Immunomodulating agents, in cancer-associated infection, 1159t, 1160
Immunoprecipitation assay
for antibody detection, 103
for antigen detection, 115
Immunosenescence, 49–50
Immunosuppression. *See also* Immunocompromised persons.
immunization and, 239t
Immunotherapy, 216–224, 217t. *See also* Immune globulin; Immunization.
Impetigo, 544–545, 545f, 545t, 546t
^{111}In scan. *See* Radionuclide scan.
In situ hybridization assay, 119–120, 121f, 122t
organism-specific, 124
Incidence, 11–12
Inclusion conjunctivitis. *See Chlamydia trachomatis* infection.
Index case, 12
India ink preparation, 69, 69f, 69t
in meningitis, 641, 642t
Indinavir, 152t, 204t, 205t
in HIV infection, 456, 457t, 459t, 460t
Indirect immunofluorescence assay, for antigen detection, 70
Indirect sandwich assay
for antibody detection, 100–101, 101f
for antigen detection, 111, 113f
Indium scan. *See* Radionuclide scan.
Infectious disease, 1. *See also specific infections.*
environment and, 13–22. *See also* Environment.
imaging in, 126–146. *See also specific imaging modalities.*
microbiology in, 57–79. *See also at* Specimen.
normal flora in, 7
parasitology in, 80–83, 81t, 82f, 83f
pathology in, 116–124. *See also* Pathology.
recurrent, 51–56. *See also* Immune response, evaluation of.
serology in, 99–115. *See also* Antibody (antibodies); Antigen(s).
subclinical, 12
virology in, 84–91, 85t–86t, 87t, 88t, 89f, 90f
vs. colonization, 6
Infectious mononucleosis, 426–435
airway obstruction in, 434
ampicillin rash in, 428
aplastic anemia in, 434
cardiac manifestations in, 434
cerebrospinal fluid examination in, 431
chronic fatigue syndrome in, 434
clinical manifestations of, 428–430, 429t
complications of, 433–435
culture in, 433
cutaneous eruptions in, 428, 536
diagnosis of, 88t, 110–111, 430–433, 431t
Infectious mononucleosis *(Continued)*
differential diagnosis of, 430
encephalitis with, 681
epidemiology of, 426–427, 427f
Epstein-Barr virus–negative, 426
etiology of, 426
fulminant, 434
hematologic manifestations of, 428–429
hemophagocytosis in, 434
hepatitis in, 429
heterophile antibody test in, 431–432
in HIV-infected children, 430
in transplant recipients, 429–430, 1176, 1179
laboratory evaluation in, 430–431, 431t
lymphadenopathy in, 612, 617
maternal, 434–435
meningoencephalitis in, 681
metamorphopsia in, 428
microbiologic evaluation in, 431–433, 431f
neurologic manifestations of, 428
pathogenesis of, 427–428
plain film radiography in, 131, 131f
pneumonia in, 434
prevention of, 435
prognosis for, 435
psychological complications of, 434
rhabdomyolysis in, 434
specific antibody test in, 432–433, 432t
splenic rupture in, 434
treatment of, 433
vs. cytomegalovirus virus infection, 430
vs. rubella, 318
X-linked lymphoproliferative syndrome in, 429
Infective endocarditis, 845–861
clinical manifestations of, 847–848, 848t
complications of, 853
congenital heart disease and, 846–847, 846t
culture in, 848–850, 849t
diagnosis of, 848–850, 849t
Duke criteria for, 849t
echocardiography in, 849–850, Plate 8D
epidemiology of, 845–846
etiology of, 845, 846t
HACEK group in, 852
incidence of, 846
pathogenesis of, 846–847, 846t
physical examination in, 848, Plate 8C
prevention of, 853–856, 854t, 855t, 856t
prognosis for, 853
purpura in, 539t, 540
serum bactericidal titer in, 852–853
surgical treatment of, 853
treatment of, 850–853, 851t–852t
Infertility, *Chalmydia trachomatis* infection and, 1019
Inflammation, 92–98
acute-phase reactants in, 96–97, 97t
cold agglutinins in, 97–98
eosinophil count in, 95–96, 95t, 96t
lymphocyte count in, 93–95
neutrophil count in, 92–93, 93t, 94f
Inflammatory bowel disease, 1182t
Influenza virus infection, 88t, 819–822
clinical manifestations of, 820
diagnosis of, 820
encephalitic, 682
epidemiology of, 819–820
etiology of, 819
Influenza virus infection *(Continued)*
immunization against, 253t, 254–255, 255t
for international travel, 1211
in HIV-infected child, 460
in AIDS, 469
pathogenesis of, 820
prevention of, 822
prognosis for, 822
transmission of, 819
treatment of, 820–821, 821t
Informed consent, for immunization, 232, 234
Innate immunity. *See* Immunity, innate.
Inoculum effect, in streptococcal toxic shock syndrome, 303
Insect repellents, 17, 1214
Insomnia, familial, 686t
β_2-Integrins, 33, 33t
Intelligence quotient (IQ), after meningitis, 648–649
Interferon, therapeutic, 221–222, 223t
Interferon-α
in human papillomavirus infection, 1030
interferon alfa-2b
in hepatitis B virus infection, 955, 955t
in hepatitis C virus infection, 956, 957f
in hepatitis D virus infection, 956
Interferon-γ, in immune response, 40t
Interleukin 1
antibodies to, in septic shock, 292
in immune response, 40t
in meningitis, 636–637, 636f
in septic shock, 284
Interleukin 2
in immune response, 40t
in septic shock, 284
Interleukin 3, 40t
Interleukin 4, 40t
Interleukin 5, 40t
Interleukin 6
in immune response, 40t
in septic shock, 284
Interleukin 7, 40t
Interleukin 8, 40t
Interleukin 10, 40t
Interleukin 12, 40t
Intermediate host, 15
International Certificate of Vaccination, 1215
International travel, 1207–1219
accident prevention for, 1217, 1217t
cholera immunization for, 1211–1212
cold in, 1217
consultation for
after trip, 1217–1218, 1218t, 1219t
before trip, 1207–1214, 1208t–1209t, 1210t
during trip, 1214–1217, 1215t, 1216t, 1217t
itinerary review for, 1207, 1210t
timing of, 1207
death of, 1217
diarrhea in, 1216–1217, 1216t
dietary precautions for, 1214–1215, 1215t
diphtheria, pertussis, tetanus immunization for, 1211
disease incubation period in, 1218t
disease risk in, 1219t
fever in, 1217
foodborne disease in, 1217
Haemophilus influenzae type b immunization for, 1211

International travel *(Continued)*
health documents for, 1215–1216
hepatitis A immunization for, 1213
hepatitis B immunization for, 1211
hepatitis E exposure and, 1213
high-altitude exposure of, 1215
HIV infection in, 1213
HIV testing of, 1207
hygiene precautions for, 1215
immunization for, 243, 243t–244t, 1207, 1209–1211, 1210t
scheduling of, 1213
influenza immunization for, 1211
information resources for, 1208t–1209t
insect repellents for, 1214
Japanese encephalitis immunization for, 1212
jet lag in, 1215
malaria chemoprophylaxis in, 1213–1214
measles immunization for, 315, 1207, 1209
medical care for, 1216
meningococcal immunization for, 1212
motion sickness in, 1215
mumps immunization for, 1209
oral rehydration for, 1216, 1216t
pneumococcal immunization for, 1211
polio immunization for, 1210–1211
posttravel evaluation of, 1217–1218, 1218t, 1219t
rabies immunization for, 1212
rash in, 1217
rubella immunization for, 320, 1209
sexual contacts of, 1215
skin-piercing procedures and, 1215
sunburn in, 1215
tick-borne encephalitis exposure and, 1213
tuberculosis exposure and, 1213
typhoid immunization for, 1212
varicella-zoster virus immunization for, 1211
website resources for, 1208t–1209t
wilderness exposure of, 1215
yellow fever immunization for, 1212–1213
International Travelers' Hotline, 243
Interstitial mononuclear reaction, 118f, 119, 120t
Interstitial pneumonitis, lymphocytic, in AIDS, 427, 430, 466, 467f
Intestinal obstruction, in ascariasis, 510
Intra-abdominal abscess, 923–929. *See also* Abscess, intra-abdominal.
Intracranial pressure, in meningitis, 637, 647
Intraocular fluid, collection of, 62t, 66
Intrauterine growth retardation, 1099
Intrauterine infection, 1099–1116. *See also* Maternal infection; Perinatal infection.
algorithm for, 1101f
cytomegalovirus, 1100t, 1107–1109, 1107f, 1108f, 1108t
diagnosis of, 1101f, 1102t
herpes simplex virus, 1100t, 1109–1110
human parvovirus B19, 1113
lymphocytic choriomeningitis virus, 1100t, 1113–1114
prevention of, 1091–1093, 1092t
rubella, 1100t, 1111–1113. *See also* Rubella, congenital.
screening for, 1101f
Toxoplasma gondii, 1100t, 1114–1116. *See also Toxoplasma gondii* infection (toxoplasmosis), congenital.

Intrauterine infection *(Continued)*
Treponema pallidum, 1100t, 1102–1107. *See also Treponema pallidum* infection (syphilis), congenital.
varicella-zoster virus, 1100t, 1110
Intubation, in bacterial tracheitis, 778
Iodine scrub, 1233
Iodine vaginal douches, in staphylococcal toxic shock syndrome, 302
Iodoquinol, 152t
in amebiasis, 892–893, 893t
in *Dientamoeba fragilis* infection, 903t
in hepatic abscess, 967t
Iron
deficiency of, in hookworm infection, 507
sequestration of, 35
Iron-overload syndrome, 1182t, 1184
Irritability, in fever evaluation, 264, 265t
Ischemia
in Kawasaki syndrome, 484
Isolation, 1233–1238
for cancer patient, 1166
in chickenpox, 340
in erythema infectiosum (fifth disease), 329–330
in measles, 315
in perinatal herpes simplex virus infection, 1140
in varicella-zoster virus infection, 1143
infection-specific, 1234t–1238t
standard precautions for, 1233, 1233t
transmission-based criteria for, 1234, 1234t
Isoniazid, 152t, 206, 206t, 207t, 208t
in latent tuberculosis, 415–416
in tuberculosis, 412–413, 414t
pyridoxine deficiency with, 417
Isoproterenol, in septic shock, 292t
Isospora belli infection, 903t, 904–906
acid-fast stains in, 82–83
clinical manifestations of, 905
diagnosis of, 905
in AIDS, 472
pathogenesis of, 904–905
treatment of, 903t, 906
Isotretinoin, in acne vulgaris, 549
Itraconazole, 152t
in histoplasmosis, 814
in sporotrichosis, 563
in tinea capitis, 558, 558t
Ivermectin
in cutaneous larva migrans, 506t
in filariasis, 518
in lice, 574
in onchocerciasis, 518
in strongyloidiasis, 514t
Ixodes dammini. See Ixodes scapularis.
Ixodes holocyclus, 17
Ixodes pacificus, 21t
in ehrlichiosis, 359
in Lyme disease, 348
Ixodes scapularis, 21t, Plate 9E
in babesiosis, 375, 376f
in ehrlichiosis, 359, 361f
in Lyme disease, 348

J

Janeway lesions, in infective endocarditis, 540, 848, Plate 8C
Japanese encephalitis, 676
immunization against, 253t, 255
for international travel, 244t, 1212
Jarisch-Herxheimer reaction
in brucellosis, 381
in leptospirosis, 387
in relapsing fever, 388
in syphilis, 1023
in trichinellosis, 516
Jaundice, in sepsis, 285
JC virus infection, progressive multifocal leukoencephalopathy in, 685
Jet lag, in international traveler, 1215
Jones criteria, in rheumatic fever, 490, 490t
Juvenile rheumatoid arthritis, fever of unknown origin and, 276t

K

Kanamycin, 151t
Kaposi's sarcoma, in AIDS, 24t, 25–26, 475
Kaposi's sarcoma-associated herpesvirus. *See* Human herpesvirus type 8.
Kaposi's varicelliform eruption, 564–565, 565f
Kasai procedure, cholangitis and, 973, 973t
Katayama fever, in schistosomiasis, 522
Kato-Katz smear, in schistosomiasis, 523
Kawasaki syndrome, 479–484
aneurysm in, 484
atypical (incomplete), 481
cardiac complications of, 483–484
clinical manifestations of, 480–481, 480f, 480t, 481f, Plate 5E
complications of, 483–484
desquamation in, 481, 481f
diagnosis of, 481–482, 482t
differential diagnosis of, 482t
echocardiography in, 482, 483
epidemiology of, 479–480
erythema of, 534t, 535, Plate 5E
etiology of, 479
gangrene in, 484
hearing loss in, 484
in Europe, 479–480
in Japan, 479
in United States, 479–480
lymphadenopathy in, 623
oral manifestations of, 480, 480f, Plate 5F
pathogenesis of, 480
prognosis for, 484
strawberry tongue in, 480, 480f
treatment of, 482–483, 482t
Keratitic precipitates, in uveitis, 1080, 1080f, 1081, 1081f
Keratitis, 1063–1068
Acanthamoeba in, 1063, 1063t, 1065, 1066f, 1067, 1068
adenovirus in, 1059, 1063, 1065, 1066f, 1067, 1068, 1068f
Chlamydia trachomatis in, 1063
clinical manifestations of, 1063t, 1064–1065, 1064f–1066f, Plate 9C
complications of, 1067
culture in, 1066
dendritic ulcer in, 1064f, 1065, Plate 9C
deprivation amblyopia with, 1067
diagnosis of, 1065–1066

Keratitis *(Continued)*
- differential diagnosis of, 1065–1066
- epidemiology of, 1064
- etiology of, 1063–1064
- fungal, 1063t, 1065, 1067
- herpes simplex virus in, 566, 1064, 1063t, 1065, 1065f, 1067, 1068
- nosocomial, 1229–1230, 1230t
- nummular, 1065, 1065f
- pathogenesis of, 1064
- prevention of, 1067–1068
- prognosis for, 1067, 1068f
- punctate, in blepharitis, 1069
- recurrence of, 1067
- ring ulcer in, 1065, 1066f
- syphilitic, 1083, 1083f
- transmission of, 1063–1064
- treatment of, 1066–1067
- ulcer in, 1065, 1064f–1066f
- varicella-zoster virus in, 1065, 1065f, 1067

Keratoconjunctivitis. *See also* Conjunctivitis; Keratitis.
- adenoviral, 1059, 1063, 1065, 1066f, 1067, 1068f
- phlyctenular, 1059, 1059f, 1070, 1070f

Keratolysis, pitted, 549, 549f, 549t
Kerion, in tinea capitis, 557, 557f
Kernicterus, sulfonamide-induced, 184
Kernig's sign, in meningitis, 639
Ketoconazole, 152t, 195–196
- in histoplasmosis, 814

Kidney
- acyclovir effects on, 198
- aminoglycoside toxicity to, 171
- amphotericin B toxicity to, 190–191
- failure of, in malaria, 372
- foscarnet toxicity to, 199, 199t
- in mumps, 422
- infection of, 983–991. *See also* Urinary tract infection.
- pentamidine toxicity to, 209
- transplantation of, 1171–1174. *See* Transplantation, renal.
- tuberculosis of, 404, 408, 413f

Killer inhibitor receptors, 36
Killing curve synergy test, in antimicrobial synergy testing, 77
Kinyoun stain, 68, 68t
- modified, 69, 69t

Kirby-Bauer disk diffusion test, in antimicrobial susceptibility testing, 75
Kissing lesions, in syphilis, 537
Klebsiella infection
- in cancer patient, 283
- in septic shock, 281
- meningeal, 630, 630t, 631t. *See also* Meningitis, bacterial.
- urinary tract, 983, 983t. *See also* Urinary tract infection.

Klebsiella pneumonia infection, intra-abdominal, 923–928. *See also* Abscess, intra-abdominal.
Koeppe nodules, in uveitis, 1080
Koilocytes, in human papillomavirus infection, 1030
Koplik's spots, 306, 308, 535, Plate 3B
Krukenberg's spindle, in uveitis, 1080, 1081f
Kupffer cells, 33–34
Kuru, 685–687, 686t

L

Labeled-antibody techniques, for antigen detection, 111, 113f–115f
Lacrimal sac, infection of, 1072–1073, 1072f
Lactate, serum, in septic shock, 287
Lactic acid, of cerebrospinal fluid, 642
Lactobacillus
- in *Clostridium difficile*–associated diarrhea, 913
- in newborn, 7
- vaginal, 1000, 1000t

Lagophthalmos, 1059
Lamivudine, 152t, 203t, 205t
- in hepatitis B virus infection, 956
- in HIV infection, 456, 457t, 458t, 460t

Lancefield carbohydrate C, of group A *Streptococcus,* 486
Langerhans cells, 31, 33–34
Language development, otitis media and, 756
Laplace's law, 1073
Larva migrans
- cutaneous, 20t, 504, 505, 506t, 569–570, 570f
- ocular, 511t, 512, 1082, 1082f, 1083, 1084
- visceral, 511–512, 511t, 512t, 1082

Laryngotracheitis, in measles, 312
Laryngotracheobronchitis, 771–774, 818–819
- clinical manifestations of, 772
- complications of, 774
- corticosteroids in, 773–774
- diagnosis of, 772–773, 773f, 774f
- epidemiology of, 771
- etiology of, 771, 772t
- imaging in, 773, 773f, 774f
- in measles, 312
- nebulized epinephrine in, 773
- pathogenesis of, 771–772
- physical examination in, 772
- prognosis for, 774
- steeple sign in, 773, 774f
- treatment of, 773–774, 774t
- vs. spasmodic (recurrent) croup, 771–772, 771t

Larynx, papilloma of, 567, 568
Laser capture microdissection assay, 122–123
Latent membrane proteins, of Epstein-Barr virus, 426
Lateral sinus thrombosis, with brain abscess, 663
Laterothoracic exanthem, unilateral, 537
Latex agglutination assay
- for antibody detection, 102
- for bacterial and fungal antigens, 70–71
- in meningitis, 641, 642t

Latex particle agglutination assay. *See* Latex agglutination assay.
Legionella micdadei infection, 805
Legionella pneumophila infection, 15, 805–807. *See also* Pneumonia, *Legionella pneumophila.*
Leiomyosarcoma, Epstein-Barr virus in, 25
Leishmaniasis
- culture in, 570
- cutaneous, 570–571, 570f
- epidemiology of, 20t
- specimen collection in, 81
- visceral, 570

Lemierre's postanginal septicemia, 736, 738t
Lentiviruses, in oncogenesis, 24t, 27
Leproma, 553–554
Lepromin test, 552
Leprosy, 552–554
- amyloidosis in, 704
- borderline, 553, 553t
- clinical manifestations of, 553–554, 553f, 553t
- complications of, 554
- diagnosis of, 554
- downgrading reactions in, 703
- epidemiology of, 552, 552f
- etiology of, 552
- indeterminate, 553
- lepromatous, 552–554, 553t, 703
- Lucio, 554
- neuritic, 554
- neuropathy of, 703–704
- pathogenesis of, 552–553
- prognosis for, 554
- reversal reactions in, 554, 703
- slit-skin smear in, 554
- transmission of, 552
- treatment of, 554, 554t
- tuberculoid, 552, 553, 553f, 553t, 703

Leptospira spp. infection (leptospirosis), 385–387
- clinical manifestations of, 386, 386t
- complications of, 387
- diagnosis of, 386–387
- epidemiology of, 18t, 386
- etiology of, 385–386
- maternal, 387
- meningitis in, 633
- pathogenesis of, 386
- prevention of, 387
- prognosis for, 387
- serologic testing in, 387
- treatment of, 387, 387t

Lethal toxin, in anthrax, 551
Leucovorin, in congenital toxoplasmosis, 1116, 1116t
Leukemia. *See also* Cancer.
- fever of unknown origin and, 276t
- lymphadenopathy in, 613, 623
- T-cell, adult, 27

Leukemoid reaction, 92
Leukocyte adhesion deficiency, 1153
Leukocyte esterase test, in urinary tract infection, 986
Leukocyte rolling, 33
Leukocytoclastic vasculitis, 539
Leukocytosis, 53, 92
Leukoencephalopathy, multifocal, progressive, 685
Leukokoria, 1083
Leukopenia
- flucytosine-induced, 193
- in AIDS, 474
- in septic shock, 287

Leukoplakia, hairy, oral, in AIDS, 470
Levofloxacin, 151t, 184–187, 185t, 186t
- dosing for, 186t

Lice, 573–574, 573f
- in day care environment, 1191

Lichen sclerosus, vs. vulvovaginitis, 1004
Lidocaine, in stomatitis, 732t
Ligase chain reaction assay, 122

Limbal flush, in uveitis, 1080
Lincomycin, 152t, 187, 187t, 188t
Lincosamide antibiotics, 187, 187t, 188t
Lindane, in lice, 574
Linezolid, 151t, 172–175, 173t, 174t, 175t
  dosing for, 174t
  drug interactions with, 175, 175t
Lipase, in acute pancreatitis, 980
Lipopolysaccharide, 3, 32
  antibodies to, in septic shock, 290, 292
Lipopolysaccharide-binding protein, 32
Lipoteichoic acid, 3t, 284
Liquid nitrogen therapy, in echinococcosis, 530
Listeria monocytogenes infection (listeriosis), 15, 16t, 908–911, 909, 910t, 911t
  epidemiology of, 18t
  in sepsis, 279
  maternal, 1088t
  meningeal, 630, 630t, 634. *See also* Meningitis, bacterial.
Liver. *See also at* Hepatitis.
  abscess of, 963–969. *See also* Abscess, hepatic.
  enlargement of, in AIDS, 472–473
  erythromycin toxicity to, 178
  isoniazid toxicity to, 206
  rifampin toxicity to, 208
  transplantation of, 1174–1176, 1174t. *See also* Transplantation, hepatic.
    cholangitis after, 973
Loaiasis, 81, 81t
Lockjaw. *See Clostridium tetani* infection (tetanus).
Löffler's syndrome, in ascariasis, 509, 509t
Log roll test, in diskitis, 1051
Lomefloxacin, 151t
  in gonorrhea, 1014t
Lone Star tick, 21t
  in ehrlichiosis, 359
  in tularemia, 382
Loperamide
  in acute enteritis, 917t, 918
  in travelers' diarrhea, 907t
Lopinavir, 152t
  in HIV infection, 456, 457t, 459t, 460t
Loracarbef, 151t
  dosing for, 164t
  formulations of, 162t
  in otitis media, 754t
  in sinusitis, 765t
  pathogen susceptibility to, 161t
  pharmacokinetics of, 163t
Louping ill disease, 676
Louseborne relapsing fever, 19t, 387–388, 388t
Louseborne typhus, 388–389, 389t
Lowenstein-Jensen medium, 73, 74t
Ludwig's angina, 582, 583, 584, 734, 736–737, 739
  treatment of, 738t
Lungs. *See also* Respiratory tract.
  abscess of, 837–840. *See also* Abscess, lung.
  transplantation of, 1177–1179, 1178t
Lung fluke infection, 522t
Lyme disease, 348–353. *See also Borrelia burgdorferi* infection (Lyme disease).
Lymph nodes, cervical, 619–621, 620f
Lymphadenitis, 610
  cellulitis with, 582–583, 583f, 584
Lymphadenitis *(Continued)*
  cervical, 619–626, 620f
    clinical manifestations of, 621–623, 622f, 622t, 623f
    complications of, 626
    diagnosis of, 623–625, 624f
    epidemiology of, 621
    etiology of, 621
    nontuberculous, 622, 622t, 626, 626t
    pathogenesis of, 621
    prevention of, 626
    prognosis for, 626
    treatment of, 625–626, 626t
    tuberculous, 400f, 402, 402f, 413–414, 414t, 622, 622t
    vs. parotitis, 423
  inguinal, 615–619, 620t
  mesenteric, vs. appendicitis, 934, 934t
  regional, cellulitis with, 582–583, 583f
Lymphadenopathy, 610
  abdominal, 611
  cervical, 610, 619–626, 620f
    clinical manifestations of, 621–623, 622f, 622t, 623f
    complications of, 626
    diagnosis of, 623–625, 624f
    epidemiology of, 621
    etiology of, 621
    in Kawasaki syndrome, 481
    pathogenesis of, 621
    prevention of, 626
    treatment of, 625–626, 626t
  chronic, 610
  epitrochlear, 611
  generalized, 611–615
    clinical manifestations of, 612–613
    complications of, 615
    diagnosis of, 613–615, 614f, 615t
    epidemiology of, 611
    etiology of, 611, 611t
    pathogenesis of, 612
    persistent, 612
    prognosis of, 615
    treatment of, 615
  iliac, 611
  in rubella, 318
  inguinal, 615–619
    biopsy of, 619
    clinical manifestations of, 616–617
    complications of, 619
    diagnosis of, 617–619
    epidemiology of, 615–616
    etiology of, 615
    needle aspiration of, 618–619
    pathogenesis of, 616
    prevention of, 619
    prognosis for, 619
    treatment of, 619, 620t
  mediastinal, 611
  pelvic, 611
  regional, 610–611
Lymphadenopathy-associated virus. *See* Human immunodeficiency virus (HIV) infection.
Lymphangitis, 579, 611, 626–628, Plate 8B
  clinical manifestations of, 627
  complications of, 627–628
  diagnosis of, 627
Lymphangitis *(Continued)*
  epidemiology of, 627
  etiology of, 626–627
  pathogenesis of, 627
  prevention of, 628
  prognosis for, 628
  treatment of, 579, 627
Lymphocutaneous syndromes, 611, 622, 622f. *See also Bartonella henselae* infection (cat-scratch disease).
Lymphocyte(s), 93–95. *See also* B cells; T cells.
  Epstein-Barr virus infection of, 427, 430, 431t. *See also* Infectious mononucleosis.
  in burn injury, 597
  in HIV infection, 444, 444t, 460–461, 461t
  in leprosy, 552–553
  normal count of, 93t
Lymphocytic choriomeningitis virus infection, 19t, 677, 1113–1114
Lymphocytic interstitial pneumonitis
  imaging in, 136, 136f, 466, 467t
  in AIDS, 427, 430, 466, 467f
Lymphocytoma, in Lyme disease, 350
Lymphocytopenia, CD4, 94–95
Lymphocytosis, 93–94
  absolute, 94
  atypical, 94
  relative, 94
Lymphocytosis-promoting factor, 94
Lymphogranuloma venereum, 1027, 1027t
  diagnosis of, 617
  groove sign of, 617
  lymphadenopathy in, 616, 617
Lymphokines, in antigen processing, 40–41, 40t
Lymphoma. *See also* Cancer.
  biopsy in, 625
  fever of unknown origin and, 276t
  Helicobacter pylori infection and, 876
  in AIDS, 465
  lymphadenopathy in, 613, 623
Lymphopenia, 94–95
  in T-cell deficiency, 53
Lymphoproliferative disease, Epstein-Barr virus in, 24t, 25, 25t
Lysozyme, 31

M

M protein, of group A *Streptococcus,* 486
MAC. *See Mycobacterium avium* complex infection.
Macaque monkey bite, 602, 605, 608
Macrolide antibiotics, 175–178, 176t
  adverse effects of, 177–178
  dosing for, 177, 178t
  drug interactions with, 178, 179t
  formulation of, 177
  mechanism of action of, 176
  metabolism of, 176–177, 177t
Macrophage, in innate immunity, 34
Macrophage inflammatory proteins, in meningitis, 636
Maculae ceruleae, 574
Macular erythema, 534–535, 534t, 535f, 536f
Macular star
  in cat-scratch disease, 344, 345f, Plate 9D
  in retinitis, 1083, Plate 9D

Macules, definition of, 533
Maculopapular rash, 535–538, 536t, 537f, 538f
Mafenide acetate, 152t
  in burn wound infection, 599t
Magnetic resonance imaging, 127t
  in brain abscess, 130f, 660, 661f
  in *Candida albicans* infection, 140, 140f
  in cellulitis, 583
  in central nervous system infection, 126–127, 128f
  in cysticercosis, 526
  in diskitis, 1052–1053, 1053f
  in echinococcosis, 529
  in meningitis, 128f, 643
  in osteomyelitis, 141, 142f, 1037
  in sinusitis, 130, 763–764, 764f
  in spinal epidural abscess, 666, 667f
  in subdural empyema, 664, 665f
  in urinary tract infection, 988
  of abdominal organs, 137, 139f, 140f
MAI. *See Mycobacterium avium* complex infection.
Major basic protein, 95
  in toxocariasis, 511
Major histocompatibility complex, in antigen processing, 37–38, 37f
Malaria, 363–374. *See also Plasmodium* spp. infection (malaria).
Malassezia furfur infection
  blood specimen collection in, 63–64
  in acne vulgaris, 547
Malathion, in lice, 574
Malnutrition, 1183t, 1185–1186
  immune response and, 49, 49t
Malta fever. *See Brucella* spp. infection (brucellosis).
Mantoux tuberculin skin test, 405–406, 405f, 406t
  in HIV-infected child, 460, 467–468
Market fever, 372
Mass spectrometry, 123
Mastitis
  maternal, 1096
  neonatal, 1129–1130, 1129t
Mastoiditis, otitis media and, 757, 757f
Maternal infection, 1085–1098, 1085t, 1086t
  asymptomatic, 1087–1089, 1088t
  breast-feeding and, 1095–1097, 1095t
  Chlamydia trachomatis, 1016t, 1018, 1019
  counseling for, 1097
  cytomegalovirus, 1096, 1107–1108, 1107f
  enterovirus, 1091
  fetal infection and, 1089–1090, 1089t
  group B *Streptococcus,* 1087, 1088t, 1091, 1093, 1093f–1095f
  hepatitis B, 1091, 1094, 1096
  herpes simplex virus, 1024, 1091, 1094, 1096, 1109–1110, 1136–1140. *See also* Herpes simplex virus infection, perinatal.
  HIV, 1087, 1088t, 1091, 1094–1095, 1096
  human papillomavirus, 1029
  human parvovirus B19, 1113
  immunization in, 238
  infectious mononucleosis, 434–435
  leptospirosis, 387
  lymphocytic choriomeningitis virus, 1113–1114
  malaria, 368
  malaria prophylaxis during, 374
Maternal infection *(Continued)*
  measles, 313
  mumps, 424
  Mycobacterium tuberculosis, 399–400, 1093–1094, 1096
  Neisseria gonorrhoeae, 1012, 1014t, 1093
  perinatal infection and, 1090–1091, 1091t. *See also* Perinatal infection.
  prevention of, 1087, 1091–1093, 1092t
  rubella, 319, 320, 1111–1113
  screening for, 1087–1089, 1088t
  Staphylococcus aureus, 1096
  symptomatic, 1089, 1089t
  Toxoplasma gondii, 1114–1116
  treatment of, neonatal sepsis treatment and, 1128
  varicella-zoster virus, 1091, 1110, 1140–1143. *See also* Varicella-zoster virus infection, perinatal.
Maxillary sinuses
  anatomy of, 760–761, 761f
  infection of. *See* Sinusitis.
  transillumination of, 762–763
McBurney's point, 932
Measles, 306–315
  atypical, 309, 535
  bacterial tracheitis with, 312
  cerebral cry with, 682
  chest x-ray in, 310–311, 311f
  clinical manifestations of, 307–309, 308f, 308t
  complications of, 312–313
  culture in, 307f, 310
  diagnosis of, 88t, 309–311, 309t, 310t
  diarrhea with, 312
  differential diagnosis of, 309–310, 309t, 310t
  enanthem of, 306, 308, 535, 536t, Plate 3B
  encephalitis with, 312–313, 681–682
  epidemiology of, 306, 307f
  etiology of, 306
  exanthem of, 308, Plate 3A
  exanthematous phase of, 307
  gestational, 313
  hospital isolation for, 315
  imaging in, 310–311, 311f
  immune globulin in, 217
  immunization against, 255–256. *See also* Measles-mumps-rubella (MMR) vaccine.
    for international travel, 244t, 1207, 1209
    postexposure, 242t
  in AIDS, 461, 469
  in immunocompromised persons, 309
  incubation phase of, 307
  international travel and, 315
  laboratory evaluation in, 310
  laryngotracheitis with, 312
  maternal, 313
  microbiologic evaluation in, 310
  modified, 308–309
    vs. rubella, 318
  otitis media with, 312
  outbreak control with, 314–315
  pathogenesis of, 306–307, 307f
  phases of, 307–308, 308f
  physical examination in, 308
  pneumonia with, 311f, 312
  postexposure prophylaxis in, 217, 314, 314t
  prevention of, 313–315, 314t
  prodromal phase of, 307
Measles *(Continued)*
  prognosis for, 313
  recovery phase of, 307–308
  serologic diagnosis of, 310
  subacute sclerosing panencephalitis with, 313
  supportive treatment of, 311–312
  treatment of, 311–312, 311t
  vitamin A in, 311, 311t
  vs. roseola, 323
  vs. rubella, 318
Measles-mumps-rubella (MMR) vaccine, 233t, 235t–236t, 253t, 313–315, 314t, 319–320
  adverse reactions to, 233t, 235t–236t
  in HIV-infected child, 460
Meatitis, 996
Mebendazole, 153t, 209–210, 209t, 210t
  in angiostrongyliasis, 517, 517t
  in enterobiasis, 515, 515t
  in hookworm infection, 506, 506t
  in trichinellosis, 516, 517t
  in trichuriasis, 508, 508t
  in visceral larva migrans, 512, 512t
Mediastinitis, 842–844
  clinical manifestations of, 842–843
  complications of, 844
  diagnosis of, 843
  epidemiology of, 842
  esophageal perforation and, 842
  etiology of, 842
  pathogenesis of, 842, 843t
  prevention of, 844
  prognosis for, 844
  treatment of, 843, 843t
Medical waste disposal, 1240
Mediterranean spotted fever, 355t
Mefloquine, 153t
  in malaria, 371t
  in malaria prophylaxis, 373t, 374
Membrane attack complex, 34, 35f
Meningitis, 630–649
  amebic, 632
  anticonvulsants in, 647
  aseptic
    etiology of, 631–632, 631t
    in Kawasaki syndrome, 481
    in varicella-zoster virus infection, 338–339
  ataxia after, 648
  bacterial
    clinical manifestations of, 637–639, 638t
    epidemiology of, 633
    etiology of, 630, 630t, 631t
    immunization against, 233t, 235t–236t, 237t, 244t, 245t, 246–248, 649
    partially treated, 643
    pathogenesis of, 635–637, 635f, 636f
    prevention of, 649
    prognosis for, 648–649
    prophylactic therapy against, 225–226, 228t
    treatment of, 643–647, 643t, 645t–646t, 1014t
  Brudzinski's sign in, 638–639
  bulging fontanelle in, 639
  cerebrospinal fluid examination in, 639–643, 640t, 642t
    acid-fast stain in, 641
    antigen detection tests in, 642
    chloride in, 642
    C-reactive protein in, 642

Meningitis *(Continued)*
cerebrospinal fluid examination in *(Continued)*
culture in, 642
glucose in, 641
Gram stain in, 641–642, 642t
India ink test in, 641, 642t
lactic acid in, 642
latex agglutination test in, 641, 642t
polymerase chain reaction test in, 642
protein in, 640t, 641, 641t
white blood cells in, 640, 640t
chronic, 630, 633
clinical manifestations of, 637–639, 638t
complications of, 647–648, 647t, 648f
computed tomography in, 643
corticosteroids in, 646–647
culture in, 642
diagnosis of, 639–643, 640t, 641t, 642t
antibiotics before, 643
differential diagnosis of, 639
eosinophilic, 517, 517t, 631, 632t
epidemiology of, 633–635
etiology of, 630–633, 630t, 631t
fever in, 647–648, 647t
fulminant, 637
fungal
epidemiology of, 634–635, 634t
prevention of, 649
treatment of, 645t–646t, 646
hearing loss after, 648
imaging in, 639, 643
in leptospirosis, 633
in Lyme disease, 633
increased intracranial pressure in, 637, 647
intelligence quotient (IQ) after, 648–649
Kernig's sign in, 639
magnetic resonance imaging in, 128f, 643
Mollaret's, 631–632, 632t
mortality for, 648
mumps, 421, 682
neonatal
clinical manifestations of, 638, 638t
epidemiology of, 633–634, 633t
etiology of, 630–631
treatment of, 644
nosocomial, 1229, 1229t
nuchal rigidity in, 638
opisthotonos in, 639
papilledema in, 639
pathogenesis of, 635–637, 635f, 636f
petechiae in, 637
plague, 384, 385, 385t
prevention of, 649
prognosis for, 648–649
recurrent, 631–632, 632t
seizures in, 638, 639, 649
subacute, 630, 632–633
subdural effusion in, 648, 648f
subdural empyema in, 648
supportive therapy in, 646–647
syndrome of inappropriate ADH secretion in, 646
syphilitic, 634, 1021, 1104
treatment of, 643–647, 643t, 645t–646t
tuberculous, 400f, 632–633, 680
clinical manifestations of, 402–403
epidemiology of, 634
Meningitis *(Continued)*
tuberculous *(Continued)*
imaging of, 408, 412f
treatment of, 414, 414t
viral
clinical manifestations of, 637–639, 638t
epidemiology of, 634
etiology of, 631, 631t
pathogenesis of, 637
prevention of, 649
prognosis for, 649
Meningococcemia
fulminant, 285
purpura in, 539–540, 539t
Meningoencephalitis, 637
amebic, primary, 632
in Epstein-Barr virus infection, 681
in infectious mononucleosis, 428, 431
in Rocky Mountain spotted fever, 357, 681
Meningomyelocele, 1182t
Meningopolyneuritis, in Lyme disease, 350
Menses, toxic shock syndrome and, 296
Mental retardation, with congenital cytomegalovirus infection, 1108
Meperidine, before amphotericin B administration, 192
Meropenem, 151t, 166–167, 166t, 167t
in acute pancreatitis, 981, 981t
in brain abscess, 661
in burn wound infection, 600t
in intra-abdominal abscess, 929t
in meningitis, 644, 645t, 646t
in neonatal sepsis, 1126t
in wound infection, 593t
Mesentery, 921
Metabolic disease, immunization in, 241t
Metagonimiasis, 522t
Metagonimus yokogawai infection, 522t
Metamorphopsia, in infectious mononucleosis, 428
Methenamine mandelate, in urinary tract infection, 991t
Methenamine silver stain, for *Pneumocystis carinii* cyst, 82
Methicillin, formulations of, 157t
Methylprednisolone, in uveitis, 1081
Metorchiasis, 522t
Metorchis conjunctus infection, 522t
Metronidazole, 152t, 187–189, 189t
dosing for, 189t
in amebiasis, 893t
in bacterial vaginosis, 1006t
in brain abscess, 661, 662t
in cholecystitis, 972, 972t
in cranial epidural abscess, 666t
in gastritis, 875–876, 876t
in giardiasis, 902, 903t
in hepatic abscess, 967t
in intra-abdominal abscess, 929t
in mediastinitis, 843, 843t
in neonatal sepsis, 1126t
in pelvic inflammatory disease, 1015t
in sepsis, 291t
in shunt-related infection, 655t
in subdural empyema, 666t
in tetanus, 694
in trichomoniasis, 1028, 1028t
Metronidazole *(Continued)*
in wound botulism, 697
in wound infection, 593t
Mezlocillin, 151t
dosing for, 159t
formulations of, 157t
in cholecystitis, 972, 972t
in hepatic abscess, 967t
in neonatal sepsis, 1126t
in sepsis, 291t
pathogen susceptibility to, 155t
Miconazole, 152t, 195–196
in *Candida* diaper dermatitis, 1006t
in vulvovaginal candidiasis, 1006t
Microhemagglutination–*T. pallidum* test (MHA-TP), 105, 108, 1021–1022, 1022t
Microsporida infection, 903t, 904–906
clinical manifestations of, 905
diagnosis of, 905
pathogenesis of, 905
treatment of, 903t, 906
Microsporum audouinii infection, 19t, 556–558, 556t, 558t
Microsporum canis infection, 558–560, 559f, 559t, 561t
macroconidia in, 75, 75f
Middlebrook-Cohn 7H10 medium, 73–74, 74t
Middlebrook-Cohn 7H11 medium, 73–74, 74t
Miliary tuberculosis, 400f, 401–402, 408, 411f
Milking sign, in rheumatic fever, 489
Minimum bactericidal concentration (MBC), 76, 148
Minimum inhibitory concentration (MIC), 76, 148
Minocycline, 151t, 180–182, 181t, 182t
adverse effects of, 182, 182t
dosing for, 181–182, 182t
drug interactions with, 182, 182t
in leprosy, 554, 554t
pathogen susceptibility to, 181t
pharmacokinetics of, 181, 181t
Mites, 571–573, 572f
Mitral regurgitation, in rheumatic fever, 488
Mixed lymphocyte reaction, 55
Molds, classification of, 59, 60t
Mollaret's meningitis, 631–632, 632t
Molluscum contagiosum, 568–569, 569f
in AIDS, 475
Monilia. *See Candida* spp. infection (candidiasis).
Monkeypox, vs. chickenpox, 334
Monobactam antibiotics, 165–166, 165t, 166t
Mononeuritis multiplex, in HIV infection, 704
Mononuclear phagocytes, 33–34
Monosodium glutamate ingestion, 16t, 912
Moon's molar, in congenital syphilis, 1104
Moraxella catarrhalis infection
conjunctival, 1058, 1058t. *See also* Conjunctivitis, bacterial.
otologic, 749. *See also* Otitis media.
sinus, 760. *See also* Sinusitis.
Morison's pouch, 923
Mortality rate, 12
Morulae, in ehrlichiosis, 355, 360f, 361
Mosquitoes, 15
in California encephalitis, 673
in Eastern equine encephalitis, 674–675
in Japanese encephalitis, 676
in St. Louis encephalitis, 673

Mosquitoes *(Continued)*
in Venezuelan equine encephalitis, 676
in West Nile virus infection, 675
in Western equine encephalitis, 673–674
protection against, 17
Motion sickness, 1215
Mouthwash, in stomatitis, 732t
Moxalactam
dosing for, 164t
pharmacokinetics of, 163t
Moxifloxacin, 152t, 184–187, 185t, 186t
Mucocele, of nasolacrimal sac, 1072–1073, 1072f
Mucocutaneous lymph node syndrome. *See* Kawasaki syndrome.
Mucor infection, 131, 134f, 812, 812t
Mucosa-associated lymphoid tissue, *Helicobacter pylori* infection and, 29, 873
Mucus, 31
Muerto Canyon virus. *See* Hantavirus cardiopulmonary syndrome.
Mulberry molar, in congenital syphilis, 1104
Multinucleated cells, 116
Multiple myeloma, human herpesvirus 8 in, 26
Multiple sclerosis, human herpes virus 6 and, 681
Multiproteinase complex, 38
Mumps, 420–425
cerebrospinal fluid examination in, 423
clinical manifestations of, 420–422, 421f, 421t
complications of, 424
culture in, 423
cutaneous eruption in, 537
diagnosis of, 88t, 422–423, 423t
encephalitis in, 421, 682
epidemiology of, 420, 421f
epididymo-orchitis in, 420–421
etiology of, 420
immunization against, 242t, 256, 424. *See also* Measles-mumps-rubella (MMR) vaccine.
for international travel, 1209
postexposure, 242t
maternal, 424
meningitis in, 421, 682
neonatal, 422
oophoritis in, 420–421
orchitis in, 995
pancreatitis in, 422
parotitis in, 420, 421, Plate 3F
pathogenesis of, 420
pathology of, 423
polyarthralgia in, 422
polyarthritis in, 422
presternal edema in, 421, 422f
prevention of, 424–425
prognosis for, 424
renal involvement in, 422
serologic testing in, 423
transmission of, 420
treatment of, 423–424
vs. lymphadenopathy, 624
Munchausen syndrome
factitious fever in, 275–276
fever of unknown origin in, 275, 276t
Munchausen syndrome by proxy
factitious fever in, 275–276
fever of unknown origin in, 275, 276t
Mupirocin, 152t, 189–190, 190t
dosing for, 190t
Mupirocin *(Continued)*
in impetigo, 545, 546t
Murine typhus, 355t, 388–389, 389t
Murmur, in rheumatic fever, 488
Muscle, postpolio atrophy of, 700
Musculoskeletal system, imaging of, 141–145, 141f–145f
Mushroom poisoning, 16t, 911–912
Mussel poisoning, 911
Mycobacteremia, blood specimen collection in, 63
Mycobacteria, classification of, 59, 59t
Mycobacterial infection. *See also specific species infections and* Tuberculosis.
antimicrobial susceptibility testing in, 76
biopsy specimen in, 66
blood specimen in, 63
body fluid specimen in, 64
culture in, 66, 73–74, 74t
urine specimen in, 66
Mycobacterium abscessus infection, 626, 626t
Mycobacterium africanum infection, 396–419. *See also* Tuberculosis.
Mycobacterium avium complex infection
in AIDS, 451t, 461, 461t, 462t, 471–472
lymphadenopathy in, 622, 622t, 623f
stool culture in, 65
treatment of, 626, 626t
Mycobacterium avium-intracellulare. See Mycobacterium avium complex infection.
Mycobacterium balnei. See Mycobacterium marinum infeciton.
Mycobacterium bovis infection, 396–419. *See also* Tuberculosis.
Mycobacterium chelonae infection
catheter-related, 66
cutaneous, 555–556, 555t
cutaneous nodules in, 542, 542f
treatment of, 626, 626t
Mycobacterium chelonei. See Mycobacterium chelonae infection.
Mycobacterium fortuitum infection
catheter-related, 66
cutaneous, 555–556, 555t
epidemiology of, 18t
treatment of, 626, 626t
Mycobacterium haemophilum infection
culture in, 73–74, 74t
lymphadenopathy in, 622
Mycobacterium kansasii infection
cutaneous, 555–556, 555t
epidemiology of, 18t
treatment of, 626, 626t
Mycobacterium leprae infection, 552–554, 552f, 553f, 553t, 554t. *See also* Leprosy.
Mycobacterium marinum infection, 588, 590
culture in, 73–74, 74t
cutaneous, 555–556, 555f, 555t
epidemiology of, 18t
of lymphatic channels, 627
treatment of, 626, 626t
Mycobacterium tuberculosis infection, 396–419. *See also* Tuberculosis.
in oncogenesis, 24t, 29
Mycobacterium ulcerans infection
culture in, 73–74, 74t
cutaneous, 555–556, 555t
Mycoplasma hominis infection, culture in, 73
Mycoplasma pneumoniae infection
cold agglutinins in, 97–98
culture in, 73
cutaneous manifestations of, 536t, 537
neurologic manifestations of, 680–681
pulmonary, 795t, 807–809. *See also* Pneumonia, *Mycoplasma pneumoniae.*
serologic testing in, 108
Myiasis, 571, 571f
Myocardial infarction, in Kawasaki syndrome, 484
Myocarditis, 857–861
chest radiography in, 860, 860f
clinical manifestations of, 858–859, 858t
complications of, 861
culture in, 859
diagnosis of, 859–860, 859t
differential diagnosis of, 859, 859t
echocardiography in, 859
electrocardiography in, 859
epidemiology of, 857
etiology of, 857, 858t
in infectious mononucleosis, 434
in rheumatic fever, 488
magnetic resonance imaging in, 860
pathogenesis of, 857–858
pathology of, 860, 860f
physical examination in, 859
polymerase chain reaction test in, 859–860
prevention of, 861
prognosis for, 861
treatment of, 860–861
with *Salmonella typhi* infection, 884
Myonecrosis, 587–595
clinical manifestations of, 591
complications of, 594
diagnosis of, 591–592
epidemiology of, 588
etiology of, 587, 588t
pathogenesis of, 589, 589t
prevention of, 595
prognosis for, 594–595
treatment of, 592–594, 592f, 593t
Myopericarditis, 863. *See also* Pericarditis.
Myringotomy, in otitis media, 756

N

Naegleria fowleri infection, 13
meningeal, 632
Nafcillin, 151t
dosing for, 158t
formulations of, 157t
in acute pericarditis, 867t
in bite-wound infection, 606, 606t, 607t
in brain abscess, 662t
in burn wound infection, 600t
in cellulitis, 580t, 585t
in cranial epidural abscess, 666t
in erysipelas, 580t
in hepatic abscess, 967t
in infectious arthritis, 1048t
in infective endocarditis, 851t–852t
in intra-abdominal abscess, 929t
in meningitis, 645t, 646t
in neonatal sepsis, 1126t
in osteomyelitis, 1040t
in sepsis, 291t

Nafcillin *(Continued)*
in shunt-related infection, 655t
in spinal epidural abscess, 667t
in staphylococcal toxic shock syndrome, 302, 302t
in subdural empyema, 666t
in tracheitis, 776t
in wound infection, 593t
pathogen susceptibility to, 155t
Nalidixic acid, 152t, 184–187
dosing for, 186t
Naloxone, in septic shock, 290
Nanophyetiasis, 522t
Nanophyetus salmincola infection, 522t
Nasolacrimal duct obstruction, 1072–1073, 1072f
bacterial conjunctivitis and, 1061
Nasolacrimal sac, mucocele of, 1072–1073, 1072f
Nasopharynx. *See also* Pharyngitis.
carcinoma of, Epstein-Barr virus in, 23
specimen collection from, 61t, 64
streptococcal infection of. *See* Streptococcal pharyngitis.
National Childhood Vaccine Injury Act (1986), 232, 234, 238
Native valve endocarditis, 847. *See also* Infective endocarditis.
Natural killer cells, 36
Natural valve endocarditis. *See* Native valve endocarditis.
Necator americanus, life cycle of, 504, 505f
Necator americanus infection, 504–507. *See also* Hookworm infection.
Neck
abscess of, 721–727. *See also* Abscess, neck.
fascial layers of, 722–723, 722f
potential spaces of, 722f, 723
stiffness of, in meningitis, 638
Necrotizing enterocolitis, 1130–1132
clinical manifestations of, 1130
complications of, 1131–1132
diagnosis of, 1130–1131, 1131f
epidemiology of, 1130
pathogenesis of, 1130, 1131f
prevention of, 1132
prognosis for, 1131–1132
short-gut syndrome in, 1132
treatment of, 1131
Necrotizing fasciitis, 587–595
clinical manifestations of, 590–591, 590f
complications of, 594
diagnosis of, 591–592
epidemiology of, 588–589
etiology of, 587, 588, 588t
mortality rate in, 594–595
pathogenesis of, 589, 589t
prevention of, 595
prognosis for, 594–595
treatment of, 592–594, 592f, 593t
Necrotizing reaction, 118f, 120t
Necrotizing ulcerative gingivitis, 734, 735–736, 737, 738t
Needle aspiration. *See also* Biopsy.
in brain abscess, 663
in cervical lymphadenopathy, 625
in cranial epidural abscess, 665
in inguinal lymphadenopathy, 618–619
in lymphadenopathy, 614
Needle-stick injury, 1241, 1241t
Neisseria catarrhalis. See Moraxella catarrhalis infection.
Neisseria gonorrhoeae infection (gonorrhea), 1010–1016
antibiotic-resistant, 1013
arthritis-dermatitis syndrome in, 1012
clinical manifestations of, 1011–1012
complications of, 1015
conjunctival, 1011, 1055–1058, 1056t, 1057f
culture in, 1012–1013, 1015
diagnosis of, 1012–1013
disseminated, 1012, 1014t, 1015, 1044, 1045, 1046t, 1049
arthritis-dermatitis syndrome in, 1045
pathogenesis of, 1045
treatment of, 1013, 1014t, 1049
epidemiology of, 1010, 1011f
etiology of, 1010
in sexual partners, 1015
lymphadenopathy in, 616
maternal, 1012, 1014t, 1088t, 1092t, 1093
molecular tests in, 124
ophthalmic, 1012, 1013–1014, 1014t, 1016, 1055–1058. *See also* Conjunctivitis, neonatal.
prophylaxis against, 1016
pathogenesis of, 1011
peritoneal, 929
pharyngeal, 1011, 1014t, 1016
prevention of, 1016
prognosis for, 1015–1016
sexual abuse and, 1012
skin lesions in, 541, 541t, 542f
specimen collection in, 65
supportive therapy in, 1015, 1016t
transmission of, 1010
treatment of, 1013–1015, 1014t
in adolescents and adults, 1013, 1014t
in children, 1013, 1014t
in neonate, 1013–1015, 1014t
vulvovaginal, 1004, 1006t, 1012, 1014t
Neisseria meningitidis infection, 630–649. *See also* Meningitis, bacterial.
CSF examination in, 288
fulminant, 285
immunization against, 245t, 247–248, 649
for international travel, 244t
in bacteremia, 270t, 272, 282t, 283
in day care environment, 1189
in primary immunodeficiency, 283
in sepsis, 279, 285, 293, 293t, 294t, Plate 5D
in septic shock, 280, 280t, 281
in sickle cell disease, 283
prognosis for, 293, 293t
prophylactic therapy against, 225–226, 228t
rapid diagnosis of, 288
Nelfinavir, 152t, 204t, 205t
in HIV infection, 456, 457t, 460t
Nematode infection, 504–518, 504t. *See also specific infections.*
Neomycin, 151t
in gastrointestinal *Escherichia coli* infection, 897, 897t
Nephritis
imaging in, 140, 140f
interstitial, penicillin-related, 156
Nephritis strain-associated protein, 594
Nephrotic syndrome, 1183t, 1185
immunization in, 241t
Nephrotoxicity
aminoglycoside-induced, 171
amphotericin B–related, 190–191
foscarnet-induced, 199, 199t
pentamindine-associated, 209
Netilmicin, 151t, 167–172, 168t
adverse effects of, 170–171
clinical indications for, 168–169
dosing for, 169–170, 169t, 170t
spectrum of activity of, 167–168, 168t
Neuralgia, postherpetic, 337, 338f
Neuritis, retrobulbar, ethambutol-induced, 206
Neuroblastoma, lymphadenopathy in, 613, 623
Neuroborreliosis, 350
Neurobrucellosis, 381
Neurocysticercosis, 526, 526t, 527, 657
Neuromuscular blockade, aminoglycoside-induced, 171
Neuroretinitis, in cat-scratch disease, 344, 345f, Plate 9D
Neurosyphilis, 633, 1020–1021, 1104, 1106
Neurotoxicity, metronidazole-induced, 189
Neurotoxins, 5
Neutralization assay, for antibody detection, 103
Neutropenia, 53, 92–93, 93t
chloramphenicol-induced, 180
in infectious mononucleosis, 428
Neutropenic colitis. *See* Typhlitis.
Neutropenic enterocolitis, 1163. *See* Typhlitis.
Neutrophil(s), 92–93, 93t, 94f
in cerebrospinal fluid, 640t
in innate immunity, 33
inclusions in, 93
margination of, 93
normal count of, 93, 93t, 94f, 640t
toxic granulation of, 93
vacuolization of, 93
Neutrophilia, 92, 93t
Nevirapine, 152t, 203t, 205t
in HIV infection, 456, 457t, 458t
New World cutaneous leishmaniasis, 570–571
Niclosamide, 153t
Niemann-Pick disease, lymphadenopathy in, 614
Nikolsky's sign, 301
in staphylococcal scalded skin syndrome, 534
in Stevens-Johnson syndrome, 538
Niridazole, 153t
Nitric oxide, in septic shock, 284–285
Nitrite test, in urinary tract infection, 986–987
Nitroblue tetrazolium test, 54
in chronic granulomatous disease, 1153
Nitrofurantoin, 152t
in urinary tract infection, 991t
Nitroprusside, in septic shock, 292t
Nits, 573
Nitzschia pungens toxin, 911
Nocardia infection, of brain, 662–663
Nodules, 542, 542f
definition of, 533
in rheumatic fever, 488, 489, 489f, 491
Noma, 730, 734
diagnosis of, 737
pathogenesis of, 736
Nonnucleoside reverse transcriptase inhibitors, 152t, 203t, 205t

Nonnucleoside reverse transcriptase inhibitors *(Continued)*
in HIV infection, 456, 457t
Nonspecific immunity. *See* Immunity, innate.
Nonsteroidal anti-inflammatory drugs
in fever, 266, 267t
streptococcal necrotizing fasciitis and, 589
Nontreponemal antibody (reagin) test, 105, 108
Norepinephrine, in septic shock, 292t
Norfloxacin, 152t
in gonorrhea, 1014t
in travelers' diarrhea, 907t
Normal flora, 6–10
barrier breakdown–related infection with, 7
body distribution of, 8t–9t, 10
direct deep inoculation of, 7
in immunity, 31–32
in infection, 7
in infection prevention, 6–7
in mucous secretions, 7
in newborn, 7, 10
translocation of, 7
North American liver fluke infection, 522t
North Asian tick typhus, 355t
North Carolina macular dystrophy, vs. toxoplasmosis, 1083
Northern blotting, in viral infection, 89
Norwalk virus infection, 16t, 898t, 900–901
Norwegian scabies, 572
Nose, foreign body in, vs. common cold, 708, 708t
Nosocomial infections, 13, 1221–1244
blood transfusion and, 1230–1231, 1231t 1232t
burns and, 1223
catheters and, 1223, 1223t
central nervous system, 1229, 1229t
cutaneous, 1227–1228, 1227t, 1228t
drugs and, 1223, 1223t
gastrointestinal tract, 1225–1227, 1226t
hepatic, 1225–1227, 1226t
host factors in, 1222–1223, 1222t, 1223t
incidence of, 1221, 1221t
ocular, 1229–1230, 1230t
organ dysfunction and, 1222–1223, 1222t
pathogens in, 1221, 1221t
peritoneal dialysis-associated, 1230, 1230t
prevention of, 1232–1240, 1232t
antibiotics for, 1238
aseptic technique for, 1233
catheter care for, 1238
cover gowns for, 1238–1239
equipment cleaning for, 1239–1240, 1239t
handwashing for, 1232–1233, 1233t
isolation for, 1233–1238, 1234t–1238t
transmission-based, 1234, 1234t
medical waste disposal for, 1240
standard precautions for, 1233–1234, 1233t
toy cleaning for, 1240
reportable, 1221–1222, 1222t
respiratory tract, 1223–1225, 1224t
diagnosis of, 1225
etiology of, 1224–1225, 1224t
negative pressure rooms for, 1225
risk for, 1222–1223, 1222t, 1223t
surgical procedures and, 1223, 1223t
transplantation and, 1230–1231, 1231t 1232t
urinary tract, 1228–1229, 1228t
Nosocomial infections *(Continued)*
vascular, 1232
viral, 1232
Novobiocin, 152t
Novy-MacNeal-Nicolle (NNN) culture medium, for leishmaniasis, 570
Nuchal rigidity, in meningitis, 638
Nuclear medicine scan, in acute myocarditis, 860
Nucleic acid hybridization, in viral infection, 89–90
Nucleoside reverse transcriptase inhibitors, 152t, 203t, 205t
in HIV infection, 456, 457t
Null reaction, 118f
Nurse cells, in trichinellosis, 516
Nutrition, in HIV infection, 460
Nystatin, 152t, 196
in candidiasis, 562, 731, 731t, 1006t

O

Observation
in bacteremia evaluation, 268–269, 269t
in fever evaluation, 264, 265t
Ocular larva migrans, 511f, 512, 1082, 1082f, 1083, 1084
Oculoglandular syndrome of Parinaud, 344, 610
Oculoglandular tularemia, 382, 382t
Odds ratio, 11
Odocoileus virginianus, in ehrlichiosis, 359
Ofloxacin, 152t
in gonorrhea, 1013, 1014t
in leprosy, 554, 554t
in pelvic inflammatory disease, 1015t
in shigellosis, 886, 886t
in travelers' diarrhea, 907t
Old World cutaneous leishmaniasis, 570–571
Omenn's syndrome, 1152, 1152t
Omentum
greater, 921, 922f
lesser, 921, 922f, 923
Omeprazole, in gastritis, 875–876, 876t
Omphalitis, 83, 588–589, 594, 1130
Onchocerca volvulus infection (onchocerciasis), 518
specimen collection in, 81
Onchocercoma, 518
Onchodermatitis, 518
Oncogenes, in cervical carcinoma, 28
Oncogenesis, 23–28. *See also* Cancer.
Oncoviruses, 24t, 27–28
Onychomycosis, 558–560, 559t, 560f, 561t
Oophoritis, mumps, 420–421
Ophthalmia neonatorum, 1012, 1013–1014, 1014t, 1016, 1055–1058. *See also* Conjunctivitis, neonatal.
Ophthalmic antibiotics, in conjunctivitis, 1060–1061, 1061t
Opisthorchis felineus infection, cholangiocarcinoma and, 29
Opisthorchis viverrini infection (opisthorchiasis), 20t, 29, 522t
Opisthotonos
in meningitis, 639
in tetanus, 693, 694, 694f
Opportunistic pathogen, 1
Opsonization, 34
Optic atrophy, in neurosyphilis, 1021
Optical immunoassay, for bacterial and fungal antigens, 71
Oral contraceptives, in menstruation-related acne, 549
Oral hairy leukoplakia, in AIDS, 427, 430, 470
Oral rehydration solution, 1216, 1216t
in acute enteritis, 916–917, 917t
Orbital cellulitis. *See* Cellulitis, head and neck.
Orbivirus infection (Colorado tick fever), 19t, 393–394, 394t, 537, 675
Orchitis, 994–995
mumps, 420–421, 424
tuberculous, 404
Organ transplantation. *See* Transplantation.
Orientia tsutsugamushi infection, 536t, 538
Ornithodoros, 21t
in relapsing fever, 387
Ornithosis, 810–811
Oropharyngeal tularemia, 382, 382t
Oseltamivir, 202, 202t
in influenza virus infection, 820–821, 821t
Osler's nodes, in infective endocarditis, 540, 848
Osp proteins, of *Borrelia burgdorferi,* 348
Osteochondritis, 1035
Osteomeatal complex, 761, 761f
Osteomyelitis, 1034–1043
chronic, 1034, 1035, 1042
clinical manifestations of, 1034–1036, 1036t
complications of, 1042
culture in, 1037
diagnosis of, 1036–1039, 1037f–1039f, 1037t
epidemiology of, 1034
etiology of, 1034, 1034t
flat bone, 1035
imaging in, 141, 141f–144f, 1037–1038, 1038f, 1039f
in sickle cell anemia, 1039f
indium radionuclide scan in, 143f
involucrum in, 1035, 1037
laboratory evaluation in, 1037
magnetic resonance imaging in, 141, 142f, 1037
microbiologic evaluation in, 1038
neonatal, 1034, 1034t, 1035, 1036, 1036t, 1040t, 1042
pathogenesis of, 1034–1035
pelvic, 1036
plain film radiography in, 141, 141f–144f
prevention of, 1042–1043
prognosis for, 1042
puncture wound, 1034, 1034t, 1041, 1042–1043
radionuclide scan in, 141, 142f, 143f, 1038, 1039f
recurrent, 1042
Schlichter titers in, 1040
sequestra in, 1035, 1037
serum bactericidal tests in, 77–78
sternal, 1034, 1034t, 1035, 1036, 1040t, 1041
subacute, 1034, 1034t, 1035, 1040t
treatment of, 1039–1042, 1040t
vertebral, 1036
Otitis externa, 745–747
clinical manifestations of, 745
complications of, 747
diagnosis of, 745–746, 746t
epidemiology of, 745
etiology of, 745
malignant, 745
clinical manifestations of, 746

Otitis externa *(Continued)*
malignant *(Continued)*
complications of, 747
treatment of, 746–747
pathogenesis of, 745
prevention of, 747
specimen collection in, 62t, 66
treatment of, 746–747, 746t
Otitis media, 748–758
acoustic reflectometry in, 752
adenoidectomy in, 756
antihistamines in, 755–756
cholesteatoma in, 756–757
clinical manifestations of, 750–751, 751f, Plate 10
complications of, 756–757
corticosteroids in, 756
decongestants in, 755–756
diagnosis of, 751–752, 752f
epidemiology of, 749–750, 750t
etiology of, 748–749, 749t
eustachian tube anatomy in, 750
Haemophilus influenzae in, 748–749
hearing loss after, 756
immunodeficiency and, 750
in immunocompromised persons, 749
in measles, 312
in neonate, 749
intracranial complications of, 757
mastoiditis with, 757, 757f
Moraxella catarrhalis in, 749
myringotomy in, 752, 756
otoscopic examination in, 750–751, 751f
pathogenesis of, 750
prevention of, 758
prognosis for, 757–758, 758f
prophylactic antibiotics in, 758
recurrent, 749–750, 750t
risk factors for, 749–750, 750t
serous, 758, 758f
silent, 750
Streptococcus pneumoniae in, 748
suppurative, chronic, 756
treatment of, 752–756, 753f, 754t, 755t
antibiotic resistance in, 755
tympanic perforation in, 756
tympanocentesis in, 752, 752f, 756
tympanometry in, 751–752, 752f
tympanostomy tubes in, 756
vaccine prevention of, 758
viruses in, 749, 758
Otitis media–purulent conjunctivitis syndrome, 755
Otoscopy
in otitis media, 750–751, 751f
pneumatic, 751, 751f
Ototoxicity
aminoglycoside-induced, 170–171
erythromycin-induced, 178
Ouchterlony double-diffusion assay, for antibody detection, 103
Ovary, tuberculosis of, 404
Owl eyes, in cytomegalovirus infection, 90
Oxacillin, 151t
dosing for, 158t
formulations of, 157t
in acute pericarditis, 867t
in bite-wound infection, 607t
Oxacillin *(Continued)*
in brain abscess, 662t
in burn wound infection, 600t
in cellulitis, 580t, 585t
in erysipelas, 580t
in hepatic abscess, 967t
in infectious arthritis, 1048t
in infective endocarditis, 851t–852t
in intra-abdominal abscess, 929t
in meningitis, 645t, 646t
in neonatal sepsis, 1125t, 1126t
in osteomyelitis, 1040t
in sepsis, 291t
in shunt-related infection, 655t
in spinal epidural abscess, 667t
in staphylococcal toxic shock syndrome, 302, 302t
in tracheitis, 776t
in wound infection, 593t
pathogen susceptibility to, 155t
Oxamniquine, 153t
in schistosomiasis, 524t
Oxantel pamoate, in trichuriasis, 508, 508t
Oxazolidinone antibiotics, 172–175, 173t, 174t, 175t
Oxygen
bacterial requirements for, 57, 58t
hyperbaric
in streptococcal toxic shock syndrome, 303
in wound infection, 594
in bronchiolitis, 788
Oxytetracycline, 151t

P

p24 protein antigen test, in HIV infection, 449
PAIR therapy, in echinococcosis, 530
Palivizumab, 152t, 218t, 220
in respiratory syncytial virus infection, 788, 788t
Pancreatic pseudocyst, 982
Pancreatitis, 977–982
amylase level in, 979–980, 980t
APACHE II score in, 979, 979f
clinical manifestations of, 978, 978t
complications of, 981–982
diagnosis of, 978–981, 979f, 979t, 980t
differential diagnosis of, 979, 979t
epidemiology of, 977–978
etiology of, 977, 977t, 978t
familial, 978
hypocalcemia with, 982
idiopathic, 977
imaging in, 980
in ascariasis, 510
in mumps, 422
interstitial, 978, 982
lipase level in, 980
necrotizing, 978, 982
needle aspiration in, 980
pathogenesis of, 978
pathologic findings in, 980–981
physical examination in, 978, 978t
prevention of, 982
prognosis for, 982
pseudocysts with, 982
Ranson's criteria in, 978–979, 979t
supportive therapy in, 981
Pancreatitis *(Continued)*
treatment of, 981, 981t
Pandemic, 12
Panencephalitis, sclerosing, subacute, 684–685, 684f
Pannus, in trachoma conjunctivitis, 1063
Panophthalmitis, 1074
Papanicolaou smear, in human papillomavirus infection, 1030
Papilledema, in meningitis, 639
Papular acrodermatitis of childhood, 536, 537f
Papular-purpuric gloves and socks syndrome, 539t, 540
Papules, definition of, 533
Paragonimus infection (paragonimiasis), 20t, 80, 522t
Paragonimus kellicotti infection, 522t
Paragonimus mexicana infection, 522t
Paragonimus pulmonalis infection, 522t
Paragonimus uterobilateralis infection, 522t
Paragonimus westermani infection, 522t
sputum examination in, 80
Parainfluenza virus infection, 88t, 818–819
in AIDS, 469
Paralysis, 1182t
Paranasal sinuses
anatomy of, 760, 761f
infection of. *See* Sinusitis.
Parapneumonic effusion, 832. *See also* Pleural effusion.
Parasites, 80–83, 81t, 504t. *See also specific helminth and protozoal infections.*
blood smear for, 83
cellophane tape collection of, 80, 82, 82f
classification of, 80, 81t
culture for, 83
molecular tests for, 124
serologic testing for, 109–110
specimen collection for, 80–81, 82, 82f
stains for, 82–83, 83f
wet mount for, 82, 82f
Paregoric, in acute enteritis, 917t, 918
Parinaud's oculoglandular syndrome, 344, 610
Paromomycin, 152t
in amebiasis, 892–893, 893t
in *Cryptosporidium parvum* infection, 903t
in *Dientamoeba fragilis* infection, 903t
in giardiasis, 902, 903t
in leishmaniasis, 571
Paronychia, *Candida,* 562
Parotitis, 741–744
clinical manifestations of, 742
complications of, 744
diagnosis of, 742–743, 743t
epidemiology of, 741, 742t
etiology of, 741, 742t
in AIDS, 470–471
mumps, 420, 421, Plate 3F
pathogenesis of, 741–742
prevention of, 744
prognosis for, 744
recurrent, 742
suppurative, 422
surgery in, 743–744
treatment of, 743–744
Parrot, pseudoparalysis of, in congenital syphilis, 1103–1104

Parrot fever, 810–811
Particle agglutination assay
 for antigen detection, 111, 115
 for bacterial and fungal antigens, 70–71
 in meningitis, 641–642
 in viral infection, 89
Particle agglutination inhibition assay, for antibody detection, 102
Parvovirus B19 virus infection. *See* Erythema infectiosum (fifth disease).
Passive agglutination assay, 102
Passive hemagglutination assay, for antibody detection, 102
Pasteurella multocida infection, 18t
 bite-wound, 602–608, 603t, 606t, 607t
Pasteurella pestis. See Yersinia pestis infection (plague).
Pasteurella tularensis. See Francisella tularensis infection.
Pastia's lines
 in scarlet fever, 534
 in staphylococcal scalded skin syndrome, 534
 in streptococcal pharyngitis, 712
Pathogen(s), 1. *See also specific infections.*
 antimicrobial resistance of, 3
 attachment factors of, 1, 3t
 attachment of, 6
 foodborne, 15, 16t, 17t
 intracellular growth of, 2–3
 soilborne, 13, 14t
 toxins of, 3–5, 4t
 transmission of, 13
 vectorborne, 15, 17, 18t–20t, 21f, 21t, 22t
 virulence factors of, 1–5, 2f, 3t, 4t
 waterborne, 13–15, 14f, 14t, 15t
 zoonotic, 15, 17, 18t–20t, 21f, 21t, 22t
Pathology, 116–124, 117f
 bacteria-specific methods in, 123–124
 cytology in, 116, 118f, 119t
 cytopathic reaction in, 118f
 direct visualization in, 116
 DNA microarrays in, 123
 electron microscopy in, 119
 exudative reaction in, 118f
 foam cell reaction in, 118f
 fungus-specific methods in, 124
 granulomatous reaction in, 118f
 immunohistochemistry in, 119, 121t
 in situ hybridization in, 119–120, 121f
 interstitial mononuclear reaction in, 118f
 laser capture microdissection in, 122–123
 ligase chain reaction in, 122
 necrotizing reaction in, 118f
 null reaction in, 118f
 polymerase chain reaction in, 120–121, 123t, 124
 protozoa-specific methods in, 124
 Qβ replicase amplification in, 122
 tissue reactions in, 116, 118f, 119, 120t
 transcription-mediated amplification in, 122
 virus-specific methods in, 124
Paul-Bunnell antibodies, 431–432, 431f
Pediculosis, 573–574, 573f
Pediculus humanus capitis infestation, 573–574, 573f
Pediculus humanus humanus infestation, 573–574
Pel-Ebstein fever, 275
Peliosis hepatitis, in cat-scratch disease, 345
Pelvic inflammatory disease, 1011
 diagnosis of, 1012
 gonorrhea and, 1011, 1012
 treatment of, 1015, 1015t
Penciclovir, in herpetic gingivostomatitis, 731, 731t
Penicillin(s), 151t, 153–157, 155t
 adverse effects of, 156, 160t
 aminoglycoside interaction with, 157, 160t
 clinical indications for, 154–155
 desensitization to, 160t
 dosing for, 156, 158t–159t
 drug interactions with, 156–157, 160t
 formulations of, 157t
 in acute pericarditis, 867t
 in anthrax, 551
 in asplenia, 1181, 1184t
 in bite-wound infection, 606, 606t, 607t
 in blistering distal dactylitis, 549
 in botulism, 697
 in brain abscess, 661, 662t
 in burn wound infection, 599, 600t
 in cellulitis, 585t
 in congenital syphilis, 1106, 1106t
 in cranial epidural abscess, 666t
 in erysipelas, 580t
 in erysipeloid, 580t
 in gonococcal vulvovaginitis, 1006t
 in group A streptococcal vulvovaginal infection, 1006t
 in infectious arthritis, 1048t
 in infective endocarditis, 851t–852t, 852
 in lymphangitis, 627
 in mediastinitis, 843, 843t
 in meningitis, 644, 645t, 646t
 in neonatal sepsis, 1126t
 in osteomyelitis, 1040t
 in perianal dermatitis, 550
 in relapsing fever, 388t
 in rheumatic fever prevention, 493, 493t
 in shunt-related infection, 655t
 in streptococcal pharyngitis, 716–717, 716t, 717t
 in subdural empyema, 666t
 in syphilis, 1022–1023, 1022t
 in tetanus, 694
 in wound botulism, 697
 in wound infection, 592, 593t
 metabolism of, 155–156, 156t
 pathogen susceptibility to, 155t
 penicillinase-resistant, 154
 pharmacokinetics of, 151t, 155–156, 156t
 probenecid interaction with, 156–157, 160t
 resistance to, 154
 spectrum of activity of, 154, 155t
Penicillin-binding proteins, 154
Pentamidine, 152t
 in *Pneumocystis carinii* infection, 826, 826t
Peptic ulcer disease, 872. *See also* Gastritis.
Peptidoglycan, 284
Peptococcus infection, 923–928. *See also* Abscess, intra-abdominal.
Perianal dermatitis, 550, 550f
Pericardial fluid, 863–864
 collection of, 60t, 64
 in pneumonia, 800
Pericardiectomy, in constrictive pericarditis, 866
Pericardiocentesis, 865, 866
Pericarditis, 863–868
 cardiac tamponade in, 864
 chest radiography in, 865
 clinical manifestations of, 864
 complications of, 866
 constrictive, 864, 866
 culture in, 865–866
 diagnosis of, 864–866, 865f, 866f
 differential diagnosis of, 865, 865t
 echocardiography in, 865, 866f
 electrocardiography in, 864, 865f
 epidemiology of, 863
 etiology of, 863, 864t
 friction rub in, 864
 in rheumatic fever, 488
 pathogenesis of, 863–864
 pericardiocentesis in, 865
 physical examination in, 864
 postoperative, 863
 prognosis for, 866, 868
 treatment of, 866, 867t
 tuberculous, 404, 863, 865–866, 867t
Pericardium, 863–864
Pericoronitis, 734–735
 clinical manifestations of, 737
 pathogenesis of, 735
 treatment of, 737
Perihepatitis, gonococcal, 1011
Perinatal infection, 1090–1091, 1091t. *See also* Intrauterine infection; Maternal infection.
 Borrelia burgdorferi, 350–351
 chickenpox, 1140–1143, 1141f, 1142t
 enterovirus, 1143–1146. *See also* Enterovirus infection, perinatal.
 group B *Streptococcus,* 1091, 1093, 1094f–1096f
 hepatitis B, 1091, 1094, 1096
 herpes simplex virus, 1091, 1094, 1096, 1135t, 1136–1140. *See also* Herpes simplex virus infection, perinatal.
 HIV, 441, 446, 1091, 1092t, 1094–1095, 1096
 Neisseria gonorrhoeae, 1011, 1012, 1013–1014, 1014t, 1016, 1056t, 1057, 1057f
 prevention of, 1092t, 1093–1095, 1093f–1095f
 varicella-zoster virus, 333–334, 1091, 1140–1143. *See also* Varicella-zoster virus infection, perinatal.
Perineal bag, for urine collection, 986
Periodic fever, aphthous stomatitis, pharyngitis, and cervical adenitis (PFAPA) syndrome, 623, 711–712, 714, 718
Periodontitis, 734
 clinical manifestations of, 737
 complications of, 738–739
 diagnosis of, 737
 pathogenesis of, 735
 treatment of, 738, 738t
Periorbital cellulitis, 581–585, 581f, 584f, 585t, Plate 7E. *See also* Cellulitis, head and neck.
Peritoneal cavity, 922f, 923
Peritoneal dialysis, infection with, 1230, 1230t
Peritoneal fluid, collection of, 60t, 64
Peritoneum, 921, 922f
Peritonitis, 924, 929–931. *See also* Abscess, intra-abdominal.
 cardiovascular evaluation in, 930–931

Peritonitis *(Continued)*
clinical manifestations of, 930
complications of, 931
culture in, 931
diagnosis of, 930–931
epidemiology of, 929–930
etiology of, 928–930
gonococcal, 929
imaging in, 931
pathogenesis of, 930
physical examination in, 930
prognosis for, 931
respiratory evaluation in, 931
treatment of, 931
tuberculous, 403
Perlèche, in candidiasis, 562, 729
Permethrin
in lice, 574
in scabies, 572
Peromyscus leucopus, in Lyme disease, 348
Pertussis syndrome, 788–792. *See also Bordetella pertussis* infection (pertussis syndrome).
Petechiae, 286, 286t
definition of, 533
in meningitis, 637
in sepsis evaluation, 286, 286t
palatal, 540
Petrolatum, in lice, 574
Phagocytes
evaluation of, 52t, 54, 56
mononuclear, 33–34
of respiratory tract, 798
Phagolysosomes, 33
Pharmaceutics, 149. *See also* Anti-infective therapy.
Pharmacodynamics, 147–149, 149t, 150f. *See also* Anti-infective therapy.
Pharmacokinetics, 149, 150f. *See also* Anti-infective therapy.
Pharyngitis, 711–719
Arcanobacterium haemolyticum in, 712t, 713, 716, 718
clinical manifestations of, 712–714, 713t, Plate 3D
complications of, 718–719
Corynebacterium diphtheriae in. *See Corynebacterium diphtheriae* infection (diphtheria), pharyngeal.
diagnosis of, 714
epidemiology of, 711–712
etiology of, 711, 712t, Plate 1E
Francisella tularensis in, 712t, 713–714, 716, 718
gonococcal, 711, 1011, 1014t, 1016
clinical manifestations of, 713
diagnosis of, 715
treatment of, 718
impetigo and, 545
pathogenesis of, 712
prevention of, 719, 719t
streptococcal, 711
clinical manifestations of, 712–713, 713t
complications of, 718
diagnosis of, 714–716, 714t, 715f
pathogenesis of, 712
rapid tests for, 714–715, 715f
recurrent, 717
Pharyngitis *(Continued)*
streptococcal *(Continued)*
serologic diagnosis of, 715
throat culture in, 714, 714t, 715f
tonsillectomy in, 717
treatment of, 716–717, 716t, 717t
vs. infectious mononucleosis, 430
treatment of, 716–718, 716t
viral, 711
clinical manifestations of, 713, 713t
diagnosis of, 714, 715
treatment of, 717–718
Pharyngoconjunctival fever, 713
Pharynx. *See also* Pharyngitis.
specimen collection from, 61t, 64
Phenobarbital, in meningitis, 647
Phenothiazine toxicity, vs. tetanus, 694
Phenylephrine, in septic shock, 292t
Phenytoin
ceftriaxone interaction with, 165
in meningitis, 647
Phlebitis, nosocomial, 1232
Phlyctenule, 1059, 1059f, 1070, 1070f
Photophobia, in keratitis, 1064
Photopsia, in retinitis, 1082
Phthirus pubis infestation, 573–574
Phthisis bulbi, 1078
Physical irritants, vs. vulvovaginitis, 1004
Physical stress, immune response and, 49
Physiotherapy, in primary immune deficiencies, 1155
Pili, 1, 3t
Pinworms. *See Enterobius vermicularis* infection (enterobiasis, pinworms).
Piperacillin, 151t
dosing for, 159t
formulations of, 157t
in acute pancreatitis, 981, 981t
in burn wound infection, 600t
in cholecystitis, 972, 972t
in ecthyma gangrenosum, 580t
in hepatic abscess, 967t
in neonatal sepsis, 1126t
in sepsis, 291t
in wound infection, 593t
pathogen susceptibility to, 155t
Piperazine citrate, 153t
Pitted keratolysis, 549, 549t
Pittsburgh pneumonia agent, 805
Pityriasis versicolor, 560, 561f
Pityrosporum obiculare. See Malassezia furfur.
Pityrosporum ovale. See Malassezia furfur.
Plague, 383–385, 385t. *See also Yersinia pestis* infection (plague).
Plain film radiography. *See* Chest radiography; Radiography.
Plaques, definition of, 533
Plasma cell pneumonia. *See* Pneumonia, *Pneumocystis carinii.*
Plasma-activating factor, in meningitis, 636
Plasmapheresis
in Guillain-Barré syndrome, 702
in septic shock, 293
Plasmodium spp., 363, 364t
life cycle of, 363, 365f
schizogony of, 363, 365f
sporogeny of, 363, 365f
Plasmodium spp. infection (malaria), 363–374
algid, 372
blood smear in, 368, 370f, Plate 2C, Plate 2D
CDC Hotline for, 369
cerebral, 372
clinical manifestations of, 366–368, 367f, 372
complications of, 372
congenital, 368
DEET prevention for, 374
diagnosis of, 368, 369t, 370f, Plate 2C, Plate 2D
differential diagnosis of, 369t
drug resistance in, 368–369
epidemiology of, 20t, 363–364, 366f, 367f
etiology of, 363, 364t, 365f, 368
geographic distribution of, 363–364, 366f
hypoglycemia in, 372
immune response in, 365–366
in international child traveler, 1213–1214
incubation period for, 366, 367f
long-term relapse in, 367, 367f
maternal, 368
pathogenesis of, 364–366
phases of, 367f
prevention of, 372–374, 373t
prognosis for, 372, 372t
prophylaxis against, 373t, 374
during pregnancy, 374
pulmonary edema in, 372
renal failure in, 372
severe, 368, 369–370, 370f, 371t, 372
short-term relapse in, 367, 367f
splenic rupture in, 372
stains in, 368
thrombocytopenia in, 372
transmission of, 363
treatment of, 368–372, 371t
supportive, 371–372
Pleconaril, in enteroviral infection, 677
Plesiomonas shigelloides infection, 909, 909t
Pleural effusion, 832–837
cells in, 835
chest radiography in, 835–836, 835f
clinical manifestations of, 834
complications of, 837
culture in, 836–837
diagnosis of, 834–837, 834t, 835t
differential diagnosis of, 834–835, 834t
epidemiology of, 833
etiology of, 832–833, 833t
pathogenesis of, 833
pH of, 835
prognosis for, 837
protein concentration of, 835, 835t
specimen collection in, 60t, 64
thoracentesis in, 837
treatment of, 837
tuberculous, 400f, 402, 406, 408, 411f
video-assisted thoracoscopic surgery in, 837
Pneumatocele, 838, 839
Pneumatosis intestinalis
in necrotizing enterocolitis, 1130, 1131, 1131f
in neonatal sepsis, 1125
Pneumococcal pneumonia. *See* Pneumonia, *Streptococcus pneumoniae.*
Pneumocystis carinii infection, 824–826
bronchoalveolar lavage in, 80

Pneumocystis carinii infection *(Continued)*
clinical manifestations of, 825
diagnosis of, 825–826
epidemiology of, 825
etiology of, 825
Giemsa stain in, 82
immunofluorescence assay in, 82
in AIDS, 453t, 454, 461, 461t, 462t, 465–466, 465f, 825
methenamine silver stain in, 82, 83f
pathogenesis of, 825
prevention of, 826, 827t
prophylaxis against, 1167
toluidine blue stain in, 82, 83f
treatment of, 826, 826t
Pneumonia, 794–830
adenovirus, 819
afebrile, 794
alveolar, 797
Aspergillus spp., 814–815
aspiration, 826–829
clinical manifestations of, 827–828
diagnosis of, 828, 828f
etiology of, 827
pathogenesis of, 827
treatment of, 828–829
atypical, 797
auscultation in, 800
biopsy in, 801
Blastomyces dermatitidis, 816–817
Bordetella pertussis, 792
bronchoalveolar lavage in, 801
bronchoscopy in, 801
Candida, 817
chest radiography in, 801
Chlamydia pneumoniae, 795t, 811–812
Chlamydia psittaci, 810–811
Chlamydia trachomatis, 795t, 809–810
clinical manifestations of, 809, 809t
diagnosis of, 810, 810f
epidemiology of, 809
etiology of, 809
prevention of, 810
treatment of, 803t, 810
clinical manifestations of, 798–800, 799t
Coccidioides immitis, 816
community-acquired, 796
Cryptococcus neoformans, 815–816, 816f
culture in, 794, 800–801
cyanosis in, 800
cytomegalovirus, in AIDS, 470
diagnosis of, 794, 800–801
imaging in, 131, 132f–134f
enterovirus, 822
etiology of, 794–796, 795t
in developed countries, 796–797
in developing countries, 796
in young infants, 794–796
foreign body, 826–829
clinical manifestations of, 827–828
diagnosis of, 828
pathogenesis of, 827
treatment of, 829
fungal, 812–817, 812t, 813f, 813t, 816f
giant cell (Hecht's), 312
group A *Streptococcus,* 803t
group B *Streptococcus,* 803t
Pneumonia *(Continued)*
Haemophilus influenzae type b, 795t, 803t
hantavirus, 822–824
clinical manifestations of, 824
complications of, 824
diagnosis of, 824
epidemiology of, 823, 823t
etiology of, 822, 823t, 824f
pathogenesis of, 823–824
prevention of, 824
prognosis for, 824
treatment of, 824
heart failure in, 800
Histoplasma capsulatum, 812–814, 813t
chest radiography in, 814
clinical manifestations of, 813, 813t
diagnosis of, 813–814, 813f
epidemiology of, 812–813
etiology of, 812
pathogenesis of, 813
prognosis for, 814
treatment of, 814
hospital-acquired, 829–830
in older infants, 796
in young infants, 795–796
host defenses against, 798
imaging in, 131, 132f–134f, 801
in burn injury patient, 601
in infectious mononucleosis, 434
in measles, 311f, 312
incidence of, 797f, 797t, 798f
influenza virus, 819–822
clinical manifestations of, 820
diagnosis of, 820
epidemiology of, 819–820
etiology of, 819
pathogenesis of, 820
prevention of, 822
prognosis for, 822
transmission of, 819
treatment of, 820–821, 821t
interstitial, 797
Legionella pneumophila, 805–807
antibody tests in, 105
clinical manifestations of, 806
culture in, 806
diagnosis of, 806–807
epidemiology of, 805–806
etiology of, 805
pathogenesis of, 806
prevention of, 807
prognosis for, 807
transmission of, 805
treatment of, 803t, 807
measles, 306–307, 310–311, 311f, 312
in AIDS, 469
Mycoplasma pneumoniae, 795t, 807–809
chest radiography in, 808, 808f
clinical manifestations of, 807–808
complications of, 809
diagnosis of, 808, 808f
epidemiology of, 807
etiology of, 807
pathogenesis of, 807
prevention of, 809
prognosis for, 809
treatment of, 803t, 808–809
Pneumonia *(Continued)*
necrotizing, 134f
diffuse, 131, 133f
nosocomial, 795–796, 829–830
parainfluenza virus, 818–819
pathogenesis of, 797–798
pericardial effusion in, 800
physical examination in, 799–800, 799t
plasma cell. *See* Pneumonia, *Pneumocystis carinii.*
pneumococcal. *See* Pneumonia, *Streptococcus pneumoniae.*
Pneumocystis carinii, 798, 824–826
clinical manifestations of, 825
diagnosis of, 825–826
epidemiology of, 825
etiology of, 825
pathogenesis of, 825
prevention of, 826, 827t
treatment of, 826, 826t
Pseudomonas aeruginosa, 803t
Q fever, 390
respiratory rate in, 799–800, 799t
respiratory syncytial virus, 795t, 818. *See also* Bronchiolitis.
round, 131, 133f
Salmonella typhi, 884
sputum culture in, 800–801
Staphylococcus aureus, 803t
Streptococcus pneumoniae, 795t, 802–805
antibiotic resistance in, 805
clinical manifestations of, 804
complications of, 805
diagnosis of, 131, 133f, 804
epidemiology of, 803–804
etiology of, 802–803, Plate 1B
imaging in, 131, 133f, 804
immunization against, 233t, 235t–236t, 245t, 249–250
pathogenesis of, 804
prevention of, 805
prognosis for, 805
transmission of, 803
treatment of, 803t, 804–805
thoracentesis in, 801
transmission of, 794
treatment of, 795t, 801–802, 801t, 803t
typical, 797
varicella, 338, 339f
in AIDS, 469–470
ventilator-associated, 829–830
viral, 817–824, 817t
imaging in, 131, 134f
Pneumonic plague, 384–385
Pneumonic tularemia, 382, 382t
Pneumonitis
hookworm, 506
hypersensitivity, 814, 815
in ascariasis, 509, 509t
interstitial, lymphocytic, 427, 430, 466, 467f
Podophyllin, in human papillomavirus infection, 1030
Podophyllotoxin, for warts, 568
pol, of HIV, 437, 439t
Poliovirus infection, 676–677, 693t, 698–701
abortive, 699
bulbar, 700

Poliovirus infection *(Continued)*
Cheyne-Stokes respiration in, 700
clinical manifestations of, 699–700
complications of, 700
culture in, 700
diagnosis of, 700
epidemiology of, 698–699, 699f
etiology of, 698
immunization against, 233t, 235t–236t, 253t, 256–257, 701
adverse reactions to, 237t
for international travel, 244t
paralytic poliomyelitis with, 257
nonparalytic, 699
pathogenesis of, 699
preparalytic, 699
prevention of, 701
prognosis for, 700–701
spinal, 699
treatment of, 700
vaccine-associated, 698–699, 700
Polyarthralgia, in mumps, 422
Polyarthritis, in mumps, 422
Polymerase chain reaction assay, 120–121, 123t
in viral infection, 89–90
organism-specific, 124
Polymyxin B, 152t
Polyomaviruses, in oncogenesis, 24t, 28
Polysplenia, 1181, 1182t, 1183
Pontiac fever, 806
Pork tapeworm infection, 530t, 531
Porphyromonas gingivalis infection, 734. *See also* Dental infection.
Postpericardiotomy syndrome, 863
Postpolio syndrome, 700
Poststreptococcal glomerulonephritis, 493–495. *See also* Glomerulonephritis, poststreptococcal.
Potassium hydroxide (KOH) examination, 69, 69t, 70f, 557
Pott's disease, 403, 1036
Pott's puffy tumor, 582, 583, 584, 585t, 767
Pouch of Douglas, 923
Povidone-iodine, in burn wound infection, 599t
Povidone-iodine scrub, 1233
Powassan virus encephalitis, 676
Powell's mouthwash, in stomatitis, 732t
Praziquantel, 153t, 210–211, 211t
in cysticercosis, 526–527, 527t
in schistosomiasis, 523, 524t
Precipitation assays, for antibody detection, 103
Predictive value, of test, 11
Prednisolone, in uveitis, 1081
Prednisone
in endophthalmitis, 1077t
in toxoplasmosis, 1116
Pregnancy. *See* Maternal infection.
Prehn's sign, in epididymitis, 994
Preseptal cellulitis, 581–585, 581f, 584f, 585t, Plate 7E. *See also* Cellulitis, head and neck.
Pressure sores, 550–551, 551f
Preterm infant
immunization in, 238
postexposure varicella-zoster virus infection prophylaxis for, 340t, 341
Prevalence, 12
Prevotella melaninogenica infection, 923–928. *See also* Abscess, intra-abdominal.
gingival, 734
Primaquine
in malaria, 370–371, 371t
in malaria prophylaxis, 373t
in *Pneumocystis carinii* infection, 826, 826t
Primaquine phosphate, 153t
Primary effusion lymphoma, human herpesvirus 8 in, 26
Prion diseases, 685–687, 686t
Probenecid, 151t
acyclovir interaction with, 198
aztreonam interaction with, 166
carbapenem interaction with, 167
cefixime interaction with, 165
penicillin interaction with, 156–157, 160t
Proctitis, 1009, 1010t. *See also* Sexually transmitted infections.
Progressive multifocal leukoencephalopathy, 28, 685
Progressive rubella encephalitis, 685
Proguanil
in malaria, 370, 371t
in malaria prophylaxis, 373t, 374
Pronator sign, in rheumatic fever, 489
Prophylactic therapy, 225–231
Propionibacterium acnes infection (acne vulgaris), 547–549, 548t
Prospective study, 11
Prostaglandins, in meningitis, 636
Prostatism, 992
Prostatitis, 992–993
Prostatodynia, 992
Prosthetic valve endocarditis, 847. *See also* Infective endocarditis.
Protease inhibitors, 152t, 204t, 205t
in HIV infection, 456, 457t
Proteasome, 38
Protein, in cerebrospinal fluid, 640t, 641, 641t
Protein C
activated, recombinant, in septic shock, 292–293
deficiency of, purpura fulminans with, 540
serum, in septic shock, 287
Protein C1 inhibitor deficiency, 1153–1154
Protein S, serum, in septic shock, 287
Proteus infection, urinary tract, 983, 983t. *See also* Urinary tract infection.
Protozoal infection, 14t, 19t–20t. *See also specific protozoal infections.*
classification of, 80, 81t
specimen collection in, 80–83, 83f
Provirus, 26
Prozone phenomenon, in brucellosis diagnosis, 381
Pruritus
in pediculosis, 574
in scabies, 572, 573
Pruritus ani, in enterobiasis, 514–515
Pseudoappendicitis syndrome, in yersiniosis, 887
Pseudomembranous colitis. *See Clostridium difficile*–associated diarrhea.
lincosamide-induced, 187
metronidazole-induced, 189
Pseudomonas aeruginosa infection, 15
bite-wound, 602–608, 603t, 606t, 607t
burn-related, 596, 597t
Pseudomonas aeruginosa infection *(Continued)*
cutaneous, 545–547
disseminated, 540
imaging in, 131, 133f
in AIDS, 474
in cancer patient, 283
in sepsis, 279
intra-abdominal, 923–928. *See also* Abscess, intra-abdominal.
meningeal, 630, 630t, 631t, 644. *See also* Meningitis, bacterial.
toxins in, 4t
Pseudoparalysis
in congenital syphilis, 1103–1104
in infectious arthritis, 1045
Psittacosis, 19t, 810–811
Psoas abscess, 938–940
clinical manifestations of, 939
culture in, 939
diagnosis of, 939
epidemiology of, 938
pathogenesis of, 939
vs. inguinal lymphadenopathy, 618
Psychological stress, immune response and, 49
Pubic lice, 573–574
Pulmonary edema, 1182t
in malaria, 372
in Rocky Mountain spotted fever, 357
Pulmonary hypertension, 1182t
Pulse-temperature deficit
in *Chlamydia psittaci* pneumonia, 811
in *Legionella pneumophilia* infection, 806
Pulsus paradoxus, in pericarditis, 864
Purified protein derivative (PPD), 405–406, 405f, 406t
Purpura, definition of, 533
Purpura fulminans, 539t, 540
Pustules, 540–541, 541f, 541t, 542f
definition of, 533
Pyelonephritis, 983–991. *See also* Urinary tract infection.
vs. appendicitis, 934, 934t
with *Salmonella typhi* infection, 884
Pyloric stenosis, hypertrophic, with erythromycin, 1057
Pyoderma gangrenosum, 540
Pyogenic infectious spondylitis. *See* Diskitis.
Pyonephrosis, vs. appendicitis, 934, 934t
Pyothorax. *See* Empyema.
Pyrantel pamoate, 153t, 211
in enterobiasis, 515, 515t
in hookworm infection, 506–507, 506t
in trichuriasis, 508, 508t
Pyrazinamide, 152t
in tuberculosis, 412–413, 414t
Pyridoxine, isoniazid administration and, 206, 417
Pyrimethamine, 153t
in congenital toxoplasmosis, 1116, 1116t
in *Isospora belli* infection, 903t
in malaria, 370
Pyrimethamine-sulfadoxine
in malaria, 371t
in malaria prophylaxis, 373t
Pyrogen, 263
Pyrogenic exotoxins, 5
Pyuria, 986. *See also* Urinary tract infection.

Q

Q fever, 13, 19t, 355t, 390–391, 390t
Qβ replicase amplification assay, 122
QT interval
  erythromycin effects on, 178
  quinolone effects on, 185
Queensland tick typhus, 355t
Quinacrine, 153t
  in giardiasis, 902, 903t
Quinidine gluconate, 153t
  in malaria, 369–370, 371t
Quinidine sulfate, in malaria, 370
Quinine, 213, 213t
  dosing for, 213t
  in babesiosis, 377, 377t
Quinine sulfate, 153t
  in malaria, 371t
Quinolones, 151t, 184–187, 185t, 186t
  in gonorrhea, 1013
  in shigellosis, 886, 886t
Quinupristin-dalfopristin, 151t, 172–175, 173t, 174t, 175t
  adverse effects of, 175
  dosing for, 174t
  drugs interactions with, 175, 175t

R

Rabbit ileal loop assay, in *Escherichia coli* infection, 72
Rabies immune globulin, 218t, 220
Rabies virus infection, 607–608, 678–680
  aerophobia in, 678
  clinical manifestations of, 678
  complications of, 680
  diagnosis of, 88t, 678, 680
  dumb, 678
  epidemiology of, 19t, 678, 679f
  etiology of, 678
  furious, 678
  hydrophobia in, 678
  immunization against, 253t, 257
    for international travel, 244t, 1212
    postexposure, 243t
  pathogenesis of, 678
  prevention of, 680
  prognosis for, 680
  transmission of, 678
  treatment of, 680
Racecadotril, in acute enteritis, 918
Radial immunodiffusion assay, for antibody detection, 103
Radiation therapy, immunosuppression with, 1149
Radiculopathy, in Lyme disease, 704
Radiography, 127t. *See also* Chest radiography.
  in amebiasis, 892
  in appendicitis, 137, 138f
  in ascariasis, 509f, 510f
  in brain calcifications, 130, 131f
  in bronchiolitis, 785, 785f
  in chickenpox, 335
  in *Chlamydia trachomatis* pneumonia, 810, 810f
  in congenital rubella infection, 1112, 1112f
  in congenital syphilis, 1103–1104, 1104f
  in dental infection, 737, 737f
  in diskitis, 1052, 1052f
  in echinococcosis, 529, 529f
Radiography *(Continued)*
  in epiglottitis, 775, 775f
  in fever of unknown origin, 277
  in infectious arthritis, 1047, 1047f
  in laryngotracheobronchitis, 773, 773f, 774f
  in measles, 310–311, 311f
  in murine typhus, 389
  in myonecrosis, 592
  in neck abscess, 725, 725f
  in necrotizing fasciitis, 592
  in neonatal sepsis, 1125
  in osteomyelitis, 141, 141f–144f, 1037–1038, 1038f
  in pertussis syndrome, 792
  in pneumonia, 801
  in sepsis, 288
  in sinusitis, 763–764, 764f
  in suppurative arthritis, 1047, 1047f
  of calcifications, 130, 131f
  of chest, 131–136, 131f–137f
  of gastrointestinal tract, 137, 137f, 138f
  of heart, 136–137
  of musculoskeletal system, 141–145, 141f–145f
  of paranasal sinuses, 130
  of respiratory tract, 131–136, 131f–137f
  of skull, 130, 131f
  of spine, 131
Radioimmunoassay
  for antibody detection, 100
  for antigen detection, 111, 115f
Radioimmunoprecipitation assay, for antibody detection, 104
Radionuclide scan, 127t
  in cat-scratch disease, 345, 345f
  in diskitis, 1052, 1052f
  in infectious arthritis, 1047
  in intra-abdominal abscess, 995
  in osteomyelitis, 141, 142f, 143f, 1037, 1038, 1039f
  in urinary tract infection, 987–988, 987f
Ramsay Hunt syndrome, 333
Ranitidine bismuth-citrate, in gastritis, 875–876, 876t
Rapid plasma reagin (RPR) card test, 105, 108, 1021–1022, 1022t
Rapid urease test, in gastritis, 874, 875, Plate 8A
Rash. *See also* Enanthem; Exanthem.
  ampicillin, in infectious mononucleosis, 428
  bacterial toxin–induced, 4t
  in erythema infectiosum, 326–327, Plage 4B, Plate 4A
  in international child traveler, 1217
  in Kawasaki syndrome, 481
  in Lyme disease, 349, 350
  in measles, 306, 308, Plate 3A
  in rat-bite fever, 605
  in Rocky Mountain spotted fever, 354, 539t, 540, Plate 5C
  in roseola, 322, Plate 3E
  in rubella, 316–317, Plate 3C
  in sepsis evaluation, 286, 286t
  in streptococcal pharyngitis, 712–713
  macular, erythematous, 534–535, 534t, 535f, 536f
  maculopapular, 535–538, 536t, 537f, 538f
Rat lungworm infection, 517
Rat tapeworm infection, 530t, 531
Rat-bite fever (*Spirillum minus* infection), 18t, 602, 605
Reactive arthritis, 1044, 1045, 1049
  clinical manifestations of, 1045, 1046t
  pathogenesis of, 1045
  treatment of, 1049
  with yersiniosis, 888
Receptors
  in innate immunity, 33, 33t
  pattern, 32
Recombinant immunoblot assay, for antibody detection, 103
Rectouterine pouch, 923
Rectovesicular pouch, 923
Red cell aplasia, in erythema infectiosum, 327–328
Red eye. *See* Conjunctivitis.
Reflectometry, acoustic, in otitis media, 752
Refugee children, 1194–1206. *See also* Foreign-born children.
Relapsing fever, 19t, 387–388, 388t
Relapsing grip, in rheumatic fever, 489
Relative risk, 11
Renal scan, 987–988, 987f
Reovirus 2 infection, cutaneous eruption in, 537
Reportable infections, 1221–1222, 1222t
Reptiles, in salmonellosis, 879, 880, 882
Reservoir, 12, 15
Residential institutions, immunization in, 238
Respiratory arrest, in bacterial tracheitis, 778
Respiratory failure, in respiratory syncytial virus infection, 785, 785f, 786
Respiratory rate, in pneumonia, 799–800, 799t
Respiratory syncytial virus immune globulin, 218t, 220, 788, 788t
Respiratory syncytial virus infection, 784–788, 818. *See also* Bronchiolitis.
  diagnosis of, 88t
  immune globulin prophylaxis in, 788, 788t
  in AIDS, 469
  in otitis media, 749, 758. *See also* Otitis media.
  nosocomial, 1223–1224
  palivizumab prophylaxis in, 788, 788t
  rapid tests for, 786
  ribavirin in, 787, 787f
Respiratory syncytial virus monoclonal antibody (palivizumab), 218t, 220
Respiratory tract
  cilia in, 798
  host defenses of, 798
  imaging of, 131–136, 131f–137f
  immune system of, 798
  lower, infection of, 794–830. *See also* Pneumonia.
  microbiological specimen collection from, 61t
  middle, infection of, 771–778. *See also* Epiglottitis; Laryngotracheobronchitis; Tracheitis.
  normal flora infection of, 7
  normal flora of, 8t
  nosocomial infection of, 1223–1225, 1224t
  phagocytes of, 798
  specimen collection from, 61t, 64
  T lymphocytes of, 798
  upper, infection of, 711–719. *See also* Pharyngitis.
Reticulate body, in *Chlamydia trachomatis* infection, 1017, 1017f

Retinal necrosis, 1083
Retinitis, 1082–1084, Plate 9D
  clinical manifestations of, 1082–1083
  complications of, 1083
  cytomegalovirus, in AIDS, 470
  diagnosis of, 1083, Plate 9D
  epidemiology of, 1082
  etiology of, 1082
  pathogenesis of, 1082, 1082f
  prevention of, 1084
  prognosis for, 1084
  syphilitic, 1083, 1083f
  treatment of, 1083
Retinoids, in acne vulgaris, 549
Retinopathy, stellate, in cat-scratch disease, 344, 345f, Plate 9D
Retrobulbar neuritis, ethambutol-induced, 206
Retroperitoneal abscess, 938–940
  clinical manifestations of, 939
  culture in, 939
  diagnosis of, 939
  epidemiology of, 938
  etiology of, 938
  pathogenesis of, 938–939, 938f
Retrospective study, 11
Retroviruses. *See also* Human immunodeficiency virus (HIV) infection.
  in oncogenesis, 24t, 26–27
Reverse class capture assay, for antibody detection, 101, 102f
Reverse transcriptase, 26
Reye's syndrome, 338t, 339, 687–688
Rhabdomyolysis, in infectious mononucleosis, 434
Rhabdomyosarcoma
  lymphadenopathy in, 623
  vs. vulvovaginitis, 1004
Rhagades, in congenital syphilis, 1104
Rheumatic fever, 486–493
  arthritis in, 488–489, 491
  Aschoff body in, 491
  brain changes in, 491
  carditis in, 488, 492
  chorea in, 488, 489, 492
  clinical manifestations of, 488–490, 488t, 489f
  complications of, 492
  culture in, 490–491
  diagnosis of, 490–491, 490t
  differential diagnosis of, 490, 490t
  epidemiology of, 486–487, 487t
  erythema marginatum in, 488, 489, 489f
  etiology of, 486
  fever of unknown origin and, 276t
  imaging in, 491
  Jones criteria in, 490, 490t
  murmurs in, 488
  nodules in, 488, 489, 489f, 491
  pathogenesis of, 487
  pathology of, 491
  prevention of, 492–493, 493t
  prognosis for, 492
  risk factors for, 487
  treatment of, 491–492, 492t
Rheumatoid arthritis, juvenile, lymphadenopathy in, 613
Rheumatoid factor, 99
Rhinitis
  allergic, vs. common cold, 708, 708t
Rhinitis *(Continued)*
  in congenital syphilis, 1104
Rhinovirus infection, 707–710. *See also* Common cold.
Ribavirin, 152t, 200–201
  in respiratory syncytial virus infection, 787, 787f
Rickettsia akari infection (rickettsialpox), 19t, 355t, 391–392, 391t
  vs. chickenpox, 334
Rickettsia felis infection, 19t
Rickettsia prowazekii infection (epidemic typhus), 388, 536t, 538
Rickettsia rickettsii infection (Rocky Mountain spotted fever), 354–357
  clinical manifestations of, 354, 356t, Plate 5C
  complications of, 357
  diagnosis of, 354–356, 356t
  differential diagnosis of, 355, 356t
  epidemiology of, 19t, 354
  etiology of, 354, 355t
  laboratory evaluation of, 355
  meningoencephalitis in, 681
  microbiologic evaluation of, 355–356
  mortality in, 357
  pathogenesis of, 354
  prevention of, 357
  prognosis for, 357
  rash in, 354, 539t, 540, Plate 5C
  serologic testing in, 108, 355–356
  treatment of, 356–357, 356t
  vs. atypical measles, 309–310
Rickettsia tsutsugamushi. See Orientia tsutsugamushi infection.
Rickettsia typhi infection (murine typhus), 19t, 108, 388–389, 389t
Rickettsialpox, 19t, 355t, 391–392, 391t
  vs. chickenpox, 334
Rickettsiosis, vesicular. *See* Rickettsialpox.
Rifabutin, 152t
Rifampin, 152t, 206–208, 206t, 207t, 208t
  in brucellosis, 381, 381t
  in ehrlichiosis, 361
  in *Haemophilus influenzae* type b infection prophylaxis, 226, 228t, 776
  in leprosy, 554, 554t
  in meningitis, 643t, 646t
  in meningococcal meningitis prophylaxis, 225, 228t
  in streptococcal pharyngitis, 717t
  in tuberculosis, 412–413, 414t
Rimantadine, 152t, 201–202, 201t, 202t
  adverse effects of, 201–202, 202t
  in influenza virus infection, 820–821, 821t
Ringworm, 558–560, 559f, 559t, 561t
Ritonavir, 152t, 204t, 205t
  in HIV infection, 456, 457t, 459t, 460t
Ritter's disease. *See* Staphylococcal scalded skin syndrome.
River blindness, 518
Rochalimaea henselae. See Bartonella henselae infection (cat-scratch disease).
Rocky Mountain spotted fever, 354–357. *See also Rickettsia rickettsii* infection (Rocky Mountain spotted fever).
Rodentborne infection, 15, 18t–20t, 21t. *See also specific infections.*
Rosacea, in *Demodex* infestation, 573
Rose spots, in typhoid fever, 537
Roseola, 321–324
  clinical manifestations of, 321–322, 322f
  complications of, 323
  culture in, 323
  diagnosis of, 322–323
  differential diagnosis of, 322–323
  encephalitic, 681
  epidemiology of, 321
  etiology of, 321
  exanthem of, 321, 322, 535–536, 536t, Plate 3E
  imaging in, 323
  in immunocompromised persons, 322
  laboratory evaluation in, 323
  neurologic disease with, 322
  pathogenesis of, 321
  physical examination in, 321–322
  prevention of, 323–324
  prognosis for, 323
  serologic testing in, 323
  transmission of, 321
  treatment of, 323
  vs. rubella, 318
Roseola infantum. *See* Roseola.
Roseola-like illness, 322
Rotavirus infection, 898–900, 898t
  clinical manifestations of, 898t, 899
  complications of, 900
  diagnosis of, 88t, 90, 90f, 899
  electron microscopy in, 90, 90f
  epidemiology of, 898t, 899, 899f
  etiology of, 898–899
  immunization against, 258
    adverse reactions to, 237t
  in day care environment, 1190
  pathogenesis of, 899
  prevention of, 900
  prognosis for, 900
  transmission of, 899
  treatment of, 899–900
Rotterdam prognostic scoring system
  in meningococcemia, 293
  in sepsis, 293
Rubella, 316–320
  clinical manifestations of, 316–317, 317f
  complications of, 318–319
  congenital, 319, 320, 1088t, 1089t, 1092t, 1111–1113
    clinical manifestations of, 1111–1112, 1111t
    diabetes with, 1112
    diagnosis of, 1112–1113, 1112f, 1112t
    epidemiology of, 1111
    hearing loss with, 1112
    pathogenesis of, 1111
    prevention of, 1113
  culture in, 318
  diagnosis of, 88t, 317–318, 318t
  differential diagnosis of, 318, 318t
  encephalitic, 682
    progressive, 685
  epidemiology of, 316, 317f
  etiology of, 316
  exanthem of, 316–317, 535, 536t, Plate 3C
  hospitalization for, 320
  imaging in, 318
  immunization against, 258, 319. *See also* Measles-mumps-rubella (MMR) vaccine.

Rubella *(Continued)*
immunization against *(Continued)*
for international travel, 320, 1209
joint manifestations of, 319
laboratory evaluation in, 318
maternal, 319, 320, 1088t, 1089t, 1092t
microbiologic evaluation in, 318
neurologic disease with, 319
outbreak control with, 319
pathogenesis of, 316
pathology of, 318
physical examination in, 317
prevention of, 319–320
prognosis for, 319
thrombocytopenic purpura with, 319
transmission of, 316
treatment of, 318
vs. erythema infectiosum, 328
vs. measles, 318
vs. roseola, 323
Rubeola. *See* Measles.
Russian spring-summer encephalitis, 676

S

Saber shins, in congenital syphilis, 1104
Sabin-Feldman dye exclusion assay, 109
Saddle nose deformity, in congenital syphilis, 1104
St. Louis encephalitis, 673, 674f
St. Vitus' dance, in rheumatic fever, 488
Salmonella infection (salmonellosis), 15, 16t, 17t, 879–882
carrier of, 879, 881
clinical manifestations of, 880–881, 880t
complications of, 881
culture in, 881
diagnosis of, 881
differential diagnosis of, 881
epidemiology of, 18t, 879–880, 880f
etiology of, 879
foodborne, 908–911, 910t, 911t
in AIDS, 471
in bacteremia, 270t, 281, 282t
in day care environment, 1190
in sickle cell disease, 283
pathogenesis of, 880
prevention of, 881–882
prognosis for, 881
reptile-associated, 879, 880, 882
sepsis with, 881
toxins of, 4t
transmission of, 879
treatment of, 881, 882t
Salmonella typhi infection (typhoid), 882–885
carrier, 884
clinical manifestations of, 883, 883t
complications of, 884
diagnosis of, 883
epidemiology of, 882
etiology of, 882
immunization against, 245t, 251–252
for international travel, 244t, 1212
heat-phenol-inactivated, 252
live-attenuated, 251–252
polysaccharide, 252
in oncogenesis, 29
Salmonella typhi infection (typhoid) *(Continued)*
pathogenesis of, 882–883
prevention of, 885
prognosis for, 884
serologic testing in, 105
skin lesions in, 537
transmission of, 882
treatment of, 883–884, 884t
Widal test in, 883
Salpingitis
Chlamydia trachomatis infection and, 1018–1019
chlamydial, 1018–1019
gonococcal, 1011
vs. appendicitis, 934, 934t
Sandwich assay
direct, for antigen detection, 101–102, 102f, 111, 113f
indirect, for antigen detection, 100, 101f, 111, 113f
Saquinavir, 152t, 204t, 205t
in HIV infection, 456, 457t, 460t
Sarcoma, fever of unknown origin and, 276t
Sarcoptes scabiei infestation, 571–573, 572f
in day care environment, 1191
Saxitoxin, 911
Scabies, 571–573, 572f
in day care environment, 1191
Scalp
abscess of, 1129
furuncular myiasis of, 571, 571f
tinea of, 556–558, 556t, 557f, 558t
Scarlet fever
erythema of, 534, 534t, Plate 3D
pathogenesis of, 712
vs. erythema infectiosum, 328
vs. roseola, 323
vs. rubella, 318
Schick test, 719
Schistosoma spp. infection (schistosomiasis), 15, 20t, 521–524
bladder cancer and, 29
clinical manifestations of, 522–523, 523t
complications of, 523–524
dermatitis in, 523
diagnosis of, 523
epidemiology of, 20t, 521, 522t
etiology of, 521
organism life cycle in, 523f
pathogenesis of, 521–522, 523f
prevention of, 524
prognosis for, 524
transverse myelitis in, 524
treatment of, 523, 524t
Schlichter titers, in osteomyelitis, 1040
Scombroid toxin, 911
Scombrotoxin, in foodborne disease, 16t
Scratch test, for animal antisera, 221, 221t
Screw worm fly infestation, 571
Scrofula, 400f, 402, 402f, 621
Scrofuloderma, 404
Scrub typhus, 355t, 536t, 538
Seafood poisoning, 911
Seborrheic vulvitis, vs. vulvovaginitis, 1004
Secondary case, 12
Seizures
after meningitis, 649
febrile, 639
Seizures *(Continued)*
fever and, 263
in brain abscess, 663
in meningitis, 638, 639
in roseola, 322
with congenital toxoplasmosis, 1116
Selective serotonin reuptake inhibitors, in chronic fatigue syndrome, 502
Selenium sulfide
in tinea capitis, 558
in tinea versicolor, 560
Sennetsu fever, 19t. *See also Ehrlichia* spp. infection (ehrlichiosis).
Sensitivity, of test, 11
Sentinel loop sign, in acute pancreatitis, 980
Sepsis, 279–294
anatomic defects and, 282
asplenia and, 282
body temperature in, 263
burn-related, 282, 597–598, 597t
catheter-related, in burn injury patient, 601
clinical manifestations of, 285–286, 285t
complications of, 293–294, 293t, 294t
culture in, 288
definition of, 279, 280t
diagnosis of, 286–288, 287t
differential diagnosis of, 286, 287t
epidemiology of, 281
etiology of, 279
fulminant, 281, 283, 285
Haemophilus influenzae type b, 285, 293
imaging in, 288
in cancer patient, 283
in hemoglobinopathy, 283
in immunocompromised host, 281–282, 282t
in sickle cell disease, 283, 293
intravenous immune globulin in, 219–220
laboratory evaluation of, 286–287, 287t
microbiologic evaluation in, 288
Neisseria meningitidis, 285, 288, 293, 293t, 294t
neonatal, 1119–1129
absolute neutrophil count in, 1123
antigen tests in, 1124
cerebrospinal fluid culture in, 1124
clinical manifestations of, 1122–1123
complications of, 1128
C-reactive protein in, 1123–1124
culture in, 1124
diagnosis of, 1123–1125
early-onset, 1120–1121, 1120t, 1121t
pathogenesis of, 1121–1122
treatment of, 1125–1127, 1125t, 1126t
epidemiology of, 1119–1121, 1120t, 1121t
erythrocyte sedimentation rate in, 1123–1124
Escherichia coli in, 1119, 1120t
etiology of, 1119, 1120t, 1122
group B *Streptococcus* in, 1119, 1120t
imaging in, 1125
intravenous hyperalimentation and, 1122
I:T ratio in, 1123
late-onset, 1121, 1121t
pathogenesis of, 1122
treatment of, 1127
leukocyte count in, 1123
pathogenesis of, 1121–1122
physical examination in, 1123

Sepsis *(Continued)*
neonatal *(Continued)*
prenatal-onset, 1120–1121, 1120t, 1121t
pathogenesis of, 1121–1122
prevention of, 1128–1129
prognosis for, 1128
screening panels in, 1124
treatment of, 1125–1128, 1125t, 1126t
duration of, 1127–1128
maternal antibiotic treatment and, 1128
supportive, 1128
urine culture in, 1124
viral culture in, 1124
pathogenesis of, 283
physical examination in, 286, 286t
postsplenectomy, 282–283
prevention of, 294
treatment of, 289–293, 289t, 290t, 291t
vs. urinary tract infection, 985
Septata intestinalis infection, in AIDS, 472
Septic arthritis. *See* Suppurative arthritis.
Septic shock, 279–294. *See also* Shock, septic.
Septicemic plague, 384–385
Serology, 99–115. *See also* Antibody (antibodies); Antigen(s).
Seroprevalence, 12
Serratia infection, in cancer patient, 283
Serum bactericidal tests, 77–78
in osteomyelitis, 1040
Serum sickness, lymphadenopathy in, 613
Seventh-nerve palsy, in Lyme disease, 350
Severe combined immune deficiency, 1152, 1152t
Sexual abuse (assault), 1030–1031, 1030t, 1031t
genital warts and, 568
HIV infection and, 476, 1031
Sexual intercourse, urethritis with, 983, 985
Sexually transmitted infections, 1009–1031, 1010t. *See also specific infections.*
clinical manifestations of, 1009
diagnosis of, 1009
epidemiology of, 1009
lymphadenopathy in, 616, 617
management of, 1009–1010
maternal. *See* Maternal infection.
prevention of, 1010
sexual assault and, 476, 568, 1030–1031, 1030t, 1031t
vs. urinary tract infection, 985
vs. vulvovaginitis, 1004
Sheep liver fluke infection, 522t
Shell vial culture, in viral infection, 89, 90f
Shellfish poisoning, 16t, 911
Shigella infection (shigellosis), 15, 16t, 17t, 885–887
clinical manifestations of, 885–886, 885t
complications of, 886–887
culture in, 886
diagnosis of, 886
differential diagnosis of, 886
ekiri with, 886
epidemiology of, 885
etiology of, 885
in AIDS, 450t, 471
in day care environment, 1190
pathogenesis of, 885
prevention of, 887
prognosis for, 887
Shigella infection (shigellosis) *(Continued)*
toxins in, 4t
transmission of, 885
treatment of, 886, 886t
vulvovaginal, 999, 1001, 1001t
treatment of, 1006t, 1007
waterborne, 908, 909, 909t
Shock
cardiogenic, vs. septic shock, 286
hypovolemic
in staphylococcal toxic shock syndrome, 302, 302t
vs. septic shock, 286
septic, 4t, 279–294. *See also* Sepsis.
anti-tumor necrosis factor antibody in, 292
clinical manifestations of, 285–286, 286t
corticosteroids in, 290
definition of, 279, 280t
diagnosis of, 286, 287, 287t
early, 285, 286t
epidemiology of, 281
etiology of, 279–281, 280t
exchange transfusion in, 293
granulocyte transfusion in, 293
ibuprofen in, 290
laboratory evaluation of, 287, 287t
late, 286, 286t
leukopenia in, 287
lipopolysaccharide antibody in, 290, 292
microbiologic evaluation in, 288
mortality rate in, 293, 294
naloxone in, 290
pathogenesis of, 283–285, 284f
physical examination in, 286
prevention of, 294
recombinant activated protin C in, 292–293
treatment of, 289–293, 290t, 291t, 292t
tumor necrosis factor-α in, 283–284
Short-gut syndrome
in necrotizing enterocolitis, 1132
infection with, 282
Shunt-related infection, 651–655
clinical manifestations of, 652
complications of, 654–655
diagnosis of, 652
epidemiology of, 651
etiology of, 651
pathogenesis of, 651
prevention of, 655
prognosis for, 655
treatment of, 652–654, 654f, 655t
Sialadenitis, 741–744
clinical manifestations of, 742
complications of, 744
diagnosis of, 742–743, 743t
epidemiology of, 741, 742t
etiology of, 741, 742t
imaging in, 743
pathogenesis of, 741–742
prevention of, 744
prognosis for, 744
recurrent, 742
suppurative, 422
treatment of, 743–744
Sialectasis, 742
Sialography, 743
Sickle cell disease, 1182t, 1183
Sickle cell disease *(Continued)*
bacteremia in, 293–294
immunization in, 240t–241t
infection in, 283
osteomyelitis in, 1039f
Siderophores, 35
Silver nitrate
conjunctivitis with, 1055, 1056t
ophthalmic prophylaxis with, 1057, 1058
Silver stain, in meningitis, 641
Silver sulfadiazine, 152t
in burn wound infection, 599t
Simian immunodeficiency virus, 437
Sin Nombre virus infection. *See* Hantavirus cardiopulmonary syndrome.
Sinus histiocytosis, lymphadenopathy in, 623
Sinusitis, 760–769
acute, 762
air-fluid level in, 763, 764f
anatomy in, 760–761, 761f
antibiotic resistance in, 766
chronic, 762
clinical manifestations of, 762–763, 762t
complications of, 766–769, 766t, 767t, 768f, 769t
cough in, 763, 763t
diagnosis of, 130, 763–764, 763t, 764f
differential diagnosis of, 763, 763t
epidemiology of, 760
etiology of, 760
imaging in, 130, 763–764, 764f
in burn injury patient, 601
intracranial complications of, 767–769
magnetic resonance imaging in, 763–764, 764f
mucociliary apparatus in, 761–762
nasal endoscopy in, 762
orbital complications of, 766–767, 767t, 768f, 769t
osteomeatal complex in, 761, 761f
pathogenesis of, 760–762, 761f, 761t
prevention of, 769
prognosis for, 769, 769t
recurrent, 769, 769t
secretory layers in, 762
sinus aspiration in, 764
subacute, 762
subdural empyema in, 767–769
supportive therapy in, 766
surgery in, 766
transillumination in, 762–763
treatment of, 764–766, 765t
vs. common cold, 708, 708t
Sixth disease. *See* Roseola.
Skin. *See also* Enanthem; Exanthem; Rash.
acne vulgaris of, 547–549, 548t
anthrax of, 551–552
bacterial infections of, 544–552. *See also specific infections.*
blistering distal dactylitis of, 549–550, 550f
Candida infection of, 560–563, 562f
carbuncles of, 545–547, 546t
color of, 534
cutaneous larva migrans of, 504, 505, 506t, 569–570, 570f
decubitus ulcers of, 550–551, 551f
dermatophyte infections of, 557–560, 559f, 559t, 560f

Skin *(Continued)*
erythematous macular rashes of, 534–535, 534f, 534t, 535f
erythrasma of, 549
examination of, 533–534
folliculitis of, 545–547, 546f, 546t
fungal infections of, 556–564. *See also specific infections.*
furuncles of, 545–547, 546t, 547f
herpes simplex virus infection of, 564–566, 564f–566f
impetigo of, 544–545, 545f, 545t, 546t
inflammation of, 578–585. *See also* Cellulitis.
leishmaniasis of, 570–571, 570f
leprosy of, 552–554, 552f, 553f, 553t, 554t
lice infestation of, 573–574, 573f
maculopapular rashes of, 535–538, 536t, 537f, 538f
microbiological specimen collection from, 61t
mite infestation of, 571–573, 572f
molluscum contagiosum of, 568–569, 569f
mycobacterial infections of, 552–556. *See also specific infections.*
myiasis of, 571, 571f
nodules of, 542, 542f
nontuberculous mycobacterial infection of, 555–556, 555f, 555t
normal flora of, 7, 8t
nosocomial infections of, 1227–1228, 1227t, 1228t
papillomavirus infection of, 566–568, 567f, 567t, 568f
parasitic infection of, 569–571, 570f
perianal, dermatitis of, 550, 550f
pitted keratolysis of, 549, 549t
purpura of, 539–540, 539t
pustular eruptions of, 540–541, 541t
scabies of, 571–573, 572f
sporotrichosis of, 563–564
target lesions of, 538–539, 539t
tinea infection of, 556–561, 556t, 557f, 558t, 559f, 559t, 560f, 561t
tinea versicolor of, 560, 561f
tuberculosis of, 404, 404f
vesicular eruptions of, 540–541, 541t
viral infection of, 564–569. *See also specific infections.*
Skin test
in cat-scratch disease, 346
in leprosy, 552
in mumps, 423
in tuberculosis, 405–406, 405f, 406t, 460, 467–468
of animal antisera, 221, 221t
Skin-piercing procedures, 1215
Skull
imaging of, 130, 131f
in congenital syphilis, 1104
SLAM-associated protein, 428
Slapped cheek appearance, in erythema infectiosum, 326, 536, Plate 4A
Slide catalase test, 57
Slit-skin smear, in leprosy, 554
Slow virus infection, 682–683
Smallpox
immunization against, 258–259
vs. chickenpox, 334, 335f
Smegma, normal flora of, 9t
Snake bite, 602–608. *See also* Bite-wound infection.
Snuffles, syphilitic, vs. common cold, 708, 708t
Sodium bicarbonate, in stomatitis, 732t
Soft chancre. *See* Chancroid.
Soft tissues
infection of. *See* Cellulitis; Necrotizing fasciitis; Wound infection.
specimen collection from, 61t, 65–66
Soilborne pathogens, 13, 14t. *See also specific infections.*
Somatization, in chronic fatigue syndrome, 502
Southeast Asian liver fluke infection, 522t
Southern blotting, in viral infection, 89
Sparfloxacin, 152t, 184–187, 185t, 186t
Specific immunity. *See* Immunity, adaptive.
Specificity, of test, 11
Specimen, 57–91
acid-fast stains of, 68, 68t
acridine orange stain of, 67, 68t
bacterial, 57–79, 58t
acid-fast stains of, 68, 68t
acridine orange stain of, 67, 68t
antimicrobial susceptibility testing of, 75–79, 75t, 78f. *See also* Antimicrobial susceptibility testing.
collection of, 59–66, 60t–62t
counterimmunoelectrophoresis of, 70
culture of, 72–75, 72f, 72t, 74t, 75f
darkfield examination of, 68, 68f
enzyme immunoassay of, 71
fluorochrome stain of, 68–69, 68t
for anaerobic culture, 62
from blood, 60t, 62–64, 62t, 63t
from body fluid, 60t, 64
from bone, 61t, 65–66
from catheter, 62t, 66
from cerebrospinal fluid, 60t, 64, 66–67
from ear, 62t, 66
from eye, 62t, 66
from gastrointestinal tract, 61t, 64–65
from genital tract, 61t, 65
from nasopharynx, 61t, 64
from pharynx, 61t, 64
from soft tissue, 61t, 65–66
from stool, 61t, 64–65
from urinary tract, 61t, 65
Gram stain of, 67, 67t
immunoassay of, 69–71, 70t
immunochromatography of, 71
immunofluorescence tests of, 70
India ink preparation of, 69, 69f, 69t
Kinyoun stain of, 68, 68t
latex agglutination assay of, 70–71
modified Kinyoun stain of, 69, 69t
optical immunoassay of, 71
processing of, 66–67, 66t
swab for, 59–62, 60t–62t
toxin detection in, 71–72
transport of, 66–67
Ziehl-Neelsen stain of, 68
calcofluor white stain of, 69, 70f, 70t
dark-field examination of, 68, 68f
fluorochrome stain of, 68–69, 68t
fungal, 59, 60t
blood culture of, 63–64
Specimen *(Continued)*
fungal *(Continued)*
calcofluor white stain of, 69, 70f, 70t
immunoassay of, 69–71, 70t
potassium hydroxide preparation of, 69, 69t, 70f
sputum culture of, 64
stool culture of, 65
susceptibility testing of, 76
Gram stain of, 67, 67t
immunoassay of, 69–71, 70t
counterimmunoelectrophoresis for, 70
enzyme immunoassay for, 71
immunochromatography for, 71
immunofluorescence for, 70
latex agglutination for, 70–71
optical immunoassay for, 71
Kinyoun stain of, 68, 68t
modified Kinyoun stain of, 69, 69t
parasite, 80–83, 81t
cellophane tape preparation for, 82, 82f
collection of, 80–81
culture of, 83
microscopic examination of, 81–83, 82f, 83f
stains for, 82–83, 83f
transport of, 81
wet mount for, 82, 82f
pathologic evaluation of, 116–125. *See also* Pathology.
potassium hydroxide preparation of, 69, 69t, 70f
serologic evaluation of, 99–115. *See also* Antibody (antibodies); Antigen(s).
viral, 84–91, 85t–86t, 87t, 88t
antigen detection for, 88t, 89
antiviral susceptibility testing of, 90–91
cell culture for, 84, 88t, 89, 89f
collection of, 84, 87t
electron microscopy for, 90, 90f
histopathologic stains for, 90
nucleic acid hybridization for, 89–90
serologic testing for, 88t, 90
shell vial culture for, 89, 90f
transport of, 84
Ziehl-Neelsen stain of, 68
Spectinomycin, 152t
in gonorrhea, 1014t
Spinal epidural abscess, 657, 665–667, 666t, 667f, 667t
Spine, imaging of, 131
Spirillum minus infection (rat-bite fever), 18t, 602, 605
Spironolactone, in menstruation-related acne, 549
Spleen
abscess of, 937–938
absence of, 282–283, 1181, 1182t
immunization and, 1181, 1184t
rupture of
in infectious mononucleosis, 434
in malaria, 372
Splenectomy
immunization and, 240t–241t
in splenic abscess, 938
infection and, 282–283
Splinter hemorrhage, in infective endocarditis, 540
Spondylitis
infectious. *See* Diskitis.
tuberculous, 403
Spongiform encephalopathy, 685–687, 686t

Sporadic case, 12
Sporothrix schenckii infection (sporotrichosis), 563–564, 627, 628
Spumaviruses, in oncogenesis, 26–27
Sputum
collection of, 61t, 64
for parasites, 80
culture of, in pneumonia, 800–801
examination of, in *Paragonimus westermani* infection, 80
Stain
acid-fast
in *Cryptosporidium parvum* infection, 82–83
in *Isospora belli* infection, 82–83
in meningitis, 641
acridine orange, 67, 68t
calcofluor white, 69, 70f, 70t
fluorochrome, 68–69, 68t
for parasites, 82–83, 83f
Gram, 67, 67t
cytocentrifugation for, 66
in meningitis, 641, 642t
in *Pneumocystis carinii* infection, 82
of cerebrospinal fluid, 641–642, 642t
Kinyoun, 68, 68t
modified, 69, 69t
methenamine silver, in *Pneumocystis carinii* infection, 82, 83f
of cerebrospinal fluid, 641, 642t
silver, in meningitis, 641
Steiner, in cat-scratch disease, 346
toluidine blue, in *Pneumocystis carinii* infection, 82, 83f
viral, 90
Warthin-Starry, in cat-scratch disease, 346
Wheatley's trichrome, for protozoa, 82, 83f
Ziehl-Neelsen, 68
Standard precautions, 1233–1234, 1233t
Staphylococcal scalded skin syndrome, 534–535, 534f, 534t, 535f, Plate 6C
Staphylococcal toxic shock syndrome, 296–304
clinical manifestations of, 299–300, 299f, 299t
complications of, 303
desquamation in, 300, Plate 6A
diagnosis of, 300, 300t
differential diagnosis of, 301
epidemiology of, 296–297
etiology of, 296
laboratory evaluation in, 301, 302t
pathogenesis of, 297–298, 298f
prevention of, 303–304
prognosis for, 303, 304t
recurrence of, 303, 304t
treatment of, 302–303, 302t
Staphylococcus aureus infection
bite-wound, 602–608, 603t, 606t, 607t
bone, 1034, 1034t. *See also* Osteomyelitis.
burn-related, 596, 597t
cardiac, 845, 846t. *See also* Infective endocarditis.
cervical lymphadenitis in, 621–626. *See also* Lymphadenitis, cervical.
conjunctival, 1055, 1056t, 1059, 1059f. *See also* Conjunctivitis, bacterial.
cutaneous, 544–547, 545f, 545t, 546f, 546t, 547f, 578–585. *See also* Cellulitis.
in AIDS, 474
Staphylococcus aureus infection *(Continued)*
in blepharitis, 1069–1070, 1070f
in cancer patient, 283
in dacrocystitis, 1072–1073
in foodborne disease, 16t
in sepsis, 279
in septic shock, 280t, 281
in toxic shock syndrome. *See also* Staphylococcal toxic shock syndrome.
maternal, 1096
meningeal, 630, 630t, 631t. *See also* Meningitis, bacterial.
of digital fat pad, 549–550
phlyctenular keratoconjunctivitis in, 1059, 1059f, 1070, 1070f
toxins of, 4t
Statistics, 11
Stavudine, 152t, 203t, 205t
in HIV infection, 456, 457t, 458t, 460t
Steeple sign, in laryngotracheobronchitis, 773, 774f
Steiner stain, in cat-scratch disease, 346
Stellate retinopathy, in retinitis, 1083, Plate 9D
Stem cell transplantation. *See* Transplantation, bone marrow.
Sterilization, 1239–1240, 1239t
Stevens-Johnson syndrome/toxic epidermal necrolysis
target lesions of, 538–539, 539t
vs. staphylococcal scalded skin syndrome, 534–535
Stomatitis, 728–733. *See also Candida* spp. infection (candidiasis), oral; Herpes simplex virus infection, oral (gingivostomatitis).
clinical manifestations of, 729–730, 730f
complications of, 732
diagnosis of, 730–731
differential diagnosis of, 730
epidemiology of, 728
etiology of, 728, 729t
gangrenous, 730, 734
diagnosis of, 737
pathogenesis of, 736
pathogenesis of, 728–729
prevention of, 733
prognosis for, 732–733
treatment of, 731–732, 731t, 732t
vesicular, 19t, 728, 730
Stool examination
Helicobacter pylori antigen in, 875
in amebiasis, 892
in ascariasis, 509
in campylobacteriosis, 890, Plate 2E
in cholera, 894
in *Clostridium difficile*–associated diarrhea, 913
in gastrointestinal *Escherichia coli* infection, 897
in giardiasis, 902
in hemolytic uremic syndrome, 915
in parasite infection, 80–81, 82–83, 82f, 83f
in salmonellosis, 883
in schistosomiasis, 523
in shigellosis, 886, Plate 2E
in strongyloidiasis, 513
in trichuriasis, 508
specimen collection for, 61t, 64–65
Straight leg raise test, in diskitis, 1051
Strawberry tongue
in Kawasaki syndrome, 480, 480f
in scarlet fever, 534, Plate 3D
in streptococcal pharyngitis, 712
Streptobacillus moniliformis infection (rat-bite fever), 18t, 602, 605
Streptococcal pharyngitis, 711
clinical manifestations of, 712–713, 713t
complications of, 718
diagnosis of, 714–716, 714t, 715f
pathogenesis of, 712
rapid tests for, 714–715, 715f
recurrent, 717
serologic diagnosis of, 716
throat culture in, 714, 714t, 715f
tonsillectomy in, 717
treatment of, 716–717, 716t, 717t
vs. common cold, 708, 708t
vs. infectious mononucleosis, 430
Streptococcal pyrogenic exotoxin A, 298
Streptococcal toxic shock syndrome, 296–304
clinical manifestations of, 300
complications of, 303
diagnosis of, 300–301, 301t
differential diagnosis of, 301
Eagle effect in, 303
epidemiology of, 297
etiology of, 296
laboratory evaluation in, 301, 302t
pathogenesis of, 298–299
prevention of, 304
prognosis for, 303
treatment of, 303
Streptococcosis syndrome, cervical lymphadenitis in, 622
Streptococcus agalactiae. See Group B *Streptococcus* infection.
Streptococcus faecalis. See Enterococcus spp. infection.
Streptococcus faecium. See Enterococcus spp. infection.
Streptococcus pneumoniae infection
conjunctival, 1058, 1058t. *See also* Conjunctivitis, bacterial.
immunization against, 233t, 235t–236t, 245t, 249–250
in AIDS, 450t, 467
in bacteremia, 269–272, 270t, 279, 281, 282t, 283, 286
in day care environment, 1189
in sepsis, 279
in sickle cell disease, 283
meningeal, 630–649. *See also* Meningitis, bacterial.
otologic, 748, 749t. *See also* Otitis media.
pulmonary, 795t, 802–805. *See also* Pneumonia, *Streptococcus pneumoniae.*
rapid diagnosis of, 288
sinus, 760. *See also* Sinusitis.
Streptococcus pyogenes. See Group A *Streptococcus* infection.
Streptogramin antibiotics, 172–175, 173t, 174t, 175t
Streptolysin O, 298, 487
Streptomycin, 151t, 152t
in brucellosis, 381, 381t
in plague, 384–385, 385t

Streptomycin *(Continued)*
in tuberculosis, 412–413, 414t
in tularemia, 383, 383t
Streptozyme test, 105
Stress, immune response and, 49
Stridor, differential diagnosis of, 771, 772t
Strongyloides fuelleborni infection, 513
Strongyloides stercoralis infection (strongyloidiasis), 512–514
agar-plate method in, 513
clinical manifestations of, 513, 513t
Enterotest (string test) in, 80–81
hyperinfection syndrome in, 514
in AIDS, 472
organism life cycle in, 512–513, 513f
pathogenesis of, 513
treatment of, 514, 514t
Strychnine poisoning, vs. tetanus, 694
Stye, 1070–1072, 1071f
Subacute bacterial endocarditis. *See* Infective endocarditis.
Subacute sclerosing panencephalitis, 306, 313, 684–685, 684f
imaging of, 311
pathogenesis of, 684, 684f
Subdural effusion, in meningitis, 648, 648f
Subdural empyema, 657, 664–665, 665f, 666t
in meningitis, 648
Subphrenic space, 921, 922f
Suckling mouse assay
in *Clostridium botulinum* infection, 71
in *Escherichia coli* infection, 72
Sucralfate, in stomatitis, 732t
Sulfacetamide, 152t
Sulfadiazine, 152t
in congenital toxoplasmosis, 1116, 1116t
in meningococcal meningitis prophylaxis, 225, 228t
in rheumatic fever prevention, 493, 493t
Sulfadoxine, 152t, 153t
Sulfadoxine-pyrimethamine, in *Isospora belli* infection, 903t
Sulfamethizole, 152t
Sulfamethoxazole, 152t. *See also* Trimethoprim-sulfamethoxazole (TMP-SMZ).
Sulfisoxazole, 152t
in urinary tract infection, 991t
Sulfonamides, 152t, 182–184, 183t, 184t
Sulfur, precipitated, in scabies, 572
Sunburn, in international child traveler, 1215
Superantigens, 1, 38
Superinfection, 6
Suppurative arthritis
clinical manifestations of, 1045, 1046t
diagnosis of, 1045–1047
differential diagnosis of, 1045–1046
etiology of, 1044, 1044t
imaging in, 1047, 1047f
neonatal, 1047, 1048
of hip, 1047, 1048
pathogenesis of, 1045
treatment of, 1047–1049, 1048t
Suppurative bursitis, 1046
Suprainfection, 6
Surgery, antibiotic prophylaxis for, 226, 228–231, 229t–230t
Surveillance culture, 10
Swab specimen, 59–62, 60t–62t
Sweat glands, infection of, 547
Swimmer's ear, 745–747, 746t. *See also* Otitis externa.
Swimmer's itch, 523
Swimming, 15, 15t
Swimming pool granuloma, 555
Swollen belly syndrome, 512, 513
Swyer-James syndrome, with adenovirus infection, 819
Sydenham's chorea, in rheumatic fever, 488, 492
Symmers' pipestem fibrosis, in schistosomiasis, 521
Sympathetic ophthalmia, 1078
Syndrome of inappropriate ADH secretion, in meningitis, 646
Synovial fluid, collection of, 60t, 64
Synovitis. *See* Reactive arthritis.
Syphilis, 1019–1023. *See also Treponema pallidum* infection (syphilis).
Systemic lupus erythematosus
fever of unknown origin and, 276t
lymphadenopathy in, 613
vs. erythema infectiosum, 328

T

T cells, 36–41, 36t, 37f, 39f, 39t, 40f, 40t, 41t
aging effects on, 49–50
CD3, 54–55, 55t
CD4, 54–55, 55t
CD8, 54–55, 55t
deficiency of, evaluation of, 53–54
evaluation of, 51, 52t, 53, 54–55
in AIDS, 444, 444t, 460–461, 461t
in burn injury, 597
in infectious mononucleosis, 427, 430
in neonate, 48–49
intraepithelial, 31
of respiratory tract, 798
properties of, 36–37, 36t, 37f
regulation of, 45–47, 46f
stimulation studies of, 55
subsets of, 41, 41f, 47
surface markers of, 36, 36t
evaluation of, 54–55, 55t
Th1, 41, 41f, 47
Th2, 41, 41f, 47
tolerization of, 45
Tabes dorsalis, in neurosphyilis, 1021
Tache noire, in scrub typhus, 538
Tachypnea, in pneumonia, 799–800, 799t
Taenia saginata infection (taeniasis), 20t, 530t, 531
Taenia solium, life cycle of, 525, 526f
Taenia solium infection (cysticercosis), 525–527
clinical manifestations of, 525, 526f, 526t
complications of, 527
diagnosis of, 525–526
epidemiology of, 525
etiology of, 525, 526f
pathogenesis of, 525
prevention of, 527
prognosis for, 527
serologic testing in, 109, 526
treatment of, 526–527, 527t
Tampons, toxic shock syndrome and, 296
Tapeworm infection, 525–531. *See also Echinococcus granulosus* infection (echinococcosis); *Taenia solium* infection (cysticercosis).
Target lesions, definition of, 533
^{99m}Tc. *See* Radionuclide scan.
T-cell receptors
in antigen processing, 38, 40f
selection of, 45–46, 46f
structure of, 40f, 44
Technetium disphosphonate scan. *See* Radionuclide scan.
Teeth, foscarnet effects on, 199
Teicoplanin, 151t, 172–175, 173t, 174t, 175t
adverse effects of, 173, 175, 175t
dosing for, 174t
Telogen effluvium, 543
Terbinafine, in tinea capitis, 558, 558t
Terconazole, 152t
in vulvovaginal candidiasis, 1006t
Testes, inflammation of, 994–995
Tetanospasmin, 589
Tetanus, 692–695, 693t. *See also Clostridium tetani* infection (tetanus).
Tetanus antitoxin, 220, 694
Tetanus immune globulin, 218t, 220
Tetanus immunization, 245t, 250–251
during pregnancy, 238
in bite-wound infection, 607
in wound infection, 594, 595t
postexposure, 242t
Tetracyclines, 151t, 180–182, 181t, 182t
adverse effects of, 182, 182t
dosing for, 181–182, 182t
drug interactions with, 182, 182t
in acne vulgaris, 548–549
in bite-wound infection, 606, 606t
in *Campylobacter jejuni* infection, 890, 890t
in cholera, 894–895, 895t
in *Dientamoeba fragilis* infection, 903t
in gastritis, 875–876, 876t
in malaria, 370, 371t
in *Yersinia pestis* prophylaxis, 385t
ophthalmic prophylaxis with, 1057, 1058
pathogen susceptibility to, 181t
pharmacokinetics of, 181, 181t
Thalassemia, immunization in, 240t–241t
Thalidomide, in erythema nodosum leprosum, 554
Therapeutics, 147, 148f, 148t. *See also* Anti-infective therapy.
Thermal injury, 1182t. *See* Burns.
Thermoregulatory center, 263
Thiabendazole, 153t, 209–210, 209t, 210t
in angiostrongyliasis, 517, 517t
in cutaneous larva migrans, 506t
in strongyloidiasis, 514t
Thomsen-Friedenreich antigen, in hemolytic uremic syndrome, 914
Thoracentesis
in pleural effusion, 837
in pneumonia, 801
Three-two-one solution, in stomatitis, 732t
Throat culture, in streptococcal pharyngitis, 714, 714t, 715f
Thrombocytopenia
chloramphenicol-induced, 180
flucytosine-induced, 193
in AIDS, 474
in disseminated intravascular coagulation, 287
in infectious mononucleosis, 428
in malaria, 372

Thrombocytopenic purpura, in rubella, 319
Thrombophlebitis, amphotericin B–related, 192
Thrombosis, with brain abscess, 663
Thrombotic thrombocytopenic purpura, vs. hemolytic uremic syndrome, 915
Thrush. *See Candida* spp. infection (candidiasis), oral.
Thyroglossal duct cyst, 624
Ticarcillin, 151t
dosing for, 159t
formulations of, 157t
in meningitis, 645t
in neonatal sepsis, 1126t
pathogen susceptibility to, 155t
Ticarcillin-clavulanate
dosing for, 159t
in bite-wound infection, 606, 606t, 607t
in ecthyma gangrenosum, 580t
in sepsis, 291t
in wound infection, 593t
Tick(s)
in Colorado tick fever, 393, 675
in ehrlichiosis, 359, 361f
in Lyme disease, 348, Plate 9E
in Rocky Mountain spotted fever, 354
Tick paralysis (toxicosis), 17
Tickborne disease, 15, 17, 18t–20t, 21t. *See also specific diseases.*
prevention of, 17, 22, 22t
Tickborne encephalitis, 676
Tickborne relapsing fever, 387–388, 388t
Ticonazole, 152t
Tinea capitis, 556–558, 556t, 557f, 558t
in AIDS, 475
Tinea corporis, 558–560, 559f, 559t, 561t
in AIDS, 475
Tinea cruris, 558–560, 559t, 561t
Tinea faciei, 558–560, 559t, 561t
Tinea incognito, 559
Tinea manuum, 558–560, 559t, 561t
Tinea pedis, 558–560, 559t, 561t
Tinea unguium, 558–560, 559t, 560f, 561t
Tinea versicolor, 560, 561f
Tinidazole, in giardiasis, 902, 903t
Tioconazole, in vulvovaginal candidiasis, 1006t
Tissue necrosis, 116
T-mycoplasma. *See Ureaplasma urealyticum.*
Tobramycin, 151t, 167–172, 168t
adverse effects of, 170–171
clinical indications for, 168–169
dosing for, 169–170, 169t, 170t
in acute pancreatitis, 981, 981t
in acute pericarditis, 867t
in burn wound infection, 600t
in cholecystitis, 972, 972t
in hepatic abscess, 967t
in infectious arthritis, 1048t
in intra-abdominal abscess, 929t
in meningitis, 646t
in neonatal sepsis, 1126t
in osteomyelitis, 1040t
in sepsis, 291t
in shunt-related infection, 655t
spectrum of activity of, 167–168, 168t
Tolerance
antimicrobial, 76
immune, in fetus, 47
Tolnaftate, 152t
Toluidine blue stain, for *Pneumocystis carinii* cyst, 82, 83f
Tonsillectomy
in otitis media, 756
in streptococcal pharyngitis, 717
quinsy, 726
TORCH syndrome, 1099. *See also* Intrauterine infection.
TORCH titers, 104
Torulopsis glabrata. See Candida spp. infection (candidiasis).
Total hemolytic complement (THC, CH_{50}), 54
Toxic shock syndrome, 296–304
clinical manifestations of, 299–300, 299f, 299t
complications of, 303
diagnosis of, 300–302, 300t, 301t
differential diagnosis of, 301, 301t
epidemiology of, 296–297, 297f
erythema of, 534t, 535, Plate 6A
etiology of, 296
laboratory evaluation of, 301, 302t
menses-related, 296
microbiologic evaluation of, 301–302
nonmenses-related, 296–297
pathogenesis of, 297–299, 298f
prevention of, 303–304
prognosis for, 303, 304t
treatment of, 302–303, 302t
Toxic shock syndrome toxin-1 (TSST-1), 5, 296, 297–298, 298f
Toxic synovitis. *See* Reactive arthritis.
Toxin(s)
anthrax, 551
bacterial, 3–5, 4t, 71–72, 115
botulinum, 911–912
Clostridium difficile, 71
Escherichia coli, 71–72
in hemolytic uremic syndrome, 914
in meningitis, 636
in rheumatic fever, 487
in septic shock, 284
in toxic shock syndrome, 297–299
mushroom, 911–912
seafood, 911–912
Toxin neutralization assay, for antigen detection, 115
Toxocara canis, life cycle of, 511f
Toxocara canis infection (toxocariasis), 20t, 511–512, 511f, 511t, 512t
retinal, 1082, 1082f, 1083, 1084
serologic testing in, 109–110
Toxoplasma gondii infection (toxoplasmosis), 20t
congenital, 1114–1116
clinical manifestations of, 1115, 1115t
computed tomography in, 1115, 1115f
diagnosis of, 1115
epidemiology of, 1114
parasite cycle in, 1114
pathogenesis of, 1114–1115
prevention of, 1116
prognosis for, 1116
treatment of, 1116, 1116t
in AIDS, 453t, 461, 461t, 462t, 465, 663
lymphadenopathy in, 612, 622–623
maternal, 1088t, 1089t, 1091–1092, 1092t
retinal, 1082, 1083, 1084
Toxoplasma gondii infection (toxoplasmosis) *(Continued)*
serologic testing in, 109
uveal, 1080
vs. infectious mononucleosis, 430
Toys, cleaning of, 1240
Tracheitis, 777–778, 777t
clinical manifestations of, 771t
treatment of, 776t
with measles, 312
Tracheotomy, in neck abscess, 725–726
Trachoma, 1063
Transcription-mediated amplification assay, 122
Transforming growth factor-β, in immune response, 40t
Transient synovitis. *See* Reactive arthritis.
Transmission, of pathogen, 13
Transplantation, 1168–1179
bone marrow, 1168–1171
antifungal prophylaxis in, 1171
antiviral prophylaxis in, 1171
enteric decontamination in, 1171
graft-verus-host disease in, 1170–1171
immunization after, 240t
immunoprophylaxis in, 1171
in primary immune deficiency, 1154
infection with, 1169–1171
bacteria in, 1169
cytokines in, 1170
fungi in, 1169
gastrointestinal tract, 1169
lower respiratory tract, 1169
prevention of, 1170–1171
susceptibility to, 1168
upper respiratory tract, 1169
viruses in, 1170, 1170t
reimmunization in, 1171
cardiac, infection with, 1176–1179, 1178t
central nervous system, 1177–1178
pathogens in, 1178–1179, 1178t
prevention of, 1179
respiratory tract, 1177
cardiopulmonary, infection with, 1177–1179, 1178t
central nervous system in, 1177–1178
pathogens in, 1178–1179, 1178t
prevention of, 1179
respiratory tract, 1177
Epstein-Barr virus infection after, 25, 429–430
hepatic, infection with, 1174–1176
bacteria in, 1175
fungi in, 1175
parasites in, 1176
prophylaxis against, 1176
site-specific, 1174–1175, 1174t
susceptibility to, 1174
viruses in, 1175–1176, 1175t
human herpes virus 6 infection after, 681
immunization and, 240t
infection after, 283, 1230–1231, 1231t 1232t
pulmonary, infection with, 1177–1179, 1178t
central nervous system in, 1177–1178
pathogens in, 1178–1179, 1178t
prevention of, 1179
respiratory tract, 1177
renal
infection with, 1171–1174

Transplantation *(Continued)*
renal *(Continued)*
infection with *(Continued)*
bacteria in, 1173
fungi in, 1173
parasites in, 1173
prevention of, 1173–1174
respiratory tract, 1172–1173, 1172t
surgical site, 1172, 1172t
susceptibility to, 1171–1172
urinary tract, 1172, 1172t
vascular aneurysm and, 1173
viruses in, 1173, 1174
vascular aneurysm with, 1173
Transverse myelitis, in schistosomiasis, 524
Trauma, immune response and, 49
Traveler. *See* International child traveler.
Travelers' diarrhea, 906–907, 906t, 907t
clinical manifestations of, 906–907
complications of, 908
diagnosis of, 907
epidemiology of, 906
etiology of, 906, 906t
prevention of, 908
prognosis for, 908
treatment of, 907, 907t
Trematode infections, 521–524, 522t, 523f, 523t, 524t
Trench fever, 344t
Trench mouth, 734, 735–736, 737, 738t
Treponema pallidum infection (syphilis), 1019–1023
cardiovascular, 1021
chancre in, 1020, Plate 7A
clinical manifestations of, 1020–1021, 1020f, Plate 7A, Plate 7B
complications of, 1023
congenital, 108, 634, 1102–1107
bone lesions in, 1103–1104, 1104f
clinical manifestations of, 1103–1104, 1103t, 1104f
CSF evaluation in, 1106
cutaneous manifestations of, 536t, 537, 538f
dental lesions in, 1104
diagnosis of, 1104–1106, 1105f
early manifestations of, 1103–1104, 1103t, 1104f
epidemiology of, 1102–1103, 1102f
late manifestations of, 1003t, 1104
meningitis in, 1104
neurologic manifestations of, 1104
ocular lesions in, 1104
pathogenesis of, 1103
periosteal inflammation of, 1104
prevention of, 1106–1107
prognosis for, 1106
rhinitis in, 1104
skin manifestations in, 1103
transmission of, 1102
treatment of, 1106, 1106t
vs. common cold, 708, 708t
copper penny lesions in, 537
corneal, 1083, 1083f
cutaneous manifestations of, 537, Plate 7B
darkfield examination in, 65, 68, 68f, 1019, 1021
diagnosis of, 65, 68, 68f, 105, 108, 1021–1022, 1022t
Treponema pallidum infection (syphilis) *(Continued)*
epidemiology of, 1019, 1020f
etiology of, 1019
gumma in, 1021
hair loss in, 542–543
imaging in, 141, 145f
immunofluorescent antigen detection in, 1021
kissing lesions in, 537
latent, 1020, 1023
lymphadenopathy in, 616, 617
maternal, 1088t, 1089t, 1090, 1091, 1092t
pathogenesis of, 1020
primary, 1020, 1021, Plate 7A
prognosis for, 1023
retinal, 1083, 1083f
satellite bubo in, 617
secondary, 1020, 1020f, 1021
lymphadenopathy in, 612
serologic testing in, 105, 108, 1021–1022, 1022t
skin rash in, 1020, Plate 7B
tertiary, 1020–1021, 1023
treatment of, 1022–1023, 1022t
Treponemal antibody test, 105, 108, 1021–1022, 1022t
Triamcinolone, in uveitis, 1081
Trichiasis, in trachoma conjunctivitis, 1063
Trichinella spp. infection (trichinellosis, trichinosis), 16t, 20t, 515–517, 516t
epidemiology of, 515–516
pathogenesis of, 516, 516t
prevention of, 517
serologic testing in, 110, 516
specimen collection in, 81
treatment of, 516–517, 517t
Trichinellosis. *See Trichinella* spp. infection (trichinellosis, trichinosis).
Trichinosis. *See Trichinella* spp. infection (trichinellosis, trichinosis).
Trichomonas vaginalis infection (trichomoniasis), 1004, 1027–1028, 1028t
diagnosis of, 1028, 1028f
specimen collection in, 81
treatment of, 1028, 1028t
wet mount for, 82, 82f, 1028, 1028f
Trichophyton rubrum infection (tinea corporis), 19t, 558–560, 559t, 560f, 561t
Trichophyton spp. infection, 19t, 556–560. *See also at* Tinea.
Trichophyton tonsurans infection (tinea capitis), 19t, 556–558, 556t, 557f, 558t
Trichuris trichiura, life cycle of, 507, 507f
Trichuris trichiura infection (trichuriasis), 507–508, 507f, 508t
wet mount in, 82, 82f
Trifluridine, 152t
Trigger sites, in fibromyalgia, 500
Trimethoprim-sulfamethoxazole (TMP-SMZ), 152t, 182–184, 183t, 184t
adverse effects of, 183–184, 184t
dosing for, 183, 183t
drug interactions with, 184
in *Aeromonas* infection, 891, 891t
in brain abscess, 661
in brucellosis, 381, 381t
in cholera, 894–895, 895t
in *Cyclospora cayetanensis* infection, 903t
Trimethoprim-sulfamethoxazole (TMP-SMZ) *(Continued)*
in donovanosis, 1026–1027
in gastrointestinal *Escherichia coli* infection, 897, 897t
in *Haemophilus influenzae* vulvovaginal infection, 1006t
in *Isospora belli* infection, 903t
in meningitis, 644, 645t, 646t
in otitis media, 754t
in *Pneumocystis carinii* infection, 466, 826, 826t
in sepsis, 291t
in shigellosis, 886, 886t, 1006t
in sinusitis, 765t
in travelers' diarrhea, 907t
in urinary tract infection, 991t
in *Yersinia enterocolitica* vulvovaginal infection, 1006t
in *Yersinia pestis* prophylaxis, 385t
in yersiniosis, 888, 888t
kernicterus with, 184
pathogen susceptibility to, 183t
precautions for, 184
Trimetrexate, in *Pneumocystis carinii* infection, 826, 826t
Triple dye, 1129
Trisomy 21, 1183t, 1185
Troleandomycin, 151t
Tropheryma whippleii disease, 916
Tropical erythrasma, 549
Tropical pulmonary eosinophilia, 506, 518
Tropical spastic paraparesis, 27, 704–705
Tropism, 1
Trousseau's sign, in acute pancreatitis, 982
Trypanosoma brucei gambiense infection (African trypanosomiasis), 19t, 81
Trypanosoma brucei rhodesiense infection (African trypanosomiasis), 19t, 81
Trypanosoma cruzi infection (American trypanosomiasis, Chagas' disease), 20t, 81, 857, 858–859
Trypanosomiasis, 19t, 81, 857, 858–859
specimen collection in, 81
TT virus infection, 944t, 945, 947, 954
Tube precipitation assay, 103
Tuberculids, papulonecrotic, 404
Tuberculin skin test, 405–406, 405f, 406t
in HIV-infected child, 460, 467–468
Tuberculoma, 403, 412f, 657
Tuberculosis, 396–419
abdominal, 403–404
adult rates of, 397–398, 397f
bacille Calmette-Guérin vaccination against, 417–418, 417t, 418f
bronchoscopy in, 406
calcification in, 408, 410f
cardiac, 404
cerebrospinal fluid examination in, 406–407
cervical lymphadenitis in, 400f, 402, 402f, 413–414, 414t, 622, 622t
childhood rates of, 398–399
clinical manifestations of, 400–405, 400f
computed tomography in, 408, 409f–412f
congenital, 399–400, 404–405, 407, 410f
corticosteroids in, 415
culture in, 73–74, 74t, 407
cutaneous, 404, 404f

Tuberculosis *(Continued)*
dactylitis in, 403
diagnosis of, 405–408, 405f, 406f
drug-resistant, 415
epidemiology of, 397–399, 397f, 397t
epididymal, 993
esophageal, 869
etiology of, 396–397, 397t
extrapulmonary, 400f, 408, 411f–413f, 413–414, 414t
clinical manifestations of, 401–405, 402f, 404f
treatment of, 413–414, 414t
follow-up for, 416–417
gastrointestinal, 403–404
genitourinary, 404
Ghon's complex in, 407
imaging in, 131, 135f, 136f, 407–408, 408f–413f
immune response to, 400
immunization against, 243, 245t, 246, 417–418, 418f
postexposure, 243t
in AIDS, 398, 405, 414–415, 450t–451t, 461, 462t, 467–468
in health care providers, 1243–1244
in international child traveler, 1213
in neonate, 399–400, 404–405, 407, 410f
inflammatory response to, 399
intravenous pyelogram in, 408, 413f
laboratory evaluation in, 406–407
latent, 415–416, 416
lymphatic, 400f, 413–414, 414t, 613, 622, 622t
clinical manifestations of, 402, 402f
lymphohematogenous, 401
maternal, 399–400, 1088t, 1092t, 1093–1094, 1096
meningeal, 400f, 632–633, 680
clinical manifestations of, 402–403
epidemiology of, 634
imaging of, 408, 412f
treatment of, 414, 414t
microbiologic evaluation in, 407
miliary, 400f, 401–402, 408, 411f
mortality from, 397
multidrug-resistant, 415
nucleic acid amplification in, 407
ocular, 404
otic, 404
papulonecrotic tuberculids in, 404
pathogenesis of, 399–400
pericardial, 863, 864, 865–866, 866, 867t
peritoneal, 930
pleural, 400f, 402, 408, 411f
pleural fluid examination in, 406
polymerase chain reaction test in, 407
prevention of, 417–418, 417t
prognosis for, 417
pulmonary, 131, 135f, 136f, 400–401, 401t, 407–408, 408f–410f
reactivation, 399, 401
renal, 404, 408, 413f
Rich focus in, 402
risk for, 397–398, 416
Simon's foci in, 401
skeletal, 400f, 403, 408, 411f, 412f
specimen collection in, 64
transport precautions and, 67

Tuberculosis *(Continued)*
supportive therapy in, 417
transmission of, 396–397, 397t
treatment of, 408–409, 412–417, 414t
compliance with, 416
follow-up for, 416–417
tuberculin skin test in, 405–406, 405f, 406f
tuberculoma in, 403, 412f
urine culture in, 65
verrucosa cutis in, 404, 404f
Tuberculosis verrucosa cutis, 404, 404f
Tubo-ovarian abscess, ultrasonography in, 140–141, 141f
Tularemia, 18t, 382–383, 382t
immunization against, 245t
oropharyngeal, 712t, 713–714, 716, 718
serologic testing in, 383, 618
treatment of, 383, 383t, 718
ulceroglandular, 615–616, 618
Tumor necrosis factor
antibodies to, in septic shock, 292
in immune response, 40t
in meningitis, 636–637, 636f
in septic shock, 283–284
TWAR strain. *See Chlamydia pneumoniae* infection.
Two-by-two table, 11
Tympanic membrane
in otitis media, 750, Plate 10
perforation of, 756
Tympanocentesis, in otitis media, 752, 752f, 756
Tympanometry, in otitis media, 751–752
Tympanostomy tube, otorrhea with, treatment of, 754t
Tympanostomy tubes, 756
Typhlitis, 1163
vs. appendicitis, 934–935, 934t
Typhoid, 882–885. *See also Salmonella typhi* infection (typhoid).
Typhoid fever, culture in, 883
Typhoidal tularemia, 382, 382t
Typhus, 355t
cutaneous manifestations of, 536t, 538
epidemic, 388, 536t, 538
murine, 19t, 388–389, 389t, 536t, 538
serologic testing in, 108, 389
Tzanck smear
in herpes simplex virus infection, 566, 566f, 1138–1139
in varicella-zoster virus infection, 335
in viral infection, 90

U

Ulcer(s)
aphthous (canker sore)
clinical manifestations of, 730
etiology of, 729
in AIDS, 470
pathogenesis of, 729
Buruli, 555
corneal, 1065, 1064f–1066f. *See also* Keratitis.
vs. endophthalmitis, 1076, 1076f
decubitus, 550–551, 551f
genital, 1009. *See also* Sexually transmitted infections.
peptic, 872. *See also* Gastritis.

Ulceroglandular tularemia, 382, 382t
Ultrasonography, 127t
in acute pancreatitis, 980
in appendiceal abscess, 137, 139f
in *Candida albicans* infection, 140, 140f
in cellulitis, 583
in central nervous system infection, 127, 130
in hip joint effusion, 144f
in intra-abdominal abscess, 925, 925f
in Kawasaki syndrome, 484
in nephritis, 140, 140f
in orchitis, 995
in tubo-ovarian abscess, 140–141, 141f
Umbilical stump
infection of, 1130
triple dye application to, 1129
Undulant fever. *See Brucella* spp. infection (brucellosis).
Unilateral hyperlucent lung, with adenovirus infection, 819
Unilateral laterothoracic exanthem, 537
Universal precautions, 1233–1234, 1233t
Upper respiratory infection. *See* Common cold.
Urea amidohydrolase, in gastritis, 872
Urea breath test, in gastritis, 874, 875
Ureaplasma urealyticum infection
culture in, 73
maternal, 1088t
serologic testing in, 108
Urethral prolapse, vs. vulvovaginitis, 1004
Urethritis, 983, 985, 989, 995–996, 1009, 1010t. *See also* Sexually transmitted infections; Urinary tract infection.
chlamydial, 1017
nongonococcal, 616
URI. *See* Common cold.
Urinalysis, in urinary tract infection, 986
Urinary tract infection, 983–991
catheter-related, 983, 985
clinical manifestations of, 984–985, 984t
complications of, 990
computed tomography in, 988
costovertebral tenderness in, 985
culture in, 987
diagnosis of, 985–988
differential diagnosis of, 985–986
enterobiasis and, 515
epidemiology of, 983–984
etiology of, 983, 983t
imaging in, 987–988, 987f
in AIDS, 473
magnetic resonance imaging in, 988
nosocomial, 1228–1229, 1228t
pathogenesis of, 984
physical examination in, 985
prevention of, 990–991, 991t
prognosis for, 990
radionuclide scan in, 987–988, 987f
rapid diagnostic tests in, 986–987
recurrence of, 990
renal scarring with, 990
supportive therapy in, 990
treatment of, 988–990, 988t
duration of, 989
response to, 990
urinalysis in, 986
urine collection in, 986

Urinary tract infection *(Continued)*
vesicoureteral reflux and, 984, 987, 987f
voiding cystourethrography in, 987, 987f, 988
Urine
collection of, 61t, 65, 986
in trichomoniasis, 1028
normal flora of, 9t
perineal bag collection of, 986
suprapubic percutaneous aspiration of, 986
Urine culture
in bacteremia, 288
in fever evaluation, 266
in urinary tract infection, 987
Urography, intravenous, 127t
URTI. *See* Common cold.
Urticaria, in hepatitis, 536–537, 536t
Uveitis, 1080–1082
clinical manifestations of, 1080–1081
complications of, 1081–1082
diagnosis of, 1081
differential diagnosis of, 1081
epidemiology of, 1080
etiology of, 1080
pathogenesis of, 1080, 1080f
physical examination in, 1081, 1081f
prevention of, 1082
prognosis for, 1082
sterile, 1078
treatment of, 1081

V

Vaccine. *See* Immunization.
Vaccine Adverse Event Reporting System, 217t, 238
Vaccinia
immunization against, 258–259
vs. chickenpox, 334, 335f
Vaccinia immune globulin, 218t
Vagina
infection of. *See* Vaginosis; Vulvovaginitis.
normal flora of, 999–1000, 1000t
physiology of, 999–1000, 999f, 1000t
Vaginal discharge, 1009, 1027–1030
in trichomoniasis, 1027–1028
Vaginitis, 998–1007. *See also* Vulvovaginitis.
in enterobiasis, 515
nonspecific, 1002
Shigella, 886
vs. urinary tract infection, 985
Vaginosis
clinical manifestations of, 1000–1001, 1001t
diagnosis of, 1004–1105, 1005f
epidemiology of, 998–999
pathogenesis of, 1000
physical examination in, 1002
treatment of, 1005, 1006t
Valacyclovir, 152t
in genital herpes simplex virus infection, 1024t
Valley fever. *See Coccidioides immitis* infection (coccidioidomycosis).
Valvular heart disease, 1182t
in Kawasaki syndrome, 484
Vancomycin, 151t, 172–175, 173t, 174t, 175t
adverse effects of, 173, 175, 175t
dosing for, 174t
drugs interactions with, 175, 175t

Vancomycin *(Continued)*
in acute pericarditis, 867t
in brain abscess, 662t
in burn wound infection, 600t
in cellulitis, 580t, 585t
in cranial epidural abscess, 666t
in ecthyma gangrenosum, 580t
in endophthalmitis, 1077t
in hepatic abscess, 967t
in infectious arthritis, 1048t
in intra-abdominal abscess, 929t
in mediastinitis, 843, 843t
in meningitis, 643t, 645t, 646t
in neonatal sepsis, 1125t, 1126t
in osteomyelitis, 1040t
in sepsis, 291t
in shunt-related infection, 655t
in spinal epidural abscess, 667t
in subdural empyema, 666t
in wound infection, 593t
Varicella gangrenosa, 587
Varicella-zoster immune globulin, 218t, 220
Varicella-zoster virus infection. *See also* Chickenpox; Zoster.
bullous, 333
cerebellar ataxia in, 681
cerebellitis in, 681
clinical manifestations of, 331–334, 332f, 333f
complications of, 337–339, 338t, 339f
corneal, 1065, 1065f, 1067
culture in, 335
diagnosis of, 88t, 334–335, 334t
encephalitic, 681
epidemiology of, 331
immunization against, 233t, 235t–236t, 253t, 259, 339–340
adverse reactions to, 237t
for international travel, 245t, 1211
in HIV-infected child, 460
in AIDS, 334, 474–475
in burn injury, 596, 598, 599
in day care environment, 1190
in hospitalized patient, 341
in immunocompromised persons, 337, 340–341, 340t, 1166–1167
laboratory evaluation of, 334–335
maternal, 333, 1088t, 1089t, 1091, 1092t
microbiologic evaluation of, 335
pathogenesis of, 331
perinatal, 333–334, 1110, 1135t, 1136t, 1140–1143
bacterial infection with, 1143
clinical manifestations of, 1141, 1141f, 1141t
complications of, 1143
diagnosis of, 1142
differential diagnosis of, 1142, 1142t
epidemiology of, 1141
isolation precautions for, 1143
pathogenesis of, 1141
physical examination in, 1141
prevention of, 341, 1143
prognosis for, 1143
supportive treatment of, 1143
treatment of, 1142–1143, 1142t
postexposure VZIG prophylaxis against, 337, 340–341, 340t, 1166–1167
prevention of, 339–341, 340t

Varicella-zoster virus infection *(Continued)*
prognosis for, 339
progressive, 332, Plate 4D
retinal, 1082, 1083
serologic testing in, 110, 335
streptococcal toxic shock syndrome and, 297
transmission of, 331
treatment of, 335–337, 336t
postexposure, 337, 340–341, 340t, 1166–1167
Variola
immunization against, 258–259
vs. chickenpox, 334, 335f
Vasculitis, leukocytoclastic, 539
Vector, 13
Vectorborne disease, 15, 17, 18t–20t, 21f, 21t, 22t. *See also specific diseases.*
Venereal Disease Research Laboratories (VDRL) test, 10, 105, 1021–1022, 1022t
Venezuelan equine encephalitis, 675–676, 676t
Ventilator-associated pneumonia, 829–830
Venting, for blood specimen collection, 63
Ventriculitis, nosocomial, 1229, 1229t
Ventriculoatrial shunt, infection of, 651–655. *See also* Shunt-related infection.
Ventriculoperitoneal shunt
infection of, 651–655. *See also* Shunt-related infection.
intra-abdominal abscess and, 923
Vero cell assay, in *Escherichia coli* infection, 72
Verruca plana, 567, 567f, 567t
Verruca vulgaris, 566–568, 567f, 567t, 568f
Vertebrae, infection of. *See* Diskitis.
Vesicles, 540–541, 541f, 541t
definition of, 533
Vesicoureteral reflux
antibiotic prophylaxis in, 990–991, 991t
urinary tract infection and, 984, 987, 987f
Vesicular rickettsiosis. *See* Rickettsialpox.
Vesicular stomatitis, 728, 730
Vibrio cholerae infection (cholera), 15, 16t, 17t, 893–895
clinical manifestations of, 894, 894t
complications of, 895
culture in, 894
diagnosis of, 894
epidemiology of, 894, 894t
etiology of, 893
immunization against, 244t, 245t, 246
for international travel, 1211–1212
pathogenesis of, 894
prevention of, 895
toxins in, 4t, 894
transmission of, 893
treatment of, 894–895, 895t
Vibrio parahaemolyticus infection, 16t
Vibrio vulnificus infection, 588, 590, 594
Vidarabine, 152t, 199–200, 200t
in herpes simplex encephalitis, 672, 672t
in perinatal herpes simplex virus, 1139
in varicella-zoster virus infection, 335–337, 336t
Video-assisted thoracoscopic surgery, in pleural effusion, 837
Vimentin, 594
Vincent's angina, 734, 735, 738t
Vincent's infection (trench mouth), 734
diagnosis of, 737

Vincent's infection (trench mouth) *(Continued)*
pathogenesis of, 735–736
treatment of, 738t
Viral inclusion, 116
Viral infection. *See also specific infections.*
bronchial, 779–788. *See also* Bronchiolitis; Bronchitis.
conjunctival, 1058–1062, 1058t, 1060f, 1060t
culture in, 84, 89, 89f
diagnosis of, 84, 88t, 89–90
antigen detection in, 89
cell culture in, 84, 89, 89f
electron microscopy in, 90, 90f
fever and, 263
histopathologic stains in, 90
nucleic acid hybridization in, 89–90
serology in, 90
shell vial culture in, 89, 90f
eosinophilia in, 95–96, 95t
fever in, 263
fever of unknown origin and, 276t
gastrointestinal, 898–901, 898t
hepatic, 943–961. *See also at* Hepatitis virus.
in burn injury, 596, 598
lymphadenopathy in, 611–615, 611t. *See also* Lymphadenopathy, generalized.
meningeal, 630–649. *See also* Meningitis, viral.
molecular tests for, 124
myocardial, 857–861. *See also* Myocarditis.
nosocomial, 1232
pericardial, 863–868. *See also* Pericarditis.
perinatal. *See at* Perinatal infection.
pharyngeal, 711
clinical manifestations of, 713, 713t
diagnosis of, 714, 715
treatment of, 717–718
pulmonary, 817–824, 817t. *See also at* Pneumonia.
purpura in, 539t, 540
retinal, 1082–1084
serologic testing in, 110–111
specimen collection in, 84, 87t
testicular, 994–995
Viridans streptococcal infection, 845, 846t. *See also* Infective endocarditis.
Virulence factors, 1–5, 2f, 3t, 4t
Virus-associated hemophagocytic syndrome, in infectious mononucleosis, 434
Viruses. *See also specific viruses.*
classification of, 84, 85t–86t
in foodborne disease, 16t
in oncogenesis, 23–28, 24t
Visceral larva migrans, 511–512, 511f, 511t, 512t, 1082
Vision, ethambutol effects on, 206
Vitamin A, in measles, 311, 311t
Vitamin B_6 deficiency, isoniazid-induced, 417
Vitamin therapy, in HIV infection, 460
Vitreitis, 1082. *See also* Retinitis.
Vocal fremitus, in pneumonia, 800
Vogt-Koyanagi-Harada syndrome, 1081
Voiding cystourethrography, 127t, 987, 987f, 988
Vomiting
bacterial toxin–induced, 4t
in appendicitis, 932
Voriconazole, 193t
Vulvitis, seborrheic, vs. vulvovaginitis, 1004
Vulvovaginitis, 998–1007
clinical manifestations of, 1000–1003, 1001t, 1002f
clue cells in, 1003, 1005f
complications of, 1007
diagnosis of, 1003–1005, 1003f, 1003t, 1005f
differential diagnosis of, 1003–1004, 1003t
epidemiology of, 998–999
etiology of, 998
gonococcal, 1004, 1006t. *See also Neisseria gonorrhoeae* infection (gonorrhea).
microbiologic evaluation in, 1004–1007, 1004t, 1005f
nonspecific, 998, 1000, 1003, 1004
treatment of, 1005, 1006t
physical examination in, 1001–1002, 1002f
prevention of, 1007
prognosis for, 1007, 1007t
treatment of, 1005–1007, 1006t
wet mount preparation in, 1003, 1003f, 1005f

W

Wakana disease, 505
Warfarin, ceftriaxone interaction with, 165
Warthin-Finkeldey cells, in measles, 306, 307f
Warthin-Starry stain, in cat-scratch disease, 346
Warts. *See also* Human papillomavirus infection.
genital, 567, 568f, 1009, 1029–1030, 1029f
nongenital, 566–568, 567f, 567t, 568f
WAS protein, 1152
Water, contamination of, 1149
Water cooling, in fever, 266
Waterborne infection, 12, 13–15, 14t, 15t, 907–911, 908–911. *See also specific infections.*
Waterhouse-Friderichsen syndrome, 285
Weil-Felix test, 108
in Rocky Mountain spotted fever, 356
Weil's disease, 386
Werdnig-Hoffmann disease, 1182t
West Nile virus infection, 675
Westergren erythrocyte sedimentation rate, 97
Western black-legged tick
in ehrlichiosis, 359
in Lyme disease, 348
Western blotting. *See* Immunoblotting.
Western equine encephalitis, 673–674, 674f
Western immunoblotting. *See* Immunoblotting.
Wet mount
for *Trichomonas vaginalis* infection, 82, 82f, 1028, 1028f
for *Trichuris trichiura* infection, 82, 82f
Wheals, definition of, 533
Wheatley's trichrome stain, for protozoa, 82, 83f
Whipple's disease, 916
Whipworm infection, 82, 82f, 507–508, 507f, 508t
White blood cell count
in bacteremia, 286–287
in cerebrospinal fluid, 640, 640t
in fever evaluation, 265, 266
in meningitis, 637–638
in occult bacteremia, 269, 271
in shunt-related infection, 652
White blood cell transfusion, 221
in septic shock, 293
White-footed mouse, in Lyme disease, 348
Whiteheads, 548
White-tailed deer, in ehrlichiosis, 359
Whooping cough, 18t, 779–780, 788–792. *See also Bordetella pertussis* infection (pertussis syndrome).
Widal test, 105
in typhoid, 883
Wimberger's sign, in congenital syphilis, 1103
Winslow, epiploic foramen of, 923
Wintrobe erythrocyte sedimentation rate, 97
Wiskott-Aldrich syndrome, 1152–1153
Wood tick *(Dermacentor andersoni),* 15, 21t
in Colorado tick fever, 393, 675
in Rocky Mountain spotted fever, 354
in tularemia, 382
Woolsorter's disease, 551
Wound infection, 587–595. *See also* Cellulitis.
bite-related, 602–608. *See also* Bite-wound infection.
burn-related, 596–601. *See also* Burns.
clinical manifestations of, 590–591, 590f
complications of, 593
diagnosis of, 591–592
epidemiology of, 588–589
etiology of, 587–588, 588t
farm injury and, 588
nosocomial, 1227–1228, 1227t, 1228t
pathogenesis of, 589–590, 589t
postoperative, 588
prevention of, 595
soilborne organisms in, 83–84
tetanus prophylaxis in, 593, 595t
treatment of, 595t
Wound myiasis, 571
Wuchereria bancrofti infection (filariasis), 20t, 518

X

X-linked agammaglobulinemia, 1150–1151
X-linked hyper IgM syndrome, 1151
X-linked lymphoproliferative syndrome, 25, 427–428, 429
X-linked severe combined immune deficiency, 1152, 1152t

Y

Yeasts, 59, 60t
Yellow fever, immunization against, 253t, 260
for international travel, 244t–245t, 1212–1213
Yersinia enterocolitica infection (yersiniosis), 16t, 17t, 887–888
clinical manifestations of, 887–888, 887t
complications of, 888
culture in, 888
diagnosis of, 888
epidemiology of, 18t, 887
etiology of, 887
foodborne, 908–911, 910t, 911t
pathogenesis of, 887
prevention of, 888
prognosis for, 888
pseudoappendicitis syndrome in, 887
reactive arthritis with, 888
toxins in, 4t
transmission of, 887
vulvovaginal, 1006t, 1007

Yersinia pestis infection (plague), 383–385, 385t
  clinical manifestations of, 384
  complications of, 385
  diagnosis of, 384
  epidemiology of, 18t, 384, 384f
  etiology of, 383–384
  immunization against, 245t
  pathogenesis of, 384
  prevention of, 21t, 385, 385t
  prognosis for, 385
  transmission of, 383–384
  treatment of, 384–385, 385t

Z

Zalcitabine, 152t, 203t, 205t
  in HIV infection, 456, 457t, 458t, 460t
Zanamivir, 202, 202t
  in influenza virus infection, 820–821, 821t
Zidovudine, 152t, 203t, 205t
  acyclovir interaction with, 198
  in HIV infection, 456, 457t, 458t, 460t
  in HIV-exposed newborn, 449, 454, 454t
Ziehl-Neelsen stain, 68
Zinc sulfate flotation technique, for parasite examination, 81
Zoonoses, 12, 15, 17, 18t–20t, 21f, 21t, 22t, 379–393. *See also specific zoonoses.*
  differential diagnosis of, 380t
Zoster, 331–341. *See also* Varicella-zoster virus infection.
  clinical manifestations of, 332–333, 332f
  diagnosis of, 334–335
Zoster *(Continued)*
  disseminated, 333
  encephalitis with, 681
  epidemiology of, 331
  in AIDS, 461, 462t
  pain in, 332, 337, 338f
  pathogenesis of, 331
  physical examination in, 333, 333f
  prevention of, 340
  prognosis for, 339
  supportive therapy in, 337
  treatment of, 336t, 337
  vesicles of, 541, 541t
Zoster ophthalmicus, 333
Zygomycosis, 131, 131f, 812, 812t

JENSON

ISBN 0-7216-8121-2